FOURTH EDITION

Merrow

Aquino | Linscott | Koch

RICHARDSON | TOWBIN | O'HARA | MEYERS | KRAUS
NAGARAJ | SMITH | BASKIN | ANTON | JONES | ORSCHELN

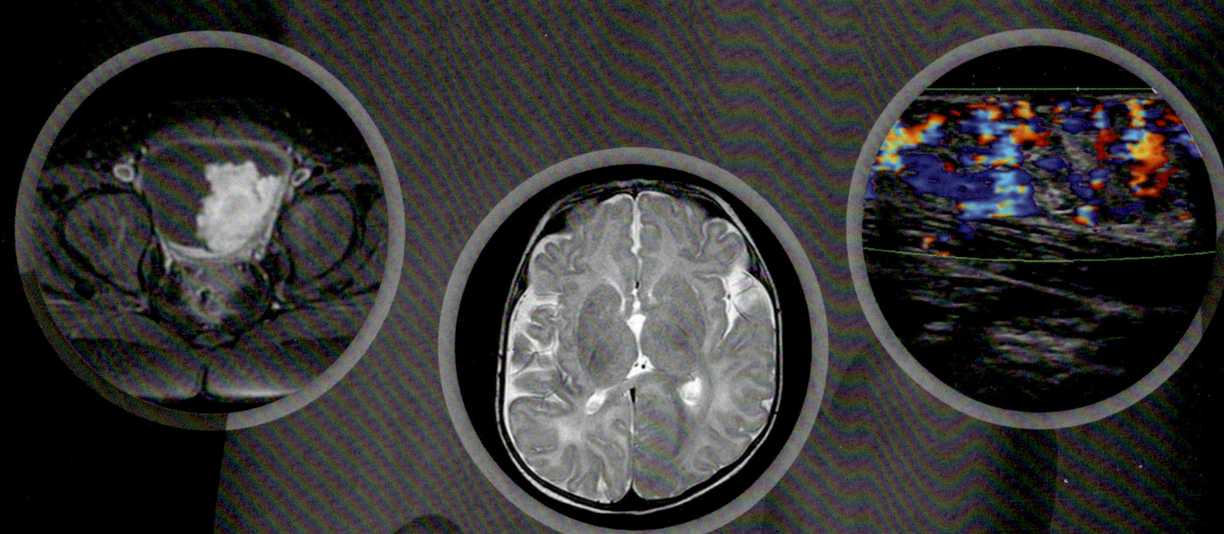

Diagnostic Imaging Pediatrics

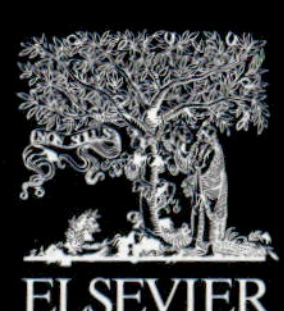

ELSEVIER

Diagnostic Imaging
Pediatrics

FOURTH EDITION

A. Carlson Merrow, Jr., MD, FAAP

Division Director, Emergency and Critical Care Imaging
Cincinnati Children's Hospital Medical Center
Associate Professor of Radiology
University of Cincinnati College of Medicine
Cincinnati, Ohio

Michael R. Aquino, MD, MHSc

Director, Pediatric Overnight Imaging
Cleveland Clinic Imaging Institute
Clinical Associate Professor of Radiology
Cleveland Clinic Lerner College of Medicine of Case Western Reserve University
Cleveland, Ohio

Luke L. Linscott, MD

Pediatric Neuroradiologist
Vice Chair, Department of Medical Imaging
Primary Children's Hospital
Salt Lake City, Utah

Bernadette L. Koch, MD

Associate Chief of Radiology (Physician Services and Education)
Cincinnati Children's Hospital Medical Center
Professor of Radiology and Pediatrics
University of Cincinnati College of Medicine
Cincinnati, Ohio

Randy R. Richardson, MD
Regional Dean
Creighton University School of Medicine
Phoenix Regional Campus
Phoenix, Arizona

Alexander J. Towbin, MD
Associate Chief of Radiology (Clinical Operations and Radiology Informatics)
Cincinnati Children's Hospital Medical Center
Professor of Radiology and Pediatrics
University of Cincinnati College of Medicine
Cincinnati, Ohio

Sara M. O'Hara, MD, FAAP
Division Director, Ultrasound
Cincinnati Children's Hospital Medical Center
Professor of Radiology and Pediatrics
University of Cincinnati College of Medicine
Cincinnati, Ohio

Arthur B. Meyers, MD
Division Director, Musculoskeletal Imaging
Cincinnati Children's Hospital Medical Center
Associate Professor of Radiology
University of Cincinnati College of Medicine
Cincinnati, Ohio

Steven J. Kraus, MD
Staff Radiologist
Section Chief of Fluoroscopy & Radiography
Department of Radiology
Texas Children's Hospital
Houston, Texas

Usha D. Nagaraj, MD
Faculty Radiologist
Cincinnati Children's Hospital Medical Center
Associate Professor of Radiology
University of Cincinnati College of Medicine
Cincinnati, Ohio

Ethan A. Smith, MD
Chair of Quality Improvement
Cincinnati Children's Hospital Medical Center
Associate Professor of Radiology
University of Cincinnati College of Medicine
Cincinnati, Ohio

Hank Baskin, MD
Pediatric Radiologist
Primary Children's Hospital
Adjunct Associate Professor
Department of Radiology
University of Utah School of Medicine
Salt Lake City, Utah

Christopher G. Anton, MD
Faculty Radiologist
Cincinnati Children's Hospital Medical Center
Associate Professor of Radiology and Pediatrics
University of Cincinnati College of Medicine
Cincinnati, Ohio

Blaise V. Jones, MD
Director, MR Safety
Division Director, Neuroradiology
Cincinnati Children's Hospital Medical Center
Professor of Radiology and Pediatrics
University of Cincinnati College of Medicine
Cincinnati, Ohio

Emily S. Orscheln, MD
Pediatric Radiologist
Children's Mercy Hospital
Assistant Professor of Radiology
University of Missouri-Kansas City School of Medicine
Kansas City, Missouri

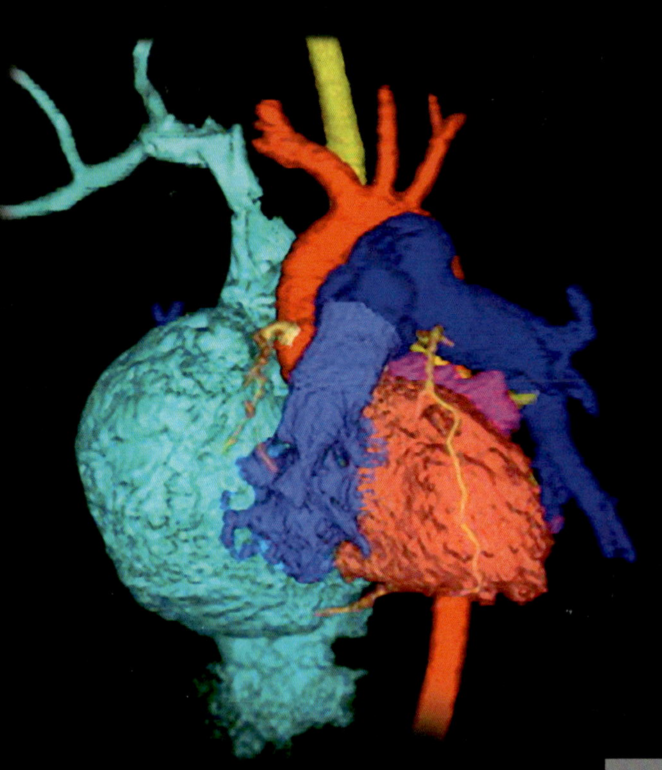

Elsevier
1600 John F. Kennedy Blvd.
Ste 1800
Philadelphia, PA 19103-2899

DIAGNOSTIC IMAGING: PEDIATRICS, FOURTH EDITION

ISBN: 978-0-323-77738-4

Notices

Practitioners and researchers must always rely on their own experience and knowledge in evaluating and using any information, methods, compounds or experiments described herein. Because of rapid advances in the medical sciences, in particular, independent verification of diagnoses and drug dosages should be made. To the fullest extent of the law, no responsibility is assumed by Elsevier, authors, editors or contributors for any injury and/or damage to persons or property as a matter of products liability, negligence or otherwise, or from any use or operation of any methods, products, instructions, or ideas contained in the material herein.

Previous edition copyrighted 2017.

Library of Congress Control Number: 2021948204

Printed in Canada by Friesens, Altona, Manitoba, Canada

Last digit is the print number: 9 8 7 6 5 4 3 2 1

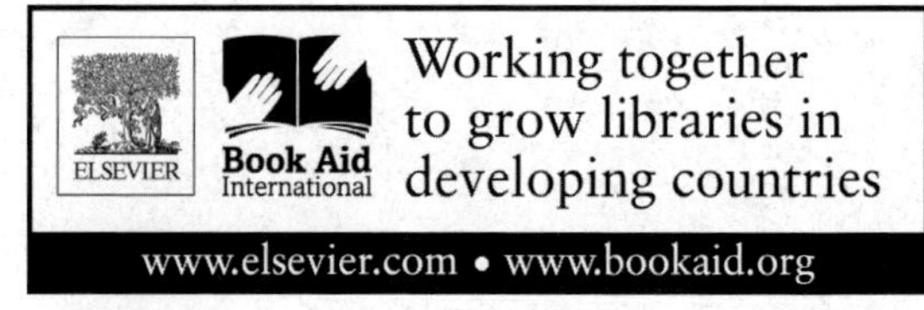

Dedication

To my wife and children: Through and through, thank you for your love and support—in this project, yes—but much more so in the everyday moments of life. You are all amazing.

To everyone who has made sacrifices to help others in the pandemic—healthcare and other frontline workers, absolutely—but also the everyday individuals who have chosen to make small but consistent sacrifices based on physician recommendations and solid scientific data (e.g., wearing masks and taking the vaccine) in order to protect yourselves and protect others: You are heroes, and individuals like you are the best hope for ending the pandemic anytime soon. Thank you for your selflessness, vision, and endurance.

ACM

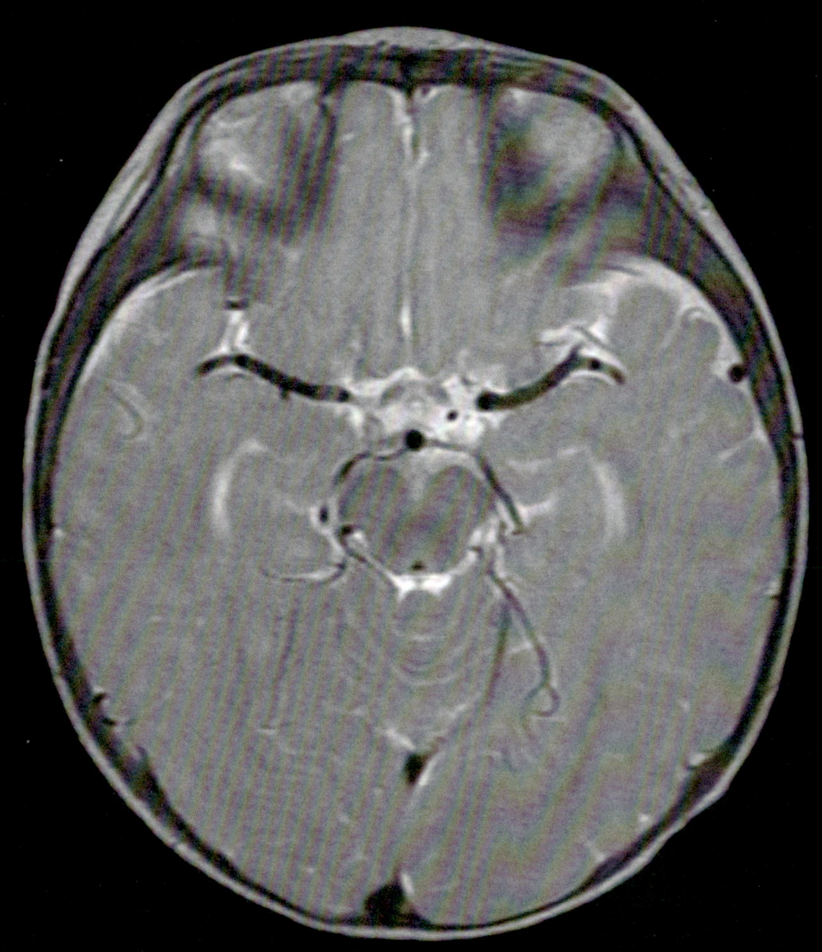

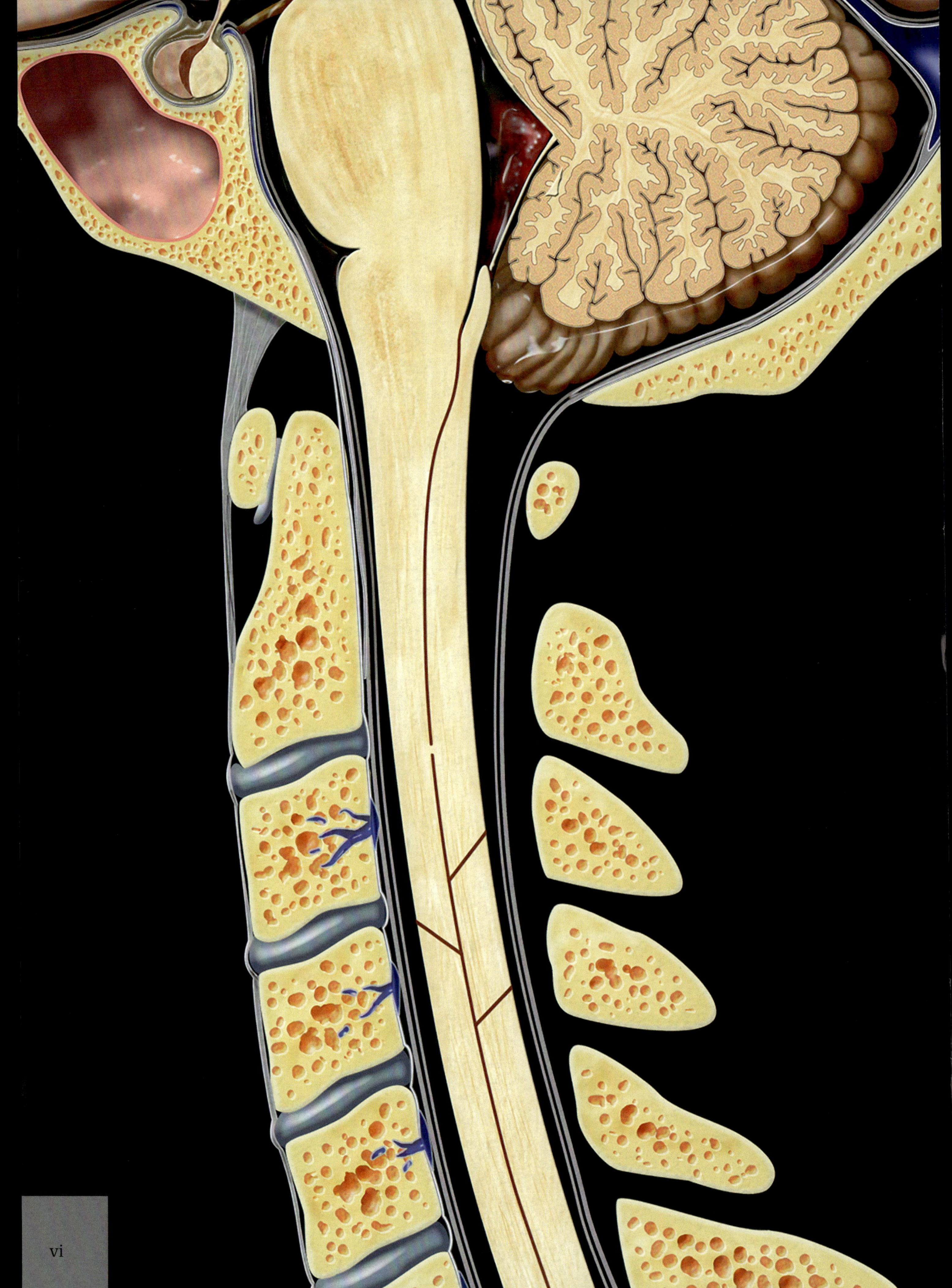

Contributing Authors

Swathi Selvam, BSc, MBBS, FRCR
Pediatric Radiology Fellow
Hospital for Sick Children
Toronto, Ontario

Additional Contributing Authors

Leila Rezai Gharai, MD
John D. Grizzard, MD
Nicholas A. Koontz, MD
Prakash M. Masand, MD
Ryan A. Moore, MD
William T. O'Brien, Sr., DO, FAOCR
Mantosh S. Rattan, MD
Caroline D. Robson, MBChB
Surjith Vattoth, MD, FRCR
Paula J. Woodward, MD

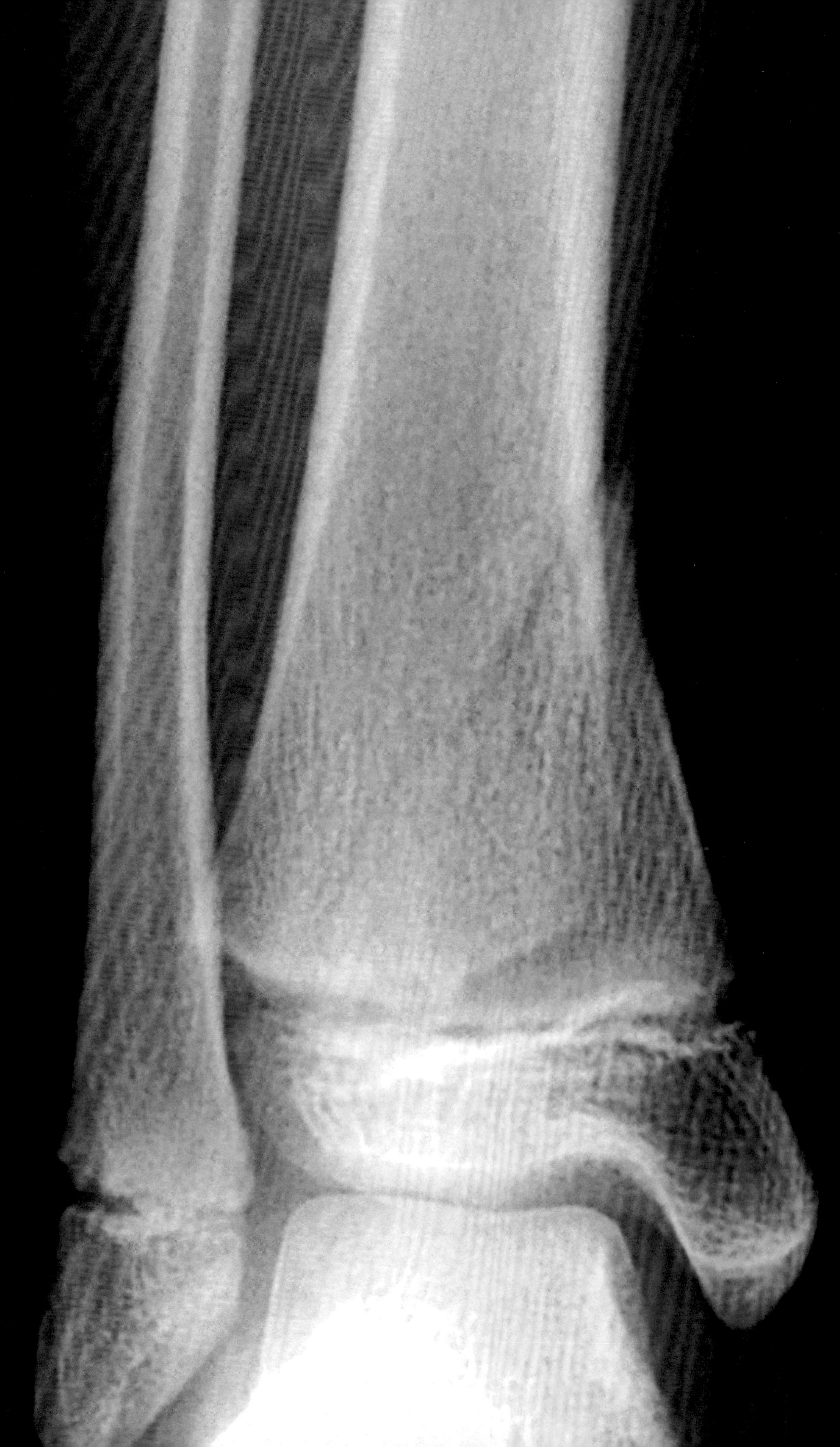

Preface

Welcome to the fourth edition of *Diagnostic Imaging: Pediatrics.* While we have made the expected updates over the third edition of the text (including new images and videos, terminology, disease classifications, and even new chapters), the events of the last 2 years have led to what I hope to be a once-in-a-lifetime occurrence: the opportunity to include a disease that did not exist 5 years ago and of which virtually the entire global population is now aware. I highly doubt that anyone reading this text has been unaffected by the COVID-19 pandemic, directly or indirectly.

So, in that context, I only have a few relevant thoughts.

I hope that each of you is truly *well.* That you've found a consistent way to refresh your soul in this trying time—that you have light, joy, purpose, and engagement—and somehow that wellness spills over into the lives of others—your patients and their families, your colleagues, your family and friends. We all need a little hope and encouragement from each other.

Finally, I must thank all who have worked on this book, especially those who helped carry my burdens when the light was dim. I am greatly indebted to you.

A. Carlson Merrow, Jr., MD, FAAP

Division Director, Emergency and Critical Care Imaging
Cincinnati Children's Hospital Medical Center
Associate Professor of Clinical Radiology
University of Cincinnati College of Medicine
Cincinnati, Ohio

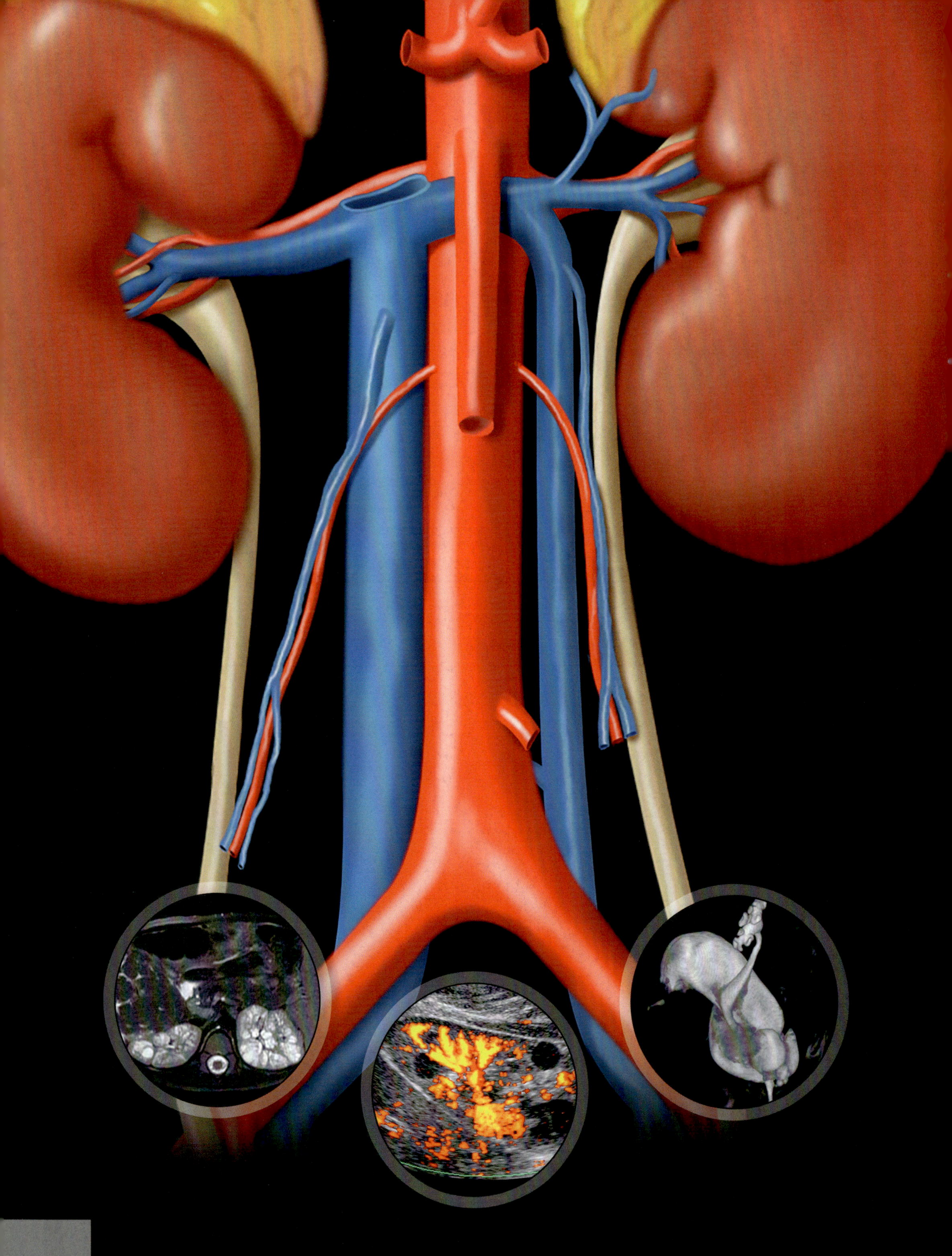

Acknowledgments

LEAD EDITOR

Nina Themann, BA

LEAD ILLUSTRATOR

Laura C. Wissler, MA

TEXT EDITORS

Arthur G. Gelsinger, MA
Rebecca L. Bluth, BA
Terry W. Ferrell, MS
Megg Morin, BA
Kathryn Watkins, BA

ILLUSTRATIONS

Richard Coombs, MS
Lane R. Bennion, MS

IMAGE EDITORS

Jeffrey J. Marmorstone, BS
Lisa A. M. Steadman, BS

ART DIRECTION AND DESIGN

Tom M. Olson, BA

PRODUCTION EDITORS

Emily C. Fassett, BA
John Pecorelli, BS

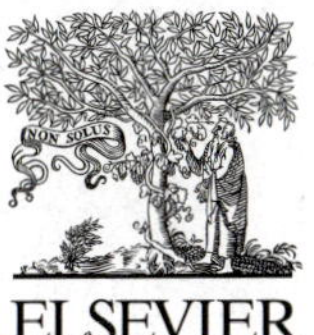

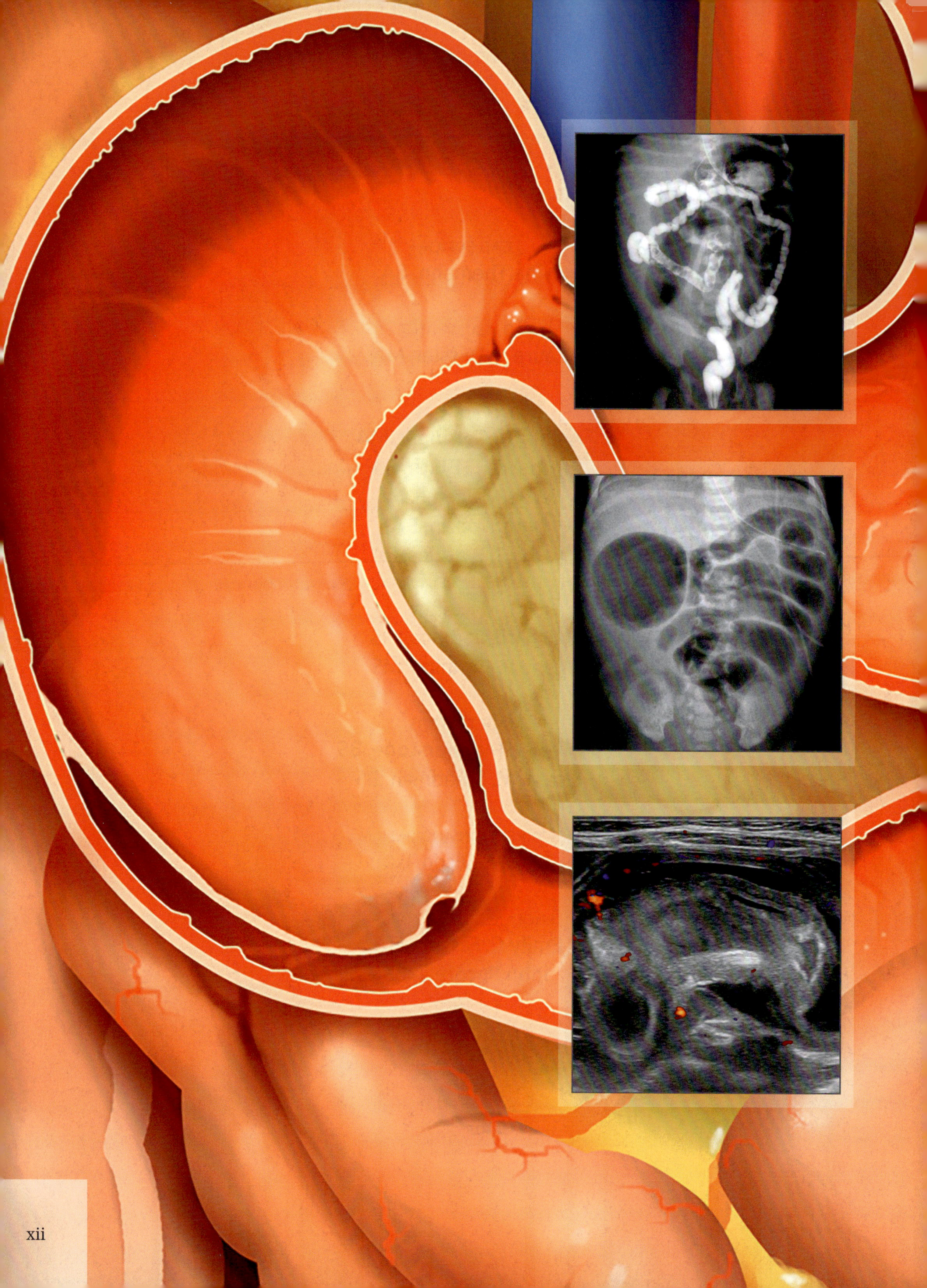

Sections

TABLE OF CONTENTS

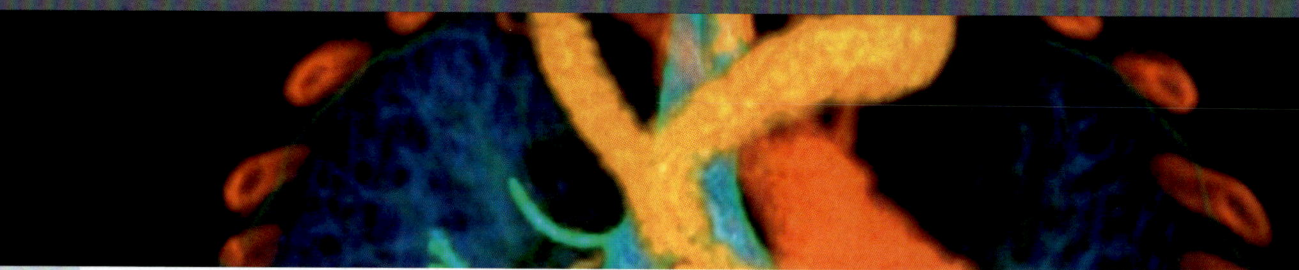

TABLE OF CONTENTS

TABLE OF CONTENTS

TABLE OF CONTENTS

TABLE OF CONTENTS

TABLE OF CONTENTS

RENAL MASSES

MISCELLANEOUS RENAL CONDITIONS

BLADDER ABNORMALITIES

ADRENAL ABNORMALITIES

UTERINE AND OVARIAN ABNORMALITIES

SCROTAL/TESTICULAR ABNORMALITIES

SECTION 6: MUSCULOSKELETAL

NORMAL DEVELOPMENTAL CHANGES

CONGENITAL ANOMALIES

TABLE OF CONTENTS

TABLE OF CONTENTS

TABLE OF CONTENTS

TABLE OF CONTENTS

FOURTH EDITION

Merrow

Aquino | Linscott | Koch

RICHARDSON | TOWBIN | O'HARA | MEYERS | KRAUS
NAGARAJ | SMITH | BASKIN | ANTON | JONES | ORSCHELN

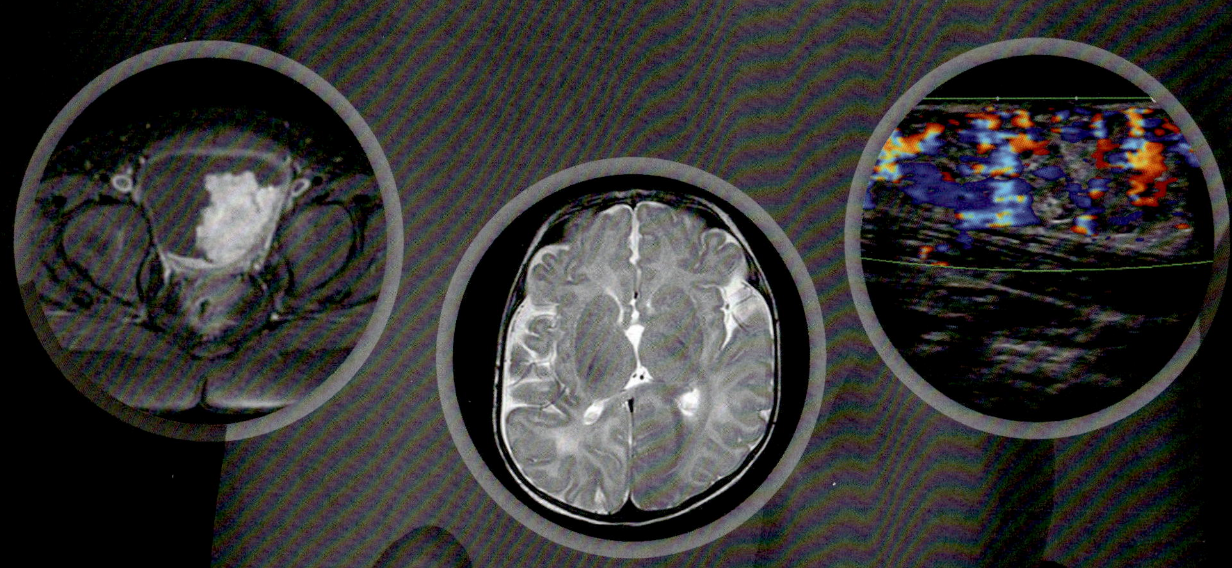

Diagnostic Imaging Pediatrics

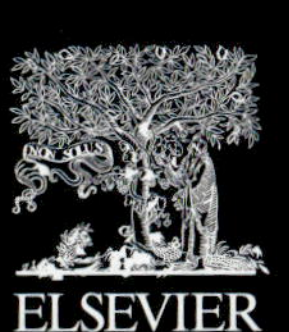

ELSEVIER

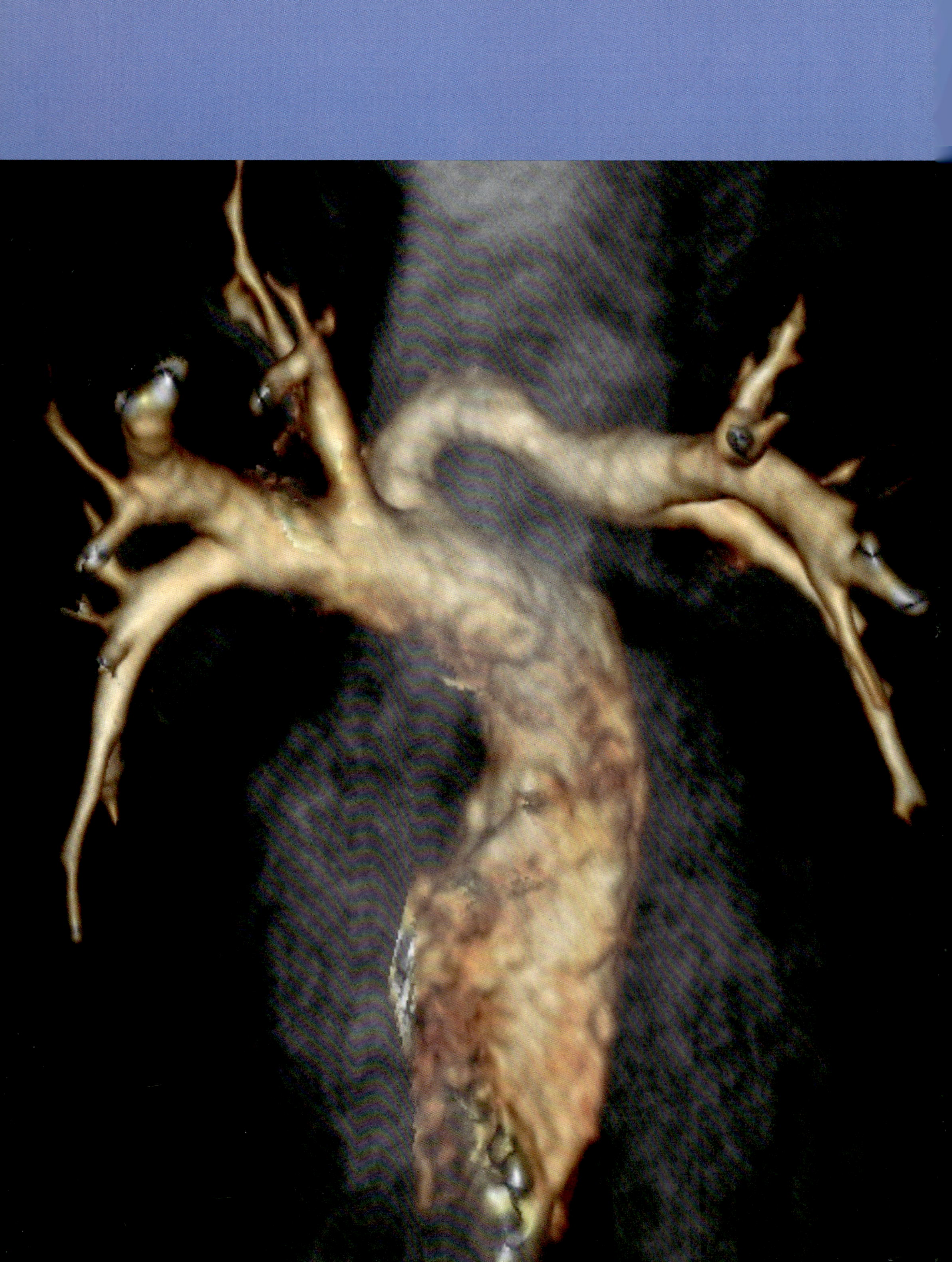

SECTION 1

Airway

Introduction

Anatomically & functionally, the pediatric airway can be divided into upper & lower segments at the glottis (larynx) or large & small airways at the transition from the cartilage-containing bronchi proximally to the distal airways that lack supporting cartilage. The superimposed disease processes may be extrinsic or intrinsic, & they may manifest as acute or chronic airway compromise at a variety of ages. Broad categories of airway compromise include congenital airway obstructions (e.g., choanal atresia), acute infectious etiologies (e.g., croup, epiglottitis), noninfectious intrinsic & extrinsic obstructions (e.g., foreign bodies, vascular rings), & obstructive sleep apnea (e.g., tonsillar hypertrophy, glossoptosis). These general categories of disease are not always distinct with some processes affecting multiple levels or presenting later in childhood despite an underlying congenital issue.

Imaging Modalities

Radiographs

Plain radiographs remain the imaging modality of choice for the initial evaluation of the pediatric airway. Two views (AP & lateral) are obtained to include the airway from the nasal passages & nasopharynx superiorly to the carina inferiorly. It is particularly important in young children to obtain the lateral view during inspiration & with the neck extended to prevent the simulation of pathology by normal tissue redundancy in these patients.

Airway radiographs are helpful in looking for ingested/inhaled foreign bodies (especially those that are radiopaque) & evaluating sites of midline pharyngeal or tracheal narrowing due to inflammation or extrinsic compression. Most extrinsic processes affecting the airway (such as peritonsillar abscesses & nodal conglomerations) will require further characterization with ultrasound or CECT.

Less acute indications for airway radiographs include infants with noisy breathing & older children with snoring (the latter of which could be obtained as a single lateral view of the upper airway).

Fluoroscopy

In the current era, fluoroscopy has a limited role in evaluating the pediatric airway. A commonly encountered circumstance is in the infant where a retropharyngeal space process is suspected clinically &/or radiographically. In this setting, the initial lateral radiograph will sometimes not be obtained with adequate extension &/or inspiration, making the retropharyngeal tissues appear abnormally thickened when they are not. Pulsed fluoroscopic visualization of such an airway during the respiratory cycle will demonstrate, in the lateral view, normal expansion & collapse of the retropharyngeal soft tissue in this age group (if there is no inflammatory change present).

Fluoroscopy may incidentally detect tracheomalacia or other sites of airway collapse in patients with obstructive sleep apnea, though it is not primarily used in the investigation of these entities.

Video swallowing studies (a.k.a. modified barium swallows) are frequently performed (in conjunction with speech pathologists) when aspiration or feeding difficulties are suspected. Another related study is the esophagram. While this exam is typically performed for dysphagia, it may have airway implications if there is a pattern of esophageal compression that suggests a vascular ring.

Computed Tomography

The applications of CT in evaluating the airway have become quite numerous. In the acute setting, CECT may be used to detail drainable abscesses of the retropharynx or peritonsillar tissues. NECT can be used to create virtual bronchoscopic images when there is concern for an aspirated foreign body that is not radiopaque. In the setting of congenital or chronic airway anomalies, CT angiography can be used to look for vascular rings causing compression of the airway (typically during a pulmonary or otolaryngology work-up). Dynamic change in the airway caliber may also be assessed, creating 4D cine images of the airway lumen during the respiratory cycle. Given these applications & its rapid acquisition, CT has taken on a significant role in the work-up of complex airway anomalies.

Magnetic Resonance

While MR has other applications in the neck, MR targeted to the airway is typically limited to the evaluation of recurrent obstructive sleep apnea after tonsillectomy. Its strengths lie in its ability to distinguish the various soft tissue components contributing to intermittent airway obstructions, allowing observation of the supraglottic airway over numerous respiratory cycles & with the application of various interventions during the scan.

The exquisite contrast resolution of MR as compared to CT makes it ideal for evaluating the relationships of slow-flow/high fluid content vascular malformations (e.g., lymphatic &/or venous malformations) to the various segments of the airway as these lesions frequently involve the oral cavity, neck, & mediastinum.

Ultrasound

Traditionally, sonography has rarely been used in the evaluation of the pediatric airway, primarily due to the artifacts associated with gas. While palpable neck masses are well characterized by ultrasound, their depth of extension & exact relationship to the airway are much better visualized by CT or MR. More recently, specific uses of airway ultrasound have been increasingly described, including the assessment of peritonsillar abscesses (using an intraoral probe), laryngeal motion (by otolaryngologists), & endotracheal tube position (during point of care ultrasound by the emergency or ICU physician).

Selected References

1. Biko DM et al: Mediastinal masses in children: radiologic-pathologic correlation. Radiographics. 41(4):E1186-207, 2021
2. Gibbons AT et al: Avoiding unnecessary bronchoscopy in children with suspected foreign body aspiration using computed tomography. J Pediatr Surg. 55(1):176-81, 2020
3. Andronikou S et al: Technique, pitfalls, quality, radiation dose and findings of dynamic 4-dimensional computed tomography for airway imaging in infants and children. Pediatr Radiol. 49(5):678-86, 2019
4. Bergeron M et al: The value of dynamic voice CT scan for complex airway patients undergoing voice surgery. Ann Otol Rhinol Laryngol. 128(10):885-93, 2019
5. Wani TM et al: The pediatric airway: historical concepts, new findings, and what matters. Int J Pediatr Otorhinolaryngol. 121:29-33, 2019
6. Liszewski MC et al: Updates on MRI evaluation of pediatric large airways. AJR Am J Roentgenol. 208(5):971-81, 2017
7. Osman A et al: Role of upper airway ultrasound in airway management. J Intensive Care. 4:52, 2016
8. Vijayasekaran S et al: Airway disorders of the fetus and neonate: an overview. Semin Fetal Neonatal Med. 21(4):220-9, 2016
9. Ciet P et al: Magnetic resonance imaging in children: common problems and possible solutions for lung and airways imaging. Pediatr Radiol. 45(13):1901-15, 2015
10. Darras KE et al: Imaging acute airway obstruction in infants and children. Radiographics. 35(7):2064-79, 2015

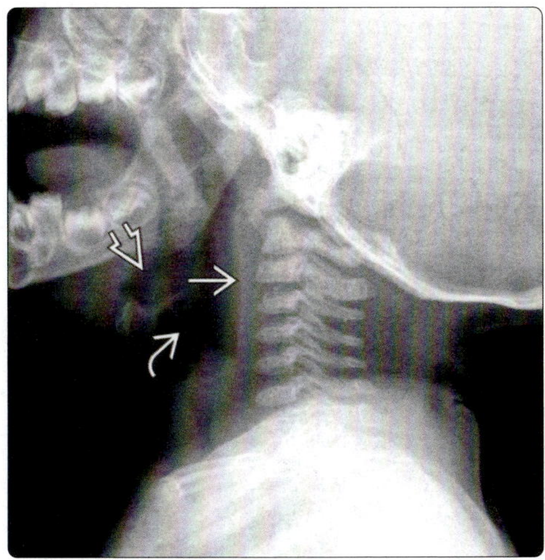

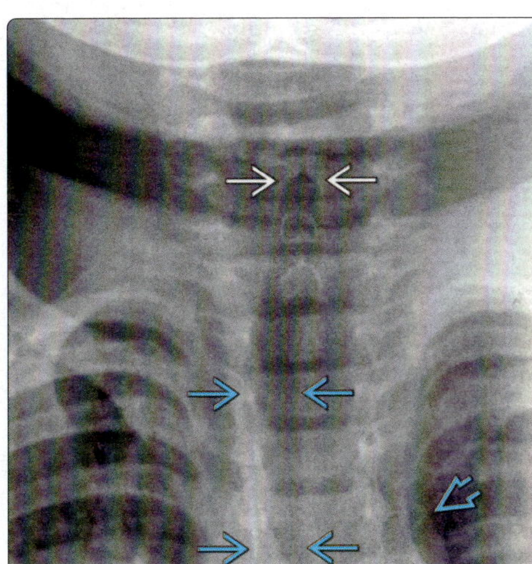

(Left) *Lateral radiograph of the normal pharynx in a young child shows a "thin" & well-defined epiglottis ➡. Note the normal retropharyngeal soft tissue width ➡ & thin aryepiglottic folds ➡.* **(Right)** *AP radiograph of a normal airway shows normal angular "shoulders" or lateral convexities ➡ in the subglottic region. The remainder of the trachea has a uniform caliber ➡ & is slightly shifted to the right by a normal left-sided aortic arch ➡.*

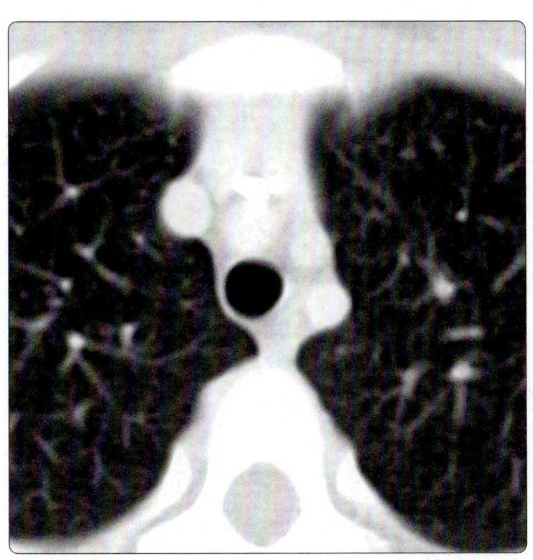

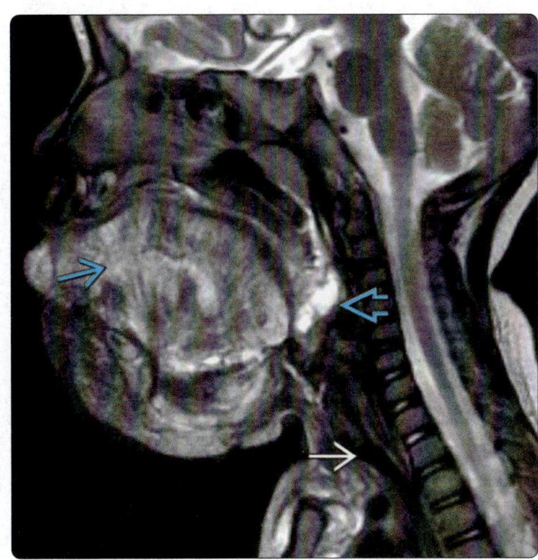

(Left) *Axial CECT of a normal trachea shows a normal round morphology of the tracheal lumen. The posterior wall may flatten slightly with expiration.* **(Right)** *Sagittal T2 MR in a 17-month-old patient with an extensive facial lymphatic malformation shows marked infiltration of the tongue ➡, floor of mouth tissues, & soft palate ➡ by the lesion, resulting in complete effacement of the oral cavity, oropharynx, & upper hypopharynx. A tracheostomy ➡ is partially visualized.*

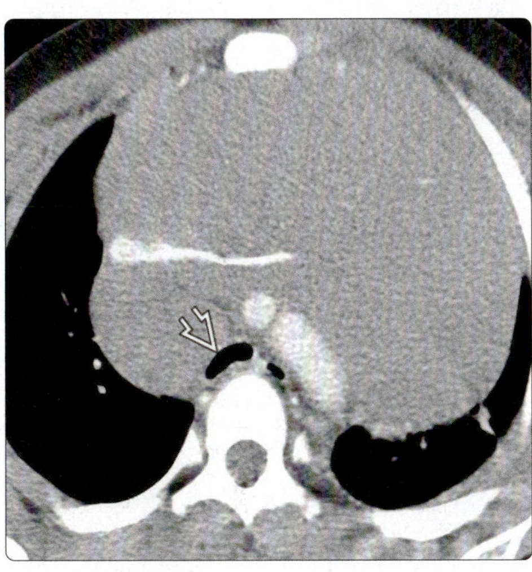

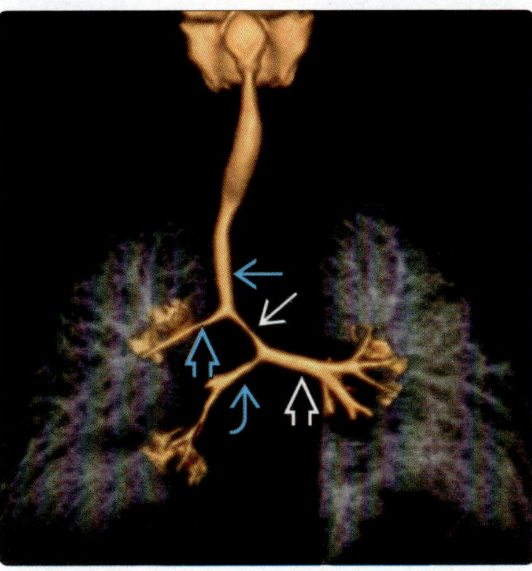

(Left) *Axial CECT in a child with lymphoma shows a large mediastinal mass with a flattened appearance of the trachea ➡ (typical of extrinsic compression).* **(Right)** *Anterior 3D NECT of the airways shows a round, narrow-caliber distal trachea ➡, typical of complete cartilage rings. There is an isolated right upper lobe bronchus ➡ arising from the trachea & leaving a narrowed intermediate left bronchus ➡, which then gives rise to the left main bronchus ➡ & a right bridging bronchus ➡.*

Expiratory Buckling of Trachea

KEY FACTS

TERMINOLOGY

- Intermittent normal change in transverse & craniocaudal configuration of trachea in infants during expiration

IMAGING

- On AP view, trachea is normally straight & of uniform caliber in older children & adults throughout respiratory cycle
- In infants, trachea is normally straight during inspiration but changes with expiration
  - Focal shortening, "crinkle," bend, or curve at/above thoracic inlet without significant caliber change
  - Directed towards right in patients with left aortic arch
    - Buckling toward left suggests right aortic arch
  - Trachea becomes straight again with inspiration
- No need to repeat radiograph

TOP DIFFERENTIAL DIAGNOSES

- Croup: Symmetric narrowing ("steeple") of subglottic trachea in young child with characteristic "barky" cough
- Infantile hemangioma: Persistent asymmetric tracheal narrowing by intraluminal, benign vascular neoplasm
  - Often associated with cutaneous infantile hemangiomas in "beard distribution"
- Tracheomalacia: Abnormal dynamic tracheal collapse in anterior to posterior dimension (not transverse)
  - Static lateral view may show caliber narrowing; dynamic change confirms tracheomalacia rather than stenosis
- Compression by extrinsic mass or aberrant vessel
  - Persistent focal airway narrowing with deviation away from mass/vessel; mass may enlarge mediastinum

CLINICAL ISSUES

- Incidental finding on chest or airway radiographs if morphology & patient age are correct
- Does not cause airway symptoms

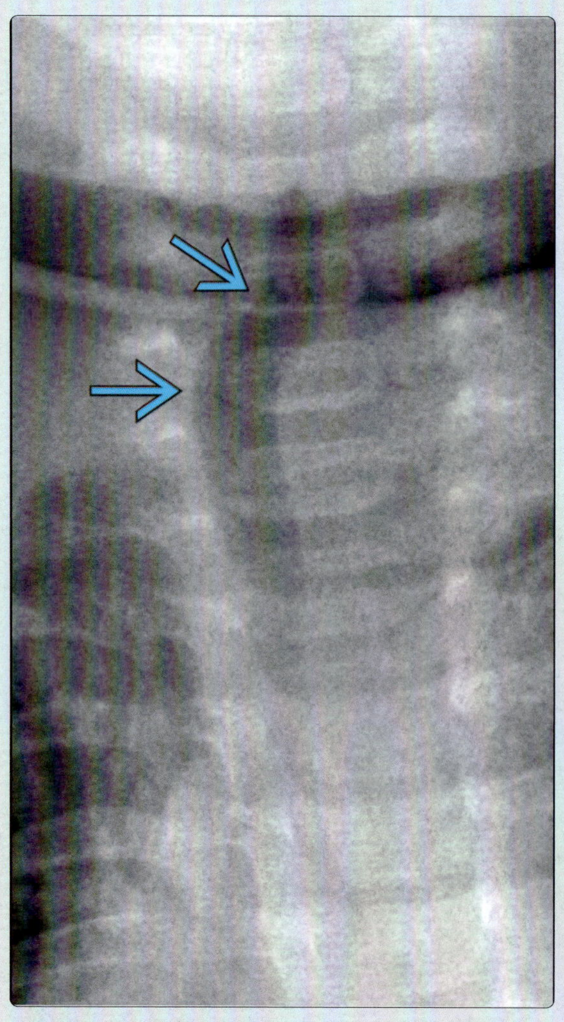

AP radiograph of the airway in an 8-month-old patient shows the typical configuration of expiratory tracheal buckling: The trachea at & just above the thoracic inlet demonstrates a focal bend toward the right ➔ but does not demonstrate narrowing.

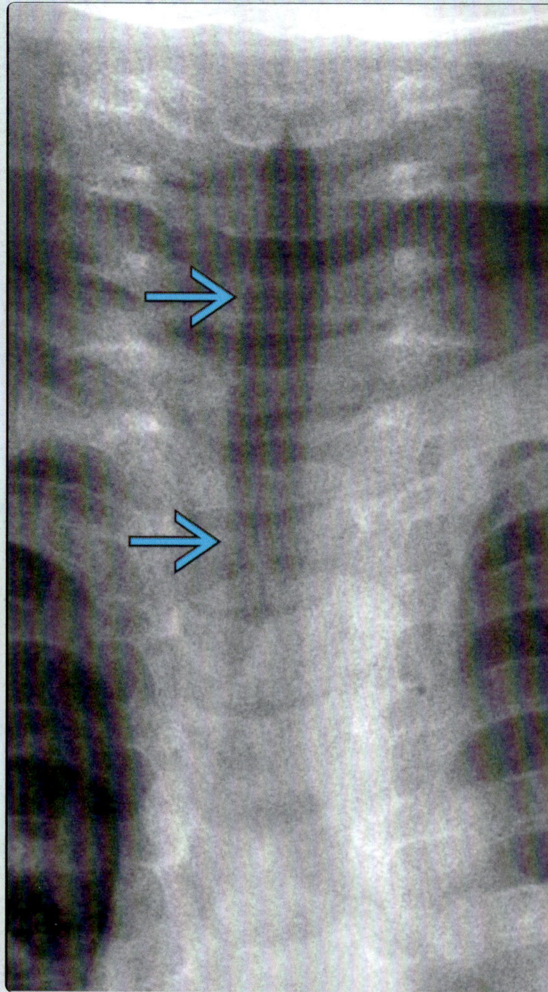

AP radiograph in an 8-month-old patient during inspiration shows a trachea that is relatively straight vertically ➔.

KEY FACTS

TERMINOLOGY

- Transient thickening of normal retropharyngeal soft tissues of infant on lateral airway radiograph
  - "Swelling" with expiration or poor extension
  - Resolution with inspiration & adequate extension
- Contributing factors to this appearance include
  - Relatively short necks of infants & young children, which lead to poor positioning for airway radiographs
  - Relatively long expiratory component of crying also challenges acquisition during maximal inspiration

IMAGING

- Generalized thickening/bulging of prevertebral soft tissues
  - ± retention of normal step-off at junction of hypopharynx & cervical esophagus
- Resolves on repeat lateral radiograph with improved inspiratory timing of exposure & ↑ neck extension
- Observation of dynamic airway changes under fluoroscopy can confirm intermittent thickening & resolution
  - Use "last image capture/image hold" for documentation
    - Thickening from expiration will recur during time required for true exposure

TOP DIFFERENTIAL DIAGNOSES

- Retropharyngeal cellulitis/abscess
  - Convex generalized bulging of prevertebral soft tissues persists despite inspiration & neck extension
  - Often lose normal step-off at hypopharyngeal-esophageal junction
- Cervical spine pathology
  - Trauma, inflammation/infection, or neoplasm → prevertebral soft tissue swelling
  - ± radiographically visible bony abnormality

CLINICAL ISSUES

- Uncommon in children > 2 years of age
- Unlike true pathology, pseudothickening does not cause characteristic signs/symptoms

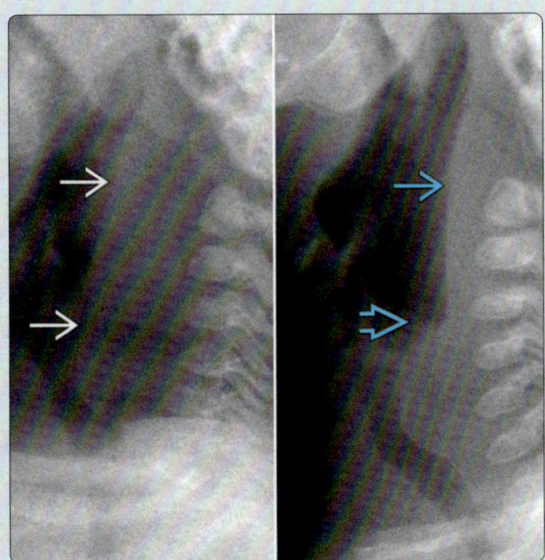

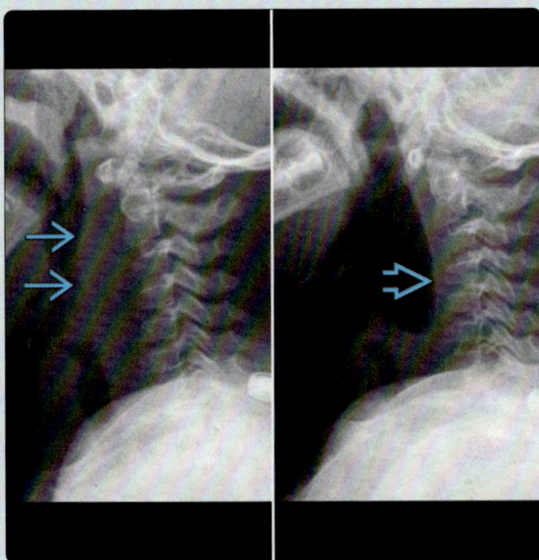

(Left) *Lateral airway radiographs in an infant show pseudothickening of the prevertebral soft tissues initially* ➡ *with improved neck extension & inspiratory timing* ➡. *Note the normal step-off at the hypopharyngeal-esophageal junction* ➡. **(Right)** *Lateral radiographs of the neck soft tissues in a 3-year-old with fever & limited neck range of motion show fullness* ➡ *& collapse* ➡ *of the prevertebral soft tissues during expiration (L) & inspiration (R), respectively.*

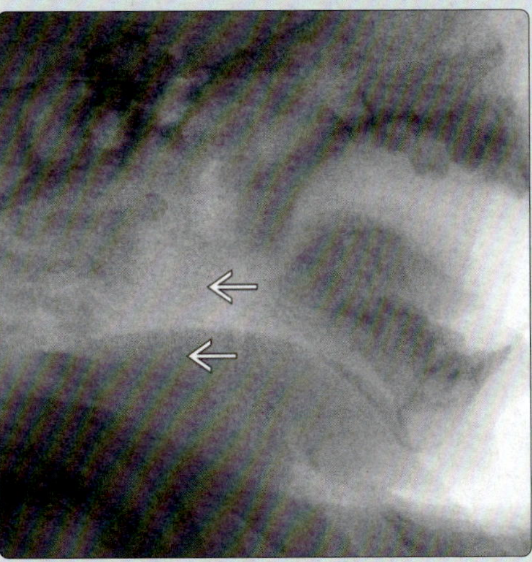

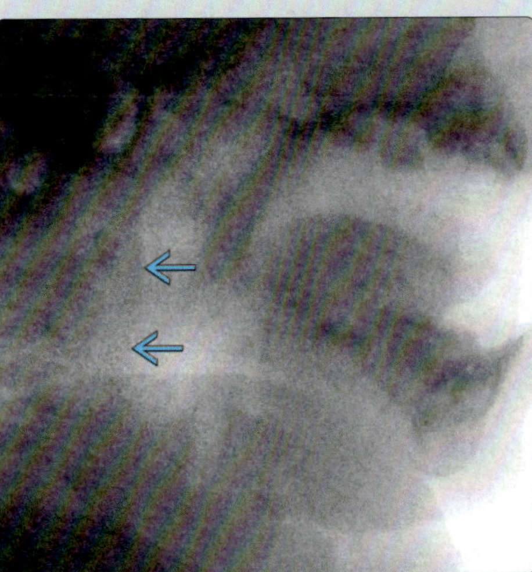

(Left) *Lateral fluoroscopic "image hold" in an 11- month-old with stridor & suggested retropharyngeal thickening on preceding radiographs (not shown) demonstrates bulging of the prevertebral soft tissues* ➡ *during expiration.* **(Right)** *Lateral fluoroscopic "image hold" in the same patient during inspiration shows normal collapse of the prevertebral soft tissues* ➡, *confirming pseudothickening on the initial image.*

KEY FACTS

TERMINOLOGY

- Congenital nasal pyriform aperture stenosis (CNPAS): Congenital narrowing of anterior bony nasal passageway

IMAGING

- Best tool: Bone CT in axial & coronal planes
  - Medial deviation of anterior maxillae ± thickening of nasal processes
  - Abnormal maxillary dentition: Solitary median maxillary central incisor (SMMCI) in up to 75%
  - Triangle-shaped palate

TOP DIFFERENTIAL DIAGNOSES

- Nasolacrimal duct mucoceles
  - Intranasal component narrows anterior nasal cavity
- Nasal choanal stenosis/atresia
  - Narrow posterior nasal passage by membrane or bone

PATHOLOGY

- CNPAS without SMMCI is almost always isolated anomaly
- Solitary maxillary central incisor in 75% of cases
  - Associated with holoprosencephaly

CLINICAL ISSUES

- Respiratory distress in newborn/infant
  - Breathing problems may be triggered by upper respiratory infection
  - Symptoms may be more pronounced with feeding
- Narrow nasal inlet on clinical exam
- CNPAS is 1/5 to 1/3 as common as choanal atresia

DIAGNOSTIC CHECKLIST

- Bone CT is recommended for diagnosis of bony narrowing & dental abnormalities
- Brain MR is recommended in cases of SMMCI to exclude midline brain anomalies

(Left) *Axial bone CT in a newborn shows the typical features of congenital nasal pyriform aperture stenosis (CNPAS). There is overgrowth & medial deviation of the anterior maxillae* ➡ *with marked narrowing of the anterior nasal passages. There is no associated choanal atresia* ➡. **(Right)** *Axial bone CT at the level of the palate in the same patient shows a classic associated finding in patients with CNPAS, a solitary median maxillary central incisor (SMMCI) or megaincisor* ➡.

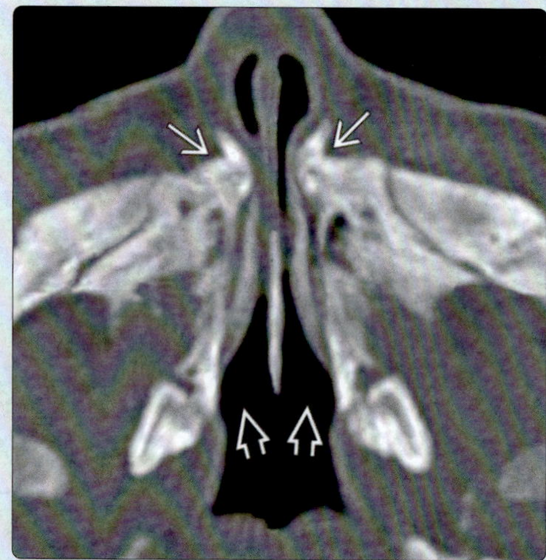

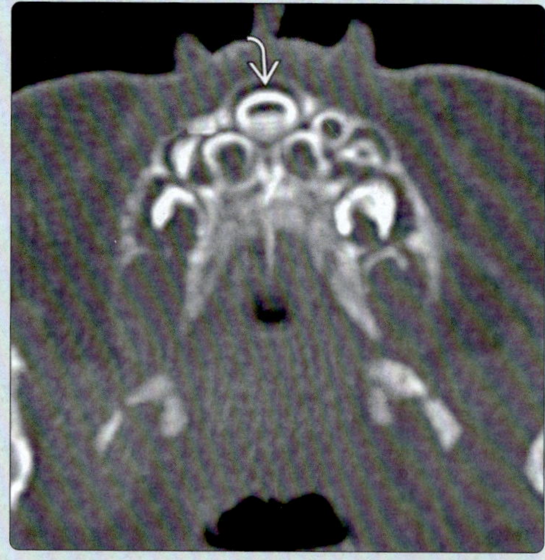

(Left) *Axial bone CT in a newborn with respiratory distress demonstrates CNPAS. The anterior & medial aspects of the maxillae are thickened* ➡*, causing narrowing of the anterior nasal airway.* **(Right)** *Coronal bone CT in the same patient demonstrates the narrowing of the anterior nasal airway bilaterally* ➡ *with an associated SMMCI* ➡.

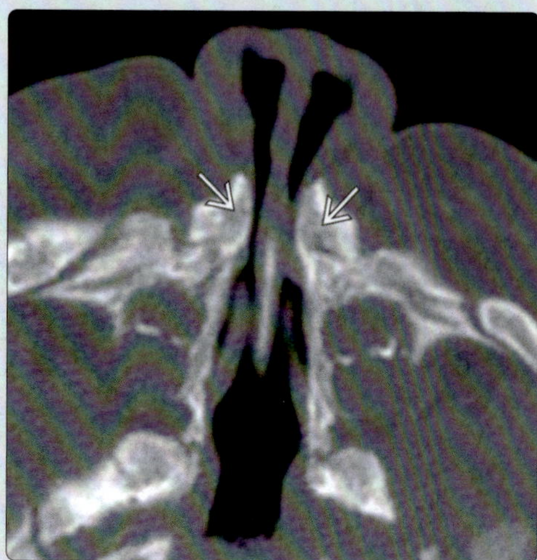

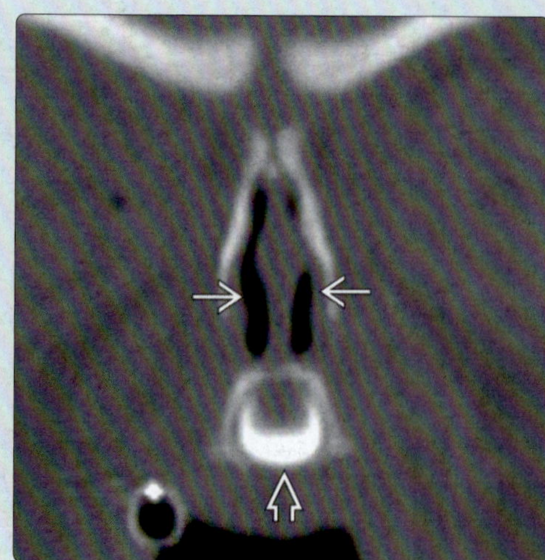

TERMINOLOGY

Abbreviations

- Congenital nasal pyriform aperture stenosis (CNPAS)

Definitions

- Congenital narrowing of anterior bony nasal passageway/nasal aperture

IMAGING

General Features

- Best diagnostic clue
  - Medialization & thickening of anterior maxillae with narrowing of nasal airway
- Location
  - Most often bilateral
- Size
  - Pyriform aperture (PA) size in CNPAS
    - PA width < 11 mm in term infant is diagnostic (normal = 13.4-15.6 mm)
    - PA area = 0.2-0.4 cm^2 (0.7-1.1 cm^2 is normal)

Imaging Recommendations

- Best imaging tool
  - Bone CT in axial & coronal planes

CT Findings

- Narrowed bony nasal inlet
  - Medial deviation of lateral wall of PA (anterior maxillae) ± thickening of nasal processes
- Triangle-shaped hard palate
  - Bony ridge along oral surface of hard palate on coronal images
- Abnormal maxillary dentition may occur
  - Fused or malaligned central & lateral incisors
  - Solitary median maxillary central incisor (SMMCI) syndrome (in up to 75%)
- Thinning of anterior nasal septum
- Posterior choanae are normal in caliber

DIFFERENTIAL DIAGNOSIS

Nasolacrimal Duct Mucoceles

- Obstruction of distal nasolacrimal ducts → cysts at bilateral inferior meatus → narrow anterior nasal cavity
- Bony aperture is normal

Nasal Choanal Stenosis/Atresia

- Narrow or occluded posterior nasal passage: Membranous, osseous, or mixed
- Anterior nasal passage is normal in caliber

PATHOLOGY

General Features

- Etiology
  - 2 theories of pathogenesis
    - Deficiency of primary palate derived from midline mesodermal tissue
      - □ Embryologically, medial maxillary swelling forms structures of primary palate, including 4 incisors
      - □ Mesoderm is thought to have inductive effect on forebrain, hence association of SMMCI syndrome with holoprosencephaly
    - Overgrowth or dysplasia of nasal processes of maxilla
  - CNPAS without SMMCI is almost always isolated anomaly
- Associated abnormalities
  - Upper teeth anomalies
    - SMMCI syndrome (75% of CNPAS cases)
  - Semilobar or alobar holoprosencephaly
  - Endocrine dysfunction: Pituitary-adrenal axis

CLINICAL ISSUES

Presentation

- Most common signs/symptoms
  - Respiratory distress, especially with feeding, as infants are obligate nasal breathers
    - Can mimic choanal atresia/stenosis
    - Breathing problems may be triggered by upper respiratory infection further compromising airway
  - Cyanosis
- Other signs/symptoms
  - Nasogastric tube is difficult to pass

Demographics

- Age
  - Newborns or infants in 1st few months of life
- Epidemiology
  - Congenital airway obstruction affects 1 in 5,000 infants
    - Majority are choanal atresia
    - CNPAS is 1/5 to 1/3 as common as choanal atresia
      - □ 1 in 25,000 live births

Treatment

- May be treated conservatively with special feeding techniques
  - Nasal cavity eventually grows & mild obstruction is relieved
- Surgical intervention in patients with persistent respiratory difficulty & poor weight gain
  - Resection of anteromedial maxilla ± anterior aspect of inferior turbinates & reconstruction of anterior nasal orifice
  - PA width < 5.7 mm in neonate may correlate with need for surgical intervention

DIAGNOSTIC CHECKLIST

Image Interpretation Pearls

- Brain MR is recommended with SMMCI to exclude midline brain anomalies

SELECTED REFERENCES

1. Ruda J et al: Radiologic, genetic, and endocrine findings in isolated congenital nasal pyriform aperture stenosis patients. Int J Pediatr Otorhinolaryngol. 128:109705, 2020
2. Shah GB et al: Congenital nasal pyriform aperture stenosis: analysis of twenty cases at a single institution. Int J Pediatr Otorhinolaryngol. 126:109608, 2019
3. Ginat DT et al: CT and MRI of congenital nasal lesions in syndromic conditions. Pediatr Radiol.45(7):1056-65, 2015
4. Wormald R et al: Congenital nasal pyriform aperture stenosis 5.7 mm or less is associated with surgical intervention: a pooled case series. Int J Pediatr Otorhinolaryngol. 79(11):1802-5, 2015

Nasolacrimal Duct Mucocele

KEY FACTS

TERMINOLOGY

- Synonym: Congenital dacryocystocele

IMAGING

- Well-defined, cystic, medial canthal mass in continuity with enlarged nasolacrimal duct (NLD) in newborn
  - Unilateral or bilateral
- Absent or minimal wall enhancement (unless infected)
- Coronal/sagittal reformatted images show continuity of proximal cyst at lacrimal sac with distal inferior meatus cyst through dilated NLD

TOP DIFFERENTIAL DIAGNOSES

- Orbital dermoid & epidermoid
- Frontoethmoidal (nasoorbital) cephalocele
- Infantile hemangioma
- Acquired dacryocystocele

PATHOLOGY

- Tears & mucus accumulate in NLD with imperforate Hasner membrane (i.e., distal duct obstruction)
- Most common abnormality of infant lacrimal apparatus

CLINICAL ISSUES

- Proximal cyst: Small, round, bluish, medial canthal mass identified at birth or shortly thereafter; ± cellulitis
- Distal cyst: Nasal airway obstruction with respiratory distress if bilateral (especially during feeding)

DIAGNOSTIC CHECKLIST

- CT or MR evaluates lacrimal apparatus lesion extent
  - Excludes other sinonasal causes of respiratory distress in newborn
- Comment on full extent of lesion from medial canthus to inferior meatus
- Exclude contralateral lesion

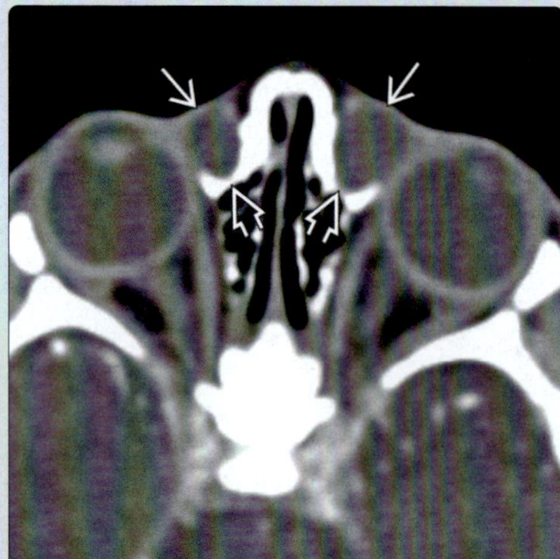

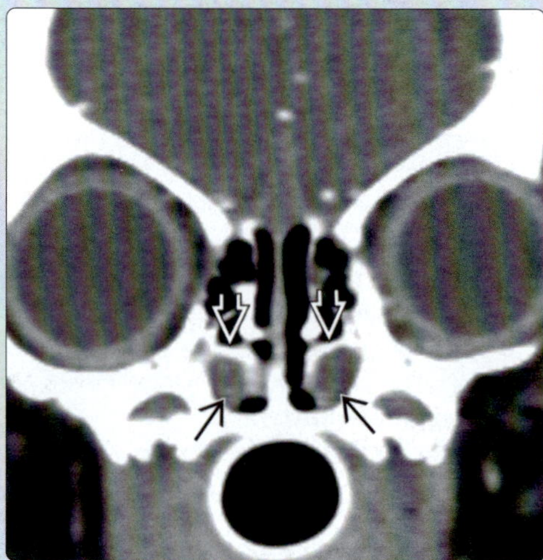

(Left) *Axial CECT in a 4-day-old with bluish, bilateral medial orbital swelling & left purulent drainage shows bilateral lacrimal sac enlargement* ➡*. Note also the bilateral lacrimal sac fossae splaying* ➡*.* **(Right)** *Coronal CECT in the same patient demonstrates the typical locations of the distal intranasal components of the nasolacrimal duct (NLD) mucoceles in the bilateral inferior meatus* ⇨ *inferior to the inferior turbinates* ➡*.*

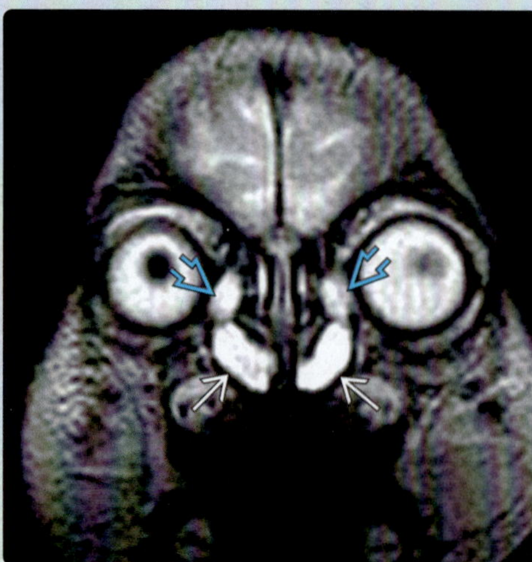

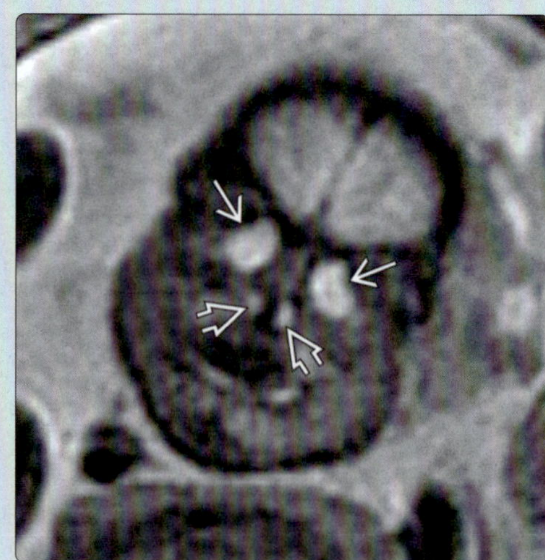

(Left) *Coronal T2 MR in an infant shows hyperintense nasolacrimal duct mucoceles extending from the dilated lacrimal sacs* ⇨ *proximally to protrude inferomedially from the inferior nasolacrimal ducts* ➡*.* **(Right)** *Coronal T2 SSFSE MR in a 2nd-trimester fetus demonstrates bilateral lacrimal sac enlargement* ➡ *with distal extension into each inferior meatus* ➡*, a typical appearance of nasolacrimal duct mucoceles.*

TERMINOLOGY

Synonyms

- Congenital dacryocystocele

Definitions

- Nasolacrimal duct (NLD) mucocele: Cystic dilation of nasolacrimal apparatus secondary to proximal & distal obstruction of NLD
- Canthus: Corner of eye where eyelids meet

IMAGING

General Features

- Best diagnostic clue
  - Well-defined, cystic, medial canthal mass in continuity with enlarged NLD in newborn
- Location
  - From lacrimal sac at medial canthus to distal aspect of NLD at inferior meatus in nasal cavity
  - Unilateral or bilateral

CT Findings

- Hypodense, thin-walled cyst at medial canthus ± bulging cystic component at inferior meatus
  - Cysts communicate through enlarged NLD
- Minimal wall enhancement; if infected, thick rim enhancement ± fluid/debris level & surrounding fat stranding

MR Findings

- T1-hypointense/T2-hyperintense, well-circumscribed mass(es)
- Signal intensity varies with protein content &/or infection
- Minimal wall enhancement normally
- If inflamed/infected → thick rim of enhancement with surrounding poorly defined soft tissue stranding

Ultrasonographic Findings

- Anechoic/hypoechoic round lesion with thin wall & ↑ through transmission at medial canthus

DIFFERENTIAL DIAGNOSIS

Orbital Dermoid & Epidermoid

- Lateral > medial canthus
- Near suture: Frontozygomatic > frontonasal/nasolacrimal
- 50% show fat density/intensity with thin rim enhancement

Frontoethmoidal (Nasoorbital) Cephalocele

- Swelling at inferomedial orbit connected to brain/meninges

Infantile Hemangioma

- Lobulated red (cutaneous) or bluish (subcutaneous) highly vascular benign neoplasm of infants
- Grows rapidly in 1st few weeks-months of life with very gradual spontaneous regression

Acquired Dacryocystocele

- Typically in adults with history of prior regional trauma
  - Other possible history
    - Post inflammatory or neoplastic stenosis
    - Previous NLD injury during Caldwell-Luc, uncinectomy, medial maxillectomy

PATHOLOGY

General Features

- Etiology
  - Tears & mucus accumulate in NLD due to imperforate Hasner membrane at distal duct
  - If bacteria enter distended sac → dacryocystitis ± cellulitis

CLINICAL ISSUES

Presentation

- Most common signs/symptoms
  - Small, round, bluish, medial canthal mass identified at or shortly after birth = distended lacrimal sac
  - Nasal airway obstruction & respiratory distress (especially during feeding) with bilateral nasal components
    - Obligate nose breathers during infancy
- Other signs/symptoms
  - Tearing & crusting at medial canthus, preseptal cellulitis, dacryocystitis
  - Small NLD mucoceles may be identified incidentally on brain MR imaging in fetus/infant

Demographics

- Epidemiology
  - Infancy: Typically 4 days to 10 weeks of age

Natural History & Prognosis

- 90% of simple distal NLD obstructions (or congenital dacryostenosis) resolve spontaneously by age 1 year
- Only 50% of those recognized on prenatal MR ultimately have postnatal symptoms
- Intervention before infection to prevent nasal airway obstruction, dacryocystitis, & permanent sequelae

Treatment

- Daily manual massage ± prophylactic antibiotics
  - Manual massage is inappropriate if NLD mucocele is infected or causing airway obstruction
- 10% require probing with irrigation ± silastic stent
- With endonasal component & no response to above → endoscopic resection with marsupialization
- Excellent prognosis with adequate early treatment
- High success rate for nasal endoscopic surgery: Cure (81.5%), improvement (18.5%), unhealed (0%)
- Theoretical risk of nasolacrimal apparatus scarring, amblyopia, & permanent canthal asymmetry if untreated

DIAGNOSTIC CHECKLIST

Image Interpretation Pearls

- Comment on full extent of lesion from medial canthus to inferior meatus, bilaterality, & signs of infection

SELECTED REFERENCES

1. Alvo A et al: Neonatal nasal obstruction. Eur Arch Otorhinolaryngol. 278(10):3605-11, 2021
2. Zhang Y et al: Selection of surgical intervention for congenital dacryocystocele. Eur J Ophthalmol. 29(2):158-64, 2019
3. Davies R et al: The presentation, clinical features, complications, and treatment of congenital dacryocystocele. Eye (Lond). 32(3):522-6, 2018
4. Rodriguez DP et al: Masses of the nose, nasal cavity, and nasopharynx in children. Radiographics. 37(6):1704-30, 2017

Choanal Atresia

KEY FACTS

TERMINOLOGY

- Congenital obstruction of posterior nasal aperture(s)

IMAGING

- Unilateral or bilateral osseous narrowing of posterior nasal cavity with complete obstruction by associated membrane &/or bony plate
  - Thickening of vomer
  - Medial bowing of posterior maxilla(e)
  - ± air-fluid level in obstructed nasal cavity
- Unilateral in up to 75% (R > L)
- Bilateral in up to 25%
  - 75% of bilateral cases have other anomalies

TOP DIFFERENTIAL DIAGNOSES

- Choanal stenosis
- Pyriform aperture stenosis
- Nasolacrimal duct mucocele

PATHOLOGY

- Choanal atresia is most common congenital abnormality of nasal cavity
- Choanal atresia types
  - Mixed bony & membranous atresia in up to 70%
  - Purely bony atresia in up to 30%

CLINICAL ISSUES

- Typical presentations include
  - Bilateral choanal atresia: Significant respiratory distress in newborn
    - Due to their physiologic obligate nasal breather status
  - Unilateral choanal atresia: Chronic, purulent unilateral rhinorrhea with mild airway obstruction in older child

DIAGNOSTIC CHECKLIST

- Respiratory distress & suspected nasal obstruction in newborn should be evaluated with thin-section bone CT

(Left) *Axial NECT (in bone windows) through the upper choanae in a child shows a complete osseous right choanal obstruction ➡ secondary to fusion of an enlarged vomer ➡ to the thickened, medially positioned posterior maxilla ➡.* **(Right)** *Axial bone CT in an infant shows significant narrowing of the choanae ➡, medialization of thickened posteromedial maxillae ➡, a wide vomer ➡, small membranes traversing the stenotic choanae, & bilateral nasal cavity air-fluid levels ➡.*

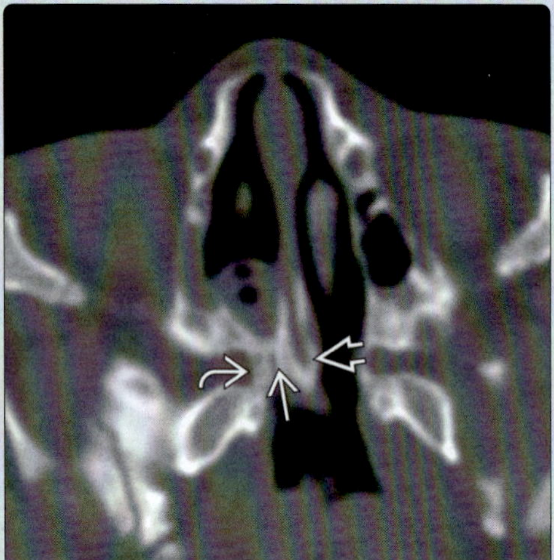

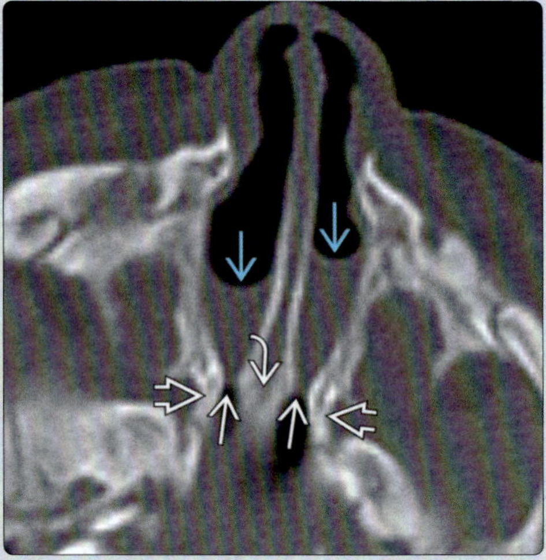

(Left) *Axial bone CT obtained at the upper aspect of the choanae in a 6-week-old with right nasal obstruction demonstrates complete obliteration of the right choana ➡ by the thickened vomer ➡ fused to the thickened posteromedial maxilla ➡.* **(Right)** *Axial bone CT 2 mm more inferior in the same patient shows a stenotic choana & crossing membrane ➡, not an uncommon appearance in patients with mixed atresia with bony (upper) & membranous (lower) components.*

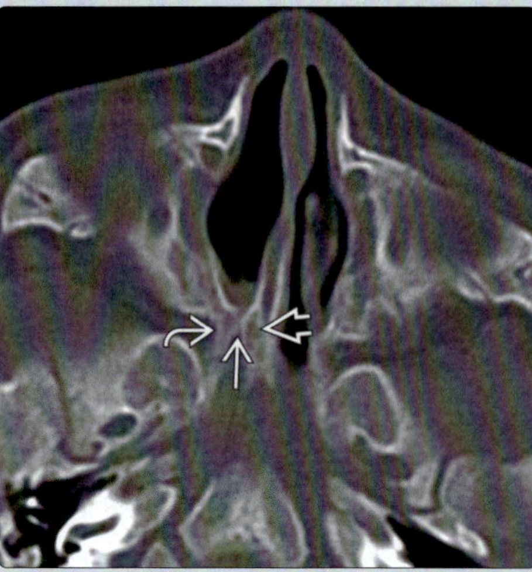

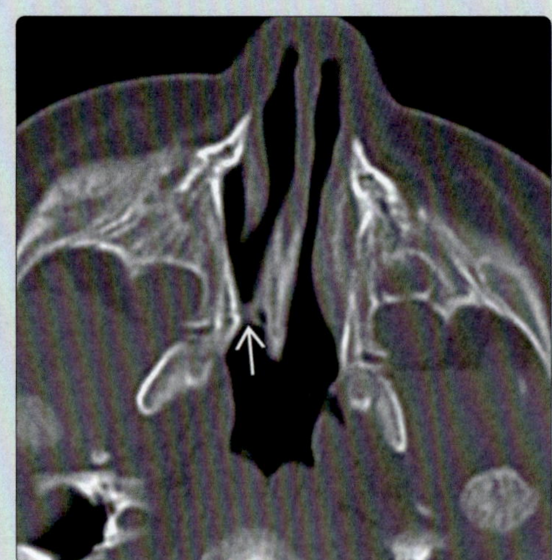

TERMINOLOGY

Definitions

- Congenital obstruction of posterior nasal aperture
  - Choana: Junction of posterior nasal cavity & nasopharynx
  - Choanal atresia: Lack of communication between nasal cavity & nasopharynx

IMAGING

General Features

- Best diagnostic clue
  - Bony narrowing of posterior nasal cavity with membranous &/or osseous obstruction of choana
- Location
  - Unilateral in ~ 75% (R > L), bilateral in ~ 25%
- Size
  - Newborn choanal opening is abnormal if < 0.34 cm wide
  - Newborn vomer is abnormal if > 0.23 cm thick
- Morphology
  - Medial bowing of posterior maxilla (lateral nasal wall) & pterygoid plate
  - Large/thickened vomer
  - Bony narrowing ± soft tissue membrane/plug or bony plate obstructing choana
    - Mixed bony & membranous atresia in up to 70%
    - Purely bony atresia in up to 30%

CT Findings

- Bone CT
  - Choanal narrowing by medially bowed posterior maxilla/pterygoid & thickened vomer
  - Narrow gap between maxilla & vomer is bridged by continuous bony plate or membrane
    - Membranous atresia may be thin/strand-like or thick/plug-like
  - Air-fluid level is frequently present in obstructed nasal passage
    - Nasal cavity may also be filled with soft tissue, hypertrophied inferior turbinates

Imaging Recommendations

- Best imaging tool
  - High-resolution unenhanced bone CT
- Protocol advice
  - Suction secretions from nasal cavity prior to scanning
  - Axial images are angled 5° cephalad to palate
    - If angle is too great, region of choanae at level of skull base creates false appearance of choanal atresia
  - Edge enhancement bone kernel helps delineate bone margins in partially ossified skull base
  - Multiplanar reformations as needed
  - 3D reconstructions may be helpful for clinical decision making & surgical planning

DIFFERENTIAL DIAGNOSIS

Choanal Stenosis

- Posterior nasal airway narrowed (not completely occluded)

Pyriform Aperture Stenosis

- Narrowed anterior inferior nasal passage(s)
- Thickened anteromedial maxilla(e)
- ± single central megaincisor
- Must evaluate brain for holoprosencephaly

Nasolacrimal Duct Mucocele

- Bilobed cystic mass extending from medial orbital nasolacrimal fossa to inferior meatus

PATHOLOGY

General Features

- Associated abnormalities
  - Syndromes are common in bilateral atresia (up to 75%)
    - CHARGE syndrome: **C**oloboma, **h**eart defect, choanal **a**tresia, **r**estricted growth, **g**enitourinary & **e**ar defects
  - Unilateral choanal atresia is more likely to be isolated

CLINICAL ISSUES

Presentation

- Most common signs/symptoms
  - Bilateral choanal atresia: Respiratory distress in newborn
    - Infants normally breathe through nose (obligate nasal breathers) until 6 months of age
    - Aggravated by feeding, relieved by crying
  - Unilateral choanal atresia or stenosis: Chronic, purulent, unilateral rhinorrhea in older child
  - Inability to pass nasogastric tube through nasal cavity beyond 3-4 cm despite aerated lungs on radiograph

Treatment

- Establish oral airway immediately for proper breathing
- Membranous atresia may be perforated upon passage of nasogastric tube
- Surgery will alleviate respiratory symptoms

DIAGNOSTIC CHECKLIST

Consider

- Once airway is established, respiratory distress with suspected nasal obstruction in newborn should be evaluated with thin-section bone CT

Image Interpretation Pearls

- Determine if choanal atresia is unilateral or bilateral
- Look for associated anomalies in head & neck

Reporting Tips

- Describe choanal atresia as
  - Unilateral or bilateral
  - Mixed membranous/bony or purely bony
    - Comment on thickness of atretic bone plate

SELECTED REFERENCES

1. Galluzzi F et al: Congenital bony nasal cavity stenosis: a review of current trends in diagnosis and treatment. Int J Pediatr Otorhinolaryngol. 144:110670, 2021
2. Messineo D et al: Radiological parameters review for choanal atresia. Pediatr Rep. 13(2):302-11, 2021
3. Moreddu E et al: International Pediatric Otolaryngology Group (IPOG) consensus recommendations: diagnosis, pre-operative, operative and post-operative pediatric choanal atresia care. Int J Pediatr Otorhinolaryngol. 123:151-5, 2019
4. Moreddu E et al: Prognostic factors and management of patients with choanal atresia. J Pediatr. 204:234-9.e1, 2019

KEY FACTS

TERMINOLOGY

- Lymphatic malformation (LM): Subtype of slow-/low-flow congenital vascular malformation composed of embryonic lymphatic sacs; not neoplastic
- Composed of macrocysts > 1 cm &/or microcysts < 1 cm

IMAGING

- Macrocystic LM: Multiloculated, cystic neck mass with imperceptible wall, thin septations, & fluid-fluid levels
- Microcystic LM: Ill-defined, infiltrative, &/or solid-appearing
- Transspatial, often crosses midline extensively
- Insinuates between vessels & other normal structures
- US: Cysts can show varying degrees of ↑ echogenicity; Doppler shows no significant internal vascularity
- T2 FS/STIR MR: Hyperintense, frequent fluid-fluid levels
    - Best defines extent, relationship to airway & vessels
- T1 FS C+ MR: No significant or minimal rim enhancement
    - Must compare with precontrast T1, as hemorrhage & protein often show hyperintensity

TOP DIFFERENTIAL DIAGNOSES

- 2nd branchial cleft anomaly
- Thyroglossal duct cyst
- Abscess
- Thymic cyst
- Teratoma
- Neurofibroma
- Soft tissue sarcoma

CLINICAL ISSUES

- Nontender, compressible mass
    - Present since birth, grows commensurate with patient
    - May not be clinically apparent until hemorrhage, infection, or hormonal stimulation → rapid ↑ in size
- Depending on size & extent, treatment options primarily include resection, sclerotherapy (for macrocysts), & sirolimus
    - Staged combination therapy is often required

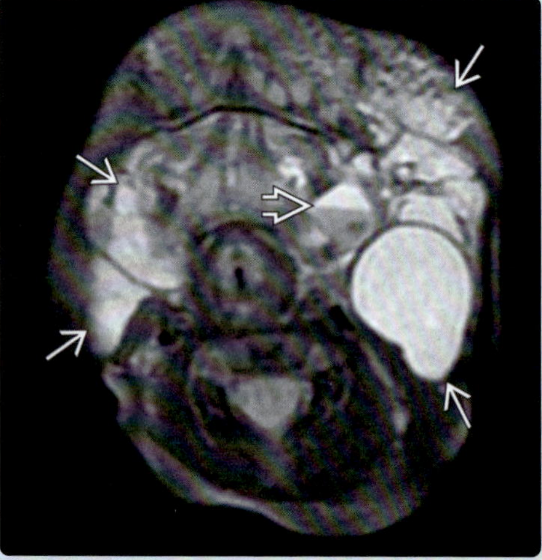

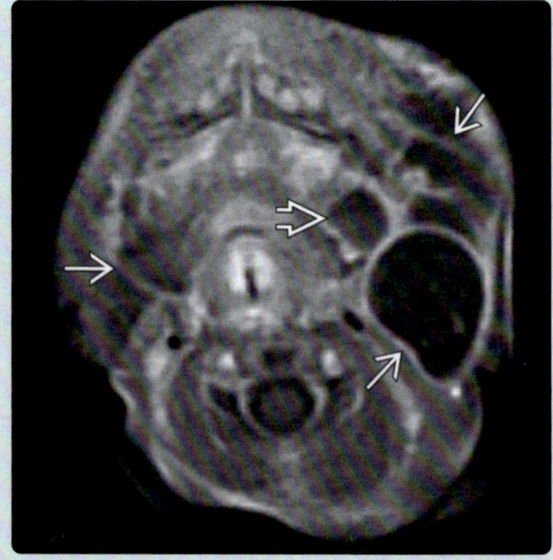

(Left) *Axial T2 FS MR in a 1-week-old infant demonstrates a multiloculated, mixed micro- & macrocystic, transspatial lymphatic malformation (LM) ➡ involving the left anterior neck more than the right. A single fluid-fluid level is present in a left-sided submandibular macrocyst ➡, typical of layering blood products.* **(Right)** *Axial T1 C+ FS MR in the same patient shows a typical appearance of an extensive LM. The macrocysts show only mild peripheral enhancement ➡, & the fluid-fluid level is much more difficult to discern ➡.*

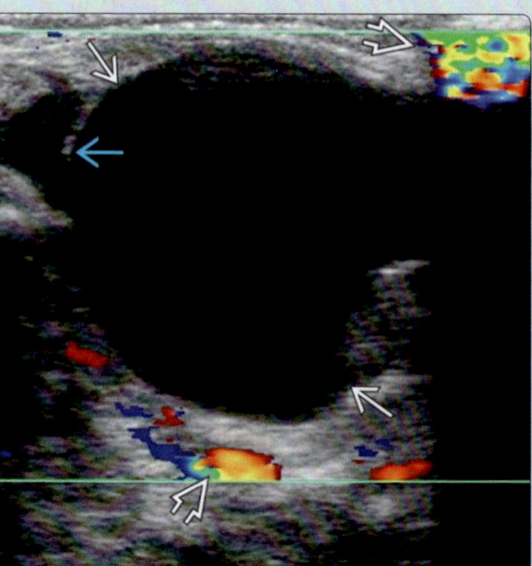

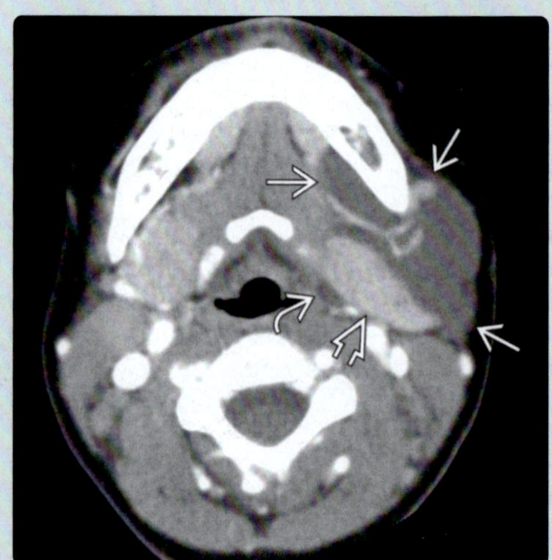

(Left) *Transverse color Doppler ultrasound in an infant with a macrocystic LM shows the typical anechoic nature of the dominant cyst ➡ with vessels ➡ identified adjacent to, but not within, the cyst. Note the thin septation ➡ peripherally.* **(Right)** *Axial CECT in a 3-year-old shows a well-defined, hypodense, macrocystic LM ➡ in the sublingual & submandibular spaces, moderately flattening the left submandibular gland ➡. There is also minimal extension deep to the left submandibular gland ➡.*

TERMINOLOGY

Definitions

- Lymphatic malformation (LM): Subtype of slow-/low-flow congenital vascular malformation composed of embryonic lymphatic sacs; not neoplastic
  - No communication with normal lymphatics
  - Composed of macrocysts > 1 cm &/or microcysts < 1 cm
- Venolymphatic malformation (VLM): Combined elements of venous malformation & LM

IMAGING

General Features

- Best diagnostic clue
  - Macrocystic LM: Multiloculated, cystic neck mass with imperceptible wall, thin septations, & fluid-fluid levels
  - Microcystic LM: More ill-defined, infiltrative, &/or solid-appearing
  - Crosses tissue planes, insinuating between vessels & other normal structures

Ultrasonographic Findings

- Unilocular vs. septated & multilocular transspatial mass
- Contents are predominantly hypo- or anechoic
  - Separate compartments in multicystic mass can show varying degrees of ↑ echogenicity
    - ± swirling debris &/or layering fluid-debris levels
- No true vascular flow in cysts by Doppler
  - ± flow (from encased normal vessels) in septations

MR Findings

- T1WI
  - Primarily hypointense fluid; hyperintense if prior hemorrhage or high protein content (± fluid-fluid levels)
- T2 FS or STIR
  - High-signal contents with thin, low-signal septa
    - Fluid-fluid levels in multiple cysts are very common
  - When transspatial, often poorly marginated
- T1WI C+ FS
  - No significant enhancement (± subtle rim enhancement)
  - Patchy enhancement suggests venolymphatic malformation (VLM) or microcystic LM

Imaging Recommendations

- Best imaging tool
  - Ultrasound is often diagnostic of superficial components
  - MR is better for defining deep extent & recognizing characteristic fluid-fluid levels
- Protocol advice
  - Fluid-sensitive sequences (T2 FS or STIR) are essential
  - T1 C+ FS is helpful to detect venous malformation component of mixed lesions: Subtraction of precontrast T1 FS improves assessment of true enhancement

DIFFERENTIAL DIAGNOSIS

2nd Branchial Cleft Anomaly

- Ovoid, unilocular cyst at angle of mandible with characteristic displacement pattern

Abscess

- Fluid collection with thick, enhancing, irregular wall
- Adjacent cellulitis > myositis, fasciitis

Teratoma

- Solid & cystic components are typical ± internal vascularity
- Frequently contain Ca^{2+}; tend to be more firm, unilateral, focal, & exophytic compared to LM

Thyroglossal Duct Cyst

- Anterior midline/paramidline unilocular cystic mass
- Anywhere from tongue base to lower anterior neck

Soft Tissue Sarcoma

- Well-defined, typically solid; rarely predominantly cystic

PATHOLOGY

General Features

- Genetics
  - ± association of anterior neck LM with Turner syndrome & trisomies; aneuploidy & high mortality in posterior midline cystic neck masses (cystic hygroma) of early gestation

Microscopic Features

- Immunohistochemical panel of PROX1, D2-40, VEGFR3, CD31, & CD34 antibodies to differentiate LM from other vascular malformations
  - PROX1 & VEGFR3 are most sensitive, specific

CLINICAL ISSUES

Presentation

- Most common signs/symptoms
  - Nontender, soft, compressible mass
  - Present since birth & grows commensurate with patient
    - May not be clinically apparent until hemorrhage, infection, or hormonal stimulation → rapid ↑ in size
  - Larger lesions are detected prenatally
- Other signs/symptoms: LMs may infiltrate upper airway or cause extrinsic compression

Treatment

- Surgical resection &/or percutaneous sclerotherapy
  - Sclerotherapy is primarily for macrocystic disease
  - Extensive disease often requires combined &/or numerous staged procedures
- Intralesional bleomycin injection for microcystic LM
- Medical therapy with sirolimus
- Tracheostomy for significant airway involvement

SELECTED REFERENCES

1. Abu Ata N et al: Neonatal vascular anomalies manifesting as soft-tissue masses. Pediatr Radiol. ePub, 2021
2. Reis J 3rd et al: Ultrasound evaluation of pediatric slow-flow vascular malformations: practical diagnostic reporting to guide interventional management. AJR Am J Roentgenol. 216(2):494-506, 2021
3. Adams DM et al: Efficacy and safety of sirolimus in the treatment of complicated vascular anomalies. Pediatrics. 137(2):1-10, 2016
4. Wassef M et al: Vascular anomalies classification: recommendations from the International Society for the Study of Vascular Anomalies. Pediatrics. 136(1):e203-14, 2015
5. Elluru RG et al: Lymphatic malformations: diagnosis and management. Semin Pediatr Surg. 23(4):178-85, 2014
6. ISSVA Classification for Vascular Anomalies. Published April 2014. Updated May 2018. Accessed May 11, 2021. https://www.issva.org/UserFiles/file/ISSVA-Classification-2018.pdf

Congenital High Airway Obstruction Syndrome

KEY FACTS

TERMINOLOGY

- Rare congenital anomaly of airway with complete intrinsic laryngeal &/or tracheal obstruction
- Results in dysfunctional & hyperexpanded lungs, everted hemidiaphragms, & cardiac/venous compression with ascites/hydrops

IMAGING

- Diffusely enlarged lungs, flattened/everted diaphragm
  - Prenatal imaging: Echogenic (US) or T2-hyperintense (MR) lungs with dilated, fluid-filled trachea inferior to obstructing lesion, ± polyhydramnios
  - Site of obstruction appears as persistent short or long segment of absent airway fluid at or below glottis
- Centralized, compressed heart
- Limited motion of abnormal diaphragm
- Abdominal distention with large volume of ascites
- Findings are lessened with stenosis, membrane perforation, or fistula (as each enables airway decompression)

PATHOLOGY

- Most commonly due to laryngeal membrane or atresia
  - Obstruction prevents clearance of fluid from lungs
  - ↑ tracheal & lung pressures cause hyperexpansion & maldevelopment
- 50% have additional anomalies

CLINICAL ISSUES

- Presentations
  - In utero: Large, bilateral, echogenic lungs + ascites
  - At birth: Respiratory distress, aphonia, & failed intubation
    - Lethal at delivery without prenatal detection
- Ex utero intrapartum therapy (EXIT) procedure: Controlled delivery with airway secured via tracheostomy while placental circulation is maintained
  - Improves survival at delivery
  - Respiratory function remains poor
  - Survival > 1 year ~ 20% with high morbidity

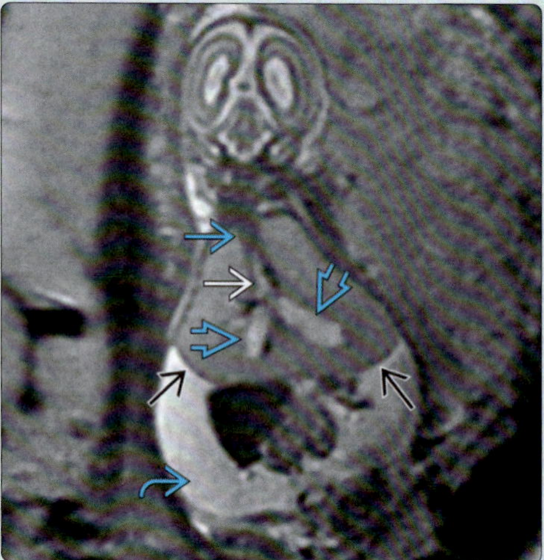

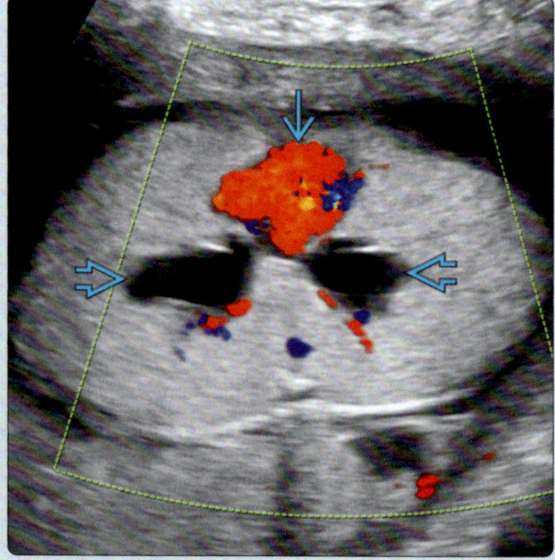

(Left) *Coronal SSFSE T2 MR of a 20-weeks-gestation fetus shows the classic features of congenital high airway obstruction syndrome (CHAOS), including uniform hyperexpansion of the lungs, everted hemidiaphragms ➡, & ascites ➡. There is a long-segment tracheal occlusion ➡ with dilation of the lower thoracic trachea ➡ & central airways ➡.* **(Right)** *Transverse color Doppler US of the same fetus at 20-weeks gestation shows compression of the heart ➡ by the enlarged hyperechoic lungs. Note the dilated central airways ➡.*

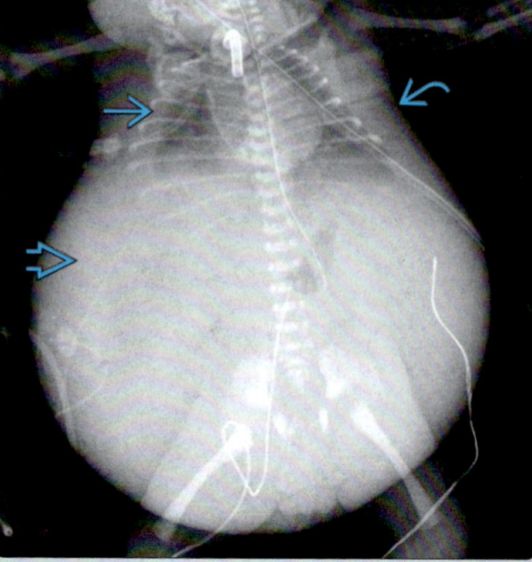

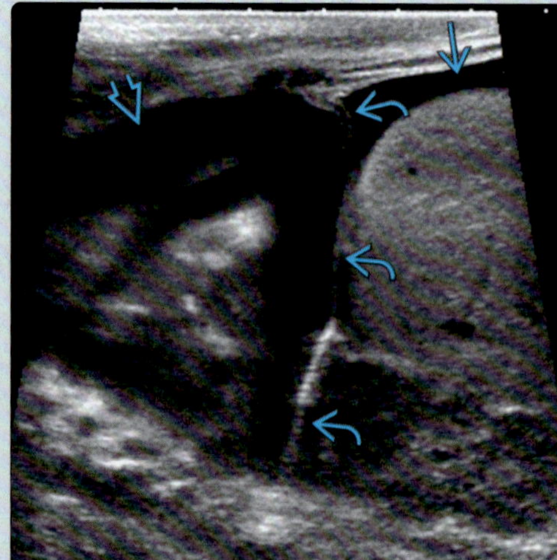

(Left) *Coronal AP radiograph of a newborn with CHAOS shows marked abdominal distention ➡ (due to ascites), a pleural effusion ➡, & chest wall edema ➡, consistent with hydrops. The hemidiaphragms are flattened. A tracheostomy was placed during an EXIT procedure.* **(Right)** *Right parasagittal US of the lower thorax/upper abdomen in the same patient shows an abnormal, everted, & lax diaphragm ➡, which did not move during the exam. The pleural effusion ➡ & ascites ➡ are noted.*

Tracheal Agenesis

KEY FACTS

TERMINOLOGY

- Rare, highly lethal anomaly with absence of majority of trachea from subglottis to main bronchi

IMAGING

- Uncommon detection prenatally, as majority of cases have fistula from residual lower airway to intact esophagus
  - Allows decompression of otherwise obstructed lungs
  - May only demonstrate polyhydramnios in utero
    - If airway anomaly is suspected, MR is performed due to superior in utero airway evaluation vs. ultrasound
  - Minority of cases have no fistula, presenting as CHAOS
    - Lacks dilated, fluid-filled trachea of CHAOS
- Postnatally, temporary ventilation occurs via fistula
  - Low lung volumes with patchy opacities of atelectasis or aspiration
  - Low origin of horizontally oriented main bronchi
  - Endotracheal tube (ETT) lies in midline esophagus, possibly below expected location of carina
  - Nasogastric tube (NGT) may curve into main bronchi

PATHOLOGY

- Classification by Floyd (most widely used): Types I-III
  - I: Absent proximal trachea; short distal trachea + TEF
  - II: Absent trachea; residual carina with main bronchi ± bronchoesophageal fistula
  - III: Absent trachea & carina; main bronchi arise from esophagus
- Associated anomalies in up to 94%

CLINICAL ISSUES

- Inability to conduct air at delivery → aphonia & insufficient ventilation; intubation is difficult
- Highly lethal due to lack of sustainable conduit for air transit from glottis to lungs
- Long-term tracheal replacement options are sparse
  - Rarely successful reconstruction with esophagus
  - Bioengineered graft material may be future therapy

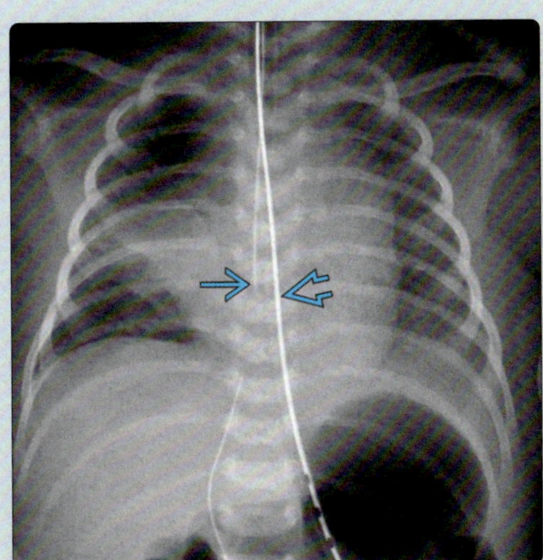

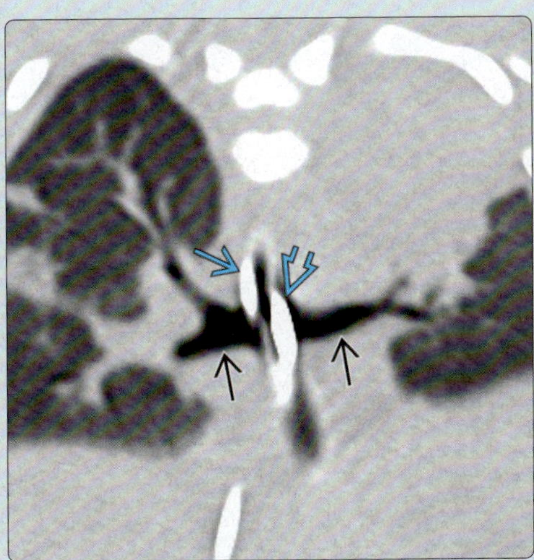

(Left) *AP chest radiograph in a 34-weeks-gestation newborn with cyanosis, aphonia, & poor ventilation at delivery shows the tip of the endotracheal tube (ETT) ➡ in the thoracic midline below the expected level of the carina. The ETT follows a similar course to the nasogastric tube (NGT) ⇨.* **(Right)** *Coronal CECT in the same patient shows horizontal orientation of low-lying main bronchi ➡ that connect to the esophagus. Note that both the NGT ⇨ & low ETT ➡ lie in the esophagus in this patient with complete tracheal agenesis.*

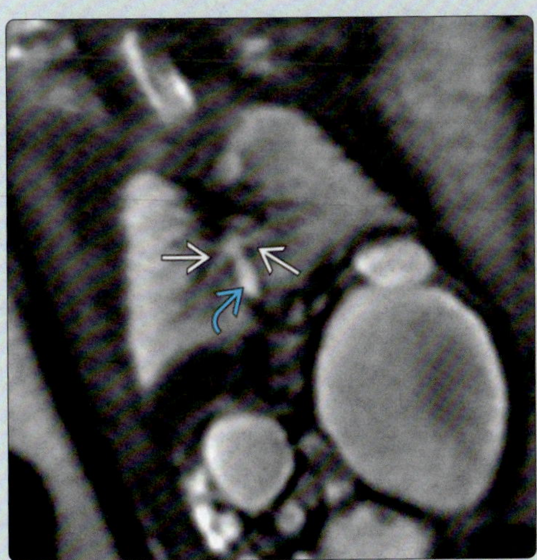

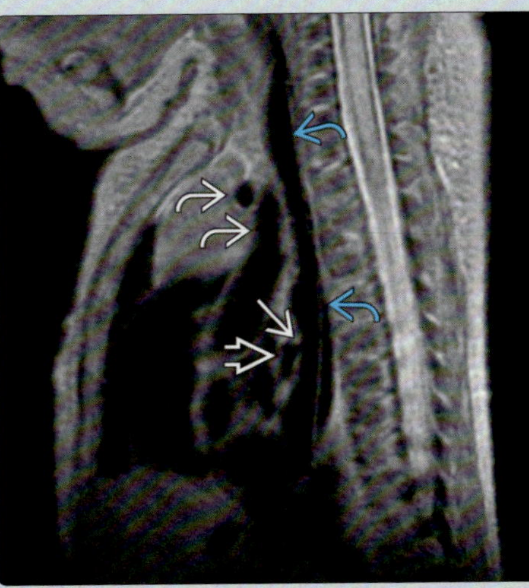

(Left) *Coronal T2 SSFSE MR in a 31-weeks-gestation fetus shows an abnormal connection of the bilateral main bronchi ➡ to the esophagus ↗. No trachea was identified. This fetus had numerous anomalies, including radial ray, genitourinary, gastrointestinal, & cardiac.* **(Right)** *Sagittal PD MR in a 34-weeks-gestation newborn shows a fistula ➡ from the carina ⇨ to the esophagus ↗. Vessels ↗ are seen anterior to the esophagus without a discernible trachea, consistent with tracheal agenesis.*

Epiglottitis

KEY FACTS

TERMINOLOGY

- Airway obstruction secondary to inflammation of epiglottis & surrounding tissues

IMAGING

- Frontal & lateral radiographs are only obtained in stable patients with questionable diagnosis
  - Child should be kept upright & comfortable
  - Patient may drool due to difficulty handling oral secretions: Should not be agitated or placed supine
- Lateral radiograph
  - Marked thickening with loss of sharp posterior margin of central epiglottis thumbprint shape/appearance
  - Thickening of aryepiglottic folds
    - Extend from epiglottis anterosuperiorly to arytenoid cartilages posteroinferiorly
    - May become thickened & convex superiorly
    - Swelling of these folds → actual airway obstruction
- Frontal radiograph
  - ± symmetric, subglottic tracheal narrowing, similar to that seen in croup
  - Swelling of epiglottis & aryepiglottic folds is often not seen on frontal view; may be visualized through foramen magnum
- CT does not play routine role in diagnosing epiglottitis

CLINICAL ISSUES

- Marked ↓ in incidence in children since vaccine for *Haemophilus influenzae* introduced
  - Mean age in children has shifted from 3.5 to 14.6 years
    - Now more common in adults than children
  - Many other infectious & noninfectious etiologies are now implicated
- Classically life-threatening if untreated; treatment includes
  - Direct laryngoscopy & bronchoscopy with intubation performed in operating room with otolaryngology present
  - Steroids & broad-spectrum IV antibiotic therapy

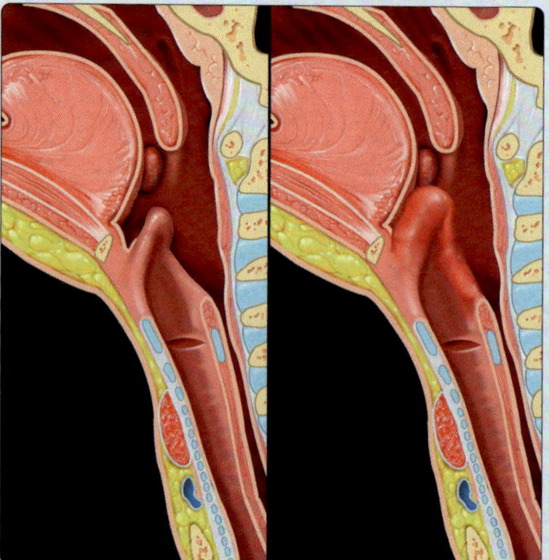

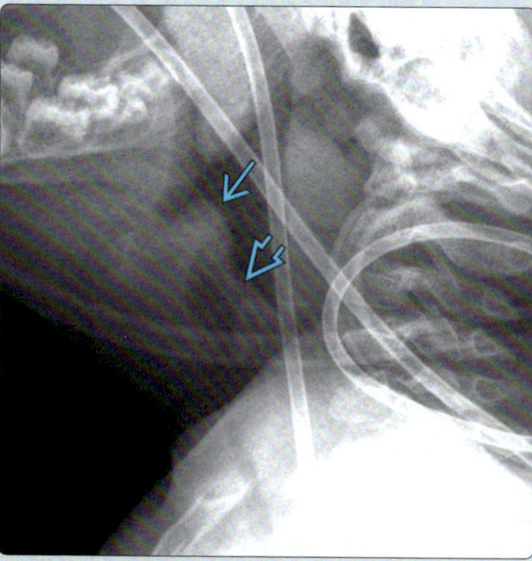

(Left) *Sagittal graphics show epiglottitis (right) as compared with a normal epiglottis (left). The epiglottis & aryepiglottic folds are swollen & diffusely enlarged (right).* **(Right)** *Lateral radiograph in a 13-month-old with stridor shows thickening of the epiglottis ➡ with loss of the normal sharp, central, posterior margin. There is thickening of the aryepiglottic folds ⇨ as well. At scope, exudates & inflammation were visualized. Cultures grew Staphylococcus aureus.*

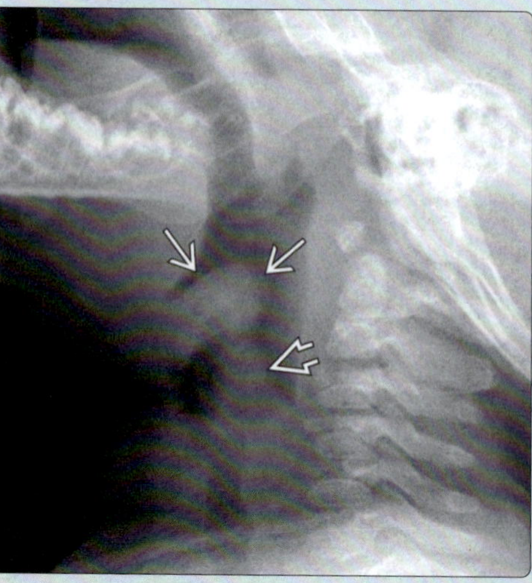

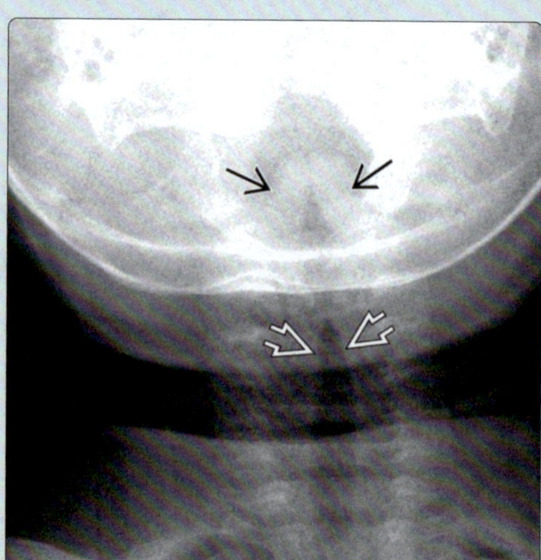

(Left) *Lateral radiograph in a 6-month-old shows marked thickening of the epiglottis ➡ & the aryepiglottic folds ⇨, typical of epiglottitis.* **(Right)** *AP radiograph in the same patient shows thickening of the epiglottis & aryepiglottic folds ➡ seen through the skull base/foramen magnum. There is mild subglottic narrowing ⇨, which can be seen in varying degrees with epiglottitis.*

TERMINOLOGY

Synonyms

- Supraglottitis

Definitions

- Airway obstruction secondary to inflammation of epiglottis & surrounding tissues

IMAGING

General Features

- Best diagnostic clue
  - Classic imaging appearance: Lateral radiograph shows enlargement/thickening of epiglottis & aryepiglottic folds
    - Epiglottis often appears like thumbprint (or frontal perspective of thumb with nail en face to x-ray beam)
  - Not to be confused with normal epiglottis
    - May appear similar to hitchhiker thumb (or lateral perspective of thumb with nail tangential to x-ray beam)
    - Epiglottis maintains sharp interfaces with well-defined, central posterior border; no thickening of aryepiglottic folds
- Location
  - Potentially life-threatening inflammation & swelling of epiglottis & surrounding tissues (i.e., aryepiglottic folds)
- Morphology
  - Swelling of epiglottitis → thumbprint appearance on lateral radiograph

Radiographic Findings

- Lateral radiograph
  - Marked thickening of epiglottis with loss of sharp, central posterior margin
  - Aryepiglottic folds
    - Extend from epiglottis anterosuperiorly to arytenoid cartilages posteroinferiorly
    - Normally thin & straight or concave (apex inferior), outlined by air
    - May become thickened & convex
    - Swelling of these folds causes actual airway obstruction
  - ± nonspecific "ballooning" (air distention) of hypopharynx
- Frontal radiograph
  - Only lateral radiograph is obtained if epiglottitis is highly suspected
    - Supine positioning of ill patient could lead to airway occlusion
  - ± symmetric, subglottic narrowing, similar to that seen in croup
  - Swelling of epiglottis & aryepiglottic folds may not be seen on frontal view
    - May see swollen epiglottis through skull base

Ultrasonographic Findings

- Limited studies describe findings on point-of-care-ultrasound (POCUS)
- ↑ AP dimension of epiglottis
  - Some overlap in measurement at midpoint between control & epiglottitis groups: 3.4 mm is upper limit of normal
  - No overlap in measurement at lateral margins between control (upper limit of normal is 3.2 mm) & epiglottitis groups (≥ 3.6 mm)

CT Findings

- CECT
  - CT has no role in diagnosing epiglottitis
  - If obtained (occasionally for other reasons), will show edematous, enlarged epiglottis with involvement of aryepiglottic folds
    - Epiglottis is slightly lower in attenuation when compared with other soft tissue
  - In rare cases, may see phlegmonous collection within adjacent soft tissues
  - May be helpful in evaluating for complications, such as deep neck space infection/abscess
    - Very rare in pediatric population as opposed to adult population where it can be seen in 2-29% of cases

Imaging Recommendations

- Best imaging tool
  - Due to potentially life-threatening airway emergency, unstable patients with classic clinical presentation undergo direct laryngoscopy & bronchoscopy with intubation in operating room by otolaryngology as indicated
  - Only lateral radiograph should be obtained in cases suspecting epiglottis
- Protocol advice
  - Child should be upright & comfortable
  - Patient may drool due to difficulty handling oral secretions; patient should not be agitated or placed supine
  - Patient with suspected epiglottitis should be accompanied by physician with readily available supportive equipment to secure airway if necessary
  - Obtaining lateral radiograph should never interfere with securing airway given potential for rapidly fatal outcome

DIFFERENTIAL DIAGNOSIS

Enlarged Lingual Tonsils

- Rounded &/or lobulated mass bulging from posterior tongue base, potentially filling vallecula & displacing epiglottis

Vallecular Mass

- Most commonly cyst but rarely sarcoma
- Fills vallecula, potentially displacing or effacing epiglottis depending on exact site of origin

Croup

- Most common acute airway condition of children
- Benign, self-limited condition with "barky" cough in patients usually < 3 years of age
- Symmetric subglottic tracheal narrowing (steeple sign)

Bacterial Tracheitis

- Children are typically older than those with croup

- Intraluminal filling defects (membranes), tracheal wall plaque-like irregularity, poorly defined tracheal margins, asymmetric subglottic narrowing

Retropharyngeal Abscess

- Pyogenic infection of retropharyngeal space
- Persistent thickening of retropharyngeal soft tissues despite inspiration & neck extension on lateral view
  - ± loss of normal step-off at junction of hypopharynx & esophagus

Ω Epiglottis

- Normal variant found in young infants, observed at scope (not on radiographs)
- Leads to laryngomalacia in association with short aryepiglottic folds & prolapsing arytenoids

PATHOLOGY

General Features

- Etiology
  - Most common agent remains *Haemophilus influenzae*
    - Dramatic changes in incidence, etiology, & patient demographics since *H. influenzae* (HiB) vaccine introduction
    - More cases of epiglottitis resulting from other bacterial, viral, or combined viral-bacterial infections are now seen since introduction of HiB vaccination
      - Other organisms include group A β-hemolytic *Streptococcus, Staphylococcus aureus, Klebsiella pneumoniae, Moraxella catarrhalis, Pseudomonas* species, *Candida albicans, Pasteurella multocida*, & *Neisseria* species, COVID-19, influenza
      - Bacterial superinfections of preceding viral infections, such as herpes simplex, parainfluenzae, varicella-zoster, & EBV
  - Can also occur from noninfectious etiologies, such as allergic reaction, angioneurotic edema, mucositis, trauma, Stevens-Johnson syndrome, caustic ingestion, & vaping

Gross Pathologic & Surgical Features

- Marked inflammation & edema of epiglottis & aryepiglottic folds
- Complete airway obstruction may occur at any time

CLINICAL ISSUES

Presentation

- Most common signs/symptoms
  - Abrupt onset of stridor (usually inspiratory), often associated with dysphagia
- Other signs/symptoms
  - High fever, sore throat, dysphonia, "hot potato voice," hoarseness, & drooling
  - Patients have toxic appearance with fever
  - Patients are described as anxious & uncomfortable
  - ↑ respiratory distress when recumbent
  - May have characteristic "tripod position" (sitting up with neck extended & leaning forward with jaw thrust out to maximize laryngeal opening)
  - Viral prodrome & cough are more likely with croup

Demographics

- Age
  - Marked ↓ in incidence in children since HiB vaccine introduced
    - 0.6-0.8 cases /100,000 persons immunized
    - Vaccine effectiveness 98%
  - Mean age in children has shifted from 3.5 years to 14.6 years since introduction of HiB vaccine
    - Significantly older than children with croup (mean age: 1 year)
  - Adult incidence has remained steady (although relatively uncommon) post vaccine
  - Now more common in adults than children (mean age: 40 years)

Natural History & Prognosis

- Classically: Life-threatening infectious disease often requiring emergent intubation
- Current era: May not be as clinically emergent given variety of non *Haemophilus influenzae* etiologies

Treatment

- In correct clinical setting: Emergent tracheal intubation to relieve/prevent airway obstruction & respiratory failure
  - Has evolved from tracheotomy to direct laryngoscopy & bronchoscopy with intubation performed in operating room with otolaryngology present
  - Intubation period is usually short (2-3 days)
- Steroids & broad-spectrum IV antibiotic therapy

DIAGNOSTIC CHECKLIST

Image Interpretation Pearls

- In current era, classic radiographic appearance must be coupled with clinical presentation to determine treatment

SELECTED REFERENCES

1. Almuzam S et al: Non-vaccine Haemophilus influenzae type a epiglottitis. J Paediatr Child Health. 57(7):1133-5, 2020
2. Bozzella MJ et al: Epiglottitis associated with intermittent e-cigarette use: the vagaries of vaping toxicity. Pediatrics. 145(3), 2020
3. Fondaw A et al: COVID-19 infection presenting with acute epiglottitis. J Surg Case Rep. 2020(9):rjaa280, 2020
4. Gottlieb M et al: Ultrasound for airway management: an evidence-based review for the emergency clinician. Am J Emerg Med. 38(5):1007-13, 2020
5. Sideris A et al: A systematic review and meta-analysis of predictors of airway intervention in adult epiglottitis. Laryngoscope. 130(2):465-73, 2020
6. Villemure-Poliquin N et al: Necrotizing epiglottitis with necrotizing fasciitis in a child: a case report and review of literature. Int J Pediatr Otorhinolaryngol. 138:110385, 2020
7. Inaguma Y et al: Thermal epiglottitis: acute airway obstruction caused by ingestion of hot food. Pediatr Int. 61(9):927-9, 2019
8. O'Bryant SC et al: Influenza A-associated epiglottitis and compensatory pursed lip breathing in an infant. Pediatr Emerg Care. 35(11):e213-6, 2019
9. Ho ML et al: The ABCs (airway, blood vessels, and compartments) of pediatric neck infections and masses. AJR Am J Roentgenol. 1-10, 2016
10. Lichtor JL et al: Epiglottitis: it hasn't gone away. Anesthesiology. 124(6):1404-7, 2016
11. Darras KE et al: Imaging acute airway obstruction in infants and children. Radiographics. 35(7):2064-79, 2015
12. Ko DR et al: Use of bedside sonography for diagnosing acute epiglottitis in the emergency department: a preliminary study. J Ultrasound Med. 31(1):19-22, 2012
13. Shah RK et al: Epiglottitis in the United States: national trends, variances, prognosis, and management. Laryngoscope. 120(6):1256-62, 2010

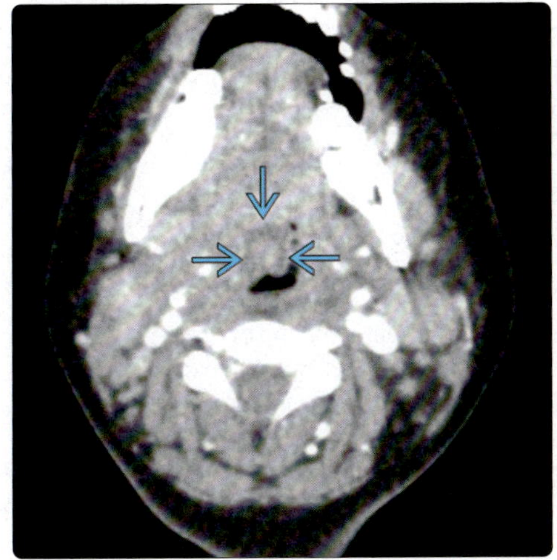

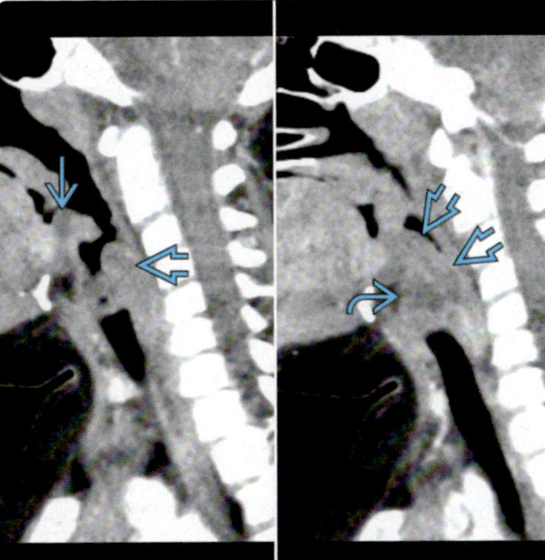

(Left) *Axial CECT in a 9-year-old with a sore throat & fever shows a thickened, edematous epiglottis* ➙. **(Right)** *Sagittal midline (left) & paramidline (right) CECT images in the same patient show the edematous epiglottis* ➙, *aryepiglottic folds* ➙, & *adjacent supraglottic tissues* ➙. *Note the upward convexity of the aryepiglottic folds. No organism was able to be cultured in this infection.*

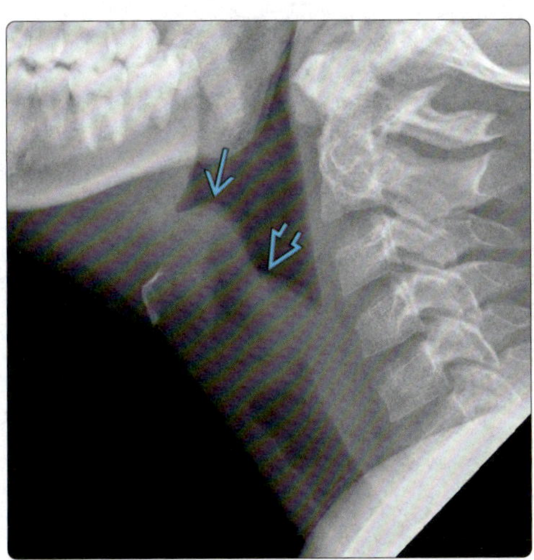

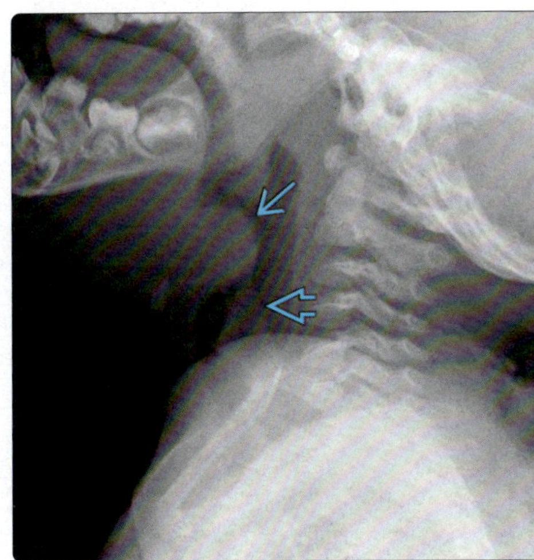

(Left) *Lateral radiograph of the airway in a 13-year-old with lymphoma shows thickening of the epiglottis* ➙ *& aryepiglottic folds* ➙, *consistent with epiglottitis, likely due to chemotherapy-related mucositis in this case.* **(Right)** *Lateral airway radiograph in an 18-month-old with epiglottitis shows a markedly enlarged epiglottis* ➙ *with poorly defined margins. The right aryepiglottic fold* ➙ *was thickened at laryngoscopy. The patient was subsequently intubated.*

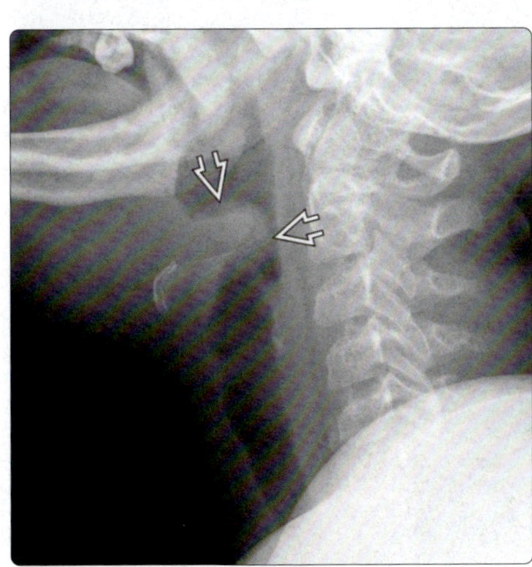

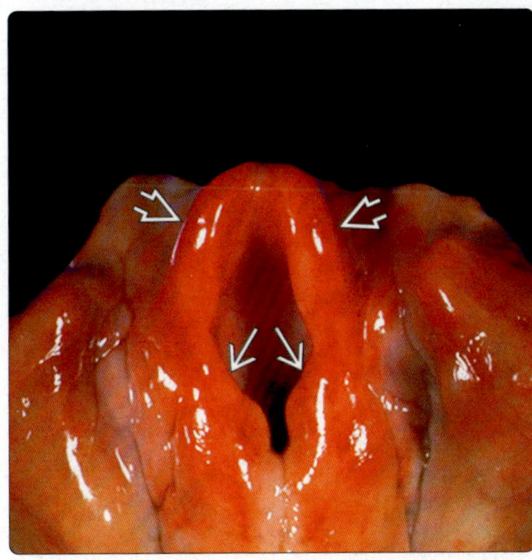

(Left) *Lateral airway radiograph shows epiglottitis as a markedly swollen & poorly defined epiglottis* ➙ *that has a thumbprint appearance in a patient with congenital insensitivity to pain.* **(Right)** *Gross pathology image from a deceased patient shows an inflamed & edematous epiglottis* ➙ *with swollen aryepiglottic folds* ➙. *It is the swelling of the aryepiglottic folds that leads to airway obstruction.*

Croup

KEY FACTS

TERMINOLOGY

- Benign, self-limited viral inflammation of upper airway
- Subglottic edema results in stridor & characteristic "barky" cough

IMAGING

- Radiographs are used to exclude more serious causes of stridor (rather than diagnosing croup)
- Frontal view: Best for typical findings of croup
  - Smooth, symmetric, long-segment narrowing of subglottic airway gradually widens to normal-caliber trachea
    - Steeple or inverted V configuration
    - Loss of normal short-segment "shoulders" of subglottic trachea secondary to edema
- Lateral view: Best for excluding other diagnoses
  - Relatively mild narrowing of AP dimension
  - Haziness with loss of subglottic tracheal wall definition
  - ± hypopharyngeal overdistention

TOP DIFFERENTIAL DIAGNOSES

- Foreign body
- Vascular ring
- Bacterial tracheitis
- Infantile hemangioma
- Epiglottitis
- Angioedema
- Iatrogenic subglottic stenosis

CLINICAL ISSUES

- Acute clinical syndrome characterized by "barky" or "seal-like" ("croupy") cough, inspiratory stridor, hoarseness
  - Age range: 6 months to 3 years; uncommon > 6 years
- ± prodrome of low-grade fever, mild cough, rhinorrhea
- Majority are due to parainfluenza viruses types 1-3
- Most cases are successfully treated with glucocorticoids ± nebulized epinephrine
- Recurrent episodes or atypical age suggest alternate diagnosis

(Left) *Lateral radiograph in a 9-month-old infant with stridor shows haziness of the subglottic airway* ⇨. *Overdistention (ballooning) of the hypopharynx is noted* ➡. *The epiglottis* ⇨ *& aryepiglottic folds* ⇨ *are normal.* **(Right)** *AP radiograph in the same patient shows symmetric narrowing of the subglottic trachea* ⇨, *typical of croup. The loss of the normal abrupt subglottic/glottic shouldering + gradual tapering of the subglottic airway lumen from inferior to superior is referred to as the steeple sign.*

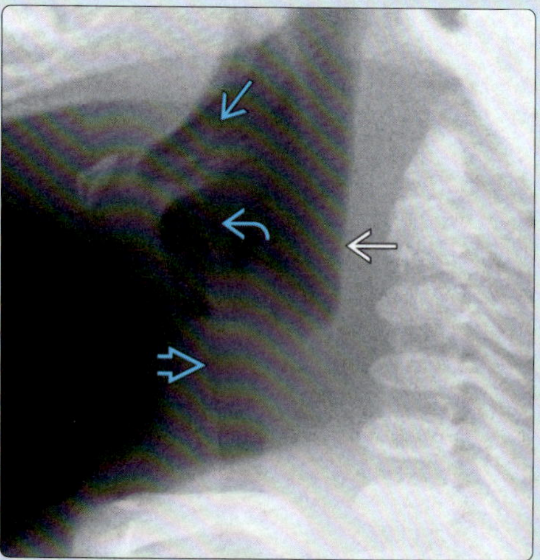

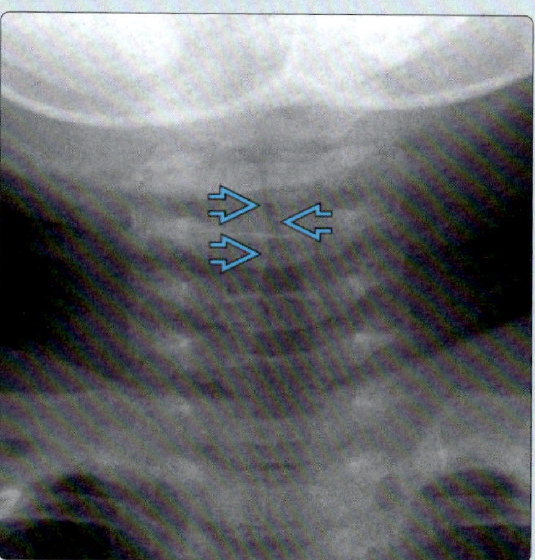

(Left) *Endoscopic photograph shows a normal appearance of the subglottic airway. The subglottis is widely patent such that the mucosa is actually hidden beneath the vocal cords.* **(Right)** *Endoscopic photograph in a child with viral croup shows edematous subglottic mucosa* ➡, *which is visualized through the vocal cords. There is marked narrowing of the subglottic airway lumen, predominantly in the transverse dimension.*

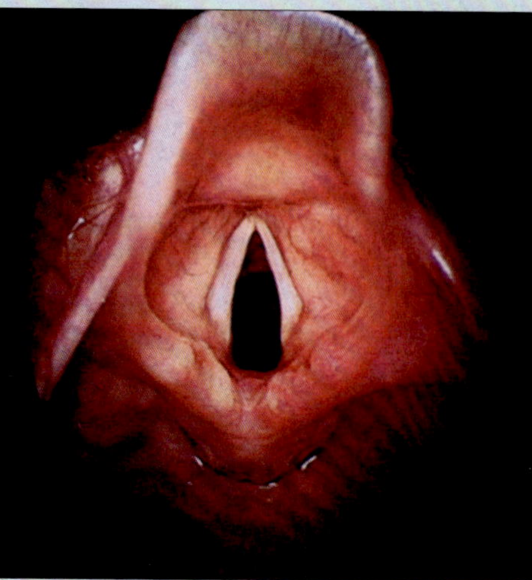

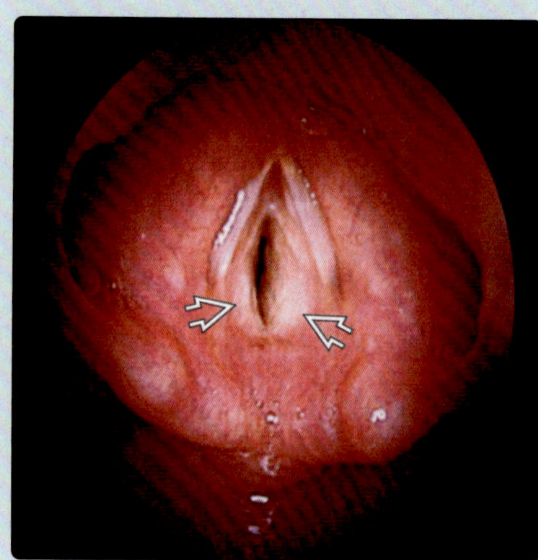

TERMINOLOGY

Synonyms

- Acute laryngotracheitis

Definitions

- Croup: Self-limited viral inflammation of subglottic airway
- Acute laryngotracheobronchitis: Croup + lower airway involvement
- Spasmodic croup: Recurrent episodes, typically without viral prodrome or fever
- Atypical croup: May refer to recurrent episodes, atypical patient age, prolonged/severe episodes, uncommon pathogen

IMAGING

General Features

- Best diagnostic clue
  - Symmetric, subglottic airway tapering/narrowing on frontal radiograph
  - Loss of normal subglottic "shoulders"
- Morphology
  - Normal
    - Uniform caliber of cervical & thoracic trachea from subglottis to carina
    - Normal subglottic "shoulders": Symmetric, focal, convex lateral margins at uppermost subglottic airway
      - Roughly 30-45° from horizontal

Radiographic Findings

- Radiography
  - AP/frontal view
    - Steeple or inverted V configuration of subglottic trachea
      - Smooth, symmetric narrowing of subglottic airway gradually widens to normal-caliber trachea
      - Loss of normal "shoulders" of subglottic trachea secondary to subglottic edema
      - Vertical length of narrowing is variable; ~ upper 1/3 of cervical trachea
  - Lateral view
    - Mild narrowing of subglottic trachea in AP dimension
      - Degree of narrowing is typically much less than narrowing of transverse dimension on frontal view
    - Haziness & poor definition of subglottic tracheal walls
    - ± hypopharyngeal overdistention
      - Also seen at end-inspiration in crying child
      - Hypopharynx may be collapsed with distention of lower cervical trachea on expiratory image
    - Normal epiglottis, aryepiglottic folds, retropharyngeal soft tissues; no foreign body

Imaging Recommendations

- Best imaging tool
  - Diagnosis of croup is primarily clinical
    - Radiographs are used to exclude more serious causes of stridor
      - Atypical or severe course, foreign body concern, recurrent episodes
    - Chest radiographs are sometimes obtained to exclude pneumonia
  - Frontal radiograph is most useful view to confirm croup
  - Lateral radiograph helps exclude other diagnoses
- Protocol advice
  - Ensure that neck is extended with adequate inspiration on lateral view
    - ↓ crowding of airway structures that may simulate disease in young child
  - Avoid image acquisition while child swallows

DIFFERENTIAL DIAGNOSIS

Airway Foreign Body

- Minority of foreign bodies are radiopaque
  - May appear as soft tissue density but with straight, irregular, or pointed margins
- Can lodge anywhere from nasal/oral cavities to bronchi
  - Right main bronchus is most common lower airway site
    - ± asymmetric lung aeration on chest radiographs
- Symptoms & imaging findings depend on location of object
- Esophageal foreign body may cause edema of adjacent trachea, especially if subacute/chronic or button battery ingestion

Vascular Ring

- Intrathoracic tracheal narrowing/deviation
- Double aortic arch, right aortic arch with aberrant left subclavian artery, pulmonary sling

Bacterial Tracheitis

- Typically occurs in older child, 6-10 years old
- May be toxic-appearing
- Intraluminal filling defects (pseudomembranes)
- Plaque-like irregularity &/or poor definition of tracheal walls
- Asymmetric subglottic narrowing

Infantile Hemangioma

- Younger child, often < 6 months
  - Develops in 1st few weeks of life → grows rapidly over 6-12 months → slow, spontaneous regression
- Asymmetric airway narrowing ± focal tracheal wall contour abnormality
- 50% have another visible hemangioma, most commonly of face/neck in "beard distribution"

Epiglottitis

- Typically occurs in older children
  - Historical mean age (pre-Hib vaccine) = 3 years
  - Now teenagers are more common
- Severe, life-threatening condition classically
- Marked enlargement of epiglottis & aryepiglottic folds
  - Loss of sharp posterior margin of central epiglottis on lateral view
- May cause symmetric, subglottic narrowing on frontal view

Thermal Injury

- History of smoke inhalation, burns

Angioedema

- Rapid swelling of facial soft tissues & upper airway
  - ± itching, pain, hives
- May be due to allergic reaction or hereditary angioedema

Iatrogenic Subglottic Stenosis

- History of prolonged or traumatic intubation
- Predisposes to recurrent croup-like episodes

PATHOLOGY

General Features

- Etiology
  - Typical croup is secondary to viral illness
    - Most cases: Parainfluenza viruses types 1-3
    - Less frequently: Respiratory syncytial virus, adenovirus, rhinovirus, enterovirus, influenza, herpes simplex, metapneumoviruses, measles, SARS-CoV-2; bacterial forms are uncommon (consider *Corynebacterium diphtheriae* & *Mycoplasma pneumoniae*)
  - Leads to inflammation & edema of subglottic airway
    - Redundant mucosa predisposes to edema & narrowing
      - Loose mucosal attachment of conus elasticus
    - Cricoid cartilage is complete ring with inability to expand
    - Swelling of vocal cords → hoarseness
    - Characteristic (but not specific) "barky" cough results from inflammation of larynx & trachea
    - Inspiratory stridor is due to proportionately small subglottic trachea in young children
      - Same viral infections & edema do not compromise older child or adult airway
- Associated abnormalities
  - Atypical or spasmodic croup
    - 20-64% incidence of large airway lesions: Subglottic hemangioma, stenosis, laryngeal cleft, laryngeal ulcer, tracheomalacia, laryngomalacia, papillomatosis, laryngeal web, or vocal cord paralysis
    - Additional common disorders in this group: Gastroesophageal reflux, asthma, sleep-disordered breathing, seasonal allergies, chronic cough, prematurity

Staging, Grading, & Classification

- Westley Croup Severity Score (clinical severity score)
  - Mild: Occasional "barky" cough, no stridor at rest, no or mild retractions
  - Moderate: Frequent "barky" cough, stridor at rest, mild to moderate retractions
  - Severe: Moderate criteria + marked retractions, distress, & agitation
  - Impending respiratory failure: Severe criteria + altered mental status, poor air entry, cyanosis or pallor

CLINICAL ISSUES

Presentation

- Most common signs/symptoms
  - Acute clinical syndrome characterized by "barky" or "seal-like" ("croupy") cough, inspiratory stridor, hoarseness, respiratory distress
- Other signs/symptoms
  - Often have prodrome of low-grade fever, mild cough, rhinorrhea
  - Typically non-toxic-appearing & able to manage secretions
  - More severe cases: Intercostal retractions, tachypnea, pallor, cyanosis, tachycardia, altered mental status
  - Symptoms worse at night or with agitation
  - May occur with other symptoms of lower respiratory tract infection (wheezing, cough, etc.)

Demographics

- Age
  - Range: Most common 6 months to 3 years
    - Uncommon > 6 years
    - Mean age of atypical croup: 2.7-4.8 years
  - If > 3 years, consider other causes of acute stridor
  - If < 6 months, consider predisposing abnormality
- Epidemiology
  - Most common cause of acute upper airway obstruction in young children
    - Affects 5% of children by age 2 years
    - Affects 3% of children per year
  - Seasonal occurrence with viral disease: Most prevalent in fall-winter; historically has shown biennial peaks

Natural History & Prognosis

- Typically benign, self-limited disease
- ~ 85% are classified as mild
- 75% of mild cases resolve within 3 days
- 11% of mild & 49% of moderate cases of croup worsen
- 5% return to emergency department within 72 hours

Treatment

- Mild: Often supportive therapy at home
  - Humidified air, antipyretics if febrile, oral fluids
  - Oral glucocorticoid
- Moderate or severe
  - Oral, IV, or IM glucocorticoid + nebulized epinephrine
  - Supportive measures (antipyretics, humidified air, oxygen, oral or IV fluids)
  - Admission for inadequate response to treatment
    - Downward trend in patients requiring inpatient treatment over last several decades
    - < 5% of patients with croup require hospitalization
  - Intubation is rarely needed, should be performed by skilled provider in controlled setting
  - Death is very rare; < 1% of patients requiring intubation

SELECTED REFERENCES

1. Lim CC et al: Croup and COVID-19 in a child: a case report and literature review. BMJ Case Rep. 14(9), 2021
2. Hanna J et al: Epidemiological analysis of croup in the emergency department using two national datasets. Int J Pediatr Otorhinolaryngol. 126:109641, 2019
3. Hanna R et al: Defining atypical croup: a case report and review of the literature. Int J Pediatr Otorhinolaryngol. 127:109686, 2019
4. Smith DK et al: Croup: Diagnosis and management. Am Fam Physician. 97(9):575-80, 2018
5. Darras KE et al: Imaging acute airway obstruction in infants and children. Radiographics. 35(7):2064-79, 2015
6. Hodnett BL et al: Objective endoscopic findings in patients with recurrent croup: 10-year retrospective analysis. Int J Pediatr Otorhinolaryngol. 79(12):2343-7, 2015
7. Petrocheilou A et al: Viral croup: diagnosis and a treatment algorithm. Pediatr Pulmonol. 49(5):421-9, 2014
8. Choi J et al: Common pediatric respiratory emergencies. Emerg Med Clin North Am. 30(2):529-63, x, 2012

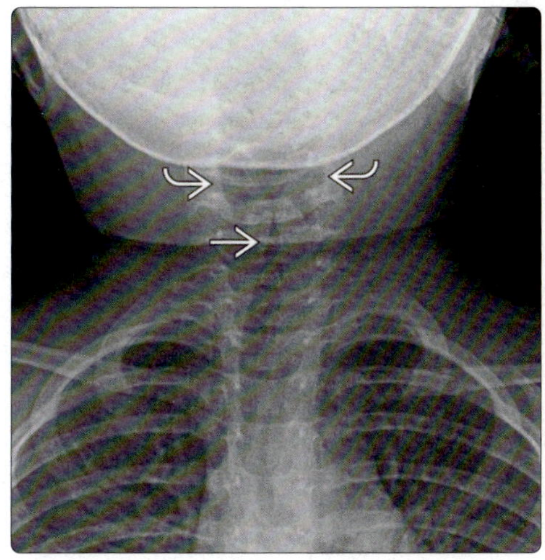

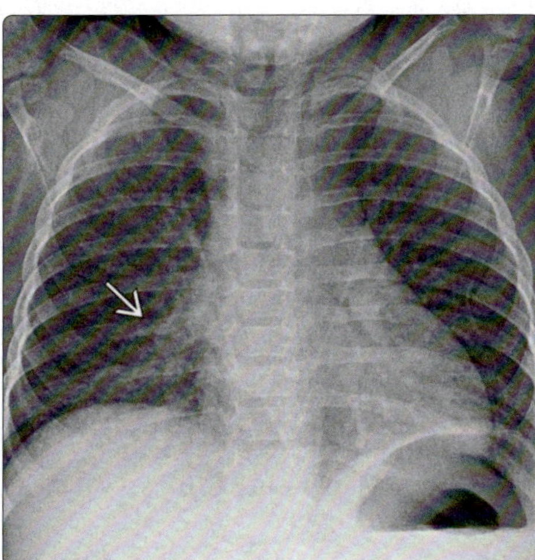

(Left) *AP radiograph in a 2-year-old with stridor shows symmetric subglottic narrowing ➡ & overdistention of the hypopharynx ➡. The trachea is otherwise normal in caliber & position.* **(Right)** *AP radiograph of the chest in the same patient shows patchy airspace opacities in the right middle lobe ➡ due to pneumonia. Chest radiographs may be obtained in children with croup if there is concern for pneumonia. Coexistent upper or lower respiratory tract infection is not uncommon.*

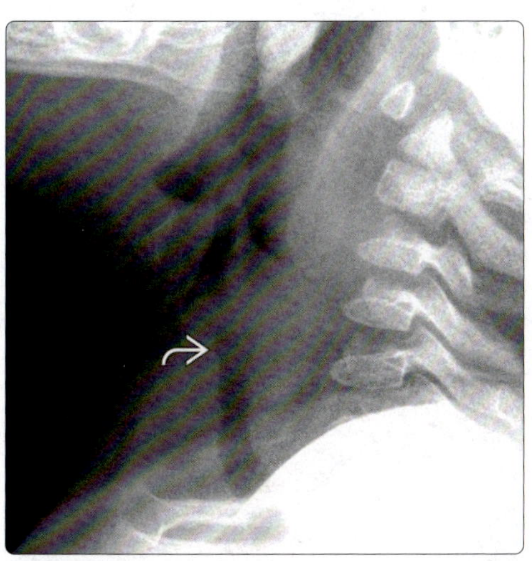

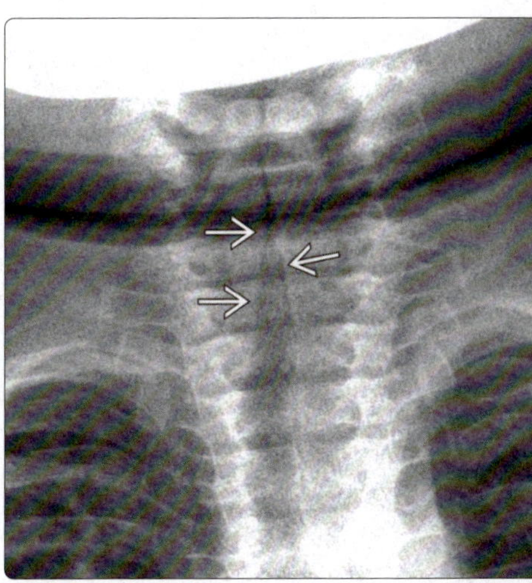

(Left) *Lateral radiograph in an 8-month-old infant with fever & a "barky" cough shows poor definition & haziness of the subglottic airway ➡, a common finding in viral croup.* **(Right)** *AP radiograph in the same patient shows severe narrowing of the subglottic trachea ➡, which gradually tapers from inferior to superior. Note the lack of a focal extrinsic mass or intrinsic filling defect.*

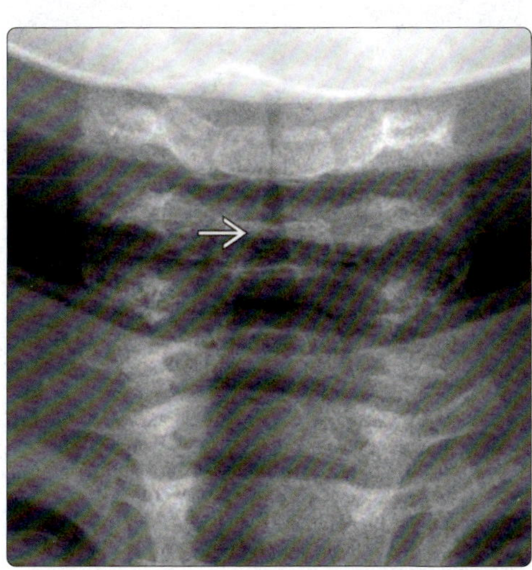

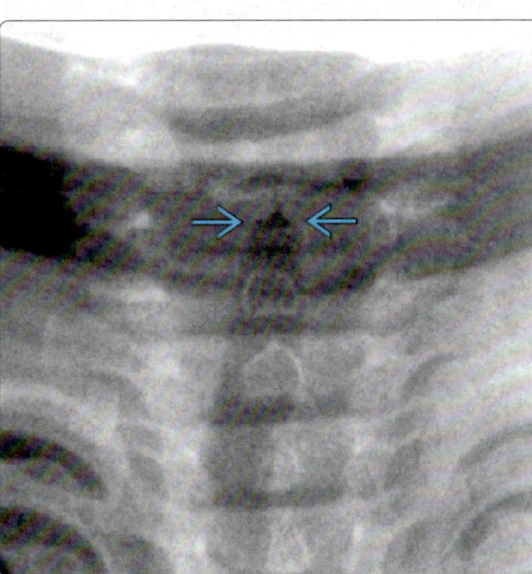

(Left) *AP radiograph in a 16-month-old child with stridor shows symmetric subglottic airway narrowing ➡, typical of viral croup. No focal mass or linear/nodular filling defect is identified.* **(Right)** *AP radiograph in a normal child shows the typical normal "shoulders" ➡ of the subglottic airway, which are more focal & horizontal than the long, gradual, vertical "steepling" seen in croup.*

Bacterial Tracheitis

KEY FACTS

TERMINOLOGY

- Synonyms: Exudative tracheitis, membranous or pseudomembranous croup, membranous laryngotracheobronchitis
- Definition: Purulent infection of trachea
    - Results in thick, adherent exudative plaques along tracheal walls
    - Plaques can slough, leading to airway obstruction
- Controversial disease
    - While many cases with significant morbidity & mortality have been confirmed, questions remain concerning overdiagnosis/overtreatment at some centers

IMAGING

- Characteristic radiographic findings
    - Thin or thick, linear or irregular soft tissue filling defects within airway (visualized pseudomembranes)
    - Loss of smooth, well-defined, parallel tracheal walls + nodular plaque-like irregularity of walls
    - Hazy or indistinct tracheal air column
    - Symmetric or asymmetric subglottic narrowing in acutely ill child older than typically seen with viral croup

TOP DIFFERENTIAL DIAGNOSES

- Epiglottitis
- Croup
- Retropharyngeal abscess
- Upper airway obstruction by foreign body
- Intraluminal secretions

CLINICAL ISSUES

- High-grade fever, cough, severe stridor, rapid onset (2-10 hours) of respiratory distress; often after viral prodrome
    - Mild symptoms are more common in recent papers
- Peak age: 3-8 years (older than classic viral croup)
- Aggressive treatment to prevent airway obstruction, death
    - Flexible laryngoscopy → rigid bronchoscopy, removal of pseudomembranes ± intubation; IV antibiotics

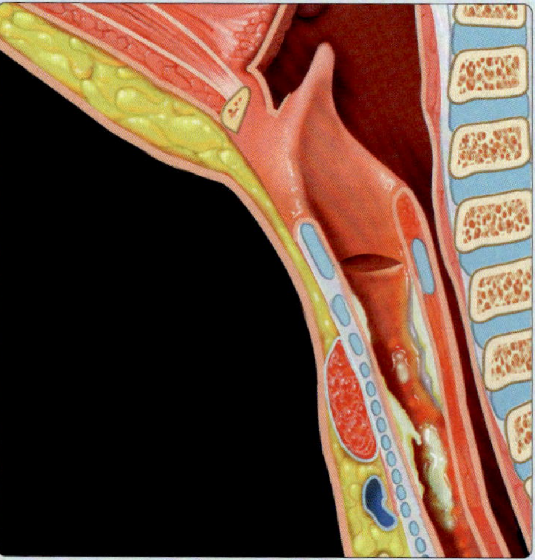

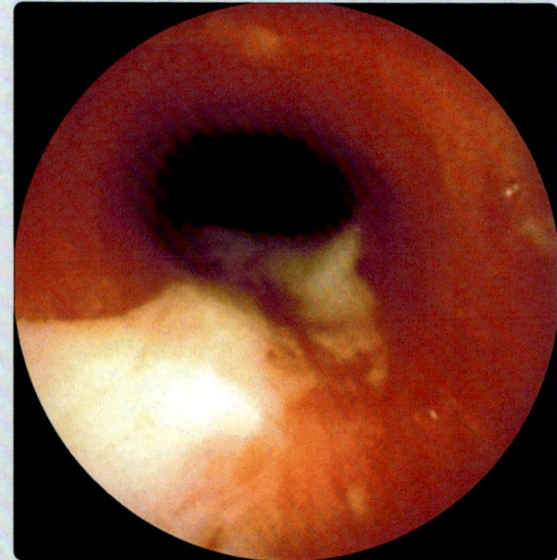

(Left) *Graphic shows inflammation of the trachea with the formation of inflammatory plaques & pseudomembranes along the tracheal walls. These plaques may detach from the tracheal wall & occlude the airway.* **(Right)** *Photograph from bronchoscopic visualization of the trachea in a child with bacterial tracheitis shows multiple purulent exudative plaques along the tracheal walls.*

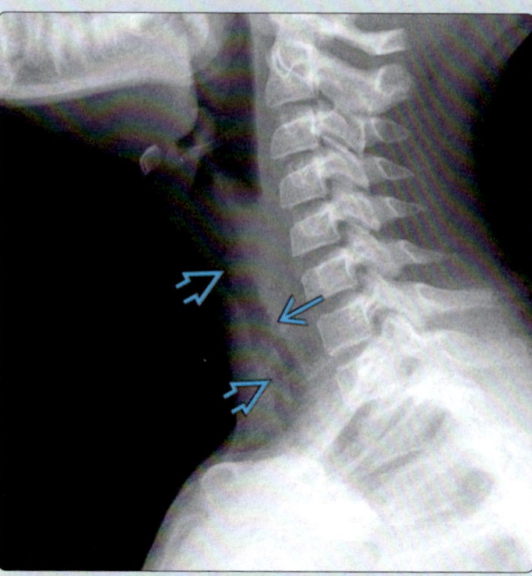

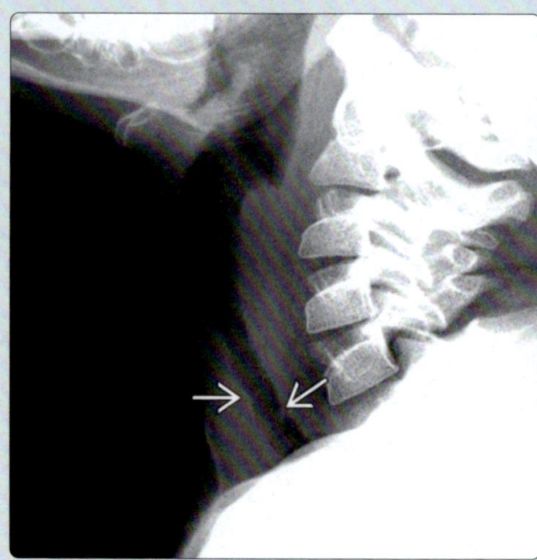

(Left) *Lateral airway radiograph in a child with fever & stridor shows multiple irregular, intraluminal filling defects* ⇨ *as well as tracheal wall irregularity* → *& moderate luminal narrowing, consistent with exudative tracheitis.* **(Right)** *Lateral radiograph in a 5-year-old boy with fever, throat pain, & cough shows mild, generalized tracheal narrowing with subtle lobular & linear filling defects* ➡ *concerning for plaques/pseudomembranes. Exudative tracheitis was confirmed at laryngoscopy.*

TERMINOLOGY

Synonyms

- Exudative tracheitis, membranous or pseudomembranous croup, membranous laryngotracheobronchitis
  - Membranous croup: Confusing term overlapping much more common benign entity of viral croup

Definitions

- Purulent infection of trachea
  - Results in thick, adherent, exudative plaques along tracheal walls with pseudomembranes extending across lumen
  - Plaques can slough & obstruct airway
- Controversial disease
  - More frequent in certain medical centers; rarely seen in other centers of similar climate
  - While many cases with significant morbidity/mortality have been confirmed, questions remain concerning overdiagnosis/overtreatment at some centers

IMAGING

General Features

- Best diagnostic clue
  - Radiography demonstrates plaque-like irregularity of tracheal walls &/or linear filling defects (pseudomembranes) within tracheal lumen
- Location
  - Purulent infection of trachea, which may extend to involve larynx & bronchi

Radiographic Findings

- Linear filling defects within subglottic airway
- Plaque-like irregularity with loss of well-defined, smooth, parallel tracheal wall contours (candle dripping sign)
  - Mucus can mimic plaques but may clear on repeat images after patient coughs
    - Coughing may be contraindicated if clinical suspicion is high (due to risk of dislodging pseudomembranes)
- Hazy, indistinct tracheal air column
- Symmetric or asymmetric subglottic narrowing in child older than typically seen with croup

CT Findings

- Not routinely used in diagnosis
- Tracheal filling defects may be detected on lung window images obtained for other clinical suspicions

MR Findings

- Not used in diagnosis

Imaging Recommendations

- Best imaging tool
  - Frontal + lateral airway radiographs

DIFFERENTIAL DIAGNOSIS

Croup

- Benign, self-limited condition classically
- Most common upper airway disease encountered in children
- Characteristic cough ("barking," "seal-like")
- Symmetric, subglottic narrowing (steepling)
- Younger age (mean: 1 year) than exudative tracheitis

Epiglottitis

- Severe, life-threatening condition
- Fever, sore throat, drooling, respiratory distress in recumbent position
- Marked enlargement of epiglottis & aryepiglottic folds
- May cause symmetric subglottic narrowing on frontal view, similar in appearance to croup (but not as isolated finding)
- Peak age has now shifted to teenage years
  - Previously 3.5 years prior to *Haemophilus influenzae* vaccine

Retropharyngeal Abscess

- True thickening of retropharyngeal soft tissues that does not change with inspiration
- CECT confirms rim-enhancing fluid collection with surrounding edema & adenopathy
- Fever, sore throat, toxic-appearing, leukocytosis
- Most often < 6 years of age

Upper Airway Foreign Body

- Rarely radiodense
- May be seen as soft tissue filling defect in oropharynx/hypopharynx
- ± recent choking episode

Intraluminal Secretions

- May cause small globular filling defect without tracheal narrowing
- May clear with coughing, though patients with suspected tracheitis should not be urged to cough (as this could theoretically dislodge plaques & obstruct airway)

PATHOLOGY

General Features

- Favored to represent bacterial superinfection following compromise of respiratory mucosa by viral illness rather than isolated primary bacterial infection
- *Staphylococcus aureus* remains most common etiology, MSSA > MRSA
  - Others: *Streptococcus* species, *H. influenzae, Moraxella catarrhalis*, & *Pseudomonas aeruginosa*
  - Polymicrobial infection is often present, supporting etiology of secondary infection
- Viral cultures are also frequently positive (up to 65%), which may be due to preceding illness
  - Parainfluenza, rhinovirus, & influenza A are common

Gross Pathologic & Surgical Features

- Endoscopy shows laryngeal & subglottic edema/erythema, ulcerations, copious secretions with adherent pseudomembrane formation
- Exudative plaques can slough & lead to obstruction of airway (much like historic airway obstructions with *Corynebacterium diphtheriae*)

CLINICAL ISSUES

Presentation

- Most common signs/symptoms

- High-grade fever, cough, severe stridor (biphasic or inspiratory), voice changes, rapid onset (2-10 hours) of respiratory distress
  - Cough may be "barky," similar to viral croup
- Usually preceded by several-day history of viral upper respiratory tract infection, low-grade fever, cough

- Other signs/symptoms
  - Initial descriptions reported patients as severely toxic in appearance
  - Many patients have only mild symptoms in more recent papers
  - Affected children are typically able to handle oral secretions & tolerate supine position, unlike epiglottitis
  - Rare reports of chronic forms
- Clinical profile
  - Preexisting intubation or tracheostomy may predispose to bacterial tracheitis
    - Presentations are more indolent
      - ↑ purulent secretions requiring more frequent suctioning of airway
      - ↓ oxygen saturations
    - Most commonly develops ~ 4 days after intubation with 2-11% incidence
      - Less predictable, lower incidence with longstanding tracheostomy
    - May be precursor to pneumonia

Demographics

- Age
  - 3 months to 14 years; peak age of 3-8 years with mean age of 5 years
    - Older than patients who present with classic viral croup
- Sex
  - No predilection
- Epidemiology
  - Incidence: 4-8 per 1 million children

Natural History & Prognosis

- Systemic complications include
  - Septic shock
  - Pulmonary edema
  - Acute respiratory distress syndrome
- Mortality historically of 20-40%, now ~ 1%
  - ↓ due to more aggressive work-up & therapy, possibly earlier presentations, & changing microbes

Treatment

- If exudative tracheitis is suspected clinically/radiographically, child is usually evaluated with flexible laryngoscopy
- If tracheal pseudomembranes/plaques are confirmed with direct visualization, patient undergoes rigid bronchoscopy with stripping of pseudomembranes ± intubation
  - Multiple debridements are usually not required
  - Intubation lasts 2-7 days
    - Less frequently required in older children
      - Close monitoring is still necessary
- IV antibiotics may be transitioned to oral antibiotics once culture sensitivities return
- Failure to respond completely to racemic epinephrine & corticosteroids is typical

DIAGNOSTIC CHECKLIST

Consider

- Bacterial tracheitis may present in
  - Young child with rapid deterioration after typical viral croup manifestations
  - Older child with croup-type symptoms

Image Interpretation Pearls

- Luminal linear filling defects (pseudomembranes) + irregularity/poor definition of tracheal walls (plaques): Very suggestive of diagnosis
- Repeat radiographs after patient coughs may aid clearance of incidental adherent mucus suspected as cause of tracheal filling defects/nodularity
  - Coughing may be contraindicated if clinical suspicion is high (due to risk of dislodging pseudomembranes)

SELECTED REFERENCES

1. Akhavan M: Ear, Nose, Throat: Beyond pharyngitis: retropharyngeal abscess, peritonsillar abscess, epiglottitis, bacterial tracheitis, and postoperative tonsillectomy. Emerg Med Clin North Am. 39(3):661-75, 2021
2. Barengo JH et al: Demographic characteristics of children diagnosed with bacterial tracheitis. Ann Otol Rhinol Laryngol. 34894211007250, 2021
3. Casazza G et al: Pediatric bacterial tracheitis-a variable entity: case series with literature review. Otolaryngol Head Neck Surg. 160(3):546-9, 2019
4. Blot M et al: Update on childhood and adult infectious tracheitis. Med Mal Infect. 47(7):443-52, 2017
5. Darras KE et al: Imaging acute airway obstruction in infants and children. Radiographics. 35(7):2064-79, 2015
6. Kuo CY et al: Bacterial tracheitis. Pediatr Rev. 35(11):497-9, 2014
7. Miranda AD et al: Bacterial tracheitis: a varied entity. Pediatr Emerg Care. 27(10):950-3, 2011
8. Sammer M et al: Membranous croup (exudative tracheitis or membranous laryngotracheobronchitis). Pediatr Radiol. 40(5):781, 2010
9. Shargorodsky J et al: Bacterial tracheitis: a therapeutic approach. Laryngoscope. 120(12):2498-501, 2010
10. Huang YL et al: Bacterial tracheitis in pediatrics: 12 year experience at a medical center in Taiwan. Pediatr Int. 51(1):110-3, 2009
11. Lee JK et al: Treatment of exudative tracheitis with acute airway obstruction under jet ventilation. Otolaryngol Head Neck Surg. 139(4):606-7, 2008
12. Salamone FN et al: Bacterial tracheitis reexamined: is there a less severe manifestation? Otolaryngol Head Neck Surg. 131(6):871-6, 2004
13. Rotta AT et al: Respiratory emergencies in children. Respir Care. 48(3):248-58; discussion 258-60, 2003
14. Stroud RH et al: An update on inflammatory disorders of the pediatric airway: epiglottitis, croup, and tracheitis. Am J Otolaryngol. 22(4):268-75, 2001
15. Damm M et al: Management of acute inflammatory childhood stridor. Otolaryngol Head Neck Surg. 121(5):633-8, 1999
16. Bernstein T et al: Is bacterial tracheitis changing? A 14-month experience in a pediatric intensive care unit. Clin Infect Dis. 27(3):458-62, 1998
17. Brody AS et al: Membranous tracheitis: how accurate is the plain film diagnosis? Pediatr Radiol (Abstr). 27:705, 1997
18. Brook I: Aerobic and anaerobic microbiology of bacterial tracheitis in children. Pediatr Emerg Care. 13(1):16-8, 1997
19. Britto J et al: Systemic complications associated with bacterial tracheitis. Arch Dis Child. 74(3):249-50, 1996
20. John SD et al: Stridor and upper airway obstruction in infants and children. Radiographics. 12(4):625-43; discussion 644, 1992
21. Han BK et al: Membranous laryngotracheobronchitis (membranous croup). AJR Am J Roentgenol. 133(1):53-8, 1979

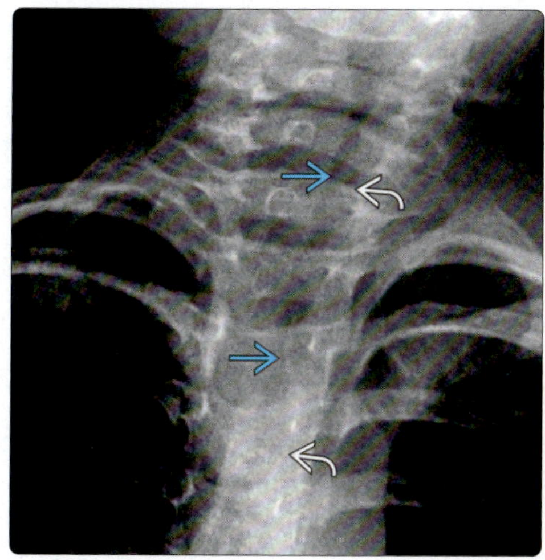

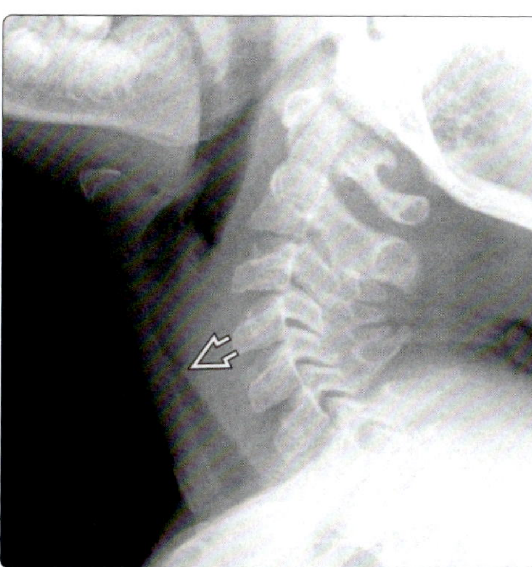

(Left) *AP airway radiograph in a 4-year-old girl with fever & rapidly progressive respiratory distress shows poor definition of the tracheal wall* ➡ *with adjacent luminal filling defects* ➡*. Extensive pseudomembranes were found at rigid bronchoscopy.* **(Right)** *Lateral radiograph in a 9-year-old boy shows moderate to marked luminal narrowing with an associated plaque* ➡ *in the cervical trachea, consistent with exudative tracheitis.*

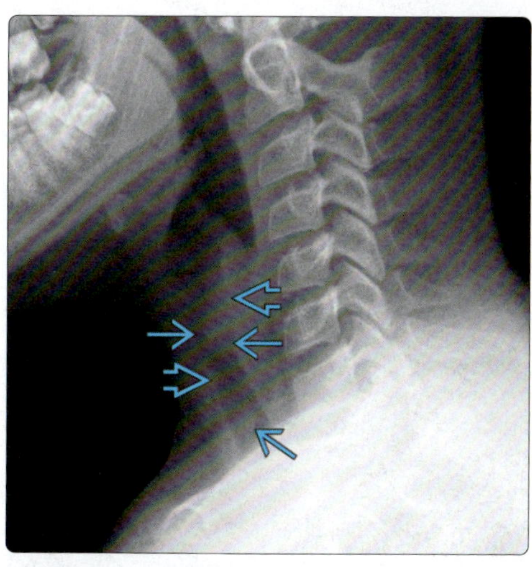

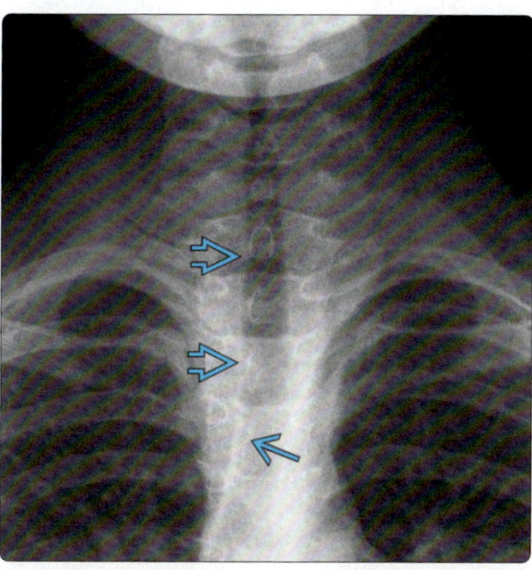

(Left) *Lateral radiograph in a 13-year-old with fever, stridor, & aphonia show multiple linear filling defects* ➡ *in the subglottic trachea as well as subtle wall irregularities* ➡*.* **(Right)** *AP radiograph in the same patient shows the linear filling defects* ➡ *& wall irregularities* ➡*, typical of exudative tracheitis. Bronchoscopy showed purulent secretions & crusting throughout the trachea. Multiple organisms, including MSSA & Streptococcus pneumoniae, grew from these cultures.*

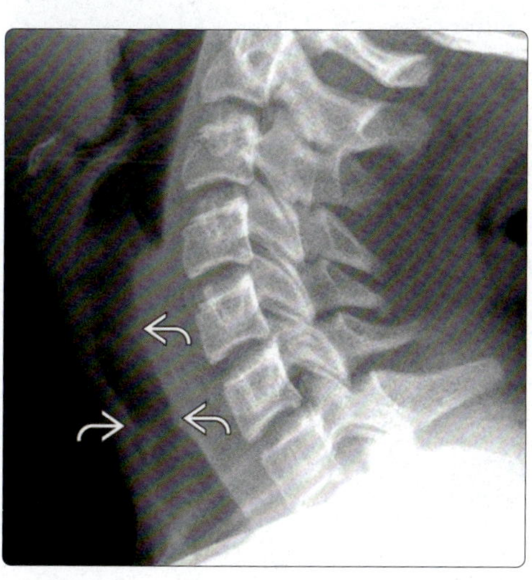

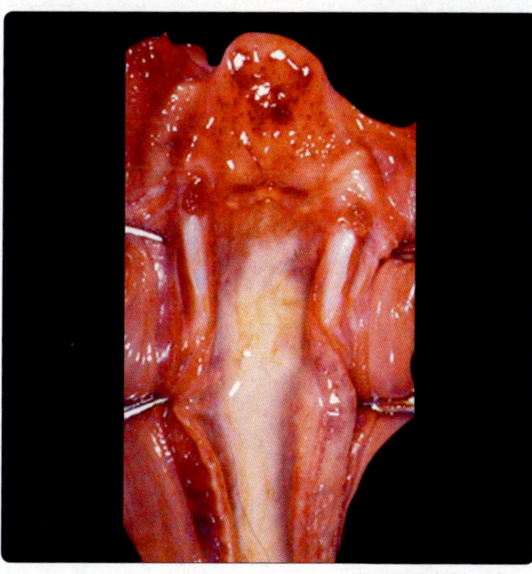

(Left) *Lateral radiograph in a 12-year-old girl with fever, throat pain, & difficulty breathing shows several linear luminal filling defects along sites of wall lobularity* ➡*, suspicious for pseudomembranes.* **(Right)** *Gross pathology image from a deceased patient shows exudative material along the entire subglottic trachea. Airway compromise & obstruction may result from sloughing of this exudative material.*

KEY FACTS

TERMINOLOGY

- Extranodal, purulent fluid collection in retropharyngeal space (RPS)

IMAGING

- Lateral radiograph: Wide prevertebral distance with loss of normal contours at hypopharynx-esophagus interface
- CECT is best tool for rapid characterization & evaluation of extent/complications
  - RPS is distended by defined, ovoid, rim-enhancing, low-density collection with convex anterior margin
  - Complications include airway compromise, jugular vein thrombosis/thrombophlebitis, mediastinal extension/mediastinitis, internal carotid artery (ICA) pseudoaneurysm (rare, suggests methicillin-resistant *Staphylococcus aureus*)

TOP DIFFERENTIAL DIAGNOSES

- Pseudothickening of retropharyngeal soft tissues
- Retropharyngeal space edema
- Necrotic/suppurative adenopathy in RPS
- Lymphatic malformation

PATHOLOGY

- Most common etiology: Rupture of suppurative RPS lymph node → abscess

CLINICAL ISSUES

- Dysphagia, sore throat, poor oral intake, dehydration
- Toxic patient: Fever, chills, ↑ WBC & ESR
- Most < 6 years old; increasing incidence in adults

DIAGNOSTIC CHECKLIST

- Distinction from RPS edema can be difficult
  - Oval-shaped collection with convex anterior margin & rim enhancement suggests drainable abscess
    - Rim enhancement may be minimal if
      - Early in disease course
      - CECT is performed with early/arterial timing

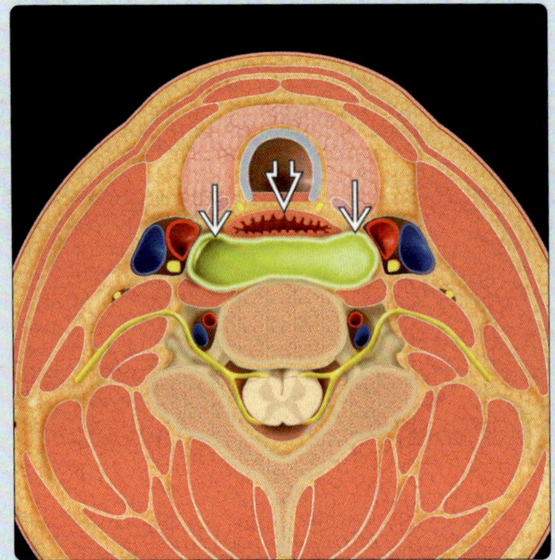

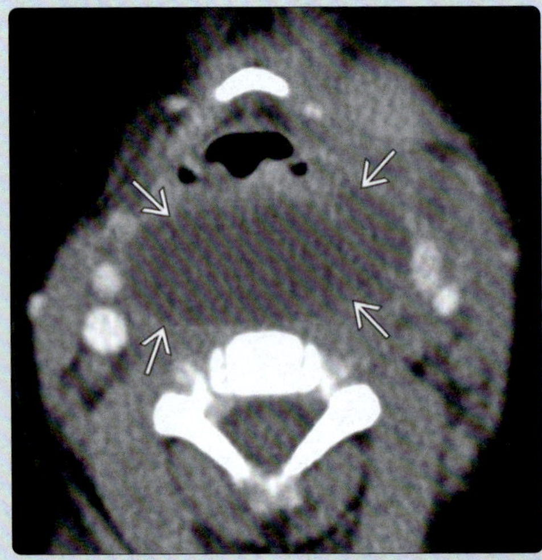

(Left) *Axial graphic illustrates the location & typical contour of a retropharyngeal space (RPS) abscess ➡ displacing the cervical esophagus ➡ anteriorly & flattening the prevertebral muscles.* **(Right)** *Axial CECT in a 10-month-old with a 5-day history of febrile illness reveals a large, low-density, ovoid collection distending the RPS ➡ with anterior displacement of the pharynx & splaying of the carotid sheaths. There is minimal enhancement of the collection wall.*

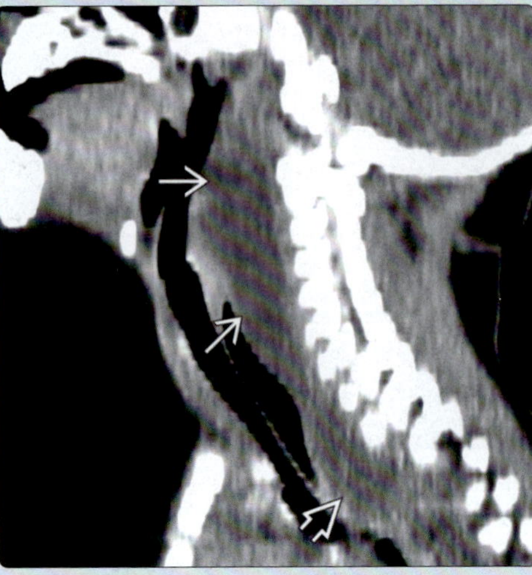

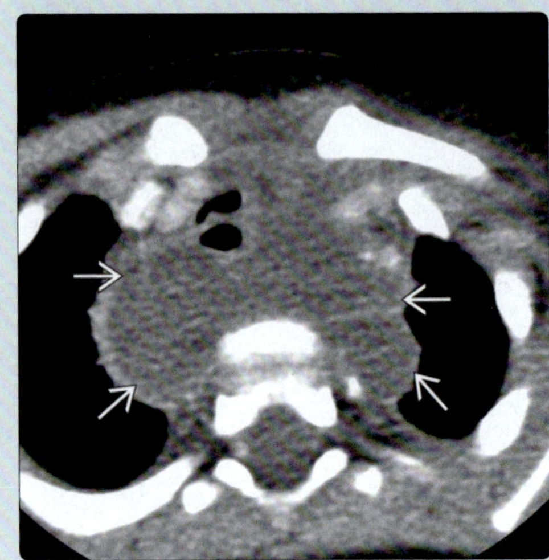

(Left) *Sagittal reformatted CECT in the same infant reveals an abscess ➡ displacing the pharynx & esophagus anteriorly & extending inferiorly to involve the superior mediastinum ➡.* **(Right)** *Axial CECT reveals the inferior extension of this methicillin-resistant Staphylococcus aureus (MRSA) abscess to the superior mediastinum ➡. This fluid was drained through a cervical approach to the collection. There was no stridor or other sign of airway compromise in this patient despite a displaced & narrowed airway.*

TERMINOLOGY

Definitions

- Retropharyngeal space (RPS): Midline space posterior to pharyngeal mucosa & cervical esophagus from skull base to T3 vertebral level in mediastinum
- RPS abscess: Extranodal, purulent fluid collection in RPS

IMAGING

General Features

- Best diagnostic clue
  - Midline rim-enhancing RPS fluid collection with mass effect in toxic-appearing patient
- Location
  - Posterior to pharynx & anterior to prevertebral muscles
- Size
  - Variable: May extend from skull base to mediastinum
- Morphology
  - Defined collection, not just infiltrative edema
  - Axial plane: Oval shape with convex anterior margin

Radiographic Findings

- Lateral view is critical
  - Normal prevertebral soft tissue thickness
    - C2 (at hypopharynx): ≤ 7 mm at any age
    - C6 (at cervical esophagus): ≤ 14 mm if < 15 years, ≤ 22 mm in adults
  - In children: Must perform lateral radiograph during inspiration with neck extension
    - Neck flexion & expiration often cause pseudothickening of prevertebral soft tissues in young children
    - Lateral fluoroscopy can distinguish persistent true thickening vs. dynamic pseudothickening
- With RPS abscess, lateral view shows widened/thickened prevertebral soft tissues
  - Convex anterior bowing ± loss of normal step-off at interface of hypopharynx & esophagus
  - Limited utility for defining extent of collection & differentiating cellulitis/phlegmon from abscess
  - RPS gas is rare but diagnostic of abscess (if no trauma)

CT Findings

- CECT
  - RPS is markedly distended by defined fluid collection with enhancing wall
    - In early stages, enhancement may be subtle
    - Thick, enhancing wall suggests mature abscess
    - Prevertebral muscles may also appear edematous
    - Gas is rarely present
  - Assess for complications
    - Airway compromise
    - Internal jugular vein (IJV) is frequently compressed/effaced, rarely thrombosed
    - Internal carotid artery (ICA) is frequently narrowed (spasm)
      - Pseudoaneurysm is rare; suggests methicillin-resistant *Staphylococcus aureus* (MRSA)
    - Mediastinal extension

Ultrasonographic Findings

- Not able to assess full craniocaudal or deep extent of disease
- Limited by operator experience & patient tolerance
- May help evaluate jugular vein patency

Imaging Recommendations

- Best imaging tool
  - CECT
- Protocol advice
  - CT from skull base to carina
  - Contrast-loading (split) bolus &/or non-CTA technique improves soft tissue contrast resolution given rapid acquisition times of CT
    - ↑ sensitivity for collections, rim enhancement

DIFFERENTIAL DIAGNOSIS

Pseudothickening of Retropharyngeal Soft Tissues

- Common radiographic mimic of retropharyngeal pathology in infants
- Adequate extension & inspiration or fluoroscopy will confirm as transient finding

Retropharyngeal Space Edema

- Poorly defined, elongated, homogeneous fluid infiltration of prevertebral soft tissues without rim enhancement
- In axial plane: Concave anterior margin
- RPS vessels may traverse infiltrated tissues
- Drainage is not required
- Etiologies include
  - Regional inflammation
    - Pharyngitis, tonsillitis, longus colli tendinitis
  - Venous or lymphatic obstruction
    - IJV thrombosis or resection, radiation

Suppurative Adenopathy in Retropharyngeal Space

- Centrally hypodense/necrotic lymph node in lateral RPS with adjacent cellulitis
- May lead to pus formation in reactive node (suppuration): Intranodal abscess
- May progress to extranodal RPS abscess with inadequate medical therapy

Lymphatic Malformation

- Multilocular, transspatial cystic neck mass with thin, nonenhancing wall (unless infected)
- Typically involves anterior & lateral neck

PATHOLOGY

General Features

- Etiology
  - Head & neck infection (pharyngitis, tonsillitis) seeds RPS lymph node
    - Reactive node → suppurative intranodal abscess → nodal rupture → RPS abscess
    - Most common organisms: *Staphylococcus aureus*, *Haemophilus*, *Streptococcus*
  - Pharyngeal penetration by foreign body
    - Child running with object in mouth
      - Lollipop/sucker, toothbrush, stick, toy

- Ventral spread of discitis/osteomyelitis & prevertebral infection
  - Uncommon in children
  - Pyogenic or tuberculous
- Mediastinal abscess spreading cranially
  - Esophageal rupture & mediastinitis with danger space (DS) abscess

CLINICAL ISSUES

Presentation

- Most common signs/symptoms
  - Dysphagia, sore throat, poor oral intake, dehydration
  - Septic patient: Fever, chills, elevated WBC & ESR
- Other signs/symptoms
  - Posterior pharyngeal wall edema or bulge
  - Reactive cervical adenopathy
- Clinical profile
  - Toxic-appearing child with marked neck pain & limited movement, especially in extension
  - Uncommonly presents with airway compromise (stridor)

Demographics

- Age
  - Most often children < 6 years old
  - Increasing frequency in adult population
    - Immunocompromised states: Diabetes, HIV, alcoholism, malignancy
    - Discitis/osteomyelitis with perivertebral infection
    - Trauma with foreign body impaction
    - Following anterior cervical spine surgery
- Sex
  - M:F = 2:1
- Epidemiology
  - ↑ frequency over last decade
  - ↓ incidence of abscess when infection is detected & treated in earlier cellulitic stage

Natural History & Prognosis

- Prognosis is generally excellent with early diagnosis & aggressive management
- Complications may result from infection spread
  - Narrowing of pharyngeal lumen → airway compromise & stridor
  - Inferior spread via DS to mediastinum → mediastinitis
    - Up to 50% mortality (much less in infants)
      - ↓ mortality rate in recent years with aggressive initial & repeat surgical intervention
    - MRSA is frequent
  - Carotid space involvement
    - Jugular vein thrombosis or thrombophlebitis
    - Narrowing of ICA caliber is often found; neurological sequelae are infrequent
    - Rarely ICA pseudoaneurysm &/or rupture; described with MRSA infection
  - Perivertebral space abscess may lead to epidural abscess
  - Aspiration pneumonia
  - Grisel syndrome is rare
    - Inflammatory, nontraumatic atlantoaxial subluxation
      - Due to distention or loosening of atlantoaxial ligaments after head & neck inflammation

Treatment

- Early ENT consultation
- IV antibiotics, airway management, fluid resuscitation
- Surgical intervention (incision & drainage) for
  - Significant or complex abscess
  - Lack of improvement/worsening with IV antibiotics

DIAGNOSTIC CHECKLIST

Consider

- Lateral radiograph: Often 1st-line screening tool
- Study of choice: CECT
  - Distinguish RPS abscess from edema
  - Evaluate full craniocaudal extent
  - Evaluate for vascular/airway complications
  - Consider contrast prebolus/split bolus or venous phase imaging to maximize wall enhancement

Image Interpretation Pearls

- Distinction from RPS edema can be difficult
  - Convex anterior margin or oval-shaped collection suggests abscess
  - Rim enhancement suggests abscess
    - May be minimal early in disease
    - May not be evident due to early arterial scanning
- Important to evaluate full extent of abscess & presence of complications
- ENT consultation is imperative

SELECTED REFERENCES

1. Donà D et al: Deep neck abscesses in children: an Italian retrospective study. Pediatr Emerg Care. ePub, 2020
2. Hansen BW et al: Infections of deep neck spaces. Semin Ultrasound CT MR. 41(1):74-84, 2020
3. Carroll W et al: Is vessel narrowing secondary to pediatric deep neck space infections of clinical significance? Int J Pediatr Otorhinolaryngol. 125:56-58, 2019
4. Ho ML et al: The ABCs (airway, blood vessels, and compartments) of pediatric neck infections and masses. AJR Am J Roentgenol. 1-10, 2016
5. Wilson CD et al: Retrospective review of management and outcomes of pediatric descending mediastinitis. Otolaryngol Head Neck Surg. 155(1):155-9, 2016
6. Novis SJ et al: Pediatric deep space neck infections in U.S. children, 2000-2009. Int J Pediatr Otorhinolaryngol. 78(5):832-6, 2014
7. Abdel-Haq N et al: Retropharyngeal abscess in children: the rising incidence of methicillin-resistant Staphylococcus aureus. Pediatr Infect Dis J. 31(7):696-9, 2012
8. Debnam JM et al: Retropharyngeal and prevertebral spaces: anatomic imaging and diagnosis. Otolaryngol Clin North Am. 45(6):1293-310, 2012
9. Maroldi R et al: Emergency imaging assessment of deep neck space infections. Semin Ultrasound CT MR. 33(5):432-42, 2012
10. Virk JS et al: Analysing lateral soft tissue neck radiographs. Emerg Radiol. 19(3):255-60, 2012
11. Hoang JK et al: Multiplanar CT and MRI of collections in the retropharyngeal space: is it an abscess? AJR Am J Roentgenol. 196(4):W426-32, 2011
12. Byramji A et al: Fatal retropharyngeal abscess: a possible marker of inflicted injury in infancy and early childhood. Forensic Sci Med Pathol. 5(4):302-6, 2009
13. Hudgins PA et al: Internal carotid artery narrowing in children with retropharyngeal lymphadenitis and abscess. AJNR Am J Neuroradiol. 19(10):1841-3, 1998

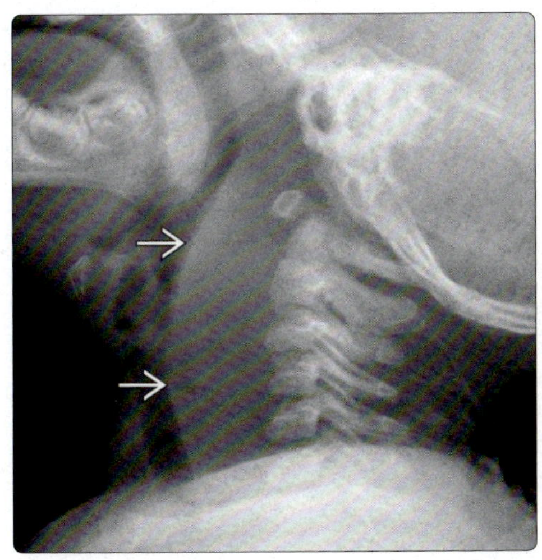

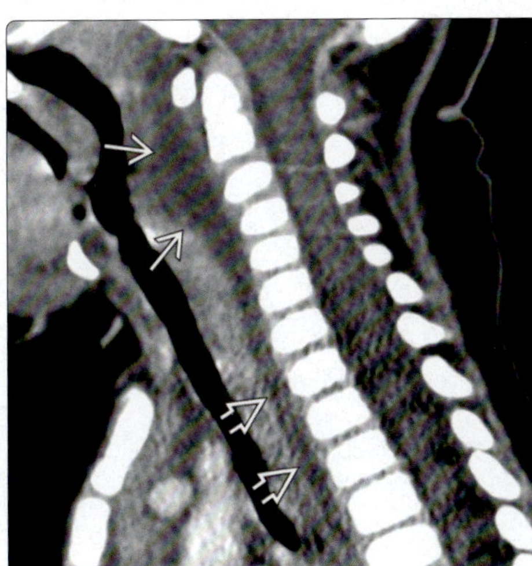

(Left) *Lateral radiograph in a 12-month-old boy with sepsis shows significant thickening of the prevertebral soft tissues* ➡. *The normal step-off at the pharyngeal-esophageal junction has been effaced.* **(Right)** *Sagittal reformatted CECT in the same child clearly shows the cause of the prominent soft tissues to be a convex anterior RPS abscess* ➡ *with extension of fluid into the posterior mediastinum* ➡. *It is important to image these children from the nasopharynx to the carina, in order to evaluate the full craniocaudad extent of the collection.*

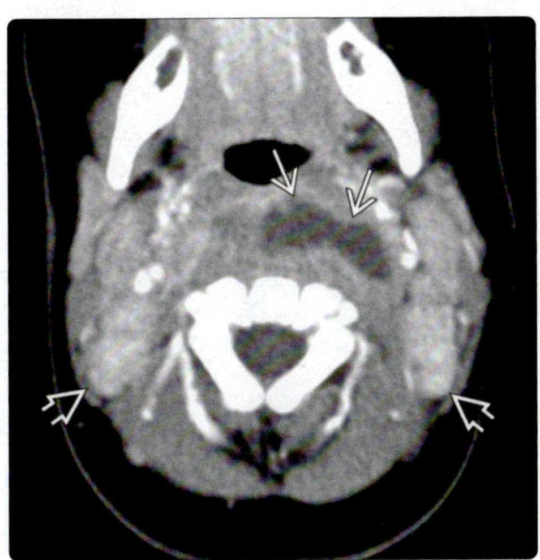

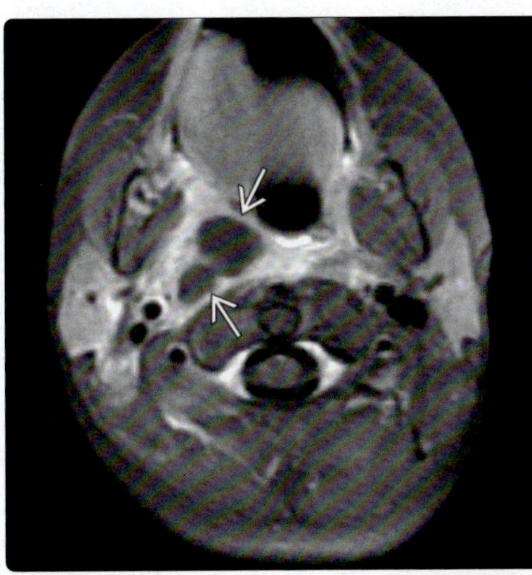

(Left) *Axial CECT in a 5-month-old boy shows an irregularly shaped RPS fluid collection* ➡ *in the midline & left paramidline soft tissues, most likely an extranodal spread of a suppurative left lateral RPS lymph node. Note the bilateral nonsuppurative cervical adenopathy* ➡. **(Right)** *Axial T1 C+ FS MR in a child allergic to iodinated contrast demonstrates a well-defined abscess* ➡ *in the right lateral RPS with significant surrounding contrast enhancement & mild extension of inflammation medial to the carotid sheath vessels.*

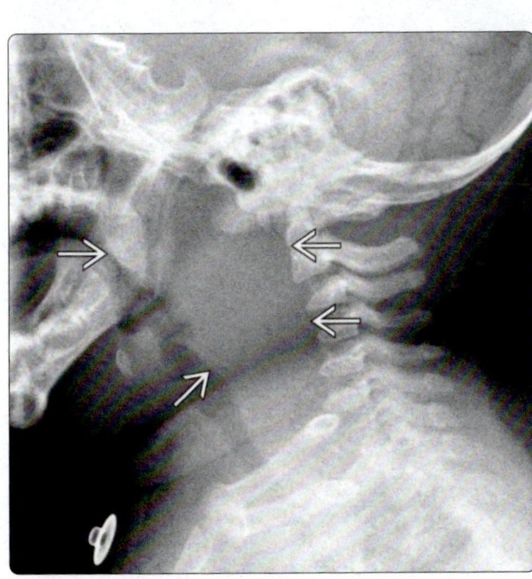

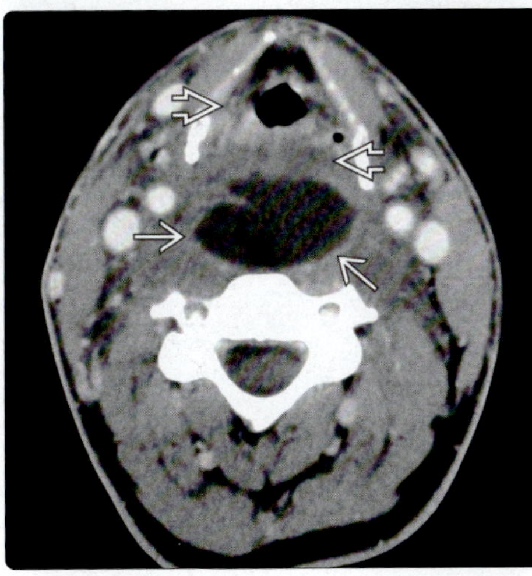

(Left) *Lateral radiograph in a 7-month-old child with fever shows marked thickening of the prevertebral soft tissues* ➡ *with ventral displacement of the pharynx & larynx. There is loss of the normal step-off at the pharyngeal-esophageal junction.* **(Right)** *Axial CECT in the same patient shows a faintly enhancing rim* ➡ *at the periphery of a large RPS abscess, which displaces the hypopharynx & larynx anteriorly* ➡. *The adjacent carotid sheath vessels are normal in position, enhancement, & caliber.*

Double Aortic Arch

KEY FACTS

TERMINOLOGY

- Congenital aortic arch anomaly related to persistence of both left & right 4th aortic arches

IMAGING

- Chest radiography is often suggestive of diagnosis
  - Bilateral tracheal indentations & midtracheal narrowing
  - Right arch indentation is commonly higher & more substantial than left ("right dominant")
- Esophagram is suggestive with characteristic bilateral & posterior indentations
- Cross-sectional imaging (CTA/MRA) for definitive diagnosis & characterization
  - Left & right arches arise from ascending aorta, encircle trachea & esophagus, & join to form descending aorta
  - Each arch gives rise to 1 ventral carotid & 1 dorsal subclavian artery (4-artery sign on axial slice)
  - Right arch is commonly larger, more superior, & more posterior extending than left (70% of cases)
    - Left descending aorta in these cases

PATHOLOGY

- Typically isolated; congenital intracardiac disease in 20%
- Dominant right arch, left descending aorta: 70-75%
- Dominant left arch, right descending aorta: 15-20%
- Arches equal in size: 5-10%
- Smaller of 2 arches may be partially atretic

CLINICAL ISSUES

- Most common symptomatic vascular ring (55%)
- Often presents < 3 years of age with stridor, wheezing, & choking that worsens with feeding
- Surgery: Left (usually) thoracotomy with division of smaller arch, atretic segment, & ligamentum arteriosum with mobilization of trachea & esophagus
  - Up to 11% require 2nd operation to relieve persistent airway symptoms

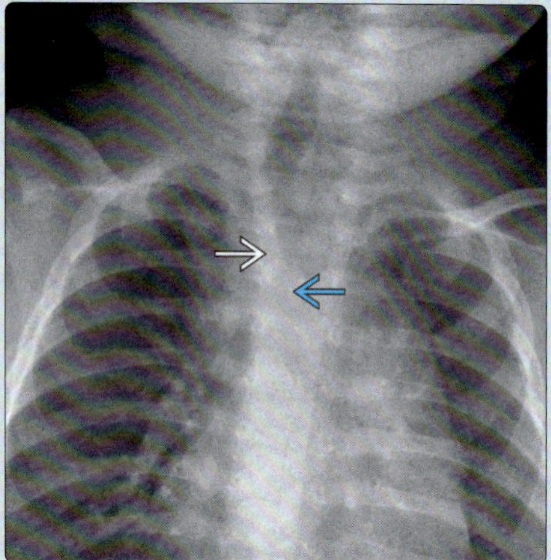

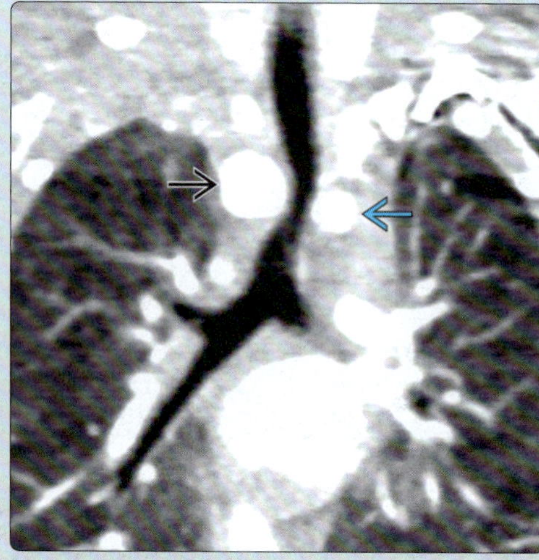

(Left) *AP radiograph of a 2-month-old with biphasic stridor shows impressions on the trachea from both the right & left with the right impression ➔ being higher than the left ➔. Radiography can be highly suggestive of a double aortic arch, though the airway morphology is often overlooked.* **(Right)** *Coronal MIP image from a chest CTA in an infant with a double aortic arch shows vascular compression of the trachea between left ➔ & right ➔ aortic arches. Note that the right arch is dominant, which is typical.*

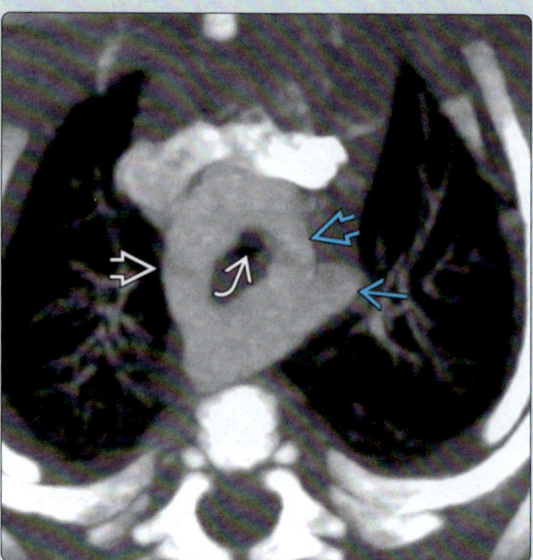

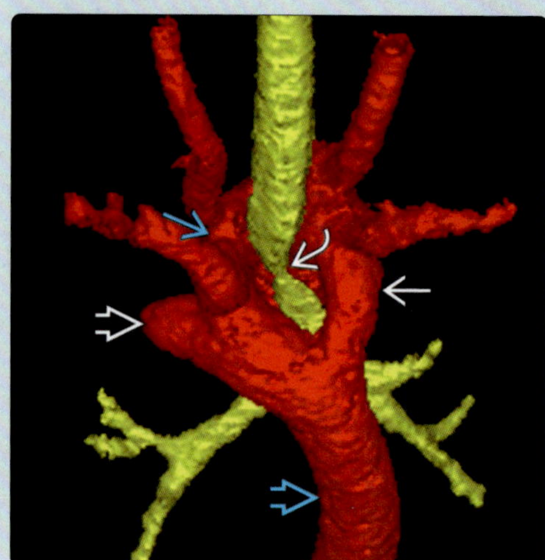

(Left) *Axial CTA MIP shows right ➔ & left ➔ aortic arches circumferentially around the compressed trachea ➔, consistent with a double aortic arch. Note the large ductal diverticulum ➔.* **(Right)** *Posterior oblique 3D image from a chest CTA shows a double aortic arch with left ➔ & right ➔ arches that converge to form a descending aorta ➔. There is severe focal compression of the trachea ➔. Note the large ductal diverticulum ➔ & the symmetric branching of the great vessels.*

TERMINOLOGY

Abbreviations

- Double aortic arch (DAA)

Definitions

- Congenital aortic arch anomaly related to persistence of both left & right 4th aortic arches

IMAGING

General Features

- Best diagnostic clue
  - Radiography: Characteristic indentations of bilateral tracheal walls
  - Cross-sectional imaging: Ascending aorta splits anterior to trachea with confluence of discrete right & left arches posterior to esophagus
- Location
  - Right arch is commonly more superior & posterior than left
  - Right arch typically runs behind esophagus to join left arch to form left-sided descending aorta
- Size
  - Right arch is commonly larger than left
- Morphology
  - Part of smaller arch (usually left) may be atretic (interrupted DAA)
    - Patent portions remain connected by fibrous band, completing compressive ring around trachea & esophagus

Radiographic Findings

- Chest radiography is often suggestive of DAA
  - Symmetric mediastinal soft tissue on either side of trachea (or R > L)
    - Typically greater on left with normal left arch
  - Trachea is deviated by dominant arch or in abnormal midline position
    - Normally, trachea is slightly deviated to right by left arch
  - Bilateral tracheal indentations with midtracheal narrowing in 47%
    - Right arch indentation is commonly higher & larger than left
  - Lateral view shows generalized tracheal narrowing ± anterior indentation
  - Symmetric aeration of lungs (no unilateral air-trapping)

Fluoroscopic Findings

- Frontal view: Bilateral indentations on contrast-filled upper esophagus, often at different levels
- Lateral view: Rounded posterior indentation on esophagus; may have anterior impression as well from left mainstem bronchus

CT Findings

- CTA
  - Ascending aorta divides anteriorly into discrete right & left arches → arches encircle trachea & esophagus → arches rejoin posteriorly to form descending aorta
    - Can cause severe midtracheal compression
    - Smaller of 2 arches may be partially atretic
      - If atresia occurs between left carotid & subclavian arteries (instead of more common atresia beyond left subclavian artery), look for superior-pointing descending aortic diverticulum to confirm atresia
      - Distorted subclavian artery sign: Proximal subclavian ipsilateral to atresia shows abnormal inferior & posterior course
  - 4-artery sign: Symmetric take-off of 4 separate aortic branches on axial image at thoracic inlet
    - 2 ventral carotid & 2 dorsal subclavian arteries
      - 1 carotid & 1 subclavian arise from each arch

MR Findings

- Findings are similar to CTA
  - Lacks airway detail of CTA
- Can be depicted with variety of conventional, flow-related, & postcontrast techniques

Ultrasonographic Findings

- Prenatal diagnosis: Trident sign of 2 arches + ductus arteriosus on transverse 3-vessel trachea view

Echocardiographic Findings

- Suprasternal notch view is most helpful: 2 separate aortic arches, each giving rise to separate carotid & subclavian arteries (with no common brachiocephalic trunk)
- Does not adequately show airway & descending aorta
- Excludes intracardiac pathologies

Angiographic Findings

- Rarely required with use of cross-sectional imaging

Imaging Recommendations

- Best imaging tool
  - Radiography remains primary diagnostic test
    - Virtually all patients receive chest radiography 1st for respiratory symptoms
      - 25% can be normal in appearance
  - Esophagram rarely obviates need for cross-sectional imaging when arch anomaly is suspected clinically & radiographically
    - However, many arch anomalies are diagnosed 1st by oral contrast studies performed for feeding difficulties
  - Cross-sectional imaging (CTA or MRA) is performed to confirm diagnosis & define anatomic variations for presurgical planning
- Protocol advice
  - Multidetector CTA is faster to perform than MR
    - Generally no need for anesthesia/intubation
  - CT shows airway details somewhat better than MR
  - Multiplanar & volume-rendered images are useful for characterization & communication with referring providers
    - Particularly helpful for understanding vascular ring relationship to airway

DIFFERENTIAL DIAGNOSIS

Right Arch With Aberrant Left Subclavian Artery

- Diverticulum of Kommerell points anteriorly toward pulmonary artery

Left Pulmonary Artery Sling

- Compression on anterior aspect of esophagus & posterior aspect of trachea on lateral radiograph or esophagram
- Often associated with tracheomalacia or complete cartilaginous tracheal rings (~ 2/3 of cases)
  - Pulmonary sling is typical vascular ring associated with asymmetric aeration

Innominate Artery Compression Syndrome

- Compression on anterior aspect of trachea without esophageal compression

Nonvascular Masses

- Variety of benign & malignant solid or cystic soft tissue masses can compress & deviate trachea

PATHOLOGY

General Features

- Etiology
  - Related to embryological persistence of right & left 4th aortic arches
- Genetics
  - 22q11 deletion in ~ 25% of all arch anomalies without intracardiac disease
    - Partial arch atresia is more likely in this setting than 2 patent arches
- Associated abnormalities
  - Typically isolated lesion without associated abnormalities
    - 20% have congenital heart disease (tetralogy of Fallot, ventricular septal defect, coarctation, patent ductus arteriosus, transposition of great arteries, truncus arteriosus)
  - Underlying tracheomalacia is frequently present
- Pathophysiology
  - Variable airway & esophageal compression by vascular ring
    - Usually severe enough to present early in life
  - No hemodynamic sequelae unless associated with congenital heart disease

Gross Pathologic & Surgical Features

- True complete vascular ring with encircled trachea & esophagus
  - Dominant right arch, left descending aorta: 70-75%
  - Dominant left arch, right descending aorta: 15-20%
  - Arches equal in size: 5-10%
  - Smaller of 2 arches may be partially atretic

CLINICAL ISSUES

Presentation

- Most common signs/symptoms
  - 0-3 years old presenting with stridor, wheezing, & choking that worsens with feeding
  - Apnea or life-threatening respiratory arrest requiring resuscitation as initial presentation in 5-10%
- Other signs/symptoms
  - Apneic attacks, noisy breathing, "seal bark" cough
  - Feeding difficulty

Demographics

- Age
  - Typically presents with respiratory symptoms soon after birth
- Epidemiology
  - Most common symptomatic vascular ring anomaly (55%)

Treatment

- Left (usually) thoracotomy with division of smaller arch, atretic segment, & ligamentum arteriosum with mobilization of trachea & esophagus
  - Postoperative complications: Chylothorax, vocal cord paralysis, transient hypertension
  - Rare complication occurring pre- or postoperatively: Aortoesophageal fistula with severe hemorrhage
- Most common persistent symptom postoperatively: Stridor in 30%
  - Persistent airway symptoms are most commonly due to
    - Tracheal stenosis
    - Tracheobronchomalacia
    - Persistent extrinsic airway compression
      - Caused by midline/circumflex descending aorta or previously ligated arch
- Up to 11% of patients require 2nd operation to relieve airway symptoms
  - Aortopexy or other vascular suspension procedures
  - Cartilaginous tracheal ring resection followed by airway reconstruction

DIAGNOSTIC CHECKLIST

Consider

- Look for atretic segment of double arch anomaly
  - Unopacified on CTA or MRA
  - No flow void on spin-echo MR
- Smaller arch by cross-sectional imaging determines side of thoracotomy

Image Interpretation Pearls

- 4-artery sign on axial CTA/MR slice at thoracic inlet

SELECTED REFERENCES

1. Priya S et al: Atretic double aortic arch: imaging appearance of a rare anomaly and differentiation from its mimics. Cureus. 12(7):e9478, 2020
2. Backer CL et al: Double aortic arch with Kommerell diverticulum. Ann Thorac Surg. 108(1):161-6, 2019
3. Mądry W et al: Non-invasive diagnosis of aortic arch anomalies in children - 15 years of own experience. J Ultrason. 19(76):5-8, 2019
4. Yang Y et al: Diagnosis and surgical repair of congenital double aortic arch in infants. J Cardiothorac Surg. 14(1):160, 2019
5. Li S et al: Congenital abnormalities of the aortic arch: revisiting the 1964 Stewart classification. Cardiovasc Pathol. 39:38-50, 2018
6. Hanneman K et al: Congenital variants and anomalies of the aortic arch. Radiographics. 37(1):32-51, 2017
7. Kaldararova M et al: Double aortic arch anomalies in children: a systematic 20-year single center study. Clin Anat. 30(7):929-39, 2017
8. Backer CL et al: Vascular rings. Semin Pediatr Surg. 25(3):165-75, 2016
9. Trobo Marina D et al: Neonatal magnetic resonance imaging in double aortic arch diagnosed prenatally by ultrasound. J Obstet Gynaecol. 36(4):526-8, 2016
10. Gould SW et al: Useful signs for the assessment of vascular rings on cross-sectional imaging. Pediatr Radiol. 45(13):2004-16, 2015
11. Iwaki R et al: Follow-up of persistent tracheal stenosis after surgery for a double aortic arch. World J Pediatr Congenit Heart Surg. 6(3):458-61, 2015
12. Trobo D et al: Prenatal sonographic features of a double aortic arch: literature review and perinatal management. J Ultrasound Med. 34(11):1921-7, 2015

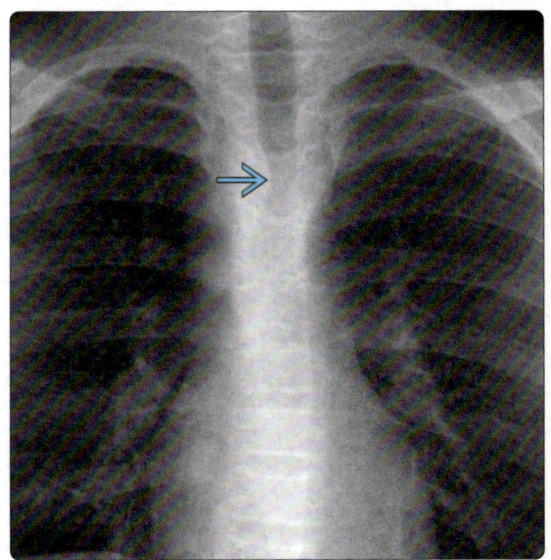

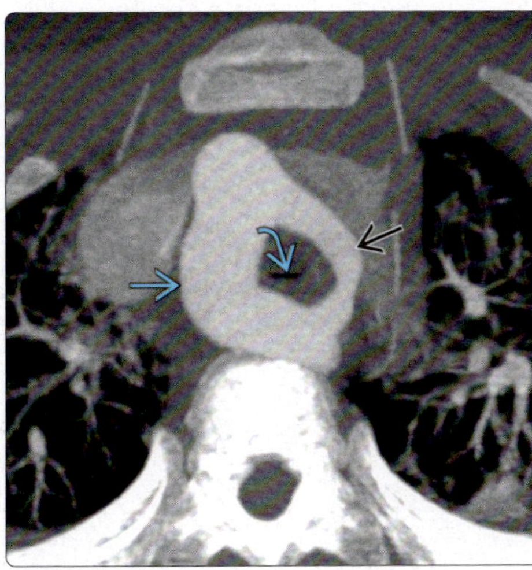

(Left) *AP radiograph of a 10-year-old with chronic stridor upon exertion shows leftward tracheal deviation* ➙. *This patient had a double aortic arch with dominant right arch.* **(Right)** *Axial CTA MIP shows a double aortic arch in a 10-year-old patient with chronic stridor. Note that the right arch* ➙ *is larger than the left arch* ➙. *Also note the tracheal compression* ➙.

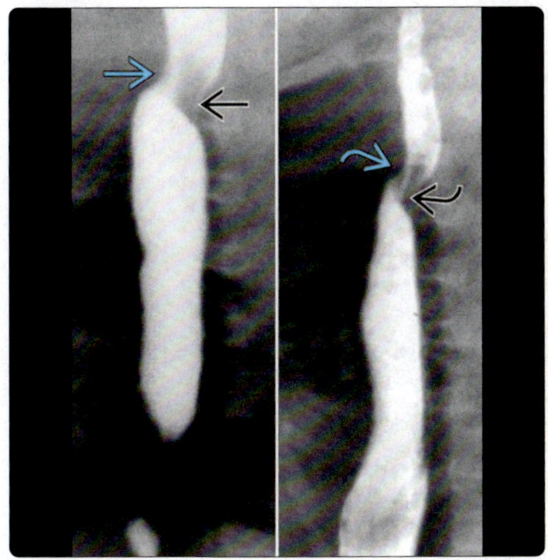

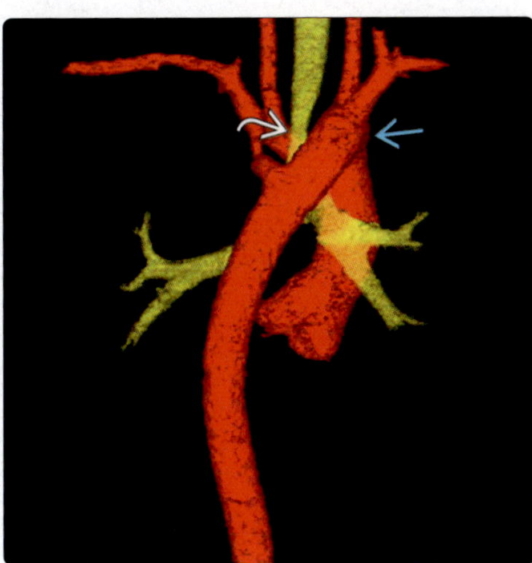

(Left) *Frontal (L) & lateral (R) views from an esophagram show vascular impressions on the right* ➙ *& left* ➙ *as well as the front* ➙ *& back* ➙ *of the esophagus in a patient with a double aortic arch.* **(Right)** *Posterior 3D image from a chest CTA shows a double aortic arch in a 10-year-old with chronic stridor. Note the dominant right arch* ➙ *& tracheal compression* ➙.

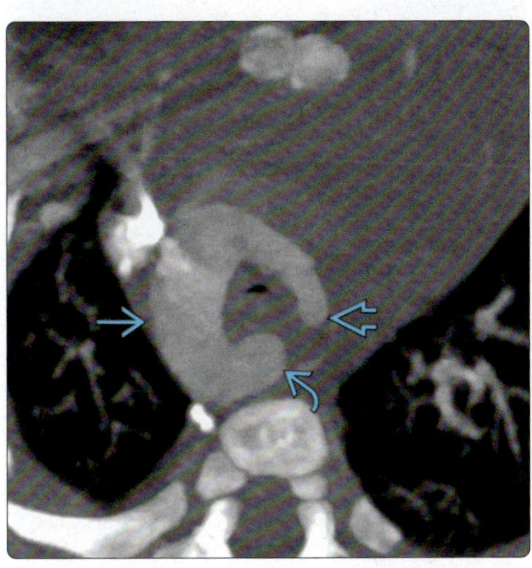

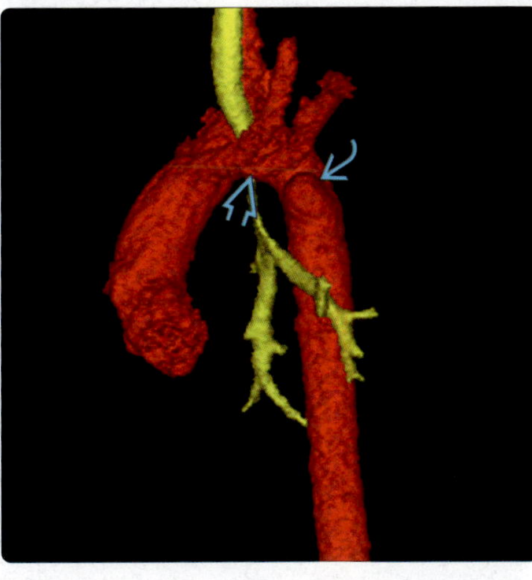

(Left) *Axial CTA MIP shows a surgically confirmed interrupted double aortic arch. The right arch* ➙ *is dominant, while the left arch is interrupted just distal to the origin of the left subclavian artery* ➙. *Note the diverticulum* ➙ *arising from the descending aorta.* **(Right)** *Left lateral 3D image from a chest CTA shows an interrupted double aortic arch. The left arch is interrupted between the origin of the left subclavian artery* ➙ *& the diverticulum* ➙ *arising from the descending aorta.*

Pulmonary Sling

KEY FACTS

TERMINOLOGY

- Left pulmonary artery (LPA) originates from posterior aspect of proximal right pulmonary artery (RPA) & forms sling around right & posterior distal tracheal walls as it passes leftward between trachea & esophagus

IMAGING

- Only vascular ring to consistently course between trachea & esophagus
  - Compresses posterior trachea & anterior esophagus
  - Lateral chest radiograph: Round opacity between distal trachea & esophagus
  - Lateral esophagram: Anterior indentation on esophagus
- CT angiography is preferred over MR to confirm diagnosis & delineate anatomy prior to surgery
  - Rapid acquisition of CTA avoids intubation
  - Exquisite 3D reconstructions of airway & vessels

PATHOLOGY

- Type I LPA sling: Carina in normal location at T4-T5 with either normal eparterial bronchus (type IA) or tracheal bronchus to right upper lobe (type IB) → hyperinflation of right lung
- Type II LPA sling: Low carina at T6 with diffuse stenosis of intermediate left bronchus by complete cartilaginous rings at multiple levels (ring-sling complex) → bilateral or left lung hyperinflation
- Many associated airway, pulmonary, & cardiac anomalies

CLINICAL ISSUES

- Typically presents in neonatal period
  - Severe stridor, hypoxia, ventilator dependency
- Surgical repair: Division of LPA from its anomalous origin with implantation to its normal origin (main PA)
  - Tracheobronchial reconstruction is required for complete cartilaginous rings or other associated tracheobronchial malformations (types IIA & IIB)

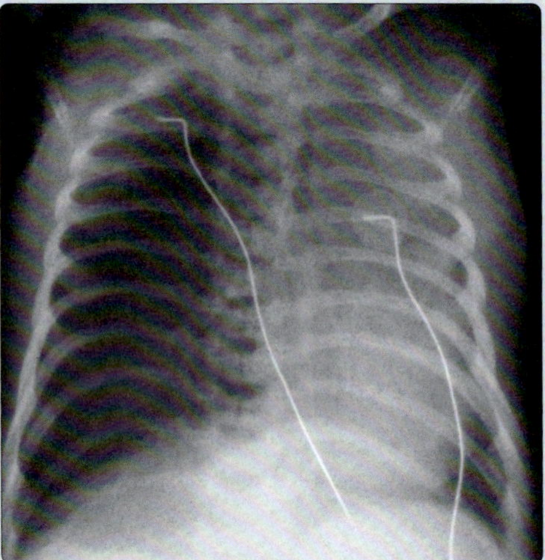

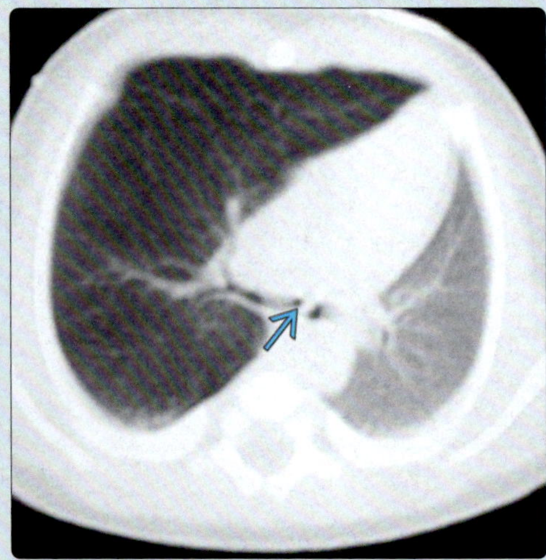

(Left) *Frontal view of the chest shows air-trapping throughout the right lung in an infant with a known pulmonary sling that is causing asymmetric compression of the right & left mainstem bronchi. Note the leftward mediastinal shift.* **(Right)** *Axial chest CT in the same infant with a pulmonary sling shows air-trapping throughout the right lung with asymmetric compression of the right mainstem bronchus ➡ & right-to-left mediastinal shift.*

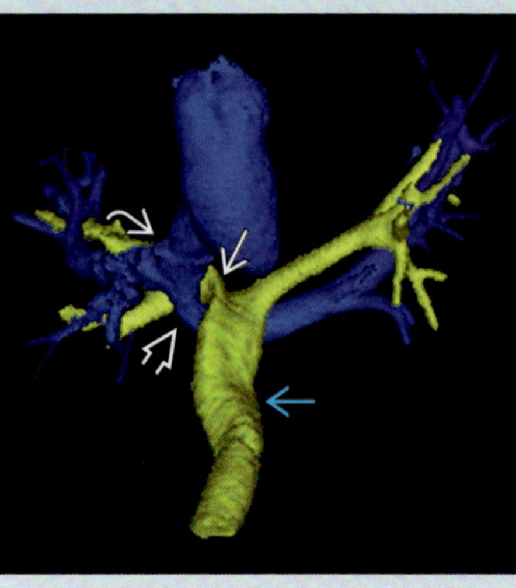

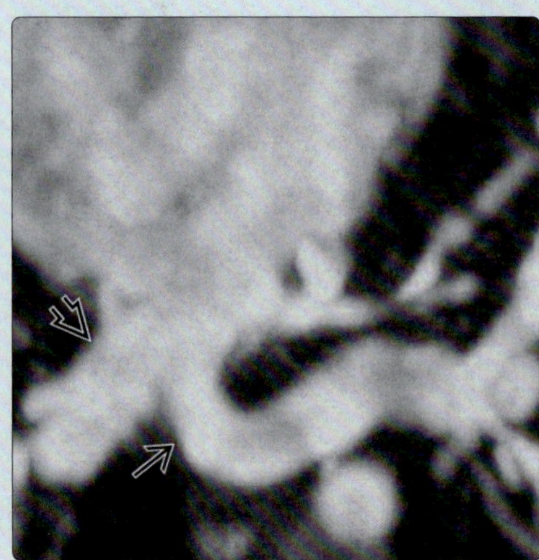

(Left) *Superior oblique 3D volume-rendered CTA in an infant with a pulmonary sling shows the left pulmonary artery (LPA) ➡ arising from the right pulmonary artery (RPA) ➡ & coursing posterior to the trachea ➡ on its way to the left lung. In this case, there was severe compression of the right mainstem ➡ bronchus causing air-trapping.* **(Right)** *Axial MR angiogram shows the classic anatomy of a pulmonary sling with the LPA ➡ arising from the RPA ➡ then coursing posterior to the trachea on its way to the left lung.*

TERMINOLOGY

Abbreviations

- Pulmonary artery sling (PAS)

Synonyms

- Aberrant left pulmonary artery (LPA), LPA sling

Definitions

- LPA originates from proximal right pulmonary artery (RPA) & wraps around right & posterior walls of distal trachea (forming sling) as it passes leftward between trachea & esophagus

IMAGING

General Features

- Best diagnostic clue
  - Classic imaging appearance: Asymmetric lung inflation, narrowed distal trachea, & focal anterior impression on midesophagus
  - Only vascular ring to course between trachea & esophagus (indenting posterior tracheal & anterior esophageal margins)
- Morphology
  - Classified by associated abnormal bronchial branching patterns
    - Type I: Carina in normal location at T4-T5 with either normal eparterial bronchus (type IA) or tracheal bronchus to right upper lobe (type IB) → right lung hyperinflation
    - Type II: Low carina at T6 with diffuse stenosis of intermediate left bronchus (ILB) by complete cartilaginous rings at multiple levels (ring-sling complex) → bilateral or left lung hyperinflation
      - Type IIA: Initial bifurcation at T4 into right upper lobe bronchus & ILB, which then bifurcates at T6 into bridging right lower lobe bronchus & left main bronchus
      - Type IIB: Absent or abortive right upper lobe bronchus

Radiographic Findings

- Lateral view is most helpful
  - Round opacity between distal trachea & esophagus
  - Posterior impression on distal trachea or carina
  - Distal trachea or right main bronchus is bowed anteriorly
- Frontal view
  - Low position of left hilum
  - Leftward displacement of narrowed distal trachea

Fluoroscopic Findings

- Esophagram: Most common vascular ring to cause anterior indentation on esophagus
  - Posterior tracheal indentation at same level

CT Findings

- CTA
  - LPA arises from posterior RPA & courses to left behind distal trachea, forming sling
    - LPA passes between trachea & esophagus
  - Tracheal stenosis or compression can be severe
    - Tracheal rings result in round, small-caliber trachea on axial images
    - May also see compression of proximal bronchi, which can result in air-trapping

MR Findings

- Spin-echo T1 or black blood sequences show dark tracheal & vascular lumens
- Contrast-enhanced angiographic techniques provide 3D rendering
- Evaluation of other congenital heart abnormalities
- Functional evaluation, including QP/QS, regurgitation, & ventricular function

Echocardiographic Findings

- Absence of normal pulmonary artery bifurcation
- Anomalous origin of LPA from proximal posterior RPA
- ± other associated cardiac anomalies

Imaging Recommendations

- Best imaging tool
  - CT angiography is preferred to confirm diagnosis & delineate anatomy prior to surgery (particularly in critically ill infants with tenuous airway)
    - Rapid acquisition avoids intubation & risks of airway manipulation
    - Provides exquisite resolution & detail obtained with 3D reconstructions of airway & vessels
      - 3D reconstruction of trachea delineates length, severity, & nature of tracheal narrowing
  - Prenatal detection is becoming more common
- Protocol advice
  - Optimize intravascular contrast bolus timing
  - Paired inspiratory/expiratory or dynamic images can demonstrate contribution of tracheobronchomalacia to airway narrowing

DIFFERENTIAL DIAGNOSIS

Middle Mediastinal Mass

- Lymphadenopathy
- Bronchogenic cyst
- Esophageal duplication cyst

Primary Bronchial Malformation

- Congenital lobar overinflation
- Bronchial atresia
- Tracheobronchomalacia
- Complete cartilaginous rings

Midline Descending Aorta-Carina Compression Syndrome

- Descending aorta lies immediately anterior to spine, leading to "crowding" of mediastinum
  - Posterior compression on carina or left main bronchus
- May be isolated or associated with right lung hypoplasia, arch anomalies

Right Arch With Aberrant Left Subclavian Artery

- Rarely courses anterior to esophagus
- More superior position than LPA sling

Double Aortic Arch

- 2 aortic arches encase trachea & esophagus (but no vessel courses between them)
- Patent ductus arteriosus (PDA) may be present
- Normal course of RPA & LPA

Arterial Tortuosity Syndrome

- Tortuous pulmonary vessels may mimic pulmonary sling
- Autosomal recessive
- ± complex congenital heart disease

PATHOLOGY

General Features

- Etiology
  - Embryology
    - Agenesis or obliteration of left 6th aortic arch, which normally forms LPA
    - Arterial supply of left lung via persistent primitive artery originating from RPA
  - Pathophysiology
    - Severe stridor secondary to
      - Compression of distal trachea, carina, & main bronchi by sling, resulting in asymmetric inflation of lungs (obstructive hyperinflation > atelectasis)
      - Associated tracheobronchomalacia
      - Associated intrinsic airway narrowing (from complete cartilaginous rings)
    - Hemodynamics are determined by associated cardiac anomalies
    - Pulmonary hypertension from severe hypoxia
- Genetics
  - No specific genetic defect identified
- Associated abnormalities
  - Intrinsic tracheobronchial anomalies: Complete rings (in 2/3), tracheomalacia, branching anomalies, tracheoesophageal fistula
    - Main bronchi have abnormal horizontal course (inverted T) with abnormal branching patterns to upper & lower lobes (types IIA & IIB)
  - Other congenital lung anomalies: Right lung hypogenesis or agenesis, horseshoe lung
  - Congenital heart disease: Aortic arch anomalies, ventricular septal defect (10%), atrial septal defect (20%), PDA (25%), single ventricle, tetralogy of Fallot, partial anomalous pulmonary venous return, persistent left superior vena cava (20%)
  - Others: Imperforate anus, Hirschsprung disease, absent gallbladder, biliary atresia, Meckel diverticulum

CLINICAL ISSUES

Presentation

- Most common signs/symptoms
  - Severe stridor, hypoxia, ventilator dependency
- Other signs/symptoms
  - Noisy breathing, "seal bark" cough, apneic spells, recurrent pulmonary infections early in life

Demographics

- Age
  - Typically presents in neonatal period

Natural History & Prognosis

- Type II is less favorable due to associated anomalies (60-80%)

Treatment

- Surgical division of LPA from its anomalous origin with implantation to its normal origin (main pulmonary artery)
- Tracheobronchial reconstruction if complete cartilaginous rings or other associated tracheobronchial malformations are present (types IIA & IIB)

DIAGNOSTIC CHECKLIST

Image Interpretation Pearls

- Anterior indentation on esophagus = LPA sling
  - Only vascular ring consistently between trachea & esophagus; other vascular rings may rarely have this course
- Round, small-caliber distal trachea on axial images = complete cartilaginous tracheal rings

SELECTED REFERENCES

1. Hong X et al: Tracheal development after left pulmonary artery reimplantation: an individual study. Sci Rep. 10(1):17702, 2020
2. Maldjian PD et al: Partial anomalous left pulmonary artery sling in an adult. J Clin Imaging Sci. 10:5, 2020
3. Porcedda G et al: Combined surgical and endoscopic approach for ring-sling complex. Thorac Cardiovasc Surg. 68(1):51-8, 2020
4. Vu HV et al: Surgical reconstruction for congenital tracheal malformation and pulmonary artery sling. J Cardiothorac Surg. 14(1):49, 2019
5. Arcieri L et al: Impact of 3D printing on the surgical management of tracheal stenosis associated to pulmonary sling: a case report. J Thorac Dis. 10(2):E130-3, 2018
6. Farkas A et al: Arterial tortuosity syndrome: an extremely rare disease presenting as a mimic of pulmonary sling. Radiol Case Rep. 13(1):295-8, 2018
7. Li X et al: Prenatal diagnosis of anomalous origin of pulmonary artery. Prenat Diagn. 38(5):310-7, 2018
8. Shi K et al: Dual-source computed tomography for quantitative assessment of tracheobronchial anomaly from type IIA pulmonary artery sling in pediatric patients. Eur J Radiol. 102:30-5, 2018
9. Yao M et al: Clinical and imaging features of pulmonary artery sling: the experience in one major medical center. Echocardiography. 35(8):1237-42, 2018
10. Fukuda H et al: 3-dimensional computed tomography imaging of the ring-sling complex with non-operative survival case in a 10-year-old female. Exp Ther Med. 14(3):2600-2, 2017
11. Ochiai D et al: Prenatal sonographic images of left pulmonary artery sling. Eur J Obstet Gynecol Reprod Biol. 211:217-8, 2017
12. Backer CL et al: Vascular rings. Semin Pediatr Surg. 25(3):165-75, 2016
13. Javia L et al: Rings, slings, and other tracheal disorders in the neonate. Semin Fetal Neonatal Med. 21(4):277-84, 2016
14. Chowdhury MM et al: Imaging of congenital lung malformations. Semin Pediatr Surg. 24(4):168-75, 2015
15. Hsieh ML et al: Single origin of right and left pulmonary arteries from ascending aorta with atretic main pulmonary artery from right ventricle and left pulmonary sling. J Cardiovasc Comput Tomogr. 9(6):599-600, 2015
16. Leonardi B et al: Imaging modalities in children with vascular ring and pulmonary artery sling. Pediatr Pulmonol. 50(8):781-8, 2015
17. Smith BM et al: Rings and slings revisited. Magn Reson Imaging Clin N Am. 23(1):127-35, 2015
18. Gundavaram MS et al: Asymptomatic pulmonary artery sling: a rare congenital vascular anomaly. Heart Lung Circ. 22(4):297-9, 2013
19. Backer CL et al: Pulmonary artery sling: current results with cardiopulmonary bypass. J Thorac Cardiovasc Surg. 143(1):144-51, 2012
20. Berdon WE et al: The triad of bridging bronchus malformation associated with left pulmonary artery sling and narrowing of the airway: the legacy of Wells and Landing. Pediatr Radiol. 42(2):215-9, 2012
21. Kir M et al: Vascular rings: presentation, imaging strategies, treatment, and outcome. Pediatr Cardiol. 33(4):607-17, 2012
22. McDonald ES et al: A rare case of horseshoe lung presenting in adulthood and associated with a pulmonary sling: case report and review of the literature. J Thorac Imaging. 25(3):W97-9, 2010

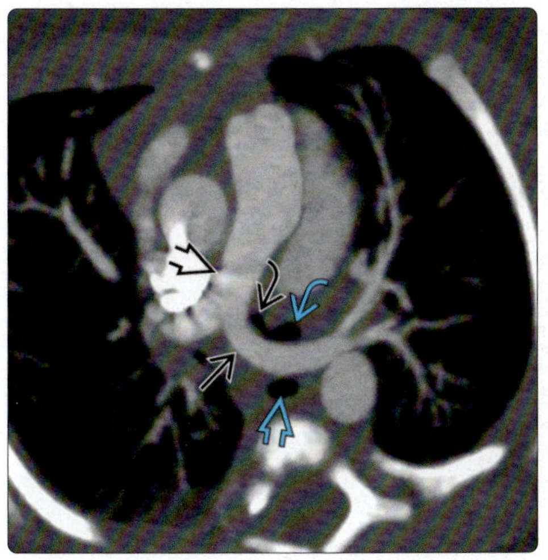

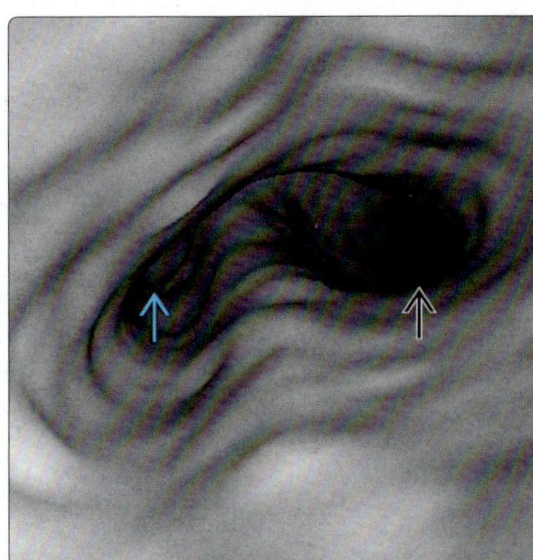

(Left) *Axial MIP CECT in an infant shows the classic pulmonary sling with the LPA ➔ arising from the RPA ➔ & coursing around the trachea on its way to the left lung. Note the asymmetric compression of the right mainstem bronchus ➔ compared to the left ➔. Also note the esophagus ➔ posterior to the LPA.* **(Right)** *Virtual bronchoscopy CT of the tracheal bifurcation in an infant with a pulmonary sling shows asymmetric compression of the left mainstem bronchus ➔ compared to the right ➔.*

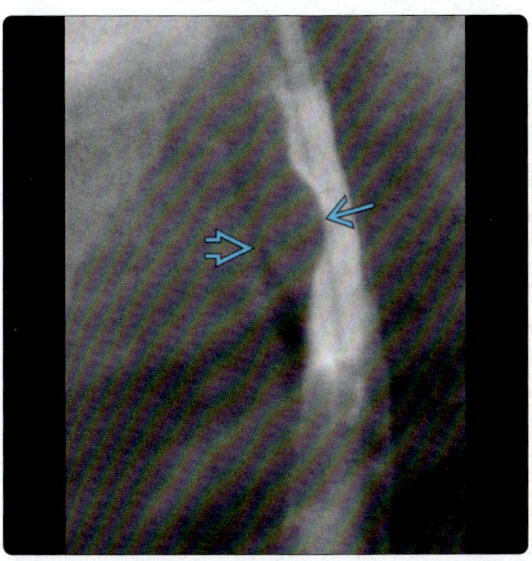

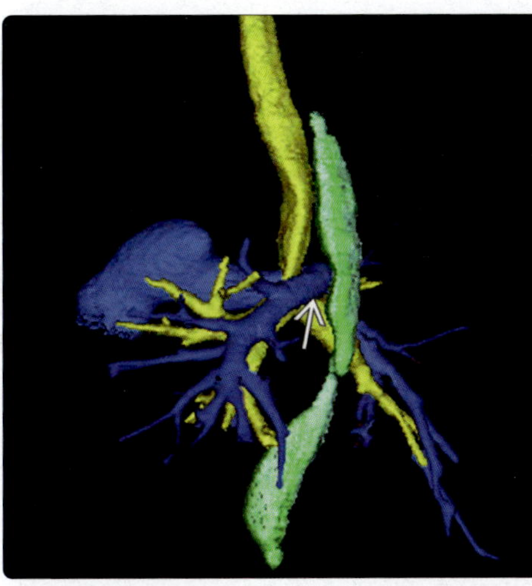

(Left) *Lateral image from an esophagram in a patient with a pulmonary sling shows a vascular impression of the aberrant course of the LPA on the anterior aspect of the esophagus ➔. Note that the LPA courses between the esophagus & trachea ➔ in this anomaly.* **(Right)** *Left posterior oblique 3D CTA of the chest in an infant with a pulmonary sling shows the LPA ➔ coursing between the esophagus (green) & the trachea (yellow). This is typical for a pulmonary sling & uncommon in other types of vascular rings.*

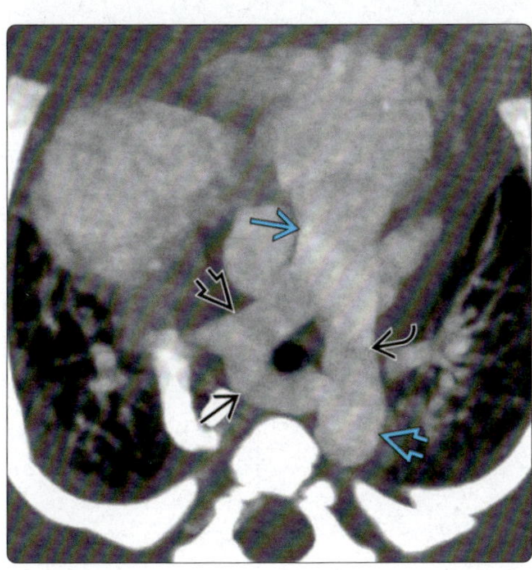

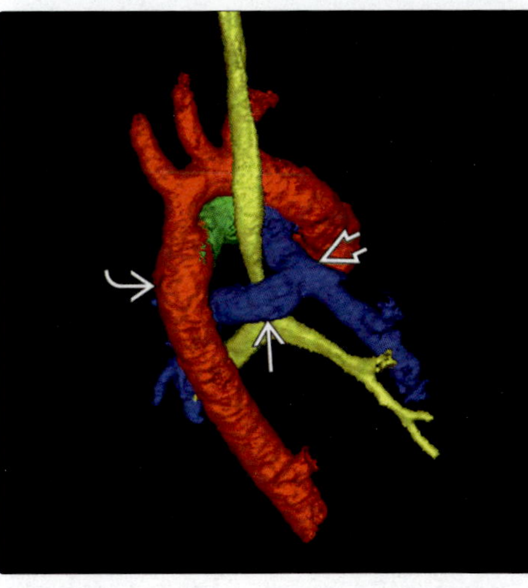

(Left) *Axial MIP image from a chest CTA in an infant with a pulmonary sling shows the LPA ➔ arising from the RPA ➔ then coursing around the trachea on its way to the left lung. Note the patent ductus arteriosus (PDA) ➔ connecting main PA ➔ with descending aorta ➔.* **(Right)** *Posterior oblique 3D CTA of the chest in an infant with a pulmonary sling shows the LPA ➔ arising from the RPA ➔ & coursing around the trachea on its way to the left lung. Note the PDA (green) connecting the main PA with the descending aorta ➔.*

KEY FACTS

TERMINOLOGY

- Symptomatic tracheal compression secondary to innominate artery traversing anterior to trachea

IMAGING

- Anterior impression on trachea from innominate artery → tracheal narrowing in AP dimension on any imaging study
  - Tracheal narrowing is confined to level at which innominate artery crosses anterior to trachea
- Detect tracheomalacia (excessive dynamic airway collapse) at level of innominate artery crossing by dynamic imaging on CT or MR
  - > 50-75% tracheal narrowing on dynamic imaging in symptomatic patient

TOP DIFFERENTIAL DIAGNOSES

- Mediastinal mass lesion causing tracheal compression
- Aberrant thyroid or ectopic thymus
- Vascular anomalies, such as vascular ring

PATHOLOGY

- Infantile trachea is relatively flaccid, lacking rigidity
- Normal innominate artery arises from left of trachea & courses across it anteriorly
  - Anomalous innominate artery syndrome is misnomer

CLINICAL ISSUES

- Presentations include stridor, apnea, dyspnea
  - History of recurrent bronchopulmonary infections in some patients with innominate artery compression syndrome
- Many asymptomatic children will have mild anterior compression (normal variant) on lateral radiographs & cross-sectional imaging studies
- Compression & resultant symptoms may ↓ over time as child grows

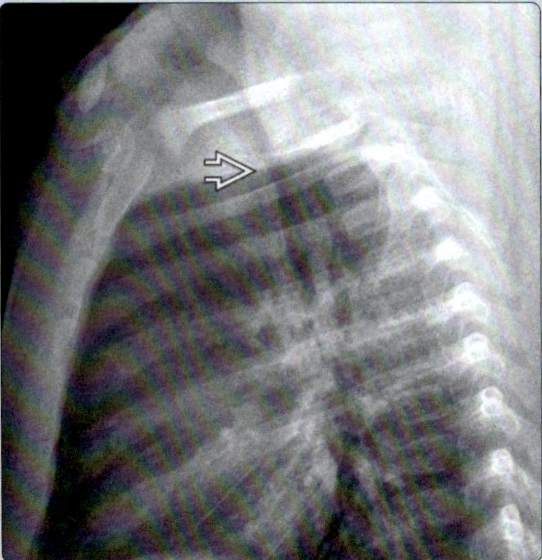

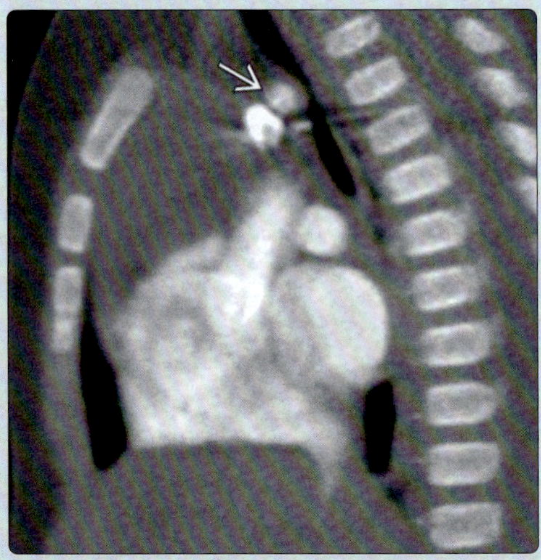

(Left) *Lateral chest radiograph shows significant narrowing of the trachea by an anterior impression ➡ just below the level of the sternal notch, compatible with innominate artery compression syndrome.* **(Right)** *Sagittal CTA in the same patient shows the relationship of the innominate artery ➡ to the trachea as it creates the anterior impression that was also seen on the lateral radiograph of the chest.*

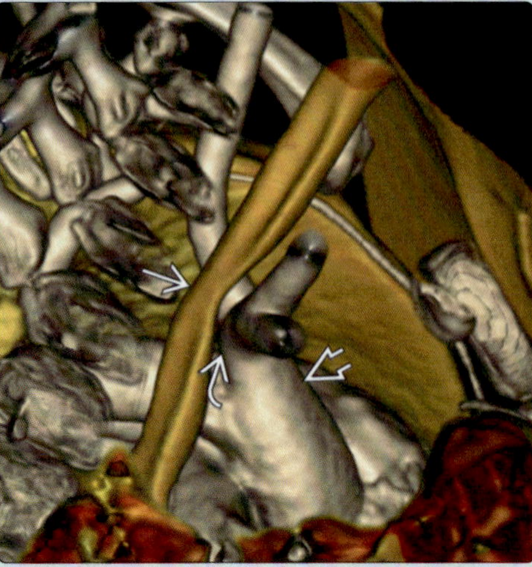

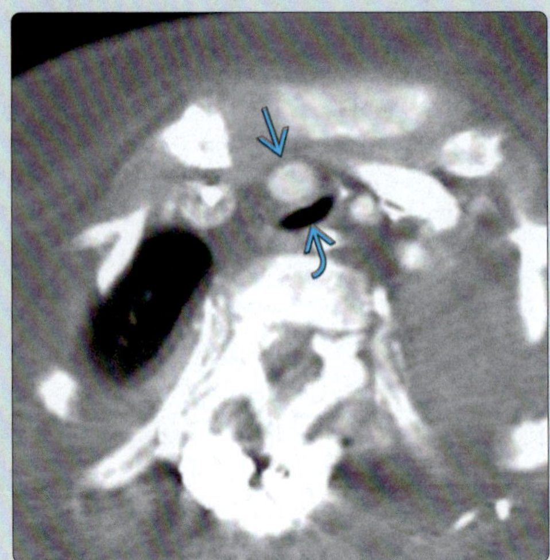

(Left) *Right lateral view of a vessel & airway 3D CTA reconstruction in a 7-month-old child demonstrates the aortic arch ➡ with the innominate artery ➡ crossing anterior to the trachea ➡ & causing compression.* **(Right)** *Axial image from a chest CTA in an adolescent patient with stridor after spine surgery shows compression of the trachea ➡ from the innominate artery ➡.*

TERMINOLOGY

Synonyms

- Anomalous innominate artery

Definitions

- Symptomatic tracheal compression secondary to innominate artery crossing anterior to trachea
  - Related to lack of rigidity in infantile trachea

IMAGING

General Features

- Best diagnostic clue
  - Anterior impression on trachea from innominate artery on any imaging study, typically at thoracic inlet

Radiographic Findings

- Radiography
  - On lateral radiography, anterior tracheal impression may be present with lack of air-trapping on frontal projection

CT Findings

- CECT
  - Tracheal narrowing is confined to level of innominate artery crossing
  - Can evaluate other etiologies in patients with tracheal compression on bronchoscopy
- CTA
  - 3D post processing shows relationship of vessels to trachea, along with virtual bronchoscopy views
  - Dynamic imaging can be performed to detect excessive dynamic airway narrowing (> 50-75% tracheal compression when compared to normal trachea)

MR Findings

- Tracheal narrowing as innominate artery crosses anteriorly

Other Modality Findings

- Endoscopy shows fixed, pulsatile compression on anterior aspect of trachea in most cases

Imaging Recommendations

- Best imaging tool
  - CT/MR defines degree of tracheal compression by innominate artery & excludes other causes
- Protocol advice
  - Endotracheal tube or positive pressure respiratory support can stent trachea & mask obstruction
  - CT evaluates vessels & relationships to airway; performance of dynamic imaging is plus
  - MR demonstrates anatomy on axial/sagittal imaging; dynamic airway imaging provides information on tracheomalacia

DIFFERENTIAL DIAGNOSIS

Masses Compressing Trachea

- Mediastinal bronchogenic cyst, duplication cyst, neurofibroma, lymphoma, thymic cyst, & teratoma

Normal Structures in Atypical Position

- Aberrant thyroid or ectopic thymic tissue

Vascular Abnormalities

- Right aortic arch + aberrant left subclavian artery, double aortic arch, & aneurysmal dilation of aorta or innominate artery

Lymphatic Malformation

- Mediastinal extension causing airway compression/infiltration

PATHOLOGY

General Features

- Etiology
  - Narrowing of trachea at thoracic inlet due to compression by innominate artery
    - Infantile trachea is relatively flaccid → crossing innominate artery accentuates tracheal narrowing

Gross Pathologic & Surgical Features

- Anterior wall of trachea demonstrates abnormal cartilage

CLINICAL ISSUES

Presentation

- Most common signs/symptoms
  - Presentations include stridor, apnea, dyspnea

Demographics

- Age
  - Young infants
- Sex
  - More common in males

Natural History & Prognosis

- Symptoms may ↓ over time as child grows

Treatment

- Most children are treated conservatively & outgrow disease
- Surgical approach is utilized in some: Aortopexy or reimplantation of innominate artery origin
  - With repeated hospitalizations due to respiratory infections
  - Symptomatic patients who fail conservative management

DIAGNOSTIC CHECKLIST

Image Interpretation Pearls

- Tracheal compression caused by innominate artery traversing anterior to trachea at thoracic inlet
- Typically detected on cross-sectional imaging, either incidentally or in patients with symptoms
- Associated tracheomalacia at site of crossing innominate artery can be elicited on dynamic airway imaging by CT or MR

SELECTED REFERENCES

1. Sainathan S et al: Median sternotomy for innominate artery compression syndrome and distal tracheal stenosis. Am Surg. ePub, 2021
2. Maddali MM et al: Real-time confirmation of tracheal decompression. J Card Surg. 35(3):666-7, 2020
3. Jennings RW et al: Surgical approaches to aortopexy for severe tracheomalacia. J Pediatr Surg. 49(1):66-70; discussion 70-1, 2014

Right Arch With Aberrant Left Subclavian Artery

KEY FACTS

IMAGING

- Right-sided aortic arch (RAA) with aberrant origin of left subclavian artery (ALSCA) from Kommerell diverticulum
- Lateral radiograph: Anterior tracheal bowing due to aberrant retroesophageal vessel
- Esophagram: Posterior indentation by aberrant vessel
  - Large posterior indentation: Diverticulum of Kommerell
- CTA or MRA with 3D reconstructions is now preferred modality for diagnosis prior to surgical intervention
  - Dynamic airway imaging can evaluate tracheomalacia at level of vascular ring

PATHOLOGY

- Related to embryologic persistence of right 4th aortic arch
- Left ductus persists as ligamentum arteriosum, which completes vascular ring
- ALSCA is typically retroesophageal; rarely it may lie anterior to esophagus (15%) or anterior to trachea (5%)

CLINICAL ISSUES

- Child presents with symptoms of stridor, apnea, cyanosis, recurrent respiratory infection, or chronic cough
  - Often referred for chest radiograph & ultimately cross-sectional imaging
- Treatment of RAA-ALSCA with constricting (symptomatic) left ligamentum arteriosum: Division of ligamentum via left thoracotomy

DIAGNOSTIC CHECKLIST

- RAA on radiograph in symptomatic child & absence of known underlying congenital heart disease (CHD) → perform further cross-sectional imaging
- RAA with airway compression & ALSCA on esophagram → perform cross-sectional imaging
- RAA, mirror image branching pattern → evaluate for underlying CHD

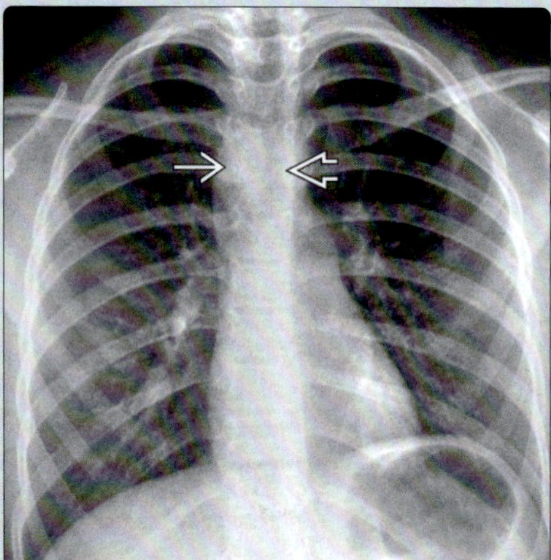

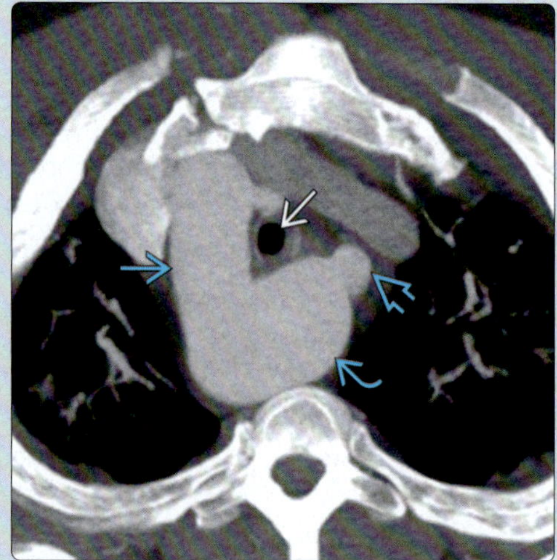

(Left) *PA radiograph of the chest shows a right aortic arch ➡ causing an impression on the right side of the trachea & displacing the trachea to the left ➡. This is an initial clue to diagnosing a right aortic arch with aberrant left subclavian artery (RAA-ALSCA) & is often overlooked.* **(Right)** *Axial MIP CTA in a child shows a right aortic arch ➡ with an aberrant left subclavian artery ➡ with mild tracheal compression ➡. Note the large diverticulum of Kommerell ➡ that often forms at the origin of the aberrant subclavian artery.*

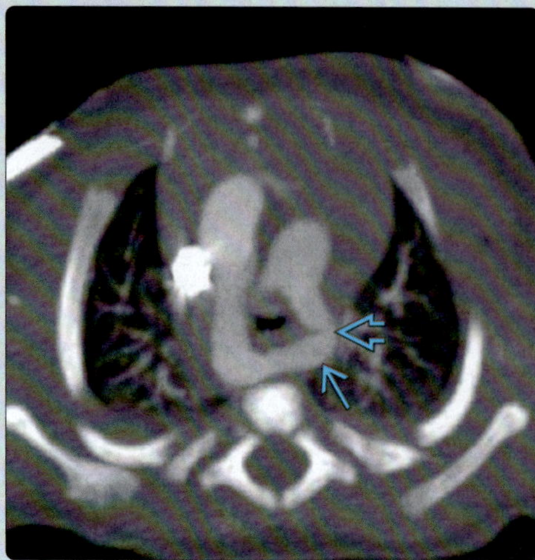

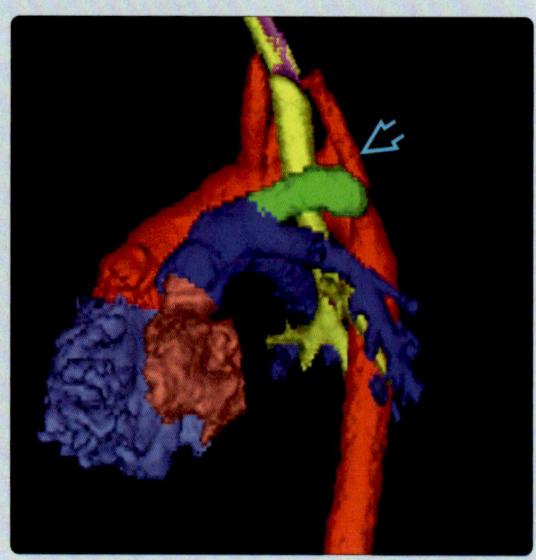

(Left) *Axial MIP cardiac CTA in an infant with stridor shows a right arch with an aberrant left subclavian ➡ & patent ductus arteriosus (PDA) ➡. This is a complete vascular ring even after the PDA closes.* **(Right)** *Lateral 3D color-coded surface-rendered CTA in an infant with stridor shows a right aortic arch (red) with an aberrant left subclavian artery ➡ & PDA (green). Note that the trachea (yellow) is completely encased by vascular structures, consistent with a complete vascular ring.*

TERMINOLOGY

Definitions

- Aortic arch lies to right of trachea [right aortic arch (RAA)], & aberrant left subclavian artery (ALSCA) originates from proximal descending aorta to course behind esophagus

IMAGING

Radiographic Findings

- Frontal view: Round soft tissue density along right side of trachea resulting in focal right-sided indentation & leftward tracheal deviation
- Lateral view: Anterior bowing of trachea

Fluoroscopic Findings

- Esophagram
  - Frontal view: Oblique filling defect at proximal 1/3 of esophagus coursing from right inferior to left superior
  - Lateral view: Large posterior indentation of esophagus caused by diverticulum of Kommerell

CT Findings

- RAA with retroesophageal ALSCA arising from bulbous diverticulum of Kommerell from proximal descending thoracic aorta
- Mass effect & airway narrowing at level of vascular ring (caused by left-sided ligamentum arteriosum)
- Reformatted 2D planes & 3D reconstructions nicely demonstrate effect on airway

MR Findings

- Black blood, bright blood, or postcontrast MRA images show abnormal branching pattern of vessels
- Black blood images show effect on tracheobronchial tree

Echocardiographic Findings

- Defines RAA & branching pattern along with origin of ALSCA

Imaging Recommendations

- Best imaging tool
  - CTA with 3D reconstruction
    - Advantages: Fast, generally no need for sedation/anesthesia; ± dynamic airway imaging for concurrent tracheobronchomalacia
    - Disadvantages: Radiation dose, use of IV iodinated contrast, & correct timing of contrast bolus
  - MRA
    - Advantages: No radiation, multiplanar technique
    - Disadvantages: May need sedation due to long exam time; need IV gadolinium contrast

DIFFERENTIAL DIAGNOSIS

Right Aortic Arch With Mirror Image Branching

- High association with cyanotic congenital heart disease (CHD), such as tetralogy of Fallot & truncus arteriosus

Double Aortic Arch With Atretic Left Arch

- Left arch is often atretic; left ligamentum arteriosum along with dominant right arch completes vascular ring
- Inferior tenting of left common carotid artery & 4-pronged branching pattern of arches at thoracic inlet

Left Aortic Arch With Aberrant Right Subclavian Artery

- Typically isolated & incidental abnormality (without airway compression)

PATHOLOGY

General Features

- Genetics
  - Right arch is often associated with 22q11 deletion
- Embryology/anatomy
  - Related to embryologic persistence of right 4th aortic arch
  - Retroesophageal (Kommerell) diverticulum: Remnant of embryonic left 4th dorsal aortic arch; connects to left ductus ligament
  - Right ductus is obliterated & left ductus persists as ligamentum arteriosum, which completes vascular ring

CLINICAL ISSUES

Presentation

- Most common signs/symptoms
  - Stridor, apnea, cyanosis, recurrent respiratory infection, chronic cough, & rarely dysphagia (lusoria) due to posterior esophageal compression
  - May be incidental finding on esophagram

Demographics

- Epidemiology
  - Aberrant subclavian artery is most common congenital anomaly of aortic arch
    - RAA-ALSCA: 0.1% of asymptomatic population
    - LAA-ARSCA: 0.5% of asymptomatic population

Natural History & Prognosis

- Prognosis is generally good after division of vascular ring
- Symptoms may persist from tracheomalacia & residual stenosis after vascular ring repair

Treatment

- RAA-ALSCA with constricting (symptomatic) left ligamentum arteriosum: Division of ligamentum via left thoracotomy
  - ± aortopexy if associated with midline descending aorta

SELECTED REFERENCES

1. Endo T et al: Right aortic arch with an aberrant left subclavian artery: sonographic features by HDlive Flow imaging. Cardiol Young. 30(6):892-3, 2020
2. Sun X et al: Prenatal diagnosis of right aortic arch and aberrant left subclavian artery in association with bilateral ductus arteriosus by two-and four-dimensional echocardiography: a case of rare vascular ring and review of literature. J Matern Fetal Neonatal Med. 1-6, 2020
3. Veger HTC et al: Right-sided aortic arch with aberrant branch vessels. Vasc Endovascular Surg. 54(7):660, 2020
4. Hanneman K et al: Congenital variants and anomalies of the aortic arch. Radiographics. 37(1):32-51, 2017
5. Tamayo-Espinosa T et al: [Right-side aortic arch with aberrant left subclavian artery and Kommerell's diverticulum. A cause of vascular ring.] Arch Cardiol Mex. 87(4):345-8, 2017

Infantile Hemangioma, Airway

KEY FACTS

IMAGING

- Asymmetric subglottic narrowing in young child on AP radiograph
- Uniform early enhancement of submucosal mass on CT/MR
  - May be circumferential, bilateral, or unilateral; usually asymmetric
- Ultrasound with Doppler may show vascular lesion

TOP DIFFERENTIAL DIAGNOSES

- Viral croup
- Tracheomalacia
- Airway papillomatosis
- Congenital subglottic tracheal stenosis
- Iatrogenic subglottic tracheal stenosis

PATHOLOGY

- Benign vascular neoplasm with predictable life cycle
  - Proliferative phase with rapid growth in 1st days-weeks after birth
  - Involuting phase with slow gradual regression over months-years
- GLUT1 positive in all phases
- Consider **PHACE(S)** syndrome: **P**osterior fossa brain malformations, segmental **h**emangiomas of face, **a**rterial anomalies, **c**ardiac anomalies, **e**ye abnormalities, **s**ternal clefts or **s**upraumbilical raphe

CLINICAL ISSUES

- Inspiratory stridor in infants < 6 months
  - Majority of lesions have progressive airway obstruction during proliferative phase
- Cutaneous infantile hemangiomas in 50%
- Treatment
  - Propranolol is 1st-line therapy; also consider corticosteroids, laser therapy, surgical excision
    - Combination used in 75%

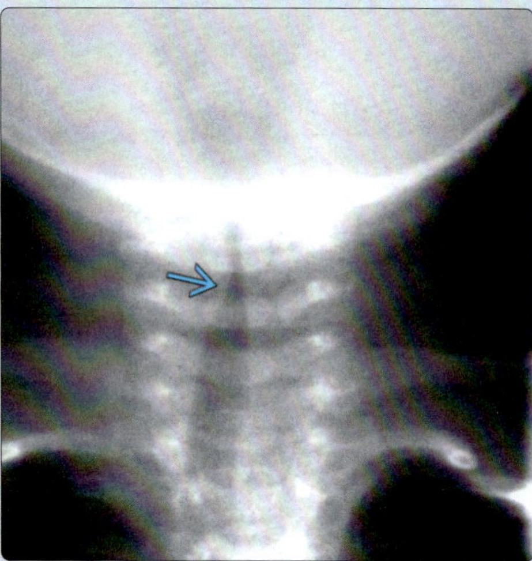

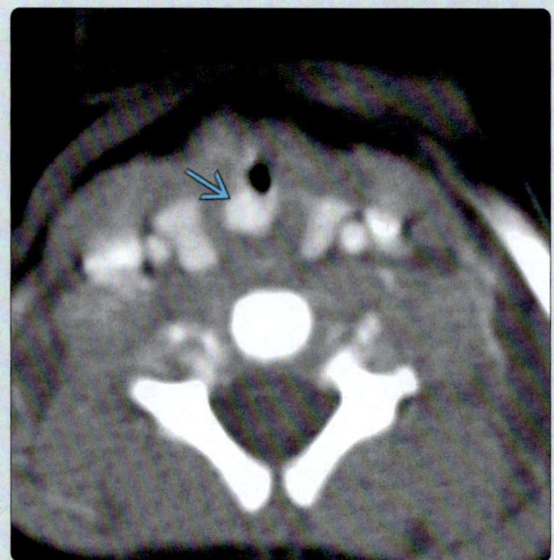

(Left) *AP radiograph shows asymmetric subglottic tracheal narrowing ➡ in a 2-week-old infant presenting with stridor. Asymmetric narrowing in this age is concerning for an infantile hemangioma (IH), as opposed to the symmetric subglottic narrowing that is typical of croup.* **(Right)** *Axial CECT in the same patient shows a well-defined, enhancing IH ➡ along the dorsolateral aspect of the subglottic airway.*

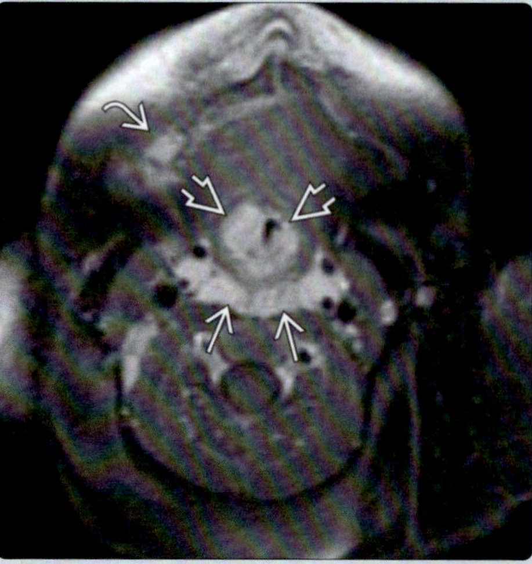

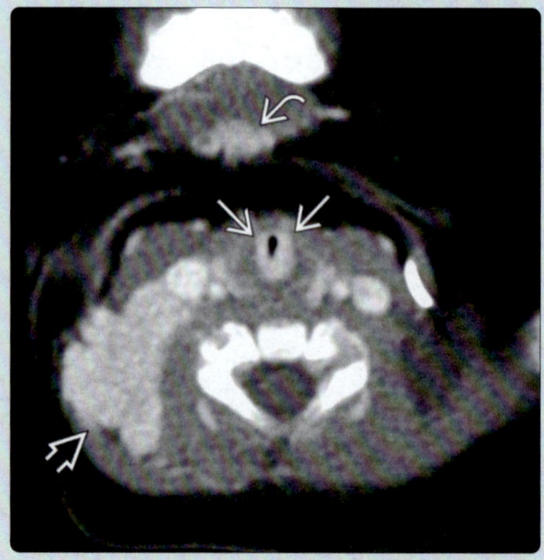

(Left) *Axial T1 C+ FS MR in a child with PHACE(S) syndrome demonstrates multiple enhancing IHs in the retropharyngeal space ➡, surrounding the subglottic trachea ➡, & in the right submental space ➡.* **(Right)** *Axial CECT in an 11-week-old girl demonstrates a circumferential, well-defined subglottic IH ➡. Note also the posterior cervical space ➡ & submental ➡ IHs, which should raise the question of PHACE(S) syndrome.*

TERMINOLOGY

Definitions

- Infantile hemangioma (IH) of subglottic airway

IMAGING

General Features

- Location
  - Classically subglottic, may be transglottic
  - Usually asymmetric or affecting only 1 side, L > R

Radiographic Findings

- Asymmetric subglottic tracheal narrowing on AP radiograph

CT Findings

- Usually solitary, homogeneously enhancing subglottic mass

MR Findings

- Intermediate T1, hyperintense T2, early homogeneous enhancement

Ultrasonographic Findings

- May show vascular subglottic mass on Doppler

Imaging Recommendations

- Best imaging tool
  - Multiplanar CECT reconstructions help define mass & tracheal compression
    - Quicker than MR & may not need sedation
  - MR is more sensitive (due to higher contrast resolution), but sedation is usually needed

DIFFERENTIAL DIAGNOSIS

Viral Croup

- Symmetric subglottic tracheal narrowing (steeple appearance on AP view)
- Most common 8 months to 3 years of age

Tracheomalacia

- Abnormal dynamic collapse of trachea

Airway Papillomatosis

- Affects entire trachea, bronchi, & lungs
- Rare in infants

Congenital Subglottic Tracheal Stenosis

- Symmetric tracheal narrowing
- Complete tracheal rings
  - Round tracheal configuration on axial images
  - ± pulmonary sling or congenital heart disease

Iatrogenic Subglottic Tracheal Stenosis

- Prior history of intubation or tracheostomy
- Secondary to scarring or granuloma formation

PATHOLOGY

General Features

- Etiology
  - Benign vascular neoplasm of proliferating endothelial cells; not vascular malformation
- Genetics
  - Majority are sporadic
- Associated abnormalities
  - **PHACE(S)** syndrome: **P**osterior fossa brain malformations, **h**emangiomas of face, **a**rterial anomalies, **c**ardiac anomalies, **e**ye abnormalities, **s**ternal clefts or **s**upraumbilical raphe
    - 7% have subglottic IHs

Staging, Grading, & Classification

- Predictable life cycle of IHs
  - Proliferative phase: ↑ size days-weeks after birth up through 9-24 months
  - Involuting phase: Gradual regression over next several years

Microscopic Features

- GLUT1 immunohistochemical marker: Positive in all phases of infantile hemangioma

CLINICAL ISSUES

Presentation

- Most common signs/symptoms
  - Inspiratory stridor in infants < 6 months
- Other signs/symptoms
  - Cutaneous IHs in 50%
  - Hoarseness or abnormal cry

Natural History & Prognosis

- Majority of lesions have progressive airway obstruction during proliferative phase
- Symptoms resolve after involution
- Benign condition but can have fatal outcome
  - With segmental bearded distribution of cutaneous IH & PHACE(S) syndrome, may have more recalcitrant & complicated natural history
- Diagnosis is confirmed at endoscopy

Treatment

- Conservative monitoring
  - Considered in children with < 30% narrowing without respiratory or feeding difficulty
- Propranolol: 1st-line treatment in recent years
- Systemic corticosteroids
  - ± rebound growth when steroids are tapered
- Intralesional corticosteroids
- CO_2 laser therapy
- Combination of therapies is used in 75%

SELECTED REFERENCES

1. Alsuwailem A et al: Vascular anomalies of the head and neck. Semin Pediatr Surg. 29(5):150968, 2020
2. Krowchuk DP et al: Clinical practice guideline for the management of infantile hemangiomas. Pediatrics. 143(1), 2019
3. McCormick AA et al: Subglottic hemangioma: understanding the association with facial segmental hemangioma in a beard distribution. Int J Pediatr Otorhinolaryngol. 113:34-7, 2018
4. Mamlouk MD et al: Arterial spin-labeled perfusion for vascular anomalies in the pediatric head and neck. Clin Imaging. 40(5):1040-6, 2016
5. Merrow AC et al: 2014 revised classification of vascular lesions from the International Society for the Study of Vascular Anomalies: radiologic-pathologic update. Radiographics. 36(5):1494-516, 2016
6. Rossler L et al: Ultrasound and colour Doppler in infantile subglottic haemangioma. Pediatr Radiol. 41(11):1421-8, 2011

Tracheobronchomalacia

KEY FACTS

TERMINOLOGY

- Excessive expiratory collapse of trachea &/or bronchi
  - May be purely intrinsic or in association with longstanding extrinsic compression

IMAGING

- > 50% ↓ in cross-sectional area of tracheal &/or bronchial lumen during expiration or coughing
  - Correlates well with bronchoscopy
  - Relatively underdiagnosed, as imaging is routinely performed only at end inspiration
- ↑ frequency & severity of air-trapping
- Dynamic 4D MDCT (real-time model of airway during respiration) vs. static inspiratory & expiratory CT scans
  - Multiplanar reconstructions & 3D volume rendering of airway are helpful
  - Intravenous contrast is useful to look for contributory adjacent mass or aberrant vessel
- Cine MR is also being used

TOP DIFFERENTIAL DIAGNOSES

- Difficult to control asthma
- Foreign body aspiration
- Extrinsic compression
- Complete tracheal rings

PATHOLOGY

- Primary (congenital): Impaired cartilage maturation or congenital absence of cartilage rings
- Secondary (acquired): Otherwise normal cartilage degenerates following infection, chronic inflammation, intubation, trauma, or longstanding extrinsic compression

CLINICAL ISSUES

- Presentations: Expiratory stridor, dyspnea, cough, sputum production, acute life-threatening events (ALTEs)

DIAGNOSTIC CHECKLIST

- Expiratory phase of imaging is necessary when evaluating for tracheobronchomalacia

(Left) *Inspiratory axial HRCT shows a normal, nearly rounded appearance of the trachea ➔. The posterior aspect is often nearly flat, as it lacks supportive cartilage. The caliber of the trachea should be uniform from the glottis to the carina & relatively unchanging between inspiration & expiration.* **(Right)** *Expiratory axial HRCT in the same patient shows marked narrowing of the trachea ➔, a substantial change from the inspiratory image that is consistent with tracheomalacia.*

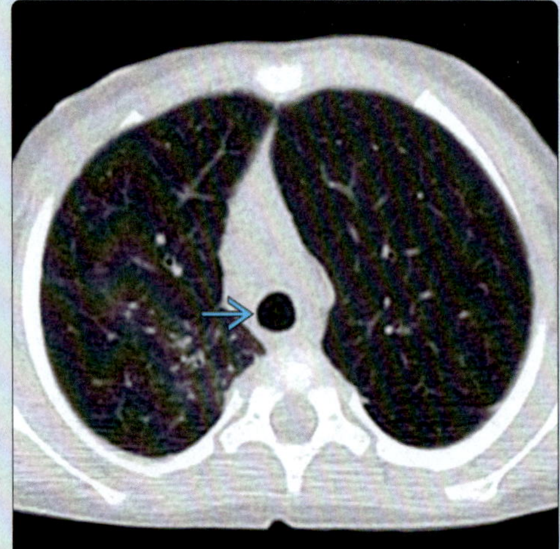

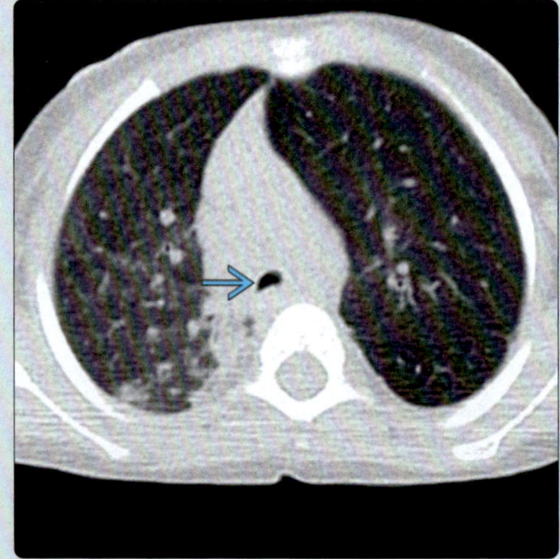

(Left) *Expiratory axial HRCT shows severe tracheomalacia, nearly obliterating the lumen, with a typical horseshoe or "frowny face" appearance ➔ of the trachea in cross section.* **(Right)** *Virtual bronchoscopy 3D surface-rendered expiratory CT shows severe tracheomalacia with a typical horseshoe or "frowny face" appearance of the trachea ➔.*

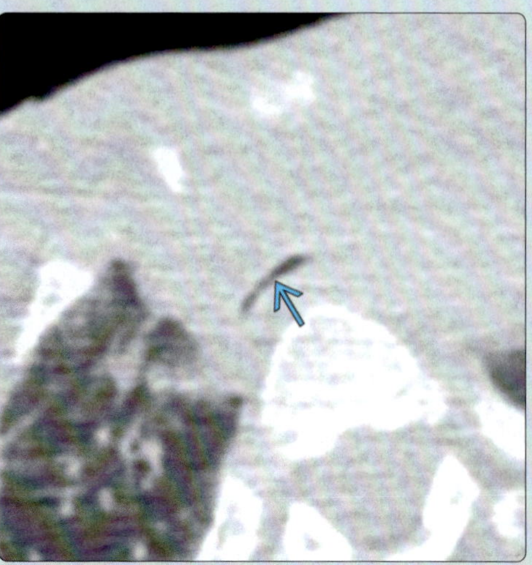

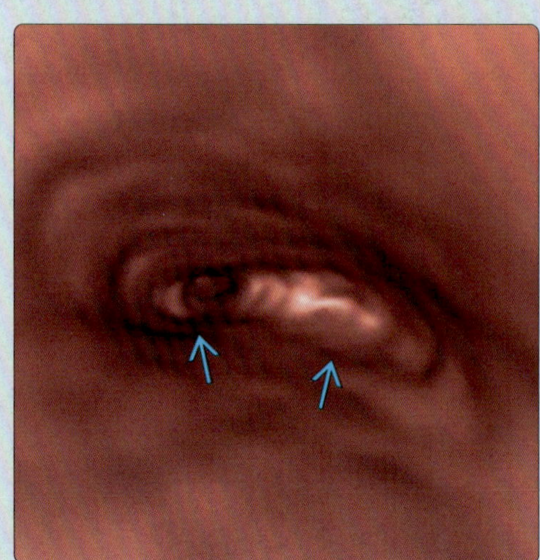

TERMINOLOGY

Synonyms

- Excessive dynamic airway collapse

Definitions

- Excessive expiratory collapse of trachea or bronchi
  - May be purely intrinsic or in association with longstanding extrinsic compression

IMAGING

General Features

- Best diagnostic clue
  - > 50% ↓ in cross-sectional area of tracheal &/or bronchial lumen during expiration or coughing
    - Correlates well with bronchoscopy, which remains gold standard for diagnosis

Radiographic Findings

- Airway radiography
  - Only 62% sensitive for tracheomalacia

CT Findings

- > 50% ↓ in cross-sectional area of tracheobronchial lumen during expiration is found to correlate well with bronchoscopy
- ↑ frequency & severity of air-trapping compared to children without tracheomalacia
- Adjacent mass or abnormal vessel (causing extrinsic compression) may contribute to collapse

MR Findings

- Cine MR: Increasingly feasible technique for assessment of tracheobronchomalacia

Imaging Recommendations

- Best imaging tool
  - CT: Dynamic airway (cine or 4D) MDCT vs. paired static inspiratory-expiratory CT
- Protocol advice
  - Intravenous contrast is helpful to define vascular anatomy as related to airway
  - Expiratory phase is necessary to evaluate dynamic large airway disease
  - Multiplanar reconstructions & 3D volume rendering are helpful

DIFFERENTIAL DIAGNOSIS

Difficult to Control Asthma

- No large airway caliber change with expiration

Foreign Body Aspiration

- Air-trapping on expiratory or ipsilateral decubitus images
- Intraluminal filling defect of airway
- ± classic history of choking episode with persistent symptoms

Extrinsic Compression

- Cystic or solid mass
- Aberrant or aneurysmal vessel, vascular ring
- Chronically dilated proximal esophageal pouch due to congenital esophageal atresia

Complete Tracheal Rings

- Completely round, small-caliber trachea
- Unchanging between inspiration & expiration
- May be associated with pulmonary sling

PATHOLOGY

General Features

- Etiology
  - Weakness of airway wall/supporting cartilage

Staging, Grading, & Classification

- Primary (congenital): Impaired cartilage maturation or congenital absence of cartilage rings
- Secondary (acquired): Otherwise normal cartilage degenerates following infection, chronic inflammation, intubation, trauma, or longstanding extrinsic compression
  - More common than primary

CLINICAL ISSUES

Presentation

- Most common signs/symptoms
  - Expiratory stridor, dyspnea, cough, sputum production, acute life-threatening events (ALTEs)

Demographics

- Epidemiology
  - Exact incidence is unknown
  - Found in up to 15% of infants & 30% of children < 3 years old who have undergone bronchoscopy for respiratory distress

Treatment

- Conservative therapy in mild cases; may improve with age
- Continuous positive airway pressure (CPAP) in moderate cases
  - ↓ energy expenditure for breathing by neonates
- Aortopexy
  - Most common initial operative approach
- Anterior tracheal suspension
  - Relief of airway symptoms in most severe & refractory cases
- Intraluminal tracheal stenting is rarely employed

SELECTED REFERENCES

1. Poore TS et al: Vascular and pulmonary comorbidities in children with congenital EA/TEF. Pediatr Pulmonol. 56(2):571-7, 2021
2. Gunatilaka CC et al: Increased work of breathing due to tracheomalacia in neonates. Ann Am Thorac Soc. 17(10):1247-56, 2020
3. Hysinger EB et al: Ultrashort echo-time MRI for the assessment of tracheomalacia in neonates. Chest. 157(3):595-602, 2020
4. Williams SP et al: Aortopexy for the management of paediatric tracheomalacia - the Alder Hey experience. J Laryngol Otol. 1-4, 2020
5. Cohen SL et al: Ultralow dose dynamic expiratory computed tomography for evaluation of tracheomalacia. J Comput Assist Tomogr. 43(2):307-11, 2019
6. Wallis C et al: ERS statement on tracheomalacia and bronchomalacia in children. Eur Respir J. 54(3), 2019
7. McInnis MC et al: Advanced technologies for imaging and visualization of the tracheobronchial tree: from computed tomography and MRI to virtual endoscopy. Thorac Surg Clin. 28(2):127-37, 2018
8. Shepard JO et al: Imaging of the trachea. Ann Cardiothorac Surg. 7(2):197-209, 2018

SECTION 2

Chest

Trauma

Pediatric Interstitial Lung Diseases

Chest Wall Issues

Miscellaneous

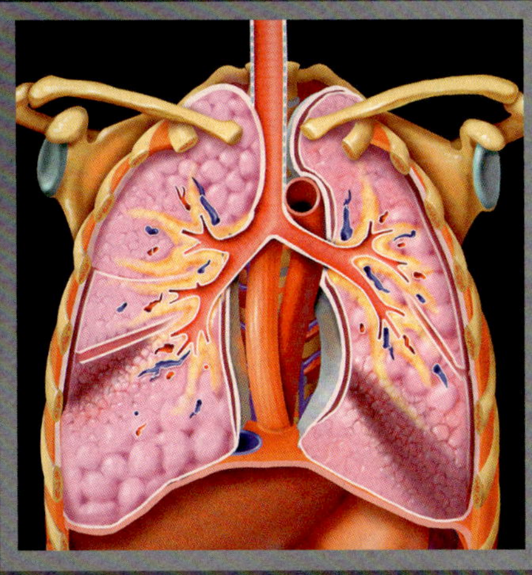

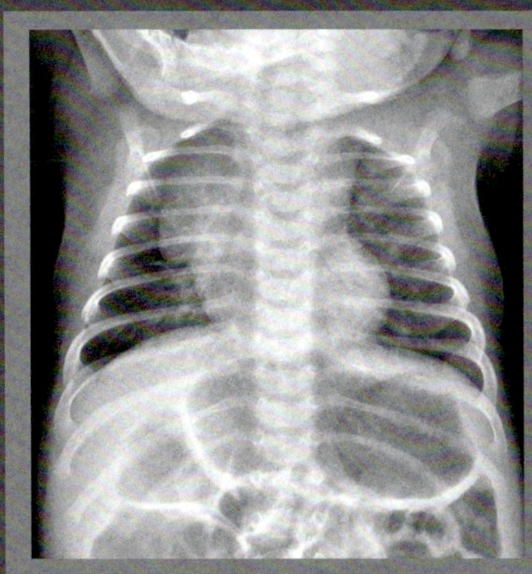

Introduction

Chest radiography is one of the most frequently performed pediatric imaging studies. The radiographic appearance of many conditions is contingent on the age & history of the patient. Additionally, there is often overlap in the radiographic appearances of very different clinical entities. Therefore, arriving at the correct diagnosis often depends on obtaining an adequate history, reviewing prior imaging, & effectively communicating with the referring clinician(s).

Pulmonary Developmental Abnormalities

With the current use of prenatal ultrasound & MR, most developmental pulmonary abnormalities have already been imaged prior to the 1st newborn chest radiograph. This has substantially improved the perinatal care for high-risk infants, particularly given that information predicting pulmonary hypoplasia & persistent pulmonary hypertension can be extracted from these exams (which allows improved planning for the delivery suite). In such lesions, postnatal imaging may be used to confirm the diagnosis & is helpful for surgical planning, particularly given that varying degrees of spontaneous regression have been reported with some entities in late gestation. Postnatal CT for prenatally diagnosed pulmonary masses should be performed as a CT angiogram because lesions can be of mixed etiology (i.e., a hybrid lesion); it is critical for the surgeons to know the vascular supply of such lesions prior to resection.

Examples

Congenital pulmonary airway malformation (CPAM) is a multicystic pulmonary mass with variable amounts of air/fluid in the lesion after birth. The mass is often seen prenatally. Postnatal CTA is always warranted, even if the radiograph appears normal.

Bronchopulmonary sequestration (BPS) is a solid lower lobe lesion that has systemic arterial supply. It is crucial to extend the CTA through the top of the kidneys to exclude an origin of the supplying artery from the upper abdominal aorta.

Components of both CPAM & BPS are present simultaneously in hybrid lesions.

A bronchogenic cyst is a fluid-density or soft tissue-density mass in the mediastinum or medial lung. These cysts can present with respiratory distress or dysphagia.

Congenital lobar overinflation presents with a hyperlucent & hyperexpanded lobe or segment in a neonate or infant. The most frequent locations are the left upper lobe > right middle lobe > right upper lobe. Do not mistake these lesions for a pneumothorax.

Bronchial atresia presents with a characteristic-appearing round or branching hilar or pulmonary mass (finger-in-glove appearance) with a hyperinflated lung distally. These lesions may be diagnosed at any age.

Congenital diaphragmatic hernia is not a primary pulmonary developmental anomaly but may appear similar to CPAM or sequestration. Congenital diaphragmatic hernia contains variable abdominal contents (stomach, small/large bowel, liver, spleen). Use abnormal support device positions as clues to this diagnosis.

Acquired Neonatal Lung Disease

Clinical history is often key in diagnosing neonatal lung disease. For example, the diagnostic dilemma of differentiating meconium aspiration from neonatal pneumonia can be solved with a brief history or a phone call to the NICU. At the very least, the radiologist should be provided with the gestational age, as this single data point often significantly narrows the differential diagnosis.

Premature Infant

- Surfactant deficiency disease is characterized by low lung volumes & diffuse, hazy granular opacities; pleural effusions are uncommon in this setting.
- Due to low pulmonary compliance & positive-pressure ventilation, patients with surfactant deficiency disease are at risk for developing pulmonary interstitial emphysema (PIE). Characterized by bubbly or linear branching lucencies, it can be difficult to differentiate PIE from the bubbly lucencies of air bronchograms & cysts; look for linear lucencies extending to the lung periphery in PIE. Also remember that air in the interstitium prevents gas exchange, similar to a pneumothorax.
- Bronchopulmonary dysplasia (or chronic lung disease of prematurity) is characterized by hyperinflation with coarse, reticular opacities & intervening lucencies (typically with > 28 days of oxygen/ventilator support). These patients are at increased risk for pulmonary infections (e.g., RSV) in the first 2 years of life.

Term Infant

- Neonatal pneumonia classically presents as patchy, asymmetric perihilar opacities, often with pleural effusions; however, the reality is that neonatal pneumonia can mimic virtually any other neonatal lung disease. Thus, clinicians are highly conservative in treating for pneumonia until proven otherwise.
- Meconium aspiration typically shows radiating, coarse, rope-like bilateral lung opacities with hyperinflation (& sometimes small pleural effusions). These patients are at risk for pneumothorax. The clinical course is highly variable. Adequate history is key as clinicians will already know whether or not meconium was present at birth.
- Transient tachypnea of the newborn (TTN), or retained fetal lung fluid, presents with streaky perihilar or granular pulmonary opacities. Infants with TTN tend to be less seriously ill, & imaging findings resolve in 24-48 hours.
- Chylothorax should be considered in infants who present with pleural fluid, especially in the setting of a lymphatic anomaly, Turner syndrome, or Noonan syndrome.
- It must also be remembered that congenital heart disease can mimic neonatal lung disease.

Pediatric Catheters & Tubes

The most common indication for ordering a NICU chest radiograph is to evaluate the positions of various indwelling support devices (such as vascular catheters, airway tubes, & enteric tubes). Neonatologists are especially meticulous in this regard, as many of them have witnessed catastrophes or near catastrophes associated with line/tube malpositions. The ubiquitous use of lines & tubes & the low frequency of complications make it disconcertingly easy to overlook line/tube malposition. Rather than simply reporting "lines & tubes unchanged," forcing oneself to report the position of each support device increases the likelihood of detecting malposition before a complication occurs.

Examples

The ideal position for the umbilical arterial catheter tip is between the T6 & T10 levels. The ideal position for an umbilical venous catheter (UVC) is at or just below the right atrium/inferior vena cava junction. Remember that a UVC that has not passed beyond the ductus venosus should generally not be used for a hyperosmolar infusate as it will be dispersed into the liver. (Note that the NICU will sometimes temporarily use a UVC below the liver margin for low-risk infusions.)

Esophageal intubation classically presents with hypoinflated lungs + gaseous distention of the esophagus & stomach.

ECMO may be performed with either arteriovenous or venovenous cannulae. Central great vessel catheters may rarely be used, particularly in the setting of complex heart disease.

Peripherally inserted central catheters are associated with rare but potentially catastrophic complications, particularly if left to dwell in the right atrium.

Common Pediatric Pulmonary Infections

"Rule out pneumonia" is one of the most common indications for outpatient pediatric imaging. The appearance of pediatric airway disease can be variable. The radiologist who finds that they are struggling with the diagnosis of airway disease should keep in mind that most pediatricians rely more heavily on clinical findings than on the radiologist's report to diagnose bronchiolitis or asthma. Clinicians are often more interested to know whether there are findings of bacterial pneumonia, or other explanations for the patient's symptoms.

Examples

Viral infection is shown by perihilar peribronchial opacities & hyperinflation, often with intermixed atelectasis.

Round pneumonia has a well-defined, mass-like appearance, typically occurring in patients under age 8 (due to poorly developed collateral pathways). If it is paraspinous in location, follow-up radiography is advised to ensure resolution of the pneumonia (thereby excluding paraspinal masses, such as neuroblastoma).

Management of parapneumonic effusion & empyema should be based on clinical findings, serial radiography, & ultrasound rather than CT.

Fungal pneumonia in immunocompromised patients classically presents as nodules, potentially with a halo of ground-glass opacity (that suggests hemorrhage).

Papillomatosis may present as multiple laryngeal, tracheal, &/or pulmonary nodules; the latter may cavitate.

Pediatric Mediastinal Masses

Simply differentiating a normal from abnormal mediastinum can be difficult in infants & young children. However, a few clues usually lead to confident radiographic differentiation.

Examples

The normal thymus can be large in children up to 5 years of age. Look for an undulating contour, the sail or wave sign, & overlying pulmonary vascular markings. There should be no mass effect on the trachea. Ultrasound can be useful to confirm thymic tissue if there is doubt radiographically.

Lymphoma often presents as a bulky anterior mediastinal mass without Ca^{2+}. Mass effect on the trachea & vascular structures is typical.

Mediastinal germ cell tumors present as anterior mediastinal masses, classically with fat & Ca^{2+} (teratoma).

Neuroblastoma typically presents as a posterior mediastinal mass. Look closely for Ca^{2+} as well as bony changes (with posterior rib splaying or erosion being particularly suggestive).

Noninfectious Pediatric Lung Masses

Metastases are by far the most common pulmonary malignancies in the pediatric age group. Primary pulmonary neoplasms are rare in children.

Examples

Lung metastases are most common with osteosarcoma, Ewing sarcoma, hepatoblastoma, soft tissue sarcomas, Wilms tumor, testicular tumors, & thyroid tumors.

Bronchial obstruction may be due to a foreign body, intrinsic airway mass, or extrinsic compression. Look for asymmetric inflation due to air-trapping.

Pediatric Chest Trauma

A very important element of chest radiography is to evaluate for evidence of child abuse, especially in infants & young children. The radiologist is obligated to immediately contact the referring clinician if there are any suspicious findings of nonaccidental trauma to ensure that the case is appropriately investigated & the child is appropriately protected.

Examples

Multiple rib fractures in a child < 3 years old are usually due to child abuse. While they can involve any portion of the rib, posterior rib fractures are most specific for child abuse.

Pulmonary contusion appears as a nonspecific opacity in the setting of trauma, often with a thin zone of peripheral lung sparing. The presence of an air-filled or fluid-filled cavity suggests pulmonary laceration.

Pediatric Diffuse Lung Disease

Diffuse lung disease is rare. A few etiologies have a characteristic appearance that may suggest a single diagnosis with reasonable confidence.

Examples

Neuroendocrine cell hyperplasia of infancy (NEHI) has a characteristic HRCT appearance of central & lingular + right middle lobe geographic ground-glass opacities.

Lymphangioleiomyomatosis presents in tuberous sclerosis as numerous bilateral, thin-walled cysts.

Selected References

1. Biko DM et al: Mediastinal masses in children: radiologic-pathologic correlation. Radiographics. 41(4):E1186-207, 2021
2. Tugwell-Allsup J et al: Mobile chest imaging of neonates in incubators: optimising DR and CR acquisitions. Radiography (Lond). 27(1):75-80, 2021
3. Frush DJ et al: Utilization of computed tomography imaging in the pediatric emergency department. Pediatr Radiol. 50(4):470-5, 2020

(Left) *Coronal chest CTA MIP in a 2-month-old infant with a prenatally diagnosed congenital lung lesion shows both the systemic arterial supply ➡ & the pulmonary venous drainage ➡ of the bronchopulmonary sequestration.* **(Right)** *Coronal SSFP fetal MR shows ↑ signal intensity of the left upper lobe of the lung ➡ due to congenital lobar overinflation (CLO). In utero, trapping of amniotic fluid results in ↑ signal intensity of the distended lung compared to the right ➡.*

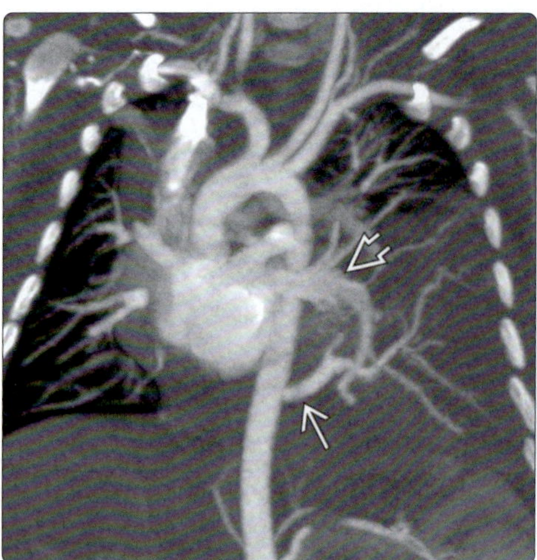

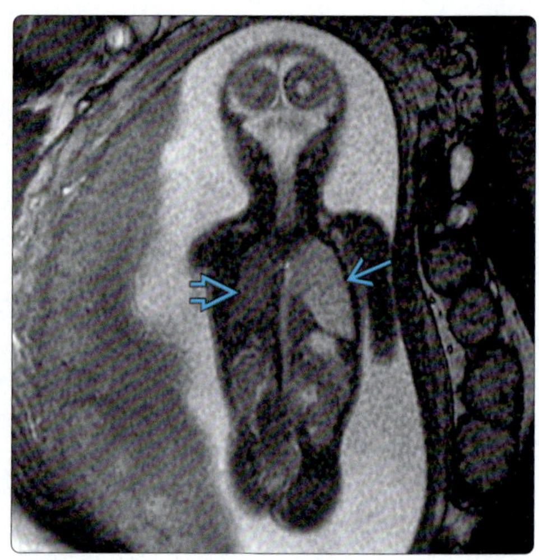

(Left) *Axial CECT in a neonate with tachypnea shows focal air-trapping ➡ in the lingula with no distortion of vessels, consistent with CLO. Note that the normal lung ➡ has comparatively higher density in the neonate.* **(Right)** *Lateral oblique 3D CT of the lungs in the same neonate demonstrates the focal air trapping of the lingula ➡ due to CLO.*

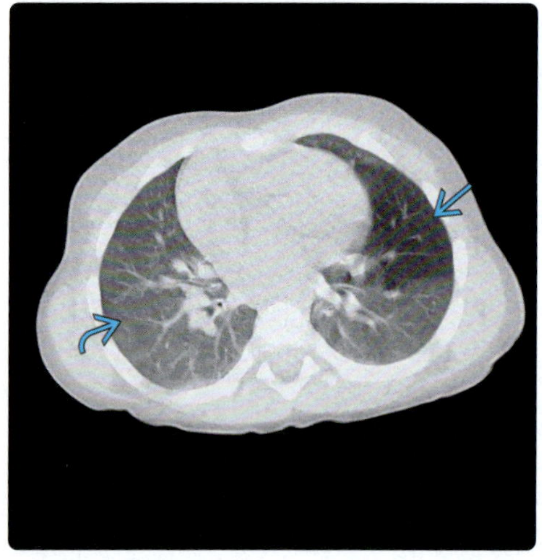

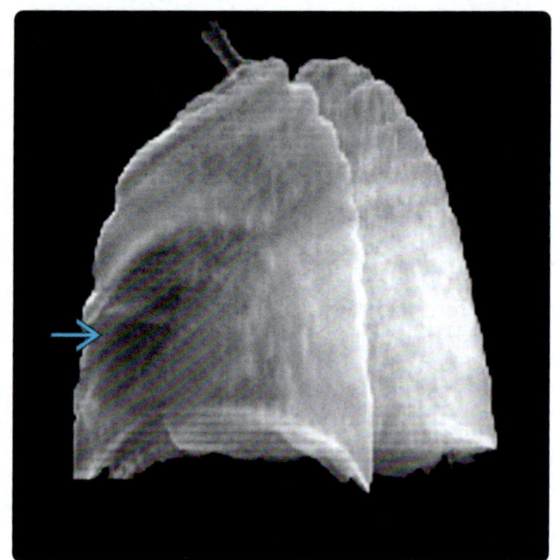

(Left) *AP radiograph in a former 25-weeks-premature girl shows bilateral bubbly & linear lucencies of pulmonary interstitial emphysema (PIE) with a large right pneumothorax. Despite the tension pneumothorax, the right lung is not collapsed (due to ↓ pulmonary compliance from surfactant deficiency & PIE).* **(Right)** *AP chest radiograph in a neonate with a left CDH shows several gas-containing bowel loops ➡ in the left upper hemithorax. The stomach is also in the chest, as confirmed by the enteric tube ➡.*

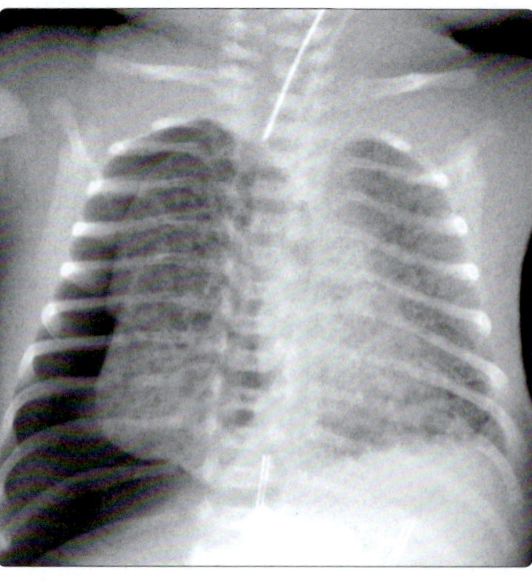

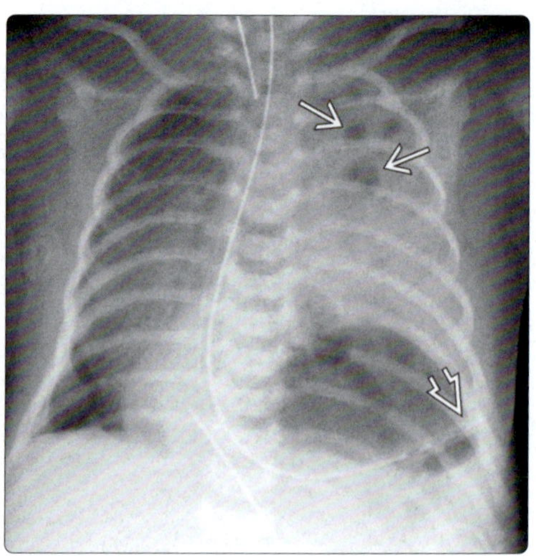

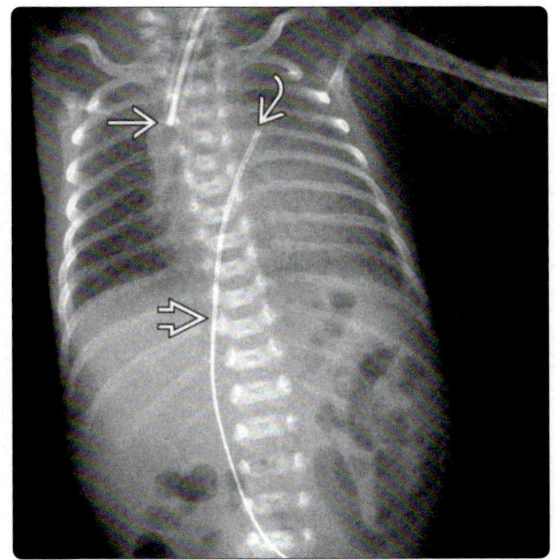

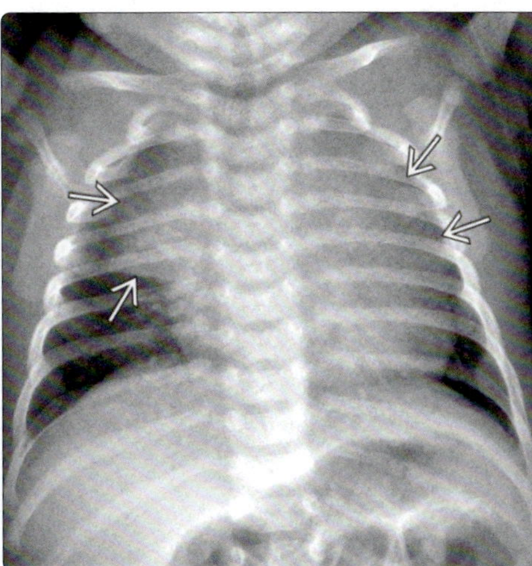

(Left) *AP radiograph following endotracheal tube & umbilical venous catheter (UVC) placement shows abnormal position of the UVC extending into the left upper pulmonary vein (having crossed a patent foramen ovale to the left atrium).* **(Right)** *AP chest radiograph in a 1-month-old boy shows a large but normal thymus that could be mistaken for a mediastinal mass. The shape, mild undulation, location, lack of mass effect, & age are normal for thymus. If uncertain, ultrasound can confirm thymic tissue.*

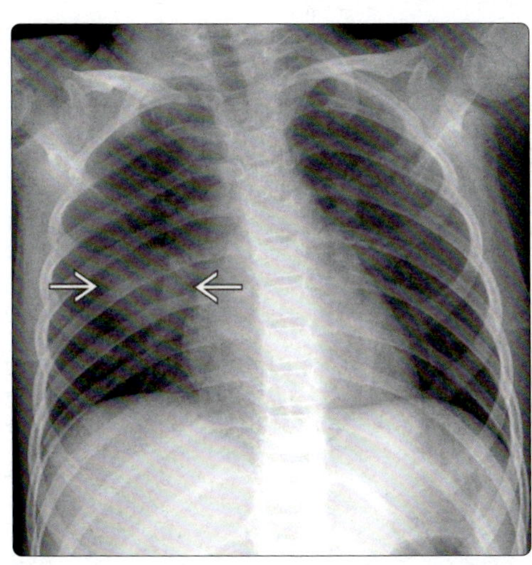

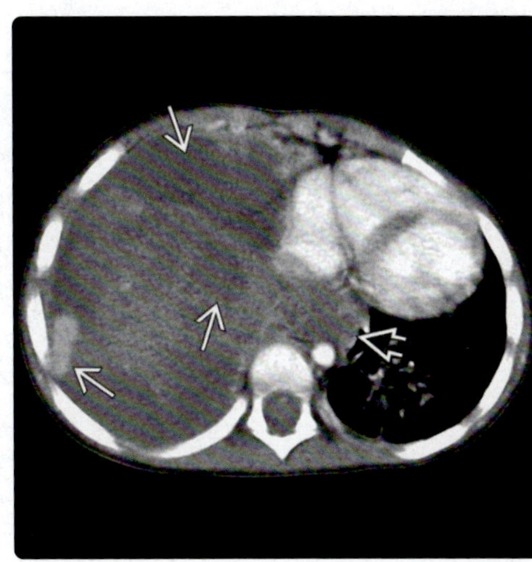

(Left) *AP chest radiograph of a 5-year-old child with cough & fever shows a round opacity with air bronchograms in the right lung, consistent with a round pneumonia.* **(Right)** *Axial CECT in a 2-year-old child with wheezing shows a heterogeneous mass filling & expanding the right hemithorax. The mass proved to be a pleuropulmonary blastoma.*

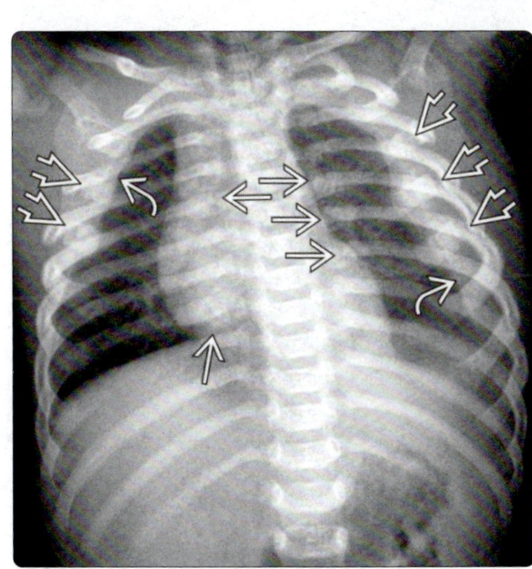

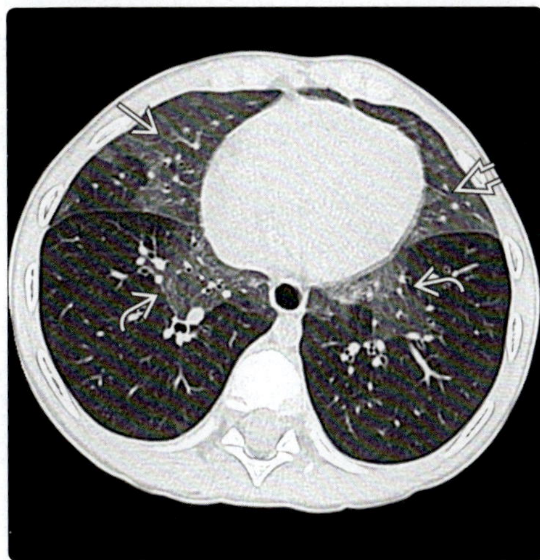

(Left) *AP chest radiograph in a 6-month-old boy who had been physically abused shows multiple posterior & anterior rib fractures with bilateral pleural effusions/pleural thickening.* **(Right)** *Axial HRCT in a 13-month-old child with dyspnea, crackles, & failure to thrive shows a characteristic distribution of ground-glass opacities in the middle lobe, lingula, & paramediastinal lower lobes, typical of neuroendocrine cell hyperplasia of infancy (NEHI).*

Normal Thymus

KEY FACTS

TERMINOLOGY

- Normal organ of anterior superior mediastinum involved in production of T cells
- Appears prominent in many young children

IMAGING

- Normal thymus is variable in size but ↓ with age
  - Moderate to large on chest radiograph up to 5 years of age, particularly in infancy
  - ↓ in relative size by end of 1st decade
  - No "mass" should be present in 2nd decade
- Normal thymus is variable in contour
  - Smooth curvilinear borders ± undulation with ribs
- Normal thymus is variable in shape & symmetry
  - Bilobed with convex margins in young children vs. concave margins in older children
  - Sail sign: Lateral triangular extension (R > L)
- Homogeneous consistency without Ca^{2+} or cysts
  - Slightly lucent: Vessels seen through thymus
- No mass effect on adjacent structures
- Normal variant locations: Cervical & retrocaval extensions
  - Keys to diagnosing normal variant thymic extensions
    - Continuous with & similar imaging appearance (on US, CT, or MR) to normally located thymus
      - US is best tool for confirmation in children
- Aberrant, ectopic thymic tissue may occur in inferior lateral neck or thyroid, ± thymic tissue in normal location
- Thymic rebound
  - Thymic volume can ↓ by > 40% with chemotherapy & other stresses
  - Volume rebounds to original (or larger) size upon stress cessation, potentially mimicking recurrent mass
    - Differentiation of recurrent lymphoma vs. thymic rebound aided by PET/CT or GRE & DWI MR
- Absent visualization on lateral neonatal chest radiograph occurs with ectopia, some immunodeficiencies, or prior sternotomy for congenital heart disease

(Left) *AP chest radiograph in a 6-month-old girl shows a normal prominent thymus ⇨ with a triangular configuration extending into the right hemithorax (sail sign). The normal thymus is lucent & "soft" with undulations at the ribs & intercostal spaces ⇨.* **(Right)** *Gross pathology (with the anterior chest wall removed) from the autopsy of a child who died of SIDS shows a normal but prominent thymus ➡ as compared to the heart ➡. (Courtesy J. Strife, MD.)*

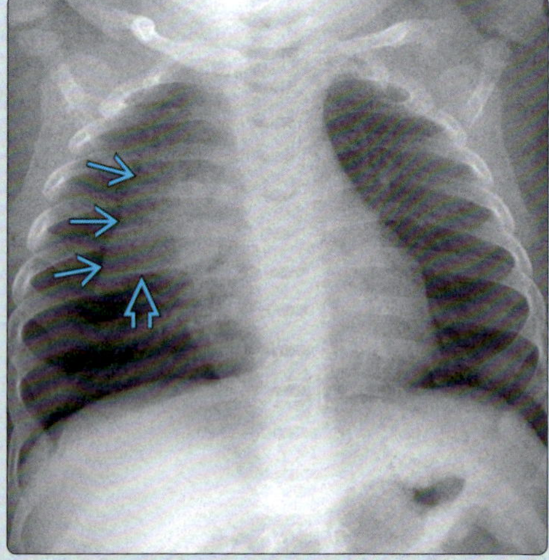

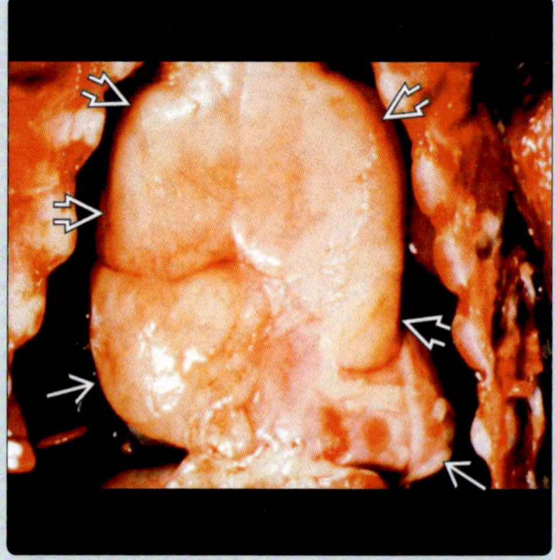

(Left) *Longitudinal US from the upper midline chest in a 7-month-old boy shows a normal thymus ⇨. Punctate & linear (dot-dash pattern) echogenic foci ⇨ are present throughout the hypoechoic parenchyma. There is cervical extension of the thymus ➡ in this child.* **(Right)** *Axial chest CECT images are shown in 2 boys of different ages. In the 2-year-old, the normal thymus is prominent with convex borders ⇨. In the 17-year-old, the normal thymus is small & relatively triangular in shape with concave borders ⇨.*

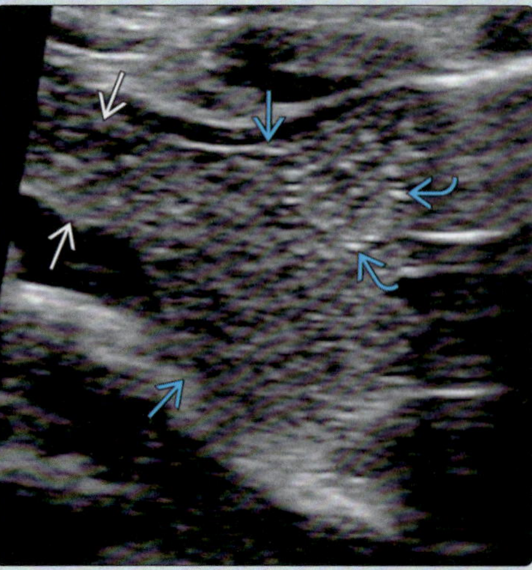

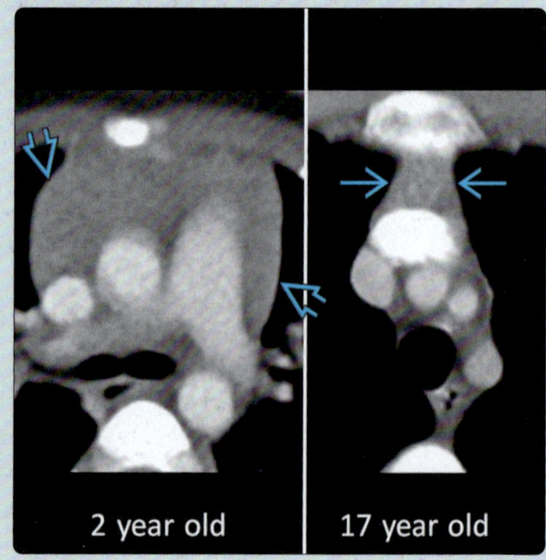

TERMINOLOGY

Synonyms

- Thymic sail sign

Definitions

- Normal organ of anterior superior mediastinum that appears prominent in many young children
  - Involved in production of T cells
- Thymos is Greek for "warty excrescence"

IMAGING

General Features

- Location
  - Normal location: Anterior superior mediastinum
    - Variable distribution of tissue (R vs. L)
  - Normal variant extensions of thymic tissue
    - Superior cervical extension
      - Tissue reaches superiorly in midline above thoracic inlet, anterior to airway
      - 65% of all children (> 80% ages 0-4 years)
      - Can mimic thoracic inlet or lower cervical mass
    - Retrocaval extension
      - Posterior extension of thymus between superior vena cava & great arteries
      - May displace (but not compress) adjacent structures (airway, vessels)
      - Can mimic mediastinal mass or right upper lobe collapse
    - Keys to diagnosing as normal variant thymic tissue extensions (rather than adenopathy or other mass)
      - Connects to normal thymus
      - Shows identical internal characteristics to normal thymic parenchyma by imaging (US, CT, MR)
  - Aberrant, ectopic thymic tissue rarely can be found discontinuous from (or in absence of) normal thymus
    - Aberrant cervical thymus
      - Arrest of normal embryologic descent along thymopharyngeal duct, anywhere from mandibular angle → thoracic inlet
      - Typically asymptomatic lateral cervical mass of normal thymic tissue
      - Retropharyngeal thymus may lead to airway compromise
      - Shows identical internal characteristics to normal thymic parenchyma by imaging (US, CT, MR)
    - Ectopic intrathyroidal thymic tissue
      - Prevalence is inversely associated with age
      - Typically detected incidentally on US & CT
      - Irregular hypoechoic intrathyroidal mass with punctate internal hyperechoic foci similar to normal thymus
      - With typical appearance, can be monitored with follow-up US until involution
  - Absence of normal retrosternal thymic tissue on lateral neonatal chest radiograph could suggest
    - Ectopic thymic tissue
    - DiGeorge syndrome
    - Severe combined immunodeficiency
    - Prior sternotomy for congenital heart disease
- Size
  - Variable, even among children of same age & size
    - May be large up until 5 years of age
    - ↓ in relative size by end of 1st decade
  - Thymic rebound
    - Thymic volume can ↓ by > 40% with chemotherapy or other stresses
    - Rebound of thymic volume occurs with cessation of stress, up to 50% > original size
      - Growing mediastinal mass in lymphoma patient after therapy could represent thymic rebound or recurrent lymphoma
      - Thymic rebound shows typical thymic characteristics
      - Recurrent lymphoma is typically more heterogeneous & nodular with lobulated contours
      - Overlap may necessitate additional imaging for differentiation: PET/CT or MR
- Morphology
  - Contour
    - Normal: Curvilinear smooth borders, mildly undulating with ribs
    - Abnormal: Irregular, lobulated, poorly defined
  - Shape
    - Bilobed ± triangular or quadrilateral configuration
    - Large with convex borders in young children
    - Relatively small with concave margins in older children

Radiographic Findings

- Radiography
  - Normal size is variable
    - ↓ in relative size by end of 1st decade
    - May be relatively large on chest radiograph up to 5 years of age, particularly in 1st year
    - Should not have prominent "mass" during 2nd decade
  - Normal shape is variable
    - Sail sign: Triangular extension laterally (R > L)
    - Not to be confused with spinnaker sail sign: Thymus is lifted off of heart by gas collection of pneumomediastinum
  - Homogeneous soft tissue density; no Ca^{2+}
    - Often slightly lucent relative to heart: Vessels are seen through thymus
  - Does not displace/compress airway or vessels
  - Drapes over cardiac silhouette; may make heart look prominent

Ultrasonographic Findings

- Current high-frequency transducers show predominantly hypoechoic, uniformly granular parenchyma with echogenic punctate & linear septa (dot-dash pattern)
  - Hyperechoic to costal/sternal cartilage
  - Hypoechoic to skeletal muscle

CT Findings

- Homogeneous soft tissue attenuation
  - No calcified or low-attenuation foci
  - Attenuation ↓ with age due to fatty replacement
- Smooth borders, not irregular
- Shape on axial imaging
  - Young children: Large, quadrilateral with convex borders

- Teenagers: Smaller triangle with concave borders
- Does not displace/compress airway or vessels
- Associated findings (such as pericardial or pleural effusion or pulmonary disease) favor pathology

MR Findings

- T1WI
  - Homogeneous signal intensity, typically isointense to skeletal muscle
  - Becomes brighter (due to fat) in later teen & adult years
- T1WI C+ FS
  - Homogeneously dark with little enhancement
- In- & opposed-phase T1 GRE
  - Can help differentiate thymic rebound vs. lymphoma
    - Children > 16 years of age: Thymic rebound ↓ in signal intensity on opposed-phase images due to microscopic fat in normal thymus
    - Children < 16 years: Less helpful, as thymus has less fatty replacement & may not drop signal
- T2 FS/STIR
  - Homogeneously intermediate to bright signal intensity
- DWI/ADC
  - Thymic rebound is less likely to show restricted diffusion & has higher ADC values vs. malignancies

Nuclear Medicine Findings

- FDG PET
  - Mildly FDG avid, much < tumor
  - Postchemotherapy thymic rebound shows ↑ FDG avidity, making differentiation from recurrent lymphoma more difficult
  - SUVmax < 3.4 suggests rebound while SUVmax > 4 suggests recurrent tumor

Imaging Recommendations

- If chest radiograph demonstrates unusual anterior/superior mediastinal prominence that is questionably normal for age, start with US

DIFFERENTIAL DIAGNOSIS

Lymphoma or Leukemia

- Most common pathologic anterior mediastinal mass in children; more common after infancy
- Confluent or nearly confluent nodular masses with mild heterogeneity
- Definite compression/displacement of vessels & airway
- Frequently causes pleural effusions

Germ Cell Tumor (Teratoma)

- Heterogeneous with Ca^{2+} & fat attenuation

Thymic Cyst

- Bilobed cyst coursing through thoracic inlet
- Left lateral neck is most common
- Typically lies near carotid sheath

Langerhans Cell Histiocytosis

- Systemic Langerhans cell histiocytosis (LCH) can manifest as thymic mass with Ca^{2+} or areas of low attenuation
- Associated findings: Lung, hepatic, or bone lesions

Neuroblastoma

- Posterior mediastinal mass (paraspinal)
- May splay/erode ribs, vertebral elements

Lymphatic Malformation

- Transspatial, multicystic mass involving variable portions of neck, chest wall, & mediastinum
- Numerous thin septations
- Cysts often contain fluid-fluid levels due to hemorrhage

Congenital Pulmonary Airway Malformation

- Solid-appearing (microcystic) vs. gas- & fluid-containing (macrocystic) mass
- Not midline

Foregut Duplication Cyst

- Well-circumscribed cyst of middle or posterior mediastinum or hilum

Thymoma

- Very uncommon in young children

PATHOLOGY

General Features

- Normal thymus is prominent relative to thoracic size in early childhood
- Thymic size is smaller relative to thorax by end of 1st decade, though largest actual size occurs in teenage years

CLINICAL ISSUES

Presentation

- Most common signs/symptoms
  - Prominent normal thymus: Asymptomatic
  - Ectopic retropharyngeal thymus rarely causes airway compromise

DIAGNOSTIC CHECKLIST

Consider

- US is best tool to confirm normal thymic tissue in young child with atypical size, shape, or location radiographically

SELECTED REFERENCES

1. Purcell PL et al: Ectopic cervical thymus in children: clinical and radiographic features. Laryngoscope. 130(6):1577-82, 2019
2. Priola AM et al: Diagnostic and functional imaging of thymic and mediastinal involvement in lymphoproliferative disorders. Clin Imaging. 38(6):771-84, 2014
3. Sams CM et al: Imaging of the pediatric thymus & thymic disorders. In Garcia-Peña P et al: Pediatric Chest Imaging, 3rd ed. Berlin: Springer-Verlag. 327-48, 2014
4. Gawande RS et al: Differentiation of normal thymus from anterior mediastinal lymphoma and lymphoma recurrence at pediatric PET/CT. Radiology. 262(2):613-22, 2012
5. Costa NS et al: Superior cervical extension of the thymus: a normal finding that should not be mistaken for a mass. Radiology. 256(1):238-42, 2010

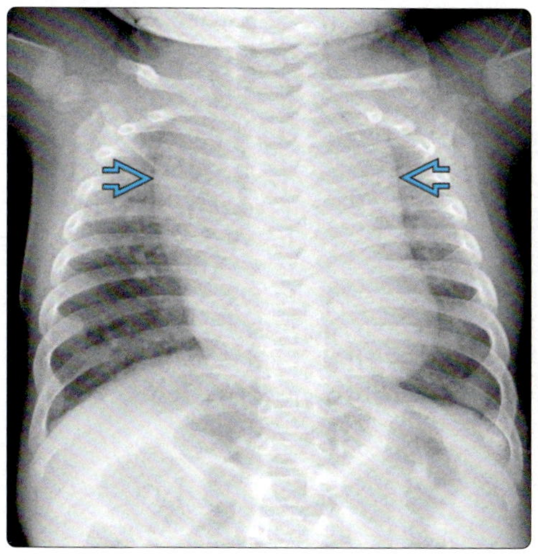

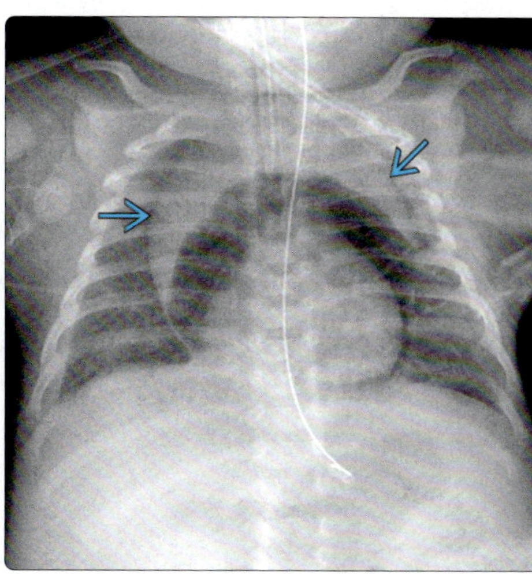

(Left) *AP radiograph in a neonate shows prominence of the superior mediastinum from L to R. This appearance of smooth convex margins is consistent with a normal thymus in a patient of this age.* **(Right)** *AP radiograph of a child in a neonatal intensive care unit shows a spinnaker sail sign, indicative of pneumomediastinum, with a lucent gas collection lifting the thymus off of the cardiac silhouette. The spinnaker sail sign should not be confused with the normal thymic sail sign.*

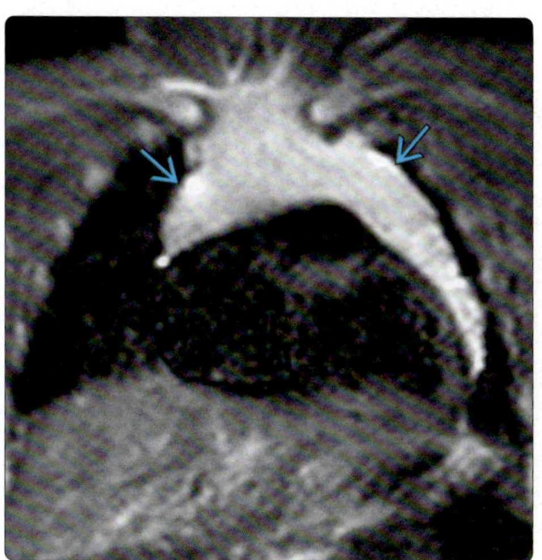

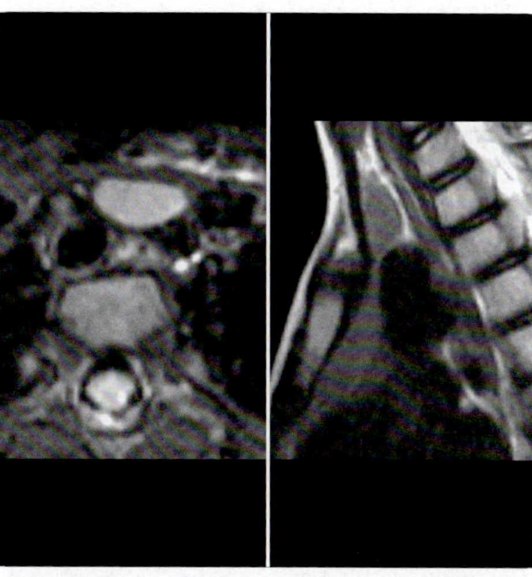

(Left) *Coronal STIR MR in a 4-month-old patient shows a common configuration of a normal thymus draped over the heart. The thymus is homogeneously hyperintense.* **(Right)** *Axial STIR (L) & sagittal T2 (R) MR images in a 6-year-old boy show a "mass" in the lower midline neck that could be mistaken for adenopathy on the axial image. The sagittal image shows a connection between the mass & the normal thymus that is isointense to both. This is cervical extension of the thymus.*

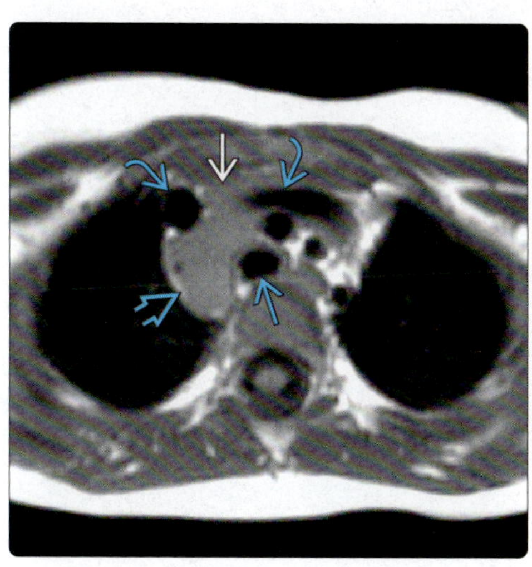

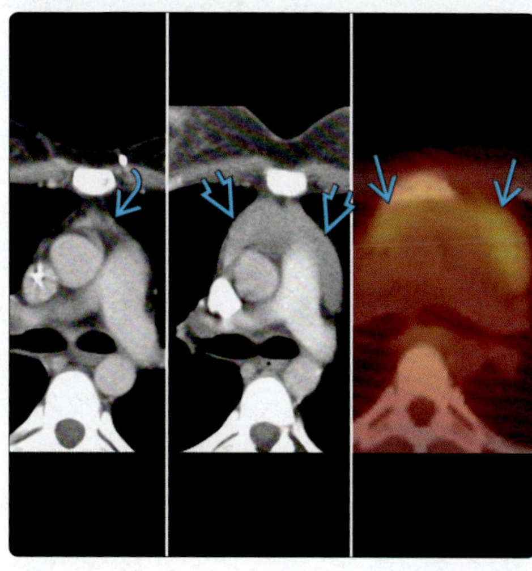

(Left) *Axial T1 MR shows a normal variant retrocaval thymus. Lobular soft tissue, equal in signal to the normal thymus, extends between the trachea & brachiocephalic veins.* **(Right)** *Axial CECT in a 16-year-old girl with lymphoma during chemotherapy (L) shows an atrophic thymus. After treatment completion (middle), thymic rebound hyperplasia is seen with convex smooth borders. FDG PET/CT (R) at this time shows ↑ FDG avidity with an SUVmax < 3.4, typical of rebound.*

Palpable Normal Variants of Chest Wall

KEY FACTS

TERMINOLOGY

- Commonly occurring normal variations of anterior chest wall that may be mistaken for pathology
- Typically isolated variant morphologies of costal cartilages, ribs, &/or sternum
  - Prominent asymmetric convexity or thickness of costal cartilage; may be isolated or due to bifid rib
  - Tilted sternum

IMAGING

- Ultrasound is best initial study for palpable mass unless bony abnormality is primarily suspected
- Radiographs are best for initial bone evaluation
  - May show bifid rib or bony sternal anomaly
  - Purely cartilaginous variants will not be seen
  - Help exclude other significant processes
    - Bone destruction by malignancy, scoliosis

TOP DIFFERENTIAL DIAGNOSES

- Vascular anomaly
- Soft tissue or bone sarcoma
- Osteochondroma
- Pectus excavatum or pectus carinatum
- Scoliosis

CLINICAL ISSUES

- Asymptomatic, palpable "mass" detected by patient, parent, or clinician; usually painless
  - History often erroneously suggests finding as newly or rapidly developed
  - Recent trauma to region may bring palpable abnormality to attention
- Typically isolated finding of little consequence
  - ~ 33% of children imaged for other causes have minor variations in chest wall configuration
  - Isolated bifid rib in 0.15-3.4% of population

(Left) *Transverse color Doppler (top) & grayscale (bottom) ultrasound images of a 2-year-old with an asymptomatic, palpable abnormality of the right chest wall show an avascular, nearly anechoic, anteriorly protuberant costal cartilage ➡ that is continuous with the anterior rib ➡. The normal comparison left side is shown at the same level ➡.* **(Right)** *AP chest radiograph in the same 2-year-old shows a bifid configuration of the right 5th rib ➡ at this same level, a normal variant.*

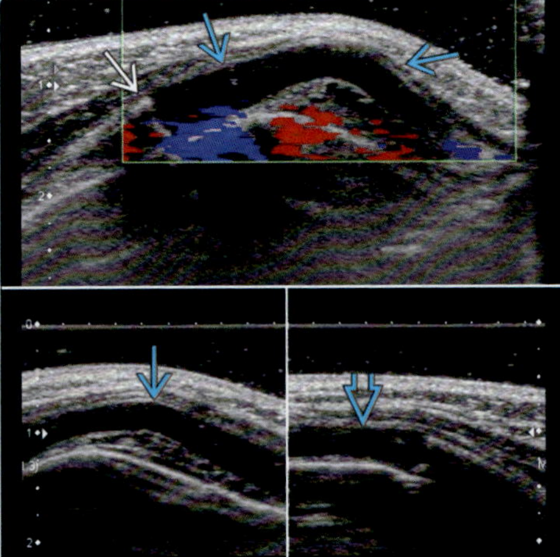

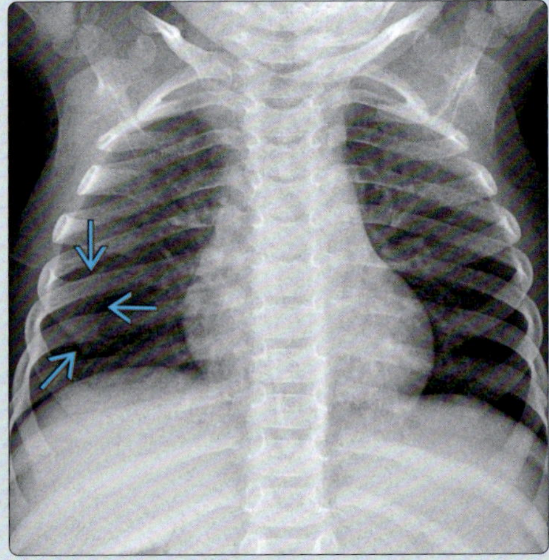

(Left) *Axial 3D T1 GRE FS MR in a teenager with a left lower anterior chest wall palpable abnormality shows focal protuberance & undulation of a costal cartilage on the left ➡, a normal variant. The normal right side is noted for comparison ➡.* **(Right)** *Axial NECT in a patient with a palpable "mass" shows tilting of the sternum with the left margin ➡ being more anterior in location as compared to the right.*

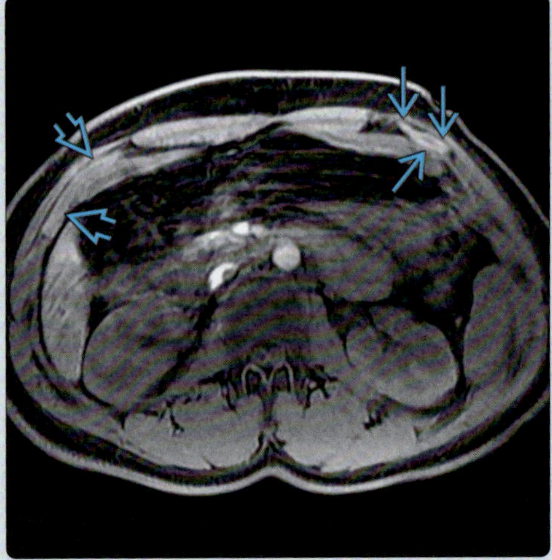

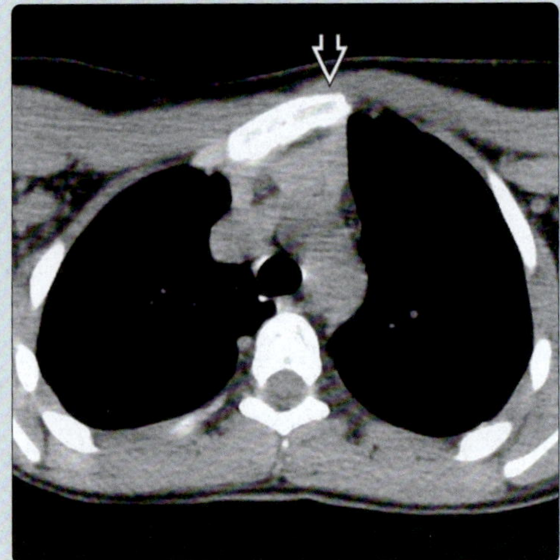

Palpable Normal Variants of Chest Wall

TERMINOLOGY

Definitions

- Commonly occurring normal variations of anterior chest wall that may be mistaken for pathology
  - Usually due to variant morphologies of otherwise normal costal cartilages, ribs, &/or sternum

IMAGING

General Features

- Morphology
  - Prominent asymmetric convexity or thickness of costal cartilage; may be isolated or due to bifid osseous or cartilaginous rib
  - Tilted sternum
    - More anterior edge of sternum is palpated as hard mass on physical examination
    - Frequently associated with prominent asymmetric convexity of costal cartilage

Radiographic Findings

- May show bifid rib or bony sternal anomaly
  - Varying degrees of anterior rib broadening/bifurcation
  - Purely cartilaginous variants will not be seen
- Help exclude other significant processes
  - Bone destruction by malignancy
  - Underlying scoliosis

Ultrasonographic Findings

- Best 1st-line modality due to
  - Lack of ionizing radiation
  - Lack of need for sedation
  - Excellent superficial spatial resolution
  - Ease of comparison to normal contralateral side
- Easily demonstrates relationship of palpable abnormality to
  - Mildly lobular, mildly echogenic subcutaneous fat
  - Striated hypoechoic muscle
  - Nearly anechoic cartilage
  - Echogenic cortical bone with posterior acoustic shadowing

MR Findings

- Excellent soft tissue contrast on variety of sequences allows for characterization of palpable soft tissue or bony mass (whether normal variation or pathology)
  - Thin section axial or coronal 3D T1 FS or 3D PD ± FS may be helpful

Imaging Recommendations

- Best imaging tool
  - Ultrasound is best initial study for palpable mass unless bony abnormality is suspected
  - Radiographs are best for initial bone evaluation

DIFFERENTIAL DIAGNOSIS

Vascular Anomaly

- Slow-flow vascular malformation: Well-circumscribed or infiltrative soft tissue mass with thin septations & fluid-fluid levels
  - Venous malformation: Channels with phleboliths & gradual patchy enhancement
  - Lymphatic malformation: Cystic compartments with rim/septal enhancement only
- High-flow vascular neoplasm
  - Infantile hemangioma
    - Well-circumscribed, lobulated, high-flow mass with many low-resistance arterial waveforms (Doppler US) & early diffuse enhancement (MR)

Soft Tissue or Bone Sarcoma

- Firm, often well-circumscribed chest wall mass ± rib destruction, pleural effusion
- Variable enhancement

Osteochondroma

- May present with hard palpable mass, local symptoms of compression/irritation, or stalk fracture
- Characteristic radiographic appearance of flowing corticomedullary continuity between osteochondroma & parent bone

Pectus Excavatum or Pectus Carinatum

- Midline sternal anomalies of concavity (former) or convexity (latter)
- May be isolated or found with many syndromes
- May have associated rib protrusions & sternal tilting

Scoliosis

- Rotary component of spinal curvature leads to protrusion of anterior chest wall on side of curve concavity

Poland Syndrome

- Unilateral absence of pectoralis musculature

CLINICAL ISSUES

Presentation

- Most common signs/symptoms
  - Asymptomatic, palpable "mass" detected by patient, parent, or clinician; usually painless
  - History often erroneously suggests finding as newly or rapidly developed
    - Recent trauma to region may bring palpable abnormality to attention

Demographics

- Frequently detected in adolescence due to changing physique & heightened awareness
- ~ 33% of children imaged for other causes have minor variations in chest wall configuration
- Isolated bifid rib in 0.15-3.4% of population

Natural History & Prognosis

- Typically isolated finding of little consequence

SELECTED REFERENCES

1. Aboughalia HA et al: Pediatric rib pathologies: clinicoimaging scenarios and approach to diagnosis. Pediatr Radiol. 51(10):1783-97, 2021
2. Jain R et al: Ultrasonography in the evaluation of pediatric chest "masses": when to consider? J Ultrasound Med. ePub, 2021
3. Mak SM et al: Imaging of congenital chest wall deformities. Br J Radiol. 89(1061):20150595, 2016
4. Kaneko H et al: Isolated bifid rib: clinical and radiological findings in children. Pediatr Int. 54(6):820-3, 2012
5. Donnelly LF et al: Abnormalities of the chest wall in pediatric patients. AJR Am J Roentgenol. 173(6):1595-601, 1999

Congenital Pulmonary Airway Malformation

KEY FACTS

TERMINOLOGY

- Heterogeneous group of cystic & noncystic congenital lung lesions resulting from maldevelopment of fetal airway
- Term congenital cystic adenomatoid malformation (CCAM) is not favored because many lesions are not obviously cystic in nature & only minority have adenomatous components

IMAGING

- Presents as cystic or solid-appearing lung mass in early life
- Appearance varies by lesion type (Stocker classification)
  - Type 1: Composed of 1 or more large (3-10 cm) cysts
  - Type 2: Numerous small & medium-sized (0.5-2 cm) cysts
  - Type 3: Microcystic (1-2 mm) or solid-appearing mass
- Even with prenatal diagnosis, initial postnatal radiographs may be normal due to phenomenon of partial or complete *in utero* regression
- CT angiogram is critical for surgical planning to identify possible systemic feeding artery (pulmonary sequestration)

TOP DIFFERENTIAL DIAGNOSES

- Bronchopulmonary sequestration (BPS)
- Congenital diaphragmatic hernia
- Bronchogenic cyst
- Pleuropulmonary blastoma
- Congenital lobar overinflation

CLINICAL ISSUES

- ~ 25% have respiratory distress at birth
- All symptomatic congenital pulmonary airway malformations (CPAMs) are resected; asymptomatic lesions are managed expectantly or with elective resection
- Overall survival > 95%; risks include recurrent infections, underlying malignancy, future malignant degeneration

DIAGNOSTIC CHECKLIST

- Low-dose postnatal chest CTA must include celiac axis to look for extrathoracic origin of systemic arterial supply to BPS component of "hybrid lesion"

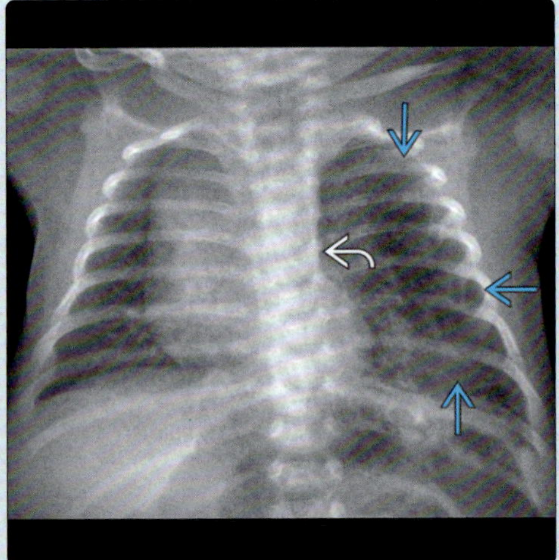

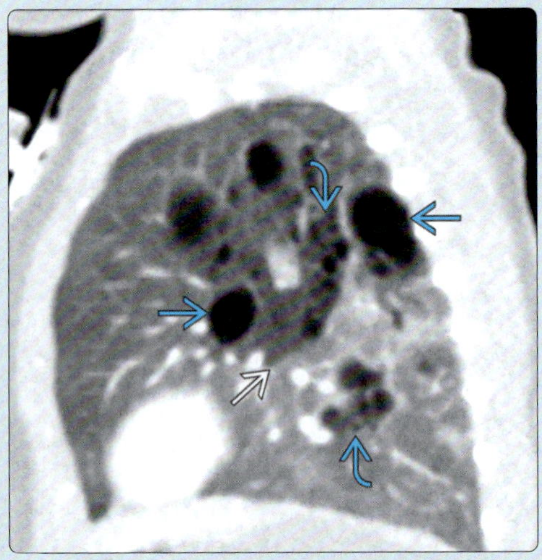

(Left) *AP radiograph in a 5-week-old with respiratory distress shows a large, multicystic lucent mass of the left lung causing mediastinal shift toward the right.* **(Right)** *Sagittal reconstruction from a CTA in the same patient reveals numerous large cysts & a few smaller cysts that blend into normal left lung. The lesion is predominantly upper lobe & has mass effect on the fissure but also extends into the lower lobe. It is unusual for CPAMs to involve > 1 lobe.*

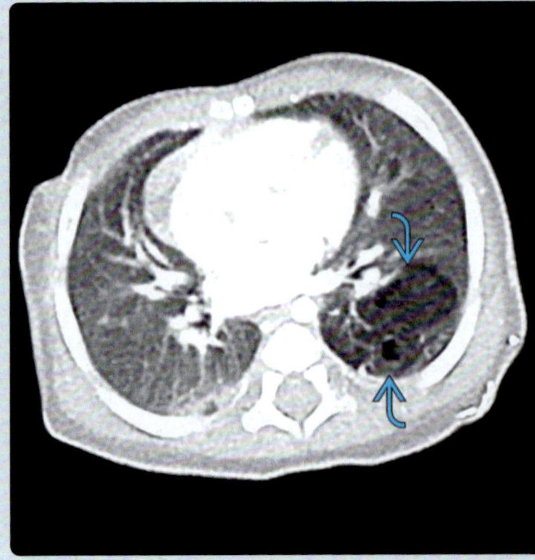

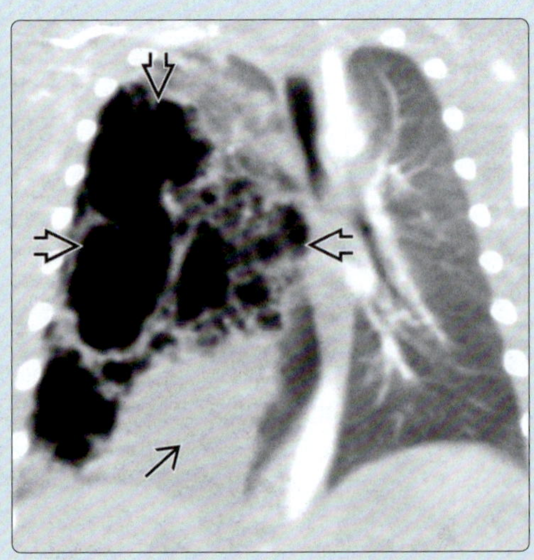

(Left) *Axial CTA in a 4-month-old with a prenatally diagnosed CPAM shows a well-defined mass composed of numerous small- & medium-sized (0.5-2 cm) cysts. Remember that ~ 50% of patients with type 2 lesions have associated anomalies.* **(Right)** *Coronal CTA in a newborn with respiratory distress shows a large mixed cystic & solid mass. Note the numerous gas-filled cysts with a solid-appearing component in the right lower lobe. Pathologic diagnosis was a mixed type 1 & 3 CPAM.*

TERMINOLOGY

Abbreviations

- Congenital pulmonary airway malformation (CPAM)

Synonyms

- Congenital cystic adenomatoid malformation (CCAM)
  - Antiquated & unsuitable term: Lesions may be noncystic, & only type 3 lesions have adenomatoid components

Definitions

- Heterogeneous group of cystic & noncystic congenital lung lesions resulting from maldevelopment of fetal airway

IMAGING

General Features

- Best diagnostic clue
  - Cystic or solid-appearing lung lesion in fetus or newborn
    - Fluid-filled cysts at birth, gradually filling with air
- Location
  - Intrapulmonary, mostly without lobar predilection
- Size
  - Depends on type of lesion: Type 0 diffusely affects both lungs; type 3 sometimes involves entire lung; types 1, 2, & 4 usually involve just 1 lobe
- Morphology
  - Appearance varies based on histopathologic type (Stocker classification)
    - Type 0 (acinar dysplasia): Small, nonaerated lungs
    - Type 1 (large cyst type): 1 or more large (3-10 cm) cysts, ± smaller cysts that blend into normal lung
    - Type 2 (small/medium cyst type): Numerous small or medium-sized (0.5-2 cm) cysts
    - Type 3 (microcyst type): Innumerable microcysts (1-2 mm) that cause marked ↑ in size of affected lobe/lung
    - Type 4 (large peripheral cyst type): Large, thin-walled, cyst in periphery of lung, often with mass effect

Radiographic Findings

- Multicystic lung mass with variable amounts of fluid & air
- Solid radiographic appearance may be due to
  - Microcystic type 3
  - Initially fluid-filled larger cysts (types 1, 2, 4)
- Mass effect is most common with types 3 & 4
- Pneumothorax may occur, especially with type 4
- Newborn chest radiographs may be normal (despite prenatal diagnosis of lesion)
  - Complete vs. partial regression in many cases
  - Occult lesions may be found by CT

CT Findings

- CTA
  - May show partial/complete regression of prenatally detected lesion
  - Performed to determine extent of residual lesion & evaluate for systemic feeding vessel prior to surgery
    - Systemic arterial supply classically suggests component of bronchopulmonary sequestration ("hybrid lesion" with CPAM)
    - Origin of arterial supply is critical for surgical planning
      - □ Must cover through celiac axis to exclude extrathoracic origin of artery
  - Mass ranges from solid/microcystic to macrocystic
    - Components of each may be present
    - Cysts of variable size; contain air &/or fluid
      - □ Intermixed microcysts may appear as air-trapping
      - □ Margins with normal lung may be difficult to define
  - May cause hyperinflation or atelectasis of adjacent lung

Ultrasonographic Findings

- Typically limited to prenatal evaluation
  - Solid-appearing echogenic mass relative to normal lung
  - Discrete anechoic cysts of variable size
  - Typically stabilizes or ↓ in size > 26-weeks gestation
    - Often regresses or "resolves" by late 3rd trimester
      - □ False-negative rate of 40% vs. postnatal CT
  - ± pleural effusion, skin edema, other findings of hydrops
    - CPAM volume ratio (CVR) > 1.6 → 80% develop hydrops
  - Systemic arterial supply on Doppler → component of BPS ("hybrid lesion")

Imaging Recommendations

- Best imaging tool
  - Chest CT angiogram that includes celiac axis (so as to exclude diagnosis of BPS)
  - Many surgeons prefer to delay surgery until child is > 6 months of age; if possible, CT angiogram should also be delayed (so as to improve quality of imaging)

DIFFERENTIAL DIAGNOSIS

Bronchopulmonary Sequestration

- Systemic arterial supply to lesion
- Solid-appearing; only becomes air-filled after infection (as it lacks communication with airway)
- Mixed CPAM/sequestration ("hybrid") lesions are common
- Left > right lower lobes

Congenital Diaphragmatic Hernia (CDH)

- Appears radiographically as multicystic, air-containing mass
  - "Cysts" are often uniform in size & morphology
- Unexpected course or position of support devices
  - Nasogastric tube has reversed J-shaped course into left lower chest if stomach is herniated (left-sided CDH)
  - Umbilical venous catheter may be deviated toward the left if liver is herniated (left-sided CDH)
- Paucity of abdominal bowel gas (due to herniation)

Bronchogenic Cyst

- Round mass lesion; typically mediastinal or perihilar location
- Fluid-attenuation mass may become air-filled if infected

Pleuropulmonary Blastoma (PPB)

- Rare in newborns, but vast majority present before age 6
- Type 1 PPB is indistinguishable from types 1 & 4 CPAM
  - Large cyst, solid soft tissue component, multilobar or bilateral involvement, lack of 2nd trimester prenatal detection, & *DICER1* mutation ↑ likelihood of PPB

Cavitary Necrosis/Abscess Complicating Pneumonia

- Older children; typically not neonates
- Typically ill with respiratory distress, fever, cough

- Thick-walled cavitary necrosis surrounded by consolidated lung
- Temporal factors favoring cavitary necrosis: Prior normal chest radiograph, progression of findings during illness, resolution after illness

Congenital Lobar Overinflation

- Progressive lobar overdistention of lung segment or lobe
- Preserved pulmonary markings without discrete cyst walls
- Strong upper & middle lobe predilection

PATHOLOGY

General Features

- Etiology
  - Congenital lung mass of various cell origins
  - Lesion development is poorly understood; related to varying degrees & levels of early airway obstruction
- Associated abnormalities
  - Type 2 lesions are associated with other congenital anomalies (50%)

Staging, Grading, & Classification

- Stocker classification is based on size of cysts & lesion's histologic resemblance to developing bronchial tree & lung
  - Type 0 (1-2%): Diffuse acinar dysplasia/dysgenesis; diffuse & bilateral → unresectable & fatal
  - Type 1 (60-65%): Large cyst type; usually presents in newborns, may be found incidentally in older children; almost always resectable
  - Type 2 (10-15%): Small & medium cyst type; presents in 1st year; outcome is often poor due to other anomalies
  - Type 3 (5-10%): Microcystic/solid type; fetal or newborn presentation, often with polyhydramnios or hydrops
  - Type 4 (10-15%): Peripheral cyst type; present in newborn period or early childhood with respiratory distress, infection, or pneumothorax from rupture

Microscopic Features

- Type 0: Contains bronchial-like structures lined with ciliated pseudostratified epithelium & goblet cells; may contain bronchiolar cartilage & muscle
- Type 1: Lined by ciliated columnar epithelium; may contain mucus-producing cells, muscle, & cartilage
- Type 2: Lined with respiratory epithelium with smooth muscle in wall; absent mucin-producing cells & cartilage
- Type 3: Adenomatoid appearance with randomly scattered, bronchiolar/alveolar, duct-like structures
- Type 4: Lined with alveolar epithelial cells &/or low columnar epithelium (hamartomatous malformation of distal acinus)

CLINICAL ISSUES

Presentation

- Most common signs/symptoms
  - Prenatal diagnosis ± symptoms at birth
  - Respiratory distress in newborn (~ 25%)
    - Depends on size of lesion, mediastinal shift, hydrops
  - Recurrent lung infections in older child

Demographics

- Age
  - Most commonly detected prenatally or during infancy
  - Can present at any age
- Epidemiology
  - Incidence: 1 per 15,000-25,000 live births

Natural History & Prognosis

- Overall survival > 95%
- ~ 13% require neonatal respiratory support
- Prenatally detected CPAM may grow until 26-weeks gestation followed by varying degrees of regression
  - ~ 20% become sonographically undetectable in 3rd trimester but with false-negative rate of 40%
  - 10% (typically microcystic with low initial CVR) show complete regression by postnatal CT &/or pathology
- Type 2 lesions are associated with other congenital anomalies (especially esophageal atresia & TE fistula, renal dysgenesis/agenesis, cardiovascular anomalies, intestinal atresias, & sirenomelia)
- Risks of unresected CPAM
  - Recurrent infections
  - Small risk that lesion actually represents PPB
  - Future malignant degeneration
    - Bronchioloalveolar carcinoma, rhabdomyosarcoma

Treatment

- Prenatally detected lesions are followed with ultrasound/MR
  - Smaller lesions without hydrops: Close follow-up ± corticosteroids
  - Larger lesions at risk for/with hydrops: Corticosteroids, consider fetal interventions
    - Aspiration/shunting of dominant cyst
    - Resection of lesion
- Symptomatic CPAM after delivery → surgical resection
- Asymptomatic CPAM management is controversial
  - Most advocate elective resection due to risks of infection & malignancy
  - Fewer complications if surgery is performed prior to development of symptoms
    - ~ 2/3 of expectantly managed patients ultimately become symptomatic

DIAGNOSTIC CHECKLIST

Consider

- Most true multicystic pulmonary masses containing air in neonatal period represent CPAM

SELECTED REFERENCES

1. Adams NC et al: Fetal ultrasound and magnetic resonance imaging: a primer on how to interpret prenatal lung lesions. Pediatr Radiol. 50(13):1839-14, 2020
2. Cortes-Santiago N et al: Pediatric cystic lung lesions: where are we now? Surg Pathol Clin. 13(4):643-55, 2020
3. Guillerman RP et al: Imaging of DICER1 syndrome. Pediatr Radiol. 49(11):1488-505, 2019
4. Maneenil G et al: Clinical presentation and outcome in congenital pulmonary malformation: 25 year retrospective study in Thailand. Pediatr Int. 61(8):812-6, 2019
5. Feinberg A et al: Can congenital pulmonary airway malformation be distinguished from type I pleuropulmonary blastoma based on clinical and radiological features? J Pediatr Surg. 51(1):33-7, 2016

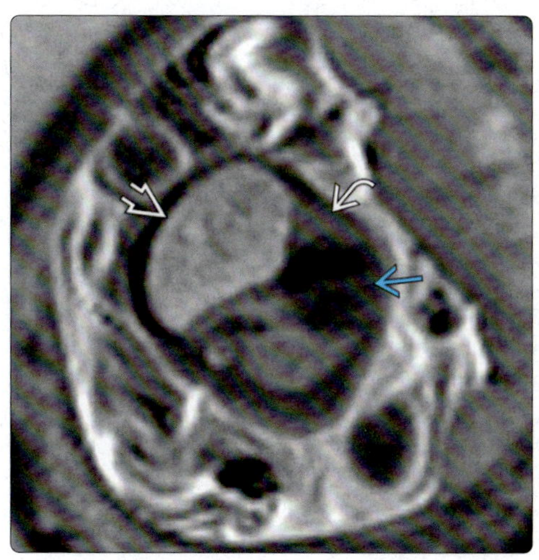

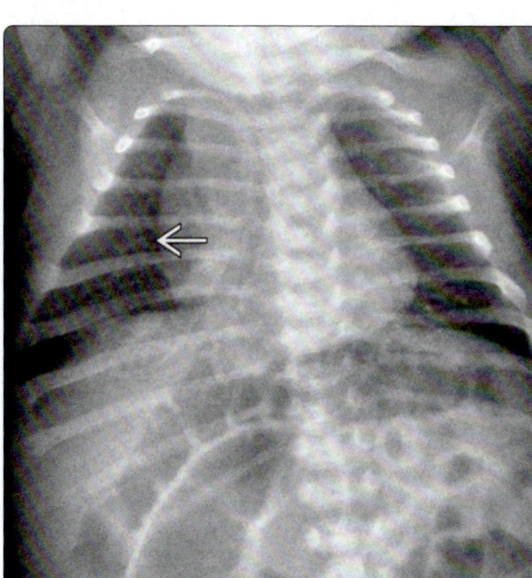

(Left) *Axial T2 SSFSE MR in a 23-weeks-gestation fetus shows a large, homogeneously hyperintense lesion ➡ occupying the majority of the right hemithorax & compressing the residual normal right lung ➡. The heart ➡ is displaced into the left chest.* **(Right)** *Newborn AP chest radiograph in the same patient shows interval regression of the lesion with only mild architectural distortion ➡ identified in the right lung. The heart now has a normal position.*

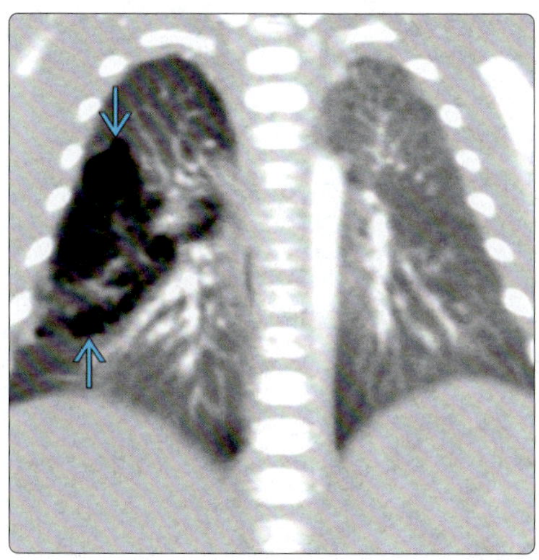

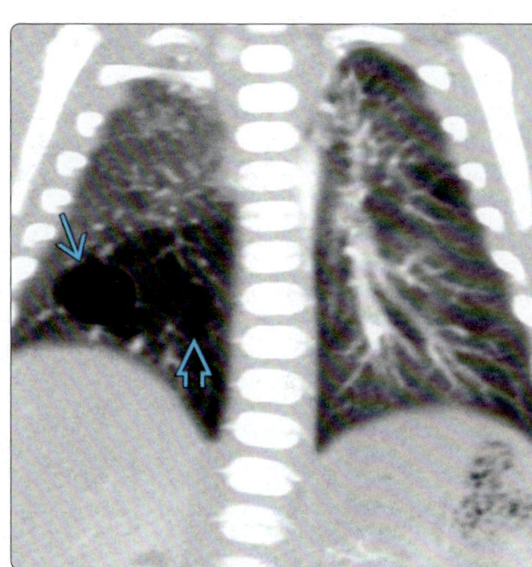

(Left) *Coronal CTA in the same patient shows a residual, predominately hyperlucent right lung lesion consisting of cysts of variable size ➡. The lesion splays normal pulmonary vessels. A mixed type 1 & type 2 CPAM was confirmed upon resection.* **(Right)** *Coronal CTA in a neonate shows a hyperlucent right lower lobe CPAM. There is a single large macrocyst ➡ laterally in the lesion. Other smaller cysts ➡ are intermixed with microcysts &/or air-trapping.*

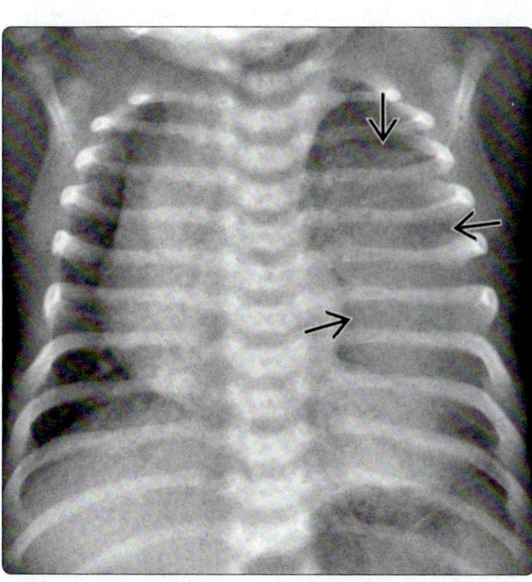

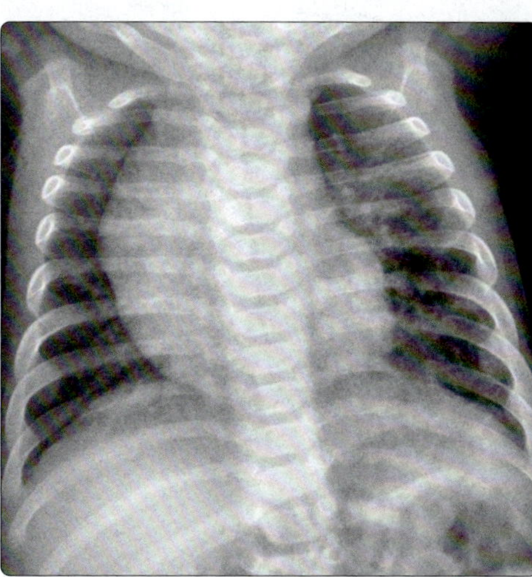

(Left) *AP chest radiograph in a 3-week-old boy shows a large dense mass ➡ of the left lung causing left to right mediastinal shift.* **(Right)** *Follow-up AP chest radiograph in the same infant 6 weeks later shows that the large left lower lobe lesion has become aerated, typical of a CPAM. The mediastinal shift has slightly ↓ in severity.*

Bronchopulmonary Sequestration

KEY FACTS

TERMINOLOGY

- Congenital focus of abnormal lung that does not connect to bronchial tree or pulmonary arteries
- Divided into intralobar (75%) & extralobar (25%) types
  - Intralobar shares pleural investment with normal lung & usually has pulmonary venous drainage
  - Extralobar has separate pleural investment from lung & usually has systemic venous drainage

IMAGING

- Lower lobe (L > R) opacity persisting over time
  - Mass may occur in mediastinum or in/below diaphragm
- Systemic arterial supply is characteristic; identification is critical for diagnosis & surgical planning
  - Postnatal CTA (vs. MR) is recommended for all congenital lung lesions (even with 3rd-trimester regression)
  - Arterial supply may be subdiaphragmatic in origin even if BPS is supradiaphragmatic
    - Chest CTA must cover through celiac axis
- Often occurs as "hybrid lesion" with congenital pulmonary airway malformation (CPAM)

TOP DIFFERENTIAL DIAGNOSES

- Depends on location & imaging features
  - Chronic lung opacity
  - Anomalous systemic blood flow to lung
  - Focal chest mass
  - Solid suprarenal mass

CLINICAL ISSUES

- Intralobar typically presents as isolated anomaly in older children/adults with recurrent pneumonia
- Extralobar is typically detected in prenatal/neonatal period, often with additional congenital anomalies
- Symptomatic is BPS resected; management of asymptomatic lesions is controversial

DIAGNOSTIC CHECKLIST

- Consider BPS with recurrent lower lobe pneumonia

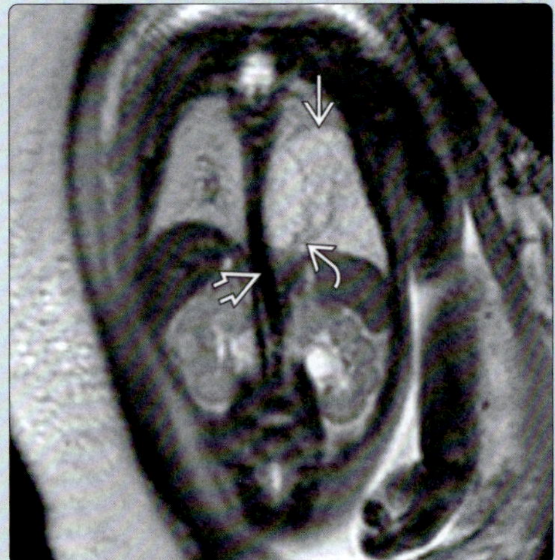

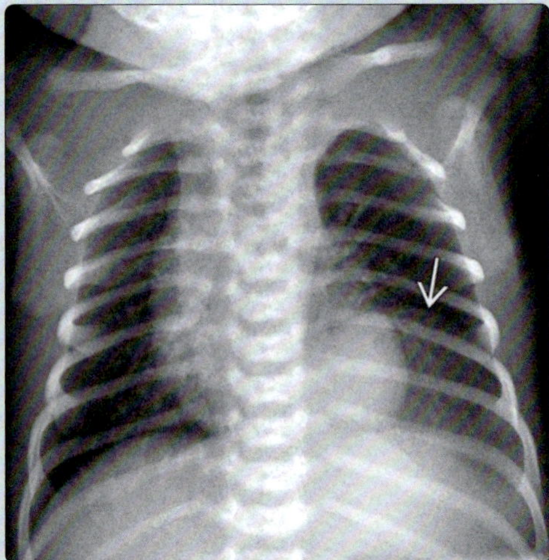

(Left) *Coronal T2 SSFSE MR of a 31-weeks-gestation fetus shows a large, homogeneously hyperintense left lower lobe mass ➡ displacing the left upper lobe & aorta ➡. Flow voids ➡ are seen extending into the mass from the aorta.* **(Right)** *AP radiograph in the same patient 5 days after birth shows mild ↓ size of the left lower lobe mass ➡.*

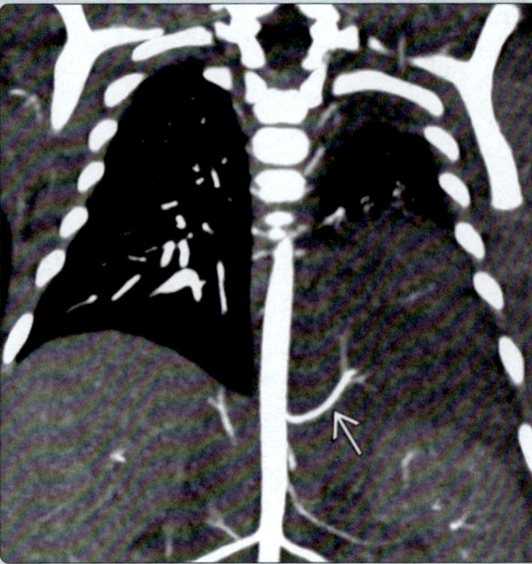

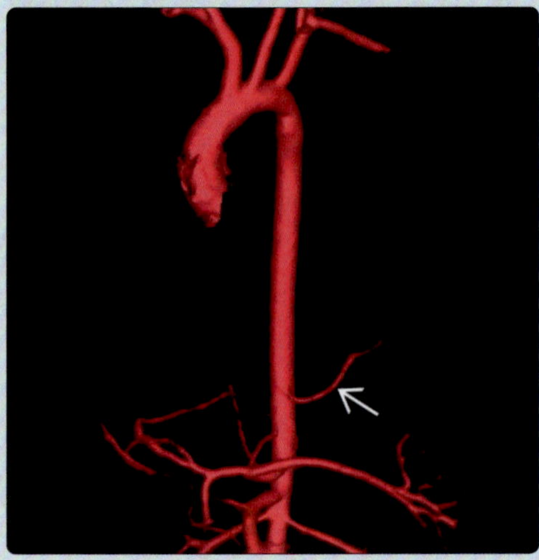

(Left) *Coronal CT angiogram in the same patient 11 days later shows an arterial feeding vessel ➡ extending into the solid mass from the upper abdominal aorta, confirming systemic arterial supply in a bronchopulmonary sequestration (BPS). Upon resection, the mass contained components of both BPS & CPAM, consistent with "hybrid lesion."* **(Right)** *3D coronal oblique reconstruction from the same CT angiogram in the same patient shows the feeding vessel ➡ relationship to other upper abdominal arterial origins.*

TERMINOLOGY

Definitions

- Bronchopulmonary sequestration (BPS): Dysplastic nonfunctional lung tissue with no connection to bronchi or pulmonary arteries
- Intralobar (75%) vs. extralobar (25%) types
  - Intralobar sequestration (ILS) typically has pulmonary venous drainage without separate pleural investment
  - Extralobar sequestration (ELS) typically has systemic venous drainage with separate pleural investment

IMAGING

General Features

- Best diagnostic clue
  - Lower lobe opacity that persists over time
  - Systemic arterial supply to lesion
- Location
  - 98% in lower lobes (L > R)
  - Up to 15% of ELS occurs below diaphragm
  - Rarely in diaphragm, mediastinum, neck
- Feeding artery usually arises from descending aorta
- ± elements of other congenital lung lesions, especially congenital pulmonary airway malformation (CPAM)
  - 17-42% of congenital lung lesions are "hybrid" or "complex"
- May be difficult to differentiate ILS vs. ELS by imaging
  - May not affect surgical management

Radiographic Findings

- Radiography
  - Persistent lower lobe opacity over time
  - May contain gas from infection, bronchial fistula (in ILS), collateral flow, or CPAM components ("hybrid lesion")
  - ELS may present as subdiaphragmatic mass displacing adjacent interfaces, such as paraspinal stripes

Ultrasonographic Findings

- Postnatal ultrasound
  - Abnormal lung may provide acoustic window
  - Doppler ultrasound may demonstrate feeding vessel
- Prenatal ultrasound
  - Homogeneous echogenic lung mass ± cystic components in hybrid lesions
  - May see systemic feeding artery with Doppler

CT Findings

- CTA
  - Recommended for all congenital lung lesions to evaluate systemic vascular supply prior to surgery
    - Descending thoracic aorta is most common source of feeding vessel
    - Other sources: Abdominal aorta; celiac, splenic, intercostal, subclavian, coronary arteries
      - Rarely aberrant pulmonary artery
    - Arterial supply may be subdiaphragmatic in origin even if sequestration is supradiaphragmatic
    - Feeding artery diameter may help predict need for resection
    - 3D reconstruction is helpful for surgical planning
  - Discrete solid mass ± cysts vs. opacification of lower lobe parenchyma
  - ± peripheral/perilesional foci of low attenuation
  - ± gas in lesion with infection, fistula, collateral alveolar communication, or hybrid lesion with CPAM
  - ELS may torse, thrombose, or hemorrhage, making diagnosis more difficult

MR Findings

- Fetal MR is often used for prenatal lung lesion assessment
- Increasing reports of postnatal utilization of MR
- Most frequently: Homogeneous, T2-hyperintense, solid-appearing mass; ± cystic components in hybrid lesions
- Feeding artery is visualized as flow void on SE/FSE sequences; may be bright GRE sequences

Imaging Recommendations

- Best imaging tool
  - Prenatal imaging
    - Ultrasound is excellent 1st-line study for detection/characterization; may not need fetal MR
  - Postnatal imaging
    - When BPS is suspected prenatally, obtain postnatal CTA for feeding vessel detection prior to surgery
- Protocol advice
  - Extend chest CTA through celiac axis to detect subdiaphragmatic arterial supply

DIFFERENTIAL DIAGNOSIS

Chronic Lung Opacity

- Chronic or recurrent pneumonia
  - Typically no systemic arterial supply
- Chronic bronchial obstruction
  - Aspirated foreign body
  - Endobronchial lesion (e.g., carcinoid)

Anomalous Systemic Blood Flow to Lung

- Hypogenetic lung syndrome (scimitar)
  - Hypoplasia of right lung & pulmonary artery
  - Partial anomalous pulmonary venous return
  - Systemic arterial supply of right lung base ± BPS
- Chronic inflammation with hypertrophied bronchial arteries
  - Cystic fibrosis, chronic pneumonia
- Pulmonary artery atresia
  - Multiple aortopulmonary collateral arteries (MAPCAs)
- Bronchial atresia may have systemic supply
  - Overlaps with ILS
- Isolated aberrant artery without lung abnormality

Focal Chest Mass

- CPAM
  - Often has cystic components filling with air postnatally
  - No systemic arterial supply unless hybrid lesion
  - May be seen in middle, upper lobes
- Bronchogenic cyst
  - Mediastinal or central pulmonary location
  - Well-defined cyst without feeding artery
  - May compress bronchus leading to overinflation lesion (mimicking BPS prenatally)
- Round pneumonia
  - Most common round lung opacity in young children

- Usually < 8 years of age
  - Should resolve/improve with antibiotics
- Pleuropulmonary blastoma (rare)
  - Type I is indistinguishable from benign lung cysts
  - Large thoracic soft tissue mass (types II & III)
- Neuroblastoma
  - Ovoid paraspinal mass displacing paraspinal stripe(s)
  - ± rib splaying, erosion
- Lymphatic malformation
  - Multicystic mass crossing multiple soft tissue planes
  - Often involves upper mediastinum, neck, chest wall

Solid Suprarenal Mass

- Adrenal hemorrhage
  - No central vascularity
  - Often diagnosed later in gestation than BPS
  - ↓ or resolves over time
- Neuroblastoma
  - Often calcifies & engulfs normal vessels

PATHOLOGY

General Features

- Abnormal dysplastic lung tissue lacking normal/functional tracheobronchial connection
- Development is likely related to caudal accessory lung bud with abnormal vascular supply from foregut
- Underlying airway obstruction likely contributes to maldevelopment
  - Foci of bronchial atresia are found in most congenital lung lesions including BPS (ELS > ILS)
- Aberrant feeding artery in all cases
  - Usually systemic (5% from pulmonary artery)
  - Single supplying artery in 80%; 2 or more in 20%
  - May not be visualized by imaging
- ELS
  - Always congenital
  - Often associated with other anomalies (65%)
    - Congenital diaphragmatic hernia, cardiac abnormalities, pulmonary hypoplasia, foregut duplication cysts, separate congenital lung lesions
  - Most common hybrid lesion: ELS + type II CPAM
  - Separate pleural investment; usually has systemic venous drainage
- ILS
  - Not all lesions are congenital; some may develop from chronic postnatal inflammation
  - Infection may lead to bronchial fistula
  - Not associated with other anomalies
  - Shares pleural investment with normal lung; usually drains into pulmonary venous system

CLINICAL ISSUES

Presentation

- Most common signs/symptoms
  - ELS: Often asymptomatic postnatally
    - May cause neonatal respiratory distress from mass effect or adjacent pulmonary hypoplasia
    - Infection is much less common than ILS
  - ILS: Recurrent pneumonia symptoms in older child/adult
- Other signs/symptoms
  - ELS: May torse, infarct
    - Prenatally can develop hydrothorax, hydrops
    - Postnatally may cause chest/abdominal pain
  - ILS: Chest pain, hemoptysis; incidental in 15%

Demographics

- Age
  - ELS: Usually detected in prenatal/neonatal period
  - ILS: Classically, late childhood/early adulthood presentation; 50% > 20 years old

Natural History & Prognosis

- High rate (up to 67%) of spontaneous in utero regression (partial or complete) of prenatal echogenic lung lesions
  - ~ 50% of prenatally detected BPS lesions

Treatment

- Surgical resection in symptomatic cases
  - Reports of preoperative vs. isolated embolization of feeding artery (with variable success as primary therapy)
- Management of asymptomatic cases is controversial
  - Elective surgical resection vs. monitoring
    - Easier surgery prior to infection
  - If no feeding artery is seen on imaging, may be excised for concern of other lesions
- High mortality if ELS leads to hydrops in utero (possibly due to torsion of lesion on vascular pedicle)
  - High success rates of minimally invasive in utero laser ablation of feeding vessel → ↓ size of mass & effusion with resolution of hydrops → up to 100% survival

DIAGNOSTIC CHECKLIST

Consider

- Raise BPS possibility with recurrent lower lobe pneumonia &/or paraspinal mass
- Postnatal CTA (or possibly MR) should be performed for prenatally detected lung lesions (even with 3rd-trimester regression)

Reporting Tips

- Imaging differentiation of ELS vs. ILS may not be possible
- Describe size, location, vascular supply/drainage, aeration, involvement of adjacent structures, associated anomalies
  - Critical to define feeding vessel origin prior to surgery

SELECTED REFERENCES

1. Alamo L et al: Revising the classification of lung sequestrations. Clin Imaging. 77:92-7, 2021
2. Lazow SP et al: Prenatal imaging diagnosis of suprarenal lesions. Fetal Diagn Ther. 48(3):235-42, 2021
3. Adams NC et al: Fetal ultrasound and magnetic resonance imaging: a primer on how to interpret prenatal lung lesions. Pediatr Radiol. 50(13):1839-54, 2020
4. Gabelloni M et al: Pulmonary sequestration: what the radiologist should know. Clin Imaging. 73:61-72, 2020
5. Hermelijn SM et al: A clinical guideline for structured assessment of CT-imaging in congenital lung abnormalities. Paediatr Respir Rev. 37:80-8, 2020
6. Kellenberger CJ et al: Structural and perfusion magnetic resonance imaging of congenital lung malformations. Pediatr Radiol. 50(8):1083-94, 2020
7. Zhang N et al: Distribution, diagnosis, and treatment of pulmonary sequestration: report of 208 cases. J Pediatr Surg. 54(7):1286-92, 2019
8. Zirpoli S et al: Agreement between magnetic resonance imaging and computed tomography in the postnatal evaluation of congenital lung malformations: a pilot study. Eur Radiol. 29(9):4544-54, 2019

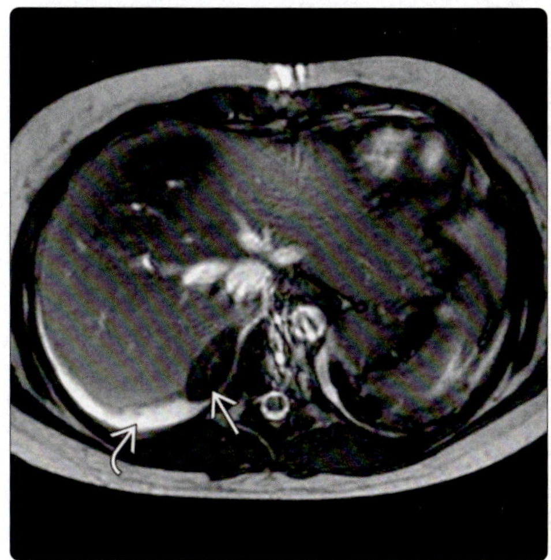

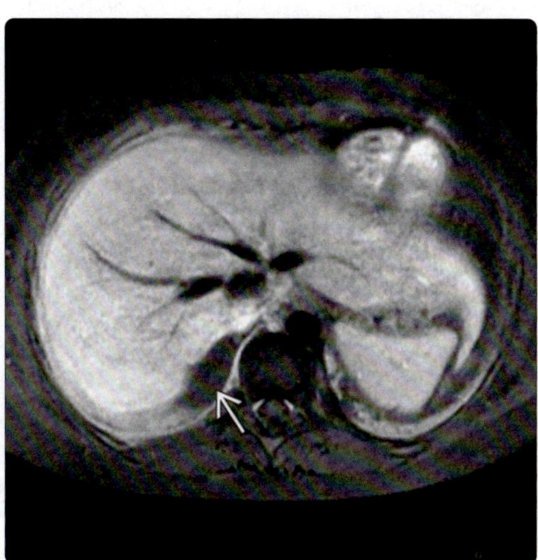

(Left) *Axial SSFP MR in a 10-year-old patient with right abdominal pain & fever shows an ovoid, hypointense mass ➡ medially in the right lower hemithorax with an adjacent pleural effusion ➡.* **(Right)** *Axial T1 C+ FS MR in the same patient shows no enhancement of the mass ➡.*

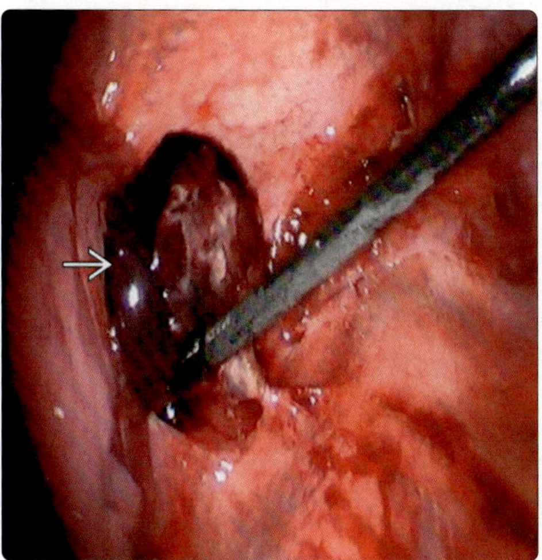

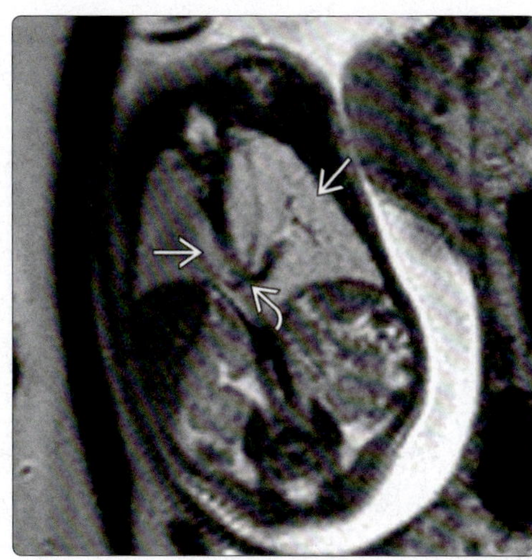

(Left) *Thoracoscopy of the right hemithorax in the same patient shows a small, hemorrhagic mass ➡ in the pleural space. Histology revealed a torsed & infarcted extralobar BPS.* **(Right)** *Coronal T2 SSFSE MR in a 27-weeks-gestation fetus shows a large, uniformly hyperintense, solid left lower lobe lesion ➡ with a large, trifurcating feeding vessel ➡ arising from the thoracic aorta, consistent with BPS.*

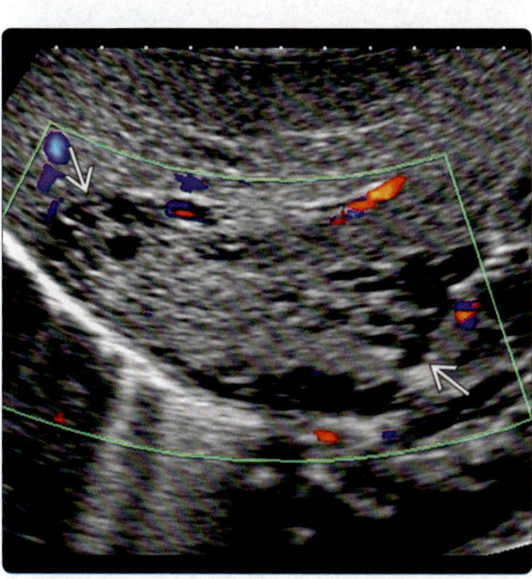

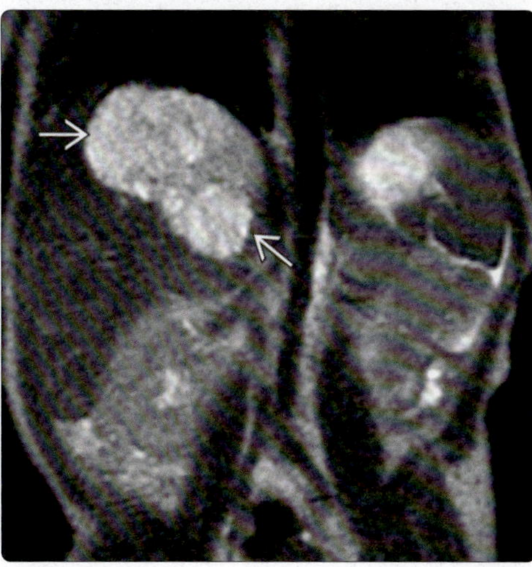

(Left) *Right upper quadrant color Doppler ultrasound in a newborn with a prenatally diagnosed suprarenal vs. hepatic mass shows an ovoid, mixed solid & cystic lesion ➡ with no significant internal vascularity or feeding vessel.* **(Right)** *Coronal T2 MR SSFSE in the same patient shows a heterogeneously hyperintense, lobular mass ➡ along the posterior liver. Upon resection, a retroperitoneal extralobar BPS was confirmed with CPAM components ("hybrid lesion"). No feeding vessel was ever seen on imaging or surgical exploration.*

Bronchogenic Cyst

KEY FACTS

TERMINOLOGY

- Congenital mass in family of foregut duplication cysts: Bronchogenic cysts, enteric cysts, neurenteric cysts
- Results from abnormal ventral budding of tracheobronchial tree between 26th & 40th days of gestation

IMAGING

- Well-defined, round to ovoid, unilocular, thin-walled cyst
- Mediastinal location >> lung (medial 1/3 of lower lobes) > extrathoracic
    - Typically subcarinal, paratracheal, or hilar
- May compress airway → adjacent atelectasis or air-trapping
- Fluid filled; gas in cyst is uncommon unless active or prior infection
- CECT: Variable attenuation of cyst contents due to protein, hemorrhage, or (rarely) calcium; minimal enhancement of thin wall
- MR: Variable T1 signal; T2 FS or STIR imaging maximizes conspicuity of high fluid signal in cyst

TOP DIFFERENTIAL DIAGNOSES

- Esophageal duplication cyst
- Neurenteric cyst
- Round pneumonia
- Neuroblastoma
- Lymphadenopathy
- Lymphatic malformation
- Congenital pulmonary airway malformation
- Bronchopulmonary sequestration

CLINICAL ISSUES

- Common presentations
    - Respiratory distress, recurrent pneumonia, chest pain, dysphagia
        - Infants are more likely to be symptomatic
    - Infection is more common in pulmonary lesions
    - Often asymptomatic in older children & adults
- Definitive treatment: Surgical resection

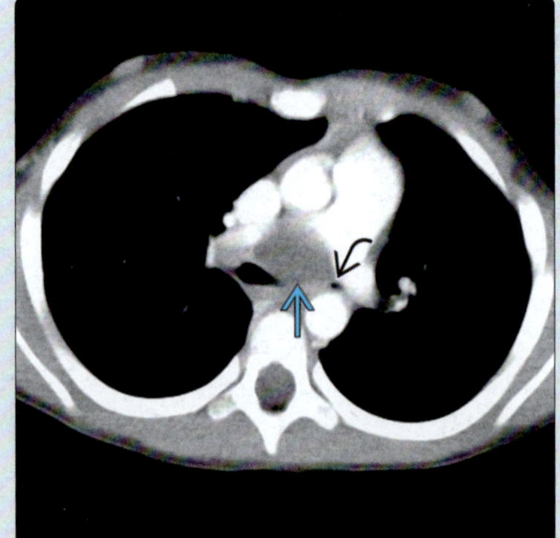

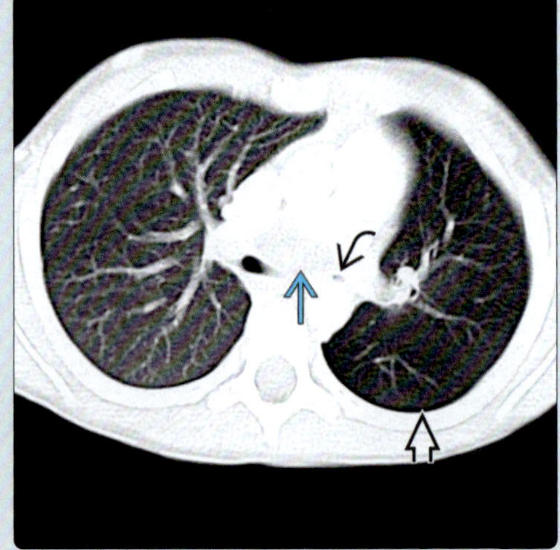

(Left) *Axial CECT of a 5-year-old girl with recurrent left lower lobe pneumonia shows a 2-cm, well-circumscribed, fluid-attenuation mass ➙ in a subcarinal location. There is marked narrowing of the adjacent left main bronchus ➘.* **(Right)** *Axial lung window in the same CECT in the same patient shows diffuse hyperlucency of the left lung ➙, indicating postobstructive air-trapping due to extrinsic compression of the left main bronchus ➘ by the bronchogenic cyst ➙ (with the cyst being poorly visualized on this setting).*

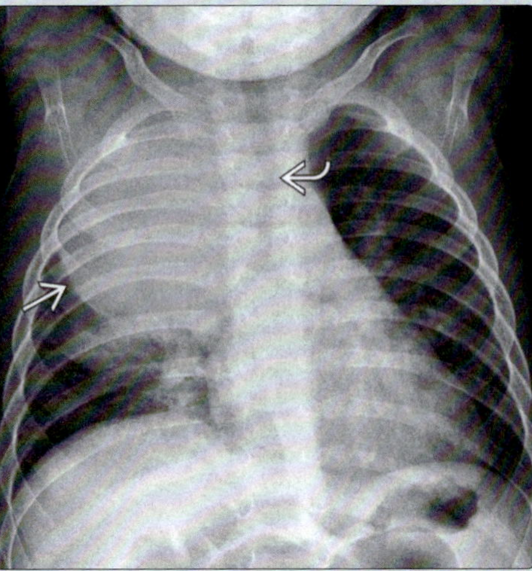

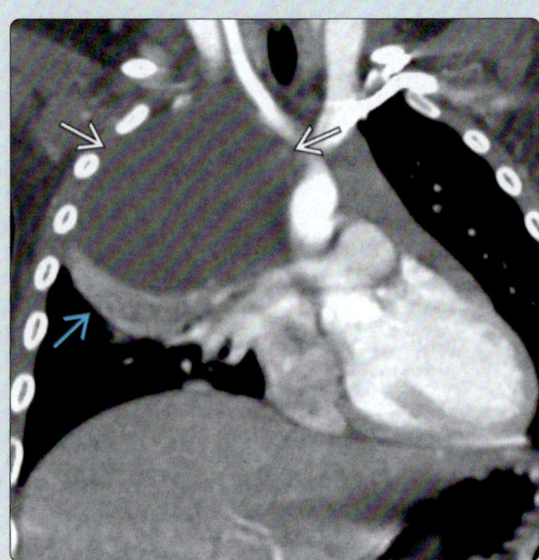

(Left) *AP chest radiograph in a 9-month-old with respiratory distress & wheezing shows a large, rounded density in the right upper hemithorax ➙ with mass effect on the airway ➘. There is patchy airspace opacity in the right lung base.* **(Right)** *Coronal CECT in the same patient shows a large, well-defined, fluid-attenuation mass ➙ arising from the right paratracheal region. The adjacent right upper lobe atelectasis ➙ is a result of mass effect on the right upper lobe airways & parenchyma. A bronchogenic cyst was confirmed at resection.*

TERMINOLOGY

Definitions

- Congenital mass in family of foregut duplication cysts: Bronchogenic cysts, enteric cysts, neurenteric cysts

IMAGING

General Features

- Best diagnostic clue
  - Well-circumscribed, round, middle mediastinal mass of soft tissue or water density
- Location
  - Mediastinal: 75-85%
    - 79% middle, 17% posterior, 3% anterior
    - Typically subcarinal, paratracheal, or hilar
  - Pulmonary: 15-25%
    - Majority in medial 1/3 of lower lobes
  - Rarely extrathoracic; can occur anywhere along foregut
    - Diaphragm, retroperitoneum, base of tongue, suprasternal or presternal soft tissues, pericardium or myocardium, subcutaneous tissues
- Size
  - 1-11 cm; average: 4.8 cm
- Morphology
  - Well-defined ovoid or round mass with smooth or slightly lobulated borders
  - Almost always unilocular
  - No communication with airway unless prior infection

Radiographic Findings

- Radiography
  - Well-defined spherical mass with smooth borders
  - Soft tissue/fluid density
  - Typically in mediastinum or central lung
  - Compression of adjacent bronchus may lead to hyperinflation or atelectasis

Fluoroscopic Findings

- Extrinsic mass effect on esophagus on esophagram or upper GI series

CT Findings

- CECT
  - Sharply marginated mass with smooth borders
  - Cyst contents are variable: Water or proteinaceous fluid, air
    - Mediastinal: 50% water attenuation, 50% soft tissue attenuation
    - May contain air if current or prior infection
  - Ca^{2+} is uncommon; may occur in wall or as layering calcium oxalate in cyst contents
  - Typically shows non- or minimally enhancing thin wall
    - Thicker enhancing wall implies infection
    - Solid nodular components favor neoplasm
  - No central enhancement
  - May see lucency in adjacent lung in pulmonary lesions indicating air-trapping

MR Findings

- T1WI
  - Well-circumscribed, thin-walled cystic mass
    - Variable internal signal, often hyperintense due to proteinaceous or hemorrhagic fluid
- T2WI FS
  - Central contents have fluid signal hyperintensity
    - Intermediate or dark T2 signal intensity could be due to hemorrhage or (rarely) Ca^{2+}
- DWI
  - Uncomplicated cyst should not restrict diffusion
- T1WI C+ FS
  - No central enhancement
  - Thin wall may mildly enhance
  - Thicker enhancing wall implies infection

Ultrasonographic Findings

- Grayscale ultrasound
  - Well-circumscribed, round mass with posterior acoustic enhancement
  - Thin wall with variable echogenicity of internal contents
- Color Doppler
  - No internal vascularity
  - With inflammation, thickened cyst wall & surrounding tissues may be hyperemic

Imaging Recommendations

- Best imaging tool
  - MR or CT is usually best for diagnosis
    - MR provides more comprehensive evaluation of lesion to exclude other diagnoses & determine full extent (particularly if paraspinal)
    - Lung parenchyma & small airways are better visualized on CT
    - May be occult or subtle on radiography
  - If mass location allows adequate acoustic window, ultrasound may demonstrate cystic nature of lesion without radiation or sedation
- Protocol advice
  - T2 FS or STIR MR to maximize contrast of cyst fluid against surrounding tissues
  - Consider additional MR sequences
    - Flow-sensitive sequence to exclude aneurysm/varix & show exact relationship to mediastinal/hilar vessels
    - Precontrast T1 FS in single plane for subtraction from postcontrast sequence (to confirm absence of true enhancement)

DIFFERENTIAL DIAGNOSIS

Esophageal Duplication Cyst

- Often has identical imaging appearance
- Duplication cyst may have thicker wall (as smooth muscle is always present)

Neurenteric Cyst

- Cyst communicates with spinal canal
- Commonly has associated vertebral anomaly

Round Pneumonia

- Well-circumscribed lung opacity in child < 8 years of age
- Air bronchograms confirm airspace disease
- No mass effect on adjacent structures
- Follow-up radiographs will show resolution after antibiotics

Neuroblastoma

- Moderately enhancing, solid paraspinal mass
- Intermediate T2 MR signal intensity; frequently calcified
- Typically restricts diffusion on MR
- ± adjacent rib & vertebral changes, intraspinal extension

Lymphadenopathy

- Generally multifocal, ovoid, solid-appearing
- Necrotic lymph nodes
  - Usually have associated pulmonary findings of infection (e.g., histoplasmosis or tuberculosis)
  - Thick, irregular rim of enhancement
  - Other nearby nodes are usually enlarged

Lymphatic Malformation

- Multilobulated, multiseptated cystic mass
- Infiltrates across multiple soft tissue compartments
  - Neck, chest wall, upper extremity
- Surrounds & displaces adjacent structures, typically without significant venous compression
- Macrocysts may contain fluid-fluid levels from hemorrhage

Congenital Pulmonary Airway Malformation

- Heterogeneous, multicystic lesion with architectural distortion of lung parenchyma
- Individual cysts in lesion vary widely in size
- Initially fluid-filled at birth with subsequent aeration

Bronchopulmonary Sequestration

- Heterogeneous cystic &/or solid mass, typically in lung bases
- Borders tend to be less well defined
- Systemic feeding vessel from aorta is pathognomonic

PATHOLOGY

General Features

- Etiology
  - Congenital lesions that develop from abnormal budding of ventral foregut between 26th & 40th days of gestation
    - Early budding results in mediastinal/tracheobronchial cysts
    - Later budding results in lung parenchymal cysts
    - Can occur anywhere along foregut (but rarely extrathoracic)
- Associated abnormalities
  - Occasional association with other congenital cardiopulmonary malformations
    - BPS, lobar overinflation, diaphragmatic hernia
    - Pericardial defect, congenital heart disease

Gross Pathologic & Surgical Features

- Well-circumscribed, unilocular cystic lesion
- Almost 50% have stalk connecting lesion to trachea/carina, pleura, or esophagus
- No communication with airway unless prior infection
- Contents usually thick or gelatinous fluid

Microscopic Features

- Lined by ciliated respiratory epithelium
- May contain bronchial glands, smooth muscle, bronchial cartilage, or (rarely) gastric mucosa

CLINICAL ISSUES

Presentation

- Most common signs/symptoms
  - Infants are more likely to be symptomatic
  - Mass effect
    - Airway: Respiratory distress, stridor, wheezing, recurrent pneumonia
    - Esophagus: Dysphagia
  - Infection is more common in pulmonary lesions
  - Often asymptomatic, incidentally discovered in older children & adults
- Other signs/symptoms
  - May be detected in utero ± mass effect
    - Can compromise airway, lead to overinflation of adjacent lung
  - Cervical & subcutaneous lesions frequently present as palpable masses

Demographics

- Age
  - May present at any age but usually in childhood
- Epidemiology
  - Frequency unknown due to asymptomatic population

Natural History & Prognosis

- Propensity for infection
- Rare case reports of malignancy arising in lesions

Treatment

- Typically surgical resection
  - Earlier resection is favored to avoid morbidity of resection after infection occurs
  - Potential for malignancy arising in lesion
- Conservative treatment may be considered in patients of high surgical risk

SELECTED REFERENCES

1. Newman B: Magnetic resonance imaging for congenital lung malformations. Pediatr Radiol. 10;1-11, 2021
2. Adams NC et al: Fetal ultrasound and magnetic resonance imaging: a primer on how to interpret prenatal lung lesions. Pediatr Radiol. 50(13):1839-54, 2020
3. Zobel M et al: Congenital lung lesions. Semin Pediatr Surg. 28(4):150821, 2019
4. Abushahin A et al: Bronchogenic cyst as an unusual cause of a persistent cough and wheeze in children: a case report and literature review. Case Rep Pediatr. 2018:9590829, 2018
5. Chowdhury MM et al: Imaging of congenital lung malformations. Semin Pediatr Surg. 24(4):168-75, 2015
6. Jiang JH et al: Differences in the distribution and presentation of bronchogenic cysts between adults and children. J Pediatr Surg. 50(3):399-401, 2015
7. Pacharn P et al: Congenital lung lesions: prenatal MRI and postnatal findings. Pediatr Radiol. 43(9):1136-43, 2013
8. Recio Rodríguez M et al: MR imaging of thoracic abnormalities in the fetus. Radiographics. 32(7):E305-21, 2012
9. Biyyam DR et al: Congenital lung abnormalities: embryologic features, prenatal diagnosis, and postnatal radiologic-pathologic correlation. Radiographics. 30(6):1721-38, 2010
10. Laberge JM et al: Asymptomatic congenital lung malformations. Semin Pediatr Surg. 14(1):16-33, 2005
11. Jeung MY et al: Imaging of cystic masses of the mediastinum. Radiographics. 22 Spec No:S79-93, 2002
12. McAdams HP et al: Bronchogenic cyst: imaging features with clinical and histopathologic correlation. Radiology. 217(2):441-6, 2000

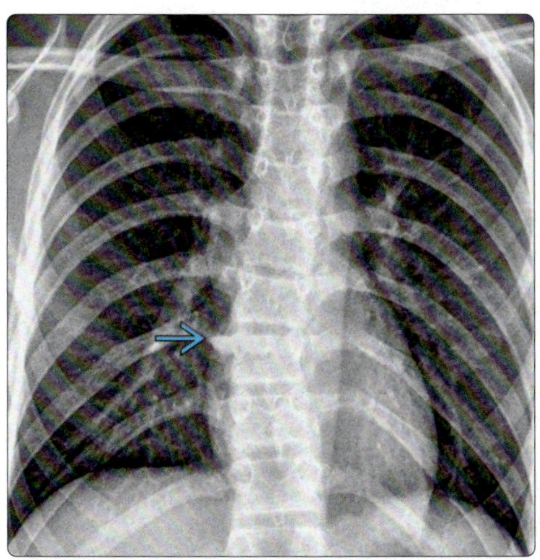

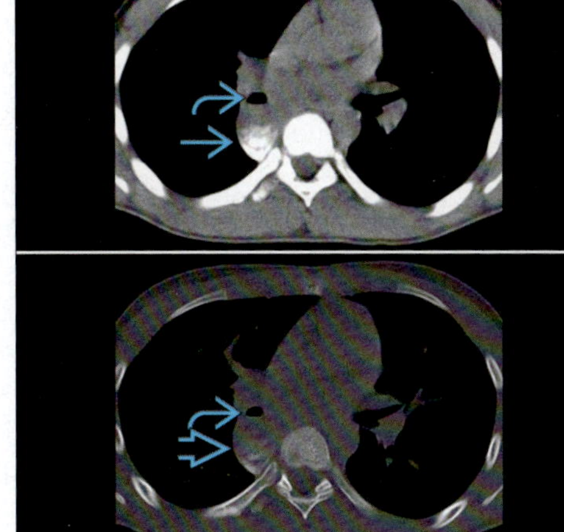

(Left) *Upright frontal radiograph in a 14-year-old boy with suspected scoliosis shows Ca^{2+} layering dependently in an otherwise occult lesion ➔.* **(Right)** *Axial NECT images in the same patient show dependent positioning of the calcium within the otherwise fluid-attenuating mass (seen here in both soft tissue ➔ & bone ➔ windows). The mass is intimately related to the bronchus intermedius ➔.*

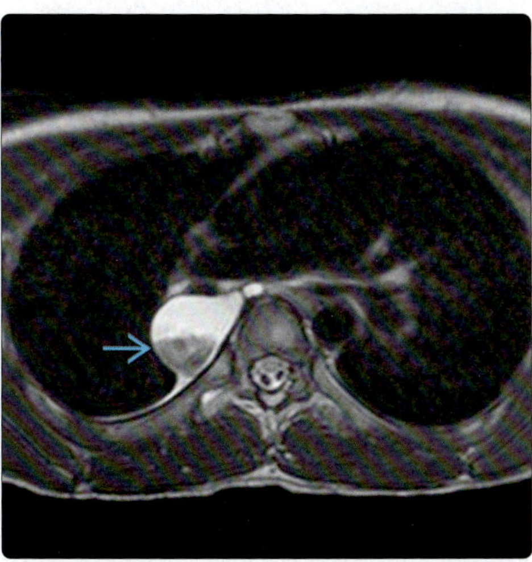

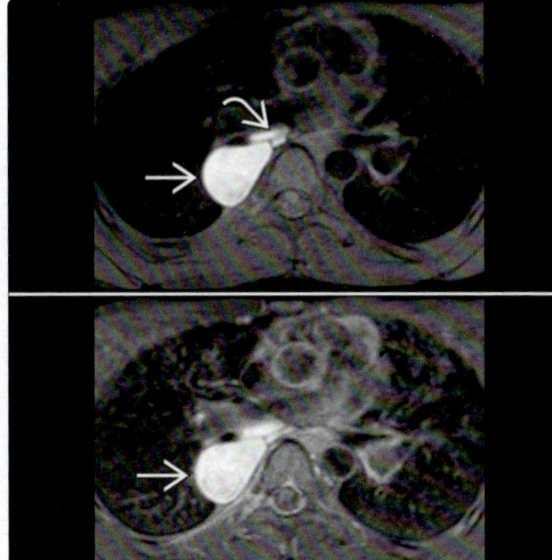

(Left) *Axial T2 MR in the same patient shows dependently layering low signal intensity material ➔ (corresponding to the known Ca^{2+}) within the rounded mass.* **(Right)** *Axial T1 FS MR images in the same patient before (top) & after (bottom) contrast administration show no significant change in the mass. Note the intrinsically bright material within the mass ➔, likely due to complex proteinaceous fluid. Small foci of the lesion ➔ extend posterior to the pulmonary artery. A bronchogenic cyst was confirmed upon resection.*

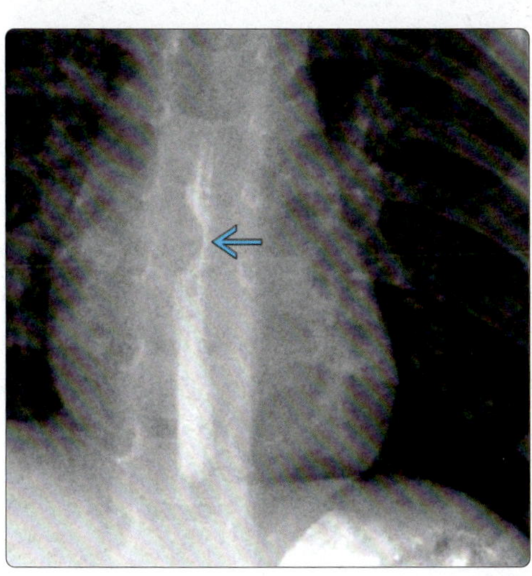

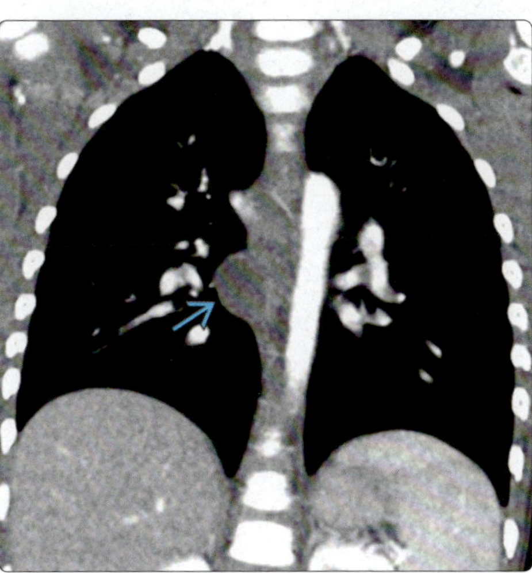

(Left) *Frontal esophagram image from a 3-year-old patient with choking episodes shows a round, relatively lucent mass extrinsically compressing the contrast-filled midesophagus ➔ from the right. The lesion was occult radiographically.* **(Right)** *Coronal CECT in the same patient shows the round mass to be of fluid attenuation with minimal rim enhancement ➔. This bronchogenic cyst was directly apposed to the bronchus intermedius.*

Congenital Lobar Overinflation

KEY FACTS

TERMINOLOGY

- Congenital lobar overinflation (CLO): Malformation of lower airways that results in overexpansion of pulmonary segment or lobe
- CLO is preferred term (vs. lobar emphysema), as microscopic analysis shows airspace overinflation, not alveolar destruction
- Considered final common pathway in various disruptions of bronchopulmonary development

IMAGING

- Progressively hyperlucent & hyperexpanded lobe in neonate → mass effect on adjacent lung, mediastinal shift
    - Lobar predilection: LUL > RML > RUL > > lower lobes
- Typically diagnosed by serial chest radiographs
- CTA is performed to confirm diagnosis, elucidate potential cause, & exclude other lung malformations (especially pulmonary sequestration)
    - No discrete cyst or feeding vessel

TOP DIFFERENTIAL DIAGNOSES

- Pneumothorax
- Bronchial atresia
- Congenital pulmonary airway malformation
- Aspirated foreign body
- Persistent pulmonary interstitial emphysema
- Swyer-James syndrome

PATHOLOGY

- Partial bronchial obstruction due to wall abnormality, luminal obstruction, or extrinsic compression leads to check-valve mechanism
- Air enters involved region but has difficulty leaving → progressive hyperinflation → mass effect

CLINICAL ISSUES

- Usually presents as neonatal respiratory distress resulting from progressive hyperexpansion & mass effect
- Treated by thoracoscopic lobectomy

(Left) *Newborn radiograph shows a large, expansile, lentiform opacity peripherally ➡. This example of CLO appears uniformly dense because it still contains retained fetal fluid. Note the malpositioned umbilical venous catheter ➡ in the right atrium & the depressed right hemidiaphragm ↗, both of which are displaced by the mass.* **(Right)** *Longitudinal US in the same patient shows that the fluid-filled CLO is hyperechoic ➡ but otherwise has normal lung architecture, giving it an appearance similar to the liver ➡ on this image.*

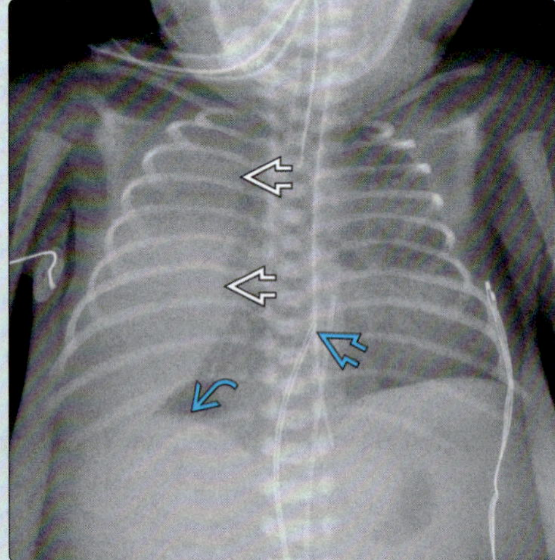

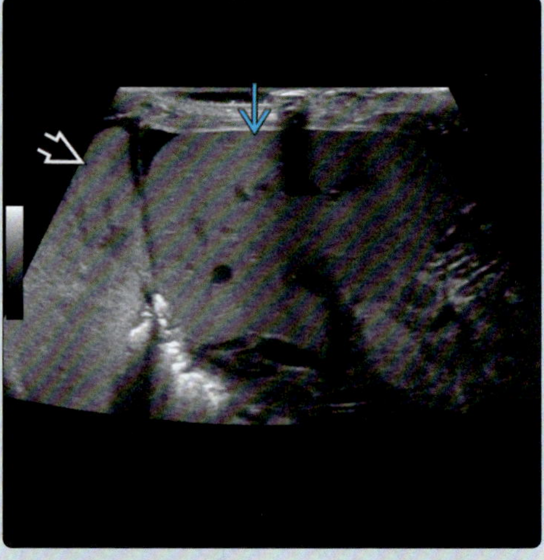

(Left) *AP radiograph obtained in the 1st few hours of life demonstrates segmental airspace opacification of the right middle lobe ↗. The opacity reflects retained fetal fluid-filling alveoli in the affected segment.* **(Right)** *Follow-up AP radiograph in the same patient the next day shows that the same segment is now gas filled, quite lucent, & hyperexpanded ↗. The retained fetal fluid has been resorbed, & the findings now reflect localized air-trapping, consistent with CLO.*

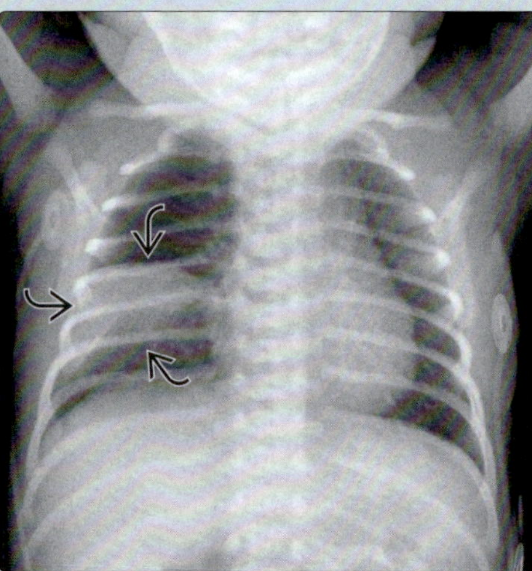

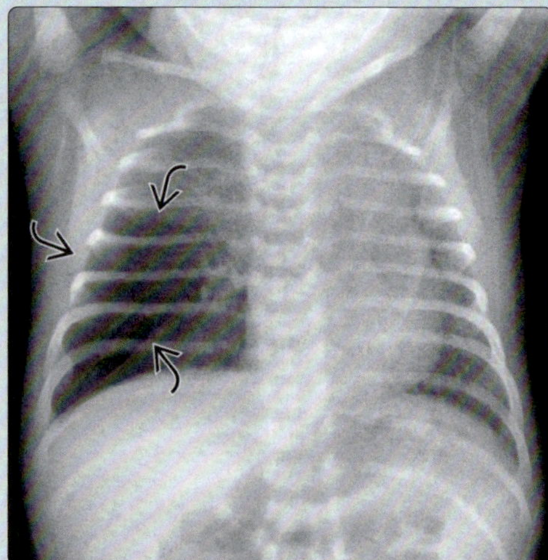

TERMINOLOGY

Abbreviations

- Congenital lobar overinflation (CLO)

Synonyms

- Congenital lobar hyperinflation
- Congenital lobar emphysema is no longer used, as microscopic analysis shows airspace overinflation, not alveolar destruction

Definitions

- Congenital lung malformation consisting of overdistended pulmonary segment or lobe; caused by partial bronchial obstruction acting as 1-way valve → air-trapping
- Considered final, common pathway of various disruptions of bronchopulmonary development
  - 50% are idiopathic
  - 25% are due to intrinsic cartilaginous abnormality
  - 25% are due to extrinsic compression

IMAGING

General Features

- Best diagnostic clue
  - Neonate with hyperexpanded lucent pulmonary lobe
    - Especially left upper lobe
    - May be fluid-filled in 1st few hours after birth
- Location
  - Lobar predilection
    - Left upper lobe: 40%
    - Right middle lobe: 35%
    - Right upper lobe: 20%
    - Lower lobes: 5%
  - May involve ≥ 1 lobe or only segment

Radiographic Findings

- Classic newborn appearance: Fluid-filled, radiopaque pulmonary segment or lobe becomes progressively hyperlucent & hyperexpanded
  - May have reticular pattern as fluid clears via distended lymphatics
- Classic appearance is uncommon
  - Usually detected as gas-filled hyperexpanded lobe beyond immediate newborn period
- Pulmonary vessels may appear attenuated & evenly splayed
- Mass effect
  - Compression of ipsilateral lung
  - Mediastinal shift with possible tracheal deviation & compression of contralateral lung
  - Deviation of anterior junction line
  - Occasional rib separation & hemidiaphragm depression
  - Persistent hyperinflation of lobe/segment despite ipsilateral decubitus positioning

CT Findings

- NECT
  - Hyperinflation with uniform hyperlucency of affected lung parenchyma (reflecting distended alveoli)
  - No discrete cysts
- CTA
  - IV contrast is used to evaluate vascular structures & aid in detecting other abnormalities (e.g., sequestration, congenital pulmonary airway malformation, bronchogenic cyst)
  - Attenuated vessels: Smaller & more widely spaced than those in adjacent lung
    - Vessels are not focally splayed (as seen with cystic mass)

Ultrasonographic Findings

- Grayscale ultrasound
  - Prenatal: Uniformly hyperechoic lung mass without macrocysts or systemic arterial supply
    - Some show hypervascularity
  - Postnatal: Useful if affected lung is still fluid-filled → homogeneous & similar to liver

MR Findings

- Fetal MR
  - Homogeneous, T2-bright pulmonary mass without architectural distortion or discrete cyst
  - Pulmonary vessels in involved segment may appear elongated
  - May see adjacent T2-bright tubular/branching structure (due to dilated, fluid-filled bronchus)
  - Mass effect with compression of ipsilateral remaining lung & mediastinal deviation
  - Location of lesion is helpful, but mass effect can make localizing lesion difficult
  - Hydrops is less common compared to CPAM
- Postnatal MR
  - Gaining interest, particularly with ultrashort TE sequences for lung parenchyma

Imaging Recommendations

- Best imaging tool
  - Diagnosis is typically made by serial chest radiographs
  - CTA is performed to
    - Confirm diagnosis
    - Exclude other neonatal hyperlucent lung lesions
    - Evaluate for causal obstructing mass
    - Define extent of disease

DIFFERENTIAL DIAGNOSIS

Pneumothorax

- Pleural line + characteristic location &/or shape confirm abnormal gas collection of pleural space
  - Look for nondependent gas collection that varies by patient position
  - No lung markings beyond pleural line
  - Lung is collapsed, not hyperexpanded

Bronchial Atresia

- Central tubular, rounded, or branching fluid- or mucus-filled mass representing atretic bronchus
- Air accumulates via collateral ventilation rather than check-valve mechanism
  - No significant mass effect from progressive hyperexpansion

Congenital Pulmonary Airway Malformation

- Composed of variable-sized, gas-filled cysts

Bronchopulmonary Sequestration

- Nonfunctioning lung tissue separated from tracheobronchial tree
- Differentiated from other lung lesions by its systemic arterial blood supply
- Unless fistulized (usually by infection), remains fluid-filled (& thus radiopaque) postnatally

Aspirated Foreign Body

- Typically older infants or toddlers with acute-onset breathing difficulties after choking/coughing episode

Persistent Pulmonary Interstitial Emphysema

- In rare cases, persistent pulmonary interstitial emphysema can present as expanding hyperlucent mass
- Pulmonary vessels & bronchi are surrounded by air as gas dissects into pulmonary interstitium

Swyer-James Syndrome

- Presents later in childhood after viral infection
- Often affects > 1 lobe

PATHOLOGY

General Features

- Etiology
  - Most likely related to bronchial obstruction with check-valve phenomenon
    - Air enters involved region but has difficulty leaving → progressive hyperinflation
  - Specific cause is found in ~ 50% of cases
    - Wall abnormality
      - Deficient, immature, or dysplastic bronchial cartilage
      - Redundant bronchial mucosal folds
      - Stenotic or kinked bronchus
    - Lumen obstruction
      - Inspissated mucus plug
      - Mucosal web or fold
    - Extrinsic compression
      - Foregut duplication cyst
      - Vascular anomaly
- Associated abnormalities
  - 15-20% have cardiac anomalies
  - May also have renal, GI, & MSK abnormalities

Staging, Grading, & Classification

- 2 forms
  - Hypoalveolar: Normal or fewer alveoli than expected
  - Polyalveolar: More alveoli than expected

Gross Pathologic & Surgical Features

- Hyperexpanded lobe is rounded
- Sponge-like appearance
- Resected lobe does not deflate
  - Compressed ipsilateral lobe will reinflate & eventually compensatorily hyperinflate

Microscopic Features

- Dilated alveoli
- Alveolar walls are thinned but intact
  - Not true emphysema (hence effort to abandon congenital lobar emphysema nomenclature)
- Defective cartilage in bronchial walls is seen in < 50%

CLINICAL ISSUES

Presentation

- Most common signs/symptoms
  - Respiratory distress in neonatal period
  - May be progressive
- Other signs/symptoms
  - Asymmetry of movement of chest with respiration
  - Use of accessory muscles of respiration
  - ↓ breath sounds on affected side
  - Hyperresonant hemithorax

Demographics

- Age
  - May be diagnosed in utero
    - Many of these are asymptomatic after birth
  - Of those developing symptoms, majority occur as neonates or infants
    - 50% present in 1st 4 weeks; 75% in 1st 6 months
  - May present with symptoms later in childhood or may be incidental finding

Natural History & Prognosis

- Fluid seen in neonatal period is removed by lymphatics & capillary reabsorption
- Lobe is subsequently filled with air by collateral air drift
- May cause progressive respiratory distress as lobe continues to expand & cause lung compression; can be fatal if not resected
- Some patients have minor symptoms & can be observed
- Over time, involved lobe becomes small with diminished markings
- No ↑ risk of malignancy or infection

Treatment

- Consider bronchoscopy to exclude endobronchial lesion, especially if presenting beyond newborn period
- Mitigate respiratory distress caused by mass effect
  - Elective intubation of opposite lung
  - Place patient in ipsilateral decubitus position
- Thoracoscopic lobectomy
  - May be needed emergently if progressive hyperinflation occurs; can be life threatening
  - Most common complications: Air leak & need to convert to open approach
- Conservative treatment has been advocated for patients with minimal symptoms

SELECTED REFERENCES

1. Newman B: Magnetic resonance imaging for congenital lung malformations. Pediatr Radiol. ePub, 2021
2. Abdel-Bary M et al: Clinical and surgical aspects of congenital lobar over-inflation: a single center retrospective study. J Cardiothorac Surg. 15(1):102, 2020
3. Bawazir OA: Congenital lobar emphysema: thoracotomy versus minimally invasive surgery. Ann Thorac Med. 15(1):21-25, 2020
4. Oliver ER et al: Congenital lobar overinflation: a rare enigmatic lung lesion on prenatal ultrasound and magnetic resonance imaging. J Ultrasound Med. 38(5):1229-39, 2019
5. Lee EY et al: Multidetector CT evaluation of congenital lung anomalies. Radiology. 247(3):632-48, 2008

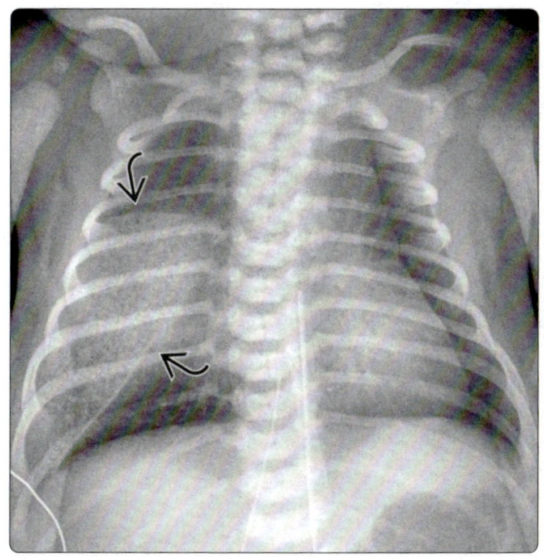

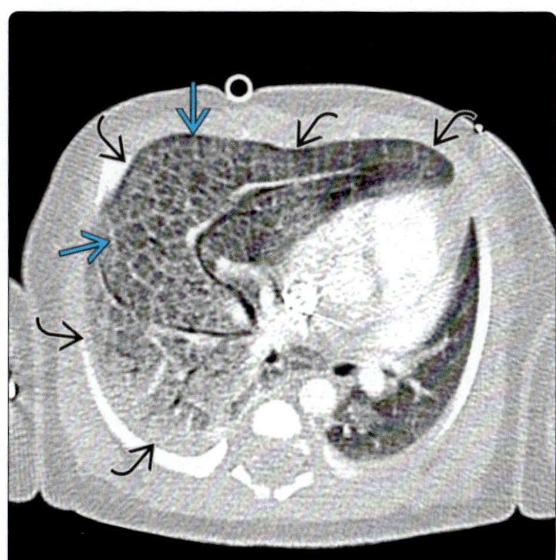

(Left) *Chest radiograph of CLO during the period when fetal fluid has not fully been resorbed, but air-trapping has already begun, shows a picture of lobar hyperexpansion with distinct reticular interstitial markings* ➲. **(Right)** *Axial CECT in the same patient shows how the right middle lobe is hyperexpanded & herniates across the midline* ➲. *The radiographic reticular pattern resulted from fluid engorgement of lymphatics causing interlobular septal thickening* ➔.

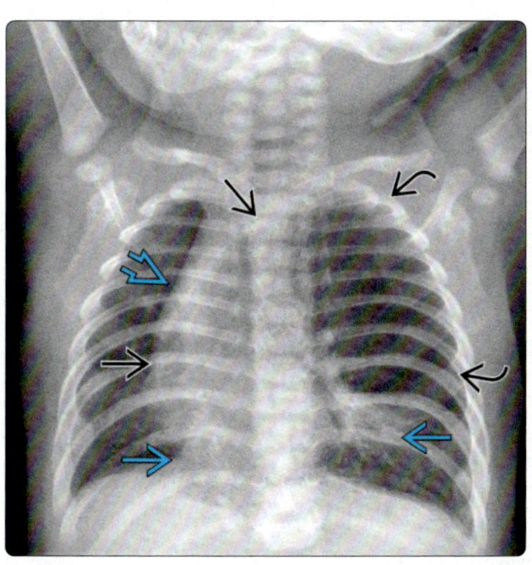

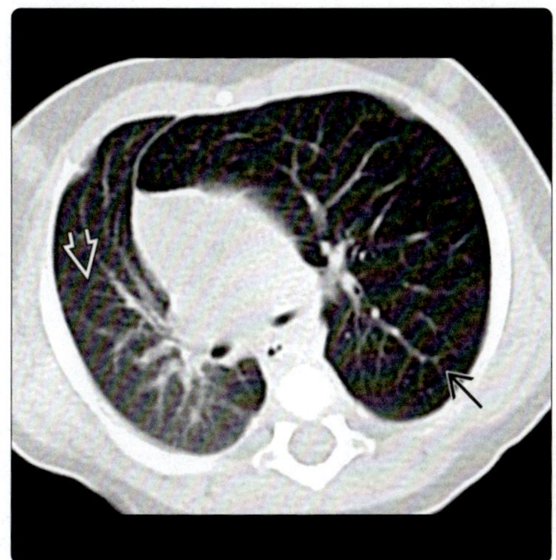

(Left) *AP radiograph of an infant with chronic wheezing shows an abnormally lucent left upper lobe* ➲ *that is so hyperexpanded that it herniates across the midline* ➔. *Note the mass effect causing mediastinal shift* ➔ *& lower lobe atelectasis* ➔. **(Right)** *Axial NECT from the same patient reveals smaller vessels in the affected hyperexpanded & hyperlucent left upper lobe* ➔ *with compressive atelectasis in the right lung* ➔. *There are no gas-filled cysts as would be seen in congenital pulmonary airway malformation (CPAM).*

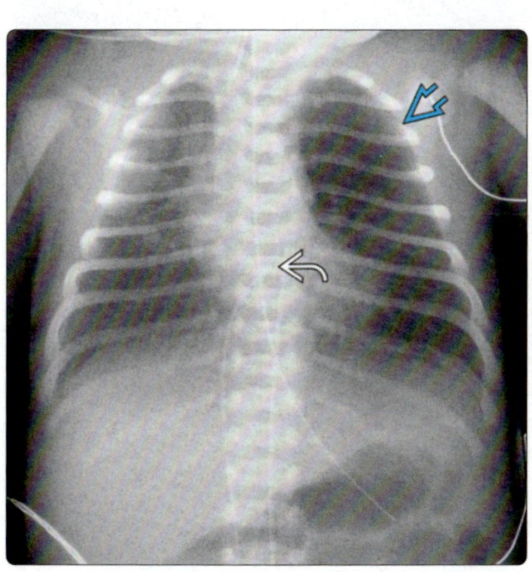

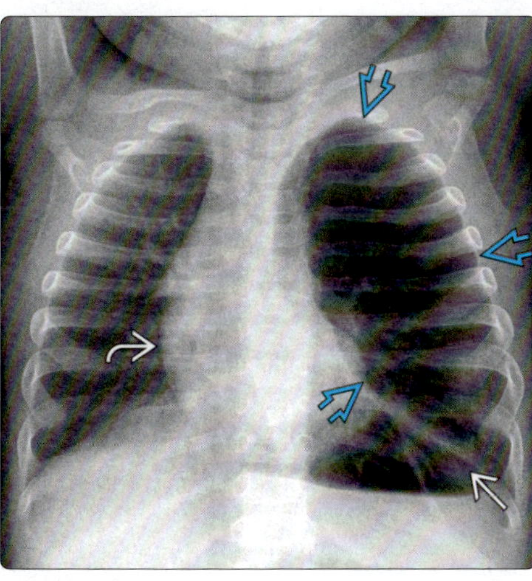

(Left) *AP radiograph shows subtle asymmetric lucency & hyperexpansion of the left upper lobe* ➔ *that went unnoticed on initial imaging. Note the malpositioned umbilical venous catheter in the right atrium* ➲. **(Right)** *AP radiograph in the same patient 9 months later, when he presented with worsening respiratory distress, shows progressive hyperexpansion & lucency in the LUL* ➔. *The resulting mass effect causes shift of the heart toward the right* ➲ *with compressive atelectasis in the LLL* ➔.

Bronchial Atresia

KEY FACTS

TERMINOLOGY

- Focal interruption of bronchus → distal mucoid impaction (bronchocele/mucocele) & hyperinflation of distal lung
  - ± hyperplasia of distal lung

IMAGING

- Classic appearance: Ovoid/round or tubular branching mass (finger-in-glove sign) with hyperinflated lung distally
  - May occur in any lobe/segment/subsegment
- Neonates & infants may present with atelectatic, fluid-filled segment that gradually fills with air
- Protocol: CTA with multiplanar reconstructions
  - Fluid-attenuation round or tubular branching mass
  - Hyperinflated distal lung + ↓ vascularity
    - Expiratory images are helpful to confirm air-trapping
  - No systemic feeding artery

TOP DIFFERENTIAL DIAGNOSES

- Congenital lobar overinflation (CLO)
- Congenital pulmonary airway malformation (CPAM)
- Bronchogenic cyst
- Bronchopulmonary sequestration (BPS)
- Allergic bronchopulmonary aspergillosis
- Scimitar syndrome (hypogenetic lung syndrome)

PATHOLOGY

- Within spectrum of other congenital lung lesions (CLO, CPAM, BPS, bronchogenic cyst)
  - Components of atretic bronchi are frequently found pathologically in other congenital lung lesions
- Aeration of distal lung occurs through collateral air drift

CLINICAL ISSUES

- Older children/adults (majority of cases) are often asymptomatic
- May present with recurrent respiratory tract infections, chronic cough, dyspnea, &/or wheezing in early childhood
- Resection is usually reserved for recurrent infections

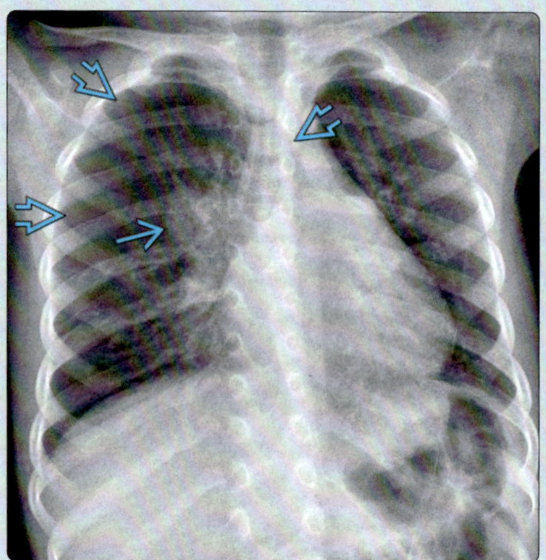

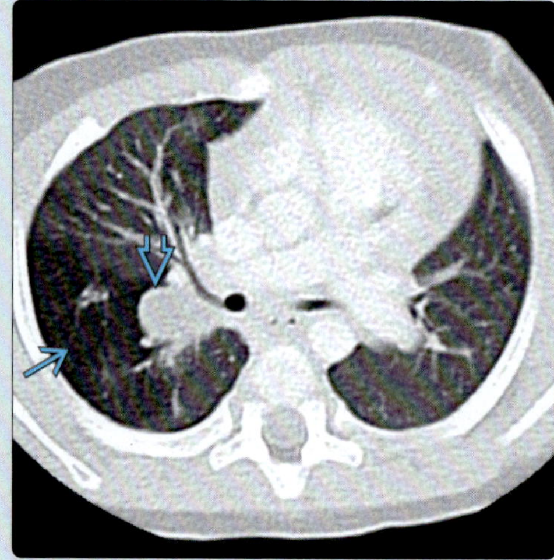

(Left) *AP radiograph in a 3-year-old with a cough & diminished breath sounds shows a round, perihilar, mass-like opacity ➡ due to a dilated, atretic right upper lobe (RUL) segmental bronchus. Note the relatively lucent & hyperexpanded RUL ➡.* **(Right)** *Axial CECT (in lung windows) in the same patient confirms the findings of segmental RUL bronchial atresia. Note the RUL hyperinflation ➡ due to collateral air drift beyond the obstructed & dilated RUL bronchus (bronchocele) ➡.*

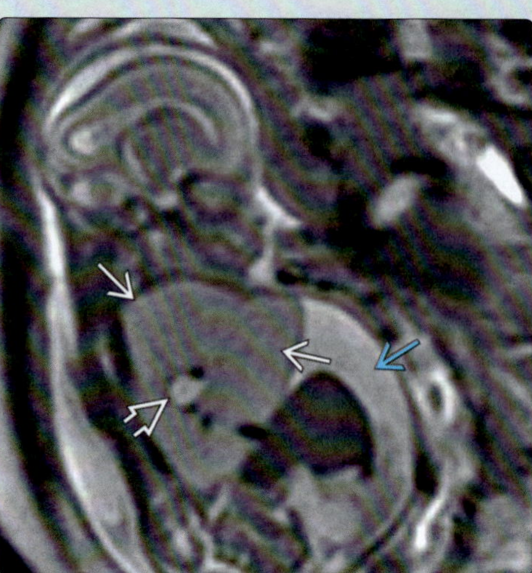

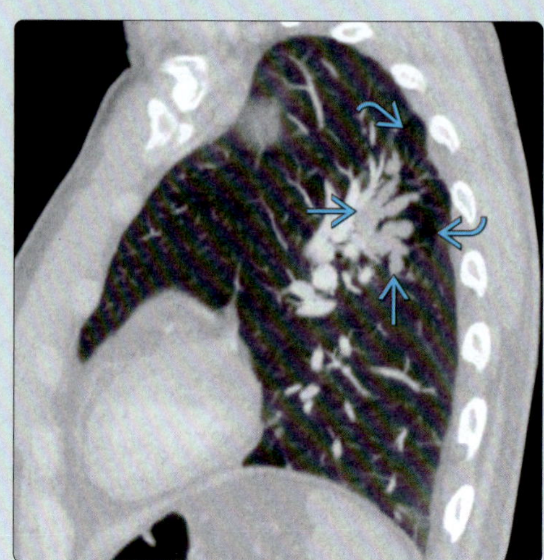

(Left) *Sagittal SSFSE T2 fetal MR shows a distended hyperintense right lung ➡. The round, fluid-signal focus ➡ in the hilum accompanying the arterial flow void represents the fluid-filled atretic right main bronchus. Note the hydropic change, including ascites ➡.* **(Right)** *Sagittal MIP CTA shows branching mucous-plugged bronchi ➡ in the posteroapical segment of the left upper lobe with distal air-trapping ➡, typical of bronchial atresia.*

TERMINOLOGY

Definitions

- Focal interruption of main, lobar, segmental, or subsegmental bronchus with associated mucoid impaction (bronchocele/mucocele) & hyperinflation of distal lung
  - ± hyperplasia of distal lung depending on level of bronchial obstruction

IMAGING

General Features

- Best diagnostic clue
  - Round or tubular branching mass (finger-in-glove sign) + hyperinflated distal lung

Radiographic Findings

- Neonates & infants
  - Presentation is more variable than in children or adults
  - Lobe or segment may be atelectatic or fluid-filled initially → gradually fills with air
  - Hyperinflation is less frequent than in children & adults
- Children & adults
  - Radiating, branching, tubular opacity (mucoid impaction of dilated airway) distal to atretic bronchus
  - More central perihilar round or ovoid mass (bronchocele)
  - Distal lung is hyperinflated with ↓ vascularity

CT Findings

- CTA
  - Fluid-attenuation round or tubular branching mass
  - Hyperinflated distal lung + ↓ vascularity
    - Expiratory images confirm air-trapping

MR Findings

- Fetal MR
  - Discrete & uniformly T2-hyperintense "solid" lung mass with varying degrees of mass effect
    - No visible cysts
  - Dilated, fluid-filled bronchus in medial/central aspect of lesion helps differentiate from other lesions

Ultrasonographic Findings

- Obstetric ultrasound
  - Homogeneously hyperechoic segment or lobe
  - May see dilated, fluid-filled bronchi

Imaging Recommendations

- Best imaging tool
  - CTA confirms that tubular opacity represents impacted atretic bronchus & not vessel
    - Expiratory images can confirm air-trapping

DIFFERENTIAL DIAGNOSIS

Congenital Lobar Overinflation

- Overlapping appearance; no mass/bronchocele
- Usually involves entire lobe with progressive hyperinflation

Congenital Pulmonary Airway Malformation

- Often heterogeneous due to macroscopic cysts with distortion/splaying of residual lung
- No associated bronchial dilation/impaction

Bronchogenic Cyst

- Discrete, round (nonbranching), fluid-filled cyst in central lung or mediastinum

Bronchopulmonary Sequestration

- Systemic arterial supply, usually from aorta
- Usually in left lower lobe
- May present beyond infancy with recurrent infections

Allergic Bronchopulmonary Aspergillosis

- FInger-in-glove sign is often present
- Frequently bilateral with widespread bronchiectasis

Scimitar Syndrome (Hypogenetic Lung Syndrome)

- Hypoplastic lung with partial anomalous pulmonary venous drainage
  - Typically right lower lobe with curvilinear opacity (vein) directed toward medial right hemidiaphragm

Slow-Growing Endobronchial Tumor

- Mass is usually smaller than mucoid impaction
- Distal lung is usually atelectatic, not hyperinflated

PATHOLOGY

General Features

- Etiology
  - Occurs between 5th-15th weeks of gestation, though exact mechanism unclear
    - Intrauterine interruption of arterial supply to bronchus → scarring of primitive bronchus
    - Disconnection of primitive bronchial cells at tip of bronchial bud with continued normal growth distally
  - Aeration of distal lung through collateral air drift
- Associated abnormalities
  - Components of atretic bronchi are frequently found pathologically in other congenital lung lesions

CLINICAL ISSUES

Presentation

- Congenital lesion but may be diagnosed at any age
  - Older children/adults (majority of diagnoses): Often asymptomatic
  - Infancy, early childhood (< 3 years): Recurrent respiratory tract infections, chronic cough, dyspnea, wheezing
  - Uncommon main bronchus atresia can be lethal in utero

Treatment

- Surgical resection is typically reserved for patients with repeated infections

SELECTED REFERENCES

1. Adams NC et al: Fetal ultrasound and magnetic resonance imaging: a primer on how to interpret prenatal lung lesions. Pediatr Radiol. 50(13):1839-54, 2020
2. Masroujeh R et al: Endobronchial treatment of bronchial atresia. Am J Respir Crit Care Med. 200(3):e25-6, 2019
3. Kozaki M et al: Fetal congenital peripheral bronchial atresia diagnosed by magnetic resonance imaging: two case reports. AJP Rep. 8(4):e201-5, 2018
4. Watanabe T et al: An investigation on clinical differences between congenital pulmonary airway malformation and bronchial atresia. J Pediatr Surg. 53(12):2390-3, 2018
5. Alamo L et al: Imaging findings of bronchial atresia in fetuses, neonates and infants. Pediatr Radiol. 46(3):383-90, 2016

Esophageal Atresia and Tracheoesophageal Fistula

KEY FACTS

TERMINOLOGY

- Atresia: Congenital occlusion of upper esophagus
- Fistula: Anomalous congenital connection(s) from esophagus to trachea

IMAGING

- 5 major anatomic variations of esophageal atresia (EA)-tracheoesophageal fistula (EA-TEF)
- Fistula level is variable depending on type of EA-TEF
  - Most commonly above/near carina
- Atretic segments are variable in length
  - Gap is often long in EA without TEF
- Radiographs
  - Air-distended upper esophageal pouch
  - Enteric tube tip near thoracic inlet in pouch, often coiled
  - EA with TEF: Gas in stomach & bowel
  - EA without TEF: Gasless stomach & bowel
- Limited indications for preoperative esophagram (except isolated TEF)
- Postoperative esophagram
  - Esophageal anastomotic leak, anastomotic stricture, recurrent/additional TEF, esophageal dysmotility, gastroesophageal reflux

TOP DIFFERENTIAL DIAGNOSES

- Tube malposition
- Laryngotracheal cleft
- Chronic respiratory issues (mimicking H-type TEF)
- Esophageal strictures of various etiologies
- Extrinsic esophageal compression

PATHOLOGY

- 47-75% have associated anomalies

CLINICAL ISSUES

- Presentation: Excessive oral secretions, cyanosis, choking, coughing during feeding
- Postsurgical survival: 75-95% (depends on associated cardiac anomalies, birth weight)

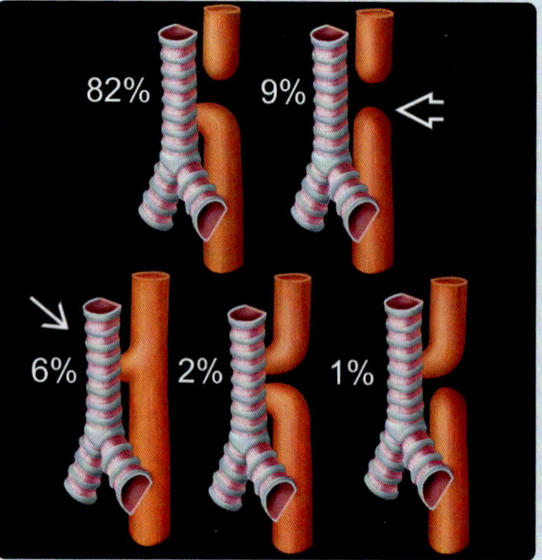

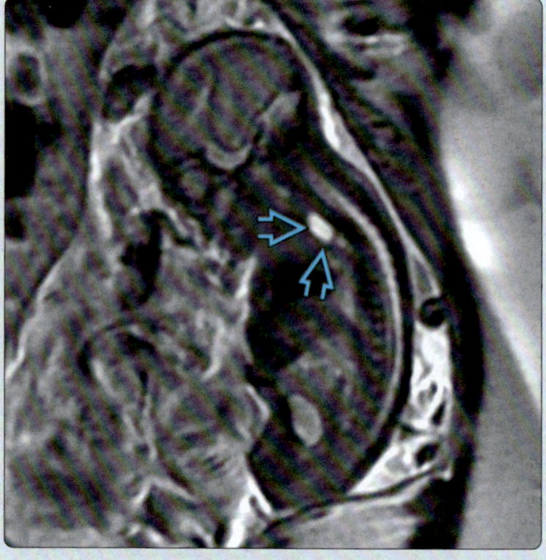

(Left) *Graphic shows the 5 main types of esophageal atresia with tracheoesophageal fistula (EA-TEF), including the isolated TEF without EA (H-type fistula)* ➡ *& the isolated EA without TEF* ➡. **(Right)** *Sagittal T2 SSFSE MR of a 26-weeks-gestation fetus imaged for polyhydramnios shows a collection of fluid in the region of the upper esophagus* ➡ *that is suggestive of an atretic esophageal pouch, which was confirmed during surgery in the newborn period.*

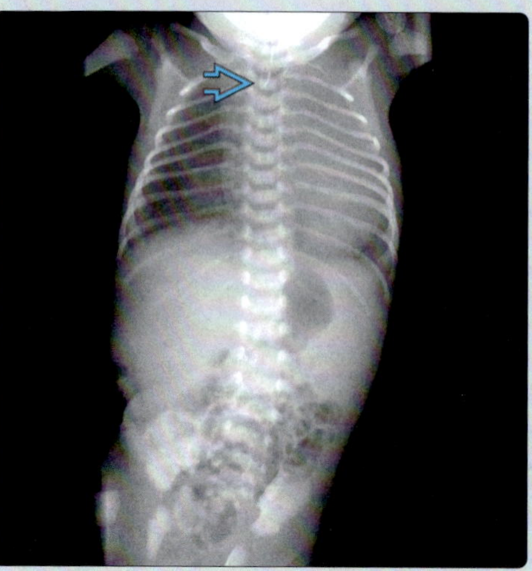

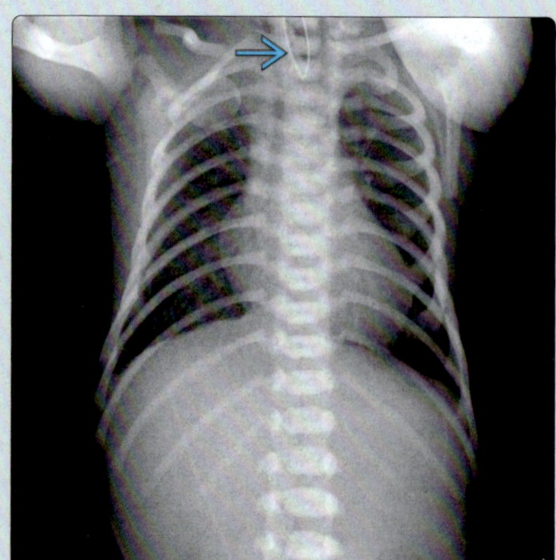

(Left) *AP radiograph of a premature newborn boy with a history of not handling secretions shows a nasogastric tube (NGT) tip* ➡ *overlying the thoracic inlet due to EA. The bowel gas confirms the presence of a distal TEF. Cardiomegaly suggests congenital heart disease.* **(Right)** *AP chest radiograph in a newborn shows an NGT coiled at the thoracic inlet* ➡, *suggesting EA. Note the lack of gas in the upper abdomen, which is typical of EA without a distal TEF.*

TERMINOLOGY

Definitions

- Esophageal atresia (EA): Congenital occlusion of upper esophagus
- Tracheoesophageal fistula (TEF): Single (less commonly multiple), anomalous, congenital connection(s) from esophagus to trachea

IMAGING

General Features

- Best diagnostic clue
  - Enteric tube tip in gas-distended proximal esophageal pouch on newborn chest radiograph
- Location
  - Fistula level is variable depending on type of EA-TEF
    - Most commonly above/near carina
    - Higher levels with multiple fistulas
    - Rarely esophagobronchial fistula
  - Atresia is usually above junction of superior & middle 1/3 of esophagus
- Size
  - TEF is usually small
  - Atretic segments of esophagus are variable in length
    - Gap is often long in EA without TEF
- Morphology
  - 5 major anatomic variations of EA-TEF

Radiographic Findings

- Radiography
  - Intermittently air-distended, dilated upper esophageal pouch
  - Enteric tube tip near thoracic inlet in pouch
  - Gas in stomach & bowel: EA with TEF
  - Gasless stomach & bowel: EA without TEF
  - Displaced, bowed, narrowed trachea due to dilated esophageal pouch & associated tracheomalacia
  - Signs of other congenital anomalies
    - Cardiomegaly, abnormal pulmonary vascularity, vertebral anomalies, dilated bowel
  - Side of aortic arch is important for surgical repair (thoracotomy performed opposite side of arch)

Fluoroscopic Findings

- Rarely needed for diagnosis of EA (clinical + radiographic diagnosis)
  - Confirm blind-ending pouch: Inject air into nasogastric tube (NGT)
- Contrast esophagram is useful preoperatively for
  - H-type TEF without EA (clinical; radiographic diagnosis is less clear in this type)
    - Oblique fistula from esophagus craniad to trachea (looks like "N")
  - EA without TEF (often long gap)
    - Often 2-stage repair if long gap
    - Preoperative measurement of gap
      - Surgical bougie into upper pouch ± contrast
      - Surgical bougie into lower pouch ± contrast via gastrostomy
      - Measure gap prior to 2nd surgery
- Esophagram/upper GI after EA-TEF repair (using iso-osmolar water-soluble contrast)
  - Esophageal anastomotic leak (early)
  - Recurrent or additional TEF
  - Esophageal dysmotility in nearly 100%
  - Gastroesophageal reflux (GER)
  - Malrotation
  - Esophageal anastomotic stricture (early or delayed)

MR Findings

- Fetal: Fluid signal in intermittently distended esophageal pouch ± decompressed stomach, associated anomalies, polyhydramnios
- Neonatal: Ultrashort echo time (UTE) sequence may allow visualization of fistula & esophageal gap length

CT Findings

- Improves surgical planning in up to 40%
  - Visualization of fistula & esophageal gap length

Imaging Recommendations

- Best imaging tool
  - Radiographs ± air injection of NGT for EA
  - Esophagram for suspected isolated TEF or postoperative complication
- Protocol advice
  - Esophagram/upper GI for isolated (H-type) TEF
    - Lateral position for H type
    - Barium by mouth in most cases (tube rarely needed)
    - If contrast injected, 5- or 8-French feeding tube sideports at mid- to distal trachea
    - Pulsed fluoroscopy in lateral position coned from pharynx to below carina
    - No exposures until convinced: Normal vs. fistula
      - ± exposures in multiple positions
    - Do not mistake aspiration for missed fistula
    - Image stomach to duodenojejunal junction to exclude malrotation, if patient stable
  - Postoperative esophagram: Evaluate for leak or other complication
    - At least 1 scout image (± other positioning)
    - By mouth vs. tube injection of iso-osmolar, nonionic, water-soluble contrast in orthogonal views
      - If by tube, position new tube just above anastomosis or retract NGT to anastomosis
      - Careful distention of esophagus to detect leak
    - If no leak with water-soluble contrast, consider using barium to ↑ detection of subtle leaks
    - Re-review images at workstation after study
      - May miss subtle leak on real-time imaging

DIFFERENTIAL DIAGNOSIS

Tube Malposition

- Traumatic pharyngeal perforation with NGT into mediastinum
  - Inject air or iso-osmolar, water-soluble contrast via NGT to differentiate air-filled pharyngeal pouch vs. pneumomediastinum

Laryngotracheal Cleft

- High fistulous connection, variable length

Chronic Respiratory Issue

- GER with aspiration
- Bronchial foreign body
- Cystic fibrosis
- Infected congenital lung lesion

Esophageal Strictures

- Caustic injury, eosinophilic esophagitis, prior foreign body, epidermolysis bullosa, mediastinal radiation

Extrinsic Esophageal Compression

- Vascular rings
- Mediastinal masses

PATHOLOGY

General Features

- Etiology
  - Likely faulty division of foregut into trachea & esophagus in 1st month of gestation
- Genetics
  - Chromosomal anomalies in 2-10%
    - Trisomy 18 & trisomy 21 are most common
- Associated abnormalities
  - 47-75% have associated anomalies
    - Musculoskeletal: 14-24%
    - Cardiovascular: 11-55%
    - GI: 8-27%
    - Genitourinary: 8-21%
    - Craniofacial: 10%
    - Neurologic: 3-15%
    - Pulmonary: 2-6%
    - VACTERL (vertebral, anal, cardiac, tracheoesophageal, renal, limb anomalies): 10-20%

Staging, Grading, & Classification

- Most widely cited surgical classification (Gross)
  - Type A: EA with no TEF (7-9%)
  - Type B: EA with proximal TEF (1%)
  - Type C: EA with distal TEF (82-86%)
  - Type D: EA with proximal & distal TEF (2%)
  - Type E: Isolated (H-type) TEF (no EA) (4-6%)

CLINICAL ISSUES

Presentation

- Most common signs/symptoms
  - Excessive oral secretions, cyanosis, choking, coughing during 1st attempts at feeding
- Other signs/symptoms
  - Enteric tube fails to reach stomach
  - Recurrent pneumonia, dysphagia (H-type TEF)

Demographics

- Age
  - Newborn or early child (isolated H type)
  - 20-35% are premature
- Epidemiology
  - 1:3,000 live births

Natural History & Prognosis

- Postoperative survival: 75-95% (depends on associated cardiac anomalies, birth weight)

Treatment

- Surgical
  - Bronchoscopy, esophagoscopy to visualize fistula(s) + extrapleural ligation of fistula + anastomosis of esophageal segments
  - If EA without TEF, proximal & distal esophagus are often widely spaced
    - 1st surgery: Place gastrostomy tube
    - 2nd surgery months later: Connect lengthened esophageal ends
    - Ultralong gap requires conduit
      - Colonic interposition vs. gastric pull-up/tube
    - Foker procedure: Actively stretches esophagus over time → primary anastomosis
    - Magnetic compression for strictures or primary repair
- Early postsurgical complications
  - Anastomotic leak (up to 15%; most small leaks resolve spontaneously)
  - Additional TEF not seen initially
- Longer term postsurgical issues
  - Anastomotic stricture (18-50%)
    - ↑ with ↑ EA gap length, anastomotic tension, GER
    - Treated with repeated balloon or bougie dilations
  - Recurrent TEF (up to 10% of cases)
  - Esophageal dysmotility (nearly 100%)
  - GER; esophagitis (51%), Barrett esophagus (6%)
    - Surgical treatment (Nissen) if medical therapy fails
  - Respiratory infections
  - Tracheomalacia (10-20%)

DIAGNOSTIC CHECKLIST

Consider

- Is there distal bowel gas?
- Are there associated anomalies?

Image Interpretation Pearls

- Always rereview postoperative fluoroscopic studies at workstation for subtle leak or fistula not seen in real time

SELECTED REFERENCES

1. Urík M et al: Videofluoroscopic swallow study in diagnostics of H-type tracheoesophageal fistula in children. Ear Nose Throat J. ePub, 2021
2. Nakayama DK: The history of surgery for esophageal atresia. J Pediatr Surg. 55(7):1414-9, 2020
3. Pardy C et al: Prenatal detection of esophageal atresia: a systematic review and meta-analysis. Acta Obstet Gynecol Scand. 98(6):689-99, 2019
4. Slater BJ et al: Use of magnets as a minimally invasive approach for anastomosis in esophageal atresia: long-term outcomes. J Laparoendosc Adv Surg Tech A. 29(10):1202-6, 2019
5. Higano NS et al: Pre- and post-operative visualization of neonatal esophageal atresia/tracheoesophageal fistula via magnetic resonance imaging. J Pediatr Surg Case Rep. 29:5-8, 2018
6. Tracy S et al: The distended fetal hypopharynx: a sensitive and novel sign for the prenatal diagnosis of esophageal atresia. J Pediatr Surg. 53(6):1137-41, 2018
7. Liszewski MC et al: Imaging of long gap esophageal atresia and the Foker process: expected findings and complications. Pediatr Radiol. 44(4):467-75, 2014

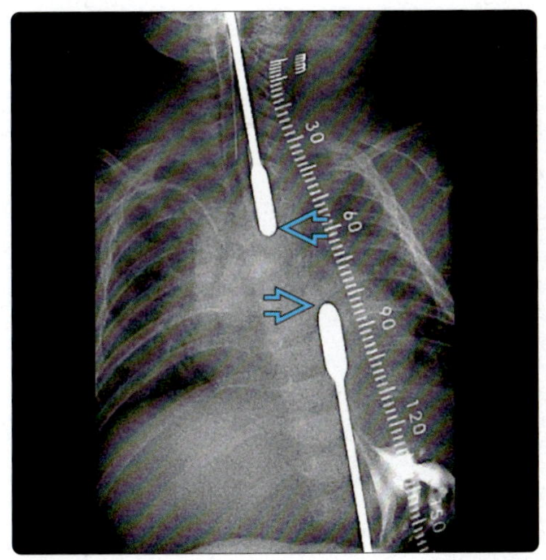

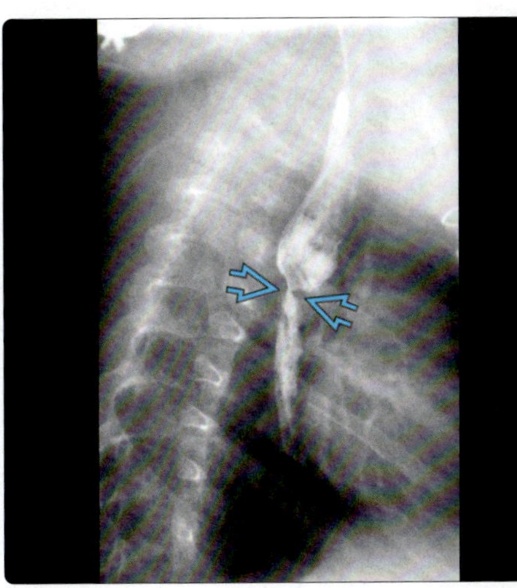

(Left) *Esophagram in an EA patient without TEF shows a long gap atresia, as measured by placing surgical bougies ➔ orally (into the upper pouch) & through the gastrostomy (into the distal atretic segment). A Foker procedure was then performed over several weeks to stretch the esophagus.* **(Right)** *Lateral esophagram in the same patient (who underwent a primary anastomosis of the esophagus in the interval) shows an anastomotic narrowing ➔ after repair. No contrast leak was seen.*

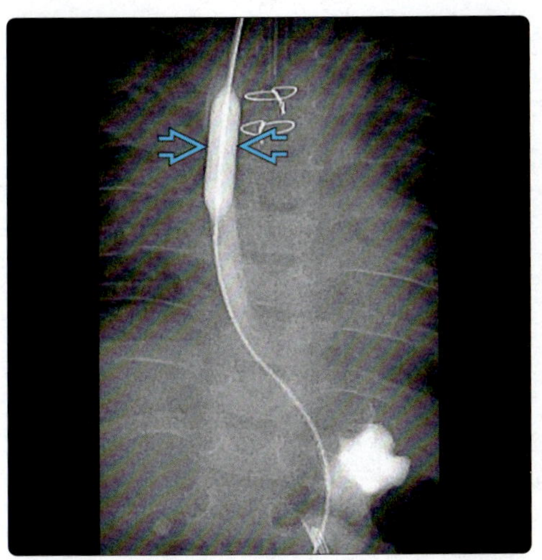

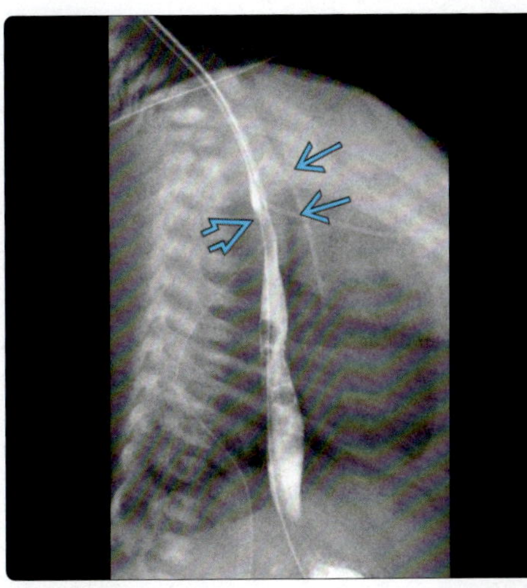

(Left) *Frontal esophagram with balloon dilation ➔ was performed on the same patient to relieve the anastomotic stricture.* **(Right)** *Lateral esophagram performed in a neonate status post EA-TEF repair shows prompt flow through the anastomosis ➔ without a leak. There is tracheomalacia ➔ in the vicinity of the atresia, a common finding in patients with EA. Note that the study was performed via an additional 5 French feeding tube above the anastomosis (instead of retracting the NGT to near the surgical site).*

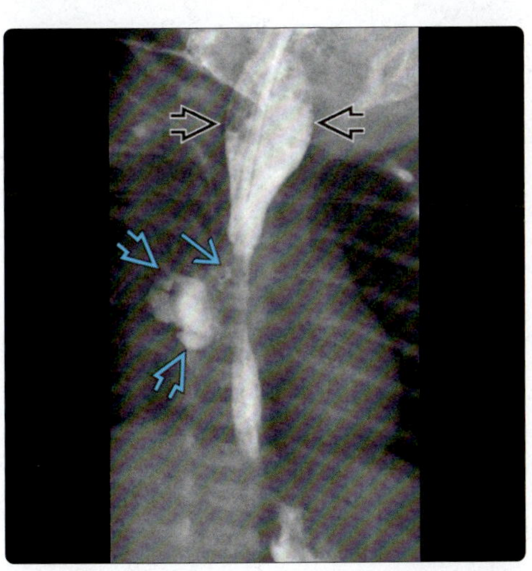

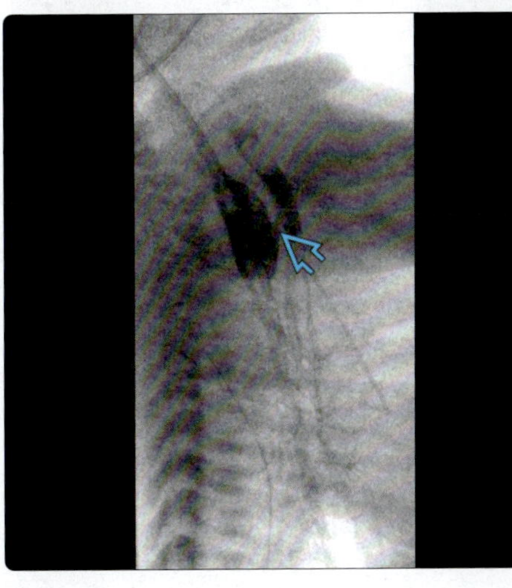

(Left) *Postoperative frontal esophagram in a neonate status post EA-TEF repair shows an extrapleural leak ➔ from a small tract ➔ next to the anastomosis. The upper esophageal dilation ➔ is likely related to residual in utero dilation rather than a postoperative obstruction.* **(Right)** *Lateral postoperative esophagram in a neonate after EA-TEF repair shows no leak; however, an additional, unsuspected proximal TEF ➔ was detected ~ 10 mm above the anastomotic site (the rare Gross type D, occurring in only 2% of all EA).*

Congenital Diaphragmatic Hernia

KEY FACTS

TERMINOLOGY

- Herniation (intrapleural in 80%, mediastinal in 20%) of abdominal contents into chest via congenital defect in diaphragm, most commonly posterior (Bochdalek type of intrapleural hernia)

IMAGING

- Best clue: Bubbly, round, or tubular, relatively uniform, air-filled lucencies in chest displacing mediastinum
- Intrathoracic herniated contents may include stomach, small & large bowel, liver, gallbladder, spleen
  - Results in paucity of bowel gas in abdomen
- Support devices are distorted in specific ways
  - Nasogastric tube due to stomach herniation
  - Umbilical venous catheter due to liver herniation
- Location of congenital diaphragmatic hernia (CDH)
  - Intrapleural: Left 85%, right 13%, bilateral 2%
  - Mediastinal: Anterior or posterior

TOP DIFFERENTIAL DIAGNOSES

- Congenital pulmonary airway malformation
- Diaphragmatic eventration
- Congenital lobar overinflation
- Bronchopulmonary sequestration

CLINICAL ISSUES

- Most are detected prenatally; respiratory distress at birth occurs in majority; delayed presentation is uncommon
- Immediate initiation of supportive postnatal care until patient can tolerate surgical repair (primary vs. patch)
- Prognosis is most related to severity of pulmonary hypoplasia, pulmonary arterial hypertension, congenital heart disease, & other anomalies
  - Various fetal ultrasound & MR parameters are used to guide prognosis & postnatal management
- Survival ↑ if diagnosis is known prenatally & patient delivers at high-volume center
- ↑ awareness of long-term morbidity in survivors

(Left) *Axial graphic shows a large left congenital diaphragmatic hernia (CDH) with portions of the liver, bowel, & stomach residing in the left hemithorax. The right lung is denoted by calipers as being measured for the prenatal LHR value that predicts lung hypoplasia.* **(Right)** *Coronal SSFSE T2 MR of a 32-weeks-gestation fetus shows herniated bowel loops ➚ filling the left hemithorax. The hypoplastic right lung ➔ overlies the aorta ➔ & herniated stomach ➔, which are shifted into the right hemithorax.*

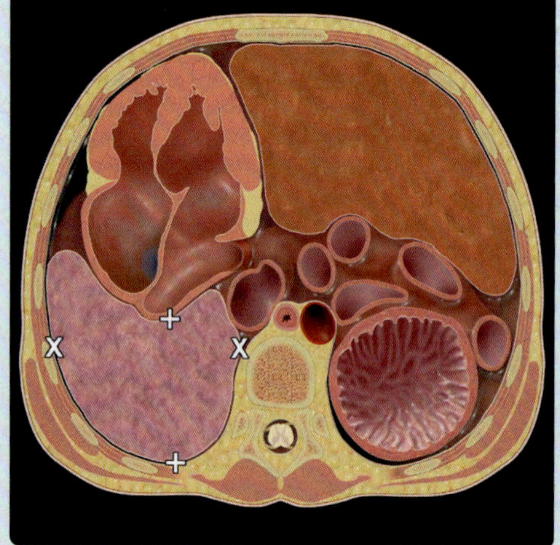

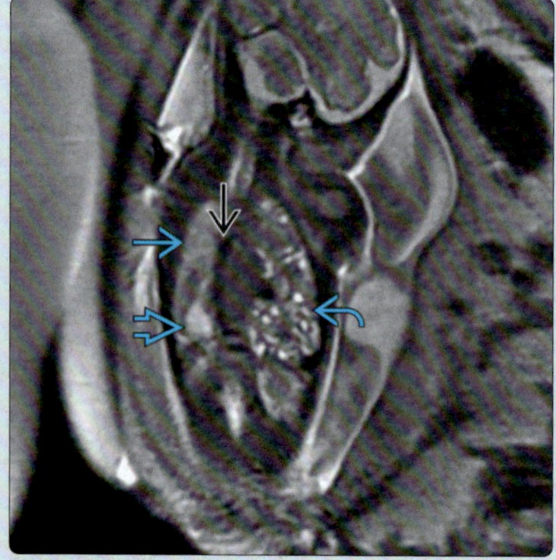

(Left) *Sagittal T1 MR in the same fetus shows a herniated left hepatic lobe ➔ separated from the remaining intraabdominal right hepatic lobe ➔ by residual anterior diaphragm ➔. Note the herniated stomach ➔ & meconium-containing bowel ➚.* **(Right)** *AP radiograph in the same patient after delivery shows gas-distended bowel ➚ filling the left hemithorax. The herniated stomach has an organoaxial rotation ➔ & overlies the herniated left hepatic lobe. Note the arterial ➚ & venous ➔ ECMO cannulae.*

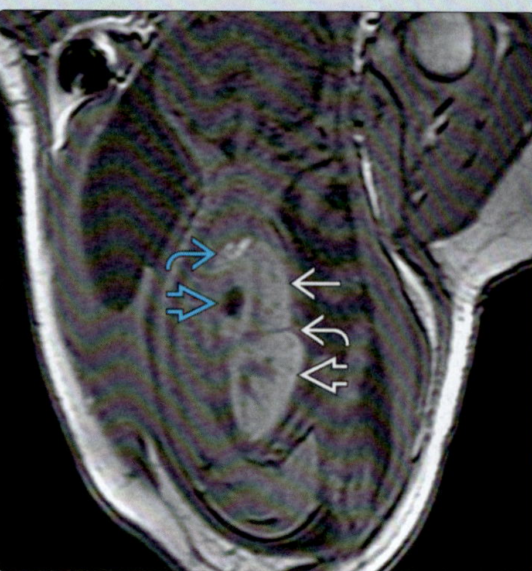

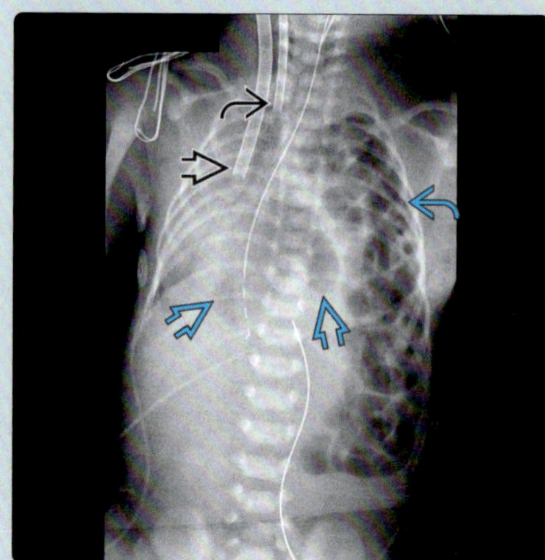

Congenital Diaphragmatic Hernia

TERMINOLOGY

Definitions

- Congenital diaphragmatic hernia (CDH): Herniation of abdominal contents into chest via developmental defect in diaphragm
  - Intrapleural hernia (80%): Worse prognosis
    - Bochdalek (posterolateral) is most common subtype
  - Mediastinal hernia (20%)
    - Anteriorly involves central tendon of diaphragm
      - Morgagni hernia: Smaller paramedian subtype
    - Posteriorly may involve hiatus of esophagus or IVC

IMAGING

General Features

- Best diagnostic clue
  - Bubbly, round, & tubular lucencies in neonatal hemithorax with contralateral mediastinal shift
- Location
  - Left 85%, right 13%, bilateral 2%
- Size
  - Degrees of diaphragmatic deficiency & herniated contents are variable
    - May contain stomach, small & large bowel, liver, gallbladder, spleen

Radiographic Findings

- Depend on hernia contents & presence vs. absence of air in herniated bowel
  - Uniform soft tissue density of herniated solid organs
  - Herniated bowel may appear solid prior to progression of swallowed air
    - Upon air entering bowel, loops appear relatively uniform in size with round & tubular morphologies
      - Degree of gaseous distention changes day to day
    - Herniated, gas-filled stomach is larger than bowel & often abnormally rotated
- Mediastinal shift away from hernia
- Low lung volumes from hypoplasia
  - Ipsilateral lung is more severe than contralateral
- Abnormal positions of support devices
  - Esophageal portion of nasogastric tube (NGT): Contralateral shift & convexity
    - NGT often descends into upper abdomen then back into left hemithorax ("reverse J")
    - NGT tip may lodge at gastroesophageal junction
  - Umbilical venous catheter (UVC) is shifted toward side of hernia (if "liver up"); may not advance to right atrium
    - If UVC extends to right atrium, catheter is typically convex toward hernia
- ↓ intraabdominal bowel gas
- Postoperative appearance
  - Resolution of herniated contents
  - Pleural fluid in 28% (typically chylothorax), eventually resolves
  - Ex vacuo negative-pressure pneumothorax: Hypoplastic lung does not fill space initially
  - Gradual expansion & growth of hypoplastic lungs
  - Repaired hemidiaphragm is often angular or laterally sloped

Ultrasonographic Findings

- Prenatal ultrasound
  - Absent crescentic hypoechoic hemidiaphragm
  - Mixed echogenicity mass in lower hemithorax with mediastinal shift into contralateral hemithorax
    - Bowel & liver are difficult to differentiate from lung lesion: Look for displacement of gallbladder & hepatic vessels
    - Herniated fluid-filled stomach helps confirm CDH
  - Lung:head ratio (LHR): Critical prognostic parameter in left CDH
    - Predictor of pulmonary hypoplasia based on residual, contralateral lung
    - LHR = Area of right lung at level of heart 4-chamber view is divided by head circumference
      - LHR < 1: Poor prognosis
- Postnatal ultrasound
  - Visualization of diaphragmatic defect size may aid in surgical planning

MR Findings

- Fetal MR
  - T2 SSFSE
    - Serpentine, fluid-filled structures (small bowel loops) fill most of hemithorax
    - Stomach is usually herniated with abnormal rotation
    - Partial herniation of low signal intensity colon
    - ± herniation of low signal intensity liver, spleen
    - Contralateral mediastinal shift
    - ↓ total, observed/expected, & predicted lung volumes
      - Lungs of lower signal intensity than normal
      - Residual ipsilateral lung is much smaller than contralateral & typically displaced superomedially
    - Sac-type hernia has better prognosis
      - Cap of lung is evenly distributed over hernia apex
    - Paucity of normal bowel in abdomen
  - T1 GRE
    - Helps localize intermediate signal intensity liver & high signal intensity meconium of small & large bowel against low signal intensity lungs
- Postnatal MR
  - Vascular density ipsilateral to CDH as assessed by time-of-flight imaging correlates with pulmonary hypertension (HTN) markers
  - Accelerated growth of hypoplastic ipsilateral lung parenchyma after repair

CT Findings

- CECT
  - Not typically used for diagnosis of CDH; may be obtained if other cystic chest mass is suspected
  - Follow-up lung CT in survivors shows variable degrees of abnormalities: Low-attenuation foci, subpleural opacities, & atelectasis
    - Severity correlates with respiratory & feeding issues

DIFFERENTIAL DIAGNOSIS

Congenital Pulmonary Airway Malformation

- Macrocystic type appears as multicystic, air-containing mass
  - Cysts are typically not uniform in size

- After gas replaces fluid in cysts (in 1st few days after birth), congenital pulmonary airway malformation (CPAM) appearance is typically static
  - CPAM is more likely to have air-fluid levels than CDH
- Support device positions are less altered by CPAM vs. CDH

Diaphragmatic Eventration

- Focal muscle aplasia of diaphragm without free protrusion of bowel into thorax
  - Abdominal contents are contained by sac of peritoneum, diaphragm tendon, & parietal pleura

Congenital Lobar Overinflation

- Progressive overdistention of single lobe
- Rarely involves lower lobes

Bronchopulmonary Sequestration

- Solid mass near diaphragm with systemic arterial supply

PATHOLOGY

General Features

- Etiology
  - Normal diaphragm development (4th-12th weeks of gestation)
    - Lateral pleuroperitoneal folds fuse with septum transversum
    - Migrating myogenic precursors reach primitive diaphragm & proliferate
    - Error in any portion of process may lead to CDH
  - Underlying cause of defective development is unknown in ~ 70-80%
    - Various chromosomal anomalies (2-35%)
      - Trisomy 18 is most common (2-5%); Down syndrome (trisomy 21) is most likely to have Morgagni type
    - Known specific genetic mutations (< 10%)
- Associated abnormalities
  - Isolated in ~ 50%
  - Cardiac malformations in 20-40%
  - Variety of other systemic anomalies described

CLINICAL ISSUES

Presentation

- Most common signs/symptoms
  - Diagnosis is known prenatally in 60-80%
  - Respiratory distress at birth
- Other signs/symptoms
  - Presence of intrathoracic bowel sounds
  - Absence of ipsilateral breath sounds
  - Scaphoid abdomen
  - < 3% present after 30 days (100% survival)
    - Gastrointestinal symptoms are more likely

Demographics

- Epidemiology
  - 1 in 2,000-4,000 live births

Natural History & Prognosis

- Prognosis is related to severity of pulmonary hypoplasia, pulmonary HTN, & other anomalies (especially heart disease)
  - Most common fetal calculations used for prognosis
    - Lung volumes: Total, observed/expected, & percent predicted by MR; LHR by ultrasound
    - Volume of thorax occupied by herniated liver by MR
  - Utility of these measurements are established for left CDH; do not clearly correlate for right CDH
- Mortality rates are variable: 10-68%
  - ↑ survival reported at single high-volume centers
  - Worse with specific syndromes, cardiac anomalies, esophageal atresia, bilateral hernias, large defects/hemidiaphragm agenesis, extracorporeal membrane oxygenation (ECMO) requirement, higher pulmonary support requirement at 30 days of life
- Long-term morbidity: Impaired lung function + recurrent respiratory infections, neurocognitive & language delays, gastroesophageal reflux disease, gastroparesis, failure to thrive, chest wall deformities, scoliosis

Treatment

- Varying degrees of supportive care are required until definitive surgery can be tolerated
  - Ventilation/oxygenation
    - Immediate intubation with gentle ventilation
    - ± ECMO
  - Pulmonary HTN: Inhaled nitric oxide or IV sildenafil
- Surgery: Primary closure of small defects vs. patch repair for larger; timing is debated
  - Complications include chylothorax, abdominal compartment syndrome, recurrent hernia; malrotation of midgut is expected but does not carry typical risk of volvulus
- Fetal tracheal occlusion (FETO) therapy: Temporary balloon occlusion of trachea in utero (to stimulate lung growth)
  - Beneficial in left CDH with severe pulmonary hypoplasia, not moderate

SELECTED REFERENCES

1. Deprest JA et al: Randomized trial of fetal surgery for moderate left diaphragmatic hernia. N Engl J Med. 385(2):119-29, 2021
2. Koh JY et al: Functional and structural evaluation in the lungs of children with repaired congenital diaphragmatic hernia. BMC Pediatr. 21(1):120, 2021
3. Mukthapuram S et al: MRI assessment of pulmonary vascularity in infants with congenital diaphragmatic hernia: a novel tool for direct assessment of severity of pulmonary hypertension and hypoplasia. J Pediatr. ePub, 2021
4. Beel E et al: Chest CT scoring for evaluation of lung sequelae in congenital diaphragmatic hernia survivors. Pediatr Pulmonol. 55(3):740-6, 2020
5. Mehollin-Ray AR: Congenital diaphragmatic hernia. Pediatr Radiol. 50(13):1855-71, 2020
6. Verla MA et al: Prenatal imaging features and postnatal factors associated with gastrointestinal morbidity in congenital diaphragmatic hernia. Fetal Diagn Ther. 47(4):252-60, 2020
7. Adaikalam SA et al: Neonatal lung growth in congenital diaphragmatic hernia: evaluation of lung density and mass by pulmonary MRI. Pediatr Res. 86(5):635-40, 2019
8. Hosokawa T et al: Postnatal ultrasound to determine the surgical strategy for congenital diaphragmatic hernia. J Ultrasound Med. 38(9):2347-58, 2019
9. Oliver ER et al: Congenital diaphragmatic hernia sacs: prenatal imaging and associated postnatal outcomes. Pediatr Radiol. 49(5):593-9, 2019
10. Victoria T et al: Right congenital diaphragmatic hernias: is there a correlation between prenatal lung volume and postnatal survival, as in isolated left diaphragmatic hernias? Fetal Diagn Ther. 43(1):12-8, 2018

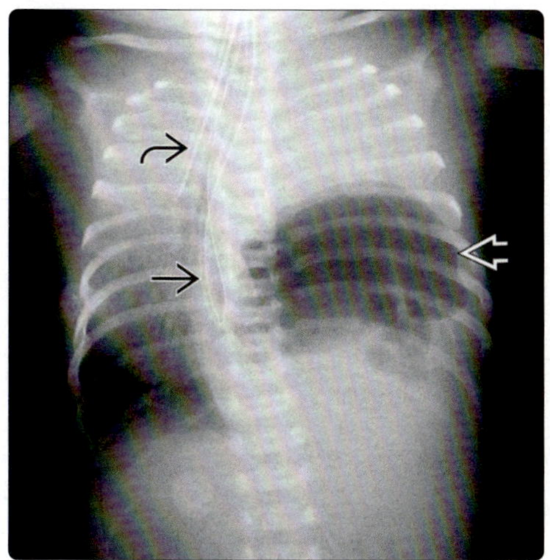

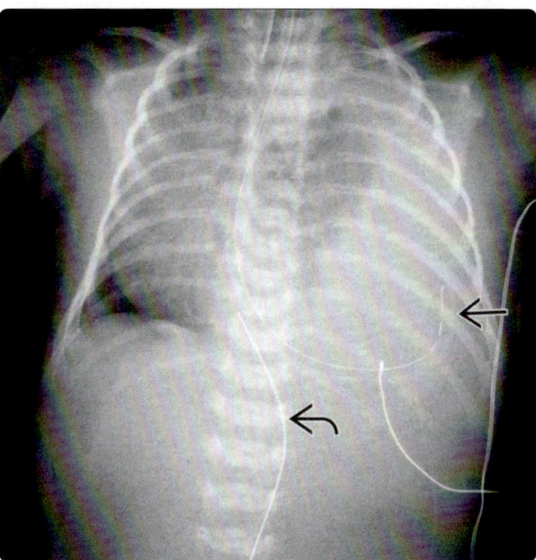

(Left) *AP radiograph shows a newborn with a left CDH. The nasogastric tube (NGT) ➡ is coiled in the distal esophagus. The heart & endotracheal tube ➡ are shifted to the right. The stomach ➡ lies in the left lower chest.* **(Right)** *Subsequent AP radiograph of the same patient shows the NGT tip ➡ decompressing the herniated stomach in the left lower chest. An umbilical venous catheter (UVC) shows convexity toward the left ➡ due to partial liver herniation. Decompressed bowel also fills the left chest.*

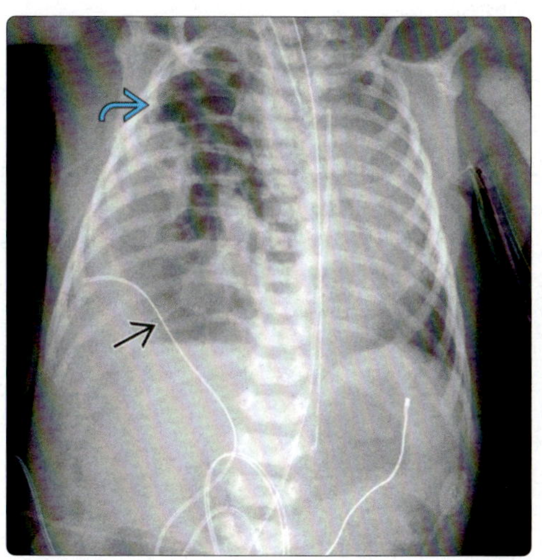

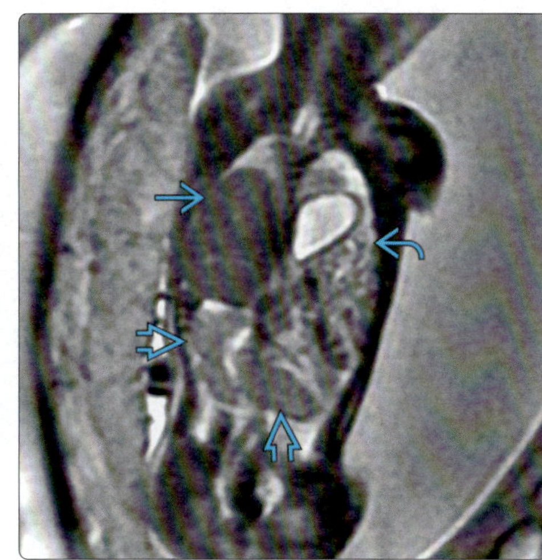

(Left) *AP radiograph shows herniated bowel ➡ filling the right hemithorax. The heart & support devices are shifted to the left. The UVC ➡ is malpositioned in the herniated right hepatic lobe.* **(Right)** *Coronal SSFSE T2 MR in a 29-weeks-gestation fetus shows bilateral diaphragmatic hernias with liver filling the right hemithorax ➡ & stomach/bowel filling the left hemithorax ➡. There is polyhydramnios + an incompletely visualized horseshoe kidney ➡ in this fetus with Cornelia de Lange syndrome.*

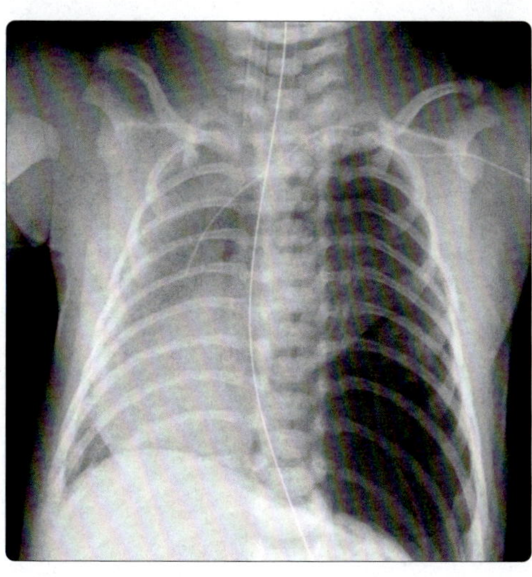

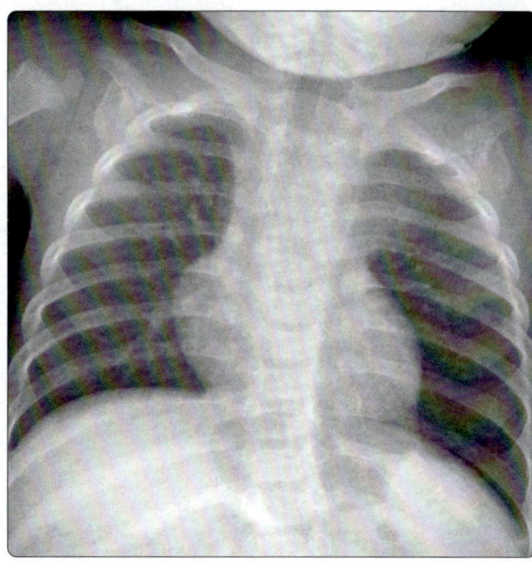

(Left) *AP radiograph in a patient after repair of a left-sided CDH shows a large ex vacuo left pneumothorax. The heart, peripherally inserted central catheter (PICC), & NGT are still shifted to the right. However, a chest tube is not required as this is a postsurgical, negative-pressure pneumothorax.* **(Right)** *AP radiograph of the same patient 8 months later shows resolution of the pneumothorax & mediastinal shift. The hypoplastic left lung is now mildly hyperexpanded & hyperlucent.*

Surfactant Deficiency Disease

KEY FACTS

TERMINOLOGY

- Surfactant deficiency disease (SDD) is favored term
- Common lung disease occurring in premature infants due to lack of surfactant
- Microatelectasis & abnormal pulmonary compliance are hallmarks of disease

IMAGING

- Premature infants < 32-weeks gestation are at risk
- Initial findings are low lung volumes & diffuse hazy/granular opacities
- High incidence of patent ductus arteriosus, which causes pulmonary edema ("whiteout" of lungs with cardiomegaly)
- Bronchopulmonary dysplasia eventually occurs in 17-55% of premature infants
- Lung ultrasound is increasingly used for diagnosis
  - Normal ultrasound findings include A & Z lines
  - SDD causes B lines (vertical lines extending from pleura); scattered in mild SDD, more confluent in severe disease

TOP DIFFERENTIAL DIAGNOSES

- Congenital heart disease: Echocardiography is gold standard for diagnosis
- Group B streptococcal pneumonia: Similar low long volumes; more common to have pleural effusions (67%)
- Meconium aspiration syndrome: Term infants with rope-like densities radiating from hila & high lung volumes
- Transient tachypnea of newborn: Findings similar to pulmonary edema but resolve by 24-48 hours of life

PATHOLOGY

- Surfactant normally coats alveoli & ↓ surface tension, allowing alveoli to stay open
- In prematurity, immature type II pneumocytes cannot produce sufficient surfactant

CLINICAL ISSUES

- Most common cause of death in live newborn infants

(Left) *Frontal radiograph in a 23-weeks-gestation triplet shows low lung volumes with severe, diffuse granular opacities of both lungs ➡ & central air-bronchograms ➡. Note the malpositioned UVC in the right portal vein ➡.* **(Right)** *Frontal radiograph in a premature newborn shows less severe granular opacities ➡ with central air-bronchograms ➡. Skin folds ➡ mimic a right pneumothorax. Note the malpositioned UAC, terminating in the left subclavian artery ➡.*

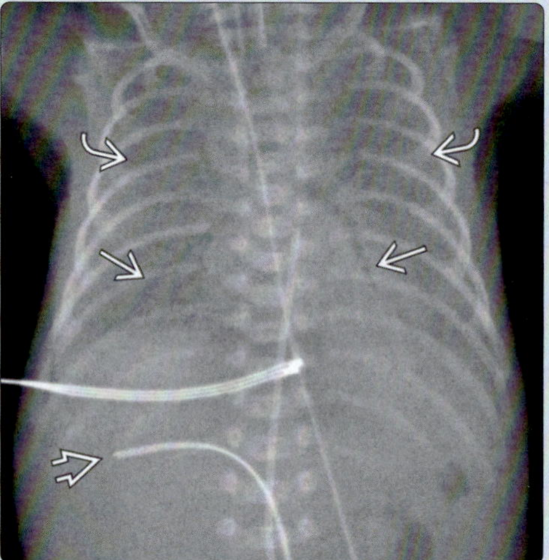

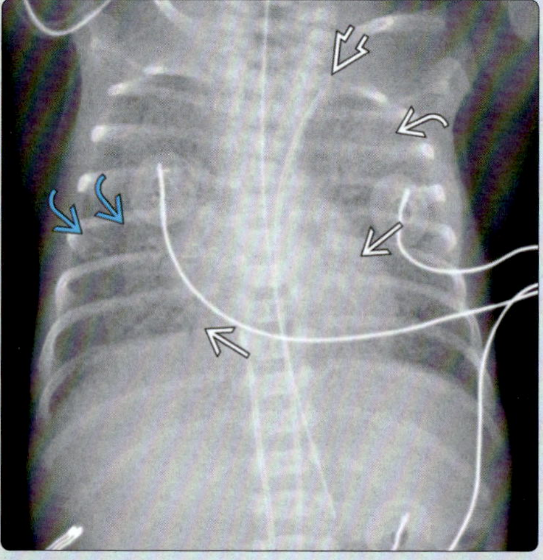

(Left) *Frontal radiograph in a premature newborn shows a more hazy pattern of SDD with patchy opacities in the central lungs ➡. The UAC is too high, at T4 ➡. As the 1st ribs in newborns commonly align with C7 ➡, malpositioned lines can be better recognized by counting from the lowest thoracic level (T12 ➡).* **(Right)** *Frontal radiograph in the same infant 4 weeks later shows evolving findings of chronic premature lung disease with diffuse, bilateral, heterogeneous, granular opacities & architectural distortion ➡.*

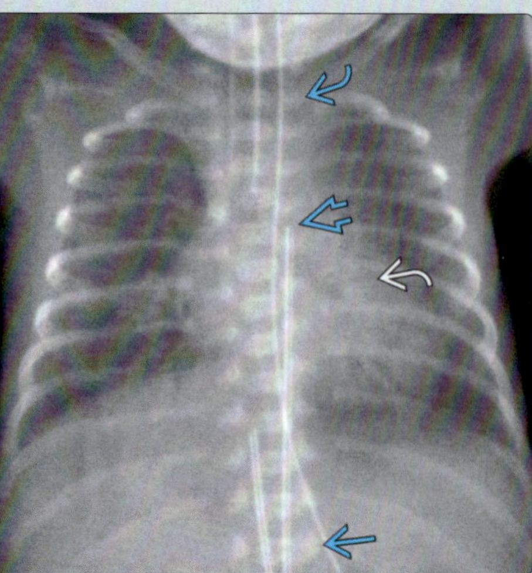

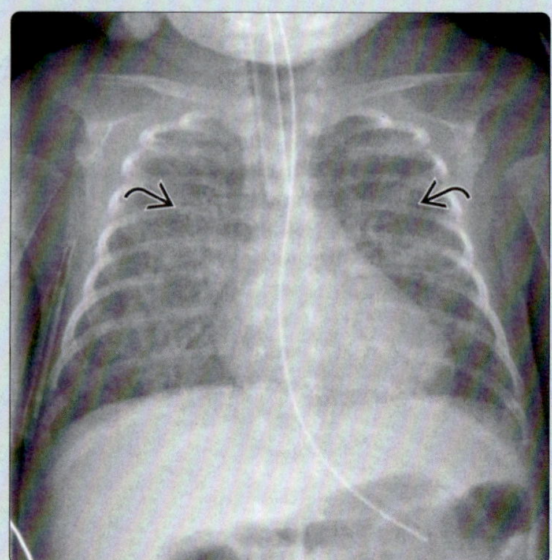

TERMINOLOGY

Abbreviations

- Surfactant deficiency disease (SDD)

Synonyms

- Lung disease of prematurity
- Respiratory distress syndrome
- Hyaline membrane disease (archaic)

Definitions

- Prematurity-related SDD (most common usage)
  - Surfactant deficiency in premature newborns
  - Lungs begin producing surfactant at ~ 24-weeks gestational age (GA); adequate amounts are usually present by 36-weeks GA
  - Lack of sufficient surfactant causes diffuse microatelectasis & abnormal pulmonary compliance
- Secondary SDD (less common usage)
  - Meconium aspiration or pneumonia can cause surfactant deactivation
  - Results are similar to those seen in prematurity, but usually heterogeneous & superimposed on other findings
- Primary SDD (least common usage)
  - Abnormal gene products adversely affect composition &/or function of surfactant
  - Often termed surfactant dysfunction disorders
  - Most well-known causes: Surfactant protein-B, surfactant protein-C, ABCA3, & TTF-1 deficiencies
  - Synergistically ↓ outcome with prematurity & 1° SDD

IMAGING

General Features

- Best diagnostic clue
  - Initial findings are low lung volumes & diffuse granular opacities
    - Air bronchograms & poor lung expansion
    - Cardiac size is normal
  - Subsequent imaging shows significant bilateral lung disease
    - Localized areas of atelectasis
    - Barotrauma leads to pneumothorax, pneumomediastinum, pulmonary interstitial emphysema (PIE)
    - Complications of patent ductus arteriosus (PDA)
    - Bronchopulmonary dysplasia (BPD) or chronic lung disease of premature infant
- Age
  - Premature infants < 32-weeks GA (or sometimes in term infants)

Radiographic Findings

- Radiography
  - Initial features
    - Low lung volumes secondary to microcollapse of innumerable alveoli
    - Diffuse granular opacities represent collapsed alveoli interspersed with open alveoli (microatelectasis)
    - Air bronchograms demonstrate patent bronchi in abnormal lung
    - Pleural effusions are very uncommon
    - Potential acute complications include PIE, pneumomediastinum, pneumothorax, superimposed pneumonia, pulmonary hemorrhage
  - Features after surfactant administration
    - Clearing of granular opacities + ↑ lung volumes
    - May have asymmetric or partial response
  - Findings after several days
    - Intubation & ventilatory support change imaging appearance
    - High incidence of PDA, which may cause pulmonary edema ("whiteout" of lungs with cardiomegaly)
  - BPD develops in 17-55% of premature infants
    - Chronic lung disease characterized by coarse interstitial opacities with focal areas of atelectasis & hyperinflation vs. diffuse hyperinflation

Ultrasonographic Findings

- Grayscale ultrasound
  - Range from scattered to completely confluent B lines
  - Severe SDD results in diffusely hyperechoic lung due to confluent B lines, a.k.a. "white lung"
  - Less severe findings include: (1) Predominance of nonconfluent B lines, or (2) mostly A lines & Z lines with scattered B lines
    - A lines: Series of horizontal lines caused by pleural reverb artifact in normally aerated lung
    - B lines: Comet-tail artifact extending from points on pleural surface into deep field, which is sign of subpleural interstitial edema &/or microatelectasis
    - Z lines: Broad-based, ill-defined, short vertical lines that do not erase A lines
  - Ultrasound is prone to missing pneumothorax, pneumomediastinum, interstitial emphysema

CT Findings

- HRCT
  - Not typically used to make diagnosis of SDD
  - Used to follow chronic lung disease

Other Modality Findings

- Premature infants have many associated diseases
  - Ultrasound: Used to detect intracranial hemorrhage
  - Abdominal radiographs/ultrasound: Used to detect necrotizing enterocolitis

DIFFERENTIAL DIAGNOSIS

Congenital Heart Disease

- Echocardiography is gold standard for diagnosis
- PDA is common in infants > 1,000 g
  - Usually closed with prostaglandin inhibitor
  - Transcatheter occlusion vs. surgery if contraindication is present

Group B Streptococcal Pneumonia

- Very common in neonates, especially premature infants
- Acquired during birth (25% of women are colonized)
- Bilateral granular opacities & low lung volumes
- Pleural effusion is common (67%): Only imaging finding that helps differentiate from SDD

Meconium Aspiration Syndrome

- Term infants
- Rope-like densities radiating from hila
- Usually have high lung volumes
- High incidence of barotrauma

Transient Tachypnea of Newborn

- Findings are similar to pulmonary edema but resolve by 24-48 hours
- Prominent interstitial markings with normal heart size
- Pleural effusions may be present

PATHOLOGY

General Features

- Etiology
  - Immature type II pneumocytes cannot produce surfactant
  - Surfactant normally coats alveoli & ↓ surface tension, allowing alveoli to stay open & improving lung compliance
  - Deficiency of surfactant results in alveolar atelectasis
  - ↓ lung compliance is associated with interstitial edema
  - Secondary surfactant insufficiency occurs due to
    - Meconium aspiration pneumonia
    - Pulmonary infections
    - Intrapartum asphyxia
- Genetics
  - Prematurity-related SDD
    - Mothers who deliver premature infants are more likely to have subsequent premature infants
    - Premature infants have many associated abnormalities
  - Uncommon primary (genetic) SDD
    - Several genetic mutations are associated with dysfunction of key surfactant components/regulators
      - Surfactant protein-B, surfactant protein-C, ABCA3, & TTF-1 deficiencies

CLINICAL ISSUES

Presentation

- Most common signs/symptoms
  - History of prematurity
  - Respiratory distress

Demographics

- Age
  - Disease of premature infants (< 36-weeks GA, < 2.5 kg)
    - 50% of premature infants will have SDD
  - Infants < 27-weeks GA have higher incidence of sequelae
- Ethnicity
  - All races are affected worldwide
- Epidemiology
  - Sex: M > F
  - Most common cause of death in live newborn infants
  - Occurs in 40,000 infants each year in USA
  - Common in all causes of premature labor & delivery
  - More common in infants of diabetic mothers

Natural History & Prognosis

- Acute complications & associations
  - Alveolar rupture with pneumothorax, pneumomediastinum, PIE
  - Sepsis & pulmonary infections
  - PDA with shunting & wide pulse pressure
  - Pulmonary hemorrhage
  - Apnea
  - Necrotizing enterocolitis ± perforation
  - Intracranial hemorrhage, periventricular leukomalacia
- Chronic complications
  - BPD is defined as ≥ 28-days oxygen (O_2) dependence in premature infant
    - Assessed by O_2 challenge at 36-weeks postmenstrual age
  - Retinopathy of prematurity
  - ↑ incidence of sudden death
  - Gastroesophageal reflux
  - Neurologic impairment in 10-70% (depending on GA)
  - Family psychodynamic complications
    - 2-year risk of parental divorce/separation is 2x higher compared to parents of term newborns
    - Maternal depression/anxiety rates are 5x higher than in mothers of term newborns

Treatment

- Prenatal prevention by treatment of mother
  - Efforts to delay delivery, allowing fetus to mature
  - Maternal steroid administration: Steroids will cross placenta & ↑ surfactant
- Surfactant administration
  - Can be given in nebulized or aerosol forms
  - Injected into trachea via endotracheal tube or via catheter inserted into trachea
  - May be given prophylactically or after symptoms develop
  - Improves oxygenation & ventilator setting requirements; ↓ rates of barotrauma, intracranial hemorrhage, BPD, & death
  - ↑ risk of PDA & pulmonary hemorrhage
- Mechanical ventilation with positive end-expiratory pressure
- High-frequency oscillatory ventilation
- Meet special needs of premature patient
  - Respiratory support
  - Monitor temperature, prevent hypothermia
  - Treat metabolic acidosis
  - IV access with fluid & caloric needs

SELECTED REFERENCES

1. Ma H et al: Diagnostic value of lung ultrasound for neonatal respiratory distress syndrome: a meta-analysis and systematic review. Med Ultrason. 22(3):325-33, 2020
2. Magnani JE et al: Persistent respiratory distress in the term neonate: genetic surfactant deficiency diseases. Curr Pediatr Rev. 16(1):17-25, 2020
3. Wu J et al: Lung ultrasound for the diagnosis of neonatal respiratory distress syndrome: a meta-analysis. Ultrasound Q. 36(2):102-10, 2020
4. Corsini I et al: Lung ultrasound for the differential diagnosis of respiratory distress in neonates. Neonatology. 115(1):77-84, 2019
5. Grimaldi C et al: Thoracic ultrasound accuracy for the investigation of initial neonatal respiratory distress. Arch Pediatr. 26(8):459-65, 2019
6. Somaschini M et al: Surfactant proteins gene variants in premature newborn infants with severe respiratory distress syndrome. J Perinatol. 38(4):337-44, 2018
7. Chen SW et al: Routine application of lung ultrasonography in the neonatal intensive care unit. Medicine (Baltimore). 96(2):e5826, 2017

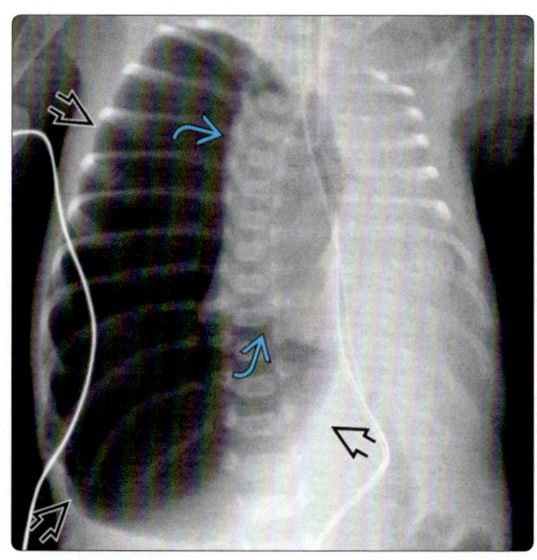

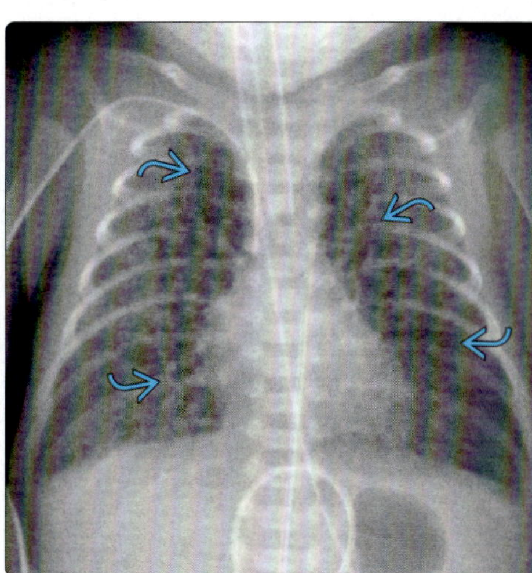

(Left) *Frontal radiograph in a 22-weeks-gestation newborn shows a massive right tension pneumothorax* ➡. *Note that despite the enormous degree of tension, the lung is not collapsed* ➡; *this is due to its lack of compliance from absent surfactant.* **(Right)** *Frontal radiograph in 23-weeks-gestation triplet shows irregular, branching lucencies in the central lungs from pulmonary interstitial emphysema* ➡. *The lack of surfactant makes premature newborns' lungs quite noncompliant & therefore more prone to barotrauma.*

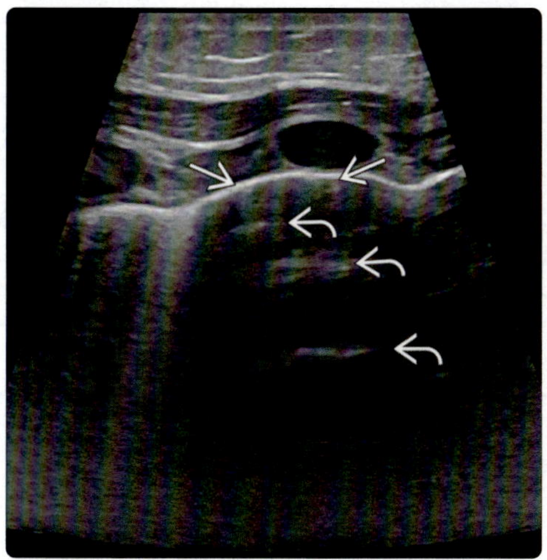

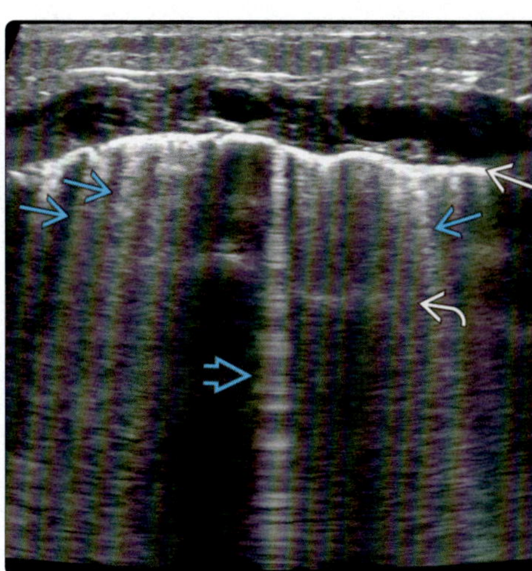

(Left) *Lung US in a near-term newborn show normal A lines, horizontal reflections from the pleural surface that extend across aerated lung* ➡. *The short, broad-based comet-tail artifacts are Z lines & are also normal* ➡; *note how they do not cross the A lines.* **(Right)** *Lung US in another premature infant, this one with mild SDD, shows scattered B lines extending from the pleural surface into the far field* ➡. *Note how closely the A line* ➡ *follows the same contour as the pleura* ➡. *Unlike Z lines, B lines* ➡ *cross A lines.*

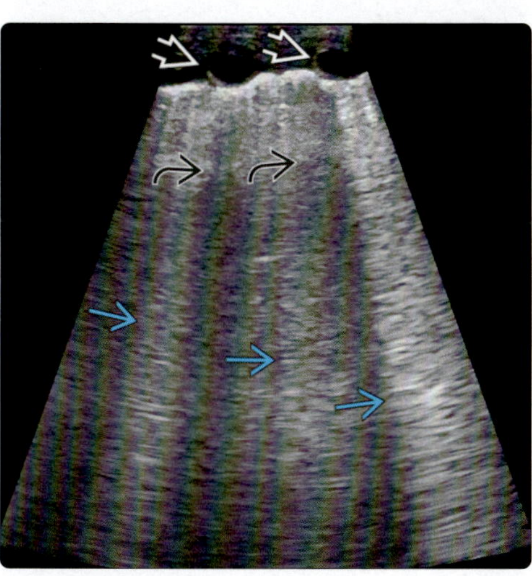

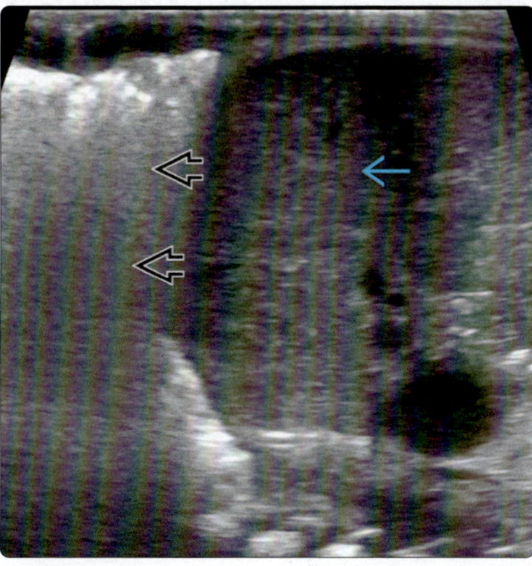

(Left) *Lung US in another premature newborn, this one with moderate SDD, shows more numerous B lines that have become almost completely confluent* ➡. *Sharp, hypoechoic shadows* ➡ *are caused from the child's ribs* ➡, **(Right)** *Longitudinal US of the lower chest in a premature newborn with severe SDD shows the appearance of lungs when B lines become completely confluent: "Total whiteout" of the lungs* ➡. *Compare the markedly echogenic lungs with the relatively hypoechoic liver* ➡.

Neonatal Pneumonia

KEY FACTS

TERMINOLOGY

- Pneumonia in first 28 days of life
- Congenital: Infection established during fetal life
- Early onset: First 7 days of life, typically within 48 hours
- Late onset: Presents in 2nd-4th weeks of life

IMAGING

- Radiographs
  - Low lung volumes & granular opacities similar to surfactant deficiency (but pleural effusion in up to 67%)
  - Confluent, patchy, reticular, &/or perihilar opacities
  - Complications: Pneumothorax, pneumomediastinum, pulmonary interstitial emphysema
- Ultrasound
  - Pleural line abnormality
  - Hepatization of parenchyma with air bronchograms
  - > 3 B lines (areas of white lung)
  - Disappearance of lung sliding
  - Pulsation of lung synchronized with heart

PATHOLOGY

- Bacterial pathogens are most common in early & late onset
- Group B *Streptococcus* (developed countries) & *Escherichia coli* (developing countries) are most common in early onset
- Transmission
  - Congenital: Ascending infection across chorioamniotic membrane or hematogenous transplacental route
  - Early onset: Perinatal exposure (intrauterine or during birth canal passage)
  - Late onset: Contaminated/colonized equipment or individuals

CLINICAL ISSUES

- Typical presentations: Respiratory distress, sepsis
- Prevention: Universal screening at 35- to 37-weeks gestation for maternal group B streptococcal (GBS) colonization
  - Intrapartum antibiotic prophylaxis with penicillin
- Treatment: Empiric antibiotics, antivirals, &/or antiparasitics

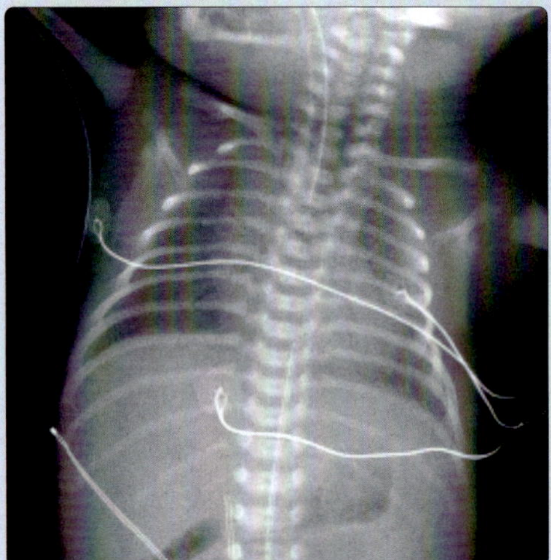
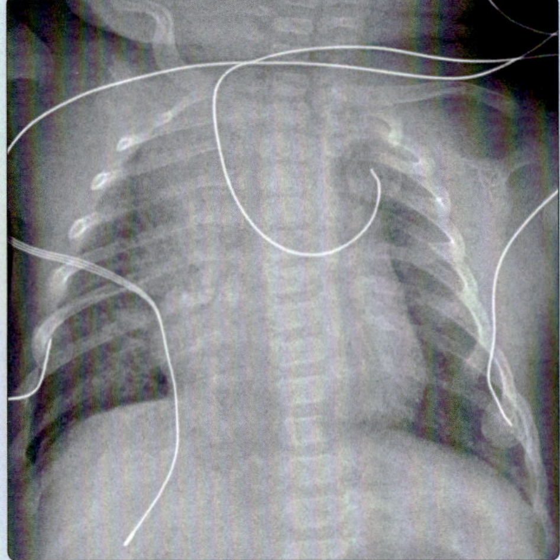

(Left) *AP radiograph of the chest in a neonate with group B streptococcal (GBS) pneumonia shows diffuse, bilateral, hazy opacities with low lung volumes. This appearance is very similar to patients with surfactant deficiency disease.* **(Right)** *AP view of the chest in a term neonate with pneumonia & a birth history of prolonged rupture of membranes, chorioamnionitis, & maternal GBS colonization shows diffuse hazy & reticular opacities bilaterally.*

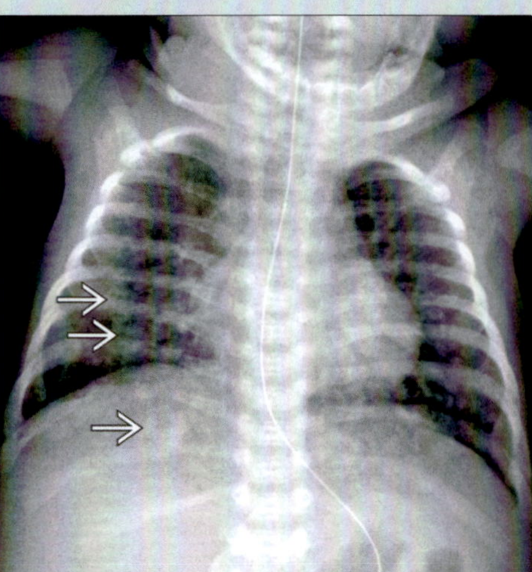
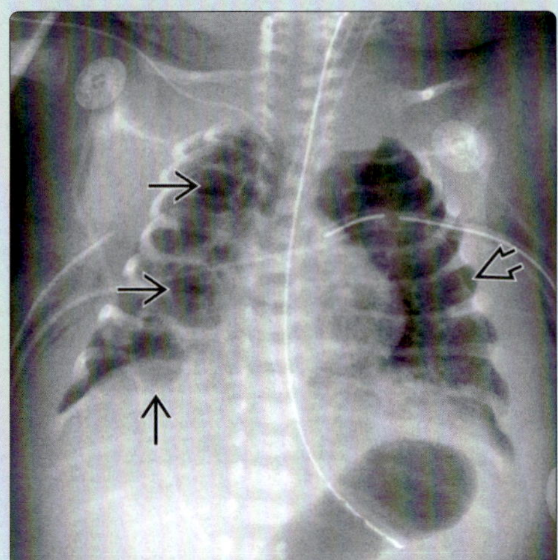

(Left) *AP radiograph in a neonate with tuberculosis shows multiple cavitating nodules in the right lung ➔ with generalized peribronchial thickening otherwise.* **(Right)** *AP radiograph in a patient with neonatal pneumonia shows a left pneumothorax ⇨ & multiple bilateral pneumatoceles →, complications that can be seen with neonatal pneumonia. Scattered hazy & coarse opacities are otherwise seen throughout.*

TERMINOLOGY

Definitions

- Pneumonia in first 28 days of life
- Congenital: Infection established during fetal life
- Early onset: First 48 hours of life; some define as < 7 days
- Late onset: 2nd-4th weeks of life

IMAGING

Radiographic Findings

- Group B *Streptococcus* (GBS)
  - Low lung volumes + granular opacities similar to surfactant deficiency
  - Pleural effusion in up to 67%
- Other appearances
  - Confluent/patchy alveolar or reticular opacities
  - Regions of hyperinflation
- Complications: Pneumothorax, pneumomediastinum, pulmonary interstitial emphysema

Ultrasonographic Findings

- Absent, irregular, disrupted, or coarse pleural line
- Parenchymal hepatization & air bronchograms (punctiform or linear hyperechogenicities)
- > 3 B lines or areas of white lung
- Disappearance of lung sliding
- Pulsation of lung synchronized with heart rate

Imaging Recommendations

- Best imaging tool
  - Chest radiography
  - ↑ use of ultrasound but role is still debated
    - Metaanalysis shows sensitivity of 96% & specificity of 93% for pneumonia in children of all ages
      - Similar findings are also seen in surfactant deficiency

DIFFERENTIAL DIAGNOSIS

Surfactant Deficiency Disease

- Premature infants < 32-weeks gestation
- Mimics GBS infection but no effusion

Congenital Pulmonary Airway Malformation

- Mixed cystic &/or solid mass

Meconium Aspiration Syndrome

- History of meconium staining with respiratory distress

Transient Tachypnea of Newborn

- Occurs in term infants delivered by C-section
- Interstitial pattern with effusions
- Resolves within 48 hours

Congenital Heart Disease

- Abnormal cardiac silhouette & vascularity ± edema
- Echocardiography for diagnosis

PATHOLOGY

General Features

- Etiology
  - GBS is most common cause of early-onset neonatal pneumonia/sepsis in developed countries
    - β-hemolysin (pore-forming cytolysin) → ↑ epithelial cell permeability → alveolar edema & hemorrhage
    - β-hemolysin is inactivated by surfactant → premature infants at ↑ risk
  - *Escherichia coli* is most common cause of early-onset neonatal pneumonia in developing countries
  - Numerous other bacterial, viral, & fungal etiologies

CLINICAL ISSUES

Presentation

- Most common signs/symptoms
  - Respiratory distress: Rapid/noisy/difficult breathing, respiratory rate > 60, chest retractions, cough, grunting
  - Sepsis: Lethargy, poor feeding, poor reflexes, temperature instability, abdominal distention
  - Abnormal WBC with > 20% bands, ↑ CRP, ↑ ESR
  - Positive cultures

Demographics

- Epidemiology
  - Congenital-onset transmission: Ascending infection across chorioamniotic membranes or hematogenous transplacental route
  - Early-onset transmission: Perinatal exposure (intrauterine or during birth canal passage)
  - Late-onset transmission: Contaminated/colonized equipment or individuals
  - GBS is leading infectious cause of infant morbidity & mortality in USA (0.34-0.37 cases/1,000 live births)

Natural History & Prognosis

- Found in up to 38% of deaths occurring in first 48 hours
- GBS case fatality rate is up to 30% if ≤ 33-weeks gestation, 2-3% if full term
- Can be associated with intraventricular hemorrhage, neurological damage, & developmental delay

Treatment

- GBS screening at 35- to 37-weeks gestation; intrapartum antibiotic prophylaxis with penicillin if positive
- Neonatal antibiotic regimen otherwise depends on pathogen, early vs. late onset, antimicrobial susceptibility

DIAGNOSTIC CHECKLIST

Image Interpretation Pearls

- Consider if effusion accompanies radiographic findings otherwise suggestive of surfactant deficiency

SELECTED REFERENCES

1. Li W et al: Quantitative assessment of COVID-19 pneumonia in neonates using lung ultrasound score. Pediatr Pulmonol. 56(6):1419-26, 2021
2. Öktem A et al: Efficiency of lung ultrasonography in the diagnosis and follow-up of viral pneumonia in newborn. Am J Perinatol. ePub, 2021
3. Liszewski MC et al: Neonatal lung disorders: pattern recognition approach to diagnosis. AJR Am J Roentgenol. 210(5):964-75, 2018
4. Liszewski MC et al: Respiratory distress in neonates: underlying causes and current imaging assessment. Radiol Clin North Am. 55(4):629-44, 2017
5. Pereda MA et al: Lung ultrasound for the diagnosis of pneumonia in children: a meta-analysis. Pediatrics. 135(4):714-22, 2015
6. Nissen MD: Congenital and neonatal pneumonia. Paediatr Respir Rev. 8(3):195-203, 2007

Meconium Aspiration Syndrome

KEY FACTS

TERMINOLOGY

- Meconium aspiration syndrome (MAS): Respiratory distress after aspiration of meconium-stained amniotic fluid (MSAF)
  - Causes ↓ lung compliance & hypoxia ± pulmonary hypertension (HTN) & air leak syndrome

IMAGING

- Coarse, rope-like, linear perihilar opacities
- Asymmetric hyperinflation
- Patchy, hazy opacities of atelectasis & pneumonitis
- ± pleural effusion
- ± air leak: Pneumomediastinum, pneumothorax, pulmonary interstitial emphysema

TOP DIFFERENTIAL DIAGNOSES

- Congenital heart disease, neonatal pneumonia, transient tachypnea of newborn, surfactant deficiency disease, pulmonary hypoplasia

PATHOLOGY

- Aspirated meconium causes injury by several mechanisms
  - Mechanical obstruction of small airways → air-trapping, air leak complications
  - Chemical pneumonitis of airways & parenchyma
  - Surfactant inactivation & ↓ production
  - Pulmonary vasoconstriction → persistent pulmonary HTN

CLINICAL ISSUES

- Disease of term & postterm neonates
- Meconium staining of amniotic fluid occurs in infants with in utero or intrapartum hypoxia or stress
  - 2-10% of patients with MSAF develop MAS
- ECMO for severe pulmonary HTN
- Mortality is up to 4%; chronic lung disease in 2.5%

(Left) *Graphic demonstrates asymmetric areas of hyperinflation & atelectasis as well as rope-like perihilar densities of aspirated meconium & inflamed airways.* **(Right)** *AP chest radiograph in a 41-weeks-gestation newborn with meconium staining of amniotic fluid & respiratory distress shows coarse, reticular, rope-like perihilar opacities ➡, typical of meconium aspiration. There are also patchy, asymmetric regions of ↑ hazy lung opacity bilaterally.*

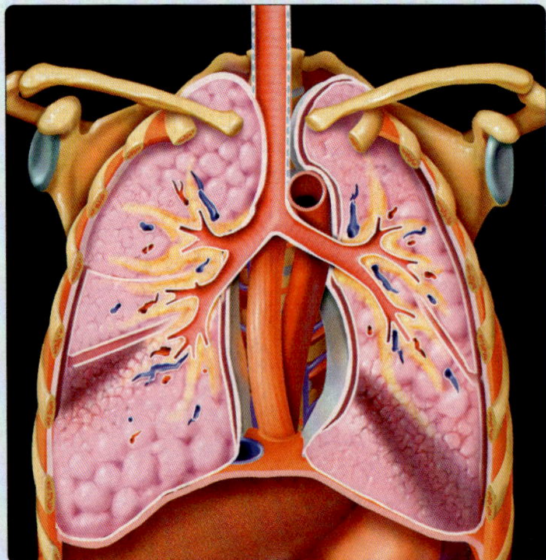

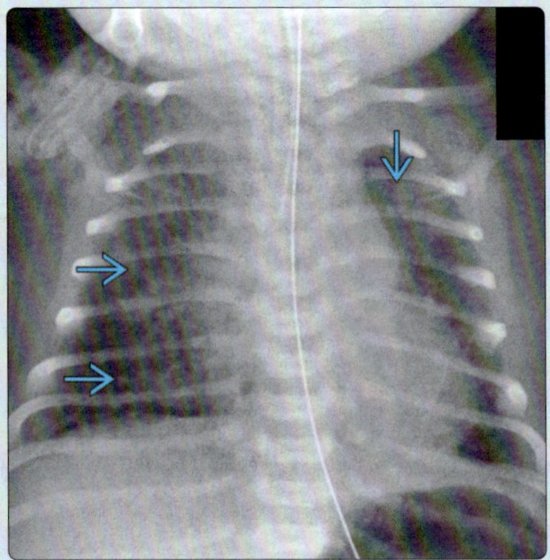

(Left) *AP chest radiograph in a term newborn with meconium aspiration shows linear perihilar opacities ➡. Small pleural effusions are present ➡.* **(Right)** *AP chest radiograph obtained 8 hours later in the same patient shows a new right pneumothorax ➡. Depression of the hemidiaphragm ➡ & leftward mediastinal shift indicate a tension pneumothorax. Pneumothorax is seen as a complication in 10-40% of patients with meconium aspiration syndrome.*

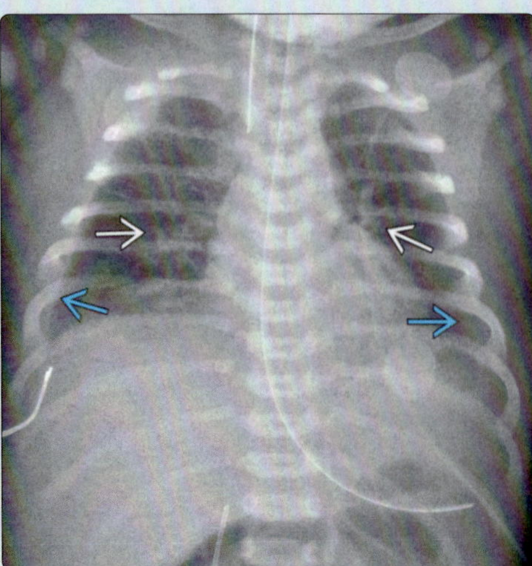

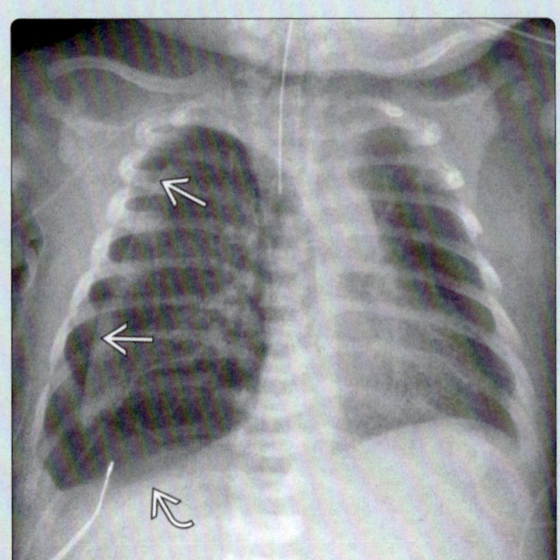

TERMINOLOGY

Definitions

- Meconium aspiration syndrome (MAS): Respiratory distress due to aspiration of meconium-stained amniotic fluid (MSAF)

IMAGING

General Features

- Best diagnostic clue
  - Coarse, rope-like perihilar opacities bilaterally + hyperinflation in term infant
  - Usually with history of MSAF

Radiographic Findings

- Linear, nodular, rope-like opacities radiating from hila
- Hyperinflated lungs, often asymmetric
- Patchy, asymmetric opacities of atelectasis & pneumonitis
- ± air leak: Pneumothorax, pneumomediastinum, pulmonary interstitial emphysema (PIE)
- ± pleural effusion

Ultrasonographic Findings

- Lung ultrasound is increasingly used at bedside of ill children: Point of care ultrasound (POCUS)
  - Findings relate to artifacts from interaction of sound with air & interstitial fluid
  - Can help predict need for mechanical ventilation
- MAS findings include: Sonographic B lines (interstitium), consolidation, bronchograms, abnormal pleural line, loss of sonographic A lines, atelectasis, airway inflammation, pleural effusion
  - Uneven & changing distribution over clinical course

DIFFERENTIAL DIAGNOSIS

Congenital Heart Disease

- Clues to underlying congenital heart disease include
  - Abnormal cardiac &/or mediastinal silhouette
  - ↑ or ↓ pulmonary vascular flow

Neonatal Pneumonia

- Patchy, asymmetric perihilar densities & hyperinflation
- Common to see pleural effusion
- Usually no history of meconium aspiration

Transient Tachypnea of Newborn

- Delayed clearance of fetal pulmonary fluid (often in cesarean section)
- ± pleural effusion or fissural thickening
- Benign, self-limited course over 24-72 hours

Surfactant Deficiency Disease

- Diffuse granular pulmonary opacities in premature infant with low lung volumes
- Pleural effusions are uncommon

Pulmonary Hypoplasia

- Pneumothoraces are common
- Bell-shaped thorax in severe cases

PATHOLOGY

General Features

- Etiology
  - Fetal distress near or beyond term → passage of meconium into amniotic fluid, which may enter lungs
- Aspirated meconium causes injury by several mechanisms
  - Mechanical obstruction of small airways → air-trapping, air leak complications
  - Chemical pneumonitis of airways & parenchyma
  - Surfactant inactivation & ↓ production
  - Pulmonary vasoconstriction leading to pulmonary hypertension (HTN)
    - Cause of pulmonary HTN is multifactorial
    - Leading cause of death in MAS

CLINICAL ISSUES

Presentation

- Most common signs/symptoms
  - Meconium staining of amniotic fluid at birth
  - Respiratory distress

Demographics

- Epidemiology
  - 0.1-1.8% of live births in resource-rich countries
  - Term or postterm infants with in utero or intrapartum hypoxia or stress
    - MSAF in up to 38% at 41 weeks; rare in preterm
  - 2-10% with MSAF develop MAS

Natural History & Prognosis

- Complications
  - Meconium injury & hypoxia
    - Respiratory support with supplemental oxygen ± mechanical ventilation, surfactant administration
  - Air leak complications in 10-40%
  - Severe pulmonary HTN in 10%
    - May be treated with inhaled nitrous oxide &/or ECMO
  - Anoxic brain injury, may be multifactorial with perinatal stress
- Outcomes have greatly improved in recent decades
  - Most recover within 72-96 hours
  - Mortality up to 4%, recently reported at 1.2%

DIAGNOSTIC CHECKLIST

Image Interpretation Pearls

- Relevant history is essential for accurate interpretation of all neonatal chest disease, particularly MAS
  - Term or postterm infant
  - MSAF at delivery

SELECTED REFERENCES

1. Dell'Orto V et al: Ultrasound-guided lung lavage for life-threatening bronchial obstruction due to meconium plug. J Clin Ultrasound. 49(4):405-7, 2021
2. Liszewski MC et al: Neonatal lung disorders: pattern recognition approach to diagnosis. AJR Am J Roentgenol. 210(5):964-75, 2018
3. Rawat M et al: Approach to infants born through meconium stained amniotic fluid: evolution based on evidence? Am J Perinatol. 35(9):815-22, 2018
4. Liu J et al: Lung ultrasonography to diagnose meconium aspiration syndrome of the newborn. J Int Med Res. 44(6):1534-42, 2016

Transient Tachypnea of Newborn

KEY FACTS

TERMINOLOGY

- Transient tachypnea of newborn (TTN), a.k.a. wet lung disease, retained fetal fluid
- Caused by delayed evacuation of fetal lung fluid that creates engorgement of pulmonary lymphatics & capillaries
- Classically seen after cesarean section due to lack of normal thoracic compression during vaginal delivery

IMAGING

- Patients are usually not intubated
- Radiograph is historically considered gold standard
  - Findings similar to pulmonary edema
  - Diffuse, bilateral, & often symmetric ↑ lung markings ± pleural effusion
- US is becoming more widely used
  - Scattered B lines separated by A lines
  - Double lung point sign
- Lungs become normal within 24-48 hours
- Diagnosis of exclusion

TOP DIFFERENTIAL DIAGNOSES

- Surfactant deficiency
  - Usually occurs in premature newborns
  - Radiograph: Low lung volumes with diffuse, hazy, or granular opacity throughout both lungs
  - US: Lungs are diffusely echogenic (confluent B lines), no preserved normal areas (lacks A lines)
- Congenital heart disease
  - Pulmonary edema from obstructed total anomalous pulmonary venous return or left-sided obstruction
  - Echocardiogram is gold standard for making diagnosis
- Meconium aspiration syndrome
  - Occurs in term infants (like TTN)
  - Rope-like perihilar markings, barotrauma

CLINICAL ISSUES

- Presents shortly after birth: Tachypnea, grunting, nasal flaring, retractions, occasional cyanosis
- Infants usually improve rapidly & are normal on follow-up

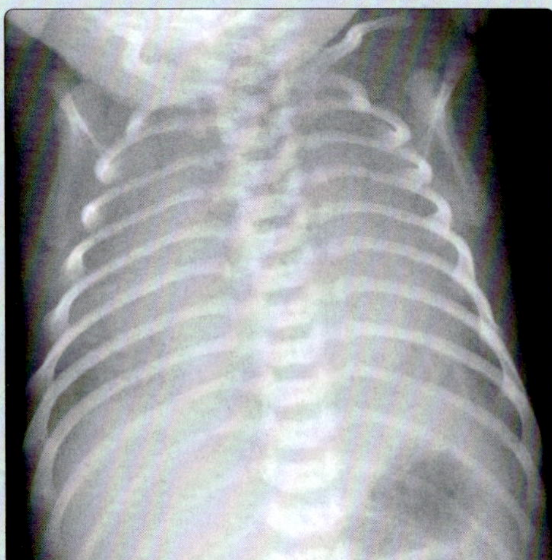

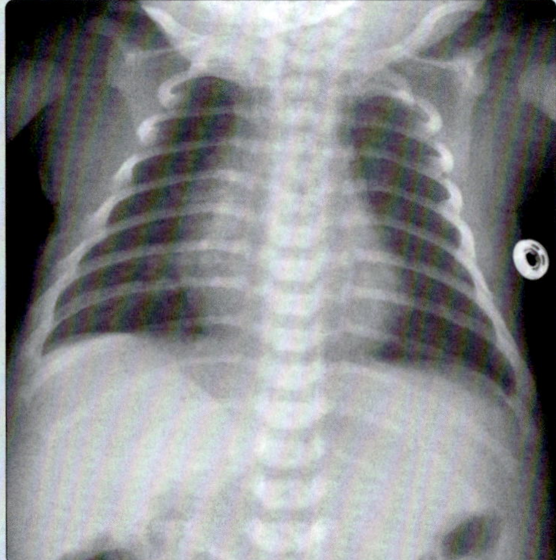

(Left) *AP radiograph of the chest in a full-term infant with tachypnea demonstrates diffuse, bilateral, hazy opacities. The findings & symptoms resolved over the 1st few days of life, & the diagnosis of transient tachypnea of the newborn (TTN) was made.* **(Right)** *Follow-up AP radiograph of the chest shows interval clearing of the previously seen diffuse opacification of the lungs. TTN is a diagnosis of exclusion & cannot be confidently diagnosed radiographically unless the findings resolve.*

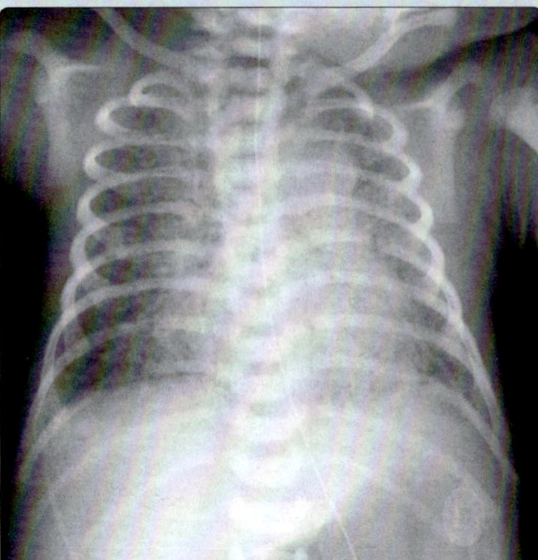

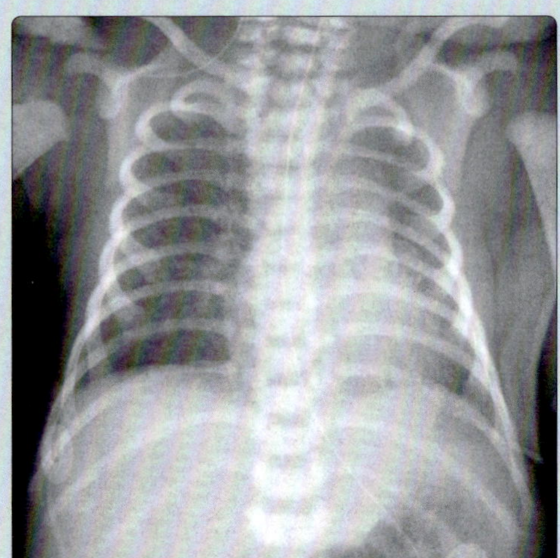

(Left) *AP radiograph of the chest in a full-term infant with tachypnea shows diffuse nodular opacities throughout the lungs. No pneumothorax or pleural effusion is seen.* **(Right)** *AP radiograph of the chest in the same patient the following day shows partial clearance of the previously seen diffuse nodular opacities, consistent with TTN.*

Transient Tachypnea of Newborn

TERMINOLOGY

Abbreviations

- Transient tachypnea of newborn (TTN)

Definitions

- TTN occurs when evacuation of fetal lung fluid is delayed, causing engorgement of pulmonary lymphatics & capillaries
  - Usually occurs in term infants
  - More common (3x) in those born by cesarean section
    - Normal thoracic compression that occurs during vaginal delivery is bypassed by cesarean section

IMAGING

General Features

- Best diagnostic clue
  - Interstitial edema on chest radiographs
  - History of cesarean section or maternal asthma
  - No signs of infection

Radiographic Findings

- Chest radiographs in first 24-48 hours of life
  - Patients are usually not intubated
  - No/minimal cardiomegaly
  - Normal to ↑ lung volumes
  - Findings are similar to pulmonary edema
    - Prominent interstitial markings
    - ± pleural effusion
      - Fluid in fissures
  - Lungs become normal within 24-48 hours
  - No consolidation or other focal lung lesion

Ultrasonographic Findings

- Scattered B lines separated by A lines
  - A lines: Series of lines horizontal to pleura, caused by reverberation artifact in normally aerated lung
  - B lines: Comet-tail artifact extending from points on pleural surface (sign of subpleural interstitial edema)
- Double point lung sign
  - In TTN, upper lungs are often normal while lower lungs reveal numerous compact or confluent B lines
  - On lung US, point where these findings are juxtaposed is termed "double lung point"
  - High sensitivity & specificity but controversial

DIFFERENTIAL DIAGNOSIS

Surfactant Deficiency

- Usually occurs in premature newborns
- Low lung volumes with diffuse, hazy, or granular opacity throughout both lungs
- US: Lungs are diffusely echogenic (confluent B lines), no preserved normal areas (lacks A lines)

Congenital Heart Disease

- Pulmonary edema from obstructed total anomalous pulmonary venous return or left-sided obstructive lesions can mimic TTN
- Echocardiogram is gold standard for making diagnosis

Meconium Aspiration Syndrome

- Occurs in term infants (similar to TTN)
- Rope-like perihilar markings
- Pneumothorax & pneumomediastinum are common

Congenital Lymphangiectasia

- Very rare, presents with persistent tachypnea
- Persistent interstitial pattern ± pleural effusions

Intrathoracic Causes of Tachypnea

- Neonatal pneumonia
- Neonatal chest masses

PATHOLOGY

General Features

- Etiology
  - During fetal life, lungs are expanded with ultrafiltrate of fetal fluid
  - During & after birth, lung fluid is replaced with air
    - Chest is normally compressed & fluid expelled during vaginal delivery: Thoracic squeeze
    - Pulmonary capillaries & lymphatics remove remaining fluid
  - Most infants with TTN are healthy & normal within 48 hours
- Associated abnormalities
  - Usually healthy infants with no other anomalies

Gross Pathologic & Surgical Features

- Not associated with any mortality or morbidity

CLINICAL ISSUES

Presentation

- Most common signs/symptoms
  - Mild to moderate respiratory distress
  - Frequent history of cesarean section delivery
  - Typically do not require intubation

Demographics

- Epidemiology
  - More common in cesarean section infants
  - High association with maternal asthma

Natural History & Prognosis

- Mild/moderate respiratory distress within 6 hours of birth
- Relatively benign clinical course
- Radiographic resolution usually by 24-48 hours

Treatment

- Exclude other causes of tachypnea in term newborn
- Normal support of infant

SELECTED REFERENCES

1. Alhassen Z et al: Recent advances in pathophysiology and management of transient tachypnea of newborn. J Perinatol. 41(1):6-16, 2021
2. Li CS et al: Prospective investigation of serial ultrasound for transient tachypnea of the newborn. Pediatr Neonatol. 62(1):64-9, 2021
3. Singh Y et al: International evidence-based guidelines on point of care ultrasound (POCUS) for critically ill neonates and children issued by the POCUS Working Group of the European Society of Paediatric and Neonatal Intensive Care (ESPNIC). Crit Care. 24(1):65, 2020

Pulmonary Interstitial Emphysema

KEY FACTS

TERMINOLOGY

- Pulmonary interstitial emphysema (PIE): Air within pulmonary interstitium & lymphatics
- Neonatal air leak syndrome: Air escapes tracheobronchial tree to spaces where it is not normally found
- Persistent PIE: Development of persistent, mass-like interstitial cysts

IMAGING

- Best clue: New small, "bubbly," cystic or linear lucencies within lung of intubated premature infant
- Ranges from single lobe to widespread involvement
- Precursor to pneumothorax or pneumomediastinum
- Persistent PIE may have mass-like cystic/multicystic lesion
  - CT shows pulmonary vessels as linear (dash) or round (dot) densities within gas collections

TOP DIFFERENTIAL DIAGNOSES

- Surfactant deficiency disease
- Air bronchograms in diffuse lung disease
- Chronic lung disease of prematurity
- Lucent or cystic congenital lung lesions
- Pleuropulmonary blastoma

CLINICAL ISSUES

- Usually secondary to barotrauma & volutrauma of positive-pressure mechanical ventilation in setting of prematurity & surfactant deficiency disease (SDD)
  - Not always on mechanical ventilation
  - May rarely be seen in older patients with underlying lung disease or after Valsalva
- Often asymptomatic, detected on NICU radiographs
- Usually occurs during first 10 days of life
- Usually transient with supportive therapy & ventilatory adjustments
  - ↓ mean airway pressure, use high-frequency ventilation

(Left) *Coronal graphic depicts round & linear foci of gas ➡ in the right lung parenchyma secondary to air escaping into the pulmonary interstitium.* **(Right)** *AP chest radiograph in an intubated 2-day-old, former 31-weeks-premature infant with surfactant deficiency disease (SDD) shows typical diffuse granular pulmonary opacities. There are mild, scattered, linear & "bubbly" lucencies of pulmonary interstitial emphysema (PIE) ➡ in the right lung.*

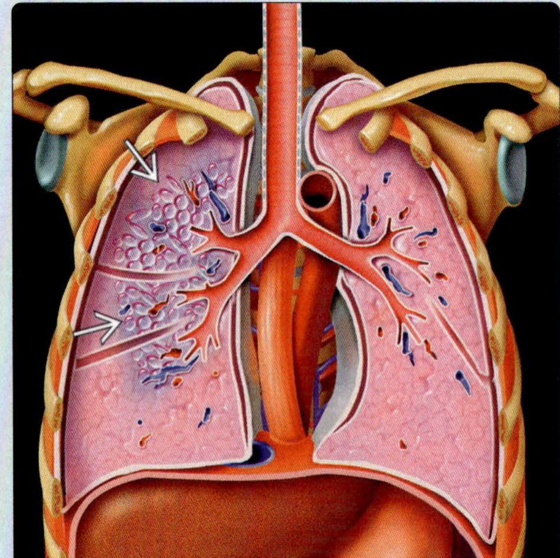

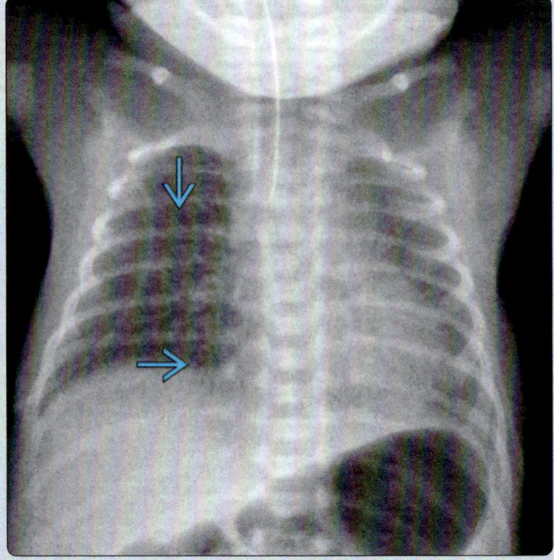

(Left) *AP chest radiograph 24 hours later in the same patient shows more extensive "bubbly" & linear lucencies throughout the right lung ➡, typical of PIE. A large, inferomedial gas collection has also developed ➡, shifting the heart leftward.* **(Right)** *Cross-table lateral radiograph in the same patient shows localized infraazygous posterior pneumomediastinum ➡. Lucencies from the right lung PIE ➡ are superimposed on the collection. Note that there is no free gas in the nondependent chest ➡ to suggest a pneumothorax.*

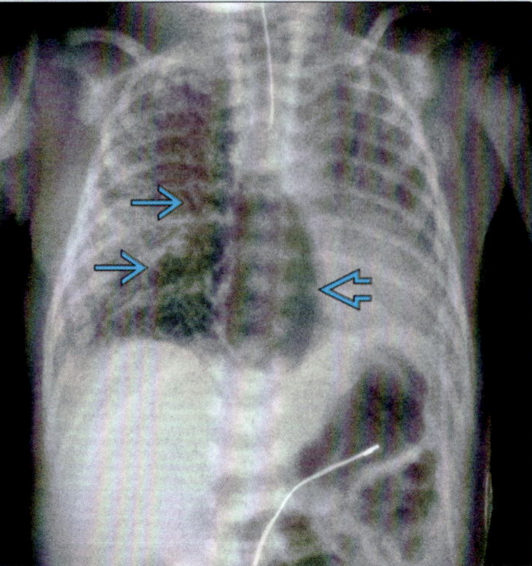

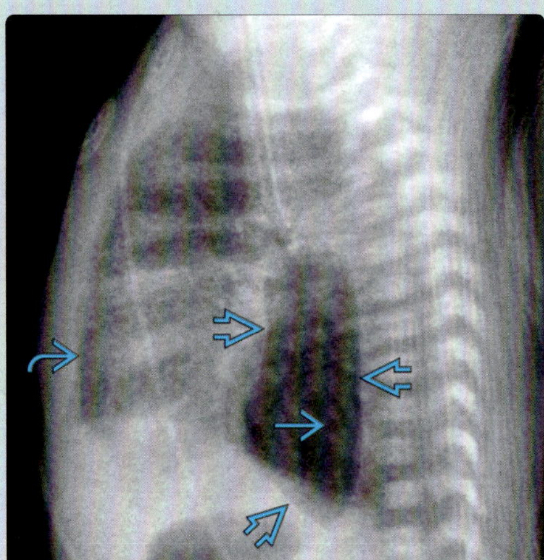

TERMINOLOGY

Abbreviations

- Pulmonary interstitial emphysema (PIE)

Definitions

- PIE: Air within pulmonary interstitium & lymphatics
- Persistent PIE: Development of persistent, mass-like interstitial cysts
- Neonatal air leak syndrome: Air escapes from tracheobronchial tree into spaces where it is not normally found
  - PIE, pneumothorax, pneumomediastinum, pneumopericardium, subcutaneous emphysema; rarely pneumoperitoneum

IMAGING

General Features

- Best diagnostic clue
  - New, "bubbly," cystic or linear lucencies within lung of intubated premature infant
- Location
  - Extent of involvement may range from single lobe to widespread bilateral PIE
- Size
  - Ranges from small interstitial lucencies to large focal/multifocal cysts

Radiographic Findings

- Radiography
  - "Bubbly," cystic or linear lucencies in lung parenchyma
    - Lucencies are typically uniform in size
    - Often radiate from hilum
  - Usually occurs on background of noncompliant lung parenchyma
    - Most commonly surfactant deficiency disease (SDD) in preterm newborn
  - Typically transient: May last days to weeks
    - Precursor to other complications: Pneumothorax, pneumomediastinum
  - Persistent PIE
    - Variable involvement from single lobe to bilateral multilobar
      - Most commonly affects left upper lobe
    - May develop mass-like cystic/multicystic lesions
      - May compress other thoracic structures to cause worsening respiratory distress

CT Findings

- Not routinely obtained to evaluate PIE
- May be utilized to evaluate persistent PIE & differentiate it from other lucent neonatal lung masses
  - Round or linear lucencies in lung interstitium
  - Lucencies do not follow normal bronchial anatomy & may widen peripherally (unlike air bronchograms)
  - With persistent PIE, pulmonary vascular branches are seen as linear (dash) or round (dot) soft tissue densities within prominent gas collections
    - Characteristic dot-dash pattern in 82% of patients with persistent PIE
    - Not seen in congenital cystic lung lesions

Ultrasonographic Findings

- ↑ use of beside ultrasound in neonatal lung disease; may detect foci of PIE

Imaging Recommendations

- Best imaging tool
  - Frontal radiograph of chest

DIFFERENTIAL DIAGNOSIS

Surfactant Deficiency Disease

- Often underlies PIE
- Uneven distribution of administered exogenous surfactant may result in heterogeneous aeration amidst granular & hazy opacities
  - Pattern of alternating distended & collapsed acini may mimic PIE

Air Bronchograms in Diffuse Lung Disease

- May be seen with pulmonary edema, hemorrhage, neonatal infections, surfactant dysfunction/deficiency, other diseases
- Follow normal bronchial course

Chronic Lung Disease of Prematurity

- "Bubbly" lucencies of developing bronchopulmonary dysplasia (BPD) can appear similar to PIE
  - On CT, vessels are not engulfed by interstitial air (unlike PIE)
- BPD is seen at > 1 month of age
- Timing of onset: PIE is abrupt, BPD is gradual

Congenital Lobar Overinflation

- Found in perinatal period; often worsens after birth
- Typically first seen as lucent neonatal lung lesion
  - May present initially as perinatal lobar opacity with gradual clearing & ↑ lobar expansion
  - Lobar architecture is preserved but uniformly splayed without discrete cysts

Congenital Pulmonary Airway Malformation

- Lung mass of cystic lucencies of varying size
- Transition from fluid-filled to air-filled mass after birth

Pleuropulmonary Blastoma

- Rare tumor of young children (but uncommon in perinatal period)
- Typically cystic in neonatal period

Meconium Aspiration

- Linear, nodular, rope-like opacities radiating from hila
- Heterogeneous lucencies related to air-trapping
- May develop air-leak complications, including PIE

PATHOLOGY

General Features

- ↑ alveolar pressure & overdistention (barotrauma + volutrauma) → disruption of alveolar basement membrane → air enters pulmonary interstitium
- Preterm infants have more abundant interstitial perivascular connective tissue, which limits further dissection relative to older infants & children

- Trapping within this space gives characteristic linear & "bubbly" lucencies of PIE
- Compresses airways & alveoli, impairing gas exchange, compliance, & possibly blood flow
- Air may further dissect, leading to pneumothorax or pneumomediastinum
- Cysts may enlarge due to ball-valve mechanism

Microscopic Features

- Air-distended lymphatics & air along vascular sheaths
  - Seen along bronchovascular bundles as well as interlobular septa & visceral pleura
- Persistent PIE
  - Fibrotic cyst walls lined by multinucleated giant cells in reaction to prolonged air trapping

CLINICAL ISSUES

Presentation

- Most common signs/symptoms
  - Often asymptomatic & detected incidentally on routine NICU radiographs
- Other signs/symptoms
  - Difficulty with ventilation secondary to pneumothorax
  - Impaired gas exchange

Demographics

- Age
  - Premature infants, most commonly occurring in first 10 days of life
  - Rarely occurs in
    - Neonates with other lung diseases (pulmonary hypoplasia, meconium aspiration, sepsis)
    - Older children due to
      - Underlying lung disease
      - Valsalva with alveolar rupture
- Sex
  - No significant sex difference
- Ethnicity
  - No significant race predilection
- Epidemiology
  - 2-3% of NICU patients
  - 20-30% of premature neonates with SDD
    - Incidence ↓ with use of surfactant in appropriate population
  - Patients on positive-pressure mechanical ventilation are most at risk
    - Rarely develops in patients not on ventilator

Natural History & Prognosis

- Usually transient with supportive therapy & careful management of ventilatory support
- Rarely develops into persistent PIE
- Complications: Pneumothorax, pneumomediastinum, pneumopericardium, ↓ pulmonary compliance, air embolus
- ↑ rates of intraventricular hemorrhage

Treatment

- Adjustments in mechanical ventilation
  - Lower mean airway pressures
  - ↑ FiO_2 to allow for dec ↓ airway pressures
  - Switch from conventional to high-frequency ventilation
- ↑ frequency of clinical & radiographic monitoring for complications, such as pneumothorax
- Heliox & steroids may be useful, evidence lacking
- Additional management options
  - Selective intubation of uninvolved lung
  - Temporary balloon blockage of main bronchus of affected side
  - Decubitus positioning with affected side down
  - Surgical resection of large cystic foci is reserved for unmanageable respiratory distress
    - ~ 53% of patients with persistent PIE in one series

DIAGNOSTIC CHECKLIST

Image Interpretation Pearls

- Age of patient & rapidity of development help differentiate PIE from BPD

Reporting Tips

- Early detection & ventilatory adjustments may help avoid complications

SELECTED REFERENCES

1. Corsini I et al: Lung ultrasound in the neonatal intensive care unit: review of the literature and future perspectives. Pediatr Pulmonol. 55(7):1550-62, 2020
2. Rocha G: Pulmonary pneumatoceles in neonates. Pediatr Pulmonol. 55(10):2532-41, 2020
3. Williams E et al: Predictors of outcome of prematurely born infants with pulmonary interstitial emphysema. Acta Paediatr. 108(1):106-11, 2019
4. Kim HR et al: Presence of subpleural pulmonary interstitial emphysema as an indication of single or multiple alveolar ruptures on CT in patients with spontaneous pneumomediastinum. Acta Radiol. 57(12):1483-9, 2016
5. Mahapatra S et al: Steroid-induced resolution of refractory pulmonary interstitial emphysema. J Matern Fetal Neonatal Med. 1-4, 2016
6. Toledo Del Castillo B et al: Diffuse persistent pulmonary interstitial emphysema secondary to mechanical ventilation in bronchiolitis. BMC Pulm Med. 16(1):139, 2016
7. Squires KA et al: High-frequency oscillatory ventilation with low oscillatory frequency in pulmonary interstitial emphysema. Neonatology. 104(4):243-9, 2013
8. Jeng MJ et al: Neonatal air leak syndrome and the role of high-frequency ventilation in its prevention. J Chin Med Assoc. 75(11):551-9, 2012
9. Srinivasan R et al: Persistent pulmonary interstitial emphysema presenting as solitary lung cyst in a preterm infant. BMJ Case Rep, 2012
10. Joseph LJ et al: Unilateral lung intubation for pulmonary air leak syndrome in neonates: a case series and a review of the literature. Am J Perinatol. 28(2):151-6, 2011
11. Gonçalves CA et al: Pulmonary lobar interstitial emphysema. Fetal Pediatr Pathol. 28(4):192-7, 2009
12. Phatak RS et al: Heliox with inhaled nitric oxide: a novel strategy for severe localized interstitial pulmonary emphysema in preterm neonatal ventilation. Respir Care. 53(12):1731-8, 2008
13. Agrons GA et al: From the archives of the AFIP: lung disease in premature neonates: radiologic-pathologic correlation. Radiographics. 25(4):1047-73, 2005
14. Donnelly LF et al: CT findings and temporal course of persistent pulmonary interstitial emphysema in neonates: a multiinstitutional study. AJR Am J Roentgenol. 180(4):1129-33, 2003
15. Cohen MC et al: Solitary unilocular cyst of the lung with features of persistent interstitial pulmonary emphysema: report of four cases. Pediatr Dev Pathol. 2(6):531-6, 1999
16. Jabra AA et al: Localized persistent pulmonary interstitial emphysema: CT findings with radiographic-pathologic correlation. AJR Am J Roentgenol. 169(5):1381-4, 1997

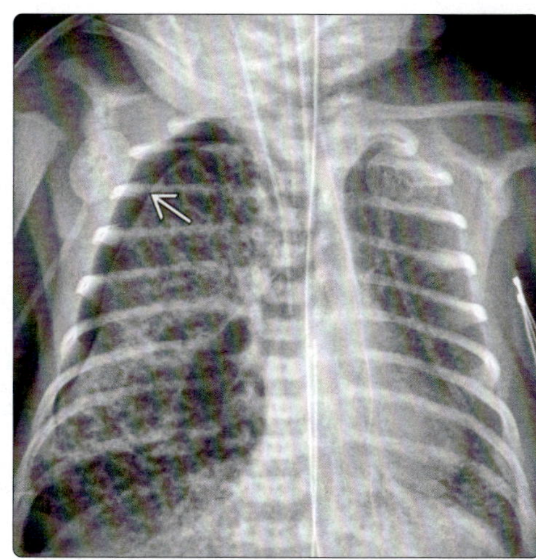

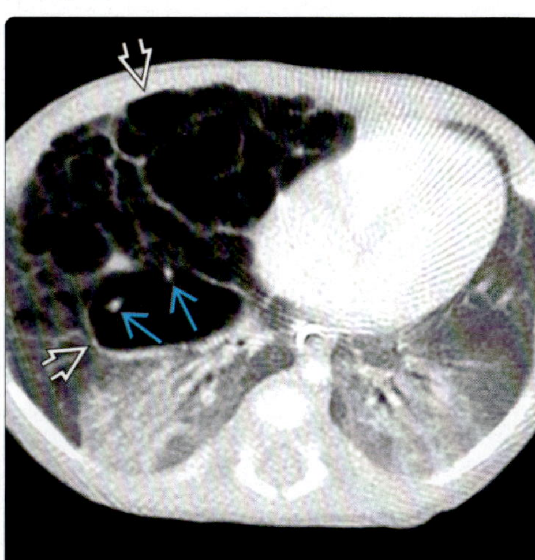

(Left) *AP chest radiograph in a 6-day-old, 27-weeks-gestation infant shows "bubbly" & linear lucencies of diffuse PIE, greater on the right. A right pneumothorax* ➡ *is also seen.* **(Right)** *Axial CECT in the same patient at 26 days of age shows development of persistent PIE with aggregate mass-like cysts* ➡*. Note the "dots" of pulmonary vascular branches* ➡ *surrounded by the interstitial cysts. There is leftward mediastinal shift indicating mass effect, commonly seen in this entity.*

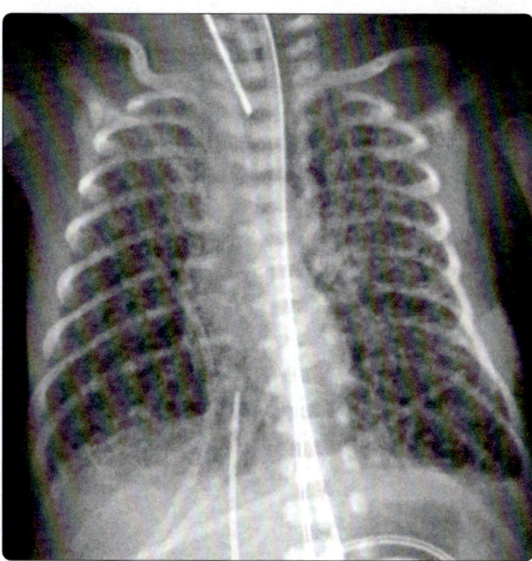

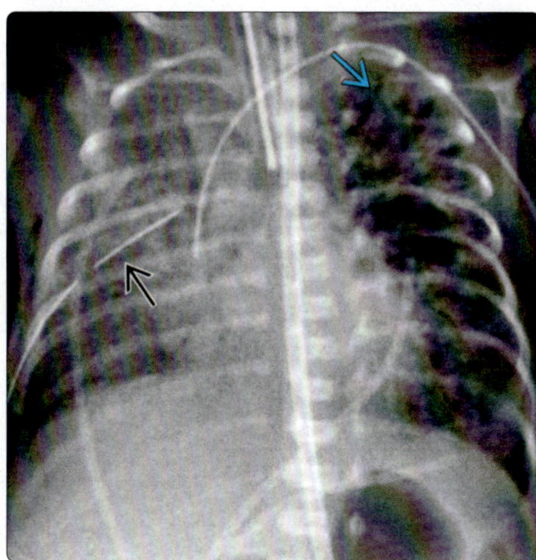

(Left) *AP chest radiograph in an intubated 4-day-old, 23-weeks-gestation premature infant shows diffuse bilateral "bubbly" lucencies of PIE intermixed with hazy opacities of surfactant deficiency.* **(Right)** *AP chest radiograph in a 4-day-old, 27-weeks-gestation infant shows linear lucencies, greatest in the left upper lobe* ➡*. Involvement in PIE may be asymmetric. A chest tube* ➡ *has been placed for a right pneumothorax.*

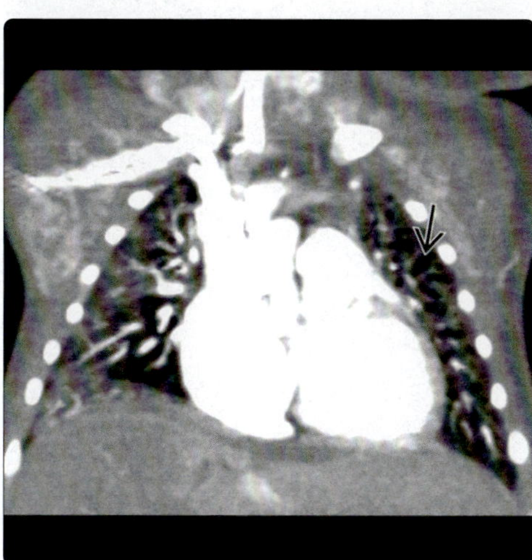

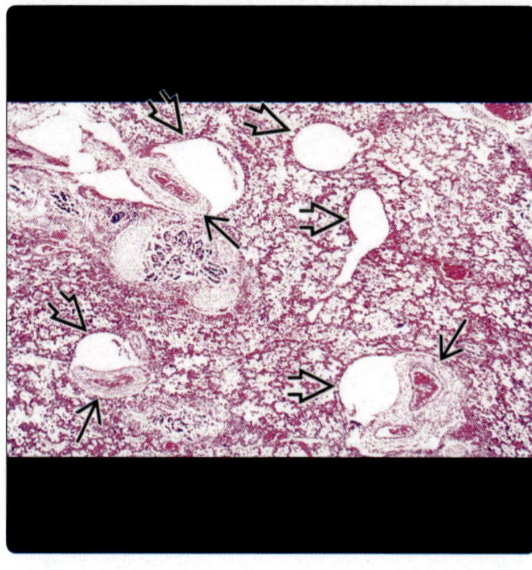

(Left) *Coronal CECT of the chest demonstrates linear lucencies in the interstitium of the left upper lobe (superimposed on a background of SDD). The lucencies in PIE do not follow the anatomy of a bronchus & may get wider* ➡ *near the periphery of the lung, helping to differentiate PIE from air bronchograms.* **(Right)** *Microscopic H&E slide shows PIE as gas collections* ➡ *in the pulmonary interstitium/lymphatics. The foci of gas abut & surround the bronchial arteries* ➡*.*

Neonatal Pneumothorax

KEY FACTS

IMAGING

- Neonatal chest radiographs are typically obtained supine
  - Clues to pneumothorax diagnosis on supine study
    - Large, hyperlucent hemithorax
    - Lucency "cloaking" diaphragm, mediastinum, &/or lung
    - Medial stripe sign: Lucency along mediastinum
    - Deep sulcus sign: Well-defined costophrenic sulcus
    - Gas-filled pleural sac herniated across midline
    - Visualization of anterior junction line if bilateral
  - Cross-table lateral view shows air anterior to lung
  - Edge enhancement on PACS may improve visibility
- Ultrasound: Absence of lung sliding & comet-tail artifact

TOP DIFFERENTIAL DIAGNOSES

- Pneumomediastinum
- Air-filled mass
- Artifact
- Recent surgical evacuation of hemithorax

PATHOLOGY

- Overdistention & rupture of alveoli
  - Directly into pleural cavity → pneumothorax
  - Into lung interstitium first → interstitial emphysema
- Risk factors: Low birth weight, premature or postmature gestation, male sex, surfactant deficiency disease, meconium aspiration, pulmonary hypoplasia, resuscitation at birth, mechanical ventilation, macrosomia

CLINICAL ISSUES

- Common signs/symptoms: Ipsilateral ↓ breath sounds, respiratory distress, cyanosis, retractions, grunting, nasal flaring, chest asymmetry (↑ on affected side), hypercapnia, hypoxemia; tension pneumothorax → hypotension, shock
- Treatment
  - Expectant/supportive management in asymptomatic patients or those with mild disease
  - Needle aspiration or chest tube drainage if symptomatic

(Left) *Supine chest radiograph in a neonate demonstrates a pneumothorax with lucency "cloaking" the right heart boarder ➡. A pleural line is seen laterally ➡ in this case, though sharp pleural lines are often not visible on supine views.* **(Right)** *Cross-table lateral view of the chest in a 1-day-old shows a circumscribed lucency anteriorly deep to the chest wall, compatible with a pneumothorax ➡. Patchy & coarse pulmonary opacities ➡ are secondary to meconium aspiration.*

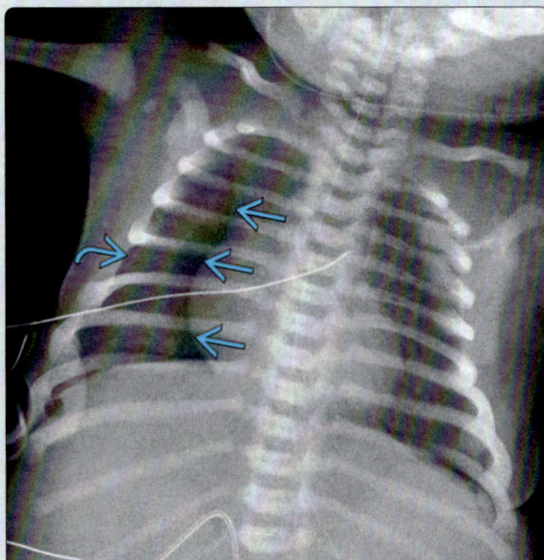

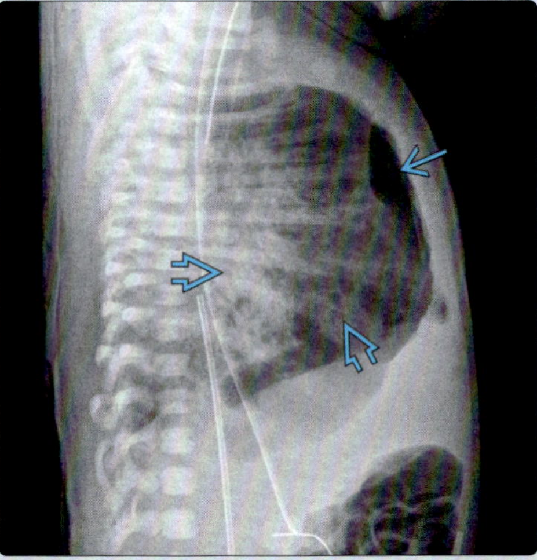

(Left) *Supine chest radiograph in a 2-day-old neonate born at 34-weeks gestation shows lucency "cloaking" the left hemithorax ➡ with a well-defined, left costophrenic angle ➡ as compared to the right. This appearance was due to a moderate left pneumothorax.* **(Right)** *Supine chest radiograph in a newborn demonstrates relative lucencies over the lungs bilaterally ➡, a pleural line on the right ➡, & the anterior junction line ➡, compatible with bilateral pneumothoraces.*

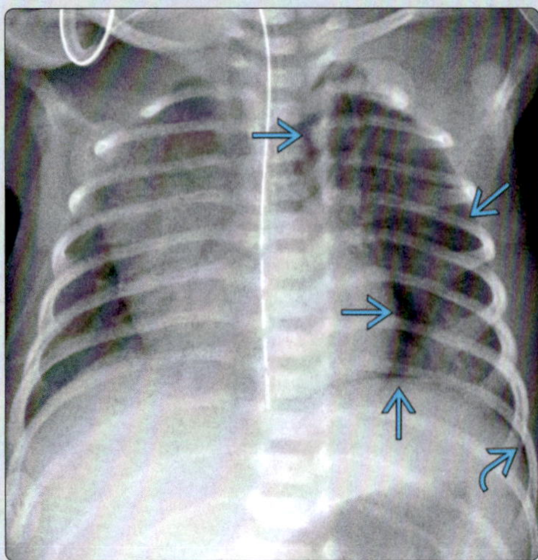

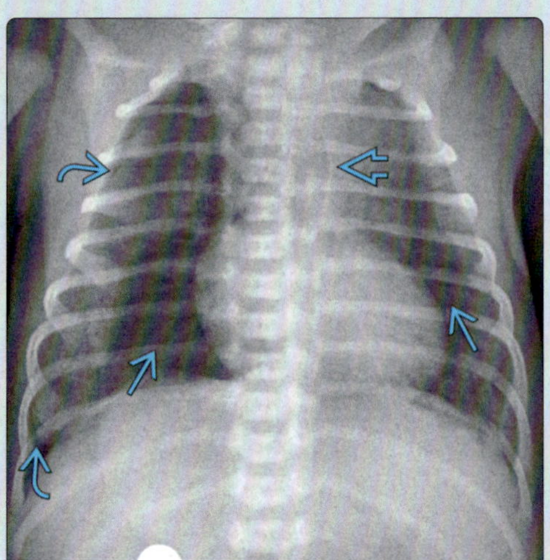

Neonatal Pneumothorax

TERMINOLOGY

Definitions

- Air in pleural space between visceral & parietal pleura

IMAGING

Radiographic Findings

- Neonatal chest radiograph is typically obtained with patient in supine position
- Air collects anterior & medial → pleural line is often not seen
- Clues to pneumothorax in supine position
  - Large, hyperlucent hemithorax
  - Lucency "cloaking" diaphragm, mediastinum, &/or lung
    - Thymus may be compressed → "pseudomass"
  - Medial stripe sign: Lucency along mediastinal edge
  - Deep sulcus sign: Well-defined costophrenic sulcus
  - Gas-filled pleural sac herniates across midline
    - Appearance is similar to pneumomediastinum
  - Bilateral anterior pneumothoraces displace thymus & allow visualization of anterior junction line
    - Anterior junction line is usually not seen in neonates
    - Uneven tension → support devices are displaced away from side of greater tension
- Cross-table lateral view
  - Intrapleural lucency anterior to lung & mediastinum
  - Minimizes neonate manipulation vs. decubitus view
- Tension pneumothorax
  - Large pneumothorax with lung collapse
    - Diseased "stiff" lungs may not collapse despite tension
  - Flattened or everted hemidiaphragm
  - Bulging intercostal spaces
  - Mediastinal shift toward/into contralateral hemithorax

Ultrasonographic Findings

- Absence of lung sliding & comet-tail artifact

Imaging Recommendations

- Best imaging tool
  - Bedside ultrasound can enable more rapid diagnosis than radiograph
  - Edge enhancement on PACS may improve radiographic visibility

DIFFERENTIAL DIAGNOSIS

Pneumomediastinum

- Air confined to upper retrosternal space
- Mediastinal shift is unlikely
- Lifting of thymus: Spinnaker sail sign

Artifact

- Skin fold
- Materials external to patient
- Mach effect

Air-Filled Mass

- Congenital pulmonary airway malformation (CPAM)
- Congenital lobar emphysema
- Congenital diaphragmatic hernia (CDH)

Recent Surgical Evacuation of Hemithorax

- Early radiographs after CDH repair or large CPAM resection demonstrate negative pressure ex vacuo pneumothorax
- Fills with fluid; ultimately ↓ in size due to lung growth

PATHOLOGY

General Features

- Uneven alveolar ventilation, air-trapping, ↑ transpulmonary pressure → alveolar overdistension → rupture into pleural cavity → pneumothorax
  - Rupture may first occur into interstitium (pulmonary interstitial emphysema) with ultimate dissection to mediastinum or pleural cavity
- Risk factors: Low birth weight, premature or postmature gestation, male sex, surfactant deficiency disease, meconium aspiration, pulmonary hypoplasia, resuscitation at birth, mechanical ventilation, macrosomia

CLINICAL ISSUES

Presentation

- Timing of pneumothorax presentation
  - Infants > 2,500 g: Median of 5.5 hours after birth
  - Infants < 2,500 g: Median of 2nd day of life
- Most common signs/symptoms: Ipsilateral ↓ breath sounds, respiratory distress, cyanosis, retractions, grunting, nasal flaring, chest asymmetry (larger on affected side), hypercapnia, hypoxemia
- Asymptomatic pneumothoraces are more common in nonlow birth weight neonates
- Tension pneumothorax may result in hypotension, shock

Natural History & Prognosis

- Incidence: 1% of term births, 6-7% of preterm births
  - ↑ morbidity & mortality in preterm infants
- High-frequency positive pressure ventilation may ↓ incidence compared to conventional mechanical ventilation

Treatment

- Expectant/supportive management in asymptomatic patients & those with mild disease
- Needle aspiration or chest tube drainage if symptomatic

DIAGNOSTIC CHECKLIST

Reporting Tips

- Unexpected or tension pneumothoraces should be communicated to clinical team immediately

SELECTED REFERENCES

1. Fei Q et al: Lung ultrasound, a better choice for neonatal pneumothorax: a systematic review and meta-analysis. Ultrasound Med Biol. 47(3):359-69, 2021
2. Liu J et al: International expert consensus and recommendations for neonatal pneumothorax ultrasound diagnosis and ultrasound-guided thoracentesis procedure. J Vis Exp. 12;(157), 2020
3. Menashe SJ et al: Pediatric chest radiographs: common and less common errors. AJR Am J Roentgenol. 207(4):903-11, 2016
4. Aly H et al: Pneumothorax in the newborn: clinical presentation, risk factors and outcomes. J Matern Fetal Neonatal Med. 27(4):402-6, 2014
5. Duong HH et al: Pneumothorax in neonates: trends, predictors and outcomes. J Neonatal Perinatal Med. 7(1):29-38, 2014
6. Cizmeci MN et al: The utility of special radiological signs on routinely obtained supine anteroposterior chest radiographs for the early recognition of neonatal pneumothorax. Neonatology. 104(4):305-11, 2013

Chylothorax

KEY FACTS

TERMINOLOGY

- Lymphatic fluid in pleural space secondary to congenital or acquired conditions, including congenital lymphatic conducting channel anomaly, ↑ pressure, impaired drainage/obstruction, or trauma to thoracic duct

IMAGING

- US, CT, MR may be done to discover underlying cause of chylothorax & evaluate treatment options
  - Persistent pleural effusion following cardiac surgery
  - Congenital chylothorax from Turner or Noonan syndrome
  - Various associated lymphatic disorders, including conducting channel anomalies, generalized lymphatic anomaly, Gorham-Stout disease, & discrete cystic lymphatic malformations
- Lymphangiogram (conventional, nuclear, or MR): Used to investigate suspected central conducting channel anomalies
  - Disorders (including atresia/absence, obstruction, disruption, or dysmotility) may show abrupt halt to visualization of normal lymphatic pathways, reflux into tissues, collaterals, delayed transit, &/or abnormal accumulations

CLINICAL ISSUES

- Symptoms may include tachypnea & dyspnea, generalized edema, chylous ascites, immunosuppression, protein-losing enteropathy (if gut involved)
- Treatment options include: Fat-restricted diet, rapamycin/sirolimus, thoracentesis or draining procedure, thoracic duct ligation or embolization, microsurgical thoracic duct repair, pleurodesis
  - Isolated neonatal chylothorax may be cured by ethiodized oil lymphangiography
- Thoracic duct injury may resolve spontaneously in 50%
- Poorer prognosis with syndromes, multiple sites of chylous fluid accumulations, prematurity

(Left) *AP radiograph shows a large pleural effusion ➡ in a neonate. Laboratory evaluation showed a chylous effusion, consistent with congenital chylothorax.* **(Right)** *Longitudinal ultrasound of the right chest in the same patient shows a right pleural effusion ➡ in a patient with known congenital chylothorax. Note the inferior aspect of the right lower lobe ➡.*

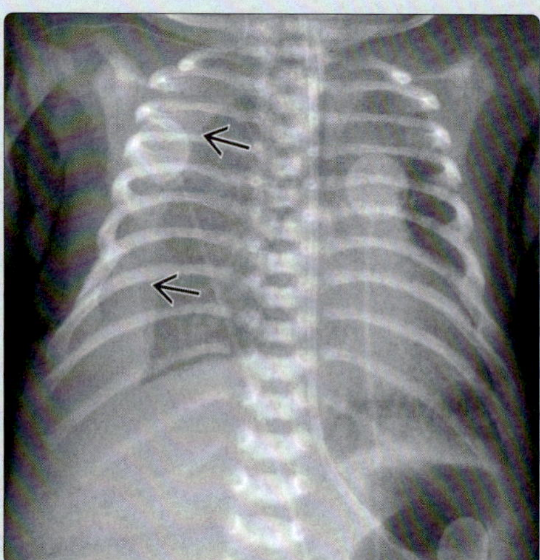

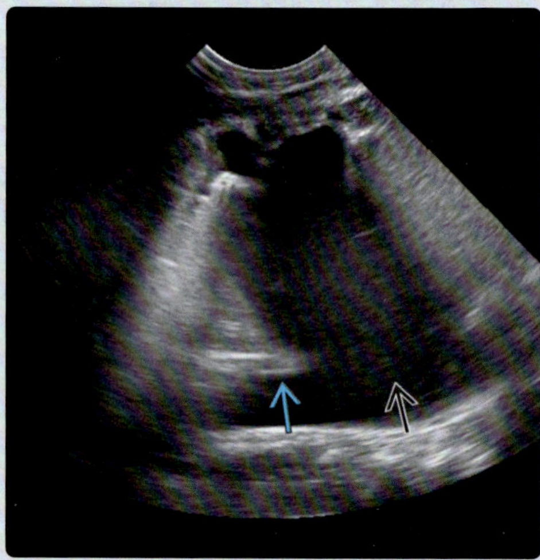

(Left) *AP radiograph in a 4-month-old infant status post surgery for congenital heart disease shows a moderate right chylothorax ➡ from a thoracic duct injury.* **(Right)** *Transverse ultrasound of the right chest in the same 4-month-old patient status post heart surgery & thoracic duct injury shows a large, mildly echogenic pleural effusion ➡. Note the compressed echogenic right lung ➡ surrounded by the effusion.*

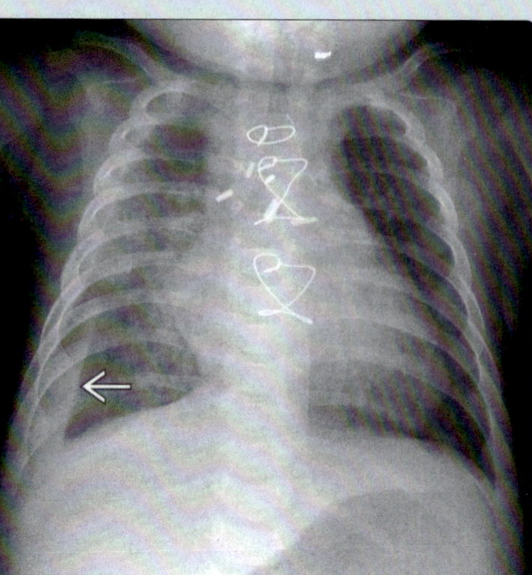

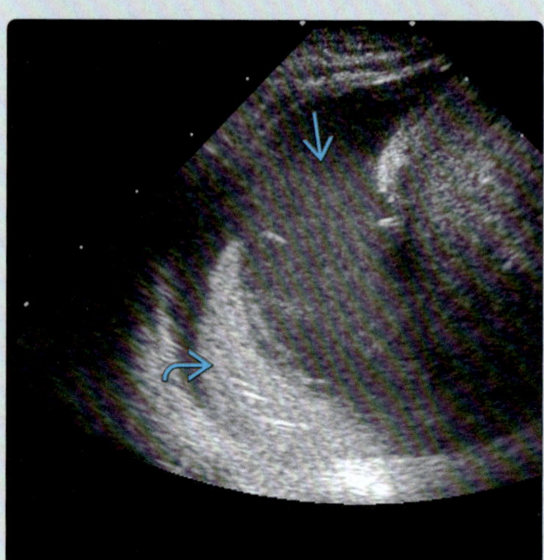

TERMINOLOGY

Definitions

- Chylothorax: Lymphatic fluid in pleural space secondary to congenital or acquired conditions, including congenital anomaly, ↑ pressure, impaired drainage/obstruction, or trauma to thoracic duct
- Lymphangiectasia: Abnormal dilation of lymphatics
  - 1°: Abnormal development of lymphatics in isolation or with genetic anomaly
  - 2°: Related to congenital heart disease (CHD) or repair
- Neonatal/congenital lymphatic flow disorders (central lymphatic conducting channel anomaly)
  - Pulmonary lymphatic perfusion syndrome: Abnormal lymphatic flow in lungs & pleura → chylothorax
  - Central lymphatic flow disorder: Abnormal flow into additional tissues/cavities → body wall, peritoneum, etc.
  - Congenital chylous ascites

IMAGING

General Features

- Best diagnostic clue
  - Isolated unilateral pleural effusion in newborn
  - Newborn with obstructive CHD or lymphatic disorders
    - ± Turner syndrome, Noonan syndrome
    - Lymphangiectasia with bilateral interstitial thickening, anasarca, protein-losing enteropathy, & chylous accumulations in body cavities
  - Persistent pleural effusion following CHD repair
  - Macroscopic lymphatic malformation of neck & chest
  - Bone disease with chylothorax: Gorham-Stout disease ("vanishing bone disease"), generalized lymphatic anomaly (GLA)

Radiographic Findings

- Persistent, nonspecific pleural effusion
  - Associated disorders dictate other findings
- ± interstitial thickening, body wall edema

Ultrasonographic Findings

- Anechoic or mildly hypoechoic fluid without septations
- Lung sonography of lymphangiectasia in setting of CHD: Surface irregularity; subpleural, cystic-appearing foci

CT Findings

- CECT
  - Lymphangiectasia with diffuse pulmonary interstitial thickening
  - ± poorly defined paraspinal soft tissue infiltration from abnormal lymphatics
  - Macro- &/or microcystic lymphatic malformation may infiltrate mediastinum & pleura
    - ± bone lesions
  - ± solid mediastinal mass obstructing vessels

MR Findings

- Fetal MR may show "nutmeg lung" (due to abnormal pulmonary lymphatics) + effusion

Lymphangiogram

- Can be performed with nuclear medicine, MR, or conventional fluoroscopy
- Depending on specific question & modality being employed, specific agent is injected into dermal or nodal lymphatics of proximal or distal lower extremity
- Extremity & body are subsequently imaged over 10-60 minutes while agent travels proximally through central lymphatic system to cisterna chyli & thoracic duct, ultimately emptying into left subclavian vein
  - MR: Gadolinium-based contrast is injected into lymph nodes, typically at groin
    - Multiple repeats of rapid T1 FS GRE
    - May also use preinjection heavily T2W 3D sequence
- Disorders (including atresia, absence, disruption, dysmotility) may show abrupt halt to visualization of normal channels
  - ± reflux of contrast into adjacent tissues, visualization of adjacent collaterals, leak into adjacent cavity, or localized extraluminal accumulation
    - Isolated abnormal flow into lungs in neonate → pulmonary lymphatic disorder, often with chylothorax

CLINICAL ISSUES

Presentation

- Most common signs/symptoms
  - Tachypnea & dyspnea
  - Classic symptoms of pleural effusion
    - ↓ breath sounds, usually with cough
- Other signs/symptoms
  - Generalized edema, chylous ascites, immunosuppression, protein-losing enteropathy (if gut is involved)

Natural History & Prognosis

- Thoracic duct injury may resolve spontaneously in 50%
- Poorer prognosis with syndromes, multiple sites of chylous fluid accumulations, prematurity

Treatment

- Conservative or medical treatment
  - ↓ chyle production
    - Fat-restricted oral diet
    - TPN
  - Rapamycin/sirolimus is of benefit with some lymphatic disorders, not clearly shown in conducting channel anomalies
  - Octreotide
- Interventions may be indicated with chyle leak > 1 L/day for 5 days or persistent leak for > 2 weeks
  - Thoracentesis or draining procedure of pleural space
  - Thoracic duct repair, lymphovenous anastomosis, ligation, or embolization
    - Ethiodized oil embolization is particularly effective in isolated neonatal chylothorax
  - Pleurodesis

SELECTED REFERENCES

1. Barrera CA et al: Imaging of fetal lymphangiectasias: prenatal and postnatal imaging findings. Pediatr Radiol. 50(13):1872-80, 2020
2. Biko DM et al: Pediatric pulmonary lymphatic flow disorders: diagnosis and management. Paediatr Respir Rev. 36:2-7, 2020
3. Chavhan GB et al: Magnetic resonance lymphangiography. Radiol Clin North Am. 58(4):693-706, 2020

Bronchopulmonary Dysplasia

KEY FACTS

TERMINOLOGY

- Bronchopulmonary dysplasia (BPD), chronic lung disease of prematurity
- Old BPD: Occurred in larger, later preterm infants with prolonged mechanical ventilation & O_2 therapy
- New BPD: Occurs in earlier, smaller preterm infants with overall milder disease
  - Alveolar simplification & dysmorphic vasculature; more uniform parenchymal inflation, less fibrosis

IMAGING

- Old BPD: Heterogeneous, hyperinflated lungs with patchy, focal lucencies + coarse, reticular, & band-like opacities
- New BPD: Diffuse, hazy opacification &/or cystic lucencies
  - Severe surfactant deficiency disease (SDD) patients may follow old imaging patterns
- Overlapping chest CT findings in old & new BPD
  - Subpleural opacities, septal thickening, air-trapping, emphysema, bronchiectasis, atelectasis, consolidation
- MR is emerging as useful modality
  - Gradient-echo & ultrashort echo time (UTE) sequences
  - Higher density lung tissues (fibrosis/inflammation) have higher signal intensity
- US may help predict progression to BPD in SDD

PATHOLOGY

- Antenatal & postnatal insults to immature lungs → impaired vascular & alveolar development
- Strongest predictors: Gestational age < 28 weeks, low birth weight, intrauterine growth restriction

CLINICAL ISSUES

- Affects 40% ≤ 28-weeks gestation, 68% of 22-26 weeks
- Most new BPD has mild/no initial respiratory disease → deterioration → slow improvement
- 16-25% develop pulmonary hypertension associated with up to 48% 2-year mortality
- Prevention: Antenatal steroids, exogenous surfactant, gentler ventilatory strategies, less aggressive oxygenation

(Left) *AP radiograph in a 1-day-old, 28-weeks-gestation infant shows hypoinflation with mild, hazy opacities, greater in the right lung than left.* **(Right)** *AP radiograph in the same infant at 3 weeks of age demonstrates hyperinflation with developing cystic & bubbly lucencies throughout the lungs. The patient was able to be managed with noninvasive positive pressure ventilation & did not require intubation.*

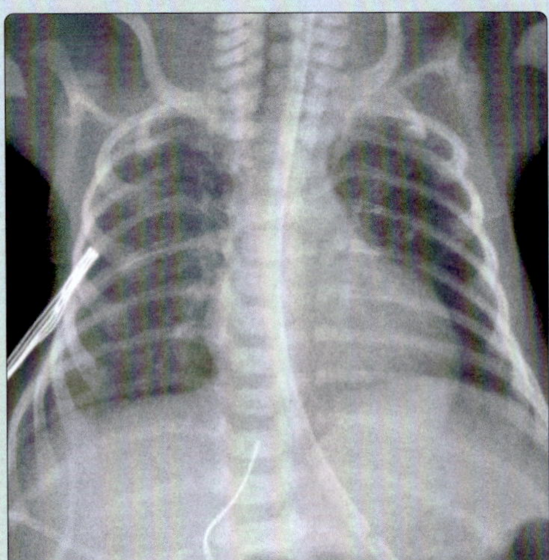

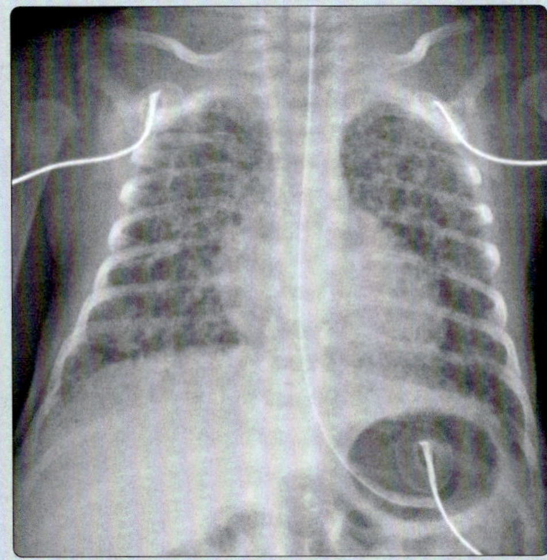

(Left) *AP radiograph in the same infant at 2 months of age demonstrates enlarging cystic spaces among coarsened, reticular opacities. The lungs demonstrate progressive hyperinflation.* **(Right)** *Axial CT of the chest in the same infant at 2 months of age shows characteristic findings of BPD, including subpleural opacities ➔, cysts ➔, air-trapping ➔, & septal thickening ➔. Due to difficulty in weaning respiratory support, CT was obtained for a more detailed characterization of the parenchymal abnormalities.*

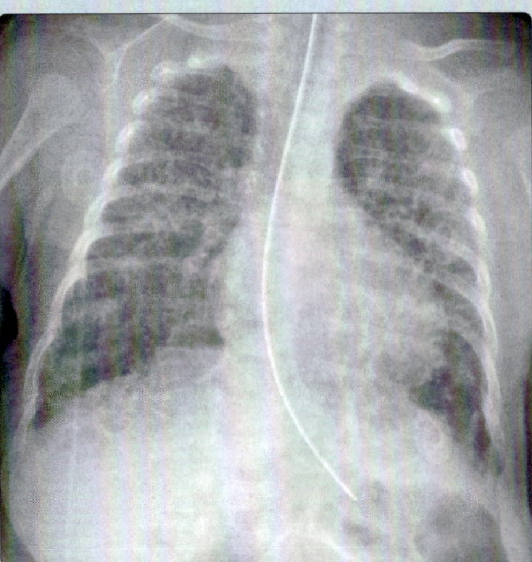

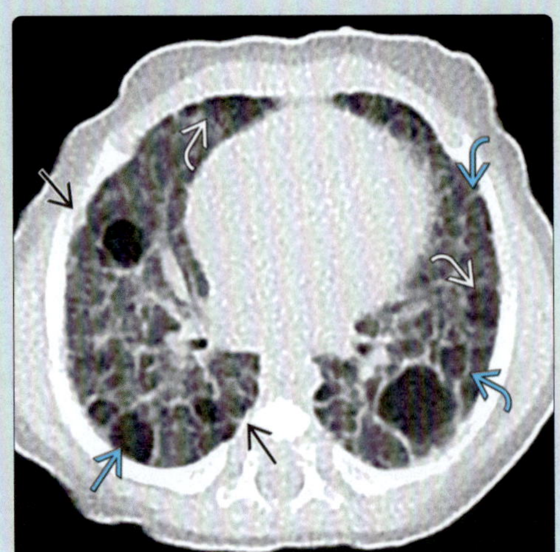

TERMINOLOGY

Abbreviations

- Bronchopulmonary dysplasia (BPD)

Synonyms

- Chronic lung disease (CLD) of prematurity

Definitions

- Definition has continually evolved over last several decades
- Initial definition (1979): 28 days oxygen (O_2) requirement + characteristic radiographic changes
- Most recent definition (2018): Born at < 32-weeks gestational age (GA) + persistent parenchymal lung disease with radiographic confirmation + requires ≥ 3 consecutive days of defined respiratory support to maintain arterial O_2 saturation 90-95% at 36-weeks postmenstrual age (PMA)
  - Grades I-III based on degree of respiratory support required
  - Grade IIIA: Early death due to persistent parenchymal lung disease (between 14 days of age & 36-weeks PMA)
- Old BPD: Larger, later preterm infants with prolonged mechanical ventilation & O_2 therapy
  - Developed severe chronic respiratory failure with heterogeneous hyperinflation & fibrosis
- New BPD: Earlier, smaller preterm infants with overall milder disease in setting of antenatal steroids, postnatal surfactant administration, & gentler methods of ventilation/O_2 support
  - More uniform parenchymal inflation, less fibrosis, characterized by alveolar simplification & dysmorphic vasculature

IMAGING

General Features

- Best diagnostic clue
  - Varying degrees of hazy opacities, cysts, hyperinflation, & coarse linear opacities diffusely in premature infant

Radiographic Findings

- Old BPD
  - Heterogeneous lung parenchyma with patchy, focal lucencies separated by coarse, reticular, & band-like opacities of fibrosis, atelectasis
- New BPD
  - Diffuse, hazy opacification &/or bubbly, cystic lucencies

CT Findings

- Overlapping chest CT findings between old & new BPD
  - Linear or triangular subpleural opacities
  - Thickening of interlobular septa
  - Air-trapping, mosaic attenuation, emphysema, bullae
    - Minimum intensity projection (MinIP) images highlight mosaic attenuation
  - Bronchiectasis, peribronchial thickening
  - Atelectasis or consolidation; architectural distortion
- Abnormalities are present on > 80% of adolescent & adult studies of former preterm infants with BPD
  - Subpleural opacities, air-trapping, bullae, & emphysema are most common
- Studies have shown CT correlation with disease severity, need for supplementary O_2 at discharge

MR Findings

- Current MR techniques can show hyperexpansion, mosaic lung attenuation, emphysema, cysts, subpleural opacities, & architectural distortion
  - Benefit of parenchymal detail without ionizing radiation
  - Sequences (GRE, UTE) can allow for nonsedated, quiet-breathing scans
- Gradient-echo (GRE) sequences depict areas of high tissue density (fibrosis, inflammation)
  - High tissue density = higher intensity
  - High contrast between high density fibrosis & remaining lung
  - Not able to differentiate hypodense lung tissue (alveolar simplification, emphysema, cysts) vs. normal lung
- Ultrashort echo time (UTE) radial/spiral acquisition sequences depict broader spectrum of tissue density
  - Higher density tissue = higher intensity; produces density-like intensity spectrum with resemblance to CT images
  - Allows differentiation of normal vs. hypodense lung tissue in addition to higher density abnormalities
- Cardiac MR may be of utility in patients with concern for pulmonary vascular disease (PVD) & pulmonary hypertension (HTN)
  - Echocardiogram can be challenging due to poor sonographic windows, hyperinflation; MR may be noninvasive alternative to gold standard cardiac catheterization
- Potential for future functional imaging utilizing hyperpolarized gas MR methods

Ultrasonographic Findings

- Investigation into lung ultrasound for diagnosis/prediction of BPD is ongoing but not yet practical vs. radiography
  - Homogenous hyperechogenicity (echogenicity = diaphragm) of lung bases is described with surfactant deficiency disease (SDD)
  - Subsequent development of streaky, irregular areas of lower echogenicity between days 9-18 may predict progression to BPD

Nuclear Medicine Findings

- V/Q scan: Ventilation/perfusion mismatch

Imaging Recommendations

- Best imaging tool
  - Chest radiography for early monitoring; CT for more detailed assessment of structural changes

DIFFERENTIAL DIAGNOSIS

Pulmonary Interstitial Emphysema

- Air in interstitium of premature neonate, usually on positive pressure ventilation
- Cystic & linear lucencies, often in background of SDD
  - May create unique dot-dash appearance of interstitial air collections surrounding pulmonary vessels
- Usually rapid onset in first 10 days of life
- Typically transient with switch to high-frequency ventilation

Meconium Aspiration

- Aspiration of meconium-stained amniotic fluid → toxic pneumonitis

- Usually in postmature infants ± distress in utero
- Rapid onset of radiographic changes
- Coarse perihilar opacities with hyperinflation ± pneumothorax, pneumomediastinum

Neonatal Pneumonia

- Often bilateral & diffuse but may be unilateral
- Pleural effusion is common, unlike BPD

Congenital Pulmonary Airway Malformation

- Often fluid-filled, multicystic mass at birth with progressive aeration due to airway communication
- Typically involves 1 lobe
- Smaller lesions may present later in life

Congenital Lobar Overinflation

- Opacified lobe with progressive aeration & expansion
- Asymptomatic until significant compression of adjacent lung &/or mediastinum occurs

PATHOLOGY

General Features

- Etiology
    - Disease of preterm low birth weight infants with (still emerging) multifactorial etiology
        - Likely result of antenatal & postnatal insults to immature/developing lungs
            - Maternal, (epi)genetic, infectious/inflammatory, & microbiome/dysbiosis factors are possible contributors
            - Mechanical ventilation & oxygen exposure
            - Disordered repair mechanisms in response to postnatal insults may play role
        - Greatest risk factors: GA < 28 weeks, lower birth weight, intrauterine growth restriction
            - 24- to 28-weeks gestation: Time of transition from canalicular through saccular stage of pulmonary development
    - Old BPD resulting from volutrauma & O_2 toxicity is less common now
        - Due to antenatal steroids, early surfactant administration, gentler ventilation, & oxygenation

Microscopic Features

- Old BPD
    - Airway injury, inflammation, & metaplasia
    - Smooth muscle hypertrophy of airways & vessels
    - Patchy atelectasis, emphysema, & septal fibrosis
- New BPD
    - Uniform inflation, less heterogeneity, less interstitial fibrosis
    - Impaired vascular & alveolar growth
        - Alveolar simplification
        - Dysmorphic vessels, abnormal capillary distribution

CLINICAL ISSUES

Presentation

- Most common signs/symptoms
    - New BPD is often mild or no respiratory disease initially followed by progressive deterioration
        - Most have subsequent slow improvement & wean respiratory support
        - Some worsen, ± development of pulmonary HTN
    - Patients with severe SDD may progress like old BPD

Demographics

- Age
    - Premature infants < 32-weeks gestation at birth
- Sex
    - M:F = 2-5:1
- Epidemiology
    - Most common chronic pulmonary disease of infancy
        - 40% of ≤ 28-weeks-gestation infants; 68% of 22- to 26-weeks gestation
        - 25% of infants weighing < 1,500 g at birth; 40% of those weighing < 1,000 g
    - Unchanged incidence of BPD since initial description
        - Due to ↑ survival of very premature infants

Natural History & Prognosis

- ↑ risk of pulmonary infections in first 2 years of life with ↑ morbidity & mortality, especially with RSV
    - Slowly improving pulmonary function with fewer respiratory infections later in childhood
    - > 50% hospital readmission rate during infancy
- Pulmonary HTN in 16-25% of BPD patients
    - Up to 48% 2-year mortality in this group
- Abnormal pulmonary function with ↑ airway hyperreactivity & obstruction may persist into adulthood

Treatment

- Many conflicting results in BPD prevention/therapy trials
- For prevention (strongest evidence)
    - Antenatal steroids
    - Exogenous surfactant
    - Gentle ventilation (noninvasive delivery, pressure limited, volume targeted)
    - Lower inspired oxygen concentrations, lower oxygenation targets
    - Vitamin A
- Less conclusive evidence: Caffeine, early PDA closure, inhaled nitric oxide, postnatal steroids (inhaled vs. systemic), sildenafil, Clara cell 10 protein

SELECTED REFERENCES

1. Higano NS et al: Modern pulmonary imaging of bronchopulmonary dysplasia. J Perinatol. 41(4):707-17, 2021
2. Vanhaverbeke K et al: Lung imaging in bronchopulmonary dysplasia: a systematic review. Respir Med. 171:106101, 2020
3. Bancalari E et al: Bronchopulmonary dysplasia: 50 years after the original description. Neonatology. 115(4):384-91, 2019
4. Higano NS et al: Neonatal pulmonary magnetic resonance imaging of bronchopulmonary dysplasia predicts short-term clinical outcomes. Am J Respir Crit Care Med. 198(10):1302-11, 2018
5. Hwang JS et al: Recent advances in bronchopulmonary dysplasia: pathophysiology, prevention, and treatment. Lung. 196(2):129-38, 2018
6. Semple T et al: Imaging bronchopulmonary dysplasia-a multimodality update. Front Med (Lausanne). 4:88, 2017
7. Jobe AH: Mechanisms of lung injury and bronchopulmonary dysplasia. Am J Perinatol. 33(11):1076-8, 2016
8. Mourani PM et al: Pulmonary hypertension and vascular abnormalities in bronchopulmonary dysplasia. Clin Perinatol. 42(4):839-55, 2015
9. Parad RB: Update on the diagnosis and management of bronchopulmonary dysplasia/chronic lung disease of infancy: what the radiologist should know. Pediatr Radiol. 42 Suppl 1:S92-100, 2012

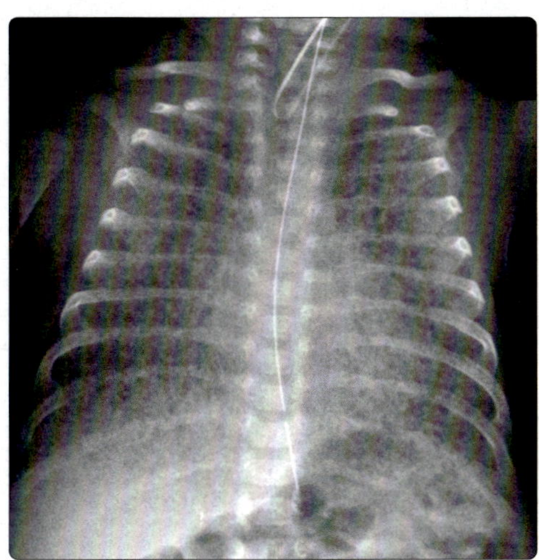

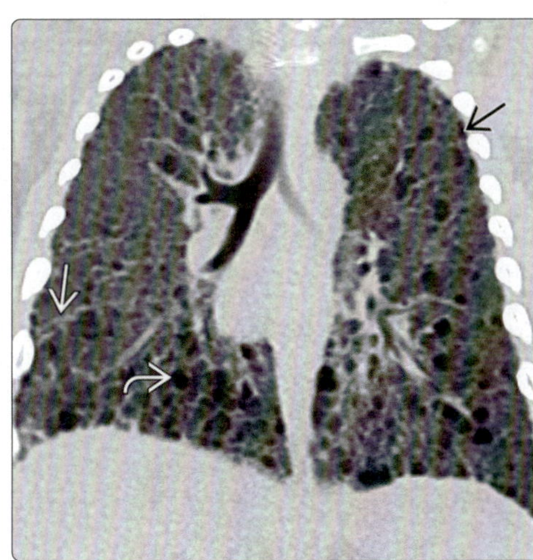

(Left) *AP radiograph in a 5-month-old, former 26-weeks-gestation premature infant with BPD shows generalized pulmonary hyperexpansion with diffuse, hazy opacities & coarse, interstitial markings.* **(Right)** *Coronal NECT during inspiration in an infant with BPD shows numerous parenchymal ➔ & subpleural ➔ cysts with generalized ground-glass opacities & parenchymal bands ➔.*

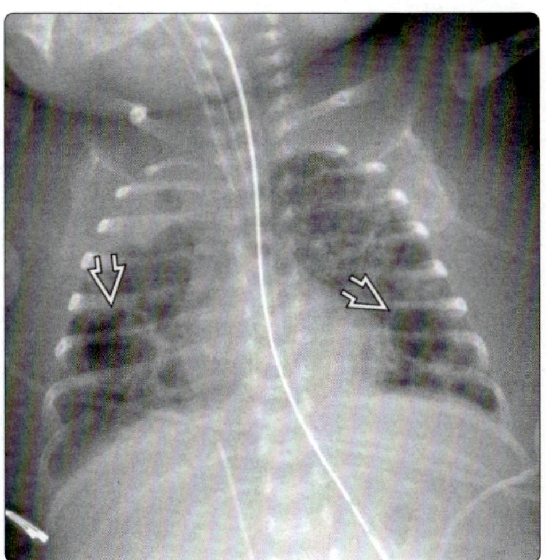

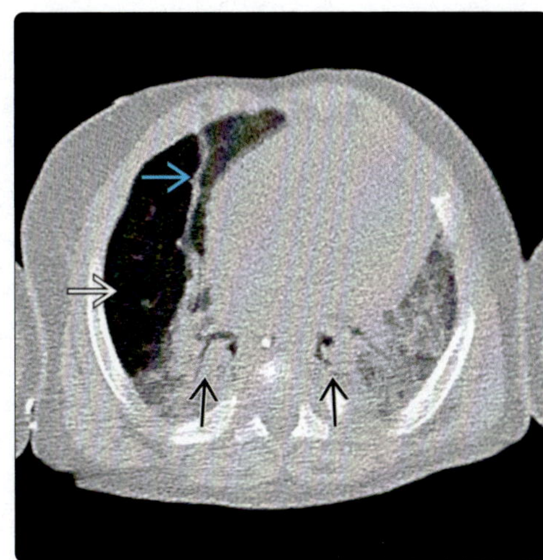

(Left) *AP radiograph in a premature patient with chronic lung disease shows bilateral cysts/pneumatoceles ➔ in the setting of coarse, linear & patchy, hazy opacities.* **(Right)** *Axial NECT shows air-trapping ➔ in the right lung with a coarse interstitial band ➔ & bibasilar consolidations ➔ in a patient with chronic lung disease of prematurity.*

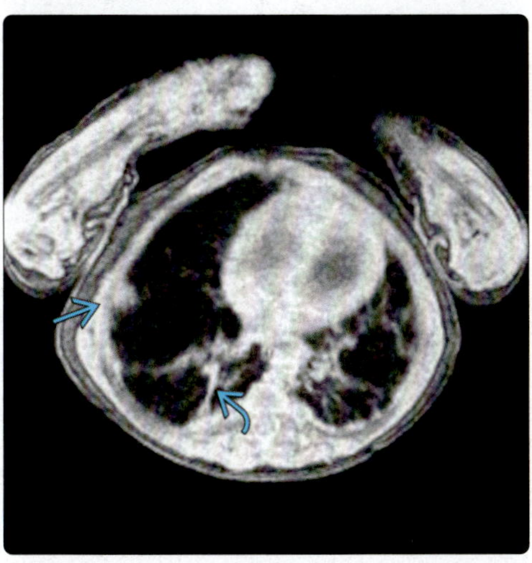

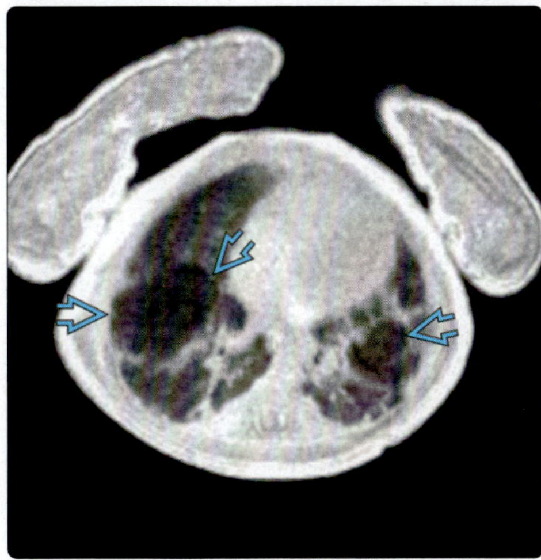

(Left) *Axial GRE MR in a patient with BPD shows areas of fibrosis or consolidation as hyperintensity with high contrast between these areas & the adjacent areas of less dense lung tissue. There are subpleural opacities ➔, linear interstitial opacities ➔, & architectural distortion.* **(Right)** *Axial UTE MR in the same patient shows the areas of higher density lung tissue, but also differentiates areas of air-trapping or emphysema ➔ within low-density lung tissue. (Courtesy N. Higano, PhD, R. Fleck, MD.)*

Umbilical Catheter Positions and Complications

KEY FACTS

TERMINOLOGY

- Umbilical venous catheter (UVC)
  - Normal course: Umbilical vein → umbilical recess → crosses left portal vein → ductus venosus → middle or left hepatic vein → inferior vena cava (IVC) → right atrium (RA)
  - Indications: Central venous access in ill/premature neonate for fluids/medications, TPN, exchange transfusion, venous pressure monitoring
- Umbilical arterial catheter (UAC)
  - Normal course: Umbilical artery → internal iliac artery → common iliac artery → aorta
  - Indications: Frequent blood sampling, monitoring of arterial pressures, angiography, exchange transfusion

IMAGING

- UVC tip optimal location: IVC-RA junction
  - At/just above diaphragm, usually T8-T9
- UAC tip optimal location
  - Ideal high line: Descending thoracic aorta (T6-T10)
  - Acceptable low line: Distal abdominal aorta (L3-L4)
- Complications include
  - UVC or UAC: Malposition, thrombosis, infection
  - UVC: Hepatic laceration, hematoma, TPN extravasation (intrahepatic or intraperitoneal), arrhythmia, atrial perforation, pericardial effusion
    - Hepatic extravasation may mimic mass
  - UAC: Aneurysm/pseudoaneurysm

DIAGNOSTIC CHECKLIST

- Correct position must be confirmed prior to use
- Umbilical catheter position is most quickly assessed by AP chest/abdomen radiograph
  - Cross-table lateral view can provide additional detail
- Ultrasound is most reliable way to confirm appropriate UVC position initially or with abnormal anatomy
- Ultrasound is best modality to assess complications

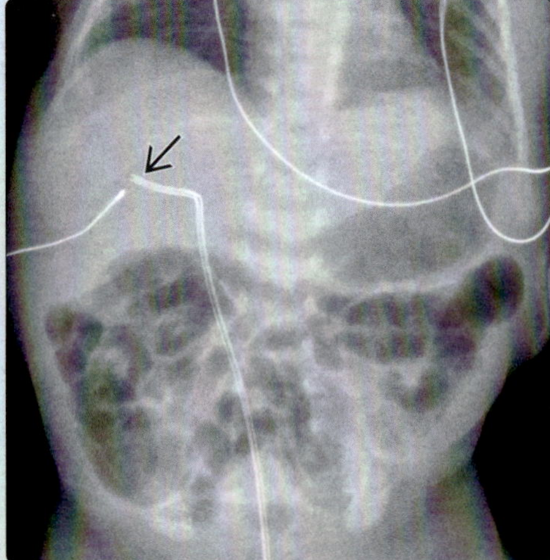

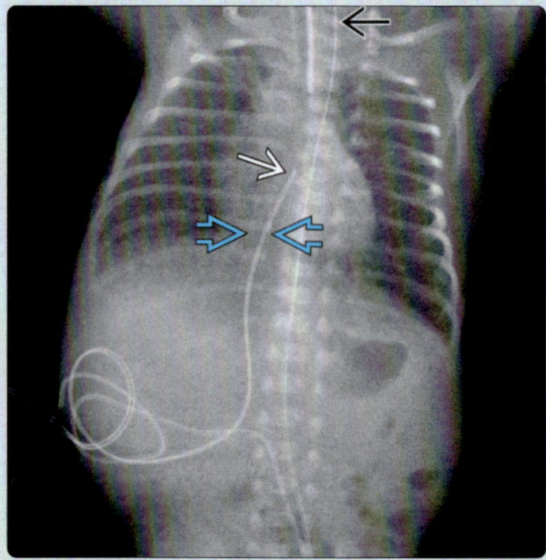

(Left) *AP radiograph shows malposition of a umbilical venous catheter (UVC) ➡, which courses laterally over the liver shadow. This catheter tip is likely within the right portal vein.* **(Right)** *AP radiograph shows malposition of a umbilical arterial catheter (UAC) ➡ into the left common carotid artery, though the tip is not included on this image. A malpositioned UVC tip ➡ courses toward the left atrium across a patent foramen ovale (PFO). Ideal radiographic position ➡ of the UVC tip would be at or just above the diaphragm.*

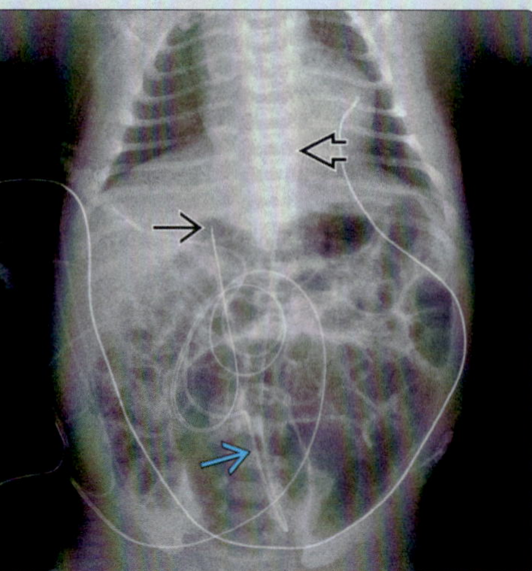

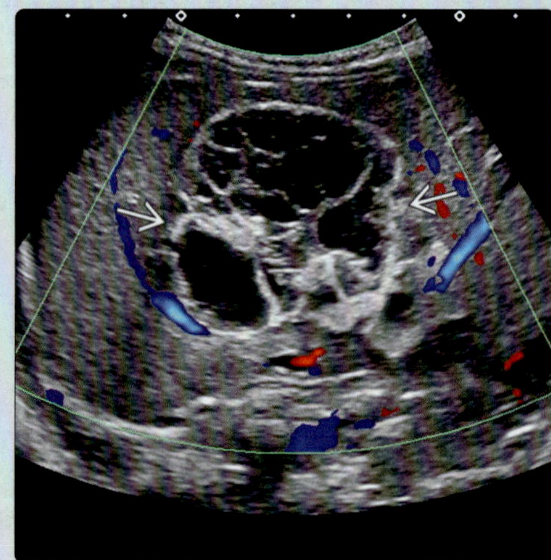

(Left) *AP radiograph of the chest & abdomen in a newborn shows a low position of the UVC ➡, which may be in the umbilical vein or recess. There is a satisfactory UAC position ➡. Note the initial caudal course of the UAC ➡, which can be useful in differentiating umbilical catheters.* **(Right)** *Transverse Doppler ultrasound of the liver in the same patient at 26 days old shows a heterogeneous, septated, avascular lesion ➡. The appearance & subsequent evolution were consistent with a hematoma complicating a malpositioned UVC.*

TERMINOLOGY

Definitions

- Umbilical venous catheter (UVC)
  - Normal course: Umbilical vein → umbilical recess → crosses left portal vein → ductus venosus → central portion of middle or left hepatic vein → inferior vena cava (IVC) → right atrium (RA)
  - Indications: Fluids/medications, TPN, exchange transfusion, venous pressure monitoring
- Umbilical arterial catheter (UAC)
  - Normal course: Umbilical artery → internal iliac artery → common iliac artery → aorta
  - Indications: Frequent blood sampling, monitoring of arterial pressures, angiography, exchange transfusion

IMAGING

Radiographic Findings

- UVC tip optimal location: IVC-RA junction
  - Best radiographic correlate is controversial
    - At/just above diaphragm; vertebral level is variable, most recommend T8-T9
  - Portal venous gas may be normal transient finding after placement
- UAC tip optimal location
  - Ideal high line: Descending thoracic aorta, T6-T10
  - Acceptable low line: Distal abdominal aorta, L3-L4
- Incorrect position in > 50% of 1st attempts
  - Common UVC malposition
    - Low: Umbilical vein or recess
    - High: RA, superior vena cava (SVC); right ventricle (via tricuspid valve); left atrium (via foramen ovale), pulmonary vein
    - Wrong vessel: Branch or main portal, splenic, or superior mesenteric vein
  - Common UAC malposition
    - Low: Internal iliac artery or branches (e.g., superior gluteal, inferior gluteal, pudendal)
    - High: Aortic arch or branch artery; pulmonary artery (via ductus arteriosus)
    - Wrong vessel: Celiac, superior mesenteric artery (SMA), renal arteries, lower extremity
- Correctly positioned catheter may be shifted or distorted with diaphragmatic hernia, large thoracic/abdominal mass, congenital heart disease, or heterotaxy

Ultrasonographic Findings

- Can be used to confirm catheter position during routine placement or if vascular anatomy is distorted/abnormal
- Normal catheter: Parallel echogenic lines surrounded by anechoic flowing blood in vessel lumen
  - Portal venous gas: Mobile echogenic foci in portal veins
- Thrombus: Lobular echogenic material surrounding catheter, often at tip
- Hepatic extravasation/hematoma/abscess (from UVC): May mimic mass
  - Multilobulated/multiseptated collection of variable echogenicity & heterogeneity
    - TPN collection/abscess may contain fat → hyperechoic rim on US, fat density on CT
  - Regresses after UVC removal, may calcify
- TPN ascites (UVC): Hypoechoic peritoneal fluid ± debris
- Aneurysm/pseudoaneurysm (UAC): Dilation or irregular outpouching of artery with turbulent flow on Doppler

PATHOLOGY

General Features

- UVC complications
  - Thrombosis: 13-30% of UVCs
    - Portal & hepatic veins are at highest risk
  - Hepatic complications: Tip proximal to ductus venosus or in portal vein
    - Vascular perforation, hepatic laceration → hematoma, extravasation of infusion
    - Infusion of hypertonic solution (often TPN) directed into portal venous rather than systemic circulation
      - Chemical irritation → parenchymal necrosis, abscess
    - May develop TPN ascites
  - Cardiac complications: Tip beyond IVC-RA junction
    - Arrhythmia, thrombotic endocarditis, atrial wall perforation with pericardial effusion ± tamponade, hemothorax
  - Up to 30% of UVCs fail prior to completion of UVC-dependent therapy
- UAC complications
  - Thrombosis, arterial aneurysm/pseudoaneurysm
    - Risk to aortic arch branches if tip above T5
    - Risk to abdominal aortic branches if tip at T12-L1
      - SMA: Gut ischemia, necrotizing enterocolitis
      - Renal arteries: Hypertension, kidney injury
    - Aortic thrombosis is more likely with low line
- Infection (UVC or UAC)
  - UVC placement is highest risk factor for neonatal sepsis

CLINICAL ISSUES

Treatment

- In general, reposition or remove malpositioned catheter
- Hepatic collections may require drainage
- Infection necessitates antibiotic therapy
- Incidental UVC or UAC thrombus may be observed (frequent spontaneous resolution)
- Symptomatic or propagating UVC or UAC thrombus: Heparinization ± thrombolytics

SELECTED REFERENCES

1. Edison P et al: Varying clinical presentations of umbilical venous catheter extravasation: a case series. J Paediatr Child Health. 57(7):1123-6, 2021
2. Sobczak A et al: Ultrasound monitoring of umbilical catheters in the neonatal intensive care unit-a prospective observational study. Front Pediatr. 9:665214, 2021
3. Chen HJ et al: Hepatic extravasation complicated by umbilical venous catheterization in neonates: a 5-year, single-center experience. Pediatr Neonatol. 61(1):16-24, 2020
4. Shahroor M et al: Complications associated with low position versus good position umbilical venous catheters in neonates of ≤32 weeks' gestation. Am J Perinatol. ePub, 2020
5. El Ters N et al: Central versus low-lying umbilical venous catheters: a multicenter study of practices and complications. Am J Perinatol. 36(11):1198-204, 2019
6. Derinkuyu BE et al: Hepatic complications of umbilical venous catheters in the neonatal period: the ultrasound spectrum. J Ultrasound Med. 37(6):1335-44, 2018
7. Mutlu M et al: Umbilical venous catheter complications in newborns: a 6-year single-center experience. J Matern Fetal Neonatal Med. 1-6, 2015

Esophageal Intubation

KEY FACTS

TERMINOLOGY

- Inadvertent placement of endotracheal tube (ETT) in esophagus

IMAGING

- Radiography
  - Esophagus normally lies posterior & left of trachea
  - Frontal view
    - Malpositioned ETT overlies esophageal air column, typically left of trachea
      - May directly overlie enteric tube
      - ± deviation of trachea to right
    - Malpositioned ETT may extend caudal to carina
    - Gaseous distention of stomach &/or esophagus
  - Lateral view
    - ETT overlies esophageal air column posterior to trachea
  - 25° right posterior oblique view with head turned right
    - Presents esophagus & trachea relationship en face
    - Facilitates visualization of esophagus to left of trachea
- Ultrasound
  - Point of care confirmation of ETT placement
  - Advantages: No radiation exposure, rapid detection of position in real-time at bedside, less handling of patient, potential for early surfactant delivery
  - Disadvantages: User dependent, lack of widespread availability
  - Technique & findings
    - High-frequency linear transducer is placed transversely on anterior neck just above suprasternal notch
    - Distortion of glottis & trachea is not observed with esophageal intubation
    - Lateral & posteriorly positioned esophagus is stented open by tube with hyperechoic curvilinear anterior wall & posterior acoustic shadowing
  - Ultrasound for esophageal intubation: Sensitivity 93%, specificity 97% in recent metaanalysis

TOP DIFFERENTIAL DIAGNOSES

- Tracheal intubation
  - ETT projects over tracheal air column
  - No significant esophageal distention
- Hypopharyngeal intubation
  - Ineffective ventilation
  - Gastric & esophageal distention
- Right main bronchus intubation
  - Left lung atelectasis
  - Right upper lobe atelectasis if ETT tip is distal to right upper lobe bronchus
- Tracheal perforation
  - Pneumomediastinum or pneumothorax
  - Aberrant lateral deviation of tube
- Tracheal intubation of tracheoesophageal fistula
  - Tip should be positioned distal to fistula
  - Tip may enter fistula, cause esophageal distention

CLINICAL ISSUES

- American College of Emergency Physicians policy for verification of endotracheal intubation
  - Confirm placement with: Direct visualization of tube passing through vocal cords, auscultation of chest & epigastrium, bilateral symmetric chest rise, fogging of ETT with respiration, pulse oximetry, chest radiography, capnography (most accurate)
- Complications of esophageal intubation
  - Hypoxemia, regurgitation, aspiration, cardiac dysrhythmia, death
- Esophageal intubation frequency in pediatrics
  - 28% of all intubation adverse events
  - Immediately recognized in 4.1% of intubations
  - Delayed recognition in 0.19% of intubations
    - Radiology may be 1st to recognize malposition

DIAGNOSTIC CHECKLIST

- Esophageal intubation is emergent finding, potentially fatal
- Immediate communication to clinical team is required

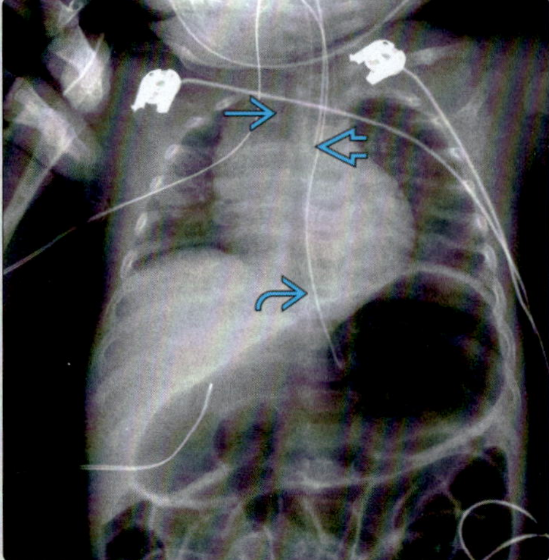

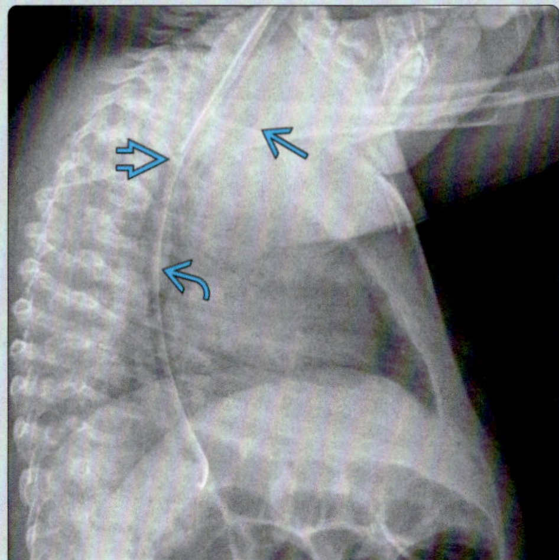

(Left) *AP radiograph in a septic 3-month-old shows the endotracheal tube ➡ to the left of the air-filled trachea ➡, compatible with esophageal intubation. There is associated gaseous distention of the stomach & upper abdominal bowel loops. An enteric tube is also present ➡.* **(Right)** *Lateral radiograph in a 3-month-old who required intubation for a sedated MR demonstrates the endotracheal tube ➡ projecting over the esophagus, posterior to the tracheal air column ➡. An enteric tube is also present ➡.*

ECMO Catheters

KEY FACTS

TERMINOLOGY

- Extracorporeal membrane oxygenation (ECMO): Modified pulmonary or cardiopulmonary bypass circuit
- Deoxygenated blood removed from venous system → oxygenated → returned to circulation via venous [venovenous ECMO (VV-ECMO)] or arterial system [venoarterial ECMO (VA-ECMO)]

IMAGING

- Radiographs to monitor catheter positions, complications
  - Most common VV-ECMO circuit
    - Internal jugular vein (dual- or triple-lumen catheter)
    - 1 or 2 lumina for venous extraction
    - 1 lumen for venous return of oxygenated blood
    - Tip in right atrium (RA) at posterior 8th or 9th rib
  - Most common VA-ECMO circuit
    - Internal jugular vein-common carotid artery (CCA)
      - Venous tip in RA at posterior 8th or 9th rib
      - Arterial tip in CCA origin at 2nd or 3rd posterior rib
  - Other circuits include
    - Femoro-femoral: VA-ECMO or VV-ECMO
    - RA-aorta/pulmonary artery: VA-ECMO
  - Right-sided vessels are favored for cannulation due to more direct central route; requires ligation of vessels
  - Expected radiographic findings
    - Generalized dense pulmonary opacification
      - Does not correlate with severity of lung disease
      - Related to low "rest" ventilator settings & systemic inflammatory response syndrome from bypass
- US to evaluate for intracranial hemorrhage or ischemia, thoracic & abdominal fluid collections
  - Benign enlargement of subarachnoid CSF spaces is common; may resolve after ECMO
- CT for suspicion of ECMO complication, underlying thoracic disease, delay in clinical improvement, &/or to identify & further characterize intracranial lesions beyond head US
- Imaging protocols vary by institution
  - Typically include head US & chest radiographs before & after ECMO is initiated & at specified intervals

PATHOLOGY

- Mechanical complications
  - General: Thrombus in circuit
    - Prevention requires adequate anticoagulation
  - Venous cannula too distal: Peripheral venous return obstruction, blocked sideholes ↓ venous extraction
  - Venous cannula too proximal: Sideholes outside lumen or dislodged → ↑ risk air of emboli, hemorrhage
  - Arterial cannula too distal: Aortic flow obstruction, ↑ left ventricle afterload
  - Arterial cannula too proximal: Inadvertent dislodgement → ↑ risk of hemorrhage
- Clinical complications
  - Intracranial hemorrhage & ischemia are most common
    - 85% of hemorrhages occur in first 72 hours
      - Common locations: Intraparenchymal (64%), posterior fossa (27%)
    - Risk of ischemia ↑ with duration of ECMO
  - Other complications: Lung consolidation, infarction, necrosis ± cavitation, barotrauma, hemothorax, pulmonary emboli; intra-/retroperitoneal hemorrhage, adrenal hemorrhage, solid organ infarct

CLINICAL ISSUES

- Indications: Severe reversible cardiac &/or respiratory failure: Meconium aspiration, congenital diaphragmatic hernia, pulmonary hypertension, sepsis, cardiomyopathy, preoperative stabilization of congenital heart disease
  - Respiratory failure + normal cardiac function → VV-ECMO
  - Cardiac or cardiopulmonary failure → VA-ECMO
- Contraindications: < 34-weeks gestation, birth weight < 2 kg, mechanical ventilation > 10-14 days, significant coagulopathy, uncorrectable congenital heart defects, lethal anomalies, major intracranial hemorrhage, irreversible brain damage

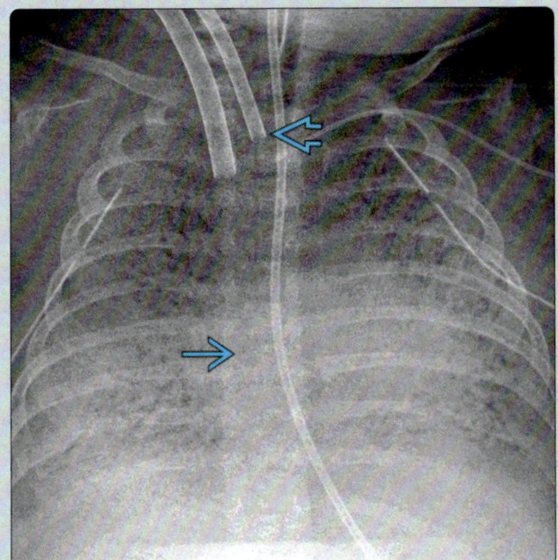

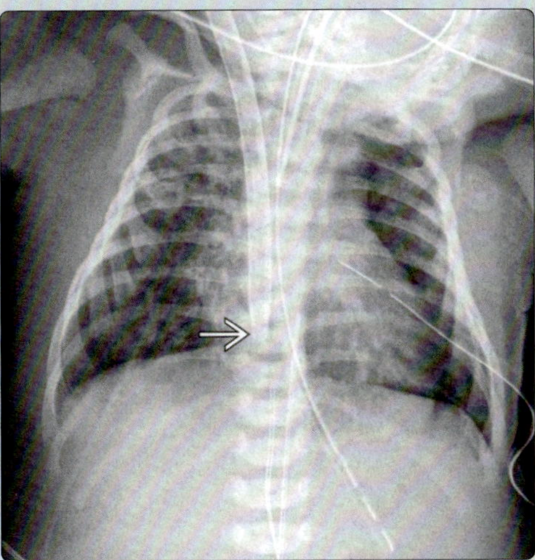

(Left) *AP chest radiograph in a 4-month-old with sepsis shows a venous ECMO cannula radiopaque marker projecting over the right atrium at T8 ➔. The arterial catheter projects over the common carotid artery origin at T2-T3 ➔. The pulmonary opacities & interstitial emphysema relate to underlying pulmonary disease.* **(Right)** *AP chest radiograph of a 5-day-old term infant with meconium aspiration shows the venovenous ECMO cannula tip in the right atrium ➔ at the T9 level.*

KEY FACTS

TERMINOLOGY

- Vascular line inserted percutaneously into peripheral vein with tip residing in central vein

IMAGING

- Optimal upper extremity tip position: Lower 1/3 of superior vena cava (SVC), near SVC-right atrial (RA) junction
  - SVC-RA junction: ~ 2 vertebral bodies + disc spaces ("vertebral units") below carina
  - Approximate SVC boundaries: Superior at right tracheobronchial angle, inferior just below right superior cardiac border
  - SVC is always to right of trachea
    - Descent left of trachea suggests venous or arterial malposition (or possibly left-sided SVC)
      - Must confirm presence of left SVC with cross-sectional imaging prior to PICC use
  - Tip is most cranial when arm is at straight 90° abduction
  - Tip appears caudal with supine position & poor inspiration
- Optimal lower extremity PICC position: IVC-RA junction
  - IVC-RA junction: ~ T8 or T9, close to level of diaphragm
  - Consider ascending lumber or inferior epigastric vein malposition with kink or bend, zigzag paraspinal course, or failure of left approach PICC to cross midline at L5

PATHOLOGY

- Risk of complications is 8x greater if tip is noncentral
- Complications include: Thrombosis, thrombophlebitis, infection, sepsis, pulmonary embolus, mechanical malfunction, extravasation, arrhythmia, myocardial perforation, arterial placement with distal tissue necrosis

CLINICAL ISSUES

- Indicated for long-term central venous access (1-8 weeks): Antibiotics, TPN, repeated transfusions, short course of chemotherapy, frequent venous sampling, central venous pressure measurements, tenuous venous access

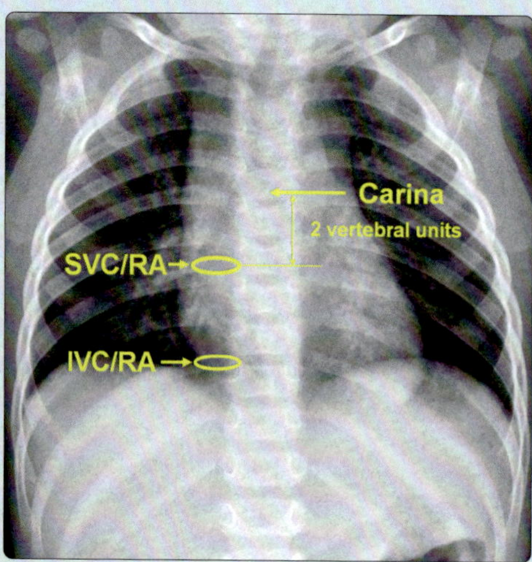

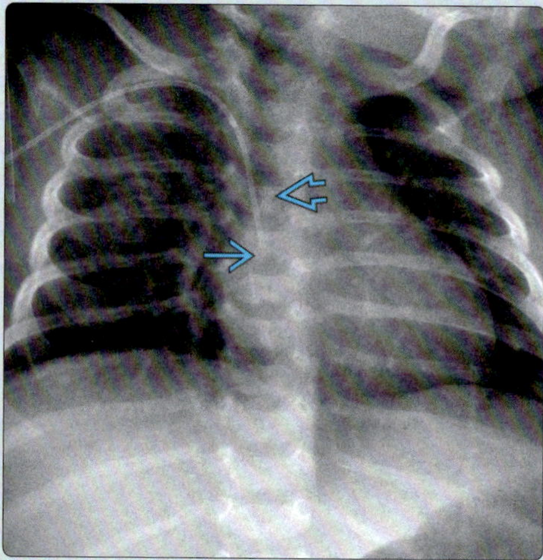

(Left) *AP chest radiograph depicts commonly used radiographic definitions of the superior vena cava (SVC)-right atrium (RA) & inferior vena cava (IVC)-RA junctions.* **(Right)** *Supine chest radiograph in a 3-month-old with meningitis shows a right upper extremity peripherally inserted central catheter (PICC) tip ➡ projecting ~ 2 vertebral bodies below the carina ➡ in the region of the SVC-RA junction.*

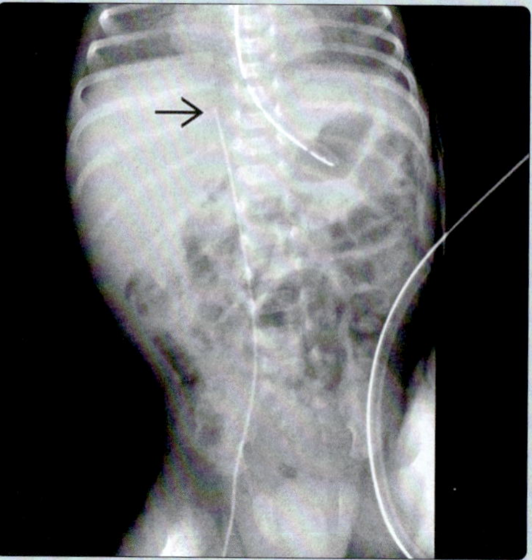

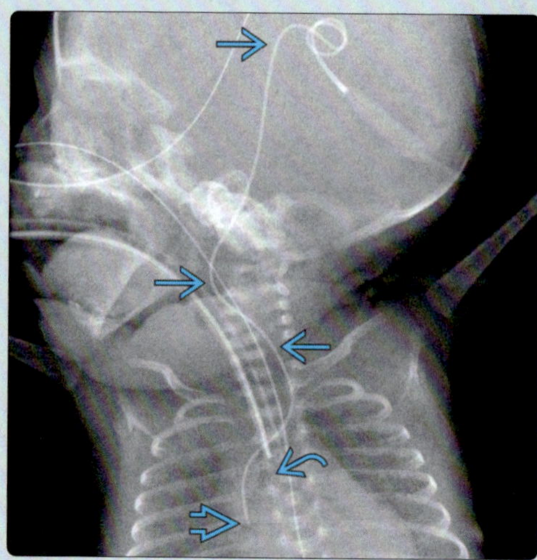

(Left) *AP abdominal radiograph shows a right lower extremity PICC tip ➡ in an appropriate position in the IVC above the level of the renal veins & below the right atrium.* **(Right)** *Supine chest radiograph in a premature infant demonstrates a scalp PICC ➡ with its tip ➡ projecting ~ 2 vertebral units below the carina ➡ in the expected region of the SVC-RA junction.*

TERMINOLOGY

Definitions

- Peripherally inserted central catheter (PICC): Vascular line inserted percutaneously into peripheral vein with tip residing in central vein

IMAGING

General Features

- Location
  - Most common insertion sites
    - Upper extremity veins: Basilic, cephalic, brachial
    - Lower extremity veins: Saphenous; occasionally deep veins used, especially in newborns
    - Scalp veins are used if extremity access is difficult
  - Tip considered central if in
    - Right atrium (RA): Not recommended due to risks of perforation & arrhythmia (specific to PICCs)
    - Superior vena cava (SVC), inferior vena cava (IVC) above renal veins
    - Brachiocephalic veins (controversial)
  - Central tip position allows for effective infusion with appropriate hemodilution given greater blood flow

Radiographic Findings

- Optimal upper extremity PICC position: Lower 1/3 of SVC, near SVC-RA junction
  - Definition of SVC on AP chest radiograph is controversial as use of landmarks varies
    - Best estimation of SVC-RA junction: 2 vertebral units (bodies + disc spaces) below level of carina
    - Superior SVC boundary: Right tracheobronchial angle
    - Inferior SVC boundary: Below right superior cardiac border
  - SVC remains right of trachea, even on rotated image
- Optimal lower extremity PICC position: IVC close to IVC-RA junction, above renal veins
  - Landmarks on supine radiograph
    - IVC-RA junction: ~ T8 or T9, close to diaphragm
    - Renal vein entrance to IVC: ~ L1
    - Common iliac vein confluence at IVC: ~ L5
- Malposition examples
  - Arterial: PICC descends left of trachea/midline (upper approach) or ascends left of midline (lower approach)
  - Internal jugular vein: Tip directed cephalad into neck
  - Left SVC: PICC descends left of trachea, typically from left upper extremity approach
    - Must be confirmed with prior or subsequent cross-sectional imaging (including echocardiography) before use
    - Acceptable except in rare circumstances of left SVC draining into left atrium
  - Ascending lumbar veins
    - Arise from common iliac veins at L5-S1
    - Left approach PICC fails to cross midline at L5
    - Bend or kink at L4-L5 with paraspinal zigzag course
    - Marked posterior deviation at L4-S1 on lateral view
  - Inferior epigastric veins
    - Arise from external iliac veins
    - Anterior course on lateral view

Imaging Recommendations

- Protocol advice
  - If position is unclear, inject contrast during fluoroscopy
    - If arterial position is being questioned, retract tip to lateral subclavian prior to injection (to avoid neck arteries)

PATHOLOGY

General Features

- Complications: 1-19 per 1,000 catheter days
  - Infection, sepsis (↑ with PICC duration)
  - Arterial placement can lead to distal tissue necrosis
  - Pulmonary embolus (air, thrombus, catheter fragment)
  - Mechanical malfunction (catheter damage, extravasation or leakage, unplanned catheter removal)
  - Thrombosis & thrombophlebitis
  - Arrhythmia or myocardial perforation if tip is in RA
  - Spinal cord injury if tip is in lumbar vein
- Risk of complications is 8x greater if tip noncentral
  - ↓ vein diameter → ↓ blood flow/hemodilution → ↑ turbulence + prolonged intimal contact of infusates → ↑ risk of endothelial injury

CLINICAL ISSUES

Indications

- Need for intermediate or long-term central venous access (1-8 weeks): Antibiotics, TPN, repeated transfusions, short course of chemotherapy, frequent venous sampling, central venous pressure measurement
- Tenuous venous access otherwise

DIAGNOSTIC CHECKLIST

Consider

- Each institution should develop standard PICC placement/verification protocols, nomenclature, & communication criteria
- PICC position varies with respiratory motion & arm position

Reporting Tips

- Avoid phrase "cavoatrial junction" as this could represent either SVC-RA or IVC-RA junction

SELECTED REFERENCES

1. Acun C et al: Peripherally inserted central cathether migration in neonates: incidence, timing and risk factors. J Neonatal Perinatal Med. 14(3):411-7, 2021
2. Dhillon SS et al: Arrhythmias in children with peripherally inserted central catheters (PICCs). Pediatr Cardiol. 41(2):407-13, 2020
3. Sertic AJ et al: Perforations associated with peripherally inserted central catheters in a neonatal population. Pediatr Radiol. 48(1):109-19, 2018
4. Concepcion NDP et al: Current updates in catheters, tubes and drains in the pediatric chest: a practical evaluation approach. Eur J Radiol. 95:409-17, 2017
5. Goldwasser B et al: Non-central peripherally inserted central catheters in neonatal intensive care: complication rates and longevity of catheters relative to tip position. Pediatr Radiol. 47(12):1676-81, 2017
6. Gnannt R et al: Variables decreasing tip movement of peripherally inserted central catheters in pediatric patients. Pediatr Radiol. 46(11):1532-8, 2016
7. Baskin KM et al: Cavoatrial junction and central venous anatomy: implications for central venous access tip position. J Vasc Interv Radiol. 19(3):359-65, 2008
8. Racadio JM et al: Pediatric peripherally inserted central catheters: complication rates related to catheter tip location. Pediatrics. 107(2):E28, 2001

Viral Chest Infection

KEY FACTS

TERMINOLOGY

- Viral infection may involve airways &/or lung parenchyma (alveoli, interstitium)
- Bronchiolitis: Acute inflammation & necrosis of epithelial cells lining small airways with ↑ mucus production
  - Classically < 2 years of age
- Other terms: Viral pneumonia, lower respiratory tract infection, peribronchial pneumonia

IMAGING

- Primary goal of chest radiography: Differentiate viral airway infection from bacterial pneumonia (which requires antibiotics)
  - 92% negative predictive value for bacterial pneumonia
- Best imaging clues for viral airway infection
  - ↑ peribronchial markings
    - Radiating coarse linear or "dirty" perihilar opacities
    - "Doughnuts" of circumferentially thickened bronchial walls (viewed in cross section)
  - Hyperinflation: Depression of hemidiaphragms with downward sloping on lateral view; ↑ AP chest diameter on lateral view; ± convex bulging of lungs between ribs
  - Subsegmental atelectasis, possibly multifocal
  - Lack of focal/lobar consolidation or pleural effusion
- Best imaging clues for viral parenchymal involvement
  - Interstitial, nodular, or patchy ground-glass opacities

CLINICAL ISSUES

- Pathogens detected in hospitalized pediatric pneumonia patients: Viral 73%, bacterial 15%
- Most common viral etiologies differ by age
  - RSV < 2 years, rhinovirus > 2 years
- Treatment
  - Antibiotics for concomitant bacterial infection
  - Nebulized hypertonic saline in hospitalized infants may shorten length of stay
  - Antiviral therapy where indicated

(Left) *Frontal chest radiograph in a 2-year-old with viral bronchiolitis shows symmetric, mild hyperinflation with ↑ perihilar peribronchial markings, as is commonly seen with small airways infection.* **(Right)** *PA view of the chest in an 11-month-old shows mildly hyperinflated lungs with ↑ perihilar peribronchial opacities, consistent with bronchiolitis secondary to known human metapneumovirus infection.*

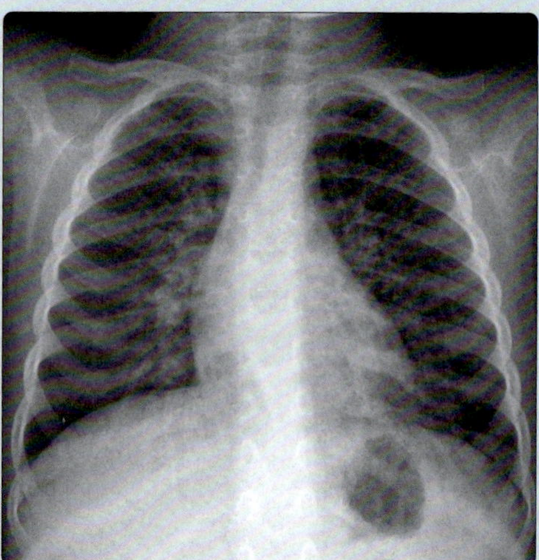

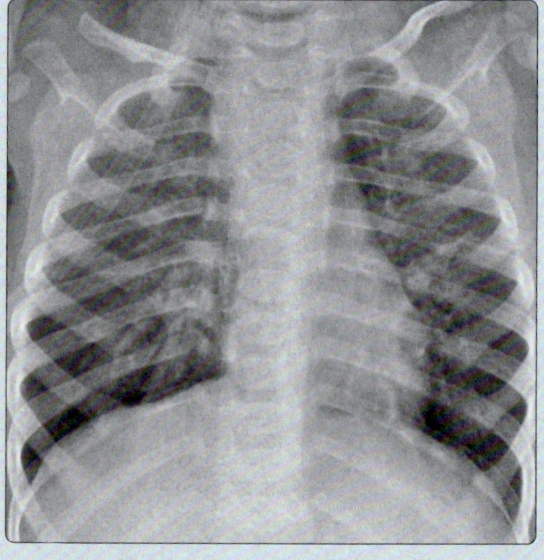

(Left) *AP radiograph in a wheezing infant shows hyperinflated lungs with ↑ rope-like perihilar markings, consistent with viral airways disease. There is no focal lung consolidation.* **(Right)** *Lateral radiograph in the same infant shows marked hyperinflation with flattening of the hemidiaphragms ➔ (much more evident than on the corresponding frontal view) & widening of the AP diameter of the chest. Also note the ↑ markings radiating from the hila.*

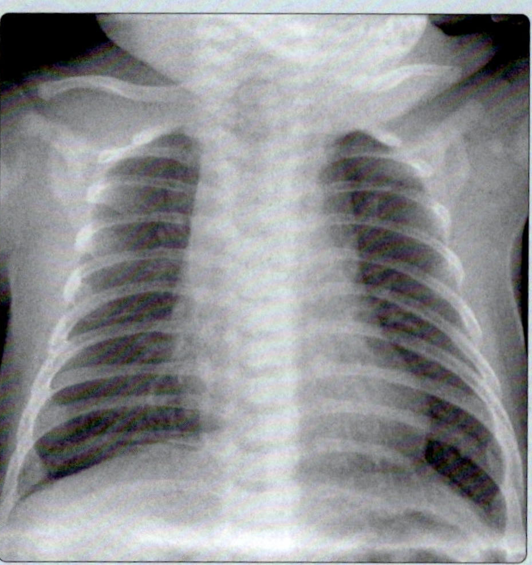

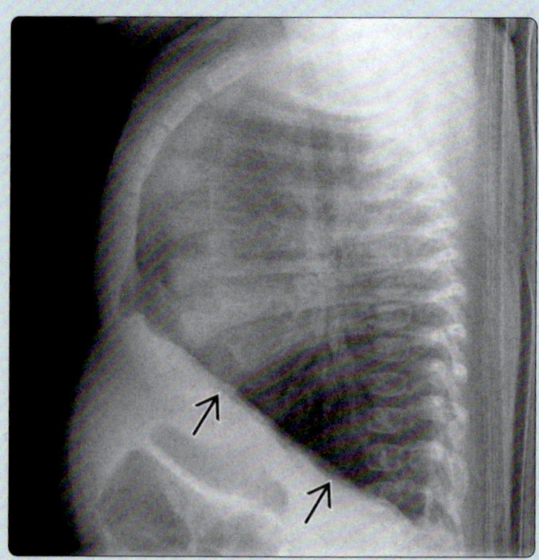

TERMINOLOGY

Definitions

- Terminology varies, can be confusing
- Bronchiolitis (per American Academy of Pediatrics): Viral lower respiratory tract infection in infants affecting small airways with inflammation, edema, & epithelial necrosis
- Lower respiratory tract infection may describe findings identical to bronchiolitis in patients ≥ 2 years old but may also refer to any infection of lower airways & parenchyma
- Viral pneumonia may refer to viral infection of lung parenchyma ± airways
- Peribronchial pneumonia is sometimes used to differentiate airways infection from parenchymal involvement
- Lower airways disease includes viral airways infection as well as asthma

IMAGING

General Features

- Best diagnostic clue
  - ↑ peribronchial markings, hyperinflation, interlobular septal thickening, & ground-glass densities
    - Dominant feature & distribution varies with pathogen
  - Lymphadenopathy, effusion, & pneumothorax are atypical

Radiographic Findings

- Primary goal: Differentiate viral airways infection from bacterial pneumonia
- Small airways viral infection
  - Lack of focal dense geographic, round, or "fluffy" lung consolidation (hallmark of bacterial infection)
  - ↑ peribronchial markings/↑ number of visible bronchi
    - Symmetric, coarse linear markings radiating from hila
    - ↑ thickness of bronchial walls appearing as "doughnuts" in cross section
    - Central lungs may appear "dirty" or "busy"
    - Hila may appear prominent on lateral view
    - Somewhat subjective finding
  - Hyperinflation
    - Hyperlucency
    - Depression of diaphragm > 10 posterior ribs or > 6 anterior ribs
    - Flattening/downward sloping hemidiaphragms
    - ↑ AP chest diameter (in infants, chest wider than tall on lateral view)
    - ± convex bulging of lungs between ribs
    - Less common > 2 years old (as bronchi are larger & less prone to narrowing or obstruction by inflammation)
  - Subsegmental atelectasis
    - Wedge-shaped or triangular opacities, often narrow
    - Commonly misinterpreted as bacterial pneumonia
- Parenchymal involvement
  - Interstitial nodular or patchy/hazy opacities
  - Lobar consolidation rarely occurs
  - Associated findings of airways infection

CT Findings

- Not used primarily to make diagnosis of viral disease but may be obtained in patient with unclear clinical/imaging presentation or concerns for complications
- Small airways viral infection
  - Prominent, ill-defined hila & peribronchial markings radiating into lung
  - Bronchial & bronchiolar wall thickening
  - Mosaic attenuation: Patchy heterogeneity of attenuation due to hypoventilation & air-trapping
- Parenchymal involvement
  - Interlobular septal thickening
  - Patchy, ill-defined consolidation
  - Ground-glass opacities (GGO)
  - Nodules, micronodules
  - ± findings of small airways infection

General Features of Epidemic & Pandemic Pathogens

- SARS-CoV-2 (COVID-19)
  - Bilateral peripheral/subpleural GGO ± consolidation with lower lung zone predominance
  - Reverse halo sign: Consolidation with rim of GGO
  - Associated with multisystem inflammatory syndrome
- SARS-CoV
  - Uni-or multifocal, peripheral or peripheral & central GGO ± consolidation with mid & lower lower lung zone predominance
- MERS
  - Bilateral peripheral GGO ± consolidation with lower lung zone predominance
  - Interstitial reticular opacities
  - Pleural effusion & pneumothorax are more common in fatal cases
- H1N1
  - Bilateral bronchovascular thickening, multifocal central GGO ± consolidation with lower lung zone predominance
  - Peribronchial thickening & peribronchovascular nodular densities
  - Pneumomediastinum is seen with some cases

Imaging Recommendations

- Best imaging tool
  - Chest radiographs (frontal & lateral)
    - Goal: Antibiotic therapy for all children with bacterial pneumonia while minimizing unnecessary antibiotic administration (for isolated viral infection)
      - Positive predictive value (PPV) for identifying bacterial pneumonia 30%
      - Negative predictive value (NPV) for excluding bacterial pneumonia 92%
    - Difficult to differentiate viral from bacterial pneumonia (i.e., lung parenchymal infection) on imaging
      - One study showed lobar infiltrate in 15% of exclusively viral pneumonia & exclusively interstitial infiltrate in 28% with bacterial pneumonia

DIFFERENTIAL DIAGNOSIS

Bacterial Pneumonia

- Focal/lobar lung consolidation > interstitial infiltrate

- Confluent geographic, round, or fluffy opacities
- Pleural effusions (more common than viral)
- Lack of ↑ peribronchial markings or hyperinflation

Asthma

- Small airways inflammation with ↑ peribronchial markings & hyperinflation (common to asthma & viral infection)
- Primary asthma diagnosis is difficult to establish in young children

Bronchial Foreign Body

- May present with wheezing very similar to viral disease
- Asymmetric hyperinflation is characteristic
  - Affected lung volume is static throughout respiratory cycle
- Foreign body is often radiographically occult

Left-to-Right Cardiovascular Shunts

- In infants, left-to-right shunts with ↑ pulmonary arterial flow may mimic ↑ peribronchial markings
- Shunts have associated cardiomegaly (& may cause air-trapping)

Miliary Tuberculosis

- Diffuse, small nodules; thickened, interlobular septa
- Lymphadenopathy (may be low in attenuation)
- History of sick contact with TB
- Very uncommon in young children

PATHOLOGY

General Features

- Etiology
  - Acute inflammation & necrosis of epithelial cells lining small airways with ↑ mucus production
  - ↓ caliber of small, relatively compliant airway lumina significantly ↑ resistance to airflow in infants
  - Occlusion of airways results in hyperinflation & foci of subsegmental atelectasis
  - Parenchymal findings vary: Interstitial pneumonitis with lymphocytic infiltration, infection of alveolar epithelium, diffuse alveolar damage, desquamation of pneumocytes, hyaline-membrane formation, alveolar hemorrhage
  - Typical pathogens
    - Bronchiolitis: RSV > rhinovirus, adenovirus, influenza > coronavirus, human metapneumovirus (hMPV), parainfluenza
      - Multiple viruses in up to 25%
    - Hospitalization-inducing, community-acquired pneumonia: RSV, rhinovirus > hMPV, adenovirus, *Mycoplasma pneumoniae*, parainfluenza, influenza, coronavirus, *Streptococcus pneumoniae*, *Staphylococcus aureus*, *S. pyogenes*

CLINICAL ISSUES

Presentation

- Signs & symptoms
  - Bronchiolitis: Rhinorrhea, cough, tachypnea, wheezing, rales, ↑ respiratory effort (grunting, nasal flaring, intercostal/subcostal retractions)
  - Community-acquired pneumonia: Cough, fever, anorexia, dyspnea, wheezing (up to 62%)
    - Difficult to differentiate bacterial from viral parenchymal infection based on physical exam or laboratory tests

Demographics

- Age
  - Typical striking radiographic findings of viral disease are more common in young children (< 5 years of age)
- Epidemiology
  - Bronchiolitis: Most common cause of hospitalization in 1st year of life
  - Viruses cause majority of chest infections in preschool children (4 months-5 years of age)
    - < 2 years old: RSV is most common
    - > 2 years old: Rhinovirus is most common
  - Pneumonia-related hospitalization from multicenter prospective study
    - Greatest in children < 5 years old
    - Viral in 73%, bacterial in 15%
  - Predisposing conditions for severe viral chest infections: Age < 6 months, prematurity, congenital heart disease, immunosuppression/immunodeficiency, asthma

Natural History & Prognosis

- Resolution of symptoms over time, typically days to weeks

Treatment

- Antibiotics only for concomitant bacterial infection
- Bronchiolitis
  - Nebulized hypertonic saline in infants may shorten hospitalization by increasing mucociliary clearance
  - Oxygen supplementation if saturations < 90%
  - Palivizumab (RSV prophylaxis, not vaccine): Given in 1st year of life to infants born before 29-weeks gestation or infants with hemodynamically significant heart disease or chronic lung disease of prematurity
  - Routine use of albuterol & nebulized epinephrine are not recommended
  - Corticosteroid use is not supported
- Clinical pneumonia with viral pathogen
  - Hospitalization for hypoxemia or respiratory distress
  - Antiviral therapy where indicated

DIAGNOSTIC CHECKLIST

Consider

- Consider aspirated foreign body if lung volumes are asymmetric

SELECTED REFERENCES

1. Foust AM et al: Pediatric SARS, H1N1, MERS, EVALI, and now Coronavirus disease (COVID-19) pneumonia: what radiologists need to know. AJR Am J Roentgenol. 215(3):736-44, 2020
2. Koo HJ et al: Radiographic and CT features of viral pneumonia. Radiographics. 38(3):719-39, 2018
3. Niles D et al: Retrospective review of clinical and chest x-ray findings in children admitted to a community hospital for respiratory syncytial virus infection. Clin Pediatr (Phila). 57(14):1686-92, 2018
4. Hilmes MA et al: Chest radiographic features of human metapneumovirus infection in pediatric patients. Pediatr Radiol. 47(13):1745-50, 2017
5. Winant AJ et al: Current updates on pediatric pulmonary infections. Semin Roentgenol. 52(1):35-42, 2017
6. Ralston SL et al: Clinical practice guideline: the diagnosis, management, and prevention of bronchiolitis. Pediatrics. 134(5):e1474-502, 2014

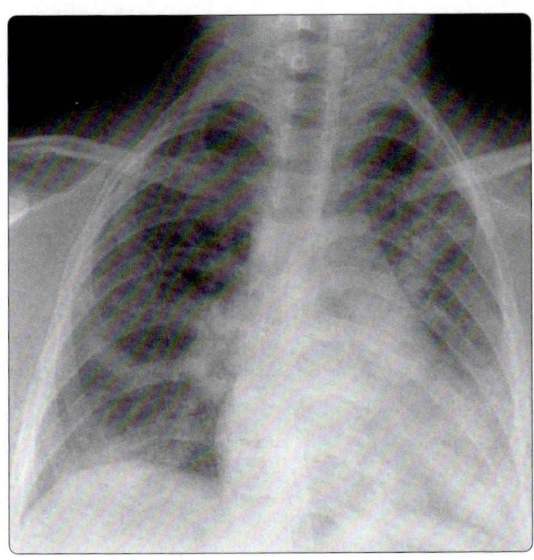

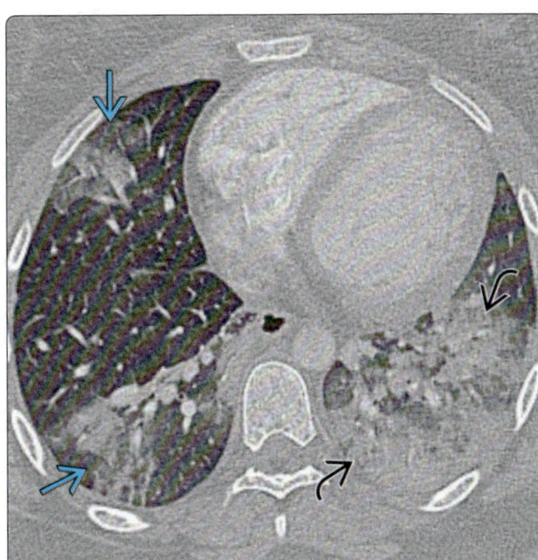

(Left) *Frontal radiograph in a 14-year-old with shortness of breath demonstrates patchy peripheral & basilar opacities.* **(Right)** *Axial CECT in the same patient depicts lower lung zone predominant peripheral patchy ground-glass densities ➡ mixed with consolidation as well as more confluent left lower lobe consolidation ➡. The patient tested positive for COVID-19.*

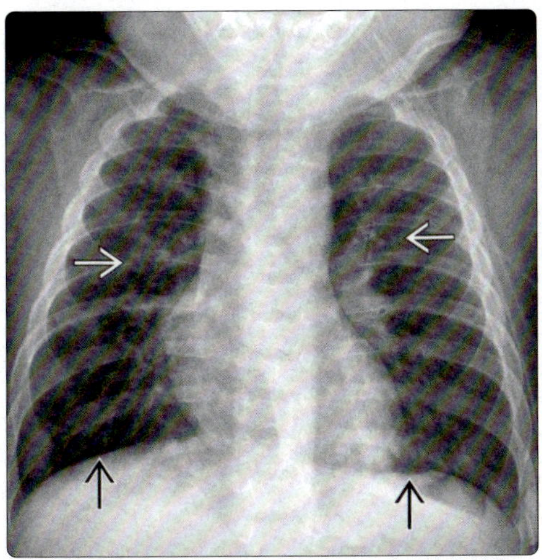

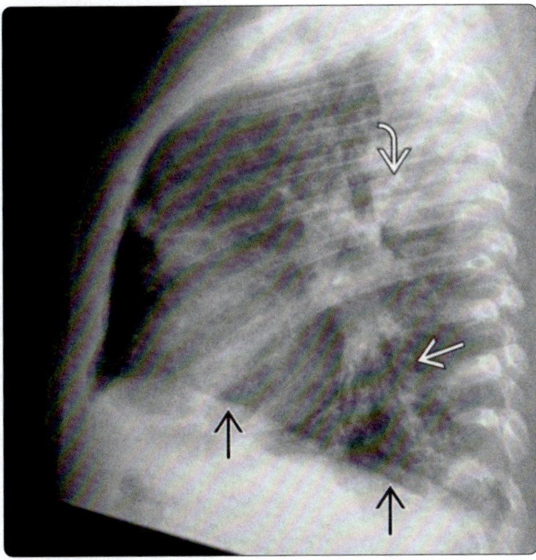

(Left) *Frontal chest radiograph in a 5-month-old patient with cough & difficulty breathing shows bilateral "dirty" perihilar peribronchial opacities ➡ & lung hyperinflation with diaphragm depression ➡, consistent with bronchiolitis.* **(Right)** *Lateral radiograph in the same patient shows linear opacities extending from the hila ➡, thickened bronchial walls ➡, & downward sloping of the flattened hemidiaphragms ➡. Note the widened AP dimension of the chest.*

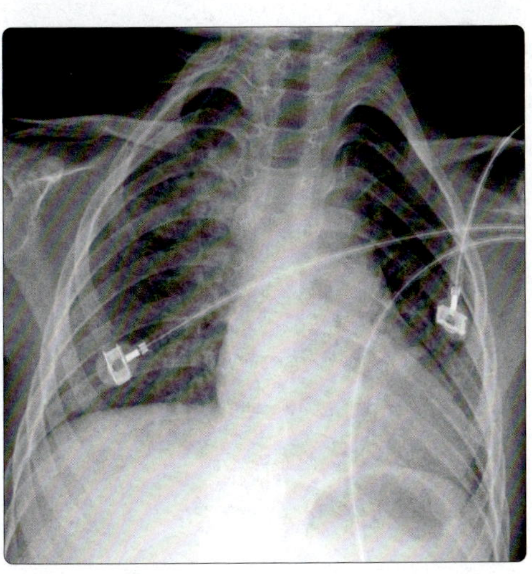

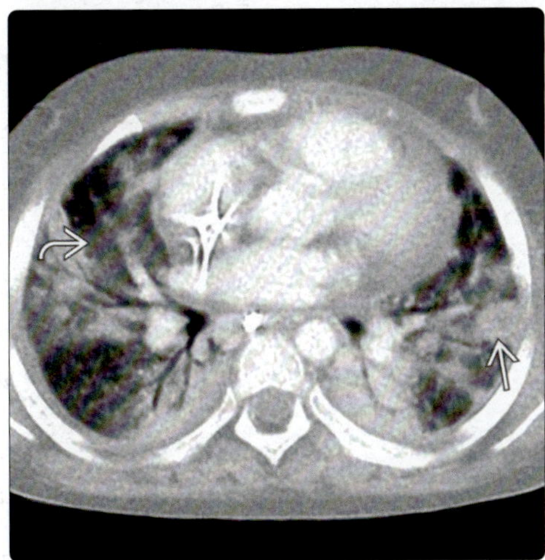

(Left) *Frontal view of the chest in a 6-year-old with known influenza infection demonstrates bilateral ↑ perihilar peribronchial & reticulonodular opacities.* **(Right)** *Axial CECT in a 7-year-old patient with influenza A shows bilateral, patchy, consolidative ➡ & ground-glass ➡ opacities.*

COVID-19/MIS-C

KEY FACTS

TERMINOLOGY

- COVID-19: Acute infection with SARS-CoV2
- MIS-C: Condition characterized by fever, inflammation, & multiorgan dysfunction that has temporal association with SARS-CoV-2 infection

IMAGING

- COVID-19
  - Chest: Bilateral or unilateral peripheral subpleural &/or peribronchial lower lobe-predominant ground-glass opacities (GGO) ± consolidation, bronchial wall thickening, halo sign
    - Uncommon features: Nodules, cavitation, pleural effusions
  - Neuro: ADEM-like imaging pattern, myelitis, neuritis, cerebrovascular complications
- MIS-C
  - Cardiac in 86.5%: Left ventricular (LV) dysfunction, shock, myocarditis, coronary artery dilatation/aneurysm
  - GI: Ascites, RLQ inflammation, bowel wall thickening, pancreatitis, hepatomegaly, splenomegaly, gallbladder sludge, pericholecystic fluid, lymphadenopathy
  - Chest: Pulmonary edema, pleural effusions, GGO related to ARDS, pulmonary embolism
  - Neuro: ↑ T2 signal lesions + restricted diffusion in corpus callosum, restricted diffusion in thalami, focal cerebral arteriopathy, ADEM-like findings, myelitis, neuritis, cerebrovascular complications, myositis of face & neck

CLINICAL ISSUES

- COVID-19
  - Initial data showed less severe disease in children overall, though rates of infection & severity of disease have been affected by newer variants & vaccination rates/eligibility
- MIS-C
  - > 60% require ICU & vasopressors, mortality 1.8%
  - LV ejection fraction normalizes in most 1-2 weeks after presentation

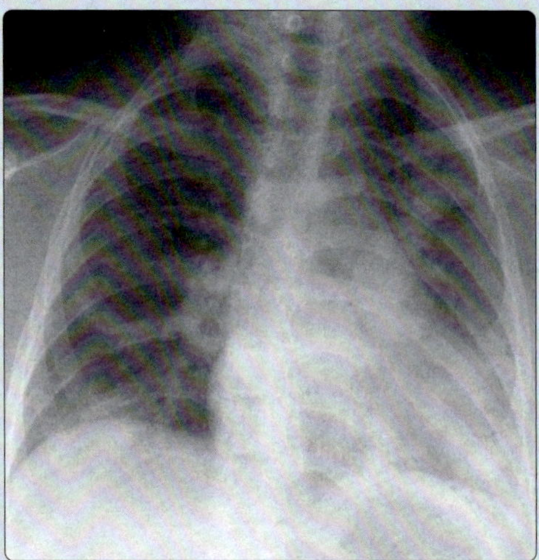

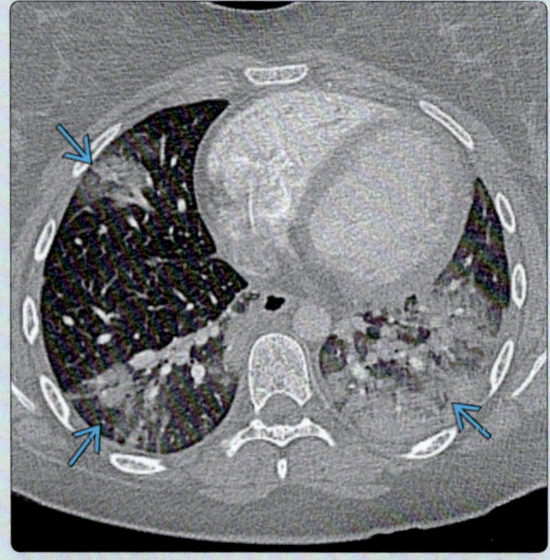

(Left) *Frontal radiograph in a 14-year-old patient with shortness of breath & fever demonstrates hazy & patchy bilateral pulmonary opacities.* **(Right)** *Axial CECT in the same patient shows bilateral lower lung zone-predominant ground-glass & consolidative densities ➔. The patient tested positive for COVID-19 on nasopharyngeal RT-PCR. Other features seen in pediatric cases of COVID-19 include bronchial wall thickening & the halo sign (not shown).*

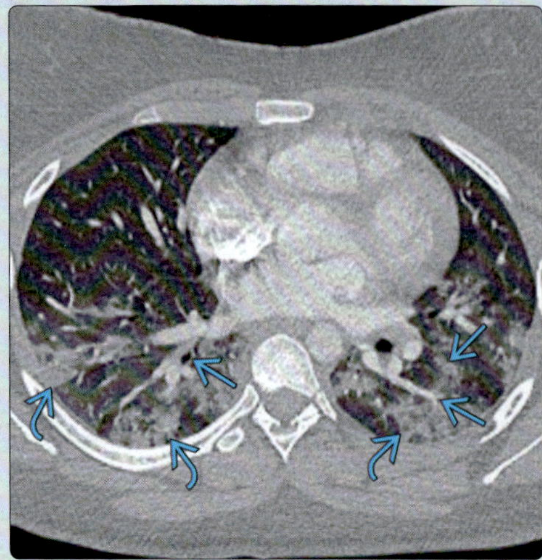

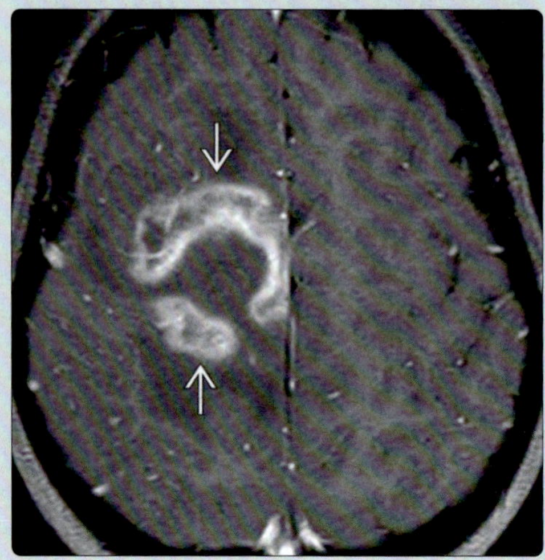

(Left) *Axial CECT in a 17-year-old demonstrates bilateral symmetric lower lung zone-predominant ground-glass & patchy densities ↷. Bronchial wall thickening ➔ is also noted.* **(Right)** *Axial T1 C+ FS MR in 9-year-old with left-sided weakness shows a right cerebral lesion with cortical enhancement ➔ & hemorrhagic necrosis (confirmed on T2 & SWI with minimal precontrast T1 shortening) due to COVID-19-associated vasculitis & infarction.*

TERMINOLOGY

Definitions

- COVID-19: Severe acute respiratory syndrome caused by SARS-CoV-2 virus
- Multisystem inflammatory syndrome in children (MIS-C): Condition characterized by fever, inflammation, & multiorgan dysfunction that has temporal association with SARS-CoV-2 infection

IMAGING

Radiographic Findings

- COVID-19
  - Bilateral or unilateral peripheral lower lobe-predominant patchy consolidation & ground-glass opacities (GGO)
- MIS-C
  - Cardiomegaly, pulmonary edema, pleural effusions, acute respiratory distress syndrome (ARDS)

CT Findings

- COVID-19
  - Bilateral or unilateral peripheral subpleural &/or peribronchial lower lobe-predominant GGO ± consolidation
  - Bronchial wall thickening (more common in children compared to adults)
  - Halo sign: Round consolidative opacity with rim of GGO
  - Uncommon: Pulmonary nodules, pleural effusions, cavitation, lymphadenopathy
- MIS-C
  - Chest: Pulmonary edema, pleural effusions, GGO related to ARDS, pulmonary embolism, lower lobe opacities
  - Cardiac: Cardiomegaly, coronary artery ectasia/aneurysm, pericardial effusion
  - GI: Ascites, right lower quadrant (RLQ) inflammation, bowel wall thickening, pancreatitis, hepatomegaly, splenomegaly, gallbladder sludge &/or wall thickening, pericholecystic fluid, lymphadenopathy

MR Findings

- COVID-19
  - Neurologic
    - Acute disseminated encephalomyelitis (ADEM)-like imaging pattern: Patchy ↑ T2 involving gray & white matter ± enhancement or diffusion restriction
    - Myelitis: Long-segment central cord ↑ T2
      - Rarely can rapidly progress to acute necrotizing myelitis with cord edema, enhancement, diffusion restriction, & hemorrhage
    - Neuritis: Enhancement of cranial/spinal nerves
- MIS-C
  - Cardiac
    - ↓ left ventricle ejection fraction (LVEF)
    - Valvular dysfunction
    - Myocarditis: Myocardial edema with ↑ T2 signal globally or at basal septal segments
  - Neurologic
    - Encephalopathy: ↑ T2 ± restricted diffusion in corpus callosum (splenium + genu), restricted diffusion in bilateral lateral thalamic nuclei
    - Focal cerebral arteriopathy: Cerebral artery stenosis, wall thickening, & concentric contrast enhancement
    - Susceptibility-induced signal drop-out due to parenchymal microthrombi
    - Myositis of neck & face musculature
    - ADEM-like imaging pattern, myelitis, neuritis

Ultrasonographic Findings

- COVID-19
  - Lung findings: Pleural irregularity, vertical artifact, confluent B lines, subpleural consolidation
- MIS-C
  - Echocardiography: Coronary artery ectasia/aneurysm, ↓ LVEF, LV diastolic dysfunction, ↑ echogenicity of interventricular septum & pericardium, valve dysfunction
  - GI: Ascites, RLQ inflammation, bowel wall thickening, pancreatitis, hepatomegaly, splenomegaly, gallbladder sludge, pericholecystic fluid, lymphadenopathy
  - Genitourinary: Echogenic kidneys

Imaging Recommendations

- COVID-19
  - Imaging is not indicated for screening or for known or suspected COVID-19 with mild disease without risk factors for progression
  - Chest radiograph is appropriate for initial imaging for pediatric patients with moderate-to-severe known/suspected COVID-19
  - Chest radiograph & CT can be considered for pediatric patients with known/suspected COVID-19 & worsening disease or lack of response to therapy
- American College of Rheumatology Clinical Guidance for Pediatric Patients with MIS-C
  - Imaging of chest, abdomen, &/or CNS as needed
  - Echocardiogram at diagnosis & during clinical follow-up & repeated at minimum of 7-14 days & 4-6 weeks after presentation; LV dysfunction & coronary artery aneurysm will require more frequent follow-up
  - Cardiac MR may be indicated 2-6 months after MIS-C diagnosis with significant transient LV dysfunction
  - Cardiac CT if suspicion of distal coronary artery aneurysm not well seen on echocardiogram

DIFFERENTIAL DIAGNOSIS

COVID-19 DDx

- **Other infectious pneumonias**
  - Bacterial: Typically focal, single segment or lobe
  - Fungal: Nodules, cavitation, air crescent sign
  - Viral (influenza): Centrilobular nodules
- **E-cigarette vaping-associated lung injury (EVALI)**
  - Subpleural sparing
  - Centrilobular nodules & GGO
  - Atoll sign
- **ADEM**
  - Similar imaging but may not meet clinical definition

Multisystem Inflammatory Syndrome in Children DDx

- **Kawasaki disease (KD)**
  - More common ≤ 5 years old
  - LV dysfunction & shock are less common in KD (~ 10%)

- Neurologic & GI findings are less common in KD
- KD is more common in patients of Asian descent, whereas MIS-C is more common in patients of African & Hispanic descent
- **Toxic shock syndrome**
  - Toxin-mediated systemic disease with shock & multiorgan failure caused by *Staphylococcus aureus* & *Streptococcus pyogenes*
- **Hemophagocytic lymphohistiocytosis (HLH)**
  - Gene-mediated or infection-/malignancy-triggered systemic hyperinflammation
  - Hemophagocytosis in liver, marrow, spleen, lymph nodes
- **Severe COVID-19 with hyperinflammation**
  - Respiratory symptoms are more prominent
  - MIS-C typically occurs 3-6 weeks after SARS-CoV2 exposure
- **Myocarditis of other etiologies**
  - Lack multisystem findings of MIS-C & temporal association with COVID-19
- **Infectious/inflammatory enterocolitis & appendicitis**
  - Lack multisystem findings of MIS-C & temporal association with COVID-19
- **ADEM**
  - Similar imaging but may not meet clinical definition
  - No temporal association with COVID-19
- **Postviral autoimmune encephalitis of other etiologies**
  - Similar encephalitis is also seen with herpes & West Nile virus infections
- **Other pediatric arteriopathies with acute stroke**
  - Moyamoya disease, arterial dissection, vasculitis

PATHOLOGY

General Features

- Single-stranded RNA virus
- Respiratory droplet transmission
- SARS-CoV2 binds ACE2 receptor & transmembrane serine protease 2 (TMPRSS2) & ↑ expression of proinflammatory cytokine IL-6, IL-8, & TNF-α
- ACE2 receptors are also found in heart, intestinal smooth muscle, liver, kidneys, neurons, & immune cells

CLINICAL ISSUES

Presentation

- Most common signs/symptoms
  - COVID-19
    - Fever, cough, sore throat, rhinorrhea, congestion, diarrhea, fatigue, dyspnea, rash, conjunctivitis
    - GI in > 50%: Diarrhea, abdominal pain, vomiting
    - ↑ CRP, ESR, LDH, D-dimer
    - Neutropenia, lymphopenia, thrombocytopenia
  - MIS-C CDC case definition
    - < 21 years old, fever, laboratory evidence of inflammation (↑ CRP, ESR, fibrinogen, procalcitonin, D-dimer, ferritin, LDH, IL-6, or neutrophils, &/or ↓ lymphocytes or albumin), & evidence of clinically severe illness requiring hospitalization with multisystem (> 2) organ involvement (cardiac, renal, respiratory, hematologic, GI, dermatologic or neurological), +
    - No alternative plausible diagnoses, +
    - (+) for current or recent SARS-CoV-2 infection by RT-PCR, serology, or antigen test; or COVID-19 exposure within 4 weeks prior to onset of symptoms
      - In largest study, 25.8% with (+) PCR test for SARS-CoV2 & 46.1% with (+) serology test for SARS-CoV2
- Other signs/symptoms
  - MIS-C
    - Neurologic in 31-47%: Headache, altered mental status, encephalopathy, seizure, coma, encephalitis, demyelinating disorder, aseptic meningitis
    - GI in 90.9%: Abdominal pain 61.9%, vomiting 61.8%, diarrhea 53.2%
    - Cardiovascular in 86.5%: Dysfunction 40.6%, shock 35.4%, myocarditis 22.8%, coronary artery aneurysm 18.6%
    - Dermatologic/mucocutaneous in 70.9%

Demographics

- Children initially accounted for ~ 6.5% of COVID-19 cases in USA
- More transmissible B.1.617.2 (Delta) variant & varying vaccination rates/eligibility may have shifted demographics
- COVID-19 & MIS-C have been more common & severe in patients of African & Hispanic descent
- Mean age of MIS-C patients: 8 years old

Natural History & Prognosis

- Children generally have milder disease with COVID-19
  - Initially accounted for ~ 1.5% of hospitalizations & 0.3% of deaths related to COVID-19 in USA
    - After vaccine development, age-matched unvaccinated populations have had greater rates of infection & severity of illness
  - Up to 1/4 of hospitalized children need ICU
- In largest study of MIS-C patients describing 570 patients
  - 63.9% required ICU care, 62% required vasopressor support, 1.8% died

Treatment

- COVID-19
  - Remdesivir is available through Emergency Use Authorization or compassionate use in pediatric patients
  - Dexamethasone may benefit patients with respiratory disease who are on mechanical ventilation
- MIS-C
  - Immunomodulatory therapy: IVIG &/or glucocorticoids, anakinra (recombinant human IL-1 receptor antagonist) for refractory disease
  - Antiplatelet/anticoagulation therapy: Low-dose aspirin until normalization of platelet count & normal coronary arteries at ≥ 4 weeks after diagnosis; enoxaparin or warfarin if coronary artery z-score > 10.0; also consider anticoagulation if moderate-severe LV dysfunction

SELECTED REFERENCES

1. Blumfield E et al: Imaging findings in multisystem inflammatory syndrome in children (MIS-C) associated with Coronavirus disease (COVID-19). AJR Am J Roentgenol. 216(2):507-17, 2021
2. Fenlon Iii EP et al: Extracardiac imaging findings in COVID-19-associated multisystem inflammatory syndrome in children. Pediatr Radiol. 51(5):831-9, 2021
3. Rostad BS et al: Chest radiograph features of multisystem inflammatory syndrome in children (MIS-C) compared to pediatric COVID-19. Pediatr Radiol. 51(2):231-8, 2021

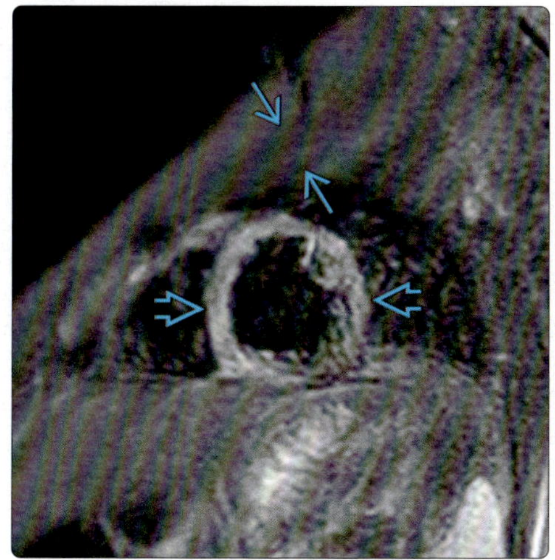

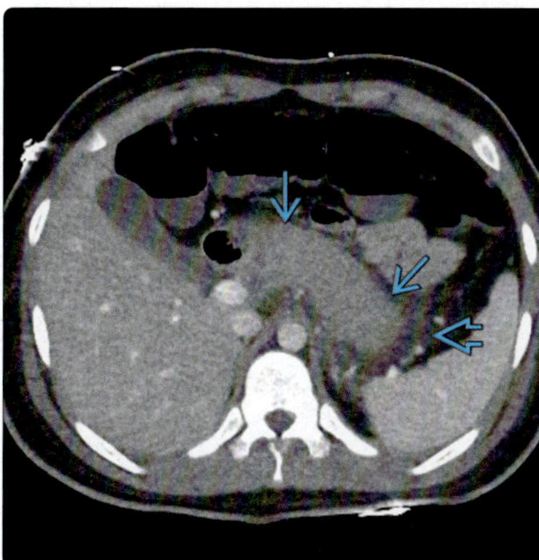

(Left) *Short-axis T2 STIR cardiac MR in a 16-year-old with 10 days of fever & abdominal pain shows high signal intensity of the left ventricular (LV) myocardium ⇨ vs. skeletal muscle ⇨ (ratio of 2.5, with > 1.9 being abnormal), consistent with edema. COVID-19 IgG was positive, consistent with MIS-C.* **(Right)** *Axial CECT in the same patient shows diffuse pancreatic thickening & homogeneous enhancement ⇨ with surrounding edema ⇨, consistent with acute interstitial edematous pancreatitis in MIS-C.*

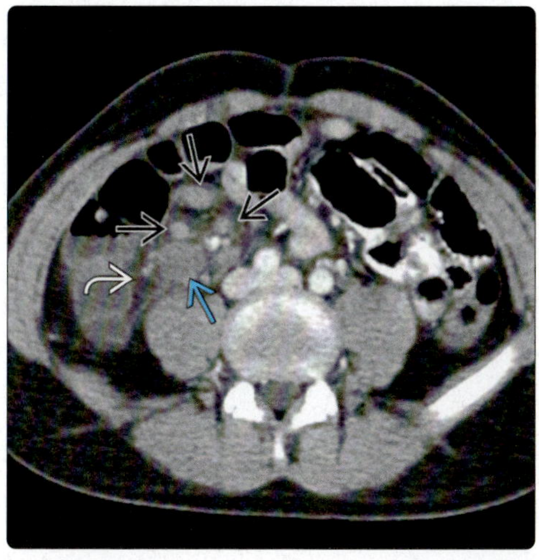

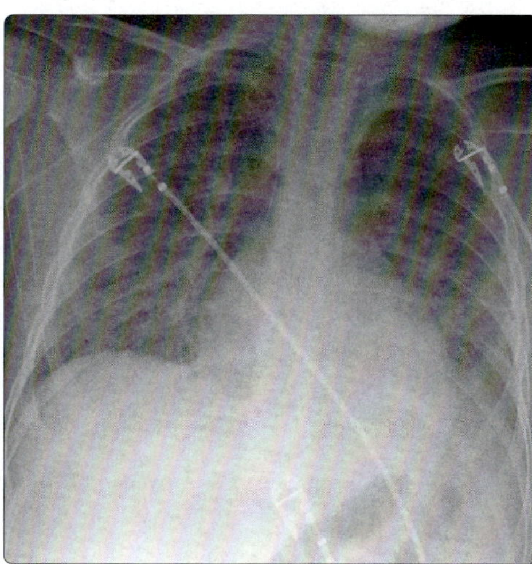

(Left) *Axial CECT of a 15-year-old with pain demonstrates inflammatory stranding at the right lower quadrant ➡ & multiple prominent lymph nodes ⇨, some with low density ⇨. The appendix was normal (not shown).* **(Right)** *Frontal radiograph in the same patient shows diffuse interstitial opacities compatible with pulmonary edema. Echocardiography showed LV dysfunction & ↓ LVEF. Inflammatory markers were elevated, & COVID-19 RT-PCR test was positive. The patient was diagnosed with MIS-C.*

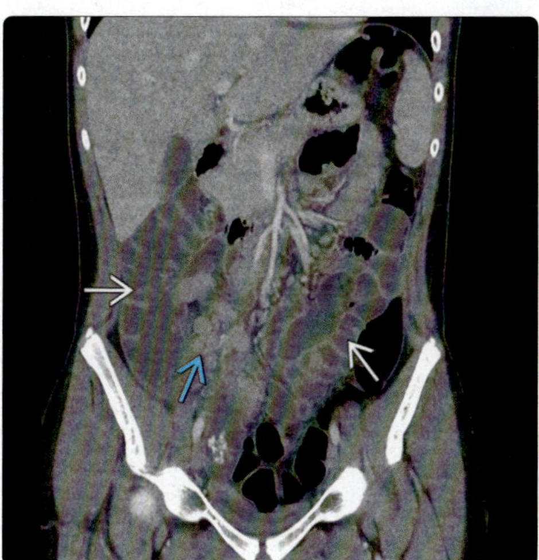

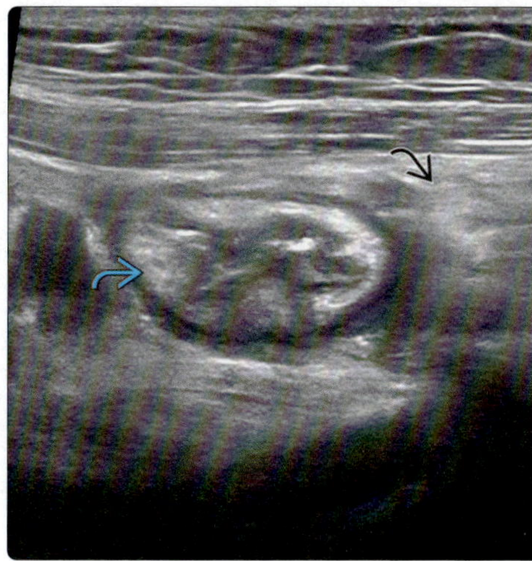

(Left) *Coronal CECT in a 10-year-old with right lower quadrant pain, fever, rash, & conjunctivitis shows multiple enlarged lymph nodes ⇨ & fluid-filled bowel ➡.* **(Right)** *Transverse US in the same patient shows distal ileal wall thickening & hyperechogenicity ➡ with adjacent fat induration ➡. Serology was positive for COVID-19 exposure. Decreased systolic LV function & coronary artery ectasia were seen on echocardiography. The patient met the criteria for MIS-C & also had elevated inflammatory markers.*

Round Pneumonia

KEY FACTS

TERMINOLOGY

- Bacterial lung infection with very round, well-defined appearance on chest radiography; simulates mass lesion
- Majority seen in patients < 8 years of age

IMAGING

- Well-circumscribed, round opacity ± air bronchograms
- Most common posteriorly in lower lobe superior segments
- No mass effect on or invasion of adjacent tissues
  - No mediastinal or vascular distortion
  - No splaying or erosion of ribs
- Margins of round lung "mass" classically create acute angles with mediastinum or chest wall but can be obtuse

TOP DIFFERENTIAL DIAGNOSES

- Bronchogenic cyst
- Neuroblastoma
- Congenital pulmonary airway malformation
- Bronchopulmonary sequestration

PATHOLOGY

- Collateral pathways of air circulation in lung are not well developed until ~ 8 years of age
  - Channels of Lambert, pores of Kohn
- Spread of bacterial infection through lung is therefore hindered in young children, predisposing to round appearance
- Typically occurs with *Streptococcus pneumoniae* infection

DIAGNOSTIC CHECKLIST

- Round lung opacity in child < 8 years of age → strongly consider round pneumonia
- With classic symptoms of pneumonia (cough, fever) in this age range, other masses do not need to be excluded
- If any doubt of diagnosis, consider
  - Targeted US or CT through lesion
  - Follow-up radiograph after completion of antibiotic course
    - Resolution of "mass" excludes other etiologies

(Left) *Frontal radiograph in a young child with cough & fever shows a round, mildly lobulated, well-circumscribed density ⇨ in the medial aspect of the right lower lobe.* **(Right)** *Lateral radiograph in the same patient confirms that the round "mass" ⇨ is located posteriorly in the right lower lobe. Note that the lesion makes acute angles with the posterior chest wall, consistent with a pulmonary origin. These findings are typical of a round pneumonia.*

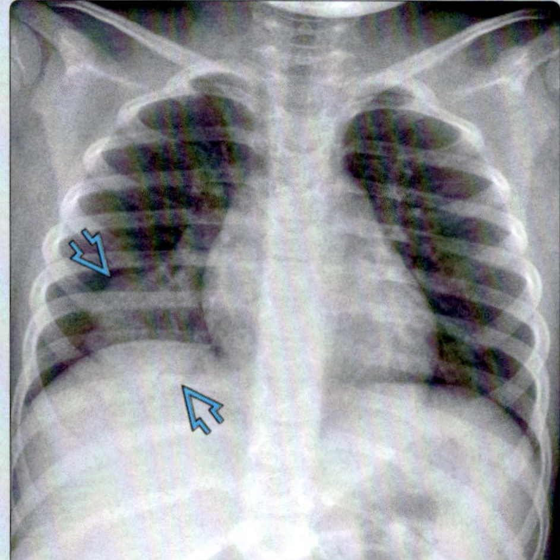

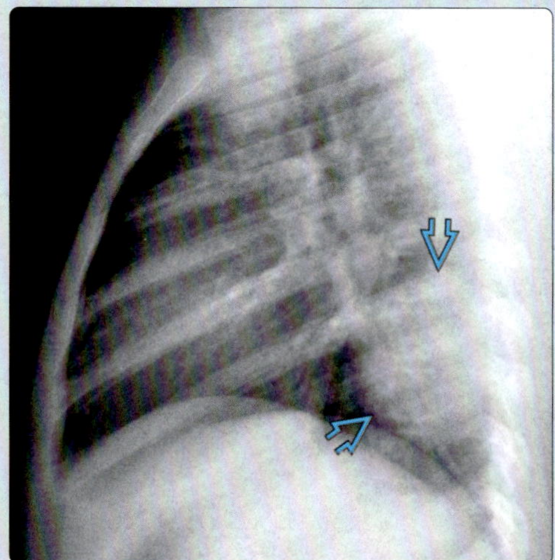

(Left) *Frontal radiograph in a 7-year-old with respiratory symptoms shows a fairly well-circumscribed, round to ovoid right middle lobe opacity ⇨.* **(Right)** *Lateral view of the chest in the same patient again shows the circumscribed round to ovoid opacity ⇨ at the right middle lobe. The radiographic findings & patient's clinical course were compatible with round pneumonia.*

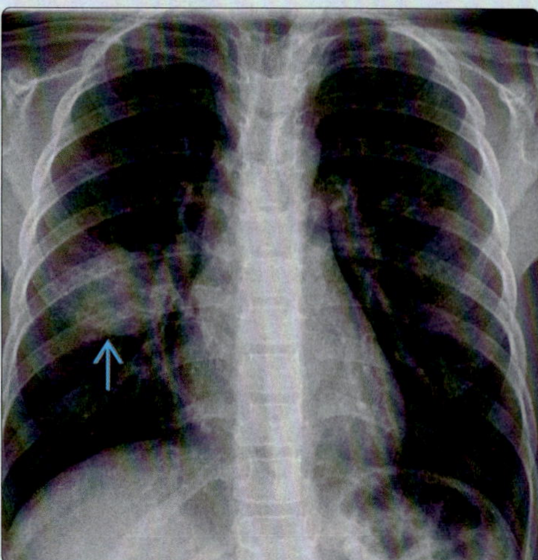

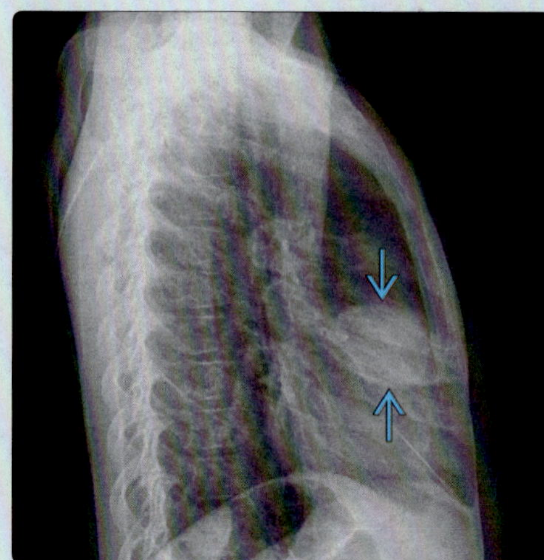

TERMINOLOGY

Definitions

- Bacterial lung infection with very round, well-defined appearance on chest radiography; simulates mass lesion
- Majority seen in patients < 8 years of age
- Typically occurs with *Streptococcus pneumoniae* infection

IMAGING

General Features

- Best diagnostic clue
  - Round lung opacity with well-defined borders in febrile child < 8 years of age
- Location
  - Most common posteriorly in superior segments of lower lobes
  - No peripheral or central predisposition
  - Single focus is most common (98%)
    - Multiple (2 or 3) foci can rarely occur
- Size
  - Ranges from 1-7 cm
  - Varies in size depending on timing of imaging relative to pneumonia development
  - With adequate treatment, usually resolves/clears (rather than progressing to lobar consolidation)
    - Resolution on follow-up imaging in 95%
- Morphology
  - Well-defined borders in 70%

Radiographic Findings

- Radiography
  - Round lung opacity typically marginated by clear lung
    - Paraspinal pneumonia may have acute or obtuse angle borders with posterior mediastinum/spine
  - Respects lobar anatomy without crossing fissures
  - Does not exert mass effect or invade adjacent tissues
    - No osseous changes (such as splaying or erosion) in adjacent ribs or spine
  - Air bronchograms help confirm airspace disease
  - Pleural effusion is uncommon
  - Rarely progresses to lobar pneumonia

CT Findings

- NECT
  - Not advocated for cases of suspected round pneumonia
    - May be obtained if mass lesion is primary concern
    - Abdominal CT may show round pneumonia in lower lobe as cause of abdominal pain
  - Homogeneous, round opacity ± air bronchograms
  - Respects lobar anatomy, does not cross fissures
  - No changes in adjacent bones
- CECT
  - Normal pulmonary vessels course through consolidated lung without mass effect
  - No enhancing rim or wall
  - No systemic arterial supply from descending aorta (as seen with bronchopulmonary sequestration)
  - Central cavity or fluid level favors alternative diagnosis

MR Findings

- Not utilized for primary suspicion of round pneumonia
- May be encountered if MR is performed to further work-up round paraspinal mass suspected to be neuroblastoma
- Round pneumonia appears as moderately high (but not fluid bright) T2 signal intensity lesion within pulmonary parenchyma ± air bronchograms
- With contrast, enhancing nondisplaced vessels course through mildly enhancing, otherwise homogeneous "mass"

Ultrasonographic Findings

- Increasingly used for diagnosis of childhood pneumonia
  - Sensitivity 96%, specificity 93% overall
    - May be lower if round pneumonia is completely surrounded by aerated lung
- Abnormality of normally echogenic pleural line: Irregular, coarse, interrupted, or absent
- "Hepatization" of subpleural parenchyma with branching mobile hyperechogenicities (air bronchograms)
- Interstitial involvement: > 3 B lines (type of comet-tail artifact in which vertical echogenic line extends from pleural surface to inferior edge of field of view)

Imaging Recommendations

- Pediatric Clinical Practice Guidelines for chest radiography in pneumonia
  - Not necessary to confirm suspected community-acquired pneumonia (CAP) in patients well enough to be treated as outpatients; exceptions include
    - Hypoxemia
    - Respiratory distress
    - Failed antibiotic therapy
  - Chest radiographs (frontal & lateral) should be obtained in all patients hospitalized for management of CAP
- If child < 8 years old has symptoms of pneumonia + round opacity on chest radiograph, additional imaging (such as CT) is not necessary
  - Look carefully at adjacent bones
- Follow-up radiograph after antibiotic therapy may be helpful to document resolution of round opacity
  - Particularly helpful for paraspinal round pneumonia that may mimic neuroblastoma
- > 8 years old: Consider evaluation for other pathologies with CECT or MR

DIFFERENTIAL DIAGNOSIS

Bronchogenic Cyst

- Round, well-defined soft tissue mass
- Most common in perihilar regions
- ± mass effect on adjacent structures
  - Airway compression may cause air-trapping/atelectasis
- Only contains air or air-fluid levels if infected
- CECT: Water-attenuation mass without air bronchograms; ± rim enhancement if infected

Neuroblastoma

- Round or elongated posterior mediastinal/paraspinal mass
- Obtuse angle borders with mediastinum
  - May only widen paraspinal stripe without focal bulge
- Rib erosion or splaying is common
- Ca^{2+} in majority by CT

Congenital Pulmonary Airway Malformation

- Round/lobulated parenchymal mass distorting adjacent lung & vessels
- Most commonly presents in utero or during newborn period
- Macrocystic type may temporarily appear solid after birth due to retained fluid
  - Quickly fills with air due to communication with airway

Bronchopulmonary Sequestration

- Lobulated or triangular parenchymal mass
- Most common in lower lobes
- Typically congenital, presenting in perinatal period; may present as recurrent pneumonia (always in same location) later in life
  - Round pneumonia almost never recurs in same location
- Characteristic systemic feeding artery arises from descending thoracic or abdominal aorta
  - May be seen prenatally or on postnatal CTA

Lung Abscess

- Round cavity containing air-fluid level
- Surrounded by irregular or poorly defined consolidation

Metastatic Disease

- Small, multifocal nodules are typical
- Rarely found incidentally in children

Pleural Pseudocyst

- Partially circumscribed, focal fluid collection within fissure
- Very uncommon as isolated finding in children without preceding history of thoracic pathology

Chest Wall Ewing Sarcoma

- Partially circumscribed, round mass with definite bony destruction (lysis, permeation)
- Associated pleural effusion is frequent
- More common in children > 8 years of age

PATHOLOGY

General Features

- Etiology
  - Collateral pathways of air circulation are not well developed until ~ 8 years of age
    - Channels of Lambert & pores of Kohn
  - Lack of well-developed collateral circulation is thought to hinder spread of bacterial infection, predisposing to round appearance on radiography

Gross Pathologic & Surgical Features

- Exudative opacification of pulmonary airspaces related to bacterial infection
  - *S. pneumoniae* is most common pathogen

CLINICAL ISSUES

Presentation

- Most common signs/symptoms
  - Cough & fever
- Other signs/symptoms
  - Abdominal pain, malaise, anorexia

Demographics

- Age
  - 75% < 8 years old; 90% < 12 years old; mean age: 5 years
  - Cases rarely reported in older children & adults
    - Sometimes leads to biopsy
    - Antibiotics & short-term follow-up may be considered if round pneumonia diagnosis is not clear

Natural History & Prognosis

- With appropriate antibiotic therapy, symptoms & opacity should resolve over days-weeks
  - Resolution of "mass" on follow-up radiograph after completion of antibiotic course confidently excludes other etiologies
- With antibiotic resistance, may progress to lobar pneumonia ± complications

DIAGNOSTIC CHECKLIST

Image Interpretation Pearls

- Round lung opacity in child < 8 years of age → strongly consider round pneumonia
  - With classic symptoms of pneumonia at presentation, other causes of radiographic mass do not need to be excluded with imaging
- > 8 years old, consider other pathologies & further work-up

SELECTED REFERENCES

1. de Benedictis FM et al: Complicated pneumonia in children. Lancet. 396(10253):786-98, 2020
2. Andronikou S et al: Computed tomography in children with community-acquired pneumonia. Pediatr Radiol. 47(11):1431-40, 2017
3. Andronikou S et al: Guidelines for the use of chest radiographs in community-acquired pneumonia in children and adolescents. Pediatr Radiol. 47(11):1405-11, 2017
4. Liszewski MC et al: Lung magnetic resonance imaging for pneumonia in children. Pediatr Radiol. 47(11):1420-30, 2017
5. Schooler GR et al: Children with cough and fever: up-to-date imaging evaluation and management. Radiol Clin North Am. 55(4):645-55, 2017
6. Stadler JAM et al: Lung ultrasound for the diagnosis of community-acquired pneumonia in children. Pediatr Radiol. 47(11):1412-9, 2017
7. Winant AJ et al: Current updates on pediatric pulmonary infections. Semin Roentgenol. 52(1):35-42, 2017
8. Jain S et al: Community-acquired pneumonia requiring hospitalization among U.S. children. N Engl J Med. 372(9):835-45, 2015
9. Pereda MA et al: Lung ultrasound for the diagnosis of pneumonia in children: a meta-analysis. Pediatrics. 135(4):714-22, 2015
10. Liu J et al: Lung ultrasonography for the diagnosis of severe neonatal pneumonia. Chest. 146(2):383-8, 2014
11. Caiulo VA et al: Lung ultrasound characteristics of community-acquired pneumonia in hospitalized children. Pediatr Pulmonol. 48(3):280-7, 2013
12. Gorkem SB et al: Evaluation of pediatric thoracic disorders: comparison of unenhanced fast-imaging-sequence 1.5-T MRI and contrast-enhanced MDCT. AJR Am J Roentgenol. 200(6):1352-7, 2013
13. Yikilmaz A et al: Evaluation of pneumonia in children: comparison of MRI with fast imaging sequences at 1.5T with chest radiographs. Acta Radiol. 52(8):914-9, 2011
14. Restrepo R et al: Imaging of round pneumonia and mimics in children. Pediatr Radiol. 40(12):1931-40, 2010
15. Kim YW et al: Round pneumonia: imaging findings in a large series of children. Pediatr Radiol. 37(12):1235-40, 2007
16. Donnelly LF: Practical issues concerning imaging of pulmonary infection in children. J Thorac Imaging. 16(4):238-50, 2001
17. Markowitz RI et al: The spectrum of pulmonary infection in the immunocompromised child. Semin Roentgenol. 35(2):171-80, 2000
18. Donnelly LF: Maximizing the usefulness of imaging in children with community-acquired pneumonia. AJR Am J Roentgenol. 172(2):505-12, 1999
19. Donnelly LF et al: The yield of CT of children who have complicated pneumonia and noncontributory chest radiography. AJR Am J Roentgenol. 170(6):1627-31, 1998

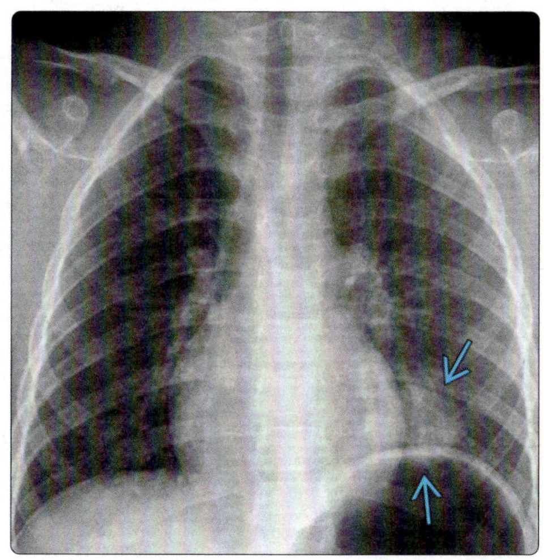

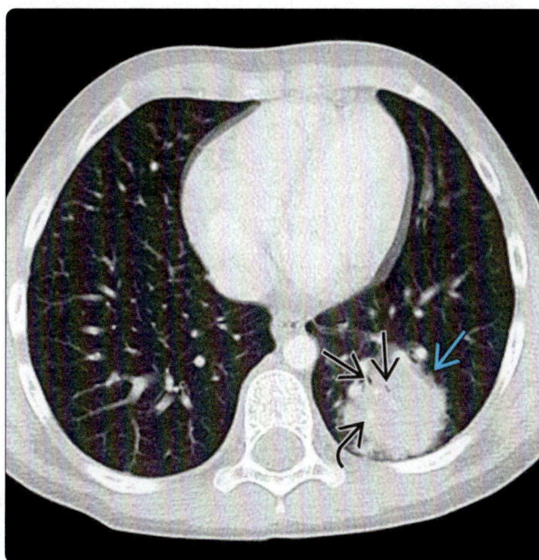

(Left) *PA view of the chest from a 7-year-old with a clinically suspected respiratory infection demonstrates a circumscribed left lower lobe density* ➔. **(Right)** *Axial CECT in the same patient shows a round left lower lobe air space opacity* ➔. *Air bronchograms* ➔ *& pulmonary vessels* ➔ *are seen coursing through the density. No mass effect is demonstrated. The findings are consistent with round pneumonia.*

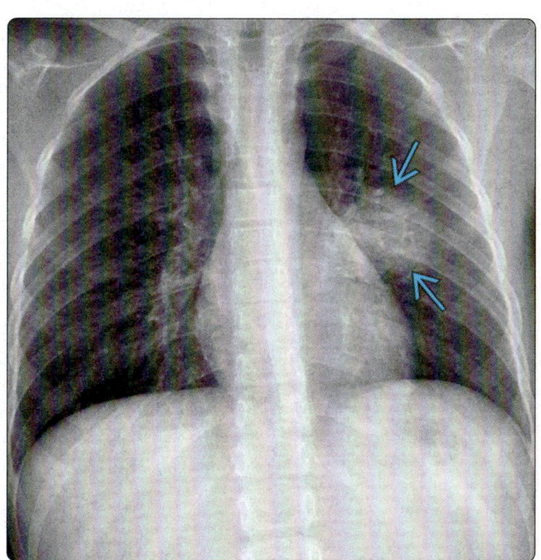

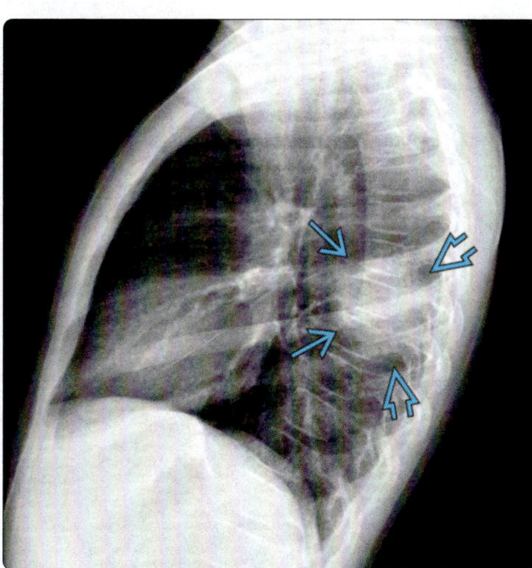

(Left) *PA chest radiograph of a 6-year-old girl with a cough demonstrates a round opacity* ➔ *projecting over the left hilum, suggesting a round pneumonia.* **(Right)** *Lateral chest radiograph in the same patient localizes the round opacity* ➔ *to the superior segment of the left lower lobe. The acute (rather than obtuse) angles* ➔ *at the interface of the opacity with the posterior chest wall are suggestive of its origin within the lung parenchyma.*

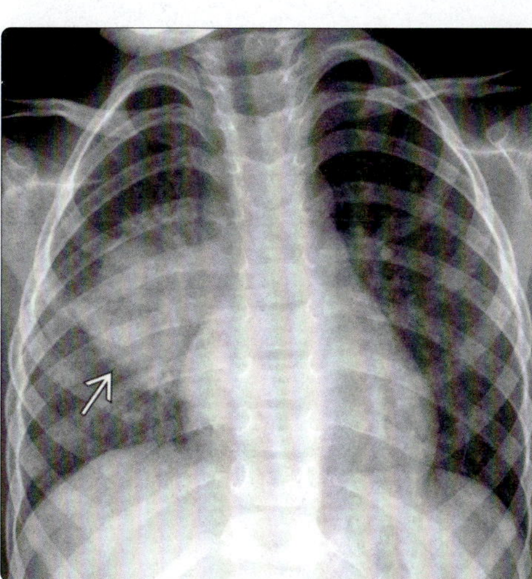

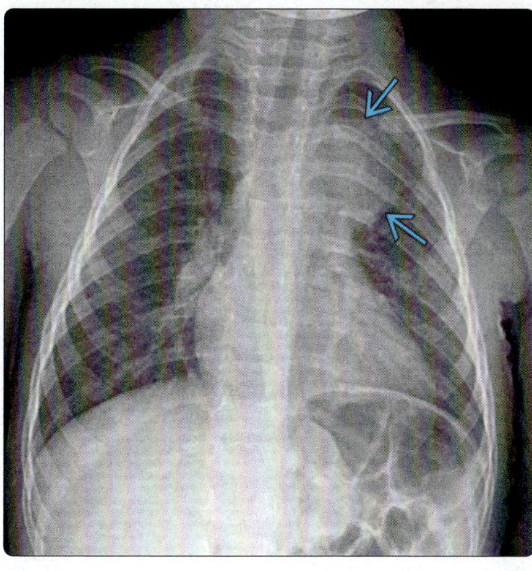

(Left) *Frontal chest radiograph from a 4-year-old with cough, fever, & chest pain shows a large, round right lower lobe opacity* ➔. *Follow-up after 2 weeks of antibiotic therapy was normal. The findings & clinical course are consistent with a round pneumonia.* **(Right)** *Frontal radiograph in a 2 year-old with fever, shortness of breath, & cough demonstrates a round opacity at the left upper lung* ➔. *Note the absence of mass effect or bone changes. The findings are compatible with round pneumonia & resolved at follow-up.*

Parapneumonic Effusion and Empyema

KEY FACTS

TERMINOLOGY

- Pleural effusions are classified as transudative or exudative
- Parapneumonic effusions are exudative secondary to adjacent lung infection & ↑ capillary permeability

IMAGING

- Upright chest radiograph
  - Flattened & elevated hemidiaphragm, lateral shift of diaphragm apex, gastric bubble > 1.5 cm from diaphragm secondary to subpulmonic fluid
  - Blunted posterior costophrenic angle (~ 50 mL)
  - Blunted lateral costophrenic angle (~ 200 mL)
  - Hemidiaphragm inversion (> 2,000 mL)
- Supine chest radiograph may require up to 500 mL
  - Homogeneous vs. gradation of hazy/dense opacification of hemithorax ± pleural cap, mass effect
- US: Effusion appears anechoic, echoic, or mixed with floating/swirling/undulating echoes
  - Floating fibrin strands attached to pleural surface, septations, &/or pleural rind/thickening; immobile lung suggests entrapment by pleural rind
  - Loculation: Nonshifting fluid with position change
- CECT: Parietal pleural enhancement & thickening, thickening of extrapleural space, & chest wall edema are seen with transudative & exudative effusions in children
- Imaging recommendations
  - US if pleural disease is suspected on chest radiograph
  - CECT for persistent/progressive illness on treatment

CLINICAL ISSUES

- American Pediatric Surgical Association recommendations
  - Antibiotics
  - Chest tube drainage if effusion is of large volume, loculated, or for worsening/persistent symptoms
  - For empyema: Chest tube + tissue plasminogen activator
    - Video-assisted thoracoscopic surgery (VATS) if no improvement

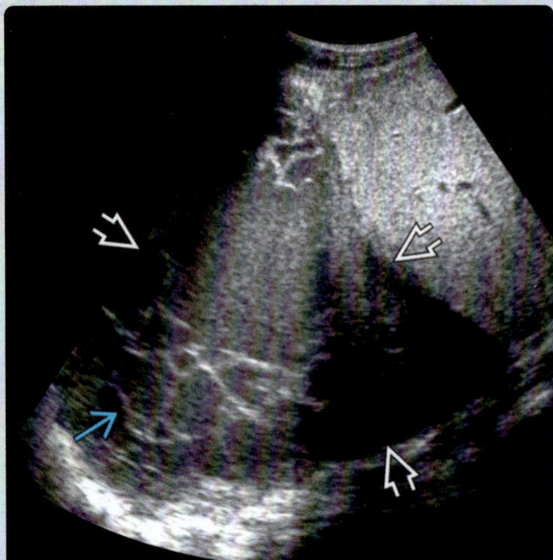
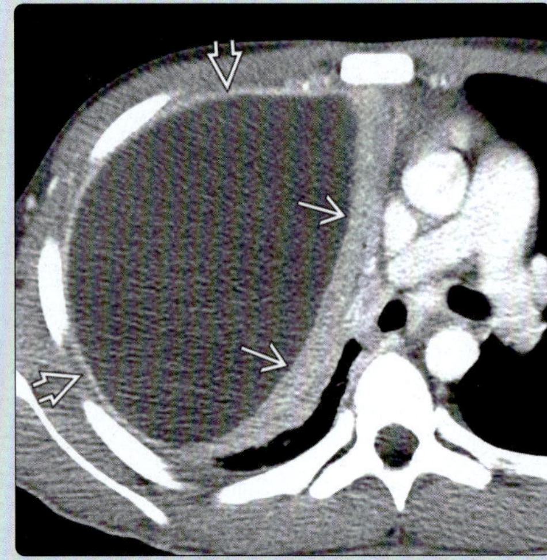

(Left) *Sagittal US in a patient with near-complete opacification of the right hemithorax on chest radiograph (not shown) shows a large pleural effusion ➡ with debris & echogenic septa ➡, consistent with a fibrinopurulent parapneumonic effusion.* **(Right)** *Axial CECT in the same patient shows the pleural effusion compressing the right lung ➡. The septations seen on the US are not visible on CT. Pleural enhancement ➡ is depicted but can be seen with transudative or exudative effusions.*

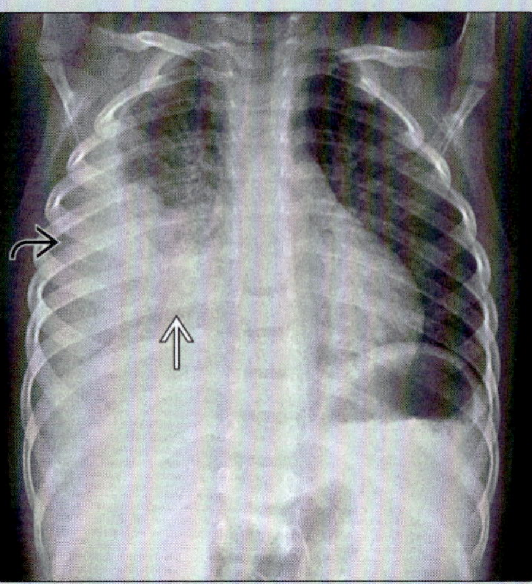
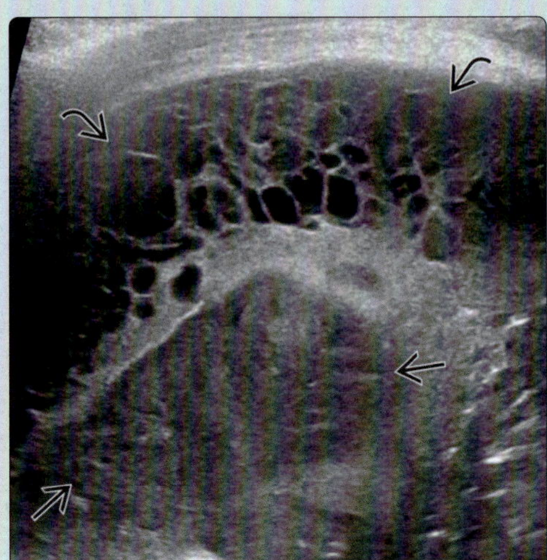

(Left) *Frontal view of the chest in a 19-month-old with pneumonia shows a large pleural effusion ➡ with basilar consolidation ➡.* **(Right)** *Transverse US in the same patient demonstrates a complex, multiloculated pleural collection ➡. A focal area of underlying lung parenchyma is heterogeneous & hypoechoic ➡, concerning for associated necrosis. An absence of flow was seen on Doppler interrogation (not shown).*

TERMINOLOGY

Definitions

- Pleural effusions are classified as transudative or exudative
  - Transudative: Due to hydrostatic & oncotic imbalances
  - Exudative: Due to ↑ capillary permeability
- Parapneumonic effusions are exudative
- Empyema is fibrinopurulent parapneumonic effusion

IMAGING

Radiographic Findings

- Pneumonia + adjacent pleural effusion
- Sequence of accumulation on upright view
  - Flattened & elevated hemidiaphragm, lateral shift of diaphragm apex, gastric bubble > 1.5 cm from diaphragm secondary to subpulmonic fluid
  - Blunted posterior costophrenic angle (~ 50 mL)
  - Blunted lateral costophrenic angle (~ 200 mL)
  - Hemidiaphragm inversion (> 2,000 mL)
- Supine images: Homogeneous vs. gradation of hazy/dense opacification of hemithorax ± pleural cap, mass effect (may require up to ~ 500 mL)
- Loculation is suggested by lenticular shape or nonshifting fluid on decubitus views but better characterized on US
- Fissural thickening or pseudotumor in minor fissure

Ultrasonographic Findings

- Effusion: Anechoic, echoic, or mixed with debris
- Fibrin deposition: Floating/flapping strands attached to pleural surface, septations, pleural rind/thickening; lack of lung mobility suggests pleural rind entrapping lung
- Loculation: Nonshifting fluid with position change

CT Findings

- Parietal pleural thickening & enhancement, thickened extrapleural space, & chest wall edema are seen with both transudative & exudative effusions in children
- Inferior to US at demonstrating fibrin strands or septations
- Loculation is inferred if air in collection separates into bubbles rather than single air-fluid level

MR Findings

- Empyema: Pleural thickening & enhancement, pleural fluid with heterogeneous signal, septation, & restricted diffusion

Imaging Recommendations

- US if pleural space disease is suspected on chest radiograph
  - Must scan dependent & nondependent pleural cavity
- CECT if persistent/progressive illness despite treatment (to evaluate for malpositioned chest tube, necrosis, abscess, purulent pericarditis)

DIFFERENTIAL DIAGNOSIS

Chylothorax

- Birth trauma, lymphangiectasia, lymphatic malformation

Lung Abscess

- Walled-off collection with pneumonia & progressive illness

Malignant Pleural Effusion

- Lymphoma, Ewing sarcoma, pleuropulmonary blastoma
- Look for nodularity/mass &/or rib destruction

PATHOLOGY

General Features

- Transudate vs. exudate classification is based on fluid analysis
- Light's criteria for exudate (≥ 1 required): Pleural fluid to serum protein ratio > 0.5 or LDH ratio > 0.6; pleural fluid LDH > 2/3 upper limit of normal serum level
- If exudative, then empyema is suggested by: pH < 7.2, lactate dehydrogenase (LDH) > 1,000 U, glucose < 40 mg/dL or < 25% blood glucose, positive Gram stain or positive culture, > 10,000 WBC/μL, loculations on imaging
- Common causes include *Streptococcus pneumoniae* & methicillin-resistant *Staphylococcus aureus*
  - Test for tuberculosis with lymphocytic exudate
- Stages of parapneumonic effusion progression
  - Precollection: Pleuritis, inflammation
  - Exudative (simple): Free fluid with low white cell count
  - Fibrinopurulent (complicated): Deposition of fibrin & purulent material
  - Organized: Thick pleural peel, which may entrap lung

CLINICAL ISSUES

Presentation

- Fever, cough, chest pain, dyspnea, tachypnea, splinting to affected side, respiratory distress if large in volume

Demographics

- Complicates 28-53% of pediatric pneumonias

Natural History & Prognosis

- Pediatric mortality < 3% in 1 study (up to 20% in adults)

Treatment

- American Pediatric Surgical Association recommendations
  - Antibiotics
  - Evacuation with chest tube for large volume &/or loculated effusion or with worsening/persistent symptoms
  - For empyema: Chest tube + intrapleural tissue plasminogen activator
    - Video-assisted thoracoscopic surgery (VATS) is required if no clinical improvement & pleural disease persists on imaging

SELECTED REFERENCES

1. de Benedictis FM et al: Complicated pneumonia in children. Lancet. 396(10253):786-98, 2020
2. Konietzke P et al: The value of chest magnetic resonance imaging compared to chest radiographs with and without additional lung ultrasound in children with complicated pneumonia. PLoS One. 15(3):e0230252, 2020
3. Liszewski MC et al: Lung magnetic resonance imaging for pneumonia in children. Pediatr Radiol. 47(11):1420-30, 2017
4. Islam S et al: The diagnosis and management of empyema in children: a comprehensive review from the APSA Outcomes and Clinical Trials Committee. J Pediatr Surg. 47(11):2101-10, 2012
5. Calder A et al: Imaging of parapneumonic pleural effusions and empyema in children. Pediatr Radiol. 39(6):527-37, 2009
6. Kurian J et al: Comparison of ultrasound and CT in the evaluation of pneumonia complicated by parapneumonic effusion in children. AJR Am J Roentgenol. 193(6):1648-54, 2009
7. Donnelly LF et al: CT appearance of parapneumonic effusions in children: findings are not specific for empyema. AJR Am J Roentgenol. 169(1):179-82, 1997

Pneumonia With Cavitary Necrosis

KEY FACTS

TERMINOLOGY

- Complication of bacterial pneumonia where dominant focus of necrosis develops in consolidated lung, resulting in variable number(s) of thin-walled cysts
- Synonyms: Necrotizing pneumonia, pulmonary gangrene
  - Abscess has thick, well-defined wall & is more commonly seen in immunocompromised children

IMAGING

- Not identified radiographically until tissue breakdown leads to communication of cavity with aerated lung/airways
- CECT shows lack of normal lung architecture, ↓ lung enhancement, & thin-walled cysts in midst of consolidation
- No clear role for percutaneous drainage in cases of cavitary necrosis in immunocompetent children

TOP DIFFERENTIAL DIAGNOSES

- Congenital pulmonary airway malformation
- Lung abscess
- Bronchopulmonary sequestration
- Bronchogenic cyst

PATHOLOGY

- Increasingly identified as pediatric pneumonia complication
- *Streptococcus pneumoniae* is most common cause
  - Other organisms: MSSA, MRSA, other *Staphylococcus* & *Streptococcus* species, *Pseudomonas*, *Fusobacterium*
- May lead to bronchopleural fistula & development of pneumothorax

CLINICAL ISSUES

- Progressive symptoms (fever, respiratory distress, sepsis) in pediatric pneumonia patient despite appropriate medical management suggest complication (such as cavitary necrosis)
- Patients with cavitary necrosis tend to be intensely ill (ICU)
- Most do recover with antibiotics & nonsurgical management

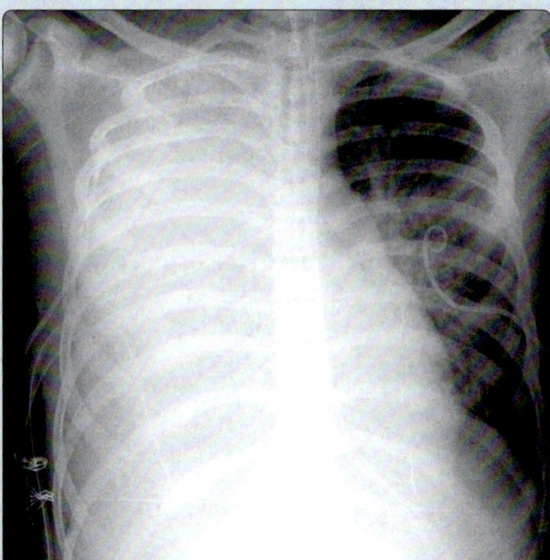

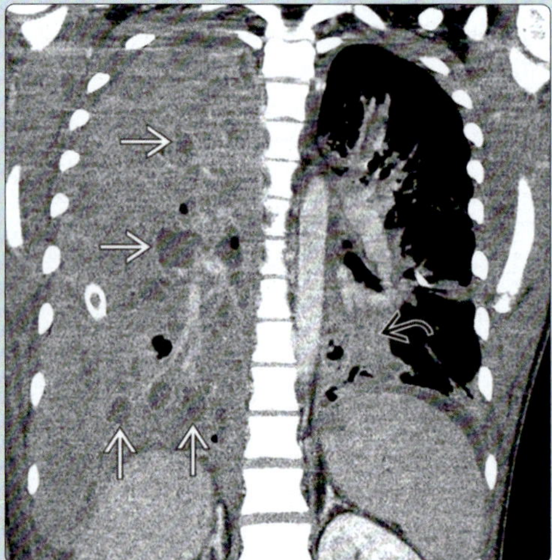

(Left) *AP chest radiograph in a child with rapidly progressive symptoms shows complete opacification of the right hemithorax & partial opacification of the medial left lower lobe (LLL). There are bilateral chest tubes in place.* **(Right)** *Coronal CECT in the same patient shows heterogeneous opacification of the right lung with multiple thin-walled, fluid-containing cystic foci ➡, consistent with cavitary necrosis. Also note the LLL opacification ↪. Development of air in foci of necrosis allows for better visualization on radiographs.*

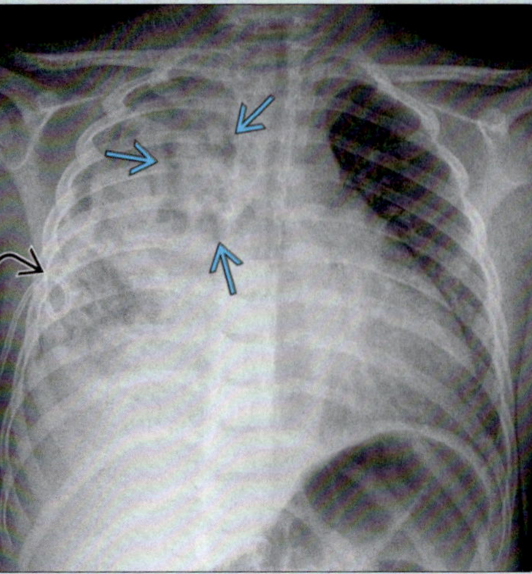

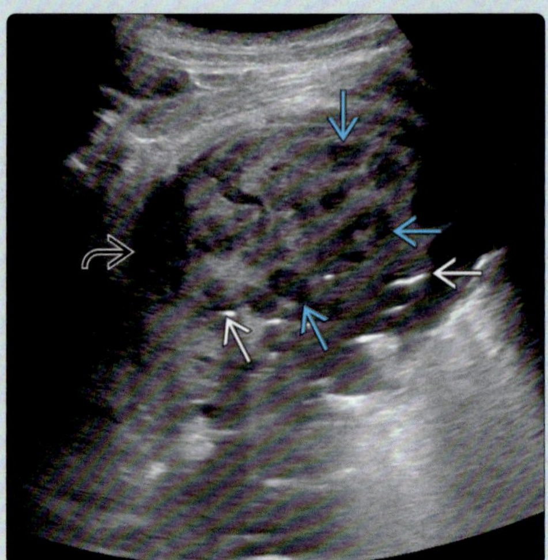

(Left) *Frontal view of the chest in a 7-year-old with MRSA pneumonia, empyema with chest tube in situ ↪, & worsening clinical course demonstrates right lung consolidation with cystic lucencies concerning for associated necrosis ➡.* **(Right)** *Longitudinal oblique ultrasound in the same patient shows consolidated lung with hypoechoic foci, compatible with areas of necrosis ➡. Hyperechoic foci ➡ within a few of the hypoechoic areas reflect air. Note residual complex pleural fluid from the empyema ↪.*

TERMINOLOGY

Synonyms

- Necrotizing pneumonia
- Pulmonary gangrene

Definitions

- Complication of bacterial pneumonia where dominant focus of necrosis develops in consolidated lung, resulting in variable number(s) of thin-walled cysts

IMAGING

General Features

- Best diagnostic clue
  - CECT of opacified lung shows loss of normal lung architecture with focally ↓ lung enhancement & development of thin-walled cysts ± air-fluid levels
- Location
  - More common in lower lobes
- Size
  - Variably sized cysts, typically 2-10 cm

Radiographic Findings

- Radiography
  - Poor sensitivity as cavitary lesions are initially fluid-filled & same density as surrounding consolidated lung
  - Cavitation is not detected radiographically until necrosis leads to communication with aerated lung or bronchi
    - Leads to introduction of air into cavity → cystic lucencies within lung opacified by pneumonia
  - ± pneumothorax related to bronchopleural fistula
  - Follow-up after antibiotics
    - Progressive ↓ in lung consolidation
    - Cystic lucencies eventually resolve
    - Radiographs obtained > 40 days later: Often normal or showing only minimal linear scarring

CT Findings

- CECT
  - Within area of consolidated lung
    - Loss of normal lung architecture
      - Breakdown of normal bronchogram pattern
    - ↓ enhancement
      - Noncompromised consolidated or atelectatic lung enhances
      - Nonenhancement suggests ischemia or developing necrosis
    - Multiple cystic foci filled with air &/or fluid
      - Not air-filled until communicating with aerated lung/airways
      - Walls of cyst: Thin, often nonenhancing

MR Findings

- Several studies on chest MR for evaluation of pulmonary infection in children show
  - ↑ sensitivity for detecting necrosis, abscess, & empyema compared to radiographs or radiographs + ultrasound
  - Comparable diagnostic characteristics to CECT for consolidation, necrosis/abscess, effusion
- Consolidation
  - Isointense T1 + hyperintense T2 signal relative to muscle
- Necrosis
  - Focus of T2 hypointensity within area of consolidation
  - Nonenhancing parenchyma
  - Signal void indicative of gas may be seen in necrotic areas or abscesses ± air-fluid levels

Ultrasonographic Findings

- Grayscale ultrasound
  - Ill-defined, heterogeneously hypoechoic foci in consolidated lung
    - Seen in 24% of cases imaged with both US & CT
  - Small, central areas may be more difficult to visualize
- Color Doppler
  - Characteristic appearance of consolidated pneumonia: Tree-like vascularity extending from center to periphery
  - ↓ or absent color Doppler flow within consolidated lung suggests perfusion impairment & correlates with severity of necrosis on CECT

Nonvascular Interventions

- Percutaneous drainage of lung abscesses is sometimes advocated, though creation of bronchopleural fistula may be problematic
- No clear role for percutaneous drainage in cases of cavitary necrosis in immunocompetent children

Imaging Recommendations

- Primary imaging modality of pneumonia: Radiographs
  - Insensitive to many complications
- CECT is used in minority of pneumonia cases
  - Typically in child who has not responded to appropriate therapy despite lack of clear radiographic explanation
- Follow-up
  - Patients with cavitary necrosis demonstrated on CECT do not typically need follow-up CT to document resolution
  - Radiographs obtained after 40 days are typically normal or near normal

DIFFERENTIAL DIAGNOSIS

Infected Congenital Lung Lesion

- Cavitary necrosis can appear similar to infection of underlying congenital pulmonary airway malformation (CPAM)
- Cavitary necrosis tends to be surrounded by consolidation
  - CPAM is often surrounded by aerated lung
- Children with cavitary necrosis tend to be more critically ill
- Temporal history is most helpful; favor cavitary necrosis if
  - Previously normal chest radiograph
  - Progression of lesion during illness
  - ↓ or resolving lesion after acute illness

Lung Abscess

- Suppurative complications of pneumonia represent spectrum; name given depends upon severity, distribution, & temporal relationship to development of pneumonia
  - Cavitary necrosis: Nonenhancing, poorly defined walls of cysts
  - Lung abscess: Fluid collection with well-defined, thick, enhancing wall
    - Lung abscesses rare in otherwise healthy, immunocompetent children

- Typically occur in immunocompromised children

Bronchopulmonary Sequestration

- L > R lower lobe lesion, typically solid
- Does not contain cavities unless superinfected or hybrid lesion with CPAM
- Systemic arterial supply from aorta

Bronchogenic Cyst

- Typically not air-filled but fluid density
- More commonly in perihilar region/mediastinum

PATHOLOGY

General Features

- Etiology
  - Increasingly identified as pediatric pneumonia complication
    - May be due to changing spectrum of causative organisms since introduction of pneumococcal vaccine, ↑ recognition of cavitary necrosis as distinct clinical entity, or ↑ use of CT
  - Causative organisms in large USA retrospective study
    - *Streptococcus pneumoniae* is most common, 22%
    - Others: Methicillin-sensitive & -resistant *Staphylococcus aureus*, *Pseudomonas* species, other *Staphylococcus* & *Streptococcus* species, *Fusobacterium*
- May lead to bronchopleural fistula & development of pneumothorax
  - In one large retrospective study, 86% had pleural effusion & 13% developed bronchopleural fistula
    - 100% of cases with bronchopleural fistula previously had chest drain in place > 7 days

Gross Pathologic & Surgical Features

- Primarily vascular process with inflammation leading to vasculitis → thrombosis of small arterioles with eventual ischemia & necrosis of consolidated lung
  - Tissue breakdown → cavity formation
  - Cavities are initially fluid-filled
  - Cavities fill with air when tissue develops communication with aerated lung
- Direct cytotoxic effects of bacterial toxins
  - Possible association with Panton-Valentine leukocidin pore-forming exotoxin & α-hemolysin seen in some strains of *S. aureus*
- Cytokine-mediated inflammatory response

CLINICAL ISSUES

Presentation

- Most common signs/symptoms
  - Lack of clinical improvement in pneumonia symptoms despite antibiotic therapy
  - Progressive sepsis
- Clinical profile
  - When children exhibit persistent or progressive symptoms (fever, respiratory distress, sepsis) despite appropriate medical management of pneumonia, suppurative complication (such as cavitary necrosis) is usually present

Demographics

- Age
  - May occur in children of all ages
  - Most common < 5 years old
- Epidemiology
  - ↑ incidence of complicated pneumonias in children since mid 1990s
  - Reason unclear
    - ↑ frequency of antibiotic resistant *S. pneumoniae*
    - ↑ viral infections (such as influenza A) that damage respiratory mucosa & render host susceptible to multiple infections
    - ↑ in antibiotic resistant bacteria

Natural History & Prognosis

- Patients with cavitary necrosis tend to be intensely ill
- Complications include: Bronchopleural fistula, empyema, abscess, empyema, tension pneumatocele/pneumothorax, hemolytic uremic syndrome
- Most do recover with nonsurgical management

Treatment

- Intensive support with IV antibodies
- Surgery reserved for minority of cases
  - Surgical therapy may have role for necrotic pneumonia in adults; natural history of recovery without surgical intervention in children should be stressed

SELECTED REFERENCES

1. de Benedictis FM et al: Complicated pneumonia in children. Lancet. 396(10253):786-98, 2020
2. Andronikou S et al: Computed tomography in children with community-acquired pneumonia. Pediatr Radiol. 47(11):1431-40, 2017
3. Liszewski MC et al: Lung magnetic resonance imaging for pneumonia in children. Pediatr Radiol. 47(11):1420-30, 2017
4. Masters IB et al: Necrotizing pneumonia: an emerging problem in children? Pneumonia (Nathan). 9:11, 2017
5. Ramgopal S et al: Pediatric necrotizing pneumonia: a case report and review of the literature. Pediatr Emerg Care. 33(2):112-5, 2017
6. Sodhi KS et al: Rapid lung MRI in children with pulmonary infections: time to change our diagnostic algorithms. J Magn Reson Imaging. 43(5):1196-206, 2016
7. Lai SH et al: Value of lung ultrasonography in the diagnosis and outcome prediction of pediatric community-acquired pneumonia with necrotizing change. PLoS One. 10(6):e0130082, 2015
8. Gorkem SB et al: Evaluation of pediatric thoracic disorders: comparison of unenhanced fast-imaging-sequence 1.5-T MRI and contrast-enhanced MDCT. AJR Am J Roentgenol. 200(6):1352-7, 2013
9. Yikilmaz A et al: Evaluation of pneumonia in children: comparison of MRI with fast imaging sequences at 1.5T with chest radiographs. Acta Radiol. 52(8):914-9, 2011
10. Hodina M et al: Imaging of cavitary necrosis in complicated childhood pneumonia. Eur Radiol. 12(2):391-6, 2002
11. Donnelly LF: Practical issues concerning imaging of pulmonary infection in children. J Thorac Imaging. 16(4):238-50, 2001
12. Markowitz RI et al: The spectrum of pulmonary infection in the immunocompromised child. Semin Roentgenol. 35(2):171-80, 2000
13. Donnelly LF: Maximizing the usefulness of imaging in children with community-acquired pneumonia. AJR Am J Roentgenol. 172(2):505-12, 1999
14. Donnelly LF et al: Cavitary necrosis complicating pneumonia in children: sequential findings on chest radiography. AJR Am J Roentgenol. 171(1):253-6, 1998
15. Donnelly LF et al: Pneumonia in children: decreased parenchymal contrast enhancement–CT sign of intense illness and impending cavitary necrosis. Radiology. 205(3):817-20, 1997

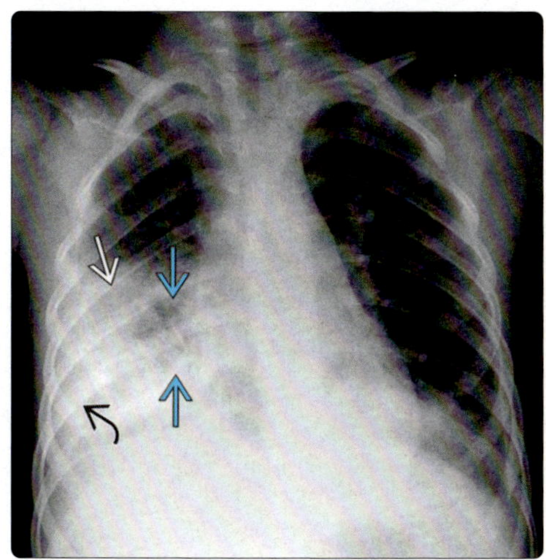

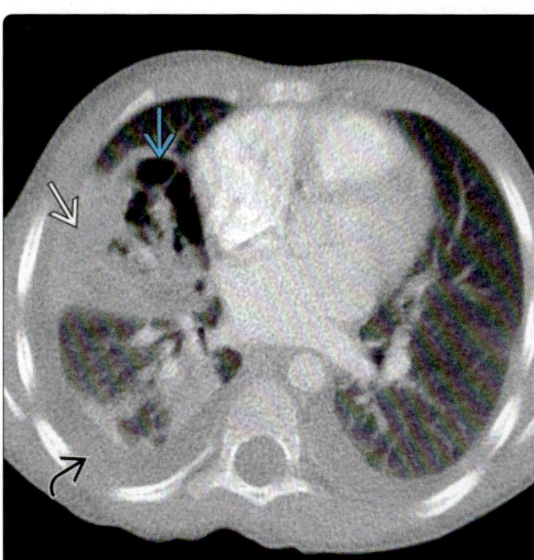

(Left) *Frontal view of the chest in a 14-year-old with pneumonia demonstrates right middle lobe consolidation* ➔ *with areas of lucency medially* ➔*, concerning for necrosis given a worsening clinical status. There is a small pleural effusion* ➔*.* **(Right)** *Axial CECT in the same patient depicts the area of right middle lobe consolidation* ➔ *as well as gas-filled cystic foci (compatible with necrosis)* ➔ *& a small right pleural effusion* ➔*.*

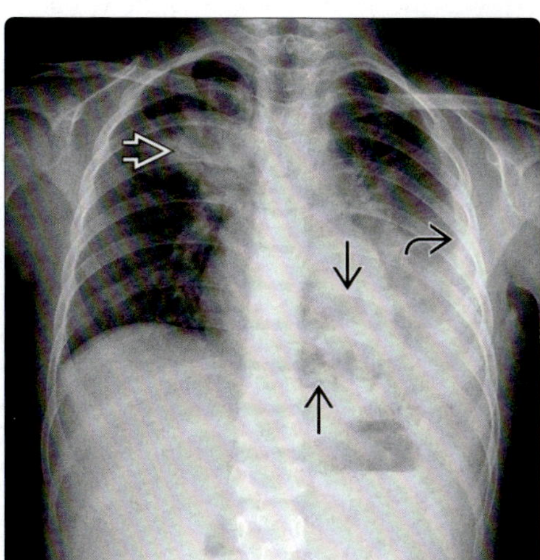

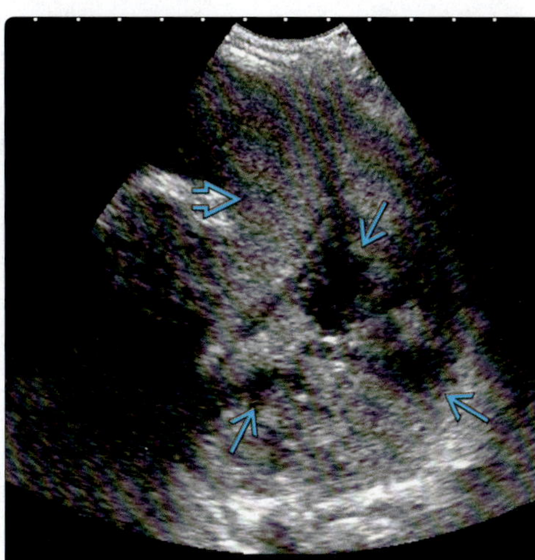

(Left) *AP chest radiograph from a 5-year-old patient demonstrates LLL consolidation with multiple foci of radiolucency* ➔ *due to cavitary necrosis. There is also right upper lobe consolidation* ➔ *& a left pleural effusion* ➔*.* **(Right)** *Transverse lung ultrasound in the same 5-year-old shows multiple hypoechoic foci* ➔ *in the consolidated left lower lobe, concerning for cavitary necrosis. The spleen is partially visualized* ➔*.*

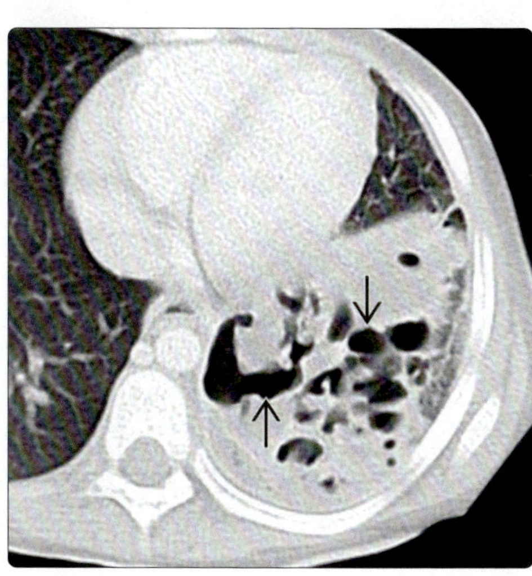

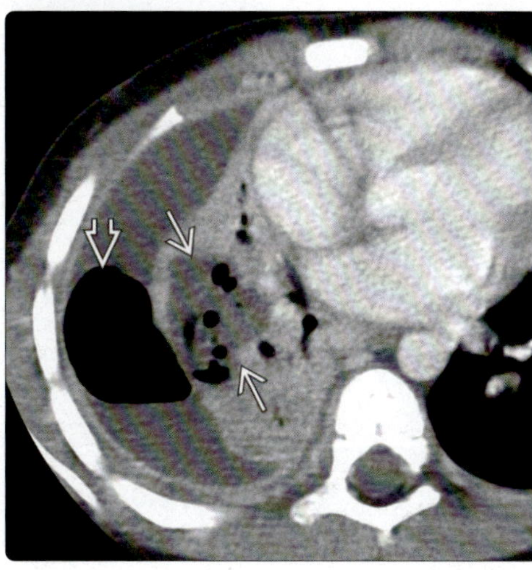

(Left) *Axial CECT in the same patient shows consolidation of the LLL with loss of the normal lung architecture & extensive tubular & cystic lucencies* ➔*, consistent with cavitary necrosis.* **(Right)** *Axial CECT in an ill child shows a consolidated right lower lobe (RLL) containing a central cavity* ➔ *with a nonenhancing wall, consistent with cavitary necrosis. Note the large pleural effusion containing gas* ➔*, suggesting an underlying bronchopleural fistula.*

Fungal Pneumonia in Immunocompromised Children

KEY FACTS

TERMINOLOGY

- Causes of immunocompromised states in children
  - Immature immune system: Premature infants
  - Primary immunodeficiency: Chronic granulomatous disease, Job syndrome, severe combined immunodeficiency, Wiskott-Aldrich syndrome, DiGeorge syndrome
  - Acquired immunodeficiency: Immunosuppression, infection, chronic illness

IMAGING

- Best clue: Pneumonia that does not respond to broad-spectrum antibiotics
- Angioinvasive pulmonary *Aspergillus:* Classic findings of halo sign, air-crescent sign, & cavitation
  - Halo sign (11% of patients): Nodule with halo of ground-glass attenuation (due to hemorrhage)
  - Air-crescent sign (2% of patients): Represents retraction of necrotic lung
  - Cavitation (~ 25% of patients): Typically occurs as neutrophil counts recover (sign of recovery)
- *Candida*: Consolidation, cannot be distinguished from bacterial pneumonia
- *Pneumocystis*: Extensive ground-glass opacity with interlobular septal thickening
- Coccidioidomycosis: Unilateral consolidation, hilar adenopathy, pleural effusion, pulmonary nodules, cavitary lesions, reticulonodular opacity
- *Cryptococcus*: Pulmonary nodules (miliary or large)
- Histoplasmosis
  - Preexisting infection: Calcified pulmonary nodule(s), calcified hilar or right paratracheal lymph nodes
  - Acute infection: Mediastinal or hilar adenopathy, miliary nodules, diffuse consolidation

CLINICAL ISSUES

- Antifungal therapy depends on type of fungus

(Left) *Axial CECT of the left lung in a child with febrile neutropenia shows a poorly defined opacity ➙ in the left lower lobe with a faint halo of ground-glass opacity. This was later confirmed to represent angioinvasive pulmonary aspergillus.* **(Right)** *Axial CECT of the chest in the same patient obtained 3 weeks later shows cavitation ➙ of the left lower lobe opacity. In patients with neutropenia & angioinvasive pulmonary aspergillus, cavitation represents a sign of recovery as the neutrophil count ↑.*

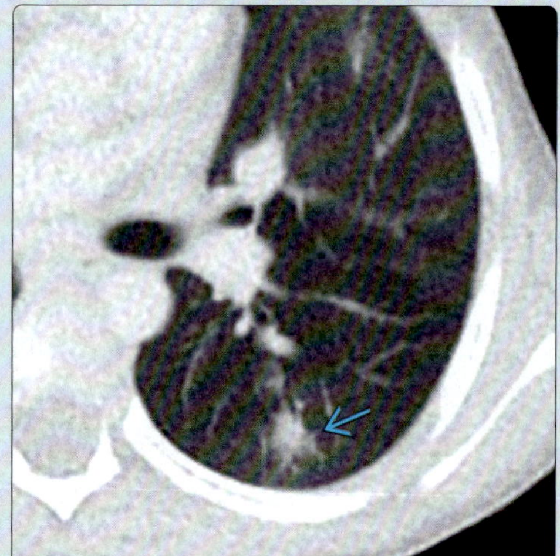

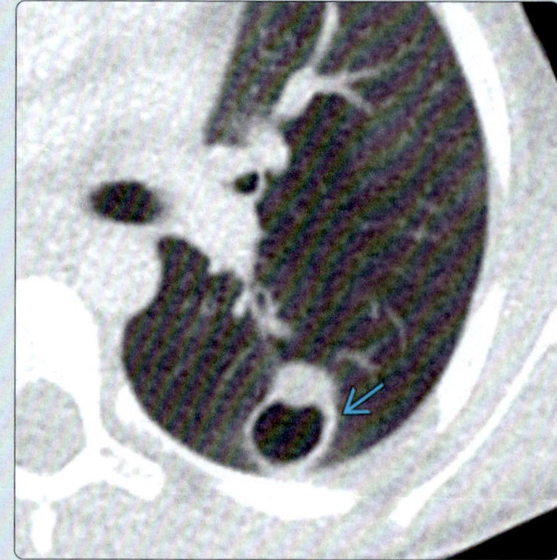

(Left) *Axial CECT of the lungs in an immunocompromised child shows diffuse, tiny pulmonary nodules in a centrilobular distribution. The patient was confirmed to have disseminated histoplasmosis.* **(Right)** *Coronal CECT of the left upper lung in a child with a history of cystic fibrosis shows mucus-impacted bronchi ➙ & a tree-in-bud pattern ➪ of pulmonary nodules, which can be secondary to allergic bronchopulmonary aspergillosis.*

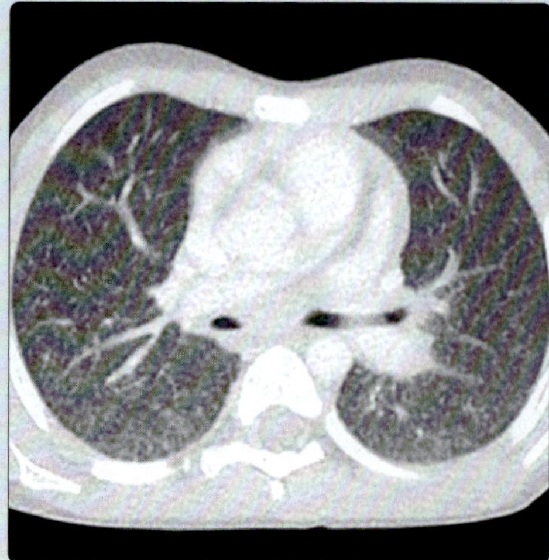

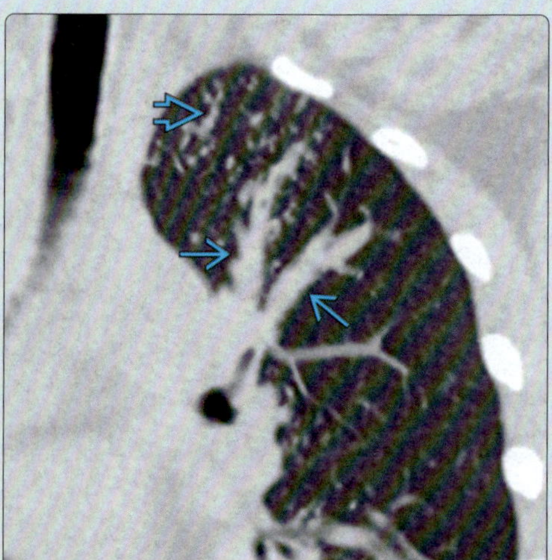

Fungal Pneumonia in Immunocompromised Children

TERMINOLOGY

Associated Syndromes

- Causes of immunocompromised states in children
  - Immature immune system: Premature infants
  - Primary immunodeficiency: Chronic granulomatous disease & severe combined immunodeficiency
  - Acquired immunodeficiency
    - Immunosuppression: After transplant or chemotherapy, chronic corticosteroid therapy
    - Infectious: HIV/AIDS
    - Chronic illness: Cystic fibrosis, burns
- 3 types of *Aspergillus* infection
  - Invasive pulmonary *Aspergillus* affects patients with neutropenia or neutrophil dysfunction
    - Subclassified as angioinvasive or airway invasive
  - Allergic bronchopulmonary aspergillosis (ABPA) represents hypersensitivity reaction to *Aspergillus*
  - Chronic airway invasive aspergillosis is rare, indolent form of *Aspergillus* infection

IMAGING

General Features

- Best diagnostic clue
  - Pneumonia that does not respond to antibiotics in immunocompromised patient

Radiographic Findings

- Angioinvasive pulmonary *Aspergillus*
  - Tree-in-bud nodules, ground-glass opacity, & consolidation
  - Cavitary lesions & air-crescent sign are uncommon
- Airway invasive pulmonary *Aspergillus:* Patchy lower lobe consolidation & poorly defined nodules
- ABPA: Tubular opacities of mucus-impacted bronchi, bronchiectasis, & atelectasis
- Chronic airway invasive *Aspergillosis:* Consolidation → cavitation → aspergilloma & pleural thickening
- *Candida*: Perivascular pulmonary opacities may coalesce into abscess or empyema
- *Pneumocystis*: Diffuse interstitial or granular opacities
- Coccidioidomycosis: Unilateral consolidation, hilar adenopathy, pleural effusion
- *Cryptococcus*: Miliary nodules, large pulmonary nodules, large areas of consolidation, or lymphadenopathy
- Histoplasmosis
  - Acute infection: Mimics tuberculosis; mediastinal or hilar adenopathy & consolidation
  - Remote infection: Ca^{2+} of pulmonary nodule & nodes

CT Findings

- Angioinvasive pulmonary *Aspergillus*
  - Halo sign: Nodule with halo of ground-glass attenuation (due to hemorrhage)
    - Appears within 5 days from fever onset
    - Lesions can ↑ in size & number for 7-10 days
  - Air-crescent sign: Retraction of necrotic lung within consolidation → crescent of air
  - Cavitation: Typically occurs as neutrophil counts recover (sign of recovery)
- Airway invasive pulmonary *Aspergillus*: Consolidation, centrilobular nodules, & ground-glass opacity
- Allergic bronchopulmonary *Aspergillosis:* Bronchial wall thickening, bronchiectasis with mucoid impaction, tree-in-bud opacities, & consolidation
- *Candida*: Multiple pulmonary nodules; may coalesce
- *Pneumocystis*: Extensive ground-glass opacity with interlobular septal thickening
- Coccidioidomycosis: Unilateral consolidation, hilar adenopathy, pleural effusion, pulmonary nodules, cavitary lesions, reticulonodular opacity
- *Cryptococcus*: Miliary or large pulmonary nodules
- Histoplasmosis
  - Acute infection: Mediastinal or hilar adenopathy, miliary nodules, diffuse consolidation
  - Remote infection: Ca^{2+} of pulmonary nodule(s) & affected lymph nodes

Imaging Recommendations

- Best imaging tool
  - Chest radiograph is best screening test for infection
  - NECT of chest is best to diagnose & characterize parenchymal infection

DIFFERENTIAL DIAGNOSIS

Bacterial Pneumonia

- Appearance is same as in immunocompetent patients

Viral Pneumonia

- Immunocompromised patients are less likely to wheeze & more likely to develop consolidation

Pulmonary Metastases

- Usually appear as discrete, round, solid nodules

CLINICAL ISSUES

Demographics

- Epidemiology
  - *Aspergillus*
    - Biggest risk for invasive aspergillosis is neutropenia
  - *Candida*
    - Major cause of morbidity & mortality in ICU/NICU
    - Risks: Central venous catheters, invasive interventions, treatment with broad-spectrum antibiotics
  - *Pneumocystis*
    - High risk in patients with lymphoid malignancies
  - Coccidioidomycosis
    - Endemic in Southwestern United States
    - Risk for exposure ↑ with storms, high winds, earthquake, & construction
  - *Cryptococcus*
    - Endemic in Southern California
  - Histoplasmosis
    - Endemic in Ohio & Mississippi river valleys

SELECTED REFERENCES

1. Katragkou A et al: Diagnostic imaging and invasive fungal diseases in children. J Pediatric Infect Dis Soc. 6(suppl_1):S22-31, 2017
2. Toma P et al: Fungal infections of the lung in children. Pediatr Radiol. 46(13):1856-65, 2016

Papillomatosis

KEY FACTS

TERMINOLOGY

- Recurrent respiratory papillomatosis (RRP): Benign tumors of aerodigestive tract caused by infection with human papillomavirus (HPV)
  - Variable lifelong morbidity; potentially fatal course

IMAGING

- Locations: Junctional sites between respiratory & squamous epithelium
  - Larynx is most common site
  - Extralaryngeal spread in ~ 30% of patients
    - Endobronchial spread → pulmonary nodules
      - Lung parenchymal involvement in 3%
- CT appearance
  - Airway: Soft tissue nodules protruding into lumen
  - Lung: Multiple solid or cavitated nodules
    - ± postobstructive atelectasis or pneumonia
    - Malignant degeneration of pulmonary disease in 0.5%
      - Squamous cell carcinoma

PATHOLOGY

- Perinatal transmission of HPV: Infected mother → child
  - ↑ risk: Vaginal delivery, firstborn, mother < 20 years of age; delivery time > 10 hours doubles risk
- Vast majority are caused by HPV-6 & HPV-11

CLINICAL ISSUES

- Most common laryngeal tumor in children
- Most common symptoms: Hoarseness, stridor, difficulty breathing
- Mean age at diagnosis: ~ 4 years
- Disease remission can occur spontaneously at any stage
- Treatment is resection using powered microdebrider
  - Need for repeated debulking is typical
- Tracheostomy is needed in 10-15% due to airway obstruction; delayed as long as possible due to ↑ risk of distal spread
- HPV 9-valent vaccine protects against strains implicated in RRP

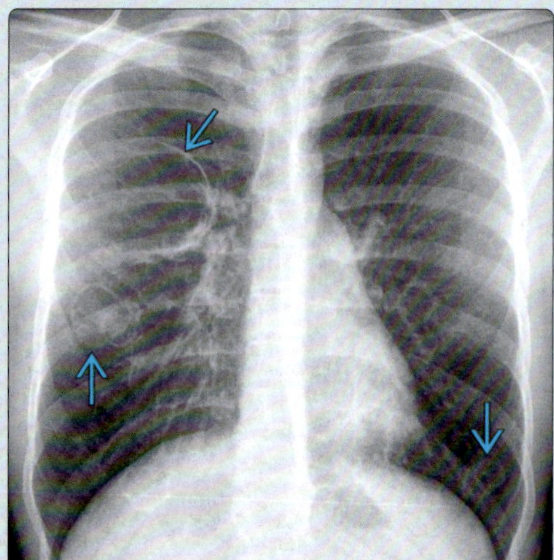

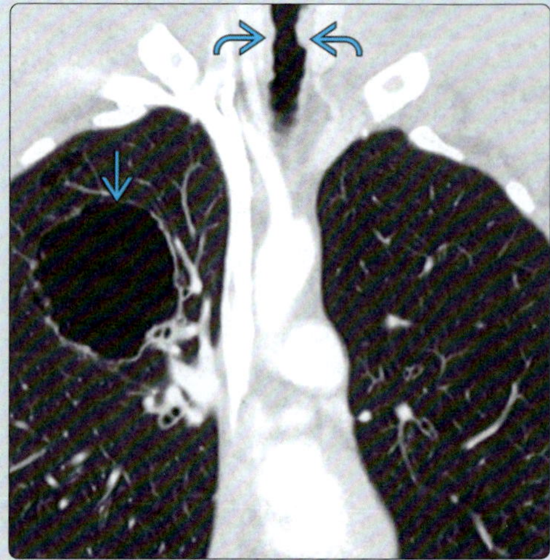

(Left) *PA radiograph of the chest in a young adult with respiratory papillomatosis shows multiple pulmonary cysts ➔ of various sizes. The cyst walls are irregular with variable thickness.* **(Right)** *Coronal CECT in the same patient shows a large cyst ➔ with varying wall thickness in the right upper lobe. Additional nodular foci in the tracheal lumen are typical of tracheal papillomas ➔.*

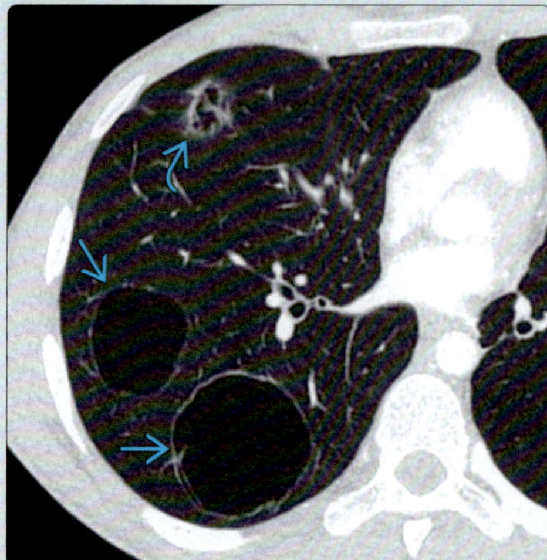

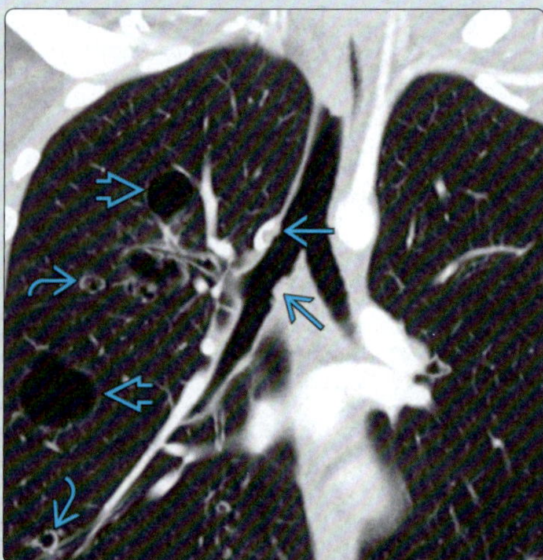

(Left) *Axial CECT in the same patient shows cysts ➔ of various sizes in the right lung. The cyst in the right middle lobe ➔ has a thick, irregular wall.* **(Right)** *Coronal CECT in the same patient shows cysts ➔ of various sizes in the right lung. Some of the smaller cysts ➔ have thickened, irregular walls. Additional nodular intraluminal tracheal & bronchial papillomas ➔ are noted.*

TERMINOLOGY

Abbreviations

- Recurrent respiratory papillomatosis (RRP)

Definitions

- Benign tumors of aerodigestive tract caused by infection with human papillomavirus (HPV)

IMAGING

General Features

- Best diagnostic clue
  - Wart-like growth in larynx
- Location
  - Occurs at junctional sites between respiratory & squamous epithelium
    - Larynx is most common
    - Extralaryngeal spread in 30%: Oral cavity, trachea, bronchi, & esophagus
    - Tracheal or central bronchial involvement in 11%
    - Peripheral airway or alveolar involvement in 3%
      - Surgical manipulation of laryngeal papillomas ↑ risk of pulmonary dissemination
- Size
  - 1-2 mm to several centimeters
- Morphology
  - Warty lesions of larynx & tracheobronchial tree
  - Solid or cavitary pulmonary nodules

Radiographic Findings

- Radiography
  - Larynx, trachea, & main bronchi: Multifocal nodular irregularity of airway wall ± luminal narrowing
  - Lung: Multiple solid or cavitated nodules
    - As nodules enlarge, more likely to cavitate
    - Cavities may be thick- or thin-walled
    - Air-fluid levels suggest superinfection
    - Atelectasis & postobstructive pneumonia are uncommon
    - Large mass suggests malignant degeneration

CT Findings

- CECT
  - Soft tissue nodules protruding into airway ± luminal narrowing
  - Pulmonary findings
    - Nodules: May have mild enhancement
    - Cavitary lesions: Thin or thick, irregular enhancing walls
    - Malignant degeneration: Suspicious findings include heterogeneous enhancement, enlarging mass, or lymphadenopathy

Nuclear Medicine Findings

- PET/CT
  - May have areas of ↑ FDG uptake ± malignant degeneration
    - Difficult to distinguish RRP from squamous cell carcinoma
    - May help target specific lesion for biopsy

Imaging Recommendations

- Best imaging tool
  - CT is most sensitive to determine extent of disease & identify complications

DIFFERENTIAL DIAGNOSIS

Subglottic Infantile Hemangioma

- Strongly enhancing tracheal nodule on CT
- Usually presents in infancy with stridor
- Lung lesions are extremely rare

Granulomatosis With Polyangiitis

- Triad of pulmonary, paranasal sinus, & renal disease
- Pulmonary nodules may form thick-walled cavities
- Circumferential subglottic tracheal wall thickening

Septic Emboli

- Cavitated pulmonary nodules, often with thick irregular walls & surrounding lung consolidation
- Common causes: Endocarditis & septic thrombophlebitis
  - Lemierre syndrome: Septic thrombophlebitis of internal jugular vein after oropharyngeal infection → septic emboli

Metastases

- Variably sized lung nodules in patient with malignancy
- Cavitation of metastases is uncommon in children

Pneumatocele

- Transient thin-walled cyst(s) of variable size
- Usually follows known insult (trauma, infection, hydrocarbon ingestion)

Lymphangioleiomyomatosis

- Scattered thin-walled cysts of variable sizes
- Occurs in women of childbearing age
- May be sporadic or related to tuberous sclerosis complex

Langerhans Cell Histiocytosis

- Nodules &/or cysts, primarily in upper lung zones of older smokers

Invasive Aspergillosis

- Nodules have ground-glass "halo" of hemorrhage
- Immunocompromised host

PATHOLOGY

General Features

- Etiology
  - Perinatal transmission of HPV from infected mother to child
    - Risks: Active condylomata, primigravid mother, prolonged vaginal delivery, prolonged rupture of membranes, & newly acquired infection
    - 1 in 400 children delivered to women with active condylomata develop RRP
    - Still questionable if elective cesarean section is protective
  - 95% of cases of RRP are caused by HPV-6 & HPV-11
    - HPV-11 is more common & causes more severe disease

- Nearly all patients with malignant degeneration have HPV-11 infection
- Malignant transformation to squamous cell carcinoma in < 1% of RRP

Staging, Grading, & Classification

- Coltera/Derkay staging system
  - Separates aerodigestive tract into 25 subsites
  - Different sites are evaluated & scored for severity of disease

Gross Pathologic & Surgical Features

- Pedunculated mass(es) with finger-like projections

Microscopic Features

- Multiple fronds with central fibrovascular core covered by stratified squamous epithelium
- Lung & laryngeal lesions are composed of squamous cells; cavities are lined with squamous epithelium
- Squamous atypia is common even in benign lesions

CLINICAL ISSUES

Presentation

- Most common signs/symptoms
  - Clinical triad: Progressive hoarseness, stridor, difficulty breathing
- Other signs/symptoms
  - Dyspnea, chronic cough, recurrent upper respiratory infections, pneumonia, respiratory distress, dysphagia, & failure to thrive
  - Symptoms are often present for ~ 1 year before definitive diagnosis is established

Demographics

- Age
  - Bimodal age distribution
    - Juvenile-onset RRP (JO-RRP): Mean age at diagnosis: ~ 4 years
      - Younger age of onset = more severe disease
    - 2nd peak in adults 20-30 years of age = adult-onset RRP (AO-RRP)
      - Etiology is most likely sexual transmission of HPV
      - AO-RRP is typically less aggressive than in children
- Sex
  - M = F
- Epidemiology
  - Most common laryngeal tumor in children
  - 2nd most common cause of chronic hoarseness in children
  - In USA, RRP affects 4.3 per 100,000 children
  - Risk factors
    - Vaginal delivery, 1stborn child, & mother < 20 years of age
    - Prolonged delivery time (> 10 hours) doubles risk for development of RRP
    - Active condylomata ↑ risk 231x

Natural History & Prognosis

- Benign disease with varying degrees of lifelong morbidity & potentially fatal course
- Papillomas show variable growth rate
  - Overall, frequent exacerbations are typical
- Disease remission can occur spontaneously at any stage
  - Duration of remission is variable & unpredictable
  - Laryngeal disease is most likely to undergo remission
- Extralaryngeal spread in ~ 30% of patients
  - Tracheobronchial involvement in 11%
    - Tracheostomy is associated with significant morbidity
      - Papillomas coalesce at tracheotomy site
      - Distal spread is more likely
      - Tracheostomy is needed in 10-15% due to airway obstruction; delayed as long as possible
  - Lung parenchymal involvement in 3%
    - Lung nodules grow very slowly, usually measured in decades
    - May cavitate & become secondarily infected
    - May get postobstructive atelectasis & pneumonia
  - Lung cancer (squamous cell carcinoma) in 0.5%
    - High suspicion needs to be maintained
    - Malignant degeneration is more common in longstanding disease with history of prior irradiation & smoking
    - Look for increasing size of nodule on imaging
- Death due to large airway obstruction or respiratory failure
  - 57% mortality associated with pulmonary disease related to respiratory failure, infection, or malignant transformation

Treatment

- Current standard of care: Surgical resection
  - Need for repeated debulking is typical
- Laser ablation is now less commonly used
- Medical therapies are used as adjunct to surgery
  - Interferon & antiviral agents (cidofovir & acyclovir) may slow growth but are not curative
  - 3-carbinol, retinoic acid, & photodynamic therapy have variable effect
- HPV 9-valent vaccine protects against strains implicated in RRP
  - Vaccines ↓ incidence of RRP

DIAGNOSTIC CHECKLIST

Consider

- Laryngeal mass or soft tissue nodules of airway should raise suspicion for RRP

Image Interpretation Pearls

- Review parenchyma & airways in soft tissue & lung windows on multiplanar CT reconstructions

SELECTED REFERENCES

1. Lawlor C et al: International Pediatric Otolaryngology Group (IPOG): juvenile-onset recurrent respiratory papillomatosis consensus recommendations. Int J Pediatr Otorhinolaryngol. 128:109697, 2020
2. Buchinsky FJ et al: Age at diagnosis, but not HPV type, is strongly associated with clinical course in recurrent respiratory papillomatosis. PLoS One. 14(6):e0216697, 2019
3. Lichtenberger JP 3rd et al: Primary lung tumors in children: radiologic-pathologic correlation from the radiologic pathology archives. Radiographics. 38(7):2151-72, 2018
4. Fortes HR et al: Recurrent respiratory papillomatosis: a state-of-the-art review. Respir Med. 126:116-21, 2017

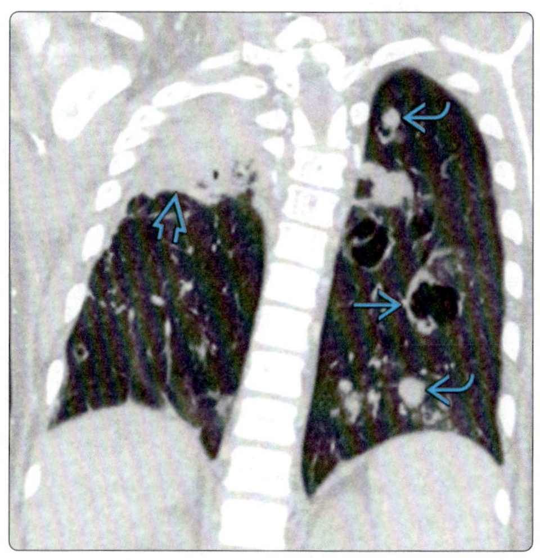

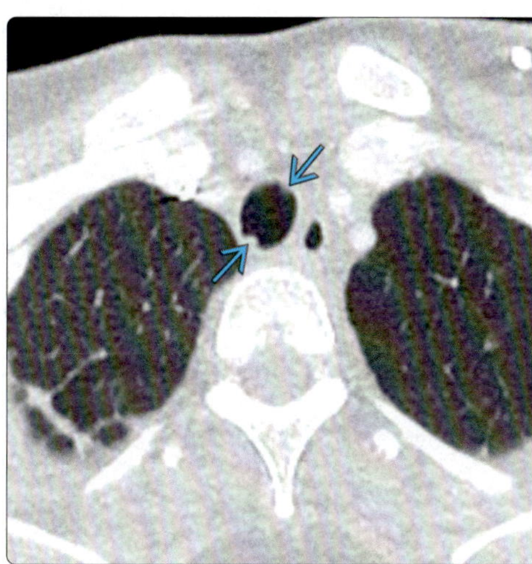

(Left) *Coronal CECT in an adolescent with respiratory papillomatosis & squamous cell carcinoma shows cysts* ➔ *& nodules* ➔ *in the left lung. The cysts have thickened, irregular walls. Consolidation* ➔ *is present in the right upper lobe.* **(Right)** *Axial CECT in an adolescent with respiratory papillomatosis shows nodular papillomas* ➔ *in the trachea.*

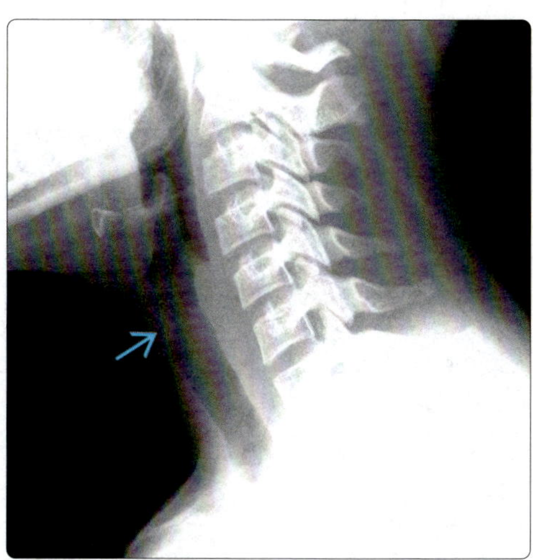

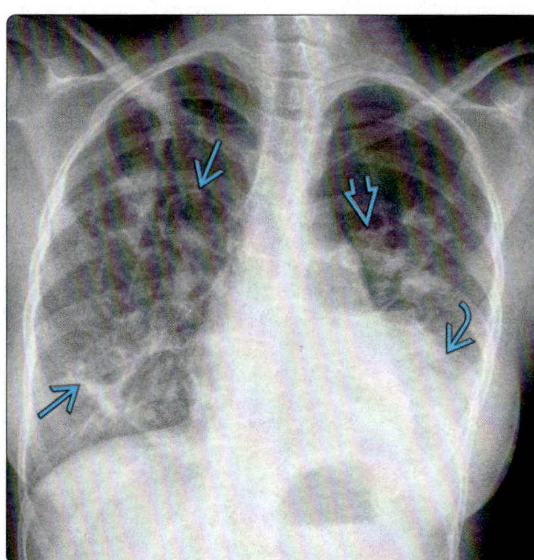

(Left) *Lateral radiograph of the airway in an adolescent with respiratory papillomatosis shows thickening & irregularity* ➔ *of the wall of the trachea, consistent with tracheal papillomas.* **(Right)** *PA radiograph of the chest in an adolescent with respiratory papillomatosis & subsequent squamous cell carcinoma shows multiple pulmonary cysts* ➔ *& nodules* ➔ *in the lungs. There is also consolidation* ➔ *in the left lower lobe.*

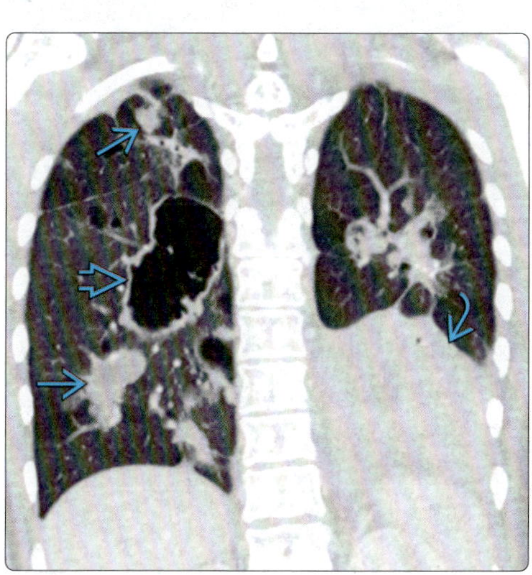

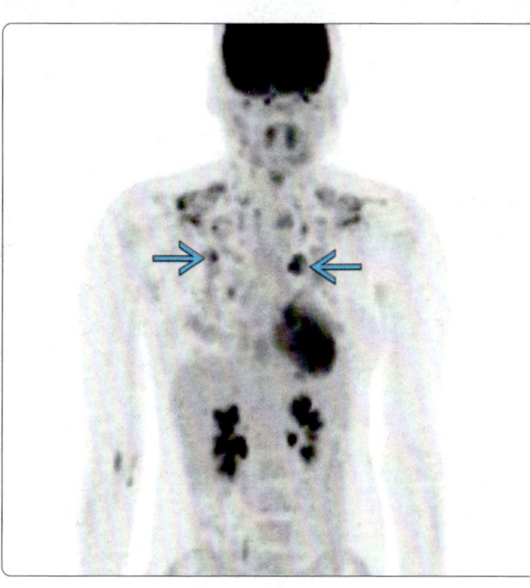

(Left) *Coronal CECT in the same patient shows multiple cysts* ➔ *& solid nodules* ➔*. The cysts have a thickened, irregular wall. There is consolidation* ➔ *of the left lower lobe.* **(Right)** *Coronal F18 FDG PET image in the same patient shows multiple areas of FDG uptake* ➔ *in the chest. FDG uptake is not specific for malignancy. However, FDG avid lesions can help to guide biopsy in this setting.*

Lymphoma

KEY FACTS

TERMINOLOGY

- Lymphoma: Malignant neoplasm arising from constituent cells of immune system or their precursors
- Hodgkin lymphoma (HL), non-Hodgkin lymphoma (NHL)

IMAGING

- Most common thoracic location: Anterior mediastinum
- US can help to distinguish normal thymus from abnormal thymus if nature of prominent anterior mediastinum is unclear radiographically
- CECT: Typically used for initial diagnosis
  - Enlarged & lobulated anterior mediastinal mass with fairly homogeneous soft tissue enhancement
    - Distorts, displaces, encases, & compresses adjacent structures
      - Airway compression: Associated with respiratory failure during induction of anesthesia
    - Other locations in thorax: Hilum, axilla, supraclavicular region, lungs, pleura, pericardium
- PET: Very sensitive & specific (96.5%, 100%) for lymphoma
  - Interpreted using Deauville criteria
  - Changes initial stage in 10-23% of patients compared to conventional imaging
  - Can distinguish active disease from residual inactive mass
  - Negative PET performed after 2 cycles of chemotherapy: Good prognostic factor

PATHOLOGY

- HL: Associated with Epstein-Barr virus in 50%
- NHL: Etiology depends on subtype, often translocation

CLINICAL ISSUES

- Lymphoma is 3rd most common pediatric malignancy
  - Accounts for 10-15% of all pediatric malignancies
- 60% of children with lymphoma have respiratory symptoms
- HL: 5-year survival = 91%
- NHL: 5-year survival = 70-76%

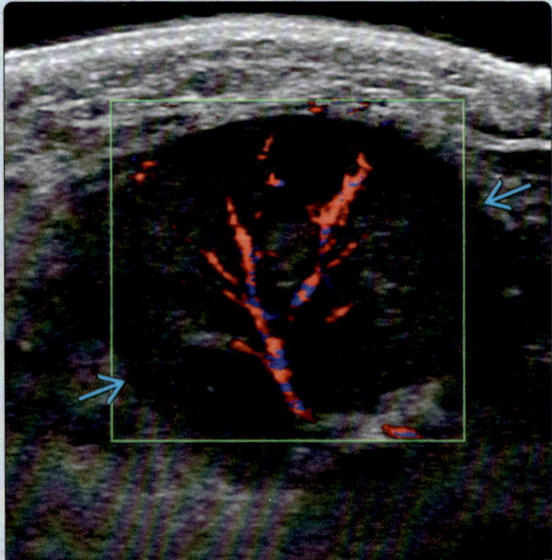

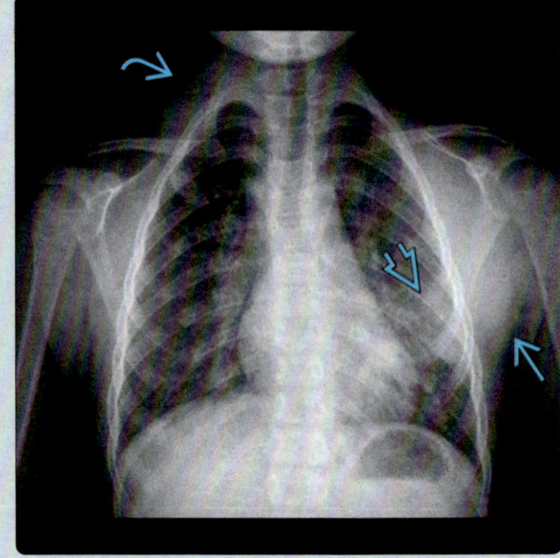

(Left) *Longitudinal color Doppler US of the left axilla in a teenager diagnosed with Hodgkin lymphoma shows an abnormally enlarged & rounded lymph node ➡ with loss of the typical nodal architecture. There is no surrounding fat edema. Multiple other enlarged axillary nodes were also visible.* **(Right)** *PA chest radiograph in the same patient shows ↑ soft tissue density & fullness in the left axilla ➡ & right neck ➡ with a patchy opacity in the left lung ➡.*

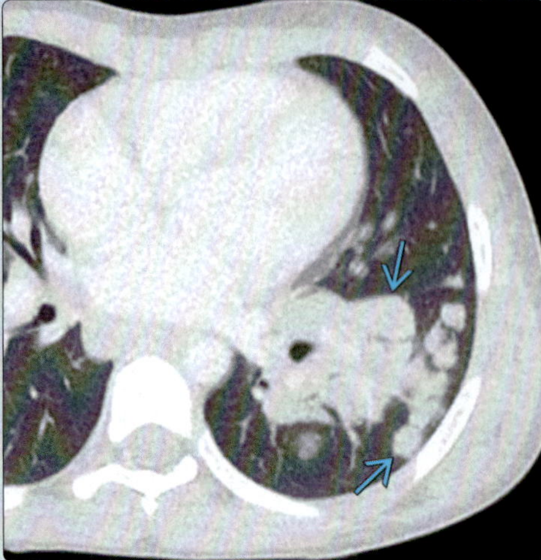

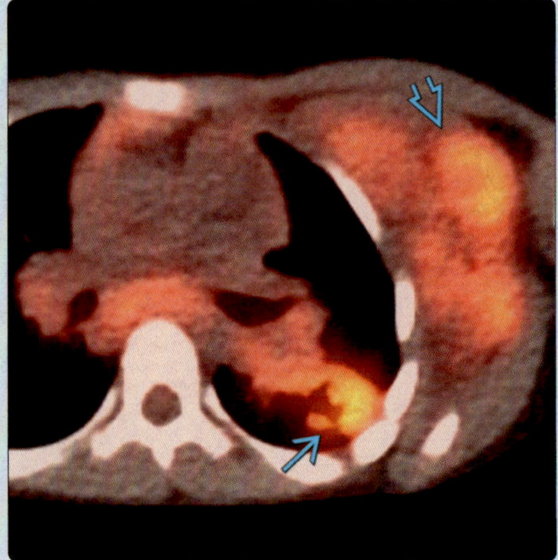

(Left) *Axial CECT of the chest in the same patient shows multiple nodular opacities ➡ in the left lower lobe extending from the hilum to the lung periphery.* **(Right)** *Axial F18-FDG PET/CT fused image in the same patient shows ↑ metabolic activity in the left axillary nodal mass ➡ as well as in the left lower lobe ➡ lymphomatous infiltrate.*

TERMINOLOGY

Abbreviations

- Hodgkin lymphoma (HL), non-Hodgkin lymphoma (NHL)

Synonyms

- Hodgkin disease

Definitions

- Lymphoma: Malignant neoplasm arising from constituent cells of immune system or their precursors
  - Classic HL subtypes: Nodular sclerosis (NS), lymphocyte rich (LR), mixed cellularity (MC), lymphocyte depleted (LD)
  - NHL subtypes: Burkitt lymphoma (BL), diffuse large B-cell lymphoma (DLBCL), anaplastic large cell lymphoma (ALCL), lymphoblastic lymphoma (LBL)

IMAGING

General Features

- Best diagnostic clue
  - Anterior mediastinal mass or dominant nodal mass
- Location
  - Most common thoracic location: Anterior mediastinum
  - Other locations in thorax: Hilum, axilla, supraclavicular region, lungs, pleura, pericardium
- Size
  - Pathologic lymph nodes are traditionally considered as > 1 cm in short axis
    - Negative & positive predictive values are not 100%
  - Bulk mediastinal disease in HL: Mediastinal tumor is > 1/3 of maximal thoracic diameter on upright PA radiograph
- Morphology
  - HL
    - Mediastinal disease in 2/3 of patients
      - Most often associated with NS subtype
    - Often associated with hilar adenopathy
  - NHL
    - Anterior mediastinum is 2nd most common primary site
    - Frequency of intrathoracic involvement depends on subtype
      - 70% with LBL have mediastinal mass
      - 25% with DLBCL have primary mediastinal disease
      - Mediastinum is common location for ALCL
- Associated findings & complications
  - Superior vena cava compression/obstruction
  - Central airway compression/obstruction
  - Pleural effusion
  - Pericardial effusion
  - Pulmonary involvement

Radiographic Findings

- Anterior mediastinal mass
- Look for evidence of complications listed previously
- Tracheal displacement or narrowing → airway compression

CT Findings

- CECT
  - Diffuse thymic infiltration: Enlarged & lobulated with fairly homogeneous soft tissue enhancement
    - Distorts, displaces, encases, & compresses adjacent structures
    - Ca^{2+} is rare in untreated disease
  - Airway compression
    - > 50% reduction in area of trachea is associated with respiratory failure during induction of anesthesia
      - Biopsy can be performed semierect with mild sedation in these patients
    - Airway compromise is predicted by orthopnea, upper body edema, great vessel compression, & mainstem bronchus compression
  - Lungs involved in 5-15% in HL & < 5% in NHL
    - Pulmonary nodules ± cavitation
    - Reticular interstitial pattern from venous or lymphatic obstruction
    - Lobar or segmental consolidation
  - ± pleural or pericardial effusions

MR Findings

- STIR
  - Sensitive for detection of bone marrow & soft tissue lesions
  - Cannot distinguish normal from abnormal lymph nodes
- Whole-body DWI with background body signal suppression (DWIBS)
  - Creates images appearing similar to PET
  - Not as specific as FDG PET; requires correlation with lymph node size
    - All lymph nodes restrict diffusion; DWIBS ↑ conspicuity of nodes compared to other MR sequences
    - Must incorporate size criteria on anatomic imaging to help determine benign vs. malignant

Ultrasonographic Findings

- Grayscale ultrasound
  - Can help assess neck & axillary nodes, potentially guiding biopsy
  - Can look for pleural or pericardial effusions
  - Can help to distinguish normal thymus from abnormal thymus
    - Normal thymus: Uniform echogenic dot-dash pattern without vessel compression
    - HL/NHL: Heterogeneously hypoechoic lobular mass encasing & distorting vessels

Nuclear Medicine Findings

- PET
  - Interpreted using Deauville criteria (5-point visual scale)
    - (1) No uptake above surrounding background
    - (2)Uptake ≤ mediastinal blood pool
    - (3) Uptake > mediastinal blood pool but ≤ liver
    - (4) Moderately ↑ compared to liver
    - (5) Markedly ↑ compared to liver
  - Very sensitive & specific (96.5%, 100%) for detection of disease
  - Changes initial stage in 10-23% of patients compared to conventional imaging
  - Can help to provide prognostic information
    - Negative PET performed after 2 cycles of chemotherapy: Good prognostic factor
  - Can distinguish active disease from residual inactive mass

- PET/MR shows promise due to combination of functional imaging, anatomic imaging, DWI, & ↓ radiation

Imaging Recommendations

- Best imaging tool
  - CECT is most commonly used for diagnosis
  - PET/CT is used for staging & follow-up
- Protocol advice
  - Beware of placing patient in prone position or using sedation if there is compression of airway

DIFFERENTIAL DIAGNOSIS

Normal Thymus

- Large normal thymus occurs in children < 5 years of age
- Undulating margins; does not displace/compress airway or vessels
- Echogenic dot-dash pattern throughout on US

Germ Cell Tumor

- Often heterogeneous with cystic, fatty, &/or calcific foci

Lymphatic Malformation

- Multicystic mass of neck & mediastinum present since birth

Neuroblastoma

- Paraspinal mass ± Ca^{2+} in child < 10 years of age

Thymoma

- Very uncommon in children

PATHOLOGY

General Features

- Etiology
  - HL: Associated with Epstein-Barr virus (EBV) in 50%
    - Other risks: Immunocompromised, ↓ socioeconomic status, small family size, early birth order
  - NHL: Etiology depends on subtype
- Associated abnormalities
  - Down syndrome has higher incidence of leukemia/lymphoma

Staging, Grading, & Classification

- HL subtypes (frequency): NS (70%), MC (20%), LR (5%), LD (5%)
- HL staging: Lugano classification
  - Stage I: Single lymph node or group of nodes
  - Stage II: 2 or more lymph node groups on same side of diaphragm
  - Stage III: Nodal involvement on both sides of diaphragm or nodal involvement in chest & splenic involvement
  - Stage IV: Extranodal involvement
  - Designations applicable to any stage
    - A: Asymptomatic
    - B: Symptoms of fever, night sweats, weight loss > 10%
- NHL subtypes (frequency): BL (30%), DLBCL (10-20%), ALCL (10%), LBL (30%)
- NHL staging: International Pediatric Non-Hodgkin Lymphoma Staging System
  - Stage I: Single nodal area outside abdomen & mediastinum
  - Stage II
    - Single extranodal tumor with regional node involvement
    - ≥ 2 nodal areas on same side of diaphragm
    - Primary gastrointestinal tract tumor that is completely resectable
  - Stage III
    - ≥ 2 extranodal tumors
    - Nodal tumor above & below diaphragm
    - Any intrathoracic tumor (mediastinal, hilar, pulmonary, pleural, or thymic)
    - Intraabdominal & retroperitoneal disease, including liver, spleen, kidney, or ovary
    - Any paraspinal or epidural tumor
    - Single bone lesion with concomitant involvement of extranodal &/or nonregional nodal site
  - Stage IV: Bone marrow or CNS disease

CLINICAL ISSUES

Presentation

- Most common signs/symptoms
  - 60% of children have respiratory symptoms
  - HL may present with painless adenopathy
- Other signs/symptoms
  - HL: B symptoms of fever, night sweats, weight loss
  - NHL: Can have life-threatening symptoms due to compression of trachea or superior vena cava or large pleural or pericardial effusion

Demographics

- Age
  - Much more common in 2nd decade of life
  - Prevalence of NHL ↑ with age
- Sex
  - HL: M > F under 15 years old; F > M over 15 years old
  - NHL: M > F
- Epidemiology
  - Lymphoma: 3rd most common pediatric malignancy
    - Accounts for 10-15% of all pediatric malignancies

Natural History & Prognosis

- HL: 5-year survival = 91%
- NHL: 5-year survival = 70-76%

Treatment

- HL: Chemotherapy ± radiation
- NHL: Chemotherapy ± bone marrow transplantation or radiation therapy

SELECTED REFERENCES

1. Biko DM et al: Mediastinal masses in children: radiologic-pathologic correlation. Radiographics. 41(4):E1186-207, 2021
2. McCarten KM et al: Imaging for diagnosis, staging and response assessment of Hodgkin lymphoma and non-Hodgkin lymphoma. Pediatr Radiol. 49(11):1545-64, 2019
3. Spijkers S et al: Imaging features of extranodal involvement in paediatric Hodgkin lymphoma. Pediatr Radiol. 49(2):266-76, 2019
4. Voss SD: Functional and anatomical imaging in pediatric oncology: which is best for which tumors. Pediatr Radiol. 49(11):1534-44, 2019
5. Voss SD et al: Surveillance imaging in pediatric lymphoma. Pediatr Radiol. 49(11):1565-73, 2019
6. Hochberg J et al: Lymphoma in adolescents and young adults: current perspectives. Cancer J. 24(6):285-300, 2018
7. Kluge R et al: Current role of FDG-PET in pediatric Hodgkin's lymphoma. Semin Nucl Med. 47(3):242-57, 2017

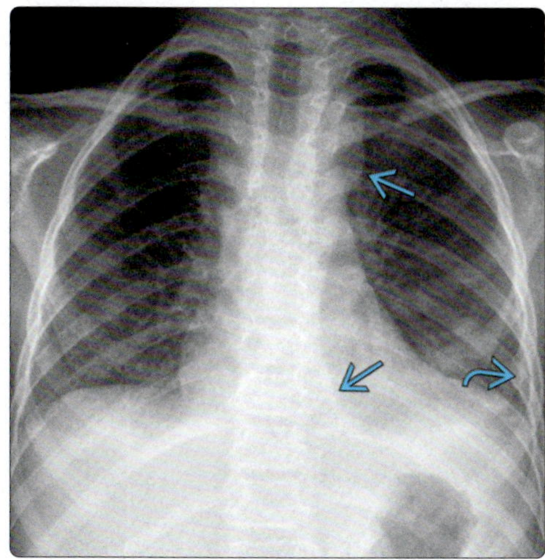

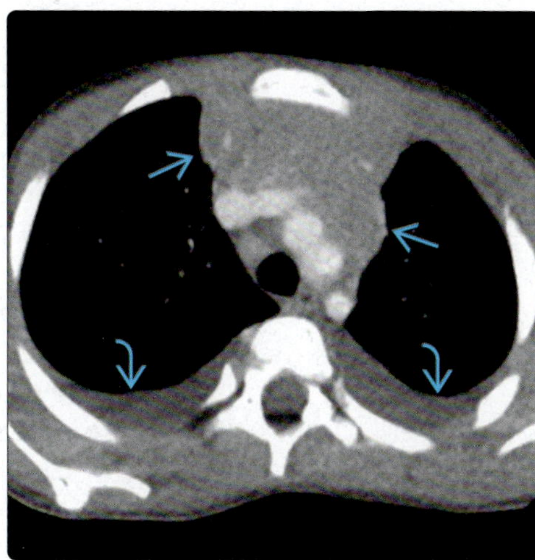

(Left) *PA radiograph of the chest in a teenager with Burkitt lymphoma shows a mediastinal mass extending from the superior mediastinum to the lower chest. A small left pleural effusion is also present.* **(Right)** *Axial CECT in the same patient shows a slightly heterogeneous anterior mediastinal mass & small bilateral pleural effusions. The volume of tissue & lobulated contours of the mass would be atypical for residual thymus in a teenage patient.*

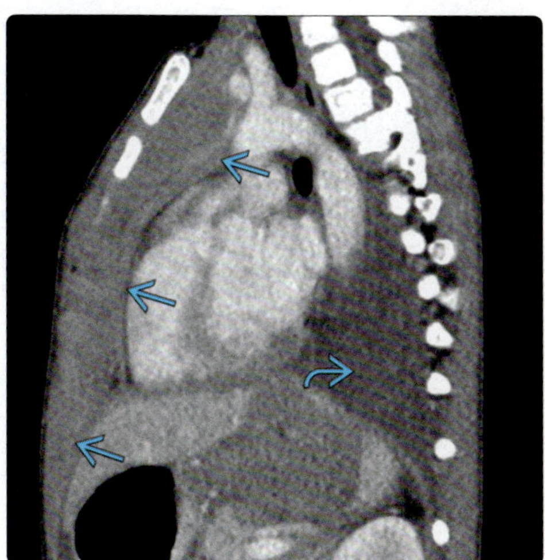

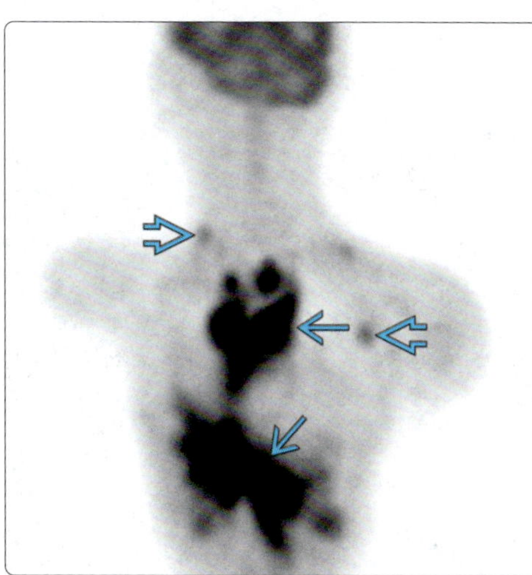

(Left) *Sagittal CECT in the same patient with Burkitt lymphoma shows the superior to inferior extent of the anterior mediastinal mass. Again note the pleural effusion.* **(Right)** *Coronal image from an F18-FDG PET in the same patient shows ↑ metabolic activity within the mediastinal mass as well as scattered lymph nodes.*

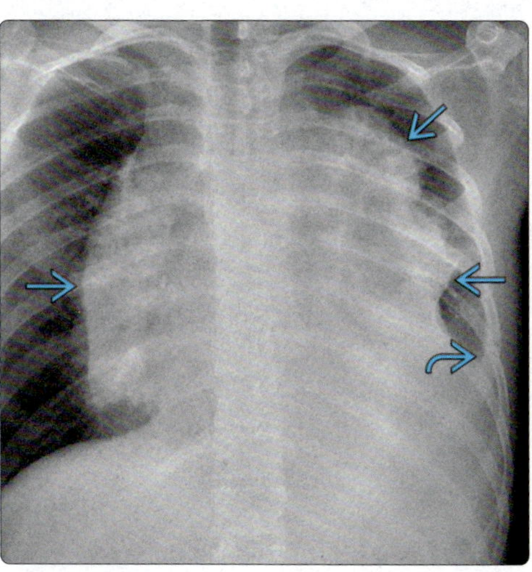

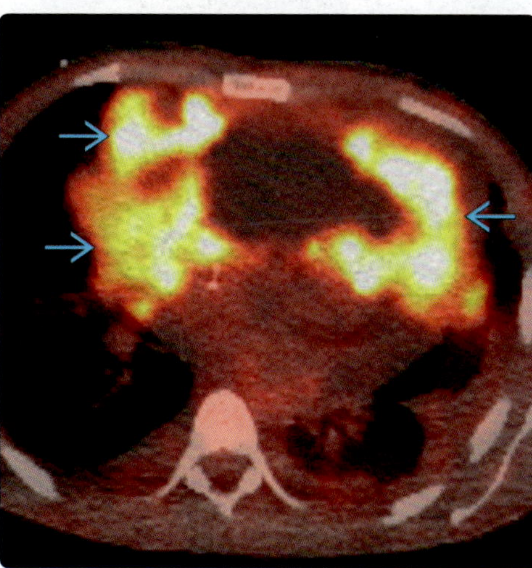

(Left) *PA radiograph of the chest in a child with Hodgkin lymphoma shows a large anterior mediastinal mass with lobulated contours. Note the left pleural effusion.* **(Right)** *Axial fused F18 FDG PET/CT in the same patient shows uptake at the periphery of the large anterior mediastinal mass. The central area without FDG uptake was necrotic.*

KEY FACTS

TERMINOLOGY

- Germ cell tumor (GCT) types: Teratoma, seminoma, nonseminomatous germ cell tumor (NSGCT)
  - Teratoma: Mature, immature, malignant
  - Seminoma: Germinoma & dysgerminoma
  - NSGCT: Embryonal cell, yolk sac tumor, choriocarcinoma, & mixed GCT
- Derived from primordial germ cells that differentiate into embryonic & extraembryonic structures

IMAGING

- Best clue: Heterogeneous anterior mediastinal mass arising within or adjacent to thymus
  - Less common locations: Posterior mediastinum, heart, pericardium
- Teratoma
  - Mostly cystic + soft tissue, fat, & calcium
    - 1 or more cysts; 20-40% calcify; 93% contain fat
    - CECT is sensitive for these components
- Seminoma
  - Homogeneous, lobulated, bulky soft tissue mass
  - Often straddles midline & has mass effect
- NSGCT
  - Heterogeneous mass with hemorrhage & necrosis
  - Irregular margins: Obliterated fat planes & lung invasion
- Pericardial lesions often cause pericardial effusion
- Beware of potential airway collapse from tumor compression during sedation/general anesthesia

PATHOLOGY

- 50-300x ↑ risk of mediastinal GCT with Klinefelter syndrome

CLINICAL ISSUES

- Dyspnea, chest pain, cough, superior vena cava syndrome, hoarseness, fever, weight loss
- Asymptomatic in 50-60% of teratomas, 38% of seminomas, & 10% of NSGCTs

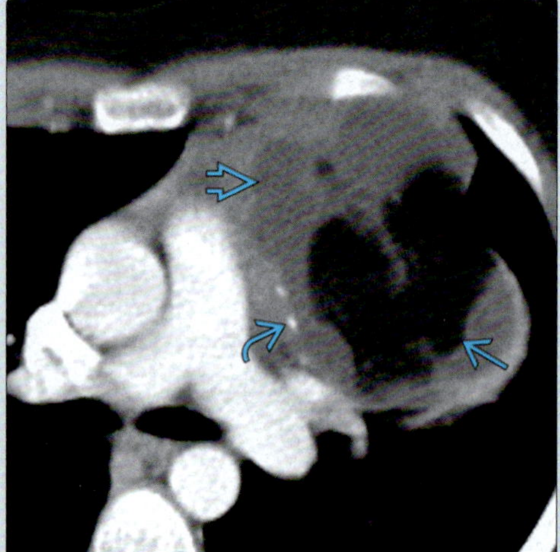

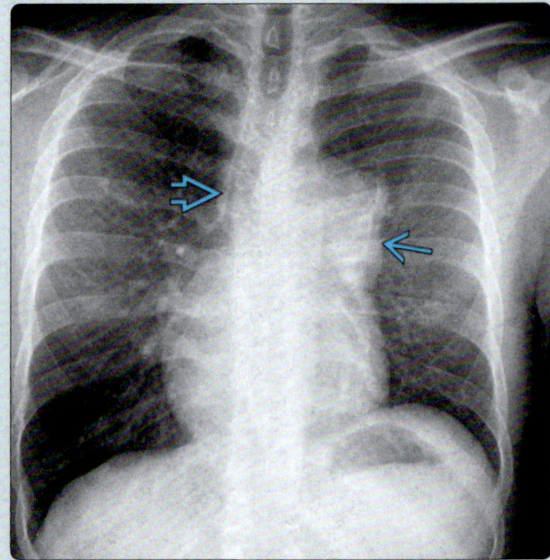

(Left) *Axial CECT shows an anterior mediastinal mass containing fat ➡, fluid ➡, & calcification ➡. This combination of densities in a mass is characteristic of a teratoma.* **(Right)** *PA chest radiograph in a young adult shows a lobulated left mediastinal mass ➡. Note the rightward tracheal deviation ➡ & the elevation of the left hemidiaphragm. This latter finding raises concern for involvement of the left phrenic nerve.*

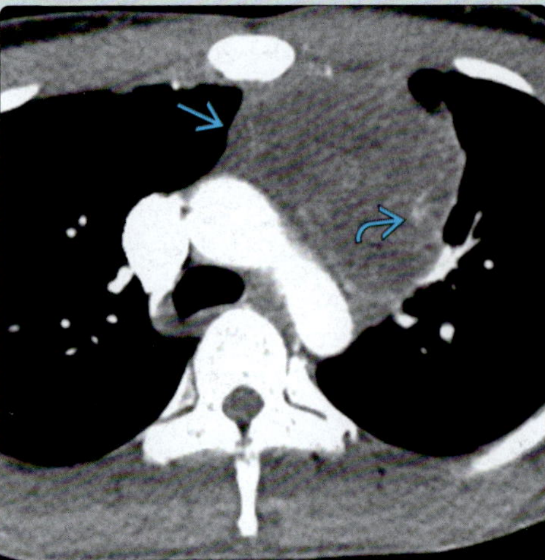

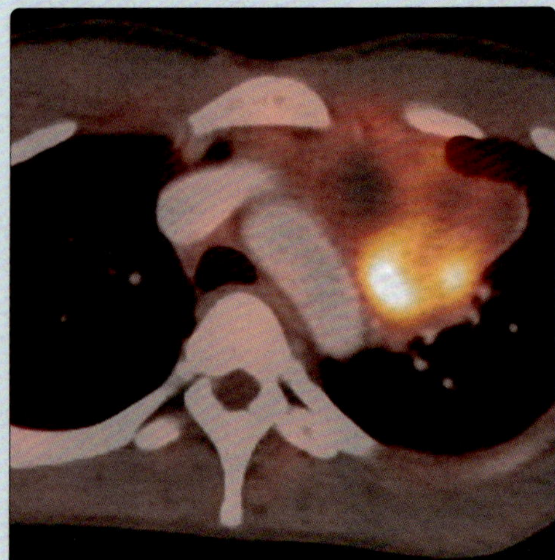

(Left) *Axial CECT in the same patient shows the soft tissue density anterior mediastinal mass ➡. Multiple small vessels ➡ extend through the mass. No fat or calcification was identified in the lesion.* **(Right)** *Axial fused F18 FDG PET/CT in the same patient shows radiopharmaceutical uptake within portions of the mediastinal mass. At pathology, this mass was confirmed to be a germ cell tumor with sarcomatous & neuroblastic components.*

TERMINOLOGY

Synonyms

- Teratoma, seminoma, nonseminomatous germ cell tumor (NSGCT)

Definitions

- Germ cell tumor (GCT): Tumor derived from primordial germ cells
- Teratoma: 3 major types
  - Mature teratoma: Characterized by mixture of adult-type tissues derived from 3 germinal layers
  - Immature teratoma: Contains embryonic or fetal tissue, often neuroepithelial structures
  - Malignant teratoma: Contains foci of malignant transformation
- Malignant GCT: Seminoma & NSGCT
  - Seminoma: Germinoma & dysgerminoma
  - NSGCT: Embryonal cell, yolk sac tumor (YST), choriocarcinoma, & mixed GCT

IMAGING

General Features

- Best diagnostic clue
  - Heterogeneous anterior mediastinal mass arising within or adjacent to thymus
- Location
  - Anterior mediastinum is most common
  - Less common locations: Posterior mediastinum, heart, pericardium
- Size
  - Average size for NSGCT: 9 cm; seminoma: 5 cm
- Morphology
  - Teratoma: Mostly cystic with soft tissue, fat, & calcium elements
  - Seminoma: Homogeneous, lobulated, bulky mass
  - NSGCT: Heterogeneous soft tissue mass with hemorrhage & necrosis

Radiographic Findings

- Teratoma: Round, sharply marginated, anterior mediastinal mass
  - 20-40% calcify
- Seminoma: Bulky, lobulated, anterior mediastinal mass
- NSGCT: Large, anterior mediastinal mass
  - Pleural or pericardial effusions may be present

CT Findings

- NECT
  - Teratoma: Sharply marginated anterior mediastinal mass
    - Extends to 1 side of midline
    - Fatty, cystic/solid soft tissue, & calcified components are often visible
      - 93% contain fat
  - Seminoma: Large solid mass with homogeneous density
    - Straddles midline; mass effect on adjacent structures
  - NSGCT: Large, heterogeneous mass
    - Central area of hemorrhage or necrosis
    - Irregular margins with obliterated fat planes
    - May invade lung, chest wall, & diaphragm
    - Metastasizes to lymph nodes, lung, & liver
- CECT
  - Better defines extent of lesion & invasion
    - Look for compression of vessels & airway
  - More clearly differentiates solid & cystic components
  - Teratoma: Enhancement of rim & septations
  - Seminoma: Mild enhancement
  - NSGCT: Enhancement of peripheral soft tissue around central necrotic region

MR Findings

- T1WI
  - Teratoma: Well-circumscribed lesion
    - Varied signal of fat, soft tissue, calcium, & fluid
      - Fluid varies in signal due to protein content
- T2WI
  - Teratoma: Signal depends on tissue types in lesion
    - Fluid has high signal
    - Look for signal drop-out on fat-saturated images

Imaging Recommendations

- Best imaging tool
  - CECT demonstrates differing tissue components, extent of disease, & complications
  - Beware of potential airway collapse from tumor compression during sedation/general anesthesia

DIFFERENTIAL DIAGNOSIS

Normal Thymus

- Large, quadrilateral-shaped, homogeneous tissue in 1st few years of life
- No mass effect on vessels or airway
- Uniform dot-dash pattern of echoes on US

Lymphoma

- Bulky, lobulated, homogeneous mass compressing & displacing airway & vessels
- Rarely calcifies before treatment

Lymphatic Malformation

- Congenital multicystic mass of neck & chest
- May have soft tissue attenuation following hemorrhage

Thymic Cyst

- Usually unilocular, may be bilobed with neck & mediastinal components
- Often asymptomatic but can compress adjacent structures

Thymoma

- Rare in children
- Associated with paraneoplastic syndromes

PATHOLOGY

General Features

- Etiology
  - Most common theory: Local transformation of primordial germ cells misplaced during embryogenesis
- Associated abnormalities
  - 50-300x ↑ risk of mediastinal GCT with Klinefelter syndrome
  - Possible relationship to Li-Fraumeni syndrome & Down syndrome

- NSGCT is associated with hematologic malignancies, most commonly acute megakaryoblastic leukemia

Gross Pathologic & Surgical Features

- Teratoma: Well-encapsulated, predominantly cystic
  - Cystic component is usually unilocular
  - May be adherent to mediastinal structures
- Seminoma: Unencapsulated, well circumscribed, large
  - Usually has solid, uniform appearance with focal areas of necrosis or hemorrhage
- NSGCT: Unencapsulated, irregularly marginated, heterogeneous large mass
  - Large areas of necrosis, hemorrhage, & cysts
  - Invades local structures

Microscopic Features

- Teratoma
  - Admixture of adult-type tissues
  - Derived from 3 germinal layers
  - Most common components: Skin & appendages, pancreatic, bronchial, neural, gastrointestinal, muscular, fatty, & cartilaginous elements
- Seminoma
  - Sheets of round or polygonal cells surrounded by septa of connective tissue infiltrated by lymphocytes
  - Prominent eosinophilic nucleoli with characteristic spiked appearance
- NSGCT
  - Embryonal: Large malignant cells arranged in sheets or tubular/acinar patterns
  - YST: Reticular pattern with cords of tumor cells embedded in myxoid stroma is most common
  - Choriocarcinoma: Mix of syncytiotrophoblast, cytotrophoblast, & intermediate trophoblast

CLINICAL ISSUES

Presentation

- Most common signs/symptoms
  - Asymptomatic in 50-60% of teratomas, 38% of seminomas, & 10% of NSGCTs
  - Dyspnea (25-85%), chest pain (10-52%), cough (10-24%), superior vena cava syndrome (6-40%), hoarseness (1-14%), fever (13%), weight loss (11%)
  - α-fetoprotein is elevated in 74% of patients with NSGCT; β-HCG is elevated in 38%
- Other signs/symptoms
  - Gynecomastia, testicular atrophy, facial fullness, precocious puberty
  - If teratoma contains endocrine pancreas, can cause hyperinsulinism & hypoglycemia
  - Rare rupture of cystic component of teratoma → erosion into tracheobronchial tree followed by expectoration of sebaceous material & hair

Demographics

- Age
  - Separated into prepubertal & postpubertal due to differences in genetics & clinical behavior
- Sex
  - Mature teratoma: M = F
  - Malignant GCTs
    - Children: M = F [except in YST where F > M (4:1)]
    - Teenagers & adults: M > F (5:1)
- Epidemiology
  - GCT is 3rd most common mediastinal tumor in children
  - Mature teratoma: 19-24% of anterior mediastinal tumors in children
    - Teratoma: 44% of mediastinal GCT
    - Seminoma: 16-37% of mediastinal GCT
    - NSGCT: 14% of mediastinal GCT
    - Mixed GCT: 13-25% of mediastinal GCT

Natural History & Prognosis

- Prognosis is dependent on multiple factors
  - Age < 30 years is associated with better prognosis
  - Histological type
    - Mature teratoma: Benign (80% of mediastinal GCT)
    - Immature teratoma: Good prognosis, no risk of recurrence or metastasis
    - Teratoma with component of malignant GCT: Prognosis depends on malignant component
    - Seminoma: 5-year survival rate = 90%
    - NSGCT: 5-year survival rate = 48%
  - Presence of metastases (most common in lungs or bone)
  - Stage: In children, prognosis is related to stage
  - Status of resection: Complete resection is strongest prognostic indicator
  - Tumor markers: α-fetoprotein > 10,000 ng/mL = worse prognosis; ↑ β-HCG = worse prognosis in adults

Treatment

- Mature teratoma: Surgery
- Seminoma: Chemotherapy followed by surgery for residual disease
- Nonseminomatous: Chemotherapy & surgery

DIAGNOSTIC CHECKLIST

Image Interpretation Pearls

- If Ca^{2+} is present, mass = teratoma until proven otherwise
- NSGCT invades surrounding structures
- Large mediastinal masses have risk of cardiopulmonary arrest at induction of anesthesia in patients with tracheal or vascular compression

SELECTED REFERENCES

1. Biko DM et al: Mediastinal masses in children: radiologic-pathologic correlation. Radiographics. 41(4):E1186-207, 2021
2. Gupta K et al: Synchronous solitary calvarial yolk sac tumor metastasis as the initial presentation of mediastinal germ cell tumor. Childs Nerv Syst. 34(2):363-6, 2018
3. Kawaguchi Y et al: Prediction of respiratory collapse among pediatric patients with mediastinal tumors during induction of general anesthesia. J Pediatr Surg. 53(7):1365-8, 2018
4. Grabski DF et al: Long-term outcomes of pediatric and adolescent mediastinal germ cell tumors: a single pediatric oncology institutional experience. Pediatr Surg Int. 33(2):235-44, 2017
5. Sudour-Bonnange H et al: Primary mediastinal and retroperitoneal malignant germ cell tumors in children and adolescents: results of the TGM95 trial, a study of the French Society of Pediatric Oncology (Société Française des Cancers de l'Enfant). Pediatr Blood Cancer. 64(9), 2017
6. Dechaphunkul A et al: Clinical Characteristics and treatment outcomes of patients with primary mediastinal germ cell tumors: 10-years' experience at a single institution with a bleomycin-containing regimen. Oncol Res Treat. 39(11):688-94, 2016
7. Olson TA et al: Pediatric and adolescent extracranial germ cell tumors: the road to collaboration. J Clin Oncol. 33(27):3018-28, 2015

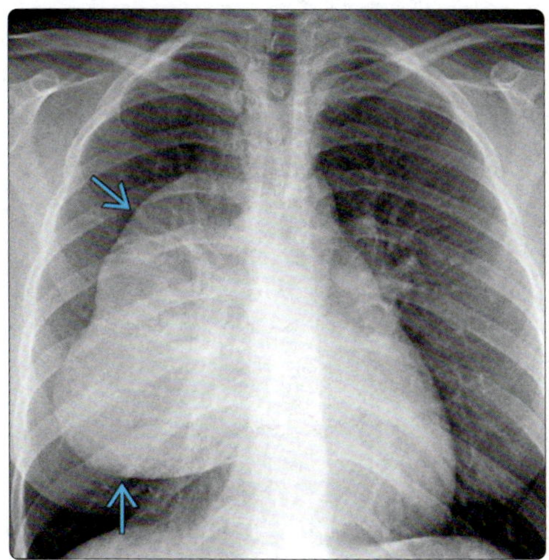

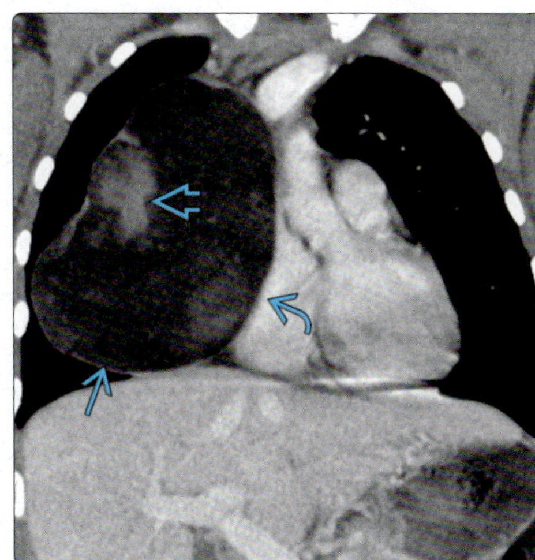

(Left) *PA radiograph of the chest shows a large, lobulated right-sided anterior mediastinal mass* ➙*.* **(Right)** *Coronal CECT in the same patient shows that the large mediastinal mass* ➙ *is mostly composed of fat. The mass compresses the right atrium* ➙*, & there is a soft tissue component* ➙ *within the mass.*

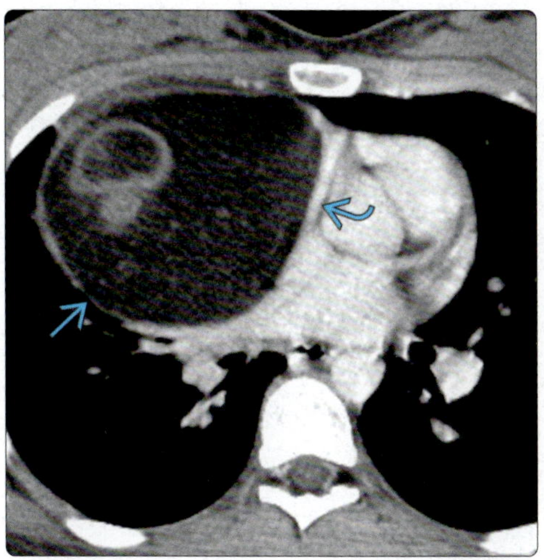

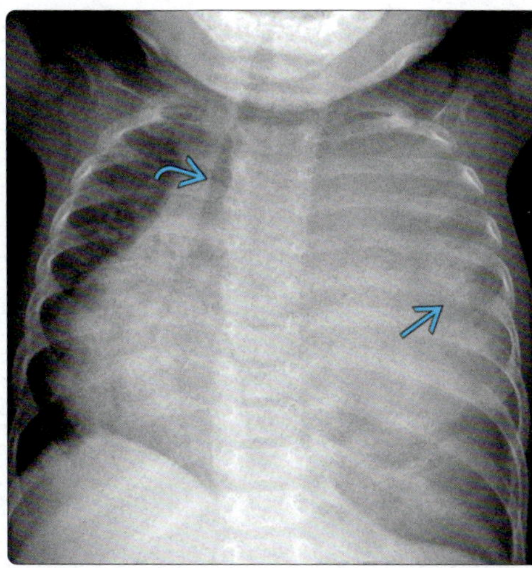

(Left) *Axial CECT in the same patient shows that the large mediastinal mass* ➙ *is mostly composed of fat. Note the marked mass effect on the superior vena cava* ➙*.* **(Right)** *PA radiograph of the chest in an infant shows a large mediastinal mass displacing the heart, trachea* ➙*, & mediastinum to the right. There are faint Ca^{2+}* ➙ *within the mass.*

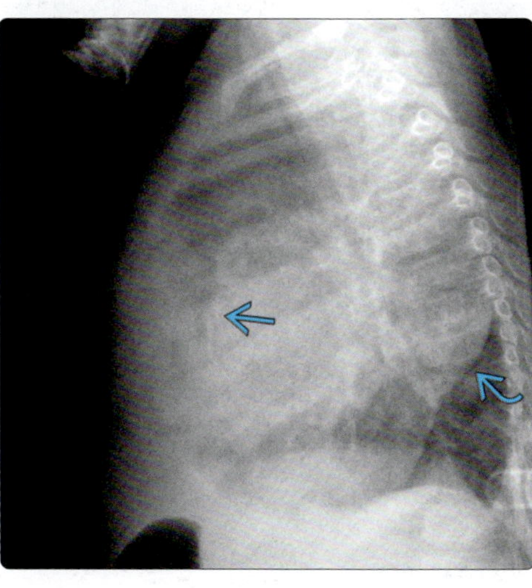

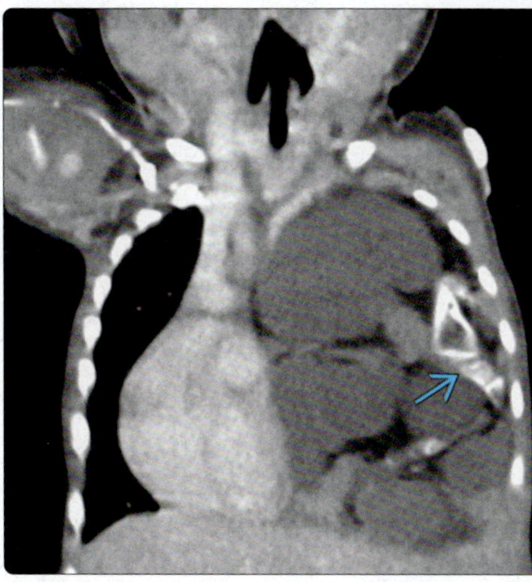

(Left) *Lateral radiograph of the chest in the same patient shows the large mediastinal mass* ➙ *extending posteriorly to the chest wall. Calcification* ➙ *is visible within the mass.* **(Right)** *Coronal CECT in the same infant shows the large mediastinal mass displacing the heart, trachea, & mediastinum to the right. The mass has fat, soft tissue, & fluid density but also contains well-formed bones* ➙ *with articulations, consistent with a teratoma.*

KEY FACTS

TERMINOLOGY

- Malignant tumor of primitive neural crest cells
- Continuous spectrum with more mature/benign counterparts: Ganglioneuroma & ganglioneuroblastoma

IMAGING

- Posterior mediastinal (paraspinal) mass with Ca^{2+}
  - Solid, elongated mass with paraspinal stripe widening ± rib splaying/erosion
- Tendency to invade spinal canal via neural foramen
- MR ± contrast is best imaging modality to assess local tumor (due to its ability to evaluate neural foraminal/intraspinal extension)
- MIBG scan is best for determining full extent of disease

CLINICAL ISSUES

- 3rd most common pediatric malignancy after leukemia & CNS tumors
  - Most common extracranial solid tumor in children
- Posterior mediastinum: 3rd most common site for neuroblastoma (NBL) (15-20% of cases)
  - Thoracic NBL is often asymptomatic & discovered incidentally
  - ± respiratory symptoms &/or neurologic symptoms (with cord compression)
- Mean age for thoracic presentation: 25 months
- 60-76% of patients with thoracic NBL have ↑ levels of urinary catecholamines (e.g., vanillylmandelic acid)
- Metastases are most commonly to liver & bone (including marrow)
- Treatment options: Surgical resection, chemotherapy, radiation, stem cell transplant, I-131 MIBG therapy
  - Based on anatomic stage, age, & histologic features
  - Stage 4S/MS: High rates of spontaneous regression
- Overall 5-year survival: 78%
  - Thoracic NBL is associated with higher survival rates than abdominal disease

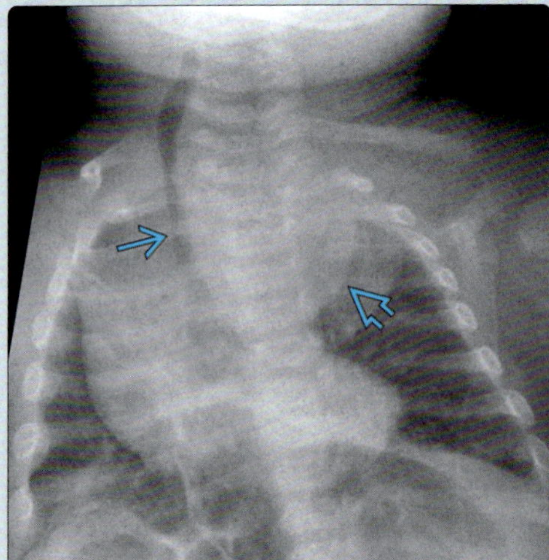

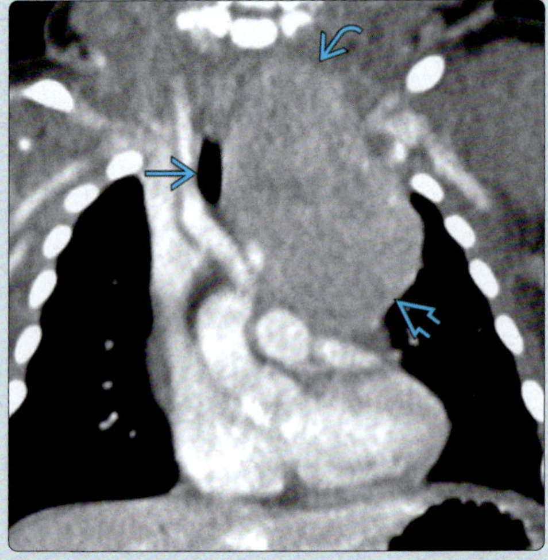

(Left) *Frontal radiograph in an infant with thoracic neuroblastoma shows a round mediastinal mass ⇨ displacing & compressing the trachea →. Lesions at the apex tend to be more rounded than the elongated lower paraspinal neuroblastomas. No obvious osseous changes are visualized.* **(Right)** *Coronal CECT in the same patient shows the large mediastinal mass ⇨ displacing the trachea → & mediastinum to the right. The tumor extends superiorly ↪ through the thoracic inlet.*

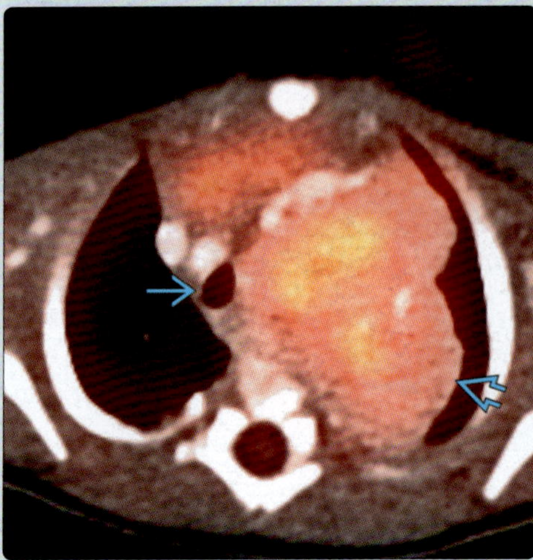

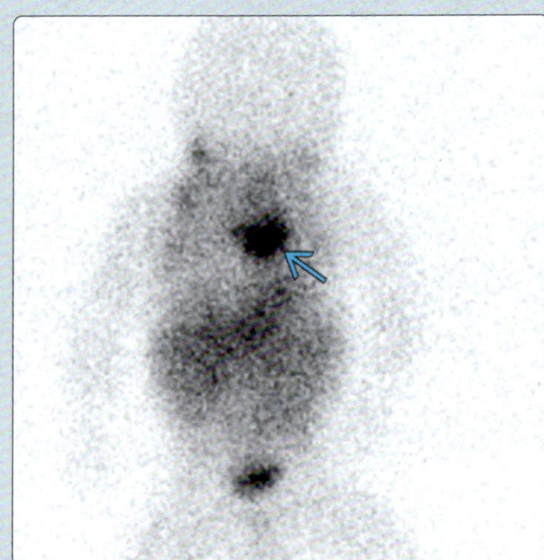

(Left) *Axial fused F-18 FDG PET/CT in the same patient shows heterogeneous FDG uptake within the mediastinal mass ⇨. The trachea → is mildly compressed & displaced to the right. Compression of the trachea is an image-defined risk factor. No intraspinal disease is identified.* **(Right)** *MIBG scan in the same patient shows uptake of the radiopharmaceutical in the mediastinal tumor ⇨. No osseous metastases were identified.*

TERMINOLOGY

Abbreviations

- Neuroblastoma (NBL)

Definitions

- Malignant tumor of primitive neural crest cells

IMAGING

General Features

- Best diagnostic clue
  - Posterior mediastinal (paraspinal) mass with Ca^{2+}
  - Invasive mass that tends to encase & displace vessels
  - Often extends into spinal canal via neural foramina
- Location
  - Posterior mediastinum arising from sympathetic chain
    - Often inferior or apical
- Morphology
  - Elongated or round solid paraspinal mass

Radiographic Findings

- Paraspinal soft tissue mass with widening of paraspinal stripe(s)
- Ca^{2+} within mass on up to 30% of radiographs
- Rib involvement is common
  - Widening/splaying of intercostal spaces
  - Mild erosion/destruction of ribs
- Neural foraminal widening from intraspinal extension
- Pleural effusion may be present
- Bone metastases are usually lucent, often subtle

CT Findings

- CECT
  - Posterior mediastinal mass, most commonly inferior
  - Mass is often heterogeneous (from necrosis & hemorrhage)
  - Ca^{2+} is seen on CT in 85-90%
  - ± local bone erosion or metastases

MR Findings

- T1WI
  - Intermediate-to-low signal paraspinal mass
- T2WI FS/STIR
  - Intermediate- to moderately high-signal paraspinal mass
  - Possible extension into neural foramen
    - Cord compression in up to 25%
  - Hyperintense bone marrow metastases
- DWI
  - May show restricted diffusion
- T1WI C+ FS
  - Variable enhancement, may be heterogeneous

Nuclear Medicine Findings

- MIBG scintigraphy
  - Avid uptake related to catecholamine production
  - 88% sensitive & 98% specific in detection of NBL
    - ~ 10% of NBL are not MIBG avid
  - Superior to PET/CT in depicting advanced disease & bone marrow metastases
  - Excellent for following therapy response
- PET/CT
  - F-18 FDG is useful in non-MIBG-avid disease
- Bone scan
  - Uptake in cortical bone metastasis &/or local bone invasion
  - Uptake in calcified primary mass (up to 74%)

Imaging Recommendations

- Best imaging tool
  - MR ± contrast: Evaluates intraspinal extension & bone marrow metastases
  - MIBG for determining full extent of disease

DIFFERENTIAL DIAGNOSIS

Widening of Inferior Paravertebral Soft Tissues

- Normal paravertebral soft tissues
  - Should not exceed adjacent pedicle in thickness or be inferolaterally oriented
  - May be more prominent in obese & supine patients
- Infectious discitis
  - Disc space narrowing, vertebral endplate irregularity
- Vertebral injury
  - Trauma & pain history are usually clear
  - Vertebral body compression or malalignment

Posterior Mediastinal Mass in Child < 3 Years of Age

- Other neuroblastic tumors
  - Ganglioneuroma
    - Most common posterior mediastinal mass in adolescents & young adults
    - Benign; similar imaging features as NBL
    - May represent mature form of NBL
  - Ganglioneuroblastoma
    - Contains both mature & immature neuroblasts
    - May represent maturing form of NBL
- Round pneumonia
  - No evidence of rib erosion or intraspinal extension
  - ± air bronchograms, parapneumonic effusion
  - Short-term follow-up radiographs after antibiotics can help confirm round pneumonia (with expected interval clearance)
- Extralobar bronchopulmonary sequestration
  - May appear similar to NBL as paraspinal mass
  - Lung relationship & feeding vessel are seen on CTA

PATHOLOGY

General Features

- Etiology
  - Malignant tumor of primitive neural crest cells
  - Continuous spectrum with more benign counterparts: NBL → ganglioneuroblastoma → ganglioneuroma
  - Most commonly arises from adrenal gland but can arise anywhere along sympathetic chain
- Genetics
  - ↑ copies of *MYCN* (n-MYC) protooncogene are associated with poor prognosis (*MYCN* amplification)
  - CD44: Glycoprotein on cell surface
    - ↑ levels: Better prognosis
- Associated abnormalities
  - Most neuroblastic tumors occur in isolation

Staging, Grading, & Classification

- International NBL Risk Group Staging System: Imaging-based staging system that requires identification of image-defined risk factors (IDRFs)
  - L1: Localized tumor confined to 1 body compartment; no IDRFs
  - L2: Local-regional tumor with ≥ 1 IDRF
  - M: Distant metastases (except stage MS)
  - MS: Metastatic disease in children < 18 months of age with metastases confined to skin, liver, &/or bone marrow
  - Thoracic-related IDRFs include
    - Tumor extension in 2 body compartments
    - Tumor encasement of carotid artery, vertebral artery, subclavian artery, aorta, celiac axis, or superior mesenteric artery
    - Tumor encasing internal jugular vein, subclavian vein, or vena cava
    - Tumor compressing trachea &/or bronchi
    - Tumor encasing brachial plexus roots
    - Lower mediastinal tumor, infiltrating costovertebral junction between T9 & T12
    - Tumor infiltrating porta hepatis
    - Tumor invading renal pedicle or touching renal vessels
    - Intraspinal tumor extension so that > 1/3 of spinal canal in axial plane is invaded, perimedullary leptomeningeal spaces are not visible, or spinal cord has abnormal signal
    - Infiltration of pericardium or diaphragm
- Bones (including marrow) in both staging systems must be clear by MIBG to qualify for stage 4S/MS (i.e., marrow disease is limited to < 10% involvement by aspiration)

Microscopic Features

- Immature, undifferentiated sympathetic cells: Small, round, blue cells
- Homer Wright rosettes: Circular groups of cells
- International NBL Pathology Classification (Shimada): Combines histiologic features & age of patient to define favorable & unfavorable histology for prognosis

CLINICAL ISSUES

Presentation

- Most common signs/symptoms
  - Thoracic NBL is often asymptomatic & discovered incidentally
  - Respiratory symptoms, including cough
  - Neurologic symptoms with cord compression
  - 60-76% of patients with thoracic NBL have ↑ levels of urinary catecholamines (vanillylmandelic acid)
- Other signs/symptoms
  - Fever, chest pain, opsoclonus-myoclonus, Horner syndrome
  - Skin mets: Blueberry muffin syndrome

Demographics

- Age
  - Mean for thoracic NBL presentation: 25 months
  - Mean for all NBL: 15-17 months
- Sex
  - F:M = 1.4:1
    - Different from other sites of NBL where M > F
- Epidemiology
  - NBL: 3rd most common pediatric malignancy after leukemia & CNS tumors
    - Most common extracranial solid tumor in children
    - 7-10% of childhood cancers
    - 10-15% of childhood cancer deaths
  - Posterior mediastinum: 3rd most common site for NBL (15-20% of cases) after adrenal & extraadrenal retroperitoneum

Natural History & Prognosis

- Thoracic NBL is associated with higher survival rates than more common NBL sites
  - Overall 5-year survival: 78%; 90% survival for stages 1, 2, 3; 29% for stage 4
- Thoracic NBL has different molecular profile than tumors of adrenal origin
  - Thoracic NBL has lower frequency of *MYCN* amplification; more likely to have numerical chromosomal alterations
- Features of NBL associated with better prognosis
  - Thoracic primary
  - Age at diagnosis < 18 months, histologic grade (Shimada system), ↓ *MYCN* amplification (copies of gene), stage MS/4S
- Metastasizes most commonly to liver, bone, & marrow
- Some lesions may spontaneously regress/mature into less malignant tumors (ganglioneuroma)

Treatment

- Options: Surgical resection, chemotherapy, radiation, stem cell transplant, biologic agents, I-131 MIBG therapy
  - Based upon stage, age, & histologic features
  - Less aggressive lesions may be treated with surgical resection alone
  - For stage 4S/MS: Some institutions advocate no treatment due to rates of spontaneous regression

DIAGNOSTIC CHECKLIST

Image Interpretation Pearls

- Look for rib splaying/erosions & soft tissue Ca^{2+} when focal paraspinal mass is seen in child

SELECTED REFERENCES

1. Biko DM et al: Mediastinal masses in children: radiologic-pathologic correlation. Radiographics. 41(4):E1186-207, 2021
2. Oldridge DA et al: Differences in genomic profiles and outcomes between thoracic and adrenal neuroblastoma. J Natl Cancer Inst. 111(11):1192-201, 2019
3. Chen AM et al: A review of neuroblastoma image-defined risk factors on magnetic resonance imaging. Pediatr Radiol. 48(9):1337-47, 2018
4. Swift CC et al: Updates in diagnosis, management, and treatment of neuroblastoma. Radiographics. 38(2):566-80, 2018
5. Brisse HJ et al: Radiogenomics of neuroblastomas: relationships between imaging phenotypes, tumor genomic profile and survival. PLoS One. 12(9):e0185190, 2017
6. Pavlus JD et al: Imaging of thoracic neurogenic tumors. AJR Am J Roentgenol. 1-10, 2016
7. Vo KT et al: Clinical, biologic, and prognostic differences on the basis of primary tumor site in neuroblastoma: a report from the international neuroblastoma risk group project. J Clin Oncol. 32(28):3169-76, 2014
8. Brisse HJ et al: Guidelines for imaging and staging of neuroblastic tumors: consensus report from the International Neuroblastoma Risk Group Project. Radiology. 261(1):243-57, 2011

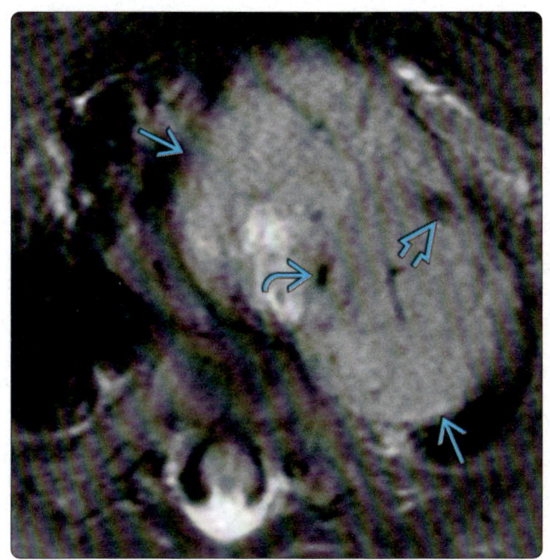

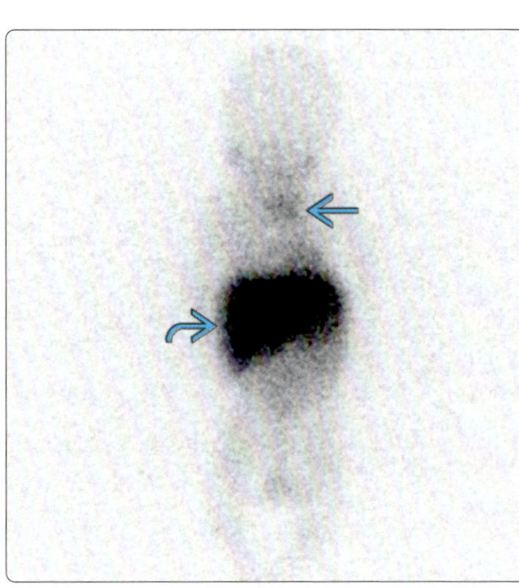

(Left) *Axial T2 FS MR in a young child with neuroblastoma shows a large solid mass in the upper chest. The tumor encases the left vertebral & subclavian arteries. Neuroforaminal extension could also be seen more superiorly (not shown).* **(Right)** *MIBG scan in the same patient shows mild uptake of the radiopharmaceutic in the cervicothoracic mass. There is considerable uptake within the liver due to hepatic metastases.*

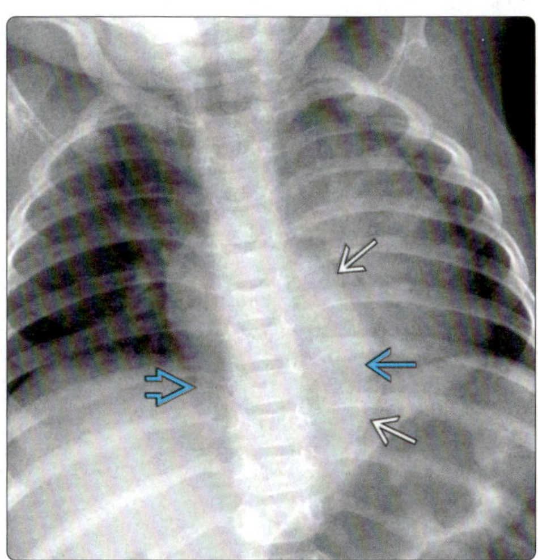

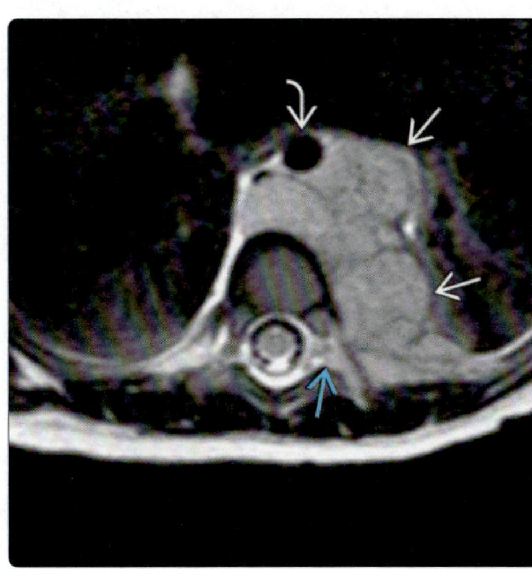

(Left) *Frontal radiograph in an infant shows an elongated left paraspinal mass with mild splaying of the left 8th-9th ribs as compared to the right intercostal space at this level.* **(Right)** *Axial T2 MR in the same patient shows a lobulated, intermediate signal intensity left paraspinal mass lifting the aorta off of the spine. The tumor surrounds 180° of the aorta but does not fully encase it. The tumor also involves the neural foramen with minimal distortion of the thecal sac.*

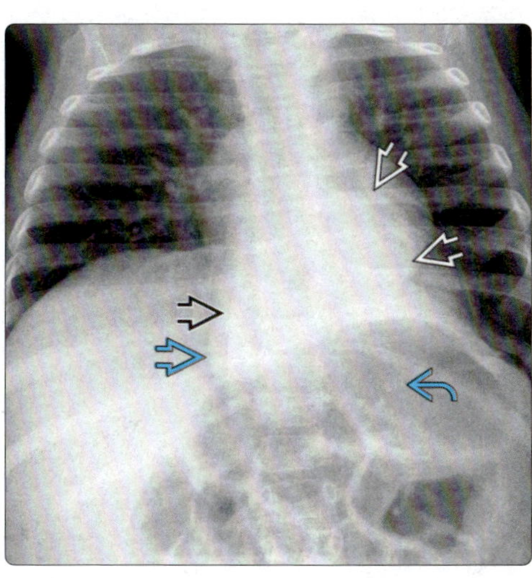

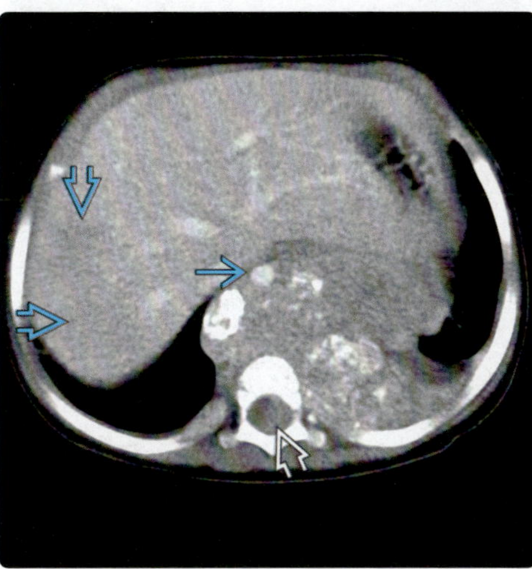

(Left) *Frontal radiograph shows widening of the right paraspinal stripe associated with a lobulated mass. A retrocardiac mass & speckled Ca^{2+} are noted on the left.* **(Right)** *Axial CECT of the same patient shows a large, heterogeneously calcified paravertebral neuroblastoma. The mass involves > 1/3 of the spinal canal diameter & lifts the aorta off of the spine, partially encasing it. Also note the poorly defined, hypoenhancing foci in the liver, consistent with distant metastases.*

Pleuropulmonary Blastoma

KEY FACTS

TERMINOLOGY

- Rare malignant embryonal mesenchymal neoplasm of lung & pleura that arises during organ development

IMAGING

- Pleuropulmonary blastoma (PPB) appearances
  - Type 1: Air-filled, multilocular cystic mass
  - Type 2: Mixed cystic (air-filled) & solid mass
  - Type 3: Soft tissue mass; opacified hemithorax with contralateral mediastinal shift
- Pleural effusion in 77% of type 2 or 3 lesions
- Spontaneous pneumothorax at presentation in 30-65%
- Multiple lesions in 35-50%; bilateral in 11-26%
- Metastases to brain, bones, & rarely liver

TOP DIFFERENTIAL DIAGNOSES

- Congenital pulmonary airway malformation
- Congenital lobar overinflation
- Mesenchymal hamartoma of chest wall
- Sarcoma
- Spontaneous pneumothorax
- Necrotizing pneumonia

PATHOLOGY

- Clear progression from type 1 → type 2 → type 3
  - Type 1r (regressed): No cancer cells found
- *DICER1* mutation: Association of PPB, cystic nephroma (CN), thyroid & ovarian tumors
  - Germline *DICER1* mutations in 65.5% with PPB
  - 10% with PPB have CN

CLINICAL ISSUES

- Most common primary pulmonary malignancy of childhood
- 94% present in children < 6 years of age
- Most common presentation: Respiratory distress

DIAGNOSTIC CHECKLIST

- Consider PPB when large chest mass is seen in young child
- Imaging cannot distinguish type 1 PPB from benign cysts

(Left) *CT scanogram in an adolescent with a DICER1 mutation & pleuropulmonary blastoma (PPB) shows a cystic lesion ➡ occupying the lower 1/2 of the right hemithorax. PPB is the most common primary lung malignancy of childhood.* **(Right)** *Coronal CECT of the chest in the same patient shows a large multiseptated cystic mass ➡ of the right hemithorax. Upon resection, a type 1r PPB was confirmed.*

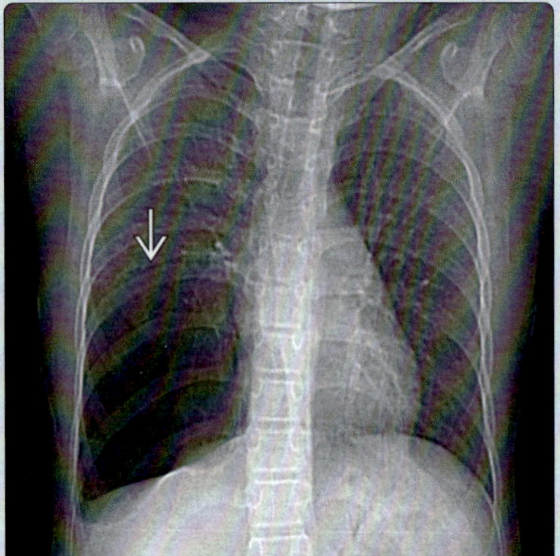

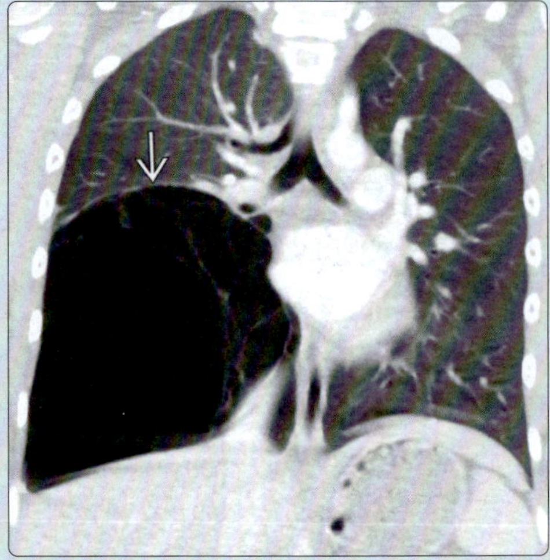

(Left) *Coronal T2 SSFSE fetal MR shows a hyperintense solid-appearing left lung mass ➡ that is most typical of a type 3 congenital pulmonary airway malformation (CPAM) but was found after postnatal resection to be a PPB.* **(Right)** *Axial CECT in the same patient 3 days after birth shows a large multicystic left lower lobe lesion ➡ containing air & fluid, most typical of a type 1 CPAM. A type 1 PPB was actually confirmed upon resection. Limited fetal reports of PPB have been of type 1 lesions indistinguishable from CPAMs.*

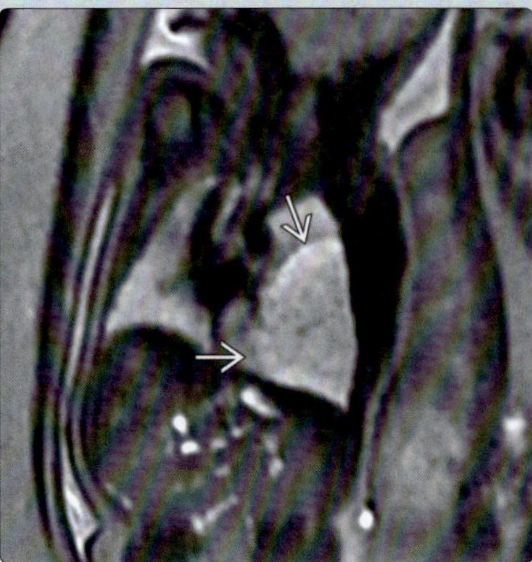

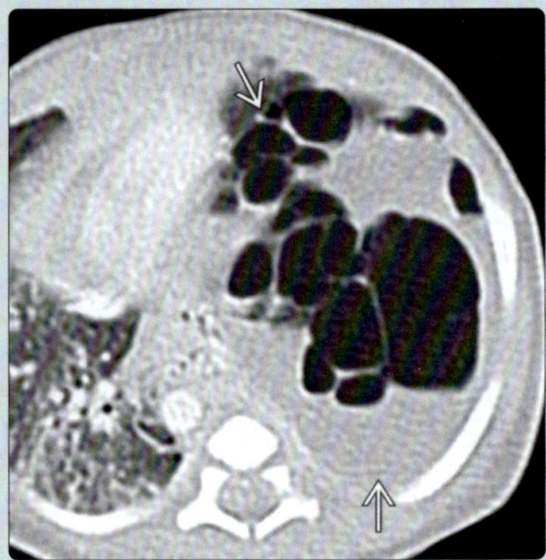

TERMINOLOGY

Abbreviations

- Pleuropulmonary blastoma (PPB)

Definitions

- Rare malignant embryonal mesenchymal neoplasm of lung & pleura that arises during organ development

Associated Syndromes

- *DICER1* mutation
  - Associated with PPB, cystic nephroma (CN), ovarian sex cord-stromal tumors (especially Sertoli-Leydig cell tumor), multinodular goiter, differentiated thyroid carcinoma, pineoblastoma, & ovarian or cervical rhabdomyosarcoma

IMAGING

General Features

- Best diagnostic clue
  - Large pulmonary cystic, solid, or mixed mass in child < 6 years old
- Location
  - Intrathoracic, located in peripheral lung adjacent to or involving visceral pleura
  - More common in right hemithorax
- Size
  - 55% of type 1 lesions are > 5 cm
  - 63% of type 2 or 3 lesions are > 10 cm
- Morphology
  - Well-defined pulmonary mass
  - 3 types
    - Type 1: Large, air-filled, multilocular cystic mass
    - Type 2: Large, air-filled, cystic & solid mass
    - Type 3: Solid pulmonary mass

Radiographic Findings

- Appearance depends on type of tumor
  - Type 1: Well-circumscribed, multilocular cystic (air-filled) mass with thin septa
  - Type 2: Cystic mass with variable soft tissue components
  - Type 3: Soft tissue mass → opacified hemithorax with contralateral mediastinal shift
- Spontaneous pneumothorax at presentation in 30-65%
- Associated with pleural effusion in 77% of type 2 or 3 lesions

CT Findings

- Type 1
  - Benign-appearing, air-filled lung cysts
  - Thin septa; no solid nodules or plaque-like thickening
  - Many different potential appearances: Unifocal (1 simple cyst), multilocular, cluster of contiguous cysts, or multifocal
- Type 2
  - Air-filled cystic mass with variable soft tissue components
- Type 3
  - Large, heterogeneous, solid mass with overall low attenuation
  - Originates from pulmonary pleura or parenchyma
  - Rarely invades chest wall
- Multiple lesions in 5-50% of patients
- Bilateral lesions in 11-26% of patients
- Metastases: Brain, bone, & rarely liver
- Imaging into upper abdomen may show associated renal tumor (i.e., CN)

Ultrasonographic Findings

- Solid heterogeneous mass (types 2 & 3)
- Pleural fluid

Imaging Recommendations

- Best imaging tool
  - Radiograph is often 1st imaging study due to respiratory symptoms
  - CECT is typically used to further characterize mass, evaluate initial extent of disease, & follow after treatment

DIFFERENTIAL DIAGNOSIS

Congenital Pulmonary Airway Malformation (CPAM)

- Type 1 CPAM: Macrocystic with large, air-filled cysts
  - ± air-fluid level on early neonatal imaging
- Type 1 CPAM is indistinguishable from type 1 PPB by imaging
  - Factors favoring CPAM: Prenatal detection (especially 2nd trimester), systemic feeding vessel (in hybrid lesion), hyperinflated lung, or asymptomatic patient

Congenital Lobar Overinflation

- Hyperinflation of affected lobe/lung
- On CT, not true cystic lesion: Lung has simplified appearance with small, widely spaced vessels

Mesenchymal Hamartoma of Chest Wall

- Intrathoracic mass of rib origin in neonate/infant
- Distortion/erosion of multiple adjacent ribs
- Ca^{2+} & fluid-fluid levels are common

Sarcoma

- Ewing/PNET, rhabdomyosarcoma, undifferentiated, others
- May be indistinguishable from type 3 PPB
- More likely to invade chest wall

Spontaneous Pneumothorax

- Should see typical patterns of lung collapse with smooth pleural line
- Septa or nodularity along suspected pleural space should suggest alternate diagnosis
  - Inserting chest tube may create bronchopleural fistula

Necrotizing Pneumonia

- Much more common than PPB
- Typically in ill child with fever

PATHOLOGY

General Features

- Genetics
  - Germline *DICER1* mutations in 70% of PPB patients
  - *DICER1* mutations are present in ~ 100% with PPB & CN
- Associated abnormalities

- Extrapulmonary lesions are identified in ~ 25% of PPB patients
- 10% are associated with CN

Staging, Grading, & Classification

- Type 1 (33%): Purely cystic
- Type 2 (35%): Cystic & solid
- Type 3 (32%): Solid

Gross Pathologic & Surgical Features

- Type 1: Cystic
- Types 2 & 3: Soft, fleshy, friable, vascular tumor

Microscopic Features

- Histologically distinct from adult pulmonary blastoma, which has malignant epithelial & mesenchymal components
  - PPB has no malignant epithelial component
- Type 1
  - Characteristic multilocular architecture with delicate septa
  - Thin cyst walls lined by alveolar-type epithelium
  - Small, primitive mesenchymal cells in stroma beneath epithelial lining
  - Focal areas of hypercellularity & hypervascularity
    - Hypercellular areas composed of hyperchromatic compact spindle cells & small round cells
  - ± foci of immature cartilage
- Type 1r (regressed): No cancer cells found
- Types 2 & 3
  - Solid components may have areas of necrosis & cystic degeneration
  - Higher grade cytologic features
    - Sheets of spindle, pleomorphic, or anaplastic cells
      - Anaplasia emerges as tumor progresses from type 1 to type 3

CLINICAL ISSUES

Presentation

- Most common signs/symptoms
  - Respiratory distress ± spontaneous pneumothorax
    - Pneumothorax is found at presentation in 30% of patients with type 1, 65% of patients with type 2, & 20% of patients with type 3 PPB
  - ± signs of upper respiratory tract infection
  - PPB may be incidental finding on prenatal US (in 3rd trimester) or postnatal chest radiograph

Demographics

- Age
  - 94% present in children < 6 years of age
  - Median age at diagnosis
    - Type 1: 8 months
    - Type 2: 35 months
    - Type 3: 41 months
- Sex
  - Type 1: 57% male
  - Types 2 & 3: M = F
- Epidemiology
  - PPB: Most common primary pulmonary malignancy of childhood
    - 15-25 cases of PPB diagnosed in USA/year
    - Incidence of PPB is estimated at 0.35-0.65 cases per 100,000 births

Natural History & Prognosis

- Clear progression from type 1 → type 2 → type 3
- Type 1
  - Presents at younger age
  - Better prognosis than types 2 & 3
  - Complete surgical resection may be curative
  - Recurrent type 1 disease frequently progresses to more malignant type (2 or 3)
- Types 2 & 3
  - Presents at slightly older age
  - Multiple patients have history of pulmonary cysts preceding diagnosis of types 2 & 3 PPB
  - Worse prognosis
- 5-year survival
  - Type 1: 94%
  - Type 2: 71%
  - Type 3: 53%
- Metastasis rate
  - Type 1: No known metastases
  - Type 2: 7%
  - Type 3: 11%

Treatment

- Type 1: Complete surgical resection ± chemotherapy
- Type 2: Surgical resection + chemotherapy
- Type 3: Surgical resection + chemotherapy; consider neoadjuvant chemotherapy
- Benefit of local radiation in types 2 & 3 PPB is controversial

DIAGNOSTIC CHECKLIST

Consider

- PPB when large chest mass is seen in young child
- Type 1 PPB is radiologically indistinguishable from benign lung cysts
  - Justification for surgical excision of all cystic lung lesions found in young children

Image Interpretation Pearls

- PPB rarely invades chest wall
- Look for other *DICER1*-associated tumors

SELECTED REFERENCES

1. Kunisaki SM et al: Pleuropulmonary blastoma in pediatric lung lesions. Pediatrics. 147(4), 2021
2. Madaan PK et al: Pleuropulmonary blastoma: a report of three cases and review of literature. Radiol Case Rep. 16(10):2862-8, 2021
3. Adams NC et al: Fetal ultrasound and magnetic resonance imaging: a primer on how to interpret prenatal lung lesions. Pediatr Radiol. 50(13):1839-54, 2020
4. Dehner LP et al: Pleuropulmonary blastoma: more than a lung neoplasm of childhood. Mo Med. 116(3):206-10, 2019
5. Guillerman RP et al: Imaging of DICER1 syndrome. Pediatr Radiol. 49(11):1488-505, 2019
6. Lichtenberger JP 3rd et al: Primary lung tumors in children: radiologic-pathologic correlation from the radiologic pathology archives. Radiographics. 38(7):2151-72, 2018
7. Waelti SL et al: Neonatal congenital lung tumors - the importance of mid-second-trimester ultrasound as a diagnostic clue. Pediatr Radiol. 47(13):1766-75, 2017

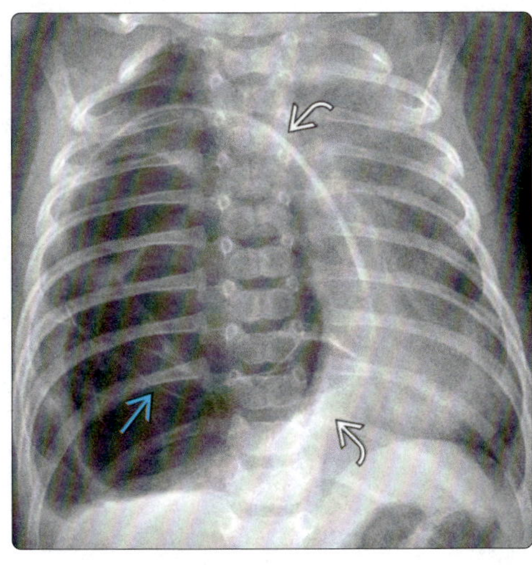

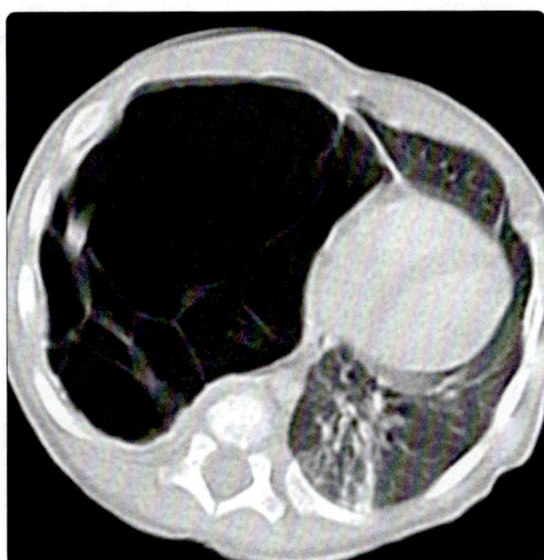

(Left) *AP radiograph of the chest shows a large, air-filled cystic mass of the right hemithorax ➦. Numerous thin septations ➔ are seen within the mass. The mass crosses the midline & displaces the heart & mediastinum to the left.* **(Right)** *Axial CECT in the same patient further details the multiseptated, cystic mass that occupies the entire right hemithorax. A multiloculated, air-filled, cystic mass without nodular or plaque-like solid tissue is typical of a type 1 PPB (but is more commonly seen with a type 1 CPAM).*

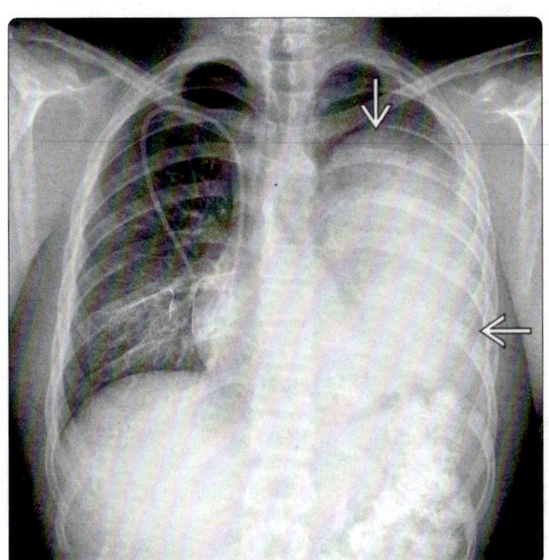

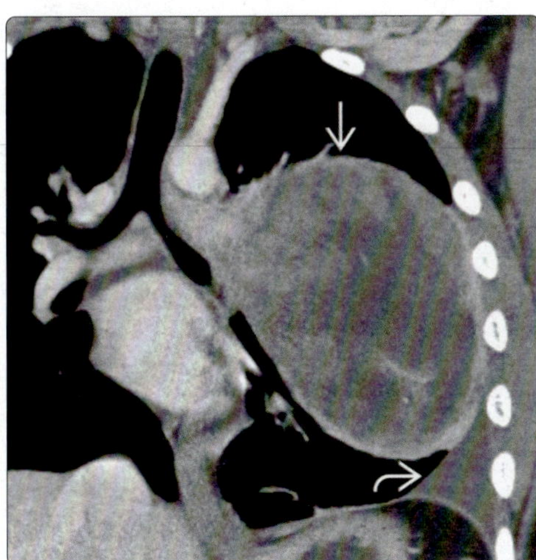

(Left) *Frontal radiograph in an adolescent boy with a PPB shows a large soft tissue mass ➔ occupying the left hemithorax, ultimately found to be a type 3 PPB. Note the lack of adjacent rib destruction that would favor a sarcoma.* **(Right)** *Coronal CECT of the chest in the same patient shows heterogeneous enhancement of the soft tissue mass ➔ in the left lung + a small left pleural effusion ➦. Pleural effusions are present in 77% of patients with type 3 PPB.*

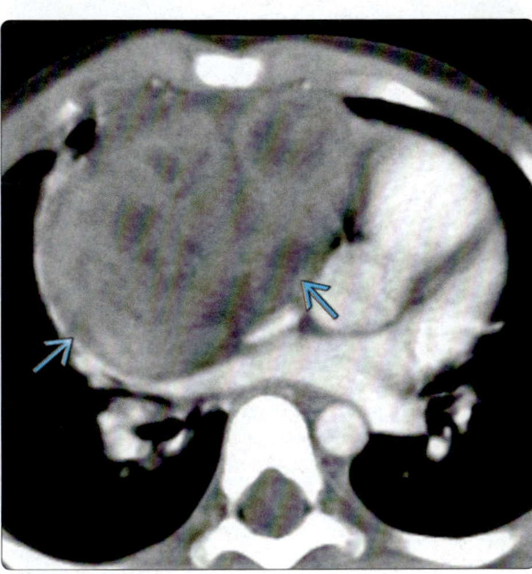

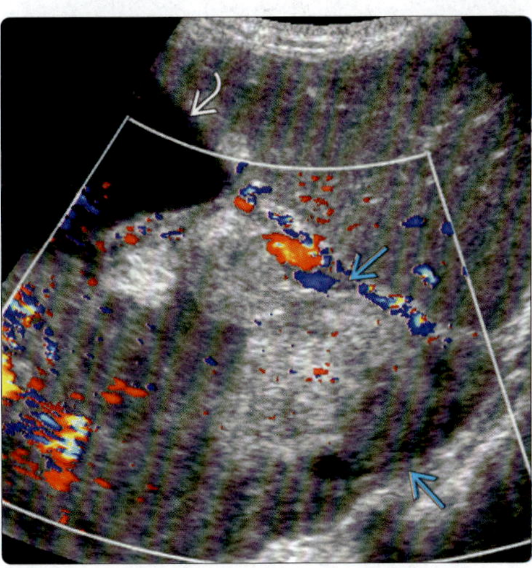

(Left) *Axial CECT of the chest shows a solid well-circumscribed heterogeneous type 3 PPB ➔ of the anterior mediastinum. The mass is displacing the heart to the left. Note that the appearance is not specific & could be seen with other malignancies, such as sarcomas.* **(Right)** *Longitudinal color Doppler ultrasound of a type 3 PPB shows a solid heterogeneous mass ➔ of the right hemithorax with mild internal vascularity. A moderate pleural effusion ➦ is present.*

Pulmonary Arteriovenous Malformation

KEY FACTS

TERMINOLOGY

- Pulmonary arteriovenous malformation (PAVM): Abnormal direct communication between pulmonary artery & vein
- Associated with hereditary hemorrhagic telangiectasia (HHT), a.k.a. Osler-Weber-Rendu syndrome

IMAGING

- Smoothly marginated, brightly enhancing nodule with feeding artery & draining vein; most occur in lower lobes
  - ± surrounding ground-glass opacity in telangiectatic subtype (more common in children)
- Multiplanar CTA reconstructions allow best depiction of PAVMs & planning for transcatheter embolization
  - Size of feeding artery (≥ 3 mm) & number of feeding vessels will impact therapy

TOP DIFFERENTIAL DIAGNOSES

- Granuloma
- Pulmonary varix
- Pulmonary metastasis

PATHOLOGY

- HHT accounts for up to 90% of patients with PAVMs
  - 50% of patients with HHT have PAVM
- Clinical triad of HHT: Epistaxis, telangiectasias, family history
  - AVMs of viscera: Lung, brain, spine, liver, &/or gastrointestinal tract

CLINICAL ISSUES

- Most HHT patients develop symptoms by age 20
- Consider referral to HHT Center of Excellence for endovascular treatment (coil, balloon, Amplatzer plug)
- Should screen family members of patient with HHT & PAVM: 35% incidence of PAVM
- Endovascular treatment allows embolization of multiple PAVMs at once; has very low morbidity & mortality with high success rate (permanent occlusion in > 90%)
- Untreated PAVMs can lead to neurologic complications (paradoxical emboli, abscess, stroke)

(Left) *Sequential inferior to superior (from left to right) lung CT images in a 12-year-old boy with hereditary hemorrhagic telangiectasia (HHT) show a large, lobulated pulmonary arteriovenous malformation (PAVM) ➔ in the right middle lobe. It is supplied by a single arterial feeder ➔ & has a larger caliber draining vein ➔ (which is typical). Note a 2nd smaller PAVM ➔ in the most superior image.* **(Right)** *Coned-down selective arteriogram in the same patient shows the lobulated PAVM ➔, arterial feeder ➔, & draining vein ➔.*

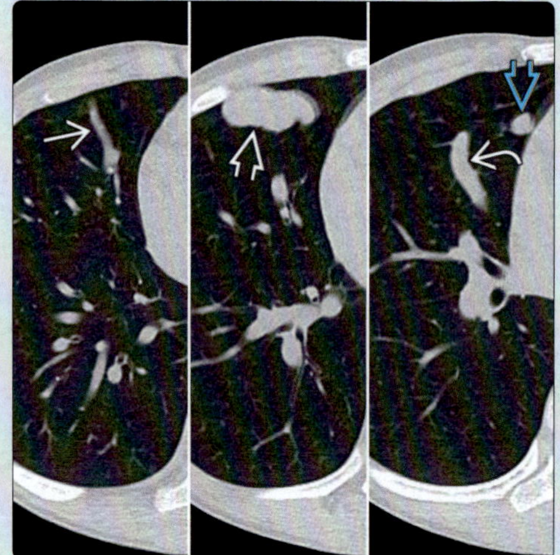

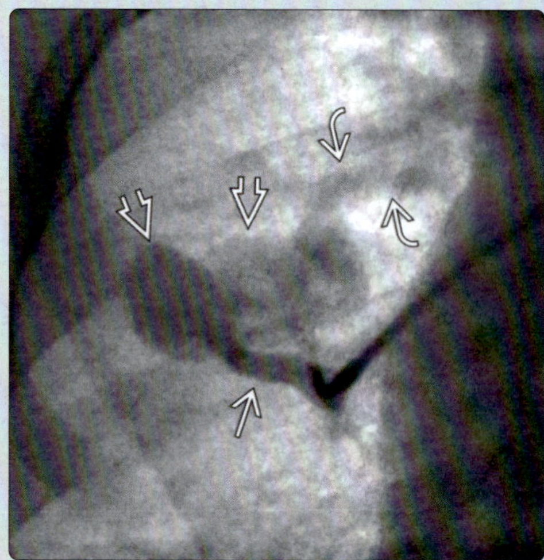

(Left) *Sequential superior to inferior axial lung CT images (labeled 1-6) demonstrate a small PAVM ➔ in the left lower lobe with a small feeding artery ➔ & adjacent draining vein ➔.* **(Right)** *Follow-up lateral radiograph in the same patient shows a small Amplatzer occlusion device ➔ used to treat the PAVM shown in the preceding CT.*

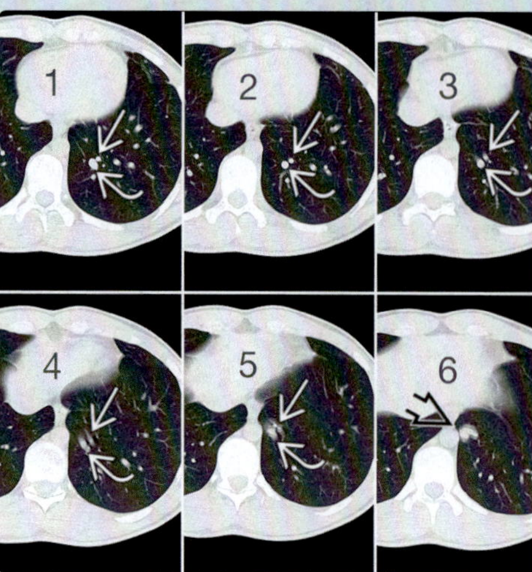

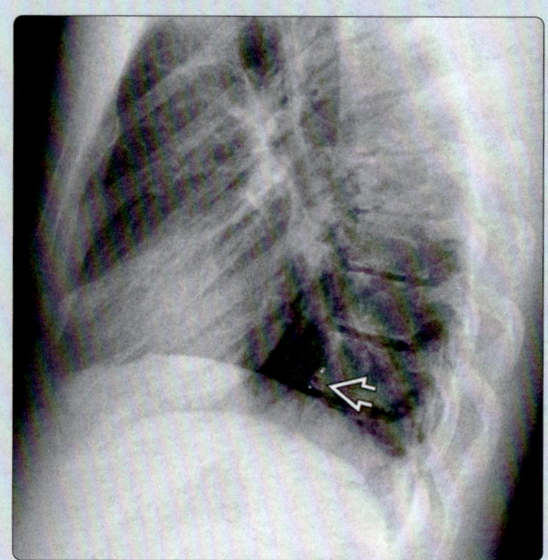

TERMINOLOGY

Abbreviations

- Pulmonary arteriovenous malformation (PAVM)

Definitions

- Abnormal, capillary-free vascular communication between pulmonary artery & vein, allowing R → L shunt

IMAGING

General Features

- Best diagnostic clue
  - Smoothly marginated, avidly enhancing nodule with enlarged feeding artery & draining vein on CECT
- Location
  - 50-70% are located in lower lobes
- Morphology
  - 3 typical appearances
    - Large single sac
    - Plexiform mass of dilated vascular channels
    - Dilated & tortuous direct arteriovenous connection
- Size: Most are 1-5 cm; may enlarge over time to > 10 cm

Radiographic Findings

- Radiography
  - Abnormal in almost all symptomatic patients
  - Sharply defined pulmonary nodule with uniform density; may have lobulated borders

CT Findings

- CTA is best to diagnose PAVMs (98% sensitivity)
  - Look for feeding artery & draining vein
  - Enhancement is similar to that of other vascular structures
  - Surrounding ground-glass opacity in telangiectatic subtype

Angiographic Findings

- DSA: Selective pulmonary angiography
  - Less sensitive but may be more specific than CT
  - Large feeder artery + large early draining vein

Imaging Recommendations

- Multidetector CTA allows best detection of PAVMs & planning for transcatheter embolization
- Catheter angiography is typically reserved for treatment

DIFFERENTIAL DIAGNOSIS

Granuloma

- No associated vessels; little to no enhancement
- Usually smoothly marginated but densely calcified or with central Ca^{2+}; ± associated calcified hilar & mediastinal lymph nodes

Pulmonary Varix

- Enlarged pulmonary vein, no large feeding artery or nidus
- DSA may be needed to differentiate from PAVM

Pulmonary Metastasis

- Typically not associated with large vessels
- Frequently multiple & seen in setting of known primary malignant tumor

PATHOLOGY

General Features

- Etiology
  - Congenital (most common)
    - Thought to form from incomplete resorption of vascular septa during embryogenesis
  - Acquired
    - Surgery for congenital cyanotic heart disease: Late complication of Glenn & Fontan procedures
    - Hepatopulmonary syndrome: 50% with end-stage liver disease acquire abnormal arteriovenous communications
- Associated abnormalities
  - Hereditary hemorrhagic telangiectasia (HHT), a.k.a. Osler-Weber-Rendu syndrome, accounts for up to 90% of patients with PAVMs
    - Autosomal dominant, variable penetrance
    - Clinical triad: Epistaxis, telangiectasias, family history
      - AVMs of viscera: Lung, brain, spine, liver, &/or gastrointestinal tract
    - 50% of patients with HHT have PAVM
    - Screen family members of HHT patients → 35% incidence of PAVM

CLINICAL ISSUES

Presentation

- Most common signs/symptoms
  - Incidental solitary pulmonary nodule on radiograph
  - Most HHT patients develop symptoms by age 20
    - Epistaxis is most common complaint
    - Findings or complications of R → L shunt: Brain abscess, embolic stroke
    - Mucocutaneous telangiectasias

Demographics

- Age: Most are congenital; 10% are detected in childhood
- Sex: M:F = 1:2
- Epidemiology: Rare, only 1:5,000

Natural History & Prognosis

- PAVMs are treated to avoid neurologic complications & heart failure
- Patients with diffuse PAVMs are almost always symptomatic

Treatment

- Options, risks, complications
  - Refer patient to HHT Center of Excellence
  - Embolization by endovascular coil, balloon, &/or Amplatzer vascular plugs
    - Traditionally reserved for feeding artery ≥ 3 mm
    - High success rate, permanent occlusion in > 98%
    - Low morbidity & mortality
    - Multiple PAVMs can be embolized at once

SELECTED REFERENCES

1. Hetts SW et al: Hereditary hemorrhagic telangiectasia: the convergence of genotype, phenotype, and imaging in modern diagnosis and management of a multisystem disease. Radiology. 300(1):17-30 2021
2. Dupuis-Girod S et al: The lung in hereditary hemorrhagic telangiectasia. Respiration. 94(4):315-30, 2017

Child Abuse, Rib Fractures

KEY FACTS

TERMINOLOGY

- Child abuse: Any act or failure to act by parent/caretaker that causes harm or imminent risk of harm to child

IMAGING

- Radiography
  - Linear lucency of acute fracture is often not visible
  - Callus/subperiosteal new bone formation may become visible 7-10 days after injury
    - Ranges from indistinct margins & broadening of rib → sharply marginated nodular/bulbous callus
  - Rib head fracture may appear fragmented with mixed sclerosis & lucency; often no subperiosteal new bone
  - Costochondral junction fractures appear like metaphyseal corner fractures with growth disturbance & sclerosis at healing
- Tc-99m MDP bone scan or F-18 NaF PET is complementary
  - Focal ↑ radiotracer activity within 24 hours
- CT is not advocated for identifying rib fractures but may be used to evaluate intrathoracic or intraabdominal injury
- Indications for initial radiographic skeletal survey
  - < 2 years old with suspicion of NAT
  - < 5 years old with suspicious fracture
  - Suspicion of NAT in any child unable to communicate
- Follow-up skeletal survey is obtained after 2 weeks

PATHOLOGY

- Posterior rib fractures are most common & specific for NAT
  - Adult hands squeeze child's chest → leverage posterior ribs on transverse processes → fractures

CLINICAL ISSUES

- Majority of rib fractures are not suspected on clinical exam
  - Overlying bruising in ~ 9%
  - ± clicking or popping sounds with crepitus
- Likely most common skeletal injury in NAT
  - Only radiographic manifestation of NAT in up to 29%

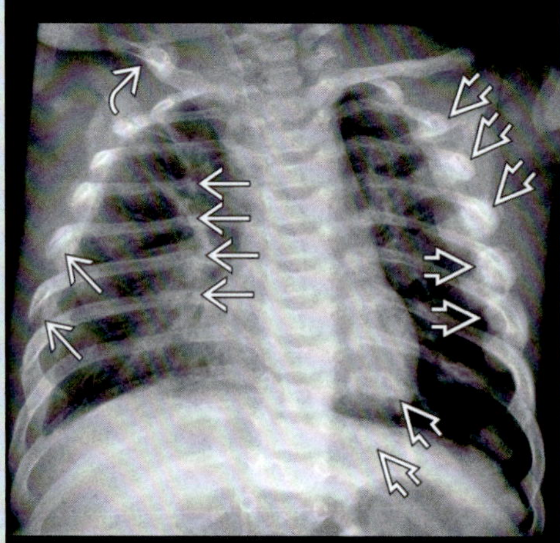

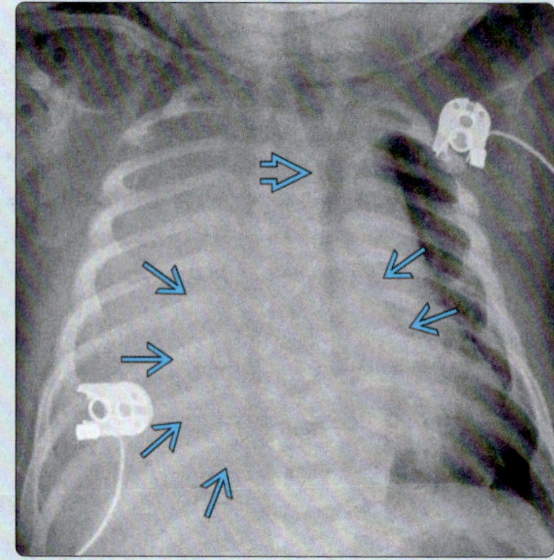

(Left) *AP radiograph in an infant with suspected abuse demonstrates multiple left lateral & posterior rib fractures with callus formation ➡ as well as more recent right-sided rib fractures without evidence of healing ➡. Also note the right clavicle fracture ➡ & right pleural effusion.* **(Right)** *AP radiograph in a 5-week-old victim of physical abuse shows complete opacification of the right hemithorax due to a large chylothorax with mediastinal shift ➡. Healing posterior rib fractures are seen bilaterally ➡.*

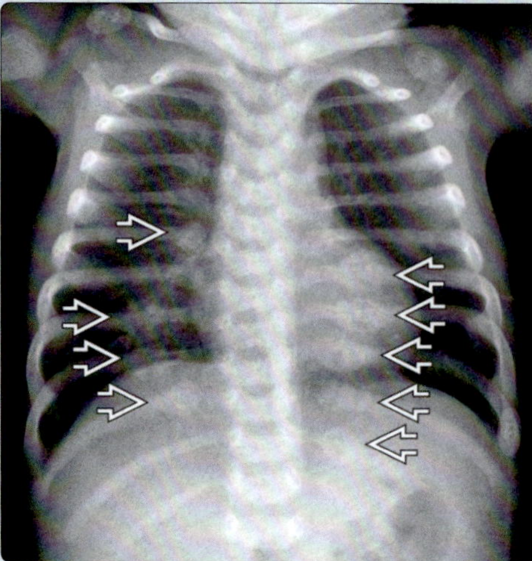

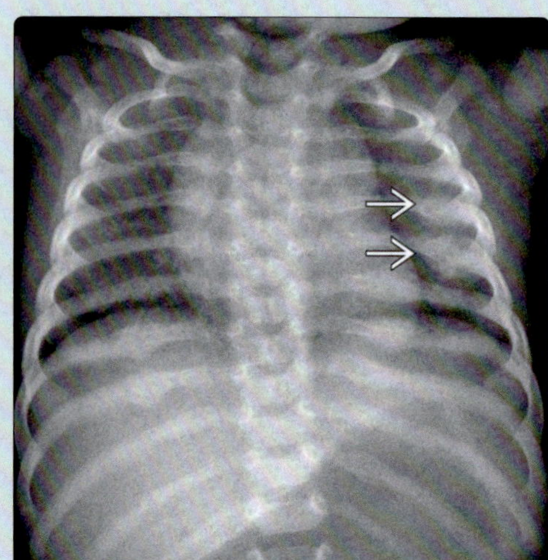

(Left) *AP radiograph in a 1-month-old shows multiple healing posterior rib fractures with bulbous callus formation ➡.* **(Right)** *AP radiograph obtained 2 weeks later in the same patient shows 2 additional healing rib fractures ➡, which, even in retrospect, are difficult to appreciate on the initial study. Follow-up skeletal surveys should be obtained at 2 weeks with persistent suspicion based on clinical or imaging findings (or if concerning fractures are seen on the initial exam).*

TERMINOLOGY

Abbreviations

- Nonaccidental trauma or injury (NAT, NAI), child abuse, & neglect

Definitions

- Child abuse: Any act or failure to act by parent/caretaker that causes harm or imminent risk of harm to child

IMAGING

General Features

- Best diagnostic clue
  - Bulbous callus/subperiosteal new bone formation of multiple adjacent posterior ribs in infant
- Location
  - Most common distribution
    - Posterior & lateral; midrib cage (ribs 5-8); L > R

Radiographic Findings

- Acute fractures are often not visualized radiographically
  - Typically vertical/oblique linear lucency in rib short axis
  - Difficult to visualize if nondisplaced & fracture plane is oriented coronal relative to x-ray beam
  - Adjacent subpleural hematoma may be clue
- Healing fractures may become visible 7-10 days after injury
  - Callus/subperiosteal new bone formation: Ranges from indistinct margins & broadening of rib → sharply marginated nodular/bulbous callus
  - "Hole-in-rib": Radiolucency (bone resorption) surrounded by sclerosis
  - Rib head: Often without subperiosteal new bone
    - May appear fragmented with mixed sclerosis & lucency
- Costochondral junction fractures
  - Disrupt physis similar to Salter-Harris injury
  - Acute appearance is dependent on projection, similar to classic metaphyseal lesion
    - Arcuate density/bucket-handle, triangular corner fragment, fissure, or transverse lucency
  - Sclerosis or growth disturbance (flaring, nodular enlargement, or cartilage invagination) with healing
- Sensitivity 73% in one study vs. follow-up radiographs
- Sensitivity 26% in one study vs. postmortem histology

CT Findings

- Performed for suspected thoracoabdominal injury
- Not advocated for identifying rib fractures alone due to radiation exposure
- Greater sensitivity than initial skeletal survey for detection of rib fractures
- Findings similar to radiography
  - Linear lucency, often in rib short axis
  - Callus & subperiosteal new bone formation with time

MR Findings

- Whole-body MR has low sensitivity (57%) for rib fractures vs. radiographs
- May see fluid signal changes in bone marrow & soft tissues ± elevation of periosteum before fracture is evident on radiographs

Ultrasonographic Findings

- Adult studies show ↑ sensitivity of US over radiography for rib fractures, particularly of cartilaginous portion
- May show occult rib fracture in children when initial skeletal survey is negative or equivocal, though patient cooperation may be issue
- Imaging findings include discontinuity of echogenic shadowing cortex, acoustic edge shadow at margin of fracture, local hematoma with elevated periosteum

Nuclear Medicine Findings

- Tc-99m MDP skeletal scintigraphy or F-18 NaF PET is complementary to initial skeletal survey
  - Focal ↑ in radionuclide activity within 24 hours, normalizes within 6 months
  - Costochondral junction fractures (metaphyseal equivalent in anterior rib) are difficult to assess due to variable physiologic uptake
- Compared to initial skeletal survey, F-18 NaF PET shows greater sensitivity for rib fractures but lower sensitivity for classic metaphyseal lesions
- Detection of bony injury by Tc-99m MDP bone scan & initial skeletal survey from one study demonstrated
  - 60 rib fractures: 63% identified on bone scan & 73% identified on skeletal survey
  - 6 cases with solitary rib fractures: 50% identified on both modalities, remaining 50% identified only on bone scan
  - Other fractures: 33% seen on both modalities, 44% seen on skeletal survey only, 25% seen on bone scan only

Imaging Recommendations

- Initial skeletal survey
  - Indications
    - < 2 years old with suspicion of NAT
    - < 5 years old with suspicious fracture
    - Concern for NAT in any child unable to communicate
  - Images include: AP & lateral skull, lateral cervical & lumbar spine, AP & lateral & both obliques of thorax, AP pelvis, AP humeri, AP forearms, PA or shallow oblique hands, AP femurs, AP lower legs, AP feet; additional views based on clinical & imaging findings
- Follow-up skeletal survey
  - Typically 2 weeks (not < 10 days) from initial evaluation
  - Indications
    - Concerning fractures on initial study
    - Normal initial study with persistent suspicion based on clinical or imaging findings
  - Used to confirm suspected fractures & identify additional fractures
  - In one study, clarified questionable fractures or identified new fractures in 48% of cases
    - Most additional fractures were of ribs
- Tc-99m MDP bone scan or F-18 NaF PET is used as complementary & problem-solving tool
- CECT for suspected intrathoracic or intraabdominal injury

DIFFERENTIAL DIAGNOSIS

Entities Associated With Multiple Fractures

- **Osteogenesis imperfecta (OI)**
  - Type IV OI is most commonly mistaken for abuse
    - Sclera is normal in color (not blue)

Child Abuse, Rib Fractures

- May see osteoporosis & wormian bones
- **Menkes syndrome**
  - Osteoporosis, metaphyseal spurs, brittle hair, tortuous intracranial vessels
  - Excessive wormian bone formation
- **Rickets**
  - Widening/lengthening of physes with loss of normal zones of provisional Ca^{2+} + metaphyseal fraying, cupping, & splaying
- **Leukemia**
  - Osteoporosis ± lucent metaphyseal bands, permeative destruction, aggressive periosteal new bone formation

Birth Trauma

- Rare but can occur with large babies & difficult deliveries
- No rib fractures in one study of 34,946 births

Trauma From Cardiopulmonary Resuscitation

- Rib fractures very rare in pediatric CPR (< 1%)
- Most such fractures involve anterior ribs

Accidental Trauma

- Age & history must be consistent with injury
- Rib fractures are more likely to be anterior & lateral
- Greater likelihood of intrathoracic injury & fewer fractures

Pseudoarthroses

- Typically in 1st rib
- No associated fractures or remodeling on follow-up images

Sternal Ossification Centers

- Normal ossification centers of sternum often project over posterior ribs on oblique views, mimicking callus

PATHOLOGY

General Features

- Assailant holds infant, wrapping hands around chest with finger tips at posterior ribs & thumbs situated anteriorly extending to midline
- AP compression while squeezing & shaking child results in fractures
  - Posterior rib fractures occur from leveraging posterior ribs on transverse processes
    - Most common location & most specific for abuse

CLINICAL ISSUES

Presentation

- Wide range of clinical presentations for NAT: Injury inconsistent with history, multiple injuries in various stages of healing, bruising in nonmobile infant, genitalia injury, cigarette burns, other injuries with high specificity for NAT (e.g., classic metaphyseal lesion/corner fracture)
  - Chest radiograph may be obtained with resuscitation for seizure, unresponsiveness, acute life-threatening event
- Rib fractures
  - Only radiographic finding of NAT in up to 29% of cases
  - Majority are not suspected based on clinical exam
    - Associated bruising at fracture site is rare, 9%
  - Clicking or popping sound from back or chest on physical exam, ± crepitus
  - Associated intrathoracic injury is less common than in accidental injury
    - 12.8% of NAT vs. 55.6% of accidental injuries
  - Rib fractures in children < 3 years of age are usually associated with abuse (61%)
  - Up to 82% of rib fractures in children < 1 year of age are from NAT

Demographics

- Epidemiology
  - 678,000 child maltreatment victims in 2018 in USA
    - Infants ≤ 1 year old are most at risk
  - Rib fractures are most common skeletal injury in NAT
    - In one study of abused children, 79% of all fractures involved rib cage
    - Rib fractures are present in 10-14% of skeletal surveys performed for suspected abuse

Natural History & Prognosis

- 1,770 fatalities from child maltreatment in 2018
  - Mortality is highest in infants < 1 year old: 46.6% of deaths

Treatment

- Multidisciplinary investigation of maltreatment allegation involves physicians, social worker, Child Protective Services, legal authorities
- Ensure "at risk" child & siblings are placed in safe environment

DIAGNOSTIC CHECKLIST

Image Interpretation Pearls

- Carefully review visible ribs on any modality in young child, regardless of study indication
  - Fractures may be incidentally noted on unrelated emergent or nonemergent exams

Reporting Tips

- Concern for child abuse based on imaging findings must be conveyed to referring clinician ASAP
- Final report represents legal document → review carefully

SELECTED REFERENCES

1. Mitchell IC et al: Identifying maltreatment in infants and young children presenting with fractures: does age matter? Acad Emerg Med. 28(1):5-18, 2021
2. Tsai A et al: Temporal pattern of radiographic findings of costochondral junction rib fractures on serial skeletal surveys in suspected infant abuse. AJR Am J Roentgenol. 216(6):1649-58, 2021
3. Kriss S et al: Characteristics of rib fractures in young abused children. Pediatr Radiol. 50(5):726-33, 2020
4. Expert Panel on Pediatric Imaging:. et al: ACR Appropriateness Criteria® suspected physical abuse-child. J Am Coll Radiol. 14(5S):S338-49, 2017
5. Barber I et al: The yield of high-detail radiographic skeletal surveys in suspected infant abuse. Pediatr Radiol. 45(1):69-80, 2015
6. Kleinman, PK. Diagnostic Imaging of Child Abuse, 3rd edition. Cambridge University Press, 2015
7. Duffy SO et al: Use of skeletal surveys to evaluate for physical abuse: analysis of 703 consecutive skeletal surveys. Pediatrics. 127(1):e47-52, 2011
8. Perez-Rossello JM et al: Whole-body MRI in suspected infant abuse. AJR Am J Roentgenol. 195(3):744-50, 2010

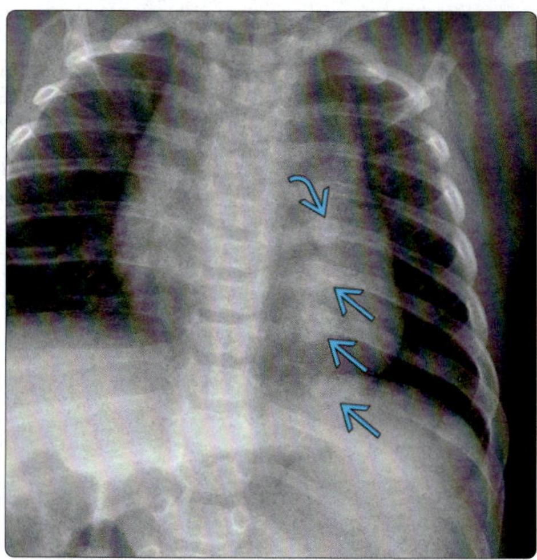

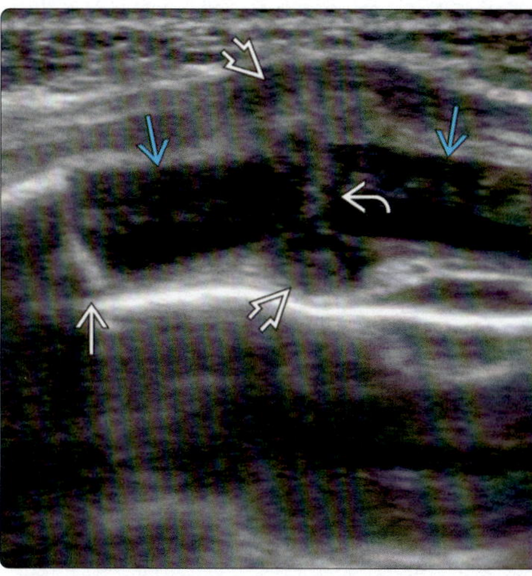

(Left) *AP chest radiograph from a follow-up skeletal survey of an infant with suspected fractures shows healing fractures of the 7th, 8th, & 9th ribs ➔. A suspected 6th rib fracture was also confirmed by visualization of callus formation ➔. The provided history was incompatible with the injuries.* **(Right)** *Transverse US demonstrates the anterior edge of an ossified rib ➔ with a fracture ➔ extending through the anterior cartilaginous rib ➔. Note the surrounding hematoma ➔.*

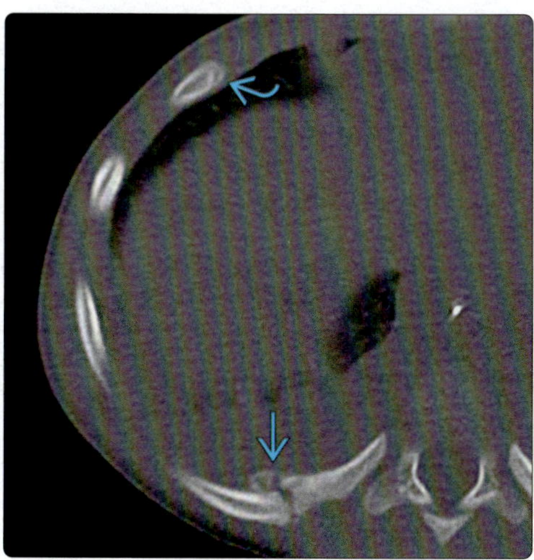

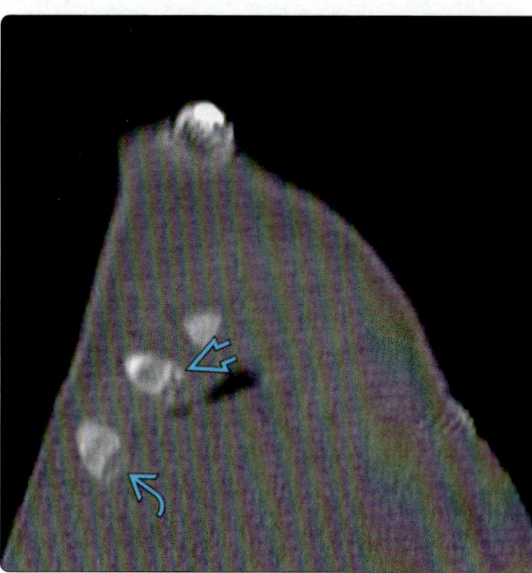

(Left) *Axial CT from a 2-year-old with blunt abdominal injuries shows a healing posterior rib fracture ➔ & an anterior rib fracture at the costochondral junction ➔.* **(Right)** *Sagittal oblique CT from the same patient demonstrates a classic metaphyseal lesion (CML)-like appearance of the costochondral junction fractures with triangular corner fragments ➔ & bucket-handle-shaped fragments ➔.*

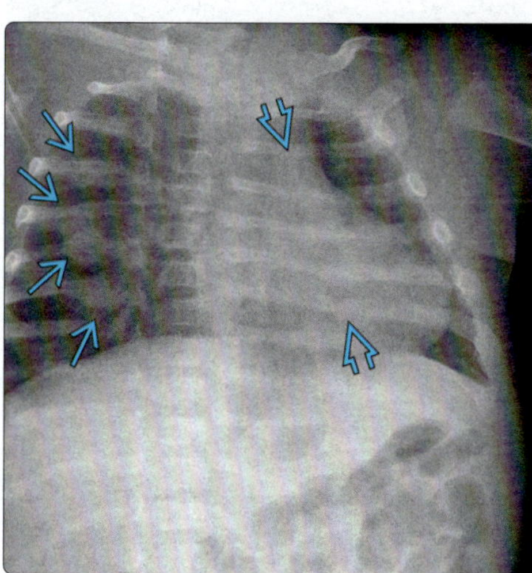

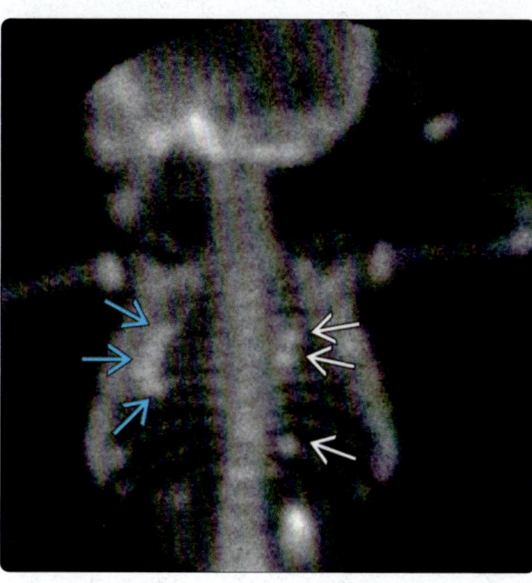

(Left) *Oblique radiograph of a 2-month-old with an unexplained femur fracture demonstrates healing fractures of the posterior right 3rd to 6th ribs ➔. Note how the rotated sternal ossification centers ➔ mimic bulbous callus of multiple left posterior ribs on this oblique view.* **(Right)** *Bone scan from the same patient confirms healing fractures at the right ribs ➔ with additional fractures identified in the medial left posterior ribs ➔.*

Lung Contusion and Laceration

KEY FACTS

TERMINOLOGY

- Lung contusion: Hemorrhage + edema in alveoli & interstitium due to traumatic alveolar capillary damage
- Lung laceration: Frank tear of lung parenchyma

IMAGING

- Radiograph: Often sufficient for blunt chest trauma evaluation
  - Contusion: Nonsegmental patchy or diffuse opacification
    - May not be radiographically evident < 4-6 hours
  - Laceration: Round lucency ± air-fluid level
    - May be obscured by contusion initially
- CECT: Performed if strong clinical or imaging findings suggest significant thoracic injury
  - ↑ sensitivity for detecting contusion & ↑ accuracy for assessing extent compared to radiographs
    - Significance of contusions seen only on CT is doubtful → may not be associated with ↑ morbidity
  - Contusion: Confluent/nodular, crescentic/amorphous consolidative or ground-glass opacities
    - Commonly peripheral with rim of subpleural sparing
  - Laceration: Air-/fluid-filled cavity surrounded by opacity

PATHOLOGY

- Associated chest injuries
  - Pneumothorax
  - Rib fractures (less common than adults)
  - Heart & great vessels (8%), diaphragm (< 5%), tracheobronchial tree (< 3%), esophagus (< 0.1%)

CLINICAL ISSUES

- Patients with lung injuries typically have ↑ overall injury severity with multisystem trauma
  - Other systems account for high morbidity & mortality
- Consider pneumonia or acute respiratory distress syndrome (ARDS) if clinical & imaging findings worsen > 48 hours

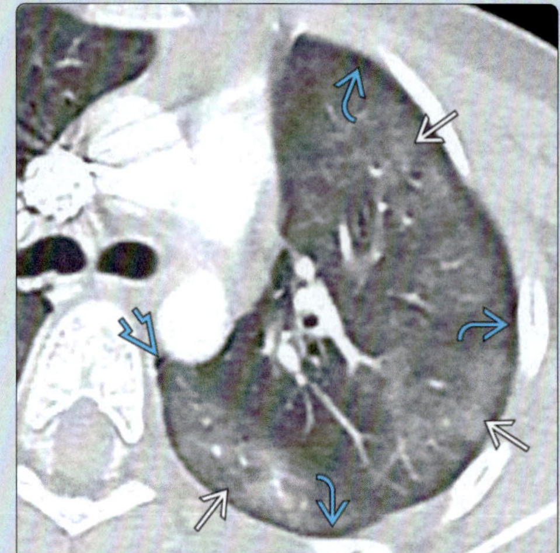

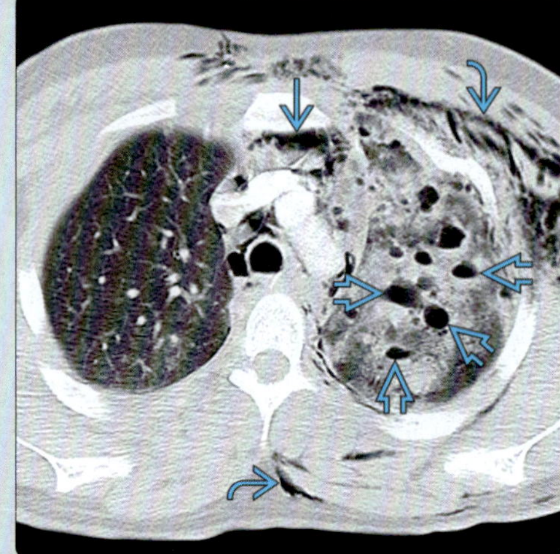

(Left) *Axial CECT from a 6-year-old who was run over by a car shows ground-glass opacities ➡ with subpleural sparing ⇨, characteristic of pulmonary contusion. A small left pneumothorax ⇨ was also present.* **(Right)** *Axial CECT of a 17-year-old after a motor vehicle accident (MVA) shows multiple air- & fluid-filled cysts ⇨ throughout the left upper lobe, consistent with lung lacerations. Also note the pneumomediastinum ⇨ & extensive subcutaneous emphysema ⇨.*

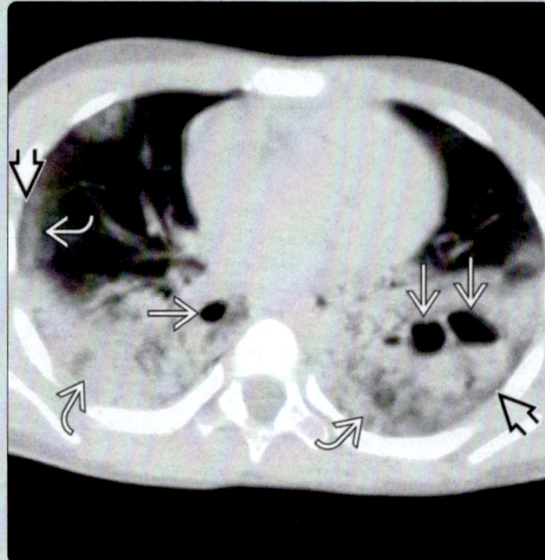

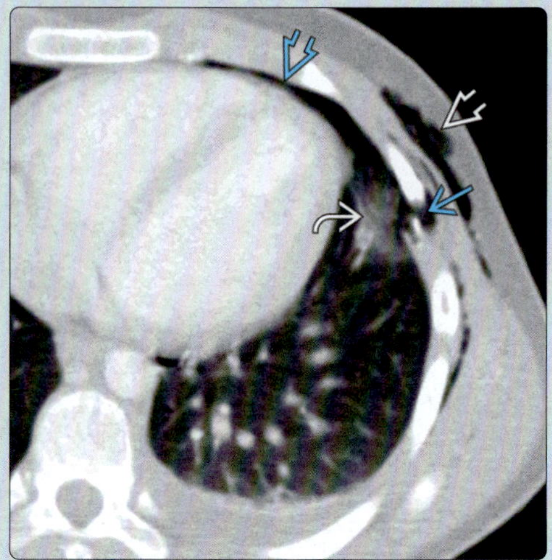

(Left) *Axial CECT in a trauma patient shows bilateral, primarily peripheral amorphous densities ➡ that do not respect lobar anatomy, consistent with lung contusions. There is associated subpleural sparing ⇨. The multiple fluid-containing cysts ➡ are typical of lacerations.* **(Right)** *Axial CECT in a 13-year-old after a bicycle collision shows a left 5th rib fracture ⇨, subcutaneous emphysema ➡, a pneumothorax ⇨, & adjacent ground-glass lung opacity ➡ that is consistent with contusion.*

TERMINOLOGY

Definitions

- Lung contusion: Blunt chest trauma → alveolar capillary damage → hemorrhage + edema in alveoli & interstitium
- Lung laceration: Chest trauma (blunt or penetrating) → frank tear of lung parenchyma

IMAGING

General Features

- Best diagnostic clue
  - Crescentic or amorphous nonsegmental pulmonary opacities of mixed confluent & nodular quality
    - Subpleural sparing of overlying lung periphery
- Location
  - Posterior lung is most common

Radiographic Findings

- Contusions
  - Irregular patchy regions of poorly defined airspace consolidation (mild) vs. diffuse homogeneous consolidation (severe)
    - Due to hemorrhage & edema in alveoli & peribronchovascular interstitium
  - Located at impaction or contrecoup lung injury sites
    - Adjacent to ribs & vertebral bodies
  - Present in 30-50% of initial chest radiographs for blunt trauma
    - Radiographs underestimate volume of contusion
  - May not be evident in first 4-6 hours after trauma
    - Radiographs are negative > 6 hours in up to 33%
  - Complete clearing within 7-10 days unless other cause of opacification develops
    - Pneumonia, acute respiratory distress syndrome (ARDS)
- Lacerations
  - Thin-walled, air-filled cysts of variable size (pneumatoceles) ± air-fluid levels
    - Single/multiple, oval/spherical, uni-/multilocular
    - May fill with hematoma & subsequently expand (uncommon)
    - May be obscured by contusion initially, appearing hours or days after trauma
  - Occur at maximum impact or contrecoup injury sites
  - Persist up to 4 months; gradually ↓ in size by 1-2 cm/week
- Bronchial injury
  - Very rare
  - Persistent pneumothorax despite chest tube
  - Fallen lung sign: Lung falls away from hilum

CT Findings

- Contusions
  - Mixed confluent & nodular lung opacities (70%)
    - Crescentic (50%) or amorphous (45%) in shape
    - Posterior location (75%); lower lobes are most common
  - Subpleural sparing in up to 95% of cases
    - Thin, 1- to 2-mm crescentic rim of uniformly nonopacified subpleural lung
      - Separates lung opacity from adjacent chest wall
    - Less likely in larger contusions
  - CT is more sensitive than radiographs for contusion & more accurately determines contused volume
    - Up to 69% of contusions are underestimated (24%) or not identified (45%) on initial radiograph vs. CT
- Lacerations
  - Air- or fluid-filled cavity/cavities surrounded by parenchymal contusion
    - Due to frank tear of parenchyma (worse injury)

Ultrasonographic Findings

- High sensitivity (> 90%) & specificity (> 90%) in adults with blunt chest trauma when 2 sonographic features are present
  - Multiple B lines (comet-tail artifacts) arising from pleural line
    - Represent interstitial edema 1-2 hours after injury
    - Other processes with alveolar/interstitial involvement can appear similar (e.g., cardiogenic pulmonary edema, ARDS)
  - Peripheral parenchymal lesion with C lines, confluent consolidations (hepatization), or parenchymal disruption with effusion
    - Represents hemorrhage & debris in alveoli

Imaging Recommendations

- Chest radiographs are usually sufficient for evaluation of blunt trauma
- CT is performed in patients with strong clinical or imaging findings of significant thoracic injury
- Differentiation of contusions from other lung opacities in blunt chest trauma has relevance to child's prognosis

DIFFERENTIAL DIAGNOSIS

Aspiration

- Segmental distribution of opacities (as aspirated materials reach lungs via airways)
  - Posterior lower lobes are most common
- Absence of subpleural sparing
- Findings develop in 24-48 hours

Pneumonia

- Focal or multifocal airspace opacification
- Absence of subpleural sparing
- May be superimposed on contusion; consider if contusion worsens after 48 hours

Atelectasis

- Triangular shape with segmental distribution
- Often dependent with lack of subpleural sparing
- Signs of volume loss

Acute Respiratory Distress Syndrome

- Extensive bilateral ground-glass opacities & consolidation
- Diffuse alveolar damage in setting of pulmonary or nonpulmonary injury

Neurogenic Pulmonary Edema

- Symmetric confluent airspace opacities; normal heart size

PATHOLOGY

General Features

- Etiology
  - Blunt trauma: 85-90% of thoracic injuries
    - Most commonly motor vehicle-related
    - Pedestrian vs. vehicle 36.5%, motor vehicle accident 31.7%, assault 11.5%, falls 9%
  - Penetrating trauma: 10-15% of thoracic injuries
    - Gunshot or stab wound, puncture from fractured rib
  - Nonaccidental trauma (NAT)
    - Thoracic injury may be more common in NAT vs. accidental trauma (17% vs. 6%)
- Associated abnormalities
  - With major chest trauma in child
    - Pneumothorax
    - Rib fractures are less common vs. adults
      - Due to elasticity of pediatric rib cage
      - Still present in 20-62% of cases
    - Uncommon injuries: Heart & great vessels (8%), diaphragm (1-5%), tracheobronchial tree (0.7-2.8%), esophagus (< 0.1%)
- Mechanism of injury
  - ↑ pliability of anterior pediatric chest wall + contrecoup forces of rapid deceleration → compression of relatively fixed posterior lung against ribs & vertebral column
  - Dispersion of forces along least mobile lung regions explains posterior location, crescentic shape, & nonsegmental distribution
  - Subpleural sparing in contusion may be due to
    - Terminal arterial branches ending prior to subpleural lung, possibly protecting this region from hemorrhage
      - Less common sign in large contusions, possibly due to extension of hemorrhage into subpleural lung
    - Compression of subpleural lung against chest wall may "squeeze" blood & edema from periphery
  - Systemic inflammatory response: ↓ surfactant production by injured alveolar tissue may lead to ARDS
  - Lung laceration: Frank tear of lung parenchyma results in cavity that fills with hemorrhage &/or air

Gross Pathologic & Surgical Features

- American Association for the Surgery of Trauma injury scale
  - Grade I: Unilateral contusion < 1 lobe
  - Grade II: Unilateral contusion of single lobe or laceration → simple pneumothorax
  - Grade III: Unilateral contusion > 1 lobe, laceration with persistent (> 72 hours) air leak from distal airway, or nonexpanding intraparenchymal hematoma
  - Grade IV: Major segmental/lobar laceration with air leak, expanding intraparenchymal hematoma, or primary branch intrapulmonary vessel disruption
  - Grade V: Hilar vessel disruption
  - Grade VI: Total uncontained transection of hilar vessel

CLINICAL ISSUES

Presentation

- ↓ breath sounds, dullness to percussion, tachypnea, chest tenderness, hemoptysis (rarely)
- May present with respiratory failure in large contusions
  - Hypercarbia, hypoxia, acidosis

Natural History & Prognosis

- Children with thoracic trauma are typically more severely injured overall than those without thoracic involvement
  - Morbidity & mortality in patients with lung contusion/laceration are usually related to severity of multisystem trauma
    - Mortality rates of pediatric patients with lung contusions & lacerations are up to 34% & 43%, respectively
    - NAT mortality with thoracic injury ↑ from 15% to 50%
  - 20-37% of children with pulmonary contusion require mechanical ventilation
    - Radiographic severity of lung contusion correlates with oxygenation impairment, carbon dioxide exchange, & duration of ventilatory support
      - Radiographically occult contusions seen by CT: No ↑ in patient morbidity
    - Contusion volume > 28% on CT is predictive of need for mechanical ventilation in one study of adult & pediatric patients
      - Not reproduced in solely pediatric population
    - Contusion volume > 20% on CT is predictive of ARDS development in adults; not reproduced in children
- Complications: Pneumonia 20%, ARDS 5-20%
- Posttraumatic ARDS
  - Rare, 0.5% of all pediatric trauma cases
  - Mortality > 18% within 1 week of injury
  - Risk factors: NAT, severe injury to head or chest, pneumonia, sepsis, thoracotomy, laparotomy, transfusion

Treatment

- Supportive therapy: Pulmonary toilet, pain control, alveolar recruitment maneuvers, noninvasive positive pressure ventilation, mechanical ventilation, rarely ECMO
- Surveillance for other major organ injuries
- Observation for complications: Infection, ARDS, tension pneumothorax, hemopneumothorax, hemoptysis
- No evidence to support prophylactic broad-spectrum antibiotics (but often used)
- No proven role for corticosteroids

SELECTED REFERENCES

1. Carson D et al: Core curriculum illustration: pulmonary laceration. Emerg Radiol. 27(2):219-20, 2020
2. Holl EM et al: Use of chest computed tomography for blunt pediatric chest trauma: does it change clinical course? Pediatr Emerg Care. 36(2):81-6, 2020
3. de Roulet A et al: Pediatric trauma-associated acute respiratory distress syndrome: incidence, risk factors, and outcomes. J Pediatr Surg. 54(7):1405-10, 2019
4. Rendeki S et al: Pulmonary contusion. J Thorac Dis. 11(Suppl 2):S141-51, 2019
5. Weerdenburg KD et al: Predicting thoracic injury in children with multitrauma. Pediatr Emerg Care. 35(5):330-4, 2019
6. Dennis BM et al: Thoracic trauma. Surg Clin North Am. 97(5):1047-64, 2017
7. Donnelly LF: Imaging issues in CT of blunt trauma to the chest and abdomen. Pediatr Radiol. 39 Suppl 3:406-13, 2009
8. Moore MA et al: The imaging of paediatric thoracic trauma. Pediatr Radiol. 39(5):485-96, 2009
9. Moore EE et al: Organ injury scaling. IV: thoracic vascular, lung, cardiac, and diaphragm. J Trauma. 36(3):299-300, 1994

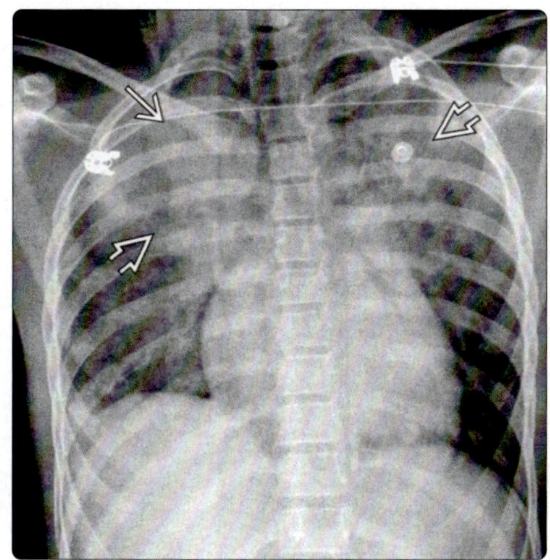

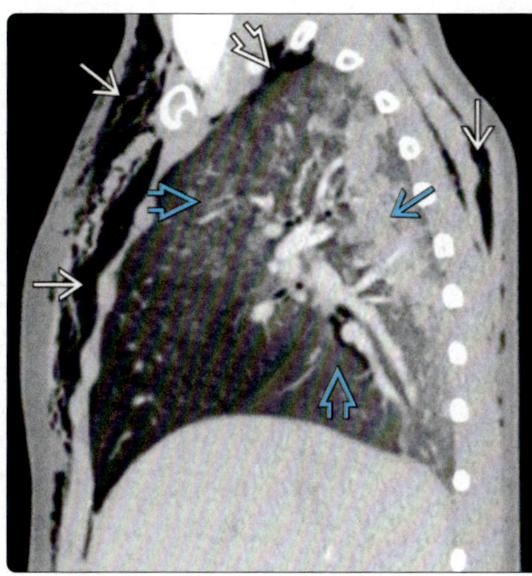

(Left) *Supine chest radiograph of an 11-year-old who was stepped on by a horse shows large areas of bilateral confluent ➡ & patchy ➡ opacities in the upper lung zones, compatible with contusions.* **(Right)** *Sagittal CECT from a 9-year-old after a bike accident demonstrates a confluent opacity ➡ with adjacent extensive ground-glass opacities ➡ in the left lung that do not respect lobar boundaries, compatible with contusions. There is extensive soft tissue emphysema ➡ & a small pneumothorax ➡.*

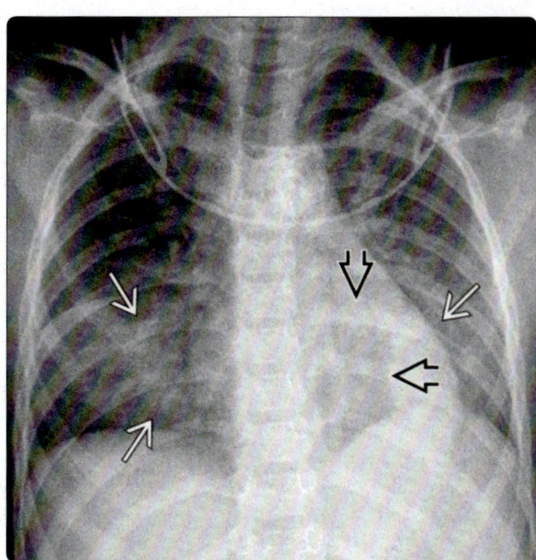

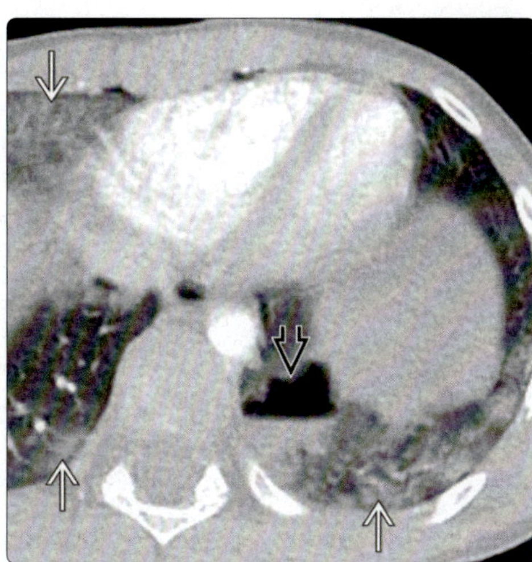

(Left) *Frontal radiograph of an 8-year-old after an all-terrain vehicle accident shows confluent right middle & bilateral lower lobe opacities ➡. The left lower lobe lucency is suspicious for a laceration ➡.* **(Right)** *Axial CECT in the same patient shows a laceration with an air-fluid level in the left lower lobe ➡. Scattered patchy & ground-glass opacities are also present in the right middle & bilateral lower lobes ➡, consistent with contusions.*

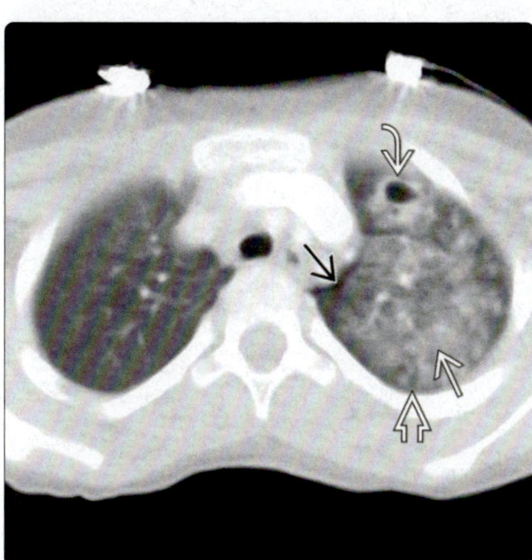

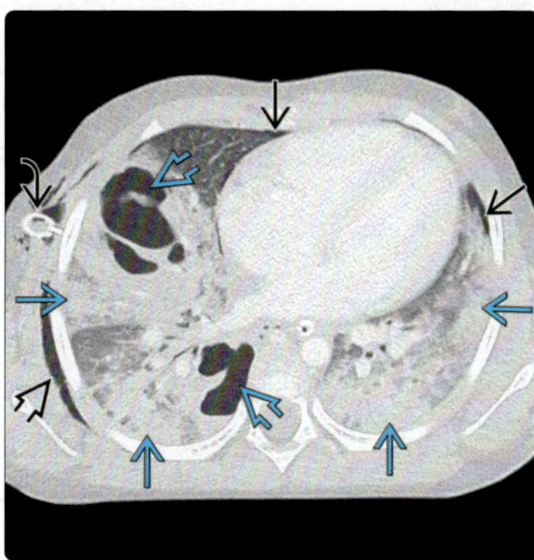

(Left) *Axial CECT of a 10-year-old who was hit by a car shows patchy densities ➡ with subpleural sparing ➡, consistent with contusion. A cavity with an air-fluid level is noted, compatible with a lung laceration ➡. There is also a left pneumothorax ➡.* **(Right)** *Axial CECT of a 3-year-old after an MVA shows consolidation & ground-glass opacities ➡ in keeping with contusions. Two lacerations are also seen ➡. In addition, there are small pneumothoraces ➡, subcutaneous emphysema ➡, & a chest tube ➡.*

Aortic Injury

KEY FACTS

TERMINOLOGY

- Blunt aortic injury (BAI) may manifest as intramural hematoma, intimal tear, larger intimal flap, contained pseudoaneurysm, or frank aortic rupture

IMAGING

- Chest radiograph: Sensitive, not specific; high NPV (> 90%)
  - Most common findings: Indistinctness of aorta, prominent aortic knob, left apical cap
- CTA: Sensitivity & specificity 90-100%; NPV nearly 100%
  - Modality of choice: Fast, accessible, accurate; has largely replaced conventional aortography
  - Most common finding: Pseudoaneurysm, followed by intimal tear; usually near aortic isthmus

TOP DIFFERENTIAL DIAGNOSES

- Normal thymus
- CT artifacts
- Ductus diverticulum

PATHOLOGY

- Majority of pediatric BAIs are due to rapid & forceful deceleration injuries (motor vehicle accidents > falls, ATV crashes, & bicyclist/pedestrian vs. automobile collisions)

CLINICAL ISSUES

- Significant change in prognosis/treatment depending on presence or absence of aortic external contour alteration
  - Absent (intimal tears & flaps): Mortality 5-15% with treatment
  - Present: Mortality 25% for pseudoaneurysm & up to 90% for aortic rupture
- Delayed endovascular treatment is becoming more common; blood pressure control is essential in interval

DIAGNOSTIC CHECKLIST

- Look for BAI in all cases of blunt, high-energy chest trauma
- Up to 50% of pediatric BAIs lack external signs of chest trauma & have obvious CNS, abdominal, or skeletal injuries

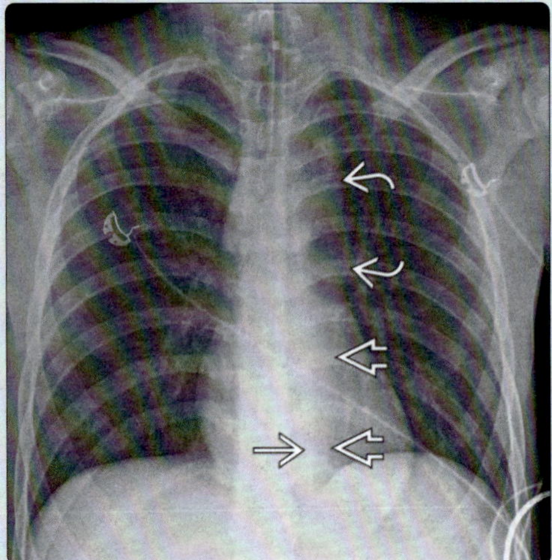

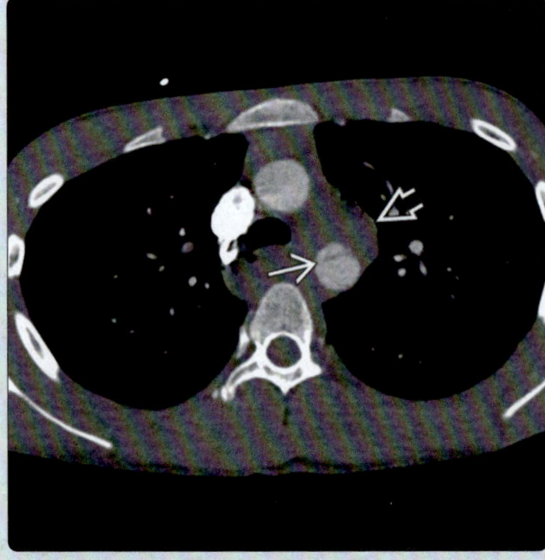

(Left) *AP radiograph in a teenager with blunt aortic injury (BAI) after a bicycle vs. car accident reveals subtle mediastinal widening from a periaortic hematoma ➡. Inferiorly, the hematoma creates an abnormal density ➡ parallel to the shadow created by descending aorta ➡. Although subtle, such findings should prompt emergent CT to exclude aortic injury.* **(Right)** *Axial CTA in the same patient better shows the periaortic hematoma ➡ & clearly identifies a linear filling defect within the aorta from an intimal tear ➡.*

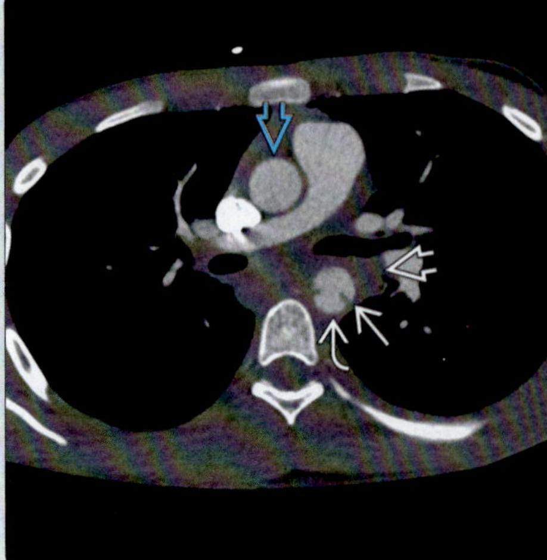

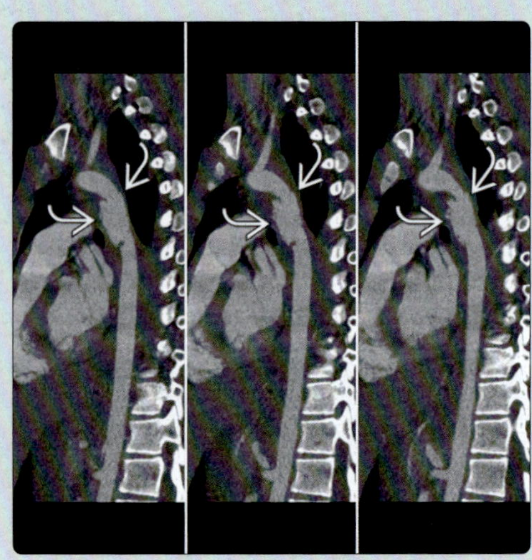

(Left) *More inferior axial CTA in the same patient shows that the mediastinal hematoma ➡ & intimal tear ➡ are associated with a focal outpouching of contrast from a pseudoaneurysm ➡. Note that the ascending aorta is normal ➡, lacking artifact from cardiac motion that can mimic an intimal injury.* **(Right)** *Sequential sagittal CTA reconstructions in the same patient better illustrate the pseudoaneurysm as a large, irregular circumferential outpouching of contrast ➡ from the aortic lumen.*

TERMINOLOGY

Abbreviations

- Traumatic aortic injury (TAI), blunt aortic injury (BAI), blunt thoracic aortic injury (BTAI)

Definitions

- Intramural hematoma: Isolated circumferential or crescentic thickening of aortic wall without intimal injury
- Intimal tear: Small, isolated injury to intimal layer of aorta without external aortic contour abnormality → linear intimal defect &/or associated thrombus < 10 mm
- Large intimal flap: Larger intimal injury than tear but still without external aortic contour abnormality → linear intimal defect &/or associated thrombus > 10 mm
- Pseudoaneurysm: Rupture contained by adventitia → focal outpouching of aortic lumen causing external aortic contour abnormality
- Rupture: Uncontained dissection causing external aortic contour abnormality with extraluminal contrast (extravasation)

IMAGING

General Features

- Location
  - Most commonly (95%) near aortic isthmus between left subclavian & 1st intercostal arteries
  - Far less common at aortic root or diaphragmatic hiatus
  - Multiple tears are seen in small number of patients
  - May occur in abdominal aorta with seat belt injury

Radiographic Findings

- Chest radiograph is sensitive but not specific; low positive predictive value (< 20%), high negative predictive value (> 90%)
- Chest radiograph may be normal with only small mediastinal hematoma
- Radiographic signs
  - Left apical cap or left hemothorax
  - Obscured outline of descending aorta
  - Obliteration of aortopulmonary window
  - Widened mediastinum (which may be mimicked by normally prominent thymus in younger children)
  - Wide paraspinal stripe
  - Rightward shift of endotracheal &/or gastric tube(s)
  - Rightward shift of trachea
  - Depressed left main bronchus
  - Fractures of 1st &/or 2nd rib(s) &/or scapula

CT Findings

- NECT
  - Low sensitivity & specificity
  - High attenuation in aortic wall: Intramural hematoma
  - Obliteration/↑ attenuation of mediastinal fat suggests hemorrhage
  - Hematoma displacing trachea & esophagus to right
  - Hemopericardium
- CTA
  - Modality of choice: Rapid, accessible, high detail of acute thoracoabdominal injuries
    - Has largely replaced conventional aortography
  - Sensitivity 90-100%, specificity 90-100%, negative predictive value nearly 100%
  - Direct signs
    - Circumferential or crescentic thickening of aortic wall due to intramural hematoma
    - Linear filling defect (intimal flap) due to dissection
    - Intraluminal thrombus
    - Well-defined external contour abnormality of pseudoaneurysm, especially at aortic isthmus
    - Aortic wall irregularity
    - Abrupt change of aortic contour or caliber
    - Irregular, uncontained extraluminal collection of extravasated contrast
  - Indirect signs
    - Periaortic hematoma (absent in up to 20% of patients)

Ultrasonographic Findings

- Point-of-care US may reveal pericardial effusion &/or left hemothorax

Echocardiographic Findings

- May be performed in operating room; especially useful when patients go immediately to surgery
- Particularly sensitive for intimal tears
- Aortic valve regurgitation, intramural hematoma, or frank aortic rupture may be seen

Angiographic Findings

- Essentially replaced by CTA
- Used in equivocal cases or if endovascular repair is planned

Imaging Recommendations

- Best imaging tool
  - Multidetector CT angiography (at least 64 slice) is less likely to show pulsation artifact & allows thin multiplanar isotropic reconstructions
- Protocol advice
  - Quarter-/half-rotation volume data reconstructions or cardiac gating can reduce pulsation artifacts

DIFFERENTIAL DIAGNOSIS

Normal Thymus

- Prominent in young children, often accentuated by rotation or low lung volumes
- May obscure aortic contour

CT Artifacts

- Cardiac motion transmitted to aorta may mimic intramural hematoma or intimal tear
  - Rapid heart beat in children ↑ chances of pulsation artifact
- Streak artifact from contrast bolus may obscure aortic lumen or mimic intimal tear
- Atelectasis or parenchymal contusion in adjacent lung may be mistaken for aortic wall thickening

Ductus Diverticulum

- Broad-based anterior outpouching of contrast with smooth contour & obtuse margins
- Like most traumatic aortic injuries, located at aortic isthmus
- Found in up to 10% of normal population
- No hematoma, contrast leak, or intimal flap

PATHOLOGY

General Features

- Etiology
  - Majority of pediatric BAIs are due to rapid & forceful deceleration injuries
    - Mostly motor vehicle accidents (MVAs)
    - Falls, ATV crashes, & bicyclist/pedestrian vs. automobile collisions are also common
  - Sudden deceleration combined with fixation of aorta at ligamentum arteriosum → shearing, stretching, & torsional forces that injure aortic wall
  - Remainder of pediatric TAIs are due to gunshot wounds, penetrating injuries, & crushing/compression forces
- Pediatric BAI is rare compared to adults, as children have
  - Greater chest wall compliance
  - Relatively elastic vascular tissues (due to lack of atherosclerotic disease)
  - Lower body mass (thus less kinetic energy on impact)
  - Lower likelihood of MVAs

Staging, Grading, & Classification

- Society for Vascular Surgery
  - Type I: Intimal tear
  - Type II: Intramural hematoma or large intimal flap
  - Type III: Contained leak or pseudoaneurysm
  - Type IV: Transection/uncontained rupture
- Harborview criteria (newer)
  - Minimal: No external contour abnormality; intimal tear or thrombus < 10 mm
  - Moderate: External contour abnormality; intimal tear > 10 mm
  - Severe: Active extravasation or left subclavian artery hematoma > 15 mm

CLINICAL ISSUES

Presentation

- Most common signs/symptoms
  - Hypotension, ↓ pulses in lower extremities, paraplegia
  - Up to 50% of children with BAI lack external signs of chest trauma
    - Often have more obvious neurologic, abdominal, or skeletal injuries
  - May have no signs/symptoms, or only nonspecific chest pain, dyspnea
- Other signs/symptoms
  - Associated thoracic cage injuries: Diaphragm rupture, pulmonary contusion, rib fractures
  - High association with other injuries, especially traumatic brain injury & solid abdominal organ injury

Demographics

- Trauma is most common cause of death in children, but vascular trauma accounts for < 1%; BAI is even more rare
  - Retrospective review of ~ 11,000 children with severe blunt trauma showed < 0.1% sustained BAI
- Associated with high-risk recreational activities
  - Most pediatric BAIs from MVAs are in older children/teenagers

Natural History & Prognosis

- Very low incidence, even in children involved in high-energy blunt chest trauma, but mortality rate is very high
  - ~ 80% die at scene of injury
- Survival depends on type of injury as well as time from injury to intervention
  - Injuries that do not alter external contour of aorta (intimal tears/flaps & intramural hematomas) have relatively good prognosis (mortality of 5-15% with treatment)
  - Injuries that do alter external contour of aorta have higher mortality (~ 25% for pseudoaneurysm & up to 90% for aortic rupture)
- Without intervention, mortality from BAI is very high (80% mortality < 1 hour & 98% mortality < 10 weeks)
- Late complications include posttraumatic pseudoaneurysm & coarctation or spinal cord ischemia → paralysis

Treatment

- Rapid recognition of diagnosis is critical
  - β-blockade for all patients if hemodynamically stable
- Society for Vascular Surgery
  - Type I: Medical management & close observation
  - Type II-IV: Surgical or endovascular repair (though II may be considered for nonoperative management)
    - Delayed endovascular repair is now favored over emergent operative treatment
      - Thoracic endovascular aortic repair (TEVAR)
    - Allows other injuries to be assessed & treated while ↓ operative complications
    - Provides time to appropriately size endograft & ensure that access sites can accommodate device
    - Short-term complications occur mainly at access site (bleeding, infection, pseudoaneurysm, etc.)
    - Long-term complications include device migration, fracture, endoleak, & arterial wall injury
    - Requires strict blood pressure control
- Harborview
  - Minimal: Follow-up
  - Moderate: Delayed repair after stabilization
  - Severe: Immediate repair

DIAGNOSTIC CHECKLIST

Consider

- Look for signs of BAI in all cases of blunt or high-energy chest trauma: Must have high index of suspicion
- Look for proxy signs of high-energy trauma, such as fractures of 1st &/or 2nd rib(s) &/or scapula
- Potential CTA pitfalls: Pulsation artifact, streak artifact, &/or periaortic focal atelectasis

SELECTED REFERENCES

1. Mouawad NJ et al: Blunt thoracic aortic injury - concepts and management. J Cardiothorac Surg. 15(1):62, 2020
2. Nicholas NW et al: Pictorial review on the endovascular management of paediatric aortic injuries. Br J Radiol. 93(1106):20190017, 2020
3. Akhmerov A et al: Blunt thoracic aortic injury: current therapies, outcomes, and challenges. Ann Vasc Dis. 12(1):1-5, 2019
4. Hasjim BJ et al: National trends of thoracic endovascular aortic repair versus open thoracic aortic repair in pediatric blunt thoracic aortic injury. Ann Vasc Surg. 59:150-7, 2019

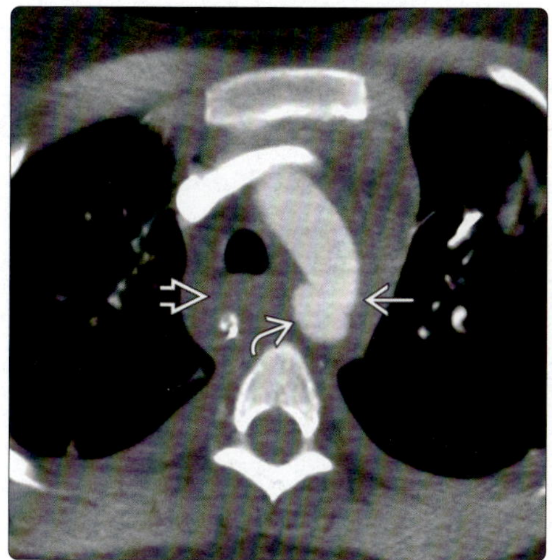

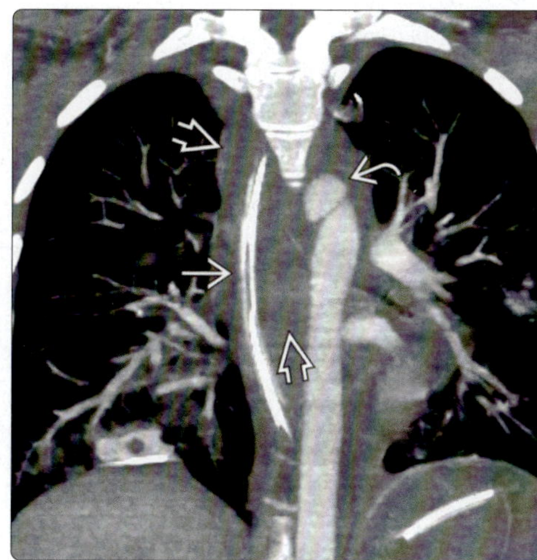

(Left) *Axial CTA in a teenager who was in an MVA shows an abnormal external contour of the aorta ➡ caused by a pseudoaneurysm ➡ near the aortic isthmus. Also note the extensive mediastinal hematoma ➡.* **(Right)** *Coronal CTA in the same patient again shows the pseudoaneurysm ➡ as a focal, rounded contour alteration of the aorta. Note how the mediastinal hematoma ➡ causes rightward deviation of the nasogastric tube ➡; this indirect finding of BAI may be the only abnormality seen on an initial trauma radiograph.*

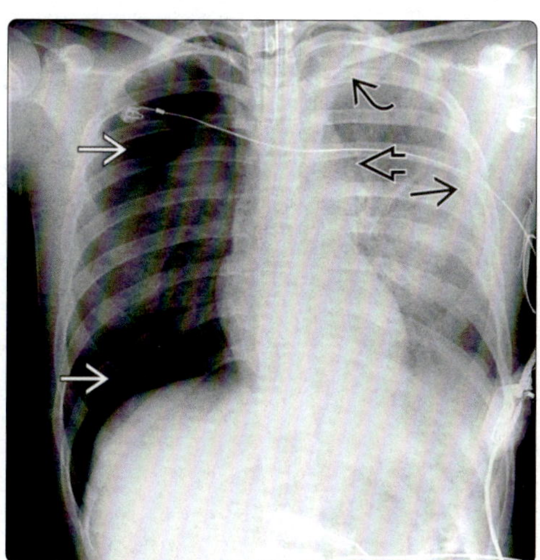

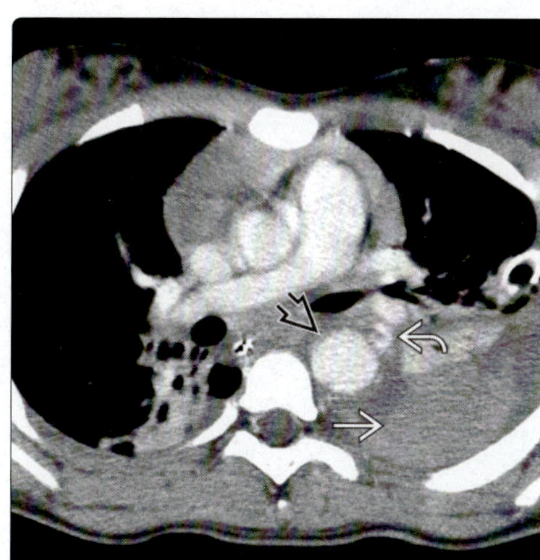

(Left) *AP radiograph of an 11-year-old patient who sustained an aortic tear during an MVA demonstrates a left apical cap ➡, obscuration of the aortic contour ➡, & a hemothorax ➡. There is also a large tension pneumothorax ➡ on the right.* **(Right)** *Axial CTA from the same study shows active extravasation ➡ from an aortic rupture as well as a large, high-attenuation hemothorax ➡. The aorta is focally enlarged & irregular ➡. This child died from aortic transection.*

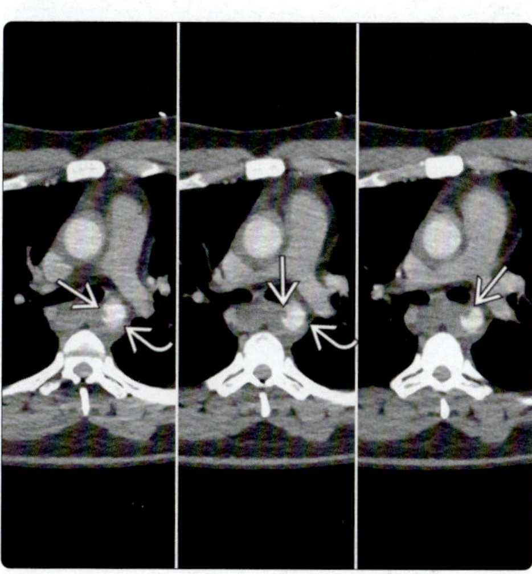

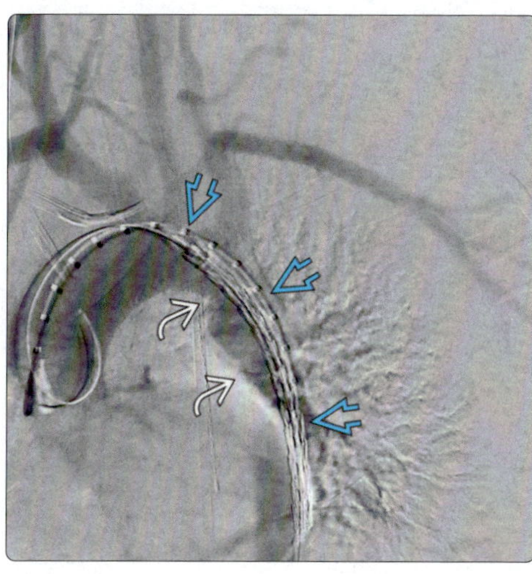

(Left) *Sequential axial CTA images in a young man who crashed his motorcycle reveal an irregular aortic filling defect ➡ as well as nonuniformity of the vessel wall ➡ caused by traumatic BAI.* **(Right)** *Oblique DSA shows placement of a conformable stent ➡ across the injury site ➡. In clinically stable patients, a delayed endovascular repair allows time for other injuries to be assessed & treated (& results in fewer complications compared to operative management).*

Pneumomediastinum

KEY FACTS

IMAGING

- Best tool for pneumomediastinum (PM): Chest radiograph
  - Pleural line lateral to main pulmonary artery & aortic arch
  - Vertical lucencies along superior mediastinum, trachea, esophagus, descending thoracic aorta
  - Continuous diaphragm sign: Air between pericardium & diaphragm results in visualization of normally obscured superior surface of central diaphragm
  - Spinnaker sail sign: Thymic elevation by mediastinal air in young child
  - Vanishing heart sign: Lucency over cardiac silhouette on supine view, posterior on lateral view
- CT or esophagram only with radiographic evidence of trauma, risk factors for aerodigestive tract injury (foreign body, surgery, mediastinitis), or respiratory distress

PATHOLOGY

- Spontaneous PM: Extension of air from ruptured alveolus into interstitium & mediastinum
  - Asthma & respiratory infection are most common
- Secondary PM: Disruption of aerodigestive tract (barotrauma, trauma, foreign body, Boerhaave syndrome), surgery, mediastinitis

CLINICAL ISSUES

- Common symptoms: Chest pain, cough, dyspnea
- Secondary PM is likely to present with rib fracture, pneumothorax, hemothorax, intracranial injury, respiratory distress, tachycardia
- Isolated spontaneous PM in stable patient: Self-limited
- Spontaneous PM with symptom progression: Further evaluate & treat underlying pulmonary cause
- Secondary PM: CT or esophagram with clinical or imaging evidence of aerodigestive tract injury
  - Widespread screening is of low yield in blunt trauma patients with otherwise normal chest radiograph
- Rarely, tension PM

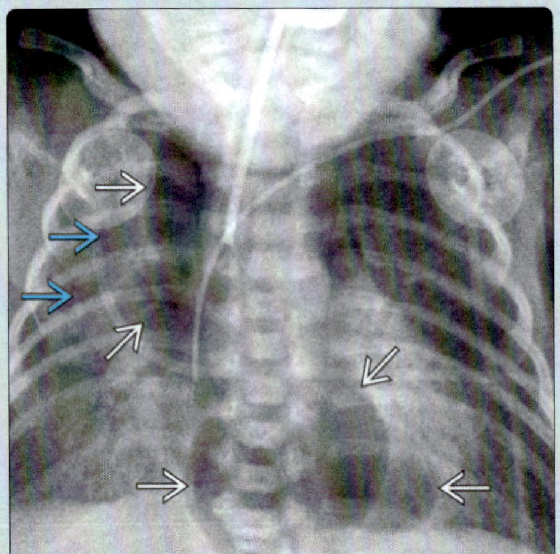

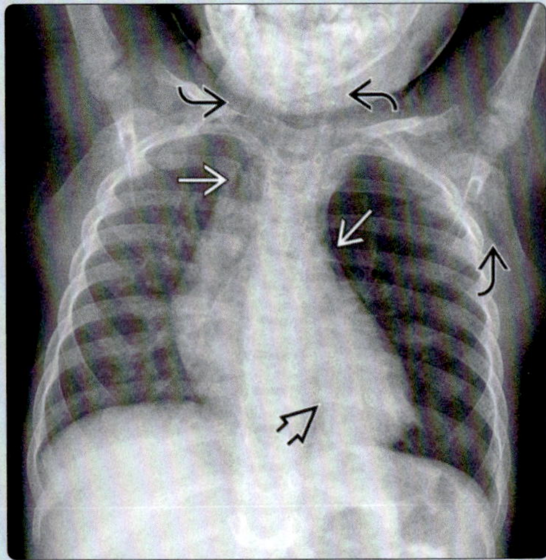

(Left) *AP radiograph of a neonate with a perforated left main bronchus demonstrates a large lucency ➔ throughout the mediastinum, consistent with pneumomediastinum. The thymic tissue ➔ is displaced to the right.* **(Right)** *AP radiograph in a 2-year-old patient shows hyperinflation of the left lung with retrocardiac atelectasis ➔ & scattered foci of pneumomediastinum ➔ & subcutaneous emphysema ➔. Subsequent bronchoscopy demonstrated an aspirated peanut in the left main bronchus.*

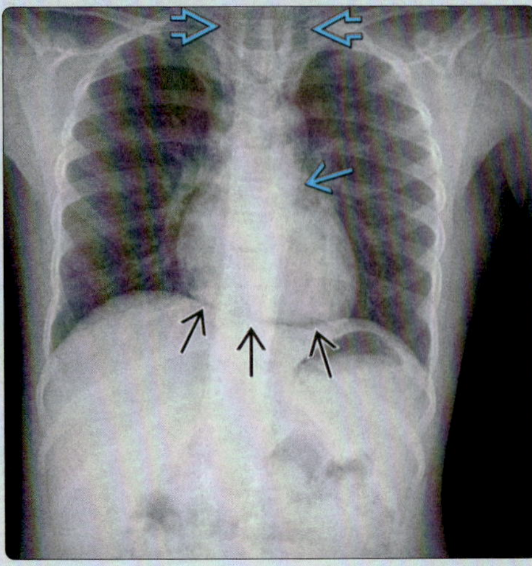

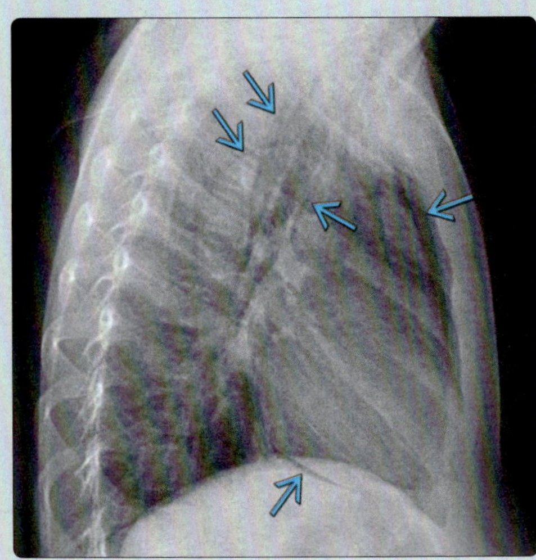

(Left) *Upright radiograph from a 6-year-old with chest pain after a fall shows a continuous diaphragm sign ➔ as well as subtle mediastinal lucencies ➔, compatible with pneumomediastinum. Soft tissue emphysema is also noted ➔.* **(Right)** *Lateral view of the chest from the same patient demonstrates lucencies ➔ surrounding the cardiac silhouette, aorta, trachea, & esophagus, compatible with pneumomediastinum.*

TERMINOLOGY

Definitions

- Pneumomediastinum (PM): Extraluminal mediastinal gas

IMAGING

Radiographic Findings

- Central lucencies with pleural line lateral to main pulmonary artery & aortic arch
- Vertical lucencies tracking on either side of superior mediastinum into neck
- Spinnaker sail sign: Elevation of thymus by mediastinal air in young child
- Vanishing heart sign: Lucency over cardiac silhouette seen on frontal view, posteriorly on lateral view due to posterior PM
- Continuous diaphragm sign: Air between pericardium & diaphragm results in visualization of normally obscured superior surface of central diaphragm
- Naclerio V sign: Air outlines lateral margin of descending aorta & extends laterally along left hemidiaphragm

Fluoroscopic Findings

- ± esophageal leakage of contrast into mediastinum

CT Findings

- Extraluminal gas in mediastinal space
- May depict underlying disruption of tracheobronchial tree

Imaging Recommendations

- Chest radiograph as initial modality
- CT or esophagram in setting of risk factors for aerodigestive tract injury (foreign body, surgery, mediastinitis, definite thoracic injury) or respiratory distress

DIFFERENTIAL DIAGNOSIS

Pneumothorax

- Upright & decubitus views can help determine whether air is localized in mediastinum vs. freely mobile in pleural space

Pneumopericardium

- Round lucency with continuous outline of heart margins; displaces pericardium outward
- Air in pericardial space changes with patient position
- Air does not extend into superior mediastinum
- Much less common than PM

Paramediastinal Pneumatocele

- ± internal fluid-fluid level or "claw" of lung parenchyma

Hernia of Stomach

- Paraesophageal or Morgagni types

PATHOLOGY

General Features

- Spontaneous PM: Pressure gradient between alveolus & surrounding tissue causes rupture with extension of air into interstices & mediastinum
  - Asthma, respiratory infection > straining against closed glottis, surfactant deficiency, meconium aspiration, inhalation drug use, forceful coughing
- Secondary PM: Disruption of aerodigestive tract (trauma, foreign body, Boerhaave syndrome, barotrauma), surgery, mediastinitis
  - Aerodigestive tract injury is rare in pediatric population (4.1% of traumatic PM)
- Extension of air from peritoneum or retroperitoneum

CLINICAL ISSUES

Presentation

- Most common: Chest pain, cough, shortness of breath
- ± crepitus in neck or chest (subcutaneous emphysema)
- Secondary PM is likely to present with rib fracture, pneumothorax, hemothorax, intracranial injury, respiratory distress, tachycardia

Natural History & Prognosis

- Spontaneous PM: Self-limited; recurrence is rare
  - Morbidity related to underlying pulmonary condition
- Secondary PM: Mortality related to other injuries
- Complications are uncommon but can include tension PM & cardiac tamponade, mediastinitis, pneumothorax

Treatment

- Isolated spontaneous PM in stable patient
  - Supportive care, emergency department observation
  - No evidence to support further studies
- Spontaneous PM with symptom progression
  - Evaluate & treat underlying pulmonary condition
- Secondary PM
  - CT or esophagram if underlying aerodigestive tract injury is specifically suspected
  - Treat underlying condition

DIAGNOSTIC CHECKLIST

Consider

- Widespread screening (especially with esophagram) is low yield in blunt trauma patients with otherwise normal chest radiograph
  - Selective investigation with high suspicion (e.g., rib fracture, effusion, pneumothorax)

Image Interpretation Pearls

- In toddler with no history of asthma or trauma, consider aspirated foreign body

SELECTED REFERENCES

1. Noorbakhsh KA et al: Management and outcomes of spontaneous pneumomediastinum in children. Pediatr Emerg Care. ePub, 2019
2. Raissaki M et al: Spontaneous pneumomediastinum in a term newborn: atypical radiographic and CT appearances. BJR Case Rep. 5(4):20180081, 2019
3. Richer EJ et al: Are esophagrams indicated in pediatric patients with spontaneous pneumomediastinum? J Pediatr Surg. 51(11):1778-81, 2016
4. Chouliaras K et al: Pneumomediastinum following blunt trauma: worth an exhaustive workup? J Trauma Acute Care Surg. 79(2):188-92; discussion 192-3, 2015
5. Bakhos CT et al: Spontaneous pneumomediastinum: an extensive workup is not required. J Am Coll Surg. 219(4):713-7, 2014
6. Kyle A et al: Barotrauma-associated posterior tension pneumomediastinum, a rare cause of cardiac tamponade in a ventilated neonate: a case report and review of the literature. Acta Paediatr. 101(3):e142-4, 2012
7. Bejvan SM et al: Pneumomediastinum: old signs and new signs. AJR Am J Roentgenol. 166(5):1041-8, 1996

(Left) *Supine frontal view of the chest in this newborn demonstrates lucency ➔ elevating the thymus ➔, compatible with pneumomediastinum. A small right pneumothorax is also present ➔.* **(Right)** *Supine chest radiograph in a neonate shows extensive lucencies of pneumomediastinum ➔ displacing the lungs laterally & outlining the descending thoracic & upper abdominal aorta ➔. Diffuse granular opacities with air bronchograms relate to the patient's surfactant deficiency ➔.*

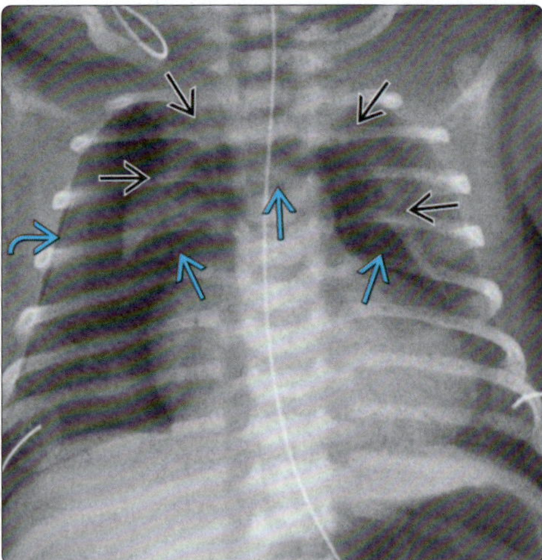

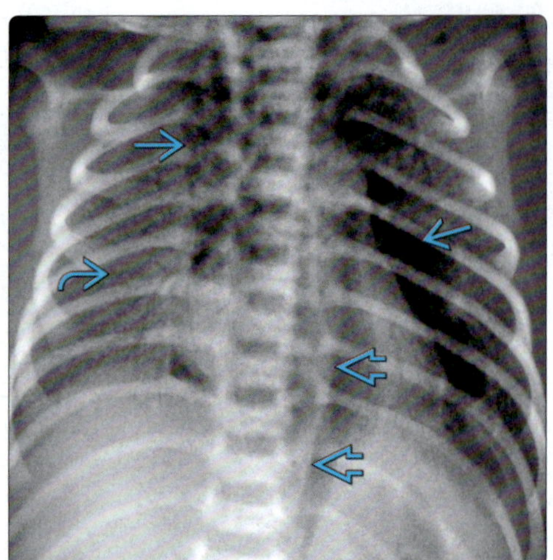

(Left) *Frontal upright radiograph of a 9-year-old who presented with shortness of breath shows curvilinear lucencies outlining the mediastinum ➔ & mildly elevating residual thymic tissue ➔. Note also the soft tissue emphysema in the neck ➔.* **(Right)** *Lateral upright view of the chest from the same patient again depicts pneumomediastinum with prominent anterior mediastinal lucencies ➔.*

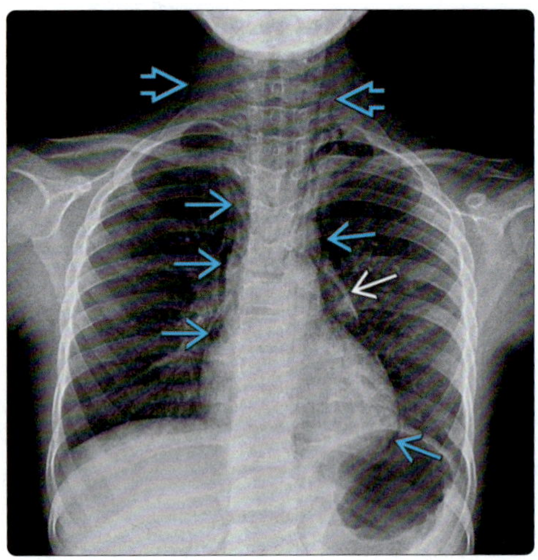

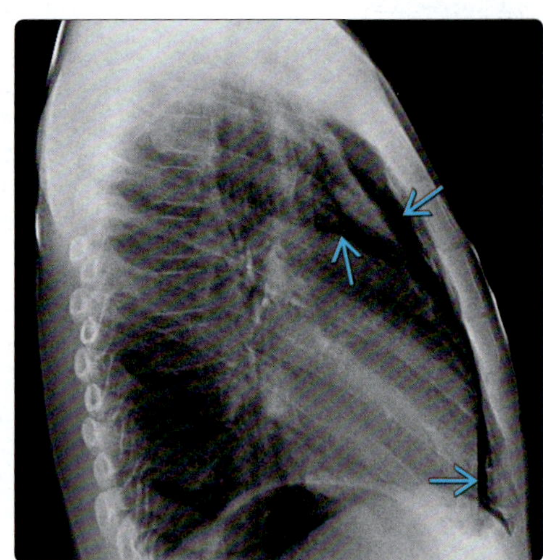

(Left) *Axial CECT in the same patient shows extensive pneumomediastinum ➔. Additionally seen are subpleural ground-glass densities ➔ & cystic changes ➔ relating to the patient's history of dermatomyositis.* **(Right)** *Supine radiograph of a 3-year-old presenting with cough, fever, & facial swelling shows extensive subcutaneous emphysema ➔ & pneumomediastinum ➔. Note the continuous diaphragm sign ➔ in this patient with RSV.*

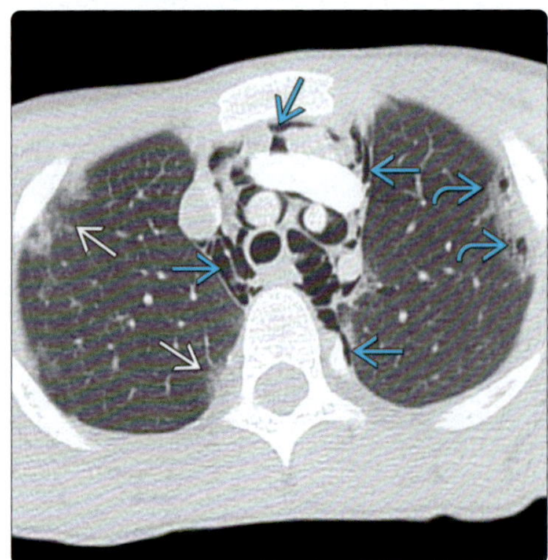

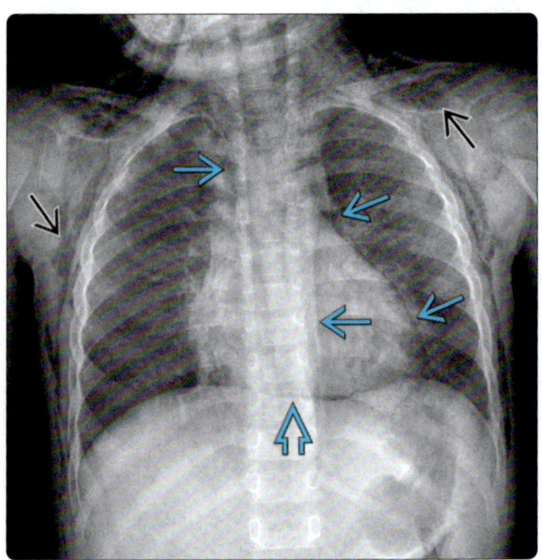

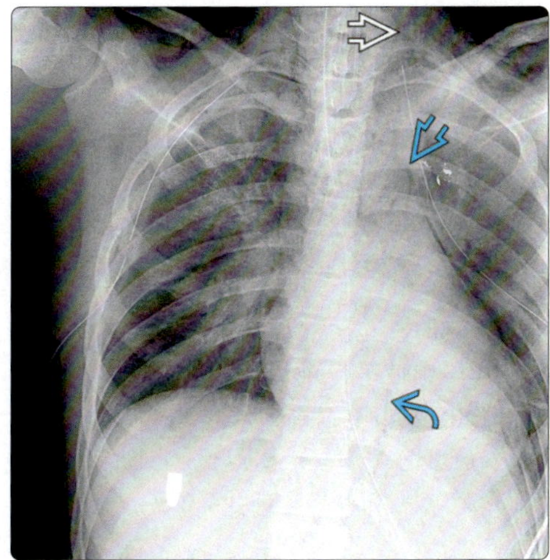

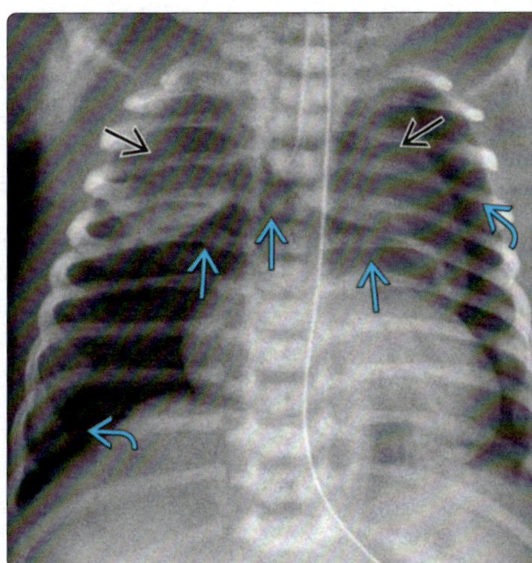

(Left) *Supine radiograph of a 17-year-old with gunshot wounds demonstrates pneumomediastinum with air outlining the aortic arch ➾ & descending aorta ➾. Also seen are scattered contusions & subcutaneous emphysema ➾.* **(Right)** *Supine radiograph from a 1-day-old shows pneumomediastinum with lucency ➾ underlying/elevating the thymus ➾. Pneumothorax is best seen at the right lung base ➾.*

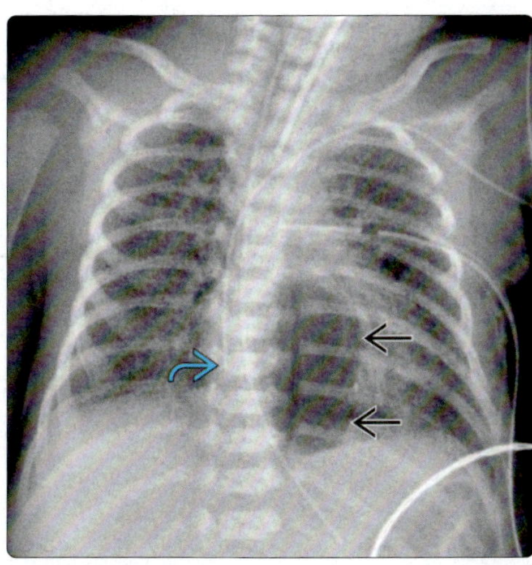

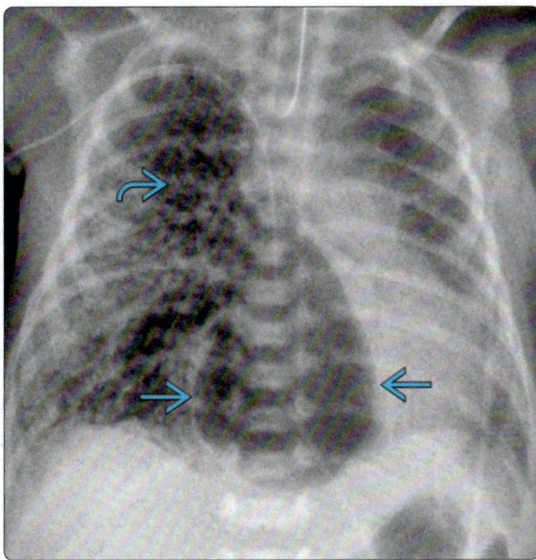

(Left) *AP radiograph in a neonate with surfactant deficiency shows a relatively large lucent collection ➾ inferiorly, typical in appearance for retrocardiac pneumomediastinum. Note also the low position of the left arm PICC in the right atrium ➾.* **(Right)** *Supine radiograph in a 2-day-old with surfactant deficiency shows a round lucent collection projecting over the inferior midline ➾, consistent with pneumomediastinum. Associated right pulmonary interstitial emphysema (PIE) is noted ➾.*

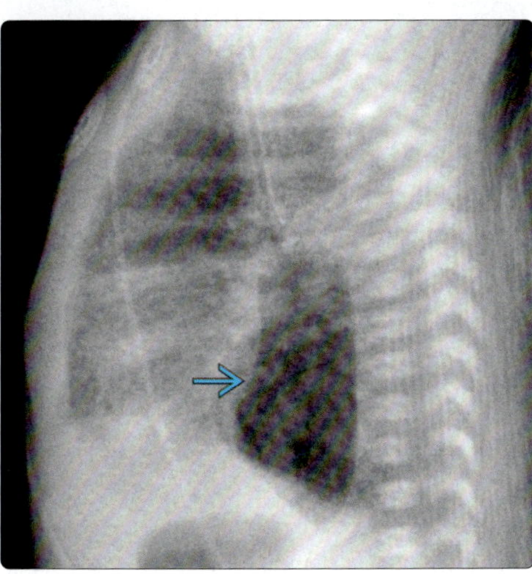

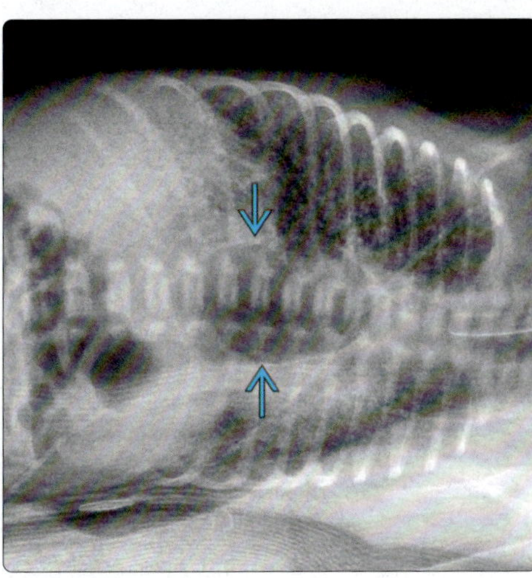

(Left) *Lateral chest radiograph in the same patient localizes the pneumomediastinum ➾ to the retrocardiac region.* **(Right)** *Left decubitus view of the chest in the same patient was obtained to assess the mobility of the lucent collection ➾ (& ensure that this did not represent mobile air from a pneumothorax). The lucency did not move & was self-limited, resolving in 5 days. These features are consistent with retrocardiac pneumomediastinum.*

Neuroendocrine Cell Hyperplasia of Infancy

KEY FACTS

TERMINOLOGY

- Neuroendocrine cell hyperplasia of infancy (NEHI): Form of childhood interstitial lung disease (chILD) associated with neuroendocrine cell hyperplasia

IMAGING

- Best test: HRCT (with inspiratory & expiratory images)
  - ~ 80% sensitive; ~ 100% specific with characteristic imaging pattern & clinical presentation
- Characteristic appearance
  - Central-predominant ground-glass opacification (GGO), especially of right middle lobe & lingula
    - Affects ≥ 4 lobes (counting lingula) in > 90% of cases
  - Diffuse mosaic air-trapping
  - No other abnormalities in 57-65% of cases

TOP DIFFERENTIAL DIAGNOSES

- Bronchiolitis obliterans (constrictive bronchiolitis)
- Asthma
- Surfactant dysfunction disorder

PATHOLOGY

- ↑ number of bombesin-immunopositive pulmonary neuroendocrine cells (PNECs) in distal respiratory bronchioles & alveolar ducts; etiology is unknown

CLINICAL ISSUES

- Typically presents in first 6-12 months of life with persistent retractions, tachypnea, crackles, hypoxemia, &/or failure to thrive
- Not responsive to steroids (unlike other chILDs)
- Does not progress to respiratory failure; gradually improves

DIAGNOSTIC CHECKLIST

- Important to suggest NEHI as diagnostic possibility
  - Immunostaining for bombesin is not routinely performed
  - If NEHI is not suggested by radiologist, diagnosis is likely to be missed by histopathology

(Left) *AP chest radiograph in a 4-month-old boy with an oxygen requirement & failure to thrive shows subtle, hazy, or ground-glass opacification (GGO) ➡ in the right middle lobe & lingula + mild overall hyperinflation.* **(Right)** *Lateral chest radiograph in the same patient shows the GGO ➡ in the middle lobe/lingula.*

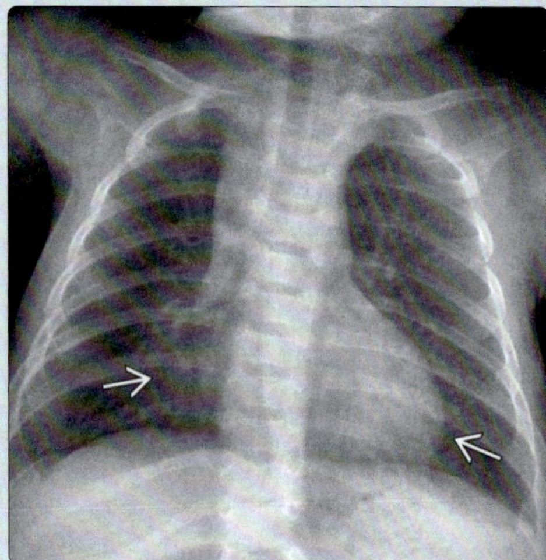

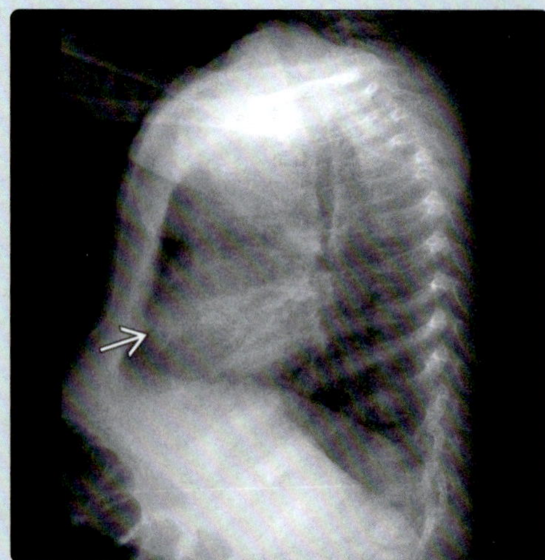

(Left) *Axial inspiratory HRCT of the chest in the same patient with an oxygen requirement & failure to thrive shows central-predominant GGO ➡ in the lower lobes, lingula, & middle lobe.* **(Right)** *Coronal inspiratory HRCT in the same 4-month-old boy shows the middle lobe & lingular distribution of GGO ➡. The imaging findings are sufficient, along with the clinical history, to make the diagnosis of neuroendocrine cell hyperplasia of infancy (NEHI) without biopsy.*

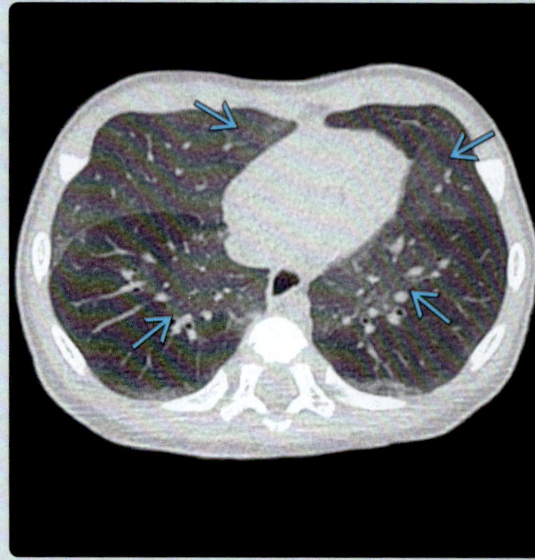

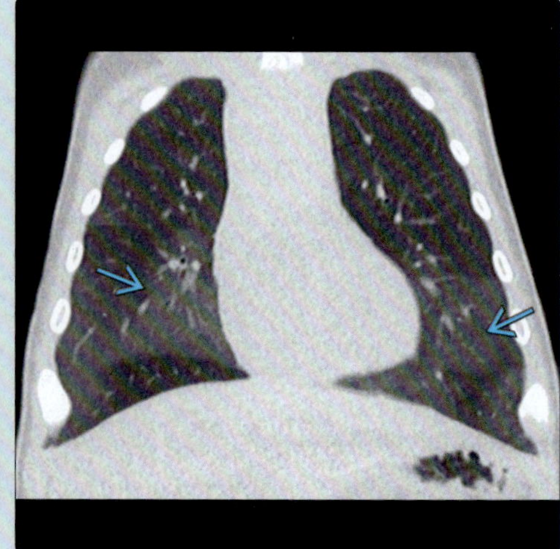

TERMINOLOGY

Abbreviations

- Neuroendocrine cell hyperplasia of infancy (NEHI)

Definitions

- Form of childhood interstitial lung disease (chILD) associated with neuroendocrine cell hyperplasia

IMAGING

General Features

- Best diagnostic clue
  - Characteristic ground-glass opacification (GGO) pattern in central lungs, especially right middle lobe & lingula, with mosaic air-trapping

Radiographic Findings

- Nonspecific radiographic findings
- Perihilar opacities & hyperinflation may be similar to viral or reactive airways disease
  - Bronchial wall thickening is typically absent

CT Findings

- HRCT
  - Geographic GGO
    - Central-predominant distribution
      - Does not change with patient position (supine vs. prone)
    - Most pronounced in right middle lobe & lingula
  - Diffuse mosaic air-trapping
  - No other abnormalities in 57-65% of cases
  - Imaging findings may confirm but do not exclude diagnosis of NEHI
    - Misdiagnosis is more likely when other abnormalities are present & distribution of GGO is not classic

Imaging Recommendations

- Best imaging tool
  - HRCT ~ 80% sensitive; specificity approaches 100% with characteristic CT pattern & clinical presentation
- Protocol advice
  - Routine HRCT, including inspiratory & expiratory images
  - May use low-dose technique (e.g., 50 mAs) if evaluation of mediastinum is not needed

DIFFERENTIAL DIAGNOSIS

Surfactant Dysfunction Disorder

- GGO is more diffuse than in NEHI
- Associated with septal thickening, unlike NEHI

PATHOLOGY

General Features

- Etiology
  - Unknown

Staging, Grading, & Classification

- Form of chILD
- Considered in class of disorders of unknown etiology
  - Pulmonary interstitial glycogenosis (PIG) is also in this category

CLINICAL ISSUES

Presentation

- Most common signs/symptoms
  - Persistent retractions, tachypnea, crackles, hypoxemia
- Clinical profile
  - Pulmonary function tests
    - ↓ forced expiratory volume (FEV), ↑ functional residual capacity (FRC), ↑ residual volume (RV)

Demographics

- Age
  - Typically diagnosed in first 12-18 months of life
    - Mean age at presentation to pulmonologist: 7 months
    - Mean age at diagnosis: 12 months
    - Age of presentation is older than other chILDs, which present in early infancy
- Sex
  - Slight male predominance in original series of 15 cases

Natural History & Prognosis

- Long-term prognosis is unclear
  - Most children gradually improve over time but may persist into adulthood
- NEHI exacerbation
  - Episodes of ↑ air-trapping in children with NEHI who had previously experienced significant clinical improvement

Treatment

- Unlike other chILDs, NEHI not responsive to steroid therapy
  - Important to differentiate NEHI from other chILDs to avoid unnecessary side effects of steroids
- Treatment supportive
  - Oxygen supplementation
  - Nutrition optimization to prevent failure to thrive

DIAGNOSTIC CHECKLIST

Consider

- NEHI in older infants with persistent tachypnea
- Expiratory images may be helpful for diagnosis (due to air-trapping)

Image Interpretation Pearls

- Characteristic CT appearance
  - Geographic GGO pattern in central lungs, especially right middle lobe & lingula
  - Mosaic air-trapping

SELECTED REFERENCES

1. Verma N et al: ChILD: A pictorial review of pulmonary imaging findings in childhood interstitial lung diseases. Curr Probl Diagn Radiol. 50(1):95-103, 2021
2. Wu M et al: Childhood interstitial lung disease: a case-based review of the imaging findings. Ann Thorac Med. 16(1):64-72, 2021
3. Liptzin DR et al: Neuroendocrine cell hyperplasia of infancy. Clinical score and comorbidities. Ann Am Thorac Soc. 17(6):724-8, 2020
4. Bush A et al: Early onset children's interstitial lung diseases: discrete entities or manifestations of pulmonary dysmaturity? Paediatr Respir Rev. 30:65-71, 2018
5. Mastej EJ et al: Lung and airway shape in neuroendocrine cell hyperplasia of infancy. Pediatr Radiol. 48(12):1745-54, 2018

Pulmonary Interstitial Glycogenosis

KEY FACTS

TERMINOLOGY

- Specific disorder of unknown etiology in childhood interstitial lung disease (chILD) classification system
- More accurate term: Neonatal pulmonary interstitial glycogen accumulation disorder

IMAGING

- Nonspecific imaging findings of diffuse or patchy hazy/ground-glass opacities, interstitial thickening, & hyperinflation
  - Appearances largely could be attributed to alveolar growth abnormalities, which pulmonary interstitial glycogenosis (PIG) often accompanies histopathologically
  - Other lung diseases, including infection & surfactant dysfunction disorders, could also show similar findings

TOP DIFFERENTIAL DIAGNOSES

- Alveolar growth abnormality (AGA)
  - PIG is commonly associated with AGA (which confounds assessment of imaging appearance of "pure" PIG)
- Diffuse lung developmental disorders
  - Profound impairment of gas exchange
  - Death usually < 1 month of age (unless ECMO bridges to lung transplantation)
- Disorders of surfactant
  - Surfactant deficiency in premature neonates & genetic disorders affecting surfactant metabolism
- Neonatal pneumonia
  - Pleural effusion is frequent

PATHOLOGY

- Infiltration & expansion of alveolar interstitium/septa by glycogen-laden immature mesenchymal cells

CLINICAL ISSUES

- PIG affects neonates & young infants
- Prognosis appears favorable without concurrent disease

(Left) *AP radiograph in a term neonate with Turner syndrome & respiratory failure reveals hyperinflation with diffuse ground-glass opacities & septal thickening.* **(Right)** *Axial HRCT from the lower lobes in the same patient with Turner syndrome shows septal thickening ➔ & areas of patchy ground-glass opacity. Biopsy revealed diffuse h pulmonary interstitial glycogenosis (PIG).*

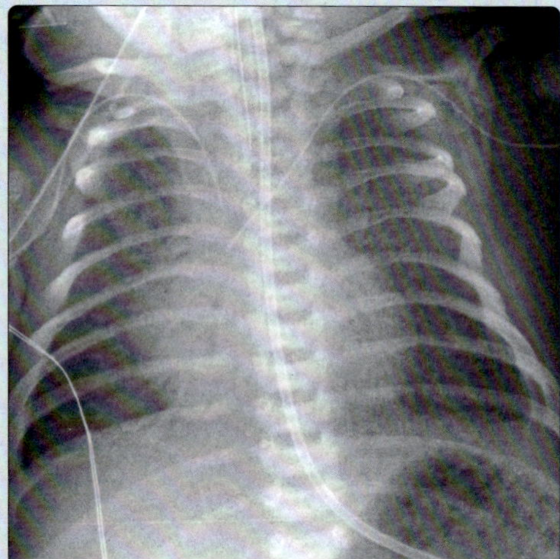

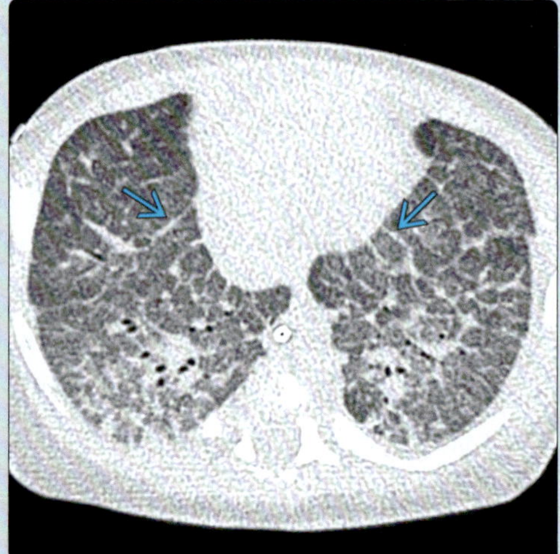

(Left) *Axial T2 FS MR shows course interstitial markings in the lungs ➔ due to PIG. Note the multiple lymphatic malformations ➔ of the mediastinum & axilla.* **(Right)** *Axial HRCT from an 11-day-old neonate at the level of the middle & lingular bronchi confirms patchy areas of ground-glass opacity ➔. Biopsy revealed a mild alveolar growth abnormality with patchy PIG.*

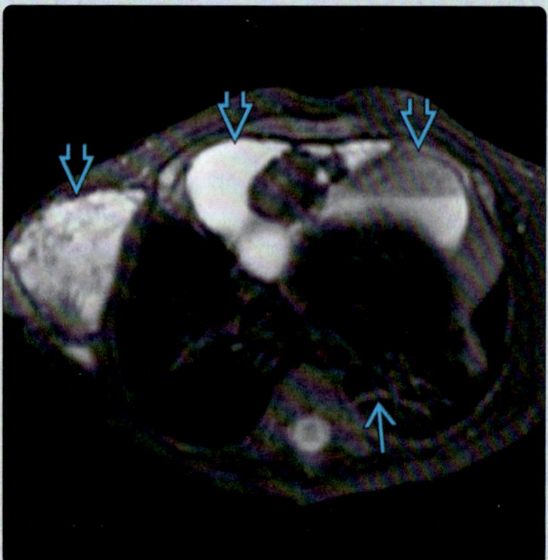

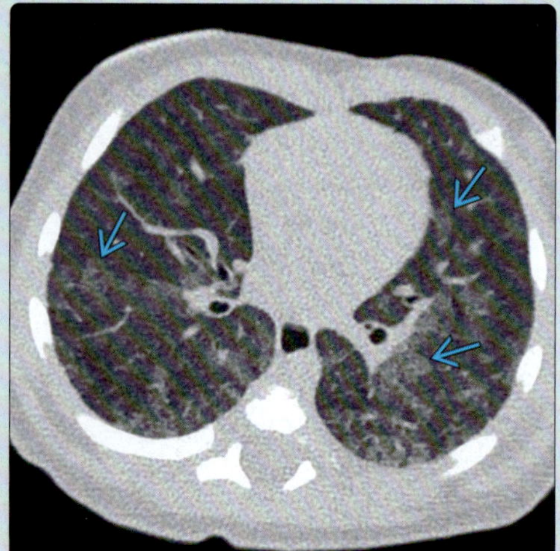

TERMINOLOGY

Abbreviations

- Pulmonary interstitial glycogenosis (PIG)

Synonyms

- Infantile cellular interstitial pneumonitis (former name)
- Neonatal pulmonary interstitial glycogen accumulation disorder

Definitions

- Specific disorder of unknown etiology in childhood interstitial lung disease (chILD) classification system
- Results from infiltration & expansion of alveolar interstitium/septa by glycogen-laden mesenchymal cells

IMAGING

General Features

- Best diagnostic clue
  - Patchy or diffuse ground-glass opacity & interstitial thickening described
  - However, coexistent lung disease (e.g., alveolar growth abnormality) likely impacts imaging appearance
- Location
  - No specific lung zonal predilection; opacities may be diffuse or heterogeneous

Radiographic Findings

- Interstitial thickening
- Diffuse or patchy hazy/ground-glass opacities
- Hyperinflation

CT Findings

- Ground-glass opacities (up to 86%)
- Hyperlucent foci ("cysts" vs. regions of alveolar simplification)
- Reticular opacities
- Architectural distortion

Imaging Recommendations

- Best imaging tool
  - HRCT

DIFFERENTIAL DIAGNOSIS

Alveolar Growth Abnormality

- PIG is commonly associated with alveolar growth abnormality (AGA), which confounds assessment of imaging appearance of "pure" PIG

Diffuse Lung Developmental Disorders

- Death usually occurs within 1st month of life without ECMO bridging to lung transplantation
- Acinar dysplasia, congenital alveolar dysplasia, alveolar capillary dysplasia with misalignment of pulmonary veins

Surfactant Dysfunction Disorders

- Abnormal proteins (SP-B, SP-C, ABCA3, & TTF-1) are important in surfactant production & function

Neonatal Pneumonia

- Pleural effusions are frequent

PATHOLOGY

Microscopic Features

- Infiltration & expansion of alveolar interstitium/septa by glycogen-laden immature mesenchymal cells, which stain positive for vimentin
  - Accumulation of glycogenated mesenchymal cells often accompanies other conditions, particularly AGA
- Little to no inflammatory change
- Diffuse or patchy involvement of pulmonary parenchyma
  - Patchy form is more common in patients with AGA

CLINICAL ISSUES

Presentation

- Most common signs/symptoms
  - Severity of presentation is highly variable
    - Respiratory failure with pulmonary hypertension
    - Tachypnea

Demographics

- Age
  - Neonates or young infants
    - Typically < 6 months of age

Natural History & Prognosis

- Most improve in absence of concurrent disease
  - Most require either no support vs. supplemental oxygen
- Mortality is reported with presence of comorbidities, such as AGA, congenital heart disease, & pulmonary hypertension

Treatment

- Possible benefits from corticosteroids

DIAGNOSTIC CHECKLIST

Image Interpretation Pearls

- No specific imaging appearance
- Published reports of PIG imaging findings describe appearances that largely could be attributed to AGA (which PIG often accompanies histopathologically)

Reporting Tips

- Caution during HRCT interpretation, as nonspecific findings of septal thickening & diffuse ground-glass opacities can overlap with other disorders, including infection or disorders of surfactant

SELECTED REFERENCES

1. Galambos C et al: Pulmonary interstitial glycogenosis cells express mesenchymal stem cell markers. Eur Respir J. 56(4), 2020
2. Bush A et al: Early onset children's interstitial lung diseases: discrete entities or manifestations of pulmonary dysmaturity? Paediatr Respir Rev. 30:65-71, 2019
3. Sardón O et al: Isolated pulmonary interstitial glycogenosis associated with alveolar growth abnormalities: a long-term follow-up study. Pediatr Pulmonol. 54(6):837-46, 2019
4. Liptzin DR et al: Pulmonary interstitial glycogenosis: diagnostic evaluation and clinical course. Pediatr Pulmonol. 53(12):1651-8, 2018
5. Seidl E et al: Pulmonary interstitial glycogenosis - a systematic analysis of new cases. Respir Med. 140:11-20, 2018
6. Still GG et al: Persistent pulmonary hypertension without underlying cardiac disease as a presentation of pulmonary interstitial glycogenosis. Fetal Pediatr Pathol. 37(1):22-6, 2018

KEY FACTS

TERMINOLOGY

- Alveolar growth abnormality (AGA): Pathologic pattern of enlargement & simplification of alveoli with concomitant underdevelopment of pulmonary vasculature
- Synonyms: Alveolar growth disorder, alveolar simplification

IMAGING

- Radiologic findings range from near normal to
  - Variably sized but often large, secondary pulmonary lobules with vascular rarefaction
  - Subpleural & perilobular reticular opacities
  - Ground-glass opacities
  - Discrete subpleural/subfissural cysts (often in trisomy 21)
  - Hyperlucent regions that can resemble cystic change

PATHOLOGY

- Enlarged alveolar spaces with few alveoli + deficient vascular & alveolar septal development
  - ± concurrent pulmonary interstitial glycogenosis
- AGA is often secondary; seen in wide variety of diseases
  - Prenatal conditions
    - Restriction of thoracic space, ↓ or absent breathing movements, cardiac anomalies limiting pulmonary blood supply, chromosomal abnormalities
  - Postnatal conditions
    - Prematurity → bronchopulmonary dysplasia
    - Term infants with early postnatal lung injury

CLINICAL ISSUES

- Most common chronic diffuse lung disease in infancy
- Respiratory difficulties occur in neonatal period but natural history variable
  - Slow improvement or worsening with time depending on underlying disorder, AGA extent, ability to develop new alveoli, & presence of pulmonary hypertension
  - Filamin A (*FLNA*) mutations: Particularly severe AGA with periventricular gray matter heterotopia, cardiovascular anomalies, & connective tissue anomalies

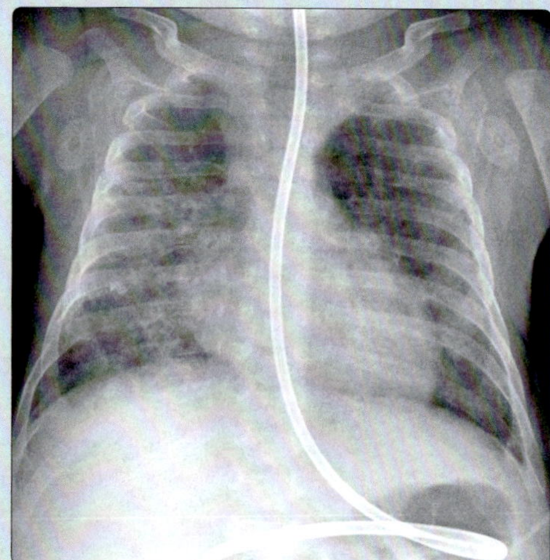

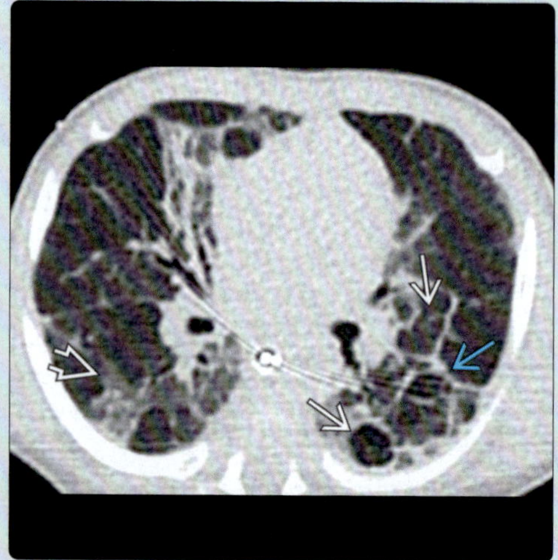

(Left) *AP chest radiograph of a former 23-weeks-premature infant at 10 weeks of age shows bilateral hyperinflation with coarse parenchymal opacities.* **(Right)** *Axial HRCT in the same infant at 10 weeks of age shows disordered, secondary pulmonary lobules ➡ of variable shape with ground-glass opacities ➡ & thick, perilobular opacities ➡, typical of chronic lung disease of prematurity with alveolar growth abnormality.*

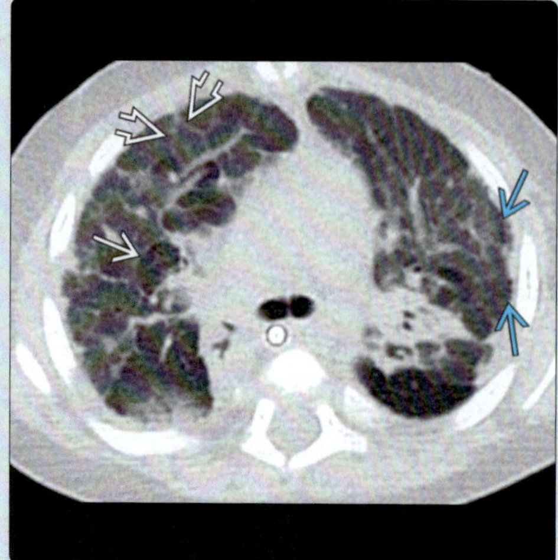

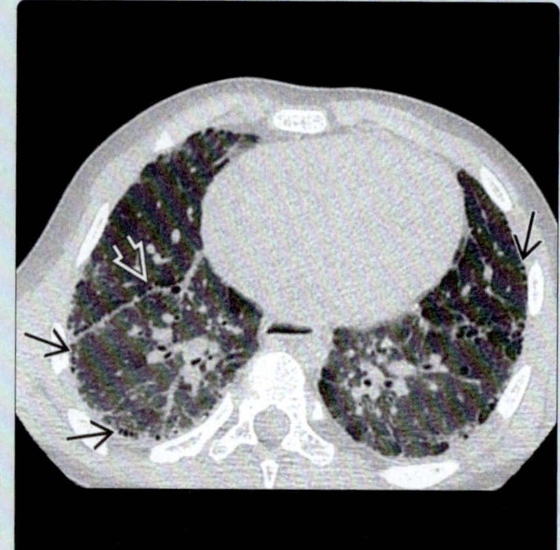

(Left) *Axial NECT in an infant with congenital heart disease (atrial septal defect & ventricular septal defect) shows large, secondary pulmonary lobules ➡, perilobular, reticular opacities ➡, & subtle, subpleural cysts ➡, typical of alveolar growth abnormality.* **(Right)** *Axial HRCT in a child with trisomy 21 shows large, secondary pulmonary lobules & subpleural/perilobular, reticular opacities with subpleural ➡ & subfissural ➡ cysts.*

TERMINOLOGY

Definitions

- Alveolar growth abnormality (AGA): Pathologic pattern of enlargement & simplification of alveoli with concomitant underdevelopment of pulmonary vasculature

IMAGING

General Features

- Best diagnostic clue
  - Large, secondary pulmonary lobules + vascular rarefaction
    - Imaging findings range from severe to near normal
- Location
  - Variable; cystic changes are often most conspicuous in subpleural & subfissural lungs
  - Unilateral in certain congenital cases with in utero ipsilateral mass effect (e.g., lung lesion, diaphragmatic hernia, chylothorax)
- Size
  - Variable ↑ size of secondary pulmonary lobule(s)

Radiographic Findings

- Hyperinflation with pulmonary vascular rarefaction & generalized lucency of parenchyma
- Coarse, reticular opacities

CT Findings

- Variably sized (but often large), secondary pulmonary lobules with vascular rarefaction
- Perilobular & subpleural linear opacities, parenchymal bands, ground-glass opacities
- Subpleural/subfissural cysts (often in trisomy 21)
- Hyperlucent regions that can appear cystic

Imaging Recommendations

- Best imaging tool: CT
  - Generally most conspicuous on inspiratory images
  - Expiratory images are helpful if clinical &/or pulmonary function test (PFT) findings suggest obstructive airways disease/air trapping
- Protocol advice: Maximize lung recruitment if patients are under sedation/anesthesia

DIFFERENTIAL DIAGNOSIS

Parenchymal Lung Diseases That May Result in Widespread Architectural Distortion

- Meconium aspiration syndrome
- Chronic aspiration
- Bronchopulmonary dysplasia (BPD)

PATHOLOGY

General Features

- Most common chronic diffuse lung disease in infancy
- AGA is often secondary; seen in wide variety of diseases
  - Prenatal conditions
    - Restriction of thoracic space, ↓ or absent breathing movements, cardiac anomalies limiting pulmonary blood supply, chromosomal abnormalities
  - Postnatal conditions
    - Prematurity (most common) with BPD
    - Term infants with early postnatal lung injury

Microscopic Features

- Reduced radial alveolar count
- Enlarged alveolar spaces with fewer alveoli & deficient vascular & alveolar septal development
- ± concurrent pulmonary interstitial glycogenosis

CLINICAL ISSUES

Presentation

- Most common signs/symptoms
  - Respiratory difficulties in neonatal period
- Other signs/symptoms
  - Filamin A (*FLNA*) X-linked genetic mutations have particularly severe AGA
    - Pulmonary hypertension & respiratory decline

Natural History & Prognosis

- Slow improvement or worsening with time depends on underlying disorder, AGA extent, ability to develop new alveoli, & presence of pulmonary hypertension
- With prematurity
  - Advances in neonatal care (improved ventilation equipment/strategies, antenatal corticosteroids, surfactant, nutrition) → shift from classic BPD (airway obstruction & fibrosis) to "new BPD" (impaired alveolar development)
    - ↓ lung injury from oxygen toxicity & barotrauma
  - Unclear how "new BPD" patients remodel alveoli & pulmonary microvasculature with age & growth
    - All extremely low birth weight infants have some degree of abnormal lung development

Treatment

- Supportive measures: Supplemental oxygen, nutrition, & prevention of RSV
- Lung transplantation in most severely affected

DIAGNOSTIC CHECKLIST

Reporting Tips

- Clinical history is important to prevent reporting all cases as chronic lung disease of prematurity/BPD
- Bilateral findings without prematurity could indicate genetic cause (trisomy 21, filamin A mutation) or peripartum condition resulting in impaired pulmonary parenchymal development

SELECTED REFERENCES

1. Wu M et al: Childhood interstitial lung disease: a case-based review of the imaging findings. Ann Thorac Med. 16(1):64-72, 2021
2. Sardón O et al: Isolated pulmonary interstitial glycogenosis associated with alveolar growth abnormalities: a long-term follow-up study. Pediatr Pulmonol. 54(6):837-46, 2019
3. Bush A et al: Early onset children's interstitial lung diseases: discrete entities or manifestations of pulmonary dysmaturity? Paediatr Respir Rev. 30:65-71, 2018
4. Toma P et al: CT features of diffuse lung disease in infancy. Radiol Med. 123(8):577-85, 2018
5. Armes JE et al: Diffuse lung disease of infancy: a pattern-based, algorithmic approach to histological diagnosis. J Clin Pathol. 68(2):100-10, 2015

Surfactant Dysfunction Disorders

KEY FACTS

TERMINOLOGY

- Group of rare lung diseases caused by mutations/deletions of genes affecting surfactant homeostasis
- Most frequent surfactant dysfunction disorders
  - Surfactant protein B (SP-B): *SFTPB* gene
  - Surfactant protein C (SP-C): *SFTPC* gene
  - ATP-binding cassette transporter A3: *ABCA3* gene
  - Receptors for GM-CSF: *CSF2RA, CSF2RB* genes
    - Congenital alveolar proteinosis
  - Thyroid transcription factor: *TTF1/NKX2-1* genes
    - Brain-lung-thyroid syndrome

IMAGING

- Radiographs: Bilateral granular opacities in term neonate
- CT: Diffuse ground-glass opacification & thickened interlobular septa: Crazy-paving pattern
  - Can progress to fibrotic changes with persistent interlobular septal thickening, cysts

TOP DIFFERENTIAL DIAGNOSES

- Surfactant deficiency related to prematurity
- Neonatal pneumonia
- Transient tachypnea of newborn
- Alveolar growth abnormalities

PATHOLOGY

- Pulmonary surfactant: Complex mixture of lipid (90% by weight) & protein lining alveolar surface
  - Prevents end-expiratory atelectasis

CLINICAL ISSUES

- Acute respiratory distress in full-term infants at birth
- SP-B: Progressive & usually fatal by 3-6 months of age with lung transplantation as only effective treatment
- SP-C, ABCA3: More commonly associated with diffuse lung disease in older infants, children, & adults
  - Onset of symptoms is highly variable

(Left) *AP radiograph in a term neonate presenting with respiratory distress secondary to an ABCA3 gene mutation shows low lung volumes with widespread granular opacities resembling surfactant deficiency of prematurity.* **(Right)** *Coronal HRCT in the same neonate with an ABCA3 mutation shows diffuse ground-glass opacification with areas of interlobular septal thickening ➔.*

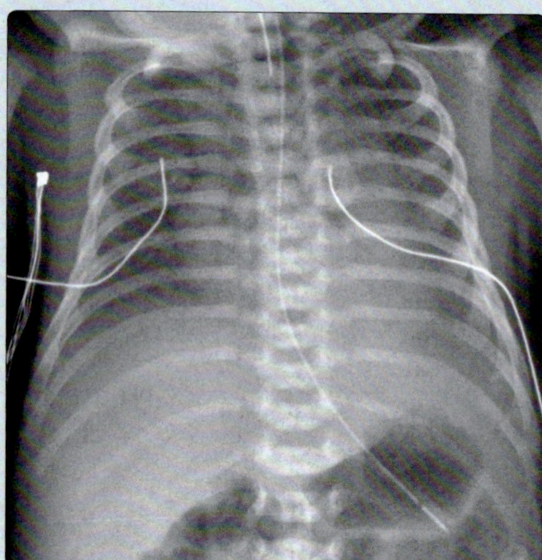

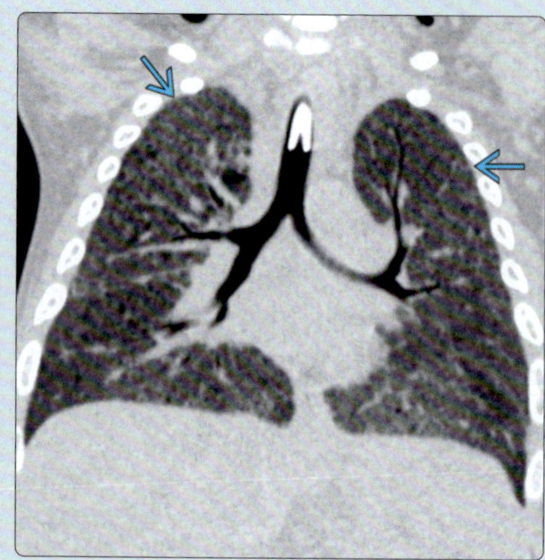

(Left) *Axial HRCT from an older infant with a surfactant protein C mutation shows areas of mild ground-glass opacity, numerous parenchymal cysts ➔, & foci of interlobular septal thickening ➔.* **(Right)** *Axial HRCT from a 17-year-old with a known ABCA3 mutation shows areas of ground-glass opacity ➔ with concomitant reticulation ➔ & traction bronchiectasis ➔, indicating fibrosis.*

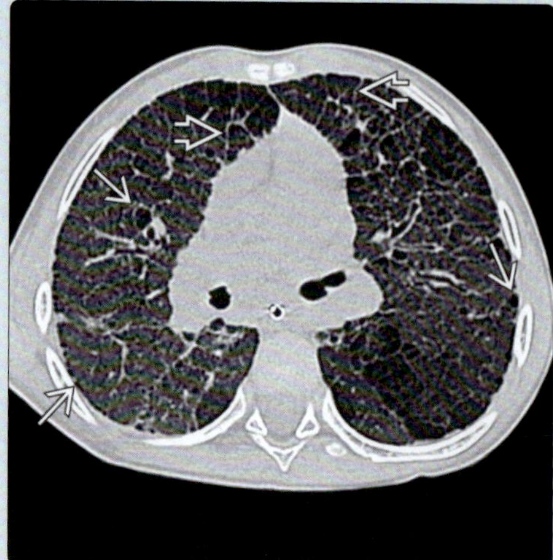

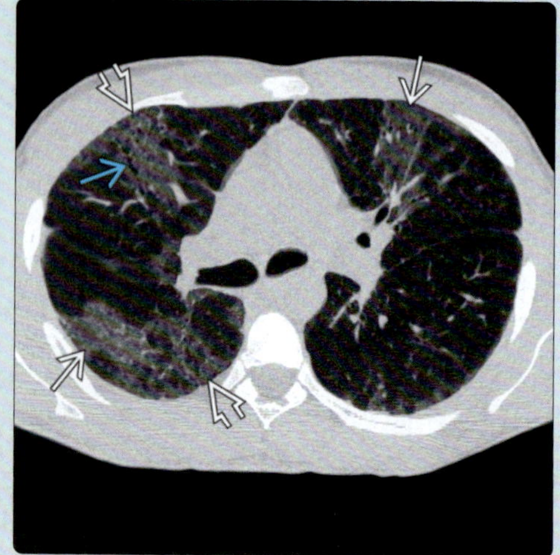

TERMINOLOGY

Definitions

- Group of rare lung diseases caused by mutations/deletions of genes affecting surfactant homeostasis
  - Differs from prematurity-related surfactant deficiency & secondary surfactant deficiency
- Most frequent surfactant dysfunction disorders
  - Surfactant protein B (SP-B): *SFTPB* gene
  - Surfactant protein C (SP-C): *SFTPC* gene
  - ATP-binding cassette transporter A3 (ABCA3): *ABCA3* gene
  - Receptors for GM-CSF: *CSF2RA*, *CSF2RB* genes
    - Congenital alveolar proteinosis
  - Thyroid transcription factor: *TTF1/NKX2-1* genes
    - Brain-lung-thyroid syndrome
- Pulmonary alveolar proteinosis of adults & older children
  - GM-CSF autoantibodies
  - Alveolar macrophage dysfunction

IMAGING

General Features

- Best diagnostic clue
  - Term infant with radiographic presentation similar to surfactant deficiency of prematurity

Radiographic Findings

- Diffuse or patchy granular opacities

CT Findings

- SP-B
  - Diffuse ground-glass opacification & thickened interlobular septa: Crazy-paving pattern
  - Can progress to fibrotic changes with persistent interlobular septal thickening
  - Rarely imaged with CT during severe neonatal presentation due to fragile clinical state
- SP-C or ABCA3
  - Infants
    - Diffuse ground-glass opacification or consolidation with interlobular septal thickening: Crazy-paving pattern
  - Older infants & children
    - Ground-glass opacities that ↓ in extent with age
    - Parenchymal cysts that ↑ in number & size with age
    - Interlobular septal thickening
    - Pectus excavatum

DIFFERENTIAL DIAGNOSIS

Surfactant Deficiency Related to Prematurity

- Differentiated clinically based on gestational age
  - Affects ~ 60% born < 28-weeks gestation
  - Affects ~ 5% born at term

Neonatal Pneumonia

- Can be acquired antenatally, perinatally, or postnatally
- Etiologies vary depending on timing of disease acquisition
- Pleural effusion is common

Transient Tachypnea of Newborn

- Self-limited illness due to delay in clearance of fetal lung fluid

Alveolar Growth Abnormalities

- Commonly due to prematurity but also observed in congenital heart disease & genetic disorders (e.g., trisomy 21)

PATHOLOGY

General Features

- Etiology
  - Pulmonary surfactant: Complex mixture of lipid (90% by weight) & protein lining alveolar surface
    - Prevents end-expiratory atelectasis

CLINICAL ISSUES

Natural History & Prognosis

- SP-B
  - Acute respiratory distress in full-term infants at birth
  - Transient or modest improvement with surfactant replacement &/or corticosteroid therapy
  - Progressive & usually fatal by 3-6 months of age with lung transplantation as only effective treatment
- SP-C
  - More commonly associated with diffuse lung disease in older infants, children, & adults
  - Onset of symptoms is highly variable: Influenced by mutation as well as environmental factors (e.g., viral infections)
    - Average onset of 2-3 months of age
      - □ 10-15% present in 1st month of life
      - □ Presentation in full-term neonates: Similar to surfactant deficiency of prematurity; may be fatal
      - □ Presentations in older infants: Tachypnea, retractions, hypoxemia, digital clubbing, & failure to thrive
  - Wide ranging long-term clinical status: From no supplemental oxygen requirement to death while awaiting transplant
  - Older adults often present with pulmonary fibrosis
- ABCA3
  - Variable: Associated with above phenotypes

Treatment

- SP-B
  - Almost always fatal without lung transplant
  - Rare cases of surviving children with partial defects in SP-B production
- SP-C & ABCA3
  - Treatment varies based on phenotypic manifestations
    - Lung transplant in infancy in severe cases

SELECTED REFERENCES

1. LeMoine BD et al: High-resolution computed tomography findings of thyroid transcription factor 1 deficiency (NKX2-1 mutations). Pediatr Radiol. 49(7):869-75, 2019
2. Toma P et al: CT features of diffuse lung disease in infancy. Radiol Med. 123(8):577-85, 2018
3. Gupta A et al: Genetic disorders of surfactant protein dysfunction: when to consider and how to investigate. Arch Dis Child. 102(1):84-90, 2017

Swyer-James Syndrome

KEY FACTS

TERMINOLOGY

- Acquired unilateral pulmonary hypoplasia thought to result from childhood viral infection [postinfectious bronchiolitis obliterans (BO)]
- Results in small, hyperexpanded lung with relative ↓ in vascularity

IMAGING

- Radiograph
  - Asymmetric hyperlucent lung with diminished number & caliber of vessels
  - May simulate pneumothorax
- HRCT
  - Air-trapping in affected lung
  - Small central & peripheral pulmonary arteries
  - Occasional bronchiectasis with minor subpleural scarring
  - Bronchial wall thickening, usually mild

TOP DIFFERENTIAL DIAGNOSES

- Foreign body aspiration
- Obstructive endobronchial lesion
- Congenital lobar overinflation
- Unilateral absence of pulmonary artery
- Poland syndrome

PATHOLOGY

- Inflammation & fibrosis of walls & contiguous tissues of membranous & respiratory bronchioles
- Do not confuse BO with bronchiolitis obliterans organizing pneumonia (BOOP)

CLINICAL ISSUES

- Frequent respiratory infections in infancy or childhood
- Chronic cough, wheezing, recurrent pneumonia
- Variable presentation depending on severity of disease
- Prognosis is usually good
- Treatment is supportive

(Left) *Frontal upright radiograph shows a 13-month -old with typical symptoms & radiographic findings of viral airway disease, a risk factor for later developing Swyer-James syndrome (SJS). Note the asymmetric geographic areas of air-space opacity & volume loss that mostly involve the right lung ➔.* **(Right)** *Follow-up CT in the same patient 8 years later shows a focal hyperlucency in the affected area of the right lung ↪; note the presence of attenuated vessels coursing through the involved area.*

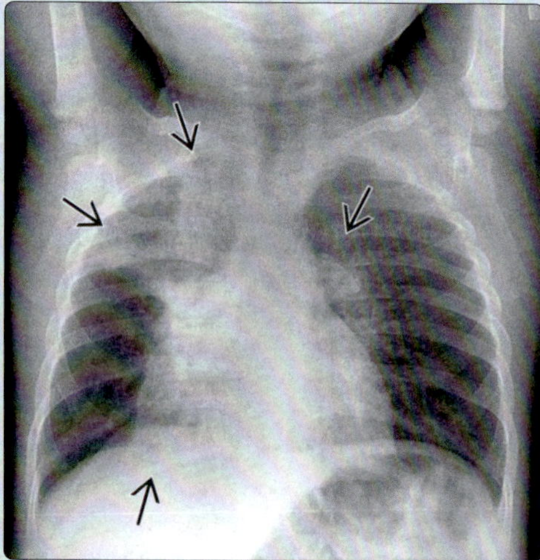

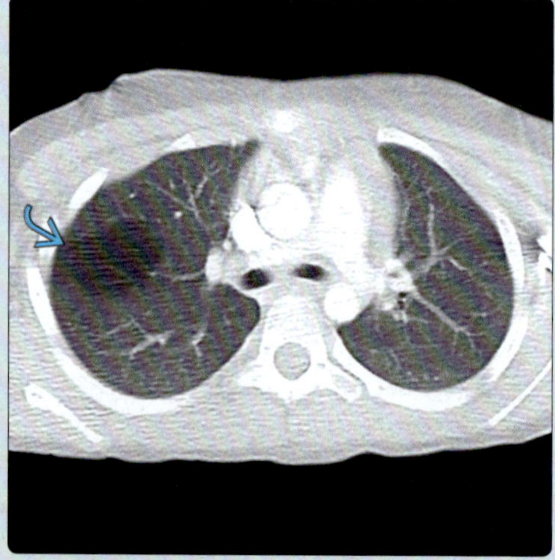

(Left) *Frontal chest radiograph in a previously healthy 8-year-old after a viral illness while traveling abroad demonstrates asymmetric lucency & mild hyperexpansion in the left upper lobe ➔.* **(Right)** *Coronal CT reconstruction in the same patient shows the presence of narrow caliber vessels ↪ in the affected area. Bronchi were normal (as opposed to bronchial atresia), & there is no mass effect (as seen with congenital lobar overexpansion, which also presents earlier in life).*

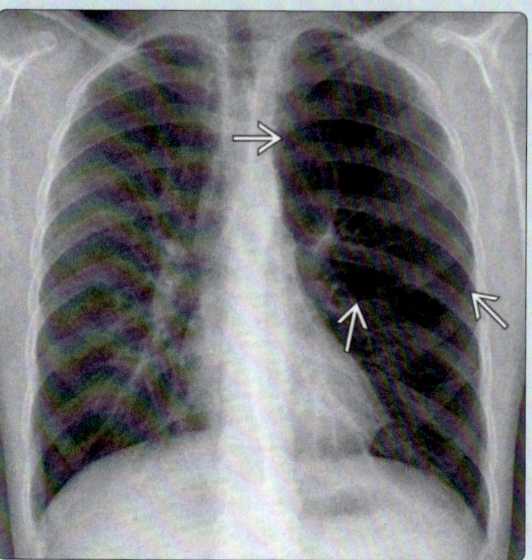

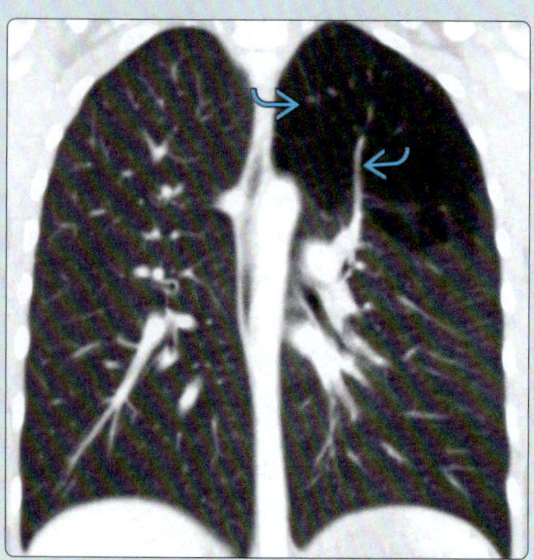

TERMINOLOGY

Abbreviations

- Swyer-James syndrome (SJS)

Synonyms

- Swyer-James-MacLeod syndrome, Brett syndrome, postinfectious bronchiolitis obliterans (BO)

Definitions

- Acquired unilateral pulmonary hypoplasia thought to result from childhood viral infection
- Results in small, hyperexpanded lung with relatively ↓ vascularity & (rarely) bronchiectasis
- Imaging findings may appear as early as 9 months after initial infectious insult

IMAGING

General Features

- Best diagnostic clue
  - Asymmetric hyperlucent lung with diminished number & caliber of vessels
  - Classically unilateral but usually multifocal

Radiographic Findings

- Radiography
  - Pronounced patchy unilateral or unilobar hyperlucency (due to oligemia of involved segments)
    - May simulate pneumothorax on radiographs
  - Possible reduced lung volume on inspiration with air-trapping on expiration

CT Findings

- HRCT
  - Mosaic pattern of attenuation
  - Inspiratory: Affected lung volume is small or normal-sized
  - Expiratory: Air-trapping in affected lung
  - Small central & peripheral pulmonary arteries
  - Bronchiectasis with minor subpleural parenchymal scarring, especially in older patients
  - Bronchial wall thickening, usually relatively mild

Imaging Recommendations

- Protocol advice
  - Important to do HRCT with expiratory images

DIFFERENTIAL DIAGNOSIS

Foreign Body Aspiration

- Acute presentation, often with supportive history (e.g., recent choking on peanuts)
- Endobronchial foreign body may be visible on CT

Obstructive Endobronchial Neoplasm

- Enhancing endobronchial filling defect on CT
- More common in older teenagers & adults

Congenital Lobar Overinflation

- Congenital abnormality of lower airways that results in progressive overexpansion of pulmonary lobe
- Most commonly presents in newborn period
- Expanding hyperlucent lung tissue exerts mass effect

Unilateral Absence of Pulmonary Artery

- Also presents as unilateral small, hyperlucent, oligemic lung
- No air-trapping on expiration (as in SJS)
- All prior chest radiographs will be abnormal (as opposed to previously normal in SJS)

Poland Syndrome

- Congenital unilateral absence of pectoralis muscles & hypoplasia of ipsilateral breast soft tissues
- Radiographs: Unilateral, hyperlucent hemithorax
- CT: Normal lung parenchyma but absent/↓ extrathoracic soft tissues on affected side

PATHOLOGY

General Features

- Inflammation & fibrosis of walls & contiguous tissues of membranous & respiratory bronchioles
  - Postobstructive hyperexpansion of terminal air sacs
  - Compensatory ↓ perfusion
- Result: Underdevelopment of alveoli & pulmonary arteries
- Main histopathological finding: Constrictive bronchiolitis

CLINICAL ISSUES

Presentation

- Most common signs/symptoms
  - Frequent respiratory infections in infancy or childhood
    - Most common infections: Adenovirus, RSV, influenza A, *Mycoplasma* pneumonia
  - Chronic cough, wheezing, recurrent pneumonia
- Other signs/symptoms
  - Variable presentations: Range from severe to asymptomatic
  - Restrictive pattern on pulmonary function tests

Demographics

- Age
  - Usually presents in infancy or childhood
  - Less severe cases may be missed until adulthood (often found incidentally on radiographs)

Natural History & Prognosis

- ~ 1% of adenovirus-induced bronchiolitis progress to BO
- If insult occurs before alveolar maturation (8 years), may affect number of alveoli & pulmonary vessels
- Prognosis is usually good

Treatment

- Pneumonectomy is reserved for intractable recurrent infections

SELECTED REFERENCES

1. Behrendt A et al: Swyer-James-MacLeod syndrome. StatPearls, 2021
2. Cherian SV et al: Lung hyperlucency: a clinical-radiologic algorithmic approach to diagnosis. Chest. 157(1):119-41, 2020
3. Gomes de Farias LP et al: Swyer-James-MacLeod syndrome: the hyperlucent lung. Radiol Cardiothorac Imaging. 2(3):e190246, 2020
4. Machado D et al: Swyer-James-Macleod syndrome as a rare cause of unilateral hyperlucent lung: three case reports. Medicine (Baltimore). 98(6):e14269, 2019
5. Hamada S et al: Swyer-James-Macleod syndrome: the differential diagnosis of unilateral hyperlucency. Intern Med. 57(17):2591-2, 2018

Lymphangioleiomyomatosis

KEY FACTS

TERMINOLOGY

- Cystic disease of lungs & thoracic/retroperitoneal lymphatics due to proliferation of lymphangioleiomyomatosis (LAM) cells
  - LAM cells: Low-grade neoplastic smooth muscle-like cells that are metastatic from unknown primary tumor
- 2 subtypes are nearly identical by histology & imaging
  - Tuberous sclerosis complex associated (TSC-LAM)
  - Sporadic (S-LAM)

IMAGING

- Chest radiograph
  - Normal to ↑ lung volumes
  - Diffuse bilateral fine reticular opacities
  - ± pneumothorax, pleural effusion
- Lung CT
  - Numerous randomly distributed, thin-walled cysts
    - Range from few scattered cysts to complete lung parenchymal replacement
    - Variable size: Usually 2 mm to 2 cm (may be larger)
      - Expiratory & minIP images are more sensitive for small cysts
  - Normal intervening parenchyma
    - Small scattered nodules in minority of patients
  - CT underestimates early functional impairment

CLINICAL ISSUES

- S-LAM: Occurs nearly exclusively in females
  - Mean age of diagnosis: 35 years
- TSC-LAM is higher in women than men (42% vs. 13% of TSC cases, respectively)
  - TSC-LAM cysts may be seen in childhood
  - 22% are affected by age 20; 80% by age 40
- Most common presentations: Dyspnea on exertion, recurrent pneumothorax
- Gradual pulmonary function deterioration from slowly advancing disease
- Treatments include mTOR inhibitors, lung transplant

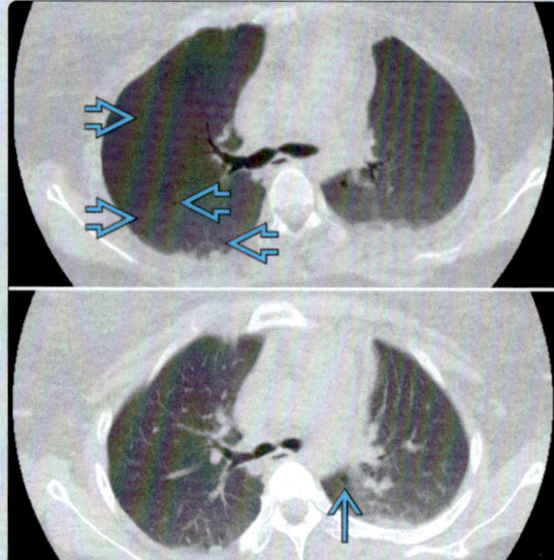

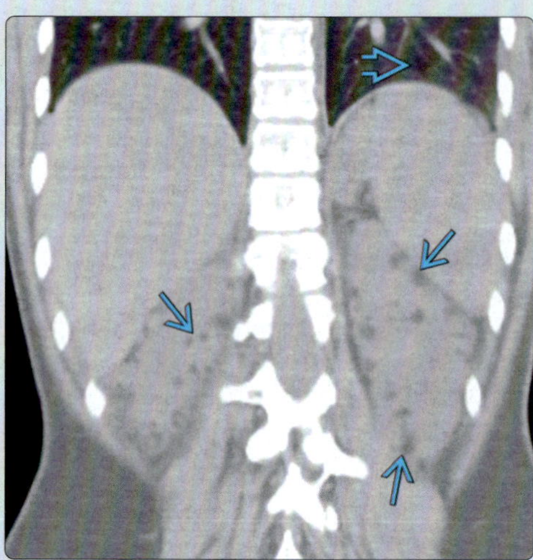

(Left) *Axial expiratory lung CT minIP (top) & standard (bottom) images in a 23-year-old woman with TSC show changes of LAM. Only a single, 4-mm cyst is visible on the standard reconstruction →, while numerous additional smaller cysts ⇨ are seen on the minIP image.* **(Right)** *Coronal NECT in a 14-year-old patient with TSC shows a small lung cyst ⇨ in the left lower lobe. Despite the lung window settings, numerous fat-containing lesions → can be seen throughout the kidneys, typical of renal angiomyolipomas.*

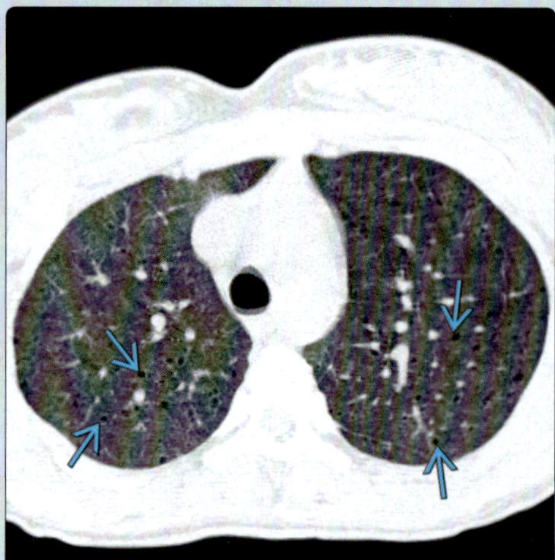

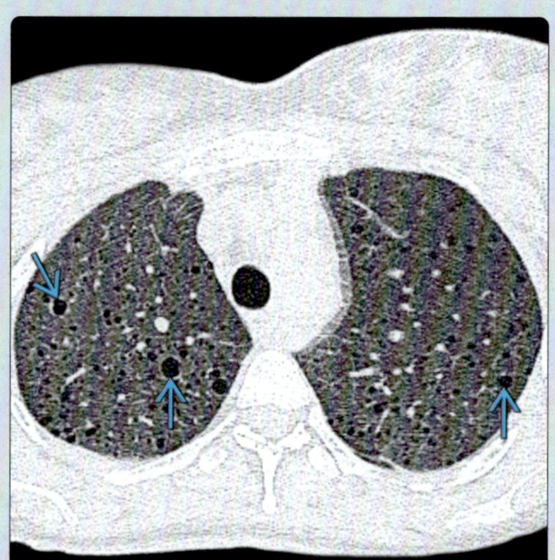

(Left) *Axial expiratory lung CT in a 22-year-old patient with TSC-LAM shows numerous scattered, 1- to 2-mm, round, thin-walled cysts → with normal intervening lung parenchyma.* **(Right)** *Axial expiratory lung CT obtained 3 years later in the same patient shows that the cysts → have ↑ in both size & number. The intervening parenchyma remains normal.*

TERMINOLOGY

Definitions

- Lymphangioleiomyomatosis (LAM): Disease characterized by abnormal proliferation of LAM cells in lungs & thoracic/retroperitoneal lymphatics
  - Occurs almost exclusively in women of childbearing age
- 2 main forms: Tuberous sclerosis complex-associated LAM (TSC-LAM); sporadic LAM (S-LAM)

IMAGING

General Features

- Best diagnostic clue
  - Bilateral, randomly distributed, thin-walled pulmonary cysts surrounded by normal intervening parenchyma

Radiographic Findings

- Chest radiograph is normal in early stages of LAM
- Eventual development of diffuse, fine reticular opacities
- Normal to ↑ lung volumes; ± pneumothorax (39-53%), pleural effusion (10-44%)
  - May precede visible parenchymal abnormalities

CT Findings

- Numerous thin-walled cysts with uniform distribution
  - Variable size: Usually 2 mm to 2 cm (may be larger)
    - Cyst sizes correlate with extent of disease
  - Variable number: From few scattered cysts to complete replacement of lung parenchyma
    - Small cysts are best seen on expiratory & minimum intensity projection (minIP) images
- Normal intervening lung parenchyma in majority
- Solid or ground-glass, 1- to 10-mm nodules in 3-20%; predominantly upper lobe & peripheral
  - Multifocal micronodular pneumocyte hyperplasia
- ± pleural effusion, pneumothorax, thoracic duct enlargement
- Quantitative CT analysis detects early emphysematous change surrounding cysts; high correlation with lung function: Threshold of -900 vs. -950 HU

MR Findings

- Hyperpolarized Xe-129 scans show ventilation defects, even with minimal cysts by CT & normal pulmonary function tests; elevated ADC values correspond to ↑ alveolar size

DIFFERENTIAL DIAGNOSIS

Langerhans Cell Histiocytosis

- Small pulmonary nodules ± cysts

Cystic Fibrosis

- Central & peripheral bronchiectasis, greatest in upper lobes

Bronchopulmonary Dysplasia

- History of prematurity + prolonged oxygen requirement

Papillomatosis

- Due to vertical transmission of human papillomavirus

PATHOLOGY

General Features

- Etiology
  - Abnormal neoplastic smooth muscle-like cell (LAM cell)
  - Evidence supports LAM cell metastases as cause for pulmonary manifestations
- Genetics
  - TSC-LAM: 2-hit Knudson hypothesis (sporadic superimposed on inherited germline) of mutations causing complete functional loss of *TSC1* or *TSC2* genes
    - *TSC1* gene product: Hamartin protein
    - *TSC2* gene product: Tuberin protein
    - Hamartin & tuberin are necessary for functioning mTOR signaling pathway
  - S-LAM: 2 sporadic somatic hits to *TSC2*

Extrapulmonary Findings

- S-LAM: Renal angiomyolipomas (AMLs) in 30% (usually small)
  - Chylous ascites, uterine leiomyomas, liver & pancreas cysts, abdominal/pelvic cystic lymphangioleiomyomas
- TSC-LAM: Renal AMLs in 80% (usually larger than in S-LAM) + renal cysts; hepatic & pancreatic lesions, PEComas
  - Cardiac rhabdomyomas (majority involute over time)
  - Cerebral > cerebellar cortical/subcortical tubers, white matter lesions, subependymal nodules, subependymal giant cell astrocytomas
  - Other: Retinal astrocytomas/hamartomas, facial angiofibromas, ash leaf spots, shagreen patches, subungual fibromas, cystic & sclerotic bone lesions

CLINICAL ISSUES

Presentation

- Most common signs/symptoms
  - Progressively worsening dyspnea on exertion in women of childbearing age
  - Spontaneous pneumothorax, often recurrent

Demographics

- Age: S-LAM mean age of diagnosis: 35 years
  - TSC-LAM lung disease can be seen on CT in childhood; 22% are affected by age 20; 80% by age 40

Natural History & Prognosis

- Progressive pulmonary function deterioration from slowly advancing lung disease; 10-year survival: 79-91%

Treatment

- Primarily symptomatic (e.g., evacuating pleural effusion, pneumothorax; bronchodilators)
- Sirolimus/rapamycin (mTOR inhibitor)
- Lung transplant

SELECTED REFERENCES

1. Daccord C et al: Effect of everolimus on multifocal micronodular pneumocyte hyperplasia in tuberous sclerosis complex. Respir Med Case Rep. 31:101310, 2020
2. Walkup LL et al: Cyst ventilation heterogeneity and alveolar airspace dilation as early disease markers in lymphangioleiomyomatosis. Ann Am Thorac Soc. 16(8):1008-16, 2019
3. Harari S et al: The changing face of a rare disease: lymphangioleiomyomatosis. Eur Respir J. 46(5):1471-85, 2015

Langerhans Cell Histiocytosis, Pulmonary

KEY FACTS

TERMINOLOGY

- Neoplastic proliferation of monoclonal Langerhans cells leading to formation of destructive granulomas

IMAGING

- Diffuse lung involvement is typical in children
  - Classic sparing of lower lungs/costophrenic sulci applies to adult pulmonary Langerhans cell histiocytosis (LCH)
    - Should not be used as diagnostic criterion in pediatrics
- Radiographs: Reticulonodular pattern of opacities
- CT: Combination of small nodules & cysts
  - Irregularly shaped nodules in centrilobular, peribronchial, or peribronchiolar locations
  - Cysts with variable wall thickness
- Chronic LCH: Fibrosis & traction emphysema
- May also see osseous, thymic, hepatic, & splenic involvement on chest imaging
  - High likelihood of multisystem LCH if lung disease is present in child

TOP DIFFERENTIAL DIAGNOSES

- Cystic fibrosis
- Papillomatosis
- Lymphangioleiomyomatosis
- Sarcoidosis

CLINICAL ISSUES

- May present at any age in childhood
- Typically occurs with multisystem disease in children
  - Lung is no longer considered risk organ for worse prognosis in LCH
- Leads to end-stage lung disease in 10-27% of cases
- HRCT is helpful to follow disease progression in young children, as pulmonary function tests are less reliable

DIAGNOSTIC CHECKLIST

- Pediatric LCH should not be confused with adult pulmonary LCH (which is typically single system disease associated with smoking)

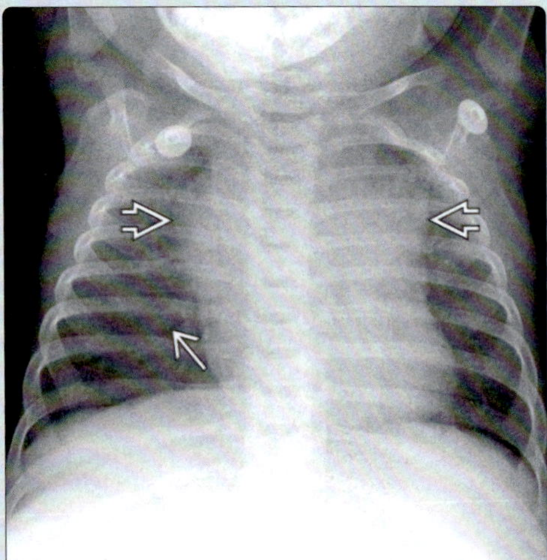

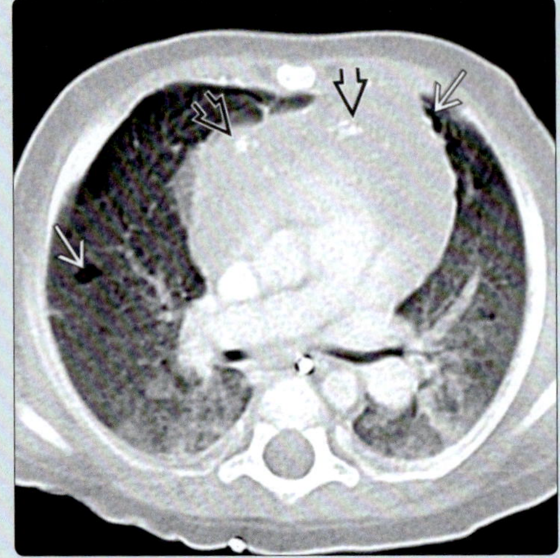

(Left) *AP chest radiograph in a 7-month-old girl shows diffuse, hazy lung opacity with areas of linear lucency ➡. The mediastinum is widened ⇨.* **(Right)** *Axial HRCT in the same patient shows bilateral pulmonary cysts ➡ within diffuse ground-glass opacities. The thymus is also involved by Langerhans cell histiocytosis (LCH), resulting in scattered thymic Ca^{2+} ⇨. Follow-up CT imaging (not shown) demonstrated clear lungs & resolved cysts after systemic therapy.*

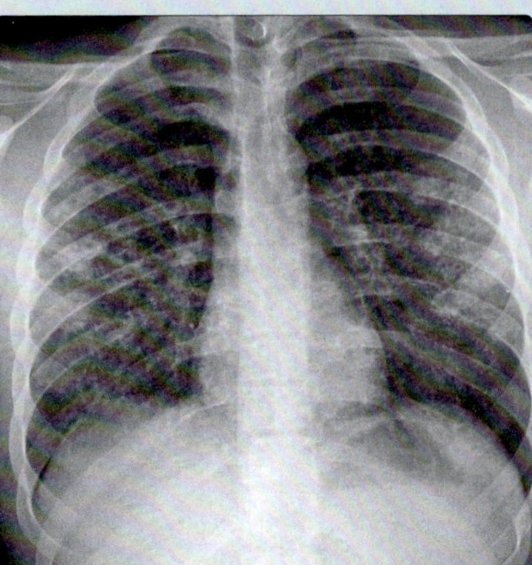

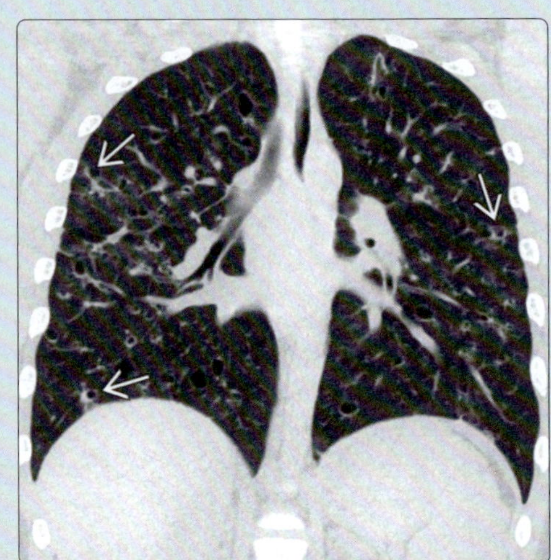

(Left) *PA chest radiograph in a 14-year-old boy with pulmonary LCH shows nodular opacities intermixed with reticulation secondary to peribronchovascular cysts.* **(Right)** *Coronal CT in the same patient with pulmonary LCH shows both nodules & cysts. Note the peribronchovascular distribution of cysts ➡, reflecting the bronchiolocentric nature of the disease.*

TERMINOLOGY

Definitions

- Langerhans cell histiocytosis (LCH): Neoplastic proliferation of monoclonal Langerhans cells in 1 or more organ systems
  - Leads to formation of destructive granulomas

IMAGING

General Features

- Best diagnostic clue
  - Combination of small pulmonary nodules & cysts

Radiographic Findings

- Early findings
  - Characteristic reticulonodular pattern (due to summation of nodules & thin-walled cysts)
  - Lung volumes are normal or ↑ (unlike many other interstitial diseases)
- Late findings
  - Honeycomb-like pattern with architectural distortion (due to summation of air-filled cysts)
- ± pneumothorax, pneumomediastinum, pleural effusion

CT Findings

- HRCT
  - Progression: Nodules → cavitary nodules → thick-walled cysts → thin-walled cysts → confluent cysts
    - Irregularly shaped nodules in centrilobular, peribronchial, or peribronchiolar locations
    - Cysts show variable wall thickness
  - Diffuse disease is common in children
    - Classic sparing of lower lungs/costophrenic sulci should not be used as diagnostic criterion in pediatrics
  - Chronic LCH: Fibrosis & traction emphysema
  - May also see osseous, thymic, hepatic, & splenic involvement on chest CT

DIFFERENTIAL DIAGNOSIS

Cystic Fibrosis

- Patchy, upper lobe-predominant disease
- Cylindrical to cystic bronchiectasis
- Bronchial wall thickening, mucous plugging

Papillomatosis

- Nodules intermixed with thick-walled cysts
- Nodules of larynx & trachea are more common than lung involvement

Lymphangioleiomyomatosis

- Small, round, thin-walled cysts with normal surrounding parenchyma
- No nodules (unless multifocal micronodular pneumocyte hyperplasia is present)

Sarcoidosis

- Apical predominant disease with ground-glass opacities, fibrotic change, subpleural honeycombing
- Hilar adenopathy is typical

PATHOLOGY

General Features

- Pulmonary LCH: Proliferation of Langerhans cells in bronchial/bronchiolar epithelium
  - Cavitating granulomas adjacent to small airways
    - Lead to airway obstruction, air-trapping, cystic change
- Diagnosed by bronchoalveolar lavage, possible biopsy
- Electron microscopy: Birbeck granule in cytoplasm of 40% of Langerhans cells
  - Classic "tennis racquet" organelle
- Immunostaining: CD1a, CD207, S100 protein positive
- Genetic mutations include *BRAF* V600E (55%), *MAP2K1*

Staging, Grading, & Classification

- Multisystem LCH
  - Pulmonary involvement in 23-50%
  - Most pediatric pulmonary LCH occurs in multisystem disease
    - Typically young children ± risk organ involvement
  - Lung disease no longer denotes risk organ involvement with worse prognosis
- Single system LCH
  - Pulmonary involvement in ~ 10% of pediatric patients
  - Typically adolescents

CLINICAL ISSUES

Presentation

- Most common signs/symptoms
  - Tachypnea, dyspnea, wheezing
- Clinical profile
  - Not associated with smoking (unlike adult LCH)

Natural History & Prognosis

- Leads to end-stage lung disease in 10-27% of patients with lung involvement
- < 65% 5-year survival if lung disease is severe

Treatment

- Corticosteroids & other chemotherapeutic agents
- Targeted: BRAF- or MEK-inhibitors (depending on underlying mutation)

DIAGNOSTIC CHECKLIST

Consider

- Pediatric LCH is not to be confused with adult pulmonary LCH
- Recommend chest radiography when LCH is discovered in any body system
- Degree of pulmonary involvement on CT correlates with functional impairment
  - HRCT is helpful to follow disease progression in young children, as pulmonary function tests are less reliable

SELECTED REFERENCES

1. Della Valle V et al: Chest computed tomography findings for a cohort of children with pulmonary Langerhans cell histiocytosis. Pediatr Blood Cancer. 67(10):e28496, 2020
2. Le Louet S et al: Childhood Langerhans cell histiocytosis with severe lung involvement: a nationwide cohort study. Orphanet J Rare Dis. 15(1):241, 2020

Pectus Excavatum

KEY FACTS

TERMINOLOGY

- Depression of sternum posteriorly → sunken appearance of midline anterior inferior chest wall

IMAGING

- Radiographs: Right heart border blurring with vertical anterior ribs; degree of depression is best seen on lateral view
- Pre-Nuss procedure evaluation with CT/MR
  - Haller index
    - Ratio of transverse (left-right) diameter divided by sagittal (anterior-posterior) diameter of chest
    - Haller index > 3.25 is considered enough deformity for surgical candidacy (by most insurance agencies)
    - Consider reporting correction & depression indices to capture patients with clinically significant deformities but possibly "normal" Haller indices
  - CT: Noncontrast, low mA images
  - MR: Single cardiac MR can replace echocardiogram & CT
    - ↓ right ventricular ejection fraction & hemodynamically insignificant pericardial effusion are common
- Post-Nuss procedure
  - Assess for complications → bar displacement/rotation, pneumothorax, pleural effusion, sternal infection

TOP DIFFERENTIAL DIAGNOSES

- Pectus carinatum
- Chest wall aggressive lesions
- Chest wall vascular malformations
- Palpable normal variants of chest wall

CLINICAL ISSUES

- Minimally invasive pectus repair (Nuss procedure)
  - Transverse curved metal bar surgically inserted internal to sternum & ribs
  - Excellent results in > 85% of patients

(Left) *Frontal radiograph shows a silhouette sign with an apparent opacity obscuring the right heart border (mimicking right middle lobe disease). Note the vertically oriented anterior ribs.* **(Right)** *Lateral radiograph in the same patient shows posterior positioning of the sternum as compared to the anterior ribs, consistent with pectus excavatum. There is no middle lobe pathology.*

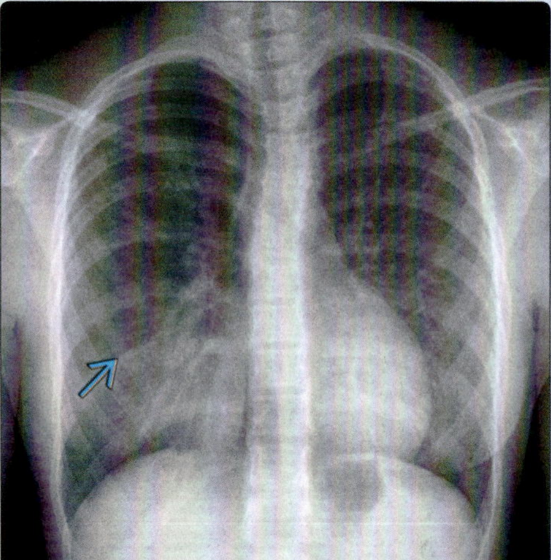

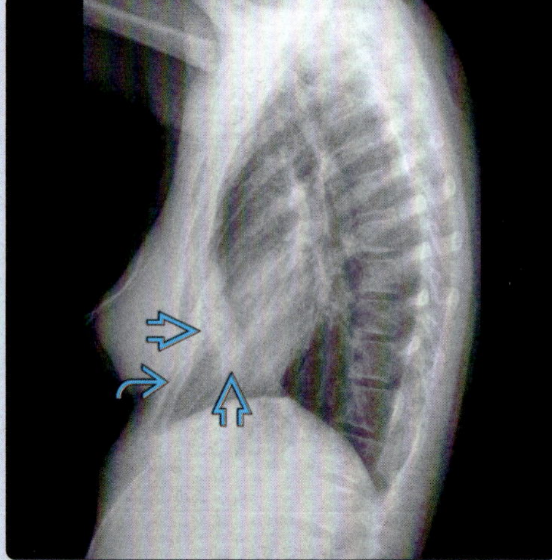

(Left) *Axial NECT of the chest shows marked pectus excavatum with posterior displacement & rotation of the sternum as compared with the anterior chest wall. Note the position of the right atrium immediately behind the sternum.* **(Right)** *Axial SSFP MR shows the landmarks used to calculate the Haller index. The left-to-right (blue line) & anterior-to-posterior (sagittal yellow line) diameters are measured, & the ratio is calculated as X/Y.*

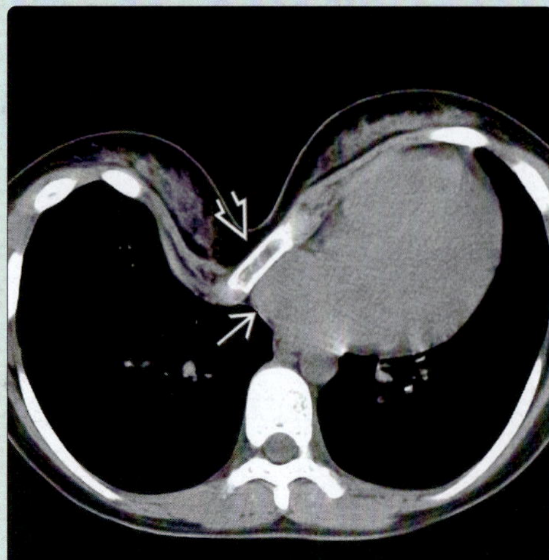

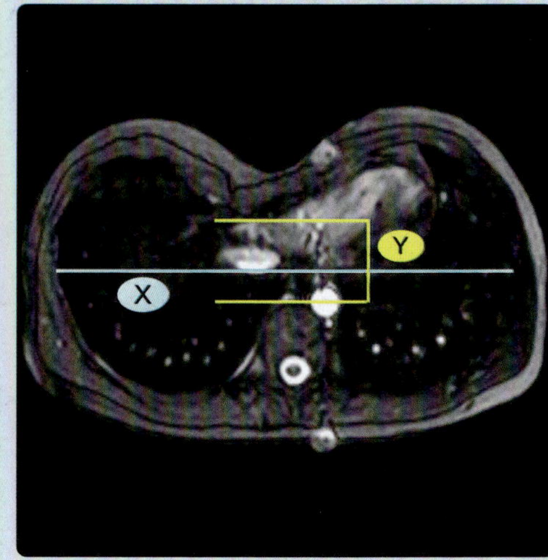

TERMINOLOGY

Definitions

- Deformity of chest wall characterized by sternal depression

IMAGING

General Features

- Imaging metrics
  - Haller index (HI)
    - Most frequently used metric to determine severity of pectus deformity; serves as indicator for Nuss procedure candidacy
    - Ratio of transverse (left-right) diameter divided by sagittal (anterior-posterior) diameter of inner aspects of osseous chest wall
    - HI > 3.25 is requirement of many insurance companies to qualify for payment of surgical correction
    - Most accurate location is caudal end of corpus sterni
  - Correction index (CI)
    - Percentage of chest depth missing from patient (i.e., percentage to be corrected by bar placement)
    - Eliminates importance of chest width
      - Narrow chest ↓ HI regardless of severity of defect
      - CI is not dependent on width; rather, CI defines distance of sternum from goal position
  - Depression index (DI)
    - Measurement of severity independent of thoracic diameters

Radiographic Findings

- Right heart border blurring with vertical anterior ribs ± obliteration of descending thoracic aortic interface
- Degree of depression is best seen on lateral radiograph
- Post-Nuss procedure
  - Nuss bar: Transverse metal bar with T-shaped stabilizer at one end
  - Potential complications: Bar displacement/rotation, pneumothorax, pleural effusion, sternal infection, cardiac injury
  - Lateral radiograph: Best view for migration of bar

CT Findings

- Pre-Nuss procedure evaluation with CT
  - Imaging metrics: HI, CI, DI, sternal tilt
  - Heart position (for surgical planning)
  - Central airway compression

MR Findings

- Expiratory axial slices with cardiac MR: Chest wall metrics + functional data (e.g., right ventricular ejection fraction, valve function)
- Right ventricle dysfunction due to extrinsic compression
- Hemodynamically insignificant pericardial effusion is common

DIFFERENTIAL DIAGNOSIS

Pectus Carinatum

- Anterior chest is convex outward: "Pigeon chest"

Chest Wall Aggressive Lesions

- Firm, painful mass ± rib destruction, pleural effusion

Chest Wall Vascular Malformations

- Soft, compressible mass; may fluctuate in size

Palpable Normal Variants of Chest Wall

- Rib anomalies may mimic sternal tilting/depression

PATHOLOGY

General Features

- Associated abnormalities
  - Connective tissue abnormalities
  - Neuromuscular disease
  - Genetic conditions
  - Pulmonary conditions

CLINICAL ISSUES

Presentation

- Most common signs/symptoms
  - Concerns about physical appearance are common
  - Exercise intolerance (82%), chest pain (68%), poor endurance (67%), shortness of breath (42%)
- Other signs/symptoms
  - Cardiac (pulmonic murmur, mitral valve prolapse, syncope, Wolff-Parkinson-White syndrome), restrictive lung disease, central airway compression
  - Palpable bony asymmetry associated with mild pectus deformity may be mistaken for soft tissue mass

Demographics

- Epidemiology: Accounts for up to 90% of anterior chest wall disorders

Treatment

- Conservative management for mild cases
- Minimally invasive repair (Nuss procedure): Transverse curved metal bar is inserted deep to sternum & rib cage
  - Excellent results in > 85% of patients

SELECTED REFERENCES

1. Daemen JHT et al: Optical imaging versus CT and plain radiography to quantify pectus severity: a systematic review and meta-analysis. J Thorac Dis. 12(4):1475-87, 2020
2. Rodríguez-Granillo GA et al: Preoperative multimodality imaging of pectus excavatum: state of the art review and call for standardization. Eur J Radiol. 117:140-8, 2019
3. Sesia SB et al: Standardized Haller and asymmetry index combined for a more accurate assessment of pectus excavatum. Ann Thorac Surg. 107(1):271-6, 2019
4. Abu-Tair T et al: Impact of pectus excavatum on cardiopulmonary function. Ann Thorac Surg. 105(2):455-60, 2018
5. Dore M et al: Advantages of cardiac magnetic resonance imaging for severe pectus excavatum assessment in children. Eur J Pediatr Surg. 28(1):34-8, 2018
6. Obermeyer RJ et al: The physiologic impact of pectus excavatum repair. Semin Pediatr Surg. 27(3):127-32, 2018
7. Sujka JA et al: Quantification of pectus excavatum: anatomic indices. Semin Pediatr Surg. 27(3):122-6, 2018
8. Abid I et al: Pectus excavatum: a review of diagnosis and current treatment options. J Am Osteopath Assoc. 117(2):106-13, 2017
9. Pilegaard H et al: Minimal invasive repair of pectus excavatum and carinatum. Thorac Surg Clin. 27(2):123-31, 2017

Minimally Invasive Pectus Repair Appearance

KEY FACTS

TERMINOLOGY

- Minimally invasive Nuss procedure has replaced open surgeries to repair pectus excavatum
  - Introducer is tunneled posterior to sternum
  - Convex stainless steel bar is passed (with convexity down) through 2 incisions, then flipped & fixed in place
    - Immediate cosmetic improvement
  - Bar remains in place 2-4 years

IMAGING

- Postoperative radiographs
  - AP & lateral views to evaluate Nuss bar position & improvement in pectus deformity
- Early postoperative complications
  - Pneumothorax, pneumomediastinum
  - Atelectasis, pneumonia
  - Hemothorax, pleural effusion
    - If lasts > 4 days, should be cultured
    - May also be due to nickel allergy
- Late postoperative complications
  - Bar displacement
    - May rotate, requiring surgical revision
    - Apex of bar may slip from deepest portion of sternal depression, causing unsatisfactory contour change
      - 2 bars may be placed in these patients
      - Typically no intervention if slippage is < 20%
    - Displacement is more likely in postpubertal patients

CLINICAL ISSUES

- Ideal age for repair: Just before puberty
  - May be performed earlier in cases of cardiac/pulmonary compression
  - Can also be performed after puberty with good outcomes

DIAGNOSTIC CHECKLIST

- Small postoperative pneumothoraces are common; may be managed conservatively

(Left) *PA chest radiograph in a 10-year-old girl following a minimally invasive pectus excavatum repair shows the stainless steel bar → in satisfactory position. Note the small left postoperative pleural effusion → & passive left lower lobe atelectasis →.* **(Right)** *Lateral chest radiograph in the same patient shows the stainless steel bar → passing posterior to the sternum at the point of maximum sternal concavity. Note the posterior pleural fluid & atelectasis →.*

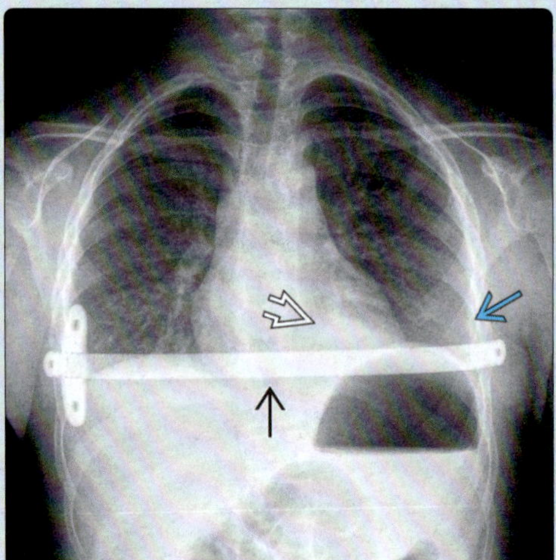

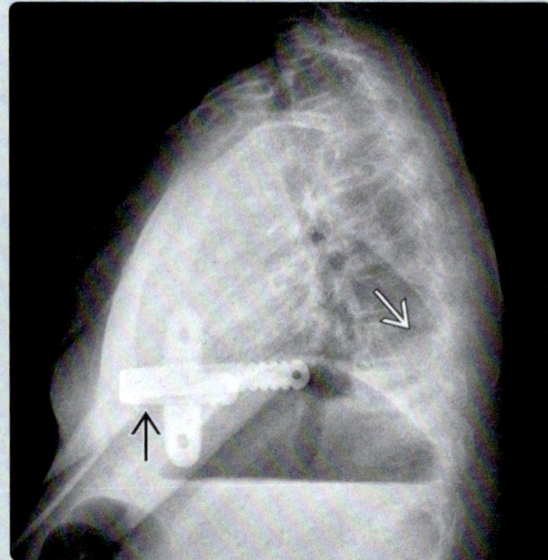

(Left) *PA chest radiograph after a Nuss procedure shows disruption at the junction of the pectus bar & left stabilizer →. The bar remains appropriately engaged with the right stabilizer.* **(Right)** *Volume-rendered axial CT in the same patient shows disruption at the junction of the pectus bar & left stabilizer →.*

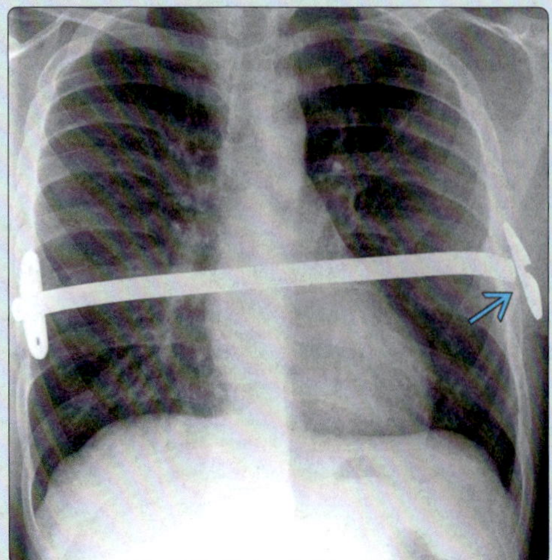

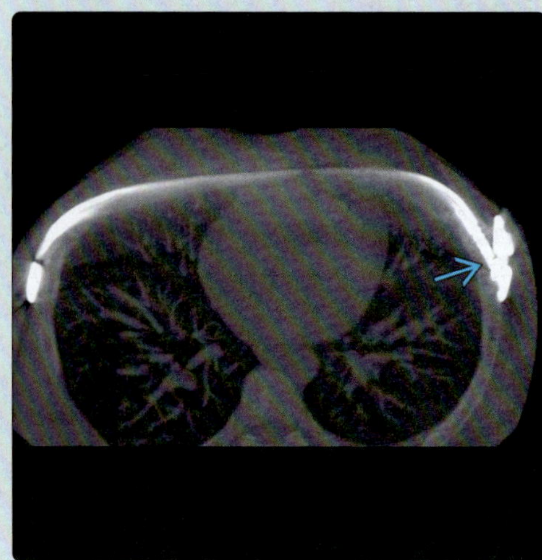

Askin Tumor/Ewing Sarcoma of Chest Wall

KEY FACTS

TERMINOLOGY

- Askin tumor: Extraskeletal Ewing sarcoma of chest
  - Ewing sarcoma & Askin tumor are closely related: Ewing sarcoma family of tumors (ESFT)
  - Soft tissue primitive neuroectodermal tumor (PNET) is now termed extraskeletal Ewing sarcoma by WHO

IMAGING

- Unilateral thoracic opacification
  - Large, lobular mass may occupy most of or entire hemithorax, especially with pleural effusion
  - Rib destruction is common (> 50%)
  - Ca^{2+} is uncommon
- Mildly heterogeneous enhancement on CT & MR
- Mass effect on mediastinal structures
  - Vessels & airway are typically compressed & shifted rather than encased or invaded
- Mediastinal lymphadenopathy: 25% at presentation
- Pulmonary metastasis: 38% at presentation
- CT & MR can be complimentary
  - CT better detects small pulmonary metastases
  - MR better evaluates involvement of chest wall

PATHOLOGY

- Identical to other Ewing sarcomas
  - Small round blue cells
  - Positive immunohistochemical stain for *CD99* (MIC2) gene product: 90%
  - Chromosomal translocation [t(11;22)(q24;q12)]: 85-95%

CLINICAL ISSUES

- Median age: ~ 15 years
- Prognosis: 5-year survival rate = 50-60%

DIAGNOSTIC CHECKLIST

- On posttherapy surveillance CT, look closely for
  - Local recurrence in chest wall
  - Mediastinal & chest wall lymphadenopathy
  - Pulmonary metastases

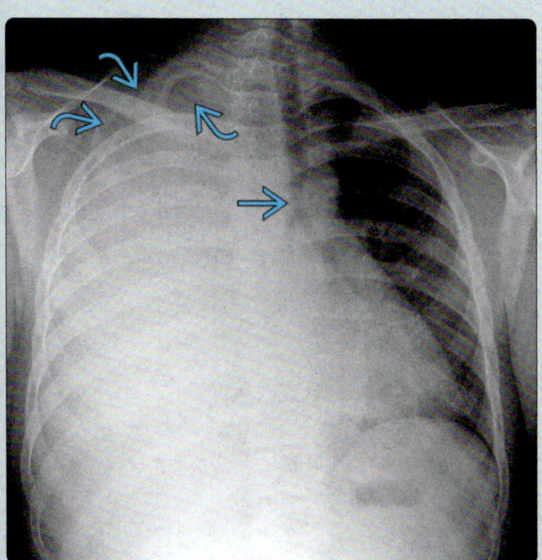

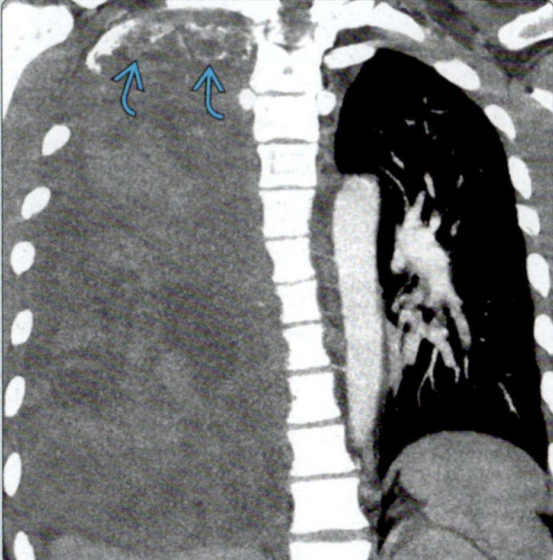

(Left) *PA radiograph in a 15-year-old girl with a chest wall Ewing sarcoma shows complete opacification of the right hemithorax with mass effect on the mediastinum ➙. Note the lucency, expansion, permeation, & erosion of the right 2nd rib ➙.* **(Right)** *Coronal CECT in the same patient shows a heterogeneous mass filling the right hemithorax with expansion & destruction of the right 2nd rib ➙.*

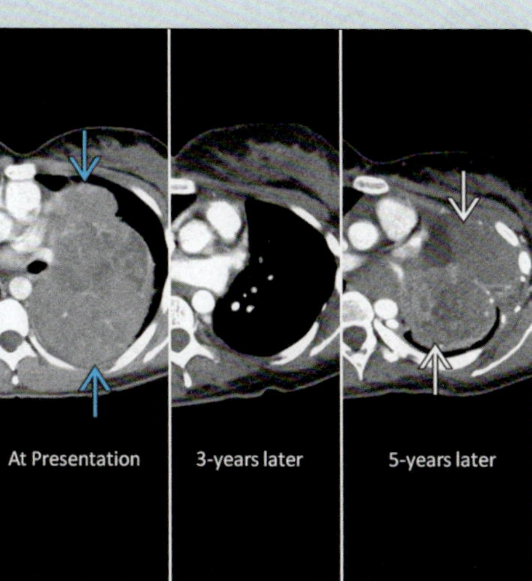

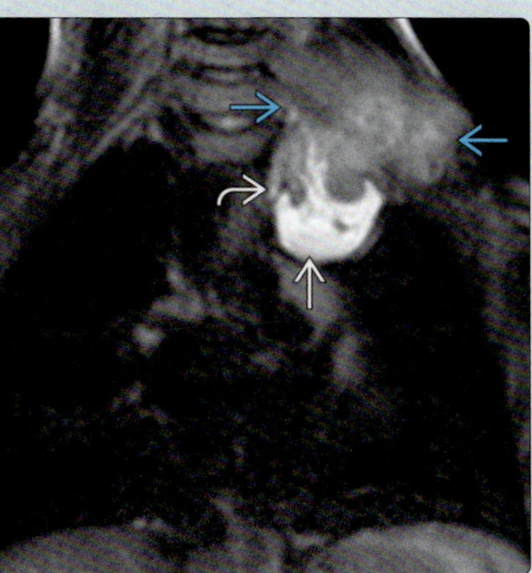

(Left) *Initial axial CECT in a girl with an Askin tumor at presentation (L) shows a large, heterogeneous mass in the left upper hemithorax ➙. After chemotherapy, resection, & radiation, no tumor was detectable on the 3-year follow-up CT (M). Tumor recurrence is present at 5 years ➙ (R).* **(Right)** *Coronal T2 FS MR shows a 3-year-old patient with an Askin tumor. A heterogeneous mass in the left upper hemithorax ➙ is partly cystic ➙ & extends into the soft tissues of the left lower neck ➙.*

Chest Wall Hamartoma

KEY FACTS

TERMINOLOGY

- Mesenchymal hamartoma of chest wall (MHCW) = benign infantile lesion of proliferating skeletal elements arising from central/internal surfaces of rib(s)

IMAGING

- Partially calcified soft tissue mass of chest wall
  - Chondroid > > osteoid mineralization (100% by CT)
- Multiple internal compartments containing fluid-fluid levels
  - Secondary aneurysmal bone cysts (60-80%, CT vs. MR)
- Bizarre remodeling/distortion & erosion of multiple adjacent ribs
- Prenatal US may show chest wall mass with echogenic rim ("capsule")
  - ± polyhydramnios, pleural effusion
- Typical locations
  - Extrapleural posterior > anterior chest wall
  - Multifocal (unilateral or bilateral) in < 20%

PATHOLOGY

- Hemorrhagic cavities intermixed with cartilage & bone

CLINICAL ISSUES

- 1 in 3,000 primary bone tumors
- Typically detected prenatally or within first 6 months of life
- Classic presentations: Congenital chest wall mass/deformity, respiratory distress
- No known risk of malignant degeneration, local invasion, or metastasis
- Many reports of spontaneous regression ≥ 2 years of age
- Observation if asymptomatic with classic age, presentation, & imaging findings
  - Potential for significant hemorrhage with disruption of blood-filled cavities during biopsy or excision
- Resection in setting of respiratory, cardiovascular, or neurologic compromise
  - Scoliosis occurs with resection of multiple posterior ribs

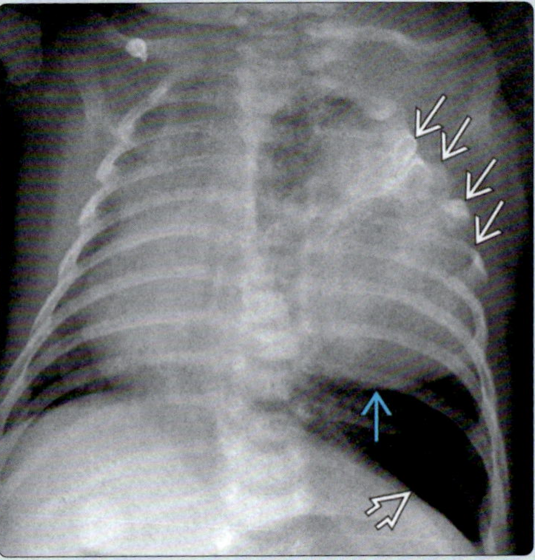

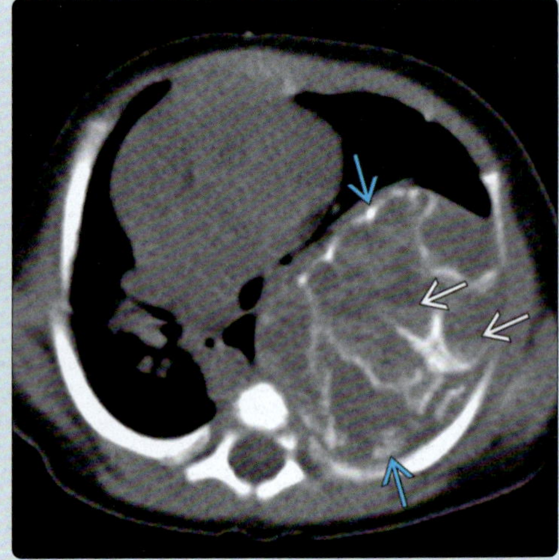

(Left) *AP radiograph in a 1-month-old with respiratory distress shows a large soft tissue mass ⇨ in the left hemithorax with bizarre remodeling & erosion of multiple adjacent ribs ➡. There is mediastinal shift & lower lobe air-trapping ➡ due to mass effect.* **(Right)** *Axial NECT in the same patient shows rim & septal Ca^{2+} ⇨ throughout the mass with numerous fluid-fluid levels ➡ due to layering blood products. Biopsy confirmed a mesenchymal hamartoma of the chest wall (MHCW).*

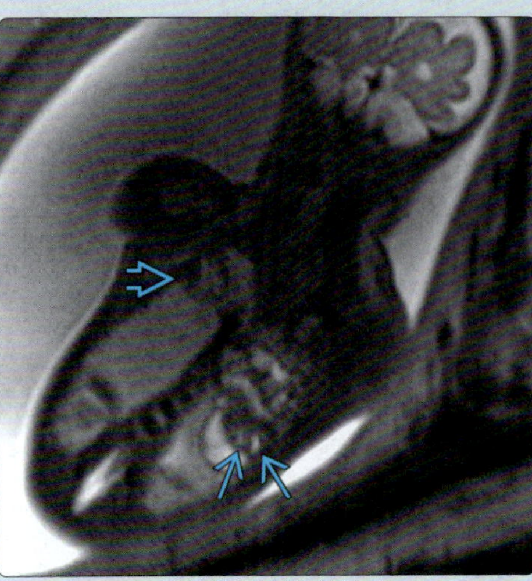

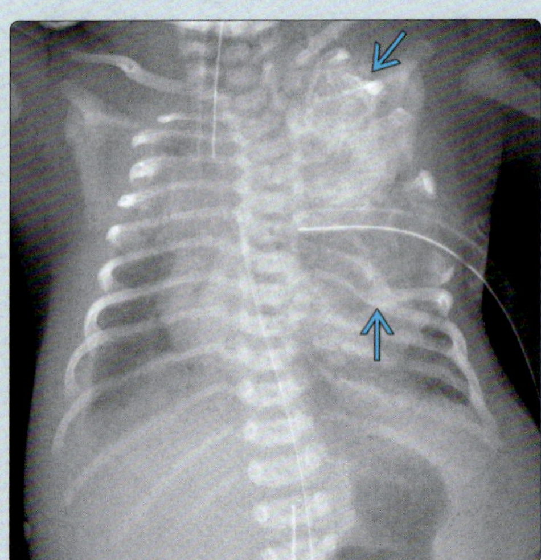

(Left) *Coronal SSFSE T2 MR in a 33-weeks-gestation fetus shows a large, heterogeneous, multicystic lesion of the left chest. Numerous fluid-fluid levels ⇨ were visible, & other images showed distortion of multiple ribs. A 2nd smaller lesion was also seen on the right ⇨. (Courtesy L. LaForest, MD.)* **(Right)** *AP radiograph in the same neonate shows distortion of numerous left ribs ⇨ by the partially calcified cystic mass, typical of an MHCW. The smaller right MHCW is much less conspicuous. (Courtesy L. LaForest, MD.)*

TERMINOLOGY

Abbreviations

- Mesenchymal hamartoma of chest wall (MHCW)

Synonyms

- Mesenchymoma, chondromatous hamartoma (antiquated terms)

Definitions

- Benign infantile lesion of proliferating skeletal elements arising from rib(s)

IMAGING

General Features

- Best diagnostic clue
  - Partially calcified soft tissue mass of chest wall in infant
    - Mineralization (100% by CT), chondroid > > osteoid
  - Multiple internal compartments containing fluid-fluid levels
    - Secondary aneurysmal bone cysts (60-80%, CT vs. MR)
  - Bizarre remodeling/distortion & erosion of multiple adjacent ribs
  - Prenatal US may show chest wall mass with echogenic rim ("capsule")
    - ± polyhydramnios, pleural effusion
- Location
  - Extrapleural posterior > anterior chest wall
    - Arises from central/internal aspect of rib
  - Multifocal (unilateral or bilateral) in < 20%
  - No invasion or metastasis

DIFFERENTIAL DIAGNOSIS

Hemangioma, Infantile or Congenital

- Solid hypervascular/high flow soft tissue mass ± characteristic cutaneous features
- Bone involvement is exceptionally rare
- Predictable life cycle

Slow-Flow Vascular Malformation, Venous or Lymphatic

- Conglomerations of multiple cysts, tubular masses, &/or abnormal vessels
- Frequently extend into multiple tissue compartments
  - May involve chest wall/ribs
- Often contain fluid-fluid levels

Infantile Myofibroma

- Soft tissue mass(es) without fluid-fluid levels or rim Ca^{2+}
- May cause chronic remodeling of subjacent bone
- May be multifocal, involving soft tissues, viscera, &/or bone; uncommonly involves thoracic cage

Congenital/Infantile Fibrosarcoma

- Uncommon solid &/or multicystic mass of infants, most common in extremities
- Bone involvement is uncommon

Teratoma

- Mixed solid & cystic mass ± Ca^{2+}
  - Multiple hemorrhagic cavities are uncommon
- Does not typically involve chest wall

Palpable Normal Variant

- Frequently due to osseous &/or cartilaginous variations of ribs (such as fusion)
  - Anterior > posterior

Ewing Sarcoma

- Older children (teenagers) with aggressive bony changes of 1 rib surrounded by large soft tissue mass, ± pleural effusion

Rib Fractures of Child Abuse

- Adjacent healing fractures can have bulbous callous
  - Ca^{2+} is not contiguous or associated with significant rib distortion or soft tissue mass

PATHOLOGY

Microscopic Features

- Hemorrhagic cavities intermixed with cartilage, bone, & fibroblasts

CLINICAL ISSUES

Presentation

- Most common signs/symptoms
  - Chest wall mass/deformity, respiratory distress

Demographics

- Age
  - Typically detected prenatally or within first 6 months of life
  - Rarely found outside of infancy, including adolescence & adulthood
- Epidemiology
  - 1 in 3,000 primary bone tumors; incidence of 1:1,000,000

Natural History & Prognosis

- Many reports of spontaneous regression
- No known risk of malignant degeneration, local invasion, or metastasis

Treatment

- Observation if asymptomatic with classic age, presentation, & imaging findings
  - Atypical age/clinical presentation, aggressive imaging features, &/or growth may require biopsy
    - Significant hemorrhage may occur with disruption of blood-filled cavities
- Resection with respiratory, cardiovascular, or neurologic compromise
  - Scoliosis is most likely with resection of multiple posterior ribs

SELECTED REFERENCES

1. Lee MYW et al: A case of mesenchymal hamartoma of the chest wall in a 4-month-old infant. Am J Case Rep. 20:511-6, 2019
2. Swaminathan A et al: Life-threatening mesenchymal hamartoma of the chest wall in a neonate. BJR Case Rep. 5(3):20190004, 2019
3. Tanaka T et al: Mesenchymal hamartoma of the chest wall in a 10-year-old girl mimicking malignancy: a case report. Skeletal Radiol. 48(4):643-7, 2019
4. Alfaraidi M et al: Bilateral mesenchymal hamartoma of the chest wall in a 3-month-old boy: a case report and review of the literature. Case Rep Pathol. 2017:2876342, 2017

Asthma

KEY FACTS

TERMINOLOGY

- Chronic, reversible, paroxysmal airway hyperresponsiveness leading to airflow obstruction
- Umbrella term for numerous phenotypes in which normally harmless environmental allergens cause airway hyperresponsiveness due to pathologic immune-mediated host response (i.e., not single disease)

IMAGING

- Usually normal; may have symmetric hyperexpansion with flattened hemidiaphragms & ↑ retrosternal airspace
- Not necessary; helpful to identify complications & mimics
  - Consider chest radiograph if poor response to therapy

TOP DIFFERENTIAL DIAGNOSES

- Viral bronchiolitis: May occur in concert with & be impossible to differentiate from asthma
- Foreign body aspiration: Static, asymmetric lung volumes on bilateral decubitus or inspiratory/expiratory imaging
- Cystic fibrosis: Focal disease with bronchiectasis & mucous plugging, most common in upper lobes
- Croup: Barky cough &/or stridor (vs. wheezing in asthma) due to subglottic airway narrowing

PATHOLOGY

- Risk factors include frequent symptoms in 1st year of life, maternal smoking or history of asthma, & signs of atopy

CLINICAL ISSUES

- Intermittent wheezing before age 6 is usually benign & typically resolves within few years
- Severity of asthma symptoms between ages 7-10 years predicts persistence into adulthood

DIAGNOSTIC CHECKLIST

- Radiographs are usually normal but are indicated to exclude suspected alternate diagnosis, complication, or poor response to therapy

(Left) *Frontal radiograph in a 17-year-old during an asthma attack shows hyperexpanded lungs, resulting in a narrow cardiac silhouette* ➔ *& flattening of the diaphragm* ➔*. Subsegmental opacity in the left lower lobe* ➔ *was favored to represent atelectasis.* **(Right)** *Lateral radiograph in the same patient reveals prominence of the retrosternal clear space* ➔ *& diaphragmatic flattening* ➔ *caused by air-trapping. Imaging is often near-normal in asthma patients & is best used to identify complications or alternative diagnoses.*

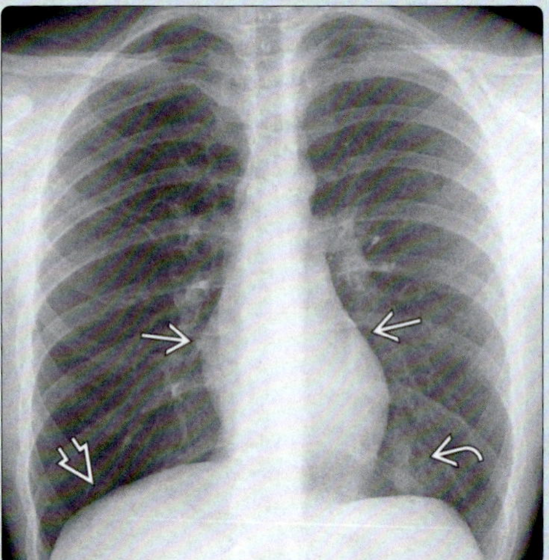

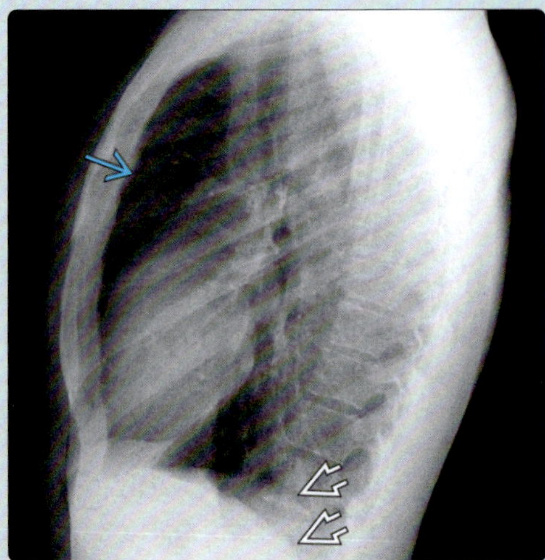

(Left) *Frontal radiograph in a 6-year-old with an asthma exacerbation caused by Mycoplasma pneumoniae shows peribronchial airway thickening* ➔ *& scattered, subsegmental opacities in the perihilar & lower lungs* ➔*. Infection from M. pneumoniae is a common cause of asthma exacerbation.* **(Right)** *Frontal radiograph in a child with shortness of breath shows a dense, triangular-shaped opacity from left lower lobe collapse* ➔*. Lobar collapse & atelectasis are common findings in patients with asthma exacerbation.*

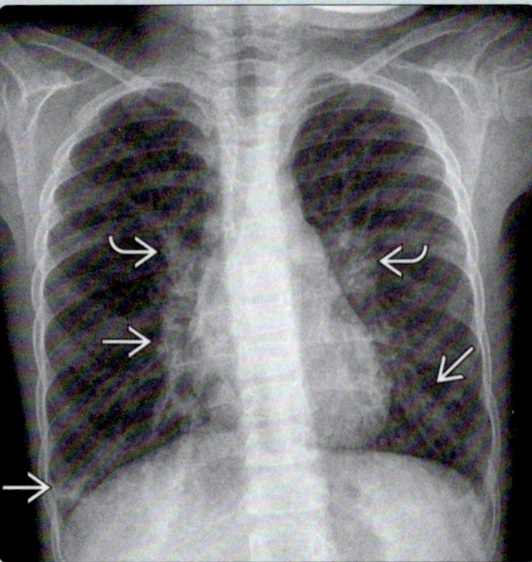

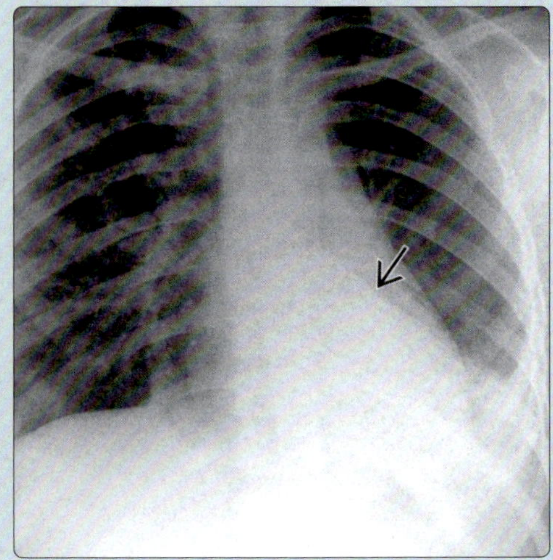

TERMINOLOGY

Synonyms

- Airway hyperreactivity
- Reactive airways disease

Definitions

- Chronic disease characterized by bronchial hyperresponsiveness, reversible airway obstruction, & chronic airway inflammation
- Umbrella term for numerous phenotypes in which normally harmless environmental allergens lead to pathologic immune-mediated host response (i.e., not single disease)
- Airway hyperresponsiveness → contraction of bronchial wall smooth muscle & cascade of inflammation → acute, reversible airway narrowing & airflow obstruction
- United airway disease (UAD): Concept that upper & lower airways function immunologically as single organ
  - Overwhelming majority of asthmatics have rhinitis; less commonly, nasal polyps & other sinonasal disorders

IMAGING

General Features

- Best imaging clue
  - Symmetric lung hyperexpansion: Flattening of hemidiaphragms, ↑ retrosternal airspace

Radiographic Findings

- Not part of most acute childhood asthma algorithms; reserved for those with fever, suspected foreign body (FB) aspiration, failure to improve with treatment, or focal findings on physical exam
- Most common finding: Normal chest radiograph
- Next most common: Subtle & nonspecific signs of hyperinflation, usually symmetric
  - Flattening of hemidiaphragms
  - ↑ AP diameter of chest & retrosternal airspace
  - ± bulging intercostal spaces
- Less common findings
  - Peribronchial thickening/cuffing
    - Irregular cardiac contour ("shaggy heart")
  - Atelectasis & lobar/partial lobar collapse
  - Peripheral oligemia
- Chronic findings
  - Bronchiectasis, mucous plugging
- Complications: More frequent in younger children as smaller bronchi are more easily narrowed or occluded & more likely to have concurrent viral bronchiolitis
  - Barotrauma (pneumomediastinum, subcutaneous emphysema, &, rarely, pneumothorax)
  - Lobar collapse, segmental & subsegmental atelectasis
  - Secondary allergic bronchopulmonary aspergillosis
  - Pneumonia

CT Findings

- HRCT
  - Signs of airway narrowing
    - Bronchial wall thickening
    - Narrowing or dilation of bronchial lumen
    - Mucous plugging
  - Signs of abnormal aeration
    - Mosaic attenuation due to combination of regional air-trapping & oligemia
    - Focal peripheral air-trapping on expiratory images
  - Signs of airspace disease
    - Segmental & subsegmental atelectasis
    - Centrilobular opacities
  - Bronchiectasis suggests asthma mimics (cystic fibrosis, ciliary dyskinesias, or immune deficiencies)
- CT is generally not indicated; quantitative studies show ↑ airway thickness & ↓ mean lung density

MR Findings

- Not used clinically; hyperpolarized noble gas MR can measure ventilation volumes
- Findings also correlate with disease severity, lung function, symptom control, & level of inflammatory marker elevation

Imaging Recommendations

- Imaging is generally not recommended except in
  - Febrile children (for possible complicating pneumonia)
  - Suspected foreign body (FB) aspiration
  - Those who fail to improve with treatment
  - Suspected barotrauma or lung collapse

DIFFERENTIAL DIAGNOSIS

Viral Bronchiolitis

- Often acts as precipitating trigger for asthma & may be impossible to differentiate radiographically or clinically
- Look for preceding or concurrent symptoms of viral upper respiratory infection (e.g., nasal congestion or fever)

Foreign Body Inhalation or Ingestion

- Vast majority of aspirated FBs are not radiopaque
- Persistent air-trapping or collapse on serial radiographs, usually unilateral
- Static lung volumes on bilateral decubitus or inspiratory/expiratory imaging
- Persistent symptoms that do not respond to bronchodilator therapy

Croup

- Stridor rather than wheezing
- Barky cough
- Narrowed subglottic trachea

Cystic Fibrosis

- Early bronchial wall thickening that progresses to bronchiectasis
- Persistent hyperinflation or recurrent consolidation
- Mucous plugging of dilated bronchi
- Focal disease, most common in upper lobes

Ciliary Dyskinesias

- Situs inversus or dextrocardia (50%), paranasal sinusitis, & bronchiectasis
- Recurrent pneumonias

Immune Deficiencies

- Recurrent pulmonary infection → bronchiectasis

Vascular Sling

- Symptoms are often present from birth
- No response to bronchodilator therapy

- Abnormal impression of left pulmonary artery coursing between trachea & esophagus
- Often has associated complete cartilage rings of trachea (appearing round & narrow in cross section)

PATHOLOGY

General Features

- Etiology
  - Exact etiology is unknown; due to interplay of environmental triggers & host factors
    - Environmental associations & triggers
      - Maternal exposure to tobacco smoke, fine (< 2.5 μm diameter) particulate matter, antibiotics
      - Antibiotic use during infancy ↑ asthma risk
      - Respiratory infections, especially Mycoplasma pneumonia
      - Poor air quality: Both indoor (tobacco smoke, cockroach & pet dander, dust mites, household chemicals, molds) & outdoor (fine & course particulate matter, pollen, ozone)
      - Changes in weather, especially cold & dry conditions
    - Host factors
      - Genetic predisposition
      - Upper respiratory tract viral illnesses
      - Exercise & strong emotional states (anger, anxiety, fear)
      - Hormonal fluctuations & menses
  - Complex response to these triggers causes release of inflammatory mediators from mast cells, macrophages, eosinophils, epithelial cells, & activated T lymphocytes
    - Bronchospasm
    - Airway edema
    - ↑ mucus production
- Risk factors
  - ↑ IgE levels; often associated with seasonal allergies & eczema (atopic triad)
  - Frequent symptoms in 1st year of life
  - Family history of asthma
  - Low birthweight
  - Male sex

Gross Pathologic & Surgical Features

- Bronchial edema & wall thickening
- Mucous plugging of airway lumen

Microscopic Features

- Inflammatory cell infiltration & edema of airway wall
- Mucous gland hyperplasia

CLINICAL ISSUES

Presentation

- Most common signs/symptoms
  - Chronic &/or recurrent cough, wheezing
  - Shortness of breath
  - Chest tightness
- Other signs/symptoms
  - ↓ peak expiratory flow rates & forced expiratory volume in 1-second (FEV_1) values
  - Symptomatic improvement with bronchodilator therapy
  - Use of accessory muscles to breathe at rest
  - Exercise limitation

Demographics

- Age
  - Prevalence peak is between 6-11 years
- Sex
  - M > F = 1.5:1.0 before puberty
  - M < F = 1.0:1.5 after puberty
- Epidemiology
  - Most common chronic disease of childhood
  - Prevalence of 1-30% worldwide
  - Positive correlation with urbanization
  - Increasing incidence worldwide with increasing mortality
  - In USA, asthma is more common in Black & Hispanic children

Natural History & Prognosis

- Prognosis is usually excellent with appropriate treatment
- Wheezing before age 6 is usually benign & typically resolves within few years
- Severity of asthma symptoms between ages of 7-10 years is predictive of persistence into adulthood
  - Small subgroup (30%) of children is characterized by signs of atopy, severe & persistent symptoms at young age, & maternal history of smoking or asthma

Treatment

- Avoid exposure to known precipitating environments
- Inhaled β-agonists for bronchospasm
- Inhaled & oral corticosteroids that dampen inflammatory response
  - Used to prevent acute exacerbations & for treatment of chronic asthma
- Inhaled mast cell stabilizers that prevent release of mediators from mast cells that cause airway inflammation & bronchospasm

DIAGNOSTIC CHECKLIST

Consider

- Radiographs are usually normal but indicated with poor response to therapy, suspected complication, or concern for alternate diagnosis
- Hyperinflation with varying degrees of atelectasis
- Difficult to distinguish from viral bronchiolitis

Image Interpretation Pearls

- Look for asthma mimics & signs of complication

SELECTED REFERENCES

1. Silva TKBD et al: High-resolution CT pulmonary findings in children with severe asthma. J Pediatr (Rio J). 97(1):37-43, 2020
2. Dharmage SC et al: Epidemiology of asthma in children and adults. Front Pediatr. 7:246, 2019
3. Wu J et al: Effects of particulate matter (PM) on childhood asthma exacerbation and control in Xiamen, China. BMC Pediatr. 19(1):194, 2019
4. Yii ACA et al: Precision medicine in united airways disease: a "treatable traits" approach. Allergy. 73(10):1964-78, 2018

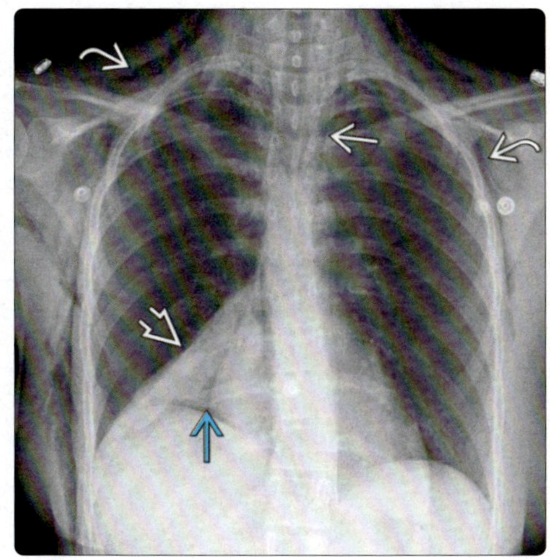

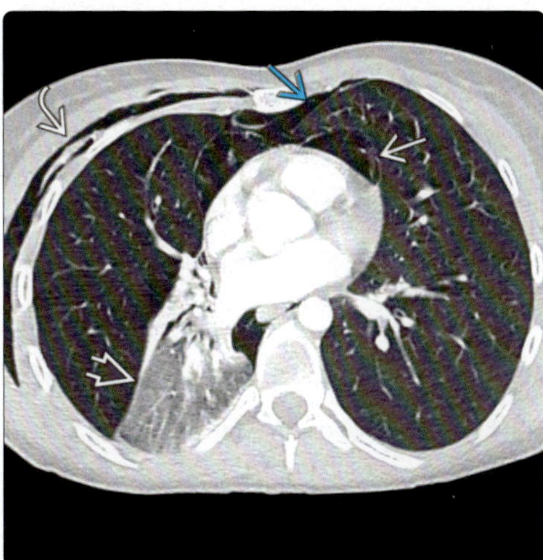

(Left) *Frontal radiograph in a 17-year-old with a severe asthma attack precipitated by rhinovirus infection shows extensive subcutaneous emphysema ➡, pneumomediastinum ➡, right pneumothorax ➡, & right lower lobe collapse ➡.* **(Right)** *Axial CECT in the same patient shows extraventilatory gas in the soft tissues ➡ & mediastinum ➡ as well as a small left pneumothorax ➡ & right lower lobe collapse ➡. Barotrauma is a common complication in asthma patients.*

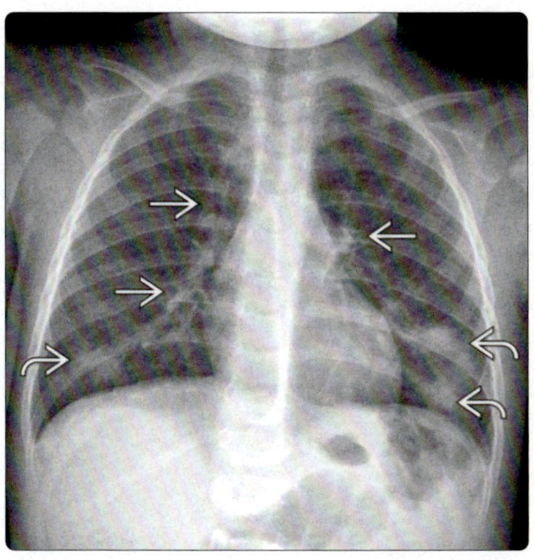

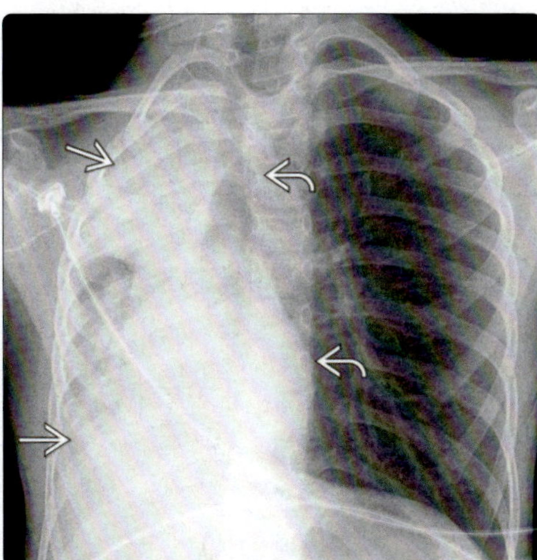

(Left) *Frontal chest radiograph in a young child with wheezing (who was later diagnosed with asthma) shows peribronchial airway thickening ➡ & multifocal atelectasis ➡ bilaterally.* **(Right)** *Frontal radiograph in a child with chronic asthma complicated by plastic bronchitis (which is the development of luminal casts, in this case due to inflammation) that caused bronchial occlusion & near total right lung collapse shows widespread opacity ➡ & shift of the mediastinum to the right ➡.*

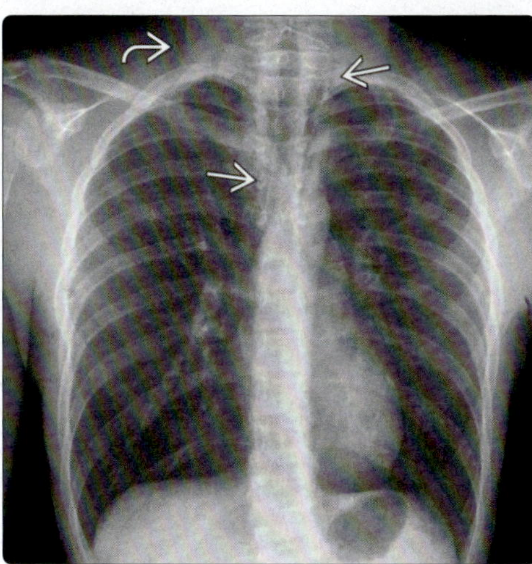

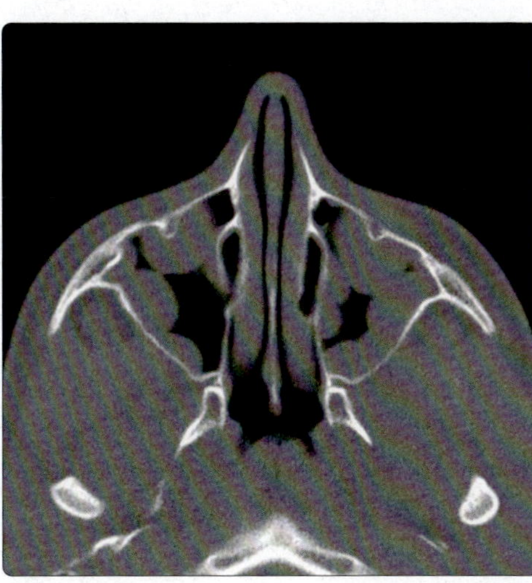

(Left) *Frontal chest radiograph in a 14-year-old with a severe asthma exacerbation shows subcutaneous emphysema in the neck ➡ & streaky lucencies in the mediastinum ➡ from pneumomediastinum.* **(Right)** *Axial sinus CT in a 14-year-old with asthma & allergic rhinitis reveals extensive sinonasal polyposis. The united airway disease hypothesis underscores how sinonasal disease & airway hyperreactivity seen in asthma are manifestations of the same inflammatory process.*

Bronchial Obstruction

KEY FACTS

TERMINOLOGY

- Complete or partial bronchial occlusion by aspirated foreign body (FB)

IMAGING

- Vast majority of aspirated FBs are **not** radiopaque
- Look for unilateral static lung/lobe volume on chest radiographs
  - In uncooperative patients (most common), obtain frontal view + bilateral decubitus images: Look for lack of passive deflation of dependent lung, suggesting air-trapping
  - In cooperative patients, radiographs can be obtained at maximum inspiration & expiration: Look for expiratory air-trapping on affected side
- Volume of affected lung segments can be normal, ↑, or ↓
- Consider CT with multiplanar reconstructions & 3D virtual bronchoscopy in cases with persistent clinical suspicion & negative chest radiographs

TOP DIFFERENTIAL DIAGNOSES

- Refractory asthma
  - Very common; ↑ peribronchial markings & symmetrically hyperexpanded lungs ± foci of atelectasis
- Viral lower respiratory tract infection
  - Very common; ↑ peribronchial markings & symmetrically hyperexpanded lungs ± foci of atelectasis
- Pulmonary sling
  - Much less common than FB; typically presents with respiratory distress at birth & asymmetric lung volumes
- Congenital lobar emphysema
  - Lobar hyperexpansion, generally since newborn period or early infancy

CLINICAL ISSUES

- Typically presents with wheezing, cough, sometimes fever
- More indolent symptoms if delayed presentation (10-25%)
- Delay in diagnosis is associated with ↑ complication rate
- Treatment: Bronchoscopic removal of FB

(Left) *Portable chest radiograph in a 3-year-old patient who aspirated glass fragments during a car crash shows 3 small radiopaque foreign bodies in the right lower lobe bronchus ➡. There is resulting airspace opacity as well as volume loss causing elevation of the right hemidiaphragm & slight mediastinal shift ➡.* **(Right)** *Axial CECT in the same child shows a square-shaped radiopaque glass foreign body in a segmental bronchus of the right lower lobe ➡.*

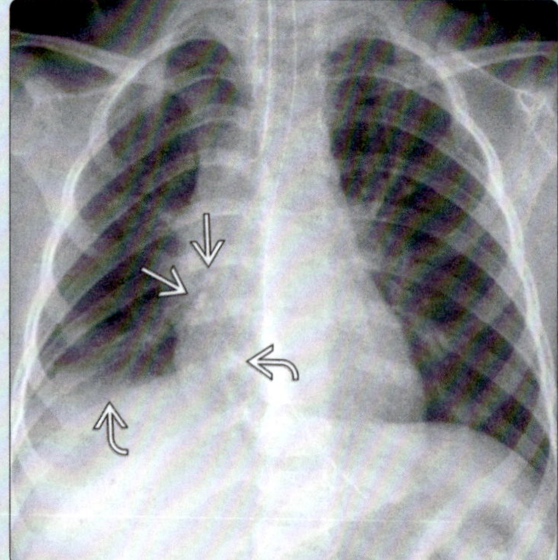

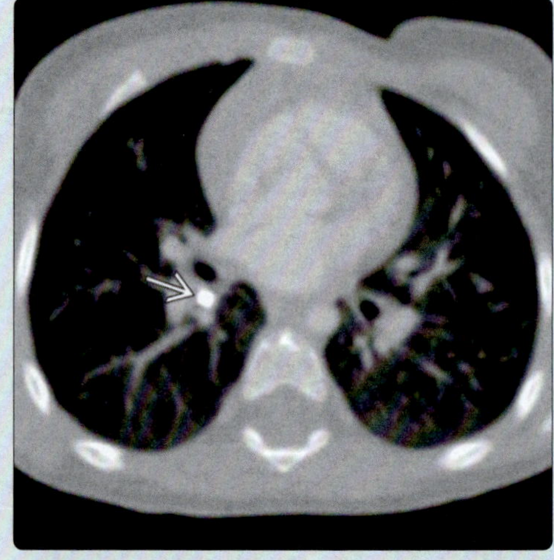

(Left) *Bronchoscopic image in the same patient shows complete occlusion of the segmental bronchus by glass fragments ➡.* **(Right)** *Portable chest radiograph of a toddler found unconscious in a debris pile after a flood shows a small, well-defined opacity in the left main bronchus ➡. The left lower lobe is relatively hyperlucent due to air-trapping ➡, & there are widespread patchy airspace opacities due to aspiration ➡. The bronchial obstruction was due to a small aspirated stone.*

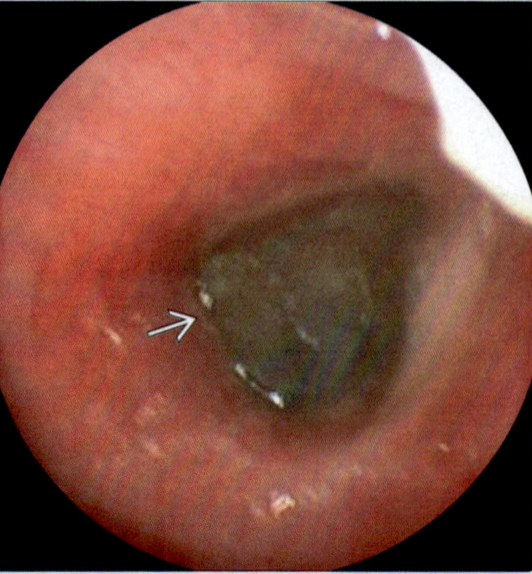

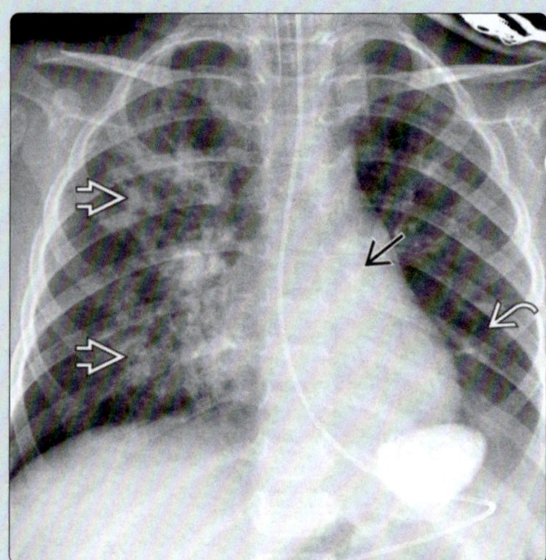

TERMINOLOGY

Synonyms

- Sometimes referred to as LEGO asthma

Definitions

- Complete or partial bronchial occlusion by aspirated foreign body (FB)

IMAGING

General Features

- Best diagnostic clue
  - Visualization of radiopaque FB in airway (rare)
  - Unilateral static lung volume on inspiratory/expiratory or bilateral decubitus chest radiographs
  - Airway filling defect on CT
- Location
  - Most FBs lodge in main bronchi
    - Bronchial (76%), laryngeal (6%), tracheal (4%)
    - Right bronchi (58%) > left bronchi (42%)
      - Due to straighter course & larger caliber of right vs. left main bronchi
- Size
  - Most FB: 5-12 mm

Radiographic Findings

- Radiography
  - Best direct evidence: Radiopaque FB
    - However, most FBs are **not** radiopaque
  - Best indirect evidence is static, unilateral lung volume on inspiration/expiration or bilateral decubitus imaging
  - Volume of affected lung segments can be normal, ↑, or ↓ (i.e., larger lung is not always abnormal)
    - Hyperinflation & oligemia from air-trapping
      - ± depressed hemidiaphragm, widening of intercostal spaces, mediastinal shift toward opposite side
    - Atelectasis from total bronchial obstruction, pneumonia from superinfection
      - ± elevation of hemidiaphragm, narrowing of intercostal spaces, ipsilateral mediastinal shift with atelectasis
  - Pneumothorax & pneumomediastinum from tracheobronchial laceration
  - Reported incidence of chest radiograph findings in FB aspiration (FBA)
    - Normal: 14-35%
    - Hyperinflation: 21-43%
    - Opacification/atelectasis: 18-29%
    - Mediastinal shift: 10-37%
    - Radiopaque FB: 3-23%
- Bilateral decubitus radiographs
  - Obtain frontal view + bilateral decubitus images
  - Normal, nonobstructed lung will become smaller & more opaque when dependent
  - Abnormal, obstructed lung will remain inflated & relatively lucent when dependent
  - Most appropriate maneuver for infants & toddlers who cannot cooperate with inspiratory & expiratory imaging
- Inspiratory/expiratory radiographs
  - In patients who are cooperative, radiographs can be obtained at maximum inspiration & expiration
    - Useful in minority of patients as this clinical scenario most often occurs from 1-2 years of age
  - Volume of nonobstructed lung diminishes significantly with expiration

Fluoroscopic Findings

- Child is fluoroscoped in supine frontal view
  - Normally, both hemidiaphragms will move superiorly & inferiorly in synchronous manner
  - With obstruction, lung volume in affected lung is static with ↓ or no motion of ipsilateral hemidiaphragm
- Fluoroscopy with forced expiration
  - Technique has been described where evaluator places gloved hand on child's abdomen & gently applies pressure immediately prior to & while obtaining image
  - Pressure drives diaphragms superiorly
  - Abnormal side with bronchial obstruction will remain static in volume
  - Normal side will show elevation of diaphragm as compared to initial neutral radiograph
  - Generally not recommended

CT Findings

- CT has not traditionally been utilized in imaging algorithm for suspected FB but used for
  - Persistent lung collapse or pneumonia
  - Work-up of suspected extrinsic airway compression
- Increasing amount of literature supporting low-dose, noncontrast chest CT with multiplanar reconstructions & 3D virtual bronchoscopy in cases with persistent clinical suspicion & negative initial chest radiograph
  - CT is nearly 100% sensitive for radiolucent objects (food, plastic, etc.)
  - May see FB as filling defect in bronchus ± focal hyperinflation or atelectasis
  - May prevent unnecessary negative bronchoscopy (& associated anesthesia)

Imaging Recommendations

- Best imaging tool
  - Initial chest radiographs
  - Traditional next step: Inspiratory/expiratory or bilateral decubitus radiographs or fluoroscopy (for air-trapping)
  - Current consideration: Low-dose noncontrast chest CT has much higher sensitivity/specificity for nonradiopaque FB than radiographs
    - Can also visualize air-trapping

DIFFERENTIAL DIAGNOSIS

Refractory Asthma

- Much more common than bronchial FB
- ↑ peribronchial markings
- Hyperinflation is typically symmetric
- Radiographs may be normal

Viral Lower Respiratory Tract Infection

- Much more common than FB
- ↑ peribronchial markings
- Hyperinflation is typically symmetric

Pulmonary Sling

- Much less common than FB
- Often presents with respiratory distress at birth
  - Due to associated congenital heart disease & complete tracheal rings
- Only vascular ring that results in asymmetric aeration
  - Either side may be larger

Extrinsic Tracheal Compression by Mass

- Bronchogenic cysts, lymphadenopathy, & other masses may compress bronchi & present with asymmetric aeration

Swyer-James Syndrome

- Postinfectious bronchiolitis obliterans
- Asymmetric lung hyperlucency: Lucent lung may be smaller than contralateral lung

Congenital Lobar Overinflation

- Gradually increasing symmetric lung hyperlucency confined to single lobe
- Generally presents in newborn period or early infancy

PATHOLOGY

General Features

- Etiology
  - Young children explore environment with their mouth, often putting discovered items in mouth
  - Young infants may be given FBs or inappropriate foods by older siblings
  - Self-feeding infants have ↑ risk of FBA because gag reflex is undeveloped before age 1
  - Lack of molars & poor swallowing coordination predisposes infants to FBA
  - Older children have tendency to talk, laugh, & be active while chewing
- Mechanism
  - Aspirated FB lodges in bronchus & leads to partial or intermittent obstruction
  - May have ball valve effect, leading to
    - Air-trapping & hyperinflation
    - Complete obstruction leading to atelectasis & collapse
- Typology of FBs
  - Vast majority of aspirated FBs are organic or plastic & therefore radiolucent
    - Most common: Peanuts, tree nuts, & seeds
    - Less common: Fruit, meat, plastic pieces (especially from toys), soil, other radiolucent items
    - Rare: Teeth, small hardware pieces, or other metallic items
  - Older children & teenagers more commonly aspirate nonfood items (pins, needles, paper clips, pen caps, small screws, etc.)

Gross Pathologic & Surgical Features

- FB lodged in tracheobronchial tree
  - Dried foods absorb water & may swell
  - Peanuts & tree nuts elicit airway irritation
  - Leukocyte infiltration & edema in adjacent bronchial wall
  - Chronic FB → granuloma formation/granulation tissue

CLINICAL ISSUES

Presentation

- Most common signs/symptoms
  - Sudden onset of coughing or choking episode
  - Classic triad of coughing, wheezing, & altered breath sounds has high sensitivity (90-95%) but low specificity (25-40%)
  - FBA may present acutely or in delayed fashion; event is often unwitnessed or not remembered until later
    - Same day (25%): Wheezing, cough, ± fever
    - Day 2-7 (45%): Indolent cough, medically refractory wheezing, dyspnea
    - Delayed by > 1 week (30%): Same as aforementioned

Demographics

- Age
  - Most common age: 1-3 years; peak: 18 months
- Sex
  - FBA is more common in boys (2:1)

Natural History & Prognosis

- High degree of suspicion is important
- Delay in diagnosis is associated with ↑ risk of major complications
  - Incidence of major complications is low if rapidly diagnosed
  - Complications: 4% at > 4 days, 91% > 30 days
- Complications of chronic FBs
  - Bronchopulmonary fistula, bronchial rupture, damage to distal lung
- Death is rare, ~ 100 per year in USA
  - In one series of 2,165 pediatric autopsies, only 10 deaths are due to FBA

Treatment

- Endobronchial removal of FB

DIAGNOSTIC CHECKLIST

Image Interpretation Pearls

- Unilateral static lung/lobe volume at different phases of respiratory cycle is suggestive

SELECTED REFERENCES

1. Chand R et al: Frequency of various foreign bodies retrieved from the airway during bronchoscopy in children: a pediatric tertiary care center experience. Cureus. 12(7):e9348, 2020
2. Ding G et al: Tracheobronchial foreign body aspiration in children: a retrospective single-center cross-sectional study. Medicine (Baltimore). 99(22):e20480, 2020
3. Gibbons AT et al: Avoiding unnecessary bronchoscopy in children with suspected foreign body aspiration using computed tomography. J Pediatr Surg. 55(1):176-81, 2020
4. Gordon L et al: Diagnosis of foreign body aspiration with ultralow-dose CT using a tin filter: a comparison study. Emerg Radiol. 27(4):399-404, 2020
5. Özyüksel G et al: Foreign body aspiration in infants: role of self-feeding. Pediatr Allergy Immunol Pulmonol. 32(2):52-5, 2019
6. Wu X et al: Fatal choking in infants and children treated in a pediatric intensive care unit: A 7- year experience. Int J Pediatr Otorhinolaryngol. 110:67-9, 2018
7. Baram A et al: Tracheobronchial foreign bodies in children: the role of emergency rigid bronchoscopy. Glob Pediatr Health. 4:2333794X17743663, 2017
8. Hanba C et al: Consumer product ingestion and aspiration in children: a 15-year review. Laryngoscope. 127(5):1202-1207, 2017

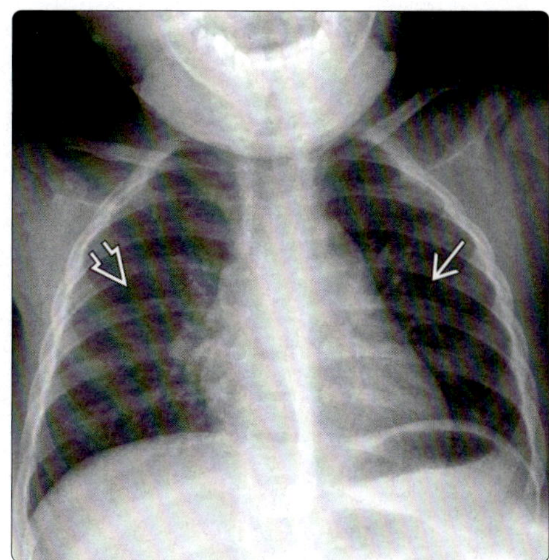

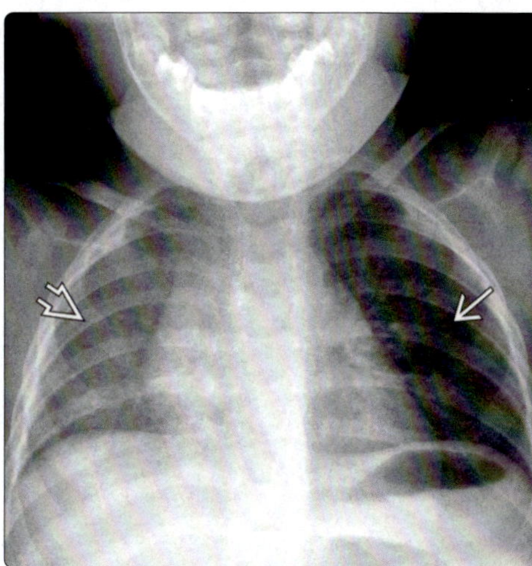

(Left) *Inspiratory upright frontal chest radiograph in a toddler with acute respiratory distress demonstrates subtle relative lucency of the left lung* ➡ *compared to the right* ➡. **(Right)** *Expiratory PA chest radiograph in the same patient demonstrates a static volume & persistent hyperlucency of the left lung* ➡ *compared to the right* ➡. *In the correct clinical setting, static lung/lobe volume on inspiratory & expiratory or bilateral decubitus chest radiographs is very suggestive of air-trapping due to foreign body aspiration.*

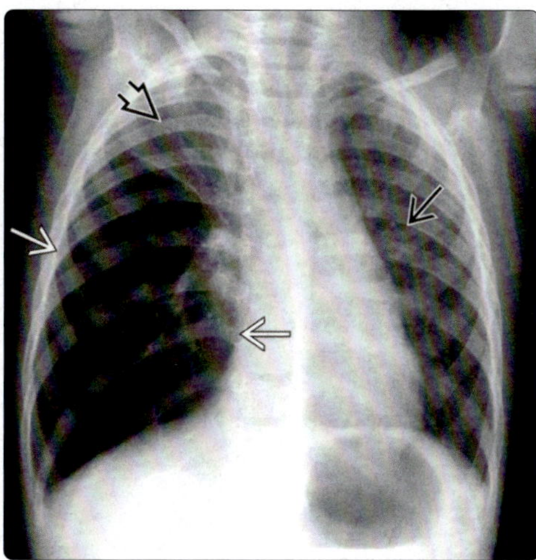

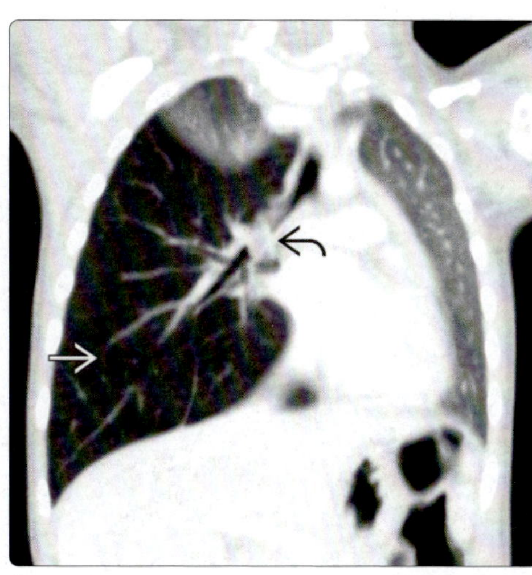

(Left) *PA chest radiograph shows asymmetric hyperexpansion & lucency in the right middle & lower lobes* ➡ *with relative ↑ opacity in the right upper lobe* ➡ *& left lung* ➡. **(Right)** *Coronal oblique CECT reconstruction in the same patient shows that the right middle lobe (RML) & right lower lobe air-trapping* ➡ *was due to a foreign body occluding the bronchus intermedius* ➡.

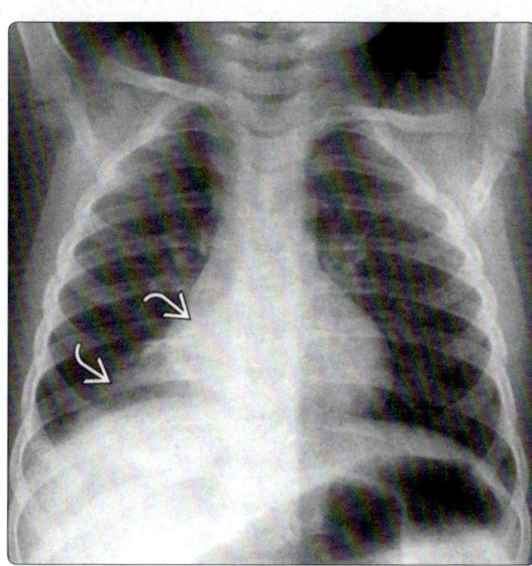

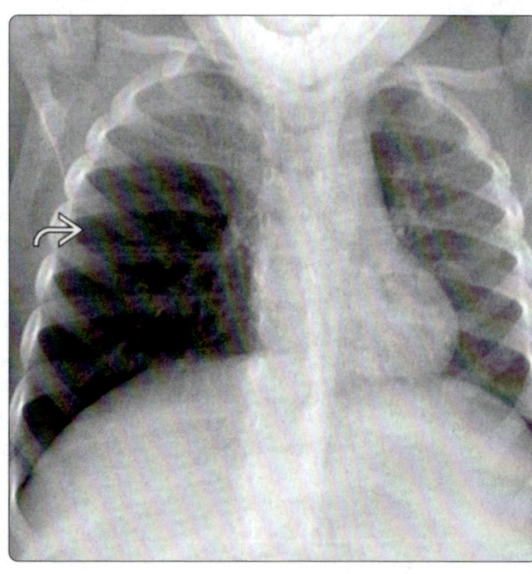

(Left) *Frontal chest radiograph in a coughing 2-year-old patient who aspirated a peanut (unrecognized at the time) shows opacity & volume loss in the RML* ➡*, presumed to be atelectasis in the setting of viral airway disease.* **(Right)** *AP radiograph in the same child 3 months later shows RML hyperlucency & oligemia due to air-trapping* ➡. *During bronchoscopy, an old peanut was found in the RML bronchus. Depending on the degree of bronchial occlusion, a foreign body may cause atelectasis, hyperexpansion, or a changing picture over time.*

Cystic Fibrosis, Pulmonary

KEY FACTS

TERMINOLOGY

- Cystic fibrosis (CF): Autosomal recessive multisystem disorder caused by dysfunctional chloride ion transport across epithelial surfaces → thickening of secretions (e.g., mucus, digestive fluids, sweat)
- In lungs, abnormal mucus & degraded WBCs → chronic airway impaction → recurrent inflammation & infections → chronic airway damage (in progressively worsening cycle)

IMAGING

- Most common in upper lobes, superior lower lobes
  - Peribronchial thickening (early finding)
  - Mosaic attenuation due to air-trapping, best seen on expiratory scan
  - Bronchiectasis with signet ring sign (bronchus larger than adjacent artery)
  - Mucus plugging within dilated bronchi (finger-in-glove appearance)
  - "Tree-in-bud" centrilobular nodular opacities

PATHOLOGY

- Most common lethal genetic disorder in White patients
  - ~ 1 in 2,500 affected
- Mutation in both copies of CF transmembrane conductance regulator (*CFTR*) gene at chromosome 7q31.2 → defective chloride transport → abnormal water regulation
- > 2,000 genetic defects can result in CF; ΔF508 mutation of *CFTR* is most common (~ 90%)

CLINICAL ISSUES

- 70% present < 1-year-old: GI symptoms are more common
- 90% by 12-years-old: Respiratory is more typical
  - Often have asthma-type symptoms
- Median survival: 41.1 years

DIAGNOSTIC CHECKLIST

- Annual chest radiograph or low-dose surveillance CT
  - CT best assesses progressive disease & predicts future exacerbations vs. pulmonary function tests, radiographs

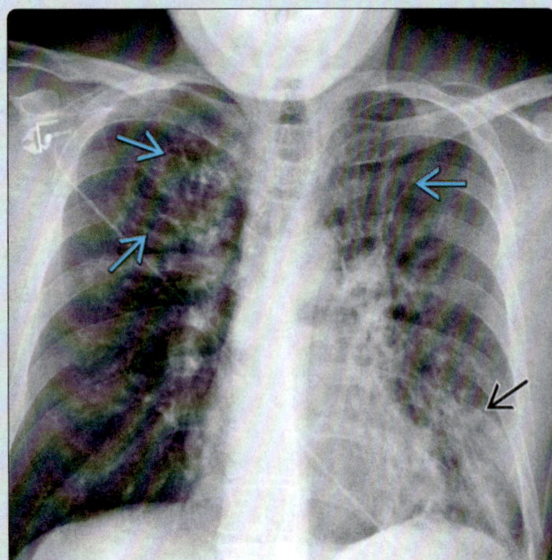

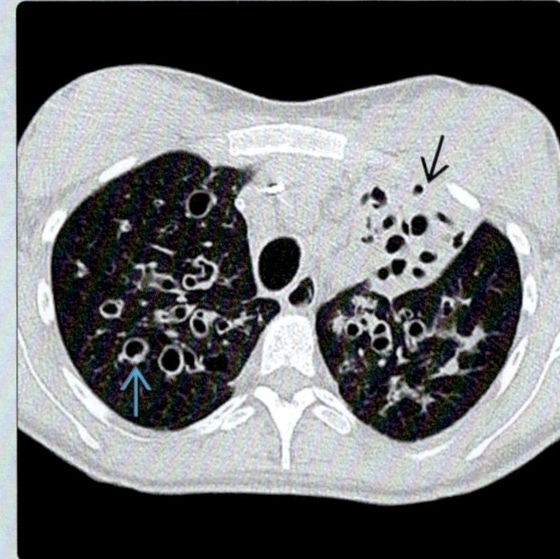

(Left) *Frontal radiograph in a patient with cystic fibrosis (CF) shows prominent bronchiectasis → in the upper lobes + left lower lobe consolidation with nodularity →.* **(Right)** *Axial NECT in a CF patient shows bilateral upper lobe bronchiectasis with consolidation → of the anterior segment of the left upper lobe. Note the signet ring sign (or pearl ring sign) → in the right upper lobe with the dilated bronchus forming the ring & the adjacent artery forming the attached jewel.*

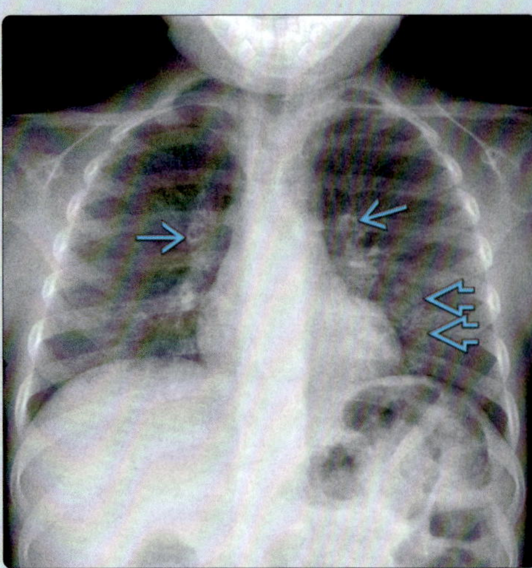

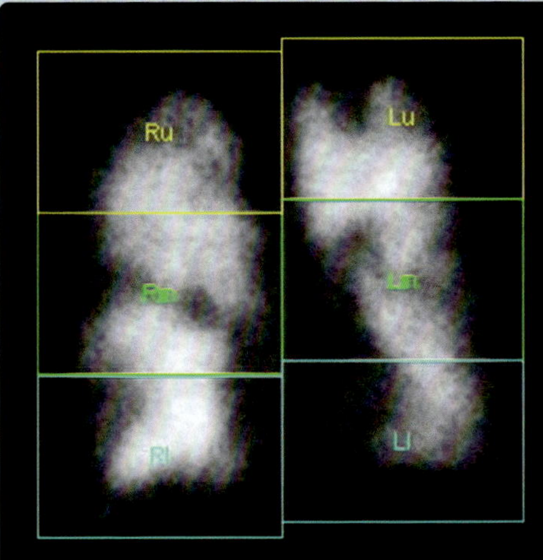

(Left) *Frontal radiograph in the chest in a 7-year-old with CF shows mild peribronchial thickening → in the perihilar regions, an early finding of CF that is indistinguishable from common viral bronchiolitis. Additional peribronchial thickening is seen in the left base →.* **(Right)** *Anterior Tc-99m MAA arterial perfusion scan in a patient with CF shows multifocal perfusion defects in the lungs bilaterally. Perfusion abnormalities may be the earliest findings in patients with CF.*

TERMINOLOGY

Abbreviations

- Cystic fibrosis (CF)

Definitions

- Autosomal recessive multisystem disorder caused by dysfunctional chloride ion transport across epithelial surfaces → thickening of secretions (e.g., mucus, digestive fluids, sweat)

IMAGING

General Features

- Best diagnostic clue
  - Upper lobe-predominant bronchiectasis & bronchial wall thickening in child with respiratory (± GI) symptoms
- Location
  - In lungs, more common in upper lobes & superior segments of lower lobes
  - Also affects sinuses, pancreas, hepatobiliary system, GI tract, & sex organs

Radiographic Findings

- Radiographs are insensitive to early changes of CF
- Late changes on radiographs include bronchiectasis, bronchial wall thickening, mucoid impaction, hyperinflation, lobar collapse, & pulmonary arterial enlargement due to pulmonary artery hypertension
- ± microcardia with chronic pulmonary hyperinflation
- ± abdominal manifestations visible on chest radiographs
  - Dilated bowel in newborn with meconium ileus
  - Ca^{2+} in newborn peritoneum if complicated meconium ileus → perforation → meconium peritonitis
  - Ca^{2+} over upper abdomen in older children & adolescents with chronic pancreatitis

CT Findings

- HRCT
  - Peribronchial thickening (early finding)
  - Bronchiectasis with signet ring sign
    - Ectatic bronchus > adjacent pulmonary artery
  - Mosaic attenuation due to air-trapping, best seen on expiratory scan
  - "Tree-in-bud" centrilobular nodular opacities
    - Bronchiolar impaction of mucus &/or infectious/inflammatory debris
  - Finger-in-glove appearance of mucus plugging within dilated bronchi
  - Other findings include: Emphysema, multifocal atelectasis, sacculations, & bullae
  - ± lymphadenopathy
- CTA
  - May show bronchial artery hypertrophy &/or aberrant/collateral arterial supply in setting of hemoptysis
  - Useful in CF patients with pulmonary hypertension to evaluate size dimensions of PA & RV

MR Findings

- Pulmonary MR ± inhaled hyperpolarized gas
  - May yield imaging results comparable to CT
  - May be able to detect early mucus plug & differentiate mucoid impaction from atelectasis
  - Phase-contrast imaging
    - Volume of flow to each lung may be calculated
    - ↑ aortopulmonary collateral flow may precede lung function decline
  - Functional cardiac information & ventricular volumes may be obtained
    - Phase-contrast imaging may be obtained to evaluate for pulmonic regurgitation from pulmonary hypertension (HTN)
    - Volumes & cine imaging to evaluate degree of RV dysfunction from pulmonary HTN

Ultrasonographic Findings

- Useful in evaluating pleural effusions
- Not helpful in lung evaluation in CF

Angiographic Findings

- Bronchial arteriography to detect (± embolize) source of pulmonary hemorrhage/hemoptysis

Nuclear Medicine Findings

- Normal chest radiograph with normal Tc-99m perfusion scan essentially excludes bronchiectasis
  - Nuclear medicine perfusion is more sensitive for detection of early disease in patients with CF
    - Multifocal perfusion defects are typically seen

Imaging Recommendations

- Best imaging tool
  - High-resolution CT with full inspiration & expiration

DIFFERENTIAL DIAGNOSIS

Asthma

- Peribronchial thickening & hyperinflation are common but without bronchiectasis

Allergic Bronchopulmonary Aspergillosis

- Findings overlap CF; allergic bronchopulmonary aspergillosis (ABPA) often complicates CF
- Other causes of ABPA include refractory asthma, tuberculosis, sarcoidosis, infectious pneumonia, Churg-Strauss syndrome

Ciliary Dyskinesia

- Abnormal ciliary movement (not abnormally thick secretions) is responsible for mucus accumulation
- Basilar predominant bronchial wall thickening, bronchiectasis
- Situs inversus & sinus disease in Kartagener syndrome

Tracheobronchomegaly (Mounier-Kuhn Syndrome)

- Rare congenital disorder with abnormal widening of upper airways

Williams-Campbell Syndrome

- Cystic bronchiectasis with bronchomalacia due to defective bronchial cartilage

PATHOLOGY

General Features

- Mutation in both copies of CF transmembrane conductance regulator (*CFTR*) gene at chromosome 7q31.2
  - > 2,000 genetic defects can result in CF; ΔF508 mutation is most common (~ 90%)
- CFTR protein malfunction → lack of chloride ion secretion → ↑ sodium retention & fluid resorption → ↑ viscosity of luminal secretions → obstruction of ducts of solid organs & hollow viscera
- In lungs, abnormal mucus & WBC degradation products (including DNA) → stasis in airways → recurrent infection & inflammation → chronic airway damage with worsening susceptibility to infection & inflammation

Gross Pathologic & Surgical Features

- Diffuse bronchiectasis & peribronchial thickening is seen on gross specimen
- Mucosal thickening of paranasal sinuses with polyposis

CLINICAL ISSUES

Presentation

- Most common signs/symptoms
  - 1st symptoms may be delayed passage of meconium with bowel obstruction ± perforation in newborn with meconium ileus
  - In childhood, patients often look similar to asthma patients, presenting with chronic cough & wheezing
- Other signs/symptoms
  - Chronic constipation
  - Recurrent pancreatitis
  - Hepatobiliary disease
  - Clubbing of fingers & toes
- Clinical profile
  - Most detected on neonatal screening
  - After symptom development, testing by sweat chloride (> 60 mEq/mL = positive for CF)

Demographics

- Age
  - 70% present < 1 year: GI symptoms are more common
  - 90% by 12 years: Respiratory is more typical
- Epidemiology
  - Most common lethal gene defect in White patients (1 in 2,500 affected)
    - Much less common in patients with African or Asian ancestry

Natural History & Prognosis

- Infancy: Often only mild or absent pulmonary symptoms
- Early childhood: Presents similar to asthma with cough, wheezing, & bronchitis
- Late childhood & adolescence: Recurrent pneumonias, bronchitis, & bronchiectasis with mucus plugging
- End-stage lung disease occurs at variable ages but often in late adolescence to early adulthood
- Exact timing of progression in CF is unpredictable
- Complications of CF lung disease
  - Recurrent infections are most common complication: > 1/2 develop infection with *Pseudomonas aeruginosa*
  - Allergic bronchopulmonary aspergillosis
  - Pneumothorax & pneumomediastinum
  - Hemoptysis
  - Bullous emphysema
  - Cor pulmonale
- Median survival: 41.1 years

Treatment

- Goal: ↓ lung damage from mucus plugging & infection
- Various internal & external airway clearance techniques
- Prophylactic antibiotics to ↓ chance of infection
- ± long-term IV (Port-a-Cath) for recurrent lung infections
- New medicines targeted at specific *CFTR* mutations
- ± lobectomy for patients with single lobe complications
- End-stage lung disease may require lung transplantation
  - Both lungs are typically transplanted to avoid infection of new lung from native lung
  - Clinical parameters typically guide transplantation

DIAGNOSTIC CHECKLIST

Consider

- Annual chest radiograph or low-dose CT surveillance of bronchiectasis complications
- Pulmonary MR is showing promise for future utility

Image Interpretation Pearls

- CT is more accurate in assessing progressive lung disease than pulmonary function tests or radiographs
- CT improves with treatment of acute exacerbations
- Brody CT score predicts future pulmonary exacerbations better than initial FEV_1; scoring is based on
  - Extent of bronchiectasis
  - Size of abnormally dilated bronchi
  - Peribronchial thickening
  - Parenchymal involvement, including consolidation, ground-glass opacity, cysts, & bullae
  - Hyperinflation

SELECTED REFERENCES

1. Bayfield KJ et al: Time to get serious about the detection and monitoring of early lung disease in cystic fibrosis. Thorax. ePub, 2021
2. Dournes G et al: The clinical use of lung MRI in cystic fibrosis: what, now, how? Chest. 159(6):2205-17, 2021
3. Joyce S et al: Computed tomography in cystic fibrosis lung disease: a focus on radiation exposure. Pediatr Radiol. 51(4):544-53, 2021
4. Serai SD et al: Pediatric lung MRI: currently available and emerging techniques. AJR Am J Roentgenol. 216(3):781-90, 2021
5. Heidenreich JF et al: Three-dimensional ultrashort echo time MRI for functional lung imaging in cystic fibrosis. Radiology. 296(1):191-9, 2020
6. Robinson TE et al: Mucus plugging, air trapping, and bronchiectasis are important outcome measures in assessing progressive childhood cystic fibrosis lung disease. Pediatr Pulmonol. 55(4):929-38, 2020
7. Strzelczuk-Judka L et al: Diagnostic value of chest ultrasound in children with cystic fibrosis - pilot study. PLoS One. 14(7):e0215786, 2019
8. Breuer O et al: Predicting disease progression in cystic fibrosis. Expert Rev Respir Med. 12(11):905-17, 2018
9. Pennati F et al: Assessment of pulmonary structure-function relationships in young children and adolescents with cystic fibrosis by multivolume proton-MRI and CT. J Magn Reson Imaging. 48(2):531-42, 2018
10. Kuo W et al: Objective airway artery dimensions compared to CT scoring methods assessing structural cystic fibrosis lung disease. J Cyst Fibros. 16(1):116-23, 2017
11. Rosenow T et al: Air trapping in early cystic fibrosis lung disease-does CT tell the full story? Pediatr Pulmonol. 52(9):1150-6, 2017
12. Scholz O et al: MRI of cystic fibrosis lung manifestations: sequence evaluation and clinical outcome analysis. Clin Radiol. 72(9):754-63, 2017

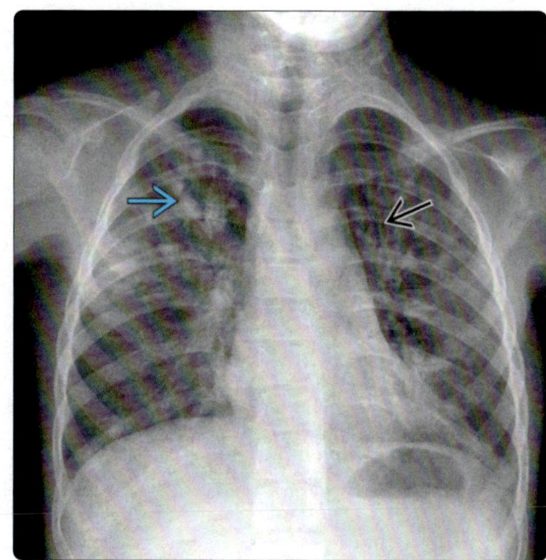

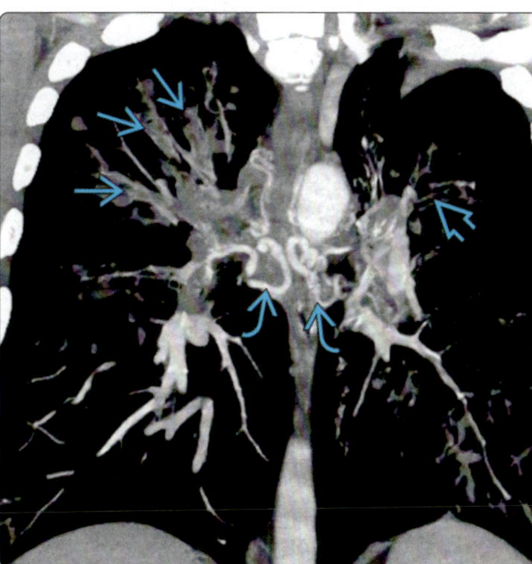

(Left) *Frontal view of the chest in a 7-year-old girl with CF shows thick tubular & nodular densities* ➔ *in the right upper lobe. Note the bronchiectasis* ➔ *in the left upper lobe. Mucus impacted in the dilated bronchi is referred to as the finger-in-glove appearance.* **(Right)** *Coronal CECT MIP in a patient with CF shows mucus impacted in the dilated bronchi* ➔ *in the right upper lobe, which is known as the finger-in-glove appearance. Also note the bronchiectasis in the left upper lobe* ➔ *as well as the dilated bronchial arteries* ➔*.*

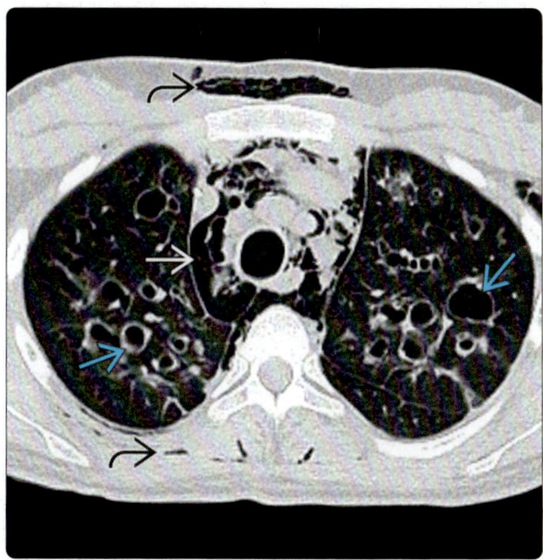

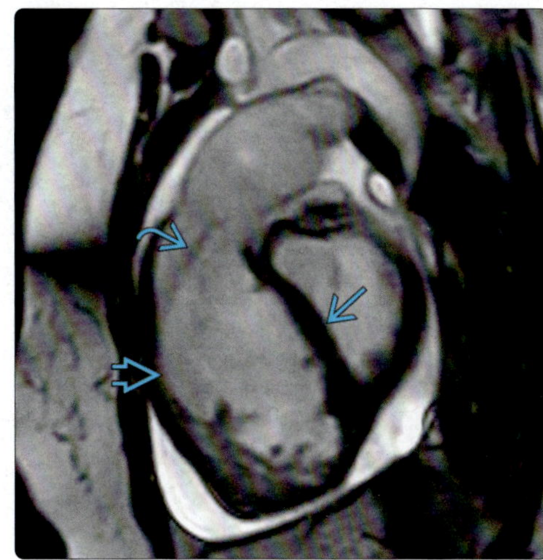

(Left) *Axial HRCT from a CF patient shows pneumomediastinum* ➔ *& subcutaneous emphysema* ➔*. Note the prominent bronchiectasis* ➔ *in the upper lobes bilaterally.* **(Right)** *Sagittal SSFP bright blood MR in a patient with CF & pulmonary hypertension shows an enlarged right ventricle (RV)* ➔ *& pulmonary artery. There is deviation/flattening* ➔ *of the interventricular septum from ↑ RV pressure. Also note the dephasing artifact from the pulmonic regurgitation* ➔*.*

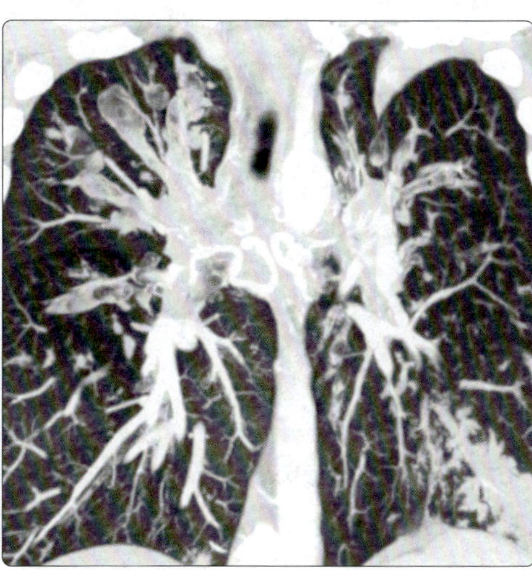

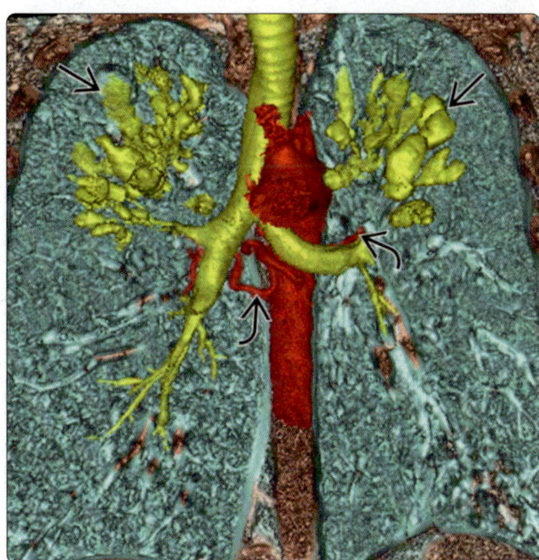

(Left) *Coronal chest CTA in a patient with CF shows bronchiectasis & mucus-filled bronchi in the upper lobes with a left lower lobe consolidation.* **(Right)** *Color-coded, volume-rendered chest CTA in a patient with CF shows upper lobe bronchiectasis* ➔*. Also note the enlarged bronchial artery collaterals* ➔ *arising from the descending thoracic aorta.*

Chronic Esophageal Foreign Body

KEY FACTS

TERMINOLOGY

- Foreign body in esophagus for prolonged period of time

IMAGING

- Foreign body may or may not be radiopaque
- Airway narrowing suggests chronicity
  - Airway displaced anteriorly
  - Proximal esophagus may be dilated
- May present with complications: Abscess, pneumomediastinum, or pneumothorax
- Most common site: Upper esophagus at thoracic inlet
  - 2nd most common site: Level of carina & aortic arch
- Coins are most commonly swallowed foreign body
  - Button batteries show characteristic double-density (2-layer) periphery
- Imaging recommendations
  - Frontal & lateral chest radiographs are best initial study; include nasal cavity on lateral airway view if respiratory symptoms present
  - Esophagram for nonradiopaque foreign bodies
  - CECT vs. MR to diagnose complications, such as abscess, mediastinitis, aortic wall injury

CLINICAL ISSUES

- Respiratory/airway or feeding symptoms are most common
  - Cough, stridor, fever, wheezing
- Removal success rate is 95-100% regardless of technique
- Use endoscopy immediately for batteries in esophagus
  - Batteries quickly cause damage by pressure against wall of esophagus, leakage of caustic alkali, & generation of electrical current
  - Aortic wall inflammation can lead to delayed rupture & exsanguination; NASPGHAN guidelines recommend serial cross-sectional imaging
- Foreign bodies present for > 24 hours have ↑ risk of esophageal perforation

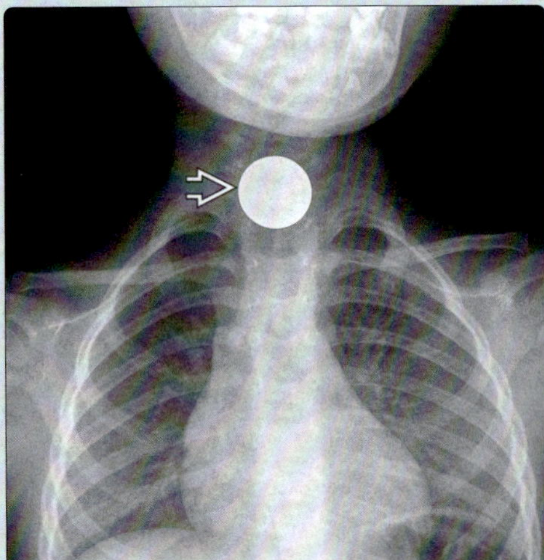

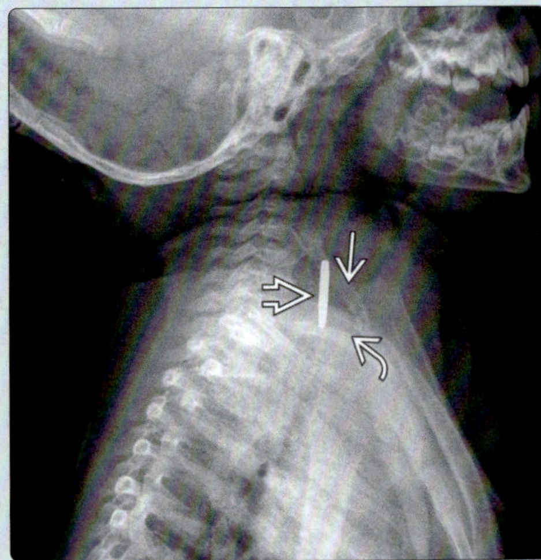

(Left) *AP radiograph of the chest shows a round, homogeneous metallic foreign body at the level of the thoracic inlet ➡, consistent with the history of a swallowed coin. This is the most common location for an esophageal foreign body.* **(Right)** *Lateral radiograph of the upper chest & neck shows an esophageal foreign body ➡. Note the narrowing of the trachea ➡ with soft tissue swelling around the metallic foreign body ➡.*

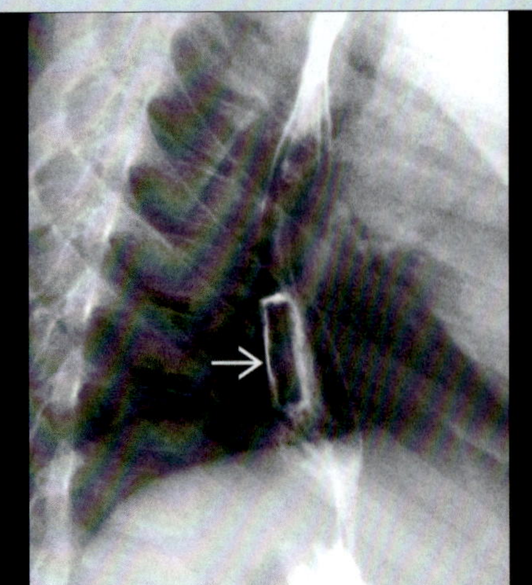

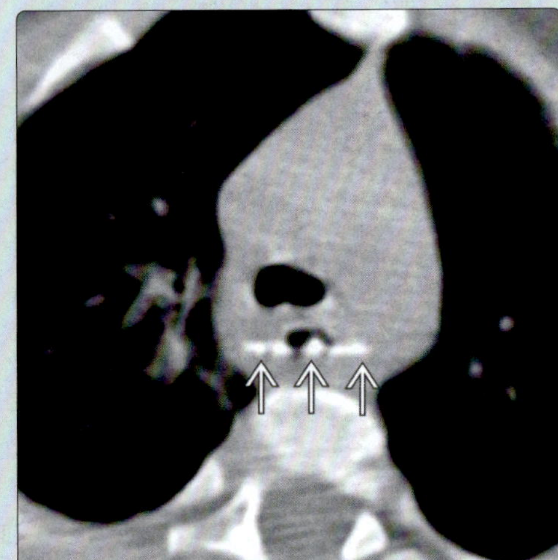

(Left) *Lateral esophagram shows a Scrabble piece ➡ outlined by barium in an 11-year-old who had symptoms of esophagitis for the past week. He denied swallowing anything.* **(Right)** *Axial NECT after a contrast esophagram demonstrates a localized leak ➡ into the mediastinum secondary to an esophageal perforation that occurred during the removal of coins in the esophagus.*

IMAGING

General Features

- Best diagnostic clue
  - Radiopaque object in region of esophagus
  - High suspicion for chronicity when airway is narrowed &/or anteriorly displaced
  - May present with complications: Abscess, pneumomediastinum, pneumothorax
- Location
  - Most common site: Upper esophagus at thoracic inlet
  - 2nd most common site: Level of carina & aortic arch from physiologic narrowing
  - 3rd most common site: Distal esophagus slightly above gastroesophageal junction
- Morphology
  - Coins are most commonly swallowed foreign body
    - Coins in esophagus will usually appear in coronal plane (en face) on frontal view
  - Button batteries show characteristic double-density (2-layer) shadow at periphery
    - Laterally, edges are rounded with step-off at junction of positive & negative terminals
    - Important to identify since batteries can cause caustic burn injury to esophagus in little time
  - Nonradiopaque foreign body
    - Hot dog & plastic toys are common

Radiographic Findings

- Radiography
  - Radiopaque foreign body in esophagus
    - Entirety or portion of foreign body may be radiolucent
  - Lateral view shows soft tissue thickening anterior to esophagus with displacement, bowing, & narrowing of trachea
    - Indicative of chronic inflammation & predictive of more difficult removal of foreign body

Fluoroscopic Findings

- Esophagram
  - Useful for detecting nonradiopaque foreign bodies
  - May diagnose stricture, fistula, or perforation

CT Findings

- CECT
  - Postremoval CT: Esophageal leak, diverticulum, mediastinitis/abscess; inflammation or injury of aorta if battery or sharp object is removed

MR Findings

- Some institutions use MR after battery removal rather than CECT/CTA

Imaging Recommendations

- Best imaging tool
  - AP & lateral chest radiograph is best initial study
    - Include nasal cavity with respiratory symptoms
  - Esophagram for nonradiopaque foreign bodies
  - CECT vs. MR to diagnose complications

DIFFERENTIAL DIAGNOSIS

Airway Obstruction/Inflammation

- May simulate foreign body in esophagus

Achalasia

- Failure of normal relaxation of lower esophageal sphincter

CLINICAL ISSUES

Presentation

- Most common signs/symptoms
  - Respiratory or airway problems are most common
    - Cough, stridor, fever, wheezing
    - Chronic upper respiratory infection or pneumonia
    - Hemoptysis, choking, cyanosis
  - GI symptoms
    - Dysphagia, drooling, vomiting, gagging
  - Chest pain when swallowing
  - Fever of unknown origin

Demographics

- Age
  - Most < 5 years; typically 8 months to 2 years

Natural History & Prognosis

- Foreign bodies present for > 24 hours have ↑ risk of esophageal perforation
- Vast majority of ingested objects pass through GI tract without problems

Treatment

- Removal success rate is 95-100% regardless of technique
- Strategy depends on type, location, & duration
- General complications prior to or without treatment
  - Most common complication: Perforation & subsequent mediastinitis
  - Rare complications include tracheoesophageal fistula & aortoesophageal fistula
- Endoscopy or surgery
  - Use urgently for sharp or irregular objects & unknown foreign bodies
    - Removal following morning after detection is acceptable
  - Use urgently for batteries in esophagus
    - Cause damage by pressure against wall of esophagus, leakage of caustic alkali, & electrical current
    - Reports of exsanguination (even delayed) due to inflammation of aortic wall by battery have led to NASPGHAN guidelines for serial cross-sectional imaging after battery removal

SELECTED REFERENCES

1. Grey NEO et al: Magnetic resonance imaging findings following button battery ingestion. Pediatr Radiol. 51(10):1856-66, 2021
2. Dipasquale V et al: Managing pediatric foreign body ingestions: a 10-year experience. Pediatr Emerg Care. ePub, 2020
3. Ergun E et al: An algorithm for retrieval tools in foreign body ingestion and food impaction in children. Dis Esophagus. 34(1), 2020
4. Esparaz JR et al: Esophageal foreign body management in children: can it wait? J Laparoendosc Adv Surg Tech A. 30(12):1286-8, 2020
5. Riedesel EL et al: Serial MRI findings after endoscopic removal of button battery from the esophagus. AJR Am J Roentgenol. 215(5):1238-46, 2020

Sickle Cell Disease, Acute Chest Syndrome

KEY FACTS

TERMINOLOGY

- New pulmonary opacity on chest radiograph + ≥ 1 additional symptom (such as fever, cough, sputum production, tachypnea, dyspnea, or hypoxia) in setting of sickle cell disease (SCD)

IMAGING

- Upper & middle lobe opacities are more common in children
- Lower lobe disease is more common in adults
- Initial chest radiograph may be normal (46%)
  - Opacity may not appear until 2-3 days after symptoms develop
- Opacities on CT may be more extensive than on radiograph

PATHOLOGY

- Potential causes: Infection (30%), pulmonary fat embolism (9%), pulmonary infarction (18%), & rib infarction

CLINICAL ISSUES

- Acute chest syndrome (ACS) is most common in patients aged 5-9 years; incidence ↓ with age
  - Fever, cough, & tachypnea are most common symptoms in patients < 10 years of age
  - Pain (chest, extremity, abdominal) is more common in adolescents & adults
- ACS is 2nd most common cause of hospitalization in patients with SCD
- ACS is most common cause of premature death in patients with SCD
  - Mortality is 4-9x higher in adults than in children
- Treatment
  - Supportive: Oxygen, antibiotics, pain control, IV fluids, incentive spirometry, & blood transfusions
  - Prevention: Pneumococcal vaccine, *Haemophilus influenzae* vaccine, & hydroxyurea

(Left) *AP radiograph of the chest in an adolescent with sickle cell disease (SCD) & acute chest syndrome (ACS) shows a poorly defined opacity in the right lower lobe ➪ with consolidation in the left lower lobe ➪. The lungs are hypoinflated, & the heart is mildly enlarged.* **(Right)** *Axial CECT in the same patient with ACS shows consolidation in the lung bases bilaterally. Note the cardiomegaly from chronic anemia.*

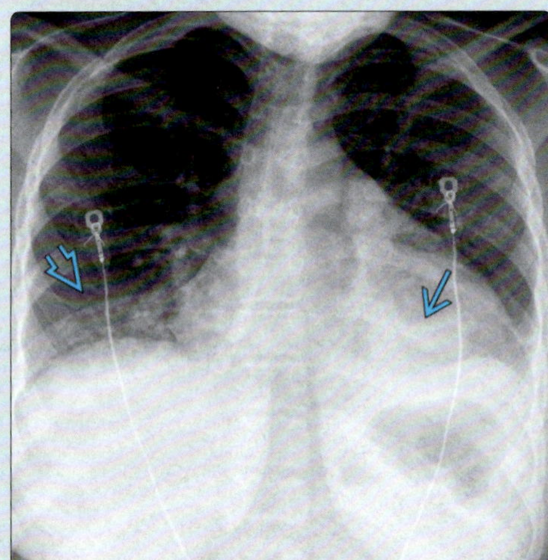

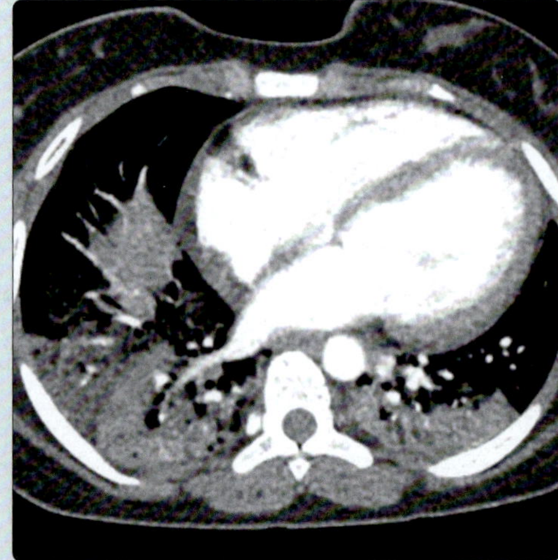

(Left) *Axial CECT in lung window in the same patient shows consolidation ➪ & ground-glass opacity ➪ in right worse than left lung bases.* **(Right)** *PA chest radiograph in an adolescent with SCD & ACS shows low lung volumes with a streaky opacity ➪ in the left lower lobe. Note the cardiomegaly, cholecystectomy clips, & absent splenic shadow (replaced by bowel gas ➪). There is also a biconcave appearance of the vertebral bodies & sclerosis of the humeral heads due to bone infarctions.*

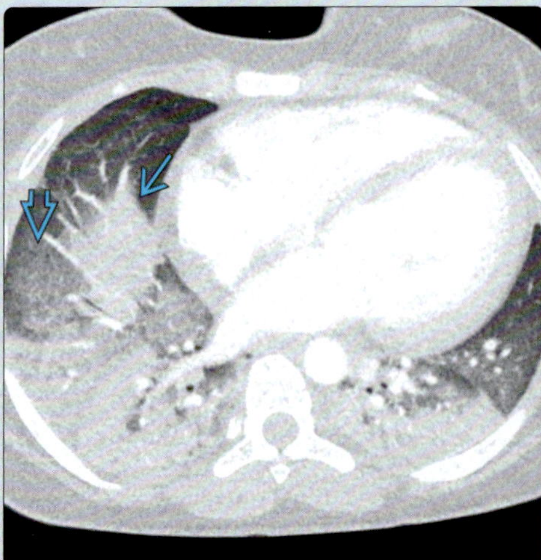

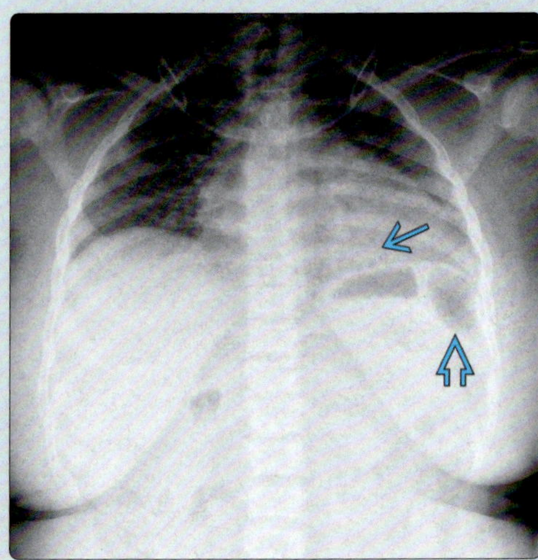

TERMINOLOGY

Abbreviations

- Acute chest syndrome (ACS)
- Sickle cell disease (SCD)

Definitions

- New pulmonary opacity on chest radiograph + ≥ 1 additional symptom (such as fever, cough, sputum production, tachypnea, dyspnea, or hypoxia) in setting of SCD

IMAGING

General Features

- Best diagnostic clue
  - Pulmonary opacity in patient with SCD who has fever & respiratory symptoms
- Location
  - Upper & middle lobe involvement is more common in children
  - Lower lobe disease is more common in adults
- Size
  - Variable: May be segmental, lobar, or multilobar consolidation

Radiographic Findings

- Radiography
  - ACS
    - Initial chest radiograph may be normal (46%)
      - Radiograph lags behind physiological changes
      - Opacity may not appear until 2-3 days after symptoms develop
    - Opacity mimics pneumonia ± volume loss
    - Pleural effusions in > 50% of patients
  - Other findings of SCD
    - Cardiomegaly due to chronic anemia
    - Avascular necrosis/sclerosis of humeral heads
    - H-shaped or biconcave vertebrae
    - Enlarged ribs due to marrow expansion
    - Small splenic shadow (autosplenectomy) with lateralization of stomach bubble
    - Cholecystectomy clips in right upper quadrant

CT Findings

- NECT
  - Limited clinical use for ACS
  - Can have consolidation or ground-glass opacity
    - Opacities may be more extensive than on radiograph
  - Simplification of lung with ↓ vascularity
  - Pleural effusion is common
  - May see healed bone infarcts
- HRCT
  - Mosaic perfusion due to microvascular occlusion
  - Sequelae of ACS
    - Parenchymal bands & interlobular septal thickening
    - Peripheral wedge-shaped opacities
    - Architectural distortion
    - Traction bronchiectasis
- CTA
  - Pulmonary embolism is 3rd most common cause of ACS
    - Accounts for 16-17% of ACS episodes
    - Occurs in segmental or subsegmental pulmonary arteries
    - No associated lower extremity deep vein thrombosis
  - Dual energy CT can be used to make pulmonary blood volume maps
    - Higher number of iodine defects in ACS vs. controls
    - More prevalent than pulmonary opacities
    - Likely due to early microvascular changes

Nuclear Medicine Findings

- Bone scan
  - Foci of abnormal radiotracer uptake in ribs
    - ↓ or ↑ uptake: Acute or subacute bone infarcts
  - May have other bone infarcts vs. osteomyelitis
- V/Q scan
  - Limited clinical use in ACS
  - Can see perfusion defect
    - May mimic pulmonary embolism
  - Defects often resolve quickly with supportive therapy

Imaging Recommendations

- Best imaging tool
  - Chest radiograph for evaluation of pulmonary opacity
  - Pulmonary CTA if concern for pulmonary embolism
- Protocol advice
  - Routine frontal & lateral chest radiographs
  - Repeat chest radiograph in 48-72 hours if clinical concern is high as initial chest radiograph is often normal

DIFFERENTIAL DIAGNOSIS

Bacterial Pneumonia

- Clinically similar to ACS with fever, leukocytosis, pleuritic chest pain, pleural effusion, & productive cough
- Multilobar involvement & recurrent opacities are more common in SCD
- Clinical symptoms & radiographic abnormalities can be prolonged, lasting 10-12 days

Viral Chest Infection

- Viral infection causes 6-8% of ACS
  - Respiratory syncytial virus (RSV) is common

Pulmonary Infarction

- ~ 50% of cases in patients with SCD are caused by fat embolism
- Vascular occlusion by sickle cells is also important cause of ACS
- Usually diagnosis of exclusion

Asthma

- Significant comorbidity in patients with SCD; may be underdiagnosed in SCD
  - 73-78% of patients with SCD have airway hyperactivity
  - Patients diagnosed with asthma have 4-6x greater risk of developing ACS

PATHOLOGY

General Features

- Etiology
  - ACS may be multifactorial

- Infection is most common cause of ACS in children
- 50% of adult patients are initially admitted with vasoocclusive crisis causing pain
- Infection
  - Documented in 38-54% of cases
  - Most common pathogens: *Chlamydia pneumoniae* (7.2%), *Mycoplasma pneumoniae* (6.6%), RSV (6.4%)
  - Pulmonary opacity persists longer than cases where infection is not documented
- Pulmonary fat embolism
  - Cause of ACS in 9-16%
  - Etiology: Vasoocclusive crisis → edema & infarction of marrow compartment → marrow necrosis → fat cells enter venous bloodstream → embolize in branches of pulmonary artery
  - Frequently have bone pain
  - Lab findings: Thrombocytopenia, anemia; ↑ LDH, lipase, phospholipase A2, & uric acid; ↓ serum calcium
  - Diagnosis is supported by lipid-laden macrophages in bronchoalveolar lavage fluid
- Pulmonary infarction
  - Cause of ACS in 16-17%
  - Occurs in segmental & subsegmental pulmonary arteries
  - No associated lower extremity deep vein thrombosis suggests in situ thrombosis
- Rib infarction with hypoventilation from pain &/or analgesics
  - High correlation between rib infarction & pulmonary opacity
  - Pain may lead to splinting & atelectasis
  - Incentive spirometry helps prevent pulmonary complications of ACS
  - Analgesics may ↓ splinting but may cause hypoventilation

CLINICAL ISSUES

Presentation

- Most common signs/symptoms
  - Fever, cough, & tachypnea are most common in patients < 10 years of age
  - Pain (chest, extremity, abdominal) is more common in adolescents & adults

Demographics

- Age
  - Most common in patients ages 5-9 years
  - Lower incidence in patients < 2 years due to higher fetal hemoglobin concentrations
  - Incidence gradually declines with age
    - Excess mortality in group with ACS
    - Fewer viral illnesses due to acquired immunity
- Sex
  - Slightly more common in males
- Ethnicity
  - In USA, almost exclusively seen in Black patients
- Epidemiology
  - Overall incidence of 12.8 episodes per 100 patient-years
  - ACS is most common cause of premature death in patients with SCD
  - ACS is 2nd most common cause of hospitalization in patients with SCD after pain crisis
    - ~ 50% of patients are admitted with diagnosis other than ACS
    - Diagnosed with ACS 2-3 days after admission

Natural History & Prognosis

- More severe in patients > 20 years
  - Mortality is 4-9x higher in adults than in children
- Features associated with poor prognosis
  - Physical exam: Altered mental status, tachycardia > 125 beats/minute, tachypnea > 30 breaths/minute, temperature > 40°C, hypotension
  - Lab findings: Arterial pH < 7.35, O_2 saturation < 88%, hemoglobin concentration ↓ by ≥ 2 g/dL, platelet count < 200,000, multiorgan failure
- Risk factors: Asthma, smoking, abdominal surgery, trauma

Treatment

- Supportive
  - Oxygen, antibiotics, pain control, IV fluids, incentive spirometry, & blood transfusions
  - Corticosteroids are controversial; may be associated with ↑ readmission rate
- Prevention
  - At higher risk for pneumonia from encapsulated organisms due to autosplenectomy
    - Pneumococcal vaccination
    - *Haemophilus influenzae* vaccination
  - Hydroxyurea
    - Reduces sickling by ↑ fetal hemoglobin level
    - Reduces incidence in patients with recurrent ACS
  - Transfusion therapy

DIAGNOSTIC CHECKLIST

Consider

- ACS in patient with SCD, chest symptoms, & pulmonary opacity

SELECTED REFERENCES

1. Dako F et al: Dual-energy CT evidence of pulmonary microvascular occlusion in patients with sickle cell disease experiencing acute chest syndrome. Clin Imaging. 78:94-7, 2021
2. Dolatkhah R et al: Blood transfusions for treating acute chest syndrome in people with sickle cell disease. Cochrane Database Syst Rev. 1:CD007843, 2020
3. El-Gohary Y et al: Acute chest syndrome after splenectomy in children with sickle cell disease. J Surg Res. 242:336-41, 2019
4. Monus T et al: Current and emerging treatments for sickle cell disease. JAAPA. 32(9):1-5, 2019
5. Rincón-López EM et al: Low-risk factors for severe bacterial infection and acute chest syndrome in children with sickle cell disease. Pediatr Blood Cancer. 66(6):e27667, 2019
6. Bou-Maroun LM et al: An analysis of inpatient pediatric sickle cell disease: Incidence, costs, and outcomes. Pediatr Blood Cancer. 65(1), 2018
7. Takahashi T et al: Acute chest syndrome among children hospitalized with vaso-occlusive crisis: a nationwide study in the United States. Pediatr Blood Cancer. 65(3), 2018
8. Takahashi T et al: Factors associated with mechanical ventilation use in children with sickle cell disease and acute chest syndrome. Pediatr Crit Care Med. 19(9):801-9, 2018
9. Subramaniam S et al: Managing acute complications of sickle cell disease in pediatric patients [digest]. Pediatr Emerg Med Pract. 13(11 Suppl Points & Pearls):S1-S2, 2016

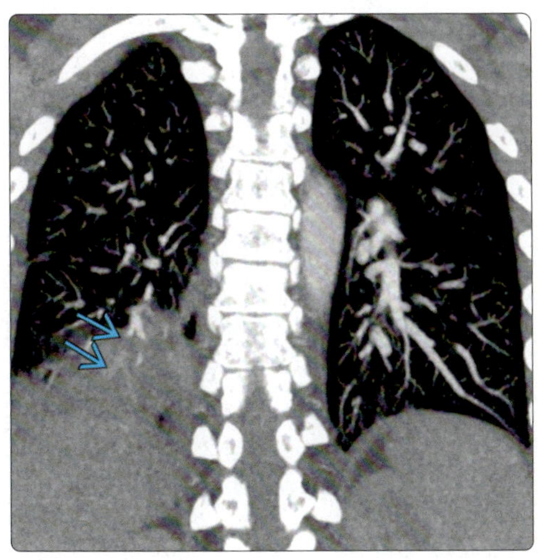

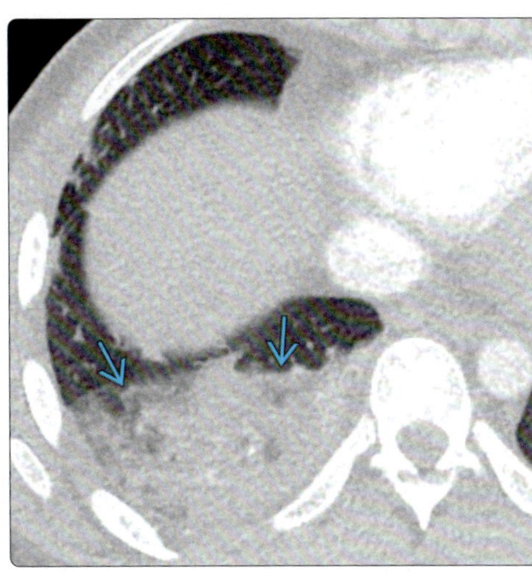

(Left) *Coronal CECT in an adolescent with SCD, acute chest pain, & ↓ right basilar breath sounds shows filling defects* → *within subsegmental branches of the right lower lobe pulmonary artery. There is adjacent consolidation of the right lower lobe.* **(Right)** *Axial CECT in lung windows in the same patient shows consolidation* → *in the right lower lobe.*

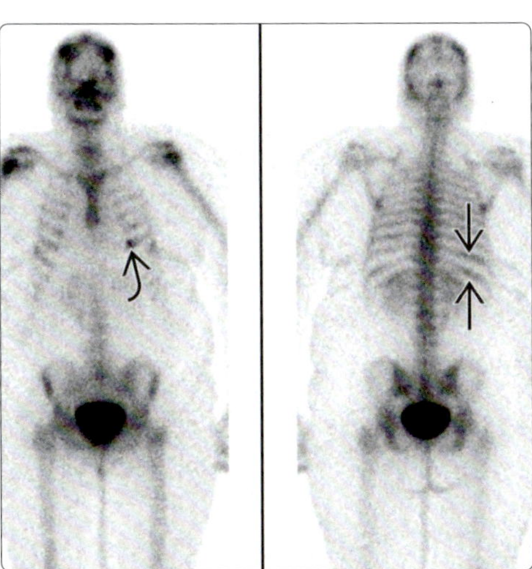

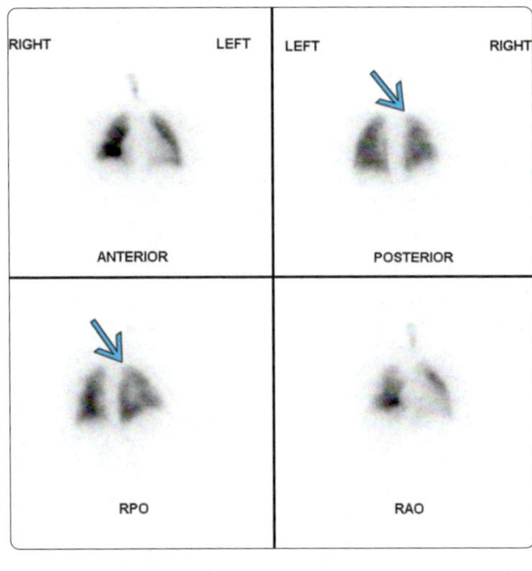

(Left) *Anterior & posterior projections from a bone scan in a patient with SCD show focally ↑ uptake in the left anterior 7th rib* → *& right posterior 10th & 11th ribs* →*, likely due to bone infarcts.* **(Right)** *Perfusion study with Tc-99m MAA in a patient with SCD shows a moderate-sized defect* → *in the right upper lobe. Perfusion defects in SCD may represent acute or chronic infarction.*

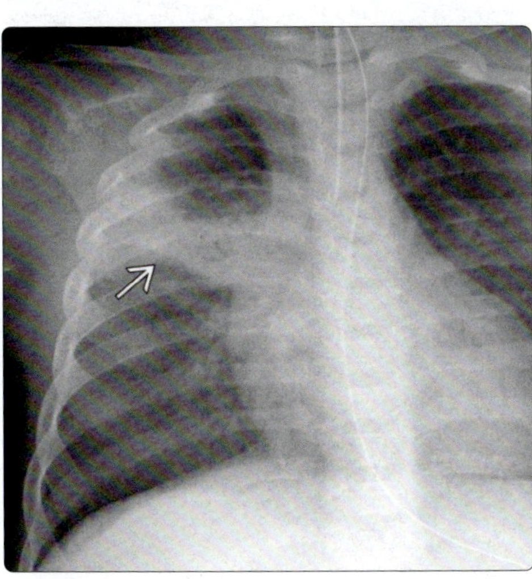

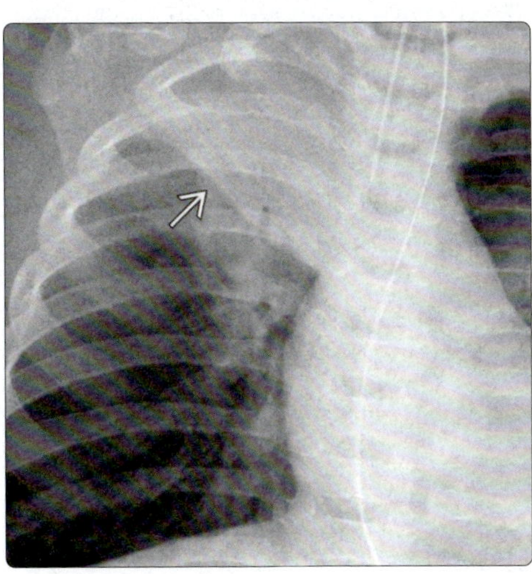

(Left) *AP radiograph of the chest shows a poorly defined opacity in the right upper lobe* → *of a 1-year-old with SCD presenting with fever & dyspnea. Note the elevation of the minor fissure, consistent with a degree of volume loss.* **(Right)** *AP radiograph of the chest in the same patient 12 hours later shows worsening opacification & volume loss of the right upper lobe* →*. ACS is defined as a new pulmonary opacity in a symptomatic patient with SCD. In children, it occurs more commonly in the upper & middle lobes.*

Kaposiform Lymphangiomatosis

KEY FACTS

TERMINOLOGY

- Kaposiform lymphangiomatosis (KLA): Uncommon but aggressive lymphatic disease with poor prognosis
  - Features of both neoplasia & malformation
- Predominantly affects thorax with progressive respiratory symptoms & hemorrhages

IMAGING

- Poorly defined, infiltrative, fluid signal intensity/attenuation soft tissue lesions of mediastinum & chest wall + peribronchial & interlobular septal thickening of lung parenchyma, ± pleural & pericardial effusions
  - Enhancement of infiltrating abnormal lymphatic tissue on T1 C+ FS MR
- Location
  - Thorax: Mediastinum (100%) > lung, pleura (80-90%)
  - Subcutaneous tissues, retroperitoneum (> 50%)
  - Bone, spleen (50-60% each, typically as discrete lesions)

TOP DIFFERENTIAL DIAGNOSES

- Generalized lymphatic anomaly (GLA)
- Gorham-Stout disease (GSD)
- Central conducting lymphatic anomaly (CCLA)
- Kaposiform hemangioendothelioma (KHE)
- Lymphoma

PATHOLOGY

- Abnormal lymphatic channels with spindled endothelial cells; stain positive for lymphatic markers PROX1, D2-40
- Intermixed extravasated RBCs, hemosiderin

CLINICAL ISSUES

- Most common presentations
  - Respiratory (50-55%): Cough, dyspnea
  - Hemorrhage from underlying coagulopathy (50%)
  - Mass (25-35%)
- Median age of presentation: 6.5 years
- 5-year survival: ~ 50%

(Left) *Axial CECT in an adolescent girl with shortness of breath shows infiltration & expansion of the peribronchial & mediastinal soft tissues by poorly defined, fluid-attenuation lesions.* **(Right)** *Axial CECT in lung windows in the same patient with kaposiform lymphangiomatosis (KLA) shows extensive peribronchial & interlobular septal thickening.*

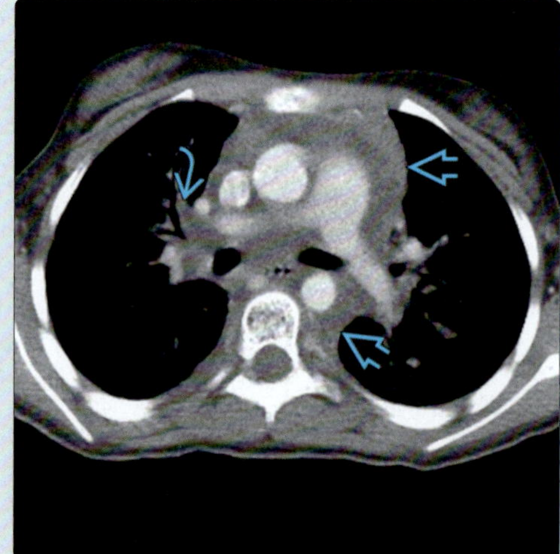

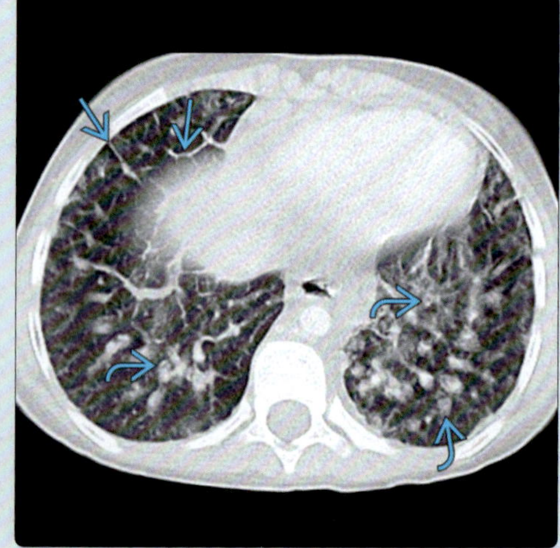

(Left) *Axial T1 C+ FS MR in the same patient several months later shows peribronchial thickening with diffuse enhancement of the infiltrating mediastinal & pleural lesions. A large left pleural effusion has developed.* **(Right)** *Sagittal T1 (left) & STIR (right) MR images show multifocal vertebral lesions in the same patient. Some lesions shows abnormal fatty deposition compared to normal (for this age & sex) vertebral marrow while other lesions show ↑ fluid signal intensity.*

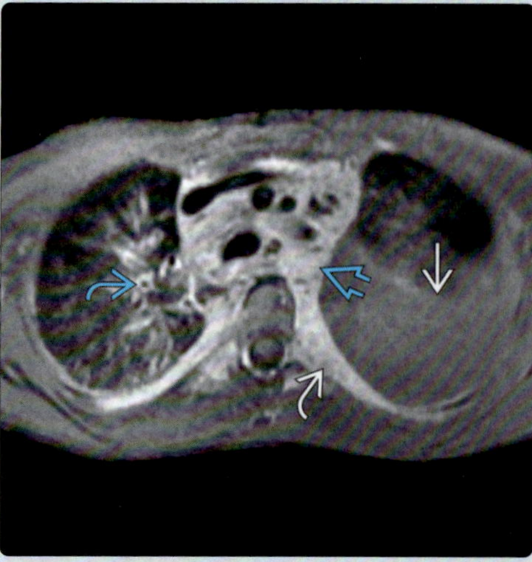

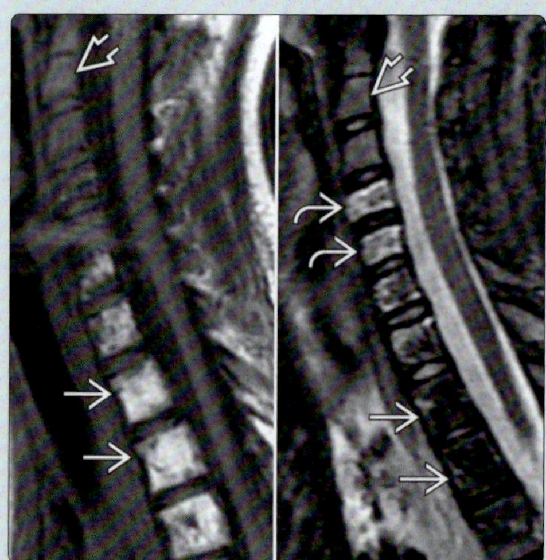

TERMINOLOGY

Abbreviations

- Kaposiform lymphangiomatosis (KLA)

Definitions

- Uncommon but distinct subtype of generalized lymphatic anomaly (GLA) with poor prognosis
  - Features of both neoplasia & malformation
- Predominantly affects thorax with progressive respiratory symptoms & hemorrhages

IMAGING

General Features

- Best diagnostic clue
  - Poorly defined, infiltrative, fluid signal intensity/attenuation soft tissue lesions of mediastinum & chest wall + peribronchial & interlobular septal thickening of lung parenchyma, ± pleural & pericardial effusions
    - Microcystic lymphatic lesions are much more common than macrocystic
    - Enhancement of infiltrating abnormal lymphatic tissue on T1 C+ FS MR
- Location
  - Thorax: Mediastinum (100%) > lung, pleura (80-90%)
    - Posterior > anterior mediastinum
  - Bone (50-60%)
    - Mainly lucent lesions of vertebral bodies without cortical destruction
    - MR signal intensity is variable
      - ↑ T1, ↓ FS T2/STIR in some lesions due to unusual fatty deposition
      - ↑ fluid signal intensity (↓ T1, ↑ FS T2/STIR) in other lesions, more typical of lymphatic anomalies of bone
      - Variable enhancement with contrast
  - Abdomen (55%)
    - Retroperitoneal &/or mesenteric enhancing infiltrative tissue
    - Spleen (50%)
      - Few discrete cysts in normal size spleen vs. innumerable cysts in enlarged spleen
      - Cystic foci may enhance with contrast
    - Pancreatic & renal cysts
  - Muscles & skin (> 50%)
  - Lymphatic channels
    - Dilation with reflux of injected lymphatic contrast at many levels
- Morphology
  - Poorly defined soft tissue infiltration, usually without macrocysts
  - Discrete splenic cysts
  - Lucent bone lesions without cortical destruction

DIFFERENTIAL DIAGNOSIS

Generalized Lymphatic Anomaly

- Osseous, splenic, & pleural disease is common
- Interstitial lung disease is uncommon
- More likely to have soft tissue macrocystic disease than KLA
- Coagulopathy is not typical

Gorham-Stout Disease

- Progressive cortical bone destruction
  - Often affects multiple bones in close proximity
- Adjacent infiltrative microcystic lymphatic anomaly
- Visceral disease is less common than GLA/KLA

Central Conducting Lymphatic Anomaly

- Major lymphatic channel obstruction, malfunction, &/or leak → lymphangiectasis & chylous effusions
- MR lymphangiography demonstrates abnormal flow patterns of contrast

Kaposiform Hemangioendothelioma

- Typically presents in infancy with purpuric skin lesion & profound coagulopathy
- Unifocal infiltrative enhancing mass with greater component of spindle cells

Cat-Scratch Disease

- Regional adenopathy & fever are common
- ± osseous & splenic disease

Lymphoma

- Bulky, confluent mediastinal & hilar lymph nodes are typical
  - Mass effect is typically > with lymphatic anomalies

Langerhans Cell Histiocytosis

- Isolated or multifocal lytic bone lesions
- Systemic involvement is uncommon, typically seen in infants
- Lung disease is more common in older children & adult smokers
  - Cysts & nodules are typical

CLINICAL ISSUES

Presentation

- Most common signs/symptoms
  - Respiratory (50-55%): Cough, dyspnea
  - Coagulopathy &/or hemorrhage (50%)
    - Thrombocytopenia is common
  - Mass (25-35%)

Demographics

- Age
  - Median age of presentation: 6.5 years

Natural History & Prognosis

- 5-year survival of ~ 50%
- Progressive symptoms over months-years

Treatment

- No established effective long-term therapy
- Limited reports of improvement with sirolimus, vincristine
- Temporary clinical improvement with drainage procedures, including thoracentesis, pericardiocentesis/pericardial window

SELECTED REFERENCES

1. Iacobas I et al: Multidisciplinary guidelines for initial evaluation of complicated lymphatic anomalies-expert opinion consensus. Pediatr Blood Cancer. e28036, 2019

EVALI

KEY FACTS

TERMINOLOGY

- Electronic cigarette (e-cigarette) or vaping product use-associated lung injury (EVALI)
- Bilateral, symmetric, ground-glass & consolidative opacities in patient with history of e-cigarette use or dabbing + negative work-up for pulmonary infection

IMAGING

- Chest radiograph
    - Bilateral, symmetric opacities
    - May not be sufficiently sensitive in detecting lung changes from EVALI; should not be used to exclude this diagnosis
- CT
    - Most common findings: Bilateral, symmetric ground-glass & consolidative opacities
    - Also seen: Atoll or reverse halo sign, interlobular septal thickening, centrilobular nodules, subpleural &/or peribronchovascular sparing
    - Pattern of injury could follow that of cryptogenic organizing pneumonia, hypersensitivity pneumonitis, acute lung injury (diffuse alveolar damage, crazy paving), acute eosinophilic pneumonia, & lipoid pneumonia

CLINICAL ISSUES

- Respiratory symptoms are common: Cough, shortness of breath
- Many patients also present with GI symptoms, including abdominal pain, nausea, vomiting, diarrhea
    - GI abnormalities may be primary presenting symptoms
- Most recover with supportive measures & glucocorticoids
- May have progressive course with respiratory failure & death

(Left) *Axial CECT in a 17-year-old who presented with right lower quadrant pain & was worked up for possible appendicitis shows bilateral, symmetric ground-glass densities that were noted at the lung bases on the abdomen & pelvis CT. Note the relative subpleural sparing.* **(Right)** *PA chest radiograph subsequently performed in the same patient shows hazy, patchy basilar opacities. The patient was diagnosed with EVALI, as he had a history of vaping & the infectious work-up was negative.*

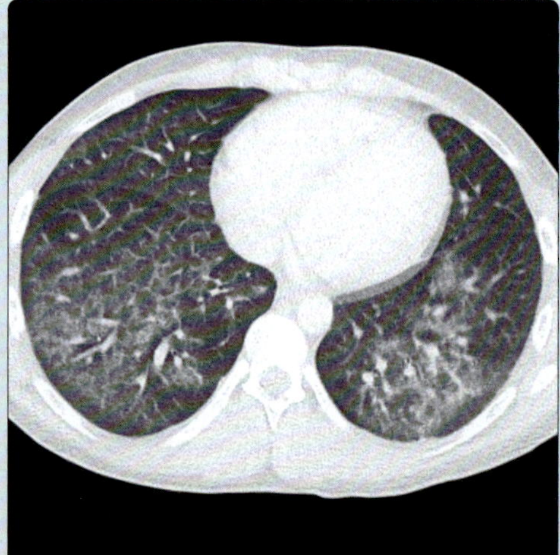

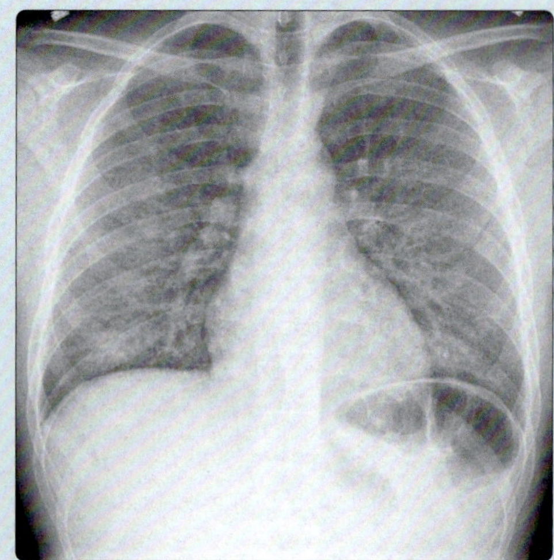

(Left) *Coronal CECT shows findings of EVALI in a 15-year-old with a history of e-cigarette use & shortness of breath, including subtle ground-glass densities ➡, patchy consolidation at the right lung base ➡, & centrilobular nodules.* **(Right)** *Axial CECT in a 16-year-old with EVALI who presented with shortness of breath & cough shows typical bilateral, symmetric opacities predominantly in the mid- to lower lung zones.*

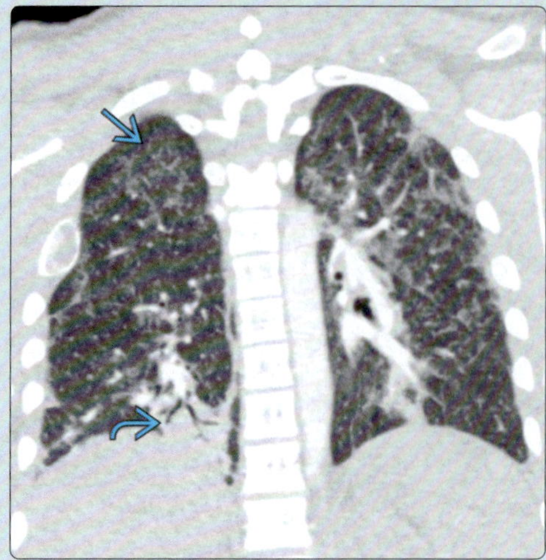

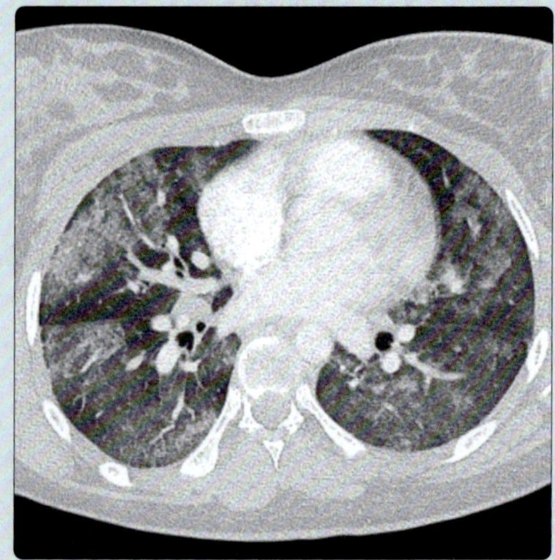

TERMINOLOGY

Abbreviations

- Electronic cigarette (e-cigarette) or vaping product use-associated lung injury (EVALI)

IMAGING

General Features

- Best diagnostic clue
  - Bilateral, symmetric ground-glass & consolidative opacities in patient with history of using e-cigarette or dabbing + negative work-up for pulmonary infection

Radiographic Findings

- Bilateral ground-glass & consolidative opacities
- Symmetric

CT Findings

- Bilateral ground-glass & consolidative opacities
- Interlobular septal thickening & centrilobular nodules
- Subpleural & peribronchovascular sparing
- Atoll or reversed halo sign: Central ground-glass opacity (GGO) surrounded by more dense ring of consolidation
- Symmetric
- Pattern/distribution of lung findings can follow that of cryptogenic organizing pneumonia, hypersensitivity pneumonitis, acute lung injury (diffuse alveolar damage), acute eosinophilic pneumonia, & lipoid pneumonia

Imaging Recommendations

- Best imaging tool
  - Radiograph is often 1st modality but may not be sufficiently sensitive in detecting lung changes from EVALI & should not be used to exclude this diagnosis
  - CT may be necessary for further characterization

DIFFERENTIAL DIAGNOSIS

Hypersensitivity Pneumonitis

- History of other inhaled antigen

Acute Eosinophilic Pneumonia

- Bronchoalveolar lavage fluid with > 25% eosinophils

Diffuse Alveolar Hemorrhage

- Etiology may be autoimmune, drug reaction, or infectious

Acute Pulmonary Infections, Including SARS-CoV2 Infection

- Positive work-up for other infectious etiology

Other Organizing Pneumonias

- Etiology may be autoimmune, drug related, infectious, or radiation related

PATHOLOGY

General Features

- Spectrum of acute & organizing lung injury: Interstitial edema, type II pneumocyte hyperplasia, vacuolated foamy macrophages, intraalveolar fibrin, acute fibrinous pneumonitis, organizing pneumonia with airway-centered micronodular lesions, & diffuse alveolar damage with hyaline membranes
- Rarely, eosinophilic infiltrate
- Lipid-laden macrophages have been reported & are not pathognomonic for exogenous lipoid pneumonia
- No histopathologic evidence of hypersensitivity pneumonitis, even in patients with hypersensitivity pneumonitis injury pattern on CT
  - GGO centrilobular nodule CT pattern is attributed to bronchiolocentric micronodular lesions of organizing pneumonia & organizing acute lung injury
- Tetrahydrocannabinol-containing e-cigarette or vaping products are linked to most EVALI cases & are suspected to play major role in reported outbreaks
- Vitamin E acetate is also strongly linked to EVALI outbreaks
  - Found in product samples tested by FDA & state laboratories & in patient lung fluid samples tested by CDC from geographically diverse states but not in lung fluid of people without EVALI

CLINICAL ISSUES

Presentation

- Most common signs/symptoms
  - Respiratory: Cough, shortness of breath
  - Majority of patients also present with GI symptoms: Abdominal pain, nausea, vomiting, diarrhea
    - GI abnormalities may be primary presenting symptoms with respiratory findings noted only during work-up
  - Constitutional symptoms: Fever, weight loss

Demographics

- Majority of patients < 35 years old, mean age of 24 years
- Patients < 18 years old account for 15% of hospitalizations

Natural History & Prognosis

- Most improve after cessation of vaping
- May have progression with respiratory failure & death

Treatment

- Supportive measures
- Glucocorticoids

DIAGNOSTIC CHECKLIST

Image Interpretation Pearls

- Evaluation of lung bases on abdominal CT is important as many patients present with gastrointestinal symptoms

SELECTED REFERENCES

1. Gonsalves CL et al: Diagnosis and acute management of e-cigarette or vaping product use-associated lung injury in the pediatric population: a systematic review. J Pediatr. 228:260-70, 2021
2. Artunduaga M et al: Pediatric chest radiographic and CT findings of electronic cigarette or vaping product use-associated lung injury (EVALI). Radiology. 295(2):430-8, 2020
3. Kligerman S et al: Radiologic, pathologic, clinical, and physiologic findings of electronic cigarette or vaping product use-associated lung injury (EVALI): evolving knowledge and remaining questions. Radiology. 294(3):491-505, 2020
4. Panse PM et al: Radiologic and pathologic correlation in EVALI. AJR Am J Roentgenol. 215(5):1057-64, 2020
5. Rao DR et al: Clinical features of e-cigarette, or vaping, product use-associated lung injury in teenagers. Pediatrics. 146(1), 2020
6. Wang KY et al: E-cigarette or vaping product use-associated lung injury in the pediatric population: imaging features at presentation and short-term follow-up. Pediatr Radiol. 50(9):1231-9, 2020

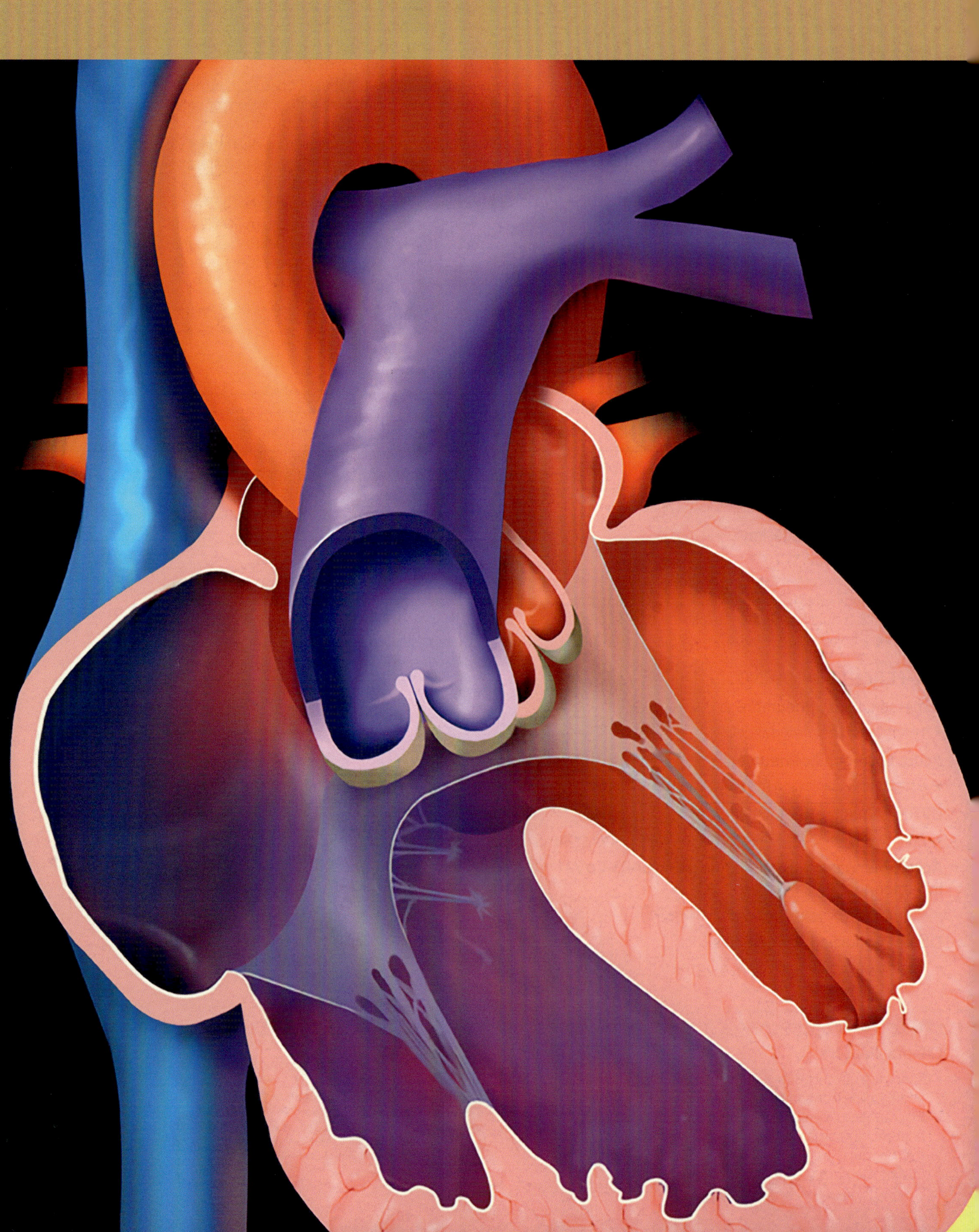

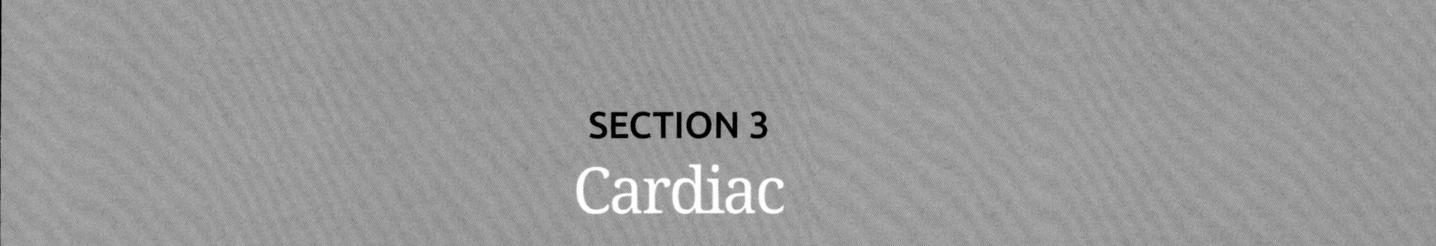

SECTION 3
Cardiac

Imaging Anatomy

The days in which congenital heart disease (CHD) was characterized by chest radiography & defined by angiography are gone. Both still play some role in the diagnosis & management of CHD. However, with echocardiography, cardiac MR, & CT, we now have robust imaging modalities that can provide detailed anatomic & functional evaluation in patients with complex heart issues. A patient who undergoes a CT or MR for CHD will often have multiple findings. For example, an asplenia heterotaxy patient with right-sided isomerism may have a long list of diagnoses, such as total anomalous pulmonary venous return (TAPVR), transposition of the great arteries (TGA), patent ductus arteriosus (PDA), atrial septal defect (ASD), ventricular septal defect (VSD), single coronary artery, situs inversus, coarctation, & tracheal stenosis. This is not out of the ordinary in a complex CHD patient referred for advanced imaging (CT or MR). A systematic approach is therefore crucial in any cross-sectional imaging modality of a patient with CHD. This introduction attempts to provide a systematic approach to cardiac CT or MR in a patient with CHD.

Situs

Evaluation of situs involves the designation of an individual as normal (situs solitus), reversed (situs inversus), or some other combination (situs ambiguous). In situs solitus, the stomach, left atrium, apex of the heart, & spleen are on the left, while the right atrium, liver, superior vena cava (SVC), & inferior vena cava (IVC) are on the right. The pulmonary veins drain to the left atrium. The tracheobronchial branching in situs solitus includes a trilobed lung & main bronchus that sits posteriorly &/or superiorly to the pulmonary artery (eparterial bronchus) on the right & a bilobed lung with a main bronchus sitting below the pulmonary artery on the left (hyparterial bronchus). Situs inversus is the exact opposite of situs solitus. There are multiple variations to the above basic designation of situs. These fall into the category of situs ambiguous. Some additional observations will often be necessary. In the abdomen, besides looking at the side of the stomach, one must look for the position of the liver, absence of the spleen or presence of multiple spleens, & presence of an intrahepatic IVC (to exclude azygous continuation of the IVC). In the heart, be aware of symmetric atria & appendages in patients with heterotaxy, as these may represent 2 right atria or 2 left atria in right or left isomerism. It is usually not difficult to differentiate the ventricles based on the prominence of the trabeculations (i.e., the more trabeculated ventricle is usually the right ventricle). The right ventricle may be identified more confidently by the presence of a moderator band (muscular fibers connecting the free wall of the right ventricle to the interventricular septum). Also, pay attention to the tracheobronchial branching relative to the pulmonary arteries: It may be abnormal, bilateral, left-sided branching (hyparterial bronchi) or bilateral, right-sided branching (eparterial bronchi).

Lungs & Airways

There is an increased incidence of airway anomalies in children with CHD. These include pig bronchus, congenital stenosis, & bilateral right- or left-sided tracheobronchial branching seen with heterotaxy syndromes. More common than congenital airway anomalies is airway compression from cardiomegaly & enlarged or anomalous vasculature. The child with CHD is also susceptible to chronic lung disease from extended mechanical ventilation as well as postoperative effusions, atelectasis, tracheobronchomalacia, & infections.

Atria & Veins

It is important to make sure the venous drainage empties into the appropriate chamber of the heart. Anomalies like TAPVR & partial anomalous pulmonary venous return can easily be missed unless specifically investigated. Always look for a left SVC & a crossing innominate vein. The unsuspected presence of a left SVC may complicate cardiac surgery & cardiopulmonary bypass unnecessarily. Also, scan the atrial septum for defects. Artifact can sometimes hide or mimic ASD. As technology advances, the ability to evaluate valvular & septal structures will also improve. The atrioventricular valves should be evaluated for position, size, & thickness, but they can be difficult to evaluate if there is motion, beam hardening artifact, or a delayed contrast bolus.

Ventricles

A VSD is any communication of the right & left ventricles. These defects are most commonly in the membranous portion of the interventricular septum. In complex congenital heart patients, defects are also frequently seen in the muscular portion of the ventricular septum. Rarely, defects can also occur along the outflow tracts. Included in the evaluation of the ventricles are the right & left ventricular outflow tracts. Outflow tract evaluation includes assuring the patency (no atresias), separation (no truncus anomaly), & connection to the appropriate great vessel (no transposition).

Great Vessels

The size, course, & position of the great vessels should be evaluated by CT & MR. Basic measurements of the size of the aorta are made at the sinuses of Valsalva, aortic valve anulus, sinotubular junction of the ascending aorta, transverse aortic arch, & descending aorta. Basic measurements are made for the main pulmonary artery at the pulmonary valve anulus, midmain pulmonary artery, & proximal & distal right & left pulmonary arteries. Any other obvious stenosis or dilation should also be measured. Vascular rings, slings, & aberrant vessels should be identified. A PDA is usually present in complex congenital heart patients, & its length & width should be measured.

Coronary Arteries

The origin, course, & termination of the coronary arteries should be evaluated when possible. Visualization of the coronaries is variable depending on the type of exam performed. Generally, the coronaries are best seen with an ECG-gated cardiac CTA. It is important to note that certain coronary anomalies will alter the surgical approach. Rarely, the left (less commonly the right) coronary artery may arise from the pulmonary artery (ALCAPA). This can lead to a steal phenomenon & cause the patient to go into heart failure. Sudden death can occur in patients (typically athletes) with an interarterial (malignant) course of the coronary arteries. This is most commonly seen when the left coronary arises from the right coronary sinus or when the right coronary artery arises from the left coronary sinus. The aberrant artery then courses between the right & left ventricular outflow tracts. Some coronary anomalies are associated with certain types of CHD. This helps focus the search for the coronary anomalies. For example, patients with TGA typically have a right coronary arising from the noncoronary sinus. If the coronary anatomy is something different from the typical pattern in TGA patients, the surgeon should be alerted, as he or she will have to translocate the coronaries during the arterial switch procedure. Coronary artery fistulas are frequently seen in patients with a hypoplastic right ventricle. It is common to see a partial interarterial course of the right coronary artery in a patient with tetralogy of Fallot since clockwise rotation of the aortic root is seen in a large percentage of these patients. Finally, for any anomaly where a coronary artery courses in front of an outflow tract, alert the surgeon so he or she can avoid severing the vessel during surgery.

Functional

Basic functional evaluation of the heart can be performed by both CT & MR cardiac exams. Routine functional evaluation includes calculating the volumes & ejection fractions of both ventricles. Indexed volumes are obtained by dividing the gross volume by the body surface area. CT & MR can also be used to evaluate the left ventricular muscle mass. Standardized data is available to compare volume & muscle mass results with other size & age matched data sets. MR has the added capabilities to evaluate & quantify flow volumes & velocities. A pulmonary to systemic flow ratio (Qp:Qs) is routinely provided by interrogating the flow from the right & left ventricular outflow tracts. In patients with pulmonic & aortic regurgitation, velocity-encoded phase-contrast imaging can be used to calculate regurgitant fractions. The regurgitant fraction is calculated by dividing the regurgitant volume by the stroke volume. Similar applications can be used to evaluate other veins, arteries, & valves as needed. Regurgitant fractions are typically followed yearly in patients with a pulmonary homograft to assess the severity of pulmonic regurgitation. When MR thresholds of end-systolic, end-diastolic, & pulmonic regurgitant fractions are met, a pulmonic valve replacement is recommended.

Anatomy-based Imaging Issues

It is crucial to know as much as possible about the patient's anatomy & postsurgical history before protocoling a cardiac CT or MR. For example, IVC (Fontan) & SVC (Glenn) shunts may introduce unopacified blood directly into the pulmonary arterial system. This can simulate a pulmonary embolism when unsuspected. Thoughtful protocoling of patients with CHD can help avoid artifacts that may simulate pathology & provide additional information to the cardiologist & cardiothoracic surgeon to better care for these patients.

Indications for Cardiac MR & CT

The routine congenital heart patient with a simple lesion (ASD, PDA, VSD) would likely never undergo an advanced imaging study, such as a cardiac CT or MR. Echocardiography provides excellent delineation of the intracardiac anatomy, great artery relationships, & function of the heart. Cardiac CT & MR are reserved for problem-solving in difficult echocardiography cases.

Extracardiac anatomy can be difficult to completely evaluate by echocardiography in complex cases. CT & MR are frequently done to evaluate the pulmonary veins, pulmonary arteries, systemic veins, & the aorta & its branches. Heterotaxy patients often have abnormalities involving the extracardiac anatomy & airways & may now routinely undergo cardiac CT or MR.

There are certain circumstances where the evaluation of the intracardiac anatomy can benefit from CT & MR. These include cardiac tumors, cardiomyopathies, ischemic heart disease, myocarditis, & coronary artery abnormalities. A more accurate volumetric analysis with CT or MR may be desirable in patients to evaluate the possibility of a 2-ventricle repair. MR has proven to be an effective tool to follow tetralogy of Fallot patients with pulmonic regurgitation to determine the timing of pulmonary valve replacement.

Cardiac MR vs. Cardiac CT

With higher temporal resolution, cardiac MR is superior to cardiac CT for functional imaging of the heart & evaluation of intracardiac anatomy. With higher spatial resolution, cardiac CT is superior to MR for extracardiac anatomy, airway evaluation, & coronary artery detail. There is significant overlap between the 2 modalities, as cardiac CT can provide volumetric functional evaluation, & MR gives adequate delineation of the extracardiac anatomy.

Cardiac MR requires longer sedation times than CT. Cardiac CT exposes the patient to ionizing radiation. Adjusting for size & using prospective gating, as well as other techniques, can significantly reduce the radiation dose.

Cardiac 3D Models

Segmentation of the anatomy in a patient with complex disease is often performed, & they can be exported to 3D printers to create physical models of the heart for surgical planning. 3D printers are now widely available & can print the models using a variety of flexible & nonflexible materials. Simple resin models of the heart can be printed & used in educating parents, patients, & health professionals. 3D congenital heart models are now used in the teaching of physicians in training at all levels. Patient-specific models can be printed in flexible material & be used to test devices on the patient's anatomy before performing the actual procedure. This method has also proven effective in decreasing procedure times. Examples include the coiling of aneurysms, sizing of devices for the closure of intramuscular VSD, & Melody valve placement along the pulmonary outflow tract.

Selected References

1. Ojha V et al: Computed tomography imaging of complications in postoperative cyanotic congenital heart diseases - A pictorial essay. Clin Imaging. 71:1-12, 2021
2. Siripornpitak S et al: CT and MRI for repaired complex adult congenital heart diseases. Korean J Radiol. 22(3):308-23, 2021
3. Sachdeva S et al: Imaging modalities in congenital heart disease. Indian J Pediatr. 87(5):385-97, 2020
4. Tian L et al: Low-dose computed tomography (CT) for the diagnosis of congenital heart disease in children: a meta-analysis. Curr Med Imaging. 16(9):1085-94, 2020
5. Roy CW et al: Fetal cardiac MRI: a review of technical advancements. Top Magn Reson Imaging. 28(5):235-44, 2019
6. Xu JJ et al: Patient-specific three-dimensional printed heart models benefit preoperative planning for complex congenital heart disease. World J Pediatr. 15(3):246-54, 2019
7. Ryan J et al: 3D printing for congenital heart disease: a single site's initial three-yearexperience. 3D Print Med. 4(1):10, 2018

(Left) *Coronal cardiac CTA shows bilateral hyparterial bronchi ➡ with multiple spleens ➡ in this patient with polysplenia syndrome (bilateral left sidedness).* **(Right)** *Posterior 3D color-coded cardiac CTA shows bilateral hyparterial bronchi ➡ with the left & right pulmonary arteries (blue) passing superior to the main bronchi (yellow).*

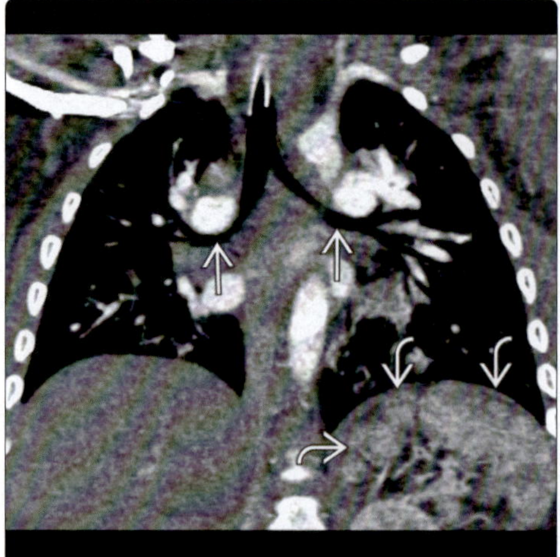

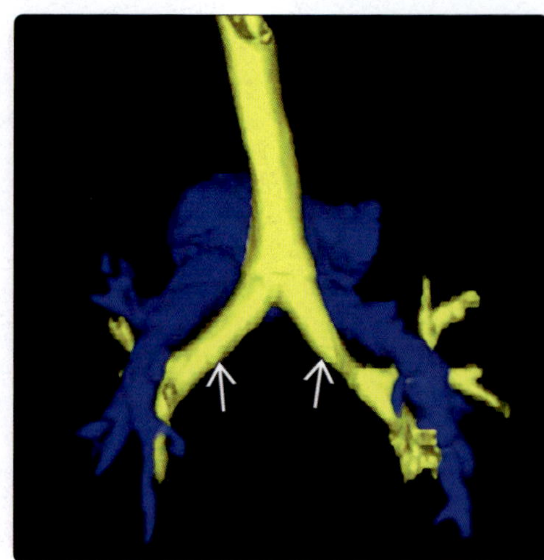

(Left) *Superior 3D surface-rendered cardiac CTA shows the left coronary artery ➡ arising from the right coronary sinus with an interarterial course between the ascending aorta (red) & the pulmonary artery (blue).* **(Right)** *3D flexible model of the proximal aorta from a CTA shows the LCA ➡ arising from the right coronary sinus ➡. The proximal course was intramural. New flexible models are being used to plan & perform procedures before the operation on the patient. Note the normal origin of the RCA ➡.*

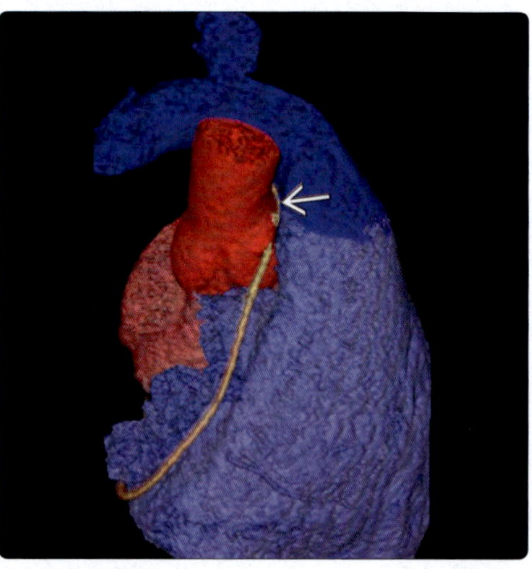

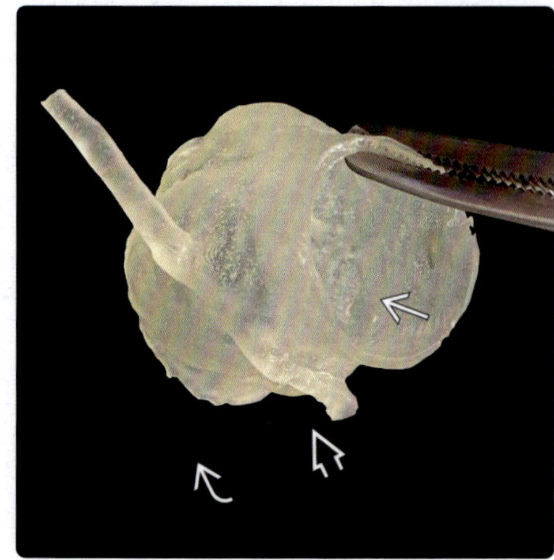

(Left) *Frontal 3D surface-rendered cardiac CTA shows the right coronary artery ➡ arising from the right side of the pulmonary artery, consistent with an anomalous right coronary artery from the pulmonary artery ➡ (ARCAPA).* **(Right)** *Frontal 3D chest CTA shows a right arch (red) with an aberrant left subclavian artery ➡. Note the tortuous patent ductus arteriosus (green) arising from the left subclavian & inserting into the left pulmonary artery ➡, completing the vascular ring.*

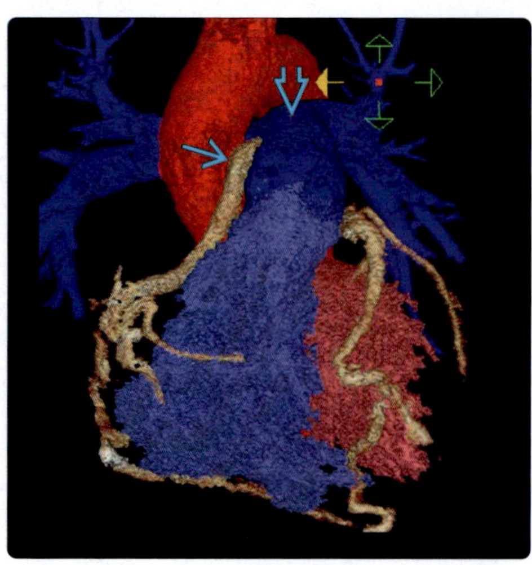

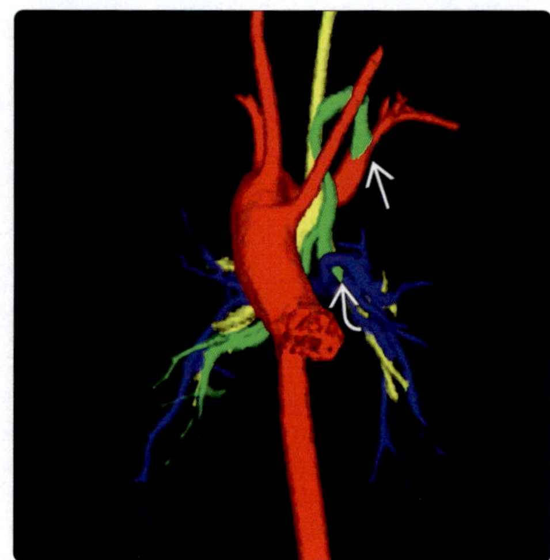

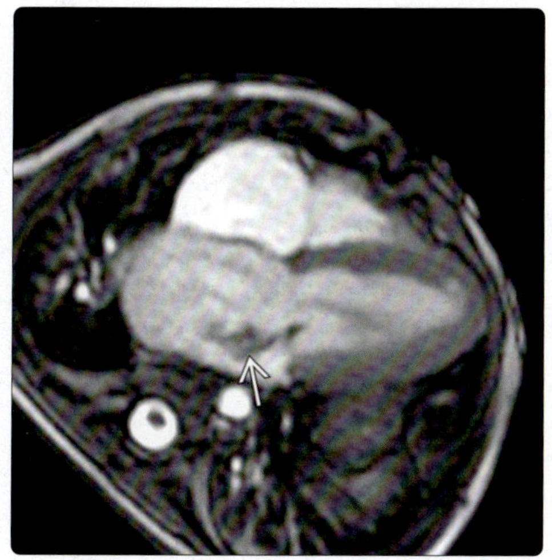

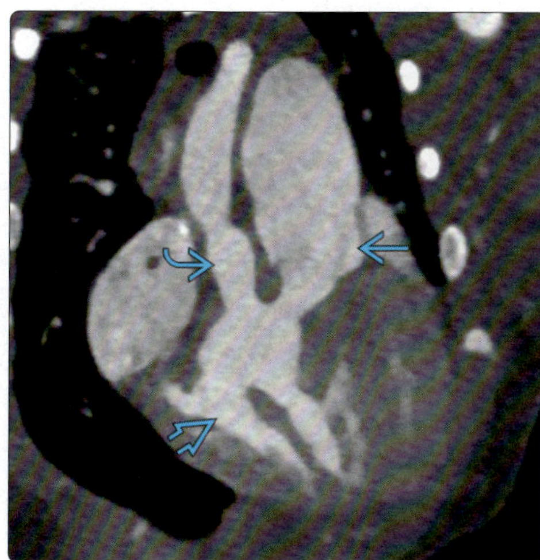

(Left) *Four-chamber SSFP cine cardiac MR shows dephasing artifact* ➡ *directed back into the left atrium from the mitral valve in this patient with mitral regurgitation.* **(Right)** *Oblique cardiac CTA shows both the pulmonary* ➡ *& aortic* ➡ *outflow tracts arising from the right ventricle (RV)* ➡ *in a patient with double-outlet right ventricle (DORV).*

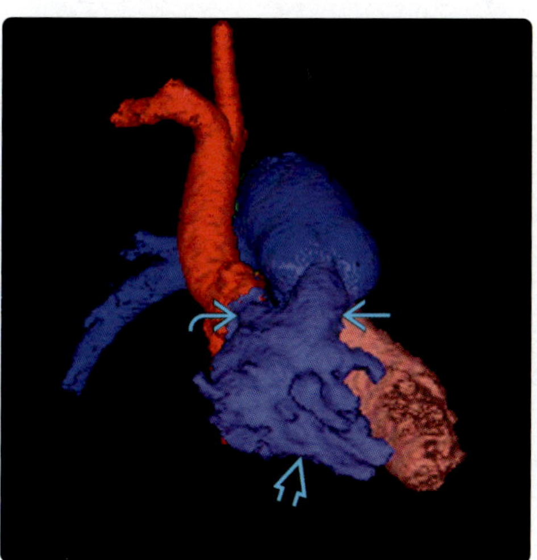

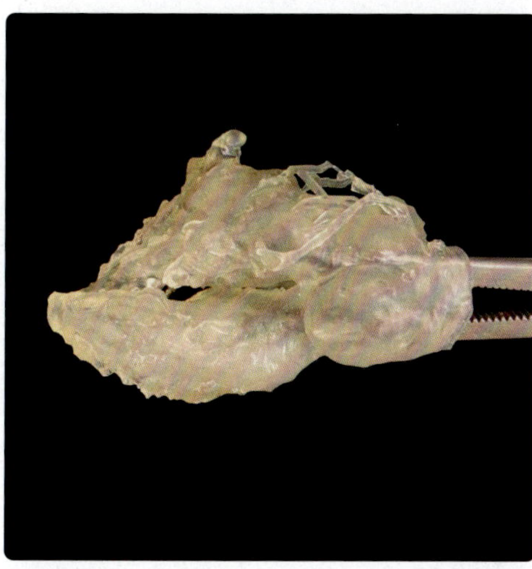

(Left) *Frontal 3D volume-rendered cardiac CTA shows both pulmonary* ➡ *& aortic* ➡ *outflow tracts arising from the RV* ➡ *in a patient with DORV.* **(Right)** *Left lateral 3D flexible model obtained from a cardiac CTA shows forceps going retrograde into the pulmonary outflow tract with one blade coursing into the RV & the other into the left ventricle (LV), consistent with a subpulmonic ventricular septal defect (VSD). Surgeons found the model useful as they closed the VSD through the pulmonary artery.*

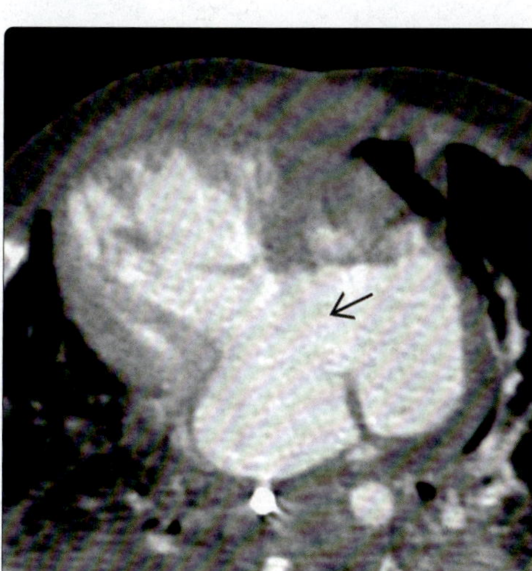

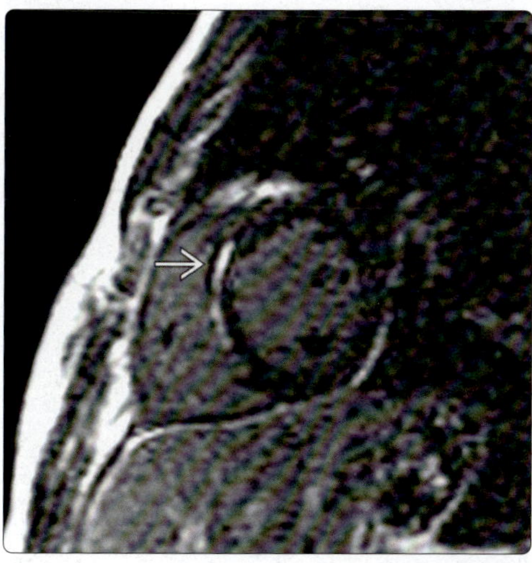

(Left) *Axial cardiac CTA shows a large defect in the atrial septum* ➡ *adjacent to the endocardial cushion in this patient with dextrocardia & a septum primum atrial septal defect.* **(Right)** *Late gadolinium-enhanced short-axis cardiac MR perfusion in a 10-year-old with acute heart failure shows ↑ uptake in the midmuscular portion of the interventricular septum* ➡*, consistent with myocarditis.*

Atrial Septal Defect

KEY FACTS

TERMINOLOGY

- ASD: Defect(s) in cardiac atrial septum; may be isolated or associated with other congenital heart disease (CHD)
- Left-to-right (LTR) shunt: Blood from left heart bypasses systemic circulation to enter right heart
  - Most ASD sequelae are related to long-term LTR shunting
- Types of ASD
  - LTR shunts: Ostium secundum (70-90%), ostium primum, sinus venosus, unroofed coronary sinus defects
  - Patent foramen ovale is normal variant & usually transient with normal atrial pressures
    - ↑ stroke risk; unclear migraine association

IMAGING

- LTR shunting leads to chronic volume overload of right heart, eventual enlargement of RA, RV, & PA
- Diagnosis of actual defect is primarily made by echocardiography
- Cardiac MR is accurate alternative for depiction of function, flow, & anatomy

CLINICAL ISSUES

- ASD: 10% of CHD in children, yet 30% of CHD in adults
- Secundum ASD: Majority of patients are asymptomatic
  - Spontaneous closure occurs in many children
  - Subtle symptoms are more likely in 2nd decade, though large defects frequently do not present until adulthood
    - Fatigue, exercise intolerance, syncope, shortness of breath, palpitations
    - ASD leading to severe pulmonary hypertension: Median age of detection is 51 years
  - Repair if shunt ratio > 1.5:1 or defect > 10 mm
  - Percutaneous closure with occlusion device
- Primum/atrioventricular septal defect is more severe; requires early surgical repair
- Sinus venosus ASDs also require surgery due to complex anatomy

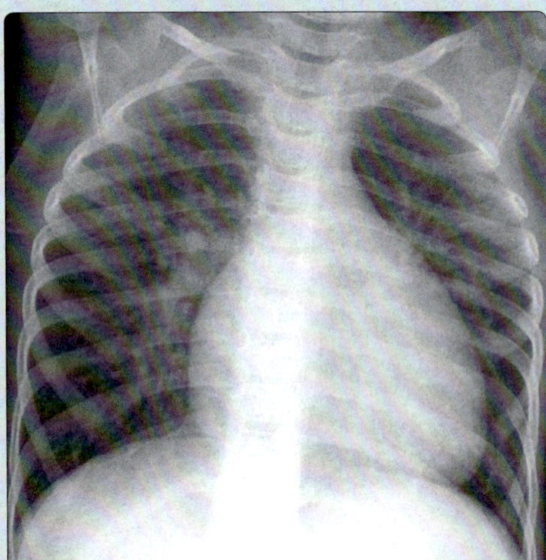

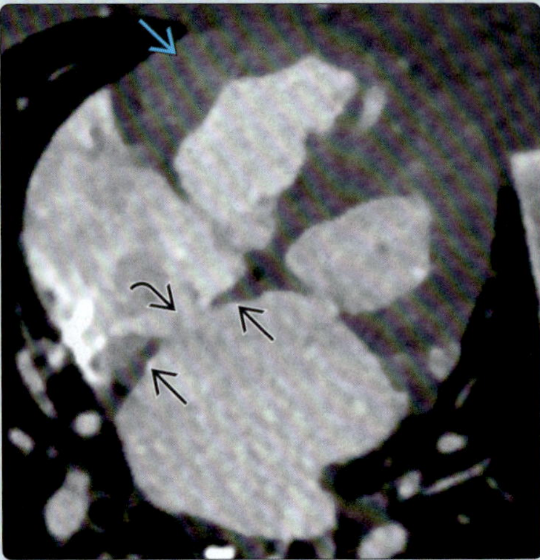

(Left) *Frontal chest radiograph in a 4-year-old child demonstrates cardiomegaly, ↑ pulmonary vascularity, & mild pulmonary edema. The patient had a large, untreated atrial septal defect (ASD).* **(Right)** *Axial cardiac CTA in an infant with other congenital anomalies shows a defect ➢ in the midportion of the atrial septum ➡, consistent with a secundum-type ASD. Note the hypertrophy of the right ventricle (RV) ➡.*

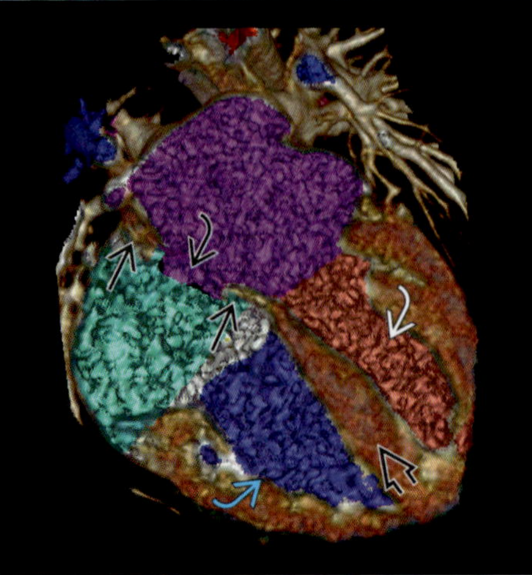

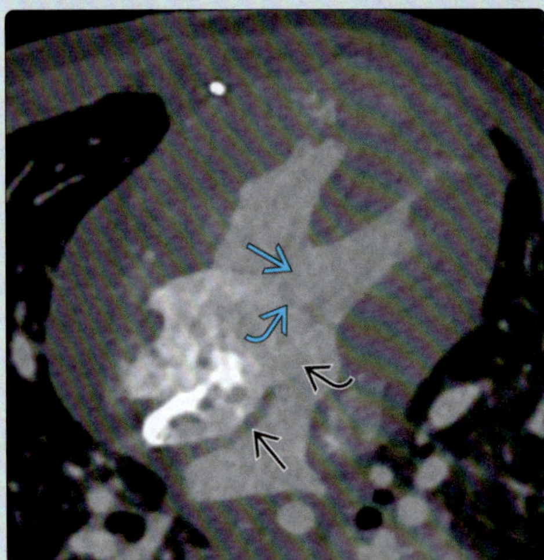

(Left) *Color-coded volume-rendered 4-chamber cardiac CTA shows a defect ➢ in the midportion of the atrial septum ➡, consistent with a secundum-type ASD. Note that the interventricular septum ➡ separates the RV ➢ & left ventricle (LV) ➢.* **(Right)** *Axial cardiac CTA in an infant with an atrioventricular (AV) canal defect shows a prominent septum primum defect ➢ of the atrial septum ➡. Note the common AV valve ➢ & the posterior ventricular septal defect (VSD) ➡.*

Atrial Septal Defect

TERMINOLOGY

Abbreviations

- Atrial septal defect (ASD)
- Congenital heart disease (CHD)

Definitions

- ASD: Defect(s) in cardiac atrial septum; may be isolated anomaly or associated with other congenital heart lesions
- Left-to-right (LTR) shunt: Blood from left heart bypasses systemic circulation to enter right heart
  - Most ASD sequelae are related to long-term LTR shunting

IMAGING

General Features

- Best diagnostic clue
  - Defect in atrial septum seen on any imaging modality
  - Sequelae of isolated ASD are uncommon in children
- Location
  - Patent foramen ovale: Persistence of normal fetal interatrial communication that allows flow from inferior vena cava (IVC) to largely bypass right atrium (RA) & freely enter left atrium (LA) in utero
    - Most common (25-30% of adults) but considered normal variant (not generally considered with other ASDs as flap only allows flow from right to left, not LTR shunting)
      - Only occurs with elevations in right heart pressures, typically transient phenomenon
      - Main concern in this population is stroke; questionable association with migraine headaches
  - Ostium secundum ASD (70-90% of LTR shunt ASDs): Defect of fossa ovalis due to defect of septum primum
  - Ostium primum ASD (2-3%): Simplest form of atrioventricular septal (endocardial cushion) defect (AVSD); this ASD lies between anterior/inferior portion of septum & AV valves
  - Sinus venosus ASD (4-11%): Posterior to fossa ovalis; superior-type (communication of cardiac superior vena cava (SVC) & at least 1 right pulmonary vein) > inferior-type (posterior inferior right atrial wall) defects
  - Unroofed coronary sinus (least common): Defect between LA & coronary sinus roof
- Size
  - Variable
- Morphology
  - Many ASDs are irregular or complex, not circular

Radiographic Findings

- Chest radiograph findings
  - Ostium secundum ASD
    - Small to moderate defects: Normal chest radiographs
    - Large defects: Mild cardiomegaly, normal to ↑ main pulmonary artery (PA) size, shunt vascularity
  - Ostium primum ASD or AVSD
    - Young child with cardiomegaly & ↑ pulmonary vascularity
    - Volume overload of RA, right ventricle (RV), & PA
  - Sinus venosus defect, superior type
    - Horizontal position of right upper lobe (RUL) pulmonary vein as it enters SVC
  - Adults with pulmonary hypertension
    - Classic enlarged, convex main PA with peripheral ↓ in size of vessels
    - RV enlargement
      - Upturned cardiac apex on frontal view
      - Diminished retrosternal clear space on lateral view

CT Findings

- CTA
  - Defect in atrial septum
    - Large shunt is suggested with unexpected equalization of contrast between atria during cardiac CTA with saline chaser
  - Enlargement of RA, RV, PA
  - Useful to look for associated congenital heart lesions
    - Partial anomalous pulmonary venous return (PAPVR) is associated with sinus venous ASD
  - Volumetric functional information can be obtained with retrospective gating

MR Findings

- SSFP cine
  - Shunt quantification using biventricular stroke volume ratio; net shunt volume = difference in stroke volumes
  - Interrupted septum is visible on 4-chamber views & short-axis stacks
    - Shunting blood may show signal loss (dephasing) on these bright-blood sequences
- Gradient-recalled echo cine with saturation band
  - Saturation band applied across 1 atrial chamber
  - Shunting from chamber of saturated blood (dark) into chamber of unsaturated blood (bright) reveals defect
- 1st-pass gadolinium perfusion
  - Rapid dynamic imaging can show ASD by
    - Dark (unenhanced) LA blood shunting into bright (enhanced) RA, followed by bright (enhanced) LA blood shunting into less enhanced RA
- Phase contrast velocity
  - Shunt ratio (Qp;Qs) is calculated by determining velocity & flow in ascending aorta & main PA
    - Qp;Qs of 1.5:1 is typically symptomatic
  - Also used to measure ASD flow directly
  - En face evaluation accurately depicts ASD size & shape as well as rim assessment
    - Critical parameters for assessing possibility of percutaneous closure
- MR angiography
  - Depiction of anomalous pulmonary veins

Angiographic Findings

- Utilized for transcatheter percutaneous treatment with closure device

Imaging Recommendations

- Best imaging tool
  - Primary diagnosis is made by echocardiography
  - Cardiac MR is accurate alternative for depiction of function, flow, & anatomy
  - Catheterization for percutaneous closure

DIFFERENTIAL DIAGNOSIS

Normal Chest Radiograph

- Main PA can be prominent normally, particularly between ages 8-12 years

Ventricular Septal Defect

- Small shunts have normal radiographs
- Moderate or large shunts have cardiomegaly & ↑ PA flow

Pulmonary Hypertension

- Variety of causes, mostly secondary to chronic lung disease
- Enlarged main & central PA with pruning distally, mosaic perfusion on CT

PATHOLOGY

General Features

- Genetics
  - Down syndrome (trisomy 21): Up to 65% have CHD
    - Up to 45% are due to AVSD; up to 42% are due to ostium secundum ASD
  - Holt-Oram syndrome (*TBX5* gene mutation on 12q24): ASD + upper extremity anomalies
  - Various other syndromes
  - Most ASDs are sporadic
    - Mutations have been found in several genes associated with cardiac septation
- Associated abnormalities
  - Sinus venosus
    - Superior: PAPVR of RUL pulmonary vein to SVC
    - Inferior: PAPVR of right lower lobe pulmonary vein to IVC or RA
  - Ostium secundum
    - Mitral valve degeneration with regurgitation in 25%
  - Unroofed coronary sinus: Persistent left-sided SVC
- Pathophysiology: Volume overload primary issue
  - ASD: Low-pressure LTR shunt
  - VSD, AVSD: High-pressure LTR shunts
  - All eventually lead to pulmonary hypertension if untreated

CLINICAL ISSUES

Presentation

- Most common signs/symptoms
  - Most children with ASDs have no symptoms
    - Detected due to murmur or other medical work-up
  - Rarely present in childhood with failure to thrive, respiratory infection, tachypnea
  - Subtle symptoms are more likely in 2nd decade, though large defects frequently do not present until adulthood
    - Fatigue, exercise intolerance, syncope, shortness of breath, palpitations
  - ASD leading to severe pulmonary hypertension: Median age of detection is 51 years
  - Ostium secundum, sinus venosus: Majority of patients are asymptomatic
  - AVSD or ostium primum defects: More likely to have early symptoms
- Other signs/symptoms
  - Abnormal heart sounds
    - Crescendo-decrescendo systolic ejection murmur of 2nd left intercostal space
      - ↑ volume through pulmonic valve
    - Widely split 2nd heart sound
      - Delayed closure of pulmonic valve

Demographics

- Age
  - Congenital defect; most ASDs are asymptomatic in infancy with symptoms developing in adulthood
  - AVSD is detected prenatally or in 1st week of life
- Sex
  - Ostium secundum defects: F:M = 2:1
- Epidemiology
  - 3rd most common CHD
  - ASD: 10% of CHD in children, yet 30% of CHD in adults
  - 56-100/100,000 live births
    - True incidence may be higher as many close spontaneously (especially ostium secundum)

Treatment

- Repair indicated: Shunt ratio > 1.5:1 or defect > 10 mm
  - Repair unless child is under 2 years of age (due to rates of spontaneous closure)
- Patients with small shunts: Monitor for right heart dysfunction
- Repair is contraindicated if pulmonary hypertension has already developed
- Ostium secundum ASD
  - Spontaneous closure occurs in many children
  - If persistent, close percutaneously with catheter-placed occlusion device
  - Large defects may need patch or direct suture closure
- Ostium primum defects are not amenable to percutaneous device closure due to relationship to AV valves
  - Surgery by 3-5 years of age
- Sinus venosus defect: More complex surgical repair is required due to pulmonary vein anatomy

SELECTED REFERENCES

1. Charisopoulou D et al: Repair of isolated atrial septal defect in infants less than 12 months improves symptoms of chronic lung disease or shunt-related pulmonary hypertension. Cardiol Young. 30(4):511-20, 2020
2. Kwon SS et al: Diagnosis of Ebstein anomaly with atrial septal defect and persistent left superior vena cava using cardiac magnetic resonance imaging. J Cardiovasc Imaging. 28(4):283-5, 2020
3. Boudoulas KD et al: Atrial septal defect sizing and transcatheter closure. Cardiology. 142(2):105-8, 2019
4. Zieliński P et al: Unroofed coronary sinus atrial septal defect. J Card Surg. 34(1):41-2, 2019
5. Chelu RG et al: Evaluation of atrial septal defects with 4D flow MRI-multilevel and inter-reader reproducibility for quantification of shunt severity. MAGMA. 32(2):269-79, 2018
6. Türkvatan A et al: Low-dose computed tomographic imaging of partial anomalous pulmonary venous connection in children. World J Pediatr Congenit Heart Surg. 8(5):590-6, 2017
7. Yamasaki Y et al: One-stop shop assessment for atrial septal defect closure using 256-slice coronary CT angiography. Eur Radiol. 27(2):697-704, 2017
8. Osawa K et al: Comprehensive assessment of morphology and severity of atrial septal defects in adults by CT. J Cardiovasc Comput Tomogr. 9(4):354-61, 2015
9. Rojas CA et al: Embryology and developmental defects of the interatrial septum. AJR Am J Roentgenol. 195(5):1100-4, 2010

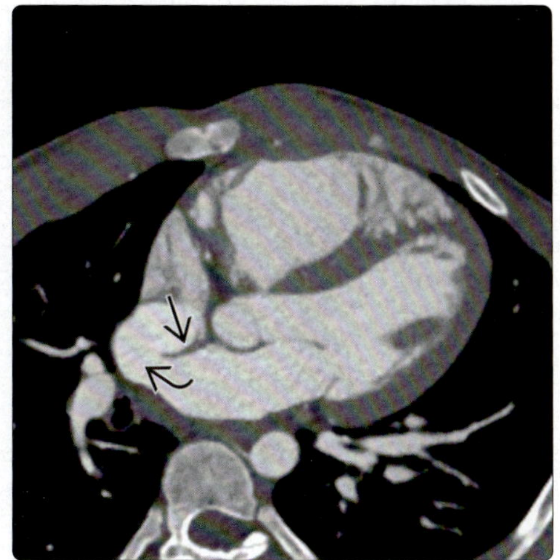

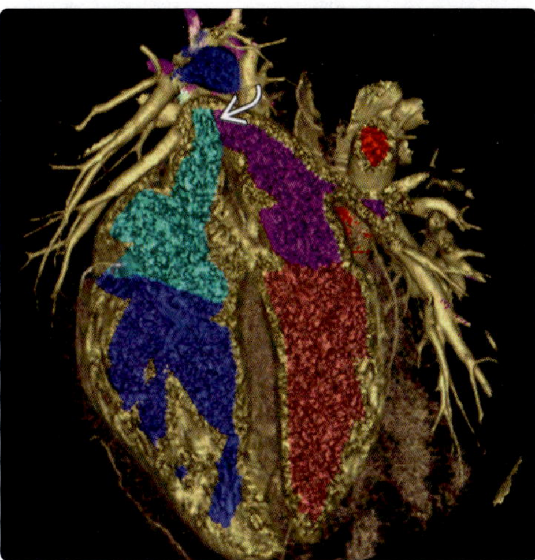

(Left) *Oblique axial cardiac CTA in a child shows a sinus venosus ASD with the defect ➔ in the superolateral aspect of the atrial septum ➔.* **(Right)** *Color-coded volume-rendered 4-chamber cardiac CTA shows the sinus venosus-type defect ➔ in the superolateral aspect of the atrial septum where the blood volume in the right atrium (teal), left atrium (magenta), right ventricle (blue), & left ventricle (salmon) are also shown.*

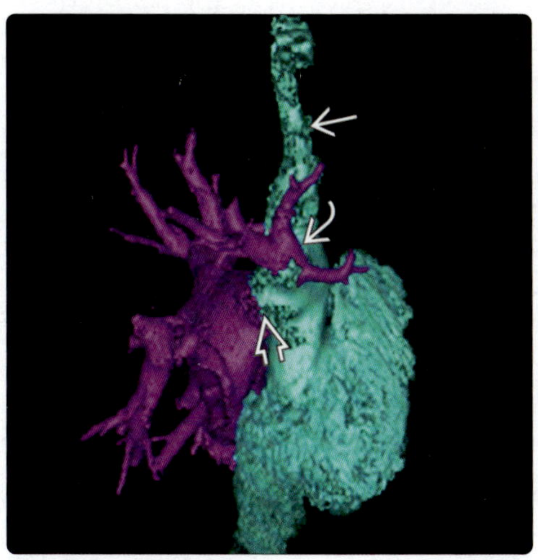

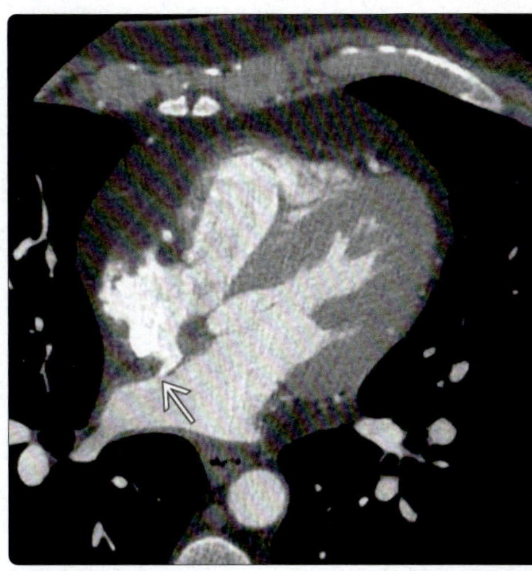

(Left) *Right lateral view of a volume-rendered cardiac CTA shows pulmonary veins ➔ draining to the SVC ➔, consistent with a right upper lobe partial anomalous pulmonary venous return (PAPVR) in a patient with a sinus venosus ASD ➔. PAPVR is common in patients with this type of ASD.* **(Right)** *Axial coronary CTA shows a patent foramen ovale ➔ with a typical oblique defect & flap in the atrial septum. This is seen in 25% of the population. Note that the size of the RA is normal as left-to-right (LTR) shunting does not occur.*

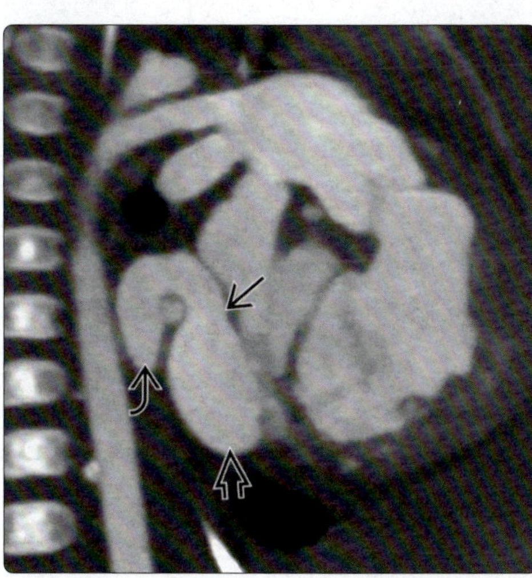

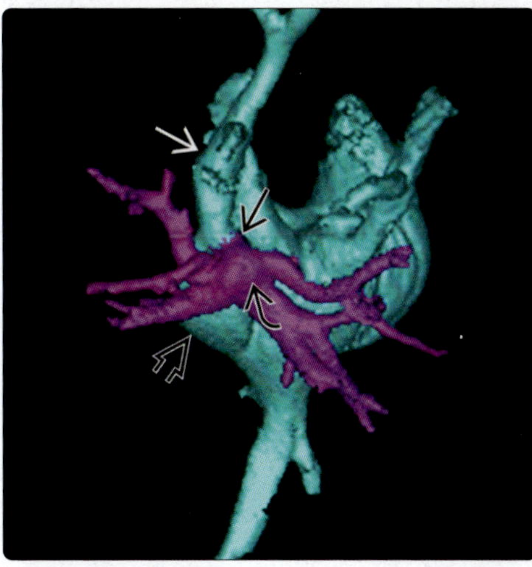

(Left) *Sagittal MIP cardiac CTA in an infant shows confluence of pulmonary veins ➔ communicating with the CS ➔, consistent with a variant of an unroofed coronary sinus ➔ type of ASD.* **(Right)** *Posterior volume-rendered cardiac CTA in an infant shows the confluence of pulmonary veins ➔ communicating with the CS ➔, consistent with a variant of an unroofed CS ➔ type of ASD. Note also that a left SVC ➔ empties into the CS.*

Ventricular Septal Defect

KEY FACTS

TERMINOLOGY

- Cardiac anomaly with communication(s) between left & right ventricles through septum
  - Perimembranous septal defect (80%)
  - Posterior or inlet defect associated with atrioventricular septal defect (AVSD) (8-10%)
  - Muscular or trabecular septal defect (5-10%)
  - Outlet septal defect or supracristal ventricular septal defect (VSD) (5%)
- Complex cardiac anomalies with VSD: Tetralogy of Fallot, truncus, double-outlet right ventricle (DORV)

IMAGING

- Cardiomegaly with ↑ size of main pulmonary artery, ↑ pulmonary artery flow, left atrial enlargement, & usually small aorta
- Hyperinflation in large shunts from abnormal lung compliance & bronchial compression by dilated pulmonary arteries
- CT & MR delineate anatomy
  - Multiple muscular VSDs: "Swiss cheese" septum
  - Shunt volume is estimated by velocity-encoded cine MR

TOP DIFFERENTIAL DIAGNOSES

- Atrioventricular canal defects
- Patent ductus arteriosus; DORV

CLINICAL ISSUES

- Small VSD: Asymptomatic but have heart murmur
  - May close spontaneously
- Moderate or large shunts are often asymptomatic early until pulmonary vascular resistance drops
  - Children develop tachypnea, tachycardia, diaphoresis, & failure to thrive
  - Treated medically with subsequent surgical approach
    - Muscular lesions require more difficult surgical approach; VSD catheter closure devices are often used

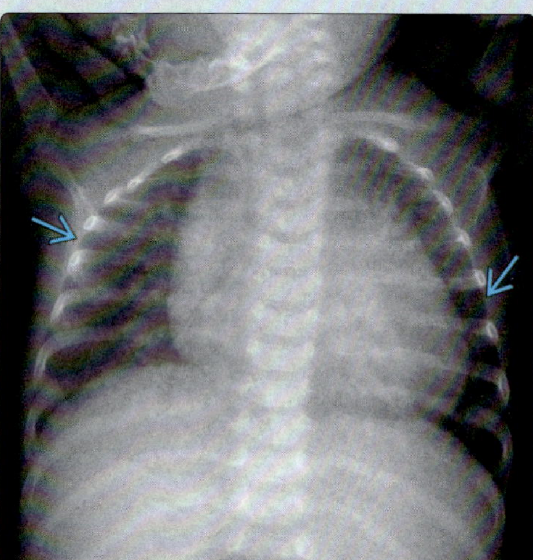

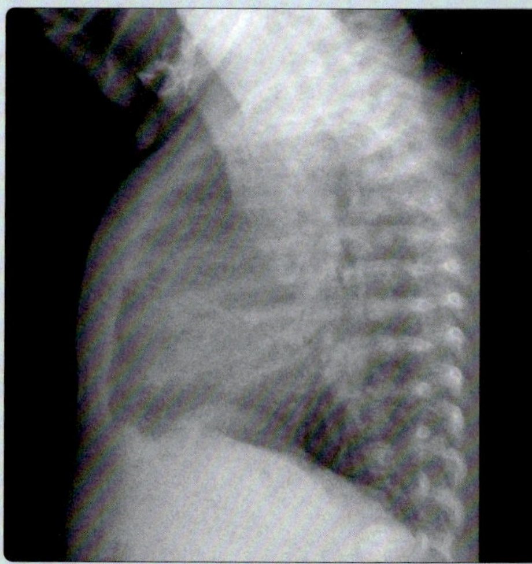

(Left) *AP radiograph in a 2-month-old with tachypnea & poor feeding secondary to a perimembranous ventricular septal defect (VSD) shows cardiac enlargement, ↑ pulmonary vascularity, & hyperinflation with bulging of the lungs between the intercostal spaces ➡.* **(Right)** *Lateral radiograph in the same patient redemonstrates these findings of cardiomegaly, ↑ vascularity, & hyperinflation. The hyperinflation is due to bronchial compression & poor lung compliance.*

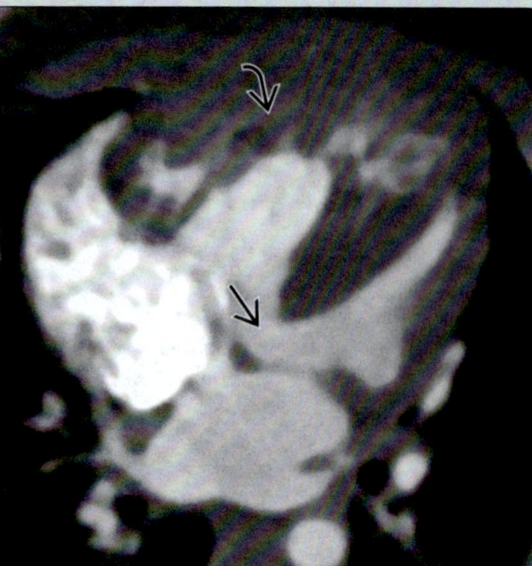

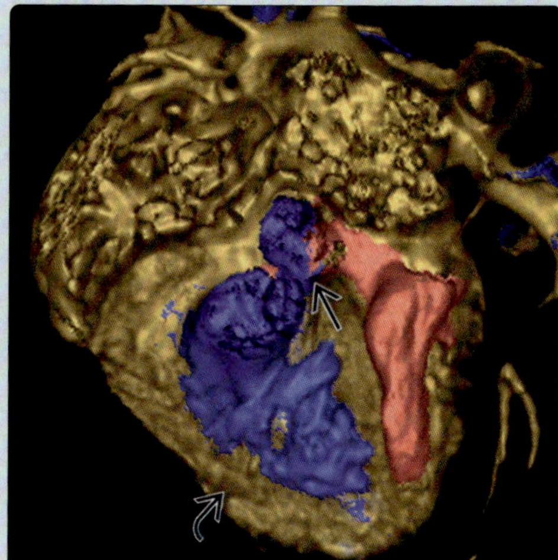

(Left) *Axial cardiac CTA in an infant shows a perimembranous-type VSD ➡. Note the right ventricular (RV) hypertrophy ➡, which is due to RV compensation from ↑ left-to-right volume.* **(Right)** *Axial image color-coded surface-rendered cardiac CTA in an infant shows a perimembranous-type VSD ➡ where the RV (purple) communicates with the left ventricle (LV) (pink). Note the right ventricular hypertrophy ➡.*

TERMINOLOGY

Abbreviations

- Ventricular septal defect (VSD)

Definitions

- Cardiac anomalies characterized by defect(s) in ventricular septum
  - Perimembranous septal defect
  - Muscular or trabecular septal defect
  - Posterior or inlet defect associated with atrioventricular septal defect (AVSD)
  - Outlet septal defect or supracristal VSD
- Complex cardiac anomalies with VSD
  - Tetralogy of Fallot, truncus arteriosus, double-outlet right ventricle
  - Associated with other congenital lesions: Coarctation, tricuspid atresia

IMAGING

General Features

- Best diagnostic clue
  - Chest radiograph with cardiomegaly (particularly left atrial enlargement) + ↑ pulmonary artery flow in small child
  - Defect in ventricular septum on any cross-sectional imaging modality
- Location
  - Membranous or perimembranous defects: 80%
    - Defects lie in outflow tract of left ventricle immediately beneath aortic valve
  - Inlet VSD: 8-10%
    - Posterior & inferior defects, beneath septal leaflet of tricuspid valve
    - Associated AVSD with usual involvement of atrioventricular valves
  - Outlet VSD occurs in 5%
    - Conal, subpulmonic, subaortic, supracristal, or infundibular
    - Malalignment defects associated with truncus arteriosus, tetralogy of Fallot, & double-outlet right ventricle
    - Supracristal defect is located about crista muscle high in ventricular outlet portion
      - May cause prolapse of aortic coronary cusp with development of aortic insufficiency & injury to aortic valve
  - Muscular or trabecular VSD occurs in 5-10%
    - Confined to muscular portion of interventricular septum
    - Central muscular, apical muscular, or marginal; may have multiple defects described as "Swiss cheese" muscular septum
- Size
  - Defects can be small, moderate, or large & involve adjacent structures

Radiographic Findings

- Small VSD
  - Normal chest radiograph does not exclude small shunt
- Moderate to large VSD
  - Cardiomegaly with ↑ size of main pulmonary artery, ↑ pulmonary artery flow, left atrial enlargement, & (usually) small aorta
    - Main pulmonary artery is high in position in infants, frequently confused with aortic knob
  - Heart failure may occur with venous edema
  - Hyperinflation is seen in large shunts due to abnormal lung compliance & possibly bronchial compression by dilated pulmonary arteries
- Supracristal VSD
  - Left-to-right shunt is usually small as anterior leaflet of aortic valve prolapses & may partially cover defect
  - May have evidence of dilated ascending aorta if aortic insufficiency is present
  - Difficult to diagnosis on chest radiographs

CT Findings

- Cardiac gated CTA
  - Delineates cardiac anatomy ± functional & volumetric evaluation
  - 3D images for planning percutaneous closure device
  - 3D printed models (made from various materials) are now occasionally used to test closure device placement before procedure
    - Simulated procedures are now performed using 3D models, virtual reality, & artificial intelligence

MR Findings

- Delineates cardiac anatomy & quantification of physiologic function
- Morphologic information is provided by ECG-gated spin-echo & cine MR imaging
- Shunt volume can be estimated by using velocity-encoded cine MR imaging
- Qp:Qs ratio (amount of blood flowing from right ventricle compared to left ventricle) may be calculated using phase-contrast imaging of right & left ventricular outflow tracts
  - Qp:Qs ratio > 1.5:1 is 1 indication for closure of VSD
- High-resolution 3D examination of vessels

Echocardiographic Findings

- Characterizes type, location, & number of septal defect(s) as well as function & hemodynamic assessment
- ECG is utilized as main diagnostic modality in infants & young children

Angiographic Findings

- Cardiac catheterization & angiography findings
  - Catheterization is utilized in complex lesions to obtain hemodynamic information & delineate anatomy

DIFFERENTIAL DIAGNOSIS

Atrioventricular Septal Defects

- Congenital defect involving atrial & ventricular septum & associated atrioventricular valves
- Chest radiograph demonstrates cardiomegaly & ↑ flow
- Presents early with clinical symptoms of large shunt
- High association with trisomy 21

Patent Ductus Arteriosus

- Persistent flow through ductus from high-pressure aorta to main pulmonary artery

- When shunt is large, chest radiograph demonstrates cardiomegaly & ↑ flow
- Presents early & has loud, continuous murmur during both systole & diastole

Double-Outlet Right Ventricle

- Both great vessels have their origins from right ventricle
- Aortic-mitral discontinuity is present with valves at similar level
- Pulmonary artery pressure is lower than systemic with significant flow into pulmonary arteries
  - Clinically & radiographically simulates large left-to-right shunt
- Complex lesion with many variants & classifications

PATHOLOGY

General Features

- Genetics
  - No specific genetic defect in majority
- Embryology
  - Complex, dependent on location of defect & associated anomalies
- Pathophysiology
  - Determinants of left-to-right shunt: Defect size, relative resistance or pressure in ventricular chambers (which may reflect systemic or pulmonary artery pressures)
  - Small defects have high resistance to flow across defect, resulting in small shunts
  - Large-sized VSDs are defined as defects that approximate size of aorta (& may have large flow)
  - ↑ flow across shunt → ↑ work of right ventricle & ↑ volume of venous return to left atrium & ventricle
  - Marked volume overload occurs → child develops tachycardia + congestive heart failure
  - Long-term ↑ in flow to pulmonary arteries is associated with vessel injury → pulmonary hypertension
    - Complex interaction between vascular endothelium & smooth muscle reaction is incompletely understood
    - May be reversible, & those with early pulmonary hypertension may need early surgical closure

CLINICAL ISSUES

Presentation

- Most common signs/symptoms
  - Dependent on size of shunt, associated lesions, & pulmonary vascular pressure
    - Small VSD: Asymptomatic but have heart murmur
    - Moderate or large VSD: Children have tachypnea, tachycardia, diaphoresis, & failure to thrive
      - Congestive heart failure may occur
- Other signs/symptoms
  - Loud systolic murmur near left heart border

Demographics

- Age
  - Although defect is present at birth, children are not symptomatic immediately due to high pulmonary vascular resistance of newborn
  - Moderate or large shunts are usually symptomatic in 1st few months of life
- Sex
  - M = F
- Epidemiology
  - Accounts for 20% of all congenital heart lesions
  - Most common congenital lesion associated with other heart lesions

Natural History & Prognosis

- Most small muscular VSDs close spontaneously
- Untreated large shunt will develop pulmonary vascular disease
  - Reversal of shunt from right-to-left with late-onset cyanosis
- Associated cardiac anomalies determine final outcome
- Lifetime risk of bacterial endocarditis

Treatment

- Small defects may close spontaneously
  - Includes many small muscular defects
  - Aneurysm of ventricular septum may be part of spontaneous closure
- Moderate & large defects are treated medically, followed by surgical approach
  - Medical therapy with diuretics & afterload reduction
  - Many infants improve & will grow
  - Poor growth &/or congestive heart failure may be indication for early surgery
- Surgical treatment depends on site of VSD
  - Perimembranous VSD: Surgical closure of shunt lesion is usually performed with right atrial approach on bypass during 1st or 2nd year if shunt is moderate or large
  - Outlet defects (such as supracristal VSD) are closed earlier to prevent aortic sinus prolapse, injury to valve leaflet, & subsequent aortic regurgitation
  - Muscular lesions require more difficult surgical approach; VSD catheter closure devices are often used

SELECTED REFERENCES

1. Maagaard M et al: Disappearance of the shunt and lower cardiac index during exercise in small, unrepaired ventricular septal defects. Cardiol Young. 30(4):526-32, 2020
2. Ojha V et al: Spectrum of changes on cardiac magnetic resonance in repaired tetralogy of Fallot: imaging according to surgical considerations. Clin Imaging. 69:102-14, 2020
3. A D et al: An unusual case of double-chambered left ventricle: a case of double-chambered left ventricle communicated with right ventricle through a ventricular septal defect presented during only in diastole and a concomitant mitral valve prolapse. J Echocardiogr. 17(3):167-8, 2019
4. Abdel Razek AAK et al: Imaging of pulmonary atresia with ventricular septal defect. J Comput Assist Tomogr. 43(6):906-11, 2019
5. Jivanji SGM et al: Novel use of a 3D printed heart model to guide simultaneous percutaneous repair of severe pulmonary regurgitation and right ventricular outflow tract aneurysm. Cardiol Young. 29(4):534-7, 2019
6. Mendez A et al: Virtual reality for preoperative planning in large ventricular septal defects. Eur Heart J. 40(13):1092, 2019
7. Alvarez A et al: Residual shunt diagnosed with 4D flow after reparation of post-infarct ventricular septal defect. Eur Heart J. 39(42):3820, 2018
8. Maagaard M et al: Biventricular morphology in adults born with a ventricular septal defect. Cardiol Young. 28(12):1379-85, 2018
9. Nicolay S et al: CT imaging features of atrioventricular shunts: what the radiologist must know. Insights Imaging. 7(1):119-29, 2016

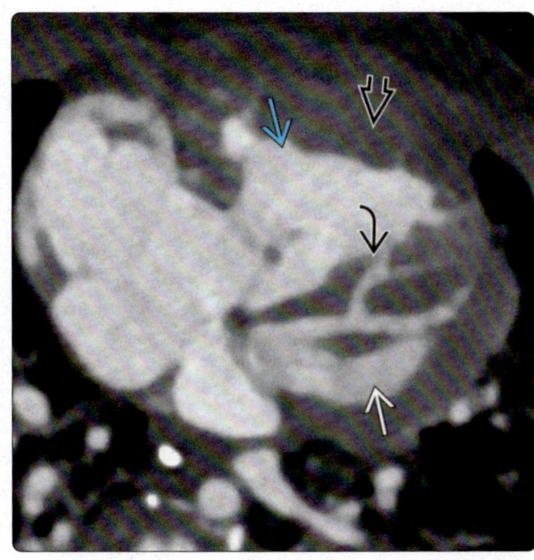

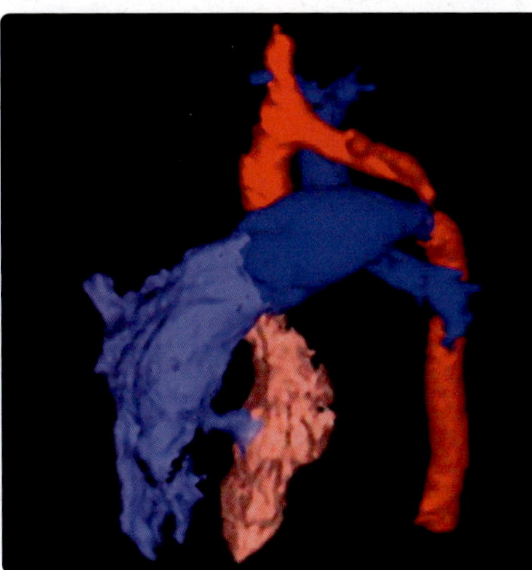

(Left) *Axial cardiac CTA in a newborn shows an intramuscular-type VSD ➔ between the RV ➔ & LV ➔. Note the significant RV hypertrophy ➔.* **(Right)** *Lateral color-coded 3D reconstruction of a cardiac CTA shows a single intramuscular-type VSD between the RV (purple) & LV (pink). Note that there is only mild enlargement of the RV (purple) as the Qp:Qs ratio was only 1.2:1.*

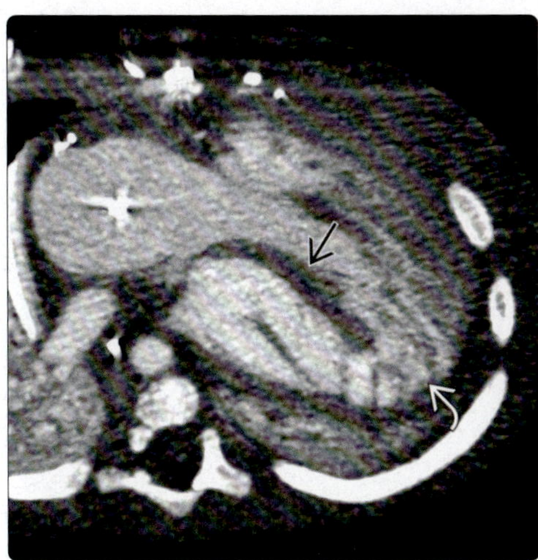

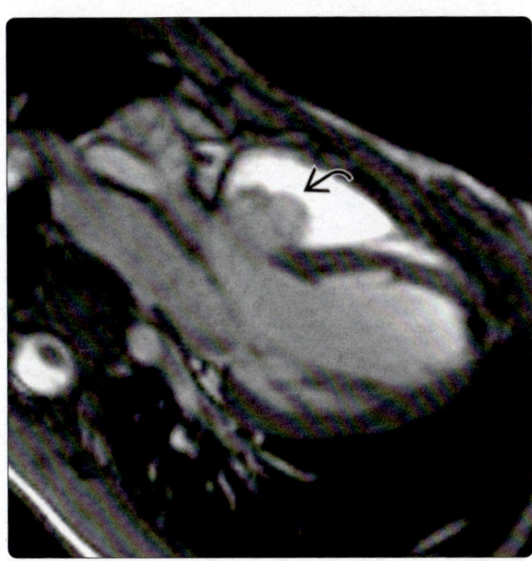

(Left) *Oblique axial cardiac CTA shows a Swiss cheese appearance of the interventricular septum ➔ near the apex in this patient with multiple muscular-type VSDs. Note the normal position of the septum ➔.* **(Right)** *Three-chamber view from a cine SSFP cardiac MR shows an aneurysm ➔ of the membranous ventricular septum protruding into the RV. This likely represents the spontaneous membranous closure of a previously patent VSD. This anomaly may cause RV outflow tract obstruction.*

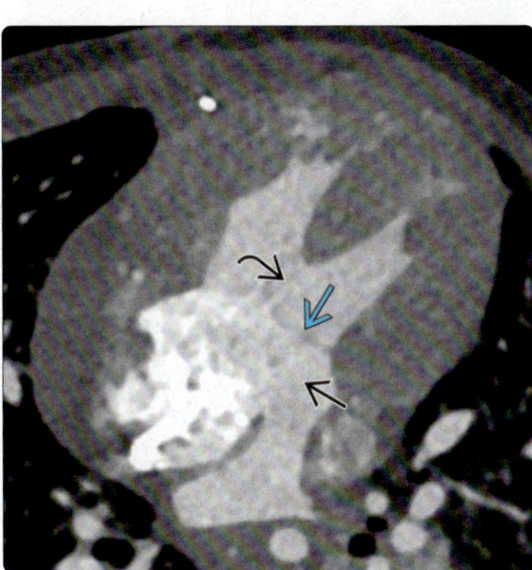

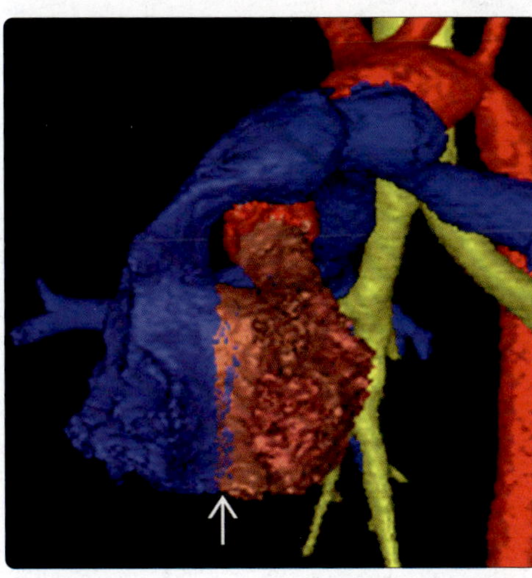

(Left) *Axial cardiac CTA in a Down syndrome patient shows a posterior-type VSD ➔. Note the septum primum atrial septal defect (ASD) ➔ in a patient with a complete atrioventricular (AV) canal defect & common AV valve ➔.* **(Right)** *Left lateral view from a color-coded 3D CTA in an infant shows a large posterior VSD ➔ typical of patients with AV canal defect.*

Atrioventricular Septal Defect

KEY FACTS

TERMINOLOGY

- Atrioventricular septal defect: a.k.a. complete atrioventricular canal (AVC) defect, endocardial cushion defect
- Broad spectrum of defects characterized by involvement of atrial septum, ventricular septum, & 1 or both atrioventricular (AV) valves
- Ostium primum defect: Considered partial AVC defect or partial AV septal defect

IMAGING

- Large right atrium, right ventricle, pulmonary artery with ↑ pulmonary artery flow
- Large defect in anterioinferior portion of atrial septum (ostium primum defect)
- Large defect in ventricular septum (posterior type is most common)
- Anterior & superior aortic position with elongation + dysplastic common 5-leaflet AV valve narrowing subvalvular LVOT → "gooseneck" deformity on angiography
- When AV valve opens toward 1 ventricle → unbalanced canal defect (right ventricular or left ventricular dominance can occur with single ventricle physiology)
- Mitral insufficiency may occur both pre- & postoperatively

CLINICAL ISSUES

- Associated with trisomy 21 in 44-48%
- Large shunts present early with tachypnea, tachycardia, & failure to thrive
- Small shunts may be well tolerated through 1st decade; children may be asymptomatic
- Single ventricle physiology may necessitate staged procedure, such as Glenn & then Fontan for unbalanced AVC
- Partial AVC is closed by pericardial patch via right atrial approach

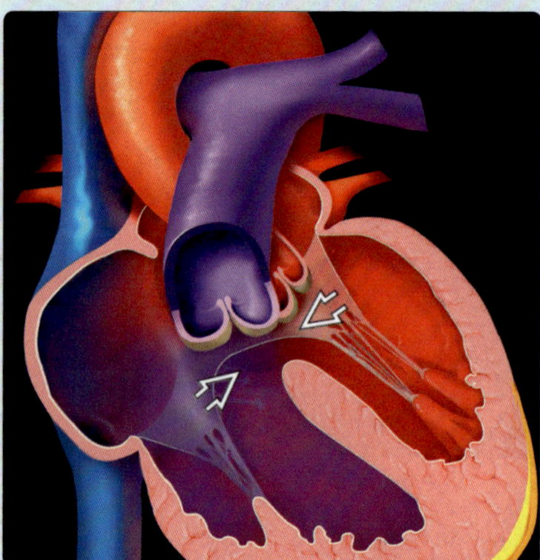

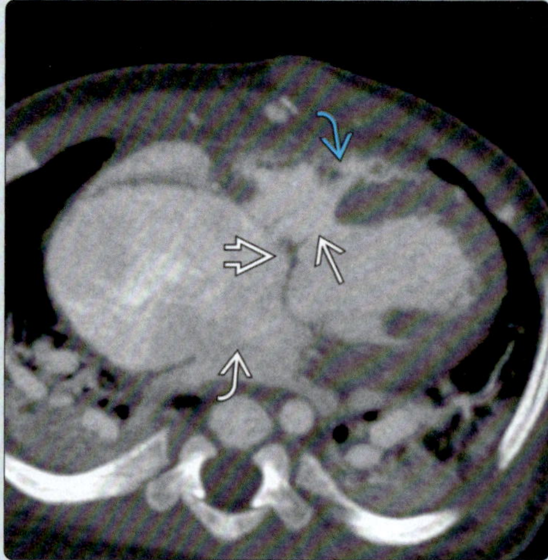

(Left) *Graphic shows a defect ➡ in the atrioventricular (AV) septum connecting the right atrium & right ventricle to the left atrium & left ventricle.* **(Right)** *Axial cardiac CTA shows an AV septal defect (AVSD). There is a common dysplastic AV valve ➡ with an inlet-type ventricular septal defect (VSD) ➡ & a septum primum atrial septal defect (ASD) ➡. Note the enlargement of the right atrium & the small right ventricle ➡ in this unbalanced AV canal defect.*

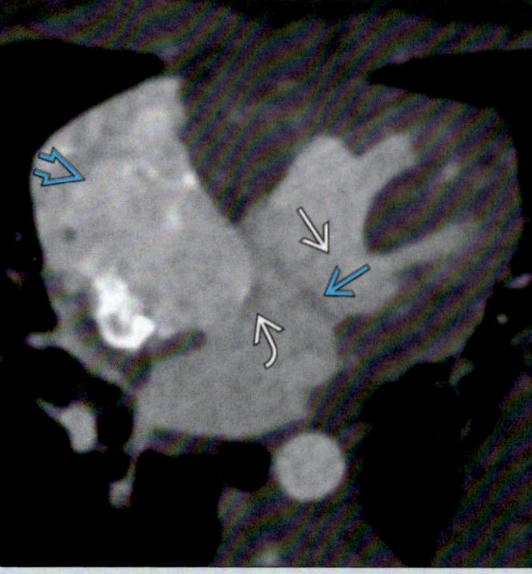

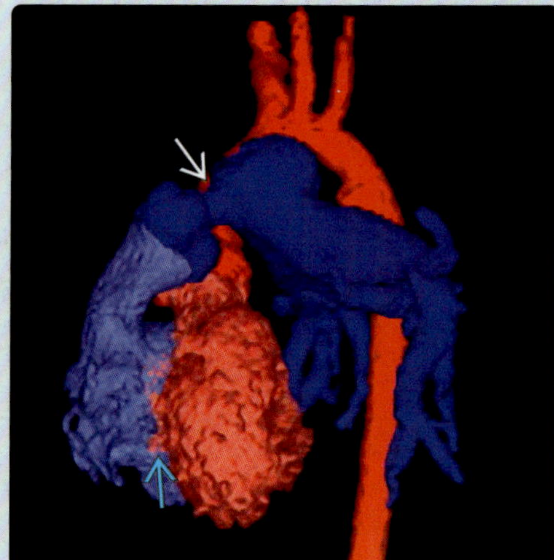

(Left) *Axial cardiac CTA in an infant with Down syndrome shows a large VSD ➡, septum primum ASD ➡, & common AV valve ➡, consistent with an AVSD. Note the large right atrium ➡.* **(Right)** *Lateral color-coded cardiac CTA shows a large posterior-type VSD ➡ in a patient with AVSD. Postoperative changes are seen from pulmonary banding ➡ to limit pulmonary flow.*

TERMINOLOGY

Abbreviations

- Atrioventricular septal defect (AVSD)

Synonyms

- AVSD
  - Atrioventricular canal (AVC) defect
  - Endocardial cushion defect
  - Complete AVC defect
- Ostium primum defect
  - Partial AVC defect
  - Partial AVSD
  - Incomplete endocardial cushion defect

Definitions

- Broad spectrum of defects characterized by involvement of atrial septum, ventricular septum, & 1 or both AV valves
  - Complete AVSD indicates presence of both atrial & ventricular septal defects with common AV valve
  - Partial AVSD indicates atrial septal involvement with separate mitral & tricuspid valve orifices
  - Unbalanced AVSD indicates 1 ventricular chamber is hypoplastic as compared to other, depending on direction of AV valve flow

IMAGING

General Features

- Best diagnostic clue
  - Chest radiograph
    - Large heart with large main pulmonary artery & ↑ pulmonary artery flow
    - Serial radiographs to evaluate for pulmonary hypertension
    - Mitral insufficiency may occur both pre- & postoperatively
      - When mitral insufficiency is severe, left atrium can be large & cause left lower lobe collapse
    - Children with large shunts have ↑ incidence of upper respiratory infections & pneumonia
    - Pulmonary hypertension patients have abnormal lung compliance: Lungs are often hyperinflated with eversion of hemidiaphragms
- Location
  - Complete AVC
    - Large defect in anterioinferior portion of atrial septum (ostium primum defect)
    - Large defect in ventricular septum (posterior type is most common)
    - Common AV valve with variable chordal attachments to ventricle
    - When AV valve opens toward 1 ventricle → unbalanced canal defect
    - Right ventricular or left ventricular dominance can occur with single ventricle physiology (or unbalanced defect)
    - Hypoplasia of inlet & outlet septum → hypoplasia of chamber with malalignment of ventricular septum
  - Ostium primum defect
    - Defect in anterioinferior aspect of atrial septum
    - ± coexistent cleft in anterior leaflet of mitral valve
    - 5-leaflet AV valve is present with separate valve orifices to right & left ventricles
- Size
  - Broad spectrum of size of defects in AV septum & respective sizes of ventricles

Echocardiographic Findings

- Echocardiogram
  - Defines lesion in infants & young children
    - Primum defects have echo dropout in lower portion of septum, cleft in mitral valve
    - Anterior & superior displacement of aorta with elongation & narrowing of left ventricular outflow tract (LVOT)
    - 3D echocardiography can better define anatomy of valve
- Color Doppler
  - Demonstration of left-to-right shunt, severity of mitral regurgitation, & tricuspid regurgitation
    - LVOT obstruction can be quantified

CT Findings

- CECT
  - Noninvasive alternative to further depict anatomy, chamber volumes, & function
  - Large right atrium, right ventricle, & pulmonary artery

MR Findings

- Excellent noninvasive alternative for depiction of function & anatomy
- Best imaging modality for calculating complex regurgitation across common AV valve
- Most accurate assessment of ventricular hypoplasia
- Qp:Qs ratio is calculated from velocity-encoded cine MR technique

Angiographic Findings

- Conventional
  - Cardiac catheterization is not usually done to evaluate anatomy but to measure pulmonary vascular resistance
    - Left ventriculogram shows cleft in mitral valve, shunts, respective sizes of ventricles, & LVOT obstruction
    - Classic "gooseneck" deformity seen on frontal projection of left ventricular angiocardiogram
      - Dysplastic common AV valve narrows subvalvular LVOT

Imaging Recommendations

- Best imaging tool
  - Echocardiography in infants & young children: Defines lesion
    - Primum defects have echo dropout in lower portion of septum, mitral valve cleft
    - Complete AVSD demonstrates varying degrees of absence of septum, size of defect, & relative size of ventricles
- 3D CT & MR reconstructions: Useful for demonstrating complex global, coronary, & extracardiac anatomy for presurgical planning

DIFFERENTIAL DIAGNOSIS

Ventricular Septal Defect

- Most common congenital heart disease (CHD) with left-to-right shunt
- Most common CHD associated with other lesions
- Cardiac enlargement with ↑ pulmonary flow

Atrial Septal Defect

- Defect in superior portion of atrial septum
- Presents in older children who are usually asymptomatic from shunt
- Left-to-right shunt is usually not large but can cause Eisenmenger physiology in adult if unrecognized

Patent Ductus Arteriosus

- Communication between high-pressure aorta & lower pressure pulmonary artery
- Left-to-right shunt usually presents in infancy
- Closed by percutaneous occlusion devices

PATHOLOGY

General Features

- Etiology
  - Malformation occurring during 5th week of gestation
  - Abnormal or inadequate fusion of superior & inferior endocardial cushion
  - Abnormal fusion of ventricular (trabecular) portion of septum
  - Iatrogenic AVSD has been described
- Genetics
  - Associated with trisomy 21 in 44-48%
- Associated abnormalities
  - Trisomy 21 children have constellation of clinical & radiographic findings
    - Chest radiograph may show 11 ribs, double manubrial ossification center in 80%
  - Heterotaxy
  - Tetralogy of Fallot

CLINICAL ISSUES

Presentation

- Most common signs/symptoms
  - Complete AVSD
    - Large shunts present early with tachypnea, tachycardia, & failure to thrive
    - Mitral insufficiency adds complexity & earlier symptoms
  - Partial AVSD
    - Small shunts may be well tolerated through 1st decade, children may be asymptomatic
    - Mitral insufficiency adds complexity & earlier symptoms
- Other signs/symptoms
  - Pathophysiology of lesions
    - Degree of left-to-right shunting is determined by size of defect & relative compliance of atria & ventricles
    - Right ventricular compliance reflects pulmonary vascular resistance
    - Infants have ↑ pulmonary vascular resistance & therefore rarely have shunts
    - As pulmonary vascular resistance ↓, left-to-right shunting ↑ with age
    - Subsequent enlargement of right atrium & right ventricle & ↑ in pulmonary vascularity
    - Cleft directs regurgitant blood through atrial defect

Demographics

- Epidemiology
  - 4-8:1,000 live births have congenital heart defects
  - 5-8% have AVSD
  - 44-48% of patients with Down syndrome or trisomy 21 have AVC defect

Natural History & Prognosis

- Complete AVC defect presents in infancy with symptoms
- Children assessed for surgical repair
  - Postoperative course may be complicated by mitral insufficiency
  - Pulmonary hypertension occurs in children without surgical intervention

Treatment

- Medical management until surgery (depending on lesion & severity)
- Surgical management: Partial AVSD
  - Closed by pericardial patch via right atrial approach
  - Percutaneous closure devices are not typically deployed as inferior attachment may injure AV valves
- Surgical management: Complete AVSD (mortality rate: 3%)
  - Elective repair in children 2-5 years of age unless mitral regurgitation is present
  - Complications include mitral insufficiency (which may require reoperation, valvuloplasty, or replacement)
  - Arrhythmias, such as sinus node dysfunction or heart block
- Surgical management: Complete unbalanced AVSD
  - Single ventricle physiology may necessitate staged procedure, such as Glenn & then Fontan

SELECTED REFERENCES

1. Nayak S et al: Echocardiographic assessment of atrioventricular canal defects. Echocardiography. 37(12):2199-210, 2020
2. Elders B et al: Altered ascending aortic wall shear stress in patients with corrected atrioventricular septal defect: a comprehensive cardiovascular magnetic resonance and 4D flow MRI evaluation. Cardiol Young. 29(5):637-42, 2019
3. Ye XT et al: Partition of common atrioventricular valve in a patient with dextrocardia and univentricular circulation. Semin Thorac Cardiovasc Surg. 31(1):113-5, 2019
4. Han J et al: Goose neck appearance: endocardial cushion defect. J Med Imaging Radiat Oncol. 62 Suppl 1:31, 2018
5. Sarısoy Ö et al: Long-term outcomes in patients who underwent surgical correction for atrioventricular septal defect. Anatol J Cardiol. 20(4):229-34, 2018
6. Zhu Y et al: Preliminary study of the application of transthoracic echocardiography-guided three-dimensional printing for the assessment of structural heart disease. Echocardiography. 34(12):1903-8, 2017
7. Davey BT et al: The natural history of atrioventricular valve regurgitation throughout fetal life in patients with atrioventricular canal defects. Pediatr Cardiol. 37(1):50-4, 2016
8. Saremi F et al: Septal atrioventricular junction region: comprehensive imaging in adults. Radiographics. 36(7):1966-86, 2016
9. Calkoen EE et al: Characterization and quantification of dynamic eccentric regurgitation of the left atrioventricular valve after atrioventricular septal defect correction with 4D flow cardiovascular magnetic resonance and retrospective valve tracking. J Cardiovasc Magn Reson. 17:18, 2015

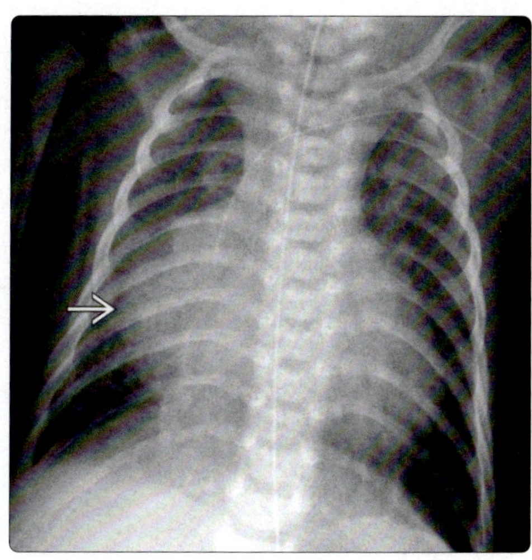

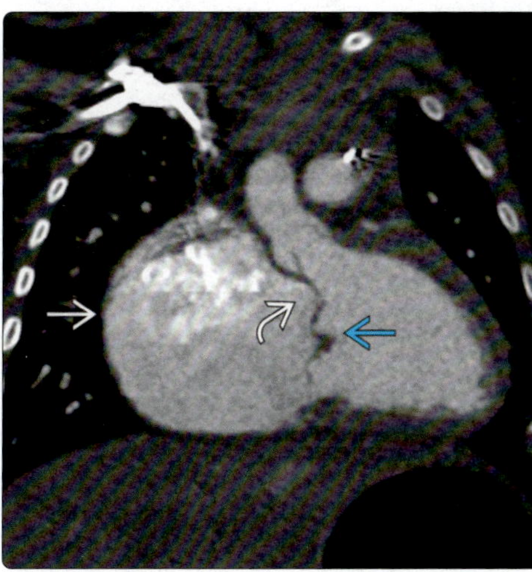

(Left) *Frontal chest radiograph in a 2-month-old with Down syndrome shows cardiomegaly, ↑ pulmonary vascularity, & venous congestion. Note the massive enlargement of the right atrium* ➡. **(Right)** *Coronal CTA shows the dysplastic common AV valve* ➡ *narrowing the subvalvular left ventricular outflow tract (LVOT)* ➡. *This is the cause of the "gooseneck" deformity seen on conventional angiography in patients with AVSD. Note the enlarged right atrium* ➡.

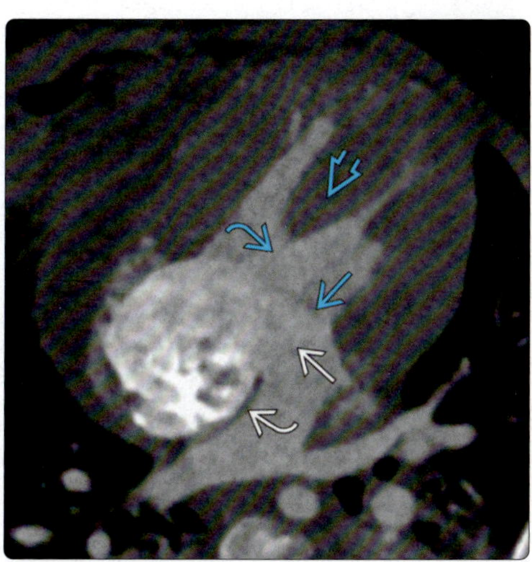

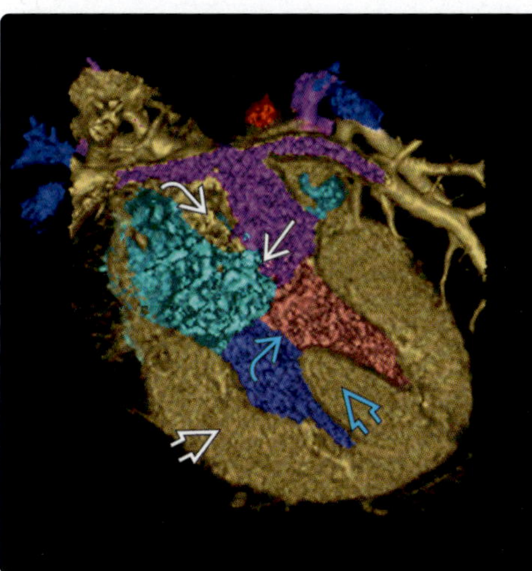

(Left) *Four-chamber cardiac CTA in an infant demonstrates an ostium primum defect* ➡ *in the atrial septum* ➡ *with a common AV valve* ➡. *There is also a defect* ➡ *in the ventricular septum* ➡ *in this patient with an AVSD.* **(Right)** *Four-chamber 3D color-coded CTA in an infant with an AVSD demonstrates an ostium primum ASD* ➡ *in the atrial septum* ➡ *with a large defect* ➡ *in the ventricular septum .* ➡. *Note the marked thickening of the right ventricle wall* ➡.

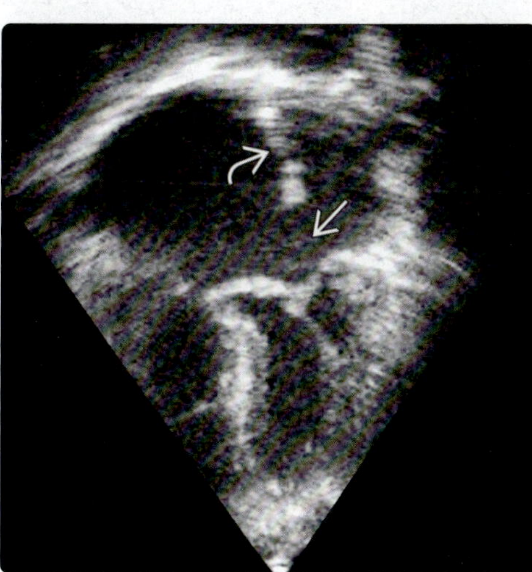

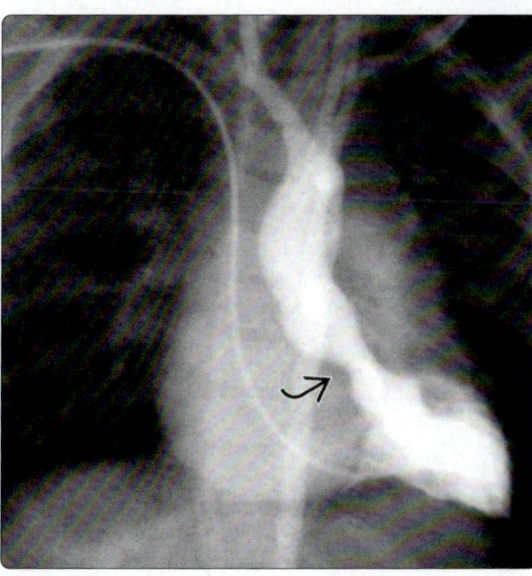

(Left) *Four-chamber view echocardiogram shows echo dropout in the inferior portion of the atrial septum* ➡, *which is characteristic of a primum ASD. Note the intact portion of the atrial septum* ➡. **(Right)** *Left ventricular angiogram shows a typical "gooseneck" deformity* ➡ *of the LVOT in a patient with AVSD. Subvalvular narrowing of the LVOT is due to the enlarged common AV valve.*

Patent Ductus Arteriosus

KEY FACTS

TERMINOLOGY

- Persistent postnatal patency of normal prenatal connection from PA to proximal descending aorta
- Hemodynamics: L-to-R shunt between aorta & PA
- PDA is frequently essential in complex congenital heart disease: L-to-R or R-to-L flow, depending on other anomalies
- PDA in persistent fetal circulation syndrome: R-to-L flow

IMAGING

- Well demonstrated by CTA & MRA: Usually linear, directed anterior to posterior, of variable size
- PDA may be tortuous vessel connecting aorta &/or innominate artery with PA
- CTA is modality of choice for showing airway compression from tortuous PDA or vascular ring

PATHOLOGY

- With normal drop of pulmonary vascular resistance, L-to-R shunt to PA through PDA: Volume overload of left-sided cardiac chambers
  - Diastolic flow reversal in aorta can lead to renal & intestinal hypoperfusion → renal dysfunction & necrotizing enterocolitis
  - Pressure overload of RV eventually causes reversal of shunt (R-to-L) → cyanosis (Eisenmenger physiology)
- When closed: Forms ligamentum arteriosum, ± Ca^{2+}
- In right arch, aberrant left subclavian artery ductus completes vascular ring

CLINICAL ISSUES

- To close ductus in premature infants: Indomethacin
- To keep ductus open in cyanotic heart disease: Prostaglandin E1
- Term infants, older children: Surgical clipping or ligation vs. endovascular closure with duct occluder devices &/or coils

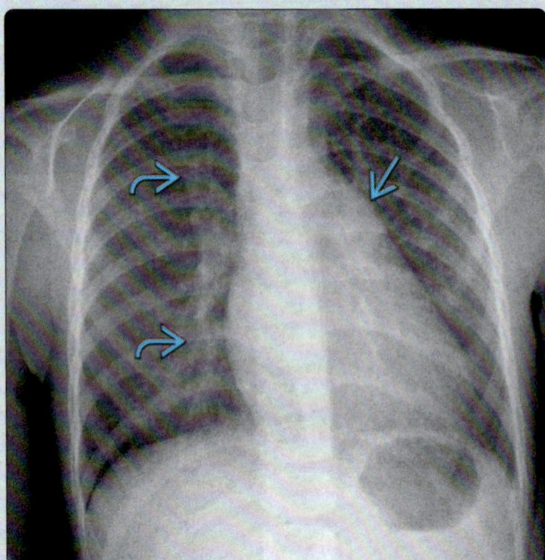

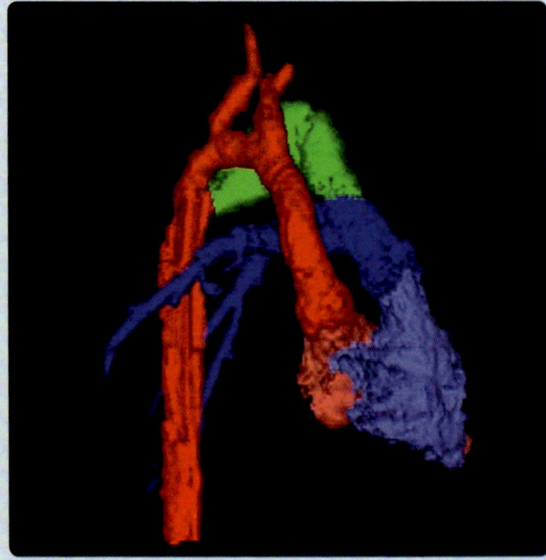

(Left) *Frontal view of the chest in an 8-year-old patient with a persistent patent ductus arteriosus (PDA) shows ↑ (shunt) vascularity ➡ with prominence of the pulmonary artery (PA) ➡. Chronic PDA can cause Eisenmenger syndrome.* **(Right)** *Frontal oblique 3D color-coded cardiac CTA shows a massively enlarged PDA (green) coursing between the main PA (blue) & the descending aorta (red). Note that the PDA can be larger than the aortic arch.*

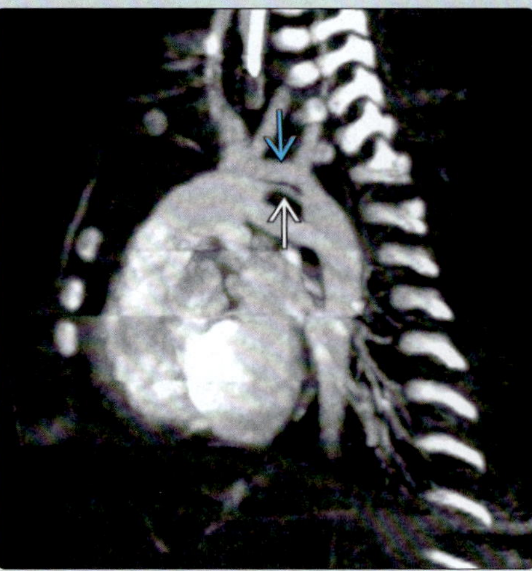

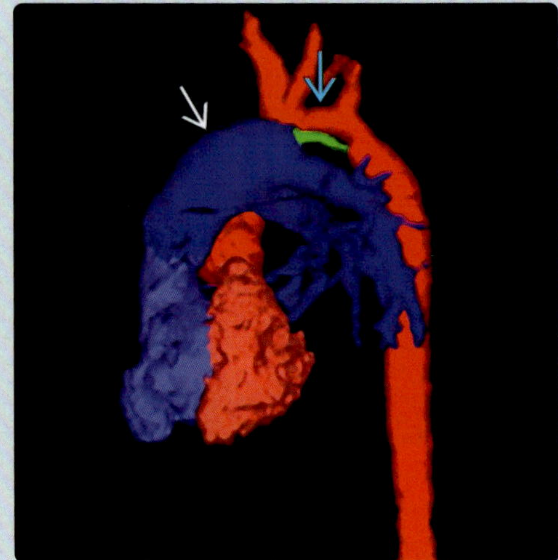

(Left) *Oblique MIP cardiac CTA shows a small PDA ➡ connecting the aorta to the main PA. Note that the transverse aortic arch is mildly hypoplastic ➡. A PDA is commonly seen in association with a left ventricular outflow tract obstruction.* **(Right)** *Oblique 3D color-coded cardiac CTA in the same patient shows a PDA (green) with a mildly hypoplastic aorta ➡. Compare this with the previous MIP image. Note the enlarged size of the main PA ➡ caused by ↑ L-to-R shunting.*

TERMINOLOGY

Abbreviations

- Patent ductus arteriosus (PDA)

Synonyms

- Persistent arterial duct, patent ductus Botalli

Definitions

- Persistent postnatal patency of normal prenatal connection from pulmonary artery (PA) to proximal descending aorta
- Category: Acyanotic, ↑ pulmonary blood flow
- Hemodynamics: Left-to-right shunt between aorta & PA
- PDA is frequently essential part of complex congenital heart disease
  - Typical ductal-dependent lesions, including hypoplastic left heart syndrome, severe hypoplastic-type coarctation, & interruption of aortic arch: Conduit for systemic perfusion (right-to-left flow)
  - D-transposition of great arteries: Necessary for admixture between systemic & pulmonary circuits (left-to-right flow)
  - Pulmonary atresia & other severe cyanotic heart diseases with right-sided obstruction: Conduit for pulmonary perfusion (left-to-right flow)
- PDA is part of persistent fetal circulation syndrome: Right-to-left flow
  - Severe lung disease (meconium aspiration, surfactant deficiency disease, neonatal pneumonia)
  - Primary pulmonary hypertension of neonate

IMAGING

General Features

- Best diagnostic clue
  - Cardiomegaly & heart failure once pulmonary vascular resistance drops in premature infant recovering from surfactant deficiency disease

Radiographic Findings

- Cardiomegaly (left atrium & left ventricle)
- ↑ pulmonary vascularity
- Wide vascular pedicle (large aortic arch with ductus bump)

CT Findings

- CTA
  - Volume renditions of aortic arch depict PDA with associated complex anatomy
  - Excellent modality for sizing of ductus prior to cardiac catheterization for placement of occluder device or prior to stenting in hybrid procedure
  - Modality of choice for showing airway compression from tortuous PDA or vascular ring
  - Valve-like structure is often identified at PA side of PDA that should not be mistaken for endarteritis

MR Findings

- SSFP bright blood cine
  - Functional right ventricular assessment in cases with Eisenmenger pulmonary hypertension
  - Dephasing artifact is depicted in direction of PDA flow
- Double inversion recovery (black blood) sequence
  - Sagittal oblique plane through aortic arch depicts ductus
- 3D gadolinium MRA with volume rendition to depict anatomy
- Velocity-encoded cine sequences are used to calculate Qp:Qs ratio
  - Closure is usually indicated for Qp:Qs ratio > 1.7

Echocardiographic Findings

- Echocardiogram
  - Suprasternal notch view: Direct visualization of ductus
  - Size & flow across ductus in early infancy have been shown to correlate with prognosis of chronic lung disease in premature infants
- M-mode
  - ↑ left atrium:aorta ratio (> 1.2:1)
- Pulsed Doppler
  - Diastolic flow reversal in descending & abdominal aorta (ductus steal)
  - Flow acceleration across constricting ductus: Transductal velocity ratio
- Color Doppler
  - For flow direction through ductus

Angiographic Findings

- Conventional
  - Cardiac catheterization is only needed for associated complex cyanotic heart disease & to determine reversibility of pulmonary hypertension
  - Placement of PDA closure device

Imaging Recommendations

- Protocol advice
  - Treatment decisions are based only on echocardiographic findings in majority of cases
  - CTA is recommended for complex anatomy with airway compression

DIFFERENTIAL DIAGNOSIS

Other Causes of Left-to-Right Shunting

- Atrial & ventricular septal defects
- Atrioventricular canal

Persistent Fetal Circulation Syndrome

- Pulmonary hypertension (primary or secondary to severe lung disease)
- Patent foramen ovale
- PDA secondary to profound irreversible hypoxia

PATHOLOGY

General Features

- Etiology
  - Prematurity: Persistent postnatal hypoxia → failure of contraction of ductus
  - Term infant: Associated with maternal rubella
- Genetics
  - No specific genetic defect is identified in most cases of isolated PDA
- Embryology
  - Ductus originates from primitive 6th aortic arch
- Pathophysiology (for simple PDA)
  - PDA is persistence of normal prenatal structure after birth

- In normal neonate, ductus arteriosus closes functionally 18-24 hours after birth, anatomically at 1 month of age
- With normal drop of pulmonary vascular resistance, left-to-right shunt occurs to PA through PDA → volume overload of left-sided cardiac chambers
- With pulmonary hypertension, pressure overload of right ventricle causes reversal of shunt (right-to-left) → cyanosis (Eisenmenger physiology)
- Diastolic flow reversal in aorta can lead to renal & intestinal hypoperfusion → renal dysfunction & necrotizing enterocolitis

Gross Pathologic & Surgical Features

- PDA is usually wider on aortic side
  - Length: 2-8 mm; diameter: 4-12 mm
  - Makes acute angle with aorta in simple PDA, blunt angle with associated congenital heart disease
- Contractile tissue is mainly on pulmonary side: Spirally arranged muscle bundles in media
  - Prostaglandin E1 (present in fetal life) maintains relaxation
  - ↑ oxygen pressure causes constriction
- Thickening of intima with mucoid degeneration
- When closed, arterial duct forms ligamentum arteriosum
- Calcified ligamentum arteriosum is often incidentally seen on radiograph or CT
- Can be right-sided & originate from base of brachiocephalic artery or from aberrant right subclavian artery
- In right arch with aberrant left subclavian artery anatomy, ductus completes vascular ring
- Rarely ducti may be bilateral with right ductus typically originating from right brachiocephalic or subclavian & left ductus originating from undersurface of aorta
  - Double ducti anatomy may be reversed with situs anomalies
  - Spontaneous closure of ductus may help differentiate from aortopulmonary collaterals

CLINICAL ISSUES

Presentation

- Most common signs/symptoms
  - Characteristic machinery-like murmur
  - Bounding peripheral pulses
  - Congestive heart failure
  - Special situation: Premature infant recovering from surfactant deficiency disease
    - ↓ in hypoxia → ↓ in pulmonary vascular resistance → ↑ shunt flow through ductus arteriosus → clinical & radiographic signs of congestive heart failure (cardiomegaly, pulmonary edema)
- Other signs/symptoms
  - Subacute bacterial endocarditis
    - Need for treatment of clinically "silent" PDA (incidentally detected with echocardiography) controversial
  - Ductal aneurysm
    - Can result from premature narrowing of ductus on pulmonary side

Demographics

- Epidemiology
  - 10-12% of congenital heart disease
  - 1/2,500-5,000 live births
  - Slightly more common in female patients
  - Associated with prematurity (21-35%)

Natural History & Prognosis

- Isolated PDA: Excellent prognosis with early closure
- When associated with complex heart disease, prognosis determined by underlying disorder
- Irreversible pulmonary hypertension (Eisenmenger physiology) → shunt reversal & development of cyanosis
- Persistent fetal circulation, pulmonary hypertension: Treatment with extracorporeal membrane oxygenation often necessary to disrupt vicious cycle
  - Hypoxia → pulmonary vasoconstriction → ↓ pulmonary flow → more severe hypoxia

Treatment

- To close ductus in premature infants: Indomethacin
  - Side effects: Renal failure, intestinal perforation, intracranial hemorrhage
- To keep ductus open (cyanotic heart disease): Prostaglandin E1
- Term infants, older children: Surgical clipping, ligation, or device closure of PDA
  - Can be performed at bedside under video-assisted thoracoscopic &/or robotic guidance
  - Complications: Inadvertent ligation of aortic isthmus or PA, recurrent laryngeal nerve injury
- Endovascular closure with duct occluder devices &/or coils
  - Small ductus (< 4 mm): Gianturco coils
  - Large ductus (> 4 mm): Ivalon plug, Rashkind & Amplatz duct occluders
  - Complications: Protrusion of occluder device into left PA orifice → ↓ left lung perfusion, peripheral embolization
  - Incomplete closure in 10-20%

SELECTED REFERENCES

1. Porayette P et al: Rare association of absent pulmonary valve with intact ventricular septum and patent ductus arteriosus: assessment in a newborn with CT angiography. J Cardiovasc Comput Tomogr. 15(1):e1-2, 2021
2. Burkett DA: Common left-to-right shunts. Pediatr Clin North Am. 67(5):821-42, 2020
3. Jadhav SP et al: Correlation of ductus arteriosus length and morphology between computed tomographic angiography and catheter angiography and their relation to ductal stent length. Pediatr Radiol. 50(6):800-9, 2020
4. Krupiński M et al: Detailed radiological study of the patent ductus arteriosus: a computed tomography study in the Polish population. Folia Morphol (Warsz). 79(3):462-8, 2020
5. Rajesh V et al: Echocardiography in adult patients with PDA: a simplified approach. Echocardiography. 37(12):2194-8, 2020
6. Hagadorn JI et al: Covariation of neonatal intensive care unit-level patent ductus arteriosus management and in-neonatal intensive care unit outcomes following preterm birth. J Pediatr. 203:225-33.e1, 2018
7. Shafi NA et al: Sizing of patent ductus arteriosus in adults for transcatheter closure using the balloon pull-through technique. Catheter Cardiovasc Interv. 91(6):1159-63, 2018
8. Xu E et al: Ductus arteriosus aneurysm: case report and review of the literature. Arch Pediatr. 25(4):283-5, 2018

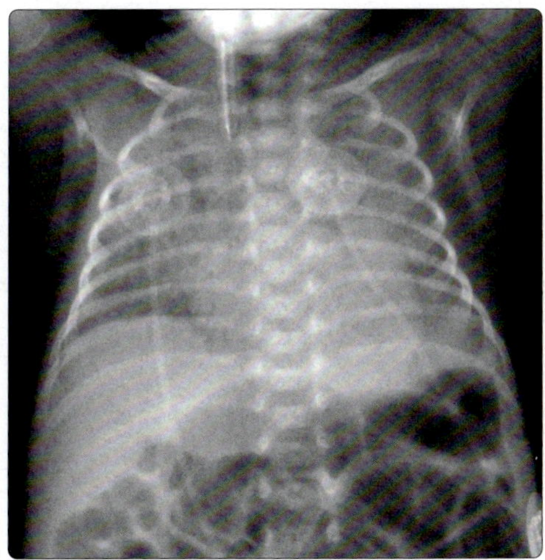

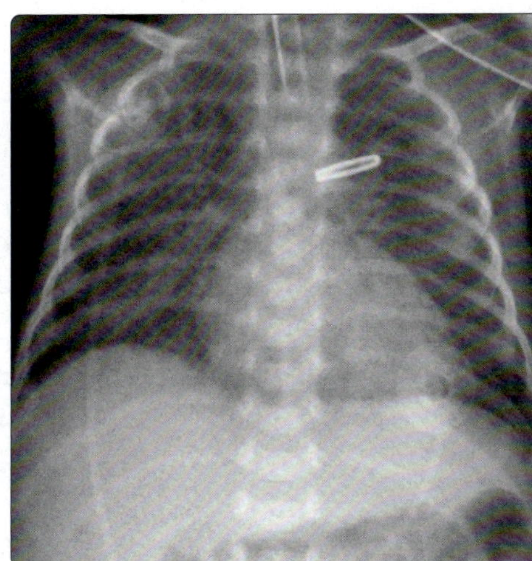

(Left) *AP chest radiograph in a 7-day-old premature infant shows diffuse, bilateral, hazy opacification of the lungs. An echocardiogram showed a PDA with left-to-right flow.* **(Right)** *AP view of the chest in the same patient shows a surgical clip from interval ligation of a PDA with ↑ aeration of the lungs & ↓ pulmonary edema.*

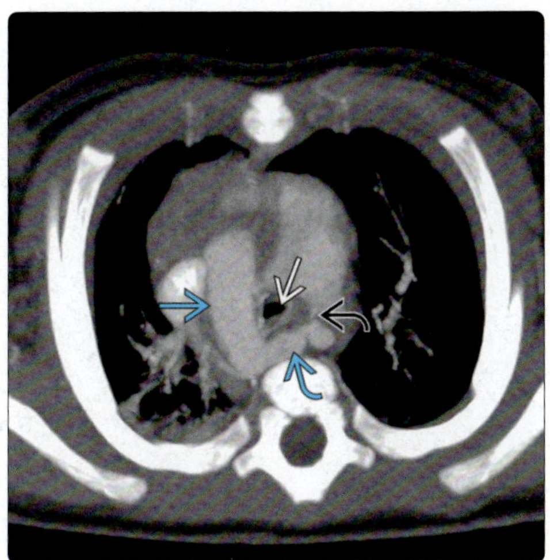

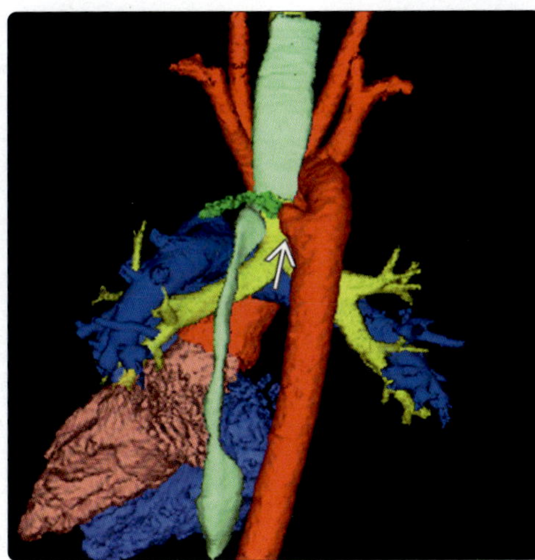

(Left) *Axial MIP CTA shows a right aortic arch ➔ with an aberrant left subclavian artery ➔ & small PDA ➔. Note that the small PDA completes the vascular ring around the trachea ➔.* **(Right)** *Posterior 3D color-coded cardiac CTA shows a PDA (green) arising from the ductus bump ➔ along the descending aorta & extending to the main PA (blue). The small PDA completes the vascular ring in this patient with a right arch. Note the impression on the esophagus (light green) at the level of the PDA.*

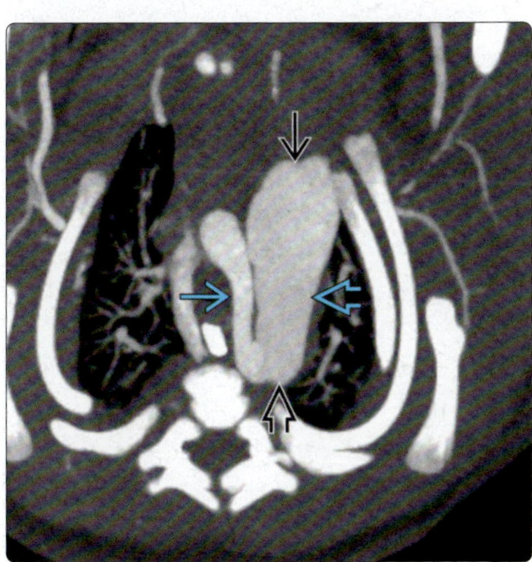

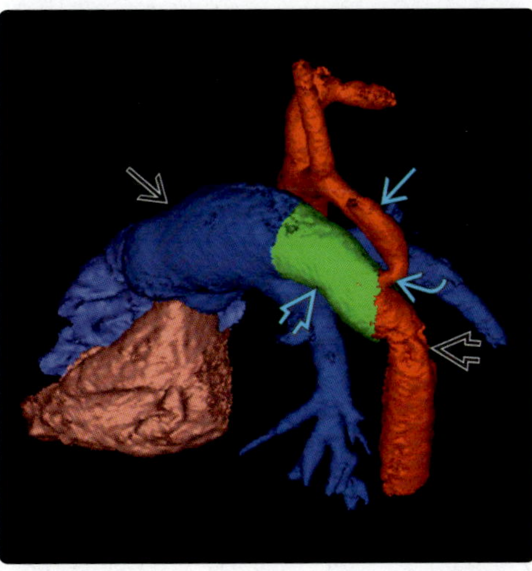

(Left) *Axial MIP cardiac CTA shows a hypoplastic aortic arch ➔ with an enlarged PDA ➔ connecting the PA ➔ to the descending thoracic aorta ➔. This constitutes a ductal-dependent lesion as the flow through the aorta is inadequate.* **(Right)** *Left posterior 3D color-coded cardiac CTA shows a hypoplastic aortic arch ➔ with an enlarged PDA ➔ connecting the PA ➔ to the descending thoracic aorta ➔. Note that there is also a focal coarctation ➔ in this ductal-dependent lesion.*

Tetralogy of Fallot

KEY FACTS

TERMINOLOGY

- Most common cyanotic congenital heart lesion
- Tetralogy: 4 heart defects from embryologic anterocephalad deviation of conoventricular septum
  - Infundibular or subpulmonary narrowing
  - Anterior malalignment ventricular septal defect (VSD)
  - Aorta overriding VSD
  - Secondary right ventricular hypertrophy (RVH)
- Spectrum of tetralogy of Fallot disease
  - "Blue tet": More subpulmonary obstruction → VSD shunts right-to-left → cyanotic appearance
  - "Pink tet": Less subpulmonary obstruction → VSD shunts left-to-right (normal) → acyanotic appearance
  - Tetralogy with pulmonary atresia & major aortopulmonary collaterals: Severe congenital heart disease
  - Tetralogy with absent pulmonary valve: To-&-fro flow in pulmonary artery (PA) leading to massively dilated branch PAs, tracheobronchial compression

IMAGING

- Radiography: Normal heart size, concave PA segment, ↓ pulmonary vascularity (oligemia)
  - RVH → upturned cardiac apex → boot-shaped heart
  - Right-sided aortic arch in 25%
- Echocardiography: Initial diagnosis, often prenatal
  - Coronary artery anomalies are important for surgical planning: Left anterior descending artery arising from right coronary & crossing RVOT (4%)
- Cardiac MR: Becoming gold standard for postoperative assessment; critical biomarker data for timing of pulmonary valve replacement (PVR)

CLINICAL ISSUES

- Typical repair within 1st year to life: VSD closure, relieve RVOT obstruction (transannular patch)
- Significant PR → RV chamber dilation over time: ↓ exercise tolerance, RV dysfunction, ventricular arrhythmias
- PVR is utilized to prevent progressive RV dilation

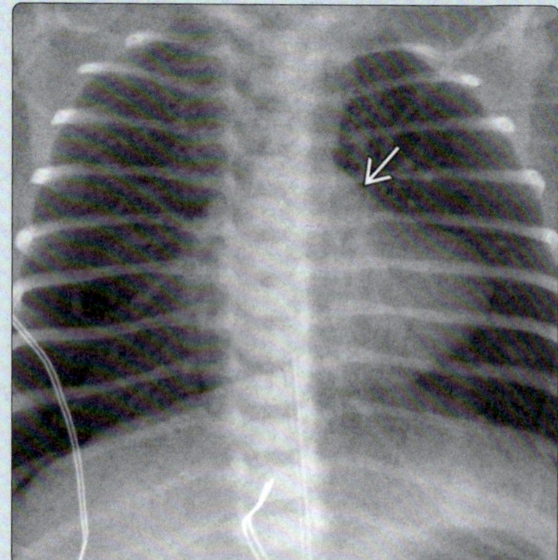

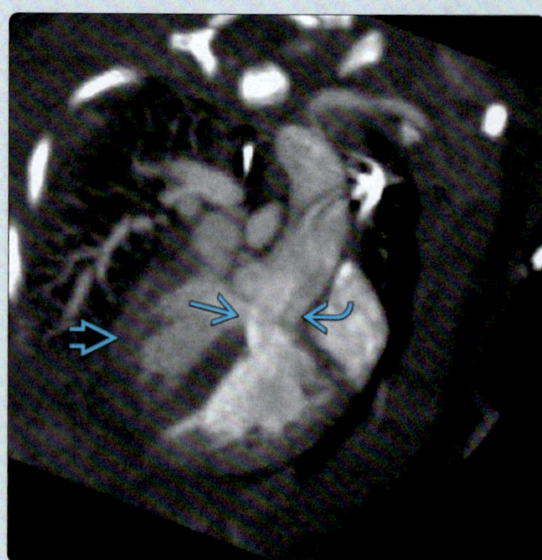

(Left) *AP radiograph shows the classic appearance of tetralogy of Fallot (TOF) with a concave pulmonary artery (PA) segment ➔ & an upturned cardiac apex creating the "coeur en sabot" (boot-shaped heart) appearance. Note the pulmonary oligemia.* **(Right)** *LVOT MIP cardiac CTA in a patient with TOF shows a ventricular septal defect (VSD) ➔ with right ventricular (RV) hypertrophy ➔ & an overriding aorta ➔ (as the aorta "overrides the VSD").*

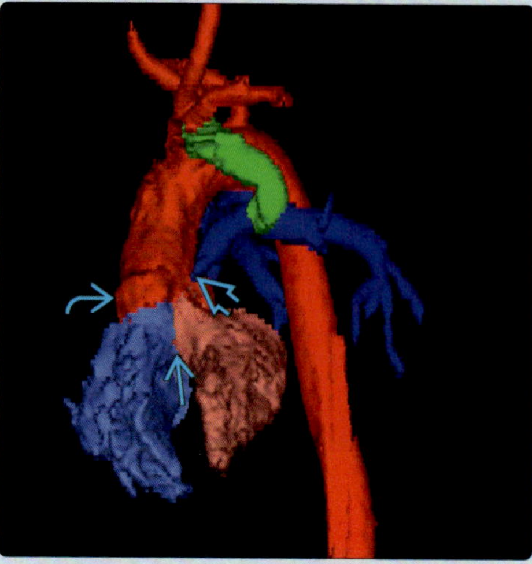

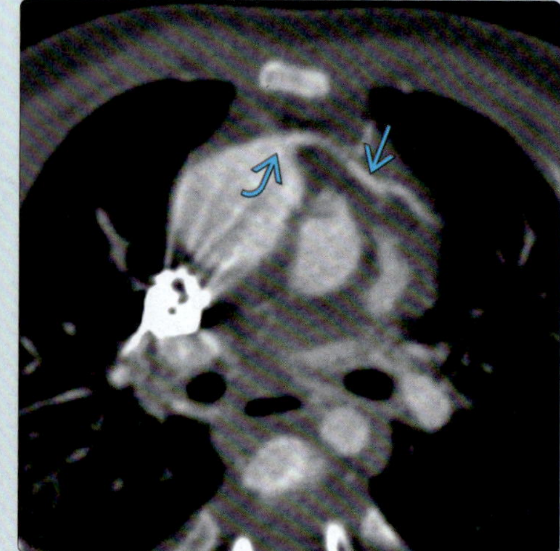

(Left) *Color-coded 3D surface-rendered cardiac CTA in an infant with TOF shows a prominent subaortic VSD ➔ with an overriding aorta ➔ & complete pulmonic atresia ➔. Note the enlarged PDA (green), which provides flow to the PAs (blue).* **(Right)** *Axial cardiac CTA in a patient with TOF shows a prepulmonic left coronary artery ➔ arising from the right coronary sinus ➔. This is critical information for presurgical planning to prevent sacrifice of the left coronary when placing a pulmonary valve homograft.*

Tetralogy of Fallot

TERMINOLOGY

Definitions

- Tetralogy of Fallot (TOF): 4 heart defects in combination
  - Obstruction to pulmonary outflow via infundibular right ventricular outflow tract (RVOT) narrowing or pulmonary valve stenosis
  - Secondary RV hypertrophy (RVH) from ↑ right ventricle (RV) pressures/fixed subpulmonary obstruction
  - Anterior malalignment ventricular septal defect (VSD)
  - Aorta overriding VSD
- Category: Cyanotic, normal heart size, ↓ pulmonary vascularity
  - Most common cyanotic congenital heart lesion
- Hemodynamics: Obstruction to pulmonary blood flow via infundibular narrowing by anterior deviation of subpulmonary conal septum
  - Spectrum: Classic "blue tet," "pink tet," TOF with pulmonary atresia & major aortopulmonary collaterals (MAPCAs), TOF with absent pulmonary valve

IMAGING

General Features

- Best diagnostic clue
  - Anterocephalad deviation of subpulmonary conoventricular septum → 4 characteristic heart defects
  - Aorta overriding large anterior malalignment VSD

Radiographic Findings

- RVH + concave pulmonary artery (PA) segment: Boot-shaped heart ("coeur en sabot")
  - RVH rotates heart, creating rounded, upturned apex
- ↓ pulmonary vascularity (oligemia) due to obstruction of pulmonary blood flow
- Normal heart size at birth
- Right-sided aortic arch (25%)

CT Findings

- CTA
  - Preoperative: Multidetector CT can diagnose coronary anomalies, obviating need for angiography
  - Postoperative: Cardiac gated cine CT can perform
    - Assessment of RV volumes & function in patients with contraindication for MR
    - CTA is also less affected by metal artifact than MR (to assess results of interventions, e.g., stents, coils)

MR Findings

- T1WI
  - Cardiac gated axial images for preoperative definition of PA anatomy, PA stenosis
  - Postoperative PA anatomy, patency of Blalock-Taussig (BT) shunts assessed by presence of flow void
- T2* GRE
  - Short-axis SSFP cine bright blood MR for RV & left ventricular (LV) volumes, ejection fraction (EF), pulmonary regurgitant fraction, branch PA differential flow
    - Functional MR: Biventricular response to exercise & recovery
    - Presence of RVOT akinesia/aneurysm & wide anulus correlates with need for pulmonary valve replacement (PVR)
- MRA
  - Gadolinium-enhanced MRA: Depiction of PA anatomy & aortopulmonary collaterals
  - Phase contrast assists with estimating RV EF & pulmonary regurgitation

Echocardiographic Findings

- Location of VSD, additional muscular VSDs
- Degree of aortic override, position of arch
- RVOT obstruction, pulmonary valve morphology
- Branch PA anatomy
- Coronary artery origin & proximal courses

Imaging Recommendations

- Best imaging tool
  - Initial diagnosis with pre- & postnatal echocardiography
- Protocol advice
  - MRA/3D whole-heart sequence or CTA for detailed PA & coronary anatomy
  - Cardiac catheterization for coronary anatomy & percutaneous interventions (RVOT or ductal stent as initial palliative procedure)
  - MR in older child/young adult with poor acoustic echocardiography windows; becoming gold standard for functional assessment of postoperative regurgitation & ventricular dysfunction prior to PVR

DIFFERENTIAL DIAGNOSIS

Double-Outlet Right Ventricle With Normally Related Great Vessels, Subaortic Ventricular Septal Defect, & Pulmonary Stenosis

- Defined as both outlets (aorta & PA) arising from RV
- Can be difficult to differentiate from TOF; therefore, secondary characteristics are often employed
  - > 50% aortic override of VSD
  - Bilateral subarterial conal septum leading to mitral-aortic fibrous discontinuity

Pulmonary Atresia With Intact Ventricular Septum

- Massive cardiomegaly with right atrial enlargement at birth

Pulmonary Valve Stenosis & Perimembranous Ventricular Septal Defect

- Significant pulmonary valve stenosis with VSD should be evaluated for conal septal deviation

Tricuspid Atresia With Normally Related Great Vessels, Subpulmonary Obstruction

- Large right atrium with obligate right-to-left atrial level shunt; subpulmonary obstruction through restricted VSD

PATHOLOGY

General Features

- Genetics
  - Chromosomal anomalies in 11% (chromosome 22)
  - Other congenital anomalies in 16%; 8% are syndromic
- Associated abnormalities
  - PA branch stenosis or hypoplasia

- Absence of pulmonary valve: Severe pulmonary regurgitation → aneurysmal dilation of PAs → tracheobronchomalacia & compression
- Pulmonary atresia & MAPCAs
  - Extreme end of TOF spectrum; severe congenital heart disease with often poor prognosis
- Patent foramen ovale vs. secundum atrial septal defect
- Right aortic arch, mirror image branching (25%)
- Coronary anomalies: Left anterior descending arising from right coronary & crossing RVOT (4%) with implications for surgical repair

- Pathophysiology: Balance between RVOT obstruction & VSD determines shunt direction
  - Classic TOF: Right-to-left shunting, ↓ pulmonary flow, cyanosis
  - "Pink" TOF: Left-to-right shunting, normal to ↑ pulmonary flow, congestive heart failure
- Embryology
  - Abnormal bulbotruncal rotation & septation
  - Primary hypoplasia of infundibular septum

Gross Pathologic & Surgical Features

- Anterior/cephalad deviation of infundibular septum, hypertrophic outlet septum, & anterior muscle bands
- Hypoplastic pulmonary valve anulus with deformed & stenosed, often bicuspid, pulmonary valve
- Large perimembranous subaortic VSD with aortic override of 15-95%

CLINICAL ISSUES

Presentation

- Most common signs/symptoms
  - Varying degrees of cyanosis at birth (most often apparent by 3 months)
  - Older child: Cyanotic spells, relieved by squatting
  - Congestive heart failure (large VSD)
- Other signs/symptoms
  - After repair: ↓ exercise tolerance, RV dysfunction
  - Severe arrhythmias, which may be fatal
    - RV chamber dilation from postoperative pulmonary regurgitation
    - Damage to conduction system during VSD closure
    - Scar from right ventriculotomy → ectopy focus
  - Bacterial endocarditis
  - Stroke due to paradoxic embolus to brain
  - Hyperviscosity syndrome due to polycythemia

Demographics

- Epidemiology
  - Incidence: 3-5 per 10,000 live births
  - 4th most common congenital heart anomaly
  - Most common cyanotic heart lesion

Natural History & Prognosis

- 10% of untreated patients live > 20 years
- Short term: Excellent results after early "complete" repair
- Long term: Determined by RV diastolic & systolic dysfunction; chronic regurgitation leading to dilation, arrhythmias, & risk of sudden death
  - Timing of PVR is determined by results of functional MR

Treatment

- Palliative shunt (needed primarily with hypercyanotic episodes or extreme desaturation)
  - Classic BT shunt: End-to-side subclavian artery to PA (opposite from aortic arch)
  - Modified BT shunt: Interposition of Gore-Tex graft
  - Central shunt: Ductus-like connection between aorta & PA
- Complete repair: Removal of RVOT obstruction, VSD closure
  - Limited transannular patch with RVOT enlargement: Postoperative pulmonary regurgitation
    - RV dysfunction, arrhythmias
  - Rastelli shunt: Valved conduit between RV & PAs in case of severe RVOT stenosis or pulmonary valve atresia
- Pulmonary valve or conduit replacement after early complete repair
  - Conduit stenosis: RV pressure overload, systolic dysfunction
  - Pulmonary regurgitation: RV volume overload, diastolic & systolic dysfunction, reciprocal left ventricle systolic dysfunction, arrhythmias
  - Timely surgery allows RV remodeling with ↓ RV size, ↑ EF, ↑ exercise capacity
- Percutaneous balloon dilation of residual pulmonary valve stenosis &/or peripheral PA stenosis (with stent placement)
- Transcatheter PVR
  - Less invasive, new option for PVR
  - Risk:benefit ratio of earlier reintervention is being evaluated compared with surgical replacement
  - Risk of bacterial endocarditis is higher compared to surgical PVR

SELECTED REFERENCES

1. Koppel CJ et al: Coronary anomalies in tetralogy of Fallot - a meta-analysis. Int J Cardiol. 306:78-85, 2020
2. Li VW et al: Ventricular myocardial deformation imaging of patients with repaired tetralogy of Fallot. J Am Soc Echocardiogr. 33(7):788-801, 2020
3. Mohamed I et al: Assessment of disease progression in patients with repaired tetralogy of Fallot using cardiac magnetic resonance imaging: a systematic review. Heart Lung Circ. 29(11):1613-20, 2020
4. Ojha V et al: Spectrum of changes on cardiac magnetic resonance in repaired tetralogy of Fallot: imaging according to surgical considerations. Clin Imaging. 69:102-14, 2020
5. Rizk J et al: Magnetic resonance imaging risk factors for ventricular arrhythmias in tetralogy of Fallot. Pediatr Cardiol. 41(5):862-8, 2020
6. Tous C et al: Ex vivo cardiovascular magnetic resonance diffusion weighted imaging in congenital heart disease, an insight into the microstructures of tetralogy of Fallot, biventricular and univentricular systemic right ventricle. J Cardiovasc Magn Reson. 22(1):69, 2020
7. Apostolopoulou SC et al: Cardiovascular imaging approach in pre and postoperative tetralogy of Fallot. BMC Cardiovasc Disord. 19(1):7, 2019
8. Egbe AC et al: Coronary artery disease in adults with tetralogy of Fallot. Congenit Heart Dis. 14(3):491-7, 2019
9. Leonardi B et al: The role of 3D imaging in the follow-up of patients with repaired tetralogy of Fallot. Eur Rev Med Pharmacol Sci. 23(4):1698-709, 2019
10. Larios G et al: Imaging in repaired tetralogy of Fallot with a focus on recent advances in echocardiography. Curr Opin Cardiol. 32(5):490-502, 2017

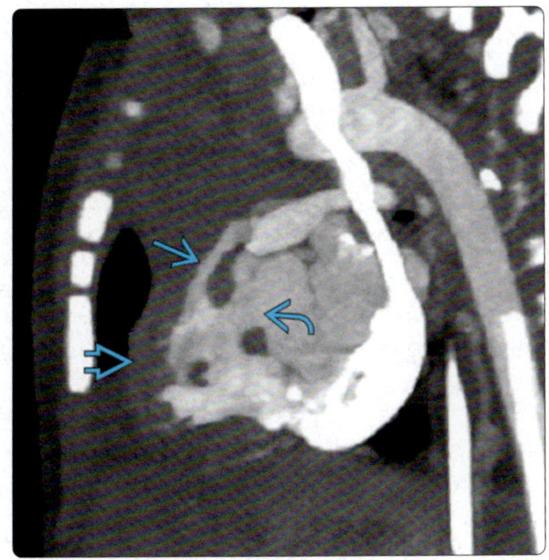

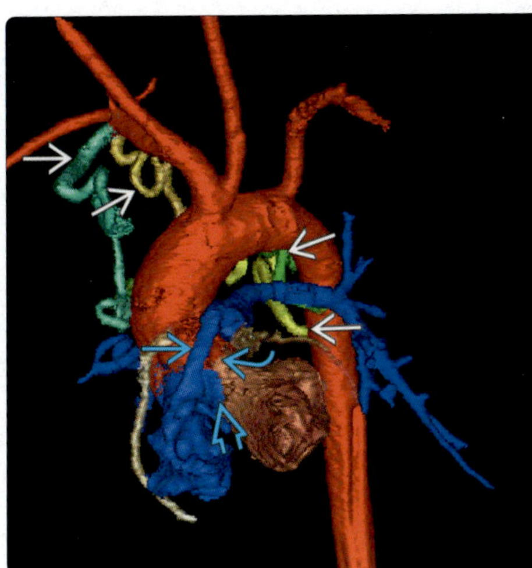

(Left) *Sagittal MIP cardiac CTA in an infant with TOF shows narrowing of the RV infundibulum ➡ with RV hypertrophy ➡ & a VSD ↪.* **(Right)** *Anterior oblique color-coded 3D surface-rendered cardiac CTA in an infant with TOF shows the narrowed RV infundibulum ➡, VSD ➡ & overriding aorta ↪. Note all the aortopulmonary collaterals ➡ feeding the PAs (blue).*

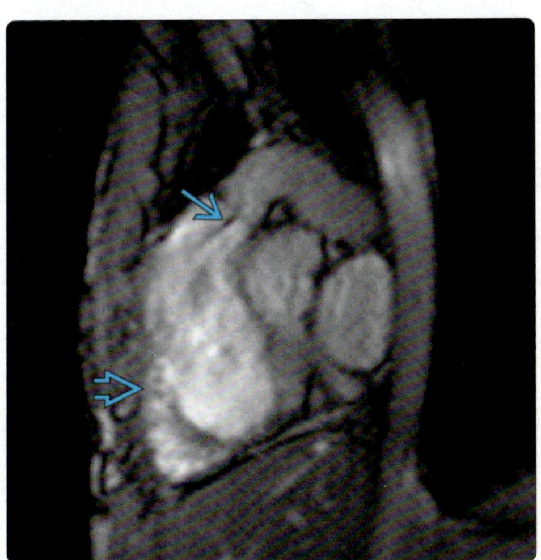

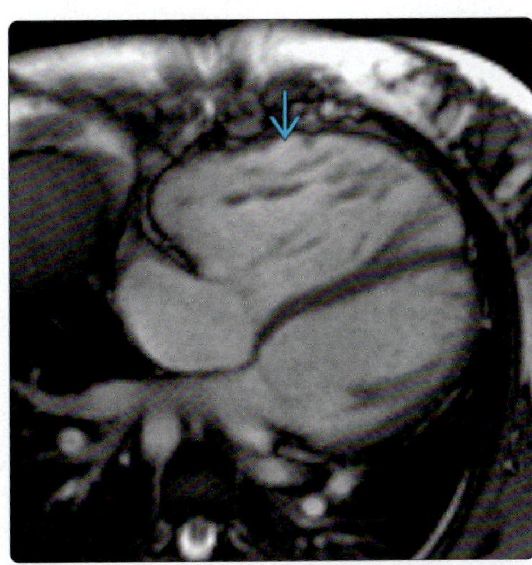

(Left) *Sagittal bright blood SSFP cardiac MR cine in a postoperative patient with TOF shows a pulmonic regurgitation signal void of dephasing artifact ➡. Also note the enlarged RV ➡. Pulmonic regurgitation is often well tolerated after primary repair.* **(Right)** *Four-chamber bright blood SSFP cine MR shows a typical appearance of the RV ➡ after "complete" repair. The RV often dilates from volume overload secondary to a large regurgitant fraction across the pulmonic valve.*

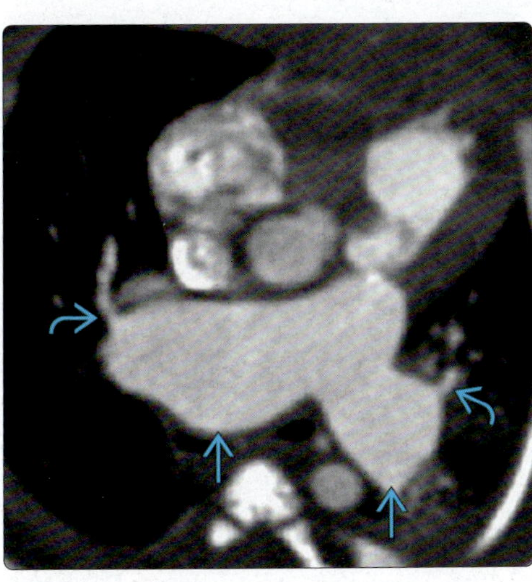

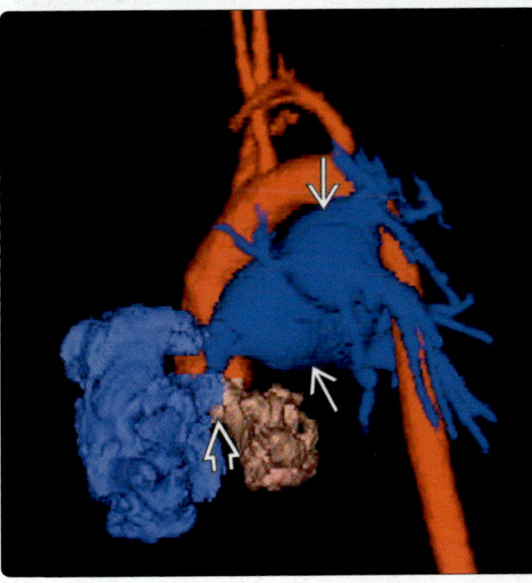

(Left) *Oblique axial MIP cardiac CTA shows massive enlargement of the central PAs ➡ in a patient with a TOF variant where there is absence of the pulmonic valve. Note the abrupt change in caliber of the secondary PAs ↪.* **(Right)** *Lateral color-coded 3D surface-rendered cardiac CTA shows massive enlargement of the central PAs ➡ in a patient with a TOF variant where there is absence of the pulmonic valve. Also note the VSD ➡.*

KEY FACTS

TERMINOLOGY

- 2 distinct entities, differentiated by presence or absence of ventricular septal defect (VSD)
  - Pulmonary atresia (PAt), intact ventricular septum (VS): Normal-sized pulmonary arteries (PAs) supplied by patent ductus arteriosus (PDA), patent foramen ovale (PFO)
  - PAt, VSD, multiple aortopulmonary collateral arteries (MAPCAs): Hypoplastic/absent PAs; MAPCAs supply 1 or both lungs
    - At extreme end of spectrum of right ventricular outflow tract (RVOT)-obstructive (Fallot-type) heart lesions with complex & highly variable PA anatomy

IMAGING

- Extreme boot-shaped appearance of heart
  - PAt, intact VS: Severe cardiomegaly from massive right atrial dilation
- Right-sided aortic arch is common
- Initial diagnosis with echocardiography
- Cardiac CTA delineates PAs, MAPCAs, & coronary artery fistulas & sinusoids
  - Provides roadmap for subsequent catheterization
- CT or MR postoperatively for shunt/conduit patency
- Cardiac catheterization for hemodynamic assessment, selective injection studies, & catheter-based interventions

CLINICAL ISSUES

- Progressive cyanosis after birth at closure of PDA
  - Prostaglandin E1 to maintain PDA
- Congestive heart failure with large unobstructed high-flow MAPCAs
- Treatment
  - PAt, VSD, MAPCAs: Unifocalization of MAPCAs & true PAs (if existent, to allow for PA growth)
  - PAt, intact VS: Type of repair depends on RV size & RV dependency on coronary circulation

(Left) *Graphic shows pulmonary atresia with an intact ventricular septum. Note the patent foramen ovale ➔, dilation of the right atrium, & right ventricular (RV) hypertrophy. The pulmonary arteries (PAs) are perfused by flow from the aorta through a patent ductus arteriosus (PDA) ➔.* **(Right)** *Frontal view of the chest in a neonate with pulmonic atresia shows cardiomegaly with ↓ pulmonary vascularity. The differential diagnosis for this appearance includes pulmonic atresia, Ebstein anomaly, & tricuspid atresia.*

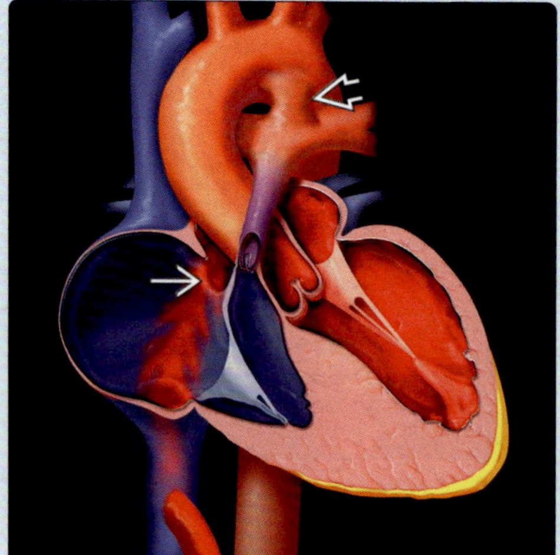

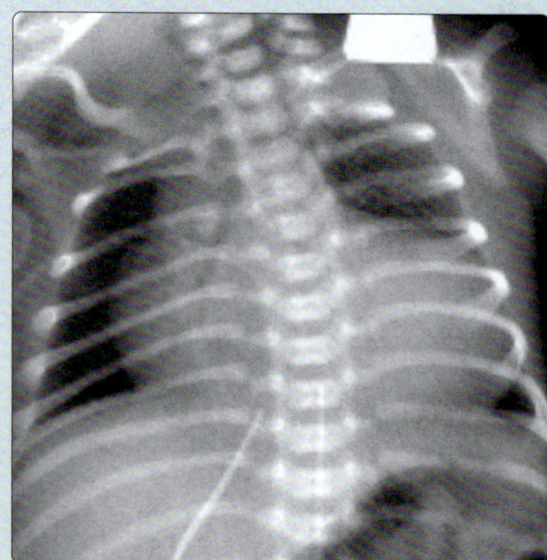

(Left) *Sagittal MIP cardiac CTA in an infant shows an atretic main PA ➔ with the PDA ➔ arising from the left brachiocephalic artery & inserting into the main PA. Also note the ventricular septal defect (VSD) ➔.* **(Right)** *Lateral 3D surface-rendered cardiac CTA in an infant shows the atretic PA ➔ & tortuous PDA (green) arising from the left brachiocephalic artery ➔ & inserting into the superior aspect of the main PA (blue). Also note the VSD ➔ between the RV (violet) & left ventricle (LV) (salmon).*

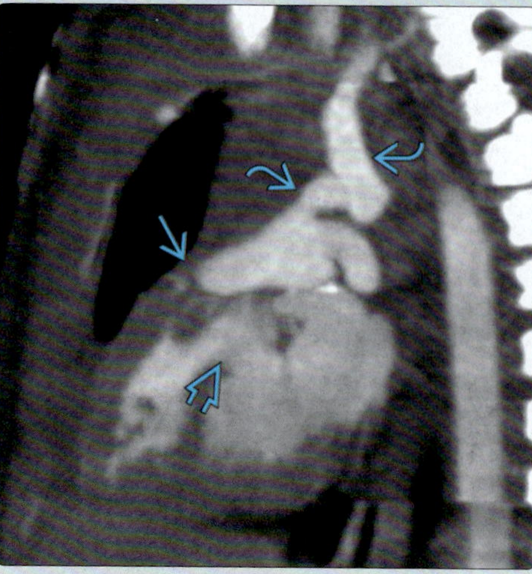

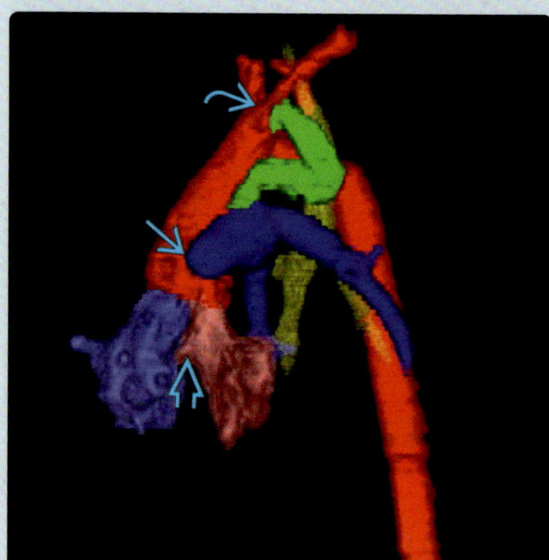

TERMINOLOGY

Abbreviations

- Pulmonary atresia (PAt)

Synonyms

- Sometimes referred to as truncus arteriosus type 4 or pseudotruncus (misnomer)

Definitions

- 2 distinct entities, differentiated by presence or absence of ventricular septal defect (VSD)
  - PAt, VSD, multiple aortopulmonary collateral arteries (MAPCAs): Hypoplastic/absent pulmonary arteries (PAs); MAPCAs supply 1 or both lungs
    - Type A: Normal-sized PAs with small aortopulmonary (AP) collaterals
    - Type B: Mild to moderate PA hypoplasia with multiple AP collaterals
    - Type C: Markedly hypoplastic PAs with pulmonary flow from numerous AP collaterals
  - PAt, intact ventricular septum (VS): Normal-sized PAs supplied by patent ductus arteriosus (PDA), patent foramen ovale (PFO)
    - Coronary sinusoids or fistulas are often present
- Both are characterized by underdevelopment of right ventricular outflow tract (RVOT) & pulmonary valve
  - PAt, VSD, MAPCAs: At extreme end of spectrum of RVOT-obstructive (Fallot-type) heart lesions with complex & highly variable PA anatomy
- Category: Cyanotic, cardiomegaly, ↓ &/or irregular pulmonary vasculature
- Hemodynamics: Extreme outflow obstruction of RV; (almost) entire cardiac output goes into dilated overriding ascending aorta

IMAGING

General Features

- Best diagnostic clue
  - Atresia of RVOT &/or pulmonary valve

Radiographic Findings

- Extreme boot-shaped appearance of heart
- Right-sided aortic arch is common
- Diminutive hilar shadows
- Irregular branching patterns of MAPCAs
- PAt, intact VS: Severe cardiomegaly from massive right atrial dilation

CT Findings

- CTA
  - Cardiac CTA provides detailed evaluation of PAs & MAPCAs
    - 3D images have proven helpful in planning for unifocalization
  - CTA is best used to provide anatomic roadmap for subsequent catheterization
    - Saves overall radiation, contrast, procedure time
    - Cardiac CTA provides delineation of coronary artery fistulas & sinusoids
  - CTA is excellent modality for unstable postoperative patients

MR Findings

- T1WI
  - PAt, VSD, MAPCAs: Cardiac gated axial images for preoperative definition of PA anatomy
- T2* GRE
  - Short- & long-axis SSFP cine MR for functional assessment, tricuspid regurgitation
- MRA
  - Coronal gadolinium-enhanced MRA for detailed analysis of PA anatomy & MAPCAs
- Phase-contrast imaging
  - Helpful in following RV volumes & regurgitant fractions in postsurgical patients

Echocardiographic Findings

- Echocardiogram
  - PAt, VSD, MAPCAs
    - Characterizes intracardiac anatomy, position, & size of VSD, aortic root override
    - Development of branch PAs & their confluence
  - PAt, intact VS
    - Morphology of interatrial septum: Identifies restriction to flow across PFO
    - Size of RV & tricuspid anulus (expressed as Z score), degree of tricuspid regurgitation: Important for planning of surgical repair

Angiographic Findings

- Conventional
  - PAt, VSD, MAPCAs
    - Selective injection with pressure recordings of all MAPCAs + imaging of true PAs
    - Pulmonary venous wedge injections for retrograde filling of diminutive PAs
  - PAt, intact VS
    - Suprasystemic pressure recordings in RV
    - Detailed imaging of coronary anatomy through RV & aortic root injections: RV to coronary communications, stenoses, interruptions

Imaging Recommendations

- Protocol advice
  - PAt, VSD, MAPCAs
    - Initial diagnosis with echocardiography
    - CT or MR for preoperative assessment of PA anatomy, postoperative assessment for shunt/conduit patency
    - Cardiac catheterization for hemodynamic assessment, selective injection studies, & catheter-based interventions

DIFFERENTIAL DIAGNOSIS

Tetralogy of Fallot

- At least partial patency of RVOT

Complex Cyanotic Heart Lesions With Component of (Sub-)Pulmonary Stenosis

- Double-outlet RV
- Transposition of great arteries with VSD
- Single ventricle
- Tricuspid atresia

Ebstein Anomaly

- May mimic PAt, intact VS with large tricuspid anulus & massive tricuspid regurgitation

PATHOLOGY

General Features

- Embryology (PAt, VSD, MAPCAs)
  - RVOT obstruction → hypoplasia of PAs
  - Persistence or hypertrophy of primitive arterial connections to lungs
  - Hypertrophy of bronchial arteries
- Pathophysiology of PAt, VSD, MAPCAs: Balance between flow through PAs & MAPCAs determines pulmonary perfusion
  - PA flow at subsystemic pressures, restricted by narrow caliber & eventual closure of ductus arteriosus
  - MAPCA flow leads to ↑ lung perfusion at systemic pressures (unless restricted by stenosis)
  - Degree of cyanosis is determined by intracardiac admixture & amount of pulmonary flow
  - Large amount of pulmonary blood flow through unrestricted MAPCAs → congestive heart failure
- Pathophysiology of PAt, intact VS: Obligatory right-to-left shunt through PFO
  - PAs are supplied by PDA
  - Small, heavily trabeculated RV with suprasystemic pressures
  - Depending on size of tricuspid valve anulus: Severe tricuspid regurgitation, leading to massive right atrial dilation (comparable to Ebstein anomaly)
  - Transmyocardial sinusoids connecting RV cavity with coronary artery system cause coronary flow reversal during diastole, leading to myocardial ischemia & infarction

Staging, Grading, & Classification

- PAt with VSD & MAPCAs
  - Type A: Majority of pulmonary flow from PAs with small MAPCAs
  - Type B: Equal pulmonary flow from PAs & MAPCAs
  - Type C: Majority of pulmonary flow from MAPCAs with markedly hypoplastic native PAs

Gross Pathologic & Surgical Features

- Hilar arteries = true PAs
- Presence & confluence of central portions of true PAs is important for surgical repair
- MAPCAs originate from
  - Ascending aorta
  - Brachiocephalic or intercostal arteries
  - Ductus arteriosus
  - Descending aorta (most common)

Microscopic Features

- Pulmonary vascular disease develops in vascular bed of high-flow MAPCAs → ↑ in cyanosis

CLINICAL ISSUES

Presentation

- Most common signs/symptoms
  - Progressive cyanosis after birth with closure of ductus arteriosus
  - Congestive heart failure with large, unobstructed, high-flow MAPCAs
- Other signs/symptoms
  - Failure to thrive, polycythemia, finger clubbing

Demographics

- Epidemiology
  - Rare, congenital cyanotic heart lesions, often classified together with tetralogy of Fallot

Natural History & Prognosis

- Progressive cyanosis due to development of pulmonary vascular disease → irreversible pulmonary hypertension
- Life expectancy when untreated: < 10 years
- Survival into adulthood is now possible: Adult congenital heart disease
  - Need for lifelong follow-up with multiple imaging tests
- Prognosis is guarded, depends on feasibility of surgery

Treatment

- Prostaglandin E1 to keep ductus arteriosus open
- Palliative: Systemic-to-PA shunt (Blalock-Taussig, central), initial banding of high-flow MAPCAs
- PAt, VSD, MAPCAs: Staged complete repair
  - Unifocalization of MAPCAs & true PAs (if existent, to allow for PA growth)
  - Early 1-stage repair in infancy with incorporation of all MAPCAs in PA conduit, may be feasible
  - Complete repair with incorporation of MAPCAs & PAs in conduit, connected to reconstructed RVOT, & closure of VSD (may not be possible due to high pressure in pulmonary system from residual stenosis/hypoplasia & pulmonary vascular disease)
  - Catheter-based interventions (balloon angioplasty with stenting of stenoses, coil embolization of small superfluous &/or bleeding MAPCAs)
- PAt, intact VS: Type of repair depends on RV size & RV dependency on coronary circulation
  - Restriction in flow across PFO: Balloon atrial septostomy
  - Catheter-based or surgical pulmonary valvotomy
  - Sudden decompression of RV through valvotomy, RVOT repair, or transannular patch may lead to myocardial ischemia/infarction
  - When RV is too hypoplastic for biventricular repair: Cavopulmonary (Glenn) shunt, staged completion of univentricular repair (Fontan)

SELECTED REFERENCES

1. Gindes L et al: Prenatal diagnosis of major aortopulmonary collateral arteries (MAPCA) in fetuses with pulmonary atresia with ventricular septal defect and agenesis of ductus arteriosus. J Matern Fetal Neonatal Med. 1-9, 2021
2. Katz JD et al: A 15-year-old with tetralogy of Fallot with pulmonic atresia, multiple aorticopulmonary collateral arteries and bilateral peripheral pulmonary stenosis. Cureus. 12(10):e11151, 2020
3. Sinha M et al: Imaging characteristics and associations in twisted atrioventricular connections on multidetector computed tomography angiography. J Card Surg. 35(11):2979-86, 2020
4. Fishbein GA et al: Tricuspid and pulmonic valve pathology. Curr Cardiol Rep. 21(7):54, 2019
5. Rato J et al: Ebstein's anomaly with 'reversible' functional pulmonary atresia. BMJ Case Rep. 12(12), 2019
6. Enaba MM et al: Multidetector computed tomography (CT) in evaluation of congenital cyanotic heart diseases. Pol J Radiol. 82:645-59, 2017

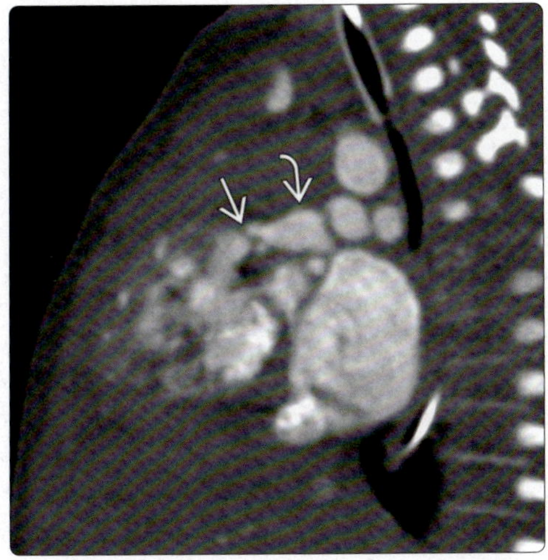

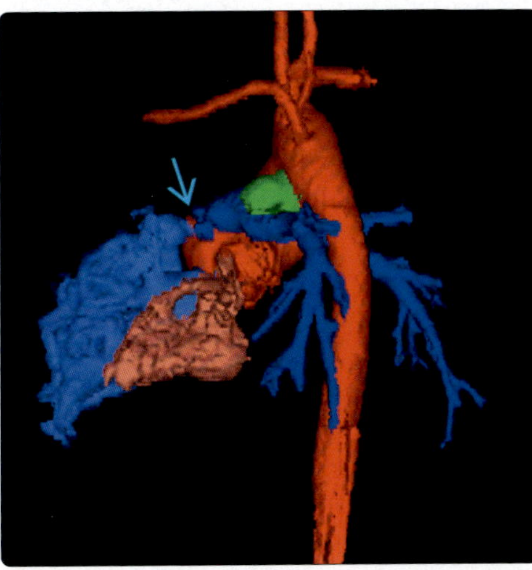

(Left) *Sagittal MIP cardiac CTA shows an atretic, thickened pulmonary valve ➡ with normal caliber PA. A PDA ➦ feeds the main PA. This patient is considered ductal dependent as survival is not possible without the PDA.* **(Right)** *Left posterior oblique 3D surface-rendered cardiac CTA shows complete pulmonic atresia with a gap ➡ seen between the RV (purple) & the PA (blue). Note the large PDA (green) that provides flow to the lungs.*

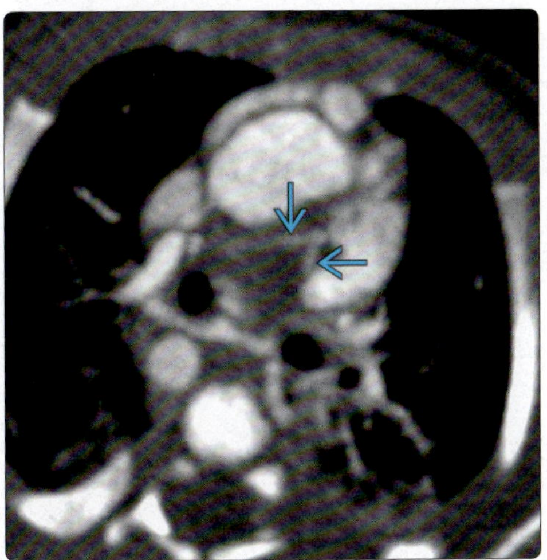

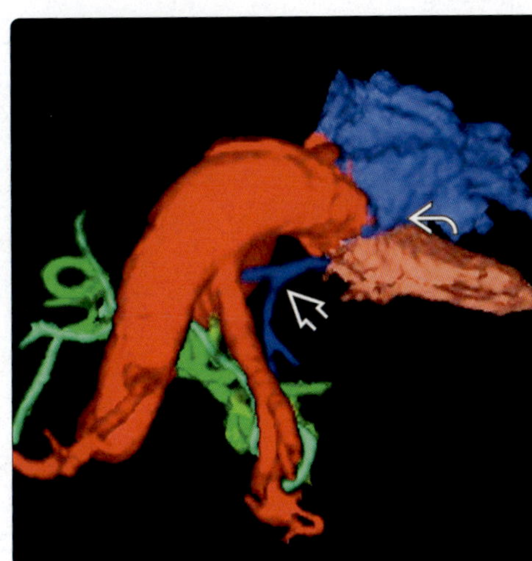

(Left) *Axial MIP cardiac CTA shows markedly hypoplastic PAs ➡ in a patient with pulmonic atresia.* **(Right)** *Superior 3D surface-rendered cardiac CTA shows markedly hypoplastic native PAs ➡ (blue). A VSD is present ➡. Multiple aortopulmonary collaterals (green) are providing the majority of the pulmonary flow (type C pulmonic atresia).*

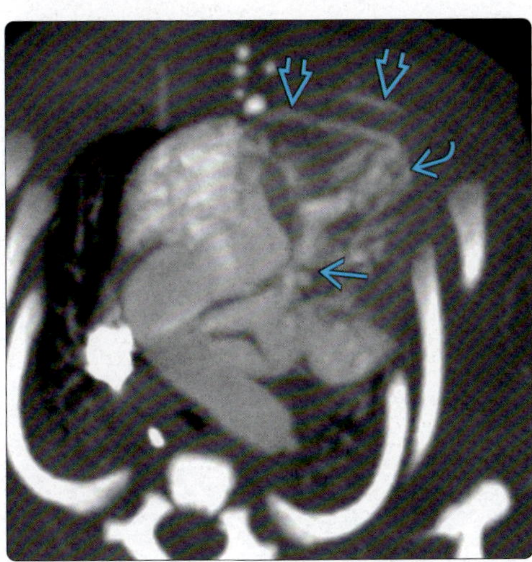

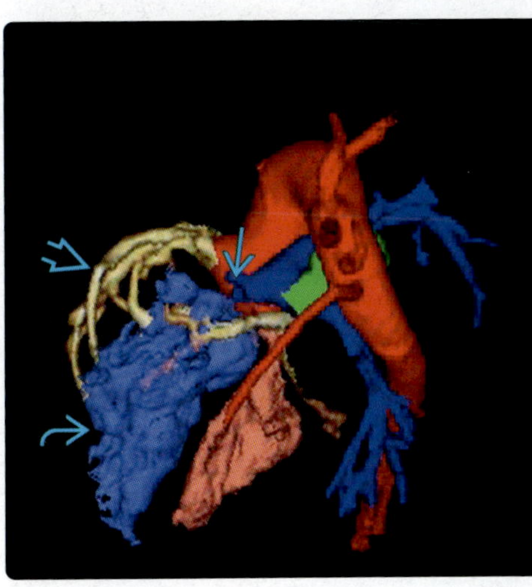

(Left) *Axial MIP cardiac CTA in an infant shows an atretic pulmonary valve ➡. There were multiple coronary artery fistulas ➡ connecting to the RV ➦ in this patient with an intact ventricular septum.* **(Right)** *Posterior oblique 3D surface-rendered cardiac CTA in an infant shows an atretic pulmonary valve ➡. There were multiple coronary artery fistulas ➡ connecting to the RV ➦ in this patient with an intact ventricular septum.*

Ebstein Anomaly

KEY FACTS

TERMINOLOGY

- Downward/apical displacement of septal & posterior leaflets of tricuspid valve with tricuspid regurgitation
- Category: Cyanotic congenital heart disease with cardiomegaly & ↓ pulmonary vascularity

IMAGING

- Classic radiographic appearance: Massive right-sided cardiomegaly (box-shaped heart)
- All cross-sectional modalities can show right atrial enlargement, apical displacement of tricuspid septal leaflet, & "atrialized" portion of right ventricle (RV)
    - Apical displacement of septal tricuspid leaflet (> 15 mm in children < 14 years; > 20 mm in adults)
- MR is excellent to evaluate ventricular volumes, ejection fraction, tricuspid regurgitant fraction

PATHOLOGY

- Patent foramen ovale (PFO), secundum atrial septal defect (ASD) in 90%

CLINICAL ISSUES

- Wide spectrum of findings & ages at 1st presentation
    - Some patients are asymptomatic
- Presence of cyanosis depends on balance between right & left atrial pressures
- Prognosis depends on hemodynamic significance of tricuspid regurgitation & presence of cyanosis, arrhythmias
- Supportive treatment in cyanotic neonate
    - Oxygen, nitric oxide ventilation to lower pulmonary vascular resistance
- Tricuspid valve replacement &/or reconstruction (valvuloplasty)
    - Definitive repair procedure

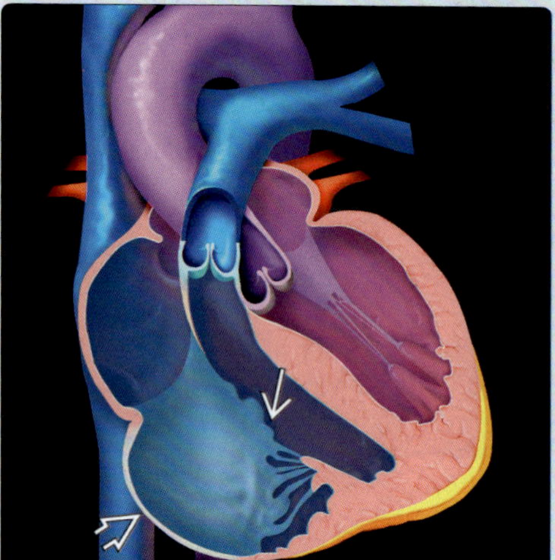

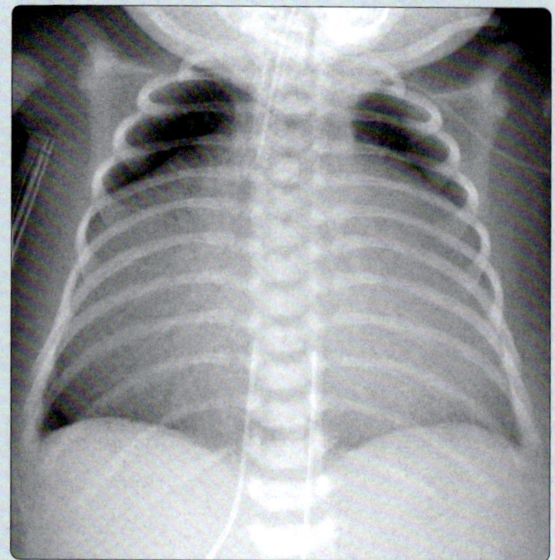

(Left) *Anterior graphic depicts downward displacement of the tricuspid posterior valve leaflet ➡, which has become incorporated into the right ventricular (RV) wall ➡, leading to "atrialization" of the inflow portion of the RV.* **(Right)** *Single frontal view of the chest in a newborn shows massive cardiomegaly (the box-shaped heart) with ↓ pulmonary vascularity, typical of patients with Ebstein anomaly.*

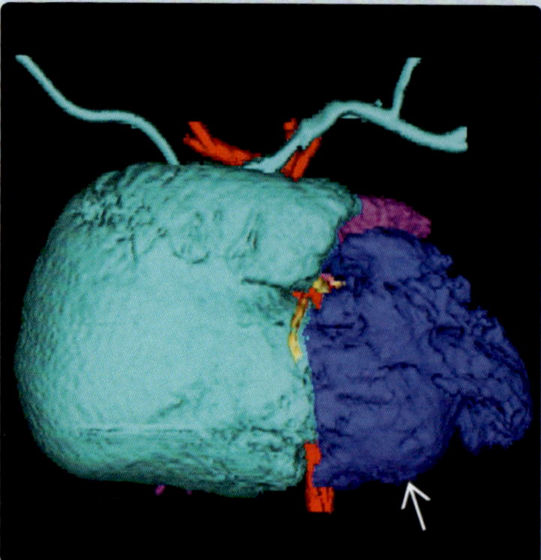

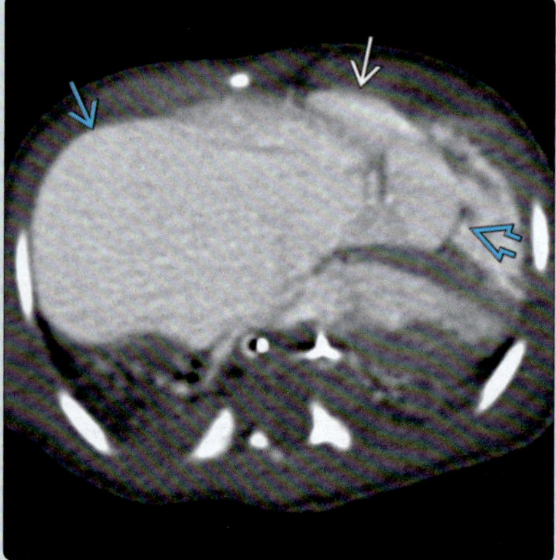

(Left) *Frontal view 3D color-coded cardiac CTA shows massive dilation of the right atrium (RA) (ight blue). Note the smooth portion of the RV wall ➡ that has become "atrialized."* **(Right)** *Axial cardiac CTA shows a massively dilated RA ➡ with the septal leaflet ➡ of the tricuspid valve deviated toward the apex of the heart. Note the atrialized (smooth) RV wall ➡.*

TERMINOLOGY

Definitions

- Downward/apical displacement of septal & posterior leaflets of tricuspid valve → tricuspid regurgitation
- Classic radiographic appearance: Massive right-sided cardiomegaly (box-shaped heart)
- Category: Cyanotic, (severe) cardiomegaly, normal or ↓ pulmonary vascularity
- Hemodynamics: Determined by severity of tricuspid valve regurgitation
  - Volume overload to right heart
  - Right-to-left shunting through patent foramen ovale (PFO) → cyanosis

IMAGING

General Features

- Best diagnostic clue
  - Downward/apical displacement of septal tricuspid leaflet (≥ 8-mm/m² body surface area)
- Location
  - Tricuspid valve

Radiographic Findings

- Severe right-sided cardiomegaly: May mimic large pericardial effusion
  - Heart size ranges from near normal in newborn period to massively enlarged
  - Heart ↑ gradually in size over time, reaching massive proportions in untreated cases during adulthood
  - Cardiothoracic ratio is used as parameter for follow-up
- Small vascular pedicle

CT Findings

- Cardiac CT can be used to obtain volumes & functional analysis of ventricular contraction
  - Also useful in defining associated complex extracardiac anomalies

MR Findings

- MR cine
  - Cardiac gated steady-state free precession bright blood MR
    - Apical displacement of septal tricuspid valve leaflet
    - Smooth "atrialized" component of right ventricle (RV)
    - Dephasing signal void from tricuspid regurgitation
    - Can calculate ventricular volumes, ejection fraction (EF), tricuspid regurgitation fraction
      - Left ventricular (LV) function is affected by RV dilation, bowing of septum, mitral valve prolapse
    - Indexed volumes & function of right heart correlate with overall prognosis
      - RV end-diastolic volume index > 200 & RV EF < 40% are helpful factors to identify ↑ perioperative risk

Echocardiographic Findings

- Echocardiogram
  - Right chamber enlargement with "atrialized" portion of RV
  - Enlarged tricuspid anulus (expressed in Z score)
  - Apical displacement of septal tricuspid leaflet (> 15 mm in children < 14 years; > 20 mm in adults)
- Color Doppler
  - Tricuspid regurgitation
  - PFO with right-to-left shunting

Angiographic Findings

- Characteristic notch at inferior RV border at insertion of displaced anterior tricuspid leaflet
- Seldom required for primary diagnosis

Imaging Recommendations

- Protocol advice
  - Anatomic & functional assessment with echocardiography in infants
  - Cardiac MR in (young) adults

DIFFERENTIAL DIAGNOSIS

Large Atrial Septal Defect

- Acyanotic
- ↑ pulmonary vascularity
- Left-to-right flow through large atrial septal defect (ASD)

Pericardial Effusion

- Acyanotic
- Easy differentiation with echocardiography

Tricuspid Insufficiency

- Primary, due to dysplastic valve
- Often secondary to pulmonary atresia with intact ventricular septum

Uhl Anomaly

- Congenital absence of RV myocardium

Arrhythmogenic Right Ventricular Dysplasia

- Fatty infiltration of RV, though fat is often not visible by imaging

Right-Sided Obstructive Cyanotic Heart Lesions With ↓ Pulmonary Vascularity

- Tetralogy of Fallot
- Pulmonary atresia
  - With ventricular septal defect & aortopulmonary collaterals
  - With intact ventricular septum
    - Causes severe cardiomegaly
- Tricuspid atresia
- Transposition of great arteries (TGA) with pulmonary stenosis
- Double-outlet RV with pulmonary stenosis

PATHOLOGY

General Features

- Genetics
  - Most often sporadic
- Associated abnormalities
  - PFO, secundum ASD in 90%
  - Ebstein anomaly frequently involves left-sided tricuspid valve in congenitally corrected (L) TGA
- Embryology

- Insufficient separation of tricuspid valve leaflets & chordae tendineae from RV endocardium
- Pathophysiology
  - 3 compartments: Right atrium, "atrialized" or noncontracting inlet portion of RV, & functional outlet portion of RV
  - Massive tricuspid regurgitation
  - Volume overload to right side of heart
  - Right-to-left shunt through PFO → cyanosis
  - LV diastolic dysfunction may result from massive right-sided cardiac enlargement
  - Arrhythmias due to conduction abnormalities

Gross Pathologic & Surgical Features

- Thickened valve leaflets, adherent to underlying myocardium
- Downward/apical displacement of septal & posterior tricuspid leaflets
- Normally placed, redundant, sail-like anterior tricuspid leaflet
- May occur on left side of heart with congenitally corrected (L) TGA

CLINICAL ISSUES

Presentation

- Most common signs/symptoms
  - Wide spectrum of findings & ages at 1st presentation; some patients are asymptomatic
  - Chronic right heart failure
    - ↓ exercise tolerance [classified as New York Heart Association (NYHA) classes I-IV]
  - Presence of cyanosis depends on balance between right & left atrial pressures
    - Physiologic ↓ in pulmonary vascular resistance in neonatal period → ↓ in right-to-left shunting through PFO → gradual improvement in cyanosis in 1st weeks of life
- Other signs/symptoms
  - Hydrops fetalis in neonatal cases
  - Severe cardiomegaly in fetal life → pulmonary hypoplasia
  - Thrombosis, paradoxic embolus
  - Arrhythmias
    - Atrial fibrillation, atrial flutter → irregular heartbeat
    - Accessory atrioventricular conduction pathways (preexcitation) → tachyarrhythmias, which can be unexpected & fatal

Demographics

- Age
  - 1st presentation can range from newborn period through old age (average: 14 years)
- Epidemiology
  - < 1% of congenital cardiac anomalies; incidence of 1/210,000 live births
  - Sex: M:F = 1:1

Natural History & Prognosis

- Sudden death due to fatal atrial arrhythmias
- Uncomplicated pregnancies are possible in women with hemodynamically well-balanced lesions
- Prognosis is highly variable, dependent on hemodynamic significance of tricuspid regurgitation, presence of cyanosis

Treatment

- Supportive treatment in cyanotic neonate: Oxygen, nitric oxide ventilation to lower pulmonary vascular resistance
- Systemic to pulmonary (Blalock-Taussig & central) shunts are ineffective
- Some patients benefit from total right-sided heart bypass procedures (Glenn → Fontan surgical treatment pathway)
- Tricuspid valve replacement &/or reconstruction (valvuloplasty): Definitive repair procedure
  - Valvuloplasty & bioprosthesis placement are preferable to mechanical valve (allow growth with no need for lifelong anticoagulation)
  - Valvuloplasty uses tissues from existing valve (redundant anterior tricuspid leaflet)
  - Bioprosthesis: Homograft or xenograft (porcine valve)
- Indications for valve repair
  - NYHA classes III & IV
  - NYHA classes I & II with cardiothoracic ratio > 0.65
  - Significant cyanosis (arterial saturation < 80%) &/or polycythemia (Hb > 16 g/dL)
  - History of paradoxic embolus
  - Arrhythmia due to accessory atrioventricular pathway
- Conal reconstruction may improve long-term RV performance & prognosis
- Arrhythmia treatments
  - Antiarrhythmic drugs
  - Permanent pacemaker implantation
  - Radiofrequency ablation

SELECTED REFERENCES

1. Qureshi MY et al: Commentary: gold or silver? Value of cardiac magnetic resonance imaging over echocardiography in Ebstein's anomaly. J Thorac Cardiovasc Surg. 161(3):1109-10, 2021
2. Rajagopal R et al: Ebstein's anomaly with imperforate tricuspid valve: an extremely rare congenital anomaly. J Cardiovasc Comput Tomogr. 14(6):e95-6, 2020
3. Holst KA et al: Ebstein's anomaly. Methodist Debakey Cardiovasc J. 15(2):138-44, 2019
4. Mrad Agua K et al: Preoperative predictability of right ventricular failure following surgery for Ebstein's anomaly. Eur J Cardiothorac Surg. 55(6):1187-93, 2019
5. Qureshi MY et al: Tricuspid valve imaging and intervention in pediatric and adult patients with congenital heart disease. JACC Cardiovasc Imaging. 12(4):637-51, 2019
6. Ciepłucha A et al: Clinical aspects of myocardial fibrosis in adults with Ebstein's anomaly. Heart Vessels. 33(9):1076-85, 2018
7. Qureshi MY et al: Cardiac imaging in Ebstein anomaly. Trends Cardiovasc Med. 28(6):403-9, 2018
8. Enaba MM et al: Multidetector computed tomography (CT) in evaluation of congenital cyanotic heart diseases. Pol J Radiol. 82:645-59, 2017
9. Kumar P et al: Ebstein anomaly with right atrial clot. Cardiol Res. 6(4-5):319-23, 2015

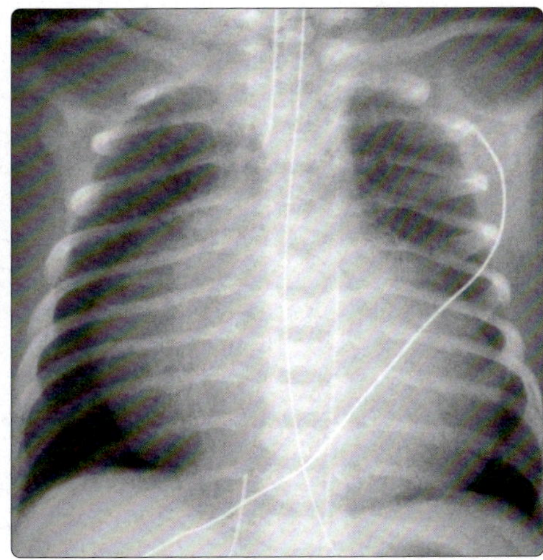

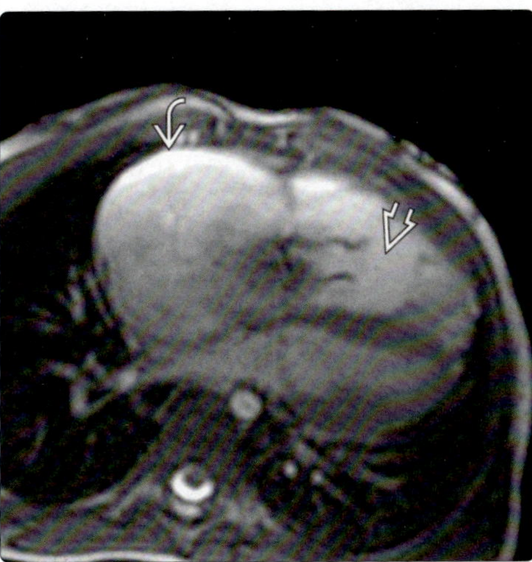

(Left) *AP radiograph of the chest demonstrates cardiomegaly with ↓ pulmonary vascularity in this patient with Ebstein anomaly. The classic differential considerations in patients with cardiomegaly & ↓ pulmonary vascularity are Ebstein anomaly, pulmonic atresia, & tricuspid atresia.* **(Right)** *Four-chamber SSFP cine of the heart shows massive dilation of the RA & RV from volume overload & "atrialization" of the RV.*

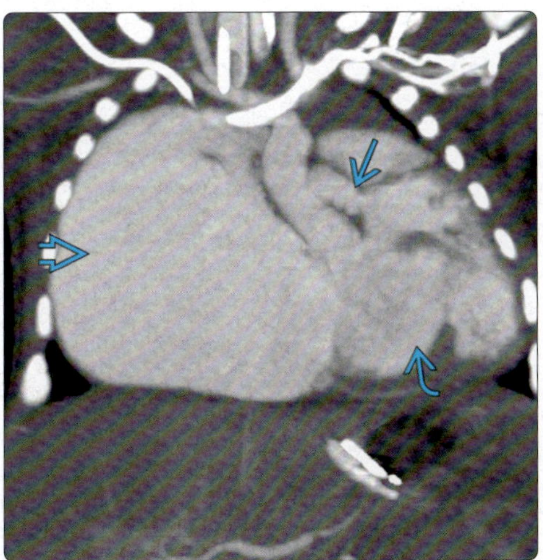

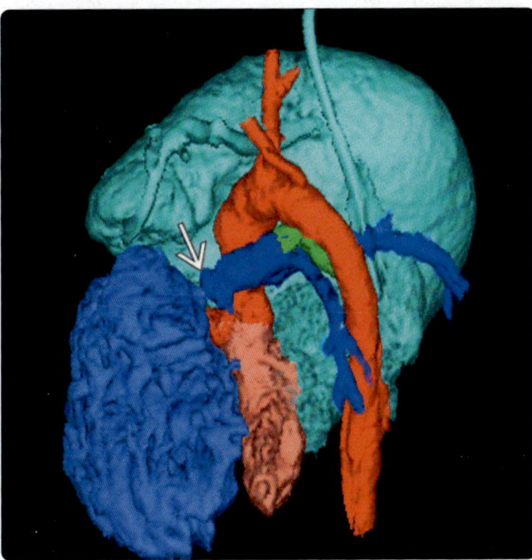

(Left) *Coronal MIP cardiac CTA shows massive dilation of the RA with enlargement of the RV in a patient with Ebstein anomaly. Note the narrowed pulmonary outflow tract.* **(Right)** *Oblique 3D reformatted cardiac CTA in an infant with Ebstein anomaly shows valvular pulmonic stenosis. Note the massively dilated RA (light blue) & the moderately dilated RV (purple).*

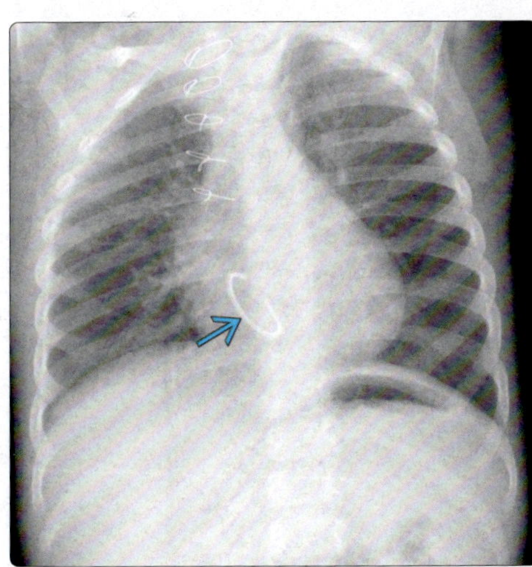

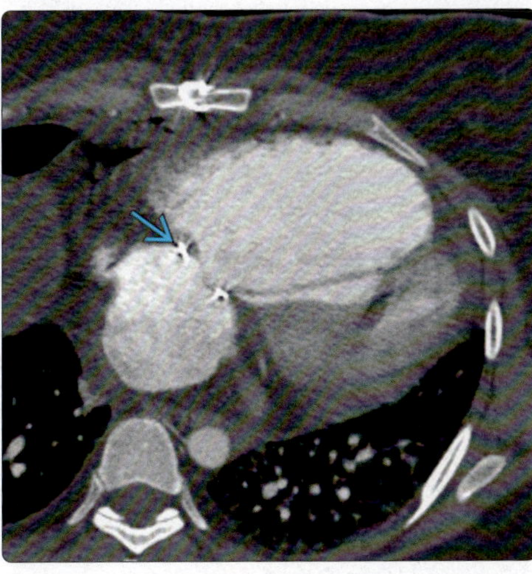

(Left) *Frontal view of the chest in a 3-year-old patient with Ebstein anomaly status post tricuspid valve replacement shows an abnormal orientation of the prosthetic valve between the RV & RA due to the underlying anomaly. Note the normal heart size & normal pulmonary vascularity.* **(Right)** *Axial CTA of the chest in patient with a history of Ebstein anomaly status post tricuspid valve replacement shows only mild RV enlargement.*

D-Transposition of Great Arteries

KEY FACTS

TERMINOLOGY

- Ventriculoarterial discordance with atrioventricular concordance: Aorta arises from right ventricle (RV) & pulmonary artery (PA) arises from left ventricle (LV)
- Complete separation of pulmonary & systemic circulations, lethal without flow admixture: Patent foramen ovale (PFO), ventricular septal defect (VSD), patent ductus arteriosus (PDA)

IMAGING

- Preoperative
  - Great vessels lie parallel & almost in same sagittal plane with aortic valve in anterior position & slightly to right (D-loop) of pulmonary valve; frequent coronary anomalies
  - Classic radiographic appearance: Narrow mediastinum with cardiomegaly ("egg on string/egg on its side" heart) + ↑ pulmonary vascularity
- Postoperative (after arterial switch/Jatene procedure)
  - Classic alterations of great vessel anatomy
    - PA is now anteriorly positioned with posterior aorta in same sagittal plane; right & left PAs now drape over ascending aorta
  - Transposed coronary arteries
  - Traction on both branch PAs may lead to stenosis

CLINICAL ISSUES

- Simple transposition: Good prognosis with early switch
- Large VSD: Congestive heart failure as neonate
- Patients with large VSD & (sub-) pulmonic stenosis have mild symptoms & may survive for years without treatment
- Long-term prognosis is determined by potential coronary abnormalities
- Potential treatments: Prostaglandin E1 to maintain PDA preoperatively; emergency balloon atrial septostomy (Rashkind); early surgery (preferred): Arterial switch with transposition of coronaries (Jatene); late surgery: Rerouting of venous flow in atria with pericardial baffle (Mustard) or reorientation of atrial septum (Senning)

(Left) *Frontal radiograph of the chest in an infant shows cardiomegaly & ↑ pulmonary vascularity in a patient with D-transposition of the great arteries (D-TGA). The superior mediastinum is narrow ➡, & the heart is globular in shape ↪. This combination is referred to as the egg-on-a-string appearance.* **(Right)** *Axial cardiac CTA in an infant shows the pulmonary artery (PA) ➡ posterior & slightly to the left of the ascending aorta ➡. This is the classic relationship of the great vessels seen with D-TGA.*

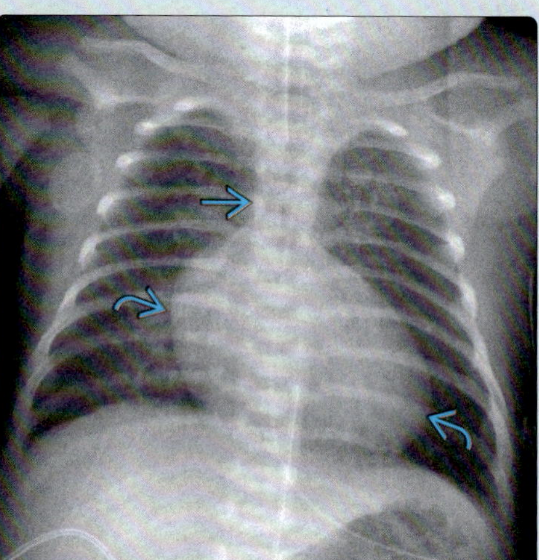

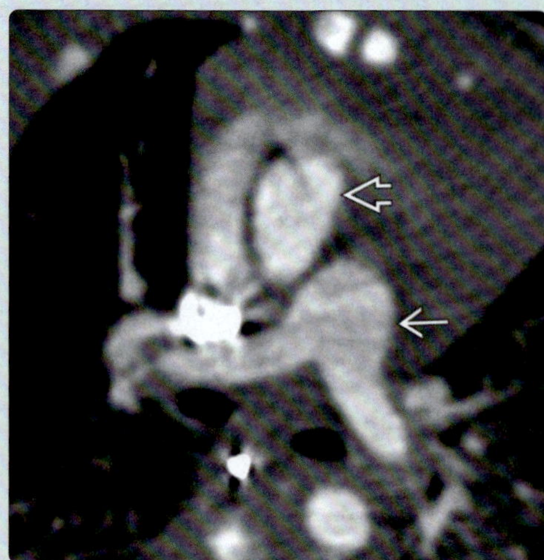

(Left) *Oblique color-coded 3D CTA in an infant with D-TGA shows that the aorta (red) arises from the right ventricle (RV) (purple) & the PA (blue) arises from left ventricle (LV) (pink). A large patent ductus arteriosus (PDA) (green) connects aortic arch to the PA (blue). Note coronary arteries (tan).* **(Right)** *Axial oblique cardiac CTA in an infant with D-TGA shows the aorta ➡ arising anterior & to the right of the base of the PA ➡. Note that the right coronary artery ↪ arises from the noncoronary sinus, which is typical for D-TGA.*

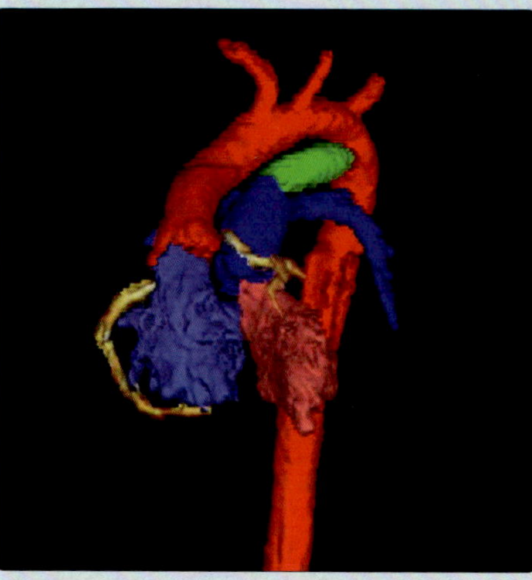

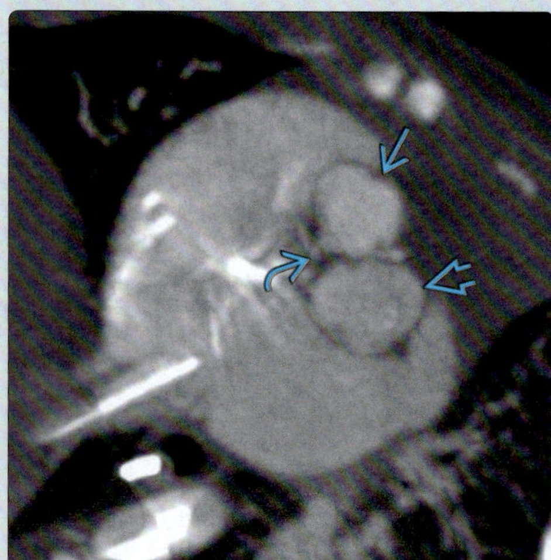

D-Transposition of Great Arteries

TERMINOLOGY

Definitions

- Aorta arises from right ventricle (RV) & pulmonary artery (PA) arises from left ventricle (LV)
- Ventriculoarterial (VA) discordance with atrioventricular (AV) concordance
- Category: Cyanotic, cardiomegaly, ↑ pulmonary vascularity
- Hemodynamics
  - RV connected with systemic circulation: Pressure overload
  - LV connected with pulmonary circulation: Volume overload
  - Lethal without flow admixture: Patent foramen ovale (PFO), ventricular septal defect (VSD), patent ductus arteriosus (PDA)

IMAGING

General Features

- Best diagnostic clue
  - Great vessels lie parallel in almost same sagittal plane: Aortic valve in anterior position & slightly to right (D-loop) of pulmonary valve

Radiographic Findings

- Radiography
  - May be normal in neonates
  - Classic appearance: Narrow mediastinum with cardiomegaly ("egg on a string" or "egg on its side" heart) + ↑ pulmonary vascularity

CT Findings

- CTA
  - Shows classic alterations of great vessel anatomy status post arterial switch procedure: PA is now anteriorly positioned with posterior aorta in same sagittal plane; right & left PAs now drape over ascending aorta
    - Traction on both branch PAs may lead to stenosis
    - Anterior tracheal or left main bronchus compression may be seen
    - Variable coronary anomalies in D-TGA; transposition is performed during surgery

MR Findings

- T1WI
  - Cardiac gated axial images for segmental cardiac analysis: AV concordance & VA discordance
    - Presence of PFO, VSD, (sub-) pulmonary stenosis
    - Postoperative assessment of PA stenosis
- T2* GRE
  - Multiplanar bright blood SSFP cine is gold standard for cardiac function evaluation & ventricular volume measurements
    - RV dysfunction following atrial switch procedures (as RV is not able to sustain systemic circulation)
- T1WI C+
  - Delayed-enhancement myocardial MR to detect ischemia complicating coronary transposition
- MRA
  - Gadolinium-enhanced MRA for postoperative PA stenosis
- Phase-contrast MR
  - Flow velocity measurements to calculate gradients across stenoses: Mustard/Senning or PA stenoses

CLINICAL ISSUES

Presentation

- Severe cyanosis not improving with oxygen with little respiratory distress

Demographics

- Epidemiology
  - Incidence: 1 in 3,000 live births
  - 5% of congenital heart disease

Natural History & Prognosis

- Early death without communicating shunt
- Large VSD: Congestive heart failure in neonatal period
- Patients with large VSD & (sub-) pulmonic stenosis have mild symptoms & may survive for years without treatment
- Simple transposition: Good prognosis with early switch
  - Long-term prognosis is determined by potential coronary abnormalities
- Complication of arterial switch: Traction on branch PAs by anteriorly transposed main PA → branch origin stenosis

Treatment

- Prostaglandin E1 to keep ductus arteriosus open preoperatively
- Emergency balloon atrial septostomy (Rashkind)
- Early surgery: Arterial switch with transposition of coronaries (Jatene)
- Late surgery (if Jatene is not performed): Rerouting of venous flow in atria with pericardial baffle (Mustard) or reorientation of atrial septum (Senning)

SELECTED REFERENCES

1. Makadia LD et al: Diagnosis of anomalous origin of the right subclavian artery from the right pulmonary artery in a patient with D-transposition of the great arteries utilizing transthoracic echocardiography. Echocardiography. 37(12):2144-7, 2020
2. Samyn MM et al: Echocardiography vs cardiac magnetic resonance imaging assessment of the systemic right ventricle for patients with d-transposition of the great arteries status post atrial switch. Congenit Heart Dis. 14(6):1138-48, 2019
3. Wu K et al: Differential myocardial mechanics in volume and pressure loaded right ventricles demonstrated by cardiac magnetic resonance. Pediatr Cardiol. 40(7):1503-8, 2019
4. Kirzner J et al: Long-term management of the arterial switch patient. Curr Cardiol Rep. 20(8):68, 2018
5. Słodki M et al: New method to predict need for Rashkind procedure in fetuses with dextro-transposition of the great arteries. Ultrasound Obstet Gynecol. 51(4):531-6, 2018
6. Khoshnood B et al: Impact of prenatal diagnosis on survival of newborns with four congenital heart defects: a prospective, population-based cohort study in France (the EPICARD Study). BMJ Open. 7(11):e018285, 2017
7. Han BK et al: Multi-institutional evaluation of the indications and radiation dose of functional cardiovascular computed tomography (CCT) imaging in congenital heart disease. Int J Cardiovasc Imaging. 32(2):339-46, 2016
8. Rickers C et al: Is the Lecompte technique the last word on transposition of the great arteries repair for all patients? A magnetic resonance imaging study including a spiral technique two decades postoperatively. Interact Cardiovasc Thorac Surg. 22(6):817-25, 2016

L-Transposition of Great Arteries

KEY FACTS

TERMINOLOGY

- Congenitally corrected transposition (misnomer)
- Inversion of ventricles & great arteries: Atrioventricular (AV) discordance & ventriculoarterial (VA) discordance
  - Right atrium connects via mitral valve to right-sided morphologic left ventricle (LV), which connects to pulmonary circulation
  - Left atrium connects via tricuspid valve to left-sided morphologic right ventricle (RV), which connects to systemic circulation
- Category: Dependent on associated anomalies
  - Ventricular septal defect (VSD) (60-70%): Acyanotic, ↑ pulmonary vascularity
  - Left ventricular (LV) outflow tract (subpulmonary) obstruction (30-50%): Cyanotic
  - Only 1% have no associated anomalies: True congenitally corrected transposition

IMAGING

- Classic radiograph: Straight upper left heart border
- CT & MR demonstrate complex anatomy

PATHOLOGY

- VSD: 80%
- LV outflow tract (subpulmonary) obstruction: 30-50%
- Left-sided tricuspid valve dysplasia, Ebstein anomaly, regurgitation: 30%

CLINICAL ISSUES

- Guarded prognosis due to progressive systemic AV valve & RV dysfunction after corrective surgery: 50% mortality after 15 years
- Patients with true congenitally corrected transposition may have normal life expectancy

(Left) *Frontal radiograph of the chest in an adolescent patient shows a straightened left upper heart border ➔ due to levo-transposition of the great arteries (L-TGA).* **(Right)** *Axial cardiac CTA shows the typical position of the great vessels in L-TGA. The aorta (Ao) ➔ is anterior & to the left of the pulmonary artery (PA) ➔.*

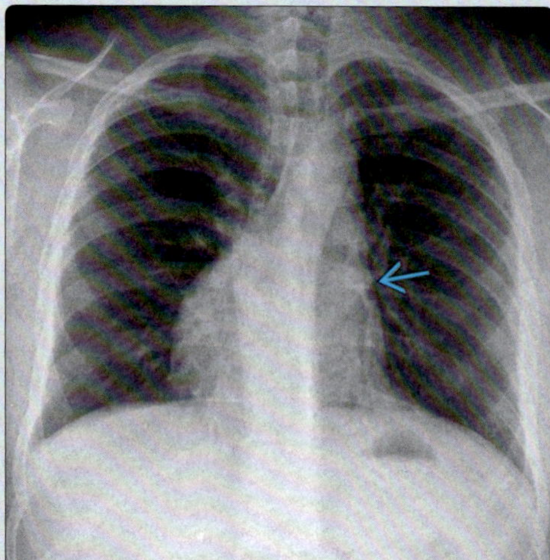

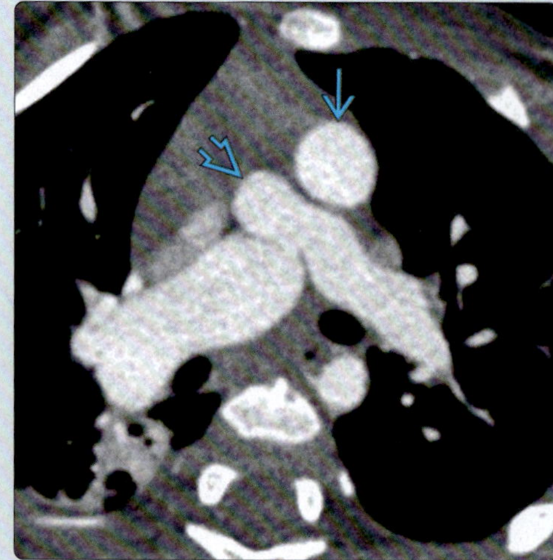

(Left) *Axial cardiac CTA in a patient with L-TGA shows a smooth-walled, morphologic left ventricle (LV) ➔ on the right. The morphologic right ventricle (RV) ➔ is on the left, demonstrating a characteristic moderator band ➔.* **(Right)** *Frontal 3D color-coded cardiac CTA shows the morphologic LV (pink) on the right giving rise to the PAs (blue) & the morphologic RV (purple) on the left giving rise to the Ao (red). The right coronary artery ➔ arises from the right coronary sinus & branches into the LAD & circumflex.*

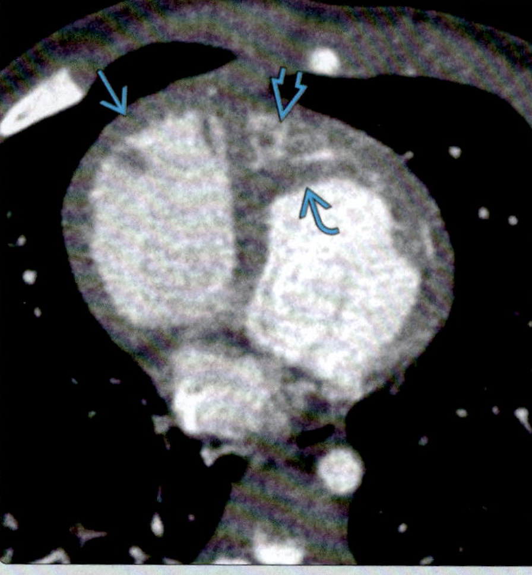

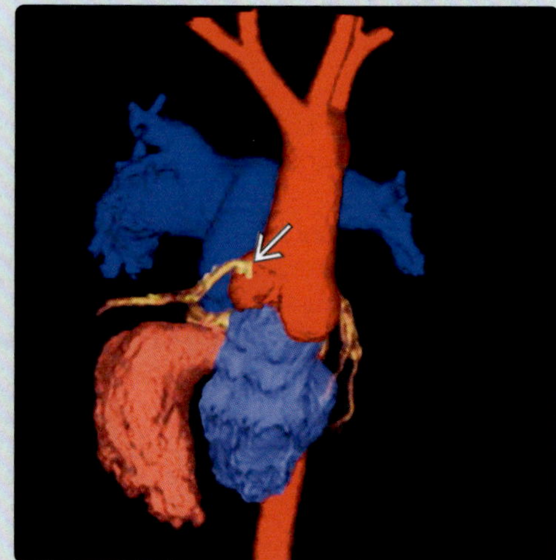

TERMINOLOGY

Synonyms

- Congenitally corrected transposition (misnomer)
- Discordant transposition

Definitions

- Inversion of ventricles & great arteries: Atrioventricular (AV) discordance & ventriculoarterial (VA) discordance
- Category: Dependent on associated anomalies
  - Ventricular septal defect (VSD) (60-80%): Acyanotic, ↑ pulmonary vascularity
  - Left ventricular outflow tract (subpulmonary) obstruction (30-50%): Cyanotic
  - Only 1% have no associated anomalies: True congenitally corrected transposition

IMAGING

General Features

- Best diagnostic clue
  - Great vessels lie parallel & almost in same coronal plane with aortic valve in anterior position & slightly to left (L-loop) of pulmonary valve
- Morphology
  - S, L, L heart: Atrial situs solitus, L-loop, L-transposed great arteries
    - Right-sided morphologic left ventricle (LV) is characterized by associated mitral valve, smooth wall, & absent outflow chamber to pulmonary valve
    - Left-sided morphologic right ventricle (RV) is characterized by associated tricuspid valve, trabeculated wall with moderator band, & infundibulum below aortic valve

Radiographic Findings

- Classic plain film appearance: Straight upper left heart border

CT Findings

- 3D CT angiography can depict abnormal AV & VA relationships
- Cardiac CTA to establish coronary artery anatomy

MR Findings

- Multiplanar cardiac gated T1 & 3D gadolinium MRA for segmental cardiac analysis & anatomic evaluation
- SSFP cine & phase contrast to evaluate function & outflow tract obstruction
  - Phase-contrast imaging is used to calculate shunt fraction (Qp:Qs)

DIFFERENTIAL DIAGNOSIS

Congestive Heart Failure, Increased Pulmonary Blood Flow

- Isolated VSD
- Double-inlet ventricle
- Tricuspid atresia with ↑ pulmonary blood flow
- Double-outlet RV + subaortic VSD

Cyanosis, Decreased Pulmonary Blood Flow

- Tetralogy of Fallot

PATHOLOGY

General Features

- Associated abnormalities
  - VSD: 60-80%
  - LV outflow tract (subpulmonary) obstruction: 30-50%
  - Left-sided tricuspid valve dysplasia, Ebstein anomaly, regurgitation: 30%
  - Coronary distribution is mirror image of normal (right-sided coronary bifurcates into circumflex & anterior descending arteries)
- Embryology: Primitive cardiac tube loops to left (L-loop) → ventricular inversion & left-sided position of ascending aorta

CLINICAL ISSUES

Presentation

- Most common signs/symptoms
  - Congestive heart failure (VSD, systemic AV valve dysfunction)
  - Cyanosis (subpulmonary stenosis)
  - Rarely completely asymptomatic, presenting as incidental finding on chest radiograph (straight upper left heart border)

Natural History & Prognosis

- Determined by presence of AV valve dysfunction
- Guarded prognosis due to progressive systemic AV valve & RV dysfunction after corrective surgery: 50% mortality after 15 years

Treatment

- Surgical treatment is focused on associated abnormalities
  - Congestive heart failure from VSD shunt: PA banding or VSD closure
  - Cyanosis from subpulmonary stenosis: Systemic to PA shunt (Blalock-Taussig) or LV to PA conduit (Rastelli)
- Double switch operation to prevent late systemic ventricular (RV) failure
  - Venous switch (Senning) reroutes atrial blood into appropriate ventricles
  - Ventricular (Rastelli) or arterial switch: Morphologic LV becomes systemic ventricle

SELECTED REFERENCES

1. Tous C et al: Ex vivo cardiovascular magnetic resonance diffusion weighted imaging in congenital heart disease, an insight into the microstructures of tetralogy of Fallot, biventricular and univentricular systemic right ventricle. J Cardiovasc Magn Reson. 22(1):69, 2020
2. Lozier MR et al: Levo-transposition of the great arteries in an adult patient: management considerations and treatment strategy. Cureus. 11(3):e4306, 2019
3. Al-Zahrani RS et al: Transposition of the great arteries: a laterality defect in the group of heterotaxy syndromes or an outflow tract malformation? Ann Pediatr Cardiol. 11(3):237-49, 2018
4. Mainwaring RD et al: An analysis of left ventricular retraining in patients with dextro- and levo-transposition of the great arteries. Ann Thorac Surg. 105(3):823-9, 2018
5. Bilal MS et al: Double switch procedure and surgical alternatives for the treatment of congenitally corrected transposition of the great arteries. J Card Surg. 31(4):231-6, 2016
6. Han BK et al: Multi-institutional evaluation of the indications and radiation dose of functional cardiovascular computed tomography (CCT) imaging in congenital heart disease. Int J Cardiovasc Imaging. 32(2):339-46, 2016

KEY FACTS

TERMINOLOGY

- Congenital absence or agenesis of tricuspid valve & inlet portion of right ventricle (RV)

IMAGING

- Type I: Normally related great arteries (70-80%)
- Type II: D-transposition of great arteries (12-25%)
- Type III: L-transposition of great arteries/malposition (3-6%)
- Small ventricular septal defect (VSD) → heart is usually normal in size, RV is hypoplastic, pulmonary flow is diminished
- Large VSD → heart is usually large with ↑ flow or transposition of great arteries
- MR: Excellent for postoperative left ventricular functional assessment & anatomy of caval-pulmonary artery anastomosis
- CTA: Useful to assess for pulmonary artery embolus & collateral vessels in children who have ↑ cyanosis
    - Knowledge of previous surgical procedure is critical to correctly prescribing protocol & interpreting imaging, particularly in Glenn anastomosis & Fontan procedures (as unopacified blood can mimic thrombus)

TOP DIFFERENTIAL DIAGNOSES

- Ebstein anomaly
- Tetralogy of Fallot

CLINICAL ISSUES

- 50% of neonates present with cyanosis in first 24 hours
- 30% present with signs of congestive heart failure
- Left axis deviation on newborn ECG is usually diagnostic
- Staged surgical approach, similar to single ventricle
    - Modified Blalock-Taussig shunt with systemic artery to pulmonary flow
    - Bidirectional Glenn anastomosis with superior vena cava to pulmonary artery
    - Modified Fontan procedure with inferior vena cava conduit to pulmonary artery

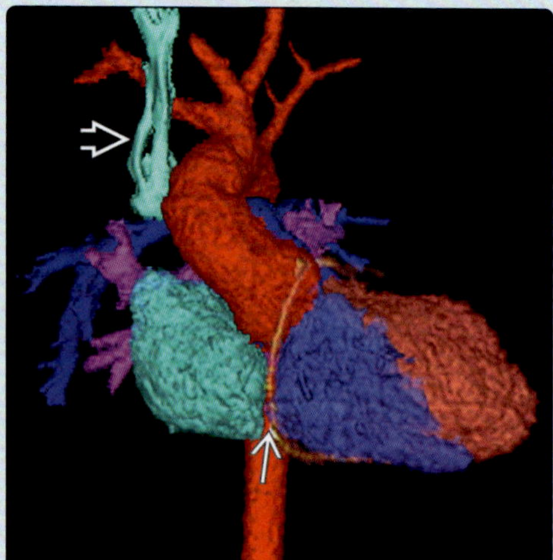

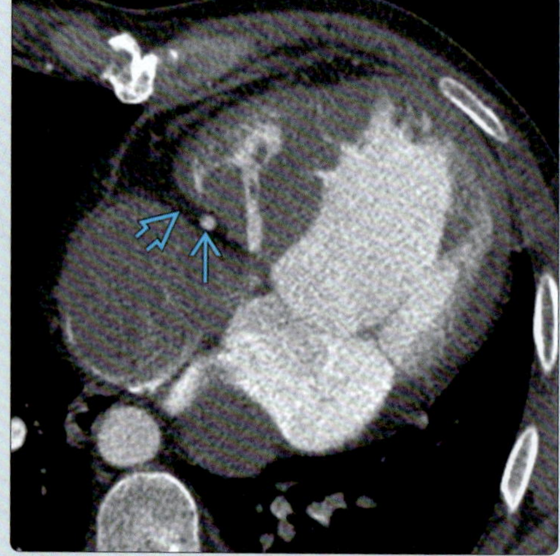

(Left) *Anterior 3D volume-rendered cardiac CTA in an infant with tricuspid atresia shows wide separation of right atrium (RA) (light blue) & right ventricle (RV) (purple). Right coronary artery ➡ lies deep in the atrioventricular (AV) groove. A Glenn shunt is seen with the superior vena cava (SVC) ➡ directly connected to pulmonary arteries (PAs) (dark blue).* **(Right)** *Axial cardiac CTA in an adolescent shows the right coronary artery ➡ & fat ➡ between the RA & RV in a patient with tricuspid atresia. Note unopacified blood in the RA from the Fontan shunt.*

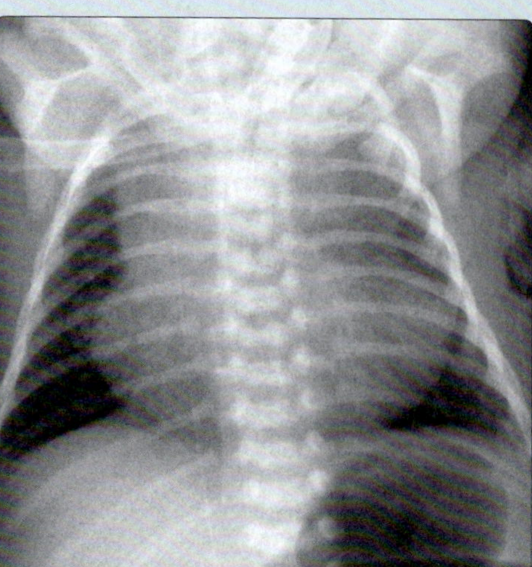

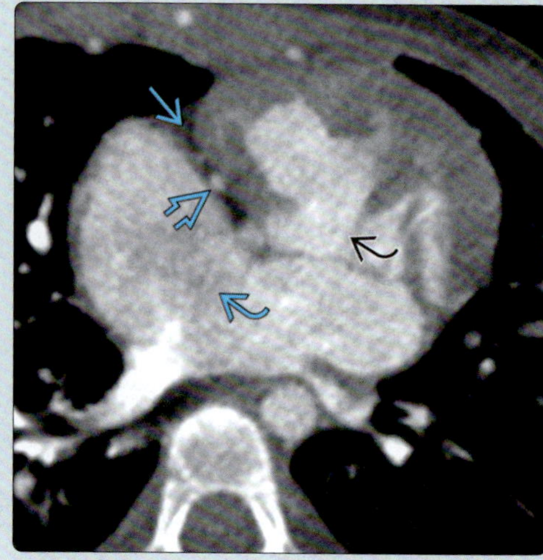

(Left) *AP radiograph of the chest shows cardiomegaly with ↓ pulmonary vascularity in an infant with tricuspid atresia.* **(Right)** *Axial cardiac CTA in an infant shows fat & soft tissue ➡ in the right AV groove where the tricuspid valve is normally located. Note the right coronary artery ➡ deep within the groove. With absence of the tricuspid valve, the coronary often sits between the RV & RA. A large atrial septal defect (ASD) ➡ & ventricular septal defect (VSD) ➡ are also seen.*

Tricuspid Atresia

TERMINOLOGY

Definitions

- Congenital absence or agenesis of tricuspid valve & inlet portion of right ventricle (RV)

IMAGING

General Features

- Best diagnostic clue
  - Absence of inflow portion of RV with atretic tricuspid valve
  - Outlet portion of RV depends on size of ventricular septal defect (VSD)
- Location
  - Tricuspid valve absent, fused, or stenotic; size of VSD & RV is variable
  - Right coronary artery & fat are seen within atrioventricular groove where tricuspid valve should be normally positioned
- Morphology
  - Type I: Normally related great arteries (70-80%)
  - Type II: D-transposition of great arteries (12-25%)
  - Type III: L-transposition of great arteries or malposition (3-6%)
  - VSD can occur with atresia, stenosis, or normal pulmonary valve

Radiographic Findings

- Neonatal chest radiograph is variable depending on size of VSD

CT Findings

- CECT
  - Demonstrates postoperative anastomosis, relative size of pulmonary arteries & systemic veins, & presence of collateral venous anatomy
  - Can be useful to assess for pulmonary artery embolus & collateral vessels in children with ↑ cyanosis
    - Must know underlying anatomy & type of surgical repair to interpret contrast studies as unopacified blood can mimic thrombus

MR Findings

- MR cine
  - Excellent for postoperative left ventricular (LV) functional assessment & anatomy of caval-pulmonary artery anastomosis
  - 3D contrast-enhanced MRA or spin-echo imaging can be used to assess connections & relations as well as size of proximal pulmonary arteries

Echocardiographic Findings

- Defines size & position of VSD, RV, & associated abnormalities

Angiographic Findings

- Cardiac catheterization prior to staged cardiac surgery repairs or for complications
  - Coiling of collateral arteries & veins to reduce workload of LV

Other Modality Findings

- Newborn pattern of left axis deviation on electrocardiography (ECG) is usually diagnostic

DIFFERENTIAL DIAGNOSIS

Tetralogy of Fallot

- Large aorta (right sided in 25%), concave left hilum, & ↓ peripheral flow

Ebstein Anomaly

- Newborn radiograph may show massive cardiomegaly
- Spectrum of disease, which involves downward displacement of septal & posterior leaflets of tricuspid valve

PATHOLOGY

General Features

- Etiology
  - Early embryologic insult with fusion of valve leaflet → stenosis (partial fusion) or atresia (complete fusion) of valves
- Genetics
  - Associated with asplenia syndromes

CLINICAL ISSUES

Presentation

- Most common signs/symptoms
  - 50% of neonates present with cyanosis in first 24 hours
  - 30% present with signs of congestive heart failure
- Other signs/symptoms
  - Extracardiac anomalies may occur in 20% of patients

Demographics

- Epidemiology
  - 3% of congenital heart lesions

DIAGNOSTIC CHECKLIST

Consider

- Knowledge of previous surgical procedure is critical to correctly prescribing protocol & interpreting imaging, particularly in Glenn anastomosis & Fontan procedures

Image Interpretation Pearls

- Hallmark is lack of direct anatomic continuity between right atrium & ventricle
- Right coronary artery & fat are seen within atrioventricular groove where tricuspid valve should be normally positioned
- Ventricular anatomy, type & size of VSD & relationship of great vessels, ventriculoarterial connections, & sources of pulmonary artery flow all need to be assessed

SELECTED REFERENCES

1. Lee C et al: Tricuspid atresia with absent pulmonary valve and intact ventricular septum: successful bidirectional cavopulmonary anastomosis with complete exclusion of the right ventricle. Cardiol Young. 30(1):126-8, 2020
2. Siddartha CR et al: Tricuspid atresia with truncus arteriosus: off-pump stage I palliation. World J Pediatr Congenit Heart Surg. 10(5):635-7, 2019
3. Enaba MM et al: Multidetector computed tomography (CT) in evaluation of congenital cyanotic heart diseases. Pol J Radiol. 82:645-59, 2017
4. Kinoshita M et al: Energetic performance analysis of staged palliative surgery in tricuspid atresia using vector flow mapping. Cardiovasc Ultrasound. 15(1):27, 2017

Truncus Arteriosus

KEY FACTS

TERMINOLOGY

- Common arterial vessel (trunk) arising from heart; gives rise to aorta, pulmonary arteries (PAs), & coronaries
- Congenital heart lesion most commonly associated with right aortic arch (30-40%)

IMAGING

- High (outlet) ventricular septal defect (VSD) immediately below truncal valve
- Classic radiograph: Cardiomegaly, ↑ pulmonary vascularity, narrow mediastinum, right aortic arch

PATHOLOGY

- Classification of Van Praagh
- Type A1: Same as Collett & Edwards type 1
- Type A2: Separate origins of branch PAs from common arterial trunk (CAT)
- Type A3: Origin of one branch of PA (usually right) from common trunk with other branch arising from aortic arch (collateral or patent ductus arteriosus)
- Type A4: Truncus with interrupted aortic arch

CLINICAL ISSUES

- Untreated: 65% 6-month & 75% 1-year mortality
- Intractable congestive heart failure → pulmonary hypertension → shunt reversal → ↑ cyanosis
- Associated thymic agenesis in DiGeorge syndrome → T-cell immunodeficiency
- Early complete repair (at 2-6 weeks of life) is favored by most surgeons: Placement of conduit between right ventricle & PA with closure of VSD
- Truncal valve dysfunction (regurgitation) is common → need for valvuloplasty, prosthesis

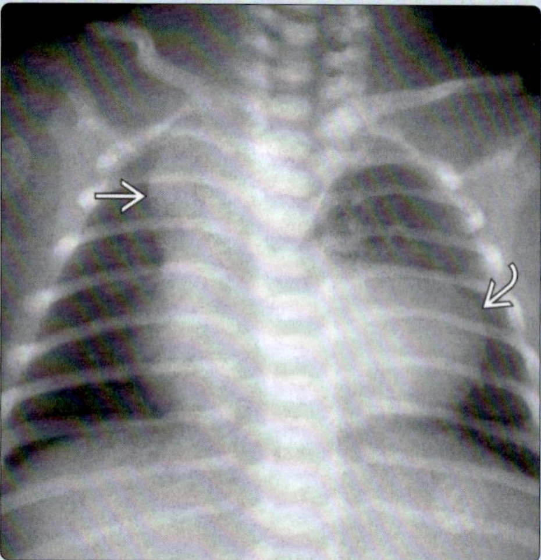
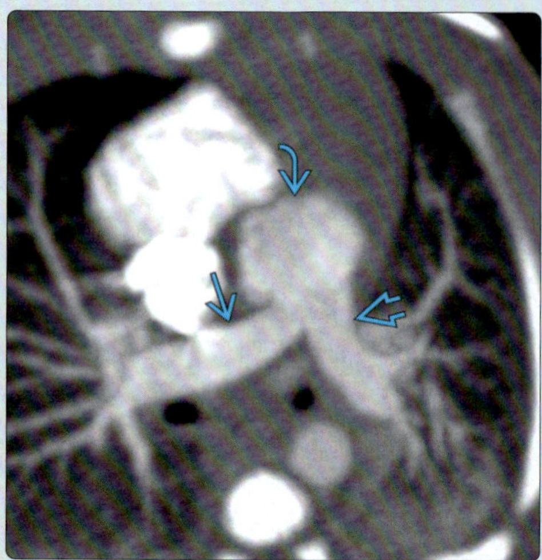

(Left) *AP radiograph shows cardiomegaly with a right aortic arch ➡ & ↑ pulmonary vascularity in an infant with truncus arteriosus. The apex of the heart is upturned ➡. This appearance is often mistaken for tetralogy of Fallot.* **(Right)** *Axial MIP cardiac CTA in an infant shows both the right pulmonary artery (PA) ➡ & left PA ➡ arising from a common trunk ➡ with the aorta. The findings are consistent with a type A2 truncus arteriosus.*

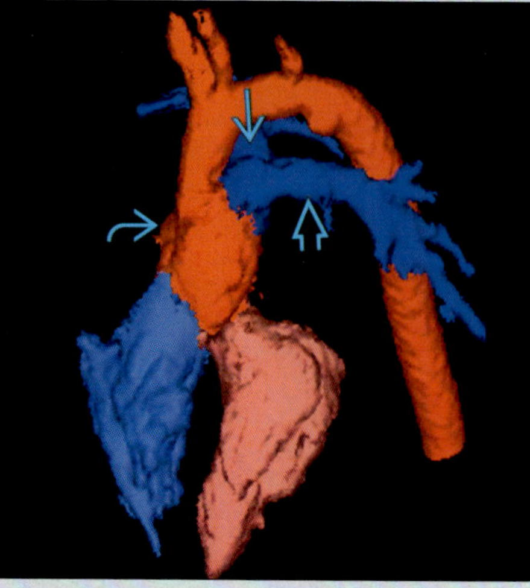
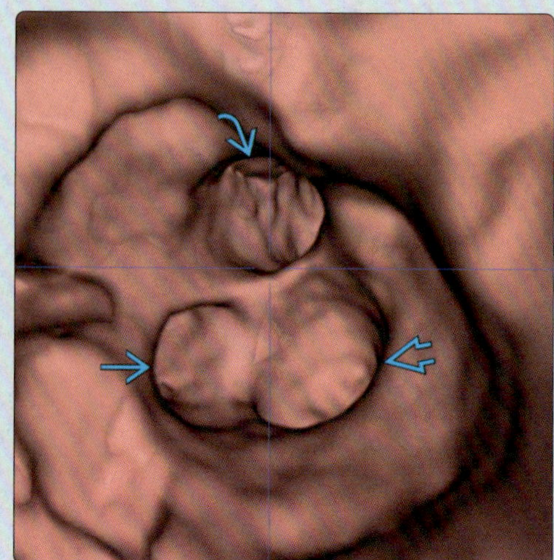

(Left) *Lateral 3D surface-rendered cardiac CTA in an infant shows both the right PA ➡ & left PA ➡ arising from a common trunk ➡ with the aorta. The findings are consistent with a type A2 truncus arteriosus.* **(Right)** *3D surface-rendered virtual angioscopy looking superiorly from inside the common trunk in an infant with truncus arteriosus shows both the right PA ➡ & left PA ➡ arising from a common trunk with the aorta ➡ seen anteriorly. The findings are consistent with a type A2 truncus arteriosus.*

TERMINOLOGY

Definitions

- Common arterial vessel arising from heart, giving rise to aorta, pulmonary arteries (PAs), & coronaries
- Classic radiographic appearance: Cardiomegaly, ↑ pulmonary vascularity, narrow mediastinum, right aortic arch
  - Truncus arteriosus is heart lesion most commonly associated with right aortic arch (30-40%)
- Category: Cyanotic, cardiomegaly, ↑ pulmonary vascularity
- Hemodynamics
  - Both ventricles are connected to pulmonary & systemic circulation
  - Flow admixture across ventricular septal defect (VSD) & within truncus → cyanosis
  - Postnatal drop in pulmonary vascular resistance → relative ↑ in pulmonary blood flow → volume overload of pulmonary circulation
- Frequently associated with absent thymus & parathyroid glands: DiGeorge syndrome

IMAGING

General Features

- Best diagnostic clue
  - Common arterial trunk (CAT) arising from both ventricles
  - Large common valve with 2-5 leaflets

Radiographic Findings

- Radiography
  - Cardiomegaly
  - Active pulmonary vascular congestion (shunt vascularity)
  - Right aortic arch is common
  - Narrow mediastinum due to thymic agenesis
  - Dilated PAs may compress neighboring bronchi → atelectasis

CT Findings

- CTA
  - Shows relationship of branch PAs with truncus
  - Coronary anatomy is well demonstrated
  - Postoperative: Patency & size of conduit, Ca^{2+}, & stenosis
  - CTA is best technique to evaluate stent placement & airway compression

MR Findings

- T1WI
  - Cardiac gated axial images for preoperative definition of PA anatomy
  - Postoperative: Conduit stenosis, anastomotic pseudoaneurysm
- T2* GRE
  - Steady-state free precession cine MR: Truncal valve regurgitation, ventricular function & volumes
- MRA
  - Gadolinium-enhanced MRA for global anatomy, patency of PA conduit
- Phase contrast
  - Velocity-encoded phase-contrast imaging to evaluate regurgitant fraction of common truncal valve or postoperative regurgitation/stenosis
  - Qp:Qs calculated with phase-contrast imaging

Echocardiographic Findings

- Echocardiogram
  - CAT originating from both ventricles
  - High (outlet) VSD immediately below truncal valve
  - Common truncal valve with 2 (5%), 3 (60%), or 4 (25%) cusps, rarely 5
- Color Doppler
  - Bidirectional flow across VSD
  - Truncal valve regurgitation

Angiographic Findings

- Cardiac catheterization with angiography
  - To define exact type of truncal anatomy
  - Visualizes truncal valve insufficiency
  - Hemodynamic study is gold standard for calculation of pulmonary vascular resistance

Imaging Recommendations

- Protocol advice
  - Primary diagnosis is made with echocardiography
  - MR/CTA for preoperative delineation of PA anatomy
  - MR/CTA for postoperative assessment of conduit regurgitation/stenosis, stent placement

DIFFERENTIAL DIAGNOSIS

Transposition of Great Arteries

- Presents earlier in life with more severe cyanosis; ductus dependent

Aortopulmonary Window

- Congenital fenestration between separate ascending aorta & PA with separate aortic & pulmonary valves

Common Atrioventricular Canal

- When unbalanced (right or left dominant), cyanosis frequently occurs due to admixture

PATHOLOGY

General Features

- Genetics
  - Strong association with deletion on long arm of chromosome 22 (22q11 syndrome)
  - Associated findings: Cardiac anomalies (truncus arteriosus), abnormal facies, thymic hypoplasia, cleft palate, & hypocalcemia with deletion of chromosome 22 (CATCH-22)
    - Includes DiGeorge syndrome, velocardiofacial syndrome, & conotruncal anomaly face syndrome
  - Theory: Abnormal migration of neural crest tissue that interferes with development of cardiac tube
- Associated abnormalities
  - Right-sided aortic arch with mirror-image branching (30-40%)
  - Persistence of primitive aortic arches
  - Absent thymus & parathyroid glands
- Embryology
  - Lack of separation of primitive bulbus cordis into aorta & main PA
  - Associated persistence of primitive aortic arches

- Pathophysiology: Congestive heart failure vs. cyanosis (degree of cyanosis is determined by balance between pulmonary & systemic vascular resistances)
  - Marked ↑ in pulmonary blood flow in early neonatal period due to drop in pulmonary vascular resistance → slight improvement in cyanosis but worsening congestive heart failure
  - Development of pulmonary vascular obstructive disease → improvement in congestive heart failure but worsening cyanosis

Staging, Grading, & Classification

- Classification of Collett & Edwards
  - Type 1: Separation of common trunk into ascending aorta & main PA
  - Type 2: Common take-off of branch PAs from trunk with no main PA
  - Type 3: Both branch PAs originate separately from posterolateral aspect of ascending aorta
  - Type 4: Pseudotruncus: Pulmonary arterial supply from major aortopulmonary collateral arteries (MAPCAs) arising from descending aorta; controversial entity (misnomer for pulmonary atresia with VSD & MAPCAs)
- Classification of Van Praagh
  - Type A1: Same as Collett & Edwards type 1
  - Type A2: Separate origins of branch PAs from CAT
  - Type A3: Origin of 1 branch of PA (usually right) from common trunk with other branch arising from aortic arch [collateral or patent ductus arteriosus (PDA)]
  - Type A4: Truncus with interrupted aortic arch

Gross Pathologic & Surgical Features

- Common outflow tract of both ventricles over nonrestrictive VSD
- Position of common trunk with respect to VSD
  - Predominantly positioned over right ventricle (42%)
  - Predominantly positioned over left ventricle (16%)
  - Equally shared (42%)
- No separate outflow portion (infundibulum) of right ventricle
- Many variations exist involving interruption of aortic arch (11-14%), absence of branch PA (hemitruncus), & PDA

CLINICAL ISSUES

Presentation

- Most common signs/symptoms
  - Progressive congestive heart failure with drop in pulmonary vascular resistance in young infant
  - ↑ cyanosis due to shunt reversal with development of pulmonary hypertension
- Other signs/symptoms
  - T-cell immunodeficiency (thymic agenesis in DiGeorge syndrome)
  - Neonatal tetany (absent parathyroid glands)

Demographics

- Epidemiology
  - 2% of congenital cardiac anomalies

Natural History & Prognosis

- Untreated: 65% 6-month & 75% 1-year mortality
- Intractable congestive heart failure
  - Marked ↑ in pulmonary flow after drop in pulmonary vascular resistance
  - Aggravated by presence of truncal valve regurgitation (in 50% of cases)
- Eventual shunt reversal with progressive cyanosis & sudden death
  - Pulmonary vascular obstructive disease with Eisenmenger physiology can develop as early as 6 months of age
- Postoperative course is determined by function of PA conduit & morbidity of conduit replacement

Treatment

- Palliative: Banding of main PA
  - Initial palliation with PA banding is often unsatisfactory with early development of pulmonary vascular disease → pulmonary hypertension
  - Early complete repair (at 2-6 weeks of life) is favored by most surgeons
- Surgical repair with placement of conduit between right ventricle & PA or creation of connection with atrial appendage & monoleaflet valve with closure of VSD
  - Conduit revisions are frequently necessary throughout patient's lifetime
    - Patient outgrows fixed conduit size
    - Ca^{2+}, stenosis, neointimal hyperplasia
    - Anastomotic pseudoaneurysm
    - Conduit valve dysfunction (regurgitation)
  - Truncal valve dysfunction (regurgitation) is common → need for valvuloplasty, prosthesis

SELECTED REFERENCES

1. Ly R et al: Multimodality imaging before persistent truncus arteriosus repair in a 36-year-old woman. Eur Heart J Case Rep. 4(6):1-2, 2020
2. Sinha M et al: Type A3 truncus arteriosus with infracardiac total anomalous pulmonary venous return and single ventricle physiology: a triad of tribulations. J Cardiovasc Comput Tomogr. 14(6):e137-8, 2020
3. Chikkabyrappa S et al: Common arterial trunk: physiology, imaging, and management. Semin Cardiothorac Vasc Anesth. 23(2):225-36, 2019
4. Fujiwara K et al: Truncus arteriosus with major aortopulmonary collateral arteries. Ann Thorac Surg. 108(2):e105-6, 2019
5. Sharma A et al: Atypical variant of truncus arteriosus: sinusal origin of pulmonary artery segment with non-confluent branch pulmonary arteries. BMJ Case Rep. 12(4), 2019
6. Naimo PS et al: Impact of truncal valve surgery on the outcomes of the truncus arteriosus repair. Eur J Cardiothorac Surg. 54(3):524-31, 2018
7. Greenhouse DG et al: Truncus arteriosus versus tetralogy of Fallot with pulmonary atresia. Cardiol Young. 27(4):801-3, 2017

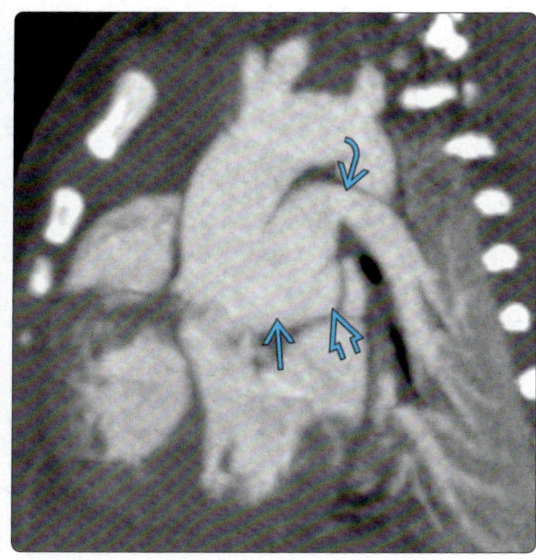

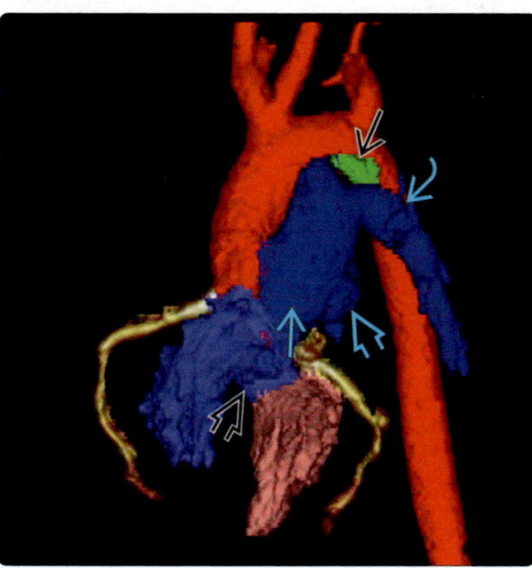

(Left) *Sagittal MIP cardiac CTA in an infant shows a truncus arteriosus with a common pulmonary trunk* ➡ *arising posteriorly before dividing into the right* ➡ *& left* ➡ *PAs. The findings are consistent with a type A1 truncus arteriosus.* **(Right)** *Lateral 3D surface-rendered image cardiac CTA in an infant shows a type A1 truncus arteriosus with a common pulmonary trunk* ➡ *arising posteriorly before dividing into right* ➡ *& left* ➡ *PAs. Note the ventricular septal defect* ➡ *& patent ductus arteriosus* ➡*.*

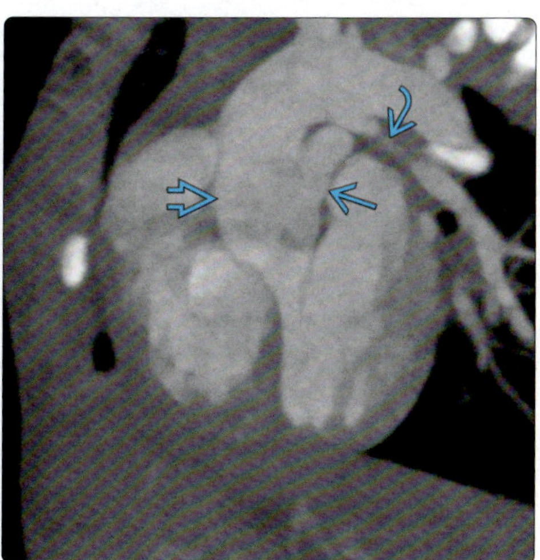

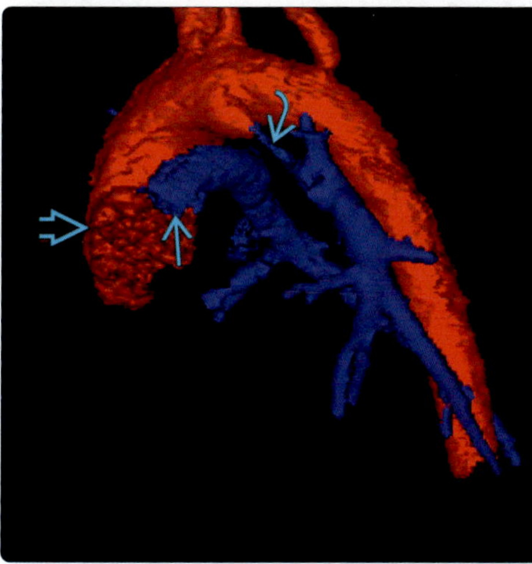

(Left) *Sagittal MIP cardiac CTA in an infant shows the origin of the right PA* ➡ *from the posterior aspect of a common trunk* ➡ *with the left PA* ➡ *arising from the undersurface of the aorta, consistent with a type A3 truncus arteriosus. Note the stenosis of the proximal left PA.* **(Right)** *Lateral 3D surface-rendered CTA shows the origin of the right PA* ➡ *from the posterior aspect of a common trunk* ➡ *with the left PA* ➡ *arising from the undersurface of the aorta, consistent with a type A3 truncus arteriosus.*

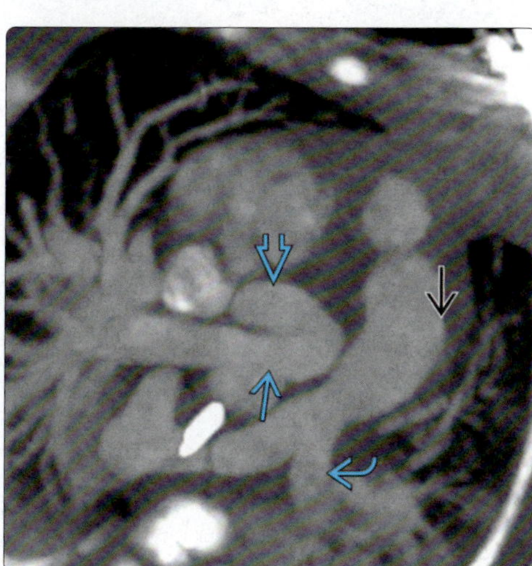

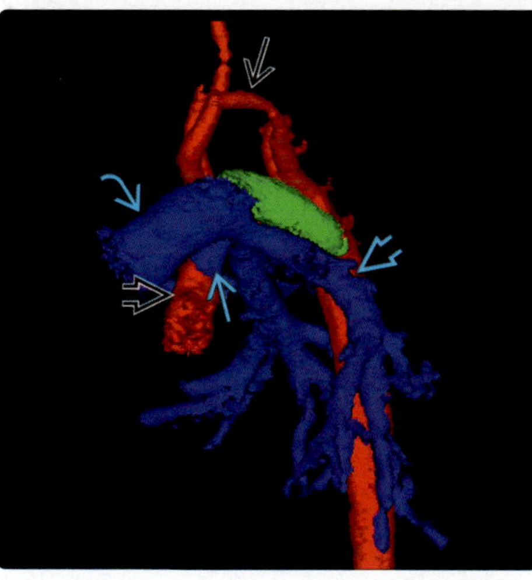

(Left) *Oblique axial MIP cardiac CTA shows the right PA* ➡ *arising from the ascending aortic trunk* ➡*. The left PA* ➡ *arises normally from the main PA* ➡*.* **(Right)** *Lateral 3D surface-rendered cardiac CTA shows a hemitruncus variation with the origin of the right PA* ➡ *from the common aortic trunk* ➡ *& the left PA* ➡ *arising normally from the main PA* ➡*. Note the large patent ductus arteriosus (green) & the hypoplastic aortic arch* ➡*.*

Total Anomalous Pulmonary Venous Return

KEY FACTS

TERMINOLOGY

- Total anomalous pulmonary venous return (TAPVR) or "drainage": Failure of connection between pulmonary veins (PVs) & left atrium
- Category: Cyanotic; heart size & pulmonary vascularity depend on type
- All pulmonary venous return goes to right heart (extracardiac left-to-right shunt)
- All types are admixture lesions
- Supracardiac TAPVR (type I, 40-50%): "Vertical" common PV joins left innominate vein
- Cardiac TAPVR (type II, 20-30%): Common PV joins coronary sinus or right atrium
- Infracardiac TAPVR (type III, 10-30%): Common PV joins portal vein, ductus venosus, or inferior vena cava

IMAGING

- Cardiomegaly (types I, II); small heart (type III)
- Shunt vascularity (types I, II); pulmonary edema (type III)
- Type I: "Snowman heart"
- Type II: Indistinguishable from atrial septal defect (ASD)
- Type III: Small heart, reticular pattern in lungs (edema)

PATHOLOGY

- All types have patent foramen ovale (PFO) to allow for obligatory right-to-left flow → varying degrees of cyanosis
- TAPVR (type III): Common PV is obstructed by diaphragmatic hiatus → pulmonary venous congestion & edema
- Left-sided cardiac chambers may be underdeveloped, especially in TAPVR type III (due to ↓ in systemic flow)

CLINICAL ISSUES

- Treatment: Early surgical anastomosis of pulmonary venous confluence to left atrium
- Anastomotic PV stenosis in up to 18% of TAPVR repairs
- Longstanding PV stenosis → irreversible pulmonary hypertension (arterial pulmonary vascular disease)
- Angioplasty of distal PVs is often required after surgery

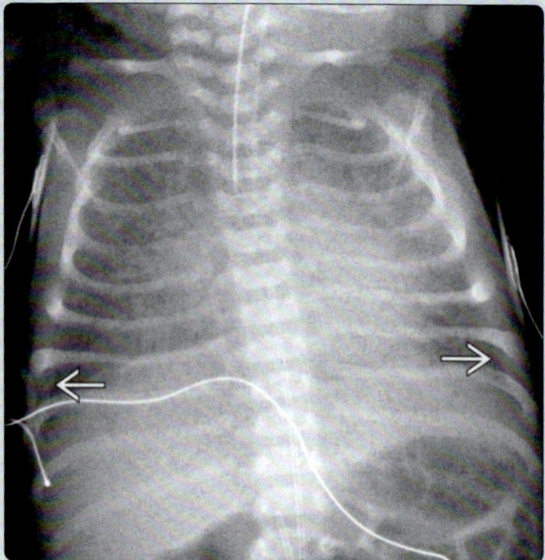

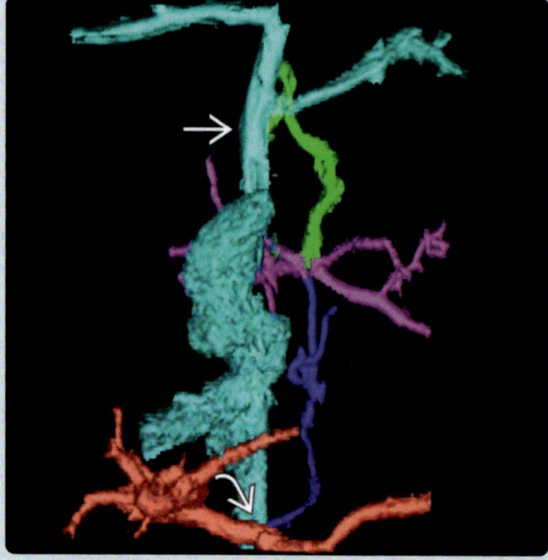

(Left) *Frontal radiograph in a newborn shows diffuse pulmonary edema with small, bilateral pleural effusions ➔. Note that the heart size is normal in this patient with a mixed type of total anomalous pulmonary venous return (TAPVR).* **(Right)** *Frontal color-coded 3D CTA in a complex TAPVR patient shows pulmonary veins (pink) draining into superior (green) & inferior (purple) vertical veins. Superior vertical vein drains to superior vena cava ➔, & the inferior vertical vein drains to the portal vein ↷.*

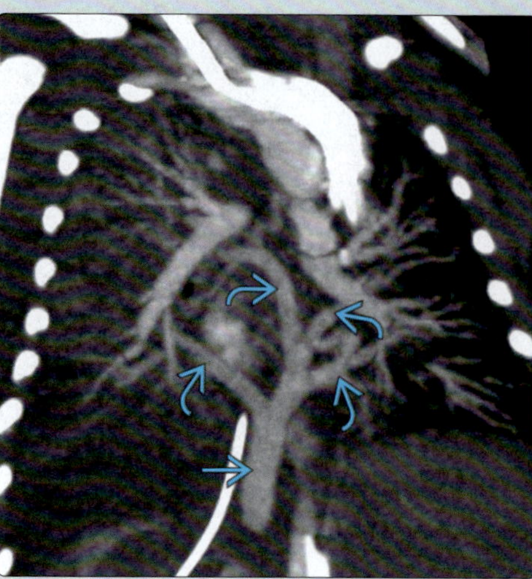

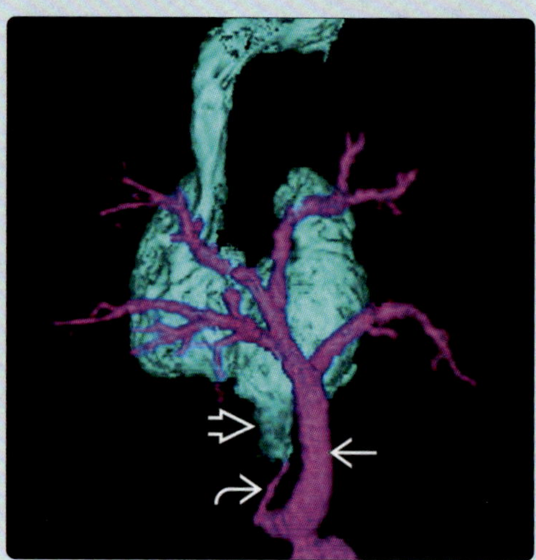

(Left) *Coronal MIP CTA of an infant with an obstructed type III TAPVR shows that the pulmonary veins ↷ connect to a large vertical vein ➔ that then drains below the diaphragm.* **(Right)** *Posterior color-coded 3D CTA shows the pulmonary veins (purple) emptying into a large inferior vertical vein ➔ in a patient with obstructed infracardiac TAPVR. Only a small venous connection ↷ was seen to the inferior vena cava ⇨. Note the symmetric atria (light blue) in this patient with heterotaxy.*

TERMINOLOGY

Synonyms

- Total anomalous pulmonary venous connection
  - Refers to anatomy: Where pulmonary veins (PVs) connect

Definitions

- Total anomalous pulmonary venous return (TAPVR) or "drainage"
  - Refers to hemodynamics: Where pulmonary venous flow returns (drain)
- Failure of connection between PVs & left atrium
- Category: Cyanotic; heart size & pulmonary vascularity depend on type
- Hemodynamics
  - All pulmonary venous return goes to right heart (extracardiac left-to-right shunt)
  - Intracardiac right-to-left shunt through patent foramen ovale (PFO)
  - All types are admixture lesions
- 3 types
  - Supracardiac TAPVR (type I, 50%): "Vertical" common PV joins left innominate vein
  - Cardiac TAPVR (type II, 20%): Common PV joins coronary sinus or right atrium
  - Infracardiac TAPVR (type III, 20%): Common PV joins portal vein, ductus venosus, hepatic veins, or inferior vena cava
  - Mixed or complex TAPVR (type IV) when there is mixture of aforementioned types (10%)

IMAGING

General Features

- Best diagnostic clue
  - No PVs connecting to left atrium
  - Supra- or infracardiac vertical vein

Radiographic Findings

- Radiography
  - Cardiomegaly (types I, II); small or normal heart size (type III)
  - Shunt vascularity (types I, II); pulmonary edema (type III)
    - Types I & II rarely may be obstructive with pulmonary edema & effusions
  - Wide mediastinum (type I → "snowman heart"), narrow mediastinum (types II & III → thymic atrophy)
  - Classic plain film appearance
    - Type I: "Snowman heart" (due to left vertical vein)
    - Type II: Indistinguishable from atrial septal defect (ASD)
    - Type III: Small heart, reticular pattern in lungs → edema

CT Findings

- CTA is useful to define anatomy in complex types of TAPVR & to define additional congenital heart lesions
  - Thickened interlobular septa, peribronchial cuffing, & ground-glass opacities suggest anastomotic PV stenosis
  - Airway compression is well visualized by CT
- Can be used postoperatively for evaluation of PV caliber & anastomoses

MR Findings

- T1WI
  - Cardiac gated black blood imaging: Anomalous connections are best seen in coronal plane
- MRA
  - Velocity-encoded phase-contrast MRA: For detection of PV anastomotic stenosis (flow velocities > 100 cm/sec are diagnostic)
    - Phase contrast
      - Qp:Qs calculation
      - Elevated velocities in distal vertical vein
      - Quantitative evaluation of cardiac valves for regurgitation
  - Dynamic time-resolved gadolinium-enhanced 3D MRA: For detailed depiction of PV anatomy
- MR cine
  - Steady-state free precession cine MR for functional assessment, flow jets, regurgitation

Echocardiographic Findings

- Echocardiogram
  - Lack of connection of PVs to normal-sized left atrium
  - Right-sided chamber enlargement in types I, II
  - PFO
  - Associated cardiac & abdominal situs abnormalities
  - Evaluation of complex types is limited by ultrasound
  - Limited assessment for postoperative anastomotic PV obstruction

Angiographic Findings

- Conventional
  - Seldom required for primary diagnosis
  - Balloon atrial septostomy when flow across ASD is restricted
  - After repair: For diagnosis & treatment of anastomotic PV stenosis

Imaging Recommendations

- Protocol advice
  - Primary diagnosis with echocardiography
  - CT, MR for postoperative PV anastomotic stenosis
  - Conventional angiography to treat postoperative PV stenosis

DIFFERENTIAL DIAGNOSIS

Cor Triatriatum

- Pulmonary venous connection is present but remains stenotic with lack of incorporation of common PV into left atrial wall

Hypoplastic Left Heart Syndrome

- PVs insert normally into left atrium with left-to-right shunting through PFO

Persistent Fetal Circulation Syndrome/Primary Pulmonary Hypertension

- Associated with
  - Severe surfactant deficiency disease
  - Meconium aspiration

Hypogenetic Lung Syndrome (Scimitar Syndrome)

- Partial anomalous pulmonary venous return to right lower lobe
- Systemic arterial supply to right lower lobe
- Hypoplastic right lung

Partial Anomalous Pulmonary Venous Return

- Majority of PVs drain normally to left atrium
- May present with volume overload to right heart

PATHOLOGY

General Features

- Genetics
  - No specific genetic defect has been found
  - Associated with heterotaxy syndromes
- Associated abnormalities
  - Single ventricle, atrioventricular septal defect, truncus arteriosus, tetralogy of Fallot, anomalous systemic venous connection
  - Asplenia syndrome with symmetric, bilateral, morphologic right atria
  - Polysplenia syndrome is less common
  - Biliary atresia
  - Thoracic lymphangiectasia & pulmonary edema are associated with infracardiac-type TAPVR
- All anomalous pulmonary venous drainage eventually flows into right atrium
- Embryology
  - Lack of normal incorporation of primitive common PV into posterior wall of left atrium
  - Persistence & enlargement of embryologic pathways for pulmonary venous return via umbilicovitteline & cardinal veins
- Pathophysiology
  - All types have PFO to allow for obligatory right-to-left flow → varying degrees of cyanosis (less severe in types I, II → pulmonary hypercirculation)
  - Nonobstructive TAPVR (types I, II): ASD physiology, pulmonary plethora, congestive heart failure
  - Obstructive TAPVR (type III): Common PV is obstructed by diaphragmatic hiatus → pulmonary venous congestion & edema
  - Left-sided cardiac chambers may be underdeveloped, especially in TAPVR type III, due to prenatal ↓ in systemic blood flow

CLINICAL ISSUES

Presentation

- Most common signs/symptoms
  - Types I, II: Congestive heart failure
  - Type III: Severe cyanosis at birth
  - Patent ductus arteriosus: Persistent fetal circulation

Demographics

- Epidemiology
  - 1-3% of congenital heart disease
  - More frequent in neonatal period

Natural History & Prognosis

- No patients survive without surgical treatment
- Natural history is highly variable
  - Types I, II: Initially asymptomatic with gradual development of congestive heart failure when pulmonary vascular resistance drops (ASD physiology)
  - Type III, obstructive forms: Death within month
- After surgical repair: Prognosis is determined by associated cardiac anomalies & development of PV anastomotic stenosis
  - Progressive distal PV stenosis is often seen → significant morbidity & mortality

Treatment

- Prostaglandin E1 to improve systemic perfusion in pulmonary hypertension (HTN)
- Preoperative extracorporeal membrane oxygenation is occasionally necessary to improve oxygenation & systemic perfusion
- Early surgical anastomosis of pulmonary venous confluence to left atrium
  - Anastomotic PV stenosis may occur in up to 18% of TAPVR repairs
  - Longstanding PV stenosis → irreversible pulmonary HTN (arterial pulmonary vascular disease)
  - Reoperation performed using sutureless technique with pericardial patch augmentation of anastomotic stenoses
- Angioplasty of distal PVs is often required after surgery due to stenosis

SELECTED REFERENCES

1. Xiang M et al: Mixed type of total anomalous pulmonary venous connection: diagnosis, surgical approach and outcomes. J Cardiothorac Surg. 15(1):293, 2020
2. Abdel Razek AAK et al: Computed tomography angiography and magnetic resonance angiography of congenital anomalies of pulmonary veins. J Comput Assist Tomogr. 43(3):399-405, 2019
3. Fuentes Rojas SC et al: Transcatheter embolization of a persistent vertical vein: a rare cause of left-to-right shunt and right-sided heart failure. Methodist Debakey Cardiovasc J. 15(1):86-7, 2019
4. Han F et al: The case of the missing pulmonary vein: a focused update on anomalous pulmonary venous connection in congenital cardiovascular disease. Echocardiography. 36(10):1930-5, 2019
5. White BR et al: Repair of total anomalous pulmonary venous connection: risk factors for postoperative obstruction. Ann Thorac Surg. 108(1):122-9, 2019
6. Seller N et al: How many versus how much: comprehensive haemodynamic evaluation of partial anomalous pulmonary venous connection by cardiac MRI. Eur Radiol. 28(11):4598-606, 2018
7. Tremblay C et al: Sutureless versus conventional pulmonary vein repair: a magnetic resonance pilot study. Ann Thorac Surg. 105(4):1248-54, 2018
8. Enaba MM et al: Multidetector computed tomography (CT) in evaluation of congenital cyanotic heart diseases. Pol J Radiol. 82:645-59, 2017
9. Kasai H et al: Adult partial anomalous pulmonary venous connection with drainage to left atrium and inferior vena cava clearly visualized on a combination of multiple imaging techniques. Circ J. 81(10):1547-9, 2017

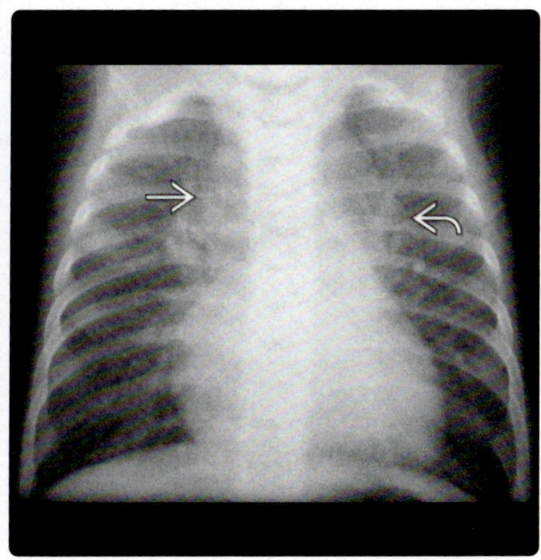

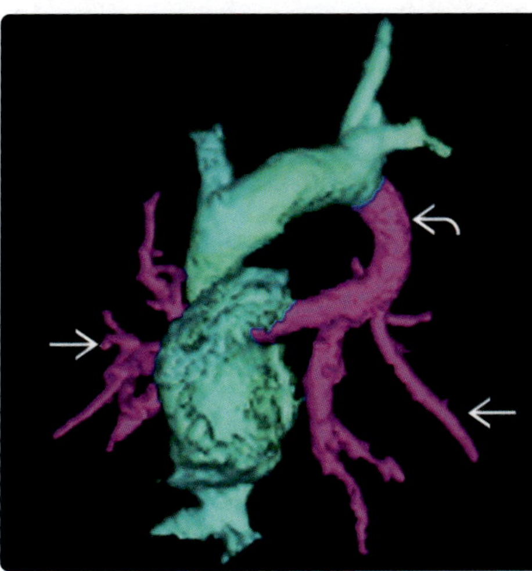

(Left) *Frontal radiograph shows a snowman appearance of the superior mediastinum in a patient with a supracardiac TAPVR. The left-sided vertical vein forms the border of the superior left mediastinum* ➡. *The dilated innominate vein & superior vena cava* ➡ *form the superior & right borders of the superior mediastinum, respectively.* **(Right)** *Frontal projection color-coded 3D CTA shows the pulmonary veins* ➡ *emptying into a large left-sided vertical vein* ➡ *in this patient with a supracardiac TAPVR.*

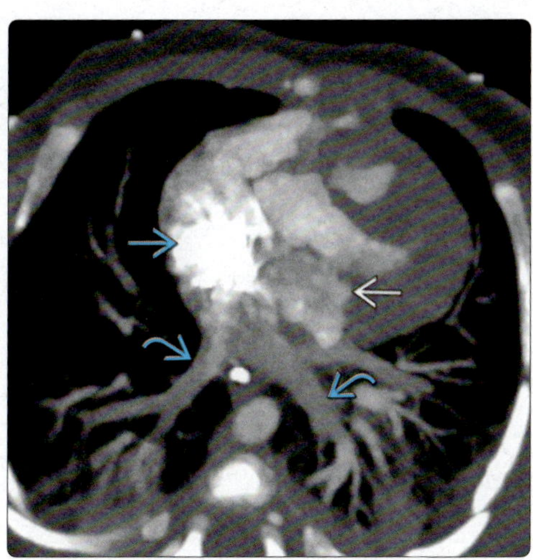

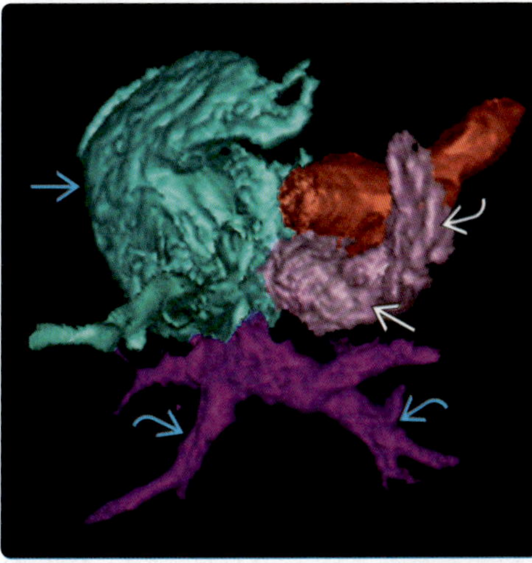

(Left) *Axial MIP cardiac CTA in an infant shows the pulmonary veins* ➡ *emptying directly into the right atrium* ➡. *Note the isolated left atrium* ➡. **(Right)** *Superior color-coded 3D CTA in an infant shows the pulmonary veins* ➡ *emptying directly into the right atrium* ➡. *Note the isolated left atrium* ➡. *The left atrial appendage is well demonstrated* ➡. *The left ventricle (salmon) is also shown.*

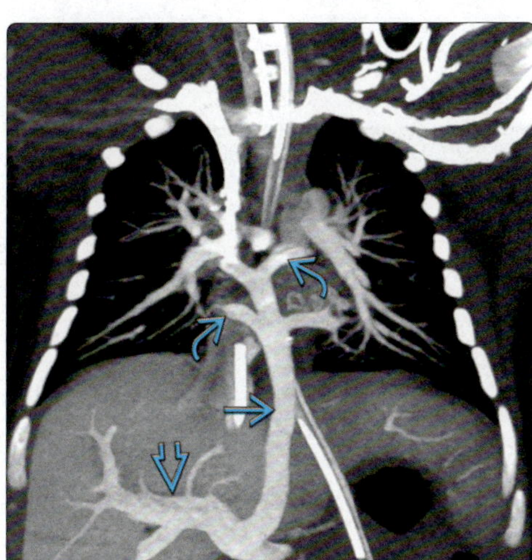

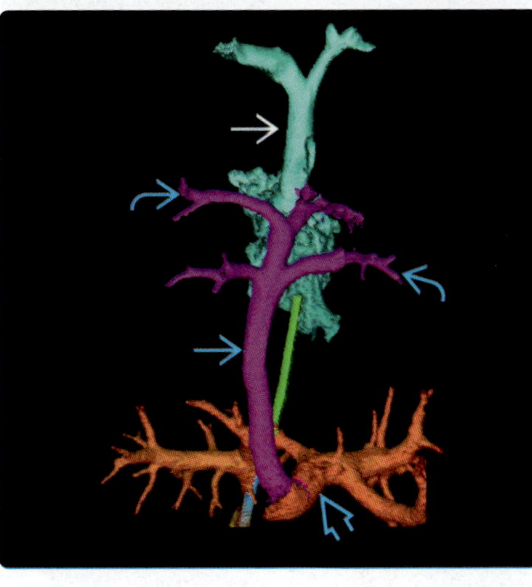

(Left) *Coronal MIP cardiac CTA in an infant shows the pulmonary veins* ➡ *draining into a large vertical vein* ➡, *which goes below the diaphragm & empties into the portal vein* ➡. **(Right)** *Frontal color-coded 3D CTA in an infant shows the pulmonary veins* ➡ *draining into a large vertical vein* ➡, *which goes below the diaphragm & empties into the portal vein* ➡, *consistent with an infracardiac type of TAPVR. The superior vena cava* ➡, *right atrium (blue), & umbilical artery catheter (green) are also shown.*

Hypoplastic Left Heart Syndrome

KEY FACTS

TERMINOLOGY

- Most severe congenital heart lesion
  - Presents in neonatal period with congestive heart failure, cardiogenic shock, & cyanosis
- Category: Cyanotic, cardiomegaly, ↑ pulmonary vascularity
- Hypoplasia/atresia of ascending aorta, aortic valve, left ventricle (LV), & mitral valve (MV)
- Secondary findings: Patent ductus arteriosus, juxtaductal coarctation

IMAGING

- Chest radiograph shows cardiomegaly, large right atrium, pulmonary venous congestion with interstitial fluid
- Postnatal echocardiogram is sufficient for treatment planning
  - Diminutive ascending aorta < 5 mm
  - Small, thick-walled LV; presence of endocardial fibroelastosis (EFE)
  - MV size is important to decide whether biventricular repair is possible in marginally hypoplastic LVs
  - Dilation of right cardiac chambers & pulmonary artery
  - Size & location of ductus arteriosus
  - Unrestricted atrial level shunt (patent foramen ovale vs. atrial septal defect) is critical for immediate postnatal care; may require emergent balloon atrial septostomy; saturations are dependent on degree of atrial level shunting
  - Abnormal ventricular wall motion (ischemic damage, EFE)
- CT can evaluate patency of aortopulmonary (Blalock-Taussig) & cavopulmonary (Glenn) shunts
- MR for functional assessment of univentricular heart to determine suitability for Fontan operation

CLINICAL ISSUES

- Mortality is high if not treated in neonatal period
- Prognosis improves substantially with surgical intervention

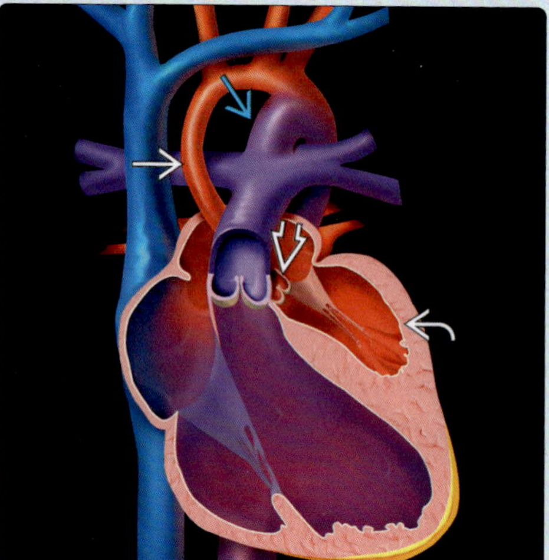

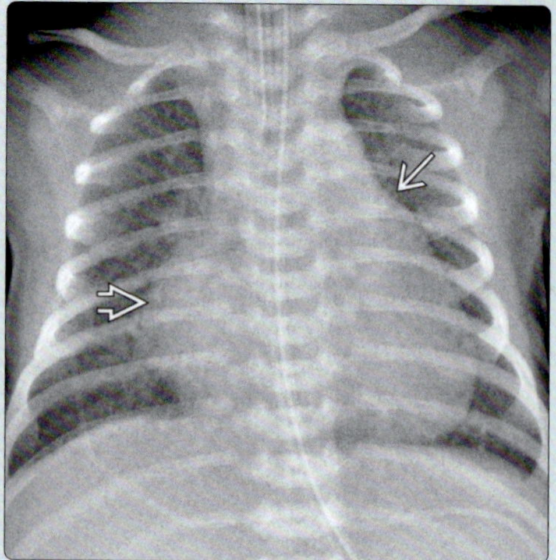

(Left) *Graphic shows hypoplasia of the left atrium (LA), mitral valve (MV), left ventricle (LV) ➡, aortic valve ➡, & ascending aorta ➡. Systemic blood flow depends on the patency of the ductus arteriosus ➡.* **(Right)** *AP radiograph in a 3-day-old shows the typically large main pulmonary artery (MPA) ➡ along the left border of the heart + an enlarged right atrium ➡ due to left-to-right shunting of blood across the atrial septal defect (ASD). Mild pulmonary edema & ↑ pulmonary blood flow characterize the vasculature.*

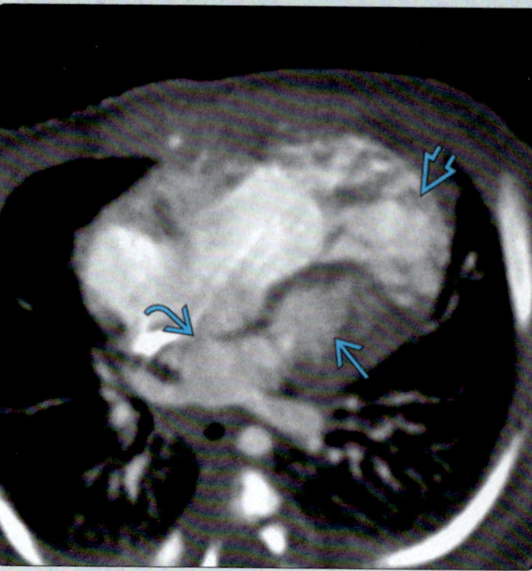

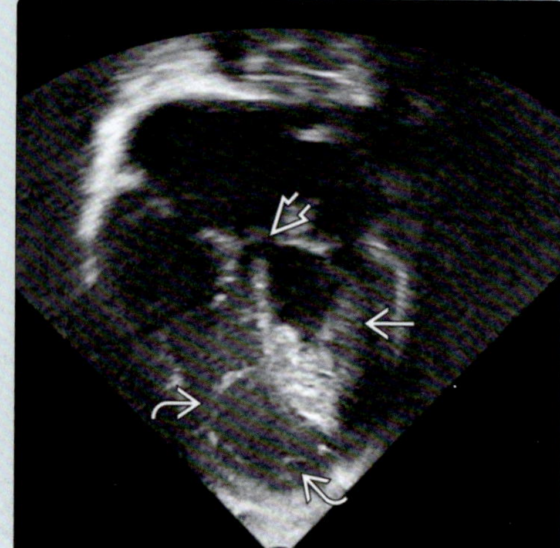

(Left) *Four-chamber cardiac CTA in an infant with hypoplastic left heart syndrome (HLHS) shows a markedly hypoplastic LV ➡. The right ventricle (RV) wraps ➡ around the smaller LV, giving the typical non-apex-forming LV seen with HLHS. Note the ASD ➡, which, if too small, may have to undergo septostomy to ↑ mixing of blood.* **(Right)** *Four-chamber echocardiogram shows a small, muscle-bound LV ➡ & small LV outflow tract (LVOT) ➡. The RV ➡ is large relative to the hypoplastic LV & wraps around the apex of the LV.*

TERMINOLOGY

Abbreviations

- Hypoplastic left heart syndrome (HLHS)

Synonyms

- 4 classic types: Mitral atresia/aortic atresia, mitral atresia/aortic stenosis, mitral stenosis/aortic atresia, mitral stenosis/aortic stenosis

Definitions

- Hypoplasia/atresia of ascending aorta, aortic valve, left ventricle (LV), & mitral valve (MV)
  - Secondary findings: Patent ductus arteriosus (PDA), juxtaductal coarctation
- Most severe congenital heart lesion
  - Presents in neonatal period with congestive heart failure, cardiogenic shock, & cyanosis
- Category: Cyanotic, cardiomegaly, ↑ pulmonary vascularity
- Hemodynamics
  - Severe obstruction of flow to systemic circulation (ductal dependent)
  - Retrograde flow in hypoplastic aortic arch & ascending aorta for cranial & coronary perfusion
  - Volume overload in pulmonary circulation
  - Obligate left-to-right shunt at atrial level via patent foramen ovale (PFO) or secundum atrial septal defect (ASD)
    - Restrictive atrial septum in neonate is highly lethal & requires emergent catheter-based balloon atrial septostomy
  - Flow admixture in right atrium → severe cyanosis

IMAGING

General Features

- Best diagnostic clue
  - Hypoplasia of ascending aorta, LV

Radiographic Findings

- Cardiomegaly, pulmonary venous congestion with interstitial fluid, hyperinflation, narrow mediastinum due to thymic atrophy

Echocardiographic Findings

- Echocardiogram
  - HLHS is often diagnosed prenatally
    - Retrograde flow in diminutive ascending aorta
    - LV growth arrest only manifests between 18-22 weeks of gestation
  - Postnatal diagnosis with echo is sufficient for treatment planning
    - Diminutive ascending aorta < 5 mm
    - Small, thick-walled LV
    - MV anulus Z score: Important parameter to decide whether biventricular repair is possible in marginally hypoplastic LVs
    - Dilation of right-sided cardiac chambers & main pulmonary artery (MPA)
    - Size & location of ductus arteriosus
    - Atrial level shunt: PFO or secundum ASD (often superior secundum defect); any degree of atrial level restriction can play significant role in decision making, pre- & post natal
    - Abnormal ventricular wall motion (ischemic damage); endocardial fibroelastosis of diminutive LV
    - Tricuspid valve regurgitation: Best marker of clinical outcomes
- Color Doppler
  - Diagnosis of HLHS subtype (mitral stenosis or atresia; aortic stenosis or atresia)
  - Left-to-right shunting through PFO/ASD: Mean diastolic gradient estimates degree of atrial-level restriction
  - Tricuspid valve regurgitation: Clinically important indicator

CT Findings

- CTA
  - Presurgical
    - Small left atrium with atretic/stenotic MV, hypoplastic LV with ascending & transverse aortic arch hypoplasia, single dilated right ventricle & MPA with large PDA continuation to descending aorta
    - Unusual anatomic variants or borderline LV volumes (mitral stenosis/aortic stenosis variants); severe single ventricle dysfunction
  - Postsurgical
    - Patency of aortopulmonary (Blalock-Taussig) & cavopulmonary (bidirectional Glenn) shunts
    - Seroma associated with Blalock-Taussig shunt
    - Airway compression (left bronchus) &/or left pulmonary artery (PA) compression by dilated neoaortic arch following Norwood repair
    - Residual stenosis of neoaortic arch, coarctation

MR Findings

- T2* GRE
  - SSFP cine MR for ventricular volume measurements in marginally hypoplastic left heart (to determine feasibility of biventricular repair)
  - Short-axis SSFP cine MR for functional assessment of univentricular heart (to determine suitability for Fontan operation)
- MRA
  - Velocity-encoded phase-contrast MRA for measurements of flow through aortic isthmus, PDA, & PFO
    - Can predict response to intraoperative test closure of ASD & PDA to determine feasibility of biventricular repair

Angiographic Findings

- Cardiac catheterization with angiography
  - Primarily interventional (as opposed to diagnostic): Obtained in case of atrial level restriction & need for early balloon atrial septostomy (BAS)
    - Delivery at pediatric care center where immediate BAS can be performed
    - Catheter & BAS can be performed via umbilical venous & arterial catheters
    - Retrograde flow in hypoplastic ascending aorta

– Catheter can be placed across ductus arteriosus to image PAs retrograde

Imaging Recommendations

- Protocol advice
  - Primary diagnosis made with pre- & postnatal transthoracic echocardiography in majority of cases
  - Postsurgical: Functional MR & interventional catheterizations for residua/sequelae of Fontan operation

DIFFERENTIAL DIAGNOSIS

Interrupted Aortic Arch

- Pressure overload of normally developed LV

Hepatic Congenital Hemangioma

- Structurally normal heart with volume overload of all chambers

Endocardial Fibroelastosis

- Globally enlarged, structurally normal heart with myocardial dysfunction

Anomalous Left Coronary Artery From Pulmonary Artery

- Left coronary originates from PA → myocardial infarction

Severe Arrhythmias: Paroxysmal Supraventricular Tachycardia

- Characteristic electrocardiogram

CLINICAL ISSUES

Presentation

- Most common signs/symptoms
  - No circulatory symptoms immediately at birth but rapid deterioration
    - Congestive heart failure (volume overload of pulmonary circulation)
    - Cardiogenic shock after closure of PDA
    - Cyanosis (flow admixture in right heart)
    - Hypoxia → pulmonary hypertension, persistent fetal circulation
- Other signs/symptoms
  - Poor systemic perfusion, metabolic acidosis
    - Acute tubular necrosis, renal failure
    - Necrotizing enterocolitis

Demographics

- Epidemiology
  - 1-3 per 10,000 live births, M:F = 2:1
  - 4th most common congenital heart lesion presenting under 1 year (7-9%)

Natural History & Prognosis

- Death within days/weeks when untreated
- Prognosis improves substantially with treatment
- Prognosis is determined by complications, residua, & sequelae of staged Norwood repair & Fontan operation (right ventricular dysfunction, venous hypertension)
- Significant tricuspid regurgitation after surgical palliation correlates with poor outcome

Treatment

- Medical: Prostaglandins initiated at birth/time of diagnosis to keep PDA open (provides right-to-left flow to descending aorta)
- Prenatal: US-guided balloon dilation of aortic valve in mid-/late fetal period is being studied
  - Change in fetal hemodynamics may enhance prenatal growth of left-sided cardiac structures
- Rashkind BAS (in case of flow restriction across PFO)
- Palliative repair: 3-stage approach
  - Norwood: Neoaorta creation from PA (with incorporation of native hypoplastic ascending aorta), atrial septectomy, & Blalock-Taussig shunt (Gore-Tex shunt from base of innominate artery to right PA) **or** Sano shunt (Gore-Tex shunt from RV to mid-PA) for controlled pulmonary blood flow (1-3 weeks of age)
  - Damus-Kaye-Stansel anastomosis: Essentially occurs with every Norwood as hypoplastic ascending aorta is filleted & incorporated into neoaorta/PA (classic description is side-to-side anastomosis between PA & aorta)
  - Conversion to hemi-Fontan: Glenn shunt between superior vena cava & right PA (4-6 months)
  - Bidirectional Glenn anastomosis: Offloads ventricle, not shunt dependent (more stable), prepares lungs for passive lung perfusion via cavopulmonary anastomosis
  - Fontan: Fenestrated venous conduit through right atrium for inferior cava flow to right PA (1.5-2 years)
- Marginally hypoplastic LV: Biventricular repair may be feasible
  - LV volume is commonly underestimated with echocardiography
  - Functional MR (SSFP cine): Ventricular volumes & mass determination are more reliable
- In some centers: Cardiac transplantation

SELECTED REFERENCES

1. Baş S et al: Ventriculocoronary fistulas with hypoplastic left heart in a neonate: imaging with cardiac CT. Case Rep Radiol. 2021:6657447, 2021
2. Bellsham-Revell H: Noninvasive imaging in interventional cardiology: hypoplastic left heart syndrome. Front Cardiovasc Med. 8:637838, 2021
3. Wang AP et al: Ventriculotomy decreases agreement between assessment of right ventricular function by echocardiography and cardiac magnetic resonance imaging in patients with hypoplastic left heart syndrome. Pediatr Cardiol. 42(4):951-9, 2021
4. Friedberg MK et al: Right ventricular failure in congenital heart disease. Curr Opin Pediatr. 31(5):604-10, 2019
5. Kovaćević-Kuśmierek K et al: Lung perfusion scintigraphy in the assessment of pulmonary circulation after completion of surgical treatment of a hypoplastic left heart syndrome (HLHS). Nucl Med Rev Cent East Eur. 22(2):81-4, 2019
6. Chen SA et al: Digital design and 3D printing of aortic arch reconstruction in HLHS for surgical simulation and training. World J Pediatr Congenit Heart Surg. 9(4):454-8, 2018
7. Salehi Ravesh M et al: Longitudinal deformation of the right ventricle in hypoplastic left heart syndrome: a comparative study of 2D-feature tracking magnetic resonance imaging and 2D-speckle tracking echocardiography. Pediatr Cardiol. 39(6):1265-75, 2018
8. Bellsham-Revell HR et al: Serial magnetic resonance imaging in hypoplastic left heart syndrome gives valuable insight into ventricular and vascular adaptation. J Am Coll Cardiol. 61(5):561-70, 2013
9. Fredenburg TB et al: The Fontan procedure: anatomy, complications, and manifestations of failure. Radiographics. 31(2):453-63, 2011
10. Valsangiacomo Buechel ER et al: Congenital cardiac defects and MR-guided planning of surgery. Magn Reson Imaging Clin N Am. 19(4):823-40; viii, 2011

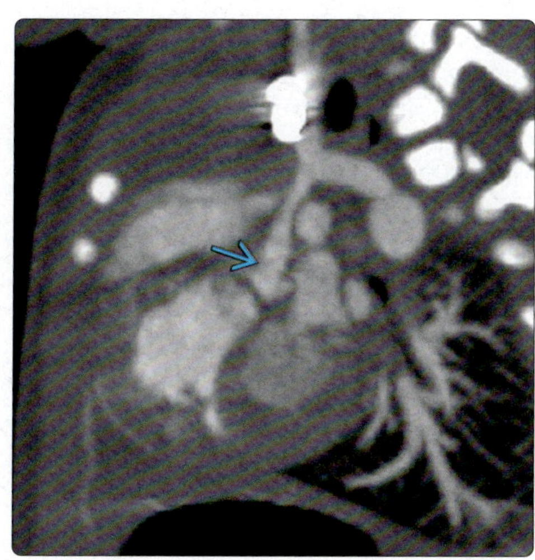

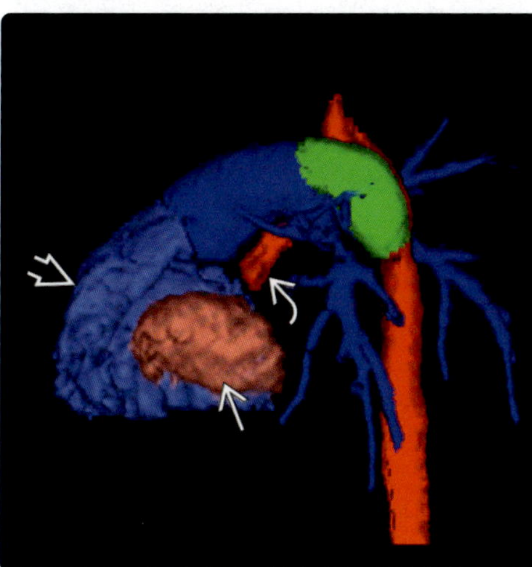

(Left) *Sagittal cardiac CTA in an infant with HLHS shows marked hypoplasia of the ascending aorta ➔ due to aortic atresia.* **(Right)** *Left lateral 3D surface-rendere cardiac CTA shows a markedly hypoplastic LV ➔ with hypoplasia of the ascending aorta ➔ due to aortic atresia. Note the enlarged RV ➔ & the large patent ductus arteriosus (PDA) (green) connecting the aorta (red) to the main PA (blue).*

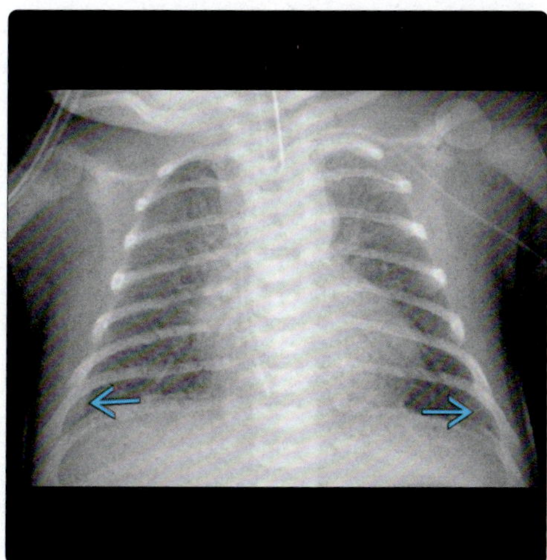

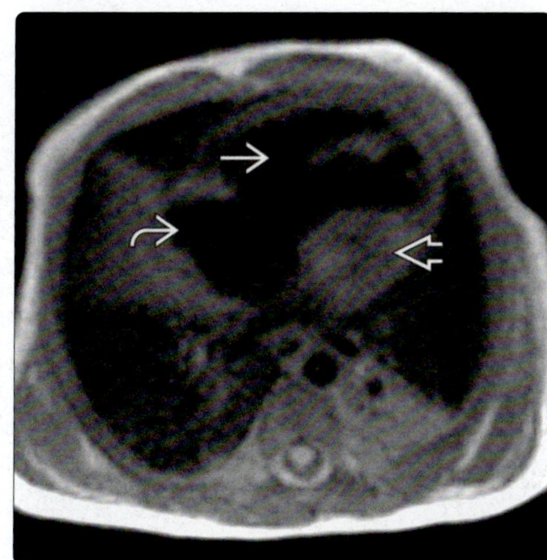

(Left) *Frontal radiograph of the chest in a patient with HLHS shows mild perihilar pulmonary edema with small, bilateral pleural effusions ➔. The findings are consistent with heart failure, which occurs when the PDA closes. Note that the tip of the PICC is abnormally deep in the right atrium.* **(Right)** *Axial T1 MR at the level of the ventricles in the same patient shows the large RV ➔ & the diminutive LV ➔. Note the large RA ➔.*

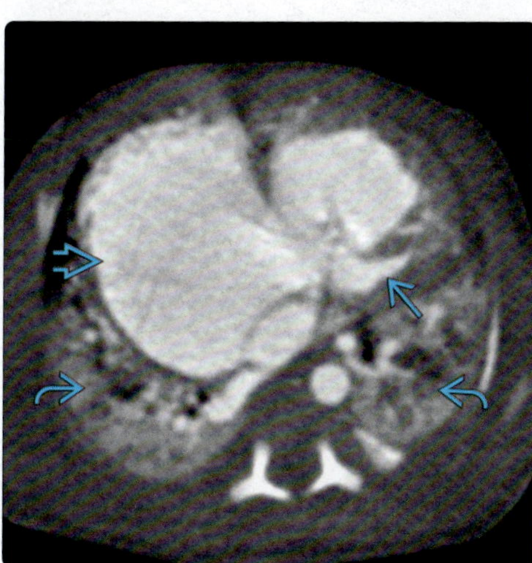

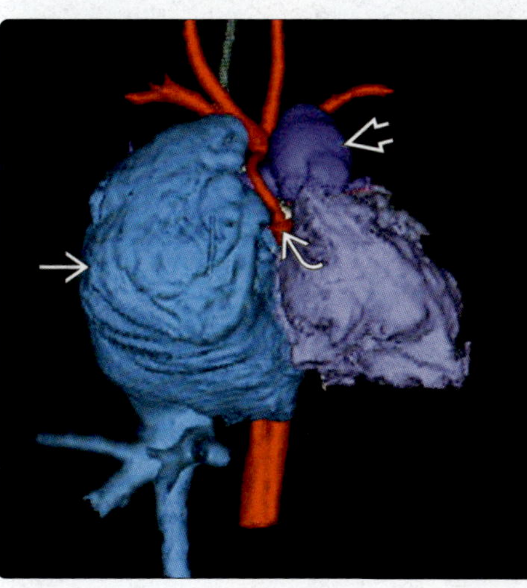

(Left) *Four-chamber cardiac CTA in an infant shows a markedly hypoplastic LV ➔ with marked enlargement of the RA ➔. Note the bilateral pulmonary edema ➔ as the PDA was closing.* **(Right)** *Anterior 3D surface-rendered cardiac CTA in an infant shows a markedly enlarged RA ➔ & hypoplastic ascending aorta ➔ in a patient with HLHS. Note the enlarged PA ➔, which is critical as this is a ductal-dependent type of congenital heart disease.*

Left Coronary Artery Anomalous Origin

KEY FACTS

TERMINOLOGY

- Anomalous origin of left coronary artery (LCA) from pulmonary artery: Most common congenital coronary artery anomaly presenting in children
- Causes cardiac ischemia & infarction, poor left ventricular (LV) systolic function, & significant mitral regurgitation

IMAGING

- Chest radiograph demonstrates cardiomegaly
- Echocardiogram (~ 90% diagnostic accuracy) demonstrates
  - Abnormal LCA ostium arising from pulmonary trunk
  - Retrograde flow in LCA toward pulmonary artery
  - Right coronary artery dilation & abundant intercoronary septal collaterals
  - Depressed LV systolic function & dilated LV chamber
  - Significant mitral regurgitation from ischemic papillary muscle dysfunction & mitral annular dilation
- CTA/MRA to identify coronary origins when echo is limited (~ 100% diagnostic accuracy)

CLINICAL ISSUES

- Rare congenital anomaly
  - Up to 90% mortality if not identified & surgically corrected
- Up to 90% present in infancy with nonspecific symptoms of irritability, failure to thrive, & wheezing (from mitral regurgitation)
  - ECG shows anterior lateral wall infarct pattern
- Older children are often asymptomatic until sudden event with syncope, dysrhythmia, & occasional sudden cardiac death
  - Surgical options include coronary reimplantation to aorta, bypass grafting with anomalous origin ligation, Takeuchi baffle
  - Simultaneous repair of mitral valve is controversial as severe regurgitation may improve with revascularization

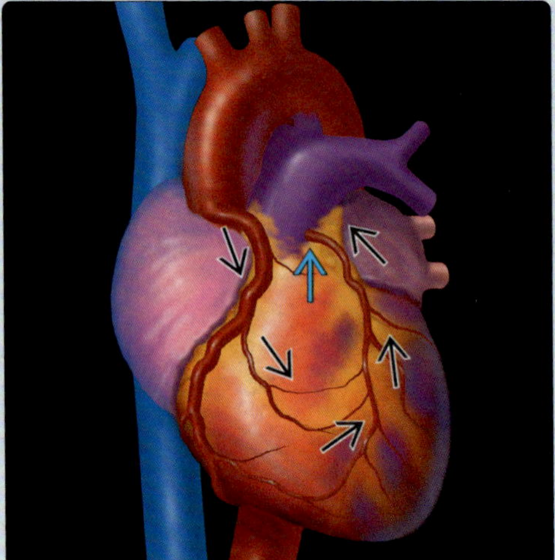

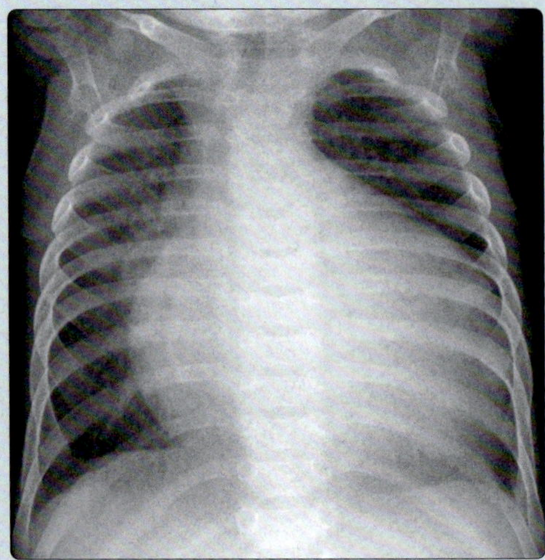

(Left) *Graphic shows an anomalous left coronary artery (LCA) origin ➙ from the main pulmonary artery (PA). Collateral flow from the normal right coronary artery (RCA) to the LCA allows retrograde flow through the LCA to the low-resistance PA (with flow direction denoted ➙). This flow bypasses the high-resistance myocardial bed of the left ventricle (LV).* **(Right)** *AP radiograph from an 8-month-old with wheezing shows a markedly enlarged cardiac silhouette. Echocardiography showed the LCA arising from the PA.*

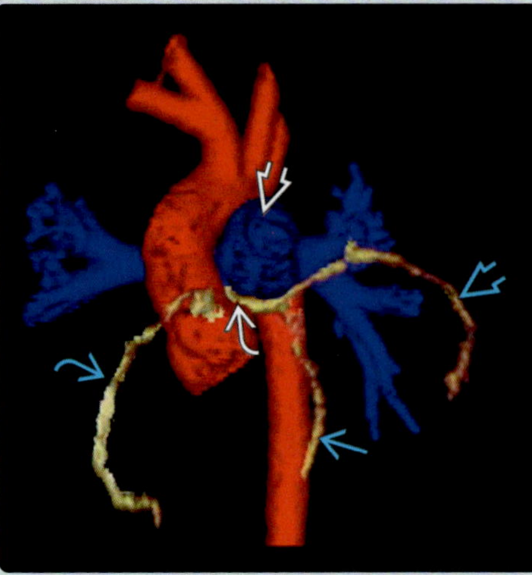

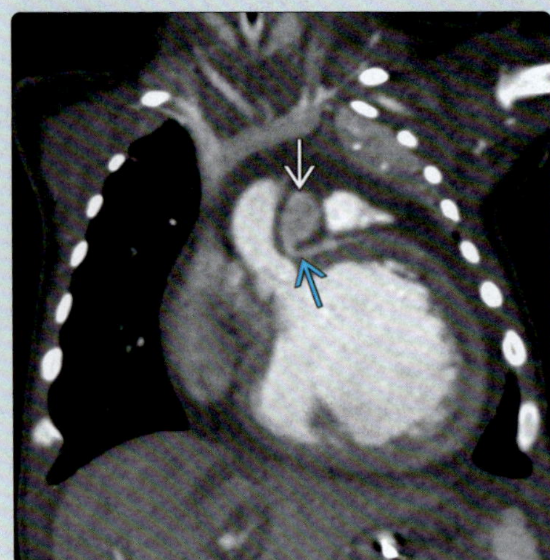

(Left) *Frontal view surface-rendered cardiac CTA shows the LCA ➙ arising from the right aspect of the main PA ➙ before bifurcating into the left anterior descending (LAD) ➙ & left circumflex (LCX) ➙. Note the normal origin of the RCA ➙ from the right coronary sinus of the ascending aorta.* **(Right)** *Coronal CTA demonstrates an anomalous LCA ➙ originating from the right inferior aspect of the main PA ➙, consistent with ALCAPA. The LV is markedly dilated due to ischemia from coronary steal.*

TERMINOLOGY

Synonyms

- Anomalous origin of left coronary artery from pulmonary artery (ALCAPA) = Bland-White-Garland (BWG) syndrome

Definitions

- ALCAPA: Most common congenital coronary artery anomaly presenting in children
  - Causes cardiac ischemia & infarction, depressed left ventricular (LV) systolic function, & significant mitral valve regurgitation

IMAGING

General Features

- Best diagnostic clue
  - Chest radiograph: Cardiomegaly in infant
  - Electrocardiogram (ECG): Deep Q waves in leads I & aVL, consistent with anterior lateral wall infarct
  - Echocardiogram: Abnormal left coronary artery (LCA) ostium arising from pulmonary trunk, retrograde LCA flow, right coronary artery (RCA) dilation, abundant intercoronary septal collaterals, significant mitral regurgitation, & depressed LV systolic function
    - ~ 90% diagnostic accuracy
  - CTA/MRA: Anomalous origin of LCA ostium; large tortuous coronary vessels with dilated RCA & significant collaterals
    - ~ 100% diagnostic accuracy

Radiographic Findings

- Radiography
  - Cardiomegaly, left atrial & LV enlargement, ↑ pulmonary vascularity or pulmonary edema (from depressed LV function & mitral regurgitation)

CT Findings

- Multidetector CTA demonstrates coronary artery anatomy & LV enlargement
  - Volume or surface 3D rendering from contrast-enhanced imaging assists with visualization

MR Findings

- T2WI
  - Myocardial edema in LV
- MRA
  - Anomalous LCA from pulmonary trunk, dilated RCA, significant intercoronary septal collaterals
- MR cine
  - Ventricular function is quantified by summation of short-axis stack
  - Wall motion abnormalities are assessed on 4-chamber & short-axis stacks, particularly LCA distribution
  - Ventricular chamber size is quantified by end-diastolic volume
- Double IR FSE
  - Thin-slice (4 mm) demonstrates excellent vessel anatomy: ALCAPA & dilated RCA
- Delayed enhancement
  - Myocardial late gadolinium enhancement (LGE) in LCA distribution is consistent with infarcted or fibrotic segments: Focal with transmural or near-transmural LGE

Echocardiographic Findings

- Abnormal origin of coronary artery recognized by retrograde flow from LCA into pulmonary artery, dilated RCA, & multiple collateral vessels
- Echocardiography demonstrates ↓ LV systolic function, segmental wall abnormalities in LCA distribution (typically representing anterolateral infarct), & significant mitral regurgitation

Angiographic Findings

- Invasive coronary angiography by cardiac catheterization: 100% diagnostic accuracy
  - Performed only when echo & cross-sectional imaging are not diagnostic
  - Pulmonary arteriogram demonstrates anomalous origin of LCA
  - Selective injection of RCA demonstrates dilated vessel & tortuous collateral vessels

Imaging Recommendations

- Best imaging tool
  - ECG in infancy: Infarct pattern with abnormal deep Q waves (particularly in leads I & aVL), ST segment depression, & T-wave inversion
  - Chest radiograph: Cardiomegaly
  - Echocardiogram: ↓ LV systolic function, anomalous origin of coronary artery, collateral vessels, significant mitral regurgitation
  - CTA/MRA when echocardiogram is not definitive
- Protocol advice
  - CTA performance is best with ECG-synchronized gating (prospective), suspended respiration (if possible), high contrast injection rate (4-5 mL/s), & contrast bolus timed or tracked to fill entire PA & aorta

DIFFERENTIAL DIAGNOSIS

Dilated Cardiomyopathy

- Most common cause of depressed LV function in infancy
  - Genetic/metabolic vs. viral origin
- Similar clinical presentation with irritability, failure to thrive, wheezing

Kawasaki Disease

- Vasculitis of medium-sized vessels leading to coronary artery ectasia or aneurysms; etiology unknown
- Myocarditis is common; aneurysms occur in < 2%
- May develop stenosis associated with aneurysm → clot → infarction

Coronary Artery Fistula

- May produce cardiac ischemia if coronary steal leads to reduced blood flow to coronary circulation

Single Coronary Artery Origin

- 40% are associated with other anomalies, including tetralogy of Fallot, transposition of great arteries, etc.
- Usually asymptomatic but occasional sudden cardiac death

PATHOLOGY

General Features

- Associated abnormalities

- Coronary artery anomalies can be isolated or associated with other defects; important to identify for surgical planning
  - Tetralogy of Fallot: Coronary anomalies include small conal branch (88%), large conal branch (6%), left anterior descending (LAD) from RCA (3%), dual LAD (2%), single RCA (0.3%), & single LCA (0.2%)
  - Transposition of great arteries: Coronary anomalies from aortic valve malposition include left circumflex from RCA (14%), single RCA (9%), LAD from RCA (6%), interarterial course of LCA or RCA (4%)
- Embryology
  - Abnormalities in signaling pathways or alterations in local factors that direct coronary development

Microscopic Features

- Signs of LV ischemia & varying degrees of reparative changes are evident on autopsy or transplant
  - Anterolateral papillary muscle is atrophic & scarred
  - Thinning & scarring of anterolateral LV wall & apex due to infarction

CLINICAL ISSUES

Presentation

- Most common signs/symptoms
  - ~ 90% present in infancy with nonspecific symptoms of irritability, fussiness, wheezing, &/or failure to thrive
- Other signs/symptoms
  - Diaphoresis or ↓ oxygenation & perfusion (severe cyanosis or grayish appearance)
- Older child or adolescent
  - Usually asymptomatic until sudden catastrophic event occurs with syncope, dysrhythmic event, occasional death
    - May occur with exercise (suggesting coronary artery or other heart disease)

Natural History & Prognosis

- Fetal life: Lungs are collapsed; normal myocardial perfusion
- Stage 1: Newborn with high pulmonary vascular resistance (PVR)
  - Preferential flow into anomalous LCA (antegrade) from pulmonary artery → normal myocardial perfusion without symptoms or ischemia
- Stage 2: PVR ↓ ~ 2-4 months of life
  - ↓ PA diastolic pressure is inadequate to provide forward flow to anomalous LCA to keep LV myocardium perfused
  - Collateral vessels develop from RCA → RCA dilation
  - Flow from RCA & collaterals meets high resistance of LV myocardial bed → preferential retrograde LCA flow into low-resistance PA
    - Retrograde flow of fully oxygenated blood into PA creates left-to-right shunt
- Later stages: Cardiac ischemia & infarct
  - Myocardial steal occurs with ↑ in collateral vessels
  - Ischemia & infarct develop in anterolateral distribution → global ventricular dilation & dysfunction + significant mitral regurgitation (secondary to papillary muscle infarction)

Treatment

- Medical therapy to stabilize patient initially
  - Mechanical ventilation with oxygen to prevent hypoxia & treat cardiogenic shock
  - Sedation to ↓ myocardial oxygen demand
    - Cardiac anesthesia team is involved due to ↑ potential for cardiac arrest or arrhythmia
- Surgical therapy: Up to 90% mortality if left unrepaired; prognosis is related to degree of preoperative LV systolic dysfunction
  - LV assist device may be utilized preoperatively
  - Surgical techniques include
    - Direct transfer of LCA to aortic root: Button of tissue around LCA ostium is transferred posteriorly to aorta
    - Bypass grafting: Proximal anomalous LCA is ligated + bypass graft to reestablish normal flow direction & tissue perfusion
    - Takeuchi repair: Intrapulmonary baffle from aorta to anomalous LCA origin
    - Simultaneous repair of mitral valve is controversial as severe regurgitation may improve with revascularization
  - Surgical mortality ~ 5-10%, usually related to poor LV function
    - Complications include bleeding, cardiac arrest, heart failure, & stroke
    - Heart transplant is warranted in cases where LV function does not improve after coronary artery surgical intervention

DIAGNOSTIC CHECKLIST

Consider

- ALCAPA in infant with abnormal ECG & unknown cause of LV systolic dysfunction
  - Readily diagnosed by imaging

SELECTED REFERENCES

1. Cavalcanti LRP et al: Anomalous origin of the left coronary artery from the pulmonary artery (ALCAPA) in adults: collateral circulation does not preclude direct reimplantation. J Card Surg. 36(2):731-4, 2021
2. De Rose C et al: Lung ultrasound in congenital cardiac abnormality: ALCAPA. Indian J Pediatr. 88(2):161-4, 2021
3. Tomoaia R et al: The role of multimodal imaging in the diagnosis of an asymptomatic patient with congenital anomaly. Med Ultrason. 23(2):231-4, 2021
4. Wen LY et al: Multimodal cardiac magnetic resonance imaging of ALCAPA syndrome. Eur Heart J. 42(7):798, 2021
5. Jinmei Z et al: Anomalous origin of the left coronary artery from the pulmonary artery (ALCAPA) diagnosed in children and adolescents. J Cardiothorac Surg. 15(1):90, 2020
6. Sadoma D et al: Anomalous left coronary artery from the pulmonary artery (ALCAPA) as a cause of heart failure. Am J Case Rep. 20:1797-800, 2019
7. Chatterjee A et al: Multimodality imaging of rare adult presentation of ALCAPA treated with Takeuchi repair. JACC Cardiovasc Interv. 11(1):98-9, 2018
8. Agarwal PP et al: Anomalous coronary arteries that need intervention: review of pre- and postoperative imaging appearances. Radiographics. 37(3):740-57, 2017
9. Heermann P et al: Coronary artery anomalies: diagnosis and classification based on cardiac CT and MRI (CMR) - from ALCAPA to anomalies of termination. Rofo. 189(1):29-38, 2017

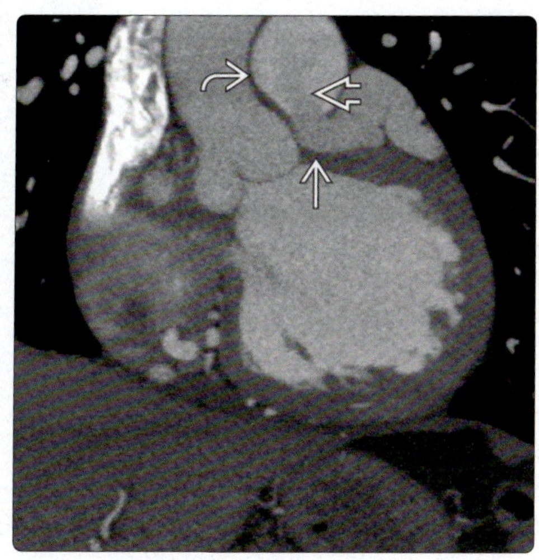

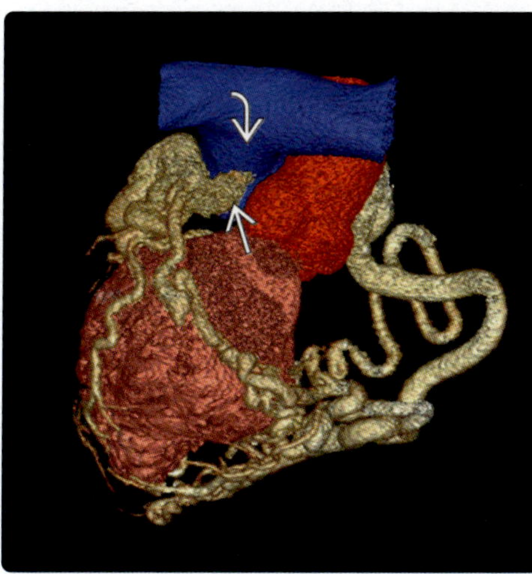

(Left) *Coronal oblique cardiac CTA in an older patient with longstanding ALCAPA shows the LCA arising from the undersurface of the main PA. Note the blush of unopacified blood extending into the main PA due to the retrograde flow in the LCA toward the PA.* **(Right)** *Posterior 3D surface-rendered cardiac CTA in an older patient with longstanding ALCAPA shows the LCA arising from the undersurface of the main PA. Note the enlarged, tortuous coronaries from chronic coronary steal.*

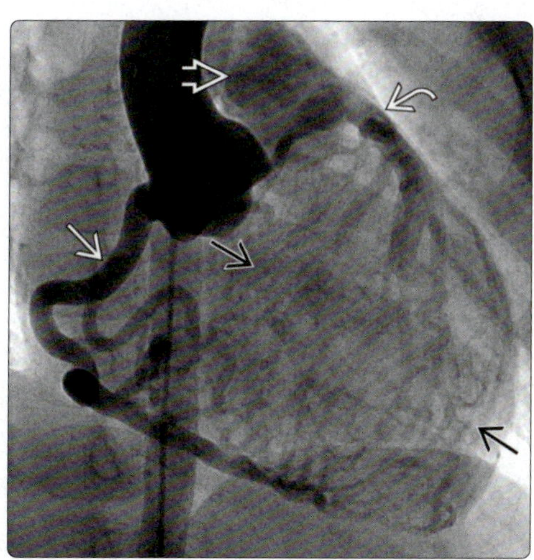

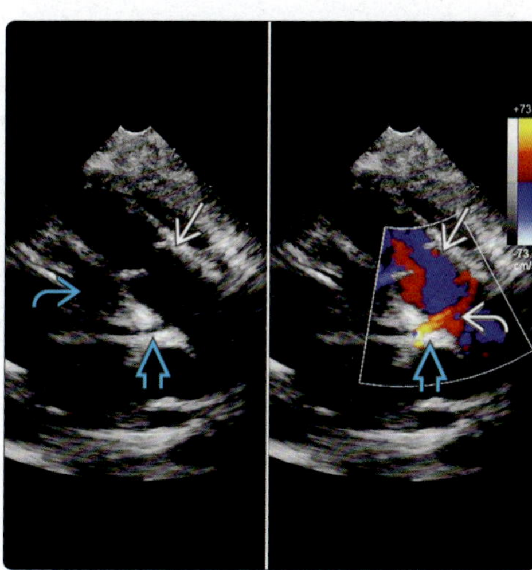

(Left) *Anterior oblique conventional angiogram shows antegrade flow through a large RCA during an injection of the ascending aorta. Retrograde flow in the LCA (which is filled by multiple collateral vessels) opacifies the PA.* **(Right)** *Echocardiogram demonstrates an ALCAPA with retrograde blood flow into the PA. While the LCA appears to arise from the aorta on grayscale imaging, the color Doppler ultrasound shows flow reversal of the LCA into the PA (demonstrated by a red jet toward the transducer).*

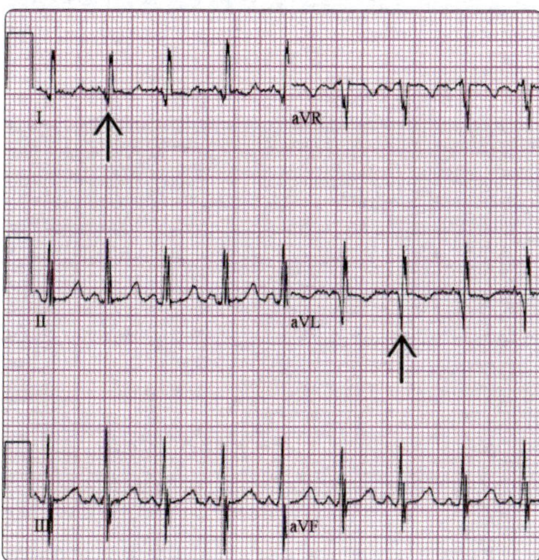

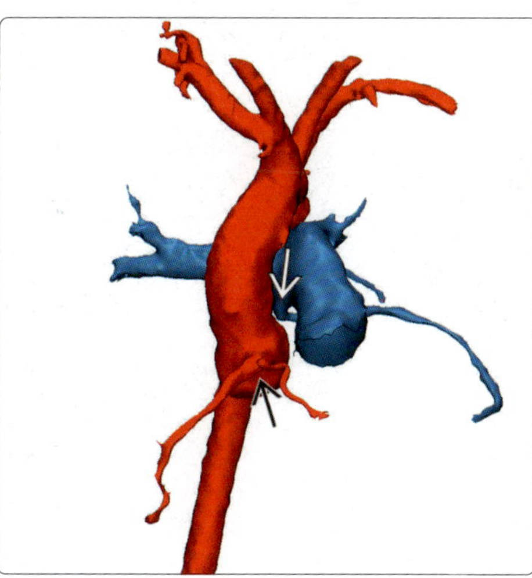

(Left) *ECG of a neonate shows pathologic deep Q waves in leads I & aVL, consistent with a diagnosis of ALCAPA & myocardial ischemia.* **(Right)** *Anterior oblique 3D-rendered CTA performed for 3D printing demonstrates a normal origin of the RCA (with acute marginal branch) from the aorta (red). An ALCAPA arises from the underside of the pulmonary trunk (blue).*

Double-Outlet Right Ventricle

KEY FACTS

TERMINOLOGY

- Double-outlet right ventricle (DORV): Form of abnormal ventriculoarterial connection in which both great arteries arise completely or predominately from morphologic right ventricle (RV)
  - 16 variants based on relationship of great arteries & position/location of ventricular septal defect (VSD)
- May be part of complex congenital heart disease coexisting with ventricular anomalies, valve stenosis or atresia, abnormal atrioventricular valve, aortic valve anomalies, coarctation, coronary anomalies, & anomalies of systemic or pulmonary venous return

IMAGING

- Opacification of both great arteries during RV injection
- Pulmonary flow is dependent on site of VSD & degree of outflow or pulmonary valve stenosis
- Side-by-side relationship of aorta & pulmonary artery with aorta on right in 50-64%
- 3D imaging can help with complex intracardiac relationships for presurgical planning

CLINICAL ISSUES

- May be diagnosed in utero; usually has clinical symptoms at birth or in 1st month
  - DORV with pulmonic stenosis: Cyanosis, failure to thrive, tachypnea
  - DORV with subaortic VSD without pulmonic stenosis: Symptoms of large left-to-right shunt & early evidence of pulmonary hypertension
- Surgery depends on anatomy
  - Closure of VSD & placement of RV to pulmonary artery conduit if 2 developed ventricles exist
  - Norwood/Fontan procedure if hypoplasia of ventricle
- 15-year survival rate for noncomplex lesions: 85-90%
  - Mortality rate is higher after operation for complex lesions

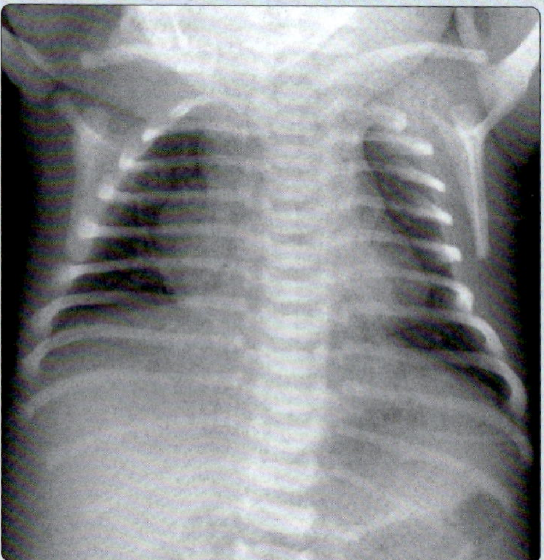

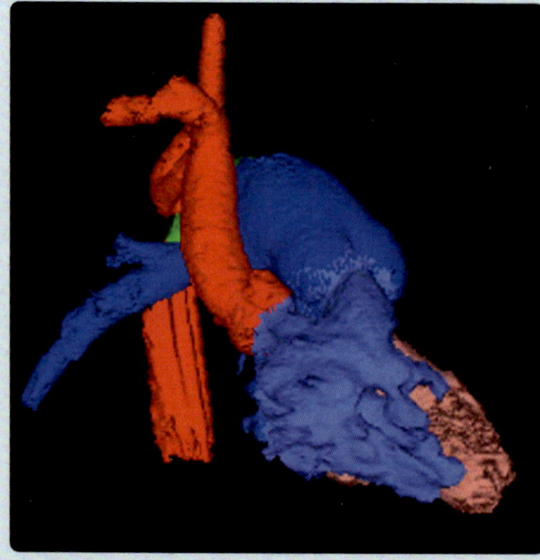

(Left) *AP chest radiograph in a patient with double-outlet right ventricle (DORV) shows ↓ pulmonary vascularity & mild cardiomegaly. Pulmonic stenosis in this patient makes the radiographic appearance similar to that of a patient with tetralogy of Fallot.* **(Right)** *Frontal 3D cardiac CTA shows both the aorta (red) & pulmonary artery (PA, blue) arising from the right ventricle (RV, purple) in a patient with DORV. Note the ↑ size of the PA (blue), reflecting ↑ left-to-right shunting.*

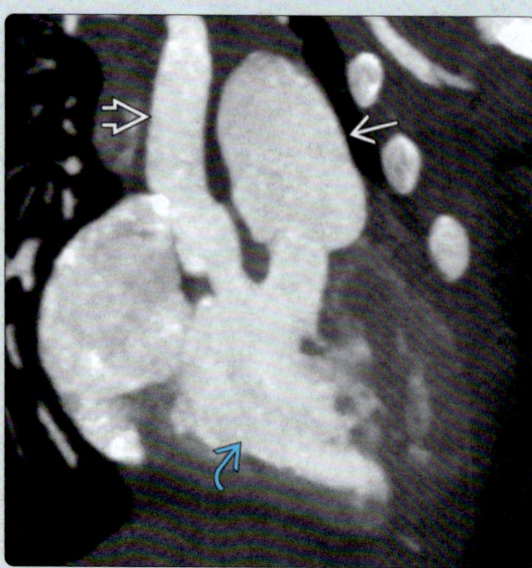

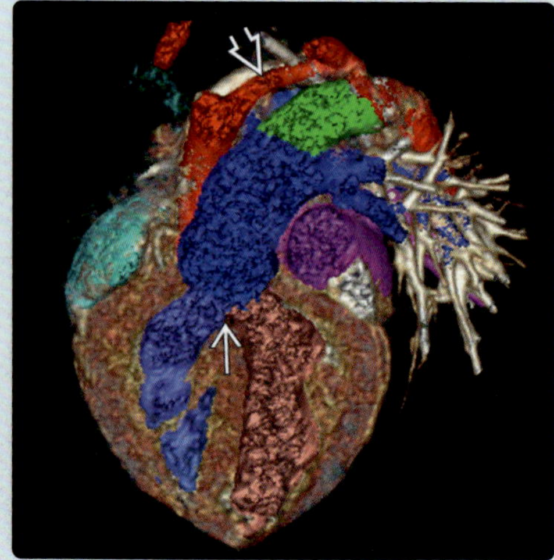

(Left) *Coronal MIP cardiac CTA in a newborn with DORV shows both the PA ➡ & aorta ➡ arising from the RV ↗. Note the enlarged PA, reflecting left-to-right shunting.* **(Right)** *Four-chamber sectioned volume-rendered cardiac CTA in an infant with DORV shows the subpulmonic position of the ventricular septal defect ➡ between the RV (light blue) & the left ventricle (salmon). Also note the patent ductus arteriosus (green) & hypoplastic aortic arch ➡.*

TERMINOLOGY

Abbreviations

- Double-outlet right ventricle (DORV)

Definitions

- Form of abnormal ventriculoarterial connection in which both great arteries arise completely or predominately from morphologic right ventricle (RV)
- 16 variants based on relationship of great arteries & position/location of ventricular septal defect (VSD)

IMAGING

General Features

- Best diagnostic clue
  - Radiologic appearance, regardless of modality, depends on physiology of lesion, which reflects variable anatomy of DORV
    - Pulmonary flow is dependent on site of VSD & degree of outflow or pulmonary valve stenosis
      - Most common VSD type is subaortic with normally related great vessels
- Morphology
  - Hallmarks of anatomy: Both great arteries originate from morphologic RV
  - Possible relationships of great vessels
    - Side-by-side relationship of aorta & pulmonary artery with aorta on right in 50-64%
  - Possible positions of VSD
    - Subaortic VSD is located anatomically closer to aortic valve than to pulmonary valve
    - Subpulmonary type of DORV: VSD is located closer to pulmonary valve; when supracristal in location, it is called Taussig-Bing anomaly
    - Doubly committed VSD is subaortic, subpulmonary type: Usually large & related to both semilunar valves
    - Remote type or noncommitted VSD is distant from both semilunar valves & may be of atrioventricular canal type or muscular VSD

Radiographic Findings

- Chest radiographs cannot reliably differentiate DORV from other forms of congenital heart disease
- DORV with subaortic VSD + severe pulmonic stenosis + normally related great vessels
  - ↓ pulmonary flow
  - Similar appearance to tetralogy of Fallot (TOF)
- DORV without pulmonic stenosis but with normally related great vessels
  - ↑ pulmonary flow
  - Appears similar to large VSD

CTA or MRA

- Shows relationships of great vessels, position of VSD, relative size of ventricles, & associated anomalies
  - Altered ventricular-great vessel relationship
  - Aortic valve & pulmonic valve may be at same level
- 3D imaging can help with complex intracardiac relationships for presurgical planning
- Postoperative assessment in older patients is useful for anatomy & functional assessment

Angiographic Findings

- Opacification of both great arteries during RV injection
- Filling defect dividing 2 outflow tracts or double conus

DIFFERENTIAL DIAGNOSIS

Ventricular Septal Defect

- Clinically presents with tachypnea, feeding problems, & failure to thrive
- DORV without pulmonic stenosis radiographically simulates large left-to-right shunt
- Distinguishing feature for VSD is normal fibrous continuity between posterior leaflet of aortic valve & anterior leaflet of mitral valve

Tetralogy of Fallot

- With severe outflow tract obstruction & VSD, aorta overrides ventricular septum & simulates DORV with pulmonic stenosis
- Physiology may be similar to DORV, but TOF has aortic-mitral continuity despite anterior position of aorta & overriding of RV

D-Transposition of Great Arteries

- Shows atrioventricular concordance & ventriculoarterial discordance (i.e., aorta arises from RV & pulmonary artery arises from left ventricle)

CLINICAL ISSUES

Presentation

- Most common signs/symptoms
  - May be diagnosed in utero; patients usually have clinical symptoms at birth or in 1st month
    - DORV with pulmonic stenosis: Cyanosis, failure to thrive, tachypnea
    - DORV with subaortic VSD without pulmonic stenosis: Symptoms of large left-to-right shunt & early evidence of pulmonary hypertension

Demographics

- DORV accounts for 1.0-1.5% of all congenital heart disease with incidence of 1 per 10,000 live births

Treatment

- Surgery depends on anatomy
  - Closure of VSD & placement of RV to pulmonary artery conduit if 2 developed ventricles exist
  - Norwood/Fontan procedure if hypoplasia of ventricle
- Survival statistics depend on specific type of DORV
  - 15-year survival rate for noncomplex lesions: 85-90%
  - Reoperation may be required for RV outflow obstruction

SELECTED REFERENCES

1. Kumar P et al: Role of computed tomography in pre- and postoperative evaluation of a double-outlet right ventricle. J Cardiovasc Imaging. 29(3):205-27, 2021
2. Young AA et al: Fetal double outlet right ventricle without heterotaxy syndrome: diagnostic spectrum, associated extracardiac pathology and clinical outcomes. Prenat Diagn. 41(9):1118-26, 2021
3. Meng H et al: Biventricular repair of double outlet right ventricle: preoperative echocardiography and surgical outcomes. World J Pediatr Congenit Heart Surg. 8(3):354-60, 2017

Aortic Coarctation

KEY FACTS

TERMINOLOGY

- Narrowing of aortic lumen with obstruction to blood flow

IMAGING

- Locations: Preductal, typically hypoplastic (infantile); juxtaductal or post ductal, typically focal (adult); abdominal, middle aortic syndrome (rare)
  - May have diffuse hypoplasia of aortic isthmus + focal coarctation (important for surgical planning)
- Can be simple (isolated coarctation in adult) or complex (additional cardiac anomalies, presenting in infancy)
- Classic radiographic findings
  - Poststenotic dilation of proximal descending aorta (figure 3 sign)
  - Rib notching (age > 5 years)
  - Left ventricular hypertrophy: Rounded cardiac apex
- Echocardiography for primary diagnosis in infancy
- CTA depicts coarctation site, percentage of stenosis, & presence/location of collaterals
- MR in older children for preoperative work-up & postoperative surveillance

PATHOLOGY

- Most common additional cardiac anomalies: Ventricular septal defect (33%), PDA (66%), bicuspid aortic valve (50%)
- Turner syndrome: 20-36% have coarctation

CLINICAL ISSUES

- Presentations include
  - Infancy: Congestive heart failure (due to aortic arch interruption, associated anomalies)
  - Older child, adult: Hypertension (HTN), diminished femoral pulses, differential blood pressure between upper & lower extremities (arm-leg gradient)
- Treatment: Resection + end-to-end anastomosis, interposition graft, patch + aortoplasty, balloon angioplasty
- Complications: Recoarctation (< 3%; ↑ if operation in infancy), postoperative aneurysms (24% after patch)
- ↓ long-term survival (HTN, coronary disease)

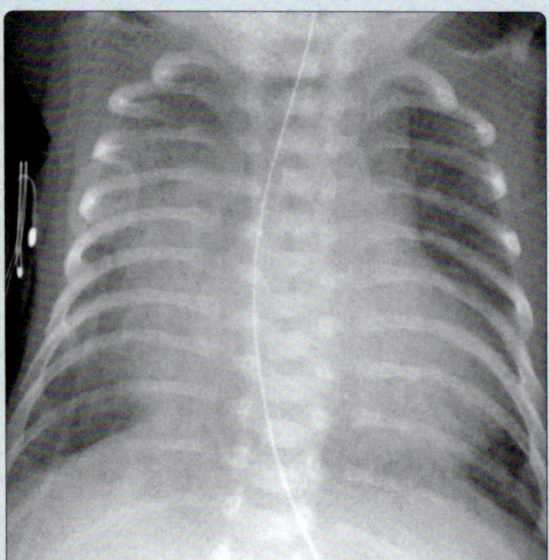

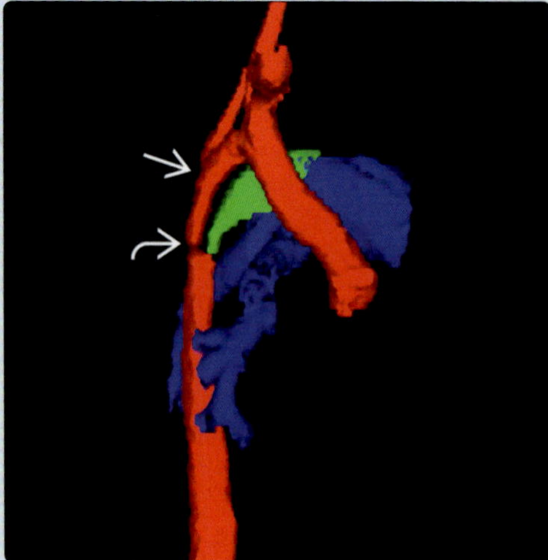

(Left) *Frontal radiograph in a 2-week-old infant with congestive heart failure & severe coarctation of the aorta shows cardiomegaly with bilateral pulmonary edema.* **(Right)** *Lateral oblique view of a 3D color-coded cardiac CTA shows a preductal hypoplastic-type coarctation ➡ of the aorta with a periductal focal coarctation ➦. Note that the patent ductus arteriosus (PDA) (green) is beginning to close with severe narrowing near the aortic connection.*

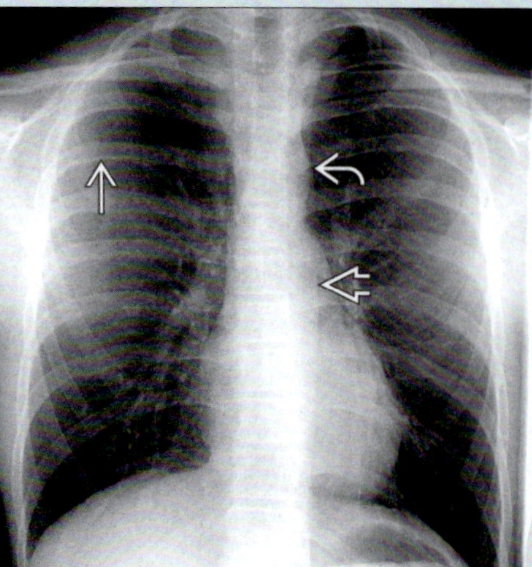

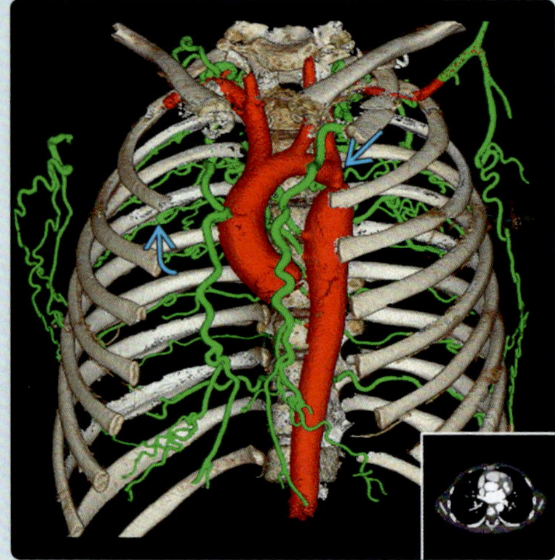

(Left) *Frontal radiograph in a teenage patient with coarctation of the aorta shows prominence of the aortic knob ➦ & descending aorta ➡ with intervening indentation, creating a figure 3 sign. Note the notching, sclerosis, & undulation of the undersurface of the ribs ➡ from collateral vessels.* **(Right)** *Frontal oblique view from a 3D color-coded CTA shows a focal coarctation ➡ of the aorta with prominent arterial collaterals (green) circumventing the obstruction. Note the dilated intercostal collaterals ➦.*

TERMINOLOGY

Definitions

- Narrowing of aortic lumen with obstruction to blood flow
- Category of congenital heart disease: Acyanotic, normal heart size (most commonly), normal pulmonary vascularity
- Hemodynamics: Left ventricular (LV) pressure overload

IMAGING

General Features

- Best diagnostic clue
  - Focal or diffuse aortic narrowing with presence of collaterals in older patients
- Location
  - Preductal: Typically hypoplastic (infantile)
  - Juxtaductal or post ductal: Typically focal (adult)
  - Abdominal: Middle aortic syndrome (rare)
    - Should be specifically looked for in patients with differential blood pressures + normal thoracic aorta
- Morphology
  - Simple (isolated coarctation in adults) or complex (associated with other cardiac anomalies, presenting in infancy)

Radiographic Findings

- Poststenotic dilation of proximal descending aorta (figure 3 sign)
- Rib notching (age > 5 years) or undulation & sclerosis of undersurface of ribs due to collaterals (Roesler sign)
  - If rib notching is unilateral & right-sided, then coarctation is likely distal to brachiocephalic artery but proximal to left subclavian artery
  - If rib notching is bilateral, then coarctation is distal to both subclavian arteries
  - If rib notching is unilateral & left-sided, then there is likely aberrant left subclavian artery
- LV hypertrophy: Rounded cardiac apex

Fluoroscopic Findings

- Esophagram: Impression by dilated descending aorta (reverse figure 3 sign)

CT Findings

- CTA
  - Cardiac CTA with prospective ECG gating is increasingly used in diagnosis
    - Advantages
      - Speed of exam
      - Highest resolution of all cross-sectional imaging modalities, provides best 3D reconstructions
      - Functional data can be obtained to evaluate ejection fraction & volumes
    - Disadvantages: Radiation dose
  - Depicts coarctation site, percentage of stenosis, & presence/location of collaterals

MR Findings

- T1WI
  - Black blood imaging (cardiac gated spin-echo or double inversion recovery)
    - Sagittal oblique ("candy cane") plane through aortic arch shows location of coarctation
    - Perpendicular views for cross-sectional diameter measurements
- T2* GRE
  - Bright blood imaging (cardiac gated steady-state free precession cine MR)
    - More reliable for diameters than black blood imaging
    - Sagittal oblique plane for anatomy
    - Length of systolic (dark) flow jet correlates with hemodynamic significance
    - ± aortic regurgitation (bicuspid aortic valve)
- MRA
  - Velocity-encoded phase-contrast MRA: For estimate of gradient, collateral flow, & aortic valve regurgitation fraction
  - 3D gadolinium-enhanced MRA: For anatomy & depiction of collaterals
- Multiple MR techniques are now available to calculate pressure gradients

Ultrasonographic Findings

- Pulsed Doppler
  - Aortic & visceral arterial waveforms distal to coarctation may show parvus et tardus morphology
    - Slowly rising & diminished systolic upstroke

Echocardiographic Findings

- Echocardiogram
  - Imaging of aortic arch & branches in suprasternal long-axis view
  - Relationship of coarctation with patent ductus arteriosus (PDA)
  - Notch in descending aorta at level of coarctation (shelf sign)
- Pulsed Doppler
  - Estimate of gradient across coarctation

Angiographic Findings

- Cardiac catheterization: Direct measurement of gradient
- Intervention: Balloon angioplasty

Imaging Recommendations

- Protocol advice
  - Echocardiography for primary diagnosis in infancy
  - Cardiac CTA with prospective ECG gating in infancy for complex anatomy
  - MR in older children for preoperative work-up & postoperative surveillance for recoarctation & aneurysms
  - Cardiac catheterization is reserved for gradient measurement & intervention

DIFFERENTIAL DIAGNOSIS

Hypoplastic Left Heart Syndrome

- Congestive heart failure in newborn
- Hypoplastic LV
- Ductus-dependent systemic perfusion
- Retrograde flow in hypoplastic ascending aorta

Interrupted Aortic Arch

- Flow reaches descending aorta via PDA

Pseudocoarctation

- Elongation & kinking of aorta without obstruction/gradient

Takayasu Arteritis

- Acquired inflammatory condition
- Acute phase: Aortic wall enhancement
- Chronic phase: Narrowing/occlusion of aorta & branch vessels

PATHOLOGY

General Features

- Etiology
  - 2 developmental theories
    - Abnormal fetal hemodynamics [when associated with cardiac lesions ↓ LV output & flow through aortic isthmus, such as hypoplastic left heart syndrome (HLHS) or large ventricular septal defect (VSD)] can lead to preductal coarctation & diffuse hypoplasia of isthmus
    - Postnatal contraction of fibrous ductal tissue in aortic wall at time of PDA closure
- Genetics
  - Usually sporadic
- Associated abnormalities
  - Cardiac: VSD (33%), PDA (66%), bicuspid aortic valve (50%), transposition, subaortic & mitral stenosis (parachute deformity: Shone syndrome), Taussig-Bing anomaly, endocardial fibroelastosis
  - Associated with Turner syndrome (20-36% have coarctation)
  - Berry aneurysms of circle of Willis
  - Scoliosis (in boys)
  - Abdominal coarctation is associated with neurofibromatosis, Williams syndrome, Alagille syndrome, fibromuscular dysplasia, mucopolysaccharidosis, fetal alcohol syndrome, & arteritis
- Pathophysiology
  - ↑ in systemic vascular resistance → ↑ in LV afterload → LV hypertrophy
  - Hypertension (HTN) due to renal hypoperfusion
  - Congestive heart failure
    - May be due to PDA closure in severe coarctation
    - May be due to associated complex heart disease
  - Arterial collaterals develop to bypass stenosis when not detected at birth
    - Internal mammary, intercostal, paravertebral, epigastric

Gross Pathologic & Surgical Features

- Focal shelf or waist lesion
- Diffuse narrowing of aortic isthmus
- Poststenotic dilation of descending aorta

CLINICAL ISSUES

Presentation

- Most common signs/symptoms
  - Frequently asymptomatic & incidentally found
  - Infancy: Congestive heart failure (due to aortic arch interruption, associated anomalies)
  - Older child, adult: HTN, ↓ femoral pulses, differential blood pressure between upper & lower extremities (arm-leg gradient)
- Other signs/symptoms
  - Bacterial endocarditis

Demographics

- Epidemiology
  - Incidence: 2-6 per 10,000 live births
  - More common in male patients (2:1), White patients

Natural History & Prognosis

- ↓ long-term survival (late HTN, coronary artery disease)

Treatment

- Resection & end-to-end anastomosis
- Interposition graft
- Prosthetic patch, subclavian flap aortoplasty
- Balloon angioplasty
- Complications
  - Recoarctation (< 3% but higher when operation occurs in infancy)
  - Postoperative aneurysms (24% after patch aortoplasty)

DIAGNOSTIC CHECKLIST

Consider

- Diffuse hypoplasia of aortic isthmus in addition to focal coarctation (important for surgical planning)

Image Interpretation Pearls

- Rib notching in asymptomatic individuals can be 1st clue to hemodynamically significant coarctation

SELECTED REFERENCES

1. Arar Y et al: 3D advanced imaging overlay with rapid registration in CHD to reduce radiation and assist cardiac catheterisation interventions. Cardiol Young. 30(5):656-62, 2020
2. Cassar MP et al: Ascending aortic dissection in a pregnant patient with neonatally repaired coarctation of aorta and bicuspid aortic valve. BMJ Case Rep. 12(12), 2019
3. Kleszcz J et al: Assessing a new coarctation repair simulator based on real patient's anatomy. Cardiol Young. 29(12):1517-21, 2019
4. Kang SL et al: Stent therapy for aortic coarctation in children
5. Rose-Felker K et al: Preoperative use of CT angiography in infants with coarctation of the aorta. World J Pediatr Congenit Heart Surg. 8(2):196-202, 2017
6. Thakkar AN et al: Imaging adult patients with coarctation of the aorta. Curr Opin Cardiol. 32(5):503-12, 2017
7. Casas B et al: 4D flow MRI-based pressure loss estimation in stenotic flows: evaluation using numerical simulations. Magn Reson Med. 75(4):1808-21, 2016
8. Chen CK et al: Left ventricular myocardial and hemodynamic response to exercise in young patients after endovascular stenting for aortic coarctation. J Am Soc Echocardiogr. 29(3):237-46, 2016
9. Nance JW et al: Coarctation of the aorta in adolescents and adults: a review of clinical features and CT imaging. J Cardiovasc Comput Tomogr. 10(1):1-12, 2016
10. Rengier F et al: Noninvasive 4D pressure difference mapping derived from 4D flow MRI in patients with repaired aortic coarctation: comparison with young healthy volunteers. Int J Cardiovasc Imaging. 31(4):823-30, 2015

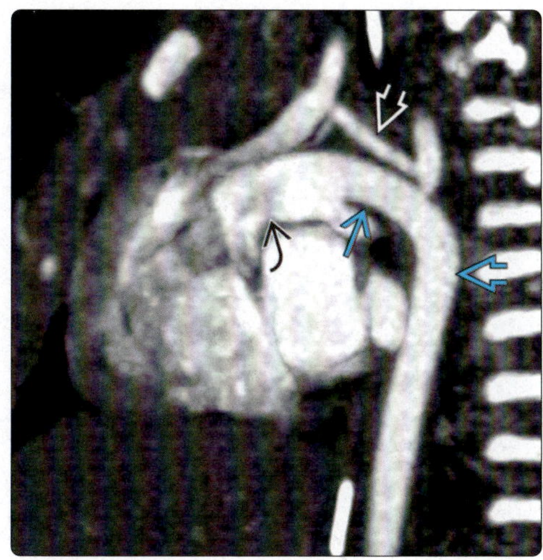

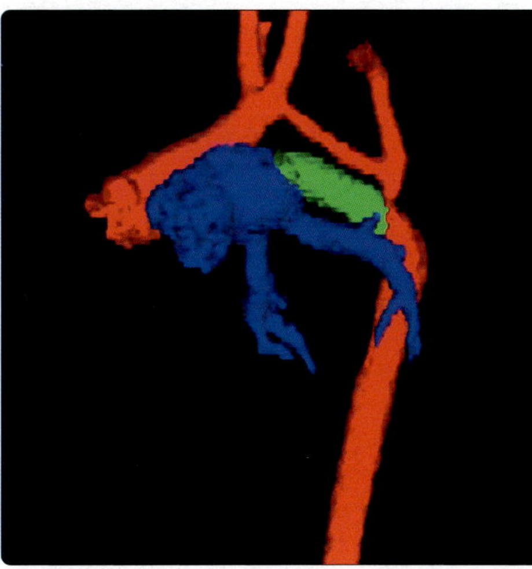

(Left) *Sagittal oblique cardiac CTA in a newborn shows a hypoplastic-type coarctation of the aorta* ➡ *with a large PDA* ➡ *connecting the main pulmonary artery* ➡ *to the descending aorta* ➡. **(Right)** *Lateral oblique 3D color-coded cardiac CTA shows a hypoplastic-type coarctation of the aorta (red) with a large PDA (green) connecting the pulmonary arteries (blue) to the descending aorta.*

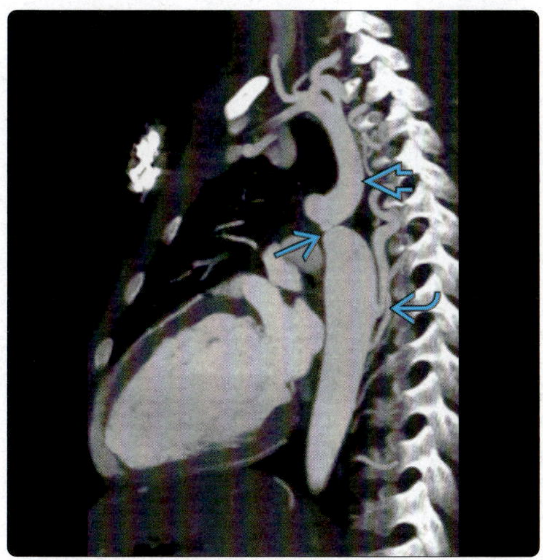

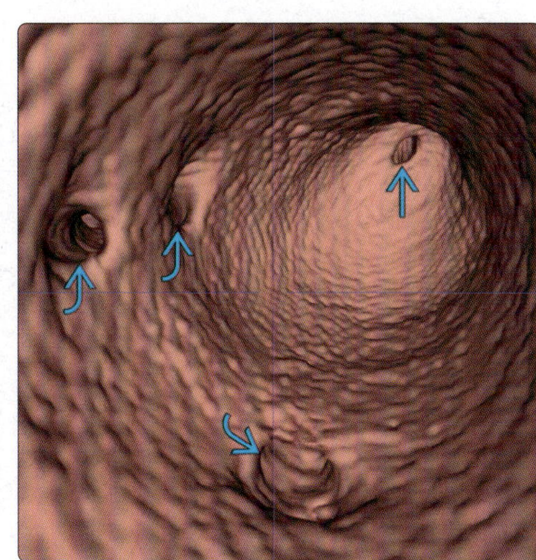

(Left) *Sagittal MIP cardiac CTA in an adolescent shows a focal coarctation* ➡ *of the aorta with dilation of the left subclavian artery* ➡. *Also note the tortuous collaterals along the descending aorta* ➡ *as flow circumvents the stenotic aorta.* **(Right)** *Endoluminal view of the descending thoracic aorta looking up at the focal coarctation* ➡ *is shown. Note the collaterals* ➡ *along the aorta as the flow circumvents the obstruction.*

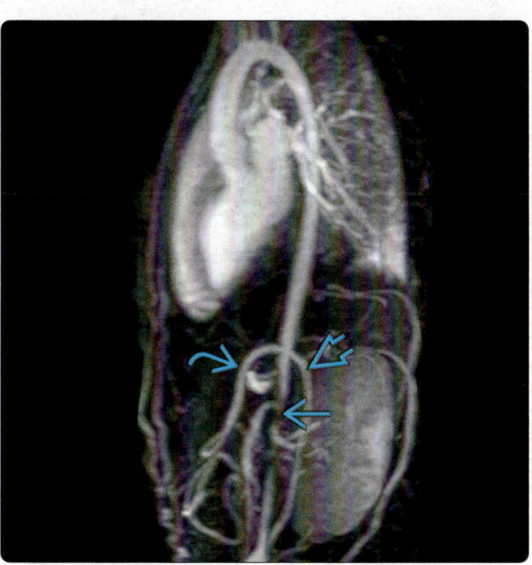

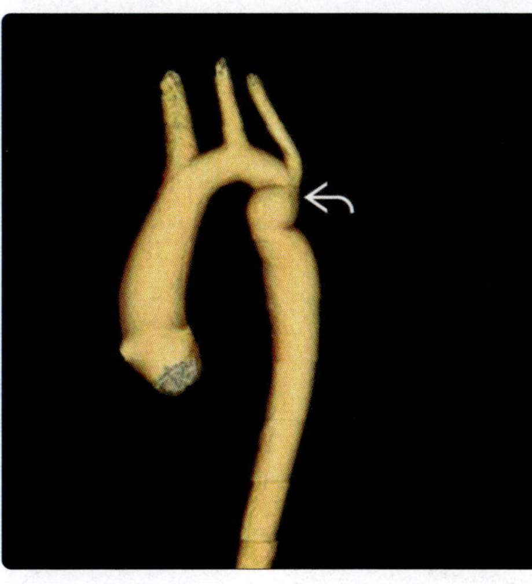

(Left) *Oblique sagittal MRA shows focal obstruction of the midabdominal aorta* ➡ *with a dilated superior mesenteric artery* ➡ *& a large collateral* ➡ *circumventing the obstruction.* **(Right)** *Lateral oblique 3D CTA shows a tortuous but normal-caliber portion* ➡ *of the descending aortic arch. No collaterals were seen, & no significant gradient was detected in this patient with pseudocoarctation of the aorta.*

KEY FACTS

TERMINOLOGY

- Spectrum of aortic valve abnormalities that ranges from asymptomatic bicuspid aortic valve to thickened & obstructed aortic valve stenosis to severe neonatal aortic atresia & hypoplastic left heart syndrome (HLHS)
- Aortic stenosis (AS) may be valvar, supravalvar, or subvalvar
  - Valvar stenosis is most common at 80%

IMAGING

- Varies by location, etiology, & severity of stenosis
- Chest radiographs range from cardiomegaly & edema in severely affected infants to normal in adolescents
- Poststenotic dilation of ascending aorta in valvar stenosis
  - Due to flow jet through stenotic valve
- Supravalvar shows hourglass shape of ascending aorta
- Subaortic stenosis may have hypertrophic cardiomyopathy
- Cardiac enlargement may not be seen in childhood
- MR & echo allow quantitative assessments
- Cardiac catheterization for interventional treatment with balloon valvotomy, leading to aortic regurgitation

PATHOLOGY

- Grading of AS: Jet velocity, gradient across valve, valve area
  - Mild has gradient < 20 mm Hg
  - Moderate has gradient from 20-40 mm Hg
  - Severe has gradient > 40 mm Hg
- Associations include Williams syndrome, HLHS, bicuspid aortic valve, hypertrophic cardiomyopathy, endocarditis

CLINICAL ISSUES

- 10-20% of AS presents in 1st year of life
- Neonatal: Signs of poor or low cardiac output with tachypnea & feeding problems
- Childhood: Usually asymptomatic but may have systolic murmur or suprasternal thrill
- 1% of sudden deaths may be related to undetected AS

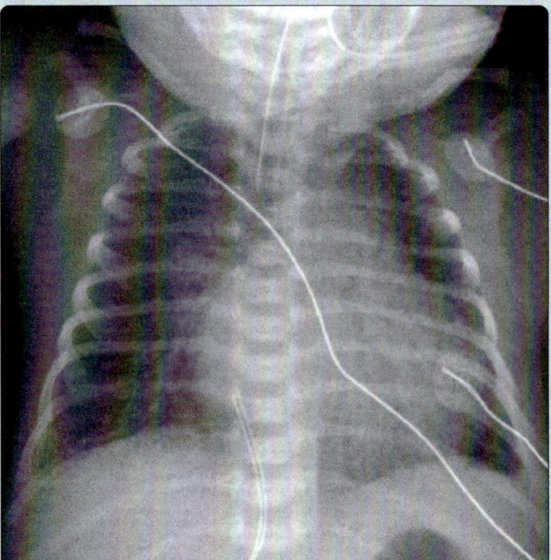

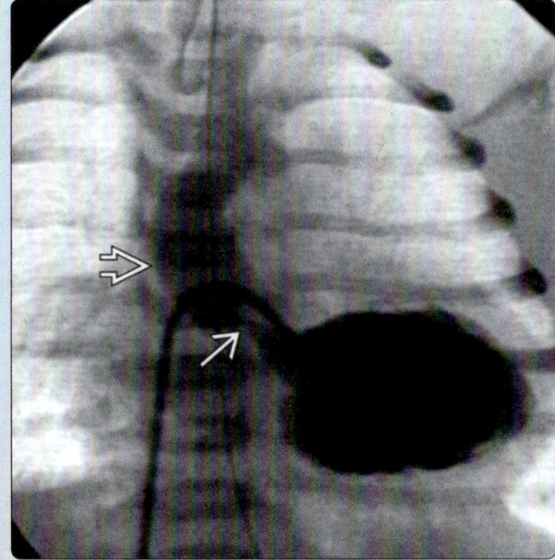

(Left) *Frontal chest radiograph shows a 2-week-old infant in heart failure with perihilar pulmonary edema & cardiomegaly. This patient had critical aortic stenosis.* **(Right)** *Single frontal left ventricular angiogram shows a jet across the aortic valve ➔ from severe aortic stenosis in a 2-week-old infant. Note the dilation of the ascending aorta ➔.*

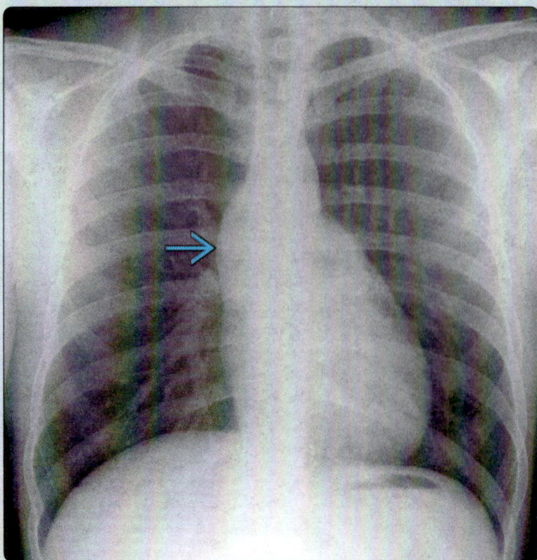

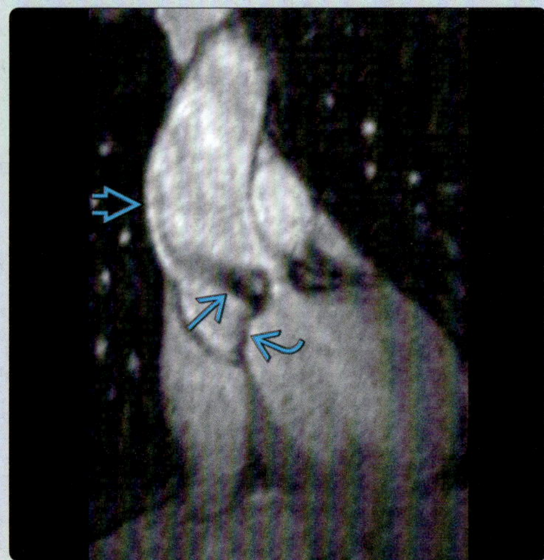

(Left) *Single frontal radiograph of the chest in an adolescent demonstrates a border-forming ascending aorta ➔ along the right mediastinum. This patient had aortic stenosis & typical poststenotic dilation of the ascending aorta.* **(Right)** *Coronal FIESTA cine MR in an adolescent with a bicuspid aortic valve shows a dephasing effect with signal void ➔ from the flow jet through the stenotic valve. Note the thickened aortic valve ➔ & dilation of the ascending aorta ➔.*

TERMINOLOGY

Abbreviations

- Aortic stenosis (AS)

Synonyms

- Aortic valvar stenosis, aortic valvular stenosis

Definitions

- Spectrum of aortic valve abnormalities that ranges from asymptomatic bicuspid aortic valve to thickened, obstructing aortic valve stenosis to severe neonatal aortic atresia & hypoplastic left heart syndrome (HLHS)
- AS may be valvar, supravalvar, or subvalvar (subaortic)
  - Valvar stenosis most common at 80%

IMAGING

General Features

- Best diagnostic clue
  - Thickened valve leaflets with fusion
    - Bicuspid aortic valve in 80% of valvar AS
    - Unicuspid aortic valve is seen in HLHS with endocardial fibroelastosis
  - High-velocity jet of blood is ejected from left ventricle during systole
  - Poststenotic dilation of ascending aorta
  - Concentric left ventricular hypertrophy
- Location
  - Stenosis may be subvalvar, valvar (most common), or supravalvar
- Size
  - Valve anulus may be small for age; valve leaflets are usually thickened; commissures may be fused
- Morphology
  - Normal valve is tricuspid & mobile; stenotic valve is usually thickened with restricted systolic motion

Radiographic Findings

- Neonates & infants may have normal chest radiograph vs. mild cardiomegaly & edema
- Children & adolescents may have normal heart size even in severe AS
  - Dilation of ascending aorta
  - Left ventricle may enlarge secondary to aortic regurgitation (AR) following balloon valvotomy for treatment
  - Ca^{2+} of valve is rare in childhood

CT Findings

- CTA
  - Used to evaluate complex anatomy
  - Can provide volumetric functional data in HLHS with AS
  - Supravalvar stenosis (as seen in Williams syndrome) shows concentric narrowing of ascending aorta (hourglass shape)
    - ± coarctation or pulmonary artery stenoses

MR Findings

- MR cine
  - Ventricular function can be qualitatively assessed on 4-chamber view & quantitatively assessed on stack of short-axis views
  - Stenosis & regurgitation evaluation
    - Flow jet: Signal loss caused by high-velocity flow & turbulence
    - Valve motion: Abnormal motion of stenotic valve is evaluated in plane parallel to anulus
    - Secondary changes in chamber size & degree of wall thickening can be measured
- Velocity-encoded (VENC) or phase-contrast MR
  - Allows quantification of transvalvular pressure gradient & valve area
  - Can quantify regurgitant fraction
  - Flow velocity maps across valve can be generated
- Delayed enhancement
  - Look for infarction or fibrosis both pre- & postablation in subaortic stenosis obstructive cardiomyopathy patients

Echocardiographic Findings

- Gold standard for making diagnosis in infants; used to assess
  - Aortic jet velocity, gradient across valve, valve area
  - Left ventricular function, aortic valve thickness & motion, & associated anomalies, such as mitral insufficiency
- Doppler echocardiography
  - Systolic high-velocity flow jet in left ventricle outflow tract

Angiographic Findings

- Cardiac catheterization for interventional treatment with balloon valvotomy
- Findings include thickened aortic valve, doming of aortic valve, systolic flow jet into ascending aorta, enlarged ascending aorta, & thickened left ventricle

DIFFERENTIAL DIAGNOSIS

Rheumatic Heart Disease

- Multisystem disease with fever, rash, carditis, & valvular disease

Marfan Disease

- Connective tissue disorder associated with aneurysmal dilation of ascending aorta

Coarctation of Aorta

- May have dilation of aorta proximal to narrowing
- 75% may have associated bicuspid valve

Systemic Hypertension

- Left ventricular hypertrophy & prominent ascending aorta, typically in older individuals

PATHOLOGY

General Features

- Genetics
  - Bicuspid aortic valve: One of most common congenital malformations
  - Williams syndrome: Due to chromosomal abnormality of 7q11.2; autosomal dominant
- Associated abnormalities
  - Endocarditis occurs in 4%
  - Williams syndrome: Associated with supravalvar AS & pulmonary artery stenosis

- Coarctation of aorta: Associated with bicuspid aortic valve & AS
- HLHS

Staging, Grading, & Classification

- Grading of AS incorporates aortic jet velocity, valve gradient, valve area
  - Mild has gradient ≤ 20 mm Hg
  - Moderate has gradient 20-40 mm Hg
  - Severe has gradient > 40 mm Hg
- Classification of AS
  - Subvalvar (left ventricular outflow tract) AS (or subaortic stenosis) due to
    - Membrane that partially obstructs left ventricular outflow
    - Thickening of interventricular septum in patients with obstructive cardiomyopathy
  - Valvar in 80% of cases, most frequently in association with bicuspid aortic valve
  - Supravalvar shows concentric narrowing in ascending aorta
    - May be isolated or associated with Williams syndrome

CLINICAL ISSUES

Presentation

- Most common signs/symptoms
  - Neonatal: Signs of poor or low cardiac output with tachypnea & feeding problems
  - Childhood: Usually asymptomatic but may have systolic murmur or suprasternal thrill
    - If prior valvotomy, there will be dilation of ascending aorta & large left ventricle secondary to AR
    - Sudden death, which usually occurs during exercise
    - Children with Williams syndrome are recognized due to multiple manifestations of disease

Demographics

- Age
  - 10-20% in 1st year of life
- Sex
  - M:F = 4:1
- Epidemiology
  - Occurs in 3-5% of children with congenital cardiac defects

Natural History & Prognosis

- Infants with critical AS may be diagnosed in utero
  - Mortality relates to degree of stenosis, presence of neonatal symptoms, & lower birth weights
    - HLHS has highest mortality
    - Endocardial fibroelastosis with ↓ left ventricular outflow
    - Coronary blood flow to subendocardium is reduced, ischemia may occur
- Children with AS constitute 3-5% of all congenital heart defects
  - Usually stenosis progresses; 20% have associated lesions
  - 1% of sudden deaths are thought to be related to undetected AS
  - Once balloon valvotomy occurs, children will have both residual AS & AR

Treatment

- In infants, AS may be part of spectrum of HLHS
  - Treated with prostaglandin to maintain ductal patency
  - May need balloon atrial septostomy or Rashkind procedure with staged Norwood procedure
  - Occasionally treated with heart transplant
- In infants with "critical" AS
  - Percutaneous balloon valvotomy urgently (but may result in AR)
  - Ross surgical procedure is performed when valvotomy is inadequate or regurgitation is moderate
    - Native pulmonary valve is placed in aortic position; homograph is placed for pulmonary valve
- In children, depends on degree of obstruction & progression
  - Mild stenosis: Monitored with echocardiogram & ECG
  - Moderate stenosis: May require valvotomy
  - Severe stenosis: Valvotomy is required
- Surgical aortic valvotomy
  - Performed for supravalvar AS, resection of subaortic membrane, & enlargement of aortic anulus
  - Mechanical valves usually need anticoagulation (undesirable for normal children)
- Replacement of aortic valve with pulmonary valve (Ross procedure)
  - Pulmonary valve is replaced with homograft or reconstruction with conduit
  - Indicated in peak-to-peak gradients > 70 mm & where valvotomy has failed
- All children need prophylaxis to prevent bacterial endocarditis

SELECTED REFERENCES

1. Antequera-González B et al: Bicuspid aortic valve and endothelial dysfunction: current evidence and potential therapeutic targets. Front Physiol. 11:1015, 2020
2. Mylonas KS et al: Rapid right ventricular pacing for balloon valvuloplasty in congenital aortic stenosis: a systematic review. World J Cardiol. 12(11):540-9, 2020
3. Correction: Diagnosis, imaging and clinical management of aortic coarctation. Heart. 105(14):e6, 2019
4. Ancona MB et al: Impact of ascending aorta dilation on mid-term outcome after transcatheter aortic valve implantation. J Invasive Cardiol. 31(10):278-81, 2019
5. De Rubeis G et al: Aortic valvular imaging with cardiovascular magnetic resonance: seeking for comprehensiveness. Br J Radiol. 92(1101):20170868, 2019
6. Lee JC et al: Evaluation of aortic regurgitation with cardiac magnetic resonance imaging: a systematic review. Heart. 104(2):103-10, 2018
7. Guner A et al: Evaluation of the congenital supravalvular aortic stenosis by different imaging modalities. Echocardiography. 34(9):1376-8, 2017
8. Opotowsky AR et al: Imaging adult patients with discrete subvalvar aortic stenosis. Curr Opin Cardiol. 32(5):513-20, 2017
9. Ren X et al: The significance of aortic valve calcification in patients with bicuspid aortic valve disease. Int J Cardiovasc Imaging. 32(3):471-8, 2016
10. Looi JL et al: Morphology of congenital and acquired aortic valve disease by cardiovascular magnetic resonance imaging. Eur J Radiol. 84(11):2144-54, 2015
11. Dusenbery SM et al: Myocardial extracellular remodeling is associated with ventricular diastolic dysfunction in children and young adults with congenital aortic stenosis. J Am Coll Cardiol. 63(17):1778-85, 2014
12. Printz BF: The 30-year road of noninvasive imaging for congenital aortic stenosis: new insights from cardiac magnetic resonance imaging. J Am Coll Cardiol. 63(17):1786-7, 2014
13. Wassmuth R et al: Cardiac magnetic resonance imaging of congenital bicuspid aortic valves and associated aortic pathologies in adults. Eur Heart J Cardiovasc Imaging. 15(6):673-9, 2014

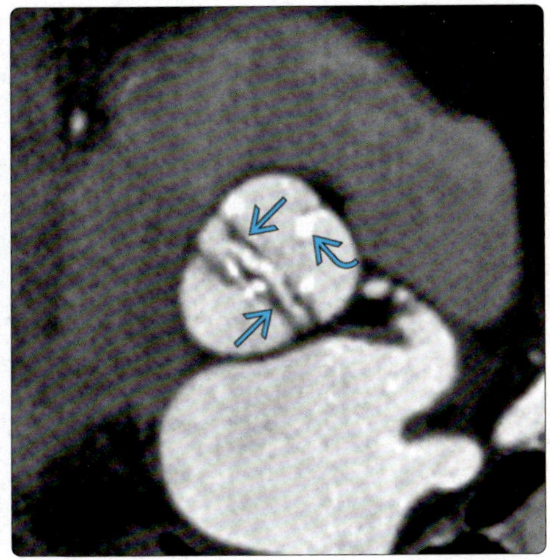

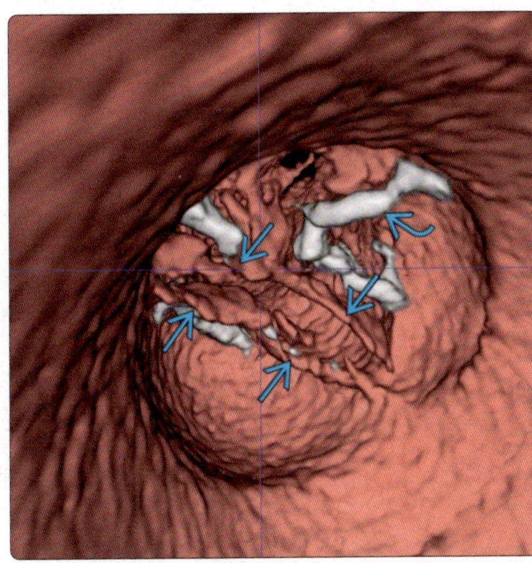

(Left) *Axial MIP cardiac CTA in an adult shows a bicuspid aortic valve forming parallel lines ➔ instead of the normal tricuspid opening. There is complete fusion of the right & left coronary cusps with Ca^{2+} ➔ forming along the fused cusps.* **(Right)** *3D surface-rendered cardiac CTA looking down on the aortic valve demonstrates a bicuspid aortic valve ➔ with a single elongated opening & complete fusion of the right & left coronary cusps with Ca^{2+} ➔.*

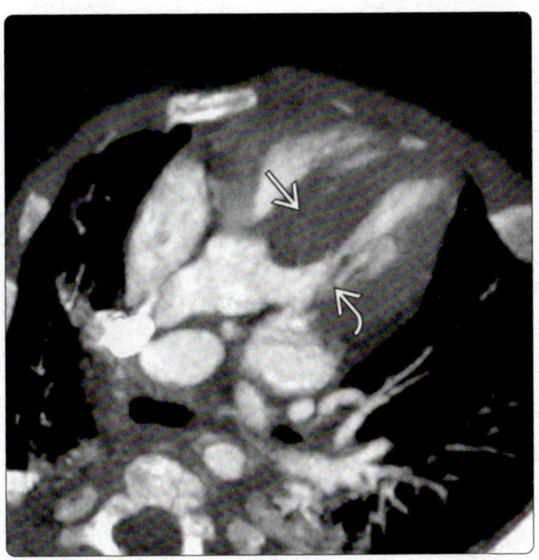

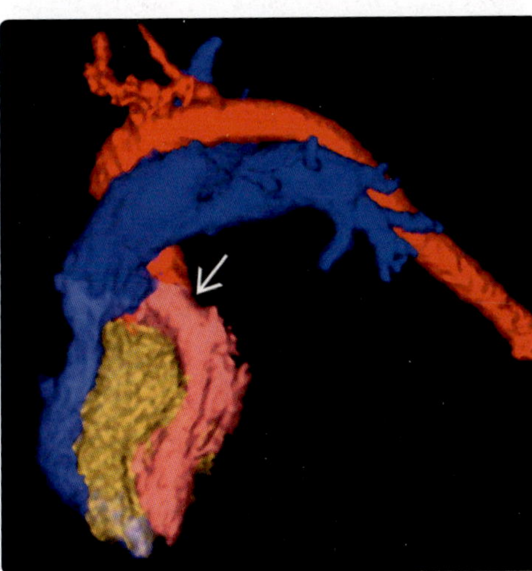

(Left) *Axial MIP cardiac CTA in an infant shows marked thickening of the interventricular septum ➔ & narrowing of the left ventricular outflow tract (LVOT) ➔ in this patient with idiopathic hypertrophic subaortic stenosis (IHSS).* **(Right)** *Oblique 3D color-coded cardiac CTA shows narrowing of the LVOT ➔ with severe contouring of the left ventricle (pink) from the thickened interventricular septum (gold) in this patient with IHSS.*

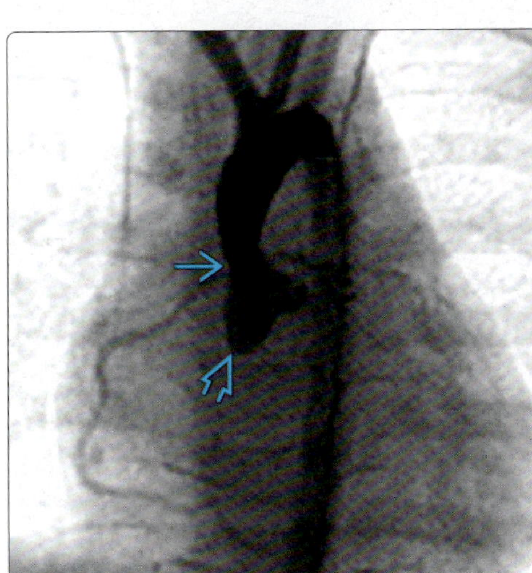

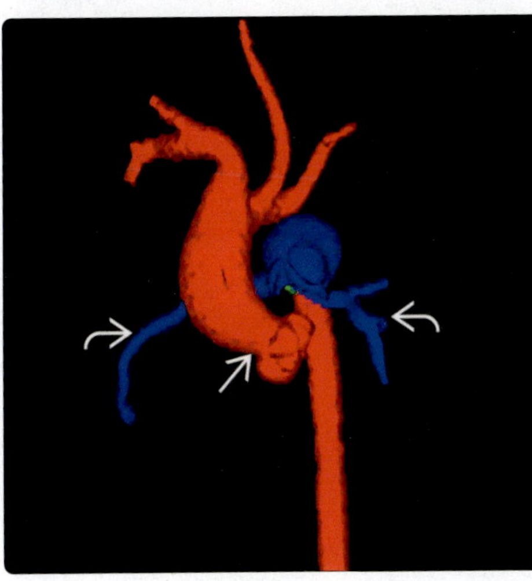

(Left) *Frontal aortogram shows a supravalvular aortic stenosis ➔ with a typical hourglass shape of the ascending aorta in a patient with Williams syndrome. Note the dilated sinuses of Valsalva ➔.* **(Right)** *Frontal 3D color-coded cardiac CTA shows supravalvular aortic stenosis ➔ in a patient with Williams syndrome. Note the hypoplastic pulmonary arteries ➔, which are often seen in this syndrome.*

Pulmonary Artery Stenosis

KEY FACTS

TERMINOLOGY

- Stenosis at level of infundibulum, pulmonary valve, supravalvar main pulmonary artery, or branches of pulmonary artery
- Pulmonary valvar stenosis is most common (> 90%)

IMAGING

- Valvar stenosis: Normal heart size with dilated main pulmonary artery segment in ~ 80%
  - Thickened valve leaflets, doming of valve, systolic high-velocity flow jet in pulmonary outflow tract
- Supravalvar pulmonary artery stenosis in Williams syndrome
- Alagille syndrome has valvar pulmonary stenosis & peripheral pulmonary artery stenosis
- Infundibular narrowing in tetralogy of Fallot & complex malformations
- Right ventricle hypertrophy occurs secondary to ↑ work

CLINICAL ISSUES

- Pulmonary stenosis is often diagnosed between 2-6 years of age during routine physical exam
- Mild stenosis: Usually asymptomatic with systolic ejection murmur
- Moderate stenosis: Exertional dyspnea, easy fatigability
- Severe stenosis: Infants may present with severe cyanosis
- Balloon valvuloplasty is treatment of choice for moderate to severe gradients > 50 mm Hg
  - Newborns with critical PS may need immediate valvotomy
    - Prostaglandin to maintain ductus arteriosus flow
    - May need surgical valvotomy or palliative Blalock-Taussig shunt
  - Not as effective in dysplastic valves (e.g., Noonan syndrome), which may require surgery

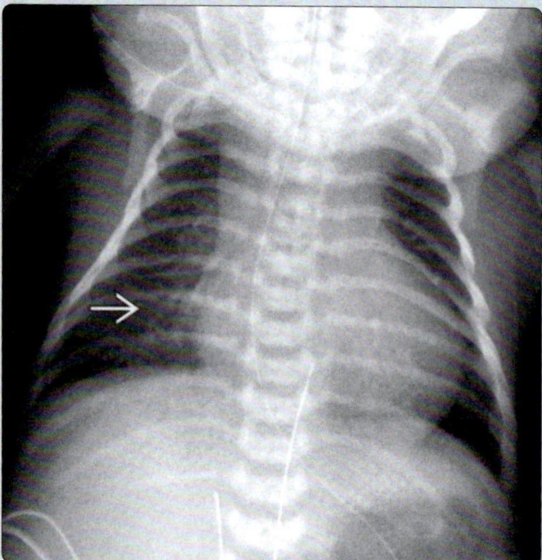

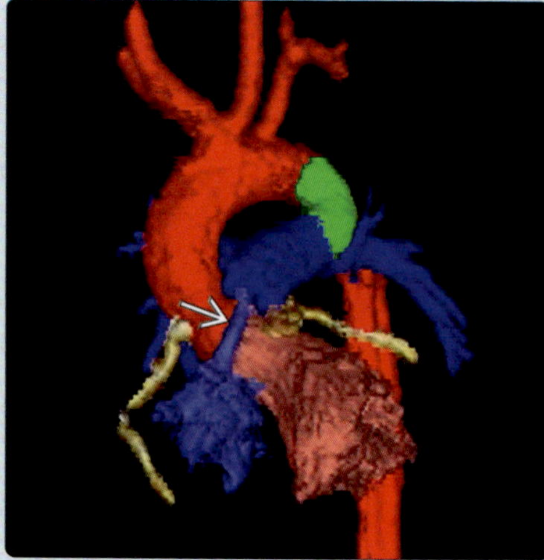

(Left) *Frontal radiograph shows mild cardiomegaly & perihilar pulmonary edema in a patient with severe pulmonary stenosis. Note how the interstitial edema makes the pulmonary vessels indistinct* ➡. **(Right)** *Anterior oblique color-coded 3D cardiac CTA in an infant shows focal pulmonary stenosis with marked narrowing of the pulmonary outflow tract* ➡. *A large patent ductus arteriosus (PDA) (green) is seen connecting the main pulmonary artery (blue) to the descending aortic arch (red).*

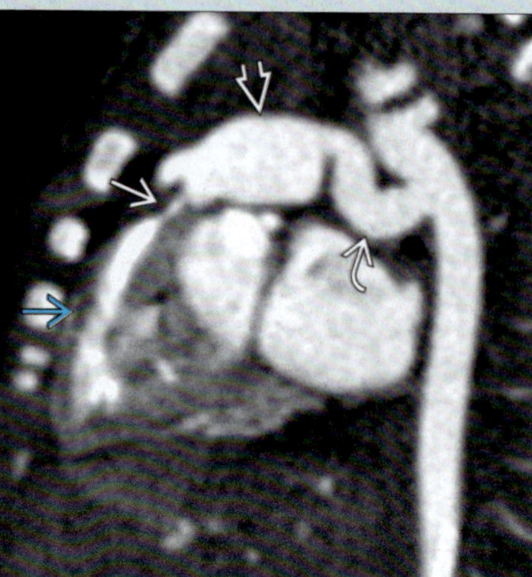

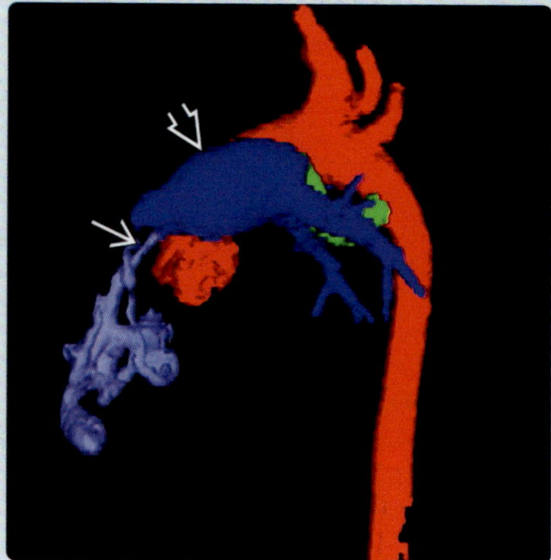

(Left) *Sagittal MIP cardiac CTA shows severe pulmonic stenosis* ➡ *with poststenotic dilation of the main pulmonary artery* ➡ *& right ventricular (RV) hypertrophy* ➡. *Note the tortuous PDA* ➡ *extending from the descending aorta to the main pulmonary artery.* **(Right)** *Lateral 3D color-coded cardiac CTA shows severe pulmonary stenosis* ➡ *with poststenotic dilation of the main pulmonary artery* ➡. *Note the large PDA (green) extending from the aorta (red) to the pulmonary artery (blue).*

TERMINOLOGY

Abbreviations

- Pulmonary stenosis (PS)

Definitions

- Stenosis at level of infundibulum, pulmonary valve, supravalvar main pulmonary artery, or branches of pulmonary artery
- Pulmonary valvar stenosis is most common (> 90%)

IMAGING

General Features

- Best diagnostic clue
  - Normal heart size & prominent main pulmonary artery segment
  - Left pulmonary artery is occasionally larger than right
  - Normal pulmonary flow
- Location
  - Infundibulum, pulmonary valve, supravalvar main pulmonary artery, &/or pulmonary artery branches
- Size
  - Orifice of valve is reduced, which creates turbulence & ↑ work of right ventricle
- Morphology
  - Thickened & stenotic pulmonary valve is most common
    - Valvar stenosis in > 90%
    - Poststenotic dilation of pulmonary artery is frequently seen
  - Dysplastic pulmonary valve in Noonan syndrome
  - Supravalvar PS in Williams syndrome
    - Also has supravalvar aortic stenosis
  - Infundibular narrowing in tetralogy of Fallot & complex malformations
  - Pulmonary artery branch stenosis in tetralogy of Fallot
  - Alagille syndrome has PS & peripheral pulmonary artery stenosis
  - Congenital rubella may have pulmonary branch stenosis
  - Right ventricle hypertrophy occurs secondary to ↑ work

Radiographic Findings

- Normal heart size with dilated main pulmonary artery segment in ~ 80%

CT Findings

- CTA
  - Most useful for supravalvar PS or peripheral PS

MR Findings

- Assessment of right ventricle function
- Can quantitate degree of pulmonary insufficiency
- MRA is useful for supravalvar & peripheral PS

Echocardiographic Findings

- Echocardiogram
  - Pulmonary valvar stenosis
    - Fusion of valve commissures
    - Thickened valve with systolic restricted motion & doming
    - Poststenotic dilation of pulmonary artery
    - Right ventricle hypertrophy
  - Dysplastic pulmonary valve
    - Thickened, irregular, redundant tissue
- Pulsed Doppler
  - Systolic high-velocity flow jet in pulmonary outflow tract
  - Can accurately determine velocity of flow, which can help predict pressure gradients

Angiographic Findings

- Conventional
  - Key features: Thickened valve, dysplastic valve, poststenotic dilation
  - Used to evaluate for coexisting abnormalities, which occur in 10-20%
  - Cardiac catheterization is utilized to measure pressures
    - Demonstrates degree of outflow tract obstruction
    - Degree of trabeculation of right ventricle relates to degree of obstruction
  - Cardiac catheterization is utilized for treatment with balloon valvotomy

Imaging Recommendations

- Best imaging tool
  - Diagnosis in infancy by echocardiography
  - Cardiac catheterization is done as part of therapeutic intervention
    - Shows thickened valve leaflets, doming of valve, & poststenotic dilation

DIFFERENTIAL DIAGNOSIS

Normal Chest Radiograph in Adolescent

- Main pulmonary artery is prominent normally
- Occasionally confused with dilation of pulmonary artery
- Patients have no murmur or symptoms

Pulmonary Hypertension

- Heart may have normal size with right ventricle enlargement
- Central pulmonary arteries are large

Congenital Heart Disease With Large Left-to-Right Shunt

- Main pulmonary artery is large with ↑ pulmonary flow

PATHOLOGY

General Features

- Etiology
  - Pulmonary valvar stenosis is congenital anomaly
    - Maldevelopment of pulmonary valve tissue & distal portion of bulbus cordis
- Genetics
  - No genetic predisposition in valvar stenosis
  - Williams syndrome is related to contiguous gene deletion of locus 7q4
    - Distinct facial features & personality, mild cognitive impairment, cardiovascular abnormalities, elastin arteriopathy
  - Noonan syndrome is autosomal dominant
    - > 50% of individuals have changes in *PTPN11* gene
    - Multiple anomalies with dysplastic pulmonary valve, growth failure, mild cognitive impairment

- Alagille syndrome is autosomal dominant, related to mutations on chromosome 20p12
  - Pulmonic valve & peripheral stenoses + cholestatic jaundice in infancy
    - Jaundice due to bile duct hypoplasia/paucity
  - Butterfly vertebrae, abnormal facies, cognitive impairment, eye & renal anomalies
- Associated abnormalities
  - Most children are normal without any other lesions
  - Can be associated with other common congenital lesions in 10%
    - Infundibular stenosis & ventricular septal defect in tetralogy of Fallot
    - Atrial septal defect, patent ductus arteriosus
    - Complex cardiac lesions
  - Williams syndrome
    - Supravalvar aortic stenosis, coarctation, supravalvar PS, peripheral pulmonary stenoses
  - Noonan syndrome
    - Dysplastic pulmonary valve
  - Alagille syndrome
    - PS with multiple peripheral artery stenoses

Staging, Grading, & Classification

- Pulmonary valvar stenosis: Mild, moderate, severe

Gross Pathologic & Surgical Features

- Valve thickened with fused commissure
- Dysplastic valves have redundant tissue & thickened leaflets

Microscopic Features

- Valve is thickened with fibrous, myxomatous, & collagenous tissue

CLINICAL ISSUES

Presentation

- Most common signs/symptoms
  - Mild stenosis: Usually asymptomatic with systolic ejection murmur
  - Moderate stenosis: Exertional dyspnea, easy fatigability
  - Severe stenosis: Infants may present with severe cyanosis
    - ↓ pulmonary flow, ↑ right ventricle pressure, tricuspid regurgitation, & shunting from right atrium to left atrium
    - Severe stenosis may appear similar to pulmonic atresia, right ventricle hypoplasia, or coronary artery fistulas
- Other signs/symptoms
  - Loud systolic ejection murmur & click at left upper heart border

Demographics

- Age
  - Critical pulmonic stenosis occurs in newborns
  - PS is often otherwise diagnosed between 2-6 years of age during routine physical exam
- Sex
  - M = F

Natural History & Prognosis

- Critical pulmonic stenosis in infancy will progress; can be fatal if not treated
- Pulmonary valvar stenosis with mild gradient does not usually progress
  - Children have normal life expectancy
- Pulmonary valvar stenosis of moderate degree will progress
  - Clinically well tolerated
  - After valvotomy, may have pulmonary insufficiency, which is usually tolerated
- Mortality depends on severity of lesions but mild to moderate degree have normal life expectancy

Treatment

- Observation, medical management for mild valvar stenosis gradients < 25 mm Hg
- Balloon valvuloplasty is treatment of choice for moderate to severe valvar gradients > 50 mm Hg
  - Balloon catheter is placed over wire
  - Balloon is dilated > estimated pulmonary valve anulus while straddling valve
  - Long-term ↓ in right ventricle pressure & estimated gradient
  - Hemodynamically insignificant pulmonary insufficiency may occur in 80%
  - Recurrence of PS occurs in 15% at 10 years
  - Excellent outcome with survival being similar to general population
  - Balloon valvotomy is not as effective in dysplastic valves, which may need surgery
- Angioplasty is done for branch stenosis
- Newborns with severe or critical pulmonic stenosis
  - Prostaglandin to maintain ductus arteriosus flow
  - May need immediate valvotomy or palliative Blalock-Taussig shunt
  - Lesion may be associated with hypoplasia of right ventricle requiring univentricular repair

DIAGNOSTIC CHECKLIST

Image Interpretation Pearls

- Normal adolescent can have mildly prominent pulmonary artery

SELECTED REFERENCES

1. Newman B et al: Congenital central pulmonary artery anomalies: part 1. Pediatr Radiol. 50(8):1022-9, 2020
2. Newman B et al: Congenital central pulmonary artery anomalies: part 2. Pediatr Radiol. 50(8):1030-40, 2020
3. Abdel Razek AAK et al: Imaging of pulmonary atresia with ventricular septal defect. J Comput Assist Tomogr. 43(6):906-11, 2019
4. Collins RT 2nd et al: Real-time transthoracic vector flow imaging of the heart in pediatric patients. Prog Pediatr Cardiol. 53:28-36, 2019
5. Escalon JG et al: Congenital anomalies of the pulmonary arteries: an imaging overview. Br J Radiol. 92(1093):20180185, 2019
6. Mouws EMJP et al: Tetralogy of Fallot in the current era. Semin Thorac Cardiovasc Surg. 31(3):496-504, 2019
7. Alkashkari W et al: Transcatheter pulmonary valve replacement: current state of art. Curr Cardiol Rep. 20(4):27, 2018
8. Pignatelli RH et al: Imaging of the pulmonary valve in the adults. Curr Opin Cardiol. 32(5):529-40, 2017
9. Roberts WC et al: Full development of consequences of congenital pulmonic stenosis in eighty-four years. Am J Cardiol. 119(8):1284-7, 2017

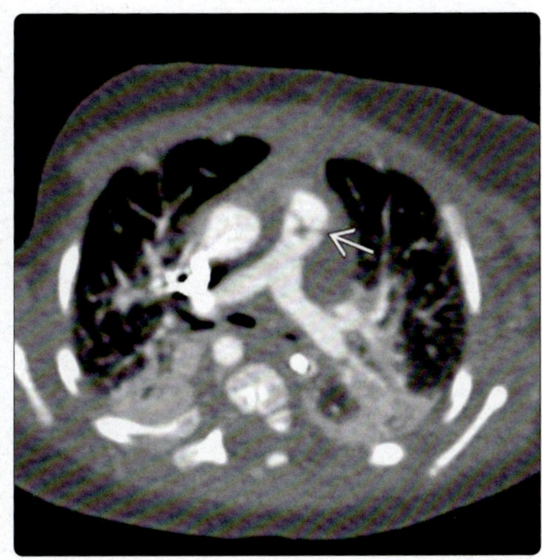

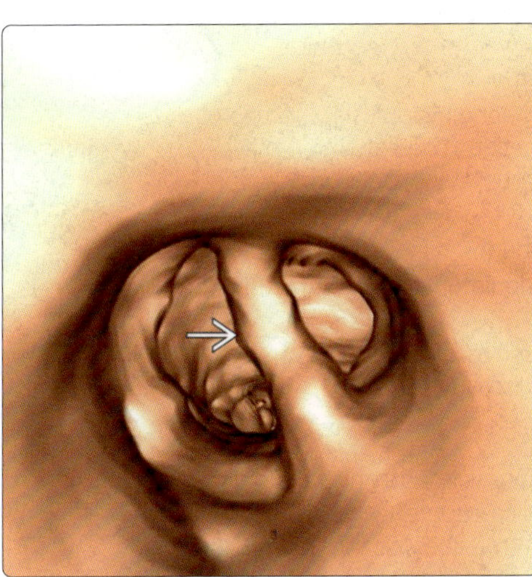

(Left) *Axial cardiac CTA shows valvular pulmonary stenosis with a markedly thickened pulmonary valve ➡.* **(Right)** *Intraluminal virtual angiography 3D cardiac CTA shows a thickened, dysplastic pulmonary valve with a thick septation centrally ➡.*

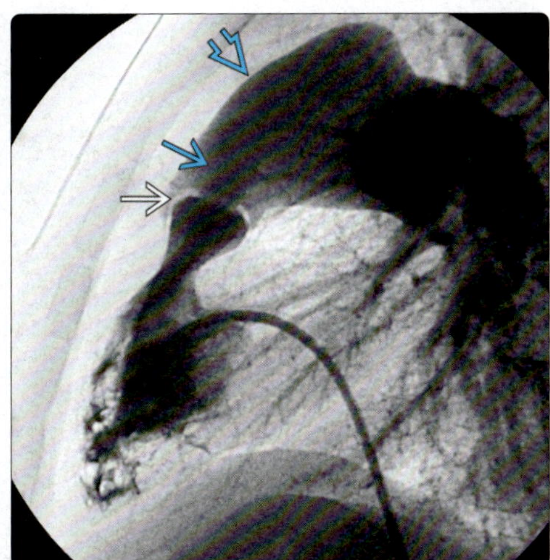

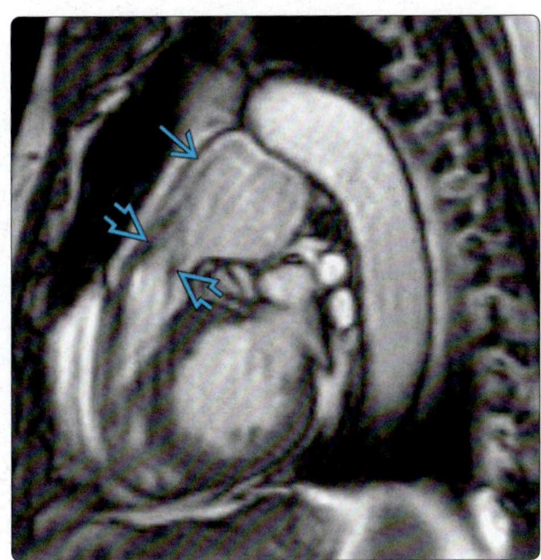

(Left) *Lateral angiography demonstrates doming of the pulmonary valve, thickening of the valve leaflets ➡, a jet created by the narrowed orifice ➡, & poststenotic dilation of the main pulmonary artery ➡.* **(Right)** *SSFP/FIESTA cine cardiac MR shows marked enlargement of the main pulmonary artery ➡ with a signal void ➡ seen from turbulent flow in a patient with valvular pulmonary stenosis.*

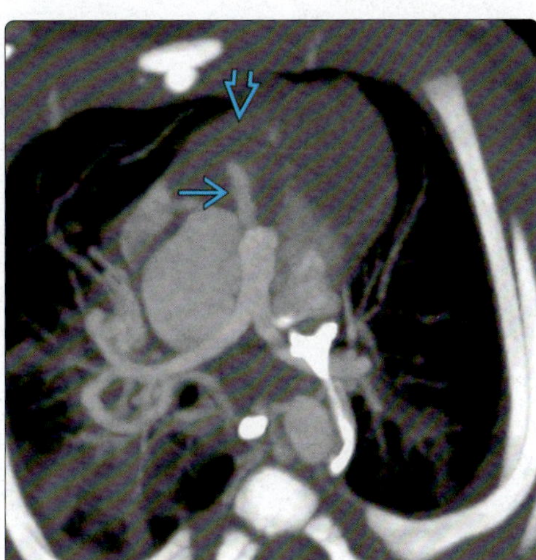

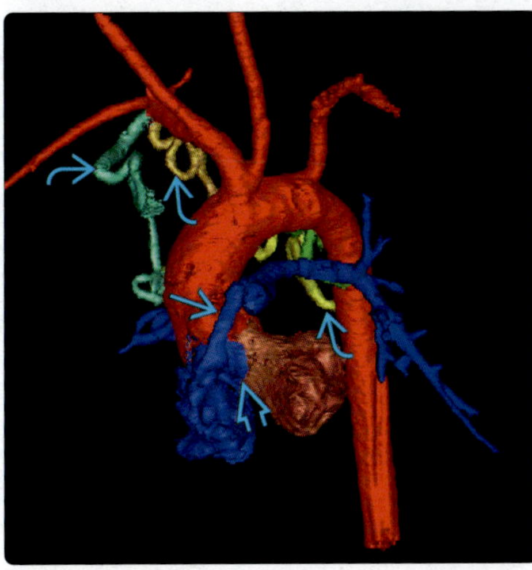

(Left) *Axial MIP cardiac CTA in an infant with severe long-segment stenosis of the pulmonary outflow tract ➡ shows marked RV muscular hypertrophy ➡.* **(Right)** *Oblique 3D surface-rendered cardiac CTA in an infant with severe long-segment stenosis of the pulmonary outflow tract ➡ shows multiple aortopulmonary collaterals ➡. Also note the ventricular septal defect (VSD) ➡ where the blood volume of the RV (violet) & left ventricle (salmon) communicate.*

Scimitar Syndrome

KEY FACTS

TERMINOLOGY

- Synonyms: Hypogenetic lung syndrome, congenital pulmonary venolobar syndrome
- Scimitar syndrome triad: Right lung hypoplasia, anomalous right pulmonary venous connection to inferior vena cava (IVC), & anomalous systemic arterial supply to right lower lobe
  - Extracardiac left-to-right shunt
  - Form of partial anomalous pulmonary venous return (PAPVR)
- Category: Acyanotic, right-sided cardiac chamber enlargement, ↑ pulmonary vascularity

IMAGING

- Scimitar sign: Curved anomalous venous trunk, resembling Turkish sword, in right medial costophrenic sulcus near right heart border; typically ↑ in caliber in caudad direction
- Right lung hypoplasia with mediastinal shift
- Dextroversion of heart (not dextrocardia as apex is still directed toward left)
- Prominent right atrium, active pulmonary vascular congestion → shunt vascularity

CLINICAL ISSUES

- Newborn: Congestive heart failure, right heart volume overload, pulmonary hypertension
- Young child: Recurrent infections in right lung base
- Older child & adult: Often asymptomatic (incidental finding on chest radiograph)
- Treatment
  - Embolization of systemic arterial supply
  - Baffling of common right pulmonary vein onto left atrium
    - Surgical repair when left-to-right shunt > 2:1

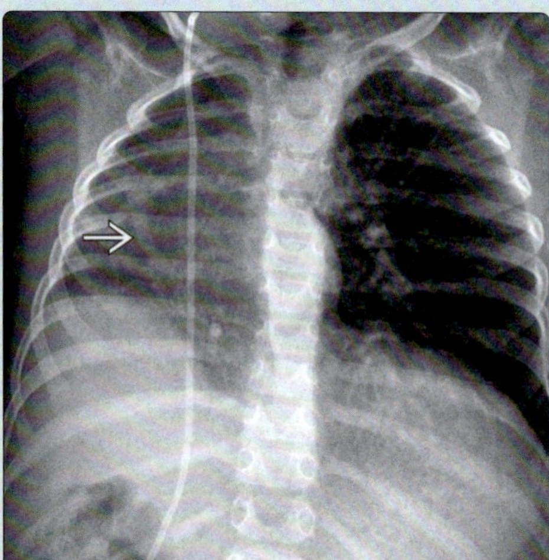

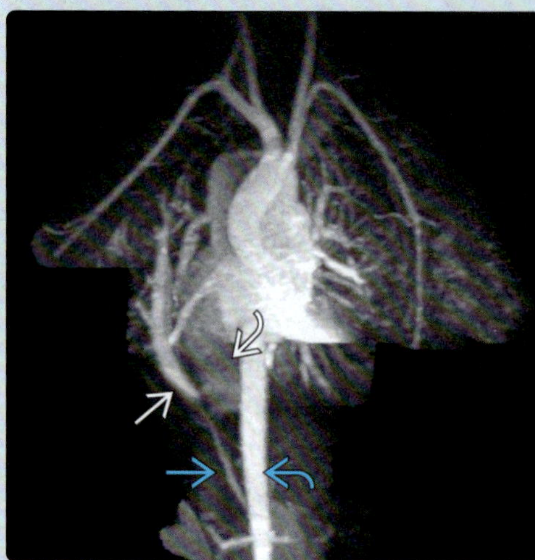

(Left) *Frontal radiograph shows mediastinal shift to the right from a hypoplastic right lung. There is an enlarged curvilinear vein ➡ in the right lower lobe from partial anomalous pulmonary venous return (PAPVR) in this patient with scimitar syndrome.* **(Right)** *Anterior MRA shows a large scimitar (pulmonary) vein ➡ draining to the inferior vena cava (IVC) ↩ with systemic arterial supply ➡ to the right lower lobe (RLL) arising from the proximal abdominal aorta ↩.*

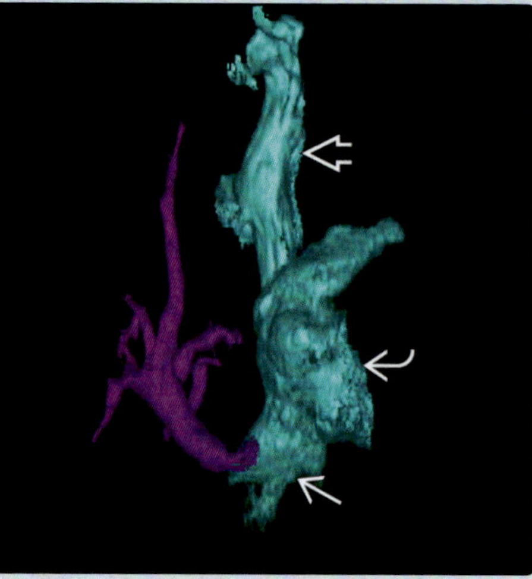

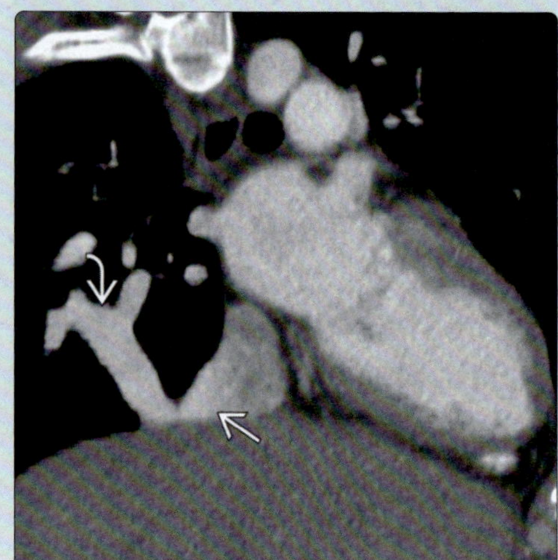

(Left) *Posterior 3D color-coded CTA shows PAPVR of the RLL with the anomalous vein (pink) draining to the IVC ➡. The superior vena cava (SVC) ⇨ & right atrium ↩ are also shown.* **(Right)** *Coronal oblique MIP CTA of the chest shows PAPVR of the RLL pulmonary vein ↩ draining into the IVC ➡.*

TERMINOLOGY

Synonyms

- Hypogenetic lung syndrome, congenital pulmonary venolobar syndrome

Definitions

- Scimitar syndrome triad: Right lung hypoplasia, anomalous right pulmonary venous connection to inferior vena cava (IVC), & anomalous systemic arterial supply to right lower lobe
  - Scimitar vein represents form of partial anomalous pulmonary venous return (PAPVR)
- Hemodynamics: Venous flow from right lung returns to right atrium → volume overload of right heart [atrial septal defect (ASD)-type physiology]

IMAGING

General Features

- Best diagnostic clue
  - Scimitar sign: Curved anomalous pulmonary vein, resembling Turkish sword, typically draining right lower & middle lobes
    - ↑ in caliber in caudad direction

Radiographic Findings

- Right lung hypoplasia with mediastinal shift
- Prominent right atrium & shunt vascularity when multiple lobes drain to IVC
- Scimitar vein may be seen in right medial costophrenic sulcus

CT Findings

- CTA with 3D reconstruction is most helpful to demonstrate venous drainage, anomalous systemic arterial supply, & right pulmonary artery & main bronchus hypoplasia

MR Findings

- Phase-contrast MRA for shunt flow calculation (Qp:Qs)
- Gadolinium-enhanced MRA coronal acquisition with 3D reconstruction for anomalous right pulmonary venous & arterial development

Echocardiographic Findings

- Echocardiogram
  - Scimitar vein connecting to IVC
  - Enlarged right atrium & ventricle with significant shunt

Angiographic Findings

- Conventional
  - Scimitar vein opacifies during venous phase of pulmonary artery injection
  - Injection of abdominal aorta: Anomalous systemic arterial supply to right lung base originating from abdominal or thoracic aorta

Imaging Recommendations

- CTA or MRA is better than echocardiography for complete assessment & can replace diagnostic angiocardiography
- Angiography is reserved for coil embolization

DIFFERENTIAL DIAGNOSIS

Other Forms of PAPVR

- Right pulmonary vein(s) to azygous vein, superior vena cava (SVC), or right atrium (with sinus venosus ASD)

True Dextrocardia With Abdominal Situs Solitus

- Other complex cardiac anomalies

Isolated Right Pulmonary Hypoplasia

- Normal right pulmonary venous connection to left atrium

Bronchopulmonary Sequestration

- Mass in lung base not connected to bronchial tree, receives systemic arterial supply

PATHOLOGY

General Features

- Embryology
  - Primary abnormality in development of right lung with secondary anomalous pulmonary venous connection
- Pathophysiology
  - Extracardiac left-to-right shunt: ASD physiology

CLINICAL ISSUES

Presentation

- Most common signs/symptoms
  - Depends on age at presentation & size of left-to-right shunt
    - Newborn: Congestive heart failure, right heart volume overload, pulmonary hypertension
    - Young child: Recurrent infections in right lung base
    - Older child & adult: Often asymptomatic (incidental finding on chest radiograph)

Natural History & Prognosis

- Large shunt → irreversible pulmonary hypertension
- Moderate to poor prognosis with neonatal presentation
- May be asymptomatic for many years with small shunt

Treatment

- Surgical repair is indicated when left-to-right shunt > 2:1
- Baffling of common right pulmonary vein into left atrium
- Embolization of systemic arterial supply

SELECTED REFERENCES

1. Diaz-Frias J et al: Scimitar syndrome. StatPearls, 2021
2. Mounir R et al: Adults forms of scimitar syndrome. J Card Surg. 35(7):1697-9, 2020
3. Trimech T et al: Scimitar syndrome with bicuspid aortic valve. A case report of cross-sectional non- invasive imaging allowing a complete anatomical and functional assessment. Ann Cardiol Angeiol (Paris). 69(5):317-22, 2020
4. Han F et al: The case of the missing pulmonary vein: a focused update on anomalous pulmonary venous connection in congenital cardiovascular disease. Echocardiography. 36(10):1930-5, 2019
5. Masrani A et al: Anatomical associations and radiological characteristics of scimitar syndrome on CT and MR. J Cardiovasc Comput Tomogr. 12(4):286-9, 2018
6. O'Byrne ML et al: Asymptomatic atresia of the anomalous pulmonary vein in a patient with scimitar syndrome presenting in childhood. Cardiol Young. 28(2):329-33, 2018
7. Althomali SA et al: Uncommon presentation of adult-form scimitar syndrome associated with single left pulmonary vein in a pregnant woman. BMJ Case Rep. 2017

Glenn Shunt

KEY FACTS

TERMINOLOGY

- Superior cavopulmonary shunt
- Goal is to direct systemic venous return from upper 1/2 of body to pulmonary circulation, directly bypassing right heart
  - Superior vena cava (SVC) is divided from right atrium at superior cavoatrial junction
  - End-to-side anastomosis between divided SVC & right pulmonary artery (PA)
  - SVC flow is directed to confluent branch PAs
- Used in patients with single ventricle physiology as staged palliative procedure prior to Fontan, ultimately resulting in total cavopulmonary connection
- Comprises stage 2 of Norwood procedure for hypoplastic left heart syndrome
- Typically performed between 3-9 months of age when pulmonary vascular resistance has ↓ sufficiently
- If 2 SVCs are present, each can be anastomosed to its respective PA, creating bilateral Glenn shunts

IMAGING

- CECT can be used to assess for shunt patency, collaterals, & branch PA stenoses
  - Delayed equilibrium-phase CTA should be performed to avoid contrast mixing artifact within branch PAs
- MR can be used in pre-Glenn & post-Glenn evaluation
  - Evaluate cardiac anatomy with ventricular & atrioventricular valve function
  - Evaluate branch PAs for stenoses along with flow differential calculation by phase-contrast imaging (PCI)
    - Velocities are picked for PCI across branch PAs typically < 100 cm/s, since venous flow occurs via Glenn shunt
  - Evaluate neoaorta
  - Quantify pulmonary-to-systemic blood flow & collaterals

TOP DIFFERENTIAL DIAGNOSES

- Hemi-Fontan operation

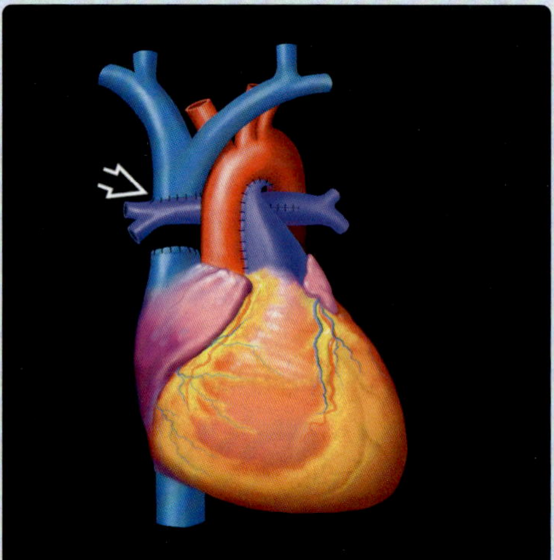

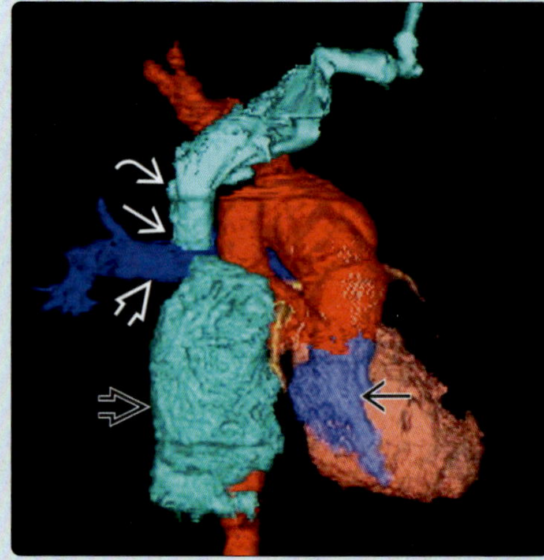

(Left) *Graphic shows a Glenn shunt ➡ as part of a stage 2 Norwood procedure. A direct connection between the superior vena cava (SVC) & the right pulmonary artery (PA) is created with deoxygenated systemic venous flow directed to both lungs.* **(Right)** *Frontal color-coded surface-rendered 3D cardiac CTA shows a bidirectional Glenn shunt ➡ connecting the SVC ➡ to the PA ➡. Note the gap between the right atrium ➡ & right ventricle ➡, consistent with known tricuspid atresia.*

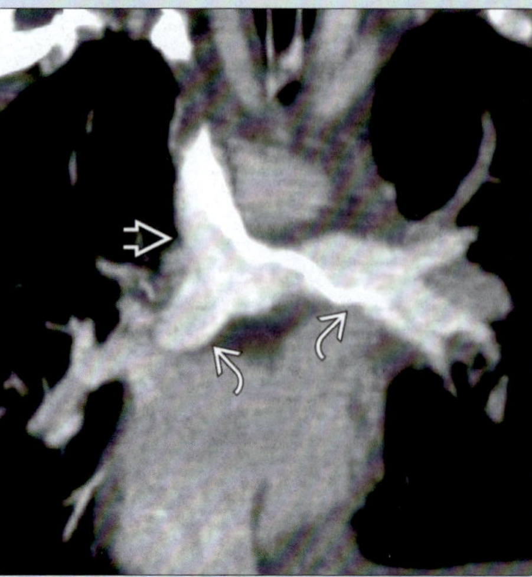

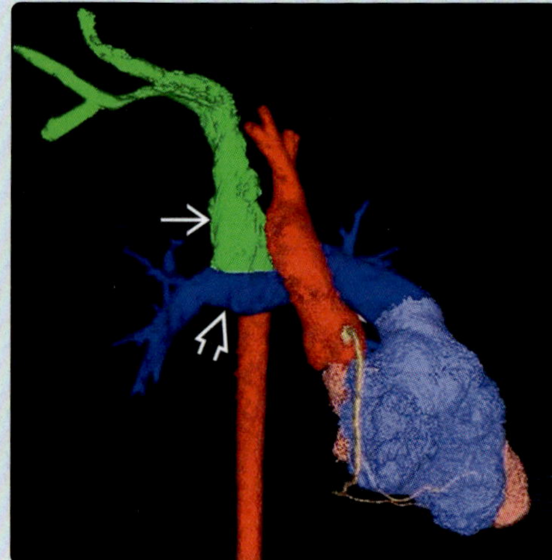

(Left) *Coronal CTA reconstruction with contrast injected via the right upper extremity demonstrates direct communication between the SVC & PAs, consistent with a right-sided bidirectional Glenn shunt ➡ with opacification of both PAs ➡.* **(Right)** *Frontal color-coded surface-rendered 3D cardiac CTA demonstrates direct communication between the SVC ➡ & PAs ➡, consistent with a right-sided bidirectional Glenn shunt.*

TERMINOLOGY

Synonyms

- Superior cavopulmonary shunt

Definitions

- Goal is to direct systemic venous return from upper 1/2 of body to pulmonary circulation, directly bypassing right heart
- Originally described by Dr. William Glenn in 1958
  - End-to-end anastomosis of divided superior vena cava (SVC) to divided right pulmonary artery (PA)
  - SVC flow is directed to right lung only
- Bidirectional Glenn shunt is more commonly used now
  - SVC is divided from right atrium at superior cavoatrial junction followed by end-to-side anastomosis between divided SVC & right PA
  - SVC flow is directed to both right & left PAs
- Performed in patients with single ventricle physiology as staged palliative procedure prior to Fontan; final result is called total cavopulmonary connection
- Glenn shunt forms stage 2 of Norwood procedure for hypoplastic left heart syndrome
- By reducing volume load, bidirectional Glenn shunt reduces single ventricle wall stress & atrioventricular valve insufficiency
- Since no synthetic graft material is used, shunt grows with child
- Typically performed between 3-9 months of age
  - By this age, pulmonary vascular resistance has ↓ to level where systemic venous return enters pulmonary circulation without assistance of right heart pump
- If 2 SVCs are present, each can be anastomosed to its respective PA, creating bilateral Glenn shunts
- Azygous & hemiazygos veins are ligated as part of procedure

IMAGING

General Features

- Complications
  - Superior-to-inferior systemic venous collaterals
    - Can be coil embolized
  - Progressive cyanosis
  - Formation of pulmonary arteriovenous malformations (AVMs)
    - Hypothesized to be secondary to exclusion of hepatic venous flow through lungs
    - Resultant lack of hepatic factor delivery to pulmonary circulation
    - Subsequent lack of inhibition of endothelial proliferation in lungs
  - Branch PA stenosis
  - Arrhythmias

CT Findings

- Can be used postoperatively to assess for shunt patency
- Useful in evaluating thoracic vasculature, including neoaorta, branch PAs, pulmonary veins, & collaterals
- Can be used for detection of pulmonary AVM
- Pre-Glenn evaluation of cardiac anatomy, including branch PAs, instead of cardiac MR
- 3D reconstructions are helpful

MR Findings

- Traditionally used in pre-Glenn evaluation instead of conventional angiography
  - Evaluate cardiac anatomy & function
  - Evaluate valvular function
  - Evaluate central PAs & veins
  - Evaluate neoaorta
  - Quantify pulmonary-to-systemic blood flow
- Useful in post-Glenn evaluation
  - Evaluate ventricular function
  - Evaluate shunt patency & flow
  - Evaluate PA narrowing
  - Evaluate collaterals & pulmonary AVMs

Ultrasonographic Findings

- Echocardiography is used for pre- & postoperative anatomic & hemodynamic assessment
- Limited evaluation of branch PAs & pulmonary veins

Angiographic Findings

- Considered gold standard in preoperative assessment of anatomic & hemodynamic suitability for Glenn shunt
- Catheter-based interventions, such as collateral embolization & aortic balloon dilation, can be performed if required

DIFFERENTIAL DIAGNOSIS

Hemi-Fontan Operation

- Similar to Glenn, except continuity of SVC & right atrium are maintained
- SVC is anastomosed to right PA
- Patch of homograft tissue is sewn across superior cavoatrial junction, preventing systemic venous return from upper body into right atrium
- Simplifies subsequent lateral tunnel Fontan completion as continuity of right atrium & SVC are maintained

SELECTED REFERENCES

1. Sethasathien S et al: Risk factors for morbidity and mortality after a bidirectional Glenn shunt in northern Thailand. Gen Thorac Cardiovasc Surg. 69(3):451-7, 2021
2. Khetan A et al: Asking bubbles for direction: assessment of a classic Glenn shunt using agitated saline contrast echocardiography. CASE (Phila). 4(6):485-9, 2020
3. Ma K et al: Effectiveness of bidirectional Glenn shunt placement for palliation in complex congenitally corrected transposed great arteries. Tex Heart Inst J. 47(1):15-22, 2020
4. Vermaut A et al: Outcome of the Glenn procedure as definitive palliation in single ventricle patients. Int J Cardiol. 303:30-5, 2020
5. Saleem K et al: Bidirectional Glenn for residual outflow obstruction in Tetralogy of Fallot. Cardiol Young. 29(5):684-8, 2019
6. Hall EJ et al: Association of Shunt type with arrhythmias after Norwood procedure. Ann Thorac Surg. 105(2):629-36, 2018
7. Sharma R: The bidirectional Glenn shunt for univentricular hearts. Indian J Thorac Cardiovasc Surg. 34(4):453-6, 2018

Fontan Operation

KEY FACTS

TERMINOLOGY

- Total cavopulmonary connection
- Used in single ventricle physiology as stage 3 of Norwood procedure
  - Tricuspid atresia
  - Hypoplastic left heart syndrome
  - Double inlet ventricle
  - Some heterotaxies
- Typically performed between 18-36 months of age
- Lateral tunnel Fontan
  - Intraatrial tunnel created in right atrium connecting inferior vena cava (IVC) to pulmonary artery
- Extracardiac conduit Fontan (typically favored)
  - Synthetic graft tube connected to IVC & right pulmonary artery
- Excellent early-, mid-, & late-term outcomes with mortality rates < 5-10%

IMAGING

- CECT can be used for detection of Fontan complications, such as thrombus, hepatomegaly, effusions, & pulmonary arteriovenous malformation
  - Delayed-phase of image acquisition during CTA eliminates contrast mixing artifacts within branch pulmonary arteries & Fontan conduit
- MR can be used in pre-Fontan & post-Fontan assessment
  - Evaluation of branch pulmonary arteries, including determination of flow differential using phase-contrast sequences
  - Evaluation of superior cavopulmonary connection (Glenn shunt)
  - Identification of collaterals
  - Evaluation of ventricular function
  - Determine patency of Fontan conduit & exclude thrombus
  - Assessment of hepatic fibrosis & lesions

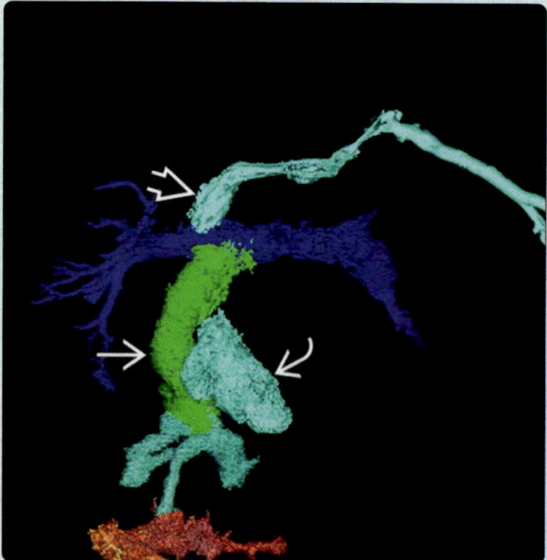

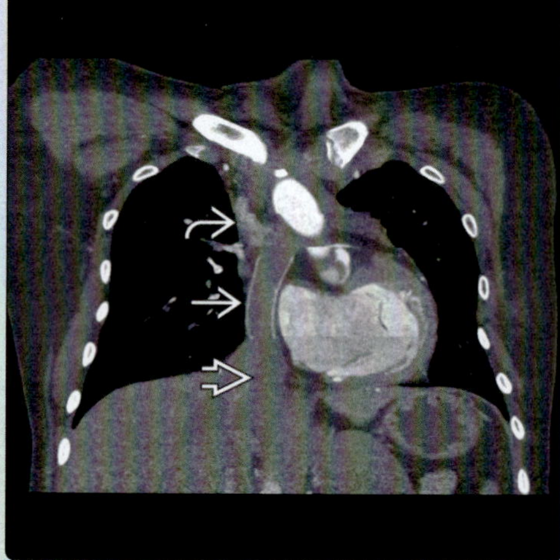

(Left) *Frontal surface-rendered chest CTA shows postoperative changes from a Fontan ➡ & Glenn ➡ shunt connecting the systemic venous return directly to the right & left pulmonary arteries (PAs) (dark blue), bypassing the right atrium (RA) ➡. Note the extracardiac course of the Fontan that bypasses the right atrium.* **(Right)** *Coronal chest CTA in a patient with a Fontan shunt shows a stent along the Fontan shunt ➡, which connects the inferior vena cava ➡ to the PAs ➡.*

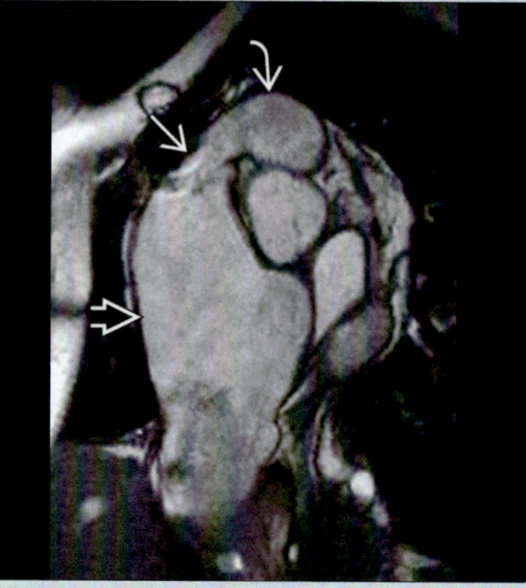

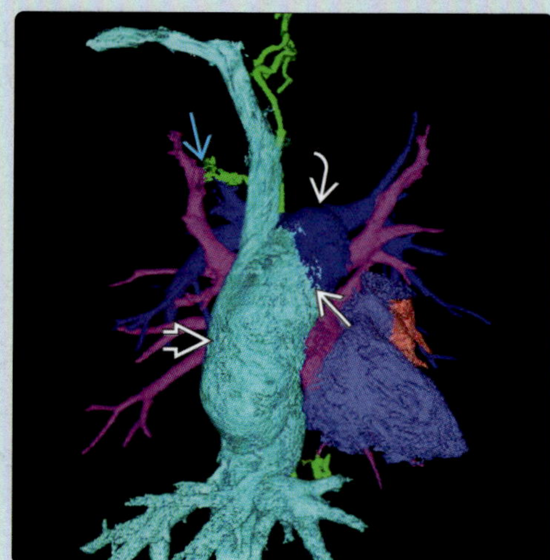

(Left) *Oblique coronal SSFP cine cardiac MR demonstrates a Fontan shunt where the RA ➡ is connected to the PAs ➡ via the atrial appendage ➡. Note the enlarged RA.* **(Right)** *Frontal surface-rendered cardiac CTA shows a Fontan shunt where the RA ➡ is connected to the PA ➡ via the atrial appendage ➡. Over time, ↑ pressure may lead to systemic venous collaterals (green) that communicate ➡ directly with the pulmonary veins (pink), leading to cyanosis.*

Fontan Operation

TERMINOLOGY

Synonyms

- Total cavopulmonary connection

Definitions

- Goal is to direct systemic venous return to pulmonary circulation directly, bypassing right heart
- Initially described by Dr. Francis Fontan in 1968
- Used in single ventricle physiology
  - Tricuspid atresia
  - Hypoplastic left heart syndrome
  - Double inlet ventricle
  - Some heterotaxies
- Stage 3 of Norwood procedure
- Typically performed between 18-36 months of age
- Originally described as extracardiac valved conduit between right atrium & left pulmonary artery
  - In combination with Glenn shunt, creates physiologic correction of blood flow
  - Superior vena cava (SVC) blood is directed to right pulmonary artery & inferior vena cava (IVC) blood is directed to left pulmonary artery
  - Complications of classic Fontan
    - Right atrial enlargement & hypertension
    - Impaired ventricular function
    - ↓ pulmonary vascular blood flow
    - Tricuspid valve insufficiency
- In order to preserve ventricular & pulmonary vascular function, modified Fontan is now favored
  - Lateral tunnel Fontan
    - Intraatrial tunnel created in right atrium using prosthetic material
    - IVC is anastomosed to caudal aspect of tunnel
    - Pulmonary artery is anastomosed to cephalad aspect of tunnel
  - Extracardiac conduit Fontan (typically favored)
    - IVC is divided from right atrium
    - Synthetic graft tube is connected to IVC inferiorly & right pulmonary artery superiorly; travels along side of right atrium
  - In either form, IVC blood directed to pulmonary circulation, bypassing right heart structures
- Small fenestration is often created between Fontan circuit & right atrium
  - Prevents volume overload to lungs
  - Buffers any ↑ in systemic venous pressure
- Excellent early-, mid-, & late-term outcomes with mortality rates < 5-10%

IMAGING

General Features

- Complications
  - Arrhythmias
  - Liver dysfunction due to fibrosis; liver lesions
  - Protein-losing enteropathy
  - Heart failure
  - Thrombus & emboli
  - Formation of pulmonary arteriovenous malformations (AVMs)
    - Hypothesized to be secondary to exclusion of hepatic veins from Fontan pathway with lack of protective hepatic factor delivery to lungs
    - Potentially reversible if hepatic venous flow can be redirected to lungs
  - Chylous pleural effusions
  - Plastic bronchitis

CT Findings

- Can be used for detection of Fontan complications, such as thrombus, hepatomegaly, effusions, & pulmonary AVM
- 3D reconstructions are very helpful

MR Findings

- Pre-Fontan evaluation
  - Can potentially obviate need for preoperative catheter angiography
  - Evaluation of superior cavopulmonary connection formed by Glenn procedure
  - Evaluation of branch pulmonary arteries
  - Identification of collaterals
  - Evaluation of ventricular function
- Post-Fontan evaluation
  - Evaluate patency of Fontan pathway
  - Evaluate ventricular function
  - Evaluate pulmonary artery stenosis
  - Identify collaterals
  - MR elastography for evaluation of hepatic fibrosis
    - ± hepatobiliary contrast agent for liver lesions
  - MR lymphangiography for chylous effusion, plastic bronchitis

DIFFERENTIAL DIAGNOSIS

Kawashima Procedure

- Used in patients with single ventricle physiology & interrupted IVC
  - Fontan not feasible
- SVC, including azygous continuation, connected to right pulmonary artery
  - All systemic venous return is directed to pulmonary artery
    - Except hepatic veins & coronary sinus

SELECTED REFERENCES

1. de Lange C: Imaging of complications following Fontan circulation in children - diagnosis and surveillance. Pediatr Radiol. 50(10):1333-48, 2020
2. Dillman JR et al: Imaging of Fontan-associated liver disease. Pediatr Radiol. 50(11):1528-41, 2020
3. Ibe DO et al: Pearls and pitfalls in pediatric Fontan operation imaging. Semin Ultrasound CT MR. 41(5):442-50, 2020
4. Udink Ten Cate FEA et al: Imaging the lymphatic system in Fontan patients. Circ Cardiovasc Imaging. 12(4):e008972, 2019
5. Files MD et al: Pathophysiology, adaptation, and imaging of the right ventricle in Fontan circulation. Am J Physiol Heart Circ Physiol. 315(6):H1779-88, 2018
6. Ginde S et al: Imaging adult patients with Fontan circulation. Curr Opin Cardiol. 32(5):521-8, 2017

Arterial Switch Procedure

KEY FACTS

TERMINOLOGY

- Surgical procedure to correct D-transposition of great arteries (D-TGA)
    - Coronary arteries are translocated to base of neoaorta
    - Ascending aorta & main pulmonary artery are transected & transposed
        - Ascending aorta is connected to left ventricular outflow tract
        - Main pulmonary artery is relocated anterior to aorta & connected to right ventricular outflow tract as part of Lecompte maneuver
- Typically performed in first 2 weeks of life
- Survival rate & freedom of reoperation at 5 years: 90% & 97%, respectively

IMAGING

- Typical postoperative appearance: Pulmonary artery arises directly anterior to ascending aorta; branch pulmonary arteries drape over either side of ascending aorta
- Complications
    - Supravalvular pulmonic stenosis & branch pulmonary artery stenoses
    - Aortic root dilation & regurgitation
    - Ischemia secondary to coronary artery stenosis/occlusion
- CTA is useful in immediate postoperative period to assess for complications & to follow status of coronary arteries & branch pulmonary arteries
- MR provides comprehensive evaluation of postoperative anatomy & function without ionizing radiation

TOP DIFFERENTIAL DIAGNOSES

- Mustard/Senning: Late atrial level repair of D-TGA with baffle
- Rastelli: Performed on subset of patients with D-TGA, ventricular septal defect, & left ventricular outflow tract stenosis/obstruction

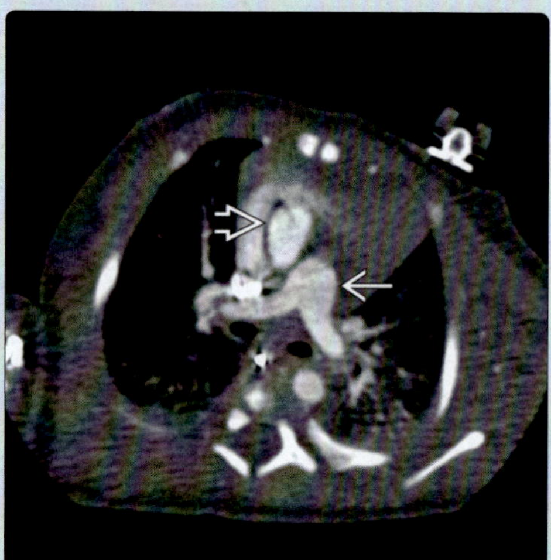

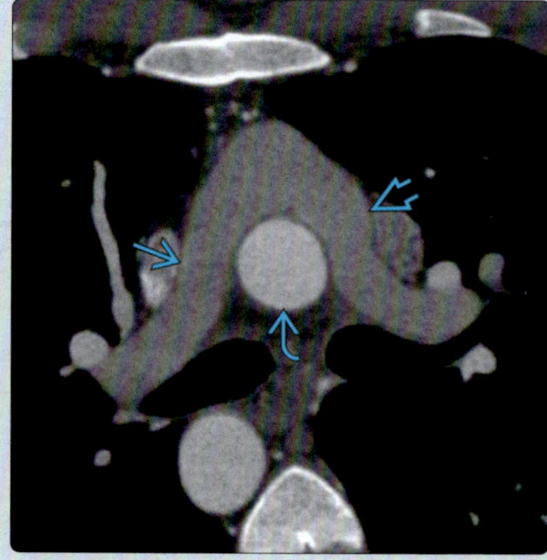

(Left) *Preoperative axial CTA in a patient with D-transposition of great arteries (D-TGA) shows abnormal positions of the great vessel origins with the ascending aorta ➡ very anterior & mildly right of the pulmonary artery ➡.* **(Right)** *Oblique axial cardiac CTA in a patient status post arterial switch procedure shows the right ➡ & left ➡ pulmonary arteries draped around the ascending aorta ➡. This is the classic postoperative appearance in a patient status post arterial switch procedure.*

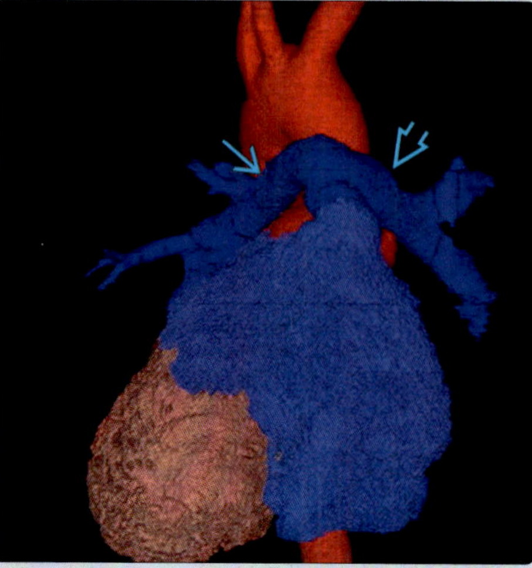

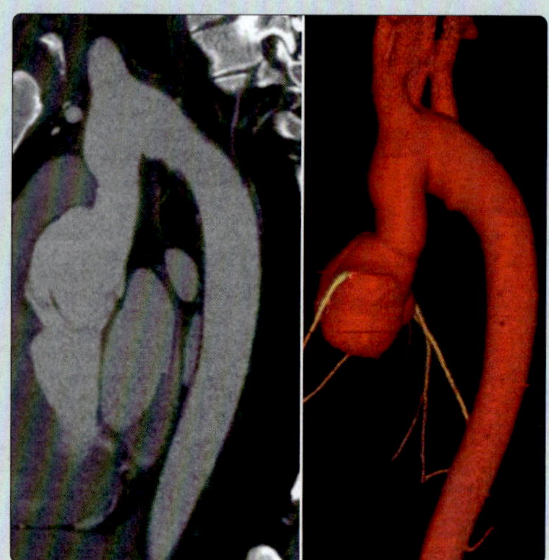

(Left) *Frontal volume-rendered cardiac CTA in a patient status post arterial switch procedure shows the right ➡ & left ➡ pulmonary arteries draped around the ascending aorta. This is the classic postoperative appearance in a patient post arterial switch procedure.* **(Right)** *Sagittal & lateral surface-rendered CTA images of the aorta status post arterial switch procedure show a posterior position of the ascending aorta & acute angle of the arch due to mass effect from the pulmonary arteries.*

TERMINOLOGY

Synonyms

- Jatene arterial switch

Definitions

- Surgical procedure to correct D-transposition of great arteries (D-TGA)
  - D-TGA involves ventriculoarterial discordance & atrioventricular concordance
    - Pulmonary trunk arises from left ventricle (LV)
    - Aorta arises from right ventricle (RV)
    - Frequently associated with ventricular septal defect (VSD) & outflow tract obstruction
- Arterial switch was 1st successfully used in 1975 by Dr. Adib Jatene
  - Coronary arteries are transposed to base of neoaorta
  - Aorta & pulmonary trunks are then sectioned, transposed, & anastomosed
    - Ascending aorta ends up being connected to LV outflow tract
    - Main pulmonary artery (PA) is relocated anterior to aorta & connected to RV outflow tract
      - This relocation of pulmonary trunk is referred to as Lecompte maneuver
      - Reduces risk of coronary artery kinking
- VSD is corrected if present
  - If no VSD is present, patient typically undergoes PA banding prior to correction to prepare LV for systemic pressures
- Arterial switch is performed in first 2 weeks of life
- If not performed early in neonatal period, PA banding ± Blalock-Taussig shunt is used to acclimate LV to systemic pressures in preparation for connection to aorta
- Arterial switch is contraindicated in presence of coronary anomalies, such as intramural course
- Arterial switch may not be feasible in presence of significant LV outflow obstruction
  - Rastelli procedure is often used instead in this situation
- Benefits of arterial switch
  - LV is used as systemic pump & mitral valve as systemic atrioventricular valve
  - Lower incidence of arrhythmias compared to atrial switch (Senning/Mustard)
  - No baffle obstructions/leaks as with atrial switch (Senning/Mustard)
  - Can be performed earlier in neonatal period than atrial switch (Senning/Mustard)
  - Survival rate & freedom of reoperation at 5 years of 90% & 97%, respectively

IMAGING

General Features

- Complications
  - Supravalvular pulmonic stenosis
    - May require angioplasty or surgical correction in small percentage of patients
  - Branch PA stenoses
  - Supravalvular aortic stenosis
  - Aortic root dilation & regurgitation
  - LV dysfunction
  - Persistent pulmonary hypertension
  - Ischemia secondary to coronary artery stenosis/occlusion, typically at ostium

CT Findings

- Useful in immediate postoperative period to assess for airway compression, branch PA stenosis, & mediastinitis
- Can be utilized to evaluate coronary artery lesions, such as ostial stenosis/kink

MR Findings

- Comprehensive evaluation of postoperative anatomy & function; excellent follow-up tool
  - Quantify RV & LV chamber sizes & function
  - Evaluate valvular function by flow quantification across vessels using phase-contrast imaging
  - Measure aortic root dilation & degree of aortic regurgitation
  - Delayed enhancement techniques are useful for evaluation of myocardial ischemia or infarction
  - 3D SSFP sequence for coronary anatomy

DIFFERENTIAL DIAGNOSIS

Mustard/Senning

- Atrial level repair of D-TGA
- Intraatrial baffle is created
  - Superior & inferior vena cava form superior & inferior limbs of systemic venous baffle, routed to morphologic LV & hence PA
  - Pulmonary veins are routed to morphologic RV & hence aorta
- Mustard procedure uses autologous or synthetic pericardium to form baffle
- Senning uses native atrial tissue to form baffle
- Complications include arrhythmias, RV dysfunction, tricuspid regurgitation, pulmonary & systemic pathway stenoses, & baffle leaks/stenoses

Rastelli

- Performed on subset of patients with D-TGA, VSD, & LV outflow tract stenosis/obstruction
- PA is divided just above valve plane, & cardiac end closed, followed by placement of extracardiac RV to PA conduit
- Intraventricular tunnel is created directing blood flow from LV through VSD into aorta

SELECTED REFERENCES

1. Fraser CD Jr: Commentary: coronary origins after the arterial switch operation: let's think of it like anomalous aortic origin of the coronaries. J Thorac Cardiovasc Surg. 161(4):1406-7, 2021
2. Casanova J: The arterial switch operation. Rev Port Cir Cardiotorac Vasc. 27(3):157, 2020
3. van Broekhoven I et al: Imaging large arteries after arterial switch operation. Heart. 106(12):891-950, 2020
4. Breinholt JP et al: Management of the adult with arterial switch. Methodist Debakey Cardiovasc J. 15(2):133-7, 2019
5. Broda CR et al: Post-operative assessment of the arterial switch operation: a comparison of magnetic resonance imaging and echocardiography. Pediatr Cardiol. 39(5):1036-41, 2018
6. Kutty S et al: Contemporary management and outcomes in congenitally corrected transposition of the great arteries. Heart. 104(14):1148-55, 2018

Norwood Procedure

KEY FACTS

TERMINOLOGY

- 3-stage procedure to palliate single ventricle physiology (most commonly hypoplastic left heart syndrome)
- Goals of Norwood procedure
  - Utilize single right ventricle as systemic pump & reconstruct systemic arterial outflow
  - Ensure pulmonary venous return to right heart
  - Reroute systemic venous return directly to lungs
- Stage 1 Norwood
  - Neoaorta is constructed using divided main pulmonary artery (PA) anastomosed to aortic root
  - Blalock-Taussig (BT) or Sano shunt is created to provide blood flow to high-resistance pulmonary arterial circulation
  - Ductus arteriosus is ligated
  - Atrial septum is resected
- Stage 2 Norwood
  - BT or Sano shunt is excised
  - Bidirectional Glenn shunt is created
- Stage 3 Norwood
  - Lateral tunnel or extracardiac Fontan procedure is performed
- ~ 70% 5-year survival of Norwood procedure
- Norwood procedure alternatives for hypoplastic left heart syndrome
  - Hybrid procedure (ductus arteriosus stenting, PA banding, & atrial septal defect ballooning in lieu of stage 1 Norwood)
  - Primary cardiac transplantation

IMAGING

- CECT can be used pre- & postoperatively to evaluate complex anatomy
- CECT is useful in evaluation of complications, such as mediastinitis, shunt thrombus, collaterals, & effusions
- MR is most commonly used between stages or after completion

(Left) *Lateral color-coded 3D CTA shows a Norwood stage 1 with a hypoplastic native ascending aorta ➡ combined with the main PA ➡ to form a neoaorta from a single ventricle (purple). A BT shunt (green) carries blood to the PAs (dark blue).* **(Right)** *Anterior color-coded 3D CTA shows a patient with a Norwood stage 3. A Fontan shunt (green) is seen carrying blood from the IVC ➡ to the PAs (dark blue). A Glenn shunt is also present connecting the SVC ➡ to the PAs. Note the hypoplastic RV (purple).*

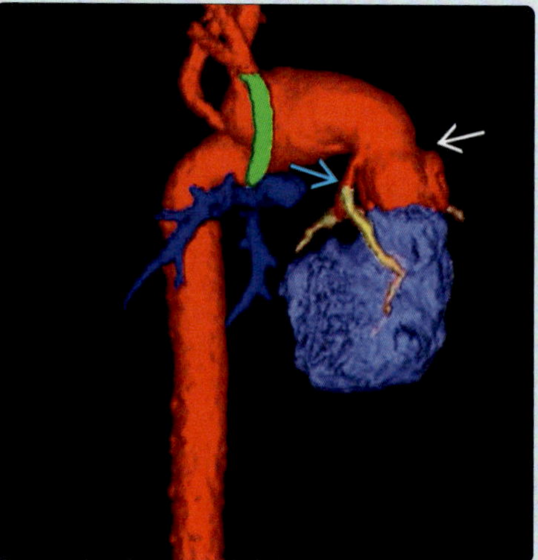

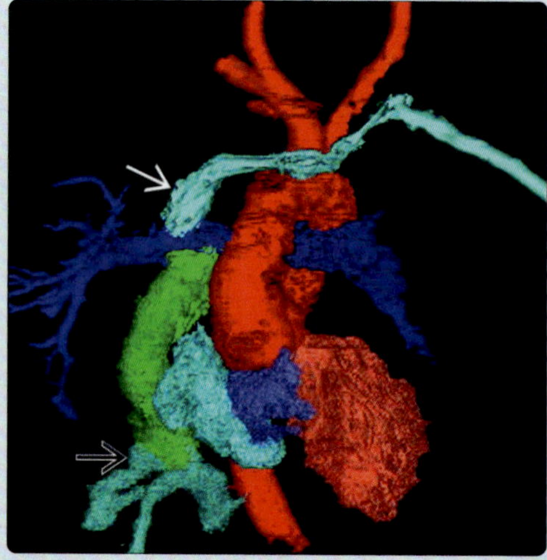

(Left) *Coronal MIP CTA shows an RA ➡ to PA ➡ (atriopulmonary)-type Fontan connection ➡. Over time, there is often ↑ venous pressure that causes systemic ➡ to pulmonary ➡ venous collaterals to develop, resulting in ↑ cyanosis.* **(Right)** *Anterior color-coded 3D CTA shows an RA ➡ to PA ➡ (atriopulmonary)-type Fontan connection ➡. Over time, there is often ↑ venous pressure that causes systemic ➡ to pulmonary ➡ venous collaterals to develop, resulting in ↑ cyanosis.*

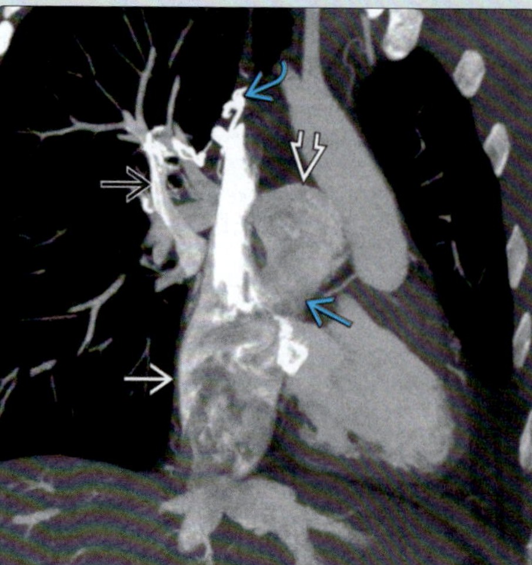

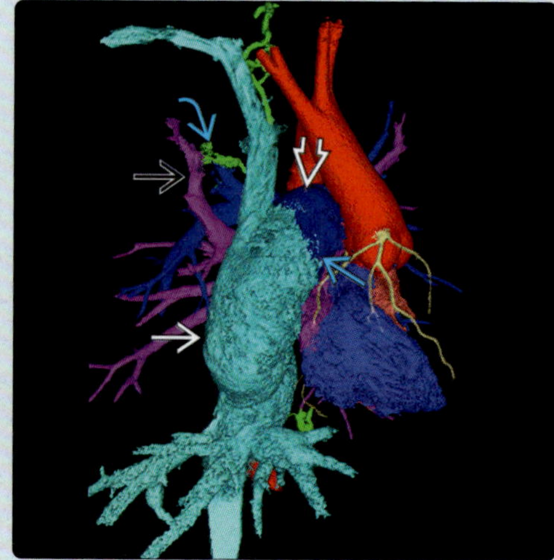

TERMINOLOGY

Definitions

- 3-stage procedure to palliate single ventricle physiology (most commonly hypoplastic left heart syndrome)
  - Staged approach is necessary due to high pulmonary vascular resistance in neonatal period
  - Developed in early 1980s, initially as 2 stages
- Goals of Norwood procedure
  - Utilize single right ventricle (RV) [or, less frequently, single left ventricle (LV)] as systemic pump & reconstruct systemic arterial outflow
  - Ensure unobstructed pulmonary venous return to right heart
  - Reroute systemic venous return directly to lungs
- Stage 1 Norwood
  - Performed within 1st few days after birth
  - Neoaorta construction: Divide main pulmonary artery (PA) & anastomose to aortic root
    - Single, unobstructed arterial trunk from RV to systemic circulation is now in place
  - Blalock-Taussig (BT) or Sano shunt is created to provide blood flow to high-resistance PA circulation
  - Ductus arteriosus is ligated
  - Atrial septum is resected
    - Common atrium receives blood from superior & inferior vena cavae (SVC & IVC) & pulmonary veins
- Stage 2 Norwood
  - Performed between 3-6 months of age
    - Pulmonary vascular resistance has ↓ by this time to normal levels
  - BT or Sano shunt is excised
  - Bidirectional Glenn shunt is created
    - End-to-side anastomosis of SVC to PAs
- Stage 3 Norwood
  - Typically performed between 18-36 months of age
  - Lateral tunnel or extracardiac type of Fontan is now performed; atriopulmonary type is not common today
    - IVC blood flow is directed to PAs

IMAGING

General Features

- Complications
  - Heart failure, pleural & pericardial effusions, arrhythmias
  - Valvular dysfunction
  - Branch PA stenoses
  - Shunt thrombosis/stenosis/obstruction
  - Liver fibrosis, liver lesions
  - Protein-losing enteropathy
  - Pulmonary arteriovenous malformation
  - Neurologic complications
  - Unexplained sudden death

Radiographic Findings

- After stage 1: Signs of RV hypertrophy, ↓ pulmonary venous congestion, & occasional new paratracheal shadow from BT shunt
- After stage 2: Normalized pulmonary vascularity & elimination of BT shunt shadow, ↑ size of head & neck (initially) from ↑ pressure in SVC
- After stage 3: ↑ pulmonary vascularity & pleural effusions

CT Findings

- CECT
  - Can be used pre- & postoperatively to evaluate patients with complex anatomy &/or for whom long anesthesia times may be difficult
  - Useful in evaluation of complications, such as mediastinitis, shunt thrombus, venous & arterial collaterals, effusions

MR Findings

- Occasionally used preoperatively in complex cases when biventricular vs. univentricular repair is being contemplated
- Used frequently after stage 1, prior to bidirectional Glenn shunt
  - Assess anatomy & ventricular/valvular function
- Can be helpful after stage 2, prior to Fontan procedure
  - Glenn pathway can be evaluated in addition to ventricular & valvular function & other anatomy
  - PA sizes & anatomy can be ascertained, which affects surgical decision making for Fontan
- Very helpful after stage 3
  - Evaluate Fontan pathway patency & for presence of thrombus
  - Evaluate for PA stenoses
  - Evaluate for venous & arterial collateral formation
- MR elastography is helpful in evaluating liver fibrosis
  - ± hepatobiliary contrast to assess liver lesions

DIFFERENTIAL DIAGNOSIS

Norwood Procedure Alternatives for Hypoplastic Left Heart Syndrome

- Hybrid procedure
  - In lieu of Norwood stage 1
  - Ductus arteriosus stenting, PA banding, & atrial septal defect ballooning
  - No cardiopulmonary bypass or thoracotomy required
  - Comparable outcomes to full Norwood
- Primary cardiac transplantation
  - ~ 70% 7-year survival
  - Lifelong immunosuppression is needed

CLINICAL ISSUES

Natural History & Prognosis

- ~ 70% 5-year survival of Norwood procedure

SELECTED REFERENCES

1. Dillman JR et al: Imaging of Fontan-associated liver disease. Pediatr Radiol. 50(11):1528-41, 2020
2. Vitanova K et al: Choice of shunt type for the Norwood I procedure: does it make a difference? Interact Cardiovasc Thorac Surg. 30(4):630-5, 2020
3. Devlin PJ et al: Intervention for arch obstruction after the Norwood procedure: prevalence, associated factors, and practice variability. J Thorac Cardiovasc Surg. 157(2):684-695.e8, 2019
4. Nakamura Y et al: The Norwood procedure with valvular pulmonary stenosis. Ann Thorac Surg. 107(1):e49-50, 2019
5. Brida M et al: Systemic right ventricle in adults with congenital heart disease: anatomic and phenotypic spectrum and current approach to management. Circulation. 137(5):508-18, 2018

Blalock-Taussig Shunt

KEY FACTS

TERMINOLOGY

- Original/classic Blalock-Taussig (BT) shunt
  - Ligation & division of subclavian artery with end-to-side anastomosis of proximal subclavian artery to pulmonary artery
  - Rarely performed today due to complications
    - Overshunting, nerve injury, & potential growth disturbance of ipsilateral upper extremity
- Modified BT shunt
  - Synthetic prosthetic graft (Gore-Tex) between subclavian artery & ipsilateral pulmonary artery
    - Contralateral to side of aortic arch
  - Up to 90% patency rate at 2 years of age
- Used as palliative procedure to ↑ pulmonary blood flow prior to definite repair
  - Tetralogy of Fallot
  - Tricuspid atresia
  - Pulmonary atresia
  - Hypoplastic left heart syndrome (part of stage 1 Norwood procedure)

IMAGING

- CTA/MRA: Linear, tubular, contrast-opacified structure connecting subclavian artery to ipsilateral pulmonary artery (usually right sided)
  - Multiplanar & 3D reformations are helpful
- Dark signal intensity within patent shunt on black blood MR sequences
- Complications
  - Stenosis/thrombosis/occlusion
  - Perigraft seroma
  - Pseudoaneurysm

TOP DIFFERENTIAL DIAGNOSES

- Other palliative shunts (Glenn, Waterston, Potts, Sano)

(Left) *Coronal graphic shows a modified Blalock-Taussig (BT) shunt ➔ extending from the right subclavian artery ➔ to the right pulmonary artery ➔. (Note that the superior vena cava has been excluded from the graphic in order to visualize the BT shunt.)* **(Right)** *Frontal conventional angiogram shows a patent BT shunt ➔ originating from the right subclavian artery ➔ & inserting into the confluence ➔ between the right & left pulmonary arteries in a patient with pulmonic atresia.*

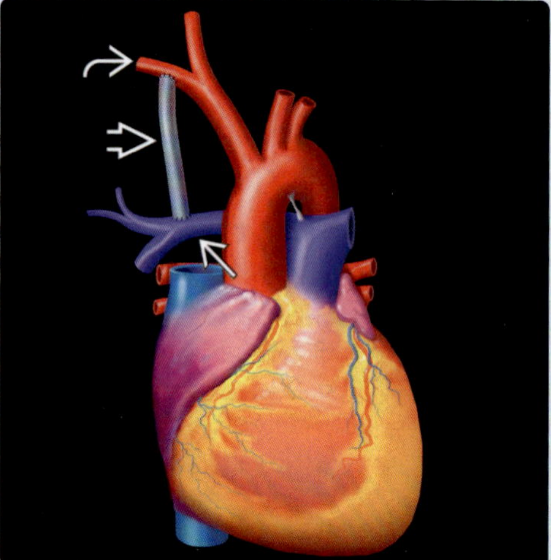

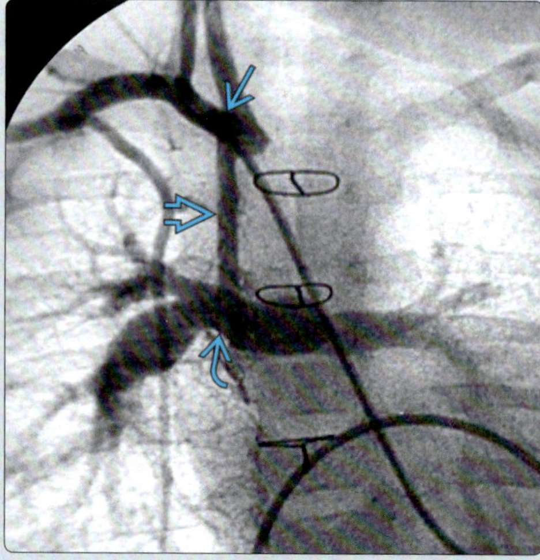

(Left) *Coronal oblique CTA MIP in an infant with tetralogy of Fallot status modified BT shunt ➔ shows the shunt extending between the right brachiocephalic artery ➔ & the proximal right pulmonary artery ➔. Flow may be ↑ to the right lung if there is any narrowing at the confluence between right & left pulmonary arteries.* **(Right)** *Frontal oblique surface-rendered CTA in an infant with tetralogy of Fallot shows a BT shunt (green) extending from the right brachiocephalic artery ➔ to the right main pulmonary artery ➔.*

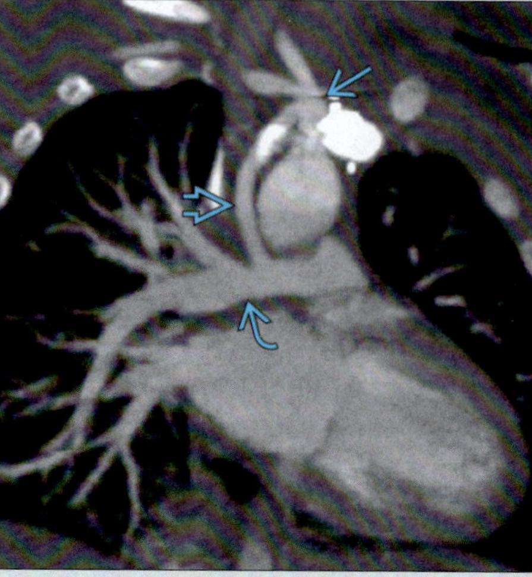

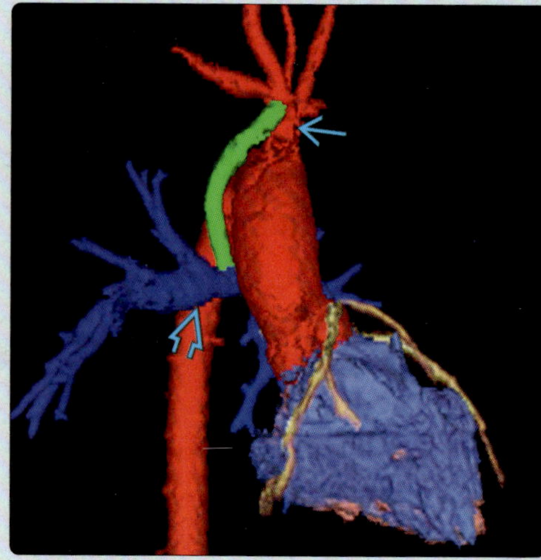

TERMINOLOGY

Abbreviations

- Blalock-Taussig (BT) shunt

Definitions

- Palliative procedure to augment pulmonary blood flow in various uni- & biventricular anatomies: Tetralogy of Fallot, tricuspid atresia, pulmonary atresia, & hypoplastic left heart syndrome (part of Norwood stage 1)
  - Original/classic BT shunt
    - Developed in 1945 by Dr. Alfred Blalock, Dr. Helen Taussig, & Vivien Theodore Thomas
    - Ligation & division of right subclavian artery with end-to-side anastomosis of proximal right subclavian artery to right pulmonary artery
    - Complications included shunt thrombosis, overshunting, nerve injury, & potential growth disturbance of ipsilateral upper extremity
    - Rarely performed today
  - Modified BT shunt
    - Synthetic graft prosthesis (Gore-Tex) between subclavian artery & ipsilateral pulmonary artery, contralateral to side of aortic arch
    - End-to-side anastomosis at each connection is performed through median sternotomy or lateral thoracotomy (with former preferred)
    - Up to 90% patency rate at 2 years of age

IMAGING

General Features

- Complications
  - Thrombosis
    - Can be early or late complication
  - Complete occlusion
    - ~ 10% of cases
    - More common in grafts < 3 mm in size
  - Stenosis, typically near proximal or distal anastomosis
  - Perigraft seroma
    - Complication secondary to leakage of fluid across Gore-Tex graft
  - Pseudoaneurysm

Radiographic Findings

- Typically ↑ pulmonary vascularity compared to pre-BT shunt radiograph
- Postthoracotomy rib changes
- Features of underlying congenital heart disease

CT Findings

- Tubular, contrast-opacified structure (synthetic graft) connecting subclavian artery to ipsilateral pulmonary artery, usually right sided
- Abrupt cut-off is consistent with occlusion or prior takedown in older child
- Filling defect within shunt compatible with thrombosis
- Evaluate for proximal or distal anastomotic stenosis
- Look for associated perigraft seroma or, rarely, pseudoaneurysm (especially if recently stented)
- In patients who have undergone classic BT shunt in past, ipsilateral subclavian artery may be absent

MR Findings

- Tubular structure connecting subclavian artery to ipsilateral pulmonary artery is seen as dark signal intensity structure on black blood sequences
- Contrast-enhanced MRA is best to confirm & characterize thrombus, occlusion, stenosis, pseudoaneurysm, or associated perigraft seroma
- Can quantify flow on phase-contrast sequences

Echocardiographic Findings

- Can evaluate BT shunt for patency & measure gradient across stenosis
- Can evaluate perigraft seroma

Angiographic Findings

- Typically performed for angioplasty with stenting of shunt stenosis or occlusion
- Pseudoaneurysm can develop around stent

Imaging Recommendations

- Best imaging tool
  - CTA/MRA with multiplanar & 3D reformations

DIFFERENTIAL DIAGNOSIS

Other Palliative Shunts

- Glenn shunt
  - Superior vena cava to pulmonary artery
  - Requires low pulmonary vascular resistance
    - Not performed under 3-6 months of age due to high pulmonary vascular resistance
- Waterston shunt
  - Ascending aorta to pulmonary artery
  - No longer performed
    - Congestive heart failure & pulmonary hypertension occur due to excessive pulmonary blood flow
- Potts shunt
  - Descending aorta to left pulmonary artery
  - No longer performed
    - Pulmonary hypertension & pulmonary artery kinking
- Sano shunt
  - Direct shunt between right ventricle & pulmonary artery
  - Performed as part of Norwood stage 1 in lieu of BT shunt in some cases of hypoplastic left heart syndrome
- PDA stent
  - PDA stent may be better tolerated than BT shunt

SELECTED REFERENCES

1. Li D et al: Modified Blalock-Taussig shunt: a single-center experience and follow-up. Heart Surg Forum. 23(1):E053-7, 2020
2. Peña-Trujillo V et al: Mediastinal mass after a Blalock-Taussig shunt: utility of CT angiography. Cardiol Young. 30(5):722-3, 2020
3. Bentham JR et al: Duct stenting versus modified Blalock-Taussig shunt in neonates with duct-dependent pulmonary blood flow: associations with clinical outcomes in a multicenter national study. Circulation. 137(6):581-8, 2018
4. Glatz AC et al: Comparison between patent ductus arteriosus stent and modified Blalock-Taussig shunt as palliation for infants with ductal-dependent pulmonary blood flow: insights from the Congenital Catheterization Research Collaborative. Circulation. 137(6):589-601, 2018
5. Sasikumar N et al: Outcomes of Blalock-Taussig shunts in current era: a single center experience. Congenit Heart Dis. 12(6):808-14, 2017

Amplatzer Occluder Device

KEY FACTS

TERMINOLOGY

- Percutaneous transcatheter occlusion of septal defect or vessel
- 4 varieties
  - Septal occluder (for secundum atrial septal defect)
  - Muscular ventricular septal defect occluder
  - Duct occluder (for patent ductus arteriosus)
  - Vascular plug (for embolization of peripheral arteries & veins)
- Device is made from nitinol mesh & polyester fabric, which provide rapid occlusion & substrate for tissue ingrowth
- Can be repositioned & recaptured during placement

IMAGING

- Requires transesophageal or intracardiac echocardiography as well as fluoroscopic imaging during implantation
- Septal occluder device: 2 radiodense dots define ends of 3- to 4-mm long waist with 2 radiodense discs on either side of waist
- Ductal occluder device: 2 radiodense dots define ends of 5- to 8-mm long waist of device with single radiodense disc on aortic side of waist
- Best visualized with bone windows on CT
- Subsequent MR scanning is safe up to 3.0 Tesla with maximum spatial gradient magnetic field of up to 720 Gauss/cm & maximum specific absorption rate of 3 W/kg for up to 15 minutes

CLINICAL ISSUES

- Very high closure rates (> 95%)
- Requires endocarditis prophylaxis & antiplatelet/anticoagulation therapy for 6 months post implantation
- Early complications: Perforation of vessel or myocardium, thrombus formation, dislodgement/embolization, & percutaneous access site complications
- Late complications: Arrhythmia (most common), thrombosis, cardiac erosion, & infection or endocarditis

(Left) *Lateral radiograph of the chest shows an atrial septal closure device ➙ in an expected location & configuration in a 4-year-old patient with a septum secundum type of atrial septal defect (ASD).* **(Right)** *Axial CECT shows a septal closure device across a secundum-type ASD. Note the 2 central metallic dots ➙ (indicating the ends of the device waist) & the discs on either side of the atrial septum.*

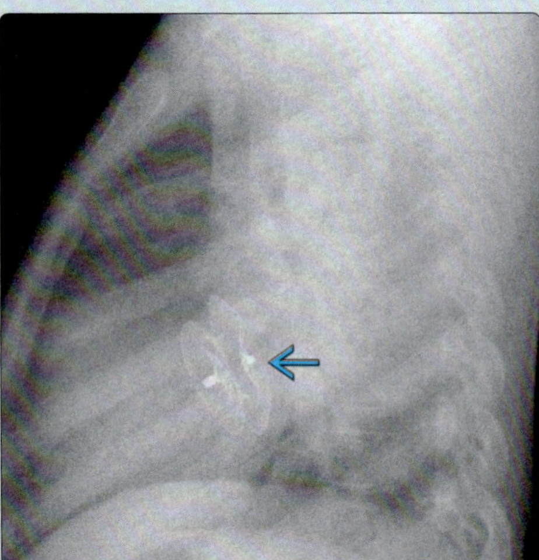

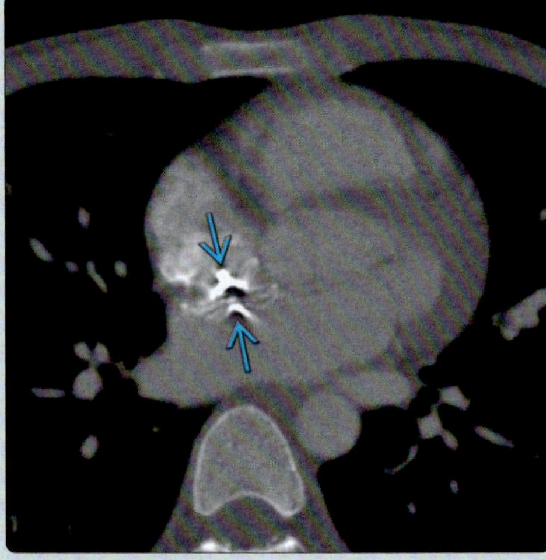

(Left) *Four-chamber cardiac GRE MR shows an atrial septal closure device ➙ in place. Note the signal void in the right atrium ➙ from a small peridevice leak. Also note the enlarged right atrium & ventricle from a longstanding left-to-right shunt in this teenage patient.* **(Right)** *AP radiograph in a 3-year-old immediately after placement of a patent ductus arteriosus (PDA) closure device shows an abnormal location of the device at the right pulmonary artery ➙ after migration (embolization) from the expected left PDA site ➙.*

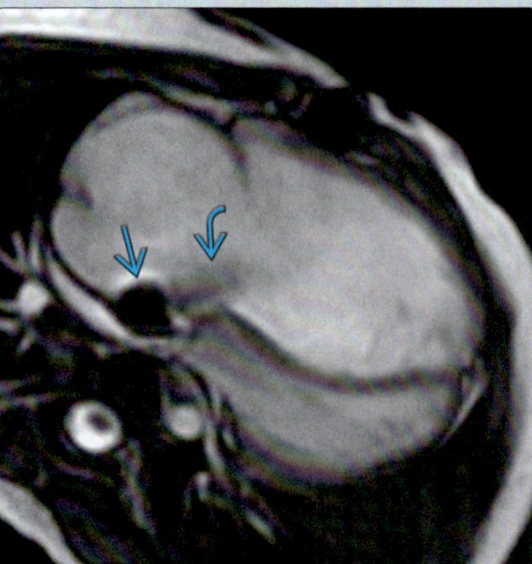

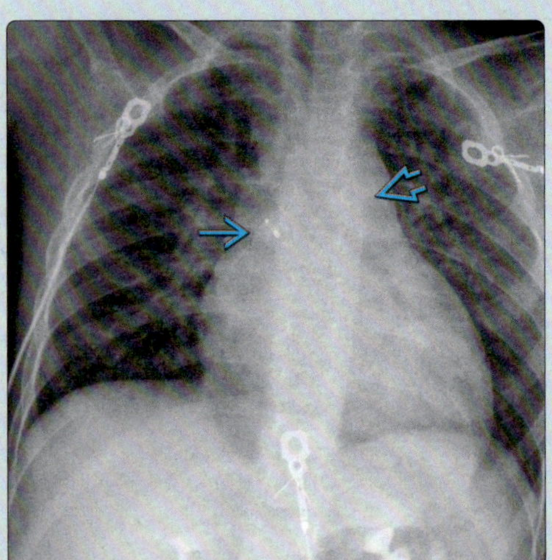

Amplatzer Occluder Device

TERMINOLOGY

Synonyms

- Septal occluder device
- Duct occluder device

Definitions

- Percutaneous, transcatheter occlusion of atrial or ventricular septal defect or vessel
- Invented by Dr. Kurt Amplatz, radiologist
- 4 varieties
  - Septal [atrial septal defect (ASD)] occluder
    - FDA approved in 2001
    - Designed to close atrial septal wall on each side of secundum defect
    - Available in 4- to 38-mm sizes in USA
    - Multifenestrated ASD requires cribriform occluder subtype
  - Muscular [ventricular septal defect (VSD)] occluder
    - Designed to close VSD on each side of defect
    - 2 discs are connected together by waist that corresponds to size of VSD
    - Available in 4- to 18-mm waist sizes
  - Duct occluder
    - Designed to seal patent ductus arteriosus (PDA)
    - Conical shape to conform to PDA
    - Available in 5- to 16-mm diameters
  - Vascular plug
    - Used for embolization of peripheral arteries & veins
    - Alternative to coils
- Device is made from nitinol mesh & polyester fabric, which provide rapid occlusion & substrate for tissue ingrowth
- Sizing balloon is used to determine correct size device
- Requires transesophageal or intracardiac echocardiography as well as fluoroscopic imaging during procedure
- Can be repositioned & recaptured during placement
- Very high closure rates (> 95%)
- Indications for ASD closure device
  - Ostium secundum ASD
  - Clinical evidence of right ventricular (RV) volume overload
    - Left-to-right shunt 1.5:1 ≥, or RV chamber enlargement
- Contraindications
  - Sepsis within 1 month prior to implantation
  - Bleeding disorder or other contraindication to aspirin therapy after device placement
  - Intracardiac thrombi
  - Septal defect location < 5 mm from coronary sinus, atrioventricular valves, or pulmonary vein orifice
  - Nickel allergy (as nitinol contains nickel)
- Follow-up
  - Requires endocarditis prophylaxis & antiplatelet/anticoagulation therapy for 6 months post implantation
  - Devices are "conditional 6" to 3.0 Tesla magnet

IMAGING

General Features

- Complications
  - Early complications include: Perforation of vessel or myocardium, thrombus formation, dislodgement/embolization, & percutaneous access site complications
  - Late complications include: Arrhythmia (most common), thrombosis, cardiac erosion, & infection or endocarditis

Radiographic Findings

- Septal occluder device
  - 2 radiodense dots define ends of 3- to 4-mm long waist of device
  - 2 radiodense flat discs on either side of waist
  - 2 dots & 2 discs may not be visualized on each view depending on projection & overlapping structures
- Ductal occluder device
  - 2 radiodense dots define ends of 5- to 8-mm long waist of device
  - 1 radiodense flat disc on aortic side of waist

CT Findings

- Best visualized on bone windows
- Radiodense dots (at either end of waist) & radiodense flat discs are easily identified

MR Findings

- Device is not evaluated/followed by MR but can be scanned immediately after placement
  - Scanned safely up to 3.0 Tesla with maximum spatial gradient magnetic field of up to 720 Gauss/cm & with maximum specific absorption rate of 3 W/kg for up to 15 minutes
- Will cause susceptibility artifact

Ultrasonographic Findings

- Transesophageal or intracardiac echocardiography is used to monitor implantation & to assess success of ASD closure

Angiographic Findings

- Catheter angiography & fluoroscopy are used to define anatomy & monitor implantation

SELECTED REFERENCES

1. Rao PS: Outcomes of device closure of atrial septal defects. Children (Basel). 7(9), 2020
2. Yasuhara J et al: Comparison of transcatheter patent ductus arteriosus closure between children and adults. Heart Vessels. 35(11):1605-13, 2020
3. Zhang X et al: Transcatheter closure of atrial septal defects with cardiac computed tomography sizing: eight-year single-center practice. Cardiology. 1-9, 2020
4. Jun JH et al: Mitral regurgitation detected during the intraoperative period after atrial septal defect closure: a case report. J Cardiothorac Surg. 14(1):140, 2019
5. Kobayashi D et al: Results of the combined U.S. multicenter postapproval study of the Nit-Occlud PDA device for percutaneous closure of patent ductus arteriosus. Catheter Cardiovasc Interv. 93(4):645-51, 2019
6. Bhatla P et al: Utility and scope of rapid prototyping in patients with complex muscular ventricular septal defects or double-outlet right ventricle: does it alter management decisions? Pediatr Cardiol. 38(1):103-14, 2017

Sano Shunt

KEY FACTS

TERMINOLOGY

- Sano shunt provides alternate source of pulmonary blood flow to modified Blalock-Taussig (BT) shunt in hypoplastic left heart patients undergoing stage 1 Norwood procedure
- Extracardiac conduit between right ventricle & pulmonary artery
  - Small ventriculotomy made in right ventricular outflow tract
  - Conduit is nonvalved, thus allowing free regurgitation
- Typically performed during 1st few days of life
- Benefits
  - Elimination of coronary steal phenomenon secondary to reversal of diastolic flow with modified BT shunt
  - Forward flow through shunt only occurs during systole
  - Improved hemodynamic stability postoperatively compared to modified BT shunt
  - Higher rate of transplantation-free survival at 12 months compared with modified BT shunt

IMAGING

- CECT is useful in immediate postoperative period to assess for complications
- CT can also be used to evaluate status of Sano shunt itself & branch pulmonary arteries
  - Evaluate shunt thrombosis or occlusion
  - Branch pulmonary artery stenoses
  - Aneurysm/pseudoaneurysm at ventriculotomy site
- MR provides comprehensive, ionizing radiation-free evaluation of postoperative anatomy & function
- 3D reconstructions of CTA/MRA are extremely helpful

TOP DIFFERENTIAL DIAGNOSES

- Modified BT shunt

(Left) *Lateral color-coded 3D surface-rendered CTA in an infant shows a Sano shunt ➚ arising from the right ventricle (RV) ➡ in an infant status post stage 1 Norwood procedure. Note the focal narrowing ➡ at the origin of the shunt from the RV. This is designed to control flow.* **(Right)** *Lateral oblique cardiac CTA shows a Sano shunt ➚ extending between the RV chamber ➡ & the pulmonary artery ➡ in a 4-month-old with a history of a Norwood operation for hypoplastic left heart syndrome.*

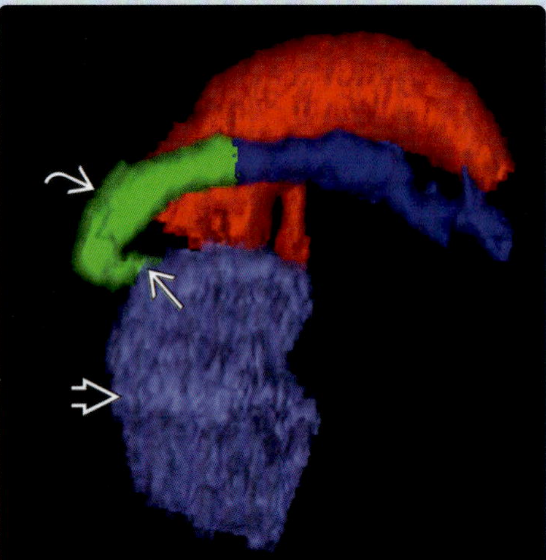

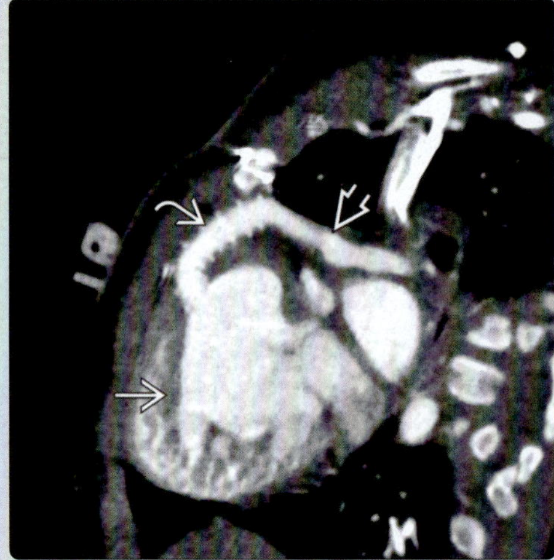

(Left) *Frontal radiographs obtained at 6 (left) & 3 (right) months of age show postoperative changes from a Sano procedure. The more recent radiograph shows a new rounded opacity ➡ along the left mediastinum, which could represent thymic rebound, round pneumonia, or pseudoaneurysm.* **(Right)** *Anterior 3D surface-rendered CTA in the same patient shows a 19-mm pseudoaneurysm ➡ arising from the left aspect of the RV outflow tract ➡. A smaller pseudoaneurysm is also noted on the right ➚.*

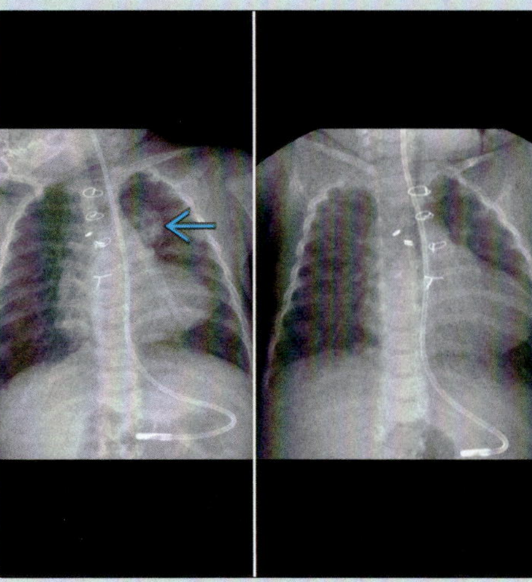

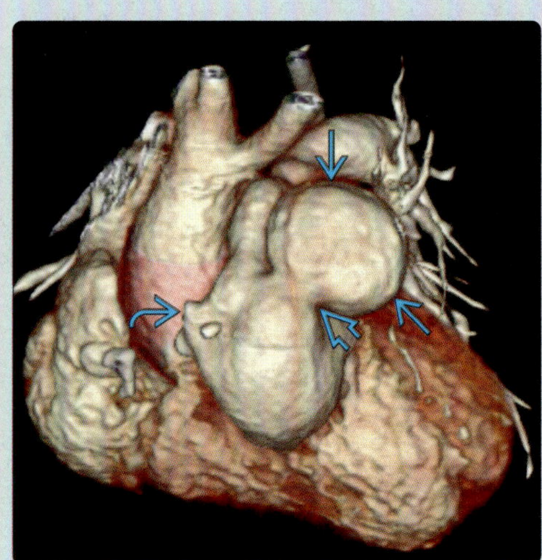

TERMINOLOGY

Synonyms

- Right ventricle-pulmonary artery (RV-PA) conduit

Definitions

- Norwood stage 1 involves using main PA to augment ascending aorta in patients with hypoplastic left heart syndrome (HLHS)
  - New source of pulmonary blood flow is required
    - Blalock-Taussig (BT) shunt provides source of pulmonary blood flow from systemic arterial system
    - BT flow is continuous in both systole & diastole
    - Because ~ 75% of coronary blood flow occurs during diastole, coronary steal phenomenon develops
      - Diastolic retrograde flow occurs in coronaries & descending thoracic aorta
      - Resultant coronary insufficiency is theorized to play major role in operative & postoperative morbidity/mortality of stage 1 Norwood with BT shunt
  - Sano conduit (extracardiac conduit between RV & PA) is alternative to modified BT shunt
    - Small ventriculotomy is made in RV outflow tract
    - 4- to 6-mm synthetic graft is anastomosed to RV & PA to left of neoaorta
    - Conduit is nonvalved, thus allowing free regurgitation
- Typically performed during 1st few days of life
- Stage 2 Norwood (Glenn anastomosis) typically needs to be performed slightly earlier after Sano shunt than with modified BT shunt in 3- to 6-month timeframe
- Benefits
  - Elimination of coronary steal phenomenon secondary to reversal of diastolic flow with modified BT shunt
    - Forward flow through shunt only occurs during systole
  - Improved hemodynamic stability postoperatively compared to modified BT shunt
  - Higher rate of transplantation-free survival at 12 months compared with modified BT shunt
  - Nonrandomized & retrospective studies have shown potential benefit in outcomes associated with RV-PA conduit when compared to modified BT shunt
- One limitation cited in available literature is poor ventricular performance in view of ventriculotomy
  - Current available evidence, although weak, does not show any adverse effects of ventriculotomy on ventricular performance in patients with Sano shunt in short & medium terms

IMAGING

General Features

- Complications
  - Arrhythmias
  - Shunt stenosis/obstruction
  - Shunt thrombosis
  - Branch PA stenoses
  - RV dysfunction
  - Aneurysm/pseudoaneurysm formation at ventriculotomy site
  - Shunt infection & pulmonary embolism
  - May require more extensive PA reconstruction at time of Glenn anastomosis (stage 2 Norwood)

CT Findings

- Useful in immediate postoperative period to assess for complications
  - Mediastinitis
  - Hemorrhage
  - Aneurysm
- Can also be used to evaluate status of Sano shunt itself & branch PAs
- Radiation exposure is concern; however, newer generation scanners can provide requisite information in sub-mSv radiation doses
- 3D reconstructions are extremely helpful

MR Findings

- Comprehensive evaluation of postoperative anatomy & function, without ionizing radiation
- Functional analysis for systemic ventricle
- Phase-contrast imaging can be used to quantify flow in
  - Sano shunt
  - Branch PAs
  - Neoaorta
- Pulmonary:systemic arterial flow ratio (Qp:Qs) can be calculated
- 3D reconstructions are extremely helpful

Echocardiographic Findings

- Duplex Doppler imaging of mid- to distal portion of Sano shunt can provide flow information & evaluation for stenosis
- Proximal anastomosis of shunt & branch PAs may not be adequately visualized in view of poor acoustic windows

DIFFERENTIAL DIAGNOSIS

Modified Blalock-Taussig Shunt

- Synthetic graft connection between subclavian artery & ipsilateral PA as part of stage 1 of Norwood

SELECTED REFERENCES

1. Çelik M et al: Alternate approach to hypoplastic left heart syndrome stage 1 surgery. Ann Thorac Surg. 111(3):e173-5, 2021
2. Gong CL et al: Impact of confounding on cost, survival, and length-of-stay outcomes for neonates with hypoplastic left heart syndrome undergoing stage 1 palliation surgery. Pediatr Cardiol. 41(5):996-1011, 2020
3. Ismail MF et al: Evolution of the Norwood operation outcomes in patients with late presentation. J Thorac Cardiovasc Surg. 159(3):1040-8, 2020
4. Carreon CK et al: Pathology of valved venous homografts used as right ventricle-to-pulmonary artery conduits in congenital heart disease surgery. J Thorac Cardiovasc Surg. 157(1):342-50.e3, 2019
5. Briceno-Medina M et al: Femoral vein homograft as Sano shunt results in improved pulmonary artery growth after Norwood operation. Cardiol Young. 28(1):118-25, 2018
6. Said SM et al: Norwood valved Sano shunt: early reward versus late penalty? J Thorac Cardiovasc Surg. 155(4):1756-7, 2018

Myocarditis

KEY FACTS

IMAGING

- Chest radiograph: Many cases are normal
  - Cardiomegaly &/or pericardial effusion in setting of cardiac dysfunction
  - Pulmonary edema in more severe cases
- Echocardiography: Often 1st imaging, identifies cardiac dysfunction &/or pericardial effusion
- Cardiac MR: Increasingly utilized for diagnostic capabilities
  - Cardiac volumes & functional assessment: ↓ ejection fraction with wall motion abnormality, ± pericardial effusion
  - Myocardial tissue characterization (edema, hyperemia, & fibrosis): ↑ T2 signal, early & late gadolinium enhancement, native T1 values > 990 ms
  - ≥ 2 positive criteria in acute phase: 80% sensitivity, 90% specificity
- Cardiac catheterization & endomyocardial biopsy: Historic gold standard (but invasive & can miss patchy inflammation)

PATHOLOGY

- Infectious etiology (typically viral) most common in otherwise healthy individuals
  - Postinfectious immune mediated: MIS-C from SARS-CoV-2, Kawasaki
- Toxins/drug reactions: Antibiotics, antiepileptics, carbon monoxide, illegal drugs (cocaine)
- Autoimmune: Lupus, sarcoidosis, Takayasu arteritis
- Ischemic: Acute coronary syndrome/myocardial infarction

CLINICAL ISSUES

- Nonspecific symptoms: Fever, fatigue, malaise, dyspnea, muscle aches, & unexplained sinus tachycardia
- May imitate acute myocardial infarction
- Rarely, fulminant with cardiovascular collapse & shock
- May account for 10% of sudden death in young
- Most cases: Mild symptoms, need only supportive care

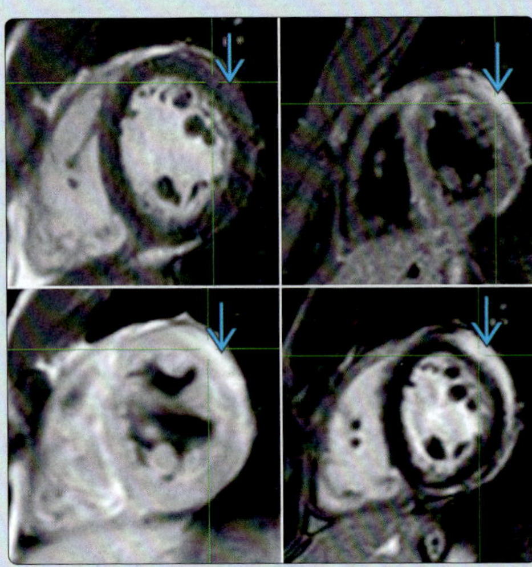

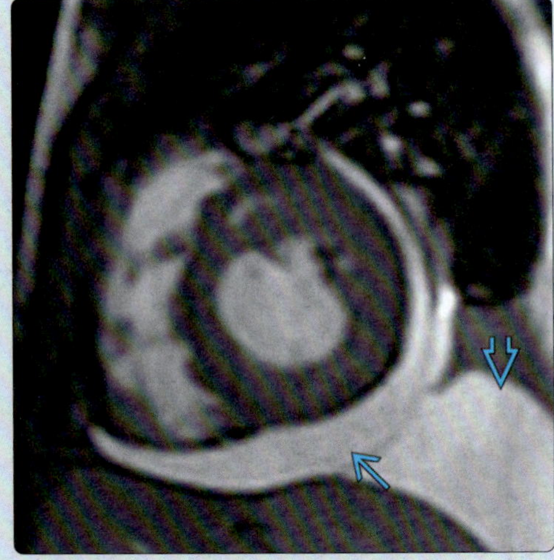

(Left) *Short-axis MR tissue characterization in myocarditis: A region of interest with ↑ signal is seen in the anterolateral segment* ➙ *on SSFP (upper left), T2 (upper right), early gadolinium (lower left), & late gadolinium (lower right) enhancement images.* **(Right)** *Short-axis SSFP cine MR in a patient with known myocarditis shows a moderate-sized pericardial effusion* ➙*. Also note the pleural effusion* ➙*.*

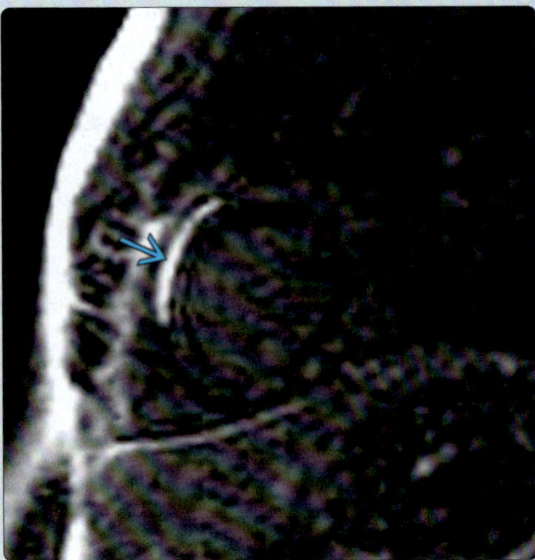

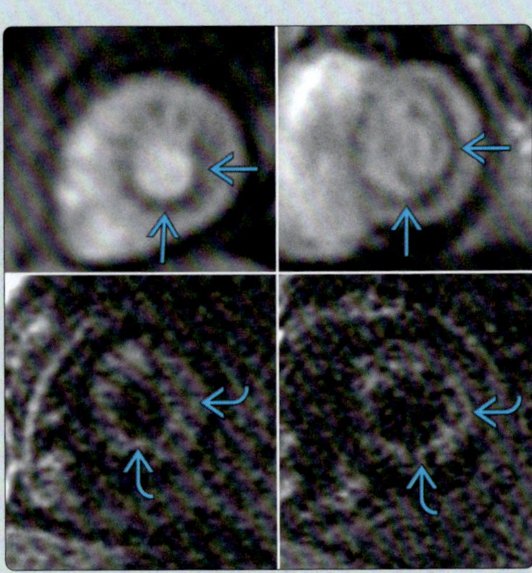

(Left) *Delayed short-axis image from a cardiac MR perfusion shows delayed enhancement* ➙ *in the midmyocardium of the interventricular septum of the left ventricle.* **(Right)** *Short-axis cardiac perfusion MR from an adolescent patient show changes of myocarditis. Immediate dynamic postcontrast images (top) show ↓ uptake* ➙ *circumferentially in the endocardium extending into the myocardium. Delayed enhancement* ➙ *is shown on delayed images (bottom) in the same distribution.*

TERMINOLOGY

Definitions

- Inflammation of myocardium with edema, hyperemia, & fibrosis, often leading to cardiac dysfunction & pericardial effusion
  - Clinical symptoms are often nonspecific

IMAGING

Radiographic Findings

- Chest radiograph findings vary based on severity
  - Many cases are normal
  - Cardiomegaly &/or pericardial effusion in setting of cardiac dysfunction
  - Severe cases show interstitial &/or alveolar pulmonary edema

MR Findings

- T2WI
  - Triple inversion recovery (with inversion pulses for fat & blood) show ↑ T2 signal
    - Quantitative analysis of signal intensity is more sensitive
      - Identification of edema throughout myocardium
    - Limited sensitivity in mild cases
- T1WI C+
  - Early gadolinium enhancement (EGE)
    - Hyperemia & capillary leak show enhancement 1 minute post gadolinium
  - Late gadolinium enhancement (LGE)
    - Fibrosis & necrosis
      - May be irreversible
    - Differentiates ischemic injury (always subendocardial) from nonischemic injury
- Native T1 mapping demonstrates location, extent, & pattern of myocarditis
  - Threshold of T1 > 990 ms (sensitivity & specificity ~ 90%) detects significantly larger areas of involvement than T2 & LGE

Echocardiographic Findings

- Often 1st imaging performed; neither sensitive nor specific
  - Mild cases: ↓ function ± wall motion abnormalities, ± pericardial effusion
  - Moderate to severe cases: ↓ function with associated wall motion abnormalities, left ventricular chamber dilation, ↑ wall thickness, ± pericardial effusion

Imaging Recommendations

- Best imaging tool
  - Cardiac MR: Functional assessment with myocardial tissue characterization
- Protocol advice
  - SSFP 2-chamber, 3-chamber, 4-chamber, & short-axis stack
  - Tissue characterization with precontrast T2 3-slice short-axis (edema) & postcontrast 3-slice short-axis EGE (hyperemia) & LGE (fibrosis)
  - Native T1 values: Most accurate detection of myocarditis

PATHOLOGY

General Features

- Etiology
  - Infectious etiology is most common if otherwise healthy
    - Direct viral infection of myocardium: Coxsackie B virus, adenovirus, parvovirus B19, echoviruses, EBV
      - May see dystrophic Ca^{2+} in neonates with enteroviral myocarditis
    - Immune-mediated postinfectious reaction
      - Kawasaki disease
      - MIS-C from SARS-CoV-2
    - Chagas disease: *Trypanosoma cruzi* (Central & South America)
  - Other causes
    - Toxins/drug reactions: Antibiotics, antiepileptics, carbon monoxide, illegal drugs (cocaine)
    - Autoimmune: Lupus, Takayasu arteritis, granulomatosis with polyangiitis, giant cell arteritis

Microscopic Features

- Endomyocardial biopsy in severe cases when definitive diagnosis is required, otherwise not recommended
  - Histopathology shows infiltration of inflammatory cells
  - Immunohistochemistry: Best sensitivity but less available
  - Viral genome analysis: PCR for most common viruses

CLINICAL ISSUES

Presentation

- Most common signs/symptoms
  - Often nonspecific with fatigue, dyspnea, muscle aches, unexplained tachycardia, or ventricular ectopy
- Other signs/symptoms
  - Many cases are asymptomatic; no medical care sought
  - May imitate acute myocardial infarction
  - Rarely fulminant with cardiovascular collapse & shock
  - Infants & small children: Dyspnea, poor feeding, & fever
    - Mistaken for reactive airway disease or pneumonia
  - ~ 10% of sudden cardiac deaths in young

Treatment

- Most cases have mild symptoms, need only supportive care
- With cardiac dysfunction, treatment is similar to other causes of heart failure
  - Drugs that stimulate heart should be avoided
  - Complete heart block requires temporary pacing
- Intravenous immunoglobulin: Variable results

SELECTED REFERENCES

1. Gottlieb M et al: Multisystem inflammatory syndrome in children with COVID-19. Am J Emerg Med. 49:148-52, 2021
2. Liguori C et al: Myocarditis: imaging up to date. Radiol Med. 125(11):1124-34, 2020
3. McMurray JC et al: Multisystem inflammatory syndrome in children (MIS-C), a post-viral myocarditis and systemic vasculitis-a critical review of its pathogenesis and treatment. Front Pediatr. 8:626182, 2020
4. Bière L et al: Imaging of myocarditis and inflammatory cardiomyopathies. Arch Cardiovasc Dis. 112(10):630-41, 2019
5. Dasgupta S et al: Myocarditis in the pediatric population: a review. Congenit Heart Dis. 14(5):868-77, 2019
6. O'Connor MJ: Imaging the itis: endocarditis, myocarditis, and pericarditis. Curr Opin Cardiol. 34(1):57-64, 2019

Left Ventricular Noncompaction

KEY FACTS

TERMINOLOGY

- Left ventricular noncompaction cardiomyopathy (LVNC): Cardiomyopathy characterized by sponge-like appearance of left ventricular (LV) myocardium
  - 2-layer appearance: Heavily trabeculated, noncompacted (NC) layer & thin, dense compacted (C) layer
  - NC:C ratio > 2.3:1 is strongly suggestive
- Controversial diagnosis due to lack of definitive criteria & variable prognostic data
  - ↑ in diagnosis has occurred with improved echocardiogram & MR imaging quality
- Primitive appearance of myocardium suggests potential arrest in fetal LV myocardial development
  - LVNC is also seen in association with other cardiomyopathies & congenital heart disease

IMAGING

- Echocardiography is widely used
- CMR defines location & extent of trabeculations, ventricular volumes & ejection fraction, fibrosis (with late gadolinium enhancement), & apical thrombus
- Multitude of imaging "criteria" have been proposed; however, varying results of imaging findings compared to prognostic data

CLINICAL ISSUES

- Highly variable clinical presentations are described, ranging from completely asymptomatic to symptomatic with heart failure, cardioembolic events, & ventricular arrhythmias
  - Mural thrombus develops within deep trabeculations of LV → significant risk factor for cardioembolic events
- Predictors of prognosis may include number of affected segments, heart failure at presentation, & ventricular arrhythmias
- Treat/prevent: Heart failure, ventricular arrhythmias, & embolic stroke

(Left) *Frontal view of the chest in a child presenting with shortness of breath shows bilateral interstitial pulmonary edema with cardiomegaly. The patient was ultimately diagnosed with left ventricular noncompaction cardiomyopathy (LVNC).* **(Right)** *Short-axis SSFP cine from a cardiac MR shows hypertrabeculated left ventricular myocardium ➲ in a patient presenting in heart failure. A thin, peripheral, compacted layer ➔ is noted.*

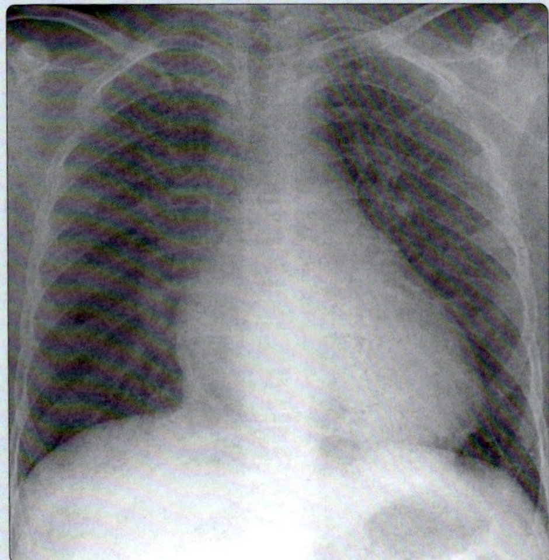

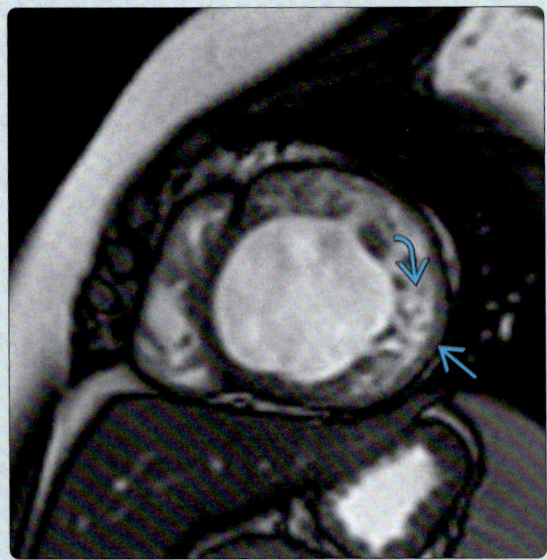

(Left) *Short-axis SSFP MR in end-diastole demonstrates marked left ventricular hypertrabeculation of the noncompacted layer ⇨ & a thin, dense appearance of the compacted layer ➔ in a patient with LVNC.* **(Right)** *Four-chamber SSFP MR shows marked left ventricular hypertrabeculation of the noncompacted layer ⇨ & a thin, dense, compacted layer ➔ in a patient with LVNC. Also note the hypertrabeculated right ventricle (RV) ➡, suggesting biventricular NC.*

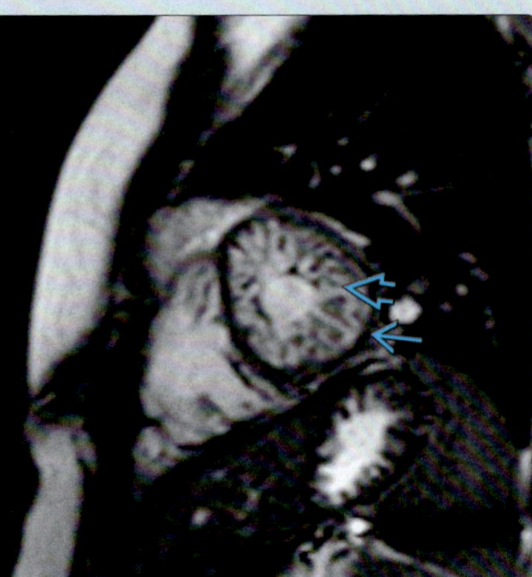

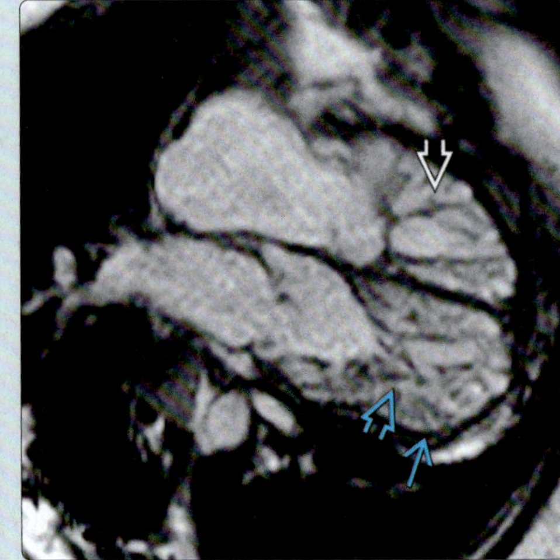

Left Ventricular Noncompaction

TERMINOLOGY

Abbreviations

- Left ventricular noncompaction cardiomyopathy (LVNC)

Synonyms

- Noncompacted left ventricle (NCLV), left ventricular hypertrabeculation, spongy myocardium

Definitions

- Inherited cardiomyopathy characterized by extensive hypertrabeculation of left ventricular (LV) myocardium
- 2-layer appearance of LV with sponge-like noncompacted (NC) inner layer & thinner, dense compacted (C) outer layer
- Primitive appearance of myocardium suggests potential arrest in fetal LV myocardial development

IMAGING

General Features

- Best diagnostic clue
  - LV myocardium in 2 layers: Thick, hypertrabeculated inner layer (NC) & thin, dense outer layer (C)
  - NC:C thickness ratio > 2.3:1 in patients with LVNC
- Location
  - Typically, LV has coalescent pattern in inferior & lateral segments of apical & midregions; rare in basal region
  - Normally RV is somewhat trabeculated; can be heavily trabeculated in severe LVNC

Radiographic Findings

- Cardiomegaly in patients with heart failure

MR Findings

- SSFP cine
  - 2-, 3-, & 4-chamber views & short-axis stacks are best sequences to locate segment distribution & extent of trabeculations
  - NC:C thickness ratio > 2.3:1 is strongly suggestive; measured in end-systole or end-diastole
  - ↑ LV end-diastolic volume (EDV): Contours performed on compacted layer in end-diastole
  - ↓ LV ejection fraction: Challenging to contour in end-systole due to heavy trabeculations coalescing
  - Can determine trabecular mass vs. total mass ratio
- Delayed enhancement
  - Myocardial fibrosis assessment by late gadolinium enhancement (LGE)
    - Difficult to accurately depict given deep trabeculations
      - Requires multiple slice planes
    - ± wall motion abnormalities if LGE is positive

Echocardiographic Findings

- Primary diagnostic modality; 3 descriptions
  - Minor trabeculation: Prominent trabeculation in posteroapical LV in noncoalescent pattern; NC:C ratio < 2.3
  - Major trabeculation: Prominent trabeculation in posteroapical LV in coalescent pattern; NC:C ratio < 2.3
  - Noncompaction: Prominent trabeculation in posteroapical LV in coalescent pattern; NC:C ratio > 2.3
- Color Doppler demonstrates flow within trabeculations & communication with ventricular cavity
- Evaluate for septal defects, apical thrombus, LV systolic &/or diastolic dysfunction

Imaging Recommendations

- Best imaging tool
  - Cardiac MR with SSFP 2-, 3-, & 4-chamber views & short-axis stack; LGE for fibrosis
- Protocol advice
  - Artifact from parallel imaging may obscure trabeculations; best images are without parallel imaging

DIFFERENTIAL DIAGNOSIS

Normal With Prominent Trabeculations

- Likely normal if NC:C ratio is < 2.3, noncoalescent trabecular pattern, normal ejection fraction & LV EDV, absence of symptoms

Dilated Cardiomyopathy

- Hypertrophy of cardiac trabeculations can imitate noncompaction; cardiac apex is not involved in dilated cardiomyopathy

Hypertrophic Cardiomyopathy

- Most commonly seen in apical hypertrophic cardiomyopathy (HCM); ↑ myocardial mass in HCM compared to LVNC

CLINICAL ISSUES

Presentation

- Most common signs/symptoms
  - Tachypnea due to low cardiac output or heart failure
    - Infants & small children with tachypnea, cyanosis, acute life-threatening event, or failure to thrive
    - Older patients with exertional dyspnea
  - Tachyarrhythmias; most have ECG abnormalities
  - Cardioembolic event

Demographics

- Familial in ~ 50%
- Sex: M > F, 3:2 ratio

Natural History & Prognosis

- Variable natural history & prognostic data → controversy in diagnosis
- Predictors of prognosis may include heart failure at presentation, systolic/diastolic dysfunction, thromboembolic events, & ventricular arrhythmias

Treatment

- Aimed at preventing/treating heart failure, ventricular arrhythmias, & stroke; new therapies target LV remodeling

SELECTED REFERENCES

1. Di Fusco SA et al: Left ventricular noncompaction: diagnostic approach, prognostic evaluation, and management strategies. Cardiol Rev. 28(3):125-34, 2020
2. Rao K et al: The role of multimodality imaging in the diagnosis of left ventricular noncompaction. Eur J Clin Invest. 50(9):e13254, 2020
3. Fennira S et al: [Left ventricular non-compaction: what should be known!.] Ann Cardiol Angeiol (Paris). 68(2):120-4, 2019
4. Wengrofsky P et al: Left ventricular trabeculation and noncompaction cardiomyopathy: a review. EC Clin Exp Anat. 2(6):267-83, 2019

Hypertrophic Cardiomyopathy

KEY FACTS

TERMINOLOGY

- Familial cardiomyopathy is characterized by thickened but nondilated LV & no identifiable systemic or cardiac cause
- Most common genetic cardiomyopathy (1 in 500)

IMAGING

- Echocardiography is primary diagnostic/screening tool
- Cardiac MR is utilized for ventricular dimensions, LVOT obstruction, & late gadolinium enhancement (LGE)
  - Asymmetric septal hypertrophy, typically of basal septum
    - Septal wall thickness > 15 mm (or > 13 mm with positive family history)
    - > 30 mm is risk factor for sudden cardiac death (SCD)
  - Dynamic LVOT obstruction
    - Severe thickening of septum during systole causes midcavitary obstruction
    - Systolic anterior motion of mitral valve
  - Systolic & diastolic dysfunction are variable
  - Patchy or focal LGE (from fibrosis) of basal & midventricle septal segments
    - Risk factor for ventricular arrhythmia & SCD

PATHOLOGY

- Primary: Typically autosomal dominant inheritance
- Secondary: Associated with syndromic, neuromuscular, & metabolic disorders
- Idiopathic: ~ 50% of affected children < 1 year old

CLINICAL ISSUES

- Typical symptoms include dyspnea, chest pain, or syncope, typically with exertion
  - Ventricular arrhythmias are common
  - Increasing intensity in systolic heart murmur with Valsalva, positional change (standing/squatting), or exercise
  - Leading cause of SCD in youth
- Treatments include β-blockers, antiarrhythmics, pacemaker, septal ablation, myomectomy

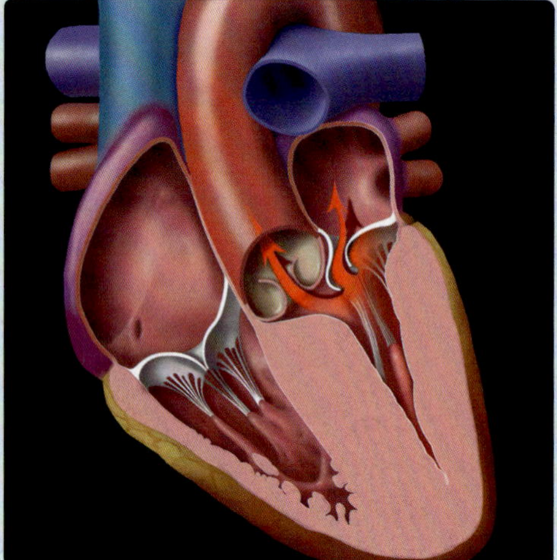

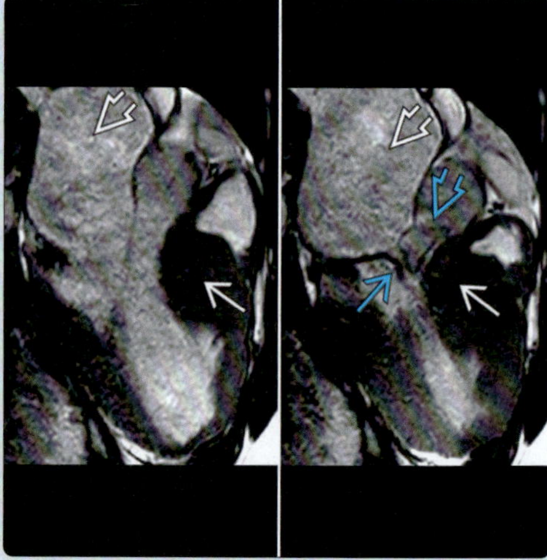

(Left) *Five-chamber graphic demonstrates concentric hypertrophic obstructive cardiomyopathy. Septal hypertrophy & systolic anterior motion (SAM) of the mitral valve leaflet combine to cause left ventricular outflow tract (LVOT) obstruction & mitral regurgitation.* **(Right)** *Three-chamber SSFP MRs during diastole (left) & systole (right) demonstrate LVOT obstruction ➱ from severe septal hypertrophy ➱ & SAM of the mitral valve apparatus ➱. Also note the left atrial enlargement ➱.*

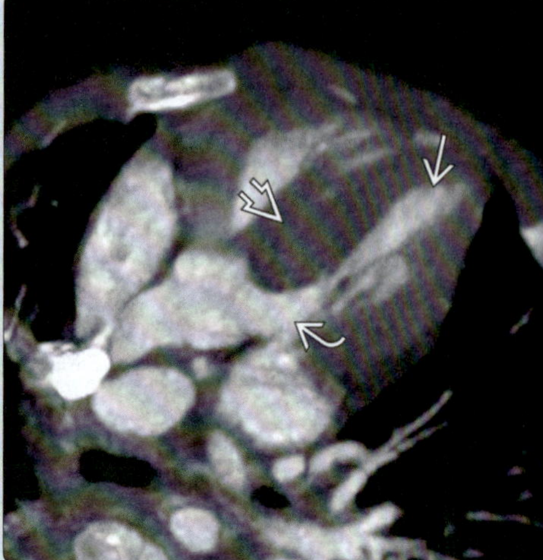

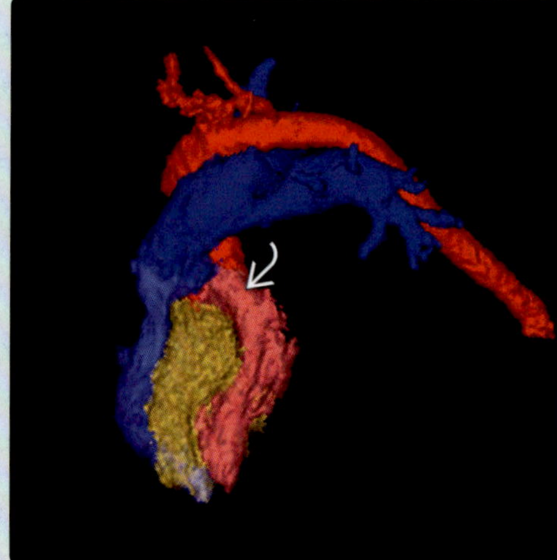

(Left) *Four-chamber view of the heart from a cardiac CTA shows a small left ventricular cavity ➔ with asymmetric septal hypertrophy ➱ & narrowing of the LVOT ➱.* **(Right)** *Lateral oblique surface-rendered color-coded image from a cardiac CTA shows a small left ventricular cavity (pink) with septal hypertrophy (gold) & mild narrowing of the LVOT ➱.*

TERMINOLOGY

Abbreviations

- Hypertrophic cardiomyopathy (HCM)

Synonyms

- Idiopathic hypertrophic subaortic stenosis, hypertrophic obstructive cardiomyopathy

Definitions

- Familial cardiomyopathy with thickening of left ventricular (LV) myocardium without other cardiac or systemic disease; typically involves ventricular septum

IMAGING

General Features

- Best diagnostic clue
  - Significant thickening of LV myocardium, typically septal
    - Diastolic wall thickness ratio: Thickest/thinnest > 2.0
- Location
  - Most common: Anteroseptal portion of basal LV
  - Less common: Concentric/symmetric or apical
- Morphology
  - 3 types: Asymmetric septal, concentric, or apical

Radiographic Findings

- Typically normal chest radiograph
- Left atrial dilation with mitral regurgitation, diastolic issues
- Cardiomegaly is evident in later stages with chamber dilation

MR Findings

- SSFP cine
  - 3-chamber, 4-chamber, & short-axis stack are best sequences for ventricular dimensions & ejection fraction
  - Asymmetric septal hypertrophy, typically basal septum
    - Septal wall thickness > 15 mm (or > 13 mm with positive family history)
    - LV thickness > 30 mm: Risk factor for sudden cardiac death (SCD)
  - Mechanism of LV outflow tract (LVOT) obstruction
    - Severe septal thickening → midcavitary obstruction
    - Systolic anterior motion of mitral valve apparatus → anterior leaflet & chordae are pulled into LVOT via Venturi effect
- Myocardial late gadolinium enhancement (LGE)
  - Patchy LGE (from fibrosis) with occasional focal areas (anteroseptal > inferoseptal)
    - Positive LGE = poor prognostic indicator

Imaging Recommendations

- Best imaging tool
  - Echocardiography: Primary diagnostic/screening tool
    - Better for diastolic dysfunction & LVOT gradient
  - Cardiac MR: Secondary diagnostic/prognostic tool
    - Better for ventricular wall dimensions & fibrosis

DIFFERENTIAL DIAGNOSIS

Secondary Left Ventricular Hypertrophy

- Typically concentric
- Due to hypertension, aortic stenosis, coarctation

Athlete's Heart (Physiologic Hypertrophy)

- LV cavity size is near normal or mildly ↑ (> 55 mm)

Left Ventricular Noncompaction

- Inner thick trabecular (noncompacted) myocardial layer + thin outer compacted layer
- Similar genetic abnormalities to HCM

PATHOLOGY

General Features

- Genetics
  - Familial form is typically autosomal dominant (AD) with de novo mutations making up small percentage of cases
  - 70% of genes involved in HCM encode β-myosin heavy chain & myosin-binding protein C; remaining in troponin T or I, α-actin, or multiple other genes

Staging, Grading, & Classification

- Primary: Familial HCM (AD inheritance)
- Secondary: Syndromic, neuromuscular, & metabolic
- Idiopathic: ~ 50% of affected children < 1 year of age

CLINICAL ISSUES

Presentation

- Most common signs/symptoms
  - Asymptomatic (often discovered via family history)
  - Physical exam: Systolic heart murmur that ↑ in intensity with position changes (squatting), Valsalva, or exercise; prominent LV apical impulse
  - Red flags: Exertional symptoms, including dyspnea, chest pain, or syncope; arrhythmias (typically ventricular)
  - SCD: Most common cause in children is HCM

Demographics

- Ethnicity
  - Black > White or Latino
- Epidemiology
  - Most common genetic heart disease (1:500)
  - Most common childhood cardiomyopathy (42%)

Natural History & Prognosis

- Variable clinical course with 1% annual mortality

Treatment

- Medical management
  - β-adrenergic blocking agents limit heart rate at baseline & with exertion
  - Antiarrhythmics reduce potential for arrhythmic events
- Invasive: Pacemaker, septal ablation, myomectomy

SELECTED REFERENCES

1. Huang G et al: Apical variant hypertrophic cardiomyopathy "multimodality imaging evaluation". Int J Cardiovasc Imaging. 36(3):553-61, 2020
2. Tower-Rader A et al: Multimodality imaging in hypertrophic cardiomyopathy for risk stratification. Circ Cardiovasc Imaging. 13(2):e009026, 2020
3. Guido V et al: [Role of multimodality imaging in the clinical evaluation of hypertrophic cardiomyopathy.] G Ital Cardiol (Rome). 20(12):746-61, 2019
4. Makavos G et al: Hypertrophic cardiomyopathy: an updated review on diagnosis, prognosis, and treatment. Heart Fail Rev. 24(4):439-59, 2019

Duchenne Muscular Dystrophy-Related Cardiomyopathy

KEY FACTS

TERMINOLOGY

- Dystrophin-associated inherited disorders with progressive muscle wasting & weakness

IMAGING

- Cardiac MR (CMR) is important for early detection of Duchenne muscular dystrophy (DMD)-associated cardiomyopathy
  - Initially, normal function with normal ejection fraction (EF)
  - Late gadolinium enhancement (LGE) from fibrosis in left ventricle (LV), typically in inferolateral segments
  - ↓ EF over time with progressive LV dilation
  - CMR allows much earlier detection of cardiac involvement than echocardiography

PATHOLOGY

- Dystrophinopathies
  - DMD: Absent dystrophin
  - Becker MD: Abnormal/reduced dystrophin
- X-linked disorders occurring in males
- Dystrophin is large, sarcolemmal glycoprotein connecting actin filaments & extracellular matrix
- Dystrophin plays role in stabilizing plasma membranes
  - Absence, reduction, or dysfunction → sarcolemmal fragility → myocyte degeneration & death
  - End result is fibrosis & myocardial dysfunction

CLINICAL ISSUES

- In past, DMD patients often died of respiratory complications; improved respiratory therapy → more cardiac complications
- Patients are often asymptomatic until late in heart failure (as immobility from skeletal muscle weakness obscures typical symptoms of heart failure)

DIAGNOSTIC CHECKLIST

- LGE is usually subepicardial in inferolateral segments
- Myocardial dysfunction is progressive

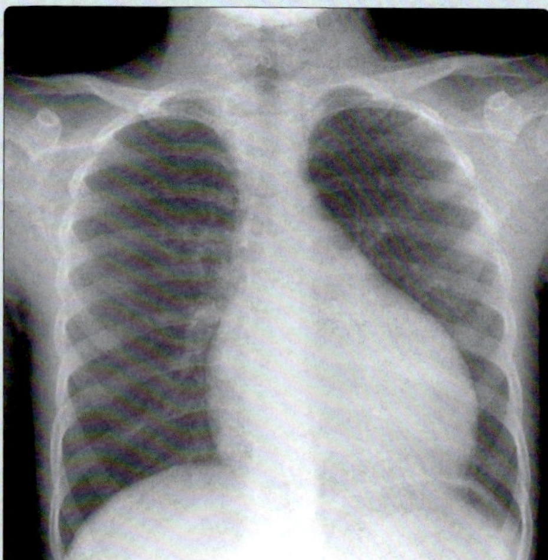

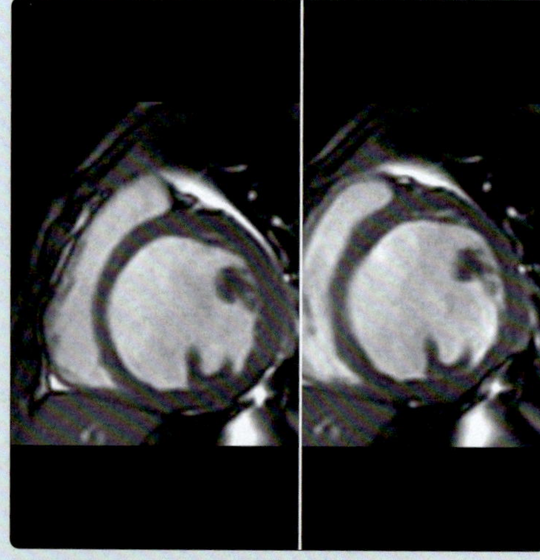

(Left) *Frontal radiograph of the chest in a patient with known Duchenne muscular dystrophy (DMD) shows moderate cardiomegaly. Patients with DMD may develop a severe dilated cardiomyopathy.* **(Right)** *Short-axis SSFP cine bright blood MR images at end-systole (left) & end-diastole (right) show a dilated left ventricle in this patient with end-stage dilated cardiomyopathy due to DMD. Findings are consistent with very poor function, as shown by the depressed ejection fraction (EF).*

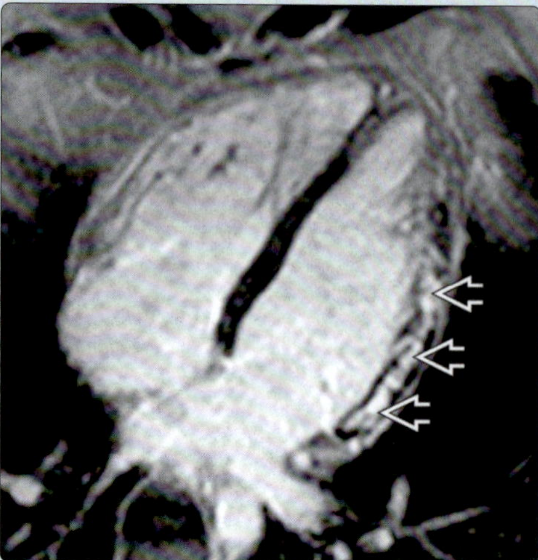

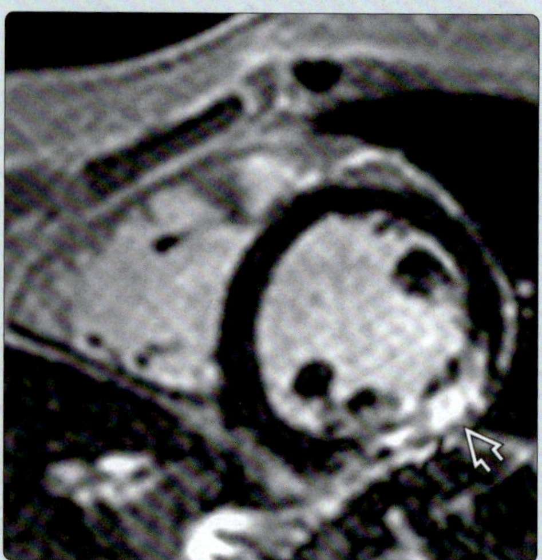

(Left) *Four-chamber late gadolinium enhancement (LGE) MR in the myocardium of a 19-year-old man with DMD shows intense, well-defined enhancement of fibrosis ➲ in the inferolateral wall. The enhancement is usually less intense & patchy.* **(Right)** *Short-axis midventricle LGE MR performed using 3D phase-sensitive inversion recovery, shows LGE ➲ of fibrosis located in the inferolateral wall, which is a typical pattern seen in DMD.*

TERMINOLOGY

Abbreviations

- Duchenne muscular dystrophy (DMD)

Definitions

- Dystrophin-associated inherited disorders with progressive muscle wasting & weakness

IMAGING

General Features

- Best diagnostic clue
  - Muscle biopsy or genetics to confirm DMD prior to presenting for cardiac imaging
  - Subepicardial late gadolinium enhancement (LGE) in left ventricle (LV) inferolateral wall
  - ↓ ejection fraction (EF)

Echocardiographic Findings

- Used to follow ventricular size & function
  - Limited due to lung artifact, pectus deformity, scoliosis, ↑ fat due to steroids

MR Findings

- Progressive LV dysfunction develops over time
  - Initially, normal function with normal EF
  - LGE in LV, typically in inferolateral segments
    - Can occur with normal EF or ↓ EF
  - ↓ EF over time with progressive LV dilation

Imaging Recommendations

- Best imaging tool
  - Cardiac MR (CMR) with LGE assessment
    - Much more reproducible than echocardiography
    - Typical short-axis cine bright blood stack for LV function & volume
    - LGE can detect areas of damaged myocardium
      - Often precursor to more rapid decline in function
    - Specialized strain analysis utilizing tracking or tagging techniques can detect LV dysfunction before EF ↓
    - CMR provides prognostic information
- Protocol advice
  - Perform standard functional analysis, which provides left ventricular end-diastolic volume, end-systolic volume, EF, & myocardial mass
  - LGE is performed in short-axis plane at minimum
    - 2-chamber, 3-chamber, & 4-chamber LGE images are very helpful

DIFFERENTIAL DIAGNOSIS

Cardiomyopathy of Other Causes

- Acute viral myocarditis
- Hypertrophic cardiomyopathy
- Noncompaction cardiomyopathy

PATHOLOGY

General Features

- Etiology
  - Dystrophinopathies: DMD with absent dystrophin; Becker MD (BMD) with abnormal/reduced dystrophin
    - X-linked disorders occurring in males
    - Dystrophin: Large, sarcolemmal glycoprotein connecting actin filaments & extracellular matrix
    - Dystrophin plays role in stabilizing plasma membranes
      - Anecdotally described as shock absorber
      - Dystrophin absence or dysfunction → sarcolemmal fragility → myocyte degeneration & death
      - End result is fibrosis & myocardial dysfunction

CLINICAL ISSUES

Presentation

- Most common signs/symptoms
  - In past, DMD patients often died of respiratory complications; improved respiratory therapy → more cardiac complications
  - Often no heart failure symptoms until later due to immobility from skeletal muscle weakness
  - Nearly all dystrophinopathy patients develop cardiomyopathy by 3rd decade
  - Death is typically related to cardiopulmonary complications in 3rd decade
  - CMR is important for early detection of DMD-associated cardiomyopathy
    - Provides prognostic information
    - CMR allows much earlier detection of cardiac involvement than echocardiography
    - Cardioprotective medical therapies slow progression

Demographics

- Age
  - Progressive muscle weakness manifests in childhood with ambulation (Gower sign)
  - Loss of ambulation by teenage years
    - 50% by 8-10 years of age
  - By 20 years of age, nearly all have dilated cardiomyopathy
- Sex
  - X-linked disorder afflicting males
- Epidemiology
  - Incidence of 1 in 3,500 males

Natural History & Prognosis

- DMD has more rapid skeletal myopathy than BMD
- BMD experience worse cardiomyopathy than DMD
- Cardiomyopathy is progressive but can be modified by medical therapies that improve quality of life & survival

SELECTED REFERENCES

1. Lee S et al: The role of imaging in characterizing the cardiac natural history of Duchenne muscular dystrophy. Pediatr Pulmonol. 56(4):766-81, 2021
2. Sanchez F et al: Cardiac MR imaging of muscular dystrophies. Curr Probl Diagn Radiol. ePub, 2021
3. Shih JA et al: Duchenne muscular dystrophy: the heart of the matter. Curr Heart Fail Rep. 17(3):57-66, 2020
4. Hor KN et al: Advances in the diagnosis and management of cardiomyopathy in Duchenne muscular dystrophy. Neuromuscul Disord. 28(9):711-6, 2018
5. Power LC et al: Imaging the heart to detect cardiomyopathy in Duchenne muscular dystrophy: a review. Neuromuscul Disord. 28(9):717-30, 2018
6. D'Amario D et al: A current approach to heart failure in Duchenne muscular dystrophy. Heart. 103(22):1770-9, 2017

Arrhythmogenic Right Ventricular Dysplasia

KEY FACTS

TERMINOLOGY

- Distinct cardiomyopathy thought to be caused by mutations in genes coding for desmosomal proteins
  - Results in apoptosis & early cell death with fibrofatty replacement
  - Predominantly affects right ventricle (RV) with variable left ventricular (LV) involvement
  - Frequently associated with arrhythmias, including sudden cardiac death

IMAGING

- Diagnosis is made using set of major & minor criteria in 6 categories (task force criteria, 2010)
- Imaging can supply only 1 major or 1 minor criterion for diagnosis
- Epicardial subtricuspid region & basal RV free wall are most commonly involved
- RV is usually dilated & shows impaired systolic function
- RV microaneurysms & thickened trabeculae are often evident
- Right ventricular outflow tract (RVOT) is commonly dilated & poorly contractile
- LV is involved in ≥ 50% of cases & may predominate in small percentage of cases
- Attempts to visualize intramyocardial fat are no longer advised since they frequently result in misdiagnosis
- May demonstrate delayed hyperenhancement of RV wall, representing fibrosis in up to 88% of cases

TOP DIFFERENTIAL DIAGNOSES

- Myocarditis
- RV volume overload
- RV infarction
- Idiopathic RVOT tachycardia

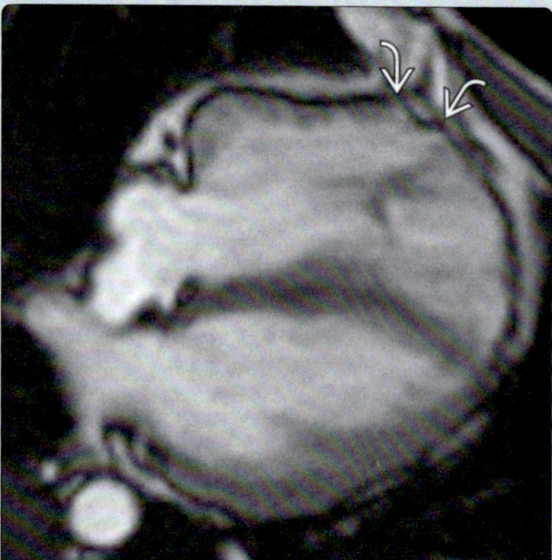

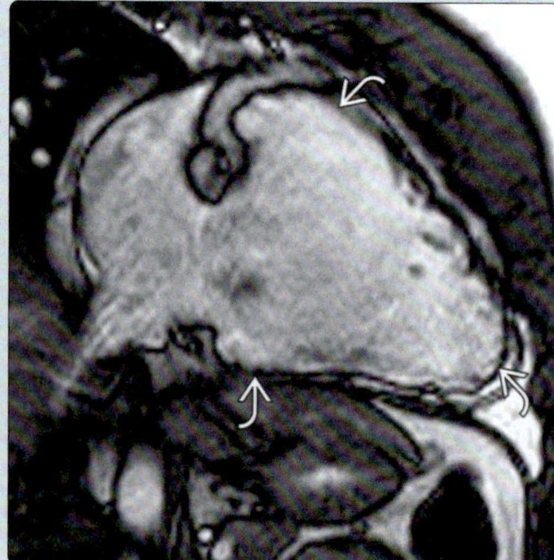

(Left) *Four-chamber SSFP bright blood cine MR in an adolescent shows a globally dilated right ventricle (RV) with severely thinned & scalloped anterior free wall ➡ in a patient who met criteria for arrhythmogenic right ventricular cardiomyopathy (ARVC).* **(Right)** *RV long-axis SSFP cine MR in a patient with ARVC shows the triangle of dysplasia ➡ extending from the subtricuspid region to the RV apex & superiorly to the infundibulum. Note the irregular outpouchings along the superior margin of the RV.*

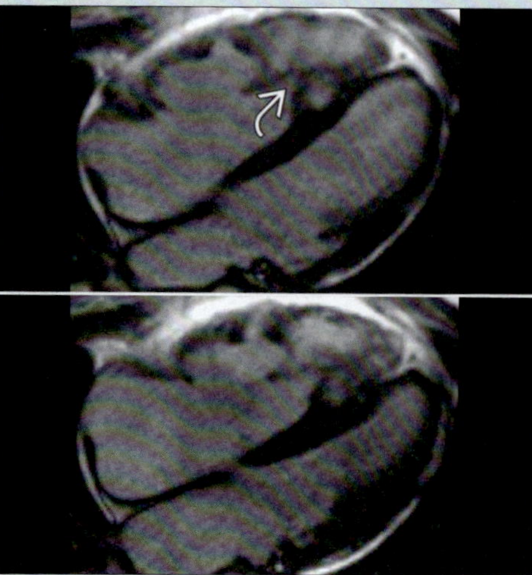

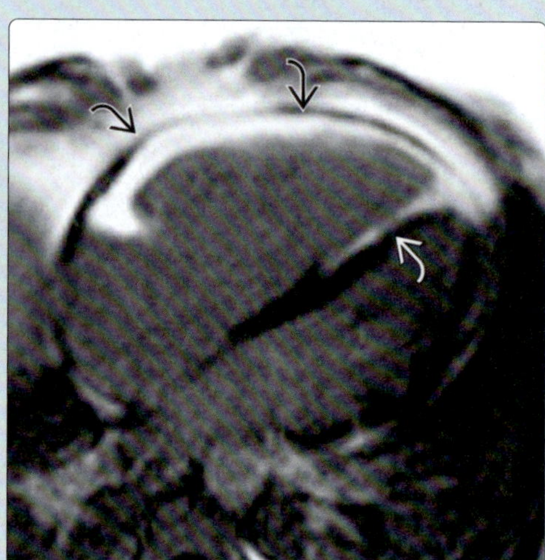

(Left) *Four-chamber cine SSFP MR images in diastole (top) & systole (bottom) in a patient with documented ARVC show dilation of the RV & prominent trabeculations ➡. Also note the poor systolic function evidenced by the lack of change in the volume of the RV from diastole to systole.* **(Right)** *Four-chamber LGE MR in the same patient demonstrates extensive enhancement of the RV free wall ➡ & the septum ➡.*

TERMINOLOGY

Abbreviations

- Arrhythmogenic right ventricular cardiomyopathy (ARVC)

Synonyms

- Formerly known as arrhythmogenic right ventricular dysplasia (ARVD)
- Term arrhythmogenic cardiomyopathy (AC) has recently been proposed to include both left ventricular (LV) & right ventricular (RV) disease

Definitions

- Distinct entity caused by mutations in genes encoding desmosomal proteins (plakoglobin, plakophilin, desmophilin, & desmocollin)
  - Result is apoptosis & early cell death with replacement by fibrofatty tissue
  - Predominantly affects RV with variable LV involvement; is associated with arrhythmias, including sudden cardiac death (SCD)

IMAGING

General Features

- Best diagnostic clue
  - Task force criteria (TFC) representing combination of clinical, pathologic, electrophysiologic, & imaging information
  - Diagnosis is considered definite when 2 major, 1 major & 2 minor, or 4 minor criteria from different categories are present; imaging can only contribute either 1 major or 1 minor or no criterion
- Location
  - Change in perception of regional structural involvement in ARVC in last decade
    - Recent studies suggest displacement of RV apex from previously accepted triangle of dysplasia (RV outflow tract, RV inflow tract, & apex)
  - Structural abnormalities are preferentially located to epicardial subtricuspid region & basal RV free wall
- Size
  - RV is commonly dilated in proven cases with wall thinning & hypertrabeculations
- Morphology
  - Often, entire RV free wall is involved, but extent of RV involvement is variable & may progress over time
    - RV free wall microaneurysms & dyskinetic segments are noted on cine imaging
    - Minimal involvement of subtricuspid RV free wall may result in accordion sign, wherein focal area of dyssynchrony results in crinkling of myocardium, resembling accordion

CT Findings

- CTA
  - Dilated RV with reduced systolic function (requires multiphase gated image acquisition)

MR Findings

- Cine steady-state free precession (SSFP) imaging
  - RV is usually dilated with impaired function & regional wall motion abnormalities (RWMA), including akinesia, dyskinesia, & contractile dyssynchrony
  - RV aneurysms, microaneurysms, & thickened trabeculae
  - Single MR diagnostic TFC includes RWMA (dyssynchronous RV contraction, dyskinesia, or akinesia) with either RV dilation or ↓ RV ejection fraction (RVEF)
    - Minor: iEDV ≥ 100 to < 110 mL/m² (male); ≥ 90 to < 100 mL/m² (female); RVEF > 40% to ≤ 45%
    - Major: iEDV ≥ 110 mL/m² (male); ≥ 100 mL/m² (female); RVEF ≤ 40%
- Black blood SE
  - May detect intramyocardial fat (not part of TFC due to high retest & interobserver variability & potential to result in misdiagnosis)
- Late gadolinium enhancement (LGE)
  - May demonstrate LGE of RV wall, representing fibrosis in 2/3 of cases, but is not TFC
  - LV involvement in ARVC may manifest as LGE, often involving inferior & lateral walls without concomitant wall motion abnormalities
    - Septal LGE is unusual in right dominant pattern

Echocardiographic Findings

- Echocardiogram
  - Hypokinetic & dilated RV with ↓ RVEF
  - Echo can supply 1 diagnostic TFC with severe (major) or moderate (minor) RV dysfunction

Imaging Recommendations

- Best imaging tool
  - MR is excellent for RV volumes & morphology
  - LGE of RV is seen in up to 88% of cases & correlates with inducibility of arrhythmias
- Protocol advice
  - Cine MR of entire RV is essential, with views of right ventricular outflow tract (RVOT) in long axis & short axis in addition to stack of 4-chamber views

DIFFERENTIAL DIAGNOSIS

Myocarditis

- Selective RV involvement is uncommon; usually LV involvement predominates
- Often patchy without predilection for "subtricuspid region"
- At follow-up, asymptomatic & free from arrhythmia (vs. 50% recurrent arrhythmia in ARVC)

Right Ventricular Dilatation in Endurance Athletes

- Marathon runners & other endurance athletes often develop RV dilation; RV function is usually preserved

Right Ventricular Volume Overload

- Pretricuspid left-to-right shunts
  - Has normal or hyperdynamic RV function
  - Shunt seen: Atrial septal defect (ASD), partial anomalous pulmonary venous return (PAPVR), unroofed coronary sinus
- Repaired tetralogy of Fallot
  - Often has significant pulmonic regurgitation with RV volume overload & failure

Right Ventricular Infarction

- Usually associated with inferior wall LV infarct (right coronary artery territory)
- Not commonly associated with localized aneurysm formation

Idiopathic Right Ventricular Outflow Tachycardia

- Benign, nonfamilial condition that may clinically mimic ARVC; usually no imaging abnormality is seen

Pitfalls

- RV free wall tether: Pericardial connective tissue joining anterior RV free wall to posterior sternum, mistaken as dyskinesia
- Apicolateral bulge: Seen in 79% as wall motion abnormality in RV at site of insertion of moderator band
- Butterfly apex: Prominent RV apex confused for aneurysm, but isolated apical aneurysm is unusual; normal systolic & diastolic motion
- Pectus excavatum: Distortion of RV; enlargement of RV apex & RVOT; restricted motion of basolateral & inferolateral walls
- Pulmonary valve sinuses: Systolic bulge due to filling with blood mimics dyskinesia; located above pulmonary valve anulus

PATHOLOGY

General Features

- Etiology
  - Mutations in genes coding for desmosomal proteins lead to early apoptosis, likely hastened by "wear & tear," which is particularly induced by repetitive exercise
- Genetics
  - Multiple mutations are now recognized, with predominantly autosomal dominant heritability with variable penetrance
    - Mutations of genes encoding plakophilin (most common), desmoglein, desmoplakin, & desmocollin
    - Cardiac ryanodine receptor defect: Calcium released from sarcoplasmic reticulum; may be responsible for adrenergically mediated arrhythmias
  - Family history may provide task force criterion if 1st-degree relative with proven (major) or suspected (minor) ARVC

Gross Pathologic & Surgical Features

- Apparent RV dilation & wall thinning
- Involves LV in 40-76% of autopsy cases

Microscopic Features

- Biopsy findings demonstrating myocyte depletion with fibrous replacement may provide TFC
- Fibrofatty infiltration of myocardium on biopsy is no longer major TFC

CLINICAL ISSUES

Presentation

- Most common signs/symptoms
  - Early ("concealed") phase: Patients are often asymptomatic but may be at risk of SCD due to arrhythmia
  - Overt ("electric") phase: Patients present with symptomatic arrhythmias & RV morphologic abnormalities, detectable with imaging
    - Characteristic arrhythmia is that of ventricular tachycardia (VT) with left bundle branch block morphology
- Other signs/symptoms
  - Palpitations are very common once symptoms develop
- Clinical profile
  - Should be considered in athletes of any age as cause of syncope or cardiovascular collapse
  - Can lead to isolated RV or biventricular heart failure
- Diagnosis
  - Made on basis of TFC representing combination of clinical, pathologic, electrophysiologic, & imaging information

Demographics

- Age
  - More clinically apparent in 2nd-4th decades of life
- Sex
  - M:F = 3:1 in younger age groups; M = F in later-onset cases
- Epidemiology
  - Estimated incidence: 1 in 2,000-5,000
  - ~ 50% of affected patients have positive family history

Natural History & Prognosis

- Annual mortality rate: ~ 0.08-3.6%

Treatment

- Avoid vigorous athletics
- Pharmacotherapy: Antiarrhythmic agents, β-blockers, & heart failure drug therapy
- Implantable cardioverter defibrillator in patients with history of VT, cardiac arrest, syncope or RV/LV dysfunction
- Catheter ablation of VT
- Heart transplant, predominantly for heart failure or untreatable arrhythmias

DIAGNOSTIC CHECKLIST

Image Interpretation Pearls

- Cine MR & volumetric analysis are often very helpful in providing diagnostic imaging

SELECTED REFERENCES

1. Conte E et al: Left-dominant arrhythmogenic cardiomyopathy diagnosed at cardiac CT. J Cardiovasc Comput Tomogr. 14(5):e7-8, 2020
2. Gomes AC et al: Arrhythmogenic right ventricular cardiomyopathy: an exuberant case affecting both ventricles. Circ Cardiovasc Imaging. 13(9):e010243, 2020
3. Khanji MY et al: Cardiovascular magnetic resonance imaging volume criteria for arrhythmogenic right ventricular cardiomyopathy: need for update? Eur Heart J. 41(14):1451, 2020
4. Towbin JA et al: 2019 HRS expert consensus statement on evaluation, risk stratification, and management of arrhythmogenic cardiomyopathy: executive summary. Heart Rhythm. 16(11):e373-407, 2019
5. Aliyari Ghasabeh M et al: Epicardial fat distribution assessed with cardiac CT in arrhythmogenic right ventricular dysplasia/cardiomyopathy. Radiology. 289(3):641-8, 2018
6. Corrado D et al: Arrhythmogenic right ventricular cardiomyopathy. N Engl J Med. 376(1):61-72, 2017
7. Haugaa KH et al: Comprehensive multi-modality imaging approach in arrhythmogenic cardiomyopathy-an expert consensus document of the European Association of Cardiovascular Imaging. Eur Heart J Cardiovasc Imaging. 18(3):237-53, 2017

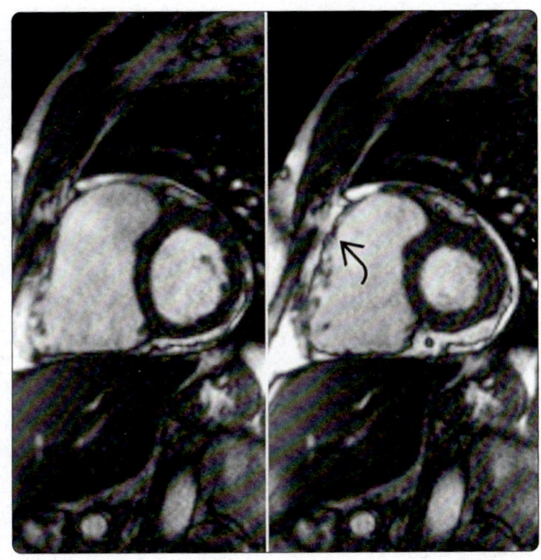

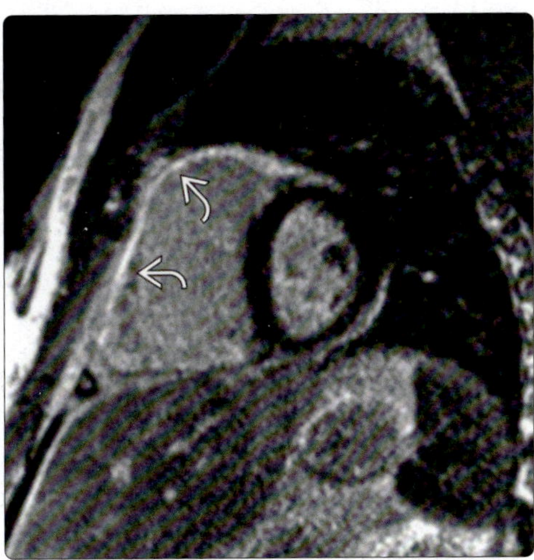

(Left) *Short-axis bright blood cine SSFP MR images in diastole (left) & systole (right) show RV dilation & ↓ function in a patient with ARVC. Note the tiny, focal outpouchings, often termed microaneurysms, along the RV free wall* ➲ *in the systolic image.* **(Right)** *Short-axis LGE MR in the same patient shows enhancement of the RV wall* ➲*, consistent with fibrosis. This finding is seen in ~ 2/3 of patients with ARVC.*

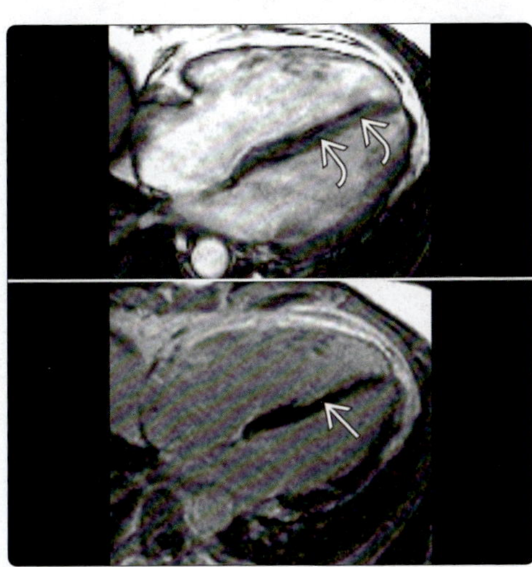

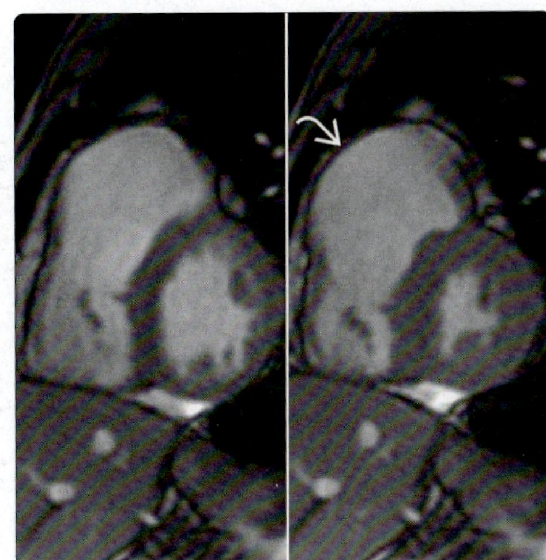

(Left) *Four-chamber cine SSFP (top) & LGE (bottom) MR images in a patient with ARVC show tiny foci of fat along the RV side of the septum* ➲*, denoted by the "etching" artifact seen in this SSFP image. Note the enhancement of the same area of the septum* ➲ *& the RV free wall on the LGE image.* **(Right)** *Sagittal cine SSFP bright blood MR in an adolescent boy through the right ventricular outflow tract (RVOT) in diastole (left) & systole (right) in a patient with ARVC shows ↑ dilation of the RVOT during systole* ➲.

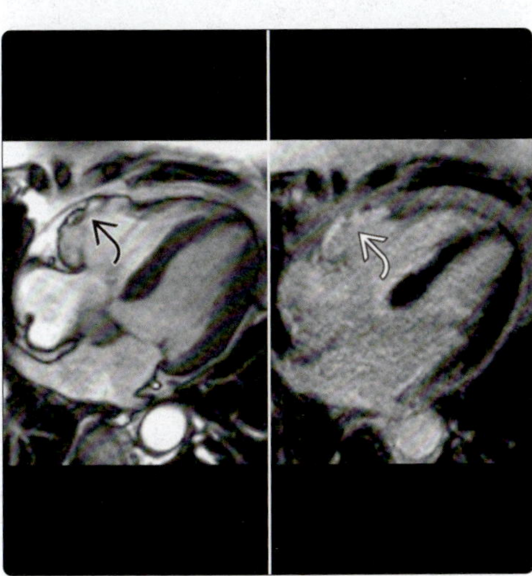

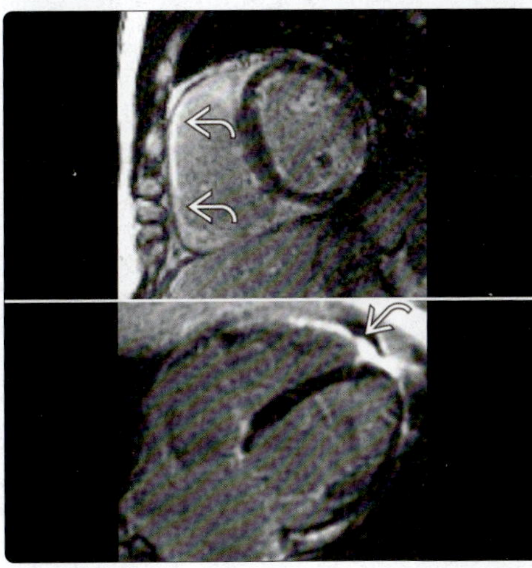

(Left) *Four-chamber cine SSFP MR (left) in a patient with minimal involvement by ARVC shows a focal systolic outpouching, termed the accordion sign, along the RV free wall in the subtricuspid region* ➲*. Note also that this is the only region with abnormal enhancement* ➲ *on the LGE image (right).* **(Right)** *Short-axis (top) & 4-chamber (bottom) LGE MR images in a patient with cardiac sarcoidosis show abnormal RV enhancement* ➲*, similar to findings seen in ARVC.*

Heterotaxy Syndromes

KEY FACTS

TERMINOLOGY

- Disturbance of normal left-right asymmetry in position of thoracic & abdominal organs
  - Typically described in terms of right atrial isomerism vs. left atrial isomerism

IMAGING

- Best diagnostic clue
  - Abnormal symmetry in chest & abdomen
- Classic radiographic appearance
  - Transverse midline liver, discrepancy between position of cardiac apex & stomach, bilateral left- or right-sidedness in chest, cardiomegaly or other findings of congenital heart disease
- Ultrasound: Easy screening of abdominal viscera
- CTA: Rapid examination of chest & abdomen for abnormalities of situs, systemic & pulmonary venous connections, tracheobronchial anatomy
- Multiplanar MR for segmental analysis of intracardiac connections & defects
  - Gadolinium-enhanced 3D MRA: Comparable to CTA
- Upper GI study: Malrotation is common

PATHOLOGY

- Any arrangement other than situs solitus or inversus is termed situs ambiguous
- Heterotaxy syndrome represents spectrum with overlap between classic asplenia & polysplenia manifestations & other anomalies

CLINICAL ISSUES

- Asplenia: Male neonate with severe cyanosis, susceptibility for infections, severe congenital heart disease
- Polysplenia: Less severe cardiac disease (i.e., systemic venous malformations, atrial septal defect), often presents later

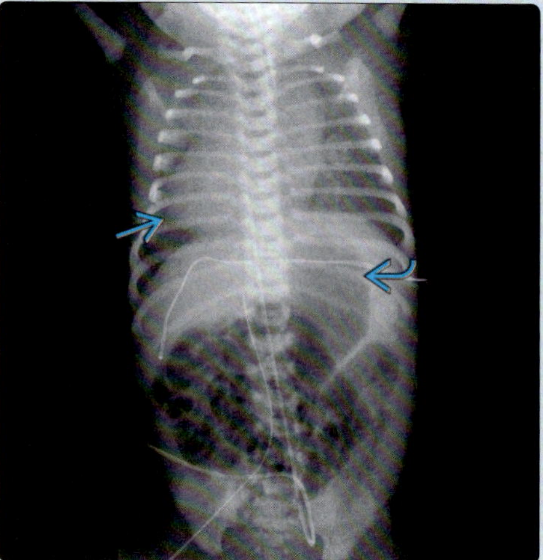

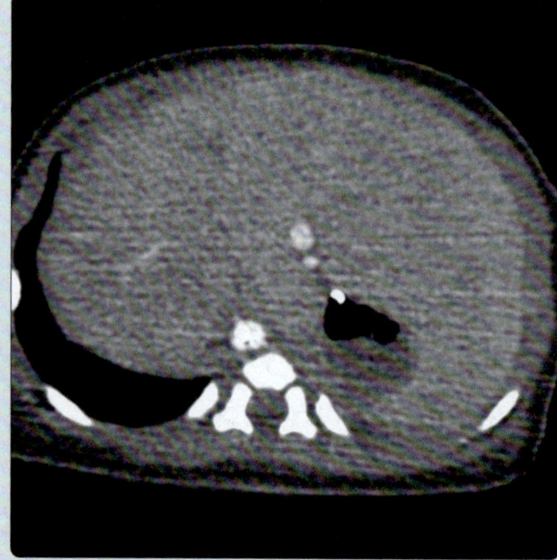

(Left) *Frontal radiograph of the chest & abdomen in a newborn demonstrates dextrocardia with a right-sided cardiac apex ➔ & a left-sided stomach ➔ in a patient with known complex congenital heart disease. The findings are consistent with heterotaxy syndrome.* **(Right)** *Axial CECT shows a midline liver with no splenic tissue seen in a patient with known heterotaxy syndrome.*

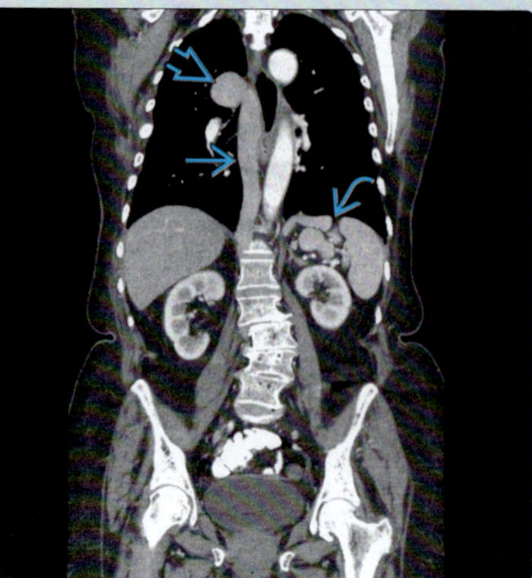

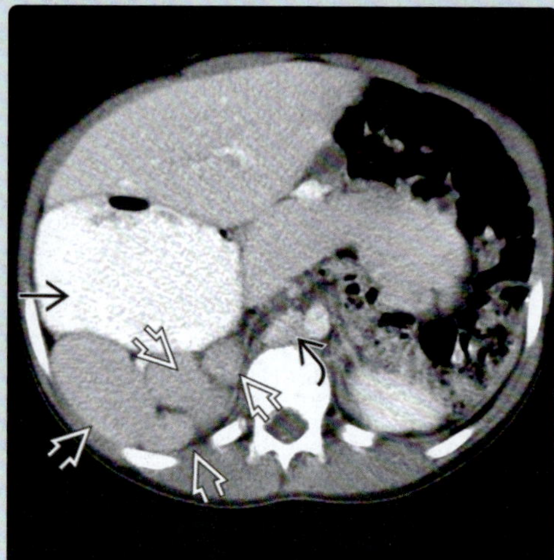

(Left) *Coronal CECT shows azygous continuation of the inferior vena cava (IVC) ➔ with polysplenia ➔ in a patient with heterotaxy syndrome. Note the enlarged distal azygous vein ➔.* **(Right)** *Axial CECT through the upper abdomen in a child with heterotaxy shows a right-sided stomach ➔ & multiple spleens ➔. An enlarged azygous vein is noted ➔, but no intrahepatic IVC is visualized, consistent with azygous continuation of the IVC.*

TERMINOLOGY

Synonyms

- Situs ambiguous, right/left isomerism, cardiosplenic syndromes, Ivemark syndrome

Definitions

- Disturbance of normal left-right asymmetry in position of thoracic & abdominal organs

IMAGING

General Features

- Best diagnostic clue
  - Abnormal symmetry in chest & abdomen

Radiographic Findings

- Radiography
  - Classic appearance: Transverse midline liver, discrepancy between position of cardiac apex & stomach, bilateral left- or right-sidedness in chest, cardiomegaly or other findings of congenital heart disease (CHD)
  - Asplenia syndrome or right atrial isomerism
    - Bilateral minor fissures
    - Symmetrical, short main bronchi with right-sided morphology (narrow carinal angle, early take-off of upper lobe bronchus)
    - Bilateral eparterial bronchi: Main bronchus is superior to branch pulmonary artery (eparterial bronchus)
    - Cardiomegaly, pulmonary edema
  - Polysplenia syndrome or left atrial isomerism
    - No minor fissure on either side
    - Symmetrical long main bronchi with left-sided morphology (wide carinal angle)
    - Bilateral hyparterial bronchi: Main bronchus is inferior to branch pulmonary artery (hyparterial bronchus)
    - Absent inferior vena cava (IVC) shadow on lateral film, prominent azygous shadow on AP
  - Both syndromes
    - Cardiac malposition (40%: Mesocardia, dextrocardia)
    - Transverse liver
    - Right-sided stomach bubble with levocardia, left-sided stomach bubble with dextrocardia, or midline stomach

Echocardiographic Findings

- Initial diagnostic test for characterization of intracardiac anomalies, abnormal systemic &/or pulmonary venous connections

Ultrasonographic Findings

- Easiest assessment of abdominal viscera
  - Look for spleen adjacent to stomach

CT Findings

- CTA
  - Rapid examination of chest & abdomen: Situs abnormalities, systemic & pulmonary venous connections, tracheobronchial anatomy
  - Best for postoperative patients with metallic coils, stents, & clips
  - Preferred modality over conventional angiography due to more detailed anatomic information

MR Findings

- T1WI
  - Multiplanar imaging for segmental analysis of intracardiac connections & defects
- T2* GRE
  - Cine MR for ventricular volumes & function to determine suitability for biventricular vs. univentricular repair
- MRA
  - Ultrafast time-resolved MRA C+ with repeated acquisitions allows for dynamic circulation study
  - Velocity-encoded phase-contrast MRA for flow quantification

Other Modality Findings

- Upper GI study: Malrotation is common

Imaging Recommendations

- Protocol advice
  - Echocardiography, followed by MR
  - CTA for anatomic study in postoperative patients

DIFFERENTIAL DIAGNOSIS

Situs Inversus Totalis (I, L, L)

- Mirror image of normal
- Low association with CHD (3-5%)
- May be associated with immotile cilia syndrome (Kartagener): Sinusitis, bronchiectasis, infertility

True Dextrocardia + Abdominal Situs Solitus or Levocardia + Abdominal Situs Inversus

- Both have high association with CHD (95-100%)

Dextroversion of Heart

- Heart positioned in right chest with apex & stomach still directed toward left
  - Right lung hypoplasia (scimitar syndrome)
  - Left-sided mass lesions
    - Diaphragmatic hernia
    - Congenital pulmonary airway malformation

PATHOLOGY

General Features

- Heterotaxy syndrome represents spectrum with overlap between classic asplenia & polysplenia manifestations & other anomalies
- Embryology: Early embryologic disturbance (5th week of gestation) leading to complex anomalies
- Pathophysiology: Determined by complexity of associated CHD
- Genetics: No specific genetic defect in majority (usually sporadic)

Staging, Grading, & Classification

- Segmental approach to analysis of complex cardiac anomalies with cardiac malposition (reported by Anderson or Van Praagh systematic descriptions)
  - Visceroatrial situs designated by S (solitus = normal) or I (inversus = mirror image of normal)
  - Always associated on same side
    - Major lobe of liver, IVC, anatomic right atrium, trilobed lung, eparterial bronchus

    - Spleen, stomach, descending aorta, anatomic left atrium, bilobed lung, hyparterial bronchus
  - Any arrangement other than situs solitus or inversus is termed situs ambiguous (heterotaxia)
  - Ventricular loop: D loop (normal) or L loop (inverted)
  - Orientation of great arteries (presence of transposition) is also designated by D or L
  - Van Praagh segmental analysis is summarized by 3-letter code describing relationships of atria, ventricles, & great arteries: S,D,D; I,L,L; S,D,L
  - Anderson connections described as concordant or discordant between atria, ventricles, & great arteries
  - Associated abnormalities: Transposition of great arteries (TGA), double-outlet right ventricle (DORV), total anomalous pulmonary venous return (TAPVR), unbalanced atrioventricular septal defects
- 2 major subtypes
  - Asplenia syndrome = right atrial isomerism or double right-sidedness
    - Absence of spleen
    - IVC & aorta are on same side
    - Bilateral superior vena cavae (~ 36%); absent coronary sinus
    - Right isomerism of atrial appendages
    - Common atrium with band-like remnant of septum crossing atria in anteroposterior direction
    - Bilateral trilobed lungs
    - Bilateral eparterial bronchi
    - Associated with severe cyanotic CHD (atrioventricular septal defect, common atrioventricular valve, DORV, TGA, pulmonary stenosis/atresia)
    - Abnormalities of pulmonary venous connections
      - TAPVR, > 80%; often obstructed, below diaphragm (type III)
      - Findings of pulmonary venous outflow obstruction may be masked when there is restriction to pulmonary arterial inflow at same time (pulmonary atresia)
  - Polysplenia syndrome = left atrial isomerism or double left-sidedness
    - Multiple spleens, anisosplenia, multilobed spleen (functional asplenia)
    - Abnormalities of systemic venous connections: Interrupted IVC with azygous continuation (> 70%), hepatic veins drain separately into common atrium
    - Bilateral superior vena cavae (~ 41%); 1 or both may connect to coronary sinus
    - Left isomerism of atrial appendages
    - Common atrium or large ostium primum atrial septal defect
    - Bilateral bilobed lungs
    - Bilateral hyparterial bronchi
    - Associated with less severe CHD (common atrium, ventricular septal defect)

CLINICAL ISSUES

Presentation

- Most common signs/symptoms
  - Asplenia: Male neonate with severe cyanosis, susceptibility for infections
  - Polysplenia: More variable, often presents later
- Other signs/symptoms
  - Malrotation, volvulus, preduodenal portal vein, absent gallbladder, extrahepatic biliary atresia, short pancreas (dorsal head agenesis)

Demographics

- Epidemiology
  - Prevalence: 1 per 22,000 to 24,000; 1-3% of CHD
  - Asplenia: M > F; polysplenia: M = F

Natural History & Prognosis

- 1st-year mortality: 85% asplenia, 65% polysplenia

Treatment

- Supportive, prostaglandins (if CHD lesion has inadequate pulmonary blood flow or if aortic arch has interruption/obstruction), antibiotic prophylaxis (functional asplenia)
- Asplenia/polysplenia with pulmonary overcirculation: Pulmonary artery banding
- Asplenia with obstructed pulmonary flow & TAPVR: Delicate balance between pulmonary arterial inflow & venous outflow
  - Placement of palliative systemic to pulmonary artery (Blalock-Taussig or central) shunt ↑ inflow
  - TAPVR repair needs to be done at same time to reduce outflow obstruction
- Early biventricular repair, if possible
- Univentricular repair, step 1: Bidirectional Glenn (superior cavopulmonary anastomosis) or hemi-Fontan
- Polysplenia: Incorporation of azygous vein to cavopulmonary anastomosis (Kawashima operation) to reduce occurrence of microscopic pulmonary arteriovenous malformation
  - Postsurgical: Development of pulmonary to systemic venous collaterals, arteriovenous malformations, pulmonary vein stenosis
- Completion of total cavopulmonary anastomosis (i.e., Fontan procedure), if possible
  - 1 or more hepatic veins may have to be excluded from Fontan shunt → venovenous collaterals
  - CTA or MRA prior to catheterization as road map for coil embolization of collaterals

SELECTED REFERENCES

1. Murat SN et al: Diagnosis of heterotaxy syndrome in a patient with multiple congenital cardiac malformations using magnetic resonance imaging. Circ Cardiovasc Imaging. 13(9):e010307, 2020
2. Broda CR et al: Outcomes in adults with congenital heart disease and heterotaxy syndrome: a single-center experience. Congenit Heart Dis. 14(6):885-94, 2019
3. Buca DIP et al: Outcome of prenatally diagnosed fetal heterotaxy: systematic review and meta-analysis. Ultrasound Obstet Gynecol. 51(3):323-30, 2018
4. Cupers S et al: Heterotaxy syndrome with intestinal malrotation, polysplenia and azygos continuity. Clin Pract. 8(1):1004, 2018
5. Mahmood K et al: Heterotaxy syndrome. J Coll Physicians Surg Pak. 28(3):252-3, 2018
6. Sanders SP et al: Classifying heterotaxy syndrome: time for a new approach. Circ Cardiovasc Imaging. 11(2):e007490, 2018
7. Moradi B et al: Fetal echocardiographic evaluation in cases of heterotaxy syndrome. J Clin Ultrasound. 45(7):436-7, 2017

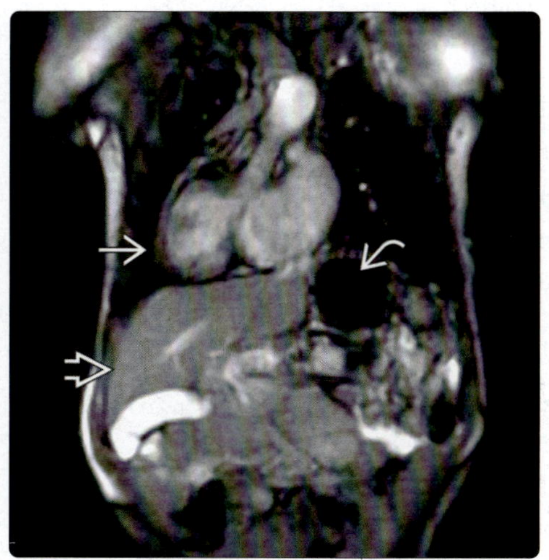

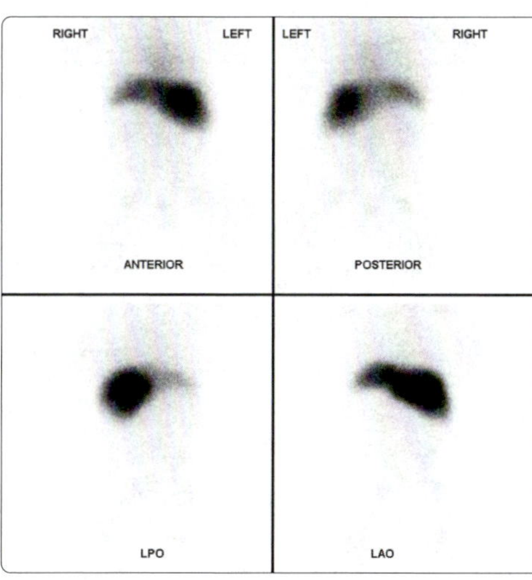

(Left) *Coronal SSFP MR in a patient with asplenia demonstrates a right-sided cardiac apex, right-sided liver, left-sided stomach, & no splenic tissue.* **(Right)** *Multiple images from a Tc-99m sulfur colloid scan in a patient with heterotaxy demonstrate normal liver uptake but no splenic tissue, confirming asplenia.*

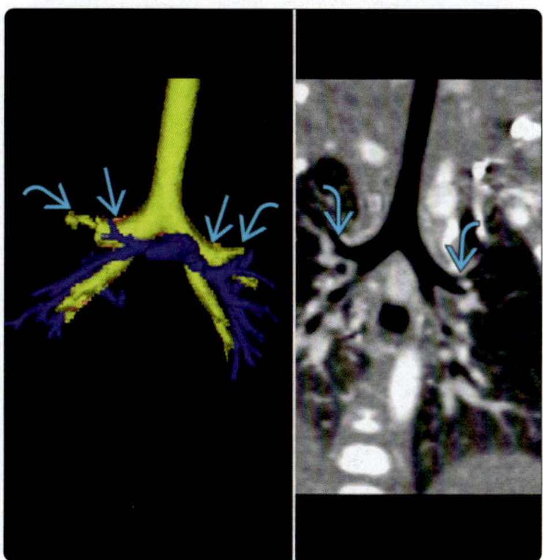

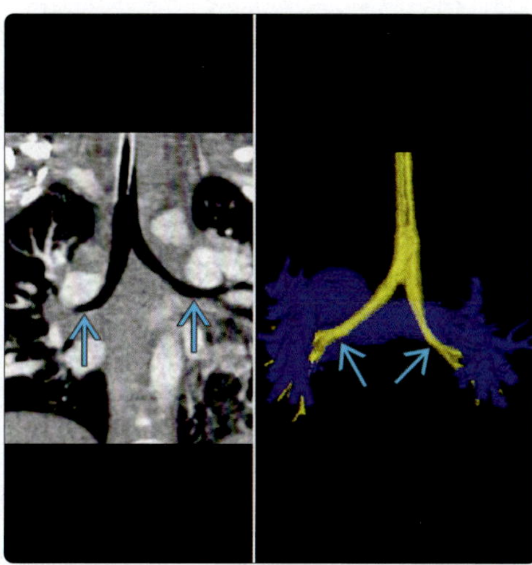

(Left) *3D surface-rendered CTA (left) & coronal CECT (right) through the airway in a patient with heterotaxy show bilateral right-sided tracheobronchial branching with eparterial bronchi [bronchi above pulmonary arteries (PAs)] & early right upper lobe branching.* **(Right)** *3D surface-rendered CTA (right) & coronal CECT (left) through the airway in a patient with heterotaxy syndrome show bilateral left-sided tracheobronchial branching with elongated hyparterial bronchi (PAs go above the bronchi).*

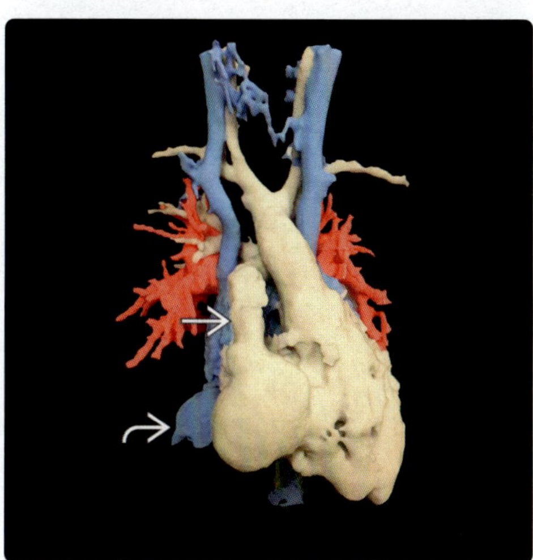

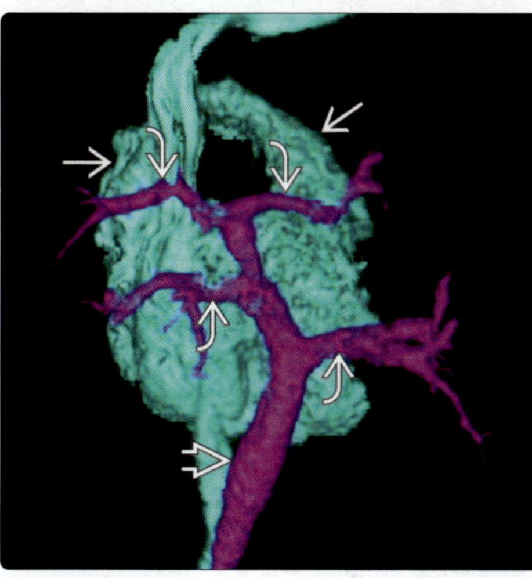

(Left) *3D-printed model of a heterotaxy patient shows bilateral SVCs (blue), interrupted IVC with azygous continuation, hepatic veins draining directly to right atrium, & complex pulmonary venous return (red). 3D model was created for surgical planning.* **(Right)** *Posterior 3D surface-rendered cardiac CTA in an infant with heterotaxy syndrome shows type 3 TAPVR with all pulmonary veins draining to a large vertical vein that courses below the diaphragm. Note the symmetric atrial appendages with 2 right-sided atria.*

Rhabdomyoma

KEY FACTS

TERMINOLOGY

- Congenital cardiac hamartoma composed of abnormal myocytes

IMAGING

- Initial diagnosis is often by fetal &/or postnatal echocardiogram
  - Homogeneous, hyperechoic mass(es) of myocardium
    - Intramyocardial: May appear as wall thickening
    - Intracavitary: Mass attached to myocardium protrudes into lumen
- MR is leading diagnostic test to delineate location, extent, & tissue characteristics of cardiac masses in children
  - T1: Iso- or mildly hyperintense to myocardium
  - T2: Hyperintense to myocardium
  - 1st-pass perfusion: Hypointense to myocardium
  - Late gadolinium enhancement: Isointense to myocardium
  - Homogeneous appearance on all sequences
- Normal chest radiograph in small masses
  - Cardiomegaly & signs of congestive heart failure in large masses
- Image brain (MR) & kidneys (US) for findings of tuberous sclerosis complex (TSC)
  - ~ 100% of patients with multiple rhabdomyomas & 50% with single rhabdomyoma have TSC

TOP DIFFERENTIAL DIAGNOSES

- Fibroma; pericardial teratoma

CLINICAL ISSUES

- Cardiac tumors are rare in children
- Rhabdomyoma is most common pediatric cardiac tumor
- 75% are diagnosed before 1 year of age
- Natural history: Up to 93% show spontaneous regression; 70% regress by 4 years of age
- Surgical excision for minority of cases with refractory arrhythmias or hemodynamic compromise

(Left) *Axial graphic shows a partially exophytic rhabdomyoma ➡ in the apex of the left ventricle (LV).* **(Right)** *Axial T1 MR was performed in an asymptomatic 8-year-old girl with tuberous sclerosis complex (TSC) after a routine screening echocardiogram showed an intracardiac mass. MR shows a round, well-demarcated, intraluminal mass ➡ originating from the free wall of the LV. It is slightly hyperintense to myocardium, a characteristic finding of rhabdomyomas.*

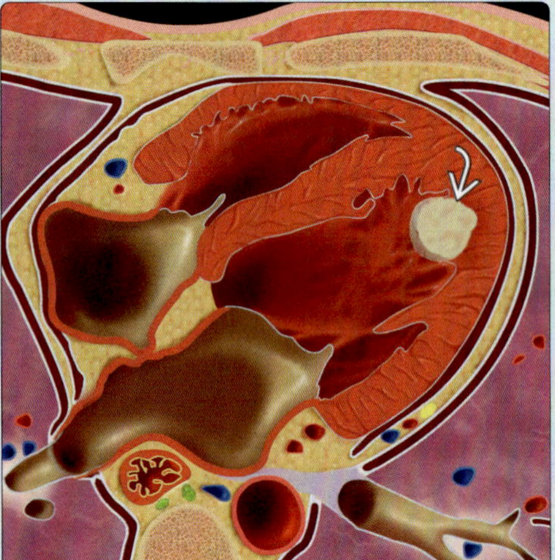

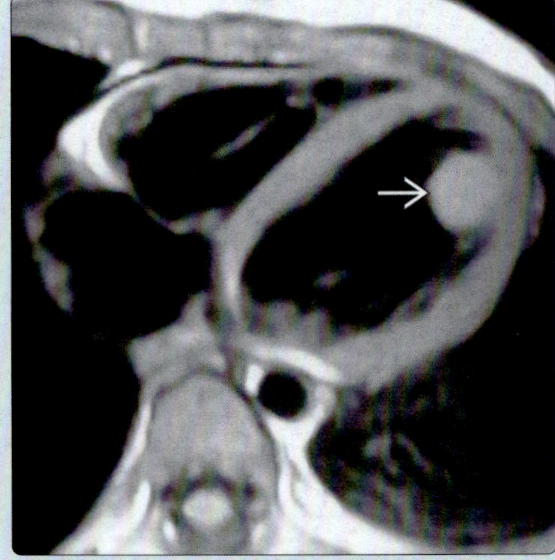

(Left) *Axial US through the fetal chest shows multiple echogenic, intracardiac masses ➡ involving both ventricles & the interventricular septum. Multiple rhabdomyomas are virtually diagnostic of TSC.* **(Right)** *Axial CECT of the heart in a 15-year-old patient with a history of multiple rhabdomyomas shows complete involution of masses with only small fatty deposits now seen along the interventricular septum, consistent with known TSC.*

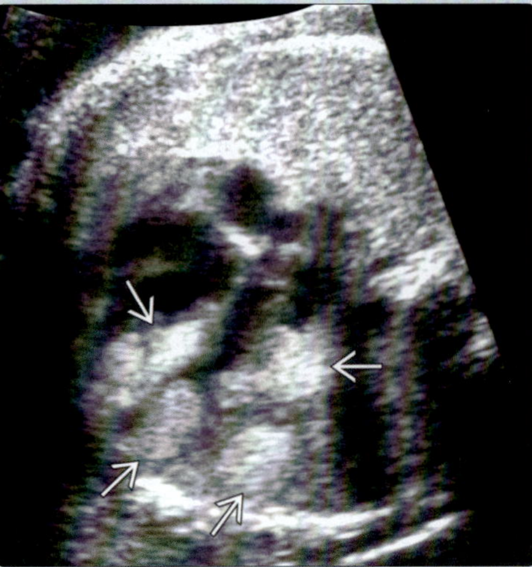

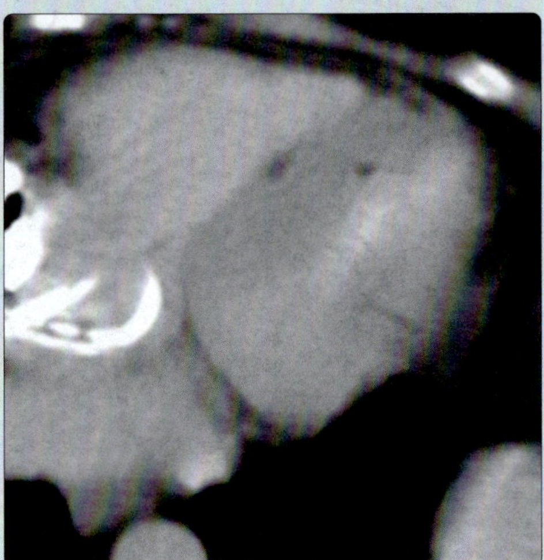

TERMINOLOGY

Definitions

- Congenital cardiac hamartoma composed of abnormal myocytes

IMAGING

General Features

- Best diagnostic clue
  - Cardiac mass within or contiguous with myocardium
- Location
  - Interventricular septum > left or right ventricular free wall > > atrium
  - Multiple in up to 90% of cases
- Size
  - < 1 mm to 10 cm; most are 3-4 cm
- Morphology
  - Well-circumscribed, nonencapsulated mass(es)
  - Intramural or exophytic
    - May involve entire wall & appear as wall thickening

Radiographic Findings

- Normal chest radiograph in small masses
- Cardiomegaly & signs of heart failure in large masses

Echocardiographic Findings

- Often superior to MR for detection of small masses
- Homogeneous, hyperechoic mass involving myocardium
- No blood flow within mass
- Most often in interventricular septum but can be anywhere
- May appear as simple wall thickening
- Intraluminal portion of mass may move across adjacent valve during cardiac cycle

CT Findings

- NECT
  - Often hypodense compared with myocardium
- CECT
  - Intraluminal component may be assessed with contrast-enhanced studies

MR Findings

- T1WI
  - Iso- or mildly hyperintense to myocardium
- T2WI
  - Hyperintense to myocardium
  - No change with fat saturation (rules out lipoma)
- T1WI C+
  - Minimal initial enhancement (1st-pass perfusion)
  - Isointense to myocardium with late gadolinium enhancement (LGE)
- SSFP cine
  - Help to differentiate tumor from contractile myocardium, evaluate hemodynamic effect of mass, & look for valvular leak

Imaging Recommendations

- Best imaging tool
  - Dedicated transthoracic echo in all cases
  - MR is helpful for diagnostic uncertainty, large masses, & surgical planning
- Protocol advice
  - If cardiac mass is identified
    - Look for additional masses
    - Assess location & quality of mass
  - Look for rhythm abnormalities
    - Premature atrial or ventricular contractions are common
    - Supraventricular tachycardia
    - Sinus bradycardia
  - Look for signs of obstruction
    - Ventricular inflow or outflow obstruction
    - May manifest as valve regurgitation or stenosis
    - ↑ cardiac work to overcome obstruction → wall hypertrophy
  - Evaluate for other findings of tuberous sclerosis complex (TSC)
  - In fetus, monitor for signs of hydrops (poor function, effusions)

DIFFERENTIAL DIAGNOSIS

Fibroma

- Benign congenital cardiac neoplasm composed of fibroblasts & collagen
- 2nd most common cardiac neoplasm in pediatric population after rhabdomyoma
- Often arises from interventricular septum or left ventricular free wall
- MR: Isointense on T1, hypointense on T2

Teratoma

- Pericardial (not myocardial) tumor
- Exophytic growth (will not be in cardiac chamber)
- Pericardial effusion is often present
- Contains all 3 germ cell layers → may be very heterogeneous on imaging with cystic, fatty, & calcified components

Lipoma

- Most arise from endocardial surface & protrude into chamber lumen
- Fat density/intensity on imaging studies allows for specific diagnosis

Myxoma

- Majority manifest in adulthood (4th-7th decades)
- 90% are solitary & atrial in location
  - 75% in left atrium, 10-20% in right atrium
  - Predilection for interatrial septum adjacent to fossa ovalis

Papillary Fibroelastoma

- > 90% involve valves
- Typically small (< 15 mm)

Cardiac Malignancies

- Extremely uncommon in children
- Sarcomas account for most (with angiosarcoma being most common)
- Usually large masses with invasive features
- Pericardial & pleural effusion are often present

PATHOLOGY

General Features

- Etiology
  - Unknown, but data suggests maternal hormones may play role in growth & development of fetal rhabdomyomas
    - Helps explain regression after delivery
- Genetics
  - Nearly 100% of patients with multiple & 50% with single rhabdomyomas have TSC
  - TSC: Autosomal dominant with variable expressivity
    - ~ 30% of cases are inherited
    - Other cases are due to new mutation
  - Caused by mutations in *TSC1* or *TSC2* genes
    - *TSC1* is located on chromosome 9q
      - Encodes for hamartin protein
      - Complexes with tuberin to regulate cell cycle
    - *TSC2* located on chromosome 16p
      - Encodes for tuberin protein
      - Participates in normal brain development & cardiomyocyte differentiation
- Associated abnormalities
  - Other findings of TSC
    - Brain: Subependymal nodules, cortical/subcortical tubers, subependymal giant cell astrocytoma
    - Lung: Lymphangioleiomyomatosis
    - Kidney: Angiomyolipomas & cysts
    - Eye: Retinal hamartomas
    - Nails: Ungual fibromas
- Pathophysiology
  - Mass may interfere with myocardial contraction
  - Exophytic masses frequently obstruct blood flow or cause valvular insufficiency

Gross Pathologic & Surgical Features

- Well-circumscribed, intramyocardial or exophytic mass(es)

Microscopic Features

- Large, vacuolated myocytes
- Glycogen-rich vacuoles stretch perinuclear cytoplasm (spider cells)

CLINICAL ISSUES

Presentation

- Most common signs/symptoms
  - Obstruction to blood flow → heart failure
  - Arrhythmias
  - Large intracavitary tumors causing turbulent flow → hemolytic anemia & thrombocytopenia
- May be seen prenatally
  - Generally incidental finding
  - Rarely presents with arrhythmia or hydrops
  - Can detect as early as 22-weeks gestation
    - May discover more masses as pregnancy progresses
    - Tend to ↑ in size prenatally & then regress after birth

Demographics

- Age
  - 75% are diagnosed before 1 year of age
- Epidemiology
  - Cardiac tumors rare (1:30,000-1:100,000)
  - Rhabdomyoma is most common pediatric cardiac tumor

Natural History & Prognosis

- Generally excellent with spontaneous regression in 70% of children by 4 years of age
- Poor prognosis for untreated large masses interfering with cardiac hemodynamics
  - Most respond well to surgical excision
  - Case reports of response to mTOR (mammalian target of rapamycin) inhibitor sirolimus
    - mTOR: Protein kinase that regulates cellular proliferation; used to treat subependymal giant cell tumors & angiomyolipomas

Treatment

- Surgical excision should be considered only for those with refractory arrhythmias or hemodynamic compromise
  - Partial resection of intraluminal component of large exophytic masses may be necessary
  - 3D printing from CT/MR data can build heart model with tumor location & extent for easy visualization; can assist with procedural planning
  - Attempts at electrophysiology testing & ablation around tumor focus have variable success rates
    - 3D printed models have been helpful
- Small, intramural masses with no hemodynamic effect typically need no treatment or surgical excision

DIAGNOSTIC CHECKLIST

Consider

- Overall prognosis is excellent
- However, rhabdomyomas may cause significant morbidity from obstruction to inflow or outflow, ventricular dysfunction, or arrhythmias

SELECTED REFERENCES

1. Tsoumani Z et al: Magnetic resonance imaging of intramyocardial fat deposition in tuberous sclerosis. Diagnostics (Basel). 10(12), 2020
2. Victoria T et al: Imaging of fetal tumors and other dysplastic lesions: a review with emphasis on MR imaging. Prenat Diagn. 40(1):84-99, 2020
3. Poterucha TJ et al: Cardiac tumors: clinical presentation, diagnosis, and management. Curr Treat Options Oncol. 20(8):66, 2019
4. Ugurlucan M et al: Giant rhabdomyoma requiring emergency resection early after birth. Ann Thorac Surg. 107(1):e65, 2019
5. Chen J et al: Fetal cardiac tumors: fetal echocardiography, clinical outcome and genetic analysis in 53 cases. Ultrasound Obstet Gynecol. 54(1):103-9, 2018
6. Dragoumi P et al: Diagnosis of tuberous sclerosis complex in the fetus. Eur J Paediatr Neurol. 22(6):1027-34, 2018
7. Palaskas N et al: Evaluation and management of cardiac tumors. Curr Treat Options Cardiovasc Med. 20(4):29, 2018
8. von Ranke FM et al: Imaging of tuberous sclerosis complex: a pictorial review. Radiol Bras. 50(1):48-54, 2017

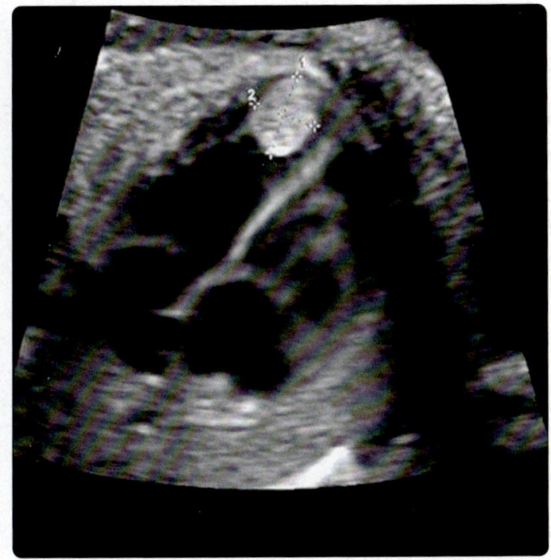

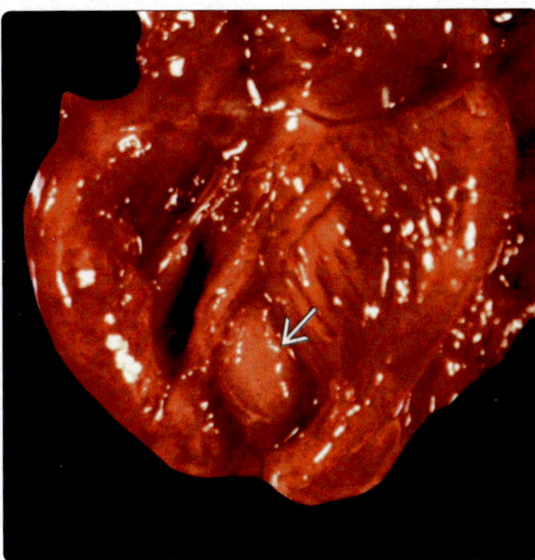

(Left) *Four-chamber view from a fetal echocardiogram shows an echogenic mass in the apex of the right ventricle (RV), most consistent with a rhabdomyoma. The patient was later diagnosed with TSC. A mass this size will likely have no physiologic effect on the cardiac function.* **(Right)** *Gross pathology of the heart shows a well-defined mass ➔ arising from the wall of the ventricle. Histology confirmed a rhabdomyoma.*

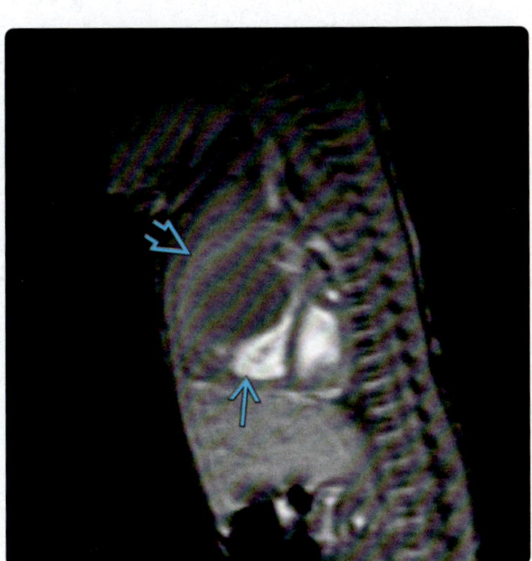

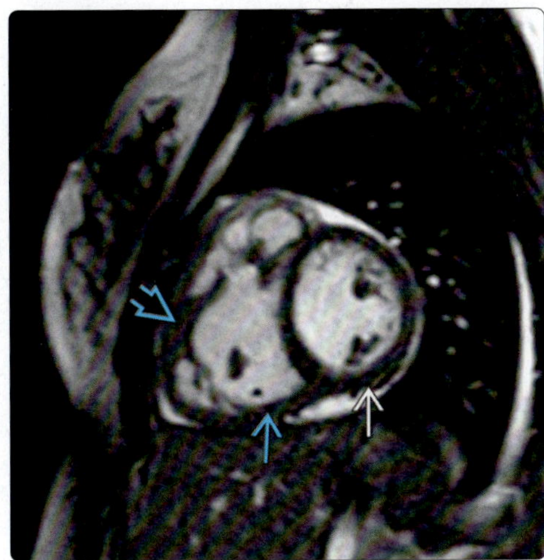

(Left) *SSFP bright blood cine short-axis MR in a neonate demonstrates a large, hypointense rhabdomyoma ➔ within the RV wall ➔.* **(Right)** *SSFP cine short-axis MR in same patient at 13 years of age demonstrates near-complete resolution of the rhabdomyoma with minimal residual tumor ➔. The RV ➔ appears borderline dilated, & the LV ➔ appears normal.*

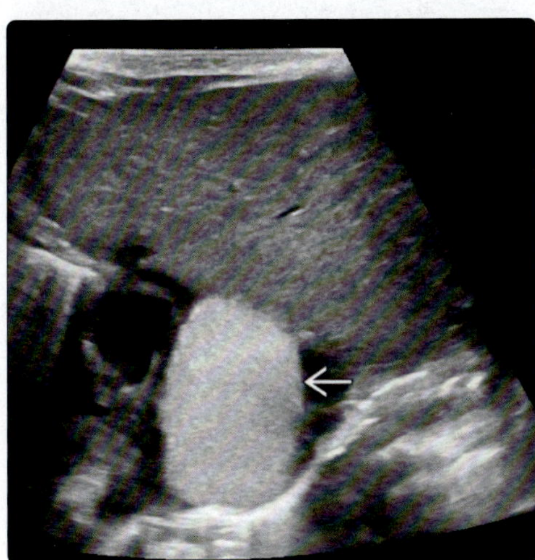

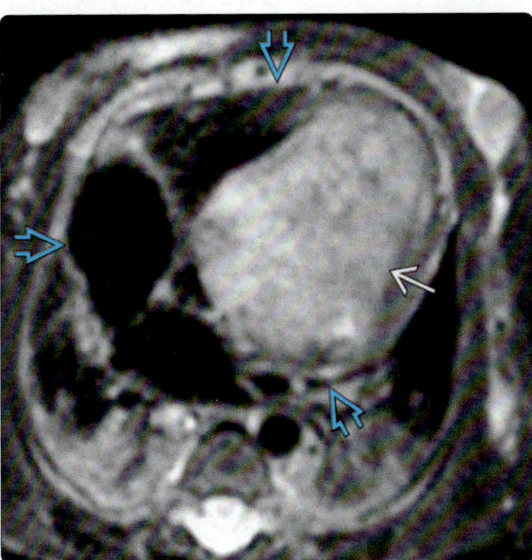

(Left) *Postnatal axial US in a patient with tuberous sclerosis shows a large echogenic mass ➔ filling the LV. Rhabdomyomas are often large at birth but usually spontaneously regress postnatally.* **(Right)** *Four-chamber view double IR image from a cardiac MR demonstrates an echogenic mass ➔ filling the LV, consistent with a rhabdomyoma. Masses of this size may have cardiac obstruction & heart failure. Note the marked enlargement of the heart ➔ in this neonate.*

KEY FACTS

TERMINOLOGY

- Inflammatory disease of small- & medium-sized blood vessels of unknown etiology, mainly in young children
  - Widespread but characteristic manifestations
  - Coronary artery aneurysms are most feared complication

IMAGING

- Chest radiography is usually normal
- Echocardiography has sufficient sensitivity & specificity in detecting proximal coronary artery aneurysms
  - Remains 1st-line modality
- CTA can demonstrate aneurysms, stenoses, & Ca^{2+} of coronary or other arteries
- Cardiac MR protocol includes function, coronary artery imaging, 1st-pass perfusion, & late gadolinium enhancement for myocardial viability
- MRA with large field of view can show aneurysms of peripheral arteries

TOP DIFFERENTIAL DIAGNOSES

- MIS-C from SARS-CoV-2 (COVID-19); exanthematous infections; allergic/hypersensitivity reactions; vasculitides

PATHOLOGY

- Etiology is unclear, but clinical & epidemiologic features suggest abnormal immune response to toxin or infection

CLINICAL ISSUES

- Acute febrile phase (days 1-11): Fever for 5 days > 104°F, bilateral, nonpurulent conjunctivitis & rash, hands, & feet develop erythema/edema, tongue & oral mucosa become red & cracked, myocarditis (36-50%) & pericarditis (16%)
- Subacute phase (days 11-21): Thrombocytosis, desquamation of digits, aneurysms develop
- Convalescent phase (days 21-60): Symptoms have resolved
- Chronic phase (> 60 days): Cardiac complications
- Favorable outcome with early recognition & treatment with intravenous γ globulin, aspirin

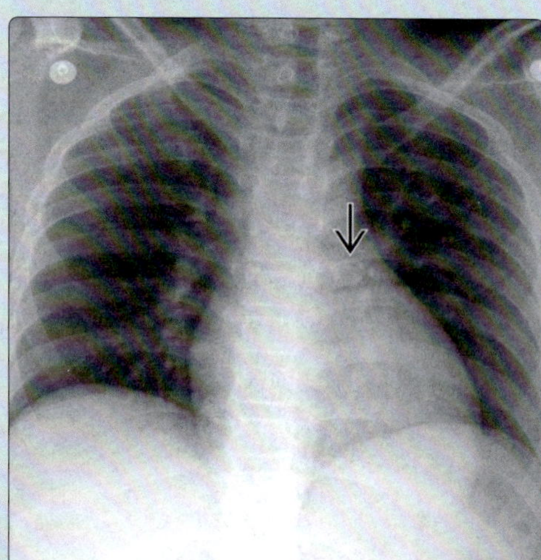

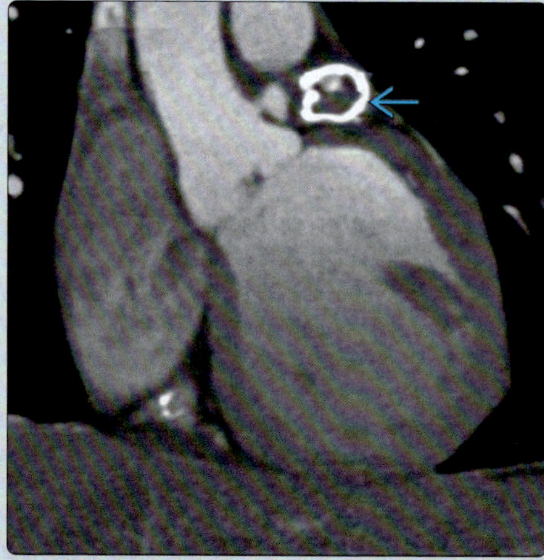

(Left) *Frontal view of the chest in an adolescent presenting with chest pain shows a left perihilar* Ca^{2+} ➔, *later shown to be a calcified left coronary artery aneurysm in a patient with undiagnosed prior Kawasaki disease.* **(Right)** *Coronal coronary CTA in the same patient shows a large calcified left proximal coronary artery aneurysm* ➔.

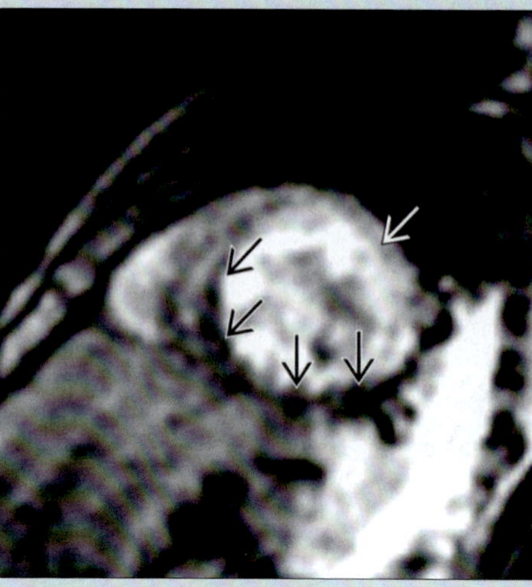

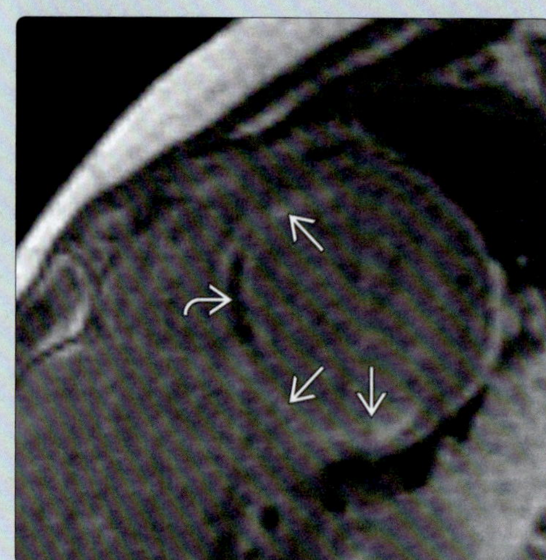

(Left) *Short-axis T2* GRE MR 1st-pass perfusion shows a large area of nonenhancing myocardium* ➔. *Note the normally enhancing myocardium* ➔ *for comparison.* **(Right)** *Short-axis late gadolinium enhanced (LGE) MR shows enhancement* ➔ *in the same distribution of myocardium that showed no 1st-pass perfusion, confirming the distribution of ischemic myocardium. The septum* ➔ *also demonstrated a no-reflow phenomenon due to continued microvascular occlusion.*

TERMINOLOGY

Synonyms

- Mucocutaneous lymph node syndrome; acute febrile mucocutaneous syndrome

Definitions

- Inflammatory disease of small- & medium-sized blood vessels of unknown etiology, occurring mainly in children
  - Manifests mainly with prolonged fever, nonsuppurative conjunctivitis, inflamed mucosal membranes of mouth & lips, cervical lymphadenopathy, maculoerythematous rash, & desquamation of hands & feet

IMAGING

General Features

- Best diagnostic clue
  - Multiple fusiform & saccular coronary aneurysms in severe cases; coronary artery ectasia in minor cases
- Location
  - Multisystem disease affecting skin, lymph nodes, mucous membranes, conjunctiva, myocardium, pericardium, coronary arteries, joints, bowel, gallbladder, kidney, urethra, & other sites

Radiographic Findings

- Chest radiography is usually normal
- Occasionally, may have large cardiac silhouette due to pericardial effusion or cardiomegaly

CT Findings

- CTA
  - Can demonstrate aneurysms, stenoses, & Ca^{2+} of coronary or other arteries

MR Findings

- T2WI
  - Can show edema secondary to myocarditis in acute phase
    - Myocarditis in up to 50%
- T2* GRE
  - MR stress imaging with quantification of regional perfusion
- MRA
  - Accurately images coronary artery aneurysms, occlusions, & stenoses
  - Used to depict & follow other aneurysms of thorax & abdomen or peripheral involvement
- MR cine
  - SSFP cine MR shows regional wall motion abnormalities
  - Can measure cardiac function with end-diastolic volumes, systolic ejection, & ejection fraction
- Delayed enhancement
  - Late gadolinium enhancement can show infarcted myocardium

Echocardiographic Findings

- Sufficient sensitivity & specificity for proximal coronary artery ectasia & aneurysms → 1st-line modality
  - Sensitivity: 80-85%
  - Evaluates ventricular function, valvar function, & pericardial effusion

Ultrasonographic Findings

- Grayscale ultrasound
  - Lymphadenopathy is usually nonsuppurative, unilateral, & in anterior triangle of neck
  - Gallbladder may be hydropic
  - ± nephromegaly
  - Aneurysms may be identified outside of chest

Angiographic Findings

- Conventional coronary angiography demonstrates aneurysm size & extent of stenosis
  - Aneurysms occur at bifurcating sites
  - Acute thrombotic occlusion of coronary artery may occur; thrombolytic therapy may be indicated

Nuclear Medicine Findings

- Thallium (Tl-201) or technetium (Tc-99m) sestamibi myocardial perfusion imaging (SPECT)
  - Pharmacologic stress testing with dipyridamole or adenosine can demonstrate myocardial ischemia

Imaging Recommendations

- Best imaging tool
  - Echocardiography for initial & sequential studies
  - Cardiac MR in older children & adults for assessing function, myocardial ischemia, myocardial viability, & aneurysms
- Protocol advice
  - Comprehensive cardiac MR protocol includes function, coronary artery imaging, 1st-pass perfusion, & late gadolinium enhancement for myocardial viability
  - MRA with large field of view can show aneurysms of peripheral arteries

DIFFERENTIAL DIAGNOSIS

MIS-C From SARS-CoV-2/COVID-19

- Occurs 2-6 weeks after COVID-19 infection
- Fever, rash, coagulopathy, gastrointestinal symptoms, hypotension
- Elevated inflammatory markers
- Higher incidence of coronary artery aneurysms than Kawasaki disease
- Mean age: 7-11 years

Exanthematous Infections: Viral or Bacterial

- Toxic shock syndrome has high fever, desquamation of hands & feet
- Rheumatic fever has skin rash, fever, arthritis, myocarditis, & pericarditis
- Mononucleosis has fever, lymphadenopathy, splenomegaly, & liver disease

Allergic or Hypersensitivity Reactions

- Drug reactions, Stevens-Johnson syndrome, & erythema multiforme have systemic signs, rash, & fever but usually do not have cardiac involvement

Vasculitides

- SLE, polyarteritis nodosa
- Takayasu may have medium- to large-vessel disease

PATHOLOGY

General Features

- Etiology
  - Remains elusive, but clinical & epidemiologic features suggest abnormal immune response to toxin or infection
- Laboratory evidence
  - C-reactive protein (CRP) is elevated
  - WBC count is elevated
  - Thrombocytosis with marked elevation of platelet counts appearing in 2nd & 3rd weeks

Gross Pathologic & Surgical Features

- Generalized systemic vasculitis involving small- & medium-sized arteries
- Late-phase fibroblastic proliferation & active inflammation replaced by progressive fibrosis & scar

Microscopic Features

- Perivasculitis involving small vessels
- Larger vessels become secondarily inflamed with aneurysm & thrombus formation

CLINICAL ISSUES

Presentation

- Most common signs/symptoms
  - Acute febrile phase (days 1-11)
    - Temperature elevated > 104°F for 5 days
    - Bilateral, nonpurulent conjunctivitis & rash
    - Hands & feet develop erythema & edema
    - Tongue & oral mucosa become red & cracked
    - Cervical lymphadenopathy, usually unilateral
    - Cardiac complications of myocarditis (36-50%) & pericarditis (16%)
  - Subacute phase (days 11-21): Fever has resolved
    - Persistent irritability, anorexia, conjunctivitis
    - Thrombocytosis develops
    - Desquamation of fingers & toes
    - Aneurysms may develop; greatest risk for sudden death
  - Convalescent phase (days 21-60): Symptoms of illness have disappeared
  - Chronic phase (> 60 days): Cardiac complications
- Other signs/symptoms
  - Dilation of gallbladder (hydrops) early in disease (15%)
  - Hepatic enlargement & jaundice can occur
  - Gastrointestinal complaints include diarrhea, vomiting, abdominal pain

Demographics

- Age
  - Peak incidence: 6 months to 2 years
  - Most are < 5 years old
- Sex
  - M:F = 5:1
- Epidemiology
  - Japan: Incidence 50/100,000 children < 4 years of age (10x incidence in USA)
  - Also prevalent in other countries, affecting mainly Asian populations
  - Minor epidemic outbursts every 3-4 years with seasonal variation

Natural History & Prognosis

- Self-limited disease in majority of cases
- Favorable outcome with early recognition, treatment with intravenous γ globulin, aspirin
- With development of coronary artery aneurysms
  - Thrombosis, arrhythmia, infarct, or delayed rupture
  - Persistent wall abnormalities after aneurysm regression
  - Chronic coronary insufficiency, premature atherosclerosis in < 4%
  - Death in > 1% due to arrhythmias

Treatment

- High-dose aspirin is used as antiinflammatory agent early in disease until fever has ↓
- Low-dose aspirin is used in children for 6-8 weeks & for prolonged period in children with confirmed aneurysms
- Intravenous γ globulin is given in acute phase to reduce coronary artery abnormalities
- Transcatheter coronary intervention if thrombosis occurs: Thrombolysis with tissue plasminogen activator (tPA)
- Long-term treatment directed by degree of coronary involvement
  - Coronary bypass surgery or cardiac transplantation may be necessary

DIAGNOSTIC CHECKLIST

Image Interpretation Pearls

- Masquerades as many common diseases in children, but distinct pattern & progression of acute illness is striking

SELECTED REFERENCES

1. Gottlieb M et al: Multisystem inflammatory syndrome in children with COVID-19. Am J Emerg Med. 49:148-52, 2021
2. Zhang QY et al: Similarities and differences between multiple inflammatory syndrome in children associated with COVID-19 and Kawasaki disease: clinical presentations, diagnosis, and treatment. World J Pediatr. 17(4):335-40, 2021
3. Lee CH et al: Coronary artery aneurysm in Kawasaki disease: from multimodality imaging. Coron Artery Dis. 31(2):193-4, 2020
4. Matsubara D et al: Echocardiographic findings in pediatric multisystem inflammatory syndrome associated with COVID-19 in the United States. J Am Coll Cardiol. 76(17):1947-61, 2020
5. McMurray JC et al: Multisystem inflammatory syndrome in children (MIS-C), a post-viral myocarditis and systemic vasculitis-a critical review of its pathogenesis and treatment. Front Pediatr. 8:626182, 2020
6. Pham V et al: Giant coronary aneurysms, from diagnosis to treatment: a literature review. Arch Cardiovasc Dis. 113(1):59-69, 2020
7. Toubiana J et al: Kawasaki-like multisystem inflammatory syndrome in children during the covid-19 pandemic in Paris, France: prospective observational study. BMJ. 369:m2094, 2020
8. Jindal AK et al: Kawasaki disease: characteristics, diagnosis, and unusual presentations. Expert Rev Clin Immunol. 15(10):1089-104, 2019
9. McCrindle BW et al: The role of echocardiography in Kawasaki disease. Int J Rheum Dis. 21(1):50-5, 2018
10. Miura M et al: Association of severity of coronary artery aneurysms in patients with Kawasaki disease and risk of later coronary events. JAMA Pediatr. 172(5):e180030, 2018
11. Singh S et al: Diagnosis of Kawasaki disease. Int J Rheum Dis. 21(1):36-44, 2018
12. Tsuda E et al: Role of imaging studies in Kawasaki disease. Int J Rheum Dis. 21(1):56-63, 2018
13. McCrindle BW et al: Diagnosis, treatment, and long-term management of Kawasaki disease: a scientific statement for health professionals from the American Heart Association. Circulation. 135(17):e927-99, 2017

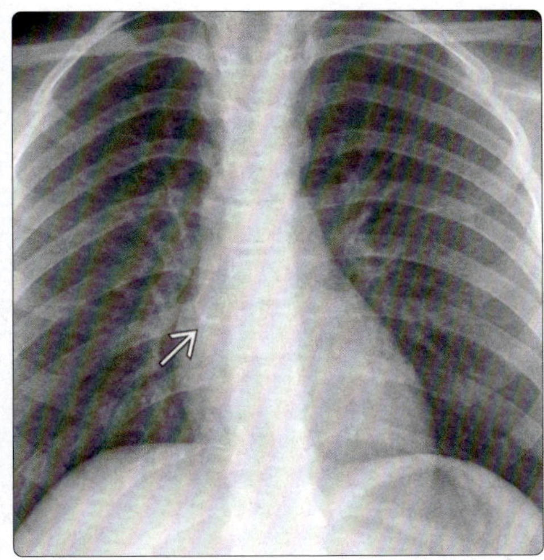

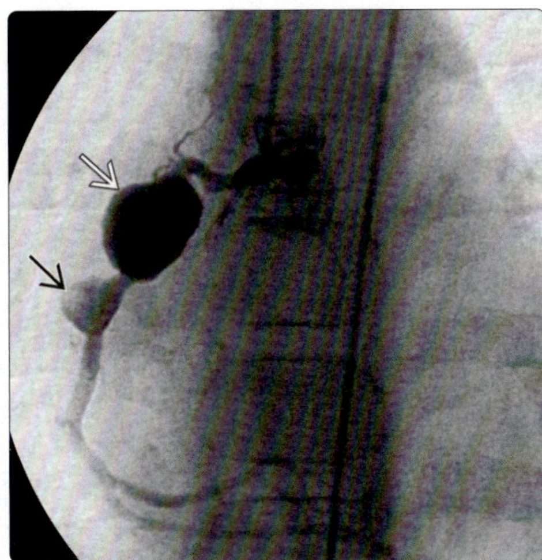

(Left) *PA radiograph shows a curvilinear* Ca^{2+} ➡ *projecting inferior to the right hilum. The patient's history revealed that the child had been diagnosed with Kawasaki disease at age 4, confirming that this abnormality is due to a calcified aneurysm.* **(Right)** *Frontal angiogram of a right coronary artery injection shows a large proximal aneurysm ➡ & a smaller, more distal aneurysm, which may contain some thrombus ➡. This patient eventually developed stenosis requiring stenting.*

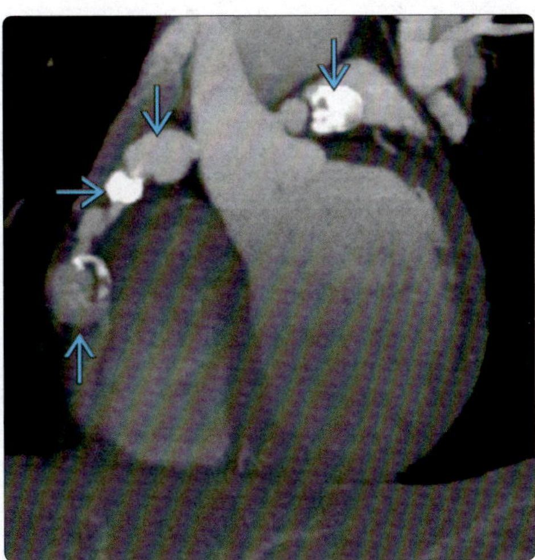

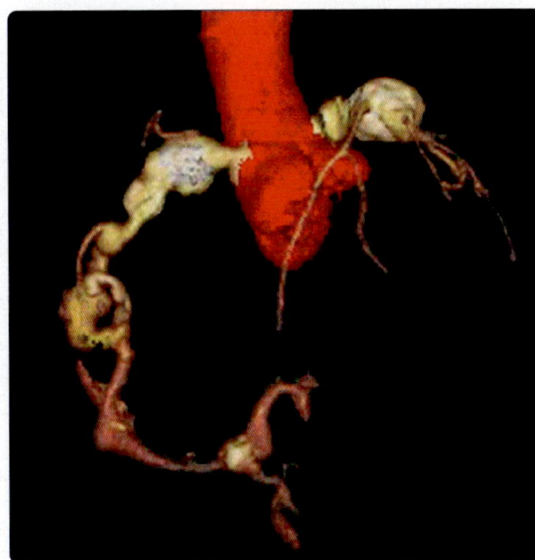

(Left) *Oblique MIP coronary CTA shows multiple bilateral calcified & noncalcified coronary artery aneurysms ➡ in a patient with Kawasaki disease.* **(Right)** *Color-coded 3D surface-rendered coronary CTA shows multiple bilateral calcified & noncalcified coronary artery aneurysms in the same patient with Kawasaki disease.*

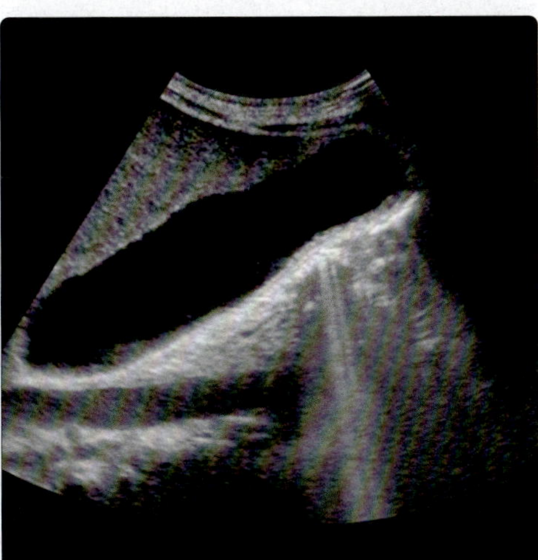

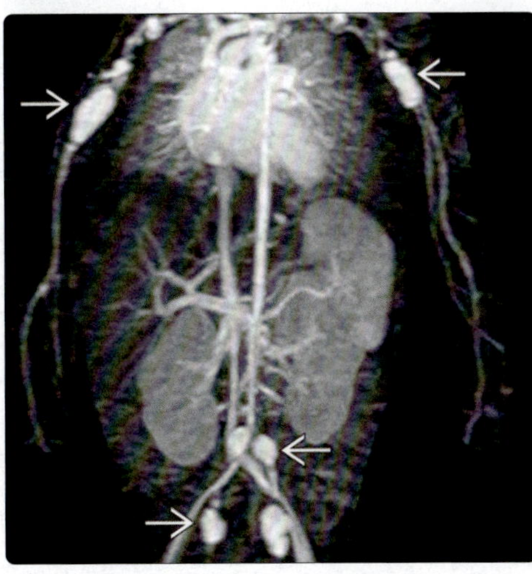

(Left) *Oblique ultrasound of the right upper quadrant in a 5-year-old with fever & pain shows an enlarged, hydropic gallbladder. This finding ultimately led to the diagnosis of Kawasaki disease.* **(Right)** *Coronal MRA in a child with Kawasaki disease shows multiple aneurysms ➡ of the peripheral arteries. This same MRA was also able to depict aneurysms of the coronary arteries (not shown). (Courtesy S. Yoo, MD.)*

Rheumatic Heart Disease

KEY FACTS

TERMINOLOGY

- Acute rheumatic fever: Multisystem disease affecting heart, joints, skin, & brain 1-5 weeks following infection with group A β-hemolytic *Streptococcus*
  - Due to autoimmune response
  - 40% of acute rheumatic fever patients develop cardiac involvement (RHD)

IMAGING

- Acute rheumatic fever: Large heart, left atrial enlargement, pulmonary edema (due to left ventricular dysfunction with mitral insufficiency)
  - Rheumatic pneumonia is rarely seen
  - Pericardial effusion
- Chronic RHD: Ca^{2+} of valves, especially mitral or aortic
- Echocardiogram during acute disease quantitates degree of mitral insufficiency & left ventricular function
- Echocardiogram in chronic disease shows progression of valve stenosis with thickened leaflets, which calcify

CLINICAL ISSUES

- Acute disease occurs in young children 3-15 years who present with streptococcal sore throat
  - RHD develops after 0.3% of such infections in USA
- Initial treatment: Therapy aimed at preventing acute rheumatic fever by treating group A streptococcal pharyngitis & eradicating reservoir for transmission
  - Disease has dramatically ↓ in USA where sore throat from *Streptococcus pyogenes* is treated
  - Disease is now most common in overcrowded areas of world where infection can spread in dry, hot climate
    - High mortality rate in malnourished populations
- Jones criteria for rheumatic fever
  - Major: Carditis, polyarthritis, chorea, subcutaneous nodules, & erythema marginatum
  - Minor: Fever, arthralgia, elevated acute phase reactants, ↑ sedimentation rate

(Left) *PA radiograph in an adult with rheumatic heart disease (RHD) shows cardiomegaly with dilation of the left atrial appendage ➡, creating a broad bump on the lateral margin of the heart below the level of the pulmonary artery. The left atrium splays the carina & creates a double shadow over the right heart border ➡.* **(Right)** *Axial CECT in a young adult shows irregular thickening of the mitral valve ➡ due to RHD.*

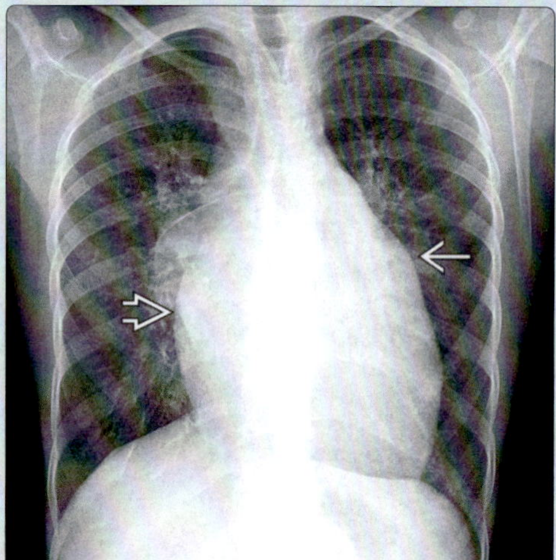

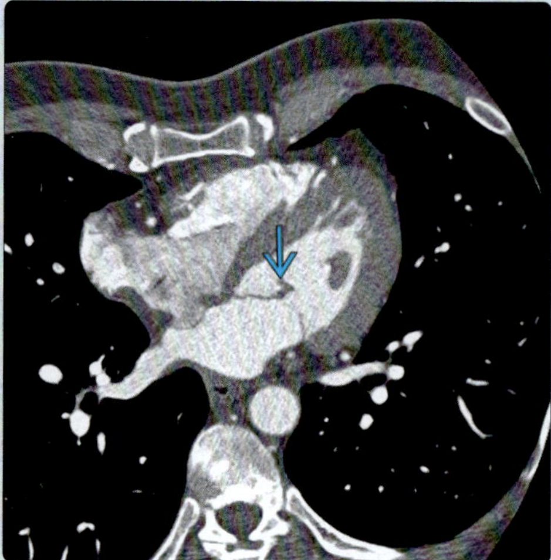

(Left) *Four-chamber SSFP cine cardiac MR in an adolescent demonstrates a dephasing jet ➡ in the left atrium due to mitral regurgitation from a damaged mitral valve in a patient with RHD.* **(Right)** *AP radiograph in a 17-year-old patient shows pulmonary edema due to progressive aortic insufficiency from acute bacterial endocarditis complicating rheumatic aortic valve disease.*

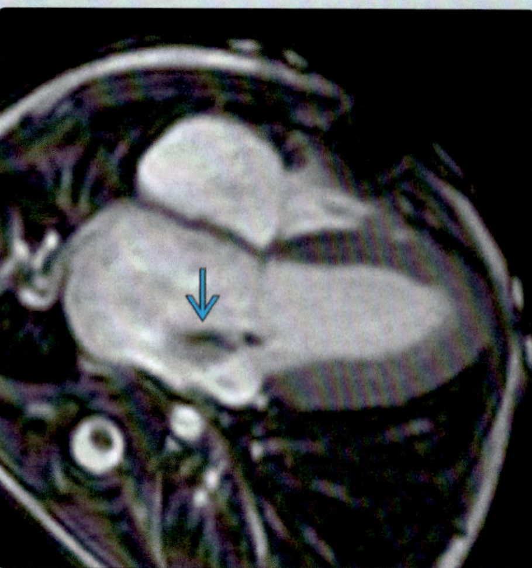

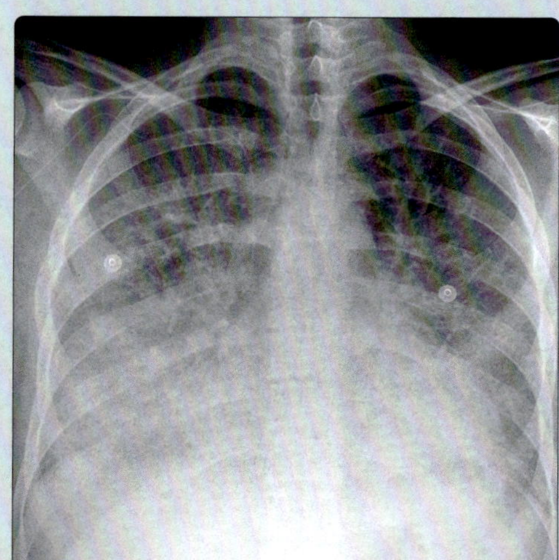

TERMINOLOGY

Abbreviations

- Rheumatic heart disease (RHD)

Definitions

- Acquired heart disease due to autoimmune response to prior group A β-hemolytic *Streptococcus* infection
- Part of multisystem disease affecting heart, joints, skin, & brain; occurs 1-5 weeks following infection

IMAGING

General Features

- Best diagnostic clue
  - Large heart, left atrial enlargement (LAE), pulmonary edema
    - Due to left ventricular dysfunction with mitral insufficiency
  - Pericardial inflammation & effusion
  - Multisystem involvement

Radiographic Findings

- Acute disease
  - Cardiomegaly & pulmonary congestion, pericardial effusion
  - LAE when mitral insufficiency or stenosis is present
  - Rheumatic pneumonia is rarely seen; various patterns have been described
- Chronic RHD
  - Ca^{2+} of valves, especially mitral or aortic
  - LAE with mitral regurgitation or stenosis

Echocardiographic Findings

- Acute disease
  - Quantitates degree of mitral insufficiency & left ventricular function
- Chronic
  - Progression of valve stenosis with thickened leaflets, which calcify
  - Fusion of commissures & chordae

MR Findings

- MR to assess cardiac function
  - Quantitates degree of valve insufficiency/stenosis

PATHOLOGY

General Features

- Etiology
  - Infection with group A *Streptococcus* is precipitating event
    - RHD develops after 0.3% of such infections in USA
  - May lead to acute rheumatic fever with inflammation of joints, heart, brain, connective tissue
    - Genetic susceptibility to rheumatic fever is related to human leukocyte antigens
    - Immune reactions with cross-reactive antibody or cell-mediated immunity

Gross Pathologic & Surgical Features

- Inflammatory reaction involves connective or collagen tissue
- Acute carditis affects endocardium & myocardium
- Pericardial serositis may later calcify
  - Pericardium is thickened & irregular
- Mitral valve involvement in 75% of cases
  - Verrucous lesions
- Arthritis does not affect cartilage, but synovial lining shows fibrinoid degeneration

CLINICAL ISSUES

Presentation

- Most common signs/symptoms
  - Cardiac symptoms
    - 39% of patients with rheumatic fever develop pancarditis with valve insufficiency
    - Pericardial friction rub: Pericardial involvement
  - Prominent noncardiac manifestations
    - Jones major criteria: Carditis, polyarthritis, chorea, subcutaneous nodules, & erythema marginatum
    - Jones minor criteria: Fever, arthralgia, elevated acute phase reactants, ↑ sedimentation rate
- Significant change in presentation over past 25 years
  - Disease has dramatically ↓ in USA where sore throat from *Streptococcus* is treated
  - Disease is now most common in overcrowded regions where *S. pyogenes* can spread in dry, hot climate

Demographics

- Age
  - Acute disease occurs in young children 3-15 years of age who present with streptococcal sore throat
  - Chronic disease can have multiple recurrences & progression
- Sex
  - Equal in numbers but prognosis is worse for females

Natural History & Prognosis

- Group A *Streptococcus* is gram-positive coccus that colonizes skin & oral pharynx
  - Acute infection may precipitate acute rheumatic fever
    - Occurs 1-5 weeks later in 0.3%
  - Chronic sequelae of acute rheumatic fever
    - 40% of patients develop cardiac involvement
    - Mitral valve is most severely affected in 65-75%, aortic valve in 25%
    - Varying degrees of arrhythmia, valve insufficiency, or ventricular dysfunction
- High mortality rate in malnourished populations
  - Mortality rate is ~ 0 in USA
  - 90,000 deaths worldwide each year

SELECTED REFERENCES

1. Aremu OO et al: Cardiovascular imaging modalities in the diagnosis and management of rheumatic heart disease. Int J Cardiol. 325:176-85, 2021
2. Atalay S et al: Echocardiographic screening for rheumatic heart disease in Turkish schoolchildren. Cardiol Young. 29(10):1272-7, 2019
3. Leal MTBC et al: Rheumatic heart disease in the modern era: recent developments and current challenges. Rev Soc Bras Med Trop. 52:e20180041, 2019
4. Baeßler B et al: The role of cardiovascular magnetic resonance imaging in rheumatic heart disease. Clin Exp Rheumatol. 36 Suppl 114(5):171-6, 2018
5. Ntusi NA: Cardiovascular magnetic resonance imaging in rheumatic heart disease. Cardiovasc J Afr. 29(3):135-6, 2018

Marfan Syndrome

KEY FACTS

TERMINOLOGY

- Inherited autosomal dominant connective tissue disorder due to *FBN1* mutation → abnormal fibrillin-1

IMAGING

- Cardiovascular: Aortic root dilation at sinuses of Valsalva (75%), ascending aortic dissection, mitral valve prolapse (MVP) (50-70%), main pulmonary artery dilation, mitral anulus Ca^{2+}, dilation of abdominal aorta
- Skeletal: Pectus excavatum, pectus carinatum, long arms & legs, arachnodactyly, joint hypermobility, scoliosis, thoracic lordosis, pes planus, protrusio acetabuli
- Pulmonary: Spontaneous pneumothorax, apical blebs
- Dural: Ectasia (enlarged nerve sleeves & posterior vertebral body scalloping)
- Postoperative complications: Pseudoaneurysm, aortic dissection, rupture
- Best imaging tools
  - CTA in acute setting to exclude dissection &/or rupture
  - Echocardiography or cardiac MR for routine follow-up of aortic root dilation & valvular disease

PATHOLOGY

- 2010 revised Ghent nosology for diagnosis
  - Based on family history, aortic root size/dissection, ectopia lentis, *FBN1* mutation, systemic score

CLINICAL ISSUES

- 90% of deaths are from cardiovascular complications (aortic dissection, congestive heart failure, & cardiac valve disease)
  - Progressive aortic dilation → highest risk of dissection
    - Chest pain radiating down back in Marfan syndrome patient → suspect aortic dissection
- Treatment
  - Medical: β-blocker or angiotensin II receptor blocker
  - Surgery: Prophylactic aortic root surgery when diameter at sinuses of Valsalva exceeds 5 cm

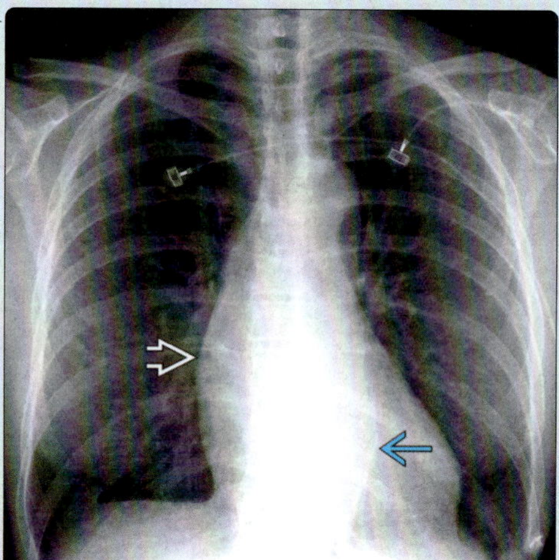
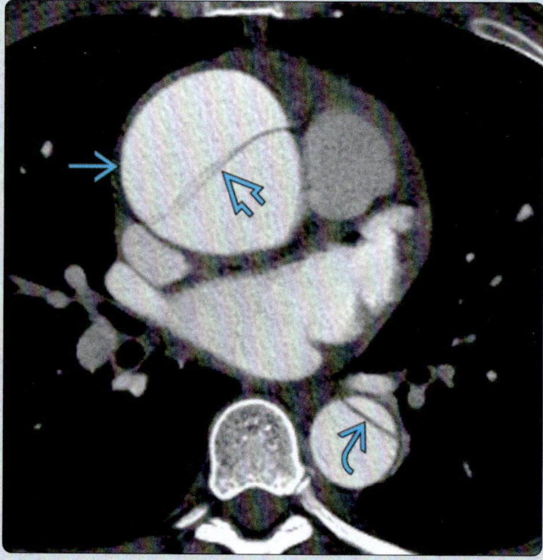

(Left) *Frontal radiograph of the chest demonstrates a right border-forming ascending aorta ➡ with a tortuous, descending aorta ➡ in this 18-year-old patient with known Marfan syndrome who presented with chest pain.* **(Right)** *Axial cardiac CTA in an adolescent patient with Marfan syndrome shows marked aneurysmal dilation of the ascending aorta ➡ with a dissection noted in the ascending ➡ & descending ➡ aorta.*

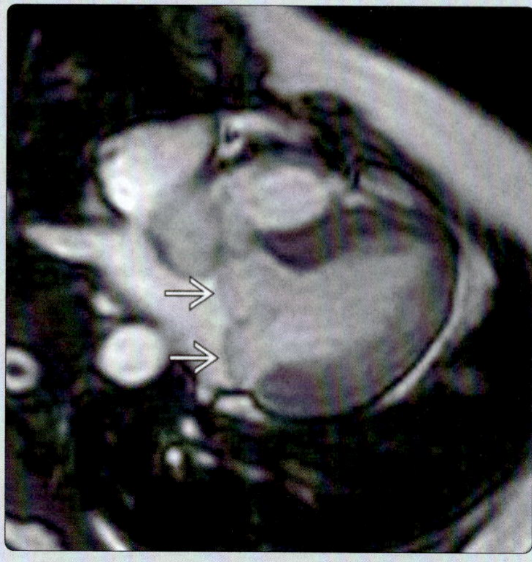
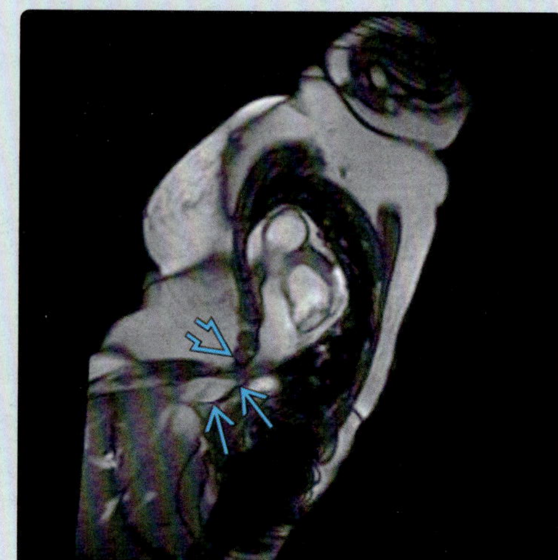

(Left) *Four-chamber cine bright blood SSFP cardiac MR demonstrates mitral valve prolapse with ballooning of the leaflets of the mitral valve ➡ into the left atrium in a Marfan syndrome patient.* **(Right)** *Short-axis FIESTA cine image from a cardiac MR in a patient with Marfan syndrome shows severe pectus excavatum ➡ deformity with compression of the upper inferior vena cava ➡.*

TERMINOLOGY

Definitions

- Inherited autosomal dominant connective tissue disorder due to *FBN1* mutation → abnormal fibrillin-1

IMAGING

General Features

- Best diagnostic clue
  - Aortic dissection in tall, thin patient with pectus deformity, scoliosis, & long fingers
- Location
  - Cardiovascular: Aortic root dilation at level of sinuses of Valsalva (75%), ascending aortic dissection, mitral valve prolapse (MVP) (50-70%), main pulmonary artery dilation, mitral anulus Ca^{2+}, dilation of abdominal aorta
  - Skeletal: Pectus excavatum, pectus carinatum, long arms & legs, arachnodactyly, joint hypermobility, scoliosis, thoracic lordosis, pes planus, protrusio acetabuli
  - Ocular: Ectopia lentis (50%), flat cornea, cataract, hypoplastic iris, nearsightedness, glaucoma (< 50 years of age), retinal detachment
  - Pulmonary: Spontaneous pneumothorax (5-10%), apical blebs
  - Skin: Stretch marks in absence of weight changes or pregnancy, recurrent hernia
  - Dural: Ectasia (widening & dilation of dural sac with enlarged nerve sleeves & posterior vertebral body scalloping)

Radiographic Findings

- Enlargement of ascending aorta creates right-sided border forming mediastinal prominence
- Enlarged main pulmonary artery
- Pectus excavatum or carinatum
- Apical bleb, spontaneous pneumothorax

CT Findings

- CTA
  - Dilation of ascending aorta (starts at sinuses of Valsalva)
  - Aortic dissection, dilated pulmonary artery, mass effect on heart or inferior vena cava from pectus excavatum
    - CTA is fast & effective way to exclude aortic dissection in acute setting
    - Coronary CTA is helpful in patients with dissection to evaluate coronary artery involvement
  - Apical blebs, pneumothorax
  - Posterior scalloping of vertebrae from dural ectasia

MR Findings

- Anatomic imaging: Ascending aortic aneurysm, dissection
- Functional cine bright blood imaging
  - Dephasing artifact from aortic & mitral regurgitation
  - MVP
  - Ventricular function is best on short-axis imaging
- Phase-contrast imaging
  - Quantify aortic & mitral regurgitant fraction
  - Pulse wave velocity measurements to evaluate aortic stiffness

Imaging Recommendations

- Best imaging tool
  - CTA in acute setting to exclude dissection &/or rupture
  - Echocardiography or cardiac MR for routine follow-up of aortic root dilation & valvular disease

PATHOLOGY

General Features

- Genetics
  - Autosomal dominant
  - Mutation in *FBN1* gene located on chromosome 15q21.1
    - Mutation causes abnormal fibrillin (major substrate for microfibrils)

Staging, Grading, & Classification

- 2010 revised Ghent nosology for diagnosis

CLINICAL ISSUES

Presentation

- Most common signs/symptoms
  - Chest pain radiating down back from aortic dissection
  - Heart murmurs from aortic & mitral regurgitation
  - Unilateral chest pain from spontaneous pneumothorax
- Other signs/symptoms
  - Visual disturbances

Demographics

- Frequency: 2-3:10,000
- Diagnosis may be made in infancy or well into adulthood

Natural History & Prognosis

- 90% of deaths are from cardiovascular complications (aortic dissection, congestive heart failure, & cardiac valve disease)
  - Progressive aortic dilation carries highest risk of aortic dissection
- Improved detection & treatment has helped prolong survival to nearly normal levels

Treatment

- Moderate restriction of physical activity
- β-blocker or angiotensin II receptor blocker
  - For prophylaxis of progressive aortic root dilation
  - Initiated at disease diagnosis
- Prophylactic aortic root surgery when diameter at sinuses of Valsalva exceeds 5 cm

SELECTED REFERENCES

1. Leidenberger T et al: Imaging-based 4D aortic pressure mapping in Marfan syndrome patients: a matched case-control study. Ann Thorac Surg. 109(5):1434-40, 2020
2. Braverman AC et al: Bicuspid aortic valve in Marfan syndrome. Circ Cardiovasc Imaging. 12(3):e008860, 2019
3. Guala A et al: Influence of aortic dilation on the regional aortic stiffness of bicuspid aortic valve assessed by 4-dimensional flow cardiac magnetic resonance: comparison with Marfan syndrome and degenerative aortic aneurysm. JACC Cardiovasc Imaging. 12(6):1020-9, 2019
4. Yuan X et al: Aortic imaging and biomechanics in Marfan syndrome: keep it simple but not too simple. Eur Heart J. 40(25):2055-7, 2019
5. Raffa GM et al: Aortic surgery in Marfan patients with severe pectus excavatum. J Cardiovasc Med (Hagerstown). 18(5):305-10, 2017
6. Thacoor A: Mitral valve prolapse and Marfan syndrome. Congenit Heart Dis. 12(4):430-4, 2017

Loeys-Dietz Syndrome

KEY FACTS

TERMINOLOGY

- Autosomal dominant connective tissue disorder due to 1 of 5 genetic mutations affecting transforming growth factor β

IMAGING

- 98% have aortic root aneurysms
- 20% have aneurysms in head & neck region
- Aneurysms also occur in coronary arteries, pulmonary arteries, & ductus arteriosus
- Recommendations
  - Baseline imaging
    - Echocardiography every 6-12 months
    - Screening CTA or MRA of head through pelvis every 2 years
  - For acute chest pain: Chest CTA for aortic dissection & aneurysms
  - For acute headache: Noncontrast head CT for intracranial hemorrhage; if positive, follow with head CTA

TOP DIFFERENTIAL DIAGNOSES

- Marfan syndrome
- Vascular Ehlers-Danlos syndrome

CLINICAL ISSUES

- Systemic involvement with craniofacial, cardiovascular, skeletal, skin, & nervous system abnormalities
- Characteristic clinical triad of hypertelorism, bifid uvula or cleft palate, & aortic aneurysms ± dissection & tortuous arteries
- Leading cause of death: Aortic dissection (67%)
  - ↑ risk for dissection or rupture at > 3.9-cm diameter
- Abdominal aortic dissection & cerebral hemorrhage from ruptured aneurysm account for 22% of deaths
- Preventative treatment with hypertension/heart rate control: β-blocker, angiotensin II receptor blocker

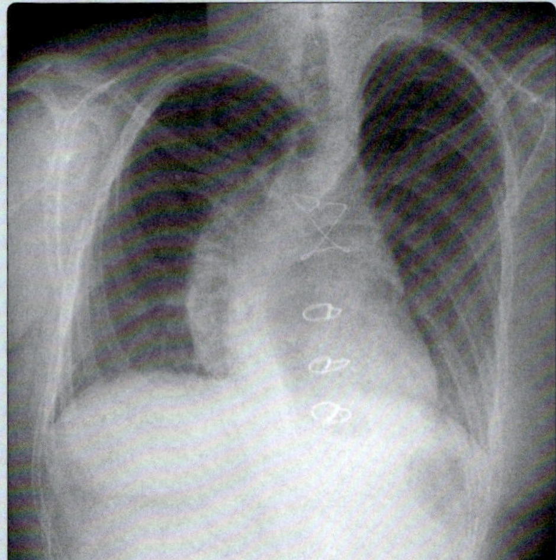

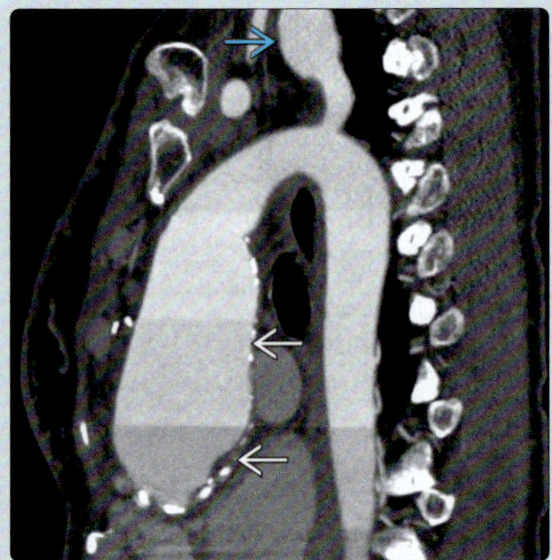

(Left) *Frontal radiograph of the chest in a 15-year-old patient with Loeys-Dietz syndrome shows severe dextroscoliosis of the thoracic spine. Note the postoperative changes of a prior sternotomy for repair of the aortic root.* **(Right)** *Oblique sagittal CTA in a 15-year-old patient with Loeys-Dietz syndrome shows an aneurysm of the left subclavian artery ➡. Note the ascending aortic aneurysm ➡ & postoperative changes.*

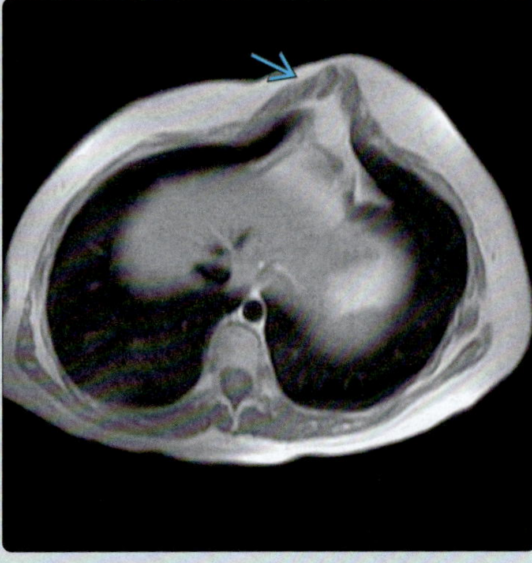

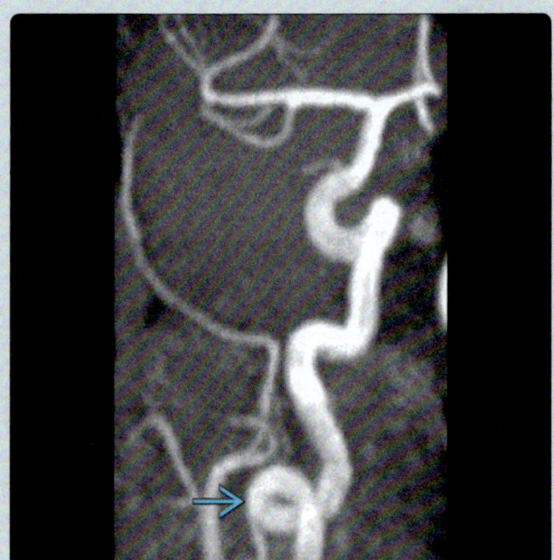

(Left) *Axial DIR cardiac MR in a 15-year-old patient with Loeys-Dietz syndrome shows a pectus carinatum deformity ➡. While this can be seen in patients with Marfan syndrome, it is more often associated with Loeys-Dietz.* **(Right)** *Anterior 3D TOF MRA in a 15-year-old patient with Loeys-Dietz syndrome shows tortuosity of the proximal right internal carotid artery ➡, which is frequently seen in this syndrome.*

TERMINOLOGY

Definitions

- Autosomal dominant connective tissue disorder with aortic/arterial abnormalities

IMAGING

General Features

- Best diagnostic clue
  - Arterial tortuosity with aortic aneurysm & dissection
  - Hypertelorism
  - Bifid uvula or cleft palate
  - Instability or malformation of spine/neck
  - Club foot
  - White sclera of eye looks blue or gray
- Location
  - 98% have aortic root aneurysms
  - 20% have aneurysms in head & neck region
  - Aneurysms also occur in coronary arteries, pulmonary arteries, & ductus arteriosus

CT Findings

- CTA
  - Evaluation of aortic aneurysm & dissection; associated coronary artery, pulmonary artery, & ductus arteriosus aneurysms

MR Findings

- MRA
  - Evaluation of aortic aneurysm & dissection
    - Phase contrast to evaluate aortic valve regurgitation, which often accompanies aortic root aneurysm
  - Tortuosity of intracranial vessels

Echocardiographic Findings

- 1st-line evaluation of aortic root, myocardial function, valve morphology (including bicuspid aortic valve)

Imaging Recommendations

- Best imaging tool
  - For acute chest pain: CTA of chest for aortic dissection & aneurysms
  - For acute headache: Noncontrast head CT for acute intracranial hemorrhage; if positive, follow with head CTA
- Baseline imaging
  - Echocardiography + screening CTA or MRA of head, neck, chest, abdomen, & pelvis
- Follow-up imaging
  - Echocardiography every 6-12 months
  - CTA or MRA of head to pelvis at least every 2 years

DIFFERENTIAL DIAGNOSIS

Marfan Syndrome

- Dissection & aortic rupture tend to occur at larger diameter & later in life than patients with Loeys-Dietz syndrome
- Lacks tortuosity, aneurysms, & dissections beyond aorta
- Lens dislocation is typical

Vascular Ehlers-Danlos Syndrome

- Aortic dissection & rupture without preceding dilation
  - Usually affects descending rather than proximal aorta
- Spontaneous carotid-cavernous fistula, bowel perforations

PATHOLOGY

General Features

- Connective tissue disorder from mutations in 1 of 5 genes

Staging, Grading, & Classification

- *TGFBR1* mutation causes Loeys-Dietz type 1
- *TGFBR2* mutation causes Loeys-Dietz type 2
- *SMAD3* mutation causes Loeys-Dietz type 3
- *TGFB2* mutation causes Loeys-Dietz type 4
- *TGFB3* mutation causes Loeys-Dietz type 5

CLINICAL ISSUES

Presentation

- Most common signs/symptoms
  - Characteristic clinical triad of hypertelorism, bifid uvula or cleft palate, & aortic aneurysms ± dissection & tortuous arteries
- Other signs/symptoms
  - Systemic involvement with craniofacial, cardiovascular, skeletal, skin, & nervous system abnormalities
    - Congenital heart problems, such as patent ductus arteriosus, bicuspid aortic valve, or atrial septal defect
    - Scoliosis or kyphosis, pectus excavatum or carinatum deformity, camptodactyly, arachnodactyly, club foot
    - Translucent skin, joint hypermobility
    - Craniosynostosis, dural ectasia
    - Strabismus from weakened eye muscles

Natural History & Prognosis

- Leading cause of death: Aortic dissection (67%)
  - ↑ risk for dissection/rupture at aortic diameter > 3.9 cm
- Abdominal aortic dissection & cerebral hemorrhage from ruptured aneurysm account for 22% of deaths

Treatment

- Preventative treatment: Hypertension/heart rate control with β-blocker, angiotensin II receptor blocker

SELECTED REFERENCES

1. Iqbal R et al: Loeys-Dietz syndrome pathology and aspects of cardiovascular management: a systematic review. Vascular. 29(1):3-14, 2021
2. Estrera AL: Loeys-Dietz syndrome: we have come a (Fur)long way. J Thorac Cardiovasc Surg. 157(2):453-54, 2019
3. Jud P et al: Vascular involvement in Loeys-Dietz syndrome. Mayo Clin Proc. 94(6):1117-9, 2019
4. Loughborough WW et al: Cardiovascular manifestations and complications of Loeys-Dietz syndrome: CT and MR imaging findings. Radiographics. 38(1):275-86, 2018
5. Gawinecka J et al: Acute aortic dissection: pathogenesis, risk factors and diagnosis. Swiss Med Wkly. 147:w14489, 2017
6. Meester JAN et al: Differences in manifestations of Marfan syndrome, Ehlers-Danlos syndrome, and Loeys-Dietz syndrome. Ann Cardiothorac Surg. 6(6):582-94, 2017

SECTION 4

Gastrointestinal

Mesenteric Abnormalities

Trauma

Abnormalities in Immunocompromised Children

Inflammatory Bowel Disease

Miscellaneous

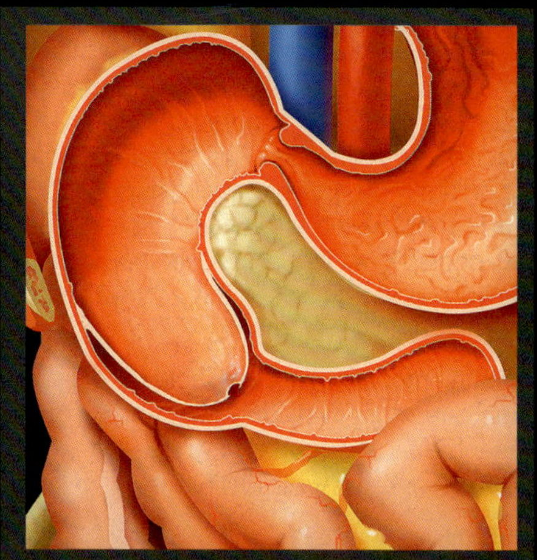

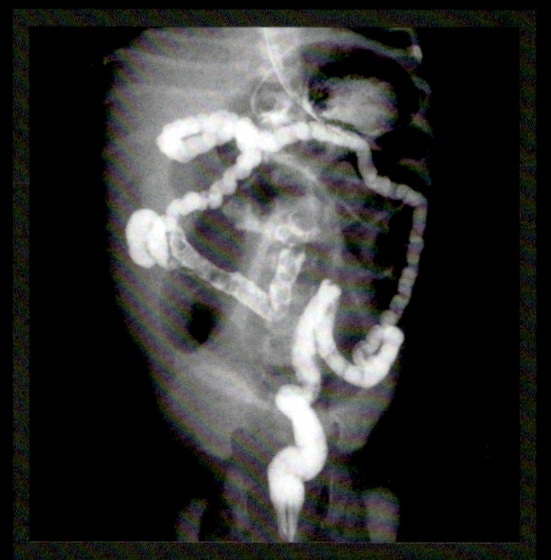

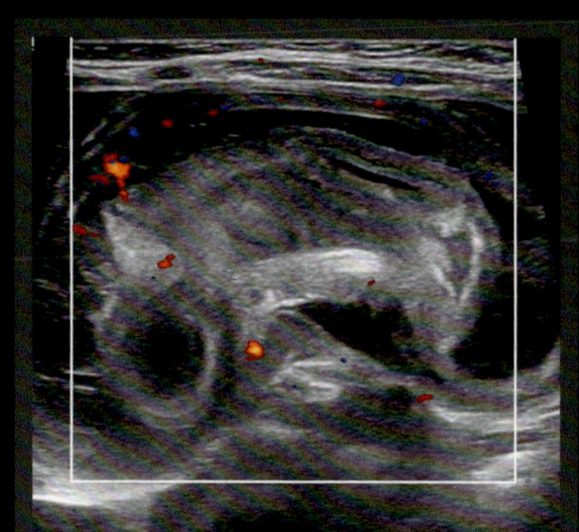

Imaging Techniques

Pediatric radiologists must have an understanding not only of the unique disorders that affect children but also the expected range of normal appearances that occur from infancy to early adulthood. The radiologist must also be able to tailor the imaging study to meet a child's needs, which includes explaining the procedure in an age-appropriate manner, distracting the child so that imaging can be performed, &, when needed, immobilizing the child safely during the procedure. In addition, radiologists must remember that children are more sensitive to the effects of ionizing radiation than adults. This should be considered when deciding on the most appropriate imaging study to diagnose a suspected condition. If the selected test requires ionizing radiation, pediatric-specific protocols should be employed to keep the dose as low as reasonably achievable (the ALARA principle).

Many imaging modalities are available for diagnosing abdominal pathology in children. Depending on the patient age, presentation, & specific clinical question, each modality has unique advantages & disadvantages.

Radiography

Constipation, pain, vomiting/bowel obstruction, & necrotizing enterocolitis are common indications for obtaining pediatric abdominal radiographs. Modifications for children include a single view for suspected constipation & the decubitus view or cross-table lateral view to look for free air in infants.

Fluoroscopy

Methods to reduce radiation exposure to the patient include minimizing fluoroscopy time, pulsed fluoroscopy, fluoroscopic image hold or clips rather than digital spot exposures, small image intensifier-to-patient distance, appropriate collimation, & low-dose fluoroscopy settings for pediatric patients based on size.

Upper GI

Common pediatric indications for the upper GI series include bilious & intractable nonbilious emesis & difficulty swallowing. A single-contrast upper GI is typically employed for these investigations, though a double-contrast study is sometimes performed in teenagers when looking for esophagitis or gastric ulcers (i.e., studies requiring fine mucosal detail). Note that evaluating the position of the duodenojejunal junction (DJJ) is crucial, especially in young vomiting infants.

The typical single-contrast upper GI technique should include the following images: A left-side-down lateral view of the esophagus while swallowing, a supine frontal view of the esophagus (which can include a fluoroscopic clip of peristalsis), a right-side-down lateral view of the 1st pass of contrast into the duodenum as it courses posteriorly in the retroperitoneum & ascends toward the DJJ, & a straight supine frontal view of the duodenum during the 1st pass of contrast to document the normal DJJ to the left of the spine at or nearly at the same level as the duodenal bulb.

Contrast Enema

Common indications for a contrast enema include the failure of a newborn to pass meconium, newborn bilious emesis (if the radiograph suggests a distal obstruction), & chronic constipation.

Enema modifications for children include selecting a rectal catheter that is appropriate for size & the use of a water-soluble contrast agent instead of barium.

The typical contrast enema technique includes the following images: An early left-side-down lateral view of the rectum through the sigmoid colon (to evaluate the rectosigmoid ratio) while contrast is flowing, a frontal view of the rectum through the sigmoid colon during active filling, an overhead frontal view of the abdomen when filled just barely to the cecum, & an overhead frontal view of the abdomen after spontaneous contrast evacuation. In newborns with a suspected distal bowel obstruction, reflux of contrast into the terminal ileum is helpful. Spot images (± oblique positioning) may be helpful at sites of suspected stricture or redundancy.

Enema Reduction of Intussusception

Various techniques can be used to reduce an ileocolic intussusception. However, air reduction is widely accepted as a safe, effective, & established method. In this procedure, air is insufflated into the colon under fluoroscopic monitoring until gas refluxes into the terminal ileum & the soft tissue mass of the intussusceptum disappears. Important points for performing this technique include: An adequate seal must be created by the rectal tube at the anus to build effective intraluminal pressure, the sustained colonic pressure must be kept below 120 mm Hg, & an 18-gauge IV-type cannula should be kept at the bedside to reduce a tension pneumoperitoneum if perforation occurs. Note that an enema reduction is contraindicated with peritoneal signs or pneumoperitoneum.

Abdominal US

US is a simple, cost-effective, noninvasive, & ionizing radiation-free method of imaging the pediatric abdomen.

Common indications for pediatric abdominal US include suspected hypertrophic pyloric stenosis (HPS), intussusception, appendicitis, a palpable mass or organomegaly, abdominal pain, hematuria, oliguria, & organ dysfunction suspected by laboratory values. US is also increasingly used for bowel abnormalities outside of intussusception, such as necrotizing enterocolitis & inflammatory bowel disease.

Sonographic modifications for children include the selection of an appropriate transducer & distraction of the patient during scanning.

Abdominal CT

Common indications for pediatric abdominal CT include trauma, abdominal pain, suspected appendicitis with an equivocal US, complications of pancreatitis, & abscess. It should be noted, however, that, outside of trauma, US & MR are increasingly replacing CT due to the concerns of ionizing radiation.

Modifications for children include the use of weight-/size-based protocols & automatic tube current modulation techniques.

The use of IV &/or oral contrast should be driven by the specific clinical indication.

Abdominal MR

MR imaging uses no ionizing radiation & provides excellent soft tissue contrast.

Common indications for pediatric abdominal MR include the further investigation of a mass, surveillance after the treatment of a cancer, assessment of inflammatory bowel disease & pancreatobiliary disorders, liver quantification (of iron, fat, &/or fibrosis), & utilization as an alternative modality for suspected appendicitis.

Specific indications will help drive the selection of the appropriate contrast agent & protocol. Diffusion-weighted imaging can be particularly helpful in increasing the conspicuity of inflammatory & neoplastic pathologies against collapsed normal bowel loops.

Modifications for children include the use of video goggles for distraction, pretest practice/simulation to prepare young patients for the noise & relatively small bore size, & the use of sedation or general anesthesia for most patients < 6 years of age.

Differential Diagnoses

Neonatal Bowel Obstruction

High or proximal intestinal obstruction (with radiographs showing a few dilated proximal loops with a paucity of distal bowel gas) should be evaluated with an upper GI, though the true double bubble sign (with bulbous distention of the stomach & proximal duodenum without any distal gas) strongly suggests duodenal atresia & requires no further imaging. Differential considerations for proximal neonatal bowel obstruction include malrotation with midgut volvulus, duodenal atresia/stenosis, duodenal web, annular pancreas, & jejunal atresia.

Low or distal intestinal obstruction (with radiographs showing many dilated loops) should be evaluated with a water-soluble contrast enema. Differential considerations in this setting will include Hirschsprung disease, meconium plug/small left colon syndrome, meconium ileus, ileal atresia, & anorectal malformation.

Specific Neonatal Disorders

Esophageal atresia with a tracheoesophageal fistula (TEF) may show a distended proximal esophageal pouch containing the tip of an enteric tube. A proximal atresia with a distal TEF is the most common type, & air is typically seen in the stomach & intestines.

Necrotizing enterocolitis typically occurs in premature neonates & presents as stagnant dilated, air-filled bowel loops & pneumatosis, ± portal venous gas & pneumoperitoneum.

Neonatal abdominal masses in the GI tract include a duplication cyst, obstructed bowel loop, meconium pseudocyst, hepatic hemangioma, hepatoblastoma, & mesenchymal hamartoma. Abdominal masses in the neonatal GU tract include severe hydronephrosis, mesoblastic nephroma, Wilms tumor, autosomal recessive polycystic kidneys, neuroblastoma, bladder outlet obstruction, hydrocolpos, & ovarian cyst.

Vomiting Infant

If bilious emesis is present, an emergent upper GI series is the study of choice to look for a proximal obstruction, such as malrotation with midgut volvulus (even though bilious emesis in a neonate is more commonly due to distal bowel obstruction). The diagnoses of malrotation & midgut volvulus are classically made on an upper GI, though they can potentially be made by other modalities, such as US.

If nonbilious emesis is present, US is an ideal test for the evaluation of suspected HPS. HPS is typically found in infants 2-12 weeks old with progressive nonbilious projectile vomiting.

Bowel Obstruction Beyond Neonates

The differential diagnosis for obstruction in this setting can be remembered by the mnemonic AAIIMM (appendicitis, adhesions, intussusception, inguinal hernia, Meckel diverticulum, malrotation/midgut volvulus), though other entities (such as foreign bodies & inflammatory bowel disease) may also cause obstruction in children.

Abdominal Pain

Common causes of abdominal pain in children include constipation, appendicitis, referred pain from pneumonia, trauma, intussusception, enteritis/colitis, & pancreatitis. The clinical history, signs, & symptoms help to focus the differential diagnosis & guide imaging options.

Radiographs & US are the most common 1st imaging choices in a child with abdominal pain. US is preferred to work-up suspected appendicitis, intussusception, or hepatobiliary abnormality, though CT remains the modality of choice in the rapid evaluation of trauma. MR imaging is preferred to diagnose inflammatory bowel disease & the potential underlying causes of pancreatitis. Either MR or CT can be used to diagnose appendicitis after an equivocal US.

Abdominal Tumors

Young children are afflicted with a unique set of tumors. The most common abdominal malignancies affecting children are Wilms tumor, neuroblastoma, & hepatoblastoma. The remaining malignancies are all considered rare tumors.

Wilms tumor is the most common pediatric malignancy of the kidney. It can invade the renal vein, uncommonly has Ca^{2+} (in ~ 15%), & rarely crosses midline.

Neuroblastoma is the most common extracranial solid tumor in children. It most commonly arises from the adrenal gland or paraspinal sympathetic ganglia. It often encases & displaces vessels, crosses the midline, & contains Ca^{2+} (~ 90%). Up to 30% of neuroblastomas arise in the neck or chest.

Hepatoblastoma is the most common pediatric hepatic malignancy. It is usually a large, heterogeneous, solid liver mass, presenting before 5 years of age. This lesion has Ca^{2+} in 50% of cases & typically causes an ↑ α-fetoprotein.

Pediatric Abdominal Trauma

Trauma is the leading cause of death in children.

Children are at ↑ risk of abdominal traumatic injury, as their visceral organs are proportionately larger compared to adult organs (leading to greater force per body surface area). Additionally, there is little fat to cushion direct blows.

Approximately 60-80% of children with seat belt contusions have intraabdominal injuries in the plane of the seat belt. Rapid deceleration in these cases causes hyperflexion with compression of the abdominal viscera. Injuries of the small & large bowel, mesentery, liver, spleen, pancreas, kidneys, aorta, & lumbar spine may occur.

Abusive abdominal trauma is the 2nd most common form of fatal child abuse. The liver & spleen are the most commonly affected organs, but pancreatic or bowel trauma without explanation should also raise suspicion.

(Left) *Lateral upper GI examination in a neonate with bilious emesis shows dilation of the stomach & proximal duodenum ⇨. There is rapid tapering, twisting, & narrowing → of the duodenum beyond this level. The findings are consistent with malrotation with midgut volvulus.* **(Right)** *Longitudinal US of the pylorus in a young infant with projectile vomiting shows findings of hypertrophic pyloric stenosis with a single pyloric wall → thickness > 3 mm & pyloric channel length > 16 mm.*

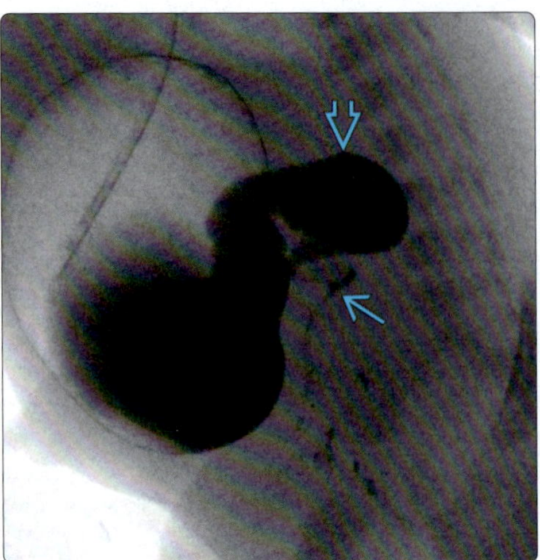

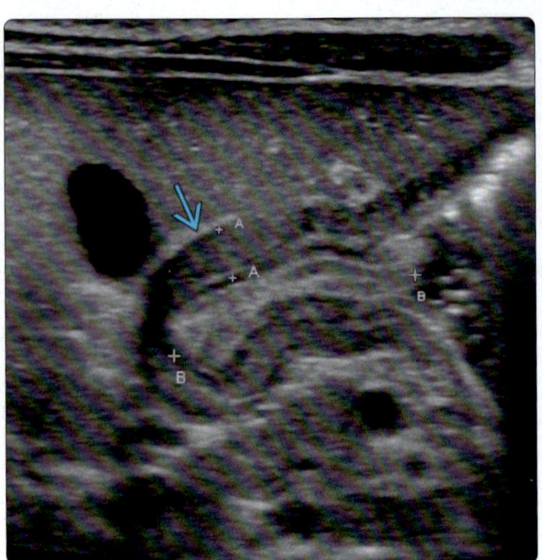

(Left) *AP water-soluble contrast enema in a newborn with a prenatal diagnosis of cystic fibrosis shows a microcolon ⇨ & filling defects within the distal ileum →, consistent with meconium ileus, which is the presenting manifestation of cystic fibrosis in up to 20% of patients.* **(Right)** *Lateral water-soluble contrast enema in an infant with difficulty stooling shows a smaller caliber of the rectum ↗ in relation to the sigmoid colon →. A rectosigmoid ratio < 1 is a classic finding of Hirschsprung disease.*

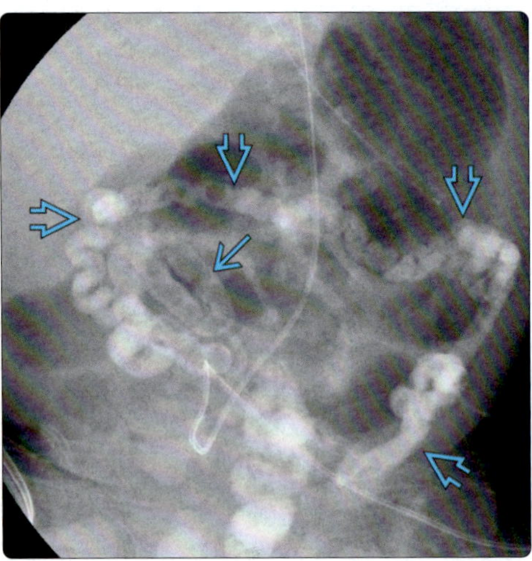

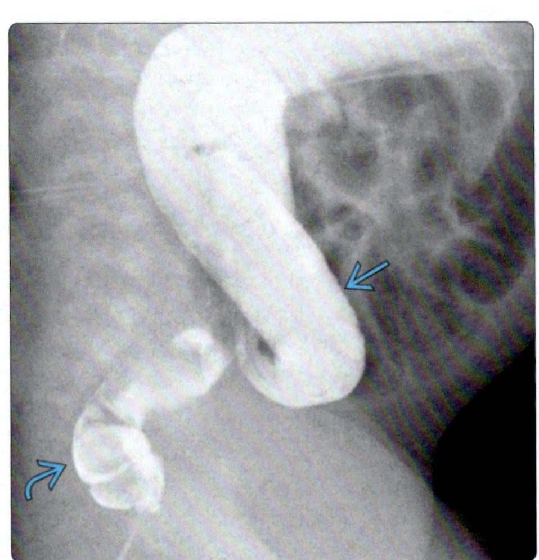

(Left) *AP radiograph of the abdomen in a premature neonate shows extensive pneumatosis intestinalis → & portal venous gas ↗. Necrotizing enterocolitis is the most common cause of pneumatosis intestinalis in neonates.* **(Right)** *AP radiograph of the abdomen in a neonate delivered after fetal distress shows a distended abdomen with Ca^{2+} → lining the peritoneal surface. This pattern of abdominal Ca^{2+} in a neonate is consistent with meconium peritonitis.*

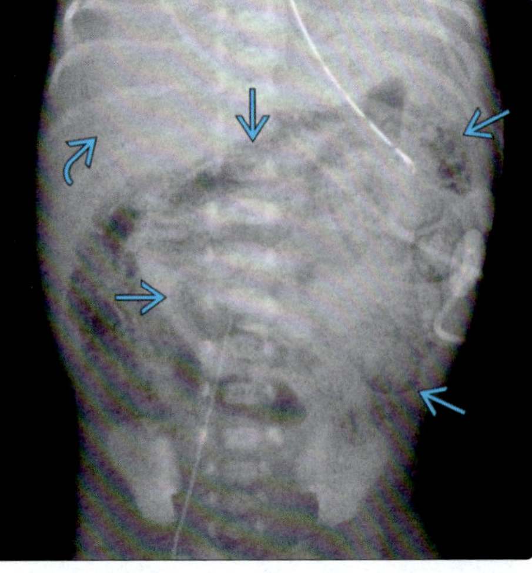

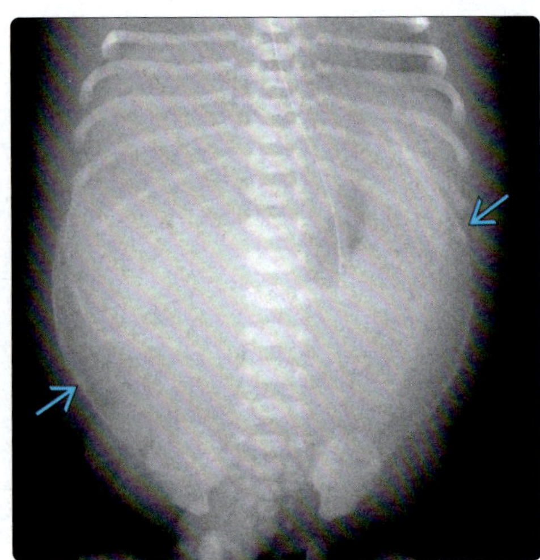

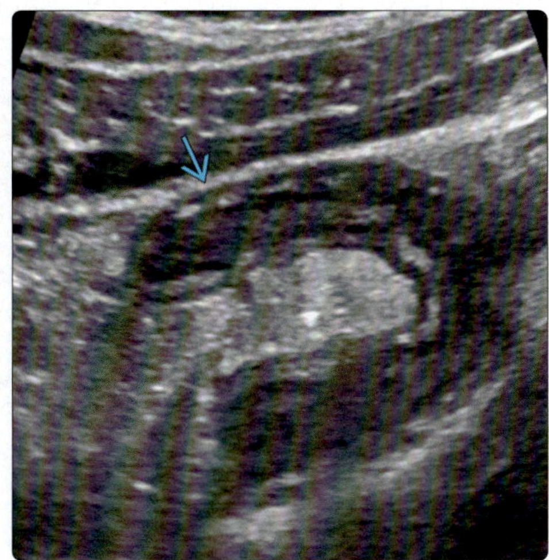

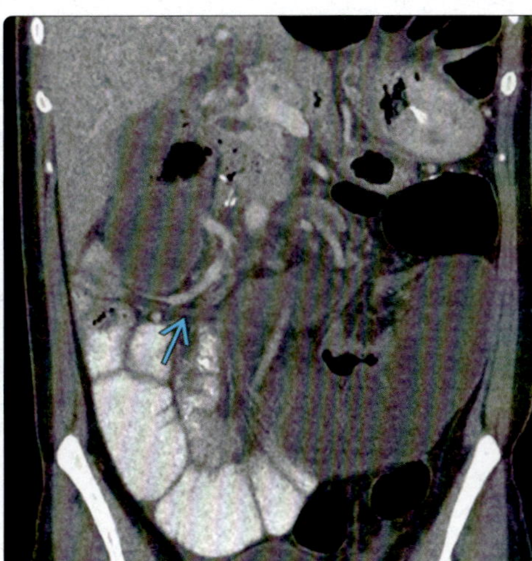

(Left) *Longitudinal US in an adolescent with right lower quadrant pain shows a dilated appendix → (> 6 mm in diameter) with echogenic periappendiceal fat. The findings are consistent with acute appendicitis.* **(Right)** *Coronal CECT in a child with prior abdominal surgery shows a thick adhesion → causing a small bowel obstruction. Bowel proximal to the adhesion is dilated & fluid filled.*

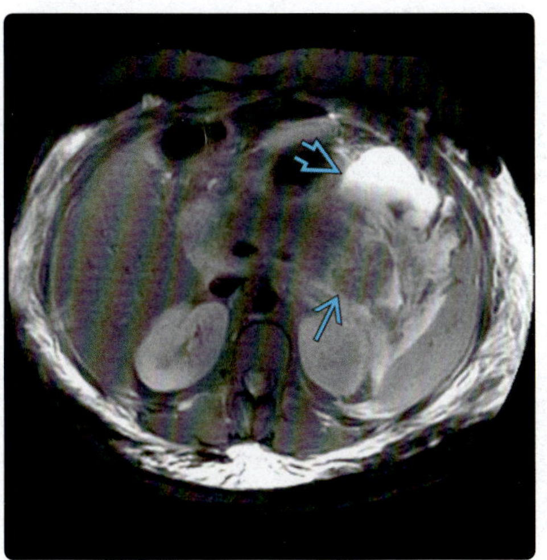

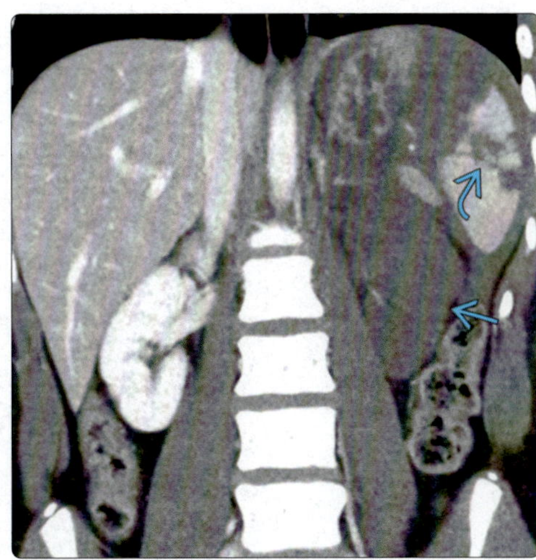

(Left) *Axial T2 FS MR in a child with severe upper abdominal pain shows findings of acute pancreatitis with edema of the tail of the pancreas →. This portion of the pancreas did not enhance with contrast (not shown). An acute necrotic peripancreatic collection → is also present.* **(Right)** *Coronal CECT in a patient status post motor vehicle accident shows devascularization of the left kidney →. Note also the adjacent splenic lacerations →.*

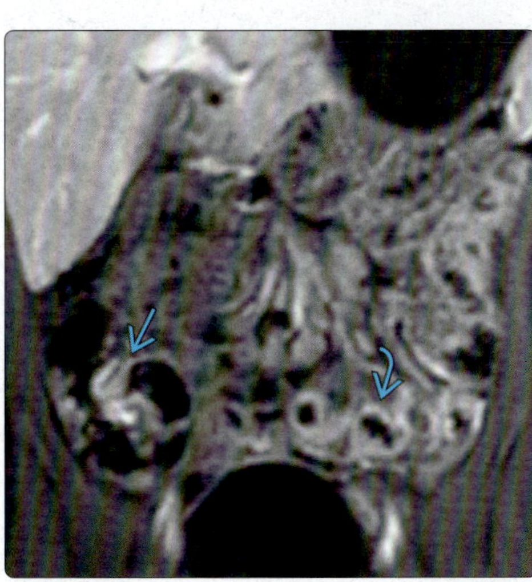

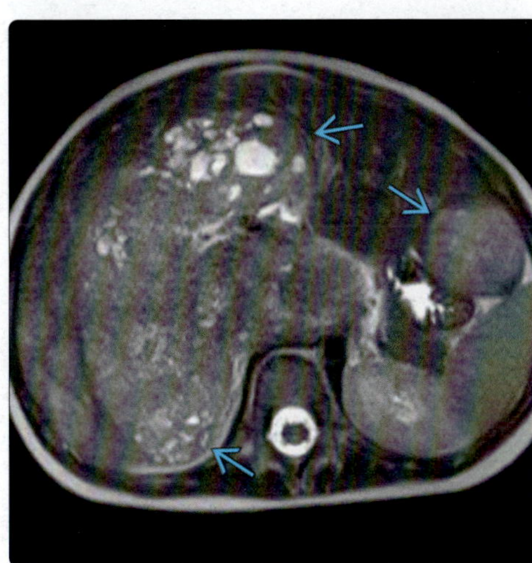

(Left) *Coronal T1 C+ FS MR in a patient with Crohn disease shows enhancement & wall thickening of the terminal ileum →. Skip lesions → are also present in the more proximal ileum.* **(Right)** *Axial T2 MR in a young child shows multifocal heterogeneous but predominantly solid masses, consistent with hepatoblastoma →. Hepatoblastoma is the most common primary hepatic malignancy in children.*

Normal Variations of Duodenojejunal Junction Position

KEY FACTS

TERMINOLOGY

- Ligament of Treitz (LOT): Combination of muscle & fibrous tissue, very pliable
  - Normal LOT position implies normal bowel rotation & fixation, low risk of midgut volvulus

IMAGING

- LOT is not directly depicted on any imaging study
- LOT position is inferred by imaging depictions of duodenum, duodenojejunal junction (DJJ), & proximal jejunum
- Guidelines for normal position of duodenum & DJJ
  - Supine upper GI: DJJ at or leftward of left vertebral pedicle & nearly as craniad as duodenal bulb
  - Lateral upper GI: D2-D4 overlap posteriorly close to spine; DJJ superimposes on or adjacent to duodenal bulb
  - US/CECT/MR: D3 crosses midline to left between superior mesenteric artery (SMA) & aorta; DJJ lies near same vertical level as duodenal bulb; SMA lies left & posterior of superior mesenteric vein

TOP DIFFERENTIAL DIAGNOSES

- True malrotation
- Artifactual displacement of normal DJJ
  - By mass or organomegaly
  - By bowel dilation
  - By enteric tube
- Redundant duodenum
- Duodenum inversum

CLINICAL ISSUES

- Treatment: None for normal variations
  - Importance lies in distinguishing normal variant from malrotation, which can predispose to life-threatening midgut volvulus

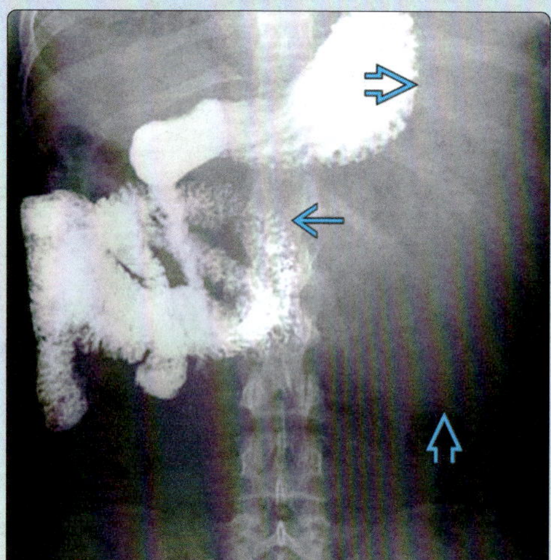

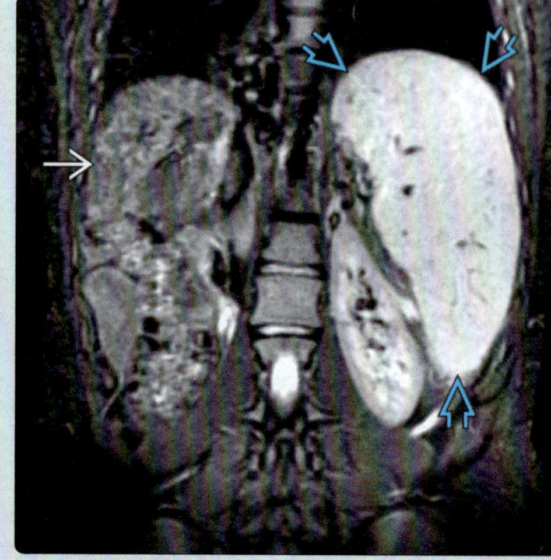

(Left) *Supine image from an upper GI shows an abnormal position of the duodenojejunal junction (DJJ) & proximal small bowel (SB)* ➡ *in the right upper quadrant, highly suggestive of malrotation. However, the child was not malrotated but had splenomegaly* ➡ *displacing the DJJ & SB.* **(Right)** *Coronal STIR MR in the same patient shows splenomegaly* ➡ *& a small, cirrhotic liver* ➡*. The combination of the large spleen & small liver has shifted the proximal bowel into the right upper quadrant, mimicking malrotation.*

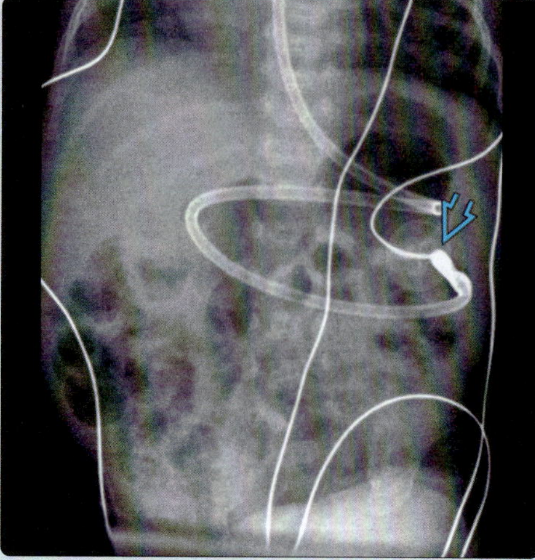

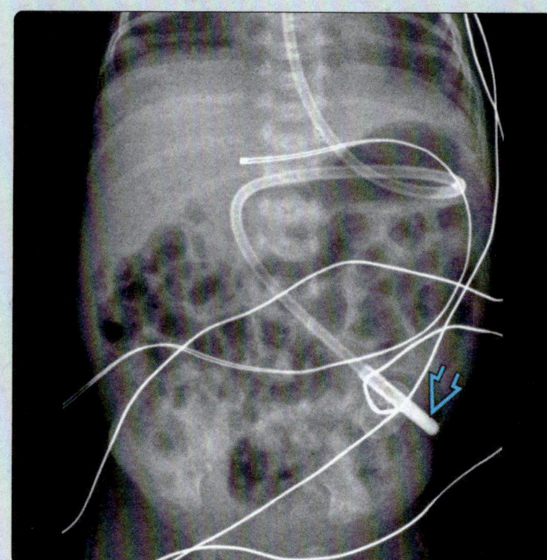

(Left) *AP radiograph in a 4-week-old infant with a nasojejunal feeding tube placed several days before this exam shows the tip of the tube at the laterally deviated DJJ* ➡*.* **(Right)** *AP radiograph several hours later in the same infant shows that the tip of the tube* ➡ *(which denotes the position of the DJJ) has moved inferiorly, not due to malrotation but likely due to the torque of the tube & the pliability of the ligament of Treitz (LOT), which has both muscular & fibrous components.*

Normal Variations of Duodenojejunal Junction Position

TERMINOLOGY

Abbreviations

- D1-D4: 1st-4th duodenal segments

Definitions

- Ligament of Treitz (LOT): Combination of muscle & fibrous tissue; normal position implies normal midgut rotation & fixation, low risk of midgut volvulus
  - Upper portion of LOT (Hilfsmuskel) is attached to diaphragmatic crus near esophageal hiatus; skeletal muscle & fibrous tissue component attaches to celiac axis
  - Lower portion of LOT (suspensory muscle of duodenum) inserts at duodenojejunal junction (DJJ) & has fibrous connection to celiac axis
  - Function
    - Involved in process of normal bowel rotation
    - With contraction, suspensory muscle of LOT widens angle of duodenojejunal flexure, allowing movement of intestinal contents

IMAGING

General Features

- Location
  - LOT is not directly depicted on any imaging study
  - LOT position is inferred by imaging depictions of duodenum, DJJ, & proximal jejunum
    - Normal DJJ is suspended by LOT: Attached craniad by diaphragmatic crus near esophageal hiatus & DJJ in left upper quadrant of abdomen
- Morphology
  - LOT is very pliable structure
    - Composed, at least partly, of muscle
    - Normal position of DJJ can be displaced by organomegaly, mass, adjacent bowel distention, or enteric tubes
  - Normal duodenum may have variant courses leading up to normal DJJ

Fluoroscopic Findings

- Upper GI
  - Supine image
    - DJJ at or leftward of left vertebral pedicle
    - DJJ nearly as craniad as duodenal bulb
  - Lateral image
    - D2-D4 course posteriorly, nearly overlap anterior to spine
      - Cannot confirm true retroperitoneal position on upper GI
    - DJJ superimposes on or adjacent to (as craniad as) duodenal bulb

Ultrasonographic Findings

- Does not visualize exact DJJ position
- Normal midgut rotation is implied if
  - D3 crosses midline to left between aorta & superior mesenteric artery (SMA)
    - Not seen with malrotation
  - Normal SMA lies to left & slightly posterior to superior mesenteric vein
    - Some false-positives & false-negatives

CT Findings

- Multiplanar CECT reconstructions can demonstrate normal retroperitoneal D3 course between aorta & SMA + appropriate height of DJJ in many cases

DIFFERENTIAL DIAGNOSIS

True Malrotation

- Abnormal DJJ position
- ± duodenal dilation/obstruction (Ladd bands or midgut volvulus)
- Cross-sectional imaging in difficult cases: Assess D3 course in relation to aorta & SMA
  - US can be reassuring, but 100% reliability is debated; requires time & expertise to demonstrate D3 relative to SMA

Artifactual Displacement of DJJ

- By gastrojejunostomy or nasojejunal tube
- By adjacent solid or cystic abdominal mass
- By organomegaly (liver, spleen, kidney)
- By adjacent dilated viscus
  - Obstructed jejunal, ileal, or colonic loops
  - Marked gastric distention can displace DJJ caudally

Redundant/Wandering Duodenum

- D2-D4 segments may be long & redundant, ultimately passing to left of spine to normal DJJ position

Duodenum Inversum

- Duodenum descends & ascends right of spine before coursing left to normally located DJJ
  - If D3-D4 traverses left above L1 level across gastric body, likely abnormal but not typical malrotation
    - Susceptible to duodenal obstruction & compression by adjacent structures, not volvulus
  - If D3-D4 courses to left below L1 level to normal DJJ, likely lies between aorta & SMA with normal rotation

CLINICAL ISSUES

Treatment

- None for normal variations
- Importance lies in distinguishing from malrotation, which can predispose to life-threatening midgut volvulus

SELECTED REFERENCES

1. Nguyen HN et al: Untwisting the complexity of midgut malrotation and volvulus ultrasound. Pediatr Radiol. 51(4):658-68, 2021
2. Strouse PJ: Ultrasound for malrotation and volvulus: has the time come? Pediatr Radiol. 51(4):503-5, 2021
3. Dumitriu DI et al: Ultrasound of the duodenum in children. Pediatr Radiol. 46(9):1324-31, 2016
4. Tang V et al: Disorders of midgut rotation: making the correct diagnosis on UGI series in difficult cases. Pediatr Radiol. 43(9):1093-102, 2013
5. Nehra D et al: Intestinal malrotation: varied clinical presentation from infancy through adulthood. Surgery. 149(3):386-93, 2011
6. Taylor GA: CT appearance of the duodenum and mesenteric vessels in children with normal and abnormal bowel rotation. Pediatr Radiol. 41(11):1378-83, 2011
7. Kim SK et al: The ligament of Treitz (the suspensory ligament of the duodenum): anatomic and radiographic correlation. Abdom Imaging. 33(4):395-7, 2008
8. Long FR et al: Intestinal malrotation in children: tutorial on radiographic diagnosis in difficult cases. Radiology. 198(3):775-80, 1996

(Left) *Supine frontal radiograph during contrast injection to check the function of a gastrojejunostomy (GJ) tube shows the tip of the tube ⇨ at the DJJ, which is in the pelvis. One might conclude that the bowel must be malrotated to create this appearance.* **(Right)** *Supine upper GI image in the same patient prior to the GJ tube placement shows a normal location of the DJJ ⇨. Tubes frequently alter the DJJ position due to the pliability of the LOT, potentially displacing the DJJ anywhere in the abdomen.*

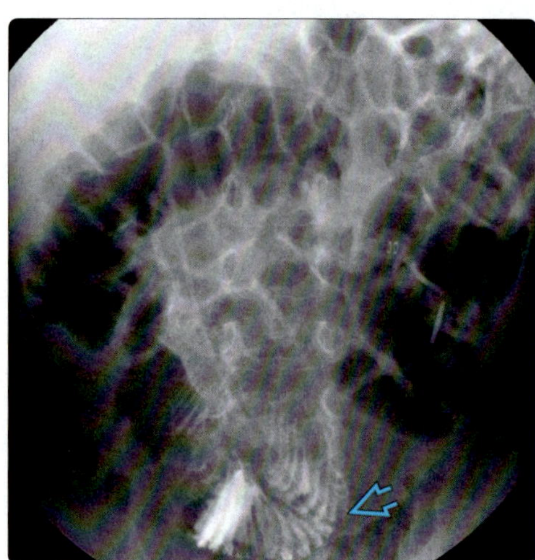

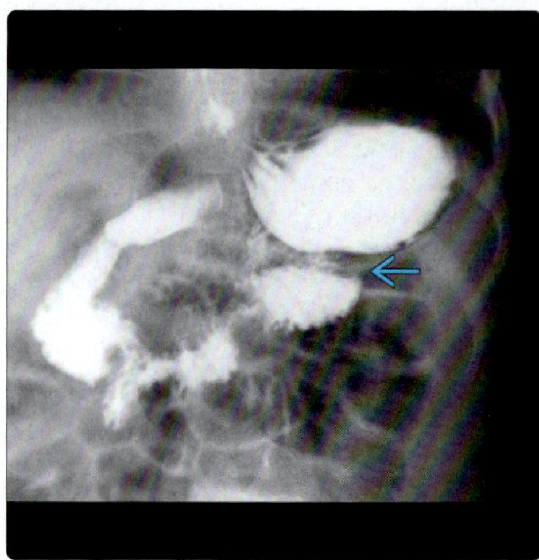

(Left) *Lateral upper GI image in a 17-year-old girl with abdominal pain & nausea shows significant redundancy of the retroperitoneal D2 & D3 segments ⇨.* **(Right)** *Supine frontal upper GI image in the same patient shows that the D2 & D3 segments ⇨ are to the right of the spine, a configuration known as duodenum inversum. Note that the remainder of the duodenum is redundant as well but courses to the left ⇨ to reach a normal DJJ ➡.*

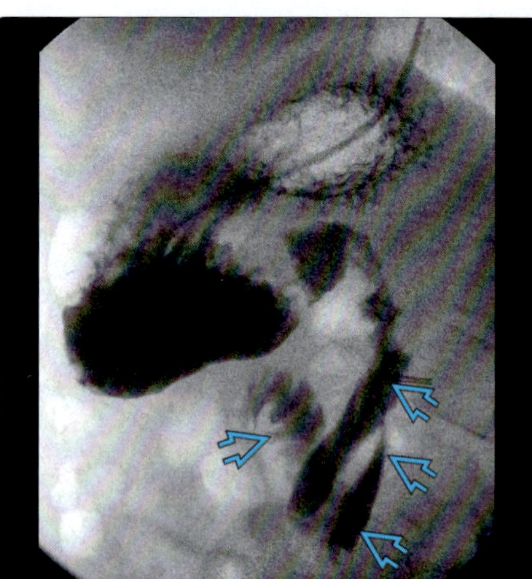

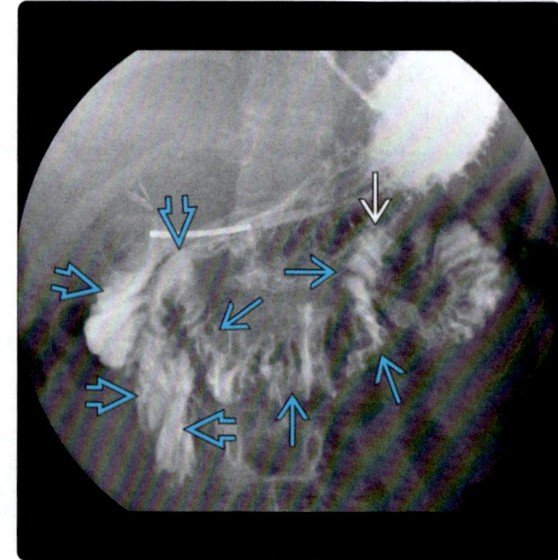

(Left) *Supine frontal upper GI image in a 2-day-old with bilious emesis shows a low position of the DJJ ⇨ compared to the duodenal bulb ⇨. This appearance is likely related to the dilated, air-filled distal bowel loops seen in the background. Such dilated loops can displace the DJJ.* **(Right)** *Supine scout fluorograph in the same patient shows the multiple, dilated, air-filled bowel loops of a congenital intestinal obstruction. Such loops can displace the DJJ & simulate malrotation.*

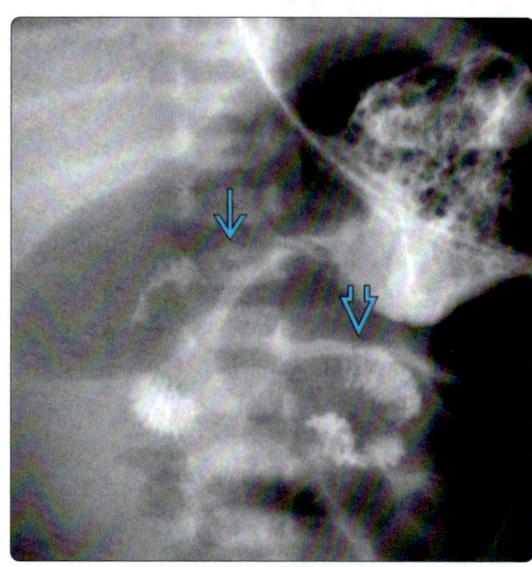

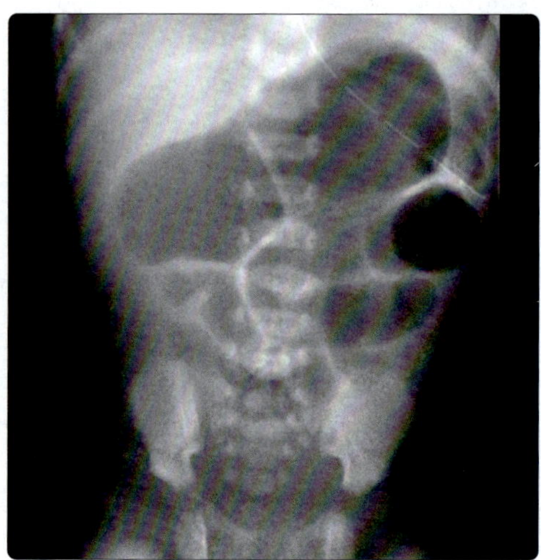

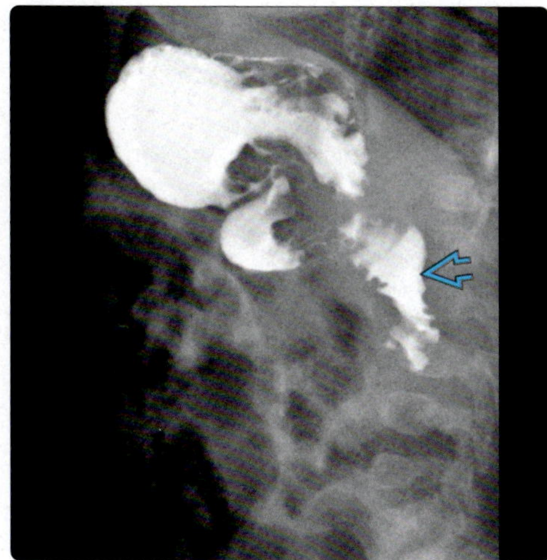

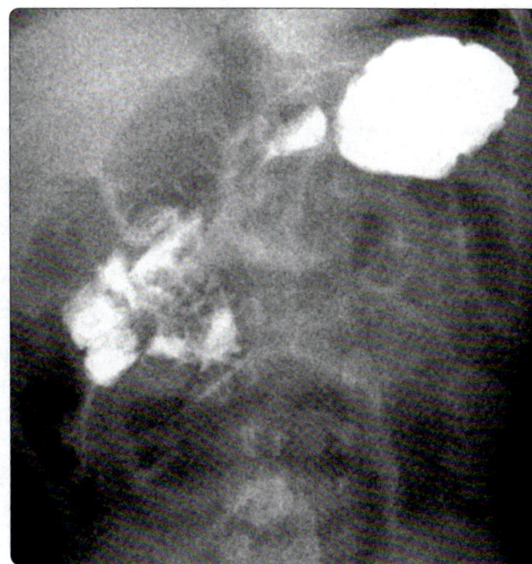

(Left) *Lateral upper GI image in a 2-month-old boy with failure to thrive & recurrent nonbilious vomiting shows the typical D2 retroperitoneal segment ⇨.* **(Right)** *Supine frontal upper GI image in the same patient shows that, as the contrast progresses, multiple redundant loops of the duodenum are seen to the right of the spine, suggestive of malrotation without obstruction.*

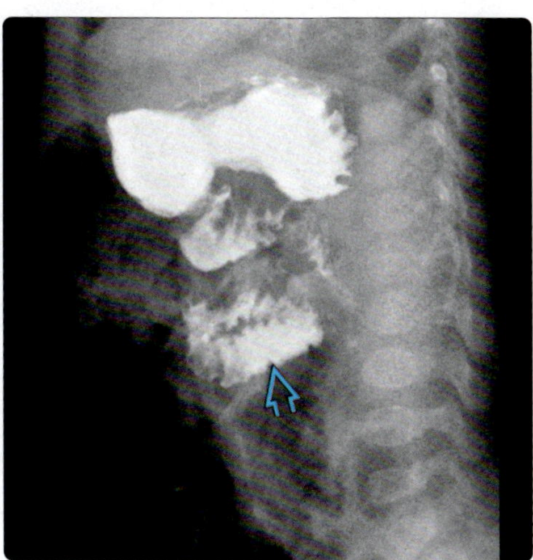

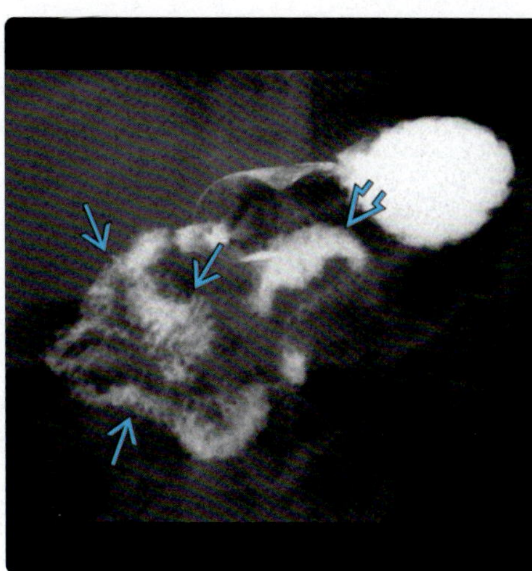

(Left) *Lateral upper GI image taken later in the same study shows the more distal loops coursing anteriorly ⇨, suggesting an intraperitoneal location of segments D3 & D4.* **(Right)** *Final supine upper GI image shows a loop of SB coursing to the expected region of the LOT ⇨. The proximal loops → appeared too long to be normal duodenum. At surgery, the duodenum was normally fixed at the LOT, consistent with a wandering duodenum.*

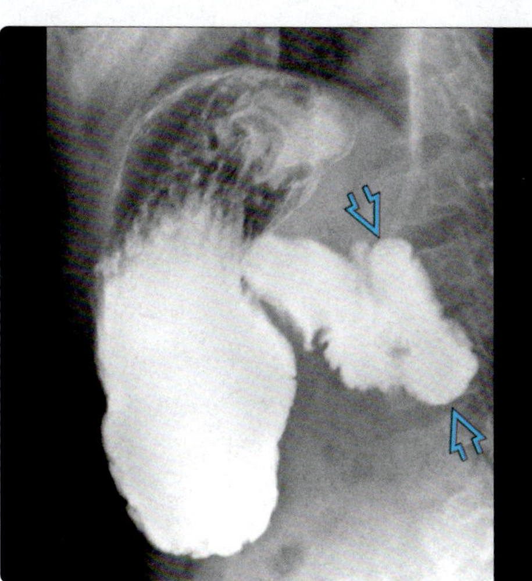

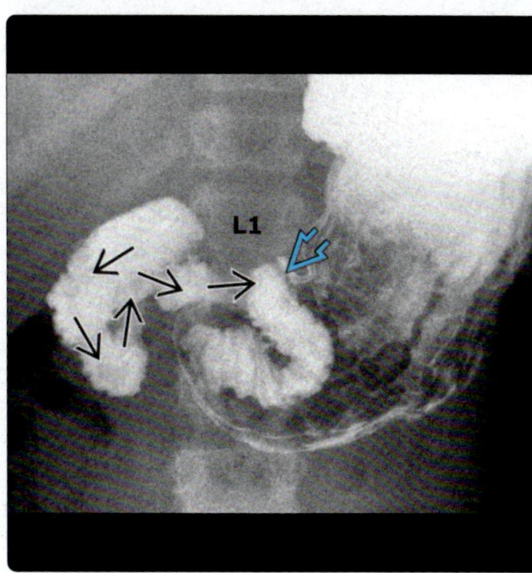

(Left) *Lateral upper GI image in a 9-year-old with recurrent nonbilious emesis, nausea, & abdominal pain shows a normal retroperitoneal duodenum ⇨.* **(Right)** *Supine frontal upper GI image in the same patient shows a redundant course → of the D2 & D3 segments to the right of the spine (duodenum inversum). The duodenum then courses to the left at the L2 level (likely between the aorta & SMA with the SMA takeoff usually at L1) to the DJJ ⇨ at the left pedicle, a normal variant course.*

Normal Variations of Cecal Position

KEY FACTS

TERMINOLOGY

- Clinical significance of cecal position
  - Often abnormal in malrotation
    - If adjacent to duodenum, suggests short mesenteric pedicle → ↑ risk of midgut volvulus (whether or not duodenal malrotation is present)
  - If air-filled, essentially excludes ileocolic intussusception
    - Best seen with left side down decubitus position
  - In evaluation for appendicitis, appendix location follows cecum
  - Inflamed cecum (due to ruptured appendicitis) deep in pelvis can mimic abscess

IMAGING

- Fluoroscopy [contrast enema or small bowel follow-through (SBFT)]
  - Cecum can be high, low in pelvis, or medially directed
    - Often above iliac fossa in young children
    - Pelvic location is common in older children
    - High & medial position raises concern for shortened mesenteric attachment
  - If sigmoid extends into right abdomen → craniad displacement of cecum
- Protocol advice
  - If questionably abnormal duodenal rotation on upper GI, get SBFT & delayed images until sure of cecal position
  - If abnormal cecal position is suggested on SBFT, evaluate entire colon with delayed images

TOP DIFFERENTIAL DIAGNOSES

- Malrotation
- Internal hernia
- Postoperative appearance of Malone appendicostomy

DIAGNOSTIC CHECKLIST

- Likely normal variation if cecum is slightly high, low, or medially directed with normal position of remaining right colon

(Left) *Supine contrast enema in a teenager with a history of constipation shows the proximal colon in the deep pelvis with the cecal tip* ⇨ *lying left of midline, such that the appendix could potentially lie on the left rather than the right. This is a variation of normal cecal position.* **(Right)** *Delayed supine small bowel follow-through (SBFT) colonic image in a 4- week-old shows a medially directed cecum* ⇨ *that was noted to be mobile in comparison to a preceding contrast enema (not shown). The full bladder* → *may also contribute.*

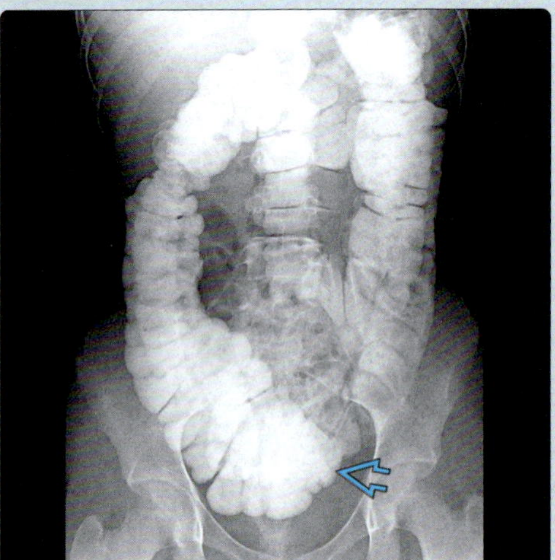

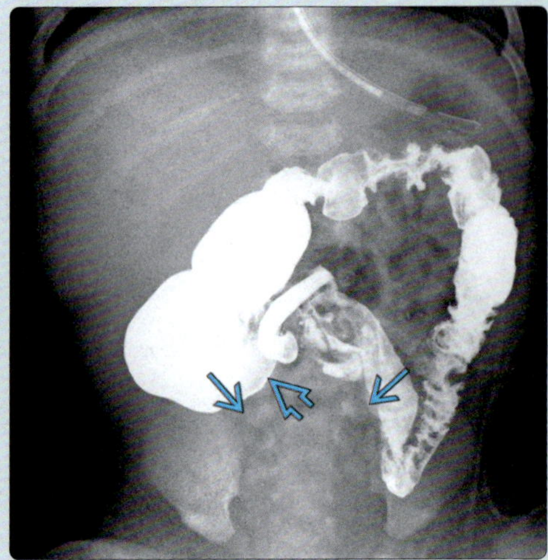

(Left) *Supine contrast enema in a teenager with a history of an anorectal malformation & a Malone appendicostomy for bowel management shows surgical mobilization of the cecum medially* ⇨ *to allow the appendix to reach the umbilicus.* **(Right)** *Supine contrast enema in a 12-year-old with chronic constipation shows a long, redundant right-sided sigmoid colon* ⇨ *with elevation of the cecum* →*, a normal variant. On postevacuation images (not shown), the cecum was more caudally located (as expected).*

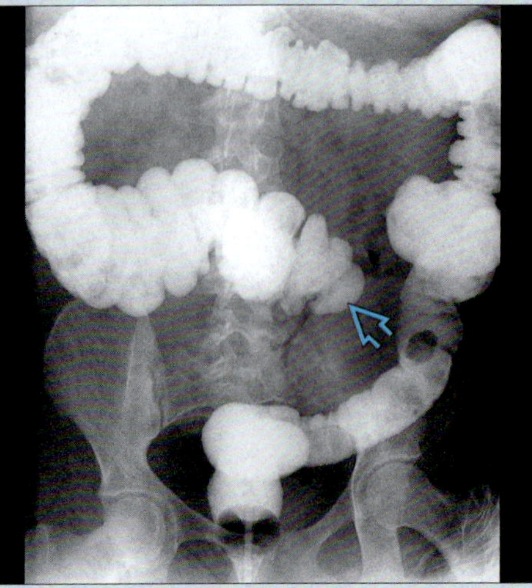

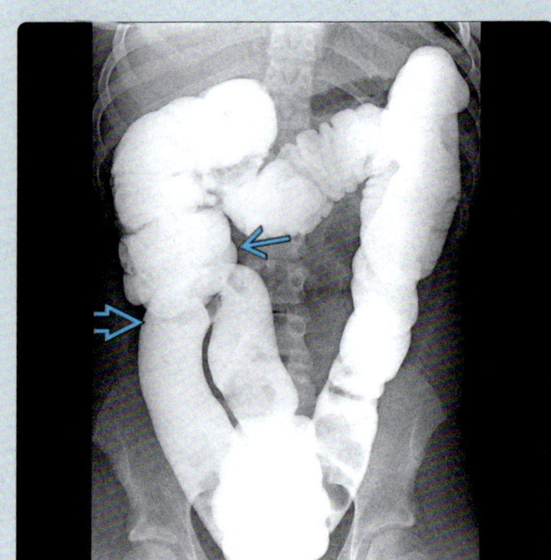

TERMINOLOGY

Definitions

- Slight mobility of fixed cecum, allowing variation in position
- Various factors can affect cecal position
- Clinical significance of cecal position
  - Often abnormal in malrotation
    - If adjacent to duodenum → short mesenteric pedicle → ↑ risk of midgut volvulus (whether or not duodenal malrotation is present)
  - If completely air-filled, excludes ileocolic intussusception
    - Best seen on left side down decubitus position
  - In imaging for appendicitis, appendix follows cecal position

IMAGING

General Features

- Best diagnostic clue
  - Mild high position of cecum on
    - Contrast enema or small bowel follow-through (SBFT)
    - US (typically when looking for appendix or terminal ileum)
- Location
  - Proximal colon, right lower quadrant (RLQ) of abdomen
  - Cecum may be high, medially directed, or deep in pelvis
    - Often mildly high (above iliac fossa) but remaining lateral in infants
- Size
  - Large in chronic illnesses
    - Myelomeningocele, cerebral palsy, other neurologic impairment; chronic constipation
    - ↑ risk of cecal volvulus
- Morphology
  - Minimally bulbous relative to ascending colon
  - Appendix emanates from inferior medial surface

Radiographic Findings

- Air- & stool-filled cecum
- RLQ extension of sigmoid colon is normal in 44%, may displace cecum craniad
  - RLQ sigmoid may mimic cecum
  - Relevant in patients with possible acute pathology
    - Misinterpreted as cecum, falsely excluding ileocolic intussusception
    - Not expecting pain from appendix in RUQ

Fluoroscopic Findings

- Cecum is located in RUQ, medially directed, or low

US/CT/MR Findings

- Find appendix or terminal ileum, trace to cecum
  - Locate relative to iliac vessels/iliac fossa
  - Stool- & air-filled proximal colon in RLQ
- Inflamed cecum deep in pelvis (due to ruptured appendicitis) can be mistaken for abscess

Imaging Recommendations

- Protocol advice
  - SBFT or contrast enema may complement evaluation for malrotation if duodenal position is unclear on upper GI: Look for abnormal cecal position (especially high & medial)
  - If cecal position is abnormal on SBFT, evaluate entire colonic position
    - With normal position of remainder of right colon, consider normal variation
    - If sigmoid extends to right, likely high normal cecum
  - If cecum lies in left abdomen or high midline → malrotation
  - Comparison with prior exams may reveal whether cecal position is fixed or mobile
    - Slight mobility can be normal variant
  - If small bowel lies along right lateral abdomen with medial right colon, consider malrotation, laxity of attachments, internal hernia, or prior surgery

DIFFERENTIAL DIAGNOSIS

Malrotation

- Look for abnormal relationships of superior mesenteric artery (SMA) to superior mesenteric vein (SMV), 3rd duodenum to SMA, duodenojejunal junction (DJJ) relative to spine & duodenal bulb

Internal Hernia

- Pericecal hernia shows small bowel loops posterior & lateral to cecum in right paracolic gutter

Postoperative Appearance of Malone Appendicostomy

- Surgical mobilization of cecum to facilitate use of appendix for catheterization for cecal irrigation

CLINICAL ISSUES

Natural History & Prognosis

- Cecal positions that are usually of no clinical significance
  - Mildly high but lateral, particularly in infant
  - Deep in pelvis
- High & medial, ± malpositioned DJJ, can predispose to volvulus
  - Short mesenteric attachment

SELECTED REFERENCES

1. Wozniak S et al: The large intestine from fetal period to adulthood and its impact on the course of colonoscopy. Ann Anat. 224:17-22, 2019
2. Soffers JH et al: The growth pattern of the human intestine and its mesentery. BMC Dev Biol. 15:31, 2015
3. Metzger R et al: Embryology of the midgut. Semin Pediatr Surg. 20(3):145-51, 2011
4. Martin LC et al: Review of internal hernias: radiographic and clinical findings. AJR Am J Roentgenol. 186(3):703-17, 2006
5. Fiorella DJ et al: Frequency of right lower quadrant position of the sigmoid colon in infants and young children. Radiology. 219(1):91-4, 2001
6. Long FR et al: Radiographic patterns of intestinal malrotation in children. Radiographics. 16(3):547-56; discussion 556-60, 1996

KEY FACTS

IMAGING

- Substantial changes occur in appearance of normal spleen during early childhood
  - Related to evolving white pulp:red pulp volume ratios
  - Normal spleen ↑ in size with age
- Normal MR signal
  - Older child & adult: T2 hyperintense vs. liver
  - Neonate: T2 iso- or hypointense vs. liver
  - Normal adult T2 appearance occurs by ~ 8 months of age
  - DWI: Restricts diffusion with ↑ signal relative to liver
    - Degree of diffusion restriction ↑ with age (↓ ADC values)
- CECT/MR
  - Transient patterns of heterogeneous enhancement occur when spleen is imaged in arterial phase
    - Should become homogeneous on more delayed phases of imaging
  - Seen in most children ≥ 1 year during arterial phase
    - Less common < 1 year of age due to white pulp:red pulp ratios
  - Patterns of normal splenic heterogeneity include
    - Archiform (alternating curvilinear & undulating bands)
    - Zebra stripe
    - Focal
    - Diffusely heterogeneous
- Ultrasound
  - Homogeneous, iso- to slightly hyperechoic relative to liver
  - Hypoechoic bands are rarely seen
  - High-resolution transducers may show reticulonodular pattern

PATHOLOGY

- Neonates & young infants have immature, small lymphoid follicles with relatively large red pulp volume
  - Accounts for changes in CT & MR appearances with age

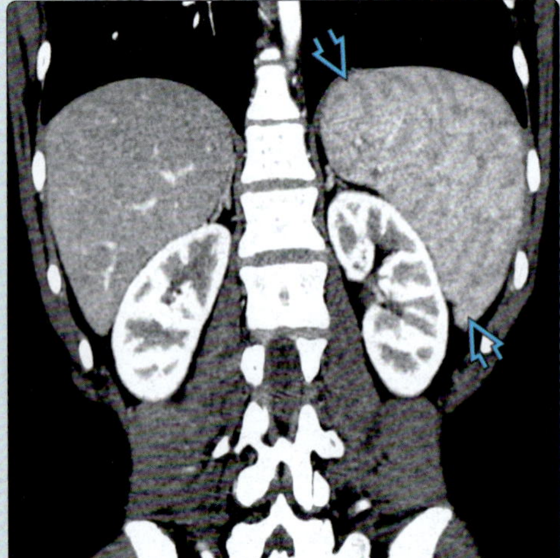

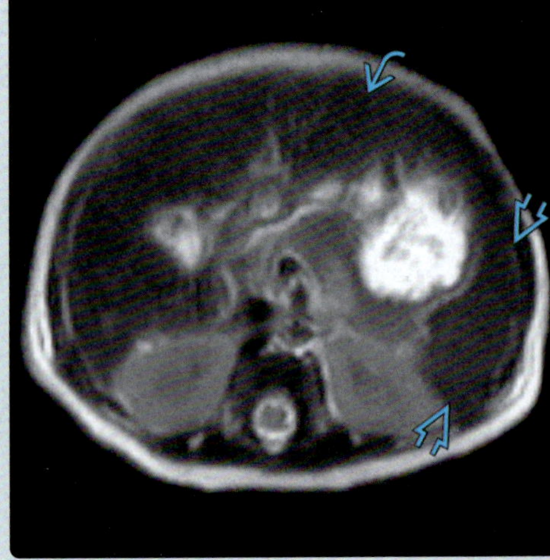

(Left) *Coronal CECT in a 15-year-old boy demonstrates a normal transient pattern of heterogeneous splenic enhancement → that is often seen when normal spleens (in children > 1 year of age) are imaged in the 1st minute after IV contrast injection (i.e., arterial or early phase).* **(Right)** *Axial T2 SSFSE MR in a 7-day-old girl being evaluated for an abdominal mass (not shown) demonstrates that the normal spleen → is nearly isointense relative to the liver →. This splenic appearance is due to a relatively high volume of red pulp at this age.*

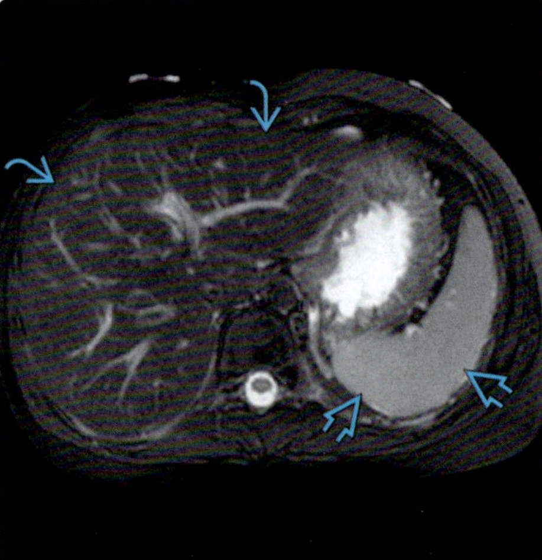

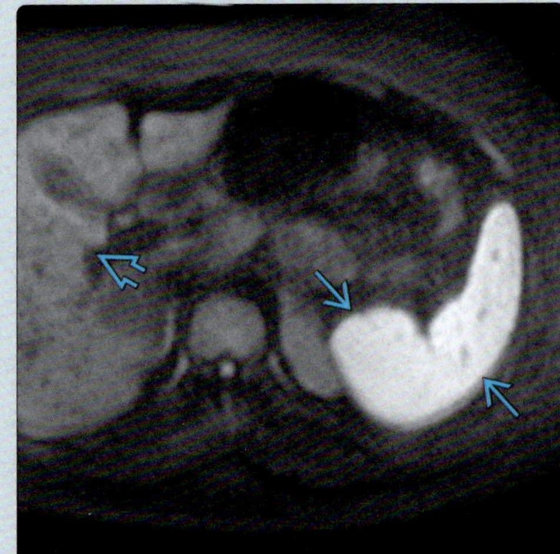

(Left) *Axial T2 FS MR in a 9-year-old patient undergoing MR enterography shows that the normal spleen → is hyperintense relative to the liver →. This change in appearance as compared to the neonate/young infant is due to an adult complement of white pulp.* **(Right)** *Axial DWI MR (b=800) of the abdomen in an 18-year-old patient undergoing MR enterography shows homogeneous hyperintense signal of the normal spleen → relative to the liver →.*

TERMINOLOGY

Definitions

- Spleen consists of red pulp & white pulp
  - White pulp: Reticuloendothelial cells organized into lymphoid follicles (or bodies)
  - Red pulp: Vascular sinusoids

IMAGING

CT Findings

- Transient patterns of heterogeneous splenic enhancement occur when patient is imaged in arterial (early) phase after IV contrast
  - Probably due to uneven blood flow through red & white pulp
  - Less commonly encountered in children < 1 year old
- Patterns of normal heterogeneous enhancement are variable
  - Archiform (alternating curvilinear & undulating bands of low & high attenuation)
  - Zebra stripe
  - Focal
  - Diffusely heterogeneous
- Enhancement becomes homogeneous on portal venous & delayed phases

MR Findings

- T1WI
  - Neonate: Spleen is isointense to liver
  - Older child & adult: Mildly hypointense to liver
  - Normal adult appearance occurs by ~ 1 month of age
- T2WI
  - Neonate: Hypointense or isointense to liver
  - Older child & adult: Hyperintense to liver
  - Normal adult appearance occurs by ~ 8 months of age
- DWI
  - Normal spleen restricts diffusion: ↑ signal relative to liver
    - Corresponding ↓ signal on ADC
  - Degree of diffusion restriction ↑ with age (↓ ADC values)
    - Spleen remains hyperintense relative to liver on DWI through adulthood
- T1WI C+
  - Heterogeneous enhancement is normal on arterial phase (similar to CECT)
    - Becomes homogeneous on later phases

Ultrasonographic Findings

- Red pulp & white pulp differences are not typically visualized
  - Normal spleen appears homogeneous in majority
    - Hypoechoic bands are rarely seen
    - High-resolution transducers may show reticulonodular pattern
  - Iso- to slightly hyperechoic relative to liver
- Age-specific normal values for spleen length are available
  - Ranges between 3.2 cm (neonate) → 12.5 cm (17-year-old boy)

DIFFERENTIAL DIAGNOSIS

Abnormal Low T2 MR Signal Intensity of Spleen

- Iron overload
  - Primary or secondary hemochromatosis; look at liver & pancreas as well
- Postchemotherapy appearance
  - Can result in low white pulp:red pulp ratio with hypointense T2 signal of spleen
- Diffuse Ca^{2+}
  - Occasionally seen in sickle cell disease with chronically infarcted spleen

Transient Heterogeneous Splenic Enhancement

- Laceration
  - Typically more focal & linear or irregular; + perisplenic hematoma & history of trauma
- Lymphoma/lymphoproliferative disorder
  - Discrete round & mass-like lesions
  - ± splenomegaly
- Infarction
  - Peripheral, wedge-shaped hypoenhancing areas
- Fungal infection
  - Numerous tiny, hypoenhancing lesions
- Sickle cell disease
  - Preserved round islands of normal splenic tissue within infarcted spleen

PATHOLOGY

General Features

- During 1st year of life, spleen undergoes histologic changes as lymphoid system matures
- Neonates have immature, small lymphoid follicles
  - ↓ white pulp & ↑ red pulp compared to adults
  - ↑ red pulp accounts for lower T2 MR signal of spleen in neonates
- By ~ 8 months of age, white pulp:red pulp ratios have ↑, giving rise to adult appearance
- Differential blood flow through cords of white & red pulp is likely reason for heterogeneous splenic enhancement on arterial-phase imaging
  - Relative lack of white pulp in neonates may explain why heterogeneous arterial enhancement is less common < 1 year of age

SELECTED REFERENCES

1. Boehnke MW et al: Imaging features of pathologically proven pediatric splenic masses. Pediatr Radiol. 50(9):1284-92, 2020
2. Di Serafino M et al: Ultrasonography of the pediatric spleen: a pictorial essay. J Ultrasound. 22(4):503-12, 2019
3. Kuint RC et al: Sonographic bands of hypoechogenicity in the spleen in children: zebra spleen. AJR Am J Roentgenol. 207(3):648-52, 2016
4. Li G et al: The effect of age on apparent diffusion coefficient values in normal spleen: a preliminary study. Clin Radiol. 69(4):e165-7, 2014
5. Clark TJ et al: Splenic trauma: pictorial review of contrast-enhanced CT findings. Emerg Radiol. 18(3):227-34, 2011
6. Donnelly LF et al: Heterogeneous splenic enhancement patterns on spiral CT images in children: minimizing misinterpretation. Radiology. 210(2):493-7, 1999
7. Donnelly LF et al: Normal changes in the MR appearance of the spleen during early childhood. AJR Am J Roentgenol. 166(3):635-9, 1996

KEY FACTS

TERMINOLOGY

- Malrotation: Any abnormal rotation of small or large bowel, which rotate separately during development
- Rotation of duodenum/small bowel & cecum/large bowel are similar but differ in timing
  - Abnormalities of rotation may be either or both

IMAGING

- Fluoroscopic GI findings
  - D3 segment never crosses midline on frontal view, often extends anteriorly on lateral view of upper GI
    - Duodenojejunal junction (DJJ) lies to right of left pedicle & below duodenal bulb on true frontal view
  - Variable degrees of colonic malrotation with abnormal cecal position on enema or small bowel follow-through (SBFT)
- Cross-sectional (US/CT/MR) findings
  - Duodenal nonrotation: D3 segment of duodenum fails to pass between superior mesenteric artery (SMA) & aorta when crossing to left of midline
  - Reversal of normal SMA/superior mesenteric vein position (not reliable)
- Best imaging tool
  - Fluoroscopic upper GI vs. US is debated

CLINICAL ISSUES

- Presentation in children: Nonbilious or bilious emesis, recurrent abdominal pain, poor weight gain, or asymptomatic

DIAGNOSTIC CHECKLIST

- If upper GI is equivocal, obtain SBFT; document cecal position & estimate length of pedicle from DJJ to cecum (which determines risk for midgut volvulus)
  - Alternatively, consider US evaluation of D3/SMA

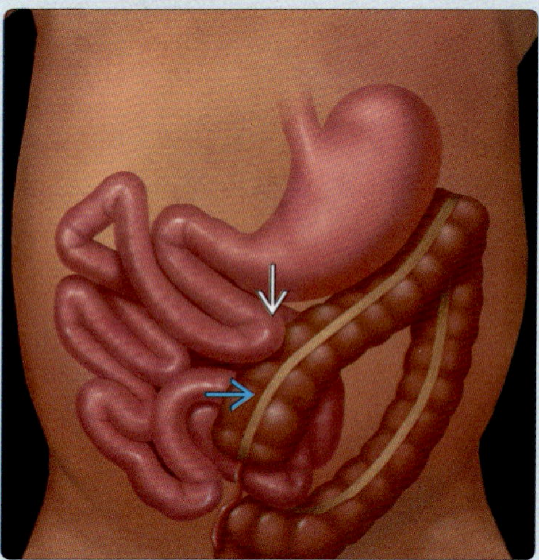

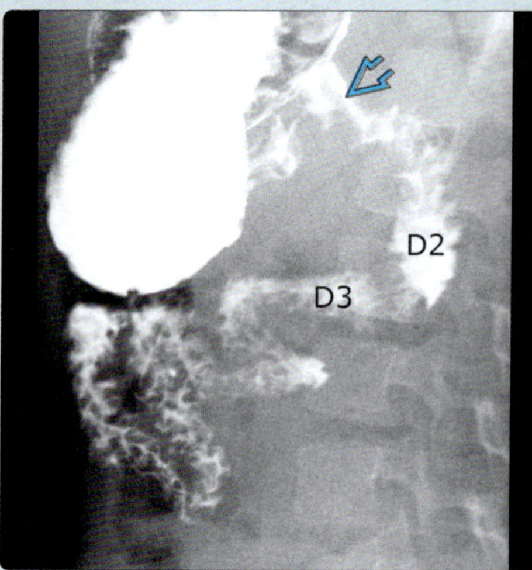

(Left) *Anterior graphic shows abnormal positions of the small & large bowel. The duodenojejunal junction (DJJ) lies low & midline ➡, very close to the malpositioned cecum ➡. This results in a short mesenteric fixation that predisposes to midgut volvulus (MGV).* **(Right)** *Lateral upper GI in a 3-year-old child with a history of nonbilious vomiting shows an anterior, intraperitoneal course of the D3 segment with a low position of the DJJ below the duodenal bulb ➡, indicating abnormal rotation.*

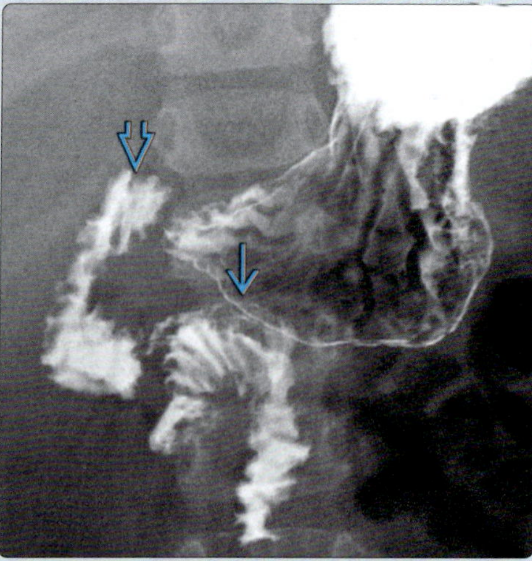

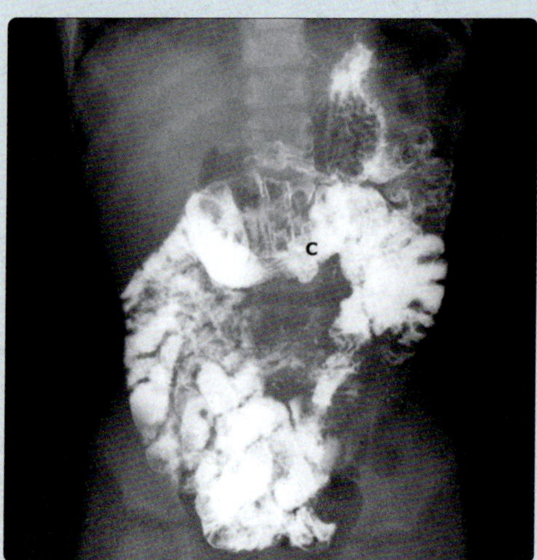

(Left) *Supine frontal view of the same patient shows a low DJJ ➡ (below the duodenal bulb ➡) that fails to adequately cross the midline, consistent with malrotation. However, there is no twisting or dilation of the duodenum to suggest MGV or obstructing Ladd bands.* **(Right)** *Supine SBFT was continued in the same patient to determine the cecal position & estimate the length of the mesenteric pedicle. The cecum (C) is high & just left of the midline, suggesting a very short mesenteric pedicle that is at high risk of future MGV.*

TERMINOLOGY

Synonyms

- Malfixation

Definitions

- Malrotation: Varying degrees of abnormal positioning of small &/or large bowel due to abnormal rotation during development
  - Small & large bowel rotate separately in utero
  - Abnormalities of rotation may affect either or both
- Malfixation: Abnormal position or length of bowel fixation by mesentery, typically associated with malrotation
  - Predisposes to midgut volvulus (MGV)

IMAGING

General Features

- Best diagnostic clue
  - Upper GI: Nonretroperitoneal position of duodenum + abnormal duodenojejunal junction (DJJ) position at or to right of midline
  - Cross-sectional imaging (US/CT/MR): Failure of D3 portion of duodenum to pass leftward between aorta & superior mesenteric artery (SMA)
  - Enema or cross-sectional imaging: Abnormal configuration of colon
- Location
  - Duodenum & right colon
- Morphology
  - Abnormal rotation of duodenum, colon, or both; degree of abnormality is quite variable (i.e., partial rotational anomalies)

Radiographic Findings

- Colon may be limited to left abdomen, small bowel in right abdomen

Fluoroscopic Findings

- Upper GI
  - D3 segment never crosses midline; often extends anteriorly on lateral view
  - DJJ to right of left pedicle on true frontal view
    - True frontal view
      - Right & left ribs are equal length
      - Base of heart lies in anatomic position
      - Vertebral pedicles appear symmetric
  - Jejunum often lies in right abdomen
  - ± abnormal cecal position
  - ± bowel obstruction due to Ladd (peritoneal fibrous) bands or MGV
- Contrast enema
  - Variable degrees of colonic malrotation
    - High &/or midline cecum of partial rotation
    - Left-sided colon of nonrotation
    - Anything in between

Ultrasonographic Findings

- D3 segment of duodenum fails to pass between SMA & aorta to left of midline
- Reversal of normal SMA/superior mesenteric vein (SMV) position (not reliable)
- Dilated proximal duodenum from Ladd bands or MGV

CT Findings

- Malposition of intestine from expected location
  - Duodenal nonrotation: D3 segment fails to pass between SMA & aorta to cross left of midline
    - Duodenal partial rotation: D3 passes between SMA & aorta but abruptly turns right, coursing anterior or posterior to SMA
  - Nonrotated colon: Right colon in left lower abdomen
  - Partially nonrotated colon: Cecum in upper abdomen
- Reversal of normal SMA/SMV position (not reliable)
- ± bowel obstruction due to Ladd (peritoneal fibrous) bands or volvulus

MR Findings

- Similar to CT findings

Imaging Recommendations

- Best imaging tool
  - Fluoroscopic upper GI through DJJ
- Protocol advice
  - If upper GI is equivocal for malrotation, perform small bowel follow-through (SBFT)
    - Determine exact location of cecum; be confident, wait for adequate filling of cecum
    - Shorter distance from DJJ to cecum → shorter mesenteric attachment → ↑ risk of volvulus
  - Normal position of DJJ can be displaced due to lax ligament of Treitz in infants
    - Adjacent dilated bowel of distal bowel obstruction
    - Adjacent masses, cysts, organomegaly
    - Enteric tube may distort duodenum

DIFFERENTIAL DIAGNOSIS

Duodenum Inversum

- Duodenum descends & ascends right of spine before coursing left to normally located DJJ
  - If D3-D4 traverses left above L1 level across gastric body, likely abnormal but not typical malrotation
    - Susceptible to duodenal obstruction & compression by adjacent structures, not volvulus

Redundant (Wandering) Duodenum

- D2-D4 segments may be long & redundant, ultimately passing to left of spine to normal DJJ position

PATHOLOGY

General Features

- Etiology
  - Failure of normal embryonic 270° counterclockwise rotation of midgut & colon, resulting in malposition of bowel to varying degrees
  - Ladd (peritoneal fibrous) bands attempt to fix abnormal duodenal &/or colonic positions
    - Potentially lead to extrinsic obstruction or volvulus
- Associated abnormalities
  - Malrotation is almost always seen with left-sided Bochdalek congenital diaphragmatic hernia, gastroschisis, & omphalocele

- Malrotation is commonly associated with duodenal atresia spectrum (including stenosis & web), small bowel atresia & stenosis, heterotaxia syndromes (asplenia & polysplenia), biliary anomalies, megacystis-microcolon-intestinal hypoperistalsis syndrome
- Less common: Intestinal pseudoobstruction, Meckel diverticulum, Hirschsprung disease, anorectal malformation, absent kidney & ureter

Staging, Grading, & Classification

- Several types of malrotation
  - Complete nonrotation
  - Nonrotated duodenum & partially rotated colon
  - Isolated nonrotated duodenum
  - Partially rotated duodenum & colon
  - Isolated partially rotated duodenum
  - Isolated partially rotated colon
- Bottom line: Length of mesenteric fixation from DJJ to cecum determines risk for MGV

Gross Pathologic & Surgical Features

- Ligament of Treitz: Actually muscle that can stretch
- Ladd bands can occur anywhere, frequently across D2 or D3 to liver hilum

CLINICAL ISSUES

Presentation

- Most common signs/symptoms
  - Children: Nonbilious or bilious emesis, recurrent abdominal pain, poor weight gain, or may be asymptomatic
  - Adults: Nonspecific → chronic vomiting, intermittent colicky abdominal pain, diarrhea
    - ± acute abdomen

Demographics

- Age
  - Majority present in 1st month of life
  - Vast majority present by 1st few years of life
  - Can present into adulthood
- 1/200 live births have asymptomatic rotational anomaly
- 1/6,000 live births have symptomatic malrotation
- M:F = 2:1
- > 33% are associated with congenital anomaly
- Patients with congenital diaphragmatic hernia, gastroschisis, & omphalocele are almost always malrotated but rarely volvulize (due to postoperative adhesions)

Natural History & Prognosis

- Complications of malrotation
  - MGV: Twisting of midgut about SMA → vascular occlusion & potential bowel ischemia
  - Bowel obstruction due to Ladd bands: Obstruction can be anywhere but can mimic MGV clinically & on fluoroscopic upper GI
  - Internal hernia: Rare, usually due to duodenal malrotation with normal colonic rotation
    - Sac-like mass of malfixed bowel herniates posterior to right colic vein into right upper quadrant

Treatment

- Ladd procedure
  - Untwist volvulus if present
  - Divide Ladd bands if present
  - Reposition small & large intestine into right & left abdomen, respectively
    - Postoperative adhesions are expected to secure bowel in place
  - ± appendectomy
  - Laparoscopy vs. laparotomy
    - Laparoscopic Ladd procedure results in ↓ perioperative complications & faster recovery but may yield ↑ risk of postoperative volvulus compared to open approach (due to fewer adhesions)

DIAGNOSTIC CHECKLIST

Consider

- Normal variants of duodenal anatomy or secondary causes of displacement resulting in fluoroscopic false-positive for malrotation
- If upper GI is equivocal for malrotation, obtain SBFT & document cecal position to estimate length of mesenteric pedicle of fixation (DJJ to cecum)
  - Alternatively, consider US to evaluate D3 position relative to SMA

SELECTED REFERENCES

1. Nguyen HN et al: Untwisting the complexity of midgut malrotation and volvulus ultrasound. Pediatr Radiol. 51(4):658-68, 2021
2. Strouse PJ: Ultrasound for malrotation and volvulus: has the time come? Pediatr Radiol. 51(4):503-5, 2021
3. Expert Panel on Pediatric Imaging. et al: ACR Appropriateness Criteria® vomiting in infants. J Am Coll Radiol. 17(11S):S505-15, 2020
4. Abbas PI et al: Evaluating a management strategy for malrotation in heterotaxy patients. J Pediatr Surg. 51(5):859-62, 2016
5. Carroll AG et al: Comparative effectiveness of imaging modalities for the diagnosis of intestinal obstruction in neonates and infants: a critically appraised topic. Acad Radiol. 23(5):559-68, 2016
6. Drewett M et al: The burden of excluding malrotation in term neonates with bile stained vomiting. Pediatr Surg Int. 32(5):483-6, 2016
7. Koch C et al: Redefining the projectional and clinical anatomy of the duodenojejunal flexure in children. Clin Anat. 29(2):175-82, 2016
8. Lesieur E et al: Prenatal diagnosis of complete nonrotation of fetal bowel with ultrasound and magnetic resonance imaging. Diagn Interv Imaging. 97(6):687-9, 2016
9. Raitio A et al: Malrotation: age-related differences in reoperation rate. Eur J Pediatr Surg. 26(1):34-7, 2016
10. Chesley PM et al: Association of anorectal malformation and intestinal malrotation. Am J Surg. 209(5):907-11; discussion 912, 2015
11. Graziano K et al: Asymptomatic malrotation: diagnosis and surgical management: an American Pediatric Surgical Association outcomes and evidence based practice committee systematic review. J Pediatr Surg. 50(10):1783-90, 2015
12. Landisch R et al: Observation versus prophylactic Ladd procedure for asymptomatic intestinal rotational abnormalities in heterotaxy syndrome: a systematic review. J Pediatr Surg. 50(11):1971-4, 2015
13. Lodwick DL et al: Current surgical management of intestinal rotational abnormalities. Curr Opin Pediatr. 27(3):383-8, 2015
14. Rajesh S et al: Malrotation of small bowel-diagnostic computed tomography (CT) signs and intraoperative findings. Indian J Surg. 77(Suppl 2):600-2, 2015
15. Shah MR et al: Volvulus of the entire small bowel with normal bowel fixation simulating malrotation and midgut volvulus. Pediatr Radiol. 45(13):1953-6, 2015
16. Yang B et al: Adult midgut malrotation: multi-detector computed tomography (MDCT) findings of 14 cases. Jpn J Radiol. 31(5):328-35, 2013
17. Jamieson D et al: Malrotation & malfixation of the midgut. In Babyn PS et al: Pediatric Gastrointestinal Imaging & Intervention, 2e. Decker. 311-32, 2000

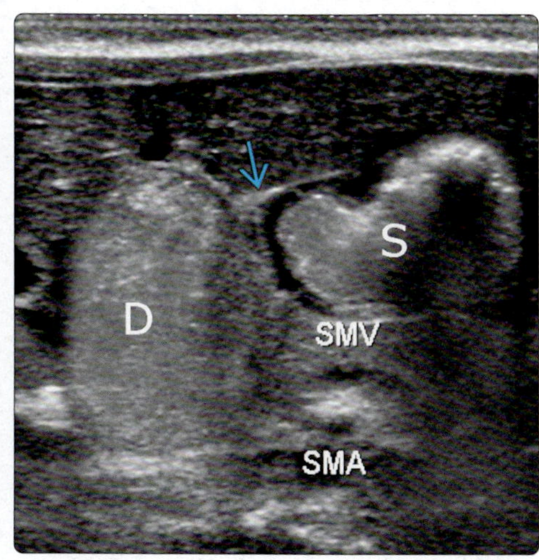

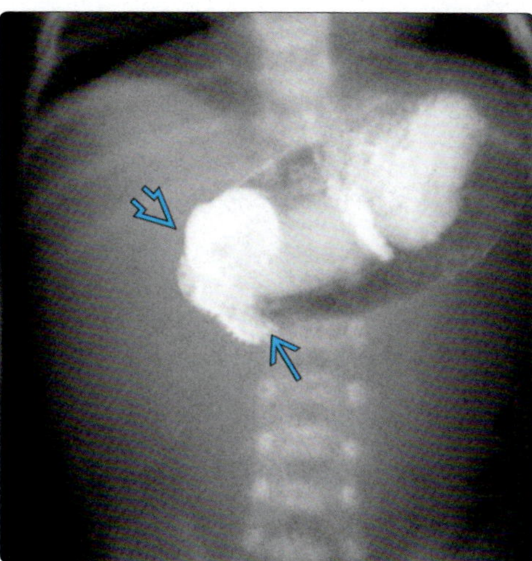

(Left) *Oblique pyloric ultrasound in an 18-day-old with projectile nonbilious vomiting shows a dilated stomach (S) with a normal pylorus ➔. There is a dilated duodenum (D), & the SMV lies directly anterior to the SMA, an abnormal configuration frequently seen in patients with malrotation.* **(Right)** *Supine upper GI in the same patient shows a dilated, obstructed duodenum ➔ up to a "beak" ➔ at D2-D3; this appearance represents MGV until proven otherwise (though only Ladd bands were found in this case).*

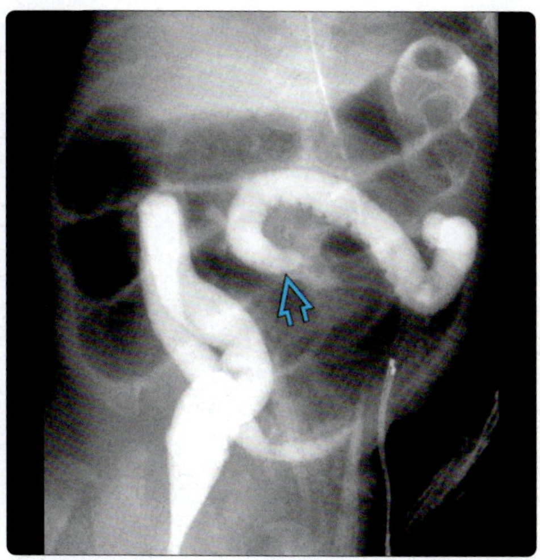

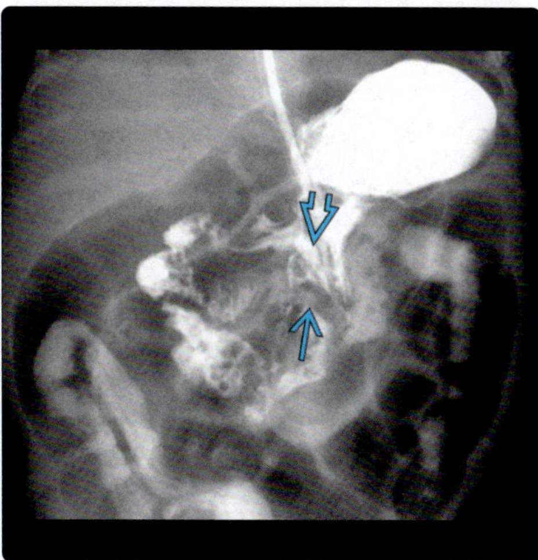

(Left) *Supine water-soluble contrast enema in a 5-week-old, former 31-weeks-gestation premature infant shows a high midline cecum ➔ with at least partial colonic malrotation. The small bowel dilation & small-caliber colon may be due to an intervening stricture from prior necrotizing enterocolitis.* **(Right)** *Supine upper GI in the same patient shows normal duodenal rotation. If a line was drawn between the DJJ ➔ & cecum ➔, the estimated mesenteric pedicle length would appear very short, ↑ the risk of future MGV.*

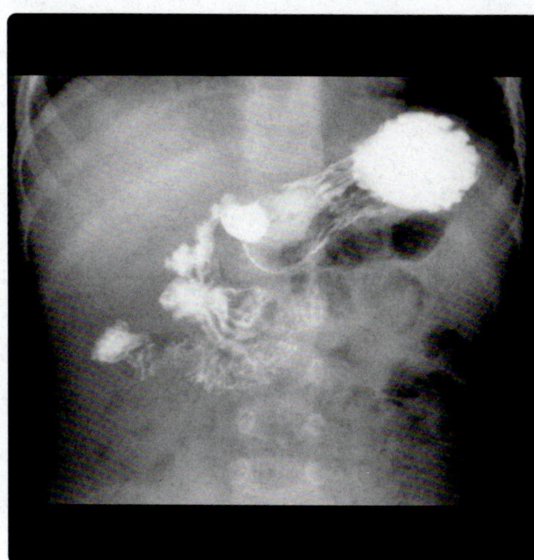

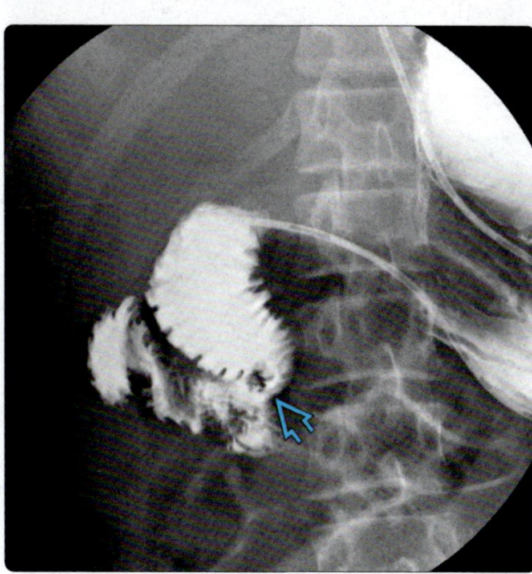

(Left) *Supine upper GI in a 2-year-old boy (who had malrotation corrected by a Ladd procedure at 6 days of age) presenting with abdominal pain & intermittent diarrhea shows malrotation without duodenal obstruction, a satisfactory postoperative appearance.* **(Right)** *Supine upper GI in a 13-year-old patient with new bilious emesis 6 days status post Ladd procedure for malrotation shows a dilated duodenum with a beak-like configuration ➔ worrisome for MGV. In the OR, incompletely lysed bands were found.*

Midgut Volvulus

KEY FACTS

TERMINOLOGY

- Malrotation: Abnormal rotation & fixation of small bowel (SB) mesentery that can lead to complications, including
  - Midgut volvulus (MGV): Abnormal twisting of SB & veins about superior mesenteric artery (SMA) that can lead to bowel obstruction & ischemia/necrosis
  - Ladd bands: Abnormal, fibrous peritoneal bands that can also cause duodenal obstruction

IMAGING

- Radiographic appearance is often normal; may show
  - Proximal obstruction with mild/moderate distention of stomach & D1/D2 with minimal distal gas
  - Ischemic ileus in very ill children
- Upper GI: Dilated duodenum to D2-D3 segment with corkscrew/spiral sign just beyond duodenal "beak"
- US or CT: Whirlpool sign with clockwise twisting of bowel & veins around SMA
  - ± cutoff of SMV/SMA, ↓ bowel perfusion/enhancement

TOP DIFFERENTIAL DIAGNOSES

- Malrotation with obstructing Ladd band
- Various congenital duodenal obstructions
- Redundant duodenum

CLINICAL ISSUES

- Classic presentation: Infant with bilious vomiting
  - Requires emergent upper GI or US by experienced sonographer
- Treatment: Ladd procedure

DIAGNOSTIC CHECKLIST

- Complete obstruction on upper GI at D2-D3 with contrast beak is considered MGV until proven otherwise
  - Different from "double bubble" of duodenal atresia
  - US can help exclude MGV; otherwise, emergent surgery is required
    - Delayed diagnosis can lead to extensive bowel necrosis or death

(Left) *Graphic of midgut volvulus (MGV) shows a corkscrew or twisting ⇨ of the distal duodenum & proximal jejunum beyond a mildly distended proximal duodenum & stomach. Note the ischemic ileus of the small bowel ⇗ & the Ladd band ⇨ attached to the 2nd duodenum.* **(Right)** *AP radiograph shows a nonobstructive bowel gas pattern in an infant with bilious emesis who was ultimately found to have MGV by upper GI. The most frequent radiographic gas pattern in MGV is normal.*

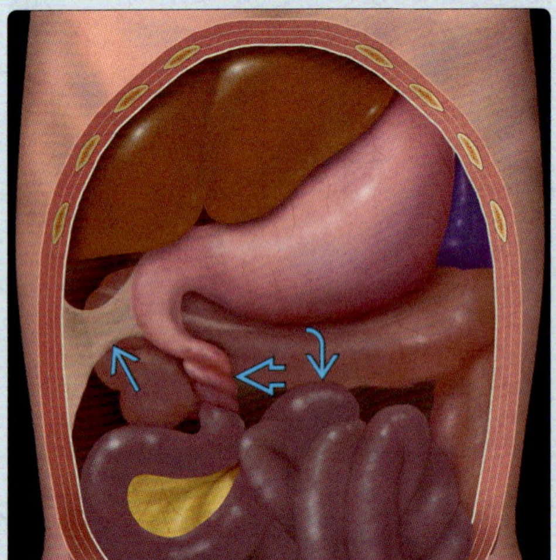

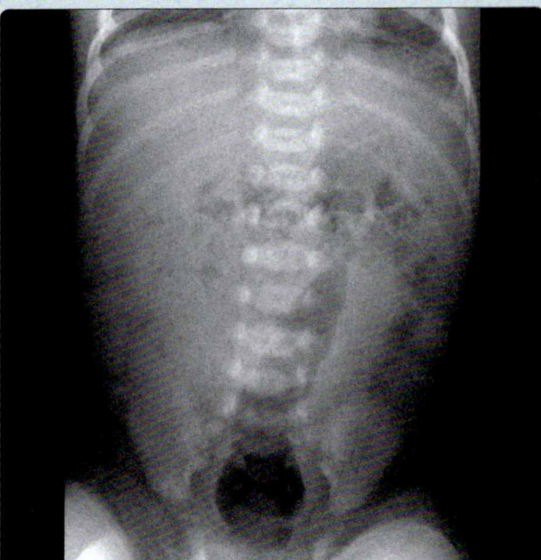

(Left) *Lateral upper GI in a 3-day-old boy with bilious vomiting shows a dilated duodenum up to D3, which ends in a beak-like configuration ⇨ with a wisp of contrast pointing anteriorly ⇨, highly suggestive of MGV.* **(Right)** *Supine frontal upper GI in the same patient (a few seconds later) shows duodenal dilation & partial obstruction at D3 ⇨ with the corkscrew/spiral sign ⇗ of MGV. Thickened bowel wall ➡ in this context suggests bowel ischemia.*

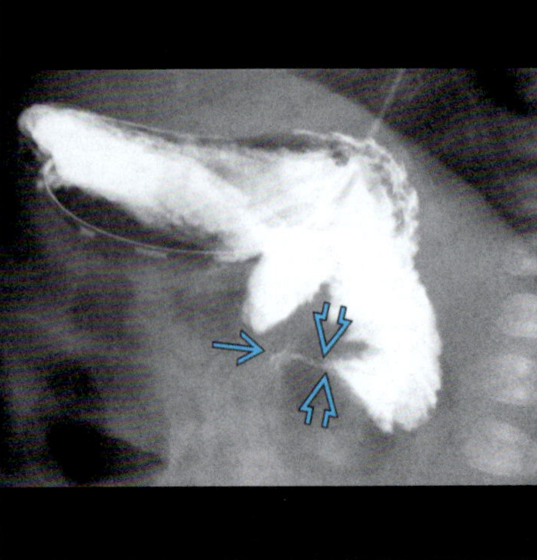

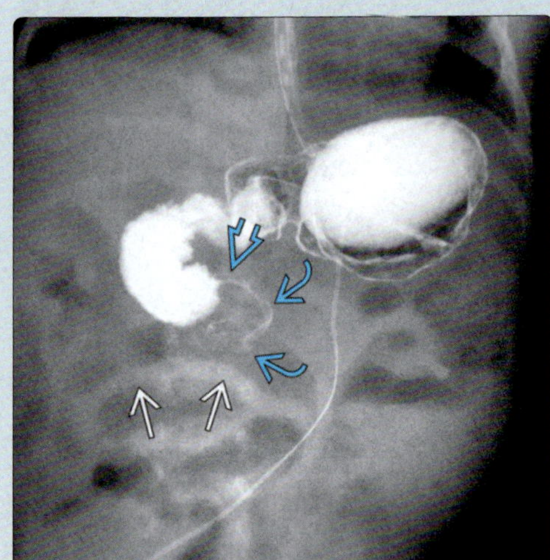

TERMINOLOGY

Definitions

- Ligament of Treitz: Suspends duodenojejunal junction (DJJ), defines normal duodenal rotation
- Malrotation: Abnormal rotation & fixation of small bowel (SB) mesentery that can lead to complications, including
  - Midgut volvulus (MGV): Abnormal twisting of SB about superior mesenteric artery (SMA) that can lead to bowel obstruction & ischemia/necrosis
  - Ladd bands: Abnormal, fibrous peritoneal bands that can also cause duodenal obstruction
- Bilious vomiting: Green/yellow vomit, typically from obstruction of duodenum distal to ampulla of Vater

IMAGING

General Features

- Best diagnostic clue
  - MGV: Upper GI shows mildly to moderately dilated duodenum (usually through D2-D3 segment) with corkscrew or spiral sign at/distal to beak of obstruction
  - Whirlpool sign on US or CECT: Wrapping of SB, mesentery, & superior mesenteric vein (SMV) around SMA
- Morphology
  - Twisting of mesentery occurs about SMA, which can lead to venous obstruction, bowel wall ischemia, & necrosis
  - Ladd bands may cause bowel obstruction, especially of duodenum

Radiographic Findings

- Radiography
  - Most common early finding: Normal abdominal radiograph
  - Distended stomach & proximal duodenum with mild distal bowel gas is very suggestive but nonspecific
    - Usually does not show classic "double bubble" (marked bulbous proximal duodenal & stomach dilation without distal gas) as seen in longstanding in utero obstruction of duodenal atresia
  - May show diffuse bowel distention/ileus (late) from ischemia/necrosis
    - Such children are often extremely ill
  - Rarely pneumatosis, portal venous gas, free intraperitoneal air

Fluoroscopic Findings

- Upper GI
  - Dilated duodenum to D2-D3, ± to-&-fro motility due to obstruction
    - Degree of proximal duodenal dilation depends on chronicity
  - Often beaked appearance at level of twist, ± complete obstruction
  - Spiral/corkscrew appearance caudally, distal to beak
  - May see malrotation without MGV
    - In patients with bilious emesis, this may reflect intermittent volvulus
- Contrast enema
  - Not typically performed if there is high level of concern for MGV
  - Colon is often abnormally rotated with cecum in upper midline abdomen, ± obstruction of ileocecal region

Ultrasonographic Findings

- Stomach & proximal duodenum are usually dilated
- Abnormal course of D3 as it tapers anterior to SMA
  - Normally courses between SMA & aorta
- Transverse superior to inferior sweep of transducer in midline shows whirlpool sign of twisting distal duodenum/proximal jejunum, mesentery, & vessels (SMV) around SMA in clockwise fashion
  - Grayscale & Doppler are complementary
- Findings of ischemia
  - Bowel wall thickening, loss of SB perfusion, ascites
  - Pneumatosis: Foci of ↑ echogenicity within bowel wall circumferentially with "dirty" shadowing posteriorly
  - Portal venous gas: Punctate echogenic foci moving in portal vein(s) from liver hilum to periphery
    - Causes random spikes on spectral tracings

CT Findings

- CECT
  - Clockwise twisting (whirlpool sign) of SMV, bowel, & mesentery around SMA
  - Potentially ↓ or no enhancement of SB due to obstruction of SMV/SMA
    - ± frank cutoff of SMV & SMA at twist
  - May have SB distention due to ischemic ileus
  - Rare: Pneumatosis, portal venous gas, free peritoneal air

Imaging Recommendations

- Best imaging tool
  - Infant with bilious vomiting → emergent upper GI vs. US
  - SB follow-through (SBFT) or contrast enema may be helpful to confirm malrotation if no volvulus is seen
    - Shorter mesenteric base (DJJ to cecal distance) ↑ risk of volvulus
- Protocol advice
  - Upper GI in infants with bilious emesis
    - Place nasogastric tube
    - Aspirate as much fluid & air from stomach as possible prior to instilling contrast
    - Inject 10 mL of contrast into stomach in right lateral decubitus position
    - If not emptying into duodenum, inject small puffs of air behind contrast to promote gastric emptying
    - If volvulus is seen, immediately notify referring clinicians
      - Longer time interval from diagnosis to operation makes intestinal ischemia & bowel loss more likely
    - Document duodenum in lateral & AP positions as per upper GI otherwise
  - US to exclude MGV in infants with bilious emesis
    - Trace course of duodenum from pylorus to D4 if possible
    - Trace superior to inferior course of SMV & SMA as far as possible
    - May need to scan at angle off of midline or alter patient position to keep bowel gas from obscuring view

DIFFERENTIAL DIAGNOSIS

Malrotation With Obstructing Ladd Bands

- May cause complete obstruction with beaking
- Cannot distinguish from MGV fluoroscopically if contrast does not pass beyond duodenal obstruction
  - US could help exclude MGV; otherwise, immediate surgery is required

Spectrum of Congenital Duodenal Obstruction

- Duodenal atresia, duodenal stenosis, annular pancreas, duodenal web
  - Atresia has double bubble sign: Marked stomach & proximal duodenal dilation with no distal gas
  - Stenosis or web usually has transition to normal distal duodenum & normal DJJ
    - Can mimic MGV fluoroscopically if contrast will not pass beyond obstruction

Redundant Duodenum

- Duodenum may make several retroperitoneal loops prior to extending leftward across spine to normal DJJ
- No duodenal dilation or obstruction

PATHOLOGY

General Features

- Etiology
  - With normal rotation, DJJ is positioned in left upper quadrant & cecum is positioned in right lower quadrant
    - Results in long, fixed mesenteric base between ligament of Treitz & cecum that keeps mesentery from twisting
  - If bowel is malrotated, DJJ to cecal length (mesenteric base) is short, predisposing to twisting (volvulus)
    - Wide range in degrees of malrotation
    - Complete nonrotation contribution is controversial; may be most common form in patients with MGV (if both DJJ & cecum lie in midline with short pedicle)
    - Isolated duodenal or colonic malrotation may also predispose to MGV
- Rarely, MGV has been reported in setting of normal rotation; some of these cases may be segmental volvulus
- Malrotation may also cause obstruction from
  - Ladd bands (abnormal fibrous peritoneal bands)
  - Paraduodenal hernias

CLINICAL ISSUES

Presentation

- Most common signs/symptoms
  - Classic presentation: Bilious vomiting in 1st month of life
    - But can occur at any age, even adulthood
- Other signs/symptoms
  - Acute abdominal pain
  - Intermittent, crampy abdominal pain
  - Failure to thrive
  - Shock

Demographics

- Age
  - 39% present within first 10 days of life
  - > 90% present within first 3 months of life
  - Can occur at any age
- Sex
  - Slightly higher incidence in boys
- Epidemiology
  - 2.86/10,000 new births

Natural History & Prognosis

- May lead to to bowel necrosis, short gut, sepsis, death

Treatment

- Surgical emergency
- Ladd procedure: Reduce volvulus, resect nonviable bowel, transect Ladd bands (if present), place SB in right & colon in left abdomen

DIAGNOSTIC CHECKLIST

Consider

- Infant with bilious vomiting → emergent upper GI vs. US by expert sonographer
- Borderline cases of DJJ location on upper GI (suspicious for malrotation) → SBFT or contrast enema to document location of cecum

Image Interpretation Pearls

- High-grade duodenal obstruction at D2-D3 with beaking & no distal contrast passage is considered MGV until proven otherwise
  - Should not be confused with classic double bubble sign of duodenal atresia in newborn
    - Markedly dilated round or ovoid proximal duodenum with no distal bowel gas
- If patient has MGV by imaging, impression should read MGV
  - Must be communicated to clinician immediately

SELECTED REFERENCES

1. Nguyen HN et al: Transition to ultrasound as the first-line imaging modality for midgut volvulus: keys to a successful roll-out. Pediatr Radiol. 51(4):506-15, 2021
2. Nguyen HN et al: Untwisting the complexity of midgut malrotation and volvulus ultrasound. Pediatr Radiol. 51(4):658-68, 2021
3. Expert Panel on Pediatric Imaging. et al: ACR Appropriateness Criteria® vomiting in infants. J Am Coll Radiol. 17(11S):S505-15, 2020
4. Hosokawa T et al: Use of ultrasound findings to predict bowel ischemic changes in pediatric patients with intestinal volvulus. J Ultrasound Med. 39(4):683-92, 2020
5. Garcia AM et al: A multi-institutional case series with review of point-of-care ultrasound to diagnose malrotation and midgut volvulus in the pediatric emergency department. Pediatr Emerg Care. 35(6):443-7, 2019
6. Drewett M et al: The burden of excluding malrotation in term neonates with bile stained vomiting. Pediatr Surg Int. 32(5):483-6, 2016
7. Horsch S et al: Volvulus in term and preterm infants - clinical presentation and outcome. Acta Paediatr. 105(6):623-7, 2016
8. Kargl S et al: Volvulus without malposition--a single-center experience. J Surg Res. 193(1):295-9, 2015
9. Mitsunaga T et al: Risk factors for intestinal obstruction after Ladd procedure. Pediatr Rep. 7(2):5795, 2015
10. Shah MR et al: Volvulus of the entire small bowel w1th normal bowel fixation simulating malrotation and midgut volvulus. Pediatr Radiol. 45(13):1953-6, 2015
11. Lampl B et al: Malrotation and midgut volvulus: a historical review and current controversies in diagnosis and management. Pediatr Radiol. 39(4):359-66, 2009
12. Strouse PJ: Disorders of intestinal rotation and fixation ("malrotation"). Pediatr Radiol. 34(11):837-51, 2004

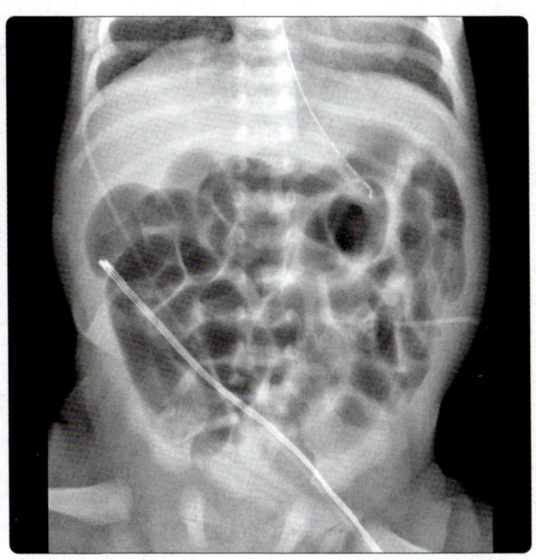

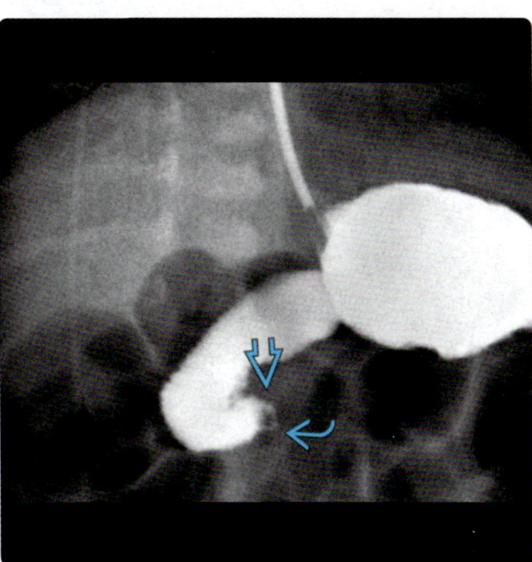

(Left) *AP radiograph in a newborn with bilious emesis shows multiple dilated, air-filled bowel loops suggestive of distal obstruction. However, prenatal imaging suggested malrotation, raising concern that this bowel dilation could be due to an ischemic ileus.* **(Right)** *LPO upper GI in the same newborn shows beaking of D3 ➡ with a subtle twist ↪ of MGV. In the OR, there was diffuse small bowel necrosis due to in utero MGV.*

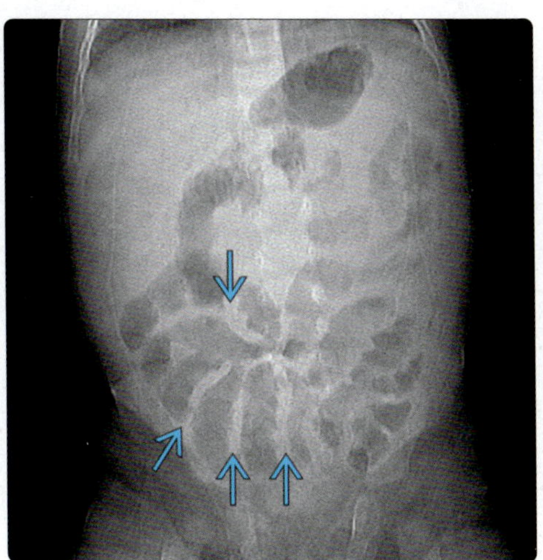

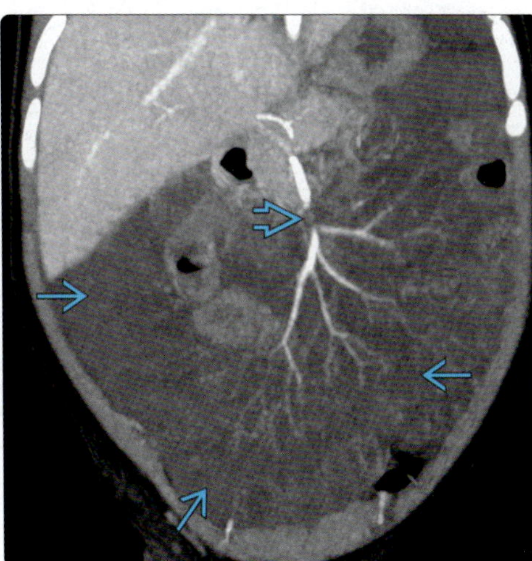

(Left) *Frontal CT scout image in a 4-month-old with shock & abdominal distention shows gaseous distention of numerous bowel loops. Separation of the loops ➡ could be due to wall thickening or interloop fluid.* **(Right)** *Coronal MIP CECT in the same patient shows absent enhancement ➡ of much of the small bowel & proximal colon. There is a focal cutoff of the superior mesenteric artery (SMA) ➡ at a site of bowel twisting. Bedside laparotomy showed MGV with ischemic bowel.*

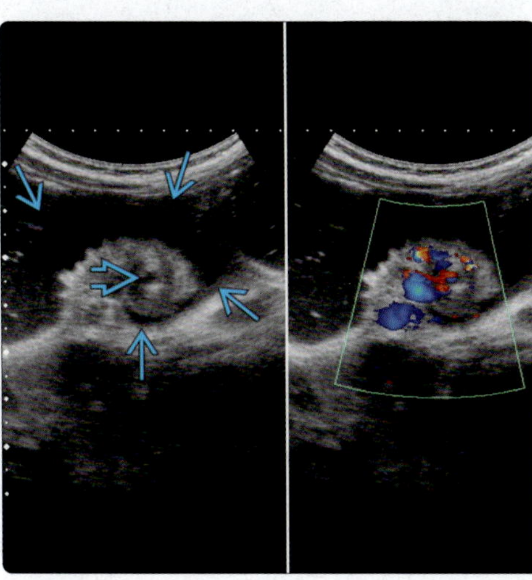

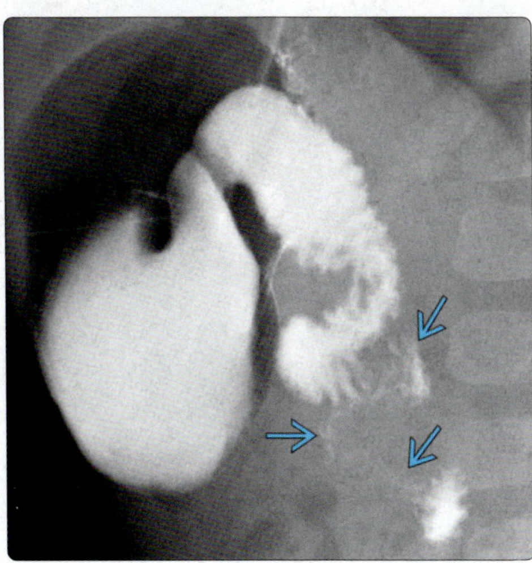

(Left) *Transverse grayscale & color Doppler ultrasounds in a 21-month-old with vomiting show clockwise tapering & twisting of fluid-distended D3 & D4 segments ➡ around the SMA ➡, highly suggestive of MGV. These findings have a whirlpool configuration when sweeping from superior to inferior with the transducer.* **(Right)** *Lateral upper GI in the same patient (requested by the surgical service) confirms narrowing & twisting of the distal duodenum in a corkscrew pattern ➡, consistent with MGV.*

Duodenal Atresia or Stenosis

KEY FACTS

TERMINOLOGY

- Most common upper intestinal obstruction in neonate
- Atresia: Congenital occlusion of intestinal lumen
- Stenosis: Fixed narrowing of intestinal lumen

IMAGING

- Newborn radiographic double bubble appearance is essentially diagnostic
  - Markedly dilated duodenum implies chronic in utero obstruction (with duodenal atresia as most common cause), especially with no distal gas
  - May not be seen on initial radiographs if stomach or duodenum is decompressed by nasogastric tube or vomiting
- If duodenum is mildly to moderately dilated with some distal gas → emergent upper GI to exclude midgut volvulus, evaluate duodenal rotation
  - US may be useful adjunct in experienced hands

TOP DIFFERENTIAL DIAGNOSES

- Midgut volvulus
- Duodenal web
- Jejunal atresia
- Gastrointestinal duplication cyst
- Annular pancreas
- Hypertrophic pyloric stenosis

PATHOLOGY

- Associated anomalies in > 50% of patients
  - 30-46% have Down syndrome (trisomy 21)

CLINICAL ISSUES

- Diagnosis is often made prenatally by US
- With surgical treatment, survival rate is > 90%
- Duodenoduodenostomy is most common operation
- Postoperative complications: Megaduodenum, motility issues, adhesions

(Left) *Axial SSFSE T2 MR in a 36-weeks-gestation fetus shows a double bubble sign of duodenal atresia with dilation of the stomach ➡, pylorus ➡, & duodenal bulb ➡. The gallbladder (GB) ➡ is noted for reference. The bowel distal to D2 is decompressed.* **(Right)** *AP radiograph immediately after delivery shows a nasogastric tube within the stomach, which can obscure the classic double bubble sign if suction is applied, as seen here. There is only minimal air in the duodenal bulb ➡. Note the lack of distal bowel gas.*

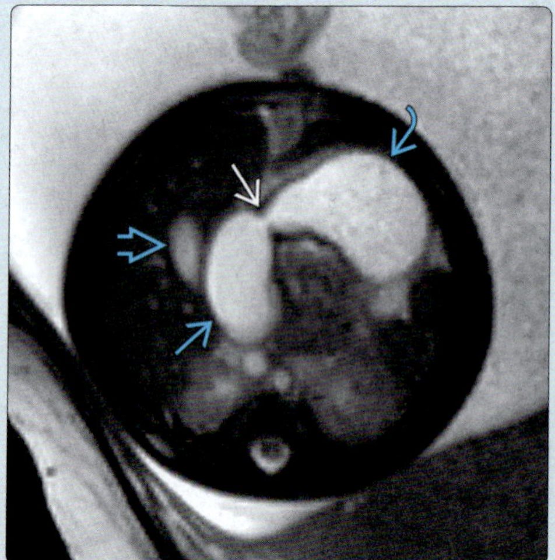

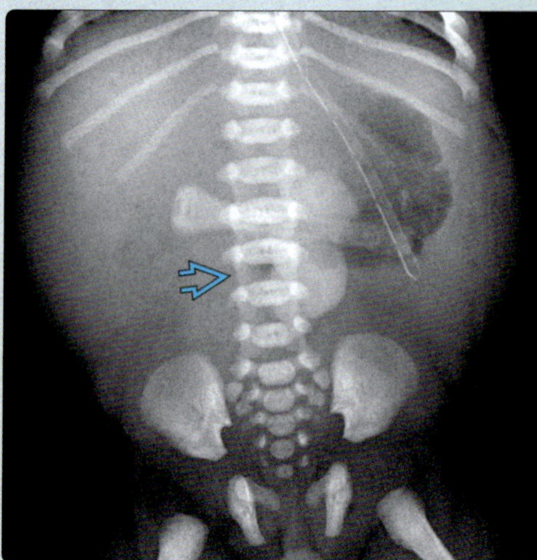

(Left) *AP radiograph performed in the same patient on day 2 of life (after turning off the nasogastric suction) shows that air is starting to collect in the duodenal bulb ➡ with no distal gas, revealing a more classic double bubble appearance of duodenal atresia.* **(Right)** *Transverse US of the abdomen in the same patient shows a portion of the dilated, fluid-filled duodenum ➡ as well as a portion of the GB ➡. Duodenal atresia was confirmed at surgery.*

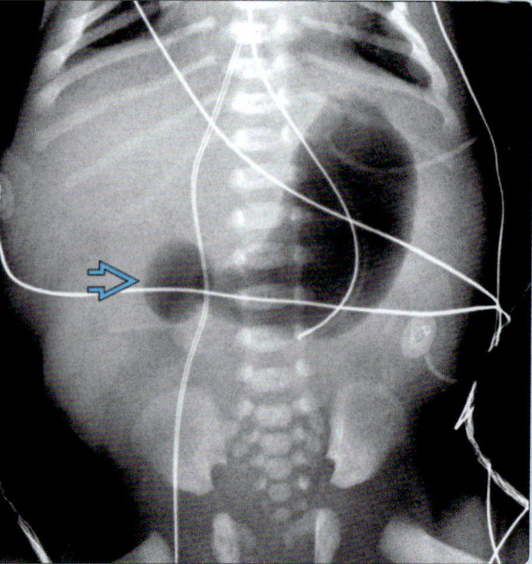

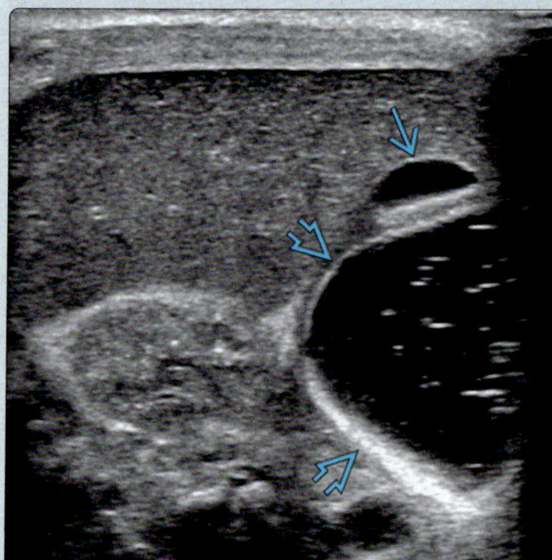

TERMINOLOGY

Abbreviations

- Duodenal atresia (DA), duodenal stenosis (DS)

Definitions

- Atresia: Congenital occlusion of intestinal lumen
- Stenosis: Fixed narrowing of intestinal lumen
- Most common neonatal upper intestinal obstruction (40-50%)

IMAGING

General Features

- Best diagnostic clue
  - Double bubble sign
- Location
  - Usually 2nd duodenum (near ampulla of Vater)

Radiographic Findings

- Radiography
  - Double bubble sign: Classic
    - Gas-distended, dilated stomach & proximal duodenum without distal bowel gas
      - In this context, markedly dilated duodenum implies chronic in utero obstruction (with DA as most common cause)
    - If dilated stomach + duodenum in newborn with distal gas, think of
      - Acute midgut volvulus (MGV) (new onset since birth), though dilation is typically less severe
      - DA spectrum (stenosis, web, ± annular pancreas, etc.)
      - Variant biliary/pancreatic anatomy (collateral pathway around atretic segment)
    - If stomach is emptied by nasogastric tube (NGT) or vomiting, double bubble may not be seen on initial radiographs
  - Free air is very uncommon
    - Rare gastric perforation; may be related to NGT placement

Fluoroscopic Findings

- Upper GI
  - Not usually performed in DA (as radiographs are typically diagnostic with no distal gas)
    - Can inject air through NGT to look for distal passage of air
  - Needed urgently with dilated duodenum in setting of distal bowel gas (particularly with less bulbous duodenal dilation)
    - Must exclude MGV
      - Can only truly be done by visualizing normal duodenojejunal junction (DJJ)
    - DS: Focal or longer segment of fixed circumferential narrowing
    - DA with biliary/pancreatic duct variations: Biliary drainage above + below atresia → distal gas in bowel

Ultrasonographic Findings

- Grayscale ultrasound
  - Dilated fluid- & gas-filled stomach & duodenum
  - ↑ thickening & echogenicity of gastric & duodenal wall
  - Can potentially be used to confirm normal position of D3 posterior to SMA & absence of twisting ("whirlpool") of MGV
  - Prenatal sonography
    - Fluid double bubble appearance; polyhydramnios in 30-40%

MR Findings

- Fetal MR: Dilated, fluid-filled stomach + proximal duodenum ± polyhydramnios

Imaging Recommendations

- Best imaging tool
  - Radiographs for double bubble sign
  - Upper GI if distal gas is present
- Protocol advice
  - If upper GI is needed for diagnosis (due to distal gas), place NGT
    - Aspirate stomach, then inject small amounts of barium in right lateral decubitus position
    - Small puffs of air to advance barium
  - Postoperative upper GI: Low-osmotic/isosmotic nonionic water-soluble contrast
    - Is there anastomotic leak, obstruction, additional web, malrotation?

DIFFERENTIAL DIAGNOSIS

Midgut Volvulus

- Proximal duodenum is usually less dilated/bulbous in acute MGV than DA
  - Chronic in utero volvulus (rare) may cause greater duodenal dilation (than acute MGV) with absent distal gas
- Abrupt beak/taper with near-complete obstruction at D2-D3 of duodenum
- Corkscrew configuration of narrowed, twisted bowel + malpositioned DJJ
  - US or upper GI may be used
- Ladd bands may also cause proximal duodenal obstruction in malrotation

Duodenal Web

- Delayed clinical presentation; distal gas is present
- ± windsock appearance of web in midduodenum

Jejunal Atresia

- Dilated stomach + duodenum + several jejunal loops without distal gas
  - Triple or quadruple bubble, classically

Gastrointestinal Duplication Cysts

- Extrinsic mass effect on bowel on upper GI
- Sonographic gut signature to cyst wall
  - With dilated stomach, may mimic double bubble sign on prenatal US

Annular Pancreas

- Circumferential narrowing of mid-2nd duodenum
- Distal gas is present
- Often with DS at level of encircling pancreas

Hypertrophic Pyloric Stenosis

- Presents at 2-12 weeks of life (not 1st week)
- Projectile, nonbilious vomiting
- US: Thick, elongated, persistently closed pyloric muscle

Less Common Newborn Upper GI Obstructions

- Preduodenal portal vein, internal hernia, pyloric atresia

PATHOLOGY

General Features

- Etiology
  - Most accepted theory: Embryologic failure of duodenal recanalization in 12th gestational week
  - Unlike other intestinal atresias (due to vascular accidents)
- Genetics
  - Typically sporadic if isolated anomaly
  - Down syndrome (trisomy 21) in 30-46%
  - Feingold syndrome (autosomal dominant)
    - Hand/foot anomalies, microcephaly, tracheoesophageal fistula, esophageal/DA, short palpebral fissures, developmental delay
- Associated abnormalities
  - > 50% of patients with DA have other anomalies
  - 30-46% have Down syndrome (trisomy 21)
    - 11 pairs of ribs, macroglossia, flat acetabular angles, cardiomegaly with shunt vascularity
  - Malrotation: 28%
  - Annular pancreas: Up to 30%
  - Additional duodenal web: 1-3%
  - Choledochal cyst, other biliary anomalies
  - Preduodenal portal vein
  - Esophageal atresia + tracheoesophageal fistula: Up to 18%
  - Imperforate anus
  - Cardiac defects: 20-30% (less frequent without trisomy 21 but more likely cyanotic)
  - Situs anomalies; renal anomalies
  - VACTERL association

Staging, Grading, & Classification

- Type I DA (69-74%)
  - Intact intestinal wall & mesentery
  - Membranous luminal obstruction
- Type II DA (1-2%)
  - 2 blind ends separated by fibrous cord
- Type III DA (5-6%)
  - 2 blind ends without intervening cord
  - Biliary anomalies
- DS (18-23%)

CLINICAL ISSUES

Presentation

- Most common signs/symptoms
  - Diagnosis is often made prenatally by US
  - Bilious > > nonbilious (80% vs. 20%) vomiting
    - Determined by site of atresia relative to ampulla of Vater
- Other signs/symptoms
  - Dehydration, weight loss, electrolyte imbalance

Demographics

- Age
  - Newborn (21-45% are premature)
- Epidemiology
  - Incidence 1:5,000-10,000 live births

Natural History & Prognosis

- Untreated: Dehydration, severe electrolyte abnormalities, death
- With surgical treatment, survival rate is > 90%
  - Mortality is largely related to associated anomalies

Treatment

- Surgical repair
  - If radiographs are diagnostic of DA (classic double bubble sign), surgical repair is urgent but not emergent
  - In setting of distal gas, failure to demonstrate normal DJJ by upper GI requires emergent exploration (as MGV cannot be not excluded)
    - US may be useful adjunct
- Duodenoduodenostomy is most common operation
  - Bypasses obstruction to preserve ampulla of Vater
  - Diamond-shaped vs. side-to-side anastomosis
  - ± tapering enteroplasty of dilated duodenum
  - Rubber catheter is passed distally in duodenum & withdrawn with balloon inflated to exclude additional distal web (1-3%)
- Surgical repair may be delayed due to
  - Electrolyte or fluid balance disturbances
  - Severe cardiac defects
  - Severe respiratory insufficiency
- Long-term complications
  - Megaduodenum, motility issues, adhesions

DIAGNOSTIC CHECKLIST

Image Interpretation Pearls

- True double bubble appearance with no distal bowel gas is essentially diagnostic for DA
- Upper GI or US is needed if distal bowel gas is present

SELECTED REFERENCES

1. Nguyen HN et al: Untwisting the complexity of midgut malrotation and volvulus ultrasound. Pediatr Radiol. 51(4):658-68, 2021
2. Tsitsiou Y et al: Diagnostic decision-making tool for imaging term neonatal bowel obstruction. Clin Radiol. 76(3):163-71, 2021
3. Bishop JC et al: The double bubble sign: duodenal atresia and associated genetic etiologies. Fetal Diagn Ther. 47(2):98-103, 2020
4. Hameed S et al: The role of sonography in differentiating congenital intrinsic duodenal anomalies from midgut malrotation: emphasizing the new signs of duodenal and gastric wall thickening and hyperechogenicity. Pediatr Radiol. 50(5):673-83, 2020
5. Chandrasekaran N et al: Prenatal sonographic diagnosis of meconium peritonitis from duodenal atresia. BMJ Case Rep. 2017, 2017
6. Rattan KN et al: Neonatal duodenal obstruction: a 15-year experience. J Neonatal Surg. 5(2):13, 2016
7. Adewole VA et al: Antenatally detected cystic biliary atresia: differential diagnoses of a double bubble. Springerplus. 3:368, 2014
8. Latzman JM et al: Duodenal atresia: not always a double bubble. Pediatr Radiol. 44(8):1031-4, 2014
9. Maxfield CM et al: A pattern-based approach to bowel obstruction in the newborn. Pediatr Radiol. 43(3):318-29, 2013
10. Mirza B et al: Multiple associated anomalies in patients of duodenal atresia: a case series. J Neonatal Surg. 1(2):23, 2012
11. Choudhry MS et al: Duodenal atresia: associated anomalies, prenatal diagnosis and outcome. Pediatr Surg Int. 25(8):727-30, 2009

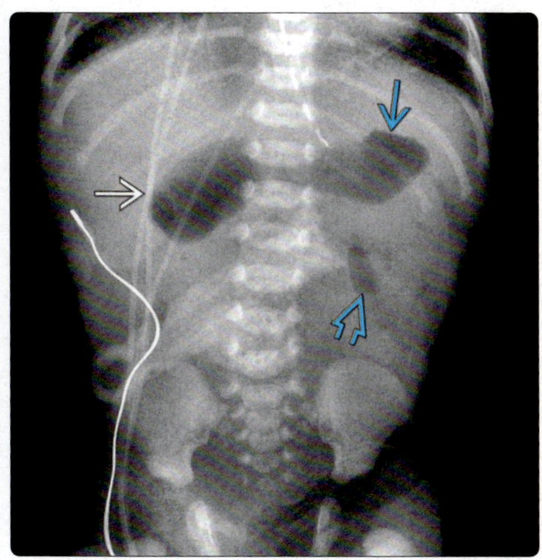

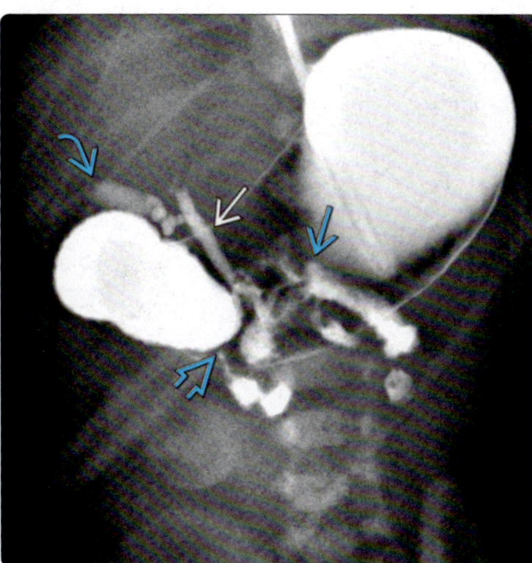

(Left) *AP radiograph in a full-term infant boy at 1 day of age shows a dilated stomach ⇨ & duodenum ➡ with a small amount of distal gas ⇨. Main surgical diagnostic considerations include midgut volvulus, annular pancreas, & duodenal stenosis or web. Immediate upper GI is indicated.* **(Right)** *Upper GI in the same patient shows dilation of the duodenum to D2 with contrast passing through a stenotic orifice ⇨ & the remaining duodenum to a normal duodenojejunal junction ⇨. Note reflux into common bile duct ➡ & GB ⇨.*

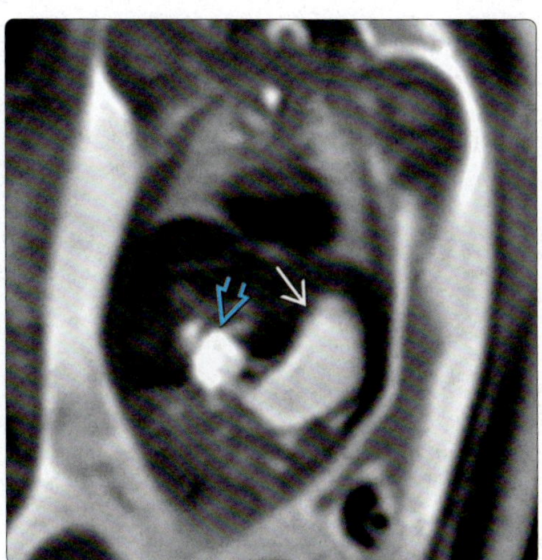

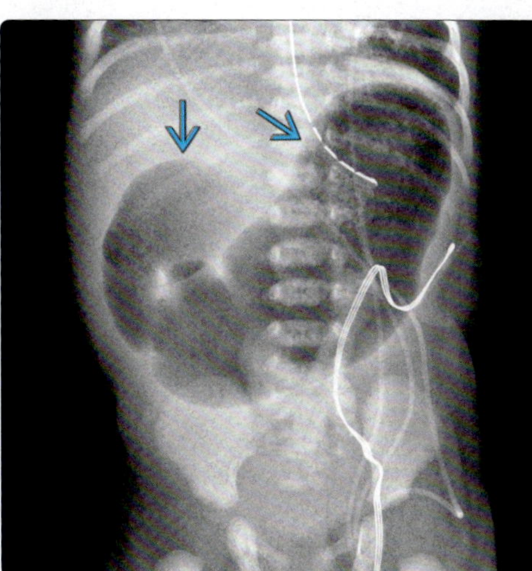

(Left) *Coronal SSFSE T2 MR in a 24-weeks-gestation fetus shows a dilated stomach ➡ & proximal duodenum ⇨ with decompressed distal bowel, the classic double bubble appearance of the duodenal atresia spectrum.* **(Right)** *AP radiograph in the same patient upon delivery shows a classic double bubble sign ⇨ of duodenal atresia with no distal bowel gas. Duodenal atresia was confirmed surgically.*

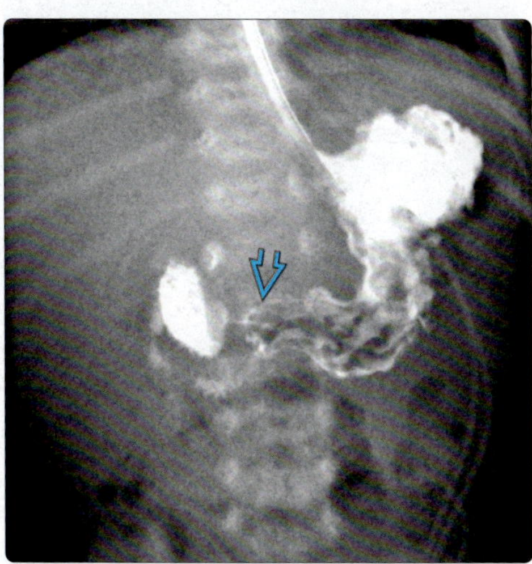

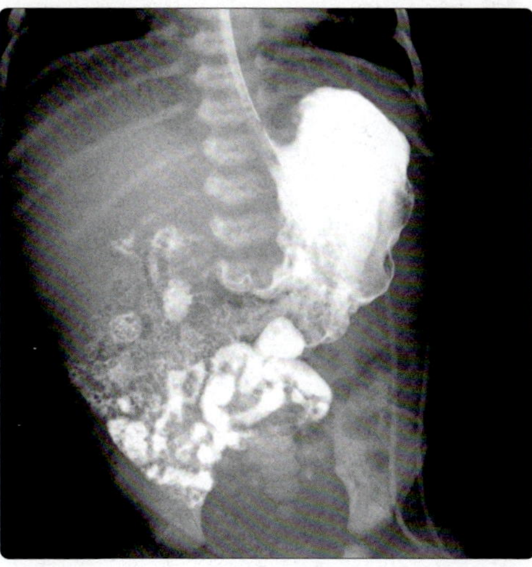

(Left) *Supine frontal upper GI was performed in the same patient following operative repair of the duodenal atresia to exclude a leak. There was a nonretroperitoneal position of the duodenum (not shown) with the duodenojejunal junction in the midline ⇨, consistent with malrotation (which is associated with duodenal atresia).* **(Right)** *Frontal upper GI (converted to a small bowel follow-through) in the same patient shows most of small bowel on the right, confirming malrotation.*

Duodenal Web

KEY FACTS

TERMINOLOGY

- Incomplete diaphragm of duodenal lumen causing partial or intermittent complete duodenal obstruction
- Duodenal atresia spectrum but with later clinical presentation

IMAGING

- Web lies at 2nd to 4th portion duodenum
  - Usually adjacent to ampulla of Vater
- Aperture size determines degree of obstruction, age of presentation, & imaging appearance
- Early presentation: Dilated stomach & proximal duodenum to D2/D3
- Late presentation: Thin, ballooned windsock in distal duodenum; variable duodenal caliber (based on orifice size)

TOP DIFFERENTIAL DIAGNOSES

- Duodenal atresia
- Midgut volvulus
- Gastrointestinal duplication cyst
- Annular pancreas
- Superior mesenteric artery syndrome

PATHOLOGY

- Failed duodenal recanalization: Spectrum of duodenal atresia
- Associated anomalies
  - Down syndrome: 30%
  - Malrotation: 28%
  - Annular pancreas: 33%

CLINICAL ISSUES

- Early presenters: Feeding intolerance, vomiting (bilious > nonbilious)
- Late presenters: Nausea, abdominal pain, progressive vomiting, acute pancreatitis
- Prognosis is excellent with treatment
  - Surgical vs. endoscopic excision

(Left) *Graphic shows a web ➡ with a windsock shape within the duodenal lumen ➡ with a pinhole ➡ opening distally. The proximal duodenum ➡ is moderately dilated from this partial obstruction.* **(Right)** *Transverse ultrasound performed for pyloric stenosis in a 3-week-old boy with recurrent emesis showed a normal pylorus. However, there is marked dilation of the duodenum ➡ to D2-D3 with no evidence of the swirl sign. Note the normal superior mesenteric artery ➡ /superior mesenteric vein ➡ relationship.*

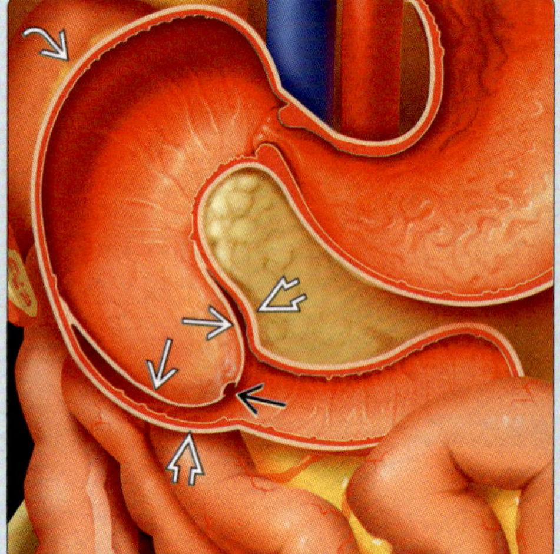

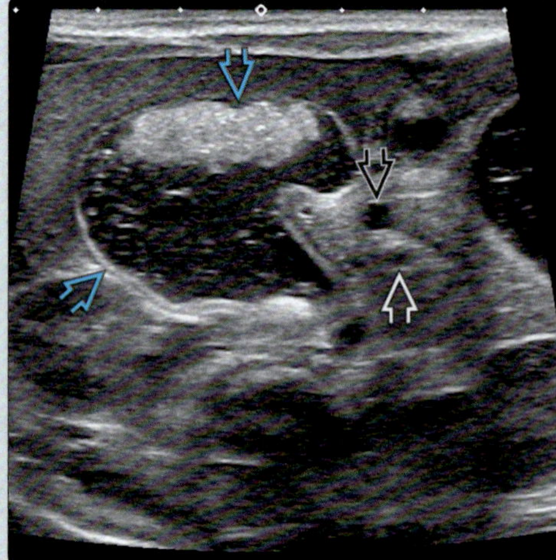

(Left) *Lateral upper GI in the same patient immediately after the ultrasound shows no barium passing beyond the dilated proximal duodenum, but distal gas is seen. A tight duodenal web was found at surgery.* **(Right)** *Supine upper GI in an older patient shows a dilated duodenum ➡ with distal gas ➡ & a tiny orifice ➡. Note also the dimple sign ➡ at the attachment of the proximal aspect of the web, which puckers when the web is stretched distally.*

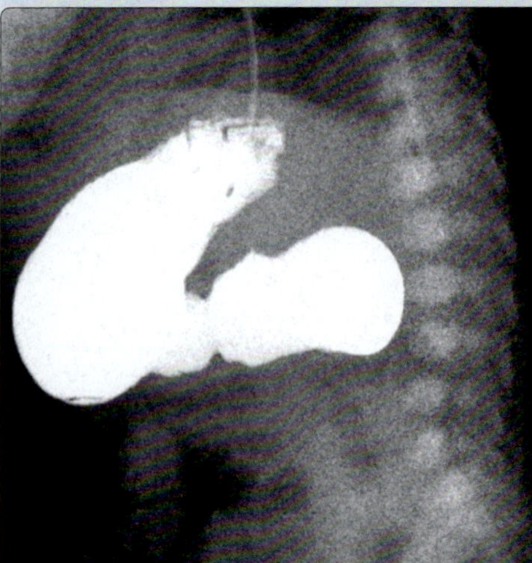

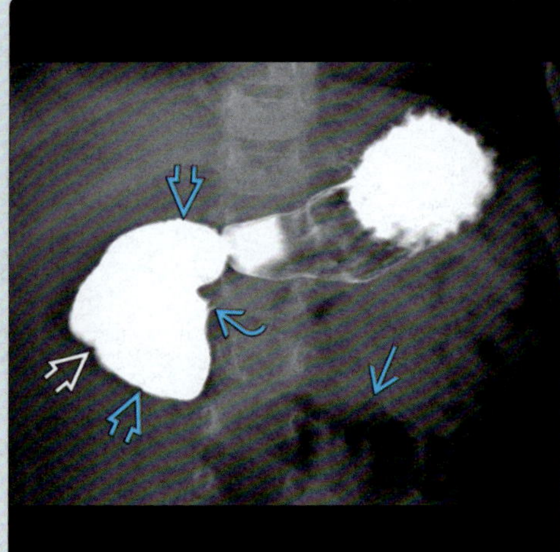

KEY FACTS

TERMINOLOGY

- Uncommon congenital gastric outlet obstruction
- Isolated vs. associated anomalies (30-50%)
  - Epidermolysis bullosa-pyloric atresia (EB-PA)
  - Hereditary multiple intestinal atresia or multiple intestinal atresia with immunodeficiency (HMIA/MIAI)

IMAGING

- Radiographs show "single bubble": Dilated, gas-filled stomach in newborn with no bowel gas otherwise
  - ± skin erosions (EB-PA)
  - ± intestinal Ca^{2+} (HMIA/MIAI)
- Ultrasound may show abnormal thin pyloric morphology + dilated gastric antrum = tennis racket appearance
  - Failure to visualize normal pyloric opening & antegrade passage of gastric contents into duodenal bulb

TOP DIFFERENTIAL DIAGNOSES

- Duodenal atresia
- Hypertrophic pyloric stenosis

PATHOLOGY

- Atresia may be web, solid cord, or discontinuous blind ends
- In MIAI: Atresias extend from pylorus to rectum (not just superior mesenteric artery territory)
  - Severe immunodeficiency → recurrent infections
- In EB-PA, clinical findings may include: Aplasia cutis, fusion/erosion/scarring with malformed protuberances (such as ears), small diameter orifices (such as nostrils), genitourinary anomalies, contractures

CLINICAL ISSUES

- Typical presentation for isolated PA: Nonbilious emesis
  - Perforated membrane may present later
- Isolated PA has excellent prognosis: Resection is curative
- Mortality approaches 100% in EB-PA or HMIA/MIAI
  - Infections & malnutrition in both

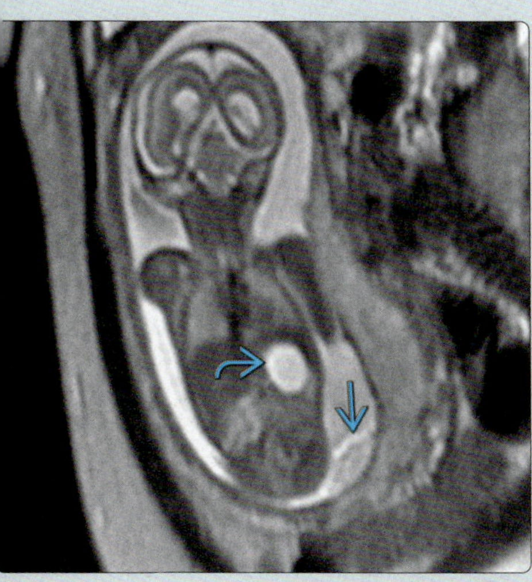

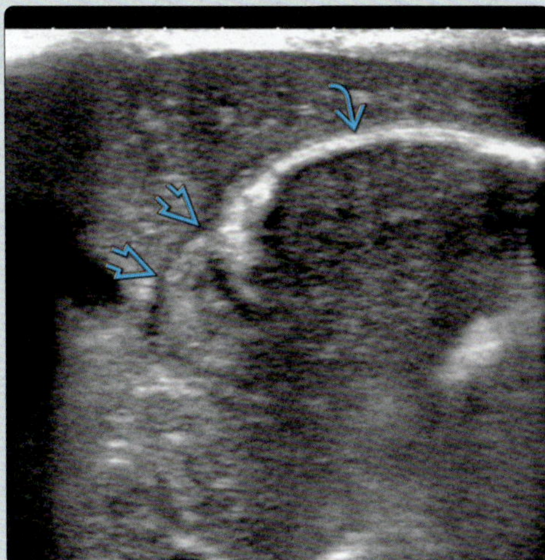

(Left) *Coronal T2 SSFSE MR at 21-weeks gestation shows dilation of the stomach ➡ (persisting throughout the exam) with no dilation of the bowel. Particulate debris ➡ was seen lying dependently in the amniotic cavity on multiple sequences, raising concern for the epidermolysis bullosa-pyloric atresia (EB-PA) association.* **(Right)** *Transverse oblique ultrasound through the newborn's right upper quadrant shows gastric distention ➡ with an abnormally thin, elongated, & persistently closed pylorus ➡. Skin biopsy confirmed EB-PA.*

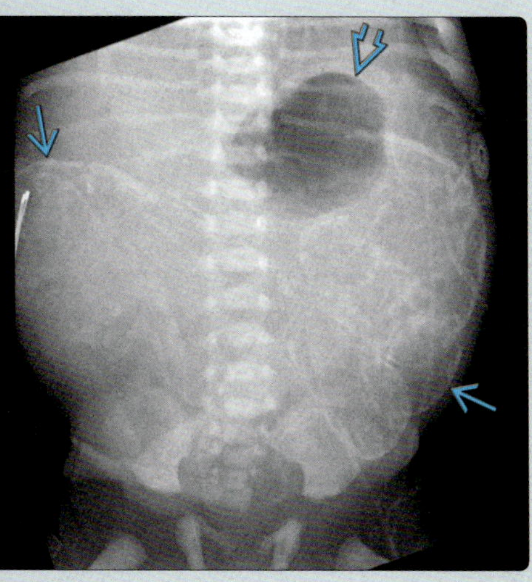

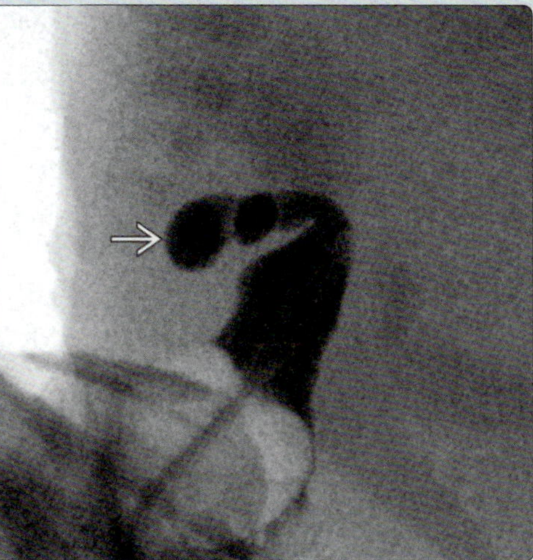

(Left) *AP abdominal radiograph in a newborn shows extensive Ca^{2+} ➡ throughout dilated bowel loops (which were fluid filled on prenatal ultrasound). The gas-filled stomach is moderately distended ➡ with no distal bowel gas identified.* **(Right)** *Lateral water-soluble contrast enema in the same patient shows a small, blind-ending rectal pouch ➡. Surgery confirmed numerous atresias from the pylorus to the rectum, consistent with MIAI/HMIA in this patient found to have immunodeficiency.*

Jejunoileal Atresia

KEY FACTS

TERMINOLOGY

- Congenital occlusion of jejunal or ileal lumen
  - Ranges from focal membrane to long-segment intestinal & mesenteric gap

IMAGING

- Site of obstruction (atresia) determines radiographic & fluoroscopic patterns
- Proximal jejunal atresia
  - Dilated stomach + duodenum + 1-2 loops of jejunum; microcolon is less likely on enema
- Midjejunal to distal ileal atresia
  - Numerous dilated loops; enema often shows microcolon
- Protocol advice
  - Water-soluble contrast enema (low osmolality, nearly iso-osmotic to body fluids)
    - Avoids fluid shifts into or out of bowel
    - Barium is not used (may impede meconium passage)
  - If microcolon is seen, reflux into small bowel up to dilated loops (if possible)

TOP DIFFERENTIAL DIAGNOSES

- Meconium ileus
- Meconium plug syndrome/small left colon
- Hirschsprung disease
- Anorectal malformation
- Inguinal hernia
- Necrotizing enterocolitis

PATHOLOGY

- Associated anomalies in 10-52% of cases
  - Gastroschisis (up to 20%), meconium ileus/cystic fibrosis (up to 10%), malrotation, volvulus

CLINICAL ISSUES

- Prognosis depends on amount of residual functional bowel post repair + associated anomalies
- Mortality: 11-14%

(Left) *AP radiograph shows the classic triple bubble sign of jejunal atresia due to a dilated stomach ➡, duodenum ➡, & proximal jejunum ➡ with no distal bowel gas.* **(Right)** *Supine upper GI in a 13-day-old girl with several days of projectile yellow emesis shows dilation of the stomach ➡, duodenum ➡, & an initial jejunal segment ➡ with transition to a normal caliber jejunum ➡ just beyond the duodenojejunal junction, most consistent with jejunal stenosis (which was found at surgery).*

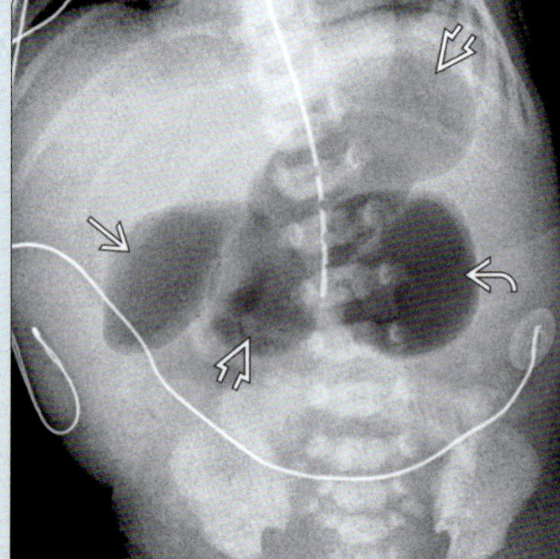

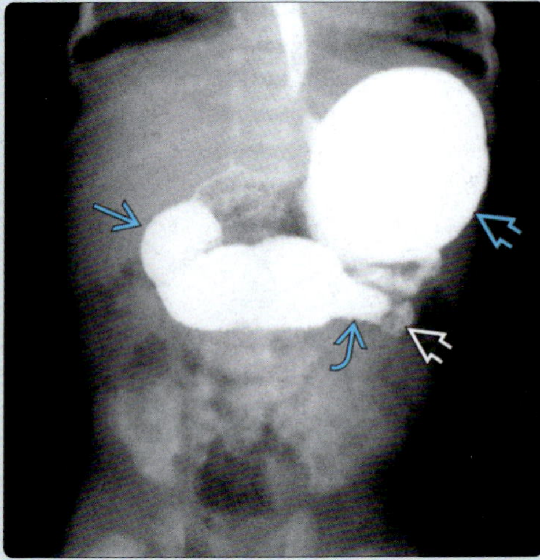

(Left) *Coronal T2 SSFSE fetal MR at 30-weeks gestation shows the triple bubble sign of jejunal atresia with a dilated, fluid-filled stomach ➡, duodenum ➡, & proximal jejunum ➡. Note the abrupt blind end of the atresia ➡.* **(Right)** *AP radiograph in the same patient upon delivery shows 3 or 4 air- & fluid-filled dilated bowel loops ➡ without other distal gas. Bilious material was aspirated from the Replogle tube. These findings are consistent with a proximal jejunal atresia, in agreement with the fetal MR.*

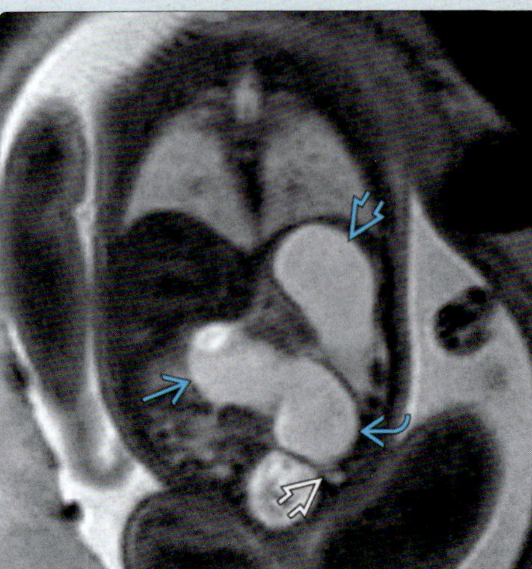

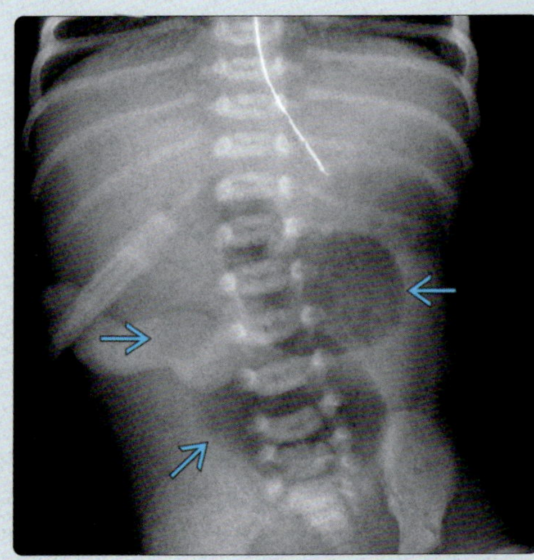

TERMINOLOGY

Definitions

- Congenital occlusion of jejunal or ileal lumen
- Ranges from focal membrane to long-segment intestinal atresia + mesenteric gap
- Stenosis, incomplete web: Forme fruste of atresia

IMAGING

General Features

- Best diagnostic clue
  - Contrast enema showing microcolon with reflux of contrast into blind-ending ileum or jejunum
- Location
  - Jejunum to distal ileum
- Morphology
  - Site of obstruction (atresia) determines radiographic & fluoroscopic patterns
    - Proximal jejunal atresia (classic high/proximal neonatal intestinal obstruction)
      - ◻ Dilated stomach + duodenum + 1-2 loops of jejunum; microcolon is less likely on enema
    - Midjejunal to distal ileal atresia (classic low/distal neonatal intestinal obstruction)
      - ◻ Numerous dilated bowel loops; enema shows microcolon
    - Multiple or long-segment intestinal atresias may have mixed imaging features
  - Appearance of microcolon on contrast enema is related to timing & level of obstruction
    - Smaller caliber colon from earlier or distal obstructions
      - ◻ Unused colon receives little succus entericus
    - Near-normal to normal-caliber colon from later or more proximal obstructions
      - ◻ Colonic succus entericus accumulation is less impaired

Radiographic Findings

- Radiography
  - Jejunal atresia: Proximal
    - Triple or quadruple bubble sign
      - ◻ Dilated stomach + duodenum + 1 (or few) proximal jejunal loop(s) without distal bowel gas
  - Ileal atresia
    - Multiple dilated bowel loops
      - ◻ Difficult to tell small bowel from colon in neonate
  - Soft tissue mass, ascites, &/or peritoneal Ca^{2+} suggest complicated obstruction
    - Perforation ± pseudocyst
    - Free intraperitoneal air is uncommon
  - Intraluminal Ca^{2+} in multiple atresias
  - Stenosis or web may have distal bowel gas beyond dilated loops

Fluoroscopic Findings

- Upper GI
  - Jejunal atresia
    - Dilated stomach, duodenum, proximal jejunum
      - ◻ Distal-most segment of bowel leading up to atresia may be very dilated & bulbous
    - Duodenojejunal junction may be displaced by dilated bowel loops in neonate (due to ↑ laxity of ligament of Treitz) despite normal rotation
  - Ileal atresia: Normal (in absence of multiple atresias)
- Water-soluble contrast enema (WSCE)
  - Jejunal atresia
    - Proximal atresia → normal or mildly small colon
    - Distal atresia → variable degrees of small colon
    - Long segment or multiple atresias → microcolon
  - Ileal atresia
    - Microcolon
    - Abrupt blind end to contrast flow at atresia
      - ◻ Contrast fails to reach dilated proximal bowel
    - Ileum distal to atresia is also small in caliber

Ultrasonographic Findings

- Grayscale ultrasound
  - Prenatal or post natal
    - Dilated, fluid-filled bowel loops
      - ◻ Echogenic, dilated loops prenatally may favor cystic fibrosis or gastroschisis ± atresia
    - Peritoneal Ca^{2+}, ascites (complex > simple), pseudocyst → suspect in utero perforation (meconium peritonitis)
    - Intraluminal Ca^{2+} is possible in multiple intestinal atresias
      - ◻ Must also consider anorectal malformation with rectourinary fistula or total colonic Hirschsprung disease
    - Whirlpool sign of twisting bowel loops has been described with "apple peel" atresia (but is classically associated with midgut or segmental volvulus)

MR Findings

- Depending on gestational age, fetal MR is better than prenatal US for detecting level of obstruction
  - Distribution of T1-bright meconium can evaluate length, caliber, & position of colon relative to abnormal small bowel loops

Imaging Recommendations

- Best imaging tool
  - For clinical + radiographic distal/low obstruction: WSCE
  - For clinical + radiographic proximal/high obstruction: Upper GI series (UGI)
    - For true triple or quadruple bubble with marked dilation & no distal gas, fluoroscopy may not be required prior to surgery
    - ± enema to exclude additional atresia preoperatively
  - If answer to obstruction site is not provided by 1st of these exams, be ready to perform 2nd
- Protocol advice
  - Enema is performed with low-osmolality, water-soluble contrast (nearly iso-osmotic to body fluids)
    - Avoids fluid shifts into or out of bowel
    - Barium is not used (may impede meconium passage)
  - If microcolon is seen, reflux contrast into small bowel until contrast reaches dilated loops or atresia

DIFFERENTIAL DIAGNOSIS

Meconium Ileus

- Microcolon on WSCE
- Meconium pellets obstruct distal ileum on enema
  - Refluxed contrast outlines ileal filling defects before passing into dilated loops

Small Left Colon/Meconium Plug Syndrome

- Small-caliber left colon up to splenic flexure on WSCE
- Normal to mildly dilated proximal colon
- ± meconium plugs in small left colon

Hirschsprung Disease

- Rectosigmoid ratio < 1 with colonic transition zone on WSCE; most of proximal colon is dilated
  - Entire colon is small in total colonic Hirschsprung disease

Anorectal Malformation

- No normal anal opening

Megacystis-Microcolon-Intestinal Hypoperistalsis

- Rare, often fatal syndrome with marked bladder dilation
- More common in female patients (4:1)

Colonic Atresia

- 1 or 2 disproportionately dilated loops on radiograph
- Small distal colon with proximal blind end on WSCE

Inguinal Hernia

- Dilated bowel with asymmetric inguinoscrotal fold
  - Gas in scrotum is essentially diagnostic

Necrotizing Enterocolitis

- Premature infants
- Uncommon in first 1-2 days of life
- Bowel separation, unchanging bowel loops, pneumatosis, portal venous gas, pneumoperitoneum
- Enema is not performed acutely

PATHOLOGY

General Features

- Etiology
  - Intrauterine vascular accident → necrosis with segmental stenosis/resorption
- Genetics
  - French Canadian ancestry was classically described in hereditary multiple intestinal atresias with immunodeficiency; has expanded
    - Specific atresias (often pyloric & sieve-like colon)
  - Autosomal recessive inheritance in some type 3b
- Associated abnormalities
  - 10-52% of jejunoileal atresia cases
    - Predisposing GI anomalies
      - Gastroschisis (up to 20%), meconium ileus/cystic fibrosis (up to 10%), malrotation, volvulus
    - Various cardiac, genitourinary, & brain anomalies

Staging, Grading, & Classification

- Atresia: Surgical grading system
  - Type 1: Membranous atresia, web/stenosis
    - No mesenteric defect, bowel is not short
  - Type 2: Blind ends are separated by fibrous cord
    - No mesenteric defect, bowel is not short
  - Type 3a: Blind ends with complete disconnection
    - V-shaped mesenteric gap, bowel is short
  - Type 3b: Apple peel or Christmas tree deformity
    - Large mesenteric defect, bowel is short
  - Type 4: Multiple small bowel atresias
    - 3-32% of jejunoileal atresias

CLINICAL ISSUES

Presentation

- Most common signs/symptoms
  - Distal ileal atresia: Failure to pass meconium + abdominal distention, bilious emesis
  - Jejunal or proximal ileal atresia: Bilious emesis
  - Stenosis or web: Early vs. delayed presentation with intermittent emesis, failure to thrive

Demographics

- Age: Atresia may present in utero or up to first 1-2 days after delivery

Natural History & Prognosis

- Prognosis depends on amount of residual functional bowel post repair + associated anomalies
  - 40 cm of normal bowel length is considered functionally adequate to avoid treatment for short gut syndrome
- Mortality: 11-14%

Treatment

- Full resuscitation prior to surgical correction (unless perforation or volvulus requires emergent intervention)
- Surgical resection of atretic segment with anastomosis
  - Tapering vs. resection of very dilated proximal segment, depending on residual bowel length
- Complications: Short gut syndrome (14%), dysmotility, adhesions

DIAGNOSTIC CHECKLIST

Consider

- Bilious emesis can occur in neonatal distal or proximal obstructions
  - Radiograph determines initial fluoroscopic study in neonatal obstruction
    - WSCE 1st for distal vs. UGI for proximal

SELECTED REFERENCES

1. Tsitsiou Y et al: Diagnostic decision-making tool for imaging term neonatal bowel obstruction. Clin Radiol. 76(3):163-71, 2021
2. Garel J et al: The role of sonography for depiction of a whirlpool sign unrelated to midgut malrotation in neonates. Pediatr Radiol. 50(1):46-56, 2020
3. Li X et al: Appearance of fetal intestinal obstruction on fetal MRI. Prenat Diagn. 40(11):1398-407, 2020
4. Hao J et al: Preliminary investigation of the diagnosis of neonatal congenital small bowel atresia by ultrasound. Biomed Res Int. 2019:7097159, 2019
5. Rubio EI et al: Prenatal magnetic resonance and ultrasonographic findings in small-bowel obstruction: imaging clues and postnatal outcomes. Pediatr Radiol. 47(4):411-21, 2017
6. Coletta R et al: Short bowel syndrome in children: surgical and medical perspectives. Semin Pediatr Surg. 23(5):291-7, 2014
7. Maxfield CM et al: A pattern-based approach to bowel obstruction in the newborn. Pediatr Radiol. 43(3):318-29, 2013

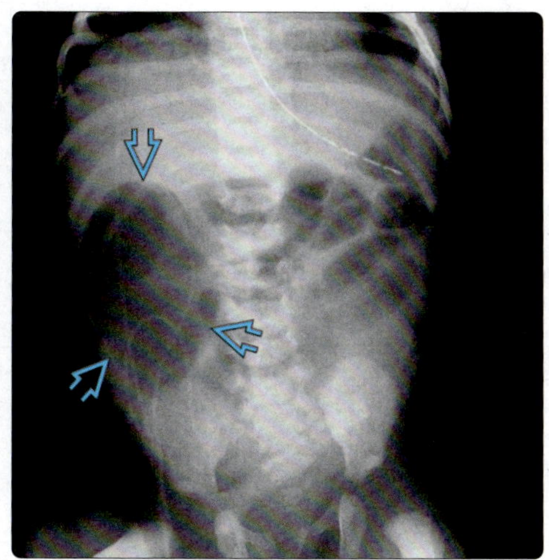

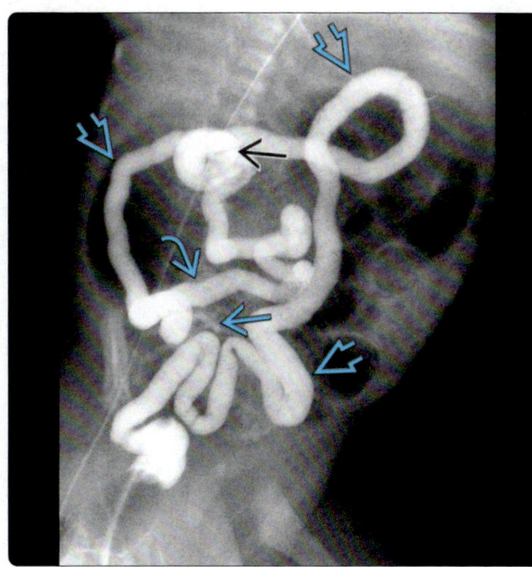

(Left) *AP radiograph in a 1-day-old term infant with abdominal distention & no meconium passage shows multiple dilated bowel loops, consistent with distal obstruction. A dominant dilated loop ➡ suggests that there may be a distal ileal or colonic atresia.* **(Right)** *Supine water-soluble contrast enema (WSCE) in the same patient shows a microcolon ➡ with reflux into the appendix ➡ & terminal ileum ➡, which curls & ends blindly ➡, consistent with ileal atresia.*

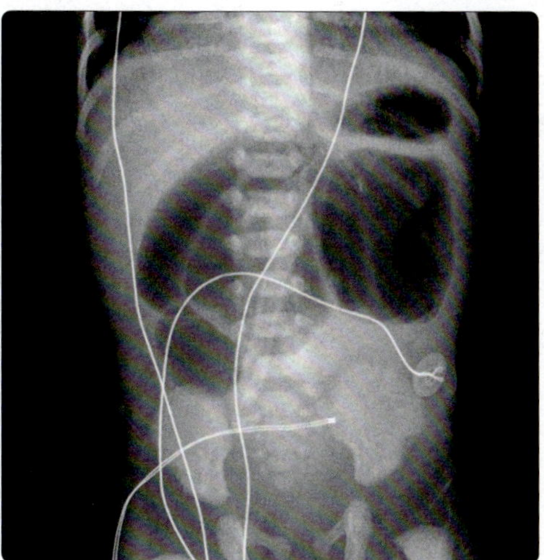

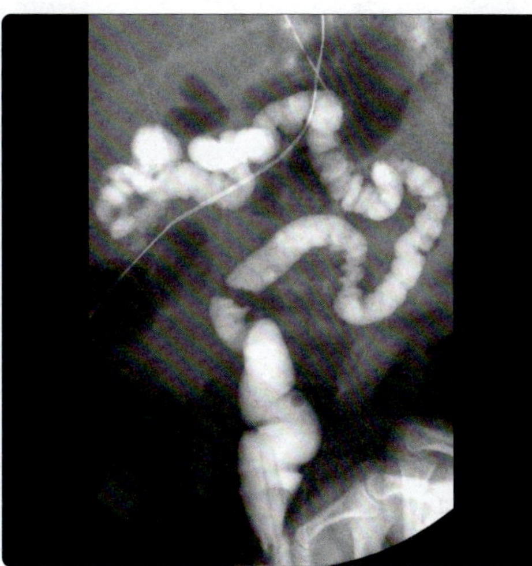

(Left) *AP radiograph in a 1-day-old boy with bilious emesis shows several dilated loops of bowel, suggestive of an upper bowel obstruction, likely jejunal atresia.* **(Right)** *Supine WSCE in the same patient shows a microcolon, suggesting that there may be an additional distal atresia or a long-segment atresia. Surgery confirmed the former.*

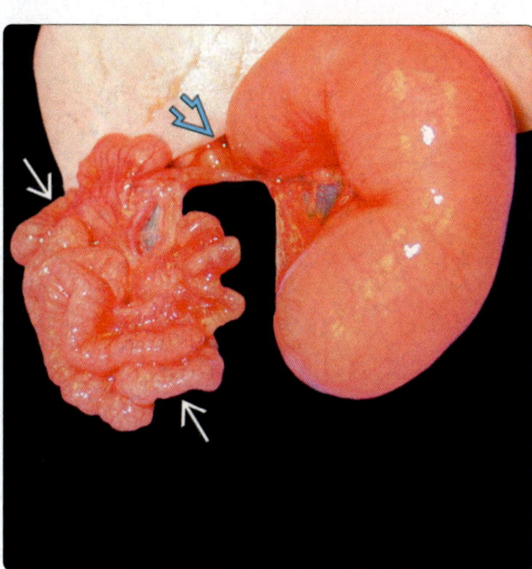

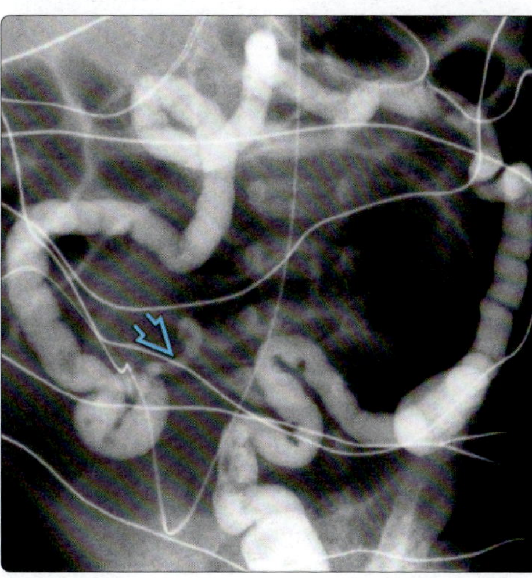

(Left) *Surgical photograph in the same patient shows the dilated jejunum to the atretic segment ➡; the distal bowel is decompressed ➡. A distal ileal atresia was also noted at surgery, explaining the microcolon.* **(Right)** *Supine WSCE in a 2-day-old shows a microcolon with reflux into appendix ➡. However, contrast would not reflux into the terminal ileum. Considerations for this appearance include meconium ileus, ileal atresia, & total colonic Hirschsprung disease. At surgery, ileal atresia was found.*

Colonic Atresia

KEY FACTS

TERMINOLOGY

- Congenital colonic obstruction due to variable forms of interruption: Membrane (type I), fibrous cord (II), or complete separation with mesenteric defect (III)

IMAGING

- Radiography: Multiple dilated, air-filled bowel loops ± 1 disproportionately dilated loop of colon proximal to atresia
- Contrast enema: Distal microcolon with abrupt termination to retrograde contrast flow proximally (at colonic blind end)
    - Contrast does not fill cecum/terminal ileum or dilated bowel loops
    - Atresia may affect any segment of colon

TOP DIFFERENTIAL DIAGNOSES

- Hirschsprung disease
- Meconium plug syndrome/neonatal small left colon
- Jejunoileal atresia
- Meconium ileus

CLINICAL ISSUES

- Presents similar to other congenital distal bowel obstructions
    - Newborn with failure to pass meconium, abdominal distention, ± bilious emesis
        - If initial abdominal radiograph shows distal bowel obstruction → water-soluble contrast enema
        - History of bilious emesis is frequent in distal obstructions; should not necessarily divert work-up to upper GI 1st (to rule out midgut volvulus) if clinical/radiologic picture suggests distal obstruction
    - May pass small amount of white or pale mucous rather than pigmented meconium
- Least common of all intestinal atresias (1.8-15%)
    - Very rare; incidence ~ 1:20,000 live births
- Treatment: Surgery to eliminate bowel obstruction & establish intestinal continuity

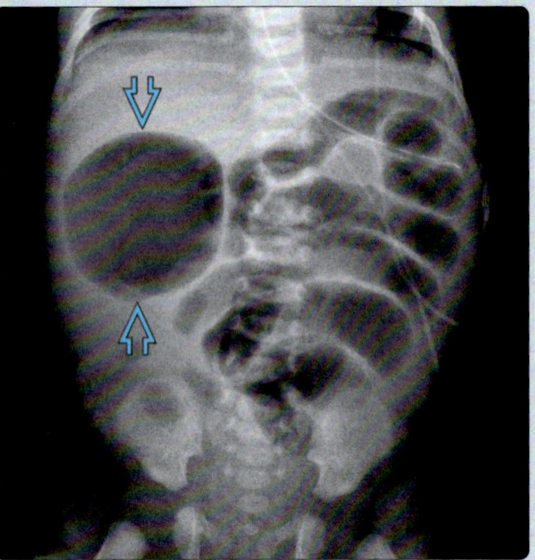

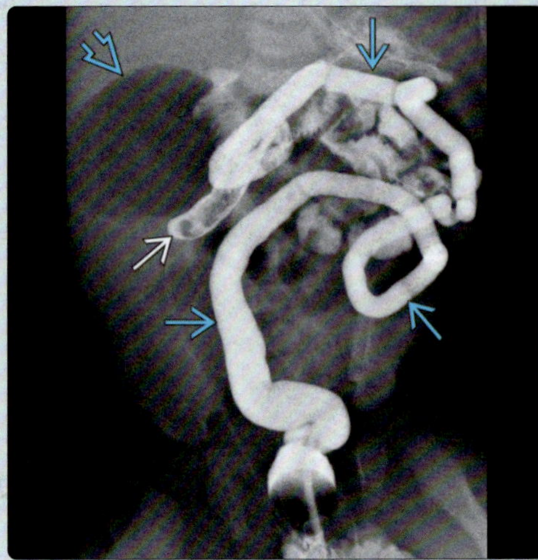

(Left) *AP supine abdominal radiograph in a 1-day-old full-term infant girl with bilious emesis shows multiple dilated gas-filled bowel loops in the left abdomen with a single, disproportionately dilated loop in the right upper quadrant ⇨, an appearance often seen in colonic atresia.* **(Right)** *Supine contrast enema in the same patient (after a normal upper GI) shows a microcolon ⇨ with a blind end ➡. The adjacent large dilated loop ⇨ was due to an atretic proximal colon.*

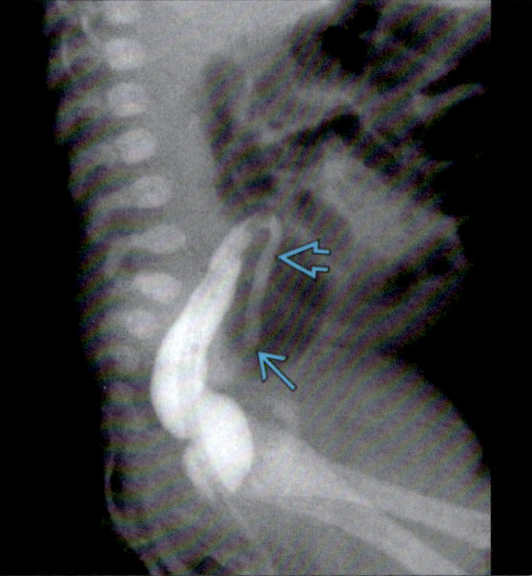

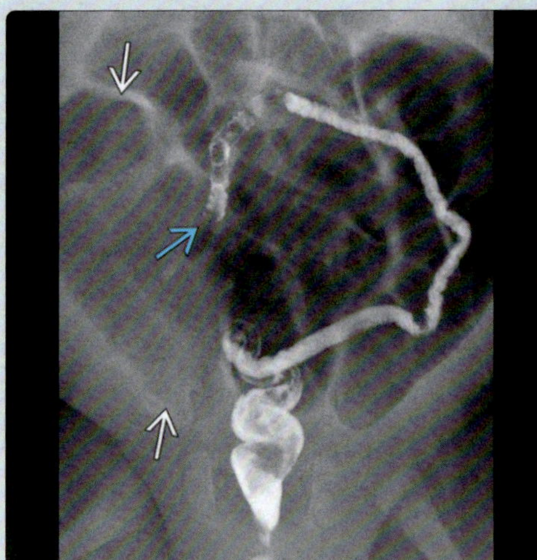

(Left) *Left-side down lateral contrast enema in a newborn with failure to pass meconium shows that the sigmoid colon is tiny ⇨ & blind ending ⇨, consistent with colonic atresia at the sigmoid level.* **(Right)** *Supine contrast enema in a newborn boy with prior fetal MR imaging that demonstrated a distal bowel obstruction shows a diffusely small colon that abruptly terminates at the ascending colon ⇨, consistent with colonic atresia. The ascending colon is displaced medially by dilated colon & ileum ➡ proximal to atresia.*

KEY FACTS

TERMINOLOGY

- Intestinal atresias are multifocal in 3-32%; 2 forms
  - Multiple intestinal atresia (MIA)
    - Atresias of types I, II, IIIa, IIIb; affects midduodenum to mid to distal transverse colon
      - Due to vascular insult to superior mesenteric artery territory (midgut)
  - Hereditary MIA (HMIA) or MIA with combined immunodeficiency (MIA-CID)
    - Atresias of types I & II only; affects pylorus to rectum, including long segments of occlusion
      - Multiple proposed etiologies
    - Develop severe infections from immunodeficiency

IMAGING

- No bowel gas beyond most proximal obstruction
- Ca^{2+} may develop in chronically obstructed, dilated closed loops of intestine
- Enema typically shows small, unused colonic segments distal to obstructions
- Ultrasound shows fluid-filled bowel ± echogenic Ca^{2+}, wall thickening; ± biliary dilation

PATHOLOGY

- Histology of HMIA/MIA-CID: Characteristic sieve-like occluded segments (multiple lumina in single cross section)
  - *TTC7A* mutations are implicated in HMIA/MIA-CID

CLINICAL ISSUES

- MIA: Operative repair is frequently curative; low mortality unless associated with gastroschisis or short gut syndrome
- HMIA/MIA-CID: Despite resection of atretic segments, patients have very high morbidity/mortality
  - Longstanding gut & biliary dysfunction
  - Immunocompromise with severe infections
    - Intestinal transplant may be curative with high level of immune system reconstitution by donor gut

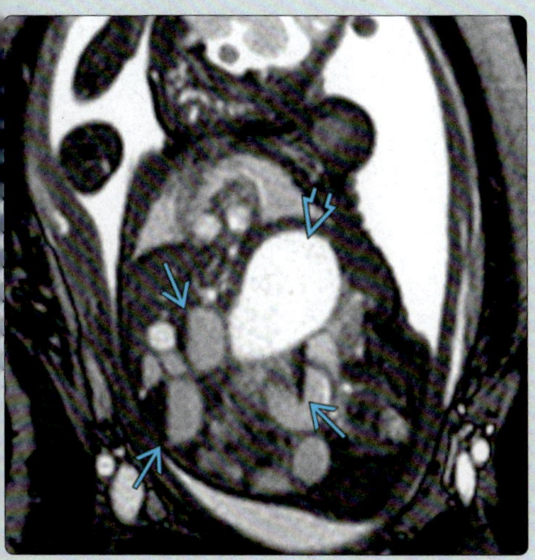

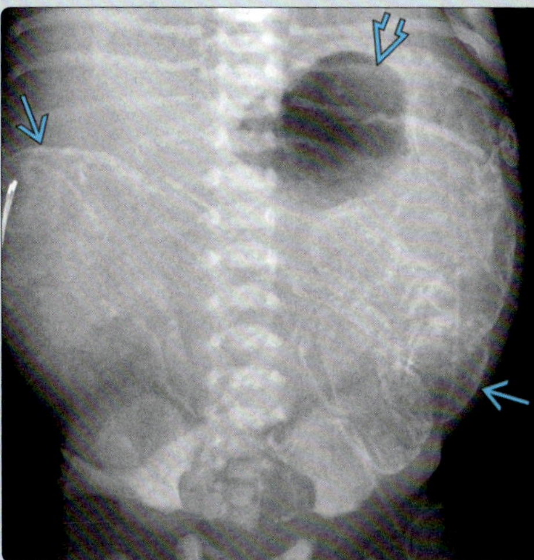

(Left) *Coronal SSFP MR in a 33-weeks-gestation fetus shows numerous dilated bowel loops containing fluid-fluid levels ➙. The distended stomach ➙ is of different signal intensity than the dilated bowel, which can suggest multiple intestinal atresias. No colonic meconium was seen on T1 MR.* **(Right)** *AP radiograph of the abdomen hours after birth shows extensive Ca^{2+} throughout the dilated bowel loops ➙. The gas-filled stomach ➙ is moderately distended with no distal bowel gas identified.*

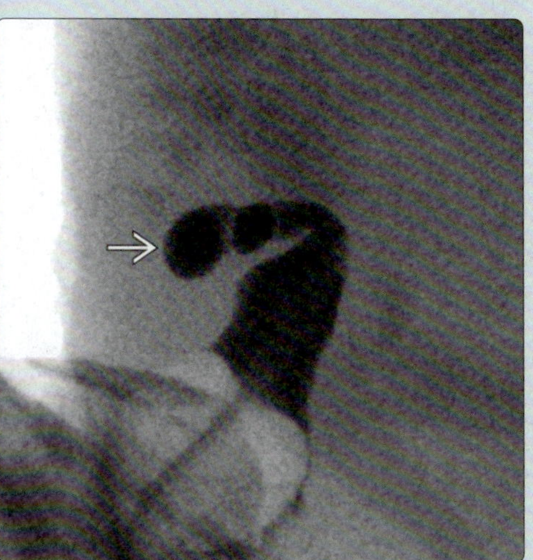

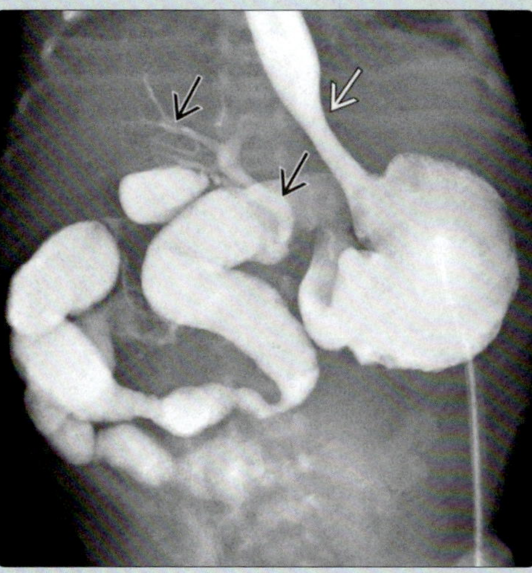

(Left) *Lateral view of a water-soluble contrast enema (with catheter balloon pressed externally against the anus) shows a small, blind-ending rectal pouch ➙. Surgery confirmed numerous atresias at the pylorus, small bowel, & colon. This patient developed infections from a severe immunodeficiency & was diagnosed with hereditary multiple intestinal atresias.* **(Right)** *After resection of the atresias (same patient), upper GI (with contrast injected through the gastrostomy tube) shows free reflux into the esophagus ➙ & bile ducts ➙.*

Meconium Ileus

KEY FACTS

TERMINOLOGY

- Neonatal obstruction of terminal ileum (TI) due to abnormally thick, tenacious meconium
- Up to 90% of meconium ileus (MI) patients have cystic fibrosis (CF)
- MI is presenting illness in 10-20% of CF patients

IMAGING

- Uncomplicated MI (50%): Numerous dilated, gas-filled bowel loops on newborn radiographs
  - Microcolon + meconium-filled pellets in TI on water-soluble contrast enema (WSCE)
- Complicated MI (50%): Due to superimposed volvulus, atresia, necrosis, ± perforation with meconium peritonitis
  - Soft tissue mass or gasless abdomen
  - ± intrauterine perforation (Ca^{2+} of meconium peritonitis)

TOP DIFFERENTIAL DIAGNOSES

- Ileal atresia
- Hirschsprung disease
- Meconium plug syndrome
- Colonic atresia
- Megacystis-microcolon-intestinal hypoperistalsis
- Anorectal malformation
- Midgut volvulus

PATHOLOGY

- Mutation of *CFTR* gene (chromosome 7)

CLINICAL ISSUES

- CF incidence: 1:3,000 live births in White patients (much less common in other races)
- Most common signs/symptoms: Failure to pass meconium, abdominal distention, bilious emesis
- Serial hyperosmotic WSCE vs. surgery for treatment of uncomplicated MI
  - Surgery is usually required in complicated MI

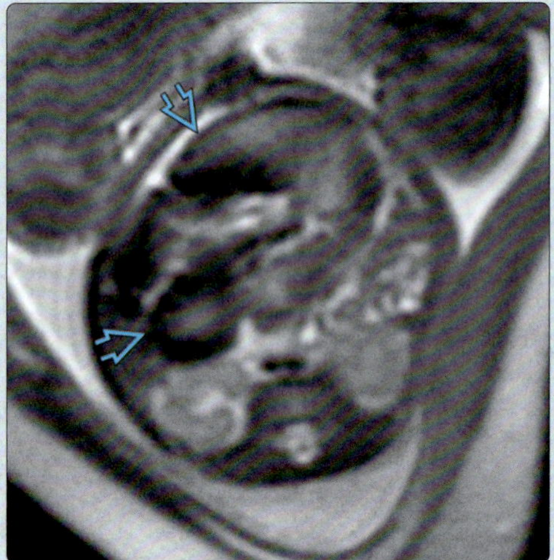

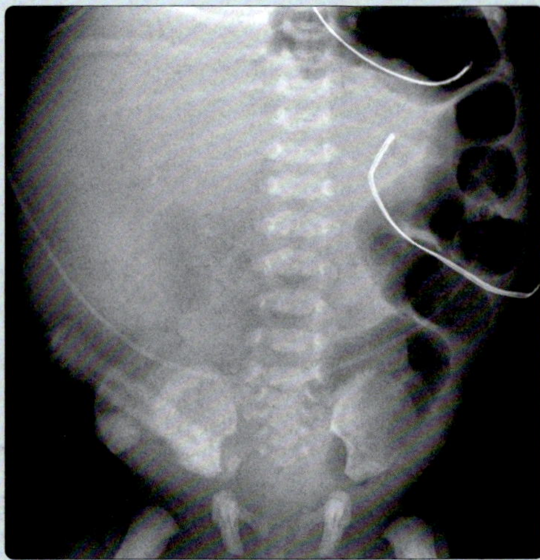

(Left) *Axial SSFSE T2 fetal MR at 33-weeks gestation shows dilated small bowel (SB) ➩ filled with intermediate to low signal intensity meconium. A tiny-caliber colon was best seen on sagittal images (not shown), consistent with a SB obstruction. The mother was noted to be a carrier of the cystic fibrosis (CF) gene.* **(Right)** *Radiograph in the same patient several hours after birth shows a large soft tissue mass displacing dilated bowel towards the left, worrisome for a complicated meconium ileus (MI).*

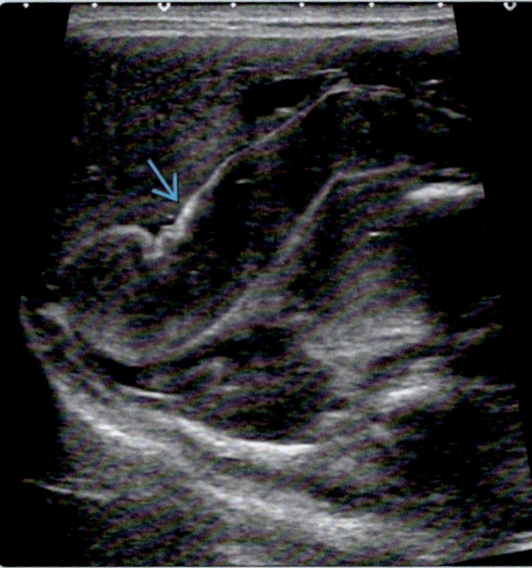

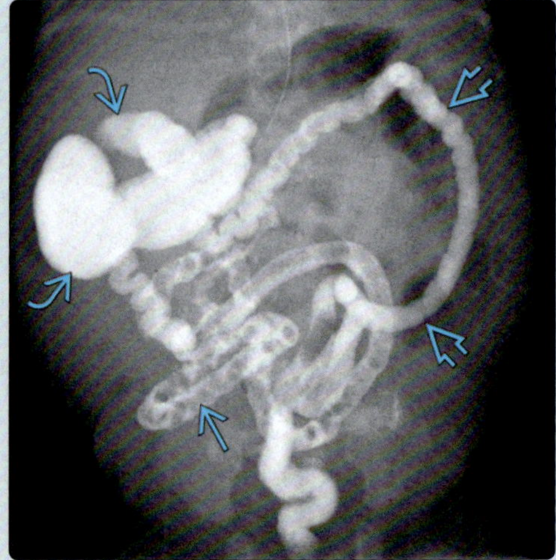

(Left) *US immediately following the radiograph in the same patient shows dilated, debris-filled bowel ➔ with echogenic walls, consistent with bowel obstruction. Ascites was scattered in the abdomen. However, no pseudocyst or other sign of perforation was seen.* **(Right)** *Supine WSCE in the same patient shows a microcolon ➩ without significant colonic meconium. Reflux into the terminal ileum (TI) shows obstructing meconium pellets ➔ before reaching dilated SB ➦, consistent with MI.*

TERMINOLOGY

Definitions

- Meconium ileus (MI): Neonatal obstruction of distal ileum due to abnormally thick, tenacious meconium
  - Up to 90% of MI patients have cystic fibrosis (CF)
  - Presenting illness in 10-20% of CF newborns
- Complicated MI: Superimposed ischemia, volvulus, atresia, &/or perforation in up to 50% of MI cases

IMAGING

General Features

- Best diagnostic clue
  - Microcolon + meconium-filled terminal ileum (TI) on water-soluble contrast enema (WSCE)
- Size
  - Microcolon (small, unused colon due to impaired passage of succus entericus through small bowel into colon in utero) varies in caliber
  - Varying degrees of proximal small bowel dilation

Radiographic Findings

- Radiography
  - Uncomplicated (or simple) MI
    - Multiple dilated bowel loops
    - ± bubbly lucencies in right lower quadrant
      - Air mixed with meconium
    - Few, if any, air-fluid levels ("sticky meconium")
    - WSCE to diagnose & treat
  - Complicated (or complex) MI
    - Soft tissue mass or gasless abdomen
    - ± intrauterine perforation → meconium peritonitis (MP)
      - Pseudocyst, Ca^{2+} lining peritoneum
    - Ultrasound &/or enema for further evaluation
      - Enema treatment usually fails (requiring surgery)

Fluoroscopic Findings

- Low osmolar WSCE for diagnosis; higher osmolar WSCE for therapy
  - Smallest of microcolons (often)
  - Contrast refluxed into TI outlines meconium pellets ("pearls on string")
    - Pellets may obstruct contrast passage proximally (mimicking ileal atresia)
    - Paucity of colonic meconium is common
  - Switching to higher osmolar WSCE can be therapeutic in uncomplicated MI
    - Up to 80% success in experienced hands
    - ± N-acetylcysteine added to WSCE for treatment

MR Findings

- Fetal MR
  - Microcolon containing little T1-bright meconium in later gestation
  - T1-bright signal is often seen in dilated, obstructed small bowel loops

Ultrasonographic Findings

- Grayscale ultrasound
  - Prenatally
    - Dilated, echogenic bowel
    - Echogenic ascites, peritoneal Ca^{2+}, pseudocyst from in utero perforation
  - Postnatally
    - Dilated, thick-walled small bowel loops containing heterogeneous meconium
      - Echogenic foci of gas in meconium
    - Echogenic ascites, peritoneal Ca^{2+}, pseudocyst from in utero perforation

Imaging Recommendations

- Best imaging tool
  - WSCE
- Protocol advice
  - With neonatal distal bowel obstruction on radiographs → WSCE for further investigation
    - Barium is not used (may impede meconium passage)
    - Nonballoon tip catheter is used (in general) due to possible risk of rectal injury
      - If using balloon-tipped Foley, inflate balloon outside & insert tip into rectum with balloon held up against anus to prevent leakage
      - Alternatively, carefully inflate balloon under fluoroscopy after visualizing normally distensible rectum with contrast (to prevent rectal injury)
      - Enema contrast gravity infusion vs. gentle pulsing of contrast by syringe injection
    - If microcolon is seen, attempt reflux into ileum
      - Visualization of meconium pellets is diagnostic
    - Switch to higher osmolality (600-900 mOsm) contrast for therapeutic enema
      - Reflux contrast up to dilated bowel if possible
      - Active fluid resuscitation during enema to balance fluid shifts into bowel: 1.5x maintenance
      - Have surgical team check electrolytes after each therapeutic enema
    - Serial enemas may be required to relieve meconium obstruction; usually 1 per day
    - Complications of enema
      - Perforation
      - Dehydration/intravascular volume depletion/hypotension
      - Electrolyte imbalances
      - Segmental volvulus of dilated proximal bowel if meconium does not clear
  - If bowel obstruction is present with soft tissue mass on radiographs (suggesting complicated MI ± MP), consider ultrasound ± enema
    - Ultrasound or MR in MP can help guide surgical management
  - If enema is normal (uncommon with numerous dilated loops), consider upper GI
    - Exclude midgut volvulus causing ischemic ileus

DIFFERENTIAL DIAGNOSIS

Ileal Atresia

- Microcolon on WSCE
- Contrast refluxing into ileum stops abruptly at atresia
- Opacified distal ileum is usually small & without meconium

Hirschsprung Disease

- Microcolon in some cases of total colonic Hirschsprung disease (HD) on WSCE
- More common: Short-segment HD
  - Low rectosigmoid (R/S) ratio (< 1), serrated mucosa
  - ± meconium plugs in colon above spasmodic rectum

Small Left Colon/Meconium Plug Syndrome

- Small distal colon; transition at splenic flexure on WSCE
- Nonobstructing meconium plugs in colon (not TI)
- Enema is often curative of this functional obstruction
- Not associated with CF

Colonic Atresia

- Microcolon up to level of atresia on WSCE
- Colon proximal to atresia is often dilated out of proportion to small bowel

Anorectal Malformation

- Distal obstruction without normal anus on exam

Megacystis-Microcolon-Intestinal Hypoperistalsis

- Microcolon on WSCE
- Very dilated bladder
- M:F = 1:4; often fatal disease

Midgut Volvulus

- Bowel loops may be dilated from ischemic ileus
- Upper GI vs. ultrasound for diagnosis

PATHOLOGY

General Features

- Genetics
  - CF: Autosomal recessive
  - Mutation of *CFTR* gene (chromosome 7)
    - > 2,000 mutations; ΔF508 mutation is most common overall & with MI
    - Faulty chloride transport across epithelium → ↓ water in luminal contents → dehydrated, thick secretions
      - ▫ Obstruction of glands & ducts
      - ▫ Pancreas, intestines, & lungs are most affected
    - Thick meconium → distal ileal obstruction
- Associated abnormalities
  - CF manifestations beyond neonatal period
    - Lung disease
    - Exocrine pancreas failure, biliary disease, chronic appendiceal dilation without inflammation, distal intestinal obstruction syndrome (DIOS)

Staging, Grading, & Classification

- Uncomplicated MI (50%)
- Complicated MI (50%): Superimposed segmental volvulus, necrosis, atresia, perforation with MP → ascites, peritoneal Ca^{2+}, pseudocyst (may be large)

CLINICAL ISSUES

Presentation

- Most common signs/symptoms
  - Failure to pass meconium, abdominal distention, bilious emesis

Demographics

- Age: Newborn
- Sex: M = F
- Epidemiology: 1:3,000 live births in White patients have CF (much less common in other races)
  - Up to 90% of patients with MI have CF
    - Some reports that up to 50% of MI patients do not have CF
      - ▫ Complicated MI rate may be higher
      - ▫ Prematurity + low birth weights are more likely
  - 10-20% of CF patients present with MI

Natural History & Prognosis

- MI patients classically have worse lung function, nutritional status, & survival vs. other CF patients
  - More recent papers show no difference
  - Earlier diagnosis of CF may be beneficial
- Recurrent bowel issues in CF
  - DIOS ("MI equivalent")
    - Older children with obstruction from thick stool in TI
  - Chronic constipation (may be 1st CF manifestation)

Treatment

- Uncomplicated MI: Serial hyperosmotic WSCE vs. surgery
  - Therapeutic enema success: Up to 83% (with experience)
    - Reported success rates vary widely (5-83%)
  - Perforation rate of enema 1-3%
    - Greatest with injection & use of rectal balloon
  - Surgery for patient decompensation, failed enemas, or perforation
    - Enterotomy, meconium removal, primary anastomosis vs. temporary enterostomy
- Complicated MI: Surgery
  - Resect abnormal bowel, meconium removal, primary anastomosis vs. temporary enterostomy
- Testing for CF

DIAGNOSTIC CHECKLIST

Consider

- Causes of distal obstruction & microcolon
- Diluted hyperosmolar WSCE for simple MI therapy
- Enema is rarely curative in complicated MI (requires surgery)

SELECTED REFERENCES

1. Tsitsiou Y et al: Diagnostic decision-making tool for imaging term neonatal bowel obstruction. Clin Radiol. 76(3):163-71, 2021
2. Galante G et al: Gastrointestinal, pancreatic, and hepatic manifestations of cystic fibrosis in the newborn. Neoreviews. 20(1):e12-4, 2019
3. Schauble AL et al: N-acetylcysteine for management of distal intestinal obstruction syndrome. J Pediatr Pharmacol Ther. 24(5):390-7, 2019
4. Gunderman PFR et al: Fetal MRI in management of complicated meconium ileus: prenatal and surgical imaging. Prenat Diagn. 38(9):685-91, 2018
5. Rubio EI et al: Prenatal magnetic resonance and ultrasonographic findings in small-bowel obstruction: imaging clues and postnatal outcomes. Pediatr Radiol. 47(4):411-21, 2017
6. Sathe M et al: Meconium ileus in cystic fibrosis. J Cyst Fibros. 16 Suppl 2:S32-9, 2017
7. Kelly T et al: Gastrointestinal manifestations of cystic fibrosis. Dig Dis Sci. 60(7):1903-13, 2015
8. Maxfield CM et al: A pattern-based approach to bowel obstruction in the newborn. Pediatr Radiol. 43(3):318-29, 2013
9. Colombani M et al: Fetal gastrointestinal MRI: all that glitters in T1 is not necessarily colon. Pediatr Radiol. 40(7):1215-21, 2010

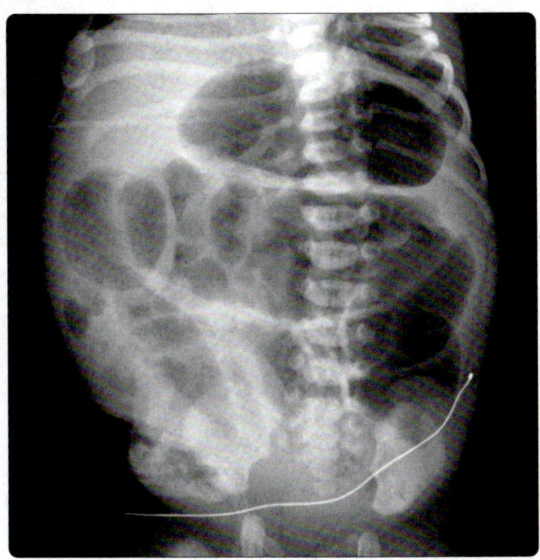

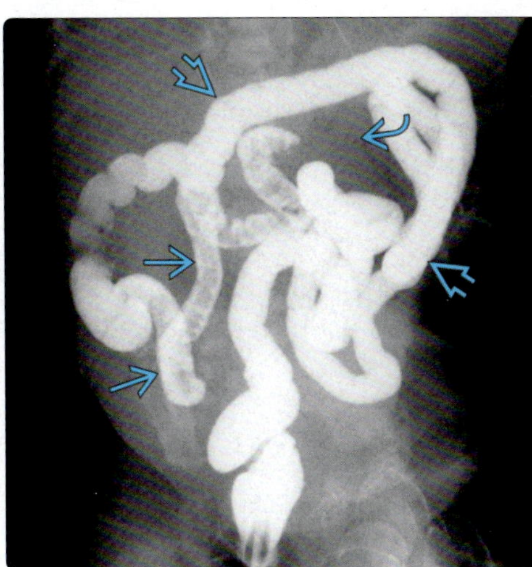

(Left) *AP radiograph in a full-term newborn with failure to pass meconium (& whose parents are CF gene carriers) shows a distal bowel obstruction without soft tissue mass effect or signs of meconium peritonitis. With this history, uncomplicated MI is the primary diagnostic consideration.* **(Right)** *Supine WSCE in the same patient shows a microcolon ➡ & reflux of contrast into the meconium-filled TI ➡, most consistent with MI. Contrast did not reach the dilated bowel ➡.*

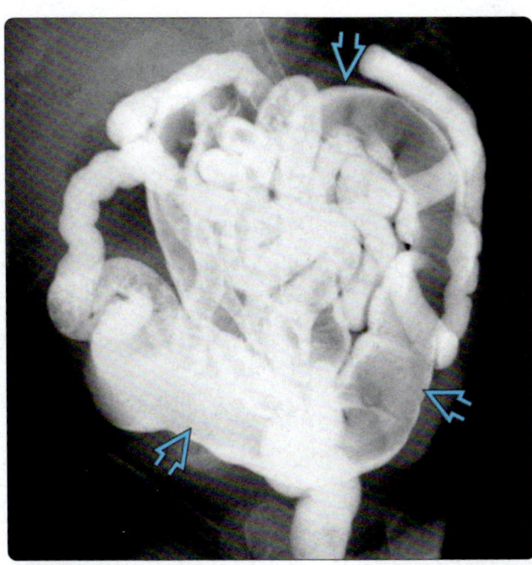

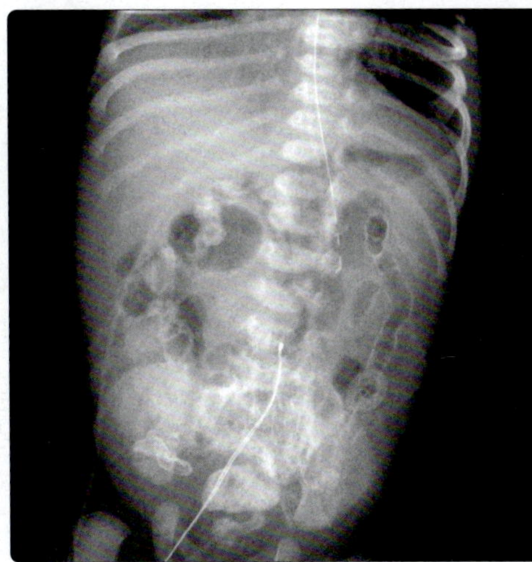

(Left) *A 2nd supine WSCE was performed in the same patient. There is now reflux of the high osmolality 1:1 diluted Gastroview contrast (950 mOsm) into multiple dilated bowel loops proximal to the obstructing meconium ➡.* **(Right)** *AP radiograph in the same patient 1 day after the 2nd enema shows much less dilation of the bowel proximal to the previously obstructed TI. There is mild residual contrast in the persistently small, unused colon. This is considered a successful treatment enema for MI.*

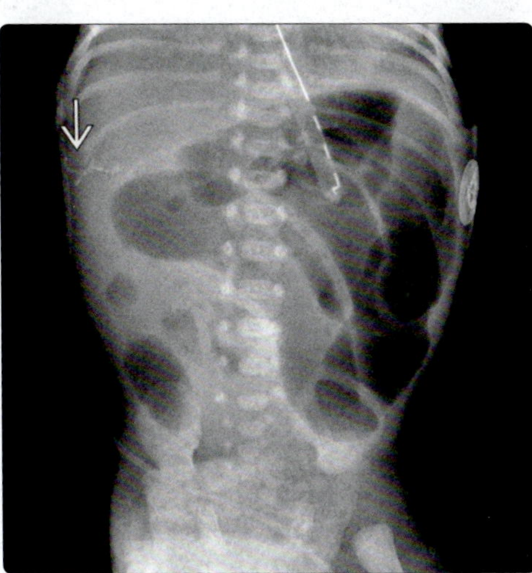

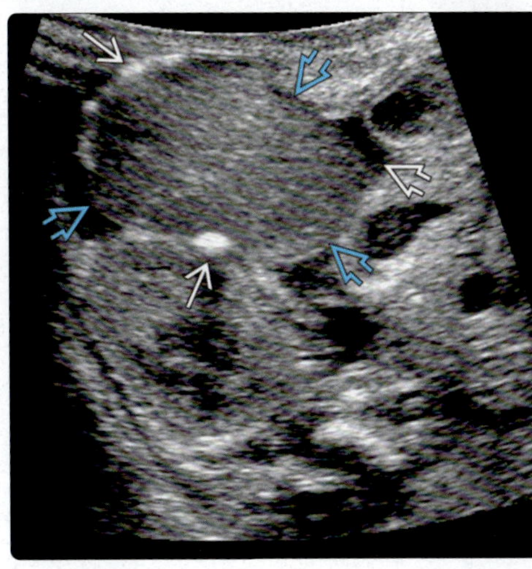

(Left) *Newborn AP radiograph shows Ca^{2+} in the right upper quadrant (RUQ) ➡, suggesting meconium peritonitis, + a distal bowel obstruction. Both parents were CF gene carriers.* **(Right)** *Transverse US shows a round fluid collection in the RUQ ➡ with punctate echogenic foci in the wall ➡, likely corresponding to the radiographic Ca^{2+}. There is also a small amount of ascites ➡. The WSCE (not shown) confirmed a microcolon with impacted TI pellets, giving a diagnosis of complicated MI.*

KEY FACTS

TERMINOLOGY

- Neonatal small left colon (NSLC): Transient functional colonic obstruction of newborn
  - Retained colonic plugs of normal meconium are secondary to functional obstruction in this scenario (not underlying cause of mechanical obstruction)
- Debate if meconium plug syndrome (MPS) is same as NSLC

IMAGING

- Numerous dilated loops of bowel on newborn radiograph
  - Difficult to radiographically distinguish small vs. large bowel in neonate
- Water-soluble contrast enema (WSCE)
  - Normal rectosigmoid ratio
  - Small-caliber distal colon (sigmoid + descending segments) up to splenic flexure with abrupt or gradual transition to normal/mildly dilated transverse colon
  - Scattered meconium filling defects in colon
    - May be proximal or distal to level of caliber change

TOP DIFFERENTIAL DIAGNOSES

- Hirschsprung disease (HD)
- Ileal atresia
- Meconium ileus
- Anorectal malformation
- Ileus secondary to midgut volvulus or necrotizing enterocolitis

PATHOLOGY

- ↑ incidence in premature infants & infants of diabetic mothers or mothers who received magnesium sulfate

CLINICAL ISSUES

- Presents with abdominal distention, delayed passage of meconium, emesis
- Temporary phenomenon: Usually resolves within several days (hastened by enemas or rectal stimulation)
- Rectal biopsy to exclude HD if symptoms persist; some advocate biopsy for all as HD is ultimately found in 13-38%

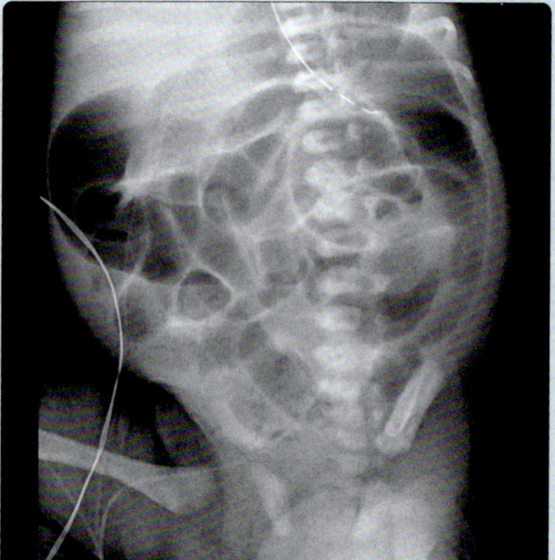

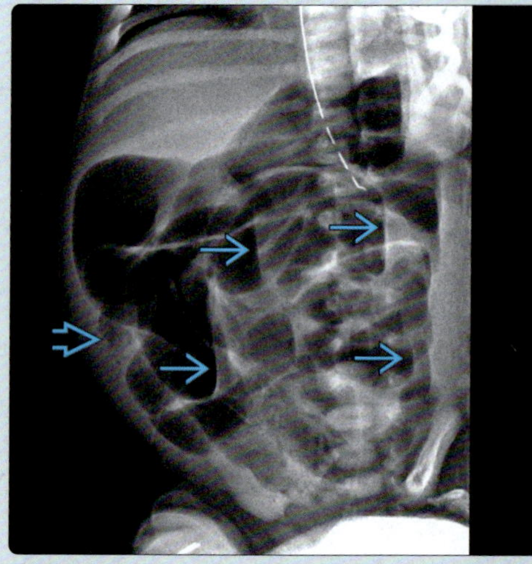

(Left) *AP radiograph in a newborn with failure to pass meconium, abdominal distention, & emesis shows numerous dilated bowel loops throughout the abdomen, typical of a distal (or low) neonatal intestinal obstruction.* **(Right)** *Left side-down decubitus radiograph obtained simultaneously shows diffuse dilation of bowel with numerous air-fluid levels ➡, consistent with a distal obstruction. There is no free air. A few bubbly lucencies ➡ are likely due to gas intermixed with retained meconium.*

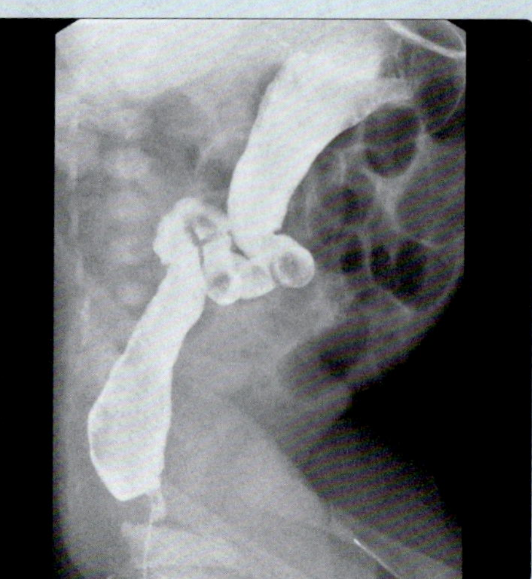

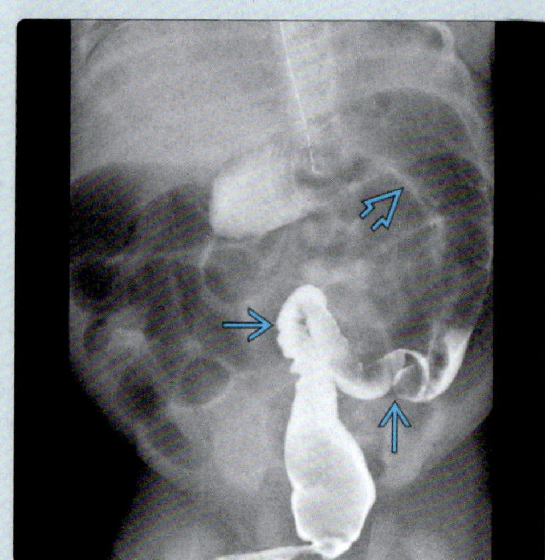

(Left) *Lateral water-soluble contrast enema (WSCE) in the same patient shows a normal rectosigmoid ratio (> 1) with a small-caliber sigmoid & tapered descending colonic segments.* **(Right)** *Supine frontal WSCE in the same patient shows gradual transition from the small-caliber sigmoid colon ➡ to a more normal colonic caliber near the splenic flexure ➡. This is a typical appearance for neonatal small left colon. A rectal biopsy ruled out Hirschsprung disease.*

TERMINOLOGY

Abbreviations

- Neonatal small left colon (NSLC)

Synonyms

- Meconium plug syndrome (MPS)
- Functional immaturity of colon

Definitions

- Transient functional obstruction of newborn colon
  - Retained colonic meconium/plug is likely secondary finding (not primary cause of mechanical obstruction)
- Debate exists if MPS & NSLC are same entity

IMAGING

Radiographic Findings

- Multiple dilated loops of bowel in newborn (i.e., neonatal distal bowel obstruction)
  - Note that dilated large & small bowel loops (from any cause) cannot be reliably differentiated in neonates by morphology or size

Fluoroscopic Findings

- Contrast enema
  - Rectosigmoid ratio is normal (> 1)
    - Rectum is of relatively normal caliber
  - Small-caliber distal colon (sigmoid & descending segments) up to splenic flexure
  - Abrupt or gradual transition to normal/mildly dilated proximal colon
  - Multiple filling defects of normal meconium may be scattered throughout colon & are often present in narrowed segment
    - May be displaced proximally during enema
  - Meconium plugs frequently pass during/after enema: Enema is often therapeutic

DIFFERENTIAL DIAGNOSIS

Hirschsprung Disease

- Distal aganglionic segment is small in caliber up to transition zone
  - Rectal caliber is typically smaller than sigmoid ± serrated mucosa/irregular contractions
  - Long-segment Hirschsprung disease (HD) with splenic flexure transition zone may mimic functional immaturity

Ileal Atresia

- Microcolon
- Contrast refluxed into ileum stops abruptly at atresia
- Cannot opacify proximal dilated small bowel

Meconium Ileus

- Microcolon
- Enema contrast outlines obstructive meconium pellets in distal ileum
- Contrast may or may not reach dilated small bowel proximal to impacted meconium
- Most have cystic fibrosis (CF)

Anorectal Malformation

- Distal obstruction with no normal anus present

Colonic Atresia

- Distal obstruction with disproportionately dilated loop
- Microcolon to level of atresia on enema

Midgut Volvulus

- Bowel loops may be diffusely dilated due to ischemic ileus in ill neonate
- Upper GI is study of choice in ill neonate with bilious emesis

PATHOLOGY

General Features

- Etiology
  - Unclear; probably due to immature ganglion cells or hormonal receptors resulting in transient functional obstruction of colon
  - ↑ incidence with
    - Infants of diabetic mothers (40-50% of MPS)
    - Infants of mothers who receive magnesium sulfate
    - Premature infants
  - Plugs of normal meconium do not cause obstruction in this diagnosis (unlike abnormal meconium in CF)

CLINICAL ISSUES

Presentation

- Most common signs/symptoms
  - Abdominal distention
  - Delayed passage of meconium (> 24-48 hours)
  - Emesis

Natural History & Prognosis

- Temporary phenomenon: Usually resolves within few days
- Excellent prognosis, though HD is ultimately found in 13-38%

Treatment

- Condition resolves over time, hastened by rectal stimulation
  - Often resolves after diagnostic contrast enema
- Suction rectal biopsy to exclude HD if symptoms persist
  - Some advocate immediate biopsy regardless of symptom resolution
  - Wide variation exists in surgical practice; higher likelihood of biopsy with
    - Neonatal intestinal perforation
    - Delayed passage of meconium > 48 hours
  - Up to 25% with both HD & MPS do not get early biopsy, which may delay appropriate management

SELECTED REFERENCES

1. Baad M et al: Diagnostic performance and role of the contrast enema for low intestinal obstruction in neonates. Pediatr Surg Int. 36(9):1093-101, 2020
2. Buonpane C et al: Should we look for Hirschsprung disease in all children with meconium plug syndrome? J Pediatr Surg. 54(6):1164-7, 2019
3. Wood K et al: Neonatal small left colon syndrome (NSLCS): rare but important complication in an infant of diabetic mother. BMJ Case Rep. 2018, 2018
4. Cuenca AG et al: "Pulling the plug"--management of meconium plug syndrome in neonates. J Surg Res. 175(2):e43-6, 2012
5. Ellis H et al: Neonatal small left colon syndrome in the offspring of diabetic mothers-an analysis of 105 children. J Pediatr Surg. 44(12):2343-6, 2009
6. Keckler SJ et al: Current significance of meconium plug syndrome. J Pediatr Surg. 43(5):896-8, 2008

Hirschsprung Disease

KEY FACTS

TERMINOLOGY

- Hirschsprung disease (HD): Congenital anomaly of enteric nervous system
  - Absence of ganglion cells in intestinal myenteric & submucosal plexus
  - Aganglionic segment extends retrograde from anus for variable length with gradual transition to normal innervation

IMAGING

- Newborn radiograph: Numerous loops of dilated bowel
- Radiograph beyond neonatal period: Large stool burden with variable colonic dilation
- Contrast enema is especially useful in neonate with distal bowel obstruction; findings suggestive of HD include
  - Rectosigmoid ratio < 1
  - Transition zone from small distal colon to dilated proximal colon
  - Mucosal irregularity

TOP DIFFERENTIAL DIAGNOSES

- Neonatal small left colon (meconium plug syndrome)
- Ileal atresia
- Meconium ileus
- Anorectal malformation
- Milk allergy colitis

CLINICAL ISSUES

- Neonate: Failure to pass meconium, abdominal distention, bilious emesis, enterocolitis
- Older child: Constipation since birth, enterocolitis
- Diagnosis is made by rectal biopsy
- Treatment: Resect affected colon & pull-through of normal bowel to anus

DIAGNOSTIC CHECKLIST

- Contrast enema cannot rule out HD (but can suggest HD or other diagnoses)
- Frank colitis in term newborn → HD until proven otherwise

(Left) *AP radiograph in a 2-day-old with failure to pass meconium shows multiple dilated loops of bowel with no air seen in the rectum. One cannot differentiate small bowel (SB) from colonic loops on this exam. A contrast enema is required to elucidate the etiology of obstruction.* **(Right)** *Lateral view of a water-soluble contrast enema (WSCE) in the same patient shows a small-caliber rectum relative to the dilated sigmoid, suggesting short-segment Hirschsprung disease (HD). This was confirmed by rectal biopsy.*

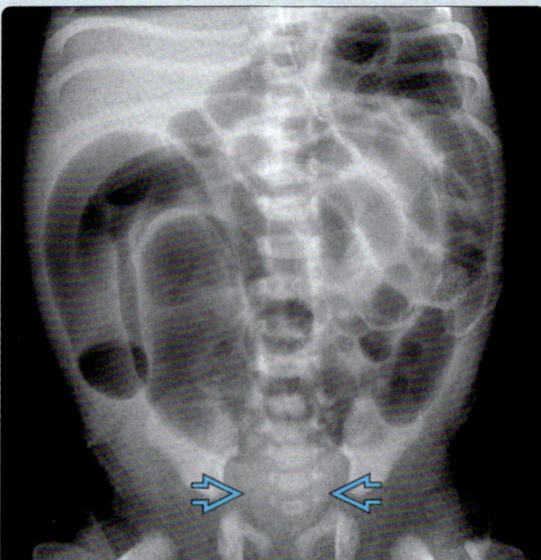

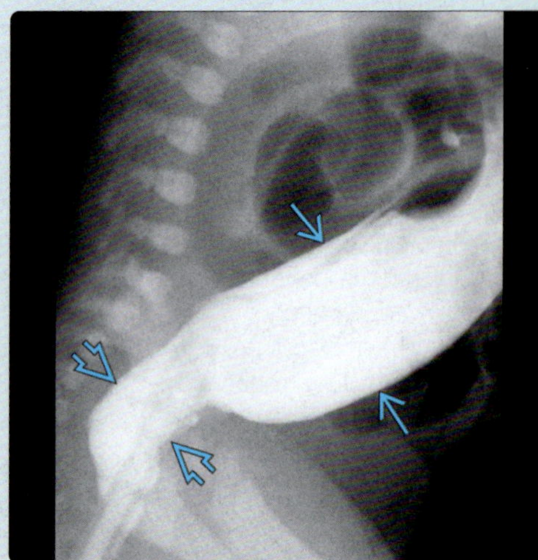

(Left) *AP radiograph in a newborn with bilious emesis shows a disproportionately dilated loop in the right abdomen distended by meconium intermixed with gas. The number of gas-filled loops overall suggests a distal obstruction.* **(Right)** *Supine WSCE in the same patient shows a narrowed sigmoid & descending colon with transition at the splenic flexure to a dilated & meconium-filled transverse & ascending colon. Note the mucosal irregularity or spasm in the left colon. Biopsy confirmed long-segment HD.*

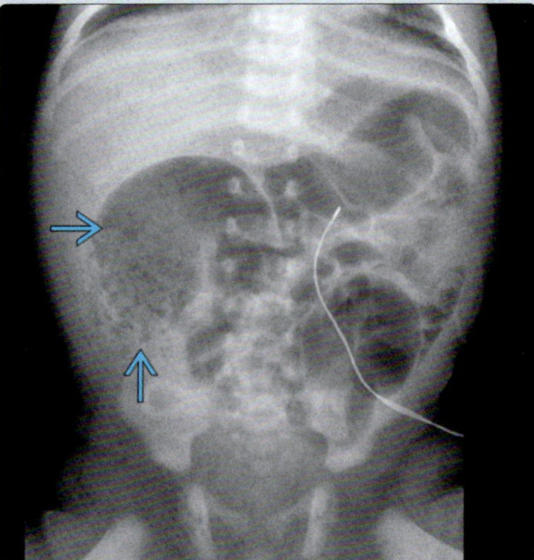

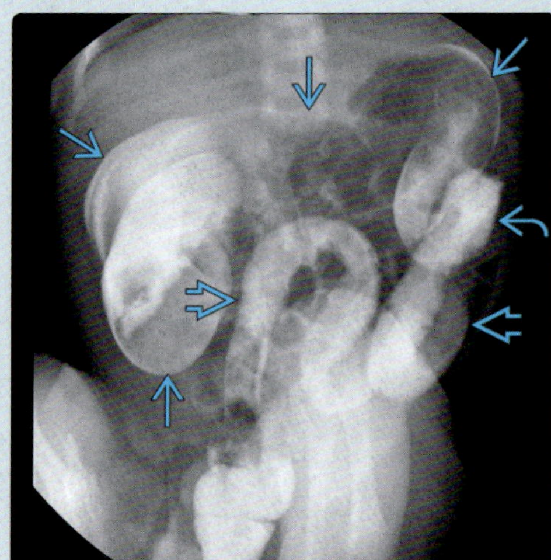

TERMINOLOGY

Synonyms

- Colonic aganglionosis

Definitions

- Hirschsprung disease (HD): Congenital anomaly of enteric nervous system
  - Absence of ganglion cells in myenteric & submucosal plexus of intestine
    - Lack of muscle relaxation → functional bowel obstruction
  - Aganglionic segment extends retrograde from anus for variable length with gradual transition to innervated proximal colon
    - Rectosigmoid: Short-segment HD (70-80%)
    - Proximal to rectosigmoid: Long-segment HD (15-25%)
    - Entire colon: Total colonic HD (4-13%)
    - Colon & small bowel (SB): Total intestinal HD (very rare)
    - Just above anorectal verge: Ultrashort-segment HD (very rare)

IMAGING

General Features

- Best diagnostic clue
  - Rectosigmoid (R/S) ratio < 1 on contrast enema
    - Requires well-distended lateral view from rectum to splenic flexure
- Morphology
  - Small caliber of aganglionic distal colon
  - Dilation of innervated proximal colon above transition

Radiographic Findings

- In newborn
  - Numerous dilated bowel loops suggesting distal obstruction
  - ± irregular, thickened bowel wall with enterocolitis
    - Rarely pneumatosis
  - Rarely intraluminal ileal Ca^{2+} in total colonic HD
- Outside neonatal period
  - Large stool burden with varying degrees of dilation
  - Paucity of gas with thick colonic wall: Question enterocolitis
  - Rarely free air from perforation in 1st year of life
    - Perforation usually at proximal colon or appendix

Fluoroscopic Findings

- Contrast enema
  - Short- or long-segment HD
    - R/S ratio is classically < 1 (but not always)
    - Transition zone: Level at which small distal colon becomes dilated proximally
    - ± sawtooth pattern of distal mucosa (spasm)
    - ± irregular mucosa/thickened wall of enterocolitis
      - Cobblestone appearance
    - Delayed (> 24-48 hours) evacuation of contrast
    - Near normal enema in ultrashort-segment HD
  - Total colonic HD
    - May appear normal vs. microcolon vs. shortened length with round flexures (question mark- or comma-shaped)
    - Rectum is often same caliber as rest of colon: R/S ratio ≤ 1
    - Ileocecal reflux is typically seen
      - Sensitivity/specificity is quite variable in isolation
    - SB proximal to colon may be dilated

Imaging Recommendations

- Best imaging tool
  - Water-soluble contrast enema (WSCE)
- Protocol advice
  - With clinical + radiographic suspicion for neonatal distal bowel obstruction → WSCE
    - Low osmolality water-soluble contrast
    - Lateral & AP views of maximally distended rectum up to splenic flexure on early images
      - Compare rectum to sigmoid + more proximal colon
      - Normal R/S ratio is > 1
    - WSCE is stopped once transition zone is reached
    - If WSCE is normal, consider upper GI to exclude midgut volvulus (MGV), as ischemic ileus can mimic obstruction

DIFFERENTIAL DIAGNOSIS

Neonatal Distal Intestinal Obstruction With Small Distal Colon

- Neonatal small left colon (meconium plug syndrome)
  - Nonpathologic transient functional obstruction
  - WSCE: R/S ratio is usually > 1 with transition at splenic flexure
  - ± rectal biopsy to exclude long-segment HD
- Colonic atresia
  - WSCE: Blind-ending, small-caliber distal colon
  - Dilated, air-filled proximal colon (larger as compared to dilated SB)

Neonatal Distal Intestinal Obstruction With Microcolon

- Ileal atresia
  - WSCE: Blind end of contrast column in ileum
- Meconium ileus
  - WSCE: Contrast outlines meconium pellets obstructing terminal ileum
- Megacystis microcolon intestinal hypoperistalsis
  - WSCE: Tiniest microcolon
  - Dilated, floppy bladder; most common in females

Neonatal Distal Intestinal Obstruction With Normal Colon

- Omphalomesenteric duct remnant
  - Various forms: Fibrous band, Meckel diverticulum
  - WSCE: May see medialization or beaking of cecum
- Inguinal hernia
  - May visualize gas in inguinal canal or scrotum
- MGV
  - Ischemic ileus in ill neonate mimics distal obstruction
  - Consider upper GI vs. ultrasound 1st in ill neonate with bilious emesis

- Necrotizing enterocolitis
  - In prematurity, most common etiology by far
  - Ischemic ileus mimics distal obstruction
  - Not typical in 1st few days after birth

Enterocolitis in Infant

- Milk allergy colitis
  - 1st weeks of life, usually with formula feeds
  - WSCE: R/S ratio < 1 ± colitis
  - Rectal biopsy: Eosinophils, normal ganglion cells

Intraluminal Calcifications

- Anorectal malformation
- Multiple intestinal atresias
- Total colonic HD

PATHOLOGY

General Features

- Etiology
  - Precise mechanism is unknown for sure
    - Defect in 1st-trimester migration of enteric ganglia
    - Normal migration but abnormal survival of ganglia
- Genetics
  - Most cases are sporadic
  - Numerous genetic mutations found
  - Familial HD in 8-10%
- Associated abnormalities
  - 5-32% of HD overall
    - Down syndrome (7-15%)
    - Neurocristopathy syndromes
    - Congenital central hypoventilation ("Ondine curse")
    - Colonic atresia
    - Other isolated anomalies

Microscopic Features

- Diagnosis by rectal biopsy
  - Suction biopsy: Bedside, less reliable
  - Full-thickness biopsy: In operating room, definitive
- Absent ganglia in myenteric & submucosal plexus
- Hypertrophic nerve fibers (acetylcholinesterase positive)
- Disease is most commonly contiguous without skip areas
  - Reported cases of segmental HD
    - May lead to incorrect diagnosis or inadequate resection/failed pull-through
- Radiologic-pathologic correlation of transition zone site
  - Short-segment (or low transition zone) HD: 75%
  - Long-segment (or high transition zone) HD: 25%

CLINICAL ISSUES

Presentation

- Most common signs/symptoms
  - Failure to pass meconium in first 24-48 hours of life (60-90%)
  - Abdominal distention (63-91%)
  - Bilious vomiting (19-37%)
  - Enterocolitis (5-44%)

Demographics

- 90% are diagnosed in newborn period
- 10% are diagnosed later, rarely adolescent or adult
- M > F = 4:1 (long-segment & total colonic HD → 1:1)

Natural History & Prognosis

- Untreated HD may lead to constipation, enterocolitis, toxic megacolon, sepsis, death
- Treated: Up to 40% have chronic soiling, constipation
  - Must assess for failure of pull-through procedure
  - Poorer outcome: Down syndrome, total colonic HD

Treatment

- Resection of aganglionic colon
- Pull-through of normal bowel to anus
  - Swenson, Soave, Duhamel procedures are most common
  - Single-stage transanal endorectal pull-through ± laparoscopy is now common
- Complications
  - Early: Leak, infection, obstruction
  - Late: Bowel adhesion/obstruction, stricture, enterocolitis, constipation, incontinence
- Common etiologies for failed pull-through
  - Soave cuff, Duhamel pouch, ischemic stricture, residual HD, twisted pull-through

DIAGNOSTIC CHECKLIST

Consider

- Contrast enema cannot rule out HD
  - With clinical suspicion, must biopsy
- Contrast enema is most useful in assessing distal obstruction in neonates
  - Only up to 80% sensitive for HD in newborns

Image Interpretation Pearls

- R/S ratio < 1 & transition zone on WSCE → HD
- Frank colitis in term newborn → HD until proven otherwise

SELECTED REFERENCES

1. Baad M et al: Diagnostic performance and role of the contrast enema for low intestinal obstruction in neonates. Pediatr Surg Int. 36(9):1093-101, 2020
2. Kapur RP et al: Postoperative pullthrough obstruction in Hirschsprung disease: etiologies and diagnosis. Pediatr Dev Pathol. 23(1):40-59, 2020
3. Vlok SSC et al: Accuracy of colonic mucosal patterns at contrast enema for diagnosis of Hirschsprung disease. Pediatr Radiol. 50(6):810-6, 2020
4. Yan J et al: Barium enema findings in total colonic aganglionosis: a single-center, retrospective study. BMC Pediatr. 20(1):499, 2020
5. Lourenção PI TA et al: Barium enema revisited in the workup for the diagnosis of Hirschsprung's disease. J Pediatr Gastroenterol Nutr. 68(4):e62-6, 2019
6. Coe A et al: Distal rectal skip-segment Hirschsprung disease and the potential for false-negative diagnosis. Pediatr Dev Pathol. 19(2):123-31, 2016
7. Frongia G et al: Contrast enema for Hirschsprung disease investigation: diagnostic accuracy and validity for subsequent diagnostic and surgical planning. Eur J Pediatr Surg. 26(2):207-14, 2016
8. Gosain A: Established and emerging concepts in Hirschsprung's-associated enterocolitis. Pediatr Surg Int. 32(4):313-20, 2016
9. Muise ED et al: A comparison of suction and full-thickness rectal biopsy in children. J Surg Res. 201(1):149-55, 2016
10. Putnam LR et al: The utility of the contrast enema in neonates with suspected Hirschsprung disease. J Pediatr Surg. 50(6):963-6, 2015
11. Garrett KM et al: Contrast enema findings in patients presenting with poor functional outcome after primary repair for Hirschsprung disease. Pediatr Radiol. 42(9):1099-106, 2012
12. Jamieson DH et al: Does the transition zone reliably delineate aganglionic bowel in Hirschsprung's disease? Pediatr Radiol. 34(10):811-5, 2004

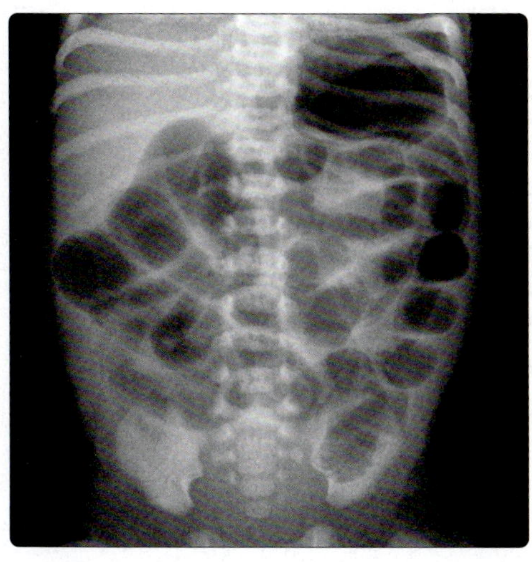

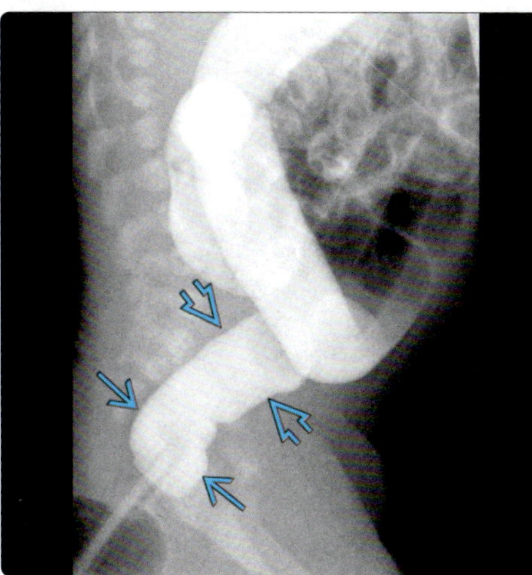

(Left) *AP radiograph of a 2-day-old with abdominal distention & failure to pass meconium shows multiple air-filled bowel loops diffusely, suggesting a distal intestinal obstruction. The next study should be a WSCE to elucidate the etiology of this obstruction.* **(Right)** *Lateral view of a WSCE in the same patient shows the rectum ➔ to be slightly smaller in caliber as compared to sigmoid ➔ & proximal colon without an abrupt transition. However, this appearance raised suspicion for HD, & biopsy was confirmatory.*

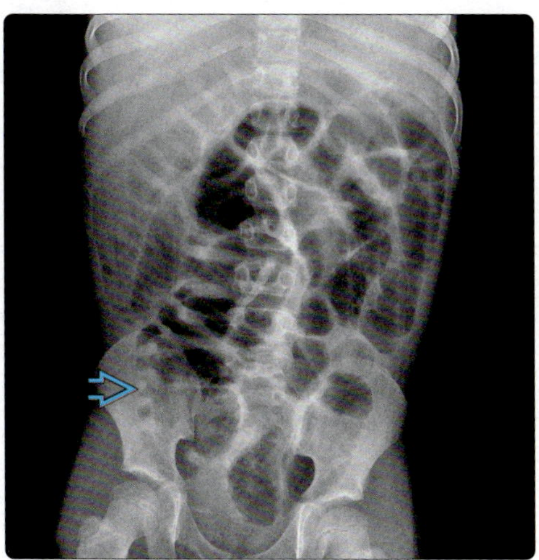

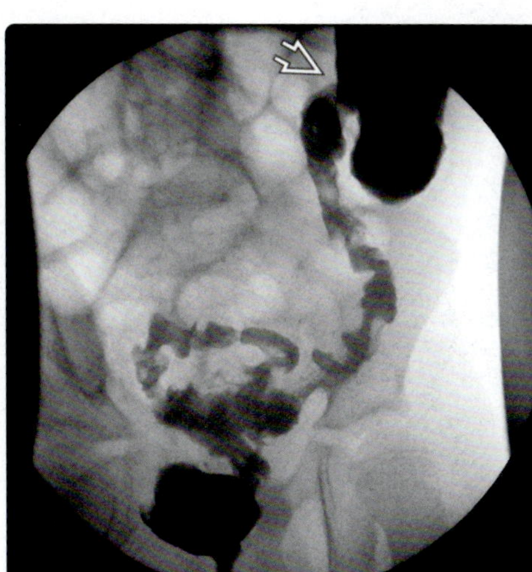

(Left) *AP radiograph in an 8-year-old with a long history of constipation & multiple episodes of colitis shows little stool after a clean out. There are dilated colonic & SB loops with possible wall thickening ➔.* **(Right)** *Frontal supine WSCE in the same patient shows a fairly distended distal rectum. However, the colon was narrow & spastic almost to the splenic flexure ➔, suggesting long-segment HD, which was confirmed at biopsy.*

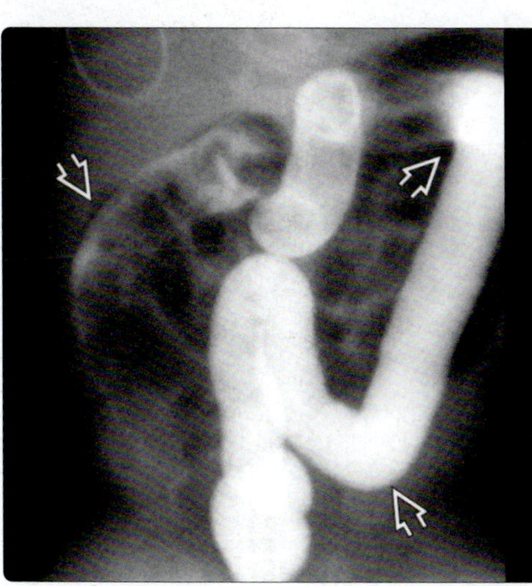

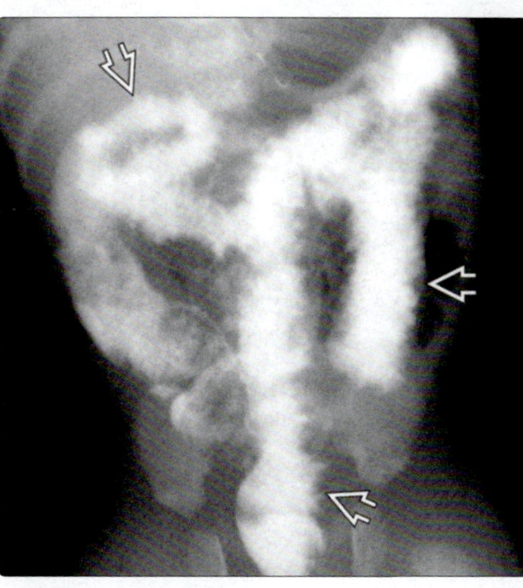

(Left) *Frontal supine WSCE in a newborn with total colonic HD shows a mildly small-caliber colon, which is fairly uniform throughout. The course of the colon is shortened with rounding of the flexures ➔.* **(Right)** *Frontal supine WSCE in a newborn with bilious emesis shows severe mucosal irregularity ➔ throughout most of the colon, suggesting colitis in HD. Biopsies showed total intestinal aganglionosis.*

KEY FACTS

IMAGING

- Neonatal clinical exam + AP abdominal radiograph
  - Many dilated bowel loops, ± rectal gas, ± bowel Ca^{2+}
  - Prone XTL view if fistula is not clinically evident (~ 5%)
- Renal, spine US; pelvic US for females with cloaca
  - Urgent drainage of hydrocolpos to prevent rupture & ureteral obstruction
- Evaluate additional anomalies (VACTERL or syndromes)
- Delayed distal colostogram for classification of ARM & preop planning: Fistula in ~ 95% of males
  - Perfect lateral view (superimposed femoral heads)
  - If bladder fills, fill until voiding; image distal colonic segment, bladder, urethra
- ± pelvic MR prior to, during, &/or after operative repair

TOP DIFFERENTIAL DIAGNOSES

- Neonatal distal bowel obstruction (with normal anus)
  - Meconium plug syndrome, Hirschsprung disease, meconium ileus, jejunoileal atresia
- Neonatal intraluminal abdominal Ca^{2+}
  - Total colonic Hirschsprung, multiple intestinal atresia

PATHOLOGY

- Imperforate anus
  - Rectoperineal fistula (male or female)
  - Rectovestibular fistula: 25% of female ARMs
  - Rectourethral fistula: 50% of male ARMs
  - Rectobladder neck fistula: 10% of male ARMs
  - No fistula: 5% of ARMs (male or female)
  - Cloacal malformation: Only females
- Rectal atresia or stenosis: 1% of ARMs

CLINICAL ISSUES

- Goals: Maximize continence of feces & urine, sexual function
- Most ARMs require
  - Diverting colostomy within days of birth
  - PSARP for definitive repair months later

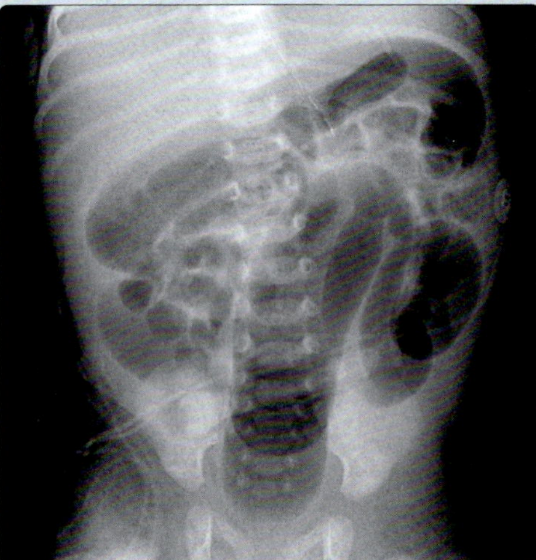

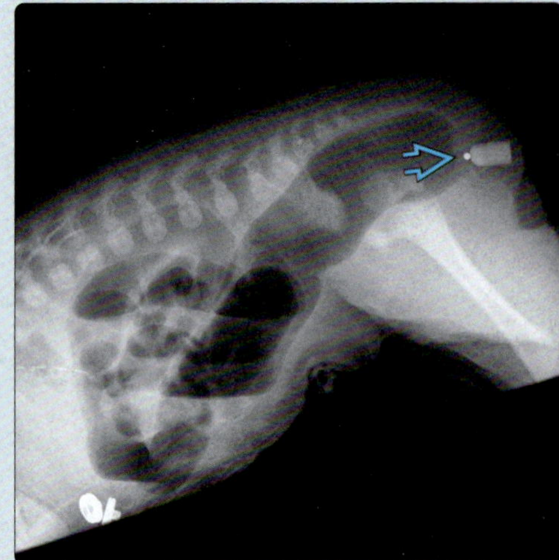

(Left) *AP radiograph in a newborn (24-hours-old) boy with imperforate anus & no clinical signs of a fistula (no meconium per urethra or perineum) shows multiple dilated bowel loops to the pelvis with a dilated rectum.* **(Right)** *Prone cross-table lateral view with a BB on the anus in the same patient shows the rectal pouch ➡ adjacent to the anus, a type of low anorectal malformation (ARM) unlikely to have a rectourinary fistula that can be repaired as a neonate without colostomy.*

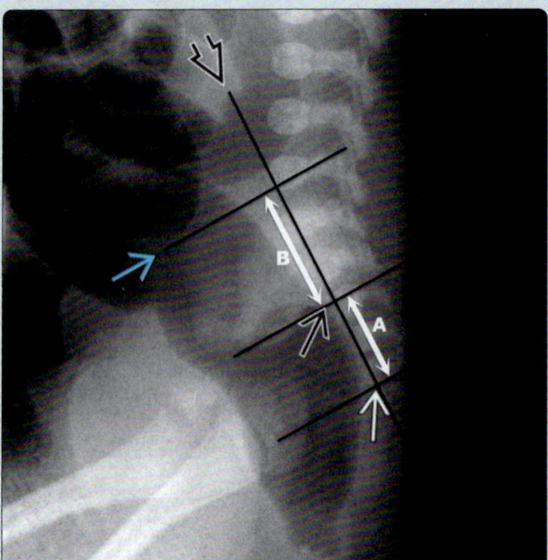

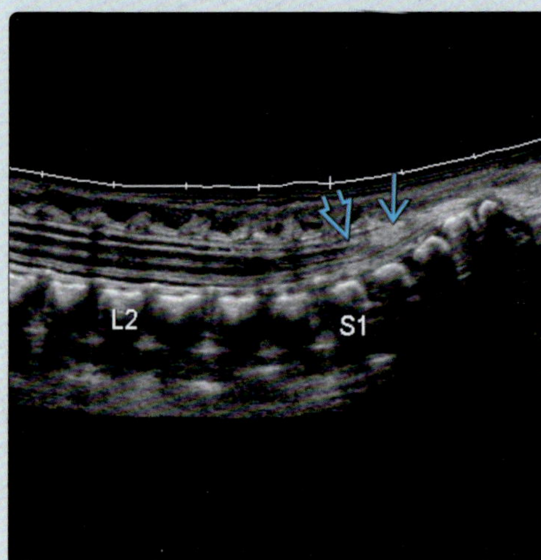

(Left) *Lateral radiograph in the same patient was taken to calculate the sacral ratio (A/B). The axis is drawn along the sacrum ➡, then lines are drawn perpendicular to the sacral axis at the iliac crest ➡, greater sciatic notch ➡, & tip of the ossified sacrum/coccyx ➡.* **(Right)** *Spinal US in a 2-day-old with a history of imperforate anus who had meconium per the urethra (clinical evidence of a rectourinary fistula) shows a low conus at the S1 level ➡ with an echogenic terminus ➡, which may represent a lipoma or lipomyelocele.*

TERMINOLOGY

Synonyms

- Imperforate anus

Definitions

- Anorectal malformation (ARM): Spectrum of congenital anomalies related to abnormal development of anorectal canal
- Diagnosis of ARM is made by clinical exam
- Imaging is used to identify associated anomalies, plan operations, & evaluate postoperative complications
- Evolution of ARM classification: Traditionally as high, intermediate, or low (relative to pubococcygeal line)
  - Current (Peña or Krickenbeck): By specific malformation with therapeutic & prognostic implications
- Cloaca: Subtype of ARM in girls; rectum, vagina, & bladder converge into common channel → single perineal orifice
- Posterior sagittal anorectoplasty (PSARP): Definitive surgical reconstruction for most ARMs

IMAGING

General Features

- Best diagnostic clue
  - Multiple dilated bowel loops in newborn without normal external anus
- Morphology
  - Rectal opening outside anal sphincter on perineum vs. no rectal opening on perineum

Radiographic Findings

- Radiography
  - Multiple dilated bowel loops of distal obstruction in newborn
  - Ca^{2+} → enteroliths (intraluminal Ca^{2+})
    - Mixing of urine & meconium via rectourinary fistula
  - Prone cross-table lateral (XTL) view of abdomen > 24-hours-old → measure pouch to anus distance
    - In ~ 5% of ARMs, fistula is **not** clinically apparent to help direct operative management
    - Rectal pouch close to anal region → neonatal repair; if not → diverting colostomy/delayed repair
  - ± hemisacrum/scimitar sacrum (different from truncated sacrum): Defect represents presacral mass
    - Teratoma, anterior meningocele, mixed lesion
  - Sacral ratio predicts potential for fecal continence; > 0.6 = normal; < 0.4 = ↓ probability of continence
  - ± esophageal atresia (EA), tracheoesophageal fistula (TEF), congenital heart disease
  - ± vertebral or radial ray anomalies

Fluoroscopic Findings

- Voiding cystourethrogram
  - Variable findings: Normal; vesicoureteral reflux (VUR); ± bladder thickening, trabecula, neurogenic bladder; fistula from bladder neck or urethra → rectum in males, reflux from urethra to vagina &/or rectum in female cloaca
- Fistulagram
  - a.k.a. augmented pressure distal colostogram using Foley catheter
    - Water-soluble contrast injection of mucous fistula
  - To be performed several weeks to months after colostomy, prior to definitive repair
    - Must opacify rectal pouch & rectourinary fistula
  - Lateral view (superimposed femoral heads) showing
    - Distal colonic segment length, fistula to bladder or urethra in boys, common channel in girls
      - Most boys (95%) have rectourinary fistula (except Down syndrome: 95% have **no** fistula)
      - **Adequate distention is needed to see fistula**
      - If bladder fills, fill until voiding; image distal colonic segment, bladder, urethra
    - Document relationship of rectal pouch to sacrum & anal sphincter (marked by BB)
    - Is presacral mass displacing rectal wall?
- ± cloacagram in females (usually performed prior to definitive repair)
  - Contrast injection of distal colostomy
  - Contrast into bladder &/or vagina via cloaca catheter
  - 3D imaging by rotational fluoroscopy, CT, or MR

MR Findings

- Prenatal: Absent T1-bright meconium posterior/inferior to bladder > 20-weeks gestation
- Post natal
  - Prerepair pelvic MR: Anal sphincter + pelvic floor musculature, rectal pouch, presacral mass, other GU anomalies
  - Intraoperative pelvic MR: Guide rectum through sphincter → novel approach
  - Postrepair pelvic MR (poor functional outcome): Look for misplaced rectum, entrapped fat, posterior urethral diverticulum
- Spine MR: Tethered cord, spinal dysraphism, sacral agenesis/dysgenesis

Ultrasonographic Findings

- Grayscale ultrasound
  - Perineal ultrasound: Assess distance of rectal pouch → perineum; not reliable
  - Assess neonate for renal + spine anomalies
  - Assess for hydrocolpos in newborn cloaca → if positive, urgent drainage is required to relieve secondary bladder/ureteral obstruction

Imaging Recommendations

- Best imaging tool
  - Neonate: Clinical exam + AP & prone XTL radiographs; renal, spine, & pelvic ultrasound (especially pelvis in cloaca)
  - Infant after colostomy: Distal colostogram for operative planning

DIFFERENTIAL DIAGNOSIS

Neonatal Distal Bowel Obstruction (Normal Anus)

- Small left colon/meconium plug syndrome
- Hirschsprung disease
- Meconium ileus
- Jejunoileal atresia

Abdominal Ca^{2+} in Newborn

- Intraluminal Ca^{2+}: ARM, total colonic Hirschsprung disease, multiple intestinal atresia

- Meconium peritonitis: Peritoneal Ca^{2+} due to in utero bowel perforation
- Visceral: TORCH, prior hemorrhage
- Mass: Teratoma, neuroblastoma, congenital hemangioma
- Vascular: Prior thrombosis

PATHOLOGY

General Features

- Etiology
  - Abnormal separation of GU system from hindgut
- Genetics
  - No responsible gene identified; ↑ risk if sibling has ARM
  - Syndromic cases
    - Trisomy 21 (Down), Currarino (ARM, sacral deformity, presacral mass), VACTERL, OEIS, caudal regression, Pallister-Hall, Townes-Brocks
- Associated abnormalities
  - GU (50% of ARMs): Solitary/horseshoe kidney, VUR, bicornuate/didelphys uterus, hydrocolpos (50% of cloacas), hemivaginas
  - Spine: Tethered cord (25% of ARM, ↑ with more complex ARM), myelomeningocele, sacral anomalies (most affected bony structure)
  - Cardiac: Tetralogy of Fallot, ventricular septal defect
  - GI: EA ± TEF, duodenal atresia, Hirschsprung disease

Gross Pathologic & Surgical Features

- Imperforate anus
  - Rectoperineal fistula (male or female) → **no** colostomy → PSARP as newborn
    - Rectum opens to small, stenotic orifice anterior to normal anal sphincter complex; normal sacrum, muscles, sphincter
  - Rectovestibular fistula: 25% of female ARMs → **no** colostomy → PSARP as newborn
    - Rectum opens between hymen & perineal skin; most patients have good sacrum, sphincter
  - Rectourethral fistula: 50% of male ARMs → divided colostomy
    - Fistula to bulbar urethra: Normal/near-normal sacrum, muscles → delayed PSARP
    - Fistula to prostatic urethra: ± deficient sacrum, muscles → delayed PSARP ± lap procedure
  - Rectobladder neck fistula: 10% of male ARMs → divided colostomy → PSARP + lap procedure
    - Only true supralevator malformation; poor sacrum, sphincter, flat bottom (poorly developed gluteal crease)
  - No fistula: 5% of all ARM patients (male or female) with normal chromosomes → divided colostomy → PSARP
    - Rectum is usually ≤ 2 cm deep to perineum (if rectum is very close to skin on XTL → ± PSARP as neonate)
    - Usually good sacrum, sphincter
    - Frequent in Down syndrome (95%)
  - Rectal atresia or stenosis: 1% of ARMs (male or female) → different operative technique → colostomy
    - Atresia between normal anus & rectum; normal sacrum & sphincter
- Cloaca: Female with single perineal orifice (genitalia are frequently ambiguous)
  - Common channel drains rectum, vagina, urethra
  - Hydrocolpos in up to 50%
    - May cause urinary obstruction at distal ureters → requires neonatal drainage
    - Undrained hydrocolpos → renal insufficiency, vaginal perforation, sepsis, even death
  - Common channel length
    - < 3 cm: Divided colostomy → delayed PSARP, good prognosis
    - > 3 cm: Divided colostomy → delayed PSARP + lap procedure, poorer prognosis (more complex malformation, more associated anomalies)
  - Urethral length predicts urinary continence after cloacal repair

CLINICAL ISSUES

Presentation

- Most common signs/symptoms
  - Absent/misplaced rectal opening, abdominal distention
- Other signs/symptoms
  - Meconium per vestibule, urethra, or abnormal perineal opening; flat bottom, poorly developed gluteal crease

Treatment

- Goals: Maximize continence of feces & urine, sexual function
- Most ARMs require diverting colostomy within days of birth, PSARP months later
  - + laparotomy/laparoscopy for bladder neck & some prostatic fistulas + long common channel cloaca
- New MR-guided repair, avoids dividing anal sphincter
- Prognosis depends on type of malformation, sacral ratio, spine anomalies, meticulous surgical technique
  - 75% of ARMs will have voluntary bowel movements
  - 25% of ARM patients suffer incontinence, bowel management enemas daily to keep clean

SELECTED REFERENCES

1. Canning DA: Re: Cloaca reconstruction: a new algorithm which considers the role of urethral length in determining surgical planning. J Urol. 204(6):1368, 2020
2. Jarboe M et al: Imaged-guided and muscle sparing laparoscopic anorectoplasty using real-time magnetic resonance imaging. Pediatr Surg Int. 36(10):1255-60, 2020
3. Hosokawa T et al: Ultrasound imaging of the anorectal malformation during the neonatal period: a comprehensive review. Jpn J Radiol. 36(10):581-91, 2018
4. Kraus SJ et al: Augmented-pressure distal colostogram: the most important diagnostic tool for planning definitive surgical repair of anorectal malformations in boys. Pediatr Radiol. 48(2):258-69, 2018
5. Bischoff A: The surgical treatment of cloaca. Semin Pediatr Surg. 25(2):102-7, 2016
6. Lee MY et al: Sonographic determination of type in a fetal imperforate anus. J Ultrasound Med. 35(6):1285-91, 2016
7. Peiro JL et al: Prenatal diagnosis of cloacal malformation. Semin Pediatr Surg. 25(2):71-5, 2016
8. Thomeer MG et al: High resolution MRI for preoperative work-up of neonates with an anorectal malformation: a direct comparison with distal pressure colostography/fistulography. Eur Radiol. 25(12):3472-9, 2015
9. Alves JC et al: Comparison of MR and fluoroscopic mucous fistulography in the pre-operative evaluation of infants with anorectal malformation: a pilot study. Pediatr Radiol. 43(8):958-63, 2013
10. Bischoff A et al: Update on the management of anorectal malformations. Pediatr Surg Int. 29(9):899-904, 2013
11. Podberesky DJ et al: Magnetic resonance imaging of anorectal malformations. Magn Reson Imaging Clin N Am. 21(4):791-812, 2013

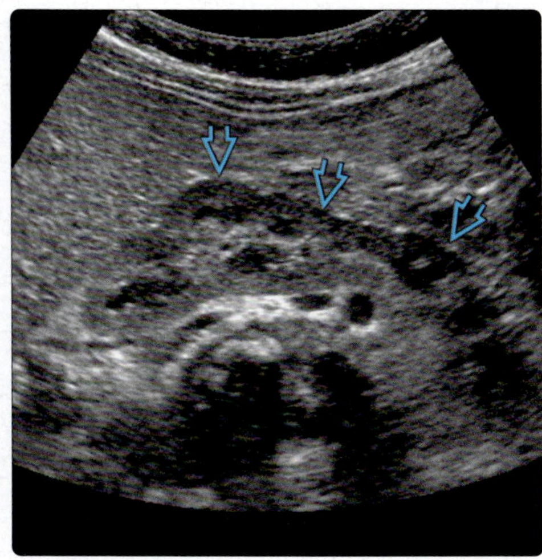

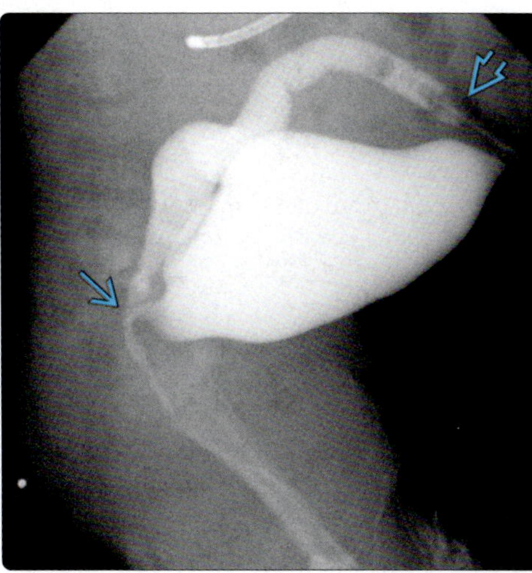

(Left) *Transverse US in a 3-day-old boy with imperforate anus shows renal tissue ➡ crossing anterior to the spine & great vessels, consistent with a horseshoe kidney.* **(Right)** *Colostogram in 3-month-old boy with an ARM shows a Foley balloon ➡ inflated in the distal colonic segment. Contrast injection shows a rectoprostatic urethral fistula ➡ located anterior to the spine, which will require laparoscopy as well as a posterior sagittal anorectoplasty (PSARP).*

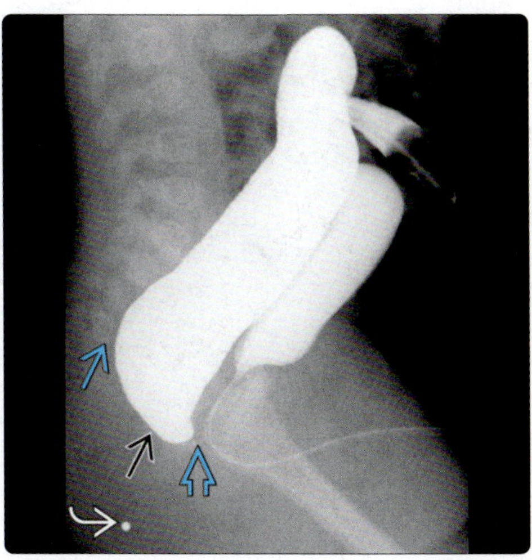

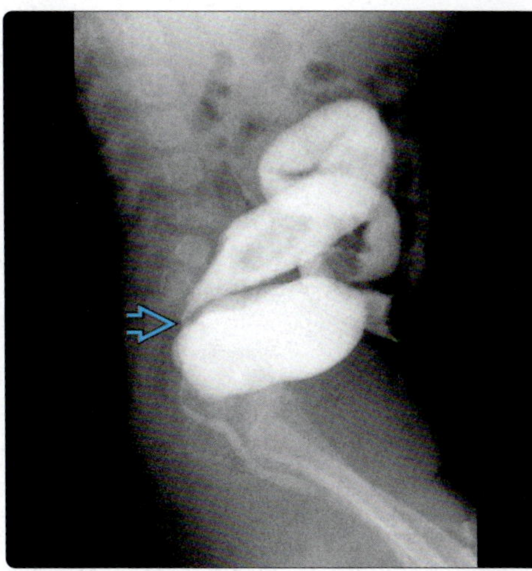

(Left) *Colostogram in a 3-month-old boy with an ARM shows a rectobulbar urethral fistula ➡ with a rectal pouch ➡ well below the tip of spine ➡. The distal colonic segment is adequate in length to bring the pouch to the anal region ➡ by a PSARP.* **(Right)** *Colostogram in a 2-month-old with an ARM & poorly developed gluteal crease shows a rectobladder neck fistula ➡. The rectal pouch lies above the spine tip at S3 & will only be reached by a laparoscopy or open abdominal approach prior to PSARP.*

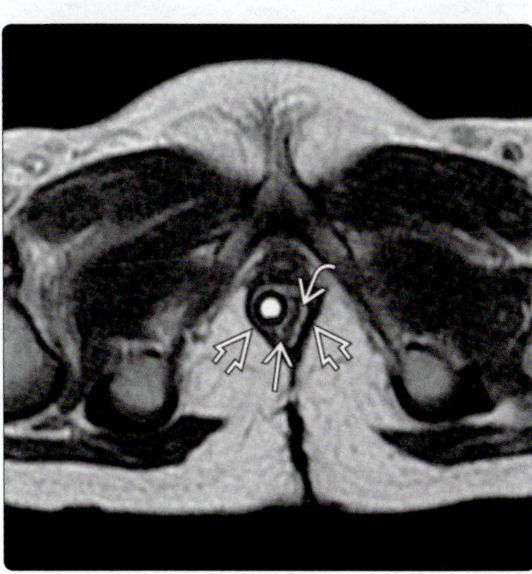

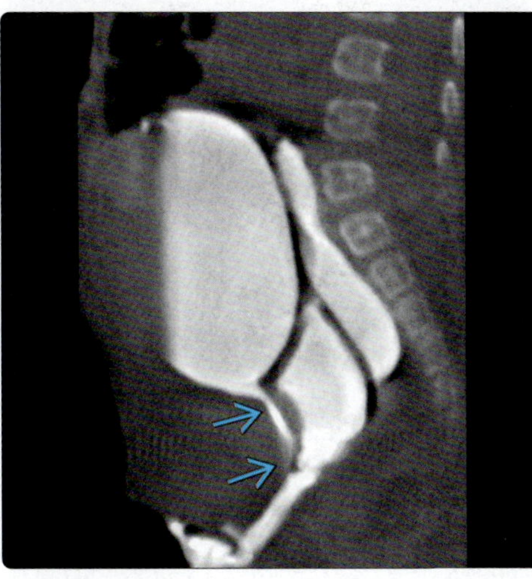

(Left) *Axial T2 MR in a repaired ARM patient shows asymmetric positioning of the rectum ➡ (containing a T2-bright catheter) within the asymmetric sphincter complex ➡. Fat ➡ is seen between the left rectal wall & sphincter muscle.* **(Right)** *Rotational fluoroscopy with 3D reconstruction was used to make this lateral view during a cloacagram in a 5-month-old girl with a history of cloaca. The urethra ➡ length, amongst other criteria, has recently been found to correlate with the potential for urinary continence.*

KEY FACTS

TERMINOLOGY

- Meconium peritonitis (MP): Chemical peritonitis from in utero bowel perforation with leakage of sterile meconium & digestive enzymes
- Meconium cyst: Meconium + fluid contained by fibrous membranes in setting of MP
- Meconium pseudocyst: Meconium + fluid contained by membranes partly derived from muscular layer of intestine

IMAGING

- Best diagnostic clue
  - Newborn abdominal radiograph showing linear, curvilinear, or punctate Ca^{2+} on peritoneal surfaces &/or cyst/mass causing bowel displacement
  - Pre- or postnatal US or prenatal MR showing peritoneal Ca^{2+}, complex ascites, dilated bowel, &/or cyst/pseudocyst
- Fluoroscopic contrast study can limit differential diagnosis

TOP DIFFERENTIAL DIAGNOSES

- Ileal atresia
- Meconium ileus
- Midgut volvulus
  - Much less common cause of MP

CLINICAL ISSUES

- Neonatal surgery is required in 50-90%
- Prenatal US prediction for neonatal surgery
  - Isolated Ca^{2+}: No surgery required
  - Ca^{2+} & 1 additional finding (ascites or pseudocyst or bowel dilation): > 50% require surgery
  - Ca^{2+} & 2-3 additional findings: 80-100% require surgery
- Newborn imaging predictors for surgery: Bowel obstruction, ascites, volvulus, pneumoperitoneum
- No treatment is required in asymptomatic patients with normal bowel function (i.e., healed perforation in utero)

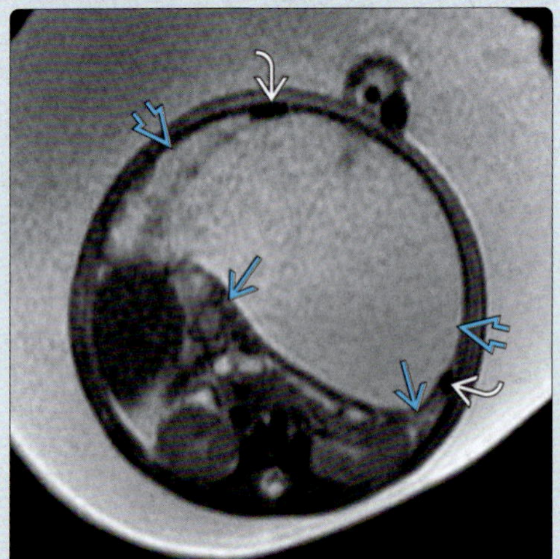

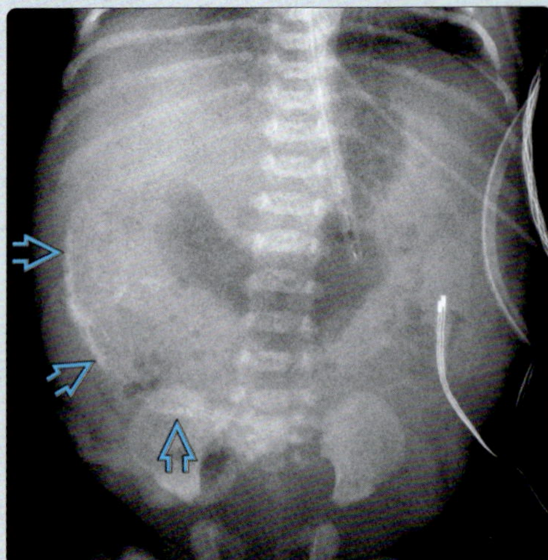

(Left) *Axial SSFSE T2 fetal MR shows a large cystic lesion of the abdomen ➯ that contains scattered foci of debris, possibly meconium, & displaces decompressed bowel ➯. Several low-signal foci ➯ suggest Ca^{2+}, raising the possibility of meconium peritonitis (MP).* **(Right)** *Newborn radiograph performed in the same patient delivered at 31-weeks gestation shows peritoneal or cyst wall Ca^{2+} ➯, consistent with MP. No free intraperitoneal air is seen.*

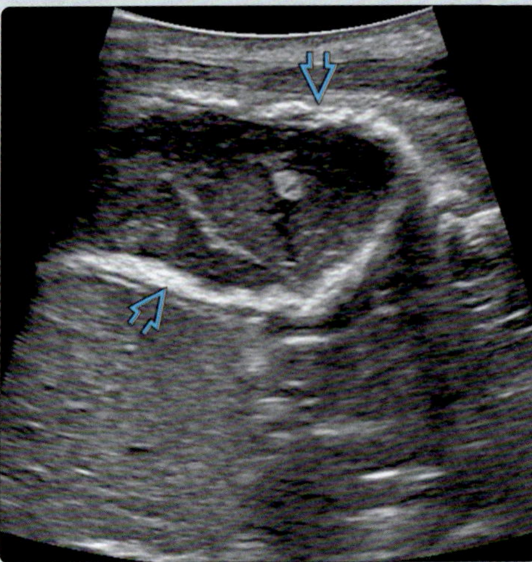

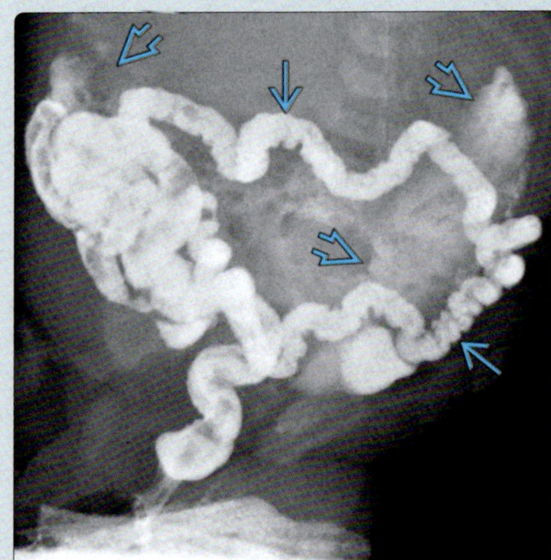

(Left) *Abdominal US in the same patient shows a complex fluid collection with a thick, echogenic, calcified wall ➯, correlating with the preceding radiograph. The bowel was decompressed (not shown).* **(Right)** *Supine WSCE was performed in the same patient to assess continuity of bowel in hopes of conservative initial management. Contrast first opacifies a microcolon ➯ & small bowel before leaking into the meconium pseudocyst ➯. Three unexplained sites of perforation were found in the OR, but no atresia or thick meconium was seen.*

TERMINOLOGY

Definitions

- Meconium peritonitis (MP): Chemical peritonitis resulting from in utero bowel perforation that leaks sterile meconium & digestive enzymes into peritoneal cavity
- Meconium cyst: Meconium + fluid contained by fibrous membranes in setting of MP
- Meconium pseudocyst: Meconium + fluid contained by membranes partly derived from muscular layer of intestine

IMAGING

General Features

- Best diagnostic clue
  - Newborn abdominal radiograph showing linear, curvilinear, or punctate Ca^{2+} along peritoneal surfaces &/or cyst wall
    - Ca^{2+} begins within hours of meconium spillage
  - Pre- or postnatal US with peritoneal Ca^{2+}, complex ascites, dilated bowel, &/or cyst

Radiographic Findings

- Radiography
  - Abdominal soft tissue mass (cyst/pseudocyst)
    - May displace bowel loops
    - May have rim or internal Ca^{2+}
    - May cause gasless abdomen
  - Amorphous, linear, or curvilinear Ca^{2+} along peritoneal surfaces
    - Parietal layer lining abdominal cavity
    - Visceral layer along organ surfaces (liver, etc.)
    - Calcified meconium in bowel loops (enteroliths) may be difficult to differentiate from MP on radiographs
      - Consider: Total colonic aganglionosis, anorectal malformation, multiple bowel atresias
  - ± centralized bowel loops due to ascites
  - Multiple dilated bowel loops of bowel obstruction; 2 possible etiologies
    - In utero obstruction → perforation
    - Spontaneously sealed in utero perforation ± adhesions &/or atresia → obstruction
  - Free intraperitoneal air may occur from persistence of in utero perforation
    - More commonly, site of perforation seals in utero
  - Ca^{2+} in scrotum (meconium orchitis)
    - Due to intraperitoneal Ca^{2+} passing through patent processus vaginalis

Ultrasonographic Findings

- Grayscale ultrasound
  - Pre- or post natal
    - Hyperechoic punctate, linear echogenic foci along abdominal surfaces ± shadowing
      - Prenatal US is more sensitive than postnatal radiographs
    - Ascites: Complex fluid (from meconium) is very suggestive
    - Dilated bowel
    - Cystic mass ± wall nodularity, Ca^{2+}, debris
      - Mass effect may mimic abdominal tumor
    - Ca^{2+}, complex fluid (hydrocele) in scrotum

MR Findings

- Prenatal MR: Similar findings to prenatal US
  - Fetal ascites or cystic collection
    - Complex ± bright T1 signal debris (meconium) vs. simple fluid
  - Dilated bowel loops
  - ± polyhydramnios

Fluoroscopic Findings

- Upper GI
  - Can be normal or show variety of anomalies
    - Malrotation ± midgut volvulus
    - Duodenal jejunal junction may be displaced by adjacent dilated bowel loops or cyst/pseudocyst despite normal rotation
      - ↑ laxity of ligament (actually muscle) of Treitz in newborn
    - Small bowel obstruction (SBO) is frequent
- Contrast enema
  - Microcolon (small colon)
    - Strongly suggests distal in utero SBO
    - Most commonly due to
      - Ileal atresia: Contrast stops at blind-ending terminal ileum (TI)
      - Meconium ileus: Numerous filling defects in TI are outlined by contrast
  - Normal colon
    - Possible proximal or late SBO
  - Colonic obstruction is uncommon (i.e., MP is uncommonly seen with Hirschsprung disease, colonic atresia)

Imaging Recommendations

- Best imaging tool
  - Prenatal &/or postnatal sonography
  - Neonatal abdominal radiographs
- Protocol advice
  - Fluoroscopic contrast study can limit differential diagnosis
    - In face of distal obstruction, water-soluble contrast enema (WSCE) is most helpful
      - Usually meconium Ileus vs. ileal atresia

DIFFERENTIAL DIAGNOSIS

Neonatal Distal Bowel Obstruction

- Ileal atresia
- Meconium ileus
- Hirschsprung disease
- Small left colon/meconium plug syndrome
- Anorectal malformation
- Malrotation
  - Midgut volvulus
    - Much less common cause of MP than distal obstructions
    - Ischemic ileus may mimic distal obstruction due to multiple dilated loops
  - Congenital bands

Neonatal Abdominal Calcifications

- Enteroliths

- Anorectal malformation
- Multiple intestinal atresias
- Total colonic Hirschsprung disease
- Liver parenchyma
  - TORCH infections
  - Vascular Ca^{2+}
- Mass
  - Sacrococcygeal teratoma
  - Neuroblastoma
  - Hepatoblastoma
  - Congenital hepatic hemangioma

PATHOLOGY

General Features

- Etiology
  - In utero bowel perforation is most commonly due to
    - Meconium ileus
      - 8-40% have meconium ileus with cystic fibrosis
    - Jejunal/ileal atresia or stenosis
    - Volvulus
      - Malrotation with midgut volvulus
      - Other segmental volvulus
  - In utero bowel perforation is less commonly due to
    - Intussusception, vascular accident, congenital bands, internal hernia, Hirschsprung disease, colonic atresia, cloaca
  - Cause is unknown in 25-50% of cases
  - Meconium & digestive enzymes leak into peritoneal cavity → intense chemical peritonitis + inflammatory response → granulomatous response + Ca^{2+} within hours-days

Gross Pathologic & Surgical Features

- Subtypes at surgery
  - Fibroadhesive: Sealed off perforation → bowel obstruction
  - Cystic or pseudocystic (fibrous vs. partially muscular/bowel wall): Perforation does not seal off → inflammation → cystic cavity
  - Generalized: Late in utero perforation → more fibrinous than fibrous

CLINICAL ISSUES

Presentation

- Most common signs/symptoms
  - Prenatal: Polyhydramnios, bowel obstruction, Ca^{2+}, abdominal cyst, ascites
  - Post natal: Abdominal distention, mass, failure to pass meconium, bilious emesis, respiratory distress

Demographics

- Age: 2nd-trimester through birth
- Epidemiology: 1:35,000 live births

Natural History & Prognosis

- Majority of cases do not resolve spontaneously in utero
- Prenatal US prediction for neonatal surgery
  - Isolated Ca^{2+}: No surgery required
  - Ca^{2+} & 1 additional finding (ascites or pseudocyst or bowel dilation): > 50% require surgery
  - Ca^{2+} & 2-3 additional findings: 80-100% require surgery
- Newborn imaging predictors for surgery: Bowel obstruction, ascites, volvulus, pneumoperitoneum
- No relation between prenatal diagnosis or type of MP & outcome
- Massive ascites or cyst may lead to hydrops, pulmonary hypoplasia in utero
  - Fetal paracentesis to ↓ fluid
  - Urinary trypsin inhibitor may ↓ inflammation
- 2-20% mortality in modern era
- Predicting factors for morbidity & mortality
  - Postnatal circulation deficiency, serum CRP, persistent ascites, persistent pulmonary hypertension

Treatment

- None in asymptomatic patients with normal bowel function (i.e., healed perforation)
- Neonatal surgery is required in 50-90%
  - Abdominal drainage
  - Relieve bowel obstruction
  - Resection of perforated &/or necrotic bowel
  - Anastomosis vs. temporizing bowel diversion with delayed anastomosis
- Cyst vs. pseudocyst may be important distinction to direct surgical treatment in recent series
  - Pseudocyst: Primary bowel anastomosis
  - Cyst: Bowel diversion with delayed anastomosis
- Complications: Sepsis, adhesions, short gut syndrome

DIAGNOSTIC CHECKLIST

Consider

- Most common causes of in utero bowel perforation
  - Complicated meconium ileus (cystic fibrosis)
  - Intestinal atresia

Image Interpretation Pearls

- Pre- or postnatal sonography: Polyhydramnios, abdominal cyst, ascites, peritoneal Ca^{2+}, dilated bowel
- Postnatal radiography: Ca^{2+} of peritoneal lining is diagnostic
  - Evaluate if Ca^{2+} could be in other locations
    - Intestinal lumen (enteroliths)
    - Hepatic, splenic parenchyma
    - Intraabdominal neoplasm

SELECTED REFERENCES

1. Lu Y et al: Fetal magnetic resonance imaging contributes to the diagnosis and treatment of meconium peritonitis. BMC Med Imaging. 20(1):55, 2020
2. Chen CW et al: Value of prenatal diagnosis of meconium peritoneum: comparison of outcomes of prenatal and postnatal diagnosis. Medicine (Baltimore). 98(39):e17079, 2019
3. Caro-Domínguez P et al: Meconium peritonitis: the role of postnatal radiographic and sonographic findings in predicting the need for surgery. Pediatr Radiol. 48(12):1755-62, 2018
4. Sciarrone A et al: Fetal midgut volvulus: report of eight cases. J Matern Fetal Neonatal Med. 29(8):1322-7, 2016
5. Lee GS et al: Calcified meconium pseudocyst: X-ray diagnosis of meconium peritonitis at birth. BMJ Case Rep, 2015
6. Veyrac C et al: US assessment of neonatal bowel (necrotizing enterocolitis excluded). Pediatr Radiol. 42 Suppl 1:S107-14, 2012
7. Jeanty C et al: Prenatal diagnosis of meconium periorchitis and review of the literature. J Ultrasound Med. 28(12):1729-34, 2009
8. Tsai MH et al: Clinical manifestations in infants with symptomatic meconium peritonitis. Pediatr Neonatol. 50(2):59-64, 2009

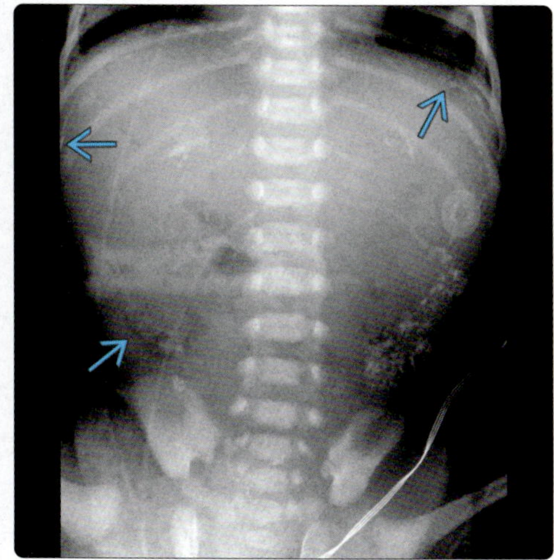

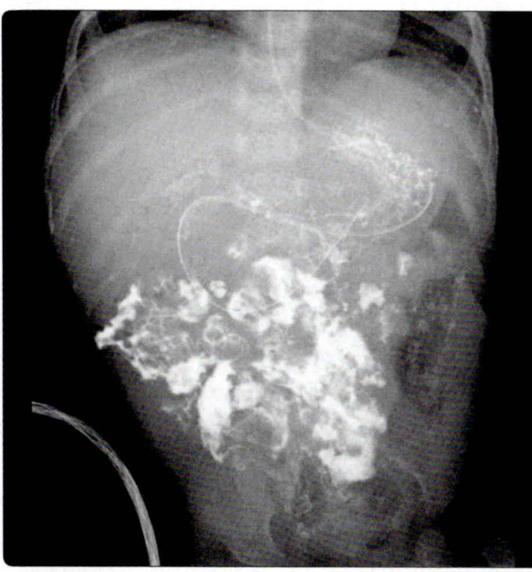

(Left) *AP radiograph in a 1-day-old girl with a prenatal concern for MP shows amorphous Ca^{2+} on peritoneal surfaces throughout the abdomen ➡, which is consistent with MP. The paucity of bowel gas is suspicious for a collection, although US showed normal bowel & no cyst.* **(Right)** *Upper GI + small bowel follow-through in the same patient shows continuous bowel & no obstruction. MP with no cystic mass, ascites, or obstruction equals a healed in utero perforation.*

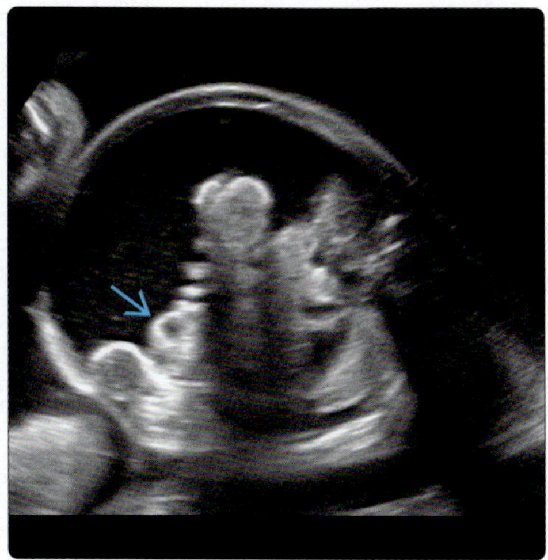

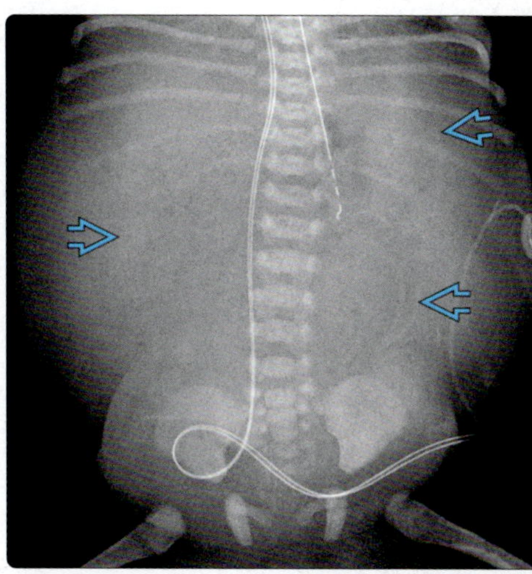

(Left) *Prenatal US shows complex ascites & somewhat thickened echogenic bowel loops ➡, suggestive of MP. Echogenic bowel is nonspecific but can be seen in cystic fibrosis.* **(Right)** *AP radiograph in the same patient at delivery shows a gasless abdomen with curvilinear & amorphous subtle Ca^{2+} ➡, suggestive of MP. The main diagnostic considerations include a bowel atresia or complicated meconium ileus, which is usually a manifestation of cystic fibrosis (CF).*

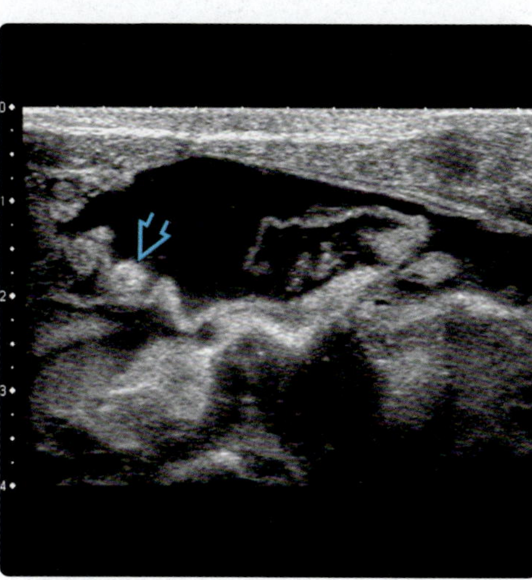

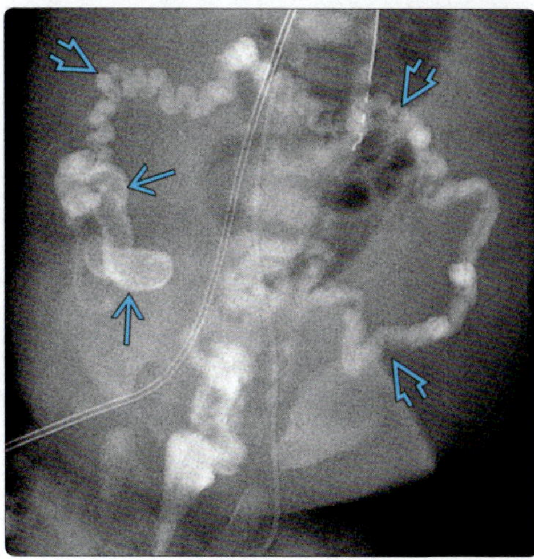

(Left) *Transverse US in the same patient confirms the presence of complex ascites, suggestive of MP (as well as echogenic bowel ➡, as seen on the prenatal US).* **(Right)** *Supine WSCE in the same patient shows a microcolon ➡ devoid of significant meconium. The normal caliber terminal ileum is filled with meconium ➡, consistent with meconium ileus, a common cause of MP. Genetic testing confirmed CF in this neonate.*

KEY FACTS

TERMINOLOGY

- Necrotizing enterocolitis (NEC): Life-threatening condition of neonatal GI tract characterized by inflammation, ischemia, & translocation of bacteria into bowel wall

IMAGING

- Diagnosis is based on clinical & imaging findings
- Radiography is mainstay of imaging for suspected NEC
  - Findings range from nonspecific (gasless abdomen) to suggestive (thickened, dilated bowel loops) to diagnostic [pneumatosis, portal venous gas (PVG), free air]
  - Duke Abdominal Assessment Scale for radiographs
    - Standard lexicon for reporting NEC findings
    - Strong intraobserver & interobserver agreement
    - ↑ scores correlate with need for surgery
- Ultrasound is excellent adjunct
  - Predictors of radiographically occult necrosis &/or perforation requiring surgery vary by study but most commonly include complex collections & free air
  - Additional findings include ↑ (early) or ↓ (late) vascularity, ↓ peristalsis, ↑ bowel wall echogenicity, intramural gas, bowel wall thickening or thinning, & PVG
- Contrast enema is not used acutely; useful to localize strictures after treatment of acute episode

CLINICAL ISSUES

- Most common in very low birth weight (< 1,500 g) &/or premature infants, usually 2-3 weeks after delivery
  - 10% in term infants (usually with underlying diseases)
- Typical history: Feeding intolerance with emesis, ↑ gastric residuals, bloody stools
- Other frequent clinical findings include abdominal distention &/or discoloration, apnea & bradycardia, lethargy, temperature instability
- Treatment: IV nutrition + antibiotics ± surgery
- Overall mortality 10-50%
  - Death is secondary to sepsis from bowel perforation
- Delayed bowel strictures in 10-20% of survivors

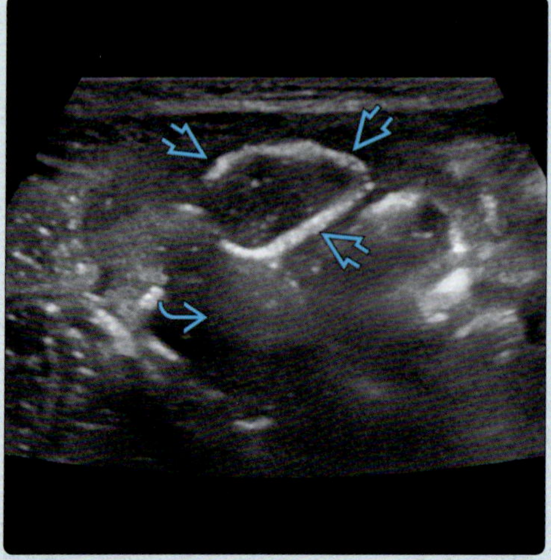

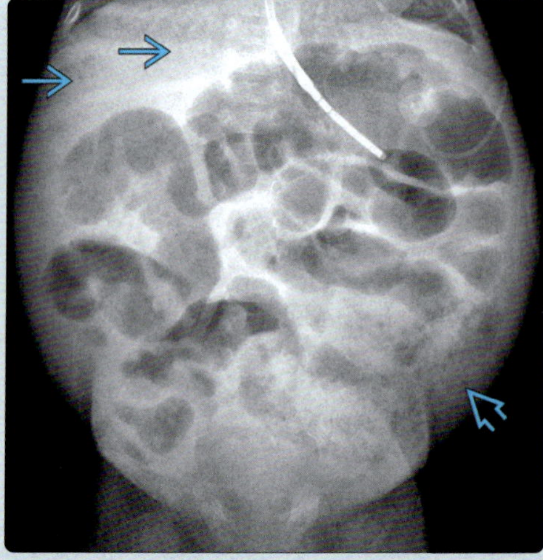

(Left) *Transverse left lower quadrant US in a 5-week-old former premature infant shows bowel wall hyperechogenicity due to pneumatosis ⇒; this can be differentiated from intraluminal bowel gas by its circumferential distribution. Note the "dirty" posterior acoustic shadowing ⇒ caused by gas in the bowel wall.* **(Right)** *Supine AP radiograph in the same patient shows "bubbly" lucencies of pneumatosis in the left lower quadrant ⇒. Subtle branching foci of portal venous gas (PVG) ⇒ are seen in the liver.*

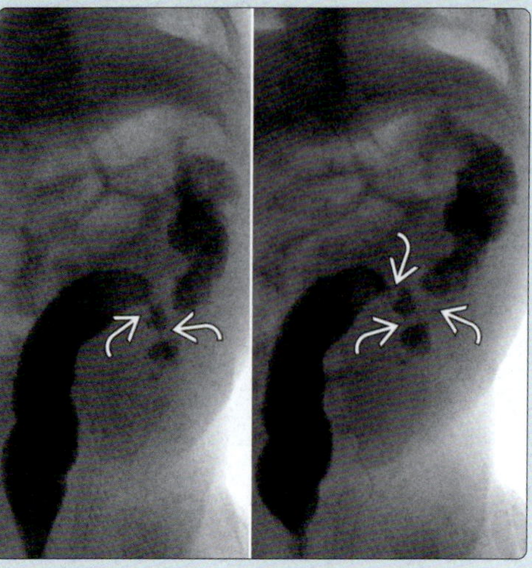

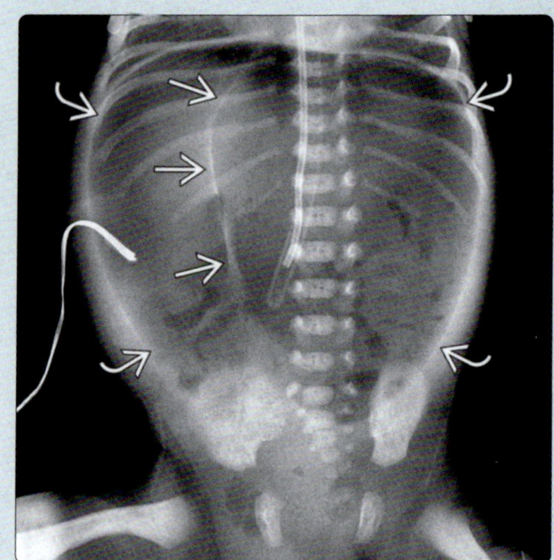

(Left) *Two weeks later, sequential frontal images from an enema in the same patient show several short-segment, high-grade colonic strictures ⇒ in the same region that was imaged with US.* **(Right)** *Supine AP radiograph in a premature infant with necrotizing enterocolitis (NEC) shows a large amount of pneumoperitoneum causing abnormal lucency ⇒. The falciform ligament ⇒ is outlined by air; this appearance resembles the laces of an American football (the football sign).*

TERMINOLOGY

Definitions

- Necrotizing enterocolitis (NEC): Poorly understood but life-threatening condition of neonatal GI tract characterized by inflammation, ischemia, & translocation of bacteria into bowel wall
- Very low birth weight (VLBW): < 1,500 g
- Extremely low birth weight (ELBW): < 1,000 g

IMAGING

General Features

- Best diagnostic clue
  - Dilated bowel loops with pneumatosis (intramural bowel gas), portal venous gas (PVG), & free intraperitoneal air
- Location
  - Affected bowel is most commonly in right lower quadrant
    - Ascending colon, terminal ileum
  - May occur anywhere from stomach to rectum

Radiographic Findings

- Nonspecific findings
  - Paucity of bowel gas
  - Loss of normal mosaic pattern of polygon-shaped bowel loops throughout abdomen
- Suggestive findings
  - Asymmetric bowel dilation
  - Fixed, "unfolded" bowel loops on serial radiographs
    - May be normal caliber or dilated
  - Separation of bowel loops
    - Due to bowel wall edema/hemorrhage or intervening collapsed or fluid-filled bowel or free fluid
- Definitive findings
  - Pneumatosis (50-75% of patients)
    - "Bubbly" (submucosal) or curvilinear (subserosal) lucencies
    - Mimics formed stool (not typically seen in unfed infants though enteric fluid may contain gas bubbles)
  - PVG
    - Branching lucencies over liver
    - Greater peripheral extension than biliary gas (with biliary gas being uncommon in newborns)
  - Free intraperitoneal air
    - Overall ↑ upper abdominal lucency on supine radiograph with liver appearing less opaque than heart
    - Football sign: Lucent, distended abdomen with gas outlining vertical falciform ligament on supine radiograph (like laces of American football)
    - Cupola sign: Gas under midline diaphragm on supine radiograph (with well-defined superior, but not inferior, borders)
    - Rigler sign: Gas outlining both sides of bowel wall
    - Crescentic lucency overlying right hepatic margin on left lateral decubitus view or anterior hepatic margin on cross-table lateral view
    - Triangles of lucency anteriorly on cross-table lateral view or peripherally on supine AP view

Ultrasonographic Findings

- Grayscale ultrasound
  - Focal fluid collections, echogenic ascites, aperistaltic bowel with thickening or thinning, & ↑ echogenicity of bowel wall all suggest NEC
    - Complex fluid collections suggest perforation
  - Pneumatosis: Nodular echogenicities around entire circumference of bowel wall ± "dirty shadowing" posteriorly
  - PVG: Branching linear & punctate echogenicities in liver periphery; may see echogenic foci coursing through portal veins in real time
  - Free intraperitoneal air: Linear echogenicities with "dirty shadowing" immediately deep to peritoneal surface
- Color Doppler
  - ↑ vascularity may be seen in earlier stages
  - ↓ vascularity indicates ischemia, potentially leading to necrosis/perforation
  - ↑ peak systolic velocity & resistive index in superior mesenteric artery
- Contrast-enhanced ultrasound
  - Can aid in assessing bowel perfusion

Fluoroscopic Findings

- Acute: Enema is contraindicated in acute NEC
- Chronic: Strictures create obstruction in "older" NICU infants; causative NEC episode not always clinically apparent
  - Single or multiple strictures found 4-8 weeks after NEC
  - Radiologically discovered strictures are usually left-sided, while most surgically discovered strictures are found in right colon (sometimes even small bowel)

Imaging Recommendations

- Best imaging tool
  - Serial radiography: Fixed, dilated loops are predictive of bowel ischemia/necrosis
  - Sonography is up to 100% sensitive & 95% specific for bowel necrosis or "surgical NEC," but specific findings vary by study

DIFFERENTIAL DIAGNOSIS

Newborn Bowel Obstruction

- Congenital bowel obstructions (e.g., atresias, meconium ileus) present within first 1-3 days after delivery, often with "bilious emesis" or "failure to pass meconium"

Newborn Spontaneous Intestinal Perforation

- Typically lacks pneumatosis & PVG
- Necrosis is focal, not extensive

Enterocolitis of Term Infants

- Milk allergy, cyanotic heart disease, maternal cocaine use, Hirschsprung disease (especially total colonic)

Nonspecific Gaseous Distention of Bowel

- Continuous positive airway pressure
- Bag ventilation at intubation

Hypertrophic Pyloric Stenosis

- Rarely associated with benign gastric pneumatosis

- Usually healthy term infants presenting with projectile vomiting at 2-12 weeks of life

Benign Pneumatosis in Older Children

- Often with complex medical history, including bone marrow transplant & steroid therapy
- Predominately colonic; may cause free air

PATHOLOGY

General Features

- Etiology
  - Different mechanisms in different newborn groups
    - Very premature: Dysregulated inflammatory response to stasis of feeds, incomplete or abnormal GI microbial colonization, & immunologic immaturity
    - Term & late preterm: Likely from hypoxia-ischemia
  - Multifactorial etiology in all patients
- Associated abnormalities
  - Lung disease of prematurity
  - Congenital heart disease
  - Intracranial hemorrhage, white matter injury

Staging, Grading, & Classification

- Duke Abdominal Assessment Scale: Standardized lexicon for reporting findings in newborns with suspected NEC
  - High intra- & interobserver agreement
  - Higher scores strongly correlate with disease severity/need for surgical intervention
    - 0: Normal gas pattern
    - 1: Mild bowel distention
    - 2: Moderate distention (or normal with nonspecific "bubbly" lucencies)
    - 3: Focal, moderate distention of bowel loops
    - 4: Separation or focal thickening of bowel loops
    - 5: Featureless or multiple separated bowel loops
    - 6: Possible pneumatosis with other abnormal findings
    - 7: Fixed or persistent dilation of bowel loops
    - 8: Pneumatosis (highly probable or definite)
    - 9: PVG
    - 10: Pneumoperitoneum

Gross Pathologic & Surgical Features

- Dilated, gray, hemorrhagic, friable bowel

Microscopic Features

- Mucosal coagulation, ulceration, submucosal hemorrhage, submucosal or subserosal gas (pneumatosis intestinalis), PVG, mesenteric gas
- Histopathologic features include coagulative & hemorrhagic necrosis, inflammation, bacterial overgrowth

CLINICAL ISSUES

Presentation

- Most common signs/symptoms
  - Signs of feeding intolerance (emesis, ↑ gastric residuals, bloody stools)
  - Abdomen may become distended, discolored, erythematous, &/or shiny
  - Apnea & bradycardia, lethargy, temperature instability
- Other signs/symptoms
  - 1/3 have fulminant course with bowel perforation
  - 1/3 develop septic shock

Demographics

- Age
  - Premature VLBW or ELBW newborns have highest incidence (90% of cases)
    - Affects 3-13% < 1,500 g; rate in ELBW is 3x that of VLBW
    - Onset of NEC peaks at 29-31 weeks postmenstrual age, especially 2-3 weeks after delivery
  - Term newborns make up 10% of cases
    - Earlier age onset of NEC (1-3 days after delivery)
    - Often have ≥ 1 risk factors
- Epidemiology
  - Overall incidence: 1 per 1,000 live births
    - Varies by nursery/ICU
    - Outbreaks frequently follow epidemic pattern; no single causative infectious agent is known

Natural History & Prognosis

- Overall mortality: 10-50%
  - Death secondary to sepsis from bowel perforation
- Morbidity in survivors includes delayed bowel strictures (10-20%), short gut syndrome, & neurodevelopmental delays

Treatment

- Prevention: Probiotics ↓ NEC incidence & mortality in VLBW infants
- When NEC is suspected: IV nutrition + antibiotics
- Indications for surgery: Clinical ± radiologic findings
  - Perforation is considered absolute indication
  - Clinical deterioration, bowel necrosis

DIAGNOSTIC CHECKLIST

Image Interpretation Pearls

- NEC can be associated with adhesions, so intraperitoneal gas may be loculated rather than "free"
  - Strongly consider left lateral decubitus &/or cross-table lateral images to look for intraperitoneal gas

SELECTED REFERENCES

1. Gokli A et al: Contrast-enhanced ultrasound of the pediatric bowel. Pediatr Radiol. ePub, 2021
2. Lazow SP et al: Abdominal ultrasound findings contribute to a multivariable predictive risk score for surgical necrotizing enterocolitis: a pilot study. Am J Surg. ePub, 2021
3. Pammi M et al: Recent advances in necrotizing enterocolitis research: strategies for implementation in clinical practice. Clin Perinatol. 47(2):383-97, 2020
4. Bazacliu C et al: Pathophysiology of necrotizing enterocolitis: An Update. Curr Pediatr Rev. 15(2):68-87, 2019
5. De Bernardo G et al: Management of NEC: surgical treatment and role of traditional x-ray versus ultrasound imaging, experience of a single centre. Curr Pediatr Rev. 15(2):125-30, 2019
6. Kim JH: Role of Abdominal US in diagnosis of NEC. Clin Perinatol. 46(1):119-27, 2019
7. Overman RE Jr et al: Necrotizing enterocolitis in term neonates: a different disease process? J Pediatr Surg. 54(6):1143-6, 2019
8. Ahle M et al: The role of imaging in the management of necrotising enterocolitis: a multispecialist survey and a review of the literature. Eur Radiol. 28(9):3621-31, 2018
9. Chen S et al: Comparison of abdominal radiographs and sonography in prognostic prediction of infants with necrotizing enterocolitis. Pediatr Surg Int. 34(5):535-41, 2018
10. Cuna AC et al: Bowel ultrasound for predicting surgical management of necrotizing enterocolitis: a systematic review and meta-analysis. Pediatr Radiol. 48(5):658-66, 2018

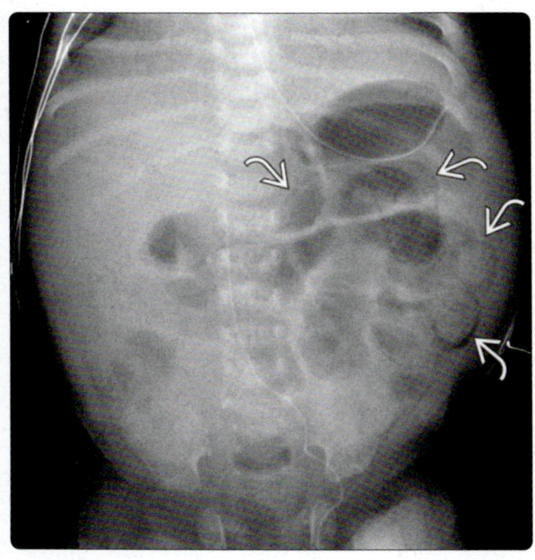

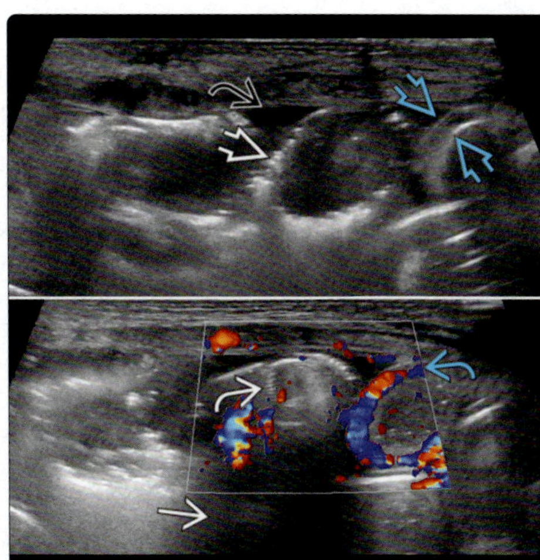

(Left) *Supine AP radiograph in a 5-week-old girl who was born prematurely shows extensive curvilinear pneumatosis* ➡ *throughout the left abdomen.* **(Right)** *Grayscale US (top) in 7-day-old premature infant shows ascites* ➡ *& segmental bowel wall abnormalities due to NEC, including pneumatosis & wall thinning* ➡ *compared to a normal bowel loop* ➡. *Doppler US (bottom) reveals ↓ blood flow* ➡ *in the affected bowel compared to the normal segment* ➡. *There is also shadowing from the pneumatosis* ➡.

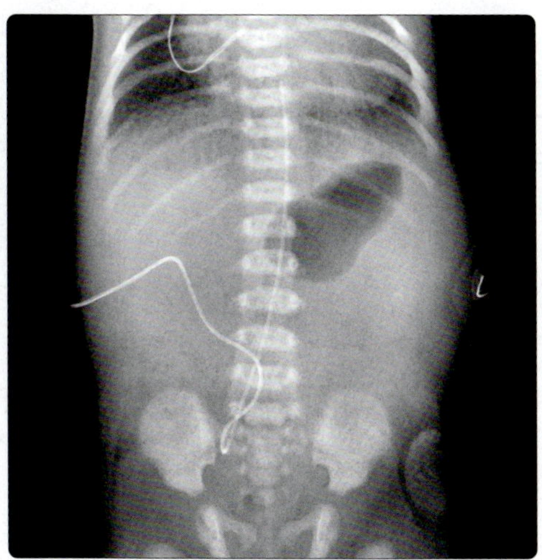

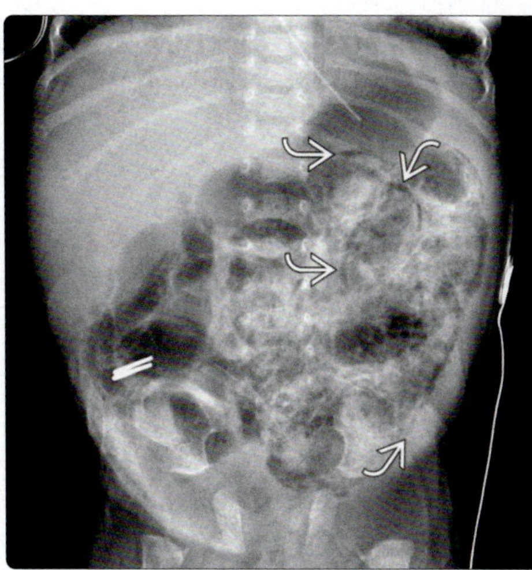

(Left) *Supine AP radiograph in a term infant with aortic coarctation, feeding intolerance, bloody stools, & spells of apnea/bradycardia shows a nearly gasless abdomen, a nonspecific finding of NEC.* **(Right)** *Supine AP radiograph shows a premature infant with NEC who has widespread pneumatosis intestinalis with curvilinear & "bubbly" lucencies seen in most of the intestinal walls* ➡, *especially on the left.*

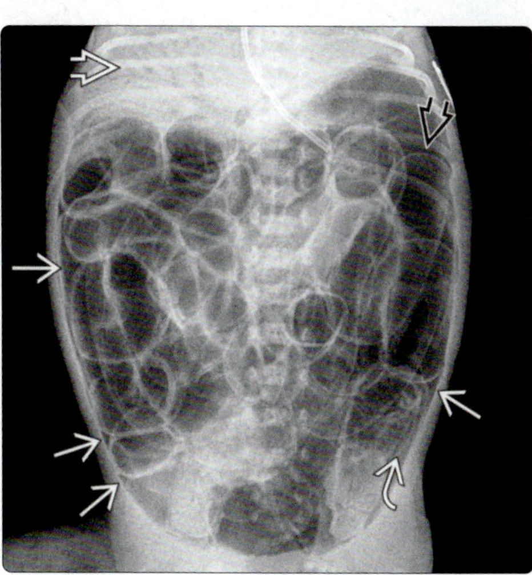

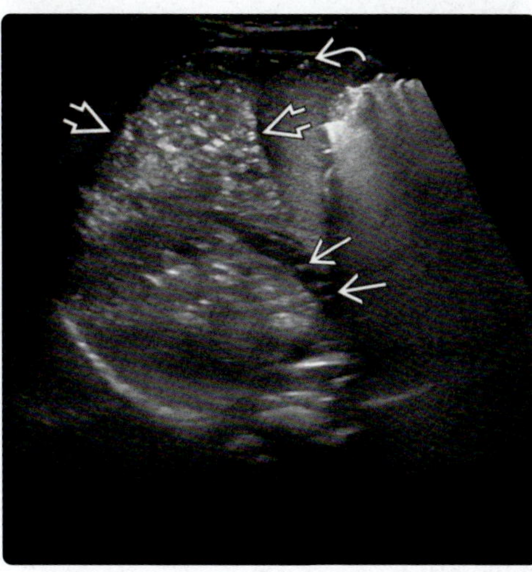

(Left) *Supine AP radiograph shows a dramatic case of NEC with PVG* ➡, *pneumatosis* ➡, *& free air causing numerous small & triangular lucencies* ➡. *Also note the Rigler sign (with gas outlining both sides of the bowel wall* ➡*), indicating pneumoperitoneum.* **(Right)** *Transverse US in a newborn with severe NEC shows extensive PVG throughout the liver parenchyma, affecting mainly the right lobe* ➡; *note scattered bubbles in the left lobe* ➡. *Gas within the main portal vein* ➡ *was much easier to see in real time.*

Spontaneous Intestinal Perforation in Neonates

KEY FACTS

TERMINOLOGY

- Spontaneous intestinal perforation (SIP)

IMAGING

- Pneumoperitoneum on radiographs
  - Small volume of free air is best seen on left lateral decubitus or cross-table lateral views
- Occasionally gasless abdomen
- Absence of pneumatosis intestinalis or portal venous gas helps differentiate from necrotizing enterocolitis (NEC)
- Free fluid with echogenic debris on ultrasound

TOP DIFFERENTIAL DIAGNOSES

- NEC: Pneumatosis intestinalis ± portal venous gas, fixed dilated bowel loops, bowel wall thickening
  - More common > 15 days of life
- Distal intestinal obstruction: Numerous dilated bowel loops, pneumoperitoneum if perforation; presents in first 1-3 days of life
- Iatrogenic perforation: Feeding tube or gastric decompression tube

PATHOLOGY

- Exact etiology unknown
  - Several associations reported, causality elusive
  - Indomethacin, postnatal steroids, inotropes, sepsis
- Localized, focal necrosis & perforation
  - Lacks extensive necrosis seen in NEC
- Ileum is most common

CLINICAL ISSUES

- Disease of premature infants; ↑ risk with lower birth weight
- Mean age of 7 days, typically < 15 days
- Treatment: Surgical repair is definitive, peritoneal drainage as definitive vs. temporizing measure
- Mortality 9-24%

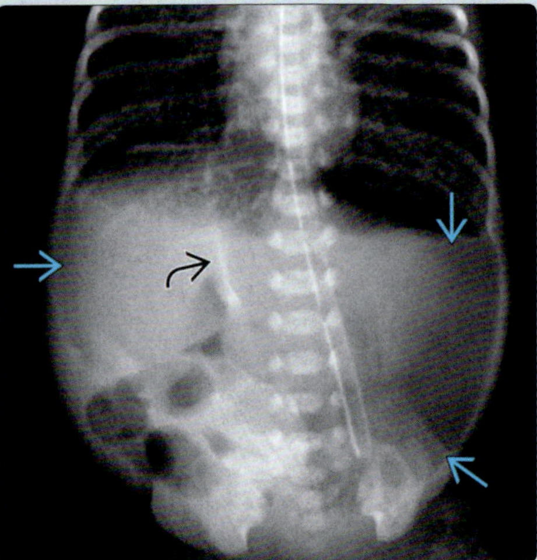

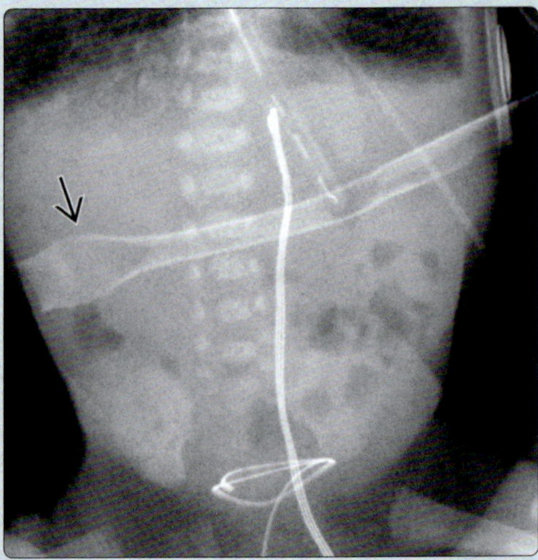

(Left) *AP radiograph in a 5-day-old, 25-weeks-gestation infant shows a large volume of pneumoperitoneum with generalized abdominal lucency ➡ & free air outlining the falciform ligament ➡. Surgery showed ileal perforation with only mild focal ischemic changes, consistent with spontaneous intestinal perforation (SIP).* **(Right)** *Postoperative AP radiograph in the same infant shows an interval ↓ in pneumoperitoneum & placement of a peritoneal drainage catheter ➡.*

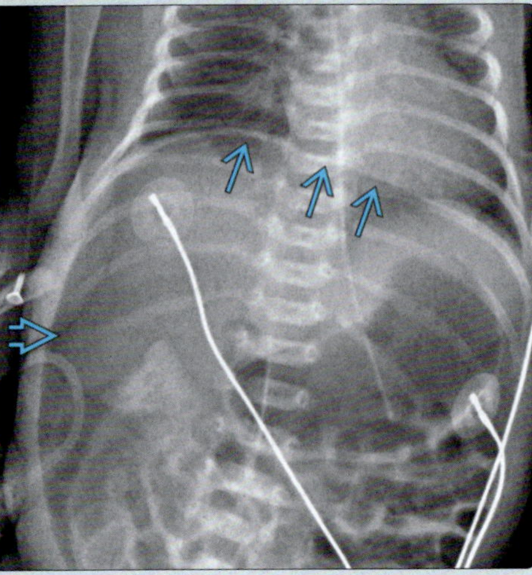

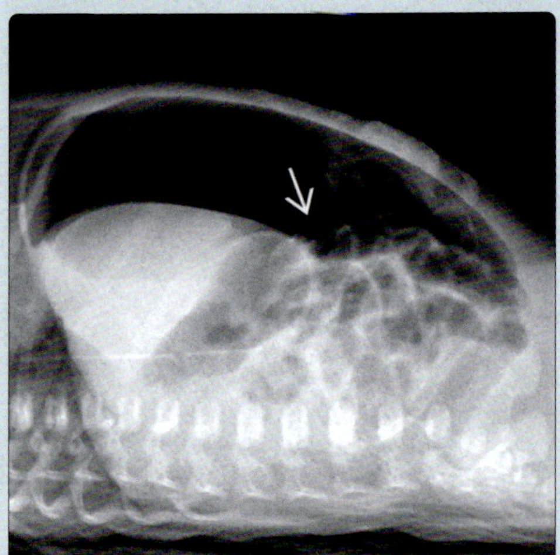

(Left) *AP radiograph in a 30-week-gestation, very low birth weight newborn (1330g) obtained for tube placement incidentally revealed pneumoperitoneum with ↑ lucency ➡ & outline of the diaphragm ➡. On pathology, a small perforation was found in the distal ileum with no significant associated inflammation, typical of SIP.* **(Right)** *Cross-table lateral radiograph in the same infant shows antidependent free air in the anterior abdomen. Note the Rigler sign with gas outlining both sides of the bowel wall ➡.*

Spontaneous Intestinal Perforation in Neonates

TERMINOLOGY

Abbreviations

- Spontaneous intestinal perforation (SIP)

Synonyms

- Focal intestinal perforation

Definitions

- Focal, isolated perforation of intestinal tract

IMAGING

General Features

- Best diagnostic clue
  - Pneumoperitoneum without pneumatosis intestinalis in premature infant in first 10 days of life

Radiographic Findings

- Absence of pneumatosis intestinalis & portal venous gas
  - Presence suggests perforated necrotizing enterocolitis (NEC) rather than SIP
- May have gasless abdomen
- Pneumoperitoneum

Ultrasonographic Findings

- Echogenic free fluid
  - Free fluid containing particulate matter
  - May precede radiographic pneumoperitoneum
- Extraluminal gas
  - Focal enhancement of peritoneal stripe with "dirty" shadowing
  - Moves with changes in patient position

Imaging Recommendations

- Best imaging tool
  - 2-view abdominal radiograph
    - Left lateral decubitus or cross-table lateral view ↑ sensitivity for pneumoperitoneum

DIFFERENTIAL DIAGNOSIS

Necrotizing Enterocolitis

- Necrosis involving large area of intestine
- Disease of premature infants
  - Tends to occur at later postnatal age vs. SIP; mean age: 15 days
- Pneumatosis intestinalis ± portal venous gas, fixed dilated bowel loops, bowel wall thickening
- Pneumoperitoneum from perforation

Distal Intestinal Obstruction

- Intestinal atresia, meconium ileus, Hirschsprung disease, etc.
  - Usually presents in first 1-3 days of life
- May present with abdominal distention, bilious emesis, &/or failure to pass meconium
- Numerous dilated bowel loops
- ± pneumoperitoneum from perforation
- Peritoneal Ca^{2+} suggests in utero perforation

Iatrogenic Perforation

- Feeding tube or gastric decompression tube ± predisposing factors affecting bowel integrity

PATHOLOGY

General Features

- Exact etiology remains unclear, may include
  - Focal ischemia
  - Altered trophism: Mucosal hyperplasia + thinned submucosa & muscularis propria
  - Impaired motility

Gross Pathologic & Surgical Features

- Localized focal necrosis & perforation
- Typically single perforation in antimesenteric bowel wall
- Ileum is most common site

CLINICAL ISSUES

Presentation

- Most common signs/symptoms
  - Pneumoperitoneum on radiograph
  - Abdominal distention ± bluish abdominal wall discoloration
  - Hypotension

Demographics

- Premature infants, especially extremely low birth weight (< 1000 g)
  - Associations with indomethacin (debated in literature), postnatal steroids, inotrope requirement, sepsis
  - Causality not clearly established
- Sex: M > F; 2-3:1
- Incidence: 1% of infants < 32-weeks-gestational age
  - 2.3% < 28 weeks in same large cohort
- Most common ~ 7 days postnatal age (range 0-15 days)
  - NEC is classically in older neonates

Natural History & Prognosis

- Recent reported mortality of 9-24%
  - Mortality lower than perforated NEC
- Coexistent comorbidities of prematurity
- Lower rates of surgical morbidity vs. NEC
  - Stricture, adhesive bowel obstruction

Treatment

- Surgical repair
  - Resection with primary anastomosis vs. temporary stoma
- Peritoneal drainage
  - Definitive therapy or temporizing measure
- Successful conservative management has been described

SELECTED REFERENCES

1. Elgendy MM et al: Spontaneous intestinal perforation in premature infants: a national study. J Perinatol. 41(5):1122-8, 2021
2. Ye N et al: Successful conservative treatment of intestinal perforation in VLBW and ELBW neonates: a single centre case series and review of the literature. BMC Pediatr. 19(1):255, 2019
3. Rayyan M et al: Risk factors for spontaneous localized intestinal perforation in the preterm infant. J Matern Fetal Neonatal Med. 31(19):2617-23, 2018
4. Houben CH et al: Spontaneous intestinal perforation: the long-term outcome. Eur J Pediatr Surg. 27(4):346-51, 2017
5. Fischer A et al: Ultrasound to diagnose spontaneous intestinal perforation in infants weighing 1000 g at birth. J Perinatol. 35(2):104-9, 2015
6. Shah J et al: Intestinal perforation in very preterm neonates: risk factors and outcomes. J Perinatol. 35(8):595-600, 2015

KEY FACTS

TERMINOLOGY

- Gastroesophageal reflux (GER): Retrograde flow of gastric contents into esophagus
- GER disease (GERD): GER that causes clinical symptoms or tissue damage

IMAGING

- Retrograde passage of gastric contents into esophagus
  - Can see on US, fluoroscopic upper GI, radionuclide scintigraphy, MR
- Reflux esophagitis (GERD)
  - Best seen fluoroscopically
  - Esophageal dysmotility is often earliest sign
  - Distal esophageal mucosal irregularity/thickening/stricture
  - Barrett esophagus (rare in children)
- Upper GI to exclude anatomic/functional abnormalities, not to identify GER
  - Esophageal dysmotility
  - Hiatal hernia
  - Gastric outlet/duodenal obstruction
  - Malrotation
- Radionuclide scintigraphy: Most sensitive imaging test to detect GER

CLINICAL ISSUES

- Symptoms
  - Recurrent vomiting/regurgitation
  - Poor weight gain/failure to thrive
  - Excessive irritability
  - Respiratory symptoms (e.g., wheezing, cough)
- Epidemiology
  - Most infantile GER resolves by 1-2 years of age
  - ~ 4% have persistent GER, 1% require surgical treatment
  - GER: 50% at 4 months, ↓ to 5-10% at 12 months
- Treatment
  - Nonsurgical: ~ 99% of refluxers
  - Surgical: Fundoplication

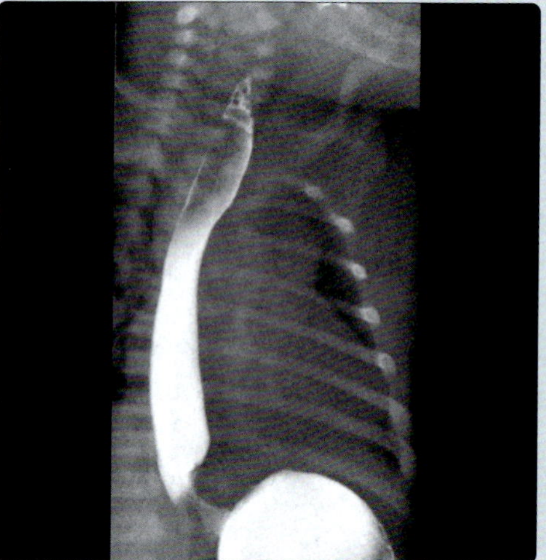

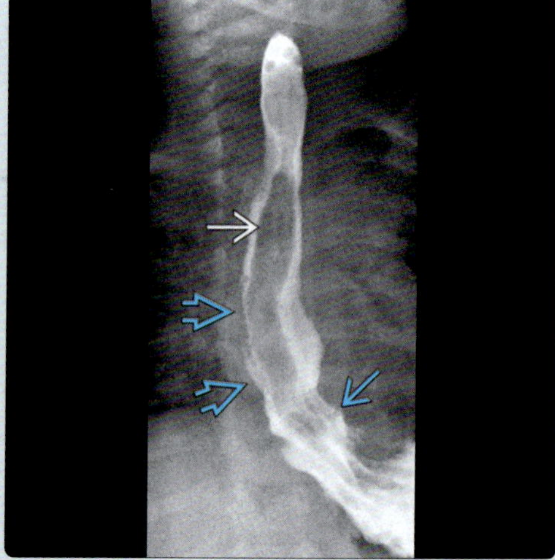

(Left) *LPO upper GI of a 3-day-old girl with severe regurgitation shows almost no peristalsis of an otherwise normal, completely distended esophagus. Hypomotility is the earliest finding in reflux esophagitis & gastroesophageal reflux disease (GERD).* **(Right)** *Upper GI in a 7-month-old with worsening GER shows a mild hiatal hernia (gastric folds above diaphragm ➨) with thickened folds of the distal esophagus ➨, consistent with reflux esophagitis & dysmotility. Note the air ➨ in the esophagus.*

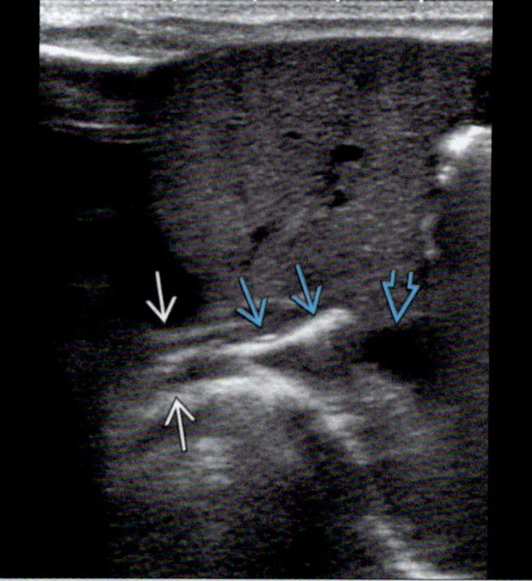

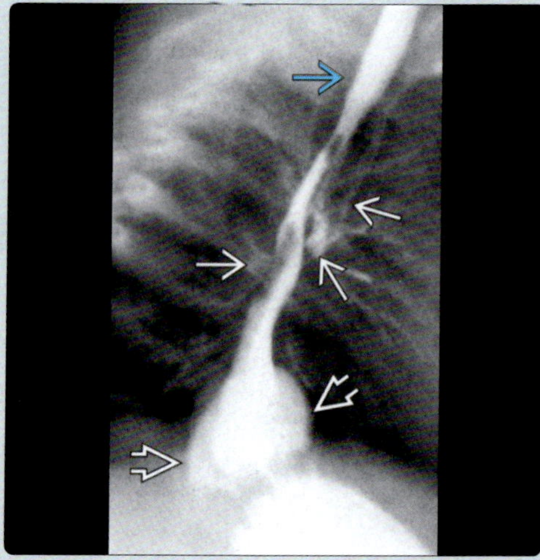

(Left) *Longitudinal US of the gastroesophageal junction in a 20-day-old with recurrent nonbilious vomiting shows a column of echogenic air ➨, which in real-time scanning was moving retrograde from the fluid-filled stomach ➨ into the esophagus ➨.* **(Right)** *Lateral upper GI in a patient with a hiatal hernia ➨ demonstrates significant reflux of contrast ➨, which the patient aspirated ➨, requiring placement of an enteric suction tube into the esophagus to prevent further aspiration of stomach contents.*

TERMINOLOGY

Abbreviations

- Gastroesophageal reflux (GER), GER disease (GERD)

Definitions

- GER: Retrograde flow of gastric contents into esophagus
  - Physiologic phenomenon, especially in young infants
- GERD: GER causes clinical symptoms or tissue damage

IMAGING

General Features

- Best diagnostic clue
  - Retrograde passage of contrast across gastroesophageal junction (GEJ) into esophagus
- Morphology
  - Normal GEJ or associated hiatal hernia, usually sliding type

Radiographic Findings

- Radiography
  - Usually normal; rarely shows round retrocardiac lucency (hiatal hernia)

Fluoroscopic Findings

- Upper GI
  - Retrograde flow of contrast into esophagus
  - Reflux esophagitis (GERD)
    - Esophageal dysmotility is often earliest sign
    - Distal esophageal mucosal irregularity/thickening/stricture
    - Barrett esophagus (rare in children)
  - Other potential findings with GER
    - Hiatal hernia, usually sliding type
    - Malrotation: Incidental in 4%
    - Gastric outlet/duodenal obstruction
      - Pyloric stenosis, gastric antral/duodenal web, etc.; delayed gastric emptying

Ultrasonographic Findings

- Retrograde flow of gastric contents at GEJ

Nuclear Medicine Findings

- Tc-99m sulfur colloid
  - Activity above GEJ during period of observation

Imaging Recommendations

- Best imaging tool
  - Tc-99m labeled sulfur colloid meal
  - Fluoroscopic upper GI evaluation for anatomic abnormality of GI tract
- Protocol advice
  - Upper GI to evaluate anatomy, not confirm reflux
    - Looking for GERD & GER causes: Evaluate swallow & motility, no provocative maneuvers
  - Radionuclide scintigraphy: Most sensitive imaging test for GER

DIFFERENTIAL DIAGNOSIS

Gastric/Duodenal Obstruction

- Pyloric stenosis, antral web, duodenal stenosis/web

Malrotation

- GER can be presenting symptom of malrotation without volvulus

Achalasia

- Rare; presents in childhood to adolescence

Esophagitis

- Many causes other than reflux

Esophageal Atresia (Repaired)

- Anastomotic stricture or GER is not uncommon after repair

PATHOLOGY

General Features

- Etiology
  - Potentially many physiologic & anatomic factors
    - Suboptimal angle of His

CLINICAL ISSUES

Presentation

- Most common signs/symptoms
  - Infants: Recurrent spit-up, irritability, feeding difficulty, poor weight gain, sleep disturbances
  - Children: Poorly localized abdominal or chest pain, heartburn, recurrent vomiting/regurgitation, dysphagia, respiratory (wheezing, cough)

Natural History & Prognosis

- Most infantile GER resolves by 1-2 years of age
- GER: 50% at 4 months, ↓ to 5-10% at 12 months
- ~ 4% have persistent GER, 1% require surgical treatment
- No treatment → pneumonia, asthma, laryngitis, otitis media, tooth decay
- Barrett esophagus, not usually seen in children

Treatment

- Nonsurgical: ~ 99% of refluxers
  - Lifestyle adjustment, diet/formula alteration
  - Prokinetic agents, antacids, & proton-pump inhibitors
- Surgical: ~ 1% of all refluxing patients
  - Fundoplication

DIAGNOSTIC CHECKLIST

Consider

- Potential anatomic causes of GER

SELECTED REFERENCES

1. Expert Panel on Pediatric Imaging. et al: ACR Appropriateness Criteria® vomiting in infants. J Am Coll Radiol. 17(11S):S505-15, 2020
2. Seif Amir Hosseini A et al: Real-time MRI for dynamic assessment of gastroesophageal reflux disease: comparison to pH-metry and impedance. Eur J Radiol. 125:108856, 2020
3. Koivusalo AI et al: Outcome of surgery for pediatric gastroesophageal reflux: clinical and endoscopic follow-up after 300 fundoplications in 279 consecutive patients. Scand J Surg. 107(1):68-75, 2018
4. Uslu Kızılkan N et al: Comparison of multichannel intraluminal impedance-pH monitoring and reflux scintigraphy in pediatric patients with suspected gastroesophageal reflux. World J Gastroenterol. 22(43):9595-603, 2016
5. Vandenplas Y et al: An updated review on gastro-esophageal reflux in pediatrics. Expert Rev Gastroenterol Hepatol. 9(12):1511-21, 2015
6. Codreanu I et al: Effects of the frame acquisition rate on the sensitivity of gastro-oesophageal reflux scintigraphy. Br J Radiol. 86(1026):20130084, 2013

Hypertrophic Pyloric Stenosis

KEY FACTS

TERMINOLOGY

- Hypertrophic pyloric stenosis (HPS): Idiopathic pyloric muscle thickening in young infants → progressive gastric outlet obstruction

IMAGING

- Near-complete gastric outlet obstruction due to abnormally elongated & thickened pyloric muscle
    - Pylorus fails to relax/open → minimal gastric emptying → gastric overdistention → emesis
- Ultrasound shows hypertrophied circumferential hypoechoic muscle & elongated pyloric canal filled with echogenic mucosa
    - Commonly accepted sonographic criteria for HPS
        - Pyloric channel length > 15-16 mm
        - Single wall thickness of pyloric muscle > 3 mm
        - Failure of thickened pylorus to change during exam
            - May still see trickle of passage of gastric contents
- Upper GI shows minimal barium traversing narrowed & elongated pyloric channel, mass effect on gastric antrum & duodenum by hypertrophied muscle, hyperperistaltic gastric contractions, & gastroesophageal reflux/emesis

CLINICAL ISSUES

- Typically seen in infants 2-12 weeks old with progressive, nonbilious projectile vomiting
    - Feedings previously tolerated (i.e., HPS is not congenital)
- Incidence of 1.5-3 per 1,000 infants; M:F = 5:1
    - HPS in 1/5 of infants imaged for vomiting
        - Gastroesophageal reflux > > HPS
- Surgical treatment: Pyloromyotomy
- Nonsurgical alternative (rarely employed): Medications & frequent small feedings

DIAGNOSTIC CHECKLIST

- Pylorospasm mimics HPS (but typically transient)
- Avoid overdistending stomach during imaging exam (which displaces/obscures pylorus)

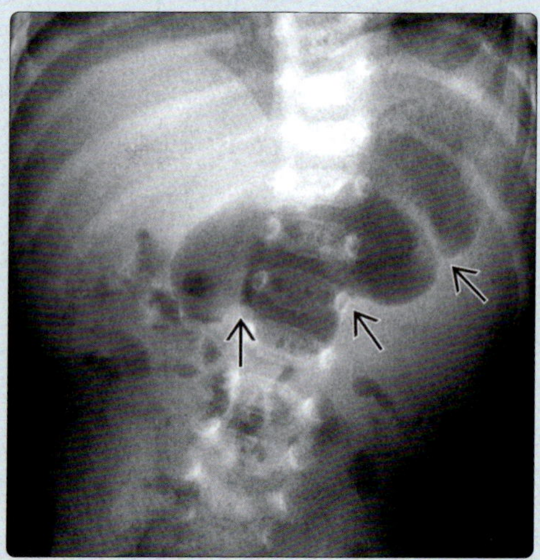

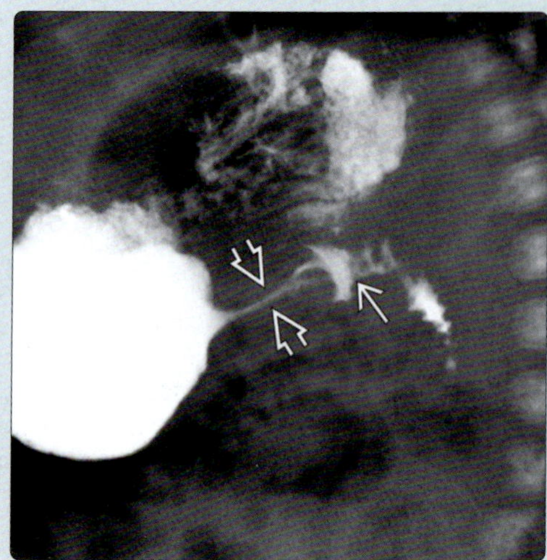

(Left) *AP radiograph in a vomiting infant with hypertrophic pyloric stenosis (HPS) shows hyperperistalsis of a gas-filled stomach with muscular contractions ⇨ attempting to push gastric contents through the narrowed, hypertrophied pylorus.* **(Right)** *Lateral upper GI shows a thin "string" of barium extending through the narrowed, elongated pyloric channel ➡, opacifying the duodenal bulb ➡. The thickened pyloric muscle creates rounded indentations on the gastric antrum & base of the duodenal bulb.*

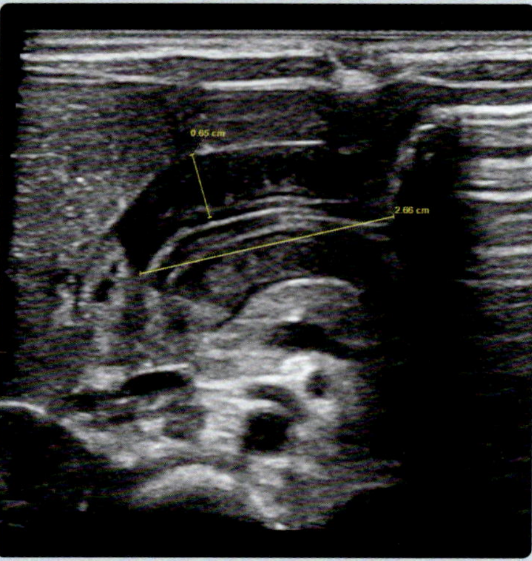

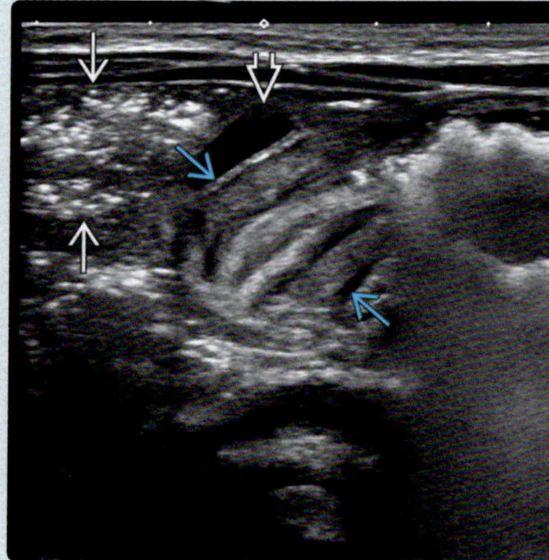

(Left) *Transverse oblique ultrasound shows yellow lines measuring the single wall thickness (6.5 mm) & length (26.6 mm) of the pyloric channel in a baby with HPS.* **(Right)** *Transverse oblique ultrasound shows echogenic foci ➡ in the left lobe of the liver, consistent with portal venous gas in a 1-month-old with HPS. The partially filled gallbladder ➡ is visible between the abnormal pylorus ⇨ & liver.*

TERMINOLOGY

Abbreviations

- Pyloric stenosis, hypertrophic pyloric stenosis (HPS)

Definitions

- Idiopathic pyloric muscle thickening → progressive gastric outlet obstruction
- Typically seen in infants 2-12 weeks old with progressive, nonbilious projectile vomiting

IMAGING

General Features

- Best diagnostic clue
  - Near-complete gastric outlet obstruction due to elongated & thickened pyloric muscle
  - Ultrasound reveals hypertrophied muscle & ↓ gastric emptying on dynamic exam
  - Upper GI shows minimal contrast traversing narrowed & elongated pyloric channel with mass effect on antrum & duodenal bulb from thickened pyloric muscle
- Location
  - Near gallbladder in RUQ by ultrasound

Radiographic Findings

- Radiography
  - Overdistended stomach with ↓ distal bowel gas
    - Enlarged stomach containing gas & retained ingested material displaces adjacent bowel
  - Stomach may be collapsed if infant has recently vomited
  - Benign gastric pneumatosis & portal venous gas are rarely reported (< 2%) in association with HPS

Fluoroscopic Findings

- Overdistended "caterpillar stomach": Undulations of wall due to exaggerated gastric motility (hyperperistalsis)
- Tram-track or string sign of contrast within narrowed & elongated pyloric channel
- Shoulders of thickened pyloric muscle create impressions on distal antrum
- "Beak" where contrast encounters narrowed pyloric canal
- Contrast in duodenal bulb (covering hypertrophied muscle impressions at base of duodenal bulb) + contrast in narrowed & elongated pyloric channel: Mushroom sign

Ultrasonographic Findings

- Grayscale ultrasound
  - Threshold for abnormal measurements of pyloric muscle & channel length varies by study
    - In general, ↑ threshold measurements ↑ specificity but ↓ sensitivity
  - Commonly accepted threshold values for HPS
    - Single wall thickness of hypoechoic pyloric muscle > 3 mm
    - Pyloric channel length > 15-16 mm
    - Pyloric diameter > 15 mm
  - Hypertrophied & redundant echogenic mucosal lining
  - Gastric hyperperistalsis & persistently obliterated pyloric lumen on dynamic exam
  - If duodenal bulb is easily identified & distended with fluid, diagnosis of HPS is unlikely
  - Echogenic foci of gas in portal veins can be visible in adjacent left lobe of liver
- Color Doppler
  - ↑ flow in pyloric muscle & mucosa with HPS
  - Microvascular flow imaging shows trickle of enteric contents in channel

Imaging Recommendations

- Best imaging tool
  - Ultrasound when HPS is suspected
    - Excellent sensitivity & specificity; no ionizing radiation
  - Barium upper GI for atypical history (including bilious emesis)
- Protocol advice
  - Begin ultrasound scan with patient rolled onto right side in order to pool gastric fluids in antrum
  - Administer glucose water in small amounts
    - Avoid overdistending stomach, which will displace pyloric channel posteriorly or into right lower quadrant
  - Watch for pyloric channel to open with thinning of muscle & passage of fluid through channel
  - Vigorous gastric contractions of body & antrum that do not open pylorus suggest diagnosis of HPS
  - Formula or glucose water will "swirl" against thickened pylorus with each wave of gastric peristalsis in HPS

DIFFERENTIAL DIAGNOSIS

Pylorospasm

- Typically seen in irritable infants; resolves with time → wait & reimage
- Rarely as thick or elongated as true HPS

Gastroesophageal Reflux

- Cause of vomiting in 2/3 of infants referred to radiology
- Presumed diagnosis when pyloric ultrasound is normal
- Gastroesophageal junction can be mistaken for pylorus on ultrasound if transducer is too high
  - Heart should not be visible on longitudinal images of pylorus

Malrotation With Midgut Volvulus

- Emesis is classically bilious (greenish) from bile
- Surgical emergency due to risk of midgut ischemia
- Upper GI: Mildly dilated proximal duodenum with abrupt beaking near junction of 2nd-3rd duodenum
  - Distal contrast passage shows "corkscrew" or swirling contrast in typically narrowed bowel
- Ultrasound: Transverse superior to inferior sweep shows twisting of SMA/SMV & bowel in clockwise "whirlpool"
  - May lose Doppler flow & grayscale lumen of SMV & SMA

Gastric Bezoar

- Caused by accumulation of undigested matter in stomach
  - Trichobezoar: Composed of hair (& sometimes nails)
  - Phytobezoar: Composed of plant or vegetable fiber
- Contrast is seen in interstices of large filling defect on upper GI

Other Causes of Proximal Obstruction

- Duodenal stenosis or antral web

- Antral polyps, antritis, annular pancreas, choledochocele, RUQ mass
- Pyloric atresia

PATHOLOGY

General Features

- Etiology
  - Idiopathic hypertrophy of circular muscle bundles in pylorus
  - Slightly ↑ incidence in preterm infants vs. full term
    - Presents at later chronologic age in preemies
  - Higher incidence in mothers < 20 years old, nulliparous, smokers, & formula-fed babies
  - May be prostaglandin or erythromycin induced, neural mediated, familial
  - Associated with erythromycin & azithromycin (macrolide) exposure prenatally & postnatally via breast milk
  - Higher incidence of HPS in patients with cystic fibrosis
  - Abnormal muscle tone/electrophysiology of gastroduodenal junction in HPS
- Genetics
  - Tends to run in families; not truly inherited
  - Discordant incidence among monozygotic twins favors environmental factors over genetic predisposition
- Associated abnormalities
  - Eosinophilic gastritis, prostaglandin-induced antral mucosal hyperplasia, hypergastrinemia, nasoenteric tubes, erythromycin, esophageal atresia

Gross Pathologic & Surgical Features

- Hypertrophy of circular muscular layers of pylorus
- Thickening of mucosa in antrum & pylorus to ~ 1/3 diameter of pylorus

CLINICAL ISSUES

Presentation

- Most common signs/symptoms
  - Progressive vomiting in infant who previously tolerated feedings
  - Palpable "olive" on physical exam: 97% specific in experienced hands
    - Less common finding due to earlier imaging diagnosis
- Other signs/symptoms
  - Weight loss
  - Alkalosis & dehydration with prolonged course

Demographics

- Age
  - 2-12 weeks or even later in premature infants
  - Peak age of 5 weeks; 80% by 8 weeks
- Sex
  - M:F = 5:1
- Ethnicity
  - Slightly more common in White patients
- Epidemiology
  - Incidence of 1.5-3 per 1,000 infants
  - Incidence is ↓ worldwide
  - Vomiting caused by HPS in 1/5 of infants referred for imaging

Natural History & Prognosis

- Weight loss & parental concerns typically prompt imaging
- Gradual progression with spontaneous remission after weeks
- Excellent prognosis following surgery or conservative medical management
  - No significant GI disturbances seen in German study of infants treated surgically or medically 16-26 years after diagnosis
- Portal venous gas has no influence on prognosis

Treatment

- Surgical: Pyloromyotomy
  - Splits thickened muscle longitudinally (without breaching mucosa), opening channel
  - Laparoscopic pyloromyotomy & open procedures have equal success rates
  - Endoscopic pyloromyotomy & balloon dilation are alternatives
- Nonsurgical alternative: Medications & frequent small feedings
  - Requires several weeks before resuming normal feeding without medications
  - Medications used include Botox, atropine
  - Withdrawal of prostaglandins after corrective cardiac surgery → muscular hypertrophy regresses
- Complications
  - Failed surgery due to inadequate pyloromyotomy
  - Gastroduodenal myotomy or enterotomy

DIAGNOSTIC CHECKLIST

Image Interpretation Pearls

- Pylorospasm mimics HPS transiently
- Avoid overdistending stomach, which displaces pylorus

SELECTED REFERENCES

1. Expert Panel on Pediatric Imaging. et al: ACR Appropriateness Criteria® vomiting in infants. J Am Coll Radiol. 17(11S):S505-15, 2020
2. Kelly MM et al: Incidence and importance of portal venous gas in children with hypertrophic pyloric stenosis. Pediatr Radiol. 50(8):1102-6, 2020
3. Donda K et al: Pyloric stenosis: national trends in the incidence rate and resource use in the United States from 2012 to 2016. Hosp Pediatr. 9(12):923-32, 2019
4. Mowrer AR et al: Low socioeconomic status and formula feeding directly correlate with increased incidence of hypertrophic pyloric stenosis. J Pediatr Surg. 54(12):2498-502, 2019
5. Tao J et al: Technical aspects of peroral endoscopic pyloromyotomy. Gastrointest Endosc Clin N Am. 29(1):117-26, 2019
6. Bakal U et al: Recent changes in the features of hypertrophic pyloric stenosis. Pediatr Int. 58(5): 369-71, 2016
7. Wu SF et al: Efficacy of medical treatment for infantile hypertrophic pyloric stenosis: a meta-analysis. Pediatr Neonatol. 57(6):515-21, 2016
8. Eberly MD et al: Azithromycin in early infancy and pyloric stenosis. Pediatrics. 135(3):483-8, 2015
9. Stark CM et al: Association of prematurity with the development of infantile hypertrophic pyloric stenosis. Pediatr Res. 78(2):218-22, 2015
10. Lund M et al: Use of macrolides in mother and child and risk of infantile hypertrophic pyloric stenosis: nationwide cohort study. BMJ. 348:g1908, 2014
11. Soyer T et al: Transient hypertrophic pyloric stenosis due to prostoglandin infusion. J Perinatol. 34(10):800-1, 2014
12. Svenningsson A et al: Maternal and pregnancy characteristics and risk of infantile hypertrophic pyloric stenosis. J Pediatr Surg. 49(8):1226-31, 2014
13. Bhargava P et al: Gastric pneumatosis and portal venous gas: benign findings in hypertrophic pyloric stenosis. Pediatr Radiol. 39(4):413, 2009

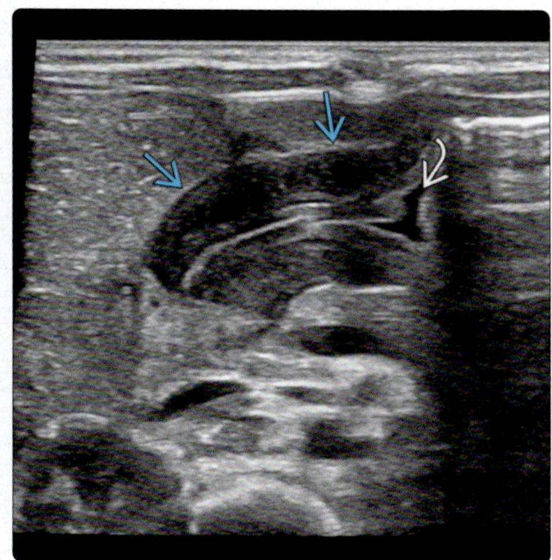

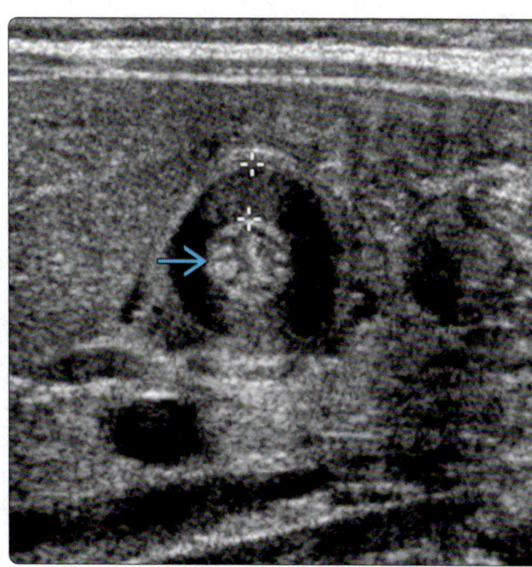

(Left) *Transverse oblique ultrasound in a 5-week-old boy with HPS shows elongation of the pyloric channel length. The hypoechoic muscle is thickened* ➡, *& there is a small amount of anechoic fluid trying to enter the channel* ➡. **(Right)** *Sonographic cross section of a hypertrophied pylorus shows the doughnut sign of HPS, consisting of a circumferentially thickened & hypoechoic muscle (calipers) + the central, redundant, echogenic mucosa* ➡.

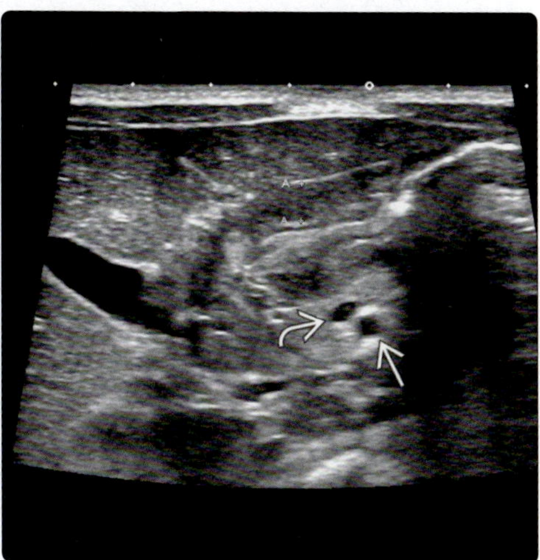

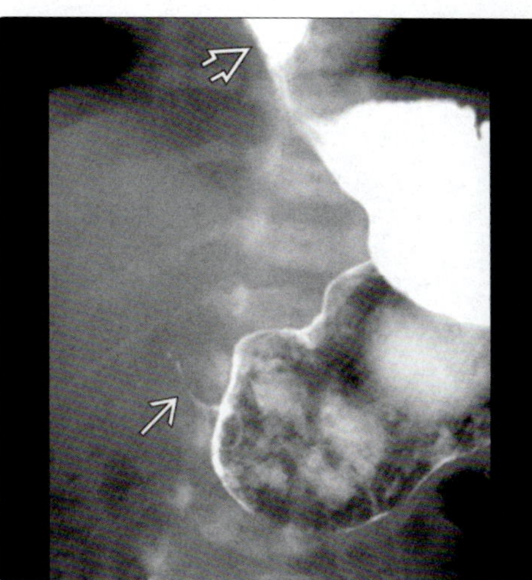

(Left) *Transverse oblique ultrasound in a different baby with HPS shows thickening of the pyloric muscle at 4.5 mm between the calipers. Note the normal relationship of the SMA* ➡ *& SMV* ➡. **(Right)** *Delayed frontal upper GI shows a string sign of barium passing through a narrowed pylorus* ➡ *with reflux into the distal esophagus* ➡. *Demonstrating barium in a tight pyloric channel requires patience & intermittent fluoroscopy.*

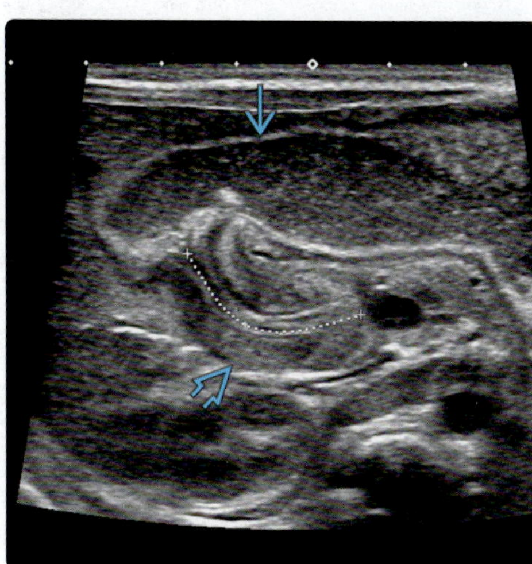

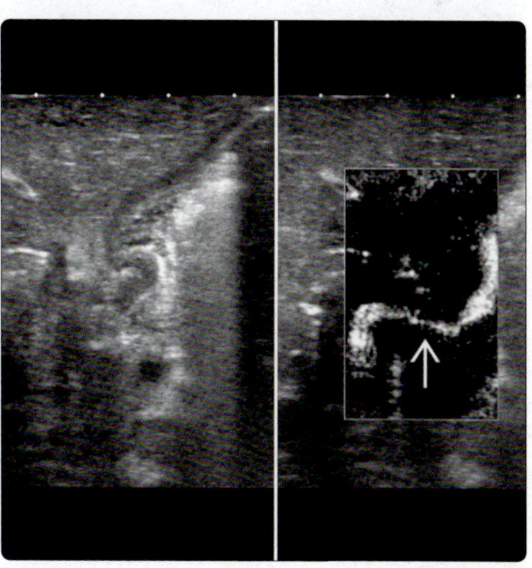

(Left) *Transverse ultrasound after a glucose water feeding in an infant with HPS shows how feeding can overdistend the stomach* ➡ *& push the pylorus* ➡ *posteriorly. The pylorus is thickened with the channel elongated at 27.6 mm.* **(Right)** *Transverse oblique postprandial ultrasound (left) shows how gas mixed with formula can interfere with visualization of structures. The insert (right) is a type of Doppler optimized for slow flow, showing a thin trickle of fluid* ➡ *passing through the hypertrophied channel.*

KEY FACTS

TERMINOLOGY

- Twisting of all or part of stomach on its axes by at least 180°
- Organoaxial volvulus (OAV): Rotation along long axis
- Mesenteroaxial volvulus (MAV): Rotation along short axis

IMAGING

- Radiographic findings
  - Round, gas-distended viscus under &/or above left hemidiaphragm that decompresses with nasogastric (NG) tube
  - Upright image may show 2 air-fluid levels
- Upper GI vs. CECT to confirm diagnosis
  - OAV
    - Horizontal stomach with pylorus directed inferiorly
    - Greater curvature superior to lesser curvature
  - MAV
    - Vertical stomach with pylorus superior to fundus
    - Pylorus lies close to or overlaps gastroesophageal junction

PATHOLOGY

- Primary volvulus: Absent, failed, or lax ligamentous fixation; chronic > acute
- Secondary volvulus: Disorder of gastric anatomy/function, often with diaphragm anomalies; acute > chronic

CLINICAL ISSUES

- 58% present within 1st year of life
- Symptoms: Retching, nonbilious emesis, pain, & distention
  - ± respiratory distress & cyanosis in acute setting
  - ± failure to thrive & colic in chronic setting
  - Complete Borchardt triad is uncommon (unproductive retching, epigastric distention, inability to pass NG tube)
- Treatment
  - Resuscitation required in 23-60% of acute presentations
  - Gastric decompression with NG tube
  - Open or laparoscopic reduction + gastropexy &/or gastrostomy tube
  - Repair of associated defects in secondary volvulus

(Left) *Left side down decubitus radiograph of a 6-month-old patient with vomiting shows 2 large air-fluid levels in the left lower hemithorax ➡ & left upper quadrant of the abdomen ⇨, respectively.* **(Right)** *Frontal upper GI in the same patient shows the stomach lying largely in the left hemithorax. The stomach is inverted with the antrum ⇨ & gastric outlet ➡ lying above the fundus ➡. Note the twisting of rugal folds ⇨ in the cardia. An acute mesenteroaxial volvulus was found at surgery with a chronic diaphragmatic hernia.*

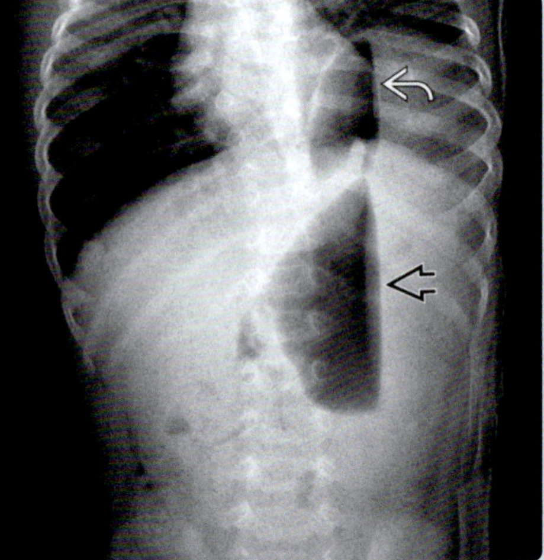

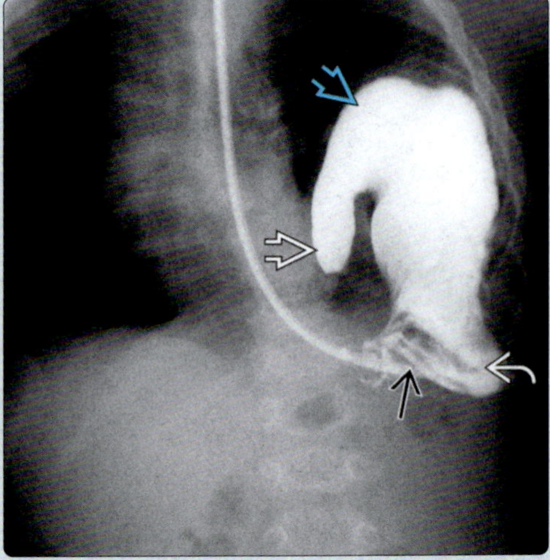

(Left) *Supine AP radiograph in a 4-month-old girl with abdominal distention & ↓ PO intake shows the stomach to be markedly distended & rounded ➡. An organoaxial gastric volvulus was found at surgery.* **(Right)** *Coronal CECT in an 11-year-old with vomiting shows a narrow pylorus ➡ above the level of the gastroesophageal (GE) junction ➡. The proximal duodenum is stretched ⇨. The abdominal contents extend abnormally into the lower left hemithorax. A mesenteroaxial gastric volvulus was found at surgery.*

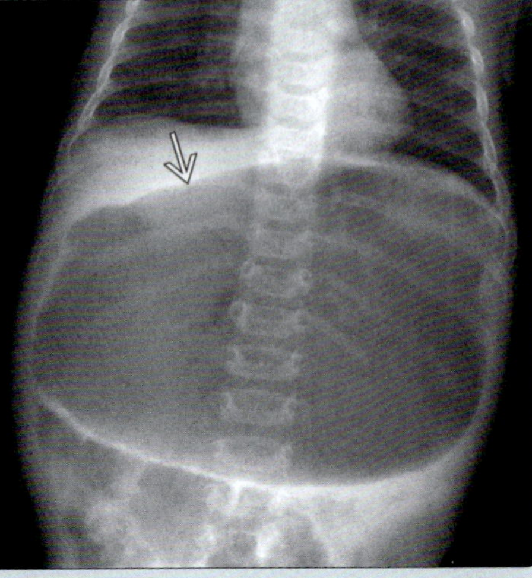

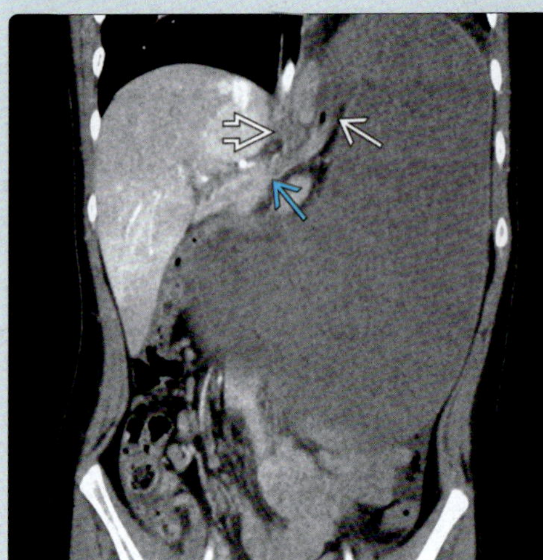

TERMINOLOGY

Definitions

- Twisting of all or part of stomach on its long or short axis by at least 180°
- Organoaxial volvulus (OAV): Twisting along long axis [i.e., line drawn from gastroesophageal (GE) junction to pylorus]
- Mesenteroaxial volvulus (MAV): Twisting along short axis (perpendicular to long axis)
- Mixed volvulus: Rotation along both long & short axes
- Twisting of stomach on axes < 180°: Gastric torsion

IMAGING

Radiographic Findings

- Round, gas-distended viscus under &/or above diaphragm
  - ↓ in size after decompression by nasogastric (NG) tube
- Stomach lies horizontally (OAV) or vertically (MAV)
- 2 air-fluid levels on upright image (in fundus & antrum)
- Inability to pass or abnormal course of NG tube
- + elevation of left hemidiaphragm
- ± paucity of bowel gas distally

Fluoroscopic Findings

- Upper GI series
  - OAV
    - Horizontal stomach with pylorus at level of gastric cardia; pylorus is directed inferiorly
    - Greater curvature lies superior to lesser curvature
  - MAV
    - Vertical stomach with pylorus superior to fundus
    - Pylorus lies close to or overlaps GE junction
  - Beaking of contrast at sites of twisting
  - Partial or complete obstruction of contrast passage into or out of stomach

CT Findings

- Findings similar to upper GI series
- Multiplanar reformatted images are helpful
- Negative oral contrast allows for optimal gastric wall evaluation on CECT (if patient can tolerate)
- Can identify associated abnormalities

MR Findings

- Fetal MR of congenital diaphragmatic hernia often shows volvulus of intrathoracic stomach ± polyhydramnios

Imaging Recommendations

- Upper GI series vs. CECT

DIFFERENTIAL DIAGNOSIS

Air-Filled Thoracic Mass ± Air-Fluid Levels

- Sliding or paraesophageal hiatal hernia
- Postoperative anatomy (e.g., esophageal atresia repair with gastric pull-up vs. colonic interposition)
- Bronchopleural fistula
- Congenital pulmonary airway malformation

Massively Dilated Abdominal Viscus

- Hypertrophic pyloric stenosis
- Toxic megacolon ± Hirschsprung disease
- Colonic volvulus

PATHOLOGY

General Features

- Stomach is relatively fixed at ends: GE junction at esophageal hiatus & pylorus to retroperitoneal duodenum
- Stomach is also normally fixed by ligaments: Gastrophrenic, gastrosplenic, gastrocolic, gastrohepatic
- Primary volvulus
  - Absent, failed, or lax ligamentous fixation
  - 74% of chronic volvulus
- Secondary volvulus
  - Disorder of gastric anatomy/function (distention, peptic ulcer, neoplasm, prior gastric surgery) or abnormality of adjacent organ (diaphragmatic hernia or eventration, splenic anomalies, intestinal malrotation)
  - 69% of acute volvulus

Gross Pathologic & Surgical Features

- Acute: OAV 54%, MAV 41%, mixed 2%
- Chronic: OAV 85%, MAV 10%, mixed 3%

CLINICAL ISSUES

Presentation

- 58% present within 1st year of life
- Acute, chronic, or acute-on-chronic symptoms include
  - Retching, nonbilious emesis, pain, & distention
  - Respiratory distress & cyanosis may be seen acutely
  - Failure to thrive & colic are also seen chronically
  - Hematemesis in late stage occurs secondary to ischemia
- Complete Borchardt triad is uncommon (unproductive retching, epigastric distention, inability to pass NG tube)

Natural History & Prognosis

- Complications: Obstruction, ischemia, perforation
- Mortality: Acute 7.1%, chronic 2.7%
- In large review, 1 in 8 chronic volvulus cases developed acute symptoms with 60% requiring resuscitation

Treatment

- Resuscitation is required in 23-60% of acute presentations
- Gastric decompression with NG tube
- Open or laparoscopic reduction + gastropexy &/or gastrostomy tube
- Repair of associated defects in secondary volvulus
  - Controversial if gastropexy is required after repair of associated anomaly

SELECTED REFERENCES

1. da Costa KM et al: Management and outcomes of gastric volvulus in children: a systematic review. World J Pediatr. 15(3):226-34, 2019
2. Mazaheri P et al: CT of gastric volvulus: interobserver reliability, radiologists' accuracy, and imaging findings. AJR Am J Roentgenol. 212(1):103-8, 2019
3. Garel C et al: Diagnosis of pediatric gastric, small-bowel and colonic volvulus. Pediatr Radiol. 46(1):130-8, 2016
4. Millet I et al: Computed tomography findings of acute gastric volvulus. Eur Radiol. 24(12):3115-22, 2014
5. Cribbs RK et al: Gastric volvulus in infants and children. Pediatrics. 122(3):e752-62, 2008
6. Oh SK et al: Gastric volvulus in children: the twists and turns of an unusual entity. Pediatr Radiol. 38(3):297-304, 2008
7. Upadhyaya VD et al: Acute gastric volvulus in neonates - a diagnostic dilemma. Eur J Pediatr Surg. 18(3):188-91, 2008

Ingested Coins

KEY FACTS

IMAGING

- Disc-shaped metallic density without circumferential beveled edge/step-off
- Most common sites of impaction
    - Upper esophagus at thoracic inlet
    - Midesophagus at aortic arch impression
    - Lower esophageal sphincter at gastroesophageal junction
- Other sites of impaction include pylorus, duodenum, ileocecal valve
- Imaging recommendations
    - Screening frontal radiographs of neck through pelvis ± lateral upper airway
    - Lateral radiograph if foreign body is identified

TOP DIFFERENTIAL DIAGNOSES

- Button battery ingestion
- Magnet ingestion
- Aspirated coin in trachea

CLINICAL ISSUES

- Majority of ingestions occur < 5 years of age
- Most common symptoms
    - Asymptomatic: Witnessed ingestion or incidental finding
    - Symptomatic: Drooling, chest/neck pain, vomiting, dysphagia, cough, respiratory distress, stridor
- Treatment of esophageal coins
    - Symptomatic: Urgent endoscopic removal
    - Asymptomatic: Endoscopic removal within 24 hours; repeat radiograph prior to endoscopy
- Treatment of coins in stomach
    - Monitor stools for passage; repeat radiograph in 2 weeks
    - Endoscopic removal if not passed in 2-4 weeks; repeat radiograph prior to endoscopy
- Treatment of small bowel coins
    - Observation
    - Enteroscopy/surgical removal if symptomatic

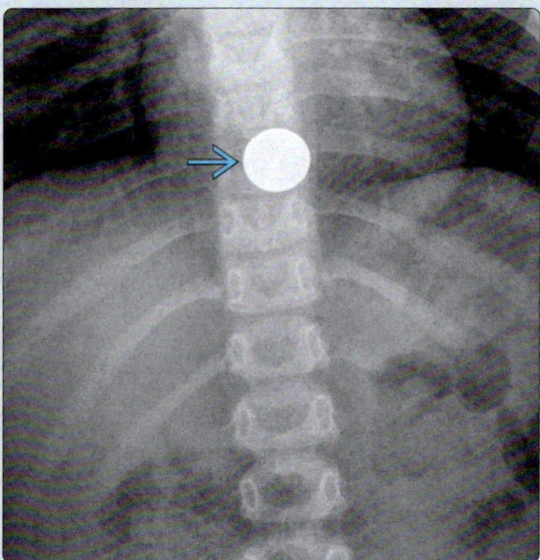

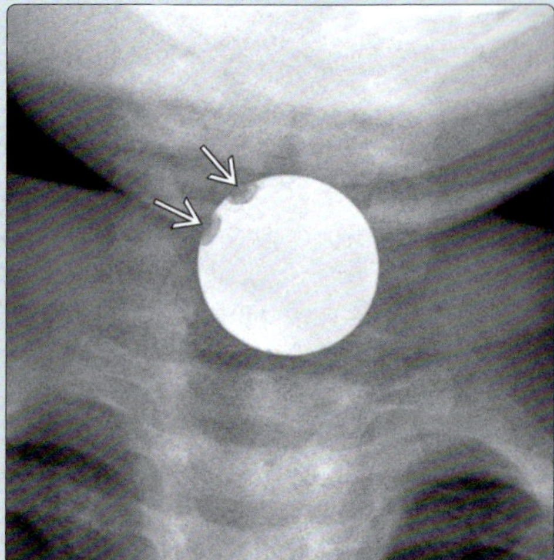

(Left) *Frontal radiograph of the upper abdomen of a 4-month-old with a witnessed ingestion of an American dime demonstrates a 19-mm metallic disc at the lower esophagus ➡. Radiographic measurements do not allow for accurate coin identification.* **(Right)** *AP radiograph shows a coin lodged in the cervical esophagus. Note that the coin is wider than the trachea, indicative of an esophageal location. The erosions ➡ are due to gastroesophageal reflux reaching a zinc-based coin.*

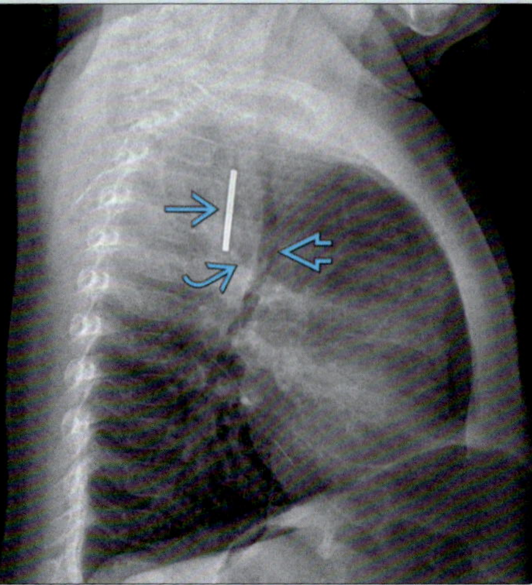

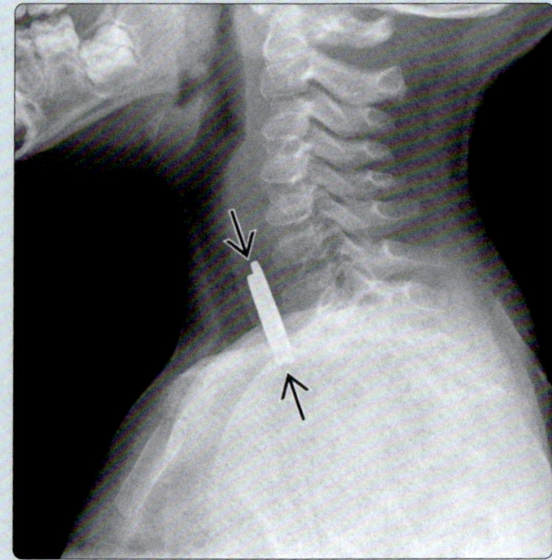

(Left) *Lateral view of the chest of a 10-month-old shows a metallic foreign body at the upper thoracic esophagus ➡ compatible with a coin. There is soft tissue thickening anteriorly ⇨, bowing the trachea ➡. Significant swelling was noted at endoscopy upon removal of a penny.* **(Right)** *Lateral airway radiograph in a 2-year-old after a witnessed ingestion shows 2 directly apposed coins ➡ projecting over the cervical esophagus at the thoracic inlet. This appearance can mimic the edge step-off of a button battery.*

IMAGING

General Features

- Location
  - Most common sites of impaction
    - Upper esophagus at thoracic inlet
    - Midesophagus at aortic arch impression
    - Lower esophageal sphincter (LES) at gastroesophageal junction
  - Other sites of impaction include pylorus, duodenum, ileocecal valve

Radiographic Findings

- Disc-shaped metallic foreign body without circumferential beveled edge/step-off/halo
- Typically seen en face (oriented in coronal plane) on frontal radiograph
- Rarely oriented in sagittal plane on frontal radiograph
- May exert mass effect on trachea secondary to size of coin or associated soft tissue swelling
- Ingestion of 2 or more coins can result in apposition that mimics button battery on tangential (usually lateral) view
  - Coins will generally be of similar density when viewed en face (usually frontal view), unlike halo margin of battery

Imaging Recommendations

- Ingested foreign body screening radiographs: Frontal views to include neck through pelvis ± lateral upper airway
- Lateral radiograph if foreign body is identified
  - Helps confirm location
    - Esophagus is much more likely than trachea
  - Helps determine type of foreign body

DIFFERENTIAL DIAGNOSIS

Button Battery Ingestion

- Disc-shaped metallic foreign body
  - Lateral view: Circumferential beveled edge/step-off
  - Frontal view: Circumferential halo or double ring sign
- Esophageal impaction requires emergent removal

Magnet Ingestion

- Metallic densities of variable shapes & sizes
- Multiple magnets or magnets with other metallic foreign bodies may attract through different bowel loops → fistulization, perforation, obstruction

Other Metallic Foreign Bodies

- Buttons, jewelry, toy parts

Aspirated Coin in Trachea

- Classic teaching that sagittally oriented coin on frontal radiograph is likely in trachea: Incorrect
  - Coin impacted in esophagus is much more likely regardless of orientation (coronal or sagittal)
  - Coin may lie in coronal or (rarely) sagittal plane in trachea or esophagus

CLINICAL ISSUES

Presentation

- Most common signs/symptoms
  - Asymptomatic: Witnessed ingestion or incidental finding
  - Symptomatic: Drooling, chest/neck pain, vomiting, dysphagia, cough, respiratory distress, stridor

Demographics

- Coin is most commonly ingested foreign body in children < 6 years old
  - Penny is most commonly ingested coin: 44%

Natural History & Prognosis

- 25-30% of esophageal coins pass spontaneously
  - Likelihood of spontaneous passage correlates with location in esophagus: Proximal 14%, middle 43%, distal 67%
- Complications are uncommon
  - Esophageal stricture, perforation, aortoesophageal or tracheoesophageal fistulas
  - Post-1982 copper-plated zinc penny is 97.5% zinc
    - Gastric acid may erode coin margins
    - Gastric acid reacts with zinc to form zinc-chloride
    - Ingestion of large number may cause zinc toxicity

Treatment

- North American Society for Pediatric Gastroenterology, Hepatology, & Nutrition (NASPGHAN) guidelines
  - Esophageal coin
    - Symptomatic: Urgent endoscopic removal
    - Asymptomatic: Endoscopic removal within 24 hours; repeat radiograph prior to endoscopy to look for interval progression
  - Gastric coin
    - Monitor stools for passage; repeat radiograph in 2 weeks
    - Endoscopic removal if not passed within 2-4 weeks
    - Repeat radiograph prior to endoscopy
  - Small bowel coin
    - Clinical observation
    - Enteroscopy/surgical removal if symptomatic
- Use of glucagon to relax LES & aid passage from esophagus is controversial: May cause vomiting & aspiration
- Fluoroscopic-guided retraction with Foley catheter may result in acute airway obstruction if coin moves into airway
- Pushing coin into stomach by dilator (bougienage) does not allow esophagus to be evaluated

SELECTED REFERENCES

1. Jacobs IN et al: Current management of aerodigestive foreign bodies in children. Semin Pediatr Surg. 30(3):151064, 2021
2. Safavi AR et al: Urgency of esophageal foreign body removal: differentiation between coins and button cell batteries. Otolaryngol Head Neck Surg. ePub, 2021
3. Orsagh-Yentis D et al: Foreign-body ingestions of young children treated in US emergency departments: 1995-2015. Pediatrics. 143(5), 2019
4. Huyett P et al: Accuracy of chest x-ray measurements of pediatric esophageal coins. Int J Pediatr Otorhinolaryngol. 113:1-3, 2018
5. Kurowski JA et al: Caustic ingestions and foreign bodies ingestions in pediatric patients. Pediatr Clin North Am. 64(3):507-24, 2017
6. Kramer RE et al: Management of ingested foreign bodies in children: a clinical report of the NASPGHAN Endoscopy Committee. J Pediatr Gastroenterol Nutr. 60(4):562-74, 2015
7. Pugmire BS et al: Review of ingested and aspirated foreign bodies in children and their clinical significance for radiologists. Radiographics. 35(5):1528-38, 2015
8. Schlesinger AE et al: Sagittal orientation of ingested coins in the esophagus in children. AJR Am J Roentgenol. 196(3):670-2, 2011
9. O'Hara SM et al: Gastric retention of zinc-based pennies: radiographic appearance and hazards. Radiology. 213(1):113-7, 1999

Ingested Button Batteries

KEY FACTS

TERMINOLOGY

- Ingestion of disc-shaped battery, typically by young child
- Esophagus is particularly susceptible to injury by lodged battery with potentially catastrophic consequences

IMAGING

- Frontal radiograph: Margin shows double halo/ring en face
- Lateral radiograph: Rim of step-off/beveled edge
- North American Society for Pediatric Gastroenterology, Hepatology, & Nutrition (NASPGHAN) imaging guidelines
  - Radiographic coverage from nasopharynx to anus
    - Lateral view at least at site of confirmed foreign body
  - After emergent removal of esophageal battery
    - CTA/MR if esophageal injury is present at endoscopy to evaluate proximity/involvement of vascular structures
      - CTA is most efficient vessel assessment
    - Esophagram to exclude leak prior to advancing diet
  - If battery is distal to esophagus, management varies based on battery size & patient age
    - Gastric location of battery at time of discovery does not exclude esophageal injury

CLINICAL ISSUES

- Caustic injury due to hydroxide radical production in tissues adjacent to negative pole (narrower side of step-off on lateral view)
- Unwitnessed ingestion is more likely to present in delayed fashion with nonspecific symptoms: Vomiting, difficulty feeding, cough, chest or abdominal pain, drooling, stridor
- ↑ risk of major complications: Unwitnessed ingestion, battery size ≥ 20 mm (majority are lithium), age < 5 years old, multiple batteries ingested
- Complications include tracheoesophageal fistula, esophageal perforation, esophageal stricture, vocal cord paralysis, aortoenteric fistula (high fatality rate)
  - Injury evolves weeks after battery removal, potentially resulting in delayed aortoenteric fistula

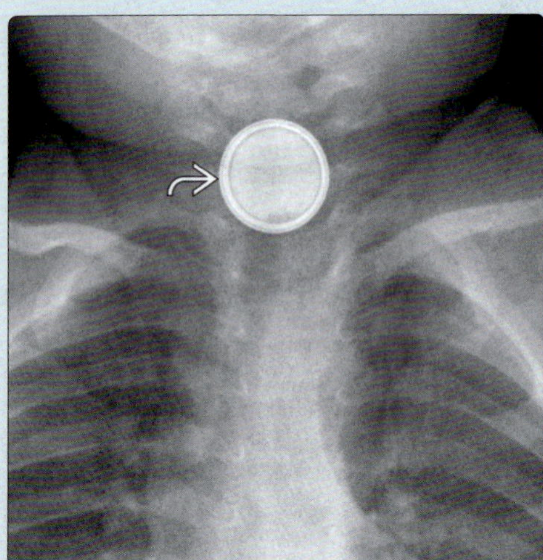

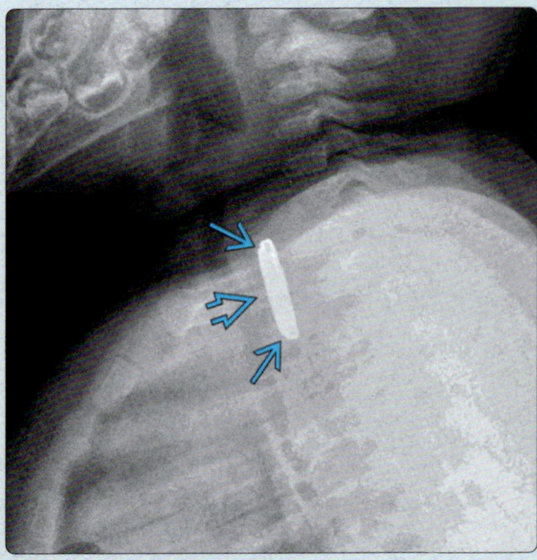

(Left) *Frontal radiograph in a 1-year-old demonstrates an ingested 23-mm, disc-shaped foreign body in the cervical esophagus above the thoracic inlet. Note the double ring/halo ➡ appearance, consistent with a button battery.* **(Right)** *Lateral radiograph in a 10-month-old with a witnessed foreign body ingestion & subsequent drooling & emesis shows the circumferential edge step-off ➡ typical of a button battery. The negative pole is the narrower anterior side ➡.*

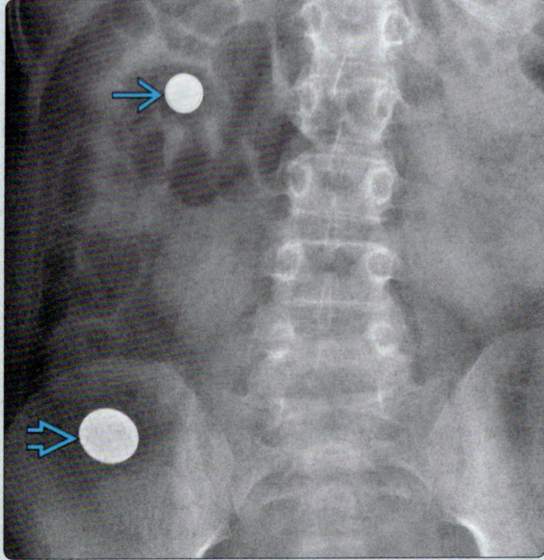

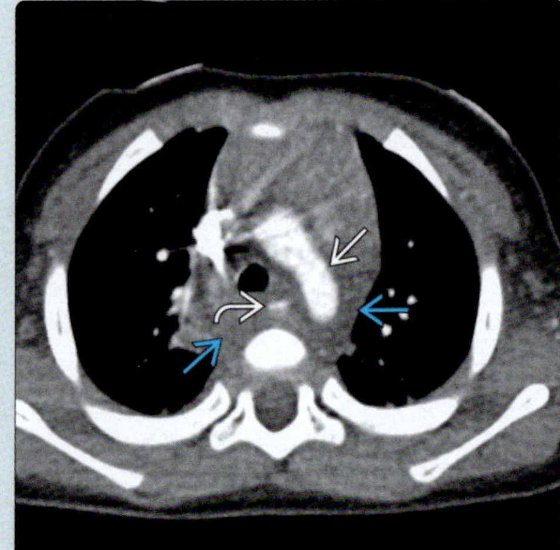

(Left) *Supine view of the abdomen in a developmentally delayed 11-year-old shows a 13-mm diameter button battery with a faint, concentric radiolucent halo ➡. Visualization of a halo is less reliable in batteries < 20 mm in size. A coin ➡ is also present.* **(Right)** *Axial CTA in a patient status post button battery removal shows marked mediastinal inflammation ➡ extending up to the aortic wall ➡ without contrast extravasation. Note the retained battery casing fragments ➡.*

IMAGING

General Features

- Most common sites of impaction in esophagus
  - Upper esophagus at thoracic inlet
  - Midesophagus at aortic arch
  - Lower esophageal sphincter at gastroesophageal (GE) junction

Radiographic Findings

- Metallic density disc of variable size
  - Size ≥ 20 mm: ↑ risk for esophageal impaction & injury
- Frontal view: Margin shows double halo/ring en face, but may not be visible if is size < 20 mm
- Lateral view: Rim of step-off/beveled edge in tangent
  - Step-off may not be visible on new thinner batteries
  - Negative pole: Narrower side on lateral view; site most likely for most severe injury
  - Soft tissue edema surrounding battery may cause anterior tracheal displacement or narrowing
- Complications may show mediastinal widening (from edema or fluid collections) &/or gas
- Metallic fragments may remain after battery removal

CT

- CTA to look for aortic/vascular injury
  - Mediastinal edema/fluid collections
  - Irregularity/outpouching or edema of aortic wall
  - Active extravasation
- No established findings are predictive of subsequent vascular catastrophes at this time

MR

- Likely more sensitive for soft tissue changes
- Multiple disadvantages relative to CTA
  - MR is not as readily available as CTA
  - MR exam time is much longer than CTA
  - Any retained metallic fragments may create MR safety &/or artifact issues

Esophagram

- Irregularity/edema of mucosa with luminal narrowing
- Leak of contrast into mediastinum or trachea
- Long-term stricturing

Imaging Recommendations

- Foreign body screening with radiographs
  - Frontal view to include neck through pelvis
  - Lateral view of upper airway with nasopharynx
  - Lateral view of foreign body site to identify negative pole & distinguish from coin
- Follow-up imaging as per NASPGHAN guidelines
  - CTA is most efficient tool to assess vessels

DIFFERENTIAL DIAGNOSIS

Coin Ingestion

- Flat metallic disc (no beveled edge or double ring sign)

Magnet Ingestion

- > 1 magnet or 1 magnet + other metallic foreign body may cause bowel injury by attraction through bowel walls

PATHOLOGY

General Features

- Lithium cell → caustic injury after impaction in esophagus
  - Mucosa contacts both poles, completes circuit
  - Electrolytic current generates hydroxide radicals in tissue adjacent to negative pole → ↑ pH
  - Injury evolves weeks after removal
- Nonlithium types injure mainly via alkaline leakage

CLINICAL ISSUES

Presentation

- Vomiting, difficulty feeding, cough, chest or abdominal pain, drooling, stridor, or asymptomatic
- Gastric location does not preclude esophageal injury
  - Gastric injury is more likely if removed > 12 hours after ingestion; may be asymptomatic

Natural History & Prognosis

- Unwitnessed ingestion accounts for 92% of associated fatalities & 56% of major outcome cases
- ↑ risk of major complications: Size ≥ 20 mm (majority are lithium), age < 5 years, multiple batteries ingested
- Major complications
  - Tracheoesophageal fistula in 48%
  - Esophageal perforation in 23%
  - Esophageal stricture in 38%
  - Vocal cord paralysis in 10%
  - Aortoenteric fistula in 46% of fatal cases (1977-2015)
    - Can occur weeks after battery removal

Treatment

- NASPGHAN guidelines are based on battery location & size, clinical stability, & patient age
  - Esophageal + stable: Immediate endoscopic removal
  - Esophageal + unstable/active bleeding: Immediate endoscopic removal in OR with surgery present
    - CTA or MR to evaluate involvement/proximity of aorta
    - Negative CTA, MR → esophagram to exclude leak
    - Injury close to aorta (≤ 3 mm) → serial CTA or MR every 5-7 days until injury recedes
  - Beyond esophagus + ≥ 20-mm battery size + < 5 years old
    - Assess for esophageal injury + endoscopic removal within 24-48 hours
    - If esophageal injury → CTA, MR
  - Beyond esophagus + < 20 mm &/or ≥ 5 years old
    - Consider outpatient observation + repeat radiograph (48 hours if ≥ 20 mm or 10-14 days if < 20 mm)
    - Endoscopic removal if GI symptoms develop or battery is not passed at time of repeat radiograph

SELECTED REFERENCES

1. Grey NEO et al: Magnetic resonance imaging findings following button battery ingestion. Pediatr Radiol. 51(10):1856-66, 2021
2. Riedesel EL et al: Serial MRI findings after endoscopic removal of button battery from the esophagus. AJR Am J Roentgenol. 215(5):1238-46, 2020
3. Pugmire BS et al: Imaging button battery ingestions and insertions in children: a 15-year single-center review. Pediatr Radiol. 47(2):178-85, 2017
4. Kramer RE et al: Management of ingested foreign bodies in children: a clinical report of the NASPGHAN Endoscopy Committee. J Pediatr Gastroenterol Nutr. 60(4):562-74, 2015

Ingested Multiple Magnets

KEY FACTS

TERMINOLOGY

- Ingestion of multiple magnets or single magnet + additional metallic foreign bodies
  - Potential for significant bowel complications
- Rare-earth magnets: 5-10x stronger than traditional magnets

IMAGING

- Metallic density foreign bodies; shapes are variable
- Magnets attract through bowel walls
  - Multiple attracted "stacked" magnets may simulate single cylindrical foreign body
- Entrapment of interposed bowel wall is suggested by
  - Gap between otherwise closely apposed magnets or magnet & adjacent metallic foreign body
  - Failure of magnet to move on sequential radiographs
- Abnormal bowel gas patterns result from complications
  - Ulceration, perforation, fistulae, obstruction, volvulus
- Foreign body ingestion radiographic series includes
  - Frontal views of neck through anus
  - ± tangential views if foreign body is identified
  - ± lateral view of upper airway

CLINICAL ISSUES

- Management depends on number of magnets, location in GI tract, & symptoms
  - Single magnet: Remove vs. follow radiographic passage
  - Multiple magnets or magnet + metal in esophagus/stomach: Endoscopic or surgical removal
  - Multiple magnets or magnet + metal beyond stomach
    - With symptoms &/or abnormal bowel gas pattern: Operative exploration with magnet removal
    - Without symptoms or abnormal bowel gas pattern: Consider careful, frequent clinical & radiographic evaluation until passage vs. removal

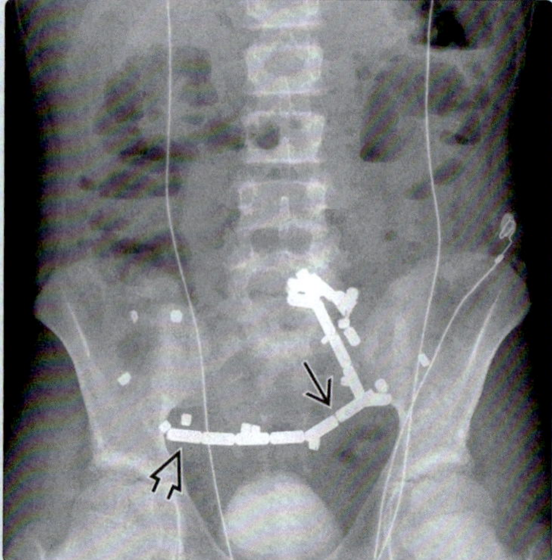

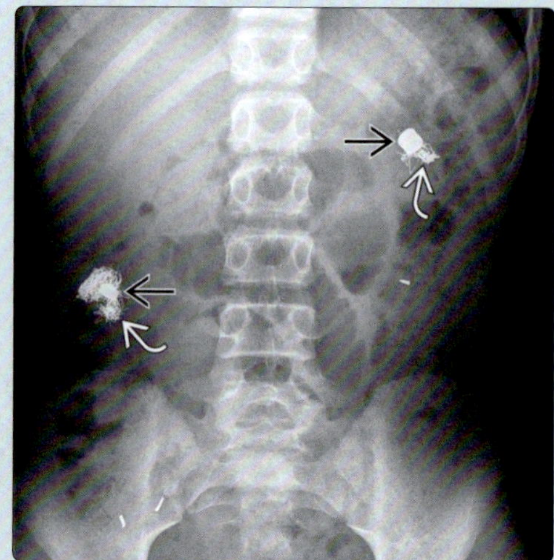

(Left) *Frontal upright radiograph of a 12-year-old autistic boy with abdominal pain & bilious emesis shows multiple rod-shaped metallic foreign bodies* ➡, *most of which appear linked. Small gaps* ➡ *between the magnets may represent entrapped intervening bowel. Numerous small bowel perforations & fistulae were found at surgery.* **(Right)** *Supine frontal radiograph shows 2 clusters of magnets* ➡, *both of which attracted additional ingested metallic foreign bodies* ➡. *Associated bowel perforations were present at surgery.*

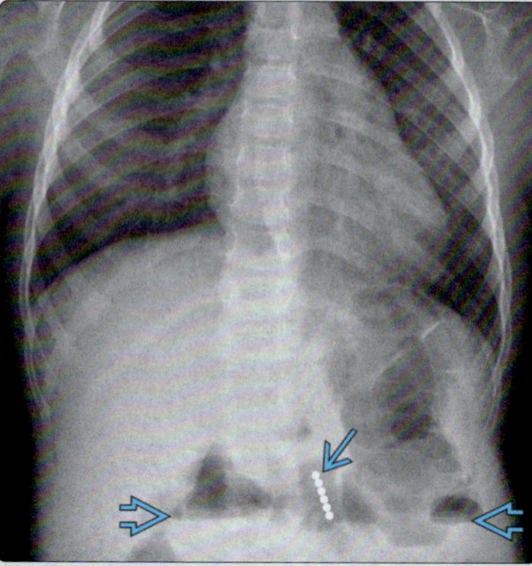

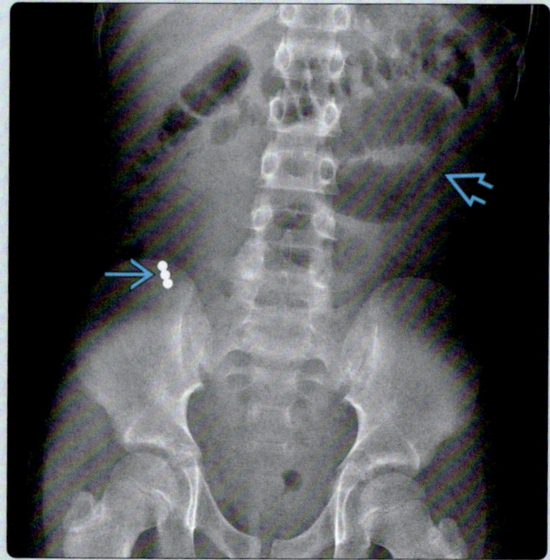

(Left) *Frontal upright radiograph in a 5-year-old shows 6 metallic densities* ➡ *in the left abdomen with scattered air-fluid levels* ➡. *The densities did not migrate over several hours. At surgery, multiple magnets were removed with identification of a jejunal perforation & a gastrojejunal fistula.* **(Right)** *Frontal supine view of a 12-year-old shows 3 metallic densities* ➡ *as well as dilated small bowel loops on the left* ➡. *A small bowel perforation caused by adherent magnets in adjacent bowel loops was seen in surgery.*

Ingested Multiple Magnets

TERMINOLOGY

Synonyms

- Postgastric magnetopathy

Definitions

- Ingestion of multiple magnets or single magnet + additional metallic foreign bodies
  - Potential for significant bowel complications due to attraction through bowel loops
- Newer rare-earth magnets are composed of iron, boron, & neodymium: 5-10x stronger than traditional magnets

IMAGING

Radiographic Findings

- Metallic density foreign bodies; variable shapes
  - Rods, discs, spheres/ball bearings, others
- May have larger nonradiopaque component
- Multiple attracted "stacked" magnets may simulate single cylindrical foreign body
  - Magnification helps delineate individual components
- Entrapment of interposed bowel wall is suggested with
  - Gap between otherwise closely apposed magnets or magnet & adjacent metallic foreign body
  - Failure of magnet to move on sequential radiographs
- Abnormal bowel gas patterns from complications
  - Ulceration, perforation, fistulae, obstruction, volvulus

Imaging Recommendations

- NASPGHAN guidelines recommend imaging if
  - Known magnet ingestion
  - Unexplained GI symptoms with rare-earth magnets in environment
- Screening foreign body ingestion radiographs
  - Frontal views from neck through anus, ± lateral view of upper airway
  - Tangential view if foreign body is identified
    - Assists in localization & characterization (such as attached metal or magnets not seen on one view)

DIFFERENTIAL DIAGNOSIS

Coin Ingestion

- Most common ingested radiopaque foreign body
- Metallic disc without beveled edge

Button Battery Ingestion

- Metallic disc with beveled edge/step-off on lateral view, double ring on frontal view
- Esophageal location requires emergent removal

PATHOLOGY

General Features

- Magnets attract to each other through bowel walls
  - Powerful rare-earth magnets attract through up to 6 bowel walls
    - Rare-earth magnets were temporarily banned from toys in USA
- Produce pressure ulcers, ischemic injury, fistulae, necrosis, perforations, &/or obstruction
  - Mucosal ulcerations may occur in < 8 hours

CLINICAL ISSUES

Presentation

- 54.7% < 5 years old
- Suspicion of magnet ingestion is critical: Only 1% of cases between 2000-2012 had witnessed ingestion [US Consumer Product Safety Commission (CPSC) data)]
- Common symptoms (single center study, 56 cases): None: 57.1%; abdominal pain/vomiting: 32.1%; choking: 10.7%

Natural History & Prognosis

- CPSC data: 72 cases in USA (2000-2012)
  - No adverse effect: 33%; > 1 perforation & necrosis: 34%; 1 perforation: 6%, ulcer: 5%, fistula: 3%, volvulus: 2%
  - Surgery: 70%; endoscopic removal: 8%; passed naturally: 21%, death: 1%

Treatment

- NASPGHAN published guideline algorithm
  - Single magnet
    - Esophagus/stomach: Remove with any risk of more ingestions or consider outpatient serial radiographs until passage is ensured
    - Beyond stomach: Removal if possible or outpatient serial radiographs until passage
  - > 1 magnet or 1 magnet + metal in esophagus/stomach
    - If < 12 hours: Pediatric GI consult for endoscopic removal
    - If > 12 hours: Consult surgery prior to endoscopic removal; surgical removal if endoscopy is unsuccessful
  - > 1 magnet or 1 magnet + metal beyond stomach
    - Consult pediatric GI & surgery
    - Symptomatic: Surgical removal
    - Asymptomatic & no obstruction/perforation on imaging
      - Entero-/colonoscopic removal or serial radiographs
      - Radiographs every 4-6 hours in emergency department
      - Progression on radiographs: Confirm passage (may educate parents & continue as outpatient)
      - No progression on radiographs: Admit → continue serial radiographs every 8-12 hours if asymptomatic or surgical/endoscopic removal
  - Parent education: No other metal or magnets near child

SELECTED REFERENCES

1. Han Y et al: Ingestion of multiple magnets in children. J Pediatr Surg. 55(10):2201-5, 2020
2. Strickland M et al: Case discussions and radiographic illustration of magnet-related injuries in children. J Emerg Med.58(6):902-9, 2020
3. Reeves PT et al: Trends of magnet ingestion in children, an ironic attraction. J Pediatr Gastroenterol Nutr. 66(5):e116-21, 2018
4. Kramer RE et al: Management of ingested foreign bodies in children: a clinical report of the NASPGHAN Endoscopy Committee. J Pediatr Gastroenterol Nutr. 60(4):562-74, 2015
5. Pugmire BS et al: Review of ingested and aspirated foreign bodies in children and their clinical significance for radiologists. Radiographics. 35(5):1528-38, 2015
6. Abbas MI et al: Magnet ingestions in children presenting to US emergency departments, 2002-2011. J Pediatr Gastroenterol Nutr. 57(1):18-22, 2013
7. De Roo AC et al: Rare-earth magnet ingestion-related injuries among children, 2000-2012. Clin Pediatr (Phila). 52(11):1006-13, 2013
8. Otjen JP et al: Imaging pediatric magnet ingestion with surgical-pathological correlation. Pediatr Radiol. 43(7):851-9, 2013

KEY FACTS

TERMINOLOGY

- Hernia: Protrusion of contents from normally encasing body cavity through normal or abnormal opening
- Inguinal hernia: Protrusion of abdominal contents through defect in inguinal region
  - Indirect inguinal hernia: Contents protrude into open deep inguinal ring, extend through patent processus vaginalis, & exit superficial inguinal ring
    - 15% of inguinal hernias are bilateral
    - In females, ovary may herniate through canal of Nuck
  - Direct inguinal hernia: Contents pass through wall of inguinal canal (due to weak abdominal musculature), exiting superficial inguinal ring
- Umbilical hernia: Contents extend into open umbilical ring
- Femoral hernia: Contents extend through femoral ring
- Littre hernia: Contains Meckel diverticulum; site varies
- Amyand hernia: Inguinal hernia contains appendix ± inflammation
- Internal hernia: Extends through defect in abdominal cavity
- Traumatic: Extends through posttraumatic abdominal wall defect
- Incarcerated hernia: Contents cannot be reduced without special maneuvers, sedation, anesthesia, or surgery
- Strangulated hernia: Contents are ischemic due to compression by hernia channel

IMAGING

- US is excellent modality to investigate palpable abnormality
  - Can characterize hernia contents & evaluate blood flow to contents & adjacent tissues
    - Bowel: Peristalsis, swirling contents, gut signature
  - Standing &/or Valsalva maneuver help reproduce reduced hernia to confirm diagnosis
- Obstructive hernia: Dilated bowel loop enters abdominal wall defect, decompressed bowel loop exits hernia defect
- Signs of strangulation: Bowel wall thickening &/or ↓ enhancement, engorged vasa recta, mesenteric stranding/fluid

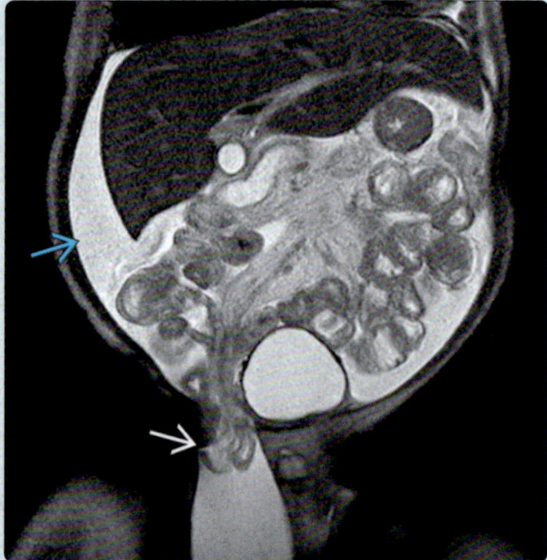

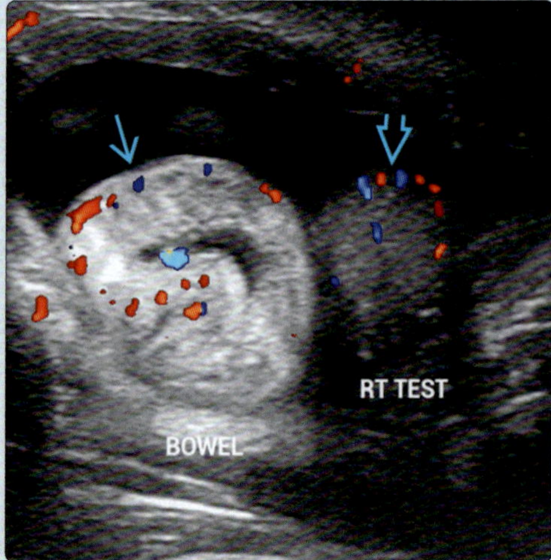

(Left) *Coronal T2 FS MR in a patient with liver failure & a large volume of ascites ➡ shows a large right inguinal hernia ➡ containing bowel & ascites.* **(Right)** *Transverse color Doppler ultrasound in the same patient shows echogenic bowel ➡ & fluid adjacent to the right testis ➡ within the scrotum. Vascular flow is visible within both the herniated bowel & the testis.*

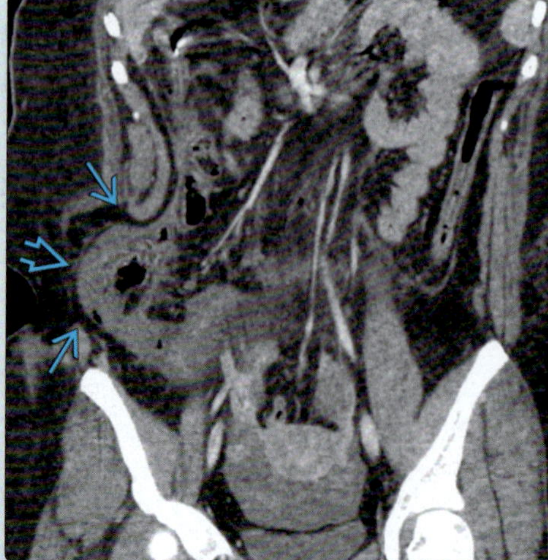

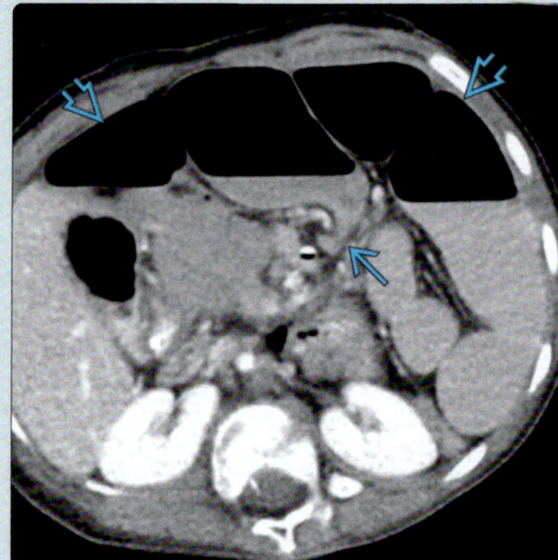

(Left) *Coronal CECT in an adolescent status post motor vehicle accident shows a large traumatic lumbar hernia ➡. The peritoneum & bowel ➡ are herniating through the defect.* **(Right)** *Axial CECT in a patient with a history of multiple surgeries shows an internal hernia with a loop of decompressed bowel ➡ extending through a small mesenteric defect. Note the multiple dilated bowel loops ➡ containing gas & fluid due to obstruction.*

TERMINOLOGY

Definitions

- Hernia: Protrusion of contents from normally encasing body cavity through normal or abnormal opening
  - Inguinal hernia: Protrusion of abdominal contents through defect in inguinal region
    - Indirect inguinal hernia: Protrusion of abdominal contents into open deep inguinal ring, through patent processus vaginalis, exiting superficial inguinal ring
      - Canal of Nuck: Term for patent processus vaginalis in females; extends into labia majoris
      - Amyand hernia: Inguinal hernia containing appendix
    - Direct inguinal hernia: Abdominal contents pass through wall of inguinal canal (due to weak abdominal musculature), exiting superficial inguinal ring
  - Umbilical hernia: Protrusion of abdominal contents through open umbilical ring
  - Femoral hernia: Protrusion of abdominal contents through femoral ring
  - Littre hernia: Hernia contains Meckel diverticulum
  - Internal hernia: Hernia through fossa or foramen within abdominal cavity
    - Defect associated with internal hernia can be congenital or acquired
  - Traumatic: Hernia through traumatic abdominal wall defect
- Incarcerated hernia: Hernia in which contents cannot be reduced without special maneuvers, sedation, anesthesia, or surgery
- Strangulated hernia: Hernia in which contents become ischemic due to vascular compression by hernia channel

Associations

- Indirect inguinal hernia: Prematurity
- Umbilical hernia: Prematurity, Down syndrome, Beckwith-Wiedemann syndrome
- Acquired internal hernia: Abdominal surgery requiring Roux-en-Y reconstruction
- Recent repair of large congenital hernia: Omphalocele, gastroschisis, diaphragmatic hernia
  - ↑ intraabdominal pressure status post reduction of abdominal contents + defect repair can lead to recurrent or new hernias

IMAGING

General Features

- Best diagnostic clue
  - Protrusion of abdominal contents through defect in abdominal wall
- Location
  - Inguinal hernia: Extends to labia or scrotum
    - 60% of inguinal hernias occur on right side
    - 15% of inguinal hernias are bilateral
  - Umbilical hernia: Extends into umbilicus
  - Femoral hernia: Extends into femoral ring, lateral to lacunar ligament
    - More common on right side
  - Littre hernia: Occurs with inguinal (50%), umbilical (30%), & femoral (20%) hernias
  - Traumatic hernia: Right lower abdomen, lateral to rectus sheath
  - Left paraduodenal hernia: To left of inferior mesenteric vein & 4th duodenum within left mesocolon
- Size
  - Abdominal wall defect can vary in size from < 5 mm to > 10 cm depending on location, size of patient, & type of hernia

Radiographic Findings

- Signs of obstruction with dilated, air-filled loops of bowel & multiple air-fluid levels
- Inguinal hernia: Soft tissue or air-filled mass extending beyond pelvis inferiorly
- Umbilical hernia: Round soft tissue or air-filled mass within umbilicus
  - Best seen on cross-table lateral view

Fluoroscopic Findings

- Small bowel follow-through
  - Contrast entering loop of bowel within hernia
  - Obstructive hernia: Dilated loop of bowel entering abdominal wall defect & decompressed loop of bowel exiting hernia defect

CT Findings

- Protrusion of abdominal contents through defect in abdominal wall
- Obstructive hernia: Dilated loop of bowel entering abdominal wall defect & decompressed loop of bowel exiting hernia defect
- Signs of impending strangulation: Free fluid within hernia, bowel wall thickening, or luminal dilation
- Signs of strangulation: Bowel wall thickening, ↓ enhancement of bowel wall, engorged vasa recta, & mesenteric stranding
- Internal hernia: Cluster of small bowel loops, stretched mesenteric vessels
  - Left paraduodenal hernia: Bowel between stomach & pancreas or transverse colon
    - Bowel may appear to be contained by sac
    - Superior/anterior displacement of inferior mesenteric vein
- Traumatic hernia: Defect in abdominal musculature with soft tissue stranding ± injury of abdominal organs

Ultrasonographic Findings

- Inguinal hernia: Abdominal contents entering scrotum or labia
  - Confirm bowel presence with peristalsis, visualization of swirling bowel contents, gut signature in bowel wall
  - Use color Doppler to confirm blood flow to bowel
  - In females, may see herniated ovary
  - In male neonates, may see ↓ to absent color Doppler flow to ipsilateral testis

Imaging Recommendations

- Best imaging tool
  - Diagnosis is often based on clinical exam
  - US is used to diagnose etiology of unknown abdominal bulges

- Standing or Valsalva maneuver helps reproduce reduced hernia (by forcing abdominal contents through abdominal defect)
- Can characterize hernia contents
- Can evaluate blood supply to hernia contents & adjacent tissues compressed by hernia
- CT is useful to diagnose etiology of obstruction or abdominal pain

DIFFERENTIAL DIAGNOSIS

Hydrocele

- Can communicate through inguinal hernia defect
- May be confined to spermatic cord or extend into scrotum
  - Fluctuant mass of inguinal canal or scrotum
  - ↑ transillumination
  - ↑ in size late in day or during viral infection

Omphalocele

- Congenital midline abdominal wall defect into base of umbilicus
- Herniated contents are covered by sac

CLINICAL ISSUES

Presentation

- Most common signs/symptoms
  - Hernia: Painless easily reducible bulge
  - Incarcerated hernia: Hernia is not easily reduced
  - Obstructed hernia: Vomiting, abdominal distention
  - Strangulated hernia: Pain, peritonitis, shock

Demographics

- Age
  - Inguinal hernia: Occurs at any age; ↑ incidence in premature infants
  - Femoral hernia: Most commonly occurs 5-10 years
  - Umbilical hernia: Most common in infants & toddlers
    - 75% of infants < 1,500 g have umbilical hernia
  - Traumatic hernia: Mean age = 9.5 years
- Sex
  - Inguinal hernia: 9-10x more common in males
  - Femoral hernia: During childhood, slightly more common in males
    - In adults, femoral hernias are more common in females
  - Traumatic hernia: More common in males due to high-risk activities
- Ethnicity
  - Umbilical hernias are more common in children of African descent
- Epidemiology
  - Indirect inguinal hernias
    - Inguinal hernias in 0.8-4.4% of children
      - 13% of infants born < 32 weeks & 30% of infants weighing < 1,000 g will have inguinal hernia
    - Risk for inguinal hernia becoming incarcerated is ↑ in early infancy
      - 10-30% become incarcerated in premature infants
      - Up to 15% become incarcerated in older children
    - Inguinal hernia repair is one of most frequently performed surgeries in children
    - Incarcerated inguinal hernia is 2nd most common cause of bowel obstruction after postsurgical adhesions
  - Direct inguinal hernia
    - Accounts for 2-5% of groin hernias in children
  - Femoral hernias
    - Rare in children
    - Accounts for 0.1-1.1% of groin hernias
    - Become incarcerated in 15-20% of patients
    - Majority contain properitoneal fat
  - Umbilical hernia
    - 10-20% of all infants are born with umbilical hernia
  - Littre hernia
    - 0.3-0.8% of all hernias contain Meckel diverticulum
  - Amyand hernia
    - Appendix found in inguinal hernia in 1% at operation
    - Accompanied by acute appendicitis in 0.1%
  - Internal hernia
    - Left paraduodenal hernia is most common type of congenital internal hernia
  - Traumatic hernia
    - May be caused by bicycle handle bar injury

Natural History & Prognosis

- Indirect inguinal hernia occurs with patent processus vaginalis
  - 40% of patent processus vaginalis close during 1st months of life
  - 20% of boys have patent processus vaginalis at 2 years of age
  - Contralateral patent processus vaginalis in ~ 20%
    - Can lead to contralateral hernia in 3-15% of patients

Treatment

- Surgery is performed to treat most types of hernia due to risk of incarceration
- Umbilical hernia has low risk of incarceration
  - 90% of umbilical hernias close spontaneously before 6 years of age
  - Surgery is performed to close large hernias or hernias that fail to spontaneously close
- Complications of inguinal hernia repair include recurrence, infection, testicular atrophy, injury to vas deferens, & infertility

SELECTED REFERENCES

1. Halleran DR et al: Association between age and umbilical hernia repair outcomes in children: a multistate population-based cohort study. J Pediatr. 217:125-30.e4, 2020
2. Almeflh W et al: A systematic review of current consensus on timing of operative repair versus spontaneous closure for asymptomatic umbilical hernias in pediatric. Med Arch. 73(4):268-71, 2019
3. Namgoong JM et al: Reliability of preoperative inguinal sonography for evaluating patency of processus vaginalis in pediatric inguinal hernia patients. Int J Med Sci. 16(2):247-52, 2019
4. Zeng K et al: Female reproductive structures found in inguinal hernia sacs: a retrospective review. J Pediatr Surg. 54(10):2134-7, 2019
5. Cigsar EB et al: Amyand's hernia: 11 years of experience. J Pediatr Surg. 51(8):1327-9, 2016
6. Orth RC et al: Acute testicular ischemia caused by incarcerated inguinal hernia. Pediatr Radiol. 42(2):196-200, 2012
7. Rathore A et al: Traumatic abdominal wall hernias: an emerging trend in handlebar injuries. J Pediatr Surg. 47(7):1410-3, 2012
8. Brandt ML: Pediatric hernias. Surg Clin North Am. 88(1):27-43, vii-viii, 2008

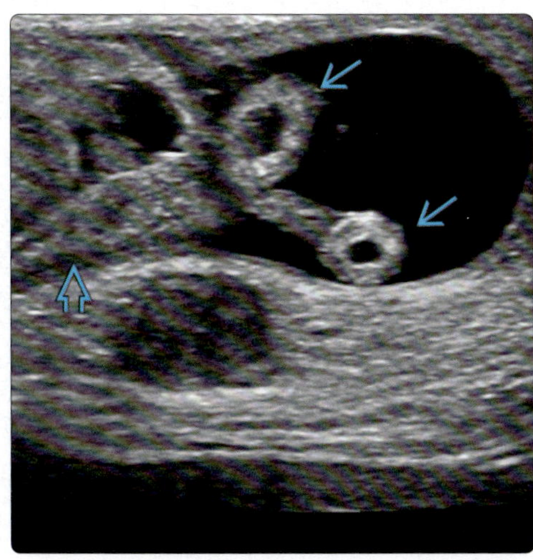

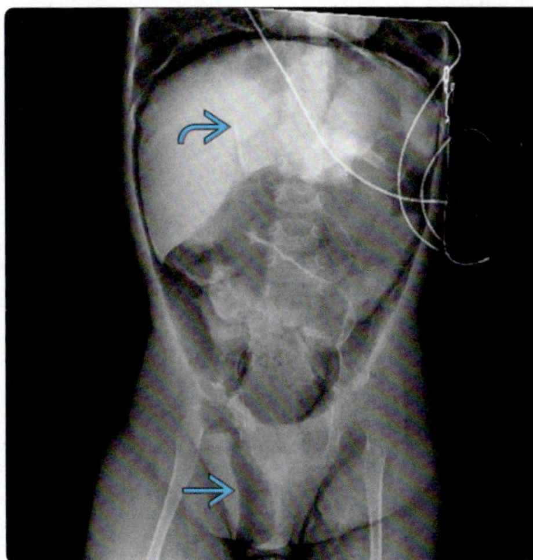

(Left) *Longitudinal ultrasound of the scrotum shows bowel ➡ & the appendix ➡ extending into the hernia, consistent with an Amyand hernia.* **(Right)** *AP radiograph of the abdomen in a young child with a large volume of intraperitoneal free air shows air extending through a right inguinal hernia ➡. Note that the falciform ligament ➡ is visible, one of the multiple different signs of intraperitoneal free air on this radiograph.*

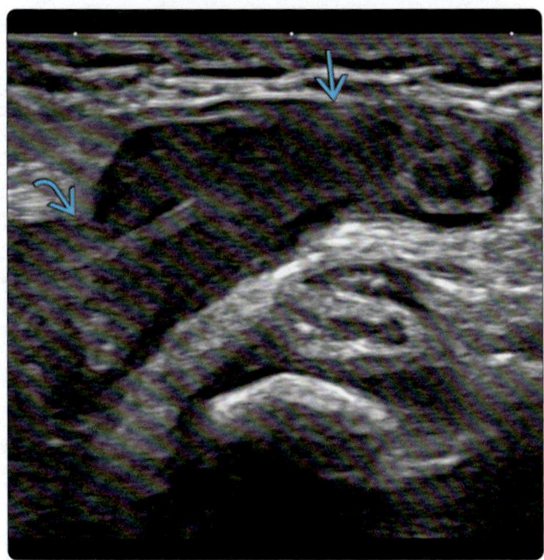

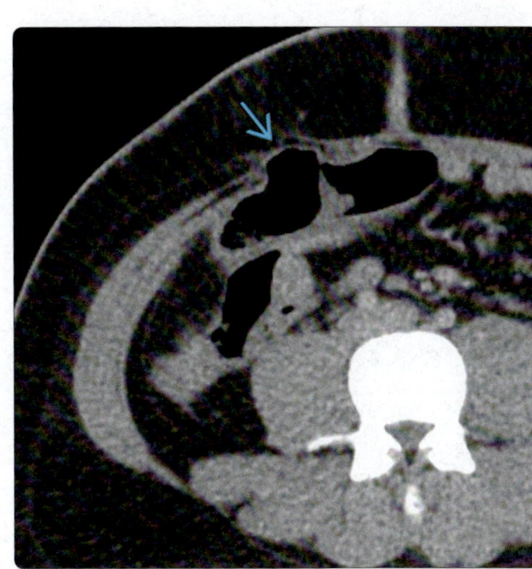

(Left) *Longitudinal ultrasound of the groin in an adolescent girl shows a left inguinal hernia ➡ containing the left ovary ➡. This is termed a hernia of the canal of Nuck. The ovary may rarely torse in this scenario.* **(Right)** *Axial NECT in a patient with a history of a prior ostomy shows a Richter hernia ➡ at the site of the prior surgical defect.*

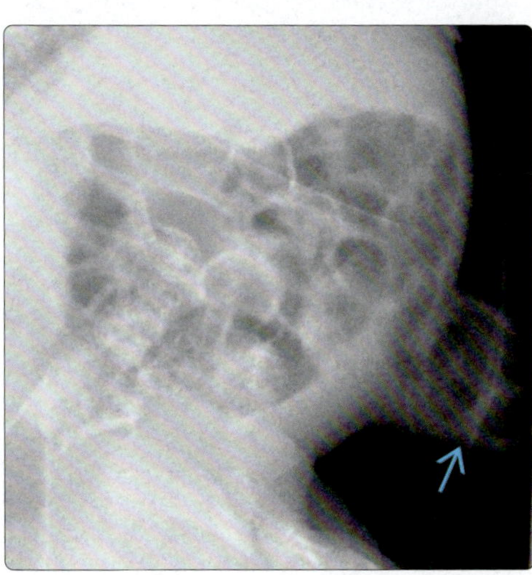

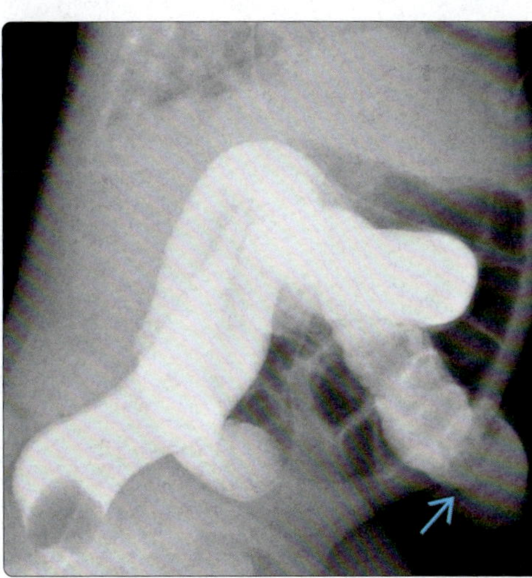

(Left) *Lateral radiograph of the abdomen shows a large umbilical hernia ➡ containing bowel.* **(Right)** *Lateral image from a water-soluble contrast enema in the same patient shows extension of the contrast-filled colon ➡ into the large umbilical hernia.*

Omphalocele

KEY FACTS

TERMINOLOGY

- Midline abdominal wall defect (AWD) with visceral extrusion into umbilical cord base
- AWD < 5 cm wide: Minor or small; > 5 cm: Giant

IMAGING

- Extruded abdominal contents are contained by round, membranous sac
  - Umbilical cord inserts on sac
- Small bowel & liver are more frequently herniated than spleen, stomach, bladder, colon, or gonads
- Bowel malrotation in virtually all cases
  - Postrepair risk of midgut volvulus is higher than gastroschisis as sac prevents bowel inflammation that incites "protective" adhesions
- Prenatal US/MR defines AWD location, size, covering, contents, & associated anomalies
- Postnatal radiographs demonstrate sac, which may contain gas-filled bowel loops

TOP DIFFERENTIAL DIAGNOSES

- Gastroschisis
- Umbilical hernia
- Bladder exstrophy
- Limb-body wall complex

PATHOLOGY

- High rates of associated structural & chromosomal anomalies: Beckwith-Wiedemann syndrome, OEIS complex, pentalogy of Cantrell, trisomy 18 > 21, 13; many others

CLINICAL ISSUES

- Repair technique & timing depend on size, contents, patient stability, & other anomalies
- With isolated omphalocele, survival of 75-95%
- Poor prognosis with
  - Associated structural &/or chromosomal abnormalities
  - Omphalocele rupture
  - Pulmonary hypoplasia

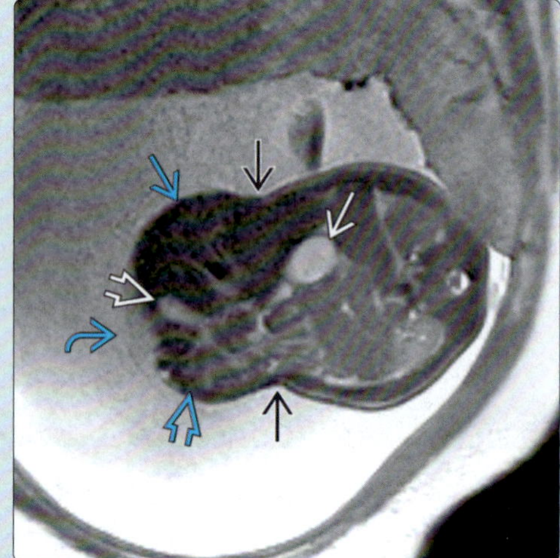

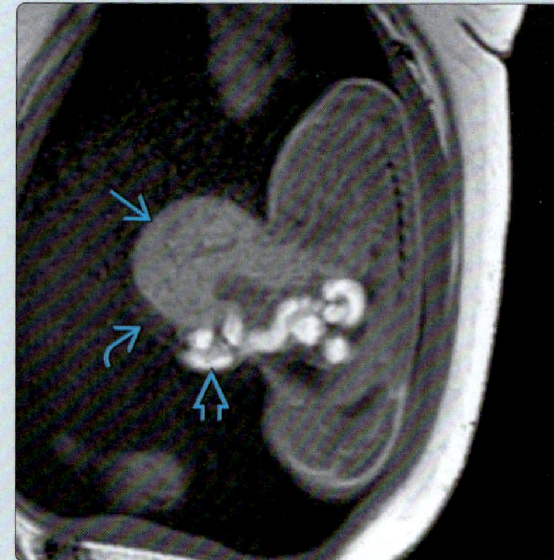

(Left) *Axial T2 SSFSE MR in a 34-weeks-gestation fetus shows a large abdominal wall defect (AWD) ➡ resulting in a giant omphalocele ➡ containing most of the liver ➡, gallbladder ➡, & bowel ➡ but not stomach ➡. The umbilical cord could be seen inserting on the sac on other images (not shown).* **(Right)** *Sagittal T1 MR in the same fetus shows the liver ➡ & meconium-containing bowel ➡ herniated through the AWD but covered by a membrane ➡.*

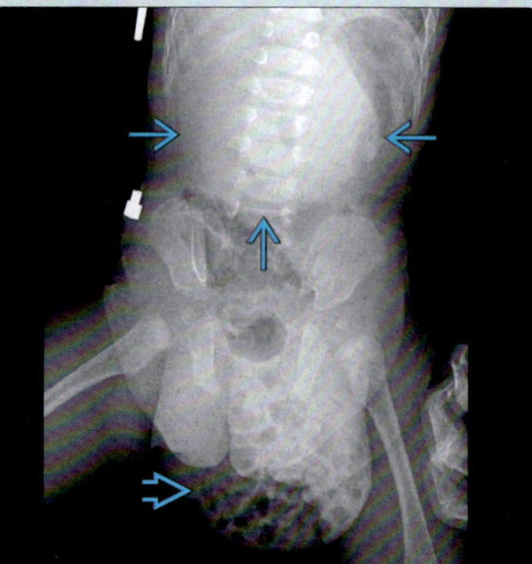

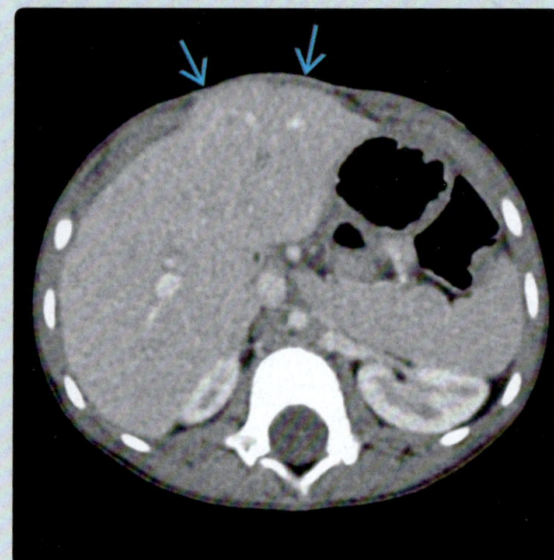

(Left) *AP radiograph in a 6-month-old shows a giant omphalocele ➡ that is undergoing sclerosis & epithelialization of the membrane ("paint & wait") after partial mesh closure. Note the large left inguinal hernia containing bowel ➡.* **(Right)** *Axial CECT in the same patient at 33 months of age shows a relatively ↓ size of the omphalocele, which is now skin-covered ➡. The liver has largely been incorporated into the abdomen at this point.*

TERMINOLOGY

Synonyms

- Exomphalos

Definitions

- Midline abdominal wall defect (AWD) with visceral extrusion into umbilical cord base

IMAGING

General Features

- Best diagnostic clue
  - Extruded abdominal contents are contained by sac
    - Small bowel & liver are more frequently herniated than spleen, stomach, bladder, colon, or gonads
  - Umbilical cord inserts on sac
- Size
  - AWD < 5 cm wide: Minor or small
    - Chromosomal abnormalities are more likely
    - Higher rate of intestinal, brain anomalies
  - AWD > 5 cm wide: Giant
    - Usually contains liver
    - Higher rate of cardiac, renal, pulmonary anomalies

Radiographic Findings

- Round mass protruding from abdominal midline
  - Gas-containing bowel may be seen in sac
- Giant omphalocele may lead to pulmonary hypoplasia
  - Pneumothorax, bell-shaped chest
- Ruptured omphalocele
  - Extruded bowel loops ± other viscera without sac
- Wide variety of associated anomalies

Fluoroscopic Findings

- Bowel malrotation in virtually all cases
  - Normal fixation never occurs for herniated bowel
  - Postrepair adhesions are not as frequent as gastroschisis (as covered/unexposed bowel not inflamed)
    - Risk of midgut volvulus may be greater

Ultrasonographic Findings

- Grayscale ultrasound
  - Prenatal scans
    - Transient physiologic bowel herniation into umbilical cord occurs before 12-weeks gestation
    - Omphalocele is confirmed with
      - Herniation of stomach or liver (not physiologic)
      - Bowel in umbilical cord > 12 weeks
    - Omphalocele circumference:abdominal circumference ratio (OC:AC) may predict type of surgical closure required
- Pulsed Doppler
  - Postnatal abdominal Doppler may be useful during reduction of abdominal viscera to evaluate flow
    - Abnormal high-resistance visceral waveforms are seen with ↑ abdominal pressures (i.e., compartment syndrome)

MR Findings

- Fetal MR is useful to
  - Characterize sac contents + associated anomalies
  - Calculate lung volumes to predict pulmonary hypoplasia

Imaging Recommendations

- Best imaging tool
  - Prenatal US detects & characterizes AWD (location, size, contents, covering)

DIFFERENTIAL DIAGNOSIS

Gastroschisis

- Small AWD to right (rarely left) of umbilical cord insertion
- No membrane covering herniated bowel loops
  - Chronic exposure to amniotic fluid → inflammation → dysmotility, adhesions
- Extruded contents are limited to bowel, stomach
  - Liver involvement is extremely rare
- Additional anomalies in < 20%
  - Intestinal atresias are most common

Umbilical Hernia

- Small (< 2 cm), skin-covered midline AWD
- May contain bowel or omentum

Bladder Exstrophy

- Lower AWD with superficial soft tissue mass (exposed bladder surface), wide pubic symphysis
- No normal bladder is visualized prenatally despite normal amniotic fluid

Limb-Body Wall Complex

- Lethal malformation complex
  - Large AWD with extruded abdominal viscera fused to placenta or uterine wall
  - Scoliosis, limb abnormalities, short umbilical cord

PATHOLOGY

General Features

- Genetics
  - Most cases are sporadic
  - Familial omphalocele is rare
    - Autosomal dominant or X-linked recessive trait
  - Chromosomal abnormalities in 30-50%
    - Trisomy 18 is most common
    - Less likely with larger, liver-containing AWD
- Associated abnormalities
  - Additional structural anomalies: 54-88%
    - More likely overall if omphalocele contains liver
    - Additional intestinal anomalies (especially Meckel diverticulum, intestinal atresias) & brain anomalies are more likely in small omphaloceles
  - Genitourinary anomalies: Up to 40%
    - Bladder exstrophy, cloacal exstrophy
    - Ureteropelvic junction obstruction, renal ectopia, solitary kidney, cryptorchidism
    - Prune-belly syndrome
  - Gastrointestinal anomalies: Up to 40%
    - Tracheoesophageal fistula, imperforate anus, absent gallbladder, enteric duplication, intestinal atresia, Meckel diverticulum
      - 7:1 likelihood of Meckel diverticulum in small vs. giant omphaloceles
  - Respiratory insufficiency

- Pulmonary hypoplasia with giant omphaloceles
  - Impaired diaphragm & thoracic cage development
  - Oligohydramnios occurs if fluid accumulates in omphalocele sac from bladder anomaly
- Congenital heart disease: Up to 50%
  - Septal defects, transposition, ectopia, tetralogy of Fallot, absent inferior vena cava
- Musculoskeletal anomalies: Up to 42%
  - Clubfoot, polydactyly, limb deficiency, rib anomalies
  - Scoliosis, vertebral abnormalities
  - Lymphatic malformation
- CNS anomalies: Up to 33%
  - Encephalocele, holoprosencephaly, cerebellar hypoplasia, myelomeningocele, anencephaly
- Specific associated syndromes
  - Beckwith-Wiedemann syndrome in 5-10%
    - Omphalocele, macroglossia, visceromegaly, hypoglycemia, embryonal tumors (hepatoblastoma, Wilms tumor)
  - OEIS complex (1:200,000 live births)
    - Omphalocele, exstrophy of cloaca/bladder, imperforate anus, spinal defects
  - Pentalogy of Cantrell
    - Cardiac anomalies, omphalocele, & defects of diaphragm, pericardium, sternum → often results in ectopia cordis
- Embryology
  - Failure of central migration of lateral mesodermal body folds in early gestation
  - Additional failure of migration of cephalic mesodermal folds: Ectopia cordis

Gross Pathologic & Surgical Features

- Omphalocele membrane is composed of peritoneum + amnion + intervening Wharton jelly
- Covered AWD protects bowel from inflammation, dilation
- Larger relative size of this AWD makes in utero vascular insults to bowel unlikely

CLINICAL ISSUES

Presentation

- Most common signs/symptoms
  - Detected by prenatal ultrasound
- Other signs/symptoms
  - ↑ maternal serum α-fetoprotein (70%)

Demographics

- Epidemiology
  - Incidence: 2-4.4/10,000
    - Multigestation:singleton pregnancies = 3:1

Natural History & Prognosis

- Premature birth in up to 42%
- Survival is 75-95% with normal chromosomes & no other anomalies
- Overall survival beyond neonatal period
  - Small/minor: Up to 92%; giant: Up to 67%
- Poor prognosis with
  - Associated structural or chromosomal abnormalities: Mortality of 80-100%
  - Omphalocele rupture
  - Pulmonary hypoplasia

Treatment

- Fetus: Amniocentesis for karyotype; no intervention
- Birth: Delivery at tertiary facility
  - C-section for giant omphalocele to prevent dystocia, rupture
  - Respiratory support in giant omphalocele patients with pulmonary hypoplasia → pneumothorax, respiratory distress
  - Sac is covered to prevent fluid & heat loss, stabilized to prevent rupture
    - Urgent repair is not indicated unless sac ruptures
- Repair goal: Return viscera to abdomen with skin & fascial coverage
  - Abdominal compartment syndrome (ACS) develops if viscera are returned too quickly, causing ↑ intraabdominal pressures with impaired visceral blood flow, hypotension, respiratory distress (↓ diaphragm motion)
- Small/minor omphalocele: Initial direct repair
  - If bladder pressure ↑ intraoperatively by visceral reduction then temporizing measures are required to prevent ACS
    - Synthetic graft; skin-only closure; silo reduction
- Giant: Treatment is controversial, more complex
  - Staged: Gradual reduction by silo with gravity vs. synthetic graft + ↑ compression
  - Nonoperative (best for unstable patients): Topical agents promote epithelialization of sac (over ~ 3 months), which gradually incorporates to abdominal cavity
    - Subsequent hernia repair is required
- Postrepair issues
  - Pulmonary dysfunction
  - Inguinal or ventral hernia
  - Gastroesophageal reflux
    - May account for associated feeding intolerance as bowel functions normally
  - Complications of malrotation
    - Midgut volvulus risk is > repaired gastroschisis patients due to lack of bowel inflammation (which incites "protective" adhesions)

DIAGNOSTIC CHECKLIST

Consider

- Omphalocele is often associated with structural &/or chromosomal anomalies

SELECTED REFERENCES

1. Revels JW et al: An algorithmic approach to complex fetal abdominal wall defects. AJR Am J Roentgenol. 214(1):218-31, 2020
2. Chock VY et al: Prenatally diagnosed omphalocele: characteristics associated with adverse neonatal outcomes. J Perinatol. 39(8):1111-7, 2019
3. Peters NCJ et al: The validity of the viscero-abdominal disproportion ratio for type of surgical closure in all fetuses with an omphalocele. Prenat Diagn. 39(12):1070-9, 2019
4. Victoria T et al: Fetal anterior abdominal wall defects: prenatal imaging by magnetic resonance imaging. Pediatr Radiol. 48(4):499-512, 2018
5. Abdelhafeez AH et al: The risk of volvulus in abdominal wall defects. J Pediatr Surg. 50(4):570-2, 2015
6. Gamba P et al: Abdominal wall defects: prenatal diagnosis, newborn management, and long-term outcomes. Semin Pediatr Surg. 23(5):283-90, 2014

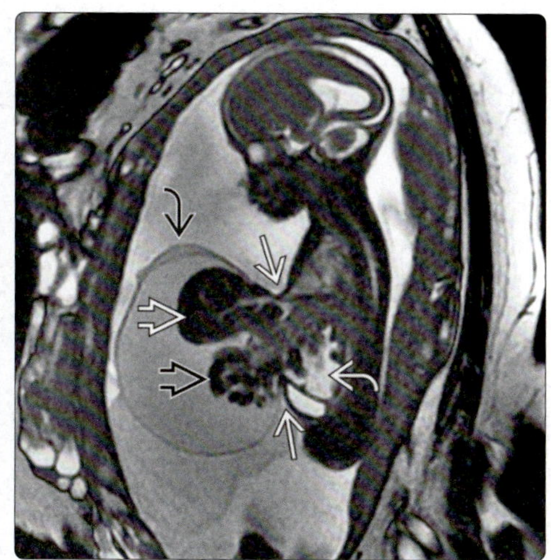

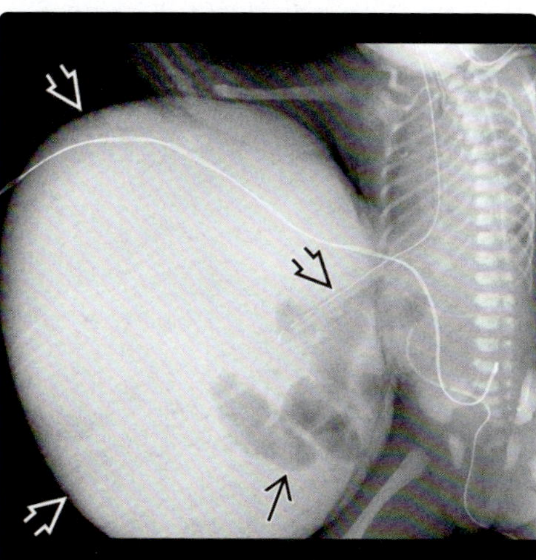

(Left) *Sagittal SSFP MR in a 23-weeks-gestation fetus shows a large midline AWD ➡ with herniation of the entire liver ➡ & much of the bowel ➡ into a large sac ➡, consistent with a giant omphalocele. Ascites is noted in the fetal abdomen ➡ as well as the sac.* **(Right)** *Oblique radiograph in the same patient after delivery shows the giant omphalocele sac ➡ containing the decompressed stomach ➡ & multiple gas-distended small bowel loops ➡.*

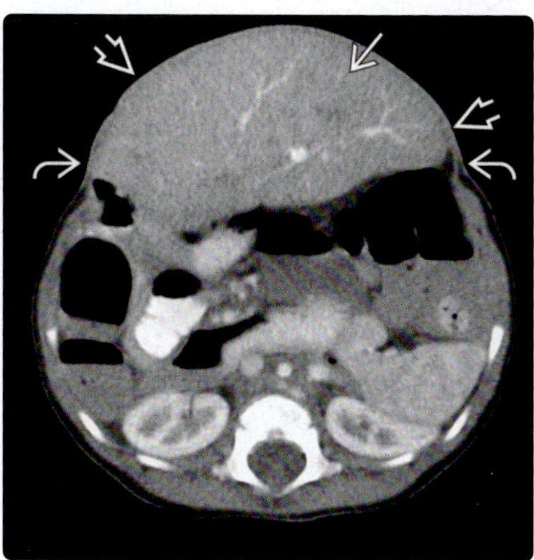

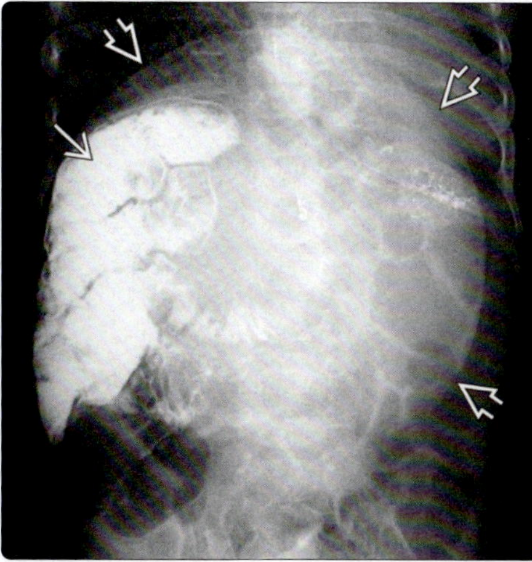

(Left) *Axial CECT of an 18-month-old shows a giant omphalocele that has been closed by epithelialization (without fascia or muscle). There is continued protrusion of the liver ➡ into the abdominal wall defect ➡ (which is covered by skin ➡).* **(Right)** *Frontal upper GI series 10-minute image in the same patient shows proximal small bowel loops in the right abdomen ➡, typical of abnormal bowel fixation (i.e., malrotation) in these patients. The large abdominal protuberance ➡ is clearly visible.*

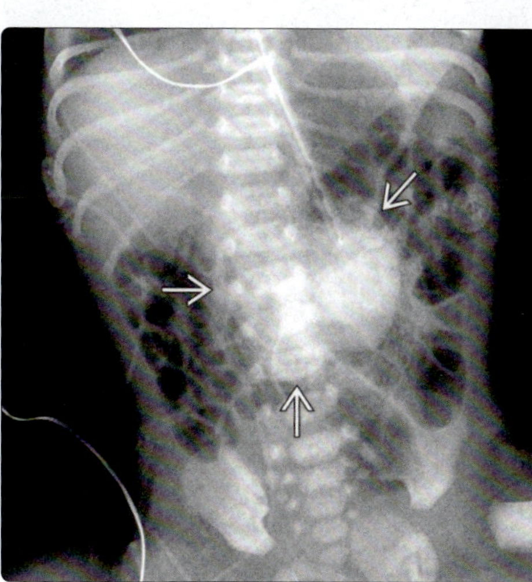

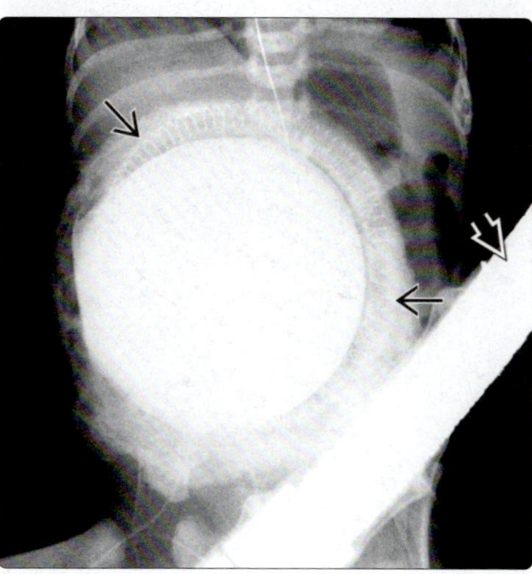

(Left) *AP radiograph in a newborn shows a lobular density ➡ overlying the central abdomen at the expected site of the umbilicus, corresponding to a small omphalocele. This protuberant mass is larger than the rounded opacity seen with an umbilical hernia.* **(Right)** *AP radiograph shows a silo enclosing a ruptured omphalocele. Note the characteristic appearances of the intraabdominal metallic coiled spring ➡ at the base of the silo as well as the overlying bar ➡ from which the silo bag is suspended.*

Gastroschisis

KEY FACTS

TERMINOLOGY

- Congenital abdominal wall defect (AWD) lateral (usually to right) of normal umbilicus
  - Bowel herniates freely into amniotic cavity without sac
- Simple gastroschisis (majority): No bowel complications
- Complex gastroschisis (10-20%): Presence of bowel atresia, necrosis, &/or perforation

IMAGING

- Prenatal: Dilated bowel & polyhydramnios in complex cases
- Postnatal: Upper GI & small bowel follow-through after repair shows malrotation ± dysmotile dilated loops, obstruction, short gut

TOP DIFFERENTIAL DIAGNOSES

- Omphalocele
- Limb-body wall complex
- Cloacal exstrophy
- Amniotic band syndrome

PATHOLOGY

- Additional anomalies in up to 20%
  - Intestinal atresias are most common
- AWD may cause prenatal bowel injury
  - Chronic irritation by exposure to amniotic fluid → dysmotility, adhesions
  - Constriction at AWD → vascular injury with atresia, volvulus, necrosis, perforation
- Postrepair bowel insults
  - Necrotizing enterocolitis, hernias, obstruction by adhesions
  - Not at risk of midgut volvulus despite malrotation

CLINICAL ISSUES

- At delivery, herniated bowel is inflamed in ~ 33%
- Treatments include immediate primary repair vs. gradual bowel reduction with preformed silo to prevent compartment syndrome
- Overall infant survival > 90% (but ↓ in complex forms)

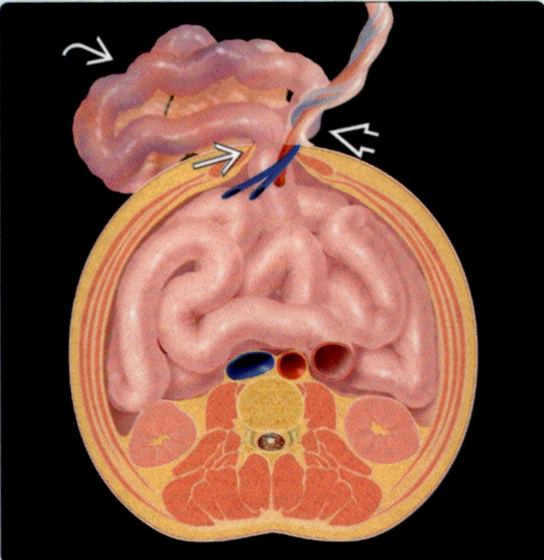

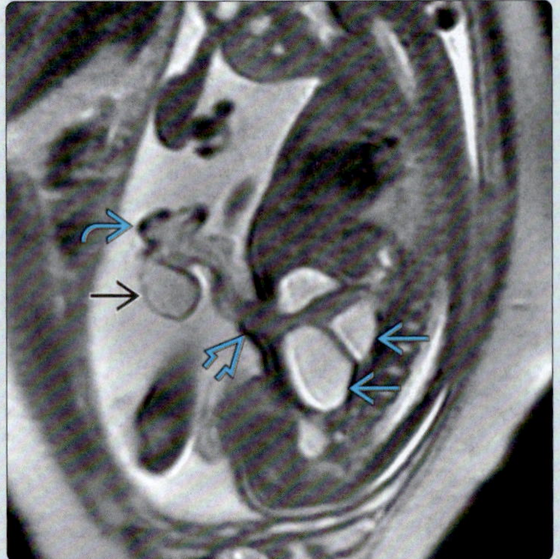

(Left) *Axial graphic shows a small abdominal wall defect (AWD) ➡ to the right of the umbilicus ➡ with herniation of bowel loops ➡. No covering membrane is seen. These features are typical of gastroschisis.* **(Right)** *Sagittal SSFSE T2 MR in a 31-weeks-gestation fetus shows a small AWD ➡ right of the umbilical cord insertion (not shown). Small-caliber, meconium-containing bowel ➡ protrudes with a cystic lesion ➡ into the amniotic fluid. Several dilated proximal small bowel loops ➡ remain in the abdomen.*

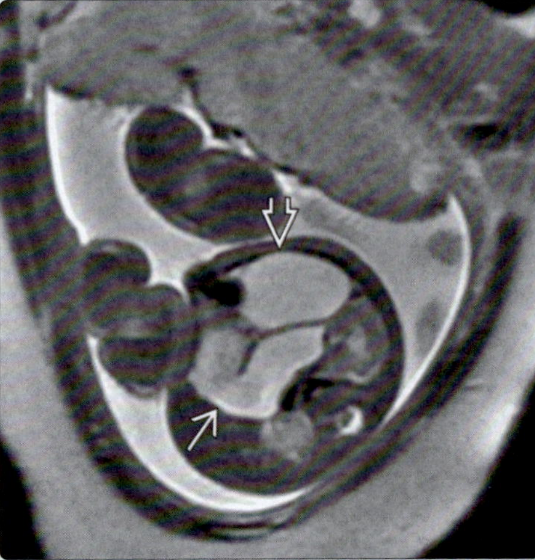

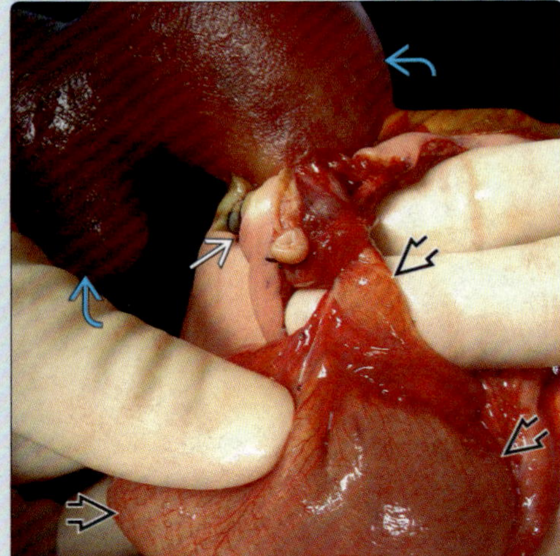

(Left) *Axial SSFSE T2 MR in the same patient shows dilated intraabdominal duodenum ➡ & proximal jejunum ➡.* **(Right)** *Intraoperative photograph of the same neonate shows a dilated atretic jejunum ➡ extending up to the AWD, which is right of the umbilicus ➡. A cystic mass of necrotic bowel ➡ protruded from the defect, consistent with a closed gastroschisis.*

TERMINOLOGY

Definitions

- Gastroschisis: Congenital abdominal wall defect (AWD) lateral to normal umbilicus
  - AWD almost always lies right of umbilical cord insertion
  - Bowel herniates into amniotic cavity without covering membrane
- Simple gastroschisis: Without bowel complications
- Complex gastroschisis: Presence of bowel atresia, necrosis, &/or perforation in ~ 10-20% of cases

IMAGING

General Features

- Best diagnostic clue
  - Prenatal ultrasound: AWD lies to right of umbilical cord with herniation of free-floating loops of bowel
    - Herniated viscera include
      - Small bowel (almost always)
      - Less frequently: Large bowel, stomach, gonads
      - Liver very rarely reported

Radiographic Findings

- Bowel loops protrude from AWD without covering sac
  - Bowel may be dilated & thick-walled
- Preformed silo: Intraabdominal metallic spring coil at base of overlying dense bag that contains herniated bowel
  - Only if utilizing gradual (rather than primary) reduction of bowel into abdomen
- Pneumatosis, portal venous gas, free air if necrotizing enterocolitis (NEC) develops

Fluoroscopic Findings

- Upper GI series + small bowel follow-through to demonstrate intestinal complications after repair
  - Malrotation (expected in all cases)
  - Dysmotility with dilated bowel loops → delayed small bowel transit time
  - Obstruction due to adhesions
  - Short gut with history of complicated gastroschisis & necrosis requiring resection

Ultrasonographic Findings

- Grayscale ultrasound
  - Prenatal ultrasound
    - Herniated bowel loops free floating in amniotic fluid without covering membrane
    - Bowel wall may be thickened, echogenic, nodular
    - Significance of bowel dilation is debated; intra- or extraabdominal loops may be dilated
      - Considerations include closing gastroschisis, volvulus, atresia, ischemia, chronic inflammation from amniotic fluid exposure
    - Oligohydramnios is more frequent than polyhydramnios
    - Intrauterine growth restriction (IUGR)
      - Overestimated by ↓ abdominal circumference due to bowel extrusion
    - Predictors of complex gastroschisis or adverse neonatal outcome: Polyhydramnios, bowel dilation, ↑ volume of herniated bowel, bowel wall thickening
      - Intraabdominal bowel dilation has been more consistently confirmed as predictive than extraabdominal dilation

MR Findings

- Fetal MR may be useful to evaluate associated anomalies
- Neonatal MR may be used to evaluate bowel motility & superior mesenteric artery (SMA) flow
  - ↑ SMA flow at time of AWD closure correlates with ↑ feeding tolerance

Imaging Recommendations

- Best imaging tool
  - Prenatal ultrasound

DIFFERENTIAL DIAGNOSIS

Omphalocele

- Viscera are herniated into base of umbilical cord with covering membranous sac
- Always contains bowel; often contains liver, other organs
- Ruptured omphalocele may mimic gastroschisis
- > 50% have associated malformations, chromosomal abnormalities

Limb-Body Wall Complex

- Lethal malformation with large AWD
- Herniated viscera are not covered by membrane
- Fetus is often fixed to placenta
- Abnormally short umbilical cord
- Scoliosis, limb anomalies

Cloacal Exstrophy

- Low AWD with nonvisualization of bladder
- Exposed bladder plates are divided by everted bowel
  - Prolapsed ileum resembles "elephant trunk"
- Low omphalocele forms upper part of AWD

Physiologic Gut Herniation

- Gut should not extend > 1 cm into cord
- Herniation is always midline
- Bowel returns to abdomen by 12-weeks gestation

Amniotic Band Syndrome

- Multiple body parts are affected (especially limbs, head)
- Random "slash" defects
- May visualize bands with extremity constriction ± distal edema/amputations

PATHOLOGY

General Features

- Etiology
  - Numerous theories
    - Incomplete lateral fold closure
    - Mesenchymal defect
    - Abnormal involution of right umbilical vein
    - Omphalomesenteric (vitelline) artery occlusion with necrosis at right side of umbilical ring
    - In utero rupture of umbilical hernia
  - Possible teratogens: Aspirin, pseudoephedrine, acetaminophen, cocaine, smoking, others
- Genetics

- No known genetic basis for gastroschisis
  - Chromosomal abnormalities in < 2%
- Familial cases are uncommon
  - 2-5% recurrence risk for siblings
- Associated abnormalities
  - Additional anomalies in up to 20%
    - Intestinal atresias in 5-20% (jejunoileal > colonic)
    - Rare
      - Gastrointestinal duplication, Meckel diverticulum
      - Hydronephrosis, bladder herniation into AWD
      - Congenital cardiac defects
      - Limb hypoplasia, arthrogryposis
      - Cryptorchidism

Gross Pathologic & Surgical Features

- Defect is usually < 2-4 cm
  - Tight, constricted defect, usually right of umbilicus
- In utero bowel injury mechanisms from AWD
  - Chronic irritation by exposure to amniotic fluid
    - Bowel thickening, coating by inflammatory fibrin peel
      - Dysmotility, ↑ risk of adhesions
    - Protein loss by bowel to amniotic fluid → IUGR
  - Constriction at AWD → complex gastroschisis (10-20%)
    - Vascular injury with necrosis, atresia, volvulus, perforation
      - Closed gastroschisis: AWD closes around prolapsed gut causing midgut infarction ± resorption (vanishing midgut); abdominal wall may be normal
    - ↑ rates of NEC, short gut
- Postrepair bowel insult
  - NEC
  - Malrotation with adhesions
    - No significant risk of midgut volvulus

CLINICAL ISSUES

Presentation

- Most common signs/symptoms
  - Recognized during prenatal ultrasound in 98% of cases in developed countries
    - ↑ α-fetoprotein in maternal serum (95%)
  - At delivery, herniated bowel is inflamed with fibrin coating ("peel") in ~ 33%; bowel is rarely necrotic

Demographics

- Epidemiology
  - 1:2,000-4,000 live births
  - Maternal risk factors: Young age, low socioeconomic status, primigravida, poor nutrition, smoking, vasoconstrictive agents

Natural History & Prognosis

- Prematurity in up to 60%
- Overall infant survival > 90% (> 95% for simple, < 70% for complex)
  - Sepsis is most common cause of death
- 10-15% with persistent disability
  - Inguinal hernias due to ↑ intraabdominal pressure
  - Short-gut syndrome with malabsorption
  - Motility disorders
    - 10% incidence of hypoperistalsis syndrome
    - 50% have gastroesophageal reflux
  - Small bowel obstruction from adhesions post repair
    - 27% in 1st year; 37% by 10 years
  - Chronic abdominal pain

Treatment

- Antenatal
  - Close monitoring in 3rd trimester due to ↑ risk of intrauterine demise
  - Delivery at tertiary care center
  - Preterm delivery is not routinely recommended
  - Without other obstetric indications, cesarean section has no advantage over vaginal delivery
- Post natal
  - Protection of herniated bowel, IV fluid replacement & nutrition, IV antibiotics, thermoregulation
  - Prior to reduction, bowel must be inspected for atresias
  - Repair of AWD: Controversy over best method
    - Operative vs. sutureless umbilical cord flap
      - Sutureless method only if bowel is not inflamed
    - Primary closure
      - Possible if intraabdominal pressure < 20 mm Hg (measured in stomach or bladder) when external contents are returned to abdominal cavity
      - Excessive intraabdominal pressure (abdominal compartment syndrome) → hypotension, renal failure, bowel necrosis, respiratory compromise
    - Staged closure
      - Preformed silo provides gradual reduction of bowel to abdomen over 1st week of life
  - Rates of reported sepsis, NEC, reoperation, days on ventilator, & days until enteral feedings vary for each closure method depending on study
  - TPN is required until intestinal function returns

DIAGNOSTIC CHECKLIST

Image Interpretation Pearls

- Prenatally: Consider ruptured omphalocele if liver is herniated into defect without covering membrane (alters prognosis)
- Postnatally: Many possible causes for vomiting + dilated bowel in repaired gastroschisis patients

SELECTED REFERENCES

1. Fisher SG et al: It is complex: predicting gastroschisis outcomes using prenatal imaging. J Surg Res. 258:381-8, 2021
2. Dewberry LC et al: Examination of prenatal sonographic findings: intra-abdominal bowel dilation predicts poor gastroschisis outcomes. Fetal Diagn Ther. 47(3):245-50, 2020
3. Revels JW et al: An algorithmic approach to complex fetal abdominal wall defects. AJR Am J Roentgenol. 214(1):218-31, 2020
4. Williams SL et al: Feeding tolerance, intestinal motility, and superior mesenteric artery blood flow in infants with gastroschisis. Neonatology. 117(1):95-101, 2020
5. Andrade WS et al: Fetal intra-abdominal bowel dilation in prediction of complex gastroschisis. Ultrasound Obstet Gynecol. 54(3):376-80, 2019
6. Oakes MC et al: Advances in prenatal and perinatal diagnosis and management of gastroschisis. Semin Pediatr Surg. 27(5):289-99, 2018
7. Victoria T et al: Fetal anterior abdominal wall defects: prenatal imaging by magnetic resonance imaging. Pediatr Radiol. 48(4):499-512, 2018
8. Abdelhafeez AH et al: The risk of volvulus in abdominal wall defects. J Pediatr Surg. 50(4):570-2, 2015

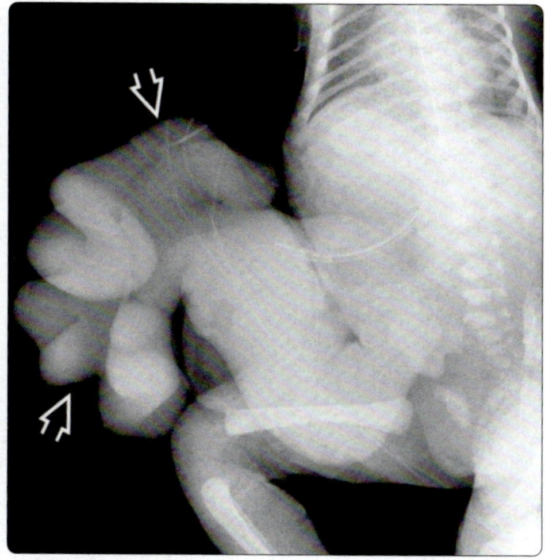

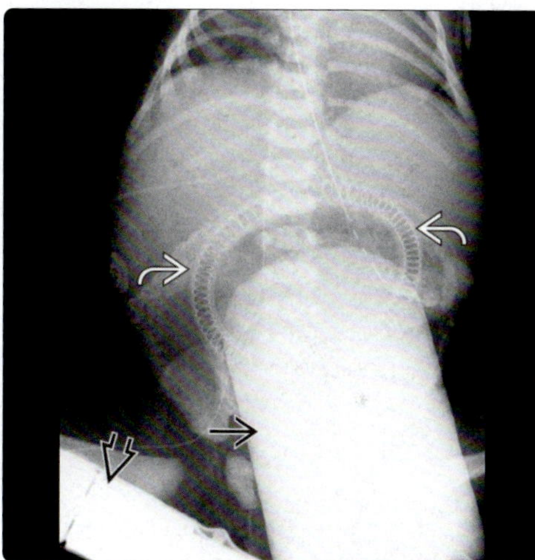

(Left) *Oblique radiograph in a newborn shows numerous dilated bowel loops* ➡ *herniated from the abdominal cavity without a covering membrane.* **(Right)** *AP radiograph in the same patient shows containment of the herniated bowel loops within a silo bag* ➡ *for gradual reduction into the peritoneal cavity. Note the characteristic metallic spring* ➡ *within the AWD as well as the overlying bar* ➡ *from which the bowel-containing silo is suspended.*

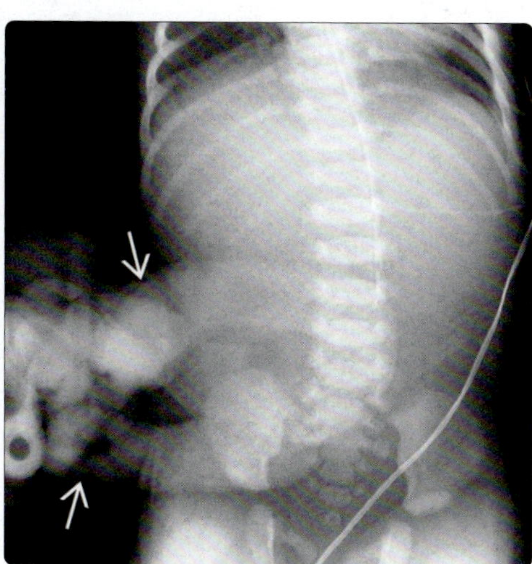

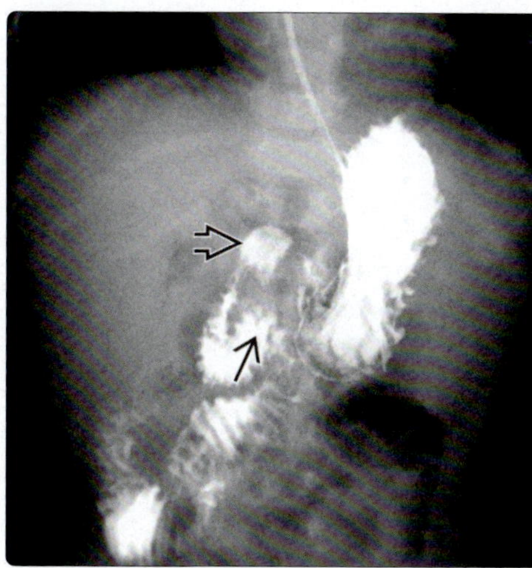

(Left) *AP radiograph in a newborn with gastroschisis shows numerous bowel loops* ➡ *herniated from the abdominal cavity without a covering membrane.* **(Right)** *Frontal upper GI in the same patient after repair of the gastroschisis shows that the duodenojejunal junction* ➡ *is abnormally positioned right of the midline & below the duodenal bulb* ➡*. This is consistent with malrotation, which is typical in gastroschisis as the herniated bowel does not undergo normal fixation in utero.*

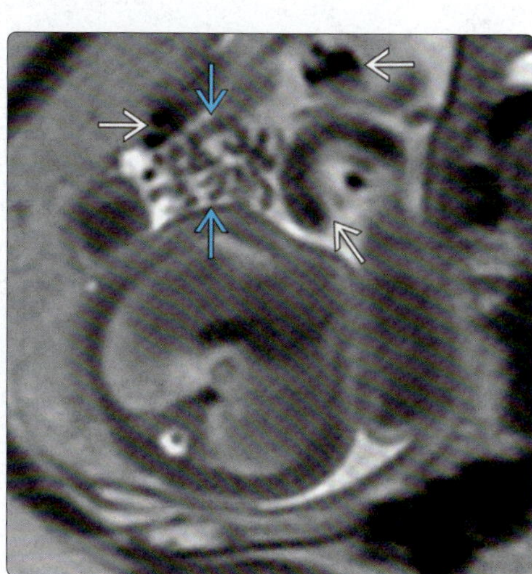

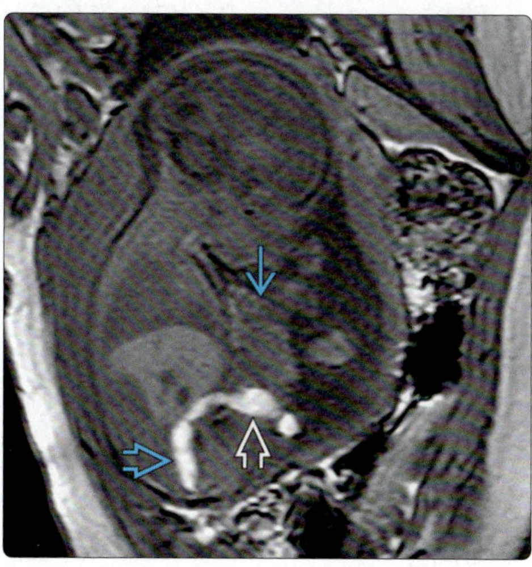

(Left) *Axial SSFSE T2 MR in a 30-weeks-gestation fetus shows numerous loops of uncovered bowel* ➡ *herniated into the amniotic cavity. The loops lie between segments of the umbilical cord* ➡ *& originated from an AWD at the right of the cord insertion (not shown). No dilated bowel is seen.* **(Right)** *Sagittal T1 MR in the same fetus with gastroschisis shows herniated meconium-containing sigmoid colon* ➡ *coursing back into the abdomen with a normal rectal appearance noted* ➡*. Herniated small bowel* ➡ *is also seen superiorly.*

Cloacal Exstrophy/OEIS

KEY FACTS

TERMINOLOGY

- Cloacal exstrophy: Complex abdominal wall defect (AWD) with exposed, abnormally persistent connection of genital, urinary, & intestinal tracts
- OEIS: Omphalocele, cloacal exstrophy, imperforate anus, spinal anomalies

IMAGING

- Prenatal/prerepair findings
  - Absence of urinary bladder with normal to ↓ amniotic fluid volume (depending on renal/ureteral anomalies)
    - Protuberant exposed hemibladder plates at lower abdominal wall
    - Stenotic ureteral orifices may lead to hydroureteronephrosis
    - Additional genitourinary abnormalities: Various renal anomalies, hemiuteri/hemivaginas, + ambiguous &/or bifid genitals
  - Everted cecum splits bladder plates
    - ± elephant trunk appearance of prolapsed terminal ileum below umbilical cord
    - Short, blind-ending microcolon remains internal
      - Lacks normal T1-bright meconium signal
      - Imperforate anus is noted clinically
  - Omphalocele above bladder plates; typically low & small
  - Splayed anterior pelvic bones with abducted thighs
  - Neural tube defects are typically closed, not open
    - Terminal myelocystocele, lipomyelomeningocele
  - ± lower limb anomalies

TOP DIFFERENTIAL DIAGNOSES

- Covered cloacal exstrophy
- Bladder exstrophy
- Limb body wall complex

CLINICAL ISSUES

- Survival is near 100%; long-term function/morbidity is related to severity of individual anomalies

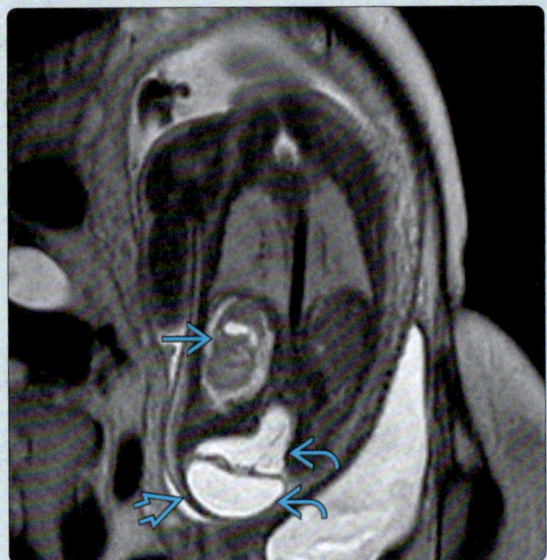

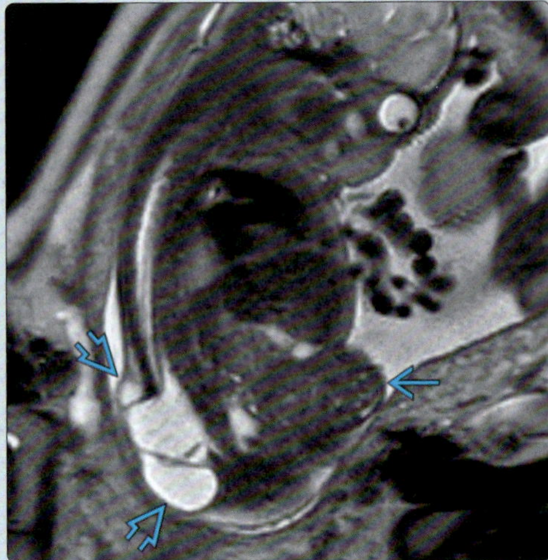

(Left) *Coronal SSFSE T2 MR in a 31-weeks-gestation fetus shows a skin-covered lumbosacral dysraphism ➔. Note the appearance of 2 fluid-containing sacs ➔, typical of terminal myelocystocele. No normal left kidney was seen, & the right kidney showed hydroureteronephrosis ➔.* **(Right)** *Sagittal SSFSE T2 MR in the same fetus shows the sac within a sac appearance ➔ of terminal myelocystocele as well as a low omphalocele ➔. No bladder or normal rectal meconium was seen, consistent with OEIS complex.*

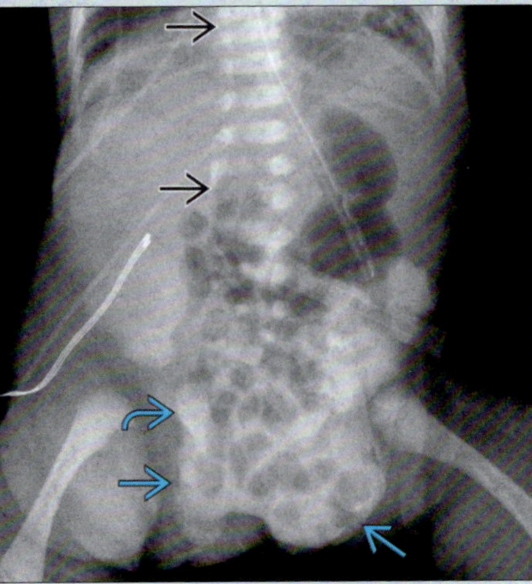

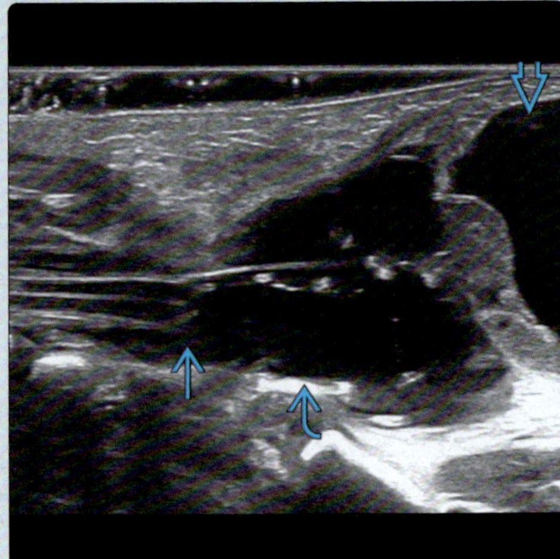

(Left) *AP radiograph in the same patient on day 1 of life shows a low omphalocele containing gas-filled bowel ➔ as well as splaying of the pelvic bones (best seen as overlap of the right pubic & ischial bones ➔). Note also the spinal anomalies ➔.* **(Right)** *Longitudinal US of the spine in the same newborn shows truncation of the lumbar spinal cord ➔ with a meningocele ➔ extending through the dysraphic bony elements into a second sac ➔. Terminal myelocystocele is most commonly associated with OEIS.*

KEY FACTS

TERMINOLOGY

- Rare lethal malformation complex with large abdominal wall defect (AWD), limb anomalies, &/or craniofacial anomalies

IMAGING

- Best imaging clue: Prenatal US/MR showing distorted fetus with AWD, fixation of extruded viscera to placenta, severe scoliosis, various limb anomalies, & short umbilical cord
- Spectrum of anomalies
  - Large AWD, may involve thorax
    - Herniated viscera include liver, bowel, stomach, bladder, ± kidney, spleen
    - Extruded organs are not contained by membrane
    - Viscera are often attached to placenta or uterine wall
  - Short or absent umbilical cord with 2 vessels
  - Severe scoliosis
  - Deformed, hypoplastic, or absent limb(s)
  - Persistent extraembryonic coelomic cavity
  - Craniofacial anomalies are considered as diagnostic component by some definitions
    - Encephalocele, exencephaly, facial clefts
  - Many other associated anomalies are reported
- Limited ex utero imaging: Typically autopsy radiographs

TOP DIFFERENTIAL DIAGNOSES

- Omphalocele
- Gastroschisis
- Amniotic band syndrome
- Pentalogy of Cantrell
- OEIS complex

PATHOLOGY

- Some classify 2 distinct LBWC phenotypes
  - Type 1: Placentocranial
  - Type 2: Placentoabdominal

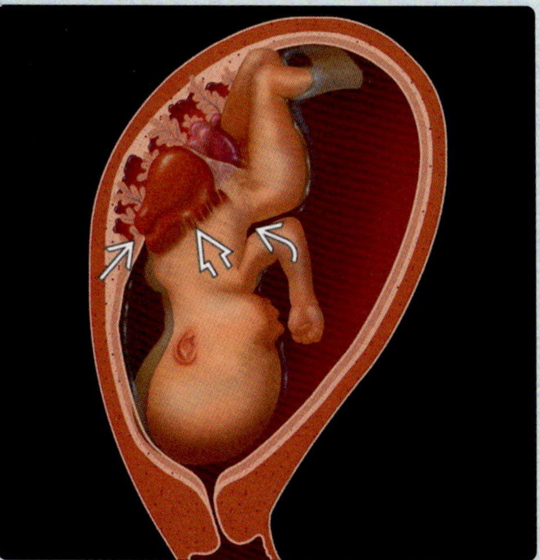

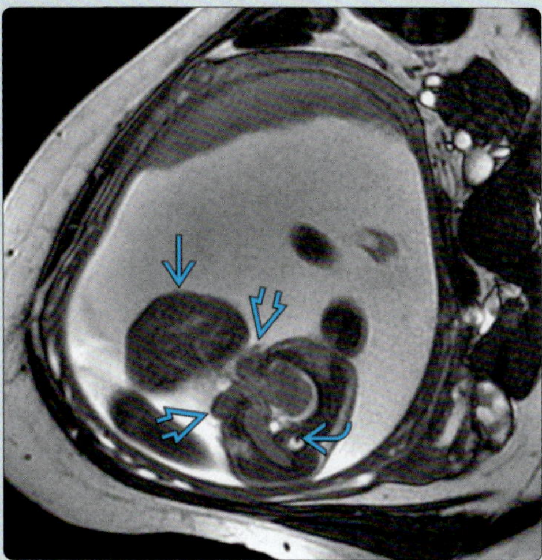

(Left) *Graphic shows a large body wall defect ➡ with fixation of the abdominal viscera to the placenta ➡. There is associated trunk distortion & scoliosis ➡. No free-floating umbilical cord is seen.* **(Right)** *Axial SSFP MR in a 24-weeks-gestation fetus shows polyhydramnios & a large thoracoabdominal wall defect with herniation of the liver ➡, lungs ➡, & heart (superior to this plane). No covering membrane was seen. Note the eccentric position of the spinal cord ➡, which was due to scoliosis.*

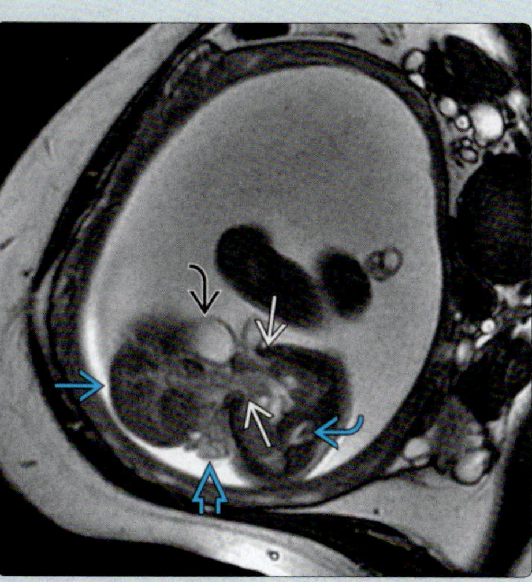

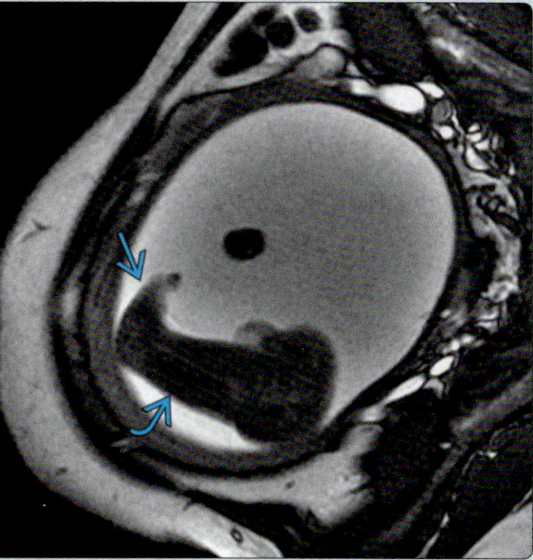

(Left) *Axial SSFP MR in the same fetus shows herniation of the liver ➡, stomach ➡, & bowel ➡ through the large thoracoabdominal wall defect ➡. Note the distortion of the spinal cord ➡ due to scoliosis.* **(Right)** *Axial SSFP MR in the same fetus shows a relatively normal right thigh ➡, while there is fixation & severe truncation of the lower leg & foot ➡. The constellation of findings is consistent with limb body wall complex (LBWC).*

KEY FACTS

TERMINOLOGY

- Acute obstruction of appendiceal lumen → distention → ↑ intraluminal pressure → venous obstruction → ischemia → superimposed infection of appendiceal wall → eventual perforation

IMAGING

- US is 1st-line modality in child with suspected appendicitis
  - Noncompressible, dilated, tubular blind-ending structure (appendix) in RLQ with induration of surrounding fat
    - ± echogenic, shadowing appendicolith
  - US diameter of appendix ≥ 6 mm (during compression)
    - Caution if seen in isolation without secondary findings
- CT diameter of appendix > 6 mm is found in 40% of normal patients; look for other inflammatory features
  - Appendiceal wall thickening & hyperenhancement
  - Periappendiceal inflammation with fat stranding ± fluid
  - RLQ focal ileus
- MR findings are similar to CECT
- Features of perforation
  - Discontinuity of appendiceal wall
  - Appendicolith surrounded by inflammatory change but no well-defined appendix
  - Adjacent bowel wall thickening, moderate free fluid, localized complex collections
    - Even free fluid may be purulent
- Staged approach: US → CT or MR if US is indeterminate or equivocal

CLINICAL ISSUES

- Classic presentation: RLQ pain, anorexia, nausea, & vomiting
  - Periumbilical pain migrating to RLQ over 12-24 hours
  - Tenderness at McBurney point
  - Fever, guarding, rebound tenderness
- Clinical presentation is nonspecific in up to 1/3
  - Especially young children
- Typically benign course with prompt diagnosis & surgery; morbidity & mortality ↑ with perforation

(Left) *AP radiograph in a 9-year-old with right lower quadrant (RLQ) pain & vomiting shows an ovoid RLQ Ca^{2+} ➡ suggesting an appendicolith. A few mildly prominent small bowel loops ➡ with air-fluid levels are noted in the left upper quadrant (LUQ), concerning for focal ileus.* **(Right)** *Transverse RLQ ultrasound in the same patient shows the round echogenic appendicolith ➡ with complete posterior acoustic shadowing (typical of Ca^{2+}). Thickening & ↑ echogenicity of the surrounding fat ➡ is noted.*

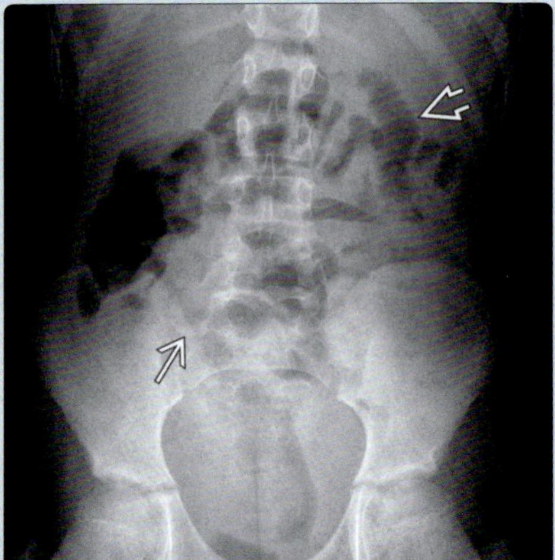

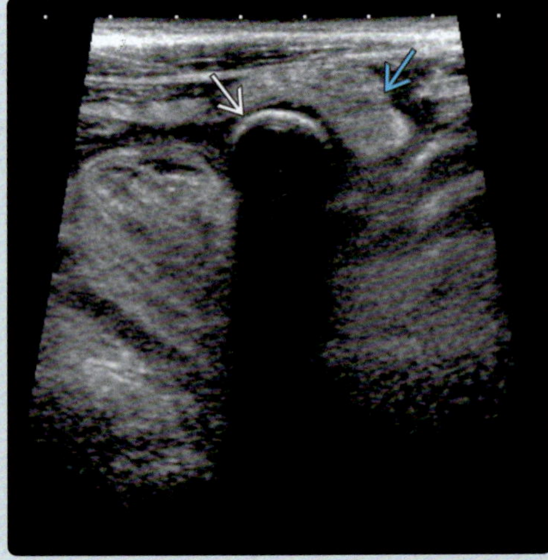

(Left) *Transverse color Doppler ultrasound in the same patient shows a poorly defined, heterogeneous RLQ fluid collection ➡ concerning for abscess.* **(Right)** *Axial CECT in the same patient shows the appendicolith ➡ & a thick-walled rim-enhancing abscess ➡ with surrounding inflammation. A similar posterior collection ➡ was also seen along the rectum. Adjacent bowel loops are displaced with wall thickening ➡. These findings are typical of perforated appendicitis.*

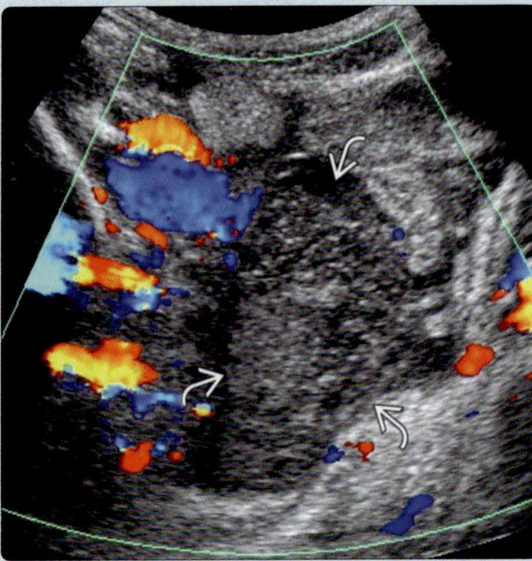

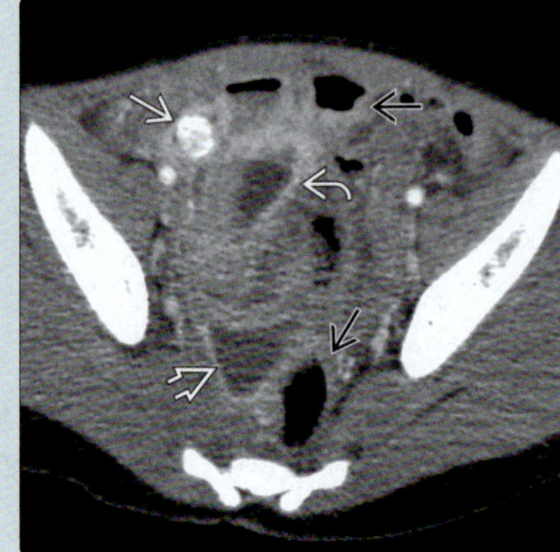

TERMINOLOGY

Definitions

- Acute obstruction of appendiceal lumen → distention → ↑ intraluminal pressure → venous obstruction → ischemia → superimposed infection of appendiceal wall → eventual perforation

IMAGING

General Features

- Best diagnostic clue
  - Noncompressible, dilated, tubular blind-ending structure (appendix) in right lower quadrant (RLQ) with surrounding inflammatory change
- Location
  - Various RLQ positions: Pelvic, retrocecal, subcecal, preileal, postileal
  - Underlying anomalies can lead to unusual locations
    - Other abdominal quadrants in setting of malrotation or situs inversus
    - Scrotum in setting of inguinal hernia (Amyand hernia)
    - Colonic lumen in setting of ileocolic intussusception (where inflamed appendix = pathologic lead point)
- Size
  - Mean diameter of normal pediatric appendix
    - ~ 4 mm on US, ~ 5.7 mm on CT, 5-6 mm on MR
  - US diameter of appendix is usually ≥ 6 mm (during compression) in acute appendicitis
    - Use with caution in absence of secondary signs
  - CT appendix diameter is > 6 mm in 40% of normal patients
  - Differences in normal appendiceal diameters between US, CT, & MR may be attributable to degree of compression normally applied during routine US
- Morphology
  - Normal
    - Smooth continuous wall with "gut signature" on US: Echogenic mucosa & serosa with intervening hypoechoic muscular layer
    - Lies dependently, minimally undulating, often collapsed; may be coiled
  - Abnormal
    - Distended, noncompressible lumen; often taut or straight configuration
    - Involvement of entire appendix vs. distal segment (tip)

Radiographic Findings

- May be normal
- ± calcified appendicolith
- Focal ileus with air-fluid levels or paucity of bowel gas in RLQ
- Loss of right psoas margin
- Abnormalities more likely with perforation
  - Obstruction or more diffuse ileus
  - RLQ extraluminal gas
  - Displacement of bowel loops from RLQ by abscess
  - RLQ bowel wall thickening

Ultrasonographic Findings

- Noncompressible blind-ending tubular structure extending from cecum; ≥ 6 mm in diameter
  - Growing evidence for 7 mm as threshold
- Echogenic thickened periappendiceal fat (may be best independent predictor)
- Echogenic appendicolith with posterior acoustic shadowing
- Free fluid in RLQ/pelvis (especially if complex) vs. localized complex phlegmon or abscess
  - Small amount of simple, anechoic fluid may be normal
- ± hyperemia of appendiceal wall on color Doppler
- Findings most suggestive of perforation include dilated or thick-walled adjacent bowel, loss of appendiceal wall integrity, fluid in at least 2 locations, complex fluid, & discrete abscess

CT Findings

- Dilated appendix (> 6-8 mm)
- Appendiceal wall thickening & hyperenhancement
- Periappendiceal inflammation with fat stranding & fluid
- Lack of appendiceal filling by enteric contrast despite contrast in cecum
- Calcified appendicolith
- RLQ lymphadenopathy
- RLQ focal ileus
- With perforation
  - Discontinuity of appendiceal wall
  - Appendicolith surrounded by inflammatory change without well-defined appendix
  - Localized phlegmon or fluid collection in RLQ or dependent pelvis ± rim enhancement to suggest abscess
  - Extraluminal gas
  - Adjacent bowel wall thickening
  - Small bowel obstruction or diffuse ileus
  - Moderate free fluid & peritoneal enhancement with generalized peritonitis
    - Even free fluid may be purulent
- Negative predictive value of normal CT with nonvisualized pediatric appendix ~ 99%

MR Findings

- Attractive alternative to CT due to lack of ionizing radiation
  - Growing use, particularly in larger pediatric centers
  - Short protocols ↓ need for sedation
- Dilated appendix ≥ 7 mm
- Appendiceal wall thickening & mural edema
- Periappendiceal edema
- Mural & periappendiceal restricted diffusion
- Mural & periappendiceal enhancement
- Appendicolith may appear as signal void
- Free fluid &/or localized phlegmon or fluid collections in RLQ or pelvis

Imaging Recommendations

- Best imaging tool
  - Staged approach with US as 1st modality
    - US is accurate in experienced hands, even if appendix is not visualized
    - No ionizing radiation exposure
    - Negative predictive value > 90% with visualized normal appendix or nonvisualization of appendix without secondary findings of inflammation
  - US → CT or MR depending on institutional or clinical factors: Similar sensitivity/specificity (> 94%)

- Protocol advice
  - US with high-frequency transducer & graded compression (to displace overlying bowel gas)
    - Must look in typical & variant locations
      - Start scanning where patient endorses pain
  - CT with IV contrast
    - ± oral contrast but may delay diagnosis without added value
    - CECT may be requested to determine extent of fluid collections prior to drainage procedure if perforation & fluid are detected by US
  - MR protocols vary
    - Multiplanar T2 ± FS, inversion recovery sequences
    - Sometimes used: DWI, pre- & postcontrast T1 + FS

DIFFERENTIAL DIAGNOSIS

Ovarian Pathology

- Hemorrhagic cyst, ovarian torsion, tuboovarian abscess

Meckel Diverticulum

- May become inflamed &/or cause obstruction

Inflammatory Bowel Disease

- Crohn disease & ulcerative colitis may primarily involve appendix (even in isolation)
- Bowel abnormalities are usually more extensive

Omental Infarct

- Focal infarction of omental fat: Nonsurgical disease
- Focal inflammatory changes in anterior RLQ near colon

Cystic Fibrosis

- Average noninflamed appendix in CF is > 8 mm, may be noncompressible
- No periappendiceal inflammation

Mucocele

- Dilated fluid-filled appendix

Fecal Impaction

- Appendiceal lumen distended by fecal material
- Nontender, no periappendiceal inflammation

Lymphoid Hyperplasia of Appendix

- Thickened hypoechoic lamina propria
- No periappendiceal inflammation

Ileocolic Intussusception

- En face ileocolic intussusception may (rarely) be difficult to distinguish from inflamed bowel & abscess in setting of perforated appendicitis
- Should be able to trace out involved bowel by US
- Tends to occur from 6 months to 3 years of age

CLINICAL ISSUES

Presentation

- Most common signs/symptoms
  - RLQ abdominal pain, anorexia, nausea, & vomiting
- Other signs/symptoms
  - Classic symptoms in older children without perforation
    - Periumbilical pain migrating to RLQ over 12-24 hours
    - Tenderness at McBurney point
    - Fever, guarding, rebound tenderness
  - Clinical presentation is nonspecific in up to 1/3
    - Delay of diagnosis, higher perforation rate
    - More common in younger children

Demographics

- Any age; ↑ incidence from ages 5-15 years
- Most common reason for emergent surgery in children

Natural History & Prognosis

- Typically benign course if classic history leads to prompt diagnosis & surgery
- Morbidity & mortality ↑ with perforation
  - Up to 40% are perforated at presentation; risk ↑ with delay in diagnosis
  - Adjacent abscesses form over days
- Delayed abscesses may present weeks to years later with retained infected appendicoliths

Treatment

- For early uncomplicated appendicitis, perform laparoscopic appendectomy
  - Nonoperative management with IV antibiotics is being increasingly studied
- For perforated appendicitis with abscess, treat with IV antibiotics, percutaneous drainage, delayed appendectomy
  - Must remove appendicolith to prevent future abscess
- Open laparotomy for peritoneal washout if frank peritonitis

DIAGNOSTIC CHECKLIST

Consider

- US 1st modality, then CT or MR if US is indeterminate/equivocal

Image Interpretation Pearls

- Caution using appendiceal diameter in isolation
- Periappendiceal inflammation is particularly useful in making diagnosis on US, CT, & MR

SELECTED REFERENCES

1. Tung EL et al: Comparison of MRI appendix biometrics in children with and without acute appendicitis. Eur Radiol. ePub, 2021
2. Expert Panel on Pediatric Imaging et al: ACR Appropriateness Criteria® suspected appendicitis-child. J Am Coll Radiol. 16(5S):S252-63, 2019
3. Swenson DW et al: Practical imaging strategies for acute appendicitis in children. AJR Am J Roentgenol. 211(4):901-9, 2018
4. Dillman JR et al: Equivocal pediatric appendicitis: unenhanced MR imaging protocol for nonsedated children - a clinical effectiveness study. Radiology. 279(1):216-25, 2016
5. Moore MM et al: Magnetic resonance imaging in pediatric appendicitis: a systematic review. Pediatr Radiol. 46(6):928-39, 2016
6. Swenson DW et al: MRI of the normal appendix in children: data toward a new reference standard. Pediatr Radiol. 46(7):1003-10, 2016
7. Tulin-Silver S et al: The challenging ultrasound diagnosis of perforated appendicitis in children: constellations of sonographic findings improve specificity. Pediatr Radiol. 45(6):820-30, 2015
8. Aspelund G et al: Ultrasonography/MRI versus CT for diagnosing appendicitis. Pediatrics. 133(4):586-93, 2014
9. Trout AT et al: Journal club: the pediatric appendix: defining normal. AJR Am J Roentgenol. 202(5):936-45, 2014
10. Dietz KR et al: Beyond acute appendicitis: imaging of additional pathologies of the pediatric appendix. Pediatr Radiol. 43(2):232-42; quiz 259, 2013
11. Trout AT et al: Reevaluating the sonographic criteria for acute appendicitis in children: a review of the literature and a retrospective analysis of 246 cases. Acad Radiol. 19(11):1382-94, 2012

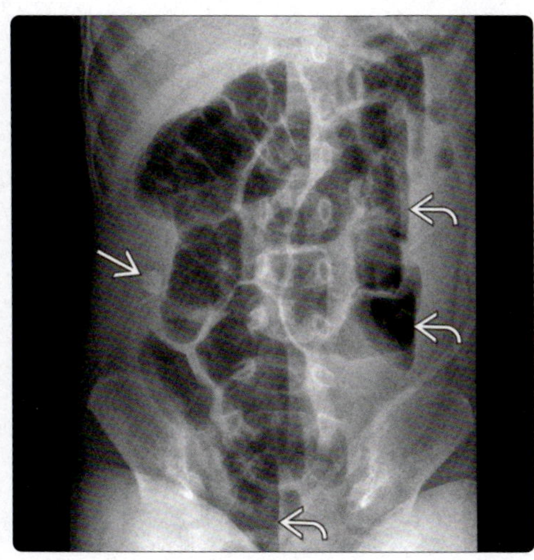

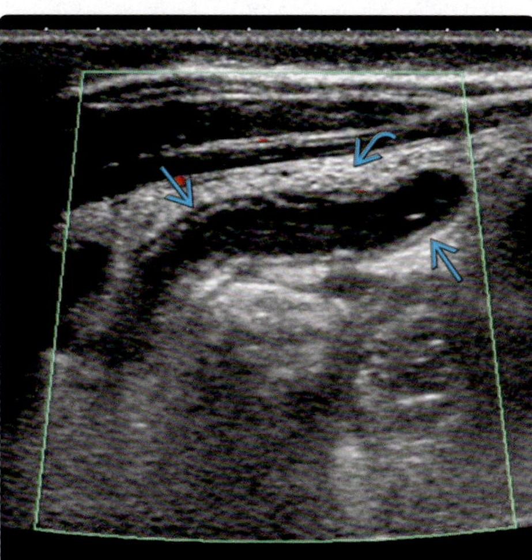

(Left) *Left side down decubitus abdominal radiograph in a 2-year-old with RLQ pain & fever shows a large appendicolith with medial displacement of adjacent bowel loops. The bowel is mildly dilated diffusely & contains numerous air-fluid levels, suggesting ileus.* **(Right)** *Longitudinal ultrasound of the RLQ in the same patient shows dilation (12 mm) of a noncompressible appendix with thickening & ↑ echogenicity of the periappendiceal fat, typical of acute appendicitis.*

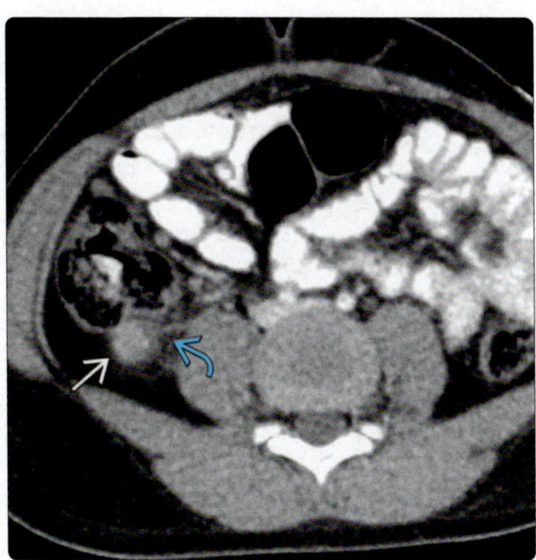

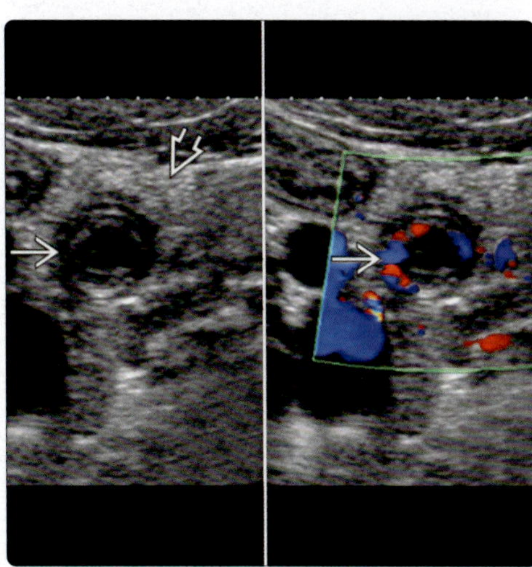

(Left) *Axial CECT in an 8-year-old with RLQ pain & nonvisualization of the appendix on US shows a thickened retrocecal appendix with surrounding fat stranding. A retrocecal appendix may be more difficult to visualize on US.* **(Right)** *Transverse grayscale & color Doppler ultrasounds in a 9-year-old with pain show a dilated appendix with a thickened, irregular, & hyperemic wall. The periappendiceal fat is indurated in this patient with acute appendicitis.*

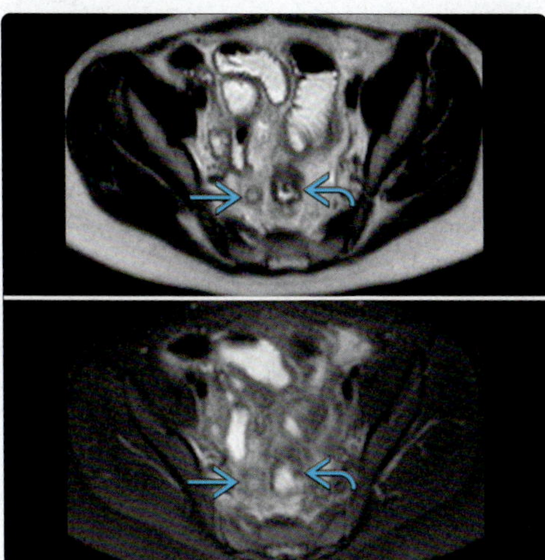

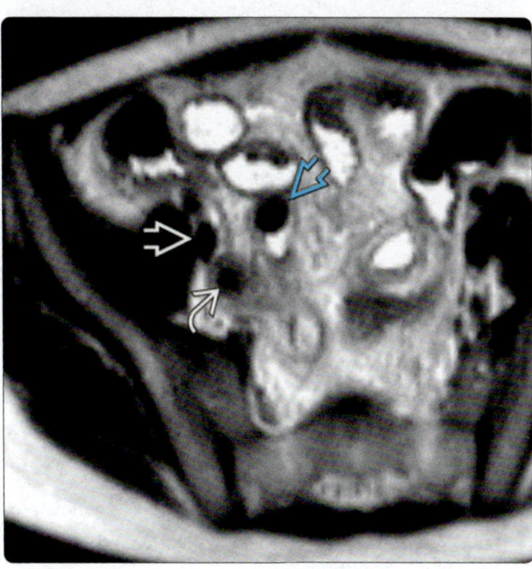

(Left) *Axial T2 SSFSE (top) & FS T2 (bottom) MR images in an 8-year-old with pain show a dilated (9-mm), thick-walled appendix with surrounding fat edema. Adjacent bowel wall thickening & a localized fluid collection (not shown) confirmed perforated appendicitis.* **(Right)** *Axial T2 SSFSE in the same patient shows a signal void in the proximal appendiceal lumen corresponding to an appendicolith. Signal voids are also seen corresponding to air within bowel loops & flowing blood in the iliac vessels.*

Ileocolic Intussusception

KEY FACTS

TERMINOLOGY

- Invagination of distal small bowel (SB) (intussusceptum) into colon (intussuscipiens) in telescope-like manner

IMAGING

- Radiography: Often abnormal, not always perceived
  - Paucity of right abdominal colonic gas ± round mass
    - ± fat density (from entrapped mesentery) in mass
  - Crescent sign: Curvilinear mass-gas interface
  - Lateralization of ileum to expected cecal location
  - ± SB obstruction
- US: Best diagnostic modality if clinically suspected
  - Round mass with target sign in right abdomen
  - Mean diameter of 2.6 cm vs. 1.5 cm for purely SB intussusceptions
  - Echogenic core contains fat, lymph nodes, & SB
    - May also see normal appendix or pathologic lead point (such as duplication cyst, juvenile polyp)
  - Sweeping transducer proximal & distal shows relationship to small & large intestine
  - Entrapped fluid: ↑ failure rate of enema reduction
  - ↓ vascularity is associated with ↑ likelihood of bowel necrosis & ↑ failure rate of reduction

PATHOLOGY

- ~ 90% are idiopathic (due to lymphoid hypertrophy)
- ~ 5-10% from pathologic lead points

CLINICAL ISSUES

- Most common from ages 3 months to 3 years
- Presents with vomiting, alternating lethargy & irritability, "currant jelly" (bloody) stools
- Treat with enema reduction (as bowel can infarct if not reduced): Air enema under fluoroscopy vs. hydrostatic with US guidance
- Intussusception recurs after reduction in ~ 5-15%
- Surgery is reserved for cases of enema reduction failure or when enema is contraindicated

(Left) *Supine (L) & left decubitus (R) radiographs in a 3-year-old with intermittent pain show a soft tissue mass partially outlined by gas in the abdominal RUQ ➡ (the crescent sign). There is a paucity of colonic gas in the right abdomen with lateralization of small bowel gas.* **(Right)** *Transverse US of the RUQ in the same patient shows the classic target sign of an ileocolic (IC) intussusception ➡, measuring > 3 cm in diameter. The echogenic core ➡ contains bowel, fat, vessels, & lymph nodes.*

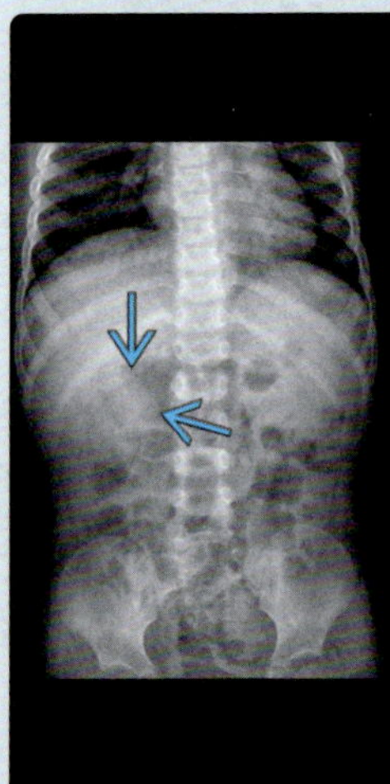

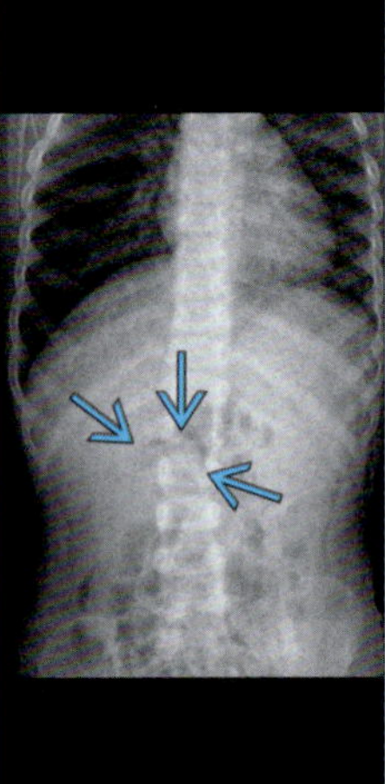

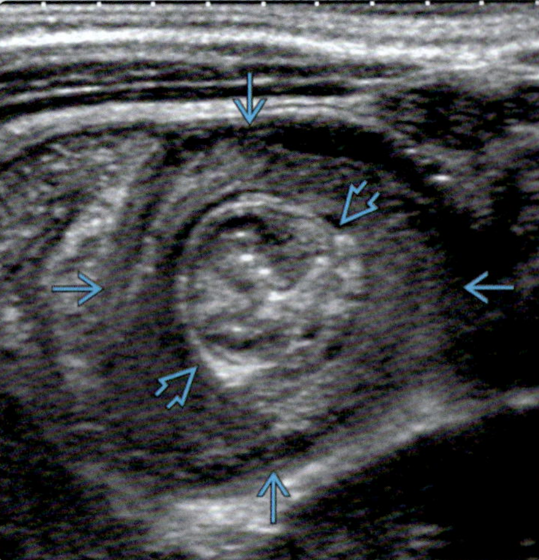

(Left) *Prone fluoroscopic image in the same patient during an air enema reduction shows gas filling the colon ➡ to the level of the cecum. Only a small component of intussusceptum ➡ remains in the cecum at this point. There is minimal small bowel gas at this time.* **(Right)** *Subsequent prone fluoroscopic image in the same patient after further air introduction shows that the intussusceptum is no longer visualized in the cecum ➡ & gas has freely refluxed into the small bowel ➡, confirming a successful reduction.*

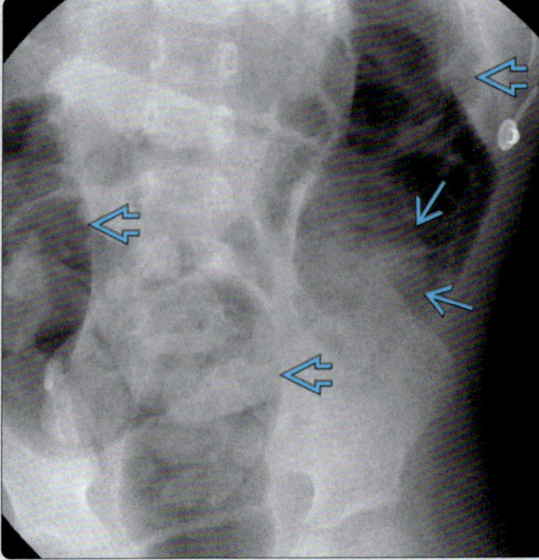

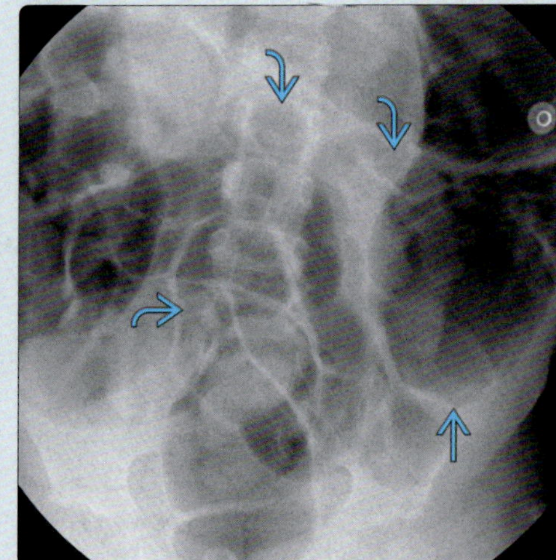

TERMINOLOGY

Definitions

- Ileocolic (IC) intussusception: Invagination of distal small bowel (SB) (intussusceptum) into colon (intussuscipiens) in telescope-like manner

IMAGING

General Features

- Best diagnostic clue
  - US: Round target sign in right abdomen at expected level of colon
  - Radiography: Paucity of colonic gas in right abdomen + gas outlining left margin of rounded soft tissue density in RUQ (crescent sign in colon)
- Location
  - Always involves right/proximal colon; extends distally to variable degrees but usually involves some length of transverse colon
- Size
  - Mean diameter of 2.6 cm (vs. 1.5 cm for purely SB intussusceptions)
    - > 3 cm strongly favors IC; < 2 cm strongly favors SB-SB

Radiographic Findings

- Paucity of colonic gas in right abdomen
- Round mass in right abdomen: May see layers of fat density (from intussuscepted mesentery)
- Crescent sign: Curvilinear gas outlining left aspect of round soft tissue mass (intussusceptum) within colon
- ± SB obstruction
- Pneumoperitoneum before air enema is extremely rare

Ultrasonographic Findings

- Grayscale ultrasound
  - Target sign: Cross section of intussusception shows round mass with alternating concentric rings of hyper- & hypoechogenicity from bowel walls & mesenteric fat
    - Mean diameter of 2.6 cm
    - Sweeping transducer proximal & distal shows relationship to small & large intestine
      - May see entrapped lymph nodes, appendix, other pathologic lead points (such as intestinal duplication cyst, juvenile polyp, or lipoma)
    - Fatty core to wall index: Never < 1.0 in IC intussusception; mean of 2.3 (vs. 0.16 for SB-SB)
      - Outer wall thickness: Mean of 0.6 cm in IC vs. 0.42 in SB-SB
      - Echogenic fat core: Mean of 1.3-1.5 cm in IC vs. 0.1-0.3 in SB-SB
  - Pseudokidney or sandwich sign: Longitudinal or oblique image showing ovoid mass with alternating layers of hyper- & hypoechogenicity
  - Often not located in right lower quadrant (RLQ) due to distal progression of intussusception (or in setting of underlying malrotation)
    - Need to scan all 4 quadrants
    - Absence of normal ileocecal region in RLQ
  - Trapped fluid within intussusception → ↑ failure rate of enema reduction
  - May be used to guide hydrostatic reduction
- Color Doppler
  - ↓ internal vascular flow → ↑ likelihood of bowel necrosis, ↑ failure rate of enema reduction

CT Findings

- CECT
  - Incidentally seen on abdominal CT performed for nonspecific abdominal pain when intussusception is not suspected or if US findings are unclear
    - Not primary modality for diagnosis
  - Abdominal mass with alternating rings of high & low attenuation (target or sandwich sign)

Fluoroscopic Findings

- Air-contrast enema
  - Apex of intussusceptum projects as round soft tissue mass against distal colonic air column
  - Multilobular intussusceptum in right colon/cecum suggests irreducibility
  - Dissection sign: Air surrounding length of intussusceptum predicts irreducibility
- Liquid contrast enema
  - Apex of intussusceptum projects as round soft tissue/lucent defect against distal colonic positive contrast column
  - Dissection or coiled spring sign: Contrast surrounding length of intussusceptum predicts irreducibility

Imaging Recommendations

- Best imaging tool
  - US for diagnosis
  - Fluoroscopic air enema vs. US-guided hydrostatic reduction for treatment

DIFFERENTIAL DIAGNOSIS

Small Bowel-Small Bowel Intussusception

- Smaller cross-sectional diameter than IC
  - Smaller or absent echogenic core lacking lymph nodes
  - Outer wall is less thick
- Location is more variable than IC
- Often able to trace SB into & out of intussusception

Appendicitis

- More common > 3 years of age
- Identification of appendicolith is helpful
- In cases of perforation, inflammatory collection can mimic soft tissue mass

Ovarian Torsion

- US may show avascular mass with peripheral cysts in midline with only 1 normal ovary visualized

Gastroenteritis

- Air-fluid levels throughout colon suggest gastroenteritis

Meckel Diverticulum

- Round or tubular, rim-enhancing mass ± surrounding inflammation
  - May also cause obstruction or GI bleed
- May serve as lead point for intussusception

PATHOLOGY

General Features

- Etiology
  - ~ 90% are idiopathic (likely secondary to reactive lymphoid hyperplasia)
    - May be preceded by viral illness
  - ~ 5-10% are caused by pathologic lead points in children
    - Meckel diverticulum > duplication cyst > polyp > lymphoma

CLINICAL ISSUES

Presentation

- Most common signs/symptoms
  - Vomiting; may be bilious
  - Alternating lethargy & irritability
  - Colic or "intermittent fussiness"
- Other signs/symptoms
  - Bloody diarrhea ("red currant jelly" stools are classic)
  - Palpable right-sided abdominal mass

Demographics

- Classic age: 3 months to 3 years
  - If < 3 months or > 3 years, question pathologic lead point
- Sex: More common in males (3:2)
- Epidemiology: ~ 56 per 100,000 children annually
  - Most common cause of pediatric SB obstruction
  - Classically reported seasonal occurrence (winter, spring) with viral illnesses

Natural History & Prognosis

- Medical urgency: Bowel can infarct if not reduced
  - Bowel necrosis → perforation → peritonitis, shock, & death
- May spontaneously reduce
- Intussusception recurs after successful reduction in ~ 5-15%
  - Most recurrences occur within 48-72 hours

Treatment

- Imaging-guided pressure reduction; options include
  - Air insufflation with fluoroscopic guidance
    - Liquid contrast under fluoroscopy is used much less commonly in current era
  - US-guided hydrostatic reduction
- Contraindications: Peritonitis (relative), pneumoperitoneum
  - In resource-rich countries, pneumoperitoneum prior to reduction attempt is rare
    - Likely due to prompt presentation to medical facility
- US findings associated with ↓ success rate of enema reduction (but not contraindications)
  - Trapped fluid within intussusception, ↓ intussusceptum vascularity, presence of pathologic lead point, SB obstruction, younger age, rectal bleeding, prolonged duration of symptoms (> 24-72 hours)
- Preparation guidelines: Adequate hydration, IV access, physical examination, surgery consultation
- Air enema guidelines
  - Good rectal seal without leak
  - Maximum of 120 mm Hg sustained colonic pressure at rest (though greater pressure spikes are usually seen during crying or Valsalva)
- Intussusception is encountered as round mass that moves retrograde toward cecum with air insufflation
- Intussusceptum is most likely to get "stuck" at ileocecal valve
- Success: Retrograde rush of gas into SB + resolution of soft tissue mass
  - Edematous ileocecal valve may protrude into cecum, mimicking persistent intussusception: Follow clinically or by US
- If mass progresses on initial attempts but does not reduce beyond ileocecal valve, period of ~ 60 minutes may ↓ edema & ↑ chance of success
  - Repeat attempts with interval of 1 hour of waiting are acceptable as long as patient is stable & head of intussusception is progressing more toward cecum with each attempt
  - Recurrences are typically treated by enema up to 5x prior to considering surgical exploration for potential pathologic lead point
- Success rates of ~ 80-90% with enema reduction
- Risk of perforation is 0.5-1.0% with air
- Surgery is reserved for cases of enema reduction failure or when enema is contraindicated

DIAGNOSTIC CHECKLIST

Image Interpretation Pearls

- Radiographs: Often abnormal, but signs of intussusception are not always perceived
  - Lateralized ileum or redundant sigmoid may mimic air in cecum with false exclusion of intussusception
    - Sigmoid colon in RLQ on radiographs 43% of time
  - Left side down decubitus radiograph can help evaluate cecum (& exclude free air)
- US: Best test if intussusception is suspected clinically

SELECTED REFERENCES

1. Delgado-Miguel C et al: Routine ultrasound control after successful intussusception reduction in children: is it really necessary? Eur J Pediatr Surg. 31(1):115-9, 2021
2. Kelley-Quon LI et al: Management of intussusception in children: a systematic review. J Pediatr Surg. 56(3):587-96, 2021
3. Zhang M et al: Accurately distinguishing pediatric ileocolic intussusception from small-bowel intussusception using ultrasonography. J Pediatr Surg. 56(4):721-6, 2021
4. Goel I et al: Evolving concepts in ultrasonography of pediatric intussusceptions: unequivocal differentiation of ileocolic, obstructive and transient small-bowel intussusceptions. Ultrasound Med Biol. 46(3):589-97, 2020
5. Ma GMY et al: Air contrast enema reduction of single and recurrent ileocolic intussusceptions in children: patterns, management and outcomes. Pediatr Radiol. 50(5):664-72, 2020
6. Patel DM et al: Radiographic findings predictive of irreducibility and surgical resection in ileocolic intussusception. Pediatr Radiol. 50(9):1249-54, 2020
7. Plut D et al: Practical imaging strategies for intussusception in children. AJR Am J Roentgenol. 215(6):1449-63, 2020
8. Shubin CE et al: Impact of a standardized clinical pathway for suspected and confirmed ileocolic intussusception. Pediatr Qual Saf. 5(3):e298, 2020
9. Flaum V et al: Twenty years' experience for reduction of ileocolic intussusceptions by saline enema under sonography control. J Pediatr Surg. 51(1):179-82, 2016
10. Lioubashevsky N et al: Ileocolic versus small-bowel intussusception in children: can US enable reliable differentiation? Radiology. 269(1):266-71, 2013

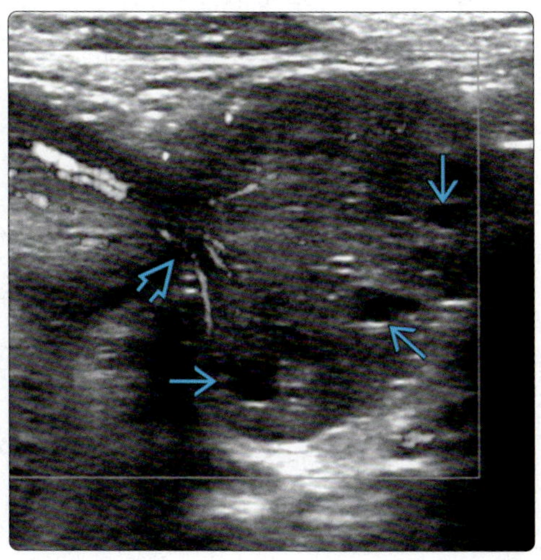

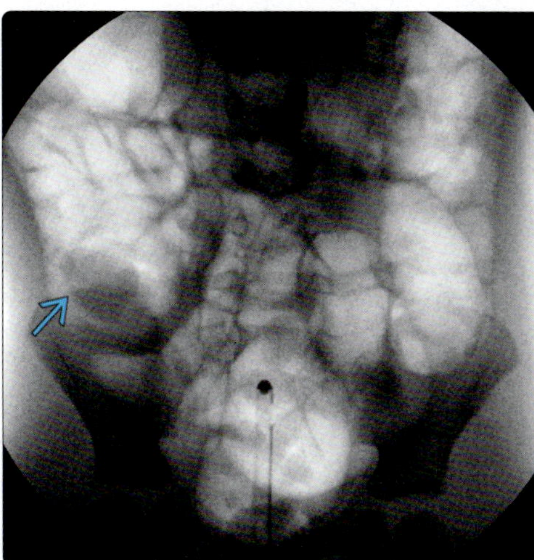

(Left) *Longitudinal US in a 3-year-old shows a pedunculated lead point mass at the head of an intussusceptum. The mostly solid mass contains peripheral cysts → & a vascular stalk →, strongly suggesting a juvenile polyp (which was confirmed upon resection).* **(Right)** *Supine air enema image in the same patient demonstrates a persistent filling defect → in the cecum status post reduction, consistent with the juvenile polyp. An edematous ileocecal valve is typically more round & medial.*

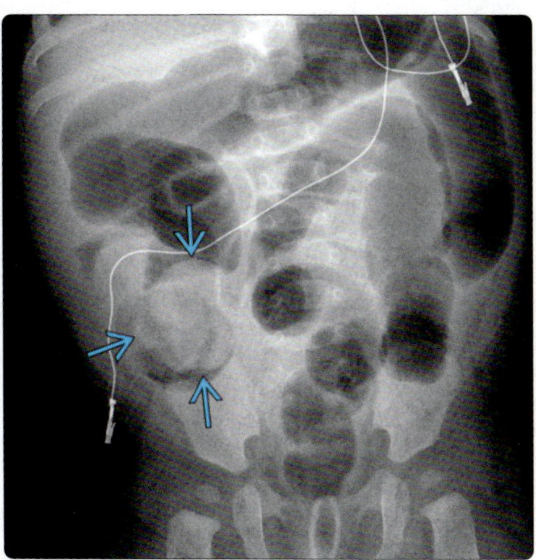

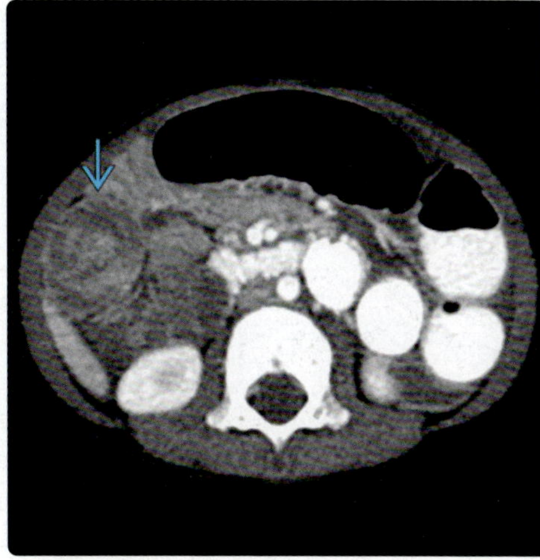

(Left) *Supine AP radiograph in a 5-month-old after multiple air enema reduction attempts shows a large, multilobular residual soft tissue mass at the cecum →. A multilobular configuration can suggest irreducibility of the IC intussusception by enema, potentially due to a lead point mass.* **(Right)** *Axial CECT of a 3-year-old child with a small bowel obstruction & clinical findings suggestive of appendicitis shows an enhancing target sign → in the right abdomen, consistent with an IC intussusception.*

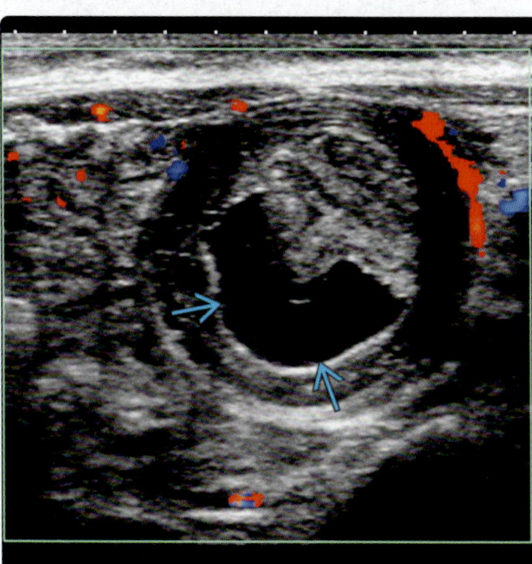

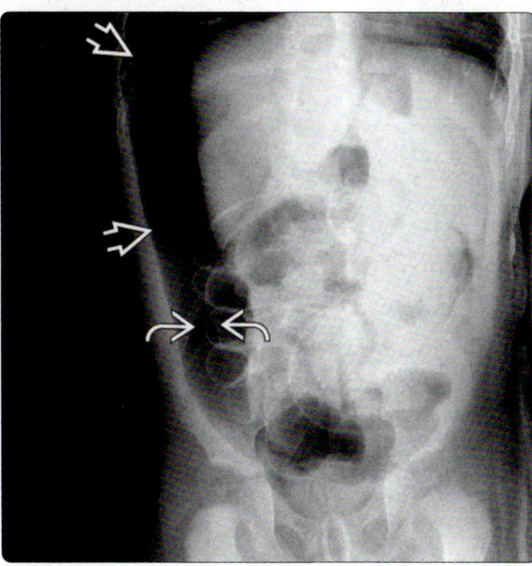

(Left) *Transverse color Doppler US in a 4-month-old with lethargy & recurrent abdominal pain shows trapped fluid → & no blood flow within the IC intussusception, suggesting that it will be more difficult to reduce without surgery.* **(Right)** *Left decubitus radiograph in a 7-month-old immediately after an unsuccessful air enema IC intussusception reduction attempt shows pneumoperitoneum →, consistent with bowel perforation. Note the Rigler sign → (with gas outlining both sides of the bowel wall).*

Meckel Diverticulum

KEY FACTS

TERMINOLOGY

- Most common omphalomesenteric duct remnant
- Presents with bleeding, inflammation, intussusception, bowel obstruction, or perforation
  - ~ 65% of symptomatic Meckel diverticula contain ectopic gastric mucosa
- Rule of 2s: 2% of general population, found within 2 feet of ileocecal valve, most have symptoms < 2 years of age

IMAGING

- Classic imaging appearance (in patient with GI bleeding): Focal persistent accumulation of radiotracer in right lower quadrant (RLQ) on nuclear pertechnetate scan
  - Coincident with & isointense to gastric uptake
  - ↑ in visibility with time
- Other modalities (US, CT, MR)
  - Blind-ending, tubular structure may be inconspicuous
  - May present as cyst, even with gut signature
  - With inflammation, findings are similar to appendicitis
    - Thick-walled, tubular structure, hyperemic bowel loops; rare perforation
  - Intraluminal mass as lead point in intussusception
  - May see bowel obstruction without obvious cause

TOP DIFFERENTIAL DIAGNOSES

- GI bleeding with positive pertechnetate scan
  - Strong accumulation in GI duplication cyst
  - Hyperemia of Crohn disease, appendicitis, or vascular lesion may cause mild accumulation
- Small bowel obstruction
  - Appendicitis, adhesions, intussusception, inguinal hernia, malrotation, + Meckel (mnemonic of AAIIMM)
- RLQ inflammation
  - Appendicitis, Crohn disease, omental infarct, mesenteric adenitis, ovarian torsion

CLINICAL ISSUES

- Treated surgically

(Left) *Axial graphic shows an inflamed Meckel diverticulum ➡ growing off of the antimesenteric border of the intestine with the obliterated remnant of the omphalomesenteric duct ➡ extending from its tip.* **(Right)** *Longitudinal US in a 14-year-old boy with right lower quadrant (RLQ) pain demonstrated a normal appendix (not shown) + a thickened, hyperemic tubular structure ➡ just above the bladder. An inflamed Meckel diverticulum was removed at surgery.*

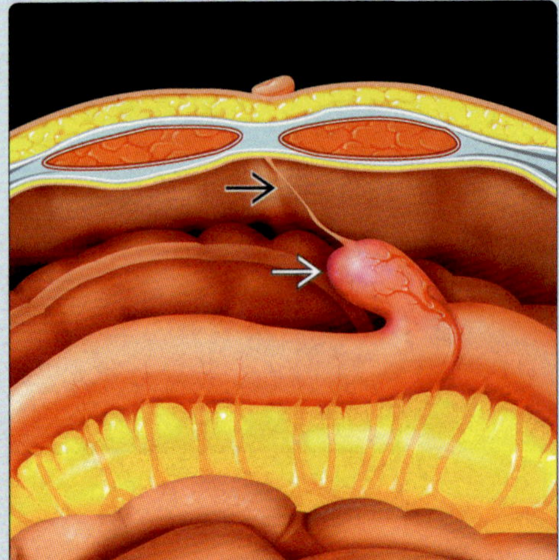

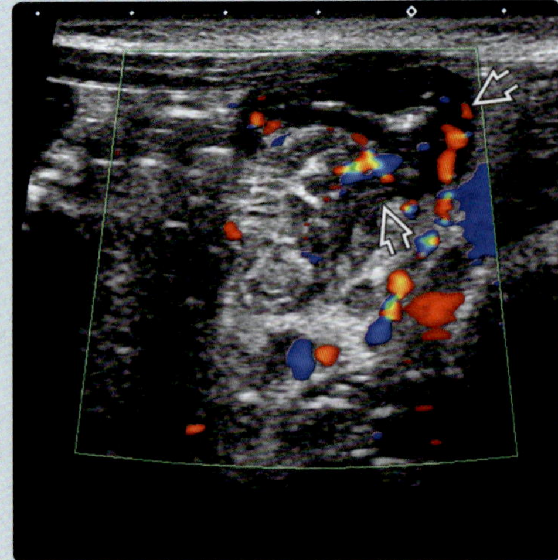

(Left) *Axial CECT in a 10-year-old boy with vague, intermittent abdominal pain shows a rim-enhancing cystic lesion ➡ just deep to the umbilicus. This cyst did not appear to communicate with the bowel.* **(Right)** *Coronal reformatted CECT in the same boy shows mild inflammation ➡ surrounding the cystic lesion ➡, which was found to be a Meckel diverticulum distended with secretions at surgery.*

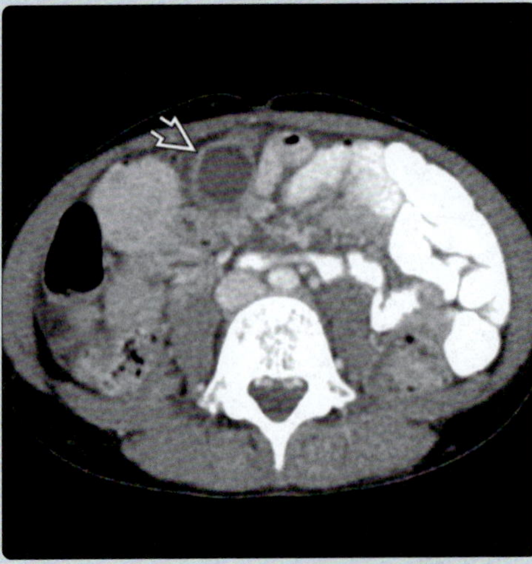

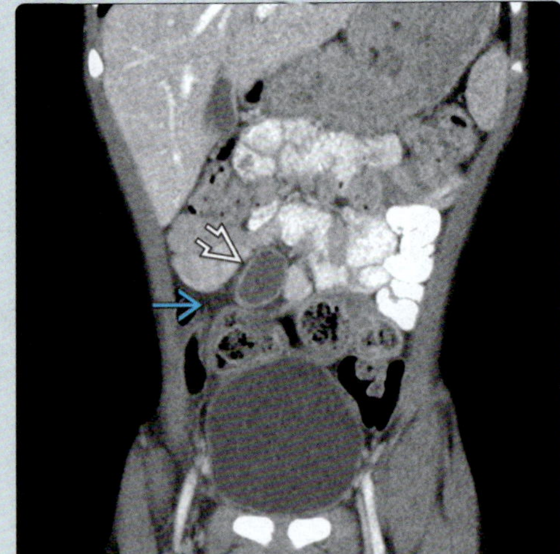

TERMINOLOGY

Definitions

- Remnant of omphalomesenteric duct
- Presents with bleeding (when containing ectopic gastric mucosa), inflammation, intussusception, bowel obstruction, or perforation
- Rule of 2s
  - Incidence: 2% of general population
  - Found within 2 feet of ileocecal valve
  - Most have clinical symptoms before 2 years of age

IMAGING

General Features

- Best diagnostic clue
  - Radiologic appearance varies by type of presentation
  - Classic imaging appearance on nuclear pertechnetate scan in patient with GI bleeding
    - Persistent, focal accumulation of radiotracer in right lower quadrant (RLQ) due to ectopic gastric mucosa in Meckel diverticulum
      - Coincident with & isointense to gastric uptake
      - Increasingly visible with time
- Location
  - RLQ or midline/periumbilical in location
  - Most within 2 feet of ileocecal valve
- Size
  - Variable; often small if uninflamed, large if inflamed or intussuscepted

Radiographic Findings

- Abdominal films may be normal or show
  - RLQ mass
  - Displacement of bowel loops
  - Small bowel obstruction
  - Enteroliths & ingested foreign bodies have been reported

Fluoroscopic Findings

- Often normal; variable communication with bowel lumen
- Contrast studies may show indirect evidence of mass & inflammatory changes in adjacent bowel
- May serve as lead point for intussusception
  - Often not reducible with air enema

Ultrasonographic Findings

- Grayscale ultrasound
  - Thick-walled, tubular structure or hyperemic bowel loops in RLQ
  - Heterogeneous echotexture mass in RLQ, may mimic appendicitis
    - Look for normal appendix
  - Meckel diverticulum may present as cyst, even with gut signature
    - Walls are more heterogeneous & thick with inflammation vs. enteric duplication cyst
  - Intraluminal mass as lead point in intussusception, inverted Meckel
- Color Doppler
  - Hyperemia related to inflammatory process

CT Findings

- CECT
  - Incidentally, may be collapsed & blind-ending or appear cystic with trapped secretions
  - CT enterography technique may be helpful
  - If inflamed, similar to appendicitis: Thick-walled blind-ending structure near cecum with surrounding inflammation
    - If perforated, may see abscess & free air
    - Normal appendix is clue to diagnosis
  - May cause small bowel obstruction with no clear explanation on imaging
  - If intussuscepted, may be occult
  - If bleeding, CTA may show ↑ flow locally

MR Findings

- Follows CECT findings; enterography may help visualize

Nuclear Medicine Findings

- Tc-99m pertechnetate scan
  - Most specific test for Meckel diverticulum: ~ 90% accuracy
  - Pertechnetate accumulates in mucous cells in acidic environment
    - Ectopic gastric mucosa of most Meckel diverticula
  - Diverticulum typically does not communicate with bowel lumen, so radiotracer does not appear to move downstream in bowel unless there is active bleeding
  - Pharmacologic enhancement of pertechnetate scans by using
    - Pentagastrin subcutaneously
    - Ranitidine or cimetidine, oral or intravenous
    - Glucagon intramuscularly
  - Given high sensitivity otherwise, additional medications may be reserved for repeat studies in patients with high clinical suspicion of Meckel diverticular disease & normal initial scans
  - False-negative pertechnetate scans
    - Lack of any or sufficient gastric mucosa to localize radiotracer
      - ~ 65% of symptomatic Meckel diverticula have ectopic gastric mucosa
    - Secondary ischemia due to volvulus or intussusception
    - ~ 50% of scans repeated for high clinical suspicion are positive on 2nd study

Imaging Recommendations

- Best imaging tool
  - Tc-99m pertechnetate scan or US for GI bleeding
    - Recent literature shows US is > 90% sensitive & specific for Meckel diverticulum in setting of GI bleeding
  - US or CECT for other presentations
- Protocol advice
  - Lateral & postvoid images should be obtained before conclusion of pertechnetate scan to look for Meckel diverticulum behind urinary bladder

DIFFERENTIAL DIAGNOSIS

GI Bleeding With Positive Pertechnetate Scan

- Strong accumulation in GI duplication cyst

- Hyperemia of Crohn disease, appendicitis, or vascular lesion may cause mild accumulation

Small Bowel Obstruction

- Appendicitis, adhesions, intussusception, inguinal hernia, malrotation
  - With Meckel diverticulum → AAIIMM mnemonic

Inflammatory Bowel Disease

- Crohn disease & other enteritis

Right Lower Quadrant Inflammation

- Appendicitis, ileitis, omental infarct, epiploic appendagitis, mesenteric adenitis, ovarian torsion

PATHOLOGY

General Features

- Form of omphalomesenteric duct remnant (OMDR) is found in 2-3% of autopsy series
  - Connection between yolk sac & primitive digestive tract in early fetal life
  - Meckel diverticulum is most common end of spectrum of OMDRs, which also include umbilicoileal fistula, umbilical sinus or cyst, & fibrous cord connecting ileum to umbilicus
- Small percentage of Meckel diverticula becomes symptomatic, typically due to presence of ectopic gastric mucosa
  - Rarely, diverticulum contains rests of pancreatic tissue
  - Can entrap fish bones, seeds, pits, ingested foreign bodies, etc.

Microscopic Features

- Composed of same layers as adjacent small bowel but with addition of heterotopic gastric or pancreatic rests
- Risk of cancer: Malignant carcinoid & adenocarcinoma in older patients

CLINICAL ISSUES

Presentation

- Most common signs/symptoms
  - GI bleeding: Bleeding can be occult or frank
- Other signs/symptoms
  - Abdominal pain with small bowel obstruction, intussusception, volvulus (including torsion of diverticulum), bowel perforation
    - Perforations reported from ingested fish bone, phytobezoar, button battery, etc.
  - Capsule endoscopy may visualize inflamed Meckel or capsule can become entrapped
  - Hemoperitoneum from necrosis & perforation is possible

Demographics

- Age
  - Most become symptomatic before 2 years of age
    - 60% come to medical attention before 10 years of age, with remainder of cases manifesting in adolescence & adulthood
    - Older patients are more likely to present with intussusception or small bowel obstruction than with GI bleeding
- Sex
  - M = F in true incidence
  - Bleeding & other symptoms/complications are more common in male patients

Treatment

- Surgical resection; incidental appendectomy is usually also performed
- Meckel diverticula are generally removed when found incidentally on imaging or in operating room
  - ↑ detection on double-balloon (push pull) endoscopy

DIAGNOSTIC CHECKLIST

Image Interpretation Pearls

- Tc-99m pertechnetate scan: Positive in Meckel diverticula containing gastric mucosa
- Consider Meckel diverticula in atypical cases of RLQ pain
- Consider some form of OMDR in small bowel obstruction otherwise unexplained on imaging & history

SELECTED REFERENCES

1. Hu Y et al: Diagnostic accuracy of high-frequency ultrasound in bleeding Meckel diverticulum in children. Pediatr Radiol. 50(6):833-9, 2020
2. Talathi S et al: Perforated Meckel diverticulum: a rare cause of acute abdomen in children. Pediatr Emerg Care. 36(5):e291-4, 2020
3. Chen Y et al: Bleeding Meckel diverticulum: a retrospective analysis of computed tomography enterography findings. J Comput Assist Tomogr. 43(2):220-7, 2019
4. McKelvie M et al: Beware the innocent presentation of a spontaneous perforated Meckel diverticulum: a rare case and review of the literature. Pediatr Emerg Care. 35(12):881-3, 2019
5. Casciani E et al: MR Enterography in paediatric patients with obscure gastrointestinal bleeding. Eur J Radiol. 93:209-16, 2017
6. Chatterjee A et al: Reminiscing on remnants: imaging of Meckel diverticulum and its complications in adults. AJR Am J Roentgenol. 209(5):W287-96, 2017
7. Rezvani M et al: Heterotopic pancreas: histopathologic features, imaging findings, and complications. Radiographics. 37(2):484-99, 2017
8. Francis A et al: Pediatric Meckel's diverticulum: report of 208 cases and review of the literature. Fetal Pediatr Pathol. 35(3):199-206, 2016
9. Ntoulia A et al: Failed intussusception reduction in children: correlation between radiologic, surgical, and pathologic findings. AJR Am J Roentgenol. 207(2):424-33, 2016
10. Sanchez TR et al: Sonography of abdominal pain in children: appendicitis and its common mimics. J Ultrasound Med. 35(3):627-35, 2016
11. Kawamoto S et al: CT detection of symptomatic and asymptomatic Meckel diverticulum. AJR Am J Roentgenol. 205(2):281-91, 2015
12. Kunitsu T et al: Neonatal Meckel diverticulum: obstruction due to a short mesodiverticular band. Pediatr Int. 57(5):1007-9, 2015
13. Vali R et al: The value of repeat scintigraphy in patients with a high clinical suspicion for Meckel diverticulum after a negative or equivocal first Meckel scan. Pediatr Radiol. 45(10):1506-14, 2015
14. Huang CC et al: Diverse presentations in pediatric Meckel's diverticulum: a review of 100 cases. Pediatr Neonatol. 55(5):369-75, 2014
15. Kotha VK et al: Radiologist's perspective for the Meckel's diverticulum and its complications. Br J Radiol. 87(1037):20130743, 2014
16. Spottswood SE et al: SNMMI and EANM practice guideline for Meckel diverticulum scintigraphy 2.0. J Nucl Med Technol. 42(3):163-9, 2014
17. He Q et al: Double-balloon enteroscopy for diagnosis of Meckel's diverticulum: comparison with operative findings and capsule endoscopy. Surgery. 153(4):549-54, 2013
18. Sinha CK et al: Meckel's scan in children: a review of 183 cases referred to two paediatric surgery specialist centres over 18 years. Pediatr Surg Int. 29(5):511-7, 2013
19. Hegde S et al: MR enterography of perforated acute Meckel diverticulitis. Pediatr Radiol. 42(2):257-62, 2012
20. Kotecha M et al: Multimodality imaging manifestations of the Meckel diverticulum in children. Pediatr Radiol. 42(1):95-103, 2012

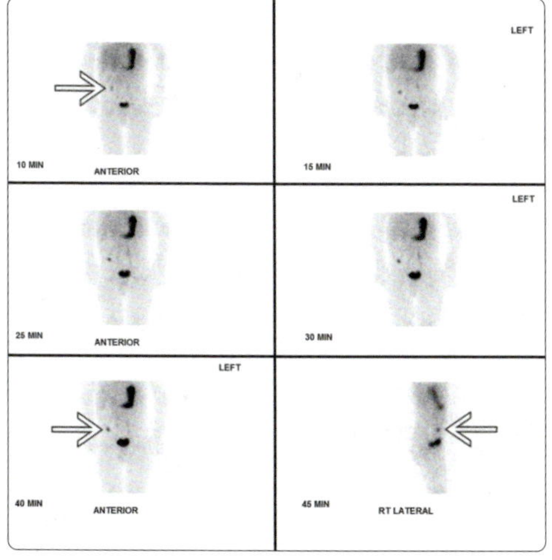

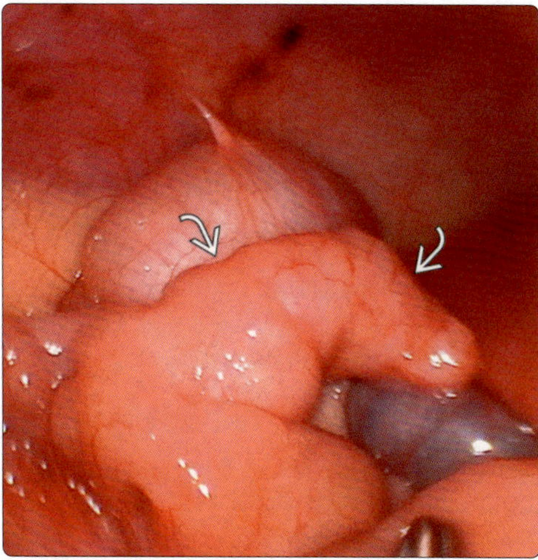

(Left) *Anterior images of a 2-year-old with intermittent bloody stools show a persistent focus of radiotracer accumulation* ➡ *in the RLQ, surgically confirmed to be a Meckel diverticulum containing gastric mucosa.* **(Right)** *Intraoperative photograph in a patient with a history of GI bleeding shows an inflamed, blind-ending Meckel diverticulum* ⤷.

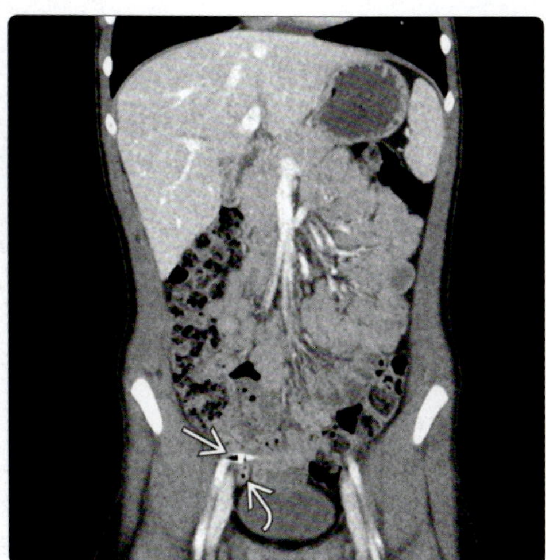

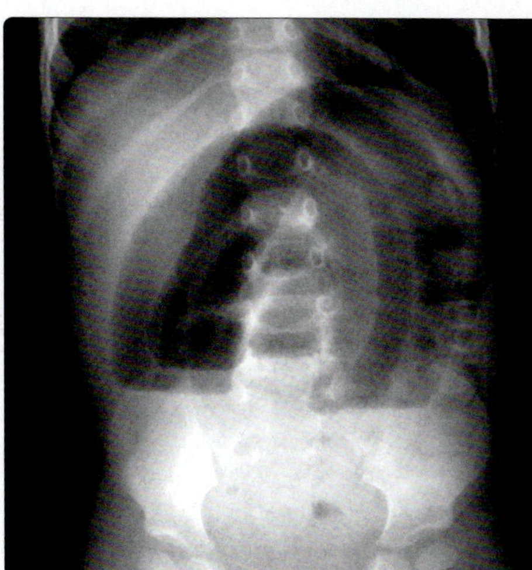

(Left) *Coronal CECT in a 10-year-old child with mild abdominal pain & no prior surgical history shows metal artifact* ➡ *in the RLQ, just superior to a normal appendix* ⤷. *At surgery, an ingested metal BB was found in a mildly inflamed Meckel diverticulum (which was resected).* **(Right)** *AP radiograph in a young child shows dilated small bowel loops with differential air-fluid levels & a paucity of colonic gas, consistent with a small bowel obstruction. An obstructing omphalomesenteric duct remnant was found at surgery.*

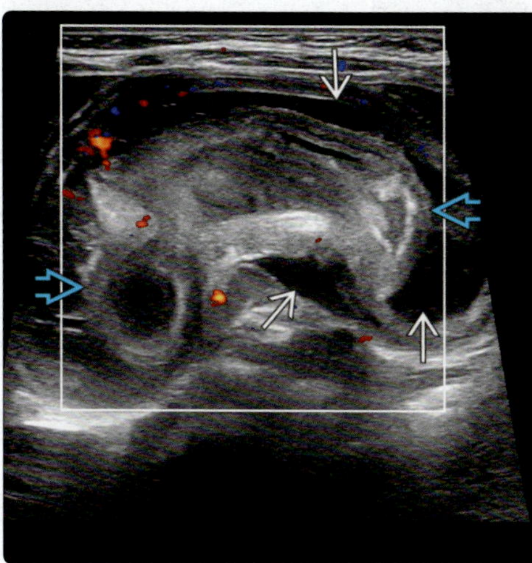

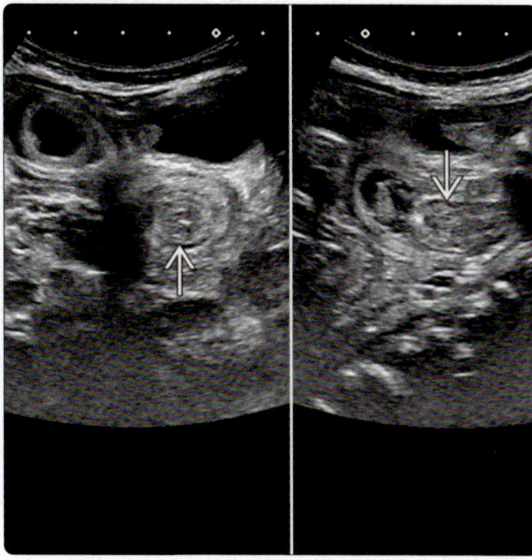

(Left) *Transverse color Doppler US shows a Meckel diverticulum* ⇨ *creating a lead point in a 5-month-old with intussusception. Note the entrapped fluid* ➡ *surrounding the Meckel diverticulum. Air reduction enema failed to reduce the intussusception; therefore, the Meckel & adjacent bowel were resected surgically.* **(Right)** *Split-screen transverse & longitudinal US images of the left lower quadrant show an intussusception containing a Meckel diverticulum* ➡ *in an 11-month-old girl.*

Colonic Volvulus

KEY FACTS

TERMINOLOGY

- Colonic volvulus: Twisting of mobile segment of colon → obstruction → vascular compromise → ischemia
  - Frequency: Sigmoid > cecum >>> transverse colon

IMAGING

- Radiographs: Upper abdominal dilated loop of unusual size & shape for small bowel
  - Cecal volvulus: Often rounded (kidney bean sign)
  - Sigmoid volvulus: Often coffee bean-shaped (1/3)
  - Paucity of distal colonic gas
- Water-soluble contrast enema (WSCE): Bird's beak shape to proximal contrast at site of colonic twisting
  - Contrast fails to pass proximal to twist
    - Does not opacify dilated loop
- CECT: Whirl sign of twisted mesocolon encircling vascular pedicle that serves affected colonic segment
  - Look for abrupt change in course & caliber of veins
  - May have ↓ enhancement of involved segment due to vascular compromise
    - ± bowel wall thickening, pneumatosis, mesenteric edema, free or trapped fluid
- Protocol advice: If initial radiographs are worrisome for colonic volvulus → WSCE for definitive diagnosis; if pneumatosis &/or ill patient → CECT

CLINICAL ISSUES

- Nonspecific abdominal distention & pain, vomiting

DIAGNOSTIC CHECKLIST

- Predisposed patients often have chronic constipation &/or chronically dilated bowel loops
- Suspicion for volvulus requires careful assessment of new radiograph for changes compared to prior radiographs that showed chronic bowel dilation

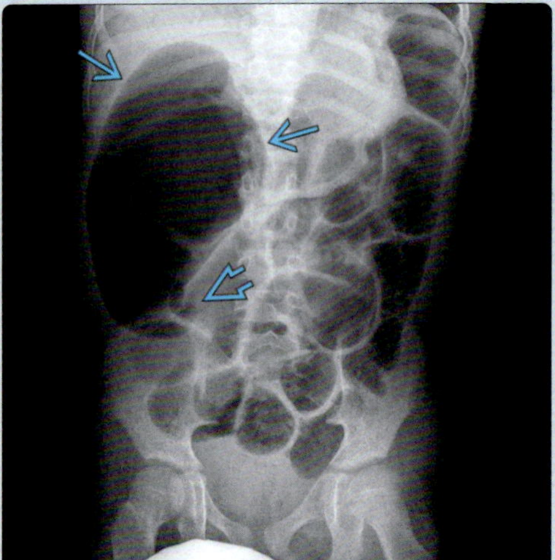

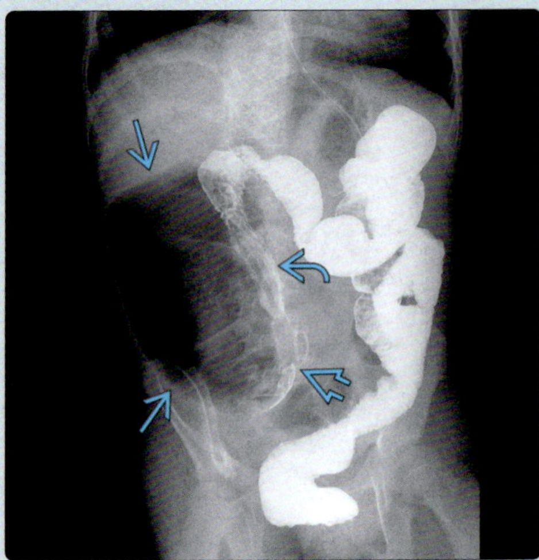

(Left) *AP radiograph in a 12-year-old developmentally delayed boy with acute abdominal pain shows a very dilated bowel loop in the right upper quadrant ➔. The loop has a beak configuration at its inferior aspect ➔, highly suggestive of a colonic volvulus. A contrast enema was recommended.* **(Right)** *Frontal radiograph in the same patient after a water-soluble contrast enema shows narrowing of the ascending colon ➔, which ends proximally in a twist ➔, leading to upstream dilation ➔ in this cecal volvulus.*

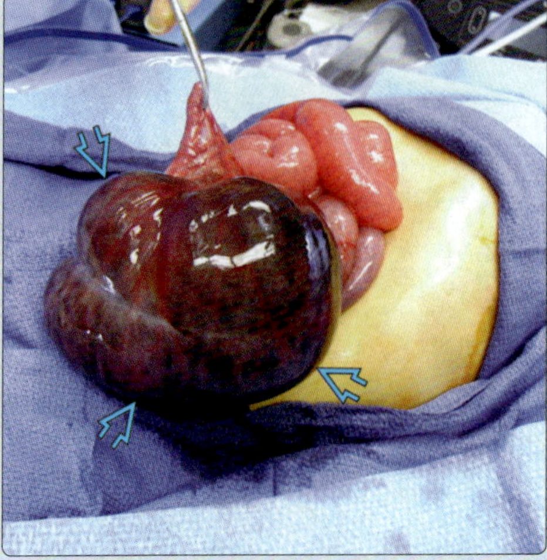

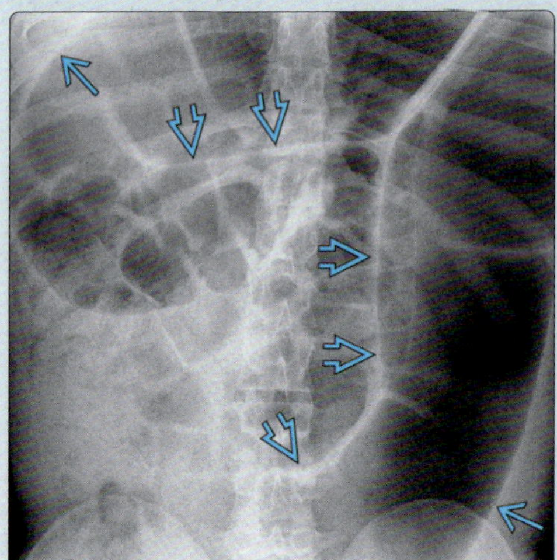

(Left) *Surgical photograph of a 2-year-old with cerebral palsy & acute abdominal pain who had a preceding enema (not shown) worrisome for cecal volvulus shows a large necrotic cecum ➔, which was extracted from the left upper quadrant & resected.* **(Right)** *AP radiograph of a 14-year-old with acute abdominal pain shows a dilated closed loop of sigmoid colon ➔. The centrally apposed colonic walls ➔ create the coffee bean sign. This appearance can be seen in almost 1/3 of sigmoid volvulus cases.*

Colonic Volvulus

TERMINOLOGY

Synonyms

- Cecal volvulus, sigmoid volvulus, transverse colon volvulus

Definitions

- Colonic volvulus: Twisting of mobile segment of colon
- Very rare in children

IMAGING

General Features

- Best diagnostic clue
  - Radiographs: Upper abdominal dilated loop of unusual size & shape for small bowel
    - Cecal volvulus is often kidney bean-shaped
    - Sigmoid volvulus is often coffee bean-shaped
  - Water-soluble contrast enema (WSCE): Bird's beak shape to proximal contrast at site of colonic twisting
- Location
  - Sigmoid colon > cecum >>> transverse colon

Radiographic Findings

- Cecal volvulus: Abnormally positioned, focally dilated & rounded cecum (kidney bean)
  - ± small bowel air-fluid levels & paucity of distal colonic gas
- Transverse colon volvulus: Gas-distended central colonic segment with paucity of distal colonic gas
- Sigmoid volvulus: Distended, twisted, ovoid closed loop; characteristic coffee bean sign in up to 1/3 of cases

Fluoroscopic Findings

- Contrast enema
  - Bird's beak shape to proximal contrast head at site of twisting on WSCE
  - Contrast fails to pass proximal to twist to opacify dilated loop

CT Findings

- CECT
  - Whirl sign: Twisted mesocolon encircling vascular pedicle that serves affected colonic segment
    - Look for abrupt change in caliber (e.g., narrowing, cut-off) or course of supplying vessels (especially veins)
      - Helpful to review in 3 planes
      - Veins beyond point of narrowing may be distended
  - Dilated & obstructed segment of colon
    - Transverse & sigmoid segments usually show closed loop obstruction
    - Cecum shows twisted tubular segment
  - Colon distal to obstruction is decompressed
  - May have ↓ enhancement of involved segment due to vascular compromise
    - ± bowel thickening, pneumatosis, mesenteric edema, free or trapped fluid

Imaging Recommendations

- Best imaging tool
  - WSCE or CECT
- Protocol advice
  - If radiographs suggest colonic obstruction with possible volvulus → WSCE for definitive diagnosis
  - If pneumatosis present, patient is ill-appearing, or diagnosis is not suggested on radiography, consider CECT

DIFFERENTIAL DIAGNOSIS

Ileosigmoid Knot

- Ileum & sigmoid become entangled, leading to knot & vascular compromise
- Acute abdominal pain & rapid shock

Colonic Pseudoobstruction

- Acutely or chronically dilated large > small bowel without identifiable mechanical obstruction

Toxic Megacolon

- Ill patient with dilated, thick-walled colon
- Infectious causes or ulcerative colitis is classic

PATHOLOGY

General Features

- Etiology
  - Predisposition in redundant & dilated mobile segments
  - ↑ risk with ↑ colonic distention, constipation, prior surgery, or malrotation
- Associated abnormalities
  - Sigmoid volvulus
    - Hirschsprung disease (18%), omphalomesenteric abnormalities, bowel malrotation, anal stenosis, chronic constipation, postoperative adhesions, prune-belly syndrome, & developmental delay

CLINICAL ISSUES

Presentation

- Most common signs/symptoms
  - Nonspecific abdominal distention & pain
- Other signs/symptoms
  - Vomiting, constipation, diarrhea

Treatment

- Endoscopic reduction success: Sigmoid > > cecal volvulus
- Even with endoscopic detorsion, affected colonic segment is typically resected to prevent recurrence
  - High recurrence rate with pexy procedures

DIAGNOSTIC CHECKLIST

Image Interpretation Pearls

- Predisposed patients often have chronic constipation &/or chronically dilated bowel loops
- Suspicion for volvulus requires careful assessment of new radiograph for changes compared to prior radiographs that showed chronic bowel dilation

SELECTED REFERENCES

1. Wortman JR et al: Pearls and pitfalls in multimodality imaging of colonic volvulus. Radiographics. 40(4):1039-40, 2020
2. Marine MB et al: Diagnosis of pediatric colonic volvulus with abdominal radiography: how good are we? Pediatr Radiol. 47(4):404-10, 2017
3. Tannouri S et al: Pediatric colonic volvulus: a single-institution experience and review. J Pediatr Surg. 52(6):1062-6, 2017
4. Garel C et al: Diagnosis of pediatric gastric, small-bowel and colonic volvulus. Pediatr Radiol. 46(1):130-8, 2016

KEY FACTS

TERMINOLOGY

- Herniation of bowel through mesenteric defect, congenital band, or normal anatomic opening
- Transmesenteric hernia: Congenital mesenteric defect, usually near ileocecal valve or ligament of Treitz
  - Most common in children
- Acquired: Post surgical (iatrogenic) or post traumatic
- Other types are more common in adults
  - Foramen of Winslow, paraduodenal, pericecal, transomental

IMAGING

- Best imaging modality: CECT
  - Dilated small bowel loops, often localized to 1 region of abdomen
    - Look for abnormal position &/or configuration
  - Closed loop obstruction is suggested by decompressed distal & proximal bowel loops
  - Vascular compromise/ischemia is suggested by
    - Mesenteric edema, free fluid (nonspecific)
    - ↓ bowel wall enhancement, pneumatosis (more specific)
    - ± swirling/twisting with narrowing &/or engorgement of vessels
- Finding exact location of obstruction is less important than recognizing signs of vascular compromise

TOP DIFFERENTIAL DIAGNOSES

- Obstruction from other causes [appendicitis, adhesions, intussusception, inguinal hernia, malrotation, + Meckel diverticulum (AAIIMM mnemonic)]
- Ileus; bowel injury

CLINICAL ISSUES

- Presents with vomiting, distention, & other clinical signs of small bowel obstruction
  - May be intermittent as bowel moves in & out of hernia
  - Vascular compromise & bowel necrosis → shock
- Treatment is surgical

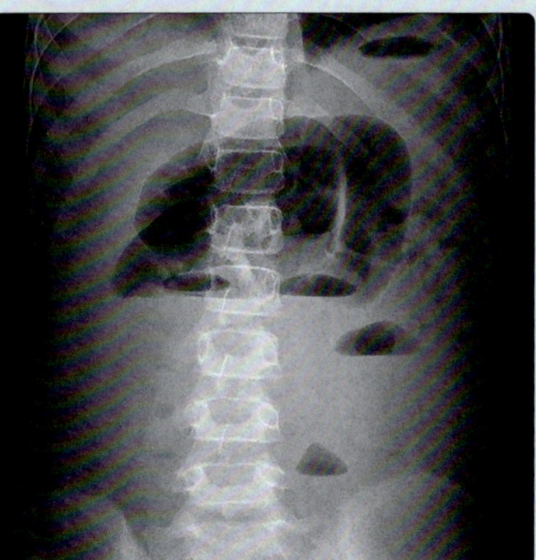
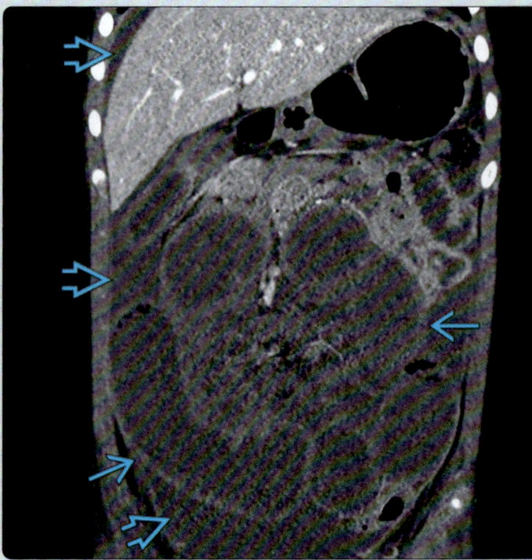

(Left) *Upright abdominal radiograph in a 7-year-old boy with vomiting shows dilated small bowel loops with air-fluid levels, consistent with a bowel obstruction.* **(Right)** *Coronal CECT in the same patient shows dilated small bowel loops with hypoenhancing walls ➾ & extensive intraabdominal free fluid ➾, consistent with a bowel obstruction complicated by ischemia. A congenital mesenteric defect with internal hernia was found at surgery.*

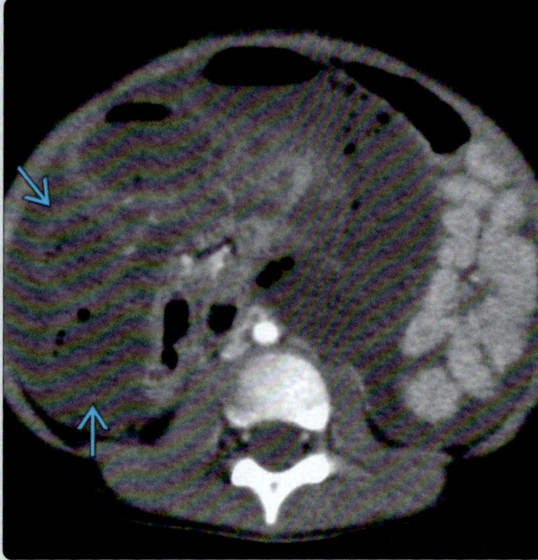
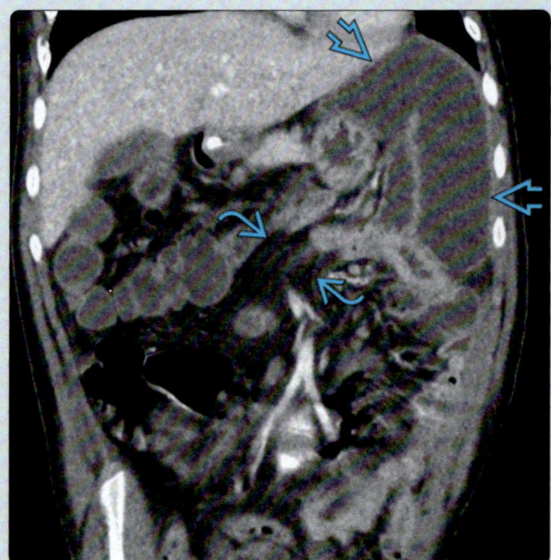

(Left) *Axial CECT in a 4-year-old girl with abdominal distention demonstrates free fluid & dilated small bowel loops (with wall hypoenhancement ➾) clustered in the right lower quadrant. These findings suggest ischemic bowel, & a transmesenteric internal hernia was found at surgery.* **(Right)** *Coronal CECT in a 13-year-old with nausea & vomiting shows dilated loops of small bowel in the left upper quadrant ➾ with fat & vessels passing through a mesenteric defect ➾.*

KEY FACTS

TERMINOLOGY

- Twisting of bowel segment (ileum > jejunum) resulting in obstruction ± ischemia
- Volvulus that is not due to malrotation
  - Can be due to bowel twisting around mesentery in neonates
  - Often from lead point or adhesions in older children

IMAGING

- Best clue: Dilated small bowel loops tapering into twist/swirl of collapsed bowel & vessels
- Radiographs
  - Dilated bowel loops with air-fluid levels
  - ± pneumatosis, pneumoperitoneum
- UGI/SBFT or water-soluble contrast enema
  - Spiral appearance of bowel loops at transition point, indicating volvulus
- CECT or ultrasound
  - Dilated proximal small bowel
  - Tapering of dilated bowel into "whirlpool" or "swirl" of collapsed small bowel & vessels
  - Bowel wall ischemia is suggested by bowel wall thickening, ↓ enhancement (CT) or color flow (Doppler), mesenteric edema, ascites, pneumatosis, pneumoperitoneum

PATHOLOGY

- Underlying lead points: Congenital band, meconium ileus, duplication cyst, Meckel diverticulum, lipoma, lymphatic malformation, postoperative adhesion, foreign body

CLINICAL ISSUES

- Presentation: Abdominal pain, distention, nausea/vomiting
- Most common in neonates but can occur at any age
- Treatment is surgical

DIAGNOSTIC CHECKLIST

- Look for signs of bowel ischemia
- Look for lead point, especially in older children

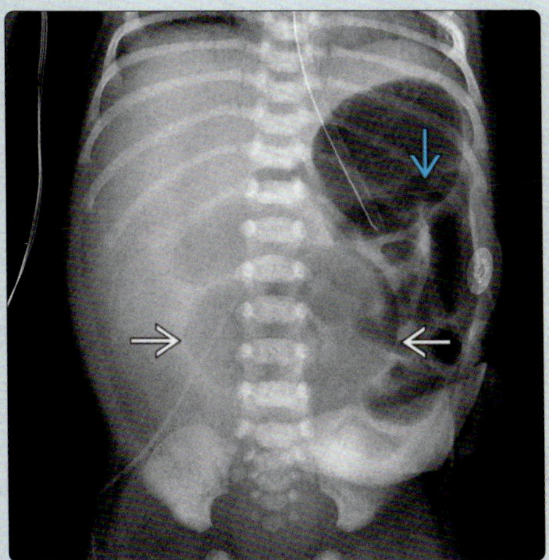

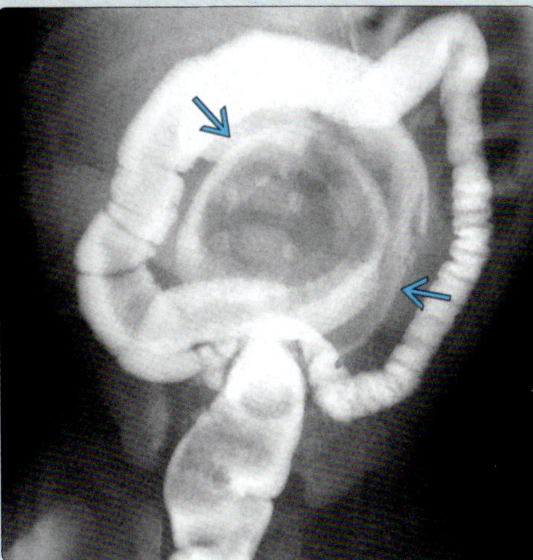

(Left) *Supine abdominal radiograph in a 3-day-old girl with vomiting shows dilated, gas-filled small bowel loops being displaced into the left abdomen ➡ by a cluster of mildly lucent dilated bowel loops in the central abdomen ➡. There is no bowel gas in the right abdomen. These features suggest a distal obstruction.* **(Right)** *Water-soluble contrast enema in the same patient shows swirling of opacified distal small bowel loops in the midabdomen ➡. Surgery confirmed an ileal volvulus around a congenital band.*

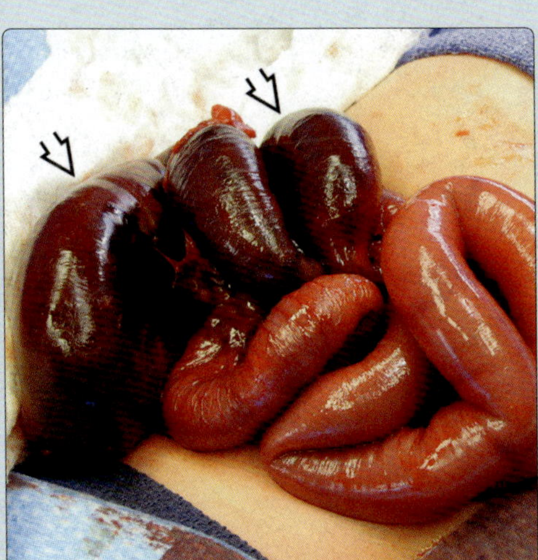

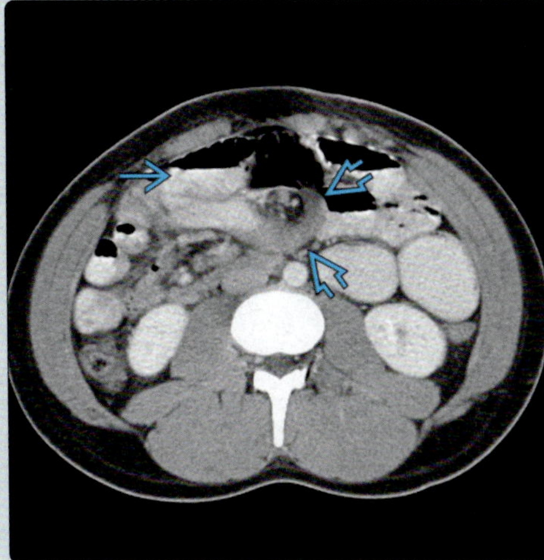

(Left) *Intraoperative photograph in the same 3-day-old girl shows twisting of the necrotic dilated small bowel loops ➡. This ileal volvulus was due to a congenital band.* **(Right)** *Axial CECT in a 17-year-old boy with a history of neonatal repair of a proximal intestinal atresia, now presenting with vomiting, shows tapering & twisting/swirling ➡ of small bowel loops at the transition point from dilated ➡ to decompressed small intestine. At surgery, this volvulus was found to be secondary to an adhesion.*

Hepatoblastoma

KEY FACTS

TERMINOLOGY

- Malignant embryonal hepatic tumor

IMAGING

- Large, well-defined, solid but heterogeneous liver mass in child < 4 years of age with high α-fetoprotein (AFP) levels
  - Heterogeneity due to hemorrhage, necrosis, Ca^{2+}, or mixed histologies
- Single round, lobulated mass (80%), usually > 10 cm
  - May be multifocal (20%)
- Displacement/compression/effacement of adjacent vessels vs. true vascular invasion
- Usually enhances less than normal liver on all phases
- Pediatric LI-RADS workgroup recommends MR with hepatobiliary contrast agent at all imaging time points
- Chest CT to evaluate for pulmonary metastases
  - Metastases in 20% at presentation

PATHOLOGY

- Risk factors: Very low birth weight, Beckwith-Wiedemann syndrome, familial adenomatous polyposis
- Epithelial type is more common than mixed epithelial & mesenchymal type
- **Pret**reatment **ext**ent of disease (PRETEXT) system is used to stage all pediatric liver tumors

CLINICAL ISSUES

- Most common primary liver tumor of childhood
- Presents as painless abdominal mass or hepatomegaly
- Median age: 19 months
  - Only 5-10% occur in children > 4 years of age
- Surgical resection ± neoadjuvant chemotherapy
  - Resection alone can be curative
  - Transplant if unresectable after neoadjuvant therapy
- Posttherapy AFP levels serve as tumor marker for surveillance

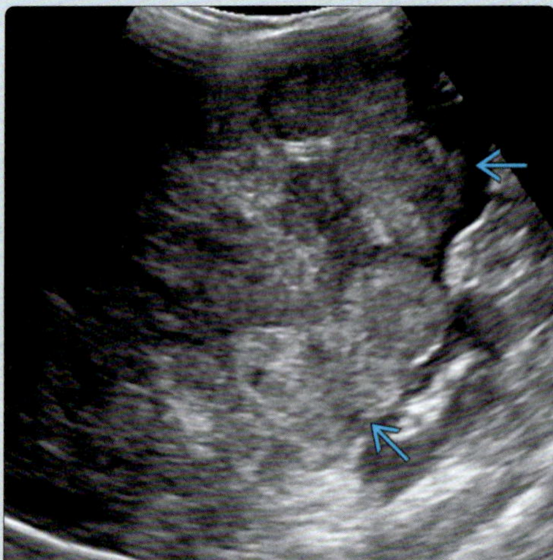

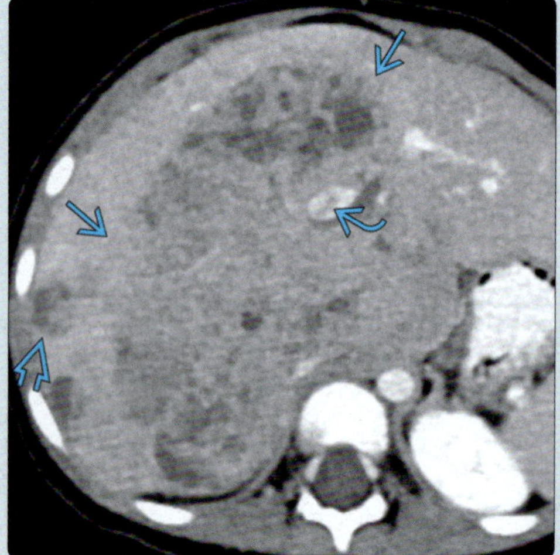

(Left) *Longitudinal US in a child with hepatoblastoma shows a large, heterogeneous, lobulated mass ➙. No normal liver parenchyma is visible.* **(Right)** *Axial CECT of the same patient obtained in the portal venous phase of imaging shows a dominant tumor ➙ occupying the right side of the liver. Thrombus ➙ is present in the adjacent left portal vein. Additional satellite lesions are also noted ➙.*

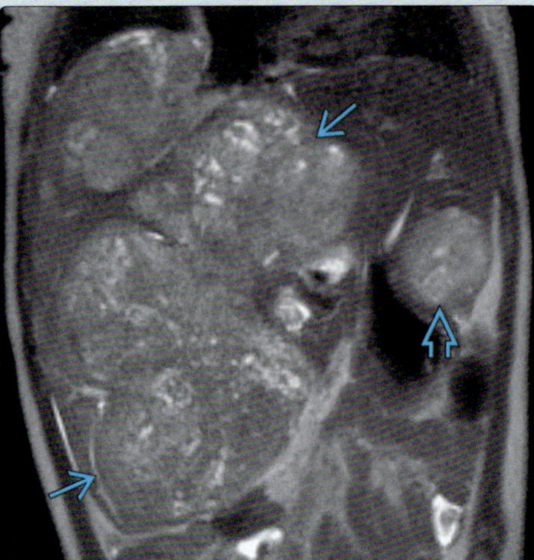

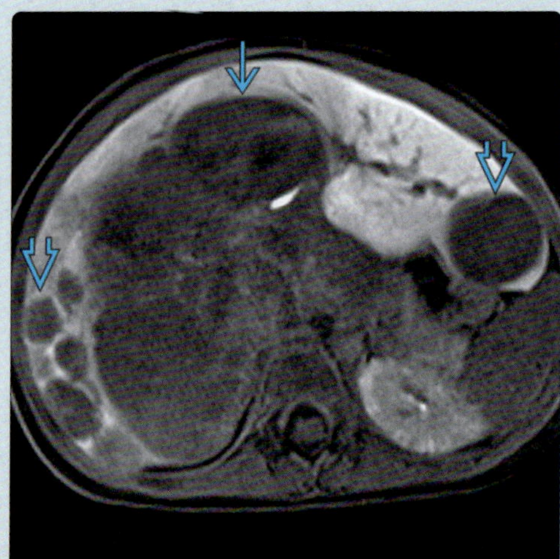

(Left) *Coronal T2 MR in the same patient shows that this tumor is multifocal with the dominant mass ➙ in the right lobe but a separate lesion ➙ in the left lateral section. Because this tumor involved all liver sections, it was considered PRETEXT IV.* **(Right)** *Axial T1 C+ FS MR during the hepatobiliary phase in the same patient highlights the multifocal tumor against the normal contrast-retaining hepatic parenchyma. The dominant mass ➙ involves the right lobe of the liver, but additional lesions are present in both lobes ➙.*

TERMINOLOGY

Definitions

- Malignant embryonal hepatic tumor

IMAGING

General Features

- Best diagnostic clue
  - Large, well-defined, solid, heterogeneous liver mass in child < 4 years of age with high α-fetoprotein (AFP) levels
    - Heterogeneity due to hemorrhage, necrosis, or mixed histologies; Ca^{2+} in 50%
- Location
  - More common in right lobe of liver
- Size
  - Usually > 10 cm
- Morphology
  - Single round, lobulated mass (80%)
    - May be multifocal (20%)
  - Displaces, compresses, & effaces adjacent hepatic structures (vessels, falciform ligament)
  - May invade portal or hepatic veins
    - Tumor thrombus is favored over bland thrombus if
      - Vessel is dilated
      - Thrombus is contiguous with mass
      - Thrombus shows enhancement with contrast or internal arterial flow on color Doppler ultrasound
  - Large unusual veins may surround tumor

Radiographic Findings

- Homogeneous soft tissue mass in right upper quadrant
  - Displaces bowel inferiorly
  - May mimic generalized hepatomegaly
- Ca^{2+} is uncommonly seen on radiographs

Ultrasonographic Findings

- Grayscale ultrasound
  - Solid, well-defined mass
  - Usually hyperechoic to liver, often heterogeneous
    - Acoustic shadowing due to echogenic Ca^{2+}
    - Hypoechoic/anechoic foci from necrosis, hemorrhage
  - May have spoke-wheel appearance
- Pulsed Doppler
  - Portal or hepatic venous tumor thrombus may show arterial waveforms in venous lumen
- Color Doppler
  - Tumor is often hypovascular
    - Variable amount of disorganized vascularity in tumor

MR Findings

- T1WI
  - Generally hypointense to normal liver
  - High signal intensity foci of intratumoral hemorrhage
- T2WI
  - Heterogeneous intermediate signal intensity but usually hyperintense to normal liver
    - ± hypointense fibrous bands, hemorrhage
    - ± internal hyperintense cystic/necrotic foci
- T1WI C+ FS
  - Pediatric LI-RADS workgroup recommends MR with hepatobiliary contrast agent at all imaging time points
  - Heterogeneous enhancement, usually less than background liver on all phases
  - Hepatobiliary phase (≥ 20-minute delay) is useful for
    - Characterizing tumor
    - Establishing relationship to biliary system & vessels
    - Detecting multifocal lesions

CT Findings

- NECT
  - Not recommended for liver mass evaluation
- CECT
  - Well-defined, heterogeneous mass
  - Most enhance < background liver
    - Pediatric LI-RADS workgroup recommends dual-phase CT with imaging during late arterial & portal venous phases
    - ± arterial phase enhancement in rim & septa

Imaging Recommendations

- Best imaging tool
  - Ultrasound is best initial imaging modality in child with palpable abdominal mass
    - Determines organ of origin, helping to protocol subsequent cross-sectional imaging study
    - ± visualization of vessel involvement
  - MR with hepatobiliary contrast agent is preferred at all imaging time points
    - Pediatric LI-RADS workgroup recommends CT only if MR is contraindicated, if pediatric anesthesia is not available, or if multiple anesthesia events would be required to image chest & abdomen
  - Chest CT to look for pulmonary metastases

DIFFERENTIAL DIAGNOSIS

Hepatocellular Carcinoma

- Most common malignant hepatic tumor in children > 10 years of age
  - Pediatric hepatocellular carcinoma (HCC) differs from adult disease
    - Underlying liver disease in 30-50%
    - Associated with glycogen storage diseases, tyrosinemia, hemochromatosis, α-1 antitrypsin deficiency, biliary atresia, hepatitis B
- AFP levels are elevated < hepatoblastoma

Mesenchymal Hamartoma

- Benign hepatic tumor, usually < 2 years of age
- Large multicystic or mixed solid-cystic mass

Undifferentiated Embryonal Sarcoma

- Rare, usually 6-10 years of age, normal AFP
- May arise from mesenchymal hamartoma
- Large mass appears solid on US but cystic at CT/MR due to myxoid stroma

Hepatic Hemangioma

- Can be congenital or infantile type
- Congenital: Typically large & solitary; may cause heart failure with shunting
  - Detected in perinatal period

- Heterogeneous mass with vigorous peripheral enhancement but central areas of persistent nonenhancement
- Often regresses in 1st few months of life
- Infantile type: Multifocal or diffuse; small to moderate size
  - Develops in 1st weeks to months of life
  - Gradual complete enhancement (periphery to center)
  - Slowly regresses after 6-24 months

Hepatic Metastases

- Most commonly caused by neuroblastoma or Wilms tumor
- Delayed hepatocyte phase MR may be most sensitive

PATHOLOGY

General Features

- Etiology
  - Unknown
  - Risk factors & predisposing conditions
    - Very low birth weight (20x risk)
    - Beckwith-Wiedemann syndrome (2,280x risk)
    - Familial adenomatous polyposis (847x risk)

Staging, Grading, & Classification

- **Pret**reatment **ext**ent of disease (PRETEXT) staging system is used to characterize pediatric liver tumors & risk stratify patients
  - Image-based system to guide surgical management
  - PRETEXT group is determined by number of contiguous hepatic sections that must be resected to remove tumor
    - PRETEXT I: Tumor only involves 1 section (left lateral or right posterior) → 3 contiguous sections free of tumor
    - PRETEXT II: 2 contiguous sections free of tumor
    - PRETEXT III: 1 section free of tumor
    - PRETEXT IV: All sections involved with tumor
  - PRETEXT annotation factors for vascular involvement (portal veins & hepatic veins), multifocality, metastases, extrahepatic spread, tumor rupture, & nodal involvement
    - Strict definitions for each annotation factor
    - Vascular invasion & metastases are most common annotation factors
    - Vascular involvement is determined by presence of thrombus, vascular encasement, or obliteration
- POSTTEXT (**postt**reatment **ext**ent of tumor) is determined using same method

CLINICAL ISSUES

Presentation

- Most common signs/symptoms
  - Painless abdominal mass
  - Hepatomegaly
  - Markedly elevated AFP levels (90%)

Demographics

- Age
  - Diagnosed in young children
    - Median age at diagnosis: 19 months
    - 4% congenital
    - Only 5-10% occur beyond 4 years of age
- Sex
  - 60% male
- Epidemiology
  - Most common primary liver tumor of childhood
    - 91% of hepatic malignancies < 5 years of age
  - Incidence
    - 10.5 cases per million in children < 1 year of age
    - 5.2 cases per million in children 1-4 years of age
  - 3rd most common pediatric abdominal malignancy after Wilms tumor & neuroblastoma

Natural History & Prognosis

- Event-free survival/overall survival
  - Standard risk: Up to 83%/95%
    - Standard risk: Tumor confined to liver, ≤ 3 sections
  - High risk: Up to 65%/69%
    - High risk: Tumor in 4 sections, metastatic disease, low AFP levels
- Metastatic disease in 20% at diagnosis
  - Lung is most common location for metastases
- Poor prognostic factors
  - Positive annotation factors, low AFP level (< 100 ng/mL), ≥ 8 years of age, PRETEXT III or IV
- Fractures present in ~18% of patients at diagnosis
  - Most common in ribs & spine
  - May be paraneoplastic effect

Treatment

- Surgical resection can be curative
  - Up to 60% are unresectable initially
- Chemotherapy
  - Neoadjuvant therapy improves resectability
- Liver transplantation for unresectable tumor
  - 75-87% disease-free survival for primary transplant
- Posttherapy AFP serves as surveillance tumor marker

DIAGNOSTIC CHECKLIST

Image Interpretation Pearls

- Large, well-defined, heterogeneous liver mass in infant
  - May have vascular invasion
    - Can be difficult initially to distinguish vascular invasion from compression

SELECTED REFERENCES

1. Schooler GR et al: Pediatric hepatoblastoma, hepatocellular carcinoma, and other hepatic neoplasms: consensus imaging recommendations from American College of Radiology Pediatric Liver Reporting and Data System (LI-RADS) Working Group. Radiology. 296(3):493-7, 2020
2. Towbin AJ et al: Fractures in children with newly diagnosed hepatoblastoma. Pediatr Radiol. 48(4):581-5, 2018
3. Towbin AJ et al: 2017 PRETEXT: radiologic staging system for primary hepatic malignancies of childhood revised for the Paediatric Hepatic International Tumour Trial (PHITT). Pediatr Radiol. 48(4):536-54, 2018
4. Meyers RL et al: Risk-stratified staging in paediatric hepatoblastoma: a unified analysis from the Children's Hepatic tumors International Collaboration. Lancet Oncol. 18(1):122-31, 2017
5. O'Neill AF et al: characterization of pulmonary metastases in children with hepatoblastoma treated on children's oncology group protocol ahep0731 (the treatment of children with all stages of hepatoblastoma): a report from the Children's Oncology Group. J Clin Oncol. 35(30):3465-73, 2017
6. Meyers AB et al: Hepatoblastoma imaging with gadoxetate disodium-enhanced MRI–typical, atypical, pre- and post-treatment evaluation. Pediatr Radiol. 42(7):859-66, 2012

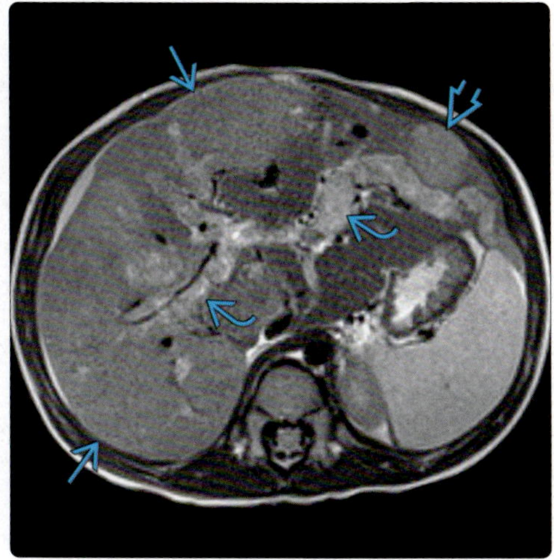

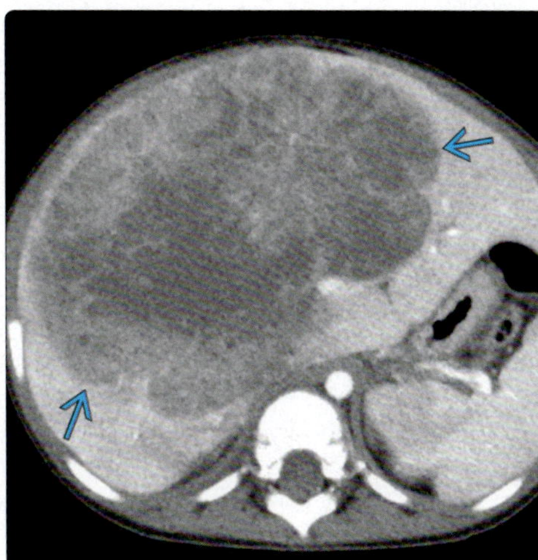

(Left) *Axial T2 MR in a child with hepatoblastoma shows a dominant tumor ➡ spanning both the right & left lobes of the liver. The tumor is multifocal with a distinct mass ➡ in the left lateral section. Tumor thrombus ➡ fills the right & left portal veins.* **(Right)** *Axial CECT in the portal venous phase shows a PRETEXT III hepatoblastoma ➡ occupying the right anterior & left medial sections of the liver. The tumor was marginated by the right hepatic vein & the umbilical segment of the left portal vein (not shown).*

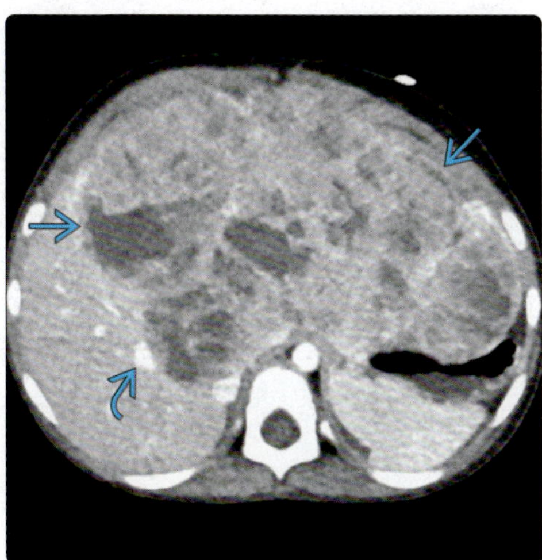

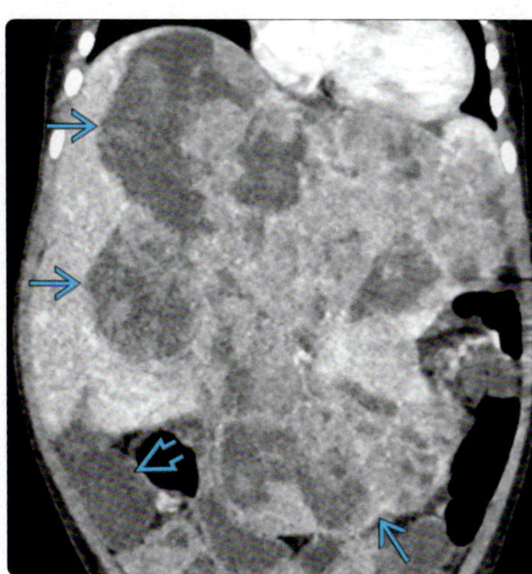

(Left) *Axial CECT obtained in the portal venous phase shows a large tumor ➡ occupying the left lobe of the liver. The tumor does not cross beyond the middle hepatic vein ➡, making this a PRETEXT II tumor.* **(Right)** *Coronal CECT obtained in the portal venous phase in the same patient shows that the large tumor ➡ of the left lobe of the liver lies entirely to the left of the middle hepatic vein & gallbladder ➡.*

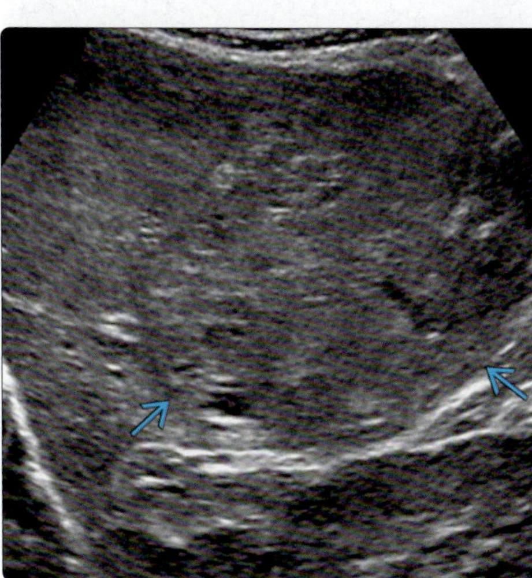

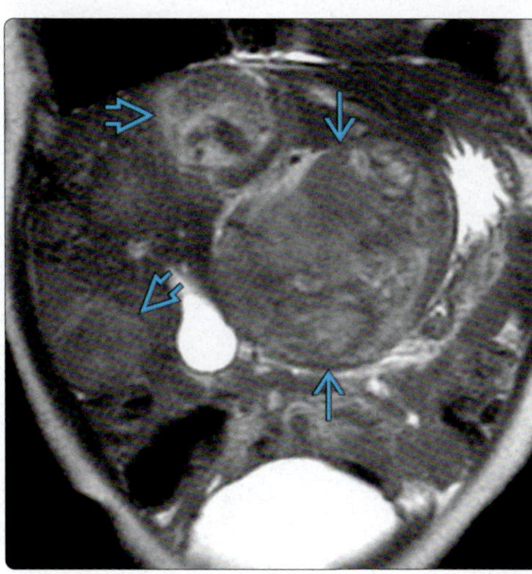

(Left) *Longitudinal US of the left lobe of the liver shows a mildly heterogeneous solid mass ➡ arising from the inferior liver.* **(Right)** *Coronal T2 MR in the same patient shows the mass ➡ arising from the inferior aspect of the left lobe of the liver. The tumor is multifocal with additional masses ➡ scattered throughout the hepatic parenchyma.*

Hepatic Hemangiomas, Infantile and Congenital

KEY FACTS

TERMINOLOGY

- Hemangioma: Benign endothelial neoplasm of neonates/infants in soft tissues or viscera (especially liver)
  - **Not** hemangioendothelioma (more aggressive tumor)
  - **Not** cavernous hemangioma (venous malformation)
- Congenital hemangioma (CH): Found in perinatal period, does not proliferate beyond birth; stains GLUT1 negative
  - Rapidly involuting subtype is more common in liver than noninvoluting
- Infantile hemangioma (IH): Develops in 1st few weeks of life with characteristic proliferating & involuting phases; stains GLUT1 positive

IMAGING

- 3 types of pediatric hepatic hemangiomas
  - Focal (CH): Solitary large heterogeneous mass
  - Multifocal (IH): Multiple small to moderate homogeneous masses
  - Diffuse (IH): Liver is enlarged & replaced by masses
- Focal hepatic CH: T2 heterogeneity; early peripheral enhancement + persistent foci of central nonenhancement
- Multifocal/diffuse IHs: T2-hyperintense lesions with gradual complete central filling after early peripheral enhancement
  - Often found in infants with ≥ 5 cutaneous IHs
- CH & IH often have enlarged feeding arteries/draining veins

CLINICAL ISSUES

- Hepatic CHs & IHs may be asymptomatic or can present with hepatomegaly, heart failure
- CHs may have anemia & mild, transient, consumptive coagulopathy (not Kasabach-Merritt phenomenon)
- Diffuse IHs may also present with hypothyroidism, liver failure, abdominal compartment syndrome
- Treatment is required if complications develop (< 10%)
  - CHs: Embolization, resection
  - IHs: Medical therapies initially (propranolol, steroids; rarely vincristine); embolization, liver transplant in extreme cases

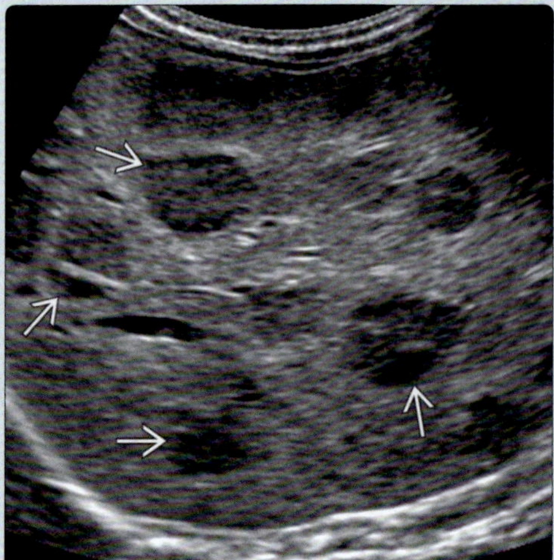

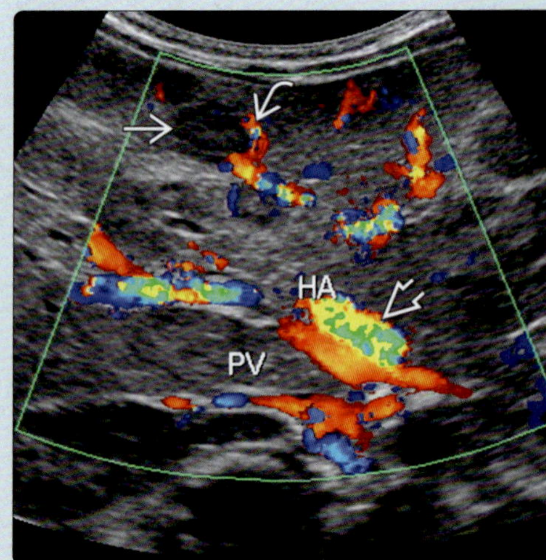

(Left) *Longitudinal US in a 7-month-old with a history of cutaneous infantile hemangiomas (IHs) shows multiple, round, well-circumscribed, hypoechoic masses ➡ throughout the liver.* **(Right)** *Transverse color Doppler US in the same patient shows ↑ vascularity ↪ along the hypoechoic masses ➡. Note the enlarged hepatic artery ➡ with color aliasing (compared to the normal color Doppler appearance of the portal vein) due to undersampling of high-velocity flow supplying the lesions.*

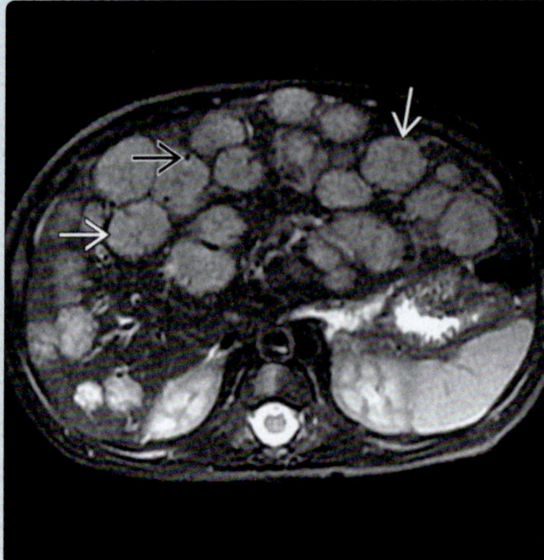

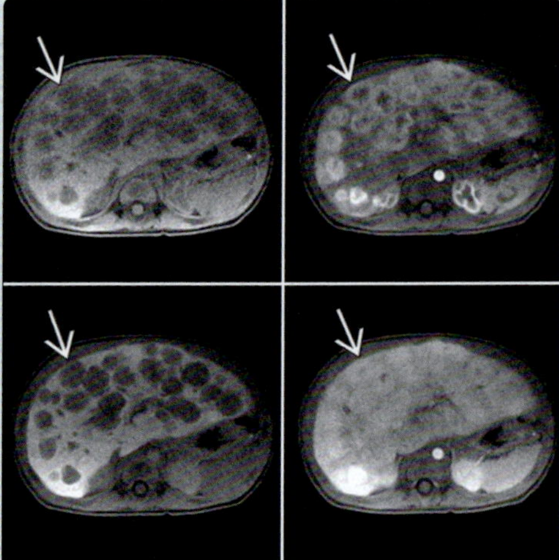

(Left) *Axial T2 FS MR in this patient shows the typical appearance of IHs: Multiple, round, well-circumscribed, small to moderate-sized, hyperintense (but not fluid-bright) lesions ➡, some of which contain flow voids ⇨.* **(Right)** *Axial dynamic T1 C+ FS MR images with a hepatocyte-specific agent in (clockwise from top left) precontrast, arterial, portal venous, & delayed hepatocyte phases show a typical appearance of IHs ➡ with early peripheral enhancement, complete venous filling, & washout.*

TERMINOLOGY

Synonyms

- **Not** hemangioendothelioma (more aggressive vascular tumor, not typically found in infantile liver)
- **Not** cavernous hemangioma (venous malformation, not typically found in infantile liver)

Definitions

- Hemangioma: Benign endothelial neoplasm occurring in soft tissues or viscera (especially liver: Most common benign hepatic tumor of infants)
  - 70% of 2009 publications used term hemangioma incorrectly
- Congenital hemangioma (CH): Found in perinatal period; does not proliferate beyond birth
  - Rapidly involuting (RICH) vs. noninvoluting (NICH) vs. partially involuting subtypes
    - Only follow-up imaging or biopsy can determine subtype
- Infantile hemangioma (IH)
  - Usually not present at birth
  - Proliferating phase: Lesion(s) develop during 1st few weeks of life with rapid growth over next few months
  - Involuting phase: Slow regression of lesion(s) over years, usually beginning by 12 months of age

IMAGING

General Features

- Best diagnostic clue
  - CH: Large, solitary, heterogeneous hypervascular hepatic mass in fetus/newborn
  - IHs: Multiple small to moderate T2-hyperintense hepatic lesions with progressive peripheral to central enhancement in infant with ≥ 5 cutaneous IHs
- Morphology
  - Hepatic hemangiomas of young children are characterized as focal, multifocal, or diffuse
    - Focal hepatic hemangioma = true CH (usually RICH)
      - Large, solitary, well-defined mass
      - Multifocal CHs are very rare
    - Multifocal/diffuse hepatic hemangiomas = IHs
      - Multifocal IHs (most common): Multiple small to moderate-sized round lesions
      - Diffuse IHs: Liver is enlarged & nearly completely replaced by lesions
      - Very rarely infiltrate along portal veins, typically in syndromic cases [e.g., PHACE(S)]
  - Enlarged feeding arteries/draining veins may be seen with either CH or IHs

Radiographic Findings

- Radiography
  - Hepatomegaly or right upper quadrant mass
    - Depends on size/number of lesions
  - Ca^{2+} can be seen in ~ 15% of CH cases
  - ± heart failure with cardiomegaly, pulmonary edema

Ultrasonographic Findings

- Grayscale ultrasound
  - Prenatal US
    - CH: Heterogeneous mass ± ↑ vascularity, hydrops
    - IHs: Not present
  - Postnatal US
    - CH: Solitary heterogeneous mass
    - IHs: Multiple, round, well-defined lesions of variable echogenicity, most frequently hypoechoic & homogeneous
- Pulsed Doppler
  - IHs: Elevated hepatic artery velocities during proliferation, ↓ with involution
- Color Doppler
  - CH: ↑ peripheral vascularity ± arteriovenous shunts; little to no central vascularity
  - IHs: Variable ↑ vascularity within/along lesions; low-resistance arterial waveforms during proliferative phase
  - Hepatic arteries & veins frequently are enlarged
- Contrast-enhanced US
  - CH: Early arterial & portal venous hyperenhancement (relative to liver); no washout
  - IHs: Early arterial hyperenhancement; isoenhancement on portal venous phase; variable washout

CT Findings

- NECT
  - Well-defined hypodense mass(es)
  - CH: ± hyperdense foci of hemorrhage, Ca^{2+}
- CECT
  - Typical enhancement patterns
    - CH: Increasingly confluent early nodular peripheral enhancement on dynamic imaging; large central areas do not fill in/enhance over time
    - IHs: Early peripheral enhancement with gradual complete central fill in

MR Findings

- T1WI
  - Hypointense mass(es) compared to unaffected liver
  - CH: Hyperintense foci of hemorrhage
- T2WI
  - CH: Very heterogeneous internally with mixed hyper-/hypointense foci
  - IHs: Relatively homogeneous, hyperintense lesions compared to unaffected liver (but not as bright as fluid); small septa; scattered prominent flow voids
- T1WI C+
  - Enhancement patterns are similar to CT
  - Washout is expected with hepatocyte-specific agents
- MRA/MRV
  - ± enlargement of
    - Upper abdominal aorta, celiac axis, hepatic arteries
    - Hepatic veins, inferior vena cava
    - Arterial & venous branches along periphery of lesions (especially CH)

Imaging Recommendations

- Best imaging tool
  - US is best screening tool for palpable abdominal mass, hepatomegaly, or infant with multiple cutaneous IHs
  - MR for further characterization, extent determination

DIFFERENTIAL DIAGNOSIS

Hepatoblastoma

- Usually large, well-defined, solitary mass
- Uncommon in newborns
- Rarely hypervascular; usually hypoenhancing
  - Peripheral enhancement is not typical
- Markedly elevated & rising α-fetoprotein (AFP)

Neuroblastoma Metastasis

- Multiple masses vs. diffuse liver heterogeneity & enlargement
- Adrenal or paraspinal mass is typically present

Mesenchymal Hamartoma

- Can be solid & highly vascular with similar enhancement to CH (but continues to grow)

Umbilical Catheter Complication

- Vascular/hepatic perforation by umbilical venous catheter may lead to hemorrhage &/or parenchymal infusion of fluid

Venous Malformation

- Uncommon in pediatric liver outside of syndromes
- Lobulated fluid-signal intensity lesions ± layering fluid-fluid levels, phleboliths
- Gradual puddling of contrast into lesion over time

Arterioportal Fistula

- Enlargement & early enhancement of portal vein branch without discrete mass

PATHOLOGY

Microscopic Features

- Clusters of thin-walled capillaries lined by plump endothelium without cellular atypia
- IH
  - Densely packed capillaries with little intervening stroma
  - Cellular proliferation is present during early stages
  - GLUT1-positive endothelium
  - Fatty infiltration is not usually seen with involution in hepatic IHs (unlike soft tissue IHs)
- CH
  - Varying-sized lobules of capillaries surrounded by dense myxoid stroma & large malformed vessels
  - Foci of hemorrhage, necrosis, fibrosis, extramedullary hematopoiesis, Ca^{2+}
  - GLUT1-negative endothelium

CLINICAL ISSUES

Presentation

- Most common signs/symptoms
  - Hepatic CH & IHs may be asymptomatic
  - CH, IHs can present with hepatomegaly, heart failure
- Other signs/symptoms
  - CH may have anemia & mild, transient consumptive coagulopathy
  - Diffuse IHs may also present with
    - Hypothyroidism (due to production of enzyme type 3 iodothyronine deiodinase)
      - 100% of diffuse IHs vs. 21% of multifocal IHs
    - Liver failure
    - Abdominal compartment syndrome
  - Cutaneous IHs are found in
    - 50-75% of multifocal/diffuse hepatic IHs
    - 15% of focal hepatic CH
  - AFP is not produced by CH or IHs
    - AFP is normally high in newborns but ↓ over 1st months of life

Demographics

- Age
  - CH is usually detected in perinatal period
  - IHs develop in 1st few weeks of life
    - More common in premature infants
- Sex
  - CH, M:F = 1:1; in IH, M:F = 1:3-4
- Ethnicity
  - IH is much more common in White patients

Natural History & Prognosis

- Focal hepatic CH
  - Can enlarge from hemorrhage
  - RICH will mostly involute by 14 months of age
  - Mortality is widely variable in literature
- Multifocal/diffuse IHs
  - May grow after detection, depending on age
  - After 1st year of life, gradually involute over years
  - Mortality: 16% overall, higher for diffuse pattern; median age of death = 115 days

Treatment

- Treatment is required if complications develop
  - < 10% of pediatric hepatic hemangiomas require therapy
- CH: Embolization, resection; medical therapies have not proven effective
- IHs: Medical therapies initially (propranolol, steroids; rarely vincristine); embolization, liver transplant in extreme cases

DIAGNOSTIC CHECKLIST

Consider

- Liver US screening in patients with ≥ 5 cutaneous IHs
- Biopsy of hepatic lesions should be performed if diagnosis is unclear by combination of clinical history/exam, initial imaging, & lesion behavior over appropriate timeframe
  - Safely performed percutaneously in experienced hands

SELECTED REFERENCES

1. Ji Y et al: Screening for infantile hepatic hemangioma in patients with cutaneous infantile hemangioma: a multicenter prospective study. J Am Acad Dermatol. 84(5):1378-84, 2021
2. El-Ali AM et al: Contrast-enhanced ultrasound of congenital and infantile hemangiomas: preliminary results from a case series. AJR Am J Roentgenol. 214(3):658-64, 2020
3. McGuire A et al: Pediatric hepatic vascular tumors. Semin Pediatr Surg. 29(5):150970, 2020
4. Iacobas I et al: Guidance document for hepatic hemangioma (infantile and congenital) evaluation and monitoring. J Pediatr. 203:294-300.e2, 2018
5. Rialon KL et al: Impact of screening for hepatic hemangiomas in patients with multiple cutaneous infantile hemangiomas. Pediatr Dermatol. 32(6): 808-12, 2015
6. Roebuck D et al: Rapidly involuting congenital haemangioma (RICH) of the liver. Pediatr Radiol. 42(3):308-14, 2012

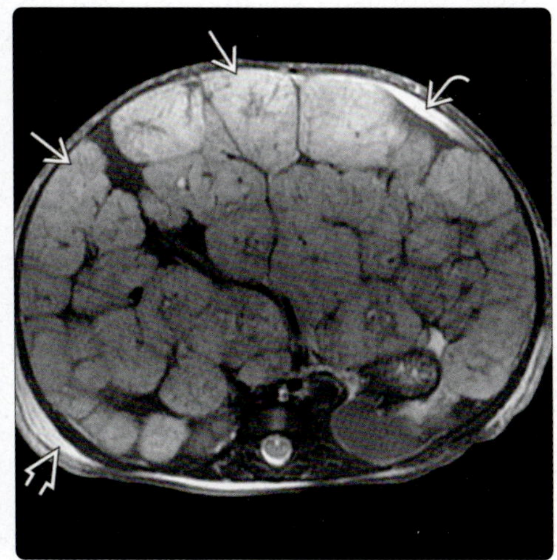

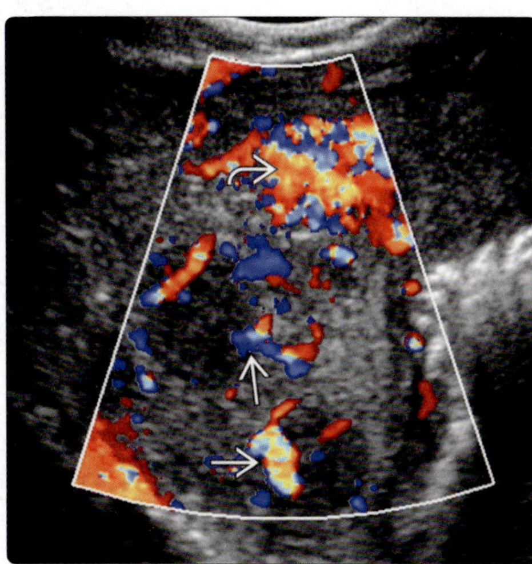

(Left) *Axial T2 FS MR in a patient with cutaneous IHs & abdominal distention shows near-total replacement of the hepatic parenchyma by innumerable hyperintense lesions ➡. Note the ascites ➡ & body wall edema ➡ secondary to liver failure.* **(Right)** *Transverse color Doppler US in a 2-month-old with cutaneous IHs shows variable vascularity within the hypoechoic hepatic lesions, ranging from moderate peripheral vascularity ➡ to diffusely ↑ internal flow ➡.*

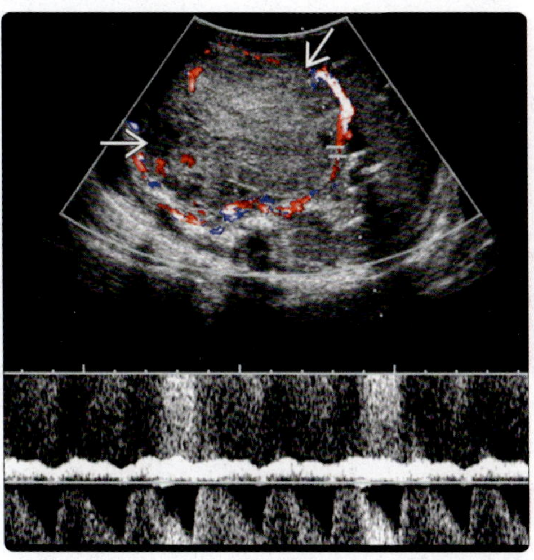

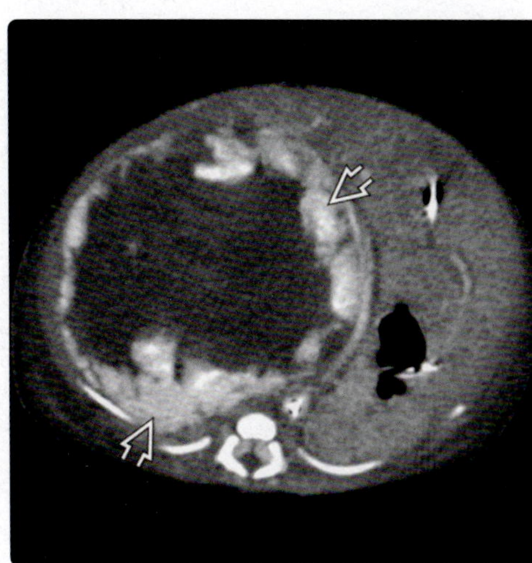

(Left) *Pulsed Doppler US in a newborn with hydrops shows a large, solid, mildly heterogeneous mass ➡ in the right hepatic lobe with ↑ peripheral vascularity. Interrogation of an enlarged artery shows elevated velocities wrapping around the scale.* **(Right)** *Axial CECT shows irregular heterogeneous enhancement ➡ of the lesion periphery on arterial phase. Central portions of the mass did not enhance on delayed images (not shown), typical of a focal hepatic congenital hemangioma (CH).*

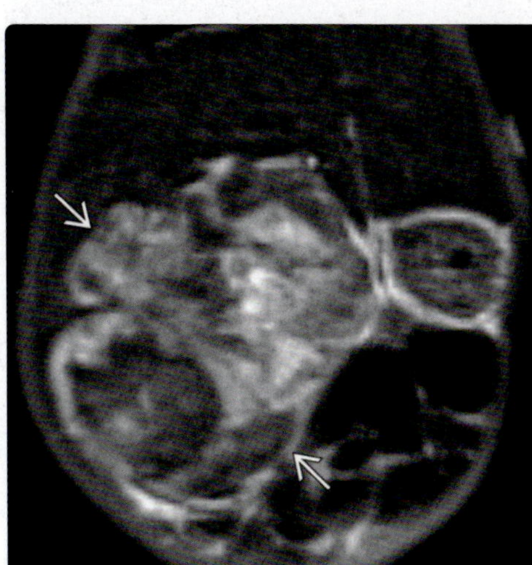

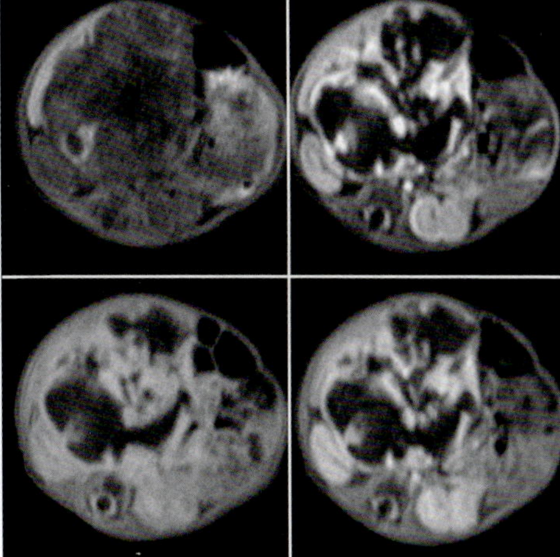

(Left) *Coronal T2 FS MR in a 4-day-old with a palpable abnormality shows a large exophytic mass ➡ arising from the inferior right hepatic lobe. The lesion shows marked internal heterogeneity.* **(Right)** *Axial T1 C+ FS MR images of the same patient at (clockwise from top left) precontrast, 90-second, 180-second, & 5-minute times show irregular peripheral enhancement with large areas of persistent central nonenhancement, typical of a focal CH of the liver.*

KEY FACTS

TERMINOLOGY

- Benign epithelial tumor composed of hepatocytes, Kupffer cells, abnormal bile ducts, & vessels
  - Central scar is present in 50-70%

IMAGING

- CECT: Homogeneous arterial enhancement ± hypoenhancing central scar
- MR with hepatobiliary-phase contrast agent (best tool)
  - T1: Iso- to slightly hypointense; ± hypointense scar
  - T2: Slightly hyperintense; ± hyperintense scar
  - Arterial phase: Hyperenhancing mass ± central scar
  - Venous phase: Iso- to slight hyperenhancement of mass ± hyperenhancing central scar
  - Hepatobiliary phase: Mild hyperenhancement but can be isoenhancing
    - Usually homogeneous (can be heterogeneous in larger lesions)
- US: ↑, ↓, or ↔ echogenicity relative to liver
  - Doppler shows spoke-wheel pattern with hypervascular central scar & radiating vessels
  - Contrast-enhanced US: Early hyperenhancement, ± spoke-wheel pattern

PATHOLOGY

- Hyperplastic response to preexisting vascular malformation within central scar
- Abnormal bile ducts → hepatobiliary phase hyperenhancement (↓ clearance of contrast agent)
- ↑ prevalence after chemotherapy &/or stem cell transplant
  - Often multiple small lesions with no central scar

CLINICAL ISSUES

- 2% of primary hepatic tumors in children
- Often asymptomatic; occasionally causes palpable mass &/or vague abdominal pain
- Managed conservatively in asymptomatic patients & surgically in symptomatic patients

(Left) *Axial arterial-phase T1 C+ FS MR in a 16-year-old girl with an incidentally discovered liver mass demonstrates a homogeneously hyperenhancing lesion ➔ typical of focal nodular hyperplasia (FNH).* **(Right)** *Axial T1 C+ FS MR 20 minutes after the injection of a hepatocyte-specific contrast agent in the same patient shows mild homogeneous hyperenhancement of the lesion ➔ relative to the normal enhancing background liver, consistent with FNH.*

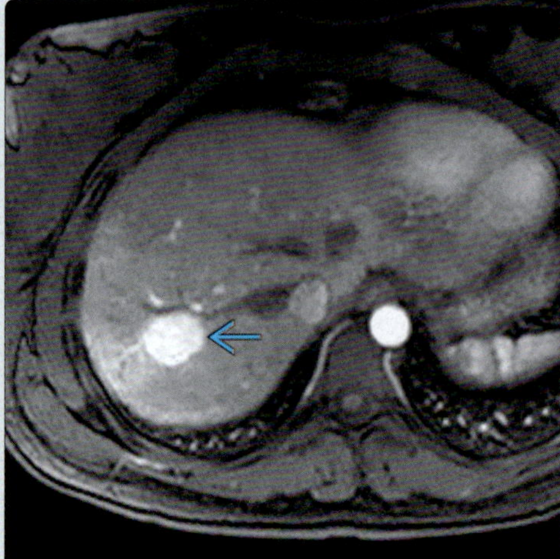

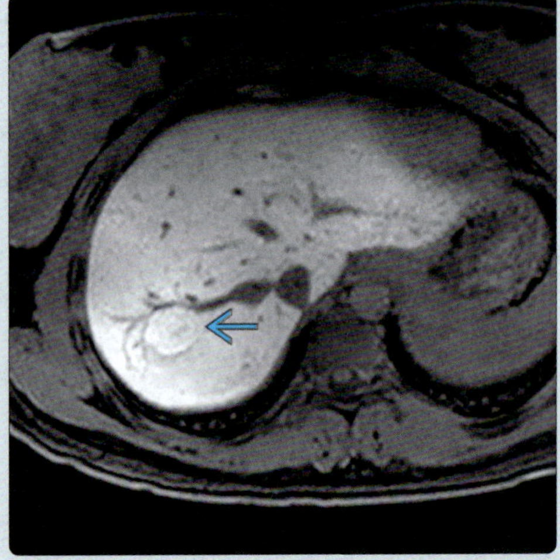

(Left) *Axial CECT in a 3-year-old boy with a palpable mass demonstrates a well-defined, homogeneously enhancing left lobe liver mass ➔ with a central hypodense scar ➔, typical of FNH. The lesion enhancement is similar to normal liver in portal venous phase.* **(Right)** *Coronal T1 C+ FS MR using a hepatocyte-specific contrast agent in a patient with a liver mass demonstrates slight hyperenhancement of the mass ➔ on the 20-minute delayed image. Note the nonenhancing central scar ➔, typical of FNH.*

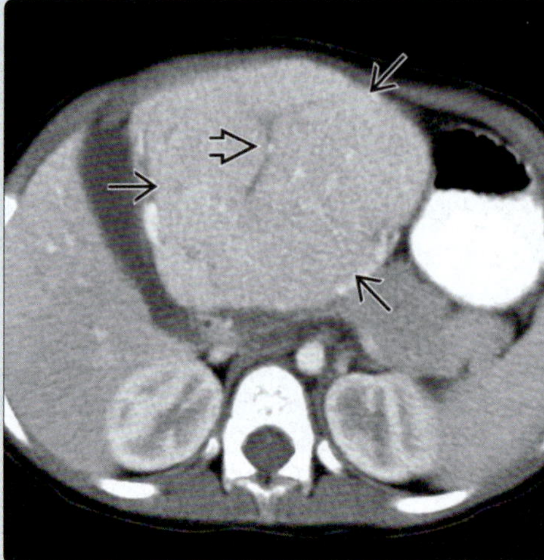

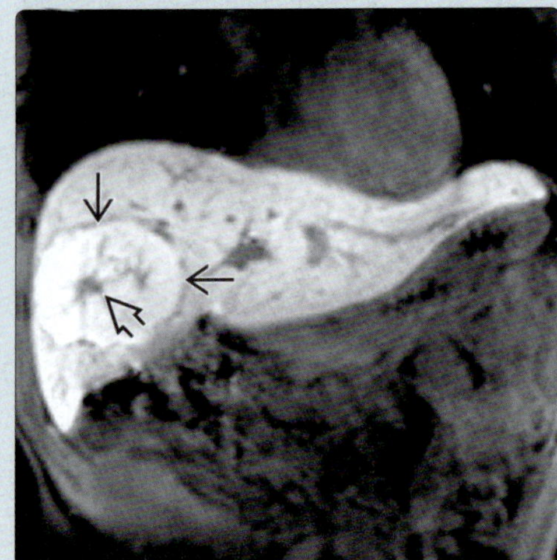

TERMINOLOGY

Abbreviations

- Focal nodular hyperplasia (FNH)

Definitions

- Benign epithelial tumor composed of hepatocytes, abnormal bile ducts, & vascular structures
- 2% of primary hepatic tumors in children

IMAGING

General Features

- Best diagnostic clue
  - Homogeneous, arterially enhancing mass on CT or MR with delayed enhancement of central scar
  - Central scar is present in 50-70%
    - Scar is more likely in larger lesions
- Morphology
  - Well-defined, round or ovoid mass
  - Smooth vs. mildly lobulated margins

Ultrasonographic Findings

- Grayscale ultrasound
  - Iso-, hypo-, or hyperechoic mass ± central scar
- Color Doppler
  - Spoke-wheel pattern with hypervascular central scar & radiating vessels extending to periphery
- Contrast-enhanced US: Early phase hyperenhancement; ↔ to ↑ on later phases
  - Can see spoke-wheel pattern of enhancement

CT Findings

- CECT
  - Arterial phase
    - Hyperenhancing hepatic lesion ± ↓ attenuation central scar
  - Portal venous & delayed phases
    - Becomes isoattenuating relative to normal liver
    - Enhancement of central scar (if present)
  - May be impossible to distinguish from normal liver on NECT or postcontrast portal venous & delayed phases

MR Findings

- T1WI
  - Iso- to hypointense lesion; ± hypointense central scar
- T2WI
  - Iso- to slightly hyperintense; ± hyperintense central scar
- T1WI C+
  - Arterial phase
    - ↑ enhancement relative to normal liver; ± ↓ enhancing scar
  - Portal venous phase
    - Becomes isointense to liver; ± ↑ enhancing scar
  - Hepatobiliary phase (e.g., gadoxetate disodium)
    - Most common: Mildly ↑ enhancement of mass relative to normal liver; ± ↓ enhancing scar
    - Different patterns of enhancement are reported: Homogeneous, heterogeneous, peripheral, or isointense to liver
      - Rare ↓ enhancement has been described

Imaging Recommendations

- Best imaging tool
  - Dynamic MR with hepatobiliary contrast agent

DIFFERENTIAL DIAGNOSIS

Fibrolamellar Hepatocellular Carcinoma

- Central scar is hypointense on both T1 & T2 MR

Hepatocellular Carcinoma

- ± underlying liver disease in children
- Typically ↓ enhancement on hepatobiliary-phase MR

Hepatic Adenoma

- Oral contraceptive use or history of liver disease

PATHOLOGY

General Features

- Hyperplastic response to preexisting vascular malformation within central scar
  - Leads to proliferation of functional hepatocytes, vascular structures, & abnormal bile ducts
    - Abnormal bile ducts → hepatobiliary-phase hyperenhancement (↓ clearance of contrast agent)
- ↑ prevalence after chemotherapy &/or stem cell transplant
  - Usually multiple & smaller lesions with no central scar

CLINICAL ISSUES

Presentation

- Most common signs/symptoms
  - Often asymptomatic; occasionally causes abdominal pain due to mass effect
- Other signs/symptoms
  - Normal lab values, including α-fetoprotein

Natural History & Prognosis

- No known malignant potential

Treatment

- Managed conservatively in asymptomatic patients vs. surgically in symptomatic patients

DIAGNOSTIC CHECKLIST

Image Interpretation Pearls

- Homogeneous, arterially enhancing mass on CT or MR, ± central scar
- ↑ enhancement relative to normal liver with delayed hepatobiliary-phase contrast MR

SELECTED REFERENCES

1. Vasireddi AK et al: Magnetic resonance imaging of pediatric liver tumors. Pediatr Radiol. ePub, 2021
2. Fang C et al: Contrast-enhanced ultrasound in the diagnosis of pediatric focal nodular hyperplasia and hepatic adenoma: interobserver reliability. Pediatr Radiol. 49(1):82-90, 2019
3. Trout AT et al: Hepatocyte-specific contrast media: not so simple. Pediatr Radiol. 48(9):1245-55, 2018
4. Smith EA et al: Incidence and etiology of new liver lesions in pediatric patients previously treated for malignancy. AJR Am J Roentgenol. 199(1):186-91, 2012
5. Towbin AJ et al: Focal nodular hyperplasia in children, adolescents, and young adults. Pediatr Radiol. 41(3):341-9, 2011

KEY FACTS

TERMINOLOGY

- Benign neoplasm arising from hepatocytes
- May hemorrhage/rupture
- Pathologic subtypes
  - Inflammatory ~ 40-50%
  - Hepatocyte nuclear factor 1α (*HNF1α*) mutated ~ 30-35%
  - β-catenin activated ~ 10-15%
    - ↑ malignant potential
  - Unclassified ~ 5-10%

IMAGING

- Variable patterns of hyperenhancement on arterial phase
  - May contain fat, hemorrhage, necrosis, Ca^{2+}
- Subtypes may have different MR features
  - Inflammatory: ↑ on T2, ↑ arterial enhancement
  - *HNF1α:* ↓ on T1 opposed phase (lipid), ↑ to ↔ arterial enhancement
  - β-catenin & undifferentiated subtypes: Variable
- Hepatobiliary-phase MR contrast agents help characterize lesions & ↑ detection of small lesions
- US: Heterogeneous, ± ↑ echogenicity due to lipid or hemorrhage
- CT: Arterial phase → typical hyperenhancement
  - ↑ attenuation subcapsular or peritoneal fluid if tumor rupture/hemorrhage occurs

TOP DIFFERENTIAL DIAGNOSES

- Focal nodular hyperplasia
- Hepatocellular carcinoma

CLINICAL ISSUES

- Adenomas are more likely with exogenous steroids, glycogen storage disease, underlying liver disease, congenital portosystemic shunts (Abernethy malformation vs. intrahepatic shunt)
- May regress if oral contraceptives are discontinued
- Surgical excision: Male (↑ β-catenin subtype), symptomatic, suspicious imaging features, or large size

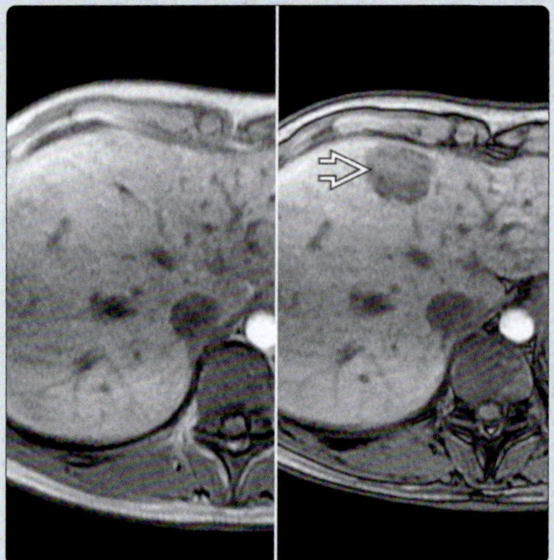

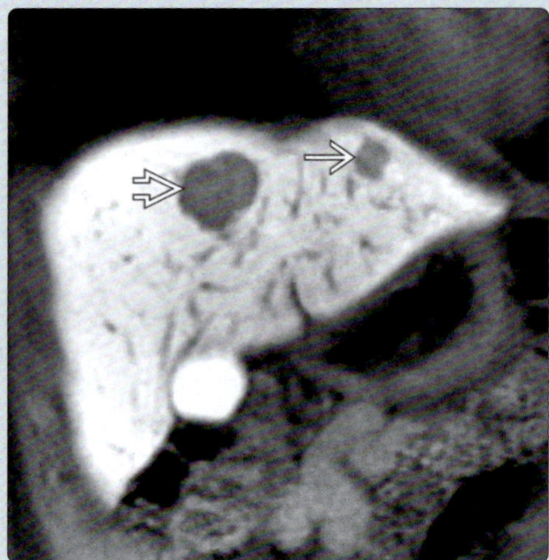

(Left) *Axial in- & opposed-phase MR images in a teenage girl with a liver mass demonstrate marked signal dropout within the mass ➡ on the opposed-phase image, indicating intracellular lipid typical of adenoma. The mass is isointense to normal liver on in-phase imaging.* **(Right)** *Hepatocyte-phase coronal T1 C+ FS MR using a hepatobiliary contrast agent (gadoxetate disodium) in the same patient shows no contrast retention by the mass ➡ relative to the surrounding normal liver. Note a 2nd similar lesion ➡ in the left hepatic lobe.*

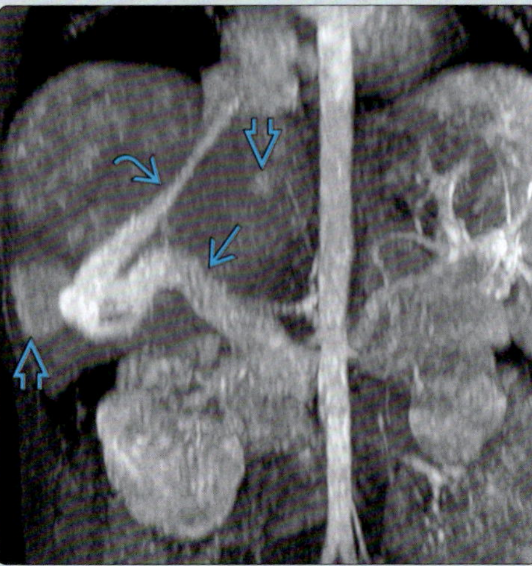

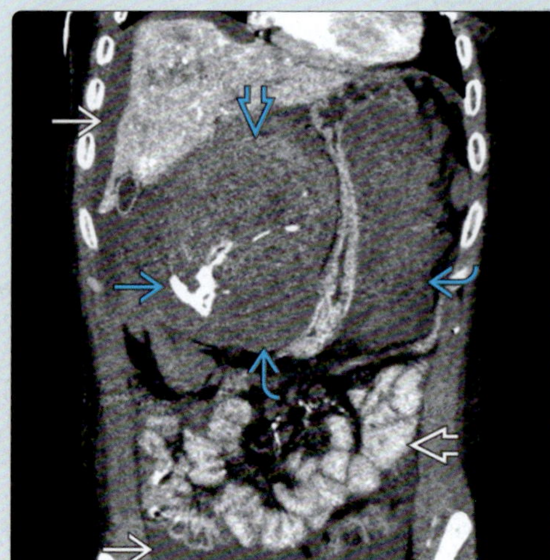

(Left) *Coronal T1 C+ FS MR MIP in a 16-year-old with an intrahepatic portosystemic shunt shows an aberrant connection of the interrupted portal vein ➡ to a hepatic vein ➡. Biopsy of the hyperenhancing lesions ➡ confirmed inflammatory adenomas.* **(Right)** *Coronal CECT in the same patient 6 months later shows active arterial extravasation ➡ from a large adenoma ➡ with hemoperitoneum ➡ & large foci of clotted blood ➡. There is profound bowel wall hyperenhancement ➡ due to hypoperfusion complex.*

TERMINOLOGY

Definitions

- Benign neoplasm arising from hepatocytes
- Different subtypes with different imaging features & clinical significance
  - Inflammatory ~ 40-50%
  - Hepatocyte nuclear factor 1α (*HNF1α*) mutated ~ 30-35%
    - More frequently have fat content
  - β-catenin activated ~ 10-15%
    - ↑ malignant potential
    - More common in males
  - Unclassified ~ 5-10%

IMAGING

General Features

- Best diagnostic clue
  - Arterial-phase enhancing liver mass in patient on oral contraceptives or with underlying liver disease

Ultrasonographic Findings

- Heterogeneous, well-defined mass; may be hyperechoic due to lipid content or hemorrhage
- Contrast-enhanced US
  - Similar enhancement to background liver on early & late phases
  - Can be heterogeneous

CT Findings

- NECT
  - Typically ↓ attenuation compared to liver (due to lipid)
  - ± ↑ attenuation due to Ca^{2+} or hemorrhage
- CECT
  - Arterial phase → variable patterns of hyperenhancement
  - Venous phase → ± heterogeneous enhancement

MR Findings

- Most common MR appearance
  - ↓ to ↔ on T1, mildly ↑ on T2
    - May be ↓ on T2 FS due to intracellular lipid
  - ± signal loss on T1 opposed-phase images due to lipid
  - ↑ arterial enhancement, ± heterogeneity
  - Most commonly hypoenhancing on hepatobiliary phase if hepatocyte specific contrast is used
- Different subtypes may have differentiating features
  - *HNF1α* subtype
    - ↑ or ↓ on T1, ↓ signal on T1 opposed phase due to lipid
    - Moderate arterial enhancement, ↓ enhancement on delayed phases
  - Inflammatory subtype
    - ↔ to mild ↑ on T1
    - Typically ↑ on T2
    - ↑ arterial enhancement, remains hyperenhancing on later phases
  - β-catenin activated & unclassified subtypes
    - Variable, can be heterogeneous
- Hepatobiliary-phase MR contrast agent
  - Variable, most commonly hypoenhancing on hepatobiliary phase
  - Can be iso- to hyperenhancing
    - Most common with β-catenin subtype

Imaging Recommendations

- Best imaging tool
  - Multiphasic MR with hepatobiliary contrast agent, in-/opposed-phase T1 imaging

DIFFERENTIAL DIAGNOSIS

Focal Nodular Hyperplasia

- Homogeneous arterial enhancement ± central scar
- No intracellular lipid
- Iso- or hyperintense to liver on hepatocyte phase with hepatobiliary contrast agent

Hepatocellular Carcinoma

- Can be indistinguishable from hepatic adenoma on imaging

Hypervascular Metastasis

- Uncommon in children
- No intracellular lipid

PATHOLOGY

General Features

- Associated with oral contraceptives, exogenous steroids, glycogen storage diseases, liver disease (e.g., cardiogenic cirrhosis), congenital portosystemic shunts (Abernethy malformation vs. intrahepatic shunt)

Gross Pathologic & Surgical Features

- ± fat, necrosis, & hemorrhage
- Can be solitary or multiple (adenomatosis)

CLINICAL ISSUES

Natural History & Prognosis

- ↑ risk of hemorrhage with ↑ size of mass
- Risk of malignant transformation to hepatocellular carcinoma ~ 5%
  - ↑ risk with β-catenin subtype

Treatment

- Discontinuation of oral contraceptives can lead to ↓ in size or even complete regression
- Surgical excision if male, suspicious/atypical imaging features, or large size

SELECTED REFERENCES

1. DiPaola F et al: Congenital portosystemic shunts in children: associations, complications, and outcomes. Dig Dis Sci. 65(4):1239-51, 2020
2. Fang C et al: Contrast-enhanced ultrasound in the diagnosis of pediatric focal nodular hyperplasia and hepatic adenoma: interobserver reliability. Pediatr Radiol. 49(1):82-90, 2019
3. Trout AT et al: Hepatocyte-specific contrast media: not so simple. Pediatr Radiol. 48(9):1245-55, 2018
4. Dhingra S et al: Update on the new classification of hepatic adenomas: clinical, molecular, and pathologic characteristics. Arch Pathol Lab Med. 138(8):1090-7, 2014
5. Katabathina VS et al: Genetics and imaging of hepatocellular adenomas: 2011 update. Radiographics. 31(6):1529-43, 2011
6. van Aalten SM et al: Hepatocellular adenomas: correlation of MR imaging findings with pathologic subtype classification. Radiology. 261(1):172-81, 2011
7. Chung EM et al: From the archives of the AFIP: pediatric liver masses: radiologic-pathologic correlation part 1. Benign tumors. Radiographics. 30(3):801-26, 2010

KEY FACTS

TERMINOLOGY

- Hepatocellular carcinoma (HCC): Malignant tumor of hepatocytes
- Hepatobiliary agent (HBA): MR contrast agent with substantial hepatocyte uptake & retention with biliary excretion

IMAGING

- Pediatric LI-RADS work group recommends MR with HBA at all imaging time points
  - CT is not recommended unless MR is contraindicated or if pediatric anesthesia is required but unavailable
- MR imaging findings
  - Variable precontrast signal intensity
  - Typically hyperenhancing on arterial phase
  - Washout on portal venous & delayed phases
  - Typically has no delayed hepatobiliary-phase contrast retention

TOP DIFFERENTIAL DIAGNOSES

- Fibrolamellar HCC
- Hepatoblastoma
- Hepatic adenoma
- Focal nodular hyperplasia
- Undifferentiated embryonal sarcoma

CLINICAL ISSUES

- 2nd most common primary hepatic malignancy in children after hepatoblastoma
- Typical age: 10-19 years
- Preexisting liver disease in 30-50% of patients
- Best therapy: Complete resection
  - 2/3 are unresectable at diagnosis due to multifocality, vascular invasion, size, or metastases (25-50%)
    - May become resectable with neoadjuvant therapy
    - Transplant may be curative for localized disease
- Overall survival rate of ~ 10-30%

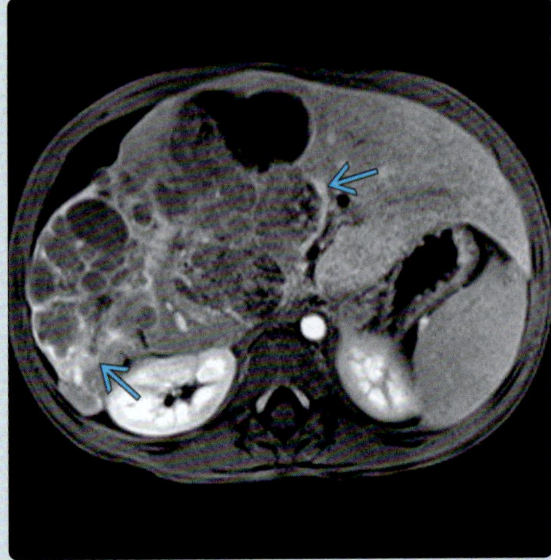
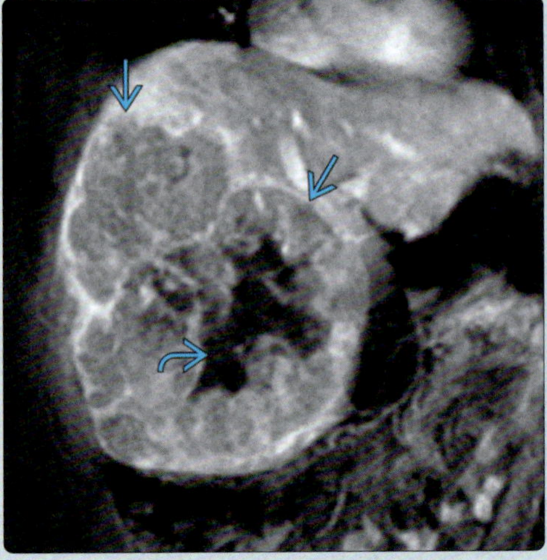

(Left) *Axial T1 C+ FS MR imaged in the hepatic arterial phase shows a large hepatocellular carcinoma (HCC) ➡ within the right lobe of the liver. The tumor is heterogeneous with some foci that enhance more than the background liver while many regions enhance less.* **(Right)** *Coronal T1 C+ FS MR during the portal venous phase shows a large HCC ➡ arising from the inferior aspect of the right lobe of the liver. The tumor has a central area of necrosis ↪.*

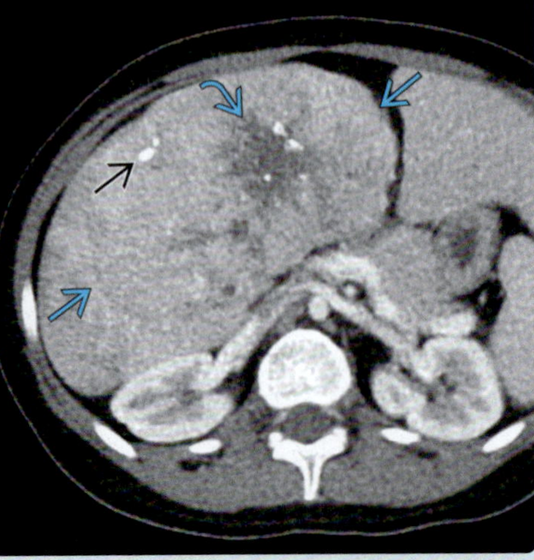
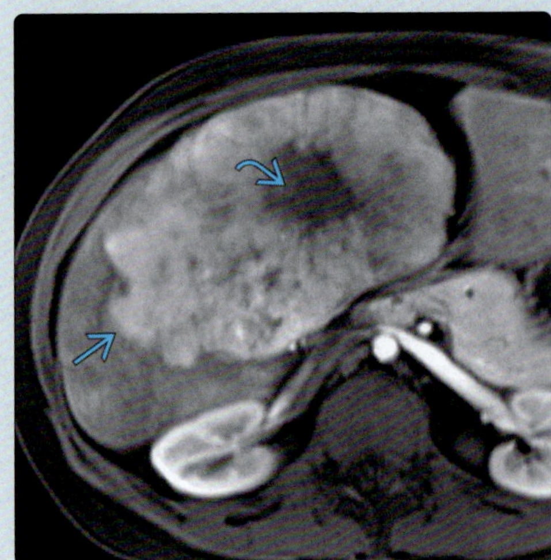

(Left) *Axial CECT in an adolescent with fibrolamellar HCC shows a large tumor ➡ with a central scar ↪ & scattered calcifications ➡. Most of the mass shows similar enhancement to the liver parenchyma.* **(Right)** *Axial T1 C+ FS MR obtained during the portal venous phase in the same patient shows the HCC ➡ to enhance more than the background liver. The central scar ↪ does not enhance, typical of the fibrolamellar variant.*

KEY FACTS

ERMINOLOGY

Malignant hepatic mesenchymal tumor with undifferentiated cells

MAGING

Well-circumscribed, solitary liver mass in 6- to 10-year-old child

Typically > 10 cm in size; mean: 14 cm

Mass appears cystic on CT/MR but solid on ultrasound due to myxoid components

- Septations & mural nodules may be present
- Minimal enhancement during arterial phase
- ± peripheral enhancement on delayed phases
- Central hyperdense foci & fluid-debris levels suggest hemorrhage; Ca^{2+} is uncommon

OP DIFFERENTIAL DIAGNOSES

Hepatoblastoma

Mesenchymal hamartoma

- Hepatocellular carcinoma
- Hepatic pyogenic abscess

PATHOLOGY

- May arise from mesenchymal hamartoma

CLINICAL ISSUES

- 3rd most common pediatric hepatic malignancy after hepatoblastoma & hepatocellular carcinoma
- Most frequently occurs between 6-10 years of age
- Most commonly presents with abdominal mass ± abdominal pain; normal α-fetoprotein (AFP) levels
    - Fever, weight loss, anorexia, vomiting, diarrhea, lethargy, constipation, & respiratory distress are less common
- 86% 5-year overall survival
    - Multimodal therapy (including chemotherapy & resection or transplant) are key for ↑ survival
- Metastases are present in 15%: Most common in lungs, pleura, & peritoneum

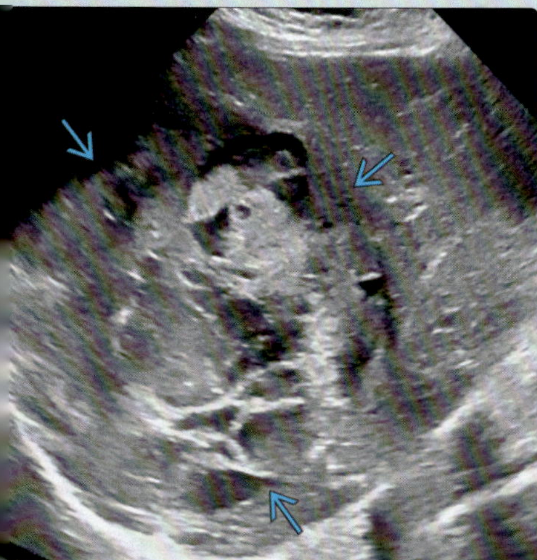

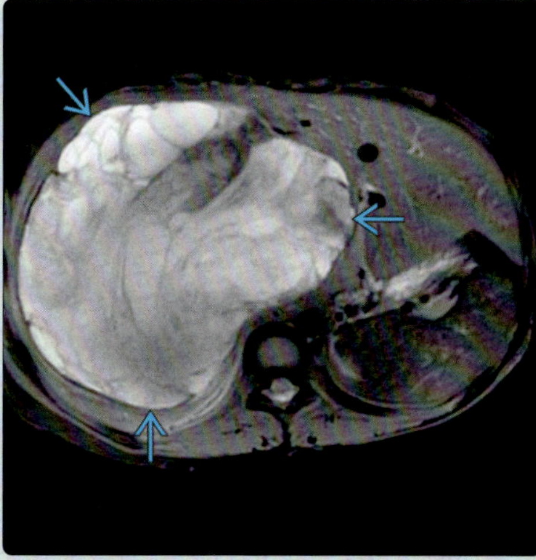

(Left) *Transverse US of the liver in an adolescent with an undifferentiated embryonal sarcoma shows a heterogeneous but predominantly solid mass* ⇨ *involving the right lobe of the liver.* **(Right)** *Axial T2 FS MR in the same patient shows a complex hyperintense mass* ⇨ *of the right lobe of the liver. Hepatic undifferentiated embryonal sarcoma often has fluid signal on MR (due to myxoid components) but is solid on ultrasound.*

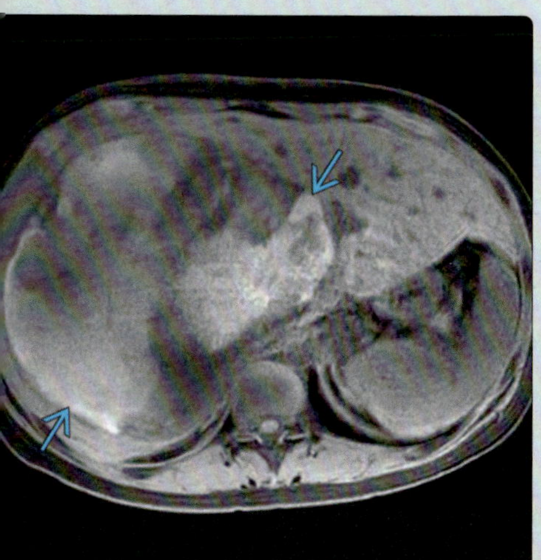

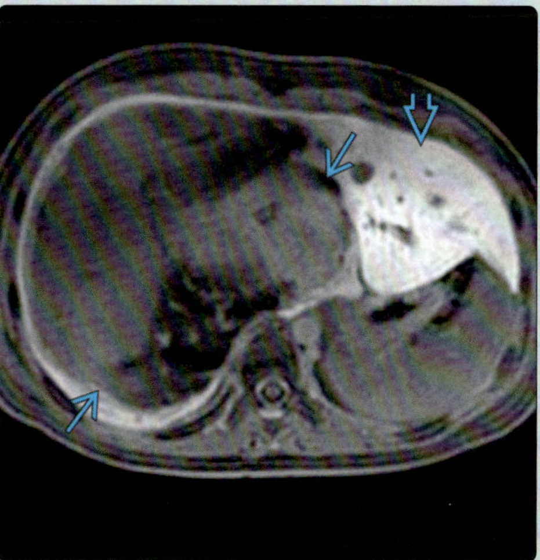

(Left) *Axial T1 FS MR in the same patient shows that the heterogeneous mass* ⇨ *has regions of hyperintense T1 signal, suggesting that internal hemorrhage has occurred.* **(Right)** *Axial T1 C+ FS MR obtained in the hepatobiliary phase (while using a hepatobiliary contrast agent) in the same patient shows that the tumor* ⇨ *does not retain the hepatobiliary contrast media. Note the retention of contrast by the normal liver* ⇨*.*

KEY FACTS

TERMINOLOGY

- Mesenchymal hamartoma (MH): Benign liver tumor of infants due to primitive mesenchymal proliferation

IMAGING

- Spectrum from mostly cystic to mostly solid masses
    - Amount of solid stromal tissue determines appearance
    - Cysts found (to some degree) in up to 85%
        - Septations may be thin or thick
- Typically unifocal; rarely multifocal or diffuse
    - Right hepatic lobe: 75%
- Up to 30 cm in size; mean: 16 cm
- Ca^{2+} & hemorrhage are uncommon

TOP DIFFERENTIAL DIAGNOSES

- Hepatoblastoma
- Congenital hemangioma (CH)
- Umbilical venous catheter (UVC) extravasation
- Undifferentiated embryonal sarcoma (UES)

CLINICAL ISSUES

- Typically < 2 years old; 5% > 5 years old
- Grow slowly or rapidly in perinatal period
    - Prenatal: May cause polyhydramnios, hydrops
    - Postnatal: May cause respiratory distress
- Subsequent stabilization vs. partial regression
- > 90% long-term survival
- Complete excision is required due to rare malignant potential: Reports of UES arising in background MH
- Cyst aspiration may be required emergently (pre- or postnatally) to alleviate compression

DIAGNOSTIC CHECKLIST

- Most likely hepatic neoplasms in young children
    - Largely cystic in neonate/infant → MH
    - Solid, hypovascular in infant/toddler → hepatoblastoma
    - Solid, heterogeneous, hypervascular in newborn → CH
- In neonate with recent UVC infusion & newly discovered "cystic hepatic mass," consider extravasation (not tumor)

(Left) *Coronal T2 FS MR in a 6-month-old shows a large multicystic mass ➡ replacing the right lobe of the liver & filling much of the abdomen. Mesenchymal hamartoma (MH) was confirmed at resection.* **(Right)** *Coronal T2 FS MR in a 13-month-old shows multiple loculated cystic masses ➡ in the liver + a small amount of ascites ➡. There was no enhancement of the lesions after contrast (not shown). Transplant was required as all hepatic sectors were involved (not shown). (Courtesy P. Masand, MD.)*

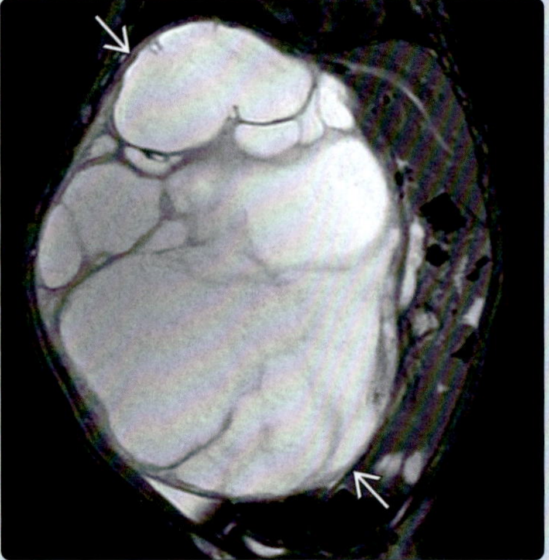

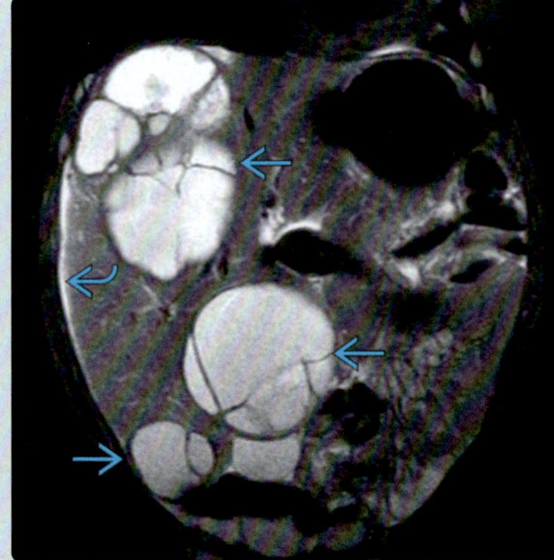

(Left) *Transverse grayscale & color Doppler US images in a 6-month-old with new-onset liver failure show numerous mixed solid & cystic masses ➡ filling the visible liver & splaying the hepatic vessels. Scant internal vascularity is seen in the lesions.* **(Right)** *Axial T1 C+ FS MR in the same patient shows heterogeneously enhancing masses replacing all but a small volume of normal liver parenchyma ➡. Note the ascites ➡ secondary to liver failure. A liver transplant was ultimately required for diffuse MHs.*

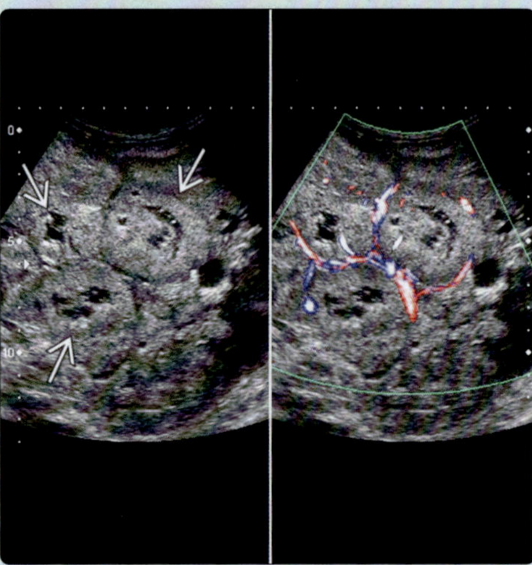

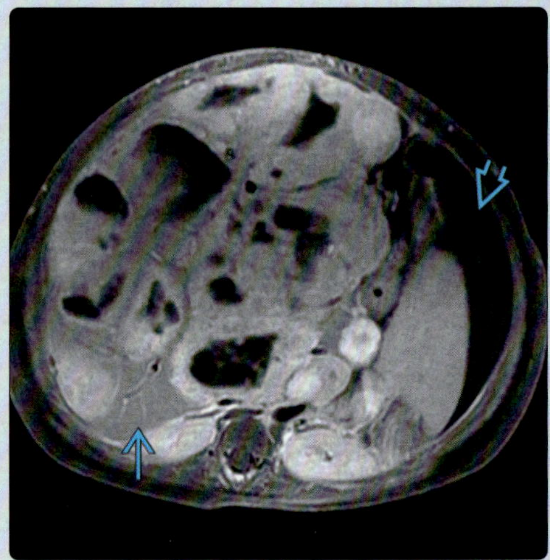

KEY FACTS

IMAGING

- Expansile intraductal biliary mass in young child
  - Most commonly arises in common bile duct
  - Dilated upstream intrahepatic bile ducts are caused by downstream biliary obstruction
  - May be difficult to distinguish tumor from dilated/obstructed bile ducts
- CT: Isodense to slightly hypodense compared to liver
- MR: Hypointense on T1, hyperintense on T2, heterogeneous enhancement, restricted diffusion
- US: Heterogeneous hypoechoic mass expanding bile duct with variable degree of internal vascularity
- ERCP: Lobulated intraductal filling defect

TOP DIFFERENTIAL DIAGNOSES

- Choledochal cyst: Spectrum of malformations involving extrahepatic & intrahepatic bile ducts
- Cholangiocarcinoma: Malignancy arising from bile duct epithelium; extremely rare in children

PATHOLOGY

- 2 subtypes: Embryonal & alveolar
- Botryoides is variant of embryonal subtype

CLINICAL ISSUES

- Most common presentation: Jaundice (60-80%)
- Other presenting signs/symptoms: Abdominal distention, fever, hepatomegaly, nausea, & vomiting
- Most common pediatric biliary malignancy
  - 75% are diagnosed before 5 years of age
  - Overall survival: 55-75%
- Metastases present in 30%

DIAGNOSTIC CHECKLIST

- Mass may follow fluid appearance on CT & MR, making it difficult to differentiate tumor from dilated ducts
- Biliary rhabdomyosarcoma may be misdiagnosed as choledochal cyst

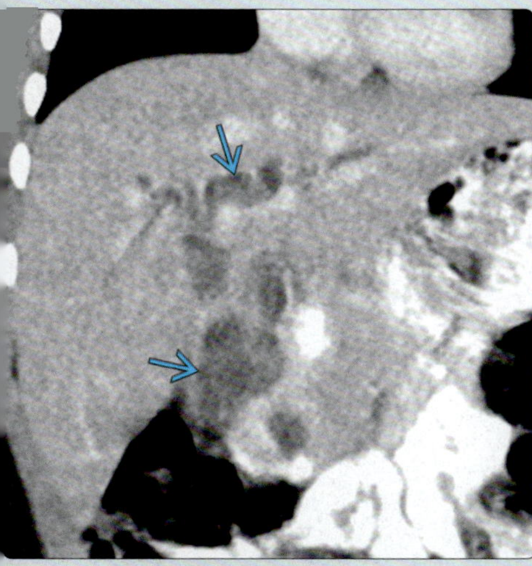

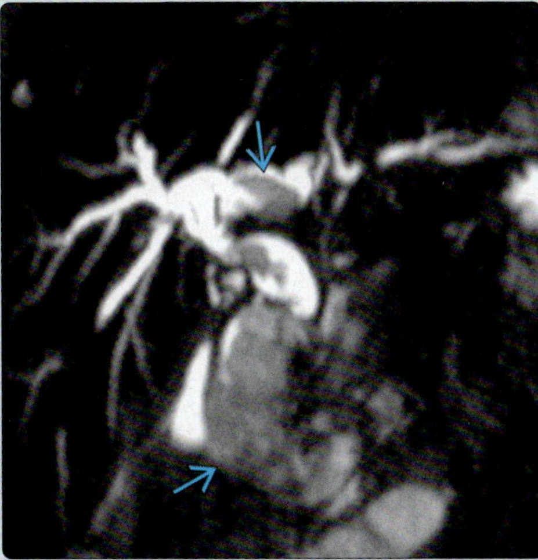

(Left) *Coronal CECT in a 3-year-old child shows a mildly enhancing solid mass ⇨ filling & distending the common & intrahepatic bile ducts. While uncommon, biliary rhabdomyosarcoma is the most common biliary mass in children.* **(Right)** *Coronal MIP image from an MRCP in a 3-year-old child shows a mass ⇨ filling & distending the common & intrahepatic bile ducts with dilation of the obstructed upstream ducts.*

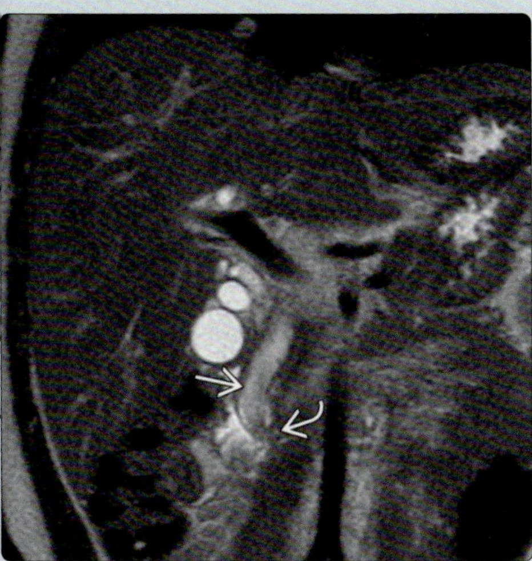

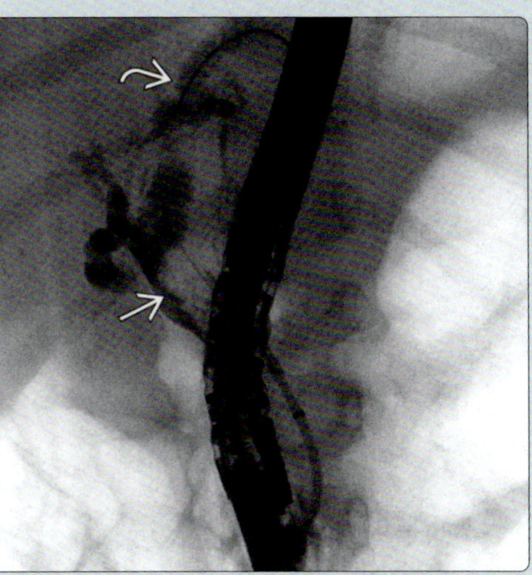

(Left) *Coronal T2 MR in another 3-year-old patient shows a heterogeneous solid mass ➡ filling & distending the common bile duct. The mass extends to the sphincter of Oddi ➦.* **(Right)** *AP image from an ERCP shows a filling defect ➡ within the common bile duct. The upstream intrahepatic ducts ➦ are dilated, suggesting that the intraductal mass is at least partially obstructive.*

KEY FACTS

TERMINOLOGY

- Biliary atresia (BA): Absent or severely deficient extrahepatic biliary tree
  - Lengths & sites of ductal involvement vary

IMAGING

- US to exclude other causes of neonatal jaundice; characteristic findings can be very suggestive of BA
  - Absent or small irregular gallbladder with discontinuous echogenic wall in vast majority (gallbladder ghost sign)
  - Echogenic fibrous tissue (triangular cord sign) anterior to right portal vein at site of obliterated bile duct
  - No biliary ductal dilation; rare hilar cyst
  - Liver echotexture is typically normal early
  - Elevated shear wave velocities on elastography
- Hepatobiliary scan: No radiotracer excretion into intestines; gallbladder is visible in up to 25%
- Intraoperative cholangiogram: Absence of contiguous extrahepatic biliary system; segments may be visualized

TOP DIFFERENTIAL DIAGNOSES

- Neonatal hepatitis
- Bile-plug syndrome
- Alagille syndrome
- Choledochal cyst

PATHOLOGY

- Associations: Preduodenal portal vein, interrupted IVC, situs anomalies, congenital heart disease, polysplenia (or asplenia), midgut malrotation in 10-20% (BASM syndrome)

CLINICAL ISSUES

- Neonatal jaundice with direct hyperbilirubinemia
  - ↑ GGT & ↑ MMP-7 are more specific for BA
- Gradual deterioration of hepatocyte function
- Kasai portoenterostomy is temporarily effective in 90% if performed < 2 months of age; ↓ to < 50% if > 3 months
- Liver transplant is ultimately required in most by adulthood, even with prompt Kasai

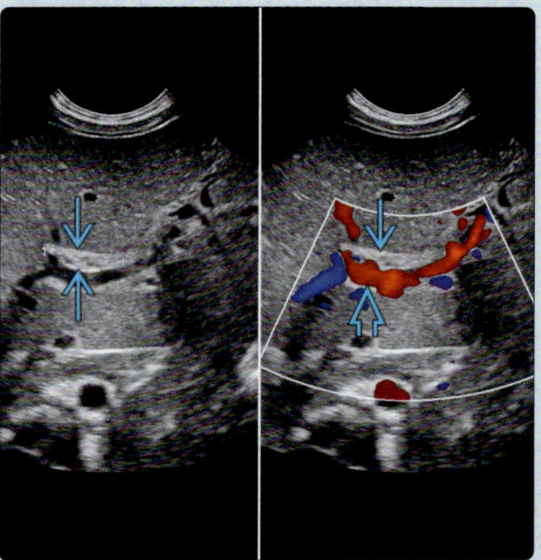

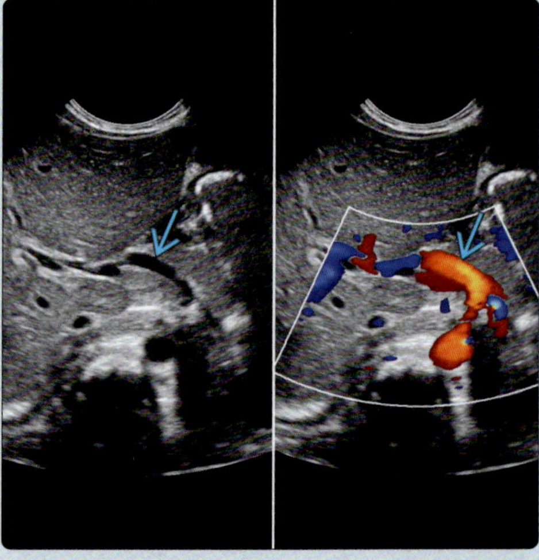

(Left) *Transverse grayscale & color Doppler liver ultrasounds in a 1-month-old with acholic stools, hyperbilirubinemia, & elevated GGT & MMP-7 show a thick (4-mm), echogenic focus anterior to the right portal vein, the classic triangular cord sign.* **(Right)** *Transverse grayscale & color Doppler ultrasounds in same neonate show enlargement of main hepatic artery at 3 mm, just above plane of partially visualized main portal vein. Biliary atresia (BA) was confirmed on biopsy.*

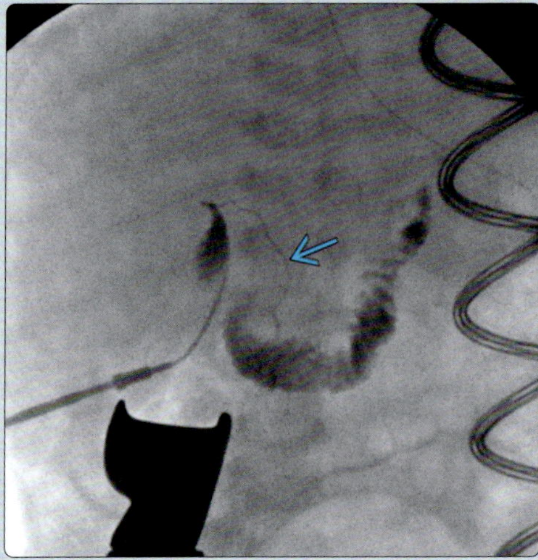

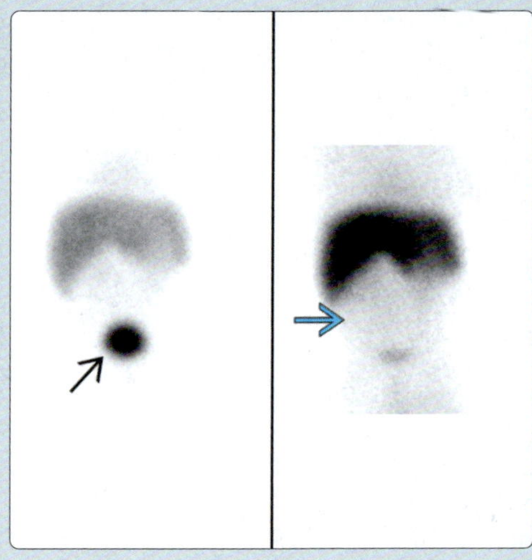

(Left) *Intraoperative cholangiogram in the same patient (through a normal gallbladder) shows a patent common bile duct to the duodenum. However, even with occlusion of this segment during injection, no hepatic ducts could be visualized, consistent with BA.* **(Right)** *Hepatobiliary scintigraphy in a jaundiced infant shows no intestinal excretion of mebrofenin. The hepatic radiotracer is slowly excreted by the kidneys into the urinary bladder. A 24-hour delayed image also shows no intestinal radiotracer, typical of BA.*

TERMINOLOGY

Definitions

- Biliary atresia (BA): Inflammatory cholangiopathy of fetal life/infancy → progressive fibrosis & obliteration of extra- & intrahepatic bile ducts
  - Variable degrees of extrahepatic involvement

IMAGING

General Features

- Best diagnostic clue
  - US shows small & irregular or absent gallbladder (GB) with obliterated/fibrosed bile duct anterior to portal vein
  - Elevated shear wave elastography velocities
  - Hepatobiliary scan shows lack of radiotracer excretion into intestines
  - Intraoperative cholangiogram shows absence of contiguous biliary system from liver to duodenum

Ultrasonographic Findings

- Grayscale ultrasound
  - Liver echotexture is typically normal in neonatal period, though liver may be enlarged
  - GB is typically absent or abnormal
    - GB ghost triad: Small (< 15-19 mm in length), irregular shape, & discontinuous echogenic wall
    - GB length to width ratio of > 5.2
  - Extrahepatic bile ducts are usually not visible
    - Triangular cord sign: Echogenic obliterated/fibrotic remnant of hepatic duct anterior to right portal vein near porta hepatis
      - Thickness of cord at 3 mm vs. 4 mm influences sensitivity/specificity of sign
    - Dilated bile ducts (intra- or extrahepatic) are not present
      - Rare cystic BA form with hilar cyst
  - Main hepatic artery diameter > 2 mm
  - Associated anomalies of BA-splenic malformation (BASM) syndrome (in 20% of BA)
    - Polysplenia
    - Preduodenal portal vein
    - Transverse liver (showing continuity of portal veins in leftward hepatic tissue)
    - Malrotation of midgut
    - Interrupted inferior vena cava (IVC)
    - Cardiac anomalies
  - Post-Kasai procedure, liver often shows gradual fibrosis/cirrhosis with portal hypertension (HTN), splenomegaly, & varices
- Color Doppler
  - Useful to demonstrate main portal vein & hepatic artery when searching for echogenic triangular cord
  - ± ↑ subcapsular flow, telangiectatic capsular/subcapsular small vessels
- Shear wave elastography
  - Evaluates liver stiffness; shear wave velocity is significantly ↑ in BA
    - Recommended cutoff values range from 1.6-2.2 m/s
    - Helps differentiate BA from other causes of neonatal jaundice

MR Findings

- MRCP
  - Technically more challenging than ultrasound
  - Features: Abnormal GB, triangular cord > 5 mm, absent common bile duct
    - Note that complete biliary tree is only visible in 60-75% of normal patients < 3 months old
- T1, T2
  - Post-Kasai procedure, liver often shows gradual fibrosis/cirrhosis with portal HTN, splenomegaly, & varices

Nuclear Medicine Findings

- Hepatobiliary scan
  - Tc-99m disofenin (DISIDA) & mebrofenin (BRIDA) have highest hepatic extraction rates & shortest transit times of hepatobiliary radiotracers
  - Pretreat with oral phenobarbital (5 mg/kg/day in divided doses x 5 days)
    - Potent inducer of hepatic microsomal enzymes: Enhances biliary excretion & improves scintigraphic accuracy
    - Ursodeoxycholic acid has also been used as choleretic prescintigraphy (20 mg/kg every 12 hours for 48-72 hours) with good results
  - Hepatocyte uptake & extraction of radiotracer from blood pool is usually preserved in first 2-3 months of life, later deteriorates
  - Lack of excretion into intestines on 24-hour delayed images highly suggestive of BA or other extrahepatic occlusion
    - Excretion into intestines effectively excludes BA
  - Visualization of GB is not helpful; seen in 25%
  - High sensitivity (~ 100%) with 87% specificity, 91% accuracy

Other Modality Findings

- ERCP: Invasive, requires general anesthesia, uses ionizing radiation, & has significant morbidity (1-7%) & failure (3-14%) rates
- Intraoperative cholangiogram: Cannulation of any GB seen by US in attempt to opacify entire biliary system
  - May show segments of extrahepatic biliary system but will not show patency from liver to duodenum in BA
- Analysis of duodenal drainage is difficult to perform, not yet standardized; sensitivity of ~ 97%, specificity of ~ 93%

Imaging Recommendations

- Best imaging tool
  - US is performed 1st
    - Traditionally to exclude other causes of jaundice
    - Combination of characteristic findings can strongly suggest BA
  - If any GB is seen by US, some surgeons proceed directly to intraoperative cholangiogram with liver biopsy; if patent ducts are not demonstrated by cholangiogram, definitive surgery is performed

DIFFERENTIAL DIAGNOSIS

Neonatal Hepatitis

- Very common entity; usually self-limited medical disease but can be caused by hepatitis A, hepatitis B, cytomegalovirus, rubella, toxoplasmosis, α-1-antitrypsin deficiency, familial recurrent cholestasis, or other metabolic disorders

Bile-Plug Syndrome

- Due to cystic fibrosis, dehydration, sepsis, hemolytic disorders, or total parenteral nutrition

Alagille Syndrome

- Intrahepatic ducts are sparse & malformed
- Pulmonic stenosis, characteristic facies, butterfly vertebra, CNS arterial anomalies

Choledochal Cyst

- Localized dilation of extrahepatic biliary tree
- ± dilated intrahepatic ducts

PATHOLOGY

General Features

- Etiology
  - Hypoplastic, atretic, or fibrosed extrahepatic ducts that worsen in perinatal period
    - Variable sites/lengths of involvement
  - May result from prenatal biliary duct inflammation of unknown etiology
  - Proposed mechanism involves initial virus-induced, progressive T-cell-mediated inflammatory obliteration of bile ducts
- Associated abnormalities
  - Preduodenal portal vein, interrupted IVC, congenital heart disease, situs anomalies, & polysplenia (or asplenia) in BASM (10-20%)
  - Another 10-25% have other anomalies, most commonly involving abdomen & genitourinary tract
  - Molecular disorders involving bile formation, canalicular transporters, tight junction proteins, & inborn errors of metabolism are increasingly recognized

Gross Pathologic & Surgical Features

- Abnormal intra- & extrahepatic ducts; cirrhosis if diagnosis is delayed
- Most common form (~ 2/3): Complete atresia of extrahepatic ducts & GB
- ~ 12% of BA patients have patent proximal ducts & can have simple reanastomosis surgery; 88% require Kasai procedure

CLINICAL ISSUES

Presentation

- Most common signs/symptoms
  - Progressive conjugated (direct) hyperbilirubinemia in neonatal period
    - Bilirubin is unconjugated in sepsis, hepatitis, & metabolic hepatocellular diseases
- Other signs/symptoms
  - ↑ gamma-glutamyl transpeptidase (GGT)
  - ↑ matrix metalloproteinase-7 (MMP-7)
    - Suggested cutoff of 52.85 ng/mL has high sensitivity/specificity

Demographics

- Affects 1 in 10,000-13,000 newborn infants
- Jaundice is evident in immediate perinatal period
- Full-term infants > premature infants
- No sex or racial predilection

Natural History & Prognosis

- Prompt diagnosis is crucial to surgical success
  - Initially, hepatocyte function is preserved; hepatocyte function gradually deteriorates
- Kasai portoenterostomy is temporarily effective in 90% if performed < 2 months of age; ↓ to < 50% if > 3 months of age
  - Poor prognosis if total bilirubin is not < 2 mg/dL within 3 months of Kasai procedure
  - Steroid treatment post Kasai hastens clearance of jaundice; long-term effects are unclear
- Most patients ultimately require liver transplantation
  - < 18% who have prompt Kasai procedures avoid liver transplantation ≥ 20 years later
  - BA is most common reason for pediatric liver transplant

Treatment

- Kasai portoenterostomy: Intestinal loop is anastomosed to dissected surface of porta hepatis
- Liver transplant

SELECTED REFERENCES

1. Napolitano M et al: Practical approach for the diagnosis of biliary atresia on imaging, part 2: magnetic resonance cholecystopancreatography, hepatobiliary scintigraphy, percutaneous cholecysto-cholangiography, endoscopic retrograde cholangiopancreatography, percutaneous liver biopsy, risk scores and decisional flowchart. Pediatr Radiol. 51(8):1545-54, 2021
2. Sandberg JK et al: Ultrasound shear wave elastography: does it add value to gray-scale ultrasound imaging in differentiating biliary atresia from other causes of neonatal jaundice? Pediatr Radiol. 51(9):1654-66, 2021
3. Chen Y et al: Three-color risk stratification for improving the diagnostic accuracy for biliary atresia. Eur Radiol. 30(7):3852-61, 2020
4. Di Serafino M et al: Ultrasound findings in paediatric cholestasis: how to image the patient and what to look for. J Ultrasound. 23(1):1-12, 2020
5. Hattori K et al: Cyst size in fetuses with biliary cystic malformation: an exploration of the etiology of congenital biliary dilatation. Pediatr Gastroenterol Hepatol Nutr. 23(6):531-8, 2020
6. Napolitano M et al: Practical approach to imaging diagnosis of biliary atresia, Part 1: prenatal ultrasound and magnetic resonance imaging, and postnatal ultrasound. Pediatr Radiol. 51(2):314-31, 2020
7. Shin HJ et al: Key imaging features for differentiating cystic biliary atresia from choledochal cyst: prenatal ultrasonography and postnatal ultrasonography and MRI. Ultrasonography. 40(2):301-11, 2020
8. Dillman JR et al: Prospective assessment of ultrasound shear wave elastography for discriminating biliary atresia from other causes of neonatal cholestasis. J Pediatr. 212:60-65.e3, 2019
9. Hwang SM et al: Early US findings of biliary atresia in infants younger than 30 days. Eur Radiol. 28(4):1771-1777, 2018
10. Yang L et al: Diagnostic accuracy of serum matrix metalloproteinase-7 for biliary atresia. Hepatology. 68(6):2069-2077, 2018
11. Koob M et al: The porta hepatis microcyst: an additional sonographic sign for the diagnosis of biliary atresia. Eur Radiol. 27(5):1812-1821, 2017
12. Cho HH et al: Ultrasonography evaluation of infants with Alagille syndrome: In comparison with biliary atresia and neonatal hepatitis. Eur J Radiol. 85(6):1045-52, 2016
13. Lee JY et al: The value of preoperative liver biopsy in the diagnosis of extrahepatic biliary atresia: a systematic review and meta-analysis. J Pediatr Surg. 51(5):753-61, 2016

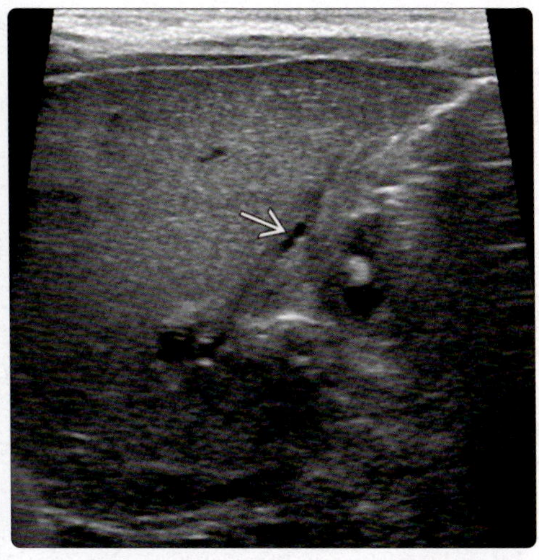

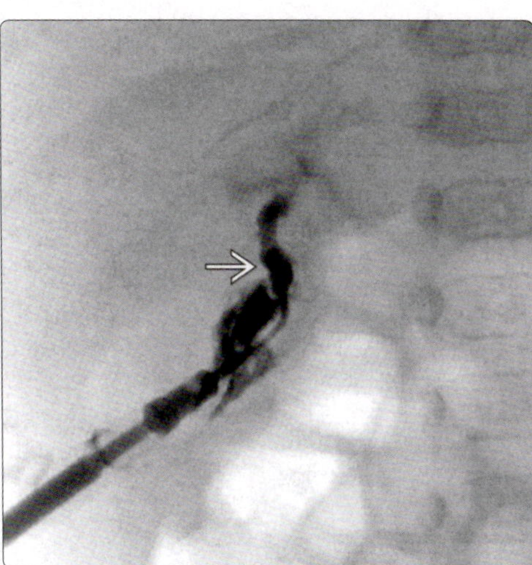

(Left) *Transverse US in a jaundiced infant shows a small, irregularly shaped gallbladder ➡ despite an adequate fast. In addition to the gallbladder ghost, this patient also had a triangular cord sign of BA (not shown).* **(Right)** *Intraoperative cholangiogram through a hypoplastic gallbladder shows a short segment of common hepatic duct ➡ but no intestinal drainage, confirming BA. A portoenterostomy (Kasai procedure) followed.*

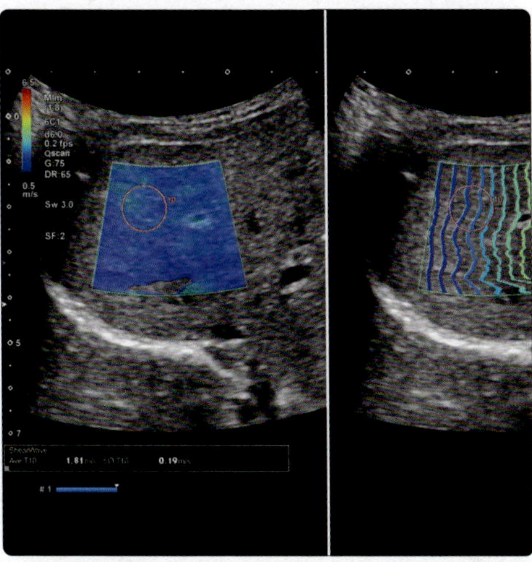

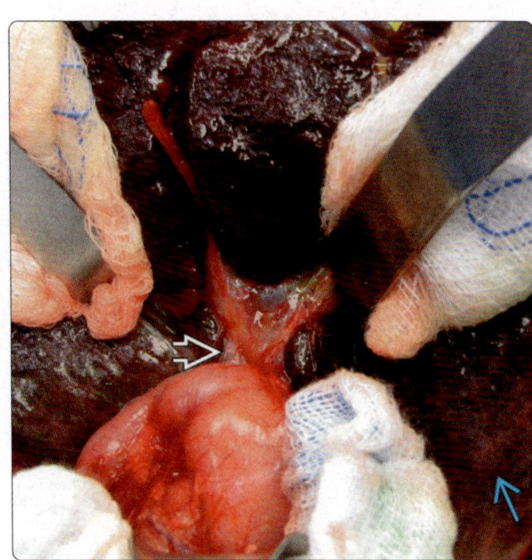

(Left) *Shear wave elastography US in an infant liver shows ↑ stiffness with a shear wave speed measuring 1.81 m/s (1 of 6-10 measurements obtained as part of the exam). Normal median values in the neonate/young infant are generally < 1.6 m/s.* **(Right)** *Intraoperative photograph during a Kasai procedure shows the discolored liver (related to chronic cholestasis), tiny spider angiomata →, & lack of a common bile duct in the porta hepatis ➡ in this patient with BA.*

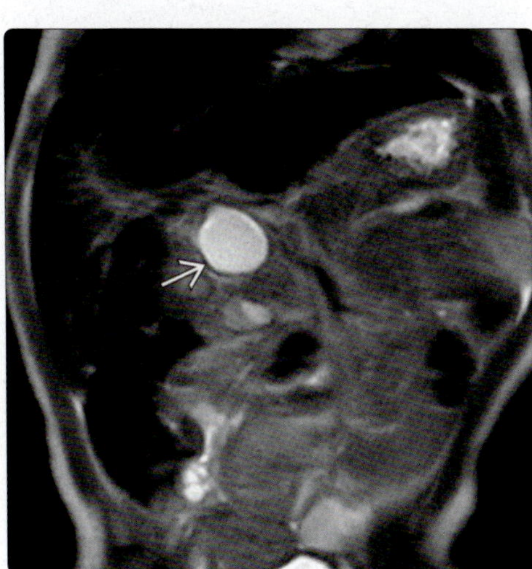

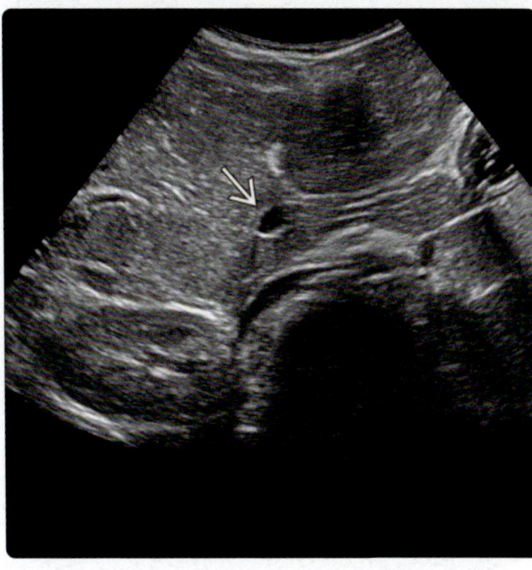

(Left) *Coronal T2 MR shows the cystic variant ➡ of BA in a 2-month-old with jaundice. No patent common bile duct or normal gallbladder was seen on MR.* **(Right)** *Paramidline US shows a preduodenal portal vein ➡ along the liver margin in an infant with BA & polysplenia, suggesting BA-splenic malformation syndrome. Look for other findings of heterotaxy in these patients, including congenital heart disease & midgut malrotation.*

Choledochal Cyst

KEY FACTS

TERMINOLOGY

- Choledochal cyst: Spectrum of malformations involving extrahepatic & intrahepatic bile ducts
- Etiology may be due to pancreaticobiliary maljunction
  - Pancreatic duct joins common bile duct (CBD) proximal to sphincter of Oddi → reflux of pancreatic enzymes
- High risk (in long term) of cholangiocarcinoma if choledochal malformation is not resected

IMAGING

- US in child with jaundice & elevated liver enzymes
  - Round or tubular, cystic right upper quadrant mass separate from gallbladder
    - CBD dilation > 10 mm is very suggestive in child
- MRCP for detailed preoperative assessment of ductal anatomy & pancreaticobiliary maljunction
  - Delayed scan with hepatobiliary contrast agent may confirm connection of cyst to biliary tree

TOP DIFFERENTIAL DIAGNOSES

- Obstructing choledocholithiasis
- Cystic biliary atresia
- Gastrointestinal duplication cyst
- Primary sclerosing cholangitis
- Pancreatic pseudocyst

CLINICAL ISSUES

- Classification modified by Todani in 1977
  - Type I: Dilated CBD; most common (75-95%)
  - Type II: Diverticulum of duct
  - Type III: Choledochocele protruding into duodenum
  - Type IV: Discontinuous extrahepatic bile duct cysts, isolated (type IVb) or with intrahepatic cysts (type IVa)
  - Type V: Intrahepatic cystic dilations (Caroli disease); not considered choledochal cyst in modern era
- General treatment: Cyst resection & biliary diversion/hepatobiliary enterostomy

(Left) *Graphic shows the choledochal malformation classification by Todani, with type V now considered a separate ductal plate malformation (Caroli disease). Note the anomalous pancreaticobiliary junction ➔ with the pancreatic duct inserting into the common bile duct proximal to the sphincter of Oddi.* **(Right)** *Transverse ultrasound of the liver in a 9-year-old shows a large, simple-appearing cyst ➔ adjacent to a normal-appearing gallbladder ➔.*

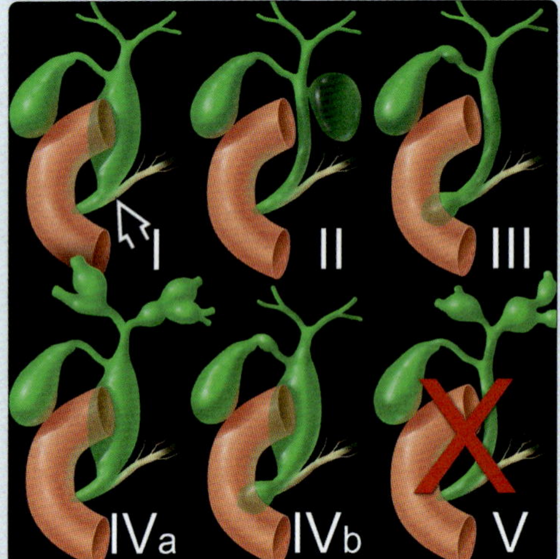

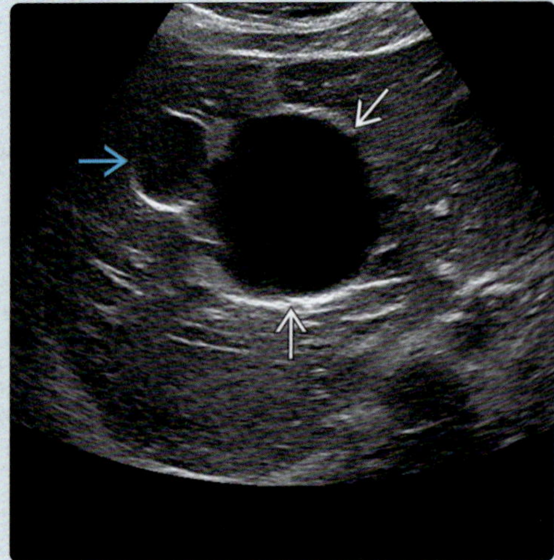

(Left) *Coronal SSFP MR in the same patient shows the elliptical cyst ➔ in the porta hepatis extending into the pancreatic head, typical of a choledochal cyst.* **(Right)** *Coronal MIP from an MRCP in the same patient shows a severely enlarged common hepatic duct ➔ & focally dilated central intrahepatic bile ducts ➔ in this case of a type IVa choledochal cyst.*

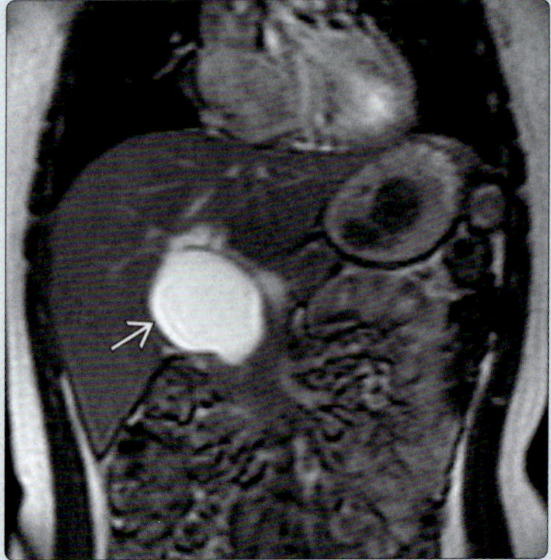

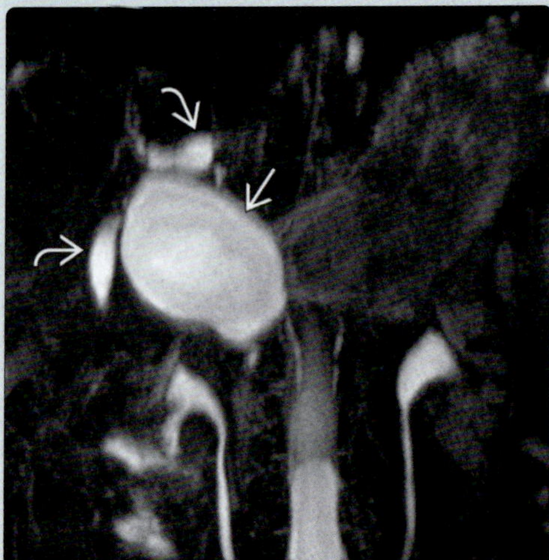

TERMINOLOGY

Synonyms

- Choledochal malformations, common bile duct (CBD) cyst or diverticulum, choledochocele, congenital biliary dilation

Definitions

- Choledochal cyst: Spectrum of malformations involving extrahepatic & intrahepatic bile ducts
- Etiology may be due to pancreaticobiliary maljunction
  - Pancreatic duct joins CBD proximal to sphincter of Oddi → biliary reflux of pancreatic enzymes
- ↑ cholangiocarcinoma risk in patients with choledochal malformations

IMAGING

General Features

- Best diagnostic clue
  - Marked dilation of biliary tree, focal or diffuse
- Location
  - May involve intrahepatic bile ducts, extrahepatic ducts, or both
- Size
  - Bile duct dilation > 10 mm is very suggestive in child
- Morphology
  - Ductal dilation may be continuous or multifocal

Ultrasonographic Findings

- Grayscale ultrasound
  - Round or tubular cystic right upper quadrant lesion separate from normal gallbladder
  - ± intrahepatic ductal dilation
- Color Doppler
  - Shows lack of flow in anechoic round/tubular mass, confirming cyst rather than abnormal vessel
  - Useful to demonstrate position & displacement of adjacent vessels

MR Findings

- T2, MR cholangiogram to show
  - Anatomy of dilated ducts & variants
  - Pancreaticobiliary maljunction
- T1 C+ with hepatocyte-specific contrast agent
  - Delayed images can confirm biliary connection of cyst

Nuclear Medicine Findings

- Hepatobiliary scan shows early photopenia at hilum with delayed filling
- Can help show bile leak after resection

Other Modality Findings

- ERCP & PTC are usually reserved for complex cases or intervention

Imaging Recommendations

- Best imaging tool
  - US in child with jaundice & elevated liver enzymes
    - Shows dilated biliary tree & extent of ductal involvement
  - MRCP for detailed preoperative assessment of ductal anatomy
    - Position/length of common channel to pancreatic duct
    - Has replaced preoperative percutaneous cholangiogram
  - Hepatobiliary nuclear scans for functional evaluation

DIFFERENTIAL DIAGNOSIS

Obstructing Choledocholithiasis

- Stone disease may cause obstruction at several levels
- Ductal dilation is typically < 10 mm

Cystic Biliary Atresia

- Uncommon biliary atresia form with hilar cyst
- No intrahepatic duct dilation
- Hypoplastic or absent gallbladder
- Echogenic cord anterior to right portal vein

Gastrointestinal Duplication Cyst

- Duodenal cyst can involve porta hepatis
- Look for wall gut signature sign & peristalsis of cyst

Primary Sclerosing Cholangitis

- Irregular beading with dilation & stenosis of bile ducts
- Look for findings of ulcerative colitis

Pancreatic Pseudocyst

- Round pancreatic head collection can mimic dilated CBD
- History/findings of recent pancreatitis

Caroli Disease

- Localized saccular ectasia of intrahepatic bile ducts
- Central dot sign of encased portal radicles

PATHOLOGY

General Features

- Etiology
  - Primary theory: Anomalous junction of common biliary & pancreatic ducts → conduit for mixing (& reflux) of pancreatic enzymes & bile
    - Dilation & structural weakness of CBD (with destruction of elastic fibers) after reflux of pancreatic secretions in animal models
    - Unclear that this leads to marked duct dilation
    - Pancreaticobiliary maljunction can occur ± congenital biliary dilation
    - Consider pancreaticobiliary maljunction in cases of pediatric pancreatitis
  - Additional theories: ↓ in ganglion cells in narrow portion of bile duct causing ↑ intraluminal pressure; preceding viral infection; familial pattern of inheritance; failure of recanalization
- Genetics
  - Autosomal recessive polycystic kidney disease is often associated with Caroli syndrome
    - Ciliopathy underlies these disorders (different etiology from remaining choledochal malformations)

Staging, Grading, & Classification

- Classification modified by Todani in 1977

- Type I: Segmental or diffuse fusiform dilation of CBD; most common variety (75-95% of cases); IA is unilocular saccular dilation of entire CBD; IB is unilocular saccular dilation of distal CBD; IC is unilocular fusiform CBD & hepatic duct dilation
- Type II: Diverticulum of duct, usually protruding from lateral wall
- Type III: Choledochocele, most often of duodenal wall (protruding into duodenal lumen)
- Type IV: Multiple discontinuous extrahepatic bile duct cysts, isolated (type IVb) or with Caroli-type intrahepatic biliary cysts (type IVa)
- Type V: Ductal plate malformation with multifocal cystic dilations of intrahepatic bile ducts (Caroli disease); **not** considered type of choledochal cyst in modern era
  - Caroli syndrome (large & small bile duct ectasia with congenital hepatic fibrosis) > > Caroli disease (large bile duct ectasia only)
- Additional proposed modifications
  - Type ID: Dilated cystic duct + dilated CBD & common hepatic duct (CHD)
  - Type VI: Isolated dilation of cystic duct
- Intrahepatic ductal dilation preoperatively may resolve postoperatively, changing cyst classification

Gross Pathologic & Surgical Features

- Range in diameter from few centimeters to > 15 cm
- Cyst wall is thickened, fibrotic, & occasionally calcified in adults

Microscopic Features

- Varying degrees of chronic inflammation
- Biliary epithelium lining cyst is often intact in infants
- Type III cysts (choledochocele) are often lined by duodenal mucosa but occasionally have biliary epithelium
- Goblet-cell metaplasia & epithelial dysplasia with nuclear hyperchromasia, irregularity, & loss of polarity have been described
  - May play role in subsequent development of carcinoma

CLINICAL ISSUES

Presentation

- Most common signs/symptoms
  - Prolonged neonatal cholestasis, so-called infantile obstructive cholangiopathy
  - Infants: Jaundice, acholic stools, hepatomegaly, & palpable abdominal mass
  - Adults: Upper abdominal pain, jaundice, cholangitis, & pancreatitis

Demographics

- Age
  - 2/3 diagnosed before 10 years of age
  - Only 20% diagnosed in adults
- Sex
  - M:F = 1:3-4
- Epidemiology
  - More common in Asian than Western countries
    - 1 in 2,000,000 live births in USA vs. 1 in 1,000 live births in Japan

Natural History & Prognosis

- Low-grade biliary obstruction may develop cirrhosis & portal hypertension (HTN)
- Complications: Bile duct perforation, biliary stone formation, bacterial cholangitis with subsequent hepatic abscess & sepsis, biliary strictures, low-grade biliary obstruction → cirrhosis & portal HTN, development of bile duct carcinomas
  - Prevalence of cancer (adenocarcinoma) in choledochal cysts: 2-18% (5-35x ↑ risk)
  - Caroli disease & Caroli syndrome are associated with risk of cholangiocarcinoma (100x that of general population)

Treatment

- Type I: Complete surgical excision + biliary drainage procedure, typically Roux-en-Y choledochojejunostomy
  - Excision with hepaticoduodenostomy has higher rate of bile reflux/gastritis
- Type II: Usually excised entirely; defect in CBD is closed primarily over T tube
  - Type II is usually diverticula of bile duct
- Type III: Choledochocele with diameter < 3 cm may be approached endoscopically with sphincterotomy
  - Cysts > 3 cm are often associated with some degree of duodenal obstruction → excised surgically using transduodenal approach
- Type IV: Dilated extrahepatic duct is completely excised + biliary-enteric drainage procedure
  - No surgery specifically directed at intrahepatic ductal disease
- Type V: Caroli disease (no longer considered type of choledochal cyst), when limited to single hepatic lobe (usually left), may be resected
  - Liver transplantation is necessary in diffuse disease with liver failure
- Internal & external drainage, without cyst excision → unacceptably high rate of cholangitis, does not alter malignant potential
- After resection of choledochal cysts
  - < 0.5% develop cancer before 18 years
  - 11% develop cancer as adult; mean age: 42 years

DIAGNOSTIC CHECKLIST

Image Interpretation Pearls

- Bile duct measuring > 10 mm in childhood is nearly always due to choledochal malformation

SELECTED REFERENCES

1. Ono A et al: Imaging of pancreaticobiliary maljunction. Radiographics. 40(2):378-92, 2020
2. Shin HJ et al: Key imaging features for differentiating cystic biliary atresia from choledochal cyst: prenatal ultrasonography and postnatal ultrasonography and MRI. Ultrasonography. 40(2):301-11, 2020
3. Banks JS et al: Choledochal malformations: surgical implications of radiologic findings. AJR Am J Roentgenol. 210(4):748-60, 2018
4. Urushihara N et al: Characteristics, management, and outcomes of congenital biliary dilatation in neonates and early infants: a 20-year, single-institution study. J Hepatobiliary Pancreat Sci. 25(12):544-9, 2018
5. Kamisawa T et al: Pancreaticobiliary maljunction and congenital biliary dilatation. Lancet Gastroenterol Hepatol. 2(8):610-8, 2017
6. Soares KC et al: Pediatric choledochal cysts: diagnosis and current management. Pediatr Surg Int. 33(6):637-50, 2017

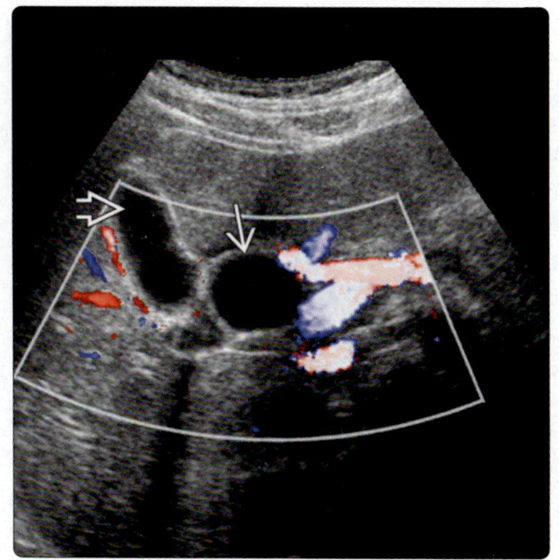

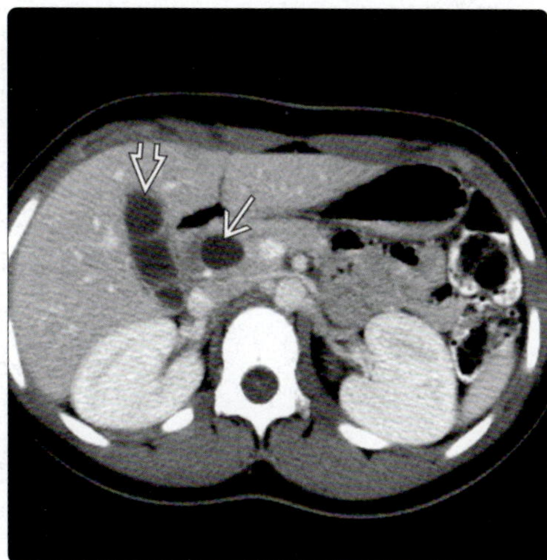

(Left) *Transverse color Doppler ultrasound through the right upper quadrant in a 12-year-old shows a normal gallbladder ➡ with diffuse, marked dilation of the common bile duct ➡.* **(Right)** *Axial CECT in the same patient shows marked dilation of the common bile duct ➡ with a normal gallbladder ➡. Mild intrahepatic ductal dilation was also noted (not shown).*

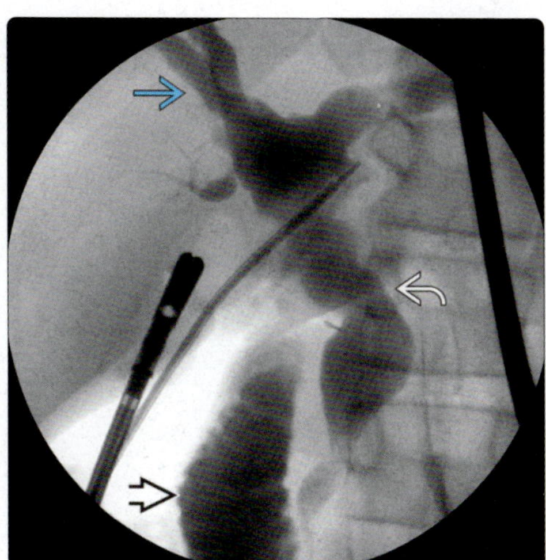

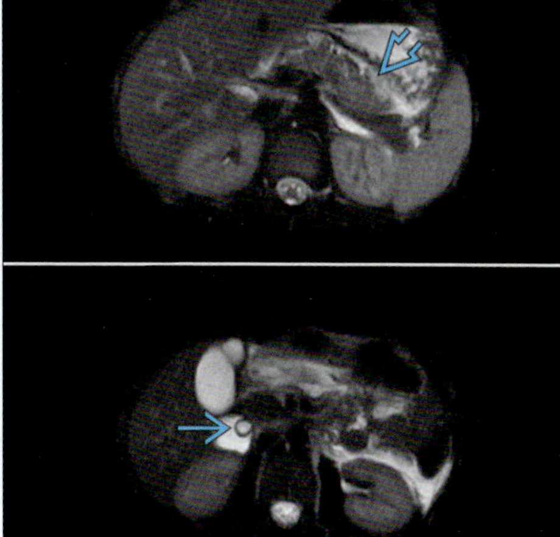

(Left) *Intraoperative cholangiogram in the same patient shows moderate intrahepatic ➡ & marked extrahepatic ➡ ductal dilation. However, the biliary tree still drained into the duodenum ➡. This patient had a type I choledochal malformation repaired surgically.* **(Right)** *Axial T2 FS MR images in a 10-year-old girl with acute pancreatitis ➡ show a type III choledochal cyst (choledochocele) ➡ protruding into the duodenal lumen.*

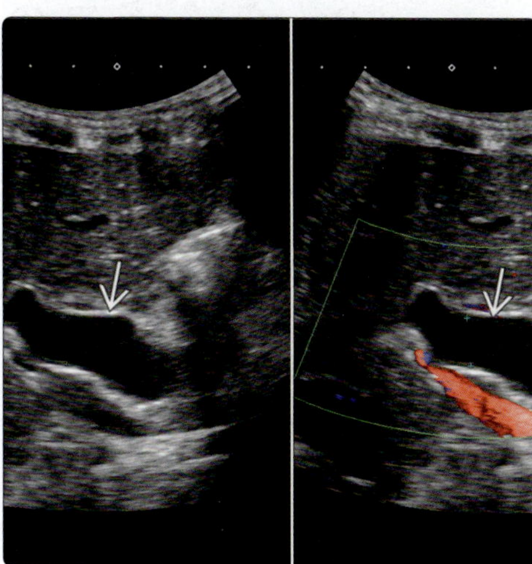

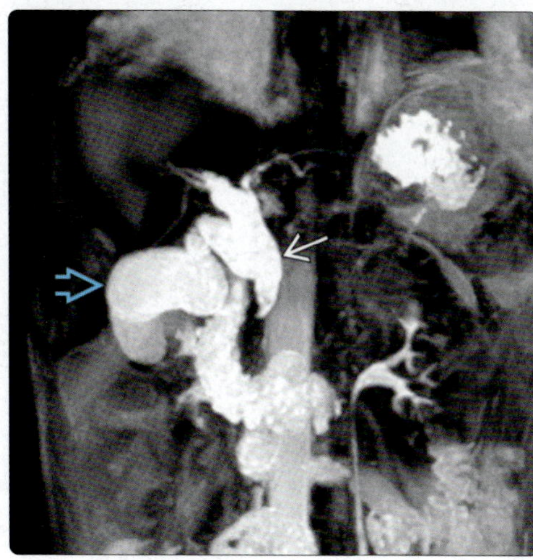

(Left) *Longitudinal split screen grayscale & color Doppler ultrasounds in a 4-year-old girl show focal dilation of the common bile duct ➡, measuring 10.6 mm, without intrahepatic biliary dilation.* **(Right)** *Coronal MIP from an MRCP in the same patient shows focal dilation of the common bile duct ➡ with a normal gallbladder ➡ & no intrahepatic biliary dilation.*

Caroli Disease

KEY FACTS

TERMINOLOGY

- Caroli disease (CD): Saccular dilation of large intrahepatic bile ducts (IHBD)
- Congenital hepatic fibrosis (CHF): Presence of fibrotic tissue between portal tracts with persistent intralobular ducts
- Caroli syndrome (CS): CD + CHF &/or autosomal recessive polycystic kidney disease (ARPKD)

IMAGING

- Multiple intrahepatic "cysts" connected to biliary tree
- Central dot sign: Cross section of dilated IHBD surrounds portal vein radicle
- Hepatic involvement can be segmental, lobar, or diffuse

TOP DIFFERENTIAL DIAGNOSES

- Choledochal cyst
- Primary sclerosing cholangitis

PATHOLOGY

- CD, CS, & ARPKD are caused by impaired ciliary function (ciliopathy)

CLINICAL ISSUES

- Rare (1:1 million of general population)
- Patients can be diagnosed at any age
- Symptoms/complications
  - RUQ pain, fever, & jaundice
  - Stone formation (95%), recurrent cholangitis
  - Hepatic fibrosis with portal hypertension → hepatosplenomegaly & gastrointestinal tract bleeding
  - Cholangiocarcinoma ultimately develops in 7% of patients (100x ↑ risk compared to general population)
- Treatment
  - Ursodeoxycholic acid to ↓ bile duct stones; broad-spectrum antibiotics for cholangitis
  - Biliary decompression
  - Resection ranging from segmentectomy to transplant

(Left) *Axial CECT shows dilated intrahepatic bile ducts. The largest dilated bile duct has a central dot characteristic of Caroli disease. This image highlights that Caroli disease may only affect a portion of the liver.* **(Right)** *Sagittal T2 SSFSE fetal MR shows abnormal dilated intrahepatic bile ducts, a markedly enlarged hyperintense kidney, & oligohydramnios. The constellation of findings is consistent with Caroli disease associated with autosomal recessive polycystic kidney disease (ARPKD).*

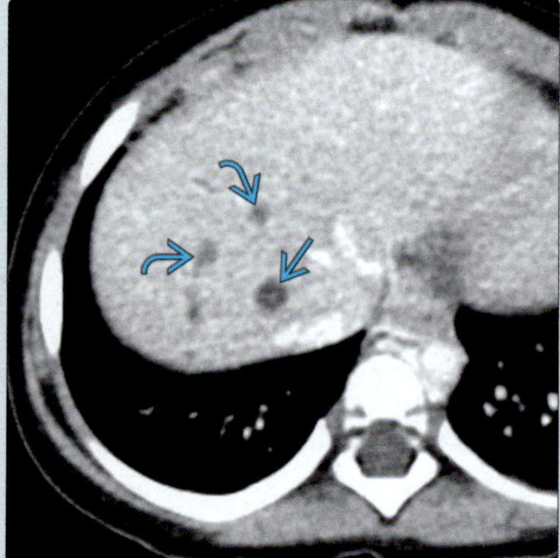

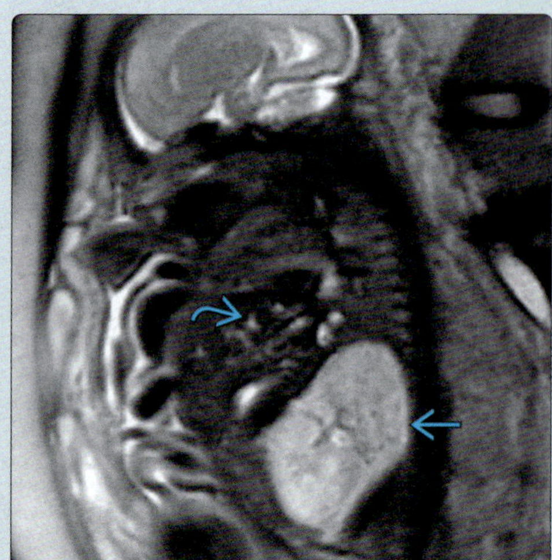

(Left) *Axial T1 FS MR in a patient with Caroli disease shows massively dilated intrahepatic bile ducts. The portal radicle is visible within the center of the dilated ducts.* **(Right)** *Axial T2 FS MR in the same patient shows massively dilated intrahepatic bile ducts. Because of the plane of imaging, the central dot of the portal radicles appears more linear.*

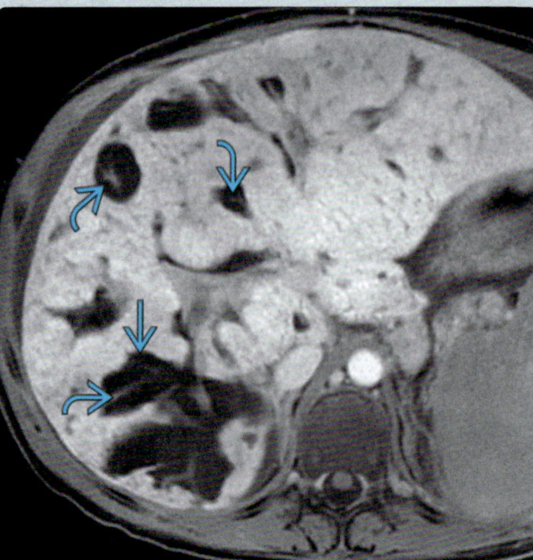

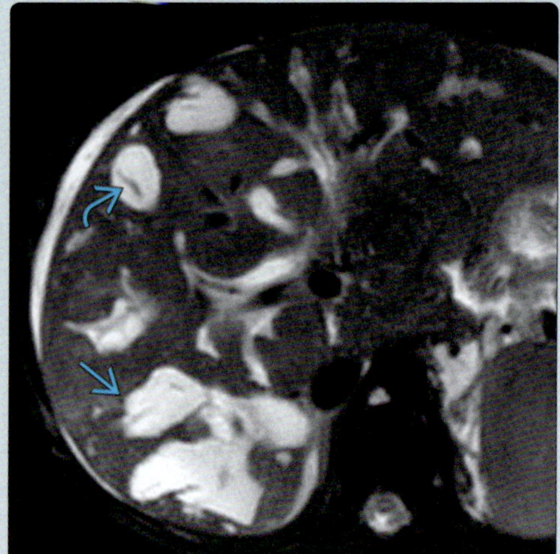

TERMINOLOGY

Definitions

- Caroli disease (CD): Saccular dilation of large intrahepatic bile ducts (IHBD)
- Congenital hepatic fibrosis (CHF): Presence of fibrotic tissue between portal tracts with persistent intralobular ducts
- Caroli syndrome (CS): CD + CHF &/or autosomal recessive polycystic kidney disease (ARPKD)

IMAGING

General Features

- Best diagnostic clue
  - Central dot sign: Portal radicle encased by dilated IHBD
  - Cholangiography confirms direct communication of segmental saccular ductal ectasia with IHBDs
- Location
  - Hepatic involvement can be segmental, lobar, or diffuse
  - Common bile duct is classically spared; dilation (in up to 50%) due to cholangitis, stones
- Size
  - Varying diameters of cystic-appearing dilated IHBDs in same patient (ranging from millimeters to centimeters)

Ultrasonographic Findings

- Grayscale ultrasound
  - Numerous "cysts" scattered throughout liver ± visible biliary communication
  - Intraluminal portal vein sign = central dot sign
    - Portal radicle surrounded by cystic-appearing IHBD
  - Intraductal bridging septa: Echogenic septa completely or incompletely traversing dilated IHBDs
- Color Doppler
  - Flow within central dot (portal vein radicle)

MR Findings

- T2WI
  - Numerous "cysts" in segmental, lobar, or diffuse distribution
  - Small, round, hypointense central dots are visible in dilated, hyperintense cystic-appearing IHBDs
    - Due to flow void of portal radicle in IHBD cross section
    - ± larger biliary filling defects from stones, sludge
  - Renal involvement in 60% with CS
    - Enlarged hyperintense kidneys
      - □ Due to diffuse medullary or corticomedullary cysts/tubular ectasia
- T1WI C+
  - Central dot of enhancement (of portal vein radicle) is surrounded by dilated IHBD
  - Heterogeneous enhancement of liver parenchyma from hepatic fibrosis
- MRCP
  - Direct communication of segmental saccular ductal ectasia with IHBDs
  - ± intraluminal filling defects of sludge or calculi within dilated IHBDs

DIFFERENTIAL DIAGNOSIS

Choledochal Cyst

- Extrahepatic bile ducts are affected in 90%
- Type IV: Cystic dilation of common bile duct ± intrahepatic ducts (type IVa has intrahepatic biliary cysts)
- Not inherited; no renal disease

Primary Sclerosing Cholangitis

- Dilation of both IHBD & extrahepatic bile ducts with multiple irregular strictures
- ± history of ulcerative colitis

PATHOLOGY

General Features

- Etiology
  - CD, CS, & ARPKD are caused by impaired ciliary function (ciliopathy)
    - Ciliopathy during fetal development leads to ductal plate malformation

Staging, Grading, & Classification

- CD is no longer considered as type of choledochal cyst

CLINICAL ISSUES

Presentation

- Most common signs/symptoms
  - Intermittent abdominal/right upper quadrant pain
- Other signs/symptoms
  - Recurrent cholangitis, fever, & jaundice
  - Hepatic fibrosis with portal hypertension → hepatosplenomegaly & GI bleeding
  - Renal failure may dominate clinical picture in infants
- Complications
  - Stone formation (95%), recurrent cholangitis, end-stage liver disease
  - Cholangiocarcinoma (ultimately) in 7% of patients
    - 100x ↑ risk compared to general population

Demographics

- Age
  - Patients can be diagnosed at any age
  - Patients diagnosed in infancy have more severe disease
- Epidemiology
  - Rare; 1:1 million of general population

Treatment

- Ursodeoxycholic acid (to ↓ biliary stones) & broad-spectrum antibiotics (for cholangitis)
- Biliary decompression: External drainage & biliary-enteric anastomosis are effective but with ↑ risk of infection
- Resection ranging from segmentectomy to transplant

SELECTED REFERENCES

1. Lewin M et al: Diffuse versus localized Caroli disease: a comparativesMRCP Study. AJR Am J Roentgenol. 216(6):1530-8, 2021
2. Moslim MA et al: Surgical management of Caroli's disease: single center experience and review of the literature. J Gastrointest Surg. 19(11):2019-27, 2015
3. Rock N et al: Liver involvement in children with ciliopathies. Clin Res Hepatol Gastroenterol. 38(4):407-14, 2014

KEY FACTS

TERMINOLOGY

- Cirrhosis: Liver disease characterized by bridging fibrosis
  - Variety of underlying disorders may lead to cirrhosis

IMAGING

- Nodular contour of liver; easiest to see along free margin
- US: Liver has coarsened echotexture
- MR: Lace-like signal of fibrosis
  - MR can detect underlying deposition (fat, iron, etc.)
  - Hepatocyte-specific contrast agents allow characterization of nodules
- MR or US elastography can determine liver stiffness as marker of fibrosis
- Progressive fibrosis leads to ↓ hepatic size
- Signs of portal hypertension: Ascites, splenomegaly, varices

CLINICAL ISSUES

- Symptoms & treatment depend on underlying condition; potential etiologies include
  - Biliary atresia
  - Choledochal cyst
  - Alagille syndrome
  - Progressive familial intrahepatic cholestasis
  - Viral hepatitis
  - α-1 antitrypsin deficiency
  - Cystic fibrosis
  - Wilson disease
  - Nonalcoholic fatty liver disease
  - Autoimmune hepatitis
  - Primary sclerosing cholangitis
  - Total parenteral nutrition cholestasis
  - Post-Fontan physiology
- Early stages of fibrosis can be reversed by treating underlying condition
- Treatment for end-stage liver disease: Liver transplant
- Cirrhotic patients are typically screened every 6 months for hepatocellular carcinoma

(Left) *Axial T2 FS MR in a patient with congenital hepatic fibrosis shows lace-like ↑ signal at the periphery of the liver, consistent with hepatic fibrosis. The spleen is enlarged, suggesting portal hypertension.* **(Right)** *Axial image from MR elastography shows abnormal ↑ thickness ➡ of the sound wave traversing the liver. The liver stiffness was measured at 8.5 kPa in this patient (normal is < 2.7).*

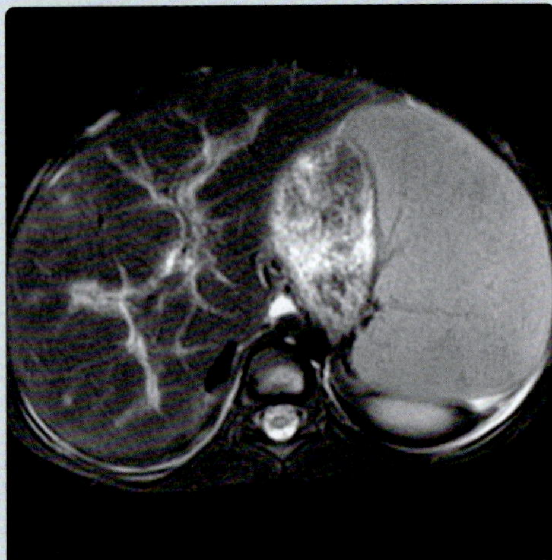

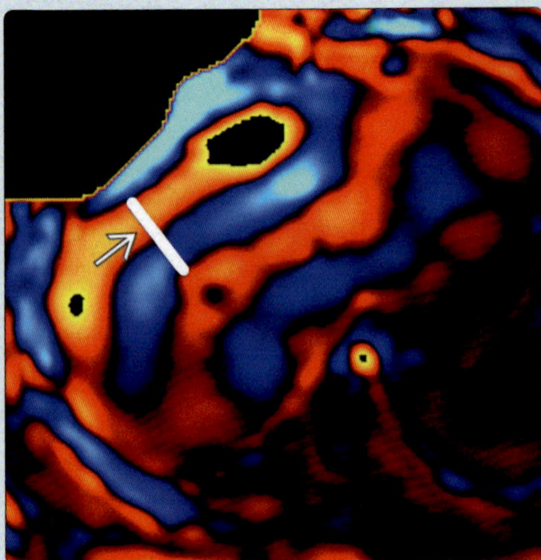

(Left) *Transverse ultrasound in an adolescent with cystic fibrosis shows a small, nodular appearance of the liver. The liver nodularity ➡ is best seen on the free edge of the liver. The underlying hepatic echotexture is coarsened.* **(Right)** *Axial T1 opposed-phase MR in an adolescent with autoimmune hepatitis shows an abnormal lace-like pattern of fibrosis throughout the liver.*

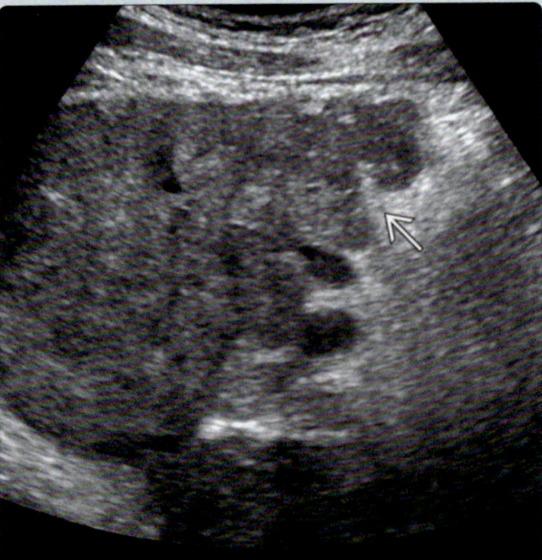

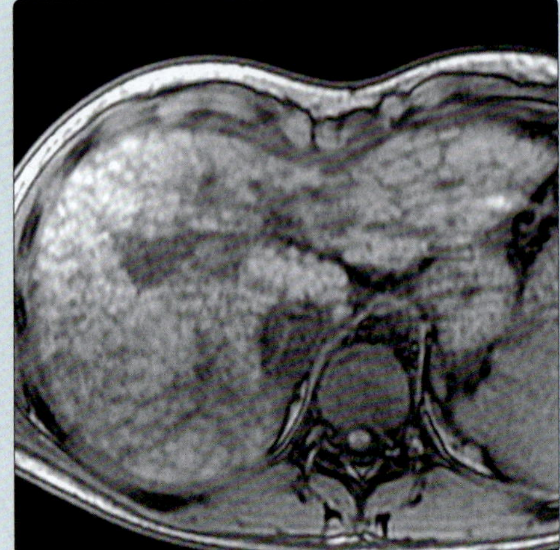

TERMINOLOGY

Definitions

- Cirrhosis: Liver disease characterized by bridging fibrosis

IMAGING

Ultrasonographic Findings

- Liver has coarsened echotexture
- Nodular contour is easier to see on free margin
- Doppler US to evaluate portal flow

CT Findings

- Morphologic changes of liver on CT or MR
  - ↓ in liver size with progressive fibrosis
  - Atrophy of right lobe & left medial section
  - Hypertrophy of caudate & left lateral section
  - Widening of porta hepatis & hepatic fissure
  - Enlargement of gallbladder fossa
  - Nodular contour of liver
  - Changes related to portal hypertension: Splenomegaly, ascites, varices

MR Findings

- Fibrosis may appear as lace-like ↓ T1 & ↑ T2 signal
- Elastography can determine liver stiffness
- Hepatocyte-specific contrast agent: Characterizes nodules
- Detects potential causes of fibrosis, such as fat or iron deposition
- MR venogram can determine portal venous flow direction & reveal varices

Imaging Recommendations

- Best imaging tool
  - MR provides complete evaluation: Fat or iron deposition, liver stiffness, vascular supply, & tumor screening

CLINICAL ISSUES

Treatment

- Depends on underlying condition
- Early stages of fibrosis can be reversed by treating underlying condition
- Treatment for end-stage liver disease: Liver transplant

SELECTED REFERENCES

1. Dillman JR et al: Imaging of Fontan-associated liver disease. Pediatr Radiol. 50(11):1528-41, 2020
2. Mojtahed A et al: Pearls and pitfalls of metabolic liver magnetic resonance imaging in the pediatric population. Semin Ultrasound CT MR. 41(5):451-61, 2020
3. Chapin CA et al: Cirrhosis and portal hypertension in the pediatric population. Clin Liver Dis. 22(4):735-52, 2018
4. Cordova J et al: An overview of cirrhosis in children. Pediatr Ann. 45(12):e427-32, 2016

Common Causes of Cirrhosis in Children

Disease	Key Facts
Biliary Obstruction	
Biliary atresia	Presents in 1st weeks of life; early diagnosis is essential; ultrasound, serum MMP7, & biopsy are replacing HIDA scan for diagnosis
Choledochal cyst	Types classified via Todani classification system
Intrahepatic Cholestasis	
Alagille syndrome	Bile ducts are malformed & reduced in number; associated with tetralogy of Fallot, vertebral anomalies, & abnormal facies
Progressive familial intrahepatic cholestasis	Autosomal recessive disorder of intrahepatic cholestasis; presents in neonatal period
Genetic	
α-1 antitrypsin deficiency	Liver disease occurs in 10-15%; onset of lung disease is usually between 20-50 years of age
Cystic fibrosis	Liver disease occurs in 25%; caused by plugging of bile ducts
Wilson disease	Caused by defect in copper transport; copper accumulates in liver, brain, & eyes
Other	
Nonalcoholic fatty liver disease	Associated with obesity & metabolic syndrome; can measure excess fat content in liver with MR
Hepatitis B	Most common cause of viral cirrhosis in children & adolescents
Autoimmune hepatitis	Hepatocellular inflammation of unknown cause; elevated levels of serum IgG
Primary sclerosing cholangitis	Associated with inflammatory bowel disease (particularly ulcerative colitis)
TPN	TPN-associated cholestasis can occur rapidly; more common in infants after bowel resection
Post-Fontan physiology	Caused by chronic passive venous congestion & volume overload

Steatosis/Steatohepatitis

KEY FACTS

TERMINOLOGY

- Hepatic steatosis: > 5% of hepatocytes with fat infiltration
- Nonalcoholic fatty liver disease (NAFLD): Steatosis with metabolic syndrome &/or abnormal liver function enzymes
- Nonalcoholic steatohepatitis (NASH): Abnormal hepatic fat content with inflammatory activity or fibrosis

IMAGING

- NECT: ↓ liver attenuation relative to spleen
  - Normally 8-10 Hounsfield units (HU) > spleen
- CECT: Difficult to assess steatosis due to variable enhancement of liver & spleen depending on phase
  - Venous/delayed images: Liver HU ≥ 35 lower than spleen
- MR: Only imaging test that can quantify hepatic fat
  - Multiple methods to measure hepatic fat content
    - MR spectroscopy
    - Chemical shift imaging
      - Signal dropout on opposed-phase vs. in-phase T1
  - Steatosis is defined as fat fraction > 5%
- Ultrasound shows diffusely ↑ hepatic echogenicity
  - Liver much more echogenic than right kidney
  - Poor through transmission of sound waves
    - ↓ visualization of echogenic portal triads & right hemidiaphragm

CLINICAL ISSUES

- Most common cause of chronic liver disease in children
  - NAFLD is present in 38-40% of obese patients
  - Most commonly presents between 11-13 years of age
- Risk factors
  - Modifiable: Obesity, sedentary lifestyle, high intake of sugar-sweetened beverages, sleep apnea
  - Nonmodifiable risk factors: Male, Hispanic origin, family history, parental obesity, intestinal microbiome, premature birth, low birth weight
- Thought to represent progression from simple steatosis → NAFLD → NASH → cirrhosis
- Treatment: Weight loss with dietary modification & exercise

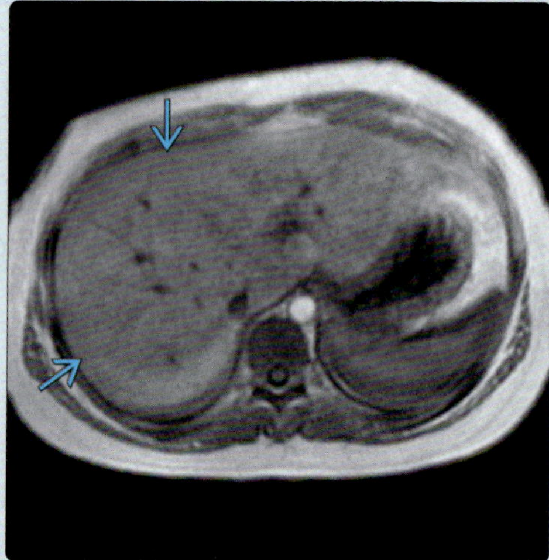

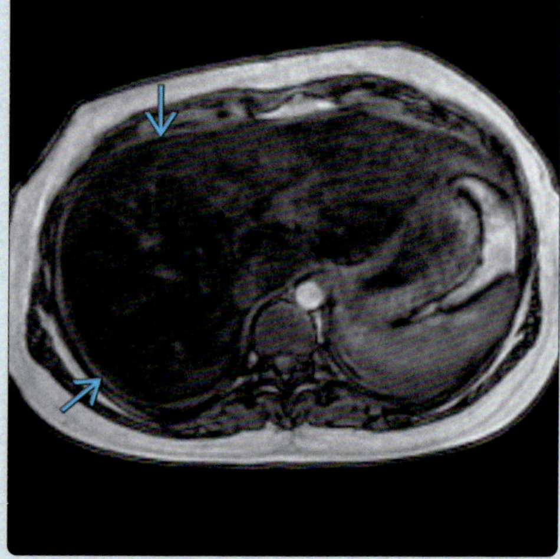

(Left) *Axial T1 in-phase MR in an 11-year-old girl with a history of obesity & steatohepatitis (confirmed with biopsy) shows a normal appearance of the liver ➡.* **(Right)** *Axial T1 opposed-phase MR in the same patient shows diffuse signal loss throughout the liver ➡ due to steatosis. The fat fraction was measured at 32% in this patient (but is normally < 5%).*

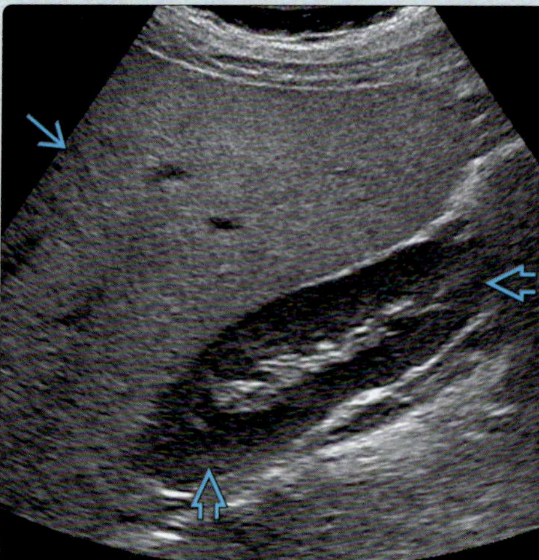

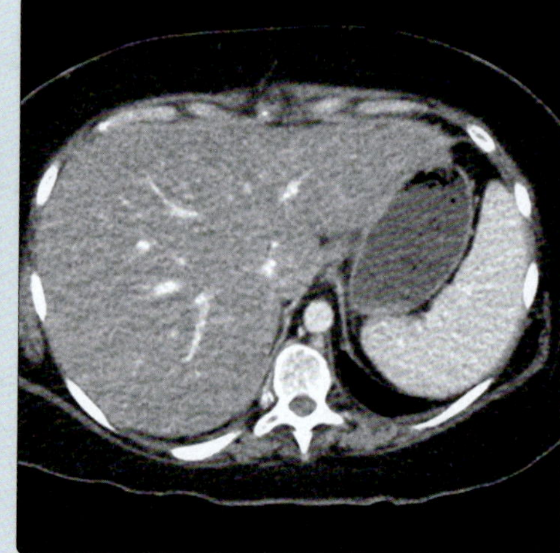

(Left) *Longitudinal ultrasound in the same patient shows diffusely ↑ echogenicity of the liver ➡ relative to the kidney ⇨ with loss of the normally visualized echogenic portal triads, typical of hepatic steatosis.* **(Right)** *Axial CECT in an adolescent status post bone marrow transplant shows diffusely low attenuation of the liver compared to the spleen. The liver measured 63 Hounsfield units (HU), while the spleen measured 119 HU, consistent with hepatic steatosis.*

TERMINOLOGY

Definitions

- Hepatic steatosis: Fatty infiltration of > 5% of hepatocytes
- Nonalcoholic fatty liver disease (NAFLD): Steatosis with metabolic syndrome &/or abnormal liver function tests
- Nonalcoholic steatohepatitis (NASH): Abnormal hepatic fat content with inflammatory activity or fibrosis

IMAGING

General Features

- Best diagnostic clue
  - Fatty infiltration of hepatic parenchyma, demonstrable by variety of modalities/techniques

CT Findings

- CT is not reliable method to identify steatosis

MR Findings

- Steatosis is defined as MR fat fraction > 5%
- Multiple methods to measure hepatic fat content
- MR spectroscopy
  - Considered imaging gold standard for quantification
    - Measures protons in acyl groups of liver tissue triglycerides
    - Able to measure fat content across spectrum of severity & confounding diseases
      - Not susceptible to effects from fibrosis, iron, or glycogen
  - Rarely performed in most clinical practices
- Chemical shift imaging
  - Spin-echo (Dixon) technique
    - By altering echo time, creates in-phase & opposed-phase images based on differing precession frequencies of protons in fat vs. water
      - Signal of fat & water protons are additive for in-phase
      - Signal cancellation for opposed-phase (if both fat & water protons are present in same voxel)
  - Modified Dixon technique: GRE images ↓ scan time
  - Multipoint Dixon technique: Adds more echo series, allowing for better fat quantification
  - Proton density fat fractionation
    - Uses spoiled gradient-recalled echo images
- MR elastography
  - ↓ liver stiffness, ↑ liver volume in hepatic steatosis
  - Liver stiffness > 2.8 kPa suggests significant fibrosis (> stage 2) in children with chronic liver disease

Ultrasonographic Findings

- Diffusely ↑ hepatic echogenicity
  - Liver much more echogenic than right kidney
- Poor through transmission of sound waves
  - Poor visualization of echogenic portal triads
  - Poor visualization of echogenic right hemidiaphragm

Imaging Recommendations

- Best imaging tool
  - MR: Currently only modality that can quantify hepatic fat

DIFFERENTIAL DIAGNOSIS

Cirrhosis

- End result of various chronic liver diseases → shrunken, nodular morphology with bridging fibrosis at histology

Cystic Fibrosis

- Steatosis occurs in 23-75% of patients, potentially due to malnutrition, oxidative stress, insulin resistance

PATHOLOGY

Staging, Grading, & Classification

- Histologic fat content measures % of cells containing fat
- MR fat fraction measures % of liver tissue made up of fat

CLINICAL ISSUES

Presentation

- Most common signs/symptoms
  - Obesity (NAFLD is present in 38-40%)
  - Vague abdominal pain, irritability, fatigue
  - Hepatomegaly

Demographics

- Age
  - Most commonly presents between 11-13 years
  - Onset may be associated with puberty
- Sex
  - More common in males
- Ethnicity
  - Affects Hispanic > White > Black patients
- Epidemiology
  - Most common cause of chronic liver disease in children
  - Affects 7-10% of all pediatric patients, 34-38% of obese children
- Risk factors
  - Modifiable risk factors: Obesity, sedentary lifestyle, ↑ fructose intake, sleep apnea
  - Nonmodifiable risk factors: Male, Hispanic origin, family history, parental obesity, intestinal microbiome, premature birth, low birth weight

Natural History & Prognosis

- Thought to represent progression from simple steatosis → NAFLD → NASH → cirrhosis
  - Unknown why some patients progress & others do not
  - Progression to NAFLD or NASH does not guarantee further progression of disease

Treatment

- Weight loss with dietary modification & exercise

SELECTED REFERENCES

1. Vittorio J et al: Recent advances in understanding and managing pediatric nonalcoholic fatty liver disease. F1000Res. 9, 2020
2. Draijer L et al: Pediatric NAFLD: an overview and recent developments in diagnostics and treatment. Expert Rev Gastroenterol Hepatol. 13(5):447-61, 2019
3. Joshi M et al: Quantitative MRI of fatty liver disease in a large pediatric cohort: correlation between liver fat fraction, stiffness, volume, and patient-specific factors. Abdom Radiol (NY). 43(5):1168-79, 2018
4. Mouzaki M et al: Assessment of nonalcoholic fatty liver disease progression in children using magnetic resonance imaging. J Pediatr. 201:86-92, 2018

Hepatic Venoocclusive Disease

KEY FACTS

TERMINOLOGY

- Occlusion of hepatic sinusoids → clinical triad of jaundice, ascites, & hepatomegaly
- Occurs after stem cell transplantation or certain tumor chemotherapy regimens
  - Usually within 2-3 weeks after stem cell transplantation
    - Late occurrences are more common in children

IMAGING

- Ultrasound with Doppler
  - Hepatomegaly, ascites
  - Reversed or to-&-fro flow in portal veins
    - Specific but not sensitive
  - Elevated resistive indices in hepatic arteries (> 0.75)
- CECT or MR
  - Enlarged, heterogeneous liver, ascites, small-caliber hepatic veins
- Newer diagnostic criteria (EBMT) are clinical & do not require imaging

TOP DIFFERENTIAL DIAGNOSES

- Graft-vs.-host disease
- Infection

PATHOLOGY

- Toxicity from chemotherapy &/or radiation therapy leads to small-vessel endothelial damage & sinusoidal occlusion

CLINICAL ISSUES

- Presents with jaundice, ascites, hepatomegaly
- May have elevated bilirubin, thrombocytopenia, ± hepatic synthetic dysfunction
- Treatment includes
  - Supportive care, withdrawal of hepatotoxic therapy
  - Defibrotide is approved to treat moderate to severe disease

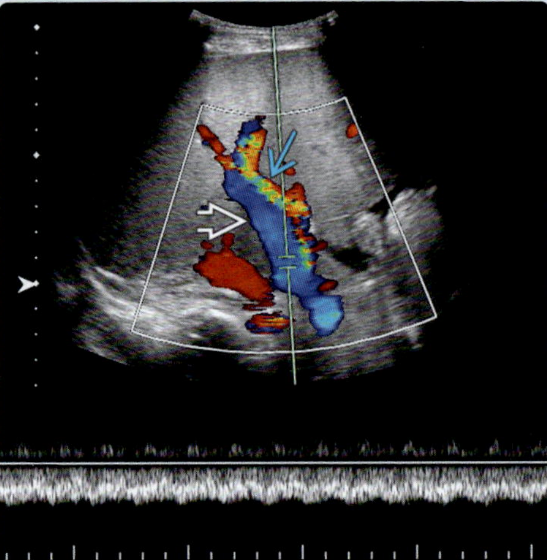

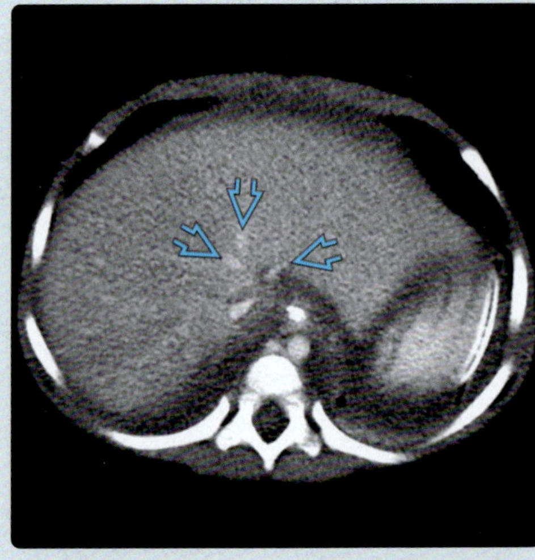

(Left) *Pulsed Doppler ultrasound in a 2-year-old girl receiving chemotherapy for neuroblastoma, now presenting with new onset of ascites & elevated bilirubin, shows that flow in the main portal vein is reversed (hepatofugal flow) ➔, typical of hepatic venoocclusive disease. Note the normal hepatopetal flow in the hepatic artery →.* **(Right)** *Axial CECT in the same patient shows small-caliber but patent hepatic veins ⇨, typical of hepatic venoocclusive disease.*

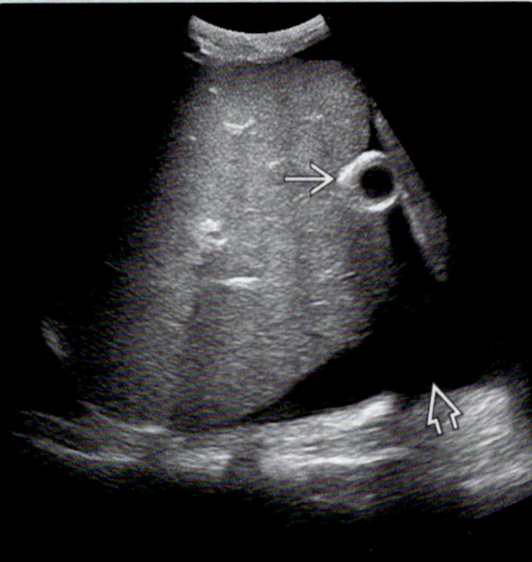

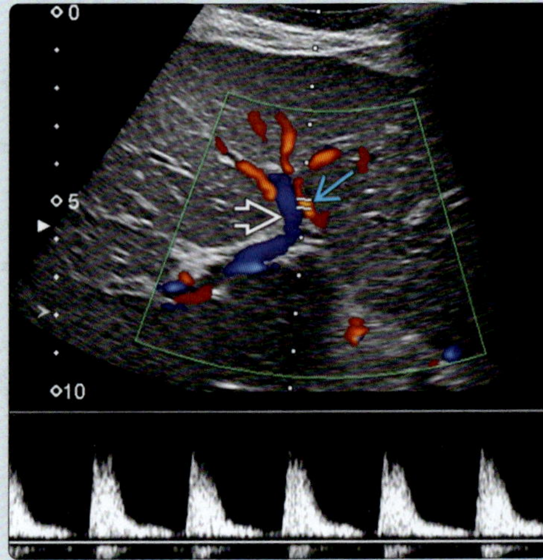

(Left) *Longitudinal grayscale ultrasound in a 13-year-old girl on chemotherapy with newly diagnosed hepatic venoocclusive disease shows ascites ⇨ & marked thickening of the gallbladder wall ➔. The portal venous flow was reversed (not shown).* **(Right)** *Transverse pulsed Doppler ultrasound in a 5-year-old patient status post stem cell transplantation shows reversed portal venous flow ➔ with high-resistance waveforms in the adjacent hepatic artery →, suggesting hepatic venoocclusive disease.*

TERMINOLOGY

Synonyms

- Sinusoidal obstruction syndrome

Definitions

- Therapy-induced occlusion of hepatic sinusoids → clinical triad of jaundice, ascites, & hepatomegaly
- Onset is typically within weeks of stem cell transplantation (SCT); later onset can occur in children
  - Secondary to myeloablative chemotherapy &/or irradiation preceding SCT
- Risk may be specific to different diseases & treatment regimens

IMAGING

General Features

- Best diagnostic clue
  - Hepatomegaly & ascites status post SCT or chemotherapy
  - Reversed flow in portal veins is specific but not sensitive

Radiographic Findings

- Displaced bowel loops due to hepatomegaly & ascites

Ultrasonographic Findings

- Grayscale ultrasound
  - Nonspecific hepatomegaly
  - Ascites
  - ± splenomegaly
- Pulsed Doppler
  - Reversed or to-&-fro flow in portal vein
  - Elevated resistive indices in hepatic artery (> 0.75)
- Color Doppler
  - Reversed portal vein flow
  - Small but patent hepatic veins
  - ± recanalized paraumbilical vein

CT Findings

- CECT
  - Enlarged, heterogeneous liver
  - ± small-caliber hepatic veins
  - Ascites

MR Findings

- Similar to CECT
  - Hepatomegaly, ascites, small-caliber hepatic veins

Imaging Recommendations

- Best imaging tool
  - Ultrasound with Doppler

DIFFERENTIAL DIAGNOSIS

Graft-vs.-Host Disease

- Affects skin, bowel, liver, lung
- Diffusely thickened, potentially featureless bowel

Infection

- Typical pathogens, particularly cytomegalovirus
- Variable imaging findings

PATHOLOGY

General Features

- Etiology
  - Toxicity from chemotherapy or radiation therapy leads to endothelial cell activation & endothelial damage
    - Sloughed endothelial lining ultimately embolizes & occludes sinusoids
  - Direct toxicity to hepatocytes also contributes

CLINICAL ISSUES

Presentation

- Most common signs/symptoms
  - Jaundice, ascites, hepatomegaly
- Other signs/symptoms
  - European Society for Bone Marrow Transplantation (EBMT) Pediatric Criteria
    - Requires 2 or more of
      - Thrombocytopenia
      - ↑ bilirubin
      - ↑ weight
      - Hepatomegaly
      - Ascites
    - Can occur any time after SCT
    - Doppler US is not part of diagnostic criteria
      - Used to evaluate ascites & hepatomegaly
  - Baltimore & Modified Seattle criteria were developed for adults
    - ↑ bilirubin, ↑ weight, ascites, hepatomegaly
      - Within 21 days of SCT

Demographics

- Age
  - Occurs in children & adults
- Epidemiology
  - Affects 8-14% of SCT patients; up to 60% of high risk

Natural History & Prognosis

- Modified EBMT severity grading
  - Mild, moderate, severe, very severe
  - Based on clinical features, lab abnormalities & multiorgan system dysfunction

Treatment

- Supportive care, withdrawal of hepatotoxic therapy
- Defibrotide is approved to treat moderate to severe disease

SELECTED REFERENCES

1. Mahadeo KM et al: Diagnosis, grading, and treatment recommendations for children, adolescents, and young adults with sinusoidal obstructive syndrome: an international expert position statement. Lancet Haematol. 7(1):e61-72, 2020
2. Albers BK et al: Vascular anomalies of the pediatric liver. Radiographics. 39(3):842-56, 2019
3. Kernan NA et al: Final results from a defibrotide treatment-IND study for patients with hepatic veno-occlusive disease/sinusoidal obstruction syndrome. Br J Haematol. 181(6):816-27, 2018
4. Mahgerefteh SY et al: Radiologic imaging and intervention for gastrointestinal and hepatic complications of hematopoietic stem cell transplantation. Radiology. 258(3):660-71, 2011
5. Erturk SM et al: CT features of hepatic venoocclusive disease and hepatic graft-versus-host disease in patients after hematopoietic stem cell transplantation. AJR Am J Roentgenol. 186(6):1497-501, 2006

Abernethy Malformation

KEY FACTS

TERMINOLOGY

- Congenital extrahepatic portosystemic shunt
  - Type 1: Absence of portal vein (PV) with extrahepatic portosystemic shunt
  - Type 2: Intact but hypoplastic PV with extrahepatic portosystemic shunt

IMAGING

- Absent or hypoplastic PV without findings of PV thrombosis or portal hypertension
- Extrahepatic portosystemic shunt, typically draining to IVC
- Small liver with multiple nodules
- Occlusion venogram is required to identify origin of very small PV branches & plan definitive shunt occlusion

TOP DIFFERENTIAL DIAGNOSES

- PV thrombosis
- Intrahepatic portosystemic shunt

PATHOLOGY

- Hepatic lesions in 65-75% of patients; 50-80% have multiple lesions
  - Most common: Focal nodular hyperplasia, nodular regenerative hyperplasia, adenoma, hepatocellular carcinoma
- Congenital heart disease in ~ 15% of patients

CLINICAL ISSUES

- F:M ratio of 3:1 in type 1 Abernethy malformation; no sex predilection in type 2
- May be diagnosed in utero or up to 7th decade of life
  - Type 1 malformations typically present at younger age with hepatic dysfunction, failure to thrive
  - Risks of hepatic encephalopathy & hepatopulmonary syndrome ↑ with age

(Left) *Digital subtraction angiography (DSA) in a 3-month-old boy with an Abernethy type 1A malformation shows the splenic vein ➡ & superior mesenteric vein ➡ joining to form the portal vein ➡. There is a connection ➡ between the portal vein & inferior vena cava ➡.* **(Right)** *Transverse color Doppler ultrasound in a 3-month-old boy with an Abernethy type 1A malformation shows a connection ➡ between the portal vein ➡ & inferior vena cava ➡.*

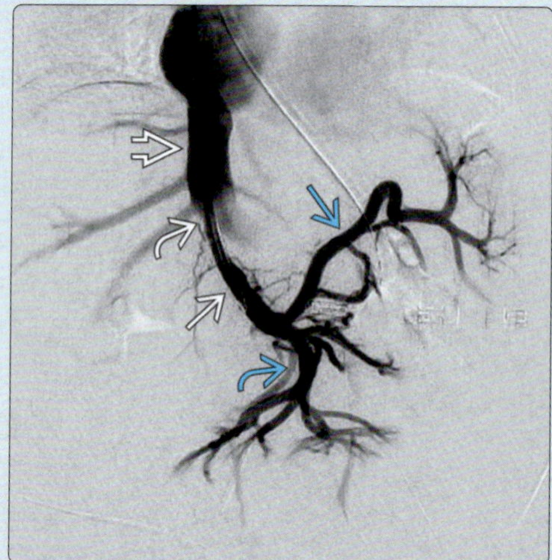

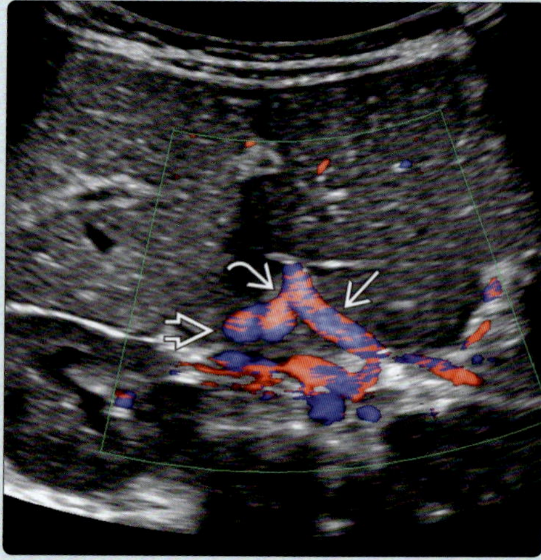

(Left) *Sagittal CECT MIP in a 3-month-old boy with an Abernethy type 1A malformation shows a connection ➡ between the portal vein ➡ & inferior vena cava ➡.* **(Right)** *Oblique noncontrast MR venogram MIP in a 7-month-old boy with Abernethy malformation shows a connection ➡ between the portal vein ➡ & inferior vena cava ➡.*

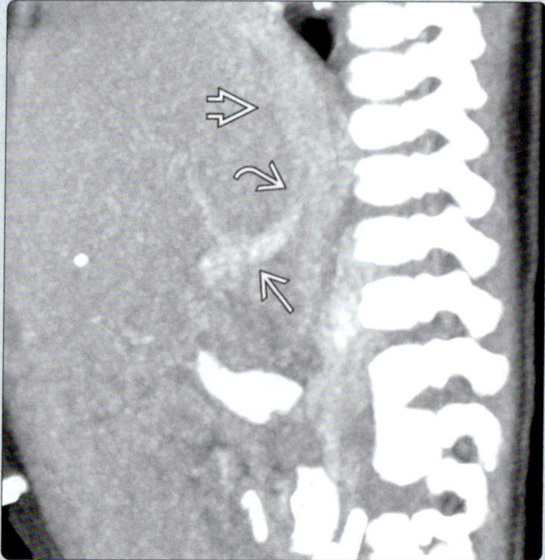

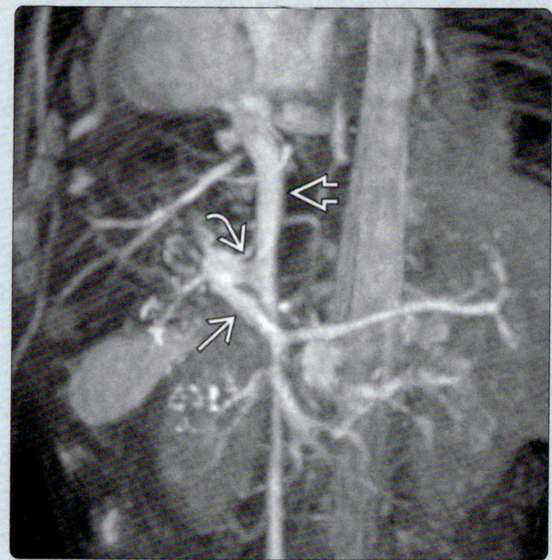

TERMINOLOGY

Synonyms

- Congenital extrahepatic portosystemic shunt

Definitions

- Congenital portosystemic shunt characterized by variable absence of intrahepatic portal vein (PV)
  - Type 1: Absence of intrahepatic PV with extrahepatic portosystemic shunt
  - Type 2: Intact but hypoplastic intrahepatic PV with extrahepatic portosystemic shunt

IMAGING

General Features

- Best diagnostic clue
  - Absent or hypoplastic intrahepatic PV without findings of PV thrombosis or portal hypertension (HTN)
    - Type 1: Absent intrahepatic PV with shunt vessel draining into inferior vena cava (IVC)
    - Type 2: Hypoplastic intrahepatic PV with partial extrahepatic drainage into IVC
  - Liver findings: Small liver with multiple nodules

CT Findings

- CECT
  - Venous phase shows portosystemic shunt ± small PV
  - Coronal plane & maximum-intensity projection images are useful to evaluate shunt & portal system

MR Findings

- T1WI C+ FS
  - Hepatocyte-specific contrast agent is helpful to delineate nodules & identify malignant degeneration
- MRV
  - Use techniques to ↑ spatial resolution to best evaluate portosystemic shunt

Ultrasonographic Findings

- Grayscale ultrasound
  - Absent PV with ↑ periportal echogenicity (related to fibrosis) in expected region of PV
  - Small liver with multiple nodules
- Color Doppler
  - Absent or ↓ PV flow without cavernous transformation
  - Enlarged hepatic artery
  - Extrahepatic shunt

Angiographic Findings

- Occlusion venogram may be required to identify origin of very small PV branches & plan definitive shunt occlusion
  - Shunt imaged via transjugular or transfemoral approach
  - Type 1: Uniform size of portal trunk; PV enters left side of IVC
  - Type 2: Dilation of portal trunk before joining IVC; PV enters anterior aspect of IVC
- Occlusion venogram can identify tiny PV branches, changing diagnosis from type 1 to type 2

Imaging Recommendations

- Protocol advice
  - Maximum-intensity projection images are useful to show small vessels or shunt vessels
  - Occlusion venogram may be required to identify origin of small PV branches

DIFFERENTIAL DIAGNOSIS

Portal Vein Thrombosis

- Filling defect with absence of portal venous flow (US) or enhancement (CECT or MR)
- Cavernous transformation with numerous small hilar venous collaterals
- Secondary findings of portal HTN

Intrahepatic Portosystemic Shunt

- Abnormal connection between branches of PV & hepatic veins or IVC
- Can spontaneously close in 1st year of life

PATHOLOGY

General Features

- Associated abnormalities
  - Hepatic lesions in 65-75% of patients; 50-80% of those have multiple lesions
    - Most common: Focal nodular hyperplasia, nodular regenerative hyperplasia, adenoma, hepatocellular carcinoma
  - Congenital heart disease in ~ 15% of patients

CLINICAL ISSUES

Presentation

- Most common signs/symptoms
  - Hyperammonemia can lead to neurocognitive deficits
  - Hepatopulmonary syndrome
  - Pulmonary arterial HTN

Demographics

- Age
  - May be diagnosed in utero or up to 7th decade of life
- Sex
  - Type 1: F:M = 3:1
  - Type 2: No sex predilection
- Epidemiology
  - Type 1 accounts for ~ 60% of all diagnoses

Natural History & Prognosis

- Risks for hepatic encephalopathy & hepatopulmonary syndrome ↑ with age
- Liver lesions are at risk for malignant transformation

SELECTED REFERENCES

1. Baiges A et al: Congenital extrahepatic portosystemic shunts (Abernethy malformation): an international observational study. Hepatology. 71(2):658-69, 2020
2. Bueno J et al: Radiological and surgical differences between congenital end-to-side (Abernethy malformation) and side-to-side portocaval shunts. J Pediatr Surg. 55(9):1897-902, 2020
3. DiPaola F et al: Congenital portosystemic shunts in children: associations, complications, and outcomes. Dig Dis Sci. 65(4):1239-51, 2020
4. Rajeswaran S et al: Abernethy malformations: evaluation and management of congenital portosystemic shunts. J Vasc Interv Radiol. 31(5):788-94, 2020
5. Sokollik C et al: Congenital portosystemic shunt: characterization of a multisystem disease. J Pediatr Gastroenterol Nutr. 56(6):675-81, 2013

Liver Transplant Complications

KEY FACTS

TERMINOLOGY

- Segmental liver transplant
  - In children, left lobe or lateral segment of left lobe of liver is usually transplanted
  - Developed to ↑ supply of liver transplants for children
    - Usually adult donor, cadaveric or living
- Vascular complications
  - Hepatic arterial thrombosis (HAT) or stenosis
  - Hepatic artery pseudoaneurysm at anastomosis
  - Portal vein stenosis or thrombosis
  - Hepatic vein stenosis
  - Anastomotic bleeding
- Biliary complications
  - Biliary stenosis or leak
- Extrahepatic fluid collection
  - Hematoma, seroma, bile leak, abscess
  - Usually found soon after surgery
- Posttransplant lymphoproliferative disorder (PTLD)
- Infection
- Organ rejection

CLINICAL ISSUES

- Treatment options
  - Vascular complications
    - Vasodilator for arterial spasm early
    - Balloon dilation ± stent for narrowing
    - Thrombectomy for early HAT
    - Surgical revision
    - Retransplant
  - Biliary complications
    - Balloon dilation
    - ± placement of percutaneous biliary drain
    - Surgery
  - PTLD
    - Reduce immunosuppression
    - ± chemotherapy

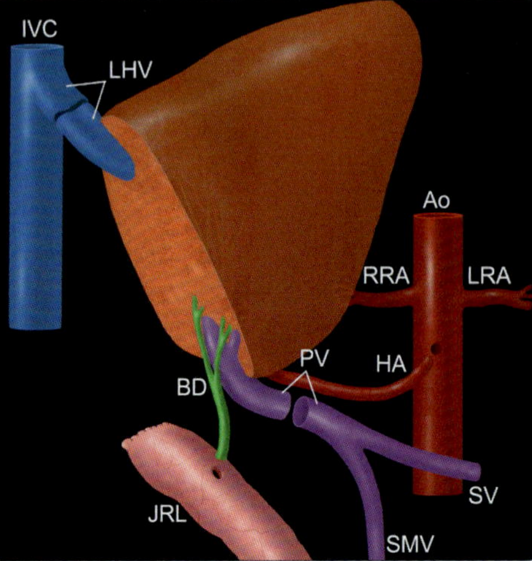

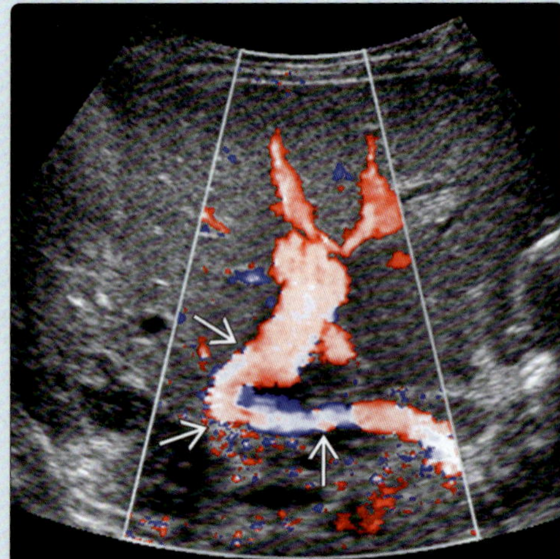

(Left) *Graphic shows segmental left lobe liver transplant anatomy: Bile duct (BD), jejunal Roux loop (JRL), portal vein (PV), superior mesenteric vein (SMV), splenic vein (SV), hepatic artery (HA), aorta (Ao), right & left renal arteries (RRA & LRA), inferior vena cava (IVC), left hepatic vein (LHV).* **(Right)** *Transverse color Doppler US shows the typical curved course of the main PV ➡ & HA following segmental liver transplant. Note how the neoporta is located along the side of the liver rather than in the center.*

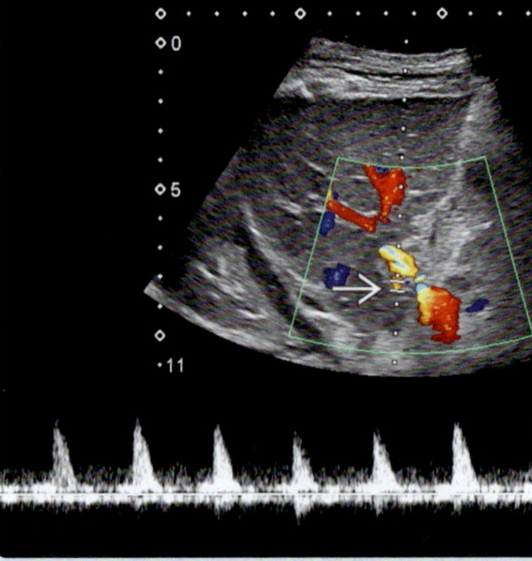

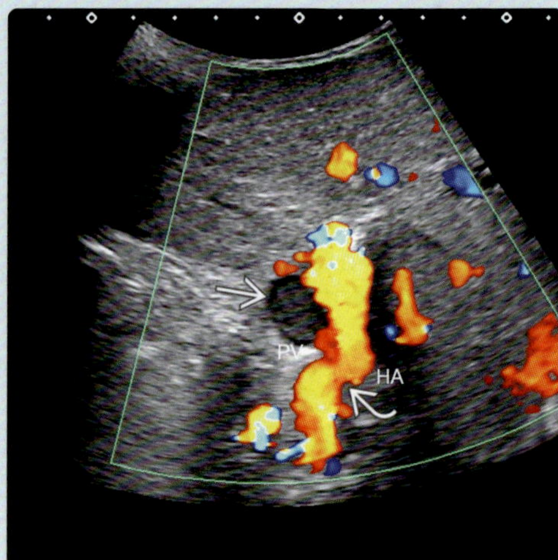

(Left) *Pulsed Doppler US of HA edema/vasospasm immediately after transplant shows a small-caliber HA ➡ with a high resistive index (RI). Elevated RIs can be seen with downstream arterial narrowing/thrombus or parenchymal edema. Sampling distal to a focus of narrowing may give a parvus et tardus waveform (not shown).* **(Right)** *Transverse color Doppler US shows acute PV thrombosis with hypoechoic clot ➡ in the main PV & robust HA flow ➦ next to the clot.*

TERMINOLOGY

Synonyms

- Segmental liver transplant = partial liver transplant, split liver transplant, reduced-size liver transplant, living donor liver transplant

Definitions

- Segmental liver transplant
  - In children, left hepatic lobe or lateral segment of left lobe is usually transplanted
    - Technique was developed to ↑ supply of liver transplants for children
  - Usually adult donor, cadaveric or living
- Vascular complications
  - Hepatic artery (HA): Vasospasm (immediate postoperative timeframe), HA thrombosis (HAT) or stenosis, pseudoaneurysm
  - Portal vein stenosis (PVS) & thrombosis
  - Hepatic vein stenosis (HVS)
  - Anastomotic bleeding
- Biliary complications
  - Anastomotic: Biliary stenosis or leak
  - Nonanastomotic: Intrahepatic biliary stenosis → dilation, biloma, intraductal sludge or stone
- Other complications
  - Extrahepatic collections: Hematoma, seroma, abscess
  - Posttransplant lymphoproliferative disorder (PTLD)
  - Infection: Abscess (hematologic spread), cholangitis (ascending route)
  - Organ rejection
  - Acute kidney injury
  - Diaphragmatic hernia post transplant

IMAGING

Ultrasonographic Findings

- Grayscale ultrasound
  - HAT: Echogenic clot within artery
  - HA pseudoaneurysm: Round, anechoic structure near HA anastomosis
  - PVS: Narrowing (usually at anastomosis), poststenotic dilation
  - PV thrombosis: Echogenic clot in PV lumen
  - HVS: Distended HVs
  - Biliary complications: Biliary dilation or collection
  - PTLD: Adenopathy, mass(es) within abdomen
- Color Doppler
  - Doppler values associated with normal graft status
    - Resistive index (RI): 0.5-0.8; some studies observe normal RI up to 0.9 in immediate postoperative period
    - HA peak systolic velocity (PSV): 50-200 cm/s is associated with normal graft status within 1st year post transplant
  - Doppler values associated with vascular complications
    - RI: < 0.5 in immediate postoperative period
    - HA PSV: > 200 cm/s or < 50 cm/s is associated with ↑ vascular & biliary complications
    - PV velocity: < 30 cm/s or HV velocity < 25 cm/s
  - HA spasm/edema/stenosis: Hours to days after transplant
    - High RI proximal to narrowing
      - ▫ Graft edema may also cause ↑ RI
    - Elevated PSV at narrowing
    - Tardus parvus waveform distal to narrowing
  - HAT: Absent or reversed flow in HA
    - ↑ RI proximal to clot
    - Distal tardus parvus waveform (if any distal flow)
    - Abundant PV flow
  - HA pseudoaneurysm: Swirling to-&-fro color flow filling hypoechoic focus along artery
  - PVS: Focal narrowing
  - PV thrombosis: ↓, absent, or reversed flow
    - May see abundant HA flow in response
  - HVS: Dampened atrial pulsations
    - May normally be dampened early from edema
  - Arteriovenous fistula: Turbulent flow with spectral broadening, low arterial RI, arterialization of veins
    - Occurs weeks-months after transplant, post biopsy
  - ↑ role for contrast-enhanced ultrasound

CT Findings

- CECT
  - HAT or stenosis
    - Peripheral, wedge-shaped, low-attenuation regions
    - Unopacified HA
    - May lead to biliary necrosis with biloma or biliary dilation due to strictures
  - HA pseudoaneurysm at anastomosis
  - PVS & thrombosis
    - Stenosis: Focal narrowing, ± poststenotic dilation
      - ▫ Note that adult donor PV is often larger
    - Thrombosis: Unopacified PV, portosystemic shunts, splenomegaly, ascites
      - ▫ Residua of pretransplant portal hypertension
  - HVS
    - Distended HVs
    - Congested liver with delayed enhancement
  - Biliary strictures from necrosis → dilation
  - Extrahepatic fluid collection
    - Hematoma, bile, abscess, or seroma
    - Aspiration is required for determination of contents
  - PTLD: Wide range of appearances; may be adenopathy or masses almost anywhere in body
  - Infection: Fluid collections, solid organ lesions, dilated bile ducts (cholangitis)
  - Organ rejection: Nonspecific, biopsy is required

MR Findings

- T1WI C+ FS
  - Hepatocyte-specific contrast agent can confirm biliary leak on delayed images
- MRA
  - HAT: Signal loss beyond thrombus due to absent flow
  - HA pseudoaneurysm: High-signal focal enlargement of artery near anastomosis
- MRCP
  - Biliary dilation: High-signal dilated bile ducts

Nonvascular Interventions

- Transhepatic cholangiography

- Biliary strictures: Anastomotic or nonanastomotic → biliary dilation proximal to stricture
- Biliary sludge/stones: Intraluminal filling defects → proximal biliary dilation

Imaging Recommendations

- Best imaging tool
  - Vasculature & biliary system
    - 1st-line screening: Ultrasound with Doppler
    - If possible arterial abnormality, may consider CTA
    - HAT: Angiogram with intervention
    - PVS/thrombosis: Percutaneous transhepatic portogram
    - HVS: Venogram with intervention
    - Biliary stenosis: Percutaneous transhepatic cholangiogram (PTC)
  - Biloma or fluid collection: MR vs. CECT
    - MR with hepatobiliary contrast agent can confirm biliary leak on delayed images
  - PTLD or infection: CECT, MR, or PET

PATHOLOGY

General Features

- Etiology
  - Biliary complications: Depends on surgical reconstruction technique, length of cold ischemia time, immunologic reactions, HAT, CMV infection, ABO incompatibility
  - PTLD: EBV related in 90%, usually EBV(-) recipient → EBV infection post transplant

CLINICAL ISSUES

Presentation

- Most common signs/symptoms
  - Depends on complication
    - HAT: Elevated liver function tests (LFTs)
    - PVS: GI bleeding, splenomegaly, ascites
    - Biliary strictures: Jaundice, cholangitis
    - PTLD: Nonspecific & variable, EBV seroconversion
    - Infection: Fever

Demographics

- Epidemiology
  - HAT
    - Most common vascular complication & cause of graft loss/retransplant (6%)
    - ↑ risk in pediatrics due to small arteries
    - Interposition grafts or anastomosis with recipient aorta may ↓ HAT incidence when arteries are < 3 mm
    - Children do better than adults because of higher rate of recruitment of collateral arteries
  - PV thrombosis
    - High risk in segmental liver transplant because of short PV segment from donor (3%)
    - Higher risk in patients with ↓ PV flow because of splenectomy, portosystemic collaterals
    - Higher risk in PV < 4 mm & weight < 7 kg
  - HVS/thrombosis or inferior vena cava (IVC) obstruction
    - Most often at anastomosis with IVC/atrium
    - Can be due to twisting when transplant moves/shifts
  - Anastomotic bleeding
    - Occurs early & usually requires surgical repair
  - Biliary complications
    - Higher incidence in segmental liver transplants
    - May lead to chronic graft failure, biliary cirrhosis
  - PTLD
    - More common in children than adults; 1-20% incidence
  - Rejection
    - Diagnosed by biopsy or acoustic radiation force impulse (ARFI) elastography
    - Acute cellular rejection is seen in up to 35% in 1st year
  - Infection: Leading cause of death (43%)

Treatment

- Vascular complications
  - HA vasospasm: Vasodilators
  - HA stenosis: Balloon dilation ± stent
    - Surgical repair if balloon resistant
  - HAT: Thrombectomy if early, HA revision, thrombolytic therapy; may require retransplantation
  - PVS: Percutaneous transhepatic portogram → balloon dilation ± stent; surgical revision if necessary
  - HVS: Balloon dilation ± stent, or surgery
- Biliary complications
  - Anastomotic biliary stricture
    - Balloon dilation ± placement of percutaneous biliary drain or surgery
    - Stents have variable long-term patency
  - Nonanastomotic biliary stricture
    - Percutaneous biliary drain & balloon dilation
  - Biliary obstruction
    - 20% have no biliary dilation despite obstruction on PTC
    - Thus, if patient is jaundiced with ↑ LFTs → PTC & possible percutaneous drain
  - Biloma: Drain if infected
  - Biliary leak: Surgery if large; heals with drain if small
  - Biliary sludge/stones: Remove percutaneously ± drain
- PTLD: Reduce immunosuppression ± chemotherapy
- Infection: Antibiotics, antifungals, ± drainage
- Rejection: Immune modulation

SELECTED REFERENCES

1. Franke D et al: Contrast-enhanced ultrasound of transplant organs - liver and kidney - in children. Pediatr Radiol. ePub, 2021
2. Lee AY et al: Non-operative management of biliary complications after liver transplantation in pediatric patients: a 30-year experience. Pediatr Transplant. e14028, 2021
3. Lim CJ et al: Clinical usefulness of T1-weighted MR cholangiography with Gd-EOB-DTPA for the evaluation of biliary complication after liver transplantation. Ann Hepatobiliary Pancreat Surg. 25(1):39-45, 2021
4. Channaoui A et al: Management and outcome of hepatic artery thrombosis after pediatric liver transplantation. Pediatr Transplant. e13938, 2020
5. Gautier S et al: Time is of the essence: a single-center experience of hepatic arterial supply impairment management in pediatric liver transplant recipients. Pediatr Transplant. e13934, 2020
6. Karmazyn B et al: Initial experience with contrast-enhanced ultrasound in the first week after liver transplantation in children: a useful adjunct to Doppler ultrasound. Pediatr Radiol. 51(2):248-56, 2020
7. Ahmad T et al: Doppler parameters of the hepatic artery as predictors of graft status in pediatric liver transplantation. AJR Am J Roentgenol. 209(3):671-5, 2017
8. Jamieson LH et al: Doppler ultrasound velocities and resistive indexes immediately after pediatric liver transplantation: normal ranges and predictors of failure. AJR Am J Roentgenol. 203(1):W110-6, 2014

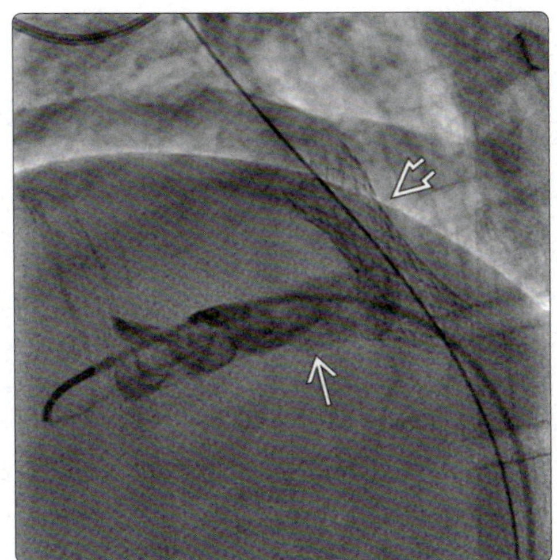

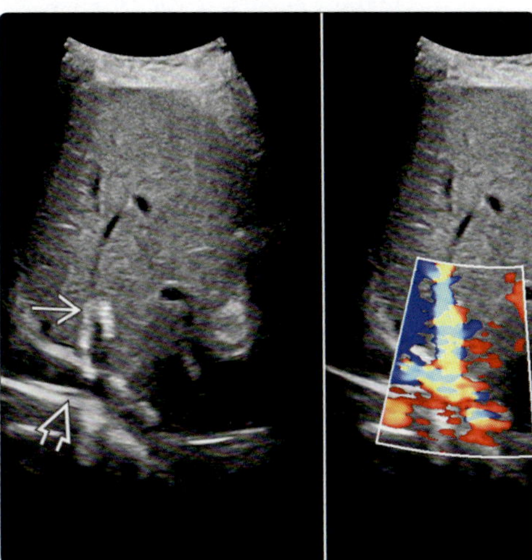

(Left) *Lateral image during a venogram shows a stent placement to treat combined hepatic vein & IVC stenoses several years after a segmental liver transplant.* **(Right)** *Tranverse split screen grayscale & color Doppler US images following venoplasty & stent placement in the same patient show a patent hepatic vein & IVC. Artifact from the metallic stent walls is minimized on live scans & dynamic clips.*

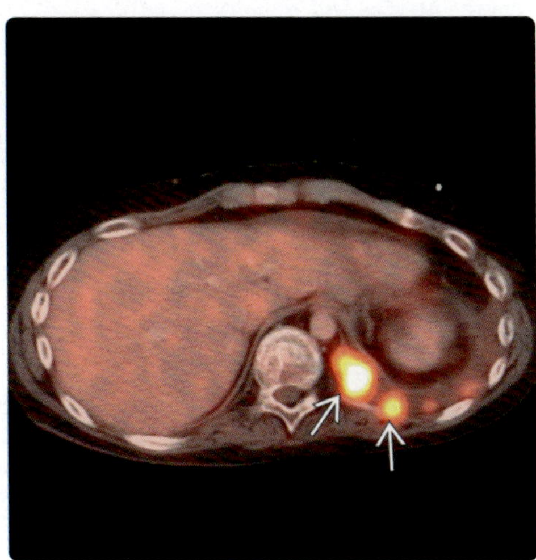

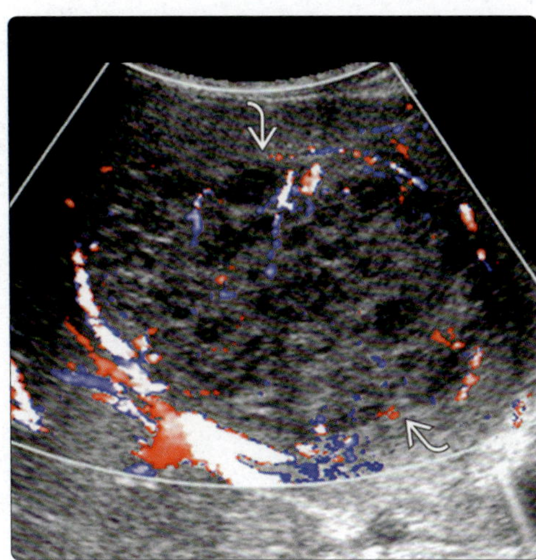

(Left) *Axial FDG PET/CT through the lung base in a liver transplant patient shows multiple FDG-avid soft tissue lesions along the pleura in this case of PTLD. Adenopathy & masses from PTLD can occur anywhere in the body.* **(Right)** *Transverse color Doppler US of the left hepatic lobe shows a heterogeneous ovoid lesion with mild surrounding hyperemia in a patient with fever & abdominal pain. This was confirmed to represent a posttransplant hepatic abscess.*

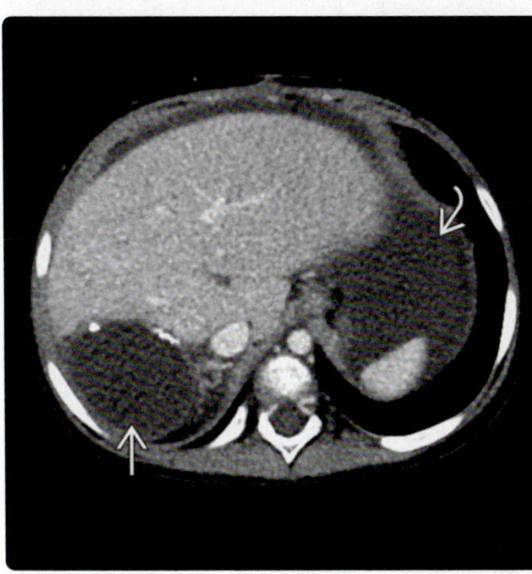

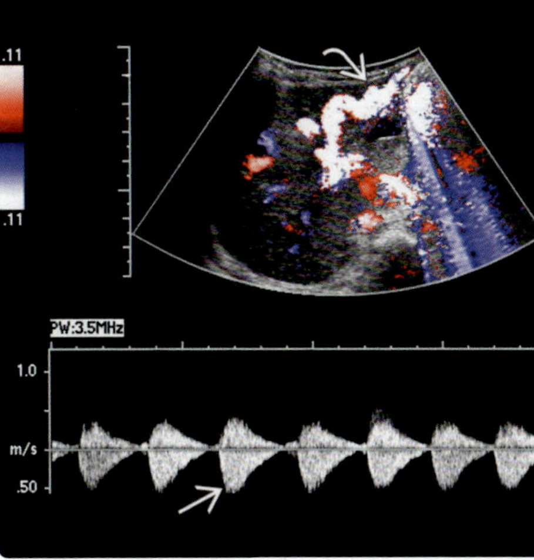

(Left) *Axial CECT through a liver transplant shows a rounded, low-density collection along the staple line in addition to abundant ascites in this case of bile leak/biloma.* **(Right)** *Transverse pulsed Doppler US shows turbulent flow (by both color & pulsed Doppler waveform) in a tortuous vessel extending to the anterior capsule, consistent with an arteriovenous fistula, likely secondary to a prior percutaneous liver biopsy.*

Wandering Spleen

KEY FACTS

TERMINOLOGY

- ↑ mobility of spleen due to abnormal ligamentous attachments (congenitally absent vs. ↑ laxity)
  - Long, vascular pedicle predisposes to acute or chronic intermittent torsion ± infarction

IMAGING

- Absence of normal spleen in LUQ
- Enlarged spleniform mass in mid lower abdomen
- With torsion: Twisted hilar vessels, fat edema, & ascites
  - CT: Globally ↓ splenic enhancement ± residual capsular/rim enhancement
  - US: Hypovascular, heterogeneous splenic parenchyma

TOP DIFFERENTIAL DIAGNOSES

- Sickle cell disease
- Heterotaxy syndromes
- Lymphoma
- Splenic trauma
- Mononucleosis

PATHOLOGY

- Due to abnormal splenic fixation by gastrosplenic, splenophrenic, splenorenal, splenocolic ligaments
  - Congenital absence of ligaments (affects young children)
  - Acquired laxity (affects women of reproductive age)
- Associated abnormalities include gastric volvulus, diaphragmatic hernia, & prune-belly syndrome

CLINICAL ISSUES

- Presentation
  - Pain, vomiting, palpable mobile abdominal mass
  - Asymptomatic (15%)
  - Rarely: Bowel obstruction, pancreatitis, bleeding varices
- Treatment
  - Without infarction: Detorsion + splenopexy
  - With infarction: Splenectomy + vaccinations, antibiotic prophylaxis for asplenia

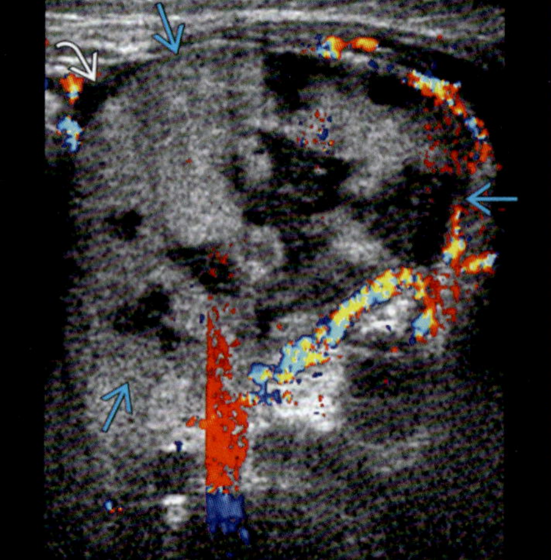

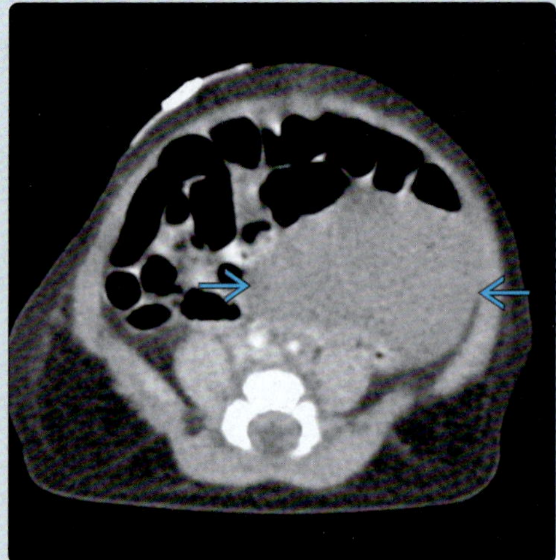

(Left) *Transverse color Doppler ultrasound in a newborn with a palpable abdominal mass shows a spleniform mass ➡ in the mid to lower left abdomen with heterogeneous internal echotexture. No internal vascular flow is seen in the mass. Mild ascites ➡ is noted. A normal spleen was not found in the LUQ.* **(Right)** *Axial CECT of the same patient shows diminished enhancement of the spleniform left abdominal mass ➡. A torsed & infarcted wandering spleen was surgically removed.*

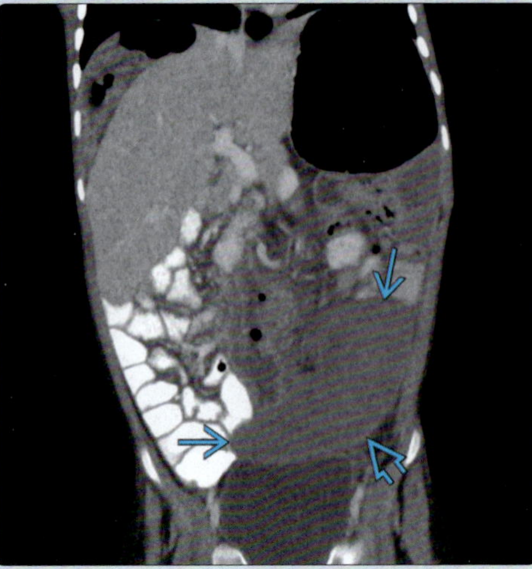

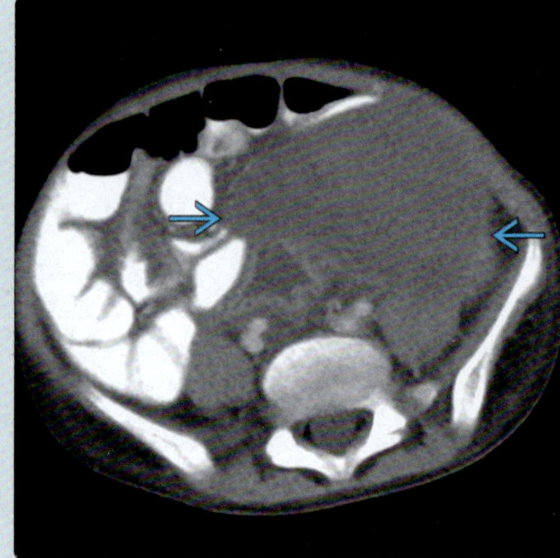

(Left) *Coronal CECT in a 9-year-old patient with abdominal pain & a history of repaired gastroschisis shows an inferiorly displaced, enlarged, & nonenhancing spleen ➡ in the mid to lower left abdomen, consistent with splenic torsion. There is a subtle residual rim of capsular enhancement ➡. No splenic tissue is seen in the LUQ.* **(Right)** *Axial CECT in the same patient shows the torsed nonenhancing spleen ➡. (Courtesy H. Baskin, MD.)*

TERMINOLOGY

Definitions

- ↑ mobility of spleen due to abnormal ligamentous attachments (absence vs. ↑ laxity)
    - Long, vascular pedicle predisposes to acute or chronic intermittent torsion ± infarction

IMAGING

General Features

- Best diagnostic clue
    - Hypoenhancing/hypovascular spleniform abdominal mass in mid to lower abdomen
    - Absence of normal spleen in high LUQ/hypochondrium

Radiographic Findings

- Splenic shadow may be enlarged or absent from LUQ
- ± mid to lower abdominal mass displacing bowel

CT Findings

- Absence of splenic tissue in normal high posterior LUQ
- Displaced, enlarged spleniform mass
- Elongated vascular pedicle
    - Chronically enlarged splenic vein ± adjacent varices
- With torsion
    - Whirl or corkscrew sign of twisted vascular pedicle
        - Swirling lucent & dense bands at hilum due to vessels surrounded by thickened folds of peritoneum & fat
    - Global nonenhancement of splenic parenchyma is more likely than heterogeneous enhancement from congestion or infarcts
        - May have preserved capsular/rim enhancement
    - Ascites + perisplenic fat edema

Ultrasonographic Findings

- Absence of splenic tissue in normal posterior LUQ
- Displaced spleniform mass with variable echogenicity
    - Heterogeneous from congestion or infarcts
- Internal vascular flow variable
    - Lack of flow confirms torsion + ischemia
- Vascular pedicle
    - Chronically dilated, tortuous vessels
    - Twisting, narrowing ± thrombosis in torsion

Imaging Recommendations

- Best imaging tool
    - Ultrasound is excellent screening modality in children with abdominal pain &/or mass
        - Altering patient position (to right decubitus) during scan can demonstrate mobility of wandering spleen
    - CECT is historically more accurate in setting of torsion

DIFFERENTIAL DIAGNOSIS

Sickle Cell Disease

- Splenic infarction
    - Heterogeneous spleen acutely
    - Calcified, small spleen chronically
- Splenic sequestration
    - Acutely enlarged, heterogeneous spleen in young patients due to blood trapping by vasoocclusion

Heterotaxy Syndromes

- Spleen may be absent (asplenia), malpositioned, or of unusual configuration (polysplenia)

Lymphoma

- Enlarged spleen with round, hypoenhancing masses

Splenic Trauma

- Broad imaging spectrum from isolated laceration to shattered, devascularized spleen

Mononucleosis

- Nonspecific splenomegaly + adenopathy
- Fever, pharyngitis, fatigue

PATHOLOGY

General Features

- Etiology
    - Abnormal splenic fixation by gastrosplenic, splenophrenic, splenorenal, &/or splenocolic ligaments
        - Congenital absence (affects young children)
        - Acquired laxity (affects women of reproductive age)
- Associated abnormalities include gastric volvulus, diaphragmatic hernia, prune-belly syndrome

CLINICAL ISSUES

Presentation

- Most common signs/symptoms
    - Without torsion: Palpable mobile mass or asymptomatic
    - With torsion: Abdominal pain, palpable mass
- Other signs/symptoms
    - Fever, vomiting ± bowel obstruction, pancreatitis (due to pancreatic tail involvement), bleeding varices

Demographics

- Bimodal distribution: < 1 year of age (M > F) or 3rd decade of life (F > > M)

Natural History & Prognosis

- Acute torsion (up to 65%): Splenic infarction, peritonitis; potentially fatal
- Chronic complications
    - Intermittent torsion: Recurrent pain, splenomegaly (rupture risk from trauma), varices
    - Functional or iatrogenic asplenia: Infections, sepsis

Treatment

- Without infarction: Detorsion + splenopexy
- With infarction: Splenectomy + vaccinations, antibiotic prophylaxis for asplenia

SELECTED REFERENCES

1. Parada Blázquez MJ et al: Torsion of wandering spleen: radiological findings. Emerg Radiol. 27(5):555-60, 2020
2. Reisner DC et al: Wandering spleen: an overview. Curr Probl Diagn Radiol. 47(1):68-70, 2018
3. Varga I et al: Anatomic variations of the spleen: current state of terminology, classification, and embryological background. Surg Radiol Anat. 40(1):21-9, 2018
4. Lombardi R et al: Wandering spleen in children: a report of 3 cases and a brief literature review underlining the importance of diagnostic imaging. Pediatr Radiol. 44(3):279-88, 2014
5. Priyadarshi RN et al: Torsion in wandering spleen: CT demonstration of whirl sign. Abdom Imaging. 38(4):835-8, 2013

Splenic Infarct

KEY FACTS

IMAGING

- CECT/MR
  - Early: Ill-defined, mottled area(s) of ↓ enhancement relative to normal spleen
  - Late: Wedge-shaped, peripheral area(s) of ↓ enhancement
  - Diffuse infarction: Global nonenhancement ± preserved cortical rim of enhancement from capsular arteries
  - ± perisplenic fluid & inflammatory changes
- Ultrasound with Doppler
  - Peripheral, wedge-shaped, hypoechoic foci ± internal, parallel echogenic lines (bright band sign)
  - Absent flow in infarcted parenchyma

PATHOLOGY

- Segmental vs. diffuse infarction
  - Segmental: Occlusion of segmental arteries, emboli, or venous occlusion
  - Diffuse: Twisting or occlusion of splenic artery
- Etiologies include
  - Hematologic: Sickle cell disease, myeloproliferative disorders, leukemia/lymphoma, hypercoagulable conditions
  - Embolic: Atrial fibrillation, endocarditis
  - Torsion: Wandering spleen, polysplenia
  - Vasculitis
  - Splenomegaly: Portal hypertension, Gaucher disease, mononucleosis

CLINICAL ISSUES

- Presents with left upper quadrant pain ± fever
- May resolve with focus of scar ± Ca^{2+} or cyst
- Acute complications: Rupture, hemorrhage, abscess formation
  - Long term: ↑ risk of infection due to asplenia
- Typically managed conservatively unless complications

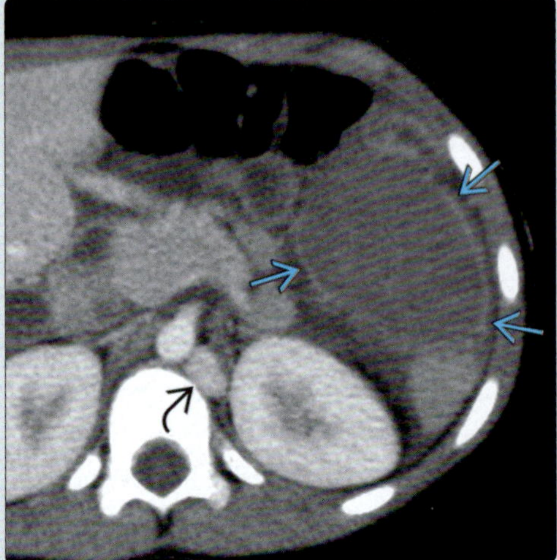

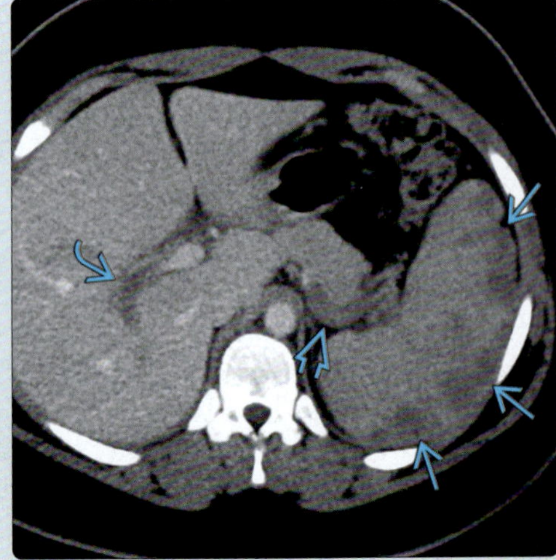

(Left) *Axial CECT in a 5-year-old girl with situs ambiguous & polysplenia who presented with abdominal pain shows a nonenhancing spleen with a rim of capsular enhancement ➙, typical of a splenic infarction. Note the left-sided inferior vena cava ➚.* **(Right)** *Axial CECT in a 17-year-old girl with a history of smoking & obesity now presenting with left upper quadrant pain shows peripheral, wedge-shaped splenic infarcts ➙, a thrombosed splenic vein ➙, & right portal vein thrombosis ➚.*

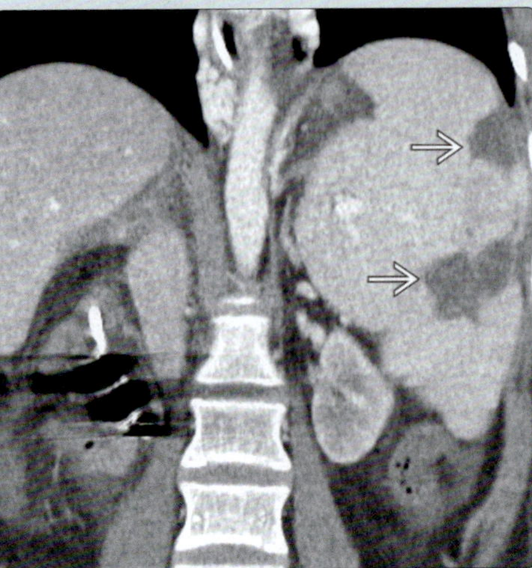

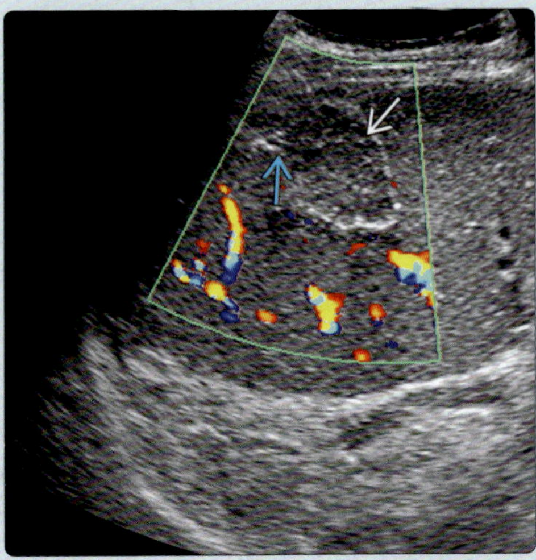

(Left) *Coronal CECT in a liver transplant patient shows splenomegaly & 2 peripheral, relatively well-demarcated areas of hypoattenuation ➡ in an enlarged spleen, consistent with splenic infarcts.* **(Right)** *Longitudinal oblique color Doppler ultrasound in a 17-year-old bone marrow transplant patient shows a well-demarcated, wedge-shaped, peripheral focus of avascular ↓ echogenicity ➡ within the spleen, consistent with infarct. Note the echogenic, parallel lines (bright band sign) ➙ in this infarct.*

TERMINOLOGY

Definitions

- Segmental or diffuse ischemia &/or necrosis caused by loss of blood supply

IMAGING

General Features

- Best diagnostic clue
  - Peripheral, wedge-shaped, hypoenhancing foci on CECT/MR
  - Heterogeneous, hypoechoic, peripheral avascular foci on ultrasound with Doppler
    - ± bright band sign: Thin, linear, echogenic foci within hypoechoic infarct
- Location
  - Peripheral, segmental, or diffuse type
- Size
  - Variable, can involve entire spleen
- Morphology
  - Typically wedge-shaped
    - Can be spherical/round or peripheral band

Ultrasonographic Findings

- Grayscale ultrasound
  - Peripheral, well-demarcated region of ↓ echogenicity
    - May see small linear parallel echogenic foci: Bright band sign
  - ± splenomegaly
  - May see islands of normal parenchyma within otherwise infarcted spleen
  - Diffuse infarction gradually results in small, calcified spleen
- Color Doppler
  - Absent flow in infarcted areas

CT Findings

- Variable appearance depending on stage
  - Early: Ill-defined, mottled area(s) of ↓ enhancement relative to normal spleen
  - Late: Wedge-shaped, peripheral area(s) of ↓ enhancement
  - Diffuse infarction: Global nonenhancement ± rim of cortical enhancement from capsular arteries
- ± associated vascular filling defects
- ± perisplenic fluid & inflammatory change

MR Findings

- Wedge-shaped, peripheral focus of nonenhancement
  - ↓ T1, ↑ T2 signal due to edema
- ↑ poorly defined edema/fluid in surrounding tissues

DIFFERENTIAL DIAGNOSIS

Laceration

- Irregular linear foci of hypoenhancement + surrounding fluid in trauma setting

Transient Heterogeneous Enhancement Pattern

- Alternating bands of ↑ & ↓ enhancement during arterial phase on postcontrast CT/MR

Lymphoma

- Focal masses throughout spleen ± splenomegaly, adjacent adenopathy

Preserved Splenic Tissue in Chronic Infarction

- Round, hypoechoic mass(es) of residual functioning splenic tissue in otherwise echogenic, chronically infarcted spleen
- Normal internal vascularity on ultrasound
- + uptake on nuclear medicine sulfur colloid scan
- Associated with sickle cell disease

PATHOLOGY

General Features

- Etiology
  - Hematologic: Sickle cell disease, myeloproliferative disorders, leukemia/lymphoma, hypercoagulable conditions
  - Embolic: Atrial fibrillation, endocarditis
  - Torsion: Wandering spleen, polysplenia
  - Vasculitis
  - Splenomegaly: Portal hypertension, infection, Gaucher disease

Staging, Grading, & Classification

- Segmental infarction
  - Occurs due to end-artery configuration of splenic arteries with ↓ collateral circulation
- Diffuse infarction
  - Due to occlusion or twisting of main splenic vessels

CLINICAL ISSUES

Presentation

- Most common signs/symptoms
  - Left upper quadrant pain
  - ± fever & constitutional symptoms
- Clinical profile
  - ↑ association with sickle cell disease & mononucleosis

Natural History & Prognosis

- Variable; often requires no treatment
- May resolve completely, leaving focus of scar ± Ca^{2+}
- May resolve & leave acquired cyst
- Complications: Rupture, abscess, intraperitoneal hemorrhage
- Functional asplenia may result from extensive infarctions
  - Predisposed to overwhelming postsplenectomy infection with encapsulated organisms

Treatment

- Typically none unless complications develop

SELECTED REFERENCES

1. Boehnke MW et al: Imaging features of pathologically proven pediatric splenic masses. Pediatr Radiol. 50(9):1284-92, 2020
2. Heo DH et al: Splenic infarction associated with acute infectious mononucleosis due to Epstein-Barr virus infection. J Med Virol. 89(2):332-6, 2017
3. Kuint RC et al: Sonographic bands of hypoechogenicity in the spleen in children: zebra spleen. AJR Am J Roentgenol. 207(3):648-52, 2016
4. Llewellyn ME et al: The sonographic "bright band sign" of splenic infarction. J Ultrasound Med. 33(6):929-38, 2014

Splenic Cysts

KEY FACTS

IMAGING

- Best clue: Well-circumscribed, round splenic mass
  - Follows fluid characteristics on all modalities
  - "Claw" of splayed splenic tissue along margin of larger cysts (confirming spleen as organ of origin)
- Typically solitary & unilocular
- Can occasionally have thin rim of Ca^{2+}
- US: Typically suffices to demonstrate cystic nature
  - Anechoic/hypoechoic with ↑ through transmission
  - Can have low-level internal echoes
  - No internal flow on color/power Doppler US
- No enhancement on CECT, MR C+, or CEUS
  - Typically hypointense on precontrast T1 MR unless proteinaceous or hemorrhagic contents

TOP DIFFERENTIAL DIAGNOSES

- Splenic lymphoma
- Splenic infection
- Splenic infarct
- Splenic perfusion artifact
- Intrasplenic pancreatic pseudocyst

PATHOLOGY

- Congenital (true) cysts: Either epidermoid or mesothelial
  - ± elevation of serum CEA, CA 125, & CA 19-9
- Acquired cysts (comprise 80% of splenic cysts)
  - Post traumatic
  - Post infarction
  - Infectious/inflammatory (pyogenic, parasitic, fungal)
  - Vascular malformation (venolymphatic)
    - Congenital but not visible early

CLINICAL ISSUES

- Most commonly incidental
- Complications may include hemorrhage, rupture, infection
- Distinction between congenital (true) & acquired cysts is not possible by imaging

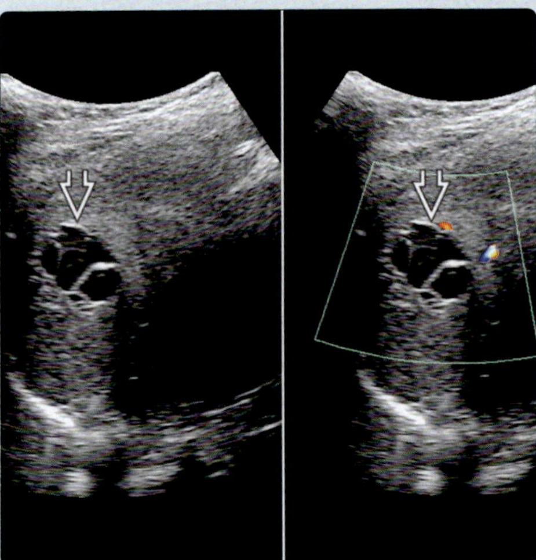

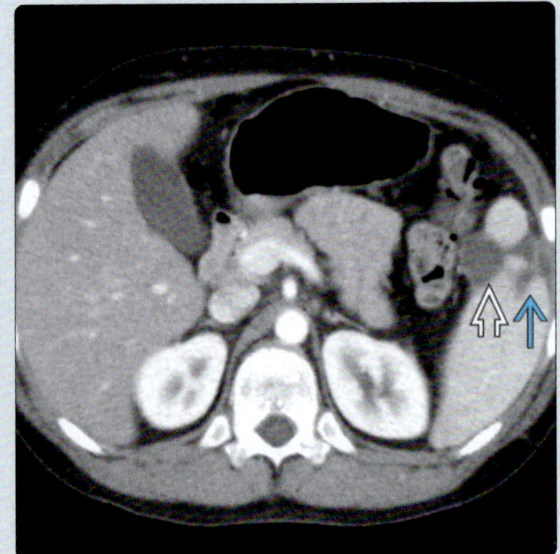

(Left) *Longitudinal grayscale & color Doppler ultrasound images show an incidentally detected, mildly complex splenic cyst ➡ with thin septations in a 10-year-old girl. Pathology confirmed a benign epidermoid cyst.* **(Right)** *Axial CECT in a teenager who was involved in a motor vehicle accident several weeks prior shows a hypoattenuating, rounded mass ➡ adjacent to a prior laceration ➡, consistent with a posttraumatic cyst.*

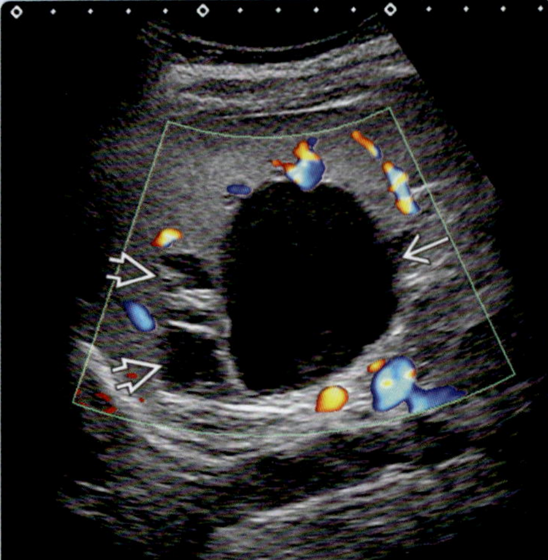

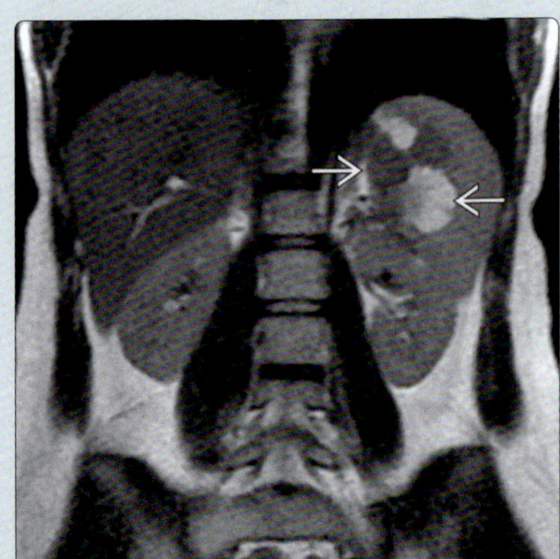

(Left) *Longitudinal color Doppler ultrasound in a 16-year-old with a posttraumatic splenic cyst shows a dominant cyst ➡ with smaller adjacent cysts ➡ in an area of ↓ perfusion related to ischemic injury.* **(Right)** *Coronal SSFSE T2 MR in a 17-year-old patient with a posttraumatic splenic cyst shows heterogeneous signal intensity ➡ in the lesion due to aging blood products.*

IMAGING

General Features

- Best diagnostic clue
  - Well-circumscribed, round mass with simple fluid characteristics
  - Distinction between congenital (true) & acquired cysts is not possible by imaging
- Size
  - Variable

Ultrasonographic Findings

- Grayscale ultrasound
  - Well-circumscribed, rounded mass
  - Typically anechoic but can have low-level internal echoes
  - ↑ posterior acoustic transmission
  - Thin wall
  - No contrast enhancement
- Color Doppler
  - No internal color flow

CT Findings

- Well-circumscribed, water attenuation mass
- Typically solitary & unilocular
- No enhancement
- Can occasionally have thin rim of Ca^{2+}

MR Findings

- Well-circumscribed, rounded mass
- Typically hypointense on T1 unless proteinaceous or hemorrhagic material is present internally
- Hyperintense on T2
- No enhancement
- No restricted diffusion (unless prior hemorrhage)

Imaging Recommendations

- Best imaging tool
  - US typically suffices to demonstrate cystic nature of splenic mass
  - Further characterization with any imaging modality is not typically possible

DIFFERENTIAL DIAGNOSIS

Splenic Lymphoma

- Can be solitary, multifocal, or diffuse
- Typically higher density/echogenicity than cysts
- Look for associated lymphadenopathy

Splenic Infection

- Numerous tiny lesions are typical for fungal microabscesses
- Look for lesions in liver, kidneys, & lungs

Splenic Infarct

- Typically well-demarcated, peripheral, wedge-shaped foci of ↓ attenuation/echogenicity/enhancement
- Higher attenuation/density than cysts
- Lacks internal blood flow
- May resolve completely or evolve into acquired cyst

Splenic Perfusion Artifact

- Focal areas of ↓ attenuation on early arterial phase of CECT or T1 C+ MR
  - Classically archiform waves of ↑ & ↓ enhancement
- Resolves on delayed phase (typically not necessary)
- US is usually normal

Intrasplenic Pancreatic Pseudocyst

- May result from tail pancreatitis
- Patient typically has clinical &/or imaging evidence of recent pancreatitis

PATHOLOGY

General Features

- Congenital (true) cysts = epidermoid or mesothelial cysts
  - Differentiated by type of epithelial lining
  - Thought to arise from defect in mesothelial migration
- Acquired cysts (comprising 80% of splenic cysts)
  - Post traumatic
  - Post infarction
  - Inflammatory/infectious (pyogenic, parasitic, fungal)
  - Vascular (venolymphatic)
    - Congenital but not visible early

CLINICAL ISSUES

Presentation

- Most common signs/symptoms
  - Typically asymptomatic & incidentally identified
- Other signs/symptoms
  - Left upper quadrant pain
  - Palpable mass
  - Splenomegaly
  - ± elevated serum CEA, CA 125, or CA 19-9
  - Large cysts predispose to splenic torsion &/or ptosis

Natural History & Prognosis

- Complications may include hemorrhage, rupture, infection

Treatment

- Small & asymptomatic masses typically require no treatment
- Larger or symptomatic masses may undergo surgical excision or splenectomy

DIAGNOSTIC CHECKLIST

Consider

- Infectious & neoplastic processes should be excluded
  - Splenic neoplasms are uncommon in children (outside of lymphoma)

SELECTED REFERENCES

1. Boehnke MW et al: Imaging features of pathologically proven pediatric splenic masses. Pediatr Radiol. 50(9):1284-92, 2020
2. Di Serafino M et al: Ultrasonography of the pediatric spleen: a pictorial essay. J Ultrasound. 22(4):503-12, 2019
3. Hassoun J et al: Management of nonparasitic splenic cysts in children. J Surg Res. 223:142-8, 2018
4. Kapatia G et al: Splenic hemangiomatosis: an uncommon vascular lesion in an infant. Fetal Pediatr Pathol. 37(5):372-6, 2018
5. Liu X et al: Successful integration of contrast-enhanced us into routine abdominal imaging. Radiographics. 38(5):1454-77, 2018
6. Li W et al: Real-time contrast enhanced ultrasound imaging of focal splenic lesions. Eur J Radiol. 83(4):646-53, 2014
7. Elsayes KM et al: MR imaging of the spleen: spectrum of abnormalities. Radiographics. 25(4):967-82, 2005

KEY FACTS

TERMINOLOGY

- Spectrum of clinical manifestations resulting from *Bartonella henselae* inoculation of skin by cat scratch
  - Typical cat-scratch disease (CSD) includes tender regional adenopathy + fever 1-3 weeks after inoculation
    - Papule at scratch site may be 1st clue
  - Self-limited in most patients; dissemination in 5-14%

IMAGING

- Numerous small, hypoechoic (US), hypodense (CT) splenic &/or hepatic lesions of variable size
- ± splenomegaly, rarely complicated by rupture
- Residual granulomas may calcify

TOP DIFFERENTIAL DIAGNOSES

- Lymphoma
- Microabscesses
- Lymphatic anomalies
- Other granulomatous diseases

CLINICAL ISSUES

- Typical CSD: Single lymph node involved in up to 85%
  - Axillary, epitrochlear > head/neck > groin, other nodes
- Disseminated disease manifestations include hepatic &/or splenic involvement, conjunctivitis, retinitis, encephalopathy, osteomyelitis, endocarditis, pneumonia
  - Adenopathy occurs in only 55% of splenic cases
- Diagnosis made by combination of cat exposure history, positive serum antibody titers or DNA PCR, hepatic/splenic lesions, positive biopsy
- Treatment
  - Most typical CSD cases in immunocompetent hosts resolve within months without antibiotics
  - Antibiotic therapy for systemic disease &/or immunocompromised states

DIAGNOSTIC CHECKLIST

- Multifocal splenic lesions → nonspecific; recent cat exposure ± focal adenopathy should raise suspicion for CSD

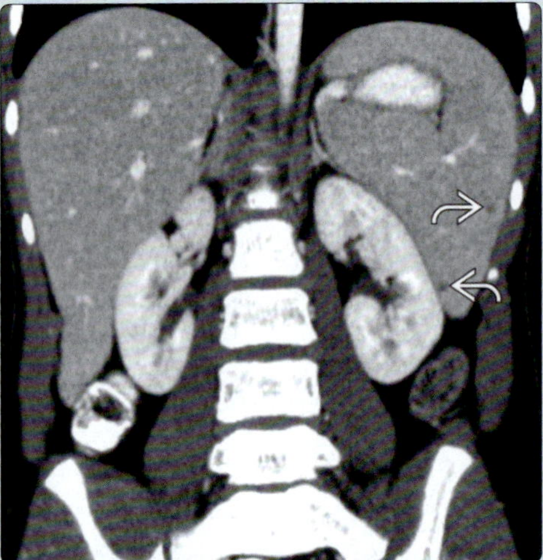

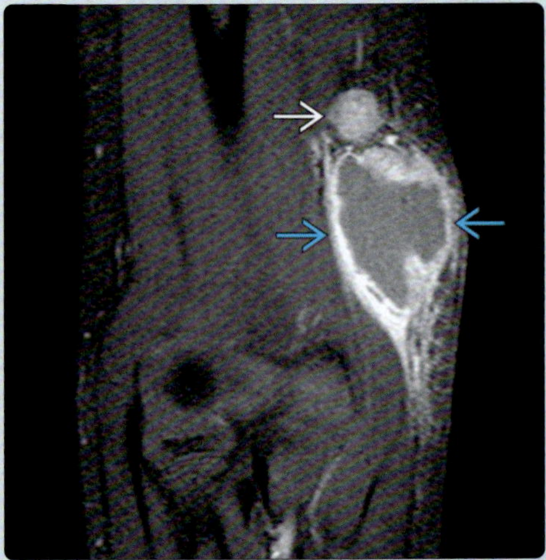

(Left) *Abdominal coronal CECT in an 11-year-old patient with 1 month of fevers + back & neck pain shows numerous tiny, hypodense lesions ➔ in the spleen. Excisional biopsy of enlarged inguinal lymph nodes showed cat-scratch disease (CSD).* **(Right)** *Coronal T1 C+ FS MR in an 8-year-old patient with arm swelling shows a suppurative medial epitrochlear lymph node with thick, irregular wall & central necrosis/fluid ⇨. Additional adjacent adenopathy is noted ➔. The patient had a history of kitten exposure & showed positive Bartonella titers.*

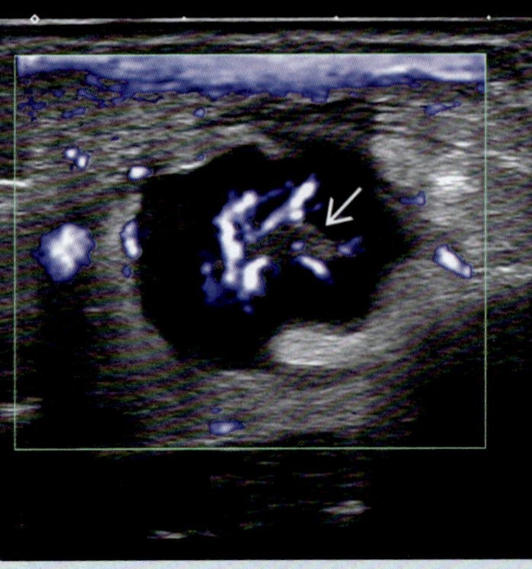

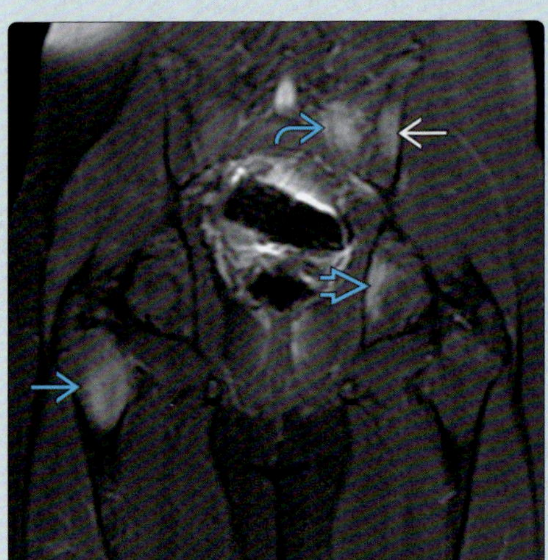

(Left) *Transverse Doppler US in a 7-year-old patient with an epitrochlear mass for weeks shows an enlarged lymph node with classic fatty hilum ➔, radiating vasculature, & surrounding subcutaneous edema. The patient had a history of kitten exposure & showed positive Bartonella titers.* **(Right)** *Coronal T2 FS MR in a 10-year-old with fever of unknown origin & leg pain shows multiple poorly defined, hyperintense lesions scattered throughout the marrow of the sacrum ⇨, iliac wing ➔, ischium ⇨, & right femur ⇨. Biopsy & titers revealed CSD.*

TERMINOLOGY

Definitions

- Cat-scratch disease (CSD): Spectrum of clinical manifestations resulting from *Bartonella henselae* inoculation of skin by cat scratch
- "Typical CSD" (most common clinical presentation): Tender regional adenopathy + fever 1-3 weeks after inoculation
  - Papule at scratch site may be 1st clue
  - Self-limited in most patients
  - Disseminated disease in 5-14%

IMAGING

General Features

- Best diagnostic clue
  - Splenic ± hepatic lesions in setting of focal extremity adenopathy & recent cat exposure
- Morphology
  - Numerous small, hypoechoic (US), hypodense (CT) splenic lesions of variable size
  - Lesions show ↑ metabolic activity on FDG PET
  - ± splenomegaly, rarely complicated by rupture
  - Residual granulomas may calcify

Imaging Recommendations

- Best imaging tool
  - US
- Protocol advice
  - Clinical history is important as many pathologies involving spleen have similar imaging appearances

DIFFERENTIAL DIAGNOSIS

Splenic Lymphoma

- Hypoechoic/hypodense, round masses of variable size
- Multifocal/confluent adenopathy ± other visceral lesions

Splenic Microabscesses

- Fungal infection (most commonly *Candida*) with numerous tiny, hypoechoic lesions
  - ± central echogenic foci (target or bull's-eye sign)

Lymphatic Anomalies

- Numerous small, hypoechoic/hypodense splenic lesions in setting of cystic soft tissue &/or bony lymphatic malformations

Other Granulomatous Diseases

- Hypoechoic splenic lesions from tuberculosis, sarcoid, histoplasmosis, Wegener granulomatosis

PATHOLOGY

General Features

- Etiology
  - Inoculation of skin by scratch (or possibly bite) of cat/kitten (less commonly guinea pig, rabbit, or dog)
    - Specific cat flea typically serves as vector with bacteria carried in flea excrement
    - Certain ticks rarely serve as vector
- Associated abnormalities
  - Lymphadenopathy (only in 55% of splenic cases), conjunctivitis, retinitis, encephalopathy, osteomyelitis, endocarditis, pneumonia

Microscopic Features

- Necrotizing granulomas + microabscesses

CLINICAL ISSUES

Presentation

- Most common signs/symptoms
  - Erythematous papule at inoculation site, regional adenopathy, fever ("typical CSD"): Up to 95% of cases
    - Adenopathy 1-3 weeks post inoculation
      - Axillary, epitrochlear > head/neck > groin, other
      - Single node involved in up to 85% of patients
- Other signs/symptoms
  - Aches, malaise, abdominal pain, fever of unknown origin (FUO), neurologic & ocular involvement
    - 3rd leading infectious cause of pediatric FUO (after Epstein-Barr virus & osteomyelitis)
- Clinical profile
  - Elevated erythrocyte sedimentation rate
  - Confirmation by serology (IgM & IgG antibodies) or tissue PCR

Demographics

- Age
  - Up to 87% of cases < 18 years old
- Epidemiology
  - 22,000 cases of CSD per year in United States
  - 50-87% report scratch by cat

Natural History & Prognosis

- Diagnosis made by combination of clinical, laboratory, &/or imaging criteria
  - Hepatosplenic lesions by imaging, cat or flea contact, positive antibody serology, positive biopsy, sterile pus aspiration

Treatment

- Most typical CSD cases in immunocompetent hosts resolve within months without antibiotics
  - Suppurative nodes require drainage in 10% of cases
- Antibiotic therapy for systemic disease &/or immunocompromised state

DIAGNOSTIC CHECKLIST

Image Interpretation Pearls

- Multifocal splenic lesions → nonspecific: Clinical history of recent cat exposure ± focal adenopathy should raise suspicion for CSD

SELECTED REFERENCES

1. Landes M et al: Cat scratch disease presenting as fever of unknown origin is a unique clinical syndrome. Clin Infect Dis. 71(11):2818-24, 2020
2. Cheslock MA et al: Human bartonellosis: an underappreciated public health problem? Trop Med Infect Dis. 4(2), 2019
3. Chang CC et al: Disseminated cat-scratch disease: case report and review of the literature. Paediatr Int Child Health. 36(3):232-4, 2015
4. Kraft KE et al: Hepatosplenic cat-scratch disease in children and the positive contribution of 18F-FDG imaging. Clin Nucl Med. 40(9):746-7, 2015
5. Rohr A et al: Spectrum of radiological manifestations of paediatric cat-scratch disease. Pediatr Radiol. 42(11):1380-4, 2012

KEY FACTS

TERMINOLOGY

- Primary exocrine epithelial malignancy of pancreas occurring in young children

IMAGING

- Most commonly arises in pancreatic head
- Mean size: 7-18 cm
  - May be difficult to determine organ of origin due to size
- Well-circumscribed mass with smooth border
- Heterogeneous appearance due to mixed cystic & solid foci
  - Predominantly hypoechoic (US), hypoenhancing (CECT)
- Speckled Ca^{2+} is common

TOP DIFFERENTIAL DIAGNOSES

- Pancreatic pseudocyst
- Solid pseudopapillary neoplasm
- Pancreatic neuroendocrine tumor
- Non-Hodgkin lymphoma

PATHOLOGY

- ↑ incidence in patients with Beckwith-Wiedemann syndrome & familial adenomatous polyposis

CLINICAL ISSUES

- Most common malignant pancreatic tumor of young children
- Mean age at presentation: 5 years
- 1.3-2.7x more common in male patients
- More common in Asian population
- Most commonly presents as asymptomatic abdominal mass
- Elevated α-fetoprotein in 33-70% of patients
- Metastases are present in 1/3 at diagnosis
  - Liver > lungs, lymph nodes
- Best treated with surgical resection ± chemotherapy
  - Recurrence is common

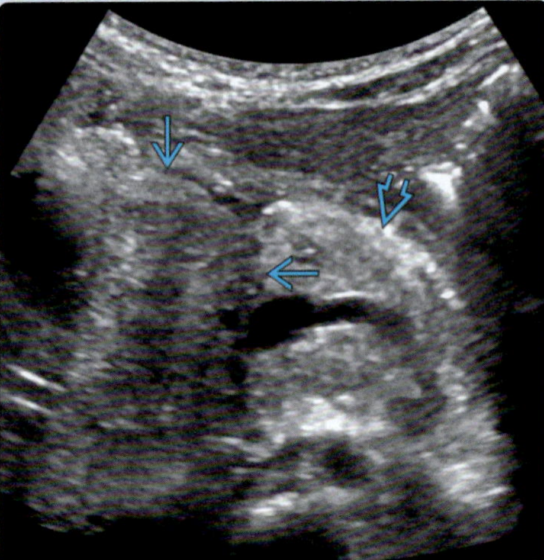

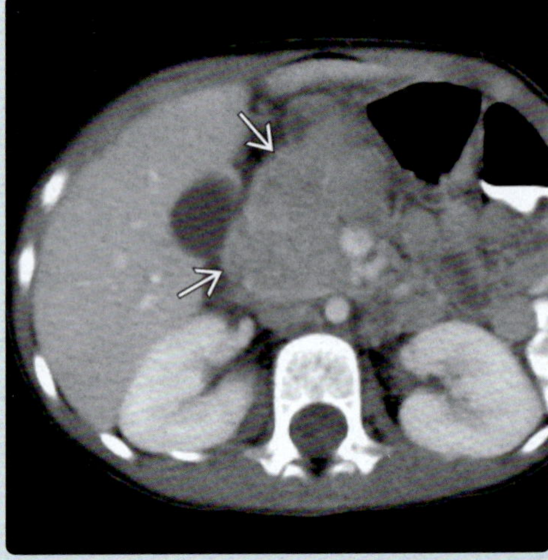

(Left) *Transverse ultrasound of the pancreas* ⇨ *in a young child with pain & a palpable mass shows a large, lobulated hypoechoic mass* ⇨ *arising from the pancreatic head.* **(Right)** *Axial CECT in the same patient shows a lobulated, nearly homogeneously enhancing mass* ➡ *arising from the head of the pancreas, which is the most common site of origin. Pancreatoblastoma usually presents in the 1st decade of life as an asymptomatic abdominal mass.*

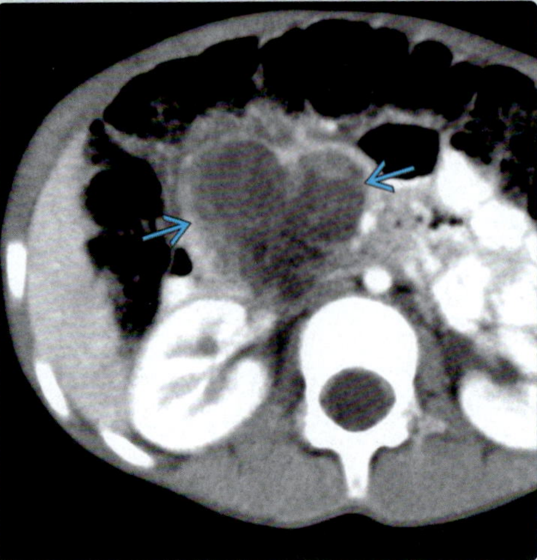

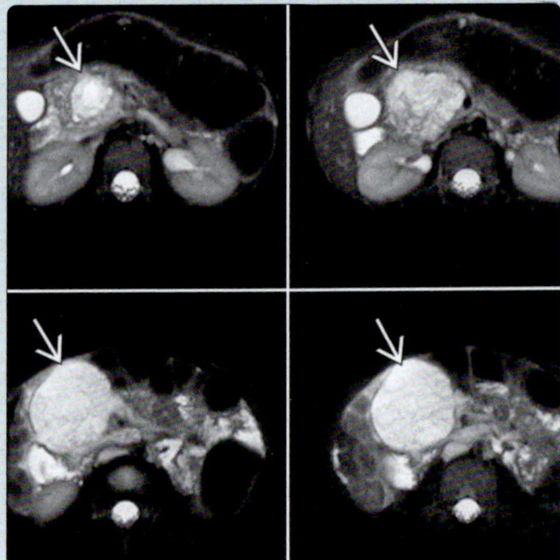

(Left) *Axial CECT in a child with pancreatoblastoma shows a heterogeneously enhancing but predominantly hypodense mass* ⇨ *arising from the head of the pancreas.* **(Right)** *Axial T2 FS MR images in the same child show a lobulated, hyperintense, cystic-appearing mass* ➡ *arising from the head of the pancreas. The internal signal intensity suggests septations.*

TERMINOLOGY

Definitions

- Primary exocrine epithelial malignancy of pancreas occurring in young children

IMAGING

General Features

- Best diagnostic clue
  - Large, heterogeneous mass of pancreas in child
- Location
  - 33-50% arise in pancreatic head
  - 13-37% arise in pancreatic tail
  - 10-25% arise in pancreatic body
- Size
  - Large tumors; average: 7-18 cm in diameter
- Morphology
  - Well-circumscribed vs. poorly defined margins; may have local/regional vascular invasion
    - May be difficult to determine organ of origin

Ultrasonographic Findings

- Well-circumscribed mass with heterogeneous echogenicity
  - Cystic & solid components
    - Cystic foci are hypoechoic with hyperechoic septa

CT Findings

- CECT
  - Well-circumscribed vs. poorly defined margins
  - Heterogeneous attenuation of mixed cystic & solid foci
    - Cystic areas represent necrosis
    - Overall hypodense vs. normally enhancing pancreas
  - Multiloculated with enhancing septa
  - Small punctate Ca^{2+} are common

MR Findings

- T1: Well-circumscribed, iso- to hypointense mass
  - Areas of lower signal correspond to necrosis
  - Areas of higher signal correspond to hemorrhage
- T2 FS: Heterogeneously hyperintense mass
- T1 C+ FS: Enhances < adjacent pancreas
  - Rim may enhance to greater degree than remainder of pancreas
- DWI: Lower ADC values than solid pseudopapillary neoplasm

DIFFERENTIAL DIAGNOSIS

Pancreatic Pseudocyst

- Collection of fluid, tissue, debris, pancreatic enzymes, & blood surrounded by fibrous capsule
- Gradually develops 4 weeks after onset of acute pancreatitis

Solid Pseudopapillary Neoplasm

- Most common pancreatic neoplasm in pediatric population
- Occurs in adolescent to young adult female patients
- Large, well-defined, solid mass of pancreas with variable cystic components
- Usually benign

Pancreatic Neuroendocrine Tumor

- Rare tumor in children, may be nonfunctioning
  - Insulinoma is most common in children
- Usually hypervascular
- Associated with von Hippel-Lindau, multiple endocrine neoplasia type 1

Non-Hodgkin Lymphoma

- Typically smaller & uniformly hypodense solid lesion
- Pancreatic involvement typically occurs in setting of other nodal &/or visceral involvement
  - Adjacent adenopathy is common

PATHOLOGY

General Features

- Associated abnormalities
  - Beckwith-Wiedemann syndrome in ~ 10%
    - Patients present earlier in life
    - More likely to have cystic tumor
  - Familial adenomatous polyposis

CLINICAL ISSUES

Presentation

- Most common signs/symptoms
  - Asymptomatic, large abdominal mass
- Other signs/symptoms
  - Abdominal pain, fatigue, lethargy, weight loss, anorexia, diarrhea, & vomiting
  - Elevated α-fetoprotein in majority of patients

Demographics

- Age: Typically occurs in 1st decade of life
  - Mean age at presentation: 5 years
- Sex: 1.3-2.7x more common in males
- Ethnicity: More common in Asian population
- Epidemiology: Most common malignant pancreatic tumor of young children

Natural History & Prognosis

- Metastases in 1/3 of patients at presentation
  - Liver > lungs, lymph nodes, brain

Treatment

- Best treated with surgical resection
- Adjuvant/neoadjuvant chemotherapy is often used

SELECTED REFERENCES

1. Qiu L et al: Pancreatic masses in children and young adults: multimodality review with pathologic correlation. Radiographics. 41(6):1766-84, 2021
2. Yang Z et al: Differential diagnosis of pancreatoblastoma (PB) and solid pseudopapillary neoplasms (SPNs) in children by CT and MR imaging. Eur Radiol. 31(4):2209-27, 2020
3. Huang Y et al: Diagnosis and treatment of pancreatoblastoma in children: a retrospective study in a single pediatric center. Pediatr Surg Int. 35(11):1231-8, 2019
4. Mylonas KS et al: Solid pseudopapillary and malignant pancreatic tumors in childhood: a systematic review and evidence quality assessment. Pediatr Blood Cancer. 65(10):e27114, 2018
5. Shet NS et al: Imaging of pediatric pancreatic neoplasms with radiologic-histopathologic correlation. AJR Am J Roentgenol. 202(6):1337-48, 2014

Solid Pseudopapillary Neoplasm

KEY FACTS

TERMINOLOGY

- Synonyms: Solid-cystic pancreatic tumor, Frantz tumor, papillary cystic tumor, solid & papillary neoplasm, solid & cystic acinar cell tumor, papillary epithelial neoplasm

IMAGING

- Large, well-defined, solid mass of pancreas with variable cystic components
  - Mean size: 6-10 cm
- Central areas of ↑ T1 & heterogeneous T2 MR signal due to hemorrhage or necrosis
- Peripheral low signal due to fibrous capsule or compressed pancreatic tissue
- Higher ADC values than pancreatoblastoma
- Ca^{2+} may be present in 30-65%
- Most common site of origin in pancreas = body & tail

TOP DIFFERENTIAL DIAGNOSES

- Pancreatic pseudocyst
- Pancreatoblastoma
- Pancreatic adenocarcinoma

CLINICAL ISSUES

- Mean age of affected pediatric patients: 17 years
- 9x more common in female patients
- Accounts for 1-3% of all pancreatic tumors but 61% of pediatric pancreatic tumors
  - Most common primary pancreatic neoplasm in pediatric population
- Patients most commonly present with large epigastric mass
  - Can present with chronic abdominal pain or acute abdominal pain after cyst rupture
- Usually benign tumor
  - > 95% overall survival
  - Local spread & metastases to liver reported in 10-20%
- Treatment: Surgical resection
  - Can rarely have local recurrence after resection

(Left) *Axial CECT in an adolescent girl with a solid pseudopapillary neoplasm (SPN) shows a well-defined, hypodense, round mass ➡ arising from the pancreatic head. SPNs occur almost exclusively in women in their 2nd or 3rd decade of life.* **(Right)** *Transverse abdominal ultrasound in a young girl with an SPN shows a cystic mass ➡ arising from the tail of the pancreas ➡. SPNs are variable in their appearance with differing solid & cystic components.*

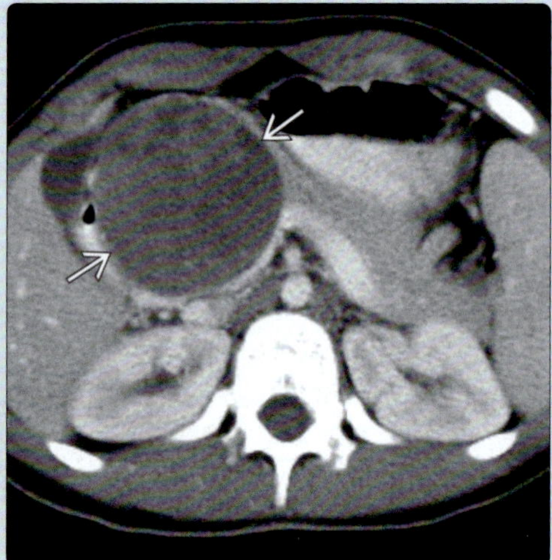

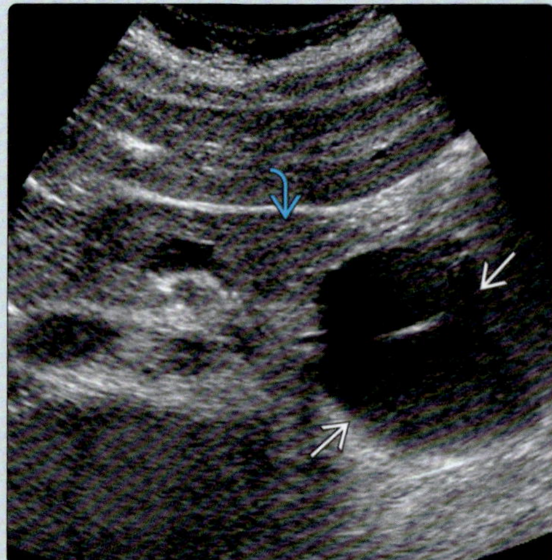

(Left) *Longitudinal ultrasound of an adolescent girl with an SPN shows a large, heterogeneous mass ➡ of the tail of the pancreas. The mass is mostly solid with a small central cystic component. There is no appreciable internal blood flow. SPNs often present as a large mass with a mean size at presentation of 6-10 cm.* **(Right)** *Axial T1 MR in a young adult woman with an SPN shows a hypointense mass ➡ arising from the tail of the pancreas. On MR, SPNs can show mildly ↑ T1 signal related to hemorrhage.*

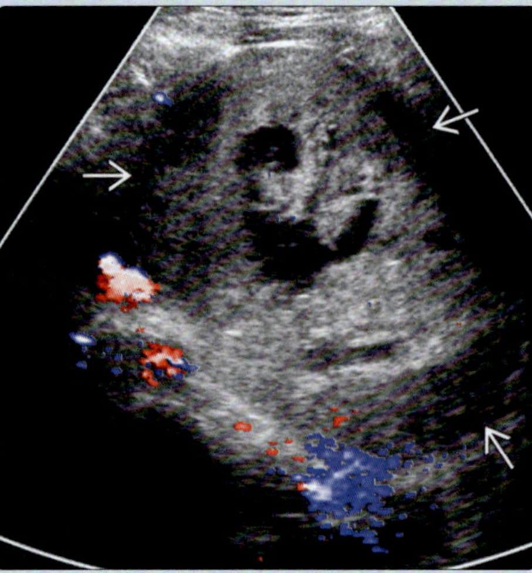

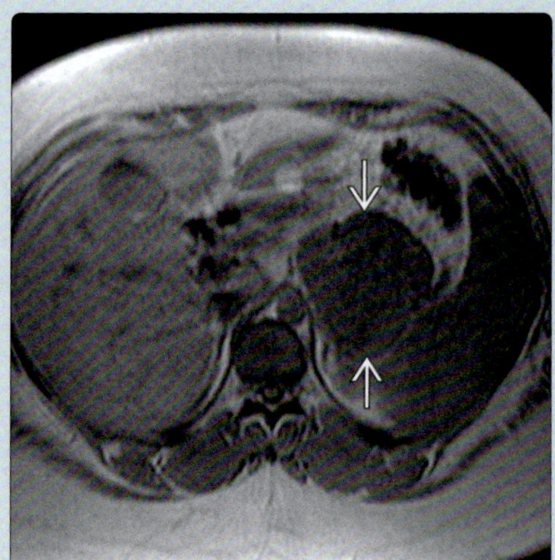

TERMINOLOGY

Definitions

- Exocrine tumor of pancreas

IMAGING

General Features

- Best diagnostic clue
  - Solid & cystic pancreatic mass in young woman
- Location
  - Most common site of origin in pancreas = body & tail
- Size
  - Mean: 6-10 cm
- Morphology
  - Well-defined pancreatic mass with variable cystic components

Radiographic Findings

- Soft tissue mass in upper abdomen displacing bowel

Ultrasonographic Findings

- Large pancreatic mass with thick capsule
- Mixed cystic & solid components
- Echogenic Ca^{2+}
- CEUS shows ↓ enhancement of tumor compared to pancreas with enhancement of fibrous capsule & intratumoral vessels

CT Findings

- Large, well-defined, solid mass of pancreas with variable cystic components
- Ca^{2+} may be present in 30-65%
  - Pattern of Ca^{2+} is variable & includes eggshell, dystrophic, or stippled
- Tumor does not enhance as much as background pancreas

MR Findings

- T1WI
  - Large, hypointense mass of pancreas
  - Central areas of ↑ signal due to hemorrhage or necrosis
  - Peripheral ↓ signal due to fibrous capsule or compressed pancreatic tissue
- T2WI
  - Heterogeneous signal due to hemorrhage & necrosis
- DWI
  - Higher ADC values than pancreatoblastoma
- T1WI C+
  - Vast majority show enhancing components

Nuclear Medicine Findings

- PET/CT: Various patterns of FDG uptake (depending on degree of cystic change)

DIFFERENTIAL DIAGNOSIS

Pancreatic Pseudocyst

- Collection of fluid, tissue, debris, pancreatic enzymes, & blood surrounded by fibrous capsule
- Gradually develops 4 weeks after onset of acute pancreatitis

Pancreatoblastoma

- Most common pancreatic malignancy in young children (mean age = 5 years)
- ~ 2x more common in male patients
- Relative to solid pseudopapillary neoplasm (SPN): Lower ADC values; higher rate of Ca^{2+}, vessel invasion, & metastases

Pancreatic Adenocarcinoma

- Extremely rare in pediatric population
- Usually originates from pancreatic duct
- Most common in head of pancreas → double duct sign of dilated biliary & pancreatic ducts

PATHOLOGY

Gross Pathologic & Surgical Features

- Pancreatic tumor with solid outer capsule
- Has solid & pseudopapillary structures, ↑ vascularization, & cellular degeneration

CLINICAL ISSUES

Presentation

- Most common signs/symptoms
  - Large epigastric mass
- Other signs/symptoms
  - Chronic abdominal pain & distention, back pain, vomiting
  - Acute abdominal pain after cyst rupture

Demographics

- Age
  - Mean age of affected pediatric patients: 17 years
- Sex
  - 9x more common in female patients
- Epidemiology
  - Accounts for 1-3% of all pancreatic tumors
  - Most common primary pediatric pancreatic neoplasm

Natural History & Prognosis

- Usually benign tumor
  - > 95% overall survival
  - Local spread & metastases to liver in 10-20%

Treatment

- Surgical resection can be curative
  - 97% 5-year survival
  - Can rarely have local recurrence after resection

SELECTED REFERENCES

1. Qiu L et al: Pancreatic masses in children and young adults: multimodality review with pathologic correlation. Radiographics. 41(6):1766-84, 2021
2. Yang Z et al: Differential diagnosis of pancreatoblastoma (PB) and solid pseudopapillary neoplasms (SPNs) in children by CT and MR imaging. Eur Radiol. 31(4):2209-17, 2020
3. Waters AM et al: Comparison of pediatric and adult solid pseudopapillary neoplasms of the pancreas. J Surg Res. 242:312-7, 2019
4. Xu M et al: Application of contrast-enhanced ultrasound in the diagnosis of solid pseudopapillary tumors of the pancreas: imaging findings compared with contrast-enhanced computed tomography. J Ultrasound Med. 38(12):3247-55, 2019
5. Mylonas KS et al: Solid pseudopapillary and malignant pancreatic tumors in childhood: a systematic review and evidence quality assessment. Pediatr Blood Cancer. 65(10):e27114, 2018

Pancreas Divisum

KEY FACTS

TERMINOLOGY

- Incomplete fusion of dorsal & ventral pancreatic ducts with persistence of 2 separate ductal systems
- 2 main types
  - Complete divisum: No connection between dorsal & ventral pancreatic ducts
  - Incomplete divisum: Rudimentary connection between dorsal & ventral pancreatic ducts

IMAGING

- Separate pancreatic ducts are seen draining dorsal & ventral pancreas on CECT, MRCP, or ERCP
  - Dorsal duct drains majority of pancreas through minor papilla
  - Short ventral duct of Wirsung drains to major papilla
    - Ventral duct does not cross midline
- Secretin may be used to ↑ diameter of pancreatic ducts

PATHOLOGY

- Dorsal anlage forms pancreatic body & tail
- Ventral anlage forms head of pancreas & uncinate process
- When dorsal & ventral ducts fail to fuse, dorsal duct drains majority of pancreas through minor papilla
  - Superior & anterior to major papilla, which drains duct of Wirsung & common bile duct
- Proposed etiology for pancreatitis: Small diameter of minor papilla causes relative obstruction to drainage of large volume from pancreatic body & tail

CLINICAL ISSUES

- Most common congenital variant of pancreatic ductal development (5-10% of general population)
- Most patients are asymptomatic
  - Children uncommonly present with pancreatitis
  - Pancreatitis is more common from 30-50 years of age
- Most symptomatic patients respond to sphincterotomy of minor papilla

(Left) *Coronal MIP MRCP shows pancreas divisum. The pancreatic duct ⇨ drains via the minor papilla ⇨, while the common bile duct ⇨ drains via the major papilla at the sphincter of Oddi ⇨.* **(Right)** *Coronal T2 MRCP shows pancreas divisum. The common bile duct ⇨ is dilated throughout its course. Its insertion at the sphincter of Oddi is not shown. The pancreatic duct ⇨ crosses the common bile duct & inserts at the minor papilla, superior to the common duct insertion.*

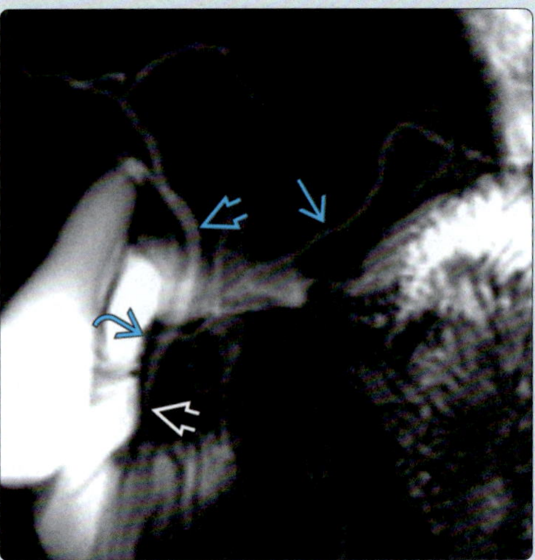

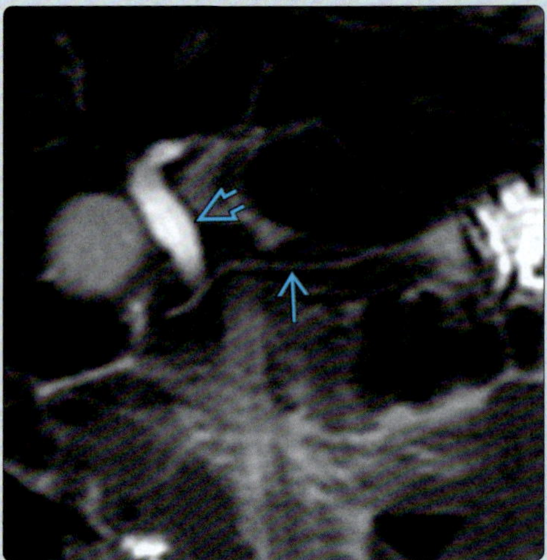

(Left) *Coronal T2 MRCP in a patient with acute-on-chronic pancreatitis & pancreas divisum shows an irregular pancreatic duct ⇨ (with areas of dilation & narrowing) that is draining to the minor papilla. There is mild peripancreatic edema ⇨.* **(Right)** *Coronal T2 MRCP in the same patient shows a focal outpouching ⇨ at the distal common bile duct. The pancreatic duct & common bile duct drain separately at the minor & major papilla, respectively, consistent with pancreas divisum.*

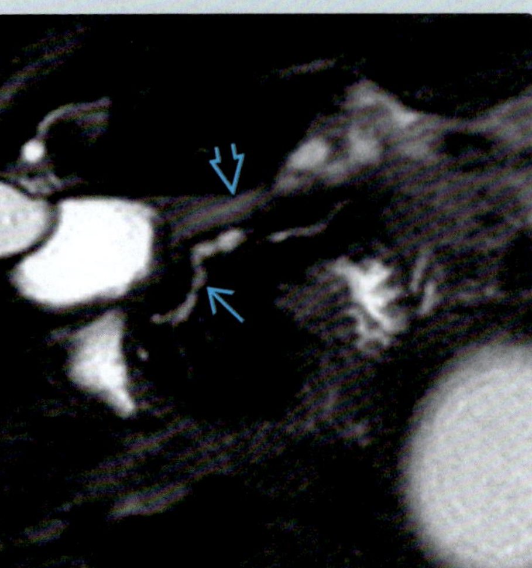

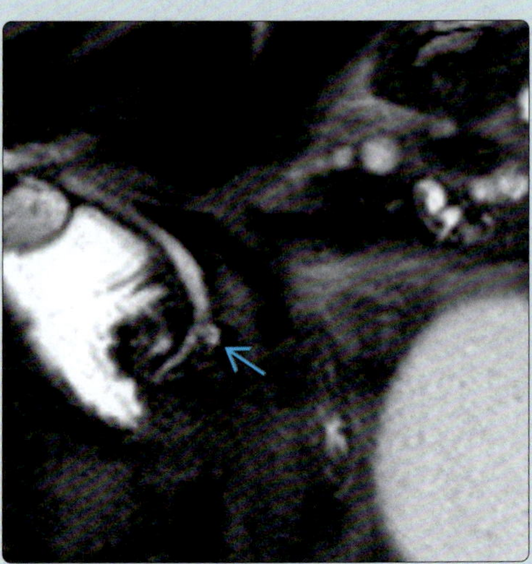

TERMINOLOGY

Definitions

- Failed fusion of dorsal & ventral pancreatic ducts with persistence of 2 separate ductal systems
- 2 main types
  - Complete divisum: No connection between dorsal & ventral pancreatic ducts
  - Incomplete divisum: Rudimentary connection between dorsal & ventral pancreatic ducts

IMAGING

General Features

- Best diagnostic clue
  - Separate pancreatic ducts draining dorsal & ventral pancreas
- Location
  - Duct of Santorini (dorsal duct) drains to minor papilla, superior & anterior to major papilla
  - Duct of Wirsung (ventral duct) joins common bile duct & drains at major papilla

CT Findings

- CECT
  - Pancreatic ducts are usually not dilated & not visible
  - May see 2 discrete pancreatic moieties separated by fatty cleft

MR Findings

- MRCP
  - Separate T2-hyperintense pancreatic ducts draining dorsal & ventral pancreas
    - Secretin may be used to ↑ diameter & visibility of pancreatic ducts

Ultrasonographic Findings

- Grayscale ultrasound
  - 2 separate pancreatic ducts do not communicate
- Endoscopic ultrasound
  - No continuity of pancreatic duct in uncinate process with duct in body & tail

Nonvascular Interventions

- ERCP
  - Cannulation of major papilla reveals short ventral duct of Wirsung
    - Ventral duct ranges from 1-4 cm in length
    - Ventral duct does not cross midline
  - Cannulation of minor papilla can be difficult
    - Located superior & anterior to major papilla

Imaging Recommendations

- Best imaging tool
  - ERCP or MRCP: Defines pancreatic ductal anatomy

DIFFERENTIAL DIAGNOSIS

Annular Pancreas

- Result of incomplete separation of dorsal & ventral pancreatic anlage
- Pancreatic tissue & duct encircle 2nd portion of duodenum
- Can cause neonatal bowel obstruction

Dorsal Agenesis of Pancreas

- Absence of pancreatic body or tail
- ERCP appearance of pancreatic duct is identical to pancreas divisum
- Associated with polysplenia

PATHOLOGY

General Features

- Etiology
  - Dorsal & ventral pancreatic anlagen normally rotate & fuse during 6th-8th weeks of fetal development
    - Ventral anlage forms head of pancreas & uncinate process
    - Dorsal anlage forms pancreatic body & tail
  - When 2 ducts fail to fuse, dorsal duct remains & drains majority of pancreas through minor papilla
  - Proposed etiology for pancreatitis
    - Small diameter of minor papilla causes relative obstruction to drainage of large volume from pancreatic body & tail
    - Thought to require 2nd hit, ↑ likelihood that pancreas divisum leads to pancreatitis
      - Most common association: Mutation in cystic fibrosis transmembrane conductance regulator (CFTR)

CLINICAL ISSUES

Presentation

- Most common signs/symptoms
  - Most patients are asymptomatic
  - Associated with acute recurrent pancreatitis &/or chronic pancreatitis

Demographics

- Age
  - Congenital anomaly that can present at any age
    - If symptomatic, patients may have recurrent abdominal pain & vomiting
    - Mean age of initial presentation in children: 6 years
- Epidemiology
  - Most common congenital variant of pancreatic ductal development
  - Occurs in 5-14% of general population

Treatment

- Most symptomatic patients respond to sphincterotomy of minor papilla

DIAGNOSTIC CHECKLIST

Image Interpretation Pearls

- Short ventral pancreatic duct does not communicate with long dorsal duct

SELECTED REFERENCES

1. Trout AT et al: Current state of imaging of pediatric pancreatitis: AJR expert panel narrative review. AJR Am J Roentgenol. 217(2):265-77, 2021
2. Li Y et al: Secretin improves visualization of nondilated pancreatic ducts in children undergoing MRCP. AJR Am J Roentgenol. 214(4):917-22, 2020
3. Wang DB et al: Pancreatitis in patients with pancreas divisum: imaging features at MRI and MRCP. World J Gastroenterol. 19(30):4907-16, 2013

KEY FACTS

TERMINOLOGY

- Pancreaticobiliary maljunction (PBM): Congenital malformation in which pancreatic duct & common bile duct (CBD) join outside of duodenal wall
- 2 types of PBM
  - PBM with congenital biliary dilation (choledochal cyst)
    - More likely to present with symptoms in childhood
  - PBM without biliary dilation
    - Often asymptomatic until cancer develops in adulthood

IMAGING

- Modalities
  - Ultrasound screening of patients with clinical/laboratory manifestations of hepatobiliary &/or pancreatic disease
  - MRCP for detailed ductal evaluation
  - ERCP to confirm diagnosis, particularly in equivocal cases
- Findings
  - Abnormal union of pancreatic duct & CBD outside of duodenal wall
  - ± visualization of fluid-filled long common channel extending from high confluence to duodenum
  - ± type I or type IV choledochal cyst
  - Associated abnormalities: Gallstones, gallbladder wall thickening, sequelae of pancreatitis

TOP DIFFERENTIAL DIAGNOSES

- Pancreas divisum
- Choledochal cyst

PATHOLOGY

- 200x ↑ risk of biliary cancer (usually in later adulthood)
  - Gallbladder is most common site

CLINICAL ISSUES

- Treated with cholecystectomy & resection of extrahepatic bile duct due to high risk of malignancy

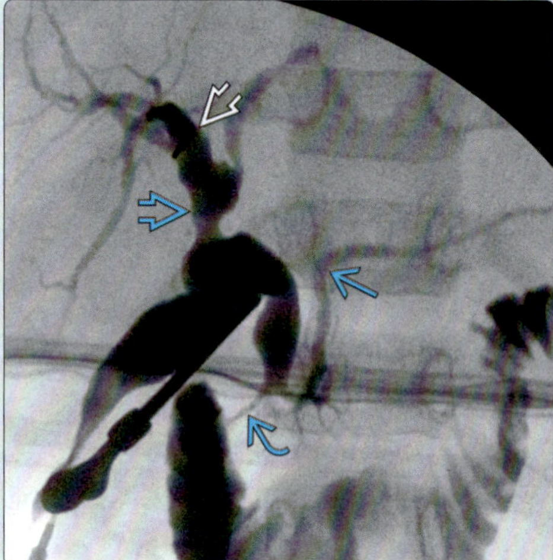

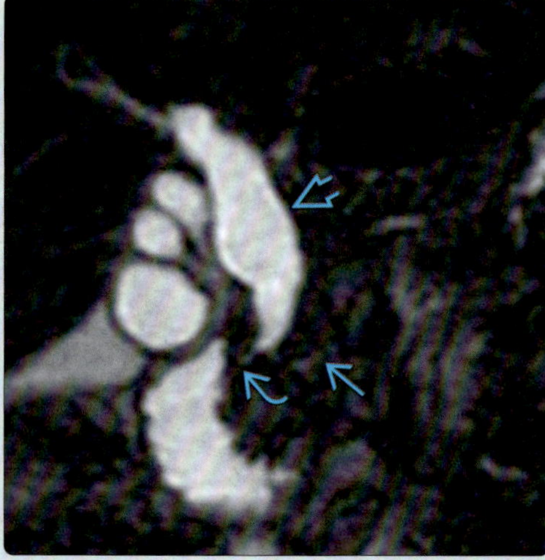

(Left) *Direct cholangiogram shows dilation & irregularity of the common bile duct ➡ & central intrahepatic bile ducts ➡, consistent with a type IV choledochal cyst. The pancreatic duct ➡ joins the common bile duct in an anomalous position, creating a long common channel ➡.* **(Right)** *Coronal MRCP in the same patient shows dilation of the common bile duct ➡. The pancreatic duct ➡ is small & joins the common bile duct in an anomalous location, creating a long common channel ➡.*

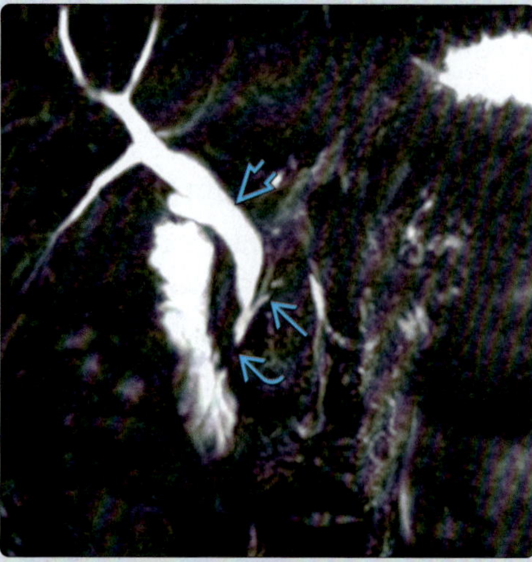

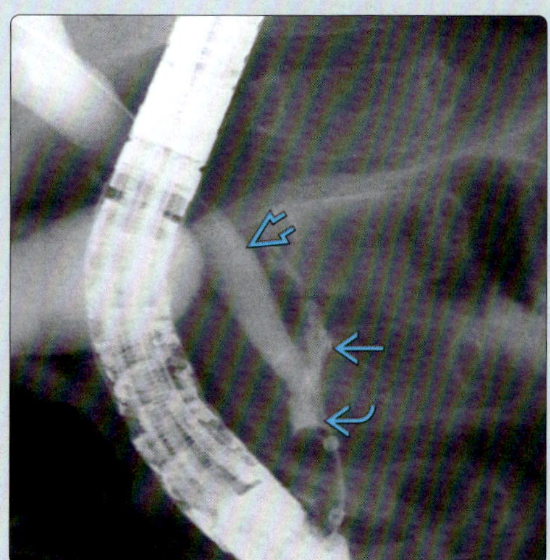

(Left) *Coronal MRCP in a patient with a choledochal cyst shows fusiform dilation of the common bile duct ➡. The pancreatic duct ➡ joins the common bile duct in an anomalous location, creating a long common channel ➡ that measured 1.8 cm in length.* **(Right)** *ERCP in the same patient shows fusiform dilation of the common bile duct ➡ + an abnormal junction with the pancreatic duct ➡, creating a long common channel ➡.*

TERMINOLOGY

Synonyms

- Long common channel

Definitions

- Pancreaticobiliary maljunction (PBM): Congenital malformation where pancreatic duct & common bile duct (CBD) join outside of duodenal wall
  - Long common channel allows pancreatobiliary & biliopancreatic reflux
  - Chronic pancreatobiliary reflux leads to high risk of gallbladder & biliary cancer
  - Biliopancreatic reflux causes acute pancreatitis
- 2 types of PBM
  - PBM with congenital biliary dilation
  - PBM without congenital biliary dilation
- Congenital biliary dilation
  - Previously referred to as type I or IVa choledochal cyst
  - Requires enlarged diameter of CBD + PBM
  - Definition for enlarged CBD depends on age

IMAGING

General Features

- Best diagnostic clue
  - Long common channel extending from abnormally high confluence of pancreatic duct & CBD to duodenum
    - Duct union lies outside of duodenal wall

Ultrasonographic Findings

- Transabdominal ultrasound may identify nonspecific gallbladder wall thickening, cholelithiasis, dilated CBD
- Endoscopic ultrasound can confirm extraduodenal union of pancreaticobiliary junction

MR Findings

- MRCP
  - Long, fluid-filled channel distal to high confluence of pancreatic duct & CBD
  - Type I or type IVa choledochal cyst may be present
  - Secretin can help to improve visualization of pancreatic duct & pancreatobiliary reflux
  - Associated findings: Gallstones, sequelae of pancreatitis

Other Modality Findings

- Endoscopic retrograde cholangiopancreatography (ERCP)
  - Only method able to evaluate location & effect of sphincter of Oddi

Imaging Recommendations

- Best imaging tool
  - Ultrasound screening of patients with clinical/laboratory manifestations of hepatobiliary &/or pancreatic disease
  - MRCP for detailed ductal evaluation
  - ERCP to confirm diagnosis, particularly in equivocal cases

DIFFERENTIAL DIAGNOSIS

Pancreas Divisum

- Incomplete fusion of dorsal & ventral pancreatic ducts with persistence of 2 separate draining ductal systems

Choledochal Cyst

- Spectrum of malformations of extrahepatic & intrahepatic bile ducts
  - Classified via system developed by Todani
  - Types I & IVa are termed congenital biliary dilation
- Associated with PBM

PATHOLOGY

Staging, Grading, & Classification

- 2 types of PBM
  - PBM with congenital biliary dilation
  - PBM without biliary dilation

CLINICAL ISSUES

Presentation

- Most common signs/symptoms
  - PBM with congenital biliary dilation
    - Presents in childhood
    - Symptoms: Pain, vomiting, jaundice, & fever
  - PBM without biliary dilation
    - Presents in adulthood
    - Most patients are asymptomatic until cancer develops
    - Up to 10% of patients present with cholangitis
- Other signs/symptoms
  - Manifestations of pancreatitis or cholelithiasis

Demographics

- More common in patients from Japan
- Congenital biliary dilation is 3x more common in female patients

Natural History & Prognosis

- Pancreatic enzymes induce chronic inflammation of biliary tree → proliferation of biliary epithelium → induction of carcinogenesis
  - 200x ↑ risk of biliary cancer
    - Gallbladder cancer is most common
  - Cancer is more common in PBM patients without biliary dilation compared to those with dilation (42.4% vs. 21.6%)
  - Cancers typically occur in 6th or 7th decade of life, 15-20 years younger than those without PBM
  - Cancer type in PBM with congenital biliary dilation: Gallbladder (62%) & bile duct (32%)
  - Cancer type in PBM without congenital biliary dilation: Gallbladder (88%) & bile duct (7%)

Treatment

- Cholecystectomy & resection of extrahepatic bile duct is recommended due to high risk of malignancy

SELECTED REFERENCES

1. Ono A et al: Imaging of pancreaticobiliary maljunction. Radiographics. 40(2):378-92, 2020
2. Kamisawa T et al: Pancreaticobiliary maljunction: markedly high risk for biliary cancer. Digestion. 99(2):123-5, 2019
3. Kamisawa T et al: Pancreaticobiliary maljunction and congenital biliary dilatation. Lancet Gastroenterol Hepatol. 2(8):610-8, 2017
4. Hamada Y et al: Diagnostic criteria for congenital biliary dilatation 2015. J Hepatobiliary Pancreat Sci. 23(6):342-6, 2016

KEY FACTS

TERMINOLOGY

- Congenital anomaly with ring of pancreatic tissue surrounding 2nd portion of duodenum (D2); results in variable degrees of duodenal obstruction

IMAGING

- Radiograph: ± newborn "double bubble" of dilated stomach & 1st portion of duodenum (D1)
  - Distal bowel gas is present
- Upper GI: Circumferential narrowing of D2
- MRCP or ERCP: Split pancreatic duct encircling D2
- MR, CT, or ultrasound: Pancreatic tissue surrounding D2
  - Water is useful as oral contrast for MR, CT, & ultrasound
- Diagnosis may be suggested on prenatal imaging

TOP DIFFERENTIAL DIAGNOSES

- Duodenal atresia
- Duodenal web
- Malrotation with midgut volvulus

PATHOLOGY

- Associations include
  - Congenital heart disease, malrotation, Meckel diverticulum, pancreas divisum, duodenal web, intestinal atresia, duplicated renal collecting system
  - Down syndrome

CLINICAL ISSUES

- 3 main presentations
  - Newborns: Signs of proximal duodenal obstruction either on prenatal ultrasound or after birth
    - Postnatal manifestations include vomiting (may be bilious), feeding intolerance, abdominal distention
  - Adults: Abdominal pain, ulcers, pancreatitis
  - Incidental imaging finding
- 51.5% diagnosed in childhood (77% of those are diagnosed by 2 days of life)
- Treatment of duodenal obstruction: Surgical duodenal bypass

(Left) *AP radiograph in a newborn with annular pancreas shows a "double bubble" appearance with a dilated air-filled stomach ➡ & a bulbous proximal duodenum ➡. However, small amounts of distal bowel gas ➡ are present, suggesting a partial obstruction rather than duodenal atresia.* **(Right)** *ERCP in a teenager shows a dilated & irregular main pancreatic duct ➡ secondary to recurrent pancreatitis. There are 2 ducts ➡ in the pancreatic head encircling the contrast in the 2nd duodenum ➡.*

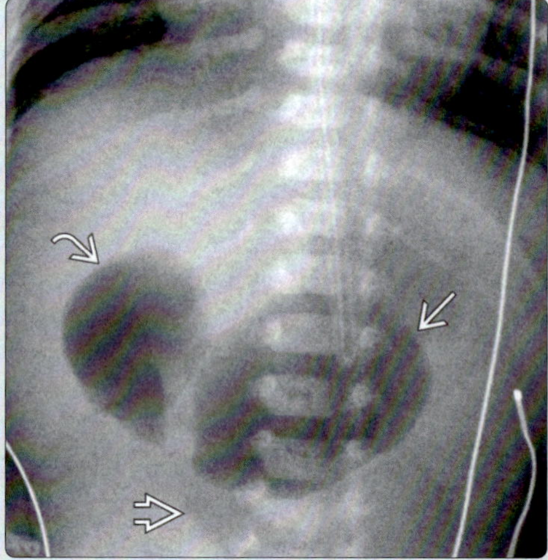

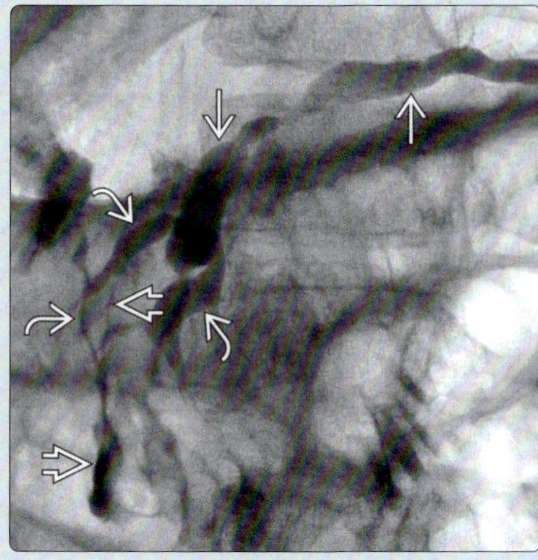

(Left) *Axial T1 FS MR shows the hypointense 2nd duodenum ➡ encircled by the hyperintense pancreatic head ➡, consistent with annular pancreas.* **(Right)** *Frontal image from an upper GI performed in the same patient shows focal moderate narrowing ➡ of the 2nd duodenum at the site of the annular pancreas. There is no significant dilation of the proximal duodenum in this case.*

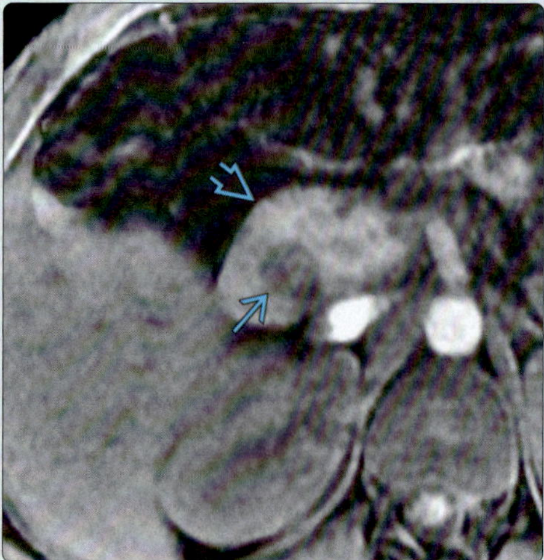

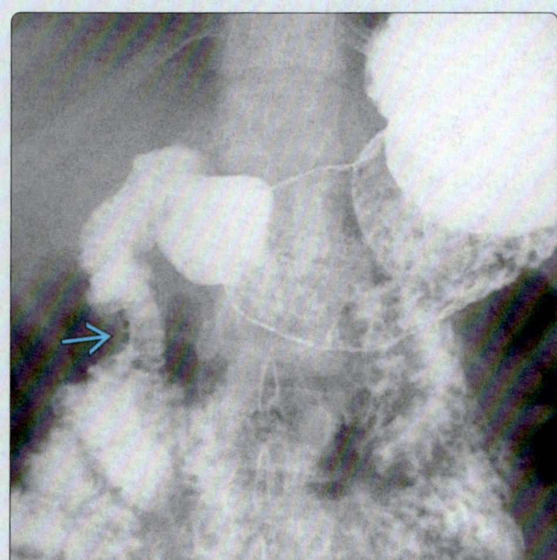

TERMINOLOGY

Definitions

- Ring of pancreatic tissue encircling 2nd portion of duodenum (D2)

IMAGING

General Features

- Best diagnostic clue
  - "Double bubble" dilation of stomach & 1st portion of duodenum (D1) on early postnatal imaging in presence of distal bowel gas
    - D1 is enlarged due to longstanding obstruction
  - Ring of pancreatic tissue encircling & narrowing D2 on cross-sectional imaging at any age

Radiographic Findings

- Newborn with partial duodenal obstruction
  - Dilated stomach & D1
  - Distal bowel gas is present (but may be diminished)

Fluoroscopic Findings

- Upper GI
  - Incomplete proximal duodenal obstruction
    - Dilation & delayed emptying of stomach + D1
  - Circumferential narrowing of D2
  - Relatively small-caliber duodenum beyond constriction
- ERCP
  - Split distal pancreatic duct encircling D2

CT Findings

- CECT
  - Pancreatic head tissue encircles D2
    - Remainder of pancreas is normal in appearance (unless patient has acute or chronic pancreatitis)

MR Findings

- Pancreatic head tissue encircles D2
  - T1 ± FS: Hypointense bowel contents pass through relatively hyperintense pancreas
  - T2 ± FS: Hyperintense bowel contents pass through relatively hypointense pancreas
- MRCP: Split distal pancreatic duct encircles D2

Ultrasonographic Findings

- Postnatal ultrasound
  - Fluid-filled proximal duodenum up to pancreatic head
  - Hyperechoic band of pancreatic tissue encircling or partially encircling duodenum at site of obstruction

Imaging Recommendations

- Protocol advice
  - Water is useful as oral contrast for MR, CT, & ultrasound
  - T1 FS MR increases conspicuity of pancreatic tissue

DIFFERENTIAL DIAGNOSIS

Duodenal Atresia

- Congenital duodenal obstruction at D2
- Radiograph (in absence of gastric decompression) shows classic large "double bubble" without distal bowel gas
- Upper GI is not necessary

Duodenal Web

- Cause of partial duodenal obstruction
- Symptoms depend on aperture of web
- ± "double bubble" appearance; distal bowel gas is present
- ± visualization of thin membrane in duodenal lumen
  - May have "windsock" configuration with distal stretching of web beyond origin at proximal duodenal wall

Malrotation With Midgut Volvulus

- Typically presents with bilious emesis in neonates/infants
- Radiograph may show distended stomach & proximal duodenum with normal to ↓ distal bowel gas
  - In acute midgut volvulus, proximal duodenum is not as bulbous as with longstanding in utero obstructions
- Upper GI shows abnormal abrupt tapering/"beaking" of distal D2/D3 with corkscrew configuration of bowel beyond taper
- Ultrasound shows abnormal anterior position of D3 with clockwise "whirlpool" twisting of bowel & mesentery
- Requires emergent surgery to prevent bowel infarction

PATHOLOGY

Associated Anomalies

- Congenital heart disease, malrotation, Meckel diverticulum, pancreas divisum, duodenal web, intestinal atresia, duplicated renal collecting system

CLINICAL ISSUES

Presentation

- Most common signs/symptoms
  - 3 main presentations
    - Newborn: High-grade duodenal obstruction either on prenatal ultrasound or after birth
      - Signs after birth include emesis (may be bilious), feeding intolerance, abdominal distention
    - Older child/adult: Abdominal pain, pancreatitis, ulcers
    - Incidental imaging finding

Demographics

- Age
  - 51.5% are diagnosed in childhood
    - 77% of children are diagnosed by 2 days of life
  - 48.5% are diagnosed in adults
- Epidemiology
  - Present in 3 of 20,000 autopsies
  - 140 cases per 100,000 patients with Down syndrome

Treatment

- Surgical duodenal bypass

SELECTED REFERENCES

1. Alkhayyat M et al: The epidemiology of annular pancreas in the United States: a population-based Study. J Clin Gastroenterol. ePub, 2021
2. Gromski MA et al: Annular pancreas: endoscopic and pancreatographic findings from a tertiary referral ERCP center. Gastrointest Endosc. 89(2):322-8, 2019
3. Yang B et al: Diagnostic value of the acute angle between the prestenotic and poststenotic duodenum in neonatal annular pancreas. Eur Radiol. 29(6):2902-9, 2019
4. Li B et al: Laparoscopic diagnosis and treatment of neonates with duodenal obstruction associated with an annular pancreas: report of 11 cases. Surg Today. 45(1):17-21, 2015

KEY FACTS

TERMINOLOGY

- Acute pancreatitis (AP): Acute inflammation of pancreas with variable involvement of local tissues/remote organs
- 2 of 3 features required for diagnosis: Abdominal pain consistent with disease, 3x rise in serum amylase or lipase, or imaging findings consistent with AP
- 2 types of AP: Interstitial edematous vs. necrotizing
- Fluid collections
  - Acute peripancreatic fluid collection: Fluid collection associated with interstitial edematous pancreatitis during first 4 weeks
  - Pancreatic pseudocyst: Fluid collection associated with interstitial edematous pancreatitis after first 4 weeks
  - Acute necrotic collection: Collection containing fluid & necrotic material during first 4 weeks
  - Walled-off necrosis: Collection containing fluid & necrotic material after first 4 weeks
- Chronic pancreatitis (CP): Relapsing or continuing inflammation with destruction of parenchyma & ducts

IMAGING

- Interstitial edematous pancreatitis: Gland enlargement with edema & homogeneous (± mildly ↓) enhancement
  - Acute peripancreatic fluid collection: Nonencapsulated collections of variable size & shape
  - Pancreatic pseudocyst: Encapsulated cystic lesion with no internal solid component, > 4 weeks from onset
- Necrotizing pancreatitis: Heterogeneous enhancement (moderately to severely ↓)
  - Acute necrotic collection: Nonencapsulated collection with heterogeneous contents
  - Walled-off necrosis: Well-circumscribed cavity containing necrotic tissue, > 4 weeks from onset
- CP: Atrophic pancreas with dilated duct & pancreatic Ca^{2+}

CLINICAL ISSUES

- Epigastric abdominal pain; ↑ amylase & lipase > 3x normal
- Therapy: Fluid resuscitation, early enteral nutrition, pain management

(Left) *Axial CECT in an adolescent with abdominal pain demonstrates acute interstitial edematous pancreatitis. Note the normal enhancement of the pancreatic parenchyma despite mild enlargement, unsharp margins, & surrounding edema ➡.* **(Right)** *Axial CECT in an adolescent with acute necrotizing pancreatitis shows a lack of enhancement ➡ of the pancreatic body & tail. There is free fluid throughout the abdomen with small amounts collecting in the parabolic gutters ➡.*

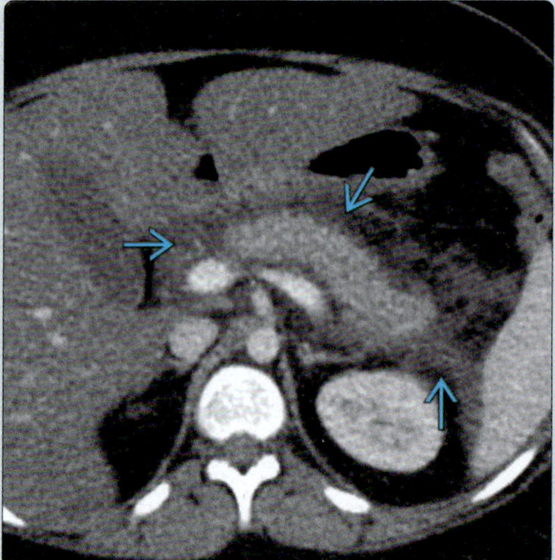

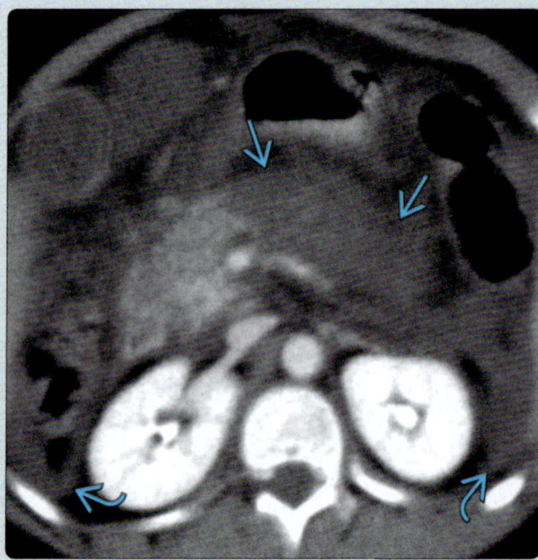

(Left) *Axial CECT in the same patient obtained 2 weeks after the prior image shows a continued lack of enhancement ➡ of the pancreatic body & tail. There is an acute necrotic collection ➡ in the lesser sac posterior to the stomach ➡.* **(Right)** *Axial CECT obtained 6 weeks after the initial imaging study in the same patient shows a conglomerate collection of walled-off necrosis ➡ in the pancreatic body & tail.*

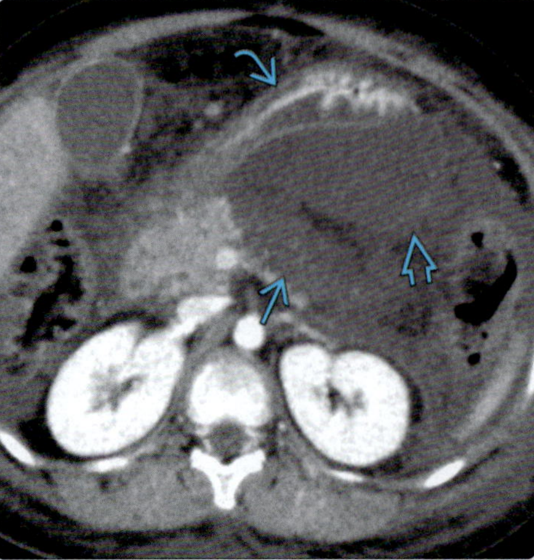

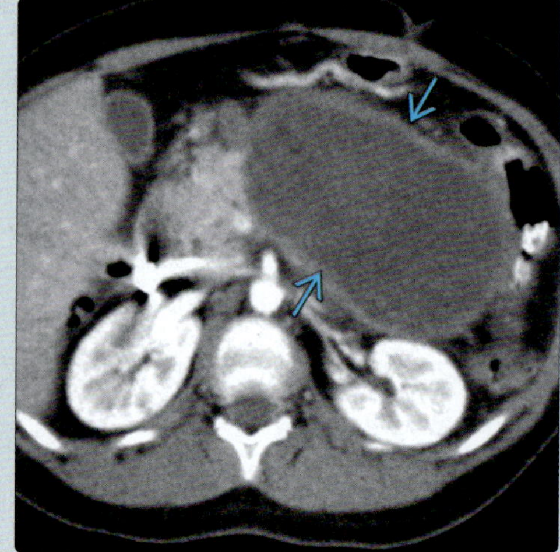

TERMINOLOGY

Definitions

- Acute pancreatitis (AP): Acute inflammation of pancreas with variable involvement of local/regional tissues
  - 2 of 3 features are required for diagnosis
    - Abdominal pain consistent with disease
    - Rise in serum amylase or lipase ≥ 3x normal
    - Imaging findings consistent with AP
  - 2 types of AP
    - Interstitial edematous pancreatitis
    - Necrotizing pancreatitis
- Acute recurrent pancreatitis (ARP): ≥ 2 distinct episodes of AP with complete resolution of pain for ≥ 1 month or normalization of enzyme levels
- Chronic pancreatitis (CP): Requires 1 or more of following clinical features or imaging findings of chronic pancreas damage
  - Abdominal pain consistent with pancreatic origin
  - Exocrine pancreatic insufficiency
  - Endocrine pancreatic insufficiency
- Fluid collections
  - Acute peripancreatic fluid collection: Fluid collection associated with interstitial edematous pancreatitis during first 4 weeks
  - Pancreatic pseudocyst: Fluid collection associated with interstitial edematous pancreatitis after first 4 weeks
  - Acute necrotic collection: Collection containing fluid & necrotic material during first 4 weeks
  - Walled-off necrosis: Collection containing fluid & necrotic material after first 4 weeks

IMAGING

General Features

- Best diagnostic clue
  - AP: Edematous pancreas & peripancreatic inflammation
    - Interstitial edematous pancreatitis: Gland enlargement, homogeneous enhancement (which may be mildly ↓ diffusely), & edema
      - Acute peripancreatic fluid collection: Nonencapsulated collections of variable size & shape
      - Pancreatic pseudocyst: Encapsulated cystic lesion with no internal solid component > 4 weeks from onset
    - Necrotizing pancreatitis: Gland enlargement, heterogeneous enhancement (with foci of moderately to severely ↓ enhancement), & edema
      - Acute necrotic collection: Nonencapsulated collection, may be single or multiple, with heterogeneous contents
      - Walled-off necrosis: Well-circumscribed cavity containing necrotic tissue, often involving pancreatic parenchyma, > 4 weeks from onset
    - Complications: Fluid collections, infection, disconnected duct, pseudoaneurysm of splenic artery, splenic vein thrombosis
  - CP: Pancreatic Ca^{2+}, glandular atrophy, duct irregularity or enlargement
- Location
  - Acute peripancreatic fluid collection/pseudocyst: Adjacent to pancreas in lesser sac or anterior pararenal space
  - Acute necrotic collection/walled-off necrosis: Peripancreatic, pancreatic, or both
- Size
  - AP: Focal or diffuse enlargement of pancreas
  - CP: Atrophy of pancreas, enlargement of pancreatic duct

Ultrasonographic Findings

- AP: Enlarged, hypoechoic, heterogeneous pancreas
  - Look for gallstones, biliary dilation, fluid collection
- CP: Atrophic pancreas with echogenic areas of Ca^{2+} & dilated pancreatic duct

CT Findings

- Interstitial edematous pancreatitis
  - Focal or diffuse pancreatic enlargement
  - Homogeneous enhancement, often mildly ↓, of edematous pancreatic parenchyma
  - ± surrounding fat inflammation
  - Acute peripancreatic fluid collection: Homogeneous fluid collection without defined capsule
  - Pancreatic pseudocyst: Fluid density cyst with well-defined capsule > 4 weeks from onset
- Necrotizing pancreatitis
  - Can affect pancreas, peripancreatic tissue, or both
  - Area of moderately to severely ↓ enhancement within pancreas or peripancreatic mesentery
  - Acute necrotic collection: Irregular hyperdense material within hypodense fluid collection
  - Walled-off necrosis: Fluid density collection in area of prior necrosis > 4 weeks from onset
    - Other findings: Paracolic or retrocolic extension, irregular border, fat attenuation debris, thick septations, pancreatic deformity
- CP
  - Atrophic pancreas
  - Dilation of pancreatic duct
  - Coarse Ca^{2+} in pancreas

MR Findings

- Interstitial edematous pancreatitis
  - T1 or T2 FS: Peripancreatic fat stranding
  - T2: Enlarged, hyperintense pancreas
    - Autoimmune pancreatitis may show striking thickening & hypointense "capsule" or rim
      - Diffuse sausage-like thickening vs. focal & mass-like
  - Diffuse enhancement
  - Acute peripancreatic fluid collection: Fluid signal on T1 & T2
  - Pancreatic pseudocyst: Fluid signal intensity on T1 or T2 with dependent debris
- Necrotizing pancreatitis
  - Portions of pancreas are hyperintense on T1, hypointense on T2, & do not enhance after contrast
  - Acute necrotic collection
    - Nonencapsulated
    - T2 hypointense material layering within hyperintense fluid
  - Walled-off necrosis: Collection with visible capsule in area of prior necrosis, disconnected duct

- MRCP
  - ARP: Look for congenital anomalies
    - Pancreas divisum
    - Pancreatobiliary maljunction
  - CP: Look for sequelae of pancreatitis
    - Pancreatic duct strictures
    - Dilated pancreatic duct
    - ↓ exocrine response to secretin administration

DIFFERENTIAL DIAGNOSIS

Pancreatic Trauma

- Can cause pancreatitis
- More common in children due to relative size of pancreas in abdomen
- Classic mechanisms include handlebar injury & nonaccidental trauma
- May cause pancreatic transection ± duct injury

Pancreatic Lymphoma

- Uncommon site of involvement
- Enlargement of pancreas can be focal or diffuse
- Hypoechoic/hypoenhancing masses + adjacent adenopathy

Shock Pancreas

- Enlarged, hyperenhancing pancreas with hypoenhancing septa in setting of hypovolemic shock
- Associated with other findings of shock
- Resolves following fluid resuscitation

Cystic Fibrosis

- Cause of CP
- Usually associated with diffuse fatty infiltration of pancreas
  - ± atrophy with speckled Ca^{2+}

PATHOLOGY

General Features

- Etiology
  - AP: Caused by acinar cell injury & premature activation of trypsinogen to trypsin in pancreas
    - Biliary obstruction: Gallstones
    - Anatomic: Pancreas divisum, pancreatobiliary maljunction, choledochal cyst, annular pancreas
    - Systemic illness: Sepsis, shock, hemolytic uremic syndrome, systemic lupus erythematosus
    - Drugs: L-asparaginase, valproic acid, azathioprine, mercaptopurine, mesalamine
    - Trauma: Motor vehicle accident, handlebar injury, nonaccidental trauma
    - Metabolic disorders: Cystic fibrosis, hyperlipidemia, hyperparathyroidism
    - Genetic/hereditary
    - Autoimmune
    - Idiopathic (up to 20%)
  - CP: Pancreatic injury followed by sustained immune activation where fibrosis dominates
    - Cystic fibrosis: Most common cause of CP
    - Hereditary pancreatitis: Autosomal dominant disorder associated with recurrent bouts of pancreatitis
    - Anatomic causes: Pancreas divisum, annular pancreas, choledochal cyst
- Genetics
  - Multiple genetic mutations are associated with ARP/CP
    - *SPINK1*, *CFTR*, *CTRC*, *PRSS1*, & *PRSS2*

CLINICAL ISSUES

Presentation

- Most common signs/symptoms
  - Epigastric abdominal pain
  - Elevated amylase & lipase to level > 3x normal
- Other signs/symptoms
  - Vomiting, anorexia, & nausea
  - Patient appears ill, irritable, & quiet
  - Physical exam findings: Tachycardia, fever, hypotension, abdominal signs

Demographics

- Epidemiology
  - Increasing in incidence over last decade
    - AP: 1 in 10:1000; CP: 2 in 100,000
  - ~ 50% of patients with hereditary pancreatitis develop CP
  - Mortality rate from AP: 2-10%

Natural History & Prognosis

- Pseudocyst is most common complication of AP
- With CP, pain may be transient & not severe
  - End-stage disease leads to endocrine & exocrine dysfunction

Treatment

- Treatment has evolved over past decade
- Current mainstays of therapy: Fluid resuscitation, early enteral nutrition, & pain management
- Fluid collections may require drainage
- Various surgical procedures in setting of chronic pain, including total pancreatectomy with islet autotransplantation (TPIAT)

SELECTED REFERENCES

1. Murati MA et al: Magnetic resonance imaging glossary of findings of pediatric pancreatitis and the revised Atlanta classification. Pediatr Radiol. ePub, 2021
2. Trout AT et al: NASPGHAN and the Society for Pediatric Radiology joint position paper on noninvasive imaging of pediatric pancreatitis: literature summary and recommendations. J Pediatr Gastroenterol Nutr. 72(1):151-67, 2021
3. Trout AT et al: Noninvasive imaging of pediatric pancreatitis: joint recommendations from the NASPGHAN and the Society for Pediatric Radiology. Pediatr Radiol. 51(1):8-10, 2021
4. Trout AT et al: Current state of imaging of pediatric pancreatitis: AJR expert panel narrative review. AJR Am J Roentgenol. 217(2):265-77, 2021
5. Grover AS et al: Updates in pediatric pancreatology: proceedings of the NASPGHAN Frontiers in Pediatric Pancreatology Symposium. J Pediatr Gastroenterol Nutr. 68(2):e27-33, 2019
6. Abu-El-Haija M et al: Pediatric chronic pancreatitis: Updates in the 21st century. Pancreatology. 18(4):354-59, 2018
7. Trout AT et al: Normal pancreatic parenchymal thickness by CT in healthy children. Pediatr Radiol. 48(11):1600-5, 2018
8. Abu-El-Haija M et al: Classification of acute pancreatitis in the pediatric population: clinical report from the NASPGHAN Pancreas Committee. J Pediatr Gastroenterol Nutr. 64(6):984-90, 2017
9. Trout AT et al: Secretin-enhanced magnetic resonance cholangiopancreatography for assessing pancreatic secretory function in children. J Pediatr. 188:186-91, 2017
10. Restrepo R et al: Acute pancreatitis in pediatric patients: demographics, etiology, and diagnostic imaging. AJR Am J Roentgenol. 206(3):632-44, 2016

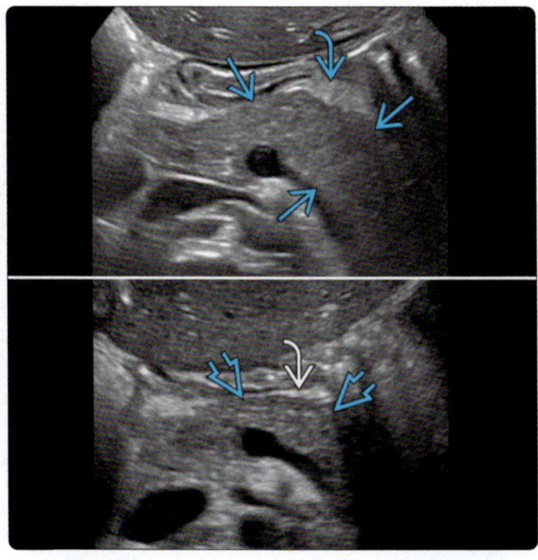

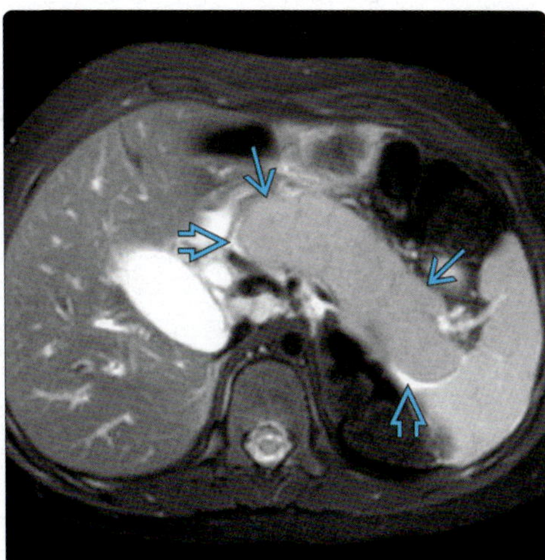

(Left) *Transverse US in a 13-year-old with abdominal pain shows that the pancreas is enlarged & heterogeneous compared to its appearance 1 year prior. Also note the induration of adjacent fat compared to the prior exam. The current findings are consistent with acute pancreatitis.* **(Right)** *Axial T2 FS MR in a 6-year-old with pain shows diffuse, sausage-like thickening of the pancreas with ↑ signal of the parenchyma + surrounding edema, a typical appearance for autoimmune pancreatitis.*

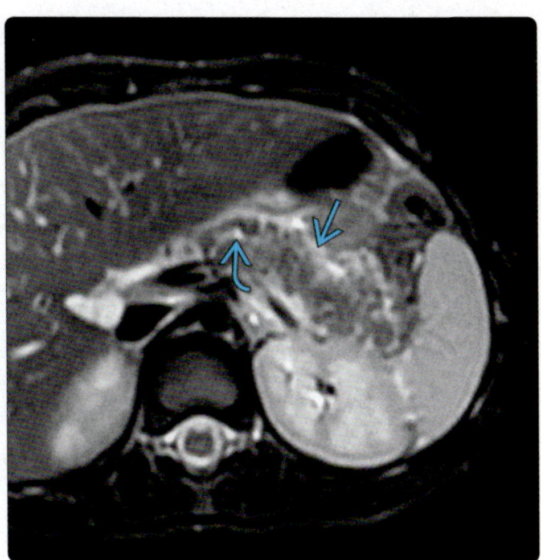

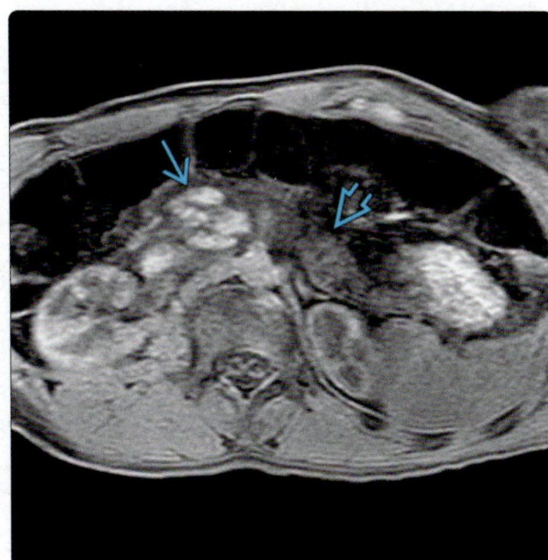

(Left) *Axial T2 FS MR in an adolescent with acute interstitial edematous pancreatitis shows enlargement & edema of the pancreatic body & tail. The pancreatic duct is mildly enlarged.* **(Right)** *Axial oblique T1 FS MR in a patient with acute interstitial edematous pancreatitis shows relatively normal ↑ T1 signal in the pancreatic head while the pancreatic body & tail have ↓ signal due to interstitial edema.*

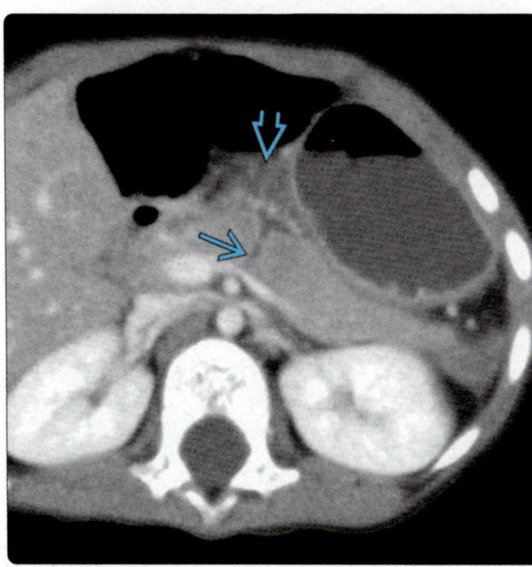

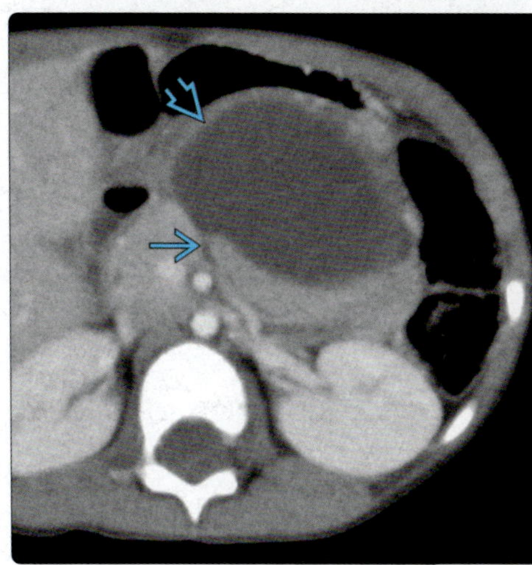

(Left) *Axial CECT in a young child with nonaccidental trauma shows a transection in the body of the pancreas. There is mild peripancreatic edema near the transection.* **(Right)** *Axial CECT in the same patient obtained 5 days later shows a large peripancreatic collection in the lesser sac arising from the transection, strongly suggesting a pancreatic duct injury.*

Primary Mesenteric Adenitis

KEY FACTS

TERMINOLOGY

- Self-limited, benign inflammation of lymph nodes in bowel mesentery; diagnosis of exclusion

IMAGING

- Best diagnostic clue
  - Cluster of ≥ 3 enlarged right lower quadrant or mesenteric lymph nodes
  - Literature on size for diagnosis varies: ≥ 5 mm in short axis vs. >10 mm in short axis vs. >10 mm in long axis
- Ultrasound
  - Enlarged hyperemic lymph nodes often retain normal nodal architecture with fatty hilum
  - Pain with compression over nodes
  - ± fat induration; no abscess or phlegmon
  - Normal appendix (< 6 mm & compressible)
- CECT findings
  - Mildly enlarged lymph nodes, most commonly anterior to right psoas muscle
  - Ileal or colonic wall thickening in < 1/3
    - More common < 5 years of age
  - Normal appendix without surrounding inflammation

TOP DIFFERENTIAL DIAGNOSES

- Appendicitis
- Omental infarction
- Crohn disease
- MIS-C
- Burkitt lymphoma

PATHOLOGY

- Majority are likely secondary to viral or bacterial infection
- Recent upper respiratory infection in up to 25%

CLINICAL ISSUES

- Most commonly occurs < 15 years of age
- Mimics appendicitis: Similar clinical presentation
  - Most frequent alternative diagnosis to appendicitis
- Conservative treatment for primary mesenteric adenitis

(Left) *Transverse ultrasound of the right lower quadrant in a 10-year-old with abdominal pain & fever shows a cluster of 3 lymph nodes →, each measuring > 5 mm in short axis, at the site of tenderness. Additional enlarged lymph nodes were also present. The appendix was not visualized.* **(Right)** *Coronal CECT in the same patient shows a cluster of 3 lymph nodes →, each measuring > 5 mm in size. The appendix was normal (not shown). The patient was diagnosed with mesenteric lymphadenitis & treated conservatively.*

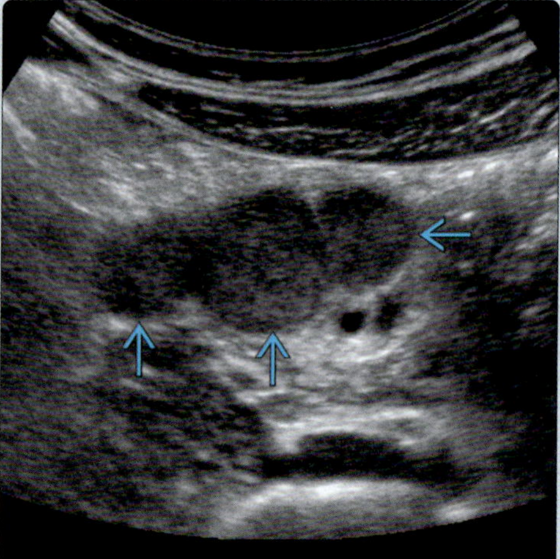

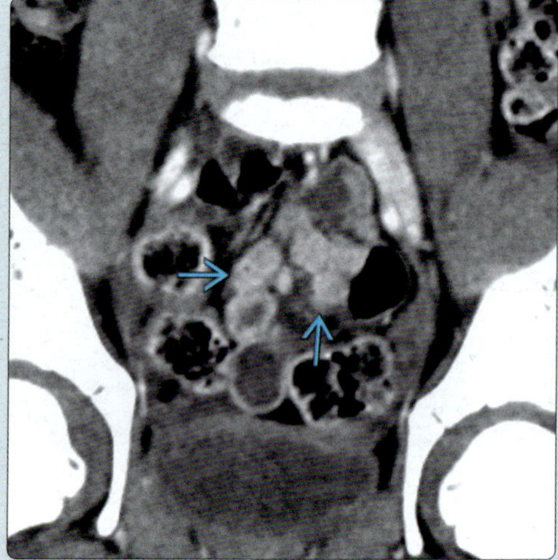

(Left) *Coronal CECT in a 9-year-old with abdominal pain depicts multiple lymph nodes that measure >5 mm → & a normal contrast opacified appendix ⇨. The patient was diagnosed with mesenteric adenitis.* **(Right)** *Longitudinal ultrasound in a 2-year-old with abdominal pain shows mildly enlarged but otherwise normal-appearing lymph nodes → in the right abdomen. No other pathology was identified. The patient's symptoms resolved with conservative therapy, typical of mesenteric adenitis.*

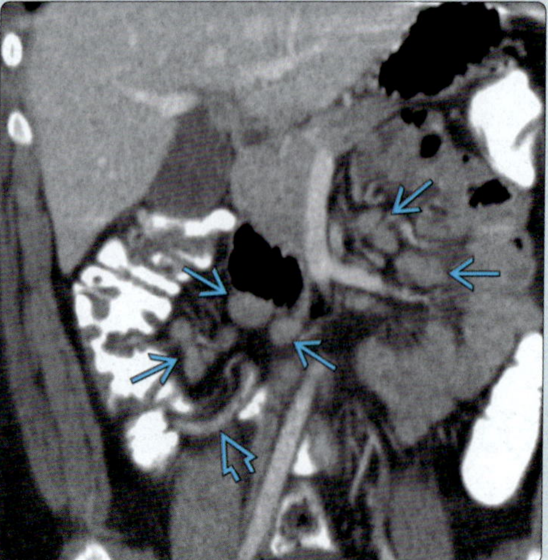

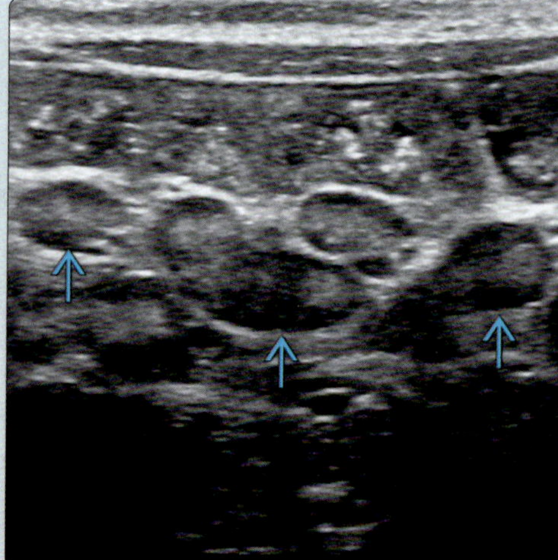

Primary Mesenteric Adenitis

TERMINOLOGY

Definitions

- Self-limited, benign inflammation of lymph nodes in bowel mesentery; diagnosis of exclusion
- Secondary mesenteric adenitis refers to lymphadenopathy associated with detectable intraabdominal inflammatory process, commonly Crohn disease or infectious ileitis
- Most frequent alternative diagnosis to appendicitis

IMAGING

General Features

- Best diagnostic clue
  - ≥ 3 clustered, enlarged right lower quadrant (RLQ) or mesenteric lymph nodes
  - Literature varies on size for diagnosis; recommendations include
    - ≥ 5 mm in short axis
    - > 10 mm in short axis
    - > 10 mm in long axis
  - Normal appendix

Ultrasonographic Findings

- Cluster of enlarged RLQ or mesenteric lymph nodes
- Nodes may be hyperemic but often retain normal sonographic architecture with echogenic fatty hilum
- May have pain with compression at nodes
- ± ↑ echogenicity of RLQ fat
- ± ileal or colonic wall thickening (especially < 5-years-old)
- Normal appendix (< 6 mm & compressible)

CT Findings

- Cluster of enlarged RLQ or mesenteric lymph nodes
  - Most commonly anterior to right psoas muscle
  - Often track along superior mesenteric artery branches
- Normal appendix
- Ileal (up to 33%) or colonic (up to 18%) wall thickening
  - More common < 5 years of age

Imaging Recommendations

- Best imaging tool
  - Graded compression ultrasound
    - No ionizing radiation
    - Confirms tenderness at lymph nodes
    - Normal appendix visualized

DIFFERENTIAL DIAGNOSIS

Appendicitis

- Noncompressible appendix ≥ 6 mm in diameter with surrounding fat induration
- Lumen is typically distended by fluid ± calcified appendicolith
- Enlarged lymph nodes in 40-82%, mean of 9 mm
  - Typically less numerous than primary adenitis
- Ileal or colonic wall thickening, particularly with appendix perforation

Omental Infarction

- Poorly defined focus of echogenic/hyperattenuating fat immediately deep to anterior right abdominal wall

Crohn Disease

- Abnormal thickening, hyperenhancement/hyperemia, & diffusion restriction of terminal ileum & cecum
- ± mesenteric fat proliferation, vasa recta engorgement, enlarged lymph nodes, fistula, abscess, small bowel feces sign (due to distal stricture)

MIS-C

- COVID-19-related pediatric inflammatory syndrome with numerous neurologic, cardiopulmonary, & abdominal manifestations
  - Gallbladder wall thickening, hepatomegaly, ascites, bowel wall thickening, mesenteric adenopathy, echogenic kidneys

Burkitt Lymphoma

- Larger conglomerate nodal masses, potentially inseparable from thickened bowel wall
- Loss of normal nodal architecture
- Rapid doubling time of tumor

PATHOLOGY

General Features

- Majority of primary mesenteric adenitis is likely infectious
  - Viral: Coxsackievirus & adenovirus
  - *Yersinia enterocolitica* is classic
  - Also *Yersinia pseudotuberculosis, Helicobacter jejuni, Salmonella, Shigella, Campylobacter, Staphylococcus*
- Recent streptococcal upper respiratory infection in up to 25% (may be reactive)

CLINICAL ISSUES

Presentation

- Diffuse or focal RLQ abdominal pain is most common
- ± nausea, vomiting, diarrhea, recent upper respiratory infection, leukocytosis

Demographics

- Most commonly < 15-years-old

Treatment

- Primary mesenteric adenitis: Conservative
- Secondary mesenteric adenitis: Treat underlying cause

DIAGNOSTIC CHECKLIST

Image Interpretation Pearls

- Bowel findings are uncommon overall in primary mesenteric adenitis & necessitate further investigation
- Appendix must be normal

SELECTED REFERENCES

1. Blumfield E et al: Imaging findings in multisystem inflammatory syndrome in children (MIS-C) associated with Coronavirus disease (COVID-19). AJR Am J Roentgenol. 216(2):507-17, 2021
2. Fenlon Iii EP et al: Extracardiac imaging findings in COVID-19-associated multisystem inflammatory syndrome in children. Pediatr Radiol. 51(5):831-9, 2021
3. Sanchez TR et al: Sonography of abdominal pain in children: appendicitis and its common mimics. J Ultrasound Med. 35(3):627-35, 2016
4. Moore MM et al: Alternative diagnoses at paediatric appendicitis MRI. Clin Radiol. 70(8):881-9, 2015

Mesenteric Lymphatic Malformation

KEY FACTS

TERMINOLOGY

- Subtype of congenital slow-flow vascular malformation due to error of lymphatic vessel formation
- Results in well-defined, cyst-like (macrocystic) &/or infiltrative, solid-appearing (microcystic) mass of abnormal lymphatic channels focally or diffusely within mesentery
  - Individual cyst size: Macrocyst > 1 cm, microcyst < 1 cm

IMAGING

- Macrocystic: Well-defined, lobulated, unilocular or multilocular, fluid-filled mass in mesentery
  - Thin septations with minimal enhancement (unless complicated by hemorrhage or infection)
  - Simple vs. complex fluid varies between cystic components
    - ± layering fluid-fluid levels (due to blood products) & fat/chylous fluid; Ca^{2+} is uncommon
- Microcystic: More solid-appearing, infiltrative
- Best imaging tool: Ultrasound or MR
  - More sensitive than CT for characteristic thin septations & fluid-debris/fluid-fluid levels

CLINICAL ISSUES

- Generally grow commensurate with patient
  - May rapidly enlarge due to hemorrhage/trauma, infection, or hormonal stimulation (puberty, pregnancy)
- Complications include bowel obstruction, volvulus, infection, hemorrhage, rupture, compartment syndrome
- Age of presentation varies widely
  - Abdominal pain, distention, vomiting, palpable mass
- Treatments include
  - Simple excision, partial bowel resection, sclerotherapy
  - Sirolimus (mTOR inhibitor) medical therapy

DIAGNOSTIC CHECKLIST

- Verify cystic mass is not actually due to distended hollow organ (such as urinary bladder)
- Look for true solid components suggesting neoplasm

(Left) Transverse ultrasound through the abdomen in a 2-year-old patient with abdominal distention shows a large, hypoechoic mass occupying the anterior peritoneal cavity & displacing bowel posteriorly. Thin septations ➔ *& swirling granular debris were seen in the mass.* **(Right)** *Sagittal STIR (left) & T1 C+ FS (right) MR images in the same patient show only mild rim & septal enhancement* ➔ *of this massive mesenteric lymphatic malformation (LM). Note the distortion of the urinary bladder* ➔ *by the mass.*

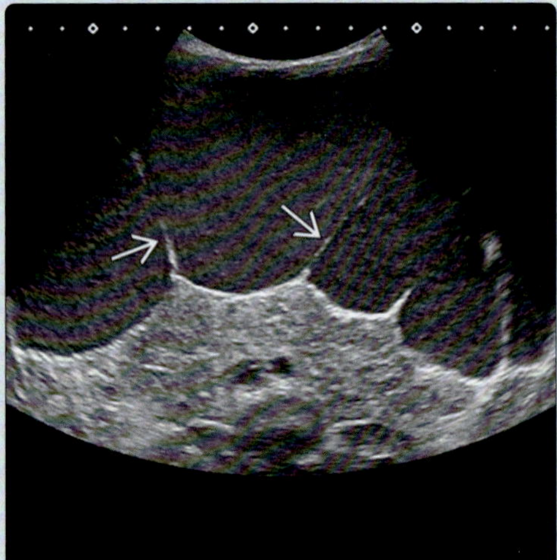

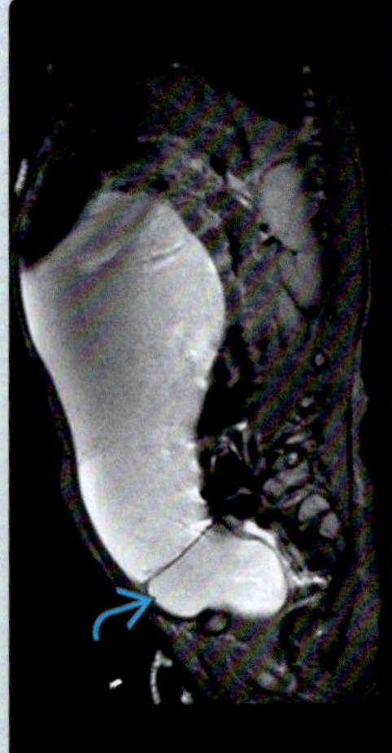

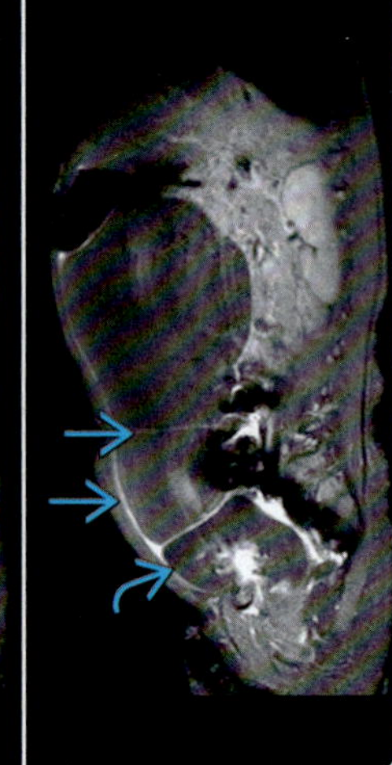

(Left) *AP radiograph in a 5-year-old with vomiting & abdominal distention shows a few dilated small bowel loops* ➔ *in the upper abdomen with a paucity of bowel gas in the lower abdomen.* **(Right)** *Coronal CECT in the same patient shows a large, fluid-attenuation mass filling the peritoneal cavity* ➔*, extending from the urinary bladder* ➔ *to the liver. This LM of the jejunal mesentery was found to be causing a segmental volvulus with proximal bowel dilation* ➔*, requiring resection.*

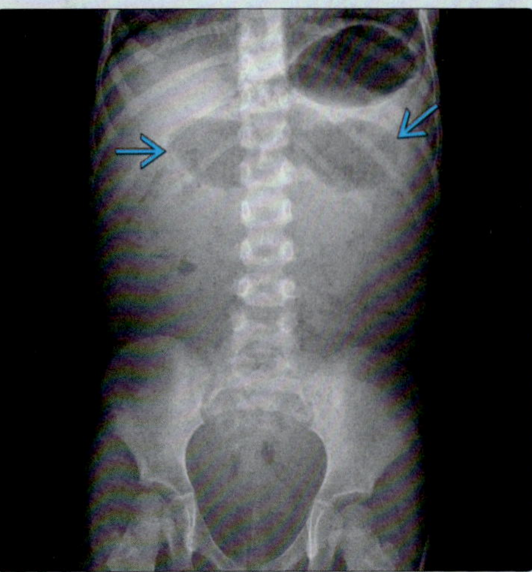

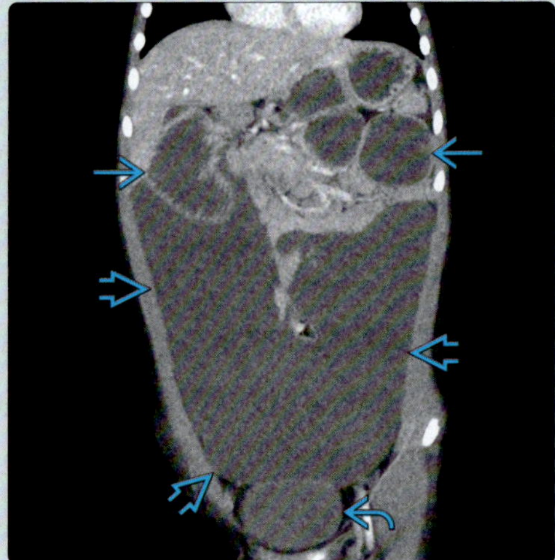

TERMINOLOGY

Synonyms

- Mesenteric or omental cyst; lymphangioma (antiquated)

Definitions

- Subtype of congenital slow-flow vascular malformation due to error of lymphatic vessel formation
- Results in well-defined, cyst-like (macrocystic) &/or infiltrative, solid-appearing (microcystic) mass of abnormal lymphatic channels focally or diffusely within mesentery
  - Individual cyst size: Macrocyst > 1 cm, microcyst < 1 cm
- Often lacks communication with normal lymphatics

IMAGING

General Features

- Best diagnostic clue
  - Multicystic mass in small bowel mesentery

Ultrasonographic Findings

- Grayscale ultrasound
  - Mostly anechoic mass with numerous thin septations
  - Can be complex with varying degrees of debris or hemorrhage within different components
    - Debris may be uniform or layer dependently
    - Contents swirl with intermittent compression
- Color Doppler
  - No significant internal vascularity, though LMs frequently encase normal vessels

MR Findings

- Unilocular or multiseptated cystic mass
  - Largely of fluid signal intensity
    - Layering fluid-fluid levels are often present (due to blood products, typical of slow-flow vascular malformations)
  - Components of T1 shortening may be due to hemorrhage or fat
  - Minimal rim/septal enhancement (unless complicated)
  - ± foci of restricted diffusion due to blood products

Imaging Recommendations

- Best imaging tool
  - Ultrasound or MR
    - More sensitive than CT for characteristic thin septations & fluid-debris/fluid-fluid levels
- Protocol advice
  - Subtracted (pre- from postcontrast) FS T1 MR images provide clearest assessment of enhancing components

DIFFERENTIAL DIAGNOSIS

Gastrointestinal Duplication Cyst

- Unilocular cyst with sonographic gut signature sign
- ± peristalsis (pathognomonic if seen)

Ovarian Cystic Mass

- Simple or complicated cyst vs. cystic neoplasm

Distended/Obstructed Viscus

- Large urinary bladder, chronically obstructed vagina (hydrocolpos), chronic focal dilation of bowel

Mesothelial Cyst

- Due to incomplete fusion of peritoneal surfaces
- Typically unilocular

Cystic Malignancy

- Infantile fibrosarcoma, primitive neuroectodermal tumor
- Typically have intermixed solid/nodular components with restricted diffusion & vascularity/enhancement

Mesenteric Lymphangiectasia

- Diffusely dilated mesenteric lymphatics/mesenteric lymphedema; difficult to discern from microcystic LM
- Due to mesenteric lymphatic flow disorder
- Protein-losing enteropathy & chylous ascites are typical
- Abnormal flow can be demonstrated on MR lymphangiography

Other Cysts/Pseudocysts

- Ventriculoperitoneal shunt pseudocyst, hepatic cyst, choledochal cyst, meconium pseudocyst, loculated ascites, peritoneal inclusion cyst, abscess, hematoma

CLINICAL ISSUES

Presentation

- Most common signs/symptoms
  - Abdominal pain, distention, vomiting, palpable mass
  - Commonly asymptomatic

Demographics

- Age of presentation varies widely

Natural History & Prognosis

- Generally grow commensurate with patient
  - May rapidly enlarge due to hemorrhage/trauma, infection, or hormonal stimulation (puberty, pregnancy)
- Complications
  - Bowel obstruction, volvulus, ischemia, infection, hemorrhage, compartment syndrome, rupture

Treatment

- Simple excision, partial bowel resection
  - Relationship to intestinal walls, mesenteric vessels, & other vital structures determines resectability
  - Recurrence: Up to 100% with incomplete resection
- Sclerotherapy (commonly used in other sites of macrocystic LM) is gaining popularity for abdominal LM
- Sirolimus (mTOR inhibitor) is now often used as medical therapy for LM

SELECTED REFERENCES

1. Dori Y et al: Intramesenteric dynamic contrast pediatric MR lymphangiography: initial experience and comparison with intranodal and intrahepatic MR lymphangiography. Eur Radiol. 30(10):5777-84, 2020
2. Gasparella P et al: Giant lymphatic malformation causing abdominal compartment syndrome in a neonate: a rare surgical emergency. J Surg Case Rep. 2020(8):rjaa252, 2020
3. Clement C et al: An acute presentation of pediatric mesenteric lymphangioma: a case report and literature overview. Acta Chir Belg. 118(5):331-5, 2018
4. Dillman JR et al: Imaging of the pediatric peritoneum, mesentery and omentum. Pediatr Radiol. 47(8):987-1000, 2017
5. Kim SH et al: Clinical features of mesenteric lymphatic malformation in children. J Pediatr Surg. 51(4):582-7, 2016
6. Malone LJ et al: Pediatric lymphangiectasia: an imaging spectrum. Pediatr Radiol. 45(4):562-9, 2015

Omental Infarction

KEY FACTS

TERMINOLOGY

- Benign, self-limited cause of acute abdominal pain due to segmental vascular occlusion of omentum

IMAGING

- General features
  - Well-demarcated, triangular/wedge-shaped or oval focus of ↑ attenuation/echogenicity within omental fat
  - Right mid to upper abdomen, deep to anterior wall
  - ± thickening of overlying peritoneal membrane
  - ± free intraperitoneal fluid &/or pleural effusion
  - No adjacent inflammatory etiologies (e.g., appendicitis)
- US: Echogenic focus with no internal color Doppler flow + tethered fat sign; painful to direct sonographic palpation
- CT: Focal fat stranding ± hyperattenuating, streaky densities due to fibrous bands or thrombosed vessels
  - ± peripheral enhancement
  - ± whirl or vascular pedicle sign with torsion
- Recommendations
  - Ultrasound: Acceptable 1st-line modality despite lower sensitivity for this diagnosis compared to CECT
    - Sensitivity is higher for surgical diagnoses (e.g., appendicitis)

TOP DIFFERENTIAL DIAGNOSES

- Epiploic appendagitis, appendicitis, slow-flow vascular malformation, mesenteric contusion, fat-containing masses

PATHOLOGY

- Etiologies: Anatomic vascular variation, hypercoagulability, torsion, systemic states prone to vascular congestion
- Majority of patients are obese

CLINICAL ISSUES

- Abdominal pain & tenderness, nausea, vomiting, fever
- Conservative treatment is typically adequate
- Occasional surgical excision if pain is intractable, symptoms worsen, or imaging is equivocal

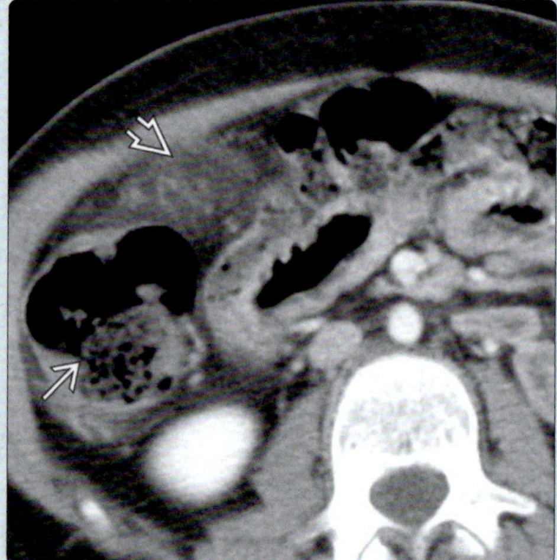

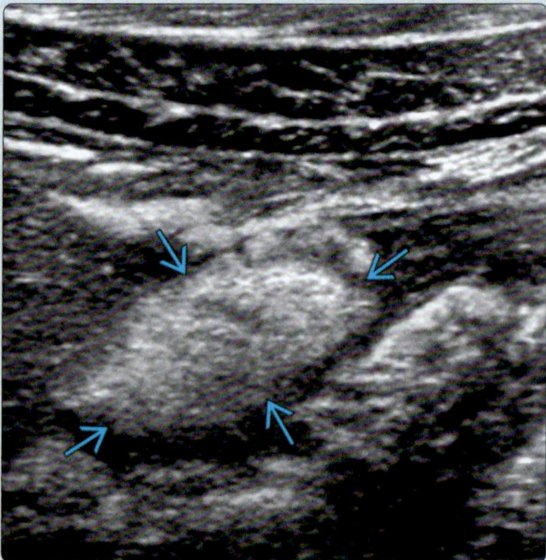

(Left) *Axial CECT in an 11-year-old with right abdominal pain depicts a focus of inflammatory stranding ➡ immediately deep to the abdominal wall & anterior to the ascending colon ➡, typical of an omental infarct.* **(Right)** *Transverse ultrasound in a 7-year-old with abdominal pain shows a well-demarcated, ovoid, hyperechoic focus ➡ deep to the right anterior abdominal wall. A normal appendix was not visualized. Omental infarct was confirmed at surgery.*

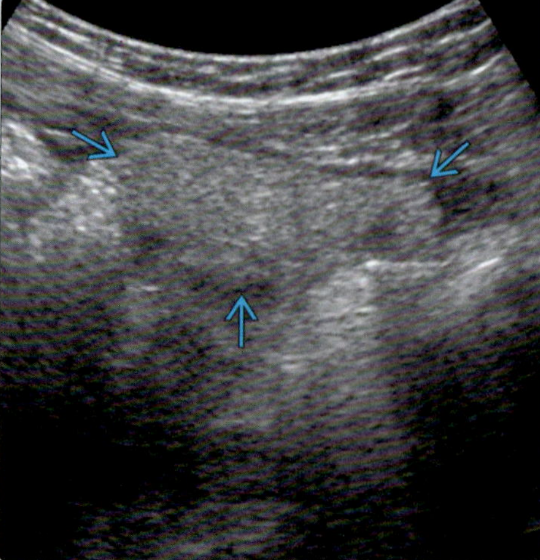

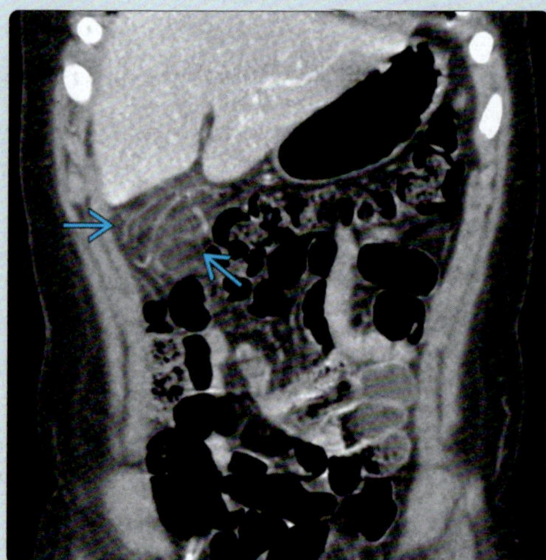

(Left) *Transverse ultrasound in an 8-year-old with right lower quadrant abdominal pain secondary to omental infarct demonstrates a triangular focus of ↑ echogenicity deep to the anterior abdominal wall at the site of palpable pain ➡.* **(Right)** *Coronal CECT from an 8-year-old with abdominal pain shows a focal area of ↑ omental attenuation at the right upper quadrant, compatible with an omental infarction ➡. Note the internal linear densities. The appendix was normal (not shown).*

TERMINOLOGY

Definitions

- Benign, self-limited cause of acute abdominal pain due to segmental vascular occlusion of omentum

IMAGING

General Features

- Best diagnostic clue
  - Well-demarcated, triangular/wedge-shaped or oval focus of omental fat stranding (CT) or hyperechogenicity (US) without other source of inflammation
    - Typically in right upper quadrant (RUQ)

Ultrasonographic Findings

- Relatively hyperechoic noncompressible, wedge-shaped, or oval focus with no color Doppler flow
- Typically in RUQ immediately deep to anterior abdominal wall
  - Tethered fat sign: Adherent to abdominal wall, no motion with respiration
- Painful to direct sonographic palpation
- ± free intraperitoneal fluid &/or pleural effusion

CT Findings

- Well-defined focus of hazy ↑ attenuation of omental fat
- Triangular/wedge-shaped or oval
- Typically in RUQ between anterior abdominal wall & transverse or ascending colon
- ± streaky/linear densities representing fibrous bands or thrombosed vessels
- ± peripheral enhancement
- ± whirl or vascular pedicle sign: Torsion of omental fat & vessels around engorged vascular pedicle
- ± thickening of overlying peritoneum
- ± free intraperitoneal fluid &/or pleural effusion
- No other source for inflammation (e.g., appendicitis, colitis, etc.)

Imaging Recommendations

- Ultrasound is typically 1st-line modality
  - Low sensitivity (60-80%) for omental infarction but higher for other diagnoses with similar presentations
- CECT has greater sensitivity (90%) for omental infarction

DIFFERENTIAL DIAGNOSIS

Epiploic Appendagitis

- Torsion & resultant inflammation of epiploic appendage along colon, typically in lower quadrants
- Oval focus of pericolonic fat inflammation
- Hyperdense central dot sign (thrombosed vessel) is classic

Appendicitis

- Enlarged, noncompressible appendix with adjacent inflammatory change

Mesenteric Lymphadenitis

- Cluster of ≥ 3 lymph nodes ≥ 5 mm each (in short axis)
- ± adjacent fat stranding

Mesenteric Contusion

- Typically preceded by clear history of trauma
- ± overlying contusion of subcutaneous fat

Slow-Flow Vascular Malformation

- ± poorly defined infiltrative components of venous or lymphatic malformations, typically in conjunction with mass-like abnormal vascular channels or cysts

Meckel Diverticulitis

- Noncompressible, blind-ending tubular structure arising from distal ileum with adjacent inflammatory change

Fat-Containing Masses

- Teratoma & lipoblastoma are uncommon in anterior abdomen in children
- More solid & heterogeneous in appearance

PATHOLOGY

General Features

- Due to anatomic vascular variation, hypercoagulability, torsion (due to scars, hernias, omental cysts), systemic states prone to vascular congestion (right heart failure)

Gross Pathologic & Surgical Features

- Venous stasis &/or thrombosis → venous congestion → omental edema & congestion (early infarct) → hemorrhagic necrosis/infarction → granulomatous infiltrate (6-7 days) → fibrosis & scar

CLINICAL ISSUES

Presentation

- Most common signs/symptoms
  - Abdominal pain & tenderness, typically right-sided
- Other signs/symptoms
  - Nausea, vomiting, mild fever, mild ↑ CRP & WBC

Demographics

- Epidemiology
  - 15% of all cases occur in children
  - M:F = ~ 2-4:1
  - Risk factors: Obesity, omental anatomic abnormalities

Treatment

- Conservative treatment, including analgesia & antibiotics
  - Complete resolution in < 2 weeks
- Occasional surgical excision if pain is intractable, symptoms worsen, &/or imaging is equivocal

SELECTED REFERENCES

1. Esposito F et al: Not only fat: omental infarction and its mimics in children. Clinical and ultrasound findings: a pictorial review. J Ultrasound. 23(4):621-9, 2020
2. McCusker R et al: Diagnosis and management of omental infarction in children: our 10 year experience with ultrasound. J Pediatr Surg. 53(7):1360-4, 2018
3. Wertheimer J et al: Radiological, clinical and histological correlations in a right segmental omental infarction due to primary torsion in a child. Diagn Interv Imaging. 95(3):325-31, 2014
4. Coulier B: Contribution of US and CT for diagnosis of intraperitoneal focal fat infarction (IFFI): a pictorial review. JBR-BTR. 93(4):171-85, 2010
5. Nubi A et al: Primary omental infarct: conservative vs operative management in the era of ultrasound, computerized tomography, and laparoscopy. J Pediatr Surg. 44(5):953-6, 2009

KEY FACTS

TERMINOLOGY

- Synonyms: Shock bowel, hypotension complex

IMAGING

- Bowel: Diffuse wall thickening, ↑ enhancement (mucosal vs. full thickness), ± fluid distention
- Vessels: ↑ enhancement but ↓ caliber
- Abnormal solid organ appearances may include
  - Adrenal glands: Prolonged enhancement > IVC
  - Kidneys: Prolonged cortical enhancement > aorta; rarely ↓ enhancement < 10 HU (poor prognosis)
  - Pancreas: Enlarged, feathery appearance due to septal edema; altered enhancement at least 20 HU > or < liver
  - Liver: Heterogeneous enhancement with ≥ 30 HU difference between highest & lowest measurements at level of portal vein
  - Gallbladder mucosal enhancement (50 HU > psoas)
  - Spleen: ↓ enhancement (20 HU < liver); ≥ 30% ↓ in volume

PATHOLOGY

- Shock: Compensated → decompensated → irreversible
- Sympathetic nervous, cardiovascular, & neuroendocrine systems help maintain arterial pressure & cardiac output in compensated state
- Pediatric patients can maintain normal/near-normal blood pressure longer than cardiac output → rapid, abrupt progression to decompensated state

CLINICAL ISSUES

- CT findings often precede clinical recognition of shock
  - In one series, hypotension developed within 10 minutes of CT in 19% of children
  - In same series, 85% mortality rate with presence of hypoperfusion complex (compared with 2% of all children who suffered blunt trauma)
- Requires prompt notification & transfer to clinical service for intense monitoring, volume replacement, supportive measures, & surgery if needed

(Left) *Coronal CECT in a 5-month-old patient in septic shock demonstrates a large volume of ascites ➡, diffuse bowel wall hyperenhancement & thickening ➡, & heterogeneity of the liver parenchyma ➡.* **(Right)** *Axial CECT in the same patient illustrates the diffuse bowel wall thickening & hyperenhancement ➡ relative to the psoas muscles ➡. A large volume of ascites is again seen ➡. The constellation of findings in this patient is compatible with hypoperfusion complex.*

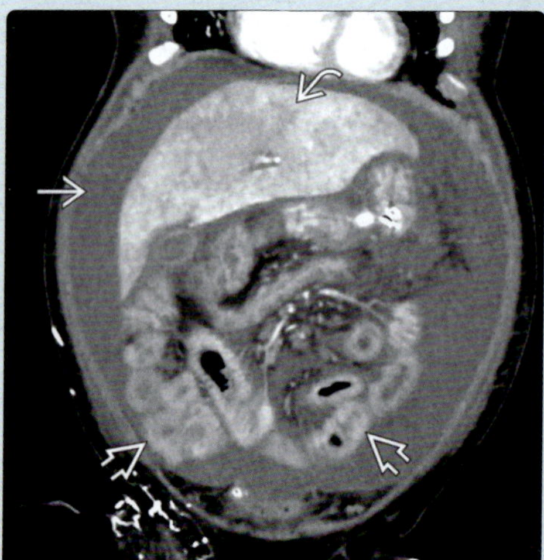

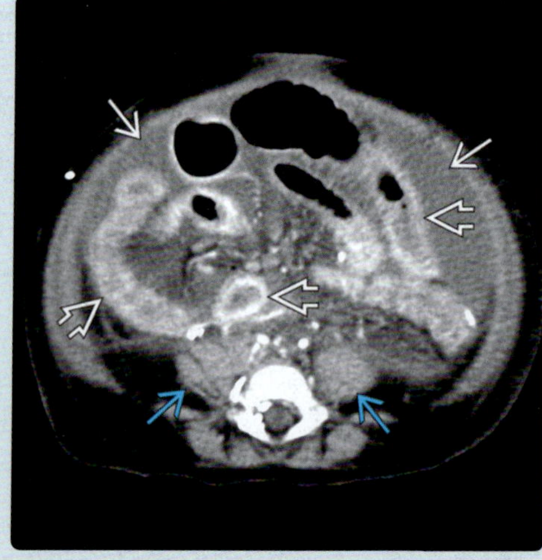

(Left) *Axial CECT in a 2-month-old boy with cardiogenic shock shows diffusely dilated & fluid-filled small bowel with mild wall thickening ➡. There is intense enhancement of the mesenteric vessels ➡.* **(Right)** *Coronal CECT in the same patient demonstrates intensely enhancing adrenal glands ➡, a characteristic finding in hypoperfusion complex. There is heterogeneous liver parenchyma ➡ & ↓ enhancement of the kidneys ➡ & spleen ➡.*

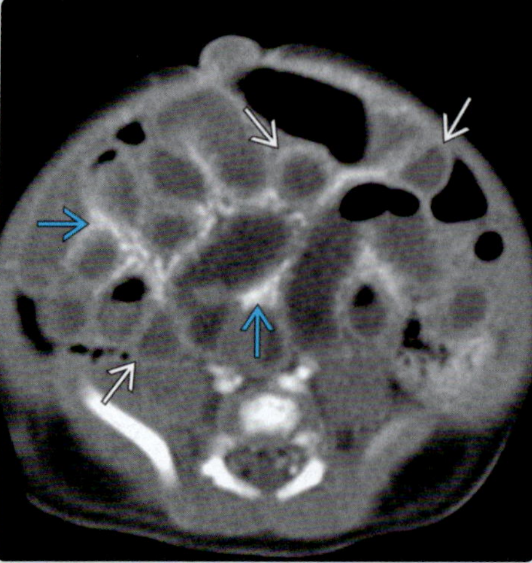

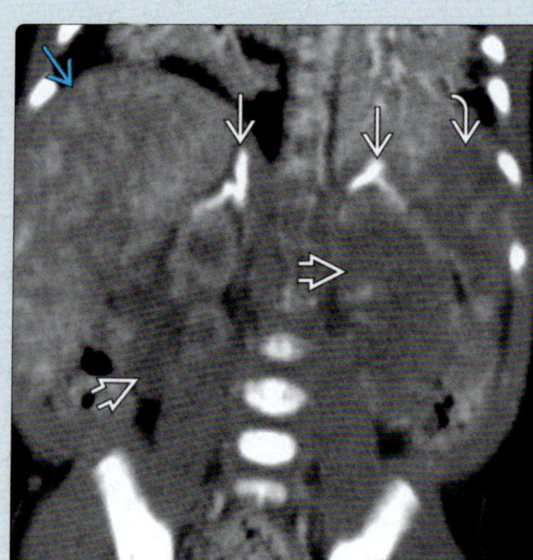

TERMINOLOGY

Synonyms

- Shock bowel, shock abdomen, hypovolemic shock complex, hypotension complex

Definitions

- Hypoperfusion complex (HC): Constellation of CT findings indicative of compensated shock

IMAGING

CT Findings

- Best imaging clues (on CECT)
  - Diffuse small bowel wall thickening with ↑ enhancement
  - Abnormal solid organ enhancement
  - ↑ enhancement of small-caliber vessels
- Bowel (predominantly small intestine)
  - Diffuse, mild dilation of fluid-filled loops
  - Diffuse mural or mucosal hyperenhancement (> psoas muscle)
  - Diffuse wall thickening > 3 mm
- Vasculature
  - Flat "pancake" inferior vena cava (IVC)
    - ± intense enhancement
    - May show normal caliber & shape with aggressive fluid resuscitation
    - Circumferential ↓ attenuation (< 20 HU) fluid halo around IVC
  - ↓ caliber of intensely enhancing aorta & mesenteric arteries
- Solid viscera
  - Adrenal glands
    - Symmetric & prolonged hyperenhancement (> IVC)
  - Kidneys
    - Symmetric hyperenhancement (> aorta), prolonged in cortex
    - May see ↓ enhancement of medulla on delayed phase
    - ↓ enhancement (< 10 HU) is rarely seen; may represent poor prognosis (black kidney sign)
  - Pancreas
    - Diffusely enlarged, feathery appearance due to edematous intervening septa
    - Altered enhancement (at least 20 HU > or < than liver)
    - Peripancreatic fluid
  - Spleen
    - ↓ enhancement (20 HU < liver)
    - Enhancement > liver is also reported in children
    - Splenic contraction: ≥ 30% ↓ in volume compared to prior study or height- & sex-corrected normal values
      - Due to adrenergic stimulation; persists after fluid resuscitation
  - Liver
    - Parenchymal heterogeneity: ≥ 30 HU difference between highest & lowest measurements at level of portal vein
  - Gallbladder
    - Wall enhancement 50 HU > psoas muscle
    - Wall thickening & surrounding edema
- Mesentery/peritoneum: Generalized edema & unexplained ascites
- Thoracic structures
  - ↓ caliber of intensely enhancing aorta & great vessels
  - ↓ caliber of superior vena cava & IVC
  - ↓ cardiac chamber volume
  - Thyroidal & perithyroidal edema (shock thyroid)
    - Enlargement with intervening septal edema

Ultrasonographic Findings

- FAST scanning of abdomen for potential injury screening
  - May show peritoneal fluid
  - Diffusely fluid-filled & dilated bowel with wall thickening
  - ↓ caliber of IVC, aorta

Imaging Recommendations

- Best imaging tool
  - CECT

DIFFERENTIAL DIAGNOSIS

Bowel Trauma

- Focal (rather than diffuse) bowel wall thickening, dilation, & enhancement abnormalities (↑ or ↓)
- Adjacent vessel extravasation, mesenteric fluid, extraluminal gas
- Extensive extraintestinal findings favor shock bowel over focal bowel injury (though these entities may coexist)

Transient Small Bowel Intussusception

- Short segment(s) of small bowel showing alternating rings of high & low attenuation (in cross section)
- Typically incidental & self-limited
- Seen with higher frequency in trauma patients

Henoch-Schönlein Purpura

- Small vessel vasculitis of unknown etiology
  - Purpuric rash, abdominal pain, arthritis, nephritis, intussusceptions
  - Typical ages of 3-7 years; boys > girls
- Bowel wall thickening with abnormal attenuation/enhancement due to intramural edema &/or hemorrhage

Graft-vs.-Host Disease

- Bone marrow transplant patient with new skin, liver, & gut abnormalities
- Diffusely hyperenhancing but featureless small bowel lumen (ribbon-like)

Other Bowel Inflammatory Processes

- Preexisting bowel conditions may rarely cause hypovolemic shock or occur coincidental with trauma
  - Pseudomembranous colitis: Pancolitis with severe bowel wall thickening but disproportionately minor pericolonic inflammatory change; related to antibiotic use
  - Crohn disease: Marked thickening & abnormal enhancement of terminal ileum & cecum with surrounding inflammation
  - Infectious enterocolitis: *Shigella*, *Escherichia coli*, etc., show abnormal bowel wall thickening & enhancement; colonic lumen is often narrowed with small bowel often being fluid filled & hyperperistaltic

Bowel Ischemia Due to Vascular Occlusion

- Iatrogenic (i.e., neonatal vascular catheter), coagulopathy, cardiovascular disease, midgut volvulus
- May present with bowel wall thickening, diffuse dilation
- Abnormal enhancement of bowel: ↓ with arterial occlusion, ↑ with venous occlusion
- Extensive extraintestinal findings favor shock bowel over primary bowel pathology

PATHOLOGY

General Features

- Shock: Clinical expression of limited oxygen supply/utilization
  - Can result from hypovolemia, head/spine injury, cardiac arrest, septicemia, diabetic ketoacidosis
- Stages of shock
  - Compensated
    - Perfusion to vital organs is maintained by response of sympathetic nervous, cardiovascular, & neuroendocrine systems
    - Children may maintain arterial pressure longer than cardiac output, thus appearing stable enough for CT
    - May abruptly transition to decompensated stage
  - Decompensated
    - Response of sympathetic nervous, cardiovascular, & neuroendocrine systems is insufficient to maintain perfusion
  - Irreversible
    - Volume replacement is unable to reverse depressed cardiac output & hypoperfusion
- Variable organ enhancement results from selective vasoconstriction mediated by ↑ sympathetic tone & renin-angiotensin axis
  - Small-caliber aorta & IVC are due to vasospasm, hypovolemia
  - Relatively intense & prolonged enhancement of adrenal glands is related to central role of adrenal in generating sympathetic response to hypovolemic shock
  - Hyperintense, prolonged enhancement of kidneys is related to vasoconstriction of renal efferent arterioles
  - Splenic arterial flow is without autoregulatory mechanism → vasoconstriction & ↓ perfusion
  - Splanchnic vasoconstriction → ↓ bowel perfusion
    - Altered, ↑ permeability of intestinal mucosa → interstitial leak of fluid & contrast → mucosal enhancement, submucosal edematous wall thickening
    - ↓ fluid reabsorption & ileus may result in fluid-distended lumen
- Associated abnormalities
  - Findings of solid organ injury: Liver, spleen, kidney
  - HC is more frequent with ↑ grades of injury, active extravasation
  - Focal bowel injury may also be present
  - In 1 review, 48% had abdominal organ injury

CLINICAL ISSUES

Presentation

- Most common signs/symptoms
  - Pediatric patients in tenuous hemodynamic state
    - Significant hemorrhage after blunt trauma
    - Less common: Neurogenic shock, septic shock, & cardiac arrest
  - Tachycardic
  - Normotensive before decompensation
  - Signs/symptoms of concomitant/causative intracranial & intraabdominal injuries
    - Low Glasgow Coma Scale: < 6 in 20%

Demographics

- Age
  - CT findings of shock are more common & more striking in young children (but can be seen at any age)

Natural History & Prognosis

- Poor prognosis in trauma patient
  - CT findings often precede clinical recognition of shock
  - Pediatric patients are able to maintain arterial pressure at or near normal levels longer than cardiac output after severe hemorrhage → stable-appearing patients can rapidly decompensate
    - In one series, progressive hypotension developed within 10 minutes of CT in 19% of children
    - In same series, 85% mortality rate occurred with presence of HC (compared with 2% of all children who suffered blunt trauma)

Treatment

- Fluid/blood volume replacement
- Intense monitoring
- Surgery when necessary for underlying injuries

DIAGNOSTIC CHECKLIST

Consider

- Diffuse small bowel wall thickening with ↑ enhancement & luminal dilation: Suspect HC & look for supporting signs
- Requires prompt notification of clinical team & transfer of patient from CT to ICU or operating room

SELECTED REFERENCES

1. Elst J et al: Signs of post-traumatic hypovolemia on abdominal CT and their clinical importance: a systematic review. Eur J Radiol. 124:108800, 2020
2. Mills A et al: Imaging of bowel wall thickening in the hospitalized patient. Radiol Clin North Am. 58(1):1-17, 2020
3. Wildman-Tobriner B et al: Hepatic heterogeneity and attenuation on contrast-enhanced CT in patients with the hypovolemic shock complex: objective classification using a contemporary cohort. Curr Probl Diagn Radiol. 48(3):224-8, 2019
4. Enslow MS et al: Splenic contraction: a new member of the hypovolemic shock complex. Abdom Radiol (NY). 43(9):2375-83, 2018
5. Sugi MD et al: CT findings of acute small-bowel entities. Radiographics. 38(5):1352-69, 2018
6. Barber JL et al: Inferior vena cava calibre on paediatric trauma CT may be a useful predictor for the development of shock. Clin Radiol. 71(6):565-9, 2016
7. Higashi H et al: Traumatic hypovolemic shock revisited: the spectrum of contrast-enhanced abdominal computed tomography findings and clinical implications for its management. Jpn J Radiol. 32(10):579-84, 2014
8. O'Hara SM et al: Intense contrast enhancement of the adrenal glands: another abdominal CT finding associated with hypoperfusion complex in children. AJR Am J Roentgenol. 173(4):995-7, 1999
9. Sivit CJ et al: Posttraumatic shock in children: CT findings associated with hemodynamic instability. Radiology. 182(3):723-6, 1992
10. Taylor GA et al: Hypovolemic shock in children: abdominal CT manifestations. Radiology. 164(2):479-81, 1987

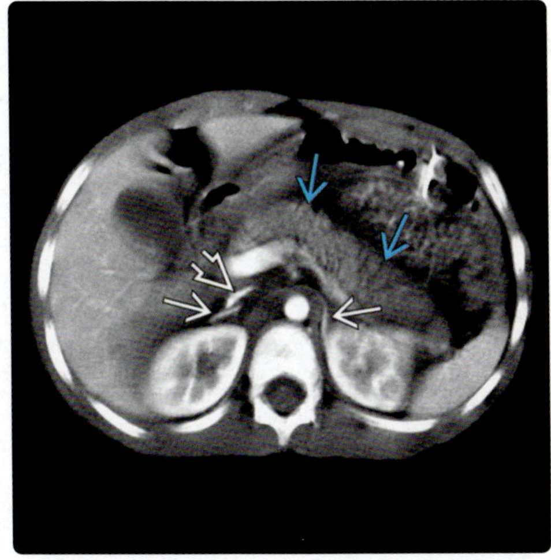

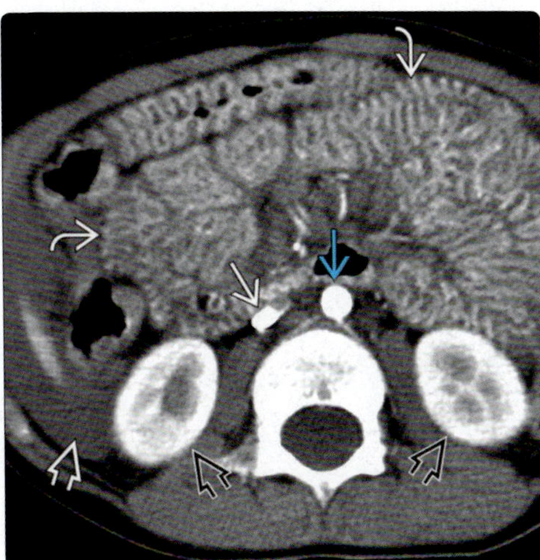

(Left) *Axial CECT shows a densely enhancing & small-caliber inferior vena cava (IVC) ➡. The pancreas ➡ is enlarged with a reticulated or feathery appearance from septal edema, typical of hypoperfusion complex. There is also hyperenhancement of the adrenals ➡ & prolonged renal corticomedullary differentiation.* **(Right)** *Axial CECT in a hypotensive patient shows diffuse small bowel wall thickening & mucosal hyperenhancement ➡, densely enhancing IVC ➡ & aorta ➡, dense renal cortical enhancement ➡, & ascites ➡.*

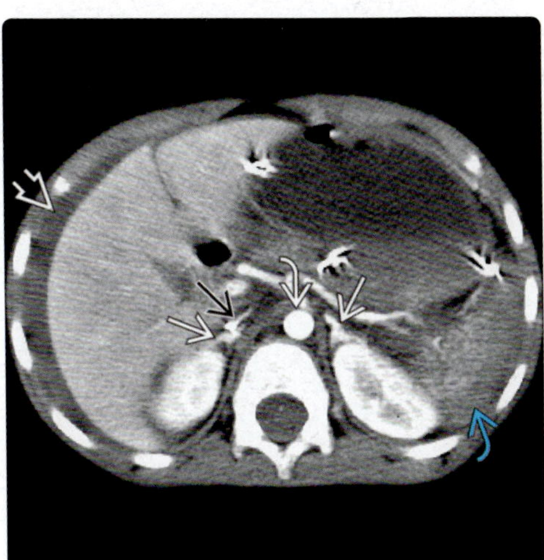

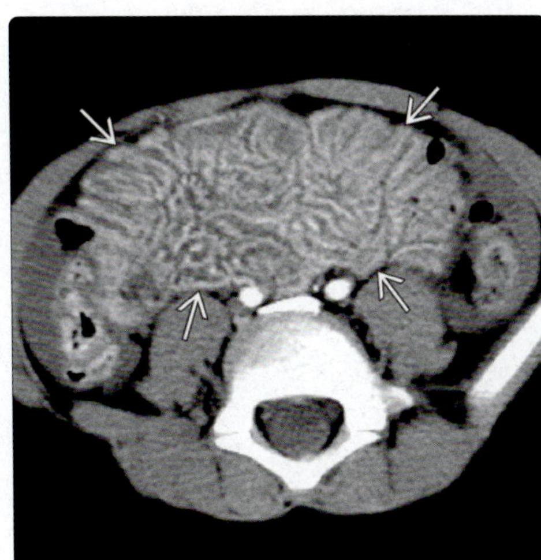

(Left) *Axial CECT shows hyperenhancement of the adrenal glands ➡ & aorta ➡. There is a dense & flattened appearance of the IVC ➡. Note the free fluid ➡ in the peritoneal cavity & the poor enhancement of the spleen ➡.* **(Right)** *Axial CECT in the same patient shows diffuse small bowel wall thickening & mucosal hyperenhancement ➡, typical of hypoperfusion complex.*

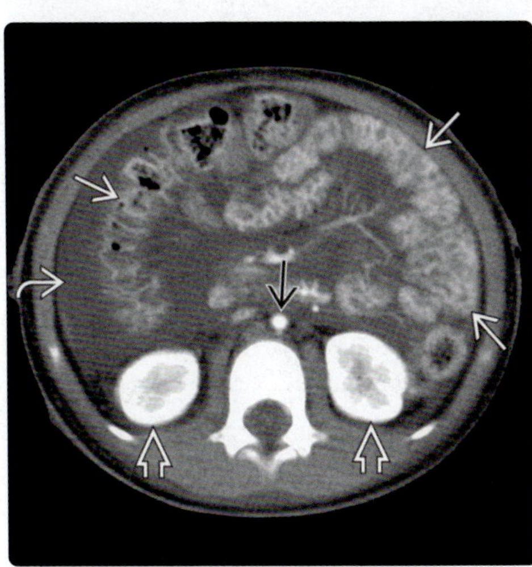

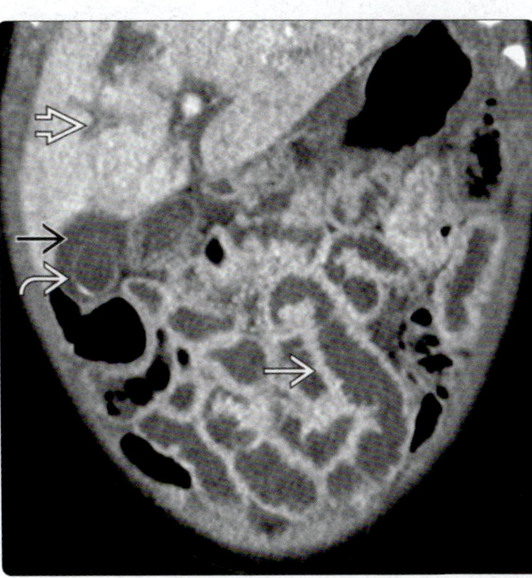

(Left) *Axial CECT in a 4-year-old patient in shock from extensive burns shows diffuse bowel wall ➡ & renal cortical ➡ hyperenhancement. The aorta is relatively small in caliber & enhances intensely ➡. A large volume of ascites is also depicted ➡.* **(Right)** *Coronal CECT from a 12-month-old nonaccidental trauma victim status post cardiac arrest shows diffuse fluid distention of the small bowel with full-thickness wall hyperenhancement ➡. Also note the periportal edema ➡ + gallbladder wall enhancement ➡ & edema ➡.*

Bowel Injury

KEY FACTS

IMAGING

- Best clue: Bowel wall discontinuity + extraluminal enteric contents + free intraperitoneal air
- Nonspecific signs: Focal bowel wall thickening, abnormal bowel wall enhancement, mesenteric fluid/stranding
- Sentinel clot sign: Localized mesenteric hematoma adjacent to bowel (40-80 HU)
- In acute blunt trauma setting, oral contrast does not significantly improve sensitivity & may result in inappropriate delay of diagnosis & treatment

TOP DIFFERENTIAL DIAGNOSES

- Hypoperfusion complex (shock bowel)
- Henoch-Schönlein purpura (HSP)
- Inflammatory bowel disease
- Air introduced by iatrogenic procedure, penetrating trauma, or from other sites (chest, genitourinary system)
- Air from extraperitoneal rectal or bladder perforation

PATHOLOGY

- 77% from blunt trauma: Motor vehicle related, nonaccidental trauma, & bicycle related are most common; mechanisms include
  - Sudden ↑ in intraluminal pressure → perforation
  - Crush injury between abdominal wall & spine
  - Shear force between fixed & mobile bowel
- 23% from penetrating trauma
  - With rectal involvement, consider sexual assault

CLINICAL ISSUES

- Signs & symptoms
  - Abdominal pain, peritoneal signs, tachycardia, ↑ WBC
  - Bowel injury in 11% of patients with seat belt sign: Relative risk of 9.4%
- Treatment
  - Perforations: Surgical management
  - Contusion/hematoma: Typically nonoperative
    - Clinical deterioration is main indicator for surgery

(Left) *Axial CECT shows extraluminal oral contrast ➡ leaking from a thickened bowel loop ➡ in a pediatric car accident victim. Ascites ➡ & soft tissue stranding ➡ are also seen. Note that oral contrast generally does not improve sensitivity for bowel perforation & delays diagnosis.* **(Right)** *Coronal CECT in a 2-year-old victim of nonaccidental trauma shows thickened bowel loops, regions of ↑ ➡ & ↓ ➡ bowel wall enhancement, & extensive free fluid ➡. Devascularized jejunum was found at surgery.*

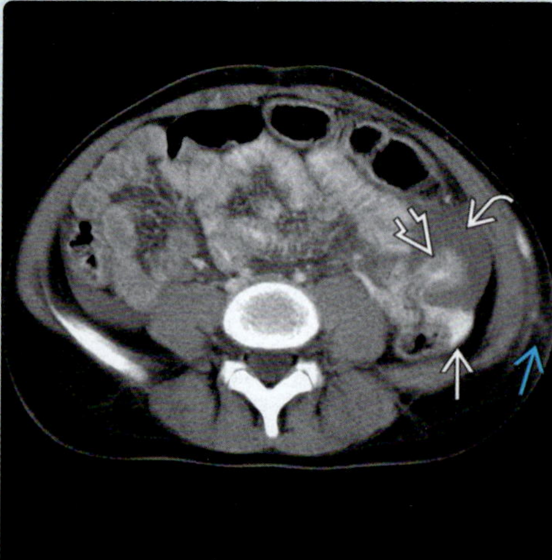

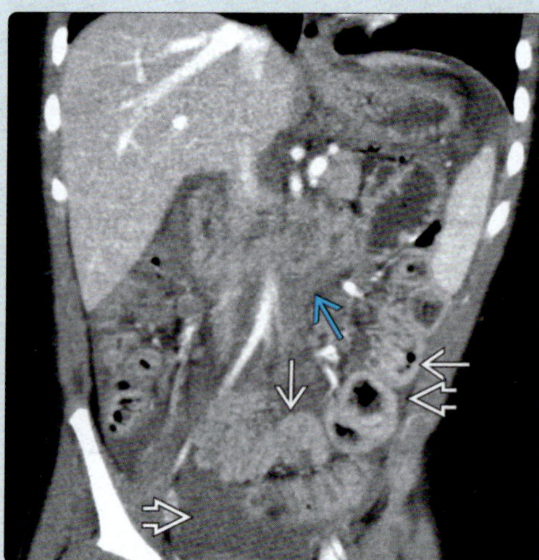

(Left) *Axial CECT in a 13-year-old after a car accident shows IV contrast extravasation ➡ from a superior mesenteric artery branch. Hyper- ➡ & hypo- ➡ enhancing segments of bowel are concerning for hypoperfusion & ischemia.* **(Right)** *Axial CECT in a 12-year-old motor vehicle accident victim shows thick-walled small bowel ➡ in the left abdomen. There is edema of the overlying subcutaneous fat with skin thickening ➡, typical of a seat belt sign. Jejunal perforations were found at surgery.*

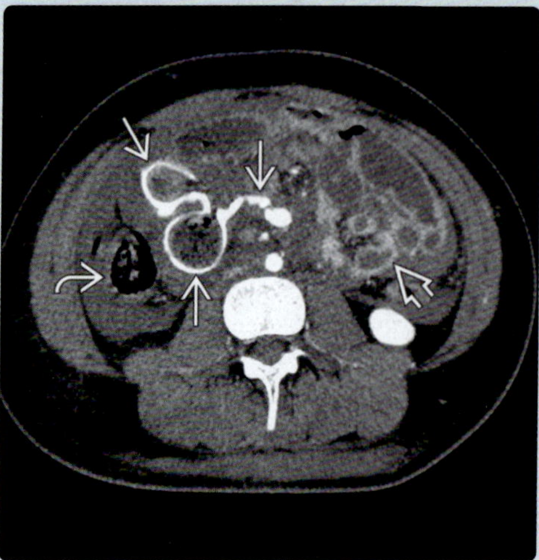

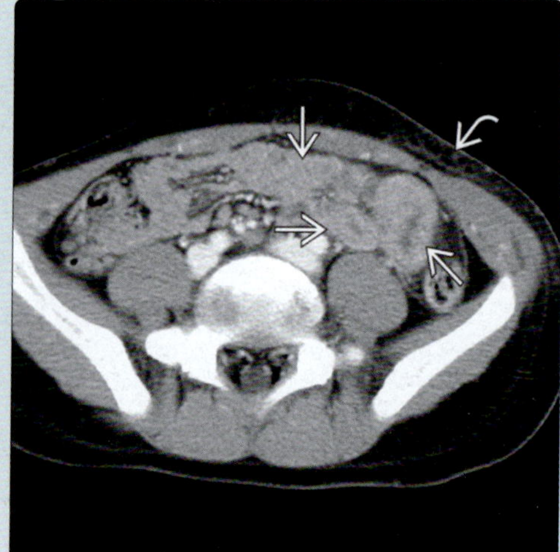

TERMINOLOGY

Synonyms

- Contusion or hematoma vs. perforation, laceration, tear, enterotomy, transection

IMAGING

General Features

- Best diagnostic clue
  - CECT: Focal bowel wall thickening with discontinuous bowel wall enhancement, extraluminal gas, & surrounding mesenteric fluid/stranding in trauma setting
- Location
  - Retroperitoneal bowel: 2nd, 3rd, & 4th duodenal segments (D2-D4) + ascending & descending colon
  - Intraperitoneal bowel: Stomach, 1st duodenal segment (D1), ileum, jejunum, cecum, transverse & sigmoid colon, upper 2/3 of rectum
  - Extraperitoneal bowel: Lower 1/3 of rectum

Radiographic Findings

- Dilated bowel loops, focal or generalized
  - Inflammation & ischemia may → ileus or obstruction
- Pneumoperitoneum (sensitivity < 30% in cases of bowel perforation due to blunt trauma)
  - Air under diaphragm: Best visualized on upright or left lateral decubitus views
  - ↑ volume of air is required for visualization on supine views
    - Rigler sign: Air outlining both sides of bowel wall
    - Falciform ligament sign: Vertically oriented linear density in medial right upper quadrant outlined by air
    - Football sign: Ovoid lucency filling abdominal cavity
    - Inverted V sign: Air outlining medial umbilical folds
- Retroperitoneal air
  - Perforation of retroperitoneal bowel segments
  - Outlines psoas, kidney, &/or hemidiaphragm crus
- Flank stripe sign: Peritoneal fluid separating ascending or descending colon from peritoneal reflection or properitoneal fat
- Dog ear sign: Pelvic fluid separating bowel from bladder
- Splinting: Scoliotic curvature concave toward injury

CT Findings

- CECT
  - Peritoneal fluid
    - Nonspecific but must consider bowel injury if > trace fluid volume is seen in absence of solid organ injury or pelvic fracture
    - Specificity 15-26%, sensitivity 90-100%
  - Bowel wall thickening of 1 or several loops
    - ≥ 3 mm or disproportionate to normal bowel wall
    - Seen in 75% of full-thickness lacerations
    - Intramural hematoma may show focal, mass-like eccentric thickening
  - Abnormal bowel wall enhancement
    - Psoas muscle is used as reference
    - ↑ enhancement
      - Patchy & irregular with full-thickness laceration
      - Seen paradoxically with hypoperfusion due to damaged vascular endothelium
    - ↓ enhancement
      - Focal contusion/hematoma, traumatic ischemia, &/or mesenteric vascular injury
  - Discontinuity of bowel wall from laceration/perforation
    - Specificity 100%, sensitivity 5-34%
  - Extraluminal enteric contents
    - Specificity ~ 100%, sensitivity 6-15% for perforation
    - Oral contrast does not ↑ sensitivity in blunt trauma; may result in unnecessary delay & aspiration
    - Oral & rectal contrast may help in stable patients with penetrating injury
  - Pneumoperitoneum
    - Angular/curvilinear gas in antidependent abdomen between anterior abdominal wall & liver surface
    - Small, round foci of gas may be confined within mesenteric sheets adjacent to disrupted bowel wall
    - Lung windows are helpful for detection
    - Specificity 95-99%, sensitivity 20-30% for surgically significant injury
    - Sensitivity for bowel perforation ~ 74%
  - Mesenteric fluid, hematoma, &/or stranding
    - Often at mesenteric root; polygonal or V-shaped
    - Sentinel clot (40-80 HU) suggests adjacent bowel injury
  - Mesenteric vessel thrombosis with partial or complete lack of vessel opacification
  - Beaded appearance of mesenteric vessels
  - Active vascular extravasation
    - Irregular, nonanatomic focus of ↑ attenuation (isodense to aorta with arterial injury) near vessel
  - Retroperitoneal gas
    - Perforation of retroperitoneal bowel segments
  - Extraperitoneal gas
    - Perforation of lower 1/3 of rectum

Ultrasonographic Findings

- FAST scan for free fluid in Morison pouch, splenorenal recess, pouch of Douglas, & paracolic gutters
  - Poor sensitivity of 35-44%; not specific for bowel injury
- Bowel wall thickening
- Intramural hematoma: Focal bowel wall thickening of varying echogenicity depending on age
- Pneumoperitoneum: Linear echogenic foci with "dirty" shadowing immediately deep to peritoneal lining

Imaging Recommendations

- Best imaging tool
  - CECT with multiplanar reformats

DIFFERENTIAL DIAGNOSIS

Hypoperfusion Complex (Shock Bowel)

- Diffuse fluid-distended bowel with wall thickening & ↑ enhancement
- ↑ enhancement of adrenals, pancreas, & mesenteric vessels
- ↓ size of aorta & inferior vena cava

Henoch-Schönlein Purpura

- Focal or multifocal bowel wall thickening from hemorrhage of vasculitis
- Purpuric rash on legs & upper extremity extensor surfaces

Inflammatory Bowel Disease

- Colicky abdominal pain, recurrent diarrhea ± blood, weight loss, perianal disease, malabsorption
- Terminal ileal & cecal involvement is most common
- Wall thickening, enhancement ± adjacent mesenteric stranding, vascular engorgement, fat proliferation

Coagulopathy

- Bleeding into bowel wall

Other Causes of Free Intraperitoneal Air

- Iatrogenic introduction of air: Diagnostic peritoneal lavage, peritoneal dialysis catheter, recent surgery
- Air extending from pneumomediastinum, pneumothorax, female genital injury, intraperitoneal bladder perforation
- Air introduced by penetrating injury
- Air from extraperitoneal rectal or bladder perforation
- Serosal rupture of benign colonic pneumatosis beyond infancy

PATHOLOGY

General Features

- Etiology
  - Blunt trauma (77%)
    - Commonly: Motor vehicle related, nonaccidental trauma, bicycle related
    - Intestinal injury in 1-15% of blunt trauma cases
  - Penetrating trauma (23%)
    - Commonly: Gunshot wound, stabbing, impalement
    - Consider sexual assault with rectal trauma
  - Incidence of iatrogenic bowel injury
    - 0.1-7.0% of esophagogastroduodenoscopies, 0.09-3.0% of colonoscopies
- Associated abnormalities
  - Spine injury (including Chance fracture) (9%)
  - Traumatic brain injury (22%)
  - Liver (16%), spleen (11%), pancreas (10%), kidney (6%)
- Injury associated with rectal impalement
  - Anterior: Bladder, uterus, bowel
  - Posterior: Retroperitoneal & vascular structures
  - Perianal: Anus, vagina, urethra

Staging, Grading, & Classification

- American Association for the Surgery of Trauma injury scale
- Grades for stomach injury
  - I: Contusion/hematoma, partial-thickness laceration
  - II: Laceration < 2 cm in gastroesophageal (GE) junction/pylorus, < 5 cm in proximal 1/3 stomach, < 10 cm in distal 2/3 stomach
  - III: Laceration > 2 cm in GE junction/pylorus, > 5 cm in proximal 1/3 stomach, > 10 cm in distal 2/3 stomach
  - IV: Tissue loss/devascularization < 2/3 stomach
  - V: Tissue loss/devascularization > 2/3 stomach
- Grades for jejunum, ileum, colon, & rectum injury
  - I: Contusion or hematoma without devascularization; partial-thickness laceration without perforation
  - II: Laceration < 50% circumference
  - III: Laceration ≥ 50% circumference without transection
  - IV: Transection (small bowel/colon) or full-thickness laceration with extension into perineum (rectum)
  - V: Transection + segmental tissue loss, devascularization

Gross Pathologic & Surgical Features

- Compression of intestinal loops at impact → sudden ↑ in intraluminal pressure → perforation
- Crush injury between anterior abdominal wall & spine
- Rapid deceleration → shear force between fixed & mobile segments of bowel
- Poor fit of seat belt contributes to injury mechanisms
  - "Submarining" under lap belt or lap belt too high on abdomen ± hyperflexion → compression + crush injuries
  - Higher center of gravity in children → shearing force

CLINICAL ISSUES

Presentation

- Abdominal pain, guarding, rigidity, absent bowel sounds, hypotension, tachycardia, elevated WBC
- Seat belt sign in 11%
- Delayed presentation of symptoms > 24 hours: 6.5%

Natural History & Prognosis

- Overall mortality of 5%, usually related to associated injuries
- In contrast to adults, delay in diagnosis & intervention by up to 24 hours does not significantly affect prognosis
- Mesenteric & vascular injury may → delayed bowel injury → ischemia, necrosis, perforation, &/or stenosis
- Can be complicated by sepsis, peritonitis, abscess, postoperative stenosis/obstruction, hernia, leak

Treatment

- Observation + serial examination if diagnosis is in question
  - Clinical deterioration is main indicator for intervention
- Contusion or hematoma typically receives nonoperative management; bowel perforations are managed surgically

DIAGNOSTIC CHECKLIST

Consider

- Unexplained free fluid with focally thickened bowel & surrounding mesenteric edema/hemorrhage is bowel injury until proven otherwise
- Relative risk of bowel injury of 9.4 with lap belt ecchymosis
- Closely analyze bowel in Chance fracture patients

SELECTED REFERENCES

1. Mills A et al: Imaging of bowel wall thickening in the hospitalized patient. Radiol Clin North Am. 58(1):1-17, 2020
2. Shin D et al: Imaging of gastrointestinal tract perforation. Radiol Clin North Am. 58(1):19-44, 2020
3. Bennett AE et al: Multidetector CT imaging of bowel and mesenteric injury: review of key signs. Semin Ultrasound CT MR. 39(4):363-73, 2018
4. Sugi MD et al: CT findings of acute small-bowel entities. Radiographics. 38(5):1352-69, 2018
5. Bates DD et al: Multidetector CT of surgically proven blunt bowel and mesenteric injury. Radiographics. 37(2):613-25, 2017
6. Schooler GR et al: Gastrointestinal tract perforation in the newborn and child: imaging assessment. Semin Ultrasound CT MR. 37(1):54-65, 2016
7. Ellison AM et al: Use of oral contrast for abdominal computed tomography in children with blunt torso trauma. Ann Emerg Med. 66(2):107-14.e4, 2015

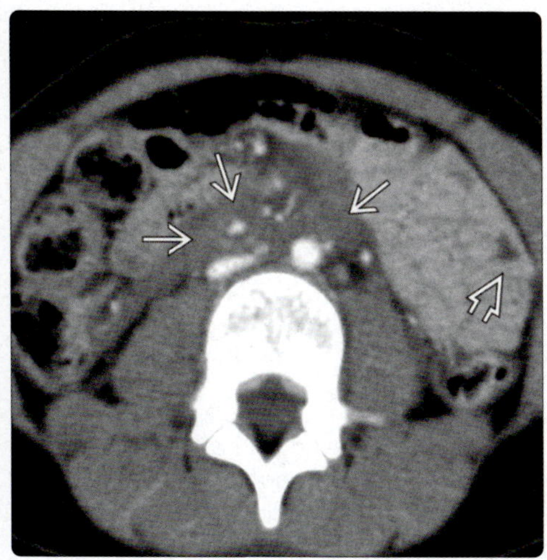

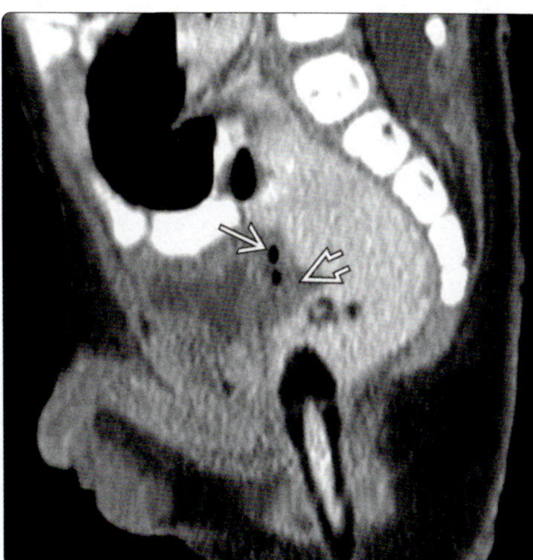

(Left) *Axial CECT in a 7-year-old with a seat belt sign shows high-attenuation fluid at the mesenteric root* → *with foci of small bowel wall thickening* →*. A mesenteric root hematoma & jejunal contusions were found at surgery.* **(Right)** *Sagittal CECT (with rectal contrast) in a 2-year-old who was rectally impaled by a pencil shows extraluminal gas* → *& high-attenuation fluid* → *anterior to the rectum in the rectovesical pouch. An intraperitoneal rectal perforation was found at surgery.*

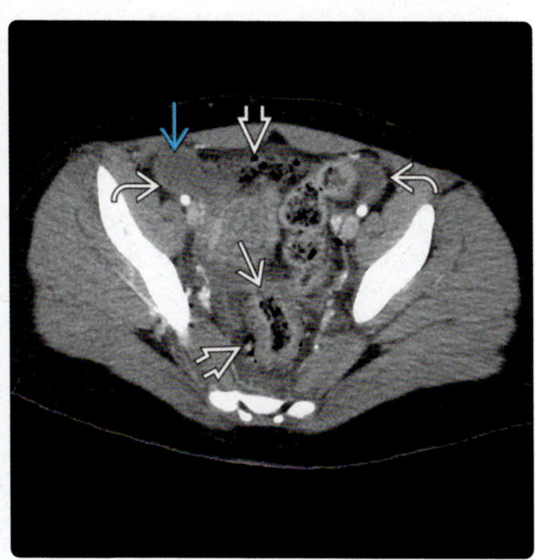

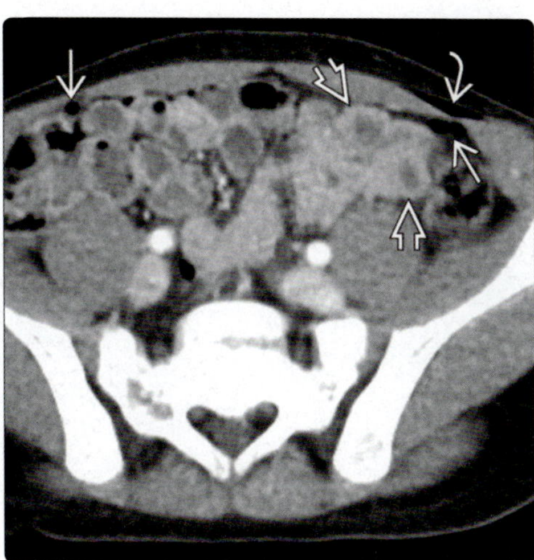

(Left) *Axial CECT in a 15-year-old after a jet ski accident shows discontinuity of the bowel wall at the rectosigmoid junction* →*. There is peritonitis with extraluminal air* →*, peritoneal enhancement* →*, & fluid* →*.* **(Right)** *Axial CECT in a 10-year-old boy shot with a pellet gun shows foci of free intraperitoneal air* → *& small bowel wall thickening* →*. Subcutaneous gas* → *was also seen in the abdominal wall near the site of penetration. Multiple jejunal perforations were discovered at surgery.*

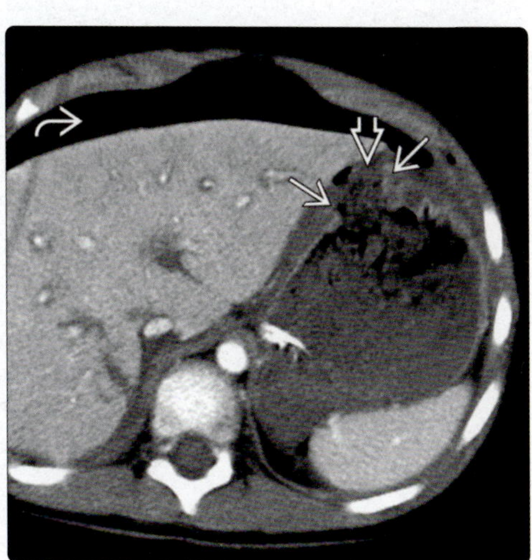

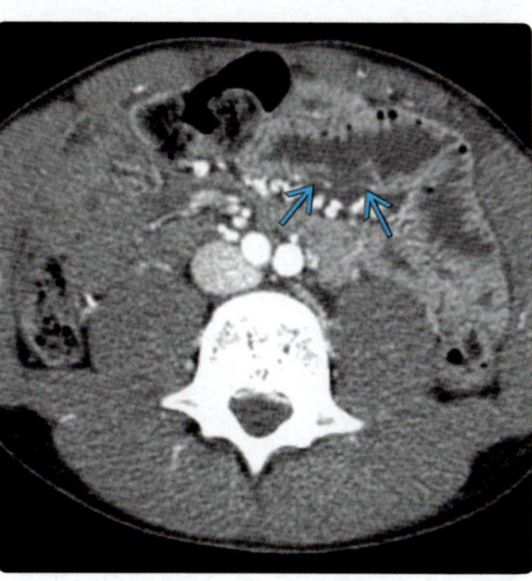

(Left) *Axial CECT in a 4-year-old boy after a motor vehicle accident demonstrates anterior gastric wall disruption* → *with extrusion of contents* →*. There is a large volume of pneumoperitoneum* →*.* **(Right)** *Axial CECT in a 12-year-old with a bicycle handlebar injury shows ↓ & discontinuous enhancement of the posterior wall of a fluid-filled jejunal loop* → *with mild adjacent mesenteric fluid. A jejunal perforation was found intraoperatively.*

KEY FACTS

IMAGING

- Gold standard exam for blunt abdominal trauma: CECT
- Parenchymal laceration
  - Irregular, linear, branching foci of fluid attenuation
  - Posterior right hepatic lobe is most commonly involved
  - Extension to bare area (segment VII) is associated with retroperitoneal hematoma
  - Risk of bile duct injury with extension to porta hepatis
- Hematoma may be intraperitoneal, retroperitoneal, subcapsular, or intraparenchymal
  - Fluid attenuation if hematoma is fresh & unclotted
  - Focal ↑ attenuation may represent clot at site of injury
  - ± hematocrit level of settling peritoneal blood in pelvis
    - ↑ density of dependent-most fluid component is due to layering cellular blood elements
- Active hemorrhage or extravasation
  - Irregular high attenuation near vessel (isodense to aorta with arterial injury); accumulates with delay
  - Majority of patients with contrast extravasation are successfully managed nonoperatively
- Generalized periportal edema
  - Frequent finding of resuscitation due to distended intrahepatic lymphatics from vigorous hydration

TOP DIFFERENTIAL DIAGNOSES

- Normal fissures
- Artifacts: Beam hardening or motion
- Hepatic abscess

CLINICAL ISSUES

- Nonoperative management of hemodynamically stable patients: > 90% successful
- Complications: Biliary injury, pseudoaneurysm, arteriovenous fistula, delayed hemorrhage, abscess
- Routine follow-up imaging is not indicated for asymptomatic patients with low-grade injury
- ↑ liver enzymes in infant warrant CECT in presence of other clinical/radiological signs of nonaccidental trauma

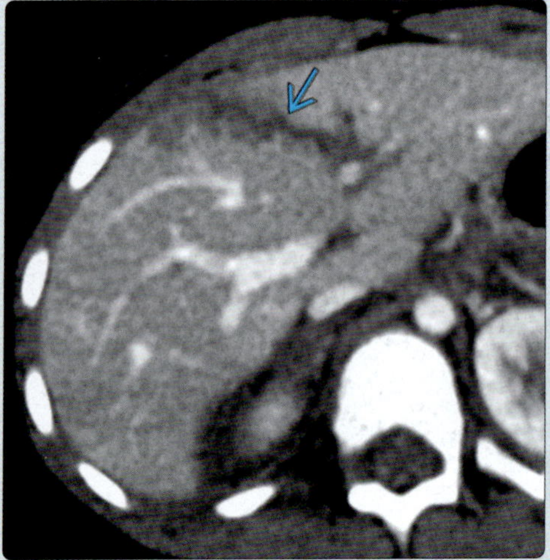

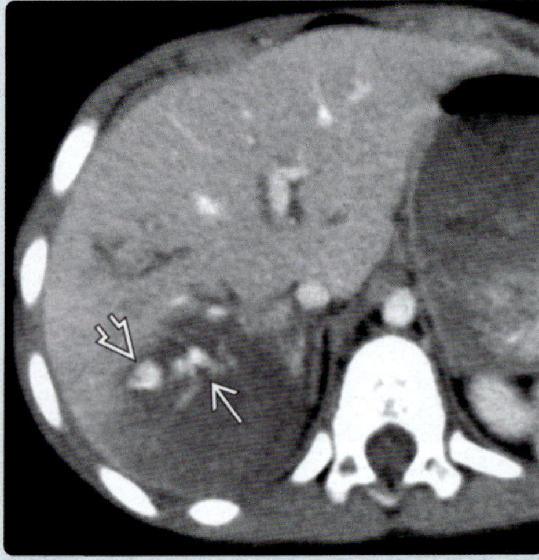

(Left) *Axial CECT in a 6-year-old girl after a motor vehicle accident depicts a laceration* ➡ *of the medial left hepatic lobe > 4 cm in depth, consistent with a grade III injury.* **(Right)** *Axial CECT in a 6-year-old car accident victim shows irregular areas of contrast extravasation contained within the parenchyma, compatible with a grade III injury* ➡*. The more rounded focus of contrast is suspicious for a pseudoaneurysm* ➡*.*

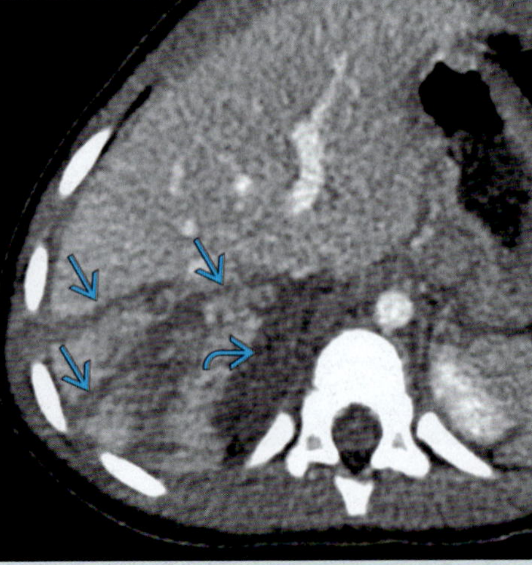

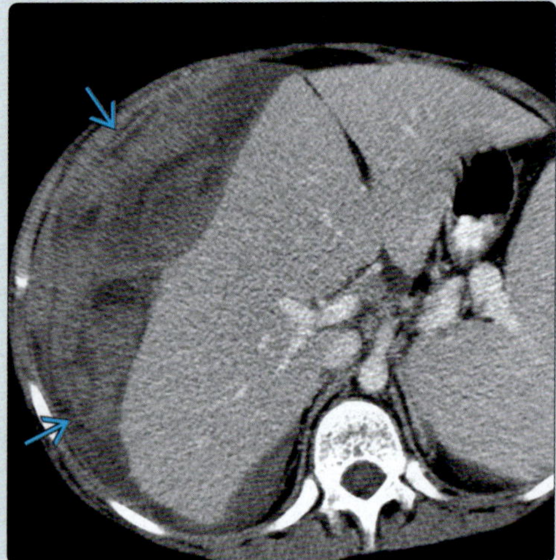

(Left) *Axial CECT in a 2-year-old boy hit by a car shows branching hypodense lacerations* ➡ *extending from the superior posterior aspect of the right hepatic lobe (bare area). This disrupted > 25% of the right lobe, consistent with a grade IV injury. There is associated retroperitoneal hemorrhage* ➡*.* **(Right)** *Axial CECT in a 12-year-old boy 1 day after liver biopsy shows a mixed attenuation, > 50% surface area subcapsular hematoma* ➡*, consistent with a grade III injury. Higher density in the hematoma represents clot.*

TERMINOLOGY

Synonyms

- Liver or hepatic laceration, fracture, or injury

IMAGING

CT Findings

- CECT
  - Laceration
    - Irregular, linear, branching foci of nonenhancement in liver parenchyma
    - May parallel hepatic or portal veins
  - Hematoma
    - Round, crescentic, or poorly defined fluid collection
    - Focal ↑ attenuation (40-70 HU) may represent clot & implicate site of injury
    - Subcapsular
      - Lentiform or crescentic peripheral collection
      - Compresses convex margin of parenchyma
    - Intraparenchymal
      - Round or irregular
    - Intraperitoneal
      - Poorly defined, tracking dependently in abdomen/pelvis vs. focal collections
      - ± hematocrit level of dependently settling peritoneal blood components in pelvis
    - Retroperitoneal
      - Surrounds inferior vena cava, right adrenal gland
      - Often occurs with lacerations of bare area (segment VII)
  - Active hemorrhage or extravasation
    - Irregular collection of high attenuation near vessel (isodense to aorta with arterial injury); accumulates on delayed images
  - Pseudoaneurysm
    - Round focus of high attenuation (isodense to aorta)
    - Will have diminished attenuation on delayed images
    - Decompression into biliary system → hemobilia, melena
  - Arteriovenous fistula (AVF)
    - Early enhancement of involved hepatic/portal vein, simultaneous with artery
  - Biliary injury (biloma, leak): Delayed, simple-appearing fluid accumulations without clinical hematocrit drop
    - Often with lacerations extending to porta hepatis + contracted gallbladder
  - Periportal edema: Generalized ↓ attenuation surrounding portal veins
    - Most commonly due to lymphatic engorgement from aggressive hydration rather than periportal blood

Ultrasonographic Findings

- Grayscale ultrasound
  - Limited for detecting hepatic injury in acute setting
    - Abdominal US: 51% sensitivity, 95% specificity
    - Abdominal CEUS: 84% sensitivity, 99% specificity
    - FAST exam: 55% sensitivity, 83% specificity for intraabdominal injury
  - Echogenicity of hematoma/laceration varies with age
    - Anechoic (initially unclotted) → hyperechoic (24 hours with fibrin & clot) → hypoechoic (2-3 days with liquefaction of blood)
  - Pseudoaneurysm
    - Anechoic, cyst-like structure near vessel
    - Yin-yang sign on color Doppler
  - AVF
    - Dilated hepatic artery with very low resistance
    - Arterialized portal/hepatic venous waveform
    - Surrounding tissue vibration
  - Biliary injury (biloma, leak)
    - Delayed appearance of intrahepatic/intraperitoneal anechoic collection ± septations
    - Continued accumulation without hematocrit drop
- CEUS
  - Laceration/contusions: Linear, round, or irregular areas of nonenhancement
  - Active bleeding: Intra- or extraparenchymal contrast pooling that ↑ in size

MR Findings

- T1 & T2 signal intensity varies with hematoma age
- MRCP can be useful in evaluation of biliary tree

Nuclear Medicine Findings

- Hepatobiliary scintigraphy
  - Bile leak: Accumulating extrabiliary collection of radiotracer around liver in peritoneal cavity
  - Biloma: Focal, contained extrabiliary radiotracer

Imaging Recommendations

- Best imaging tool: CECT

DIFFERENTIAL DIAGNOSIS

Normal Fissures

- Isolated thin, smooth, linear hypodense foci in characteristic locations for ligamentum venosum or falciform ligament

Artifacts

- Beam hardening: ↓ density streaks extending from ribs
- Excessive patient motion: Random throughout whole image ± adjacent images
- Both artifacts extend beyond liver

Hepatic Abscess

- Round or irregular discrete lesion(s) in ill patient
- Central fluid attenuation with thick, irregular rim & septal enhancement ± surrounding edema

Primary Tumor or Metastatic Disease

- Neoplasm may rupture or bleed, ± trauma

Liver Infarction

- Peripheral, wedge-shaped focus of nonenhancement
- Uncommon in children, occasionally results from trauma

PATHOLOGY

General Features

- Etiology
  - Blunt vs. penetrating trauma: 90% vs. 10%
    - Blunt trauma causes deceleration or shearing injury
      - Motor vehicle-related injuries are most common

- Falls & recreational accidents
- Hepatic injury is seen in 25% of blunt trauma cases & 3% of nonaccidental trauma (NAT) cases overall
- Associated abnormalities
  - Concomitant splenic injury: 45%

Staging, Grading, & Classification

- American Association for the Surgery of Trauma (AAST)
  - Grade I
    - Hematoma: Subcapsular, < 10% surface area
    - Laceration: < 1-cm parenchymal depth
  - Grade II
    - Hematoma: Subcapsular, 10-50% surface area; intraparenchymal, < 10 cm in diameter
    - Laceration: 1- to 3-cm parenchymal depth & ≤ 10 cm in length
  - Grade III
    - Hematoma: Subcapsular, > 50% surface area or ruptured subcapsular or parenchymal hematoma; intraparenchymal, > 10 cm
    - Laceration: > 3-cm parenchymal depth
    - Vascular injury (defined as pseudoaneurysm or AVF) or active bleeding contained within parenchyma
  - Grade IV
    - Laceration: Parenchymal disruption involving 25-75% of 1 hepatic lobe
    - Active bleeding extending beyond liver parenchyma into peritoneum
  - Grade V
    - Laceration: Parenchymal disruption involving > 75% of hepatic lobe
    - Vascular: Juxtahepatic venous injuries (i.e., retrohepatic vena cava/central major hepatic veins)
  - ↑ 1 grade for multiple injuries up to grade III

Gross Pathologic & Surgical Features

- Pattern of injury
  - Posterior segment of right lobe is most common
    - Greatest volume of liver & surrounded by ribs, spine
    - Fixation by coronary ligaments enhances effect of acceleration-deceleration injury
  - Left lobe is most commonly injured in NAT

CLINICAL ISSUES

Presentation

- Most common signs/symptoms
  - Right upper quadrant pain, guarding, rebound tenderness, hypotension, lap belt ecchymosis (seat belt sign); elevated LFTs

Natural History & Prognosis

- Hemodynamic stability is primary determinant of nonoperative success
  - > 90% are successfully managed nonoperatively
- Contrast extravasation
  - Associated with more severe overall injury & transfusion
  - Association with delayed hemorrhage is debated
  - Nonoperative management is successful in 83% of patients with contrast extravasation
- Complications
  - Typically occur with higher grade injuries (> grade III)
  - Biliary: Biloma (most common), bile leak, hemobilia
  - Vascular: Pseudoaneurysm, AVF, delayed hemorrhage
  - Abscess

Treatment

- Nonoperative management if hemodynamically stable
- 2019 updated American Pediatric Surgical Association guidelines for hemodynamically stable isolated liver injury
  - Length of stay is based on clinical presentation
  - Activity restriction = injury grade + 2 weeks
    - Imaging may not correlate with organ integrity
    - Return to full-contact sports at discretion of surgeon
  - Arterial embolization
    - May be useful in patients with arterial contrast extravasation + hemodynamic compromise from ongoing bleeding
    - Prophylactic embolization is not indicated if hemodynamically stable
  - Follow-up imaging
    - Routine reimaging of asymptomatic, uncomplicated, low-grade injuries is not indicated
    - Limited data support reimaging of high-grade injuries
    - Symptomatic patients may benefit from reimaging
- ATOMAC+ guidelines outline clinical parameters to define end point for nonoperative management
- Laparotomy & surgical hemostasis in unstable patients
- Consider ERCP + sphincterotomy &/or stent for bile leak

DIAGNOSTIC CHECKLIST

Consider

- In infants, CECT is warranted with ↑ liver enzymes + clinical/radiological signs of NAT

Image Interpretation Pearls

- Describe hepatic injuries & seek out additional injuries that may be less obvious but of greater clinical significance

Reporting Tips

- AAST grade guides management

SELECTED REFERENCES

1. Di Renzo D et al: Contrast-enhanced ultrasonography (CEUS) in the follow-up of pediatric abdominal injuries: value and timing. J Ultrasound. 23(2):151-5, 2020
2. Gates RL et al: Non-operative management of solid organ injuries in children: an American Pediatric Surgical Association Outcomes and Evidence Based Practice Committee systematic review. J Pediatr Surg. 54(8):1519-26, 2019
3. Katsura M et al: Association between contrast extravasation on computed tomography scans and pseudoaneurysm formation in pediatric blunt splenic and hepatic injury: a multi-institutional observational study. J Pediatr Surg. 55(4):681-7, 2019
4. Notrica DM et al: Reimaging in pediatric blunt spleen and liver injury. J Pediatr Surg. 54(2):340-4, 2019
5. Trinci M et al: Contrast-enhanced ultrasound (CEUS) in pediatric blunt abdominal trauma. J Ultrasound. 22(1):27-40, 2019
6. Armstrong LB et al: Contrast enhanced ultrasound for the evaluation of blunt pediatric abdominal trauma. J Pediatr Surg. 53(3):548-52, 2018
7. Kozar RA et al: Organ injury scaling 2018 update: spleen, liver, and kidney. J Trauma Acute Care Surg. 85(6):1119-22, 2018
8. The American Association for the Surgery of Trauma: Injury Scoring Scale. Update 2018. Accessed October 3, 2021. https://www.aast.org/resources-detail/injury-scoring-scale#liver
9. Temiz A et al: Management of traumatic bile duct injuries in children. Pediatr Surg Int. 34(8):829-36, 2018
10. Ingram MC et al: Hepatic and splenic blush on computed tomography in children following blunt abdominal trauma: Is intervention necessary? J Trauma Acute Care Surg. 81(2):266-70, 2016

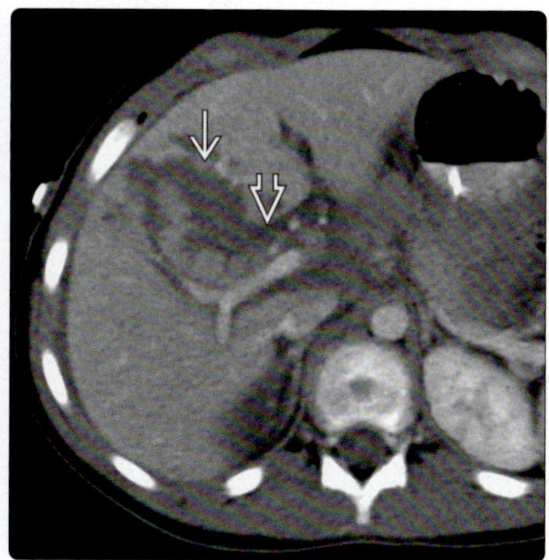

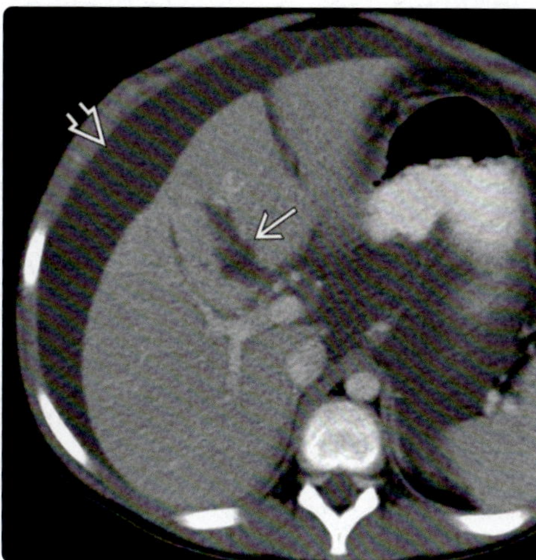

(Left) *Axial CECT in an 11-year-old with right upper quadrant pain after a roller skating accident shows a grade IV liver laceration ➡ that extends to the porta hepatis ➡.* **(Right)** *Axial CECT in the same patient was performed 9 days later for increasing jaundice & distention. While the laceration is again seen ➡, there is new moderate to large volume of free fluid ➡.*

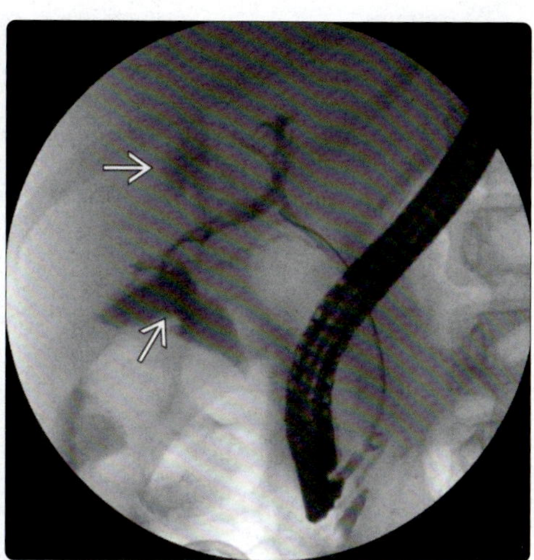

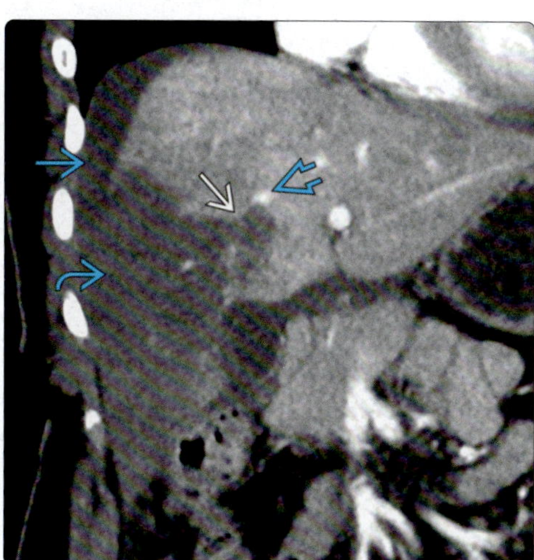

(Left) *ERCP in the same patient demonstrates irregular pools of contrast ➡ collecting along the biliary system during injection, compatible with biliary injury.* **(Right)** *Coronal CECT in a 14-year-old girl after an all-terrain vehicle accident shows a laceration ➡ extending to the right hepatic vein ➡ with devascularization of the inferior right hepatic lobe ➡. Injuries to the retrohepatic inferior vena cava or central major hepatic veins are grade V injuries. Hemoperitoneum ➡ is also shown.*

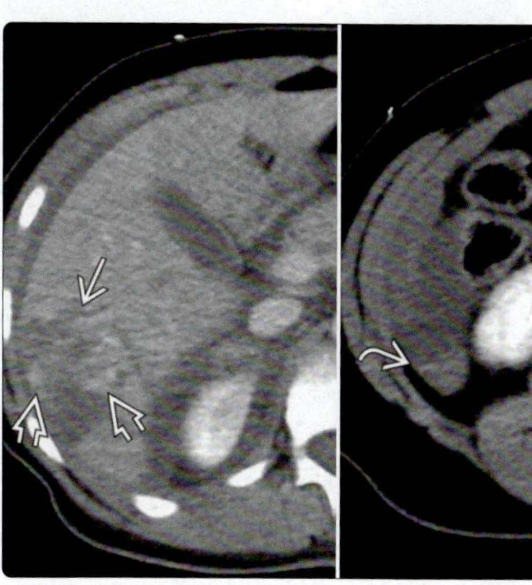

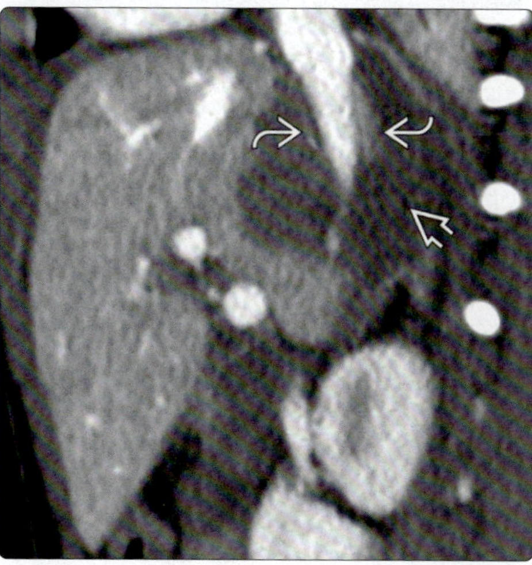

(Left) *Axial CECT images obtained in an 11-year-old that was hit by a bus demonstrate a laceration ➡ with ill-defined vascular contrast extravasation ➡ that extends inferior ➡ to the liver parenchyma, compatible with a grade IV injury.* **(Right)** *Right parasagittal CECT in a 3-year-old trauma patient with a laceration that extends to the inferior vena cava demonstrates contrast extravasation ➡ & retrohepatic hematoma ➡, compatible with a grade V injury.*

Splenic Trauma

KEY FACTS

IMAGING

- CECT: Gold standard for blunt abdominal trauma
- Laceration: Irregular, linear, branching foci of fluid density
- Hematoma: Intraperitoneal, retroperitoneal, subcapsular, &/or intraparenchymal collection(s)
  - Fluid attenuation (0-30 HU) if fresh, unclotted blood; ↑ attenuation (40-80 HU) suggests clotted blood, may implicate site of injury by proximity (sentinel clot)
- Active extravasation: Irregular, nonanatomic focus of ↑ density (isodense to adjacent artery); accumulates on delayed images
- Pseudoaneurysm: ↑ density outpouching of arterial lumen (isodense to adjacent artery); washes out with delay
- Complications: Pseudocyst, pseudoaneurysm, arteriovenous fistula, delayed rupture (hemorrhage > 48 hours after trauma), venous thrombosis, abscess

TOP DIFFERENTIAL DIAGNOSES

- Splenic cleft
- Artifacts: Beam hardening, early bolus, patient motion
- Hypoperfusion complex
- Splenic infarct
- Splenic abscess

PATHOLOGY

- Typical etiologies: Blunt trauma, motor vehicle accident
- ± additional injuries: Left lower rib fractures, other viscera

CLINICAL ISSUES

- Presentations: LUQ pain & tenderness, hypotension
- Treatment
  - Nonoperative management of isolated blunt splenic injury in stable patients: > 95% success rate
  - Routine follow-up is not indicated in asymptomatic patients with low-grade injury
  - Prophylactic arterial embolization is not indicated in hemodynamically stable patients with contrast extravasation

(Left) *Axial CECT in an 8-year-old after a motor vehicle accident shows a grade V splenic injury. There is contrast extravasation ➡ that extends outside the fractured spleen ➡ with high-density fluid ➡ (i.e., blood) throughout the abdomen.* **(Right)** *Coronal CECT in a patient injured while playing basketball shows a grade III splenic injury with lacerations > 3 cm in depth ➡. A subcapsular hematoma > 50% of the splenic surface area ➡ scallops the splenic margin ➡.*

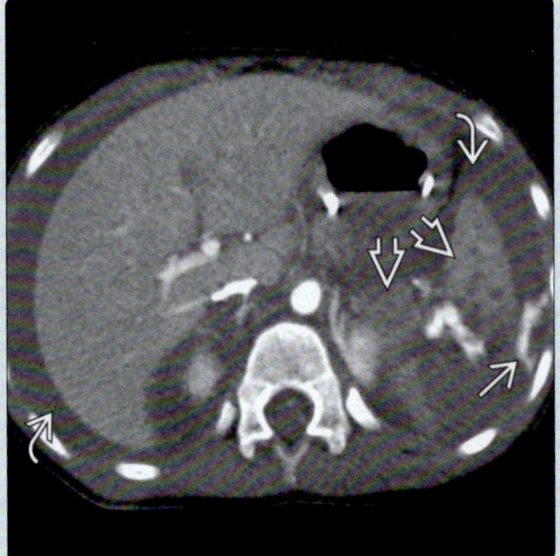

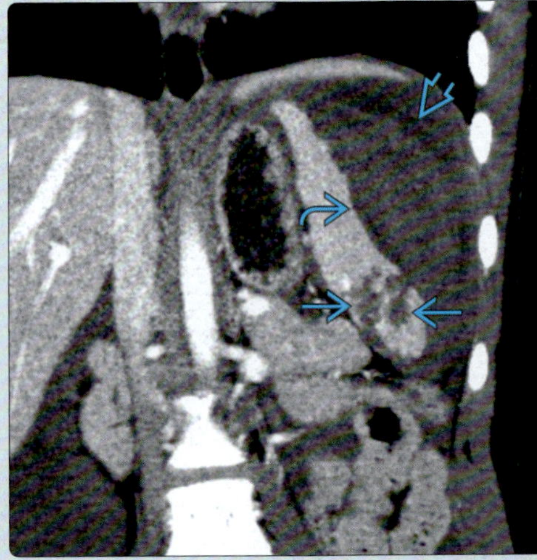

(Left) *Coronal CECT in a 14-year-old after a fall from a bike shows a grade IV splenic injury involving hilar vessels ➡ with major devascularization of the spleen (> 25%) as represented by the hypoattenuating parenchyma ➡. A perisplenic hematoma ➡ is also noted.* **(Right)** *Coronal CECT in a 14-year-old injured while skiing shows a grade III splenic injury. Branching linear & jagged hypodensities > 3 cm in depth ➡ & extending to the splenic capsule are consistent with lacerations. A small perisplenic hematoma ➡ is also seen.*

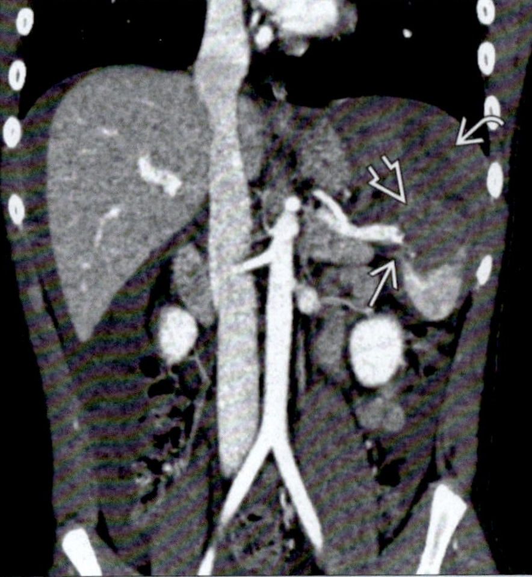

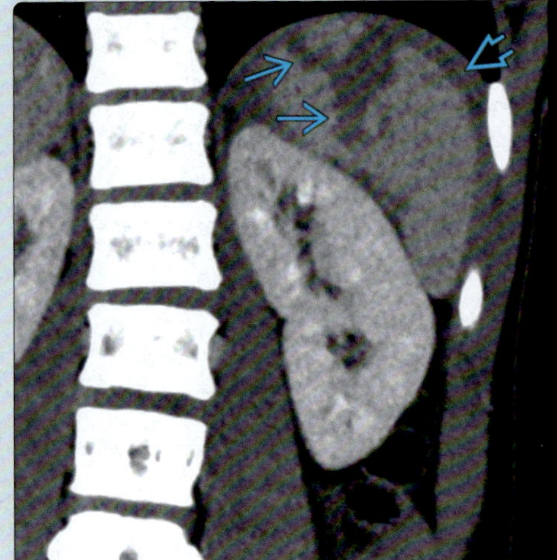

TERMINOLOGY

Synonyms

- Splenic laceration, fracture, or injury; blunt injury to spleen

Definitions

- Parenchymal injury to spleen ± capsular disruption

IMAGING

General Features

- Best diagnostic clue
  - Jagged, linear, fluid-density foci in splenic parenchyma ± intraparenchymal or subcapsular fluid collection
  - Perisplenic hematoma > 40 Hounsfield units (HU)

Radiographic Findings

- Triad: Elevated left hemidiaphragm, left lower lobe atelectasis/collapse, left pleural effusion
- Left lower rib fractures are common (44% of patients)
- Medial displacement of gastric bubble
- Inferior displacement of splenic flexure, bowel gas
- Hemorrhage may obscure contours of intraperitoneal/retroperitoneal structures: Psoas margin, flank stripe, renal contour, splenic margin

CT Findings

- CECT
  - Accuracy 98%, sensitivity 95%
  - Laceration: Irregular, fluid-attenuation, linear/branching foci within parenchyma; may extend to capsule
  - Fracture: Laceration extending from one capsular surface to another
  - Rupture: Multiple fractures with discontinuous splenic fragments
  - Hematoma: Fluid-attenuation (0-30 HU) collection; ↑ attenuation (40-80 HU) may represent clotted blood
    - Parenchymal: Round or irregular collection in spleen
    - Subcapsular: Peripheral crescentic or lenticular collection compressing parenchymal margin
    - Perisplenic: Collection in adjacent peritoneal spaces
      - Sentinel dense clot adjacent to spleen: Sensitive predictor for splenic injury
    - Hemoperitoneum: Layering, dense hematocrit level in dependent pelvis (may be subtle)
    - Retroperitoneal: Typically if splenic hilum is injured
      - Involves splenorenal ligament, anterior pararenal space, pancreas
  - Active arterial hemorrhage (extravasation)
    - Irregular, nonanatomic contrast collection; isodense to aorta; accumulates on delayed images
  - Pseudoaneurysm
    - ↑ attenuation outpouching of arterial lumen; isodense to aorta
    - ↓ attenuation on delayed images without ↑ size
    - Almost 75% are not seen on initial CECT
  - Arteriovenous fistula (AVF)
    - Early enhancement of involved vein, simultaneous with artery
  - Venous thrombosis: Focal or diffuse lack of splenic vein enhancement despite visualization of other veins

Ultrasonographic Findings

- Grayscale ultrasound
  - Linear or branching hypoechoic foci
  - Subcapsular or perisplenic collection with variable echogenicity
  - Free intraperitoneal fluid (absent in 25% of splenic injury)
- Color Doppler
  - Splaying or compression of vessels by hematoma
  - Yin-yang appearance of pseudoaneurysm
  - Lack of splenic vein flow with venous thrombus
  - Lack of parenchymal flow with devascularizing injury
- CEUS: 93% sensitivity, 99% specificity
  - Laceration/contusions: Linear, round, or irregular areas of nonenhancement
  - Active bleeding: Intra- or extraparenchymal contrast pooling that ↑ in size
- FAST exam: 37-85% sensitivity, 99-100% specificity

Angiographic Findings

- Blush from active arterial extravasation of contrast
- Distortion of vessels & enhancing parenchyma by hematoma
- Pseudoaneurysm: Arterial outpouching
- Venous thrombosis: Filling defect

Imaging Recommendations

- Best imaging tool
  - CECT rapidly covers entire abdomen & pelvis

DIFFERENTIAL DIAGNOSIS

Splenic Cleft

- Congenital variant in contour of spleen
- Smooth, thin, curvilinear ↓ attenuation focus without other evidence of hemorrhage

Artifacts

- Beam hardening: Linear hypodense streaks from ribs/arms
- Motion: Blurring or discontinuity of structures across image
- Early bolus: Specific pattern of enhancement
  - Parallel, archiform, "corrugated" waves of ↓ splenic enhancement on early arterial-phase CECT
    - 95% resolve by 70 seconds
    - Due to enhancement differences of red & white pulp

Hypoperfusion Complex

- ↓ splenic enhancement; fluid-filled bowel with ↑ wall enhancement diffusely
- ± flattened inferior vena cava, intensely enhancing small-caliber aorta

Splenic Infarct

- Wedge-shaped focus of ↓ density with apex towards hilum
- Associated with splenomegaly & systemic disorders

Splenic Abscess

- Fluid attenuation with enhancing rim, surrounding edema
- Clinical history/findings of infection, immunodeficiency, trauma, emboli, travel, or cat-scratch disease

PATHOLOGY

General Features

- Etiology
  - Blunt trauma
    - Motor vehicle accident is most common
    - Bicycle-related, falls, sports-related injuries
    - Iatrogenic injury is rare (thoracentesis, biopsy, intraoperative)
    - Nonaccidental trauma (NAT) is rare cause (1%)
      - Seen in up to 26% of NAT patients
  - Preexisting splenic enlargement (EBV, hematologic disorders) predisposes to injury

Staging, Grading, & Classification

- American Association for the Surgery of Trauma (AAST)
  - Grade I
    - Hematoma: Subcapsular, < 10% surface area
    - Laceration: Capsular tear, < 1-cm parenchymal depth
  - Grade II
    - Hematoma: Subcapsular, 10-50% surface area; intraparenchymal, < 5 cm in diameter
    - Laceration: 1- to 3-cm parenchymal depth
  - Grade III
    - Hematoma: Subcapsular, > 50% surface area; ruptured subcapsular or parenchymal hematoma; intraparenchymal hematoma ≥ 5 cm or expanding
    - Laceration: > 3-cm parenchymal depth
  - Grade IV
    - Laceration: Involving segmental or hilar vessels producing > 25% devascularization
    - Vascular injury (defined as pseudoaneurysm or AVF) or active bleeding confined within capsule
  - Grade V
    - Laceration: Completely shattered
    - Active bleeding extending beyond spleen into peritoneum
  - Advance 1 grade for multiple injuries up to grade III

Gross Pathologic & Surgical Features

- Forceful flexion of spleen along axis
- Laceration is typically intersegmental, extending towards hilum

CLINICAL ISSUES

Presentation

- Most common signs/symptoms
  - Left upper quadrant (LUQ) tenderness, pain
  - Hypotension (25-30%); lap belt ecchymosis, seat belt sign
- Other signs/symptoms
  - Rib pain: Left lower posterior rib fractures
  - Kehr sign: Pain radiating to left shoulder by phrenic nerve; abdominal rigidity, shock in neonates
  - Not clinically apparent (10-20%)

Natural History & Prognosis

- Nonoperative management of isolated blunt splenic injuries in stable patients: > 95% success rate
  - Hemodynamic stability is important for nonoperative success
- Contrast extravasation
  - Associated with more severe overall injury & transfusion
  - Pseudoaneurysm may result in delayed hemorrhage; many spontaneously resolve
    - Some data suggest association with contrast extravasation on initial CT
  - Nonoperative management is successful in 83% of patients with contrast extravasation
- Complications: Pseudocyst, pseudoaneurysm, AVF, delayed rupture (hemorrhage > 48 hours after trauma), venous thrombosis, abscess

Treatment

- 2019 updated American Pediatric Surgical Association (APSA) guidelines for hemodynamically stable patient with isolated splenic injury
  - Length of stay is based on clinical presentation
  - Activity restriction = injury grade + 2 weeks
    - Imaging may not correlate with organ integrity
    - Return to full-contact sports at discretion of surgeon
  - Arterial embolization
    - May be useful in patients with arterial contrast extravasation + hemodynamic compromise from ongoing bleeding
    - Prophylactic embolization is not indicated if hemodynamically stable
  - Follow-up imaging: Routine reimaging of asymptomatic, uncomplicated, low-grade injuries is not indicated
    - Limited data support reimaging of high-grade injuries
    - Symptomatic patients may benefit from reimaging
- ATOMAC+ guidelines outline clinical parameters to define end point for nonoperative management
- Splenectomy or splenorrhaphy when surgery is required
  - ↑ hospital stay, ↑ transfusions, ↑ infections
- Vaccination (pneumococcal, *Haemophilus influenzae* type b, meningococcal, influenza) if no functional spleen
- Daily prophylactic antibiotics in patients < 5 years old without functional spleen

DIAGNOSTIC CHECKLIST

Reporting Tips

- Injury grade assists with management decisions

SELECTED REFERENCES

1. Di Renzo D et al: Contrast-enhanced ultrasonography (CEUS) in the follow-up of pediatric abdominal injuries: value and timing. J Ultrasound. 23(2):151-5, 2020
2. Gates RL et al: Non-operative management of solid organ injuries in children: an American Pediatric Surgical Association Outcomes and Evidence Based Practice Committee systematic review. J Pediatr Surg. 54(8):1519-26, 2019
3. Notrica DM et al: Reimaging in pediatric blunt spleen and liver injury. J Pediatr Surg. 54(2):340-4, 2019
4. Stylianos S: To save a child's spleen: 50years from Toronto to ATOMAC. J Pediatr Surg. 54(1):9-15, 2019
5. The American Association for the Surgery of Trauma: Injury Scoring Scale, Updated 2018. Accessed October 3, 2021. https://www.aast.org/resources-detail/injury-scoring-scale#spleen
6. Armstrong LB et al: Contrast enhanced ultrasound for the evaluation of blunt pediatric abdominal trauma. J Pediatr Surg. 53(3):548-52, 2018
7. Durkin N et al: Post-traumatic liver and splenic pseudoaneurysms in children: diagnosis, management, and follow-up screening using contrast enhanced ultrasound (CEUS). J Pediatr Surg. 51(2):289-92, 2016
8. Ingram MC et al: Hepatic and splenic blush on computed tomography in children following blunt abdominal trauma: is intervention necessary? J Trauma Acute Care Surg. 81(2):266-70, 2016

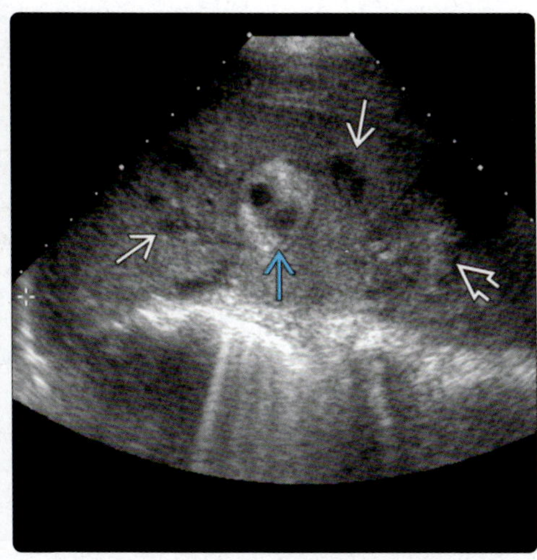

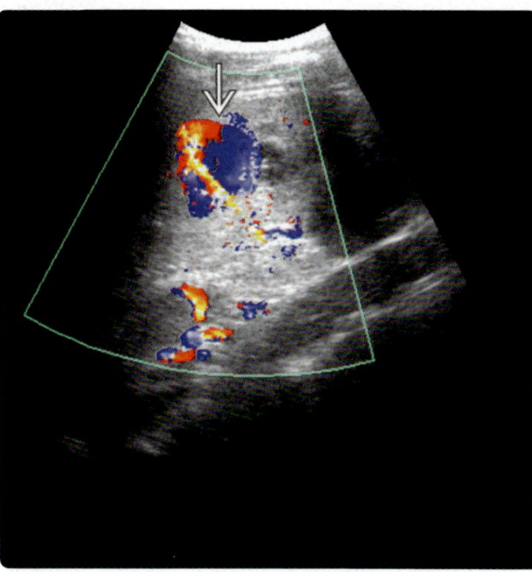

(Left) *Longitudinal ultrasound of the spleen in a pediatric trauma patient shows multiple irregular, hypoechoic lacerations & an ill-defined heterogeneous region of hematoma. A rounded, heterogeneously hyper- & hypoechoic focus centrally is suspicious for pseudoaneurysm.* **(Right)** *Color Doppler ultrasound in the same patient shows the characteristic yin-yang sign of bidirectional flow in the round, heterogeneous lesion, consistent with a traumatic pseudoaneurysm.*

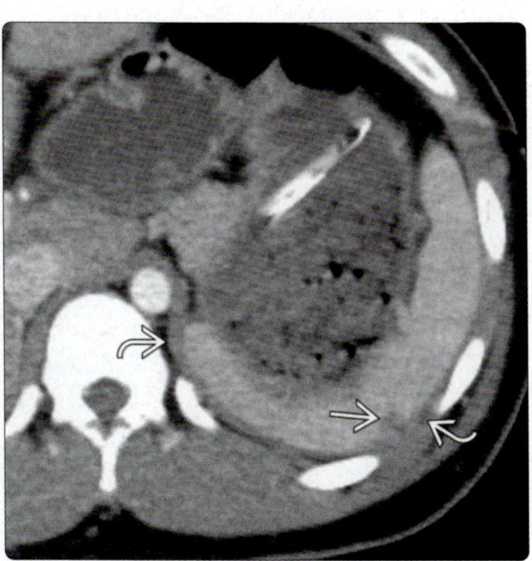

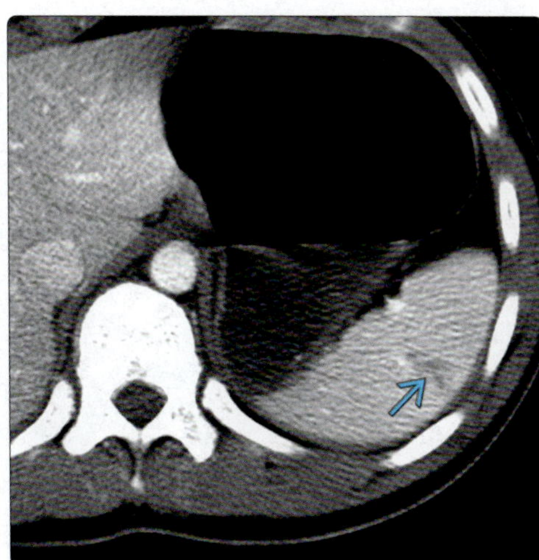

(Left) *Axial CECT obtained in a 14-year-old after a skiing accident shows an irregular parenchymal hypodensity < 1 cm in depth, compatible with a grade I injury. Trace perisplenic fluid is also seen.* **(Right)** *Axial CECT shows a small, irregular, linear, hypodense band within the spleen. This was categorized as a grade II splenic injury given that it was between 1-3 cm in length.*

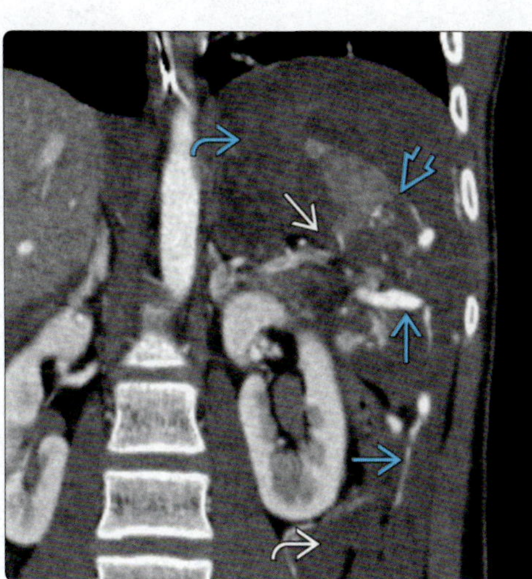

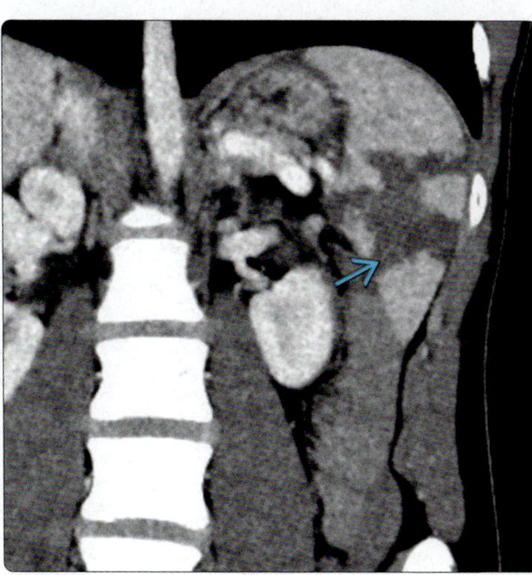

(Left) *Coronal CECT in a patient hit by a train shows a grade V splenic injury. The spleen is shattered & devascularized due to hilar avulsion. There is contrast extravasation from active arterial hemorrhage extending beyond the spleen. Note the large perisplenic hematoma & hemoperitoneum.* **(Right)** *Coronal CECT in a 15-year-old trauma patient depicts a jagged, stellate hypodensity representing a branching laceration, consistent with a grade III splenic injury.*

Duodenal Trauma

KEY FACTS

IMAGING

- CECT is best imaging tool in acute trauma setting
- Injuries classified as hematoma vs. laceration
  - Hematoma: Nonenhancing intraluminal, intramural, &/or paraduodenal collection of ↑ attenuation
    - Intraluminal: Expansile ovoid or tubular filling defect
      - Coiled-spring appearance on upper GI series
    - Intramural: Mass-like focal wall thickening ± intramural gas; eccentric narrowing of displaced lumen
  - Duodenal laceration/perforation
    - Interruption of bowel wall, extravasation of intraluminal contents, & free retroperitoneal air: Specific but not sensitive
    - Duodenal wall thickening > 3 mm & ↑ attenuation fluid + stranding in retroperitoneum: Sensitive but not specific
- Associated pancreatic trauma in up to 42% of cases

PATHOLOGY

- Blunt trauma in > 70%, penetrating trauma in > 20%
  - Motor vehicle accident, fall, bicycle handlebar injury, assault
  - Consider nonaccidental trauma in young patients (particularly < 2 years old with delayed presentation)
- Also consider with bleeding disorders, anticoagulation, Henoch-Schönlein purpura, recent endoscopic procedures

CLINICAL ISSUES

- Common symptoms: Abdominal pain, nausea, vomiting
- Delay in diagnosis & treatment: ↑ morbidity & mortality
- Treatment
  - Intramural/intraluminal hematoma: Initial management is nonoperative (bowel rest, TPN, nasogastric decompression); drainage in refractory cases
  - Perforation: Primary surgical repair & drainage vs. more complex procedures in severe cases

(Left) *Axial CECT in a 17-year-old boy with abdominal pain after being kicked shows retroperitoneal air ➡ posterior to the 2nd & 3rd portions of the duodenum (D2 & D3) & posterior to the right kidney ⇨. Adjacent fluid is also noted ↪. A duodenal laceration was found at surgery.* **(Right)** *Coronal CECT in a 16-year-old with perforation from an ERCP shows active contrast extravasation ➡ into a large hematoma that distends the duodenum ➡. Note the adjacent pneumoperitoneum ⇨.*

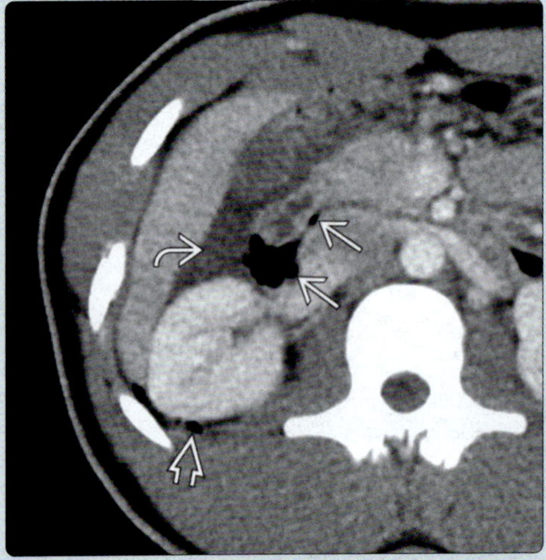

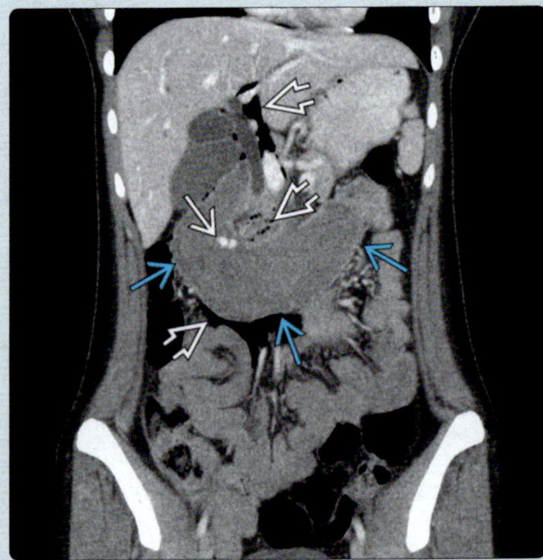

(Left) *Supine AP radiograph shows gas outlining the right kidney ➡ & underlying the medial right diaphragm ⇨ in this 11-year-old nonaccidental trauma victim.* **(Right)** *Axial CECT in the same patient demonstrates discontinuity of the hyperenhancing duodenal wall at D2, compatible with perforation ➡. There is free retroperitoneal ➡ & intraperitoneal air ⇨. A laceration involving intra- & retroperitoneal portions of the duodenum was discovered at surgery.*

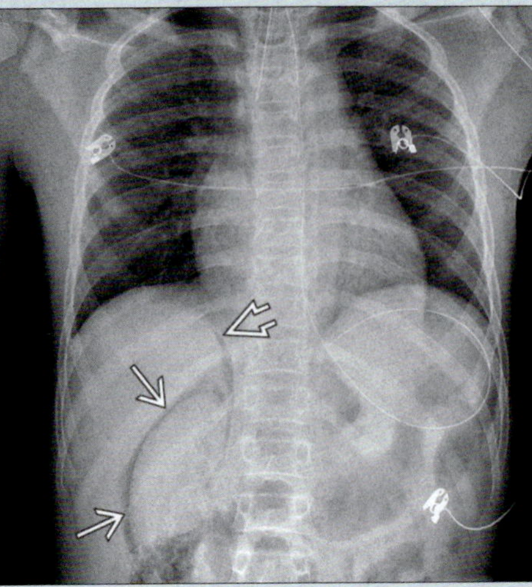

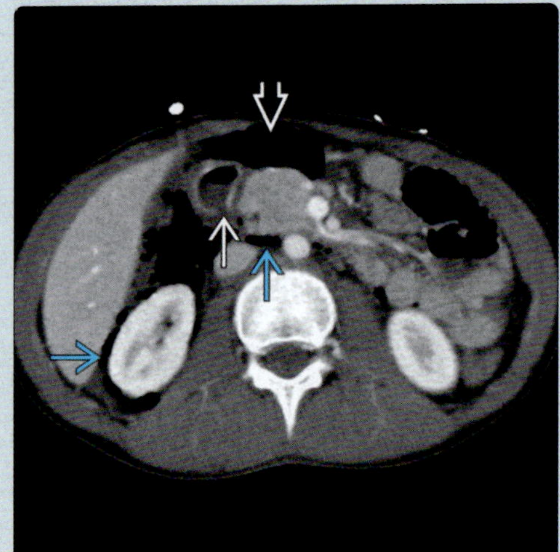

Duodenal Trauma

TERMINOLOGY

Abbreviations

- D[x] = segment of duodenum (e.g., D1 = 1st segment of duodenum)

IMAGING

General Features

- Location
  - Most commonly involves D2 (46%) or D3 (63%)

Radiographic Findings

- Mass effect of hematoma may lead to
  - Dilated stomach &/or duodenal bulb
  - Displaced bowel gas in right upper quadrant (RUQ)
- Laceration may lead to
  - Retroperitoneal air (from D2-D4 injury)
    - Outlines kidneys, psoas muscles
  - Intraperitoneal air (from D1 injury)
    - Upright or left-side down (i.e., left lateral decubitus) view: Air under diaphragm overlying liver
    - Supine
      - Rigler sign: Air on both sides of bowel wall
      - Falciform ligament sign: Vertical linear density in RUQ outlined by air lucency
      - Football sign: Ovoid lucency of whole abdomen

Fluoroscopic Findings

- Upper GI
  - Typically not performed in acute trauma setting
  - Intramural hematoma
    - Displaced lumen with eccentric or circumferential narrowing/obstruction
    - Wall/fold thickening
  - Intraluminal hematoma
    - Ovoid clot expands duodenal lumen
    - Coiled-spring appearance due to contrast tracking between mucosal folds & intraluminal clot

CT Findings

- CECT
  - Hematoma: Well-circumscribed, ovoid, heterogeneous, or homogeneous mass with ↑ attenuation of 40-80 HU
    - Occurs in lumen, bowel wall, or paraduodenal tissues
      - Dense sentinel clot may localize injury site
  - Contusion: Focal duodenal wall thickening/edema
    - > 3 mm or disproportionate to normal bowel wall
  - Vascular insult vs. response to wall injury: Abnormal bowel wall enhancement
    - Judged relative to psoas muscle
    - ↑ enhancement: Paradoxically found with hypoperfusion due to damaged vascular endothelium
    - ↓ enhancement: Suggests traumatic ischemia, vascular compromise
  - Specific signs of duodenal laceration/perforation
    - Interruption of enhancing bowel wall
    - Extraluminal contrast &/or air
      - Retroperitoneal (if D2-D4) or intraperitoneal (if D1)
      - Sensitivity of free air for traumatic bowel injury: 30-60%
      - Lung windows ↑ sensitivity for free air

MR Findings

- Not generally performed in acute trauma setting
- T1, T2: Hematoma signal varies with age
- T1 C+: Nonenhancing mass; may have enhancing rim

Ultrasonographic Findings

- Grayscale ultrasound
  - Hematoma
    - Focal intramural/intraluminal/paraduodenal mass, wall thickening, or collection
    - Variable echogenicity based on age; ↓ with time
  - Retroperitoneal air: May see linear hyperechogenicity with "dirty" posterior acoustic shadowing
- Color Doppler
  - No vascularity within hematoma

Imaging Recommendations

- Best imaging tool: CECT
  - In blunt trauma setting, oral contrast does not significantly improve sensitivity for duodenal injury → delay in imaging & treatment
  - In cases with persistent clinical symptoms, consider follow-up with ultrasound or upper GI every 7 days

DIFFERENTIAL DIAGNOSIS

Enteric Duplication Cyst

- 12% occur in gastroduodenal location
- Well-circumscribed, cystic mass
- US: Cyst wall frequently has trilaminar gut signature; may demonstrate peristalsis

Duodenal Ulcer/Duodenitis

- Uncommon in young patients
- Poorly defined proximal duodenal wall edema with interruption of enhancing mucosa
- May perforate → extraluminal gas
- May cause duodenal stricture & gastric outlet obstruction

Crohn Disease

- Involves duodenum in 5-20% of patients
- Wall thickening, hyperenhancement, or stricture
- May form fistula with adjacent bowel

Small Bowel Neoplasm

- Rare in children; Burkitt lymphoma is most common
- Typically enhances & demonstrates internal vascularity, unlike hematoma
- May cause duodenal luminal narrowing or (rarely) paradoxical dilation

Pancreatitis

- Enlarged, edematous pancreas with peripancreatic stranding & fluid
- Duodenum may have secondary inflammatory change

Pancreatic Trauma

- Concomitant pancreatic & duodenal injuries are common
- Enlarged, edematous pancreas with peripancreatic stranding & fluid
- Linear transversely oriented focus of ↓ attenuation due to parenchymal laceration

Annular Pancreas

- Commonly presents in neonatal period
- Ring of pancreatic tissue surrounding D2 results in duodenal stenosis, obstruction

PATHOLOGY

General Features

- Etiology
  - Blunt trauma accounts for > 70% of duodenal injuries
    - Duodenal injury in 2-10% of children with blunt abdominal trauma
    - Common causes: Motor vehicle accidents, falls, bicycle-related accidents, nonaccidental trauma (NAT)
      - Consider NAT in younger patients (particularly < 2 years of age) with delayed presentation to emergency department
  - Penetrating trauma in > 20%
  - Iatrogenic
    - Upper endoscopy with biopsy: Hematoma in 0.1-7.0%
      - ↑ risk in bone marrow transplant patients
    - ERCP: Hematoma in 1.3%, perforation in 0.1-0.6%
  - Spontaneous intramural hematomas occur with bleeding disorders, anticoagulation therapy, vasculitis, Henoch-Schönlein purpura
- Associated abnormalities
  - Abdominal injuries: Pancreas 42%, liver 29%, spleen 17%
  - Duodenal hematoma may obstruct papilla of Vater → cholestasis & pancreatitis

Staging, Grading, & Classification

- American Association for the Surgery of Trauma Organ Injury Scale
  - I: Hematoma involving single portion of duodenum; partial-thickness laceration without perforation
  - II: Hematoma involving > 1 portion of duodenum; laceration disrupting < 50% of circumference
  - III: Laceration disrupting 50-75% of circumference of D2 or 50-100% D1/D3/D4
  - IV: Laceration disrupting > 75% of circumference of D2 or involving ampulla or distal common bile duct
  - V: Laceration with massive disruption of duodenopancreatic complex; duodenum devascularized
  - Advance 1 grade for multiple injuries up to grade III

Gross Pathologic & Surgical Features

- 3 mechanisms act in isolation or in combination
  - Compression of intestinal loops at impact
    - Sudden ↑ in intraluminal pressure → perforation
  - Direct force crush-injury between anterior abdominal wall & spine
  - Rapid deceleration → tear at junction of mobile intraperitoneal & fixed retroperitoneal segments

Microscopic Features

- Duodenal hematoma typically develops in submucosal &/or subserosal layers

CLINICAL ISSUES

Presentation

- Most common signs/symptoms
  - Nausea, vomiting, abdominal pain

Natural History & Prognosis

- Overall morbidity 48%, mortality 19%
- Delay in diagnosis & treatment → ↑ length of hospitalization, ICU time, need for TPN, complication rates
- Mortality is usually secondary to associated injuries, most commonly traumatic brain injuries
- Stricture may rarely occur as long-term complication
- Postoperative complications: Postoperative ileus 19%, wound infection 9%, traumatic pancreatitis 5%, abscess 3%, pancreatic fistula 2%, enterocutaneous fistula 2%

Treatment

- Nonoperative
  - Hemodynamically stable patients
  - Bowel rest, nasogastric decompression, TPN
  - Progressive symptoms, worsening imaging findings, or unresolved obstruction due to hematoma after 14 days may indicate nonoperative management failure
    - Consider operative management or percutaneous drainage of hematoma
    - Nonoperative failure rate for hematoma: 5-10%
- Operative
  - Hemodynamically unstable & patients with definite evidence of perforation
  - Duodenal primary repair/resection, nasogastric decompression, drain
  - Ancillary pyloric exclusion ± gastrojejunostomy & biliary diversion considered for grades III, IV, & V
- Disruption of duodenopancreatic complex
  - May require antrectomy & gastrojejunostomy or other Roux-en-Y reconstructions depending on level of injury
  - Staged pancreaticoduodenectomy for extensive duodenopancreatic complex injury

DIAGNOSTIC CHECKLIST

Image Interpretation Pearls

- Duodenal injury is suggested by wall thickening &/or intraluminal mass + air, fluid, or stranding in retroperitoneum
  - Bowel wall interruption & extravasation are rarely seen
- Evaluate pancreas closely for concomitant injury
- Consider NAT in younger patients (especially patients < 2 years old with delayed presentation)

SELECTED REFERENCES

1. Shin D et al: Imaging of gastrointestinal tract perforation. Radiol Clin North Am. 58(1):19-44, 2020
2. Coccolini F et al: Duodeno-pancreatic and extrahepatic biliary tree trauma: WSES-AAST guidelines. World J Emerg Surg. 14:56, 2019
3. Niehues SM et al: Intramural duodenal hematoma: clinical course and imaging findings. Acta Radiol Open. 8(4):2058460119836256, 2019
4. Bennett AE et al: Multidetector CT imaging of bowel and mesenteric injury: review of key signs. Semin Ultrasound CT MR. 39(4):363-73, 2018
5. The American Association for the Surgery of Trauma: Injury Scoring Scale. Updated 2018. Accessed October 3, 2021. https://www.aast.org/resources-detail/injury-scoring-scale#duodenum
6. Sugi MD et al: CT findings of acute small-bowel entities. Radiographics. 38(5):1352-69, 2018
7. Zhou H et al: Evolution of intramural duodenal hematomas on magnetic resonance imaging. Pediatr Radiol. 48(11):1593-9, 2018
8. Melamud K et al: Imaging of pancreatic and duodenal trauma. Radiol Clin North Am. 53(4):757-71, viii, 2015

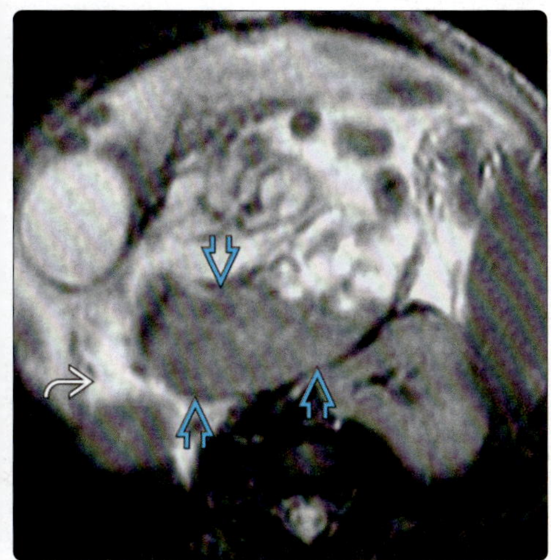

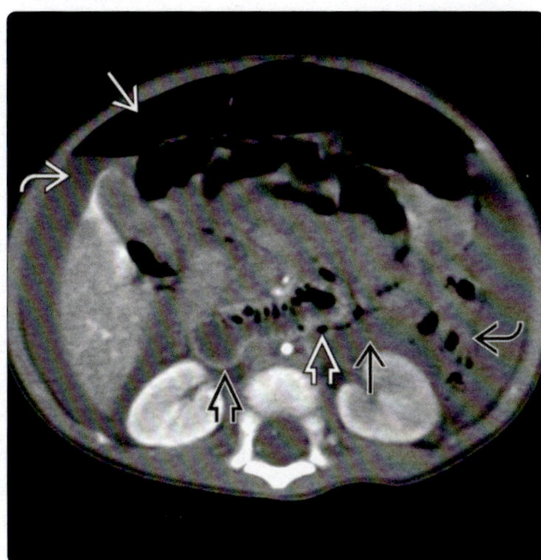

(Left) *Axial T2 FS MR shows an intermediate signal intensity hematoma filling D3* ⇨ *in this patient with liver disease & a preceding endoscopic biopsy. Note the adjacent fluid* ➨. **(Right)** *Axial CECT in a 9-year-old with nonaccidental trauma shows free intra-* ➨ *&* *retroperitoneal* ➨ *air as well as intra-* ➨ *& retroperitoneal* ⇨ *fluid. Mucosal hyperenhancement* ⇨ *& small bowel wall thickening* ⇨ *are also noted. Perforations of the duodenum & jejunum were repaired surgically.*

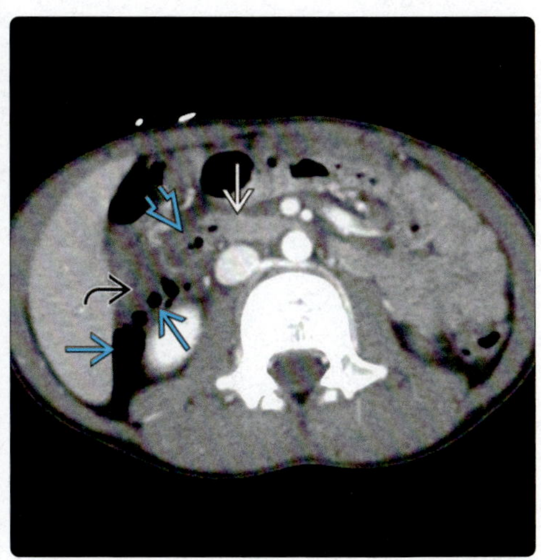

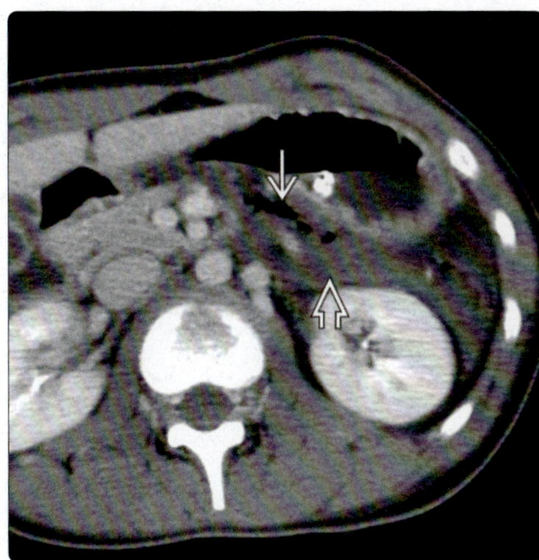

(Left) *Axial CECT in an 8-year-old with a handlebar injury shows hyperenhancement of the D3 wall* ➨ *with retroperitoneal air* ⇨ *& fluid* ⇨. *There is poor definition of the bowel wall* ⇨ *at the junction of D2 & D3 with perforations confirmed at this level at surgery.* **(Right)** *Axial CECT in a 16-year-old girl after a motor vehicle accident shows free air* ➨ *& fluid* ➨ *in the anterior pararenal space near D3 & D4. A perforation was found at this site during surgery.*

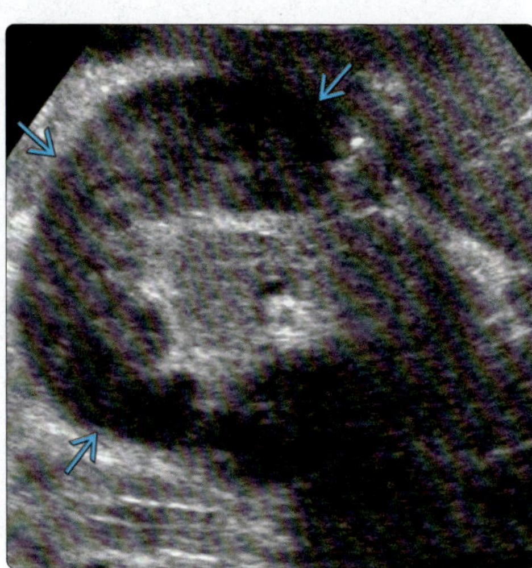

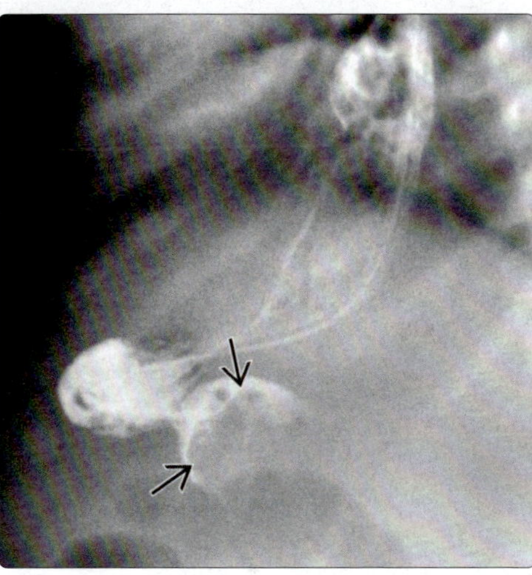

(Left) *Transverse ultrasound in a 2-year-old girl with pancytopenia & hematemesis after endoscopy with biopsy shows a bulky, C-shaped, heterogeneous mass of D1-D3* ⇨*, consistent with an intraluminal duodenal hematoma.* **(Right)** *Lateral view from an upper GI series in the same patient demonstrates a large, obstructive filling defect* ⇨ *expanding D1, consistent with an intraluminal duodenal hematoma.*

Pancreatic Trauma

KEY FACTS

IMAGING

- Modality of choice: CECT
  - Caveat: 20-40% false-negative rate in first 12 hours
- Classic imaging findings
  - Contusion/inflammation: Focal or diffuse ↓ enhancement & ↑ size relative to normal parenchyma
  - Laceration: Linear fluid-attenuation parenchymal defect
    - Usually of short axis; most common at junctions of pancreatic head-neck or body-tail
    - Depth > 50% suggests pancreatic duct disruption
  - Hematoma: Irregular or round fluid collection in/around pancreas; ↑ attenuation (40-80 HU) if clotted
  - Varying degrees of peripancreatic fluid tracking along/within fascial planes & adjacent compartments
- MRCP or ERCP to assess main pancreatic duct injury

PATHOLOGY

- Blunt trauma in 93%, penetrating trauma in 7% of cases
- Pancreatic injury in 17% of nonaccidental trauma patients

CLINICAL ISSUES

- Epigastric pain out of proportion to physical findings
- ↑ serum amylase (may be normal initially)
- Management of American Association for the Surgery of Trauma grades
  - I & II: Typically nonoperative
    - TPN, serial abdominal exams, bowel rest, nasogastric tube, ± percutaneous/endoscopic collection drainage, ± endoscopic duct stenting
    - Failure is more likely with pancreatic duct injury
  - III-V: No consensus on management strategy
    - Hemodynamic stability is important determinant
    - Nonoperative management is successful in 89% of those attempted; risk of pseudocyst formation
    - Operative management: Pancreaticojejunostomy, operative drainage, spleen-sparing partial/distal pancreatectomy

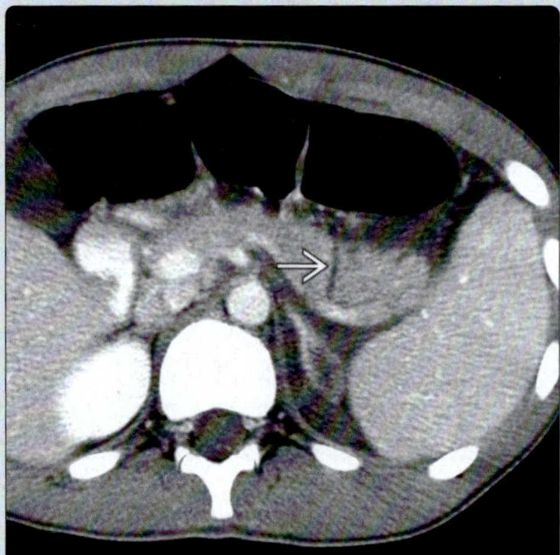

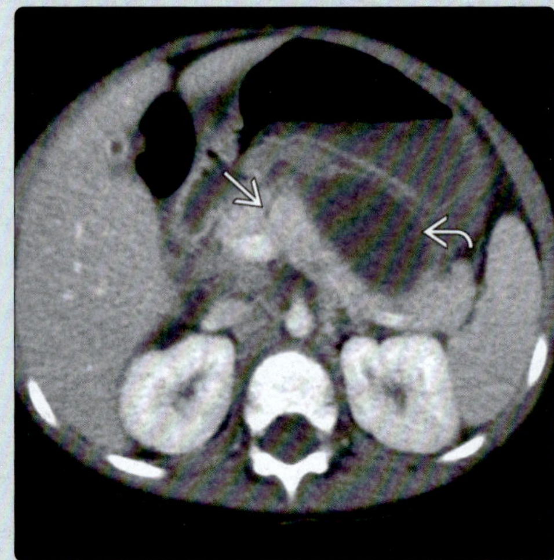

(Left) *Axial CECT in a 14-year-old patient who sustained an elbow injury to the abdomen shows a linear, fluid-density laceration ➔ through the pancreatic body near the tail. A left adrenal injury was also noted on contiguous images.* **(Right)** *Axial CECT in a 2-year-old nonaccidental trauma victim with elevated serum amylase shows a laceration at the pancreatic neck-body junction ➔. The > 50% depth of the laceration is concerning for duct injury, & a large pancreatic bed fluid collection is noted anteriorly ➔.*

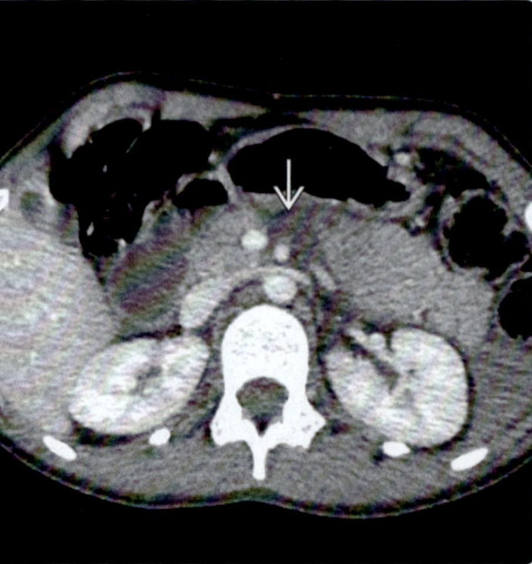

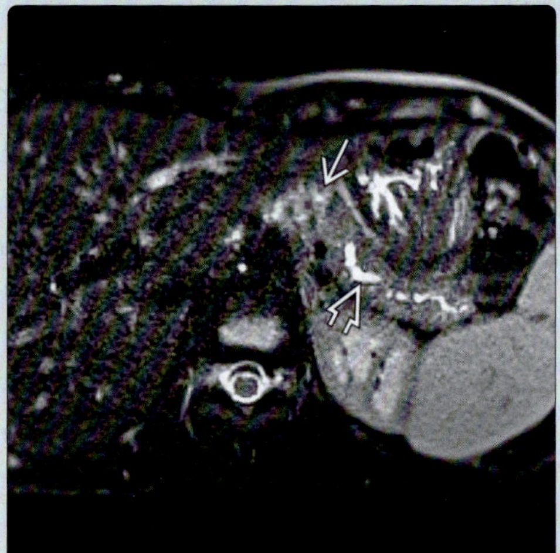

(Left) *Axial CECT in a 12-year-old patient after a motor vehicle accident shows a fluid-attenuation laceration ➔ through the body of the pancreas with depth > 50% of the parenchyma.* **(Right)** *Axial STIR MR in the same patient from a follow-up study performed 6 months later shows high signal at the site of the laceration ➔ as well as dilation & irregularity of the upstream pancreatic duct ➔, suggesting a duct stricture.*

IMAGING

General Features

- Best diagnostic clue
  - Linear, fluid-attenuation cleft through short axis of enhancing pancreas + peripancreatic fluid

CT Findings

- CECT
  - Contusion/inflammation
    - Focal or diffuse ↓ attenuation relative to normally enhancing parenchyma
    - Focal or diffuse enlargement of pancreas
  - Laceration
    - Linear fluid-attenuation cleft; ↑ attenuation with clotted blood (40-80 HU)
    - Usually involves short axis of organ
      - Most common at junctions of pancreatic head-neck or body-tail
    - Depth > 50% suggests pancreatic duct disruption
  - Hematoma
    - Irregular or round parenchymal/peripancreatic fluid-attenuation collection; ↑ attenuation with clotted blood (40-80 HU)
  - Fluid collections adjacent to & tracking away from pancreas
    - Separating splenic vein & pancreas
    - Surrounding superior mesenteric & portal veins
    - Separating pancreas & duodenum
    - Intraperitoneal: Lesser sac, paracolic gutters
    - Retroperitoneal: Anterior & posterior pararenal spaces
      - Thickening of fascial planes
  - Pseudocyst
    - Well-circumscribed peripancreatic fluid collection (in absence of pancreatic necrosis)
      - < 4 weeks = acute peripancreatic fluid collection
      - ≥ 4 weeks + enhancing rim = pseudocyst
    - Components are essentially all liquefied

MR Findings

- T2WI
  - ↑ signal intensity in & around pancreas: Edema, hemorrhage, pancreatic enzymes, inflammation
  - Focal or diffuse pancreatic enlargement
  - Linear discontinuity of parenchyma in short axis: ↑ intensity fluid within defect or separating 2 fragments of fractured parenchyma
- T1WI C+
  - Heterogeneous enhancement of pancreas
  - Nonenhancing fluid collections
  - Pseudocyst (≥ 4 weeks post trauma)
    - Nonenhancing, low signal intensity fluid collection
      - Hyperintense signal may indicate hemorrhage (with precontrast T1 shortening)
    - May have enhancing capsule
- MRCP
  - Allows better visualization of duct vs. CT
  - Signs of pancreatic duct injury
    - Disruption of duct continuity ± dilation
    - Signal intensity difference proximal vs. distal to injury
    - Continuity of pseudocyst with pancreatic duct
  - May be difficult to distinguish disruption vs. compression by extrinsic collection

Ultrasonographic Findings

- Grayscale ultrasound
  - Hematoma
    - Poorly marginated fluid collection in/around pancreas; variable echogenicity
  - Laceration
    - Linear hypoechoic defect in parenchyma; hyperechoic with clot
  - Contusion
    - Focal/diffuse enlargement of hypoechoic gland ± peripancreatic fluid
  - Pseudocyst (≥ 4 weeks post trauma)
    - Anechoic collection ± septations, thick rim
    - Internal echoes may indicate infection or hemorrhage
- For acute pancreatic injury, abdominal US sensitivity is 44-71%, specificity 100%

Fluoroscopic Findings

- ERCP
  - Definitive pancreatic duct evaluation
    - Duct may be normal, deviated, or narrowed with contusion or laceration
    - Duct obstruction: Disruption vs. compression
    - Duct laceration is confirmed with irregular pooling of contrast adjacent to main/branch duct (extravasation)
      - ± continuity of duct with fluid collection, pseudocyst
      - ± extension of contrast into retroperitoneal spaces
  - At risk for post-ERCP pancreatitis, infection, stricture
  - Not always readily available

Imaging Recommendations

- Best imaging tool
  - CECT
    - Caveat: 20-40% false-negative rate in first 12 hours
  - MRCP or ERCP if main pancreatic duct injury is suspected

DIFFERENTIAL DIAGNOSIS

Shock Pancreas

- Diffusely enlarged & heterogeneous pancreas
  - Low-attenuation septa throughout enhancing parenchyma
- Typical constellation of findings in hypoperfusion complex
  - Diffuse fluid distention of small bowel with thickened, hyperenhancing walls
  - Intense enhancement of adrenal glands
  - ↓ caliber of hyperenhancing aorta; collapsed inferior vena cava
  - Free fluid & mesenteric stranding

Duodenal Trauma

- Hematoma/contusion
  - Wall thickening, ↓ enhancement, &/or ovoid intramural/intraluminal mass
- Duodenal perforation
  - Retroperitoneal contrast, extraluminal gas, discontinuity of enhancing duodenal wall
- Luminal narrowing, edema/fluid in retroperitoneum

- High association with pancreatic injuries

Pancreatitis

- Focal/diffuse pancreatic enlargement with mildly ↓ enhancement
- Peripancreatic fluid & fat stranding
- Fluid in lesser sac &/or anterior pararenal space
- Areas of nonenhancement represent necrosis

PATHOLOGY

General Features

- Etiology
  - Blunt trauma: 93% of pancreatic injuries
    - Motor vehicle related 36%, bicycle injury 24%, nonaccidental trauma 10%, other assault 8%, fall 7%, other blunt injury 15%
  - Penetrating trauma: 7% of pancreatic injuries
    - Gunshot wound: 88% of penetrating injuries
- Pancreatic injury found in
  - 0.4% of abdominal trauma patients; 0.3% of blunt & 0.1% of penetrating trauma patients
    - 15% involve pancreatic duct
  - 17% of patients admitted for nonaccidental trauma
- Mechanism of injury
  - AP force compresses pancreas against spine
  - Children at greater risk than adults

Staging, Grading, & Classification

- American Association for the Surgery of Trauma (AAST)
  - Grade I: Minor contusion without duct injury; superficial laceration without duct injury
  - Grade II: Major contusion, no duct injury or tissue loss; major laceration, no duct injury or tissue loss
  - Grade III: Distal transection or parenchymal injury with duct injury
  - Grade IV: Proximal (right of superior mesenteric vein) transection or parenchymal injury involving ampulla
  - Grade V: Massive disruption of pancreatic head
  - Advance 1 grade for multiple injuries up to grade III

CLINICAL ISSUES

Presentation

- Clinical triad
  - Epigastric pain out of proportion to physical findings
  - Leukocytosis
  - ↑ serum amylase
    - May be normal initially
    - Trend may help identify injury or complications
    - Magnitude is not predictive of injury severity
    - Not specific to pancreatic injury
- Isolated injuries are rare (< 30%); average of 3-4 coexisting injuries per patient
  - Hepatic: 46.8%; major vascular: 41.3%; splenic: 28%; renal: 23.4%; duodenal: 19.3%
- Subtle imaging findings may lead to delay in diagnosis & treatment with ↑ morbidity & mortality

Natural History & Prognosis

- Pancreatic duct injury: Critical prognostic factor
  - ↑ morbidity, more likely to fail nonoperative management
- Complications
  - Pancreatitis: 3-26%; pseudocyst: 15-35%; fistula: 2-15%; abscess 10-25%

Treatment

- Grades I & II
  - Nonoperative management if hemodynamically stable
    - Successful in 96% of cases
    - TPN ± percutaneous or endoscopic fluid drainage
    - Serial abdominal exams, bowel rest, nasogastric tube
- Grades III-V
  - No consensus regarding nonoperative vs. early operative management; hemodynamic stability is important determinant
  - Nonoperative management
    - Attempted in 46% of patients; successful in 89%
    - ↑ rates of pseudocyst formation & repeat IR or endoscopic drainage procedures
    - At risk for post-ERCP pancreatitis, infection, stricture
    - US if symptoms progress/persist or if patient is unable to tolerate oral diet after 7 days
  - Operative management
    - Options include: Pancreaticojejunostomy, operative drainage (open cystogastrostomy, Roux-en-Y), spleen-sparing partial/distal pancreatectomy
    - Complications include: Bowel obstruction, fistula, leak/dehiscence, pancreatitis, infection
- With penetrating trauma, operative exploration is often necessary to manage associated injuries
- US, CEUS, or MR is recommended for follow-up of fluid collections, pseudocysts, pancreatic disruption

SELECTED REFERENCES

1. Ibrahim A et al: CT and MRI findings in pancreatic trauma in children and correlation with outcome. Pediatr Radiol. 50(7):943-52, 2020
2. Coccolini F et al: Duodeno-pancreatic and extrahepatic biliary tree trauma: WSES-AAST guidelines. World J Emerg Surg. 14:56, 2019
3. Rosenfeld EH et al: Management and outcomes of peripancreatic fluid collections and pseudocysts following non-operative management of pancreatic injuries in children. Pediatr Surg Int. 35(8):861-7, 2019
4. Rosenfeld EH et al: Comparison of diagnostic imaging modalities for the evaluation of pancreatic duct injury in children: a multi-institutional analysis from the Pancreatic Trauma Study Group. Pediatr Surg Int. 34(9):961-6, 2018
5. Koh EY et al: Operative versus nonoperative management of blunt pancreatic trauma in children: a systematic review. Pancreas. 46(9):1091-7, 2017
6. Naik-Mathuria BJ et al: Proposed clinical pathway for nonoperative management of high-grade pediatric pancreatic injuries based on a multicenter analysis: a pediatric trauma society collaborative. J Trauma Acute Care Surg. 83(4):589-96, 2017
7. Englum BR et al: Management of blunt pancreatic trauma in children: review of the National Trauma Data Bank. J Pediatr Surg. 51(9):1526-31, 2016
8. Garvey EM et al: Role of ERCP in pediatric blunt abdominal trauma: a case series at a level one pediatric trauma center. J Pediatr Surg. 50(2):335-8, 2015
9. Melamud K et al: Imaging of pancreatic and duodenal trauma. Radiol Clin North Am. 53(4):757-71, viii, 2015
10. Iqbal CW et al: Operative vs nonoperative management for blunt pancreatic transection in children: multi-institutional outcomes. J Am Coll Surg. 218(2):157-62, 2014
11. Westgarth-Taylor C et al: Paediatric pancreatic trauma: a review of the literature and results of a multicentre survey on patient management. S Afr Med J. 104(11 Pt 2):803-7, 2014

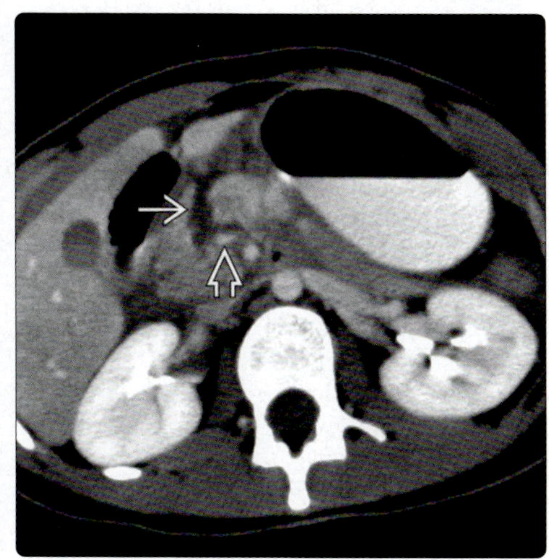

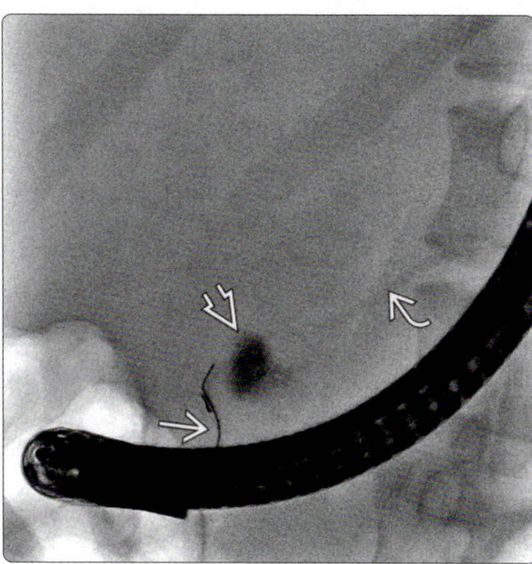

(Left) *Axial CECT in a 14-year-old girl with a soccer injury shows a deep grade IV proximal transection of the pancreas ➡ to the right of the superior mesenteric vein ⇨, raising concern for an associated main duct disruption.* **(Right)** *Oblique frontal view from an ERCP in the same patient shows cannulation ➡ of the major papilla. There is irregular pooling of contrast at the site of pancreatic neck injury ⇨, consistent with main duct disruption. The distal duct is opacified ↪, & a stent was subsequently placed.*

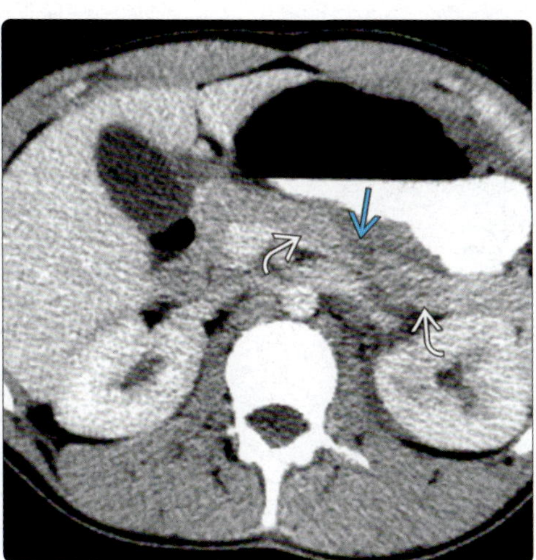

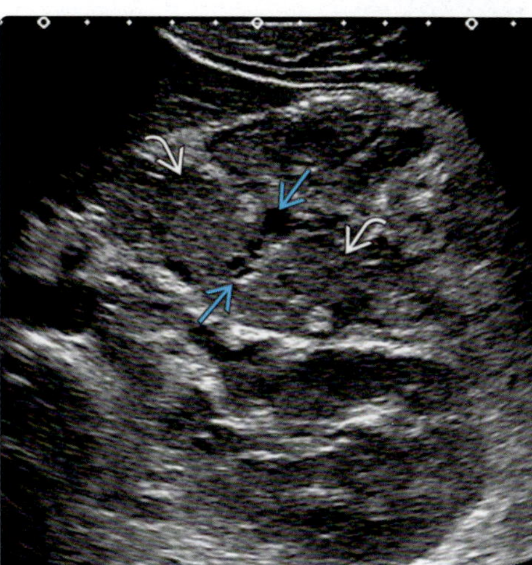

(Left) *Axial CECT in a 15-year-old patient after blunt abdominal trauma during a baseball game shows a fluid-attenuation focus ➡ interrupting the pancreatic parenchyma ↪, consistent with laceration.* **(Right)** *Axial oblique US through the pancreatic body & tail in the same patient shows the fluid-filled cleft ➡ separating the pancreatic parenchyma ↪.*

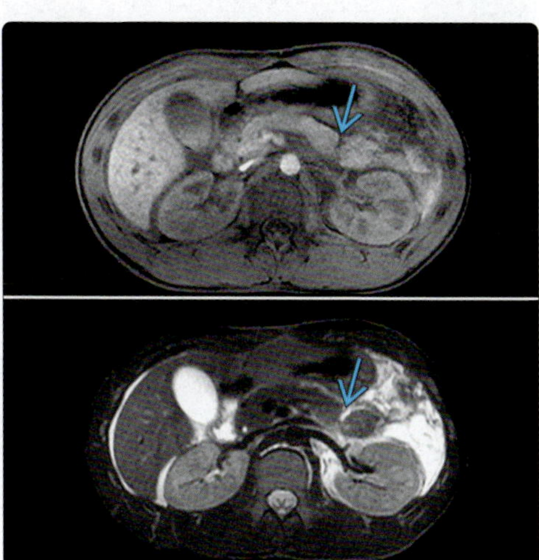

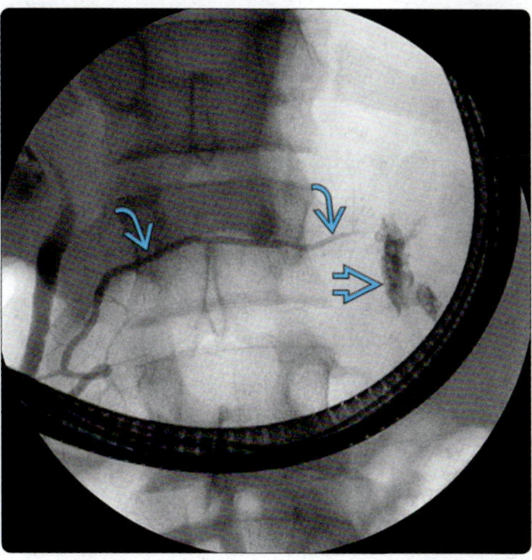

(Left) *Axial 3D T1 GRE FS (top) & T2 FS (bottom) MR images in the same patient show the site of parenchymal transection ➡ with surrounding intraperitoneal & retroperitoneal fluid.* **(Right)** *ERCP in the same patient shows retrograde opacification of the main pancreatic duct ↪ with a contrast leak ⇨ occurring at the site of parenchymal transection, consistent with ductal disruption. This patient ultimately required a spleen-preserving distal pancreatectomy.*

Posttransplant Lymphoproliferative Disease

KEY FACTS

TERMINOLOGY

- Posttransplant lymphoproliferative disease (PTLD): Spectrum of abnormal lymphoid proliferation in transplant patients

IMAGING

- Any organ system can be affected
- Abdominal region is most commonly involved by PTLD, including
  - Gastrointestinal: Bowel wall thickening & dilation, eccentric mass, luminal ulceration, mesenteric stranding, & intussusception
  - Liver: Low-attenuation nodules, periportal infiltration, heterogeneous porta hepatis mass
  - Spleen: Splenomegaly, multiple low-attenuation lesions
  - Kidney: Nephromegaly, multifocal parenchymal masses, heterogeneous renal or pararenal mass
  - Chest: Pulmonary mass, parenchymal nodules, pleural effusion, adenopathy
- Imaging: Lesions are often detected by US, CT, or MR
  - DWI MR ↑ conspicuity of nodes against soft tissues
  - PET/CT is useful for staging & therapy response

PATHOLOGY

- Risk factors for PTLD: EBV status, young age, type of transplanted organ (& degree of immunosuppression)
  - Greatest risk: Donor EBV positive, recipient EBV negative
  - 50-80% of PTLD biopsies are positive for EBV
  - Small bowel transplant is at highest risk (20%)
  - Kidney transplant is at lowest risk (2%)
- WHO classification: Early lesions, polymorphic, monomorphic, classic Hodgkin lymphoma-like

CLINICAL ISSUES

- Most common malignancy in pediatric transplant patients
- Universally fatal if not treated
- Treatment: Reduce immunosuppression, add chemotherapy for lymphoma

(Left) *Coronal CECT in an adolescent with a history of renal transplant & a new diagnosis of posttransplant lymphoproliferative disorder (PTLD) shows abnormal thickening of the bowel wall ➔ centered near the ileocecal valve & cecum. The right lower quadrant transplanted kidney ⇒ is also visible.* **(Right)** *Coronal F-18 FDG PET/CT in the same adolescent shows FDG uptake within periportal & mesenteric lymph nodes ➔. The right lower quadrant renal transplant ⇒ is partially included in this image.*

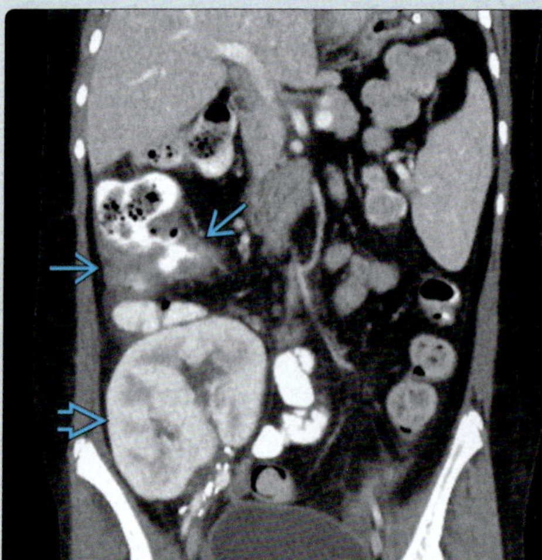

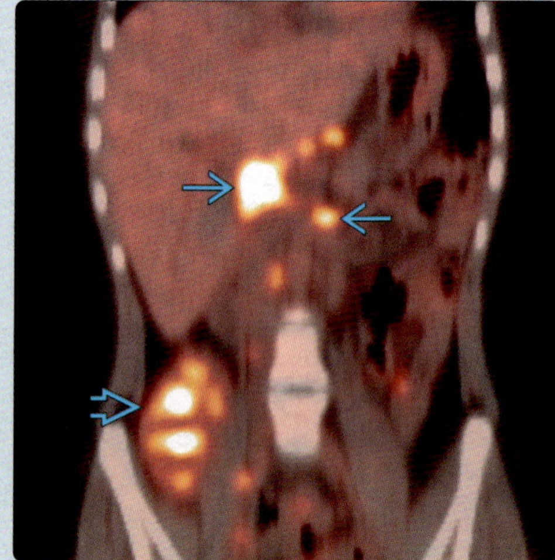

(Left) *Transverse ultrasound in an adolescent with a history of small bowel transplant shows multiple small, hypoechoic nodules ➔ scattered throughout the liver. These nodules were later confirmed to represent PTLD.* **(Right)** *Coronal CECT in the same patient shows multiple hypodense PTLD nodules ➔ in the liver.*

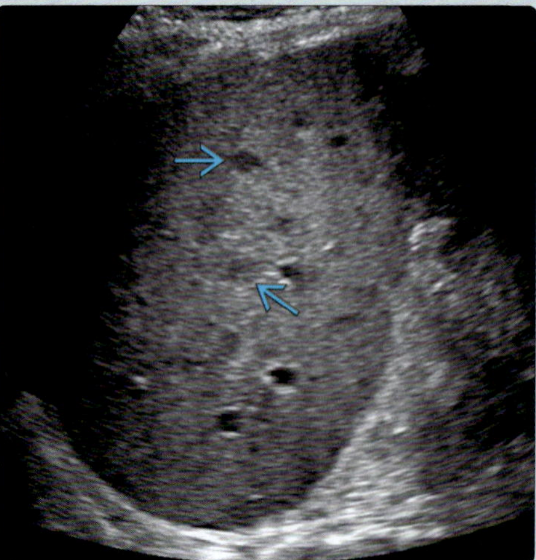

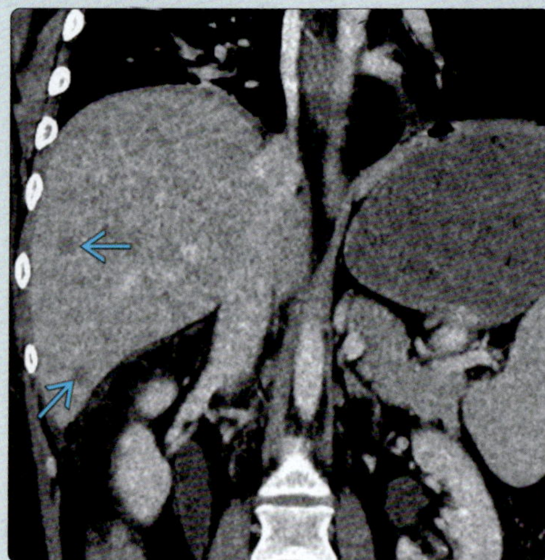

TERMINOLOGY

Abbreviations

- Posttransplant lymphoproliferative disease (PTLD)

Definitions

- Spectrum of abnormal lymphoid proliferation in transplant patients

IMAGING

General Features

- Best diagnostic clue
  - Lymphadenopathy or solid mass occurring virtually anywhere in organ transplant patient
- Location
  - Any organ system can be affected
  - Abdomen is most commonly involved by PTLD
    - Transplanted organ, gastrointestinal (GI) tract, & liver are most commonly affected
  - Other sites: Tonsils, lungs, kidneys, brain, muscle

Radiographic Findings

- Airway: Enlargement of adenoids & palatine tonsils
- Chest: Pulmonary nodule(s), adenopathy, consolidation, pleural effusion

CT Findings

- CECT
  - Abdomen
    - GI tract
      - Focal or uniform bowel wall thickening, bowel dilation, eccentric bowel wall mass, luminal ulceration, mesenteric stranding, & intussusception
      - More common in distal small bowel & proximal colon
    - Liver
      - Hepatomegaly, low-attenuation nodules, infiltrative pattern along portal vessels, heterogeneous porta hepatis mass
    - Spleen
      - Splenomegaly, multiple low-attenuation lesions
    - Kidney
      - Nephromegaly, multifocal parenchymal masses, heterogeneous renal or pararenal mass
  - Lymph nodes
    - Discrete, homogeneous, enlarged lymph node or conglomeration of enlarged lymph nodes
  - Chest
    - Pulmonary mass, parenchymal nodules, pleural effusion, adenopathy
    - Parenchymal nodules usually have homogeneous density but can have halo of ground-glass opacity
  - Neck
    - Nonspecific adenopathy & enlarged tonsils
  - Brain
    - High-attenuation, ring-enhancing parenchymal lesions surrounded by vasogenic edema

MR Findings

- Abdomen
  - Liver
    - Multiple lesions are hypointense on T1 & slightly hyperintense on T2 with mild peripheral enhancement
  - Spleen
    - Splenomegaly, lesions hypointense to spleen on T1 & iso- to hypointense on T2
  - Kidney
    - Discrete renal mass or diffuse, infiltrative lesion causing renal enlargement
      - T1: Isointense to kidney
      - T2: Slightly hypointense
      - T1 C+: Hypoenhancing relative to kidney
    - Unilateral or bilateral
    - Hydronephrosis if mass is obstructive
  - Discrete or conglomerate nodal masses, often isointense to bowel wall
    - Hyperintense on DWI → stand out against bowel
- Brain
  - Solitary or multiple periventricular mass(es) with vasogenic edema
    - T1: Heterogeneously hypo- to isointense with foci of hyperintense hemorrhage
    - T2: Mostly hyperintense
    - T1 C+: Peripheral enhancement

Ultrasonographic Findings

- Solid masses with variable echogenicity & internal vascularity

Nuclear Medicine Findings

- PET
  - ↑ FDG uptake in lesions
  - PET/CT is useful for staging & to determine response to therapy

Imaging Recommendations

- Best imaging tool
  - Body: Disease is often detected on US, CT, or MR; PET/CT to stage & follow-up disease
  - Brain & spine: MR ± contrast
  - Airway: Radiograph to assess tonsils; CECT is more sensitive
- Protocol advice
  - DWI is helpful in identifying body lesions on MR

DIFFERENTIAL DIAGNOSIS

Graft-vs.-Host Disease

- Allogenic bone marrow transplant patients
- Lymphocytes from donor attack recipient tissues
- Often involves bowel, liver, & skin
  - May have similar symptoms, including abdominal pain & diarrhea
  - CECT classically shows featureless, ribbon-like hyperenhancing bowel
- Treatment: ↑ immunosuppression

Colitis

- Types: Inflammatory, pseudomembranous, neutropenic, infectious
- Symptoms: Fever, diarrhea, abdominal pain

- CECT: Circumferential colonic wall thickening (accordion sign)
- Abdominal radiograph: Thumbprinting of colonic wall

Fungal Infection

- *Candida* is most common type to infect GI tract, liver, & spleen
- Microabscess in liver, spleen, or kidneys
  - US: Multiple small, hypoechoic lesions, some with hyperechoic centers → target or bull's-eye appearance
  - CT: Numerous low-attenuation lesions
  - MR: Hypointense on T1 & hyperintense on T2

Abscess/Septic Emboli

- Visceral &/or soft tissue lesion(s) with irregular, thick rim enhancement, surrounding edema

PATHOLOGY

General Features

- Risk factors for PTLD
  - Ebstein-Barr virus (EBV) status at time of transplant
    - Greatest risk: Donor is EBV positive, recipient is EBV negative
    - 50-80% of PTLD biopsies are positive for EBV in tumors cells
      - In immunocompromised host, EBV can lead to uncontrolled B-cell expansion
  - Young age
    - Patients is more likely to be EBV negative
    - Patients will have longer exposure to immunosuppression
  - Type of transplanted organ
    - Small bowel transplant at highest risk (14-19%)
    - Kidney transplant at lowest risk (0.005-9%)
  - Extent of immunosuppression
  - Time from transplantation < 1 year
  - Previous history of PTLD

Staging, Grading, & Classification

- WHO classification
  - Early lesions
    - Includes 3 subtypes: Plasmacytic hyperplasia, florid follicular hyperplasia, & infectious mononucleosis
    - Similar to infectious mononucleosis
    - Reactive plasmacytic hyperplasia without destruction of normal lymph node or tissue architecture
  - Polymorphic
    - Mixture of monoclonal B-cell lymphocytes & polyclonal T-cell lymphocytes
    - B-lymphocytes are EBV positive
  - Monomorphic
    - Exclusively monoclonal
    - Divided into diffuse large B-cell lymphoma, Burkitt lymphoma, & plasma cell myeloma
    - Usually EBV positive
  - Classic Hodgkin lymphoma-like
    - Rare in childhood

CLINICAL ISSUES

Presentation

- Most common signs/symptoms
  - Lymphadenopathy, fever, weight loss, tonsillitis, transplant dysfunction
- Other signs/symptoms
  - Depends on location of mass
    - Airway: Noisy breathing, snoring, changes in voice
    - Gastrointestinal: Secretory diarrhea, hematemesis, hematochezia, intussusception
    - General abdominal: Abdominal pain, distention, multisystem organ failure
    - Chest: May be asymptomatic with incidental opacity on chest radiograph, fever, ↓ pulmonary function tests
    - Head & neck: Mononucleosis-like symptoms, including fever, malaise, adenopathy, & pharyngitis
    - Neurologic: Seizure, focal neurological deficit

Demographics

- Age
  - Children > adults
- Epidemiology
  - Most common malignancy in pediatric transplant patients (52%)
  - Incidence of PTLD in children is 4x higher than adults
  - Incidence ↑ with ↑ immunosuppression
  - Incidence ↑ in transplants that require more immunosuppression
    - Highest in small bowel transplant & heart-lung transplant; lowest in kidney & liver transplants

Natural History & Prognosis

- Early-onset is more likely to be due to EBV infection
- Universally fatal if not treated
- Prognosis depends on degree of immunosuppression
  - More immunosuppressed = poorer prognosis

Treatment

- Reduced immunosuppression
  - Upon EBV seroconversion or ↑ EBV viral load
  - Works best in early lesions & polymorphic PTLD
  - Must balance with risk of transplant rejection
- Chemotherapy
  - For overt malignancy (Burkitt lymphoma)
  - If inadequate response to reduced immunosuppression

SELECTED REFERENCES

1. Song H et al: 18F-FDG PET/CT for evaluation of post-transplant lymphoproliferative disorder (PTLD). Semin Nucl Med. 51(4):392-403, 2021
2. Dembowska-Bagińska B et al: Non-Hodgkin lymphoma after liver and kidney transplantation in children. Experience from one center. Adv Clin Exp Med. 29(2):197-202, 2020
3. White ML et al: Primary central nervous system post-transplant lymphoproliferative disorders: the spectrum of imaging appearances and differential. Insights Imaging. 10(1):46, 2019
4. Absalon MJ et al: Post-transplant lymphoproliferative disorder after solid-organ transplant in children. Semin Pediatr Surg. 26(4):257-66, 2017
5. Borhani AA et al: Imaging of posttransplantation lymphoproliferative disorder after solid organ transplantation. Radiographics. 29(4):981-1000; discussion 1000-2, 2009

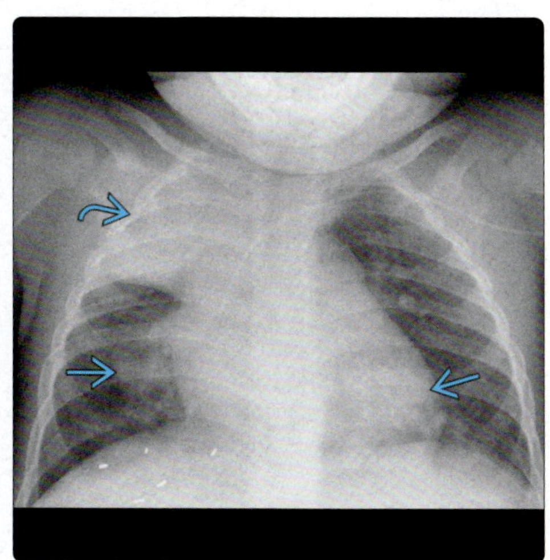

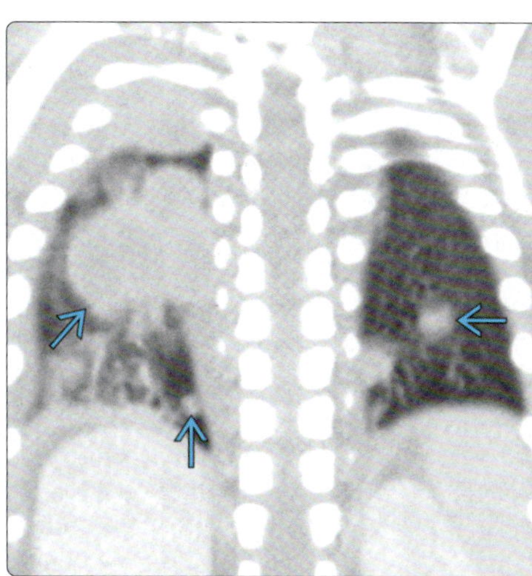

(Left) *Frontal chest radiograph in a young child with liver transplant shows multiple rounded pulmonary opacities ➔ bilaterally as well as consolidation ➔ in the right upper lobe.* **(Right)** *Coronal CECT in the same patient shows multiple rounded opacities ➔ in both lungs. This was confirmed to represent pulmonary PTLD at biopsy.*

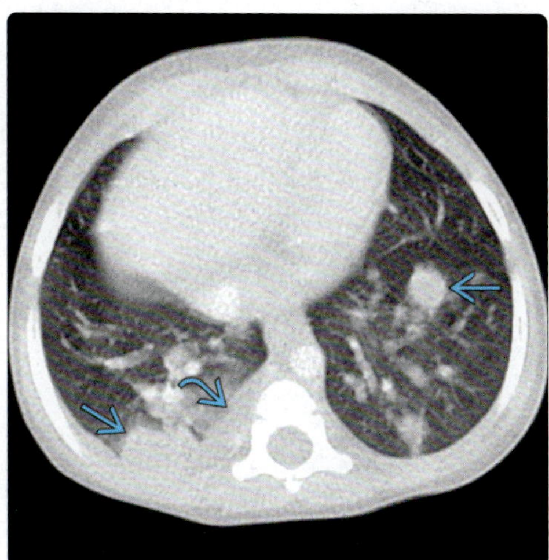

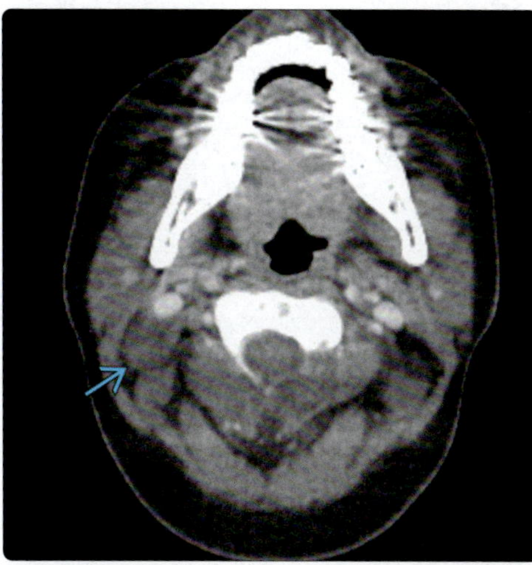

(Left) *Axial CECT in the same patient shows multiple well-defined, rounded opacities ➔ in both lungs. These nodules were confirmed to represent pulmonary PTLD at biopsy. A small pleural effusion ➔ is also present.* **(Right)** *Axial CECT in an adolescent with a palpable cervical mass status post small bowel transplant shows an enlarged cervical lymph node ➔ posterior to the right jugular vein. This was confirmed to represent PTLD at biopsy.*

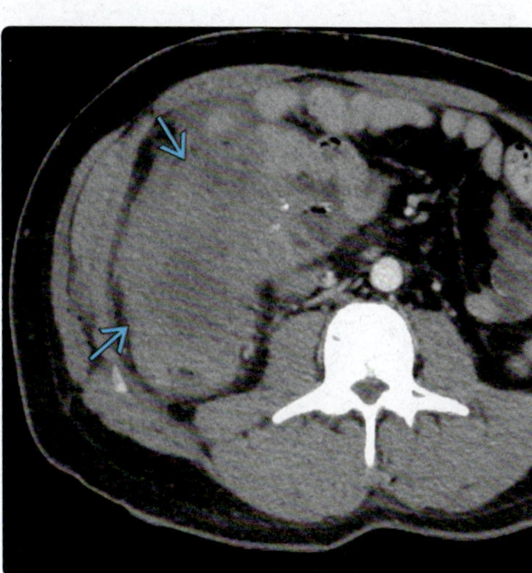

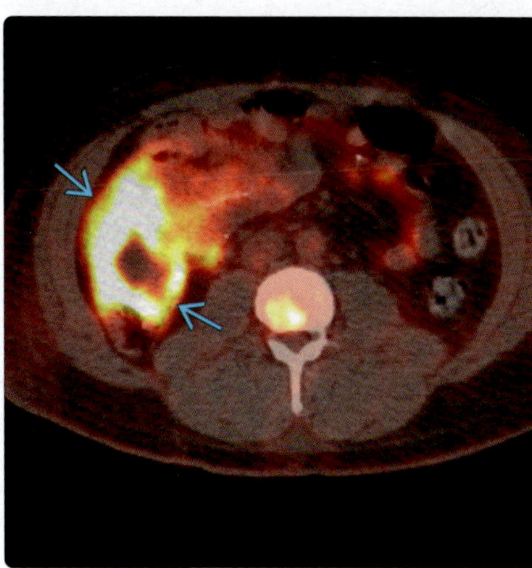

(Left) *Axial CECT in a young adult with a prior history of renal transplant shows a large soft tissue mass ➔ arising from bowel in the right lower quadrant.* **(Right)** *Axial F-18 FDG PET/CT in the same patient shows marked FDG uptake in the right lower quadrant mass ➔, confirmed to represent PTLD.*

KEY FACTS

TERMINOLOGY

- Colonic inflammation due to *Clostridium difficile* & its toxins A & B → epithelial necrosis & pseudomembranes

IMAGING

- Classic appearance: Pancolitis with marked wall thickening
- Radiographs
  - Thumbprinting ± colonic or small bowel ileus
- CECT
  - Accordion sign: Alternating bands of ↑ & ↓ attenuation of colon due to oral contrast interdigitating between edematous haustra
    - Lumen appears stellate in cross section
  - Target sign: Rings of hyperenhancing mucosa & lower attenuation submucosal/muscular edema
  - Pericolonic stranding is usually very mild, ± ascites
- Ultrasound
  - Accordion sign: Echogenic bowel contents between hypoechoic, thickened wall
  - Pseudomembranes: Linear hyperechogenicity
  - ± ascites
- Paucity of colonic gas with luminal narrowing

PATHOLOGY

- *C. difficile* overgrowth (usually due to antibiotic therapy) → toxin A & B release
- Inflamed colon with discrete or confluent, raised, yellow-white plaque pseudomembranes on endoscopy

CLINICAL ISSUES

- Most common presentations: Watery or bloody diarrhea, dehydration, abdominal pain, leukocytosis, fever
- Primary treatments include cessation of inciting antibiotic with addition of metronidazole or vancomycin
- Severe *C. difficile* infections are less common in children compared to adults
- If treated early, full recovery is expected
  - Up to 25% recurrence rate

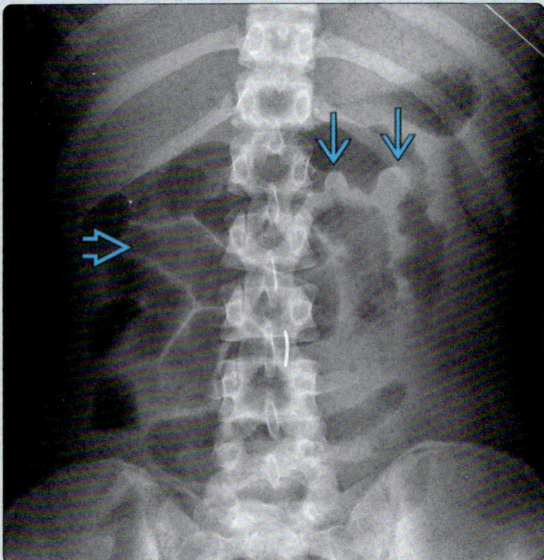

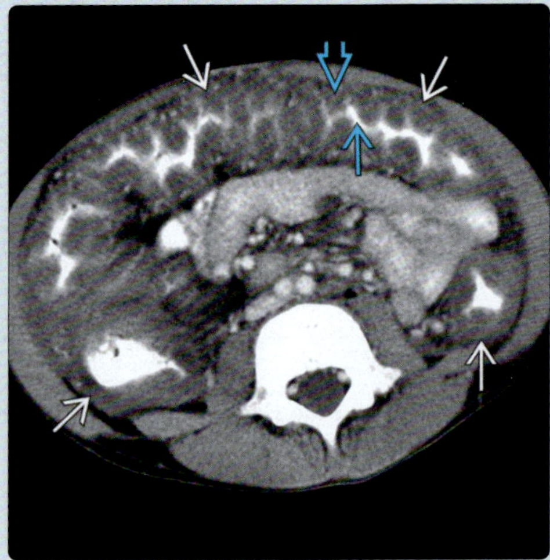

(Left) *Supine abdominal radiograph in a 15-year-old with known pseudomembranous colitis (PMC) demonstrates thumbprinting along the colon due to haustral thickening ➔. A small bowel ileus ➔ is also present.* **(Right)** *Axial CECT in a 10-year-old child with fever, abdominal pain, & diarrhea demonstrates findings of PMC with pancolonic marked wall thickening ➔. The alternating bands of hyperdense contrast ➔ between the thickened, fluid-density haustra ➔ create the accordion sign.*

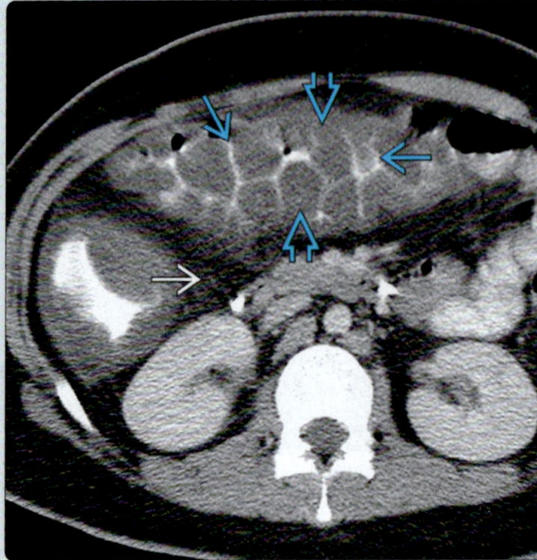

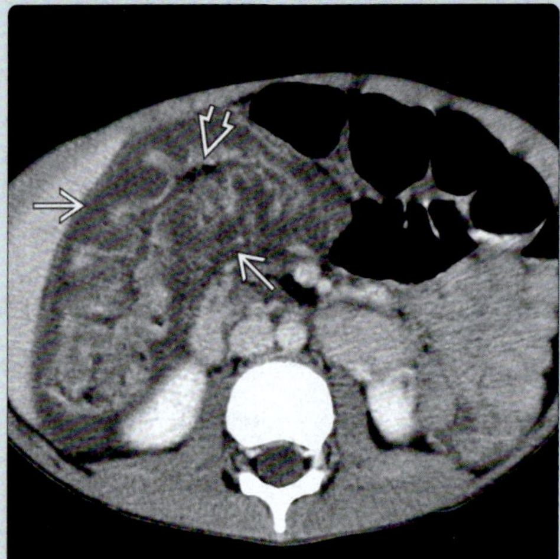

(Left) *Axial CECT shows marked pancolitis with enteric contrast ➔ trapped between thickened haustral folds ➔ (the accordion sign). Note the minimal pericolonic fat infiltration ➔, which is typical with PMC.* **(Right)** *Axial CECT demonstrates asymmetric pancolitis with the greatest colonic wall thickening ➔ & mucosal enhancement ➔ seen in the right & transverse colon. Involvement limited to the proximal colon can be seen in 10-20% of PMC cases.*

TERMINOLOGY

Definitions

- Inflammation of colon by *Clostridium difficile* toxins A & B

IMAGING

General Features

- Location
  - Pancolitis is typical
  - Rectum & sigmoid colon: Up to 90% of cases
  - Proximal colon only: 10-20%

Radiographic Findings

- Low sensitivity: Up to 68% can be normal
- Paucity of colonic gas with luminal narrowing
  - Small amounts of gas in lumen outline thickened haustra (thumbprinting)
    - En face view of affected loop may show stellate lucency of gas in narrowed lumen outlining haustra
  - Haustral thickening may be nodular
- ± colonic & small bowel ileus
- ± separation & centralization of bowel loops by ascites
- Toxic megacolon in fulminant cases
  - Colonic dilation, R > L, usually > 6 cm
  - Loss of haustral pattern
  - Pneumoperitoneum if perforation occurs

Ultrasonographic Findings

- Marked colonic wall thickening effacing lumen
  - Hypoechoic mural edema
  - ± loss of wall stratification (gut signature)
  - Ultrasound accordion sign: Echogenic bowel contents between less echogenic but thickened walls
- Pseudomembranes may appear as linear hyperechogenicity
- ± ascites

CT Findings

- CECT
  - Colonic wall thickening
    - Usually marked; average > 10 mm
    - Smooth, plaque-like, nodular or polypoid
  - Accordion sign: Small amounts of oral contrast (or hyperenhancing mucosa) interdigitate between very thick/edematous haustra → alternating bands of ↓ & ↑ attenuation when viewed in long axis
    - Narrowed lumen may appear stellate in cross section
  - Target sign: In cross section/short axis, thickened colonic wall shows rings of hyperenhancing mucosa, lower attenuation submucosal/mural edema, & possible outer layer of serosal enhancement
  - Pericolonic stranding is usually mild due to mucosal & submucosal nature of disease; ± ascites
  - ± pneumatosis &/or pneumoperitoneum if severe

Imaging Recommendations

- CECT with IV & oral contrast

DIFFERENTIAL DIAGNOSIS

Infectious Colitis

- May be indistinguishable from pseudomembranous colitis

Crohn Disease

- Skip lesions; ileocolic involvement is typical
- Strictures, fistulas, abscesses, "creeping fat"

Ulcerative Colitis

- Contiguous colitis extending variable distances retrograde from rectum
- Symmetric wall thickening < 10 mm

Typhlitis (Neutropenic Colitis)

- History of neutropenia & immunosuppression
- Usually isolated to right colon

Benign Pneumatosis in Older Children

- History of steroids or bone marrow transplant is typical
- Often lacks wall thickening or free fluid

PATHOLOGY

General Features

- *C. difficile* colonization, overgrowth, & toxin production
  - Overgrowth is usually due to antibiotic therapy but can be due to chemotherapy, abdominal surgery, obstruction, uremia, hypotension, bowel hypoperfusion
  - Toxins A & B (enterotoxin & cytotoxin) mediate disease

Gross Pathologic & Surgical Features

- Inflamed colon with discrete or confluent, raised, yellow-white plaques (pseudomembranes) on endoscopy

CLINICAL ISSUES

Presentation

- Most common: Watery or bloody diarrhea, dehydration, abdominal pain, leukocytosis, fever

Natural History & Prognosis

- If treated early, full recovery is expected
- All-cause mortality in children with *C. difficile* infection: 4%
- Severe forms of *C. difficile* infection (pseudomembranous colitis, toxic megacolon, death) are less common in children
  - 8% in recent population surveillance study, with 0 deaths
- 12-25% recurrence rate in pediatric population

Treatment

- Cessation of inciting antibiotic & starting replacement if needed
- 1st-line therapy with metronidazole or vancomycin
- Fecal microbiota transplantation may be considered for refractory/recurrent cases
- Surgery for severe disease resulting in toxic megacolon or perforation, or if rapidly progressing or refractory

SELECTED REFERENCES

1. Concepcion NDP et al: Imaging assessment of complications from transplantation from pediatric to adult patients: part 2: hematopoietic stem cell transplantation. Radiol Clin North Am. 58(3):569-82, 2020
2. Duffin C et al: Radiologic imaging of bowel infections. Semin Ultrasound CT MR. 41(1):33-45, 2020
3. Guerri S et al: Clostridium difficile colitis: CT findings and differential diagnosis. Radiol Med. 124(12):1185-98, 2019
4. Borali E et al: Clostridium difficile infection in children: a review. J Pediatr Gastroenterol Nutr. 63(6):e130-40, 2016
5. Choi HH et al: Fecal microbiota transplantation: current applications, effectiveness, and future perspectives. Clin Endosc. 49(3):257-65, 2016

KEY FACTS

TERMINOLOGY

- Necrotizing inflammatory process of bowel most commonly affecting right colon of neutropenic patients (with absolute neutrophil count < 500 cells/μL)

IMAGING

- Right colon is most commonly affected, but distal colon, appendix, & small bowel can be involved
- Bowel wall thickening: Circumferential & symmetric, typically low attenuation on CECT
  - Radiographs may show thumbprinting of thickened haustra &/or paucity of right lower quadrant bowel gas
    - ± stellate appearance of narrowed, gas-containing bowel lumen
- Mucosal hyperenhancement is less common than in graft-vs.-host disease (GVHD)
- Pericolic fluid & fat stranding/hyperechogenicity
- Pneumatosis is more common than other colitides & GVHD
- ± small bowel ileus; ± pneumoperitoneum with perforation
- Modality of choice: US vs. CECT
  - US is more accurate for measurement of bowel wall thickness & uses no ionizing radiation
    - Sufficient for diagnosis & follow-up in most cases
  - CECT may be more sensitive for early changes & complications (necrosis, perforation, abscess)

TOP DIFFERENTIAL DIAGNOSES

- Other colitides: Infectious, pseudomembranous, ischemic
- Acute graft-vs.-host disease
- Appendicitis
- Benign pneumatosis of older children

CLINICAL ISSUES

- Clinical triad: Neutropenia, abdominal pain, fever
- Uncomplicated cases: Bowel rest, broad spectrum IV antibiotics (including antifungal), ± granulocyte colony-stimulating factor
- Surgery for perforation, peritonitis, GI bleeding, obstruction

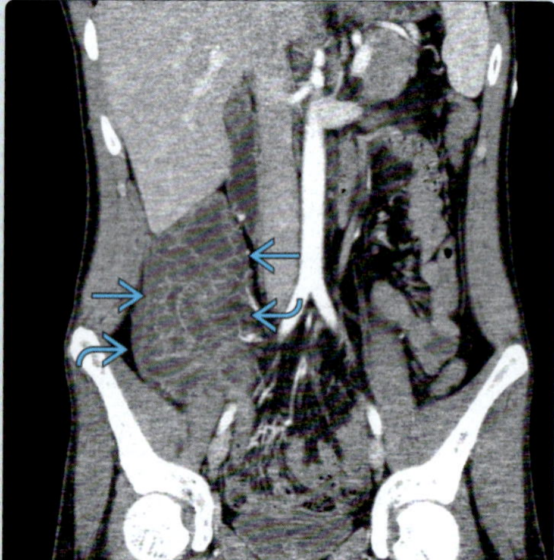

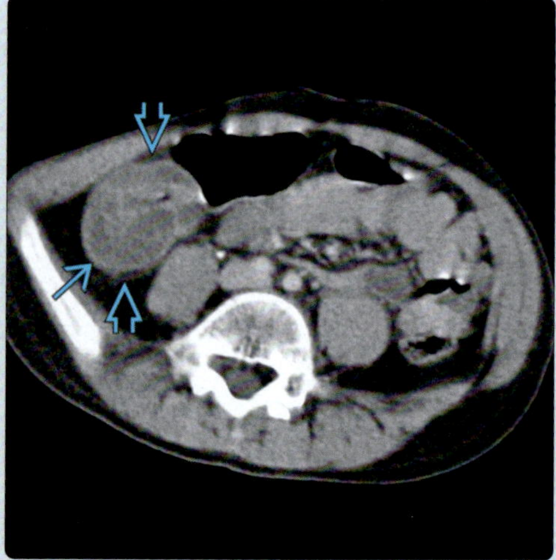

(Left) *Coronal CECT shows marked wall thickening of the cecum & ascending colon ➡ in a patient with a history of osteosarcoma status post chemotherapy. Mild surrounding fluid/edema ↪ is also noted. The patient presented with neutropenia, vomiting, nausea, & abdominal pain.* **(Right)** *Axial CECT in a 7-year-old neutropenic patient demonstrates marked thickening & edema of the cecal wall ➡ & mild adjacent fat stranding ⇨, compatible with neutropenic colitis.*

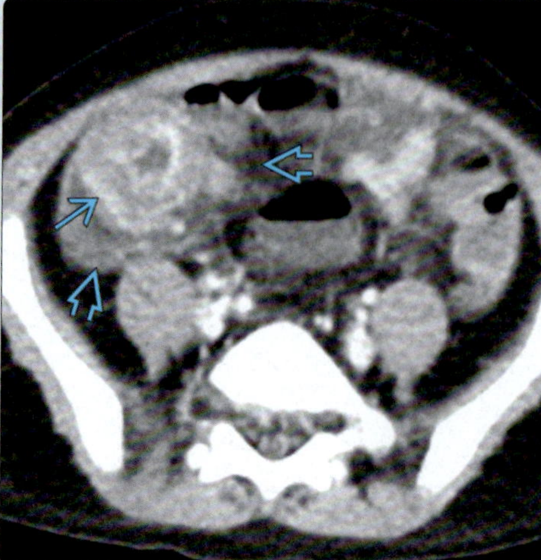

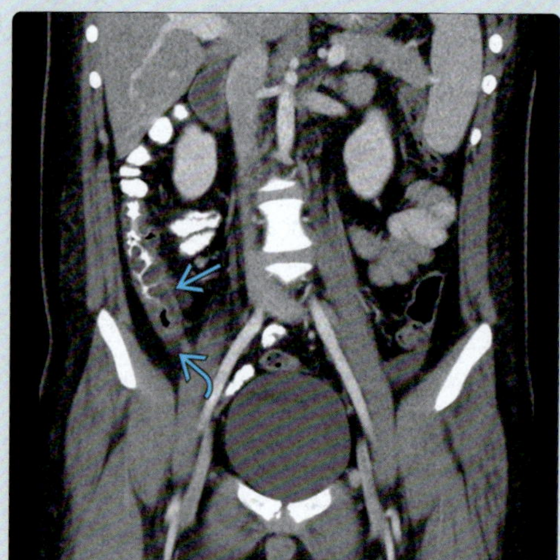

(Left) *Axial CECT in a 3-year-old with acute lymphocytic leukemia presenting with fever, abdominal pain, & neutropenia shows findings typical of neutropenic colitis, including wall thickening ➡ in the cecum & ascending colon + moderate associated pericolonic stranding ⇨. Note mucosal & serosal hyperenhancement.* **(Right)** *Coronal CECT in an 18-year-old with acute lymphocytic leukemia, neutropenia, & abdominal pain shows edematous wall thickening ➡ at the cecum with pericolonic inflammatory change ↪.*

TERMINOLOGY

Definitions

- Necrotizing inflammatory process of bowel most commonly affecting right colon of neutropenic patients (with absolute neutrophil count < 500 cells/μL)

IMAGING

General Features

- Best diagnostic clue
  - Wall thickening of right colon + pericolic stranding & fluid in neutropenic patient with abdominal pain &/or fever without other etiology identified
  - Pneumatosis > compared to other colitides & graft-vs.-host disease (GVHD)
- Location
  - Most common: Cecum & ascending colon
  - ± other colonic segments, appendix, & small bowel

Radiographic Findings

- Paucity of bowel gas in right lower quadrant
- "Soft tissue mass" in right lower quadrant
- Thumbprinting (thickened haustra)
  - May create stellate appearance of narrowed, gas-containing bowel lumen
- ± pneumatosis; ± small bowel ileus

CT Findings

- Circumferential & symmetric bowel wall thickening > 3 mm, predominantly of ↓ attenuation due to muscularis edema
- ± mucosal & serosal hyperenhancement
- Cecal luminal distention or narrowing
- Pericolic fluid & fat stranding
- ± pneumatosis
- ± dilated adjacent small bowel loops (ileus)
- Pneumoperitoneum if perforation occurs

Ultrasonographic Findings

- Bowel wall thickening > 3 mm
  - Hypoechoic muscularis layer & echogenic mucosal layer
- Pericolic fluid & echogenic fat
- ± echogenic pneumatosis tracking circumferentially in wall

DIFFERENTIAL DIAGNOSIS

Crohn Disease

- Mouth to anus may be affected but ileocolic region is most common
- Skip lesions (up to 90%) with transmural inflammation
- Strictures, sinus tracts, fistulas, perianal disease

Appendicitis

- Dilated, noncompressible appendix
- Inflammatory changes are centered at appendix

Infectious Colitis

- Nonspecific imaging findings; many possible organisms

Pseudomembranous Colitis

- Clinical history of recent antibiotic therapy
- Typically pancolitis; isolated to right colon in 10-20%
- Marked wall thickening (mean > 10 mm) & nodularity

Acute Graft-vs.-Host Disease

- Classic triad of dermatitis, hepatitis, & enteritis
- Typically < 100 days from bone marrow transplant
- Mucosal hyperenhancement & fluid-filled bowel are common
  - Small bowel is classically featureless & ribbon-like

Benign Pneumatosis of Older Children

- Patients on steroids or after bone marrow transplant
- Extensive colonic involvement is common
- Bowel wall thickening & free fluid are uncommon

Ischemic Colitis

- Uncommon in children but must be considered in ill, complex patients with pneumatosis
- Bowel wall thickening with ↓ enhancement + free fluid

PATHOLOGY

General Features

- Multifactorial etiology: Immunocompromise, therapy toxicity, bowel ischemia, intramural hemorrhage, neoplastic cell infiltration of bowel wall
- Mechanism: Chemotherapy-related mucositis & mucosal injury → bacterial/fungal invasion of bowel wall → inflammation, hemorrhage, edema → ulceration, transmural necrosis, & perforation

CLINICAL ISSUES

Presentation

- Most common signs/symptoms: Neutropenia, abdominal pain, fever, diarrhea
- Risk factors: Leukemia, hematologic & solid malignancies, solid organ & bone marrow transplant, immunocompromised state, recent chemotherapy
- Incidence: 0.4-6% in pediatric oncology patients

Natural History & Prognosis

- Early diagnosis & treatment are essential to reduce risk of transmural necrosis & perforation
- Mortality ↓ over last 3 decades, recently 0-2.5%

Treatment

- Medical management for uncomplicated cases
  - Bowel rest & decompression
  - Broad spectrum IV antibiotics (including antifungal)
  - ± granulocyte colony-stimulating factor
- Surgery for perforation, peritonitis, active GI bleeding, obstruction

SELECTED REFERENCES

1. Concepcion NDP et al: Imaging assessment of complications from transplantation from pediatric to adult patients: part 2: hematopoietic stem cell transplantation. Radiol Clin North Am. 58(3):569-82, 2020
2. Handa A et al: Pediatric oncologic emergencies: clinical and imaging review for pediatricians. Pediatr Int. 61(2):122-39, 2019
3. Pelletier JH et al: Neutropenic enterocolitis (typhlitis) in a pediatric renal transplant patient. A case report and review of the literature. Pediatr Transplant. 21(6), 2017
4. Chavhan GB et al: Imaging of acute and subacute toxicities of cancer therapy in children. Pediatr Radiol. 46(1):9-20; quiz 6-8, 2016
5. Rizzatti M et al: Neutropenic enterocolitis in children and young adults with cancer: prognostic value of clinical and image findings. Pediatr Hematol Oncol. 27(6):462-70, 2010

Graft-vs.-Host Disease

KEY FACTS

TERMINOLOGY

- Disease of allogenic bone marrow transplant (BMT) or stem cell transplant (SCT) recipients
- Donor T lymphocytes cause damage to epithelial cells lining recipient target organs
    - Can involve skin, GI tract, liver, lung

IMAGING

- Diffuse bowel wall thickening, hyperenhancement & featureless bowel (↓ folds)
- Radiography
    - May see findings of ileus
    - ± evidence of bowel wall thickening, pneumatosis
- Fluoroscopy/SBFT
    - Separation of bowel loops & luminal narrowing due to bowel wall thickening, featureless bowel wall
- CECT
    - Diffusely abnormal bowel with wall thickening & hyperenhancement; featureless bowel
    - ± hepatomegaly, ascites
    - Lungs: Typically bilateral ground-glass opacities

CLINICAL ISSUES

- Affects 30-70% of patients with allogenic BMTs or SCTs
- Older children have ↑ likelihood of graft-vs.-host disease (GVHD)
- Acute GVHD (< 100 days post transplant)
    - Most commonly involves skin
        - Maculopapular rash, itching, ± pain
    - GI tract & liver are also commonly involved
    - Differentiate from infection, drug toxicity, hepatic venoocclusive disease
- Chronic GVHD (> 100 days post transplant)
    - Can affect muscles/joints, lungs, eyes, kidneys
- Treatment: ↑ immunosuppression, steroids
- Overall prognosis is good: 80-85% survival

(Left) *Low-power H&E stain of the intestine shows an ulcerated mucosal surface ⇨. Note the underlying blood vessels ➔, which may predispose to bleeding.* **(Right)** *Axial CECT shows fluid-filled loops of bowel with central hyperenhancement ➔ & infiltration of the mesentery ↪. The mucosal surface is relatively smooth & featureless without typical folds (as this layer actually represents vascular granulation tissue replacing destroyed mucosa), a classic appearance of graft-vs.-host disease (GVHD).*

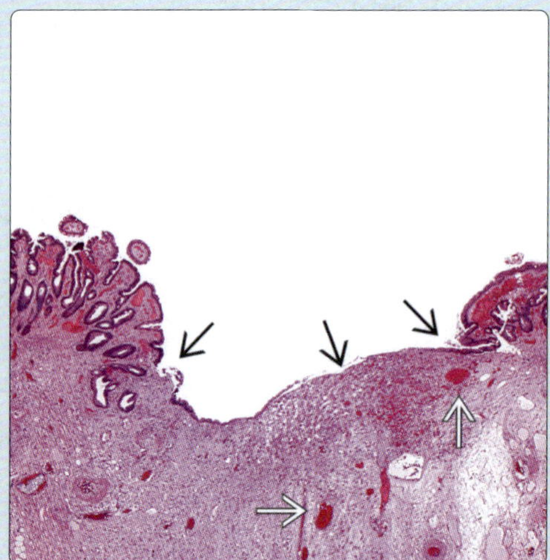

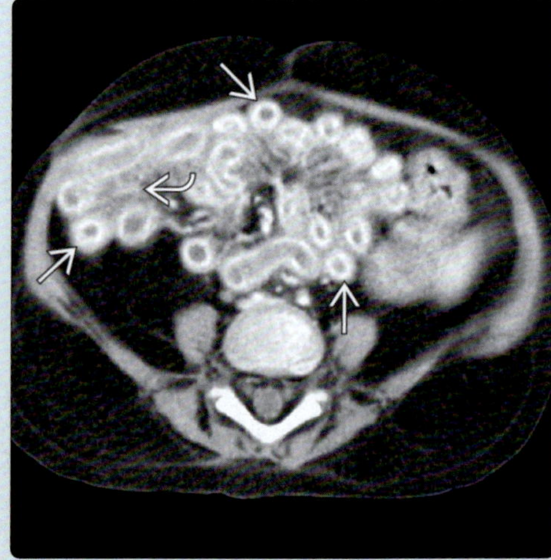

(Left) *Coronal CECT shows multiple fluid-filled loops of abnormal small bowel throughout the abdomen. Note the mildly thickened bowel walls ➔ with smooth central hyperenhancement that is typical of GVHD.* **(Right)** *Axial CECT in the same child shows multiple loops of fluid-filled small bowel with mild wall thickening ➔ & smooth, central hyperenhancement, which is due to granulation tissue replacing destroyed mucosa.*

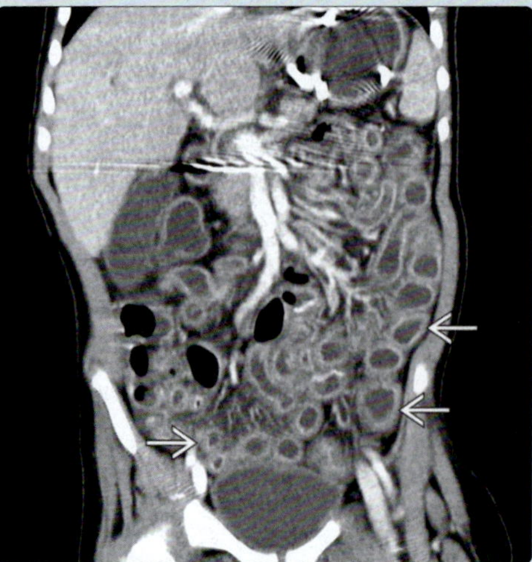

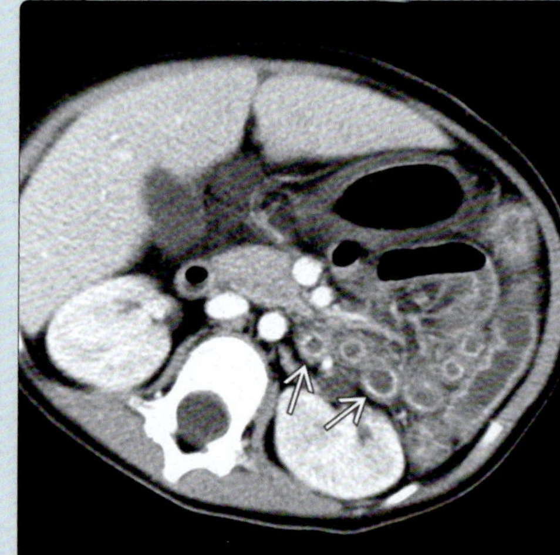

TERMINOLOGY

Abbreviations

- Graft-vs.-host disease (GVHD)

Definitions

- Disease of allogenic bone marrow transplant (BMT) or stem cell transplant (SCT) recipients
- Donor T lymphocytes cause damage to epithelial cells lining recipient target organs

IMAGING

General Features

- Best diagnostic clue
  - Diffuse bowel wall thickening with central, smooth (featureless) hyperenhancement
    - Enhancing layer represents vascular granulation tissue replacing destroyed mucosa
- Location
  - Skin, GI tract, liver, lung

Radiographic Findings

- May resemble adynamic ileus
- ± evidence of bowel wall thickening, pneumatosis

Fluoroscopic Findings

- SBFT: Small bowel wall thickening with luminal narrowing & separation of loops; may be featureless & "ribbon-like"

Ultrasonographic Findings

- Fluid-filled loops of thick-walled bowel ± ascites
  - ↑ blood flow due to inflammation
  - Contrast & elastography of bowel may provide additional detail

CT Findings

- CECT
  - Diffuse bowel abnormality
    - Bowel wall thickening/edema ± loss of folds
    - Hyperenhancement of bowel wall, especially centrally
  - ± hepatomegaly, ascites, bilateral ground-glass pulmonary opacities

MR Findings

- Similar to CECT: Bowel wall thickening, hyperenhancement

DIFFERENTIAL DIAGNOSIS

Infectious Colitis

- Nonspecific wall thickening, inflammation

Typhlitis

- Severely immunocompromised patients
- Most commonly right-sided

Radiation Enteritis

- Thickened bowel wall & adhesions

Posttransplant Lymphoproliferative Disease

- Associated with Epstein-Barr virus infection
- Bowel wall thickening ± aneurysmal dilation, solid organ lesions, lymph node enlargement

Shock Bowel (Hypoperfusion Complex)

- Relevant clinical history; bowel wall thickening, hyperenhancement

PATHOLOGY

General Features

- Complication of allogenic transplants
  - Histocompatibility is major predictor of incidence & severity of GVHD
- Development of GVHD requires
  - Immunocompetent cells (T cells) within graft
  - Recipient (host) tissue antigens
    - Donor T cells react to mismatched host antigens & attack host tissues

Microscopic Features

- Extensive crypt cell necrosis
- In severe cases, diffuse large & small bowel ulceration & mucosal destruction
- Mucosal replacement with thin layer of highly vascular granulation tissue

CLINICAL ISSUES

Presentation

- Most common signs/symptoms
  - Skin is most commonly affected; usually 1st site of involvement
    - Typical maculopapular rash, ± pain, pruritus
  - GI tract: Diarrhea, anorexia, vomiting, pain, rarely, GI bleed
  - Liver: Cholestatic hyperbilirubinemia, hepatomegaly
- Other signs/symptoms
  - Chronic GVHD: More diverse manifestations
    - Often affects skin, mucosal surfaces

Demographics

- Age
  - Older children have ↑ likelihood of GVHD
- Epidemiology
  - Affects 30-70% of patients with allogenic transplant of immunocompetent lymphocytes
- Sex: M = F

Natural History & Prognosis

- Overall prognosis is good: 80-85% survival

Treatment

- Typically steroids, ↑ immunosuppression

SELECTED REFERENCES

1. Concepcion NDP et al: Imaging assessment of complications from transplantation from pediatric to adult patients: part 2: hematopoietic stem cell transplantation. Radiol Clin North Am. 58(3):569-82, 2020
2. Yan Y et al: Pulmonary acute graft-versus-host disease and infections after allogeneic hematopoietic stem cell transplantation in pediatric recipients: a comparative study on CT. Transpl Infect Dis. 22(4):e13285, 2020
3. Weber D et al: Non-invasive diagnosis of acute intestinal graft-versus-host disease by a new scoring system using ultrasound morphology, compound elastography, and contrast-enhanced ultrasound. Bone Marrow Transplant. 54(7):1038-48, 2019
4. Derlin T et al: Magnetic resonance enterography for assessment of intestinal graft-versus-host disease after allogeneic stem cell transplantation. Eur Radiol. 25(5):1229-37, 2015

Chronic Granulomatous Disease

KEY FACTS

TERMINOLOGY

- Primary immunodeficiency characterized by recurrent infections at epithelial surfaces & organs with large numbers of reticuloendothelial cells

IMAGING

- Recurrent infections with catalase-positive organisms such as *Aspergillus* or *Staphylococcus aureus*
- Chronic granulomatous disease (CGD) can affect any organ system
- Pneumonia: Consolidation, nodules, reticulonodular opacities, & scarring
  - Complicated by abscess or empyema in 20%
- Lymph nodes
  - Lymphadenopathy in ~ 100% of patients
  - Suppurative adenitis is most common in neck
  - Calcified lymph nodes as sequelae of prior infection
- Osteomyelitis
  - Common locations: Lower & upper extremities
  - Chest wall & vertebral body involvement in up to 1/3 from contiguous spread of *Aspergillus* pneumonia
- Hepatic abscess(es)
- Gastrointestinal
  - CGD involvement mimics Crohn disease

PATHOLOGY

- Defect in 1 of 5 genes encoding for NADPH-oxidase
  - Defect prevents phagocytic cells from producing respiratory burst used to kill pathogens
- 2 types: X-linked > autosomal recessive

CLINICAL ISSUES

- 76% of patients are diagnosed before 5 years of age
- 85% of patients with CGD are male
- Pneumonia is most common infection in CGD (80%)
- Suppurative adenitis is 2nd most common infection (60%)
- Hepatic abscesses occur in 1/3 of patients

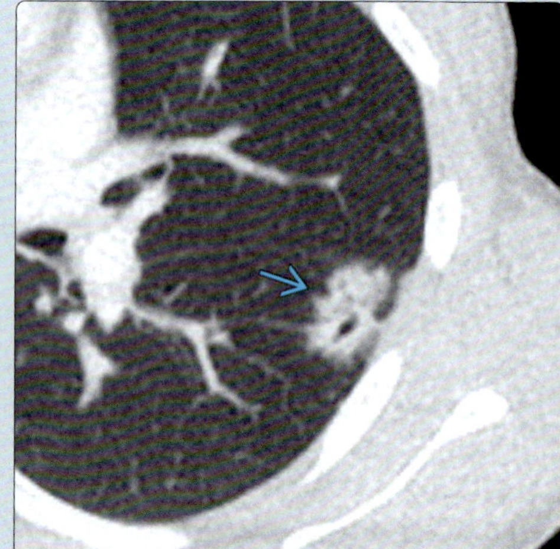

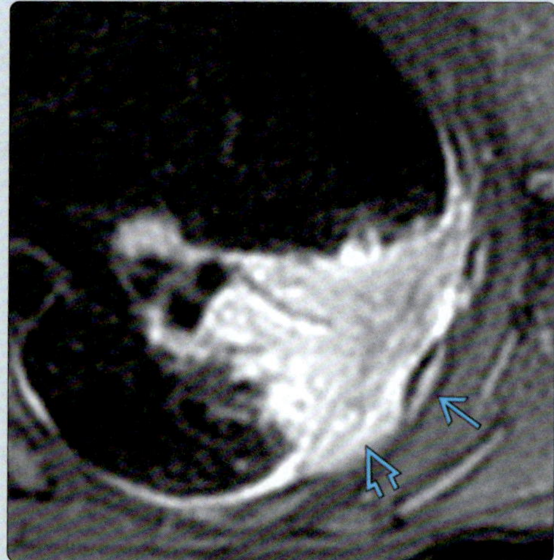

(Left) *Axial NECT of the chest in a patient with chronic granulomatous disease (CGD) shows cavitary pneumonia ➡ in the left lower lobe. Aspergillus is the most common cause of pneumonia in patients with chronic granulomatous disease.* **(Right)** *Axial T2 FS MR shows focal consolidation in the left lower lobe with edema of the adjacent rib ➡ & intervening pleural thickening & fluid ⇨. Aspergillus pneumonia can cause osteomyelitis of adjacent ribs.*

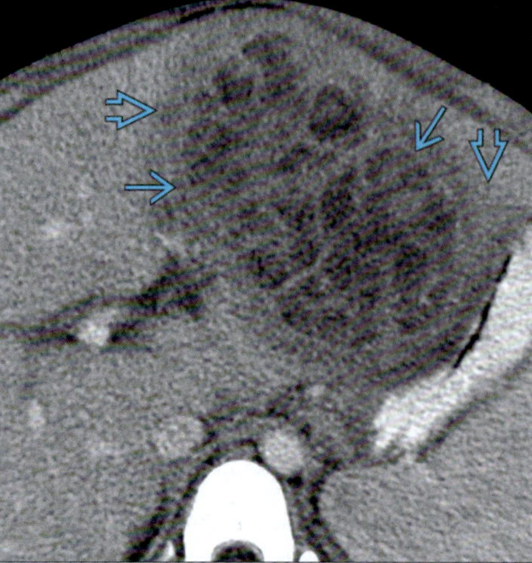

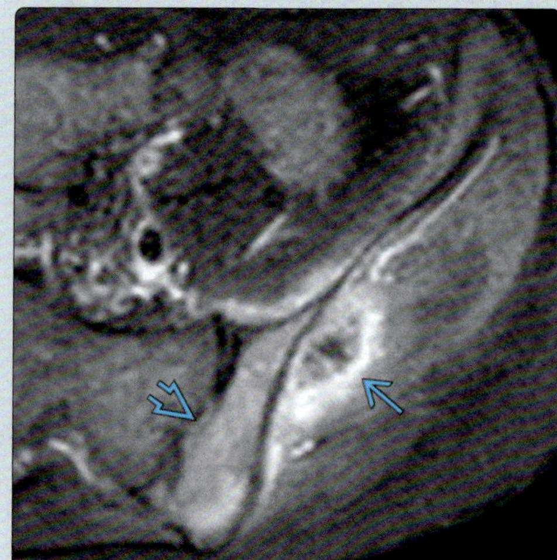

(Left) *Axial CECT of the abdomen shows a multiseptated abscess ➡ in the left lobe of the liver. Note the surrounding parenchymal edema ⇨. Up to 33% of patients with CGD develop a hepatic abscess, & 60% of these patients will have multiple abscesses at diagnosis.* **(Right)** *Axial T1 C+ FS MR in a patient with CGD shows enhancement of the iliac bone ⇨ consistent with osteomyelitis. There is an intramuscular abscess ➡ in the adjacent gluteal musculature.*

TERMINOLOGY

Abbreviations

- Chronic granulomatous disease (CGD)

Definitions

- Primary immunodeficiency characterized by recurrent infections at epithelial surfaces & organs with large numbers of reticuloendothelial cells

IMAGING

General Features

- Best diagnostic clue
  - Recurrent infections with catalase-positive organisms such as *Aspergillus* or *Staphylococcus aureus*
- Location
  - CGD can affect every organ system

Radiographic Findings

- Chest
  - Consolidation, nodules, reticulonodular opacities, & scarring
- Skeletal
  - Osteomyelitis
    - Common locations: Extremities, chest wall
      - Chest wall & vertebral involvement in up to 1/3 from contiguous spread of *Aspergillus* pneumonia

Fluoroscopic Findings

- Upper GI
  - Gastrointestinal
    - Esophagus: Dysmotility & strictures
    - Stomach: Narrowing of gastric antrum
      - Gastric outlet obstruction, delayed gastric emptying, thickened rugae
    - Bowel: Can mimic Crohn disease

CT Findings

- NECT
  - Chest
    - Pneumonia
      - Consolidation, ground-glass opacity, tree-in-bud opacity, centrilobular or random nodules, bronchiectasis, air trapping, septal thickening, or scarring
      - ± cavitation, mycetoma
      - Abscess or empyema in 20%
    - Prolonged course may lead to chronic findings
      - Mediastinal or hilar adenopathy, pulmonary fibrosis, honeycomb lung, pulmonary arterial hypertension, & pleural thickening
      - Adenopathy can be calcified related to granuloma formation
- CECT
  - Lymph nodes
    - Lymphadenopathy in nearly all patients with CGD
    - Suppurative adenitis occurs most commonly in neck
      - Enlarged, enhancing lymph node with central hypodensity ± thick, enhancing septations
    - Calcified lymph nodes as sequelae of prior infection
  - Liver
    - Hepatic abscess occurs in 1/3
      - Multiple in 60% of patients
      - Recurrence in 40% of patients
      - Abscesses < 1 cm in size enhance homogeneously
      - Abscesses between 1-3 cm have incomplete central enhancement
      - Abscesses > 3 cm have heterogeneous enhancement with thick, irregular loculations
      - Ca^{2+} can occur at site of prior infection
    - Hepatomegaly
  - Spleen
    - Splenic abscesses occur in up to 1/3 of patients with hepatic abscess
      - Splenic Ca^{2+} can occur after abscess has healed
    - Splenomegaly
  - Gastrointestinal tract
    - CGD involvement mimics Crohn disease
      - Can affect mouth to anus
      - Stomach: Narrowing of gastric antrum with wall thickening
      - Bowel: Wall thickening, mucosal hyperenhancement, skip lesions, luminal narrowing, fistulas, & perirectal abscess
  - Kidneys
    - Renal findings occur in 3% of patients
    - Pyelonephritis ± renal abscess
      - Ca^{2+} can occur after renal abscess
  - Sinuses
    - Sinusitis has similar appearance to that in immunocompetent patients (i.e., mucosal thickening, air-fluid levels)
      - Fungal sinusitis can appear hyperdense
      - ± bone destruction

MR Findings

- Liver
  - Abscess
    - T1: Hypointense
    - T2: Heterogeneously hyperintense with irregular, hypointense septations/rim ± surrounding edema
    - T1 C+: Thick rim with enhancing septations
    - DWI: Central diffusion restriction
  - Hepatosplenomegaly
- Gastrointestinal
  - Stomach: Wall thickening
  - Bowel: Wall thickening, mucosal hyperenhancement, skip lesions, luminal narrowing, fistulas, & perirectal abscess
- Brain
  - Encephalitis
  - Brain abscess
    - T2-hypointense rim with surrounding vasogenic edema
    - Irregular rim enhancement with central diffusion restriction
    - Typically occur at gray-white matter junctions
  - Meningitis: Thickened, enhancing meninges
- Sinuses
  - Sinusitis

- Similar appearance to sinusitis in immunocompetent patients
- Fungal sinusitis: Hypointense on T1/T2

Ultrasonographic Findings

- Grayscale ultrasound
  - Lymph nodes
    - Suppurative adenitis: Hypoechoic internal contents ± swirling internal debris, thickened septa; absent central vascularity, ↑ peripheral vascularity
    - Late: Hyperechoic foci with posterior shadowing (Ca^{2+}) after prior infection
  - Liver
    - Hepatic abscess: Solid or complex-appearing, hypo- to isoechoic mass
    - Absent or only septal central vascularity, ↑ peripheral vascularity
  - Bladder
    - Urinary tract infection with wall thickening
    - Inflammatory pseudotumors: Focal bladder wall thickening
      - Can mimic rhabdomyosarcoma

Imaging Recommendations

- Best imaging tool
  - Depends on site of infection: US or MR are preferred modalities due to frequent imaging in affected patients
    - Patients often receive multiple CECT scans over course of life due to rapid scan time & ease of scheduling
  - PET/CT (or potentially whole-body MR + DWIBS) can be used if site of infection cannot be identified

DIFFERENTIAL DIAGNOSIS

Recurrent Bacterial Pneumonia

- May be indistinguishable from pneumonia in CGD
- Look for underlying congenital lung lesion

Severe Combined Immunodeficiency

- Primary immunodeficiency with severe T- & B-cell dysfunction
- Infants present with infections due to lack of T cells

Crohn Disease

- Chronic, recurrent, segmental, granulomatous inflammatory bowel disease
- Differentiated from CGD by absence of pigmented histiocytes
- CGD should be considered in all patients with early-onset inflammatory bowel disease

PATHOLOGY

General Features

- Etiology
  - Defect in 1 of 5 genes encoding for NADPH-oxidase
    - Defect prevents phagocytic cells from producing respiratory burst used to kill pathogens
    - Neutrophils are able to phagocytose catalase-positive organisms but not kill them
    - Organism lives inside neutrophil causing chronic inflammatory response & granuloma formation
- Genetics
  - Transmitted in X-linked or autosomal recessive patterns
    - X-linked transmission in 65-70% of cases
    - Incidence of autosomal recessive transmission is higher in countries with higher rates of consanguinity

CLINICAL ISSUES

Presentation

- Most common signs/symptoms
  - Pneumonia is most common infection in CGD, occurring in 80% of patients
    - Most commonly caused by *Aspergillus*
  - Suppurative adenitis is 2nd most common infection in CGD, occurring in 60% of patients
    - Most commonly caused by *S. aureus*
  - Hepatic abscesses occur in 1/3 of patients with CGD
    - Most commonly caused by *S. aureus*
  - Osteomyelitis occurs in up to 25% of patients with CGD
    - Most commonly caused by *Serratia marcescens*

Demographics

- Age
  - 76% are diagnosed before 5 years of age
  - 15% diagnosed in 2nd decade
- Sex
  - 85% of patients with CGD are male
- Epidemiology
  - Occurs in 1 in 200,000-250,000 live births

Natural History & Prognosis

- X-linked disease typically presents at younger age with more severe manifestations
- Recurrent infections are typical
  - CGD has highest prevalence of invasive fungal infections among primary immunodeficiencies (20-40%)
- Historically high mortality rate: In 1967, only 21% of patients survived beyond 5 years of age
  - Currently 90% survive to 10 years of age
  - Median age of death: 30-40 years of age
  - Pneumonia or sepsis is most common cause of death

Treatment

- Stem cell transplant is only known cure for CGD
  - CGD is 3rd most common indication for stem cell transplant in patients with primary immunodeficiency

DIAGNOSTIC CHECKLIST

Consider

- Consider CGD in patients with hepatic abscess, recurrent pneumonia, or other unusual infections

SELECTED REFERENCES

1. Marsh RA et al: Chronic granulomatous disease-associated ibd resolves and does not adversely impact survival following allogeneic HCT. J Clin Immunol. 39(7):653-67, 2019
2. Rider NL et al: Chronic granulomatous disease: epidemiology, pathophysiology, and genetic basis of disease. J Pediatric Infect Dis Soc. 7(suppl_1):S2-5, 2018
3. Arnold DE et al: A review of chronic granulomatous disease. Adv Ther. 34(12):2543-57, 2017
4. Towbin AJ et al: Chronic granulomatous disease. Pediatr Radiol. 40(5):657-68; quiz 792-3, 2010

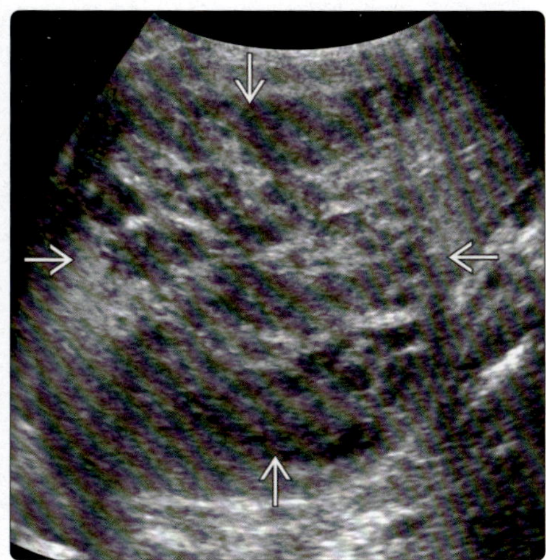

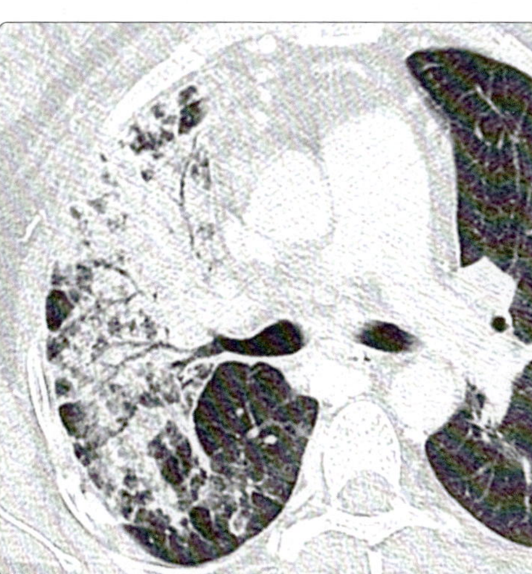

(Left) *Transverse ultrasound of the liver shows a heterogeneous, multiseptated abscess ➡. No significant internal vascularity was identified on color Doppler imaging (not shown) to suggest a solid mass.* **(Right)** *Axial CECT of the chest in a patient with CGD shows pneumonia throughout the right lung. Pneumonia is the most common type of infection & the most common cause of death in patients with CGD.*

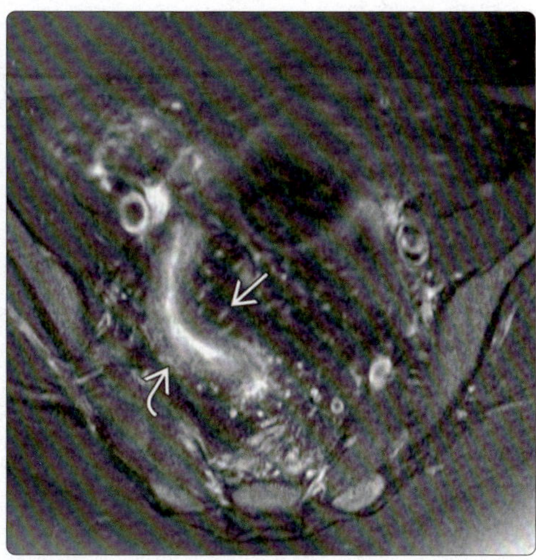

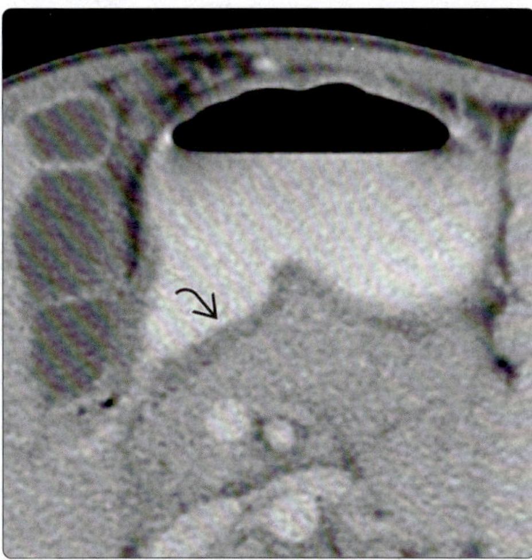

(Left) *Axial T2 FS MR of the pelvis shows diffuse wall thickening ⮫ & ↑ signal intensity of the sigmoid colon with associated engorgement of the vasa recta ➡. Inflammatory bowel disease in patients with CGD can mimic Crohn disease.* **(Right)** *Axial CECT of the stomach shows thickening ⮫ of the gastric antrum, a typical location of inflammation in chronic granulomatous disease.*

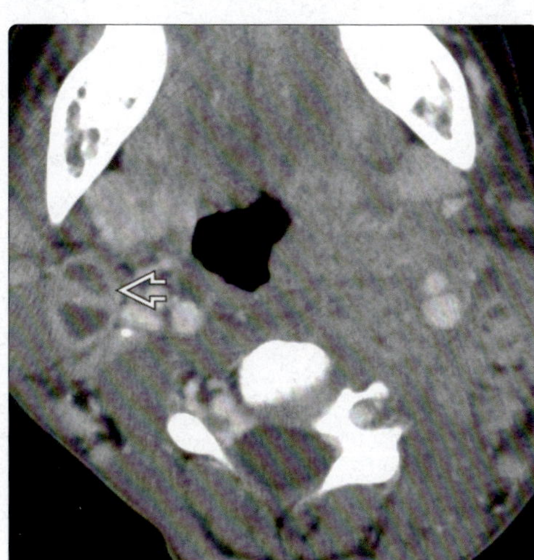

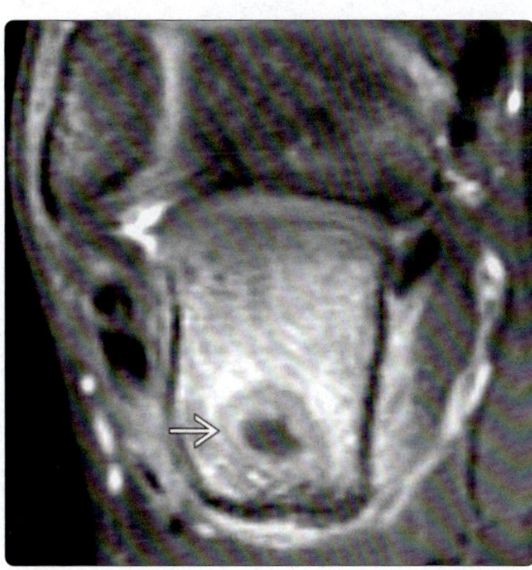

(Left) *Axial CECT of the neck shows a suppurative lymph node ⇨ in the right cervical chain. All patients with CGD have lymphadenopathy, & up to 60% of patients develop suppurative adenitis.* **(Right)** *Coronal T1 C+ FS MR shows a targetoid focus of abnormal enhancement of the calcaneus. The center of this lesion does not enhance, typical of pus. There is a moderately thick rim of enhancing granulation tissue ➡ + marked surrounding marrow edema.*

Pneumatosis in Older Children

KEY FACTS

TERMINOLOGY

- Presence of gas within walls of gastrointestinal tract
- In older children, more frequently benign & associated with variety of underlying conditions & medications

IMAGING

- Radiography is 1st-line imaging modality
  - CT is more sensitive but often not needed
- Curvilinear or round gas collections within bowel wall
  - Colon > small bowel > > stomach
  - Benign pneumatosis can be extensive
- ± free intraperitoneal air
  - Not necessarily due to intestinal perforation
- CT findings concerning for clinically significant causes: Bowel wall thickening or ↓ enhancement, adjacent inflammatory stranding, free fluid

TOP DIFFERENTIAL DIAGNOSES

- Benign causes: Medications (corticosteroids), systemic or pulmonary diseases, solid organ or bone marrow transplant
- Significant causes: Ischemia, bowel obstruction, severe infection, trauma

PATHOLOGY

- Multiple proposed mechanisms for gas dissecting into bowel wall; likely multifactorial
  - Mucosal damage &/or ↑ intraluminal pressure allows gas to dissect into wall

CLINICAL ISSUES

- Without worrisome clinical features → managed conservatively
  - Observation, bowel rest, alter medications, treat underlying conditions
- Worrisome clinical features → frequently require surgical management

(Left) *AP radiograph in a 3-year-old boy with multiple medical problems shows extensive curvilinear lucencies separating layers of the colonic wall ➡. This pneumatosis extends all the way to the rectum. The patient was clinically stable, & the pneumatosis was thought to be benign & due to corticosteroid use.* **(Right)** *Axial CECT in a different child shows diffuse pneumatosis throughout the visualized colonic wall ➡.*

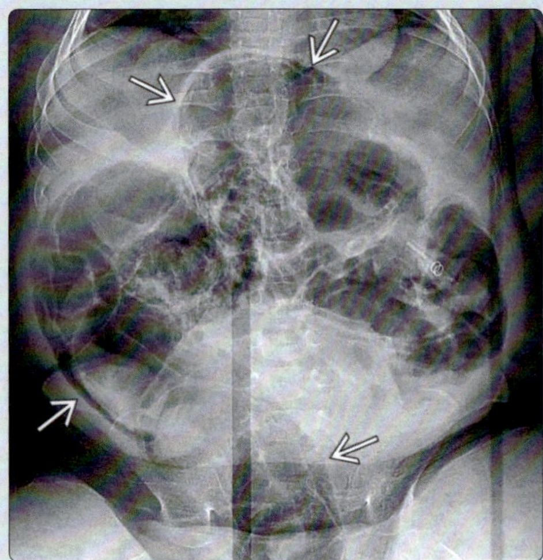

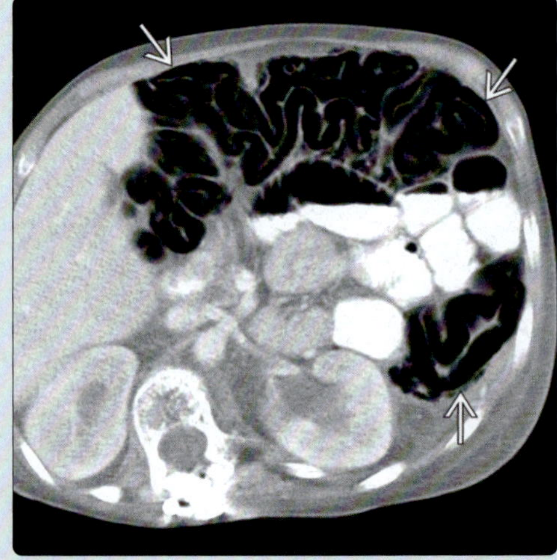

(Left) *AP radiograph in a 2-year-old boy with a seizure disorder & multiple medical problems shows colonic pneumatosis, mostly in the ascending colon & proximal transverse colon ➡.* **(Right)** *Coronal CECT in the same 2-year-old boy shows extensive pneumatosis ➡ throughout the colon. There is also a small amount of free intraperitoneal gas ➡. Despite the presence of free air, the patient was treated conservatively due to his clinical status & lack of other imaging features to suggest ischemia or obstruction.*

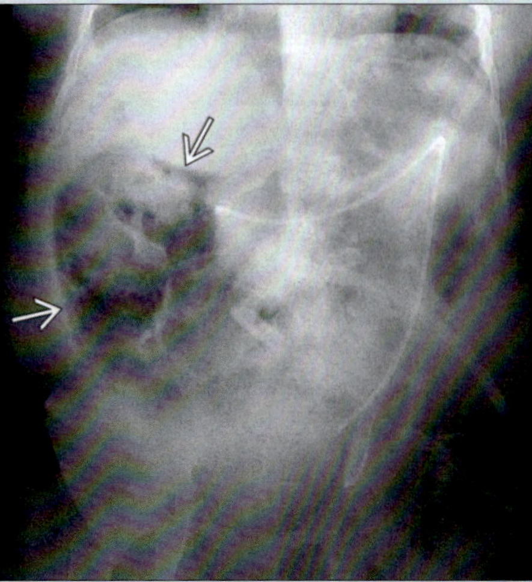

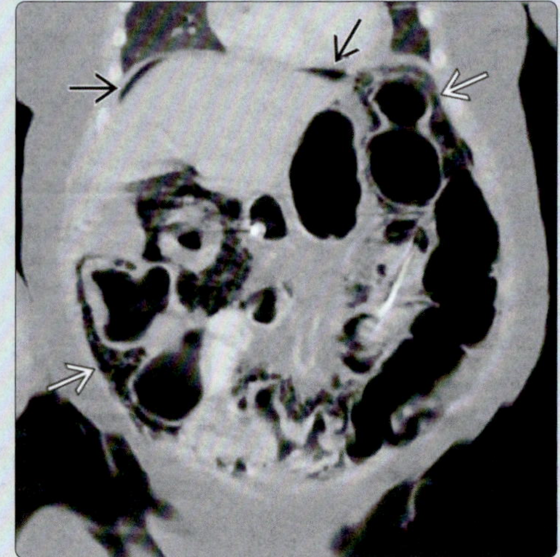

TERMINOLOGY

Synonyms

- Pneumatosis intestinalis; pneumatosis coli (confined to colon); pneumatosis cystoides intestinalis

Definitions

- Presence of gas within walls of gastrointestinal tract
  - Associated with necrotizing enterocolitis in
    - Premature infants
    - Term newborns with congenital heart disease & other cardiovascular abnormalities
  - In older children, more frequently benign & associated with variety of underlying conditions & medications

IMAGING

General Features

- Best diagnostic clue
  - Curvilinear or rounded gas collections within bowel wall
    - Colon > small bowel > > stomach
  - Extensive colonic pneumatosis is most frequently due to benign causes

Radiographic Findings

- Curvilinear or rounded foci of gas outlining bowel wall
  - Can have mottled appearance
- ± dilated bowel or evidence of bowel wall thickening
- ± free intraperitoneal air

CT Findings

- CECT
  - Gas collections within wall of bowel
    - Foci of gas in posterior bowel wall may help differentiate from intraluminal gas or gas-containing fecal debris
  - CT findings helpful in differentiating benign from clinically significant causes
    - Extensive pneumatosis: More commonly benign
    - Bowel wall thickening: Usually significant
    - ↓ bowel wall enhancement: Typically significant
    - Adjacent inflammatory stranding: Typically significant
    - Moderate to large free fluid: Typically significant
  - Some CT findings **not** helpful in differentiating benign from clinically significant causes
    - Curvilinear vs. cystic pattern
    - Distribution in small vs. large bowel
    - Portal venous gas
    - Free intraperitoneal air

Ultrasonographic Findings

- Look for echogenic gas tracking within bowel wall, particularly lateral & posterior aspects
  - Posterior acoustic shadowing & ring-down artifact
  - ± twinkling artifact with color Doppler

DIFFERENTIAL DIAGNOSIS

Benign Causes of Pneumatosis Intestinalis

- Medications
  - Corticosteroids, certain chemotherapy agents
- Transplant patients
  - Bone marrow/stem cell transplants
    - May be associated with graft-vs.-host disease
  - Solid organ transplants
- Pulmonary disease
  - Mechanical barotrauma
- Autoimmune/rheumatologic diseases
  - ↑ in conditions associated with vasculitis

Clinically Worrisome Causes of Pneumatosis Intestinalis

- Intestinal ischemia
- Severe enterocolitis
- Bowel obstruction
- Trauma

PATHOLOGY

General Features

- Etiology
  - Multiple proposed mechanisms; may be multifactorial
    - Mucosal injury ± limited ability to repair mucosa due to medications (e.g., corticosteroids) or vascular abnormalities (e.g., vasculitis)
    - Abnormal bowel wall lymphatics from medications (chemotherapy, corticosteroids), allowing gas to dissect into wall
    - ↑ intraluminal pressure pushing gas or gas-forming bacteria into bowel wall
    - Dissection of gas from mediastinum → mesentery → bowel wall

Gross Pathologic & Surgical Features

- Gas within submucosal & subserosal spaces
  - May represent gas within dilated intramural lymphatics

CLINICAL ISSUES

Treatment

- Managed conservatively if clinically stable
  - Bowel rest, removal of offending medications, treatment of underlying conditions
- If worrisome by clinical or laboratory features → surgical or more aggressive medical management

SELECTED REFERENCES

1. Ryan JL et al: Conservative management of pneumatosis intestinalis and portal venous gas after pediatric liver transplantation. Transplant Proc. 52(3):938-42, 2020
2. Gui X et al: Is pneumatosis cystoides intestinalis gas-distended and ruptured lymphatics? Reappraisal by immunohistochemistry. Arch Pathol Lab Med. 138(8):1059-66, 2014
3. Lee KS et al: Distinguishing benign and life-threatening pneumatosis intestinalis in patients with cancer by CT imaging features. AJR Am J Roentgenol. 200(5):1042-7, 2013
4. Korhonen K et al: Incidence, risk factors, and outcome of pneumatosis intestinalis in pediatric stem cell transplant recipients. Pediatr Blood Cancer. 58(4):616-20, 2012
5. Olson DE et al: CT predictors for differentiating benign and clinically worrisome pneumatosis intestinalis in children beyond the neonatal period. Radiology. 253(2):513-9, 2009
6. McCarville MB et al: Clinical and CT features of benign pneumatosis intestinalis in pediatric hematopoietic stem cell transplant and oncology patients. Pediatr Radiol. 38(10):1074-83, 2008

Crohn Disease

KEY FACTS

TERMINOLOGY

- Chronic, recurrent, segmental, granulomatous inflammatory bowel disease; etiology is unknown

IMAGING

- CD occurs anywhere in GI tract from mouth to anus
  - Disease distribution in children varies with age & differs from adults
- US: Thickened bowel wall with loss of gut signature, ↑ perienteric fat echogenicity, ± bowel wall & perienteric hyperemia
- CT/MR enterography
  - Bowel findings
    - Mural hyperenhancement & thickening: Most sensitive findings
    - Mural stratification of bowel wall enhancement
    - Strictures showing upstream effects (dilation & small bowel feces sign)
    - Ulcers/fistulas/sinus tracts
  - Mesenteric findings
    - Engorged vasa recta (comb sign & dot sign)
    - Fat stranding, fibrofatty proliferation
    - Inflammatory mass/abscesses
    - ↑ size & number of lymph nodes
  - Perianal disease
    - Tract/collection extending from anus/skin

PATHOLOGY

- Skip lesions of transmural inflammation occur anywhere from mouth to anus: Ileocolic is most common

CLINICAL ISSUES

- Prevalence: 58 cases/100,000 children
- 25-30% of patients are diagnosed in 1st 2 decades of life
- Extraintestinal manifestations in 17-28% at diagnosis

DIAGNOSTIC CHECKLIST

- Penetrating &/or stricturing disease alters management

(Left) *Delayed image from a small bowel follow-through in a patient with CD shows isolation, narrowing, & irregularity of the terminal ileum ➡ & cecum ⇨. It is inferred that the separated loops are caused by bowel wall thickening & "creeping fat."* **(Right)** *Axial T1 C+ FS MR in an adolescent shows multiple findings of Crohn disease. The affected bowel ⇨ is thickened with diffuse wall enhancement. There is stranding ⇨ of the adjacent mesenteric fat. The loops of bowel are clumped together at the site of a fistula ⇨.*

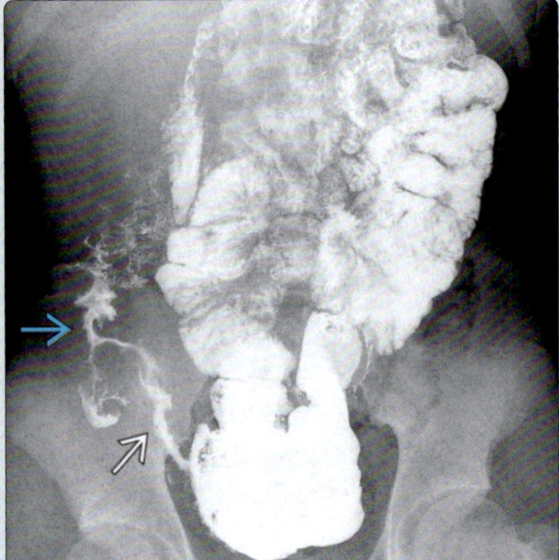

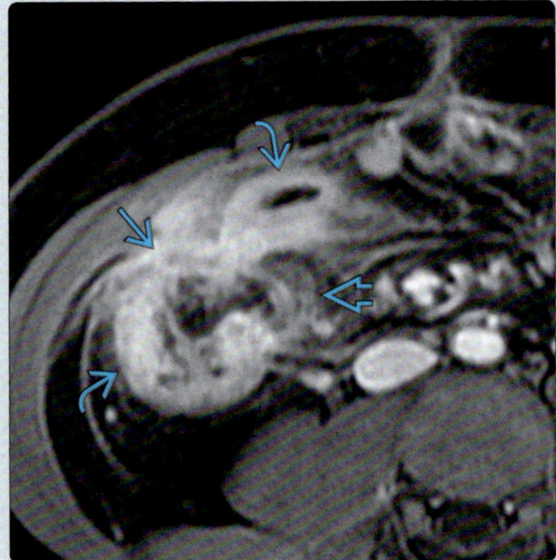

(Left) *Coronal T1 FS MR shows inflammation & wall thickening ⇨ of the terminal ileum. The affected bowel has a bulging nonthickened focus ⇨ along the antimesenteric border, typical of a pseudosacculation.* **(Right)** *Axial DWI MR of the pelvis shows a segment of bowel with restricted diffusion ⇨, which is a sign of active inflammation in patients with Crohn disease.*

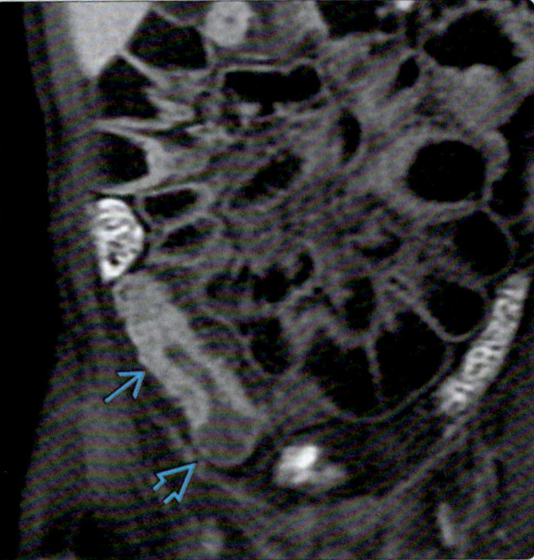

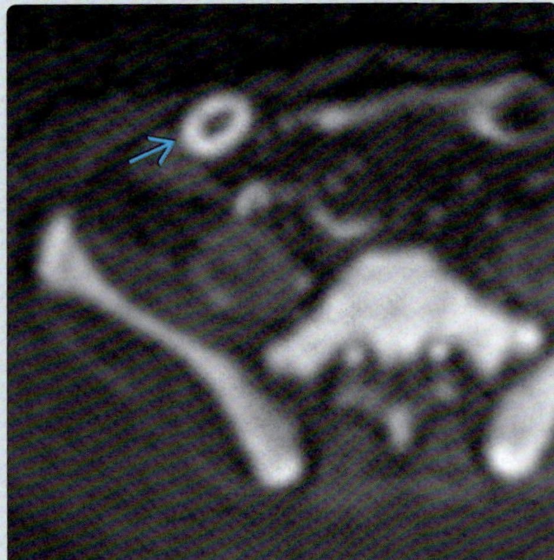

TERMINOLOGY

Abbreviations

- Crohn disease (CD)

Definitions

- Chronic, recurrent, segmental, granulomatous inflammatory bowel disease (IBD)

IMAGING

General Features

- Best diagnostic clue
  - CT/MR enterography
    - Bowel wall thickening & mucosal hyperenhancement with associated perienteric inflammatory changes
- Location
  - Anywhere in gastrointestinal (GI) tract from mouth to anus
  - Disease distribution in children varies with age & differs from adults
    - Very early onset IBD (age < 6 years)
      - More likely to present with isolated colonic disease
    - Older children/adolescents
      - Most common location: Ileocolonic region
      - Isolated terminal ileum (TI) disease is uncommon, occurring in < 10%
      - Small bowel involvement proximal to TI in > 50%
      - Upper GI involvement occurs in 1/3-1/2 of patients
      - Gastric involvement is more common than in adults
      - Appendix may be involved, even in isolation

Fluoroscopic Findings

- Upper GI with SBFT
  - Separation of bowel loops due to wall thickening & "creeping" proliferative fat
  - Irregular appearance of bowel mucosa
    - Cobblestone pattern: Longitudinal + transverse ulcers
    - Thickened mucosal folds & featureless mucosa
  - String sign of narrowed bowel lumen
    - Up to 20%, most commonly in TI
  - Skip lesions (90%)
  - Sacculations at antimesenteric border

CT Findings

- CT enterography
  - Technique
    - Low-density oral contrast material maximizes bowel luminal distention
    - IV contrast with imaging in enteric phase (~ 45 s) or portal venous phase (~ 70 s)
  - Bowel findings
    - Mural hyperenhancement
    - Bowel wall thickening (lower attenuation edema)
    - Mural stratification: Layers of bowel wall show differential enhancement
    - Luminal narrowing or stricture
    - Sacculations
  - Mesenteric findings
    - Engorged vasa recta (comb sign if tangential or dot sign in cross section)
    - Fat stranding ± fibrofatty proliferation
    - Prominent lymph nodes (↑ in size & number, often not > 1 cm in short axis)
  - Penetrating disease
    - Ulceration/fistula/sinus tract
    - Inflammatory mass/abscess
    - Perianal disease
  - Stricturing disease
    - Luminal narrowing with proximal dilation ± proximal small bowel feces sign or stuck pill/enterolith

MR Findings

- MR enterography
  - Technique
    - Biphasic enteric contrast agent to maximize bowel luminal distention
      - Bright on T2, dark on T1
    - Glucagon may be used to slow/stop bowel peristalsis
    - SSFSE T2 ± FS
    - DWI (particularly helpful if IV contrast is not possible)
    - Rapid 3D GRE T1 C+ FS sequences
    - Targeted axial & coronal oblique images of anus for suspicion of perianal disease
  - Findings are similar to those seen with CT enterography
    - Additional findings
      - Restricted diffusion of inflamed segment
      - Focally ↓ peristalsis
  - Benefits of MR enterography over CT enterography
    - Improved visualization of penetrating/fistulizing disease, particularly in perianal region
    - Visualization of bowel at multiple timepoints
    - Lack of ionizing radiation
    - Improved visualization of extraintestinal manifestations of CD

Ultrasonographic Findings

- Grayscale ultrasound
  - High-resolution, high-frequency linear transducer with graded compression
  - Findings are similar to those seen on CT/MR
    - Thickened bowel with loss of normal gut signature
    - ↓ or absent peristalsis
    - ↑ perienteric fat echogenicity & volume
    - Lymphadenopathy
    - Fluid collections
- Color Doppler
  - Bowel wall & perienteric hyperemia

Other Modality Findings

- Direct visualization with upper & lower endoscopy
  - Allows contemporaneous biopsy
  - Cannot view jejunum & ileum
  - Cannot visualize extraintestinal manifestations
- Capsule endoscopy
  - 11- x 27-mm capsule camera
  - Direct visualization of mucosal lesions
  - Risk of capsule not passing beyond area of stricture
  - Retained capsule camera is not MR compatible

Imaging Recommendations

- Protocol advice

- CT & MR enterography: High accuracy for detection of active IBD & associated complications
  - MR enterography lacks ionizing radiation exposure
  - CT enterography may be more sensitive in detecting early/mucosal disease & has less interrater variation
- Ultrasound is less sensitive but may be useful in initially suggesting CD or following diseased segment

DIFFERENTIAL DIAGNOSIS

Ulcerative Colitis

- Contiguous colitis extending proximally from anus
  - No skip lesions
- Most common cause of IBD in children < 6 years of age
- ± backwash ileitis
- Not transmural: No strictures, sinuses, or fistulas
- Pseudopolyps, ↑ risk of colon cancer

Indeterminate Colitis

- Term used when there are histologic features of CD & ulcerative colitis (UC)
- Accounts for 5-33% of IBD in pediatric population
- Up to 30% are later reclassified as CD or UC

Appendicitis

- Dilated, thick-walled, noncompressible appendix with induration of surrounding fat
  - ± hyperemia, appendicolith, abscess
- Adjacent bowel is typically normal in absence of appendiceal perforation

Infectious Enterocolitis

- Nonspecific imaging findings of ileocecal infection; resolves with appropriate treatment

Chronic Granulomatous Disease

- Primary immunodeficiency characterized by recurrent infection with catalase-positive organisms
- Bowel is affected in 30-50% of patients
  - Mimics CD with involvement from mouth to anus

PATHOLOGY

General Features

- Etiology
  - Idiopathic IBD with prolonged & unpredictable course

Gross Pathologic & Surgical Features

- Skip lesions, edema, inflammation, fibrosis, & strictures

Microscopic Features

- Transmural inflammation, lymphoid aggregates, & noncaseating granulomas
- Dilation & sclerosis of lymphatic channels

CLINICAL ISSUES

Presentation

- Most common signs/symptoms
  - Pain, diarrhea, & weight loss
    - Weight loss is presenting feature in 85% of children
- Laboratory findings
  - Anemia, leukocytosis, ↑ C-reactive protein, & ↑ erythrocyte sedimentation rate
  - ↑ fecal calprotectin
  - p-ANCA(-), ASCA(+): Favors CD over UC
    - UC is suggested when p-ANCA(+) & ASCA(-)

Demographics

- Age
  - Bimodal age distribution with main peak at 18-25 years, smaller peak at 60-80 years
  - 25-30% of patients are diagnosed in 1st 2 decades of life
- Sex
  - 1.5:1 male predominance in prepubertal patients
- Epidemiology
  - ↑ incidence in developing world
  - Prevalence: 58 cases/100,000 children

Natural History & Prognosis

- Recurrence: 30-53% after resection; only 10-20% lead symptom-free lives
- Complications
  - Stricturing/penetrating
    - Penetrating complications almost always occur in setting of stricture
    - Potential complications: Ulceration, sinus tracts, fistulas, & abscesses
  - Extraintestinal manifestations in 17-28% at diagnosis
    - Stones: Cholelithiasis, urolithiasis (oxalate)
    - Arthropathy: Enthesis-related arthritis
    - Hepatobiliary: Autoimmune hepatitis, primary sclerosing cholangitis
    - Skin: Erythema nodosum, pyoderma gangrenosum
    - Other: Thromboembolism, pancreatitis, episcleritis, uveitis
  - Malignancy
    - Adenocarcinoma: Latency of 25-30 years
    - Lymphoma

Treatment

- Medical
  - Bowel rest, steroids, azathioprine, mesalamine, metronidazole
  - Biologic agents: Infliximab
- Surgical
  - Resection of diseased bowel, strictureplasty, & primary fistulotomy

DIAGNOSTIC CHECKLIST

Image Interpretation Pearls

- Penetrating/stricturing disease: Alters clinical management

SELECTED REFERENCES

1. Bruining DH et al: Consensus recommendations for evaluation, interpretation, and utilization of computed tomography and magnetic resonance enterography in patients with small bowel crohn's disease. Radiology. 286(3):776-99, 2018
2. Orscheln ES et al: Penetrating Crohn disease: does it occur in the absence of stricturing disease? Abdom Radiol (NY). 43(7):1583-9, 2018
3. Dillman JR et al: MR enterography: how to deliver added value. Pediatr Radiol. 46(6):829-37, 2016
4. Dillman JR et al: Pediatric small bowel crohn disease: correlation of us and mr enterography. Radiographics. 35(3):835-48, 2015
5. Towbin AJ et al: CT and MR enterography in children and adolescents with inflammatory bowel disease. Radiographics. 33(7):1843-60, 2013

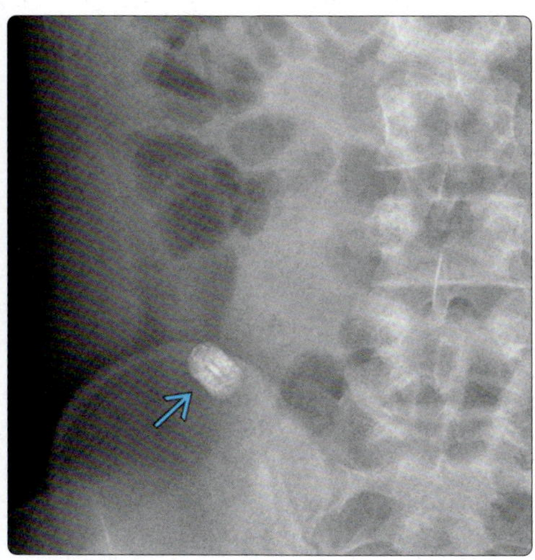

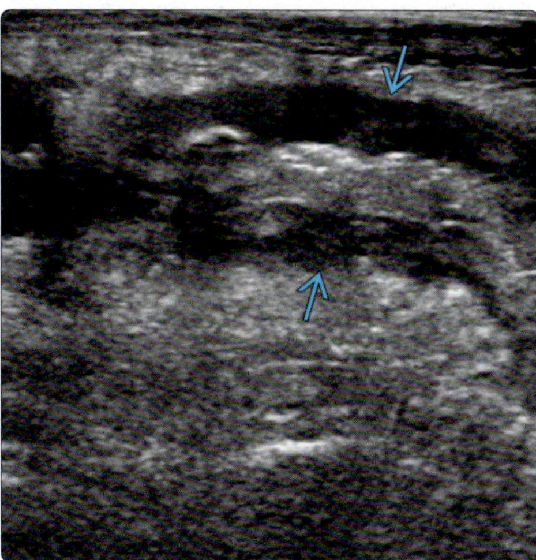

(Left) *AP abdominal radiograph shows a patency capsule ➔ in the right lower quadrant. Patency capsules are used to identify a bowel stricture prior to capsule endoscopy as a stricture is a contraindication to this procedure.* **(Right)** *Transverse ultrasound of bowel in the right lower quadrant shows diffuse wall thickening ➔ of the imaged segment. There is proliferation of echogenic fat deep to this loop of bowel.*

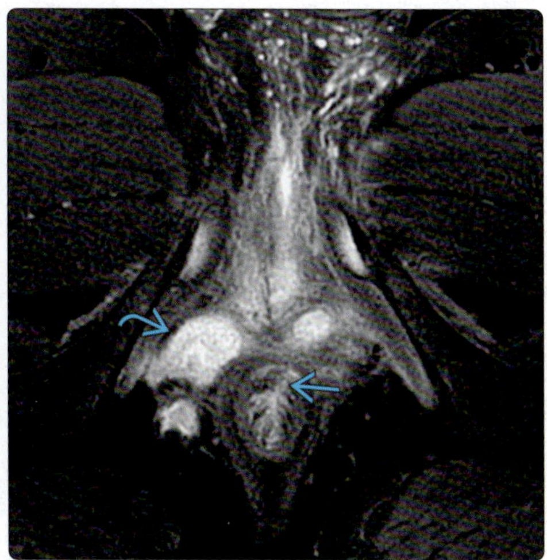

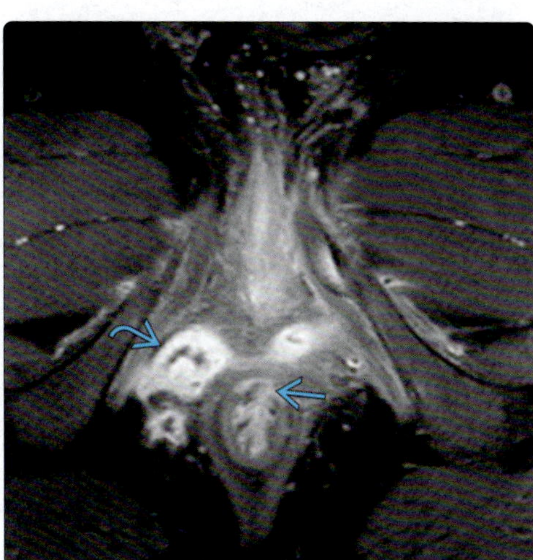

(Left) *Axial T2 FS MR shows a fistula ➔ arising from the 12:00-1:00 position of the rectum. There is a large abscess ➔ in the ischiorectal fossa.* **(Right)** *Axial T1 C+ FS MR in the same patient shows a fistula ➔ arising from the 12:00-1:00 position of the anus. There is a large abscess ➔ in the ischiorectal fossa. An abscess can be differentiated from an inflammatory mass by the lack of central enhancement in the collection.*

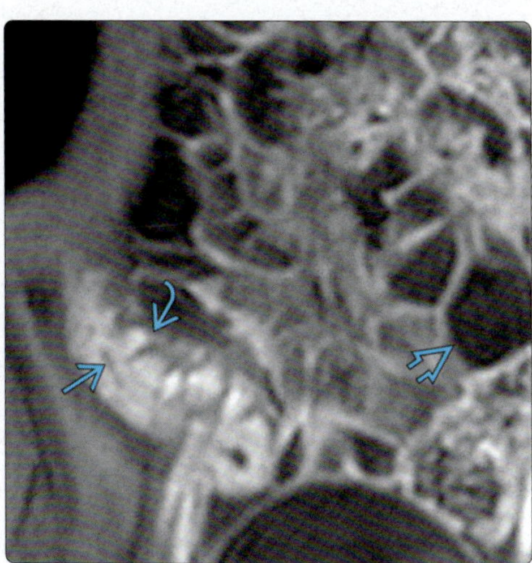

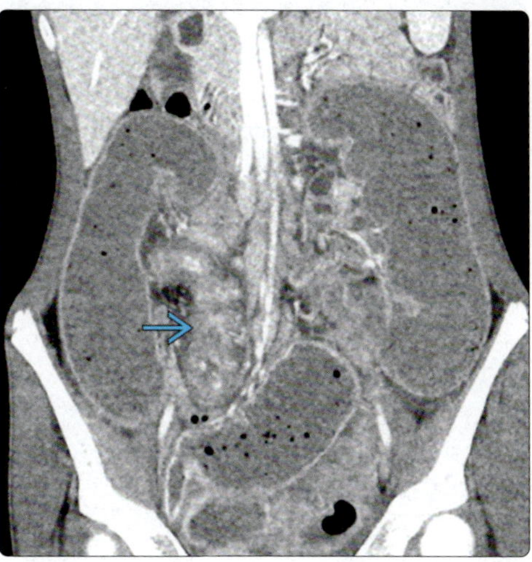

(Left) *Coronal T1 C+ FS MR shows the terminal ileum to be inflamed with wall thickening, enhancement, & sinus tracts ➔ extending perpendicular to the bowel. The bowel lumen ➔ is severely narrowed, causing a stricture. Upstream small bowel loops ➔ are dilated.* **(Right)** *Coronal CECT shows severe inflammation with stricture of the terminal ileum ➔. Upstream loops of small bowel are markedly dilated with their luminal contents appearing as feces, a sign that the stricture has been longstanding.*

Ulcerative Colitis

KEY FACTS

TERMINOLOGY

- Chronic, idiopathic inflammatory disease that primarily involves colorectal mucosa & submucosa
  - Extends retrograde from rectum
  - No skip lesions or transmural involvement

IMAGING

- CT/MR enterography findings
  - Continuous colonic inflammation extending proximally from rectum for variable distance
  - Mucosal hyperenhancement & wall thickening
  - Thickened, edematous haustra (thumbprinting)
  - Luminal narrowing
  - Mural stratification: More common in ulcerative colitis than Crohn disease
  - DWI MR can aid in detecting inflammation, particularly if IV contrast is not available
  - In later disease, dilation or narrowing of colon with loss of haustra

TOP DIFFERENTIAL DIAGNOSES

- Crohn disease
- Pseudomembranous colitis
- Infectious colitis

CLINICAL ISSUES

- Majority of patients are diagnosed in 4th-5th decades
- Annual incidence: 5-10 cases/100,000 population
  - More common than Crohn disease in preschool age
- Most common presenting symptom: Bloody diarrhea
- Complications
  - Toxic megacolon: 5-10%
  - Stricture: 10%
  - Colorectal cancer risk: ↑ 30x
- Common extraintestinal manifestations: Arthralgias, primary sclerosing cholangitis, uveitis

(Left) *Axial T1 C+ FS MR enterography in an adolescent with ulcerative colitis shows inflammation of the ascending ➡, descending ➡, & sigmoid ➡ colon with wall thickening & hyperenhancement. There is mild stranding of the adjacent fat & engorgement of vasa recta at several levels.* **(Right)** *Axial DWI MR in the same patient shows restricted diffusion ➡ of the sigmoid colon, consistent with active inflammation.*

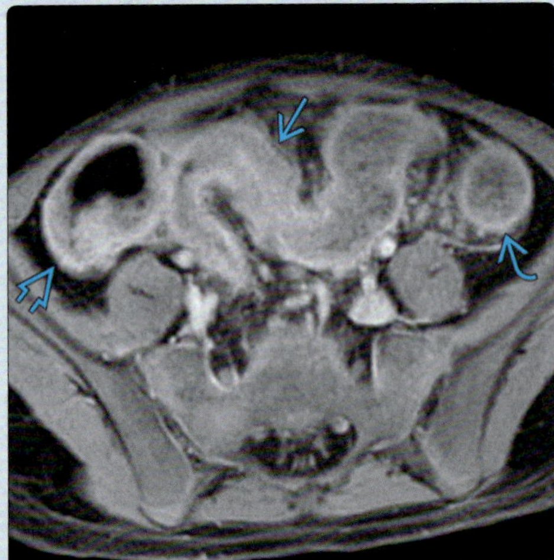

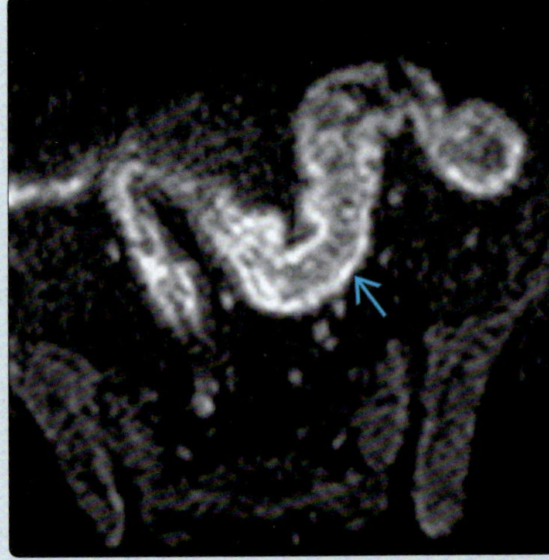

(Left) *Axial CECT in an adolescent with ulcerative colitis shows inflammation of the sigmoid colon ➡, demonstrating mild wall thickening & enhancement. The vasa recta ➡ are engorged.* **(Right)** *Coronal T2 FS MR in a patient with ulcerative colitis shows an abnormal, featureless appearance of the descending colon ➡ with associated wall thickening. The featureless or lead pipe appearance of the colon is a classic description in the setting of ulcerative colitis.*

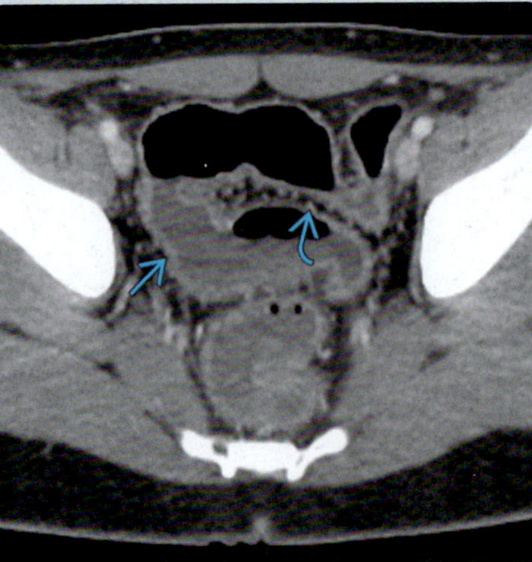

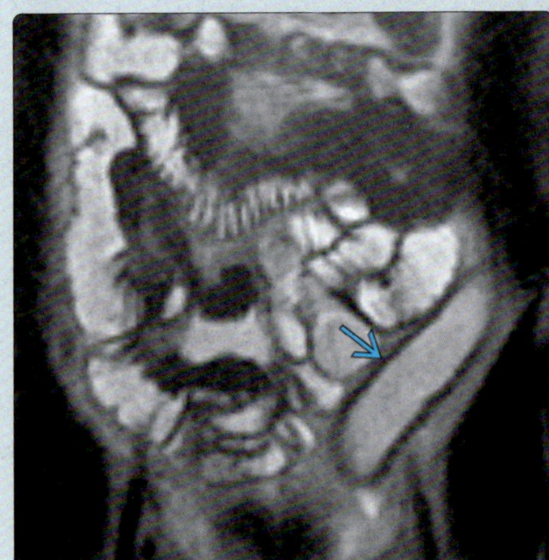

TERMINOLOGY

Abbreviations

- Ulcerative colitis (UC)

Definitions

- Chronic, idiopathic diffuse inflammatory disease that primarily involves colorectal mucosa & submucosa

IMAGING

General Features

- Best diagnostic clue
  - CT/MR enterography: Mucosal hyperenhancement & wall thickening of colon/rectum
- Location
  - Continuous colonic inflammation extending proximally from rectum for variable distance
  - Pancolonic disease is present in 60-90% of children at diagnosis

Radiographic Findings

- Thickened, edematous haustra (thumbprinting) with narrowing of gas-filled lumen
- In later disease, dilation of colon with loss of haustra

Fluoroscopic Findings

- Contrast enema is not routinely used for UC evaluation in current practice
- Classic findings on contrast enema: Mucosal irregularity, ulceration, thickened haustra, luminal narrowing
  - Chronic phase: Featureless, foreshortened colon ("lead pipe" colon)

CT Findings

- CECT
  - Continuous, symmetric wall thickening of colon
  - Luminal narrowing
  - Mucosal islands or inflammatory pseudopolyps
  - Mural stratification: More common in UC than Crohn disease
  - Inflammatory pericolonic stranding
  - No penetrating disease (fistula, abscess) due to lack of transmural inflammation

MR Findings

- Findings similar to those seen with CT
- DWI can aid in detecting inflammation

Ultrasonographic Findings

- Degree of colonic wall thickening & loss of colonic wall stratification may predict failure of steroids

Other Modality Findings

- Ileocolonoscopy
  - Allows contemporaneous biopsy
  - Cannot visualize extraintestinal manifestations

Imaging Recommendations

- Relatively low sensitivity for detecting colonic inflammation with CT/MR enterography due to colonic nondistention

DIFFERENTIAL DIAGNOSIS

Crohn Disease

- Anywhere from mouth to anus may be involved
- Noncontiguous skip lesions are characteristic
- Transmural eccentric sinuses, fissures, fistulas

Pseudomembranous Colitis

- Pancolitis related to antibiotic use & overgrowth of *Clostridium difficile*

Infectious Colitis

- Nonspecific wall thickening & hyperenhancement
- Distribution varies depending on organism

CLINICAL ISSUES

Presentation

- Most common presentation: Bloody diarrhea
- Less common presenting symptoms: Anemia, poor growth, perianal symptoms
- Complications
  - Toxic megacolon: 5-10%
  - Stricture: 10%
  - Colorectal cancer risk: ↑ 30x
- Extraintestinal manifestations
  - Occur in 16-30% of patients
  - Common: Arthralgias, primary sclerosing cholangitis, uveitis
  - ↑ likelihood of colectomy
- Laboratory finding
  - p-ANCA(+) & ASCA(-) favors UC over Crohn disease

Demographics

- Age
  - Majority of patients are diagnosed in 4th-5th decades
  - More common than Crohn disease in preschool age
  - UC accounts for 25-30% of pediatric inflammatory bowel disease (IBD)

Treatment

- Medical: Sulfasalazine, steroids, azathioprine, methotrexate, LTB4 inhibitors
- Surgical: Total colectomy

DIAGNOSTIC CHECKLIST

Image Interpretation Pearls

- Continuous involvement of colon extending proximally from rectum for variable length
- UC is more common than Crohn disease in patients with sclerosing cholangitis

SELECTED REFERENCES

1. Scarallo L et al: Bowel ultrasound scan predicts corticosteroid failure in children with acute severe colitis. J Pediatr Gastroenterol Nutr. 71(1):46-51, 2020
2. Schooler GR et al: MR imaging evaluation of inflammatory bowel disease in children:: where are we now in 2019. Magn Reson Imaging Clin N Am. 27(2):291-300, 2019
3. Yu YR et al: Clinical presentation of Crohn's, ulcerative colitis, and indeterminate colitis: symptoms, extraintestinal manifestations, and disease phenotypes. Semin Pediatr Surg. 26(6):349-55, 2017

Esophageal Strictures

KEY FACTS

TERMINOLOGY

- Acquired narrowing of esophagus, caused by variety of entities; congenital stenosis is considered here as well

IMAGING

- Focal or diffuse narrowing of esophagus, associated with proximal dilation & altered peristalsis
- Particular segment affected as well as length & degree of narrowing depend on etiology & severity of initial esophageal injury
- Different causes of stricture have different imaging characteristics
- Esophagram findings
  - Esophageal atresia repair: Focal stricture at junction of upper & middle 1/3
  - Peptic stricture: Stricture in distal esophagus
  - Eosinophilic esophagitis: Most commonly normal; may be diffusely narrow
  - Caustic strictures: Most common in proximal & mid esophagus
    - Multiple strictures can occur
  - Epidermolysis bullosa: Stricture is most common in cervical esophagus
  - Infective esophagitis: May progress to strictures
  - Congenital stenosis
    - Membranous web: Upper or middle 1/3
    - Fibromuscular thickening: Middle or distal 1/3
    - Tracheobronchial cartilage remnant/foregut malformation: Distal 1/3

CLINICAL ISSUES

- Infants present with feeding difficulties; food bolus impaction occurs in older children with drooling, vomiting, pain, sensation of food getting stuck
  - ± airway symptoms (e.g., wheezing, recurrent coughing)
- Balloon dilation is used for many conditions; stricture resection or esophageal replacement for refractory cases

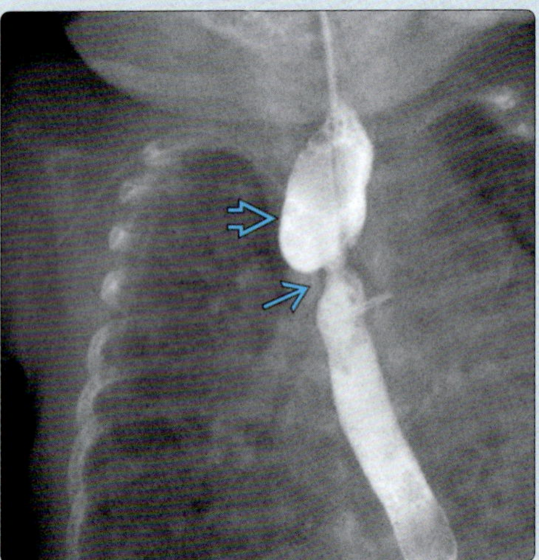

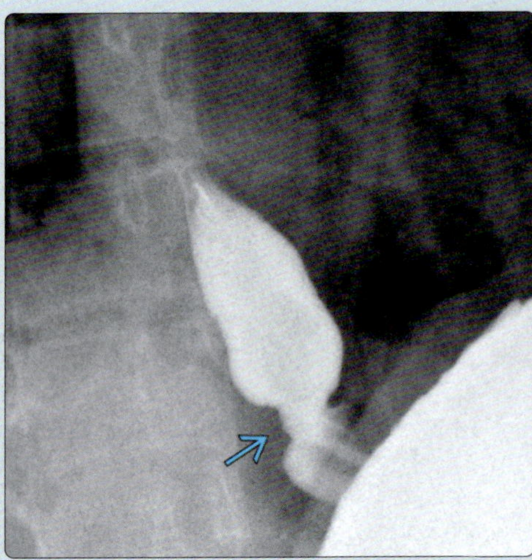

(Left) *Frontal image from an esophagram in an infant status post esophageal atresia repair shows a focal stricture ➡ at the esophageal anastomosis. The proximal esophagus ➡ remains dilated due to longstanding obstruction prior to repair.* **(Right)** *Frontal image from an esophagram in an adolescent with a history of food getting stuck & eosinophilic esophagitis shows a stricture ➡ in the distal esophagus, confirmed at endoscopy.*

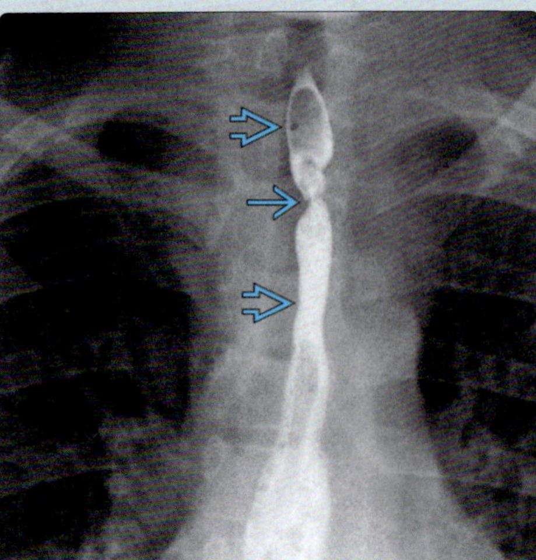

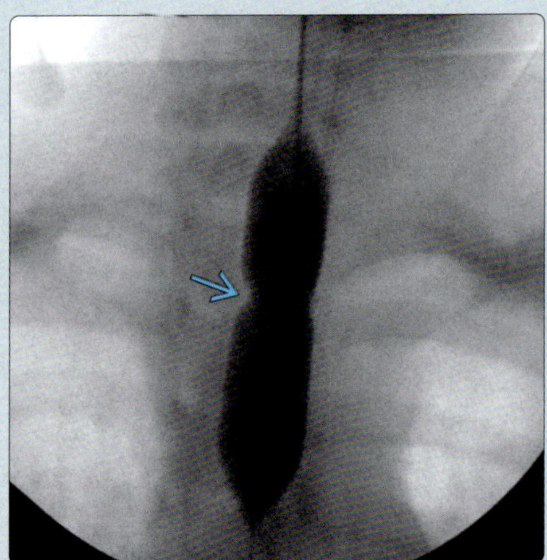

(Left) *AP image from an esophagram in a child with epidermolysis bullosa shows a focal stricture ➡ at the thoracic inlet, which is superimposed on more generalized narrowing ➡.* **(Right)** *Frontal fluoroscopic image in the same patient shows balloon dilation of the proximal esophageal stricture. The waist ➡ in the mid balloon corresponds to the site of stricture.*

TERMINOLOGY

Definitions

- Acquired narrowing of esophagus from variety of entities
- Congenital causes of stenosis considered here as well

IMAGING

General Features

- Best diagnostic clue
  - Narrowing of esophagus, associated with proximal dilation & altered peristalsis
  - Particular segment affected as well as length & degree of narrowing depend on etiology & severity of esophageal injury

Radiographic Findings

- Search for radiopaque foreign body
- Search for acute or chronic complications of foreign body or caustic ingestion
  - Perforation of esophagus with pneumomediastinum or pleural effusion
  - Chronically dilated esophagus with air-fluid level on upright view

Fluoroscopic Findings

- Esophagram
  - Focal or diffuse narrowing of esophagus; dysmotility is common
  - Different causes of stricture have different imaging characteristics
    - Congenital stenosis
      - Membranous web: Upper or middle 1/3
      - Fibromuscular thickening: Middle or distal 1/3
      - Tracheobronchial cartilage remnant/foregut malformation: Distal 1/3
    - Prior esophageal atresia repair
      - Focal stricture at site of prior anastomosis between dilated proximal esophageal pouch & remaining mid to distal esophagus
    - Peptic stricture
      - Stricture in distal esophagus from chronic gastroesophageal reflux (GER)
    - Caustic strictures
      - Esophagram may not be helpful in acute phase as it delays endoscopy & may not reveal mucosal injury
      - Subsequent strictures can be focal, multifocal, or long segment, depending on ingested substance
      - Most common in proximal & mid esophagus
    - Eosinophilic esophagitis
      - Most common finding: Normal esophagus
      - ± GER, irregular contractions, esophageal strictures or rings, generally small-caliber esophagus, & food bolus impaction
    - Epidermolysis bullosa
      - Stricture is most common in cervical esophagus
    - Infective esophagitis
      - Severe esophageal infections may progress to strictures
  - Useful to identify complications (e.g., food impaction, leak after dilation or repair)

CT Findings

- CECT may be used in concert with esophagram to identify complications
  - Esophageal injury ± perforation → mediastinitis, abscess
    - Look for extraluminal oral contrast or gas
  - Enhancement pattern of esophagus may be able to predict future stricture in setting of caustic ingestion
- Esophageal thickening & periesophageal stranding during acute inflammation
- CECT is important to evaluate for aortic injury in setting of button battery ingestion

Ultrasonographic Findings

- Endoscopic US may visualize congenital cartilage rings

Imaging Recommendations

- Best imaging tool
  - Esophagram
- Protocol advice
  - Barium is used for chronic strictures
  - Water-soluble contrast is used for initial imaging if leak is suspected
    - Iso-osmolar contrast if concerned for aspiration
  - Double contrast technique is not commonly used in children

DIFFERENTIAL DIAGNOSIS

Achalasia

- Failure of relaxation of lower esophageal sphincter
- Neuromuscular abnormality with thickening of circular & longitudinal muscles
- Dilated esophagus + air-fluid levels in upright position

Vascular Ring/Sling

- Smooth, round impression on esophagus
  - Pulmonary sling: Impression on anterior wall
  - Double aortic arch: Impression on posterior wall with reverse S appearance of esophagus on AP view
  - Right arch with aberrant left subclavian artery: Oblique impression upon posterior esophagus

Extrinsic Compression by Mass

- Neoplastic: Neuroblastoma, plexiform neurofibromas
- Congenital: Foregut duplication cyst, thymic cyst, lymphatic malformation

PATHOLOGY

General Features

- Etiology
  - Postoperative esophageal atresia anastomotic stricture
    - Probably most frequent cause in children; occurs in up to 80% of esophageal atresia repairs
    - May present with retained foreign bodies in proximal pouch
  - Esophageal foreign body
    - Button batteries cause caustic burn injuries in esophagus within hours of ingestion, may lead to perforation or subsequent stricture
    - Chronic foreign bodies in esophagus can cause esophageal edema
  - Peptic strictures

- Caused by acidic injury due to GER
- Eosinophilic esophagitis
  - Allergic response to food
- Postoperative Nissen fundoplication
  - Complication of procedure occurs when wrap is too tight
  - Proximal esophagus dilates secondary to stricture or tight wrap
- Caustic esophagitis & strictures
  - Ingestion of household cleaners, lye, or acid cleaning substance
    - Ingestion is usually accidental in younger children, purposeful in teens
  - Type of ingested material affects depth of injury
    - Alkali ingestion causes liquefactive necrosis, destroying cell architecture, & leading to deeper tissue injuries
    - Acid ingestion causes coagulation necrosis leading to eschar of burnt tissue
  - Type of ingested material can affect appearance of stricture
    - Alkali ingestion typically causes long-segment stricture, more commonly injures esophagus
    - Acid ingestion typically causes short-segment stricture, more commonly injures stomach
  - Strictures can occur as early as 3 weeks after ingestion
- Infective esophagitis
  - Higher risk in immunocompromised
  - *Candida albicans* is most common
- Epidermolysis bullosa
  - Hereditary disorder with > 100 distinct genotypes
    - Mutations in genes expressed at dermal-epidermal junction
  - Numerous bullous lesions, sloughing, then healing/scarring
  - Patients develop blisters & erosions after minor mechanical trauma
    - Repeated blistering → scar formation
- Associated abnormalities
  - Peptic strictures are more common in patients with associated comorbidity
    - 25% of patients have neurologic impairment

Microscopic Features

- Eosinophilic esophagitis is characterized by esophageal mucosal biopsy with > 15 eosinophils per HPF
- Specific diagnosis of infectious esophagitis is made by biopsy or culture

CLINICAL ISSUES

Presentation

- Most common signs/symptoms
  - Difficulty swallowing, pain, drooling, vomiting, or sensation of food stuck due to bolus impaction
    - Common symptoms in eosinophilic esophagitis, esophageal atresia repair, & tight Nissen fundoplication
  - Airway symptoms, such as wheezing, recurrent coughing episodes
    - Postoperative esophageal atresia patients have tracheomalacia
    - As esophagus dilates, it imprints posterior wall of trachea
  - Systemic diseases (such as scleroderma, dermatomyositis, epidermolysis bullosa) have multiorgan involvement
    - Many systemic diseases have skin findings
  - Feeding difficulties &/or choking in infants

Demographics

- Ethnicity
  - Eosinophilic esophagitis is more common in White population
- Age: Depends on disease process
- Sex: Eosinophilic esophagitis is 4x more common in male patients

Natural History & Prognosis

- Strictures may occur at site of prior injury or surgery
- Can progress to obliteration of esophageal lumen
- Recurrent strictures may occur in similar site
- Patients with caustic ingestion are at risk of developing esophageal squamous cell carcinoma
- Patients with GER & Barrett esophagitis have higher risk of developing esophageal adenocarcinoma

Treatment

- Balloon dilation is used for many conditions
  - Preferred over dilation using bougie as balloons dilate strictures in radial direction rather than longitudinal direction
  - Children often require multiple dilations depending on symptoms
  - Complications of balloon dilation
    - Perforation, mediastinitis
  - Endoscopic US can be used to triage congenital strictures
- Stricture resection or esophageal replacement is reserved for cases where dilation fails
  - Tracheobronchial cartilage remnant classically fails dilation

SELECTED REFERENCES

1. Hoffman RS et al: Ingestion of caustic substances. N Engl J Med. 382(18):1739-48, 2020
2. Alterio T et al: Eosinophilic esophagitis in children: current knowledge to open new horizons. Scand J Gastroenterol. 54(7):822-9, 2019
3. Bruzzi M et al: Emergency computed tomography predicts caustic esophageal stricture formation. Ann Surg. 270(1):109-14, 2019
4. Anderson BT et al: Approach and safety of esophageal dilation for treatment of strictures in children with epidermolysis bullosa. J Pediatr Gastroenterol Nutr. 67(6):701-5, 2018
5. Ghiselli A et al: Endoscopic dilation in pediatric esophageal strictures: a literature review. Acta Biomed. 89(8-S):27-32, 2018
6. Krom H et al: Serious complications after button battery ingestion in children. Eur J Pediatr. 177(7):1063-70, 2018
7. Macchini F et al: Classification of esophageal strictures following esophageal atresia repair. Eur J Pediatr Surg. 28(3):243-9, 2018
8. Mahawongkajit P et al: Risk factors for esophageal stricture in grade 2b and 3a corrosive esophageal injuries. J Gastrointest Surg. 22(10):1659-64, 2018
9. Arnold M et al: Caustic ingestion in children-A review. Semin Pediatr Surg. 26(2):95-104, 2017
10. Diniz LO et al: Fluoroscopic findings in pediatric eosinophilic esophagitis. Pediatr Radiol. 42(6):721-7, 2012
11. Diniz LO et al: Causes of esophageal food bolus impaction in the pediatric population. Dig Dis Sci. 57(3):690-3, 2012

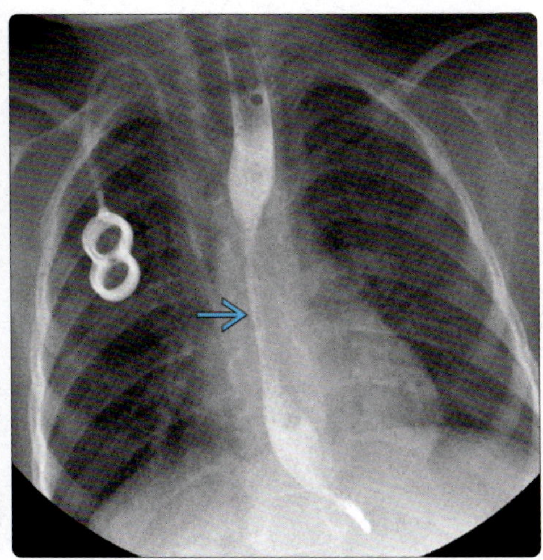

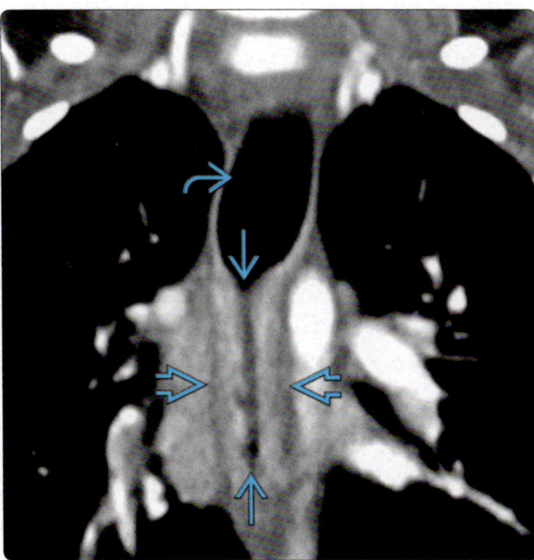

(Left) *Frontal image from an esophagram in a child who has received radiation therapy for thoracic neuroblastoma shows a long-segment stricture* ➙ *in the mid esophagus.* **(Right)** *Coronal CECT in the same patient shows the long segment esophageal stricture* ➙ *with associated wall thickening* ➙. *Note the gaseous esophageal distention* ➙ *above the level of the stricture.*

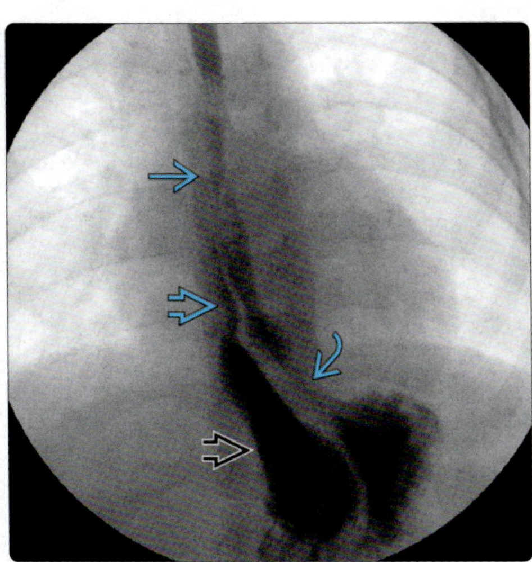

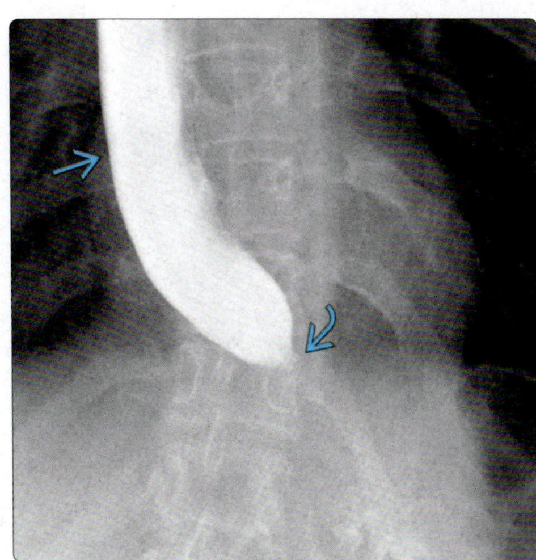

(Left) *Frontal image from an esophagram in a child with a recent caustic ingestion shows a long segment of narrowing* ➙ *of the esophagus, starting in its mid portion. The most severe narrowing is at the gastroesophageal junction* ➙. *Contrast also extends through a false tract* ➙ *into a collection* ➙ *in the upper abdomen.* **(Right)** *Frontal image from an esophagram in an adolescent with achalasia shows diffuse dilation of the esophagus* ➙, *which extends to a stricture* ➙ *at the gastroesophageal junction.*

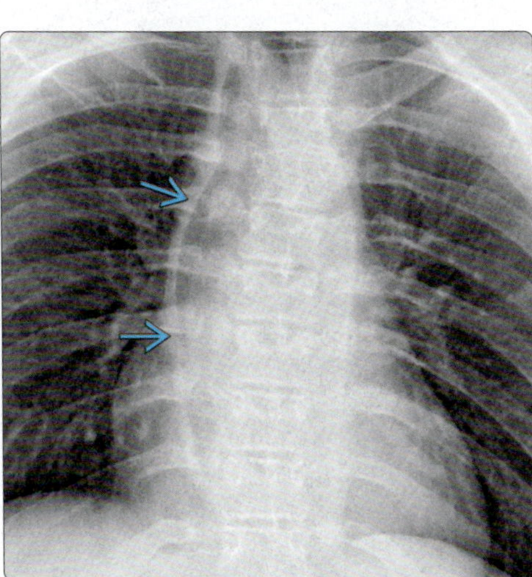

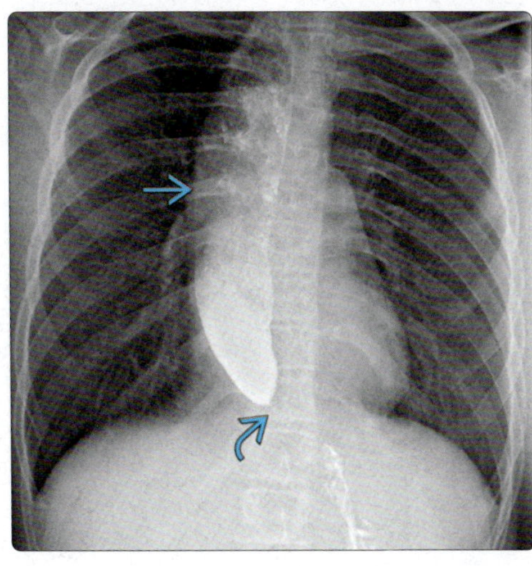

(Left) *PA radiograph of the chest in an adolescent with achalasia shows dilation of the air-filled esophagus* ➙. *The esophageal wall is visible as an undulating interface along the right mediastinal border.* **(Right)** *Frontal esophagram in the same patient shows a dilated esophagus* ➙ *with flocculation of the barium, suggesting that it has mixed with other ingested material. There is a focal narrowing* ➙ *at the distal esophagus near the gastroesophageal junction.*

Bezoars

KEY FACTS

TERMINOLOGY

- Specific ingested materials accumulate to form indigestible & potentially obstructive mass in GI tract
- Classified based on ingested material, including
  - Trichobezoar: Hair
  - Phytobezoar: Indigestible food components
  - Lactobezoar: Concretion of milk & mucous proteins

IMAGING

- Radiographs: Round/ovoid/tubular mass with mottled appearance due to air in interstices
  - Distention of affected lumen ± frank obstruction
- Fluoroscopy: Filling defect with contrast in interstices
- US: Echogenic, arc-like surface & posterior shadowing
- CT: Concentric architecture & air/contrast in mass
  - ↑ sensitivity for gastric bezoars with window level setting of -100 HU
  - Small bowel bezoars are located at transition point in cases presenting with obstruction
  - Floating fat density debris sign & relatively short length help distinguish from small bowel feces sign

CLINICAL ISSUES

- Presentation: Palpable abdominal mass, abdominal pain, vomiting, distention, dysphagia, bowel obstruction
- Trichobezoar
  - Most common in young female patients with alopecia, trichotillomania, trichophagia
  - Treatment: Surgical removal by laparotomy
- Lactobezoar
  - Most common in premature neonates
  - Treatment: NPO, IV fluids, ↓ caloric intake ± gastric lavage & saline dissolution; surgery if necessary
- Phytobezoar
  - Most common in adults
  - Treatment: Endoscopic fragmentation ± suction; gastric lavage with enzymatic dissolution; surgery if necessary

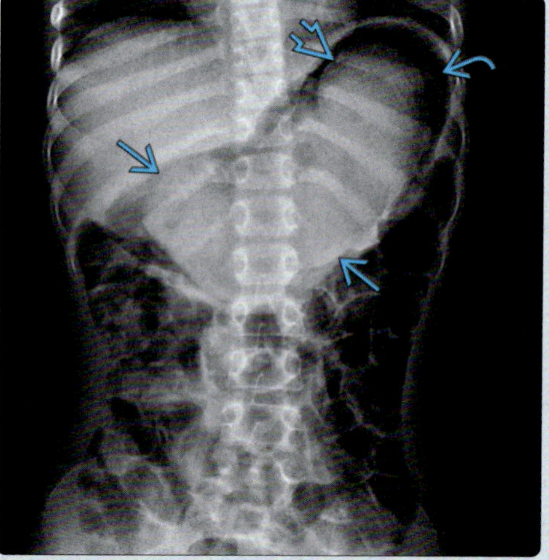

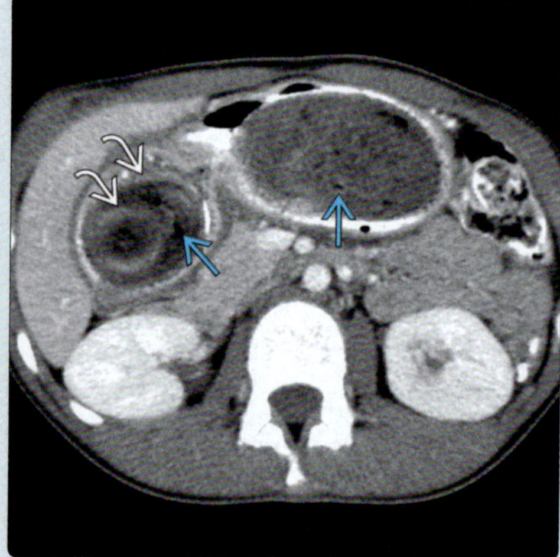

(Left) *Abdominal frontal radiograph in an 8-year-old girl with trichotillomania shows a circumscribed mass ➡ in the stomach that is outlined by a crescent of air ➡, compatible with a trichobezoar. Note the mottled appearance ➡ due to entrapped air.* **(Right)** *Axial CECT in a 13-year-old girl with abdominal pain & a palpable mass shows concentric rings ➡ & trapped air ➡ in the interstices of the mass. The mass conforms to the stomach & is surrounded by contrast. A trichobezoar was removed surgically.*

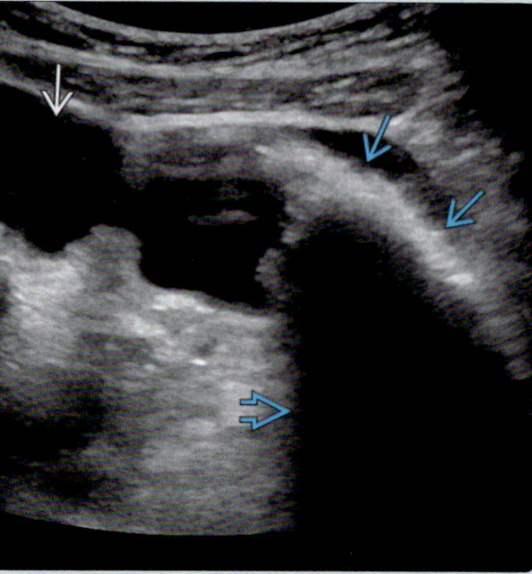

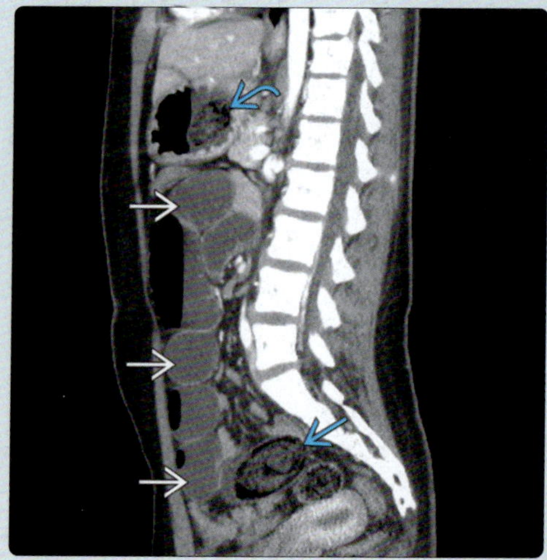

(Left) *Longitudinal US in a 12-year-old with pain & vomiting demonstrates a mass with a broad, echogenic, arc-like surface ➡ & posterior acoustic shadowing ➡. Proximal small bowel loops are fluid filled & dilated ➡.* **(Right)** *Sagittal CECT in the same patient shows a small bowel obstruction with dilated, fluid-filled bowel ➡. An obstructing mass with an appearance similar to feces ➡ is seen distally & was confirmed to be a bezoar at surgery. Another bezoar ➡ is seen in the stomach.*

TERMINOLOGY

Definitions

- Specific ingested materials accumulate to form indigestible & potentially obstructive mass in GI tract
- Classified based on ingested material, including
  - Trichobezoar: Hair
  - Phytobezoar: Indigestible food components, typically vegetable or fruit fibers
  - Lactobezoar: Concretion of coagulated milk & mucous proteins
- Rapunzel syndrome: Gastric trichobezoar that extends distally through pylorus

IMAGING

Radiographic Findings

- Mottled appearance of solid matter in (typically proximal) GI tract due to lucencies of gas in interstices of accumulated ingested material
  - Nonspecific appearance: Abscess, stool, or recently ingested food can have similar appearance
- Bezoars are rarely identified on radiographs alone
- ± evidence of small bowel obstruction: Dilated proximal bowel with air-fluid levels

Fluoroscopic Findings

- Upper GI
  - Round, ovoid, or tubular filling defects
  - May have mottled appearance due to contrast within interstices of accumulated ingested material
  - Gastric bezoars
    - Majority are freely mobile
    - Gastric dilation with ↓ or absent peristalsis
  - Small bowel bezoars commonly present with obstruction
    - Impacted filling defect
    - Dilated, air-/fluid-filled loops of proximal bowel

Ultrasonographic Findings

- Intraluminal mass with broad, hyperechoic, arc-like surface & posterior acoustic shadowing
  - "Dirty" shadowing due to intermixed air
  - Lactobezoar lacks posterior acoustic shadowing
- Dilated, fluid-filled bowel in cases of obstruction
  - Compression of bowel loops may show fluid shifting around intraluminal mass
- Color Doppler twinkling artifact at hyperechoic surface
  - No true internal vascularity in mass
- Low sensitivity to detect multiple bezoars & gastric bezoars
  - Only 2/5 cases with multiple intestinal bezoars were identified as such in 1 study
  - Same study identified only 2/8 gastric bezoars associated with intestinal bezoars

CT Findings

- Circumscribed intraluminal mass with interstitial air
- Mass may have concentric ring architecture
- Persimmon fruit seeds appear as hyperdense foci in mass
- Gastric bezoars
  - May float or fill lumen
  - May not be identified on soft tissue windows: Window level setting of -100 HU may improve sensitivity
- Small bowel bezoars are located at bowel transition point in cases presenting with obstruction
  - Appearance strongly mimics small bowel feces sign
    - Bezoars may extend distally into nondilated bowel
    - Floating fat densities in dilated bowel loops proximal to obstruction help distinguish from small bowel feces
      - Floating fat density debris sign reported using window level of -50 HU & width of 500 HU
    - Mean attenuation < -11.75 HU & length < 9.5 cm have also been reported to help differentiate from small bowel feces
- Up to 97% sensitivity for GI bezoars

Imaging Recommendations

- Abdominal radiographs are typically obtained due to presenting symptoms
- CECT
  - Advantages
    - High sensitivity
    - Can identify multiple bezoars
    - Allows evaluation of entire abdomen
  - No consensus on use of oral contrast
  - Often ordered in setting of suspected small bowel obstruction
- Upper GI
  - Dynamic study allows evaluation of intraluminal mass mobility
  - Can identify mucosal injuries to gastric & bowel wall
  - Ideally performed after fasting

DIFFERENTIAL DIAGNOSIS

Small Bowel Feces

- Classically seen in dilated bowel just proximal to transition point of obstruction
- Longer length, greater density, & lack of encapsulated appearance is more likely than bezoars

Ingested Material

- Recently ingested food in stomach can simulate bezoar on radiographs
- Food & gas in stomach show "dirty" shadowing on US
  - Gastric food should be minimal with adequate NPO ("nothing by mouth") status for exam

Neoplasm

- Intraluminal & adjacent extraluminal masses: Juvenile polyp, lymphoma, neuroblastoma, etc.
- Solid mass with visible internal vascularity by color Doppler
- Calcified masses may simulate US features of bezoars
  - True Ca^{2+} is not typical of bezoars
- Intraluminal neoplasm has connection to gastric/bowel wall

Duodenal Hematoma

- ↑ attenuation nonenhancing mass in duodenal wall or lumen
- History of trauma, endoscopy/biopsy, bleeding disorder, Henoch-Schönlein purpura

Gallstone Ileus

- Gallstone may have similar appearance to bezoar on US
- Pneumobilia is classic feature in gallstone ileus
- Extremely uncommon in children

PATHOLOGY

General Features

- Trichobezoar
  - Hair is resistant to digestion & peristalsis
  - Forms concretion with mucus + food
- Lactobezoar
  - GI tract capacity becomes overwhelmed
    - Caloric & protein intake > age-related dietary reference (erroneous preparation of formula, low-birth-weight formula)
    - Medication-induced antagonization of gastric secretion & motility
    - Likely multifactorial as also seen with breast milk & cow's milk
  - GI tract capacity overload → vomiting & diarrhea → dehydration → excessive water reabsorption → lactobezoar
- Phytobezoar
  - Indigestible fruit & vegetable fibers: Cellulose, tannin, lignin
    - Persimmon is common culprit
  - Gastroparesis/↓ gastric peristalsis: Major risk factor; may be due to
    - Gastric surgery
    - Medical conditions: Hypothyroidism, diabetes, cystic fibrosis

CLINICAL ISSUES

Presentation

- Most common signs/symptoms
  - Palpable abdominal mass, abdominal pain, vomiting, distention, dysphagia, small bowel obstruction
- Other signs/symptoms
  - Trichobezoar: Alopecia, psychiatric conditions (anxiety, trichotillomania, trichophagia, depression)
  - Lactobezoar: Dehydration, diarrhea, respiratory distress, weight loss/failure to thrive, feeding intolerance
  - Phytobezoar: Small bowel obstruction is most common presentation
  - Lamerton sign: Mobile, palpable, & indentable mass in upper abdomen

Demographics

- Trichobezoar
  - Most common bezoar in pediatric population
  - Almost all documented cases are in female patients
- Lactobezoar
  - > 70% of documented cases: Patient ≤ 30 days old
  - > 75% of documented cases: Patient born prematurely
- Phytobezoar
  - Most common in adult population
  - Prevalence varies among ethnic groups & geographic locations relating to food preferences

Natural History & Prognosis

- Complications
  - Obstruction, mucosal erosion/ulceration, GI bleeding, perforation
  - Less common: Intussusception, jaundice, protein-losing enteropathy, pancreatitis

Treatment

- Trichobezoar
  - Laparotomy is typically required due to bezoar size; allows evaluation of GI tract
    - Laparoscopy has been reported
  - Endoscopy is valuable for diagnosis
    - Poor therapeutic option: No success in series of 40 reported cases due to obstruction
      - Large size of bezoars
      - Bezoars resistant to fragmentation
      - With fragmentation, components may impact distally
  - Psychiatric referral is critical to prevent recurrence
- Lactobezoar
  - Conservative management: NPO, IV fluids, ↓ caloric density
  - Gastric lavage with saline + N-acetylcysteine if conservative management fails
  - Surgery for perforation or failure of conservative management & gastric lavage
- Gastric phytobezoar
  - Endoscopic fragmentation ± suction retrieval
  - Gastric lavage with enzymatic or biochemical dissolution
    - N-acetylcysteine, papain, metoclopramide, cellulase, Coca-Cola

DIAGNOSTIC CHECKLIST

Consider

- Trichobezoar in patients with psychiatric conditions, alopecia
- Phytobezoar in patients with prior gastric surgery, ↓ or absent gastric peristalsis, or ↓ gastric acid secretion/acidity
- Lactobezoar in premature infants

Image Interpretation Pearls

- Adjust CT window level & width: ↑ sensitivity to bezoars

SELECTED REFERENCES

1. Shah M et al: Gastric bezoar: retrieve it, leave it, or disbelieve it? J Pediatr Gastroenterol Nutr. 72(2):e31-6, 2021
2. Soon YQA et al: Clinics in diagnostic imaging (198). Small bowel obstruction secondary to a bezoar. Singapore Med J. 60(8):397-402, 2019
3. García-Ramírez BE et al: Small-bowel obstruction secondary to ileal trichobezoar in a patient with Rapunzel syndrome. Case Rep Gastroenterol. 12(3):559-65, 2018
4. Lalith S et al: Rapunzel syndrome. J Clin Diagn Res. 11(9):TD01-2, 2017
5. Marilina D et al: A non-occlusive bezoar of caecum in a 7-year-old child: ultrasound detection and multimodality imaging management. J Ultrasound. 19(3):223-6, 2016
6. Castle SL et al: Management of complicated gastric bezoars in children and adolescents. Isr Med Assoc J. 17(9):541-4, 2015
7. Chen YC et al: Imaging differentiation of phytobezoar and small-bowel faeces: CT characteristics with quantitative analysis in patients with small-bowel obstruction. Eur Radiol. 25(4):922-31, 2015
8. Iwamuro M et al: Review of the diagnosis and management of gastrointestinal bezoars. World J Gastrointest Endosc. 7(4):336-45, 2015
9. Lee KH et al: Ultrasonographic differentiation of bezoar from feces in small bowel obstruction. Ultrasonography. 34(3):211-6, 2015
10. Park SE et al: Clinical outcomes associated with treatment modalities for gastrointestinal bezoars. Gut Liver. 8(4):400-7, 2014
11. Fallon SC et al: The surgical management of Rapunzel syndrome: a case series and literature review. J Pediatr Surg. 48(4):830-4, 2013
12. Gorter RR et al: Management of trichobezoar: case report and literature review. Pediatr Surg Int. 26(5):457-63, 2010
13. Hewitt AN et al: Gastric bezoars: reassessment of clinical and radiographic findings in 19 patients. Br J Radiol. 82(983):901-7, 2009

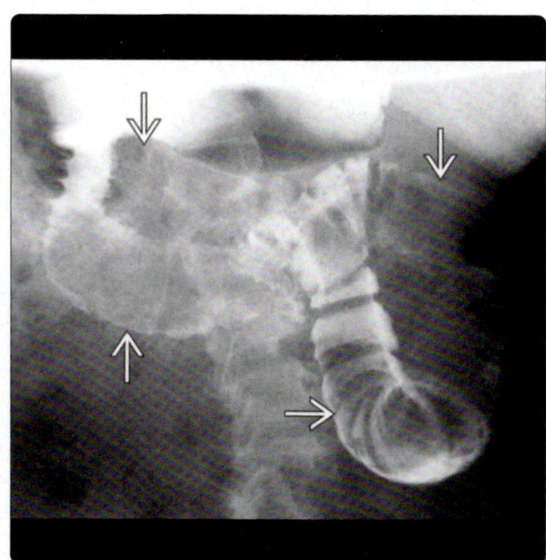

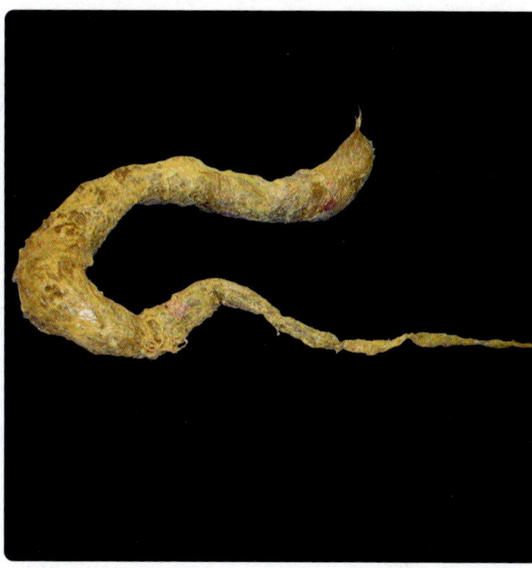

(Left) *Supine frontal upper GI series shows an elongated filling defect ➡ in the duodenum & proximal jejunum that is surrounded by contrast & conforms to the bowel contour.* **(Right)** *Surgical photograph of the specimen removed from the proximal small bowel in the same patient shows an elongated trichobezoar.*

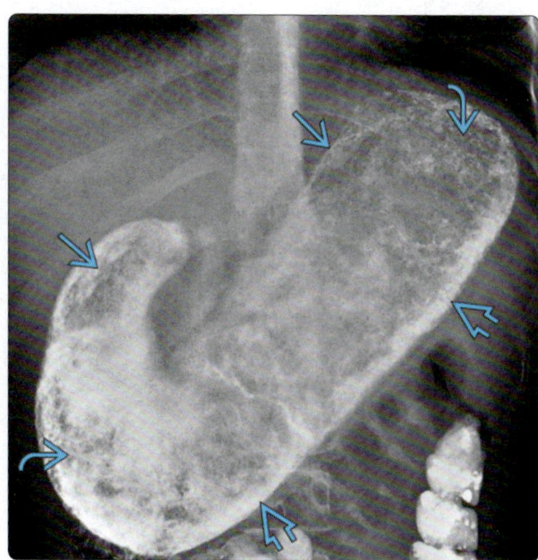

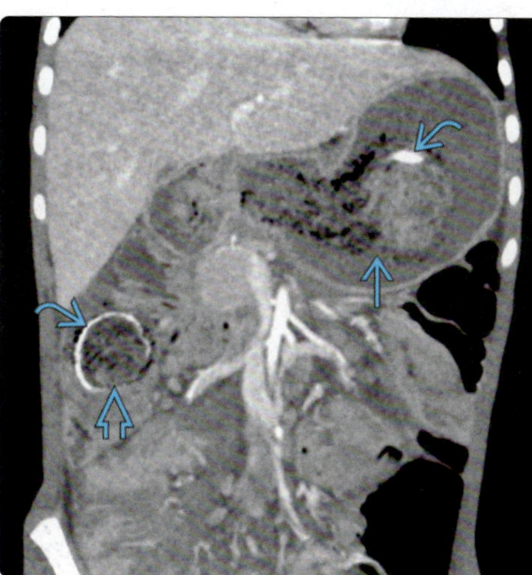

(Left) *Supine frontal upper GI in a 14-year-old girl with vomiting & abdominal pain shows a large filling defect ➡ in the stomach. Contrast surrounds the mass ➡ & fills the interstices ↪, giving it a mottled appearance compatible with a known trichobezoar.* **(Right)** *Coronal CECT demonstrates bezoars in the stomach ➡ & small bowel ➡ of a 10-year-old girl with abdominal pain. The bezoars appear as mottled masses with areas of rim-like calcification ↪.*

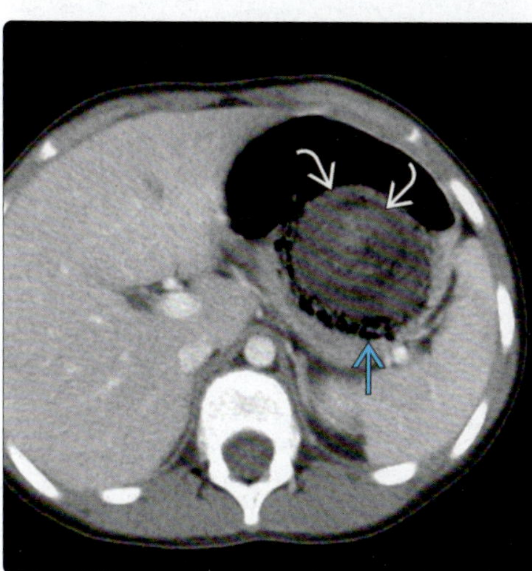

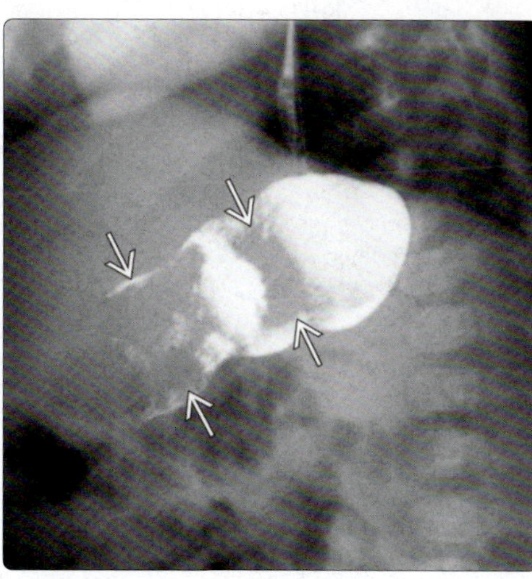

(Left) *Axial CECT in an 8-year-old girl with a history of trichotillomania, trichophagia, & episodes of epigastric pain shows an intraluminal mass with concentric architecture ↪. Air is trapped within the peripheral interstices ➡ of the mass, consistent with a bezoar.* **(Right)** *Lateral view from an upper GI series in a 3-month-old boy with failure to thrive & emesis shows fragmented filling defects ➡ in the stomach. A lactobezoar was confirmed at endoscopy.*

Gastrointestinal Duplication Cysts

KEY FACTS

TERMINOLOGY

- GI duplication cysts have 3 defining characteristics
  - Well-developed coat of smooth muscle
  - Epithelial lining representing some part of GI tract
  - Attachment to (± communication with) GI tract
    - Rarely: Isolated cyst with no persistent attachment

IMAGING

- Cystic (80-90%) vs. tubular (10-20%) lesions with well-defined wall
  - Can occur anywhere along GI tract; most frequently associated with ileum (>30%) & esophagus (18-20%)
- Contiguous (but not necessarily communicating) with adjacent GI tract
- Ultrasound is best modality to visualize key features, though findings with highest specificity have lowest sensitivity
  - Gut signature sign: Trilaminar appearance of wall is less specific than 5-layered wall
  - Y sign: Hypoechoic muscularis propria divides at point of attachment between cyst & adjacent bowel
  - Peristalsis of cyst wall is pathognomonic (if visualized)

TOP DIFFERENTIAL DIAGNOSES

- Mesenteric lymphatic malformation
- Ovarian cyst
- Meconium pseudocyst
- Urachal cyst
- Hydrometrocolpos
- Choledochal cyst
- Aneurysm

CLINICAL ISSUES

- Congenital lesions, most often presenting < 2 years of age
  - Pain, mass, rectal bleeding; may be incidental
  - Small bowel obstruction is most frequent presentation for ileal duplications
- Complete surgical resection is ideal

(Left) *Axial graphic shows an enteric duplication cyst ➡ between sectioned bowel loops. Note that the muscular layer of the bowel is continuous with that of the duplication cyst, creating a Y ➡ as the muscle splits.* **(Right)** *Transverse ultrasound of the upper abdomen in a 15-month-old with intermittent pain & vomiting shows an ileocolic intussusception extending to the transverse colon & terminating in a complex cystic mass with a trilaminar wall ➡. The mass was initially mistaken for fluid trapped around the intussusceptum.*

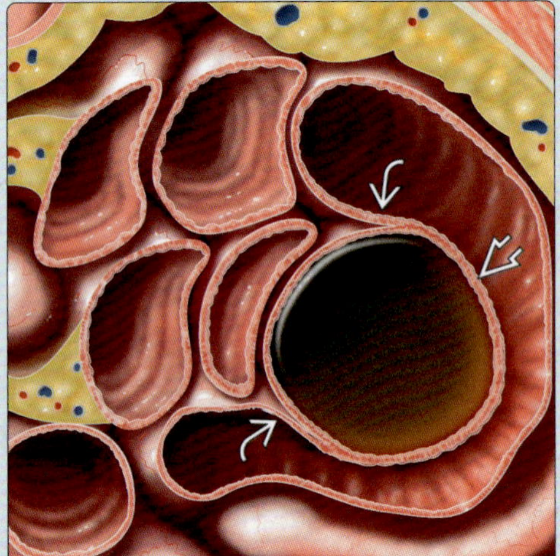

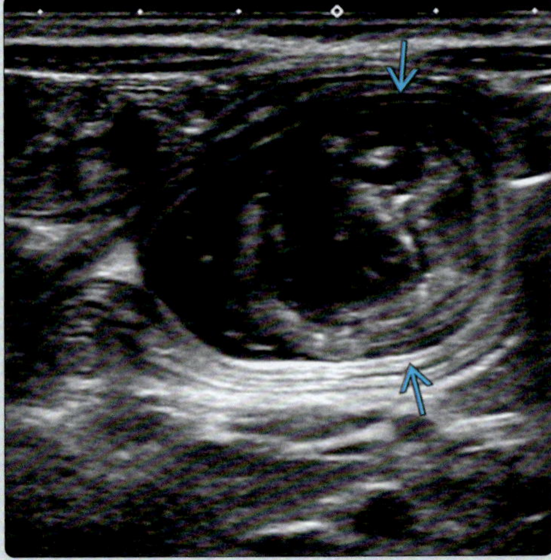

(Left) *Frontal radiograph in the same patient after successful air-enema reduction (confirmed by free reflux of air into the small bowel) shows a persistent, round mass ➡ outlined by air in the midright abdomen, concerning for a lead point.* **(Right)** *Transverse grayscale (left) & color Doppler (right) ultrasound images in the same patient after the air-enema reduction show the residual complex cystic mass with no internal vascularity. This mass was found to be an ileocecal duplication cyst with internal debris upon resection.*

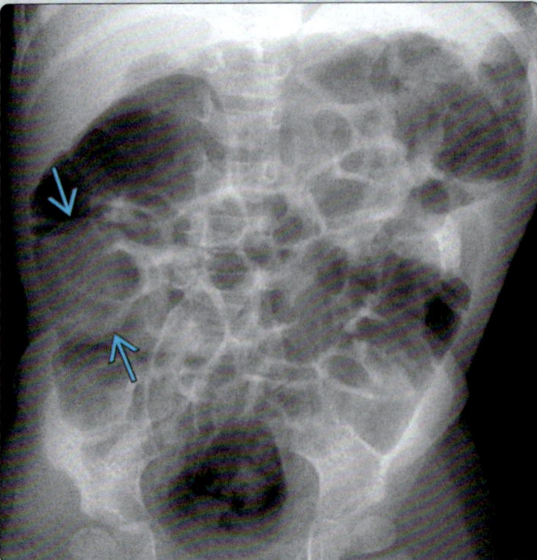

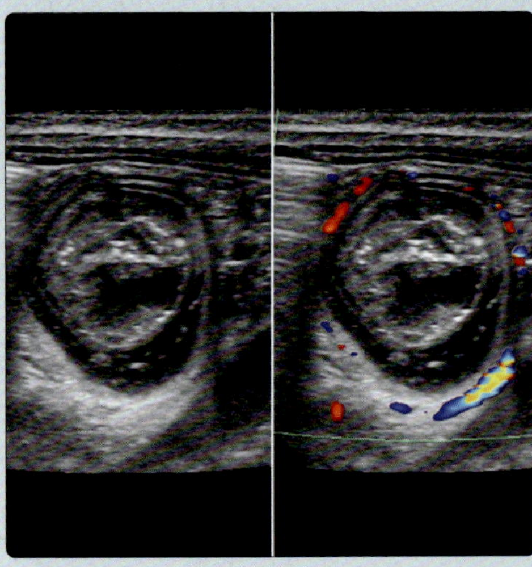

TERMINOLOGY

Synonyms

- Foregut/midgut/hindgut malformation or duplication, enteric cyst, enterocyst, enterocystoma, enterogenous cyst, dorsal enteric cyst, alimentary tract duplication (ATD)

Definitions

- GI duplication cysts have 3 defining characteristics
  - Well-developed coat of smooth muscle
  - Epithelial lining representing some part of GI tract
  - Attachment to (± communication with) GI tract
    - Isolated cysts: No longer attached (extremely rare)
  - Neurenteric cysts often have associated vertebral & intraspinal anomalies
    - Most frequent with esophageal duplications

IMAGING

General Features

- Best diagnostic clue
  - Cystic lesion with well-defined wall; contiguous (but not necessarily communicating) with adjacent GI tract
  - Cyst wall has similar appearance to bowel (gut signature sign) on ultrasound
  - Peristalsis is pathognomonic (but often not visualized)
- Location
  - Can occur anywhere along alimentary tract
    - 75% abdominal, 20% thoracic
  - Most frequently associated with ileum (> 30%) & esophagus (18-20%)
  - Less common: Colon (13%), jejunum (10%), stomach (7%), duodenum (6%), retrorectal (4%), floor of mouth (1%), retroperitoneal (< 1%), intrapancreatic (< 1%)
  - Esophageal duplications
    - R > L; inferior > superior
  - Gastric duplications
    - Typically occur at greater curvature or posterior wall
  - Duodenal duplications
    - 2nd or 3rd portions are most common
  - Tubular duplications
    - Can be short or very long
      - Rarely, complete duplication of GI tract segment
    - Tubular form is more likely to extend above & below diaphragm
  - Multiple cysts: 1-20%
    - Single GI segment is affected more frequently than different segments
  - Isolated cyst (separated from GI tract): Extremely rare
- Morphology
  - Cyst (80-90% of duplications)
    - Spherical, ovoid, or dumbbell in shape
    - Sharing bowel wall > > isolated cyst in peritoneum with mesenteric stalk
  - Tubular duplication (10-20%)
    - Perpendicular branch of bowel with solitary communication vs. parallel tube (double-barrel configuration) communicating at both ends

Radiographic Findings

- Abdomen
  - Displacement of bowel gas (depending on size of cyst)
  - ± bowel obstruction
- Chest: Middle or posterior mediastinal/paraspinal mass

Fluoroscopic Findings

- Contrast by mouth or rectum may demonstrate continuity of duplication with normal GI tract

CT Findings

- CECT
  - Ovoid, round, or tubular lesion
  - ± thick, enhancing wall, especially if inflamed
  - ± fluid-debris levels
  - Duplication may be difficult to separate from adjacent normal bowel, especially if no oral contrast has been given

MR Findings

- Best for intraspinal extension of neurenteric cysts
- MR enterography may have increasing role

Ultrasonographic Findings

- Grayscale ultrasound
  - Gut signature sign of cyst wall
    - Trilaminar appearance is classically described but not specific
      - Deep → superficial layers: Hyperechoic mucosa, hypoechoic muscle, hyperechoic serosa
    - Described 5-layered wall is difficult to visualize but more specific
      - Deep → superficial layers: Hyperechoic mucosa, hypoechoic muscularis mucosa, hyperechoic submucosa, hypoechoic muscularis propria, hyperechoic serosa
    - Wall signature may be disrupted by inflammation, ulceration, or perforation
  - Y sign (specific): Split hypoechoic muscularis propria at point of attachment between cyst & adjacent bowel
  - Peristalsis is uncommon but specific
  - Variable cystic contents
  - Wall Ca^{2+} is rare
  - May shift locations slightly in abdomen between exams
- Color Doppler
  - ± vascularity in wall

Nuclear Medicine Findings

- Tc-99m pertechnetate uptake in duplications containing ectopic gastric mucosa

Imaging Recommendations

- Best imaging tool
  - Ultrasound for pediatric abdominal cyst
  - CT or MR for intrathoracic lesions

DIFFERENTIAL DIAGNOSIS

Mesenteric Lymphatic Malformation

- Cystic, often with fluid-fluid levels from hemorrhage
- Unilocular vs. multiseptated
- Round, well-defined vs. irregular, infiltrating
- Microcystic components may appear solid

Ovarian Cyst

- Simple vs. hemorrhagic vs. mixed cystic & solid
- Follicles may be visible in distorted ovary

Meconium Pseudocyst

- Localized complex collection (debris, Ca^{2+}) secondary to in utero bowel perforation
- Bowel obstruction is usually present

Urachal Cyst

- Lies along midline tract from bladder dome to umbilicus

Hydrometrocolpos

- Moderate to marked vaginal distention in neonate or teenager
- Relatively small uterus projects off superior aspect of obstructed vagina

Choledochal Cyst

- Right upper quadrant cyst, often elongated, communicating with biliary system

Aneurysm

- Uncommon in children but may appear as cystic mass
- Fills with color flow on Doppler

PATHOLOGY

General Features

- Etiology
  - Pathogenesis remains unclear; theories include
    - Split notochord theory
    - Possible early embryologic error in branching/diverticularization
    - Error in epithelial recanalization
    - Fusion of longitudinal folds along bowel
    - Result of vascular compromise

Gross Pathologic & Surgical Features

- Attachment ± communication with parent bowel is much more common than complete isolation

Microscopic Features

- GI duplication cysts are lined with either stratified squamous or columnar epithelium
- Supported by muscular & serosal layers
- 50-60% contain gastric mucosa or pancreatic tissue
- Duplications secreting alimentary tract substances (gastric acid, pancreatic enzymes, mucus) are predisposed to rupture & hemorrhage

CLINICAL ISSUES

Presentation

- Most common signs/symptoms
  - Pain, palpable mass, rectal bleeding
  - Intussusception or volvulus causing small bowel obstruction (most frequent presentation for ileal duplications)
  - May be incidental
- Other signs/symptoms
  - Ulceration, perforation, hemorrhage
  - Vascular compromise & urinary retention have been reported from mass effect
  - Respiratory symptoms in thoracic & oral cavity lesions
  - May be detected on prenatal sonography

Demographics

- Age
  - Congenital lesions, most often presenting < 2 years of age (up to 85%)
  - Up to 30% present in adulthood
- Epidemiology
  - Prevalence of 1 per 4,500 fetal/neonatal autopsies

Natural History & Prognosis

- Very good prognosis overall
- Complications include ulceration, perforation, hemorrhage, volvulus, intussusception
- Pancreatitis, acute or chronic, if cyst lies near pancreas
- Rare reports of malignant transformation
  - Most common with colonic duplications

Treatment

- Complete surgical resection is ideal
- Partial excision with removal of lining or marsupialization may be required in difficult regions

DIAGNOSTIC CHECKLIST

Image Interpretation Pearls

- Look for sonographic gut signature sign of cyst wall (5-layered wall is more specific than trilaminar appearance)
  - Trilaminar wall may also be seen with
    - Fluid-distended hollow organs (bowel, vagina, urinary bladder) or Meckel diverticulum
    - Alternate histologies occurring in layers (pseudogut signature)
    - Artifact

SELECTED REFERENCES

1. Gourishankar A et al: Acute painless lower gastrointestinal bleed that mimics meckel diverticulum. Pediatr Emerg Care. 35(10):e188-9, 2019
2. Arshad M et al: Duplication cyst of the pylorus: a rare cause of gastric outlet obstruction. BMJ Case Rep. 2018, 2018
3. Khanna V et al: Total midgut duplication: a ticking time bomb. BMJ Case Rep. 2018, 2018
4. Sangüesa Nebot C et al: Enteric duplication cysts in children: varied presentations, varied imaging findings. Insights Imaging. 9(6):1097-106, 2018
5. Catania VD et al: Fetal intra-abdominal cysts: accuracy and predictive value of prenatal ultrasound. J Matern Fetal Neonatal Med. 1-9, 2015
6. Kumar D et al: Education and imaging. Gastroenterology: revisiting the forgotten sign: five layered gut signature and Y configuration in enteric duplication cysts on high resolution ultrasound. J Gastroenterol Hepatol. 30(7):1111, 2015
7. Kumar K et al: Synchronous thoracic and abdominal enteric duplication cysts: accurate detection with (99m)Tc-pertechnetate scintigraphy. Indian J Nucl Med. 30(1):59-61, 2015
8. Sharma S et al: Enteric duplication cysts in children: a clinicopathological dilemma. J Clin Diagn Res. 9(8):EC08-11, 2015
9. Tritou I et al: The sonographic multilaminar appearance is not enough for the diagnosis of enteric duplication cyst in children. AJR Am J Roentgenol. 204(2):W222-3, 2015
10. Liu R et al: Duplication cysts: diagnosis, management, and the role of endoscopic ultrasound. Endosc Ultrasound. 3(3):152-60, 2014
11. Cheng G et al: Sonographic pitfalls in the diagnosis of enteric duplication cysts. AJR Am J Roentgenol. 184(2):521-5, 2005

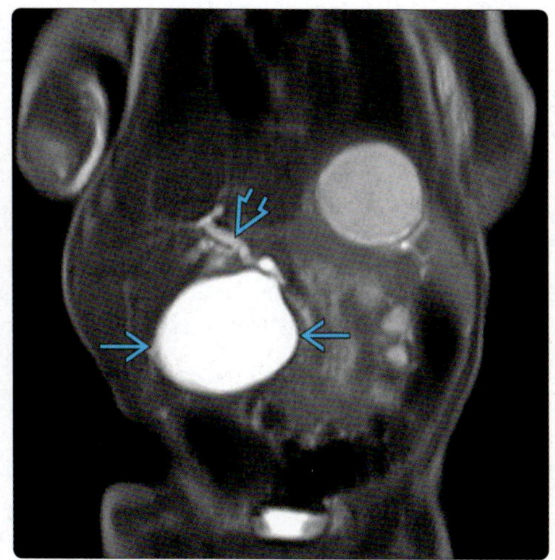

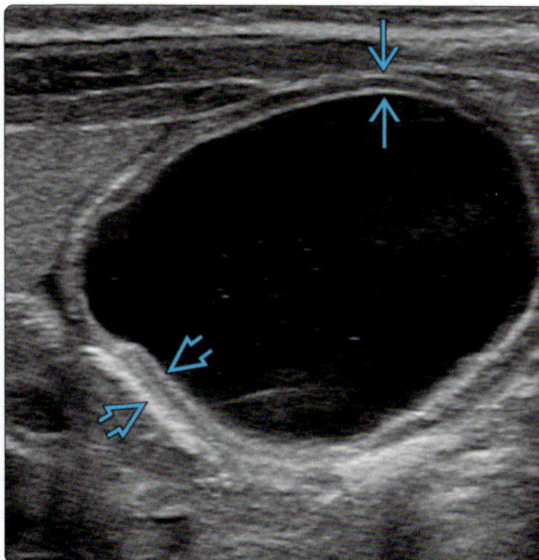

(Left) *Coronal SSFSE T2 MR in a 1-week-old with a prenatally detected anomaly shows a 3.5-cm cystic mass ➡ inferior to the liver & immediately lateral to the dilated common bile duct (CBD) ➡. A duodenal duplication cyst compressing the CBD was confirmed at surgery.* **(Right)** *Longitudinal ultrasound in a 1-month-old shows a well-circumscribed, round cyst of the right upper quadrant with a trilaminar gut signature wall ➡, confirmed to be an enteric duplication cyst at surgery. Five layers can be seen in portions of the wall ➡.*

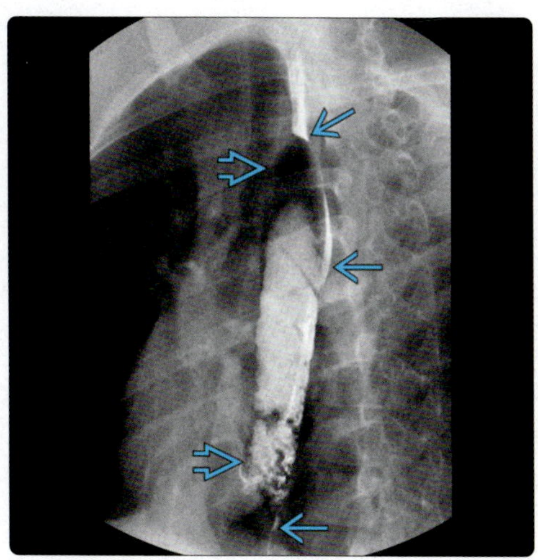

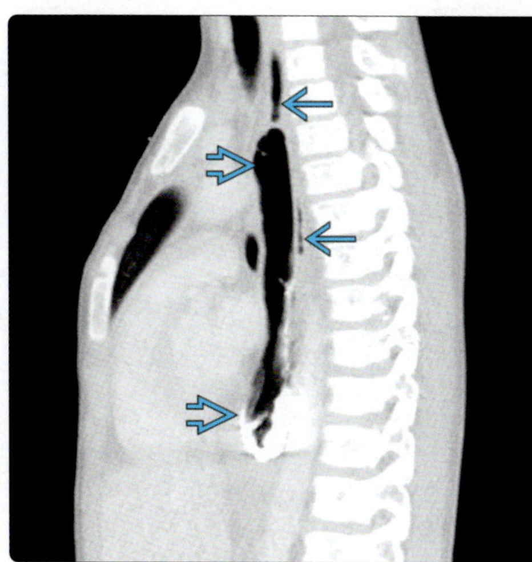

(Left) *Right posterior oblique esophagram in a 12-year-old with dysphagia shows a tubular mediastinal mass ➡ that filled with air & contrast during the exam. Note the compression & posterior displacement of the esophagus ➡.* **(Right)** *Sagittal CECT in the same patient immediately after the esophagram demonstrates posterior displacement of the esophagus ➡ by the air- & contrast-filled mass ➡, consistent with a communicating tubular esophageal duplication that was 15 cm long.*

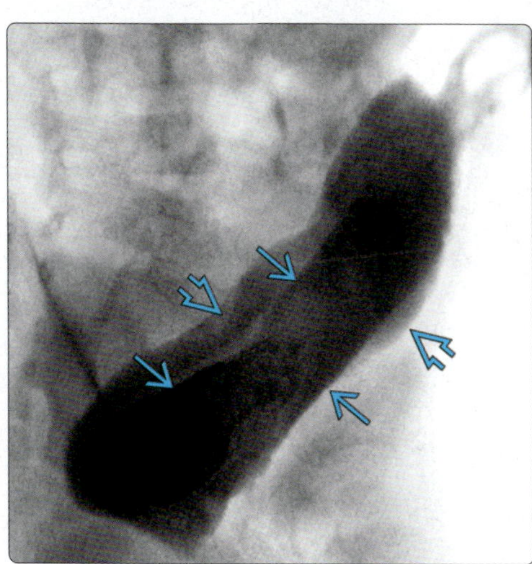

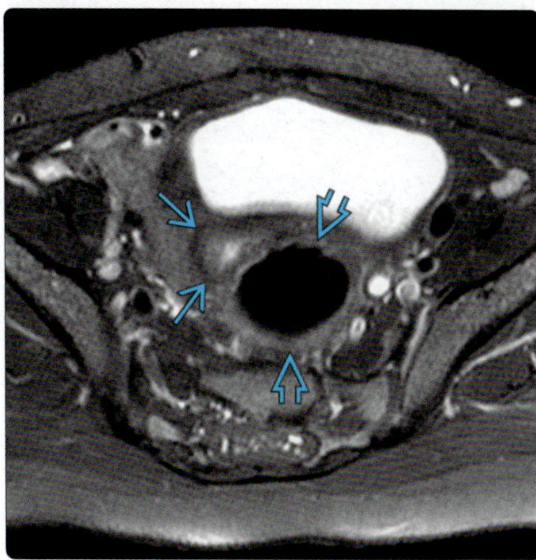

(Left) *Left posterior oblique high-pressure distal colostogram in an anorectal malformation patient shows overlapping opacification of parallel functional ➡ & nonfunctional ➡ limbs of a rectosigmoid tubular duplication.* **(Right)** *Axial T2 FS MR of the pelvis in the same patient shows the collapsed nonfunctional limb ➡ of the tubular duplication adjacent to the gas-distended functional rectosigmoid colon ➡.*

Small Bowel Intussusception

KEY FACTS

TERMINOLOGY

- Telescoping of proximal small bowel segment (intussusceptum) into contiguous distal small bowel segment (intussuscipiens)

IMAGING

- US or CECT show bowel within bowel appearance of round or tubular mass
  - Alternating layers of bowel wall ± mesenteric fat
  - Target appearance in cross section
- Continuity of central trapped fat with mesenteric fat
- Mesenteric vessels extend into or out of mass
- Normal terminal ileum up to ileocecal valve
- Small bowel intussusception (SBI) features that differentiate it from ileocolic intussusception (ICI)
  - Smaller diameter (mean of 1.5 vs. 2.6 cm)
  - Less hyperechoic mesenteric fat centrally
  - Entrapped lymph nodes are less common
  - More commonly periumbilical or in left abdomen

PATHOLOGY

- Lead points (uncommon): Lymphoid hyperplasia, Meckel diverticulum, duplication cyst, adhesions, polyps, intramural hematoma, foreign body, enteric tubes, lipoma
- Associated pathology: Henoch-Schönlein purpura, malabsorption syndromes (celiac), cystic fibrosis
- May occur postoperatively

CLINICAL ISSUES

- Majority are self-limited & spontaneously reduce
- Sonographic findings that may indicate need for surgery
  - Length > 3.5 cm
  - Findings of small bowel obstruction (SBO) & ascites
  - Pathologic lead point (but US has low sensitivity)
- Postoperative SBI is typically surgically reduced
- Complications are more likely with delayed presentation & diagnosis: SBO, ischemia, necrosis

(Left) *Transverse US in an 11-month-old with vomiting shows a target appearance of the bowel in the left abdomen. A small amount of hyperechoic mesenteric fat* ➡ *is interposed between the intussuscipiens* ➡ *& intussusceptum* ➡*. The location & diameter are typical of a small bowel intussusception (SBI). This resolved during the exam.* **(Right)** *Transverse US in a 1-year-old shows the target appearance of a SBI* ➡ *caused by a nasojejunal tube* ➡ *that has an echogenic shadowing rim.*

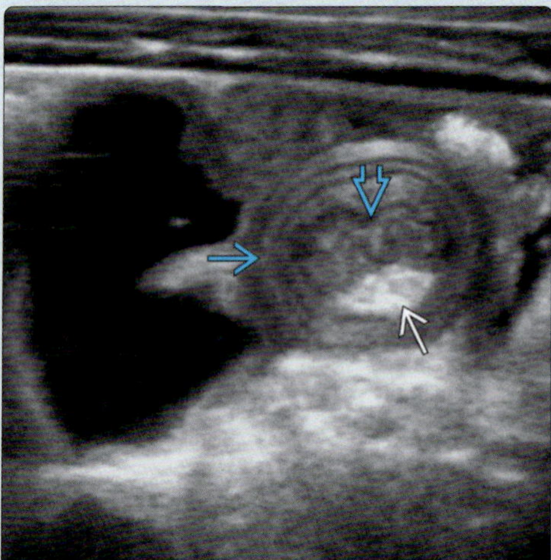

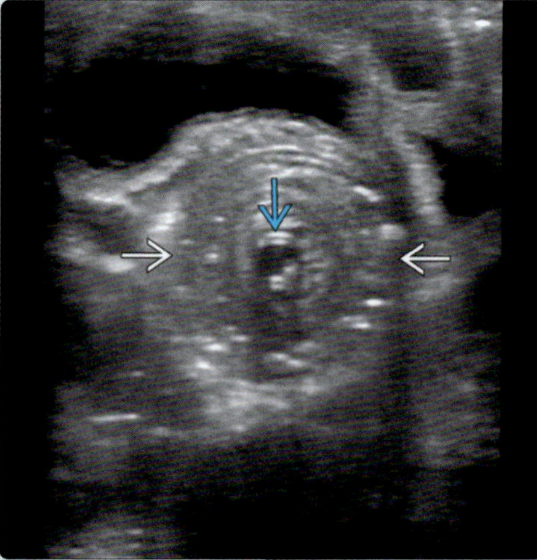

(Left) *Longitudinal US in a 12-year-old demonstrates an SBI that measures > 5 cm in length* ➡*. An echogenic lipoma* ➡ *(discovered at surgery) served as a lead point. Note the lack of entrapped mesenteric fat or lymph nodes, typical of an SBI.* **(Right)** *Axial CECT in a child with pancreatitis shows an incidental left lower quadrant SBI* ➡ *without entrapped fat or lymph nodes. Most SBIs are asymptomatic & resolve without intervention.*

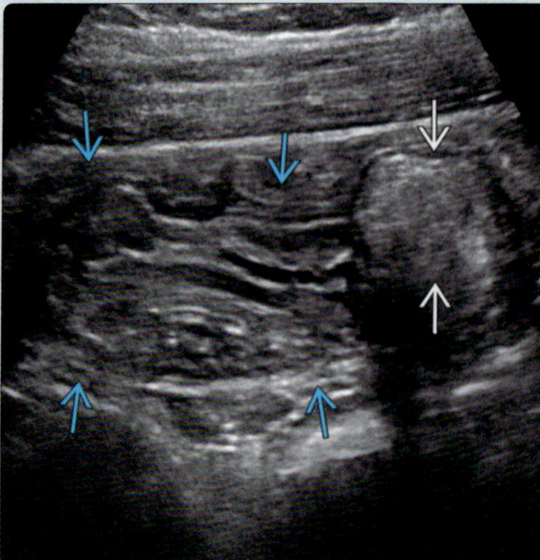

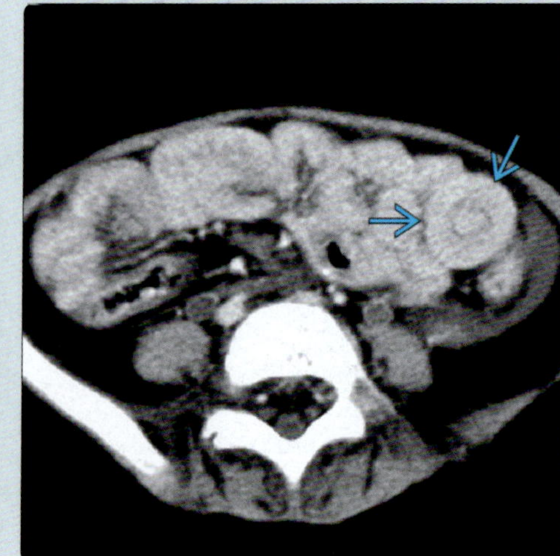

TERMINOLOGY

Definitions

- Telescoping of proximal small bowel segment (intussusceptum) into contiguous distal small bowel segment (intussuscipiens)

IMAGING

General Features

- Best diagnostic clue
  - US or CECT: Round or tubular "mass" with alternating layers of bowel wall (bowel within bowel appearance)
    - Target appearance in cross section
  - Continuity of fat trapped in mass with mesenteric fat
    - Relatively little fat compared to ileocolic intussusception (ICI)
  - Mesenteric vessels extend into or out of mass
  - Normal terminal ileum insertion into ileocecal valve
  - ± proximal bowel dilation
  - ± pathologic lead point

Ultrasonographic Findings

- Focal mass demonstrating multiple internal layers of bowel wall, each with characteristic gut signature
  - Inner hyperechoic mucosa, middle hypoechoic muscular layer, outer hyperechoic serosa
  - ± trapped echogenic mesenteric fat
- Target appearance in cross section
- Features that differentiate small bowel intussusception (SBI) from ICI
  - Smaller diameter
    - Mean diameter of 1.5 cm (range: 1.1 cm-2.5 cm)
      - Size may ↑ with age, edema, hemorrhage or intramural mass
  - Less hyperechoic mesenteric fat centrally
    - Thin crescent or no visible fat
    - Ratio of central fat core diameter to outer wall thickness > 1.0 in all ICI & < 1.0 in all SBI
  - SBI is more commonly periumbilical or in left abdomen
  - Entrapped lymph nodes are less common in SBI
- Majority of SBIs are transient & spontaneously reduce during exam
- Sonographic findings that may indicate need for surgery
  - Length of SBI > 3.5 cm
    - Sensitive (93%) & specific (100%) independent predictor of need for surgery by one paper
  - Findings of small bowel obstruction (SBO) & ascites
  - Pathologic lead point (but US has low sensitivity)

CT Findings

- Layered, alternating bands of ↑ (enhancing bowel wall) & ↓ (mesenteric fat ± fluid) attenuation
- Target appearance in transverse plane

Imaging Recommendations

- US for initial imaging evaluation
  - Should be able to clearly trace small bowel into & out of intussusception (further differentiates SBI vs. ICI)
- CECT is occasionally used to further investigate if
  - Patient is symptomatic
  - Findings are present that may indicate need for surgery

DIFFERENTIAL DIAGNOSIS

Ileocolic Intussusception

- ICI extends from right lower quadrant into right upper quadrant (& possibly beyond into/through transverse colon)
- ICI has mean diameter of 2.6 cm in cross section
- Entrapped lymph nodes are more likely with ICI
- Vomiting, bloody stool, & leukocytosis are more likely

Meckel Diverticulum

- Tubular mass (± gut signature on US)
- Complications (20%): Obstruction, bleeding, inflammation, perforation, & intussusception

Henoch-Schönlein Purpura (IgA Vasculitis)

- Hypersensitivity reaction with small vessel vasculitis
- Purpuric rash on legs or extensor surfaces of arms
- Mural bleed predisposes to intussusceptions

Ruptured Appendicitis

- May have target appearance with walled-off perforation

PATHOLOGY

General Features

- Etiology
  - Abnormal peristalsis → invagination of proximal bowel & mesenteric fat into contiguous bowel segment
  - Lead points (uncommon): Lymphoid hyperplasia, Meckel diverticulum, duplication cyst, polyps, intramural hematoma, foreign body, enteric tubes, lipoma
  - Associated pathology: Henoch-Schönlein purpura, malabsorption syndromes (celiac), cystic fibrosis
  - Prior abdominal or nonabdominal procedures
    - > 85% of postoperative intussusceptions are SBIs

CLINICAL ISSUES

Presentation

- 65% are asymptomatic in one study
- May lead to pain, distention, vomiting, blood in stool

Natural History & Prognosis

- Majority are self-limited & spontaneously reduce

Treatment

- Asymptomatic patient without concerning imaging features: Conservative management (often spontaneously reduces during study)
- Symptomatic patient or concerning imaging features: Surgical consult ± CECT/follow-up US

SELECTED REFERENCES

1. Binkovitz LA et al: Pediatric ileocolic intussusception: new observations and unexpected implications. Pediatr Radiol. 49(1):76-81, 2019
2. VanHouwelingen LT et al: Use of ultrasound in diagnosing postoperative small-bowel intussusception in pediatric surgical oncology patients: a single-center retrospective review. Pediatr Radiol. 48(2):204-9, 2018
3. Lioubashevsky N et al: Ileocolic versus small-bowel intussusception in children: can US enable reliable differentiation? Radiology. 269(1):266-71, 2013
4. Munden MM et al: Sonography of pediatric small-bowel intussusception: differentiating surgical from nonsurgical cases. AJR Am J Roentgenol. 188(1):275-9, 2007

Henoch-Schönlein Purpura

KEY FACTS

TERMINOLOGY

- Immune complex-mediated small vessel vasculitis commonly affecting skin, GI tract, urologic system, joints

IMAGING

- GI features (up to 75%)
  - Circumferential bowel wall thickening of discontinuous segments of variable lengths
    - Due to intramural hemorrhage &/or edema
    - Thumbprinting sign on radiographs
  - Intussusception, commonly ileoileal
- Urologic features (up to 60%)
  - Henoch-Schönlein purpura (HSP) nephritis
    - Normal or bilaterally enlarged & echogenic kidneys
  - Stenosing ureteritis
    - Hydroureteronephrosis & thick urothelium
  - Scrotal wall thickening, edema, & hyperemia
- Arthritis/arthralgias (up to 82%)
- Neurologic features (up to 2%)
  - Cerebral edema, intracranial hemorrhage, cerebral vein thrombosis, posterior reversible encephalopathy syndrome
- Pulmonary features (up to 5%)
  - Diffuse alveolar hemorrhage (DAH)
    - Alveolar infiltrates & ground-glass opacities
    - Pleural effusions, often large & requiring drainage

CLINICAL ISSUES

- Most common primary pediatric vasculitis at 49%
- Purpura or petechiae ultimately in 100%
- Peak age: 7 years
- Typically self-limited, resolves in 3-4 weeks
  - Treatment is largely conservative & directed to specific systems involved
  - Recurrence in up to 1/3 of cases
  - HSP nephritis: 20% develop nephritic/nephrotic syndrome
  - DAH: Up to 28% mortality

(Left) *Transverse ultrasound of the abdomen in a 7-year-old with intermittent pain shows relatively homogeneous thickening of multiple small bowel loops ⇨. The patient was ultimately diagnosed with Henoch-Schönlein purpura (HSP).* **(Right)** *Transverse ultrasound of the scrotum in the same patient shows scrotal wall edema ⇨ in the setting of HSP. Note the small hydrocele ➡ around the normal testicle.*

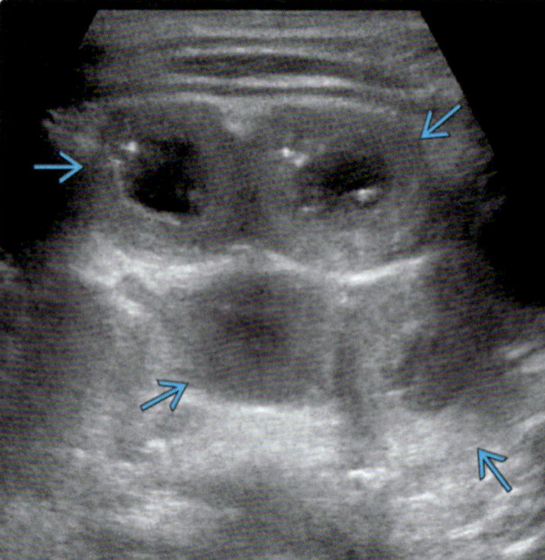

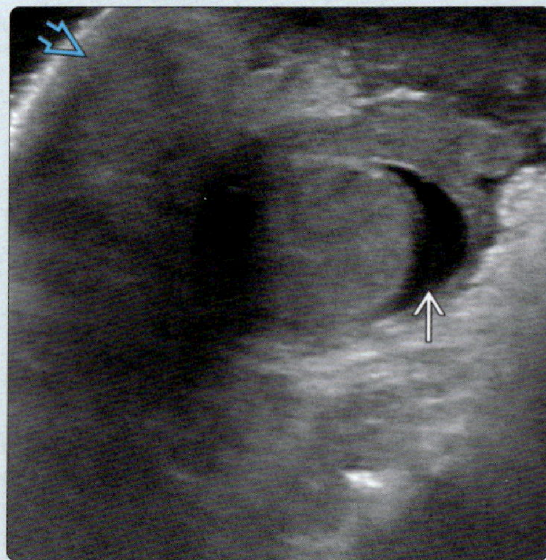

(Left) *Axial CECT in a 9-year-old with HSP, vomiting, & abdominal pain demonstrates a thick-walled loop of small bowel ➡ with mucosal hyperenhancement & mild surrounding mesenteric inflammation.* **(Right)** *Longitudinal ultrasound in a 4-year-old with HSP & abdominal pain shows a small bowel-small bowel intussusception with well-delineated intussuscipiens ⇨ & intussusceptum ⇨. There is no significant entrapped fat. This intussusception was > 5 cm long & required surgical reduction.*

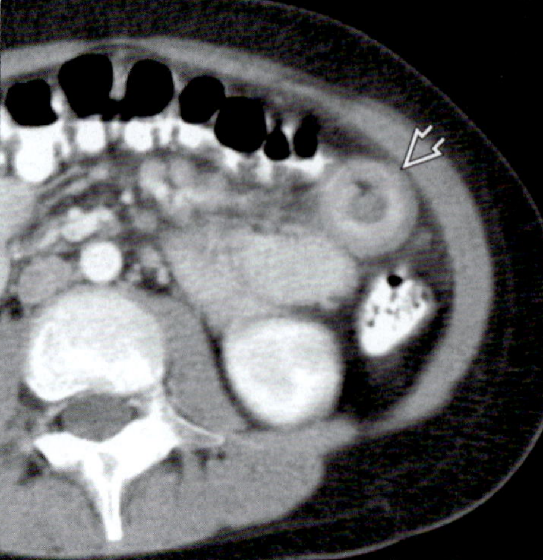

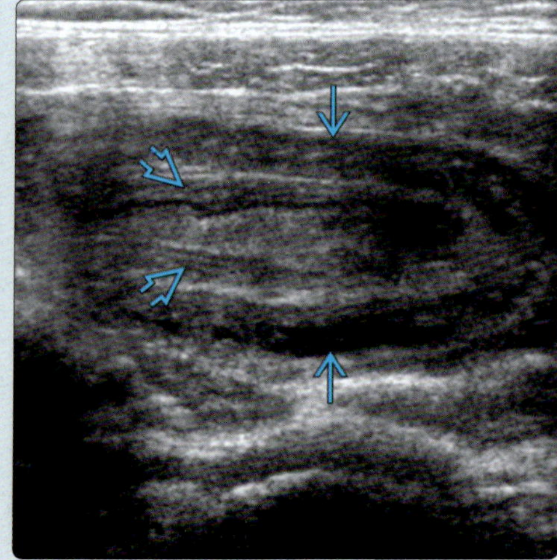

TERMINOLOGY

Abbreviations

- Henoch-Schönlein purpura (HSP)

Synonyms

- IgA vasculitis

Definitions

- Systemic nonthrombocytopenic immune complex-mediated small vessel vasculitis

IMAGING

General Features

- Multisystem diffuse vasculitis most commonly affecting GI tract, urologic system, joints, & (to lesser extent) nervous system & lungs
- Imaging findings are nonspecific & must be considered in context of clinical & laboratory findings to make diagnosis

GI Findings

- Bowel wall edema with submucosal & intramural hemorrhage
  - Circumferential bowel wall thickening involving discontinuous segments of variable lengths
  - Thumbprinting sign from fold thickening on radiographs
  - Hypo- or hyperattenuating bowel wall on CECT
  - Hypomotility of involved bowel loops
- Mesenteric vascular engorgement
- ↑ attenuation or echogenicity of mesenteric fat
- Ileus or obstruction
- Intussusception occurs in up to 14% of HSP cases
  - Ileoileal most common (~ 50%)
- Rarely, ischemia, pneumatosis, & spontaneous bowel perforation
- Nonspecific lymphadenopathy
- Hydropic gallbladder

Urologic Findings

- HSP nephritis in 30-50% of HSP cases
  - Normal or bilaterally enlarged kidneys
  - Diffusely ↑ echogenicity of renal cortex
- Stenosing ureteritis
  - Secondary to ureteral/periureteral vasculitis
  - Hydroureteronephrosis, urothelial thickening
- Bladder & ureteral wall hematomas
- Acute scrotum
  - Scrotal wall edema & hyperemia ± hydrocele
  - Normal or slightly hyperemic testicles & epididymis
  - ± spermatic vein thrombosis
- Penile HSP
  - Diffuse edema of shaft & foreskin
  - Penile purpura may precede extremity rash
    - Hypoechoic avascular lesion
  - Thrombosis & priapism

Joint Findings

- Arthritis with synovitis & effusion, soft tissue swelling

Neurologic Findings

- Cerebral edema
- Intracranial hemorrhage
- Cerebral vein thrombosis
- Posterior reversible encephalopathy syndrome
  - Patchy cortical & subcortical white matter lesions are most pronounced in posterior circulation distribution (parietal, occipital, cerebellar)
    - Hypodense on CT; ↓ T1, ↑ T2 & FLAIR on MR, most without diffusion restriction
  - Due to hypertension or cerebral vasculitis

Pulmonary Findings

- Edema related to kidney failure
- Diffuse alveolar hemorrhage (DAH) in 0.8-5%
  - Alveolar infiltrates & ground-glass opacities
  - Reticulonodular opacities are less common
  - Pleural effusions, often large & requiring chest tube

DIFFERENTIAL DIAGNOSIS

Idiopathic Thrombocytopenic Purpura

- Life-threatening multisystem disorder with disseminated microvascular thrombi
- ↓ platelets (whereas HSP may have ↑ platelets)
- Anemia, petechiae, microscopic hematuria

Hemolytic Uremic Syndrome

- Microvascular lesions with platelet aggregation
- Caused by enterohemorrhagic strains of *Escherichia coli*, especially *E. coli* 0157:H7
- Transient, severe, crampy abdominal pain with bloody diarrhea; precedes renal failure by 3-14 days

Infectious or Inflammatory Colitis

- Abdominal pain & bloody diarrhea
- Pseudomembranous colitis is characterized by fever, diarrhea, & diffuse colonic mucositis, typically while on antibiotics
  - Toxin produced by *Clostridium difficile* is most important cause of antibiotic-associated colitis
- Crohn disease most commonly has ileocecal involvement

Child Abuse

- Bruising on extremities may simulate HSP rash
- Bowel hematomas can be seen in both HSP & child abuse

Juvenile Idiopathic Arthritis

- Arthralgias involving 1 or more joints: Knee (90%), ankle (70%), wrist (70%)
  - Joint effusion, synovial thickening/hyperemia, bone marrow changes ± erosions
- ± rash

Leukemia

- Numerous possible symptoms & signs, including petechiae, pain, swelling, adenopathy

Testicular Torsion

- Doppler demonstrates ↓ or absent blood flow of acutely painful testicle

Scrotal Cellulitis

- Lacks other features of HSP
- May have history of insect bite

PATHOLOGY

General Features

- Etiology
  - Inflammatory disorder of unknown cause; characterized by specific immune complexes in venules, capillaries, & arterioles

Gross Pathologic & Surgical Features

- HSP nephropathy demonstrates mesangial hypercellularity, endocapillary proliferation, necrosis, cellular crescents, & leukocyte infiltration
- HSP has no specific diagnostic laboratory markers
  - Serum IgA levels ↑; ± platelets high

Microscopic Features

- Leukocytoclastic angiitis initiated by deposition of immune complexes
- Renal biopsy is indistinguishable from IgA nephropathy
  - Changes range from minimal mesangial proliferation to severe necrotizing glomerulonephritis
  - Glomerular crescents associated with poor renal outcome & development of end-stage renal disease
- Pulmonary involvement
  - DAH is predominant finding

CLINICAL ISSUES

Presentation

- Consensus criteria for HSP
  - Purpura or petechiae with lower limb predominance & at least 1 of following
    - Abdominal pain
    - Arthritis or arthralgia
    - Renal involvement
    - IgA deposition on biopsy
- Purpura or petechiae (100%)
  - Lower limb predominance
  - May develop bullous lesions
  - May not be initial manifestation
- Arthralgia & arthritis (up to 82%)
  - Typically oligoarthritis of lower limbs
  - May precede rash in 25% of cases
- GI disturbances (50-75%)
  - Abdominal pain, vomiting, GI bleeding (which may be massive), intussusception, pancreatitis, hydropic gallbladder, protein-losing enteropathy
  - GI symptoms can precede rash in up to 43% of cases
- Renal (20-60%)
  - Hematuria, hypertension, proteinuria, acute renal failure
  - HSP nephritis may develop up to 6 months after acute presentation
- Urogenital (up to 27%)
  - Scrotal swelling, priapism, ureteral stenosis
  - 3% of all acute scrotal cases
- Neurological (2%)
  - Seizure, intracranial hemorrhage, headache, focal deficit, polyradiculopathy
- Pulmonary (0.8-5.0%)
  - Hemoptysis, dyspnea, chest pain
- Conditions associated with or preceding HSP include
  - Upper respiratory infection
  - Vaccinations with measles, yellow fever, typhoid
  - Environmental exposures, such as drugs, cold temperature exposure, insect bites

Demographics

- Most common primary pediatric vasculitis (49%)
- Majority occur between 3-15 years of age
  - Peak age: 7 years
- Annual incidence: 20 per 100,000
- Seasonal variation, most occur in winter

Natural History & Prognosis

- Typically self-limited, resolves in 3-4 weeks
- Recurrence in up to 1/3 of cases
- 20% of HSP nephritis cases develop nephritic or nephrotic syndrome
  - Long-term renal impairment in 20-44% of patients that develop nephritic or nephrotic syndrome
  - End-stage renal disease < 1%
- DAH is often severe: 50% require mechanical ventilation; 28% mortality

Treatment

- Conservative management of symptoms
  - Steroids for severe skin lesions
  - Oral prednisolone for GI disease is controversial
- Reduction of ileocolic intussusceptions
- Hemodynamic monitoring with possible endoscopy for GI bleeding
- HSP nephritis
  - No evidence-based treatment
  - Current therapeutic approach includes
    - Angiotensin-converting enzyme inhibitors
    - IV or oral corticosteroids
    - Cyclophosphamide if severe
    - Early-onset plasmapheresis

SELECTED REFERENCES

1. Du L et al: Multisystemic manifestations of IgA vasculitis. Clin Rheumatol. 40(1):43-52, 2020
2. Singhal M et al: Imaging in small and medium vessel vasculitis. Int J Rheum Dis. 22 Suppl 1:78-85, 2019
3. Fink AZ et al: Imaging findings in systemic childhood diseases presenting with dermatologic manifestations. Clin Imaging. 49:17-36, 2018
4. Dalpiaz A et al: Urological manifestations of Henoch-Schonlein purpura: a review. Curr Urol. 8(2):66-73, 2015
5. Kasahara K et al: Stenosing ureteritis in Henoch-Schönlein purpura: report of two cases. Pediatr Int. 57(2):317-20, 2015
6. Khanna G et al: Pediatric vasculitis: recognizing multisystemic manifestations at body imaging. Radiographics. 35(3):849-65, 2015
7. Lim Y et al: Henoch-Schonlein purpura: ultrasonography of scrotal and penile involvement. Ultrasonography. 34(2):144-7, 2015
8. Pohl M: Henoch-Schönlein purpura nephritis. Pediatr Nephrol. 30(2):245-52, 2015
9. Stefek B et al: Henoch-Schönlein purpura with posterior reversible encephalopathy Syndrome. J Pediatr. 167(5):1152-4, 2015
10. Rajagopala S et al: Pulmonary hemorrhage in Henoch-Schönlein purpura: case report and systematic review of the english literature. Semin Arthritis Rheum. 42(4):391-400, 2013
11. McCarthy HJ et al: Clinical practice: Diagnosis and management of Henoch-Schönlein purpura. Eur J Pediatr. 169(6):643-50, 2010
12. Nchimi A et al: Significance of bowel wall abnormalities at ultrasound in Henoch-Schönlein purpura. J Pediatr Gastroenterol Nutr. 46(1):48-53, 2008
13. Jeong YK et al: Gastrointestinal involvement in Henoch-Schonlein syndrome: CT findings. AJR Am J Roentgenol. 168(4):965-8, 1997

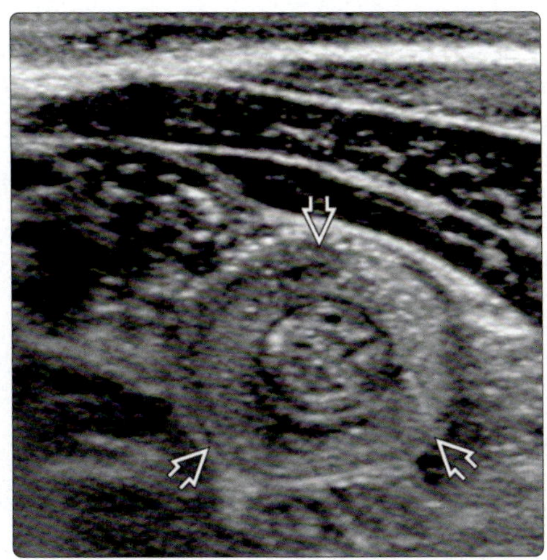

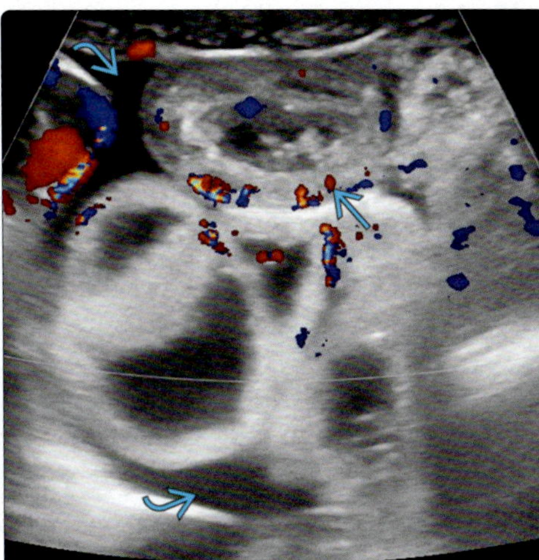

(Left) *Transverse ultrasound in a 5-year-old with HSP & abdominal pain demonstrates a small bowel intussusception in cross section with a target appearance ⮚. Multiple small bowel intussusceptions were encountered during the exam (not shown).* **(Right)** *Transverse ultrasound in an 8-year-old with a history of HSP & abdominal pain shows small bowel wall thickening & hyperemia ⮕ with a small volume of ascites ⮣.*

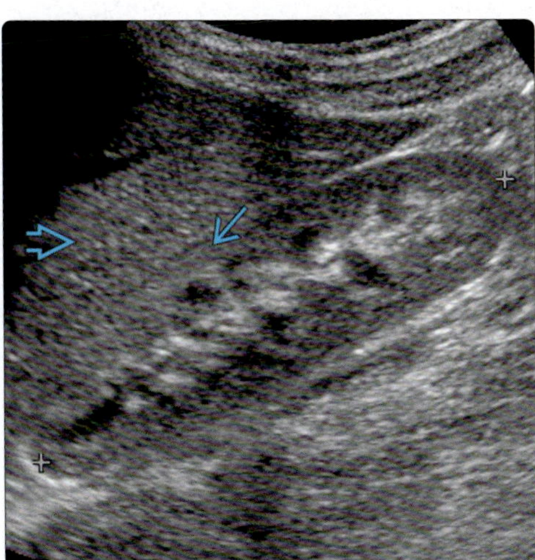

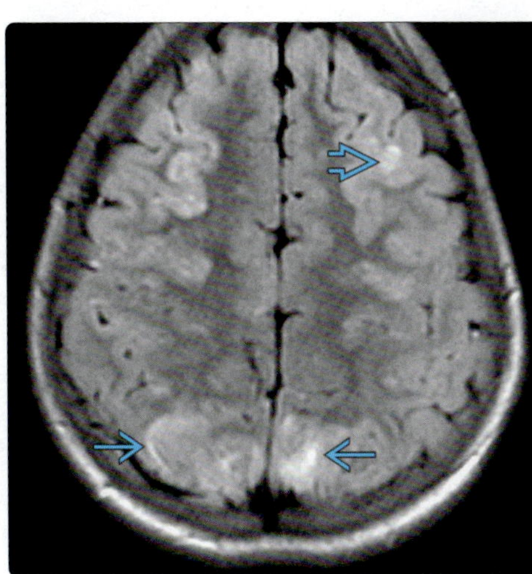

(Left) *Longitudinal ultrasound in an 11-year-old with known HSP shows ↑ echogenicity of the renal cortex ⮕ that is equivalent to or slightly greater than the adjacent liver ⮚. The patient presented with worsening hypertension (HTN).* **(Right)** *Axial FLAIR MR in the same patient with HSP nephritis & HTN (who developed seizures) shows superficial foci of ↑ signal intensity in the parietal ⮕ & frontal ⮚ lobes. The findings are consistent with posterior reversible encephalopathy syndrome (PRES).*

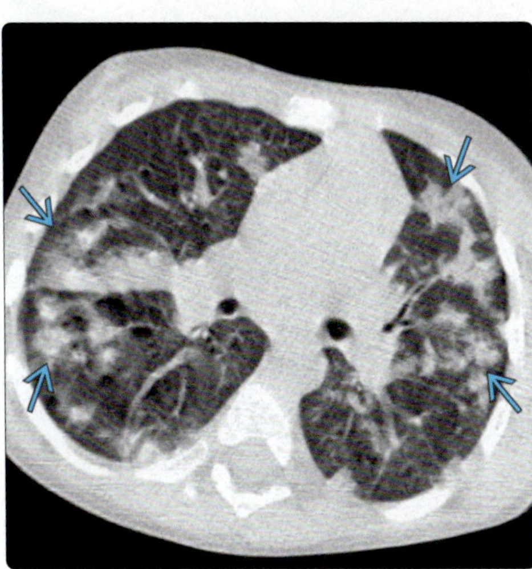

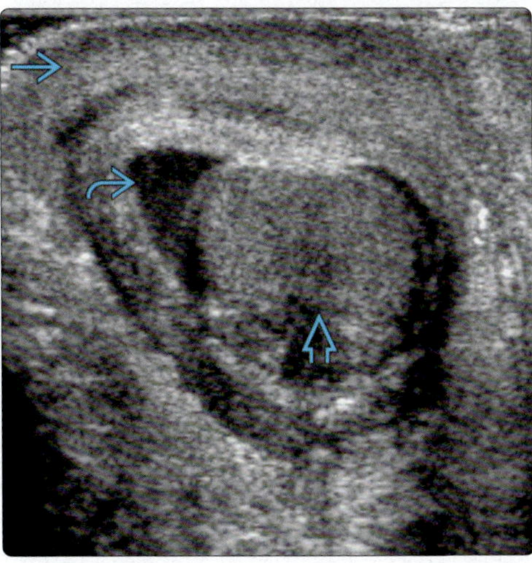

(Left) *Axial NECT in a 2 year-old with HSP, shortness of breath, & a drop in hemoglobin demonstrates bilateral patchy opacities ⮕, compatible with diffuse alveolar hemorrhage.* **(Right)** *Transverse ultrasound demonstrates marked scrotal wall thickening ⮕, a small hydrocele ⮣, & a normal testicle ⮚ in a 21-month-old with HSP. Scrotal swelling can be the presenting symptom in HSP.*

KEY FACTS

TERMINOLOGY

- Cystic fibrosis (CF): Autosomal recessive multisystem disorder caused by dysfunctional chloride ion transport across epithelial surfaces

IMAGING

- Pancreas: Abdominal organ most commonly involved in CF
  - Pancreatic insufficiency: Affects 85-90%
  - Pancreatitis: Can be acute or chronic
    - Acute: More common in patients with pancreatic sufficiency
    - Chronic: May appear as lipomatous hypertrophy, Ca^{2+}, &/or gland atrophy
  - Pancreatic cystosis: Rare sequela caused by occlusion of small ductules
- Intestinal
  - Gastroesophageal reflux disease: Prevalence is 6-8x higher than general population
  - Meconium ileus: Congenital bowel obstruction caused by tenacious meconium occluding terminal ileum
  - Distal intestinal obstruction syndrome (DIOS): Meconium ileus equivalent in older children
  - Constipation: Excess stool throughout colon
  - Intussusception: 10x higher than general population
  - Appendix: Enlarged without inflammation
    - Appendicitis rates are lower in CF patients
- Hepatobiliary: Most common cause of CF mortality after pulmonary complications
  - Hepatic fibrosis/cirrhosis: Occurs in 5-15% of children/adolescents with CF
  - Focal biliary cirrhosis: Most common cause of liver pathology in patients with CF
  - Microgallbladder: Caused by atresia/stenosis of cystic duct

(Left) *Frontal image from a water-soluble contrast enema in a neonate with distal obstruction shows a microcolon ⇨. The ileum is dilated & contains multiple filling defects ➔, consistent with meconium ileus. In the absence of superimposed complication, this obstruction may respond to treatment with serial enemas to break up the impacted meconium.* **(Right)** *Axial T2 FS MR in a patient with cystic fibrosis shows diffuse fatty replacement of the pancreas ➔.*

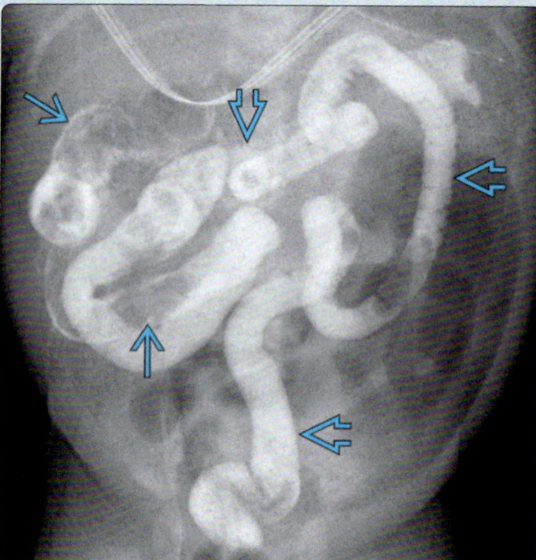

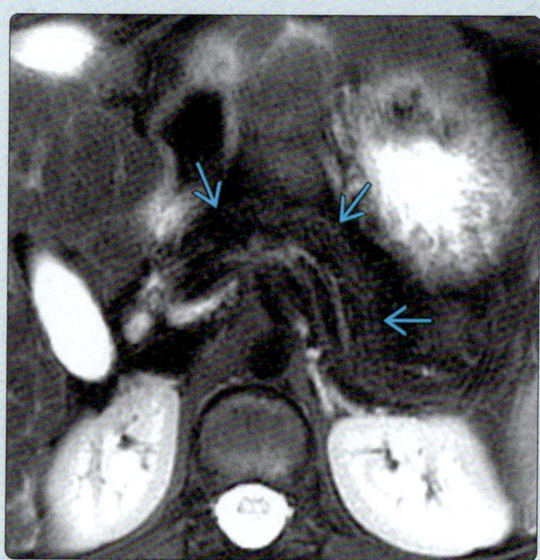

(Left) *Axial T2 FS MR in a patient with cystic fibrosis shows that the liver is enlarged with a nodular contour with linear regions of ↑ T2 signal. In addition, the spleen is enlarged. The findings are typical of advanced cystic fibrosis liver disease with portal hypertension.* **(Right)** *Axial T1 opposed-phase MR in a patient with cystic fibrosis shows diffuse loss of signal in the liver, consistent with steatosis. The measured fat fraction in this patient was 38% (normal is < 5%).*

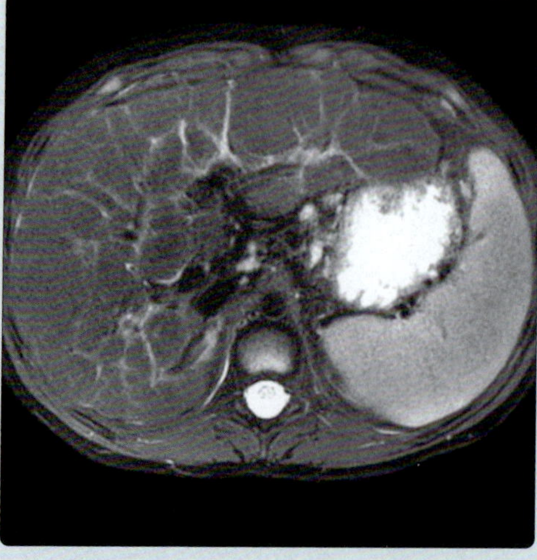

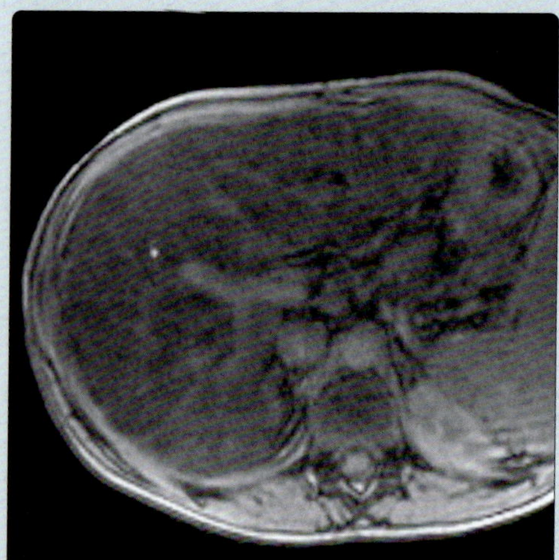

TERMINOLOGY

Definitions

- Cystic fibrosis (CF): Autosomal recessive multisystem disorder caused by dysfunctional chloride ion transport across epithelial surfaces
  - Presenting symptoms of CF in infants & young children are most commonly GI related

IMAGING

General Features

- Associated conditions in CF patients
  - Pancreas: Abdominal organ most commonly involved
    - Pancreatic insufficiency: Affects 85-90%
    - Pancreatitis: Can be acute or chronic
      - Acute: Occurs in 10% of patients with pancreatic sufficiency
      - Chronic: May appear as lipomatous hypertrophy, Ca^{2+}, &/or gland atrophy
    - Pancreatic cystosis: Rare sequela caused by occlusion of small ductules
  - Intestinal
    - Gastroesophageal reflux disease (GERD): Prevalence is 6-8x higher than in general population
    - Meconium ileus: Congenital bowel obstruction (not ileus) caused by tenacious meconium occluding terminal ileum
      - Simple: Meconium causes bowel obstruction
      - Complex: Obstruction leads to complication, such as volvulus, perforation, pseudocyst, or atresia
    - Distal intestinal obstruction syndrome (DIOS): Meconium ileus equivalent occurring in all ages
      - Complete: Causes vomiting & complete obstruction
      - Incomplete: Causes abdominal pain & distention but not complete obstruction
    - Constipation: Excess stool throughout colon
    - Appendicitis: Occurs less commonly than in general population
      - Normal appendix is enlarged in CF: Mean diameter of 8.3 mm
    - Intussusception: 10x more common than general population
    - Malignancy: Intestinal malignancies occur 23x more commonly in CF patients (typically adults)
  - Hepatobiliary: Most common cause of mortality after pulmonary complications
    - Steatosis: Occurs in up to 2/3 of children & adolescents
    - Hepatic fibrosis/cirrhosis: Occurs in 5-15% of children/adolescents
    - Focal biliary cirrhosis: Most common cause of liver pathology
    - Microgallbladder: Caused by atresia/stenosis of cystic duct

Radiographic Findings

- Radiography
  - Meconium ileus: Distal obstruction bowel gas pattern occurring in newborn
    - Complication by in utero perforation may lead to peritoneal Ca^{2+} (meconium peritonitis) &/or fluid collection (meconium pseudocyst)
  - DIOS: Dilated small bowel loops with stool mass in right lower quadrant of older child
    - Complete: Fluid levels in dilated proximal small bowel, stool mass in distal small bowel
    - Incomplete: Stool mass in terminal ileum but no findings of bowel obstruction
  - Constipation: Large amount of stool throughout colon (not just confined to cecal region)
  - Chronic pancreatitis: Occasionally see scattered Ca^{2+}

Fluoroscopic Findings

- Upper GI
  - GERD: Retrograde propulsion of contrast from stomach to esophagus
  - Duodenal fold thickening
- Contrast enema
  - Meconium ileus
    - Microcolon with filling defects of abnormal meconium in terminal ileum
    - Complicated by ischemia, atresia, volvulus, or perforation in up to 50% of cases
    - Enema can be therapeutic in uncomplicated cases
      - Performed with N-acetylcysteine & Gastrografin
  - DIOS
    - Normal colon with filling defects in terminal ileum
    - Enema can be therapeutic
      - Performed with N-acetylcysteine & Gastrografin

CT Findings

- Acute pancreatitis: Appears as pancreatitis in patients without CF
- Chronic pancreatitis: Varying amounts of fatty replacement, pancreatic atrophy, Ca^{2+}
- Pancreatic cystosis: Multiple cysts of varying sizes in pancreas
- DIOS: Mass of stool in terminal ileum
- Appendix: Larger than in normal patients & often filled with inspissated secretions despite lack of inflammation
- Steatosis: Diffuse or patchy areas of low attenuation in liver
- Hepatic fibrosis/cirrhosis: Small liver with nodular contour; may have findings of portal hypertension
- Microgallbladder: Gallbladder < 2-3 cm long x 0.5-1.5 cm wide

MR Findings

- Steatosis: Loss of hepatic signal on opposed-phase images
- Hepatic fibrosis/cirrhosis: MR elastography to assess for liver fibrosis

Ultrasonographic Findings

- Meconium ileus: May create stool ball equivalent in dilated bowel
  - ± complex ascites &/or meconium pseudocyst from in utero bowel perforation
- Appendix: Larger than in normal patients & often filled with inspissated secretions without inflammation
- Intussusception: Target sign or pseudokidney sign
- Pancreatic lipomatosis: Echogenic pancreas (compared to kidney)

- Pancreatic cystosis: Multiple cysts of varying size in pancreas
- Steatosis: Hyperechoic liver (compared to right kidney) with poor visualization of portal triads & right hemidiaphragm

Imaging Recommendations

- Best imaging tool
  - Depends on patient symptoms
    - Neonate with vomiting or failure to pass meconium
      - Radiograph with distal obstruction pattern → contrast enema
    - Abdominal pain in older child
      - DIOS, constipation: Radiograph
      - Pancreatitis: Ultrasound followed by MR/MRCP
      - Intussusception: Ultrasound followed by air-reduction enema
    - Liver disease
      - US or MR can assess hepatic fat content, fibrosis, & findings of portal hypertension

DIFFERENTIAL DIAGNOSIS

Neonate With Failure to Pass Meconium

- Hirschsprung disease
- Meconium plug/small left colon
- Ileal atresia

PATHOLOGY

General Features

- Genetics
  - Autosomal recessive
  - CF transmembrane conductance regulator (*CFTR*) gene mutation (chromosome 7q31.2)
    - > 2,000 genetic defects can result in CF; ΔF508 is most common
      - Genotypes with less severe lung disease may have more severe extrapulmonary disease
- Etiology
  - *CFTR* gene mutation → lack of chloride ion secretion → ↑ sodium retention & fluid absorption → ↑ viscosity of luminal secretions → obstruction
  - CFTR protein is located in epithelial cells of airway, GI tract, sweat glands, & GU system
  - Most GI manifestations are due to combination of disordered motility, thickened secretions, pancreatic insufficiency, & medications
- Associated abnormalities
  - Pulmonary disease

CLINICAL ISSUES

Presentation

- Most common signs/symptoms
  - Meconium ileus: Failure to pass meconium ± emesis in newborn
  - Intussusception: Colicky abdominal pain, intermittent fussiness
  - Pancreatic insufficiency: Greasy stools, flatulence, bloating, failure to thrive
  - GERD: Heartburn, dysphagia, dyspepsia
  - DIOS: Crampy abdominal pain, distended abdomen, palpable right lower quadrant mass, anorexia, weight loss, flatulence
  - Constipation: Frequent or chronic abdominal pain, palpable mass of stool

Demographics

- Age
  - Meconium ileus occurs in neonates
  - Other findings can be found throughout life; patients may not manifest until later in childhood
  - Most patients are diagnosed with CF in 1st year of life during neonatal screening
- Epidemiology
  - CF is most common lethal genetic defect in White population
    - 1 in 2,500 White live births; 1 in 20 White = CF carriers
    - 1 in 17,000 Black live births

Natural History & Prognosis

- Most common cause of death: Progressive lung disease
- Median survival: 41.1 years
  - Survival has ↑ > 10 years since 2002

Treatment

- CFTR modulators: New class of therapy designed to help CFTR protein function
  - Improves pulmonary function
  - Uncertain effect on extrapulmonary manifestations
- Meconium ileus
  - Simple: Dilute N-acetylcysteine & Gastrografin enema + patient hydration
  - Complicated: Surgery
- DIOS: N-acetylcysteine & Gastrografin enema + patient hydration
- Intussusception: Air-contrast enema
- Pancreatic insufficiency: Pancreatic enzyme replacement

DIAGNOSTIC CHECKLIST

Consider

- CF in neonate with distal bowel obstruction
- Abdominal manifestations of CF cause significant morbidity & can contribute to pulmonary complications

SELECTED REFERENCES

1. Levitte S et al: Clinical use of shear-wave elastography for detecting liver fibrosis in children and adolescents with cystic fibrosis. Pediatr Radiol. 51(8):1369-77, 2021
2. Konrad J et al: Changing paradigms in the treatment of gastrointestinal complications of cystic fibrosis in the era of cystic fibrosis transmembrane conductance regulator modulators. Paediatr Respir Rev. ePub, 2020
3. Toledano MB et al: The emerging burden of liver disease in cystic fibrosis patients: a UK nationwide study. PLoS One. 14(4):e0212779, 2019
4. Dos Santos ALM et al: cystic fibrosis: clinical phenotypes in children and adolescents. Pediatr Gastroenterol Hepatol Nutr. 21(4):306-14, 2018
5. Assis DN et al: Gastrointestinal disorders in cystic fibrosis. Clin Chest Med. 37(1):109-18, 2016
6. Demeyer S et al: Beyond pancreatic insufficiency and liver disease in cystic fibrosis. Eur J Pediatr. 175(7):881-94, 2016
7. Kelly T et al: Gastrointestinal manifestations of cystic fibrosis. Dig Dis Sci. 60(7):1903-13, 2015
8. Lavelle LP et al: Cystic fibrosis below the diaphragm: abdominal findings in adult patients. Radiographics. 35(3):680-95, 2015
9. Leung DH et al: Baseline ultrasound and clinical correlates in children with cystic fibrosis. J Pediatr. 167(4):862-868.e2, 2015

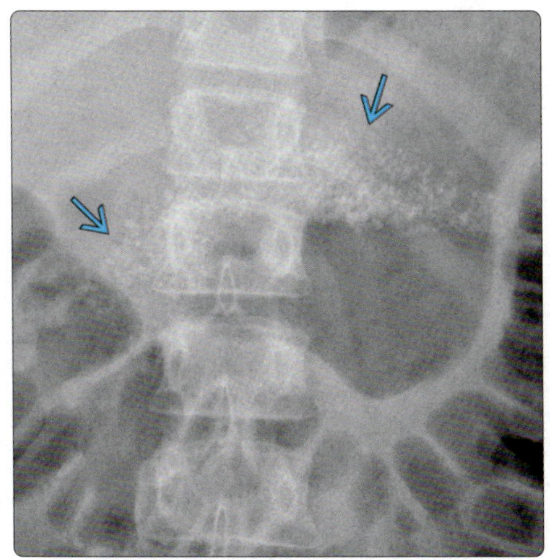

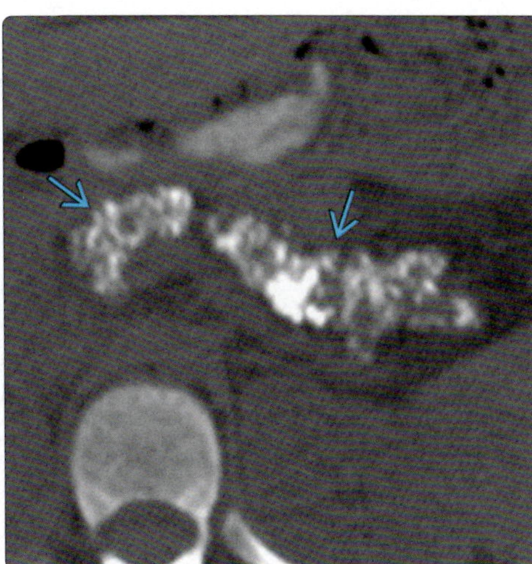

(Left) *AP radiograph of the upper abdomen in a patient with cystic fibrosis shows diffuse speckled calcifications* → *of the pancreas due to chronic pancreatitis.* **(Right)** *Axial NECT in the same patient shows diffuse calcification* → *of the atrophied pancreas. Up to 90% of patients with cystic fibrosis demonstrate pancreatic insufficiency.*

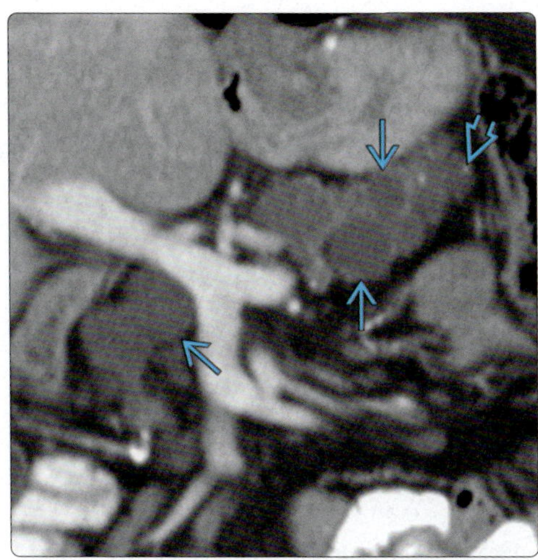

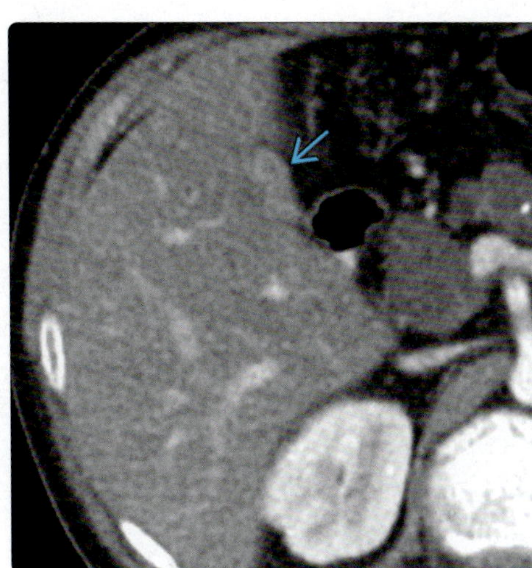

(Left) *Coronal CECT in a patient with cystic fibrosis shows numerous cysts* → *replacing the pancreatic parenchyma. The finding is typical of pancreatic cystosis. Scattered calcifications are also noted* ⇨. **(Right)** *Axial CECT in a patient with cystic fibrosis shows a microgallbladder* →, *which is defined as smaller than 2-3 cm long x 0.5-1.5 cm wide.*

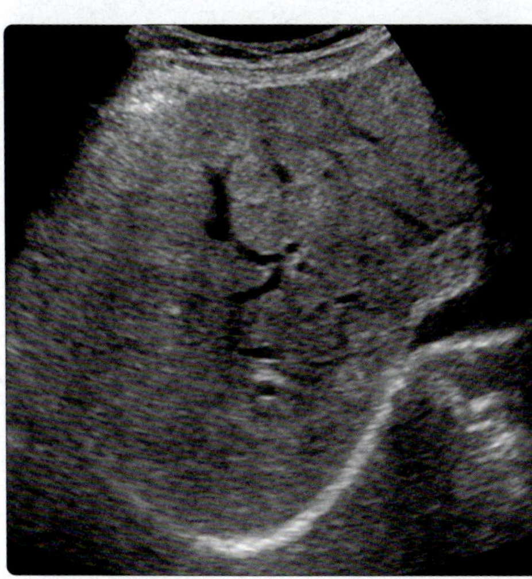

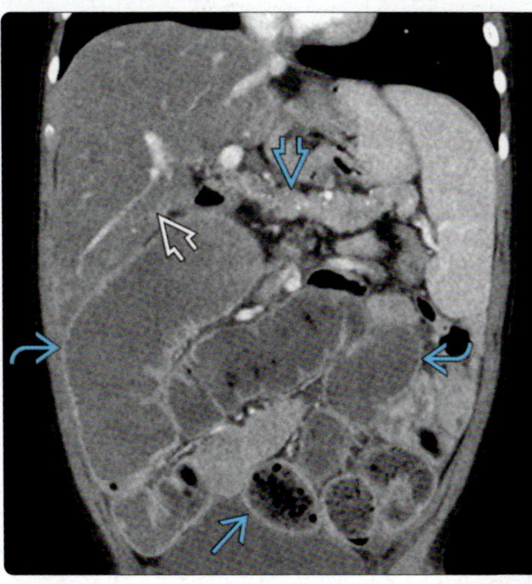

(Left) *Transverse ultrasound of the liver shows findings of cystic fibrosis liver disease. The liver has a heterogeneous appearance with ↑ echogenicity around portal triads.* **(Right)** *Coronal CECT in a cystic fibrosis patient with abdominal distention & pain shows dilated fluid-distended small bowel loops* ↪. *Fecal material* → *is present in some loops of small bowel, consistent with DIOS. Also note other sequelae of cystic fibrosis with atrophy & calcification of the pancreas* ⇨ *as well as hepatic steatosis* ➡.

Hemophagocytic Lymphohistiocytosis

KEY FACTS

TERMINOLOGY

- Rare disorder of pathological immune activation resulting in systemic hyperinflammation
- Likely to represents wide spectrum, divided into 2 types
  - Genetic/primary/familial: Inherited genetic abnormalities
  - Acquired/secondary: Environmental or acquired mechanisms, such as infection, malignancy, autoimmune conditions, & immunocompromise

IMAGING

- Nonspecific findings, used to assess & monitor disease activity & response to treatment
- Chest radiograph, abdominal US, & brain MR are often obtained during work-up based on signs & symptoms
- Recent paper suggests consideration of PET to detect occult lymphoma; no standard protocol exists
- Thoracic findings: Alveolar opacities, interstitial thickening, atelectasis, volume loss, pleural effusions, pneumothorax
  - Can show rapid evolution & resolution
- Abdominal findings: Hepatosplenomegaly, nephromegaly, ↑ periportal echogenicity, hyperechoic kidneys, gallbladder wall thickening, ascites
- CNS findings: Multiple T2-hyperintense lesions ± contrast enhancement, edema, volume loss
- Generalized lymphadenopathy

CLINICAL ISSUES

- Diagnostic criteria: Known hemophagocytic lymphohistiocytosis (HLH) genetic defect or 5/8 of
  - Fever; splenomegaly; cytopenia ≥ 2 cell lines; hypertriglyceridemia; hypofibrinogenemia; soluble CD25 > 2,400 U/mL; hemophagocytosis in bone marrow, spleen, liver, or lymph nodes; low or absent NK-cell cytotoxicity
- Diagnostic criteria in setting of juvenile idiopathic arthritis (JIA)
  - Ferritin > 684 ng/mL & 2 of: Platelets ≤ 181 x 10^9/L, aspartate aminotransferase > 48 U/L, triglycerides > 156 mg/dL, fibrinogen ≤ 360 mg/dL

(Left) *Axial FLAIR MR in a 9-year-old boy presenting with progressive headache, vomiting, & unsteadiness over the past 3 months shows numerous hyperintense cortical, subcortical, & deep lesions ➡ within the brain parenchyma. He was subsequently found to have familial HLH.* **(Right)** *Axial FLAIR MR in the same patient shows numerous hyperintense, confluent lesions in the supra- ➡ & infratentorial ➡ parenchyma. Mass effect is demonstrated by effacement of the 4th ventricle ➡.*

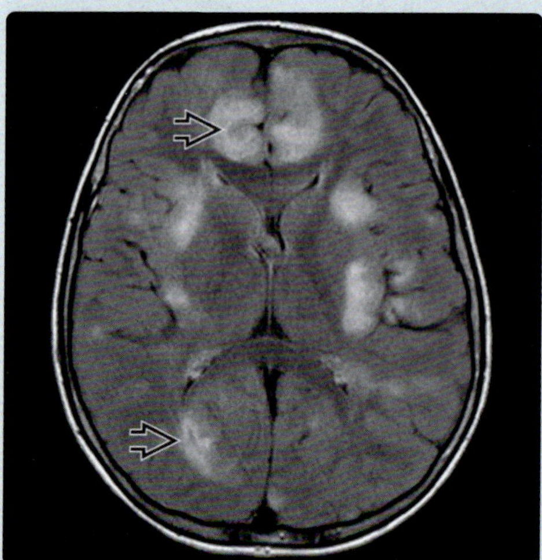

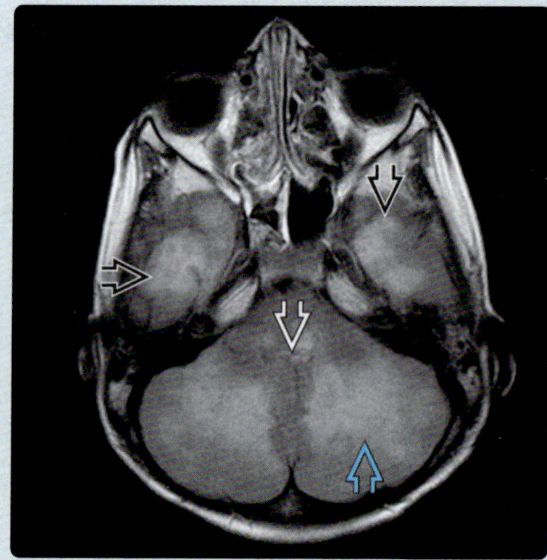

(Left) *Frontal chest radiograph in an ill child with HLH shows ill-defined perihilar opacities ➡, right worse than left.* **(Right)** *Longitudinal grayscale ultrasound in a child with HLH shows the right lobe of the liver ➡ extending far below the inferior pole of the right kidney ➡, suggesting hepatomegaly, a common but nonspecific finding in this disorder.*

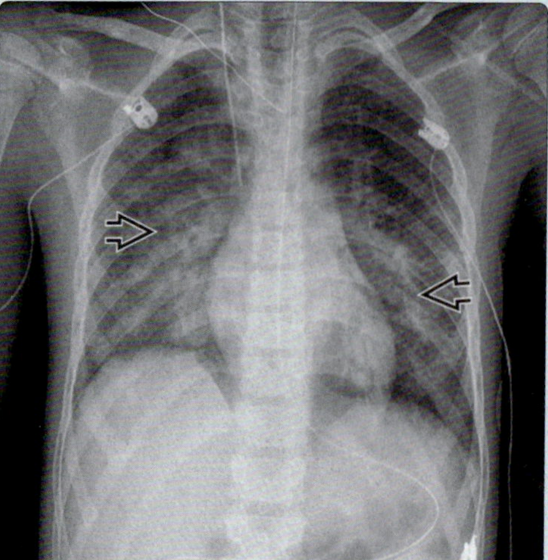

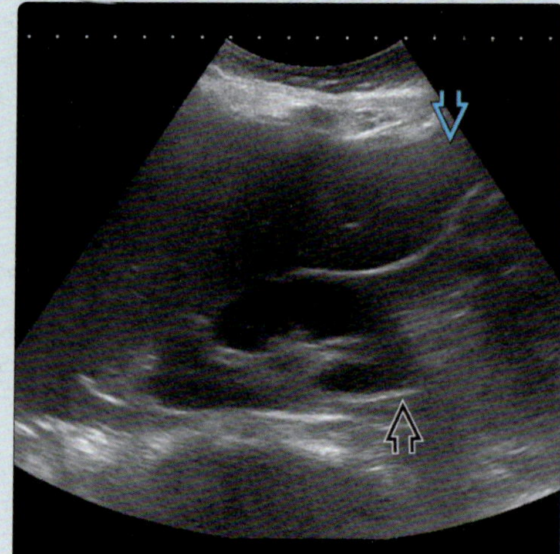

TERMINOLOGY

Abbreviations

- Hemophagocytic lymphohistiocytosis (HLH)

Synonyms

- Hyperferritinemic inflammation
- Macrophage activation syndrome (MAS) when occurring in those with underlying rheumatologic or autoimmune syndrome
- Cytokine release syndrome (CRS) if related to iatrogenic immunosuppression therapy

Definitions

- Rare, life-threatening disorder of pathological immune activation resulting in extreme systemic hyperinflammation
- Despite name, hemophagocytosis is not required for diagnosis
- Likely to represent wide spectrum, divided into 2 types
  - Genetic/primary/familial
  - Acquired/secondary
- Genetic/primary or familial HLH
  - Inherited genetic abnormalities
  - Familial HLH: Autosomal recessive pattern, commonly associated with familial HLH genes
  - Primary HLH: Associated with immune deficiency syndromes, such as X-linked lymphoproliferative disease, Griscelli type 2, & Chediak Higashi
- Acquired/secondary HLH
  - Environmental or acquired mechanisms, such as infection, malignancy, autoimmune conditions, immunocompromise

IMAGING

General Features

- Best diagnostic clue
  - Nonspecific; imaging is not included in diagnostic criteria
  - Imaging is used to assess & monitor disease activity & response to treatment

Radiographic Findings

- Chest: Alveolar opacities, interstitial thickening, atelectasis, volume loss, pleural effusions, pneumothorax
  - Can show rapid evolution & resolution
- Bone: Rib fractures, diaphyseal periosteal reaction of long bones

CT Findings

- CNS
  - Edema, low-attenuation parenchymal lesions, foci of Ca^{2+}, volume loss
- Abdominal
  - Hepatosplenomegaly, nephromegaly, gallbladder wall thickening, ascites
- Thoracic
  - Alveolar opacities, interstitial thickening, atelectasis, pneumatoceles, pleural effusions, pneumothorax
- Lymphadenopathy

MR Findings

- CNS
  - Multiple T2-hyperintense lesions (supra- & infratentorial) ± contrast enhancement
  - Edema, intracranial hemorrhage
  - Brain parenchymal volume loss ± Ca^{2+}, associated enlargement of ventricles & extraaxial spaces
  - Rarely, leptomeningeal enhancement, foci of parenchymal restricted diffusion, extraaxial collections

Ultrasonographic Findings

- Hepatosplenomegaly, gallbladder wall thickening, ↑ periportal echogenicity, hyperechoic kidneys, ascites
- Lymphadenopathy

Imaging Recommendations

- Best imaging tool
  - Chest radiograph, abdominal US, & brain MR are often obtained during work-up as indicated by clinical signs & symptoms
  - Recent paper suggests consideration of PET to detect occult lymphoma
- Protocol advice
  - No agreed standard protocol exists

DIFFERENTIAL DIAGNOSIS

Acute Respiratory Distress Syndrome

- Can occur with HLH, making it difficult to separate these processes

Malignancy (Lymphoma, Leukemia, Solid tumors)

- More likely to present with large nodal mass/solid tumor

Infection (Viral, Bacterial, Parasitic)

- Difficult to differentiate on imaging alone

Autoimmune Disorders

- Difficult to differentiate on imaging alone

Langerhans Cell Histiocytosis

- More likely to present in combination with destructive bone lesion

Child Abuse

- Injuries of varying age incompatible with described mechanism

PATHOLOGY

General Features

- Gene-mediated &/or infection/malignancy-triggered defect of lymphocyte cytotoxicity or inflammasome activity
- Cycle of abnormal activation of mononuclear phagocytes & type 1 lymphocytes with overproduction of inflammatory cytokines

Staging, Grading, & Classification

- Diagnostic criteria for HLH
  - Genetic defect consistent with HLH or 5 of 8 clinical & laboratory criteria
    - Fever
    - Splenomegaly
    - Cytopenia in ≥ 2 cell lineages
    - Hypertriglyceridemia or hypofibrinogenemia
    - Hyperferritinemia

- Soluble CD25 > 2,400 U/mL
- Hemophagocytosis in bone marrow, spleen, lymph nodes, or liver
- Low or absent NK-cell cytotoxicity

- Diagnostic criteria for HLH/MAS in setting of known juvenile idiopathic arthritis (JIA)
  - Ferritin > 684 ng/mL & 2 of 4 criteria
    - Platelet count ≤ 181 x 10^9/L
    - Aspartate aminotransferase > 48 U/L
    - Triglycerides > 156 mg/dL
    - Fibrinogen ≤ 360 mg/dL

CLINICAL ISSUES

Presentation

- Most common signs/symptoms
  - Can be multisystemic & show wide variation
  - Difficult to differentiate from more common diseases
  - Infections are often triggers, especially herpes & Epstein Barr virus groups
  - When associated with malignancies, they are most commonly hematologic in nature
    - In adults, malignancy is thought to be most common trigger but is much less common in pediatrics
  - Immunosuppression is also recognized as predisposition to HLH
  - When HLH is related to autoimmune disease (most commonly systemic onset JIA &SLE), it is referred to as MAS
  - Systemic
    - Fever, coagulopathy, cytopenia, multiorgan failure, lymphadenopathy, hyperferritinemia
  - CNS
    - Tends not to precede systemic findings but are present in > 1/2 of patients with HLH
    - Wide range: Headache, vomiting, psychiatric symptoms, dystonia, hemiparesis, visual disturbance, cognitive decline, seizures, cranial nerve palsies, encephalopathy, ataxia, gait disturbance, ↑ intracranial pressure, coma
  - Abdominal
    - Jaundice, hepatitis, liver dysfunction/failure, hepatosplenomegaly
  - Musculoskeletal
    - Skin rash, edema

Demographics

- Primary HLH usually presents within 1st few years of life; some cases of adult onset have been reported
- Secondary HLH can occur at any age; initial presentation is usually associated with infection, autoimmune condition, or malignancy
- Majority of adult HLH patients do not demonstrate underlying immune defect
- Incidence is likely underestimated
  - Retrospective study performed in Sweden estimated incidence of ~ 1.2/1 million children/year
  - More recent retrospective study performed in Texas suggests prevalence of 1/100,000 with median age at diagnosis of 1.8 years

Natural History & Prognosis

- Untreated disease is essentially fatal; with treatment, survival has ↑ significantly over last few decades
- Overall, current 5-year survival ~ 62%

Treatment

- Goal is to dampen cytokine storm & eliminate activated T cells & macrophages
  - Immunosuppressive chemotherapeutic drugs & biologics
    - Dexamethasone, etoposide, & cyclosporine A
    - Intrathecal methotrexate for CNS involvement
- Treatment of underlying trigger
- Allogenic stem cell transplantation is only cure for primary/familial HLH

SELECTED REFERENCES

1. Bergsten E et al: Stem cell transplantation for children with hemophagocytic lymphohistiocytosis: results from the HLH-2004 study. Blood Adv. 4(15):3754-66, 2020
2. Canna SW et al: Pediatric hemophagocytic lymphohistiocytosis. Blood. 135(16):1332-43, 2020
3. Shieh AC et al: Hemophagocytic lymphohistiocytosis: a primer for radiologists. AJR Am J Roentgenol. 214(1):W11-9, 2020
4. Benson LA et al: Pediatric CNS-isolated hemophagocytic lymphohistiocytosis. Neurol Neuroimmunol Neuroinflamm. 6(3):e560, 2019
5. Al-Samkari H et al: Hemophagocytic lymphohistiocytosis. Annu Rev Pathol. 13:27-49, 2018
6. Bergsten E et al: Confirmed efficacy of etoposide and dexamethasone in HLH treatment: long-term results of the cooperative HLH-2004 study. Blood. 130(25):2728-38, 2017
7. Emile JF et al: Revised classification of histiocytoses and neoplasms of the macrophage-dendritic cell lineages. Blood. 127(22):2672-81, 2016
8. Allen CE et al: Pathophysiology and epidemiology of hemophagocytic lymphohistiocytosis. Hematology Am Soc Hematol Educ Program. 2015:177-82, 2015
9. Lehmberg K et al: Malignancy-associated haemophagocytic lymphohistiocytosis in children and adolescents. Br J Haematol. 170(4):539-49, 2015
10. George MR: Hemophagocytic lymphohistiocytosis: review of etiologies and management. J Blood Med. 5:69-86, 2014
11. Guandalini M et al: Spectrum of imaging appearances in Australian children with central nervous system hemophagocytic lymphohistiocytosis. J Clin Neurosci. 21(2):305-10, 2014
12. Rosado FG et al: Hemophagocytic lymphohistiocytosis: an update on diagnosis and pathogenesis. Am J Clin Pathol. 139(6):713-27, 2013
13. Zhang K et al: Hypomorphic mutations in PRF1, MUNC13-4, and STXBP2 are associated with adult-onset familial HLH. Blood. 118(22):5794-8, 2011
14. Niece JA et al: Hemophagocytic lymphohistiocytosis in Texas: observations on ethnicity and race. Pediatr Blood Cancer. 54(3):424-8, 2010
15. Janka G: Hemophagocytic lymphohistiocytosis: when the immune system runs amok. Klin Padiatr. 221(5):278-85, 2009
16. Henter JI et al: HLH-2004: Diagnostic and therapeutic guidelines for hemophagocytic lymphohistiocytosis. Pediatr Blood Cancer. 48(2):124-31, 2007
17. Janka GE: Hemophagocytic syndromes. Blood Rev. 21(5):245-53, 2007
18. Histiocyte Society: HLH-2004 Study Group. Published January, 2004. Accessed November 20, 2020. https://www.skion.nl/workspace/uploads/HLH-2004-protocol1.pdf
19. Fitzgerald NE et al: Imaging characteristics of hemophagocytic lymphohistiocytosis. Pediatr Radiol. 33(6):392-401, 2003
20. Rooms L et al: Hemophagocytic lymphohistiocytosis masquerading as child abuse: presentation of three cases and review of central nervous system findings in hemophagocytic lymphohistiocytosis. Pediatrics. 111(5 Pt 1):e636-40, 2003

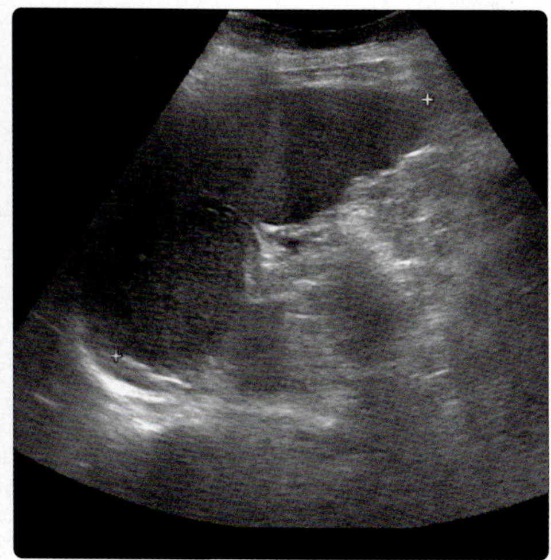

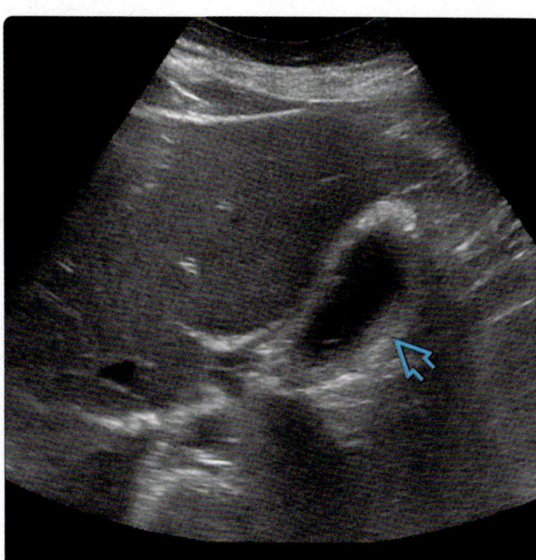

(Left) *Longitudinal grayscale ultrasound in a 9-year-old patient with HLH shows splenomegaly, measuring 13.9 cm (with the upper limit of normal for age at 10.5 cm). While nonspecific, this is a common finding in HLH.* **(Right)** *Transverse grayscale ultrasound shows diffuse nonspecific gallbladder wall thickening ➡ in a child with HLH.*

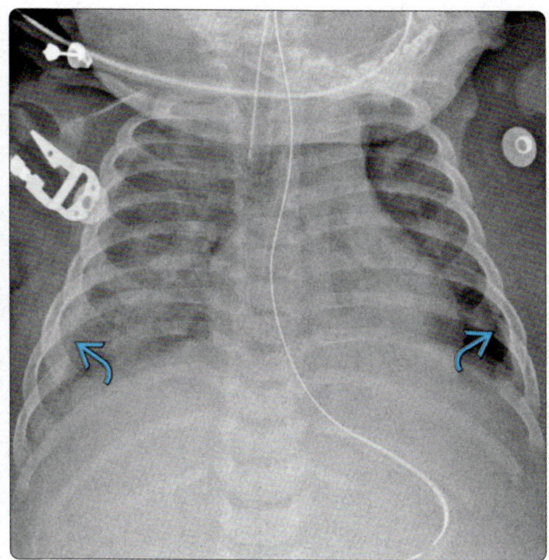

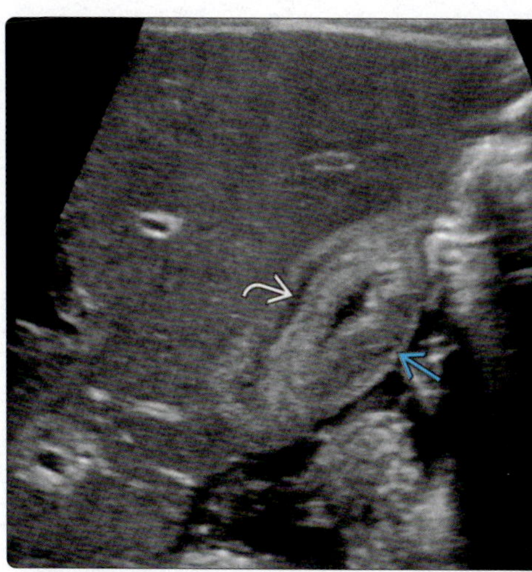

(Left) *Frontal chest radiograph in a 4-month-old that met diagnostic criteria for HLH shows bilateral pulmonary opacities & small pleural effusions ➡.* **(Right)** *Longitudinal ultrasound in the same patient with HLH demonstrates marked gallbladder wall thickening ➡ & pericholecystic edema ➡. Also noted is mildly ↑ periportal echogenicity.*

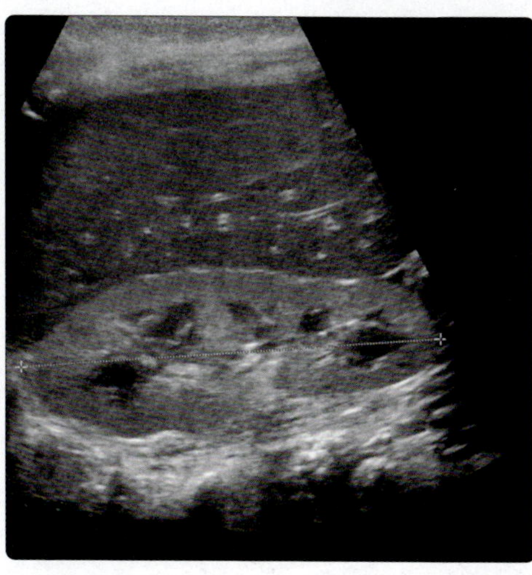

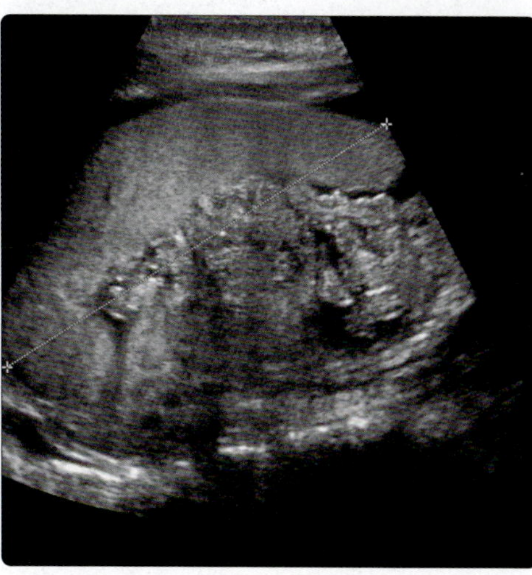

(Left) *Longitudinal ultrasound in the same patient shows an enlarged kidney with ↑ echogenicity of the renal cortex & ↑ hepatic periportal echogenicity.* **(Right)** *Longitudinal ultrasound in the same patient shows splenomegaly, measuring up to 9.3 cm. The pulmonary opacities, gallbladder wall thickening, nephromegaly with ↑ cortical echogenicity, splenomegaly, & ↑ periportal echogenicity are nonspecific, but this patient met criteria overall for HLH.*

KEY FACTS

TERMINOLOGY

- Aggressive B-cell non-Hodgkin lymphoma (NHL)
- Most common form of NHL in children ≤ 15 years of age

IMAGING

- Most common imaging appearance depends on type
  - Sporadic: Abdominal soft tissue mass &/or bowel wall thickening; may involve solid organs
    - Discrete or conglomerate masses &/or infiltrating, encasing, poorly defined lesions
  - Endemic: Head & neck soft tissue mass
- Ultrasound: Homogeneous, hypoechoic soft tissue mass(es)
  - Irregular bowel wall thickening; ± intussusception
- CT/MR
  - Moderately enhancing homogeneous mass(es) &/or thickened bowel wall (ileocecal region)
    - Hypoenhancing relative to involved organs
  - Enlarged lymph nodes
  - ± peritoneal thickening or nodularity

PATHOLOGY

- 3 distinct subtypes
  - Endemic
    - Commonly involves head & neck (mandible)
    - Almost always associated with EBV
    - More common in Africa & other sites along equator
  - Sporadic
    - Most commonly involves abdomen (60-80%)
      - Bowel, mesentery, solid organs, gonads
      - May involve head & neck, chest, superficial sites
    - Less commonly associated with EBV (15%)
    - More common in North America, Europe
  - Immunodeficiency related

CLINICAL ISSUES

- Mean age: 8 years
- Short doubling time of neoplasm (~ 24 hours) may lead to rapid growth, acute presentations
- With appropriate treatment, survival ~ 90%

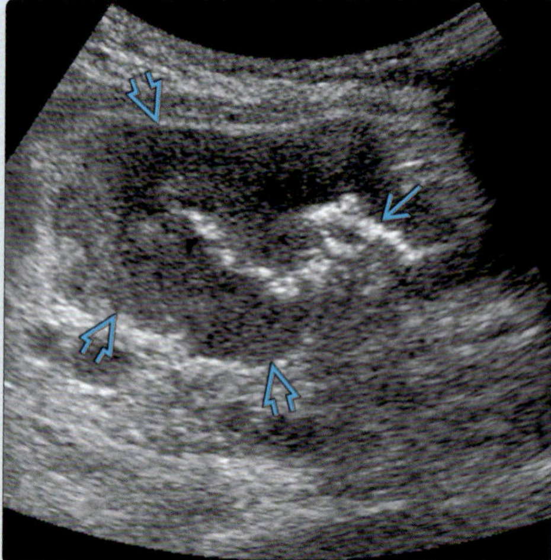

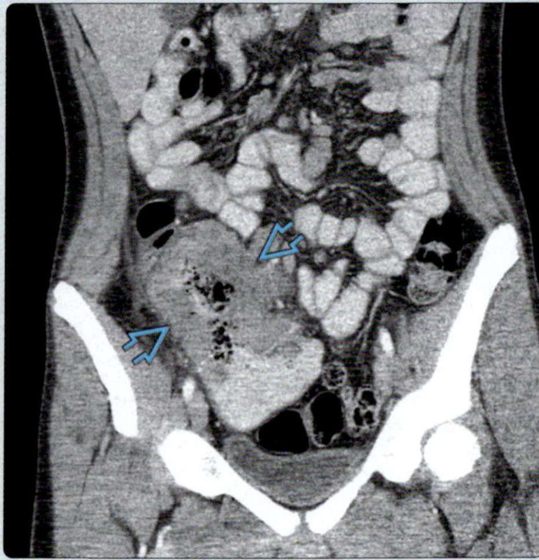

(Left) *Transverse abdominal ultrasound in a 12-year-old boy with abdominal pain shows markedly hypoechoic & somewhat irregular bowel wall thickening ⇨ in the right lower quadrant. The central echogenic foci ⇨ represent gas within the compressed bowel lumen.* **(Right)** *Coronal CECT in the same patient shows marked nodular bowel wall thickening ⇨. Biopsy confirmed Burkitt lymphoma.*

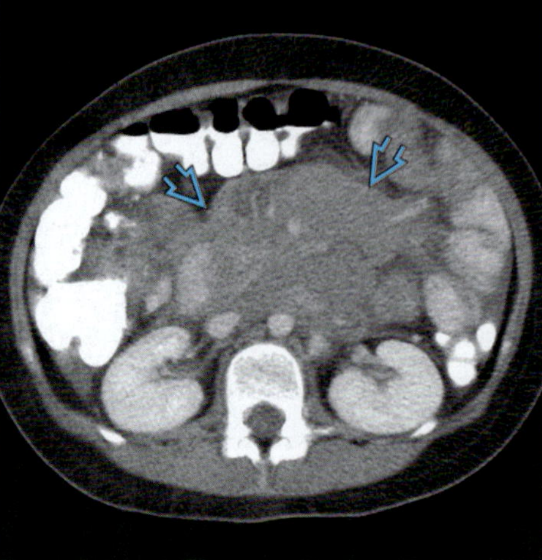

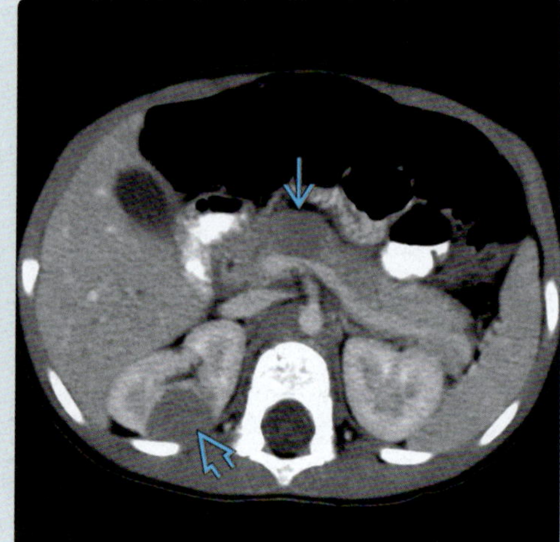

(Left) *Axial CECT in a 9-year-old girl with abdominal pain shows a large, conglomerate lymph node mass ⇨ engulfing bowel loops & multiple vessels. Biopsy confirmed Burkitt lymphoma.* **(Right)** *Axial CECT in a 5-year-old boy with Burkitt lymphoma shows a homogeneous, low-attenuation mass in the right kidney ⇨. A similar focus of tumor is visualized in the pancreatic neck ⇨. Additional lesions were also present in the left kidney (not shown).*

TERMINOLOGY

Synonyms

- Small non-cleaved-cell lymphoma

Definitions

- Aggressive B-cell non-Hodgkin lymphoma (NHL)
- Most common form of NHL in children ≤ 15 years of age
  - 40% of childhood NHL

IMAGING

General Features

- Location
  - Sporadic
    - Abdominal involvement is most common (60-80%)
      - Bowel wall, most commonly ileocecal region (including appendix)
      - Mesentery & peritoneal lining
      - Can involve solid organs, including kidneys & gonads
    - Head & neck
    - Others: Mediastinum, bone marrow, CNS
  - Endemic
    - Head & neck are most common
      - Classically involves mandible

Radiographic Findings

- Displacement or separation of bowel loops, narrowing of bowel lumen, organomegaly

Ultrasonographic Findings

- Grayscale ultrasound
  - Irregular bowel wall thickening
    - Thickened bowel wall is usually hypoechoic
    - May cause ileocolic intussusception
  - Solid, hypoechoic mass or enlarged lymph nodes
    - May be confluent with abnormal bowel
- Color Doppler
  - Internal blood flow due to tumor vascularity &/or vessel encasement
  - Thickened bowel wall causes less hyperemia than infectious or inflammatory etiologies

CT Findings

- CECT: Homogeneous, solid soft tissue mass
  - Moderate to marked irregular bowel wall thickening involving ileocecal region
  - Conglomerate mesenteric nodal masses encasing vessels
  - Nodular or mass-like peritoneal thickening

MR Findings

- T2 FS: Intermediate-signal soft tissue mass
  - Bowel wall thickening
  - Enlarged lymph nodes
- T1 C+ FS: Hypoenhancing relative to involved organ (e.g., kidney, spleen)
- DWI: Restricts diffusion

Nuclear Medicine Findings

- ↑ uptake on FDG PET

DIFFERENTIAL DIAGNOSIS

Other Potentially Extensive Abdominal Neoplasms

- Hodgkin lymphoma
- Rhabdomyosarcoma
- Ovarian neoplasm
- Desmoplastic small round cell tumor

Other Causes of Bowel Wall Thickening

- Inflammatory bowel disease
- Infectious enterocolitis

PATHOLOGY

General Features

- Translocation t(8:14)(q24:q32) in 70-80% of patients
  - Linked to deregulated expression of *MYC* oncogene

Staging, Grading, & Classification

- Classified into 3 distinct subtypes
  - Endemic
    - Africa, Papua New Guinea, & other locations clustered around equator
      - Linked to malaria
    - Almost always associated with EBV
  - Sporadic
    - North America, Europe
    - Less commonly associated with EBV (15%)
  - Immunodeficiency related
    - Associated with HIV infection

CLINICAL ISSUES

Presentation

- Most common signs/symptoms
  - Sporadic: Abdominal pain, distention, obstruction
  - Endemic: Head & neck mass, usually mandible
- Other signs/symptoms
  - Recurrent ileocolic intussusception
- Short doubling time of neoplasm (~ 24 hours) may lead to rapid growth, acute presentations

Demographics

- Mean age: 8 years; most common between 5-9 years
- Boys > > girls

Natural History & Prognosis

- With appropriate treatment, survival ~ 90%

Treatment

- Chemotherapy ± surgery, radiation therapy

SELECTED REFERENCES

1. Gillman J et al: PET in pediatric lymphoma. PET Clin. 15(3):299-307, 2020
2. Tannenbaum MF et al: Imaging musculoskeletal manifestations of pediatric hematologic malignancies. AJR Am J Roentgenol. 214(2):455-64, 2020
3. Kalisz K et al: An update on Burkitt lymphoma: a review of pathogenesis and multimodality imaging assessment of disease presentation, treatment response, and recurrence. Insights Imaging. 10(1):56, 2019
4. McCarten KM et al: Imaging for diagnosis, staging and response assessment of Hodgkin lymphoma and non-Hodgkin lymphoma. Pediatr Radiol. 49(11):1545-64, 2019
5. Chung EM et al: Solid tumors of the peritoneum, omentum, and mesentery in children: radiologic-pathologic correlation: from the radiologic pathology archives. Radiographics. 35(2):521-46, 2015

Castleman Disease

KEY FACTS

TERMINOLOGY

- Nonmalignant lymphoproliferative disorder
  - Also termed angiofollicular lymph node hyperplasia
- Can be unicentric (most common) or multicentric/systemic
  - Multicentric is more common in adults
    - Idiopathic or associated with HIV & human herpesvirus-8 infections, autoimmune disorders
- Most common location: Mediastinum
  - Can occur in abdomen & other nodal sites

IMAGING

- Radiographs: Soft tissue mass ± punctate Ca^{2+}
- Ultrasound: Hypoechoic, sometimes hypervascular mass
- NECT/CECT
  - Well-circumscribed, homogeneously enhancing mass
    - ± Ca^{2+} in branching (arborizing) pattern
- MR
  - Low to intermediate T1; intermediate to high T2
  - Homogeneous enhancement is most common
  - Typically restricts diffusion
- FDG PET
  - FDG avidity is typically < lymphoma

TOP DIFFERENTIAL DIAGNOSES

- Lymphoma
- Granulomatous infection
- Neurogenic tumor
- Inflammatory myofibroblastic tumor

PATHOLOGY

- Hyaline-vascular type
  - Most common, usually unicentric asymptomatic mass
  - Typically in adolescents & young adults
- Plasma cell type
  - Rare in children

CLINICAL ISSUES

- Unicentric form: Excellent prognosis with surgical excision
- Multicentric form: Systemic treatment; worse prognosis

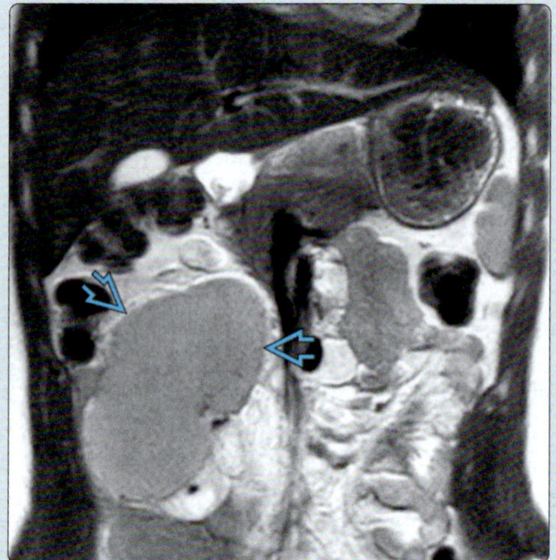

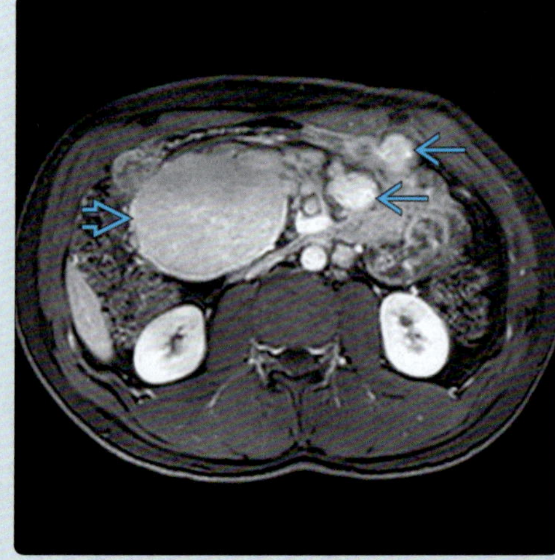

(Left) *Coronal T2 SSFSE MR in a 16-year-old with abdominal pain shows an abdominal mass ⇨ of homogeneous intermediate signal intensity centered in the mesentery.* **(Right)** *Axial T1 C+ FS MR in the same patient again shows moderate homogeneous enhancement of the right mesenteric mass ⇨ as well as several enlarged mesenteric lymph nodes →.*

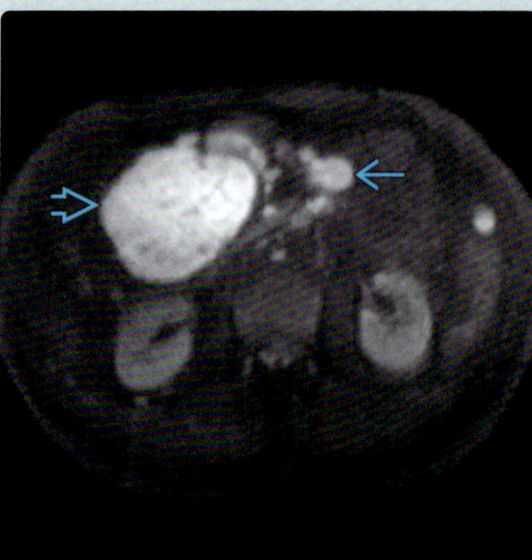

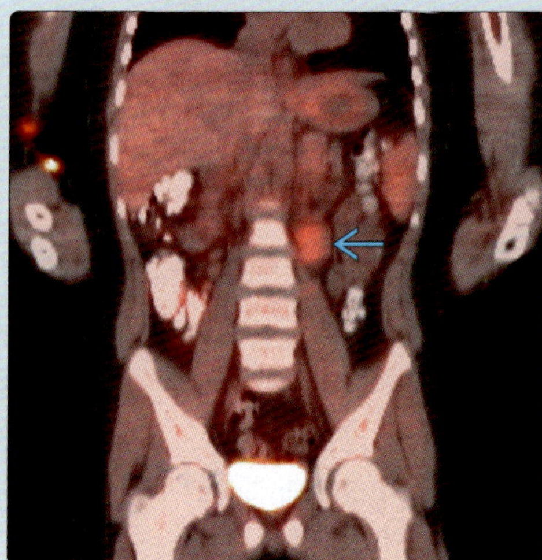

(Left) *Axial DWI MR in the same patient shows marked hyperintense signal throughout the mass ⇨ & adjacent lymph nodes →. The corresponding ADC map (not shown) confirmed restricted diffusion. Biopsy revealed Castleman disease.* **(Right)** *Coronal FDG PET/CT in a different patient shows moderate FDG avidity within a retroperitoneal mass → (maximum SUV of 3). Biopsy revealed Castleman disease.*

KEY FACTS

ERMINOLOGY

Spindle cell neoplasm with intermediate malignant potential in children & young adults

Synonyms: Inflammatory pseudotumor; plasma cell granuloma

MAGING

Locations: Lung, abdominal solid organs, bowel, mesentery, urinary bladder
- Most common primary lung neoplasm in children

Typically well-defined, round or lobulated mass
- May be discrete & bulky or infiltrative & ill-defined in mesentery & bowel

Heterogeneously enhancing on CT/MR
- ± delayed enhancement, central necrosis, or central Ca^{2+}

May be T2 hypointense on MR with ↑ fibrous stroma

OP DIFFERENTIAL DIAGNOSES

Other fibrous lesions
- Soft tissue sarcomas
- Lymphoma
- Castleman disease
- Desmoplastic small round cell tumor

PATHOLOGY

- Spindle cell proliferation + inflammatory cells
- *ALK* gene mutation in ~ 60%

CLINICAL ISSUES

- Symptoms due to local mass effect ± nonspecific constitutional symptoms
- Low risk of distant metastases (~ 5%) with local/regional recurrence being more common
  - Most morbidity/mortality from local invasion/mass effect
- Excellent prognosis with complete surgical resection
  - If resection not feasible → chemotherapy ± steroids, targeted ALK or COX2 inhibitors

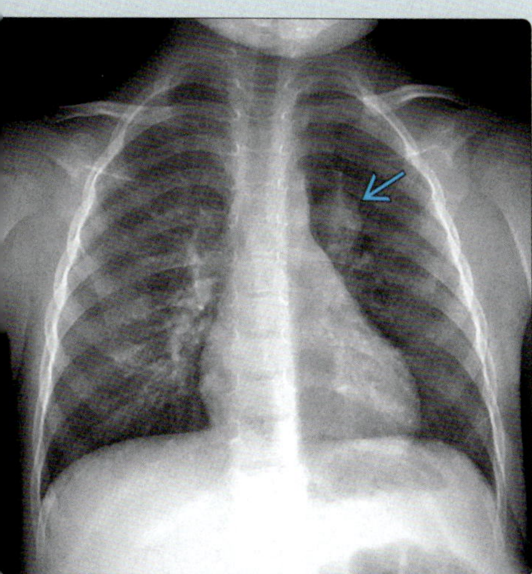

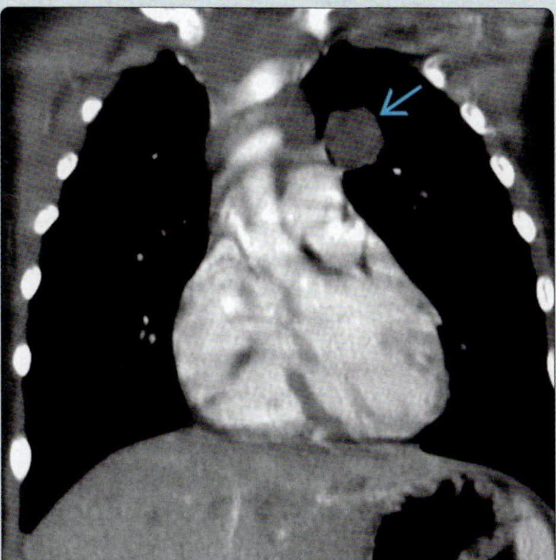

(Left) *Frontal chest radiograph in a 3-year-old boy with a cough shows a well-defined perihilar left upper lobe mass ⇒, ultimately confirmed to be an inflammatory myofibroblastic tumor (IMT).* **(Right)** *Coronal CECT in the same patient demonstrates a well-defined, nearly homogeneous, relatively hypoenhancing mass situated in the left upper lobe ⇒. IMT should be remembered as the most common pediatric lung neoplasm.*

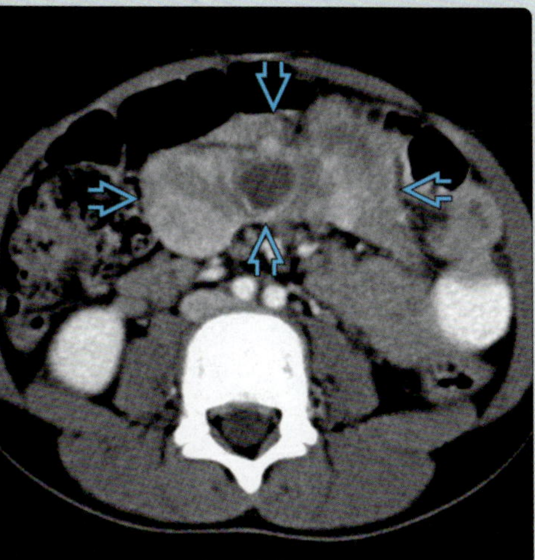

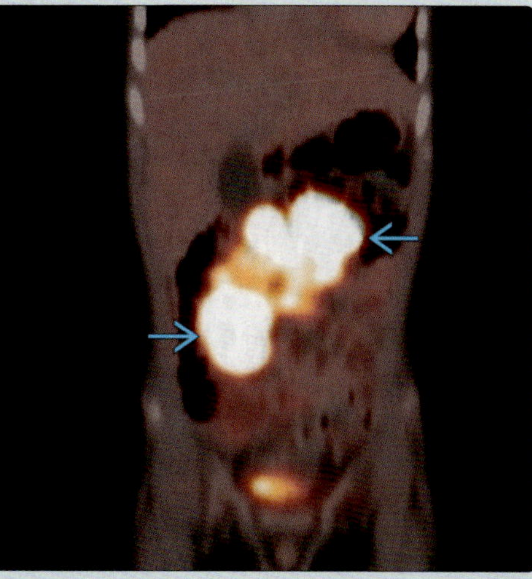

(Left) *Axial CECT in an 8-year-old boy shows a lobulated, heterogeneously enhancing mass ⇒ centered in the mesentery, found to be an IMT at surgical resection. Central necrosis is suggested in this lesion, a finding of variable frequency in these tumors.* **(Right)** *Coronal fused FDG PET/CT in the same patient shows nearly uniform, intense FDG avidity by the mesenteric IMT ⇒ except for the central focus of necrosis.*

Abdominal Aneurysms

KEY FACTS

TERMINOLOGY

- Dilation of abdominal aorta &/or major arterial branches
- Often idiopathic, other etiologies include
  - Syndromic: Tuberous sclerosis, neurofibromatosis type 1, connective tissue disorders
  - Inflammatory arteritides: Takayasu, Kawasaki, Behçet
  - Infectious: Bacterial, mycobacterial, fungal
  - Traumatic: Iatrogenic (umbilical arterial catheter, etc.), blunt trauma

IMAGING

- Any portion of aorta & branches may be affected
  - ± dilation &/or stenosis of visceral branches
  - Normal aortic diameter varies with patient age & size
- Ultrasound for initial investigation of pediatric abdominal mass (± pulsation)
  - Layers of clot may mimic heterogeneous neoplasm
  - Color Doppler is essential to exclude aneurysm upon visualization of any "cystic" lesion
- Best imaging tool to define extent & branch involvement: CTA or MR angiography
  - Fusiform or saccular dilation of aorta &/or branches
  - Vessel wall enhancement in inflammatory etiologies
- Digital subtraction angiography (DSA) excellently depicts aneurysms & stenoses
  - Invasive, ↑ risk of complications

CLINICAL ISSUES

- Presentations include
  - Asymptomatic ± pulsatile abdominal mass
  - Stenosis &/or thromboembolism of branch vessels
    - End-organ hypoperfusion; renin-mediated hypertension if renal arteries are involved
  - Rupture (rarely) with abdominal pain & shock
  - Signs/symptoms of underlying systemic disease
- Treatment: Surgical repair vs. endovascular stent grafting
  - Medical therapy to ↓ inflammation, control blood pressure; IV antibiotics for infection

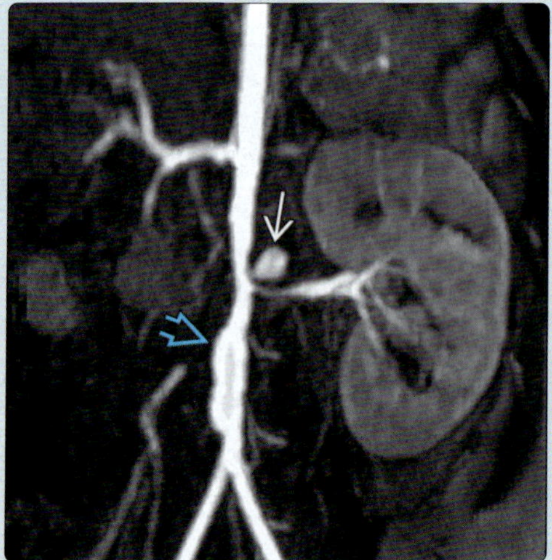
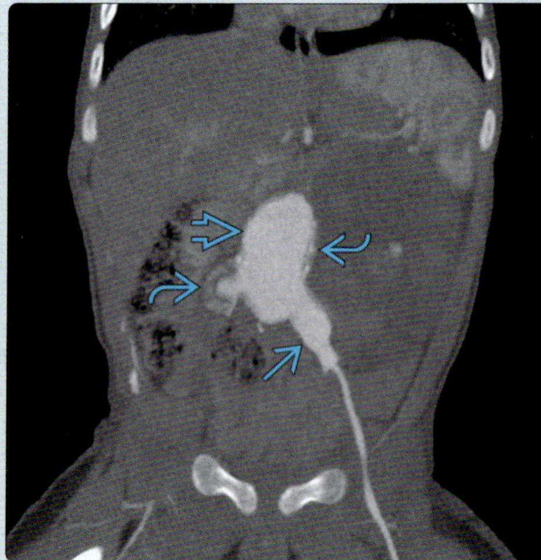

(Left) *Coronal oblique MIP image from a contrast enhanced MR angiogram in a 5-year-old child with neurofibromatosis type 1 & hypertension shows a saccular pseudoaneurysm ➔ arising from the abdominal aorta. There is also a fusiform aneurysm ➔ in the infrarenal aorta.* **(Right)** *Coronal MIP image from a CT angiogram in a 7-month-old boy shows aneurysmal dilation of the aorta ➔ with extension into the bilateral iliac arteries ➔. Calcifications are present in the wall of the aortic & iliac aneurysms ➔.*

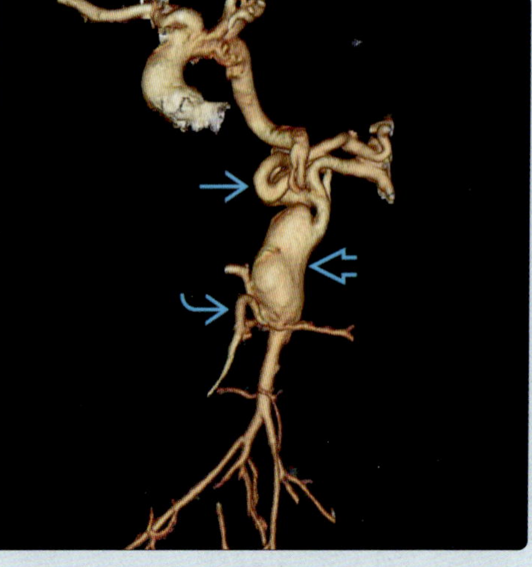
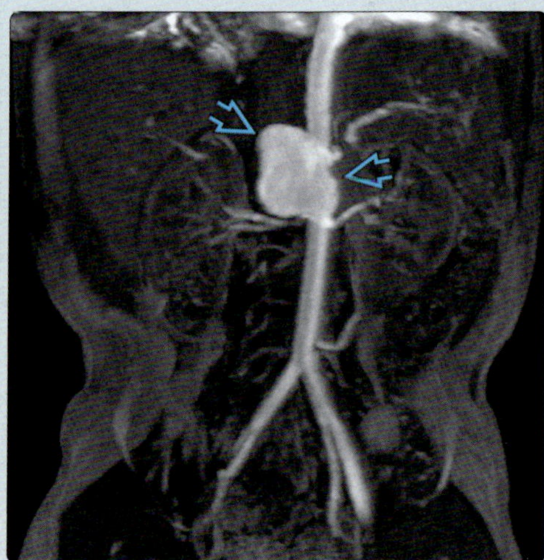

(Left) *Oblique CTA 3D reconstruction in a 3-month-old with congenital anomalies & hypertension shows an aneurysm of the abdominal aorta ➔ with involvement of the celiac trunk & superior mesenteric artery (SMA) ➔. The patient also had occlusion of the lower thoracic aorta with resultant formation of multiple collateral vessels ➔.* **(Right)** *Coronal MIP MR angiogram in a 7-year-old boy shows a large saccular abdominal aortic aneurysm ➔. The origins of the celiac axis & SMA were involved (not shown).*

TERMINOLOGY

Definitions

- Dilation of abdominal aorta &/or its major branches
  - True aneurysm: All layers of arterial wall are expanded
  - Pseudoaneurysm: Focal rupture contained by adventitia

IMAGING

General Features

- Best diagnostic clue
  - Focally dilated aorta &/or visceral branches
    - Normal aortic dimensions vary with patient age & size
      - > 2.5-cm diameter is enlarged for any age
- Location
  - Can affect any portion of aorta & branches
  - Aortic aneurysm is associated with dilation &/or stenosis of visceral branches
    - Can also extend into iliac arteries
  - Distant aneurysms are often found with systemic diseases & idiopathic aneurysms
- Morphology
  - Aneurysm can be fusiform or saccular

Ultrasonographic Findings

- Grayscale ultrasound
  - Dilation of aorta/artery: Well-defined, pulsatile, anechoic round or tubular mass (cystic appearing)
  - Heterogeneous mural thrombus due to layers of clot ± Ca^{2+}; may compose majority of aneurysm
- Color Doppler
  - Confirms vascular nature of round or tubular anechoic structure (rather than cyst or fluid-filled tube)
  - ↑ velocity at stenosis; turbulent flow, parvus et tardus waveforms, & spectral broadening beyond stenosis

CT Findings

- CTA: ↑ luminal diameter of aorta
  - Look for associated aneurysms in visceral branches
  - Also associated with vascular stenoses
  - May see vessel wall thickening or enhancement if due to inflammatory causes (e.g., Takayasu arteritis)

MR Findings

- Pulsation artifact in phase-encoding direction
- ± layers of T1/T2 heterogeneous thrombus surrounding flow void in lumen
- ± vessel wall thickening & abnormal signal with inflammatory causes
  - T2 FS, T1 C+ FS, DWI
- MRA for luminal dilation ± associated stenoses

Imaging Recommendations

- Best imaging tool
  - CT angiography or MR angiography
  - Catheter-based digital subtraction angiography (DSA) may be employed in therapy
- Protocol advice
  - MR angiography ± gadolinium
  - Vessel wall imaging: Thin-section T1 C+ FS MR (spin-echo based with dark lumen)
    - Used with suspected inflammatory arteritis

DIFFERENTIAL DIAGNOSIS

Abdominal Cyst

- Well-defined cysts, such as ovarian, gastrointestinal duplication, mesenteric lymphatic malformation
- Color Doppler will show no significant internal flow

Solid Abdominal Mass

- Large, heterogeneous, partially thrombosed aneurysm may mimic neoplasm, such as Wilms or ovarian tumor

PATHOLOGY

General Features

- Etiology
  - Syndromes: Connective tissue disorders (Ehlers-Danlos, Marfan), tuberous sclerosis, neurofibromatosis type 1
  - Traumatic: Iatrogenic (umbilical artery catheter), blunt abdominal trauma (uncommon)
  - Inflammatory arteritides: Takayasu (most common), Kawasaki, polyarteritis nodosa, Behçet disease
  - Infectious: Bacterial, mycobacterial, fungal
  - Idiopathic
- Associated abnormalities
  - Various features of underlying syndromes
  - Multifocal abdominal &/or distant aneurysms are not uncommon, even in idiopathic setting

CLINICAL ISSUES

Presentation

- Most common signs/symptoms
  - Asymptomatic vs. pulsatile abdominal mass
  - Hypertension due to renal artery stenosis/compression → renin-mediated (renovascular) hypertension
- Other signs/symptoms
  - Abdominal pain & shock due to rupture (rare)
  - Signs/symptoms of associated syndromes or septic emboli in infectious setting

Natural History & Prognosis

- Rupture can lead to life-threatening hemorrhage
- Visceral organ hypoperfusion due to associated arterial stenoses or thromboses

Treatment

- Surgery vs. endovascular stent grafting
  - May require operative reimplantation of branches
- Medical therapy to ↓ inflammation, treat infection, control blood pressure

SELECTED REFERENCES

1. Subbaraj L et al: Congenital superior mesenteric artery aneurysm in a 6-week-old infant presenting with upper gastrointestinal bleeding. J Vasc Surg. 71(4):1391-4, 2020
2. Tanga CF et al: Ruptured abdominal aortic aneurysm in an 11-year-old with multiple peripheral artery aneurysms. J Vasc Surg Cases Innov Tech. 6(4):539-42, 2020
3. Akturk Y et al: Normal abdominal aorta diameter in infants, children and adolescents. Pediatr Int. 60(5):455-60, 2018
4. Min SK et al: Pediatric vascular surgery review with a 30-year-experience in a tertiary referral center. Vasc Specialist Int. 33(2):47-54, 2017
5. Eliason JL et al: Surgical treatment of abdominal aortic aneurysms in infancy and early childhood. J Vasc Surg. 64(5):1252-61, 2016

SECTION 5

Genitourinary

Bladder Abnormalities

Adrenal Abnormalities

Uterine and Ovarian Abnormalities

Scrotal/Testicular Abnormalities

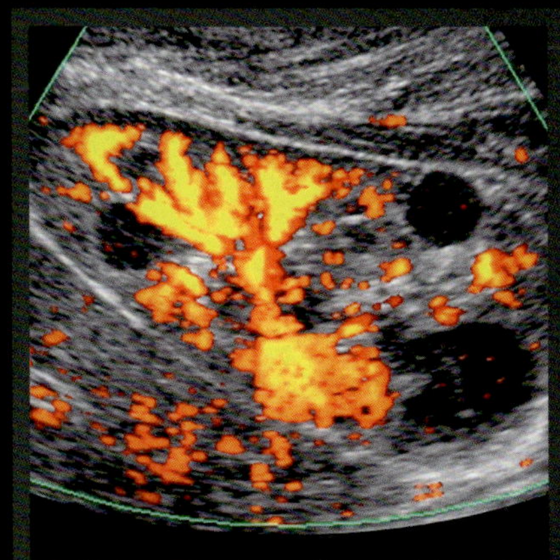

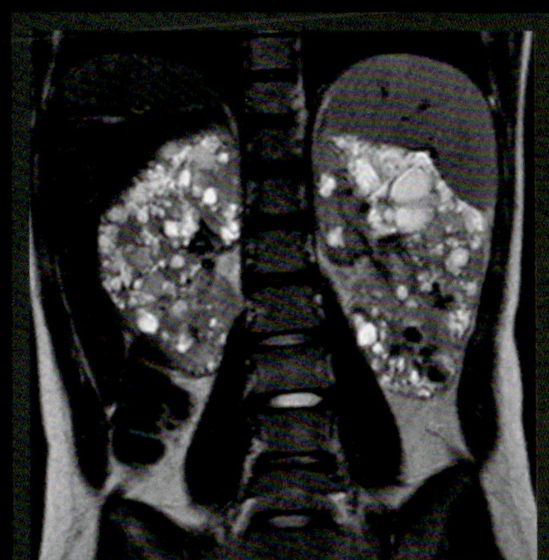

Embryology

A basic understanding of developmental anatomy will help explain the spectrum of congenital anomalies seen in the pediatric genitourinary tract.

During the 5th week of gestation, the mesonephric duct develops a budding tube (the ureteric bud) near its attachment to the cloaca. As this ureteric bud elongates, it reaches the metanephric blastema & undergoes a series of branchings to form the major & minor calyces, the renal pelvis, & the ureter. Signals from the ureteric bud induce changes in the metanephric blastema to form renal tubules, collecting tubules, & glomeruli of individual renal lobules. By 16- to 18-weeks gestation, the fetal kidneys are the major source of amniotic fluid for the fetus. The induction of mature renal lobules is complete by 32- to 36-weeks gestation.

While the kidney is forming, it migrates cephalad & rotates so that the renal pelves, which are initially directed anteriorly, are ultimately directed medially. At week 6, the kidneys lie in front of the primitive sacrum in the pelvis. By weeks 10-12, the kidneys have relatively ascended to their expected location along the upper lumbar spine. As the kidneys migrate, they pick up & discard nearby vascular attachments to both the aorta & inferior vena cava. This accounts for accessory vessels in normally located kidneys & for multiple vessels seen with ectopic & crossed fused kidneys.

Pediatric Genitourinary Tract Disorders

Congenital Abnormalities

Congenital anomalies of the kidney & urinary tract (CAKUT) are commonly discovered during the evaluation of pediatric patients. In fact, the urinary tract is the most common organ system affected by congenital anomalies. Many of these abnormalities are found incidentally, while others become symptomatic, causing infections, stone disease, pain, hematuria, renal failure, or, in severe bilateral cases, respiratory distress (due to pulmonary hypoplasia at birth).

The most commonly seen anomalies are ureteropelvic duplications, vesicoureteral reflux (VUR), ureteropelvic junction obstruction, & renal ectopia ± fusion anomalies.

Renal Cystic Disease in Pediatrics

Pediatric renal cystic diseases range from the often lethal autosomal recessive polycystic kidney disease (ARPKD) to simple cortical cysts. A myriad of other diagnoses fall in between these 2 extremes with variable degrees of symptoms & clinical impact. Some of the renal cystic diseases are due to ciliopathies, helping explain their multisystem organ involvement in many cases.

Multicystic dysplastic kidneys (MCDKs) are often diagnosed prenatally & confirmed with imaging in the newborn period. Anatomic imaging shows contiguous cysts of variable sizes in the renal fossa with no discernible renal parenchyma. The lack of renal function on nuclear studies can confirm the diagnosis. Typically unilateral, the rare bilateral form is classically fatal.

ARPKD is a rare disorder in which the renal parenchyma is virtually replaced by microscopic cysts & occasional macrocysts. In severe cases, the kidneys are massively enlarged, function only minimally, & cause oligohydramnios in utero, leading to lung hypoplasia. There is a variable degree of hepatic involvement in this disorder.

Autosomal dominant polycystic kidney disease (ADPKD) is characterized by macroscopic cysts that typically ↑ in both size & number over years. Patients are often aware of the family history of cystic renal disease in relatives with hypertension or renal insufficiency. Scattered cysts can be seen in very young children, but ADPKD typically presents in the teenage years, either incidentally or during the evaluation of hematuria.

Other renal cysts found in the pediatric population include simple cortical cysts, calyceal diverticula, cystic renal dysplasia (secondary to chronic obstruction), syndromic cysts (such as those seen with tuberous sclerosis, von Hippel-Lindau, Meckel-Gruber, & others), & cystic neoplasms (such as pediatric cystic nephroma).

Renal "Masses"

Hydronephrosis is by far the most common cause of an enlarged kidney in pediatric patients & can present as a palpable mass on physical exam, prompting imaging.

Wilms tumor is the most common pediatric renal malignancy with a peak incidence between 2 & 3 years of age. These tumors are heterogeneous on imaging, but their origin from the kidney provides an important clue to their diagnosis. Renal vein thrombus & vascular invasion are common.

Nephroblastomatosis is a rare entity often associated with syndromes & chromosomal abnormalities. It is defined as the persistence of primitive nephrogenic rests in the kidney after birth. The rests fail to differentiate into functional renal tissue & do not enhance like normal parenchyma on imaging. Its importance lies in its frequent degeneration into Wilms tumor.

Mesoblastic nephroma is the most common renal tumor in neonates. It has a peak age of 3 months as opposed to the 3-year range for Wilms. Mesoblastic nephroma is classically solid, but it can be cystic or have mixed solid & cystic components.

Pediatric cystic nephroma, previously known as multilocular cystic nephroma, is distinct from adult cystic nephromas, which are now classified as mixed epithelial & stromal tumors. Pediatric cystic nephromas are almost entirely cystic with many thin septations, occasionally herniating into the central renal pelvis. They have an important association with the *DICER1* mutation (resulting in predisposition to various other tumors).

Angiomyolipoma is a benign tumor of mixed cellularity, typically with prominent fatty components & vascularity that can result in hemorrhage. The fatty component provides the key to the imaging diagnosis. In children, these lesions are most often seen in association with tuberous sclerosis.

Renal medullary carcinoma is a very rare & highly aggressive tumor associated with sickle cell trait.

Uncommon renal masses in pediatrics include renal lymphoma (typically multifocal), clear cell sarcoma, ossifying renal tumor of infancy, renal cell carcinoma, & rhabdoid tumor.

Other Renal Processes

Pyelonephritis is imaged very frequently in pediatrics with the goal of identifying predisposing anatomic variants & complications of infection that require intervention.

Renal vein thrombosis may be seen in newborn infants & other ill children, particularly in the setting of dehydration &/or systemic disorders.

Renal stones are increasingly diagnosed in pediatric patients by ultrasound & CT.

Adrenal Abnormalities

The most important adrenal abnormality in children is neuroblastoma. This tumor typically is seen in children < 2 years of age. Imaging commonly shows a mass with Ca^{2+} encasing the adjacent aorta & inferior vena cava; the mass may also extend into the spinal canal. Venous tumor thrombus is rare, unlike in Wilms tumors. Bony metastases are more common in neuroblastoma vs. lung metastases in Wilms.

Uterine & Ovarian Abnormalities

Congenital abnormalities often present either in the newborn period (due to the influence of maternal hormones) or in adolescence at menarche. Imaging should always include a search for associated renal anomalies, which are frequently coincident.

Testicular Abnormalities

Torsion, infection, & inflammation are the most common reasons for testicular/scrotal imaging in pediatric patients. Congenital anomalies may predispose to inflammatory conditions or spermatic cord twisting that leads to ischemia. Tumors are less frequent & typically present as palpable masses without pain.

Bladder Abnormalities

Neurogenic bladder is the most common genitourinary entity imaged. Children typically show an evolution from a high-compliance, large-capacity bladder in new neurogenic bladders to a poorly distensible, low-capacity bladder in chronic neurogenic bladders. Bulking agents, such as Deflux, may be used to treat VUR & will be visible on follow-up imaging. Cloaca & other anorectal malformations are rarely imaged (except at dedicated centers). Bladder rhabdomyosarcoma is also uncommon but should be considered when a solid or heterogeneous mass is visualized in the bladder.

Imaging the Pediatric Genitourinary Tract

Ultrasound

Ultrasound is the mainstay of imaging in the pediatric genitourinary tract. Infants & children typically have excellent sonogenic body habitus. The advantages of ultrasound include that it is painless, noninvasive, portable, relatively inexpensive, & does not involve ionizing radiation or require sedation. Although ultrasound is user dependent, assessments of renal lengths & hydronephrosis should be reproducible from exam to exam. With the approval of ultrasound contrast agents, ultrasound is increasingly utilized for VUR evaluation. It is important to know that renal ultrasound may be normal in cases of pyelonephritis & VUR, a point that referring clinicians also need to recognize.

Instillation of ultrasound contrast into the bladder can be used in lieu of a conventional fluoroscopic cystogram for the evaluation of VUR.

Fluoroscopic Voiding Cystourethrogram

Fluoroscopic VCUGs are most often performed to exclude VUR but can also evaluate voiding dysfunction, enuresis, urethral abnormalities, & predisposing causes of infections. The study requires bladder catheterization by experienced health care providers, education of parents & children, optimal environmental distractions, & age-appropriate communication.

The VCUG is performed after aseptic bladder catheterization (with urine specimen collection optional). Standard views include a scout image of the pelvis & kidney regions, an early filling image of the bladder to exclude intraluminal abnormality, oblique views of the fully distended bladder to detect ureterovesical junction abnormalities, voiding images of the urethra, postvoid images of the pelvis & kidney regions, & spot views of any reflux or other abnormality.

Tips to aid with patient cooperation include the following: Providing distractions during the exam (such as videos, music, & toys; a child life specialist can be invaluable for both the physician & patient), pouring warm water over the perineum or toes if the patient has difficulty voiding, running water in the sink to provide an audible cue, or continuing to fill the bladder to 2x the estimated capacity, causing overflow incontinence (though this is not recommended in high spinal cord injury patients or postsurgical bladders).

Nuclear Medicine

Nuclear imaging is 2nd only to ultrasound in terms of utility in working up pediatric genitourinary abnormalities. Nuclear imaging studies examine the physiologic function of the urinary tract, not just the anatomy. All nuclear exams require an injection or catheterization, making patient & parental acceptance < that for ultrasound.

Diuretic renal scans are widely used to monitor obstructive progression of hydronephrosis or surgical success.

Nuclear cystograms are widely used to follow VUR, though historically lower radiation exposures (compared to VCUG) are now less substantial due to current fluoroscopic equipment & techniques.

DMSA renal cortical scans are still more sensitive & specific than ultrasound for documenting pyelonephritis & renal scarring.

Glomerular filtration studies are indispensable in patients on chemotherapy & with chronic renal insufficiency.

Magnetic Resonance Imaging

MR provides exquisite detail of genitourinary anatomy, & MR urography is able to quantify renal uptake & excretion rates. In fact, MR urography has the capacity for complete anatomic & physiologic assessment during a single exam, which may be useful in complex disorders. MR studies are motion sensitive, often requiring sedation, & are more costly compared to the other modalities. Although contrast-enhanced studies or sedation require intravenous access, MR does not utilize ionizing radiation.

Computed Tomography

Due to the risks of ionizing radiation, CT use is limited in pediatrics, most often for trauma & stone disease.

Selected References

1. Houat AP et al: Congenital anomalies of the upper urinary tract: a comprehensive review. Radiographics. 41(2):462-86, 2021
2. Expert Panel on Interventional Radiology et al: ACR Appropriateness Criteria® radiologic management of urinary tract obstruction. J Am Coll Radiol. 17(5S):S281-92, 2020
3. Expert Panel on Pediatric Imaging: ACR Appropriateness Criteria® antenatal hydronephrosis-infant. J Am Coll Radiol. 17(11S):S367-79, 2020
4. Expert Panel on Pediatric Imaging: ACR Appropriateness Criteria® hematuria-child. J Am Coll Radiol. 15(5S):S91-103, 2018
5. Chow JS et al: Classification of pediatric urinary tract dilation: the new language. Pediatr Radiol. 47(9):1109-15, 2017
6. Expert Panel on Pediatric Imaging: ACR Appropriateness Criteria® urinary tract infection-child. J Am Coll Radiol. 14(5S):S362-71, 2017
7. Ramanathan S et al: Multi-modality imaging review of congenital abnormalities of kidney and upper urinary tract. World J Radiol. 8(2):132-41, 2016

(Left) *Graphic shows early kidney formation as the ureteric bud extends from the primitive bladder/cloaca to the metanephric blastema & induces the formation of renal lobules. Note the low starting position of the kidneys, in front of the sacrum, & the anterior position of the renal pelves.* **(Right)** *Graphic shows early ascent of the kidneys up from the fetal pelvis with rotation of the renal pelves medially. The renal axis is still vertical, but this will become oblique along the psoas muscle with further ascent.*

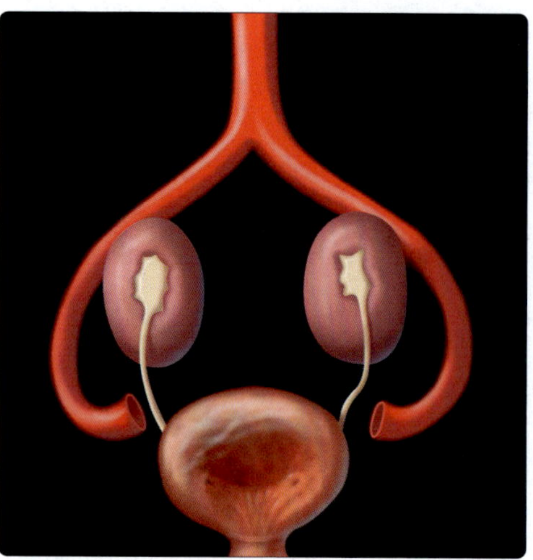

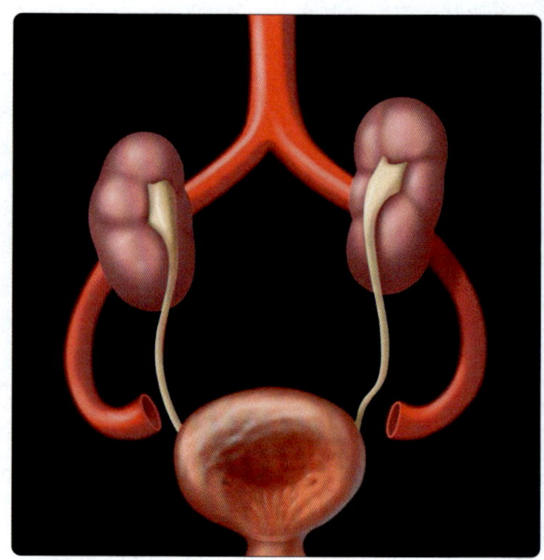

(Left) *Graphic from a lateral perspective of an early fetus shows the interrelated development of the genital & urinary organs. The mesonephric duct has differentiated into the ureteric bud ➔ & müllerian ducts budding from a common urogenital sinus ➔ in this female fetus. The hindgut lies posterior ➔.* **(Right)** *Graphic depicts a later developmental stage with separate urinary & genital tracts, ascent & rotation of the kidneys, & development of the uterus & fallopian tubes. The colon is seen posteriorly.*

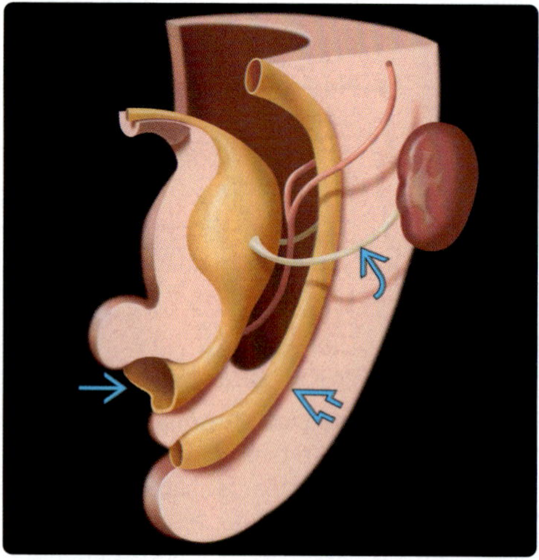

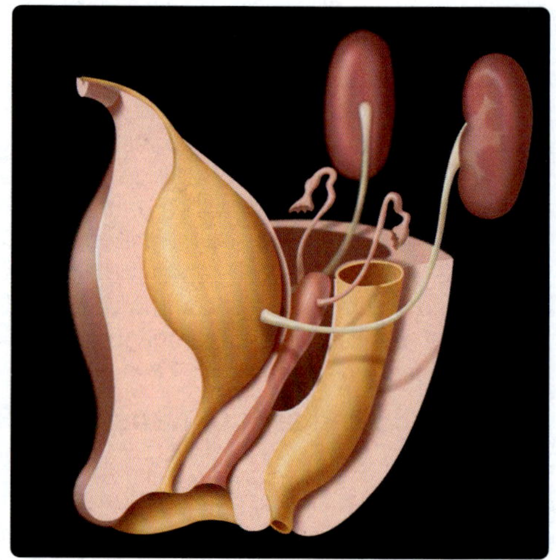

(Left) *Graphic illustrates the spectrum of renal ascent & fusion anomalies: (A) Pelvic kidney, (B) thoracic kidney, (C) crossed fused ectopia, & (D) horseshoe kidney. Note the aberrant blood supply to the ectopically located kidneys.* **(Right)** *Graphic shows typical normal anatomy with kidneys in the upper lumbar region & renal pelves directed medially with single ureters & single renal arteries.*

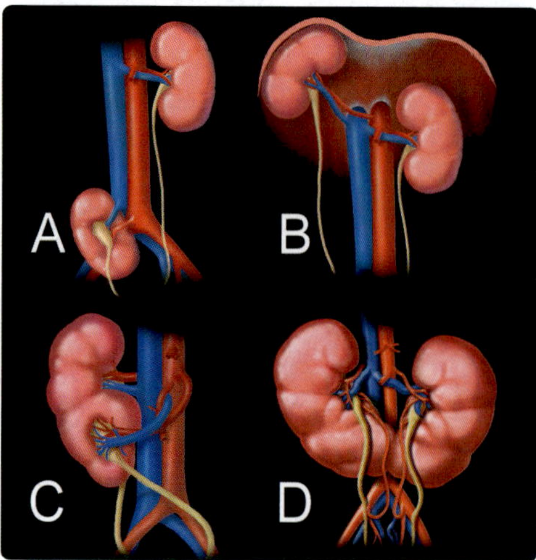

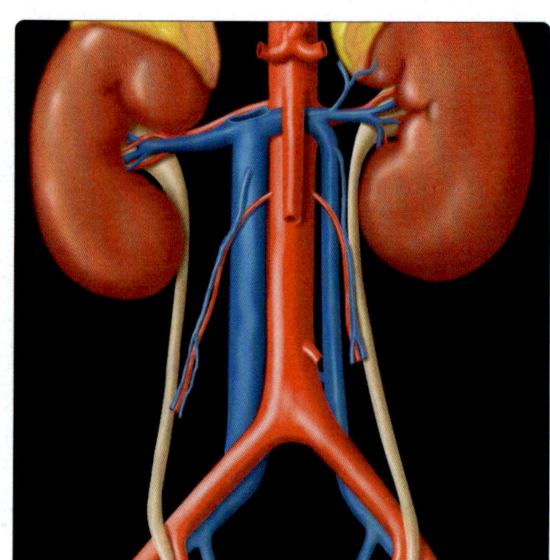

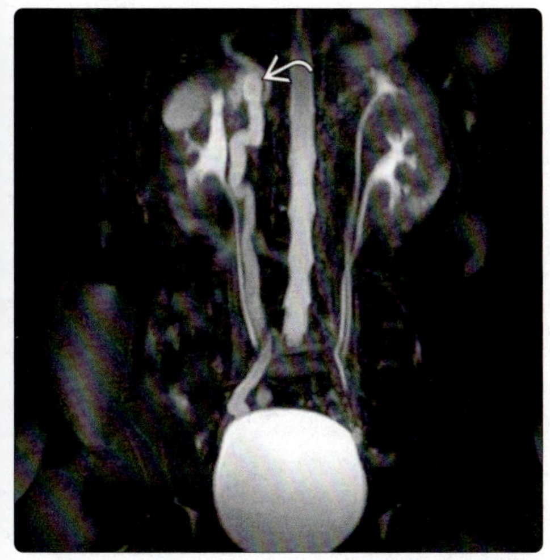

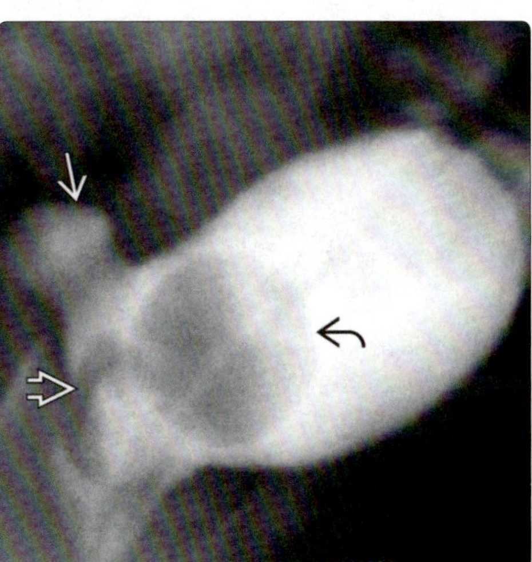

(Left) *Coronal MR urogram shows bilateral duplicated collecting systems & ureters in a teenager with flank pain & "giggle incontinence," likely related to the dilated right upper pole moiety inserting ectopically in the vagina (not shown).* **(Right)** *Voiding cystourethrogram shows an unusual case of a prolapsing ureterocele below the Foley catheter balloon. The ureterocele was causing intermittent bladder outlet obstruction. This patient also has a periureteral diverticulum.*

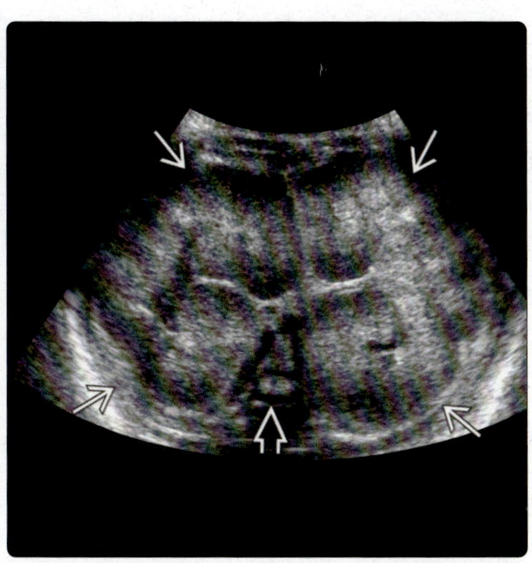

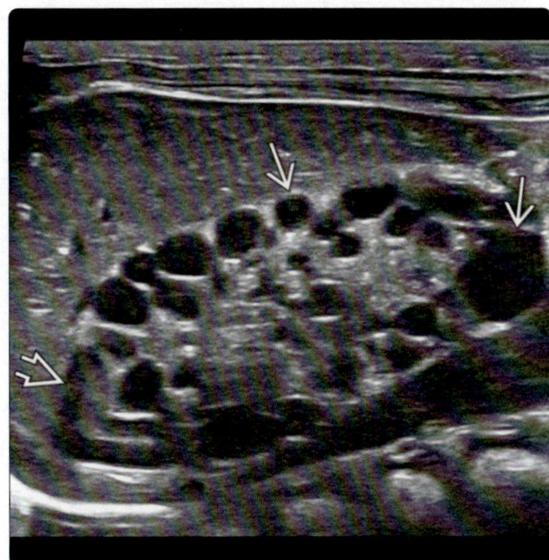

(Left) *Transverse anterior abdominal ultrasound in a newborn shows massively enlarged echogenic kidneys in a patient with autosomal recessive polycystic kidney disease. The spine is visible in the midline posteriorly.* **(Right)** *Longitudinal ultrasound in a newborn shows cysts of varying sizes completely replacing normal renal parenchyma in a case of multicystic dysplastic kidney. Note the normal newborn adrenal gland between kidney & liver.*

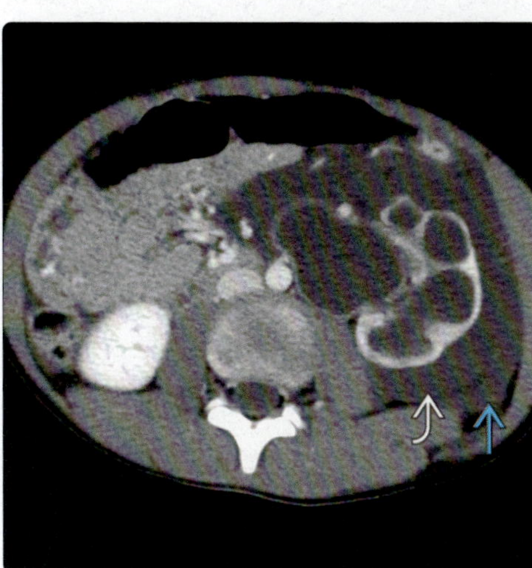

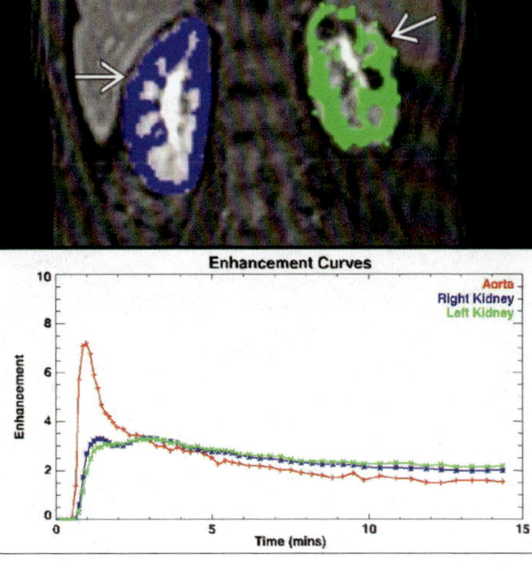

(Left) *Axial CECT shows marked hydronephrosis of the left kidney with a perinephric collection in a teenager following blunt abdominal trauma. The perinephric & paracolic gutter fluid are due to rupture of a previously undiagnosed ureteropelvic junction obstruction.* **(Right)** *Coronal contrast-enhanced MR urography illustrates the color-coded regions of interest for each kidney & the corresponding enhancement curves compared to the aorta in this normal study.*

Normal Neonatal Kidney

KEY FACTS

IMAGING

- Renal cortical echogenicity of normal term infant is often same as adjacent normal liver
  - Cortical echogenicity is ↑ in very premature infants compared to liver/spleen
- Medullary pyramids are large & hypoechoic
  - Renal cortex is thin relative to medullary pyramids
- Corticomedullary differentiation of infants & children is > adults
  - Partially due to differences in cellular composition
  - Partially due to ↑ resolution of higher frequency transducers penetrating less overlying tissue
- Central echo complex is less hyperechoic than adults
  - Less peripelvic fat in infants than adults
- Transient ↑ in echogenicity of pyramidal tips is commonly seen in neonates; etiology uncertain
  - Self-limited: Usually resolves within few days
- Fetal lobulation ("lobation") of kidneys persists into newborn period & sometimes into childhood/adulthood
  - Not to be mistaken for scarring
- Arterial resistive indices ↓ over 1st year of life

TOP DIFFERENTIAL DIAGNOSES

- Urinary tract obstruction
  - Pyramids do not interconnect as dilated calyces would
- Cystic renal disease
  - Normal pyramids line up around central echo complex
- Medical renal disease
  - Normal hyperechogenicity of neonatal renal cortex can mimic medical renal disease
  - Corticomedullary differentiation persists in normal kidneys of young children
- Renal scar
  - Fetal lobulation: Indentations between lobes/pyramids
  - Scars: Indentations within lobes/pyramids with dilated subtending calyces

(Left) *Longitudinal US of a newborn right kidney ➡, adrenal gland ➡, & liver ➡ shows echogenic cortex overlying each hypoechoic pyramid ➡. The renal cortical echogenicity is similar to the adjacent liver.* **(Right)** *Longitudinal color Doppler US of a normal kidney in a 35-weeks-gestational age newborn shows normal branching vessels ➡ extending to the corticomedullary junctions, confirming that the hypoechoic foci ➡ are renal pyramids, not cysts or dilated calyces.*

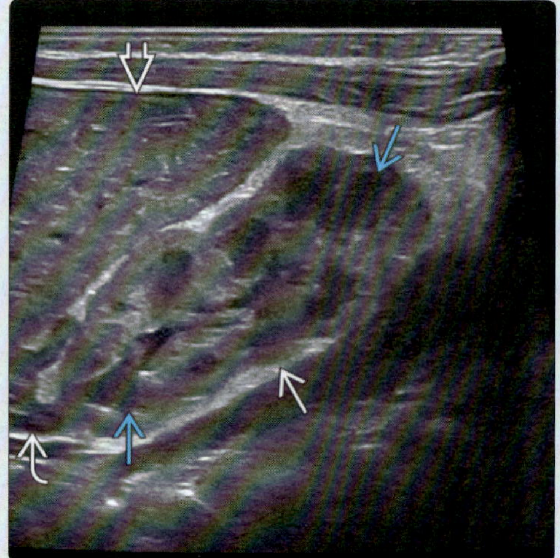

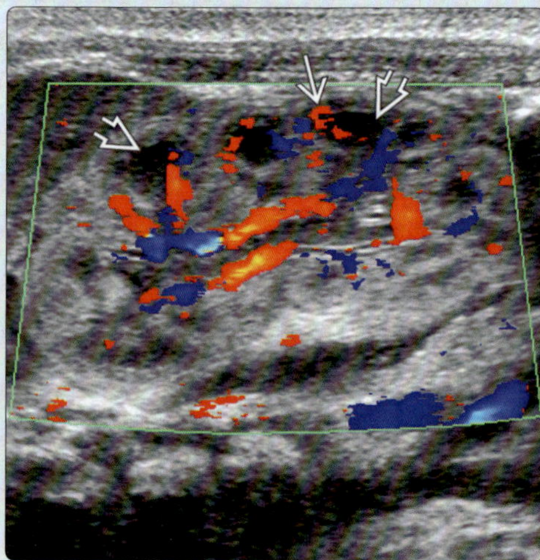

(Left) *Longitudinal prone US of the left kidney with a high-frequency linear transducer shows relatively echogenic cortex & underlying hypoechoic pyramids ➡. Cortical indentations ➡ are seen between each pyramid ("fetal lobation").* **(Right)** *Prone longitudinal US of a newborn kidney shows hyperechoic bands ➡ at the tips of several pyramids, related to solutes or proteins, a common transient phenomenon. This case also shows a junctional cortical defect ➡ between lobules of renal parenchyma.*

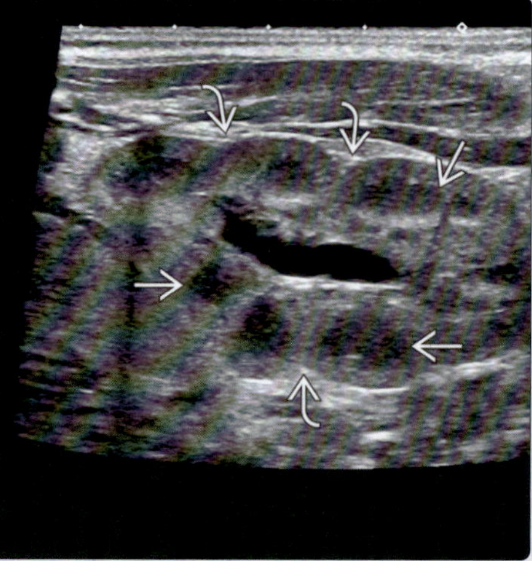

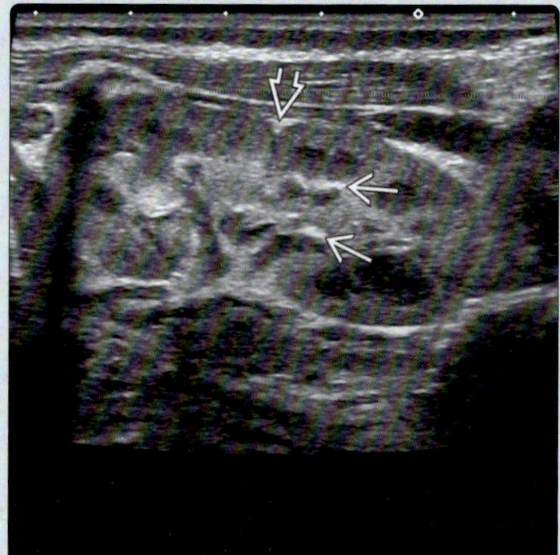

IMAGING

Ultrasonographic Findings

- Echogenicity of renal cortex in healthy term infant is often equal to adjacent normal liver
  - Renal cortex is less echogenic than liver in older children & adults
- Renal cortex echogenicity is typically ↑ in very premature infants compared to liver/spleen
  - May see striations in cortex & medulla
    - Due to vasculature in cortex & collecting ducts in medulla
- Corticomedullary differentiation of infants & children > adults
  - Partially due to differences in cellular composition of renal parenchyma
    - Greater density of glomeruli in renal cortex in neonates
  - Partially due to better resolution from higher frequency transducers with less tissue overlying kidney
  - If renal cortical echogenicity is much > adjacent liver, suspect underlying renal parenchymal disease
- Renal cortex is thin relative to medulla
- Medullary pyramids are large & hypoechoic
  - ↑ echogenicity at tips of pyramids is common in neonates, typically transient
    - Zone of maximal echogenicity at apex of pyramids with ↓ in echogenicity towards base of pyramids
      - Base of pyramids typically spared
    - Usually affects multiple pyramids but can range from 1 to all
    - Self-limited: Usually resolves within days as glomerular filtration rate ↑
      - May require 10 ≥ days, especially in premature infants
    - Historically attributed to transient precipitation of Tamm-Horsfall proteins
      - Proteins & other solutes passing out of developing nephrons likely contribute to ↑ echoes
      - Exacerbated by hypernatremic dehydration (similar to reversible appearance of hypernatremic dehydration with oliguria in older patients)
- Central echo complex is less hyperechoic than in adults
  - Less peripelvic fat in infants than in adults
- Neonatal kidneys are often more spherical than kidneys in older children & adults
- Fetal lobulation ("lobation") of kidneys persists into newborn period (& sometimes into childhood/adulthood)
  - Not to be mistaken for scarring
- Sulcation: Interrenicular junction line, Odonno sulcus, junctional parenchymal defect
  - Commonly occurring hyperechoic sulcus in upper pole; controversial etiology
  - Not to be mistaken for scarring
- Rapid growth of kidney in 1st few months
  - Mainly due to disproportionate growth of cortical renal tubules
- Doppler shows gradual ↓ of intraparenchymal renal arterial resistive indices (RI) during early life
  - RI in preterm neonate: Up to 0.9 is normal
  - RI < 1 year of age: 0.6-0.8 is normal
  - RI > 1 year of age: 0.5-0.7 is normal

Imaging Recommendations

- Best imaging tool
  - Ultrasound with high-frequency linear transducer
    - 14-6 MHz
  - Posterior or lateral decubitus approach

DIFFERENTIAL DIAGNOSIS

Urinary Tract Obstruction

- Normal hypoechoic pyramids in neonatal kidney can mimic dilated calyces (resulting in misinterpretation as hydronephrosis)
  - Pyramids are especially prominent due to hyperechoic cortex
- Normal pyramids line up around central echo complex
  - Pyramids do not interconnect as dilated calyces would
- Position of arcuate artery at corticomedullary junction can help identify hypoechoic structure as pyramid

Cystic Renal Disease

- Normal hypoechoic pyramids in neonatal kidney can mimic cysts
- Normal pyramids line up around central echo complex
- Position of arcuate artery at corticomedullary junction can help identify hypoechoic structure as pyramid

Medical Renal Disease

- Normal hyperechogenicity of neonatal renal cortex can mimic medical renal disease
  - Cortical echogenicity in newborn is same as or slightly > liver or spleen
- If echogenicity is much > liver/spleen, consider other causes
  - Look for loss of corticomedullary differentiation

Renal Scar

- Normal fetal lobulation/"lobation" of neonatal kidney with relatively thin cortex can mimic scarring
- Fetal lobulation: Indentations between lobes/pyramids
- Scars: Indentations within lobes/pyramids, often with dilated subtending calyces

SELECTED REFERENCES

1. Brennan S et al: The effect of diabetes during pregnancy on fetal renal parenchymal growth. J Nephrol. 33(5):1079-89, 2020
2. Paltiel H et al: The pediatric kidney & adrenal glands. In Rumack CM et al: Diagnostic Ultrasound. 5th ed. Elsevier Mosby. 1775-832, 2017
3. Hansen KL et al: Ultrasonography of the kidney: a pictorial review. Diagnostics (Basel). 6(1), 2015
4. Hemachandar R et al: Transient renal medullary hyperechogenicity in a term neonate. BMJ Case Rep. 2015, 2015
5. Daneman A et al: Renal pyramids: focused sonography of normal and pathologic processes. Radiographics. 30(5):1287-307, 2010
6. Chavhan GB et al: Normal Doppler spectral waveforms of major pediatric vessels: specific patterns. Radiographics. 28(3):691-706, 2008
7. Swischuk LE: Genitourinary tract & adrenal glands. In Swischuk LE: Imaging of the Newborn, Infant, & Young Child. 5th ed. Lippincott Williams & Wilkins. 590-724, 2004
8. Currarino G et al: The Oddono's sulcus and its relation to the renal "junctional parenchymal defect" and the "interrenicular septum". Pediatr Radiol. 27(1):6-10, 1997
9. Riebel TW et al: Transient renal medullary hyperechogenicity in ultrasound studies of neonates: is it a normal phenomenon and what are the causes? J Clin Ultrasound. 21(1):25-31, 1993
10. Hricak H et al: Neonatal kidneys: sonographic anatomic correlation. Radiology. 147(3):699-702, 1983

KEY FACTS

IMAGING

- Ultrasound nicely shows newborn adrenal gland
  - Doppler is useful in setting of neonatal adrenal lesions
- Normal outer hypoechoic fetal adrenal cortex & inner echogenic adrenal medulla have layered arrangement with mildly undulating margins
- Shape of newborn adrenal varies: Described as capital letters A, Y, V, X, or Z, or λ
- Flat shape when ipsilateral kidney is absent/ectopic
  - Lying down adrenal sign
- Appearance evolves during infancy
  - Newborn adrenal gland is quite large (5g), almost 2x weight of adult adrenal gland
  - Mainly due to prominent fetal cortex, which functions in utero & grows until term
    - Adrenal cortex is initially much thicker than medulla; overall contour convex outward
  - Fetal cortex starts to involute after delivery; gradually ↓ until almost inapparent by 6 months of age
    - After 2-3 months, cortex & medulla are equivalent in thickness; contour starts to flatten

TOP DIFFERENTIAL DIAGNOSES

- Neonatal adrenal hemorrhage
- Congenital adrenal hyperplasia
- Neuroblastoma
- Extralobar bronchopulmonary sequestration
- Adrenal cyst
- Adrenal insufficiency
- Wolman disease

CLINICAL ISSUES

- Prominent newborn adrenal gland is typically noted incidentally on spinal or renal ultrasound
- Awareness of normal newborn adrenal appearance avoids inappropriate work-up

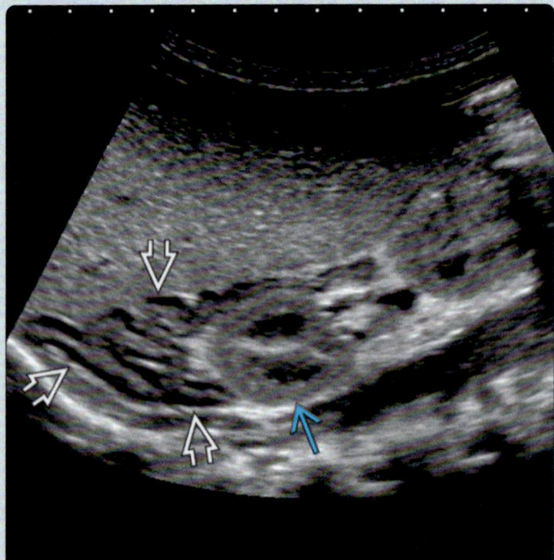

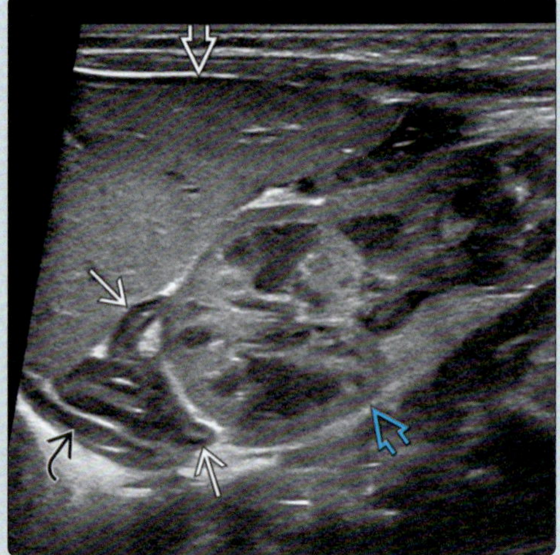

(Left) *Longitudinal ultrasound of the right upper quadrant shows the folded, alternating layers of a normal newborn adrenal gland ➡ draped over the right kidney ➡. The outer fetal adrenal cortex is hypoechoic compared with the inner echogenic medulla.* **(Right)** *Longitudinal ultrasound of the left upper quadrant shows a coiled snake shape of the normal newborn adrenal gland ➡ situated between the spleen ➡, left kidney ➡, & diaphragmatic crus ➡.*

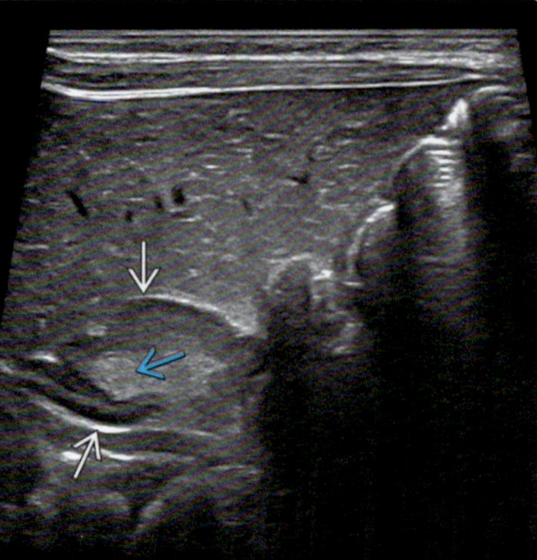

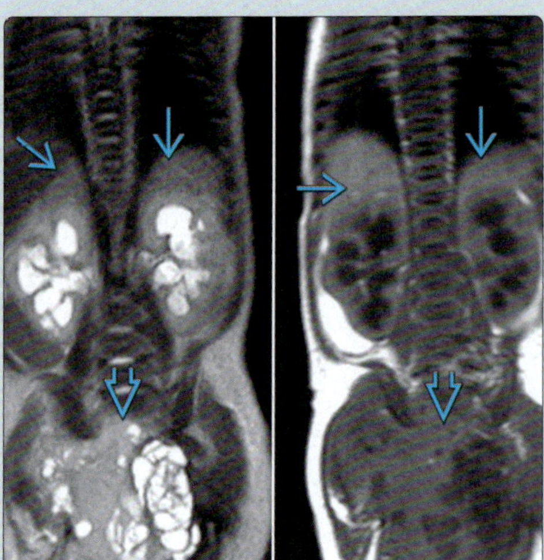

(Left) *Transverse ultrasound of the right suprarenal region shows echogenic fat ➡ between the limbs ➡ of the normal newborn adrenal gland.* **(Right)** *Coronal SSFSE T2 (left) & T1 (right) MR images in a newborn with a sacrococcygeal teratoma ➡ show an undulating trilaminar appearance of normal neonatal adrenal glands ➡. Note the bilateral hydronephrosis from obstructions of the distal ureters by the teratoma.*

Normal Neonatal Adrenal Gland

TERMINOLOGY

Synonyms

- Suprarenal gland

Definitions

- Part of hypothalamic-pituitary axis that regulates many body functions & responds to stress
- **Adrenal cortex**: Largest part of adrenal gland; 3 layers produce different hormones (described below from superficial to deep)
  - **Zona glomerulosa**: Aldosterone (mineralocorticoid)
    - Retains sodium & wastes potassium; regulates fluid & electrolyte balance, helps maintain BP
  - **Zona fasciculata**: Cortisol (glucocorticoid)
    - Regulates metabolism of glucose, protein, & fat; responds to stress by ↑ blood glucose levels & cardiac output
  - **Zona reticularis**: Dehydroepiandrosterone
    - Sex hormone that works much like testosterone
- **Adrenal medulla**: Makes & stores epinephrine, norepinephrine

IMAGING

General Features

- Best diagnostic clue
  - Layered arrangement of outer hypoechoic fetal cortex & central echogenic medulla
  - Shape described as capital letters A, Y, V, X, or Z, or λ
  - Sandwich or flat shape when ipsilateral kidney is absent/ectopic
- Location
  - Cephalad to kidney
- Size
  - 0.9- to 3.6-cm length, 0.2- to 0.3-cm thick
- Morphology
  - Newborn adrenal cortex is much thicker than medulla; overall contour convex outward
    - Margins are mildly undulating throughout
    - Small (< 5-mm) round focus of accessory adrenal tissue (with similar layered echogenicity) is described in < 6% of neonates; typically not visible on follow-up
  - After 2-3 months, cortex & medulla are equivalent in thickness; contour starts to flatten
  - ~ 6 months, corticomedullary differentiation is lost on imaging; contours flatten
  - After 1 year, resembles adult gland with thin limbs & flat or concave margins

Imaging Recommendations

- Best imaging tool
  - Ultrasound nicely shows newborn adrenal gland
- Protocol advice
  - Doppler is helpful in evaluating adrenal lesions

DIFFERENTIAL DIAGNOSIS

Neonatal Adrenal Hemorrhage

- Perinatal bleeding into normal gland, leading to avascular mass distorting adrenal tissue; gradually resolves
- Associated with perinatal stress: Asphyxia, sepsis, labile blood pressure, birth trauma, coagulopathy
- Hemorrhage is bilateral in 10% → ↑ risk of adrenal insufficiency

Congenital Adrenal Hyperplasia

- Enlarged, bilateral adrenal glands with redundant folds of cortex & medulla resembling sulci & gyri of brain (cerebriform appearance)
- Length > 2 cm & width > 4 mm suggests diagnosis (gland weight may reach 15g)
- Due to deficiency in 1 of 5 enzymes necessary to produce hormones cortisol & aldosterone, leading to overproduction of androgen
  - Females manifest with ambiguous genitalia; males manifest with salt-wasting crisis

Neuroblastoma

- Most common malignancy in infancy
- Congenital/neonatal neuroblastoma tends to have good prognosis, even with disseminated disease (stage 4S/MS)
  - May spontaneously involute
- Neonatal neuroblastomas can be more cystic than tumors in older children

Extralobar Bronchopulmonary Sequestration

- Solid or mixed cystic & solid mass; can be in or below diaphragm above kidney

Adrenal Cyst

- Sequelae of prior hemorrhage or in association with Beckwith-Wiedemann syndrome

Adrenal Insufficiency

- Congenital aplasia is very rare; found in 10% with unilateral renal agenesis

Wolman Disease

- Rare autosomal recessive lipid storage disorder
- Deficiency of lysosomal acid lipase → triglycerides & cholesterol esters build up in liver, spleen, adrenal glands
- Markedly enlarged adrenals with dystrophic Ca^{2+}

CLINICAL ISSUES

Presentation

- Most common signs/symptoms
  - Prominent newborn adrenal gland is usually noted incidentally on renal or spine ultrasound
  - Awareness of normal newborn adrenal appearance avoids inappropriate work-up

SELECTED REFERENCES

1. Aderotimi TS et al: Ultrasound of the adrenal gland in children. Ultrasound. 29(1):48-56, 2021
2. Hanafy AK et al: Imaging features of adrenal gland masses in the pediatric population. Abdom Radiol (NY). 45(4):964-81, 2020
3. Alonso V et al: Conservative management of scrotal hematoma secondary to adrenal hemorrhage in newborns. Urology. 133:e1-2, 2019
4. Iijima S: Sonographic evaluation of adrenal size in neonates (23 to 41 weeks of gestation). BMC Pediatr. 18(1):60, 2018
5. Majmudar A et al: "Lying-down" adrenal sign: there are exceptions to the rule among fetuses and neonates. J Ultrasound Med. 36(12):2599-603, 2017
6. Paltiel H et al: The pediatric kidney and adrenal glands. In Rumack CM et al: Diagnostic Ultrasound. 5th ed. Elsevier Mosby. 1775-832, 2017

Normal Prepubertal Uterus and Ovaries

KEY FACTS

TERMINOLOGY

- Thelarche: Onset & progress of breast development
- Adrenarche: Onset & progress of pubic/axillary hair development
- Menarche: 1st episode of vaginal bleeding

IMAGING

- Uterus & cervix
  - Neonatal
    - Cervix larger than uterus, ~ 2:1 ratio
  - Prepubertal
    - Cervix & uterus are equivalent
  - Pubertal
    - Uterus enlarges > cervix, 2:1 or 3:1 ratio
- Ovaries
  - Volumes
    - Neonatal ovarian volume is generally < 1 mL
    - Prepubertal up to 3 mL (age 1-6 years)
    - Pubertal 3-20 mL
  - Morphology
    - Cysts can be seen in any age
    - If 3-5 cm, consider repeat scan in 6-8 weeks
    - Cysts can predispose to ovarian torsion
- **Best imaging tool**
  - Ultrasound screening
  - MR in complex cases

TOP DIFFERENTIAL DIAGNOSES

- Ambiguous genitalia
- Amenorrhea
  - Turner syndrome
  - Müllerian anomalies
  - Hypothalamic pituitary abnormalities
  - Constitutional/familial/other
- Prepubertal vaginal bleeding
  - Foreign body/abuse
- Ectopic ovary

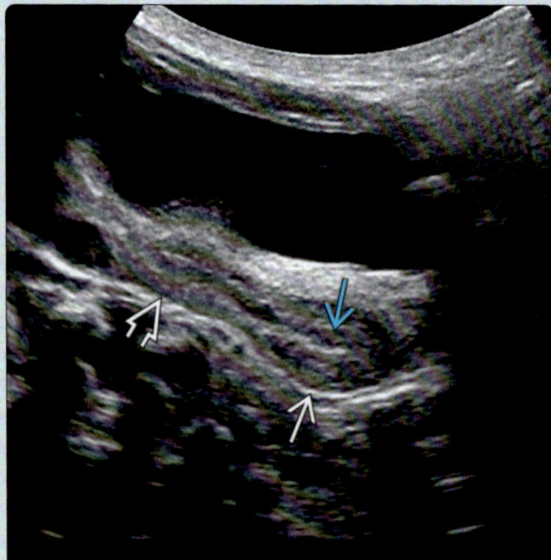

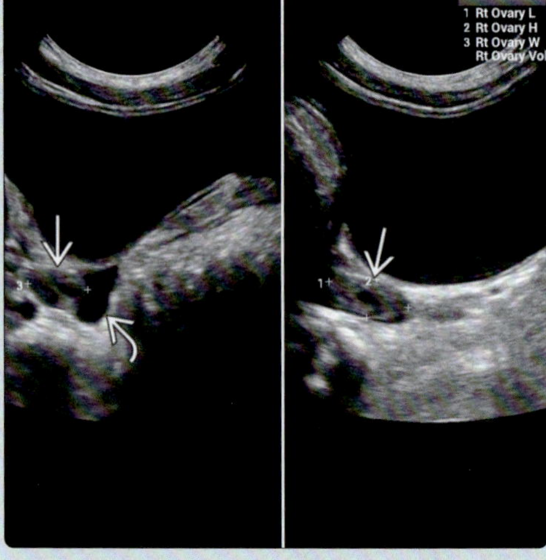

(Left) *Midline longitudinal pelvic ultrasound in a newborn girl shows a relatively large cervix compared to the uterus due to maternal hormones. A thin ellipse of fluid is present in the lower uterine segment/upper cervical os.* **(Right)** *Transverse & longitudinal ultrasound just right of midline in a 2-year-old girl shows small follicles in the right ovary. The ovarian volume measures ~ 1 mL. A minimal amount of physiologic free fluid is present next to the ovary.*

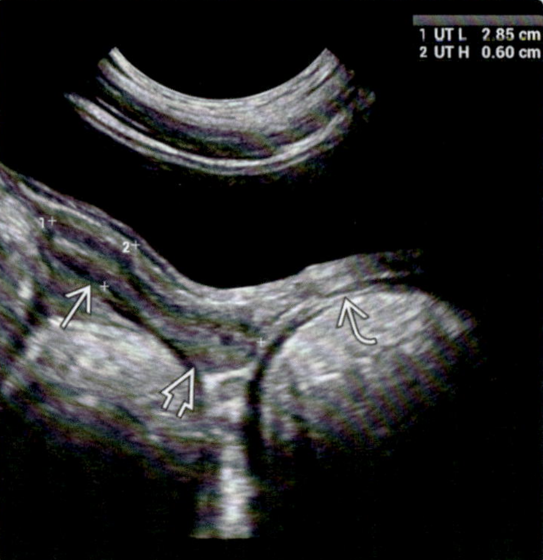

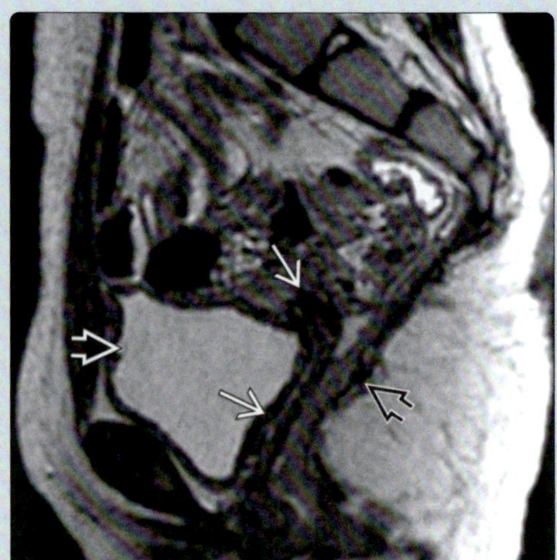

(Left) *Midline longitudinal ultrasound through a distended urinary bladder in a 2-year-old girl shows a thin, tubular cervix & uterus above a collapsed vaginal vault. Note the lack of fundal broadening in this prepubertal girl.* **(Right)** *Midline sagittal T2 MR in a 6-year-old girl being followed for a sacrococcygeal tumor shows a typical tubular appearance of the vaginal vault, cervix, & uterus (all blending together) between the bladder & collapsed rectosigmoid colon.*

Normal Prepubertal Uterus and Ovaries

TERMINOLOGY

Definitions

- Varied appearance of uterus & ovaries with age
  - Prominence in newborns due to maternal hormones
  - Small, quiescent stage in ages 1-8 years
  - Growth with hormonal surge during puberty
- Thelarche: Onset & progress of breast development
- Adrenarche: Onset & progress of pubic & axillary hair development
- Menarche: 1st episode of vaginal bleeding

IMAGING

General Features

- Best diagnostic clue
  - Female genital organs are best imaged with ultrasound or MR
- Size
  - Uterus & cervix
    - Neonatal
      - Cervix larger than uterus, ~ 2:1 ratio
      - Uterus ~ 3.5 cm long x 1.5 cm thick
    - Prepubertal
      - Cervix & uterus are equivalent in size
      - Uterus ~ 2.5-4 cm long x 1 cm thick
    - Pubertal
      - Uterus enlarges > cervix, 2:1 or 3:1 ratio
      - ~ 5-8 cm long x 1.5 cm thick x 3 cm transverse
  - Ovaries
    - Neonatal volume generally < 1 mL
    - Prepubertal up to 3 mL (age 1-6 years)
    - Pubertal 3-20 mL
- Morphology
  - Uterus
    - Neonatal: Endometrial echoes visible, fluid possible
    - Prepubertal: Very thin endometrial line
    - Pubertal: Measurable endometrial stripe
  - Ovaries
    - Ovarian cysts can be seen at any age
    - If 3-5 cm, consider 4- to 6-week follow-up
    - Cysts can predispose to torsion

Ultrasonographic Findings

- Primary diagnostic modality for uterus & ovaries
- Bladder sonographic window may be problematic for patients not yet toilet trained
  - Repeat scanning often yields diagnostic exam
  - Alternatively, bladder filling by catheter

MR Findings

- Useful in complex anatomy or when ultrasound is indeterminate
- Multiplanar & 3D images are possible

CT Findings

- Genital findings may be seen incidentally in trauma/pain evaluation
- May be used in staging & follow-up of tumors

Imaging Recommendations

- Best imaging tool
  - Ultrasound; MR for complex cases
- Protocol advice
  - Endovaginal scanning is avoided until adolescents are sexually active or using tampons (postpubertal patients)
  - Transabdominal
    - Adequate hydration prior to exam as well-distended urinary bladder is needed for sonographic window
      - Use gentle transducer pressure on bladder to avoid inducing micturition
    - Alternatively, use Foley catheter to fill bladder
  - Limited need for Doppler

DIFFERENTIAL DIAGNOSIS

Ambiguous Genitalia

- Pelvic ultrasound in neonatal period searching for gonads: Include scrotum/labia
  - Female pseudohermaphroditism due to congenital adrenal hyperplasia
  - True hermaphroditism

Amenorrhea

- Turner syndrome
  - Typical prepubertal uterus & streak ovaries
  - 5-15% have normal pubertal onset: Mosaicism
- Müllerian anomalies
  - Müllerian agenesis
  - Obstructive müllerian anomalies
  - Nonobstructive müllerian anomalies
- Hypothalamic pituitary abnormalities
- Constitutional/familial/other

Prepubertal Vaginal Bleeding

- Foreign body/abuse
- Vaginal rhabdomyosarcoma
- Precocious puberty

Ectopic Ovary

- Canal of Nuck hernia containing ovary

SELECTED REFERENCES

1. Calle-Toro JS et al: Incidental findings during ultrasound of thyroid, breast, testis, uterus and ovary in healthy term neonates. J Ultrasound. 22(3):395-400, 2019
2. Dao KA et al: Pediatric ovarian volumes measured at ultrasound after contralateral unilateral oophorectomy. Pediatr Radiol. 49(5):632-7, 2019
3. Kaplan SL et al: Size of testes, ovaries, uterus and breast buds by ultrasound in healthy full-term neonates ages 0-3 days. Pediatr Radiol. 46(13):1837-47, 2016
4. Bhagwat NM et al: Asymmetrical ovarian enlargement: caught timely before the cut! J Pediatr Adolesc Gynecol. 28(3):e83-5, 2015
5. Bumbuliene Z et al: Uterine size and ovarian size in adolescents with functional hypothalamic amenorrhoea. Arch Dis Child. 100(10):948-51, 2015
6. Otero HJ et al: Ovary and testicle and everything in between: lesions and imaging in the newborn. Semin Ultrasound CT MR. 36(2):178-92, 2015
7. Asăvoaie C et al: Ovarian and uterine ultrasonography in pediatric patients. Pictorial essay. Med Ultrason. 16(2):160-7, 2014
8. Heo SH et al: Review of ovarian tumors in children and adolescents: radiologic-pathologic correlation. Radiographics. 34(7):2039-55, 2014
9. Tinggaard J et al: Ovarian morphology and function during growth hormone therapy of short girls born small for gestational age. Fertil Steril. 102(6):1733-41, 2014

Ureteropelvic Junction Obstruction

KEY FACTS

TERMINOLOGY

- Ureteropelvic junction (UPJ) obstruction is most common form of urinary tract obstruction in children

IMAGING

- Marked pelvocaliectasis that ends abruptly at UPJ with normal-caliber ureter downstream
- Dilated calyces are relatively uniform in size & distribution; all connect centrally to disproportionately dilated renal pelvis
- Thinned but otherwise intact renal parenchyma
- Doppler US shows ↑ renal resistive indices with obstruction
- Severity of delayed nephrogram, excretion, & collecting system drainage (on IVP, CECT, MRU, or nuclear renal scan) depends on degree of obstruction
- Contrast entering dilated collecting system (by excretion, retrograde injection, or vesicoureteral reflux during VCUG) may be very diluted due to mixing with retained urine
- ± crossing vessel at obstruction site on CECT, MRU, or US
- Nuclear medicine renal scan is well established for initial assessment & follow-up of renal function & obstruction
- MR urography may provide optimal combination of anatomic & physiologic assessment

PATHOLOGY

- Theoretical etiology of obstruction at UPJ
  - Abnormal smooth muscle arrangement impairs distensibility; abnormal innervation of proximal ureter (Hirschsprung equivalent)
  - Crossing vessel or fibrous scar at UPJ
- UPJ obstruction is associated with contralateral multicystic dysplastic kidney (MCDK)

CLINICAL ISSUES

- May be diagnosed antenatally or in infancy/childhood with urinary tract infection, intermittent abdominal/flank pain, vomiting, or hematuria
- Treatment: Pyeloplasty, ureteroureterostomy, or endoureteral balloon plasty/stenting (infants)

(Left) *Longitudinal US of an infant with prenatal hydronephrosis shows dilated central & peripheral calyces ➡ & a large renal pelvis ➡ (incompletely visualized). No ureteral dilation was seen, & a ureteropelvic junction (UPJ) obstruction was subsequently diagnosed. Note that hypoechoic renal pyramids ➡ are normal in infants.* **(Right)** *Frontal fluoroscopic image during cystoscopy & retrograde ureterography shows a dilated right renal collecting system & abrupt caliber change at the UPJ ➡.*

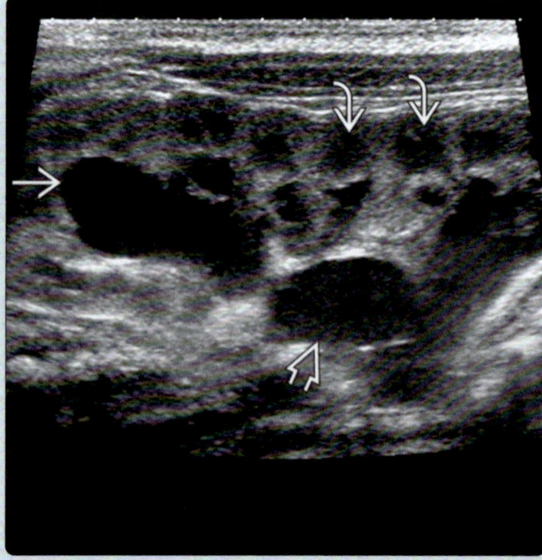

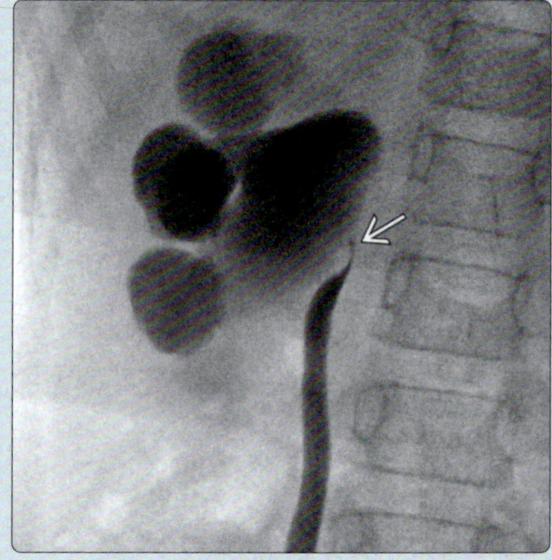

(Left) *Posterior Tc-99m MAG3 diuretic renal scintigraphy shows minimal uptake in a dilated right kidney ➡ with central photopenia. The time activity curve for the right kidney shows progressive accumulation of counts ➡ with no washout during the exam, typical of a UPJ obstruction.* **(Right)** *Coronal MIP from heavily T2-weighted MR urography in a 2-month-old shows left worse than right collecting system dilation in a typical configuration of UPJ obstructions (with no ureteral dilation seen).*

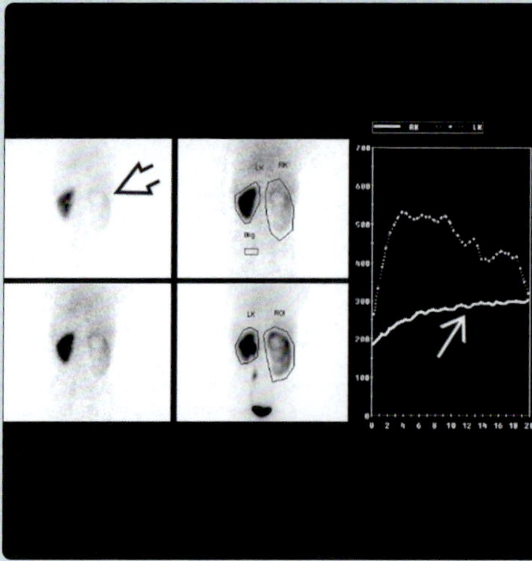

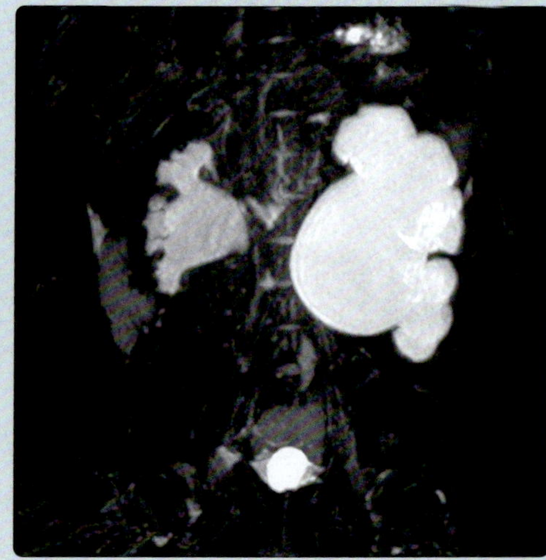

TERMINOLOGY

Synonyms

- Pelviureteric obstruction

Definitions

- Ureteropelvic junction (UPJ) obstruction: Variable degree of blockage to urine flow at level of UPJ
- Most common urinary tract obstruction in pediatrics
- May be diagnosed antenatally with sonography or present in infancy or later childhood with urinary tract infection, intermittent abdominal pain, vomiting, &/or hematuria
  - Occasionally found incidentally during trauma work-up

IMAGING

General Features

- Best diagnostic clue
  - Marked pelvocaliectasis that ends abruptly at UPJ with normal-caliber ureter
  - Disproportionate enlargement of renal pelvis
  - Severity of delayed nephrogram, excretion, & collecting system drainage depends on degree of obstruction
- Morphology
  - UPJ obstruction has been likened to Hirschsprung disease with focal transition zone & aperistaltic segment
  - Obstruction may be extrinsic rather than intrinsic
    - Crossing vessel at UPJ in 25% of infants

Radiographic Findings

- Radiography
  - May see mass effect from enlarged hydronephrotic kidney; ± scoliosis/splinting with pain
- IVP
  - Delayed nephrogram
  - Delayed contrast excretion into dilated collecting system
    - Contrast gradually opacifies distended renal pelvis, which tapers abruptly
    - Contrast may be very diluted due to mixing with retained urine
  - Delayed ureteral visualization

Ultrasonographic Findings

- Grayscale ultrasound
  - Moderate to severe pelvocaliectasis without hydroureter
  - Dilated calyces are relatively uniform in size & distribution; all connect centrally to disproportionately dilated renal pelvis
  - Abrupt tapering of renal pelvis at UPJ
  - Thinned but otherwise intact renal parenchyma
- Pulsed Doppler
  - ↑ resistive indices (RIs) with obstruction
    - RIs may correlate with degree of obstruction (when contralateral kidney is normal & can serve as internal standard)
      - As normal RIs change with age, strict cutoff value for obstruction is not applicable in pediatrics
- Color Doppler
  - Search for crossing aberrant vessel at site of obstruction
  - Ureteral jets (in urinary bladder) are useful in excluding complete obstruction
- Shear wave elastography
  - May help discriminate degree of obstruction

Fluoroscopic Findings

- Voiding cystourethrogram
  - With ≥ grade 2 vesicoureteral reflux (VUR), contrast may be seen entering disproportionately dilated renal pelvis (relative to ureter)
    - Chronically dilated ureter may kink at UPJ, creating additional etiology for pelvocaliectasis
    - Look for delayed drainage of high-grade VUR
  - May see contralateral VUR
- Intraoperative retrograde ureterogram is variably used to confirm focal narrowing, identify crossing vessels (by negative impression), & search for intraluminal polyp or stone
  - Shows abrupt transition of normal-caliber ureter to dilated renal pelvis
  - Contrast entering renal pelvis becomes very diluted by retained volume of urine

CT Findings

- CECT
  - Delayed nephrogram in enlarged kidney
  - Marked renal pelvic > calyceal dilation with normal or nonvisualized ureter
  - May demonstrate crossing vessel at UPJ
  - Delayed contrast excretion into collecting system

MR Findings

- MR urography ± contrast is particularly helpful in visualizing crossing vessels
- Drainage curves & differential function can be used to guide timing of surgery

Nuclear Medicine Findings

- Renal scans show delayed uptake, excretion, & drainage of radiotracer
  - Early central photopenia of affected kidney
  - Gradual & progressive accumulation of radiotracer replacing central photopenia
  - Little to no ureteral activity; variable change with diuretic administration
- Time activity curve provides quantified assessment of radiotracer distribution throughout scan
  - Time to half of peak activity (T½) can measure severity of obstruction
    - T½ < 10 min is normal
    - T½ > 20 min is obstructed
    - T½ between 10-20 minutes is indeterminate
- Nuclear studies are used for initial assessment & follow-up of function & obstruction
  - Should be performed in standardized fashion with adequate hydration, bladder drainage, & diuretic administration

Imaging Recommendations

- Best imaging tool
  - Sonography is usually performed 1st
  - Nuclear renal scan is then used to grade degree of obstruction & determine if surgical intervention or percutaneous drainage is required
  - MR urography may be viable single test alternative, optimizing anatomic & physiologic assessment

- Protocol advice
  - Obstruction is often partial & can ↑ or ↓ over time
  - Affected children typically undergo serial exams every 6-12 months (if they remain asymptomatic) to determine when to intervene

DIFFERENTIAL DIAGNOSIS

Multicystic Dysplastic Kidney

- No discernible normal renal parenchyma
- Cysts do not interconnect
- Largest cyst is not usually located centrally

Ureteral Fibroepithelial Polyp

- Found in 5% of UPJ obstructions
- Increasing awareness with pediatric ureteroscopy

Megacalycosis or Congenital Megacalyces

- Idiopathic dilation & ↑ number of calyces without enlarged renal pelvis
- Drainage in megacalycosis is normal or minimally delayed
- Often presents with hematuria after minor trauma

Hydronephrosis of Other Etiologies

- VUR
- Urinary tract calculus
- Ureterovesical junction obstruction
- Ureterocele

Megaureter

- Dilated ureter with narrowed distal aperistaltic segment
- Obstructed or nonobstructed, refluxing or nonrefluxing

PATHOLOGY

General Features

- Etiology
  - At surgical resection, massively dilated pelvis is often too distorted to confirm any single theory
  - Theoretical etiology of obstruction at UPJ
    - Abnormal smooth muscle impairs distensibility
    - Abnormal innervation of proximal ureter (Hirschsprung equivalent)
    - Crossing vessel or fibrous scar at UPJ
- Associated abnormalities
  - UPJ obstruction is associated with contralateral multicystic dysplastic kidney (MCDK)
    - Requires prompt intervention since MCDK is nonfunctional & UPJ may compromise remaining renal function

Staging, Grading, & Classification

- Anteroposterior pelvic diameter > 10 mm in 3rd-trimester fetus or newborn suggests obstruction

Microscopic Features

- Obstructive nephropathy leads to tubulointerstitial fibrosis & loss of renal function
- Nerve fibers are depleted in muscular layer in ureteric walls
- Denervation results in dysfunction/atrophy of muscle fibers & ↑ collagen fibers within muscle layers
- Deficiency of Cajal cells (pacemaker cells in smooth muscles), which enhance ureteral peristalsis
- Abnormal accumulations of intercellular & interstitial collagen are also seen pathologically

CLINICAL ISSUES

Presentation

- Most common signs/symptoms
  - Antenatally detected on fetal sonogram or MR
- Other signs/symptoms
  - Infants & children: Urinary tract infection, intermittent abdominal pain, flank pain, or hematuria
  - In older children who present with symptomatic UPJ obstruction, crossing vessel is causative in ~ 50%
  - Dietl's crisis: Episodic abdominal pain & UPJ obstruction

Demographics

- Males are affected 2-4x more than females
- L > R; bilateral in 10-15%
- Incidence of 1 in 75-1500 births

Natural History & Prognosis

- May improve or deteriorate spontaneously
- Prognosis is excellent if renal function has not been compromised by longstanding, high-grade obstruction
- Following successful surgery, pelvocaliectasis persists for years on sonography
- Appropriate renal growth & adequate drainage on nuclear scans help quantify surgical success

Treatment

- Pyeloplasty (open or laparoscopic surgery)
  - Tapered, dismembered pyeloplasty has been classic surgery for UPJ obstruction
  - Narrowed segment is resected, or crossing vessel is rerouted
  - Ureteral stents are often left in place (crossing surgical anastomosis) for several weeks postop
  - Open or laparoscopic procedures are preferable when crossing vessels or aberrant vessels are recognized
- Endoscopic incision (a.k.a. endopyelotomy)
- Endopyeloplasty (horizontal percutaneous suturing of conventional longitudinal endopyelotomy incision)
- Ureterocalicostomy, which is reconstructive option in rare patient with surgically failed UPJ or difficult anatomy due to fibrosis or other concurrent problems
- Endoureteral balloon plasty/stenting
- Percutaneous drainage, temporizing, if infected

SELECTED REFERENCES

1. Houat AP et al: Congenital anomalies of the upper urinary tract: a comprehensive review. Radiographics. 41(2):462-86, 2021
2. Expert Panel on Interventional Radiology et al: ACR Appropriateness Criteria® radiologic management of urinary tract obstruction. J Am Coll Radiol. 17(5S):S281-92, 2020
3. Gnech M et al: Pyeloplasty vs. nephrectomy for ureteropelvic junction obstruction in poorly functioning kidneys (differential renal function < 20%): a multicentric study. J Pediatr Urol. 15(5):553.e1-3.e8, 2019
4. Sertorio F et al: Non-contrast-enhanced magnetic resonance angiography for detecting crossing renal vessels in infants and young children: comparison with contrast-enhanced angiography and surgical findings. Pediatr Radiol. 49(1):105-13, 2019
5. Wong MCY et al: Surgical validation of functional magnetic resonance urography in the study of ureteropelvic junction obstruction in a pediatric cohort. J Pediatr Urol. 15(2):168-75, 2019
6. Morin CE et al: Use of MR urography in pediatric patients. Curr Urol Rep. 19(11):93, 2018

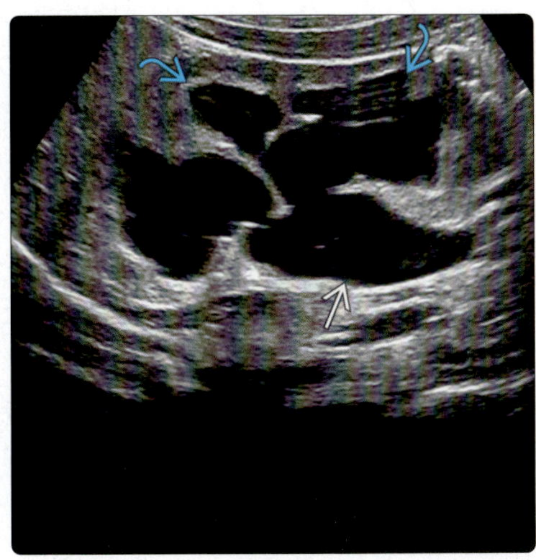

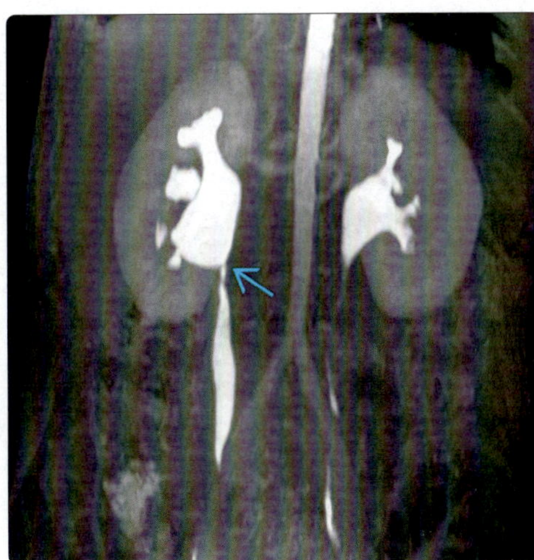

(Left) *Longitudinal US in a 10-day-old shows moderate peripheral & central caliectasis* ⇨ *with an enlarged renal pelvis* ➡ *that rapidly tapers without hydroureter.* **(Right)** *Coronal delayed postcontrast MRU MIP in the same patient shows focal narrowing at the UPJ* ⇨ *but without a crossing vessel identified. This case was followed with imaging to monitor for progression vs. resolution.*

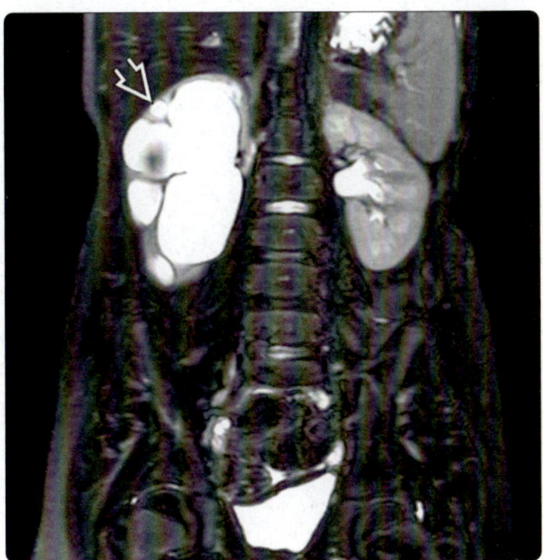

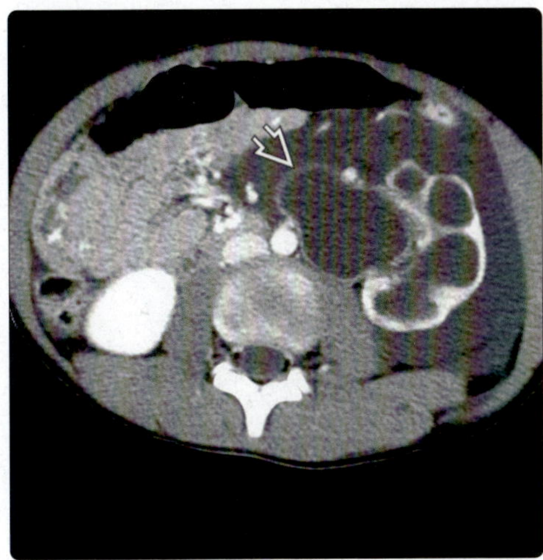

(Left) *Coronal T2 FS MR shows marked right pelvocaliectasis* ➡ *in this teenager with intermittent flank pain caused by a UPJ obstruction. A crossing vessel was not identified.* **(Right)** *Axial CECT shows marked hydronephrosis of the left kidney with an enlarged renal pelvis* ➡*, cortical thinning, & marked perinephric fluid in a 12-year-old involved in a motor vehicle accident. This left UPJ obstruction ruptured in the collision.*

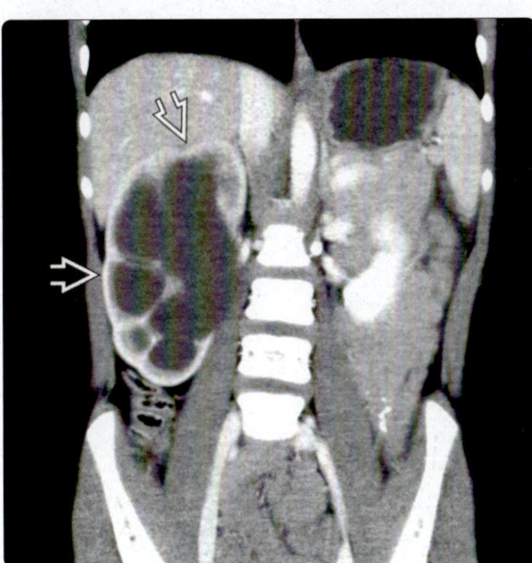

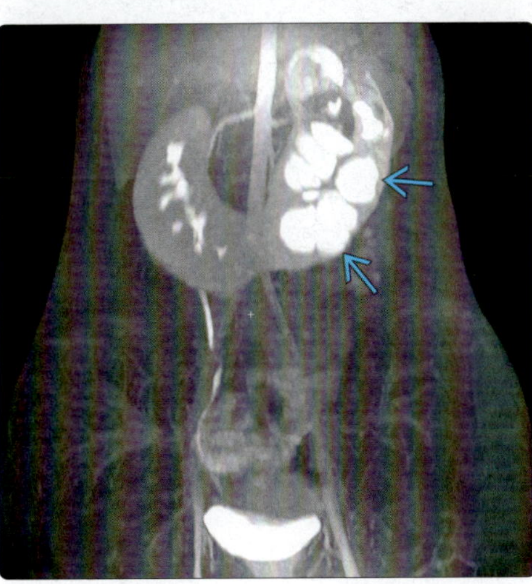

(Left) *Coronal CECT shows a markedly hydronephrotic right kidney* ➡ *with delayed enhancement. On adjacent images (not shown), the renal pelvis appeared dilated, but no ureter was visualized, consistent with UPJ obstruction.* **(Right)** *Coronal delayed postcontrast MRU MIP in a 14-year-old with a horseshoe kidney & left UPJ obstruction shows marked dilation of partially contrast-filled calyces* ⇨ *& no visualization of a left ureter.*

Vesicoureteral Reflux

KEY FACTS

TERMINOLOGY

- Retrograde urine flow from bladder toward kidney(s)

IMAGING

- International Reflux Study Committee grading system of vesicoureteral reflux (VUR)
  - I: Reflux into ureter but not reaching renal pelvis
  - II: Reflux reaching pelvis without blunting of calyces
  - III: Mild calyceal blunting
  - IV: Progressive calyceal & ureteral dilation
  - V: Very dilated & tortuous collecting system
  - ± intrarenal reflux as modifier to grade
- Voiding cystourethrogram has been preferred when anatomic detail of upper tracts/urethra is needed
- Nuclear cystogram has been preferred when anatomy is known (e.g., renal ultrasound is normal) &/or for follow-up studies
- Use of renal US alone for screening is controversial: Variable sensitivity & specificity for scar as compared to DMSA
- US contrast agent can be instilled into bladder for sonographic voiding cystogram

CLINICAL ISSUES

- Present in up to 2% of general population
- VUR is seen in 25-40% of children with acute pyelonephritis
- VUR is seen in 5-50% of asymptomatic siblings of children with documented reflux
- 80% outgrow VUR before puberty
- ↑ grade or longstanding VUR, more numerous urinary tract infections, & subsequent renal scarring → ↑ incidence of renal insufficiency, hypertension, & end-stage renal disease
- Treatment options
  - Prophylactic antibiotic therapy (medical management)
  - Ureteral reimplantation surgery (surgical management)
  - Endoscopic periureteral injections (minimally invasive endoscopic management)

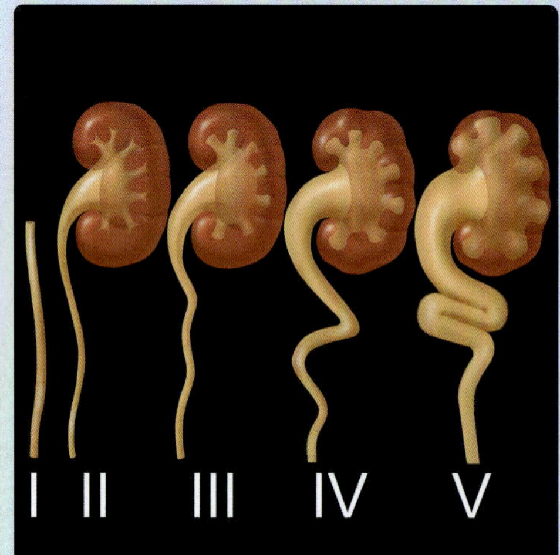

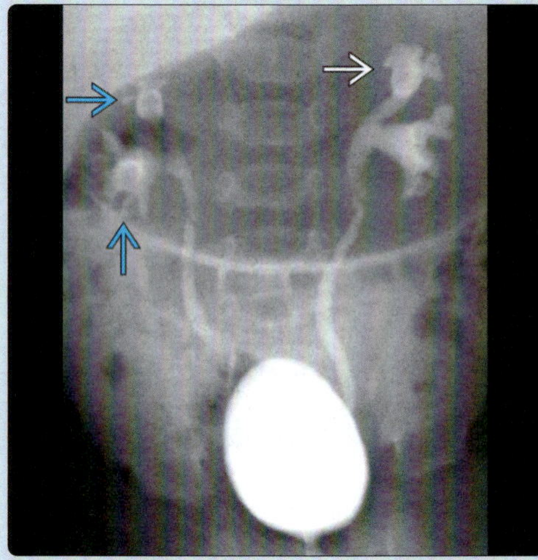

(Left) *Graphic of the International Reflux Study Committee grading system is shown. Note the progressive level of reflux, dilation, calyceal blunting, & ureteral tortuosity from grade I on the left to grade V on the right.* **(Right)** *Voiding cystourethrogram (VCUG) in an infant shows bilateral vesicoureteral reflux (VUR). The calyces are sharp ➜ on the right (grade II). On the left, the calyces are slightly blunted ➜, & the ureter is mildly dilated & tortuous, making this grade III VUR.*

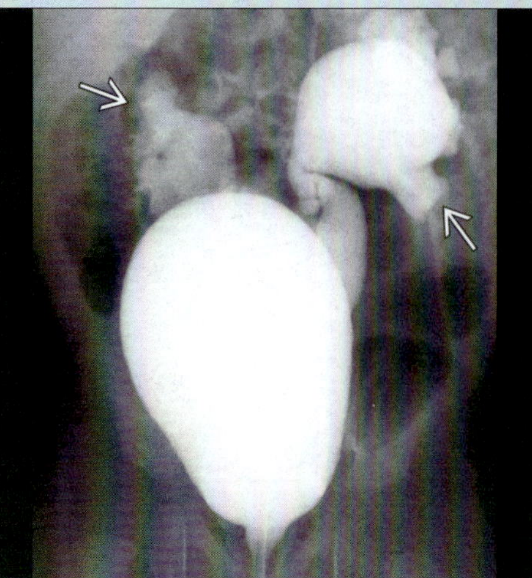

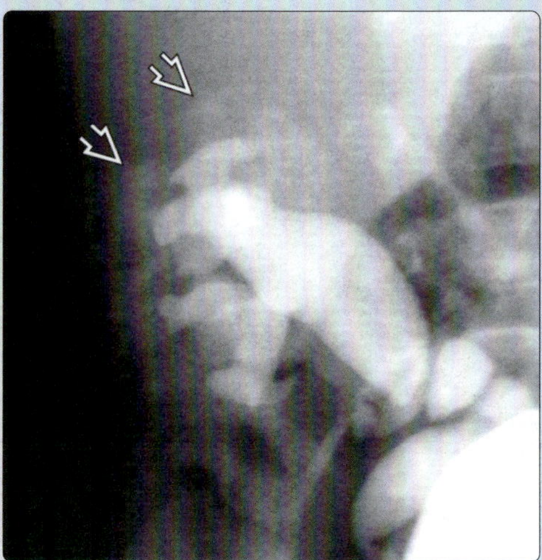

(Left) *VCUG shows large-volume VUR into both kidneys, which have very dilated collecting systems ➜. Grade V reflux was diagnosed in this infant with prenatal hydronephrosis.* **(Right)** *Frontal VCUG shows high-grade VUR into the right kidney with a dilated tortuous ureter, blunted calyces, & intrarenal reflux into the tubules ➜. These findings constitute grade V VUR with intrarenal reflux. Intrarenal reflux is associated with cortical scarring.*

TERMINOLOGY

Abbreviations

- Vesicoureteral reflux (VUR)

Definitions

- Retrograde urine flow from bladder toward kidney(s)

IMAGING

General Features

- Best diagnostic clue
  - Contrast instilled into urinary bladder opacifies at least 1 ureter
  - Contrast may reach intrarenal collecting system
  - Findings are often seen only transiently

Fluoroscopic Findings

- Voiding cystourethrogram
  - Requires bladder catheterization for contrast installation
  - Preliminary scout film can be useful, especially when there has been prior surgery or urolithiasis
  - Early filling image of bladder is best to show intraluminal abnormalities: Ureterocele, polyp, mass
  - Contrast seen in ureter &/or renal collecting system confirms VUR
    - Estimated bladder volume/timing of VUR should be reported
  - Oblique views of distended bladder are helpful to show periureteral diverticula & ureteric insertion site
  - Ectopic ureters that insert below bladder neck only reflux during voiding (if they do drain to bladder)
    - May not visualize ectopic ureters unless they are inadvertently catheterized
    - In such cases, separate catheter should also be passed into urinary bladder to study other ureters for VUR
  - Voiding images of urethra are performed to exclude distal pathology, which may contribute to back pressure
    - Obtain voiding images without catheter in place
  - In cases of high-grade VUR, delayed upright image is used to assess drainage from upper tract & exclude concomitant ureteropelvic junction or ureterovesical junction obstruction
    - Note that contrast refluxed into obstructed, dilated system may become very diluted
- PIC during cystoscopy [positional instillation of contrast at ureteral orifice (PIC) during cystoscopy]
  - Higher positive results in laterally positioned & patulous ureteral orifices

Ultrasonographic Findings

- Varying degrees of renal collecting system &/or ureteral dilation ± urothelial thickening
  - Normal US without dilation does not exclude VUR, even high grade
- Look for signs of scarring: Globally small kidney or polar foci of cortical thinning subtended by dilated calyces
- Contrast-enhanced retrograde urosonography (CEUS cystogram)
  - US contrast agent can be instilled into bladder for sonographic cystogram
  - Bladder catheterization is still required; no ionizing radiation used
  - Urethral evaluation is possible with US probe on perineum
- Doppler optimized for low velocity (SMI/microvascular imaging) has been used to show retrograde flow in ureter without contrast or bladder catheterization

Nuclear Medicine Findings

- Nuclear cystogram
  - Study is performed with posterior gamma camera
  - Tc-99m pertechnetate is instilled into bladder via catheter
  - Imaging is performed continuously throughout bladder filling & voiding
  - With VUR, radiotracer activity extends cephalad from bladder in varying amounts
  - Grade I VUR is harder to see on nuclear cystogram due to bladder activity
  - Nuclear cystogram gives no information about urethral abnormalities
- Renal cortical scan
  - Study is performed with posterior pinhole imaging
  - Radiotracer: Tc-99m DMSA or MAG3
  - Photopenic renal cortical foci due to acute pyelonephritis or chronic scarring

Imaging Recommendations

- Best imaging tool
  - Controversial
  - American Academy of Pediatrics & National Institute for Health & Care Excellence (United Kingdom) guidelines advocate less imaging than historically performed
  - Traditionally
    - Voiding cystourethrogram (VCUG) is preferred when anatomic detail of upper tracts & urethra is needed
    - Nuclear cystogram is preferred when anatomy is known &/or for follow-up studies
    - CEUS cystography requires proficiency with exam & ultrasound contrast agents
  - Historic "bottom-up" approach to urinary tract infection (UTI) work-up
    - VCUG + renal US; DMSA if 1st-line studies are abnormal or with febrile UTI
  - Current "top-down" approach to UTI work-up
    - Renal US ± DMSA; VCUG if 1st-line studies are abnormal
  - Use of renal US alone for screening is controversial due to variable sensitivity (37-100%) & specificity (65-99%) for scar as compared to DMSA
  - DMSA is therefore advocated by some as better test for scarring, which serves as surrogate for high-grade VUR requiring treatment (with scarring in 50% of grades IV-V but < 10% of grades I-III VUR)
    - RIVUR trial showed no difference in progressive scarring on antibiotic prophylaxis vs. placebo
    - ↑ scars in older patients, higher-grade VUR, & those with recurrent febrile UTI
  - Though anatomic detail is < VCUG, continuous imaging of nuclear medicine ↑ detection of transient VUR so that nuclear cystogram is more sensitive for VUR

DIFFERENTIAL DIAGNOSIS

Fluoroscopic Mimics of Vesicoureteral Reflux

- Normal bowel wall contrasted by intraluminal air, enteric contrast or stool, or bony iliopectineal line can mimic contrast in ureter
  - Clarify with oblique views & comparison to scout image
- Ventriculoperitoneal tubing & other intraabdominal catheters can resemble contrast-filled ureter

Urolithiasis, Especially Staghorn Calculus

- Density may simulate contrast in renal pelvis
- Check scout image & watch for drainage; correlate with US

Sonographic Mimics of Vesicoureteral Reflux

- Normally peristalsing ureter or renal pelvis
- Distended distal ureter in patients with very full bladders
- Pathologies causing obstruction of ureter or renal pelvis

PATHOLOGY

General Features

- Etiology
  - Shortened or abnormally angulated insertion of ureter into bladder is theorized to result in primary VUR
  - Vast majority (80%) of pediatric patients outgrow primary VUR, presumably due to changes at level of ureterovesical junction
  - VUR may also be secondary to periureteral (Hutch) diverticulum, ureterocele, bladder outlet obstruction, voiding dysfunction, duplicated collecting system, or neurogenic bladder
  - Probable association of sterile reflux with renal scarring
    - Antibiotic prophylaxis after 1st UTI reduces febrile UTI recurrences, not scarring
  - Risk factors: Family history, sex, age at presentation, duplication, & other voiding dysfunctions
- Associated abnormalities
  - Multicystic dysplastic kidney
  - Ectopic kidney
    - Note that VUR most commonly involves contralateral orthotopic kidney
  - VUR is present in 25-40% with acute pyelonephritis
  - Duplicated collecting system: Upper pole moiety obstructs, lower pole moiety refluxes

Staging, Grading, & Classification

- International Reflux Study Committee grading system
  - I: Reflux into ureter but not reaching renal pelvis
  - II: Reflux reaching pelvis without blunting of calyces
  - III: Mild calyceal blunting
  - IV: Progressive calyceal & ureteral dilation
  - V: Very dilated & tortuous collecting system
  - ± intrarenal reflux as modifier to grade

Gross Pathologic & Surgical Features

- Deficiency or immaturity of longitudinal muscle in submucosal ureter
- Abnormal angle of ureteral insertion through bladder wall, which tends to correct as ureter grows & elongates
- Distortion of ureteral insertion by adjacent bladder anomaly

CLINICAL ISSUES

Presentation

- Most common signs/symptoms
  - Usually discovered during work-up of febrile UTI

Demographics

- Age
  - VUR is most common in children < 2 years old
  - 0.5x as likely in those 3-6 years old
  - 0.3x as likely in those 7-11 years old
  - 0.15x as likely in those 12-21 years old
- Sex
  - F:M = 2:1
- Epidemiology
  - Up to 2% of general population
  - VUR in 5-50% of asymptomatic siblings of children with documented reflux

Natural History & Prognosis

- 80% outgrow VUR before puberty
- ↑ grade or longstanding VUR, more numerous UTIs, & subsequent renal scarring → ↑ incidence of renal insufficiency, hypertension, & end-stage renal disease
- Intrarenal reflux is associated with ↑ renal scarring

Treatment

- Prophylactic antibiotic therapy (medical management)
  - Reduces febrile UTI recurrences, not scarring
- Ureteral reimplantation surgery (surgical management)
- Endoscopic periureteral injections (minimally invasive endoscopic management) utilizing inert material to alter shape of abnormal/refluxing ureterovesical junction
  - Treatment-induced hydroureteronephrosis following endoscopic procedures is uncommon & usually self-limited

SELECTED REFERENCES

1. Kim D et al: Contrast-enhanced voiding urosonography for the diagnosis of vesicoureteral reflux and intrarenal reflux: a comparison of diagnostic performance with fluoroscopic voiding cystourethrography. Ultrasonography. 40(4):530-7, 2021
2. Ntoulia A et al: Contrast-enhanced voiding urosonography, part 1. vesicoureteral reflux evaluation. Pediatr Radiol. ePub, 2021
3. Ji D et al: Accuracy of subjective vesicoureteral reflux timing assessment: supporting new voiding cystourethrogram guidelines. Pediatr Radiol. 50(7):953-7, 2020
4. Arlen AM et al: New trends in voiding cystourethrography and vesicoureteral reflux: who, when and how? Int J Urol. 26(4):440-5, 2019
5. Garin EH: Primary vesicoureteral reflux; what have we learnt from the recently published randomized, controlled trials? Pediatr Nephrol. 34(9):1513-9, 2019
6. Kosmeri C et al: An update on renal scarring after urinary tract infection in children: what are the risk factors? J Pediatr Urol. 15(6):598-603, 2019
7. Schneider KO et al: Intrarenal reflux, an overlooked entity - retrospective analysis of 1,166 voiding cysturethrographies in children. Pediatr Radiol. 49(5):617-25, 2019
8. Kim HK et al: Feasibility of superb microvascular imaging to detect high-grade vesicoureteral reflux in children with urinary tract infection. Eur Radiol. 28(1):66-73, 2018
9. Ntoulia A et al: Contrast-enhanced voiding urosonography (ceVUS) with the intravesical administration of the ultrasound contrast agent Optison™ for vesicoureteral reflux detection in children: a prospective clinical trial. Pediatr Radiol. 48(2):216-26, 2018
10. Wang ZT et al: A reanalysis of the RIVUR trial using a risk classification system. J Urol. 199(6):1608-1614, 2018

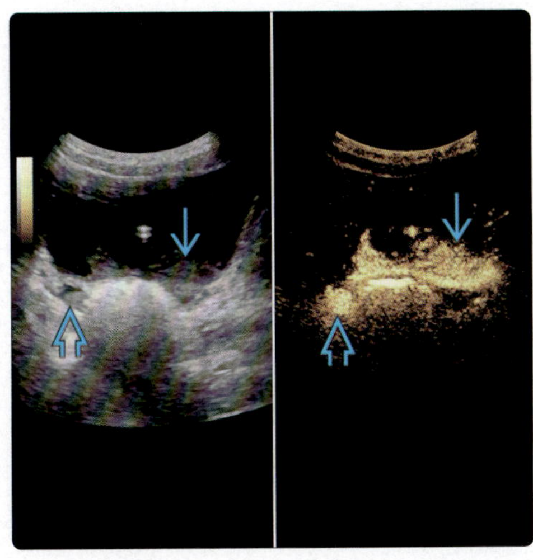

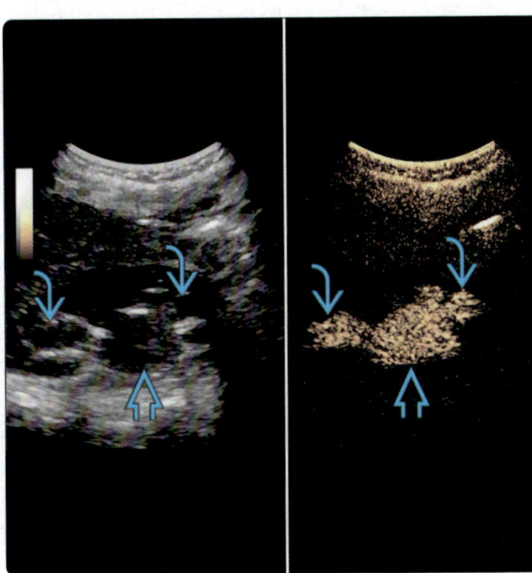

(Left) *Transverse grayscale & contrast-only images from a contrast-enhanced ultrasound (CEUS) in a 4-year-old girl with recurrent UTIs show contrast filling the bladder* ➡ *& refluxing into the right ureter* ➡. *(Courtesy S. Back, MD.)* **(Right)** *Longitudinal grayscale & contrast-only images from a CEUS in the same patient show refluxed contrast distending the right renal pelvis* ➡ *& calyces* ➡*, which are mildly blunted (grade III VUR). (Courtesy S. Back, MD.)*

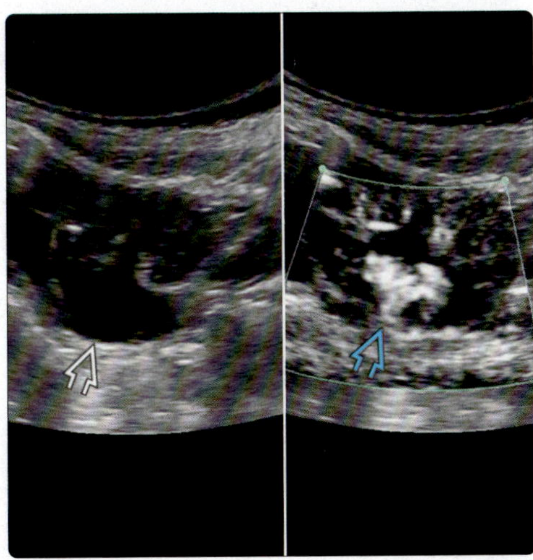

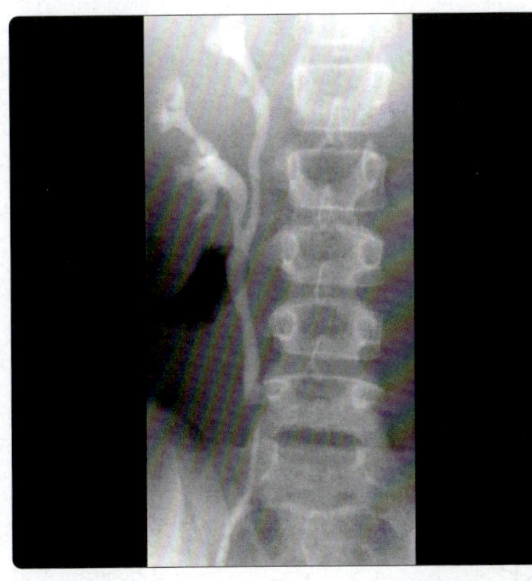

(Left) *Prone posterior US shows the anechoic renal pelvis* ➡ *(left) with swirling echogenic urine refluxing into the pelvis* ➡ *(right) by using Doppler SMI to detect slow velocity flow.* **(Right)** *VCUG shows VUR into a partially duplicated collecting system, which resembles the letter y. VUR can sometimes be seen fluoroscopically entering one limb of the y first, receding, & then filling the other limb, the so-called "yo-yo" reflux.*

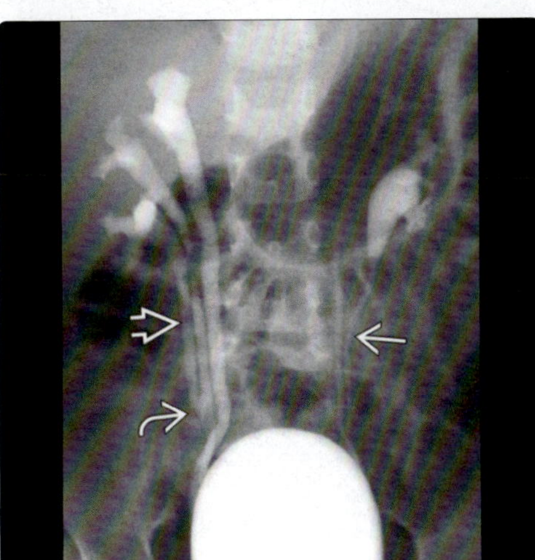

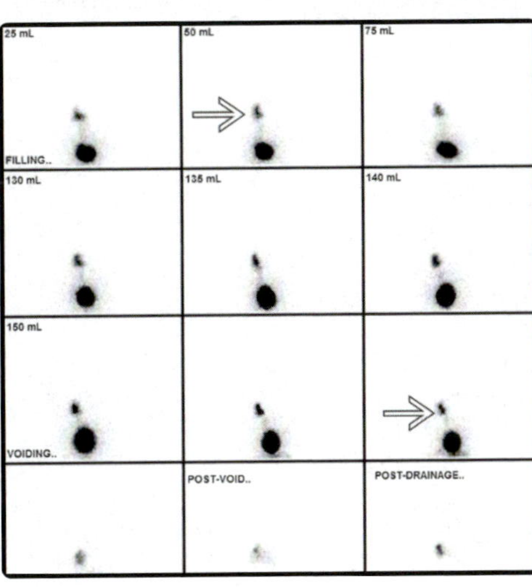

(Left) *Frontal VCUG shows high-grade VUR into a triplicated ureter* ➡ *on the right + lower grade reflux into a duplicated ureter on the left* ➡. *Two of the 3 right ureters join inferiorly* ➡. **(Right)** *Posterior nuclear cystogram images show radiotracer extending into the left ureter & reaching the intrarenal collecting system* ➡*, likely corresponding to fluoroscopic grade II VUR. Note that reflux occurs early during bladder filling in this 2-year-old girl.*

Ureteropelvic Duplications

KEY FACTS

TERMINOLOGY

- Presence of 2 separate pelvicalyceal collecting systems in 1 kidney; 2 draining ureters may
  - Join above bladder: Partial duplication (most common, often of no consequence)
  - Insert into bladder separately: Complete duplication

IMAGING

- Central renal sinus fat is separated by bar of cortical tissue
  - Renal parenchyma is otherwise normal unless complications of vesicoureteral reflux (VUR) &/or obstruction are present
- Separate renal pelves are often visible on either side of this tissue, ± separate proximal ureters
- Duplicated kidneys tend to be larger than nonduplex kidneys, even without hydronephrosis
- With complete duplication, ureter draining upper pole (UP) of kidney inserts in bladder inferior & medial to ureter draining lower pole (LP) of kidney (Weigert-Meyer rule)
  - LP ureter inserts orthotopically in trigone
  - UP ureteral orifice is ectopic in location & often associated with ureterocele
- Corollary to Weigert-Meyer rule
  - UP tends to obstruct
  - LP tends to have VUR: Lack of dilation of ureter & collecting system in no way excludes VUR
- Drooping lily sign: Classic appearance of opacified LP collecting system on IVP or VCUG, displaced by mass-like UP hydronephrosis
  - Correlation with US is critical to confirm UP obstruction rather than other mass lesion

CLINICAL ISSUES

- Incidence of 12-15% in general population
- Treatment depends on extent of anomalies & complications
- Chronic obstruction, VUR, infection, &/or scarring may lead to secondary hypertension & renal insufficiency

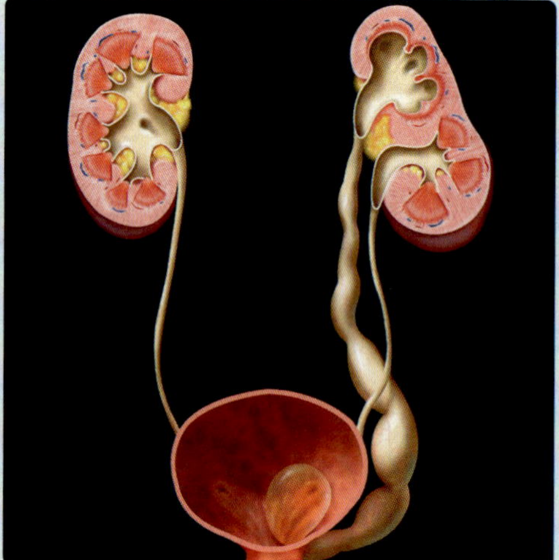

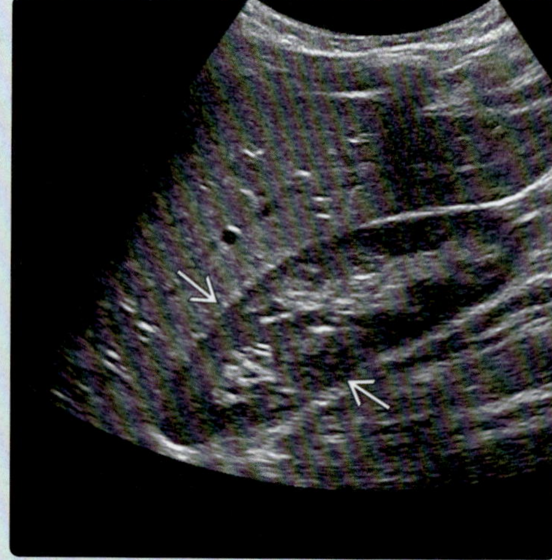

(Left) *Coronal graphic shows a normal right kidney & completely duplicated left kidney with a poorly draining upper pole (UP) ectopic ureterocele seen in the bladder medial & inferior to the lower pole (LP) ureteral orifice. The LP ureter on the left inserts into bladder orthotopically at the trigone.* **(Right)** *Longitudinal ultrasound in a child shows a band of cortex ➡ separating the central sinus fat & other medullary structures in this duplicated kidney without any evidence of obstruction or hydronephrosis.*

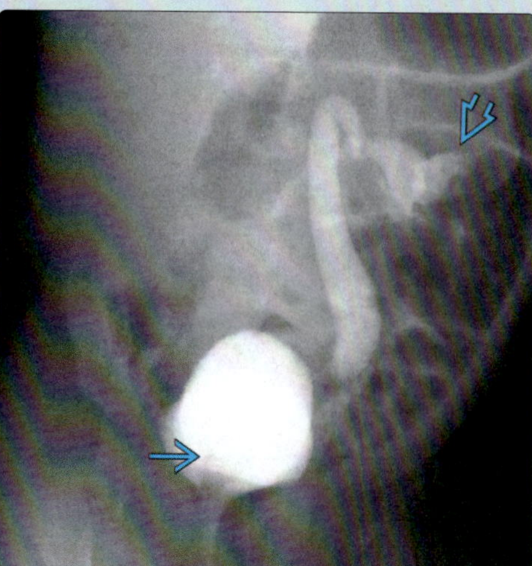

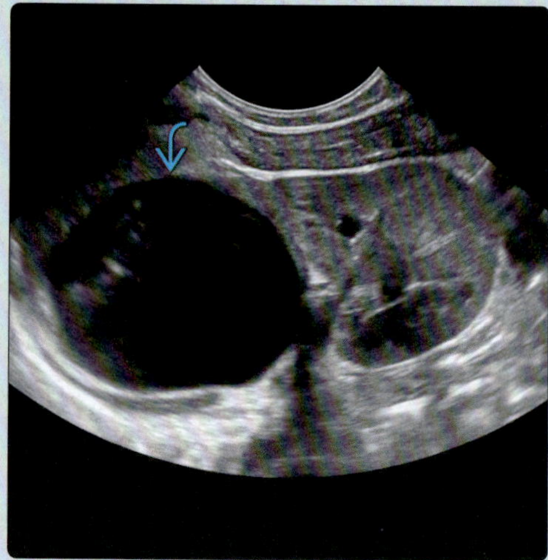

(Left) *Frontal VCUG in a 1-month-old girl shows grade 4 vesicoureteral reflux (VUR) into an LP moiety ➡, which is directed inferiorly by a nonvisualized obstructed UP system (the drooping lily sign). The UP moiety terminates as a ureterocele ➡ (poorly seen due to the degree of bladder filling).* **(Right)** *Longitudinal ultrasound in the same patient shows the obstructed left UP moiety with severe thinning of the surrounding renal parenchyma ➡. The LP appears normal despite the degree of VUR.*

TERMINOLOGY

Synonyms

- Duplicated kidney, duplex collecting system, partial/incomplete/complete duplication, bifid pelvis

Definitions

- Presence of 2 separate pelvicalyceal collecting systems in 1 kidney
  - 2 draining ureters may
    - Join above bladder (partial duplication)
    - Insert into bladder separately (complete duplication)

IMAGING

General Features

- Best diagnostic clue
  - Identification of 2 renal pelves or proximal ureters on any imaging modality
- Location
  - Duplication can involve any length of urinary tract (from renal parenchyma to urethra)
  - L > R
- Size
  - Duplicated kidneys tend to be larger than nonduplex, even without hydronephrosis
- Morphology
  - Central renal sinus fat is completely separated by bar of renal cortex; renal parenchyma is often otherwise normal
    - Unless vesicoureteral reflux (VUR) has led to scarring or obstruction has led to thinning/dysplasia
  - Duplex system has > 10 calyces, 2 renal pelves, & 1 or 2 ureters
  - > 1 renal artery & vein is very common
  - If duplication is complete, ureter draining upper pole (UP) of kidney inserts in bladder inferior & medial to ureter draining lower pole (LP) of kidney (Weigert-Meyer rule)
  - Corollary to Weigert-Meyer rule
    - UP tends to obstruct
    - LP tends to have VUR
  - UP ureteral orifice is, by definition, ectopic in location & may be associated with ureterocele

Ultrasonographic Findings

- Grayscale ultrasound
  - Band of renal cortex splits echogenic sinus fat
  - Separate renal pelves are often visible, ± separate proximal ureters
  - Distal ureters are more difficult to identify due to bowel gas near bladder
    - While dilated distal ureter may be suggestive of VUR, remember that
      - Lack of dilation of ureter & collecting system in no way excludes VUR
      - Severe VUR may not show dilation at US
  - Look for thin-walled ureterocele protruding into urinary bladder; assess for presence & location of ureteral jets
  - Remember to survey for concomitant genital anomalies, especially of uterus
- Color Doppler
  - May show elevated resistive indices (RIs) in obstructed moiety
  - Useful to define arterial anatomy
  - Used to confirm lack of blood flow in renal pelves & tubular ureters
  - Can show foci of hypoperfusion from superimposed infection (pyelonephritis)

Fluoroscopic Findings

- Voiding cystourethrogram
  - Look for VUR (LP > > UP)
  - Saddle VUR or yo-yo VUR is unique to partial duplications, which have single distal ureter
    - VUR contrast first enters 1 component of upper tract collecting system, drains, & then refluxes into 2nd component
  - Ectopic ureter may only be visualized when inadvertently catheterized (e.g., intersphincteric ureter)
    - If this occurs, contrast opacification can help delineate anatomy
    - However, catheterization of urinary bladder must also occur to look for VUR into other ureters

CT Findings

- CECT can demonstrate course of ureters (particularly with delay) & locate renal arteries
- Presence of supernumerary calyces & bifid pelvis can be more challenging to detect on axial imaging; multiplanar reformats are helpful

MR Findings

- MR urography
  - Anatomy: 3D T2 images (conventional vs. heavily T2-weighted/MRCP type) capitalize on fluid signal in urinary tract
  - Physiology: Dynamic postcontrast imaging (with quantitative processing) is used to guide surgical interventions
  - Often best test when ectopic ureter cannot be demonstrated with other imaging

Nuclear Medicine Findings

- Occasionally, nuclear study can be 1st to suggest renal duplication
- Renal scans are used to show differential function, drainage, & scarring
- Results help guide surgical intervention

Multimodality Findings

- Obstructed hydronephrotic UP moiety of duplicated system exerts mass effect on LP moiety, displacing/rotating it inferiorly
  - Drooping lily sign: Classic appearance of inferiorly displaced/rotated opacified LP collecting system on IVP or VCUG
  - Can be seen on coronal CT, MR, & US
  - Beware that UP or suprarenal masses can also create this fluoroscopic appearance, necessitating correlation with cross-sectional investigation (typically US)

Imaging Recommendations

- Best imaging tool
  - US is usually 1st-line study for suspected GU abnormality

- VCUG & nuclear studies generally complete imaging work-up if duplicated system is causing problems
- MR is useful in complex cases; can provide complete anatomic & physiologic work-up
- Protocol advice
  - When searching for ectopic ureter from poorly functioning &/or chronically obstructed UP, consider MR urography
  - MRU feed & sleep technique had 90% success rate in infants < 10 months old in one study

DIFFERENTIAL DIAGNOSIS

Column of Bertin

- Normal variant of junctional parenchyma, typically in midkidney; looks like focally thickened cortex

Segmental Multicystic Dysplastic Kidney

- UP dysplasia of duplicated system can mimic obstructed, hydronephrotic moiety

Adrenal Mass

- Can mimic drooping lily sign by displacing collecting system inferiorly

Other Suprarenal Mass

- Pulmonary sequestration, duplication cyst, etc.

PATHOLOGY

General Features

- Etiology
  - Early branching of ureteric bud or 2 ureteral buds arising from wolffian duct
  - Each bud induces formation of its own nephrons when it meets metanephric blastema
  - Abnormal branching of ureteric bud can also give rise to supernumerary kidney or triplicate collecting system (both very rare)
- Associated abnormalities
  - Duplications of bladder, urethra, & genital structures are associated with renal duplication
    - Genital anomalies in 50% of affected females
  - Ureteropelvic junction obstruction is more common in duplicated kidneys

Gross Pathologic & Surgical Features

- Almost always has 2 renal arteries & veins, often with separate renal artery orifice from aorta
- In absence of complications, renal parenchyma & collecting system tissue are normal

Microscopic Features

- Depends on complications: Scarring, hydronephrosis, fibrosis

CLINICAL ISSUES

Presentation

- Most common signs/symptoms
  - Most often discovered antenatally or incidentally on imaging studies performed for other reasons
- Other signs/symptoms
  - Symptomatic duplications may lead to infection, obstruction, calculi, scarring, hematuria, abdominal or flank pain, voiding dysfunction, urinary retention

Demographics

- Age
  - Congenital; usually discovered early in life
- Sex
  - Complete duplications are much more common in women
  - Partial duplications have no sex predilection
- Epidemiology
  - Incidence of 12-15% in general population, but only 1% are found de novo in cadaveric renal donors

Natural History & Prognosis

- Prognosis varies with type of duplication & severity of complications
- Chronic obstruction, VUR, infection, &/or scarring may lead to secondary hypertension & renal insufficiency

Treatment

- Depends on extent of anomalies & complications
  - Associated ureteroceles are incised, unroofed, resected, or reimplanted
  - Ectopic ureter may be reimplanted if kidney it subtends retains good function; otherwise resected
  - Hydronephrosis is treated surgically to improve drainage
    - Cortical thinning & relative function are used to determine surgical course: Salvage vs. resection
  - Infections are treated with antibiotics & evaluated for urine stasis & VUR
  - VUR may be managed conservatively (medically) or treated surgically, depending on grade & associated anomalies
  - Calculi are removed, fragmented, or monitored
  - Voiding dysfunction is assessed to exclude ectopic ureter/ureterocele, prolapsing cecoureterocele, & bladder dyskinesia

SELECTED REFERENCES

1. Houat AP et al: Congenital anomalies of the upper urinary tract: a comprehensive review. Radiographics. 41(2):462-86, 2021
2. Chan KKC et al: Unusual ureteric duplication abnormality in a child with pelvoureteric junction obstruction. BMJ Case Rep. 13(3), 2020
3. Ji H et al: Prenatal diagnosis of renal duplication by magnetic resonance imaging. J Matern Fetal Neonatal Med. 33(14):2342-7, 2020
4. Abdelhalim A et al: Ipsilateral ureteroureterostomy for ureteral duplication anomalies: predictors of adverse outcomes. J Pediatr Urol. 15(5):468.e1-6, 2019
5. Damasio MB et al: Comparative study between functional mr urography and renal scintigraphy to evaluate drainage curves and split renal function in children with congenital anomalies of kidney and urinary tract (CAKUT). Front Pediatr. 7:527, 2019
6. Tsiflikas I et al: Functional magnetic resonance urography in infants: feasibility of a feed-and-sleep technique. Pediatr Radiol. 49(3):351-7, 2019
7. Didier RA et al: The duplicated collecting system of the urinary tract: embryology, imaging appearances and clinical considerations. Pediatr Radiol. 47(11):1526-38, 2017
8. Expert Panel on Pediatric Imaging:. et al: ACR Appropriateness Criteria® urinary tract infection-child. J Am Coll Radiol. 14(5S):S362-71, 2017
9. Mendichovszky I et al: Nuclear medicine in pediatric nephro-urology: an overview. Semin Nucl Med. 47(3):204-28, 2017
10. Michaud JE et al: Upper pole heminephrectomy versus lower pole ureteroureterostomy for ectopic upper pole ureters. Curr Urol Rep. 18(3):21, 2017

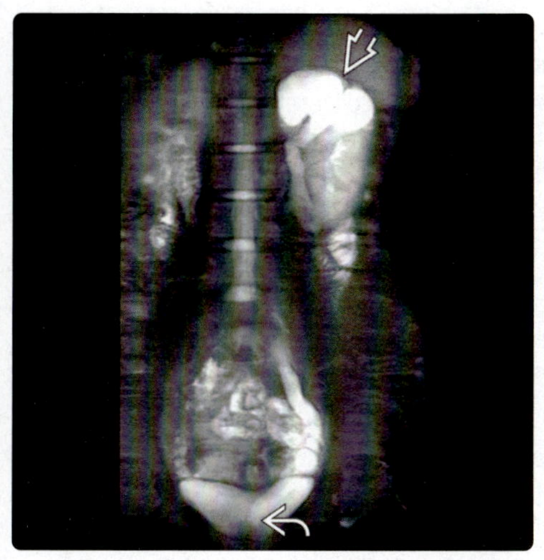

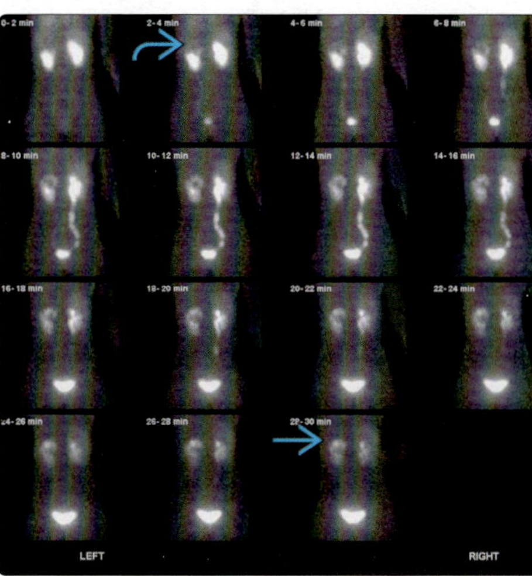

(Left) *Coronal MIP MR urogram in a teenager shows a duplicated left kidney & obstructed UP moiety, which drains ectopically into the vagina. Note the cortical thinning of the left UP from chronic injury.* **(Right)** *Posterior images from a Tc-99m MAG3 renogram in the same patient show delayed uptake by the UP of the left kidney with poor function & excretion. The postdiuretic washout curve for the left UP showed no drainage (not shown).*

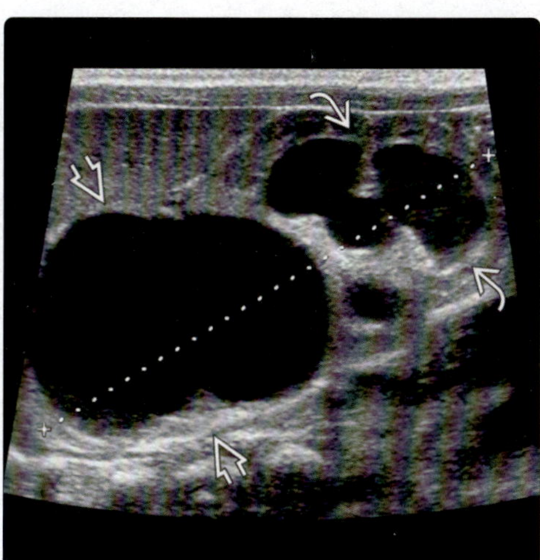

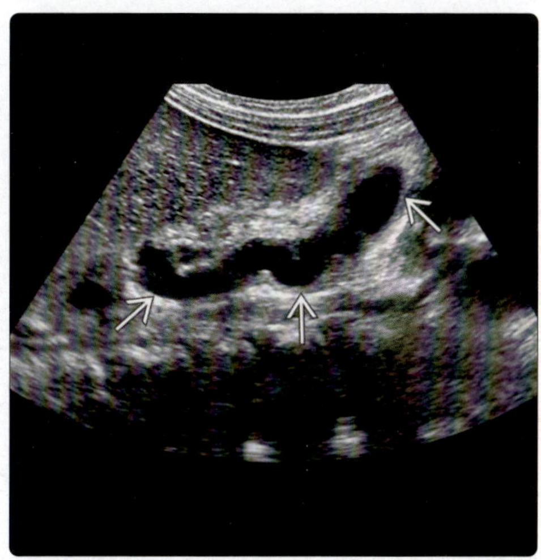

(Left) *Longitudinal oblique ultrasound in a patient with a duplicated right kidney shows severe dilation of the UP moiety with marked parenchymal thinning. There is also mild to moderate dilation of the LP moiety. Cursors mark the length of the kidney.* **(Right)** *Longitudinal oblique ultrasound in the same patient shows the tortuous course of the dilated right UP ureter.*

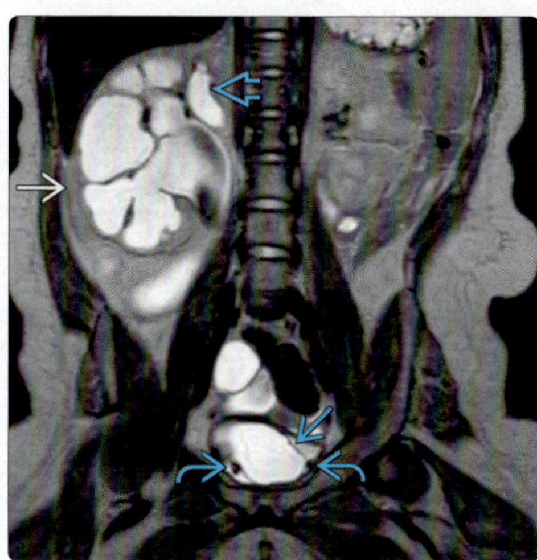

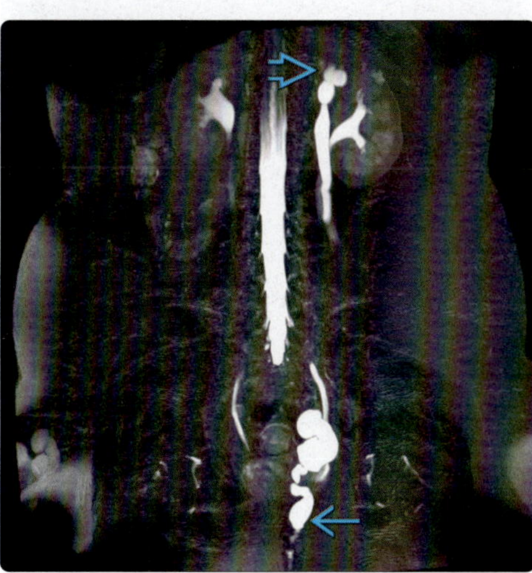

(Left) *Coronal 3D T2 MR urogram in a 10-month-old girl shows a UP moiety ureterocele outlined by a catheter in the bladder. The UP moiety is small relative to the ureterocele (ureterocele disproportion). Marked dilation of the LP moiety with parenchymal thinning was due to obstruction by the adjacent UP ureterocele.* **(Right)** *Coronal MIP MR urogram in a 17-year-old with giggle incontinence shows a small dysplastic left UP moiety with ectopic insertion of the ureter into the vagina.*

Ureterocele

KEY FACTS

TERMINOLOGY

- Congenital cystic dilation of distal submucosal portion of 1 or both ureters within urinary bladder
- Categorized according to ureterocele position
  - Intravesical: Completely contained within bladder
  - Extravesical: Partially extends to bladder neck, urethra, vagina, prostate, seminal vesicles, or perineum
- Categorized according to ureterocele insertion
  - Orthotopic (simple): Orifice is located in normal anatomic position in bladder trigone
  - Ectopic: Orifice is located anywhere else
- Categorized according to type of kidney drained
  - Single system vs. duplicated system with 2 ureters
  - 1 ureter of duplicated system must be ectopic
- Weigert-Meyer rule: Ureter from upper pole (UP) moiety of duplicated kidney inserts inferior & medial to normal lower pole (LP) moiety insertion site at trigone
- Any ureterocele may obstruct & cause hydronephrosis

IMAGING

- Round/ovoid filling defect in urinary bladder
  - Thin-walled & cystic-appearing on US, MRU
    - Wall appears thicker, collapsed after surgery
- ± visualization of associated dilated distal ureter
- In duplicated system, UP moiety (associated with ureterocele) typically obstructs, & LP moiety typically refluxes
  - Varying degrees of hydronephrosis & parenchymal dysplasia of UP moiety
  - Vesicoureteral reflux into LP moiety classically shows drooping lily sign
    - Due to rotation of LP system by obstructed UP

CLINICAL ISSUES

- Ectopic variety > orthotopic variety by 3-4:1 ratio
- Typical treatment: Endoscopic incision of ureterocele, especially if infected or obstructed in neonate

(Left) *Longitudinal ultrasound of the urinary bladder in an 18-day-old with prenatally detected hydronephrosis shows a large, thin-walled cyst ➡ filling much of the bladder lumen, typical of a ureterocele. The cyst connects to a dilated distal left ureter ⇨.* **(Right)** *Longitudinal ultrasound of the duplicated left kidney in the same patient shows severe pelvocaliectasis & parenchymal thinning of the left upper pole (UP) moiety ⇨. The lower pole (LP) moiety shows mild pelvocaliectasis with more normal-appearing renal parenchyma ➡.*

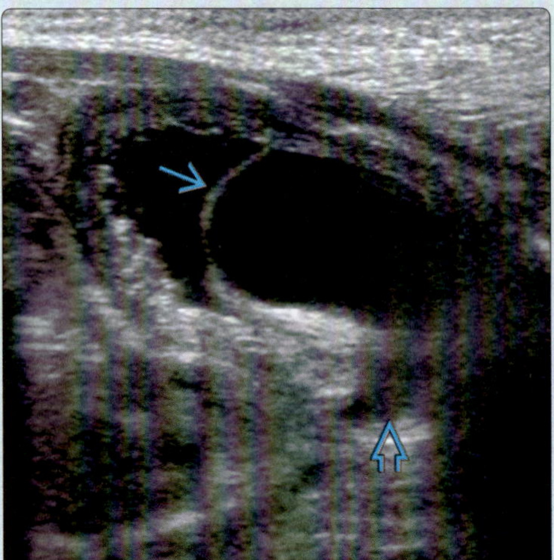

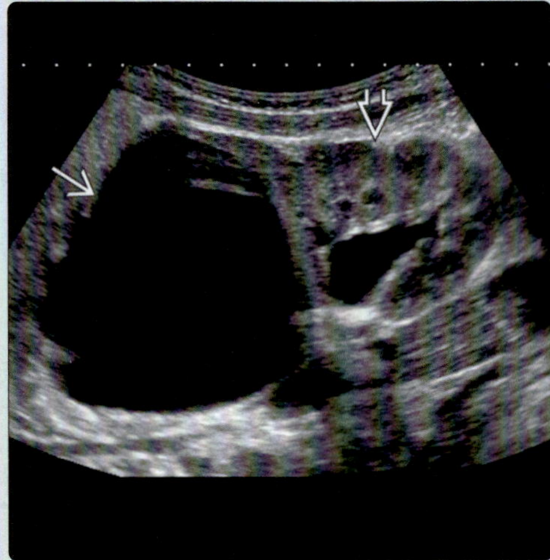

(Left) *Frontal early filling image from a VCUG in the same patient shows the ureterocele as a large, ovoid filling defect ➡ partially outlined by contrast in the urinary bladder.* **(Right)** *Postvoid VCUG in the same patient shows grade 2-3 vesicoureteral reflux (VUR) into the LP collecting system ↷. The drooping lily configuration of contrast within the LP strongly suggests obstruction of a UP moiety (as confirmed on the ultrasound). The UP ureterocele ➡ remains visible in the contrast-filled bladder.*

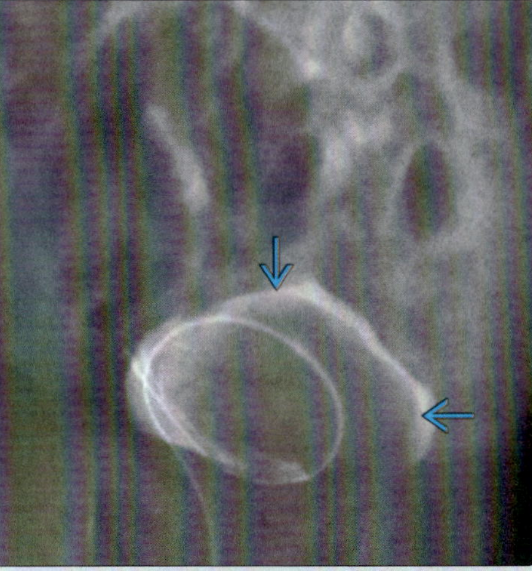

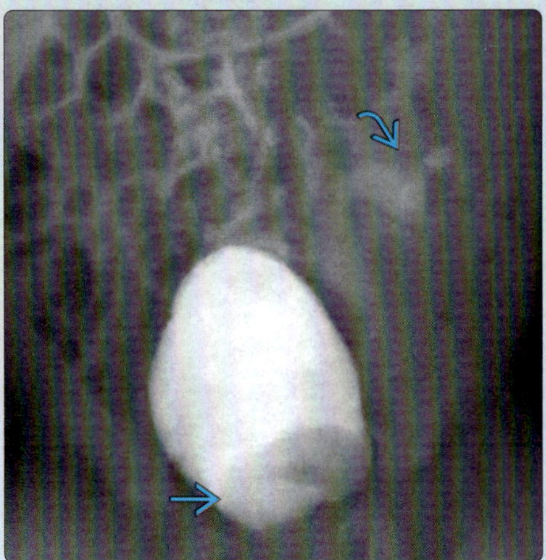

TERMINOLOGY

Definitions

- Congenital cystic dilation of distal submucosal portion of 1 or both ureters within urinary bladder
- Categorized according to ureterocele position
    - Intravesical: Completely contained within urinary bladder
    - Extravesical: Partially extends into bladder neck, urethra, or perineum
- Categorized according to ureterocele insertion
    - Orthotopic (simple): Orifice located in normal anatomic position in bladder trigone
    - Ectopic: Orifice located anywhere else
        - Ectopic ureter may drain to other genitourinary locations without ending as ureterocele
- Categorized according to type of kidney drained
    - Single-system ureterocele: Kidney gives rise to single collecting system with solitary ureter
        - Typically simple, intravesical ureterocele
    - Duplex-system ureterocele: Kidney has completely duplicated collecting system with 2 complete ureters
        - 1 ureteral insertion must be ectopic by definition (often extravesical)
- Cecoureterocele: Unique subtype elongated beyond ureteral orifice by tunneling under trigone & urethra
- Any type of ureterocele may become obstructed or prolapse into bladder neck & cause hydronephrosis

IMAGING

General Features

- Best diagnostic clue
    - Round or ovoid cystic filling defect in bladder
- Location
    - L > R; bilateral in 10%
    - Ectopic variety > orthotopic variety by 3-4:1 ratio
    - Weigert-Meyer rule: Ureter from upper pole (UP) moiety of duplicated kidney inserts inferior & medial to normal insertion site of LP moiety in bladder trigone
        - UP moiety typically obstructs, LP typically refluxes
    - Ureterocele may prolapse in & out of bladder

Fluoroscopic Findings

- Voiding cystourethrogram (VCUG)
    - Best seen on early bladder-filling image before contrast is too dense & intravesical pressure compresses ureterocele
    - Vesicoureteral reflux (VUR) is frequently seen in LP moiety
        - May create drooping lily sign where nonopacified obstructed UP moiety distorts opacified refluxing LP moiety
            - Long axis of opacified LP moiety collecting system points toward ipsilateral shoulder
    - If ureterocele everts, creates appearance of diverticulum & may cause VUR

Ultrasonographic Findings

- Grayscale ultrasound
    - Anechoic, thin-walled cyst inside urinary bladder
    - Ureteral jet & connection to dilated distal ureter may be demonstrated
    - ± duplicated kidney with hydroureteronephrosis
        - Single system kidney typically shows uniform degree of pelvocaliectasis
        - Obstructed UP moiety of duplex kidney is variable in morphology
            - Often shows worse pelvocaliectasis than LP
            - Variable degrees of UP parenchymal thinning ± cystic dysplasia
            - Variable size of UP moiety: Enlarged with severe pelvocaliectasis vs. small with dysplastic parenchyma in setting of large ureterocele (ureterocele disproportion)
    - After incision (to relieve obstruction), residual partially or totally collapsed ureterocele often has thick, undulating wall
- Color Doppler
    - Ureteral jet is useful to exclude complete obstruction of ureterocele
- 3D
    - "Virtual sonocystoscopy" may be useful preop tool
- Contrast-enhanced ultrasound
    - Round filling defect in contrast-filled bladder
    - Contrast may reflux after ureterocele incision

MR Findings

- MR urography
    - 3D T2-weighted sequences emphasize fluid-filled urinary tract anatomy
    - Dynamic postcontrast images can evaluate function & drainage of urinary tract
        - Can be processed for quantitative data
    - Associated gynecologic anomalies in 50% of females with duplication

Nuclear Medicine Findings

- Nuclear cystogram
    - Ureterocele is difficult to see on nuclear cystogram unless very large or prolapsing
- Nuclear renal scan
    - Used to assess function of obstructed or poorly functioning UP moiety
    - Poor function on nuclear scan is predictive of severe histologic changes in renal parenchyma; helps justify heminephrectomy

Imaging Recommendations

- Best imaging tool
    - VCUG & ultrasound are best 1st-line studies
    - Nuclear renal scan is most established technique for evaluating differential function in duplicated kidney
    - MRU & IVP have been reserved for difficult or complex cases; increasing use of MRU as comprehensive study of anatomy & function
- Protocol advice
    - VCUG is best test to assess dynamic nature of ureterocele: Everting, refluxing, prolapsing, &/or causing bladder outlet obstruction
        - Fluoroscopic vs. contrast enhanced

DIFFERENTIAL DIAGNOSIS

Bladder Mass

- Lacks communication with distal ureter; typically solid
  - Rhabdomyosarcoma, neurofibroma, polyp: Nonmobile with variable internal vascularity
  - Focal cystitis: Variety of infectious & noninfectious causes
  - Fungus ball, hematoma: Often mobile; no internal vascularity

Mass Effect From Sigmoid Colon

- Can appear as filling defect on VCUG: Get oblique views

Bladder Hutch Diverticulum

- Periureteral diverticulum; separate from distal ureter
- May mimic everted ureterocele; does not usually prolapse into bladder to cause filling defect

Ovarian Cyst

- May deform but does not typically bulge into bladder

PATHOLOGY

General Features

- Etiology
  - Embryology/anatomy
    - Thought to result from delayed canalization of Chwalla membrane during embryogenesis → obstruction of ureteral orifice
      - Chwalla membrane: Primitive separation of ureteral bud from developing urogenital sinus
- Associated abnormalities
  - VUR into lower pole of duplicated system: 50%
  - VUR in contralateral kidney: 25%

Microscopic Features

- In heminephroureterectomy specimens, histologic changes include chronic interstitial inflammation, fibrosis, tubular atrophy, glomerulosclerosis, & dysplasia
- Normal urothelium in dilated intramucosal or submucosal segment

CLINICAL ISSUES

Presentation

- Most common signs/symptoms
  - Prenatal detection of hydronephrosis is typical
  - Febrile urinary tract infection (UTI) is most common postnatal presentation
- Other signs/symptoms
  - Simple ureterocele may not be diagnosed until adulthood
  - Ectopic ureterocele is usually diagnosed in infancy or shortly after toilet training: Presents with hematuria, UTI, chronic enuresis, or hydronephrosis
  - Rarely presents with prolapse & acute bladder outlet obstruction
  - Other rare presentations: Failure to thrive, cyclic abdominal pain, ureteral calculus

Demographics

- Age
  - Detected antenatally & in infancy
- Epidemiology
  - 1 in 4,000 children; less frequently diagnosed in adults
- Sex: Ectopic ureterocele F:M = 4-7:1

Natural History & Prognosis

- Prognosis is excellent if nonobstructing & nonrefluxing
- Prognosis is variable if prolonged obstruction or high-grade VUR has compromised renal function
- Antenatal diagnosis is reported to improve overall course: Fewer infections, fewer surgical procedures
- Ureteroceles diagnosed antenatally should be treated surgically within 1st weeks of life since rate of UTI exceeds 50% despite prophylactic antibiotics

Treatment

- Endoscopic incision (puncture or unroofing) of ureterocele, especially if infected or obstructed in neonate
  - Following incision, ureterocele wall appears thickened, irregular, even mass-like
  - Endoscopic incision may convert obstructed ureterocele into refluxing ureterocele
    - LP dilation may improve with UP ureterocele incision
  - Double-puncture technique: Double-J stent inserted into 2 punctured sites at poles of ectopic ureterocele, & tissue is fulgurated
- Ureteral reimplantation surgery: Extravesical reimplantation, ureteroureterostomy, ureteropyelostomy
  - Patients undergoing bilateral ectopic ureterocele repair are at ↑ risk for postoperative voiding dysfunction
    - Unclear if risk is present preoperatively or due to trigonal surgery
- Heminephroureterectomy if UP moiety is very poorly functioning
- Antenatal fetoscopic laser ablation of ureteroceles
  - Performed in fetuses with severe bilateral hydronephrosis, bladder outlet obstruction, & oligohydramnios with good results
- Success after single procedure is higher in single ureters; many require > 1 surgical procedure
- Best surgical management remains controversial

SELECTED REFERENCES

1. Benya EC et al: Assessment of distal ureteral and ureterovesical junction visualization on contrast-enhanced voiding urosonography. Pediatr Radiol. 51(8):1406-11, 2021
2. Houat AP et al: Congenital anomalies of the upper urinary tract: a comprehensive review. Radiographics. 41(2):462-86, 2021
3. Kim J et al: The fate of lower pole hydronephrosis after transurethral incision of upper pole ureteroceles in children with duplex systems. J Pediatr Urol. 16(6):847.e1-7, 2020
4. Calle-Toro JS et al: Morphologic and functional evaluation of duplicated renal collecting systems with MR urography: a descriptive analysis. Clin Imaging. 57:69-76, 2019
5. Nabavizadeh B et al: A novel approach for an old debate in management of ureterocele: long-term outcomes of double-puncture technique. J Pediatr Urol. 15(4):389.e1-5, 2019
6. Nabavizadeh B et al: Three-dimensional virtual sonographic cystoscopy for detection of ureterocele in duplicated collecting systems in children. J Ultrasound Med. 37(3):595-600, 2018
7. Chalouhi GE et al: Prenatal incision of ureterocele causing bladder outlet obstruction: a multicenter case series. Prenat Diagn. 37(10):968-74, 2017
8. Chowdhary SK et al: Ureterocele in newborns, infants and children: ten year prospective study with primary endoscopic deroofing and double J (DJ) stenting. J Pediatr Surg. 52(4):569-73, 2017
9. Timberlake MD et al: Minimally invasive techniques for management of the ureterocele and ectopic ureter: upper tract versus lower tract approach. Urol Clin North Am. 42(1):61-76, 2015

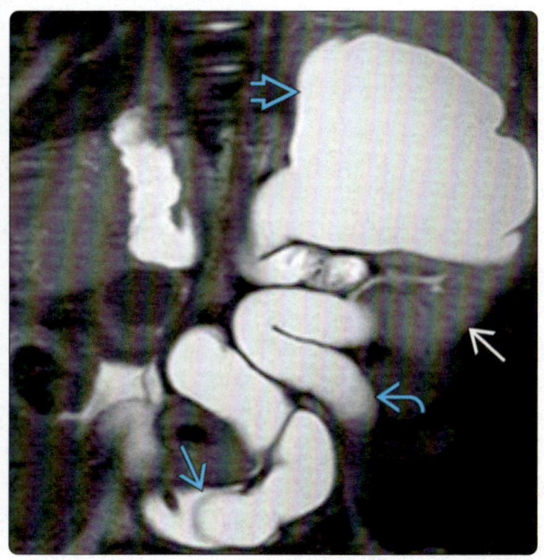

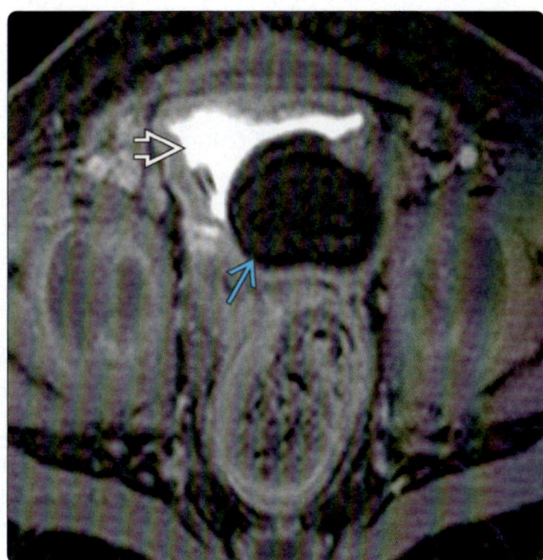

(Left) *Coronal T2 FS MR in an infant shows an ectopic ureterocele ⇨ partially filling the urinary bladder & connecting to a markedly dilated UP ureter ↷. There is severe UP hydronephrosis ⇨ due to obstruction. Note the normal LP moiety ➡.* **(Right)** *Delayed axial T1 C+ FS MR in the same patient shows no contrast in the ureterocele ⇨ due to the longstanding UP obstruction with ↓ function. Contrast has filled the surrounding bladder ➡ by excretion from the remaining urinary tract. (Courtesy J.R. Dillman, MD.)*

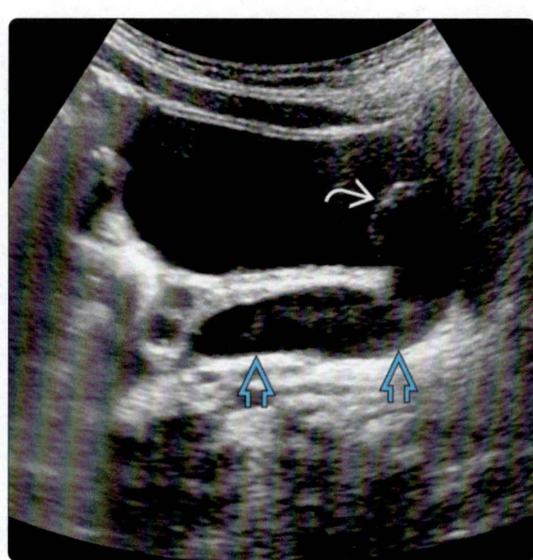

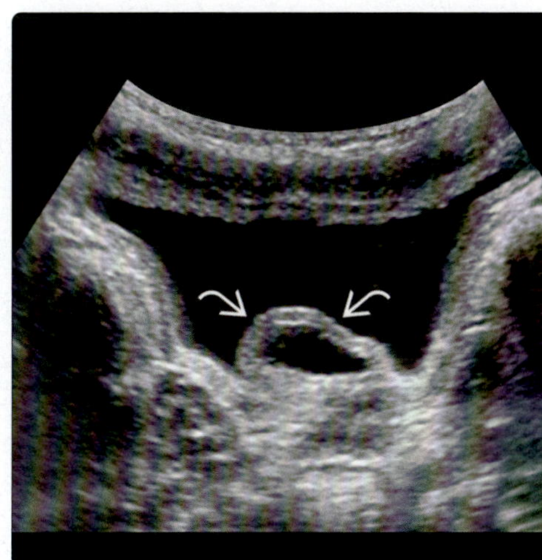

(Left) *Longitudinal ultrasound shows a dilated distal ureter ⇨ entering the bladder & forming a thin-walled bulbous end, typical of a ureterocele ↷. This ureterocele is inserting low in the bladder base & is likely ectopic.* **(Right)** *Transverse ultrasound through the bladder base in a patient after a ureterocele incision shows a partially collapsed, relatively thick-walled ureterocele ↷. After endoscopic incision, ureteroceles tend to decompress & may show wall thickening with an undulating contour, as in this case.*

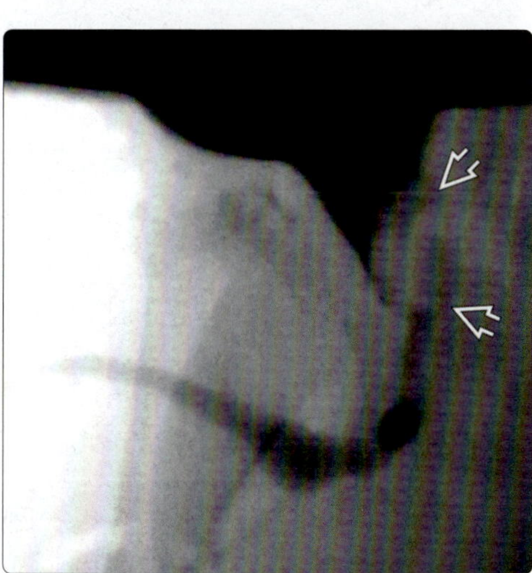

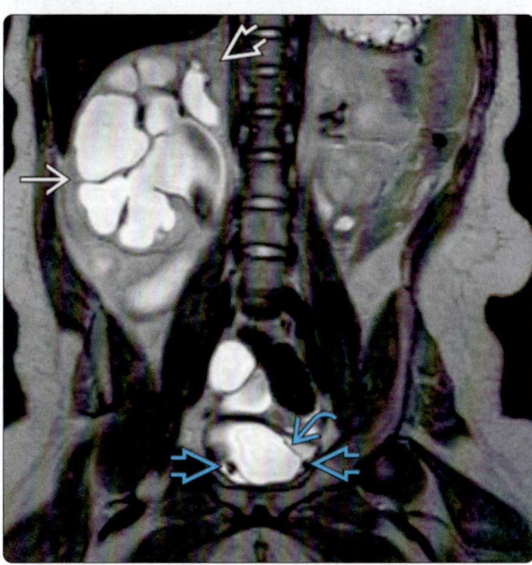

(Left) *Oblique VCUG shows prolapse of a ureterocele into the posterior urethra ➡ as voiding starts & the catheter is expelled. Voiding stopped seconds later due to urethral obstruction.* **(Right)** *Coronal 3D T2 MR urogram in a 10-month-old girl shows a UP moiety ureterocele ↷ outlined by a catheter in the bladder ⇨. The UP moiety is small ➡ relative to the ureterocele (ureterocele disproportion). Marked dilation of the LP moiety with parenchymal thinning ➡ was due to obstruction by the adjacent UP ureterocele.*

Primary Megaureter

KEY FACTS

TERMINOLOGY

- Megaureter: General term for ureteral dilation
  - Can be due to vesicoureteral reflux (VUR), obstruction, both, or neither
- Primary obstructive megaureter: Functional obstruction at juxtavesical segment of ureter due to absent peristalsis

IMAGING

- Best imaging clues
  - Variable degree of hydroureteronephrosis with transition to nondilated distal ureter
    - Nondilated aperistaltic segment involves terminal 0.5-4 cm of ureter
    - Most commonly unilateral: 67% on left
  - VUR: Ipsilateral in 5%, contralateral in < 10%
  - ± debris, calculi in dilated ureter
  - Long-term obstruction can lead to parenchymal thinning & lack of renal growth
- Best imaging modalities
  - Ultrasound is best screening exam for urinary tract anomalies (pre- or postnatally)
  - Diagnostic & treatment considerations are refined with
    - Fluoroscopic VCUG (to assess for VUR &/or bladder outlet obstruction)
    - Nuclear medicine diuretic renography to assess for renal function & delayed ureteral drainage
    - MR urography can assess anatomy & physiology

CLINICAL ISSUES

- M:F = 4:1
- Diagnosed prenatally in nearly 50%; remaining cases present over wide range of ages
- May be asymptomatic but can present with urinary tract infections (UTIs), abdominal/flank pain, hematuria ± calculi, renal failure
- 70% regress spontaneously by 7 years of age
- Surgery is considered for worsening renal function or recurrent UTIs

(Left) *Longitudinal ultrasound at the left ureterovesical junction (UVJ) in a male infant shows a dilated left ureter ➡ tapering distally to a normal-caliber aperistaltic juxtavesical segment ⇨ that shows urothelial thickening. The urinary bladder ⇨ is seen anteriorly.* **(Right)** *Oblique fluoroscopic image from a voiding cystourethrogram in the same patient shows vesicoureteral reflux into the normal-caliber juxtavesical segment ⇨ with transition to the proximally dilated ureter ➡.*

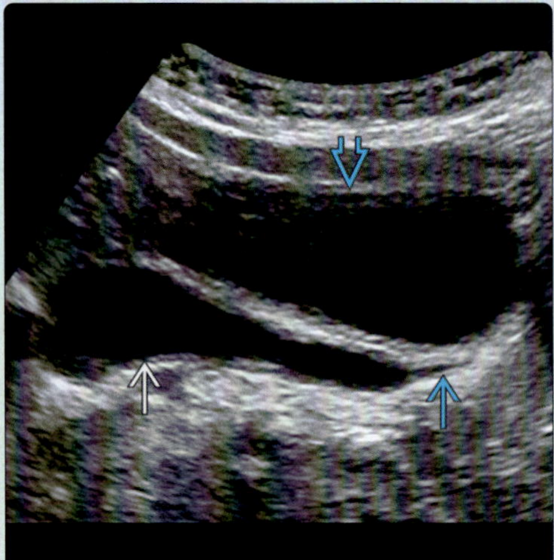

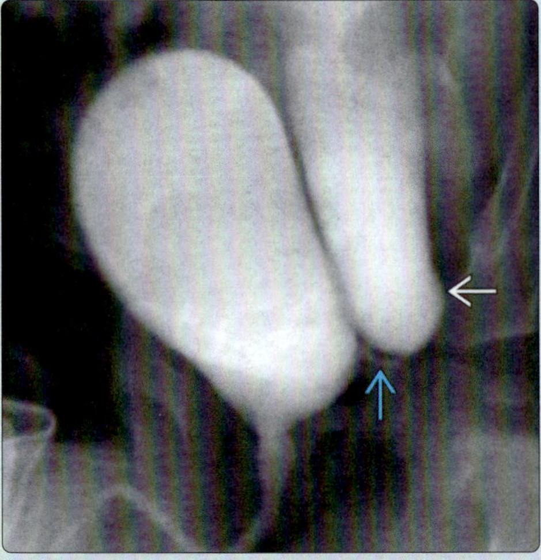

(Left) *Dynamic posterior view postdiuretic images from a Tc-99m MAG3 renogram in the same patient show qualitatively slow drainage of the left dilated ureter. The T1/2 for drainage of the left ureter was > 20 minutes on the quantitative evaluation, consistent with obstruction.* **(Right)** *Oblique MIP from an MR urogram in a patient with a primary obstructive megaureter shows a narrow juxtavesical segment of the left ureter ➡ with proximal hydroureteronephrosis ⇨.*

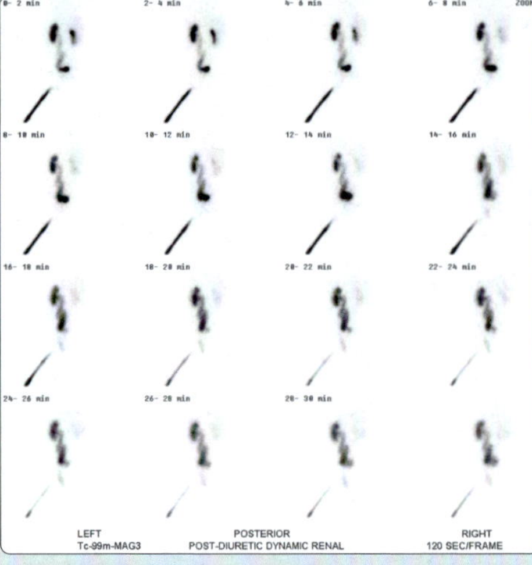

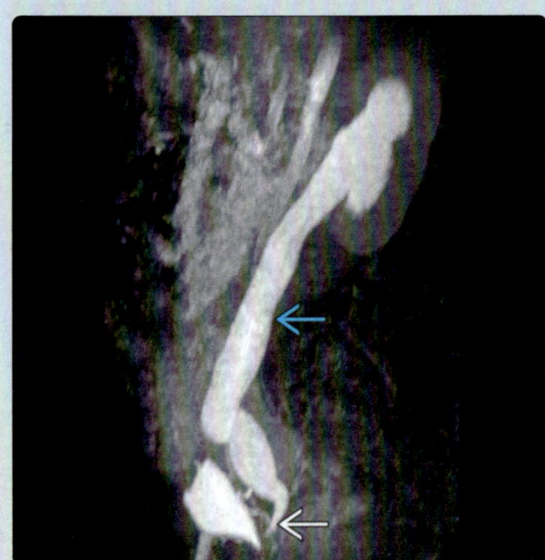

TERMINOLOGY

Definitions

- Megaureter: Ureteral diameter ≥ 7 mm
- 4 types classified by presence of vesicoureteral reflux (VUR) &/or obstruction
  - Nonrefluxing obstructed (NR, O)
  - Refluxing obstructed (R, O)
  - Refluxing nonobstructed (R, NO)
  - Nonrefluxing nonobstructed (NR, NO)
- Primary obstructive megaureter: Congenital functional obstruction at juxtavesical segment of ureter
  - Presumably due to absent peristalsis in normal-caliber distal segment, though exact etiology is unclear

IMAGING

General Features

- Best diagnostic clue
  - Hydroureteronephrosis (HUN) with short segment of normal-caliber distal ureter
- Location
  - Transition from normal-caliber distal ureter to proximal dilation ~ 0.5-4 cm above ureterovesical junction (UVJ)
  - 60% are unilateral (of which 67% involve left ureter)

Ultrasonographic Findings

- Grayscale ultrasound
  - Unilateral or bilateral HUN
  - ± renal parenchymal thinning & lack of renal growth
  - Hyperperistalsis of dilated ureter down to distal aperistaltic normal-caliber segment
  - ± intraluminal debris (proteinaceous or infectious)
  - ± calculus formation

Fluoroscopic Findings

- Voiding cystourethrogram
  - If no VUR, study may appear normal
  - Ipsilateral VUR in 5%, contralateral in < 10%
  - When VUR is present, assess for obstruction
    - Delayed drainage of dilated ureter
    - Short segment of normal-caliber distal ureter
- Retrograde ureterogram (by urology service)
  - More reliably demonstrates distal adynamic ureter

Nuclear Medicine Findings

- Diuretic renography (Tc-99m MAG3 or DTPA)
  - Delayed clearance of radiotracer from dilated ureter & collecting system after furosemide administration
    - Prolonged ureteral ± renal $T_{1/2}$ (> 20 minutes)

MR Findings

- MR urography
  - Comprehensive anatomic & functional evaluation
    - Can assess renal parenchymal function & urinary clearance, similar to nuclear medicine renal scan

DIFFERENTIAL DIAGNOSIS

Refluxing Nonobstructive Megaureter

- Usually high-grade VUR; drains into bladder at end of VCUG
- Much more common than primary obstructive form
- May be idiopathic or seen with neurogenic bladder, posterior urethral valves, prune belly syndrome, megacystis-megaureter, duplicated ureters, incised ureterocele

Nonrefluxing Nonobstructive Megaureter

- Idiopathic aperistaltic distal ureter may occur without quantitative obstruction
- Polyuria (diabetes insipidus) may cause general ureteral dilation

Mechanical Obstruction

- Unilateral (ureteral obstruction)
  - Stricture, ureterocele, urolithiasis, retrocaval ureter, extrinsic mass, ureteral valve (rare)
- Bilateral (bladder outlet or urethral obstruction)
  - Bladder outlet: Posterior urethral valves, cloaca with hydrocolpos, extrinsic mass
  - Urethral: Stricture, polyp, anterior valve, atresia, primary megalourethra; unclear: Prune belly syndrome

PATHOLOGY

General Features

- Etiology is unclear: Possibilities include ↑ collagen deposition, muscle hypertrophy, ↓ number of interstitial cells of Cajal

CLINICAL ISSUES

Presentation

- Most common signs/symptoms
  - Asymptomatic vs. febrile urinary tract infections (UTIs), abdominal/flank pain, hematuria ± calculi, gradual renal failure

Natural History & Prognosis

- 70% resolve spontaneously by 7 years of age
  - Initial ureteral diameter < 8.5 mm: Likely to resolve
  - Initial ureteral diameter > 15 mm: Likely to persist
- May develop renal dysfunction or recurrent UTIs

Treatment

- Conservative management
  - Prophylactic antibiotics; imaging every 6-12 months
- Surgical management: Temporary double J stent, various ureteral reimplantation options
  - Consider with worsening renal function or recurrent UTIs

SELECTED REFERENCES

1. Torino G et al: High-pressure balloon dilatation for the treatment of primary obstructive megaureter: is it the first line of treatment in children and infants? Swiss Med Wkly. 151:w20513, 2021
2. Dekirmendjian A et al: Primary non-refluxing megaureter: analysis of risk factors for spontaneous resolution and surgical intervention. Front Pediatr. 7:126, 2019
3. Teklali Y et al: Endoscopic management of primary obstructive megaureter in pediatrics. J Pediatr Urol. 14(5):382-7, 2018
4. Emad-Eldin S et al: Diagnostic value of combined static-excretory MR Urography in children with hydronephrosis. J Adv Res. 6(2):145-53, 2015
5. Kart Y et al: Altered expression of interstitial cells of Cajal in primary obstructive megaureter. J Pediatr Urol. 9(6 Pt B):1028-31, 2013
6. Gimpel C et al: Complications and long-term outcome of primary obstructive megaureter in childhood. Pediatr Nephrol. 25(9):1679-86, 2010
7. Meyer JS et al: Primary megaureter in infants and children: a review. Urol Radiol. 14(4):296-305, 1992

Megaureter-Megacystis

KEY FACTS

TERMINOLOGY

- Megaureter-megacystis syndrome (MMS): Marked vesicoureteral reflux (VUR) leads to large bladder due to repetitive recycling of urine

IMAGING

- On voiding cystourethrogram (VCUG)
  - Large urinary bladder with smooth, thin wall
    - > 2x estimated normal bladder capacity
  - Unilateral or bilateral high-grade VUR
    - VUR may occur (during filling &/or voiding) into single system or lower pole of duplex system
    - Usually grade IV or V VUR
  - Voiding demonstrates complete bladder emptying
  - However, bladder rapidly refills (almost to capacity) by drainage of retained refluxed contrast from dilated ureters & collecting systems
    - Termed aberrant micturition, though bladder neck & urethra are normal

TOP DIFFERENTIAL DIAGNOSES

- Mechanical bladder outlet obstruction
  - Posterior urethral valves
  - Extrinsic/intrinsic mass
  - Obstructing ureterocele
- Functional bladder outlet obstruction
  - Neurogenic bladder
- Megacystis of unclear etiology
  - Prune belly (Eagle-Barrett) syndrome
  - Megacystis-microcolon-intestinal hypoperistalsis
  - Megalourethra

PATHOLOGY

- Ureter(s) & bladder act as common chamber

CLINICAL ISSUES

- Most commonly presents with urinary tract infections or abnormal prenatal ultrasound
- Bladder function may deteriorate if VUR is not improving

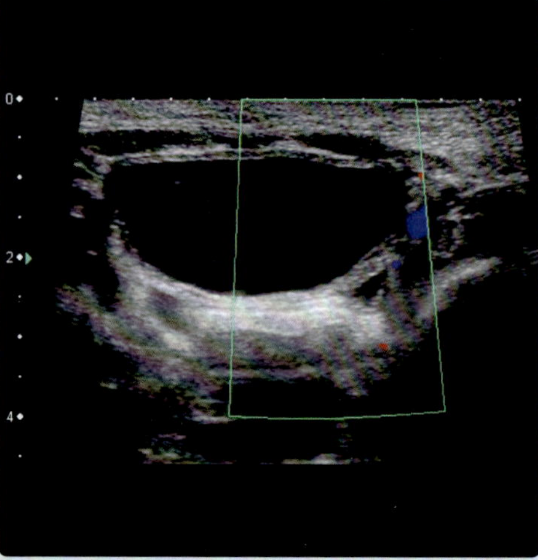

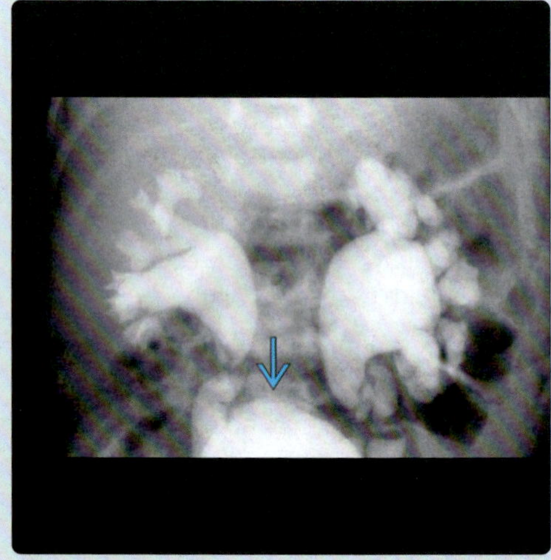

(Left) *Transverse ultrasound in a 5-day-old boy shows a well-distended urinary bladder with a dilated left distal ureter with moderate urothelial thickening, a nonspecific finding that can be seen in megaureter ± vesicoureteral reflux or could be related to infection.* **(Right)** *Frontal view of the kidneys during a voiding cystourethrogram (VCUG) in the same patient shows bilateral high-grade vesicoureteral reflux (VUR), L > R. Note the dome of a large thin-walled urinary bladder* ➙.

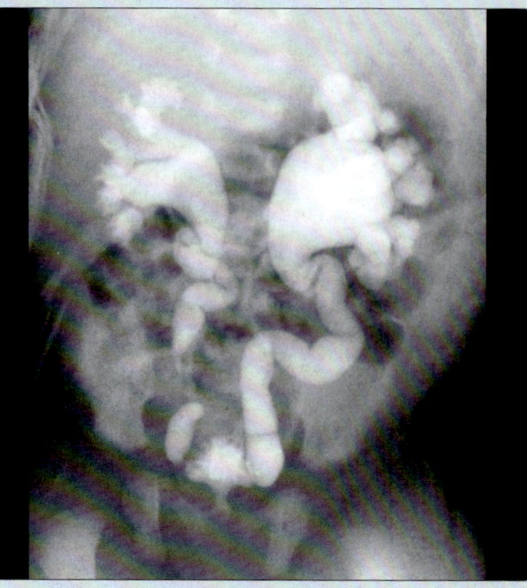

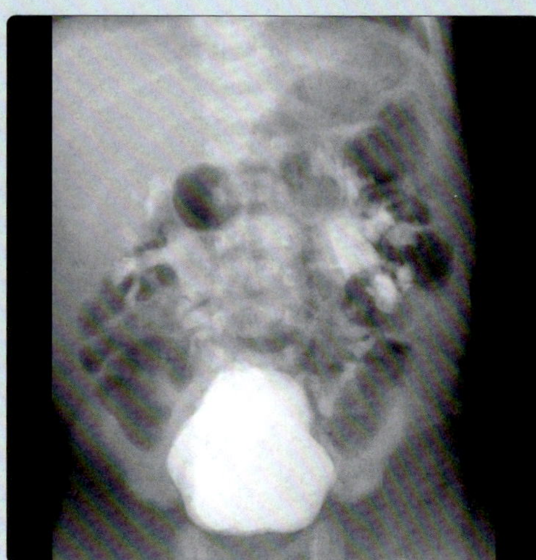

(Left) *Frontal VCUG in the same patient immediately after voiding shows complete bladder emptying. However, the ureters & collecting systems are full of contrast.* **(Right)** *Frontal VCUG in the same patient 5 minutes after voiding shows that the refluxed contrast from the ureters & collecting systems have completely refilled the bladder. This is seen in patients with high-grade VUR & is consistent with megaureter-megacystis physiology. If the VUR does not improve, this physiology can cause bladder dysfunction.*

KEY FACTS

TERMINOLOGY

- Megacystis-microcolon-intestinal hypoperistalsis syndrome (MMIHS): Rare disease of smooth muscle dysfunction resulting in poor motility of GI & GU tracts
- Synonyms: Berdon syndrome (described by Berdon et al. in 1976), familial visceral myopathy

IMAGING

- Variably dilated, featureless small bowel
    - Poor/absent peristalsis
- Colon is not dilated: Unused microcolon, no haustrations
- Abnormal bowel fixation: Malrotation
- Variable pelvocaliectasis & hydroureter
- Bladder is very dilated with poor or no emptying
    - Nonobstructive urinary tract dilation
        - Polyhydramnios in utero with megacystis in female fetus is suggestive
    - Bladder aspiration improves urinary tract dilation
- Severe abdominal distention → pulmonary compromise

TOP DIFFERENTIAL DIAGNOSES

- Posterior urethral valves
- Prune-belly syndrome
- Congenital megalourethra
- Cloacal malformation
- Hirschsprung disease

PATHOLOGY

- Mutation in *ACTG2* gene → abnormal smooth muscle actin
- Autosomal dominant, often sporadic
- *MYH11*, *MYL9*, & other genes reported

CLINICAL ISSUES

- Sex: F > > M
- Clinical triad: Abdominal distention, bilious emesis, failure to pass meconium or urine
- Previously lethal within 1 year
- Survival has improved with TPN & multivisceral transplant

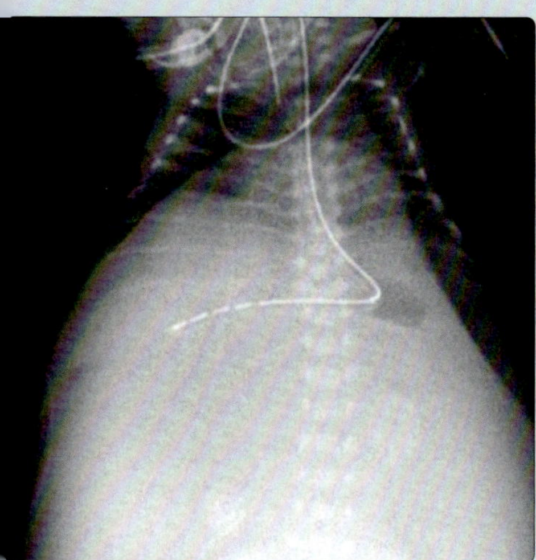

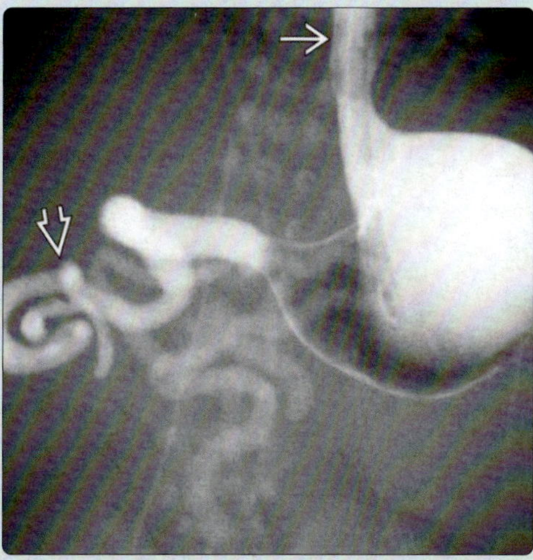

(Left) *Frontal view of the chest in a newborn with MMIHS shows massive abdominal distention impressing on the lung bases. Pulmonary function & development are compromised by mass effect both in utero & postnatally in MMIHS.* **(Right)** *Frontal upper GI through a nasogastric tube shows full-column gastroesophageal reflux into the mildly dilated esophagus ➡ with distal passage of contrast into the featureless tubular small bowel ➡ malpositioned in the right upper abdomen, consistent with malrotation.*

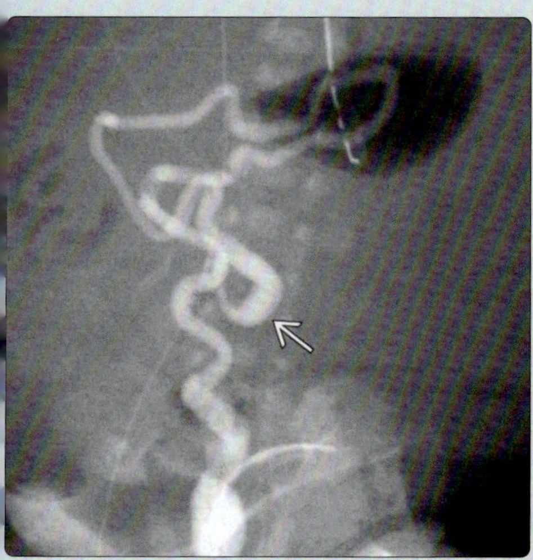

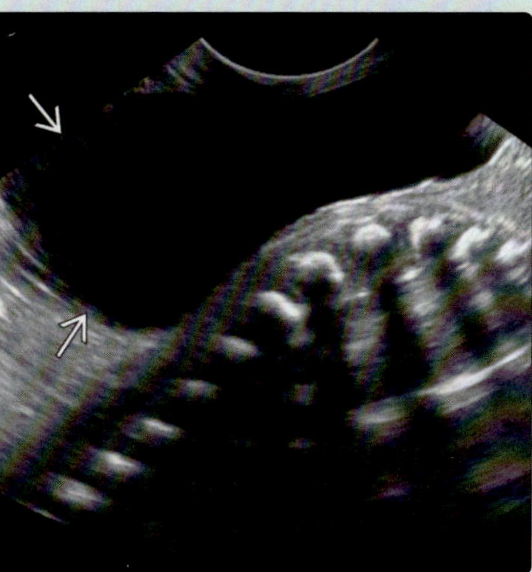

(Left) *Frontal contrast enema in a newborn with MMIHS shows a very small-caliber, unused microcolon without haustrations positioned in the midline abdomen. The cecum ➡ is overlying the spine. Marked hydronephrosis is displacing the bowel.* **(Right)** *Longitudinal ultrasound in a newborn with MMIHS shows a massively distended bladder ➡ extending toward the umbilicus, consistent with megacystis. A markedly enlarged bladder in utero is often the 1st clue to this diagnosis.*

KEY FACTS

TERMINOLOGY

- Prune-belly syndrome (PBS): Congenital triad of
  - Urinary tract dilation
  - Cryptorchidism
  - Abdominal wall muscle deficiency/laxity (with thin, wrinkled skin resembling prune)

IMAGING

- Radiographs: Enlarged abdomen with laterally bulging flanks
  - ± undulation or wrinkling of redundant skin
  - ± centralization of bowel gas due to markedly dilated ureters &/or renal collecting systems
  - Small, bell-shaped thorax ± pneumothorax
- VCUG: Marked bilateral vesicoureteral reflux
  - Dilated posterior urethra, but true mechanical obstruction is uncommon
- US: Dilated bladder & ureters; ± caliectasis, cystic renal dysplasia, urachal anomalies
  - Empty scrotum (cryptorchidism)
- MR urography can help delineate complex anatomy & assess renal drainage & dysplasia

TOP DIFFERENTIAL DIAGNOSES

- Posterior urethral valves
- Severe vesicoureteral reflux
- Primary megaureter
- Cloacal anomaly

CLINICAL ISSUES

- Large flaccid abdomen with redundant skin, cryptorchidism, ± Potter facies
- 1 in 30,000-40,000 live births
- 95-99% male
- Variable renal impairment & pulmonary hypoplasia determine prognosis
- Many survivors but with chronic health issues
  - Dialysis or renal transplant in 10-20%

(Left) *Frontal babygram in a newborn with prune-belly syndrome (PBS) shows an enlarged abdomen ➡ with bulging flanks & a small thorax. The massively distended urinary bladder shadow ➡ is seen in the lower abdomen.* **(Right)** *Longitudinal US in the same newborn with PBS shows numerous cysts ➡ scattered through the echogenic renal parenchyma with poor corticomedullary differentiation. The findings are typical of cystic dysplasia of the kidneys, likely due to longstanding bladder outlet obstruction.*

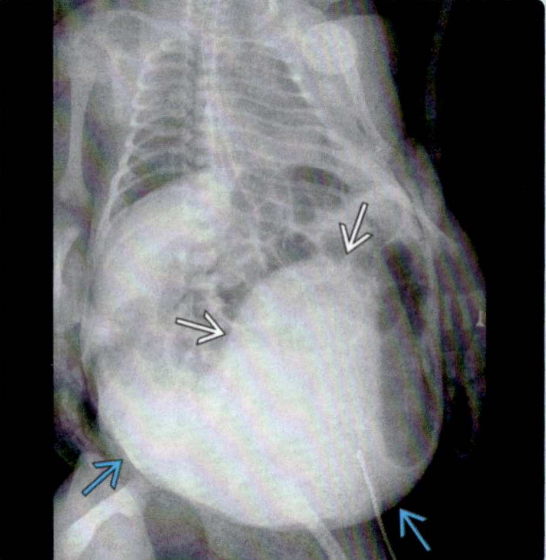

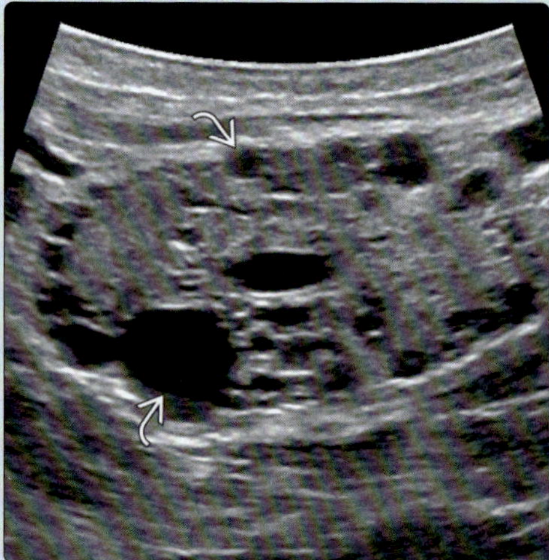

(Left) *Transverse US of the pelvis in a newborn with PBS shows an enlarged urinary bladder with markedly dilated ureters surrounding the rectum ➡.* **(Right)** *Frontal VCUG in a patient with PBS shows infused contrast filling the bladder & rapidly refluxing into markedly dilated, tortuous ureters bilaterally ➡. The ureters hold several times the volume of the bladder ➡. Note the wrinkled abdominal wall ➡.*

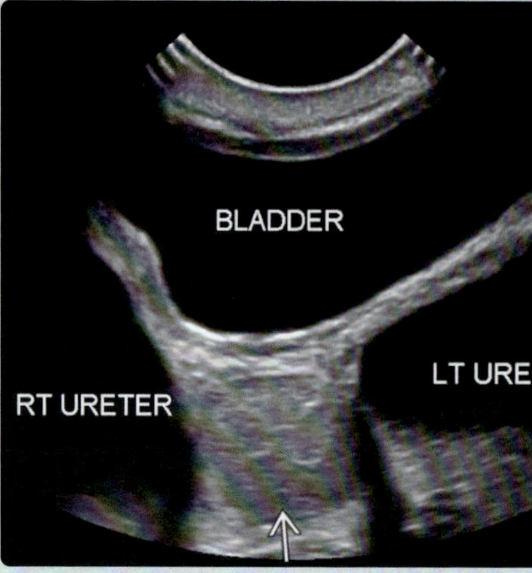

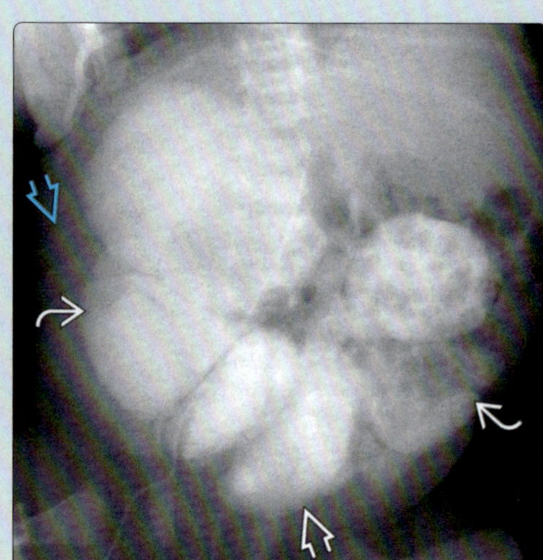

TERMINOLOGY

Synonyms

- Eagle-Barrett syndrome, abdominal muscle deficiency, triad syndrome

Definitions

- Prune-belly syndrome (PBS): Congenital triad of
  - Urinary tract dilation
  - Cryptorchidism
  - Abdominal wall muscle deficiency/laxity (with thin, wrinkled skin resembling prune)

IMAGING

General Features

- Best diagnostic clue
  - Urinary tract dilation with abdominal distention & laxity

Radiographic Findings

- Enlarged abdomen with laterally bulging flanks
  - ± undulation or wrinkling of redundant skin
- ± centralization of bowel gas due to markedly dilated ureters &/or renal collecting systems
- Small, bell-shaped thorax ± pneumothorax
  - Longstanding oligohydramnios → pulmonary hypoplasia

Fluoroscopic Findings

- Dilated bladder with lobulation, elongation, wall thickening, diverticula, ± urachal anomaly
- Marked bilateral vesicoureteral reflux
- Dilated posterior urethra; true mechanical obstruction is uncommon

Ultrasonographic Findings

- Dilated bladder & ureters, ± caliectasis & cystic renal dysplasia (echogenic kidneys with small peripheral cysts)
- Urachal anomalies are common
- Empty scrotum (cryptorchidism)
- Deficient abdominal wall musculature

MR Findings

- MR urography can help sort through complex anatomy, assessing renal function & drainage

Nuclear Medicine Findings

- Delayed drainage of ureters is common

DIFFERENTIAL DIAGNOSIS

Posterior Urethral Valves

- "Keyhole" bladder with high-grade obstruction of posterior urethra by valve tissue in males

Severe Vesicoureteral Reflux

- May be associated with megacystis but is typically isolated

Primary Megaureter

- Adynamic distal ureter with proximal dilation

Cloacal Anomaly

- Failure of separation of distal genitourinary & gastrointestinal tracts → single perineal orifice
- Hydrocolpos can cause bladder outlet obstruction

Megacystis-Microcolon-Intestinal Hypoperistalsis Syndrome

- Prognosis is worse in megacystis-microcolon-intestinal hypoperistalsis syndrome (MMIHS)
- MMIHS is more common in females

Congenital Megalourethra

- Findings of bladder outlet obstruction, but entire urethra is dilated

Urethral Atresia

- Very rare; anhydramnios → pulmonary hypoplasia

PATHOLOGY

General Features

- Etiology
  - Controversial: Mesodermal defect vs. early obstruction of bladder outlet
  - Pseudo PBS: Unilateral/incomplete triad, or females
  - Debated whether PBS is truly unique entity vs. phenotype of various bladder outlet pathologies

CLINICAL ISSUES

Presentation

- Large, flaccid abdomen with wrinkled, redundant skin
- Cryptorchidism
- Potter facies if oligohydramnios

Demographics

- 95-99% male
- 1 in 30,000-40,000 live births

Natural History & Prognosis

- Variable renal impairment & pulmonary hypoplasia determine prognosis
  - Perinatal mortality 10-25%
  - Respiratory complications dominate in infancy
  - Renal complications dominate in childhood
- Many survivors but with chronic health issues
  - Genitourinary: 100%
  - Cardiovascular: 10%
  - Orthopedic: 20%
  - Gastrointestinal

Treatment

- Bladder outlet: Vesicostomy, cystoplasty, Mitrofanoff
- Dialysis or renal transplant in 10-20%
- Orchiopexy
- Abdominoplasty, rectus femoris grafts

SELECTED REFERENCES

1. Loganathan AK et al: Unusual variant of pseudo prune belly syndrome. BMJ Case Rep. 13(10):e236611, 2020
2. Meyers ML et al: Imaging of fetal cystic kidney disease: multicystic dysplastic kidney versus renal cystic dysplasia. Pediatr Radiol. 50(13):1921-33, 2020
3. Arlen AM et al: Prune belly syndrome: current perspectives. Pediatric Health Med Ther. 10:75-81, 2019
4. White JT et al: Vesicoamniotic shunting improves outcomes in a subset of prune belly syndrome patients at a single tertiary center. Front Pediatr. 6:180, 2018
5. Yalcinkaya F et al: Outcomes of renal replacement therapy in boys with prune belly syndrome: findings from the ESPN/ERA-EDTA Registry. Pediatr Nephrol. 33(1):117-24, 2018

Posterior Urethral Valves

KEY FACTS

TERMINOLOGY

- Varying degrees of chronic urethral obstruction due to fusion &/or prominence of plicae colliculi (which are normal concentric folds within posterior urethra)
- Occurs exclusively in males

IMAGING

- Voiding cystourethrogram (VCUG)
  - Abrupt transition from dilated posterior urethra to small bulbar urethra at level of valvular tissue; actual valve tissue may not be visible
  - Bladder dilation, wall trabeculation, muscular hypertrophy, diverticula, ± patent urachus
  - Vesicoureteral reflux (50-70%)
- Ultrasound
  - Bilateral hydroureteronephrosis
  - Echogenic, dysplastic kidneys with poor corticomedullary differentiation ± cortical cysts, urinomas, ascites
  - Thickened, irregular bladder wall ± diverticula; dilated posterior urethra may be visible
  - Contrast-enhanced US (with transducer on perineum) can evaluate urethra during voiding

CLINICAL ISSUES

- Severity & duration of obstruction determine age of presentation & clinical symptoms, which include
  - Perinatal: Anuria, pulmonary hypoplasia → pneumothorax
  - Infancy: Urinary tract infection, sepsis, urinary retention, poor urinary stream, failure to thrive
  - Childhood: Abnormal voiding patterns, hesitancy, straining, poor stream, large postvoid residual, renal insufficiency/failure
- Catheterization at birth to relieve obstruction, followed by urgent endoscopic valve ablation
- 30-40% will eventually develop end-stage renal disease
- 75% have long-term urinary bladder dysfunction

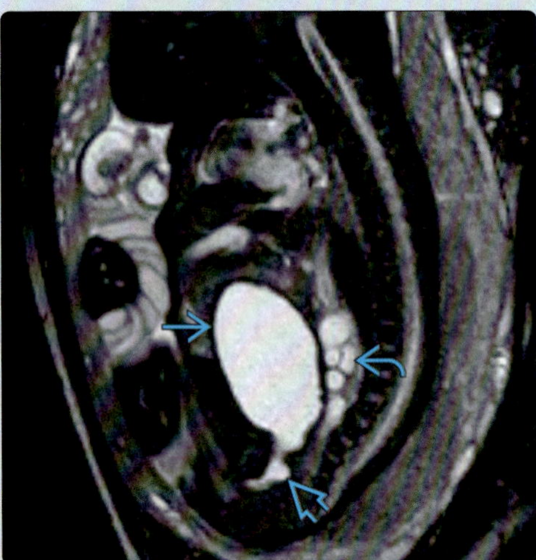

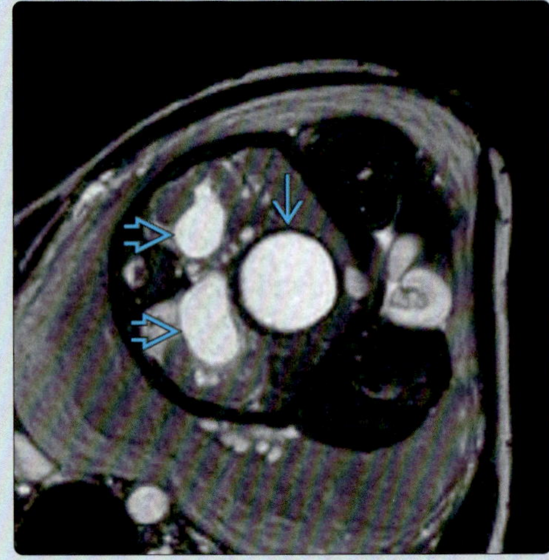

(Left) *Sagittal SSFP MR in a 33-weeks-gestation male fetus shows a dilated bladder ➡ with wall thickening & irregularity. Note the dilated posterior urethra ➡ & ureteral dilation ➡. There is also oligohydramnios with a small chest, suggesting pulmonary hypoplasia.* **(Right)** *Axial SSFP MR in the same fetus shows the dilated, thick-walled urinary bladder ➡ & oligohydramnios. Note the marked dilation of the bilateral renal pelves ➡.*

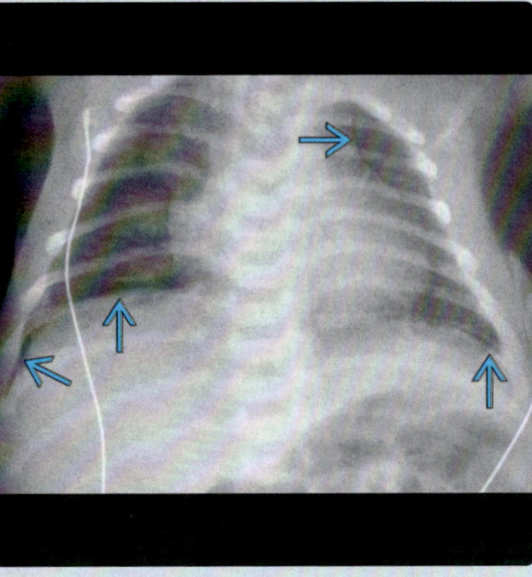

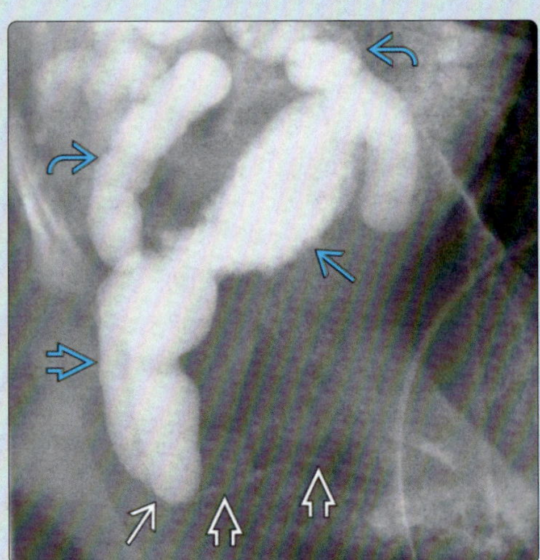

(Left) *AP radiograph in the same patient after delivery shows small bilateral pneumothoraces ➡ due to pulmonary hypoplasia.* **(Right)** *Oblique VCUG 3 days later in the same patient shows marked dilation of the posterior urethra ➡ with thin valve tissue ➡ visualized at the transition to a small-caliber anterior urethra ➡. The urinary bladder is trabeculated ➡, & there is bilateral grade V vesicoureteral reflux (VUR) ➡, incompletely visualized on this image.*

TERMINOLOGY

Abbreviations

- Posterior urethral valves (PUV)

Definitions

- PUV: Varying degrees of chronic urethral obstruction due to fusion &/or prominence of plicae colliculi (which are normal concentric folds within posterior urethra)
- Valve bladder: Varying degrees of urinary bladder dysfunction secondary to chronic bladder obstruction

IMAGING

General Features

- Best diagnostic clue
  - Dilated posterior male urethra with distinct caliber change at level of valves
    - Actual valve tissue is very thin, may not be visible
  - Diagnosis is made on voiding cystourethrogram (VCUG), cystoscopy, or cystosonography
- Location
  - PUV lie just distal to prostatic urethra

Radiographic Findings

- Dilated urinary bladder creates pseudomass in pelvis, displacing bowel loops superiorly
- Perinephric urinoma, dilated ureters, & dilated renal collecting systems may cause additional mass effect
- ± small, bell-shaped thorax of pulmonary hypoplasia, ± pneumothorax & pneumomediastinum

Fluoroscopic Findings

- Voiding cystourethrogram
  - Hallmark: Abrupt caliber change in posterior urethra
    - Dilated posterior urethra gives rise to small-caliber bulbar & penile urethra
    - Actual valve tissue need not be seen on imaging to make diagnosis
    - Note that leaving urethral catheter in place during voiding may "stent" valve tissue, obscuring caliber change & pushing valve tissue against urethral wall
      - Removal of catheter for diagnostic purposes should be approved by clinical service (if bladder outlet obstruction is suspected prior to test)
  - Associated findings
    - Bladder dilation, wall trabeculation, muscular hypertrophy, diverticula
    - Vesicoureteral reflux (VUR) in 50-70%
    - Urinary ascites
    - Urinoma/perinephric urine collection
    - Reflux into utricle, vas deferens, or other ducts
    - Patent urachus

Ultrasonographic Findings

- Grayscale ultrasound
  - Bilateral or unilateral hydroureteronephrosis
  - Echogenic, dysplastic kidneys with poor corticomedullary differentiation ± cortical cysts, urinomas, ascites
  - Lobular bladder with thickened, irregular wall ± diverticula
  - Angling transducer toward bladder neck (or placing on perineum) may reveal dilated posterior urethra
- Cystosonography or contrast-enhanced US
  - Eliminates radiation of fluoroscopic VCUG
  - Exam is performed from transperineal approach
  - Catheterization (to instill bladder contrast) & voiding during imaging are still required

MR Findings

- Fetal MR
  - Shows bladder outlet obstruction with dilated posterior urethra as well as hydroureteronephrosis & cystic renal dysplasia
  - May be used to measure lung volumes in setting of oligohydramnios
- MR urogram
  - Anatomic findings mirror US, though dilated ureteral course is more discernible by MR
  - Physiologic study can be performed with dynamic contrast evaluation of renal function & drainage
    - Caution is required with low glomerular filtration rate due to concerns of gadolinium retention & nephrogenic systemic fibrosis

Nuclear Medicine Findings

- Cortical imaging for scarring & differential renal function
- Diuretic renogram to evaluate additional obstructing lesion of ureter or renal pelvis

Other Modality Findings

- At direct cystoscopy, valve tissue is translucent & may be pushed back against outer walls of urethra by inflowing irrigation fluid
- Similar drawbacks to fluoroscopic retrograde urethrogram, which may not show dynamic change in urethral caliber

Imaging Recommendations

- Best imaging tool
  - Fluoroscopic VCUG vs. cystosonography with contrast

DIFFERENTIAL DIAGNOSIS

Prune-Belly Syndrome (Eagle-Barrett)

- Hydroureteronephrosis
  - Posterior urethra is dilated but nonobstructed
  - Entire urethra may be dilated
- Absence/hypotonia of abdominal wall musculature
- Cryptorchidism

Anterior Urethral Valves

- Very rare entity where prominent semilunar fold obstructs anterior urethra

Voiding Dysfunction

- Detrusor external sphincter dyssynergia can resemble PUV transiently (due to opening of bladder neck with bulging posterior urethra & contracted external sphincter)
- Appearance is not persistent

Ureterocele

- Prolapse into posterior urethra can cause obstruction

Megalourethra

- Rare entity where entire length of urethra is markedly dilated due to absence of corpus spongiosum

Urethral Stricture

- Post surgical, post traumatic, or post infectious
- History is key to making this diagnosis

Megacystis-Microcolon-Intestinal Hypoperistalsis Syndrome

- M:F = 1:4
- Dilated hypoperistaltic bowel with malrotation
- Nonobstructive megacystis

Megacystis-Megaureter Association

- Large-volume VUR cycling between dilated upper tracts & bladder

PATHOLOGY

General Features

- Associated abnormalities
  - Longstanding oligohydramnios leads to pulmonary hypoplasia, which may not be survivable

Staging, Grading, & Classification

- Type I (most common): Anterior fusion of plicae colliculi
- Type II (rarest): Longitudinal folds from verumontanum to bladder neck
- Type III (rare): Disc, ring, or windsock-type tissue distal to verumontanum

Gross Pathologic & Surgical Features

- Valve tissue is typically very thin but functions like sail, causing near complete obstruction to antegrade flow of urine

Microscopic Features

- Valve tissue is thin, normal urothelium
- Bladder wall will show muscular hypertrophy & fibrosis
- Kidneys may show tubulointerstitial fibrosis & dysplasia

CLINICAL ISSUES

Presentation

- Most common signs/symptoms
  - Severity & duration of obstruction determine age of presentation & clinical symptoms, which include
    - Perinatally: Oligohydramnios, hydronephrosis ± renal dysplasia & renal failure, anuria, urinary ascites, urinoma, pulmonary hypoplasia
    - In infancy: Urinary tract infection, sepsis, urinary retention, poor urinary stream, failure to thrive
    - In childhood: Abnormal voiding patterns, hesitancy, straining, poor stream, large postvoid residual, renal insufficiency/failure
  - Classically 1/3 present at each age: Perinatal, infancy, childhood
    - Up to 1/2 of all cases are now diagnosed in utero

Demographics

- Sex
  - Males only
- Epidemiology
  - Incidence: 1 in 4,000-5,000 births

Natural History & Prognosis

- Varies with degree of renal dysplasia related to chronic obstruction & VUR
- Unilateral reflux & urinary ascites are protective for contralateral kidney (relieve pressure)
- Renal insufficiency has bimodal peak, developing in 1st months of life vs. adolescence after initial improvement
  - Lowest creatinine in 1st year of life (nadir Cr) has some prognostic value
- 17-40% will eventually develop end-stage renal disease
- 75% have long-term urinary bladder dysfunction
  - Poor bladder compliance, overactivity, & myogenic failure (incomplete bladder emptying, overflow incontinence)

Treatment

- Catheterization at birth to relieve obstruction
- Urgent endoscopic valve ablation
  - VUR ↓ by 30% after valve ablation
  - Improved renal function with early treatment
- Long-term follow-up is necessary to monitor renal function & bladder compliance
  - Urodynamics to assess bladder capacity, overactivity, contractility
  - Treated with anticholinergics, alpha-adrenergic blockers, bladder neck incision
- Secondary bladder surgeries are often needed: Bladder augmentation or continent diversion (Mitrofanoff)
  - ↑ risk of malignancy decades after bowel augmentation
- Dialysis, renal transplant for end-stage renal disease
  - 10-15% of pediatric renal transplants are due to PUV
  - Comparable transplant survival rates in PUV patients vs. patients with nonobstructive etiologies
- Fetal intervention is performed in cases of severe oligohydramnios; conflicting data on long-term renal function benefit, though procedures may ↑ "pulmonary survivors" needing renal replacement therapy
  - Serial amnioinfusions to restore normal amniotic fluid volume (to promote lung development)
  - Serial bladder taps vs. vesicoamniotic shunt
  - In utero cystoscopy with valve fulguration

SELECTED REFERENCES

1. Expert Panel on Pediatric Imaging et al: ACR Appropriateness Criteria® antenatal hydronephrosis-infant. J Am Coll Radiol. 17(11S):S367-79, 2020
2. Manyevitch R et al: Adolescent presentation of posterior urethral valves. Urology. 136:e1-2, 2020
3. Shekar PA et al: "When ablation goes wrong"- urethral strictures after ablation of posterior urethral valves-characteristics, management and outcomes". J Pediatr Urol. 16(6):843.e1-9, 2020
4. Vinit N et al: Fetal cystoscopy and vesicoamniotic shunting in lower urinary tract obstruction: long-term outcome and current technical limitations. Fetal Diagn Ther. 47(1):74-83, 2020
5. Brownlee E et al: Current epidemiology and antenatal presentation of posterior urethral valves: outcome of BAPS CASS National Audit. J Pediatr Surg. 54(2):318-21, 2019
6. Lundar L et al: Prenatal extravasation of urine seems to preserve renal function in boys with posterior urethral valves. J Pediatr Urol. 15(3):241.e1-7, 2019
7. Farrugia MK et al: Report on The Society for Fetal Urology panel discussion on the selection criteria and intervention for fetal bladder outlet obstruction. J Pediatr Urol. 13(4):345-51, 2017
8. Fernbach SK et al: Pediatric voiding cystourethrography: a pictorial guide. Radiographics. 20(1):155-68; discussion 168-71, 2000

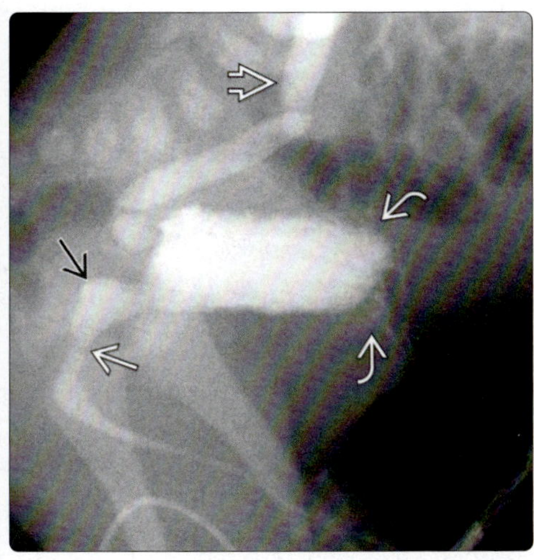

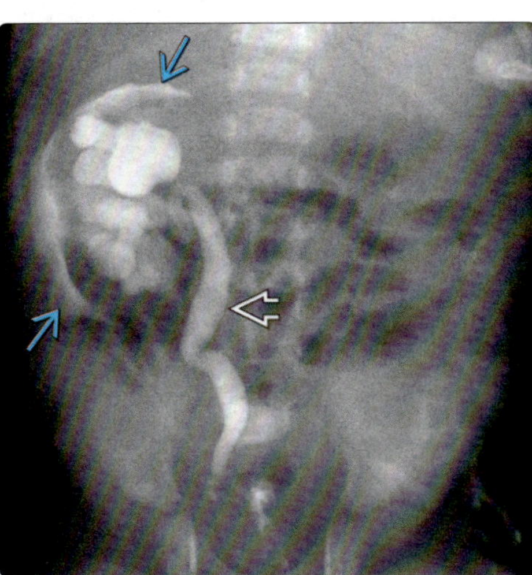

(Left) *Lateral VCUG in a newborn with PUV shows the thin valvular tissue* ➡ *at the inferior margin of the dilated posterior urethra* ➡*. The urinary bladder wall is markedly thickened with contrast extending between the trabeculations* ➡*. High-grade unilateral VUR* ➡ *is noted.* **(Right)** *Frontal VCUG in the same patient after voiding shows contrast pooling around the right kidney* ➡*. This urinoma is due to high-pressure VUR* ➡ *causing a forniceal rupture in the setting of a chronic bladder outlet obstruction.*

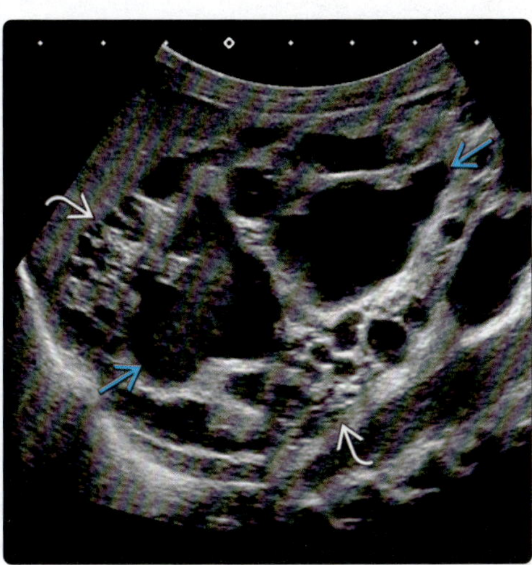

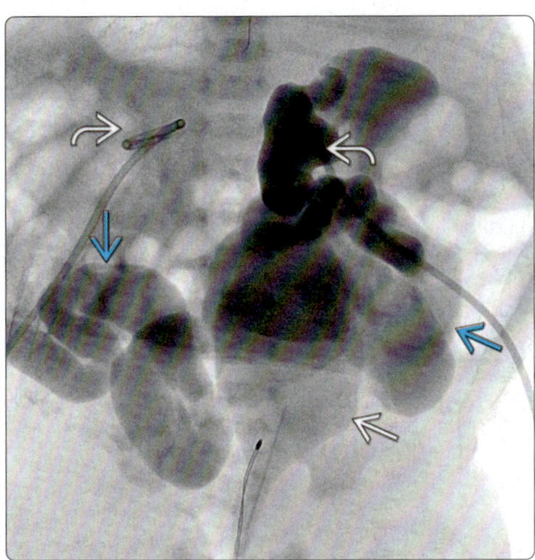

(Left) *Longitudinal ultrasound of the left kidney in a newborn with PUV shows marked pelvocaliectasis* ➡ *& cystic dysplastic changes of the renal cortex* ➡ *due to chronic obstruction in utero.* **(Right)** *Frontal prone radiograph during bilateral percutaneous nephrostomy tube placements* ➡ *shows contrast filling severely dilated ureters* ➡ *& a lobulated urinary bladder* ➡*.*

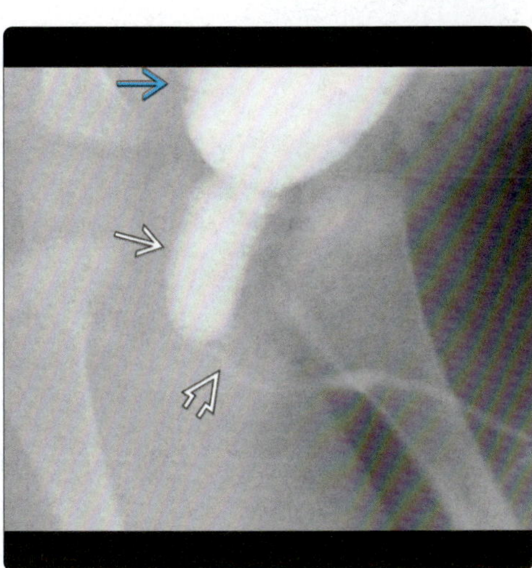

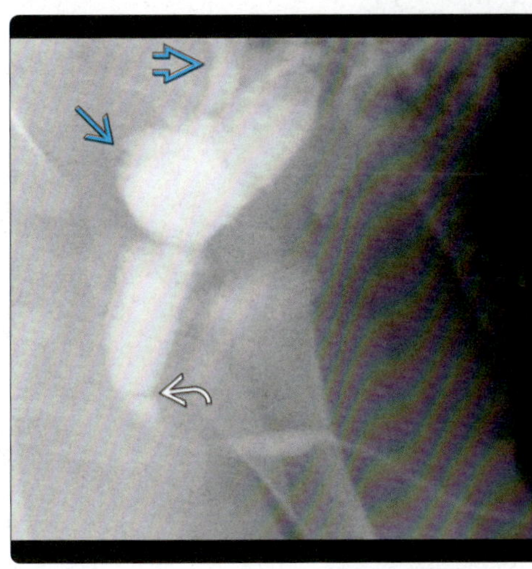

(Left) *Fluoroscopic image in a 4-month-old during VCUG voiding phase shows marked dilation of the posterior urethra* ➡ *with an abrupt change in urethral caliber* ➡*. Note the bladder wall hypertrophy* ➡ *visible at the bladder base.* **(Right)** *Additional fluoroscopic spot image in the same infant just moments later shows contrast surrounding the valve tissue* ➡*, illustrating the dynamic nature of the VCUG findings in PUV. Bladder wall hypertrophy* ➡ *& VUR* ➡ *are also visible.*

Urachal Abnormalities

KEY FACTS

TERMINOLOGY

- Persistence of all or portion of connection between bladder dome & umbilicus; remnant of fetal allantoic stalk

IMAGING

- Patent urachus or urachal fistula
  - Open channel from bladder to umbilicus through which urine can leak
- Urachal sinus
  - Persistence of superficial segment of channel opening onto skin surface
- Urachal diverticulum
  - Persistence of deep segment of tract, creating point or diverticulum off of anterior-superior bladder wall
- Urachal cyst
  - Persistence of intermediary segment with fibrous attachments to bladder & umbilicus
- Size & shape depend on type of remnant, location, & presence of inflammation
- Helpful hints for US scanning
  - Bladder should be fairly full
  - Patient should be relaxed as Valsalva maneuver can squeeze fluid out of patent tract
  - Begin scanning at inferior bladder level & sweep transducer upward toward umbilicus
  - Gentle pressure on bladder dome can push fluid into patent tract to aid visualization

CLINICAL ISSUES

- Incidence of patent urachus: 1 in 40,000
  - Other urachal anomalies are more common
  - More cases are now recognized with ↑ cross-sectional imaging
- Generally, prognosis is excellent
  - Urachal tract is resected; no further follow-up is needed
    - Open surgery previously, now laparoscopic
- Risk of malignancy in adults if not resected
  - Urachal malignancies: < 1% of all bladder cancers

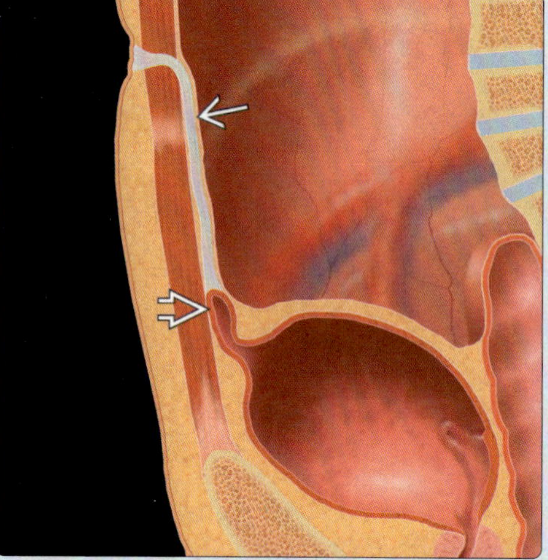

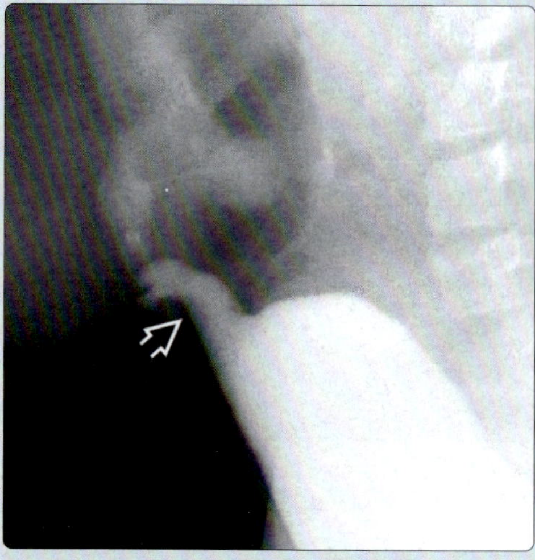

(Left) *Sagittal graphic shows a urachal diverticulum ➡ & fibrotic tract ➡ to the umbilicus. When the entire tract remains open, it is called a patent urachus. The urachal sinus & urachal cyst are additional variations along this spectrum.* **(Right)** *Lateral voiding cystourethrogram (VCUG) in an infant with a history of umbilical drainage shows a tubular, contrast-filled connection ➡ between the bladder dome & the umbilicus, consistent with a patent urachus.*

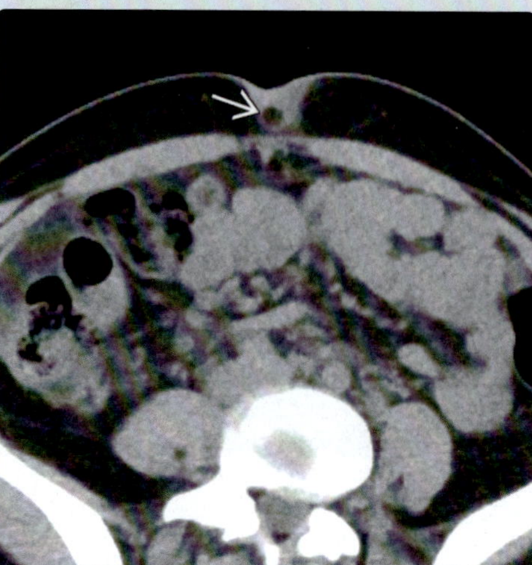

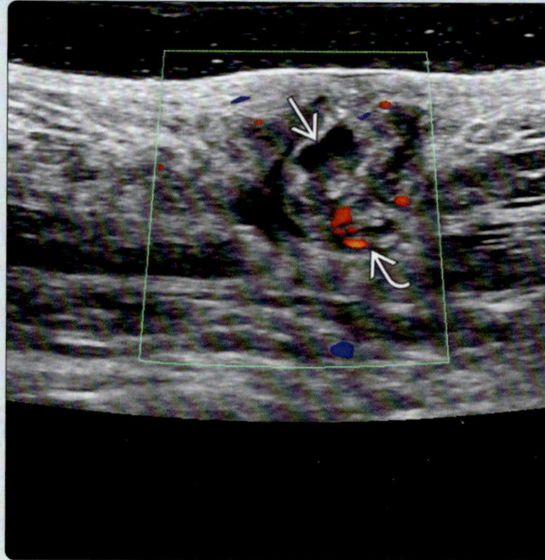

(Left) *Axial NECT in a teenager shows a low-density cyst ➡ at the base of the umbilicus with thickening of the periumbilical tissues.* **(Right)** *Longitudinal US in the same patient shows mild hyperemia ➡ & heterogeneity of the periumbilical tissues with a small fluid collection centrally ➡. A small urachal cyst was resected. Additional considerations for this appearance could include an evolving hematoma, abscess, inflamed dermoid, or other lesions.*

TERMINOLOGY

Synonyms

- Patent urachus, urachal fistula, urachal remnant, urachal cyst, urachal sinus, urachal diverticulum

Definitions

- Partial or complete persistence of connection between bladder dome & umbilicus; remnant of fetal allantoic stalk

IMAGING

General Features

- Best diagnostic clue
  - Fluid or cyst along tract between bladder dome & umbilicus ± umbilical drainage
- Location
  - Midline between dome of bladder & umbilicus
- Size
  - Variable
- Morphology
  - Patent urachus or urachal fistula
    - Open channel from bladder to umbilicus through which urine can leak
  - Urachal sinus
    - Persistence of superficial segment of channel opening onto skin surface
  - Urachal diverticulum
    - Persistence of deep segment of channel creating point or diverticulum off of anterior-superior bladder wall
  - Urachal cyst
    - Localized, fluid-containing intermediary segment with fibrous attachments to bladder & umbilicus
    - Case reports of intravesical urachal cysts along anterior superior bladder wall

Ultrasonographic Findings

- Grayscale ultrasound
  - Size & shape depend on type of remnant, location, & presence of inflammation
    - Diverticulum of fully patent urachus is contiguous with anterior superior aspect of bladder
  - Often has thick, well-defined wall (especially if inflamed)
  - Wall may have layered appearance mimicking gut signature sign
  - Remnant may or may not contain fluid
  - Fluid-debris level may be present in urachal cyst
- Color Doppler
  - Doppler is useful in
    - Assessing degree of hyperemia when infected
    - Excluding vascular anomaly
- Helpful hints when scanning for urachal remnants
  - Bladder should be fairly full
  - Patient should be relaxed as Valsalva maneuver can squeeze fluid out of patent tract
  - Begin scanning at bladder level & sweep transducer upward toward umbilicus
  - Gentle pressure on bladder dome can push fluid into patent tract to aid visualization

Fluoroscopic Findings

- Voiding cystourethrogram (VCUG)
  - Best test to document patency of urachus
  - Tends to underestimate length or extent of remnant
  - Inflammation along tract can intermittently block lumen
  - True lateral views are necessary (with full bladder)
  - Radiopaque marker on umbilicus can be helpful

CT Findings

- Occasionally recognized incidentally on CT scans performed for other reasons
  - Infected urachal cyst may present with "rule out abscess" manifestations
- Look for round, triangular, or tubular, fluid-filled structure extending along anterior aspect of peritoneal cavity between urinary bladder & umbilicus
  - Lies superficial to parietal peritoneal layer
- Localized cyst may be seen when proximal & distal segments of tract are fibrotic
- Surrounding inflammation is common

MR Findings

- Similar findings as CT
- Often incidental finding on MR scan

Nuclear Medicine Findings

- Flow of renally excreted radiotracers into tract from urinary bladder may mimic other pathology
  - FDG PET could falsely suggest malignancy

Imaging Recommendations

- Best imaging tool
  - Ultrasound defines static anatomy well
  - VCUG will show flow dynamics & confirm patency

DIFFERENTIAL DIAGNOSIS

Granulation Tissue of Umbilical Stump

- Hypoechoic tissue often confused with urachal remnants, especially urachal sinus
- No deeper discrete fluid-filled tract is visible

Omphalitis

- Poorly defined, heterogeneous inflammation of anterior abdominal wall just deep to umbilicus
- Can be present in conjunction with urachal remnant
- In severe cases, may need to treat with antibiotics & reevaluate

Obliterated Median Umbilical Ligament

- Normally closed urachus may remain visible as nondistensible tract

Umbilical Hernia

- Usually readily discerned by physical exam & imaging
- Hernia may contain peristalsing bowel or omentum
- Helpful to scan patient upright & with Valsalva

Hemangioma of Umbilical Cord

- Doppler ultrasound will show high volume of low-resistance arterial blood flow in lobulated mass rather than stagnant fluid

PATHOLOGY

General Features

- Etiology
  - In embryos, allantois
    - Forms from caudal end of yolk sac
    - Functions as primitive bladder as well as blood-forming organ
    - Normally involutes by 12th week of gestation
    - Obliteration forms median umbilical ligament
    - Segments may persist as urachal remnants
  - Urachus lies in space of Retzius
    - Between transversalis fascia anteriorly & peritoneum posteriorly
- Associated abnormalities
  - Periumbilical associations
    - Omphalocele
    - Omphalomesenteric remnant
  - Bladder outlet associations
    - Posterior urethral valves
    - Urethral atresia
    - Cloacal anomalies
    - Urogenital sinus malformation
  - Miscellaneous associations
    - Myelomeningocele (perhaps because of neurogenic bladder)
    - Unilateral kidney & other renal anomalies
    - Vaginal atresia

Gross Pathologic & Surgical Features

- Well-defined stalk with mucosal lining & varying degrees of fibrosis/lumen obliteration

Microscopic Features

- Cellular histology varies, not simple urothelium
  - Transitional cell epithelium
  - Columnar epithelium
  - Glandular epithelium
  - Squamous epithelium
- Varied cell types explain variety of malignant cell lines found in adults with urachal tumors
- Fibrostromal histology has low risk of malignant transformation, while epithelial histology has higher risk
  - Imaging & symptoms do not differentiate between histologic subtypes

CLINICAL ISSUES

Presentation

- Most common signs/symptoms
  - Varies with type of urachal remnant
    - Patent urachus presents with drainage from umbilicus, urinary tract infection, & relapsing periumbilical inflammation
    - Occasionally, urachus remains patent in response to bladder outlet obstruction (posterior urethral valves, pelvic mass, etc.) & will close when outlet is repaired
    - Urachal sinus presents with periumbilical tenderness, wet umbilicus, or nonhealing granulation of umbilicus
    - Urachal cyst presents in childhood or adolescence with suprapubic mass, fever, pain, & voiding issues
    - Urachal diverticula are often asymptomatic & discovered incidentally; rarely, they enlarge, fail to drain during urination, & become predisposed to infection or stone formation

Demographics

- Age
  - Patent urachus is seen primarily in newborns
  - Urachal sinus is also typically diagnosed within 1st few months of life
  - Urachal cysts may go undetected until childhood or adulthood
  - Urachal diverticulum often goes undetected (autopsy finding)
- Epidemiology
  - Incidence of patent urachus: 1 in 40,000
  - Other urachal anomalies are more common, though reliable statistics are not available

Natural History & Prognosis

- Generally excellent prognosis
  - Urachal tract is resected; no further follow-up needed
- Risk of malignancy without resection: Adenocarcinoma, mucinous cystadenocarcinoma, villous adenoma, yolk sac carcinoma
  - Urachal malignancies: < 1% of all bladder cancers
  - Typically occur in patients 40-70 years of age
  - Majority of cancers occur in men (~ 75%)
  - Present with pain, hematuria, or mucinous micturition
  - Local tumor invasion is common at diagnosis of urachal cancer
  - Tumor rupture → pseudomyxoma peritonei
- Reports of using urachal remnant instead of appendix for Mitrofanoff

Treatment

- Resection of entire tract
  - Open surgery previously, now laparoscopic
- Often performed in staged fashion
  - Inflammation & infection are treated, allowed to heal
  - Definitive surgery is delayed
- When accompanied by bladder outlet obstruction
  - Surgery to fix outlet obstruction must be performed 1st
    - Patent urachus serves as pop-off valve in these cases
  - Following correction of bladder outlet problems, allow ~ 1 year for patent urachus to close independently
  - If drainage persists, reassess bladder outlet; if functioning well, resect tract

SELECTED REFERENCES

1. Keçeli AM et al: Are urachal remnants really rare in children? An observational study. Eur J Pediatr. 180(6):1987-90, 2021
2. Das JP et al: The urachus revisited: multimodal imaging of benign & malignant urachal pathology. Br J Radiol. 93(1110):20190118, 2020
3. Tsai IS et al: An infected urachal cyst presenting as acute abdominal pain in a child: a case report. Medicine (Baltimore). 99(5):e18884, 2020
4. Buddha S et al: Imaging of urachal anomalies. Abdom Radiol (NY). 44(12):3978-89, 2019
5. Parada Villavicencio C et al: Imaging of the urachus: anomalies, complications, and mimics. Radiographics. 36(7):2049-63, 2016
6. Yu JS et al: Urachal remnant diseases: spectrum of CT and US findings. Radiographics. 21(2):451-61, 2001

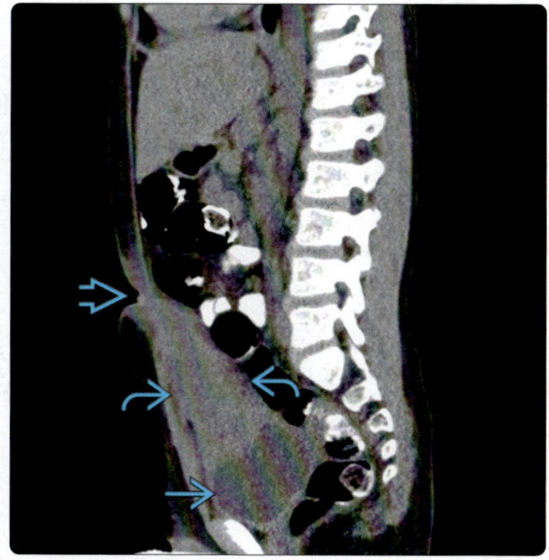

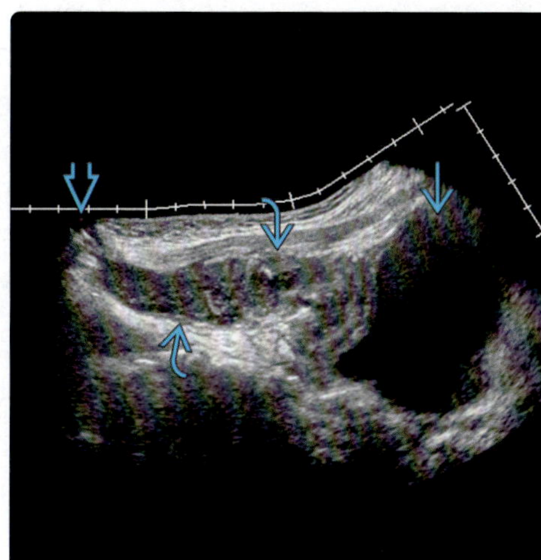

(Left) *Sagittal NECT in a 7-year-old boy with abdominal pain & fever shows mildly heterogeneous soft tissue density ➢ between the bladder ➞ & umbilicus ⇨. The appendix was normal (not shown), & US was ordered for further evaluation.* **(Right)** *Sagittal US in the same patient shows a complex collection ➢ extending from the bladder ➞ to the umbilicus ⇨. No flow of internal mobile contents to the bowel, bladder, or skin was demonstrated. At surgery, an infected urachal remnant was resected.*

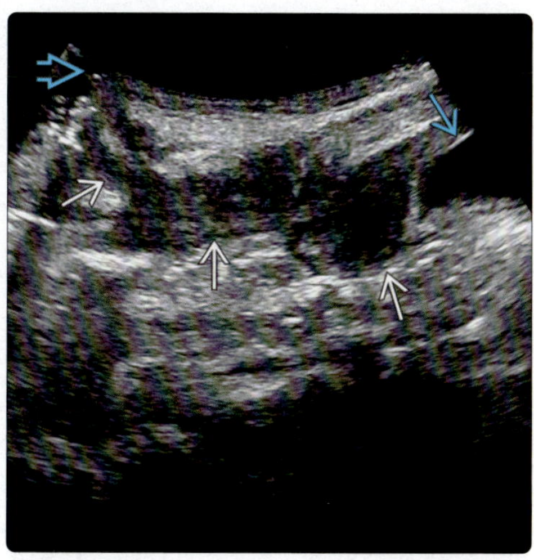

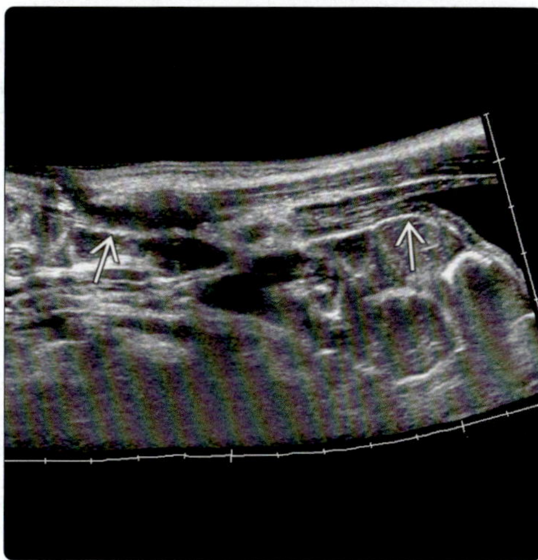

(Left) *Longitudinal US in a 6-year-old boy with fever & periumbilical pain shows an irregularly shaped hypoechoic tract ➔ between the bladder ➞ & umbilicus ⇨. Foul smelling fluid/urine was expressed from the tract during the scan, consistent with an infected patent urachus.* **(Right)** *Longitudinal US in the same patient after a course of antibiotics shows a ↓ caliber of the patent urachus ➔, which was subsequently surgically excised. Note the pointed shape of the bladder dome (which is usually round).*

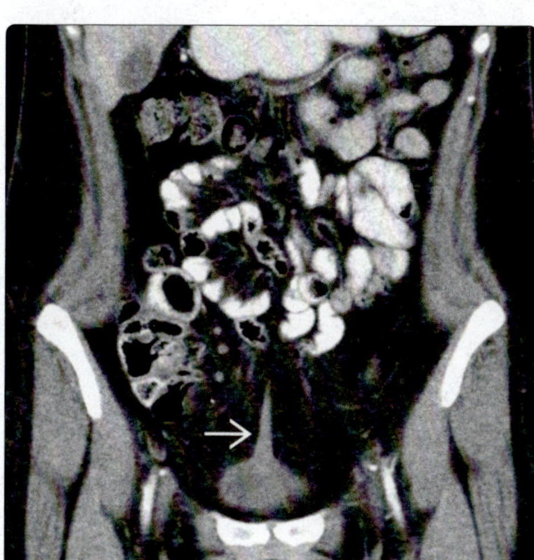

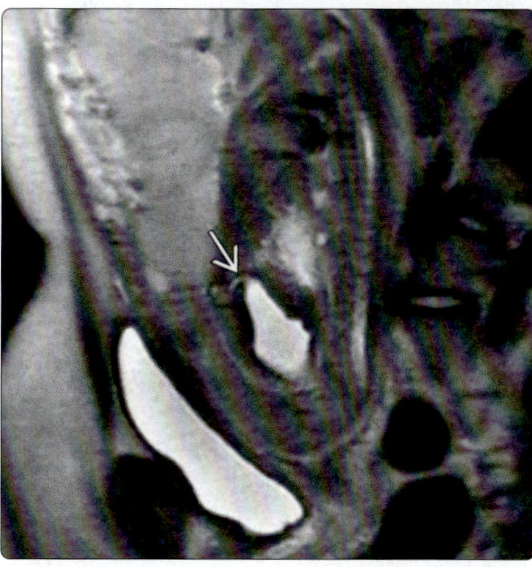

(Left) *Coronal CECT performed for suspected appendicitis in a patient with pain shows a thin, triangular soft tissue lesion extending from the dome of the bladder ➔ toward the umbilicus, either a urachal remnant or bladder diverticulum.* **(Right)** *Sagittal SSFSE T2 MR of a fetus with bladder outlet obstruction shows high signal intensity fluid in a small-caliber patent urachus ➔ helping to decompress the thick-walled urinary bladder. Note the lack of amniotic fluid surrounding the fetus.*

Cloacal Malformation

KEY FACTS

TERMINOLOGY

- Anorectal malformation of female patients in which rectum, urethra, & vagina converge to form common channel draining to single perineal orifice (which allows clinical diagnosis)
- Imaging is performed for operative planning & to evaluate associated malformations

IMAGING

- Radiographs: Multiple dilated bowel loops, ± bowel Ca^{2+}
- US: Renal, pelvic, & spine
  - Cystic pelvic mass: Most commonly hydrocolpos (> 30% of all cloaca patients)
    - Rarely dilated bladder, meconium pseudocyst
  - ± hemivaginas/hemiuteri (40%)
  - ± hydroureteronephrosis
  - ± echogenic calcified meconium in dilated bowel or bladder
  - ± spinal anomalies
- Postcolostomy distal colostogram/cloacagram prior to definitive repair
  - Fluoroscopy, MR, or contrasted US

TOP DIFFERENTIAL DIAGNOSES

- Anorectal malformation
- Other low/distal neonatal bowel obstructions
- Isolated hydrocolpos
- Megacystis-microcolon-intestinal hypoperistalsis syndrome

CLINICAL ISSUES

- Hydrocolpos → ↓ renal function without urgent drainage
- Prognosis is based on common channel length
  - < 3 cm: Most common type (56%), less complex repair, better functional prognosis
  - > 3 cm: Less common type (44%), more complex repair, worse functional prognosis

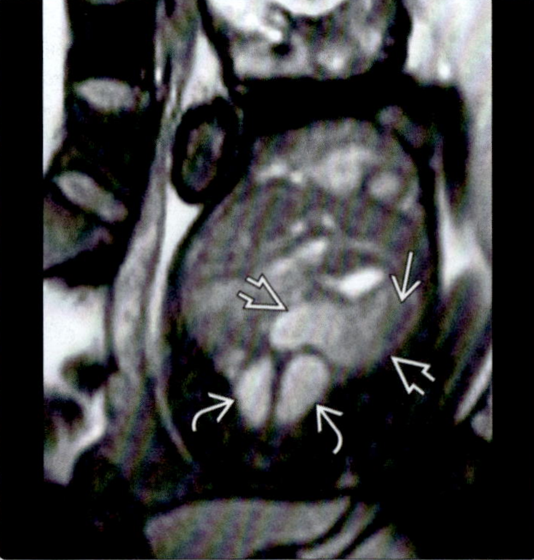

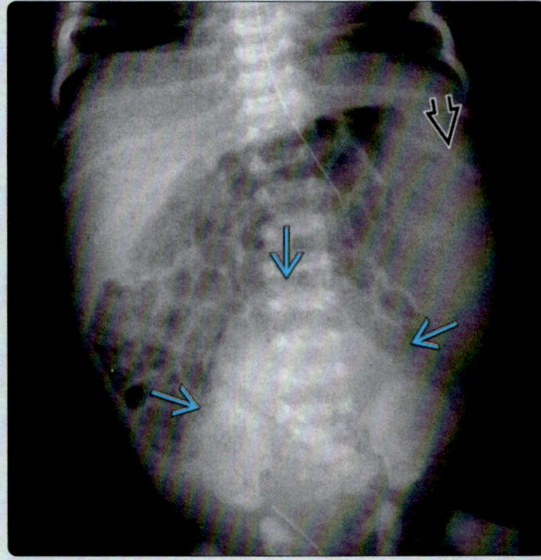

(Left) *Coronal SSFP MR in a 31-weeks-gestation female fetus with a cloaca shows 2 dilated hemivaginas (HVs) ➡ & a dilated but tapering distal colon ➡. The heterogeneous, low-signal material ➡ within the dilated colon suggests meconium ± calcification.* **(Right)** *AP abdominal radiograph in a 1-day-old girl with a cloaca shows a large soft tissue mass arising from the pelvis ➡, displacing bowel superiorly & laterally, likely representing hydrocolpos. The left flank soft tissue mass is likely due to a meconium-filled colon ➡.*

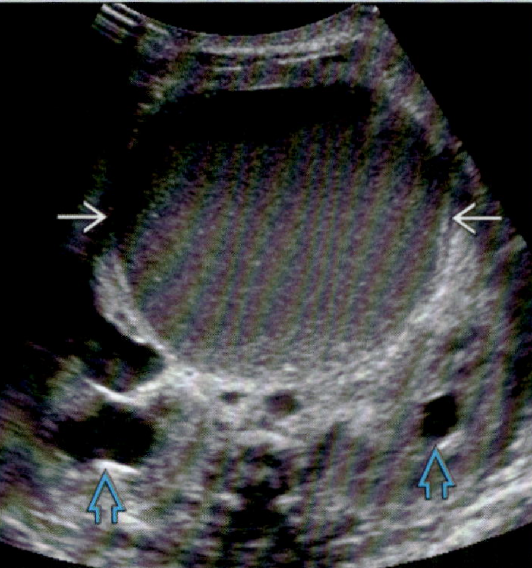

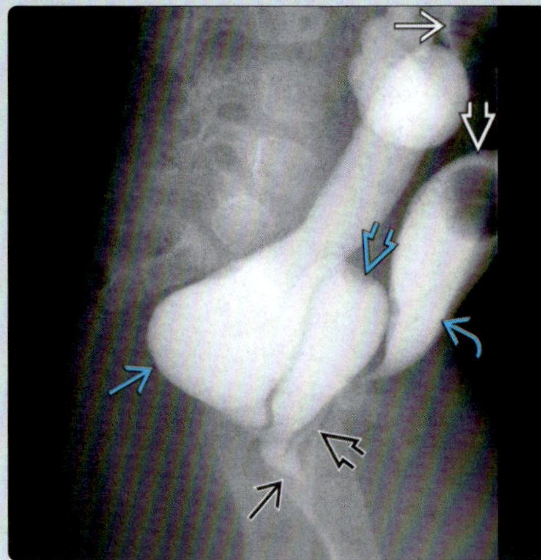

(Left) *Transverse ultrasound in the same patient shows a markedly distended vagina ➡ filled with echogenic fluid. There is moderate hydronephrosis ➡ of both kidneys. The urinary bladder & distal ureters (not shown) were compressed by the hydrocolpos.* **(Right)** *Injection of a mucous fistula ➡ & vesicostomy ➡ shows filling of the rectum ➡, vagina (with cervical impression ➡), & bladder ➡ + urethra ➡. All of these structures drain into a common channel (or cloaca) ➡.*

TERMINOLOGY

Definitions

- Anorectal malformation in female patients in which rectum, urethra, & vagina converge to form common channel (CC) that drains to single perineal orifice (which allows clinical diagnosis)

IMAGING

General Features

- Best diagnostic clue
  - Dilated bowel + hydrocolpos in female fetus (or neonate with single perineal orifice)

Radiographic Findings

- Neonatal intestinal obstruction
  - Multiple dilated bowel loops with variable degree of rectal distention
  - Displacement of gas-filled bowel by dilated structures
    - Hydrocolpos (> 30% of all patients)
    - ± meconium filled colon
  - ± bowel or bladder Ca^{2+} from mixing of urine & meconium
  - ± curvilinear peritoneal Ca^{2} (if bowel perforation)
  - Additional findings
    - ± spinal/radial ray anomalies
    - ± cardiomegaly, pulmonary edema → congenital heart disease
    - ± proximal esophageal pouch → esophageal atresia
    - ± double bubble → duodenal atresia

Ultrasonographic Findings

- Grayscale ultrasound
  - Neonatal cystic pelvic mass: Commonly hydrocolpos
    - Dilated vagina(s) mimics bladder
  - Hemivaginas/hemiuteri (40%)
  - ± hydroureteronephrosis (HUN); other GU anomalies (renal agenesis, cross-fused ectopia, horseshoe kidney)
  - ± echogenic calcified meconium in dilated bowel or bladder
  - ± ascites
  - ± spinal cord anomalies
- Contrast-enhanced ultrasound
  - Catheterization of CC can be used to study cloaca after colostomy: Genitosonography & colosonography

Fluoroscopic Findings

- Voiding cystourethrogram
  - Not often helpful precolostomy; difficult bladder catheterization
  - Usually postrepair to check for vesicoureteral reflux, neurogenic bladder
- Fistulagram
  - Postcolostomy: Inject mucous fistula → opacify distal colon ± bladder, single/hemivagina(s), CC
    - Length of CC & urethra are important to operative planning, prognosis
  - ± cloacagram by rotational fluoroscopy or MR

DIFFERENTIAL DIAGNOSIS

Anorectal Malformation

- Other types in female patients: Imperforate anus + rectovestibular fistula, rectoperineal fistula, or no fistula
  - Isolated rectovaginal fistula is rare
  - > 1 perineal orifice is present clinically

Other Low/Distal Neonatal Bowel Obstructions

- Anus is present on physical exam
- Contrast enema to differentiate
  - Meconium ileus
  - Ileal atresia
  - Hirschsprung disease
  - Small left colon/meconium plug syndrome
  - Colonic atresia

Isolated Hydrometrocolpos

- Vaginal septum or imperforate hymen; anus is present on physical exam

Megacystis-Microcolon-Intestinal Hypoperistalsis Syndrome

- Large bladder may mimic hydrocolpos; anus is present on physical exam

CLINICAL ISSUES

Presentation

- Most common signs/symptoms
  - Single perineal orifice; abdominal distention

Natural History & Prognosis

- Hydrocolpos → ↓ renal function in neonate (due to bladder outlet obstruction) without urgent drainage
- Prognosis is based on CC length
  - < 3 cm: Most common (56%), less complex repair, better functional prognosis
  - > 3 cm: Less common (44%), more complex repair, worse functional prognosis

Treatment

- Surgical repair depends on length of CC
  - < 3 cm: Posterior sagittal anorectoplasty (PSARP) + urogenital mobilization
  - > 3 cm: PSARP ± laparotomy/oscopy + complex surgical reconstruction

SELECTED REFERENCES

1. Chow JS et al: Contrast-enhanced genitosonography and colosonography: emerging alternatives to fluoroscopy. Pediatr Radiol. ePub, 2021
2. Wood RJ et al: Cloacal malformations: technical aspects of the reconstruction and factors which predict surgical complexity. Front Pediatr. 7:240, 2019
3. Wood RJ et al: Cloaca reconstruction: a new algorithm which considers the role of urethral length in determining surgical planning. J Pediatr Surg. S0022-3468(17)30644-9, 2017
4. Bischoff A: The surgical treatment of cloaca. Semin Pediatr Surg. 25(2):102-7, 2016
5. Kraus SJ: Radiologic diagnosis of a newborn with cloaca. Semin Pediatr Surg. 25(2):76-81, 2016

KEY FACTS

TERMINOLOGY

- Classic bladder exstrophy (CBE): Low midline abdominal wall defect with exposure of bladder plate & urethra + low-set umbilicus
  - Split lower abdominal skin & rectus abdominis + pubic symphysis diastasis
  - Bifid clitoris in females, epispadias in males
  - Deficient genitalia & pelvic floor muscles
- Epispadias: Abnormal dorsal urethral opening
  - With CBE, entire dorsal urethra is open with abnormal bladder sphincter

IMAGING

- Absent urinary bladder by prenatal sonography with normal amniotic fluid
- Pubic symphysis diastasis
- Lobular soft tissue at lower abdominal wall
- High rates of vesicoureteral reflux & dysfunctional bladder prior to ureteral reimplants & bladder neck reconstruction

TOP DIFFERENTIAL DIAGNOSES

- Cloacal exstrophy/OEIS complex
- Omphalocele
- Gastroschisis
- Impaired urine production (absent bladder)

PATHOLOGY

- Cloacal membrane rupture due to failed mesodermal ingrowth

CLINICAL ISSUES

- Incidence of 1:10,000-1:50,000 live births
- 2.3-6:1 = M:F
- Modern staged repair vs. complete primary repair
  - Continence is achieved in up to 81%
  - Most perform clean intermittent catheterization

(Left) *AP pelvic radiograph in a neonate with bladder exstrophy shows lobular soft tissues of the open bladder plate ➔ with splayed pubic ➔ & ischial ➔ bones. Note the normal sacrum. This can help differentiate this entity from cloacal exstrophy in which the sacrum is dysplastic or hypoplastic.* **(Right)** *Frontal VCUG in a 3-year-old girl after bladder exstrophy repair shows a small lobulated bladder ➔ with elevated bladder base ➔, J-shaped ureterovesical junctions ➔, & bilateral high-grade vesicoureteral reflux (VUR) ➔.*

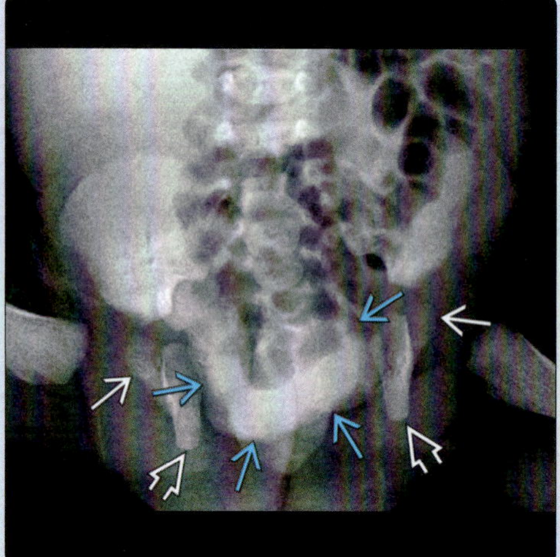

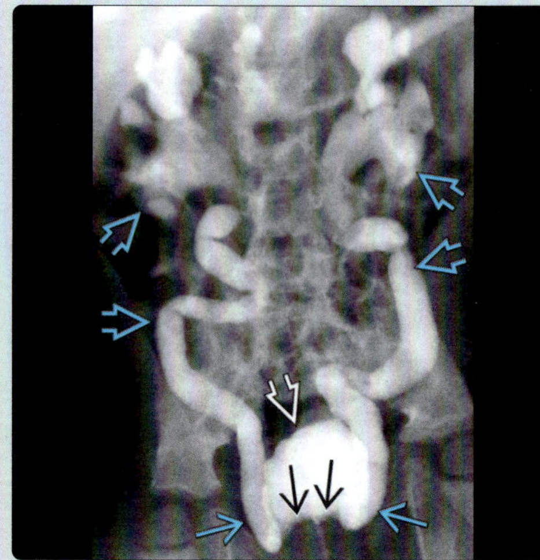

(Left) *Transverse US of the bladder in an adolescent with a history of bladder exstrophy shows a large echogenic stone ➔ with posterior shadowing at the dependent portion of the bladder. These may be treated by extracorporeal shock wave lithotripsy. Note the irregular bladder morphology.* **(Right)** *Coronal CECT in a 17-year-old boy with a history of repaired bladder exstrophy shows multifocal renal scars ➔ bilaterally with a globally scarred small left kidney ➔ secondary to VUR of infected urine after bladder closure.*

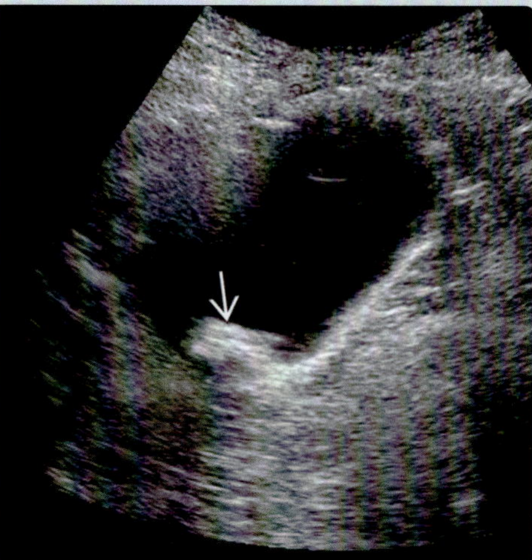

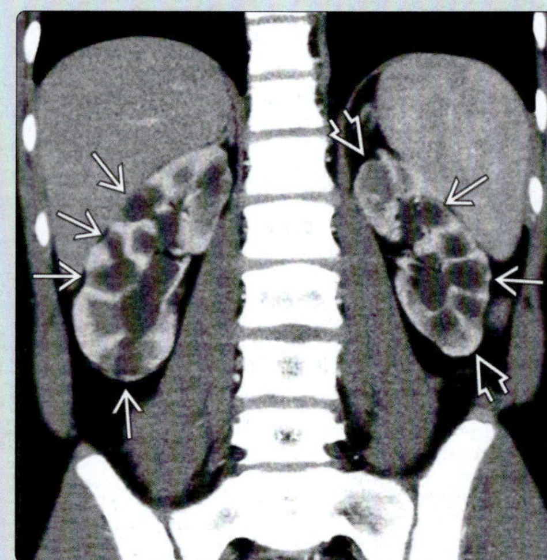

TERMINOLOGY

Synonyms

- Exstrophy-epispadias complex

Definitions

- Classic bladder exstrophy (CBE): Low midline abdominal wall defect (AWD) with exposure of bladder plate & urethra + low-set umbilicus
  - Split lower abdominal skin & rectus abdominis + pubic symphysis diastasis
  - Bifid clitoris in girls, epispadias in boys
- Epispadias: Abnormal dorsal urethral opening
  - In CBE, entire urethra is open with abnormal bladder sphincter

IMAGING

General Features

- Best diagnostic clue
  - Absent urinary bladder on prenatal US but normal amniotic fluid
  - Pubic symphysis diastasis on postnatal radiographs

Radiographic Findings

- Pubic symphysis > 1 cm
- Lobular soft tissues of lower abdominal wall from everted bladder
- ± inguinal hernias (with gas-filled bowel within hernia)

Fluoroscopic Findings

- Voiding cystourethrogram
  - Performed after bladder closure
  - High rate of vesicoureteral reflux (VUR)
  - Variable bladder capacity, shape
  - Postop findings: Potential bladder rupture, urethral stricture/fistula

Ultrasonographic Findings

- Prenatal
  - Nonvisualized urinary bladder but normal amniotic fluid
  - Low position of umbilicus
  - Lobular soft tissue at infraumbilical abdominal wall
  - Diminutive genitalia
  - Splayed echogenic pubic & iliac bones
- Postnatal
  - Variable bladder size, shape, & wall thickness post repair
  - VUR → pelvocaliectasis ± pyelonephritis & scarring

CT Findings

- External rotation of pubic & iliac bones, pubic bone shortening, acetabular retroversion

Nuclear Medicine Findings

- DMSA to evaluate renal split function & scarring

MR Findings

- Assessment of pelvic floor musculature deficiencies

Imaging Recommendations

- Best imaging tool
  - Prenatal ultrasound/MR, postnatal clinical exam

DIFFERENTIAL DIAGNOSIS

Cloacal Exstrophy/OEIS Complex

- Low midline AWD
- Absent bladder with normal amniotic fluid
- Exposed bladder halves divided by everted cecum
  - ± elephant trunk appearance of prolapsed ileum
- Omphalocele, imperforate anus, spine anomalies

Omphalocele

- Central AWD
- Bowel & other viscera herniate into umbilical cord base
  - Contents are covered by sac
- Lower abdominal wall & urinary bladder are intact

Gastroschisis

- Off-midline AWD: Bowel herniated right of umbilicus
  - No covering membrane
- Lower abdominal wall & bladder are intact

Impaired Urine Production (Absent Bladder)

- Bilateral renal abnormalities (same or combination) → oligo-/anhydramnios → pulmonary hypoplasia
  - Multicystic dysplastic kidney
  - Ureteropelvic junction obstruction
  - Polycystic renal disease, recessive
  - Renal agenesis

CLINICAL ISSUES

Demographics

- Sex
  - M:F = 2.3-6:1
- Epidemiology
  - 1:10,000-1:50,000 live births

Natural History & Prognosis

- Continence in up to 81%: Most perform clean intermittent catheterization, especially after augmentation

Treatment

- Modern staged repair
  - Stage I, newborn: Close AWD, bladder, & posterior urethra + iliac osteotomy
  - Stage II, age 6-12 months: Epispadias repair
  - Stage III, age 4-5 years: Reconstruct bladder neck + ureteral reimplants
- Complete primary repair ± ureteral reimplant

SELECTED REFERENCES

1. Weiss DA et al: Key anatomic findings on fetal ultrasound and MRI in the prenatal diagnosis of bladder and cloacal exstrophy. J Pediatr Urol. 16(5):665-71, 2020
2. Szymanski KM et al: Probability of bladder augmentation, diversion and clean intermittent catheterization in classic bladder exstrophy: a 36-year, multi-institutional, retrospective cohort study. J Urol. 202(6):1256-62, 2019
3. Victoria T et al: Fetal anterior abdominal wall defects: prenatal imaging by magnetic resonance imaging. Pediatr Radiol. 48(4):499-512, 2018
4. Pierre K et al: Bladder exstrophy: current management and postoperative imaging. Pediatr Radiol. 44(7):768-86; quiz 765-7, 2014

Renal Ectopia and Fusion

KEY FACTS

TERMINOLOGY

- Includes horseshoe or pancake kidney; crossed fused ectopia; pelvic, iliac/pelvic (ptotic/mobile), & thoracic kidneys
- Results from abnormal ascent & rotation of fetal kidney
- Found anywhere from presacral to intrathoracic; may be bilateral or unilateral; may cross midline
- Malpositioned kidneys are more susceptible to trauma, iatrogenic injury, obstruction, infection, & stones

IMAGING

- US is typically sufficient to document location & gross morphology of ectopic & fused kidneys
  - Accurate lengths are difficult to obtain due to more globular, less reniform shape & poor definition of margin with contralateral fused kidney
- Other modalities are used to answer specific questions (as needed): Drainage, stones, vascular supply, ureteral course
- Isthmus of horseshoe kidney may contain functioning renal tissue or fibrotic nonfunctional tissue
- Ureteral insertion site in bladder provides clue to site where kidney initially formed (i.e., lower pole ureter of crossed fused ectopia inserts into trigone on contralateral side)
- Colon typically occupies empty renal fossa

PATHOLOGY

- Horseshoe kidneys are associated with genital anomalies, VACTERL, Turner & other syndromes
- Adrenal ectopia is reported in association with renal ectopia
- Vesicoureteral reflux (20-30%), contralateral renal dysplasia (4%), cryptorchidism (5%), hypospadias (5%)

CLINICAL ISSUES

- Horseshoe kidney is most common: 1 in 400 births
- All types of ectopia are more common in boys than girls
- Primary concern: Avoidance of iatrogenic injury to renal parenchyma & supplying vessels during routine surgery
- Treat complications of obstruction, reflux, & stones

(Left) *Graphic shows variations of renal ectopia & fusion: (A) Pelvic kidney, (B) subdiaphragmatic/thoracic kidney, (C) crossed fused renal ectopia, & (D) horseshoe kidney.* **(Right)** *Longitudinal US shows a crossed fused renal ectopia in the left abdomen with a relatively normal upper moiety & a malrotated, globular lower moiety. Note that the long axis of each moiety is different, which helps distinguish this entity from a duplication. Also, no renal tissue will be seen in the contralateral renal fossa in this setting.*

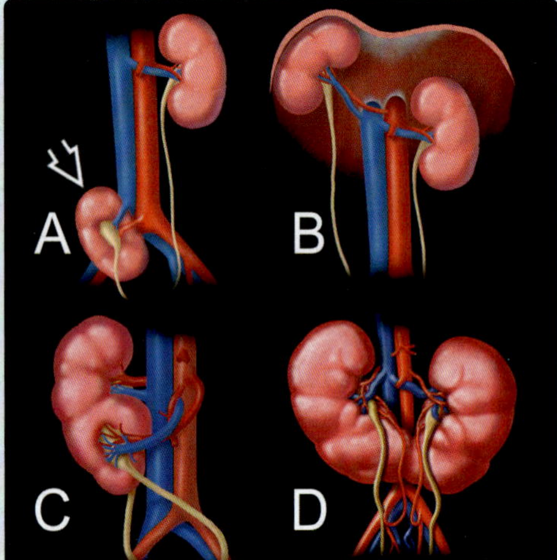

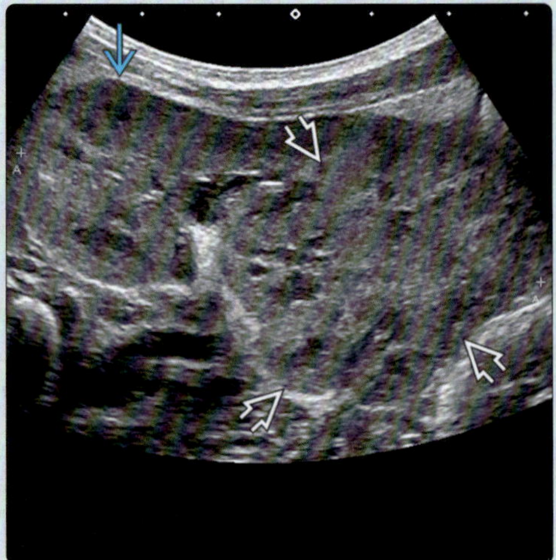

(Left) *Longitudinal US shows a pelvic kidney (between cursors) abutting the bladder dome in the right lower quadrant. It is easy to imagine this kidney being injured during a laparoscopic appendectomy.* **(Right)** *Coronal oblique T2 FS MIP from an MR urogram in a 14-year-old with a horseshoe kidney shows marked left hydronephrosis secondary to a left moiety ureteropelvic junction (UPJ) obstruction. Note the bridging isthmus of renal tissue at the midline.*

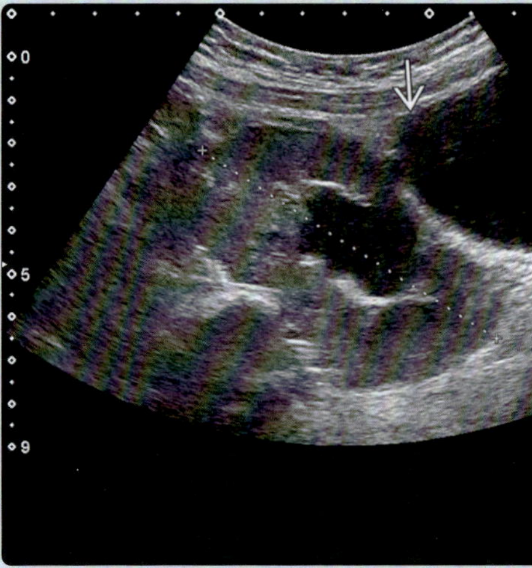

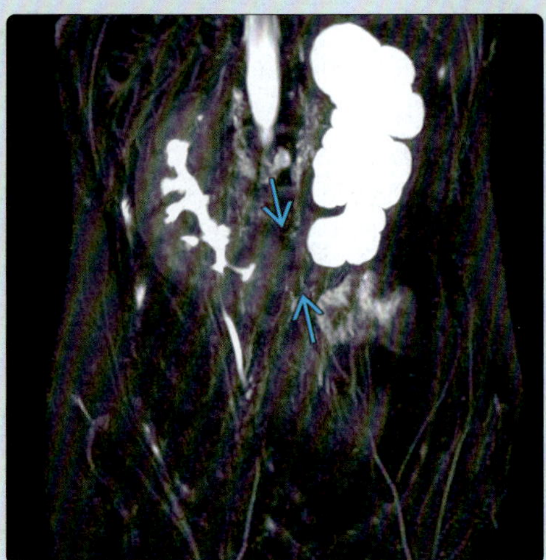

TERMINOLOGY

Synonyms

- Includes horseshoe or pancake kidney; crossed fused ectopia; pelvic, iliac/pelvic (ptotic/mobile), & thoracic kidneys

Definitions

- Normal renal tissue in abnormal location
- Results from abnormal ascent & rotation of fetal kidney
- Kidneys form at sacral level & ascend to L1 by term; renal pelvis is initially directed anteriorly but rotates 90° medially as it ascends
- Malpositioned kidneys are more susceptible to trauma, iatrogenic injury, obstruction, infection, & stones
- High incidence of multiple renal arteries & veins

IMAGING

General Features

- Best diagnostic clue
  - Normal renal parenchyma with abnormal location, axis of orientation, or position of renal pelvis
- Location
  - Anywhere from presacral to intrathoracic, bilateral or unilateral; may cross midline
- Size
  - Overall renal parenchyma volume is similar to orthotopic kidneys; longitudinal measurements vary based on ectopic kidney shape
- Morphology
  - Normal cortex, pyramids, & collecting system; however, pelvocaliectasis is commonly associated
  - Isthmus or midline junctional zone of horseshoe kidney may contain functioning renal tissue or fibrotic nonfunctional tissue

Radiographic Findings

- Radiography
  - Renal shadows are altered from expected positions
  - May simulate midline or pelvic mass
  - Bowel gas may be
    - Displaced by ectopic kidney
    - Occupying renal fossa (with repositioning of splenic & hepatic flexures of colon most commonly)
- IVP
  - Functional renal parenchyma in atypical location; pelvocaliectasis is commonly associated
  - Ectopic kidneys, especially thoracic & horseshoe varieties, may appear mass-like on initial scout view
    - Expect bowel to occupy empty renal fossa
  - Early nephrogram may be missed on tightly coned films (not included in field of view)
  - Abnormalities of vasculature & ureter are also common
    - Ureteral insertion site in bladder provides clue to where kidney initially formed (i.e., lower pole ureter of crossed fused ectopic kidney inserts into trigone on contralateral side)
  - Oblique views are often helpful to profile abnormally rotated collecting system
  - May require fluoroscopic spot views to capture ureteral course
  - Pelvic compression devices should be avoided

Fluoroscopic Findings

- Renal ectopia may be noted incidentally during other fluoroscopic procedures: Gastrointestinal tract studies, voiding cystourethrogram (VCUG), or genitograms

Ultrasonographic Findings

- Grayscale ultrasound
  - Normal echotexture of abnormally positioned renal parenchyma
    - Hydronephrosis & scarring may alter echotexture & architecture
  - Accurate length measurements are difficult to obtain due to more globular & less reniform shape as well as poor definition of margin with fused contralateral kidney
    - Volumes can be helpful
  - May be difficult to see pelvic kidneys due to adjacent bowel gas
  - Colon typically occupies empty renal fossa
- Color Doppler
  - Useful in detecting aberrant vessels & localizing urinary bladder ureteral jets
- Power Doppler
  - Pyelonephritis has ↓ parenchymal perfusion in infected segments

CT Findings

- NECT
  - May initially be seen on renal stone CT
  - Soft tissue "mass" identified along with absence of renal tissue in renal fossa
  - Associated hydronephrosis or stone disease can be clue to aberrant renal position
    - Look for aberrant ureteral course during stone assessment
- CECT
  - Look for abnormal location, rotation, axis, & ureteral course
  - Expect normal renal enhancement & excretion of contrast, except in obstruction
  - Delayed imaging may be useful, depending on study indication
    - To assess parenchyma & collecting system for laceration in trauma setting
    - To localize distal ureters
- CTA
  - Occasionally used for mapping vessels preoperatively

MR Findings

- Similar to other modalities: Abnormal location, axis, & rotation

Nuclear Medicine Findings

- May be found incidentally on renal imaging studies or whole-body exams performed for unrelated reasons
- Nuclear renal studies are sometimes requested specifically to document presence of pelvic kidney that could not be appreciated on US due to intervening bowel gas
- Ectopic kidneys show normal uptake of radiopharmaceutical with variable degrees of pelvocaliectasis

Imaging Recommendations

- Best imaging tool
  - US is typically sufficient to document location & gross morphology of ectopic & fused kidneys
  - Other modalities are used to answer specific questions (as needed): Drainage, stone disease, vascular supply

DIFFERENTIAL DIAGNOSIS

Mass in Typical Ectopic Location

- Renal tissue is still visible in normal locations
- Thoracic considerations
  - Bronchopulmonary sequestration
  - Neuroblastoma
  - Hernia/eventration
- Abdominal
  - Lymphoma
  - Any large neoplasm or cyst of solid organ, viscus, or mesentery
- Pelvis
  - Ovarian tumors
  - Sacrococcygeal teratoma
  - Pelvic rhabdomyosarcoma

Pseudokidney of Intussusception

- Depending on image orientation, ileocolic intussusception can mimic reniform shape & architecture on US
- Real-time cross-sectional sweep or cine through entire length of intussusception will reveal nature of "mass"

Simulated Ectopia Related to Severe Kyphoscoliosis

- Mimics horseshoe kidney or crossed fused ectopia but lacks connection between right & left kidneys
- Cross-sectional imaging or orthogonal views clarify difference

Transplant Kidney

- Often located in pelvis adjacent to iliac vessels
- Native kidneys are often atrophic bilaterally

PATHOLOGY

General Features

- Genetics
  - Horseshoe kidney is associated with genital anomalies, VACTERL (vertebral, anorectal, cardiac, tracheoesophageal, renal, limb abnormalities), Turner & other syndromes
  - Other abnormalities of ascent & rotation are less frequently associated with syndromes
  - Geographic "hot spots" for ectopia suggest either common exposure to teratogenetic factors or hereditary condition with variable penetrance
- Associated abnormalities
  - Urologic abnormalities associated with simple ectopia
    - Vesicoureteral reflux (20-30%)
    - Contralateral renal dysplasia (4%)
    - Cryptorchidism (5%)
    - Hypospadias (5%)
  - Adrenal ectopia is reported in association with renal ectopia
  - Cardiac & skeletal anomalies are common
  - 25% of external ear malformations also have renal anomalies
- Parenchyma is developmentally normal, though secondary changes of obstruction, scarring, & nephrolithiasis are not uncommon
- Embryology/anatomy
  - Results from abnormal ascent & rotation of metanephric blastema after induction by ureteric bud
  - Multiple supplying vessels & draining ureters are common

CLINICAL ISSUES

Presentation

- Most common signs/symptoms
  - Often discovered incidentally
  - May be suspected on antenatal US
  - Can present later in infancy as palpable mass or with urinary tract infection (UTI) or obstruction

Demographics

- Sex
  - All types of ectopia are more common in boys than girls
- Epidemiology
  - Horseshoe kidney incidence: 1 in 400 births; most common fusion anomaly
  - Crossed fused ectopic kidney is less common
    - 10% are crossed but not "fused"
  - Simple ectopia is seen in 1 in 900 (autopsy series)
  - Agenesis & pelvic kidney L > R

Natural History & Prognosis

- Aside from complications of obstruction, stone formation, UTI, & injury, most ectopic kidneys function normally
- Primary concern: Avoidance of iatrogenic injury to renal parenchyma & supplying vessels during routine surgery, especially laparoscopic surgery
- Slightly ↑ risk of Wilms & carcinoid tumors reported in horseshoe kidneys
- Prognosis is generally excellent
  - 1/3 of patients with horseshoe kidney are asymptomatic throughout life

Treatment

- Treat complications of obstruction, reflux, & stones

SELECTED REFERENCES

1. Asanad K et al: Grade IV renal laceration in a 13-year-old boy with cross-fused renal ectopia. Urology. 145:243-6, 2020
2. Sarhan O et al: Crossed fused renal ectopia: diagnosis and prognosis as a single-center experience. J Pediatr Surg. 56(9):1632-7, 2020
3. Lomoro P et al: Pancake kidney, a rare and often misdiagnosed malformation: a case report and radiological differential diagnosis. J Ultrasound. 22(2):207-13, 2019
4. Taghavi K et al: The horseshoe kidney: surgical anatomy and embryology. J Pediatr Urol. 12(5):275-80, 2016
5. Ratola A et al: Crossed renal ectopia without fusion: an uncommon cause of abdominal mass. Case Rep Nephrol. 2015:679342, 2015
6. Szmigielska A et al: Rare renal ectopia in children - intrathoracic ectopic kidney. Dev Period Med. 19(2):186-8, 2015
7. Schreuder MF: Unilateral anomalies of kidney development: why is left not right? Kidney Int. 80(7):740-5, 2011

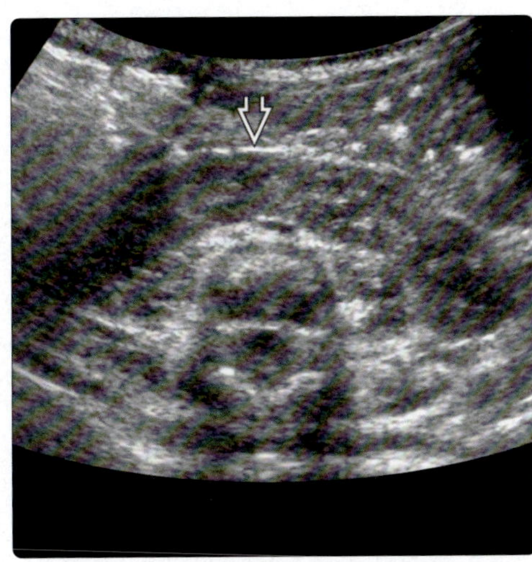

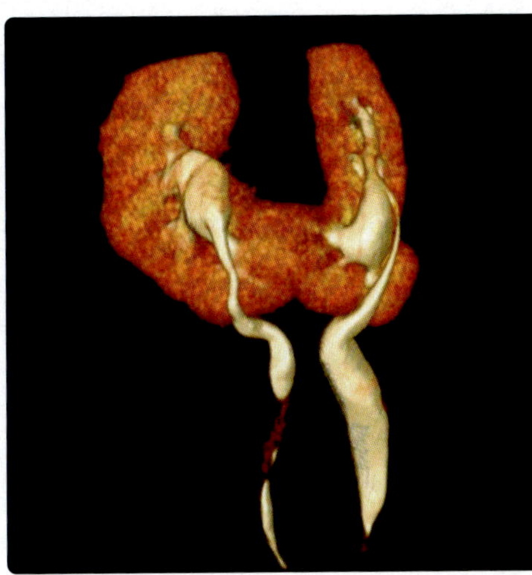

(Left) *Transverse US in a patient with a horseshoe kidney shows a band of renal parenchyma crossing over the spine.* **(Right)** *Anterior view 3D reformation from a CECT scan in a patient with multiple congenital anomalies shows a horseshoe kidney with fused lower poles & anteriorly directed renal pelves.*

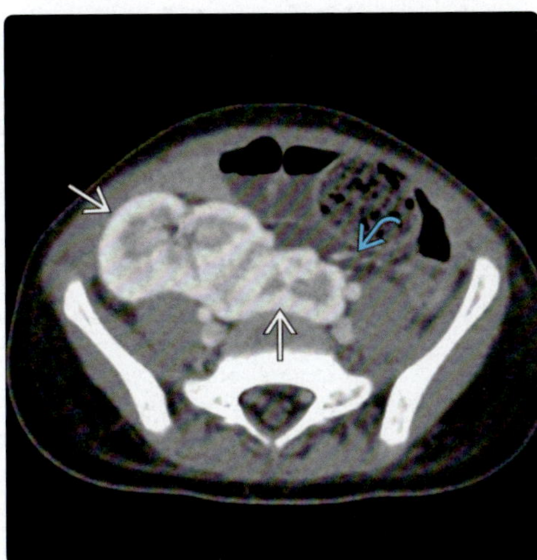

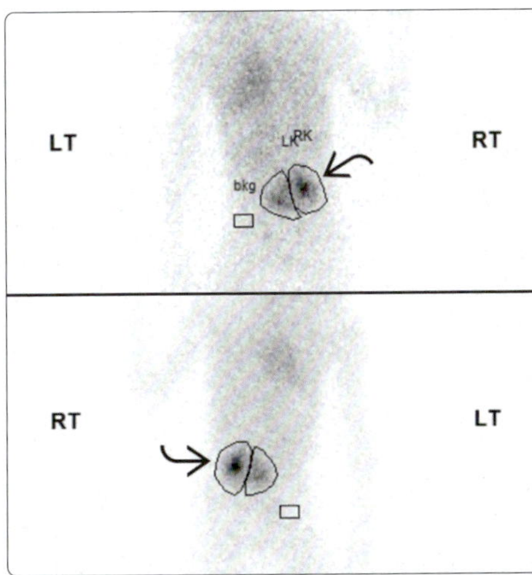

(Left) *Axial CECT in the pelvis of a 3-year-old shows a crossed fused pelvic kidney, lower in position than a typical horseshoe kidney. Several small vessels on the left may reflect accessory vessels, which are commonly seen.* **(Right)** *Posterior (top) & anterior (bottom) Tc-99m DTPA images in the same patient, performed to assess differential function & GFR, show slightly greater contribution of the right moiety. Knowledge of ectopic renal position helps to appropriately position gamma cameras for nuclear studies.*

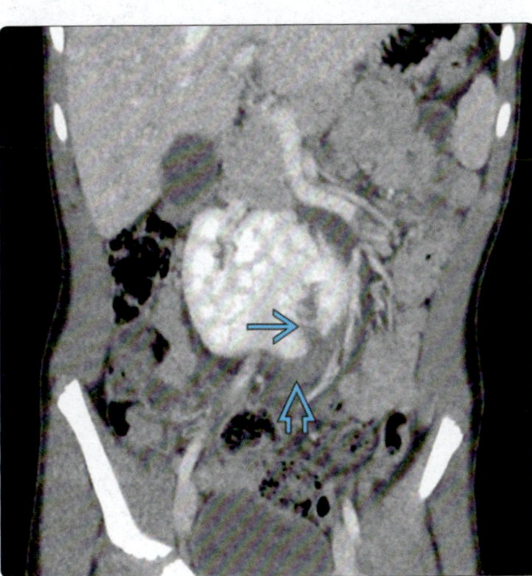

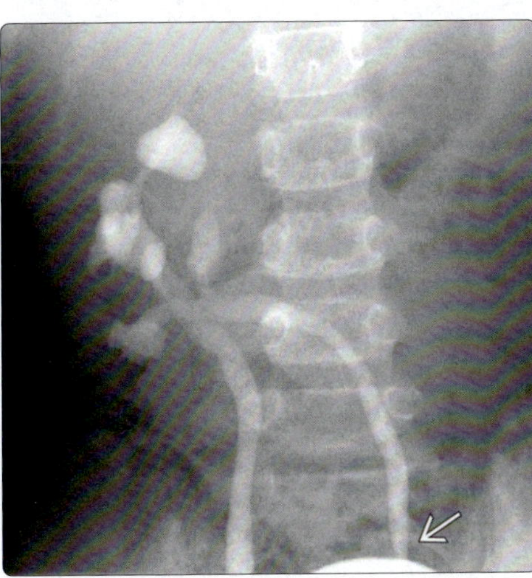

(Left) *Coronal CECT in a 9-year-old after a motor vehicle accident shows a grade III laceration of the left inferior moiety of a horseshoe kidney, which is incompletely visualized on this image. A small perinephric hematoma is noted, but no urine extravasation was seen on delayed images (not shown).* **(Right)** *Frontal fluoroscopic image during a VCUG shows a crossed fused kidney with the lower moiety ureter crossing the midline to the left side of the bladder (since this kidney initially formed as a left kidney).*

Renal Agenesis

KEY FACTS

TERMINOLOGY

- Congenital absence of functioning renal tissue
- **C**ongenital **a**bnormality of **k**idney & **u**rinary **t**ract (CAKUT)

IMAGING

- Complete absence of 1 or both kidneys
  - No ectopia or fusion anomaly
- Bowel fills renal fossa
- Linear/flat configuration of ipsilateral adrenal gland
- ± compensatory hypertrophy of remaining kidney
- Best modality: Ultrasound (prenatal or post natal)

TOP DIFFERENTIAL DIAGNOSES

- Involuted multicystic dysplastic kidney
- Ectopic kidney
- Crossed fused renal ectopia
- Prior nephrectomy

PATHOLOGY

- Due to abnormal interaction between ureteric bud of mesonephric duct & metanephric mesenchyme
- Unilateral renal agenesis is associated with
  - Müllerian abnormalities
    - **O**bstructed **h**emi**v**agina, **i**psilateral **r**enal **a**genesis (OHVIRA syndrome)
  - Contralateral renal anomalies are common
  - Extrarenal anomalies in up to 30%
- Bilateral agenesis → Potter sequence: Oligo-/anhydramnios, lung hypoplasia, dysmorphic facies, ± fetal demise

CLINICAL ISSUES

- Unilateral: Usually asymptomatic; associated with medical renal disease later in life
- Bilateral: Classically fatal due to pulmonary hypoplasia & anuria
  - Serial amnioinfusions in utero may allow for "pulmonary survivor" needing dialysis & renal transplant

(Left) *Longitudinal ultrasound of the right renal fossa in a 1-day-old girl with right renal agenesis shows absence of the kidney in the expected location along the right psoas muscle ➡. There are normal, fluid-filled bowel loops in the right renal fossa ➡.* **(Right)** *Oblique ultrasound of the right renal fossa in a 1-day-old boy with right renal agenesis shows an elongated, linear adrenal gland ("lying down adrenal") ➡.*

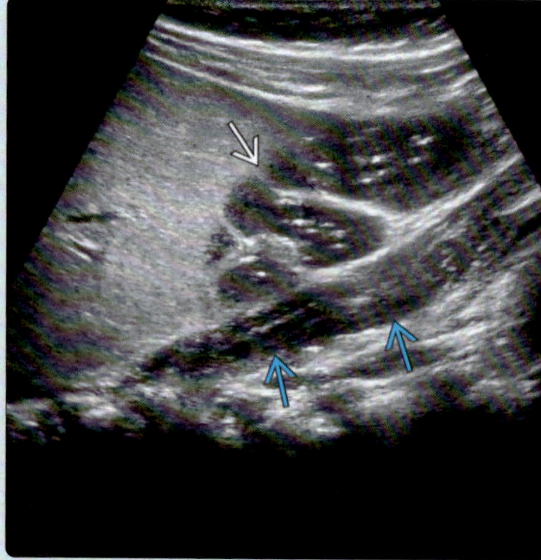

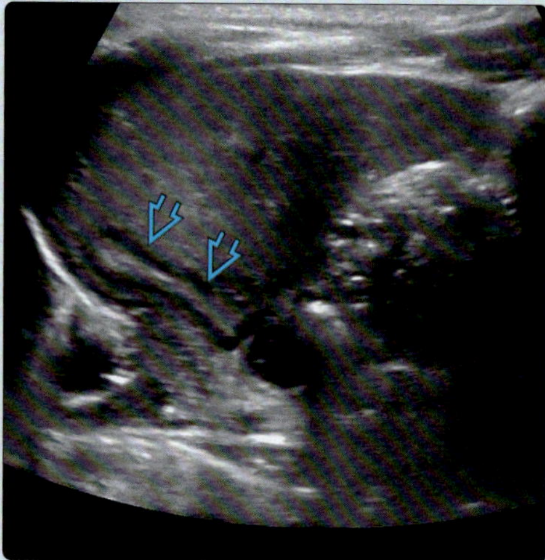

(Left) *Coronal T1 C+ FS MR in a 3-year-old with left renal agenesis shows absence of renal tissue in the left renal fossa (which is filled with decompressed bowel ➡). The right renal collecting system is dilated secondary to a ureteropelvic junction obstruction ➡.* **(Right)** *Posterior coronal image from a Tc-99m DTPA renal scan in a 2-year-old with left renal agenesis shows normal radiotracer uptake in the right kidney ➡ with no radiotracer uptake on the left.*

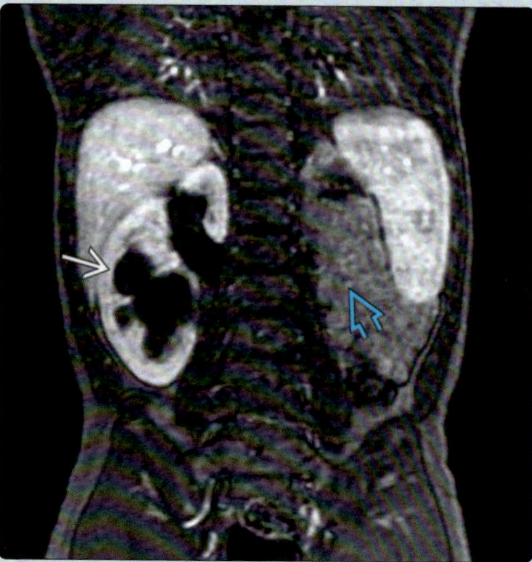

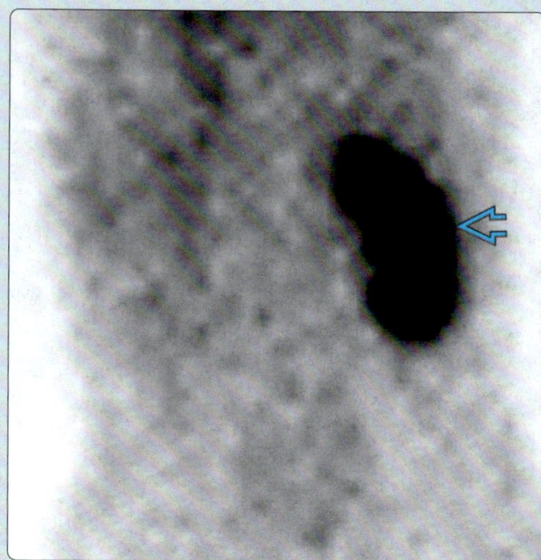

TERMINOLOGY

Synonyms

- **C**ongenital **a**bnormality of **k**idney & **u**rinary **t**ract (CAKUT)
- Solitary kidney

Definitions

- Congenital absence of functioning renal tissue

IMAGING

General Features

- Best diagnostic clue
  - Ultrasound, CT, MR: Absence of kidney in renal fossa without fusion anomaly or ectopia

Radiographic Findings

- Radiography
  - Unilateral: Absence of normal renal shadow
  - Bilateral: ± Potter sequence due to oligohydramnios
    - Abnormal facies, ears
    - Pulmonary hypoplasia with small thorax
    - Respiratory distress, pneumothorax ± pneumomediastinum

Ultrasonographic Findings

- Absent kidney(s) without fusion anomaly or ectopia
- Ipsilateral elongated linear/flat adrenal gland ("lying down adrenal")
- Unilateral: ± compensatory hypertrophy of remaining kidney
- Bilateral: Typically detected by prenatal ultrasound
  - Oligo-/anhydramnios + lack of urinary bladder distention
  - No renal arteries by Doppler

Nuclear Medicine Findings

- Renal scans show lack of renal uptake & excretion

Imaging Recommendations

- Best imaging tool
  - Ultrasound (prenatal or post natal)
  - Nuclear medicine renal scan, CT/MR will demonstrate lack of renal tissue
    - Rarely required for confirmation
- Protocol advice
  - Consider pelvic imaging in girls due to association with müllerian abnormalities

DIFFERENTIAL DIAGNOSIS

Involuted Multicystic Dysplastic Kidney

- Gradual atrophy of reniform collection of cysts

Ectopic Kidney

- Often located in pelvis

Crossed Fused Renal Ectopia

- Contralateral kidney is normally positioned with ectopic kidney lying across midline & fused to lower pole
- Separate ureters insert normally into urinary bladder

Prior Nephrectomy

- Due to renal tumor, severe trauma, obstructed nonfunctioning kidney

PATHOLOGY

General Features

- Etiology
  - Renal development begins in 5th week of gestation
  - Agenesis results from abnormal interaction between ureteric bud of mesonephric duct & metanephric mesenchyme
- Associated abnormalities
  - Unilateral renal agenesis
    - Müllerian abnormalities in girls
      - **O**bstructed **hemiv**agina, **i**psilateral **r**enal **a**genesis (OHVIRA syndrome)
      - May be due to ectopic insertion of ureter with resultant obstruction & renal aplasia
      - Typically with uterine didelphys configuration
    - Contralateral renal abnormalities are common
      - Vesicoureteral reflux most common
      - Others: Contralateral ureteropelvic junction obstruction, megaureter, collecting system duplication
    - Extrarenal abnormalities present in up to 30%
  - Bilateral agenesis → Potter sequence: Oligohydramnios, lung hypoplasia, dysmorphic facies

CLINICAL ISSUES

Presentation

- Most common signs/symptoms
  - Unilateral agenesis is usually asymptomatic
  - Bilateral agenesis typically presents in utero with oligohydramnios & pulmonary hypoplasia ± clubfeet, fetal demise
    - At delivery → respiratory distress, abnormal facies, anuria

Demographics

- Epidemiology
  - Overall incidence ~ 1/2,000

Natural History & Prognosis

- Unilateral renal agenesis is associated with medical renal disease later in life
  - ↑ incidence of hypertension, impaired glomerular filtration rate, & proteinuria
    - May be due to hyperfiltration by remaining kidney
- Bilateral is classically fatal due to pulmonary hypoplasia
  - Can perform serial amnioinfusions in utero for oligohydramnios to create "pulmonary survivor" with need for dialysis & renal transplant; controversial

SELECTED REFERENCES

1. Kirkpatrick J et al: Side predilection in congenital anomalies of the kidney, urinary and genital tracts. J Pediatr Urol. 16(6):751-9, 2020
2. Sugarman J et al: Ethical considerations concerning amnioinfusions for treating fetal bilateral renal agenesis. Obstet Gynecol. 131(1):130-4, 2018
3. Laurichesse Delmas H et al: Congenital unilateral renal agenesis: prevalence, prenatal diagnosis, associated anomalies. Data from two birth-defect registries. Birth Defects Res. 109(15):1204-11, 2017
4. Bienstock JL et al: Successful in utero intervention for bilateral renal agenesis. Obstet Gynecol. 124(2 Pt 2 Suppl 1):413-5, 2014
5. Westland R et al: Unilateral renal agenesis: a systematic review on associated anomalies and renal injury. Nephrol Dial Transplant. 28(7):1844-55, 2013

Multicystic Dysplastic Kidney

KEY FACTS

TERMINOLOGY

- Congenital, nonfunctional kidney is composed of numerous cysts & dysplastic tissue
- Tends to involute with time: Cysts shrink & residual tissue may lose reniform shape

IMAGING

- Reniform-shaped, multicystic mass occupying renal fossa
  - ± lobulated outer contour (due to cysts of variable size)
  - Wide range of sizes: Up to 15 cm in length in newborn period; may be only 1-2 cm after years of involution
- Cysts of varying size do not connect
  - Largest cyst typically peripheral, not central
- Poorly defined, intervening, echogenic parenchyma without normal corticomedullary architecture
- Can be segmental in duplicated kidneys or partially involve fused/horseshoe kidney
- Nuclear scintigraphy documents lack of renal function in MCDK (multicystic dysplastic kidney disease)

PATHOLOGY

- Probably due to atresia of ureter or ureteropelvic junction (UPJ) during metanephric stage of intrauterine development
- Up to 40% of patients with MCDK have contralateral renal abnormality
  - UPJ obstruction & vesicoureteral reflux most common

CLINICAL ISSUES

- ~ 70% are discovered antenatally or in infancy as palpable mass
- Unilateral MCDK with normal contralateral kidney: Excellent prognosis
  - Vast majority involute with time & remain asymptomatic
  - Rare reports of Wilms tumor developing in MCDK
- Unilateral MCDK with abnormal contralateral kidney: May develop renal insufficiency
- Bilateral MCDK: Lethal from pulmonary hypoplasia or absence of functioning renal tissue

(Left) *Frontal graphic of the right kidney shows multiple cysts of varying size replacing the renal parenchyma. There is minimal intervening dysplastic renal tissue. A ureter may or may not be recognizable at the renal hilum on imaging studies, but no renal pelvis should be seen.* **(Right)** *Coronal SSFSE T2 fetal MR shows a multicystic mass in the left renal fossa ➡ with no discernible normal left renal tissue, most consistent with a left multicystic dysplastic kidney (MCDK). The right kidney ➡ & volume of amniotic fluid appear normal.*

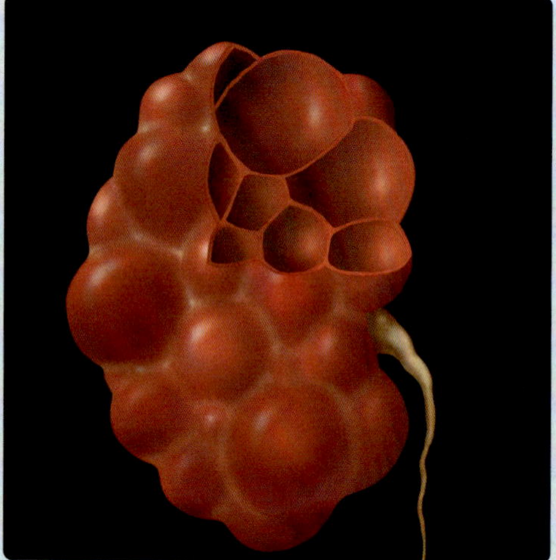

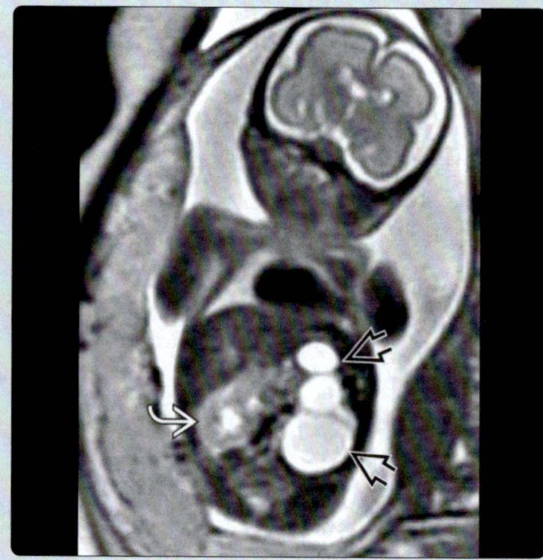

(Left) *Prone postnatal US of the left flank in the same patient shows multiple cysts ➡ of varying size replacing the left kidney. A reniform shape is retained, but no normal left renal parenchyma is seen.* **(Right)** *Posterior images in the same infant during a Tc-99m MAG3 renal scan show normal function of the right kidney ➡ but no function on the left side ➡, confirming a left MCDK. Early transient activity in MCDK on nuclear scans merely reflects that the tissue is being perfused, but continued images show no function.*

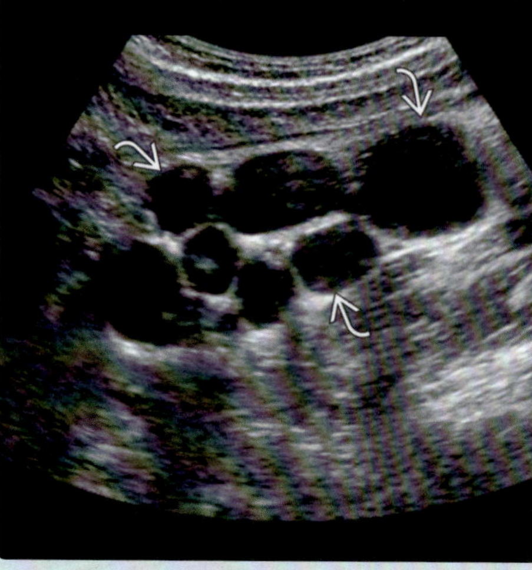

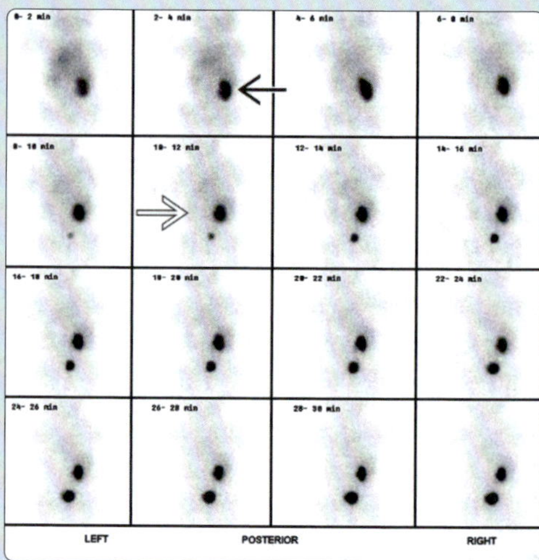

TERMINOLOGY

Definitions

- Multicystic dysplastic kidney (MCDK): Congenital, nonfunctional kidney replaced by multiple cysts & dysplastic tissue
- 2 forms of MCDK are classically recognized
  - Pelvoinfundibular (more common): Theoretically results from atresia of ureter or renal pelvis; cysts are remnants of dilated calyces
  - Hydronephrotic (occurs less frequently): Results from atretic segment of ureter; cysts replace entire pelvocalyceal system
- Tend to involute with time: Cysts shrink & residual tissue may lose reniform shape

IMAGING

General Features

- Best diagnostic clue
  - Cysts & dysplastic, echogenic tissue replace entire kidney
  - Nuclear scintigraphy documents lack of renal function
    - If some delayed excretion is present, consider poorly functioning hydronephrosis
- Location
  - Renal fossa is most common but can occur ectopically from pelvis to chest
- Size
  - Wide range: Up to 15 cm in length in newborn period; may be only 1-2 cm after years of involution
- Morphology
  - Numerous cysts of varying size with dysplastic intervening parenchyma
  - No recognizable normal corticomedullary architecture
  - Renal shape is typically preserved, though cysts may result in lobulated contour
  - Can be segmental in duplicated kidneys

Radiographic Findings

- Radiography
  - Indirect evidence: Space-occupying lesion in flank
- IVP
  - No enhancement of or excretion from MCDK
  - May see transient blush during contrast bolus infusion due retained vascularity

Ultrasonographic Findings

- Grayscale ultrasound
  - Reniform-shaped multicystic mass occupying renal fossa
    - ± lobulated outer contour (due to cysts of variable size)
  - Cysts of varying size do not connect
  - Largest cyst is typically peripheral rather than central
  - Poorly defined, intervening, echogenic parenchyma without normal corticomedullary architecture
- Color Doppler
  - Minimal, if any, vascularity in parenchyma; central hilar vessels tend to be small
- Often followed with annual US scans to
  - Assess growth of contralateral kidney
  - Confirm involution of MCDK
    - Wilms tumor arising in < 0.1% of MCDK

CT Findings

- NECT
  - Low-attenuation cysts (though some may contain debris) replacing normal renal parenchyma
- CECT
  - No parenchymal contrast enhancement
  - No contrast excretion on delayed images
  - No hydronephrosis

MR Findings

- Cysts replace normal renal parenchyma
- May be noted incidentally on MR performed for other indications or may follow abnormal 2nd trimester US

Nuclear Medicine Findings

- MAG3 scintigraphy
  - Initial blood flow images may show slight perfusion of MCDK but sequential images show lack radiotracer uptake or excretion
- Tc-99m DMSA renal cortical scan
  - Radiotracer may localize to scattered tubular cells in dysplastic parenchyma

Other Modality Findings

- Retrograde ureterogram will show blind-ending ureter
  - Different from rapid change in caliber of ureter & communication with calyces seen in ureteropelvic junction (UPJ) obstruction or other causes of hydronephrosis

Imaging Recommendations

- Best imaging tool
  - Ultrasound for initial identification
  - Nuclear scan to confirm nonfunction of suspected MCDK & assess drainage of contralateral kidney

DIFFERENTIAL DIAGNOSIS

Hydronephrosis

- "Cysts" (dilated calyces) are relatively uniform in size & connect centrally
- Largest "cyst" (renal pelvis) lies central

Congenital Obstructive Uropathy

- Bladder outlet obstruction often leads to echogenic kidneys with small, peripheral cysts (cystic renal dysplasia)
- May rarely appear similar to MCDK
  - Presence of renal pelvis makes MCDK unlikely

Congenital Mesoblastic Nephroma

- Solid or mixed solid & cystic neonatal/infantile renal mass
- "Claw" of renal tissue splayed along tumor margin

Wilms Tumor

- Typically large, solid, heterogeneous round mass with "claw" of renal tissue splayed along tumor margin

Pediatric Cystic Nephroma

- Round renal mass in males 3 months to 4 years of age
- Numerous thin-walled cysts throughout mass with central herniation of cysts
- "Claw" of renal tissue splayed along tumor margin

Tuberous Sclerosis

- Numerous cysts &/or angiomyolipomas bilaterally
- Look for cardiac rhabdomyomas & brain manifestations

Autosomal Recessive Polycystic Kidney Disease

- Enlarged, echogenic bilateral kidneys with striated parenchyma & intermixed small cysts

HNF1B/TCF2 Mutations

- Can mimic bilateral MCDK

End-Stage Renal Disease

- Bilateral kidneys tend to be small & echogenic, resembling involuted MCDK
- Cysts may be present from underlying disease or secondary to dialysis

PATHOLOGY

General Features

- Etiology
  - Probably due to atresia of ureter or UPJ during metanephric stage of intrauterine development
- Genetics
  - Generally considered sporadic; reported familial cases of autosomal dominant inheritance with variable expression & penetrance
- Associated abnormalities
  - Genitourinary abnormalities in 25-40%
    - Up to 40% of patients have contralateral abnormality
      - UPJ obstruction & vesicoureteral reflux (VUR) are most common (VUR in 12-26%)
    - Megaureter
    - Cystic dysplasia of testis
    - Case reports of Zinner syndrome: Seminal vesicle cysts, ejaculatory duct obstruction, unilateral renal agenesis (vs. involuted MCDK)
  - Nonurologic abnormalities in 15%
    - Cardiac & musculoskeletal are most common
  - Associated syndromes: Turner, trisomy 21, chromosome 22 deletions, Waardenburg, others

Gross Pathologic & Surgical Features

- Walls of cysts vary in thickness; fibrotic dysplastic tissue replaces normal renal stroma; may be quite large & nonreniform in shape

CLINICAL ISSUES

Presentation

- Most common signs/symptoms
  - ~ 70% are discovered antenatally or in infancy as palpable mass
  - Can have delayed presentation as incidental finding when
    - Symptoms of contralateral UPJ obstruction are evaluated
    - Patient is evaluated for urinary tract infection
    - Patient is imaged for traumatic injury or spine abnormality

Demographics

- Age
  - Congenital abnormality, usually presents in infancy
- Incidence
  - 0.03% in autopsy series
  - 1 in 4,300 live births

Natural History & Prognosis

- Unilateral MCDK with normal contralateral kidney: Excellent prognosis
  - Vast majority involute with time & remain asymptomatic
    - ~ 50% involute in 1st decade
    - MCDK > 5 cm in newborn is less likely to involute
  - Can have complications of infection or mass effect
  - Rare reports of hypertension with unilateral MCDK
    - Less common than cystic renal dysplasia
    - In patients treated with nephrectomy for hypertension, blood pressure normalized in only 50%, suggesting other cause of hypertension
  - Wilms tumor developing in < 0.1% of MCDK
  - Reports of hyperfiltration in solitary kidney → renal insufficiency
  - Contralateral compensatory hypertrophy in 60%
- Unilateral MCDK with abnormal contralateral kidney
  - If contralateral kidney has delayed diagnosis of UPJ or ureterovesical junction obstruction or VUR, renal insufficiency can be problem
  - VUR into contralateral kidney is associated with smaller renal size during 1st year of life; may lead to recurrent pyelonephritis, scarring, hypertension (HTN)
- Bilateral MCDK: Lethal without dialysis/renal transplant; pulmonary hypoplasia (secondary to anhydramnios) may be lethal at delivery

Treatment

- Surgical excision when complicated by focal enlargement, mass effect, recurrent infections, HTN
- Otherwise, serial ultrasounds for 3-5 years to monitor

SELECTED REFERENCES

1. Choi SM et al: Renal growth slope in children with congenital and acquired solitary functioning kidneys. Ultrasonography.40(3):357-65, 2020
2. Gilad N et al: Multicystic dysplastic kidney: prenatal compensatory renal growth pattern. J Ultrasound Med. 40(10):2165-71, 2020
3. Meyers ML et al: Imaging of fetal cystic kidney disease: multicystic dysplastic kidney versus renal cystic dysplasia. Pediatr Radiol. 50(13):1921-33, 2020
4. Pettit SM et al: Multicystic dysplastic kidney with mass effect in a neonate treated with nephrectomy: case Report. Urology.149:e11-4 2020
5. Takemura K et al: Seminal vesicle cysts with upper urinary tract abnormalities: a single-center case series of pediatric Zinner syndrome. Urology. 149:e11-4, 2020
6. Brown CT et al: Trends in surgical management of multicystic dysplastic kidney at USA children's hospitals. J Pediatr Urol. 15(4):368-73, 2019
7. Brown C et al: Knowledge of vesicoureteral reflux obtained by screening voiding cystourethrogram in children with multicystic dysplastic kidney does not change patient management or prevent febrile urinary tract infection. J Pediatr Urol. 15(3):267.e1-5, 2019
8. Gimpel C et al: Imaging of kidney cysts and cystic kidney diseases in children: an International Working Group consensus statement. Radiology. 290(3):769-82, 2019
9. Gaither TW et al: Natural history of contralateral hypertrophy in patients with multicystic dysplastic kidneys. J Urol. 199(1):280-6, 2018
10. Kara A et al: Clinical features of children with multicystic dysplastic kidney. Pediatr Int. 60(8):750-4, 2018
11. Matsumura K et al: Trajectory of estimated glomerular filtration rate predicts renal injury in children with multicystic dysplastic kidney. Nephron. 140(1):18-23, 2018
12. Iscaife A et al: Segmental multicystic dysplastic kidney: a rare situation. J Pediatr Urol. 7(4):491-4, 2011

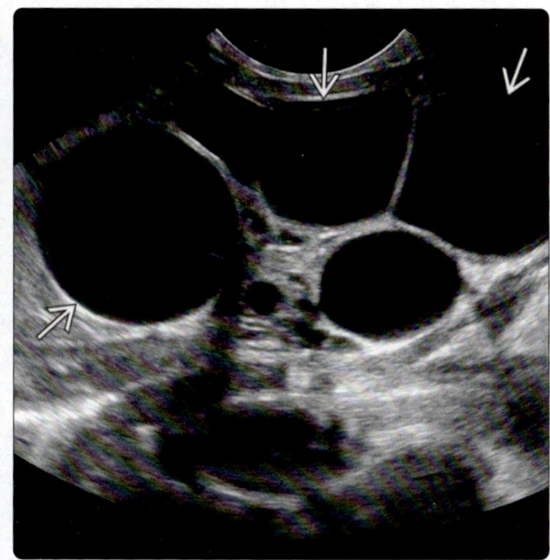

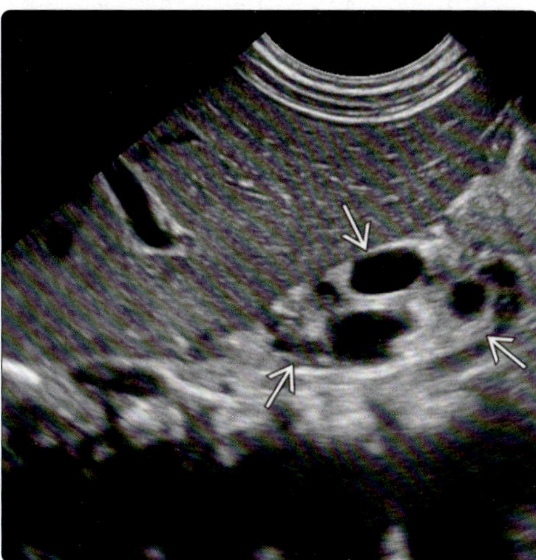

(Left) *Longitudinal US in a newborn shows a massive group of cysts ➔ measuring 8.8 cm in length occupying the left flank. This MCDK caused abdominal distention but no respiratory compromise & was managed conservatively.* **(Right)** *Longitudinal US shows only a few cysts in a 7-month-old with MCDK ➔. Note that the largest cysts are in the midkidney but do not connect (which helps to differentiate MCDK from hydronephrosis). Echogenic dysplastic tissue between the cysts becomes more evident as the cysts involute over months/years.*

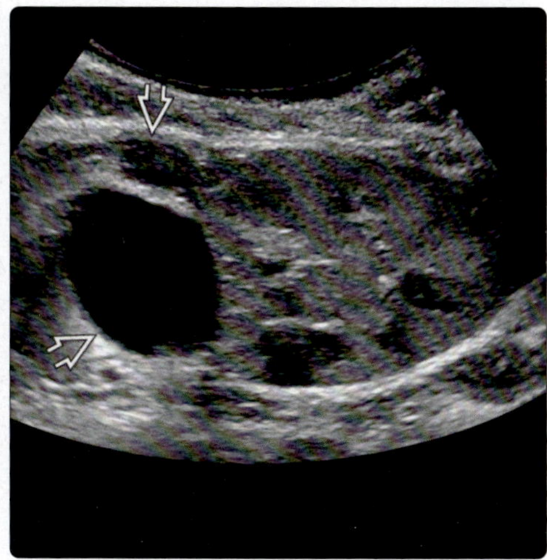

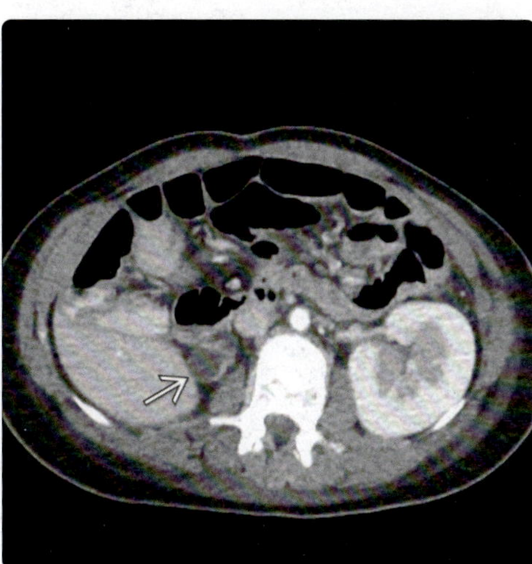

(Left) *Longitudinal US shows an unusual case of a segmental MCDK in an infant with cysts on a prenatal scan. The 2 cysts in the upper pole of the kidney ➔ do not communicate, & there is echogenic, solid parenchyma between the cysts. The lower pole is normal. The contralateral kidney in this infant was congenitally absent.* **(Right)** *Axial CECT performed for trauma in this 19-year-old patient shows an involuted right MCDK ➔, discovered incidentally. The left kidney demonstrated compensatory hypertrophy.*

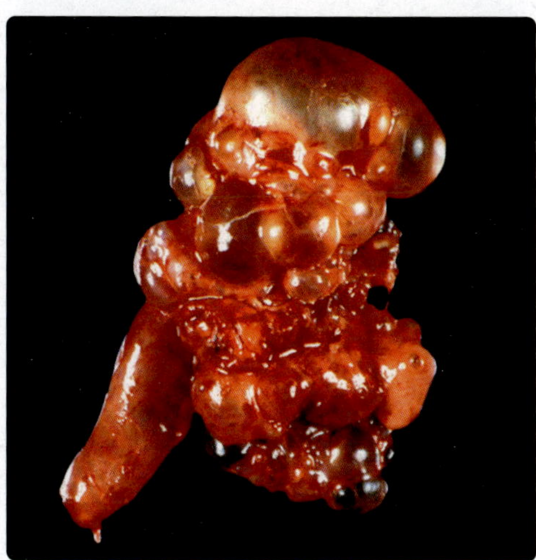

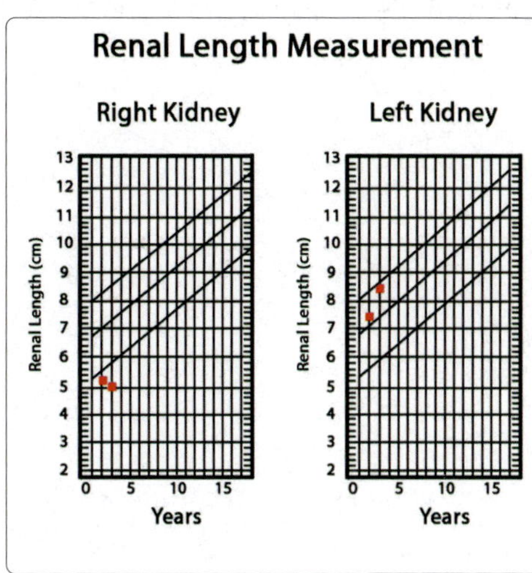

(Left) *Gross pathology shows numerous cysts replacing the renal parenchyma & distorting the contour of this MCDK. Note that the largest cyst in this specimen is in the upper pole, not in the renal hilum.* **(Right)** *This chart measures renal growth over serial exams in children. This particular patient has a shrinking right-sided MCDK & a rapidly growing normal left kidney, which would be expected to show compensatory hypertrophy.*

Polycystic Kidney Disease, Autosomal Recessive

KEY FACTS

TERMINOLOGY

- Single gene ciliopathy with marked bilateral renal enlargement due to dilated, distal tubules & collecting ducts
- Synonyms: Infantile polycystic kidney disease

IMAGING

- Radiographs: Bilateral flank "masses" bulging lateral abdominal contours & displacing bowel gas centrally
  - Pulmonary hypoplasia with history of oligohydramnios
    - Bell-shaped thorax ± pneumothorax, pneumomediastinum
- US: Bilaterally enlarged, echogenic kidneys in newborn with loss of corticomedullary differentiation
  - 2-6 standard deviations (SD) above mean size for age
  - Dilated, radially arranged tubules on high-resolution linear transducers ± small cysts (< 1 cm)
  - Tiny, punctate, hyperechoic foci (likely calcium deposits) develop with time & correlate with renal failure
- MR: Large kidneys of diffusely high signal intensity on T2
  - Intervening low-signal septa
- Variable degrees of liver disease

PATHOLOGY

- Autosomal recessive, due to mutations of polycystic kidney & hepatic disease 1 gene (*PKHD1*) on chromosome 6p12.2
  - Risk of recurrence in subsequent pregnancies: 25%

CLINICAL ISSUES

- Perinatal presentation: More severe renal disease with pulmonary hypoplasia
  - Renal replacement therapy (dialysis or transplant)
- Juvenile presentation: Less renal disease, more hepatic issues
  - Portal hypertension & fibrosis develop in 50%
- Severity & outcomes vary within affected families
- Survival rate for milder forms is up to 82% at age 3 years & 79% at 15 years

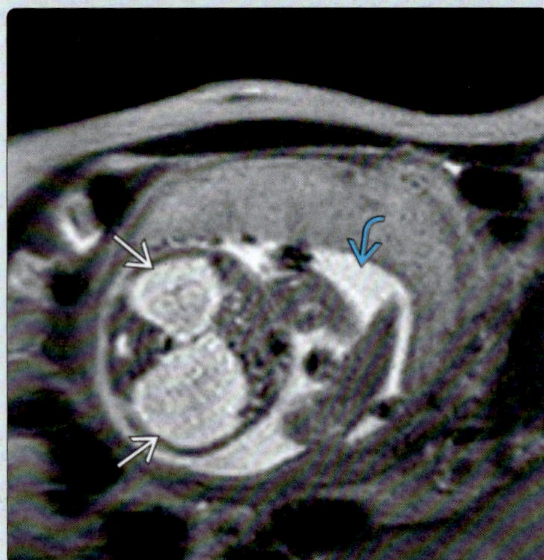

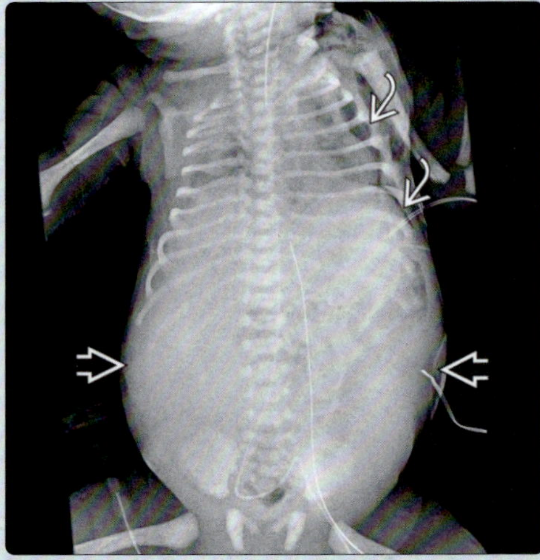

(Left) *Axial SSFSE T2 MR of a 2nd-trimester fetus shows massively enlarged, hyperintense kidneys ➡ with absent corticomedullary differentiation & low amniotic fluid volume ➡, typical of autosomal recessive polycystic kidney disease (ARPKD).* **(Right)** *Frontal radiograph in a newborn with a history of oligohydramnios shows bowel loops displaced centrally by bilateral flank "masses" ➡ (due to markedly enlarged kidneys). Note the bell-shaped thorax & left pneumothorax ➡.*

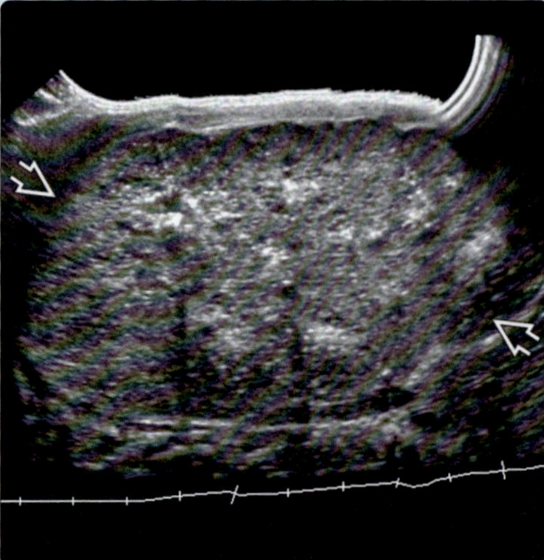

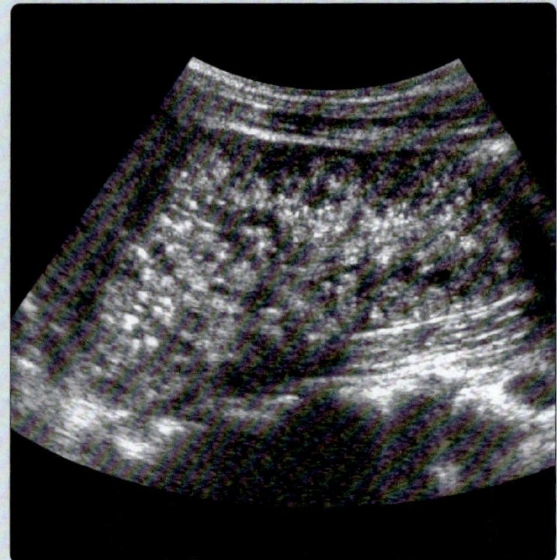

(Left) *Extended field-of-view longitudinal US shows a newborn kidney measuring > 10 cm in length ➡ (usually is between 4-6 cm). There is loss of corticomedullary differentiation with replacement of the renal parenchyma by microscopic cysts & dilated tubules with hyperechoic walls.* **(Right)** *Longitudinal US in a patient with ARPKD shows nephromegaly with numerous punctate echogenic foci throughout the kidney. The echogenic foci likely represent calcium deposits & correlate with worsening renal function.*

TERMINOLOGY

Synonyms

- Infantile polycystic kidney disease

Definitions

- Autosomal recessive polycystic kidney disease (ARPKD): Single gene ciliopathy characterized by dilated, distal, convoluted tubules & collecting ducts

IMAGING

General Features

- Best diagnostic clue
  - Bilaterally enlarged kidneys, > 2-6 standard deviations (SD) above mean with loss of intrarenal architecture
  - Massive kidneys fill flanks & displace adjacent organs
  - Pulmonary hypoplasia with history of oligohydramnios further supports diagnosis
- Variable degrees of liver disease
  - Caroli syndrome, hepatic fibrosis, portal hypertension (HTN)

Radiographic Findings

- Radiography
  - Bilateral flank "masses" bulging lateral abdominal contours & displacing bowel gas centrally
  - Pulmonary hypoplasia with bell-shaped thorax ± pneumothorax, pneumomediastinum

Ultrasonographic Findings

- Enlarged, hyperechoic kidneys
  - Renal size is maximal by 1-2 years old
- Poor or absent corticomedullary differentiation
- Dilated, radially arranged tubules seen in 2/3 of affected kidneys by high-resolution linear transducers
  - Creates striated appearance
- Focal rosettes consisting of clusters of radially oriented, dilated collecting tubules also reported
- Small cysts may be present, generally < 1 cm in diameter; seen in ~ 1/2 of patients
  - Cysts > 1 cm only in minority of cases
- Diffuse microcystic appearance also described
- Tiny, punctate, hyperechoic foci develop with time & correlate with renal failure
  - Do not cause posterior acoustic shadowing but may cause ring-down artifact
  - Calcium citrate & oxalate crystals found histologically
- Doppler suggests random arrangement of intrarenal vessels rather than typical branching pattern
- Prenatal ultrasound findings
  - Renal size & renal circumference to abdominal circumference ratio > 2 SD above mean for gestational age
  - Enlargement may not occur until mid 2nd trimester
  - Cysts may be visible but do not predominate
  - Abnormal corticomedullary differentiation in variable patterns
  - Oligohydramnios
    - In 1st or 2nd trimester, carries poor prognosis
  - Fetal bladder is not visible
  - Associated musculoskeletal abnormalities due to mechanics: Oligohydramnios limits movement
- Liver involvement
  - Enlargement, ↑ or coarse echogenicity, periportal fibrosis with ↑ periportal echogenicity, ↑ parenchymal stiffness on elastography, intrahepatic bile duct dilation, cysts
  - Portal HTN: ↓ or reversed portal flow, splenomegaly, ascites
  - Caroli syndrome: Cystic dilation of intrahepatic ducts with central echogenic dot of portal radicles

MR Findings

- Large kidneys of diffusely high signal intensity on T2
  - May have striated appearance of dilated tubules ± small, discrete cysts with low-signal septa
- Uniform or grainy intermediate to low signal on T1
- MRU: Radially arranged, dilated tubules throughout kidney
- No urine in bladder
- Liver involvement
  - Caroli syndrome
    - Cystic intrahepatic biliary dilation: Delayed enhancement on hepatobiliary phase with hepatobiliary contrast agents
    - Central dot sign: Portal radicle enhancement on T1 C+ or flow void on T2/MRCP centrally in dilated intrahepatic duct
  - Hepatic fibrosis
    - ↓ T1 & ↓ T2, ↑ parenchymal stiffness on elastography
  - Portal HTN
    - Abnormal portal flow on MR venogram, splenomegaly, ascites

Nuclear Medicine Findings

- Hepatobiliary scintigraphy
  - Delay in maximal hepatocyte uptake & tracer excretion into biliary tree & gut; cystic foci of hepatic photopenia early with gradual & prolonged tracer accumulation
- Tc-99m DMSA renal cortical scans
  - Loss of kidney outline & internal structure; patchy tracer uptake with focal defects throughout kidneys

Imaging Recommendations

- Best imaging tool
  - Ultrasound
    - Fetal US with serial renal measurements if at risk
    - Diagnostic infant US with ↑ frequency linear transducer
    - Annual abdominal ultrasound
      - No clear prognostic value of kidney size on function
      - Kidney imaging mainly for decision making prior to nephrectomy/transplant
      - Evaluate for signs of portal HTN & fibrosis
  - MRCP if complications of liver disease

DIFFERENTIAL DIAGNOSIS

Bilateral Multicystic Dysplastic Kidney

- Macroscopic cysts of varying size with no normal renal parenchyma
- Essentially lethal disorder

Autosomal Dominant Polycystic Kidney Disease

- Renal enlargement is < autosomal recessive polycystic kidney disease (ARPKD), may be asymmetric
- Few small cysts may be visible in 3rd trimester; renal echogenicity is normal or with echogenic cortex; amniotic fluid is normal
  - Check family history & scan kidneys of parents
- Rare phenotype reported with homozygous mutations, resulting in enlarged echogenic kidneys similar to ARPKD

Cystic Renal Dysplasia

- Small with numerous cysts (frequently peripheral) & echogenic parenchyma
- Most commonly due to chronic obstruction
  - May be unilateral or asymmetric

Meckel-Gruber Syndrome

- Encephalocele, large polycystic kidneys, & polydactyly

Tuberous Sclerosis

- Rhabdomyoma: Echogenic cardiac mass
- Tubers & subependymal nodules in brain: May be difficult to detect in newborn
- Renal cysts: May be seen in utero
- Angiomyolipomas: Not usually seen in newborn

HNF1B/TCF2 Mutation

- Variable renal cystic disease, potentially mimics bilateral multicystic dysplastic kidney (MCDK)
- Early-onset diabetes mellitus

Joubert Syndrome & Related Disorders

- Ciliopathy with molar tooth malformation brainstem & cerebellum; variable renal cystic disease

PATHOLOGY

General Features

- Genetics
  - Autosomal recessive
  - Polycystic kidney & hepatic disease 1 gene (*PKHD1*)
    - Chromosomal locus 6p12.2
  - Carrier frequency: 1 in 70 of general population
- Associated abnormalities
  - Musculoskeletal abnormalities due to oligohydramnios
  - Pulmonary compromise due to oligohydramnios & elevation of diaphragm by enlarged kidneys

Microscopic Features

- Ectatic distal convoluted tubules & collecting ducts
- Tubules described as saccular or cylindrically enlarged

CLINICAL ISSUES

Presentation

- Most common signs/symptoms
  - Bilateral renal enlargement, renal insufficiency ± respiratory distress
    - Pulmonary hypoplasia may be life-limiting
- Other signs/symptoms
  - Fetal presentation: Enlarged kidneys at imaging
    - Majority detected > 24 weeks
    - Poor prognosis with fetal diagnosis
  - Marked nephromegaly may cause dystocia at birth

Natural History & Prognosis

- Perinatal presentation
  - Severe renal disease; pulmonary hypoplasia
  - Worst prognosis; high mortality in 1st month of life
  - Nephrectomy is common due to mass effect
- Perinatal survivors
  - Require renal replacement therapy (dialysis or transplant)
  - If prolonged survival, liver disease becomes relevant
- Juvenile presentation
  - Milder renal disease
  - Liver disease is more relevant in survivors
    - Portal HTN & fibrosis develop in ~ 1/2 of patients
  - Survival rate has ↑ for milder form to 82% at age 3 years & 79% at 15 years
- Severity & outcomes vary within affected families
  - Systemic HTN in 75%
  - Chronic ventilatory support in 30-50%

Treatment

- With fetal detection
  - Monitor fetal abdominal circumference for risk of dystocia
  - Counsel on outcomes, interventions (serial amnioinfusions, postnatal pulmonary & renal support) vs. comfort care options
  - Deliver at tertiary center
- With survivors
  - As needed, dialysis (peritoneal in infants) as bridge to renal transplant
    - Dialysis or transplant in 25-60% by 10 years old
  - Nephrectomy when renal size compromises respiratory status or peritoneal dialysis
  - Liver transplant when associated with progressive hepatic fibrosis
    - Combined liver kidney transplant (CLKT)
    - Kidney after liver transplant (KALT)

SELECTED REFERENCES

1. Benz EG et al: Predictors of progression in autosomal dominant and autosomal recessive polycystic kidney disease. Pediatr Nephrol. 36(9):2639-58, 2021
2. Hartung EA et al: Magnetic resonance elastography to quantify liver disease severity in autosomal recessive polycystic kidney disease. Abdom Radiol (NY). 46(2):570-80, 2020
3. Meyers ML et al: Imaging of fetal cystic kidney disease: multicystic dysplastic kidney versus renal cystic dysplasia. Pediatr Radiol. 50(13):1921-33, 2020
4. Overman RE et al: Early nephrectomy in neonates with symptomatic autosomal recessive polycystic kidney disease. J Pediatr Surg. 56(2):328-31, 2020
5. Thomas CC et al: Ultrasound Imaging of Renal Cysts in Children. J Ultrasound Med. 40(3):621-35, 2020
6. Wicher D et al: Occurrence of portal hypertension and its clinical course in patients with molecularly confirmed autosomal recessive polycystic kidney disease (ARPKD). Front Pediatr. 8:591379, 2020
7. Garel J et al: Prenatal ultrasonography of autosomal dominant polycystic kidney disease mimicking recessive type: case series. Pediatr Radiol. 49(7):906-12, 2019
8. Gimpel C et al: Imaging of kidney cysts and cystic kidney diseases in children: an International Working Group consensus statement. Radiology. 290(3):769-82, 2019
9. Dillman JR et al: Hereditary renal cystic disorders: imaging of the kidneys and beyond. Radiographics. 37(3):924-46, 2017

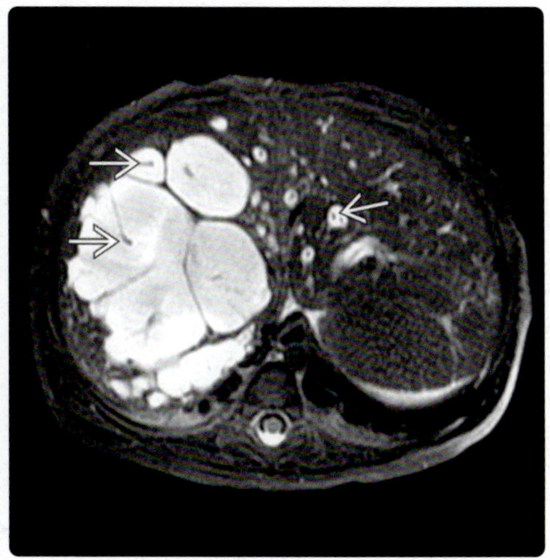

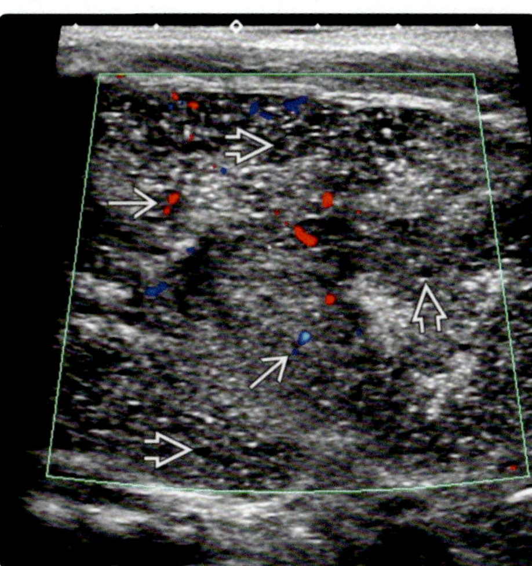

(Left) *Axial T2 FS MR in a patient with ARPKD & Caroli disease shows the dilated intrahepatic biliary tree affecting the right lobe of the liver more than the left. The central dots within these fluid-filled spaces are tiny portal vein branches ➡.* **(Right)** *Color Doppler US in an infant with ARPKD demonstrates cysts & dilated tubules ➡ replacing the normal renal parenchyma. Also seen are small vessels ➡ coursing randomly in the replaced renal parenchyma (rather than in the organized pattern of normal interlobular & arcuate branches).*

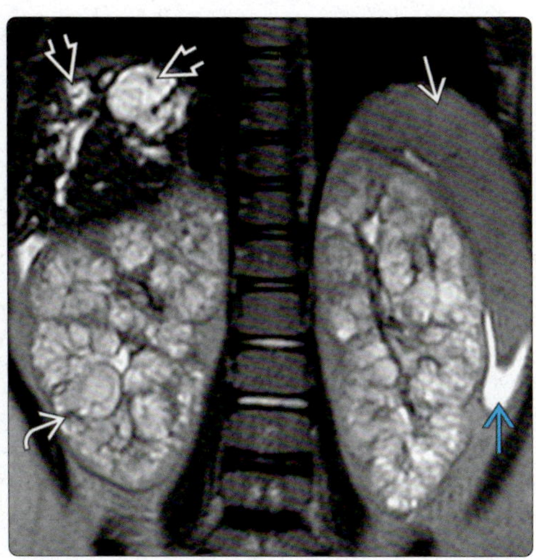

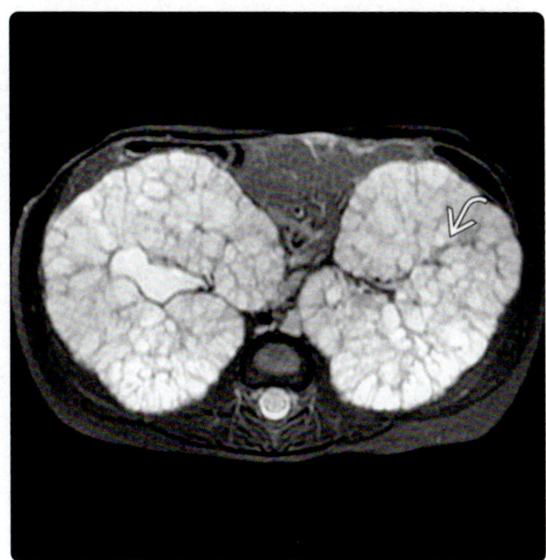

(Left) *Coronal T2 FS MR in a 4-year-old with ARPKD & Caroli disease shows the enlarged, hyperintense kidneys replaced with tiny cysts & lace-like fibrous septa ➡. A central dot pattern of biliary ductal dilation ➡ is noted. The progressive hepatic fibrosis has led to splenomegaly ➡ & ascites ➡ from portal hypertension (HTN).* **(Right)** *Axial T2 FS MR in a child with ARPKD & Caroli disease shows complete replacement of the kidneys with cysts & lace-like fibrous septa ➡. The kidneys are markedly enlarged & hyperintense.*

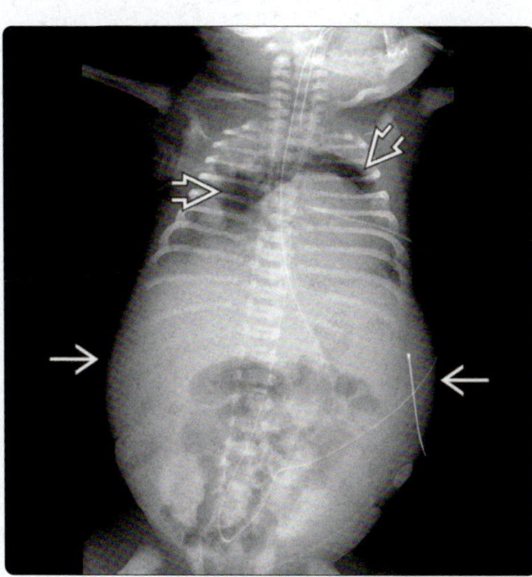

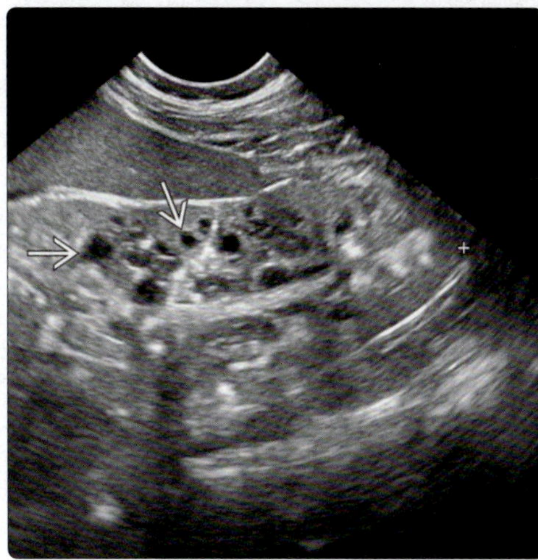

(Left) *AP radiograph shows bulging flanks ➡ in a newborn with severe respiratory distress & pneumomediastinum ➡. The patient has ARPKD with the massively enlarged kidneys causing the bulging flanks & displacing the bowel gas centrally.* **(Right)** *Longitudinal US of the left kidney in an 8-year-old with ARPKD & portal HTN shows the cursor (+) on the lower pole of this 13-cm long kidney. Note the presence of a few macrocysts ➡ in the kidney.*

Polycystic Kidney Disease, Autosomal Dominant

KEY FACTS

TERMINOLOGY

- Autosomal dominant polycystic kidney disease (ADPKD)
- Hereditary ciliopathy characterized by multiple renal cysts & various other systemic manifestations
- Cystic organ involvement: Kidneys (100%), liver (50%), pancreas (9%), brain/ovaries/testis (1%)
- Cerebral berry aneurysms (5-10% in adults)

IMAGING

- Renal size within 2 standard deviations above normal at time of diagnosis in 1/2 of pediatric patients
- Scattered renal cysts of variable number & size
  - ↑ throughout life: 54% of ADPKD cysts appear in 1st decade; 72% occur within 2nd decade
  - ± complication by hemorrhage, infection, or rupture
- Renal parenchyma is often otherwise normal
- Rare phenotype appearing like ARPKD (enlarged, echogenic kidneys) with variant homozygous mutations

PATHOLOGY

- 90% autosomal dominant; 10% spontaneous mutations
- Types of ADPKD is based on gene location
  - *PKD1*: Short arm of chromosome 16 (90%)
  - *PKD2*: Long arm of chromosome 4 (10%)
- Family history lacking in almost 1/2 of patients

CLINICAL ISSUES

- Typically asymptomatic in childhood
  - Discovered incidentally or when screening children of affected adults
  - Flank pain, hematuria, hypertension (HTN), & renal failure are also reported in children
- Prognosis is excellent in childhood
- Prognosis in adulthood is variable: Hemorrhage, infection, rupture; renal failure; HTN; rarely malignancy

(Left) *Longitudinal ultrasound in a 17-year-old patient undergoing treatment for lymphoma shows an incidental simple cyst ➡ in the midkidney. The patient developed additional cysts over time & had a family history of renal failure.* **(Right)** *Axial CECT in the same patient several years later shows multiple low-density, nonenhancing cysts ➡ in both kidneys, consistent with autosomal dominant polycystic kidney disease (ADPKD).*

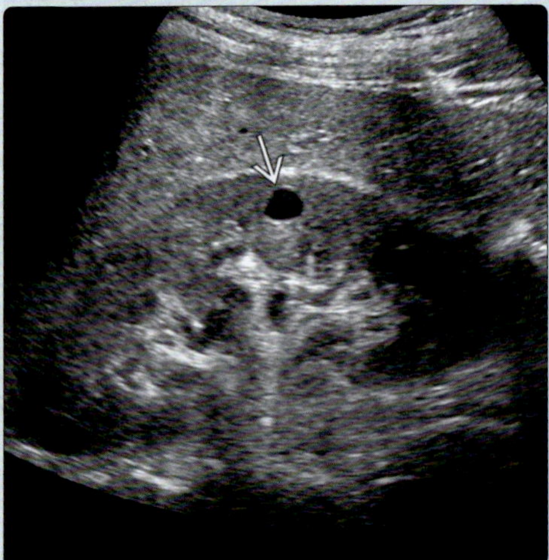

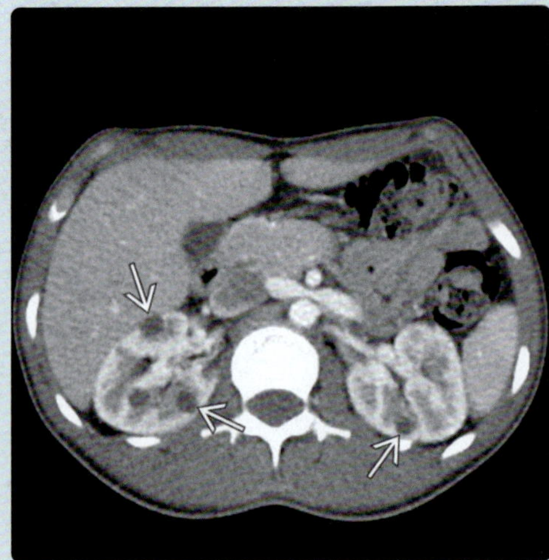

(Left) *Coronal T2 MR in a 13-year-old patient with a family history of ADPKD shows numerous high signal intensity cysts ➡ of varying size.* **(Right)** *Longitudinal power Doppler ultrasound shows normal blood flow in normal-appearing renal parenchyma between multiple simple-appearing cysts ➡. Vascular compression by the enlarging cysts is one theory to explain progressive renal insufficiency in ADPKD.*

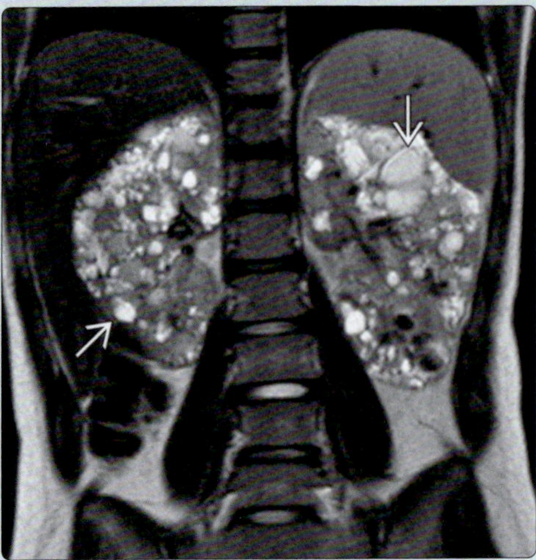

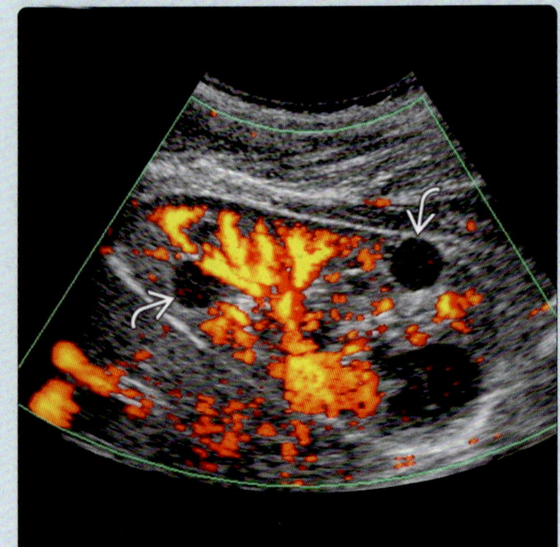

TERMINOLOGY

Synonyms

- Autosomal dominant polycystic kidney disease (ADPKD), adult polycystic kidney disease

Definitions

- Hereditary ciliopathy characterized by multiple renal cysts & various other systemic manifestations
  - Pei Ravine criteria: ≥ 3 uni- or bilateral cysts if ≥ 15-years-old; <15-years-old with positive family history, ≥ 1 kidney cyst &/or renal enlargement is considered highly suggestive of ADPKD
- Cystic organ involvement
  - Kidneys (100%), liver (50%), pancreas (9%), brain/ovaries/testes (1%)
- Noncystic manifestations
  - Cardiac valve (26%), hernias (25%), colonic diverticula
  - Aneurysms: Cerebral berry aneurysms (5-10%); aortic or coronary aneurysms are less common

IMAGING

Ultrasonographic Findings

- Grayscale ultrasound
  - Multiple well-defined, round, anechoic cysts bilaterally
  - Renal contour, size, & echotexture are typically normal early in life
  - Renal contour may become lobulated as more cysts form
  - Rare phenotype: Appears more like ARPKD (enlarged echogenic kidneys in fetus/neonate) with variant homozygous *PKD1* mutations

MR Findings

- T1WI
  - Uncomplicated cysts: Hypointense
  - Complicated (hemorrhagic cysts)
    - Signal intensity varies with age of hemorrhage
    - Classic appearances suggesting blood products: Hyperintense, fluid-fluid levels
- T2WI
  - Uncomplicated cysts: Hyperintense contents, thin wall
  - Complicated: Variable signal intensity, blood products may be hypointense & layering; mural thickening

Imaging Recommendations

- Best imaging tool
  - Ultrasound (sensitivity, specificity, accuracy 97+%)

DIFFERENTIAL DIAGNOSIS

Autosomal Recessive Polycystic Kidney Disease

- Very enlarged newborn kidneys
- Echogenic parenchyma with dilated tubules & loss of corticomedullary differentiation; few small cysts

Isolated Simple Cysts

- Very few in number, normal renal function

Tuberous Sclerosis

- Fat-containing renal angiomyolipomas + cysts
- Characteristic brain & cutaneous findings

Multicystic Dysplastic Kidney

- Congenital, nonfunctioning mass of cysts replacing kidney
- Rarely bilateral (fatal)

Acquired Cystic Disease of Dialysis

- Early stage: Small kidneys with multiple cysts
- Advanced stage: Indistinguishable from ADPKD

PATHOLOGY

General Features

- Genetics
  - 50% chance of child inheriting mutant gene from parent
  - Types of ADPKD based on gene location
    - *PKD1*: Short arm of chromosome 16 (90%)
    - *PKD2*: Long arm of chromosome 4 (10%)
- Associated abnormalities
  - Cystic changes in other organs, including liver, pancreas, spleen, thyroid, lung, brain, gonads, & bladder
  - Cardiac & aortic abnormalities include valvular disease, coarctation, & aneurysms
    - 10% of adults with ADPKD die from rupture of intracranial berry aneurysm
  - Slightly ↑ risk of renal cell carcinoma
  - Up to 3% of tuberous sclerosis patients have ADPKD
    - *TSC2* gene is adjacent to *PKD1* on chromosome 16

CLINICAL ISSUES

Presentation

- Typically asymptomatic in childhood
  - Discovered incidentally or when screening children of affected adults
- Flank pain, hematuria, hypertension (HTN), & renal failure

Demographics

- Variable age at diagnosis: in utero to 8th decade
  - Prevalence of cysts ↑ with age
    - 54% appear in 1st decade of life
    - 72% occur within 2nd decade
- Incidence: 1 in 400 to 1,000 live births

Natural History & Prognosis

- Prognosis is excellent in childhood
- Prognosis in adulthood is variable
  - Hemorrhage, infection, rupture, renal failure, HTN, rarely malignancy

SELECTED REFERENCES

1. Benz EG et al: Predictors of progression in autosomal dominant and autosomal recessive polycystic kidney disease. Pediatr Nephrol. 36(9):2639-58, 2021
2. Meyers ML et al: Imaging of fetal cystic kidney disease: multicystic dysplastic kidney versus renal cystic dysplasia. Pediatr Radiol. 50(13):1921-33, 2020
3. Thomas CC et al: Ultrasound imaging of renal cysts in children. J Ultrasound Med. 40(3):621-35, 2020
4. Garel J et al: Prenatal ultrasonography of autosomal dominant polycystic kidney disease mimicking recessive type: case series. Pediatr Radiol. 49(7):906-12, 2019
5. Chung EM et al: From the radiologic pathology archives: pediatric polycystic kidney disease and other ciliopathies: radiologic-pathologic correlation. Radiographics. 34(1):155-78, 2014

Wilms Tumor

KEY FACTS

TERMINOLOGY

- Malignant tumor of primitive metanephric blastema in younger child

IMAGING

- Ultrasound is frequently 1st study performed
  - Large, heterogeneous but predominantly solid hypoechoic mass
  - Can have cystic foci, rarely Ca^{2+}
- Contrast-enhanced CT/MR: Characterizes tumor, extent, multifocality → staging
  - Hypoenhancing solid mass, often heterogeneous; restricts diffusion
    - Purely cystic form is rare
  - Look for local extension, tumor thrombus (renal vein, IVC), & lymph node enlargement
    - Moderate/complex ascites may indicate tumor rupture
  - Assess contralateral kidney for synchronous masses
- Chest CT: Lung metastases in 10-20% at presentation

TOP DIFFERENTIAL DIAGNOSES

- Neuroblastoma: Extrarenal, more often calcified
- Congenital mesoblastic nephroma: < 3-12 months
- Clear cell sarcoma: May have bone metastases
- Renal cell carcinoma: Older child, adolescent

PATHOLOGY

- Associated predisposing syndromes in 10%

CLINICAL ISSUES

- 80% occur in children < 5 years old
- Typical presentation: Incidentally discovered palpable mass
- Preferred treatment: Up front complete surgical resection
  - Preoperative chemotherapy for unresectable tumors, bilateral tumors, or extensive tumor thrombus
  - Postoperative chemotherapy ± radiation
- > 90% 5-year-survival for localized abdominal disease

(Left) *AP radiograph in a 3-year-old child with a firm, palpable mass shows leftward & inferior displacement of bowel loops ➡ by a right-sided soft tissue mass ➡. CT was performed next in this child due to suspicion for a Wilms tumor.* **(Right)** *Coronal CECT in the same patient confirms a large, heterogeneous, solid mass ➡ arising from the right kidney. A residual "claw" of normal renal tissue ➡ is splayed along the upper pole of this Wilms tumor. No contralateral lesions or venous invasion were identified.*

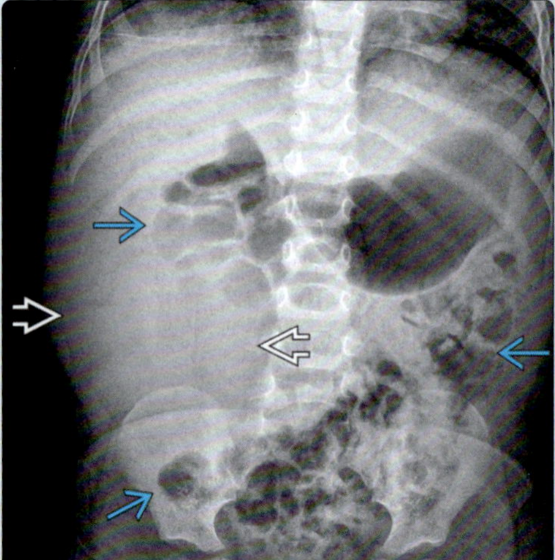

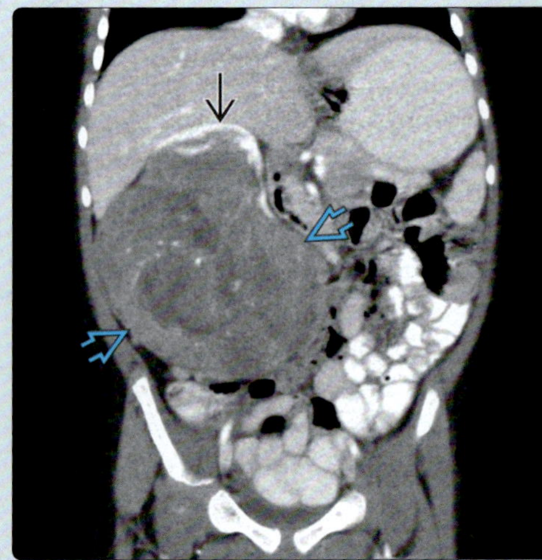

(Left) *Longitudinal US in a 5-year-old with hypertension & abdominal fullness shows a round, heterogeneous mass ➡ extending out of the lower pole of the left kidney ➡. Wilms tumor was confirmed upon surgery.* **(Right)** *Axial CECT shows a large, poorly defined, heterogeneous Wilms tumor ➡ arising from the left kidney in a 4-year-old girl. Note the enlarged lymph node ➡ displacing the aorta anteriorly & to the right ➡.*

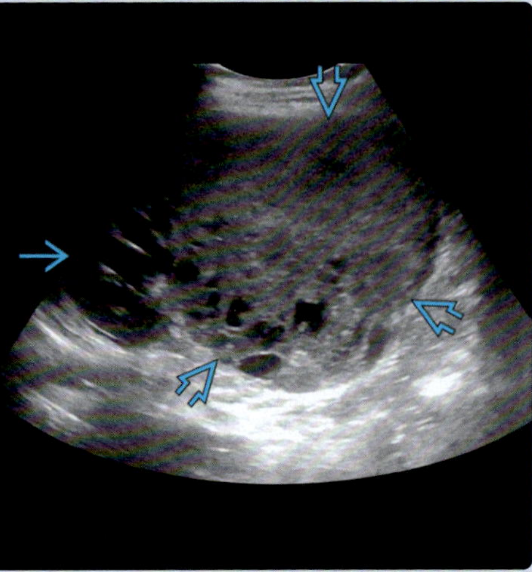

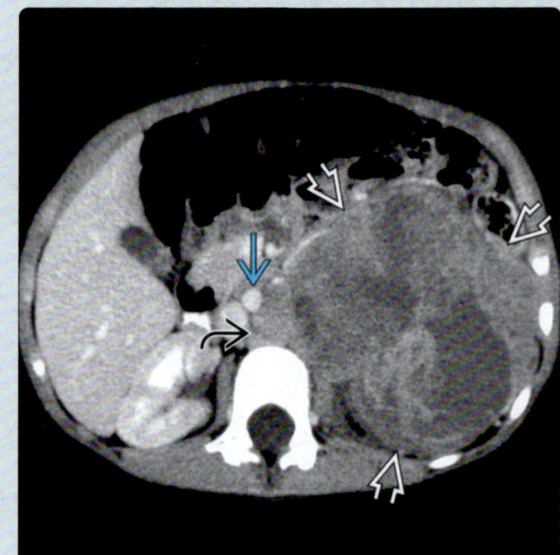

TERMINOLOGY

Synonyms

- Nephroblastoma

Definitions

- Malignant tumor of primitive metanephric blastema
- Most common abdominal neoplasm ages 1-8 years

IMAGING

General Features

- Best diagnostic clue
  - Large, heterogeneous renal mass in young child ± tumor thrombus in renal vein/inferior vena cava (IVC)
- Location
  - > 90% unilateral, 5-10% bilateral
- Size
  - Typically large (mean diameter: 5-10 cm)
- Morphology
  - Usually spherical; sometimes lobulated or multicentric
  - Usually smooth contours; may have local extension

Radiographic Findings

- Mass displacing adjacent bowel
- Ca^{2+} visible in 10%

Ultrasonographic Findings

- Grayscale ultrasound
  - Large, typically hypoechoic but heterogeneous mass
    - May see adjacent enlarged lymph nodes
  - Look for "claw" of splayed residual kidney surrounding mass
- Color Doppler
  - Evaluate renal vein/IVC for tumor thrombus

CT Findings

- NECT
  - Ca^{2+} in 15%
  - Lung metastases in 10-20% at time of diagnosis
    - Well-defined, solid nodules
- CECT
  - Large, poorly enhancing, heterogeneous mass
    - "Claw" of residual renal tissue splayed along tumor margin
  - Often has well-defined margins or pseudocapsule
  - Displaces adjacent organs, especially bowel
  - ± enlarged retroperitoneal lymph nodes
  - ± tumor thrombus in renal vein, IVC, right atrium
  - May have local extension into perirenal fat or gross tumor rupture with ascites

MR Findings

- T1: Typically heterogeneous, predominantly intermediate to low signal; may have foci of high signal due to blood products
- T2: Typically heterogeneous, solid, & predominantly of high signal
  - Purely cystic lesions are uncommon
- T1 C+: Heterogeneous & hypoenhancing relative to normal renal parenchyma
- DWI: Solid portions restrict diffusion
- Multiphase postcontrast imaging may be helpful to evaluate for tumor thrombus

Nuclear Medicine Findings

- PET
  - Problem-solving tool in selected cases
    - May be helpful in suspected recurrences
  - Tumor &/or metastatic lesions are typically FDG avid

Imaging Recommendations

- Best imaging tool
  - Ultrasound to confirm presence of renal mass
  - Contrast-enhanced CT/MR to further characterize tumor, local extent, staging
    - MR is typically preferred in suspected bilateral Wilms
  - Chest CT for staging
- Protocol advice
  - Contrast-enhanced CT/MR is adequate to evaluate for tumor thrombus
    - Doppler ultrasound if needed in specific cases

DIFFERENTIAL DIAGNOSIS

Neuroblastoma

- Suprarenal (adrenal gland) or paraspinal (sympathetic chain)
  - Typically displaces rather than invades kidney
- Much more likely than Wilms to contain Ca^{2+}, cross midline, & engulf or "lift" adjacent vessels

Congenital Mesoblastic Nephroma

- Solid or mixed solid & cystic tumor of infants
  - > 90% diagnosed in 1st year of life

Multilocular Cystic Renal Tumor

- Entirely cystic mass with numerous thin septations
- Classically herniates into renal pelvis
- Associated with *DICER1* mutation

Renal Cell Carcinoma

- Solid renal mass typically seen in 2nd decade of life

Renal Rhabdoid Tumor

- Nonspecific solid renal mass in young child
- Subcapsular fluid collection is suggestive
- May have synchronous intracranial rhabdoid tumor

Clear Cell Sarcoma

- Solid renal mass ± bone metastases

Pyelonephritis

- Developing abscess can mimic cystic neoplasm (but is typically more infiltrative)
- Patients often have clinical & laboratory features of upper urinary tract infection

Renal Medullary Carcinoma

- Poorly defined, infiltrating renal mass
- Typically adolescent/young adult; associated with sickle cell trait or disease

Nephroblastomatosis

- Multiple nonenhancing foci of residual primitive nephrogenic rests in infant, usually bilateral
- Individual lesions are relatively small & homogeneous

Lymphoma

- Multifocal, solid, hypoenhancing renal masses, typically with other evidence of lymphoma

PATHOLOGY

General Features

- Etiology
  - Primitive metanephric blastema differentiates by 34-weeks gestation
  - Persistence of metanephric blastema is termed "nephrogenic rests" (NRs)
    - Found in 1% of infant autopsies; most spontaneously regress
    - Multiple NRs = nephroblastomatosis
    - Perilobar NRs = multifocal, peripheral
      - Associated with hemihypertrophy, Beckwith-Wiedemann syndrome
    - Intralobar NRs = central, often solitary, ↑ risk of Wilms
      - Associated with WAGR syndrome, Denys-Drash
    - NRs are present in 30-40% of unilateral Wilms tumors
    - NRs are present in 94% of patients with metachronous contralateral Wilms tumors
      - 1% of unilateral Wilms tumor patients develop metachronous disease
    - NRs are present in 99% of patients with synchronous bilateral Wilms tumors
      - Represent 4-7% of all Wilms tumors
      - Present at slightly younger age than unilateral Wilms tumor (2.6 vs. 3.3-3.6 years)
- Genetics
  - Numerous somatic & germline mutations described
    - 10-20% have 11p13 (*WT1*) gene mutation
  - Only 2% of Wilms tumors are familial
- Associated abnormalities
  - Genitourinary anomalies
  - Overgrowth syndromes (Beckwith-Wiedemann syndrome, isolated hemihypertrophy, CLOVES)
  - WAGR syndrome: Wilms tumor, aniridia, genitourinary anomalies, mental retardation
  - Sporadic aniridia
  - Denys-Drash syndrome
  - Trisomy 18
  - Sotos syndrome
  - Bloom syndrome

Staging, Grading, & Classification

- Similar systems used by Children's Oncology Group (COG)/National Wilms Tumor Study Group (NWTSG) or Socièté Internationale d'Oncologie Pediatrique (SIOP)
  - I: Confined to kidney, completely excised
  - II: Local extension, completely resected
  - III: Incomplete resection, no distant metastases
  - IV: Distant metastases to lung, liver, brain, or bone
  - V: Bilateral synchronous tumors

Microscopic Features

- 4-10% have unfavorable (anaplastic) histology

CLINICAL ISSUES

Presentation

- Most common signs/symptoms
  - Asymptomatic palpable mass, abdominal pain, rarely hematuria
- Other signs/symptoms
  - Hypertension (vascular compression), fever (tumor necrosis), anemia

Demographics

- Age
  - 80% of cases occur in children < 5 years old
  - Peak: 3.6 years
    - Syndromic tumor occurrence is typically younger

Natural History & Prognosis

- Prognosis is based on stage, histology
- 5-year survival for localized abdominal disease > 90%

Treatment

- Up front complete surgical resection (nephrectomy) is preferred
  - Partial nephrectomy is rarely feasible in unilateral cases
- Preoperative chemotherapy for unresectable tumors, bilateral tumors, or extensive tumor thrombus
- Bilateral tumor undergoes partial nephrectomies after chemotherapy, if feasible
- Postoperative chemotherapy ± radiation
- Bone marrow transplant is usually reserved for relapses

DIAGNOSTIC CHECKLIST

Consider

- Children with predisposing syndromes require ultrasound screening every 3 months until 8 years of age

Image Interpretation Pearls

- Careful assessment of renal vein & IVC, adjacent soft tissues & lymph nodes, contralateral kidney, & lungs
  - Doppler assessment of renal vein/IVC is not needed if CT/MR images are normal
- Moderate or complex ascites may suggest tumor rupture

SELECTED REFERENCES

1. Sandberg JK et al: Imaging characteristics of nephrogenic rests versus small wilms tumors: a report from the Children's Oncology Group Study AREN03B2. AJR Am J Roentgenol. 214(5):987-94, 2020
2. Servaes SE et al: Imaging of Wilms tumor: an update. Pediatr Radiol. 49(11):1441-52, 2019
3. Chung EM et al: Renal tumors of childhood: radiologic-pathologic correlation part 1. The 1st decade: from the Radiologic Pathology Archives. Radiographics. 36(2):499-522, 2016
4. Kieran K et al: Current surgical standards of care in Wilms tumor. Urol Oncol. 34(1):13-23, 2016
5. Servaes S et al: Comparison of diagnostic performance of CT and MRI for abdominal staging of pediatric renal tumors: a report from the Children's Oncology Group. Pediatr Radiol. 45(2):166-72, 2015
6. Gawande RS et al: Role of diffusion-weighted imaging in differentiating benign and malignant pediatric abdominal tumors. Pediatr Radiol. 43(7):836-45, 2013
7. Khanna G et al: Detection of preoperative wilms tumor rupture with CT: a report from the Children's Oncology Group. Radiology. 266(2):610-7, 2013
8. Khanna G et al: Evaluation of diagnostic performance of CT for detection of tumor thrombus in children with Wilms tumor: a report from the Children's Oncology Group. Pediatr Blood Cancer. 58(4):551-5, 2012

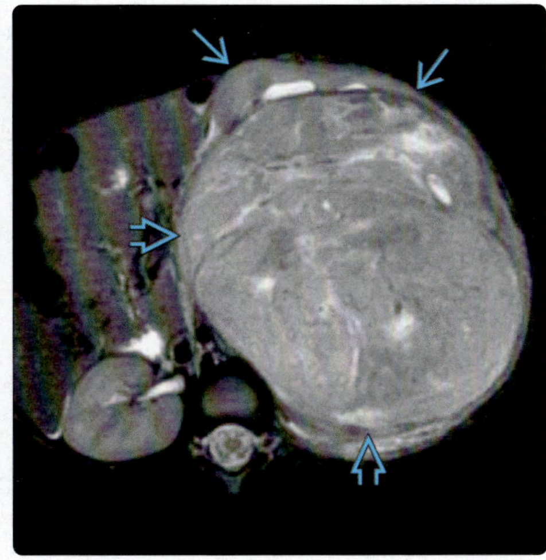

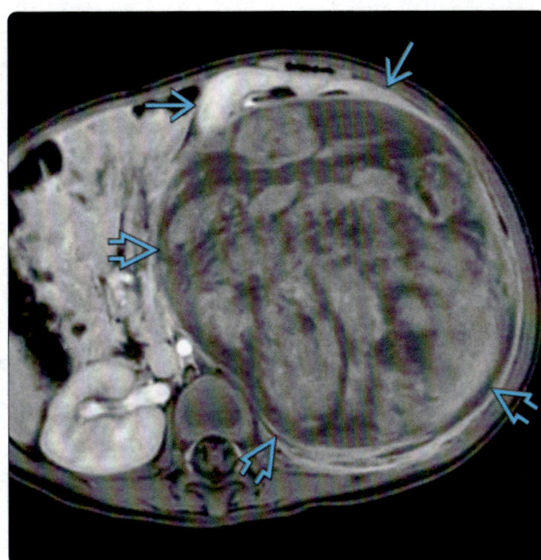

(Left) *Axial T2 FS MR in a 2-year-old with a palpable left abdominal mass shows a large, heterogeneous, solid Wilms tumor ➡ arising from a splayed "claw" of residual left kidney ➡.* **(Right)** *Axial T1 C+ FS MR in the same patient with Wilms tumor shows a large, heterogeneously hypoenhancing left renal mass ➡ with residual distorted kidney & collecting system displaced anteriorly ➡.*

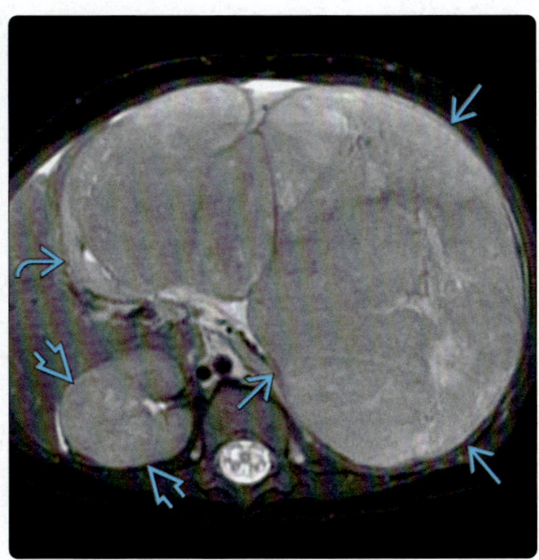

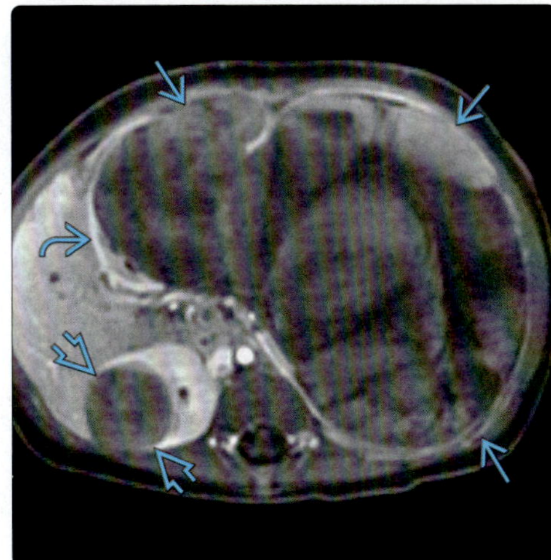

(Left) *Axial T2 FS MR in a 5-month-old shows a very large solid mass ➡ displacing the splayed left kidney anteriorly to the right ➡. There is a smaller round, mildly T2-hyperintense mass in the right kidney ➡, consistent with bilateral (stage V) Wilms tumor.* **(Right)** *Axial T1 C+ FS MR in the same child with bilateral Wilms tumors shows ↑ conspicuity to the hypoenhancing right renal mass ➡. The large, lobulated left renal mass ➡ is also heterogeneously hypoenhancing relative to normal kidney ➡.*

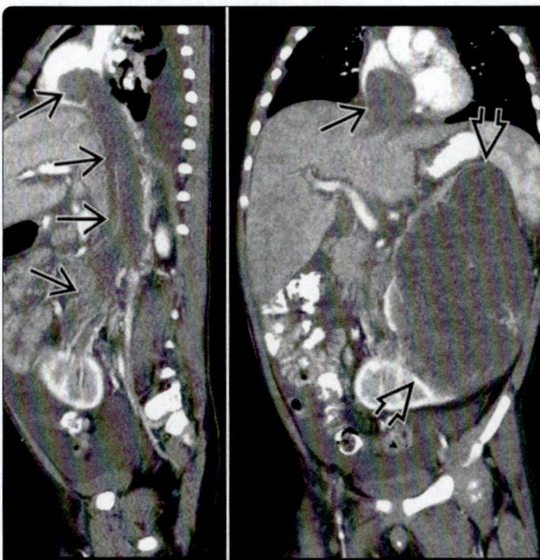

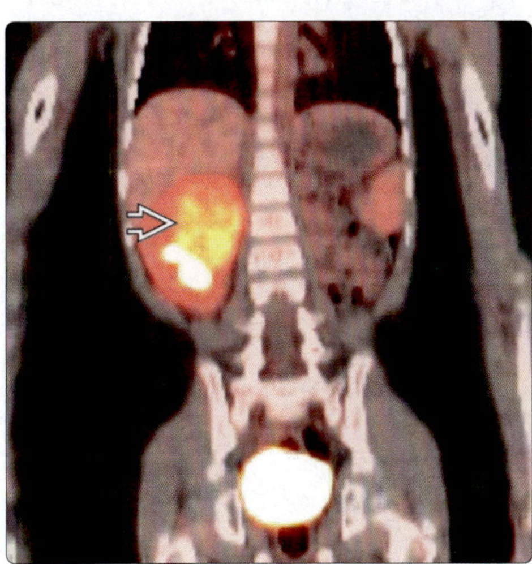

(Left) *Sagittal (left) & coronal (right) CECT images show tumor thrombus ➡ extending through the left renal vein, up the inferior vena cava, & into the right atrium from a Wilms tumor ➡ in the left kidney.* **(Right)** *Coronal FDG PET/CT in a child with a history of left nephrectomy for Wilms tumor shows a contralateral recurrence with metabolically active tumor ➡ in the right upper kidney.*

KEY FACTS

TERMINOLOGY

- Nephrogenic rests (NR): Persistent metanephric blastema; precursor to Wilms tumor
  - Perilobar NR: Occur at periphery of kidney
  - Intralobar NR: Occur within kidney
- Nephroblastomatosis: Multiple or diffuse NR

IMAGING

- Homogeneous multifocal ovoid or subcapsular rind-like renal masses that enhance less than normal kidney on CT/MR
  - Diffuse disease: Thick, uniform, homogeneous rind of hypoenhancing abnormal tissue
  - Multifocal disease: Scattered nodules resembling normal renal cortex on precontrast imaging
- Differentiating NR from Wilms tumor
  - NR: Cutoff measurement of 1.75 cm has 100% negative predictive value & 81% positive predictive value
  - Wilms tumor is usually spherical in shape & more likely to be exophytic
- Imaging findings suggesting conversion of NR to Wilms
  - Rapid ↑ in size
  - Stable or ↑ size while on chemotherapy
  - Nodule within initial lesions
  - New heterogeneous appearance of mass

PATHOLOGY

- Biopsy to distinguish NR from Wilms tumor; tumor/parenchymal border is most helpful for accurate distinction

CLINICAL ISSUES

- Most NR spontaneously regress
  - Currently, no specific treatment protocol is advocated
- Common associated syndromes: Beckwith-Wiedemann syndrome, hemihypertrophy, sporadic aniridia, & WAGR syndrome

(Left) *Longitudinal US of the left kidney in a 4-day-old shows a centrally located, ovoid, isoechoic nephrogenic rest ➡. Intralobar nephrogenic rests are less common than the perilobar form but have a higher risk of malignant transformation to Wilms tumor.* **(Right)** *Coronal CECT of the abdomen in the same patient shows a homogeneously hypodense intralobar nephrogenic rest ➡. Intralobar rests are associated with the WT1 gene, sporadic aniridia, & Drash syndrome.*

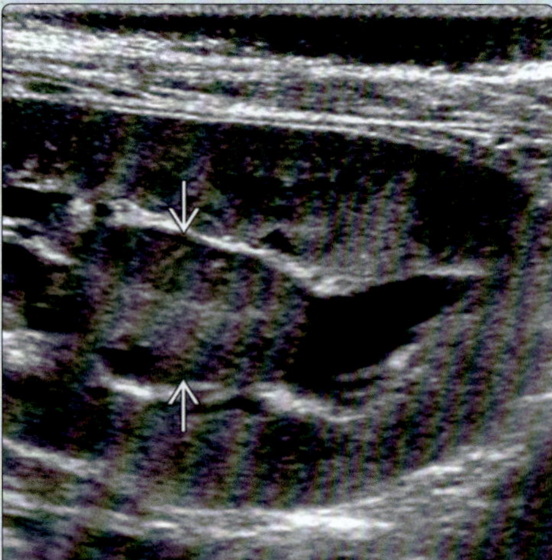

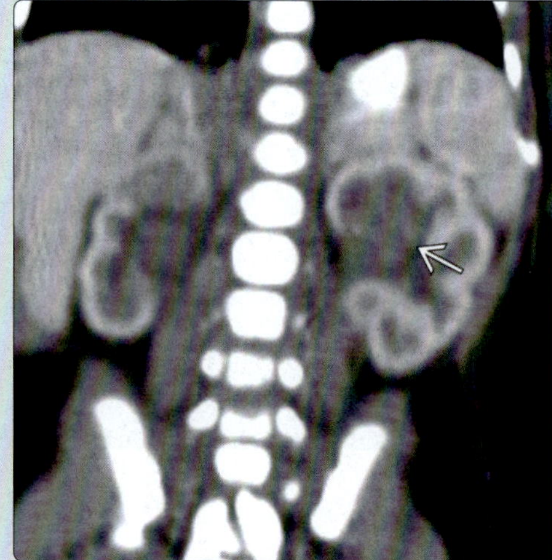

(Left) *Axial CECT in a neonate shows unilateral diffuse perilobar nephrogenic rests as a thin rind of homogeneously hypodense tissue ➡ surrounding the left kidney.* **(Right)** *Coronal CECT in the same patient shows the unilateral diffuse perilobar nephrogenic rests ➡ of the left kidney. Perilobar nephrogenic rests are more common than the intralobar form & are associated with the WT2 gene, Beckwith-Wiedemann syndrome, & hemihypertrophy.*

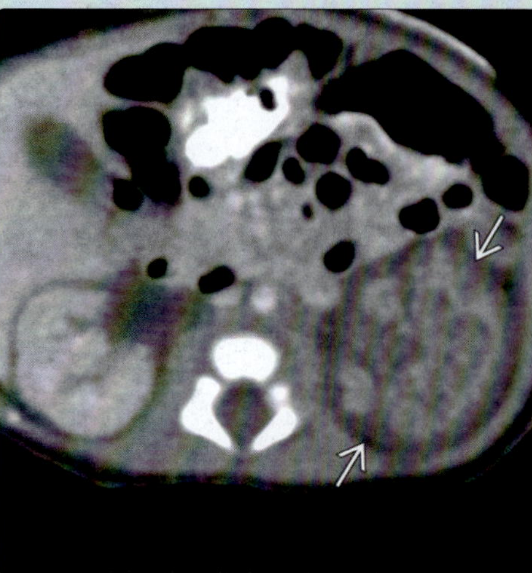

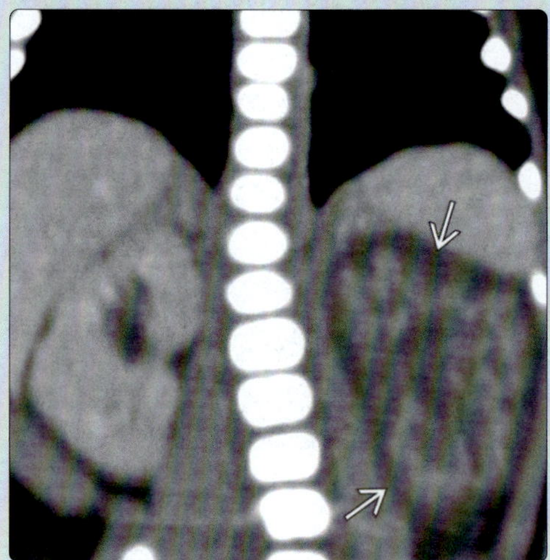

TERMINOLOGY

Definitions

- Nephrogenic rests (NR): Metanephric blastema that persists after 36-weeks gestation; precursor to Wilms tumor
- Nephroblastomatosis: Presence of multiple or diffuse NR
- Intralobar NR: Occur anywhere in renal parenchyma
- Perilobar NR: Occur in peripheral cortex

Associated Syndromes

- Perilobar NR: Beckwith-Wiedemann syndrome, hemihypertrophy, Perlman syndrome, trisomy 18
- Intralobar NR: Drash syndrome, sporadic aniridia, WAGR syndrome

IMAGING

General Features

- Best diagnostic clue
  - NR: < 1.75 cm nonspherical mass
  - Nephroblastomatosis: Multifocal ovoid vs. subcapsular rind-like homogeneous renal masses that enhance much less than normal kidney
    - ↓ enhancement due to hypovascularity
  - 2 main patterns of disease, similar on all modalities
    - Diffuse disease: Thick, uniform, homogeneous rind of hypoenhancing abnormal tissue
    - Multifocal disease: Scattered nodules resembling normal renal cortex on precontrast imaging
  - Perilobar rests are more likely to have homogeneous imaging appearance
- Location
  - Intralobar: Occur within kidney
  - Perilobar: Occur at periphery of kidney
- Size
  - Microscopic to several centimeters (usually < 3 cm)
- Morphology
  - Kidneys are enlarged in diffuse disease
    - May lose normal corticomedullary differentiation
  - NR may deform renal surface, creating nodular or lobulated appearance
  - In diffuse perilobar NR, interfaces between hypoenhancing NR & centrally located normal parenchyma can be jagged or irregular

Ultrasonographic Findings

- Grayscale ultrasound
  - Homogeneously hypoechoic or isoechoic to renal parenchyma
    - May not be able to distinguish NR from background kidney
  - Enlarged, distorted kidneys in diffuse disease
    - Poor renal corticomedullary differentiation
- Color Doppler
  - Hypovascular lesions

CT Findings

- NECT: Isodense to slightly hyperdense to renal cortex
- CECT: Homogeneous hypodense lesions enhancing < normal renal tissue

MR Findings

- T1WI
  - Homogeneous masses isointense to slightly hypointense to renal parenchyma
- T2WI
  - Homogeneous masses isointense to renal parenchyma
- DWI
  - Can restrict diffusion
- T1WI C+
  - Homogeneous, hypointense masses that enhance < renal parenchyma

Nuclear Medicine Findings

- PET
  - Avid FDG uptake in Wilms tumor

Imaging Recommendations

- Best imaging tool
  - MR is equivalent to CT in evaluation of single Wilms tumor
    - However, MR is more likely to identify additional lesions
  - Intravenous contrast administration is essential
    - Most sensitive method to identify NR

Differentiation From Wilms Tumor

- Best differentiator: NR is < 1.75 cm
  - Has 100% negative predictive value & 81% positive predictive value
- Other differentiators
  - Wilms tumor is more likely to have spherical shape & be exophytic
  - Homogeneous imaging appearance is more likely to be perilobar NR
  - Wilms tumor is surrounded by fibrous pseudocapsule (not visible on imaging)
- Imaging findings suggesting conversion from NR to Wilms tumor
  - Rapid ↑ in size
  - No change or growth while patient on chemotherapy
  - Nodule within initial lesions
  - Newly heterogeneous appearance of mass

DIFFERENTIAL DIAGNOSIS

Wilms Tumor

- Solid mass with heterogeneous enhancement
- Bilateral in 4-13% of patients
- NR: Precursor to Wilms tumor
  - NR is present in 30-40% of unilateral Wilms tumor cases
  - NR is present in 94% of patients with metachronous contralateral Wilms tumor
    - 1% of unilateral Wilms tumor patients develop metachronous disease
    - ↑ risk in children < 12 months of age with NR at diagnosis
  - NR is present in 99% of patients with synchronous bilateral Wilms tumors
    - Represent 4-7% of all Wilms tumors
    - Present at slightly younger age than unilateral Wilms tumor (2.6 vs. 3.3 years)

Renal Lymphoma

- Multifocal, homogeneous, hypodense lesions on CECT
- Other manifestations of disease are typically present
  - Multifocal &/or confluent adenopathy
  - Splenomegaly
- Unusual in infants & young children

Pyelonephritis

- Wedge-shaped foci of renal parenchymal hypoenhancement (CT/MR) or hypoperfusion (color Doppler US)
- Can cause striated nephrogram

PATHOLOGY

General Features

- Etiology
  - Metanephric blastema that persists beyond 36-weeks-gestational age

Staging, Grading, & Classification

- 2 pathologic subtypes
  - Perilobar rests (90%): In renal cortex or at corticomedullary junction
    - Associated with 1-2% risk of developing Wilms tumor
  - Intralobar rests (10%): Deeper in renal parenchyma
    - Associated with 4-5% risk of developing Wilms tumor
- 3 patterns of distribution: Unifocal, multifocal, & diffuse
- 4 developmental phases
  - Incipient/dormant
    - Contains primitive epithelial cells
    - Rarely progresses to Wilms tumor
  - Regressing/sclerosing
    - Cells show signs of maturation or sclerosis
    - Rarely progresses to Wilms tumor
  - Hyperplastic
    - Adenomatous benign neoplasms that ↑ in size
  - Neoplastic

Gross Pathologic & Surgical Features

- Diffuse nephroblastomatosis
  - White plaques or whorls of tissue replacing renal parenchyma
    - ± peripheral rind
    - ± small cysts
    - ± masses of hyperplastic or neoplastic (Wilms) tissue

Microscopic Features

- Biopsy is helpful in distinguishing NR from Wilms tumor; important to look at tumor/kidney border
  - Wilms tumor has pseudocapsule separating tumor from kidney
  - Perilobar nephrogenic rests have abrupt interface with adjacent kidney & lack pseudocapsule
  - Intralobar nephrogenic rests intermingle with renal parenchyma at periphery of lesion

CLINICAL ISSUES

Presentation

- Most common signs/symptoms
  - Asymptomatic vs. flank mass
  - Incidental finding of ipsilateral or contralateral kidney in setting of Wilms tumor

Demographics

- Age
  - Most common in infancy
    - May not be detectable on initial imaging study
  - Incidence ↓ with age
- Sex
  - M = F
- Epidemiology
  - NR are present in 1% of perinatal autopsies
    - Incidence ↓ significantly in 1st months of life
  - Most are sporadic, but ↑ risk with some syndromes

Natural History & Prognosis

- Risk for developing Wilms tumor
  - Only small percentage of patients with NR will develop Wilms tumor
  - NR are present in 30-40% with unilateral Wilms tumor
  - Found in up to 99% of bilateral Wilms tumors
  - Risk for developing Wilms tumor is highest in younger children; ↓ with age
  - 35% of diffuse hyperplastic perilobar NR develop Wilms tumor (highest risk group)

Treatment

- Most NR spontaneously regress
- Currently, no specific treatment protocol is advocated
  - Can be treated empirically with chemotherapy
- Children with syndromes at risk for Wilms tumor are typically screened regularly with imaging for development of nephroblastomatosis/Wilms tumor
  - Screening renal sonography at 3-month intervals up to 8 years of age
  - US is more useful to identify Wilms tumor than NR
    - On US, look for new/enlarging spherical mass
- MR C+ or CECT if renal ultrasound shows mass → follow-up with MR > CECT to minimize radiation
- ↑ size of nephroblastomatosis is sometimes treated empirically as stage 1 Wilms tumor without biopsy

DIAGNOSTIC CHECKLIST

Image Interpretation Pearls

- Nephroblastomatosis enhances much less than surrounding kidney
- Wilms tumor tends to be heterogeneous

SELECTED REFERENCES

1. Sandberg JK et al: Imaging characteristics of nephrogenic rests versus small Wilms tumors: a report from the Children's Oncology Group Study AREN03B2. AJR Am J Roentgenol. 214(5):987-94, 2020
2. Chung EM et al: Renal tumors of childhood: radiologic-pathologic correlation part 1. the 1st decade: from the radiologic pathology archives. Radiographics. 36(2):499-522, 2016
3. Littooij AS et al: Intra- and interobserver variability of whole-tumour apparent diffusion coefficient measurements in nephroblastoma: a pilot study. Pediatr Radiol. 45(11):1651-60, 2015
4. Servaes S et al: Comparison of diagnostic performance of CT and MRI for abdominal staging of pediatric renal tumors: a report from the Children's Oncology Group. Pediatr Radiol. 45(2):166-72, 2015
5. Cox SG et al: Magnetic resonance imaging versus histopathology in Wilms tumor and nephroblastomatosis: 3 examples of noncorrelation. J Pediatr Hematol Oncol. 36(2):e81-4, 2014

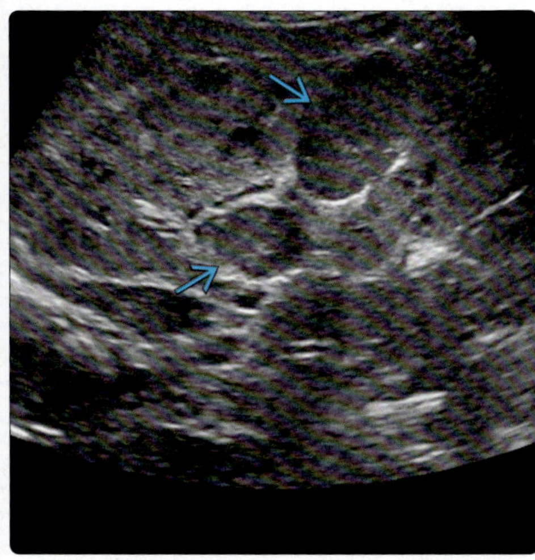

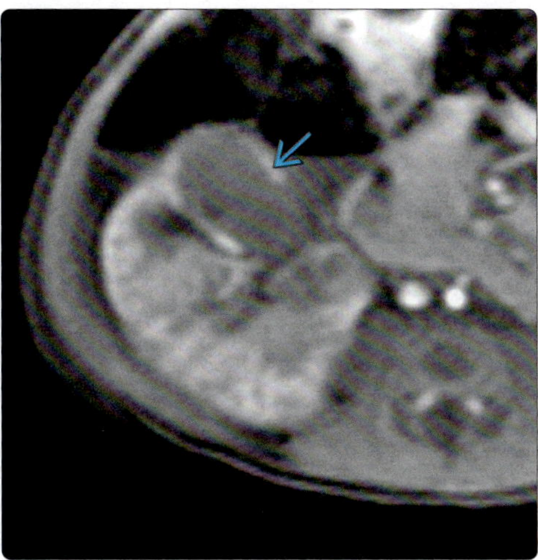

(Left) *Longitudinal US in a newborn with Beckwith-Wiedemann syndrome shows multiple hypoechoic nephrogenic rests* ➔ *within the right kidney.* **(Right)** *Axial T1 C+ FS MR in the same patient shows the large perilobar nephrogenic rest* ➔*. Note how the nephrogenic rest shows typical hypoenhancement relative to the renal cortex. Multiple other small nephrogenic rests were visible on the remainder of the MR.*

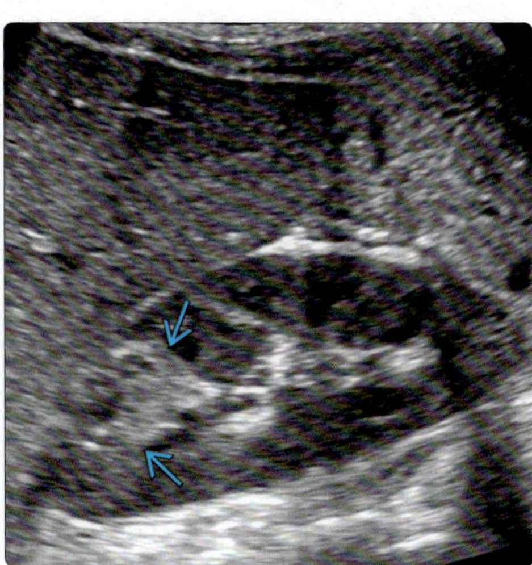

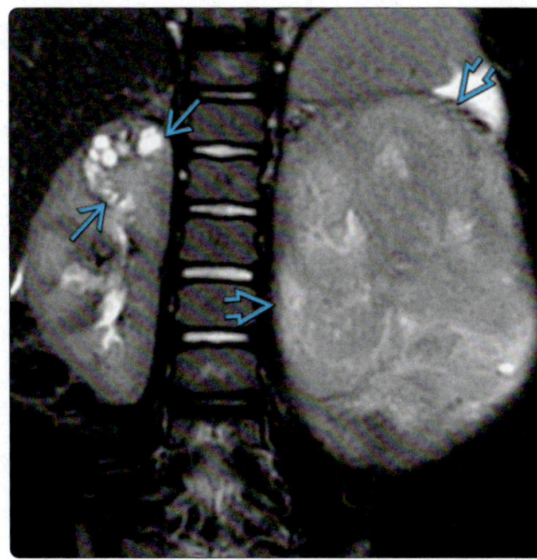

(Left) *Longitudinal US in a child with a left Wilms tumor shows a poorly defined echogenic nephrogenic rest* ➔ *in the superior pole of the right kidney.* **(Right)** *Coronal T2 FS MR in the same patient shows a large left Wilms tumor* ➔*. A multilocular mixed cystic & solid mass* ➔ *in the superior pole of the right kidney corresponds to the prior US findings. At resection, this right upper pole mass was confirmed to be a perilobar nephrogenic rest.*

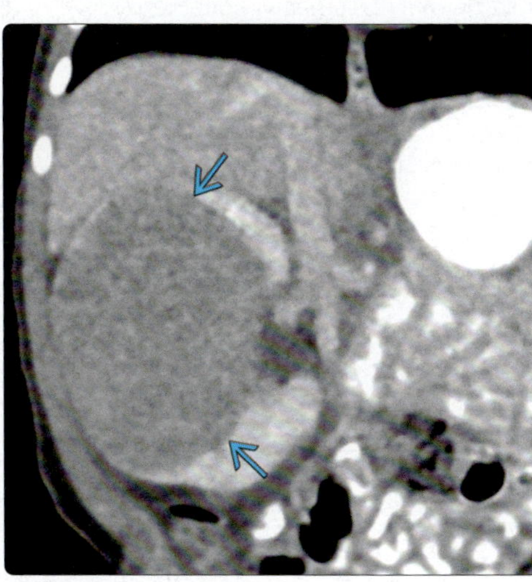

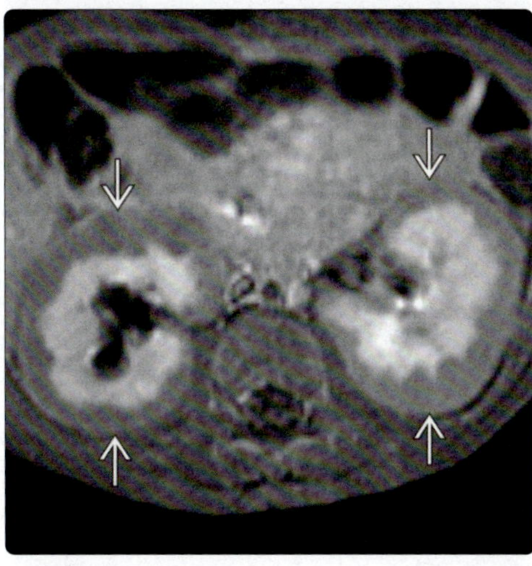

(Left) *Coronal CECT in a young child shows a large hypoenhancing mass* ➔ *occupying the mid-portion of the right kidney. At resection, this was confirmed to be a large hyperplastic nephrogenic rest. Multiple other small perilobar nephrogenic rests were not visible on imaging. Typically nephrogenic rests are not spherical in shape & are smaller than 1.75 cm.* **(Right)** *Axial T1 C+ FS MR of the kidneys in a young patient shows diffuse bilateral hypoenhancing perilobar nephrogenic rests* ➔*.*

Multilocular Cystic Nephroma

KEY FACTS

TERMINOLOGY

- Multilocular cystic nephroma (MLCN): Benign mixed mesenchymal & epithelial renal neoplasm

IMAGING

- Large, multilocular, cystic renal mass in young child
- Cystic components generally follow imaging characteristics of simple fluid on all modalities
- Septa show variable enhancement
  - No excretion of contrast into cysts
- Mass may herniate into renal hilum
- "Claw" of normal, splayed/compressed renal tissue at periphery of mass

TOP DIFFERENTIAL DIAGNOSES

- Cystic Wilms tumor
- Multicystic dysplastic kidney
- Mesoblastic nephroma
- Renal cyst

PATHOLOGY

- > 70% of MLCNs have *DICER1* gene mutation
  - Tumor predisposition syndrome at risk for pleuropulmonary blastoma & other malignancies
  - Anaplastic sarcoma of kidney may arise in *DICER1*-associated MLCN
- Cystic partially differentiated nephroblastoma (CPDN): Indistinguishable at imaging from cystic nephroma, but septa contain blastema
  - *DICER1* mutations are not present in CPDN

CLINICAL ISSUES

- M:F = 2-3:1; occurs between 3 months & 2 years
- Presentation
  - Painless abdominal/flank mass
  - Hematuria & urinary tract infection are less frequent in children
- Benign mass with excellent prognosis overall
  - Resection is usually curative

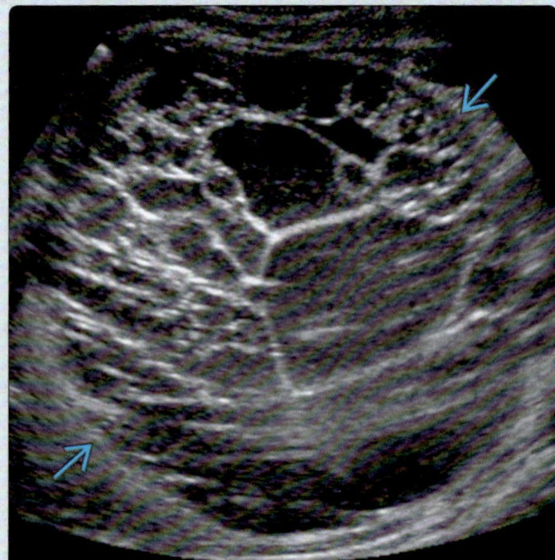

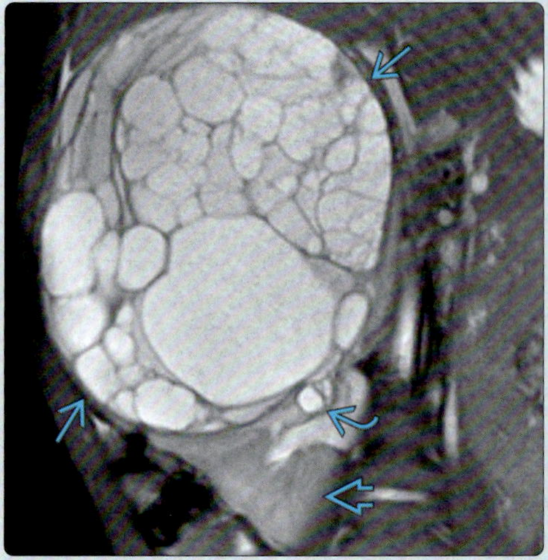

(Left) *Longitudinal ultrasound through the right renal fossa in a young child shows a multiloculated mass ➡ with innumerable thin septations & no visible nodular component or renal tissue.* **(Right)** *Coronal 2D SSFP MR in the same child shows that the multiloculated mass ➡ involves the upper pole of the right kidney, the remainder of which is displaced inferiorly ⇨. A portion of the mass ↪ herniates into the renal collecting system, a specific sign of multilocular cystic nephroma.*

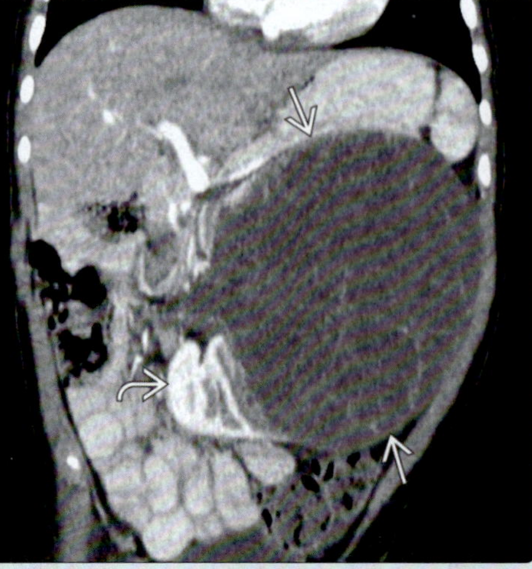

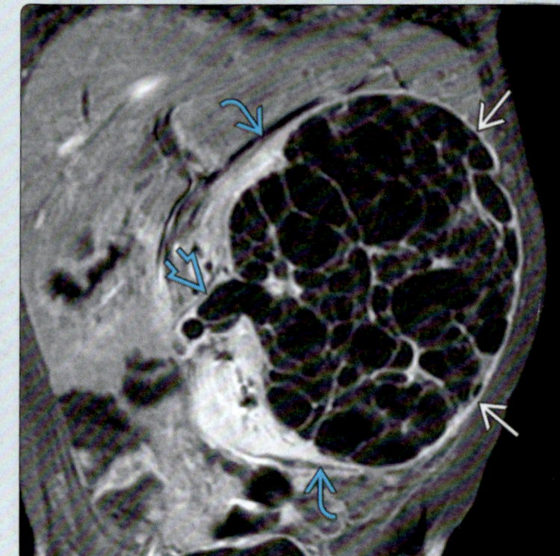

(Left) *Coronal CECT shows a large cystic mass occupying the upper pole of the left kidney in a young child. The normal lower pole of the kidney is displaced inferiorly & medially ↪ by the mass ➡.* **(Right)** *Coronal T1 C+ FS MR in the same patient shows only septal enhancement of the large multicystic renal mass ➡, which otherwise followed fluid signal on all sequences. There is a "claw" of renal tissue ↪ along the medial border of the mass, & a portion of the cystic nephroma herniates into the renal pelvis ⇨.*

TERMINOLOGY

Definitions

- Multilocular cystic nephroma (MLCN): Benign mixed mesenchymal & epithelial renal neoplasm

IMAGING

General Features

- Best diagnostic clue
  - Large, multilocular, cystic renal mass in young male

CT/MR/US

- Large, well-defined, multiloculated cystic mass
- Splayed "claw" of normal, compressed renal tissue stretched along mass periphery
- Mass may herniate into renal hilum
  - Can distort collecting system & cause obstruction
- Cystic components have attenuation/signal/echogenicity equal to or slightly > water
  - Small locules with closely packed septa may appear as solid mass
  - Cyst contents may vary due to hemorrhage or protein
- Septa have variable enhancement
  - Fibrous septa & capsule are hypointense on T1 & T2 MR
- No excretion of contrast into cystic components of mass

Imaging Recommendations

- Best imaging tool
  - US: Excellent for investigating palpable mass in child
  - CT or MR with contrast: Further characterize mass & define extent

DIFFERENTIAL DIAGNOSIS

Wilms Tumor

- Most common renal neoplasm of childhood
- Predominantly cystic form is uncommon

Multicystic Dysplastic Kidney

- Presents in utero/neonate, unlike MLCN
- Involves entire kidney (no normal renal parenchyma), unless duplicated

Mesoblastic Nephroma

- Presents < 1 year of age, often 0-3 months
  - Most common renal neoplasm of infancy
- Can be mixed cystic & solid (cellular subtype)

Renal Cyst

- Sharply marginated round/ovoid lesion with water density/echogenicity & imperceptible wall
- Uncommon in young children
- Septated cyst can mimic multicystic renal tumor

PATHOLOGY

General Features

- Etiology
  - May arise from metanephric blastema
    - Old hypothesis: Continuum of degeneration from MLCN to cystic partially differentiated nephroblastoma (CPDN) to Wilms tumor
    - New hypothesis: MLCN & CPDN are different lesions
      - *DICER1* mutations are present in MLCN, not CPDN
- Genetics
  - *DICER1* (14q32.13) mutation inactivates tumor suppressor gene → autosomal dominant tumor predisposition syndrome, at risk for
    - Pleuropulmonary blastoma (PPB)
    - MLCN: > 70% have *DICER1* mutation
      - > 80% of these patients develop PPB
    - Ovarian sex cord-stromal tumor
    - Embryonal rhabdomyosarcoma of urinary bladder or uterine cervix
  - Low penetrance (15%) → no tumors in most carriers

Microscopic Features

- Septa are lined by flattened or cuboidal epithelium with areas of eosinophilic cuboidal cells protruding into lumen
- MLCN & CPDN are differentiated by septa
  - MLCN: No undifferentiated elements
  - CPDN: Contain blastemal ± other embryonal elements

CLINICAL ISSUES

Presentation

- Most common signs/symptoms
  - Painless abdominal/flank mass
- Other signs/symptoms
  - Hematuria & urinary tract infection are less frequent in children

Demographics

- 3 months to 2 years of age: 2-3x more common in males
- *DICER1*-associated MLCN: < 4 years of age
- Adult lesion also previously referred to as MLCN is now known as mixed epithelial & stromal tumor of kidney

Natural History & Prognosis

- MLCN: Benign mass with excellent prognosis in isolation
- Reports of *DICER1*-associated anaplastic sarcoma of kidney (ASK) arising in MLCN

Treatment

- Complete or partial nephrectomy is usually curative

DIAGNOSTIC CHECKLIST

Consider

- *DICER1* genetic testing, annual chest radiographs (for PPB)

SELECTED REFERENCES

1. Guillerman RP et al: Imaging of DICER1 syndrome. Pediatr Radiol. 49(11):1488-505, 2019
2. Stanescu AL et al: Pediatric renal neoplasms: MR imaging-based practical diagnostic approach. Magn Reson Imaging Clin N Am. 27(2):279-90, 2019
3. Kurian JJ et al: Multiloculated cystic renal tumors of childhood: has the final word been spoken. J Indian Assoc Pediatr Surg. 23(1):22-6, 2018
4. Chung EM et al: Renal tumors of childhood: radiologic-pathologic correlation part 1. The 1st decade: from the radiologic pathology archives. Radiographics. 36(2):499-522, 2016
5. Faure A et al: DICER1 pleuropulmonary blastoma familial tumour predisposition syndrome: what the paediatric urologist needs to know. J Pediatr Urol. 12(1):5-10, 2016
6. Granja MF et al: Multilocular cystic nephroma: a systematic literature review of the radiologic and clinical rindings. AJR Am J Roentgenol. 205(6):1188-93, 2015

Congenital Mesoblastic Nephroma

KEY FACTS

TERMINOLOGY

- Congenital mesoblastic nephroma (CMN): Hamartomatous renal tumor of young infants
- Composed predominantly of elongated spindle cells
- Classic benign vs. more aggressive cellular type vs. mixed
  - Studies vary on which type is more common

IMAGING

- Solitary renal mass in fetus or young infant
- Oval/round mass which may have poorly defined margins
  - Classic type is usually solid, smaller
  - Cellular type is usually larger with cystic/necrotic/hemorrhagic foci

PATHOLOGY

- Classic type (33-50%) is similar to infantile myofibroma
- Cellular type (40-63%) is similar to infantile fibrosarcoma
  - Local recurrence, metastases
- Mixed (< 15%)

CLINICAL ISSUES

- 3-6% of childhood renal tumors
- Presentations include
  - Palpable abdominal mass in young infant
  - Hypertension, hypercalcemia, hematuria
  - Prenatally detected renal mass with polyhydramnios, preterm labor
- Most CMNs are diagnosed < 1-3 months of age
  - Classic type is more common in this time frame
- After 1-3 months
  - Wilms tumor becomes more common
  - Remaining CMNs are more likely to be cellular
- Nephrectomy with wide margins is usually curative
  - 5-year survival of 94-100%

DIAGNOSTIC CHECKLIST

- Preoperative feature for best differentiating solid renal masses in children: Age

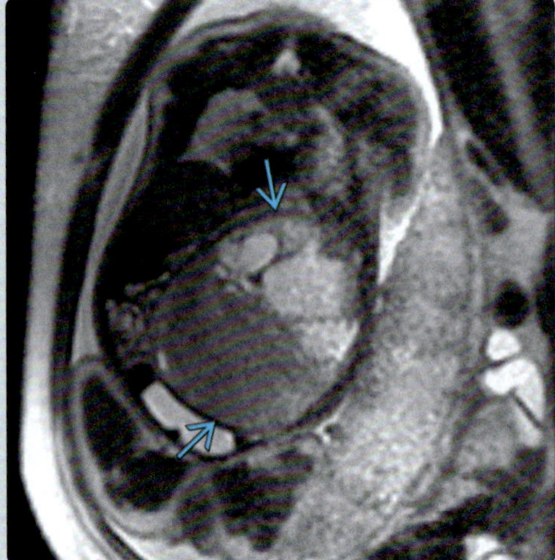

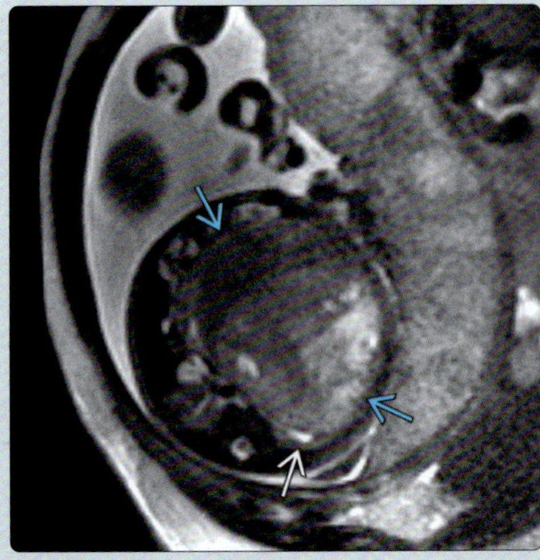

(Left) *Coronal T2 SSFSE MR in a 37-weeks-gestation fetus shows a large mixed cystic & solid mass ⇨ in the left fetal abdomen.* **(Right)** *Axial T2 SSFSE MR in the same fetus shows the relationship of the large mass ⇨ to the residual left kidney ➡, though it is difficult to tell if the kidney is splayed over the mass or merely compressed by it. Additionally, the amniotic fluid volume is > typically seen for this gestational age.*

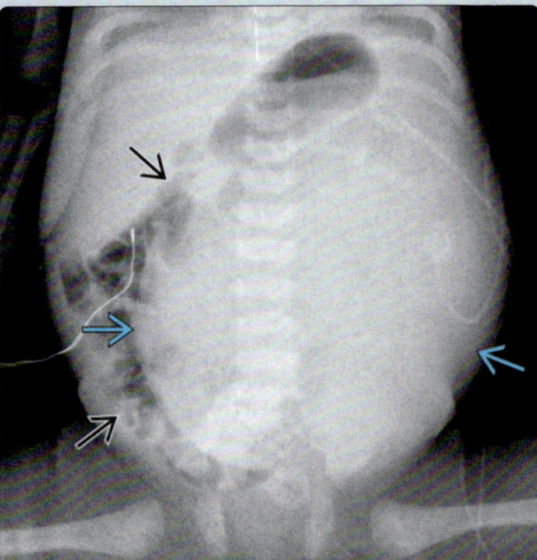

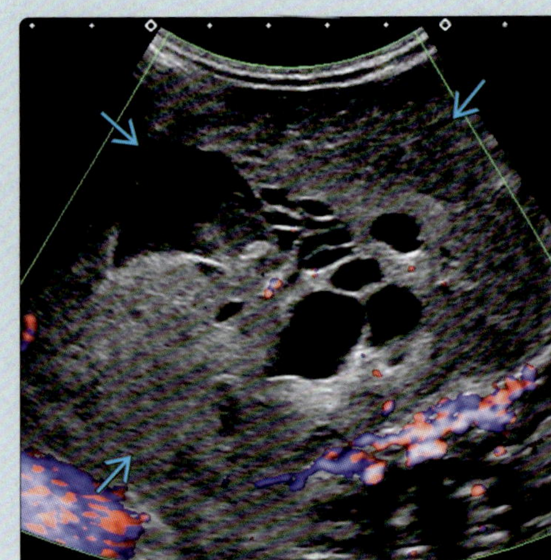

(Left) *Postnatal AP radiograph of the abdomen in the same patient shows displacement of gas-filled bowel loops ⇨ into the right abdomen by a large round mass ⇨.* **(Right)** *Longitudinal color Doppler US of the abdomen in the same patient shows the 11-cm mixed cystic & solid mass ⇨ with little detectable internal vascularity. The cellular subtype of mesoblastic nephroma was confirmed upon resection.*

TERMINOLOGY

Synonyms

- Congenital mesoblastic nephroma (CMN), fetal renal hamartoma, Bolande tumor
  - Bolande described CMN as histologically distinct from Wilms tumor in 1967

Definitions

- Hamartomatous renal tumor of young infants composed predominantly of elongated spindle cells
  - Types: Classic benign CMN vs. more aggressive cellular variant vs. mixed

IMAGING

General Features

- Best diagnostic clue
  - Solitary renal mass in fetus or neonate
- Location
  - Intrarenal but may replace entire kidney & cross midline when large
  - Metastases are very uncommon
- Size
  - Variable, from < 1 cm diameter to > 15 cm
    - Cellular variant is often much larger than classic type
- Morphology
  - Oval/round mass, which may have poorly defined margins with kidney
    - Usually solid
    - Cystic/necrotic/hemorrhagic foci imply more aggressive cellular variant
  - Claw of residual renal parenchyma splayed along tumor margin helps confirm renal origin
  - Hydronephrosis & vascular invasion are not typical
  - Irregularity/discontinuity of margins, infiltration of adjacent soft tissues, surrounding fluid &/or free pelvic fluid suggest tumor rupture
    - More common with cellular type

Ultrasonographic Findings

- Grayscale ultrasound
  - Smaller masses leave renal shape largely intact
    - Smooth contours to mass by imaging
  - Larger masses may fill abdomen & cross midline
  - Variable internal echogenicity
    - Greater heterogeneity & large cystic components are more typical of cellular type
  - Hyper- & hypoechoic ring pattern at periphery more common in classic type
    - Corresponds to CECT double layer sign
  - Prenatal findings include polyhydramnios, rarely hydrops
- Color Doppler
  - Vascular invasion is not seen

CT Findings

- NECT
  - Ca^{2+} is not typically seen
  - Pockets of high attenuation correspond to hemorrhage in cellular type
- CECT
  - Heterogeneous enhancement of solid components
    - Hypoenhancement is typical in classic type
  - Cystic/necrotic/hemorrhagic foci of nonenhancement are typical of cellular type
  - Double layer sign: 2 enhancing rims at margin of classic type
  - Intratumor pelvis sign: Portion of renal pelvis encapsulated by tumor in classic type

MR Findings

- T1WI
  - Intermediate to dark
  - Hemorrhage may be bright
- T2WI
  - Variable for solid components
  - Bright cystic foci ± fluid-fluid levels from hemorrhage
- T1WI C+
  - Heterogeneous enhancement of solid components
  - Rim/septal enhancement of cystic foci

Imaging Recommendations

- Best imaging tool
  - US best initial tool for investigating palpable abdominal mass in child
  - MR will better define local extension, adenopathy

DIFFERENTIAL DIAGNOSIS

Wilms Tumor

- Most common pediatric renal tumor
- Imaging appearance may be identical to CMN
- Best preoperative discriminator from CMN: Age
  - Average presentation of Wilms: 3-4 years of age
  - Rare in utero

Neuroblastoma

- Suprarenal/paraspinal mass displacing (or rarely invading) kidney
- Often contains Ca^{2+}
- Frequently engulfs & displaces vessels, crosses midline

Adrenal Hemorrhage

- Avascular cystic or heterogeneous suprarenal mass in newborn
- ↓ size over time
- No claw of surrounding renal tissue

Multicystic Dysplastic Kidney

- Cysts of varying size completely replace renal parenchyma
  - Not cysts within well-defined round mass

Ossifying Renal Tumor of Infancy

- Extremely rare tumor characterized by ossification/Ca^{2+}

Rhabdoid Tumor

- Aggressive rare solid renal tumor of infancy
- Association with CNS atypical teratoid-rhabdoid tumors

Clear Cell Sarcoma of Kidney

- 2nd most common pediatric renal tumor
- Classically causes bone metastases
- Average presentation: 1-4 years of age

Multilocular Cystic Nephroma

- Large multicystic mass herniating into central collecting system
- Average presentation: 3 months to 2 years of age

PATHOLOGY

General Features

- Genetics
  - Sporadic
  - No recurrence risk in siblings
  - Cellular subtype of CMN shares t(12;15)(p13;q25) chromosomal translocation with infantile fibrosarcoma (IFS)
    - Fusion of genes *ETV6* & *NTRK3*
    - Trisomy 11 occurs less frequently

Staging, Grading, & Classification

- 3 histologic subtypes: Reports vary regarding most common
  - Classic (33-50%): Similar features to infantile myofibroma/fibromatosis
  - Cellular (40-63%): Similar features to IFS
  - Mixed (< 15%)
- Staging by Wilms tumor criteria

Gross Pathologic & Surgical Features

- Classic: Infiltrative without capsule ± entrapped renal parenchymal islands
- Cellular: Cystic, hemorrhagic foci

Microscopic Features

- Classic: Bundled spindle cells, entrapped tubules & glomeruli, few mitoses
- Cellular: Sheets of randomly arranged spindle cells with few bundles, high mitotic rate, nuclear atypia

CLINICAL ISSUES

Presentation

- Most common signs/symptoms
  - Palpable abdominal mass in young infant
  - Prenatally detected renal mass with polyhydramnios, preterm labor
- Other signs/symptoms
  - Hypertension, hypercalcemia, hematuria

Demographics

- Age
  - Most CMNs are diagnosed before 3 months of age; 16% are found prenatally
    - Classic type is most likely in this period
  - After 1-3 months
    - Wilms tumor becomes more common
    - Remaining CMNs are more likely to be cellular variants
- Ethnicity
  - No ethnic predisposition
- Epidemiology
  - 3-6% of childhood renal tumors
  - 93% of renal tumors detected in utero
  - 90% are diagnosed before 1 year of age

Natural History & Prognosis

- Can show rapid growth despite benign histology
- Large abdominal circumference may result in dystocia at delivery
- Excellent prognosis for classic subtype
  - Complete surgical resection is curative
- Cellular subtype is more aggressive
  - 10% relapse with local recurrence or metastases
    - Most common metastatic site: Lung
    - Liver, heart, brain, & bone metastases are also reported

Treatment

- Amnioreduction for polyhydramnios
- Referral to pediatric surgeon/urologist
- Resection in neonatal period
  - Nephrectomy with wide margins is usually curative
  - Adjuvant chemotherapy for patients > 3 months of age with stage III (incomplete resection/positive margins) cellular type
- 5-year event-free survival of 94-100%

DIAGNOSTIC CHECKLIST

Consider

- Best differentiating factor for solid renal masses in children: Age

Image Interpretation Pearls

- Look for incomplete splayed rim of renal parenchyma along tumor margins (claw sign)
  - Helps confirm renal origin
  - Inferiorly displaced, distorted kidney with concave but intact cortex suggests suprarenal lesion
- Look for findings related to rupture
  - Surrounding soft tissue findings & free fluid may suggest preoperative tumor rupture
  - Cysts predispose to intraoperative rupture

SELECTED REFERENCES

1. Li Y et al: Imaging manifestations of congenital mesoblastic nephroma. Clin Imaging. 72:91-6, 2021
2. Sze SK: Neonatal renal tumors. Clin Perinatol. 48(1):71-81, 2021
3. Stanescu AL et al: Pediatric renal neoplasms: MR imaging-based practical diagnostic approach. Magn Reson Imaging Clin N Am. 27(2):279-90, 2019
4. Chen Y et al: Specific computed tomography imaging characteristics of congenital mesoblastic nephroma and correlation with ultrasound and pathology. J Pediatr Urol. 14(6):571.e1-6, 2018
5. Gooskens SL et al: Congenital mesoblastic nephroma 50 years after its recognition: a narrative review. Pediatr Blood Cancer. 64(7), 2017
6. Jehangir S et al: Recurrent and metastatic congenital mesoblastic nephroma: where does the evidence stand? Pediatr Surg Int. 33(11):1183-8, 2017
7. Lamb MG et al: Renal tumors in children younger than 12 months of age: a 65-year single institution review. J Pediatr Hematol Oncol. 39(2):103-7, 2017
8. Chung EM et al: Renal tumors of childhood: radiologic-pathologic correlation part 1. The 1st decade: from the Radiologic Pathology Archives. Radiographics. 36(2):499-522, 2016
9. Bayindir P et al: Cellular mesoblastic nephroma (infantile renal fibrosarcoma): institutional review of the clinical, diagnostic imaging, and pathologic features of a distinctive neoplasm of infancy. Pediatr Radiol. 39(10):1066-74, 2009
10. Chaudry G et al: Imaging of congenital mesoblastic nephroma with pathological correlation. Pediatr Radiol. 39(10):1080-6, 2009

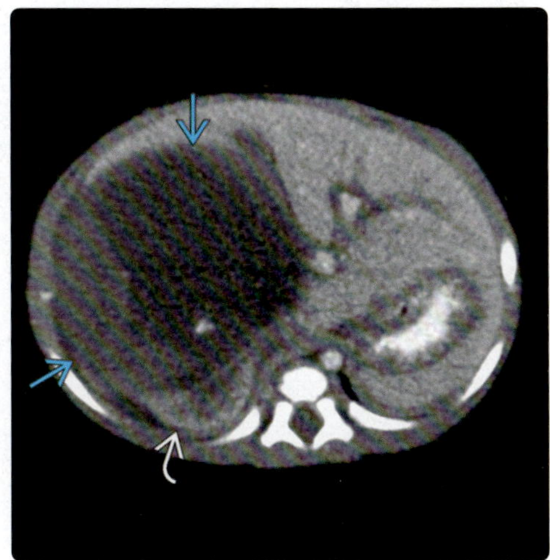

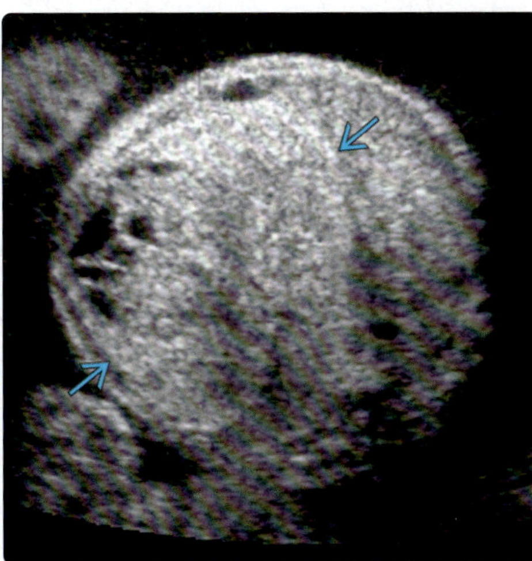

(Left) *Axial CECT in a patient with cellular mesoblastic nephroma shows a crescent of residual right kidney ➡ splayed along the posterior margin of the heterogeneous mass ➡. This claw sign helps to identify the kidney as the organ of origin for the tumor.* **(Right)** *Transverse US in a 2nd-trimester fetus with polyhydramnios shows a large, predominantly solid mass ➡ in the right abdomen. No right kidney could be identified. Mesoblastic nephroma was confirmed postnatally at resection.*

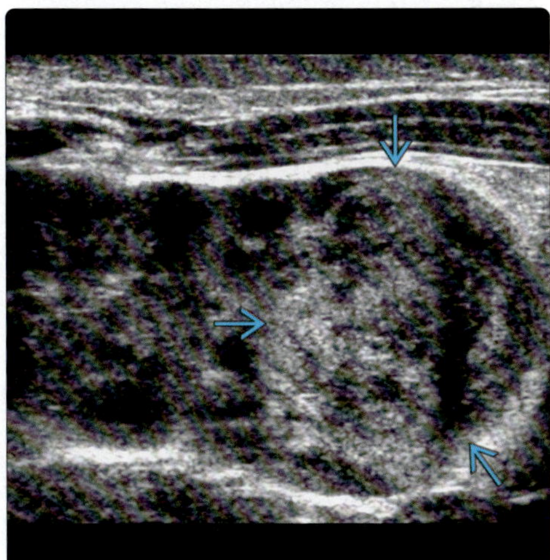

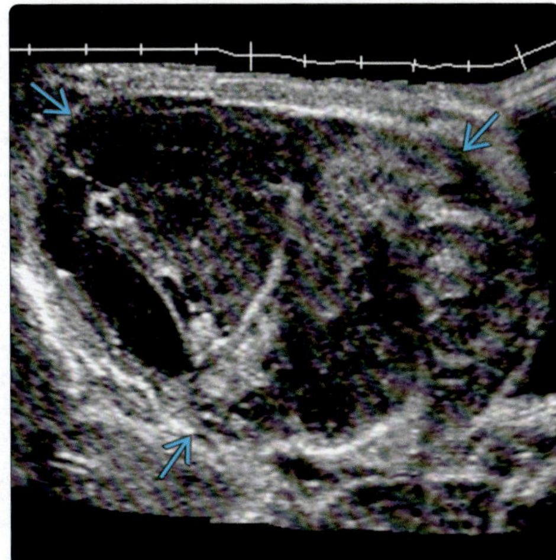

(Left) *Longitudinal US in a newborn shows a relatively small, solid (but heterogeneous) mass ➡ involving only the lower pole of this kidney. The patient age, tumor size, & imaging features are typical for the classic type of mesoblastic nephroma.* **(Right)** *Longitudinal panoramic US in a 5-day-old with abdominal fullness shows a large, heterogeneous mass ➡ in the left flank replacing most of the left kidney.*

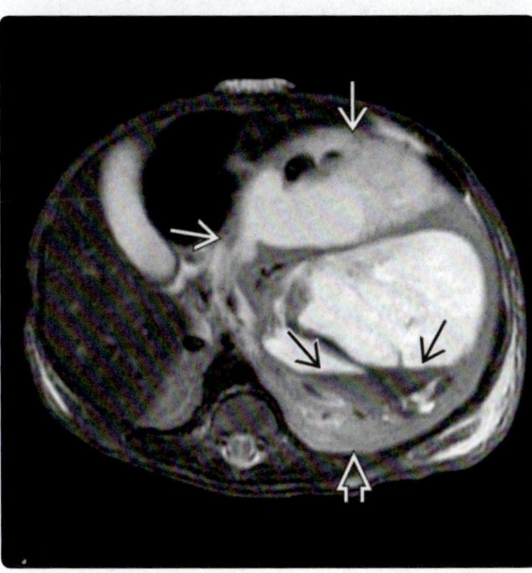

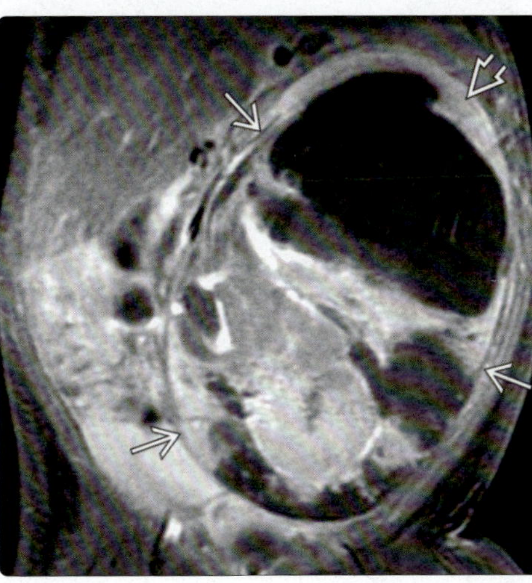

(Left) *Axial T2 FS MR in the same patient shows a heterogeneous mass ➡ in the left flank. The layering fluid-fluid levels ➡ are typical of hemorrhage within cysts. A claw of the splayed residual left kidney is seen posteriorly ➡.* **(Right)** *Coronal T1 C+ FS MR in the same patient shows heterogeneous enhancement of the tumor ➡ with large foci of nonenhancement. A claw of residual renal parenchyma is seen superiorly ➡. Resection of this cellular mesoblastic nephroma was complicated by intraoperative rupture/spill.*

Renal Rhabdoid Tumor

KEY FACTS

TERMINOLOGY

- Rare, highly aggressive neoplasm in young children
- Commonly arises from kidney
- Extrarenal sites include CNS, soft tissues > liver, lung

IMAGING

- Contrast-enhanced CT or MR is most useful
  - Large, heterogeneous renal mass
    - Foci of hemorrhage, necrosis, &/or Ca^{2+} separating tumor lobules
      - Ca^{2+} is more common than Wilms
  - Crescentic subcapsular fluid collection is characteristic
  - Sinus/hilar, local, & vascular invasion are common
  - Metastasizes most frequently to lungs

PATHOLOGY

- ~ 2% of pediatric renal tumors
- Associated with inactivation or deletion of *SMARCB1* (*INI1*) gene on chromosome 22q11

CLINICAL ISSUES

- Mean age of presentation: ~ 11 months
  - Younger than mean age for Wilms tumor
- Signs/symptoms
  - Most common: Palpable abdominal mass, hematuria (gross or microscopic)
  - Others include fever, anemia, hypercalcemia
- Aggressive neoplasm with poor prognosis
  - Patients often present with advanced disease
    - Stages 3-4 in ~ 70% at presentation
  - Overall 5-year survival ~ 20%
  - Prognosis is worse in younger patients (< 6 months of age)

DIAGNOSTIC CHECKLIST

- Consider brain MR to evaluate for synchronous or metachronous CNS neoplasm

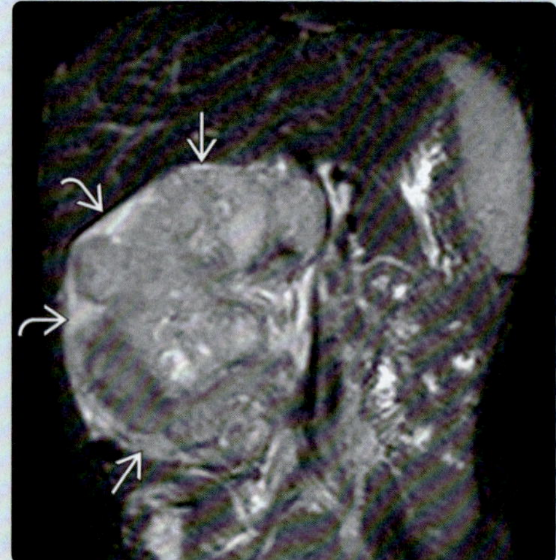

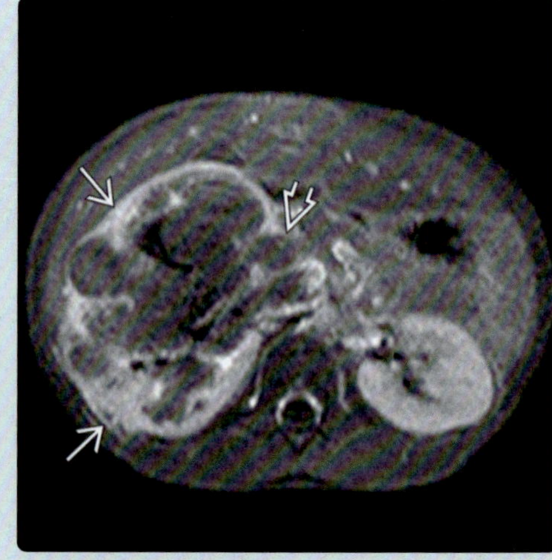

(Left) *Coronal T2 FS MR in an 11-month-old boy ultimately diagnosed with a rhabdoid tumor shows a large, heterogeneous, lobulated mass ➔ replacing the right kidney. A subcapsular fluid collection ➔ is noted at the periphery of the mass.* **(Right)** *Axial T1 C+ FS MR in the same patient demonstrates heterogeneous enhancement of the large right renal rhabdoid tumor ➔. Note the hilar invasion by the tumor lobules ➔.*

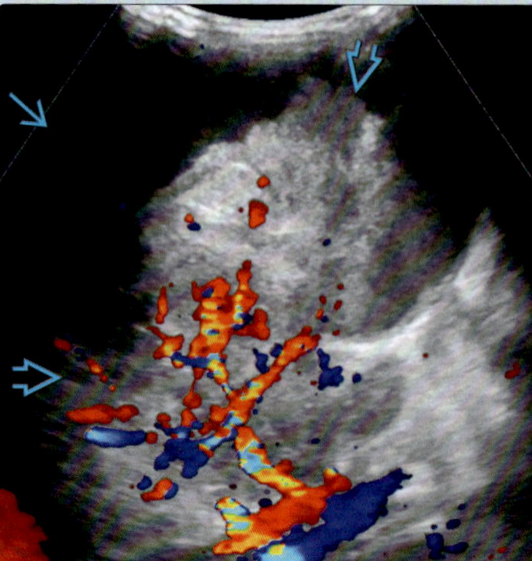

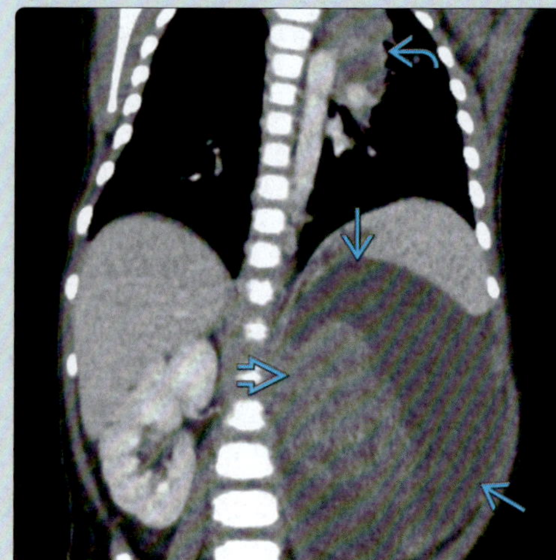

(Left) *Longitudinal color Doppler ultrasound in a 1-year-old shows a large subcapsular fluid collection ➔ overlying a lobulated & highly vascular mass ➔ that replaces the left kidney. The patient age & findings favor a malignant rhabdoid tumor.* **(Right)** *Coronal CECT in the same patient shows the solid mass ➔ & large subcapsular collection ➔ replacing the left kidney. Multiple lung metastases ➔ were present in this patient with a renal rhabdoid tumor, but no intracranial lesions were found.*

KEY FACTS

TERMINOLOGY

- "Bone metastasizing tumor of childhood"
- Rare malignant renal neoplasm in young children
  - 5% of pediatric renal tumors

IMAGING

- CECT or MR is best for characterizing tumor & evaluating local extension
  - Best clue: Large, solid renal mass in young child
    - Most commonly heterogeneous, well-circumscribed mass
      - Can be homogeneous
    - Ca^{2+}: 25%
    - Vascular invasion: 5%
    - Regional lymph node involvement: Up to 30%
    - Delayed recurrence in brain, bones
- Metastatic work-up: Chest CT & nuclear medicine (FDG PET)

PATHOLOGY

- Variable histological patterns
  - Most have *BCOR* gene duplications
- Staging similar to Wilms tumor
  - Most present with stage II or higher

CLINICAL ISSUES

- Most common presentation: Palpable abdominal mass ± hematuria
  - Rarely presents with pain from osseous metastases
- Mean age at presentation: 36-45 months
- Male predominance of 2:1
- 5-year survival = 73-86%
  - Up to 98% for stage I disease
  - ~ 50% for stage IV disease
- Treatment: Combination chemotherapy, surgery, & radiation (depending on stage)

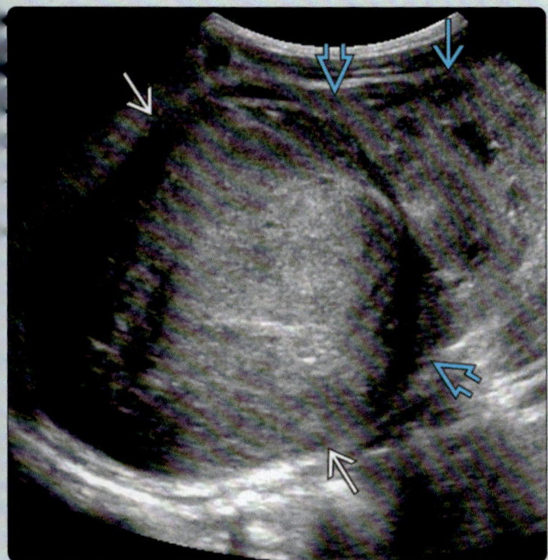

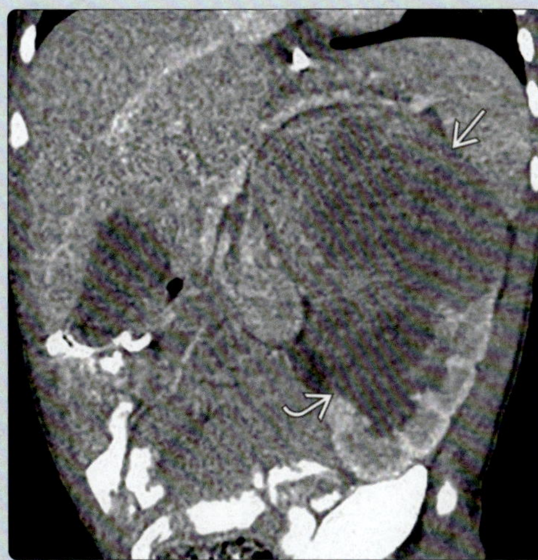

(Left) *Longitudinal ultrasound in a 2-year-old boy with a palpable abdominal mass shows a solid mass ➡ arising from the upper pole of the left kidney ⇨. Note the splayed residual left renal parenchyma ⇨ forming the claw sign.* **(Right)** *Coronal CECT in the same patient shows a large, hypoenhancing mass ➡ arising from the upper pole of the left kidney. The mass is causing obstruction of the lower portion of the left renal collecting system ➡. Clear cell sarcoma was confirmed at resection.*

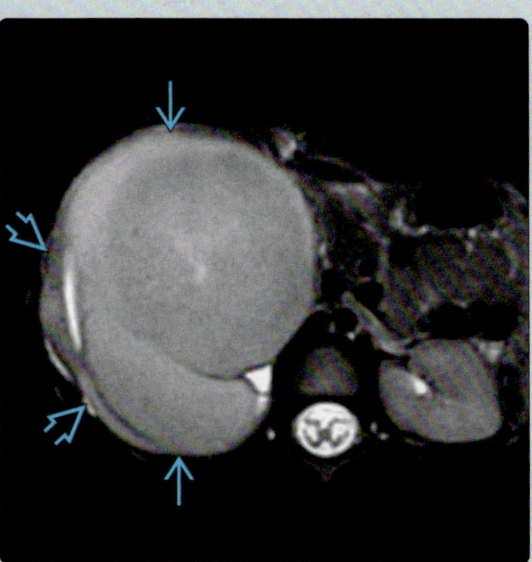

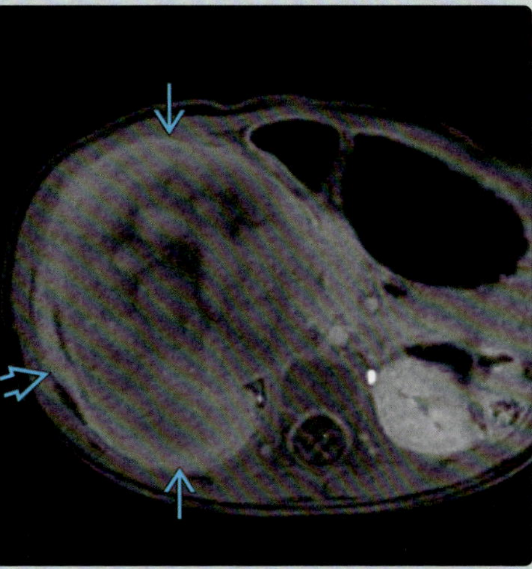

(Left) *Axial T2 FS MR in a 16-month-old girl with a palpable abdominal mass shows a relatively homogeneous, well-circumscribed T2-hyperintense mass ➡ arising from the right kidney ⇨.* **(Right)** *Axial T1 C+ FS MR in the same patient shows heterogeneous enhancement of the right renal mass ➡ with central areas of nonenhancement likely representing necrosis. Note the splayed "claw" of residual enhancing renal parenchyma ⇨.*

Renal Cell Carcinoma

KEY FACTS

TERMINOLOGY

- Malignant renal tumor that is more common in adolescents & young adults
  - 2-6% of renal malignancies in children
  - > 50% of renal tumors > 14 years of age
- tRCC or TFE RCC = translocation subtype (most common)

IMAGING

- Best clue: Solid or mixed solid/cystic renal mass in adolescent/young adult
  - Metastases to lymph nodes, lung, liver, bone
- NECT: Can be mildly ↑ attenuation due to hemorrhage
  - Ca^{2+} in 40-60%
- CECT: Heterogenous enhancement but ↓ vs. adjacent normal kidney
  - Usually well-defined margins, may see enhancing capsule
  - Enlarged retroperitoneal lymph nodes are common
- T2: Heterogeneous, ± foci of ↓ signal from hemorrhage
- T1 C+: Heterogeneous enhancement is typical
  - ± enhancing capsule on delayed images

TOP DIFFERENTIAL DIAGNOSES

- Wilms tumor, clear cell sarcoma, rhabdoid tumor, angiomyolipoma, renal medullary carcinoma

PATHOLOGY

- Translocation subtype (tRCC) is most common
  - Xp11.2 translocation → *TFE3* gene overexpression
- Papillary subtype is 2nd most common
- TMN staging is similar to adult RCC

CLINICAL ISSUES

- Clinical presentation: Abdominal/flank pain, palpable mass
  - Rarely hematuria
  - Frequently incidental
- Treatment: Radical nephrectomy & lymph node sampling &/or dissection
  - Targeted therapies > cytotoxic chemotherapy
  - XRT limited role, palliative

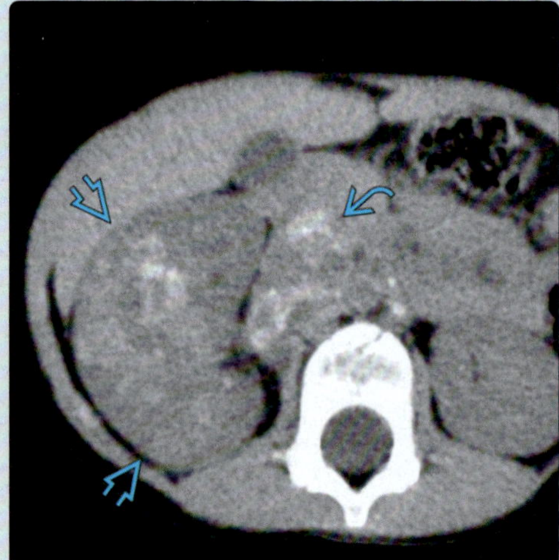
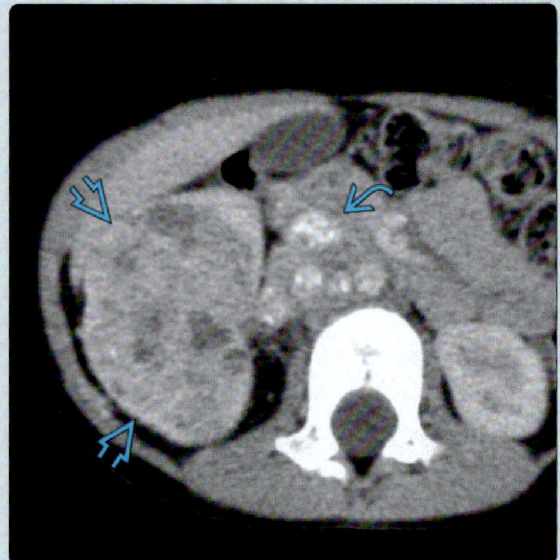

(Left) *Axial NECT in a 9-year-old girl with flank pain, found to have renal cell carcinoma (RCC), shows a right renal mass ➡ with high-attenuation foci. Note the enlarged retroperitoneal lymph nodes, which also contain heterogeneous high-attenuation ➡, likely due to Ca^{2+}.* **(Right)** *Axial CECT in the same patient shows heterogeneous enhancement of the right renal mass ➡ with multiple enlarged retroperitoneal lymph nodes ➡.*

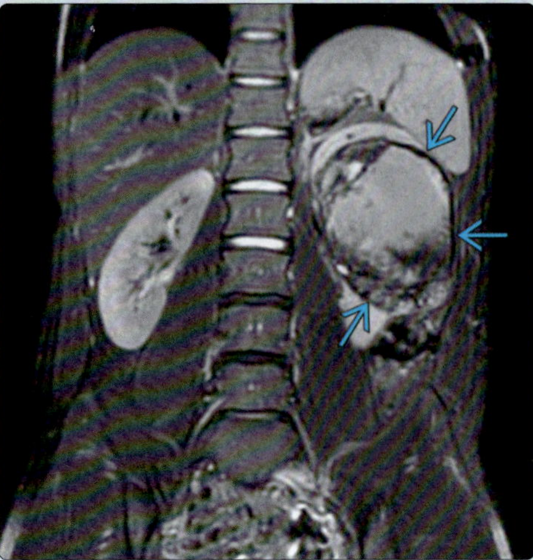
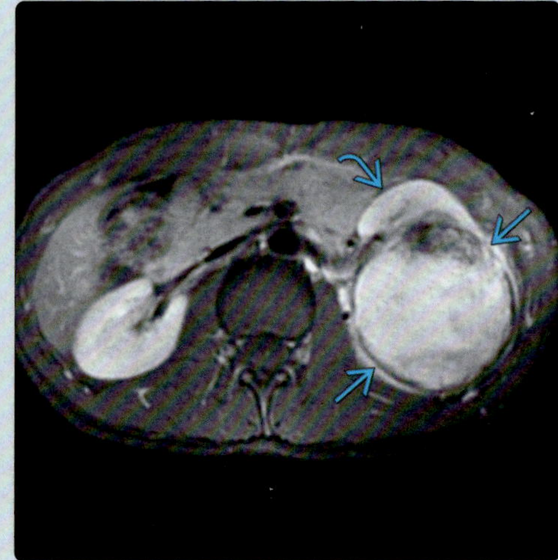

(Left) *Coronal T2 FS MR in a 15-year-old with shoulder pain (due to metastatic RCC in the humerus, not shown) demonstrates a heterogeneous left renal mass with a rim of low signal ➡ due to hemosiderin from prior hemorrhage.* **(Right)** *Axial T1 C+ FS MR in the same patient shows a hyperintense solid mass in the left kidney with a low-signal rim ➡. Note the residual left kidney anteriorly ➡. The majority of the mass showed precontrast T1 shortening due to internal blood products.*

TERMINOLOGY

Abbreviations

- Renal cell carcinoma (RCC)

Synonyms

- tRCC or TFE RCC = translocation subtype (most common) of RCC

Definitions

- Malignant renal tumor that is more common in adolescents & young adults
  - 2-6% of renal malignancies in children

IMAGING

General Features

- Location
  - tRCC is typically located in renal medulla
- Size
  - Mean size of tRCC = 6-7 cm
- Morphology
  - Usually round, well circumscribed

Ultrasonographic Findings

- Heterogeneous mixed solid/cystic mass
  - Can have hyperechoic foci due to Ca^{2+}

CT Findings

- NECT
  - Can be mildly ↑ in attenuation relative to normal kidney
  - Ca^{2+} in 40-60%
- CECT
  - Heterogenous but ↓ enhancement vs. normal kidney
  - Usually well-defined margins, may see enhancing capsule
  - Enlarged retroperitoneal lymph nodes are common
  - Metastases to lymph nodes, lung, liver, bone

MR Findings

- T1WI
  - Iso- to mildly hyperintense due to hemorrhage, Ca^{2+}
- T2WI FS
  - Heterogeneous, ± foci of ↓ signal from hemorrhage
- DWI
  - Typically hyperintense, can be heterogeneous
- T1WI C+ FS
  - Heterogeneous enhancement is typical
  - May have nonenhancing necrotic areas
  - ± enhancing capsule in tRCC

DIFFERENTIAL DIAGNOSIS

Wilms Tumor

- Most common pediatric renal malignancy
- 80% present < 5 years of age
- Typically large

Clear Cell Sarcoma

- 2nd most common renal malignancy < 10 years of age
- Bone metastases are classic

Malignant Rhabdoid Tumor

- Uncommon aggressive renal malignancy
- 80% present < 2 years of age
- Subcapsular fluid collection may be present

Angiomyolipoma

- Typically contains macroscopic fat
- Usually seen with tuberous sclerosis complex

Renal Medullary Carcinoma

- Heterogeneous infiltrating malignancy in adolescents & young adults with sickle cell trait

PATHOLOGY

General Features

- Translocation subtype (tRCC) is most common
  - Xp11.2 translocation; *TFE3* gene overexpression
- Papillary subtype is 2nd most common
- Clear cell RCC (most common in adults) is rare; may be seen with von Hippel Lindau syndrome

CLINICAL ISSUES

Presentation

- Most common signs/symptoms
  - Abdominal/flank pain, palpable mass
  - Hematuria is less common
  - Often found incidentally

Demographics

- Age
  - Older children, adolescents, young adults
    - > 50% of renal tumors ≥ 14 years of age
- Epidemiology
  - ↑ risk with history of treatment for prior malignancy

Natural History & Prognosis

- More advanced stage (III or IV) is common at presentation
- Stage I, II = > 90% survival
- Stage IV = < 30% survival

Treatment

- Radical nephrectomy & lymph node sampling &/or dissection; rarely partial nephrectomy
- Targeted therapies > cytotoxic chemotherapy
- XRT has limited role, usually palliative

DIAGNOSTIC CHECKLIST

Image Interpretation Pearls

- Remember to look for abnormal lymph nodes
- Metastatic disease to lung, liver, bone

SELECTED REFERENCES

1. Geller JI et al: A prospective study of pediatric and adolescent renal cell carcinoma: a report from the Children's Oncology Group AREN0321 study. Cancer. 126(23):5156-64, 2020
2. Ray S et al: Pediatric and young adult renal cell carcinoma. Pediatr Blood Cancer. 67(11):e28675, 2020
3. Chen X et al: Renal cell carcinoma associated with Xp11.2 translocation/TFE gene fusion: imaging findings in 21 patients. Eur Radiol. 27(2):543-52, 2017
4. Chung EM et al: Renal tumors of childhood: radiologic-pathologic correlation part 2. The 2nd decade: from the Radiologic Pathology Archives. Radiographics. 37(5):1538-58, 2017
5. Downey RT et al: CT and MRI appearances and radiologic staging of pediatric renal cell carcinoma. Pediatr Radiol. 42(4):410-7; quiz 513-4, 2012

Renal Medullary Carcinoma

KEY FACTS

TERMINOLOGY

- Rapidly growing tumor of renal medulla

IMAGING

- Best clue: Infiltrating, poorly defined renal mass in young adult with sickle cell trait
  - Tumor arises in renal medulla with extension toward renal sinus & cortex
  - Heterogeneous tumor enhancement due to necrosis
    - Can mimic abscess
  - Kidney may maintain reniform shape
  - Central masses may cause caliectasis
  - Extension to perinephric tissues is common
- 60% occur in right kidney
- Mean size: 6.5 cm
- Lung metastases & lymph node involvement are common
  - Lung metastases often have lymphangitic pattern with clustered or diffuse poorly defined nodules intermixed with interstitial thickening

TOP DIFFERENTIAL DIAGNOSES

- Pyelonephritis with developing abscess
- Renal cell carcinoma
- Wilms tumor

PATHOLOGY

- 88% occur in patients with sickle cell trait
  - May be related to sickling blood & local renal environment

CLINICAL ISSUES

- Most common presenting symptoms: Hematuria & pain
- Other symptoms: Weight loss, respiratory symptoms, nausea, & vomiting
- 3.2x more common in males
- Therapy has not not been effective
  - Typically treated with nephrectomy & chemotherapy
  - Poor prognosis with median overall survival of 5 months

(Left) *Axial CECT in a young adult with sickle cell trait & renal medullary carcinoma (RMC) shows a poorly defined infiltrative & heterogeneous mass ➡ of the right kidney with perinephric extension ➦.* **(Right)** *Axial CECT in the same patient shows extensive lung metastases with nodular opacities intermixed with interstitial thickening ➡, typical of lymphangitic spread. Metastases are common in RMC, with the most common sites being lymph nodes, lungs, & liver.*

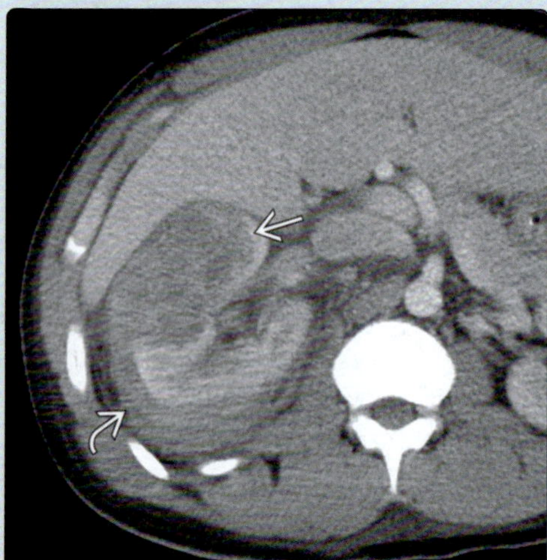

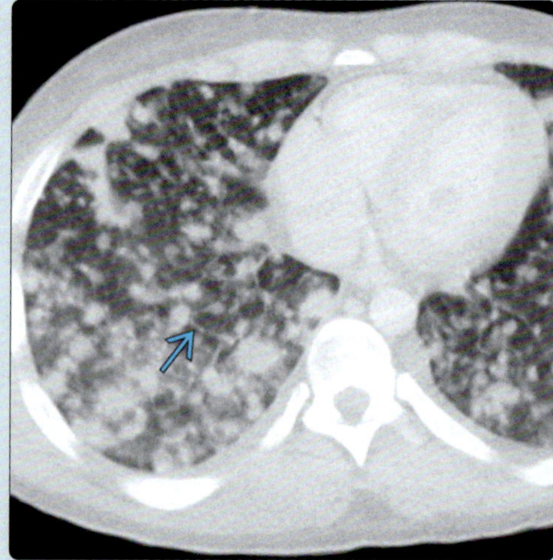

(Left) *Axial CECT in an adolescent with RMC shows an infiltrative, poorly defined mass ➡ in the upper pole of the right kidney. An enlarged right retroperitoneal lymph node ➡ is also present.* **(Right)** *Axial CECT in the same patient shows multiple pulmonary metastases ➡. Many of the lesions demonstrate a spiculated border.*

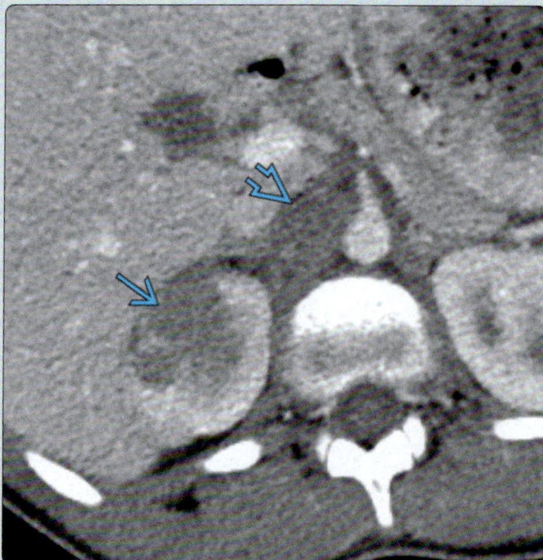

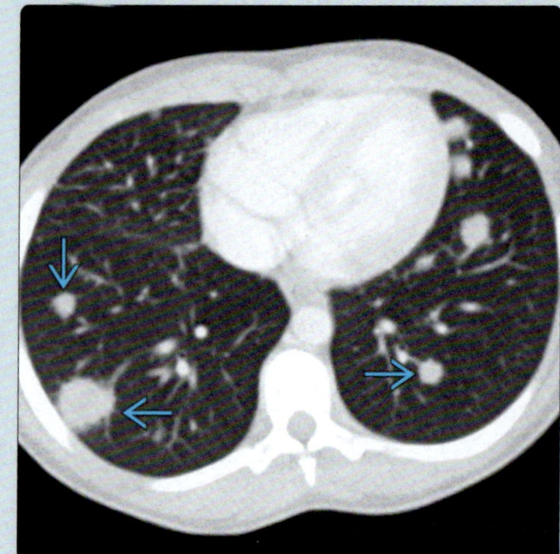

TERMINOLOGY

Definitions

- Rapidly growing tumor of renal medulla

IMAGING

General Features

- Best diagnostic clue
  - Infiltrating renal mass in adolescent/young adult with sickle cell trait
  - Kidney may maintain reniform shape
- Location
  - Arises in renal medulla with extension toward renal sinus & cortex
  - 60% occur in right kidney
- Size
  - Mean size: 6.5 cm

Radiographic Findings

- IVP
  - Mass distorts renal collecting system

CT Findings

- Infiltrative, poorly defined mass growing from renal medulla toward cortex
- Central masses may cause caliectasis
- ↓ enhancement compared to renal parenchyma
  - Necrotic components can mimic abscess
- Extension to perinephric tissues is common
- Lung metastases & lymph node involvement are common
  - Lung metastases often have lymphangitic pattern with clustered or diffuse nodules intermixed with interstitial thickening

MR Findings

- Similar imaging findings as on CT
- Hemorrhagic products may be conspicuous on gradient-echo images

Imaging Recommendations

- Best imaging tool
  - CECT to evaluate lungs & kidney

DIFFERENTIAL DIAGNOSIS

Renal Cell Carcinoma

- 2nd most common renal malignancy in children
- Typically occurs in adolescents
- Well-defined, heterogeneous, small- to moderate-sized mass; often superficial (distorting renal contour)

Wilms Tumor

- Most common renal malignancy in children; 80% < 5 years of age
- Well-defined, typically large, round heterogeneous mass replacing most of kidney
  - "Claw" of residual renal parenchyma is splayed around tumor margin

Pyelonephritis With Developing Abscess

- Relatively uncommon complication of commonly occurring renal parenchymal infection
- Poorly defined, heterogeneous parenchymal mass with retained reniform shape
- ± systemic features of infection, positive urinalysis

PATHOLOGY

General Features

- Etiology
  - 88% of cases occur in patients with sickle cell trait
  - Thought to be related to sickling blood & local renal environment

CLINICAL ISSUES

Presentation

- Most common signs/symptoms
  - Hematuria & pain
- Other signs/symptoms
  - Weight loss, respiratory symptoms, nausea, & vomiting

Demographics

- 3.2x more common in males

Natural History & Prognosis

- Poor prognosis; median overall survival: 5 months
- Metastases at presentation in 88%
  - Most common sites: Lymph nodes, lungs, & liver

Treatment

- Typically treated with nephrectomy & chemotherapy
- No known effective therapies

SELECTED REFERENCES

1. Jia L et al: Distinctive mechanisms underlie the loss of SMARCB1 protein expression in renal medullary carcinoma: morphologic and molecular analysis of 20 cases. Mod Pathol. 32(9):1329-43, 2019
2. Cajaiba MM et al: The classification of pediatric and young adult renal cell carcinomas registered on the Children's Oncology Group (COG) protocol AREN03B2 after focused genetic testing. Cancer. 124(16):3381-9, 2018
3. Chung EM et al: Renal tumors of childhood: radiologic-pathologic correlation part 2. The 2nd decade: from the Radiologic Pathology Archives. Radiographics. 37(5):1538-58, 2017
4. Sandberg JK et al: Imaging of renal medullary carcinoma in children and young adults: a report from the Children's Oncology Group. Pediatr Radiol. 47(12):1615-21, 2017
5. Alvarez O et al: Renal medullary carcinoma and sickle cell trait: a systematic review. Pediatr Blood Cancer. 62(10):1694-9, 2015

Angiomyolipoma

KEY FACTS

TERMINOLOGY

- Angiomyolipoma (AML): Benign hamartomatous tumor consisting of abnormal blood vessels, smooth muscle, & fat
  - Vast majority of AMLs occur in kidneys
- Almost always associated with tuberous sclerosis complex (TSC) in children

IMAGING

- Renal masses showing variable amounts of fat
  - Fat-containing renal mass is diagnostic of AML in child
    - Signal dropout on opposed-phase MRs
    - Contrast is not needed for diagnosis with known TSC
      - Potentially useful for vascular evaluation
- Bilateral in 85-95% of TSC patients with AMLs
- Tortuous vessels ± aneurysms in larger AML
  - Vessels may be splayed by fatty components or cysts
- Benign renal cysts are also common in TSC

PATHOLOGY

- 2 patterns of disease: Sporadic vs. TSC-associated AML
  - Sporadic lesions are extremely rare in children
- Underlying mutations of tumor suppressor genes *TSC1* or *TSC2* → dysregulation of mammalian target of rapamycin (mTOR) → ↑ cell growth & division
- Frequency, severity, & risk of bleeding are higher in patients with *TSC2* mutation

CLINICAL ISSUES

- Pediatric AMLs are usually asymptomatic
  - Children typically have clinical (especially cutaneous & neurologic) manifestations of TSC
- Conservative symptomatic management for AMLs in TSC
  - mTOR inhibitors are used for lesions > 3 cm
- Possible life-threatening spontaneous hemorrhage
  - Hemorrhage rare if AML ≤ 4 cm or aneurysm < 5 mm
  - Treated with arterial embolization

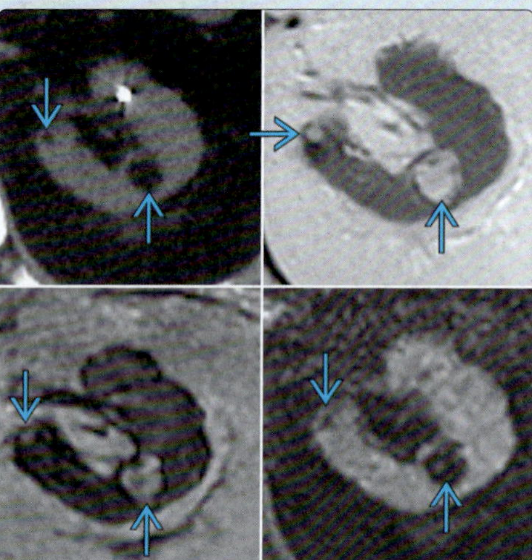

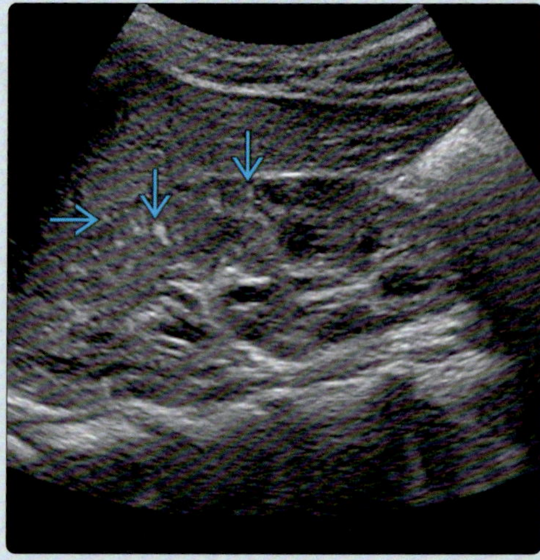

(Left) *Axial (clockwise from upper left) NECT, T1 MR, T1 FS MR, & opposed-phase MR images show a fat-containing angiomyolipoma (AML) ⇨ in a patient with tuberous sclerosis complex (TSC). Note that the signal drop is only seen at the margins of these lesions containing macroscopic fat on the opposed-phase images.* **(Right)** *Longitudinal ultrasound in a child with TSC shows multiple tiny echogenic lesions ⇨ of the right renal parenchyma, consistent with AMLs.*

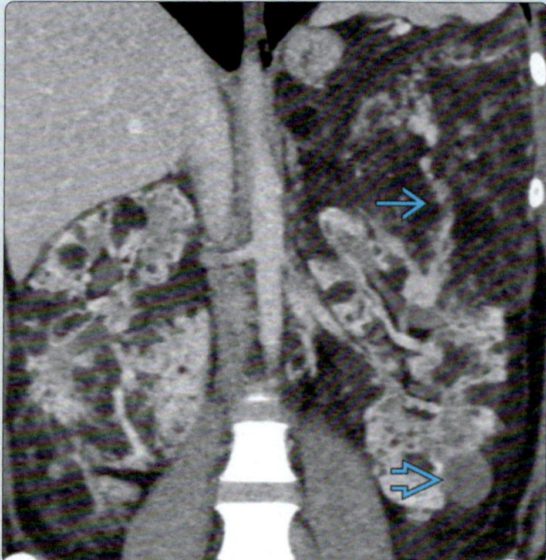

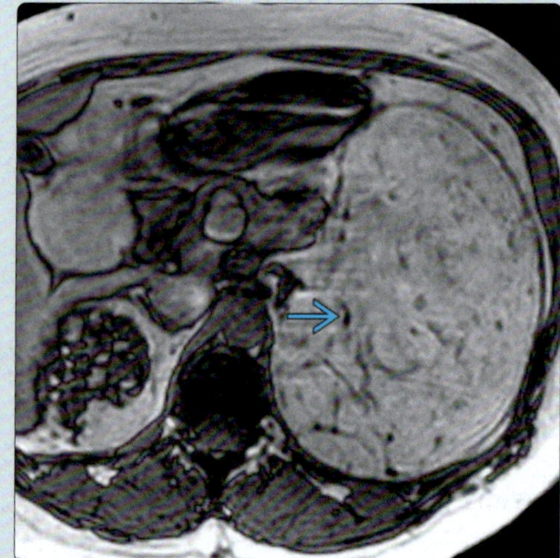

(Left) *Coronal CECT in a patient with TSC shows AMLs replacing both kidneys. The largest AML is in the upper pole of the left kidney & extends to the top of the image. The large AML contains multiple tumoral vessels ⇨. A cyst ⇨ is also present in the lower pole of the left kidney.* **(Right)** *Axial opposed-phase MR in the same patient shows signal dropout ⇨ where the fat-containing tumor & tumoral vessels share the same imaging voxel.*

TERMINOLOGY

Abbreviations

- Angiomyolipoma (AML)

Definitions

- Benign hamartomatous tumor consisting of abnormal blood vessels (angio), smooth muscle (myo), & fat (lipoma)

Associated Syndromes

- Almost always associated with tuberous sclerosis complex (TSC) in children

IMAGING

General Features

- Best diagnostic clue
  - Renal masses containing variable amounts of fat
  - Benign renal cysts are also common in patients with TSC
    - Variable signal depending on proteinaceous content
    - Cysts do not contain fat or enhance
- Location
  - Vast majority of AMLs occur in kidneys
    - Can occur in liver, pancreas, & other abdominal organs
    - Hepatic AMLs occur in 15-30% of TSC patients with renal AMLs
      - Hepatic AMLs are typically small; median of 1 cm
      - Renal AMLs are typically diffuse in this setting
- Size
  - Variable: Range from tiny (mm) to large (many cm)
- Morphology
  - Variable shape, fat content, & number in kidneys
  - Bilateral in 85-95% of TSC patients with AMLs

CT Findings

- NECT
  - Renal mass with tumoral fat → diagnostic of AML in children with TSC
  - Fat-poor lesions are isodense to slightly hyperdense compared to kidney
- CECT
  - Contrast is not needed in setting of known TSC
  - Lesions may significantly enhance with contrast (depending on extent of vascular component)
  - Fat-poor AMLs show homogeneous & prolonged enhancement
- CTA
  - ± aneurysmal renal vessels in large AMLs

MR Findings

- T1WI
  - Mass contains variable amounts of high-signal fat
  - Low signal in fatty portion on fat-saturated images
  - Fat-poor lesions are hypointense compared to renal parenchyma
- T2WI
  - Mass contains variable amounts of high-signal fat
  - Low signal in fatty portion on fat-saturated images
  - Fat-poor AMLs are hypointense compared to renal parenchyma
- T1WI C+
  - Contrast is not needed for diagnosis in setting of known TSC
  - Variable enhancement
    - With high fat content, may show minimal enhancement
    - With high vessel content, may show marked enhancement
- In phase/opposed phase
  - Signal dropout when fat & water share same voxel on opposed-phase images
    - Small lesions have complete signal dropout
    - Large lesions have signal dropout at border with vessels & normal renal parenchyma
  - No signal dropout for fat-poor AMLs
  - Opposed phase is useful to identify extrarenal AMLs

Ultrasonographic Findings

- Grayscale ultrasound
  - Hyperechoic mass relative to normal kidney & liver
  - Fat-poor AMLs are usually isoechoic compared to kidney
- Color Doppler
  - Can detect aneurysms in larger lesions

Angiographic Findings

- Characteristic tortuous vessels with multiple aneurysms
- Vessels may be splayed by larger fatty lesions or cysts

Imaging Recommendations

- Best imaging tool
  - MR is recommended at diagnosis of TSC to evaluate potential renal lesions
    - Minimize CT as these patients will undergo many studies during their lifetimes
    - Renal MR is performed at same time as brain MR
    - Surveillance MR is performed every 1-3 years depending on imaging findings & patient symptoms
  - Routine US is not preferred in children with known TSC
    - Fat-poor AMLs are not visible
    - Tumor & cyst measurements are not reproducible
- Protocol advice
  - MR with in-phase/opposed-phase sequences is most sensitive for detecting small lesions
  - T1 & T2 MR performed with & without fat saturation
  - IV contrast is not necessary for diagnosis in patients with known TSC

DIFFERENTIAL DIAGNOSIS

Renal Cell Carcinoma

- Rare in children
- Rarely reported to contain fat
  - Fat-poor AML may mimic renal cell carcinoma (RCC)
- Ca^{2+} in mass is highly suggestive of RCC
  - Ca^{2+} is extremely rare in AML
- Association of RCC with TSC is controversial
  - Even if risk is ↑, RCC remains very rare in TSC
  - Fat-poor AMLs are much more common

Renal Cyst

- Commonly seen in patients with TSC
- Fat-saturated MRs help differentiate fat from proteinaceous fluid

Wilms Tumor

- Most common pediatric renal malignancy
- Solid mass that rarely contains fat
- ± invasion of renal vein & inferior vena cava
- Metastases to lymph nodes, liver, lung
- ↑ frequency in certain syndromes
  - Beckwith-Wiedemann
  - Hemihypertrophy
  - Congenital aniridia
  - WAGR syndrome

Retroperitoneal Teratoma

- Heterogeneous, fat-containing mass; ± Ca^{2+}
- Displaces/compresses kidney rather than arising from it

PATHOLOGY

General Features

- Etiology
  - Benign renal tumor with mixed vessel, muscle, & fat elements
  - 2 main patterns of disease
    - Sporadic AML
      - ~ 80% of AMLs overall; however, sporadic AMLs are extremely rare in children
      - Usually solitary
      - More common in females due to stimulation by estrogen/progesterone
      - Risk of hemorrhage in lesions ≥ 4 cm in size
    - TSC-associated AML
      - Occur in 55-80% of patients with TSC
      - Multiple, bilateral tumors
      - Typically larger than sporadic AML
      - ± ↓ risk of hemorrhage vs. sporadic lesions
- Genetics
  - 2 tumor suppressor genes are associated with TSC
    - *TSC1*, band 9q34, encodes for hamartin
    - *TSC2*, band 16p13.3, encodes for tuberin
  - Hamartin & tuberin help inhibit activation of mammalian target of rapamycin (mTOR)
    - Mutations lead to uncontrolled cell size & division
  - Frequency, severity, & risk of bleeding are higher in patients with *TSC2* mutation
- Associated abnormalities
  - LAM: Numerous thin-walled cysts throughout lungs
    - Likely represent metastatic AMLs

CLINICAL ISSUES

Presentation

- Most common signs/symptoms
  - Characteristic skin & neurologic stigmata of TSC
  - AMLs are usually asymptomatic
- Other signs/symptoms
  - Renal failure (usually not until adulthood)

Demographics

- Age
  - Frequency of renal lesions ↑ with age
  - Small AMLs in TSC patients in early childhood
    - 45% have renal cysts or AMLs by 6 years of age
- Sex
  - TSC-associated AMLs are slightly more common in females
  - Sporadic AMLs are much more common in females
- Epidemiology
  - Sporadic AML in 0.3-3% of population at autopsy
  - AMLs are present in 55-80% of TSC patients

Natural History & Prognosis

- Untreated TSC-associated AMLs enlarge into adulthood
- Possible life-threatening spontaneous hemorrhage
  - Presents with flank/abdominal pain, hematuria
  - Bleeding occurs in up to 15% of TSC patients with AML
  - Risk factors for spontaneous hemorrhage
    - AML size > 4 cm
    - Aneurysm size > 5 mm
    - Age between 20 & 30 years
    - Risk ↓ with mTOR inhibitor therapy

Treatment

- Conservative, symptomatic management for patients with TSC-associated AMLs
  - Lesions can ↓ in size with mTOR inhibitors; reserved for lesions > 3 cm in size

DIAGNOSTIC CHECKLIST

Image Interpretation Pearls

- Classic appearance: Well-circumscribed, fatty renal mass
- 3 renal lesion types are seen on MR in patients with TSC
  - Classic AML: Bright on T1 & T2; ↓ signal with fat saturation; signal dropout on opposed phase
  - Fat-poor AML: Isointense to muscle on T1 & T2; no change with fat saturation or opposed phase
  - Cyst (typical): Dark on T1, bright on T2; no change with fat saturation
    - Hemorrhage/protein in cyst may alter internal signal

SELECTED REFERENCES

1. Kingswood JC et al: Renal angiomyolipoma in patients with tuberous sclerosis complex: findings from the TuberOus SClerosis registry to increase disease Awareness. Nephrol Dial Transplant. 34(3):502-8, 2019
2. Jóźwiak S et al: Liver angiomyolipomas in tuberous sclerosis complex-their incidence and course. Pediatr Neurol. 78:20-6, 2018
3. Morin CE et al: Thoracoabdominal imaging of tuberous sclerosis. Pediatr Radiol. 48(9):1307-23, 2018
4. Chung EM et al: Renal tumors of childhood: radiologic-pathologic correlation part 2. The 2nd decade: from the Radiologic Pathology Archives. Radiographics. 37(5):1538-58, 2017
5. Cockerell I et al: Prevalence of renal angiomyolipomas and spontaneous bleeding related to angiomyolipomas in tuberous sclerosis complex patients in France and Norway: a questionnaire study. Urology. 104:70-6, 2017
6. Manoukian SB et al: Comprehensive imaging manifestations of tuberous sclerosis. AJR Am J Roentgenol. 204(5):933-43, 2015
7. Kingswood JC et al: The effect of everolimus on renal angiomyolipoma in patients with tuberous sclerosis complex being treated for subependymal giant cell astrocytoma: subgroup results from the randomized, placebo-controlled, phase 3 trial EXIST-1. Nephrol Dial Transplant. 29(6):1203-10, 2014
8. Krueger DA et al: Tuberous sclerosis complex surveillance and management: recommendations of the 2012 International Tuberous Sclerosis Complex Consensus Conference. Pediatr Neurol. 49(4):255-65, 2013

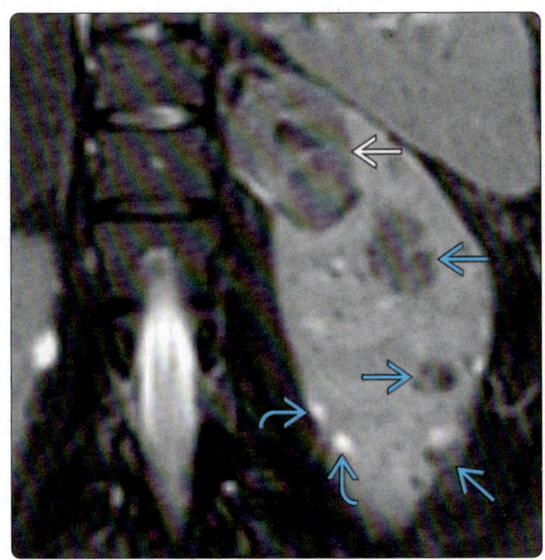

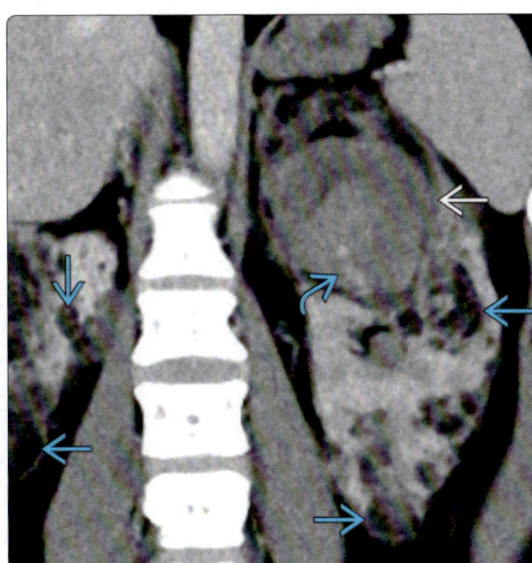

(Left) *Coronal T2 FS MR in a patient with TSC shows multiple renal AMLs ➙ & small cysts ➙ with a dominant heterogeneous AML ➙ in the upper pole of the kidney.* **(Right)** *Subsequent coronal CECT in the same patient shows that the dominant upper pole AML ➙ has ↑ in size due to hemorrhage. A blush of contrast ➙ at the base of the tumor represents active bleeding of the AML. Note the numerous fat-containing AMLs bilaterally ➙.*

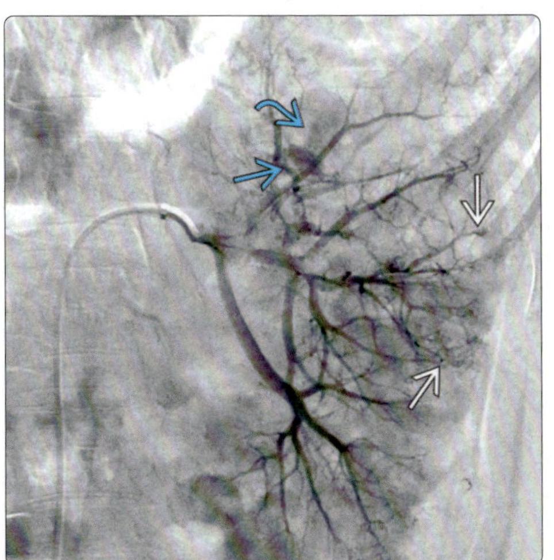

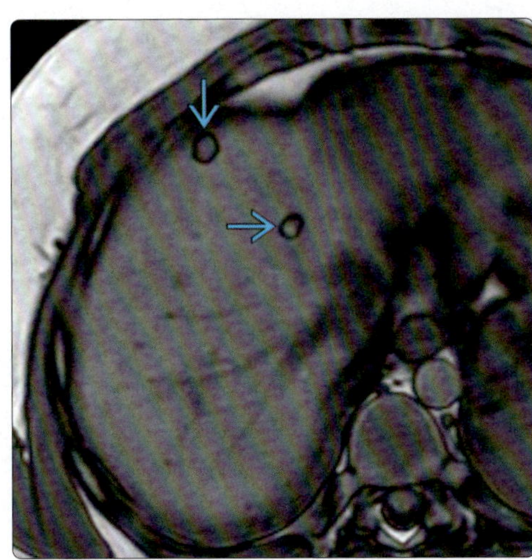

(Left) *AP projection from a left renal artery DSA in the same patient shows multiple tiny aneurysms ➙ & tumoral vessels. The largest aneurysm ➙ shows active hemorrhage ➙.* **(Right)** *Axial T1 opposed-phase MR in a patient with TSC shows signal dropout ➙ at the periphery of 2 hepatic AMLs. Hepatic AMLs occur in 15-30% of TSC patients with renal AMLs.*

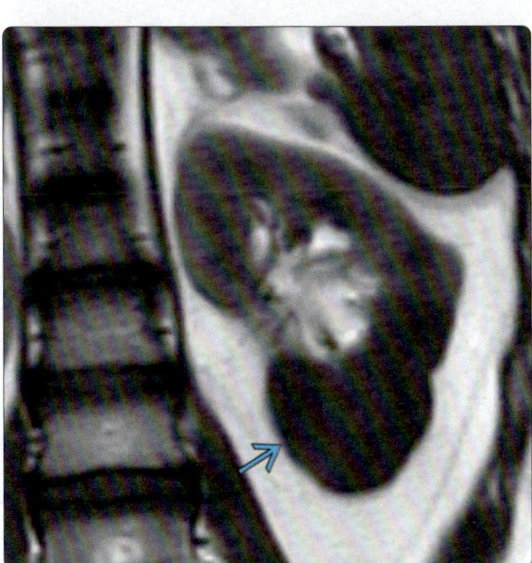

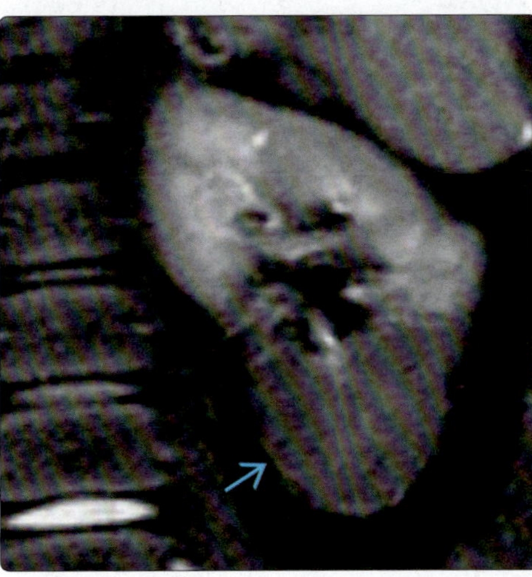

(Left) *Coronal T1 MR in a patient with TSC shows a hypointense lipid-poor AML ➙ of the lower pole of the left kidney. The AML maintains the normal reniform shape of the kidney.* **(Right)** *Coronal T2 FS MR in the same patient with TSC redemonstrates a hypointense lipid-poor AML ➙ in the lower pole of the left kidney. The AML maintains the normal reniform shape of the kidney.*

KEY FACTS

TERMINOLOGY

- Acute infection of renal parenchyma; often difficult to clinically distinguish from lower urinary tract infection (UTI)
- Classic imaging appearance: Focal swelling & ↓ perfusion of affected parenchyma visible on nuclear scintigraphy, US, CECT, MR, & IVP
  - Imaging work up of is UTI controversial
    - See professional society guidelines

IMAGING

- Marked inflammatory response to infection causes swelling that alters normal tissue properties & effectively ↓ radiologic contrast agent delivery to site, which results in
  - Photopenic focus on nuclear cortical scan
  - ↓ perfusion on Doppler imaging with altered echotexture on grayscale US
  - Striated or wedge-shaped foci of ↓ enhancement on CECT/MR/IVP
  - Developing abscess may be mass-like, ± cystic foci
- US with Doppler is least invasive & readily available but less sensitive than nuclear renal cortical scans, CT, & MR
- US is frequently performed to search for associated complications (abscess, stones, scarring), congenital anomalies, & hydronephrosis

CLINICAL ISSUES

- Symptoms nonspecific: Malaise, irritability, fever, abdominal/flank pain, vomiting, hematuria, dysuria, change in urinary habits/enuresis
- Treatment: 7- to 14-day course of antimicrobial therapy; may be started IV & changed to oral
- Imaging work-up for VUR & congenital anomalies
- Complications: Perirenal abscess, necrotizing papillitis, pyonephrosis (obstruction), & cortical scarring
- Permanent scarring is more likely < 2 years old
- Recurrent infections & subsequent scarring lead to end-stage renal disease in small but significant percentage of pediatric patients

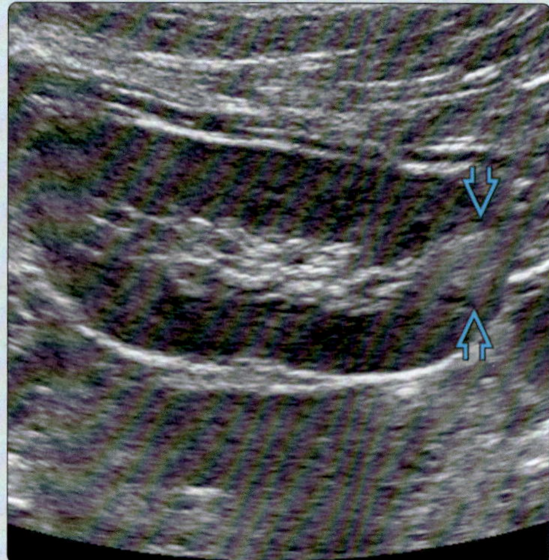

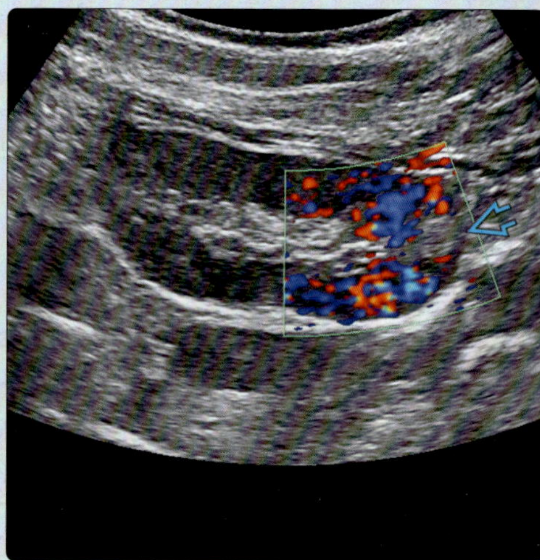

(Left) *Longitudinal US of the left kidney in a 4-year-old girl with fever & abdominal pain shows a focus of ↑ echogenicity in the lower pole ⇨.* **(Right)** *Color Doppler US of the left renal lower pole in the same patient shows ↓ blood flow ⇨ in the echogenic focus, consistent with pyelonephritis. US findings of pyelonephritis can be subtle, & color (especially power) Doppler is useful to localize an abnormality.*

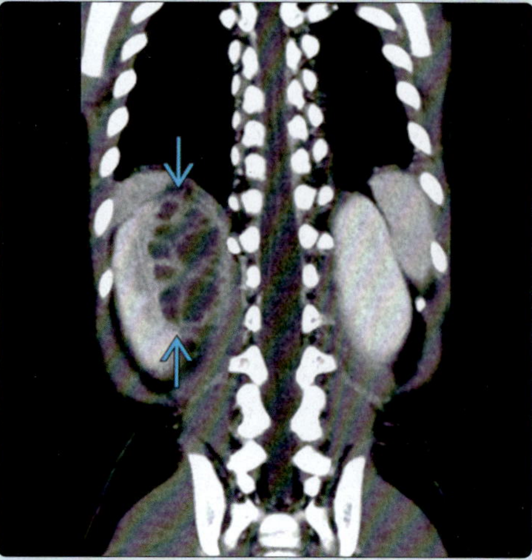

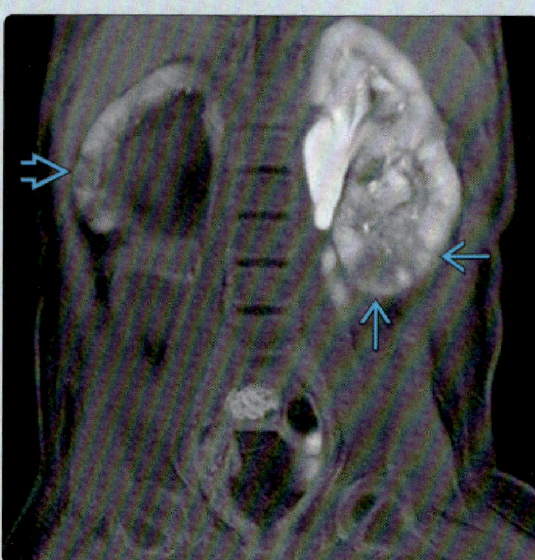

(Left) *Coronal CECT in a 5-month-old with fever shows a predominantly fluid-attenuation, multiseptated mass → with irregular walls & adjacent parenchymal & perinephric edema, consistent with pyelonephritis with abscess. Antibiotic therapy led to resolution without requiring drainage.* **(Right)** *Coronal T1 C+ FS MR in a 32-month-old with a history of urinary anomalies shows swelling, ↓ enhancement, & perinephric edema in the left lower pole → due to acute pyelonephritis. Scarring was noted on the right ⇨.*

TERMINOLOGY

Synonyms

- Acute lobar nephronia, focal bacterial nephritis

Definitions

- Acute infection of renal parenchyma
- Overview
  - Classic imaging appearance: Focal swelling & ↓ perfusion of affected parenchyma visible on nuclear scintigraphy, US, CT, & MR
  - Associated vesicoureteral reflux (VUR) in ~ 1/3 of cases
  - Permanent scarring is more likely in children < 2 years old
  - Variable presentation: Fever, lethargy, irritability, vomiting, abdominal/flank pain, hematuria, or dysuria
- Imaging work-up of urinary tract infection (UTI) is controversial; professional society guidelines vary internationally

IMAGING

General Features

- Best diagnostic clue
  - Inflammatory response to infection causes swelling that alters normal tissue properties & effectively ↓ radiologic contrast agent delivery to this site, which results in
    - Photopenic area on nuclear cortical scans
    - ↓ perfusion on Doppler imaging & altered echotexture on grayscale US
    - Striated or wedge-shaped areas of ↓ enhancement on CT or IVP
    - Focal ↓ contrast enhancement on MR
- Morphology
  - Areas of infection tend to be peripheral & wedge-shaped; can be more rounded & mass-like when inflammation is more severe

Radiographic Findings

- IVP
  - Striated nephrogram is classic, though IVPs are rarely performed in pediatric patients

Ultrasonographic Findings

- Grayscale ultrasound
  - Localized or generalized swelling; unilateral renal enlargement may be only clue to pyelonephritis
  - Poor corticomedullary differentiation & focal areas of ↑ or ↓ echogenicity
  - Occasionally rounded or mass-like areas of altered echotexture are noted, particularly with developing abscess
- Color Doppler
  - ↓ perfusion in areas of pyelonephritis
    - Adding power Doppler improves accuracy & sensitivity
  - Nonspecific ↑ resistive indices with parenchymal edema
- Contrast-enhanced ultrasound & microvascular imaging
  - ↓ perfusion noted in areas of pyelonephritis

CT Findings

- CECT
  - Wedge-shaped or round areas of poor enhancement
  - May have streaky enhancement, striated nephrogram
  - Inflammatory changes in perirenal fat
  - Occasionally mass-like; may distort normal renal contour & appear as partially cystic neoplasm during abscess development

MR Findings

- T1WI
  - Loss of corticomedullary differentiation
- T2WI
  - High signal intensity in affected renal parenchyma, potentially heterogeneous
  - May also see inflammatory changes in perirenal fat
  - Fat suppression techniques are more sensitive
- DWI
  - ↑ sensitivity for acute parenchymal inflammation
- T1WI C+ FS
  - Similar to CECT: Foci of ↓ enhancement

Nuclear Medicine Findings

- Nuclear scintigraphic findings
  - ↓ accumulation of renal cortical agents, typically wedge-shaped with apex pointed toward renal hilum
    - Tc-99m DMSA or glucoheptonate
    - Pinhole collimation & SPECT imaging improve diagnostic sensitivity & accuracy
  - No volume loss until scarring ensues
  - Findings persist for up to 6 weeks after acute infection

Imaging Recommendations

- Best imaging tool
  - Ultrasound with Doppler is least invasive & readily available but less sensitive than nuclear renal cortical scans, CECT, & MR
  - Ultrasound is frequently performed to search for associated complications (abscess, stones, scarring), underlying congenital anomalies, & hydronephrosis
- American Academy of Pediatrics Clinical Practice Guidelines
  - Renal & bladder US in febrile infants with UTI
  - VCUG is not performed routinely for 1st febrile UTI
    - Performed if US shows hydronephrosis, scarring, or other findings of high-grade VUR or obstructive uropathy as well as in other atypical or complex clinical circumstances

DIFFERENTIAL DIAGNOSIS

Renal Infarction

- Wedge-shaped pattern of ↓ perfusion
- Retained thin rim of capsular enhancement
- May see Doppler abnormalities of vessels

Renal Scarring

- Typically more superficial than pyelonephritis
- Associated cortical volume loss & dilated calyx

Renal Mass

- Heterogeneous, well-circumscribed mass, typically round
- Large masses (Wilms tumor, mesoblastic nephroma, etc.) may only show "claw" of residual splayed renal parenchyma along margin of tumor
  - Usually solid ± foci of necrosis; rarely entirely cystic or hemorrhagic

- Extremely rare but aggressive renal medullary carcinoma (RMC) can be very poorly defined & infiltrative, mimicking pyelonephritis/abscess & surrounding inflammatory change; check for history of sickle trait

Renal Contusion/Laceration

- Focal ↓ enhancement (often jagged or linear) with surrounding fluid in setting of trauma

PATHOLOGY

General Features

- Infection may occur via ascending route (VUR), hematogenous spread, or recent instrumentation
- Vast majority of urine cultures grow gram-negative bacilli, typically normal inhabitants of intestinal tract (*Escherichia coli is* most common)

CLINICAL ISSUES

Presentation

- Most common signs/symptoms
  - Often nonspecific: Malaise, irritability, fever, abdominal/flank pain, vomiting, hematuria, dysuria, change in urinary habits/enuresis
- Other signs/symptoms
  - Strong smelling urine in any age
- Laboratory studies
  - Urine dipstick for nitrite, leukocyte esterase; both are associated with higher likelihood of positive urine culture
  - Urine for Gram stain; *E. coli* is causative in > 80% of 1st-time UTIs, *Klebsiella* is 2nd most common
    - Urine specimen for culture: Catheter specimen, clean-catch midstream, or suprapubic aspirate
    - Urine culture is considered positive when single organism grows as follows
      - > 1,000 colony-forming units (cfu)/mL for suprapubic aspirate
      - Or > 10,000 cfu/mL for catheter specimen
      - Or > 100,000 cfu/mL for clean-catch midstream specimen
  - Bloodwork: Leukocytosis, occasionally positive blood cultures as well
- Complications
  - Perirenal abscess, necrotizing papillitis, pyonephrosis (obstruction), & cortical scarring
  - Recurrent infections & subsequent scarring lead to end-stage renal disease in small but significant percentage of pediatric patients
  - Recent study found that 1/2 of all patients with acute pyelonephritis went on to develop scarring
  - Some studies have found risk of scarring to be greater in younger patients
  - Xanthogranulomatous pyelonephritis is unusual, rare form of chronic renal suppuration often associated with renal stone disease

Demographics

- Epidemiology
  - Associated with VUR in ~ 25-40%
  - Higher incidence in obstruction, duplicated kidneys, other anomalies
- Sex: At least 2x as common in girls vs. boys

Natural History & Prognosis

- Generally excellent, unless there are complications or recurrent infections
- Potential sequelae of renal scarring, chronic renal failure, hypertension, & pregnancy-related complications

Treatment

- 7- to 14-day course of antimicrobial therapy; may be started IV & changed to oral
- Imaging work-up for VUR & congenital anomalies
- Prophylactic antibiotics for VUR & other predisposing conditions is controversial

DIAGNOSTIC CHECKLIST

Consider

- May be difficult clinically to distinguish lower UTI (cystitis) from pyelonephritis

Image Interpretation Pearls

- Partially cystic renal mass could be abscess, particularly if small to moderate in size with surrounding inflammation
  - Pyelonephritis is much more common than tumor
  - Abscess does not always cause positive urine testing
  - In correct clinical setting, consider short-term follow-up after antibiotics
- Conversely, very uncommon RMC is often poorly defined & infiltrative, mimicking pyelonephritis/abscess
  - Check for history of sickle trait (associated with RMC) if clinical history of pyelonephritis is not apparent

SELECTED REFERENCES

1. 't Hoen LA et al: Update of the EAU/ESPU guidelines on urinary tract infections in children. J Pediatr Urol. 17(2):200-7, 2021
2. Buettcher M et al: Swiss consensus recommendations on urinary tract infections in children. Eur J Pediatr. 180(3):663-74, 2020
3. Pleniceanu O et al: Acute pyelonephritis in children and the risk of end-stage kidney disease. J Nephrol. ePub, 2020
4. Warner J et al: Unenhanced MRI of the abdomen and pelvis in the comprehensive evaluation of acute atraumatic abdominal pain in children. AJR Am J Roentgenol. 215(5):1218-28, 2020
5. Zhu H et al: Semiquantitative analysis of power doppler ultrasonography versus Tc-99m DMSA scintigraphy in diagnostic and severity assessment of acute childhood pyelonephritis. Transl Pediatr. 9(4):487-95, 2020
6. Bahat H et al: Predictors of grade 3-5 vesicoureteral reflux in infants ≤2 months of age with pyelonephritis. Pediatr Nephrol. 34(5):907-15, 2019
7. Kosmeri C et al: An update on renal scarring after urinary tract infection in children: what are the risk factors? J Pediatr Urol. 15(6):598-603, 2019
8. Bosakova A et al: Diffusion-weighted magnetic resonance imaging is more sensitive than dimercaptosuccinic acid scintigraphy in detecting parenchymal lesions in children with acute pyelonephritis: a prospective study. J Pediatr Urol. 14(3):269.e1-7, 2018
9. Palmer LS et al: Cost-effectiveness of antimicrobial prophylaxis for children in the RIVUR trial. World J Urol. 36(9):1441-7, 2018
10. Chung EM et al: Imaging of the pediatric urinary system. Radiol Clin North Am. 55(2):337-57, 2017
11. Expert Panel on Pediatric Imaging:. et al: ACR Appropriateness Criteria® Urinary Tract Infection-Child. J Am Coll Radiol. 14(5S):S362-71, 2017
12. Reaffirmation of AAP Clinical Practice Guideline: The Diagnosis & Management of the Initial Urinary Tract Infection in Febrile Infants & Young Children 2–24 Months of Age. American Academy of Pediatrics. Published December, 2016. Accessed March 2021. https://pediatrics.aappublications.org/content/138/6/e20163026
13. Urinary tract infection in children: diagnosis, treatment & long-term management. National Collaborating Centre for Women's & Children's Health. Commissioned by the National Institute for Health & Clinical Excellence. Published August 2007. Updated 2017. Accessed March 2021. https://www.nice.org.uk/guidance/cg54/evidence/full-guideline-pdf-196566877

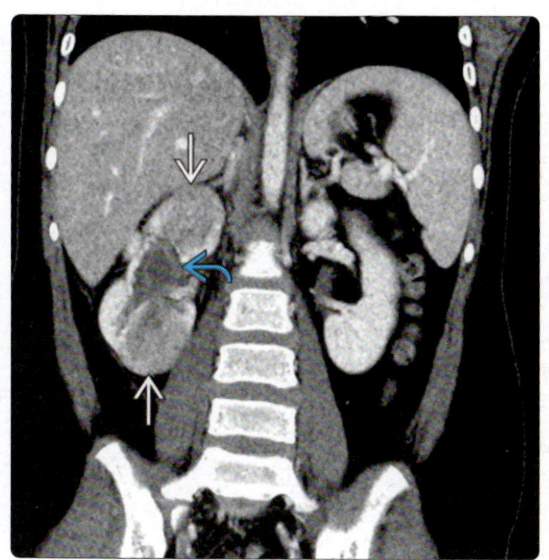

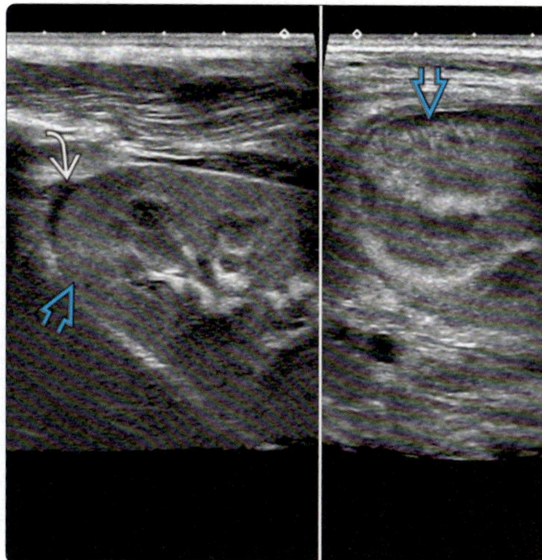

(Left) *Coronal CECT in a 9-year-old with pain shows foci of swelling & ↓ contrast enhancement → in both the upper & lower poles of the right kidney. Note the urothelial thickening & enhancement → of the renal pelvis in this case of pyelonephritis.* **(Right)** *Longitudinal US images of the kidneys with a high-frequency linear transducer show areas of altered cortical echogenicity → + a crescent of fluid → adjacent to the right renal upper pole in this patient with bilateral pyelonephritis.*

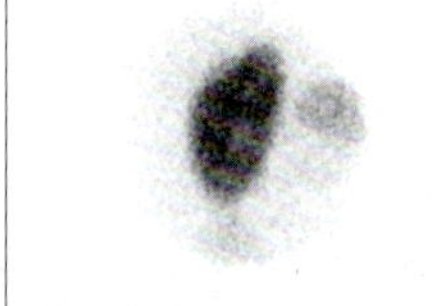

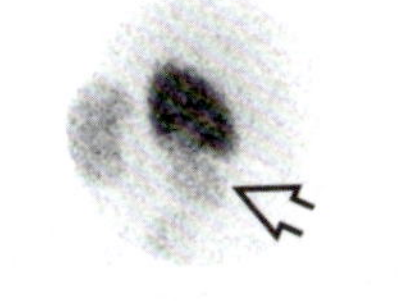

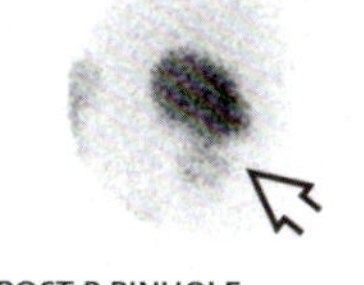

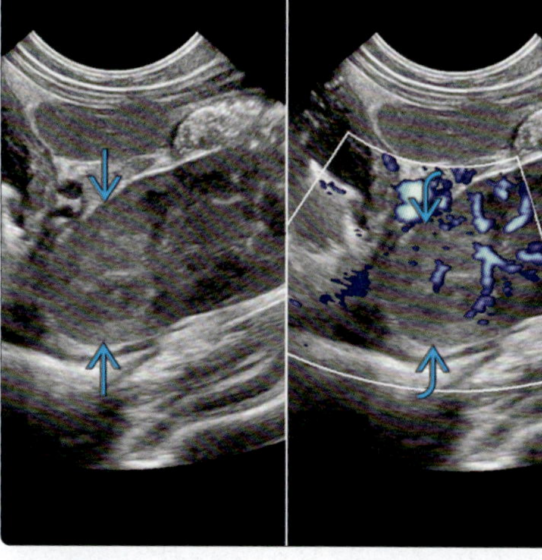

(Left) *Posterior pinhole images from Tc-99m DMSA renal cortical scintigraphy show absent radiotracer in the lower pole of the right kidney →, consistent with acute pyelonephritis. Large, wedge-shaped photopenic areas suggest pyelonephritis, while smaller, crescent-shaped cortical defects suggest scarring.* **(Right)** *Longitudinal US images of the left kidney in an 8-week-old girl show altered echotexture → in the upper pole with associated ↓ perfusion → on a microvascular Doppler image.*

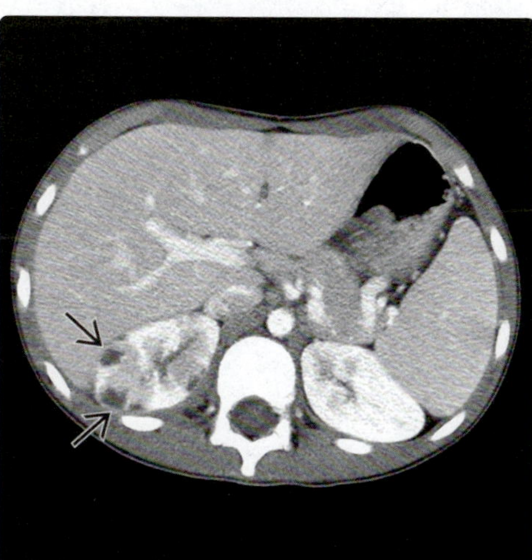

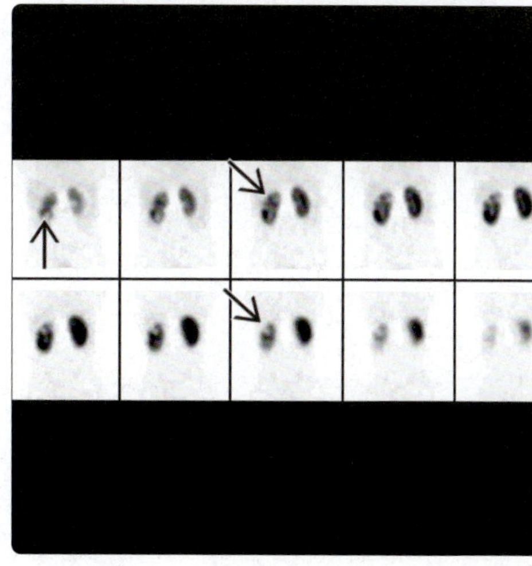

(Left) *Axial CECT in a patient with immune compromise shows multiple fluid-density foci in the right kidney →, suggesting developing abscesses. With subsequent ↑ size & confluence, drainage was ultimately required.* **(Right)** *Coronal anterior SPECT images from a Tc-99m DMSA cortical scan in the same patient show multiple defects in the right kidney →, consistent with pyelonephritis & developing abscesses seen on the patient's CECT scan. The left kidney was normal.*

Renal Injury

KEY FACTS

IMAGING

- Protocol
  - CECT in late cortical or early nephrographic phase
  - Obtain delayed images to detect ureteral injury or collecting system injury (if parenchymal laceration or perinephric fluid is present on initial images)
- Imaging findings
  - Renal parenchymal contusion, laceration
  - Subcapsular or perinephric/perirenal hematoma
  - Collecting system/ureteropelvic junction (UPJ) laceration
    - Fluid attenuation of 0-40 HU: Unclotted blood &/or urine
    - Intermediate attenuation of 40-80 HU: Clotted blood &/or urine
    - High attenuation of > 150-200 HU on delayed images only: Urinary contrast leak
  - Complete UPJ avulsion: Unopacified ipsilateral ureter distal to injury on delayed images
  - Active hemorrhage: High attenuation (isodense to vessel) nonanatomic collection on initial images; accumulates on delayed images
  - Vascular thrombosis or avulsion: Delayed or persistent renal enhancement vs. subtotal or global nonenhancement (± preservation of thin, enhancing rim due to capsular arterial supply)

PATHOLOGY

- Etiology: Blunt trauma 90%, penetrating trauma 10%

CLINICAL ISSUES

- Most common presentations: Flank pain, hematuria
- Successful nonoperative management in hemodynamically stable patients: 85%
  - Most common complication: Urinoma
- Possible predictors of intervention: Vascular contrast extravasation, collecting system clot, interpolar urinoma, urinoma > 4.3 cm, perirenal hematoma > 3.5 cm, dissociated renal fragments, > 25% devitalized fragments

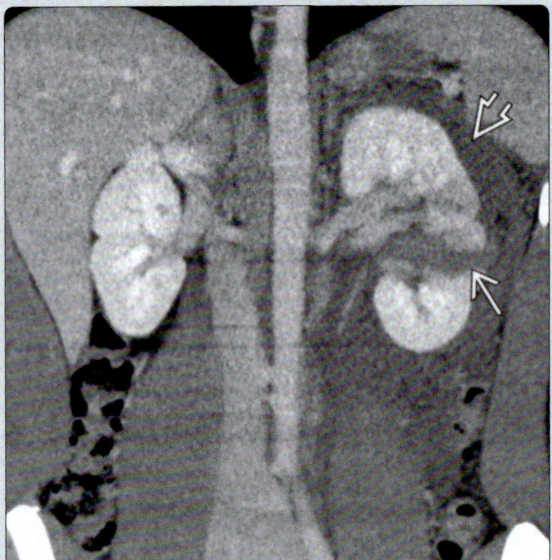

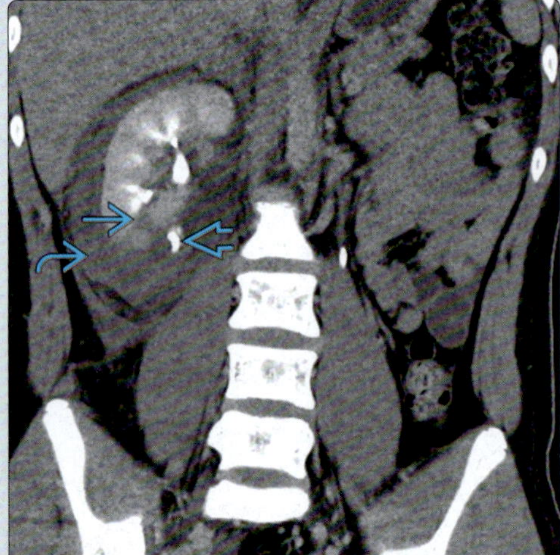

(Left) *Coronal CECT in a 17-year-old with an American football injury shows a grade III laceration ➡ that extends to the renal pelvis with a subcapsular hematoma ➡. No urinary extravasation was seen on delayed images.* **(Right)** *Delayed coronal CECT from a follow-up study in a 14-year-old after a skiing accident shows a grade IV laceration ➡ with urinary contrast extravasation ➡ from the lower pole collecting system. The perinephric urinoma ➡ had ↑ in size since the initial study. A ureteral stent was required.*

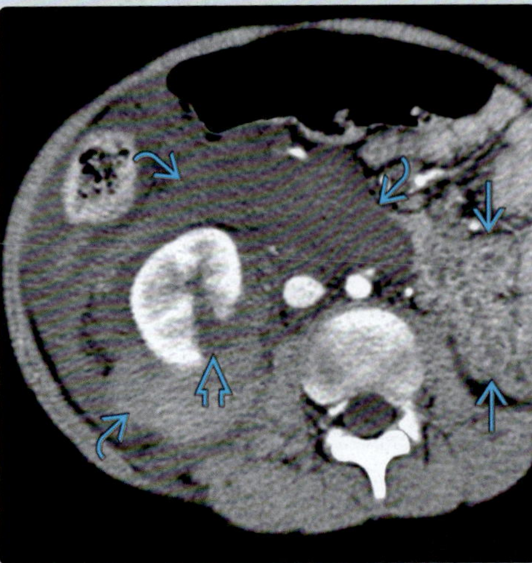

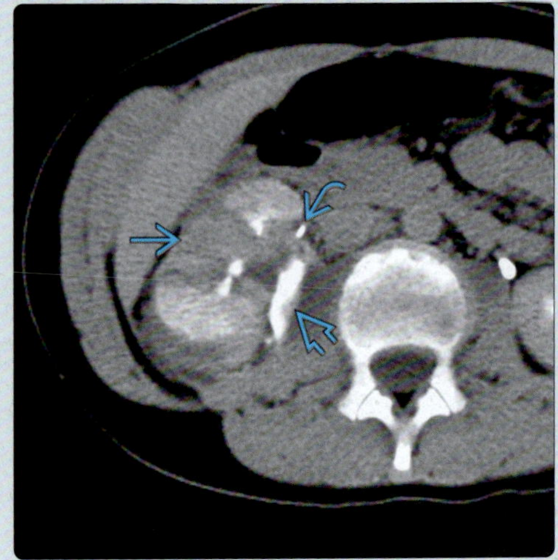

(Left) *Axial CECT in a 5-year-old hemodynamically unstable child after a bike accident shows a renal laceration ➡ & a large surrounding hematoma ➡. Note the shock bowel appearance ➡ due to hypoperfusion.* **(Right)** *Delayed axial CECT in a 15-year-old boy after a snowmobile accident shows a right renal grade IV laceration ➡ that extends to the ureteropelvic junction (UPJ). Extravasation of contrast-opacified urine is noted ➡. The ureter distal to the injury is opacified with contrast ➡, indicating that the UPJ tear is incomplete.*

TERMINOLOGY

Definitions

- Trauma to parenchyma &/or collecting system of kidney

IMAGING

General Features

- Best diagnostic clue
  - Defect of renal parenchymal enhancement + perirenal hematoma on CECT
    - ± extravasation of contrast-opacified urine or blood

CT Findings

- CECT
  - Contusion
    - Region of ↓ parenchymal enhancement with ↑ attenuation on delayed images (persistent nephrogram); may be radiologically occult
  - Hematoma
    - Fluid-attenuation collection; ↑ density of 40-80 HU upon clot formation
    - Subcapsular
      - □ Peripheral crescentic or lentiform collection
      - □ Flattening/indentation of underlying parenchyma
    - Perinephric/perirenal
      - □ Between renal parenchyma & Gerota fascia
      - □ Thickened, lateral conal fascia
      - □ May displace (but not indent) kidney; may have mass effect on colon
  - Parenchymal laceration
    - Irregular, linear fluid-attenuation defect; 40-80 HU if clotted blood is present
  - Collecting system/ureteropelvic junction (UPJ) laceration
    - Perinephric collection of fluid attenuation or higher
      - □ Urine or urine mixed with hematoma
    - Collection attenuation & size ↑ on delayed images
    - Delayed images with UPJ/proximal ureter injury show
      - □ Opacification of ureter distal to injury: Partial tear
      - □ Unopacified ureter distal to injury: Complete tear/avulsion
  - Main renal artery thrombosis
    - Partial or complete lack of arterial enhancement
    - Subtotal/global renal nonenhancement: Infarction
      - □ Cortical rim sign: Rim of enhancing peripheral cortex remains perfused by collateral flow from renal capsular artery; may be absent in first 8 hours
    - Retrograde opacification of renal vein from inferior vena cava
  - Segmental vascular infarct
    - Triangular, nonenhancing, parenchymal focus
    - Injury due to accessory, capsular, or intrarenal segmental arterial branches
  - Pseudoaneurysm
    - ↑ density of round focus (isodense to aorta) directly adjacent to artery
    - Stable size with contrast washout on delayed images
  - Active hemorrhage
    - Irregular ↑ density collection (isodense to adjacent vessel) on initial images; ↑ in size on delayed images
  - Main renal vein thrombosis
    - Enlarged vein with filling defect of thrombus
    - Nephromegaly with delayed nephrogram & excretion
    - Less common than main renal artery thrombosis

Ultrasonographic Findings

- Grayscale ultrasound
  - Hematoma
    - Parenchymal, subcapsular, or perinephric collection
    - Echogenicity varies with age of blood products
    - Can be difficult to differentiate from urinoma
  - Laceration
    - Hypoechoic linear/branching defect interrupting renal architecture; hyperechoic if contains clot
- Color Doppler
  - Thrombosis: Various aberrant waveforms are possible depending on extent & location of thrombus
    - Tardus-parvus waveform distal to proximal nonocclusive arterial thrombus/stenosis
    - Reversal of diastolic flow with thrombosis of renal vein or distal artery
    - Absence of flow in occluded vessel
  - Parenchymal ischemia/infarct: Focally or globally ↓ or absent color Doppler signal
- CEUS
  - Improved detection of segmental & subcapsular infarcts
  - Improved confidence for diagnosing renal artery & vein occlusion as well as differentiating complete vs. partial occlusion
  - Allows visualization of hyperechoic active extravasation
  - Lack of microbubble urinary excretion limits evaluation
- Sensitivity & specificity vary widely across multiple studies
  - FAST US: Sensitivity 23-100%, specificity 98-100%
  - Abdominal US: Sensitivity 36-90%, specificity 98-100%
  - CEUS: Sensitivity 69%, specificity 99%

Imaging Recommendations

- American Urological Association (AUA) recommends
  - CECT for initial evaluation
    - Portal venous phase (late cortical or early nephrographic phase)
    - Delayed (5-15 minutes) images to evaluate for urinary contrast leak in stable patient with suspicion for ureteral injury or renal laceration &/or perinephric fluid on initial images
  - Follow-up CECT in 48 hours for
    - Grade IV or V injuries (due to ↑ complication rates)
    - Injury grade < IV with clinical signs of complication
- American Association for the Surgery of Trauma (AAST)
  - Recommends CECT but notes US may be used for
    - Initial evaluation & follow-up if hemodynamically stable
    - In those with mild symptoms, minimal clinical findings, hematuria < 50 RBC/HPF & no other CT indications

DIFFERENTIAL DIAGNOSIS

Normal Variant Contour

- Dromedary hump, column of Bertin, fetal lobation

Pyelonephritis

- Enlarged kidney with delayed or striated nephrogram in patient with flank pain, fever, abnormal urinalysis

- Abscess can mimic multicystic mass with irregular rim/septal enhancement

Renal Neoplasm

- Most pediatric renal tumors
  - Present with distention, palpable mass, &/or hematuria
  - Have overlapping imaging features
    - Differential is best determined by patient age & history
  - Can rupture or hemorrhage (causing pain)
- Angiomyolipoma (AML) is unique
  - Fat-containing renal masses typically associated with tuberous sclerosis in children
  - AML > 4 cm or aneurysm > 5 cm is prone to spontaneous hemorrhage (uncommon in children)

PATHOLOGY

General Features

- Etiology
  - Blunt trauma in 90%, penetrating trauma in 10%
  - Common causes: Falls, sports related, motor vehicle related, bicycle accidents, assault, child abuse
  - Rapid deceleration: ↑ risk of vascular pedicle & UPJ injury
  - Children are at ↑ risk compared to adults due to ↑ organ mobility & relative size, ↓ perirenal fat, low renal position, elastic rib cage with ↓ renal coverage, & fetal lobations (which may act as cleavage plane)
  - Preexisting renal abnormalities predispose to injury
- Associated abnormalities
  - Other organ injuries: Liver: 22%, lungs: 19%, spleen: 16%

Staging, Grading, & Classification

- AAST
  - Grade I: Subcapsular hematoma &/or parenchymal contusion without laceration
  - Grade II: Perirenal hematoma confined to Gerota fascia; laceration ≤ 1 cm depth without urine extravasation
  - Grade III: Laceration > 1 cm depth without collecting system rupture/urine extravasation; vascular injury (pseudoaneurysm or arteriovenous fistula) or active bleeding contained in Gerota fascia
  - Grade IV: Laceration extending into collecting system with urine extravasation; renal pelvis laceration or ureteropelvic disruption; segmental renal vein/artery injury; segmental or complete kidney infarction due to thrombosis without active bleeding; active bleeding beyond Gerota fascia
  - Grade V: Main renal artery/vein laceration or hilar avulsion; devascularized kidney with active bleeding; shattered kidney (loss of identifiable renal anatomy)
  - Advance 1 grade for bilateral injuries up to grade III

CLINICAL ISSUES

Presentation

- Most common signs/symptoms
  - Flank pain/tenderness, hematuria, ecchymosis
    - Hematuria may be absent, even in high-grade injury

Natural History & Prognosis

- Majority are low-grade injuries (I-III): 79%
- Of all renal injuries, 85% are managed conservatively
- 50% of grade V & 44% of penetrating injuries are managed operatively
- Findings associated with nonoperative management failure
  - Vascular contrast extravasation, medial urinary extravasation/urinoma, collecting system clot, interpolar contrast urinoma, urinoma > 4.3 cm, dissociated renal fragments, > 25% devitalized fragments, perirenal hematoma > 3.5 cm, lack of ureteral opacification
- Early complications (< 4 weeks)
  - Urinoma: Most common; most reabsorb
  - Delayed bleeding: Due to arteriovenous fistula/pseudoaneurysm, usually 2-3 weeks after injury
  - Perinephric abscess, sepsis, infected urinoma
- Late complications (> 4 weeks)
  - Hypertension due to Page kidney
  - Hydronephrosis, calculi, chronic pyelonephritis

Treatment

- Nonoperative management is generally recommended in hemodynamically stable patients with grade I-V injuries
  - UPJ or proximal ureteral avulsion warrants prompt intervention, endoscopic or operative
- Ureteral stent ± percutaneous urinoma drain &/or percutaneous nephrostomy for complications of ↑ urinoma, ↑ pain, ileus, fistula, or infection
- Renal artery thrombosis: Thrombolysis, stent
- Angioembolization in hemodynamically stable patients to control ongoing/delayed bleeding (if readily available)
- Surgery in hemodynamically unstable patients or those failing nonoperative management

DIAGNOSTIC CHECKLIST

Image Interpretation Pearls

- View CECT in multiple planes (as transverse lacerations may be occult on axial images)

SELECTED REFERENCES

1. Bowen DK et al: Does contrast-enhanced ultrasound have a role in evaluation and management of pediatric renal trauma? A preliminary experience. J Pediatr Surg. 55(12):2740-5, 2020
2. Redmond EJ et al: Contemporary management of pediatric high grade renal trauma: 10 year experience at a level 1 trauma centre. J Pediatr Urol. 16(5):656.e1-5, 2020
3. Coccolini F et al: Kidney and uro-trauma: WSES-AAST guidelines. World J Emerg Surg. 14:54, 2019
4. Gates RL et al: Non-operative management of solid organ injuries in children: an American Pediatric Surgical Association Outcomes and Evidence Based Practice Committee systematic review. J Pediatr Surg. 54(8):1519-26, 2019
5. Hagedorn JC et al: Pediatric blunt renal trauma practice management guidelines: collaboration between the Eastern Association for the Surgery of Trauma and the Pediatric Trauma Society. J Trauma Acute Care Surg. 86(5):916-25, 2019
6. Armstrong LB et al: Pediatric renal injury: which injury grades warrant close follow-up. Pediatr Surg Int. 34(11):1183-7, 2018
7. Kozar RA et al: Organ injury scaling 2018 update: spleen, liver, and kidney. J Trauma Acute Care Surg. 85(6):1119-22, 2018
8. Bryk DJ et al: Guideline of guidelines: a review of urological trauma guidelines. BJU Int. 117(2):226-34, 2016
9. Dangle PP et al: Evolving mechanisms of injury and management of pediatric blunt renal trauma–20 years of experience. Urology. 90:159-63, 2016
10. LeeVan E et al: Management of pediatric blunt renal trauma: a systematic review. J Trauma Acute Care Surg. 80(3):519-28, 2016
11. Dahlstrom K et al: Blunt renal trauma in children with pre-existing renal abnormalities. Pediatr Radiol. 45(1):118-23; quiz 115-7, 2015
12. Grimsby GM et al: Demographics of pediatric renal trauma. J Urol. 192(5):1498-502, 2014

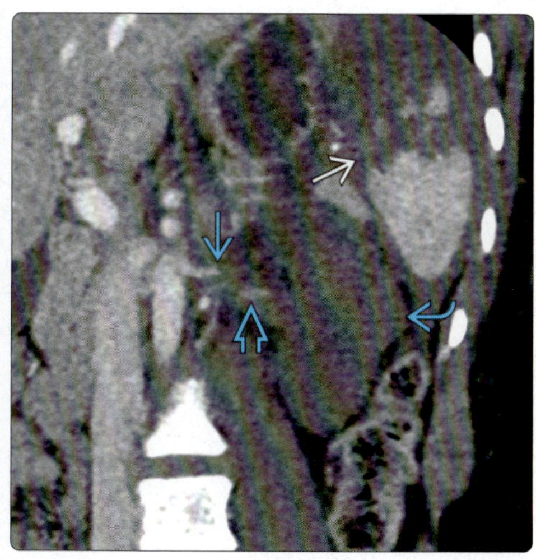

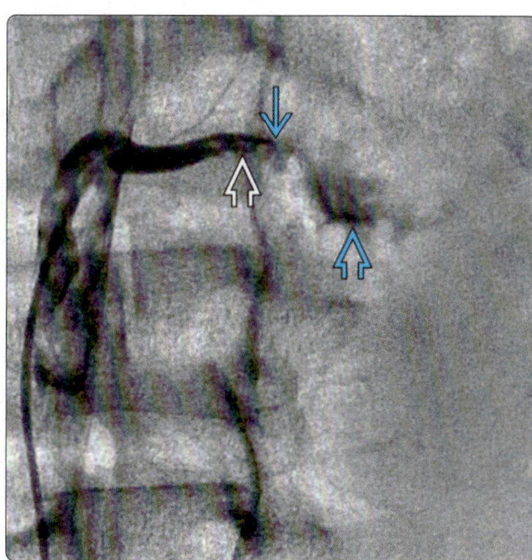

(Left) *Coronal oblique CECT in a 13-year-old girl with a grade V renal injury shows truncation of the left renal arterial opacification ➔ with adjacent contrast extravasation ➔. The left kidney is devascularized ➔. A grade IV splenic injury ➔ is also noted.* **(Right)** *Frontal view from a catheter angiogram of the same left renal artery shows complete left renal artery avulsion ➔ with proximal vessel thrombosis ➔ & distal contrast extravasation ➔. A revascularization attempt failed.*

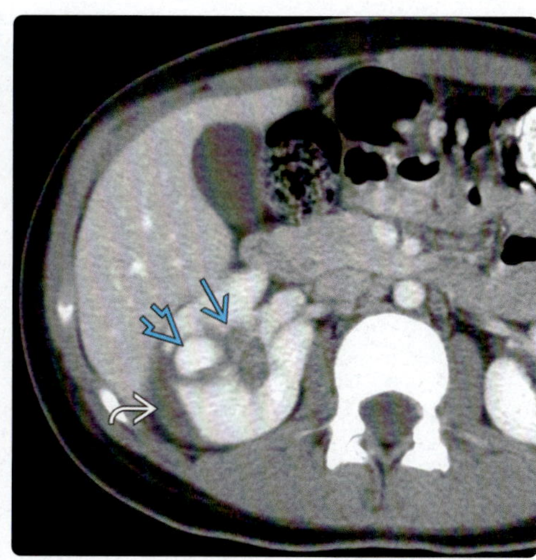

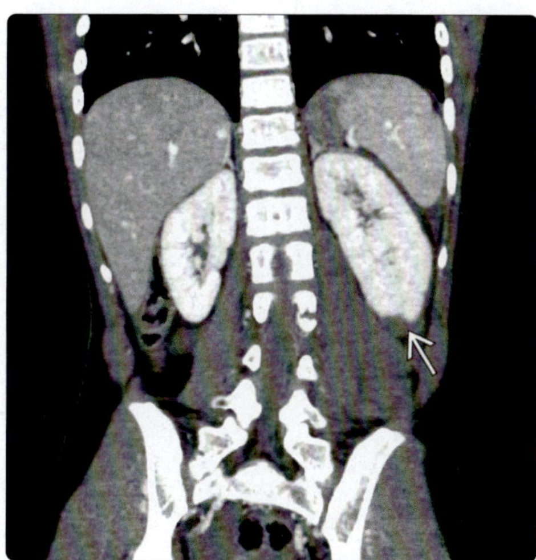

(Left) *Axial CECT in a 14-year-old that fell off of a horse demonstrates a grade III injury. There is a laceration that extends to the renal hilum ➔ with an associated subcapsular hematoma ➔. The focal rounded area of contrast is compatible with a traumatic pseudoaneurysm ➔.* **(Right)** *Coronal CECT in a 14-year-old after a motor vehicle accident (MVA) shows a laceration < 1 cm with associated small subcapsular hematoma, compatible with a grade II injury ➔.*

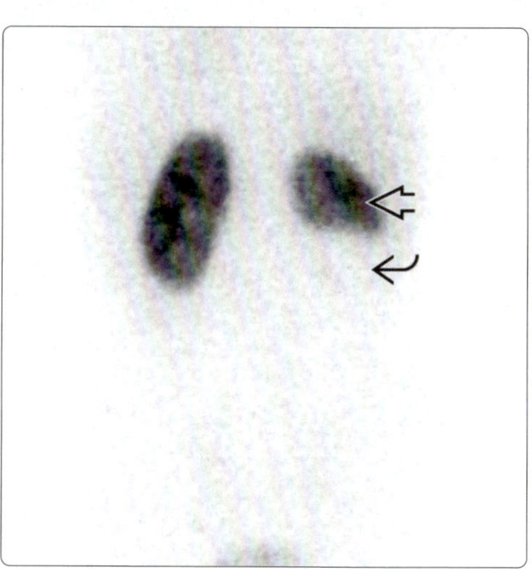

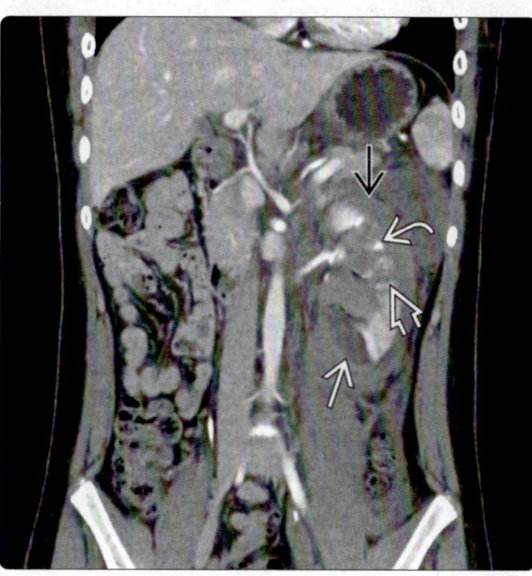

(Left) *Posterior view from a 2-month follow-up Tc-99m DMSA scan in a 15-year-old with a right grade V renal injury from a sledding accident shows that the right kidney has normal uptake in the upper pole ➔ but none in the lower pole ➔. The split renal function was 60% left & 40% right.* **(Right)** *Coronal CECT in a 13-year-old after a skiing accident shows a grade IV injury with a left kidney lower pole segmental infarction ➔. Also seen are lacerations ➔, active bleeding ➔, & a perinephric hematoma ➔.*

KEY FACTS

TERMINOLOGY

- Concretion in urinary system

IMAGING

- Most stones are seen in kidneys & upper urinary tract
- Range in size from 1-2 mm to > 1 cm
- NECT is most sensitive modality to detect stones
  - Calcified density in urinary system
- Ultrasound shows hyperechoic urinary tract focus with posterior acoustic shadowing &/or twinkling artifact
- Important to report signs of obstruction
  - Hydroureteronephrosis
  - Nephromegaly
  - Perinephric/periureteral edema
  - Lack of ureteral jet in urinary bladder on Doppler ultrasound
  - High-resistance renal artery flow on Doppler ultrasound
  - Delayed renal enhancement & excretion after IV contrast administration

TOP DIFFERENTIAL DIAGNOSES

- Fecal material
- Phleboliths
- Nephrocalcinosis
- Ureteropelvic junction obstruction

PATHOLOGY

- 75-85% of children have identifiable metabolic predisposition

CLINICAL ISSUES

- Presentations
  - 94% of adolescents have colicky flank pain
  - Nonspecific symptoms (abdominal pain, nausea, vomiting, & irritability) in younger children
  - Microscopic hematuria in up to 90% of patients
- Treatment depends on stone size, location, presence of obstruction, & underlying etiology

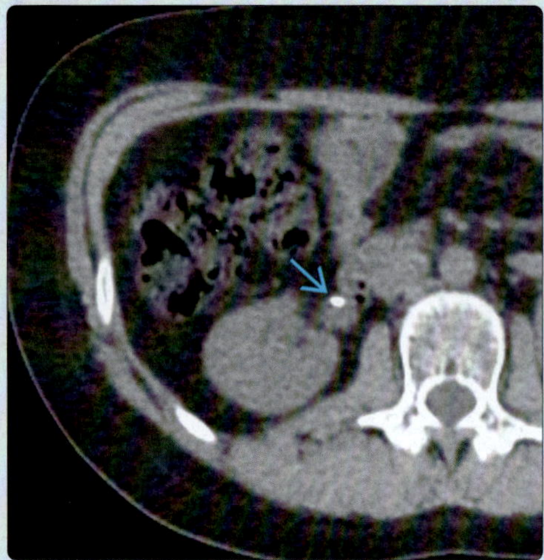

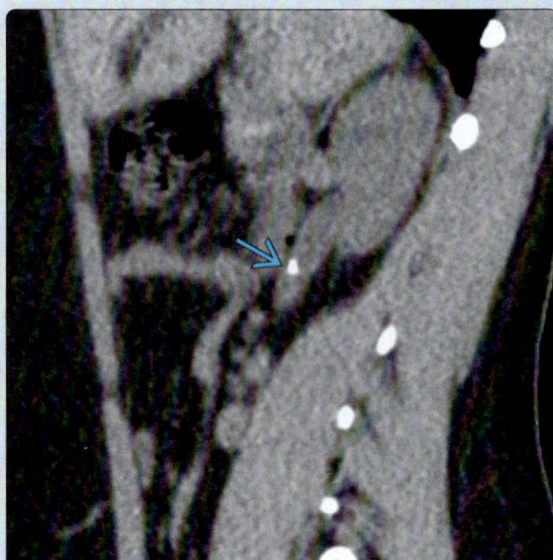

(Left) *Axial NECT shows a calcified urinary stone ➡ in the right ureter near the ureteropelvic junction. While the proximal ureter is dilated, there is no hydronephrosis or perinephric stranding.* **(Right)** *Sagittal NECT in the same patient shows the urinary stone ➡ in the proximal ureter. The renal collecting system is not dilated, & there is no perinephric or periureteral stranding to suggest obstruction.*

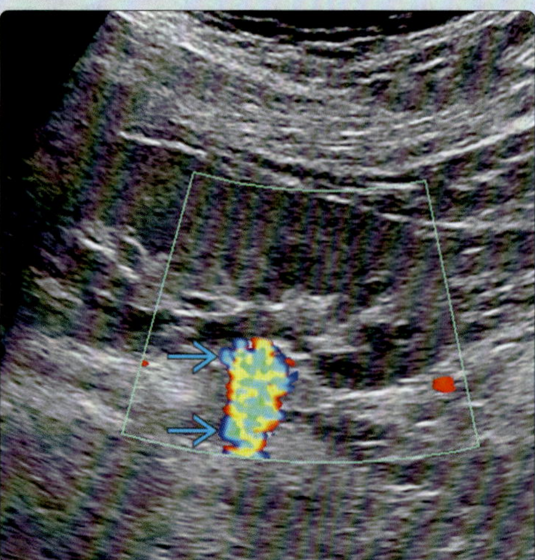

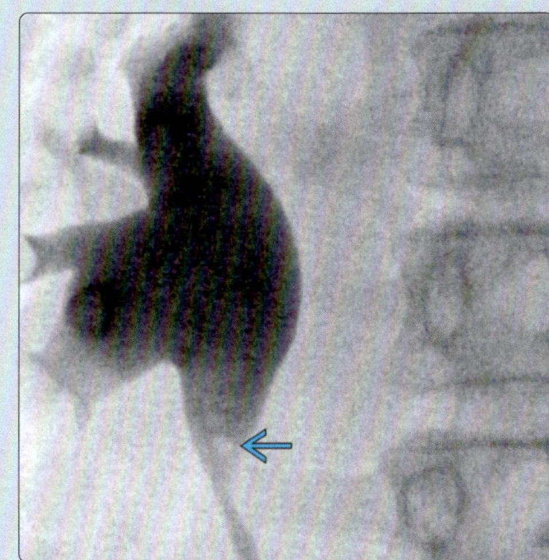

(Left) *Longitudinal color Doppler ultrasound of the right kidney in the same patient shows considerable twinkling artifact ➡ in & deep to the stone. Note the lack of renal collecting system dilation.* **(Right)** *Retrograde ureterogram in the same patient shows a filling defect ➡ from a urinary stone at the ureteropelvic junction. The mild dilation of the collecting system is secondary to the injection pressure.*

TERMINOLOGY

Synonyms

- Nephrolithiasis, nephrolith, urolithiasis, urolith, urinary stone, kidney stone, renal calculi

Definitions

- Concretion in urinary system

IMAGING

General Features

- Best diagnostic clue
  - Calcific density in renal collecting system, ureters, or urinary bladder
- Location
  - Usually seen at renal collecting system, ureteropelvic junction (UPJ), or ureterovesical junction (UVJ)
    - Most stones are seen in kidneys & upper urinary tract
- Size
  - Range in size from 1-2 mm to > 1 cm

Radiographic Findings

- Radiography
  - Irregular, calcified density over region of kidneys, ureters, or bladder
  - If stone is seen on radiograph, can be used to follow disease
- IVP
  - Uncommonly used modality to identify obstructive calculi in known stone formers
  - Often modified for children to ↓ radiation dose
  - Signs of urinary obstruction
    - Enlarged kidney
    - Hydronephrosis
    - Hydroureter up to stone
    - Filling defect at level of calculus
    - Delayed & prolonged nephrogram with delayed collecting system excretion

Ultrasonographic Findings

- Grayscale ultrasound
  - Considered as 1st-line imaging study due to lack of radiation; however, overall sensitivity & negative predictive value are low (66% & 79%, respectively)
  - Hyperechoic focus with posterior acoustic shadowing
    - Shadow artifact may not be present on machines with harmonic or spatial compounding
    - Shadow artifact is considered as specific finding
  - Stones are usually visible in renal collecting system (at UPJ, UVJ, or bladder)
    - Midureteral stones are difficult to find due to bowel gas
  - Ultrasound can be used to identify obstruction of urinary system
    - Grayscale signs of obstruction
      - □ Hydronephrosis
      - □ Hydroureter to level of urinary stone
      - □ Enlarged kidney
      - □ Perinephric fluid
- Color Doppler
  - Twinkling artifact: Rapidly changing random mixture of color in/posterior to stone
    - Thought to be due to rough but strongly reflective surface of stone
    - Twinkle artifact has high specificity but low sensitivity for detecting stones
  - Signs of obstruction
    - High-resistance renal artery flow
    - Lack of ureteral jet in urinary bladder

CT Findings

- NECT
  - Most sensitive modality to detect urinary stones
  - Stone appears as calcified density in renal collecting system, ureters, or bladder
  - Stones can obstruct urinary system
    - Most stones are not obstructive
    - Signs of obstruction
      - □ Hydronephrosis
      - □ Hydroureter
      - □ Enlarged kidney
      - □ Perinephric or periureteral stranding
      - □ Loss of slightly hyperattenuating pyramids
- CECT
  - Not primarily used for detection of urinary tract calculus
  - Findings are similar to IVP

Imaging Recommendations

- Best imaging tool
  - Ultrasound as 1st test; NECT if ultrasound is negative & suspicion for stones remains high
  - NECT is most sensitive modality to detect stones
    - Many perform CT in prone position to better distinguish UVJ vs. bladder stone
    - Beware of multiple CTs due to radiation dose
  - In known stone formers, presence or absence of obstruction may be only imaging question
    - Ultrasound detects urinary obstruction without radiation

DIFFERENTIAL DIAGNOSIS

Fecal Material

- Colonic contents may overlie kidneys, ureters, or bladder on radiographs & mimic nephrolithiasis

Phleboliths

- Round Ca^{2+} with lucent center in abnormal stagnant vein
- Most common in pelvis, near bladder

Nephrocalcinosis

- Ca^{2+} within renal parenchyma
- ± cortical, medullary, or diffuse

Ureteropelvic Junction Obstruction

- Chronically dilated renal collecting system due to intrinsic or extrinsic process; no visible stone

Transient Neonatal Renal Medullary Hyperechogenicity

- Evenly distributed echogenic renal pyramid tips
- Incidental, benign finding lasting up to 3 weeks
- Not clearly due to Tamm-Horsfall proteinuria

PATHOLOGY

General Features

- Etiology
  - 75-85% of children with stones have identifiable predisposition
    - Metabolic cause of stones in 75-90% of patients
    - Infection in 4% of patients
- Metabolic causes of pediatric stone disease
  - Calcium stones
    - Hypercalciuria: Most common metabolic abnormality causing pediatric stones
      - Accounts for 34-50% of children with identifiable metabolic cause of stones
    - Hyperuricosuria: Can be caused by excess purine production or ingestion, renal tubular disorders, medications, or juvenile gout
      - Present in 2-20% of children with stones
    - Hypocitruria: Can be caused by renal tubular acidosis
      - 10% of children with stones
    - Hyperoxaluria: Can be caused by primary hyperoxaluria or ↑ intestinal absorption due to bowel disease
      - Found in 10-20% of children with stones
  - Uric acid stones: Seen with excessively acidic urine, such as in diarrheal states or diet high in animal protein
    - Radiolucent stones
  - Struvite stones: Caused by infection with urease-splitting bacteria
    - Often appear as staghorn calculi
- Hereditary causes of pediatric stone disease
  - Adenine phosphoribosyltransferase deficiency
    - Autosomal recessive inborn error of adenine metabolism
    - Most common manifestation: Radiolucent stones
    - Pathognomonic round/brown DHA crystals in urine
  - Cystinuria
    - Most common cause of inherited kidney stones
    - Accounts for up to 25% of pediatric stones
    - Defect in proximal tubular resorption of filtered cystine
    - Average age of 1st stone: 12-13 years
    - Pathognomonic hexagonal crystals in urine

CLINICAL ISSUES

Presentation

- Most common signs/symptoms
  - Depends on age
    - 94% of adolescents present with colicky flank pain
    - Nonspecific symptoms (abdominal pain, nausea, vomiting, & irritability) in younger children
  - Microscopic hematuria in up to 90% of patients
- Other signs/symptoms
  - Gross hematuria in 14-32%
  - Concomitant urinary tract infection in 8-20%

Demographics

- Age
  - Can occur at any age
  - Median age of nephrolithiasis onset: 4.4 years for boys, 7.3 years for girls
- Ethnicity
  - More common in White patients
- Epidemiology
  - Incidence of stones in kids is increasing 6-10% annually
    - 18 per 100,000 patients in 1999; 50 per 100,000 in 2018
    - Overall incidence ↑ 5x over last 2 decades
  - Potential causes for ↑ prevalence
    - ↑ obesity & related poor dietary habits
    - ↓ water intake coupled with ↑ sodium & protein intake
    - ↓ dietary calcium (from milk)
    - ↑ use of CT (improved detection)
    - Global warming: ↑ incidence with ↑ temperatures

Natural History & Prognosis

- Higher morbidity of stone disease in children
  - Longer hospital stay
- Stones < 5 mm may pass spontaneously
- Residual stones can act as nidus for more stones

Treatment

- Treatment depends on underlying etiology
- ↑ fluid intake
  - Poor long-term compliance
- Expectant management
  - Up to 60% of stones < 5 mm pass spontaneously
- Medical treatment depends on underlying cause
  - Hypercalciuria: ↑ fluid intake, ↓ dietary sodium, & ↓ dietary calcium to recommended levels
    - Thiazide diuretics can ↓ urinary calcium
  - Hyperoxaluria: Potassium citrate & calcium supplements may ↓ intestinal oxalate absorption
  - Hyperuricosuria: Urinary alkalinization
- Surgical management is required in 22%
  - Extracorporeal shock wave lithotripsy (ESWL)
    - Used for treatment of proximal ureteral calculi & mid or upper pole stones < 2 cm
  - Ureteroscopy: Currently most commonly used option for children
    - Improved stone-free rates (88-100%) compared to ESWL for ureteral stones
    - Similar stone-free rates compared to ESWL for intrarenal stones (58-62%)
  - Percutaneous nephrolithotomy
    - Reserved for larger stone burden/treatment failure

SELECTED REFERENCES

1. Tekgül S et al: European Association of Urology and European Society for Paediatric Urology Guidelines on paediatric urinary stone disease. Eur Urol Focus. ePub, 2021
2. Verhagen MV et al: Acoustic shadowing in pediatric kidney stone ultrasound: a retrospective study with non-enhanced computed tomography as reference standard. Pediatr Radiol. 49(6):777-83, 2019
3. Bowen DK et al: Pediatric stone disease. Urol Clin North Am. 45(4):539-50, 2018
4. Roberson NP et al: Comparison of ultrasound versus computed tomography for the detection of kidney stones in the pediatric population: a clinical effectiveness study. Pediatr Radiol. 48(7):962-72, 2018
5. Scoffone CM et al: Pediatric calculi: cause, prevention and medical management. Curr Opin Urol. 28(5):428-32, 2018

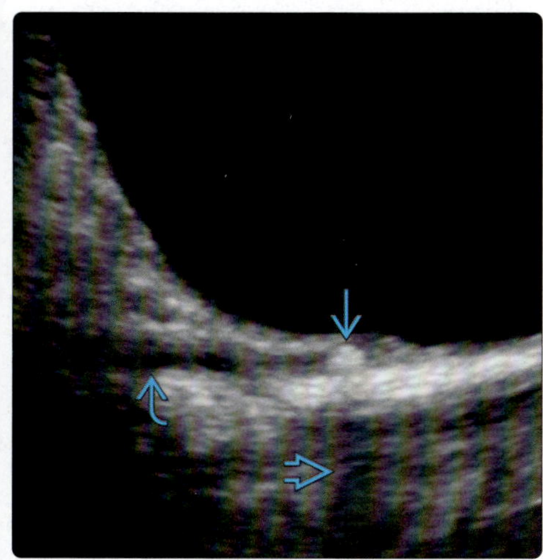

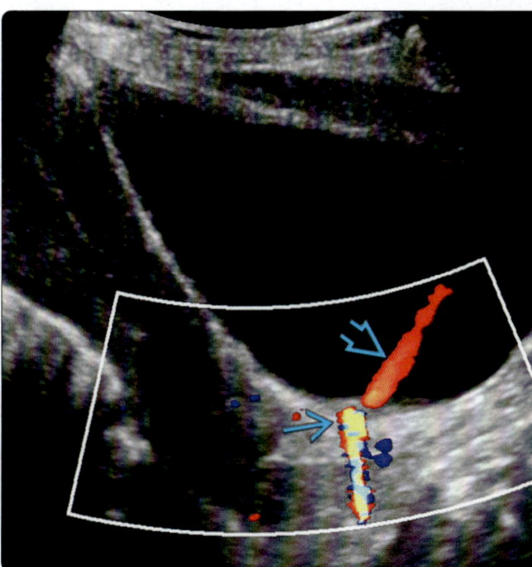

(Left) *Longitudinal ultrasound of the bladder in an adolescent shows an echogenic stone* ➙ *at the ureterovesical junction. The stone causes mild posterior acoustic shadowing* ➙*, & the distal ureter is mildly dilated* ➙*.* **(Right)** *Longitudinal color Doppler ultrasound in the same patient shows twinkling artifact* ➙ *from the stone at the ureterovesical junction. The presence of a ureteral jet* ➙ *in the urinary bladder confirms that the stone does not cause complete obstruction.*

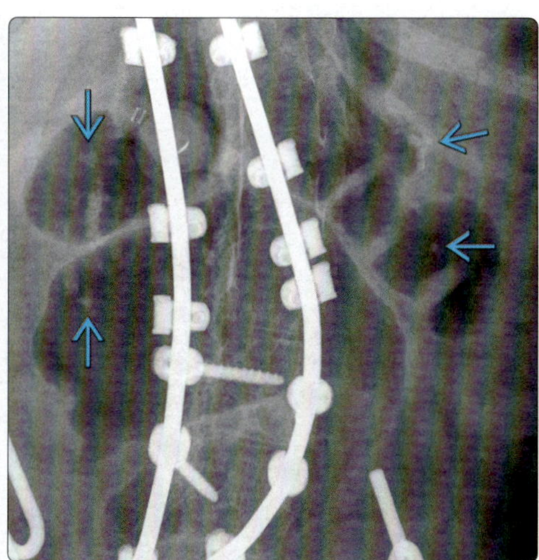

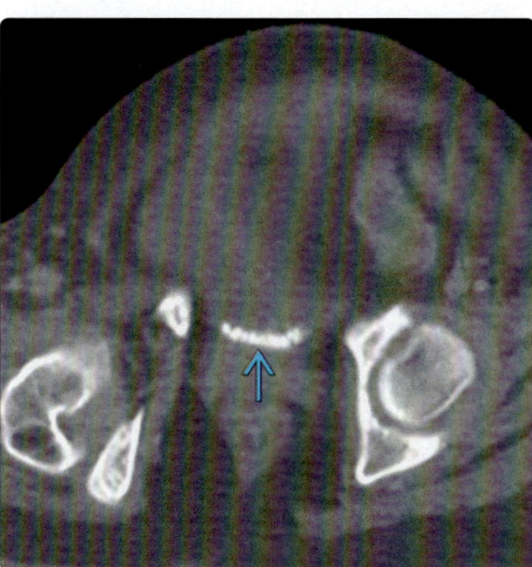

(Left) *AP radiograph of the abdomen in a child with cerebral palsy shows numerous calcified stones* ➙ *within the bilateral renal collecting systems.* **(Right)** *Axial CECT in bone windows in the same patient shows numerous calcified stones* ➙ *layering dependently within the urinary bladder.*

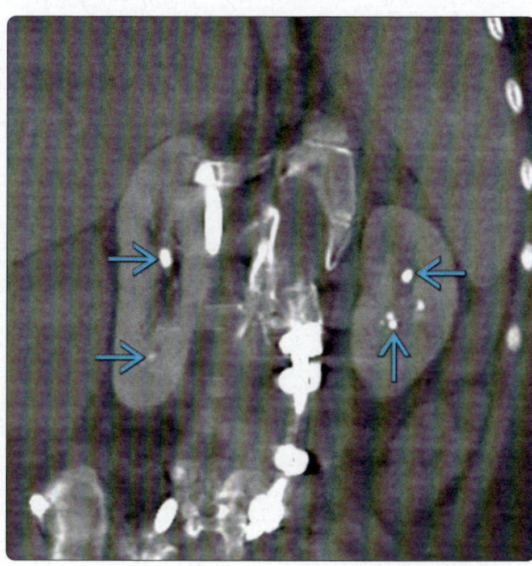

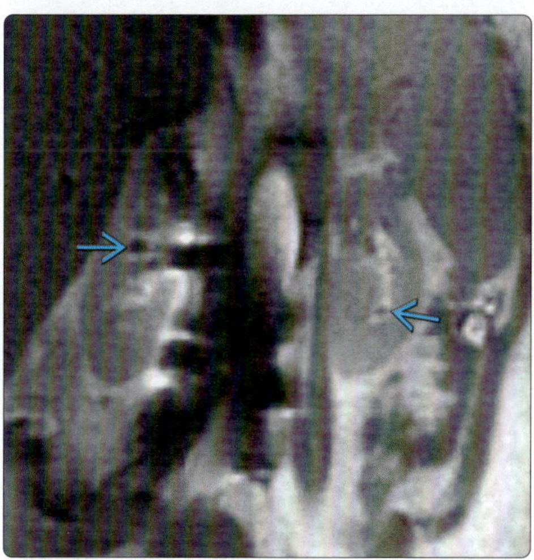

(Left) *Coronal CECT in the same patient shows numerous stones* ➙ *within the nondilated right & left renal collecting systems. Note that IV contrast was administered on this exam for other reasons, not the investigation of urinary tract calculi.* **(Right)** *Coronal T2 MR in the same patient shows multiple hypointense stones* ➙ *in the nondilated right & left renal collecting systems.*

Transient Neonatal Renal Medullary Hyperechogenicity

KEY FACTS

TERMINOLOGY

- Temporary sonographic appearance of hyperechoic renal medullary pyramids in some normal neonates
  - Neonatal renal pyramids are usually hypoechoic to renal cortex on US
- Etiology unclear: Not linked to ↑ concentration of normal Tamm-Horsfall glycoproteins in neonatal urine
  - Though appearance previously has been termed "Tamm-Horsfall proteinuria"
  - Therefore, recent literature uses descriptive term "transient renal medullary hyperechogenicity"

IMAGING

- Renal US shows ↑ echogenicity of medullary pyramids in neonate with normal renal function
  - Usually involves tips & central portions of pyramids
  - Bases of pyramids typically remain hypoechoic
  - Diffuse involvement of entire medullary pyramid is uncommon
  - May appear as layering gradient of ↑ echogenicity, brightest at tips of pyramids
  - Posterior acoustic shadowing is typically absent
  - Bilateral > unilateral renal involvement
  - Segmental involvement (sparing of some medullary pyramids) > diffuse (involvement of all pyramids)
  - Normal renal cortical echogenicity & size
- ↑ echogenicity of renal medullary pyramids usually resolves spontaneously by 10 days

CLINICAL ISSUES

- If renal insufficiency/failure is present, consider pathologic causes for ↑ echogenicity

DIAGNOSTIC CHECKLIST

- Normal finding up to 10th day of life; repeat US is not indicated
- If hyperechoic medullary pyramids are seen beyond 10-14 days or in setting of renal dysfunction, then another diagnosis should be considered

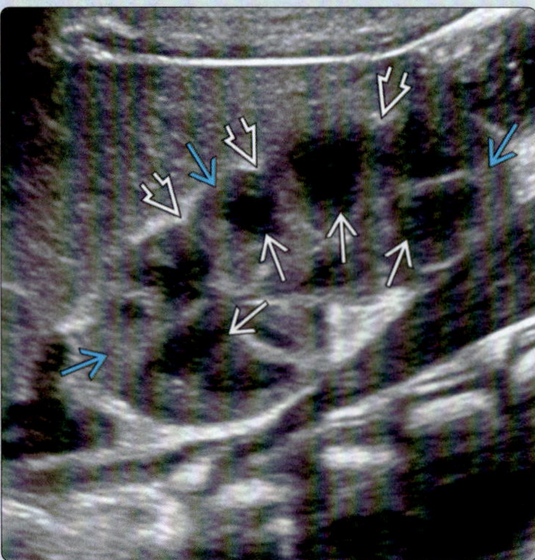

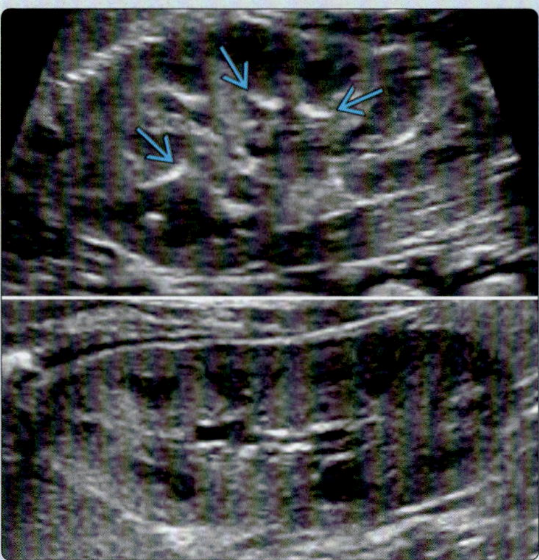

(Left) *Longitudinal US shows a normal right kidney in a 1-day-old girl. In the neonatal period, the medullary pyramids are normally hypoechoic ➡ compared to the renal cortex ➡. Also note the normal fetal lobations ➡.* **(Right)** *Longitudinal US of the left kidney in a neonate on the 1st day of life (top) shows ↑ echogenicity at the tips of multiple renal pyramids ➡. The medullary ↑ echogenicity has resolved on the repeat US 1 month later (bottom).*

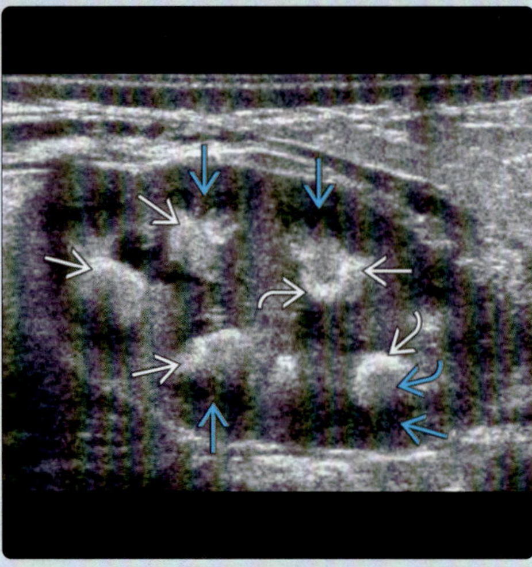

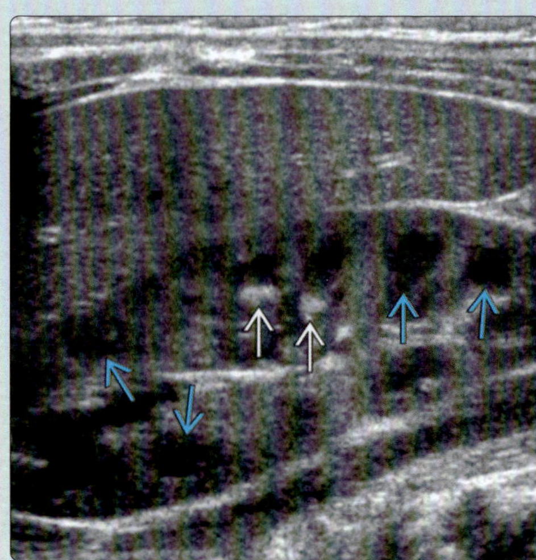

(Left) *Longitudinal US in a newborn shows ↑ echogenicity ➡ in all renal pyramids. Note the extensive involvement of individual pyramids with a gradient of echogenicity that is most pronounced at the tips ➡ & less so in the central portions ➡. Only the bases of the pyramids have a normal hypoechoic appearance ➡.* **(Right)** *Longitudinal US in a newborn shows discrete foci of ↑ echogenicity at the tips of 2 medullary pyramids ➡, while other pyramids have a normal hypoechoic appearance ➡.*

Transient Neonatal Renal Medullary Hyperechogenicity

TERMINOLOGY

Synonyms

- Transient renal medullary hyperechogenicity
  - Descriptive term used in recent literature because etiology is unknown
- Tamm-Horsfall proteinuria (THP)
  - Older term devised because of theory that THP precipitates in renal tubules → transient ↑ echogenicity
  - Theory has not been substantiated

Definitions

- Temporary sonographic appearance of hyperechoic renal medullary pyramids in some normal neonates
- Etiology is unclear (not linked to THP)

IMAGING

General Features

- Best diagnostic clue
  - ↑ echogenicity of medullary pyramids in neonate with normal renal function
    - Neonatal renal medullary pyramids are usually hypoechoic relative to cortex
- Location
  - Bilateral > unilateral
  - Segmental involvement (sparing of some medullary pyramids) > diffuse (involvement of all pyramids)
- Morphology
  - Usually involves tips & central portions of pyramids
  - Typically spares bases of pyramids

Ultrasonographic Findings

- ↑ echogenicity of medullary pyramids
  - Usually involves tips & central portions of pyramids
  - Bases of pyramids typically remain hypoechoic
  - Diffuse involvement of entire medullary pyramid is uncommon
  - Discrete, hyperechoic foci may be seen with denser precipitates
  - May demonstrate layering gradient of ↑ echogenicity, brightest at tip of pyramid
  - Posterior acoustic shadowing is usually absent
- Normal renal cortical echogenicity & size
- ↑ echogenicity of pyramids usually resolves by 10 days
  - Rarely persists several days longer

Imaging Recommendations

- Best imaging tool: US
  - Commonly found incidentally on US performed for other reasons
  - Generally considered normal up to 10 days of life; repeat US is not indicated
  - Another diagnosis should be considered if
    - Hyperechoic pyramids are seen beyond 10-14 days
    - Renal dysfunction is present

DIFFERENTIAL DIAGNOSIS

Medullary Nephrocalcinosis

- Loop diuretics (e.g., furosemide)
- Distal renal tubular acidosis
- Williams syndrome: Supravalvular aortic stenosis & hypercalcemia
- Bartter syndrome: Ion transport channel mutation → ↓ Ca^{2+} resorption & hypercalciuria
- Neonatal primary hyperparathyroidism

Hypernatremic Dehydration

- Seen in some solely breastfed neonates due to poor milk production or inadequate intake
- More common in 2nd week of life

Perinatal Ischemia

- More common in premature infants

Neonatal Renal Vein Thrombus

- Pyramids can be echogenic in acute phase, ± linear echogenic striations of kidney
- Associated renal enlargement & Doppler abnormalities

PATHOLOGY

General Features

- Etiology
  - Classic theory: Reversible precipitation of THP in renal tubules → transient ↑ echogenicity of medullary pyramids seen by US in some neonates
  - Not proven: Some suggest urate crystal deposition may account for transient ↑ echogenicity
  - Resolution by ~ 10th day of life may be due to physiologic ↑ in glomerular filtration

CLINICAL ISSUES

Presentation

- Most common signs/symptoms
  - Asymptomatic
  - Renal insufficiency/failure warrants search for alternative cause of ↑ medullary echogenicity

Demographics

- Age
  - Early neonatal period
  - Full-term infants > premature infants
- Epidemiology
  - Incidence in neonates without renal impairment: 3.9–37%

Natural History & Prognosis

- Should resolve by 10th day of life
  - Rarely seen several days beyond this

Treatment

- None

SELECTED REFERENCES

1. Walawender L et al: Diagnosis and imaging of neonatal UTIs. Pediatr Neonatol. 61(2):195-200, 2020
2. Hemachandar R et al: Transient renal medullary hyperechogenicity in a term neonate. BMJ Case Rep. 2015, 2015
3. Daneman A et al: Renal pyramids: focused sonography of normal and pathologic processes. Radiographics. 30(5):1287-307, 2010
4. Elsaify WM: Neonatal renal vein thrombosis: grey-scale and Doppler ultrasonic features. Abdom Imaging. 34(3):413-8, 2009
5. Khoory BJ et al: Transient hyperechogenicity of the renal medullary pyramids: incidence in the healthy term newborn. Am J Perinatol. 16(9):463-8, 1999

Renal Vein Thrombosis

KEY FACTS

TERMINOLOGY

- Obstruction of renal vein(s) by thrombus

IMAGING

- Ultrasound with Doppler
  - Enlarged, echogenic kidney with ↓ corticomedullary differentiation
  - ± visualization of main renal vein thrombus
  - High-resistance renal arterial waveforms (RI > 0.9)
    - May see complete diastolic flow reversal
- CECT/MR
  - Heterogeneous or delayed renal enhancement
  - ± filling defect in renal vein, ± inferior vena cava extension
- Chronic appearance: Renal atrophy ± Ca^{2+}
- Associated adrenal hemorrhage may be present

TOP DIFFERENTIAL DIAGNOSES

- Acute tubular necrosis
- Pyelonephritis
- Transient neonatal renal medullary hyperechogenicity
- Tumor thrombus

PATHOLOGY

- In neonates, thrombosis begins in small intrarenal veins → proximal extension to main renal vein
  - ↑ renal venous pressure & ↓ arterial flow
- Etiologies: Dehydration, sepsis/infection, iatrogenic

CLINICAL ISSUES

- Most commonly diagnosed in neonatal period
  - Renal dysfunction, hematuria, hypertension (HTN)
  - Classic triad: Palpable flank mass, hematuria, & thrombocytopenia in 13-22%
- Irreversible damage occurs in 70%
  - Up to 20% will have persistent HTN
- Treatment: Supportive, ± anticoagulation, rarely thrombolysis

(Left) *Longitudinal oblique US in a newborn shows an enlarged, hyperechoic right kidney with poorly defined, hypoechoic medullary pyramids in the upper pole ➡. Corticomedullary differentiation is lost in the lower pole ➡.* **(Right)** *Longitudinal US obtained 2 days later in the same patient shows progressive ischemia in the upper pole with a new, large, hypoechoic focus involving the medulla & cortex ➡. A thin rim of echogenic peripheral cortex ➡ remains in this neonate with renal vein thrombosis.*

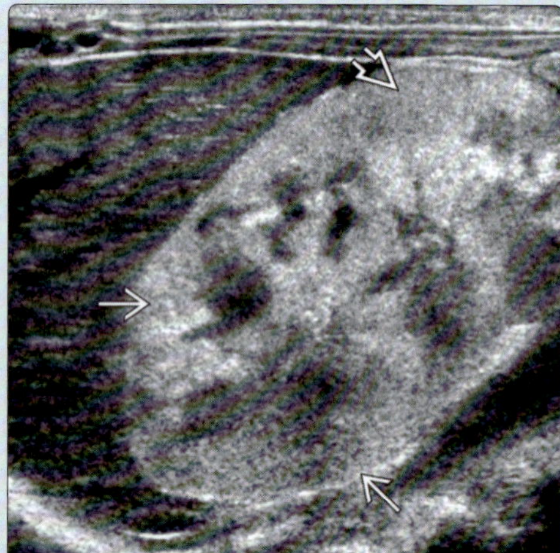

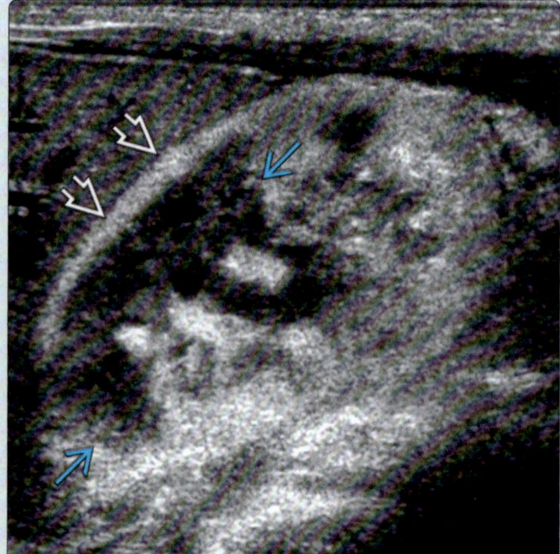

(Left) *Longitudinal US in a newborn with oliguria shows diffusely ↑ echogenicity of the right kidney ➡ with diminished corticomedullary differentiation due to renal vein thrombosis. Scattered echogenic striations ➡ are noted.* **(Right)** *Pulsed Doppler US in the same newborn with renal vein thrombosis shows a high-resistance renal arterial waveform with complete reversal of diastolic flow ➡.*

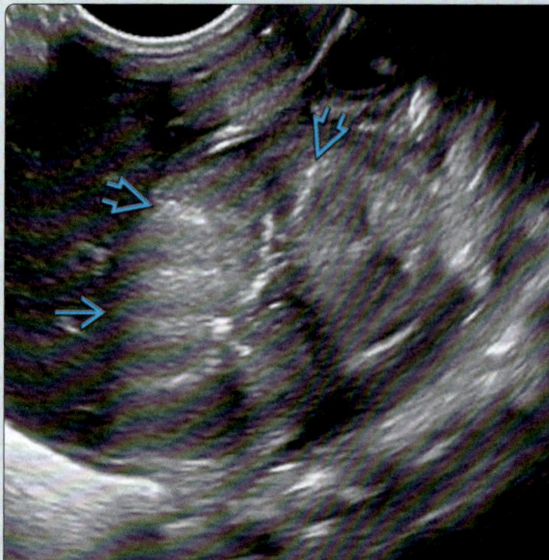

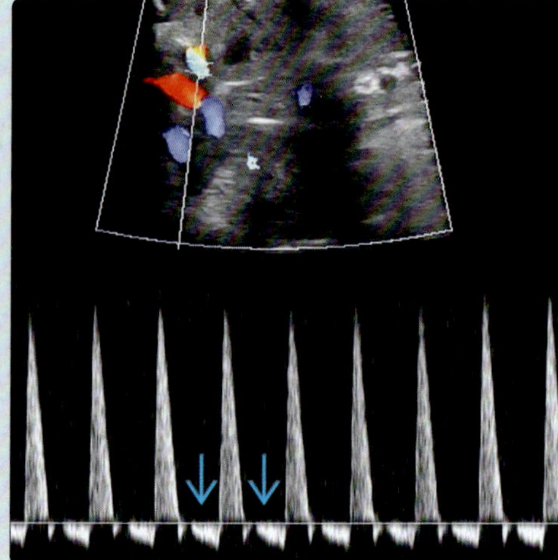

TERMINOLOGY

Definitions

- Obstruction of renal vein(s) by thrombus

IMAGING

General Features

- Best diagnostic clue
  - Enlarged, echogenic kidney with ↓ corticomedullary differentiation
    - Cannot rely on visualization of main renal vein thrombus for diagnosis in neonates
- Location
  - Unilateral (L > R) is more common than bilateral
- Size
  - Enlarged kidney in acute stage
  - Normal size or atrophy in later stages

Ultrasonographic Findings

- Grayscale ultrasound
  - Acute phase
    - Echogenic parenchyma, predominantly cortex
      - May see echogenic striations
    - ↓ corticomedullary differentiation
    - Enlarged kidney(s)
  - Chronic phase
    - Parenchymal Ca^{2+}; renal size may be normal or atrophied
  - Other findings
    - Visualization of thrombus in main renal vein
      - May or may not be identified in neonates
    - Medullary pyramids can be hypo- or hyperechoic
      - Profoundly hypoechoic pyramids → poorer outcome
    - Associated adrenal hemorrhage may be present
- Color Doppler
  - High-resistance renal arterial waveforms (RI > 0.9) or complete reversal of diastolic flow

CT Findings

- CECT
  - Generally not indicated in neonates
  - Enlarged kidney ± perinephric stranding
  - Delayed or heterogeneous nephrogram
  - Low-attenuation thrombus within main renal vein (± inferior vena cava extension); ± collateral vessels if chronic

MR Findings

- T1WI C+
  - Delayed enhancement (most prominent in medullary pyramids)
- MRV
  - Filling defect in main renal vein (also seen on T1/T2)

Imaging Recommendations

- Best imaging tool
  - Renal US with Doppler

DIFFERENTIAL DIAGNOSIS

Acute Tubular Necrosis

- Both kidneys are typically affected; causes include shock, ischemia, infection, hemolytic-uremic syndrome

Pyelonephritis

- Patchy ↓ in perfusion & corticomedullary differentiation

Transient Neonatal Renal Medullary Hyperechogenicity

- Echogenic central renal medullary pyramids
- Normal renal size, cortical echogenicity, & vascularity

Autosomal Recessive Polycystic Kidney Disease

- Markedly enlarged & echogenic kidneys with extensive, fine striations from dilated tubules

Tumor Thrombus

- Clot continuous with renal mass (most commonly Wilms)

PATHOLOGY

General Features

- Etiology
  - In neonates, thrombosis begins in small intrarenal veins → proximal extension to main renal vein
    - ↑ renal venous pressure & ↓ arterial flow
  - Large number of potential causes dehydration, sepsis/infection, iatrogenic

CLINICAL ISSUES

Presentation

- Most common signs/symptoms
  - Renal dysfunction, oliguria, hypertension (HTN)
  - Classic clinical triad of palpable flank mass, hematuria, & thrombocytopenia; complete triad is seen in only 13-22%
  - ± signs of renal dysfunction

Demographics

- Age: Most commonly diagnosed in neonatal period

Natural History & Prognosis

- Irreversible damage occurs in 70%; up to 20% will have persistent HTN

Treatment

- Unilateral: Supportive care ± anticoagulation
- Bilateral &/or inferior vena cava extension: May require thrombolysis

SELECTED REFERENCES

1. Kayemba-Kay's S: Spontaneous neonatal renal vein thrombosis, a known pathology without clear management guidelines: An overview. Int J Pediatr Adolesc Med. 7(1):31-5, 2020
2. Niada F et al: Spontaneous neonatal renal vein thromboses: should we treat them all? A report of five cases and a literature review. Pediatr Neonatol. 59(3):281-7, 2018
3. Kumar R et al: Thrombosis of the abdominal veins in childhood. Front Pediatr. 5:188, 2017
4. Bidadi B et al: Neonatal renal vein thrombosis: role of anticoagulation and thrombolysis–an institutional review. Pediatr Hematol Oncol. 33(1):59-66, 2016
5. Kraft JK et al: Sonography of renal venous thrombosis in neonates and infants: can we predict outcome? Pediatr Radiol. 41(3):299-307, 2011

Renal Artery Stenosis

KEY FACTS

TERMINOLOGY

- Renovascular or renin-mediated hypertension (HTN)
  - Arterial stenosis → ↓ renal parenchymal blood flow → activation of renin-angiotensin system → HTN

IMAGING

- Arterial stenoses may be extrarenal (aorta, main renal artery), intrarenal, or both
  - Intrarenal are more common in children
- Pulsed/spectral Doppler shows abnormal renal arterial waveforms
  - Distal to stenosis: Parvus et tardus, prolonged acceleration index, low resistive index (< 0.5)
  - At stenosis: ↑ peak systolic velocity
  - Evaluate aorta if waveforms are abnormal bilaterally
- CT & MR angiography
  - Focal arterial narrowing ± poststenotic dilation or aneurysm formation
  - Useful to evaluate aorta & main renal arteries; ↓ sensitivity for intrarenal abnormalities
- Digital subtraction angiography (DSA)
  - Most sensitive & specific imaging modality

TOP DIFFERENTIAL DIAGNOSES

- Reflux nephropathy
- Essential HTN
- Pheochromocytoma

PATHOLOGY

- Common cause: Idiopathic developmental arteriopathy
  - Similar to but distinct from fibromuscular dysplasia
- Associations include neurofibromatosis type 1, Williams syndrome, tuberous sclerosis, & Marfan syndrome
- Other causes: Vasculitis, extrinsic compression, iatrogenic

CLINICAL ISSUES

- Severe HTN refractory to multiple medications
- Endovascular or surgical treatment

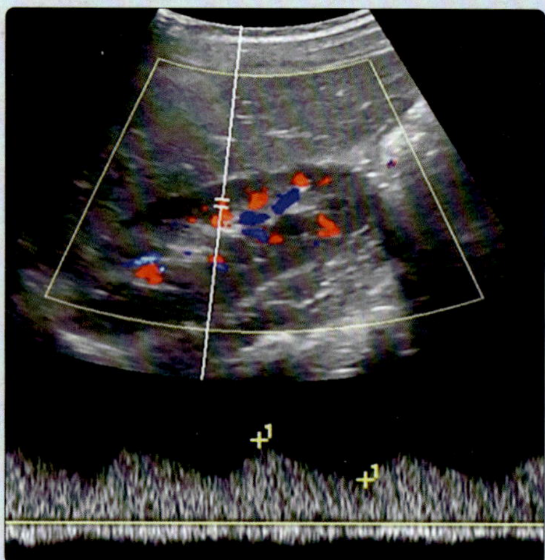

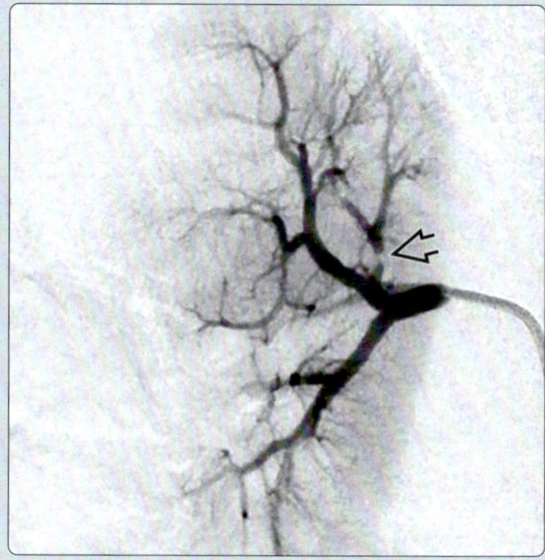

(Left) *Pulsed Doppler ultrasound of the right kidney in a 7-year-old with refractory hypertension (HTN) demonstrates an abnormal, intrarenal arterial waveform with a diminished & delayed arterial upstroke (parvus et tardus) & an abnormally low resistive index (RI = 0.41).* **(Right)** *Anterior oblique digital subtraction angiogram (DSA) of the right kidney in the same patient reveals a tight stenosis of an intrarenal arterial branch ⇨.*

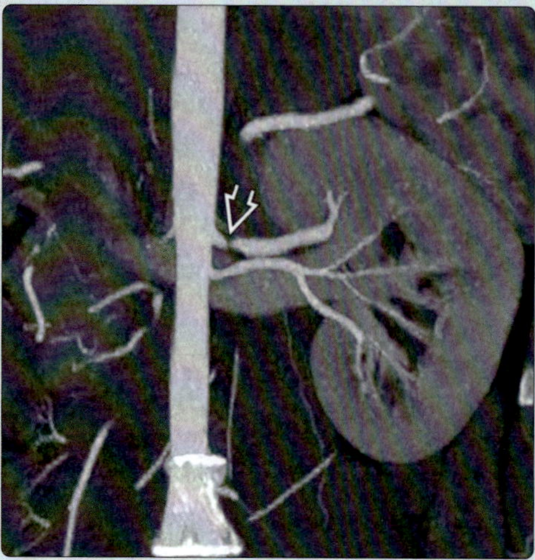

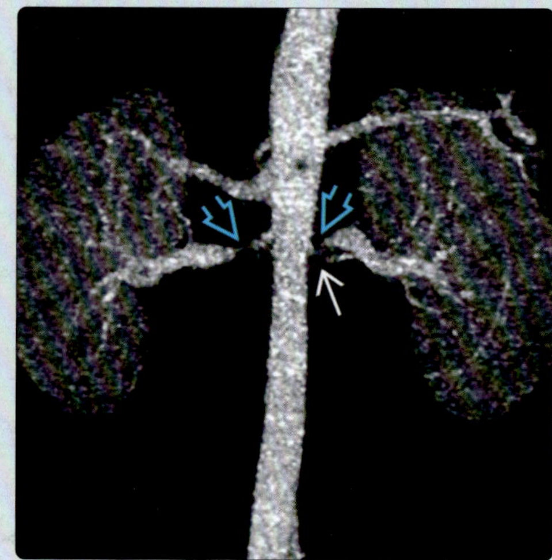

(Left) *Maximum intensity projection CTA in an 8-year-old with severe HTN shows a focal narrowing of a left upper pole accessory renal artery ➡.* **(Right)** *Coronal 3D surface rendering of a CTA in an 11-year-old boy with HTN demonstrates ostial narrowing of both main renal arteries ⇨. There is also a stenosis of an accessory left renal artery ➡.*

KEY FACTS

TERMINOLOGY

- Typical hemolytic uremic syndrome (HUS): Thrombotic microangiopathy occurring after diarrheal illness (hemorrhagic colitis) from Shiga toxin-producing bacteria (classically *Escherichia coli* O157:H7)
  - Clinical triad of hemolytic anemia, thrombocytopenia, & acute renal failure
  - Affected organ systems: Kidneys > CNS (20-50%) > gastrointestinal tract, heart, lungs
- Atypical HUS: Due to dysregulation in alternative complement pathway
  - Diarrhea is less common; higher mortality

IMAGING

- Bowel: Fluid-filled loops with wall thickening
- Kidneys: ↑ renal cortical echogenicity, ↓ vascular perfusion of parenchyma early with high resistance arterial flow; perfusion improves in 2nd-4th weeks
  - Improved diastolic flow precedes urine production
- Brain: Potentially reversible, frequently symmetric lesions
  - Restricted diffusion & T2, FLAIR MR signal abnormalities
    - Deep gray nuclei, deep white matter > cortex, pons
    - Foci of T1 MR shortening due to hemorrhage, necrosis

CLINICAL ISSUES

- 1 in 100,000 children affected annually
- Most patients are 3-5 years of age
- Gastrointestinal illness precedes renal failure by 3-14 days
- With onset of HUS: Fatigue, pallor, ↓ urine output, body/extremity edema, bruising ± seizures, altered mental status, visual disturbances
- Full recovery in 70%; 1-5% mortality
- Long-term sequelae: Renal, neurologic
- Typical HUS treatment: Supportive therapy (including dialysis), packed RBCs; ± plasma exchange; no direct treatments
- Atypical HUS treatment: As above, + C5 antibody eculizumab for terminal complement blockade

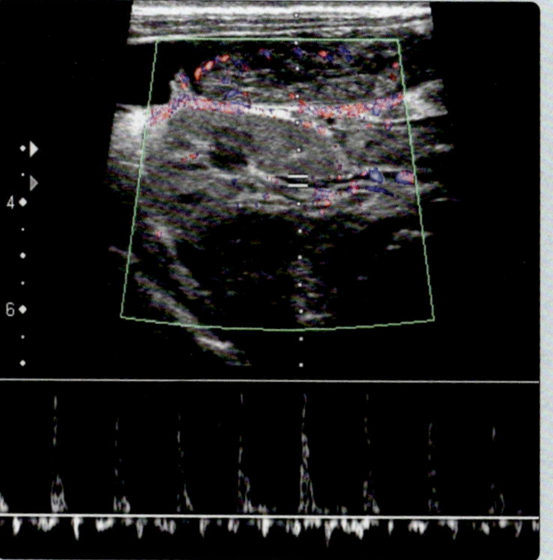

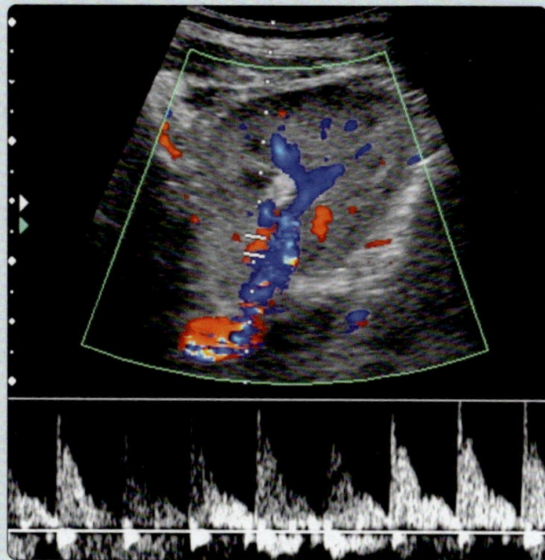

(Left) *Transverse spectral Doppler US in a 15-month-old with vomiting & ↓ urine output shows an echogenic right kidney with complete reversal of diastolic flow in the main renal artery. The left main renal artery showed similar findings. Aortic waveforms were normal.* **(Right)** *Transverse spectral Doppler US in the same patient with HUS 9 days later shows improved flow in the right renal parenchyma with return of diastolic flow in the main renal artery. The patient began producing urine the following day.*

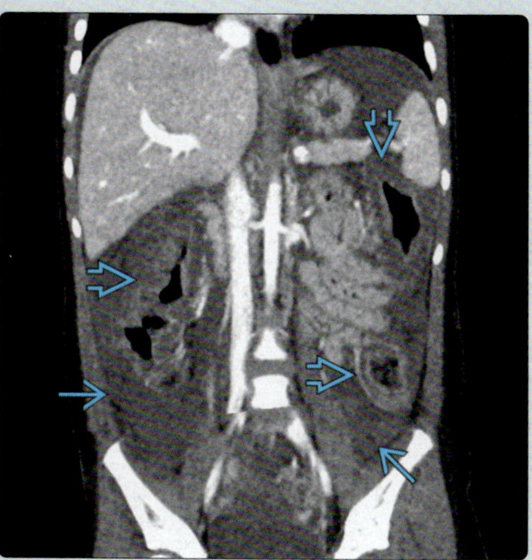

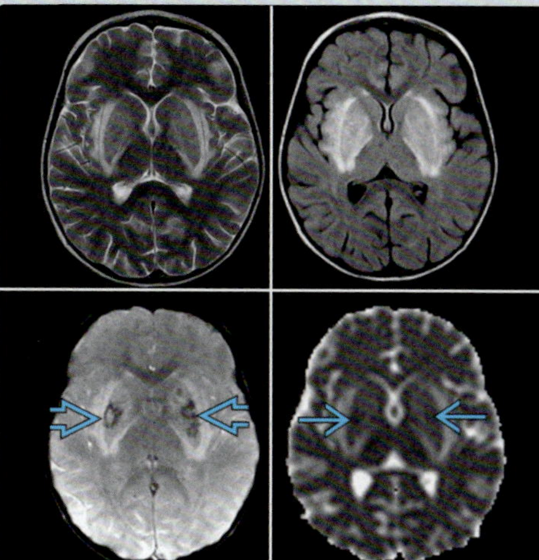

(Left) *Coronal CECT in a 3-year-old with fever & bloody diarrhea (due to Escherichia coli O157:H7) shows diffuse, marked colonic wall thickening ➡ with regions of hyper- & hypoenhancement. There is marked surrounding inflammatory change ➡.* **(Right)** *Axial T2, FLAIR, ADC map, & SWI (clockwise from top left) MR images in the same patient after a seizure show foci of microhemorrhage ➡ & restricted diffusion ➡ in the putamen & globus pallidus, a pattern consistent with HUS. Surrounding edema extends to the insula.*

Neurogenic Bladder

KEY FACTS

TERMINOLOGY

- Bladder dysfunction secondary to neurologic disorder

IMAGING

- Voiding cystourethrogram &/or US
  - Towering, contracted bladder with thickened trabeculations
  - Bladder volume is variable, ranging from small & contracted to large & atonic
  - Involuntary, uninhibited detrusor contractions
  - High filling pressure
    - Results in ↓ rate of filling or spontaneous cessation of contrast infusion
  - Voiding dysfunction: Inhibited micturition reflex
  - ↑ postvoid residual
  - Secondary bladder & upper tract abnormalities
    - Dilated upper tracts: Vesicoureteral reflux, functional obstruction, scarring

PATHOLOGY

- Classification
  - Contractile bladders (hyperreflexive detrusor)
  - Intermediate (mixed) bladders
  - Acontractile bladders (detrusor areflexia)

CLINICAL ISSUES

- Frequency, nocturia, urgency, incontinence
- Urinary tract infection, epididymitis in boys with detrusor-sphincter dyssynergia who are allowed to void
- Upper tract deterioration & chronic renal failure related to ↑ bladder pressure
- Without intervention, 50% show upper urinary tract deterioration in first 5 years of life

(Left) *Frontal voiding cystourethrogram (VCUG) in a teenage girl with a cloacal exstrophy variant & a neurogenic bladder (NGB) who catheterizes 4x/day shows a small, hypertonic bladder with trabeculation & multiple diverticula/pseudodiverticula ➙, the so-called "Christmas tree" bladder. Note the pubic symphysis diastasis ➙ & sacral truncation ➙ of cloacal exstrophy.* **(Right)** *Transverse US of the bladder shows a trabeculated, thickened bladder wall in the same patient with cloacal exstrophy variant.*

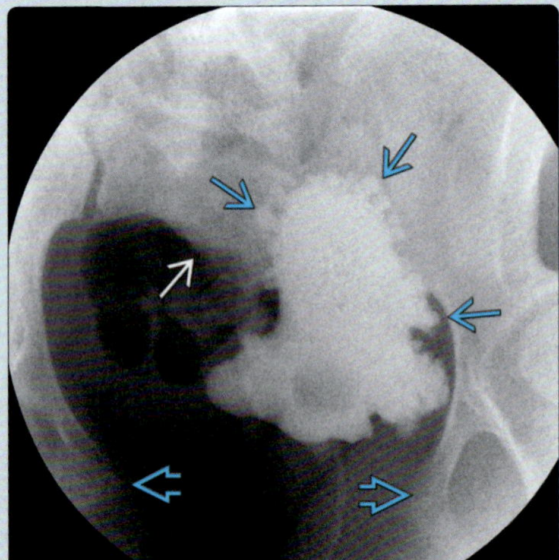

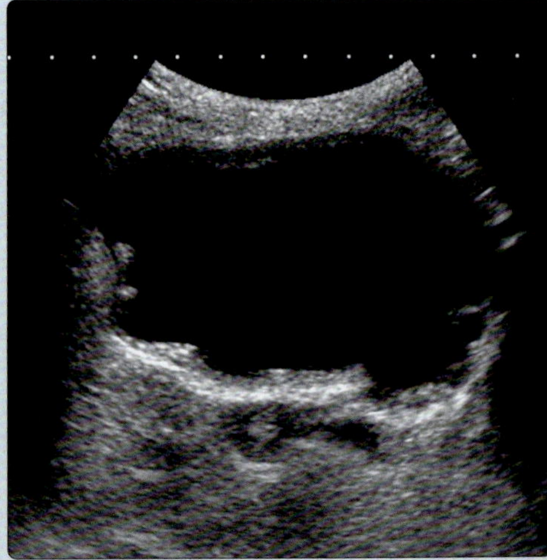

(Left) *Oblique cystogram in a 7-day-old status post myelomeningocele (MMC) repair shows a mildly lobular, large capacity bladder with no wall thickening, an open bladder neck ➙, left vesicoureteral reflux ➙, & no significant bladder emptying due to an atonic detrusor, consistent with NGB. Note the ventriculoperitoneal shunt catheter ➙.* **(Right)** *Transverse US in the same patient after MMC repair shows a large, mildly lobular bladder without significant bladder wall thickening in an atonic-type NGB.*

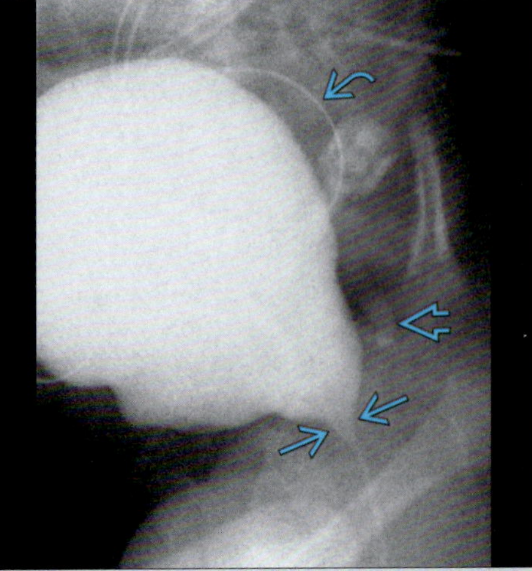

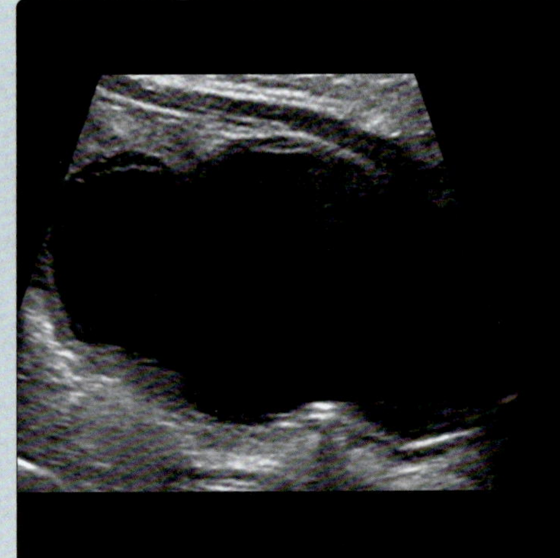

TERMINOLOGY

Definitions

- Neurogenic bladder (NGB): Bladder dysfunction due to neurologic disorder

IMAGING

General Features

- Best diagnostic clue
  - Small, contracted bladder with thickened trabeculations ("Christmas tree" bladder)
  - Vertical, large, smooth, borderline thick atonic bladder
  - Abnormal filling & emptying phases of modified voiding cystourethrogram (VCUG)
- Size
  - Bladder volume is variable; small & contracted to large & atonic
- Morphology
  - Taller than wide, trabeculated, thickened ± diverticula

Radiographic Findings

- Sacral anomalies, spinal dysraphism, pubic symphysis diastasis, scoliosis, obstipation
- Urinary tract calculi
- Can be normal

Fluoroscopic Findings

- VCUG
  - Noncompliant bladder
    - Involuntary, uninhibited detrusor contractions
      - Thickened, trabeculated bladder wall (hypercontractile & intermediate bladders): Grading scale of trabeculations may have clinical implications for altering therapy
    - Serrated mucosa with prominent interureteric ridge (hypercontractile bladder)
    - High filling pressure
    - Results in ↓ rate or spontaneous cessation of contrast infusion
    - Relatively low bladder capacity
    - Leakage around catheter at low volume/high pressure
  - Acontractile bladders (detrusor areflexia)
    - Little, if any, detrusor contraction
    - Relatively high bladder capacity
    - Relatively little bladder thickening
    - Bladder leaks but does not empty spontaneously
      - Large bladder residual, incomplete emptying
  - May or may not sense need to void (inhibited micturition reflex) or have physiologic urination, depending on level of lesion
  - Voiding dysfunction
    - Detrusor-sphincter dyssynergia: Seen with contractile bladders
      - Sudden opening of bladder neck at ↑ pressure
      - Reflexive contraction of external sphincter: Functional obstruction
      - Ejaculatory duct reflux → epididymitis in boys
      - Bulging of posterior urethra
    - Gradual bladder neck opening: Intermediate (mixed) bladders
      - Bladder neck is incompetent but closed on early filling
      - Opens with ↑ volume/pressure
      - Funnel-like appearance: No bulging of posterior urethra
    - Persistent bladder neck opening: Acontractile bladder
      - Incompetent, open throughout filling phase
  - Secondary bladder & upper tract abnormalities
    - Diverticula/pseudodiverticula
    - Vesicoureteral reflux (VUR) in 20-25% cases
    - Dilated upper urinary tracts
    - ↑ postvoid residual
  - Complication of VCUG in NGB
    - Autonomic dysreflexia
      - Life-threatening condition
      - Typically occurs with spinal lesions above T6
      - Sympathetic discharge in response to bladder distention or urethral catheterization
      - Severe paroxysmal hypertension, anxiety, sweating, piloerection, headaches, bradycardia
      - Treatment: Evacuate bladder & catheter, elevate head of table, check blood pressure, pharmacologic intervention if necessary

Ultrasonographic Findings

- Grayscale ultrasound
  - Small contracted/large atonic bladder; ± wall thickening; ↑ postvoid residual
  - Diverticula, pseudodiverticula
  - ± urinary tract dilation, unilateral or bilateral
  - ± VUR or functional obstruction
  - ± renal scarring

Imaging Recommendations

- Best imaging tool
  - Modified VCUG
- Protocol advice
  - VCUG: Follow-up yearly
    - ± videourodynamics (if available)
  - Renal & bladder sonography: Follow-up every 6 months

DIFFERENTIAL DIAGNOSIS

Congenital Bladder Outlet Obstruction

- Including posterior urethral valves, prune belly syndrome, urethral atresia
- Prior to ablation of valves, severity of bladder findings is dependent on VUR
  - ↑ grade of VUR → less severe bladder findings

Pelvic Mass

- ± extrinsic mass or filling defect at bladder base; may lead to degree of obstruction/voiding difficulties
  - Bladder, prostatic, ovarian, or vaginal rhabdomyosarcoma
  - Sacrococcygeal teratoma
  - Neuroblastoma
- No trabeculation; features do not change with voiding

Multiple Diverticula

- Williams syndrome
- Menkes syndrome

- Cutis laxa or Ehlers-Danlos

PATHOLOGY

General Features

- Etiology
  - Myelodysplasia (e.g., myelomeningocele)
  - Sacral agenesis
  - Cerebral palsy
  - Traumatic spinal cord lesions
- Associated abnormalities
  - Anorectal malformations
  - Caudal regression
  - Closed congenital spinal dysraphism
  - Spinal cord tethering

Staging, Grading, & Classification

- Multiple classification schemes
- Type of bladder dysfunction
  - Contractile bladders (hyperreflexive detrusor)
    - Upper motor neuron lesion
    - Uninhibited detrusor contraction, sudden bladder neck opening
    - Detrusor-sphincter dyssynergia → potential epididymitis in boys allowed to void
    - Functional obstruction; deterioration of upper tracts, especially with VUR
  - Intermediate (mixed) bladders
    - Lesions overlap neural pathways
  - Acontractile bladders (detrusor areflexia)
    - Lower motor neuron lesion
    - No detectable detrusor contractions
    - Sphincter weakness incontinence: Leakage of contrast around catheter, especially during coughing
- Bladder function
  - Inability to store urine properly
  - Inability to evacuate urine properly
- Level of neurologic disorder
  - Upper motor neuron lesion
  - Lower motor neuron lesion

CLINICAL ISSUES

Presentation

- Most common signs/symptoms
  - Failure to empty bladder
  - Frequency, nocturia, urgency, retention, incontinence
  - Urinary tract infection (UTI)
  - Bladder stones, hematuria
  - Epididymitis

Natural History & Prognosis

- Complications
  - Pyelonephritis
  - Hydronephrosis
  - Urolithiasis
  - Epididymitis
  - Sexual dysfunction
  - Autonomic dysreflexia
- Upper tract deterioration, UTI, & chronic renal failure are related to ↑ bladder pressure
  - Without bladder management, 50% develop nephropathy in first 5 years of life
  - Predictive indicators for nuclear medicine renal cortex DMSA defects &/or deterioration of renal function vary by study but often include
    - VUR
    - Trabeculations
    - Bladder wall thickness
    - High bladder-filling pressure
    - Detrusor-sphincter dyssynergia
    - Poor bladder compliance
    - High leak point pressure
    - Large postvoid residual volume

Treatment

- Treatment goals
  - Preservation of renal function
  - Avoidance of UTI, epididymitis
  - Achieve appliance-free, social continence
- Therapeutic maneuvers to achieve goals
  - Clean, intermittent catheterization
  - Medications: Antibiotics, anticholinergics, etc.
  - Surgical procedures
    - Operation for continence
    - Bladder augmentation
    - Artificial sphincters
- Hyperreflexia
  - ↑ volume: Cystoplasty, muscular or fascial slings, parasympatholytic drugs, botulinum A toxin
  - ↑ voiding: Catheter, transurethral sphincterotomy
- Hyporeflexia
  - Bladder training, intermittent catheterization, bladder neck resection/denervation, parasympathomimetic drugs

DIAGNOSTIC CHECKLIST

Image Interpretation Pearls

- During VCUG
  - Monitor contrast flow
  - Evaluate bladder contour, degree of trabeculations, sphincter function, bladder filling volume, VUR, & degree of emptying

SELECTED REFERENCES

1. Bagińska J et al: Non-invasive markers in the management of pediatric neurogenic bladder over the last two decades - a review. Adv Med Sci. 66(1):162-9, 2021
2. Selby B et al: Development and validation of a bladder trabeculation grading system in pediatric neurogenic bladder. J Pediatr Urol. 16(3):367-70, 2020
3. Timberlake MD et al: Streamlining risk stratification in infants and young children with spinal dysraphism: vesicoureteral reflux and/or bladder trabeculations outperforms other urodynamic findings for predicting adverse outcomes. J Pediatr Urol. 14(4):319.e1-7, 2018
4. Prakash R et al: Predictors of upper tract damage in pediatric neurogenic bladder. J Pediatr Urol. 13(5):503.e1-7, 2017
5. Sripathi V et al: Management of neurogenic bladder. Indian J Pediatr. 84(7):545-554, 2017
6. Helmy TE et al: Vesicouretral reflux with neuropathic bladder: studying the resolution rate after ileocystoplasty. Urology. 82(2):425-8, 2013
7. Gormley EA: Urologic complications of the neurogenic bladder. Urol Clin North Am. 37(4):601-7, 2010
8. Vidal I et al: Severe bladder dysfunction revealed prenatally or during infancy. J Pediatr Urol. 5(1):3-7, 2009

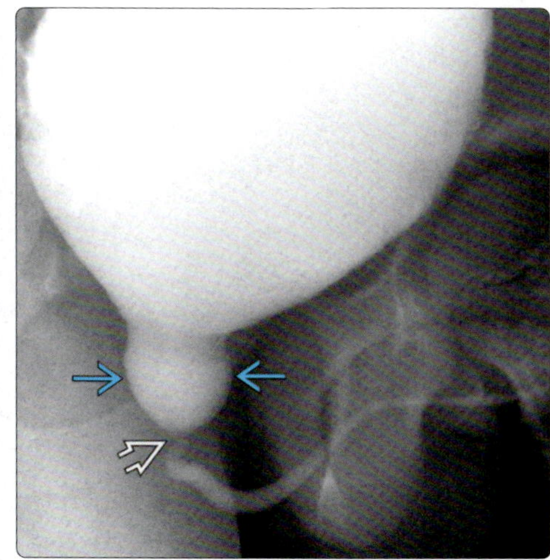

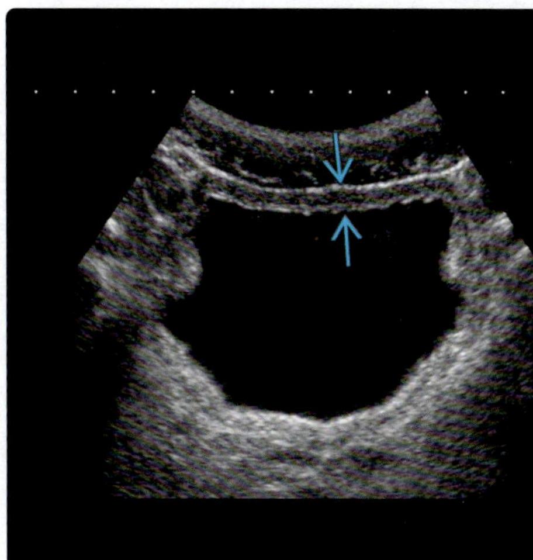

(Left) *Frontal VCUG in an 11-year-old boy with NGB on intermittent catheterization shows a caliber change of the proximal urethra ➡ with dilation of the posterior urethra ➡. Considerations include detrusor-sphincter dyssynergia & catheter-related urethral stricture.* **(Right)** *Transverse US in the same patient with NGB & VCUG findings suggestive of detrusor-sphincter dyssynergia or urethral stricture shows a diffusely thickened bladder wall ➡, which is characteristic of NGB or bladder outlet obstruction.*

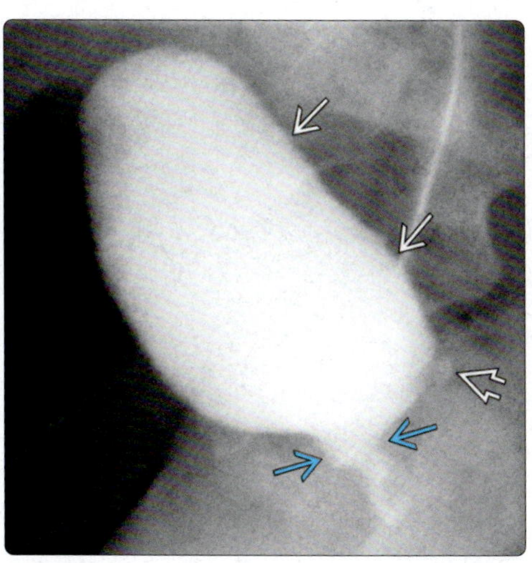

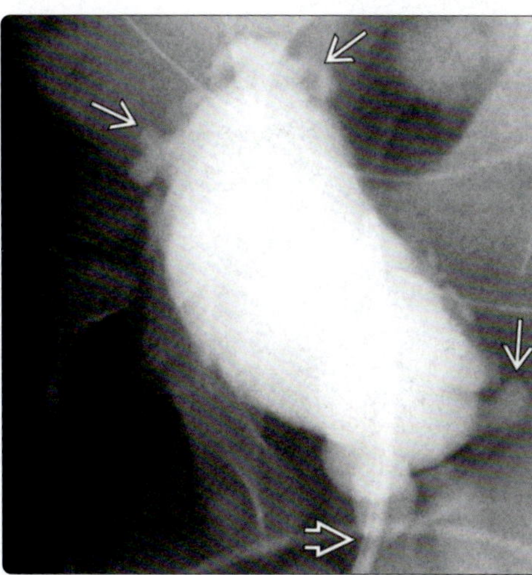

(Left) *Oblique VCUG of an infant with a history of MMC repair shows a towering bladder with wall thickening ➡, a small diverticulum at the bladder base ➡, & a lax bladder neck sphincter ➡.* **(Right)** *Oblique VCUG obtained several years later in the same patient without appropriate follow-up shows the development of additional diverticula ➡. Also note the bulging bladder neck with contracted external sphincter ➡ on this nonvoiding image (due to detrusor-sphincter dyssynergia).*

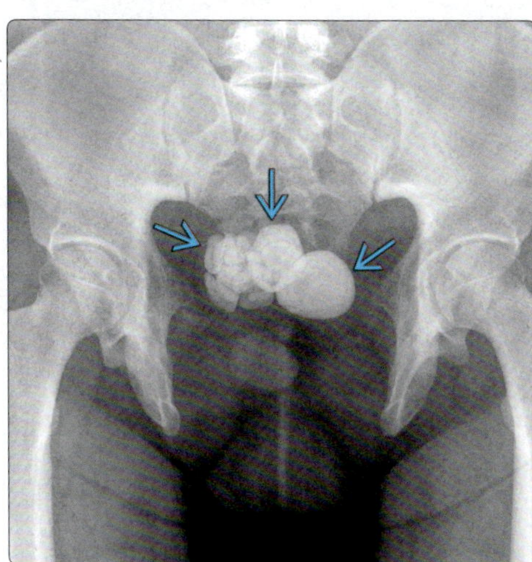

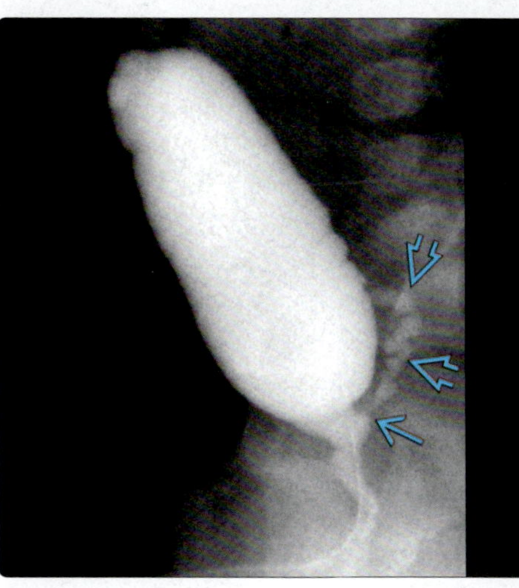

(Left) *AP radiograph in a young adult man with a history of bladder exstrophy (suggested by pubic symphysis diastasis & a normal sacrum) who had bladder augmentation shows multiple variable-sized, lamellated bladder calculi ➡.* **(Right)** *Oblique VCUG in an 8-month-old boy status post anorectal malformation repair shows a tall, trabeculated NGB. During voiding, there is reflux into the left ejaculatory duct ➡ & seminal vesicle ➡, suggesting high posterior urethral pressures & ↑ the risk of left epididymitis.*

Bladder Diverticula

KEY FACTS

TERMINOLOGY

- Herniation of urinary bladder mucosa through bladder detrusor muscle
  - Primary (congenital): Poor muscular backing near ureterovesical junction (UVJ)
    - Periureteral (Hutch): Most common congenital diverticulum (90%)
  - Secondary (acquired)
    - Chronically elevated bladder pressures
    - Weak bladder wall in connective tissue disorders
    - Iatrogenic/traumatic causes (prior surgery/catheter)

IMAGING

- Best diagnostic clues
  - Round, cystic focus directly adjacent to bladder
    - Changes size with bladder filling &/or voiding
    - Anechoic on ultrasound; ± jet of urine into bladder
    - Fills with contrast on voiding cystourethrogram (VCUG)
- Diverticula with narrow neck may be small or absent during bladder filling & only seen with voiding
  - Contrast may remain after bladder emptying
- Vesicoureteral reflux (VUR) in 50%
  - Large diverticulum incorporates & distorts UVJ → VUR
- Without history of neurogenic bladder or bladder outlet obstruction, multiple diverticula should suggest syndromes
  - Williams, Menkes, Ehlers-Danlos, cutis laxa

TOP DIFFERENTIAL DIAGNOSES

- Everting ureterocele, ureteral stump, ovarian/paraovarian cyst, gastrointestinal duplication cyst

CLINICAL ISSUES

- Asymptomatic vs. urinary tract infection, hematuria, voiding dysfunction
- Surgery for complications: Resection of diverticulum ± ureteral reimplantation

(Left) *Transverse color Doppler ultrasound of the urinary bladder shows not only a jet of urine → draining from a diverticulum → but also a jet of urine → emanating from the adjacent ureteral orifice → in this patient with a periureteral (Hutch) diverticulum.* **(Right)** *Oblique fluoroscopic voiding cystourethrogram (VCUG) was performed tangential to the neck → of a moderate to large bladder diverticulum →. A projection demonstrating the neck should be acquired when a diverticulum is encountered.*

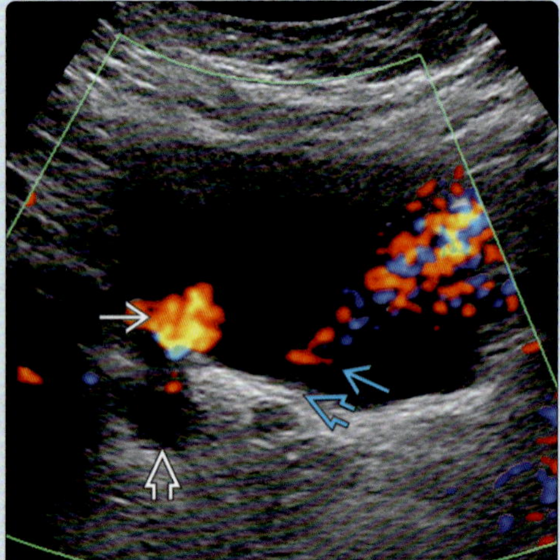

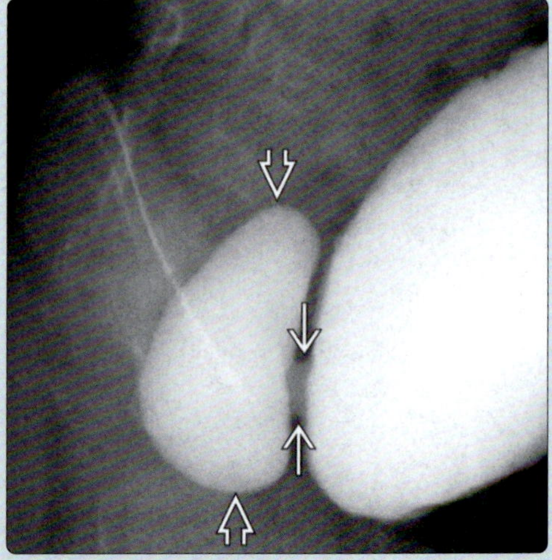

(Left) *Lateral fluoroscopic VCUG shows vesicoureteral reflux (VUR) → accompanying a periureteral diverticulum. Ureter → inserts directly into the diverticulum →, which is important information for the urologist making management decisions.* **(Right)** *Frontal VCUG in a 3.5-year-old with Menkes disease shows multiple moderate to large diverticula → about the bladder, characteristic of this connective tissue (CT) disease. Other CT diseases with this appearance include Williams syndrome, cutis laxa, & Ehlers-Danlos syndrome.*

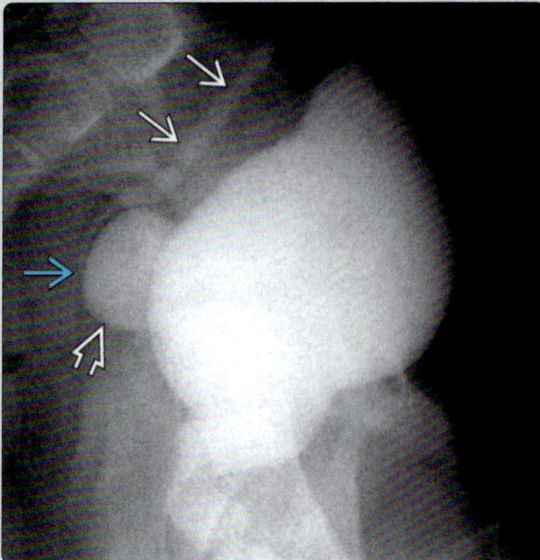

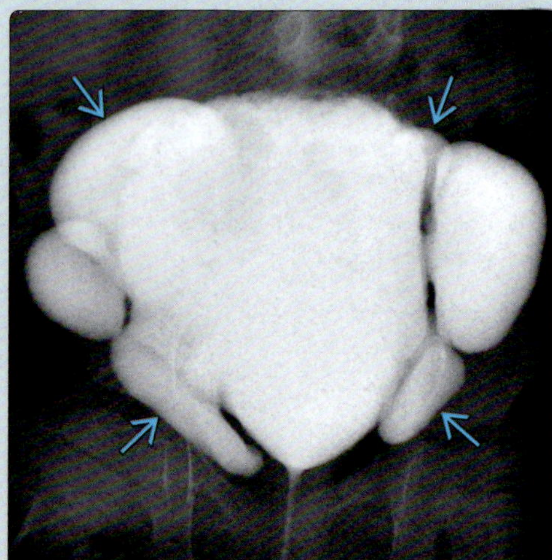

TERMINOLOGY

Definitions

- Herniation of urinary bladder mucosa through bladder detrusor muscle
  - Primary (congenital) due to poor muscular backing near ureterovesical junction (UVJ)
  - Secondary (acquired) due to
    - Chronically elevated bladder pressures
    - Weak bladder wall in various connective tissue disorders
    - Iatrogenic/traumatic causes (prior surgery/catheter)

IMAGING

General Features

- Best diagnostic clue
  - Focal round or ovoid outpouching of urinary bladder
- Location
  - Periureteral (Hutch): Most common primary diverticulum (90%)
  - Nonperiureteral: Usually secondary

Ultrasonographic Findings

- Grayscale ultrasound
  - Normal: Diverticulum may be decompressed & not visible
  - Focal bladder wall thickening adjacent to ureteral orifice
  - Round, anechoic structure adjacent to bladder
    - ± echogenic shadowing calculus
  - Ureteral dilation if ipsilateral vesicoureteral reflux (VUR) is present
- Color Doppler
  - Turbulence within diverticulum
  - Color jet of urine into bladder lumen
    - Especially helpful when communication with bladder is not apparent on grayscale images

Fluoroscopic Findings

- Voiding cystourethrogram
  - Outpouching of contrast at any bladder location
    - Periureteral is most common
    - Oblique images help visualize neck of diverticulum
  - Can enlarge during voiding due to ↑ bladder pressure
  - Contrast persists in diverticulum after bladder emptying
  - VUR in 50%: Larger diverticula predispose to VUR due to UVJ distortion
    - Ureter may appear to insert into diverticulum
    - Diverticula rarely obstruct ureter
  - Urethral obstruction from large diverticulum (uncommon)
  - Multiple diverticula are seen with syndromes
    - Williams, Menkes, cutis laxa, Ehlers-Danlos

Imaging Recommendations

- Protocol advice
  - Bladder sonography including kidneys
    - Scan bladder in full & postvoid states
  - Fluoroscopic VCUG
    - Be sure to image during & after voiding
      - ▫ Diverticulum may only fill during voiding
      - ▫ Document drainage pattern of diverticulum
    - Oblique images help visualize diverticulum neck & site of UVJ relative to diverticulum (if VUR occurs)

DIFFERENTIAL DIAGNOSIS

Everting Ureterocele

- Round, smooth-walled cyst within bladder at UVJ
- Everts near bladder capacity; inverts postvoid
- Duplex kidney ± obstructed upper pole, lower pole VUR

Ureteral Stump

- Often associated with ipsilateral multicystic dysplastic kidney/nephrectomy

Urachal Diverticulum

- Located at bladder dome pointing toward umbilicus

Ovarian or Paraovarian Cyst

- No communication of cyst with bladder
- Ovarian parenchyma/vascularity may surround cyst

Gastrointestinal Duplication Cyst

- Sonographic trilaminar wall may appear similar to bladder
- No communication of cyst with bladder
- Peristalsis strongly suggests duplication cyst

PATHOLOGY

General Features

- Associated abnormalities
  - Williams syndrome
  - Menkes syndrome
  - Cutis laxa
  - Ehlers-Danlos syndrome

CLINICAL ISSUES

Presentation

- Most are found incidentally (asymptomatic)
- Other cases: Urinary tract infection, hematuria, voiding dysfunction, pain

Natural History & Prognosis

- Complications determine need for operative treatment
  - Stagnant urine: Infection, hematuria, calculi
  - Deformed UVJ: VUR or obstruction
  - Urethral obstruction: Uncommon

Treatment

- Conservative: Observation ± chemoprophylaxis
- Surgery: Resection of diverticulum ± ureteral reimplant

SELECTED REFERENCES

1. Chen J et al: Multiple bladder diverticula with Williams-Beuren syndrome: a case report. Transl Pediatr. 9(6):863-6, 2020
2. Saruggia M et al: A rare case of bladder diverticulosis. Clin Imaging. 65:33-6, 2020
3. Marte A et al: Vesicoscopic treatment of symptomatic congenital bladder diverticula in children: a 7-year experience. Eur J Pediatr Surg. 26(3):240-4, 2016
4. Celebi S et al: Current diagnosis and management of primary isolated bladder diverticula in children. J Pediatr Urol. 11(2):61.e1-5, 2015
5. Im YJ et al: Implications of paraureteral diverticulum for the management of vesicoureteral reflux. Int J Urol. 22(9):850-3, 2015
6. Psutka SP et al: Bladder diverticula in children. J Pediatr Urol. 9(2):129-38, 2013

Post-Deflux Procedure Appearance

KEY FACTS

TERMINOLOGY

- Bulking agent injected near ureterovesical junction (UVJ) to prevent vesicoureteral reflux (VUR)
  - Deflux is dextranomer-hyaluronic acid copolymer
    - Biodegradable, does not migrate
  - Other brand agents: Dexell, Macroplastique, etc.
- Deflux procedure
  - Injected submucosally near UVJ
  - Techniques: STING, hydrodistention implantation technique (HIT), double HIT injections
  - Sufficient agent is used to create mass effect
  - Effectively alters angle of intramural ureter
  - Favors detrusor muscle creating effective 1-way valve

IMAGING

- Focal, round mass at UVJ in patient with history of antireflux procedure; uniformly echogenic on US
- Ca^{2+} can be seen months to years after injection
- Follow-up fluoroscopic VCUG or nuclear cystogram weeks to months later to assess change in VUR

TOP DIFFERENTIAL DIAGNOSES

- Urinary tract calculus
- Rhabdomyosarcoma
- Ureterocele
- Fungus ball
- Bladder clot

CLINICAL ISSUES

- Hydroureteronephrosis may be seen transiently following Deflux procedure
- Ultrasound is useful to confirm ureteral jet/patency
- Overall success rates of procedure are high
- Rare complications include obstruction, urosepsis, acute renal failure
- Recovery time is shorter than with open procedures

(Left) *Transverse US through a well-filled urinary bladder shows 2 echogenic mounds at the bladder base. The right mound is rounded ➡, while the left is bilobed ⮌. Both represent Deflux material injected at the ureterovesical junctions (UVJ).* **(Right)** *Voiding cystourethrogram (VCUG) in the same patient following Deflux injections shows expected filling defects at the UVJ on the right ➡ & left ⮌. A VCUG or nuclear cystogram is often performed several weeks after the procedure to confirm successful treatment.*

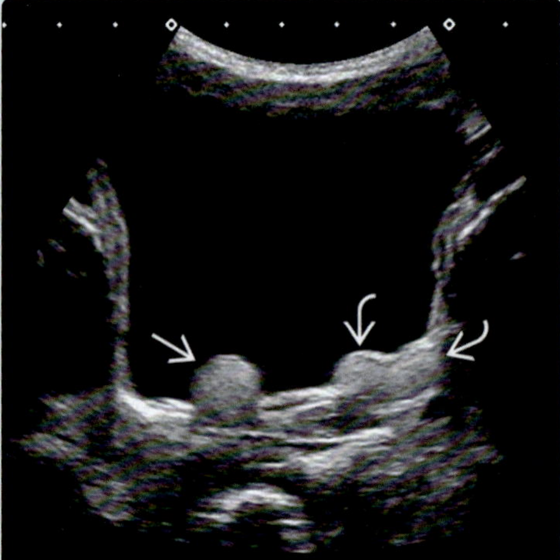

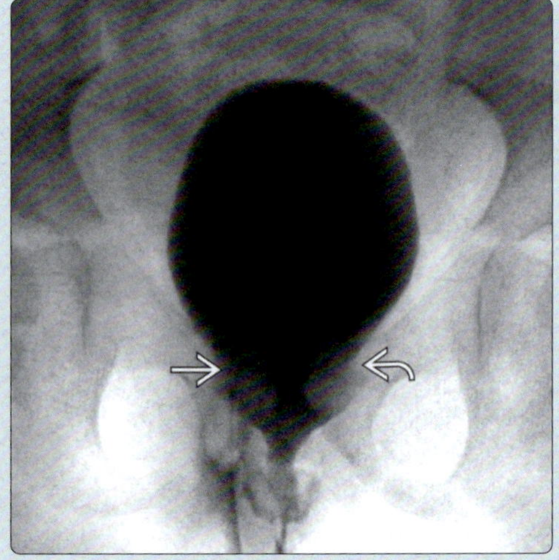

(Left) *Split screen grayscale & color Doppler ultrasounds of a Deflux mound ➡ at the right UVJ, 5 years after injection, show irregular Ca^{2+} with shadowing ⮌ & twinkle artifact ➡.* **(Right)** *KUB radiograph in the same patient shows the irregular Ca^{2+} in the lower right pelvis ➡ that can form months to years after Deflux procedures.*

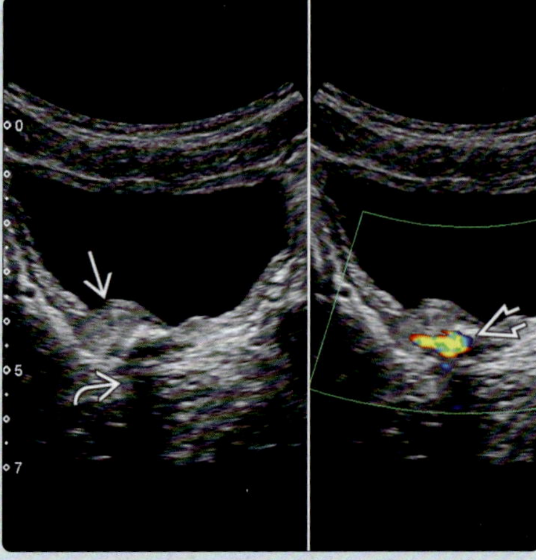

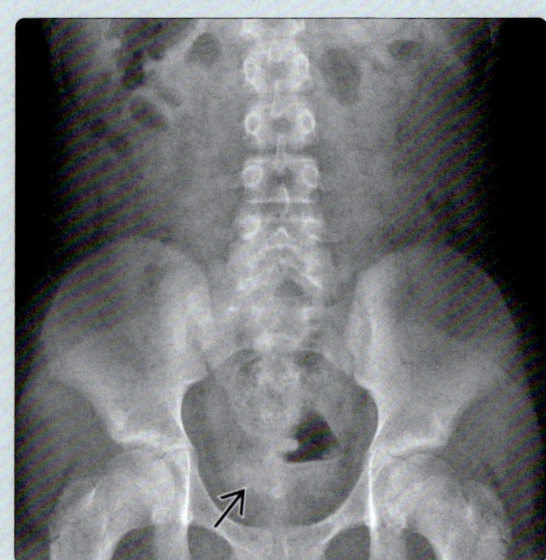

TERMINOLOGY

Definitions

- Bulking agent injected near ureterovesical junction (UVJ) to alter UVJ orientation & prevent vesicoureteral reflux (VUR)
  - Deflux (Q-Med; Uppsala, Sweden): Dextranomer-hyaluronic acid copolymer (DHA, DxHA); most commonly used in USA
    - In use clinically since 1995, FDA approved 2001
    - Relatively large particle size inhibits migration
    - Biodegradable, stable in vivo
  - Dexell (Istem Medical; Ankara, Turkey); most commonly used in Europe
    - Manufactured since 2007
    - Polycationic derivative of Dextran & cross-linked hyaluronic acid
    - Similar size & biologic profile to Deflux
  - Macroplastique (Congentix; Geleen, Netherlands)
    - FDA approved in 2006
    - Polydimethylsiloxane (solid silicone elastomer)
    - Suspended in bioexcretable polyvinylpyrrolidone gel
  - Vantris (Promedon; Cordoba, Argentina)
    - Manufactured since 2005
    - Polyacrylate-polyalcohol copolymer not biodegraded
    - Induces fibrotic response → difficult revision

IMAGING

General Features

- Best diagnostic clue
  - Focal mass at UVJ in patient with history of anti-VUR procedure
- Location
  - Periureteral at UVJ
  - Submucosal location is desired
    - Subureteral transurethral injection: STING technique initially widely used
    - Hydrodistention implantation technique [(HIT) intraluminal submucosal ureteral injection] developed
    - Double HIT (proximal & distal intraluminal submucosal injection) is now most often used
  - Intramuscular & subserosal spread is common
- Size
  - 1-2 mL per ureter
- Morphology
  - Round or ovoid
  - Bilobed appearance is common, may be due to
    - Intramuscular or subserosal spread
    - 2 injections in tandem (double HIT)
  - Can calcify after years: 2% after 4 years

Radiographic Findings

- Dystrophic calcium is occasionally seen in mound

Ultrasonographic Findings

- Round or ovoid
- Homogeneously echogenic
- Posterior shadowing if calcified, mimics UVJ stone
- Avascular on Doppler imaging; twinkle artifact if calcified

Imaging Recommendations

- Best imaging tool
  - Ultrasound encounters these "masses" most often
  - Also seen by VCUG, MR, CT, & possibly radiograph (if calcified)
  - VCUG or nuclear cystogram is performed several weeks following procedure to document success
    - ↓ in grade of VUR, even if not completely resolved, is considered procedural success

DIFFERENTIAL DIAGNOSIS

Urinary Tract Calculus

- Most are smaller, less round, & more uniformly echogenic (with posterior shadowing or twinkle artifact)
- Typically with renal colic history ± hematuria

Rhabdomyosarcoma

- More lobulated & heterogeneous than Deflux mound
- Doppler flow is expected in bladder neoplasm

Ureterocele

- Cystic protrusion of distal ureter into bladder on cross-sectional modalities

Fungus Ball

- Typically in immunocompromised patients
- Mobile & more heterogeneous on imaging

Bladder Clot

- Expect history of hematuria & mobile debris in bladder
- Doppler should not show flow in clot

Inflammatory Myofibroblastic Pseudotumor

- Nonspecific lobulated mass with internal vascularity

Fibrovascular Polyp

- Vascular pedunculated mass

CLINICAL ISSUES

Presentation

- Most common signs/symptoms
  - History of Deflux procedure
- Other signs/symptoms
  - Hydronephrosis & hydroureter is seen transiently 1-6%
  - Ultrasound is useful to confirm ureteral jet/UVJ patency

Natural History & Prognosis

- Success rates
  - ~ 70-80% for VUR grades 2-3
  - ~ 50-60% for VUR grades 4-5
- Reinjection vs. reimplantation if initial injection fails
- Delayed failure rates 15-20%

SELECTED REFERENCES

1. Kirsch AJ et al: Non-animal stabilized hyaluronic acid/dextranomer gel (NASHA/Dx, Deflux) for endoscopic treatment of vesicoureteral reflux: what have we learned over the last 20 years? Urology. ePub, 2021
2. Steinborn M et al: The color Doppler twinkling artifact of implants after endoscopic treatment of vesicoureteral reflux in children: a common finding with high potential for misdiagnosis. J Pediatr Urol. ePub, 2021
3. Friedmacher F et al: Ureteral obstruction after endoscopic treatment of vesicoureteral reflux: does the type of injected bulking agent matter? Curr Urol Rep. 20(9):49, 2019

Rhabdomyosarcoma, Genitourinary

KEY FACTS

TERMINOLOGY

- Malignant tumor of striated muscle originating from any pelvic organ (but paratesticular is discussed separately)

IMAGING

- Best clue: Large, heterogeneous, predominantly solid pelvic mass in child with symptoms of urinary tract obstruction
  - Variable cystic components
  - Botryoid variety resembles "bunch of grapes" with cysts protruding into lumen of vagina or urinary bladder
- May originate from bladder, vagina, cervix, uterus, pelvic side walls, prostate, & paratesticular tissues
  - May also occur in adjacent non-GU soft tissues
- Tumors spread by local extension as well as lymphatic & hematogenous routes, sending metastases to lungs, liver, & bone
  - 15-20% have metastases at diagnosis
- Work-up typically includes
  - US for initial investigation of urinary tract symptoms or palpable mass
  - CECT or MR for further tumor characterization & localization
  - Staging with chest CT & PET

PATHOLOGY

- Small round blue cell tumor of primitive muscle cells
- Major histologic types: Embryonal (majority, especially in GU sites), alveolar, & undifferentiated (adults)
- Bladder & prostate sites are unfavorable, automatically at least stage II

CLINICAL ISSUES

- Peak incidence: 2-6 years old
  - 75% < 5 years old at diagnosis
- Surgery, chemotherapy, & radiation therapy combined
- 5-year survival: Stage I (93%) vs. stage IV (~ 30%)
  - Embryonal type has better prognosis than alveolar

(Left) *AP radiograph of a 6-year-old boy shows displacement of bowel by a soft tissue mass ➡ in the pelvis, initially suspected to be due to urinary retention but not relieved by bladder catheterization.* **(Right)** *Axial CECT in the same patient with urinary retention shows a large, heterogeneously enhancing mass ➡ displacing the urinary bladder (with Foley balloon in place ⤻) anteriorly.*

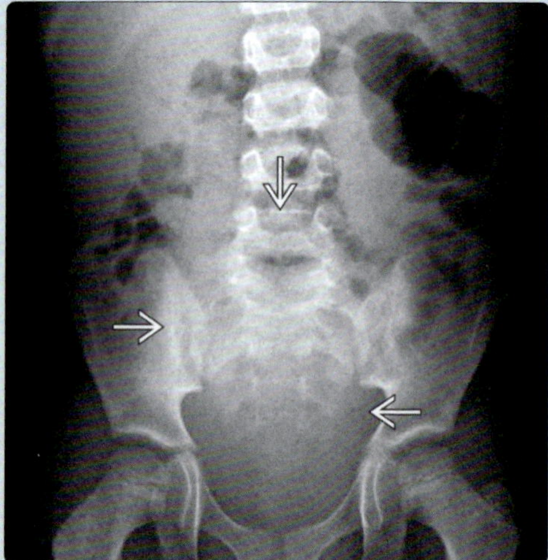

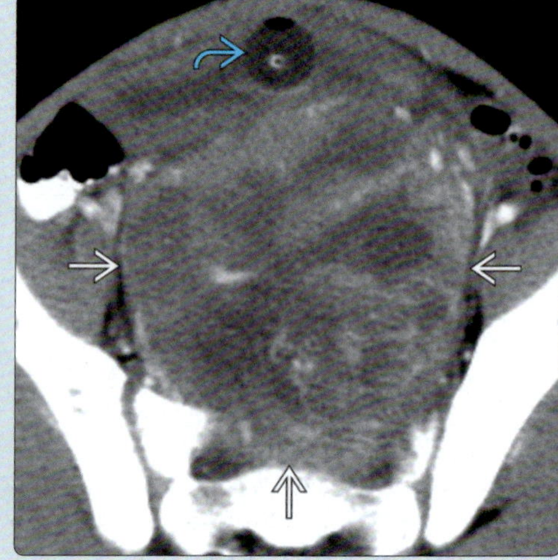

(Left) *Coronal FDG PET/CT in the same patient shows predominantly peripheral uptake in the pelvic tumor ➡ but no evidence of metastatic disease. Biopsy confirmed a rhabdomyosarcoma (RMS) originating from the bladder base/prostate.* **(Right)** *Sagittal T2 FS MR in a 7-year-old boy shows a large, heterogeneous, high signal intensity RMS ➡ arising from the prostate. Note the superior displacement of the bladder ⤻ & the altered course of the catheter ➡.*

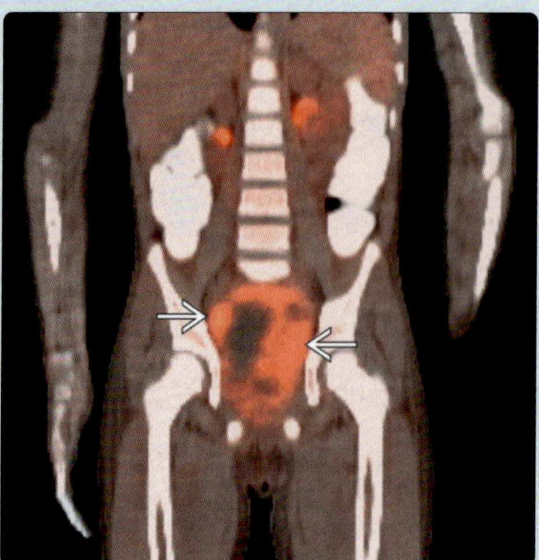

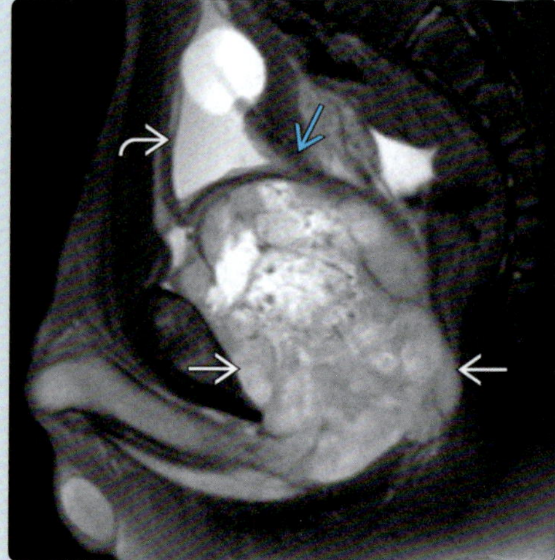

TERMINOLOGY

Abbreviations

- Rhabdomyosarcoma (RMS), genitourinary (GU)

Synonyms

- Botryoid tumor, sarcoma botryoides, embryonal RMS

Definitions

- Malignant tumor of striated muscle originating from any pelvic organ (but paratesticular site is discussed separately)

IMAGING

General Features

- Best diagnostic clue
  - Large, heterogeneous, predominantly solid pelvic mass in child with symptoms of urinary tract obstruction
- Location
  - May originate from urinary bladder, vagina, cervix, uterus, pelvic side walls, prostate, & paratesticular tissues
    - RMS may also occur in adjacent non-GU soft tissues
  - Tumors spread by local extension as well as lymphatic & hematogenous routes, sending metastases to lungs, liver, & bone
- Morphology
  - Heterogeneous, round or lobulated, solid tumor
  - Botryoid variety resembles "bunch of grapes" protruding into lumen of vagina or urinary bladder

Radiographic Findings

- Radiography
  - Soft tissue mass displacing bowel out of pelvis; can mimic distended urinary bladder

Ultrasonographic Findings

- Grayscale ultrasound
  - Round or lobulated tumor distorting &/or extending into urinary bladder
  - Mass is typically large & heterogeneous
    - Most commonly solid with variable cystic components
  - Look for evidence of urinary tract obstruction & adenopathy
- Color Doppler
  - Internal vascularity is variable in degree; presence of internal flow helps confirm solid neoplasm
  - Useful to trace displaced & compressed vessels
  - Vascular invasion is unusual

Fluoroscopic Findings

- Voiding cystourethrogram
  - Distortion of urinary bladder lumen by intrinsic or extrinsic mass
  - Filling defect may be round, lobulated, or irregular

CT Findings

- CECT
  - Heterogeneously enhancing, predominantly solid mass
  - Frequently locally invasive; look for disruption of fat planes
  - Search for adjacent adenopathy
  - Include liver due to frequency of metastatic disease

MR Findings

- Intermediate to low T1, intermediate to high T2 signal intensity
- Variable degrees of enhancement, ranging from mild & heterogeneous to intense & uniform
- DWI
  - Solid portions of tumor typically restrict diffusion
  - DWI ↑ conspicuity of all lymph nodes (normal & pathologic), helping draw attention to mildly enlarged nodes that might otherwise go unnoticed

Nuclear Medicine Findings

- Bone scan
  - Traditionally used for bony metastatic disease
- PET/CT
  - Improves staging with ↑ sensitivity for nodal spread & distant metastases
  - May improve assessment of therapeutic response

Imaging Recommendations

- Best imaging tool
  - US is typically used for initial investigation of urinary tract symptoms or palpable mass
    - Must include inferior bladder & confirm normal position of bladder
  - CECT or MR for further tumor characterization & localization
  - Staging with chest CT & PET

DIFFERENTIAL DIAGNOSIS

Ureterocele

- Cystic protrusion of distal ureter into bladder; ureteral jet &/or continuity with dilated ureter can help confirm

Bladder Hematoma/Debris

- Clinical history of instrumentation, augmentation, trauma, cystitis, or chemotherapy
- Heterogeneous mobile filling defect(s); no Doppler flow

Pelvic Neuroblastoma

- Younger age, Ca^{2+}, & encasement of vessels

Burkitt Lymphoma

- Look for bowel, splenic, & renal involvement

Ovarian Tumor

- Identifying organ of origin may be difficult
- Ovarian malignancies are often larger with higher likelihood of peritoneal spread (nodules, ascites)

Hematometrocolpos

- Markedly distended vagina posterior to bladder
- Look for layering or swirling debris on US
- Blood products are often bright on T1 MR

Sacrococcygeal Teratoma

- Heterogeneous solid &/or cystic presacral mass associated with coccyx
- Most commonly exophytic from perineum in newborn with variable size of internal components

Pelvic Inflammatory Disease/Abscess

- Complex fluid-filled mass with peripheral hyperemia, internal debris
- ± MR T2-hypointense rim; thick, irregular peripheral enhancement; central diffusion restriction of abscess

Other Solid Bladder Mass

- Inflammatory myofibroblastic tumor, plexiform neurofibromas, eosinophilic cystitis

PATHOLOGY

General Features

- Etiology
  - RMS can occur virtually anywhere in body
  - Thought to arise from primitive muscle cells
- Associated abnormalities
  - ↑ incidence of RMS in
    - Neurofibromatosis type 1
    - Li-Fraumeni syndrome
    - Rubinstein-Taybi syndrome
    - Beckwith-Wiedemann syndrome
    - *DICER1* mutation
  - Environmental factors linked to RMS
    - Parental use of marijuana & cocaine
    - In utero radiation exposure
    - Exposure to alkylating agents

Staging, Grading, & Classification

- Based on tumor invasiveness, tumor size, nodal disease, & metastases
  - Stage I* = T1 or T2; T size a or b; nodes N0, N1, or NX; M0
  - Stage II = T1 or T2; T size a; nodes N0 or NX; M0
  - Stage III = T1 or T2; T size a with nodes N1 or T size b with N0, N1, or NX; M0
  - Stage IV = T1 or T2; T size a or b; nodes N0 or N1; & M1
    - *GU site excluding bladder & prostate
      - Bladder & prostate are unfavorable sites, automatically at least stage II
    - T (tumor): T1 = confined to organ of origin; T2 = local extension
    - T size: a ≤ 5 cm diameter; b > 5 cm diameter
    - N (regional nodes): N0 = not clinically involved; N1 = involved; NX = unknown
    - M (metastases): M0 = no distant metastases; M1 = distant metastases

Gross Pathologic & Surgical Features

- Botryoid subtype has cysts of mucosanguineous fluid
  - Can have transparent, gelatinous appearance

Microscopic Features

- Small round blue cell tumor
- Rhabdomyoblasts are hallmark
  - Not always present, especially if poorly differentiated
- Histochemical markers for muscle cells are helpful: Desmin, myoglobin, actin
- Disseminated rhabdomyoblasts in bone marrow mimic leukemia
- 4 major histologic types
  - Embryonal (majority, especially in GU sites)
    - Botryoid variant of embryonal type (5%)
  - Alveolar
  - Undifferentiated (adults)

CLINICAL ISSUES

Presentation

- Most common signs/symptoms
  - Large pelvic mass
  - Urinary symptoms, such as dysuria, hematuria, frequency, urinary retention
  - Pain variably present
- Other signs/symptoms
  - Vaginal discharge/bleeding or constipation

Demographics

- Age
  - Peak incidence: 2-6 years old
  - 75% < 5 years old at diagnosis
  - Paratesticular tumors are more common in adolescents
- Sex
  - M:F = 2-3:1 for GU tumors
  - M = F for head, neck, & extremity tumors
- Epidemiology
  - 250 new cases per year in USA
  - 4.5 cases per million

Natural History & Prognosis

- 5-year survival rates
  - Stage I (93%)
  - Stage II (81%)
  - Stage III (~ 50%)
  - Stage IV (~ 30%)
- Embryonal cell type has better prognosis than alveolar
- RMS of paratesticular tissues & vas deferens have best prognoses
- 15-20% have metastases at diagnosis

Treatment

- Surgery, chemotherapy, & radiation therapy
  - Initial surgery includes wide margins (when possible) & lymph node sampling
  - Pelvic exenteration-type surgeries are now rejected
    - Organ sparing surgery is now performed
    - Gonads are often moved out of radiation field temporarily
  - Secondary cancers in XRT field are not uncommon 10-20 years later

SELECTED REFERENCES

1. Rogers TN et al: Management of rhabdomyosarcoma in pediatric patients. Surg Oncol Clin N Am. 30(2):339-53, 2021
2. Harrison DJ et al: PET with 18F-fluorodeoxyglucose/computed tomography in the management of pediatric sarcoma. PET Clin. 15(3):333-47, 2020
3. Guillerman RP et al: Imaging of DICER1 syndrome. Pediatr Radiol. 49(11):1488-505, 2019
4. Jawad N et al: The clinical and radiologic features of paediatric rhabdomyosarcoma. Pediatr Radiol. 49(11):1516-23, 2019
5. Bueno MT et al: Pediatric imaging in DICER1 syndrome. Pediatr Radiol. 47(10):1292-301, 2017
6. Kim JR et al: Rhabdomyosarcoma in children and adolescents: patterns and risk factors of distant metastasis. AJR Am J Roentgenol. 209(2):409-16, 2017
7. Shelmerdine SC et al: Pearls and pitfalls in diagnosing pediatric urinary bladder masses. Radiographics. 37(6):1872-91, 2017

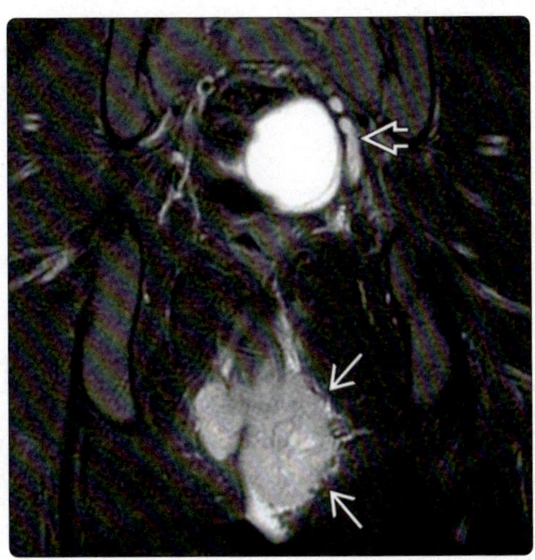

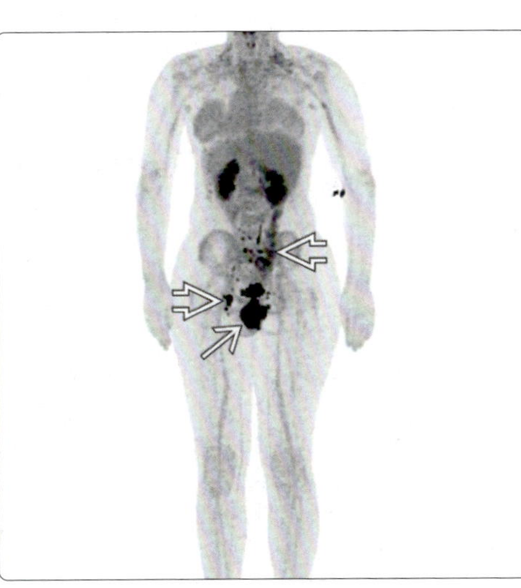

(Left) *Coronal T2 FS MR shows irregular high signal intensity mass in the left labia ➡ of this 15-year-old girl, initially treated as infection. Subsequent biopsy showed RMS. Suspicious left-sided lymph nodes ➡ are seen in the iliac chain.* **(Right)** *Posterior view 3D MIP FDG PET in the same patient shows that the primary tumor is FDG avid ➡ & that FDG-avid lymph nodes are present bilaterally in the groin & pelvis ➡.*

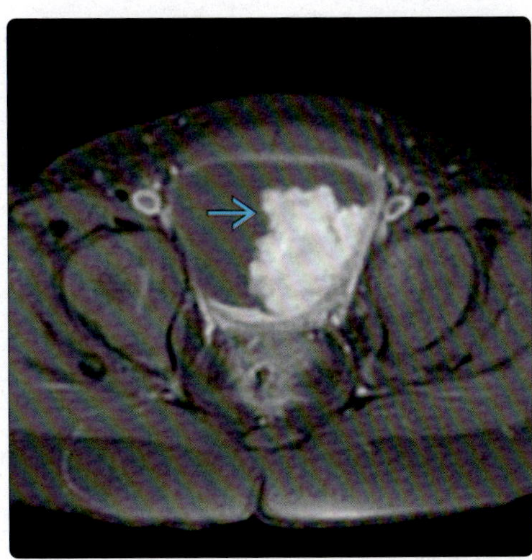

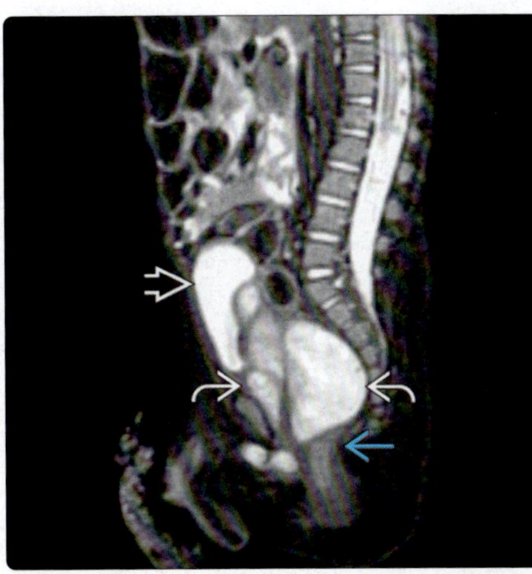

(Left) *Axial T1 C+ FS MR in a 2-year-old with hematuria shows an enhancing, lobulated mass ➡ in the bladder, confirmed as RMS by biopsy. The preceding US (not shown) only visualized the superior components of this mass in a well-distended bladder, but Doppler confirmed its likely neoplastic nature.* **(Right)** *Sagittal STIR MR in a young boy shows a RMS ➡ growing up & out of the pelvis between the urinary bladder ➡ & rectum ➡. The mass likely originated from the prostate or bladder base.*

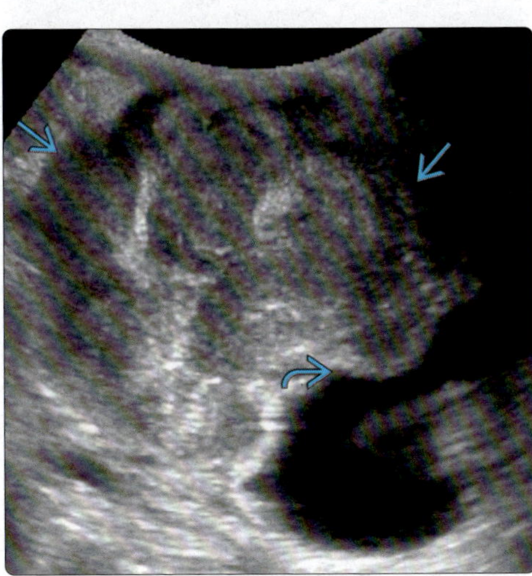

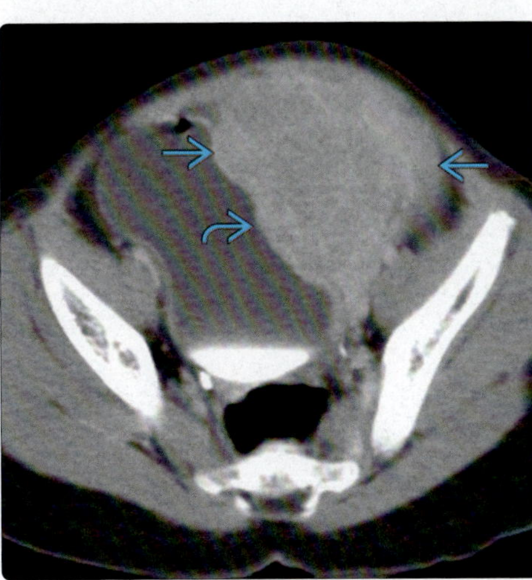

(Left) *Longitudinal US in a 4-year-old girl shows a lobulated, heterogeneous mass ➡ distorting the anterior wall ➡ of the urinary bladder. Vascularity in the mass on color Doppler (not shown) confirmed a solid lesion.* **(Right)** *Axial CECT of the pelvis in the same patient shows the enhancing mass ➡ involving the lateral wall ➡ of the urinary bladder. Biopsy confirmed RMS.*

Neonatal Adrenal Hemorrhage

KEY FACTS

TERMINOLOGY

- Perinatal bleeding into normal adrenal gland
  - Associated with many perinatal stressors: Asphyxia, sepsis, birth trauma, coagulopathies

IMAGING

- R > L; bilateral in 5-10%
- Ultrasound: Echogenic, avascular mass replacing or expanding newborn adrenal gland
  - Appearance varies with timing of imaging
    - Acute: Hemorrhage appears echogenic & mass-like
    - Subacute: Blood products liquefy & contract, creating mixed echotexture mass
    - Chronic: Adrenal resumes normal size, ± Ca^{2+} or cyst
- CT, MR: Nonenhancing ± rim of enhancing adrenal
  - MR may show high T1 signal intensity &/or blooming on GRE, depending on age of blood products
- Radiographs (months to years later): Small unilateral or bilateral adreniform Ca^{2+}

TOP DIFFERENTIAL DIAGNOSES

- Neuroblastoma
- Congenital adrenal hyperplasia
- Extralobar bronchopulmonary sequestration

CLINICAL ISSUES

- Newborns may present with anemia, dropping hematocrit, jaundice, palpable mass, or adrenal insufficiency
  - Medical therapy for adrenal insufficiency is rarely needed

DIAGNOSTIC CHECKLIST

- In neonate: Follow-up ultrasound in 2-3 weeks to confirm expected evolution with ↓ size
  - Alternatively, determine catecholamine levels &/or characterize lesion with MR (to exclude neuroblastoma)
- In older child with incidental radiographic paraspinal Ca^{2+}
  - If morphology & extent are unclear, start with abdominal ultrasound to exclude neuroblastoma

(Left) *Longitudinal ultrasound in a 13-day-old with multiple medical problems shows a large heterogenous collection in the right adrenal ➡ with intermixed isoechoic & hypo- to anechoic regions. The adrenal is almost as large as the right kidney, which is duplicated ➡.* **(Right)** *Transverse color Doppler ultrasound in the same patient shows mass effect from the avascular subacute adrenal hemorrhage flattening the adjacent inferior vena cava (IVC) ➡ at the level of the portal vein & hepatic artery ➡.*

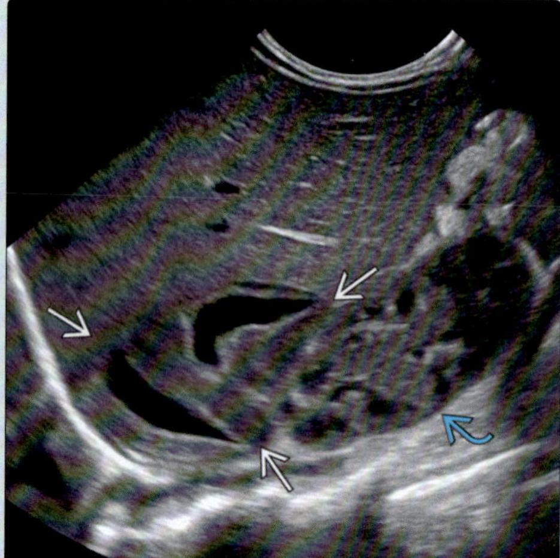

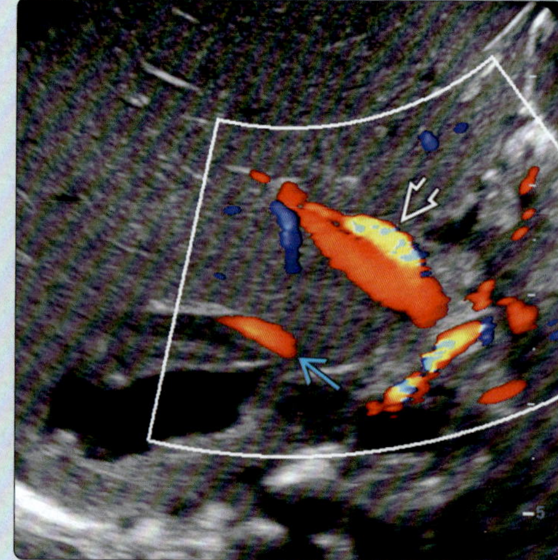

(Left) *Longitudinal oblique power Doppler ultrasound in a neonate with subacute, liquefying adrenal hemorrhage shows an absence of blood flow in the lesion ➡ with normal perfusion of the adjacent kidney & spleen.* **(Right)** *Transverse oblique color Doppler ultrasound performed 2 months later shows partial resorption of the same hematoma ➡ with improved blood flow in the adrenal gland ➡. Mass effect on the left renal upper pole ➡ has resolved.*

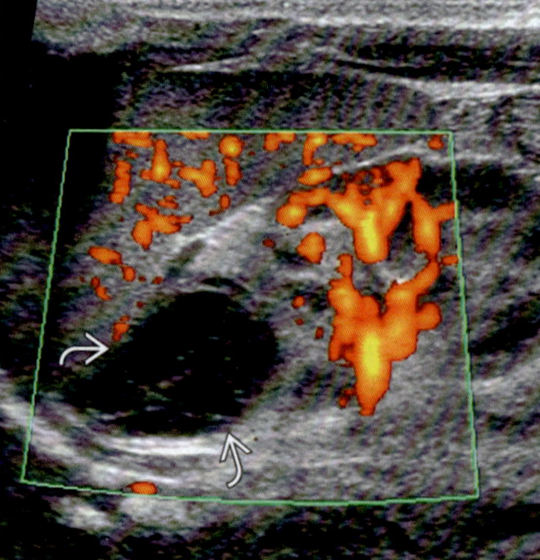

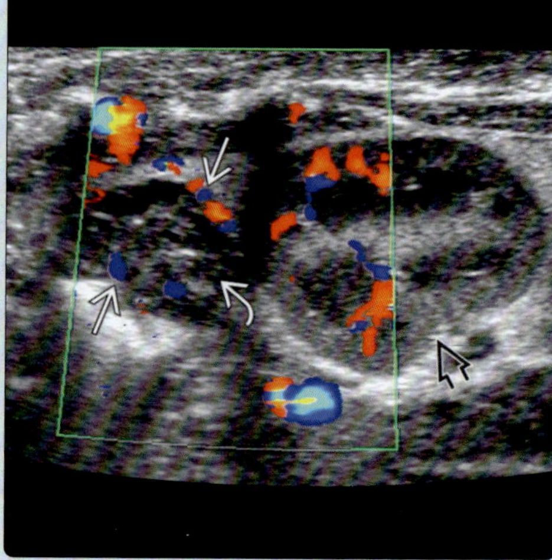

TERMINOLOGY

Synonyms

- Adrenal hemorrhage, adrenal cortical hematoma

Definitions

- Perinatal bleeding into normal adrenal gland
- Associated with many perinatal stressors
  - Asphyxia, sepsis, birth trauma, coagulopathies

IMAGING

General Features

- Best diagnostic clue
  - Heterogeneous, avascular, well-defined mass replacing or expanding newborn adrenal gland
  - Bleeding seldom extends outside of adrenal
    - Case reports of concurrent scrotal hematoma
- Location
  - Suprarenal; R > L; bilateral in 5-10%

Radiographic Findings

- Radiography
  - May see Ca^{2+} months to years after hemorrhage

Ultrasonographic Findings

- Grayscale ultrasound
  - Imaging appearance varies with timing of exam
    - Acute: Hemorrhage appears echogenic & mass-like
      - Acute hemorrhage may be less echogenic in patients on anticoagulants, ECMO, etc.
    - Subacute: Blood products liquefy & contract, creating mixed echotexture mass ± internal septations
    - Chronic: Gland resumes normal size; may calcify
- Color Doppler
  - Avascular hematoma
  - Doppler is useful to assess adjacent renal veins & inferior vena cava (IVC)
    - Renal vein thrombosis is associated with adrenal hemorrhage
      - Causal relationship not established
      - Similar stressors are associated with renal vein thrombosis

CT Findings

- CECT
  - Dense (if acute) or hypodense (if subacute) mass enlarging/splaying/compressing adrenal gland
    - No enhancement of hematoma
    - Residual rim of compressed adrenal enhances
  - May see Ca^{2+} months to years after hemorrhage

MR Findings

- Variable signal intensity depending on age of blood products
  - T1 hyperintensity suggests hemorrhage
  - ± blooming of hemosiderin on GRE
  - Blood products may restrict diffusion
- Enhancing residual adrenal surrounds nonenhancing hematoma

Nuclear Medicine Findings

- MIBG or PET may show photopenic focus in adrenal
- ± nonspecific flattening of ipsilateral renal upper pole

Imaging Recommendations

- Best imaging tool
  - Ultrasound for initial diagnosis & follow-up
  - MR & MIBG are useful if lesion shows internal flow or interval ↑ in size (concerning for neuroblastoma)
    - MR documents characteristic signal intensity of aging blood products
    - MIBG shows lack of uptake
- Protocol advice
  - Doppler ultrasound confirms lack of vascular flow in mass-like hematoma

DIFFERENTIAL DIAGNOSIS

Neuroblastoma

- Most common malignancy in 1st month of life
- More likely to be cystic in neonates than older children
- Ca^{2+} in ~ 85-90% of all neuroblastomas
- May extend beyond adrenal
  - Paraspinal mass crossing midline, invading spine, encasing vessels
  - Distant metastases to liver, bone, skin
- Doppler shows internal tumor vascularity
  - Can have concurrent avascular hemorrhage
- Many cases of spontaneous regression in congenital neuroblastoma

Congenital Adrenal Hyperplasia

- Various enzyme deficiencies → lack of aldosterone & cortisol production → low cortisol triggers pituitary to secrete corticotropin → enlarged adrenal gland
- Bilateral "cerebriform" adrenal enlargement
  - Single limb thickness > 4 mm; length of gland > 20 mm
- Autosomal recessive inheritance
  - 1 in 15,000-20,000 live births
- Females: Present at birth with ambiguous genitalia
- Males: Usually present at 5-14 days of life with severe electrolyte abnormalities

Wolman Disease

- Rare autosomal recessive disorder of lipid metabolism
  - ↓ levels of lysosomal acid lipase → bilateral adrenal Ca^{2+}
- Occurs in infancy; historically fatal in most cases before 1 year of age
- Bone marrow transplant & enzyme replacement have changed prognosis
- Affected infants show signs of lipid storage in most tissues, causing
  - Hepatosplenomegaly
  - Abdominal distention
  - Vomiting
  - Steatorrhea
  - Failure to thrive
- Case reports of isolated fetal ascites in Wolman disease

Extralobar Bronchopulmonary Sequestration

- Congenital anomaly of lung formation
  - No connection to tracheobronchial tree
- May be intra- or subdiaphragmatic above kidney
- Homogeneous solid mass ± systemic vessel feeding

- Cystic components with "hybrid" CPAM lesion

Adrenal Cysts

- Well-defined, round, anechoic, avascular mass
- Associated with Beckwith-Wiedemann syndrome
  - May have hypertrophied adrenal

Lymphatic Malformation

- Multicystic congenital mass crossing soft tissue planes
- May have suprarenal components

PATHOLOGY

General Features

- Etiology
  - Several proposed mechanisms
    - Fetal compression during birth causes ↑ venous pressure & rupture of small venules
      - Does not explain in utero/fetal adrenal hemorrhages
    - Transient hypoxia or hypotension causes hemorrhage
    - Normal involution of fetal cortex & vacuolization ↑ tendency for bleeding
- Genetics
  - Not inherited
- Embryology & anatomy
  - Relative size of neonatal adrenal glands is large compared to adults
    - Fetal adrenal cortex functions in utero to produce corticosteroids
      - Quite thick at birth, creating convex borders
    - Central medullary portion of gland is brightly echogenic in comparison to cortex
    - Fetal cortex & overall size of gland ↓ after birth: Almost inapparent by 6 months

Gross Pathologic & Surgical Features

- Hemorrhage into otherwise normal adrenal
- More common on right side; up to 85% in one study
  - One theoretic risk for greater right-sided incidence: Relatively short right adrenal vein

Microscopic Features

- Ischemic necrosis, supporting theory of involuting fetal cortex as predisposing factor

CLINICAL ISSUES

Presentation

- Most common signs/symptoms
  - Anemia, dropping hematocrit, jaundice, adrenal insufficiency, or palpable mass in perinatal period
- Other signs/symptoms
  - Occasionally discovered incidentally during work-up of
    - Unrelated antenatal hydronephrosis
    - Unrelated abdominal pain in older child
      - Incidental paraspinal Ca^{2+} from remote hemorrhages
- Clinical profile
  - Occurs more often in full-term infants
  - Macrosomic, large for gestational age (LGA) babies
  - Perinatal asphyxia

Demographics

- Age
  - Newborn infants
- Epidemiology
  - 1-2 per 1,000 births

Natural History & Prognosis

- Blood products gradually retract & liquefy
- Cysts or dystrophic Ca^{2+} may develop
- Adrenal function is typically preserved
  - Especially in unilateral cases
- Involutes/resorbs in weeks to months
- Prognosis is excellent

Treatment

- Observation in most cases
- Adrenal insufficiency is extremely rare, requires damage to > 90% of adrenal tissue
  - Medical therapy may be required transiently
    - Exogenous steroid support of hypotension
- Case reports of adrenal abscess formation

DIAGNOSTIC CHECKLIST

Image Interpretation Pearls

- Localized avascular suprarenal mass in neonate
  - Follow-up ultrasound in 2-3 weeks to confirm liquefaction & smaller size, **or**
  - Correlate with catecholamines, **or**
  - Evaluate with MR for solid mass (neuroblastoma)
- Incidental radiographic detection of paraspinal adrenal Ca^{2+} in older child
  - If clearly adreniform & not crossing midline, no further work-up required
  - If morphology & extent unclear, start with abdominal ultrasound to exclude neuroblastoma

SELECTED REFERENCES

1. Birkemeier KL: Imaging of solid congenital abdominal masses: a review of the literature and practical approach to image interpretation. Pediatr Radiol. 50(13):1907-20, 2020
2. Schwab ME et al: Imaging modalities and management of prenatally diagnosed suprarenal masses: an updated literature review and the experience at a high volume Fetal Treatment Center. J Matern Fetal Neonatal Med. 1-8, 2020
3. Tognato E et al: Neonatal adrenal hemorrhage: a case series. Am J Perinatol. 37(S 02):S57-60, 2020
4. Alonso V et al: Conservative management of scrotal hematoma secondary to adrenal hemorrhage in newborns. Urology. 133:e1-2, 2019
5. Angelis D et al: Neonatal adrenal findings: significance and diagnostic approach. Description of two cases. Clin Case Rep. 6(4):658-63, 2018
6. Wang L et al: Clinical value of serial ultrasonography in the dynamic observation of foetal cystic adrenal lesions. Prenat Diagn. 38(11):829-34, 2018
7. Zessis NR et al: Severe bilateral adrenal hemorrhages in a newborn complicated by persistent adrenal insufficiency. Endocrinol Diabetes Metab Case Rep. 2018:17-0165, 2018
8. Bhatt S et al: Neonatal adrenal hemorrhage presenting as "acute scrotum"-looking beyond the obvious: a sonographic insight. J Ultrasound. 20(3):253-9, 2017
9. Mandelia A et al: Non-surgical management of bilateral adrenal abscess in neonates: report of two cases. J Neonatal Surg. 6(2):31, 2017
10. Gyurkovits Z et al: Adrenal haemorrhage in term neonates: a retrospective study from the period 2001-2013. J Matern Fetal Neonatal Med. 1-4, 2014
11. Lai LJ et al: Neonatal adrenal hemorrhage associated with scrotal hematoma: an unusual case report and literature review. Pediatr Neonatol. 53(3):210-2, 2012

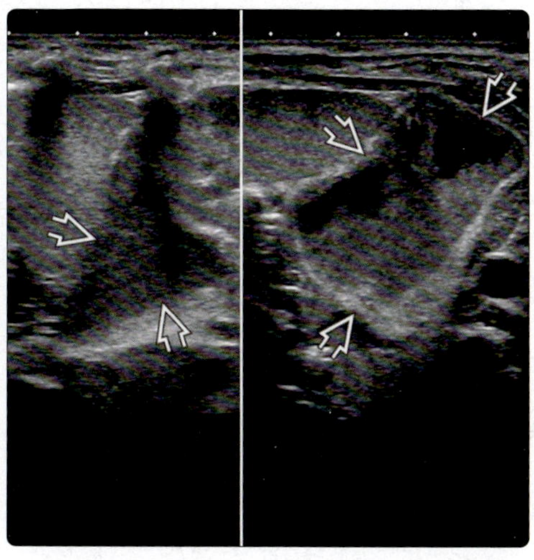

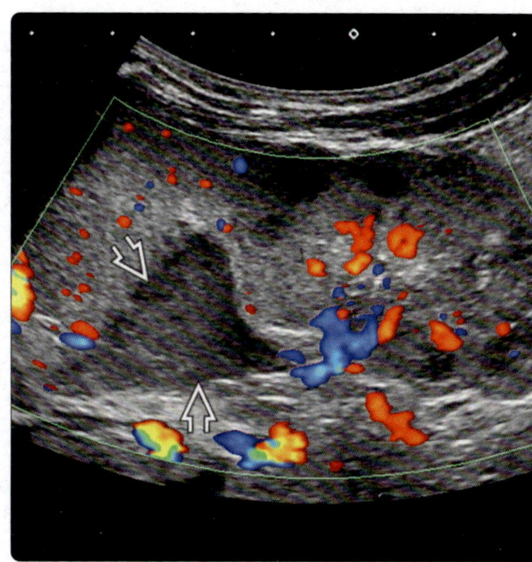

(Left) *Longitudinal (left) & transverse (right) ultrasound images of the left suprarenal region in a 9-day-old infant with congenital heart disease show a mixed-echogenicity lesion ➡ with well-defined margins between the spleen & kidney.* **(Right)** *Color Doppler ultrasound in the same patient shows an absence of blood flow in the lesion ➡, typical of adrenal hemorrhage.*

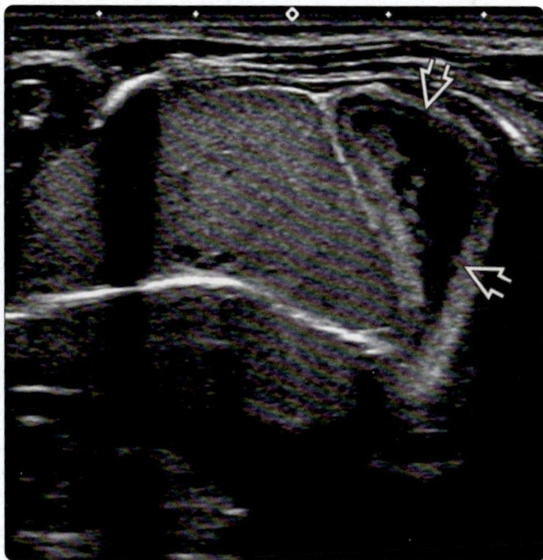

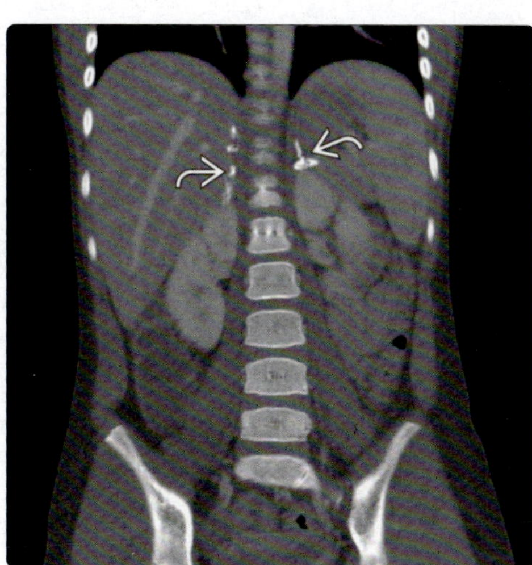

(Left) *Transverse ultrasound of the same lesion 1 week later shows progressive liquefaction ➡, consistent with evolving hemorrhage & confirming the benign nature of the "mass."* **(Right)** *Coronal CECT in an elementary school-aged patient (who had been a premature infant) shows adreniform Ca^{2+} bilaterally ➡, likely due to remote neonatal adrenal hemorrhages.*

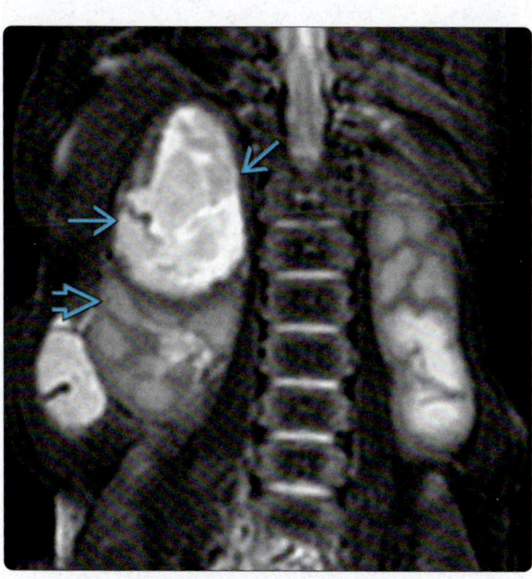

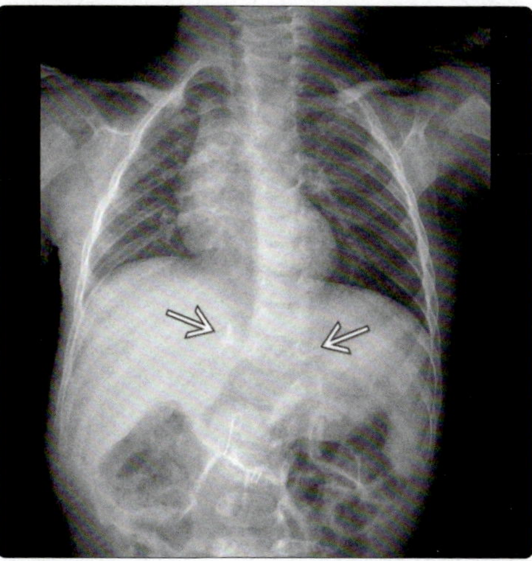

(Left) *Coronal T2 FS MR in a 20-day-old with left prenatal hydronephrosis shows a heterogeneous right suprarenal mass ➡ deforming the right kidney ➡. The mass was T1 bright with a few foci blooming on GRE (not shown). Serial ultrasound images showed progressive ↓ in size of the mass over the next 5 weeks.* **(Right)** *AP chest radiograph in a 3-year-old with cerebral palsy shows bilateral adrenal Ca^{2+} ➡, the long-term sequela of neonatal hemorrhages due to neonatal stresses.*

Congenital Adrenal Hyperplasia

KEY FACTS

TERMINOLOGY

- Congenital adrenal hyperplasia (CAH): Inherited disorder of cortisol (± aldosterone) biosynthesis, which leads to hypertrophy of adrenal glands & excess androgen production
- Classic & nonclassic CAH, based on presentation
  - Classic: Presents as neonate with salt-wasting or virilization
  - Nonclassic: Presents as child with premature puberty or findings related to androgen production

IMAGING

- Adrenal glands
  - Bilateral enlargement with cerebriform morphology
- Females
  - Ambiguous genitalia in neonates
    - US is used to identify normal female uterus
      - Excess androgen stimulation may make ovaries small & difficult to find on US
  - Polycystic appearance of ovaries in nonclassic CAH
- Males
  - Testicular adrenal rests occur in ~ 95% of adult males with CAH
    - Hypoechoic mass in each testis with ↑ vascularity, often adjacent to mediastinum testis

PATHOLOGY

- Caused by deficiency in 1 of 5 enzymes required to synthesize cortisol from cholesterol in adrenal cortex
  - 21-hydroxylase deficiency is most common

CLINICAL ISSUES

- Most common cause of ambiguous genitalia in females
- Males with classic CAH usually present at 5-14 days of life with acute salt-wasting crisis
- Neonatal screening panels test for severe forms of CAH
- Treated with lifelong glucocorticoids to replace cortisol & suppress androgen production

(Left) *Photograph of the perineum shows ambiguous genitalia in a genetic female (XX) with congenital adrenal hyperplasia (CAH). There is clitoromegaly & masculinization of the labioscrotal folds.* **(Right)** *Longitudinal oblique US shows a very enlarged adrenal gland with a characteristic wrinkled or cerebriform appearance ➙. The adrenal gland has lost its normal adreniform shape but maintains corticomedullary distinction.*

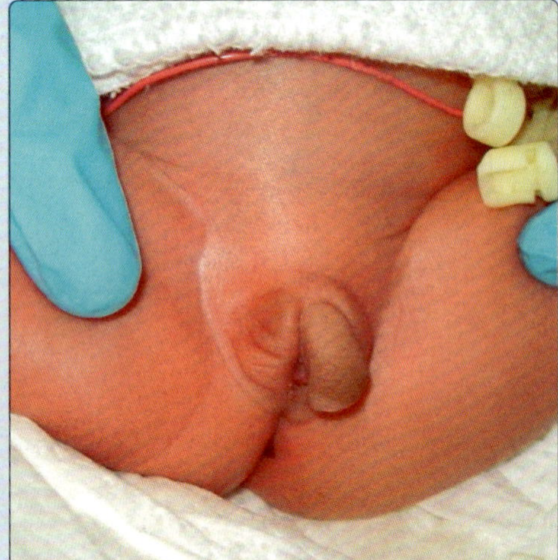

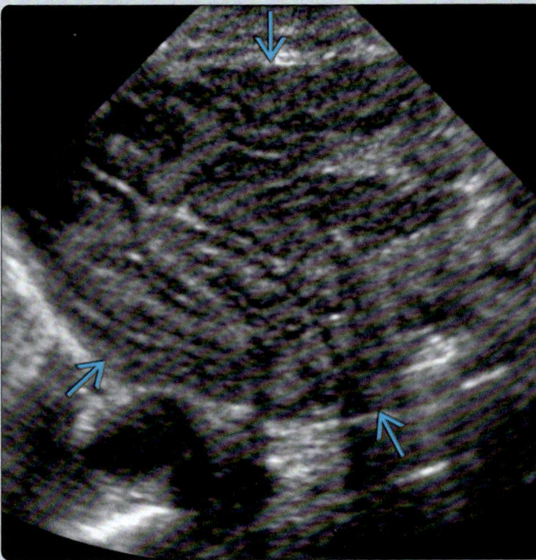

(Left) *Transverse US of the scrotum in a patient with CAH shows round masses in both testes, consistent with congenital testicular adrenal rests. The lesion in the right testis ➙ is smaller & more uniformly hypoechoic compared to the lesion in the left testis ➙.* **(Right)** *Transverse color Doppler US of the testes in the same patient shows hyperemia of the testicular adrenal rests ➙, a typical finding in CAH. The vessels are not distorted as they pass through the lesions (as would be expected with testicular neoplasms).*

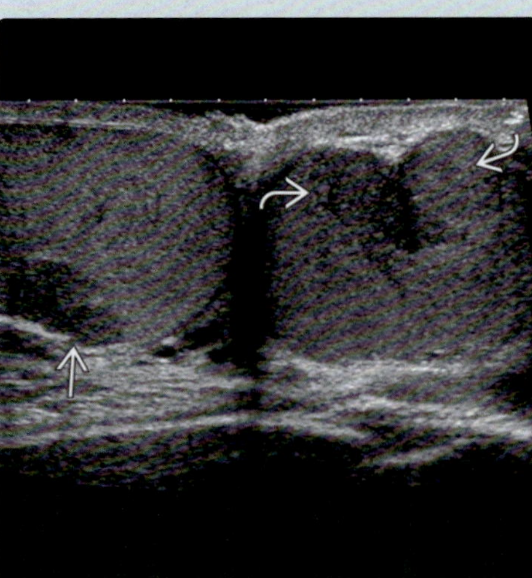

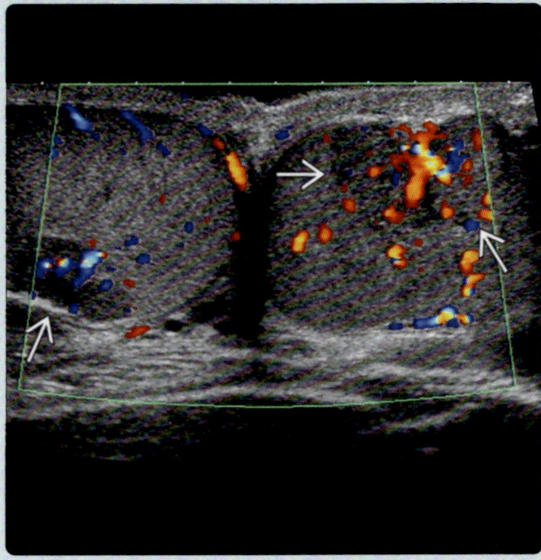

TERMINOLOGY

Abbreviations

- Congenital adrenal hyperplasia (CAH), 21-hydroxylase deficiency (21-OHD)

Definitions

- Inherited disorder of cortisol (± aldosterone) biosynthesis, which leads to hypertrophy of adrenal glands
- 2 types of CAH: Classic & nonclassic based on presentation
  - Classic CAH: Presents as neonate with salt-wasting or virilization
  - Nonclassic CAH: Presents as child with premature puberty or in adolescence/adulthood with hirsutism, irregular menses, chronic anovulation, acne, or infertility
- Classification of classic & nonclassic is artificial as disease severity is continuum determined by enzyme activity

IMAGING

General Features

- Best diagnostic clue
  - Enlarged, wrinkled appearance of adrenal glands in neonate with ambiguous genitalia
- Morphology
  - Markedly enlarged adrenal glands folded back upon themselves, giving characteristic wrinkled or cerebriform appearance

Ultrasonographic Findings

- Adrenal glands
  - Diffuse enlargement of both adrenal glands with wrinkled, cerebriform appearance
    - Single limb of adrenal gland ≥ 4 mm
    - Cerebriform appearance is caused by hypertrophied adrenal gland folding back upon itself
      - Hypoechoic cortex & hyperechoic medulla are usually maintained
      - Creates appearance similar to cerebral gyri & sulci
  - Left adrenal gland is usually larger than right
    - Potential space for right adrenal gland is smaller due to liver
  - Normal adrenal glands do not exclude CAH
  - Adrenal myelolipomas may develop in adults with CAH who have poor adherence to medical therapy
- Female reproductive organs
  - Neonatal findings
    - Classic CAH presents with ambiguous genitalia
      - Potential findings: Enlarged clitoris, partly fused labia majora with rugae, common urogenital sinus, & development of male urethra
    - US is used to identify normal female uterus
      - Excess androgen stimulation may make ovaries small & difficult to find on US
      - Hydrocolpos or hydrometrocolpos may be present
    - US confirms absence of testes in masculinized labioscrotal folds
      - Undescended testes may be present in genetic females
  - Postpubertal findings
    - Ovaries may be enlarged with polycystic appearance
    - ± ovarian adrenal rest tumors appearing as small, hypoechoic nodules
- Male reproductive organs
  - Neonatal findings
    - Normal appearance of testes at birth
    - Hyperpigmented scrotum
  - Postpubertal findings
    - Testicular adrenal rests occur in ~ 95% of adolescent & adult males with CAH
      - Ovoid hypoechoic foci within each testis; often adjacent to mediastinum testis
      - Often bilateral
      - Variable echogenicity
      - ↑ vascularity on color Doppler

Radiographic Findings

- If untreated or undertreated, can have advanced bone age

Fluoroscopic Findings

- Voiding cystourethrogram
  - High prevalence of upper tract genitourinary malformations in girls, including vesicoureteral reflux, hydronephrosis, & duplex collecting systems
- Genitography can be performed with ambiguous genitalia
  - Females with CAH & ambiguous genitalia may have common urogenital sinus
  - Genitography shows urethra, external sphincter, presence or absence of vagina, urethrovaginal confluence, & cervix

CT Findings

- Bilateral, symmetric enlargement of adrenal glands
  - Usually maintains normal adreniform shape
  - Occasionally, adrenal gland has ovoid mass-like configuration
- Adrenal myelolipomas & adenomas may occur in adults

MR Findings

- Used to identify anatomy & morphology of female reproductive organs in setting of ambiguous genitalia
- Adrenal myelolipomas & adenomas may occur in adults
- Testicular adrenal rests
  - T1: Isointense to normal testicle
  - T2: Hypointense to testicle with well-defined margins
  - T1 C+: Homogeneous enhancement with well-defined margins
- MR is used to evaluate brain during acute adrenal crisis
  - May help to detect changes related to acute encephalopathy vs. stroke
  - MR is also used to detect chronic changes, including white matter abnormalities, smaller amygdala, & temporal lobe atrophy

Imaging Recommendations

- Best imaging tool
  - US for neonates with ambiguous genitalia or salt-wasting crisis
    - US confirms cerebriform appearance of enlarged adrenal glands
    - US can confirm presence of uterus & absence of testes
  - MR can be used for problem solving & to image brain during adrenal crisis

DIFFERENTIAL DIAGNOSIS

Normal Neonatal Adrenal Gland

- Normally enlarged due to hyperplasia of adrenal cortex

Neonatal Adrenal Hemorrhage

- Variably echogenic, heterogeneous, or cystic avascular mass due to perinatal bleeding into adrenal gland from stress

Neuroblastoma

- Most common adrenal mass in children
- Well-circumscribed & confined to adrenal vs. large lobulated & invasive mass that often calcifies, encases vessels, & crosses midline
- Internal vascularity is variable

Beckwith-Wiedemann Syndrome

- Disorder characterized by omphalocele, macroglossia, & hemihypertrophy
- ± adrenal enlargement with normal configuration

Wolman Disease

- Rare, autosomal recessive lipid storage disorder
- Enlarged adrenal glands with dystrophic Ca^{2+}

Polycystic Ovary Syndrome

- Polycystic ovarian morphology with clinical & endocrinologic dysfunction
- Significant overlap in imaging findings & clinical presentation with nonclassic CAH
  - Women with nonclassic CAH have higher hydroxyprogesterone & progesterone concentrations than women with polycystic ovary syndrome (PCOS)
  - Women with PCOS may have undiagnosed CAH

PATHOLOGY

General Features

- Etiology
  - Caused by deficiency in 1 of 5 enzymes required to synthesize cortisol from cholesterol in adrenal cortex
    - Deficiency of 21-hydroxylase is most common cause of CAH
      - Accounts for > 90% of cases of CAH
      - Caused by mutation in *CYP21A2* gene
      - Aldosterone & cortisol cannot be produced
      - Adrenal gland is chronically stimulated, leading to enlargement
    - Deficiency of 11β-hydroxylase is next most common enzyme affected
- Genetics
  - Autosomal recessive disorder

Gross Pathologic & Surgical Features

- Enlarged adrenal gland appears folded on itself
- Adrenal gland weighs 2-4x more than normal
- Glands are darker than normal due to depletion of lipid-rich cells of zona fasciculata

CLINICAL ISSUES

Presentation

- Most common signs/symptoms
  - CAH is part of normal neonatal screen in USA
  - 2 main types: Classic or nonclassic
  - Classic type: Presentation varies by sex
    - Females: Present at birth with ambiguous genitalia
      - Clitoromegaly, posterior fusion of labia majora, & masculinization of labioscrotal folds
      - May mimic penis with hypospadias
    - Males: Usually present at 5-14 days of life with acute salt-wasting crisis
      - Vomiting, weight loss, lethargy, severe dehydration, electrolyte imbalance, hypoglycemia, hypovolemia, & anion gap acidosis
      - May be misdiagnosed as hypertrophic pyloric stenosis
  - Nonclassic type most commonly presents with precocious puberty or hirsutism

Demographics

- Epidemiology
  - Classic type occurs in 1 in 5,000-15,000 live births
    - Most common cause of ambiguous genitalia in females
  - Nonclassic type occurs in 1 in 1,000

Natural History & Prognosis

- Adrenal crisis is most common cause of early death
- Quality of life scores are ↓ compared to population
  - Major factors related to ↓ quality of life: Sexual function & ↓ fertility
- High prevalence of adrenal tumors in adults (73-83%)
  - Most common: Adenomas & myelolipomas

Treatment

- Treated with lifelong glucocorticoids to suppress secretion of corticotropin-releasing hormone + ACTH as well as to reduce androgen levels
- Patients require hydrocortisone in times of stress, such as illness or surgery
- Ongoing ethical debate regarding timing of genitoplasty in girls

SELECTED REFERENCES

1. Hanafy AK et al: Imaging features of adrenal gland masses in the pediatric population. Abdom Radiol (NY). 45(4):964-81, 2020
2. Goncalves LF et al: Prenatal and postnatal imaging techniques in the evaluation of disorders of sex development. Semin Pediatr Surg. 28(5):150839, 2019
3. Harris RM et al: Ethical issues with early genitoplasty in children with disorders of sex development. Curr Opin Endocrinol Diabetes Obes. 26(1):49-53, 2019
4. Ma L et al: Sonographic features of the testicular adrenal rests tumors in patients with congenital adrenal hyperplasia: a single-center experience and literature review. Orphanet J Rare Dis. 14(1):242, 2019
5. Podgórski R et al: Congenital adrenal hyperplasia: clinical symptoms and diagnostic methods. Acta Biochim Pol. 65(1):25-33, 2018
6. White PC: Update on diagnosis and management of congenital adrenal hyperplasia due to 21-hydroxylase deficiency. Curr Opin Endocrinol Diabetes Obes. 25(3):178-84, 2018
7. Sargar KM et al: Imaging of nonmalignant adrenal lesions in children. Radiographics. 37(6):1648-64, 2017
8. Witchel SF: Congenital adrenal hyperplasia. J Pediatr Adolesc Gynecol. 30(5):520-34, 2017
9. Teixeira SR et al: The role of imaging in congenital adrenal hyperplasia. Arq Bras Endocrinol Metabol. 58(7):701-8, 2014

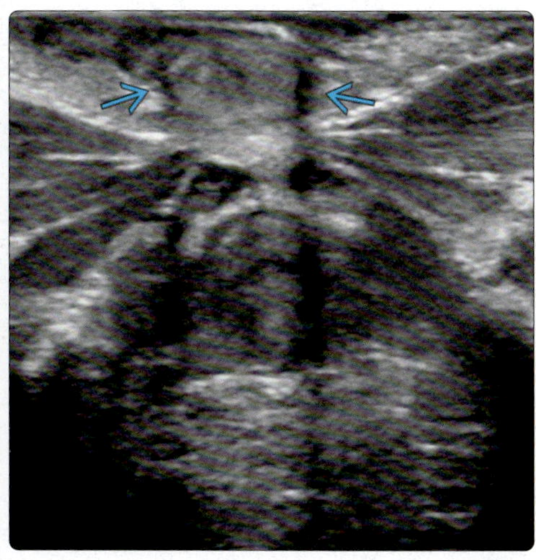

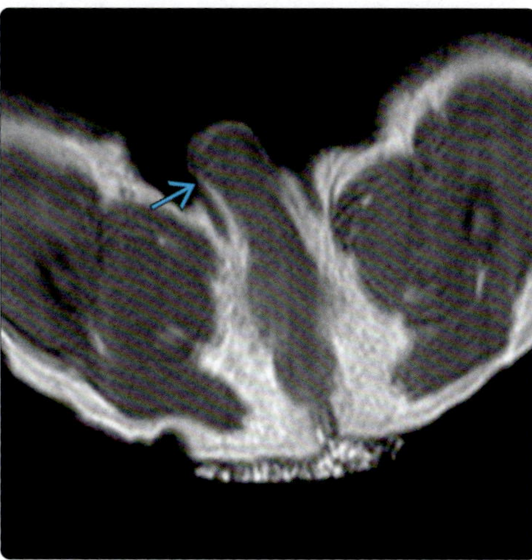

(Left) *Transverse US of the labia in a newborn with ambiguous genitalia caused by CAH shows clitoromegaly ➞.* **(Right)** *Axial T1 MR of the pelvis in the same patient shows clitoromegaly ➞. Determining the infant's sex was not possible via imaging as gonadal structures were not visible. Ultimately, genetic testing confirmed 2 X chromosomes.*

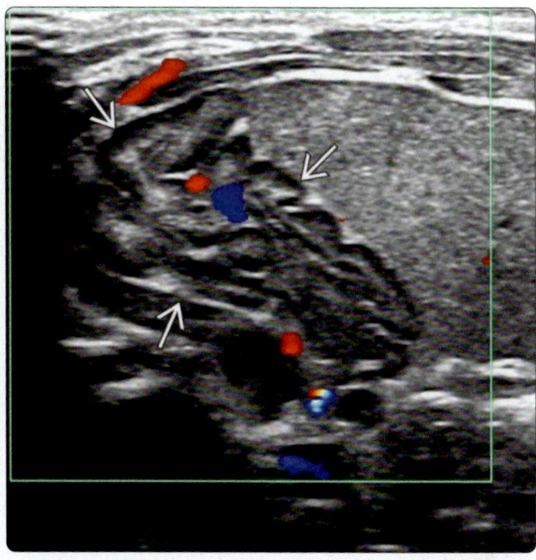

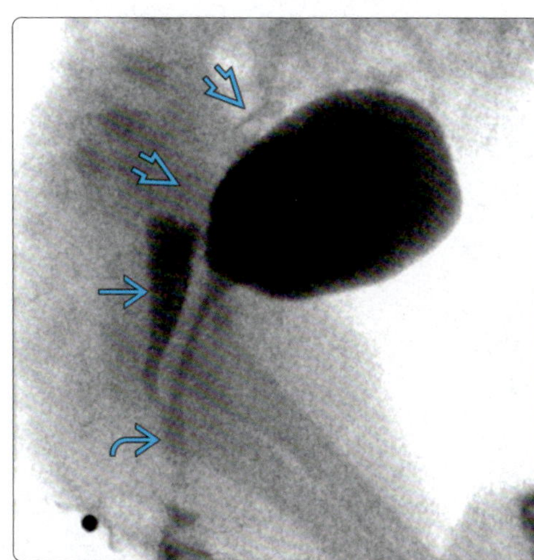

(Left) *Color Doppler US of the left adrenal gland in a patient with CAH shows an enlarged gland ➡ with a cerebriform appearance & mild hyperemia.* **(Right)** *Lateral voiding cystourethrogram in a 1-week-old girl with CAH & ambiguous genitalia shows a genitourinary sinus ➚ with reflux of voided contrast into the vagina ➞ & uterus ⇨.*

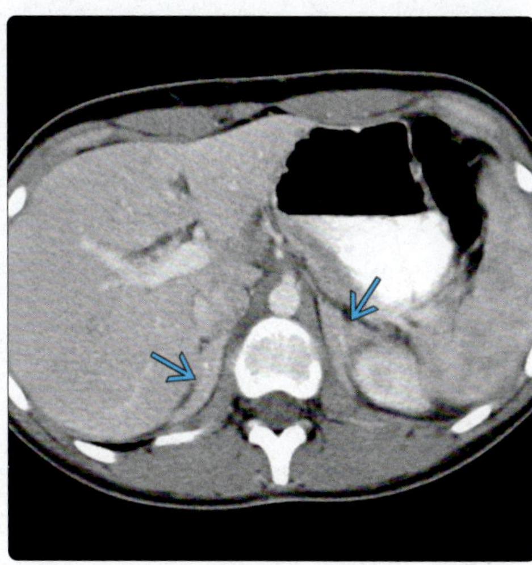

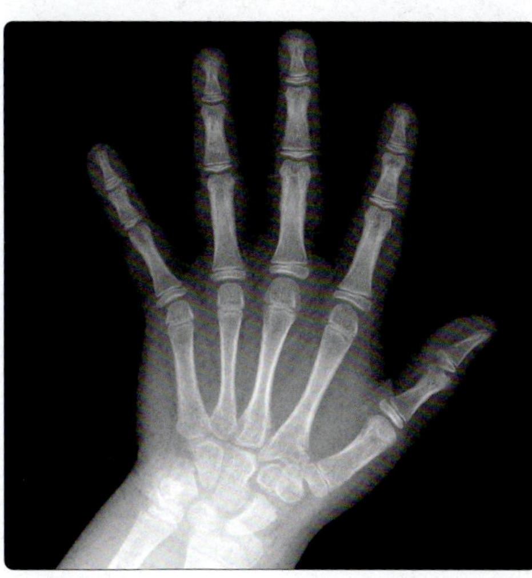

(Left) *Axial CECT (performed after a motor vehicle accident) in a 14-year-old girl with CAH shows mild persistent enlargement & homogeneous enhancement of the bilateral adrenal glands ➞.* **(Right)** *PA bone age radiograph of the left hand & wrist in an 8-year-old boy with CAH shows an advanced bone age of 13 years.*

KEY FACTS

TERMINOLOGY

- Malignant tumor of sympathetic chain primitive neural crest cells
- Increasing degrees of cellular differentiation/benignity along spectrum: Neuroblastoma (malignant) → ganglioneuroblastoma → ganglioneuroma (benign)

IMAGING

- Location
  - Adrenal (35-48%)
  - Extraadrenal retroperitoneum (18-35%)
  - Posterior mediastinum (14-20%)
  - Less common: Neck, pelvis, unknown primary
- Small round solitary mass vs. large multilobulated lesion
- Aggressive tumor with tendency to invade adjacent tissues
- Frequently engulfs & displaces adjacent vascular structures
- Ca^{2+} in up to 90% by CT
- Metastases in 50-60% at diagnosis, most commonly to bone/marrow, lymph nodes, liver, soft tissues

TOP DIFFERENTIAL DIAGNOSES

- Wilms tumor
- Neonatal adrenal hemorrhage
- Less common adrenal tumors
  - Adrenal cortical neoplasms
  - Pheochromocytoma
- Other cystic/solid suprarenal lesions

CLINICAL ISSUES

- Most common extracranial solid malignancy in children
- Median age at diagnosis: 15-19 months
- Wide variety of clinical presentations; most commonly presents as palpable abdominal mass
- Features associated with better prognosis
  - Age at diagnosis < 18 months
  - Stage 4S/MS
  - Localized tumor not involving vital structures
  - Absent *MYCN* (*N-myc*) oncogene amplification

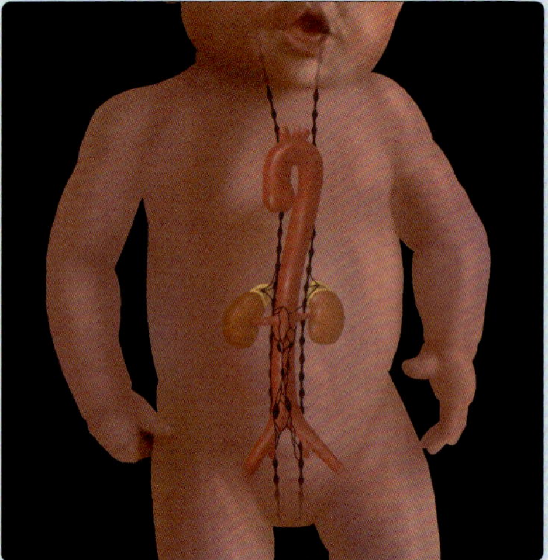

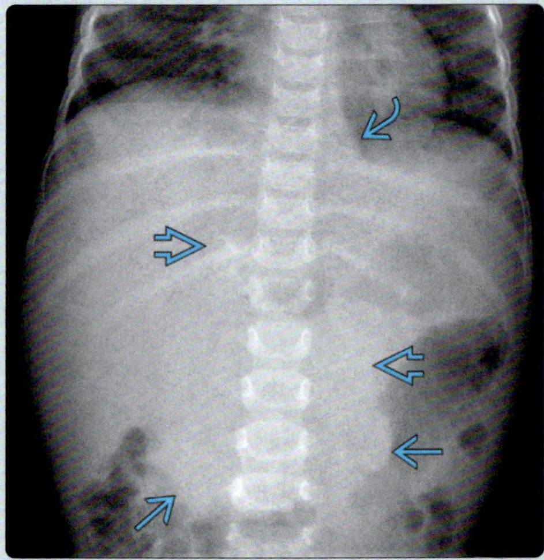

(Left) *Graphic shows the anatomic extent of the sympathetic chain ganglia (including the adrenal glands) from the cervical region to the pelvis. Neuroblastoma (NBL) can arise anywhere along the sympathetic chain.* **(Right)** *AP radiograph in a 2-year-old with abdominal distention & pain shows displacement of bowel loops by a lobulated ➡, partially calcified ⇨ mass in the mid to upper abdomen. Note the widened left paraspinal stripe ⇨.*

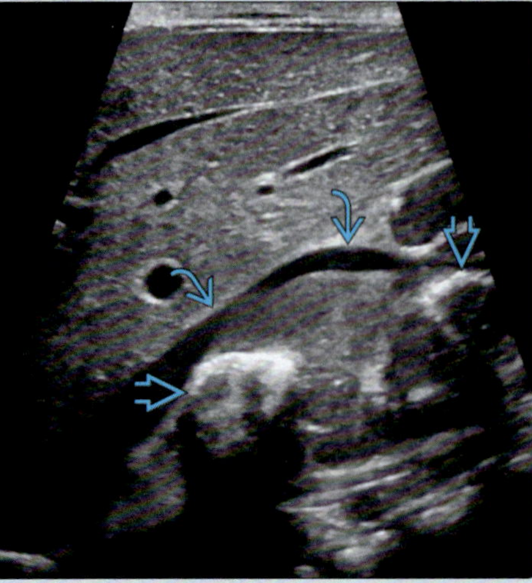

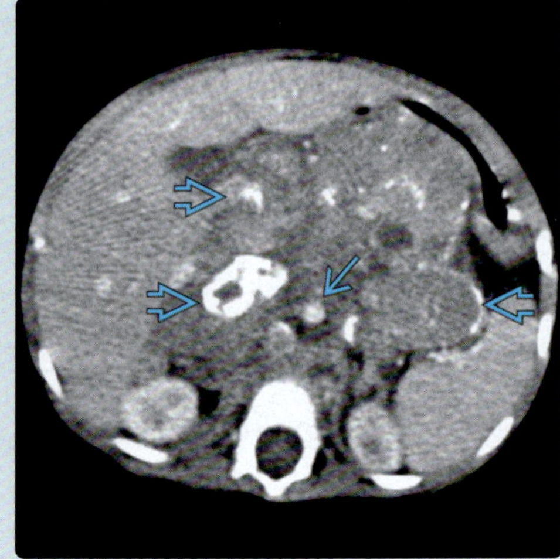

(Left) *Longitudinal ultrasound in the same patient shows anterior displacement & narrowing of the inferior vena cava (IVC) ⇨ by a partially calcified retroperitoneal mass ⇨.* **(Right)** *Axial CECT in the same patient shows elevation & encasement of the aorta ➡ by a large, lobulated, heterogeneous mass that crosses the midline & contains numerous calcifications ⇨, typical of NBL. The patient also had extensive bony metastases.*

TERMINOLOGY

Definitions

- Malignant tumor of sympathetic chain primitive neural crest cells
- Increasing degrees of cellular differentiation/benignity along spectrum: Neuroblastoma [(NBL), malignant] → ganglioneuroblastoma (GNBL) → ganglioneuroma [(GN), benign]

IMAGING

General Features

- Best diagnostic clue
  - Partially calcified, lobulated suprarenal/paraspinal mass in infant
- Location
  - Anywhere along sympathetic chain from neck to pelvis
    - Adrenal (35-48%)
      - 90% adrenal in prenatally detected cases
    - Extraadrenal retroperitoneum (18-35%)
    - Posterior mediastinum (14-20%)
    - Pelvis (2-5%)
    - Neck (1-5%)
    - Metastatic disease with no primary identified (1%)
  - 35% involve regional lymph nodes
  - 50% have distant metastases at diagnosis
    - May involve distant lymph nodes
- General imaging features
  - Small, round, solitary suprarenal/paraspinal mass vs. large, lobulated lesion crossing midline
  - Aggressive tumor; may invade adjacent tissues
    - Intraspinal invasion via neural foramina (~ 15%)
    - Kidney, muscle
  - Frequently engulfs & displaces adjacent vascular structures (rather than just displacing/compressing)
    - Aorta & inferior vena cava (IVC) are frequently lifted off of spine
  - Ca^{2+} in up to 90% by CT
  - Metastases in 50-60% at diagnosis, most commonly to bone/marrow, lymph nodes, liver, soft tissues
    - Liver: Well-defined focal vs. extensive, poorly defined lesions with hepatomegaly
    - Bone: Focally destructive, cortical &/or well-defined or confluent intramedullary lesions
    - Soft tissues: Cutaneous/subcutaneous lesions may be visible on physical exam & imaging

Radiographic Findings

- Often occult or subtle by radiographs
- Ca^{2+} in only 30% by radiography
- Displacement of bowel by soft tissue mass
- Widening of inferior thoracic paraspinal soft tissues
  - May be only finding of retrocrural extension of upper abdominal mass
- Subtle bony clues of soft tissue mass
  - Splaying/remodeling of adjacent ribs
  - Vertebral body scalloping, small pedicle
- Bone metastasis
  - May be extensive with little radiographic presence (especially marrow disease)
  - May be only presenting clinical/imaging finding

CT Findings

- Mass is often heterogeneous from necrosis, hemorrhage
- Ca^{2+} in up to 90% by CT

MR Findings

- Generally intermediate to high T2/intermediate to low T1 signal intensity
  - Heterogeneity from Ca^{2+}, hemorrhage, necrosis
- Variable enhancement from none to diffuse
- Typically restricts diffusion due to high cellularity
- Excellent depiction of intraspinal extension
- High sensitivity/specificity for marrow disease (but ↓ specificity posttherapy)

Ultrasonographic Findings

- Mass is often heterogeneous
  - Ca^{2+} causing echogenic foci ± posterior shadowing
- Suprarenal location displaces/distorts kidney
- Variable internal tumor vascularity on Doppler
- Vessels are often engulfed/lifted by tumor

Nuclear Medicine Findings

- MIBG scintigraphy
  - I-123 MIBG for diagnosis, staging, follow-up imaging
  - MIBG is related to norepinephrine → avid uptake in catecholamine production process
  - ↑ uptake at any site of active NBL
    - Sensitivity & specificity ~ 90% in NBL
  - Evaluates bony cortical & marrow disease
  - In MIBG-avid tumors, posttherapy evaluation is more specific than MR or FDG PET
- PET
  - 18-F FDG remains primary radiotracer
    - High sensitivity for soft tissue & bony NBL, though generally < MIBG
      - Select populations may benefit from PET, particularly non-MIBG-avid disease
  - DOTATATE
    - Somatostatin receptor analog, typically bound with Ga-68
      - May lead to targeted therapies
- Bone scan
  - Tc-99m MDP
    - Uptake in primary mass in up to 74% of cases
    - ↑ uptake in bony metastasis (cortical > marrow)
  - Limited role in current era

DIFFERENTIAL DIAGNOSIS

Wilms Tumor

- Mean age: 3 years; Ca^{2+} is uncommon
- Usually grows like ball, displacing vessels
- Arises from kidney: Claw sign of residual renal parenchyma splayed along tumor
- Lung metastases in 20%
- Invasion of renal vein + IVC

Neonatal Adrenal Hemorrhage

- Cystic &/or solid-appearing avascular suprarenal mass
- Serial US exams show gradual ↓ in size with ↑ Ca^{2+}

Less Common Adrenal Tumors

- Pheochromocytoma (uncommon in young children)
- Adrenal cortical neoplasms (usually hormonally active)

Other Cystic/Solid Suprarenal Lesions

- Congenital adrenal hyperplasia
- Extralobar bronchopulmonary sequestration
- Foregut duplication cyst
- Lymphatic malformation

PATHOLOGY

General Features

- Genetics
  - ↑ copies of *MYCN* oncogene (*MYCN* or *N-myc* amplification): Unfavorable prognosis (even stage MS)
  - *ALK* mutation/amplification: Unfavorable
  - Segmental chromosome aberrations (loss at 1p, 3p, 11q, 14q): Unfavorable
  - DNA index (measure of ploidy)
    - Diploidy or tetraploidy: Unfavorable
    - 1.26-1.76 (near triploid): Favorable
  - Only 1-2% of cases are familial, often with multiple primary tumors in infants
- Associated abnormalities
  - Neurofibromatosis type 1, Beckwith-Wiedemann syndrome, Hirschsprung disease, congenital central hypoventilation syndrome, Turner syndrome
  - Most NBL cases occur in children without associations

Staging, Grading, & Classification

- International NBL Staging System (INSS)
  - Original 1-4S system based on resection & pathology (1988, 1993)
  - Traditionally used by Children's Oncology Group (COG) to risk stratification as low, intermediate, or high
- International NBL Risk Group Staging System (INRGSS)
  - More comprehensive, imaging-based system (2009)
  - Utilizes modifying image-defined risk factors
    - L1: Tumor in 1 body compartment, no vital structures involved
    - L2: Tumor in 2 body compartments **or** encasing/invading major structures; rarely resectable at diagnosis
    - M: Distant metastases
    - MS: Age < 18 months; metastases confined to skin, liver, bone marrow
      - ▫ Bones (including marrow) must be clear by MIBG to qualify for stage 4S/MS (with marrow disease limited to < 10% involvement by biopsy)
  - Used to stratify as very low, low, intermediate, or high risk in conjunction with age, genetics, histology
    - High risk: *MYCN* amplification, metastases if ≥ 18 months of age; additional criteria by some systems
    - "Ultra high risk": Potential, evolving category

CLINICAL ISSUES

Presentation

- Most common signs/symptoms
  - Painless abdominal mass
- Other signs/symptoms
  - Malaise, irritability, weight loss, limping, opsoclonus-myoclonus, Horner syndrome, cerebellar ataxia, neurologic symptoms related to compression, hypertension, watery diarrhea with hypokalemia
  - Classic presentations
    - Skin metastases: Blueberry muffin syndrome
    - Skull base metastases: "Raccoon eyes"
    - Massive liver metastases: Pepper syndrome
  - 90-95% of NBL patients have elevated levels of catecholamines/metabolites (VMA, HVA) in urine

Demographics

- Age
  - Median age at presentation: 15-19 months
  - 95% diagnosed by 7 years
  - May be diagnosed prenatally
- Epidemiology
  - Most common extracranial solid malignancy in children
    - Most common malignancy of infancy

Natural History & Prognosis

- Risk stratification: Criteria vary by cooperative groups & trials; COG version includes
  - Low risk (30% of all NBL, 70% of neonatal NBL): 5-year survival > 95% with observation (select cases) or surgery
    - Spontaneous regression most likely in
      - ▫ Infants < 6 months of age with small adrenal lesions
      - ▫ Non-*MYCN* amplified infants with localized disease or asymptomatic 4S/MS disease
  - Intermediate risk (20% of all NBL): 5-year survival > 90% with surgery + chemotherapy
  - High risk (36-50% of all NBL): 5-year survival of 30-40% with intensive multimodality therapy
    - May also use radiation therapy, myeloablative therapy with stem cell rescue, molecular inhibitors, antibodies, &/or I-131 MIBG therapy, especially for refractory/recurrent disease
- Risk stratification by INRGSS
  - Very low risk: 5-year event-free survival (5y EFS) of > 85%
  - Low risk: 75-85%
  - Intermediate risk: 50-75%
  - High risk: < 50%
  - Ultra high risk: Evolving category that typically includes
    - Anything < very good partial response to induction chemotherapy
    - 5y EFS of < 15%; death < 18 months from diagnosis

SELECTED REFERENCES

1. Morin CE et al: Imaging for staging of pediatric abdominal tumors: an update, from the AJR Special Series on Cancer Staging. AJR Am J Roentgenol. 217(4):786-99, 2021
2. Morgenstern DA et al: The challenge of defining "ultra-high-risk" neuroblastoma. Pediatr Blood Cancer. 66(4):e27556, 2019
3. Newman EA et al: Update on neuroblastoma. J Pediatr Surg. 54(3):383-9, 2019
4. Sznewajs A et al: Congenital malformation syndromes associated with peripheral neuroblastic tumors: a systematic review. Pediatr Blood Cancer. 66(10):e27901, 2019
5. Aygun N: Biological and genetic features of neuroblastoma and their clinical importance. Curr Pediatr Rev. 14(2):73-90, 2018
6. Chen AM et al: A review of neuroblastoma image-defined risk factors on magnetic resonance imaging. Pediatr Radiol. 48(9):1337-47, 2018
7. Swift CC et al: Updates in diagnosis, management, and treatment of neuroblastoma. Radiographics. 38(2):566-80, 2018

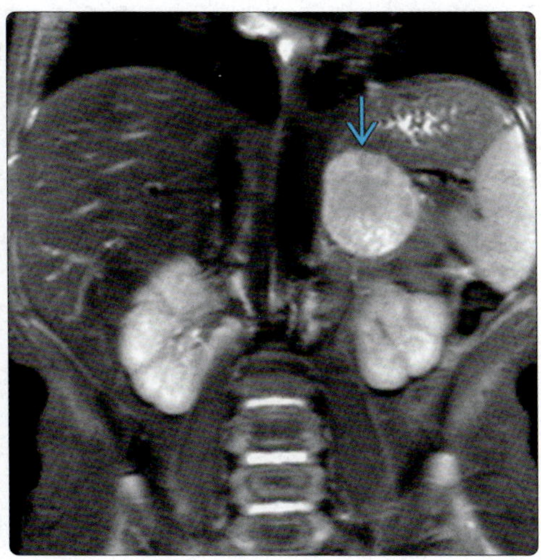

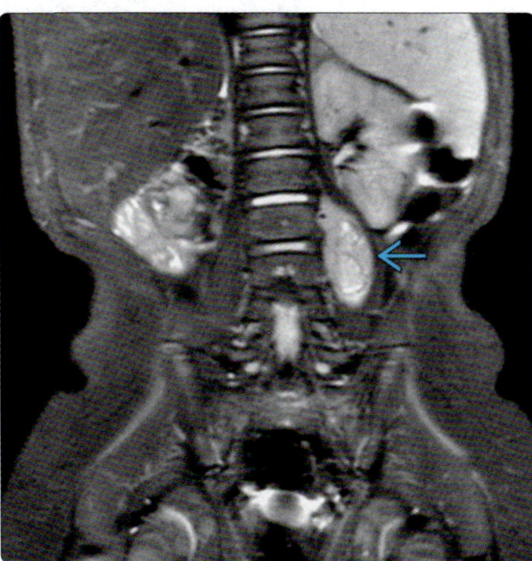

(Left) *Coronal STIR MR in a 4-month-old shows a hyperintense, round, well-circumscribed left suprarenal mass ➡ that was incidentally detected on a renal ultrasound & ultimately confirmed as NBL.* **(Right)** *Coronal STIR MR in an 11-month-old shows a mildly heterogeneous mass ➡ in the left psoas muscle, subsequently confirmed as NBL. The mass was incidentally detected as a region of heterogeneous paraspinal echogenicity on a renal ultrasound.*

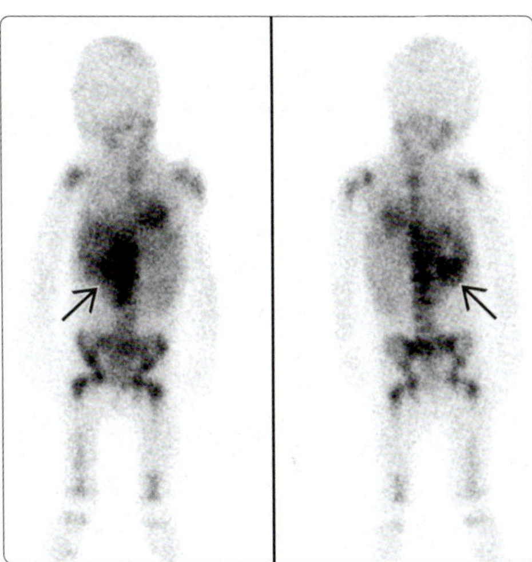

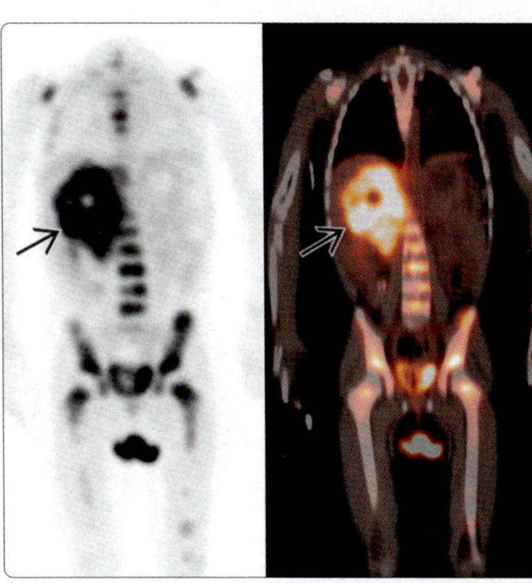

(Left) *Anterior & posterior I-123 MIBG scans in a 2-year-old NBL patient show uptake throughout the primary tumor ➡ in the right abdomen as well as numerous foci of skeletal metastases. Note that the skeleton is not normally visualized with MIBG, making all foci of bony uptake in these images consistent with metastatic disease.* **(Right)** *F-18 FDG PET & fused PET/CT images in the same patient show ↑ metabolic activity within the primary tumor ➡ as well as numerous sites of skeletal disease.*

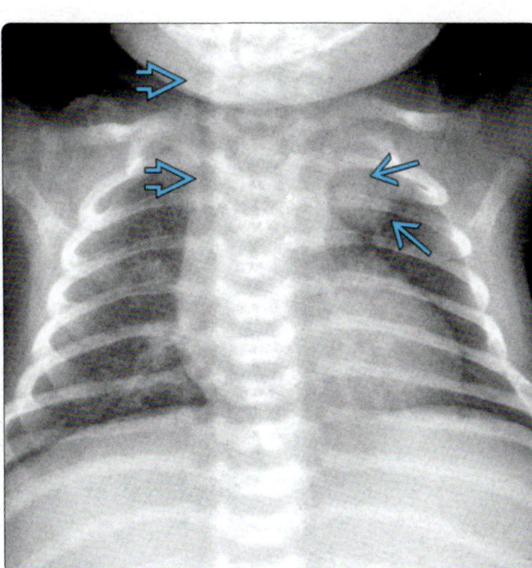

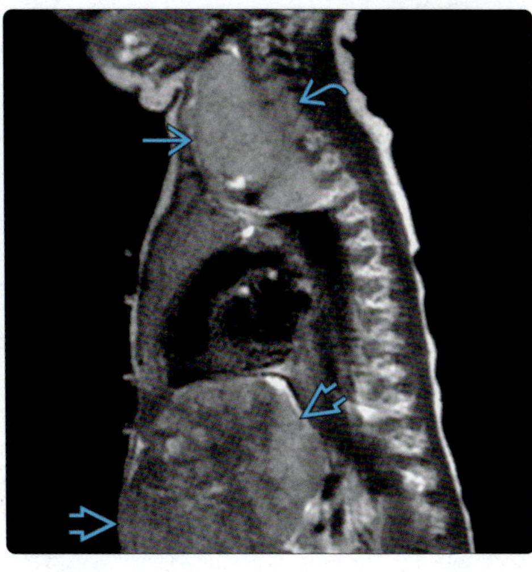

(Left) *AP radiograph in a 7-week-old with abdominal distention shows a lobulated left apical mass ➡ with marked rightward shift of the trachea ⇨. Note that no stomach bubble is seen in the upper abdomen.* **(Right)** *Sagittal SSFSE T2 MR in the same patient shows a primary cervicothoracic NBL ➡ with multilevel neuroforaminal involvement ↗. The liver is enlarged & heterogeneous ⇨ due to hyperintense metastases.*

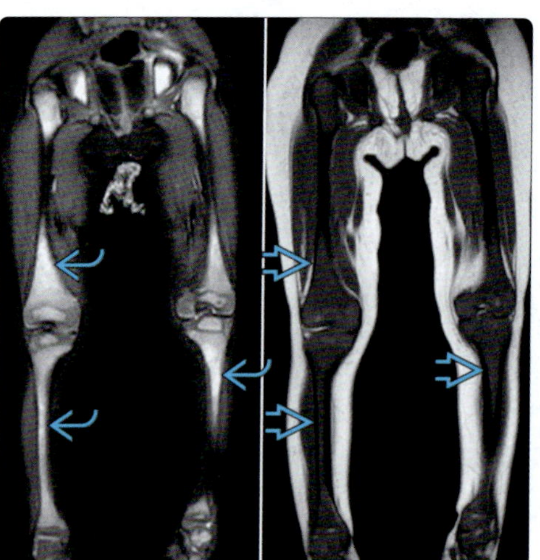

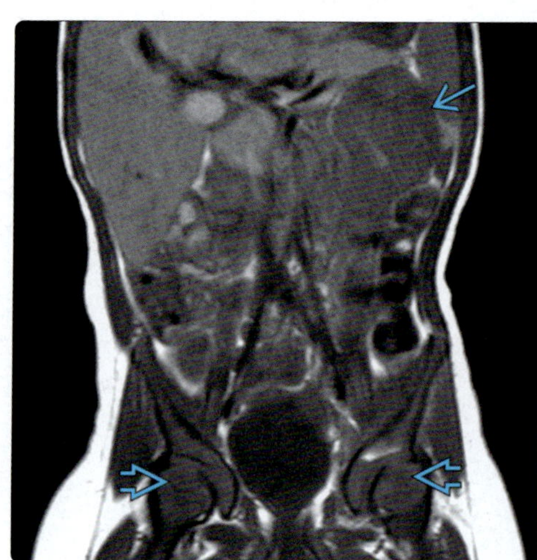

(Left) *Coronal STIR (left) & T1 (right) MR images in a 19-month-old with limping for 5 weeks show extensive confluent marrow signal abnormalities that are diffusely bright ➔ & dark ➔, respectively.* **(Right)** *Coronal T1 MR in the same patient shows loss of the normal yellow marrow bright signal in the femoral heads ➔ due to metastases. Portions of the primary tumor are visualized in the left upper quadrant ➔.*

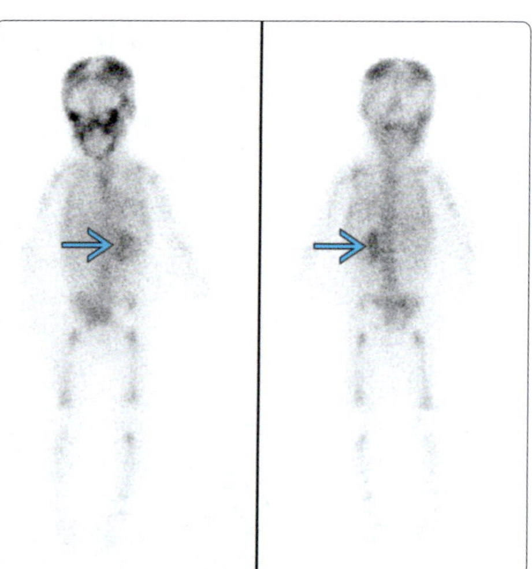

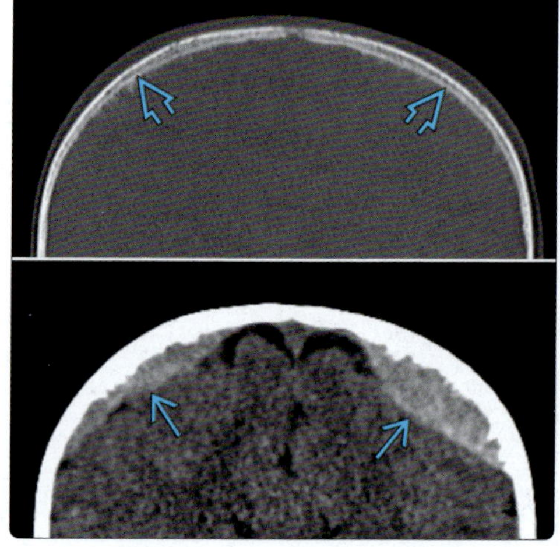

(Left) *Anterior (left) & posterior (right) I-123 MIBG images in the same patient show uptake in the primary left upper quadrant neuroblastoma ➔. As the bones should not be visualized on an MIBG scan, the osseous activity is due to metastases, most pronounced in the skull.* **(Right)** *Coronal NECT images in the same patient in bone (top) & brain (bottom) windows show a spiculated pattern of new bone formation ➔ within the soft tissue masses ➔. This appearance is typical of metastatic NBL in the skull.*

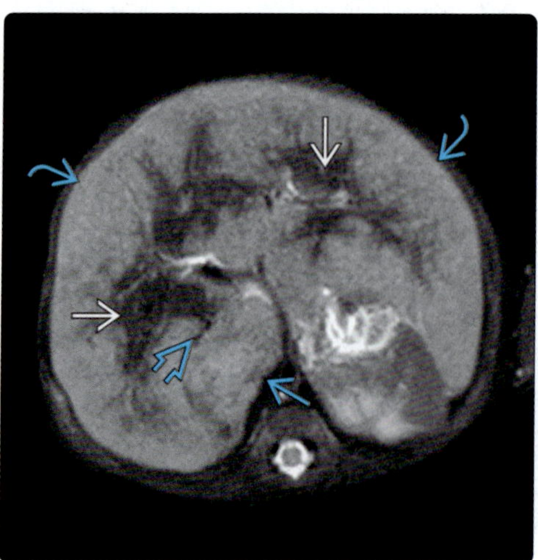

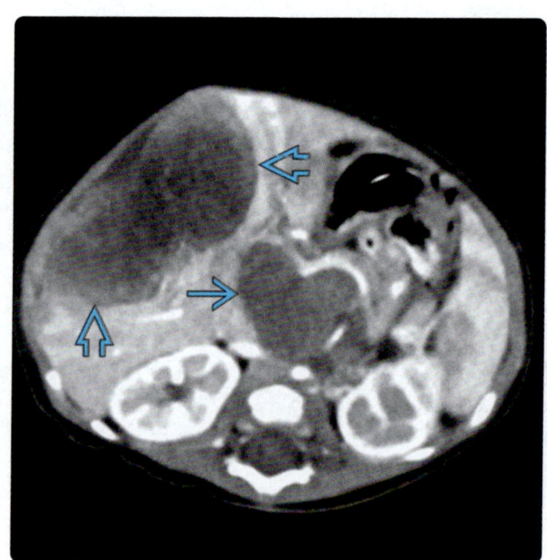

(Left) *Axial T2 FS MR in a newborn with abdominal distention shows a confluent rind of hyperintense tissue ➔ encasing small residual islands of normal liver parenchyma ➔. The IVC is effaced ➔ between the liver & a right adrenal NBL ➔ that is otherwise inseparable from the liver metastases.* **(Right)** *Axial CECT in a 4-month-old with abdominal distention shows the largest of several well-circumscribed hepatic metastases ➔ from a retroperitoneal NBL ➔.*

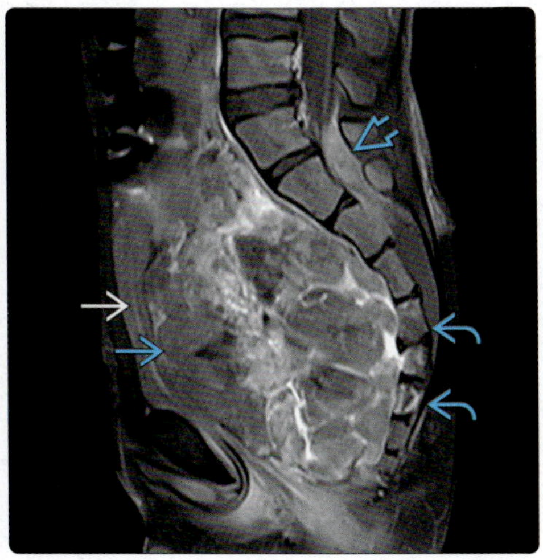

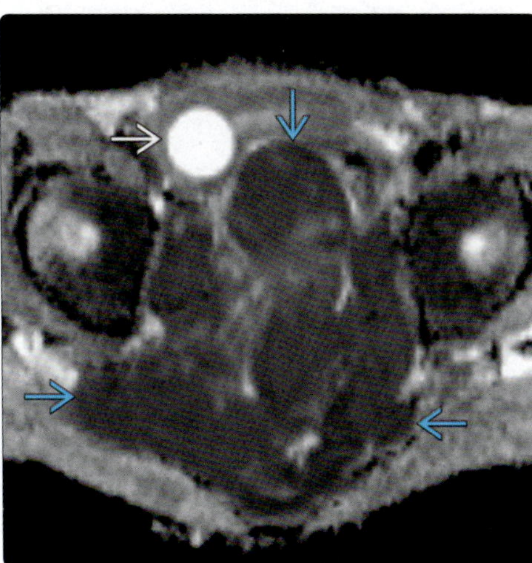

(Left) *Sagittal T1 C+ FS MR in a 7-year-old with back pain & urinary symptoms shows a heterogeneously enhancing presacral mass ➔ with bone involvement ➔ & intraspinal extension ➔. The urinary bladder is anteriorly displaced & decompressed around a Foley catheter ➔.* **(Right)** *Axial MR ADC map in the same patient at the level of the hips shows restricted diffusion throughout the NBL ➔. The Foley catheter balloon ➔ is displaced anteriorly.*

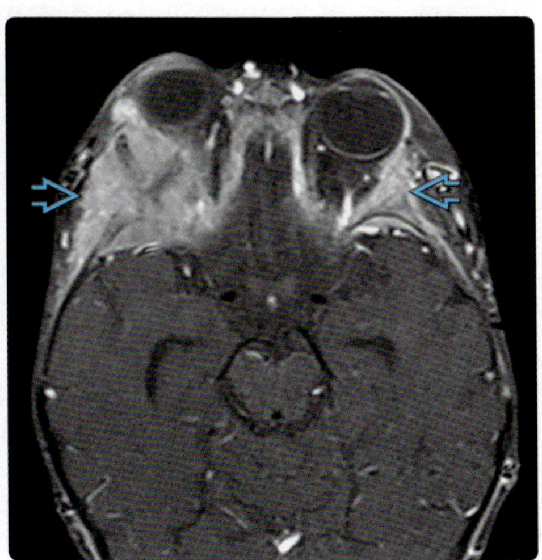

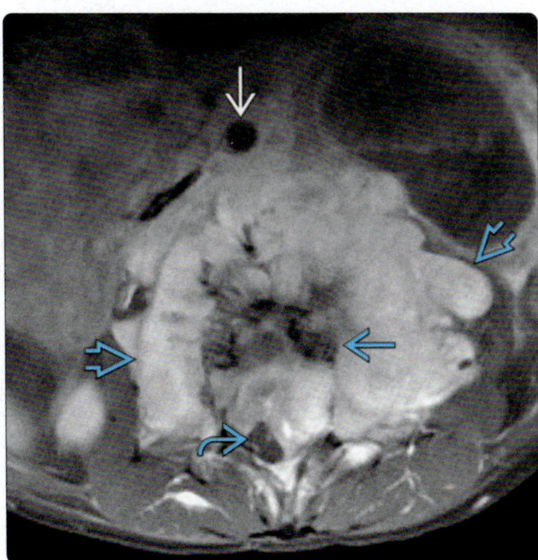

(Left) *Axial T1 C+ FS MR in a 2-year-old with proptosis shows homogeneously enhancing soft tissue masses ➔ of the R > L greater sphenoid wings secondary to NBL metastases.* **(Right)** *Axial T1 C+ FS MR in 4-year-old with an abnormal gait shows a large, lobulated enhancing mass ➔ emanating from a permeated vertebral body ➔, displacing the aorta ➔ & compressing the thecal sac ➔. NBL was proven at biopsy.*

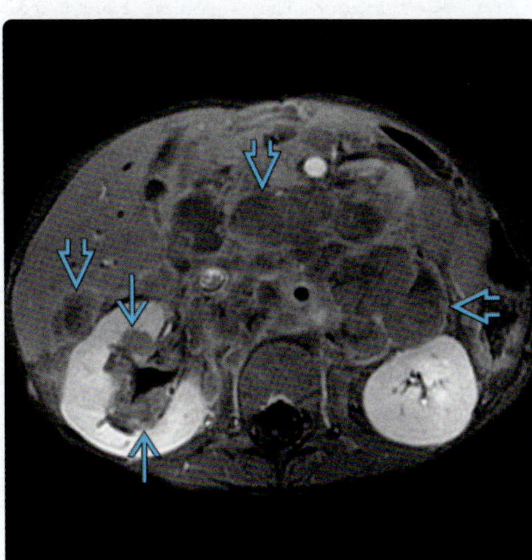

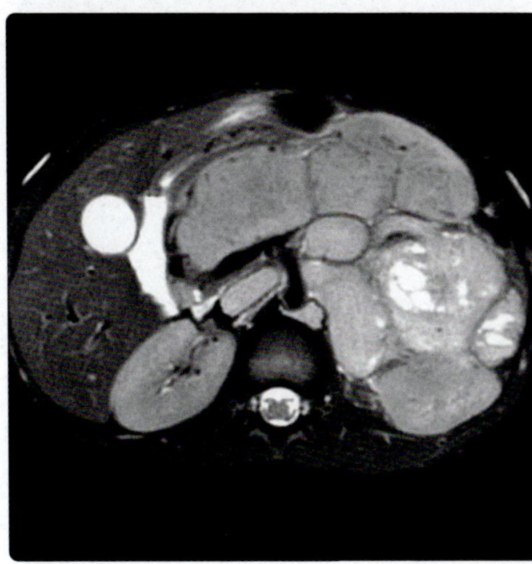

(Left) *Axial T1 C+ FS MR in a 5-year-old with constipation & weight loss shows numerous hypoenhancing retroperitoneal & peritoneal NBL nodules ➔ with invasion of the right kidney ➔.* **(Right)** *Axial T2 FS MR in a 7-year-old with NBL shows complete replacement of the pancreatic parenchyma by confluent nodular masses. Pancreatic NBL lesions may occur from direct local invasion or distant metastases.*

Adrenocortical Carcinoma

KEY FACTS

TERMINOLOGY

- Malignant adrenal cortical neoplasm

IMAGING

- Best clue: Suprarenal mass in young child with virilization or Cushing syndrome
- Average size: 7-10 cm (median: 9.5 cm)
- Well-defined mass with thin, enhancing rim
- Heterogeneous internal enhancement
- Central stellate focus: Low attenuation (CT) or high signal (T2 FS MR) without enhancement after contrast
- Ca^{2+} in ~ 70% of masses
- May invade IVC
- Sites of metastasis: Liver, lungs, lymph nodes
  - Occur in ~ 80% of patients older than 4 years of age

TOP DIFFERENTIAL DIAGNOSES

- Neuroblastoma
- Adrenal hemorrhage
- Adrenal adenoma
- Pheochromocytoma

PATHOLOGY

- Associated with Li-Fraumeni & Beckwith-Wiedemann syndromes
- Up to 80% have mutation of *TP53* gene
- Wienecke criteria: Best predictor of clinical outcomes in children

CLINICAL ISSUES

- Median age of 4 years; bimodal distribution in children
  - < 4 years of age vs. 2nd peak in adolescence
- Hormonally active
  - Virilization in 75-95% of patients
  - Cushing syndrome in up to 60%
- Prognosis is better than in adults
- Treatment of choice: Complete surgical excision

(Left) *Axial CECT of the abdomen shows a large mass ➡ arising from the left adrenal gland. The mass is typical of adrenocortical carcinoma (ACC) with a heterogeneous enhancement pattern & a thin rim of tissue that enhances more than the central components.* **(Right)** *Axial T2 FS MR of the abdomen in the same patient with ACC shows a heterogeneous mass ➡ that is hyperintense to the liver. The tumor has a poorly defined central stellate focus ➡ that is hyperintense to the remainder of the tumor.*

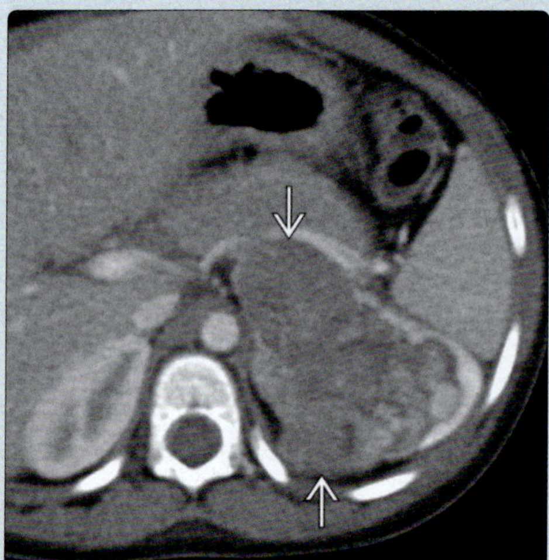

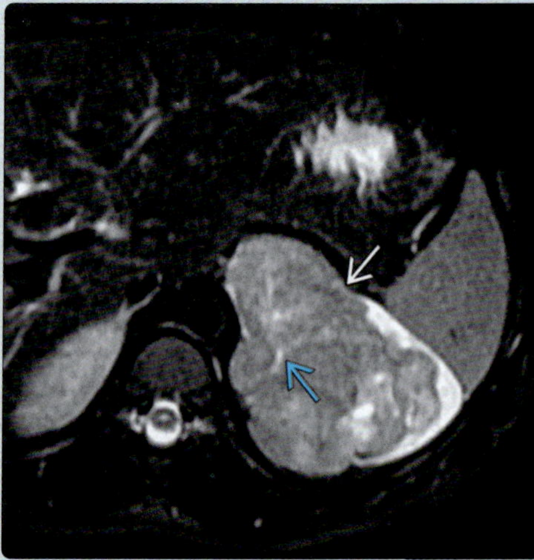

(Left) *Longitudinal color Doppler ultrasound in the same patient with ACC shows a large left suprarenal mass ➡ that is isoechoic to the adjacent spleen ⇨. There is a subtle central stellate focus ↪ that is hypoechoic compared to the remainder of the tumor.* **(Right)** *Coronal PET/CT in a toddler with virilization shows intense FDG uptake throughout the majority of a left suprarenal mass ➡ that is displacing the left kidney inferiorly ⇨. Histology confirmed an ACC.*

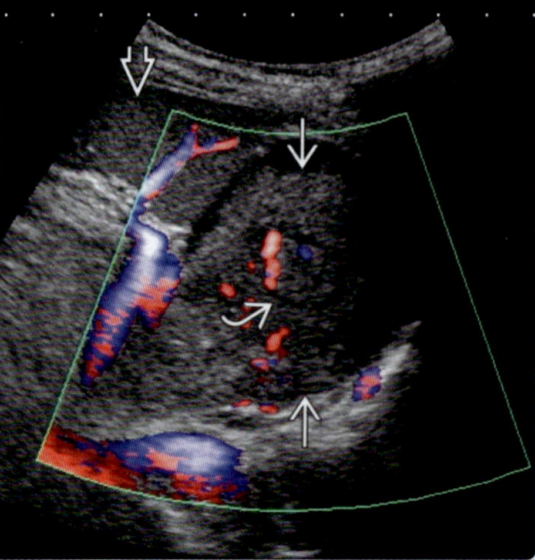

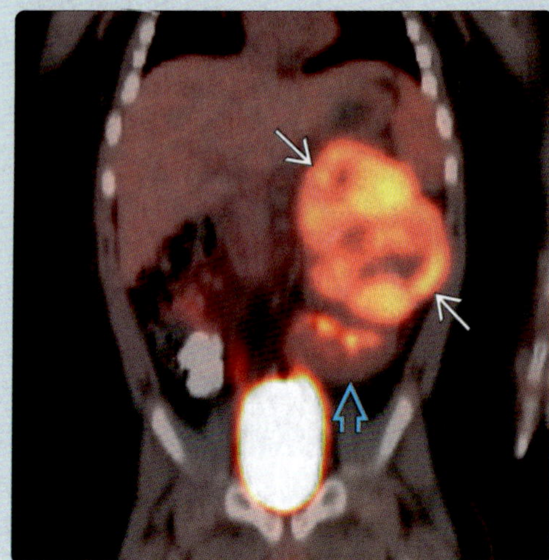

TERMINOLOGY

Abbreviations

- Adrenocortical carcinoma (ACC)

Definitions

- Malignant adrenal cortical neoplasm

IMAGING

General Features

- Best diagnostic clue
  - Suprarenal mass in young child with virilization or Cushing syndrome
- Location
  - Adrenal cortex
  - Metastasis to liver, lungs, lymph nodes
    - Occur in ~ 80% of patients > 4 years of age
- Size
  - At presentation: 7-10 cm (median: 9.5 cm)

CT Findings

- Well-defined mass with thin, enhancing rim
- Heterogeneous internal enhancement
  - Central stellate focus of low attenuation is common
- Ca^{2+} in ~ 70%

MR Findings

- T1WI
  - Heterogeneous mass, isointense to muscle
- T2WI FS
  - Variable signal intensity: Iso-/hyperintense to fat
  - ± central stellate focus: Hyperintense to fat
- T1WI C+
  - Heterogeneous enhancement pattern
  - Central stellate focus does not enhance

Ultrasonographic Findings

- Slightly hyperechoic suprarenal mass
- Central stellate focus is often hypoechoic
- Inferior vena cava (IVC) compression or invasion

DIFFERENTIAL DIAGNOSIS

Neuroblastoma

- Most common pediatric adrenal neoplasm
  - Arises from medulla, not cortex
- No hormonal changes
- Uptake on I-123 MIBG scans

Adrenal Hemorrhage

- Most common in neonatal age group (due to birth stress)
- No internal vascularity
- Regresses with time

Adrenal Adenoma

- Benign cortical neoplasm; uncommon in children
- Pathologic/radiologic spectrum with ACC; malignancy is favored with
  - Larger, heterogeneously enhancing tumors with Ca^{2+}
  - Distant metastases
  - FDG avidity on PET/CT

Pheochromocytoma

- Uncommon in younger children
- Typically causes hypertension
- Small, round suprarenal mass; hyperintense on T2 MR
- Uptake on I-123 MIBG scans

PATHOLOGY

General Features

- Associated abnormalities
  - Li-Fraumeni syndrome
  - Beckwith-Wiedemann syndrome
  - Other syndromes associated with ACC: Carney complex, congenital adrenal hyperplasia, McCune-Albright syndrome, & multiple endocrine neoplasia type 1

Staging, Grading, & Classification

- Various pathology-based systems for determining benignity vs. malignancy of adrenal cortical neoplasm
  - Weiss & Wienecke criteria are most commonly used
    - Wienecke criteria has shown to be better predictor of clinical outcomes in children

CLINICAL ISSUES

Presentation

- Most common signs/symptoms
  - Virilization occurs in 75-95%
- Other signs/symptoms
  - Cushing syndrome: ~ 60% (less common than in adults)
  - Other symptoms: Abdominal mass, hypertension

Demographics

- Epidemiology
  - 0.2% of all childhood cancers
    - 15x incidence in Southern Brazil due to higher frequency of *TP53* germline mutation
  - Median age: 4 years; bimodal distribution in children
    - < 4 years of age vs. 2nd peak in adolescence

Natural History & Prognosis

- 5-year survival rates: ~ 50%
- Factors improving prognosis
  - Age < 4 years
  - Tumor size < 10 cm
  - Tumor weight < 400 g
  - Lack of distant metastases

Treatment

- Complete surgical excision
- Chemotherapy if complete resection is not possible

SELECTED REFERENCES

1. Al-Sarhani H et al: Screening of cancer predisposition syndromes. Pediatr Radiol. ePub, 2021
2. Hanafy AK et al: Imaging features of adrenal gland masses in the pediatric population. Abdom Radiol (NY). 45(4):964-81, 2020
3. Gupta N et al: Adrenocortical carcinoma in children: a clinicopathological analysis of 41 patients at the Mayo Clinic from 1950 to 2017. Horm Res Paediatr. 90(1):8-18, 2018
4. Bulzico D et al: Recurrence and mortality prognostic factors in childhood adrenocortical tumors: analysis from the Brazilian National Institute of Cancer experience. Pediatr Hematol Oncol. 33(4):248-58, 2016
5. Flynt KA et al: Pediatric adrenocortical neoplasms: can imaging reliably discriminate adenomas from carcinomas? Pediatr Radiol. 45(8):1160-8, 2015

Pheochromocytoma

KEY FACTS

TERMINOLOGY

- Paraganglioma arising from catecholamine-producing chromaffin cells of adrenal medulla
- Associated with
  - Mutations in succinate dehydrogenase
  - von Hippel-Lindau syndrome
  - Multiple endocrine neoplasia syndrome type 2
  - Neurofibromatosis type 1

IMAGING

- Best diagnostic clue: Suprarenal mass in child with hypertension
- CECT: Avidly enhancing adrenal mass
- MR
  - T1: Isointense to muscle
  - T2: Mildly to moderately hyperintense vs. "light bulb bright"
  - T1 C+: Avidly enhancing mass
- MIBG: ↑ uptake in tumor

TOP DIFFERENTIAL DIAGNOSES

- Neuroblastoma
- Adrenocortical carcinoma
- Adrenal adenoma

CLINICAL ISSUES

- Responsible for ~ 1.5% of pediatric hypertension
  - Sustained hypertension in 63%
  - Headache, sweating, flushing, palpitations, blurred vision, syncope, panic attacks, tremor, & weight loss
- Mean age: 11-13 years
- Diagnostic test of choice: Plasma or urine metanephrine
- Bilateral tumors in 19-38% of patients
- Malignant in up to 50% of pediatric patients
  - No histologic criteria for malignancy
- Treatment: Surgical excision of primary mass
  - α- & β-blockers to block effect of catecholamines

(Left) *Coronal Ga-68 DOTATATE PET in a young adult with multiple endocrine neoplasia (MEN) 2a shows intense uptake of the radiopharmaceutical in a right adrenal pheochromocytoma ➔. This agent is useful for neuroendocrine tumors, which generally have ↑ somatostatin receptors.* **(Right)** *Axial DWI MR in the same patient shows restricted diffusion ➔ in the small pheochromocytoma of the right adrenal gland.*

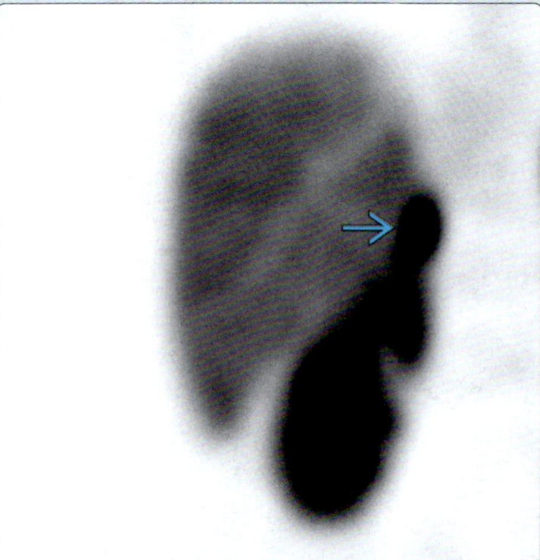

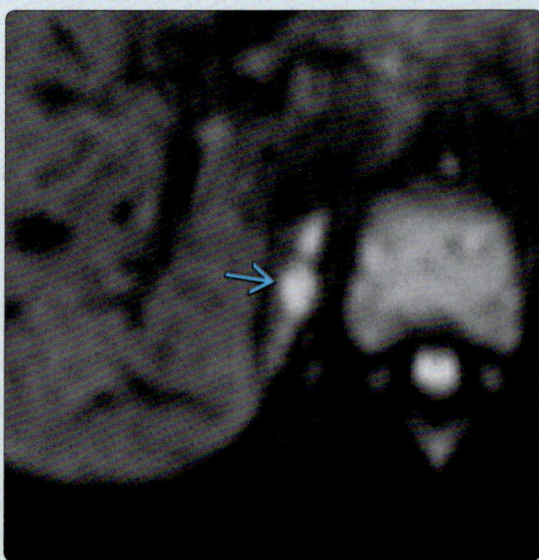

(Left) *Axial CECT in an adolescent with pheochromocytoma shows a heterogeneously enhancing mass ➔ at the inferior aspect of the right adrenal gland.* **(Right)** *Coronal fused MIBG SPECT CT in the same patient shows MIBG uptake ➔ within the right suprarenal pheochromocytoma. MIBG scans are used to identify tumors that manufacture catecholamines.*

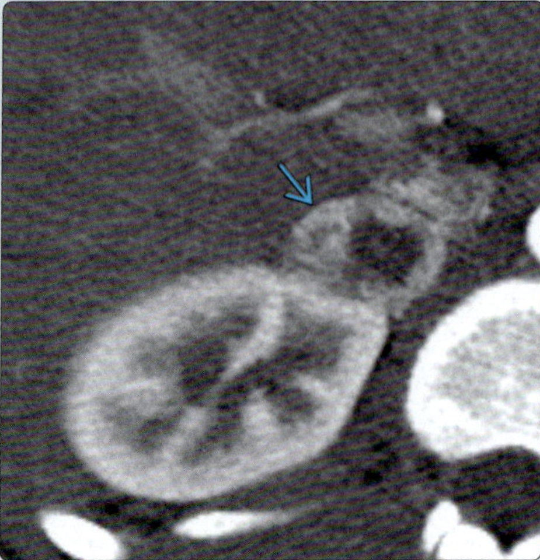

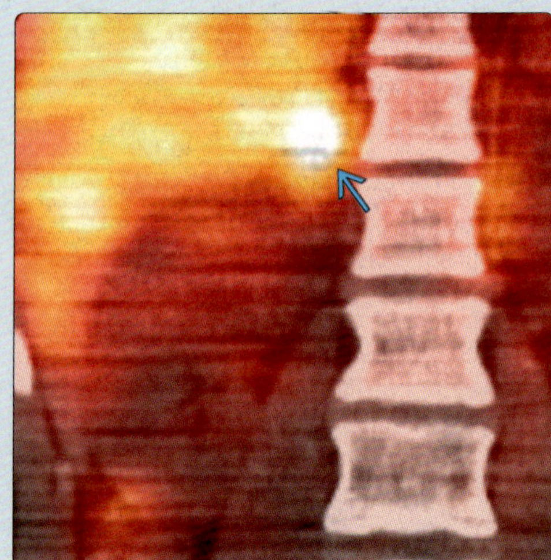

TERMINOLOGY

Definitions

- Paraganglioma arising from catecholamine-producing chromaffin cells of adrenal medulla

Associated Syndromes

- Hereditary predisposition in up to 40%
  - Mutations in succinate dehydrogenase (SDH), von Hippel-Lindau syndrome, multiple endocrine neoplasia type 2, & neurofibromatosis type 1
- Identifiable germline mutation in 70-80% of patients

IMAGING

General Features

- Best diagnostic clue
  - Suprarenal mass in child with hypertension
- Location
  - Adrenal gland

Ultrasonographic Findings

- Suprarenal soft tissue mass
- Iso- to hypoechoic to liver

CT Findings

- CECT
  - Homogeneously enhancing adrenal mass
  - Nonionic contrast material does not incite hypertensive crisis → premedication is not required

MR Findings

- T1: Isointense to muscle
  - No signal drop on opposed-phase images
- T2: Mildly to moderately hyperintense vs. "light bulb bright"
- T1 C+: Avid enhancement, prolonged washout
  - May have salt & pepper appearance with enhancing tumor & vascular flow voids
  - Larger lesions are more likely heterogeneous

Nuclear Medicine Findings

- PET/CT
  - Useful in searching for extraadrenal tumors or metastases
  - F-18 FDG PET is less sensitive & specific than MIBG scintigraphy
  - Ga-68 DOTATATE PET/CT is more sensitive than F-18 FDG PET
    - Identifies neuroendocrine tumors with somatostatin receptors
- MIBG scintigraphy
  - I-123 is used in children
  - ↑ uptake in tumors that produce catecholamines
  - Very specific but less sensitive than CT or MR
  - Useful in searching for extraadrenal tumors or metastases

Imaging Recommendations

- Best imaging tool
  - MR due to lack of ionizing radiation
  - MIBG or whole-body MR to identify extraadrenal tumor

DIFFERENTIAL DIAGNOSIS

Neuroblastoma

- Most common adrenal tumor in children
- Median age of presentation: 15-17 months
- Often large, multilobulated mass crossing midline; displaces & encases vessels; Ca^{2+} in ~ 85-90%
- MIBG for diagnosis & staging

Adrenocortical Carcinoma

- Large, heterogeneous adrenal mass causing virilization or precocious puberty in young child; ± inferior vena cava invasion

Adrenal Adenoma

- Smaller homogeneous mass with intracellular lipid
  - Signal drop-out on opposed-phase MR imaging

CLINICAL ISSUES

Presentation

- Most common signs/symptoms
  - Sustained hypertension in 63%
  - Symptoms of mass effect in up to 30%
- Other signs/symptoms
  - Headache, sweating, flushing, palpitations, blurred vision, syncope, panic attacks, tremor, & weight loss
  - Paroxysmal episodes: Headaches, palpitations, diaphoresis
  - Complications: Cardiomyopathy, hypertensive crisis, cardiovascular accidents, & seizures
- Laboratory tests
  - Diagnostic test of choice: Plasma or urine metanephrine

Demographics

- Age
  - Mean age: 11-13 years
- Epidemiology
  - Most common pediatric endocrine tumor
  - Responsible for ~ 1.5% of pediatric hypertension
  - Bilateral tumors in ~ 19-38% of patients

Natural History & Prognosis

- Malignant in up to 50% of pediatric patients
- No histologic criteria for malignancy
  - Malignancy determined by local tumor invasion or metastases (bones, lungs, liver)

Treatment

- Surgical excision of primary mass
  - Pretreatment with α- & β-blockers is required to block effect of catecholamines

SELECTED REFERENCES

1. Jochmanova I et al: Clinical characteristics and outcomes of SDHB-related pheochromocytoma and paraganglioma in children and adolescents. J Cancer Res Clin Oncol. 146(4):1051-63, 2020
2. Peard L et al: Pediatric pheochromocytoma: current status of diagnostic imaging and treatment procedures. Curr Opin Urol. 29(5):493-9, 2019
3. Jha A et al: Superiority of 68Ga-DOTATATE over 18F-FDG and anatomic imaging in the detection of succinate dehydrogenase mutation (SDHx)-related pheochromocytoma and paraganglioma in the pediatric population. Eur J Nucl Med Mol Imaging. 45(5):787-97, 2018
4. Sargar KM et al: Imaging of nonmalignant adrenal lesions in children. Radiographics. 37(6):1648-64, 2017

Hydrometrocolpos

KEY FACTS

TERMINOLOGY

- Dilation of vagina ± uterus secondary to distal stenosis, atresia, transverse vaginal septum, or imperforate hymen
  - Prefix: "Hydro-" meaning fluid, "hemato-" meaning blood
  - Suffix: "-metra" meaning uterine cavity
  - Suffix: "-metrocolpos" meaning uterus & vagina

IMAGING

- Well-defined, cystic or debris-filled mass in female pelvis between urinary bladder & rectum
- Vertically oriented in sagittal plane, round in axial plane
- Uterus is frequently visible arising from dome of collection; may be normal or mildly distended (much less than vagina)
- US may show trilaminar appearance of vaginal wall, swirling internal debris, lack of internal vascularity
- MR often shows aging blood product signal intensities (↑ T1, ↓ T2); can help discern uterine & vaginal anomalies
- Urinary bladder or ureters may be obstructed
- Check for associated renal anomalies: Unilateral renal agenesis or secondary hydronephrosis
- Primary imaging modality for female genitourinary (GU) anomalies: US
- MR is used when uterine & complex GU anomalies cannot be clearly defined with US

PATHOLOGY

- Imperforate hymen is more common cause of obstruction than vaginal septum
- ± associated anal, renal, vertebral, & cardiac anomalies

CLINICAL ISSUES

- Bimodal age of presentation
  - Infants (due to maternal hormonal stimulation): Pelvic mass, sepsis, or urinary tract obstruction
    - Vaginal contents are more likely mucous, fluid
  - Adolescent girls (pubertal onset): Delayed menarche, cyclic pelvic pain, mass, &/or urinary tract obstruction
    - Vaginal contents are more likely blood

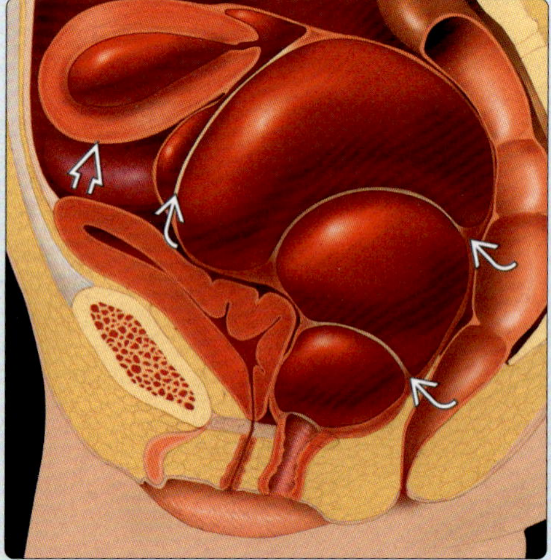

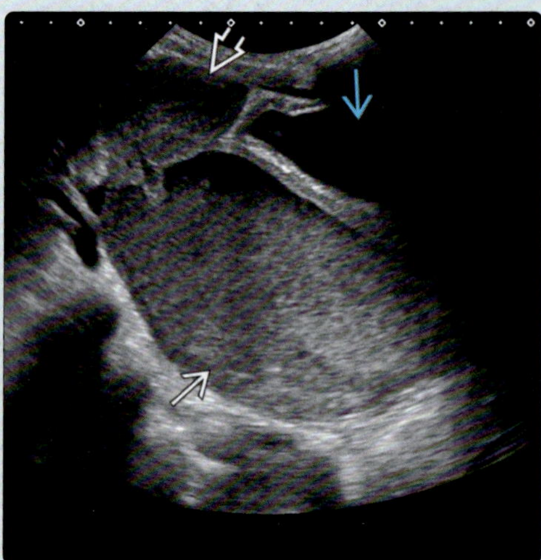

(Left) *Lateral graphic shows potential levels of vaginal septa ➔ causing obstruction & hydro-/hematometrocolpos. Note that the vagina distends to a much greater degree than the uterus ➔.* **(Right)** *Longitudinal transabdominal US through the pelvis of a 12-year-old girl with urinary retention, cramping, & no history of menses shows a large, well-marginated, heterogeneous collection ➔ posterior to the urinary bladder ➔, suggestive of hematometrocolpos. The uterus ➔ is slightly anteflexed but not distended.*

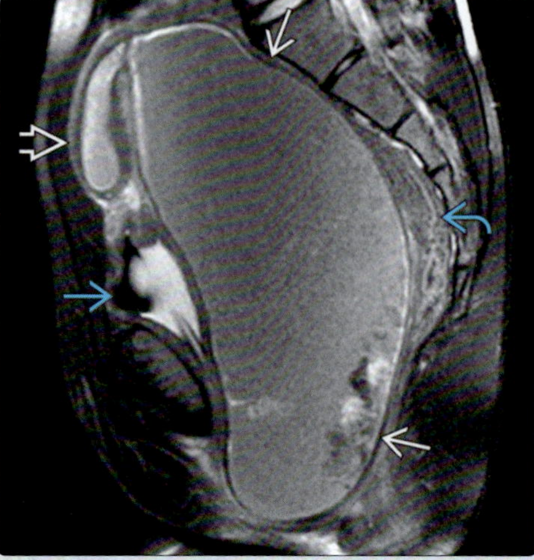

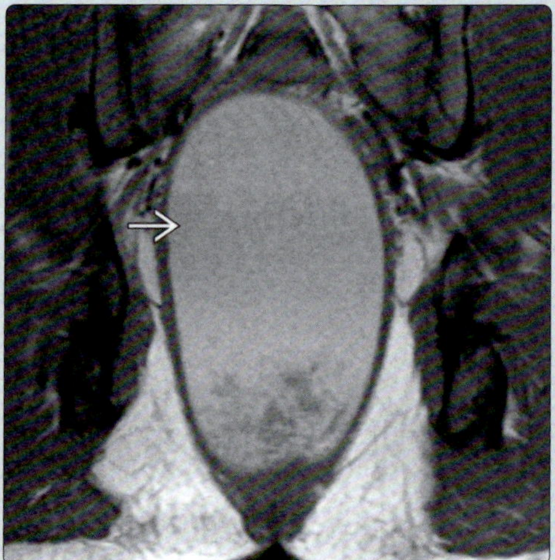

(Left) *Sagittal T2 FS MR in the same patient shows a markedly distended vagina ➔ containing heterogeneous fluid & layering debris. The uterus ➔ projects anteriorly & is much less distended than the vagina, findings typical of hematometrocolpos. Note the mass effect on the urinary bladder ➔ & rectum ➔.* **(Right)** *Coronal T1 MR in the same patient shows that the fluid in the vagina is predominantly hyperintense ➔, typical of blood products. A vaginal septum was resected, relieving the obstruction.*

TERMINOLOGY

Abbreviations

- Hydrometrocolpos (HMC)

Synonyms

- Hematometrocolpos, hydrometra, hematometra

Definitions

- Dilation of vagina or vagina & uterus secondary to distal stenosis, atresia, transverse vaginal septum, or imperforate membrane
  - Prefix: "Hydro-" meaning fluid, "hemato-" meaning blood
  - Suffix: "-metra" meaning uterine cavity
  - Suffix: "-metrocolpos" meaning uterus & vagina

IMAGING

General Features

- Best diagnostic clue
  - Well-defined, cystic or debris-filled vertically oriented mass in pelvis, between bladder & rectum
  - Can cause secondary bladder outlet obstruction with hydronephrosis
- Location
  - Between bladder & rectum
- Size
  - Variable; can be very large & simulate mass or early pregnancy in teenage girls
- Morphology
  - Vertically oriented on sagittal & coronal images, round on axial images
- Classic imaging appearance: Echogenic debris filling dilated vagina & (to lesser extent) uterus, creating mass effect in pelvis
  - Vagina has elastic walls & can dilate more than uterus
- Can be associated with müllerian duct fusion anomalies, particularly uterus didelphys

Radiographic Findings

- Soft tissue mass in pelvis displacing bowel loops
- Case reports of peritoneal Ca^{2+}, presumably from debris spilling out of fallopian tubes

Ultrasonographic Findings

- Grayscale ultrasound
  - Echogenic, layering debris in large, well-defined cavity between urinary bladder & rectum
    - Distended vaginal walls may have trilaminar appearance, mimicking gut signature sign
    - Fluid in vagina will typically swirl with mild compression
  - Relatively small uterus is frequently visible arising from dome of collection
    - Look for variable uterine distention (typically much less than vagina)
    - Look for associated müllerian duct fusion anomalies
  - Urinary bladder & ureters may be dilated from secondary bladder outlet or ureteral compression
  - Also confirm presence of both kidneys, look for secondary hydronephrosis
- Color Doppler
  - Useful to confirm lack of blood flow within debris-filled cavities, as complex blood (especially acute) may appear solid on US

CT Findings

- CECT
  - Vertically elongated, fluid-filled cavity with enhancing walls originating deep in pelvis
    - Appears round on axial images
  - Displaces bladder, rectum, & small bowel
  - Enhancing uterus extends from cephalad aspect of collection
    - Scrutinize uterus for associated malformations

MR Findings

- MR findings are similar to CECT
- Aging blood components may have characteristic signal intensity (↑ T1, ↓ T2)
- Multiplanar imaging is useful to optimally profile uterine & cervical anomalies
  - Consider planes oriented to uterus

Other Modality Findings

- Percutaneous/transvaginal drainage if septic or complex care
- Rarely, hysterosalpingography or sonohysterography is performed in convalescent phase to reevaluate uterine morphology

Imaging Recommendations

- Best imaging tool
  - US is best initial imaging modality for suspected genitourinary (GU) pathology in female
  - MR is used when uterine & complex GU anomalies cannot be clearly defined with US
    - Consider delaying MR exam to convalescent phase, after fluid & debris have been drained

DIFFERENTIAL DIAGNOSIS

Perforated Appendicitis

- Poorly defined inflammatory collection of right lower quadrant
- May visualize appendiceal remnant, appendicolith

Meconium Pseudocyst

- Heterogeneous peritoneal collection (± Ca^{2+}) in newborn, typically secondary to in utero bowel perforation
- Dilated bowel is usually still present

Lymphatic Malformation

- Infiltrative multicystic mass with thin septations
- Individual compartments show varying complexity, typically due to hemorrhage

Pelvic Abscess

- Heterogeneous adnexal collection with surrounding inflammation
- Unlikely in newborn
- In adolescents, consider pelvic inflammatory disease

Fallopian Tube Torsion, Cyst, or Obstruction

- Tubular fluid collection with folds

Pelvic Rhabdomyosarcoma

- Sarcoma botryoides protrudes into vagina ("cluster of grapes")

Other Pelvic Masses

- Sacrococcygeal teratoma
- Burkitt lymphoma
- Pelvic neuroblastoma

PATHOLOGY

General Features

- Etiology
  - Embryology-anatomy: Failure of canalization with stenosis or atresia along lumen
  - In infancy, maternal hormone effects stimulate neonatal uterus & vagina
- Genetics
  - Generally sporadic; not inherited
  - McKusick-Kaufman syndrome
    - Rare multiple autosomal recessive syndrome
      - HMC
      - Postaxial polydactyly
      - Congenital heart malformation
  - Bardet-Biedl syndrome, a.k.a. Laurence-Moon syndrome
    - Also has HMC & postaxial polydactyly with retinitis pigmentosa, obesity, & learning disability becoming apparent by early school age
    - Inherited as autosomal recessive trait
- Associated abnormalities
  - Associated anal, renal, vertebral, & cardiac anomalies are most common
  - Also associated with intestinal aganglionosis, imperforate anus, urogenital sinus, cloacal anomalies
  - Can be associated with müllerian duct fusion anomalies, particularly uterus didelphys
    - Obstructed hemivagina & ipsilateral renal anomaly (OHVIRA), a.k.a. Herlyn-Werner-Wunderlich syndrome
      - Uterus didelphys, cervicovaginal obstruction, unilateral renal agenesis
  - Iatrogenic cases have been reported due to malposition of artificial urinary sphincter in prepubertal girls
- Site of obstruction can be
  - Imperforate hymen
  - Vaginal stenosis or atresia
  - Cervical stenosis or atresia
  - Mass effect from duplications of uterus & vagina (didelphys)
  - Transverse vaginal septum
    - Most common location: Between middle & upper 1/3 of vagina
    - These patients have functional uteri, though fertility can be compromised
- Secondary urinary obstruction can occur at level of
  - Urethra, ureterovesical junction, ureter

Gross Pathologic & Surgical Features

- Debris contents
  - In fetal life & infancy, contents are primarily of cervical mucus (mucocolpos or hydrocolpos)
    - Maternal estrogen stimulates cervical mucus production & causes swelling of labia minora
  - Peripubertal contents are typically blood, sloughed endometrial lining, & cervical/vaginal mucus

CLINICAL ISSUES

Presentation

- Most common signs/symptoms
  - In infancy: Presents as pelvic mass, sepsis, or urinary tract obstruction
  - In adolescent girls: Presents as delayed menarche, cyclic pelvic pain, mass, &/or urinary tract obstruction
- Other signs/symptoms
  - Occasionally presents as prolapsing interlabial mass
  - In utero urinary tract obstruction from massive HMC can lead to fetal anuria, oligohydramnios with pulmonary hypoplasia, & renal dysplasia with renal failure in newborn
    - Intrauterine aspiration of obstructed bladder or vagina may be attempted

Demographics

- Age
  - Bimodal age presentation: Infancy or peripubertal
- Epidemiology
  - Transverse vaginal septum incidence: 1 in 80,000
  - Imperforate hymen is more common

Natural History & Prognosis

- Immediate prognosis is excellent
- Compromised fertility & endometriosis can be long-term complications

Treatment

- Typically drained with septum or stenotic segment excised from inferior approach; minimal tissue is resected
- Stenoses & focal atresias may require primary anastomosis & perioperative stenting
- Secondary hydronephrosis typically resolves spontaneously without additional intervention

SELECTED REFERENCES

1. Liu M et al: New consideration of Herlyn-Werner-Wunderlich syndrome diagnosed by ultrasound. J Ultrasound Med.40(9):1893-900, 2020
2. Goncalves LF et al: Prenatal and postnatal imaging techniques in the evaluation of disorders of sex development. Semin Pediatr Surg. 28(5):150839, 2019
3. Xu S et al: MRI features and differential diagnoses of congenital vaginal atresia. Gynecol Endocrinol. 35(9):777-81, 2019
4. Garcia Rodriguez R et al: Fetal hydrometrocolpos and congenital imperforate hymen: prenatal and postnatal imaging features. J Clin Ultrasound. 46(8):549-52, 2018
5. Simonetti I et al: A rare case of hydrometrocolpos from persistent urogenital sinus in patient affected by adrenogenital syndrome. J Ultrasound. 21(3):249-52, 2018
6. Veiga VF et al: Pelvic pain in young girls: not only dysmenorrhoea! BMJ Case Rep. 2018, 2018
7. Iraha Y et al: CT and MR imaging of gynecologic emergencies. Radiographics. 37(5):1569-86, 2017
8. Naffaa L et al: Imaging of acute pelvic pain in girls: ovarian torsion and beyond. Curr Probl Diagn Radiol. 46(4):317-29, 2017
9. Saleh R et al: Hematometrocolpos disguised as abdominal pain. J Emerg Med. 53(5):e97-9, 2017
10. Zhang H et al: MRI in the evaluation of obstructive reproductive tract anomalies in paediatric patients. Clin Radiol. 72(7):612.e7-15, 2017
11. Kraus SJ: Radiologic diagnosis of a newborn with cloaca. Semin Pediatr Surg. 25(2):76-81, 2016

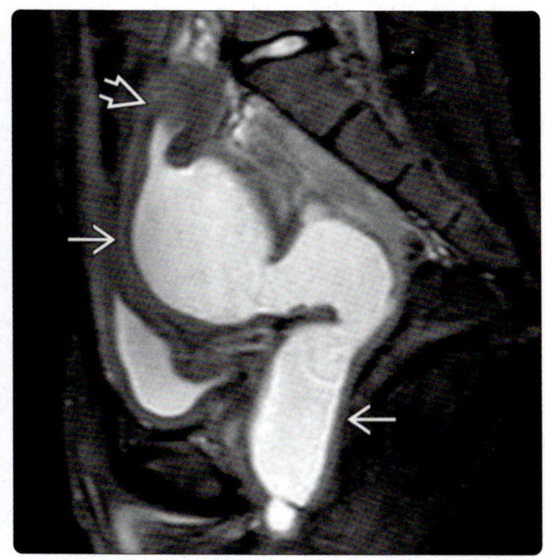

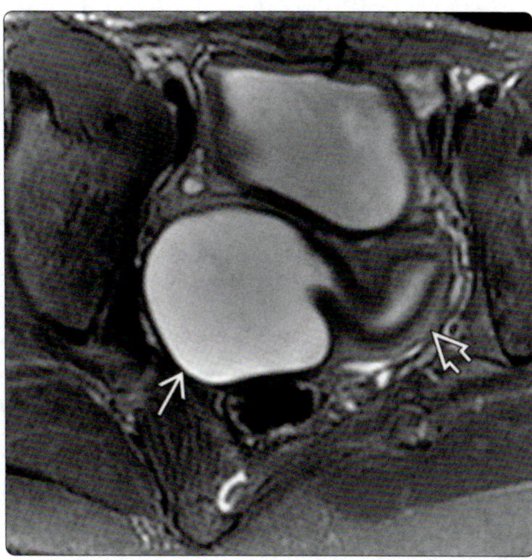

(Left) *Sagittal STIR MR in a 14-year-old who had a cloacal repair in infancy shows fluid distending her tortuous neovagina ➡ &, to a lesser degree, her endometrial cavity ➡. This was due to a stricture at the introitus.* **(Right)** *Axial T2 FS MR in a 12-year-old with pelvic pain shows a very distended vagina ➡ with high-signal fluid extending into the uterus ➡, consistent with hydrometrocolpos.*

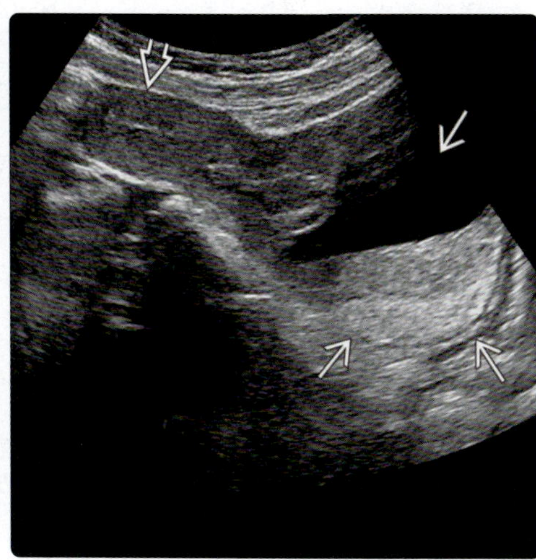

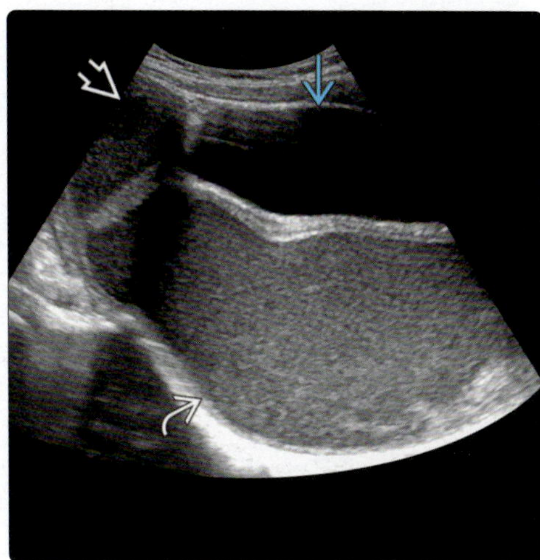

(Left) *Longitudinal US in a teenage girl with right lower quadrant & pelvic pain shows heterogenous material distending the vagina ➡ in layers, from anechoic anteriorly to hyperechoic posteriorly in this case of hematocolpos. The uterus ➡ is not distended.* **(Right)** *Longitudinal oblique US in a case of hematometrocolpos in a teenager with cyclic pain shows marked distention of a debris-filled vagina ➡ posterior to the bladder ➡. Note the mildly distended uterus ➡.*

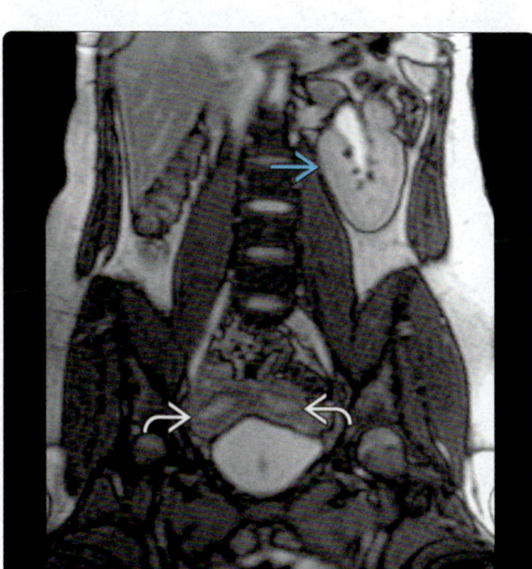

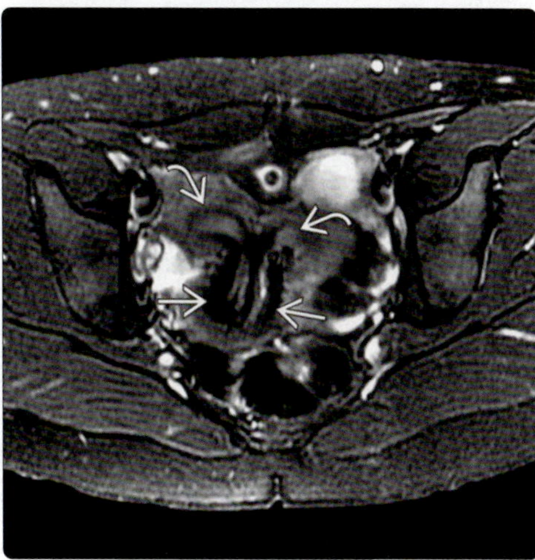

(Left) *Coronal SSFP localizer MR in a patient who had a "vaginal collection" drained at an outside hospital shows 2 endometrial cavities ➡ draped over the bladder. A solitary left kidney ➡ is noted, a commonly associated abnormality.* **(Right)** *Axial T2 FS MR shows the paired cervices ➡ & endometrial cavities ➡ in the same patient with uterine didelphys & an obstructing septum of a hemivagina (that led to hematometrocolpos). This combination of findings is typical of Herlyn-Werner-Wunderlich syndrome.*

Müllerian Duct Anomalies

KEY FACTS

TERMINOLOGY

- Abnormal development, improper fusion, or failure of resorption of müllerian (paramesonephric) duct structures

IMAGING

- Abnormal contour of uterus &/or structural abnormality of endometrial cavity or vagina
- Septate uterus is most common müllerian duct anomaly (MDA): 55%
- MR is best for definitive diagnosis
- Always image kidneys to look for renal anomaly

PATHOLOGY

- MDAs occur in 1 of 3 phases
  - Organogenesis: Agenesis, hypoplasia, unicornuate
  - Fusion: Didelphys, bicornuate
  - Septal resorption: Septate, arcuate
- Renal anomaly is present in ~ 30%
  - Renal agenesis is most common (~ 2/3)

CLINICAL ISSUES

- Asymptomatic
- Symptoms may develop at menarche
  - Primary amenorrhea
  - Dysmenorrhea
  - Cyclic abdominal pain
- Incidence is estimated at 1%
- Critical to differentiate septate vs. bicornuate uterus
  - Septate is treated with hysteroscopic resection of septum
  - Bicornuate rarely requires surgery
- Treatment
  - Surgery to remove rudimentary horn, resect septum, or relieve obstruction

DIAGNOSTIC CHECKLIST

- Outer fundal contour is important for differentiating bicornuate from septate uterus

(Left) *Graphic of a septate uterus shows minimal indentation of the uterine fundus ➔. There is myometrium in the superior aspect of the septum, though normal zonal anatomy is not present in this portion ➔.* **(Right)** *Axial T2 MR of a septate uterus shows that the outer fundal contour is smooth ➔, & the intercornual angle is < 75°. There is a low-signal fibrous septum extending along the length of the endometrial cavity ➔ to a single cervix.*

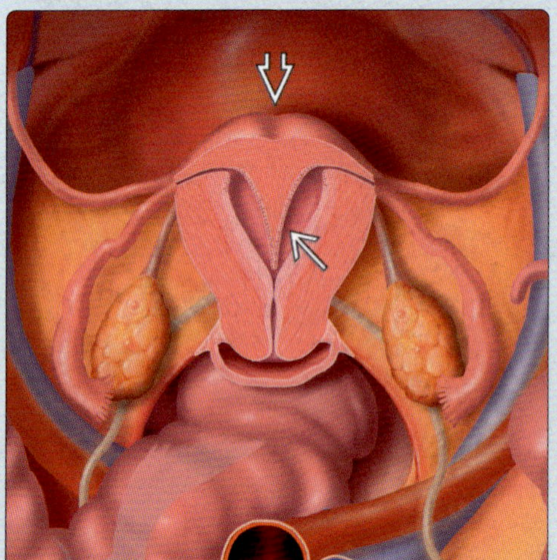

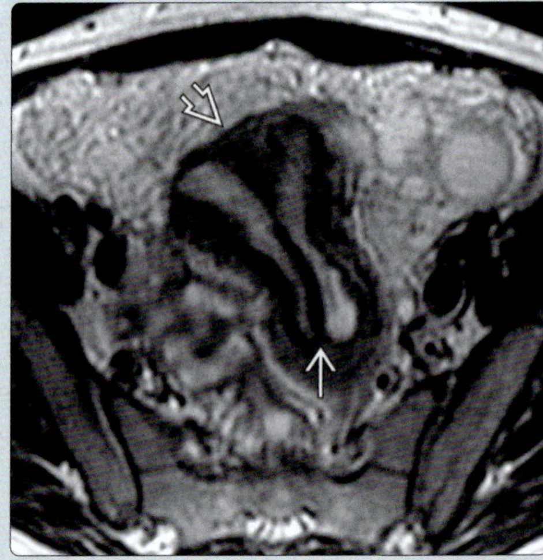

(Left) *Graphic of a bicornuate uterus demonstrates a deep external fundal cleft ➔ & 2 symmetric cornua ➔ that are fused inferiorly.* **(Right)** *Transverse US shows the outer contour/notch ➔ of this bicornuate uterus due to a small amount of free fluid in the pelvis. The 2 endometrial cavities ➔ are separated by myometrium.*

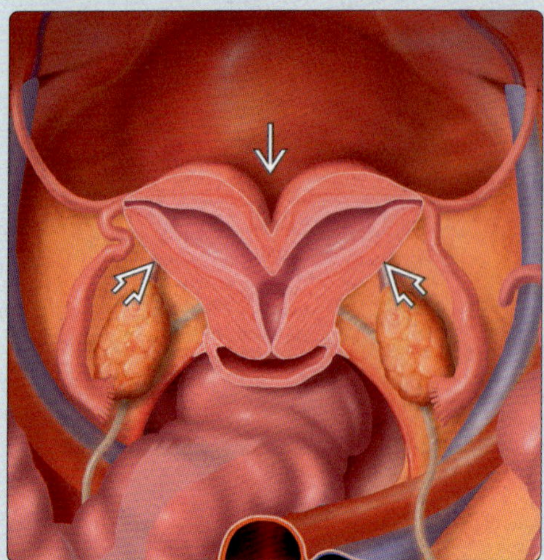

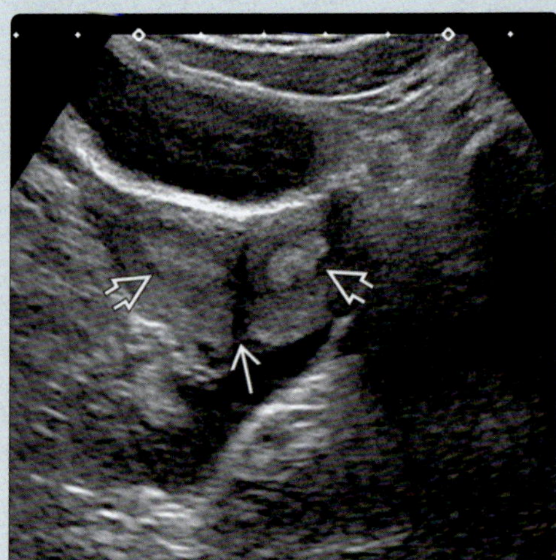

TERMINOLOGY

Abbreviations

- Müllerian duct anomalies (MDA)

Synonyms

- Uterine fusion anomalies
- Subtype: Obstructed hemivagina & ipsilateral renal agenesis (OHVIRA syndrome)

Definitions

- Abnormal development, improper fusion, or failure of resorption of müllerian (paramesonephric) duct structures
  - Müllerian agenesis or hypoplasia (class I in American Fertility Society classification system)
    - Complete or segmental agenesis or variable degrees of uterovaginal hypoplasia
  - Unicornuate uterus (class II)
    - Partial or complete unilateral hypoplasia
  - Uterus didelphys (class III)
    - Duplication of uterus
  - Bicornuate uterus (class IV)
    - Incomplete fusion of superior uterovaginal canal
  - Septate uterus (class V)
    - Incomplete resorption of uterine septum
  - Arcuate uterus (class VI)
    - Near-complete resorption of uterine septum

IMAGING

General Features

- Best diagnostic clue
  - Abnormal contour of uterus &/or structural abnormality of endometrial cavity or vagina
- **Müllerian agenesis or hypoplasia**
  - Mayer-Rokitansky-Kuster-Hauser syndrome
    - Aplasia of upper 2/3 of vagina
    - 90% have uterine agenesis
    - 10% have rudimentary uterus
    - Incidence of 1 in 4,500 women
    - 2nd most common cause of primary amenorrhea (gonadal dysgenesis is 1st)
  - ± hydrometrocolpos
- **Unicornuate uterus**
  - 20% of MDAs
  - Single-horned uterus
  - Asymmetric curved & elongated (banana-shaped)
  - Hypoplastic uterine horn of variable size is usually present
    - May be cavitary or noncavitary
      - Cavity may communicate with contralateral endometrium
  - ± hydrometrocolpos with obstruction
- **Uterus didelphys**
  - 5% of MDAs
  - Bilateral hemiuteri with noncommunicating endometrial cavities
  - Divergent uterine horns with deep fundal cleft
    - Each horn has normal zonal anatomy
  - 2 cervices
  - Vaginal septum is present in 75%
  - Herlyn-Werner-Wunderlich syndrome (OHVIRA): Uterus didelphys, blind hemivagina, ipsilateral renal agenesis
  - ± hematometrocolpos with obstruction
- **Bicornuate uterus**
  - 10% of MDAs
  - 2 symmetric cornua are fused inferiorly
    - Normal zonal anatomy is maintained
    - ± septum of fibrous tissue (low signal on T2)
  - External fundal cleft
    - Must be at least 1 cm in depth
      - Differentiates bicornuate from septate uterus
    - Extends to internal cervical os in complete bicornuate uterus
  - Intercornual angle is variable
    - > 105° is suggestive of bicornuate (not septate) uterus
  - Usually single cervix though variations exist
    - Bicornuate bicollis: Duplicated cervix, though there is some degree of communication between horns
  - ± hydrometrocolpos with obstruction
- **Septate uterus**
  - Most common MDA (55%)
  - Persistent uterovaginal septum of variable length
    - Septum extends into upper vagina in 25%
    - Inferior portion of septum is composed of fibrous tissue (low signal on T2)
    - Cervical duplication is rare
  - External fundal contour is usually mildly convex or flat though can be indented < 1 cm
  - Intercornual angle is variable
    - < 75° is suggestive of septate (not bicornuate) uterus
  - Overall uterine size is normal though each endometrial cavity is smaller than normal
  - ± hydrometrocolpos with obstruction
- **Arcuate uterus**
  - Mild convex indentation on fundal endometrium
  - Normal external fundal contour
  - No fibrous component
- **Vaginal septum**
  - Can be associated with any MDA
  - ± transverse or longitudinal

Ultrasonographic Findings

- Usually 1st imaging test performed, so important to recognize abnormality
- Altered uterine contour & endometrial cavity as above
- Limitations
  - Uterine characterization is limited from 2-3 months until puberty due to small size
    - Some anomalies can be seen prenatally & in neonate under influence of maternal hormones
  - Can be difficult to image outer fundal contour
    - Need transverse view of fundus in orthogonal plane
  - Demonstrating communication between endometrial cavities can also be challenging
  - 3D can be helpful
- Always image kidneys when MDA is identified

MR Findings

- T1WI
  - When obstructed, high signal intensity contents indicate hemorrhagic byproducts

- T2WI
  - Normal zonal anatomy
    - High-signal endometrium & intermediate-/high-signal myometrium
    - Junctional zone is seen as low-signal line separating endometrium & myometrium
  - Imaging parallel to long axis of uterus is best for determining uterine morphology
  - In unicornuate & uterine hypoplasia, hypoplastic uterine remnant is best seen on sagittal or axial T2
    - Usually intermediate or low signal intensity myometrium with small endometrial cavity
  - Fibrous septum is low signal intensity (septate, bicornuate)

Radiographic Findings

- Hysterosalpingography
  - Classification is based on contour/morphology of endometrial cavity or cavities
  - Outer fundal contour is not visible

Imaging Recommendations

- Best imaging tool
  - Ultrasound as initial screening exam
  - MR for definitive diagnosis
- Protocol advice
  - Image kidneys when MDA is identified on ultrasound
  - MR
    - Combination of T1/T2 for external contour & endometrial cavity
    - Image parallel to long axis of uterus for fundal contour
    - T2 is best for distinguishing zonal anatomy
    - Obtain at least 1 coronal series to cover renal fossa

DIFFERENTIAL DIAGNOSIS

Imperforate Hymen

- Not associated with MDA
- Differentiation from low transverse vaginal septum can be difficult by imaging

Cervical Stenosis

- ± inflammatory, iatrogenic, or secondary to mass effect
- Mimics MDA if obstructed & endometrium is distorted

PATHOLOGY

General Features

- Etiology
  - Müllerian duct structures
    - Fallopian tubes
    - Uterus
    - Cervix
    - Upper 2/3 of vagina
  - MDAs occur in 1 of 3 phases
    - Organogenesis: Agenesis, hypoplasia, unicornuate
    - Fusion: Didelphys, bicornuate
    - Septal resorption: Septate, arcuate
- Associated abnormalities
  - Renal anomaly is present in ~ 30%
    - Renal agenesis is most common (~ 2/3)
    - Ectopic kidney
    - Horseshoe kidney
    - Renal dysplasia
    - Duplicated collecting system

CLINICAL ISSUES

Presentation

- Most common signs/symptoms
  - Asymptomatic
  - Symptoms may develop at menarche
    - Primary amenorrhea, dysmenorrhea, cyclic abdominal pain

Demographics

- Epidemiology
  - Incidence is estimated at 1%

Natural History & Prognosis

- Fertility issues
- Spontaneous abortions
- Ectopic pregnancy
- Endometriosis is postulated to result from retrograde menstruation

Treatment

- Septate vs. bicornuate uterus is important
  - Septate treated with hysteroscopic resection of septum
  - Bicornuate rarely requires surgery
- Medical: Suppression of menses
- Surgical
  - Removal of rudimentary horn
  - Relieve obstruction
  - Resection of uterine septum

DIAGNOSTIC CHECKLIST

Image Interpretation Pearls

- Outer fundal contour is important for differentiating bicornuate from septate uterus
- Define endometrial cavity & presence of communication when there are 2 uterine horns
- 1 or 2 cervices: Complete bicornuate vs. bicornuate bicollis vs. didelphys
  - Differentiate low-signal septum extending through single cervical os from 2 separate cervices

SELECTED REFERENCES

1. Habiba M et al: The development of the human uterus: morphogenesis to menarche. Hum Reprod Update. 27(1):1-26, 2021
2. O'Flynn O'Brien KL et al: The prevalence of müllerian anomalies in women with a diagnosed renal anomaly. J Pediatr Adolesc Gynecol. 34(2):154-60, 2020
3. Pitot MA et al: Müllerian duct anomalies coincident with endometriosis: a review. Abdom Radiol (NY). 45(6):1723-40, 2020
4. Yen CF et al: Laparoscopic metroplasty: reconstructive surgery for unicornuate uterus with noncommunicating, functional uterine horn. Fertil Steril. 114(5):1119-21, 2020
5. Ludwin A et al: Septate uterus according to ESHRE/ESGE, ASRM and CUME definitions: association with infertility and miscarriage, cost and warnings for women and healthcare systems. Ultrasound Obstet Gynecol. 54(6):800-14, 2019
6. Jegannathan D et al: Magnetic resonance imaging of classified and unclassified Müllerian duct anomalies: comparison of the American Society for Reproductive Medicine and the European Society of Human Reproduction and Embryology classifications. SA J Radiol. 22(1):1259, 2018

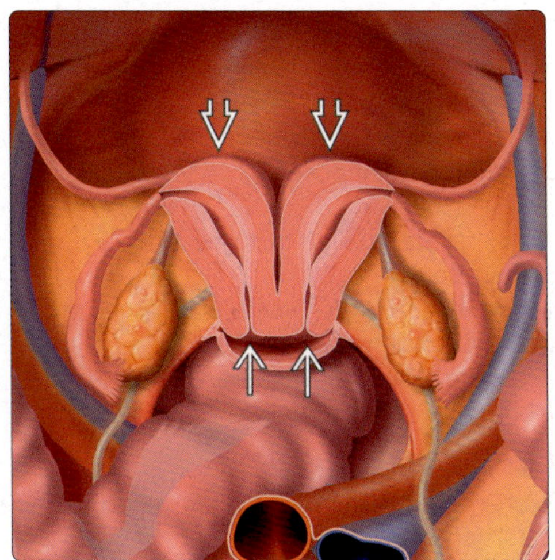

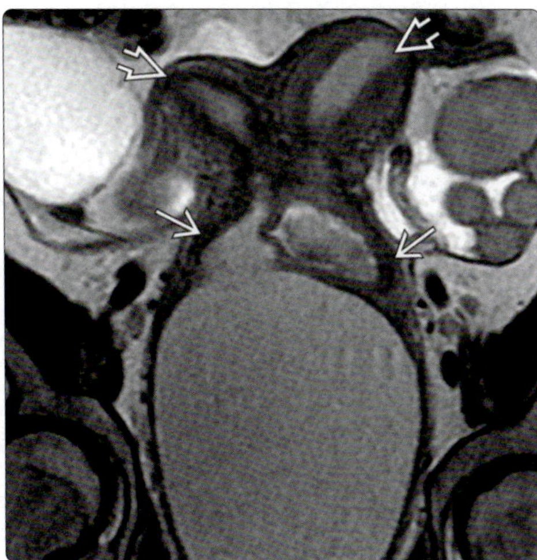

(Left) *Graphic of uterus didelphys shows 2 separate uterine horns ➩, each with normal zonal anatomy as well as 2 cervices ➩.* **(Right)** *Coronal oblique T2 MR shows 2 separate uterine horns ➩, 2 cervices ➩, & a massively distended vaginal vault in this patient with hydrometrocolpos & obstructed didelphys.*

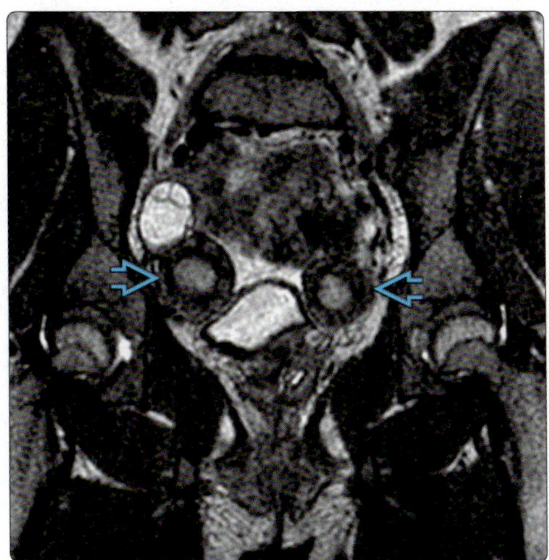

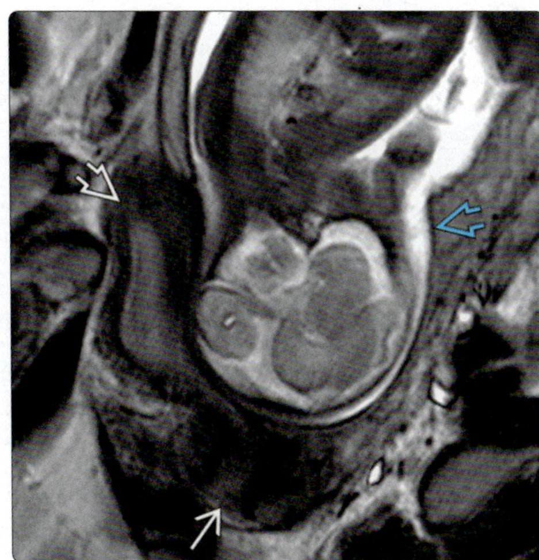

(Left) *Coronal T2 MR shows 2 uterine horns ➩ that are widely separated in the pelvis in a patient with didelphys & an anorectal malformation.* **(Right)** *Coronal oblique T2 MR shows a uterus didelphys with a 25-week fetus in the left uterine horn ➩ as compared to endometrial proliferation in the right horn ➩. Both cervices are closed ➩.*

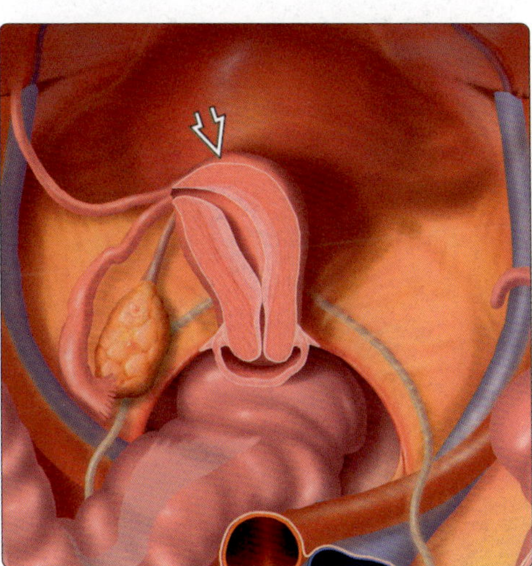

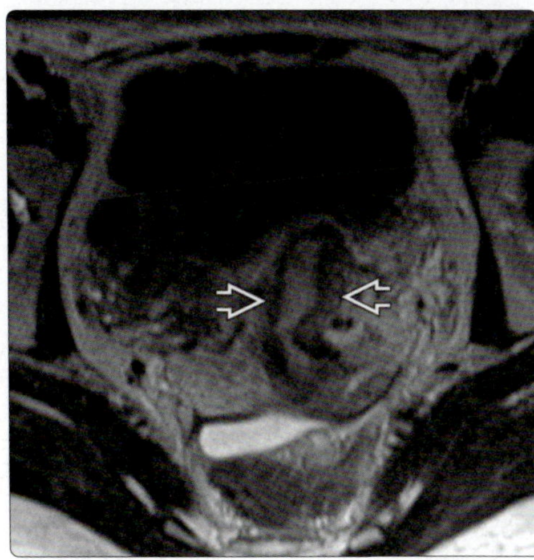

(Left) *Graphic of a unicornuate uterus ➩ illustrates the typical banana shape. There is complete absence of left-sided müllerian duct structures, although this is not always the case.* **(Right)** *Axial T2 MR from an 18-year-old demonstrates a unicornuate uterus ➩ to the left of midline. A right uterine horn was present (not shown). No renal anomalies were observed.*

KEY FACTS

TERMINOLOGY

- Follicle: Normal physiologic cyst < 1 cm in diameter
  - Dominant follicle may measure up to 3 cm
- Functional cysts: Can measure up to 3-10 cm
  - Corpus luteal cyst: Dominant follicle after ovulation
  - Follicular cyst: Normal mature follicle fails to involute
- Hemorrhagic cyst: Hemorrhage into functional cyst

IMAGING

- Ultrasound is mainstay of ovarian imaging; MR in limited circumstances
- Well-marginated, round or ovoid structure within borders of ovary with no solid component
  - Thin wall (< 3 mm)
  - No internal septa, nodule, fat, Ca^{2+}, or vascularity
  - ↑ heterogeneity with hemorrhage: Internal reticulations (or lace-like pattern) of clot mixed with tiny cystic spaces vs. layering debris

CLINICAL ISSUES

- Usually asymptomatic; pain if large or complicated by rupture, hemorrhage, or torsion
- Treatment/prognosis
  - > 90% of all functional cysts resolve spontaneously
  - Cysts < 3 cm should be considered physiologic in pre- & postmenarchal children
  - Cysts up to 4-5 cm are usually monitored with surveillance ultrasound
  - Surgery vs. further imaging is considered in larger cysts due to risk of torsion or neoplasm
    - For resection, ovarian sparing approach is preferred if benign etiology is suspected

DIAGNOSTIC CHECKLIST

- With cystic ovarian lesion in child, radiologist must consider: Could this be torsion, neoplasm, or other pathology?
- Follow-up ultrasound of asymptomatic cyst in 4-6 weeks if initial study is unclear (due to size or mild complexity)

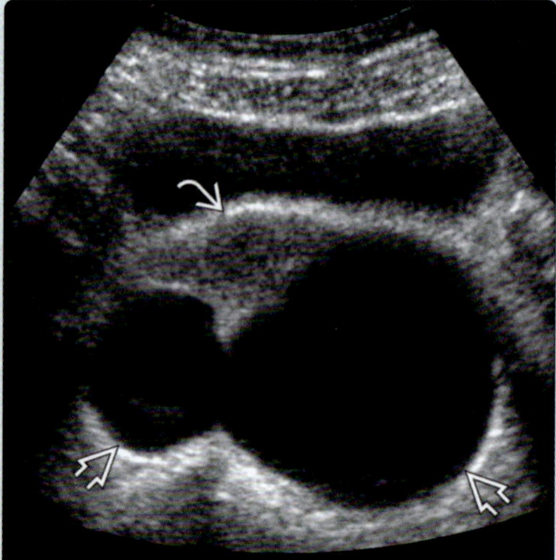

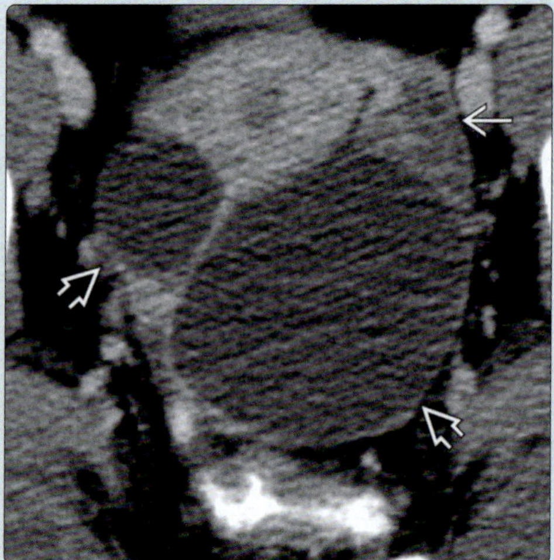

(Left) *Transverse ultrasound shows 2 well-defined, round, anechoic structures ➔ abutting the uterus ➔, both of which have imperceptible walls & ↑ through transmission, consistent with simple cysts.* **(Right)** *Axial CECT obtained in the same patient also demonstrates typical characteristics of simple cysts ➔. The normal-appearing left ovary ➔ lies directly adjacent to the larger cyst on this image. Both cysts resolved by the time of a follow-up ultrasound obtained several weeks later, consistent with follicular cysts.*

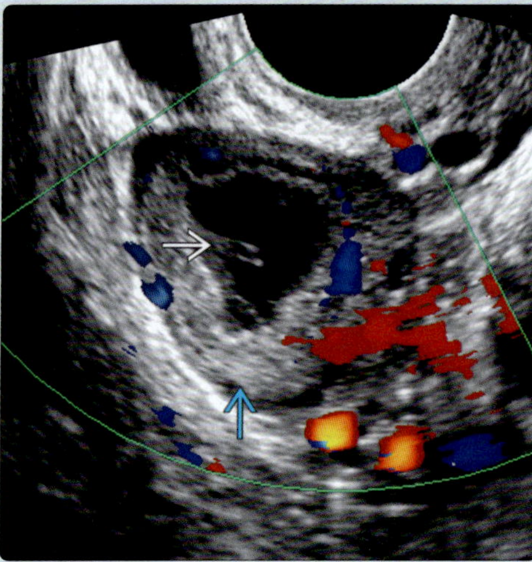

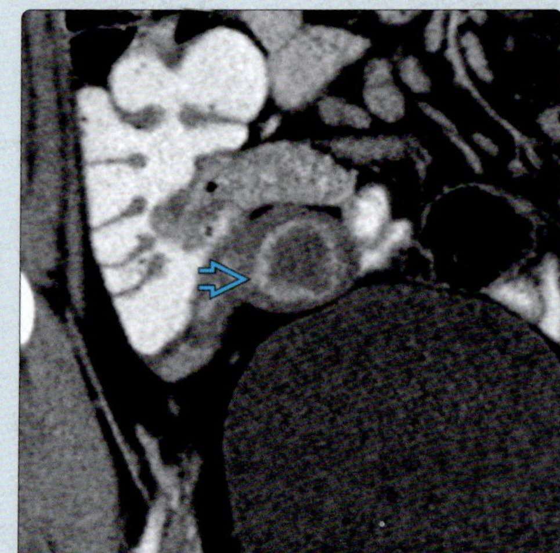

(Left) *Transverse endovaginal color Doppler ultrasound shows a hypoechoic structure within the right ovary ➔ that has an irregular contour, a hyperechoic rim, & a small amount of echogenic material centrally ➔. There is mild adjacent hyperemia. The findings are characteristic of a corpus luteal cyst.* **(Right)** *Coronal CECT of the same patient on the same day shows the typical mildly thickened, irregular, hypervascular wall indicative of a corpus luteal cyst ➔.*

TERMINOLOGY

Definitions

- Well-marginated, round or ovoid structure within or at borders of ovary; no solid component
  - No fat, Ca^{2+}, or septa
  - Thin, imperceptible wall (< 3 mm thick)
  - May appear more complex after internal hemorrhage
  - No internal vascularity on color Doppler imaging
- Definitions of different cyst types & their sizes vary
  - Follicle
    - Generally < 1 cm in diameter
    - Dominant follicle may measure up to 3 cm
  - Functional cysts
    - Corpus luteal cyst
      - After ovulation, dominant follicle becomes corpus luteal cyst
      - Usually < 3 cm, though can be much larger
    - Follicular cyst
      - Occurs when normal mature follicle fails to ovulate/involute
      - Usually 3-10 cm
  - Hemorrhagic cyst
    - Hemorrhage occurs into one of above

IMAGING

General Features

- Best diagnostic clue
  - Simple cyst: Unilocular with imperceptible wall & near water echogenicity/attenuation/signal intensity internally with no central complexity or vascularity
- Size
  - Cysts < 3 cm should be considered physiologic in pre- & postmenarchal children
  - Cysts > 4-5 cm may require additional consideration
- Morphology
  - Round or ovoid with well-defined margins

Ultrasonographic Findings

- Differentiation of follicle & functional cyst is mainly by size
- Follicles & follicular cysts without hemorrhage
  - Unilocular with smooth margin
  - No internal septations, though adjacent follicles can sometimes simulate septations
  - Anechoic with ↑ through transmission
    - May have minimal internal debris
- Corpus luteal cysts
  - Unilocular but with irregular contour
  - Range from anechoic to isoechoic
  - Wall thickness is variable due to vascularization
  - Classically have ↑ peripheral vascularity ("ring of fire")
  - Appearance can be identical to follicular cyst
- Hemorrhagic cysts
  - Contain heterogeneously echogenic debris, which becomes more hypo- or anechoic as clot lysis occurs
  - Reticular or lace-like pattern of internal echoes is classic
  - Fluid-debris level is sometimes present
  - ↑ through transmission is maintained despite echogenicity

CT Findings

- CECT
  - Hypoattenuating, well-marginated mass within ovary without enhancement
  - Ovarian stroma is usually low density, though normal tissue surrounding cyst can simulate soft tissue rim
    - Punctate hypodense follicles may be visualized in mildly enhancing ovarian parenchyma
  - Fat density or Ca^{2+} is always pathologic
  - Corpus luteal cysts
    - Unilocular
    - Thicker wall, usually 2-4 mm, often hyperenhancing & crenulated (irregular), especially if ruptured
  - Hemorrhagic cysts are more dense than simple cysts
    - Most commonly arise in follicular or corpus luteal cysts
    - Fluid-fluid level is rarely seen on CT
    - Cyst rupture can cause free peritoneal fluid, which may be hyperdense if due to hemorrhage
      - Corpus luteal cysts more commonly result in hemoperitoneum due to their vascular wall

MR Findings

- May be performed if ultrasound diagnosis is unclear
  - Accuracy for MR in characterizing sonographically indeterminate lesions ranges from 83-93%
  - Findings more indicative of neoplasm include
    - Thick, enhancing wall or septations > 3 mm
    - Enhancing mural nodule, papillary projections, or other solid components
    - Size > 5 cm
- Functional cysts: Homogeneously low T1, high T2 signal
- Hemorrhagic cyst: Typically high T1 & T2 signal
  - Fluid-debris level is sometimes seen on T2
  - No loss of high T1 signal with fat suppression
  - Hemorrhagic components may restrict diffusion
- T1 FS & in-/opposed-phase GRE sequences aid in looking for fat of dermoid
- Mild rim enhancement with hemorrhagic or corpus luteal cyst on T1 C+ FS
  - Subtracted pre- from postcontrast T1 FS images are helpful to confirm true enhancement rather than pseudoenhancement of blood products

Imaging Recommendations

- Best imaging tool
  - Ultrasound is mainstay for evaluation of ovaries
    - Characterization of cyst wall & internal components
    - Color Doppler gives additional information, especially in evaluating for presence of solid component
  - MR is considered when ultrasound is indeterminate or if neoplasm is suggested but full extent is not discernible by ultrasound
  - CT use is minimized due to radiation concerns

DIFFERENTIAL DIAGNOSIS

Dermoid/Teratoma

- 10-15% may appear as entirely cystic by imaging
- MR is much more sensitive/specific (due to fat component)

Ovarian Malignancy

- Enlarging, mildly complex cyst or higher degrees of complexity (solid nodular components, internal vascularity) should raise concern
- MR if question of hemorrhage vs. solid components

Ovarian Torsion

- Asymmetric, edematous ovarian parenchyma with peripheral follicles, ± midline/contralateral location of ovary
- ± twisted vascular pedicle (whirlpool), ↓ or absent blood flow
- Frequently associated with cysts > 5 cm

Paraovarian Cyst

- Long list of potential causes, including
  - Enteric duplication cyst
  - Peritoneal inclusion cyst
  - Lymphatic malformation
- Resected paratubal cysts recur in ~ 11% of girls

Tuboovarian Abscess

- Wide range of appearances from relatively simple-appearing cyst to complex, heterogeneous, cystic mass
- Clinical history & exam findings are crucial

Ectopic Pregnancy

- History & pregnancy test results are critical

PATHOLOGY

General Features

- Etiology
  - Infancy
    - In fetus, follicular stimulation occurs from maternal estrogen, placental hCG, & fetal gonadotropins
    - More common in maternal diabetes, toxemia, or Rh isoimmunization during pregnancy
    - Small cysts may be seen as early as 28-weeks gestation
    - Newborn estrogen & hCG levels fall but serum LH & FSH levels ↑, peaking at 3-4 months
  - Premenarchal
    - Cysts > 1 cm are least common in this age group due to low hormone levels
    - Follicle maturation occurs at low rate
  - Postmenarchal
    - Hormone levels approach adult levels & cysts become more common
    - Usually result of dysfunctional ovulation

CLINICAL ISSUES

Presentation

- Most common signs/symptoms
  - Usually asymptomatic; pain if large or complicated by rupture, hemorrhage, or torsion
  - Corpus luteal cyst is more commonly symptomatic, even without significant hemorrhage

Demographics

- Epidemiology
  - Neonates: Small cysts are present in up to 98% at birth
    - ~ 20% ≥ 1 cm
  - Premenarchal: Cysts > 1 cm in 2-5%
  - Postmenarchal: Cysts are very common
    - Nonfunctional cysts & malignant ovarian neoplasms also occur at greater rate

Natural History & Prognosis

- Over 90% of all functional cysts resolve spontaneously
  - Larger cysts may take longer to resolve
  - 91-94% of pediatric ovarian cysts are benign

Treatment

- Cysts < 4-5 cm are usually monitored with surveillance US
- Surgery is considered in larger cysts due to risk of torsion or neoplasm
  - Options include aspiration, fenestration, & resection
  - For resection, ovarian sparing approach is preferred if benign etiology suspected

DIAGNOSTIC CHECKLIST

Consider

- 3 main concerns for radiologist when cystic ovarian lesion is encountered in child
  - Could this be torsed?
  - Could this be neoplastic?
  - Could this be other pathology (e.g., tuboovarian abscess, ectopic pregnancy, ruptured appendicitis, etc.)?

Image Interpretation Pearls

- Superimposed torsion is more likely with cysts > 5 cm
- Clinical judgment overrides imaging: Simple or hemorrhagic cyst with otherwise normal-appearing ovarian parenchyma (by grayscale & Doppler US) can still be torsed
  - Does not give license to use phrase "cannot rule out torsion" in every report
  - Strong clinical suspicion + any ovarian abnormality on imaging may require laparoscopy

Reporting Tips

- Close follow-up if complexity/size of asymptomatic cyst is not typical of most simple or hemorrhagic cysts
  - Repeat US in 4-6 weeks; subsequent MR &/or gynecology referral if questions persist

SELECTED REFERENCES

1. Abdelmeguid Y et al: Huge ovarian cyst in a neonate with classical 21-hydroxylase deficiency. Clin Pediatr Endocrinol. 30(1):57-60, 2021
2. Kitami M et al: "Follow the fallopian tube": a technique to improve sonographic identification of ovaries in children. J Clin Ultrasound. 49(1):33-7, 2021
3. Xac MC et al: Benign, borderline, and malignant pediatric adnexal masses: a ten-year review. J Pediatr Adolesc Gynecol. 34(4):454-61, 2021
4. Magistrado L et al: Paratubal cyst recurrence in children and adolescents. J Pediatr Adolesc Gynecol. 33(6):649-51, 2020
5. Peeraully R et al: Effect of surgical specialty on management of adnexal masses in children and adolescents: an 8-year single-center review. J Pediatr Adolesc Gynecol. 33(1):89-92, 2020
6. Caprio MG et al: Ultrasonographic and multimodal imaging of pediatric genital female diseases. J Ultrasound. 22(3):273-89, 2019
7. Schallert EK et al: Physiologic ovarian cysts versus other ovarian and adnexal pathologic changes in the preadolescent and adolescent population: US and surgical follow-up. Radiology. 292(1):172-8, 2019
8. Gonzalez DO et al: Management of benign ovarian lesions in girls: a trend toward fewer oophorectomies. Curr Opin Obstet Gynecol. 29(5):289-94, 2017
9. Trotman GE et al: Rate of oophorectomy for benign indications in a children's hospital: influence of a gynecologist. J Pediatr Adolesc Gynecol. 30(2):234-8, 2017

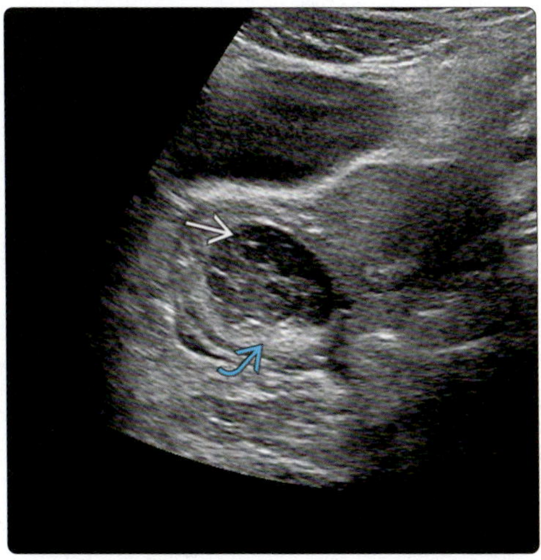

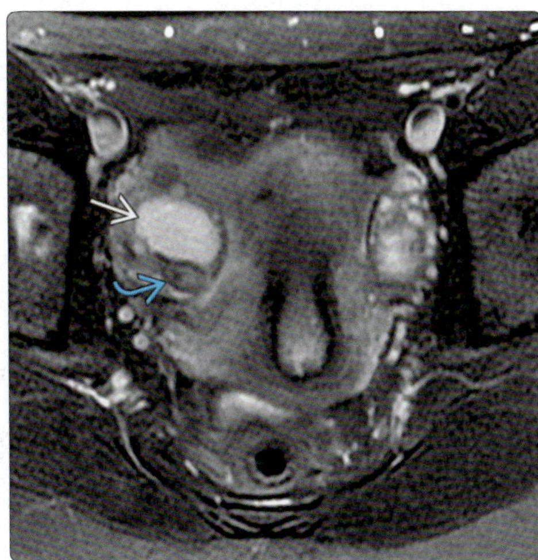

(Left) *Transverse ultrasound of the right ovary in a 17-year-old with pelvic pain shows a complex cystic lesion with lacy septations ➡ in the near field & more echogenic contents ➡ dependently.* **(Right)** *Axial T2 FS MR in the same patient a few days later (imaged for persistent pain) shows liquefying cyst contents anteriorly ➡ & hemorrhagic debris dependently ➡ in this case of a hemorrhagic ovarian cyst.*

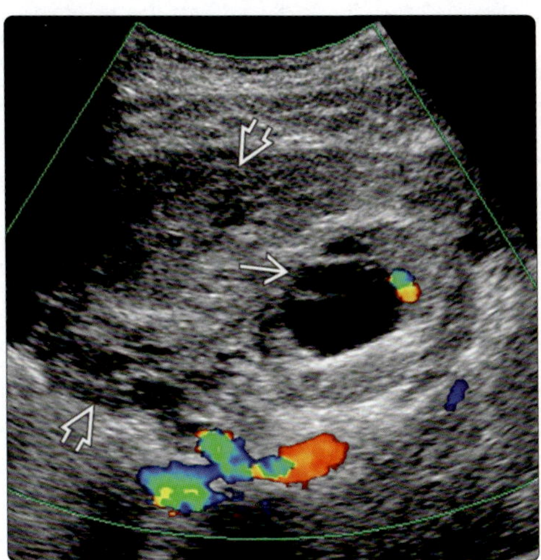

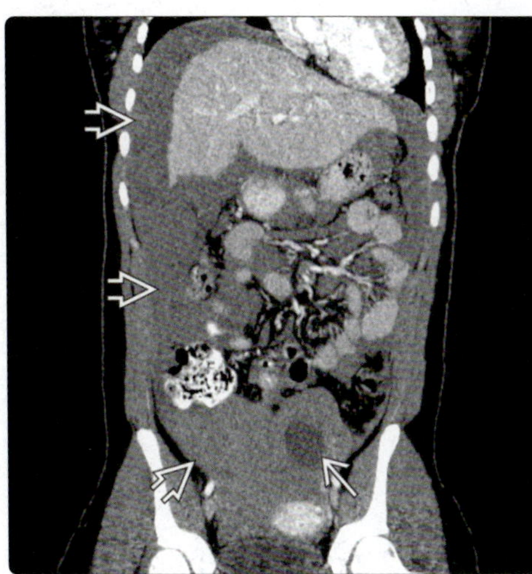

(Left) *Transverse color Doppler ultrasound shows an irregular cystic structure containing septations ➡ within the left ovary. The ovary is surrounded by a large amount of heterogeneously echogenic material ➡, which was mobile in real time. The findings are indicative of a ruptured hemorrhagic cyst.* **(Right)** *Coronal CECT in the same patient also demonstrates the left adnexal cyst ➡ surrounded by a large volume of hemoperitoneum ➡ that extends to the subdiaphragmatic region.*

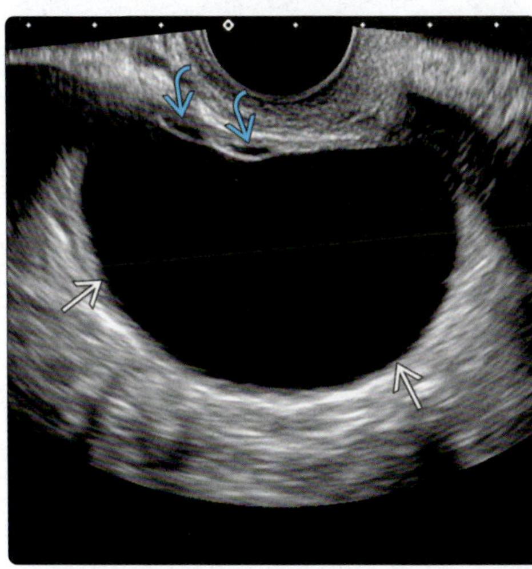

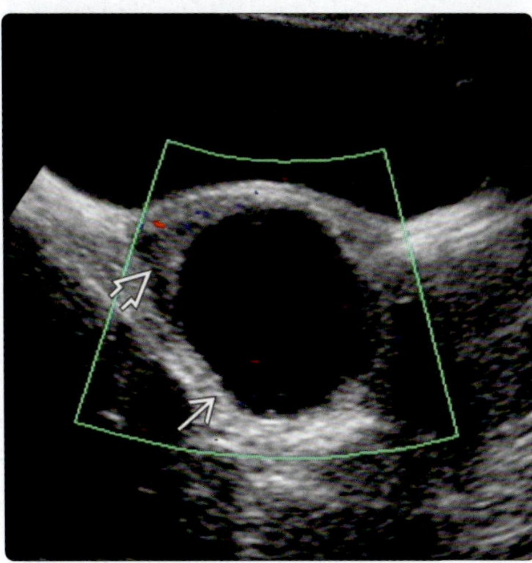

(Left) *Transvaginal ultrasound in an 18-year-old with pain shows a large simple cyst ➡ with thin wall & ↑ through transmission, volume of ~ 100 mL, stretching the ovarian tissue in the near field where 2 tiny follicles ➡ are seen.* **(Right)** *Transverse color Doppler ultrasound in a patient with a simple cyst ➡ shows eccentric but otherwise normal-appearing ovarian tissue ➡ splayed along the cyst. Despite the unalarming sonographic appearance, the patient's symptoms warranted laparoscopy, where the ovary was found to be torsed.*

Ovarian Teratoma

KEY FACTS

TERMINOLOGY

- Dermoid tumor, dermoid cyst, mature cystic teratoma
- Teratomas are made up of variety of parenchymal cell types from > 1 germ cell layer, usually all 3

IMAGING

- Best clue: Heterogenous pelvic mass containing Ca^{2+}, hair, fat, & cystic components
- Typically well-defined margins without surrounding inflammatory changes
- US: 1st-line modality for female pelvic pain &/or mass
  - Multiple classic signs described for teratoma
    - Dermoid plug: Echogenic nodule protruding into cyst
    - Dermoid mesh: Linear/punctate echogenic foci of hair
    - Tip of iceberg sign: Echogenic superficial interfaces obscure deeper components of mass
- Radiographs: Tooth-like Ca^2 is strongly suggestive
- MR & CT: Best demonstrate fat, confirming teratoma

PATHOLOGY

- Complications of ovarian teratoma include
  - Ovarian torsion
  - Rupture, causing chemical peritonitis
    - May lead to severe adhesions
  - Anti-NMDA receptor encephalitis
  - Malignancy (2%)

CLINICAL ISSUES

- Teratoma is most common ovarian germ cell tumor
- Teratoma is most common ovarian neoplasm < 20 years old
  - Found in any age; mean age of presentation: 30 years
- Often incidental finding on physical exam or during imaging for unrelated symptoms
  - With torsion or rupture, acute onset of pain is typical
- Treatment: Surgical resection, ovary-sparing surgery
  - Laparoscopic surgery is preferred

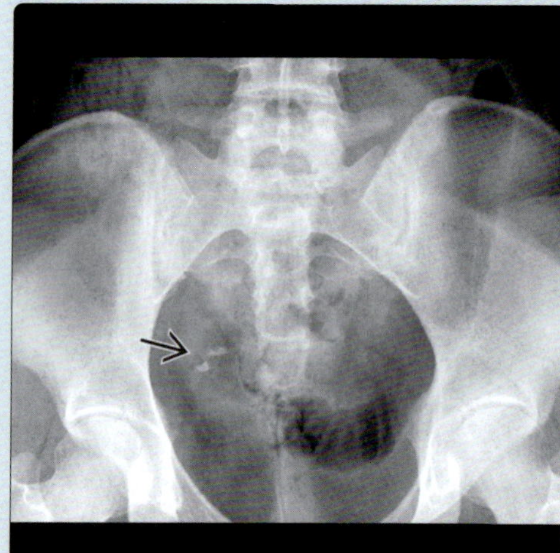

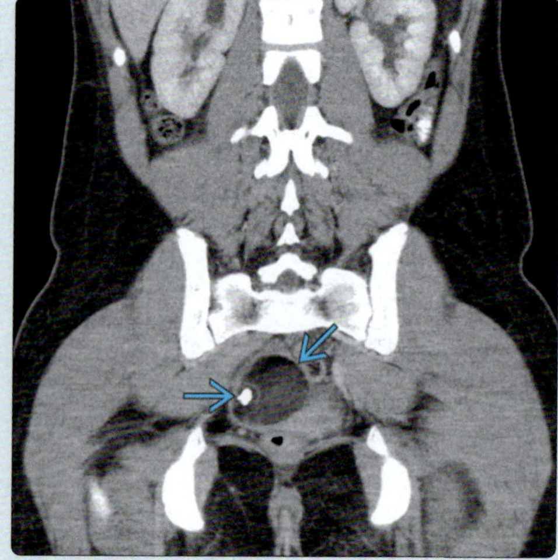

(Left) *AP radiograph in a teenage girl with pelvic pain & normal menstrual cycles shows chunky Ca^{2+} in the pelvis ➔ that are suspicious for an ovarian teratoma (or possibly appendicoliths).* **(Right)** *Coronal CECT in the same patient shows a heterogeneous mass ➔ in the right adnexa containing Ca^{2+}, fat, fluid (not shown), & nonlayering debris. The presence of all these tissues confirms ovarian teratoma as the diagnosis.*

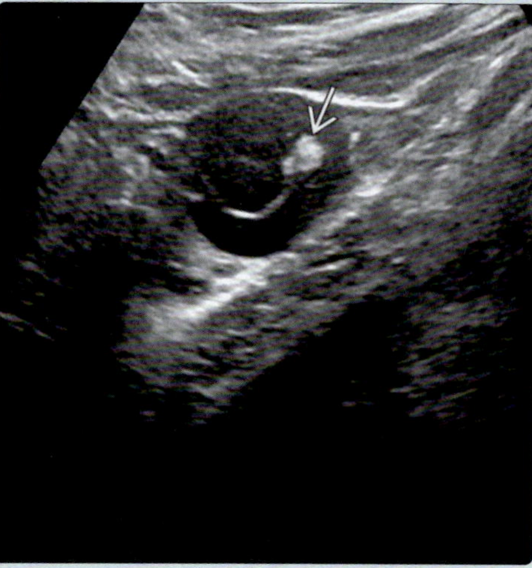

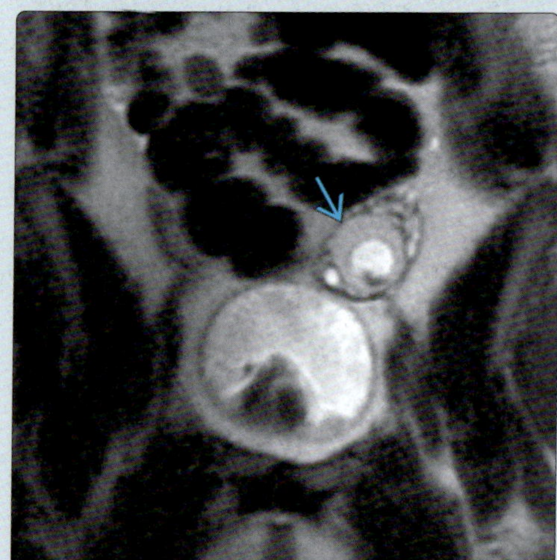

(Left) *Longitudinal US of the left ovary in a 14-year-old girl shows a mixed cystic & solid mass with hyperechoic foci ➔ & curvilinear septations.* **(Right)** *Coronal SSFSE T2 MR in the same patient (performed for other medical issues) shows fat & fluid centrally ➔ within the left ovary. The lesion was subsequently surgically shelled out of the ovary (i.e., an ovarian-sparing resection) & found to be a mature teratoma.*

TERMINOLOGY

Synonyms

- Dermoid tumor, dermoid cyst, cystic teratoma

Definitions

- Teratomas are made up of various parenchymal cell types from > 1 germ layer, usually all 3
- Teratomas generally lie in midline or paraxial & arise from totipotential cells
- Term dermoid comes from skin-like lining found in many of these tumors

IMAGING

General Features

- Best diagnostic clue
  - Heterogeneous pelvic mass containing calcium, fat, fluid, & other internal debris
  - Typically well-defined margins without surrounding inflammatory changes
- Location
  - Pelvis & lower abdomen
- Size
  - Variable, from 1-45 cm in diameter
  - Mean diameter: 6 cm
- Morphology
  - Mixed tissue types surrounded by capsule

Radiographic Findings

- May be occult
- ± Ca^{2+}; those resembling teeth or bone strongly suggest teratoma
- ± mass effect on bowel

Ultrasonographic Findings

- Grayscale ultrasound
  - Heterogeneous mass with cystic & solid components
  - Ca^{2+} may show posterior shadowing or ring-down artifact when very small
  - Fat & hair appear echogenic; hair may appear reticular
  - ± fluid-fat-debris levels &/or floating debris within cysts
  - Dermoid mesh sign: Linear & punctate hyperechoic foci (due to hair) within cystic mass
  - Dermoid plug (Rokitansky nodule): Echogenic solid focus bulging into lesion from cyst wall
  - Tip of iceberg sign: Strong echogenic interface at leading edge of teratoma blocks deeper components from view
    - May be caused by Ca^{2+}, hair, fat, etc.
- Color Doppler
  - Flow is useful in differentiating solid perfused tissue from solid avascular hair, teeth, etc.

CT Findings

- Exquisite for identifying fat & Ca^{2+}
- Otherwise heterogeneous tissue components with septations & fluid-debris levels
- Residual ovarian tissue giving rise to teratoma may be difficult to identify if tumor is large

MR Findings

- Heterogeneous signal due to mix of elements
  - Low signal intensity foci with blooming on T2* GRE suggests Ca^{2+}
  - Identification of fat is key to diagnosis
    - T1 ± FS
      - Signal loss upon FS application confirms presence of macroscopic fat (vs. other T1-bright material, such as blood, protein, etc.); may show fat-fluid level
    - In-/opposed-phase GRE sequences assess for microscopic fat
      - Signal loss on opposed-phase confirms fatty lesion

Imaging Recommendations

- Best imaging tool
  - US is primary investigative tool for female pelvic pain or palpable mass
  - MR is reserved for complex cases or patients ill-suited to sonography
  - CT is minimized due to radiation concerns
- Protocol advice
  - Scan mass in orthogonal planes looking for variable tissue & cyst contents
  - Endovaginal scanning is optimal when tolerated
  - Larger masses may require transabdominal scanning & extended field of view

DIFFERENTIAL DIAGNOSIS

Other Ovarian Neoplasms

- Benign
  - Simple/follicular cysts
  - Cystadenomas
    - Mucinous
    - Serous
  - Gonadoblastoma
- Malignant
  - Germ cell tumors
  - Sex cord-stromal tumors
  - Epithelial tumors
  - Malignant teratomas

Perforated Appendicitis With Appendicolith

- Heterogeneous collection in lower abdomen, ± Ca^{2+} & shadowing foci

Tuboovarian Abscess

- Fever, cervical tenderness, & vaginal discharge is typical

Ovarian Torsion

- May require surgical exploration to distinguish
- May coexist with ovarian teratoma

Ectopic Pregnancy

- Correlate with β-hCG

Stool Impaction

- Stool & gas in rectum can mimic tip of iceberg sign

Bladder Calculi

- Ca^{2} in pelvis could reside in urinary bladder
  - Especially in patients with Mitrofanoff, other bladder surgeries, & those performing bladder catheterization

Endometrioma

- Cyclic pain history is useful

Peritoneal Inclusion Cyst

- Lacks complex contents seen in teratomas

PATHOLOGY

General Features

- Etiology
  - Arise from primordial germ cells, which migrate during embryogenesis from yolk sac to gonads
- Associated abnormalities
  - Complications of ovarian teratoma include
    - Ovarian torsion
    - Rupture, causing chemical peritonitis
      - Severe adhesions can result from perforation of teratoma
    - Infection
    - Hemolytic anemia
    - Malignancy in ~ 2%
- 3 types of ovarian teratomas
  - Mature cystic teratoma (dermoid cyst)
  - Monodermal teratomas (struma ovarii, carcinoid tumors, & neural tumors)
  - Immature teratomas
    - Associated with growing teratoma syndrome (peritoneal recurrence)
- Teratoma distribution
  - Sacrococcygeal (57%)
  - Gonadal (29%), ovarian > testicular
  - Mediastinal > retroperitoneal > cervical > intracranial
- Cells differentiate along various germ lines, essentially recapitulating any tissue of body
- Ectoderm, mesoderm, & endodermal elements may all be present
  - Because ectodermal components tend to predominate, term dermoid cyst has been applied
  - Tissues include hair, teeth, fat, skin, muscle, & endocrine tissue

Gross Pathologic & Surgical Features

- Heterogeneous mass surrounded by well defined capsule
- Cyst contents may be oily, milky, or have serous fluid, hair, teeth, cartilage, etc.

Microscopic Features

- Variable well-differentiated tissues, including bone, cartilage, muscle, thyroid follicles, gastrointestinal lining, respiratory epithelium, etc.
- Immature teratomas are graded from 0 to 3 based on amount of immature neural tissue found in tumor specimen
  - Higher grades are more likely to have yolk sac tumor components

CLINICAL ISSUES

Presentation

- Most common signs/symptoms
  - Often incidental finding on physical exam or during imaging for unrelated symptoms
  - With torsion or rupture, acute onset of pain is typical
- Other signs/symptoms
  - Abdominal pain, abdominal mass, or swelling
  - Abnormal uterine bleeding
  - Urinary symptoms
  - Gastrointestinal complaints
  - Back pain is less common
  - Elevated α-fetoprotein or hCG is more likely with germ cell tumors/immature teratomas
  - Rarely associated with anti-NMDA encephalitis
  - Opsoclonus-myoclonus syndrome/ataxia association

Demographics

- Age
  - Any; mean of 30 years
- Sex
  - Females only for ovarian lesions
- Epidemiology
  - Teratoma is most common ovarian germ cell tumor
  - Also most common ovarian neoplasm in patients < 20 years old
  - 10% of teratomas are diagnosed during pregnancy
  - Bilateral in up to 15%
    - Right-sided teratomas are slightly more common than left

Natural History & Prognosis

- Teratomas enlarge, spontaneously hemorrhage, or twist
- Prognosis is generally excellent following resection
  - Prognosis is poor in small minority with malignant foci
  - Malignant teratomas tend to metastasize widely
  - 5-year survival for malignant teratomas is < 30%
- Fertility issues may arise
  - When entire ovary is removed
  - When chemical peritonitis impairs ovulatory function

Treatment

- Treatment is surgical resection, ovary-sparing surgery
- Laparoscopic surgery is preferred
- Malignant teratomas are treated with surgery, hyperthermic intraperitoneal chemotherapy, neoadjuvant chemotherapy

SELECTED REFERENCES

1. Brind'Amour A et al: Recurrent high-grade ovarian immature teratoma with peritoneal dissemination. J Pediatr Adolesc Gynecol. 33(5):586-9, 2020
2. Hanafy AK et al: Imaging in pediatric ovarian tumors. Abdom Radiol (NY). 45(2):520-36, 2020
3. Imran H et al: Growing teratoma syndrome after chemotherapy for ovarian immature teratoma. J Pediatr Hematol Oncol. 42(7):e630-3, 2020
4. Park C et al: Pediatric whole body MRI detects causative ovarian teratoma in opsoclonus myoclonus syndrome. Radiol Case Rep. 15(3):204-9, 2020
5. Szymon O et al: Ovarian sparing surgery in mature ovarian teratomas in children: a 20-year single-center experience. Eur J Pediatr Surg. 31(1):2-7, 2020
6. Lala SV et al: Ovarian neoplasms of childhood. Pediatr Radiol. 49(11):1463-75, 2019
7. Faure-Conter C et al: Immature ovarian teratoma: when to give adjuvant therapy? J Pediatr Hematol Oncol. 39(7):487-9, 2017
8. Gonzalez DO et al: Management of benign ovarian lesions in girls: a trend toward fewer oophorectomies. Curr Opin Obstet Gynecol. 29(5):289-94, 2017
9. Salvucci A et al: Pediatric anti-NMDA (N-methyl D-aspartate) receptor encephalitis. Pediatr Neurol. 50(5):507-10, 2014
10. Park SB et al: Imaging findings of complications and unusual manifestations of ovarian teratomas. Radiographics. 28(4):969-83, 2008

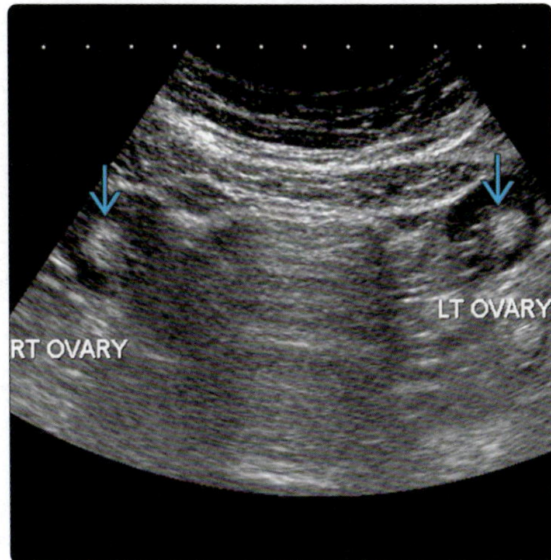

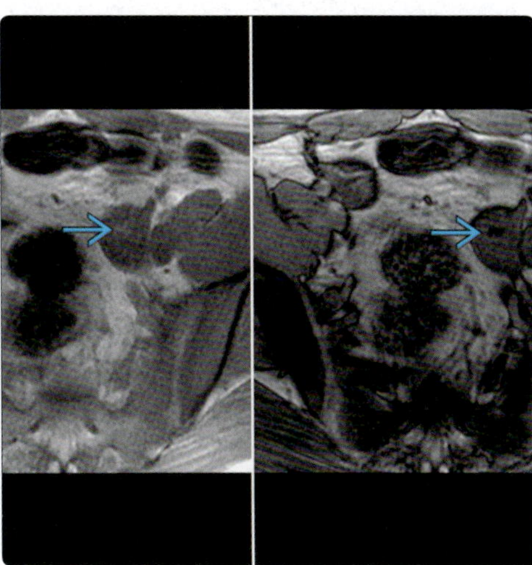

(Left) *Tranverse US in an 11-year-old girl with anti-NMDA receptor encephalitis shows bilateral 1-cm echogenic ovarian lesions* ➔*, potentially teratomas.* **(Right)** *Axial in- (left) & opposed- (right) phase T1 GRE MR images in the same patient show a left ovarian lesion* ➔ *containing macro- & microscopic fat with signal drop on the opposed-phase image. A similar finding was seen in the right ovary. T1 FS images (not shown) also confirmed fat in both lesions. Ovarian-sparing teratoma resection was performed bilaterally.*

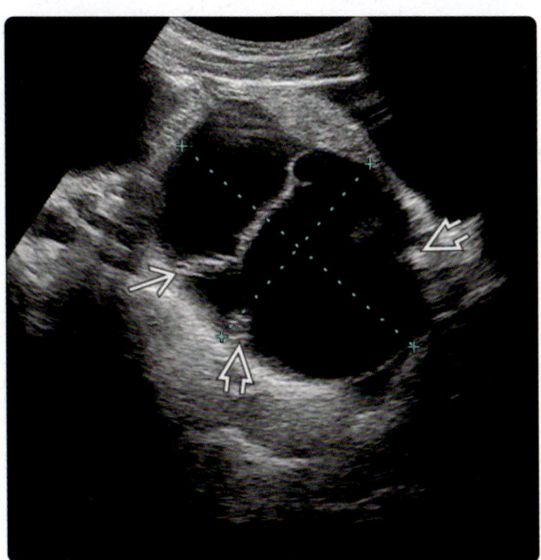

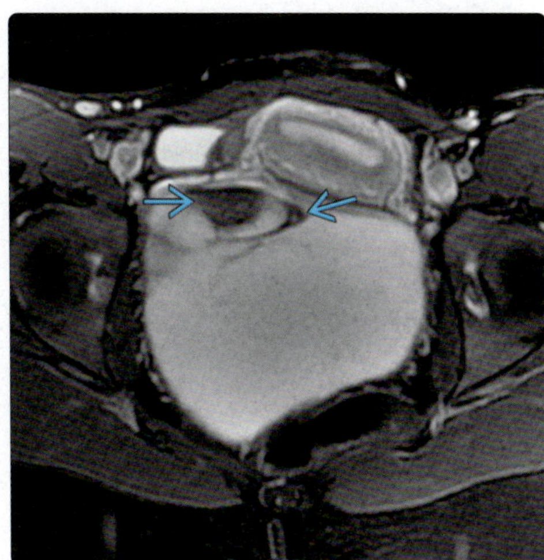

(Left) *Longitudinal US of a 7 x 10 cm complex cystic mass in right pelvis of a 17-year-old girl with vague pelvic pain & fullness shows an echogenic septation* ➔ *& echogenic nodules* ➔ *in this right ovarian lesion.* **(Right)** *Axial T2 FS MR in the same patient shows dark fat* ➔ *within this complex ovarian mass, pathologically proven to be a mature ovarian teratoma.*

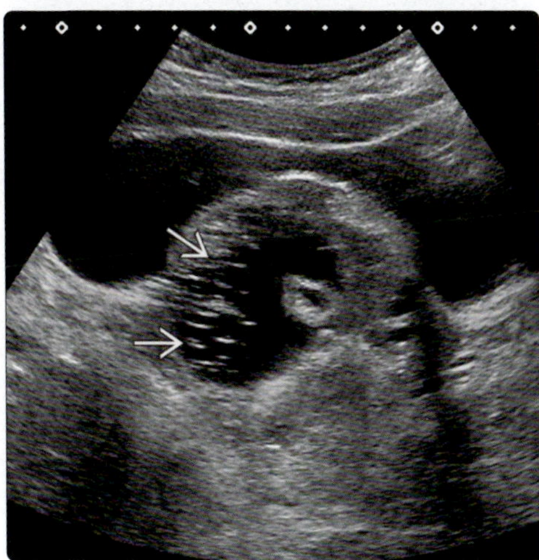

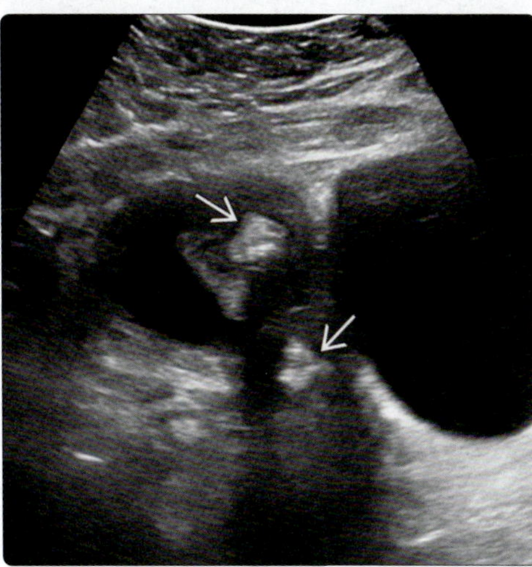

(Left) *Transverse US in a 12-year-old girl shows a complex cystic adnexal lesion with linear bright echoes* ➔*, fluid, & solid components. The linear echoes corresponded to hair at gross pathology in this case of mature ovarian teratoma.* **(Right)** *Transverse oblique US in this 11-year-old scanned for incidental Ca^{2+} seen on a radiograph shows echogenic chunks of Ca^{2+}* ➔ *in this right ovarian teratoma. At pathology, poorly formed bone & teeth were found.*

Ovarian Malignancies of Childhood

KEY FACTS

IMAGING

- **Germ cell tumors**
  - Mature ovarian teratoma: Cystic mass with fat & Ca^{2+}
  - Immature ovarian teratoma: Cannot differentiate from mature teratoma on imaging
  - Ovarian dysgerminoma: Multilobulated, solid mass with Ca^{2+}
  - Yolk sac tumor: Large, complex cystic & solid mass that extends into abdomen
  - Choriocarcinoma: Solid, hypervascular mass in female with elevated β-hCG
- **Sex cord-stromal tumors**
  - Juvenile granulosa-theca cell tumor: Large, multilocular mass with septations & solid component
  - Sertoli-Leydig cell tumor: Heterogeneous cystic & solid mass
- **Epithelial tumors**
  - Serous tumor: Homogeneous cystic mass with thin walls & no mural nodule
  - Mucinous tumor: Large, heterogeneous, multilocular cystic mass
- **Miscellaneous**
  - Small cell carcinoma of ovary, hypercalcemic type
    - May represent aggressive malignant rhabdoid tumor

CLINICAL ISSUES

- Abdominal pain &/or distention, mass, ↓ appetite
- Hormonally active tumors
  - Juvenile granulosa-theca cell tumor: 80% present with pseudoprecocious puberty due to hyperestrogenism
  - Sertoli-Leydig cell tumor: ~ 30% virilizing
- Torsion is more likely with benign neoplasms
- Current treatment: Unilateral salpingo-oophorectomy
- Chemotherapy for stage II disease & higher

DIAGNOSTIC CHECKLIST

- Look for signs of tumor rupture/peritoneal seeding

(Left) *Longitudinal color Doppler ultrasound of the ovary in an adolescent diagnosed with an ovarian immature teratoma shows a mixed cystic & solid ovarian mass* ⇨*. The solid portion* ⇨ *of the tumor contains a focus of* Ca^{2+} ⇨ *with posterior acoustic shadowing.* **(Right)** *Coronal CECT in the same patient shows the ovarian mass* ⇨ *containing fat* ⇨ *&* Ca^{2+} ⇨*. While the findings are consistent with a teratoma, the designation of tumor maturity can only be made at histology.*

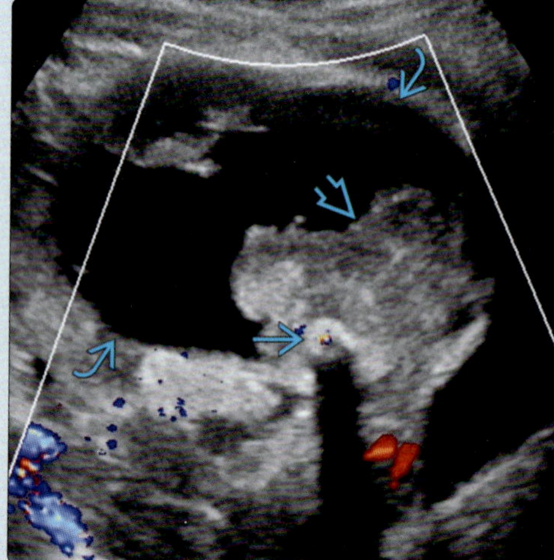

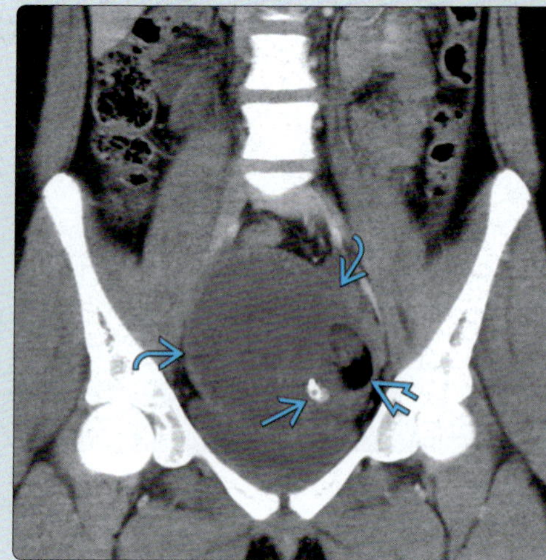

(Left) *Transverse transvaginal ultrasound of the left ovary in an adolescent diagnosed with a borderline serous cystadenoma shows a large cystic mass* ⇨ *with no internal complexity.* **(Right)** *Coronal T2 MR in the same patient shows the large cystic left ovarian mass* ⇨ *extending to the left upper abdomen. The mass is attached to the fallopian tube* ⇨*, stretching the tube & pulling the uterus* ⇨ *to the left.*

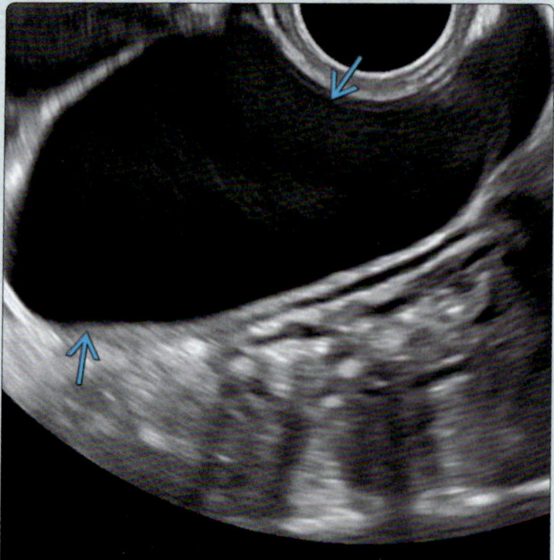

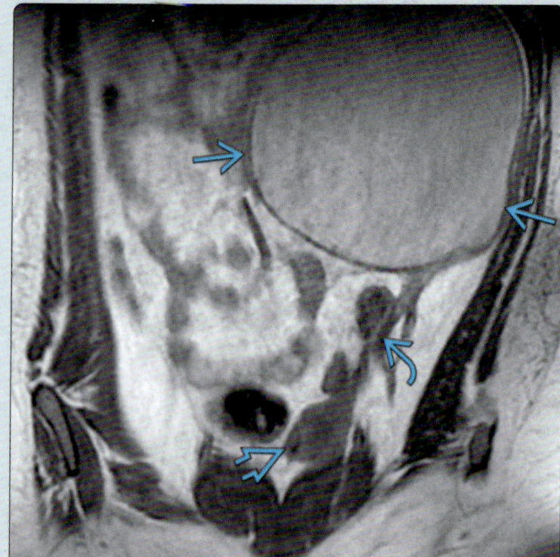

IMAGING

General Features

- Best diagnostic clue
  - Germ cell tumors
    - Mature ovarian teratoma: Cystic mass with intratumoral fat & Ca^{2+}
    - Immature ovarian teratoma: Cannot differentiate from mature teratoma on imaging; immature teratomas tend to be larger, have smaller, speckled Ca^{2+}, & have more prominent solid components
    - Dysgerminoma: Multilobulated, solid mass with speckled Ca^{2+}
    - Yolk sac tumor: Large, complex cystic & solid mass that extends into abdomen
    - Choriocarcinoma: Solid, hypervascular mass with elevated β-hCG
  - Sex cord-stromal tumors
    - Juvenile granulosa-theca cell tumor: Large, multilocular mass with septations & solid component
    - Sertoli-Leydig cell tumor: Heterogeneous, cystic, & solid
  - Epithelial tumors
    - Serous tumor: Homogeneous cystic mass with thin walls & no mural nodule
    - Mucinous tumor: Large, heterogeneous, multilocular cystic mass
- Location
  - Most ovarian tumors are unilateral
    - Slightly more common on right
    - Bilateral tumors in 5-15%, depending on tumor type
      - More common with borderline malignant potential epithelial tumors, immature teratomas, & dysgerminomas
- Size
  - Variable; small (< 1 cm) to very large (> 20 cm)

Radiographic Findings

- Mature teratoma: May see tooth-like Ca^{2+}
- Other ovarian tumors: If large enough, tumor can cause mass effect upon bowel, displacing it superiorly & laterally

Ultrasonographic Findings

- International Ovarian Tumor Analysis (IOTA) group rules to distinguish benign from malignant ovarian tumors
  - Not validated in children
  - Factors that favor malignancy: Size > 10 cm, solid tumor, presence of ascites, ≥ 4 papillary structures, hyperemia, irregular borders
  - Factors that favor benign lesion: Unilocular cyst, solid components < 7 mm, presence of acoustic shadows, smooth borders, size < 10 cm, absent blood flow
- Germ cell tumors
  - Ovarian teratoma: Cystic mass with echogenic nodule that shadows (Rokitansky nodule)
    - May have multiple thin, echogenic bands from intratumoral hair
    - May have fat-fluid level
  - Ovarian dysgerminoma: Multilobulated mass with anechoic areas representing hemorrhage or necrosis
  - Yolk sac tumor: Large, heterogeneous mass with cystic & solid components
  - Choriocarcinoma: Mostly solid mass with cystic areas of hemorrhage or necrosis
- Sex cord-stromal tumors
  - Juvenile granulosa-theca cell tumor: Large, multilocular mass with septations & solid component
  - Sertoli-Leydig cell tumor: Heterogeneous mass with cystic & solid components
- Epithelial tumors
  - Serous: Simple cystic mass
  - Mucinous: Large cystic mass with multiple loculations

MR Findings

- Germ cell tumors
  - Mature ovarian teratoma: Intratumoral fat confirmed with fat-saturated images
  - Immature ovarian teratoma: Mass with prominent solid component, cystic areas, & intratumoral fat
  - Dysgerminoma: Multilobulated, septated mass
    - Septa are low signal intensity on all sequences but enhance intensely
  - Yolk sac tumor: Large, heterogeneous cystic & solid mass
  - Choriocarcinoma: Solid enhancing tumor with areas of hemorrhage or necrosis
- Sex cord-stromal tumors
  - Juvenile granulosa-theca cell tumor: Large, multilocular mass with septations & solid component
    - Foci of ↑ T1 signal due to intratumoral hemorrhage
    - Sponge-like appearance with solid areas interspersed with many cystic areas on T2
  - Sertoli-Leydig cell tumor: On T2, mass is predominantly low signal with scattered foci of ↑ signal
- Epithelial tumors
  - Serous: Unilocular cystic mass with homogeneous signal intensity & thin wall
  - Mucinous: Multilocular cystic mass with locules containing fluid of differing signal intensity
- Small cell carcinoma
  - Solid & enhancing mass with cystic or hemorrhagic foci

CT Findings

- MR is preferred to CT for evaluation of ovarian mass
- CT findings similar to MR findings
- CT is more likely to visualize Ca^{2+}
  - Mature ovarian teratoma: Cystic mass + fat & Ca^{2+}
  - Immature ovarian teratoma: Ca^{2+} can be scattered rather than confined to mural nodules
  - Dysgerminoma: May have speckled Ca^{2+}

Imaging Recommendations

- Best imaging tool
  - Ultrasound: 1st-line imaging modality
  - MR for further characterization & localization
    - DWI & T1 C+ FS images can help detect peritoneal tumor deposits
    - ADC values overlap in benign & malignant pediatric ovarian tumors

Tumor Markers Associated With Pediatric Ovarian Tumors

Tumor Markers	Tumor Type
Alpha feto-protein (AFP)	Yolk sac tumor Immature teratoma Embryonal carcinoma Mixed germ cell tumor Sertoli-Leydig cell tumor
Beta-human chorionic gonadotropin (ß-hCG)	Choriocarcinoma Embryonal carcinoma Dysgerminoma
Lactate dehydrogenase (LDH)	Dysgerminoma
CA-125	Epithelial tumors
Inhibin A	Juvenile granulosa cell tumor
Calcium	Sex cord stromal tumor Small cell carcinoma

DIFFERENTIAL DIAGNOSIS

Functional Cyst

- Occurs during follicular phase of menstrual cycle
- Simple ovarian cyst (usually < 3 cm) that resolves over time

Hemorrhagic Cyst

- Variable internal complexity depending on age of blood products
  - Layering debris, lace-like septations, retracting clot
- No internal vascularity

Ovarian Torsion

- Presentation: Acute pain & asymmetric ↑ in ovarian size
- Torsion may occur secondary to mass acting as lead point
  - Tumor is present in 26% of cases of torsion
  - Best suggested by size of lesion & new onset pain

PATHOLOGY

Microscopic Features

- Epithelial serous & mucinous tumors can be differentiated into benign, borderline, & malignant, depending on histology
- Small cell carcinoma of ovary, hypercalcemic type, likely represents malignant rhabdoid tumor

CLINICAL ISSUES

Presentation

- Most common signs/symptoms
  - Abdominal pain &/or distention
- Other signs/symptoms
  - Palpable mass, fever, ↓ appetite
  - Torsion is uncommon presentation for ovarian malignancy
    - Torsion is more likely with benign neoplasms
    - Tumor is present in 26% of cases of torsion; only 3.5% of these tumors are malignant
  - Teratomas may present with N-Methyl-D-aspartic acid or N-Methyl-D-aspartate (NMDA) encephalitis
  - Hormonally active tumors
    - Juvenile granulosa-theca cell tumor
      - 80% present with pseudoprecocious puberty due to hyperestrogenism
    - Sertoli-Leydig cell tumor: ~ 30% virilizing; associated with *DICER1* mutation

Demographics

- Epidemiology
  - Incidence of ovarian masses in childhood: 2.6 cases per 100,000 girls per year
  - 16-55% malignant; account for < 3% of all pediatric cancers

Natural History & Prognosis

- Most tumors are FIGO stage I at diagnosis
- Different tumors have different markers (see Table)

Treatment

- Current treatment: Fertility-sparing surgery if possible
- Chemotherapy for stage II disease & higher

DIAGNOSTIC CHECKLIST

Image Interpretation Pearls

- Fat-containing ovarian mass: Teratoma
- Other ovarian masses are often diagnosed at resection
  - More important to suggest neoplasm & evaluate for complication than name specific tumor type
- Complications include
  - Ovarian torsion (typically in benign lesions)
  - Tumor rupture/peritoneal seeding
    - Irregular or discontinuous tumor margins
    - Ascites ± dependently layering debris
    - Smooth or nodular peritoneal thickening
    - Nodularity & abnormal enhancement of omentum
  - Distant metastases

SELECTED REFERENCES

1. Janssen CL et al: The diagnostic value of magnetic resonance imaging in differentiating benign and malignant pediatric ovarian tumors. Pediatr Radiol. 51(3):427-34, 2021
2. van Nimwegen LWE et al: MR imaging in discriminating between benign and malignant paediatric ovarian masses: a systematic review. Eur Radiol. 30(2):1166-81, 2020
3. Lala SV et al: Ovarian neoplasms of childhood. Pediatr Radiol. 49(11):1463-75, 2019

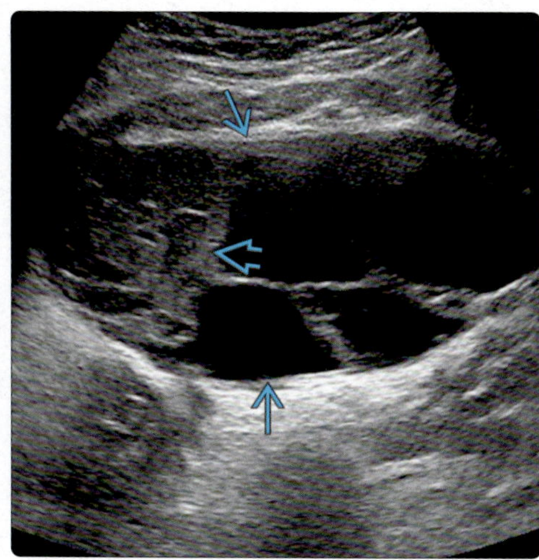

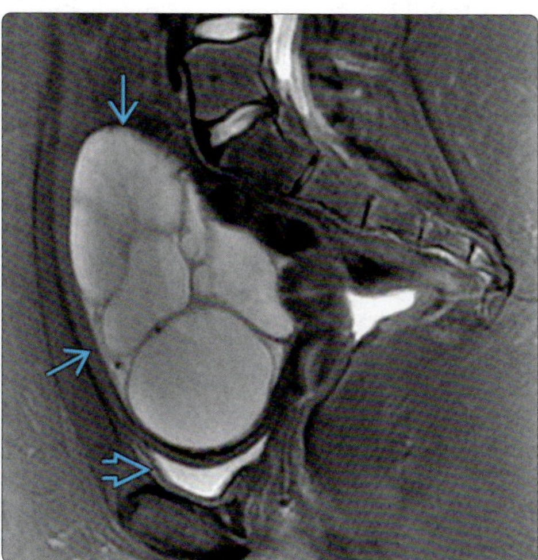

(Left) *Longitudinal ultrasound of the ovary in an adolescent diagnosed with a granulosa cell tumor shows a mixed cystic & solid mass ➡. The cystic component has multiple septations. A solid component ➡ is present in the superior aspect of the mass.* **(Right)** *Sagittal T2 FS MR in the same patient shows the multiseptated granulosa cell tumor ➡ superior to the urinary bladder ➡.*

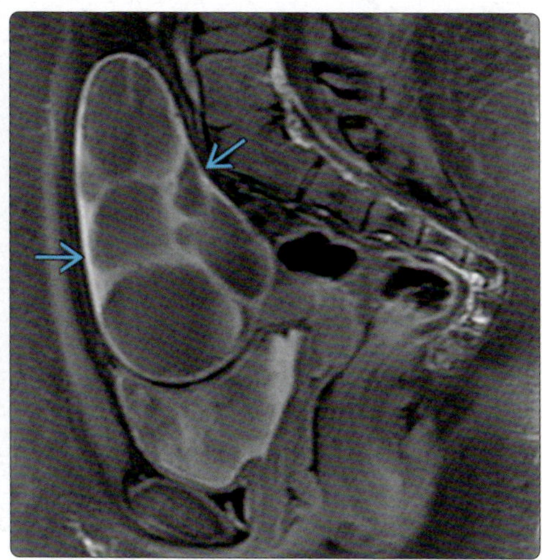

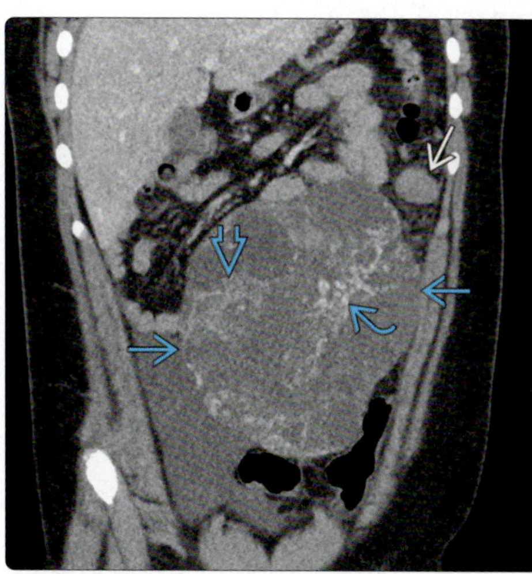

(Left) *Sagittal T1 C+ FS MR in the same patient shows the multiseptated ovarian mass ➡ superior to the bladder. The wall & septations of the mass enhance.* **(Right)** *Coronal CECT in an adolescent diagnosed with a metastatic ovarian germ cell tumor shows a large mass ➡ extending to the midabdomen. The mass has multiple aggressive features, including septations or nodularity ➡ & large internal tumor vessels ➡. A large peritoneal deposit ➡ is also present.*

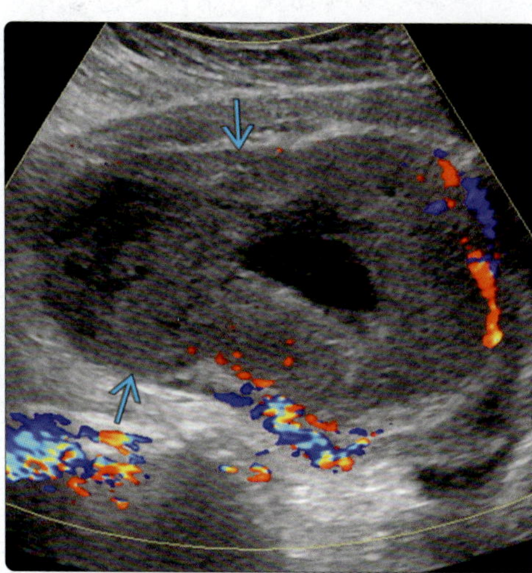

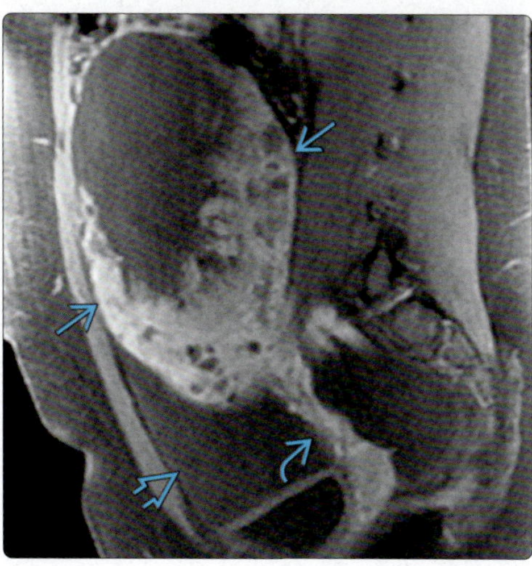

(Left) *Transverse color Doppler ultrasound of the pelvis in an adolescent diagnosed with a small cell ovarian carcinoma shows a mostly solid mass ➡ of the left ovary.* **(Right)** *Sagittal T1 C+ FS MR performed in the same patient shows the large ovarian mass ➡. The superior aspect of the mass does not enhance. The inferior aspect of the mass is connected to the fallopian tube ➡. Note the ascites ➡ superior to the urinary bladder.*

Ovarian Torsion

KEY FACTS

TERMINOLOGY

- Definition: Twisting of vascular pedicle of ovary, fallopian tube, or both → venous obstruction → edema → arterial compromise → ischemia → hemorrhagic infarction

IMAGING

- Unilaterally enlarged ovary
  - Ovarian volume > 100 mL is highly suggestive of torsion
  - Ovarian volume < 20 mL in postpubertal patient was never torsed in one series
  - Ratio of abnormal to normal ovarian volumes ≥ 5:1 strongly correlated with torsion in same series
- Scattered mostly peripheral follicles, often 8-12 mm
- Torsed ovary is often displaced to midline
  - May extend into abdomen or contralateral pelvis
- Sonographic whirlpool sign of twisted vascular pedicle
- Variable patterns of Doppler flow within twisted ovary ranging from normal to completely absent
- Pelvic free fluid or hemoperitoneum
- Hemorrhagic cyst in fetal/neonatal ovary suggests torsion

CLINICAL ISSUES

- Urgent surgical detorsion
  - Conservation of ovarian tissue if not frankly necrotic
  - > 90% salvage rate of ovarian function
- Variable rates of retorsion; oophoropexy is controversial

DIAGNOSTIC CHECKLIST

- Painful midline pelvic mass may represent torsed ovary if both normal ovaries are not confidently visualized
- Doppler exam of ovarian parenchyma may be normal despite true adnexal torsion → grayscale findings & high clinical suspicion are more predictive
- Presence of underlying ovarian cyst/mass can create diagnostic dilemma
  - Experienced clinical evaluation is key in these cases
- Normal symmetric grayscale & Doppler appearance of ovaries makes ovarian torsion highly unlikely

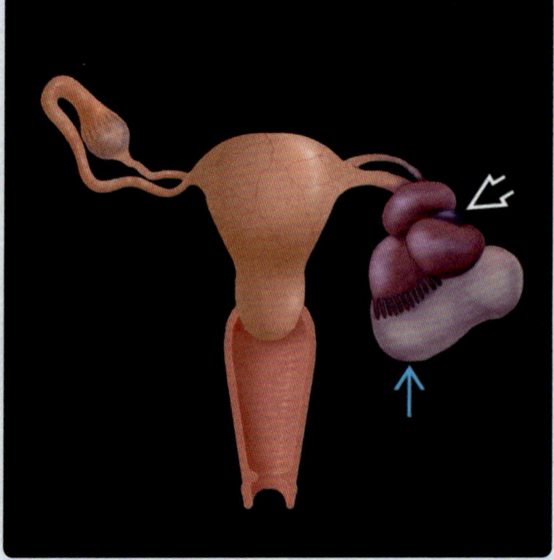

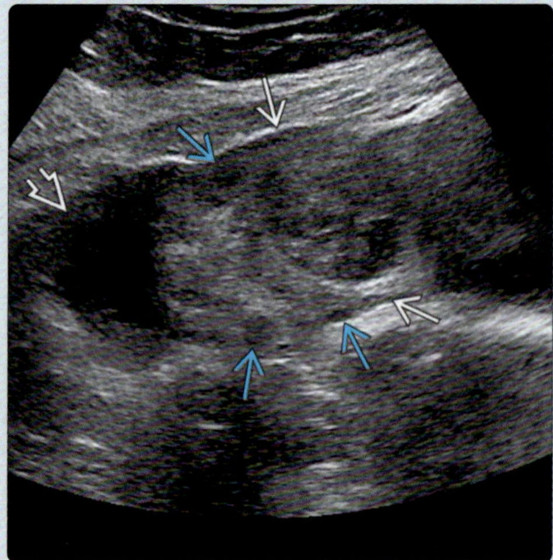

(Left) *Graphic shows torsion ➔ of the ovarian vascular pedicle & fallopian tube, which results in ischemia of the ovary ➔ & distention of the distal segment of the fallopian tube.* **(Right)** *Transverse pelvic ultrasound for acute pain in a 13-year-old girl shows a large 6- to 7-cm heterogeneous mass ➔ with adjacent free fluid ➔. A few cysts ➔ are present at the outer margin of the mass. No normal right ovary was visualized.*

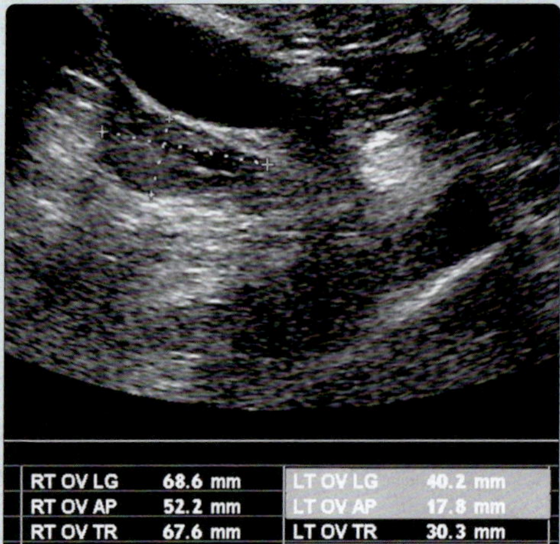

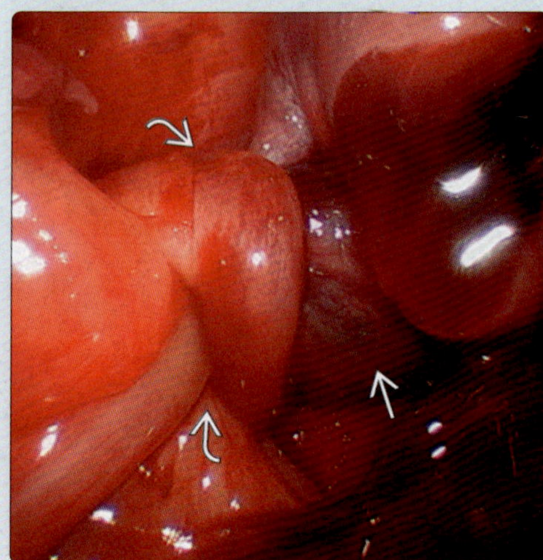

(Left) *Comparison ultrasound of the left adnexa in the same patient shows the normal left ovary between the cursors, with a volume of 11 mL. The painful right-sided mass (her right ovary) was over 10x as large & was torsed 3x at laparoscopy.* **(Right)** *Intraoperative photograph during laparoscopy shows the typical twisting & spiral appearance ➔ of adnexal-supporting structures. The darker structure deep to the twisted tissue is the torsed ovary ➔.*

TERMINOLOGY

Synonyms

- Adnexal torsion, twisted ovary

Definitions

- Twisting of vascular pedicle of ovary, fallopian tube, or both → venous obstruction → edema → arterial compromise → ischemia → hemorrhagic infarction

IMAGING

General Features

- Best diagnostic clue
  - Unilateral ovarian enlargement with scattered peripheral follicles ± discrete cyst or tumor in setting of acute pain
  - Painful midline pelvic mass with failure to identify ipsilateral normal ovary is also very suspicious
  - Doppler exam is not sensitive for ovarian torsion
    - Abnormal flow can be useful adjunct to grayscale
- Location
  - Ovaries usually lie on either side of uterus; torsed ovary is often displaced to midline
    - May extend into abdomen or contralateral pelvis
  - Right ovary is affected slightly more often than left
- Size
  - Twisted adnexa: 7- to 200-mL volume (mean of 24 mL in recent series); rarely > 2,000 mL
  - Twisted ovary is generally > 2x size of contralateral ovary
    - Can be much larger, especially with underlying mass

Ultrasonographic Findings

- Grayscale ultrasound
  - Unilateral ovarian enlargement
    - Ovarian volume > 100 mL suggests torsion
    - Ovarian volume < 20 mL in postpubertal patient was never torsed in one series
      - Ratio of abnormal to normal ovarian volumes ≥ 5:1 strongly correlated with torsion in same series
      - Median torsed to normal ovarian volume ratio of 12:1 in another series
  - Scattered, predominantly peripheral follicles of 8-12 mm in enlarged ovary
    - Moderately sensitive, highly specific for torsion in adolescents
      - Different than numerous "string of pearls" peripheral follicles bilaterally in polycystic ovarian syndrome patient without pain
    - ± fluid-debris levels in follicles; variable size of follicles
    - Follicular ring sign: ↑ echogenicity surrounding follicles in torsion (38%)
  - Variable ovarian parenchymal echotexture depending on presence of
    - Edema vs. hemorrhage/infarction
    - Underlying cystic or solid mass
      - Consider normal vs. abnormal appearance of residual ovary surrounding lesion
  - Failure to confidently visualize bilateral normally positioned ovaries
  - Fallopian tube thickening > 10 mm
  - Pelvic free fluid or hemoperitoneum
  - In neonate, hemorrhagic cyst also suggests torsion
    - Fluid-debris level, retracting clot, lace-like contents
- Color Doppler
  - Sonographic whirlpool sign of twisted vascular pedicle
    - Round, swirling bull's-eye or target appearance of hyper- & hypoechoic rings or stripes ± Doppler flow
    - May only be achieved with endovaginal scanning
  - Variable patterns of flow within twisted ovary ranging from normal to completely absent
    - View any asymmetry in flow with suspicion

MR Findings

- Tubal thickening, enlargement of ovarian stroma
- Scattered T2-hyperintense peripheral follicles
- ± T2 hyperintensity of ovarian stroma
- ± foci of T1 hyperintensity from hemorrhage
- ↓ or absent enhancement of ovarian parenchyma
- Surrounding soft tissue edema & fluid
- Whirlpool sign of twisted vessels & adnexal supporting structures

CT Findings

- Not recommended for evaluation of ovarian torsion but may be 1st modality obtained for other clinical suspicions
- Bland, rounded, soft tissue density mass ± cyst
  - Smooth thickening of wall suggests torsion
- Uterine deviation toward twisted adnexa
- Tubal thickening (> 10 mm) + surrounding edema/fluid
- Ascites, which may be hemorrhagic

Imaging Recommendations

- Best imaging tool
  - Ultrasound: Grayscale findings are more reliable (92% sensitive, 96% specific) than Doppler (50% sensitive)
    - Doppler exam of ovary may be normal despite true adnexal torsion
  - MR offers greater sensitivity & specificity but delays surgical treatment as secondary exam
  - Overall sensitivity: 79-92% for ultrasound; > 95% for MR, 42% for CT
- Protocol advice
  - Endovaginal scanning in patients who are sexually active
  - Transabdominal scanning via well-distended urinary bladder in patients who are not sexually active
    - May need to fill bladder via Foley if patient is vomiting & dehydrated

DIFFERENTIAL DIAGNOSIS

Appendicitis

- Noncompressible, thick-walled, blind-ending tubular structure in right lower quadrant originating from cecum & measuring > 6 mm in diameter with surrounding fat induration; more difficult to define with perforation

Ovarian Cyst

- Simple or hemorrhagic cyst may cause pain without torsion
  - In fetus/neonate, hemorrhagic cyst should suggest torsed ovary
- Avascular internally by Doppler
- Hemorrhagic cyst has reticular septations, debris, nodular clot
- Cyst > 5 cm is more likely to be associated with torsion

Isolated Fallopian Tube Torsion

- Dilated fluid-filled tube or paraovarian cystic mass, often with normal adjacent ovary

Pelvic Inflammatory Disease

- Complex tuboovarian fluid collection in setting of cervical tenderness, discharge, & generalized pain is typical of pelvic inflammatory disease

Ovarian Tumor

- Discrete heterogeneous cystic &/or solid mass
- Painful rarely from rupture or necrosis vs. superimposed torsion (always painful)

Ectopic Pregnancy

- Cystic tubal mass ± yolk sac, extrauterine embryonic cardiac activity, surrounding hyperemia, free fluid
- Serum β-hCG result is crucial

Distal Ureteral Calculus

- Echogenic stone ± Doppler twinkle artifact, posterior acoustic shadowing, thick-walled hydroureter, abnormal ureteral jet, variable hydronephrosis

PATHOLOGY

General Features

- Etiology
  - Usually spontaneous twist of ovary & fallopian tube
    - Torsion of normal adnexal structures is more common in children than adults
  - Developmental abnormalities of fallopian tubes or mesosalpinx (such as excessively long tube or absent mesosalpinx) can precipitate torsion
  - Intrinsic ovarian or tubal disease, tumors, cysts, trauma, or recent surgery also predispose to torsion
    - ~ 50% of pediatric cases have dominant cyst or tumor
      - Torsion is most likely if mass > 5 cm

Microscopic Features

- Peripheral cysts reflect ovarian congestion & transudation of fluid into follicles

CLINICAL ISSUES

Presentation

- Most common signs/symptoms
  - Acute, severe unilateral lower abdominal/pelvic pain, constant or intermittent
  - Nausea & vomiting (often synchronous with pain)
- Other signs/symptoms
  - Low-grade fever
  - Tender palpable mass
  - Incarcerated inguinal hernia

Demographics

- Age
  - Mean: 10-11 years
  - 50% of cases occur in premenarchal girls
    - Tend to have delayed diagnosis & longer duration of ovarian ischemia
  - ~ 10% occur in perinatal period
- Epidemiology
  - Annual incidence: 1 in 20,000 females ages 1-20 years

Natural History & Prognosis

- Infarction → nonfunctioning ovary → infertility risk
- Risk of autoamputation of infarcted ovary → mobile calcified ovary
- Variable retorsion rate after detorsion
  - Higher retorsion rate in prepubertal girls
- Asynchronous bilateral ovarian torsion in 5-10%

Treatment

- Urgent surgical detorsion
  - Conservation of ovarian tissue
    - Oophorectomy is now uncommon, even if necrotic-appearing
  - Oophoropexy (to prevent retorsion) is controversial
- Salvage rates are better for ovarian than testicular torsion
  - > 90% salvage rate for ovarian function
  - Length of symptoms prior to surgery does not always predict viability
  - Appearance at surgery is also not predictive of salvage
- Aspiration ± biopsy vs. resection of cyst or solid lesion

DIAGNOSTIC CHECKLIST

Consider

- Painful midline pelvic mass may represent torsed ovary if 2 normal ovaries are not confidently visualized

Image Interpretation Pearls

- Documenting normal arterial & venous flow in adnexa does not exclude torsion
  - Grayscale findings & high clinical suspicion are more predictive
- Presence of underlying ovarian cyst/mass can create diagnostic dilemma
  - Hemorrhagic cyst may be painful in absence of torsion despite causing overall ↑ ovarian volume
  - However, cyst/mass also predisposes to torsion & may obscure other classic imaging findings of torsion
  - Experienced clinical evaluation is key in these cases
- Completely normal & symmetric grayscale & Doppler appearance of ovaries makes ovarian torsion highly unlikely

SELECTED REFERENCES

1. Alberto EC et al: Variations in the management of adolescent adnexal torsion at a single institution and the creation of a unified care pathway. Pediatr Surg Int. 37(1):129-35, 2021
2. Dawood MT et al: Adnexal torsion: review of radiologic appearances. Radiographics. 41(2):609-24, 2021
3. Hartman SJ et al: Ovarian volume ratio is a reliable predictor of ovarian torsion in girls without an adnexal mass. J Pediatr Surg. 56(1):180-2, 2021
4. Strachowski LM et al: Pearls and pitfalls in imaging of pelvic adnexal torsion: seven tips to tell it's twisted. Radiographics. 41(2):625-40, 2021
5. Lipsett SC et al: Variation in oophorectomy rates for children with ovarian torsion across US children's hospitals. J Pediatr. 231:269-72., 2020
6. Rougier E et al: Added value of MRI for the diagnosis of adnexal torsion in children and adolescents after inconclusive ultrasound examination. Diagn Interv Imaging. 101(11):747-56, 2020
7. Prieto JM et al: Premenarchal patients present differently: a twist on the typical patient presenting with ovarian torsion. J Pediatr Surg. 54(12):2614-6, 2019
8. Shapira-Zaltsberg G et al: Non-visualization of the ovaries on pediatric transabdominal ultrasound with a non-distended bladder: Can adnexal torsion be excluded? Pediatr Radiol. 49(10):1313-9, 2019

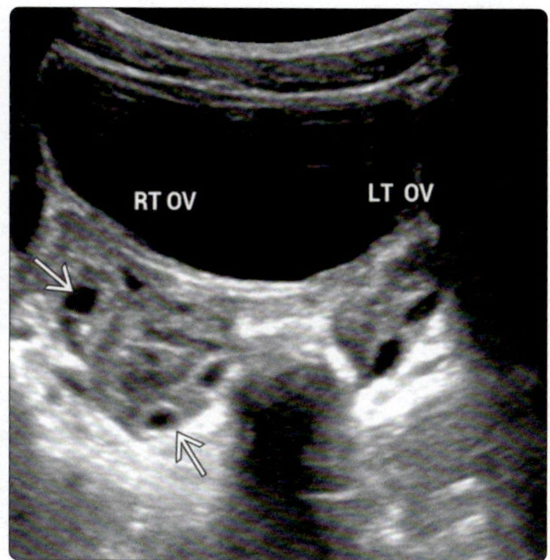

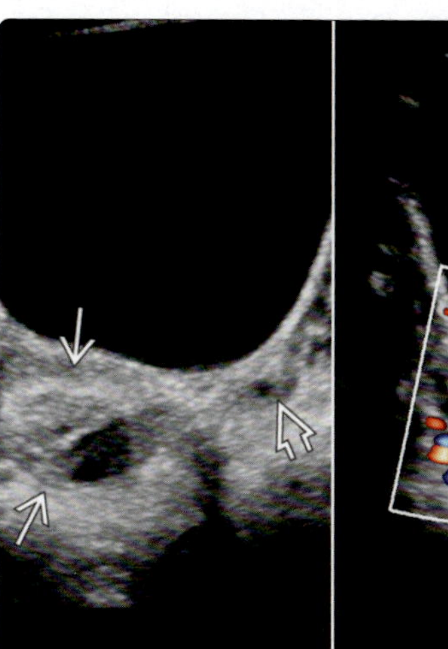

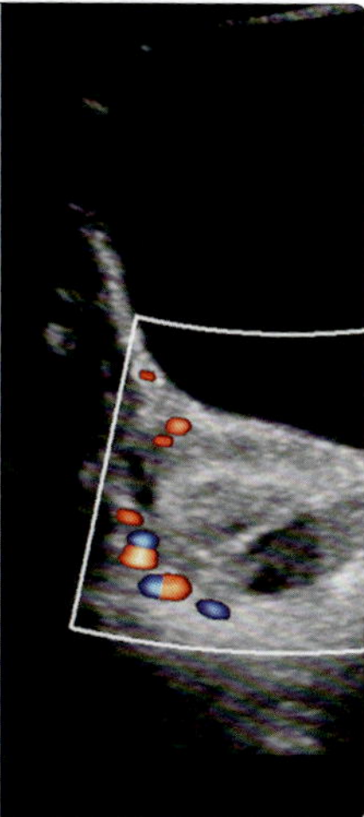

(Left) *Transverse ultrasound in a 6-year-old premenarchal girl shows an enlarged right ovary with peripheral cysts ➔. The right ovarian volume was 4.5x the left ovarian volume in this case of surgically confirmed right ovarian torsion.* **(Right)** *Transverse grayscale & color Doppler ultrasound images show an asymmetrically enlarged & heterogeneous right ovary ➔ in this 11-year-old premenarchal girl with a volume of 22 mL (compared to 4 mL on the left side ➔) in another case of ovarian torsion.*

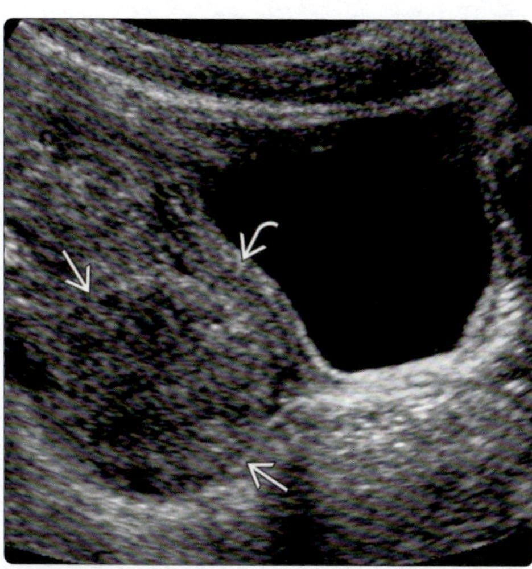

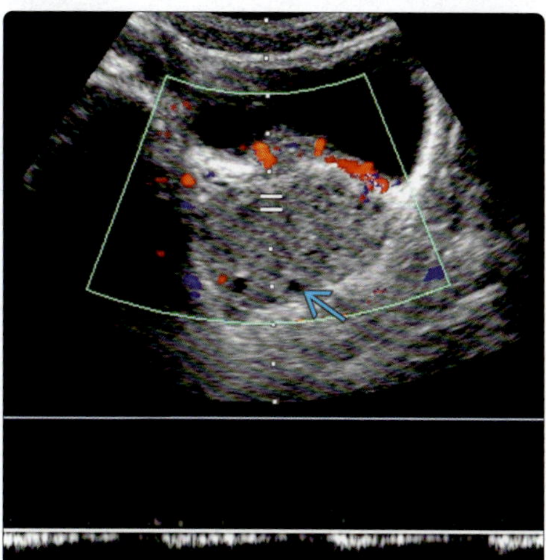

(Left) *Midline longitudinal ultrasound in a 7-year-old girl with acute pain shows a round, solid mass ➔ posterior to the uterus ➔. No normal right ovary was identified.* **(Right)** *Transverse color Doppler ultrasound in the same patient shows numerous small peripheral follicles ➔ & minimal blood flow within this displaced edematous right ovary. Ovarian torsion was confirmed at surgery.*

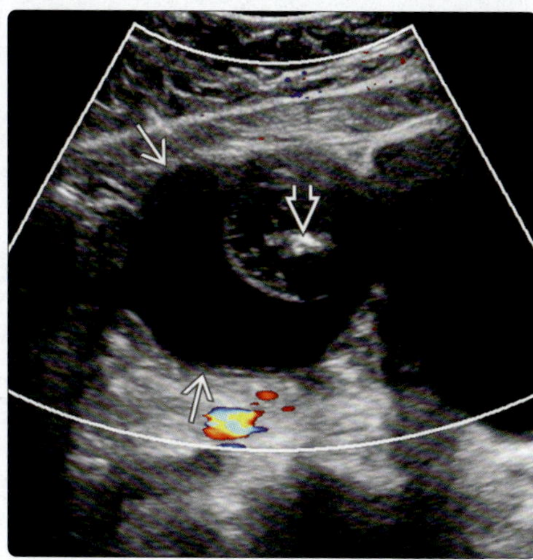

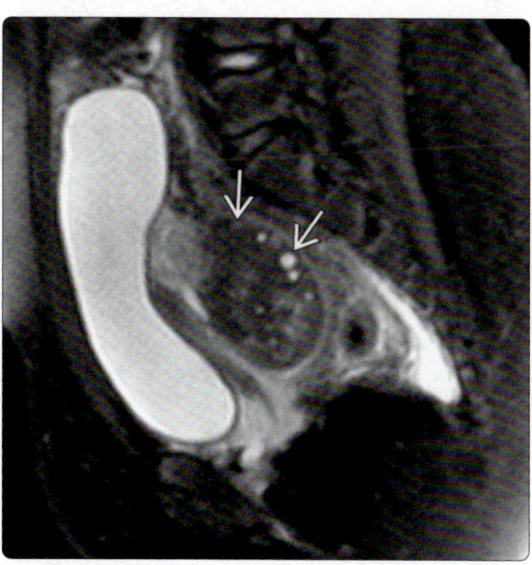

(Left) *Transverse ultrasound in an adolescent girl shows a large, heterogenous, complex cystic lesion ➔ in the right ovary with shadowing Ca^{2+} ➔ corresponding to her point of maximal pain. A mature teratoma with torsion was found at surgery.* **(Right)** *Sagittal T2 FS MR in a 12-year-old girl with pain & a reported "uterine mass" shows an enlarged, displaced, low signal intensity ovary with peripheral follicles ➔ & surrounding soft tissue edema, consistent with torsion.*

Ectopic Ovary

KEY FACTS

TERMINOLOGY

- Ectopic ovary: Abnormally located ovary
  - Inguinal ovarian hernia (95%): Presents as labial mass
    - Canal of Nuck hernia
  - Intraabdominal ectopia may be incidental or iatrogenic
  - Retroperitoneal location is extremely rare

IMAGING

- Labial/groin soft tissue mass with numerous follicles
  - R > L (60% vs. 30%); 10% bilateral
- US is study of choice for palpable inguinal mass (± specific suspicion for ovarian herniation)
  - Use highest frequency transducer available
  - Step-off pad improves visualization of superficial structures (including herniated ovarian follicles)

TOP DIFFERENTIAL DIAGNOSES

- Abscess
- Inguinal lymphadenopathy
- Bowel-containing inguinal hernia
- Mesothelial cyst of round ligament
- Ovarian torsion

PATHOLOGY

- Canal of Nuck is analogous to processus vaginalis in boys
  - May remain patent in up to 10% of term newborns
- Up to 20% with ovarian herniation also have herniation of salpinx, urinary bladder, bowel, &/or uterus
- ~ 20% of herniated ovaries develop strangulation or torsion
- Small association of ovarian herniation with müllerian anomalies

CLINICAL ISSUES

- Inguinal ovarian hernia should be top consideration in any newborn/infant girl with labial or groin mass
- Little morbidity without superimposed strangulation/torsion

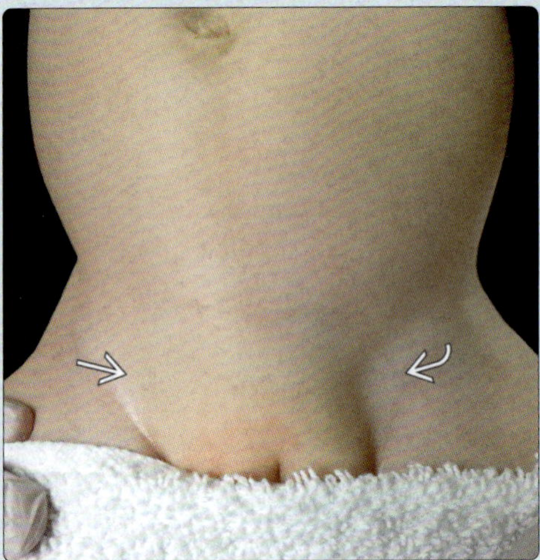

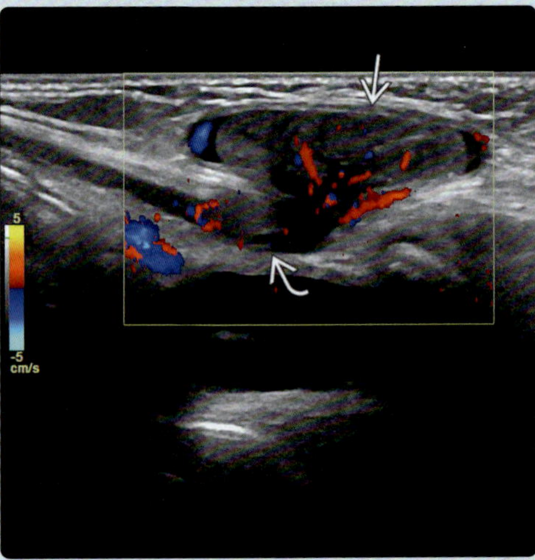

(Left) *Clinical photograph shows an 8-month-old girl with a new, nonpainful right inguinal mass ➡ due to herniation of the right ovary through the canal of Nuck. Note the relative concavity on the normal, contralateral side ⮰.* **(Right)** *Longitudinal color Doppler US of the right groin in the same patient shows a normal-appearing ovary ➡ in the superficial soft tissues. Note the adnexal vessels extending through the canal of Nuck ⮰. Transverse US (not shown) better demonstrated anechoic follicles, confirming that this was the ovary.*

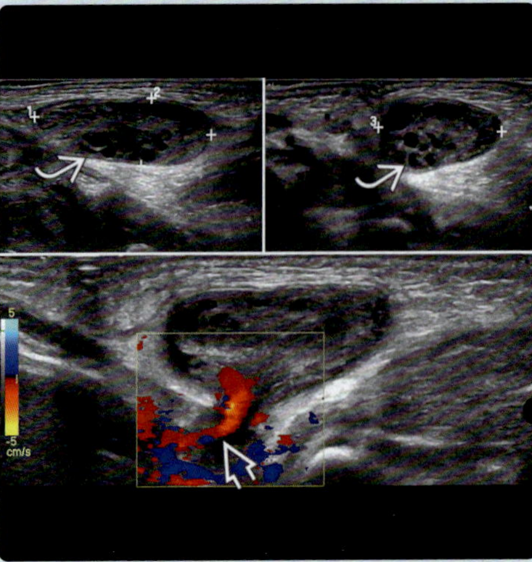

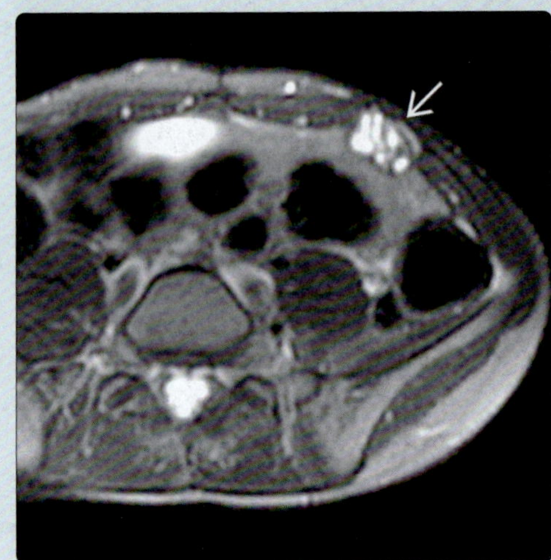

(Left) *Longitudinal (top left) & transverse (top right) US images of a palpable labial mass in a newborn show a normal-appearing ovary (calipers) with numerous anechoic follicles ⮰. Oblique longitudinal color Doppler US (bottom) better shows the adnexal vessels of the herniated ovary extending though the canal of Nuck ⮰.* **(Right)** *Axial T2 FS MR in a 12-year-old girl with several prior surgeries for an anorectal malformation shows an ectopic left ovary positioned in a prior ostomy site ➡.*

TERMINOLOGY

Definitions

- Ectopic ovary: Abnormally located ovary
  - Inguinal ovarian hernia (95%): Presents as labial mass
  - Intraabdominal ectopia: Incidental or iatrogenic
    - Nonstandard ovarian location is common & usually incidental (due to long ovarian ligaments)
    - Nonpelvic location is sometimes seen after numerous or complex abdominopelvic surgeries
    - Ovarian transposition is sometimes performed to preserve fertility prior to radiation therapy
  - Retroperitoneal location is extremely rare

IMAGING

General Features

- Best diagnostic clue
  - Oval soft tissue mass with numerous follicles in unexpected location for ovary
- Location
  - Inguinal, groin, or labial mass (95%)
    - R > L (60% vs. 30%); 10% bilateral
- Size
  - Ovarian size remains normal for age (0.5-3.0 cm)

Ultrasonographic Findings

- Grayscale ultrasound
  - Typical ovarian morphology: Oval soft tissue mass with multiple round anechoic follicles scattered throughout
- Color Doppler
  - Look for ↓, absent, or otherwise abnormal blood flow as sign of ovarian torsion/strangulation
    - Grayscale findings are actually more sensitive

MR Findings

- T2-bright follicles are easily recognized on MR

Imaging Recommendations

- Protocol advice
  - Newborn or infant with groin or labial mass
    - US: Use highest frequency transducer available
    - Step-off pad further ↑ visualization of superficial structures (such as herniated ovarian follicles)
- Suspected intraabdominal ovary in older child
  - Multiplanar T2 MR through pelvis
  - Preceding ovarian stimulation aids identification

DIFFERENTIAL DIAGNOSIS

Abscess

- Complex fluid collection without internal blood flow
- Look for other signs of inflammation/infection: Cellulitis, erythema, exquisite pain, fever, etc.

Lymphadenopathy

- Usually multiple hypoechoic ovoid/reniform masses
- Look for hilar vessels & echogenic fatty hilum
  - May be absent with necrosis or infiltration

Bowel-Containing Inguinal Hernia

- Most common labial mass, often easily reducible
- Look for classic bowel wall US signature & peristalsis

Mesothelial Cyst of Round Ligament

- Benign cyst of round ligament within inguinal canal
- Simple, unilocular cystic mass; may be complex if infected
- Rare; analogous to hydrocele of spermatic cord in boys

Ovarian Torsion

- Swollen, torsed ovary (without herniation) may be displaced to midline or contralateral pelvis
- Failure to visualize 2 normal ovaries in patient with pain & "pelvic mass" → torsion until proven otherwise

PATHOLOGY

General Features

- Canal of Nuck is analogous to processus vaginalis in boys
  - Evagination of parietal peritoneum into inguinal canal
  - Normally loses connection with peritoneal cavity but may remain patent in up to 10% of term newborns
  - Up to 20% with ovarian herniation also have herniation of salpinx, urinary bladder, bowel, &/or uterus

Gross Pathologic & Surgical Features

- Small association with müllerian anomalies
- ~ 20% of herniated ovaries are strangulated or torsed

CLINICAL ISSUES

Presentation

- Most common signs/symptoms
  - Painless, palpable, mobile mass in groin or labia majora
  - Pain & vomiting are common with superimposed strangulation or torsion

Natural History & Prognosis

- Good prognosis with little morbidity if not strangulated

Treatment

- Relatively urgent reduction, hernia repair, & oophoropexy
- Emergent reduction for ovarian strangulation/torsion

DIAGNOSTIC CHECKLIST

Consider

- Always consider ectopic ovary in girls with labial/groin mass
- ~ 10% of term newborns have metachronous hernias

Image Interpretation Pearls

- Look for rare associated müllerian duct anomalies (solitary or pelvic kidney, uterine anomalies, etc.)

SELECTED REFERENCES

1. Rosa F et al: How embryology knowledge can help radiologists in the differential diagnosis of canal of Nuck pathologies. Radiol Med. 126(7):910-24, 2021
2. Morabito G et al: A young girl with right ovarian torsion and left ovarian ectopy. Ital J Pediatr. 46(1):51, 2020
3. Jedrzejewski G et al: Nuck canal hernias, typical and unusual ultrasound findings. Ultrasound Q. 35(1):79-81, 2019
4. Thomas AK et al: Canal of Nuck abnormalities. J Ultrasound Med. 39(2):385-95, 2019
5. Castro AD et al: Ectopic ovary with torsion: uncommon diagnosis made by ultrasound. Radiol Bras. 50(1):60-1, 2017
6. Moawad NS et al: Laparoscopic ovarian transposition before pelvic cancer treatment: ovarian function and fertility preservation. J Minim Invasive Gynecol. 24(1):28-35, 2017

Epididymoorchitis

KEY FACTS

TERMINOLOGY

- Infectious inflammation of epididymis, testicle, or both
- Orchitis alone is much less common than epididymoorchitis

IMAGING

- Enlargement of affected tissues (i.e., testicle, epididymis, or both) with accompanying ↑ blood flow
  - ↑ blood flow is best demonstrated on transverse side-by-side comparison view
  - Arterial waveforms typically remain low resistance
- Echotexture may be ↑ or ↓, often heterogeneous
- Reactive hydrocele
- Scrotal wall is also thickened

TOP DIFFERENTIAL DIAGNOSES

- Torsion of appendage testis/epididymis
- Testicular torsion
- Scrotal cellulitis
- Hernia

PATHOLOGY

- Bacterial infections may be due to ascending infection (in sexually active adolescents), direct seeding of infected urine with genitourinary (GU) anomalies (especially in young children), or hematogenous seeding
- Can also be viral (typically mumps) or posttraumatic
- Some cases of epididymitis are likely due to unrecognized appendage torsion

CLINICAL ISSUES

- Gradual onset of painful scrotum, swelling, erythema ± dysuria, enuresis, frequency
  - Prehn sign: Elevation of affected hemiscrotum relieves pain of epididymitis & exacerbates pain of torsion
- Primary therapy: Antibiotics
- Bedrest, scrotal support & elevation, ice packs, antiinflammatory agents, & analgesics are also used
- Consider work-up for GU anomalies in younger children & recurrent cases

(Left) *Graphic shows epididymitis with an inflamed, hyperemic epididymal body ➔ draped over a normal-appearing testicle. In epididymoorchitis, the testicle would also be inflamed.* **(Right)** *Longitudinal oblique color Doppler US shows marked hyperemia of the left testis ➔ & epididymis ➔ in a teenager with acute pain, consistent with epididymoorchitis.*

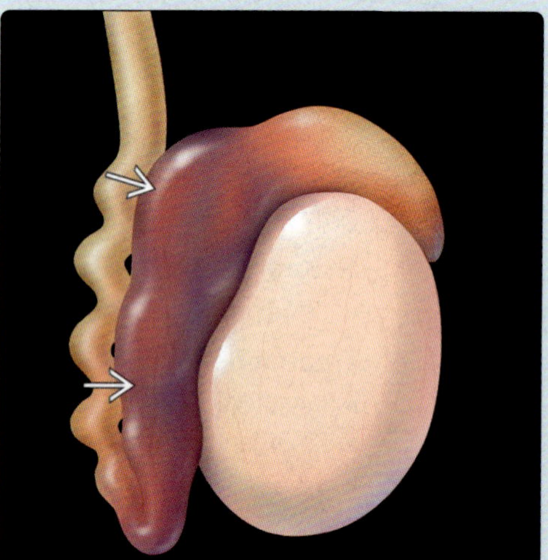

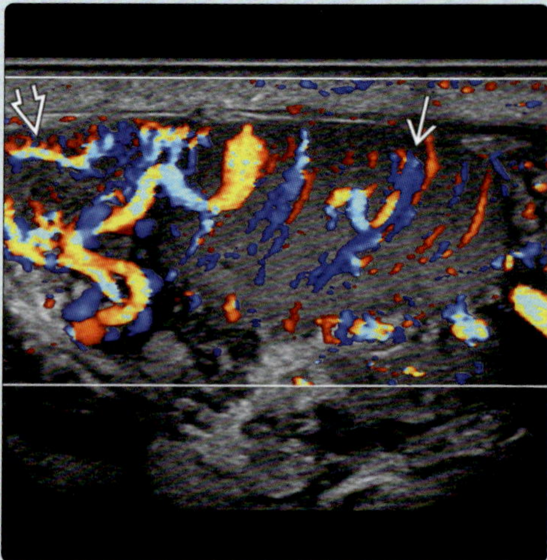

(Left) *Transverse grayscale US in a 5-year-old boy with acute right scrotal swelling shows asymmetric enlargement & heterogeneous echotexture of the epididymis ➔. The testicle has ➔ normal echotexture but was larger than the contralateral side. A small, simple hydrocele ➔ is also present.* **(Right)** *Color Doppler US in the same patient shows marked hyperemia ➔ of the right epididymis, testicle, & surrounding scrotal tissues, consistent with epididymoorchitis.*

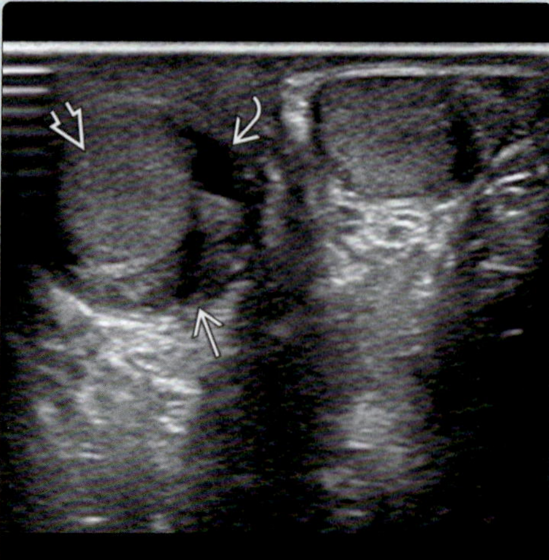

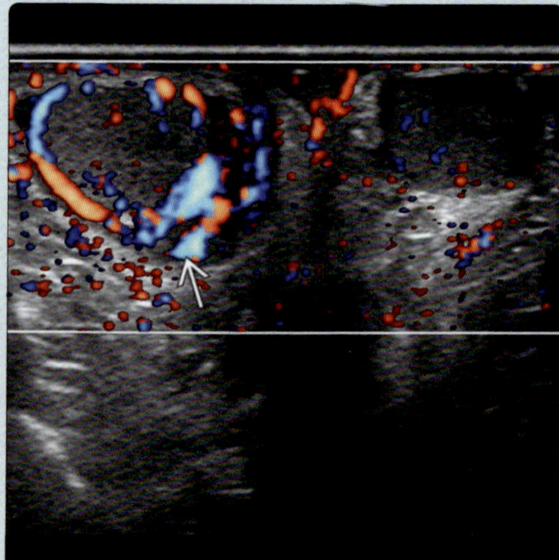

TERMINOLOGY

Synonyms

- Acute scrotum, epididymitis, orchitis, mumps

Definitions

- Infectious inflammation of epididymis, testicle, or both
- Orchitis alone is much less common than epididymoorchitis

IMAGING

General Features

- Best diagnostic clue
  - Enlargement of affected tissues (i.e., testicle, epididymis, or both)
  - Accompanying ↑ blood flow
  - Small reactive hydrocele
- Location
  - Entire hemiscrotum may show inflammatory changes
  - Acute epididymitis is bilateral in 5-10% of patients

Ultrasonographic Findings

- Grayscale ultrasound
  - Inflamed organs typically show ↑ size when compared to asymptomatic side
  - Echotexture may be ↑ or ↓ from normal, often heterogeneous
  - Reactive hydrocele is common
  - Scrotal wall is also thickened
- Color Doppler
  - Hyperemia of involved tissues
    - Flow in testis typically remains low resistance
  - ↑ blood flow is often best demonstrated on transverse side-by-side comparison view
  - Testicular blood flow can sometimes be difficult to demonstrate in very young males
    - Flow is easy to see in cases of epididymoorchitis
- Power Doppler
  - Doppler flow dramatically ↑

Fluoroscopic Findings

- Voiding cystourethrogram
  - May be performed in infants & nonsexually active boys to exclude underlying genitourinary (GU) anomaly
    - Ectopic ureter, vesicoureteral reflux
    - Urethral abnormality with reflux into vas deferens
    - Voiding dysfunction/high-pressure voiding pattern
  - Trend toward less imaging work-up with presumed viral etiology

Nuclear Medicine Findings

- Nuclear scintigraphy
  - Historical interest only (now replaced by US)
  - Radiotracer of choice: Tc-99m pertechnetate
  - Scan shows hyperemia with ↑ radiotracer accumulation & enlargement; occasional cold rim of large hydrocele

MR Findings

- MR urography if complex GU anomalies are suspected & not fully elucidated by US & VCUG

Radiographic Findings

- No role for radiography except in cases of penetrating injury or suspected foreign body

Imaging Recommendations

- Best imaging tool
  - Ultrasound with Doppler
- Protocol advice
  - High-frequency linear transducer is best
  - Supporting scrotum on towel(s) may be helpful

DIFFERENTIAL DIAGNOSIS

Torsion of Appendage Testis

- Nodular hypo- or hyperechoic avascular mass adjacent to testis with surrounding hyperemia
- Likely is most common cause of acute scrotum in childhood
  - Some cases of epididymal hyperemia are likely reactive from unrecognized appendage torsion

Testicular Torsion

- Unilateral testicular blood flow is diminished or absent (on side of pain)
- May see twist or knot of spermatic cord above testis
- Surgical emergency
- Note that intermittent torsion may show hyperemia; look for other clues, including
  - Abnormal lie of testis
  - Hydrocele completely surrounding testis (suggesting bell-clapper deformity)
  - High-resistance arterial waveforms in setting of "improved pain"

Traumatic Rupture of Testicle

- Focal parenchymal heterogeneity with contour deformity & interruption of echogenic tunica albuginea
- History is typically obvious

Scrotal Cellulitis

- Generalized wall thickening & hyperemia
- Normal testicle & epididymis
- May be infectious, allergic, related to insect bite, or Henoch-Schönlein purpura

Scrotal Hernia

- Herniated abdominal contents are continuous with peritoneal cavity through inguinal canal
- Look for bowel wall signature & peristalsis
- Herniated bowel displaces normal testis & epididymis
  - May cause ↓ blood flow of ipsilateral testis in young infants

Leukemia

- Unilateral or bilateral enlargement
- Parenchyma may be hypoechoic diffusely with palisading vessels

PATHOLOGY

General Features

- Etiology
  - Ascending GU tract infection in sexually active adolescents

- In males 14-35 years of age, disease is most frequently caused by *Neisseria gonorrhoeae* & *Chlamydia trachomatis*
- Retrograde passage of infected urine from prostatic urethra to epididymis via ejaculatory ducts & vas deferens
    - Bacterial seeding may also occur
        - Directly in cases with GU anomaly
        - Hematogenously in cases without demonstrable anomaly
    - Most often caused by *Staphylococcus aureus*, *Escherichia coli*, or viruses, especially mumps
        - Mumps orchitis often has fever, malaise, & myalgia
        - Parotiditis precedes onset of orchitis by 3-5 days
        - Subclinical infections occur in 30-40% of patients
        - Outbreaks of mumps have been reported in school age children, despite mumps, measles, & rubella (MMR) vaccination
        - Mumps epididymoorchitis most often has focal swelling of epididymal head with head:tail ratio > 2
        - Mumps orchitis is typically unilateral & seen in only 1/3 of all mumps cases
- Associated abnormalities
    - When seen in infants & young children, search for predisposing GU anomaly
        - Ectopic ureter
        - Ectopic vas deferens
        - Prostatic utricle
        - Urethral duplication
        - Posterior urethral valves
        - Urethrorectal fistula
        - Detrusor sphincter dyssynergia
        - Vesicoureteral reflux
        - Neurogenic bladder
        - Anorectal malformation

CLINICAL ISSUES

Presentation

- Most common signs/symptoms
    - Gradual onset of painful scrotum, swelling, erythema
    - Systemic symptoms of fever, nausea, vomiting
    - Urinary symptoms of dysuria, enuresis, frequency
- Other signs/symptoms
    - Prehn sign: Elevation of affected hemiscrotum relieves pain of epididymitis & exacerbates pain of torsion
    - Instrumentation & indwelling catheters are common risk factors for acute epididymitis
    - Association with clean intermittent catheterization
    - Urethritis or prostatitis can also coexist

Demographics

- Age
    - Adolescents beginning sexual activity
    - In infants & children, consider work-up for underlying urinary tract anomalies
- Sex
    - Males
- Ethnicity
    - No ethnic or racial predilection
- Epidemiology
    - MMR vaccine has reduced incidence of mumps orchitis
    - 1 in 1,000 men are affected yearly; frequency in pediatric patients is lower
    - Torsion of testicular/epididymal appendage is more common than epididymoorchitis or testicular torsion
        - Some cases of epididymitis are likely due to unrecognized appendage torsion

Natural History & Prognosis

- Prognosis is generally excellent
- Can lead to abscess if not treated
- Can recur in ~ 25%
    - Recurrent episodes can lead to long-term fertility problems
- Term "chronic epididymitis" refers to patients with symptoms lasting ≥ 6 months
- Reports of secondary thrombosis of pampiniform plexus

Treatment

- Antibiotics are mainstay of therapy
    - Antibiotics are reserved for culture positive cases; otherwise, viral etiology is presumed
    - Bedrest, scrotal support & elevation, ice packs, antiinflammatory agents, & analgesics are also used
    - Follow-up scans to exclude abscess if not improving
- Work-up for GU anomalies in younger children & recurrent cases
- Surgical exploration is only performed
    - If testicular torsion cannot be ruled out
    - If complications occur from acute epididymitis & orchitis
        - Abscess, pyocele, testicular infarction

SELECTED REFERENCES

1. Alshubaili HM et al: Acute right epididymo-orchitis complicated by pampiniform plexus thrombosis. Urol Case Rep. 31:101171, 2020
2. Devlies W et al: Case report on secondary testicular necrosis due to fulminant epididymitis: ultrasonographic evaluation and diagnosis. BMC Urol. 20(1):115, 2020
3. Gagliardi L et al: Orchiepididymitis in a boy With COVID-19. Pediatr Infect Dis J. 39(8):e200-2, 2020
4. Expert Panel on Urological Imaging et al: ACR Appropriateness Criteria® acute onset of scrotal pain-without trauma, without antecedent mass. J Am Coll Radiol. 16(5S):S38-43, 2019
5. Afsarlar CE et al: Ultrasonographic findings in the epididymis of pediatric patients with testicular torsion. J Pediatr Urol. 13(4):393.e1-6, 2017
6. Alkhori NA et al: Pediatric scrotal ultrasound: review and update. Pediatr Radiol. 47(9):1125-33, 2017
7. Hester AG et al: The prostatic utricle: an under-recognized condition resulting in significant morbidity in boys with both hypospadias and normal external genitalia. J Pediatr Urol. 13(5):492.e1-5, 2017
8. Chang CD et al: Acute epididymo-orchitis-related global testicular infarction: clinical and ultrasound findings with an emphasis on the juxta-epididymal string-of-bead sign. Ultrasound Q. 32(3):283-9, 2016
9. Cordeiro E et al: Mumps outbreak among highly vaccinated teenagers and children in the central region of Portugal, 2012-2013. Acta Med Port. 28(4):435-41, 2015
10. Park SJ et al: Distribution of epididymal involvement in mumps epididymo-orchitis. J Ultrasound Med. 34(6):1083-9, 2015
11. Gkentzis A et al: The aetiology and current management of prepubertal epididymitis. Ann R Coll Surg Engl. 96(3):181-3, 2014
12. Redshaw JD et al: Epididymitis: a 21-year retrospective review of presentations to an outpatient urology clinic. J Urol. 192(4):1203-7, 2014
13. Rizvi SA et al: Role of color Doppler ultrasonography in evaluation of scrotal swellings: pattern of disease in 120 patients with review of literature. Urol J. 8(1):60-5, 2011
14. Baldisserotto M: Scrotal emergencies. Pediatr Radiol. 39(5):516-21, 2009
15. Karmazyn B et al: Duplex sonographic findings in children with torsion of the testicular appendages: overlap with epididymitis and epididymoorchitis. J Pediatr Surg. 41(3):500-4, 2006

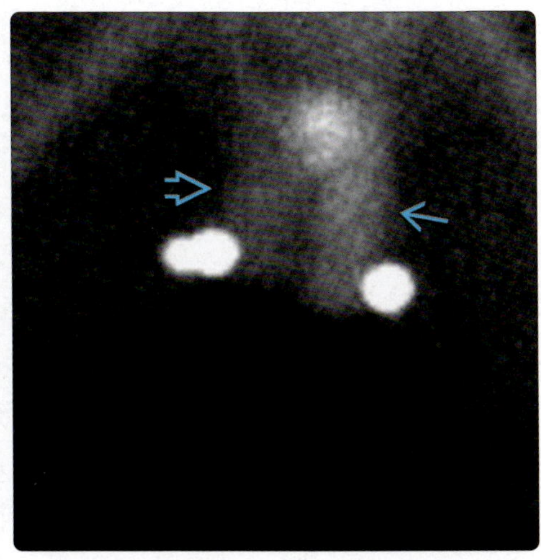

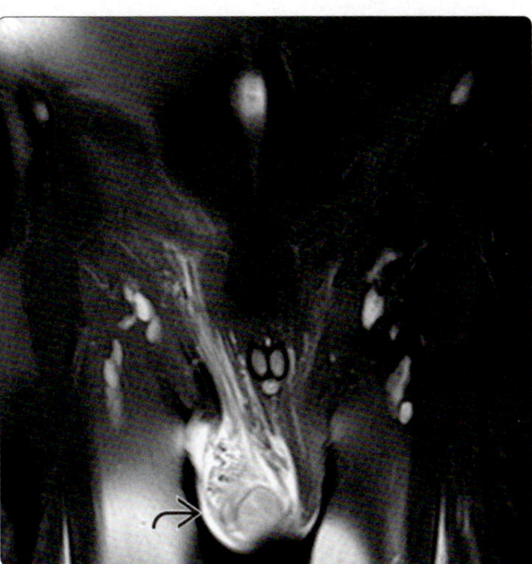

(Left) *Anterior 5-minute image from a Tc-99m pertechnetate scan in a 17-year-old with left scrotal pain demonstrates ↑ radiotracer uptake at the left testicle ➔ compared to the right ➔, which can be seen with epididymoorchitis.* **(Right)** *Coronal T2 FS MR in a 12-year-old with 1 week of right hip pain shows marked high signal intensity throughout the right hemiscrotum ➔, suspicious for epididymoorchitis or subacute torsion given the duration of his symptoms.*

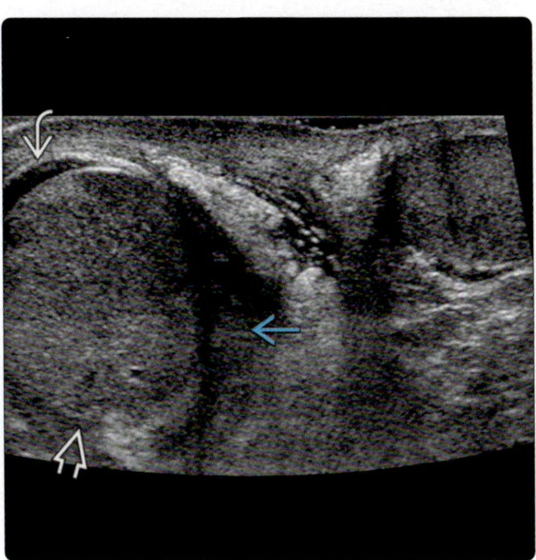

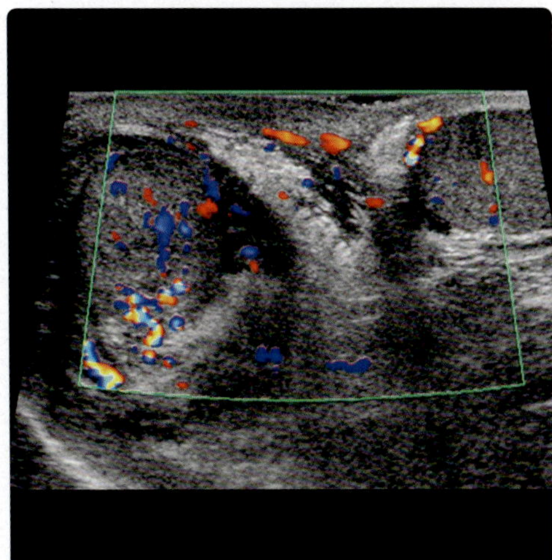

(Left) *Transverse side-by-side US performed following the MR shows an enlarged right testicle ➔, enlarged heterogeneous epididymis ➔, hydrocele ➔, & right-sided scrotal wall thickening.* **(Right)** *Transverse side-by-side color Doppler US in the same patient shows hyperemia in all of the right-sided scrotal structures compared to the left, confirming right epididymoorchitis. There was no evidence of testicular torsion.*

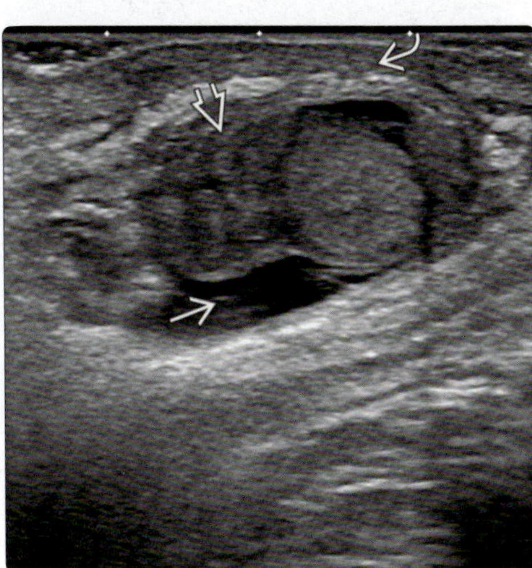

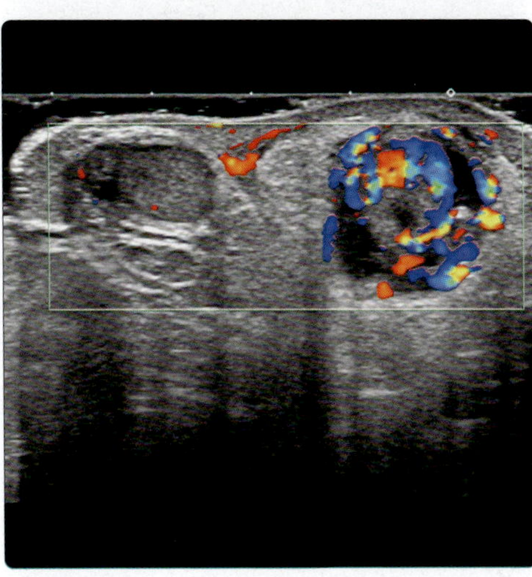

(Left) *Transverse US in a 6-year-old boy who had marked scrotal swelling on the left shows a hydrocele ➔, enlarged heterogeneous epididymis ➔, & scrotal wall thickening ➔.* **(Right)** *Transverse side-by-side color Doppler US in the same patient shows marked hyperemia of all the left-sided scrotal contents, consistent with epididymoorchitis.*

Testicular Torsion

KEY FACTS

TERMINOLOGY

- Spontaneous or traumatic twisting of testis & spermatic cord within scrotum → vascular occlusion/infarction

IMAGING

- ↓ or absent blood flow in testicle on Doppler US
    - Transverse side-by-side comparison image of asymptomatic & symptomatic testicles is very helpful
- "Spiral" twist of spermatic cord just above testis
- ± abnormal lie of testicle within scrotal sac
- Enlarged testis ± altered echotexture
- May see hyperemia after detorsion

TOP DIFFERENTIAL DIAGNOSES

- Epididymoorchitis or orchitis
- Torsion of testicular or epididymal appendage
- Testicular trauma
- Hernia complications

PATHOLOGY

- Intravaginal torsion of spermatic cord
    - Abnormally high attachment of tunica vaginalis → bell clapper deformity
- Extravaginal torsion of spermatic cord
    - Occurs proximal to attachments of tunica vaginalis
    - More common in neonates; rarely salvageable

CLINICAL ISSUES

- Presents with acute scrotal &/or inguinal pain
- Surgical emergency to prevent testicular infarction
- Surgical exploration with detorsion & bilateral orchiopexy if testicle is viable
    - Nonviable testicle is usually removed
- Salvage rates
    - 80-100% within 6 hours of pain onset
    - Virtually 0% after 12 hours of pain onset

(Left) *Anatomic drawing of testicular torsion shows a twisted cord (resembling a snail shell) ➡ & an enlarged epididymis ➡.* **(Right)** *Longitudinal power Doppler US at the inguinal-scrotal junction shows a twisted spermatic cord ➡ ("cord knot") surrounded by a hydrocele in a teenager with several hours of left-sided scrotal pain. The epididymis is enlarged & heterogeneous ➡, & no flow was seen in the testicle (not shown), consistent with torsion.*

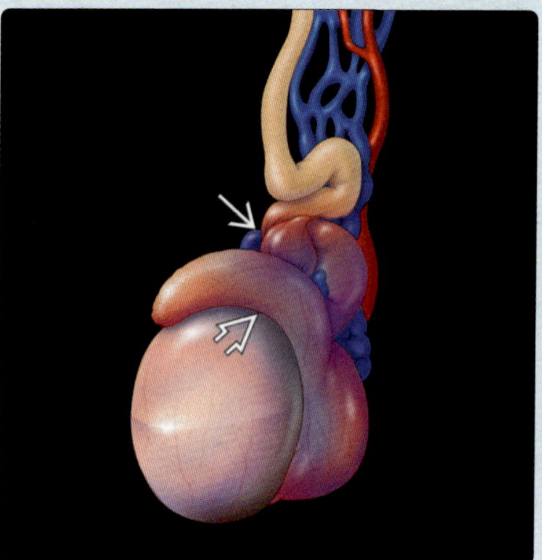

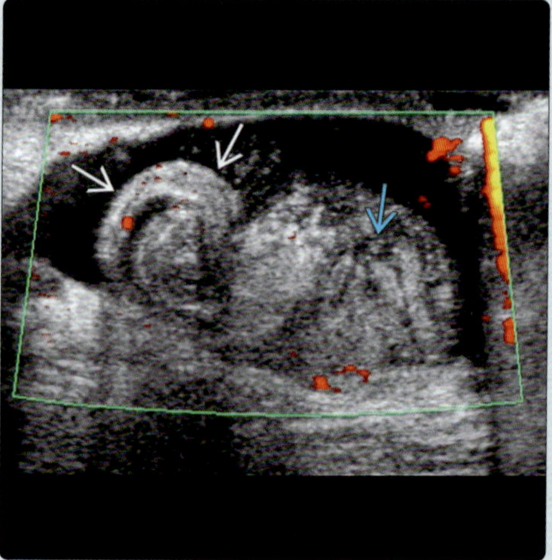

(Left) *Transverse side-by-side US of the testes in a 3-year-old with scrotal pain & swelling shows a mildly enlarged left testis ➡ with no color Doppler flow & a small hydrocele. Left testicular torsion was found at surgery.* **(Right)** *Transverse side-by-side view of the scrotum in a teenager awakened from sleep by left-sided pain shows a mildly enlarged & avascular left testis ➡, confirmed as torsion at surgery.*

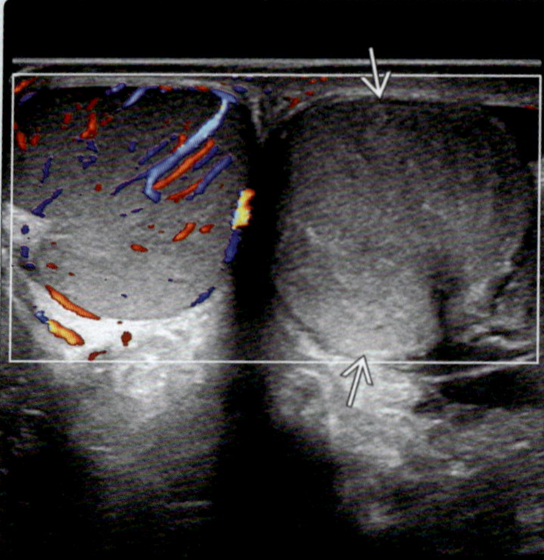

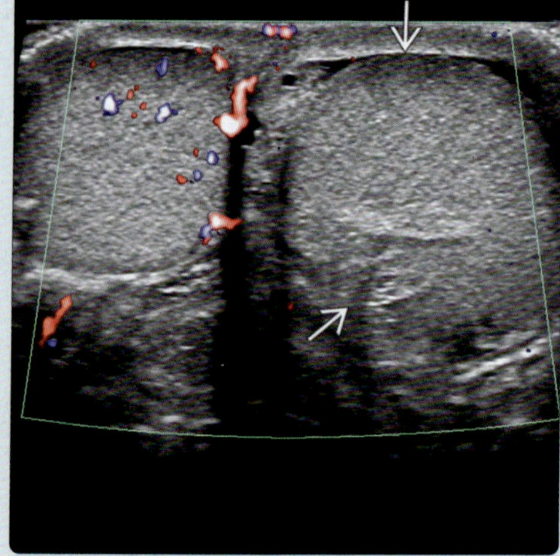

TERMINOLOGY

Synonyms

- Torsion, late or "missed" torsion, acute scrotum

Definitions

- Spontaneous or traumatic twisting of testis & spermatic cord within scrotum → vascular occlusion/infarction
- Testicle twists medially in 2/3 of cases, so manual detorsion laterally is more likely to be effective
  - Direction of manual detorsion is described as "opening book"

IMAGING

General Features

- Best diagnostic clue
  - ↓ or absent blood flow in testicle on color Doppler US
    - Easiest to appreciate when compared side by side to normal flow in asymptomatic testicle
- Location
  - Unilateral in 95% of patients
  - Caution: Undescended testes can also torse!
    - Look for avascular inguinal testis & empty hemiscrotum
- Size
  - Normal testicular volume
    - 1 mL in newborn
    - 15-20 mL in postpubertal males
  - Volume may ↑ in torsion depending on severity & length of ischemia

Ultrasonographic Findings

- Grayscale ultrasound
  - Testicular parenchyma may be normal early
    - Gradual development of hypoechoic &/or heterogeneous testicular parenchyma
    - Intratesticular necrosis, hemorrhage, or fragmentation is seen with delayed diagnosis
  - Enlarged testicle & epididymis
    - Remote torsion shows small testicle ± Ca^{2+}
  - Testicle may lie in abnormal plane
  - Spiral, whirlpool, or knot twist of spermatic cord just above testicle (below inguinal canal)
    - Snail shell-shaped mass measuring 11-33 mm
  - Reactive or secondary hydrocele
  - Scrotal wall thickening
- Color Doppler
  - Absent or ↓ blood flow throughout testicle
    - Compare side by side with asymptomatic testicle
    - Small percentage of patients with early or partial torsion have normal exam
  - ± high-resistance residual flow in partially or intermittently torsed testicle
  - Peripheral capsular & scrotal wall hyperemia
  - Hyperemia may be seen in testicle after detorsion
- Microvascular Doppler imaging is helpful in neonates & prepubertal testes
- Sensitivity of 86%, specificity of 100%, accuracy of 97% in diagnosis of testicular torsion when presence of intratesticular flow is sole criterion for diagnosis
- Contrast-enhanced ultrasound is seldom indicated

Nuclear Medicine Findings

- Tc-99m pertechnetate: Sensitivity 80-90%
  - Technique
    - Dynamic flow imaging at 2- to 5-second intervals for 1 minute (vascular phase)
    - 5-minute intervals for tissue phase
    - Pinhole collimation is useful, especially in young patients
    - Penis should be positioned out of field of view, usually secured to anterior abdominal wall
    - Scrotum is supported symmetrically on towels
  - "Cold" spot of torsed testicle with surrounding hyperemia

Imaging Recommendations

- Best imaging tool
  - US with high-frequency linear transducer & color Doppler
- Protocol advice
  - Power Doppler with comparison to contralateral normal testis
    - Particularly helpful in neonates & young boys
  - Transverse superior to inferior sweep of spermatic cord from distal inguinal canal through testis will help demonstrate "cord knot"

DIFFERENTIAL DIAGNOSIS

Epididymoorchitis or Orchitis

- Enlarged hypoechoic epididymis with ↑ flow on color Doppler
- Swollen heterogeneous epididymis may mimic cord knot of torsion

Torsion of Testicular or Epididymal Appendage

- Look for round, devascularized, enlarged, heterogeneous appendix with surrounding hyperemia

Inguinal Hernia

- Incarcerated/strangulated hernia can mimic testicular torsion
- Can cause ↓ blood flow in testis in neonate/infant

Testicular Trauma

- Hematocele, irregular contours, heterogeneous parenchymal echogenicity, ± interruption of echogenic capsule

Testicular Tumor

- Focal intratesticular mass with abnormal flow

PATHOLOGY

General Features

- Etiology
  - Most occur spontaneously; occasionally due to trauma
- Embryology/anatomy
  - Intravaginal torsion of spermatic cord
    - Abnormally high attachment of tunica vaginalis → bell clapper deformity
      - Testicle rotates freely within scrotum → spermatic cord twists → venous flow occludes → arterial flow occludes

- Bell clapper deformity is present in 12% of male population at autopsy
  - ◻ Much higher than testicular torsion
- Extravaginal torsion of spermatic cord
  - Occurs proximal to attachments of tunica vaginalis
  - More common in neonates
  - Accounts for only 5% of all cases of testicular torsion
  - Bilateral in 20%

Staging, Grading, & Classification

- Previously classified as acute, subacute, or delayed based on duration of symptoms
  - Duration of symptoms is not always predictive of salvage rate, especially in partial or intermittent torsion

Gross Pathologic & Surgical Features

- Purple, edematous, ischemic testicle; may rapidly reperfuse when manually untwisted
- Varying degrees of ischemic necrosis & fibrosis depending on duration of symptoms

CLINICAL ISSUES

Presentation

- Most common signs/symptoms
  - Acute scrotal &/or inguinal pain; occasionally referred pain in abdomen
  - Swollen erythematous hemiscrotum without recognized trauma
  - Physical exam findings highly predictive of testicular torsion include
    - Elevation of affected testicle
    - Transverse position of testicle
    - Anterior rotation of epididymis
    - Absence of cremasteric reflex
    - Pain relief with successful manual detorsion
    - TWIST score 0-6
  - In neonates, purple discoloration of swollen scrotum may indicate extravaginal testicular torsion
    - More common in high birth weight babies
    - Can be confused with scrotal hematoma due to birth trauma
- Other signs/symptoms
  - Nausea & vomiting
  - Incomplete/intermittent torsion may be tolerated for long periods
  - Almost 1/2 of patients have history of similar symptoms previously that resolved spontaneously
    - Indicates spontaneous torsion & detorsion

Demographics

- Age
  - Bimodal peak: Teenagers during puberty vs. neonates
- Sex
  - Males only
- Epidemiology
  - Epididymoorchitis & torsion of testicular appendage > testicular torsion
  - 4.5/100,000 males < 25 years of age per year

Natural History & Prognosis

- Surgical emergency: Testicular infarction if not treated promptly
- Testicular viability depends on
  - Degree of torsion: > 540° twist is worse
  - Duration of symptoms & time to surgical intervention
    - ~ 1/3 of testes are not salvageable at operation
- Unilateral testicular loss typically does not lead to infertility problems

Treatment

- Surgical exploration + detorsion + bilateral orchiopexy if testicle is viable
  - Nonviable testicle is usually removed (due to antisperm antibody theory)
  - Higher risk of subsequent torsion on contralateral side justifies contralateral pexy
- Salvage rates
  - 80-100% within 6 hours of pain onset
  - Virtually 0% after 12 hours
  - Only 9% salvage rate in neonates
- Neonatal torsion: Asynchronous contralateral torsion in 5%; prompt surgery & orchiopexy are recommended
- Bilateral pexy is advocated in children with intermittent scrotal pain
  - Risk of testicular loss approaches 80% in patients with intermittent torsion
- Orchiopexy does not 100% guarantee against future torsion
  - Case reports of torsion postpexy → twisted hammock appearance
- Antioxidant medications, heparin, & steroids are being tested to ↓ ischemia-reperfusion injury

DIAGNOSTIC CHECKLIST

Consider

- Early/partial/intermittent torsion may not show complete absence of flow

Image Interpretation Pearls

- Heterogeneity of avascular testicular parenchyma on US ↓ likelihood of salvageability

SELECTED REFERENCES

1. Dupond-Athénor A et al: A multicenter review of undescended testis torsion: a plea for early management. J Pediatr Urol. 17(2):191.e1-6., 2020
2. O'Kelly F et al: Delaying urgent exploration in neonatal testicular torsion may have significant consequences for the contralateral testis: a critical literature review. Urology. 153:277-84, 2020
3. Taghavi K et al: The bell-clapper deformity of the testis: the definitive pathological anatomy. J Pediatr Surg. 56(8):1405-10, 2020
4. Zvizdic Z et al: Duration of symptoms is the only predictor of testicular salvage following testicular torsion in children: a case-control study. Am J Emerg Med. 41:197-200, 2020
5. Expert Panel on Urological Imaging et al: ACR Appropriateness Criteria® acute onset of scrotal pain-without trauma, without antecedent mass. J Am Coll Radiol. 16(5S):S38-43, 2019
6. Vasconcelos-Castro S et al: Abdominal pain in teenagers: beware of testicular torsion. J Pediatr Surg. 55(9):1933-5, 2019
7. Wang M et al: Testicular torsion postorchiopexy: a case of twisted hammock. Urology. 125:202-4, 2019
8. Alkhori NA et al: Pediatric scrotal ultrasound: review and update. Pediatr Radiol. 47(9):1125-33, 2017

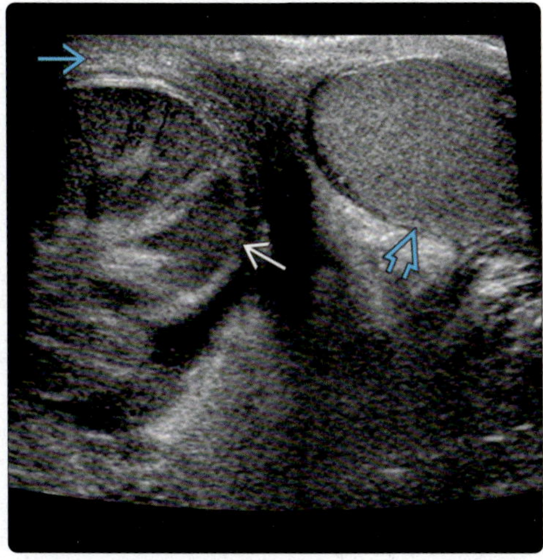
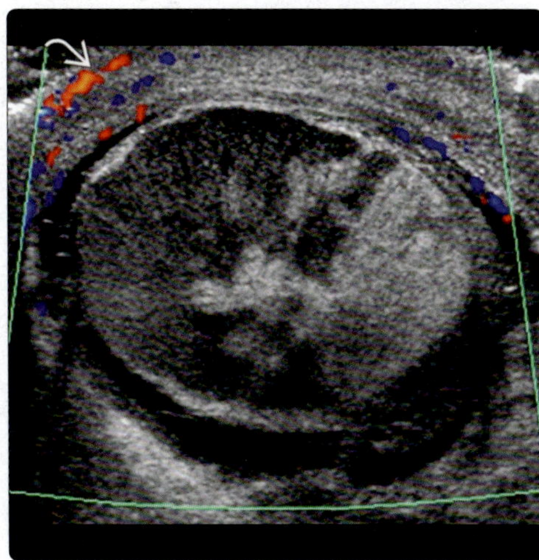

(Left) *Transverse US in a 13-year-old boy with 2 weeks of waxing & waning pain in the right scrotum shows an enlarged right testis with heterogeneous echotexture. There is also a small right hydrocele with scrotal wall thickening. The left testis has a normal homogeneous echotexture.* **(Right)** *Transverse color Doppler US of the symptomatic right testicle shows absent blood flow within the testicle, confirming subacute testicular torsion. Note the mild hyperemia in the thickened scrotal wall.*

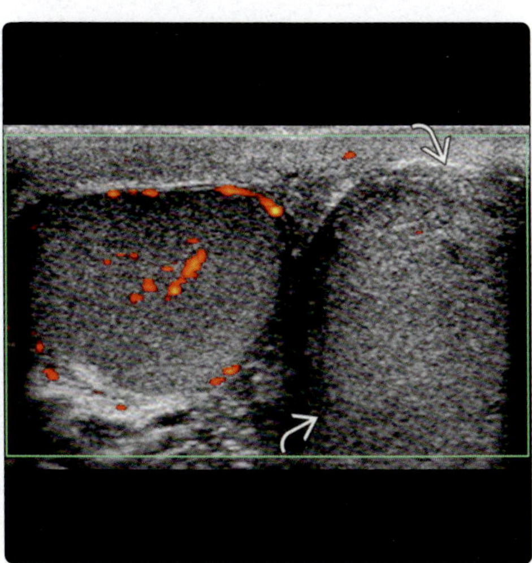
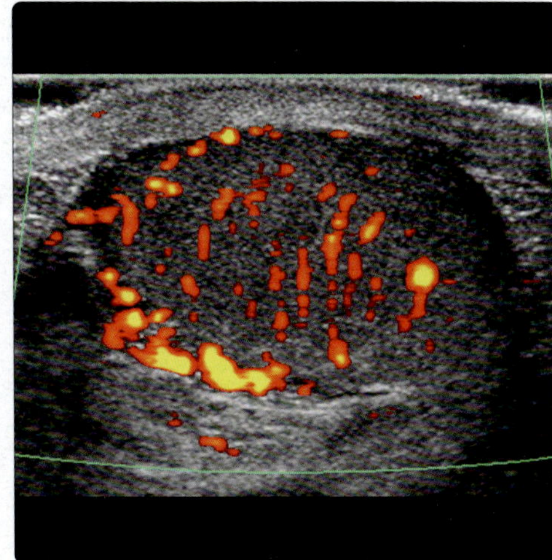

(Left) *Transverse power Doppler US in a 14-year-old boy with acute left-sided pain shows absent blood flow in the left testicle, consistent with testicular torsion. After the patient repositioned his scrotal contents on the exam cushions, he exclaimed that he felt much better.* **(Right)** *Repeat power Doppler US in the same patient shows hyperemia in the previously avascular symptomatic testicle, indicating spontaneous/manual detorsion. This testicle remains at risk for retorsion & requires orchiopexy.*

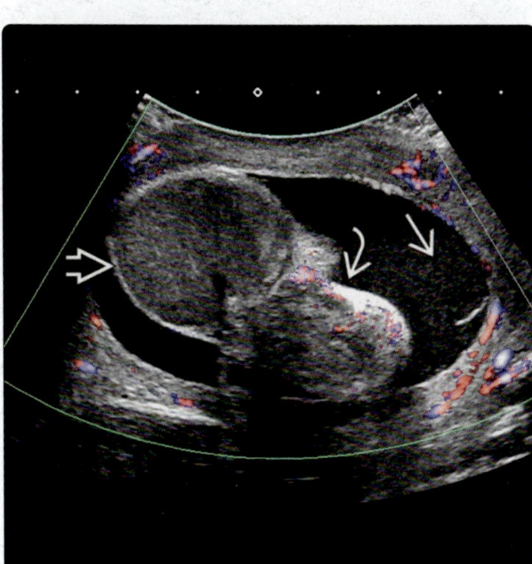
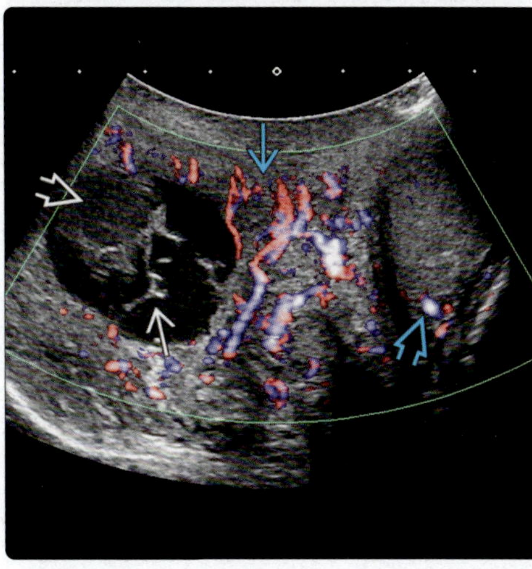

(Left) *Longitudinal color Doppler US in a teenage boy with several hours of right-sided pain & swelling shows a large hydrocele with mobile debris & an avascular enlarged right testis. Note the enlarged epididymis.* **(Right)** *Transverse color Doppler US of both testes in the same teenager shows a complex hydrocele, avascular right testis, hyperemia of the thickened scrotal wall, & blood flow in the left testicle. At surgery, the right testis was necrotic & could not be salvaged.*

Torsion of Testicular Appendage

KEY FACTS

TERMINOLOGY

- Synonyms: Twisted appendage, torsed appendix testis, torsion of appendix epididymis, appendiceal torsion
- Definitions
  - Spontaneous twisting of pedunculated vestigial remnant along testicle or epididymis, causing ischemia & pain
  - Acute scrotal pain in children: Torsed appendage is most common (62%)
    - Testicular torsion 25%, epididymoorchitis 10%, trauma 2%

IMAGING

- Ultrasound with Doppler: Best imaging modality
- Appendage size is best indicator of torsion (> 5-6 mm acutely)
- Spherical shape suggests swelling (normally vermiform)
- Duration of symptoms determines echogenicity
  - < 24 hours: Hypoechoic with salt & pepper pattern
  - > 24 hours: Hypo-, iso-, or hyperechoic
- Classically ↓ or absent internal vascularity of torsed appendix with periappendiceal hyperemia
- Reactive hydrocele & scrotal wall edema are common

TOP DIFFERENTIAL DIAGNOSES

- Testicular torsion
- Epididymoorchitis or orchitis
- Isolated scrotal wall edema
- Inguinal hernia complications
- Testicular or paratesticular tumor
- Testicular trauma

CLINICAL ISSUES

- Acute scrotal pain, swelling
- ± small, tender, mobile lump at upper pole of testis
- ± blue dot sign of ischemic appendage seen through scrotal wall in minority of patients (< 30%)
- 80% of cases are 7-14 years old; mean age: 9 years
- Self-limited illness, excellent prognosis

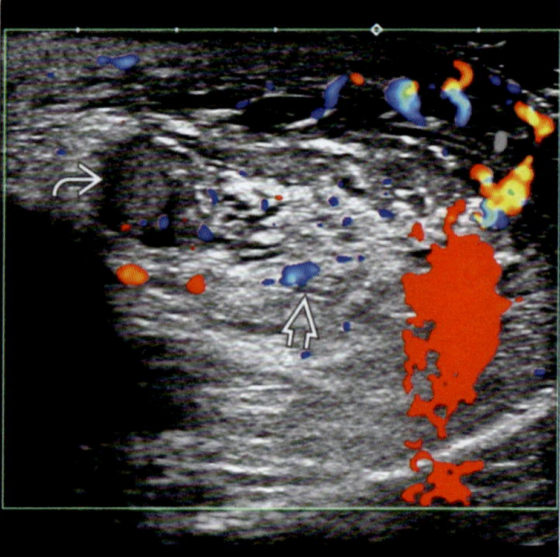

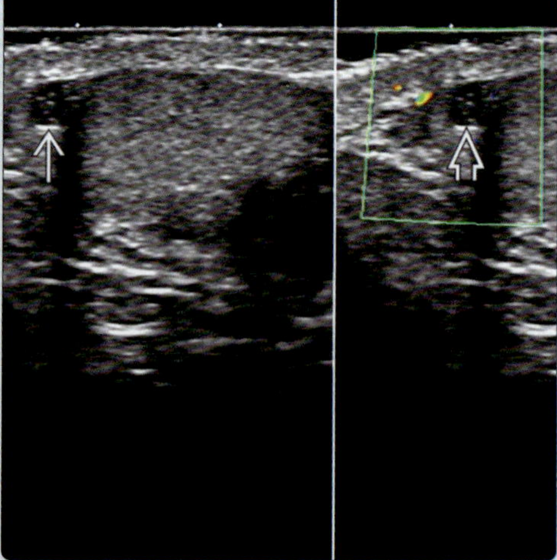

(Left) *Longitudinal color Doppler US in 7-year-old with scrotal pain & swelling shows lack of blood flow in a small round nodule ➡ adjacent to an inflamed epididymis ➡. Testicular blood flow (not shown) was normal. The findings are consistent with a torsed appendage.* **(Right)** *Longitudinal US images of epididymis in a 6-year-old show a hypoechoic nodule ➡ (superior to the testis) that is avascular ➡ on Doppler. This was the point of maximal discomfort & likely represented a torsed appendage.*

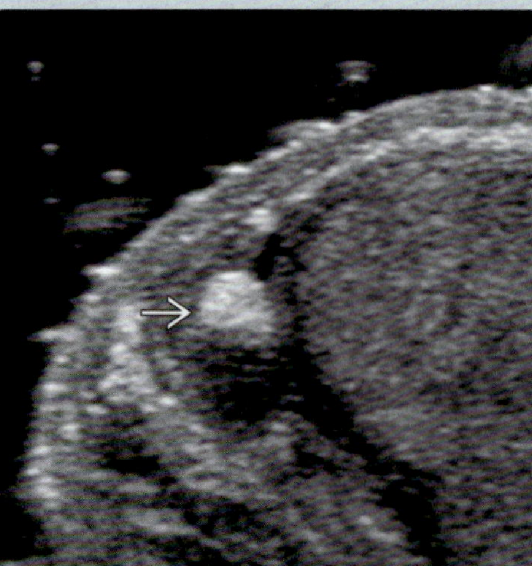

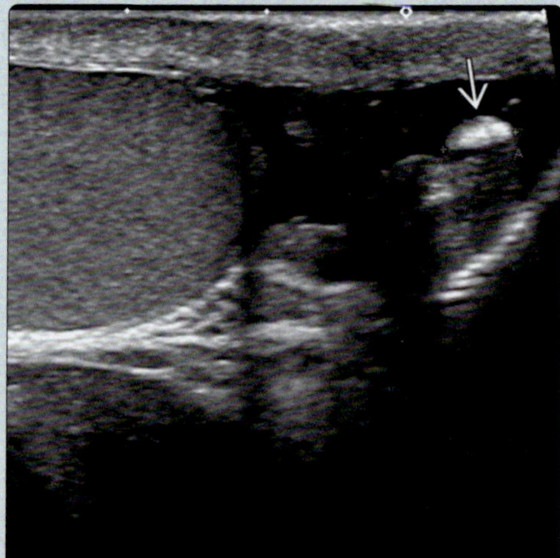

(Left) *Oblique scrotal US shows an echogenic appendage ➡ in a patient with a subacute history of pain. The ↑ echogenicity may reflect acute hemorrhage vs. more chronic fibrotic change or Ca^{2+} in a torsed appendage.* **(Right)** *Longitudinal US shows a hyperechoic ovoid focus ➡ surrounded by a small hydrocele, consistent with a partially calcified, chronically torsed appendage. At this point in time, the patient was asymptomatic.*

Torsion of Testicular Appendage

TERMINOLOGY

Synonyms

- Twisted appendage, torsed appendix testis, torsion of appendix epididymis, appendiceal torsion

Definitions

- Spontaneous twisting of pedunculated vestigial remnant along testicle or epididymis, causing ischemia & pain
- Most common etiology of acute scrotal pain in children
  - Incidence > > epididymoorchitis & testicular torsion

IMAGING

General Features

- Best diagnostic clue
  - Enlarged, spherical, hypoechoic, avascular nodule along testis or epididymis at site of patient pain + hyperemia of surrounding tissues
    - Reactive hydrocele is very common
- Location
  - Most common appendage to twist: Testicular remnant of paramesonephric (müllerian) duct
    - Located between superior pole of testis & epididymis
  - Appendix epididymis is remnant of mesonephric (wolffian) duct
    - Most often seen projecting from head of epididymis
  - Other minor appendages of testicle & epididymis have variable locations & may also twist
  - Can be difficult to differentiate testicular vs. epididymal appendage (not clinically relevant)
- Size
  - Appendage > 5.6 mm in size: Diagnostic of acute torsion
    - Enlarged appendage sensitivity of 68.2% & specificity of 100%
    - Normal appendix is usually tubular, pedunculated, & ≤ 4 mm
  - Chronically torsed appendage is also small
- Morphology
  - Spherical shape & enlargement are most reliable indicators of appendiceal torsion
  - Echotexture is not predictive of torsion, but ↑ echotexture is associated with longer chronicity

Ultrasonographic Findings

- Grayscale ultrasound
  - Appendix size is best indicator of torsion (> 5-6 mm acutely)
  - Spherical shape suggests swelling (normally vermiform)
  - Duration of symptoms determines echogenicity
    - < 24 hours: Hypoechoic with salt & pepper pattern
      - Echogenic dots & septa
    - > 24 hours: Hypo-, iso-, or hyperechoic
  - Reactive hydrocele
  - Scrotal wall edema
  - Epididymal head enlargement
- Color Doppler
  - Classically ↓ or absent internal vascularity of torsed appendix with periappendiceal hyperemia
    - Findings can be variable
  - Testicular blood flow may be normal or ↑
- Power Doppler
  - Useful in younger, uncooperative patients
    - Sensitive for low flow; no directional information
- Contrast-enhanced ultrasound
  - May be useful in equivocal exams but delays surgery if there is testicular torsion

MR Findings

- Reserved for complex cases or to clarify abnormal anatomy

Nuclear Medicine Findings

- Tc-99m pertechnetate scan
  - Historic interest only: Replaced by ultrasound
  - Normal testicular uptake, excluding diagnosis of testicular torsion
  - May show focal ↑ or ↓ uptake in region of superior testicle at site of twisted appendix
    - Focal "hot" spot is equivalent to blue dot sign seen on physical exam
  - Technique is same as scan for testicular torsion
    - Pinhole or low-energy, high-resolution collimator
    - Scrotum supported on towels; penis secured up & out of field of view
    - Dynamic acquisition during blood flow or perfusion phase
    - Static delayed imaging ± markers

Imaging Recommendations

- Best imaging tool
  - Ultrasound with Doppler
    - More sensitive & specific for diagnosing appendage torsion than
      - Clinical signs alone
      - Imaging in other causes of acute scrotal pain (i.e., testicular torsion or epididymoorchitis)
- Protocol advice
  - High-frequency linear transducer
  - Thick layer of ultrasound gel ↓ discomfort during scan
  - Support scrotum on towels
  - Compare with asymptomatic side

DIFFERENTIAL DIAGNOSIS

Testicular Torsion

- Abnormal Doppler (absent, diminished, or high-resistance flow) in painful testis compared to asymptomatic side
- Whirlpool or knot sign of twisted spermatic cord above testis
- Normal grayscale appearance of testicular parenchyma early with subsequent changes of frank infarction

Epididymoorchitis/Orchitis

- Hyperemia & enlargement of affected side ± tissue heterogeneity
- Global tenderness on physical exam

Isolated Scrotal Wall Edema

- Thickening, heterogeneity, & hyperemia of scrotal wall
- May be isolated & self-limited or due to cellulitis, insect bite, allergic reaction, or Henoch-Schönlein purpura

Inguinal Hernia Complications

- Normal peristalsing bowel vs. abnormal, thick-walled ischemic bowel tracking from peritoneal cavity through inguinal canal into scrotum
- Pressure effects may cause testicular ischemia in young infants

Testicular or Paratesticular Tumor

- Distortion of normal sonographic anatomy by focal intratesticular or paratesticular mass
- Scrotal tumors range from small & homogeneous to large & heterogeneous
- Usually manifest with gradual swelling or palpable mass, not pain

Testicular Trauma

- Hematocele, altered testicular echotexture, irregular testicular contour with capsular disruption
- History of trauma is usually known

PATHOLOGY

General Features

- Etiology
  - Spontaneous twisting of appendage is most common; occasionally associated with trauma or tumor
  - Rising levels of estrogen & androgens early in puberty may account for appendiceal enlargement & predisposition to appendiceal torsion in this age group
    - Testicular appendage contains variable numbers of both androgen & estrogen receptors
  - Metachronous contralateral testicular appendage torsion is reported in < 5%
- Associated abnormalities
  - Rare case reports of tumors arising in scrotal appendages
    - Appendix testis contains müllerian epithelium
    - May produce epithelial tumors similar to those occurring in female genital tract
  - Paratesticular tumors (e.g., rhabdomyosarcoma) are likely arise from stromal tissues rather than appendages

Microscopic Features

- Variable degrees of interstitial edema, hemorrhage, & necrosis

CLINICAL ISSUES

Presentation

- Most common signs/symptoms
  - Acute scrotal pain & swelling
  - ± small, tender, mobile lump at upper pole of testis
  - ± blue dot sign of ischemic appendage seen through scrotal wall in minority of patients (< 30%)
- Other signs/symptoms
  - Metachronous & bilaterally synchronous cases of appendiceal torsion are rarely reported

Demographics

- Age
  - 80% of cases occur between ages 7-14 years
  - Mean age: 9 years
    - Mean age of 14 years for testicular torsion & epididymoorchitis
- Sex
  - Males only
- Epidemiology
  - Most common cause of acute scrotal pain in children
    - Torsion of testicular or epididymal appendage: 62%
    - Testicular/spermatic cord torsion: 25%
    - Epididymoorchitis: 10%
    - Trauma: 2%
  - Incidence of 1 in 2,000 males

Natural History & Prognosis

- Self-limited illness, excellent prognosis
- Pain usually resolves within 1 week
- Consider repeat imaging if symptoms persist
  - Rare reports of secondary infection in infarcted, necrotic tissue

Treatment

- Analgesics & antiinflammatory agents for symptom relief
  - Antibiotics are not indicated in routine cases
- Reports of manual detorsion with ultrasound guidance
  - Reduction by pulling or squeezing appendage
  - Success if pain relieved, appendix size ↓, Doppler flow restored
- Resection of torsed appendage if scrotum is explored due to concern for testicular/spermatic cord torsion
  - Surgery is not indicated if torsed appendix diagnosis is clear

DIAGNOSTIC CHECKLIST

Image Interpretation Pearls

- Can be difficult to distinguish from epididymitis if no discrete nodule is visualized
  - Appendage torsion is more common, especially in prepubertal population
  - Treatment for both entities is nonsurgical

SELECTED REFERENCES

1. Gopal M et al: Emergency scrotal exploration in children: is it time for a change in mindset in the UK? J Pediatr Urol. 17(2):190.e1-7, 2020
2. Koh YH et al: Testicular appendage torsion-to explore the other side or not? Urology. 141:130-4, 2020
3. Expert Panel on Urological Imaging et al: ACR Appropriateness Criteria® acute onset of scrotal pain-without trauma, without antecedent mass. J Am Coll Radiol. 16(5S):S38-43, 2019
4. Lala S et al: Re-presentations and recurrent events following initial management of the acute paediatric scrotum: a 5-year review. ANZ J Surg. 89(4):E117-121, 2019
5. Sweet DE et al: Imaging of the acute scrotum: keys to a rapid diagnosis of acute scrotal disorders. Abdom Radiol (NY). 45(7):2063-81, 2019
6. Hart J et al: Chronic orchalgia after surgical exploration for acute scrotal pain in children. J Pediatr Urol. 12(3):168.e1-6, 2016
7. Pogorelić Z et al: Management of acute scrotum in children: a 25-year single center experience on 558 pediatric patients. Can J Urol. 23(6):8594-601, 2016
8. Lev M et al: Sonographic appearances of torsion of the appendix testis and appendix epididymis in children. J Clin Ultrasound. 43(8):485-9, 2015
9. Boettcher M et al: Differentiation of epididymitis and appendix testis torsion by clinical and ultrasound signs in children. Urology. 82(4):899-904, 2013
10. Yusuf GT et al: A review of ultrasound imaging in scrotal emergencies. J Ultrasound. 16(4):171-8, 2013
11. Sung EK et al: Sonography of the pediatric scrotum: emphasis on the Ts–torsion, trauma, and tumors. AJR Am J Roentgenol. 198(5):996-1003, 2012

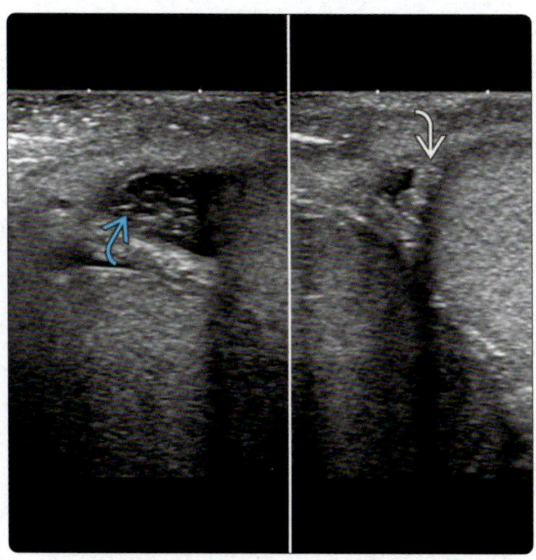

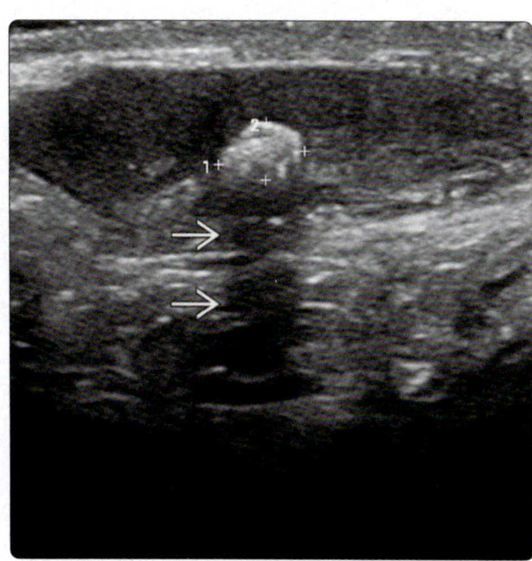

(Left) *Transverse US views of the scrotum show asymmetric size & shape of small appendages along the testes. The right appendage* ↪ *is enlarged, ovoid, & hypoechoic compared to the isoechoic & vermiform left appendage* ↪*. Pain at this site on the right confirmed acute torsion of the appendage.* **(Right)** *Longitudinal US in the lateral aspect of the scrotum shows a hyperechoic nodule between cursors with posterior shadowing* ➔*, consistent with a calcified, autoamputated remotely torsed appendage.*

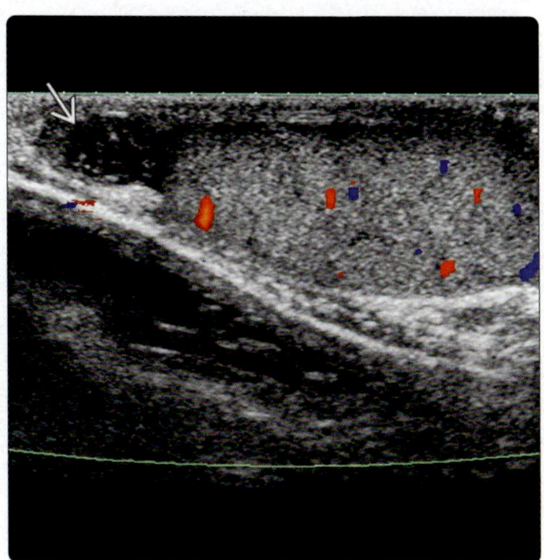

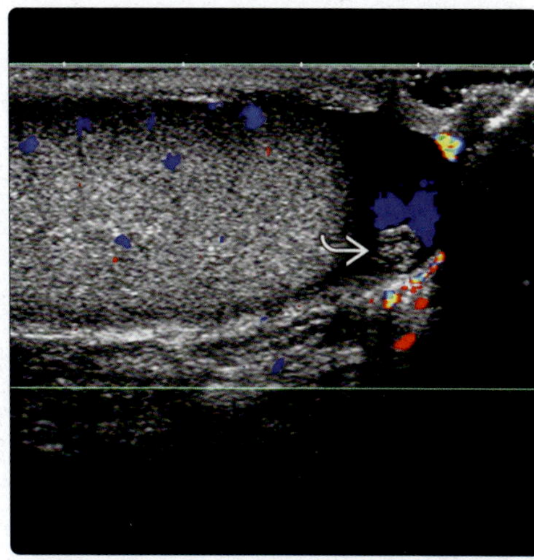

(Left) *Longitudinal color Doppler US in a 12-year-old boy with acute right-sided scrotal pain shows an ovoid, heterogeneously hypoechoic, avascular nodule* ➔ *along the superior pole of the testis, consistent with a torsed appendage.* **(Right)** *Longitudinal color Doppler US of the scrotum in a 15-year-old boy with acute left-sided scrotal pain shows a small discrete avascular nodule* ↪ *at the lower pole of the left testis. There is surrounding hyperemia & an adjacent hydrocele, consistent with appendage torsion.*

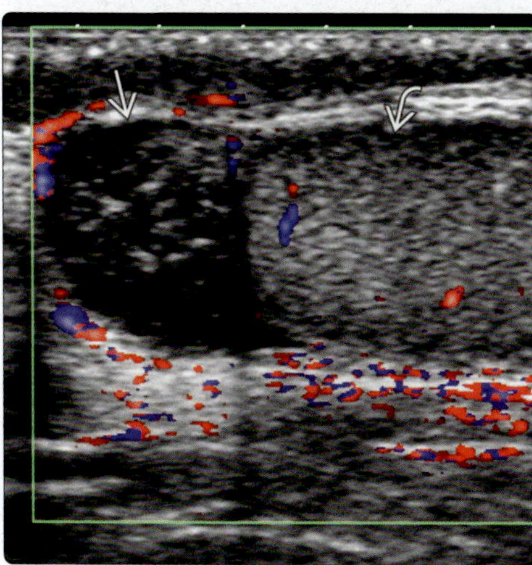

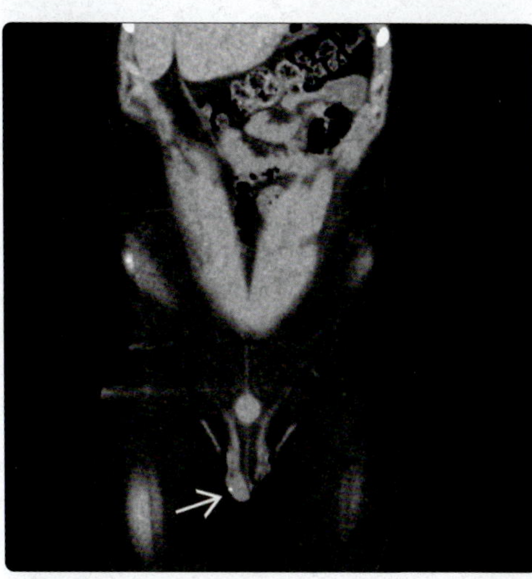

(Left) *Longitudinal color Doppler US in a 5-year-old boy with scrotal pain shows a round, heterogeneously hypoechoic nodule* ➔ *along the superior pole of the testicle* ↪*. Note the internal salt & pepper appearance with surrounding hyperemia but no internal vascularity, consistent with a torsed appendage.* **(Right)** *Coronal localization PET/CT shows a tiny Ca^{2+} in the right scrotum* ➔ *in this teenage boy having oncologic imaging. The Ca^{2+} is most likely due to the remote torsion of a testicular appendage.*

Paratesticular Rhabdomyosarcoma

KEY FACTS

TERMINOLOGY

- Malignant solid tumor of mesenchymal origin; arises from skeletal muscle precursors
- Paratesticular rhabdomyosarcoma (PT-RMS) refers only to intrascrotal rhabdomyosarcoma (RMS), not other genitourinary sites

IMAGING

- Large, lobulated paratesticular mass with variable echogenicity; often heterogeneous & hypervascular compared to testis
  - Usually arises in epididymis; may arise from or invade tunica, testis, or spermatic cord
  - Can be ill defined or well defined; may encase testicle
- Look for retroperitoneal adenopathy

TOP DIFFERENTIAL DIAGNOSES

- Epididymitis: Usually painful swelling; no discrete mass
- Inguinal hernia: Peristalsing bowel loop in inguinal canal
- Hematoma: Avascular, associated with trauma
- Lipoma: Usually homogeneously hyperechoic
- Polyorchidism: Identical appearance to testis
- Testicular adrenal rests: Multiple, bilateral, intratesticular

PATHOLOGY

- Most PT-RMS are embryonal RMS subtypes
- Most cases are sporadic; ↑ risk with *TP53* mutations, *DICER1* mutations, RASopathies

CLINICAL ISSUES

- Gradual, painless scrotal swelling, ± palpable mass
- 2 age peaks: < 5 years vs. 2nd decade
- Most common extratesticular solid mass in boys
- PT-RMS accounts for ~ 5% of childhood RMS but has much better prognosis than other forms of genitourinary RMS
  - > 90% survival rate for localized (nonmetastatic) PT-RMS
  - Age < 1 or > 10 years, tumor size ≥ 5 cm, & lymph node involvement portend worse prognosis

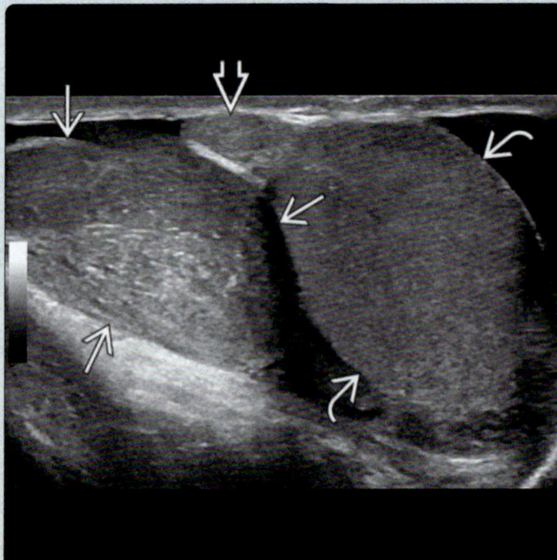

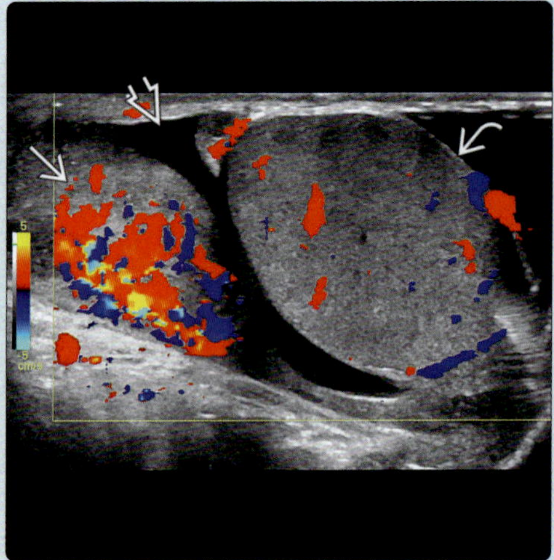

(Left) *Longitudinal oblique US through the left hemiscrotum shows a slightly heterogeneous & hyperechoic paratesticular soft tissue mass. Note the normal testis & epididymis.* **(Right)** *Color Doppler US in the same patient reveals markedly ↑ blood flow within the mass compared to the testis. Also note the small hydrocele. This mass was a localized paratesticular rhabdomyosarcoma (PT-RMS).*

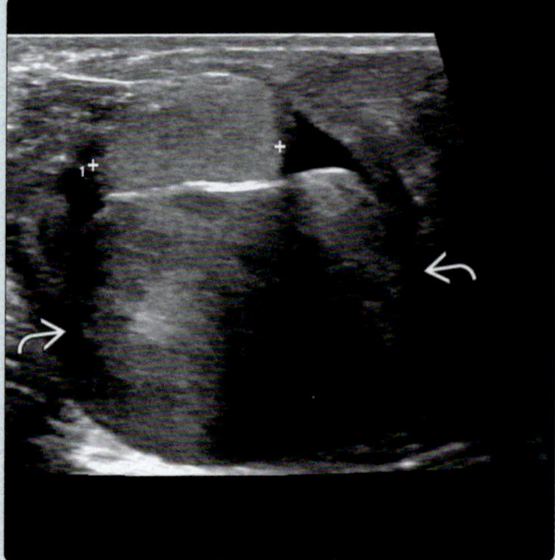

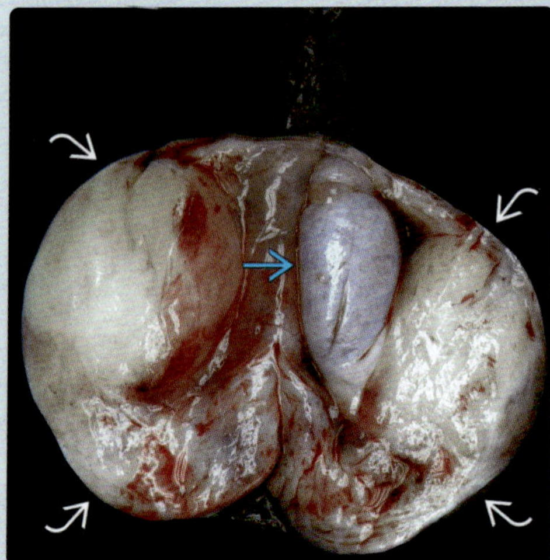

(Left) *Scrotal US in a 5-year-old with 1 week of right scrotal swelling shows a large, slightly heterogeneous paratesticular mass, ultimately proven to be a PT-RMS. Real-time imaging showed the mass to almost completely surround the testis (shown with calipers).* **(Right)** *Gross pathologic bivalved specimen in the same patient status post orchiectomy shows a large, bland, tan-white PT-RMS almost completely surrounding, but not invading, the testis.*

TERMINOLOGY

Abbreviations

- Paratesticular rhabdomyosarcoma (PT-RMS)

Definitions

- Malignant solid tumor of mesenchymal origin arising from skeletal muscle precursors

IMAGING

General Features

- Best diagnostic clue
  - Large, vascular paratesticular soft tissue mass
- Location
  - PT-RMS refers only to intrascrotal RMS; other genitourinary locations of RMS are considered separately
  - Usually arises within epididymis but can occur within testicular tunica, testis, or spermatic cord
- Morphology
  - Can be ill defined or well defined, may encase testicle, & may invade tunica or testis itself

Ultrasonographic Findings

- Lobulated paratesticular mass with variable echogenicity, often heterogeneous
- Doppler shows ↑ blood flow compared to testes
- May have associated hydrocele

CT Findings

- Chest/abdomen/pelvis CT used to evaluate for lung metastases & retroperitoneal lymphadenopathy (LAD)
- PET/CT improves sensitivity for nodal disease

MR Findings

- Generally not indicated for PT-RMS (vs. RMS) but may be used to evaluate retroperitoneal LAD

DIFFERENTIAL DIAGNOSIS

Epididymitis

- Enlarged, hypervascular epididymis; no distinct mass
- History usually involves painful scrotal swelling

Inguinal Hernia

- Peristalsing bowel loops, omental fat
- Continuity with peritoneal cavity through inguinal canal

Lipoma

- Most common benign paratesticular neoplasm
- Usually within spermatic cord; homogeneously hyperechoic on US & of fat attenuation/signal on CT/MR

Adenomatoid Tumor

- Most common benign tumor of epididymis
- Usually affects young adult men aged 20-30 years
- Typically well-circumscribed, round to oval, homogeneous mass with variable echogenicity

Polyorchidism

- Well-defined mass resembling normal testicle
- Ipsilateral testis is often small, may be contiguous
- Identical appearance to testis on all imaging modalities

Testicular Adrenal Rest Tumors

- Multiple, bilateral (usually peripheral) intratesticular masses with ↑ vascularity; typically hypoechoic
  - Intermixed with echogenic mediastinum testis
- Adrenal rests are trapped in developing fetal testis
  - 10-15% of newborns; < 1% of adults
  - Enlarge if exposed to ↑ ACTH; otherwise, regress

Splenogonadal Fusion

- Extremely rare, almost always left sided; occurs in association with limb deficiency & micrognathia
- May be in continuity with spleen (through inguinal canal)
- Splenic scintigraphy can be diagnostic

PATHOLOGY

General Features

- Etiology
  - Primitive skeletal muscle precursors within testes, epididymis, & spermatic cord
- Associated abnormalities
  - Most cases are sporadic
  - Several genetic diseases have predisposition for RMS

Staging, Grading, & Classification

- RMS consists of 6 histologic subtypes; most PT-RMS are of embryonal subtypes
- Staging is complex: PT-RMS is stratified into 1 of 4 risk groups based on TNM stage, histologic subtype, extent of postoperative residual tumor, & age at diagnosis

Gross Pathologic & Surgical Features

- Tumor spreads mostly by lymphatics → retroperitoneal LAD
- Hematogenous spread is less common: Liver, lungs, & bones
- Direct invasion of tunica or testicle is rare

CLINICAL ISSUES

Presentation

- Most common signs/symptoms
  - Gradual, painless scrotal swelling, ± palpable mass

Demographics

- 2 age peaks: < 5 years vs. 2nd decade

Natural History & Prognosis

- Most common extratesticular solid mass in boys
- PT-RMS accounts for ~ 5% of childhood RMS but has much better prognosis than other forms of genitourinary RMS
  - > 90% survival rate for localized (nonmetastatic) PT-RMS
  - Age < 1 or > 10 years, tumor size ≥ 5 cm, & lymph node involvement portend worse prognosis

Treatment

- Multimodal treatment based on local control & assessment of any distant involvement: Radical orchiectomy, chemotherapy, ± radiation

SELECTED REFERENCES

1. Rogers TN et al: Surgical management of paratesticular rhabdomyosarcoma: a consensus opinion from the Children's Oncology Group, European Paediatric Soft Tissue Aarcoma Study Group, and the Cooperative Weichteilsarkom Studiengruppe. Pediatr Blood Cancer. 68(4):e28938, 2021

KEY FACTS

TERMINOLOGY

- Testicular neoplasms: Germ cell vs. nongerm cell tumors
  - Germ cell tumors: ~ 2/3 of pediatric tumors
  - Nongerm cell tumors: ~ 1/3 of pediatric tumors
  - Lymphoma & leukemia can also involve testes

IMAGING

- Intratesticular mass of variable echogenicity & vascularity
- Vary widely in size, from imperceptible to testis-replacing
- Teratomas characteristically have extremely complex appearance with cystic areas, Ca^{2+}, solid components, & punctate or linear echogenic hairs
- Epidermoids (true cysts, not neoplasms) appear solid, targetoid, or "onion skin" from laminations of keratinizing stratified squamous epithelium
- Regressed MGCTs may appear as subtle architectural distortion with ill-defined microcalcification
- Sex cord-stromal tumors are often small & well defined

CLINICAL ISSUES

- Presentations: Asymptomatic or painless mass
- ↑ risk with microlithiasis or cryptorchidism
- Most prepubertal intratesticular masses are benign (teratoma, epidermoid), though YSTs are 2nd most common tumor
  - YSTs: 90% have ↑ AFP, used as tumor marker
- Most postpubertal intratesticular masses are malignant: Embryonal carcinoma & MGCT most common
- Standard of care: Orchiectomy; testis-sparing enucleation is increasingly performed in newborns & prepubertal boys without ↑ AFP; ± adjuvant chemotherapy depending on tumor type & stage

DIAGNOSTIC CHECKLIST

- Use high-frequency linear-array US transducer
  - With other diagnostic considerations (e.g., hematoma, focal orchitis), short-term follow-up can help clarify
- MR for problem-solving or questionable masses

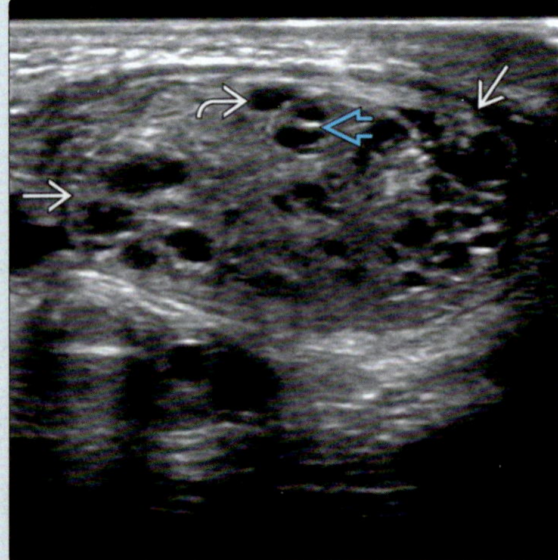

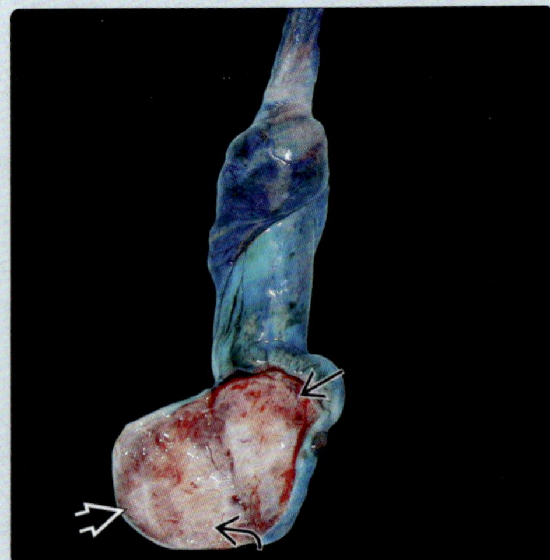

(Left) *Longitudinal US of a juvenile granulosa cell tumor in a newborn with firm testicular enlargement shows a heterogeneous mass replacing the testis ➡. There are numerous hypoechoic foci ➡ separated by thin septations ⇨, a classic appearance for this rare tumor.* **(Right)** *Gross pathologic photograph status post orchiectomy in the same patient shows complete replacement of the testis by a gray-white tumor ➡ with scattered cystic spaces ⇨ & foci of hemorrhagic staining ⇨.*

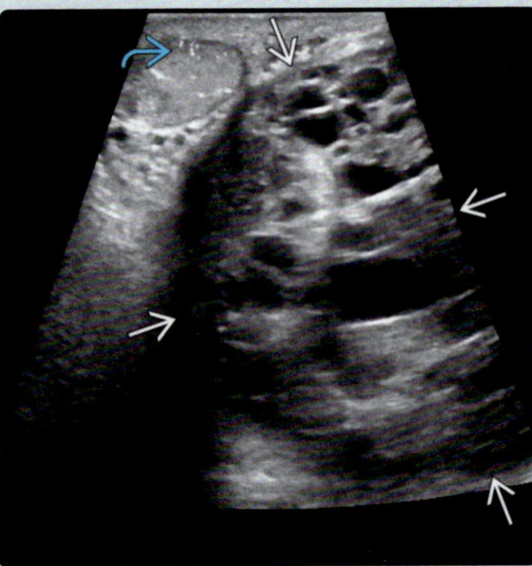

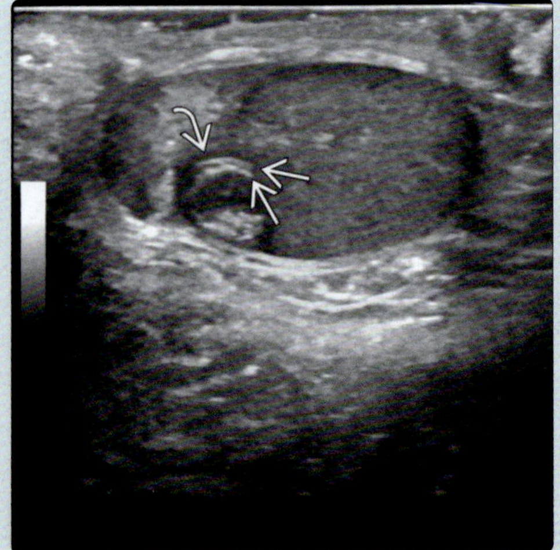

(Left) *Transverse US shows a large left-sided testicular teratoma ➡ in a 15-year-old with 12 months of painless scrotal swelling. The 8-cm partially cystic mass is quite heterogeneous & complex, as is typical of this common pediatric testicular tumor. Note right-sided microlithiasis ⇨.* **(Right)** *Longitudinal US shows an intratesticular epidermoid ➡ incidentally discovered in a child with contralateral epididymitis; note its multilaminated onion skin appearance ➡, a classic finding in epidermoids.*

TERMINOLOGY

Synonyms

- Yolk sac tumor (YST): Endodermal sinus tumor, orchioblastoma
- Teratoma: Differentiated or mature teratoma, undifferentiated or immature teratoma
- Mixed germ cell tumor (MGCT): Polyembryoma
- Leydig cell tumor: Interstitial cell tumor
- Sertoli cell tumor: Androblastoma

Definitions

- Primary testicular tumors: Germ cell tumors (GCTs) vs. non-GCTs
- GCTs: ~ 2/3 of pediatric testicular tumors
  - YST: Histologically recapitulates yolk sac, allantois, & extraembryonic mesenchyme
  - Teratoma: Contains elements of all 3 germinal layers (endoderm, mesoderm, & ectoderm)
    - Mature contains only well-differentiated tissues; immature adds fetal elements
    - Epidermoids: Monodermal cysts (not neoplasms) filled with keratinizing stratified squamous epithelium
  - Embryonal carcinoma: Malignant tumor of anaplastic undifferentiated cells similar to those seen in very early embryo
  - Choriocarcinoma: Rare, highly malignant tumor composed of placenta-like tissues
  - Mixed GCTs: Malignant tumor of 2 or more germ cell types
  - Seminoma: Malignant tumor of germ cell origin lacking any embryonic elements
- Non-GCTs: ~ 1/3 of pediatric testicular tumors
  - Leydig cell tumors: Recapitulate normal development of Leydig cells (stromal cells that produce androgens)
  - Sertoli cell tumors: Recapitulate normal development of Sertoli cells (sex cord cells that support spermatogonial stem cells)
  - Juvenile granulosa cell tumors: Extremely rare stromal tumor that resembles ovarian graafian follicles
- Lymphoma & leukemia can also involve testes

IMAGING

General Features

- Best diagnostic clue
  - Intratesticular mass ± internal vascularity
- Morphology
  - Epidermoids, YSTs, & sex cord-stromal tumors tend to be well defined; others tend to be ill-defined

Ultrasonographic Findings

- Nonspecific appearance for most testicular masses, necessitating surgery
  - Most nonseminomatous GCTs have variable echogenicity
    - ± hypo-, iso-, or hyperechoic; homogeneous vs. heterogeneous
    - Commonly have cystic areas from necrosis & echogenic areas from Ca^{2+}, fibrosis, or hemorrhage
    - More aggressive tumors (especially embryonal carcinoma) may invade tunica albuginea
    - YSTs are often well defined; may simply enlarge testis without discernible mass
  - Teratomas characteristically have extremely complex appearance with cystic areas, Ca^{2+}, solid components, & punctate or linear echogenic hairs
  - Epidermoids (true cyst, not neoplasm) appear solid, targetoid, or "onion skin" from laminations of keratinizing stratified squamous epithelium
  - Regressed MGCTs may appear as subtle architectural distortion with ill-defined microcalcification
  - Seminomas are usually hypoechoic, homogeneous, well-defined intratesticular masses with lobulated margins
  - Sex cord/stromal tumors may be small & well defined
    - Most (2/3) juvenile granulosa cell tumors are multicystic, multiseptated; remaining 1/3 appear solid
    - Leydig cell tumors are usually small (< 1-cm diameter) & very well defined; markedly hypervascular on color Doppler & contrast-enhanced US; stiffer than surrounding parenchyma by elastography

MR Findings

- Nonseminomatous GCTs are usually heterogeneous, T1 iso- or hyperintense, T2 hypointense
- Regressed MGCTs have ill-defined areas of low T2 signal or architectural distortion without visible mass
- Seminomas are usually homogeneous, T1 isointense, & T2 hypointense
- Look for pelvic & retroperitoneal adenopathy

Imaging Recommendations

- Best imaging tool
  - US ~ 100% sensitive; MR for problem-solving
  - Chest (CT) + abdomen & pelvis (CT or MR) screening for metastases, depending on tumor type
- Protocol advice
  - US: Supine positioning with warm folded towel between thighs to support scrotum; use highest frequency linear-array transducer available; color Doppler setting should be sensitive to low-velocity flow
  - MR: Large field-of-view (FOV) axial T2 FS & DWI from kidneys through pelvis; small FOV high-resolution T2 FS images in 3 planes + axial GRE & T1 FS pre- & post gadolinium of scrotum

DIFFERENTIAL DIAGNOSIS

Hematoma

- History is crucial, but trauma does not exclude hemorrhage of preexisting neoplasm
- Can be multifocal & any size; color Doppler demonstrates no internal vascularity
- Hyperacute/acute → isoechoic to parenchyma; chronic → becomes hypoechoic/anechoic; 24-hour repeat US can be useful to document evolution

Focal Orchitis

- Presents with acute scrotal pain & swelling; concomitant epididymitis is common
- Altered echotexture, swelling, hypervascularity
- Appearance improves with short-term follow-up

Epidermoid Cyst

- Ectodermal inclusion cyst; most common benign intratesticular mass
- Laminated, concentric rings of low & high echogenicity or signal, a.k.a. onion skin pattern; no blood flow
- Surgeon may remove by enucleation, not orchiectomy

Testicular Adrenal Rest Tumors

- Adrenal rests (not neoplasm) trapped in developing fetal testis, found in 10-15% of newborns
- Enlarge if exposed to ↑ adrenocorticotrophic hormone; otherwise, regress; seen in < 1% of adults
- Multiple bilateral intratesticular nodules; usually near mediastinum or peripheral
- Usually hypoechoic but may be hyperechoic; may have homogeneous or heterogenous echogenicity
- Characteristic low T2 signal; hypo- or isointense on T1
- Variable vascularity (often hypervascular) but do not distort vessels passing through lesion

Dilated Rete Testes

- Benign dilation of tubules near mediastinum, rare in boys
- Often bilateral; associated with spermatoceles; geographic margins, no mass effect

Segmental Infarction

- Uncommon, may see in sickle cell disease
- Wedge-shaped hypoechogenicity with absent or diminished flow; MR may show hemorrhagic signal around avascular region

PATHOLOGY

Staging, Grading, & Classification

- No universal staging system for pediatric testicular tumors
- Children's Oncology Group stages GCTs
  - Stage I: Limited to testis; complete resection, normal tumor markers
  - Stage II: Invasion of scrotum or spermatic cord, incomplete resection (microscopically), persistent elevation of tumor markers
  - Stage III: Incomplete resection (macroscopically); retroperitoneal lymph node involvement but no visceral or extraabdominal metastases
  - Stage IV: Distant metastases

CLINICAL ISSUES

Presentation

- Most common signs/symptoms
  - Asymptomatic; painless (rarely painful) testicular mass; mild discomfort or pain in abdomen, groin, or testicle; perceived scrotal heaviness
- Other signs/symptoms
  - YST: 90% have ↑ α-fetoprotein, used as tumor marker
  - Choriocarcinoma: Most have ↑ β-hCG; diagnosis is usually due to result of hematogenous metastasis
  - Sertoli cell tumors: Painless mass in infants; may have gynecomastia
  - Leydig cell tumors: Boys aged 5-10 years; may elaborate testosterone or have ↑ estrogen & estradiol levels → precocious puberty or gynecomastia
  - Juvenile granulosa cell tumors: Most frequent congenital testicular neoplasm

Demographics

- Represent 1-2% of childhood solid tumors
- ~ 1 per 100,000 boys; most common malignancy in postpubertal young men (15-34)
- 2 age peaks: First 2 years of life & late adolescence
  - Most prepubertal masses are benign (teratoma, epidermoid), though YSTs are 2nd most common tumor
    - YST: Most common pure GCT
    - Teratoma: Increasingly reported as most common prepubertal tumor; most present in 1st year of life
      - Prognosis depends on age rather than presence of mature or immature histologic features
  - Most postpubertal masses are malignant: Embryonal carcinoma & MGCT are most common
    - Embryonal carcinoma: Very rare prior to puberty
    - Seminoma: Extremely rare prior to puberty; usually men
- 10% are associated with cryptorchidism
  - If orchiopexy occurs before puberty → relative risk is 2x that of general population
  - If orchiopexy after puberty → relative risk is 5x that of general population
- ↑ risk in patients with microlithiasis

Natural History & Prognosis

- YST: Most in infants are stage I → orchiectomy only, > 80% are disease free at 6 years; recurrence has excellent response to platinum therapy
- Teratoma: Age predicts prognosis → benign in prepubertal testes, even if immature; 1/3 are malignant in postpubertal teratomas, even if mature
- Choriocarcinoma: Seen in older adolescents & young men, usually with advanced disease
- Juvenile granulosa cell tumors: Benign & hormonally inactive; 20% are associated with Y-chromosomal &/or urogenital abnormalities

Treatment

- Standard of care: Orchiectomy; testis-sparing enucleation may be performed in newborns & prepubertal boys without ↑ AFP
- YST & teratomas in prepubertal boys may need no further treatment beyond orchiectomy

SELECTED REFERENCES

1. Davis JT et al: Imaging of childhood urologic cancers: current approaches and new advances. Transl Androl Urol. 9(5):2348-57, 2020
2. Yu CJ et al: Incidence characteristics of testicular microlithiasis and its association with risk of primary testicular tumors in children: a systematic review and meta-analysis. World J Pediatr. 16(6):585-97, 2020
3. Wu D et al: Prepubertal testicular tumors in China: a 10-year experience with 67 cases. Pediatr Surg Int. 34(12):1339-43, 2018
4. Alkhori NA et al: Pediatric scrotal ultrasound: review and update. Pediatr Radiol. 47(9):1125-33, 2017
5. Trout AT et al: Association between testicular microlithiasis and testicular neoplasia: large multicenter study in a pediatric population. Radiology. 285(2):576-83, 2017
6. Yılmaz R et al: Sonography and magnetic resonance imaging characteristics of testicular adrenal rest tumors. Pol J Radiol. 82:583-8, 2017

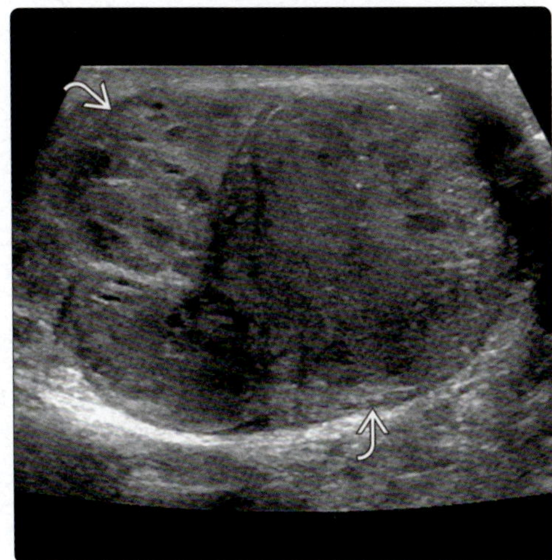

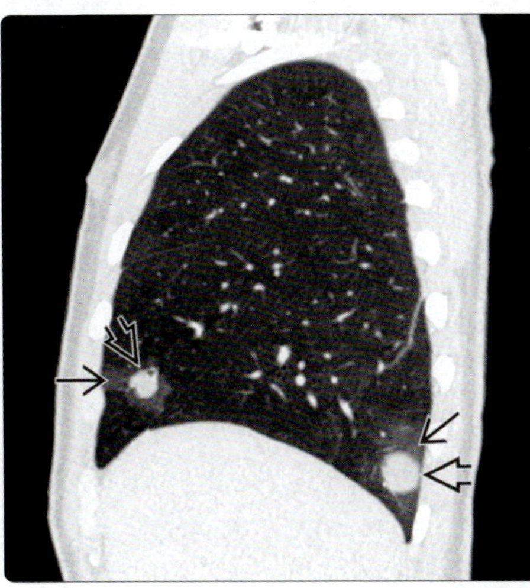

(Left) *Longitudinal US in a 17-year-old boy who presented with chronic fatigue & a large, firm testicular mass shows a lobulated, complex, & heterogeneous lesion ➡ replacing the right testis. Blood tests revealed anemia & elevated levels of LDH & β-hCG. Metastatic choriocarcinoma was ultimately diagnosed.* **(Right)** *Sagittal lung CECT in the same patient with choriocarcinoma demonstrates well-defined pulmonary metastases ➡ with surrounding areas of ground-glass attenuation ➡ due to hemorrhage.*

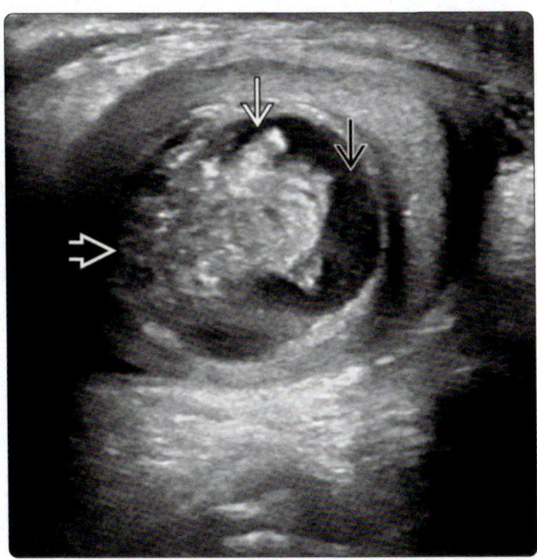

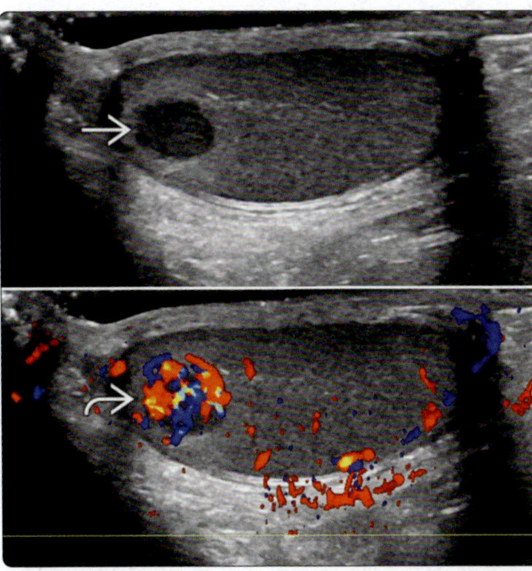

(Left) *Transverse US in an infant with nonpainful testicular swelling shows a well-defined, complex testicular mass ➡. Note the echogenic, solid component ➡ surrounded by fluid ➡. A mature teratoma was found at resection.* **(Right)** *Longitudinal grayscale & color Doppler US images in a 7-year-old with precocious puberty, ↑ testosterone, & a bone age 8 standard deviations above the mean show a well-defined, hypoechoic testicular mass ➡ with marked hypervascularity ➡, ultimately proven to be a Leydig cell tumor.*

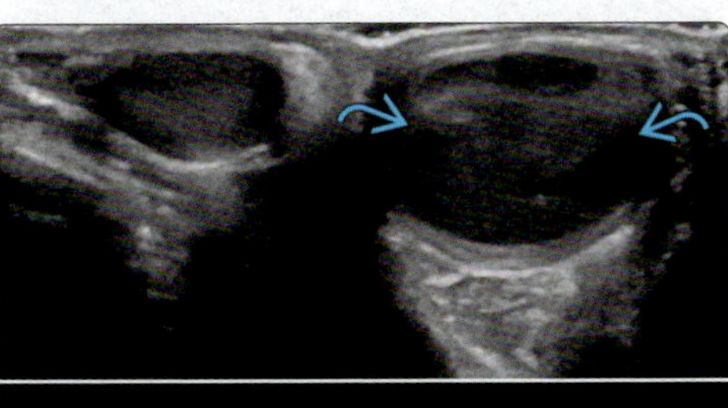

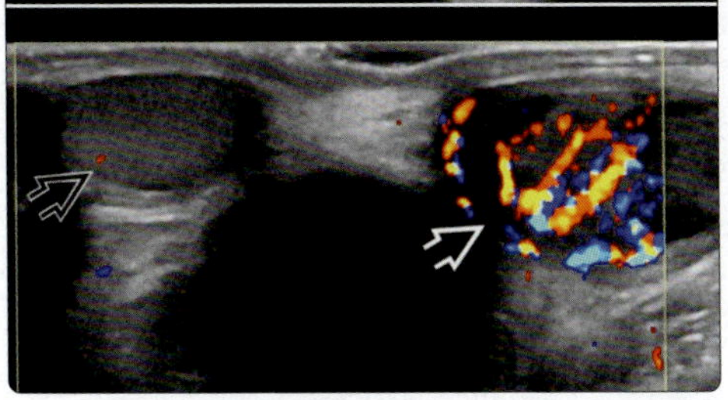

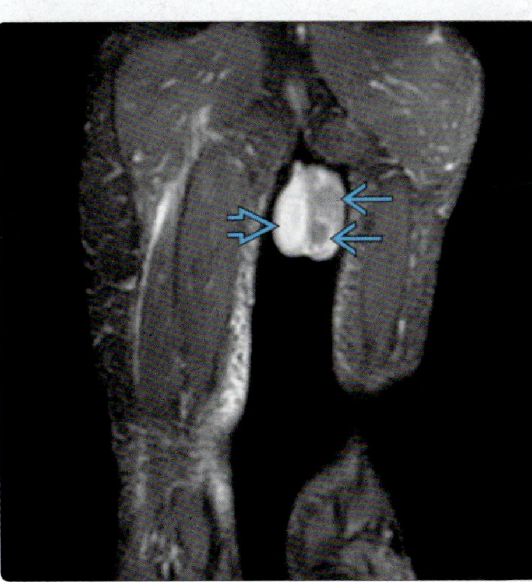

(Left) *Transverse grayscale US (top) shows asymmetric enlargement of the left testis ➡ due to leukemic infiltration. Color Doppler US (bottom) shows marked asymmetric hyperemia of left testis ➡ compared to the normal right side ➡, a common finding in leukemic infiltration.* **(Right)** *Coronal STIR MR in a teenager with a thigh hematoma shows 2 incidental hypointense masses ➡ in the left testis. Note the normal homogeneously hyperintense appearance of the right testis ➡. Seminoma was found at biopsy.*

Testicular Trauma

KEY FACTS

TERMINOLOGY

- Hydrocele: Simple fluid between layers of tunica vaginalis
- Hematocele: Blood between tunica vaginalis layers
- Hematoma: Contained collection of blood products within testis, epididymis, or scrotal wall; may involve ≥ 1 site
- Testicular fracture: Disruption of testicular parenchyma
- Testicular rupture: Disruption of tunica albuginea, often with extrusion of testicular parenchyma
- Devascularization: Vascular pedicle injury causing absent or diminished blood flow without true torsion (twisting)
- Traumatic epididymitis: Epididymal contusion causing inflammation, enlargement, & hypervascularity
- Traumatic testicular ectopia: Traumatic dislocation of testis into inguinal canal, abdominal cavity, or perineum

IMAGING

- Look for alteration of normal testicular echotexture, disruption of tunica albuginea, absent or diminished blood flow, complex hydrocele, &/or scrotal wall thickening

TOP DIFFERENTIAL DIAGNOSES

- Infectious epididymitis
  - Epididymal enlargement, heterogeneity, & hyperemia
  - Imaging is indistinguishable from trauma without history
- Testicular torsion
  - No blood flow to testis; twisting of spermatic cord
  - May occur spontaneously or after minor trauma
- Torsion of testicular appendage
  - Leading cause of acute scrotum in boys
  - Enlarged, spherical, echogenic, pedunculated remnant of tissue, ± periappendiceal hyperemia, reactive hydrocele
- Neoplasm
  - Rare, but 10-15% are found during US for scrotal trauma
  - Intratesticular mass with vascular flow (vs. testicular hematoma, which will not have blood flow)

CLINICAL ISSUES

- Testicular fracture/rupture → urologic emergencies → prompt treatment reduces infection, atrophy, necrosis

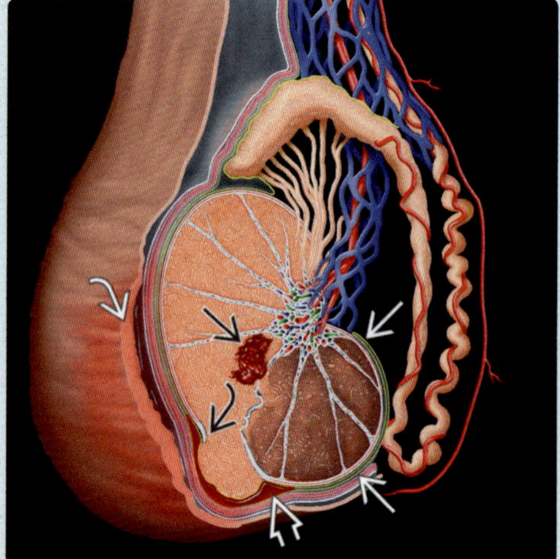

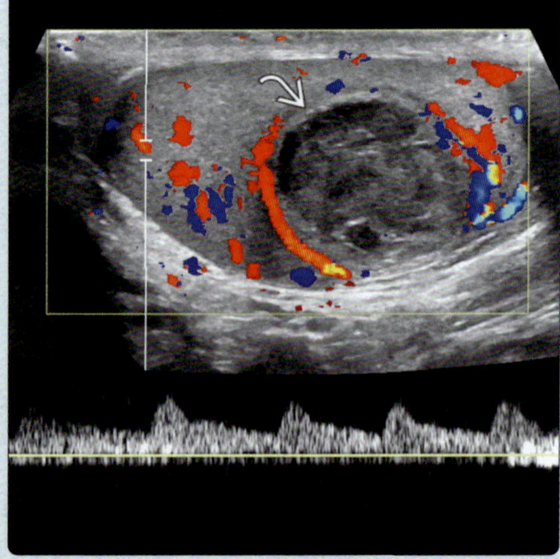

(Left) *Graphic shows various manifestations of scrotal trauma, including a scrotal wall hematoma ➔, rupture of the tunica albuginea ⇨, segmental testicular infarction ➔, parenchymal hematoma ⇨, & a small hematocele ➔.* **(Right)** *US in a teenager with hemophilia A who hit a tree while skiing shows a well-defined, heterogeneous, avascular intratesticular hematoma ➔, which was smaller on follow-up US (not shown). Note that a neoplasm would have internal blood flow & would not be smaller on follow-up.*

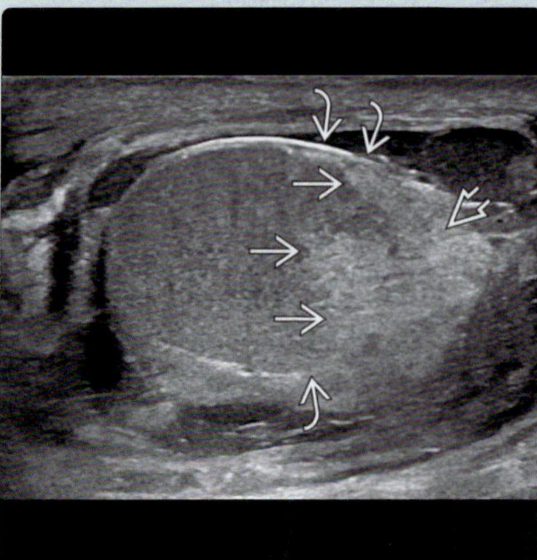

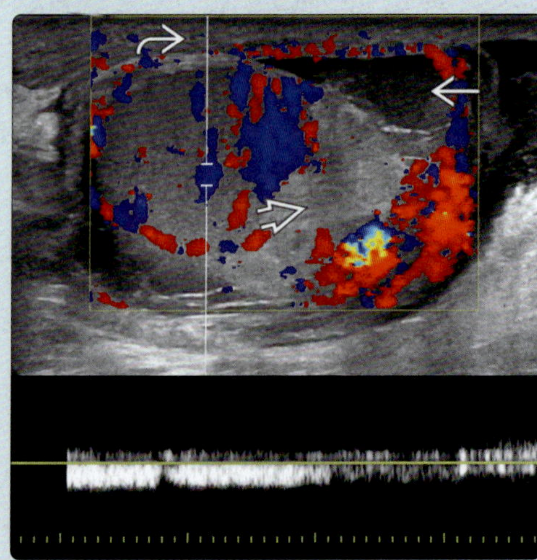

(Left) *US in an 11-year-old who was kneed during a basketball game shows a sharp, jagged demarcation through the parenchyma ➔, representing a testicular fracture & hyperechogenicity in the lower pole due to segmental infarction ➔. Tunica albuginea ➔ is interrupted.* **(Right)** *Doppler US in the same boy shows no vascularity in lower testis due to segmental infarction ➔ (with reactive hypervascularity of adjacent parenchyma). Note the surrounding hematocele ➔ & adjacent scrotal wall edema ➔.*

TERMINOLOGY

Definitions

- Hydrocele: Simple fluid between layers of tunica vaginalis
- Hematocele: Blood products between layers of tunica vaginalis
- Hematoma: Contained collection of blood products within testis, epididymis, or scrotal wall; can be multifocal
- Testicular fracture: Disruption of testicular parenchyma
- Testicular rupture: Disruption of tunica albuginea, often with extrusion of testicular parenchyma
- Devascularization: Vascular pedicle injury causing absent or diminished blood flow without true torsion (twisting)
- Traumatic epididymitis: Epididymal contusion causing inflammation, enlargement, & hypervascularity
- Traumatic testicular ectopia: Traumatic dislocation of testis into inguinal canal, abdominal cavity, or perineum

IMAGING

Ultrasonographic Findings

- Hydrocele, hematocele, epididymitis, scrotal hematoma
  - Echogenic/complex fluid of hematocele is most common finding (after hydrocele)
- Fracture: Hypoechoic line through testicular parenchyma with focally altered echotexture ± disruption of echogenic tunica albuginea
  - Testicular parenchyma may extrude through tunica (resulting in contour deformity)
- Hematoma
  - Scrotal: Echogenic thickening of scrotal wall ± focal areas of complex fluid
  - Epididymal: Mixed echogenicity, nonvascular mass
  - Testicular: Mixed echogenicity, nonvascular mass
- Devascularization: Absent/diminished testicular blood flow
- Testicular dislocation: Rare; consider if testis not in scrotum
- If available, contrast-enhanced ultrasound improves delineation of testicular fractures; also has ↑ sensitivity for devascularization & hematomas

Imaging Recommendations

- Best imaging tool: Grayscale & color Doppler ultrasound with highest frequency (10- to 14-MHz) linear-array transducer available
  - Sensitivity & specificity > 95%
  - Compare echotexture, size, & vascularity of testis to asymptomatic side in transverse side-by-side view

DIFFERENTIAL DIAGNOSIS

Infectious Epididymitis

- Epididymal enlargement, heterogeneity, & hyperemia
- Indistinguishable from traumatic cause without history

Testicular Torsion

- Absent or diminished vascularity in testis
- Look for twisting of spermatic cord just above testicle
- May occur spontaneously or after minor trauma

Torsion of Testicular Appendage

- Echogenic or salt & pepper appearance of enlarged nodular tissue along margin of testis, usually with periappendiceal hyperemia
- May cause reactive hydrocele & scrotal wall thickening
- Leading cause of acute scrotum in boys

Neoplasm

- Intratesticular mass with internal vascular flow
- 10-15% are found during ultrasound for trauma

CLINICAL ISSUES

Presentation

- Most common signs/symptoms
  - Intense scrotal pain in setting of recent trauma
  - Ecchymosis, swelling, skin abrasion, or laceration

Natural History & Prognosis

- Possible complications: Infarction, infection, atrophy, ↓ sex hormones & spermatogenesis, infertility

Treatment

- Physical exam has poor correlation to degree of injury; therefore, ultrasound is important to guide management (conservative vs. surgical repair or debridement)
- Fracture & rupture = urologic emergency
- Salvage rate for rupture: 90% → 45% after 72 hours
- Testis can usually be repaired to avoid orchiectomy
- Large hematocele or hematoma may require evacuation

DIAGNOSTIC CHECKLIST

Consider

- Ultrasound helps exclude testicular fracture or rupture (injuries which usually require urgent surgery)
- In cases of penetrating trauma, ultrasound may be limited by air artifact but can be helpful to identify possible foreign body

Image Interpretation Pearls

- Testicular rupture may violate tunica vasculosa → high rate of devascularization
- Do not confuse testicular hematoma with neoplasm; do remember that hemorrhagic neoplasms can cause false-positive ultrasound for trauma
- Hematoceles have high association with rupture (but lack of hematocele does not rule out testicular rupture or fracture)
- Testicular dislocation is extremely rare, but do not assume cryptorchism in cases of trauma with missing testicle

Reporting Tips

- Patients with large, expanding hematocele may need surgery secondary to pain or possible compromise to testis
- Large hematomas may need follow-up to exclude superinfection or testicular necrosis

SELECTED REFERENCES

1. Choi HH et al: How common are traumatic injuries to the epididymis? A study of prevalence, imaging appearance, and management implications. Emerg Radiol. 28(1):31-6, 2020
2. Yusuf GT et al: The role of contrast-enhanced ultrasound (CEUS) in the evaluation of scrotal trauma: a review. Insights Imaging. 11(1):68, 2020
3. Blok D et al: Testicular rupture following blunt scrotal trauma. Case Rep Emerg Med. 2019:7058728, 2019
4. Rebik K et al: Scrotal ultrasound. Radiol Clin North Am. 57(3):635-48, 2019
5. Wang A et al: A review of imaging modalities used in the diagnosis and management of scrotal trauma. Curr Urol Rep. 18(12):98, 2017

Ectopic Testicle

KEY FACTS

TERMINOLOGY

- Undescended testis (UDT): Found along normal pathway of descent but outside scrotum
- Ectopic testis: Found outside normal pathway of descent
  - Very rare, < 5% of boys worked up for UDT
- Testicular retraction: Physiologic, reducible retraction of testis out of scrotum due to hyperactive cremasteric reflex
- Ascending testis: Nonphysiologic, nonreducible retraction of testis out of scrotum (acquired UDT)

IMAGING

- Many pediatric urologists prefer to skip imaging for UDT
- UDT: Empty hemiscrotum, ± testis along pathway of descent; no history of testis having been within scrotum
- Ectopic testes: Empty hemiscrotum & testis abnormally located in perineum, femoral canal, superficial inguinal pouch, suprapubic area, or contralateral hemiscrotum

TOP DIFFERENTIAL DIAGNOSES

- Inguinal lymphadenopathy
- Female with congenital adrenal hyperplasia

PATHOLOGY

- Pathogenesis of testicular ectopia & UDT is influenced by hormonal, genetic, environmental, & anatomic factors
- UDT: Testis is intrinsically abnormal with altered spermatogenesis
- Ectopic: Testis is normally developed with normal spermatogenesis (if treated)

CLINICAL ISSUES

- UDT: Most spontaneously descend in 1st year of life; testis will not descend after 12 months; ↑ risk of infertility, testicular tumors, torsion, inguinal hernia if not treated
- Ectopic: ↑ risk of trauma, ± altered spermatogenesis
- Testicular retraction is very common in 1st decade but may herald ascending testis (↑ risk of infertility, trauma, tumor)

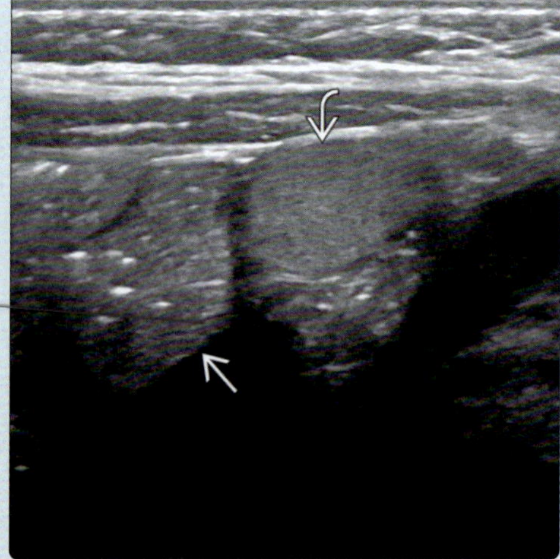

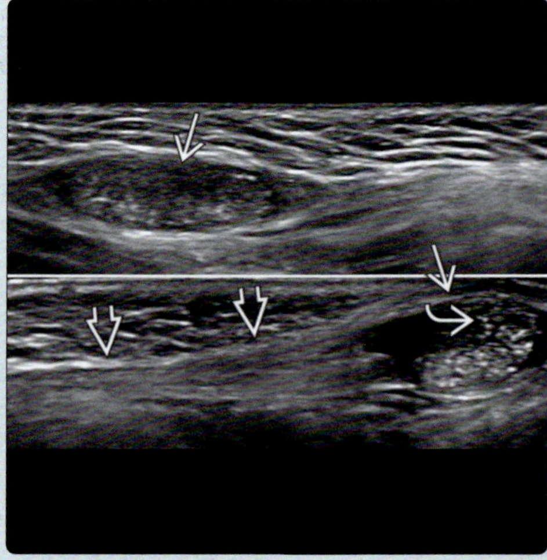

(Left) *RLQ US in an infant with cryptorchidism shows a normal-appearing testis ➦ next to bowel ➡ in the abdomen. Testes located outside the normal pathway of descent are termed ectopic testes.* **(Right)** *Trans (top) & long (bottom) US in a boy with cryptorchidism show the right testis ➡ in the inguinal canal. Normal spermatic cord course ➡ implies that it followed a normal pathway of descent. Unlike ectopic testes, undescended testes (UDTs) are intrinsically abnormal & have a higher rate of microlithiasis ➦.*

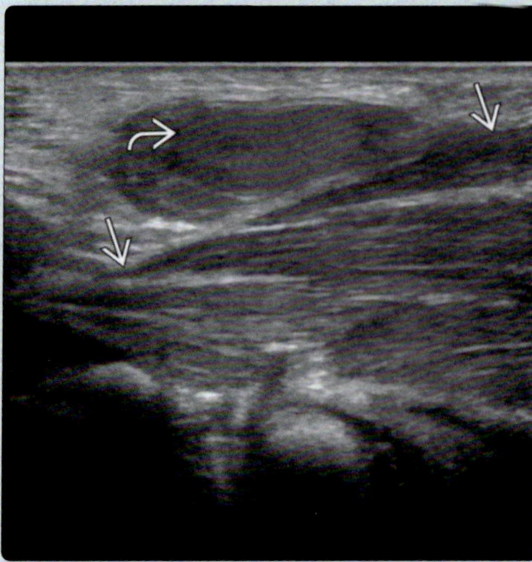

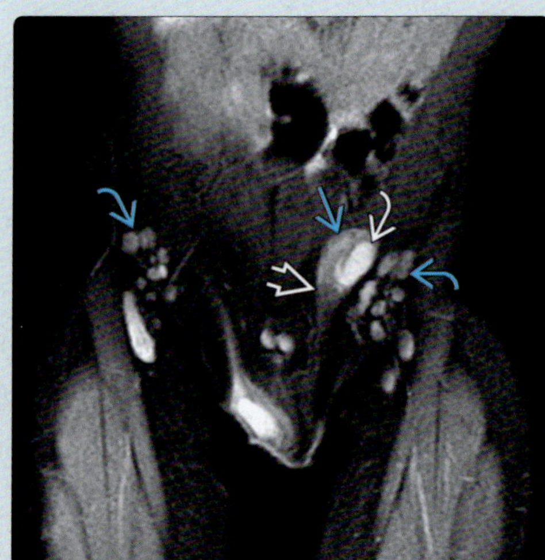

(Left) *Oblique US of the left perineum in a 1-week-old with a persistent bulge lateral to the inguinoscrotal crease shows an otherwise normal testis ➡ within the perineal subcutaneous fat. Note adductor muscles ➡ deep to the testis. Treatment in such cases is elective orchiopexy.* **(Right)** *Coronal STIR MR in a toddler shows a retracted testis ➡ next to inguinal lymph nodes ➦. The spermatic cord ➡ & epididymis ➡ help distinguish the testis from lymph nodes, which have vessels entering at the hilum.*

TERMINOLOGY

Synonyms

- Undescended testis (UDT), cryptorchidism

Definitions

- UDT: Along normal route of descent but outside scrotum
- Ectopic testis: Outside normal pathway of descent
- Testicular retraction: Physiologic, reducible retraction of testis out of scrotum due to hyperactive cremasteric reflex
- Ascending testis: Nonphysiologic, nonreducible retraction of testis out of scrotum (acquired UDT)

IMAGING

General Features

- UDT: Empty hemiscrotum with testis along pathway of descent in 80% (or not found); no history of testis ever in scrotum
  - Differentiation of UDT from testicular retraction & ascending testis is based on history & physical exam
- Ectopic testes: Empty hemiscrotum with testis abnormally located in perineum, femoral canal, superficial inguinal pouch, suprapubic area, or contralateral hemiscrotum

Ultrasonographic Findings

- Ectopic testis is usually normal-appearing; UDTs may be normal or small with hydrocele ± microlithiasis

CT Findings

- Testicular retraction is often noted on CT as 1 or both testes "riding high" in inguinal canal(s)

MR Findings

- Useful problem-solving tool for ambiguous genitalia or ectopic testes; no added value for UDT

Points to Consider

- Many pediatric urologists prefer to skip imaging for UDT

DIFFERENTIAL DIAGNOSIS

Lymphadenopathy

- Look for typical hilar fat & vessels + classic reniform shape
- Lymph nodes will be lateral to inguinal canal

Female With Congenital Adrenal Hyperplasia

- Ambiguous external genitalia with normal ovaries & uterus
- Abnormal electrolytes & endocrinologic studies

PATHOLOGY

General Features

- Pathogenesis of testicular ectopia & UDT is multifactorial
  - Hormonal factors (hypothalamic-pituitary dysfunction, low androgens) & genetics play major role in UDT
  - Environmental & anatomic factors (short vas deferens, ventral wall defects, etc.) play role in ectopia & UDT
- Associated abnormalities
  - Boys with UDT have higher rates of inguinal hernia, other GU abnormalities, & endocrine abnormalities
  - Prader-Willi syndrome, Kallmann syndrome, pituitary hypoplasia, ventral wall defects → high rates of UDT

Staging, Grading, & Classification

- Testicular ectopia can be congenital or posttraumatic
  - Congenital: Femoral canal, base of penis, or perineum
    - Crossed testicular ectopia: Rare anomaly of aberrant migration into opposite hemiscrotum
      - a.k.a. transverse testicular ectopia
  - Posttraumatic: Dislocation into inguinal canal, abdominal cavity, or perineum
- UDT: Classified based on location
  - 80% are superficial & palpable (upper scrotum, superficial inguinal pouch, or inguinal canal)
  - 20% are not palpable (intraabdominal)

Gross Pathologic & Surgical Features

- UDT: Testis is intrinsically abnormal with altered spermatogenesis; ↑ risk of inguinal hernia, testicular neoplasm, torsion, & infertility
- Ectopic: Testis is normally developed with normal spermatogenesis (if treated); no ↑ risk of inguinal hernia, testicular neoplasm, torsion, or infertility

CLINICAL ISSUES

Presentation

- Most common signs/symptoms
  - UDT: Empty hemiscrotum, ± palpable testis along pathway of descent; right 50%, left 30%, bilateral 20%
  - Ectopic testes: Unilateral empty scrotal sac & palpable mass in location characteristic for ectopic testis

Demographics

- UDT is most common gonadal abnormality in boys; incidence is 30% if preterm, 5% if term, & 1% by 1 year
- Ectopic testis is very rare (< 5% of boys worked up for UDT)

Natural History & Prognosis

- UDT: Most spontaneously descend in 1st year of life; testis will not descend after 12 months; ↑ risk of infertility, testicular tumors, torsion, inguinal hernia if not treated
- Ectopic: ↑ risk of trauma ± altered spermatogenesis
- Testicular retraction is very common in 1st decade but may herald ascending testis (↑ risk of infertility, trauma, tumor)

Treatment

- Orchiopexy by 1 or 2 years of age; reduces (but does not remove) risk of testicular cancer

DIAGNOSTIC CHECKLIST

Image Interpretation Pearls

- Make sure inguinal "mass" is not actually testicle prior to biopsy of "enlarged node"

SELECTED REFERENCES

1. Zhou G et al: Clinical characteristics, ultrasonographic findings, and treatment of pediatric transverse testicular ectopia: a 10-year retrospective review. Urology. 154:249-54, 2021
2. Punwani VV et al: Testicular ectopia: why does it happen and what do we do? J Pediatr Surg. 52(11):1842-7, 2017

Variations of Hydroceles

KEY FACTS

TERMINOLOGY

- Hydrocele: Abnormal fluid in scrotal tunica vaginalis &/or spermatic cord/inguinal canal
- Communicating hydrocele: Fluid connects freely between scrotum & peritoneal cavity via patent processus vaginalis
- Noncommunicating hydrocele: No connection between scrotum & peritoneal cavity
  - Implies closed processus vaginalis
- Encysted hydrocele: Loculated fluid in inguinal canal with no connection to scrotum or peritoneal cavity
- Funicular hydrocele: Fluid in inguinal canal with connection to peritoneal cavity (via open internal ring)
- Abdominoscrotal hydrocele: Loculated, dumbbell-shaped fluid collection with abdominal & scrotal components
- Hydrocele of canal of Nuck: Females only → localized fluid collection in groin &/or labia majora
- Complex hydrocele: Complicated fluid, which may be due to blood (hematocele) or pus (pyocele)

IMAGING

- Simple, anechoic fluid surrounding testicle
  - Sparing of "bare area": Site of testicular attachment to epididymis; lacks tunica vaginalis
- ± connection to inguinal canal & peritoneal cavity
- ± mild debris or thin septations

TOP DIFFERENTIAL DIAGNOSES

- Indirect inguinal hernia
- Paratesticular rhabdomyosarcoma
- Lymphatic malformation
- Enlarged lymph nodes

CLINICAL ISSUES

- Most common < 1 year of age
  - ↑ incidence in premature infants & children with peritoneal dialysis, ventriculoperitoneal shunts, or ascites
- Patent processus vaginalis often spontaneously closes ≤ 2 years of age; surgery is often required > 2 years

(Left) *Transverse ultrasound in an 18-month-old boy with scrotal swelling demonstrates simple fluid isolated to the tunica vaginalis surrounding the left testicle, consistent with a noncommunicating hydrocele.* **(Right)** *Axial T2 FS MR in a 3-year-old girl undergoing pelvic MR for early-onset inflammatory bowel disease shows well-circumscribed fluid in the right labia majora, consistent with a canal of Nuck hydrocele.*

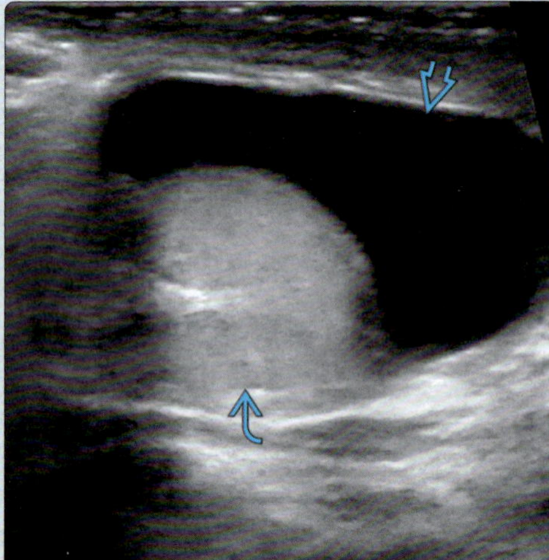

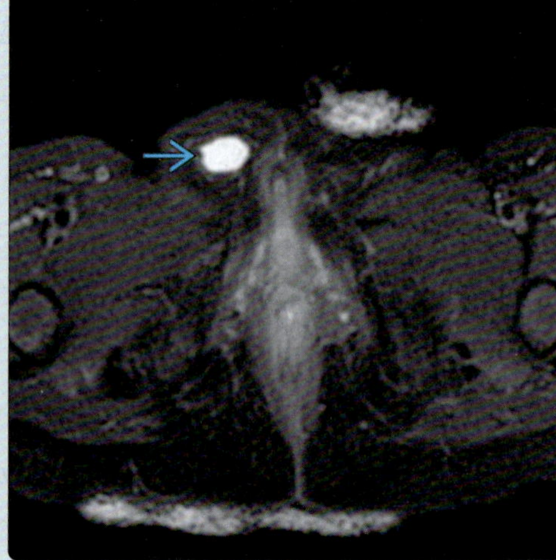

(Left) *Longitudinal ultrasound of the left inguinal canal in a 5-year-old boy with groin swelling shows fluid in the inguinal canal above the left testicle. The fluid ↑ when the patient was upright, indicating a connection to the peritoneal cavity (i.e., a funicular hydrocele of the spermatic cord).* **(Right)** *Coronal T2 FS MR in 12-year-old boy with a history of hernia & hydrocele repair shows a large amount of simple fluid surrounding the right testicle, consistent with a recurrent noncommunicating hydrocele.*

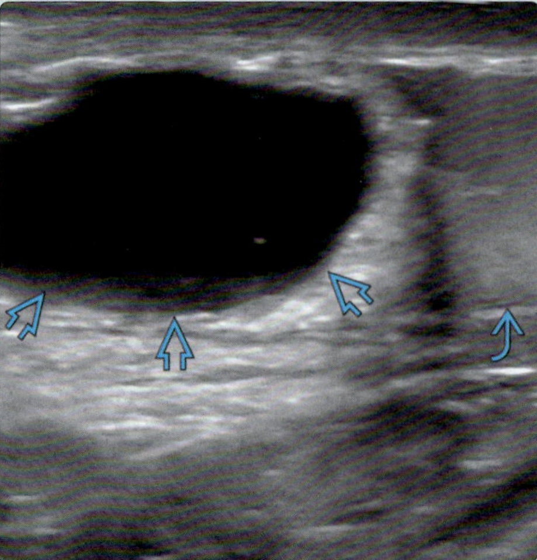

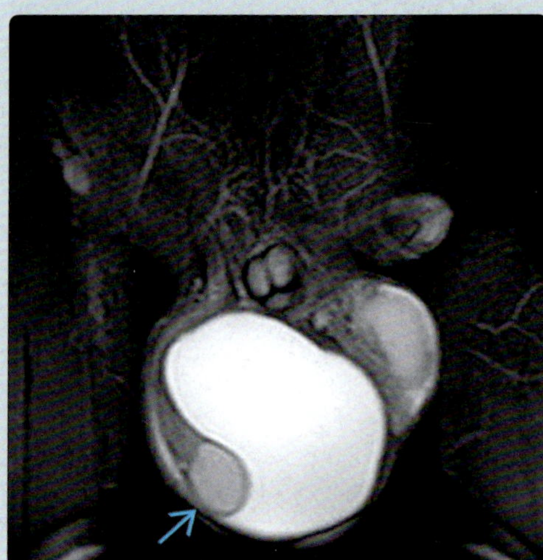

TERMINOLOGY

Definitions

- Hydrocele: Abnormal fluid in scrotal tunica vaginalis &/or spermatic cord/inguinal canal
- Communicating hydrocele: Fluid connects freely between scrotum & peritoneal cavity via patent processus vaginalis
- Noncommunicating hydrocele: No connection between scrotum & peritoneal cavity
  - Implies closed processus vaginalis
- Encysted hydrocele: Loculated fluid in inguinal canal with no connection to scrotum or peritoneal cavity
- Funicular hydrocele: Fluid in inguinal canal with connection to peritoneal cavity (via open internal ring)
- Abdominoscrotal hydrocele: Loculated, dumbbell-shaped fluid collection with abdominal & scrotal components
  - More frequent in adolescents & adults
- Hydrocele of canal of Nuck: Females only → localized fluid collection in groin &/or labia majora
- Complex hydrocele: Complicated fluid, which may be due to blood (hematocele) or pus (pyocele)
  - Older children, usually with history of trauma, infection, testicular torsion, or malignancy

IMAGING

General Features

- Best diagnostic clue
  - US showing simple fluid around testicle with extension into inguinal canal
- Size
  - Variable size; can be quite large
  - Canal of Nuck hydroceles tend to be smaller (< 3 cm)

Ultrasonographic Findings

- Grayscale ultrasound
  - Simple, anechoic fluid surrounding testicle
    - Except for "bare area" (site of testicular attachment to epididymis; lacks tunica vaginalis)
  - ± connection to inguinal canal & peritoneal cavity
  - ± mild debris or thin septations
  - Hydrocele may deform or resolve with compression

MR Findings

- T2WI
  - High fluid signal surrounding testes
  - May extend into inguinal canal
  - Canal of Nuck hydrocele: High-signal fluid collection in inguinal canal & labia majora

Imaging Recommendations

- Best imaging tool
  - Grayscale ultrasound
- Protocol advice
  - Must image inguinal canal to determine communication with peritoneal cavity
  - Consider imaging with different positions (upright, supine) & Valsalva maneuver

DIFFERENTIAL DIAGNOSIS

Indirect Inguinal Hernia

- Dynamic protrusion of bowel &/or echogenic mesenteric fat into inguinal canal ± scrotum

Paratesticular Rhabdomyosarcoma

- Solid, heterogeneous, extratesticular malignant mass with variable internal vascularity

Lymphatic Malformation

- Multicystic slow-flow vascular malformation infiltrating different tissue compartments
- Rarely isolated to scrotum (though scrotum is often involved by more extensive lymphatic malformations)

Enlarged Lymph Nodes

- Inguinal adenopathy is common; usually benign, reactive
  - Enlarged, reactive nodes with normal architecture
  - Necrotic/suppurative adenitis with cellulitis → abscess
  - Malignant infiltration with loss of architecture, round morphology, & distorted internal vascularity

PATHOLOGY

General Features

- Etiology
  - Failure of involution of normal developmental peritoneal fold extending into scrotum during testicular descent → patent processus vaginalis
  - Occurs at labia majora in girls along round ligament

CLINICAL ISSUES

Presentation

- Most common signs/symptoms
  - Scrotal or inguinal swelling, typically painless
  - May change with position & Valsalva (if communicating)

Demographics

- More common in infants
- Boys > > girls
- ↑ incidence in premature babies & children with peritoneal dialysis, ventriculoperitoneal shunts, or ascites

Natural History & Prognosis

- Patent processus vaginalis often spontaneously closes ≤ 2 years of age → observation considered
- > 2 years of age, spontaneous resolution is unlikely → surgery usually required
  - Closure of patent processus vaginalis + opening or drainage of hydrocele sac

SELECTED REFERENCES

1. Funatsu Y et al: Laparoscopic abdominoscrortal hydrocele: a case series. Urology. 145:236-42, 2020
2. Alkhori NA et al: Pediatric scrotal ultrasound: review and update. Pediatr Radiol. 47(9):1125-33, 2017
3. Costantino E et al: Abdominoscrotal hydrocele in an infant boy. BMJ Case Rep. 2017, 2017
4. Williamson ZC et al: Imaging of the inguinal canal in children. Curr Probl Diagn Radiol. 42(4):164-79, 2013
5. Khanna PC et al: Sonographic appearance of canal of Nuck hydrocele. Pediatr Radiol. 37(6):603-6, 2007

SECTION 6

Musculoskeletal

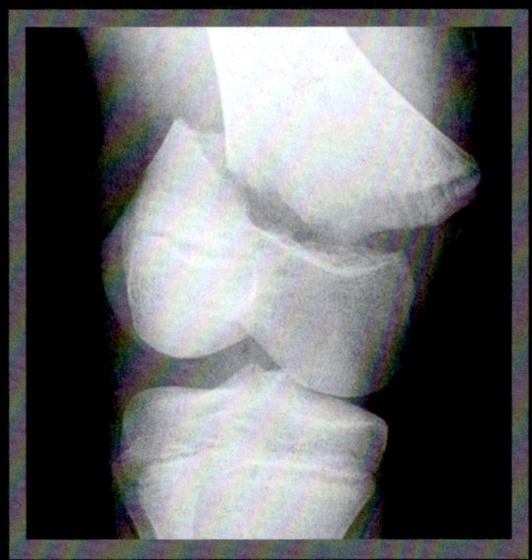

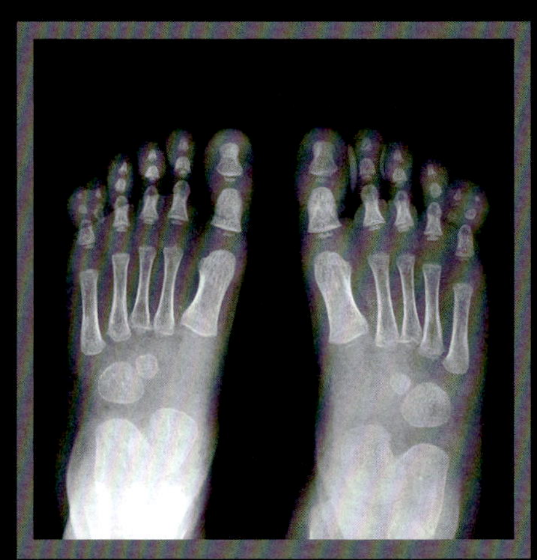

Soft Tissue Masses

Focal, Multifocal, and Diffuse Bone Lesions

Abnormalities of Hip

Constitutional Disorders of Bone

Miscellaneous

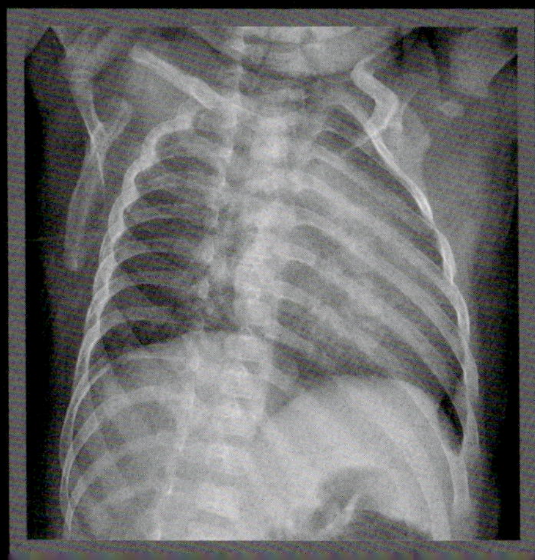

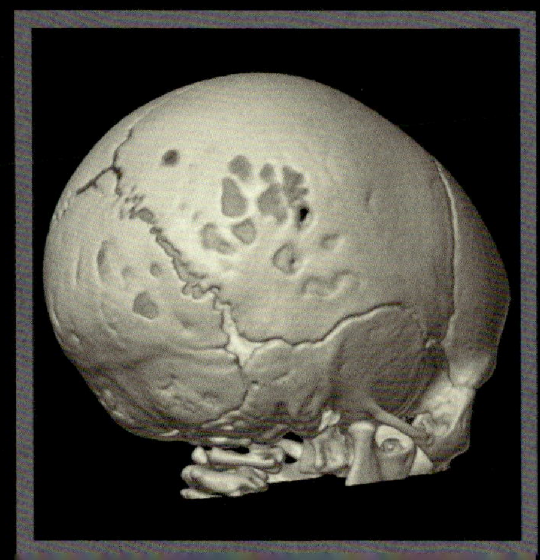

Musculoskeletal Imaging Modalities

Radiography

Although there have been great advances in imaging technology, radiography remains the most important imaging test in most circumstances of suspected musculoskeletal pathology. With appropriate techniques, the associated radiation exposure is usually minimal, & radiography is less expensive than other more advanced imaging studies. Most cases of trauma require radiographs & no other imaging. With suspicion of nonaccidental trauma (or an underlying skeletal dysplasia), a full skeletal survey should be performed.

Computed Tomography

CT is fast but utilizes ionizing radiation & must be employed judiciously. It allows multiplanar assessments & provides better soft tissue contrast than radiographs. Cortical bone detail is excellent by CT, though marrow evaluation is limited. CT is helpful in the detection & characterization of specific fractures that are intraarticular or complex, or for fractures that are often subtle but risk significant consequences if the diagnosis is delayed. Additional CT indications include the evaluations of osteoid osteoma, sequestra of osteomyelitis, tarsal coalitions, & union of complicated fractures.

Ultrasound

Ultrasonography uses no radiation, is relatively inexpensive, requires no sedation, & provides excellent superficial spatial resolution. It also enables dynamic assessments, differentiates cystic vs. solid masses, & characterizes vascular flow. Specific indications include the evaluations of developmental dysplasia of infant hips, retained nonradiopaque foreign bodies, soft tissue masses & fluid collections, & tendon injuries.

Magnetic Resonance

MR imaging uses no ionizing radiation; however, it is costly, has a relatively long exam time, & may require sedation & IV contrast agents. MR provides excellent soft tissue contrast & is multiplanar. When there is a high suspicion of pathology at a targeted musculoskeletal site, MR is the primary tool for investigation. Such indications include joint trauma, infection, soft tissue masses, & bone tumors. Other indications are stress injuries, physeal osseous bridges, & myopathy/myositis. Whole-body MR imaging has seen increased use in the last decade for several indications, including detecting occult or multifocal infection & screening for childhood malignancies in the setting of a tumor predisposition syndrome.

Nuclear Medicine

In isolation, nuclear medicine scans have excellent sensitivity (but low specificity) for whole-body screening of bone pathology. Traditional bone scan indications include the detection of osteomyelitis, metastatic disease, nonaccidental trauma, stress fracture, spondylolysis, osteoid osteoma, & osteonecrosis, though MR imaging has replaced many of these routine uses. Sensitivity can be ↑ by using bone scan SPECT, & excellent anatomic localization is achieved in combination with bone CT (e.g., for the detection of spondylolysis). FDG PET indications are most commonly centered on cancer staging.

Congenital Abnormalities

These abnormalities are typically discovered prenatally, at birth, or within the 1st few months of life. The diagnosis of such entities mainly relies on radiographs.

Proximal focal femoral deficiency (PFFD) is a malformation in which complete growth & development of the upper femur fails to occur. The Aitken classification, from class A (the least severe form with a short femur & common subtrochanteric varus deformity) to class D (in which both the femoral head & acetabulum are absent with a short, distal femoral segment), guides treatment in PFFD. However, classification can be difficult with radiographs at an early age (due to unossified segments).

Tarsal coalition is the congenital or acquired fusion of 2 or more tarsal bones & is most commonly found at the calcaneonavicular or talocalcaneal levels.

Congenital tibial dysplasia is a congenital pseudoarthrosis with anterolateral tibial bowing or fracture. Seventy percent of patients will eventually be diagnosed with neurofibromatosis type 1 (NF1).

Congenital tibial bowing is otherwise typically convex posteromedially & due to in utero positioning. It tends to resolve.

Other malformations include syndactyly, radial clubhand, radioulnar synostosis, arthrogryposis, & amniotic band syndrome.

Trauma

Pediatric fractures may be complete (i.e., all the way through the bone from one surface to the opposite surface) or incomplete. The elastic properties of the developing pediatric skeleton ↑ the potential for incomplete fractures, including plastic deformation (bowing), buckle, or greenstick fractures. It is important to obtain orthogonal views for a complete evaluation of the fracture. When describing the fracture, remember to include the location, extension, translation, & angulation.

Salter-Harris Classification

Approximately 1 in 5 pediatric fractures involves an adjacent growth plate.

In a type I fracture, the fracture is purely through the growth plate or physis (e.g., slipped capital femoral epiphysis).

In a type II fracture [the most common type of Salter-Harris (SH) fracture], the physeal fracture extends through a portion of the metaphysis.

In a type III fracture, the physeal fracture extends through the epiphysis (e.g., juvenile Tillaux fracture).

In a type IV fracture, the fracture extends across the physis & involves both the epiphysis & metaphysis (e.g., triplane & lateral condylar fractures).

In a type V fracture, there is a crush injury of the physis. This is rarely seen in actual practice.

Common Elbow Fractures

The supracondylar fracture is the most common pediatric elbow fracture, most frequently occurring at 5-7 years of age. An elbow effusion may suggest an occult, nondisplaced supracondylar fracture.

The medial epicondyle avulsion comprises 10% of elbow fractures in pediatrics. The avulsed fragment may become entrapped in the elbow joint.

The lateral condylar fracture is typically a SH type IV fracture with the distal component extending through the unossified distal humeral cartilage.

The radial neck fracture accounts for 5% of pediatric elbow fractures with an average age of 10 years. Ninety percent are SH type II fractures.

Important Ankle Fractures

The juvenile Tillaux fracture is a SH type III fracture through the anterolateral distal tibial epiphysis. Mortise or oblique imaging views are helpful, but bone CT with coronal & sagittal reformation helps determine the degree of articular displacement & required therapy (e.g., when there is > 2 mm of articular surface displacement, operative treatment is employed).

The triplane fracture is typically a SH type IV fracture in 3 planes (transverse physeal, sagittal epiphyseal, & coronal metadiaphyseal planes). Bone CT has similar implications as for the juvenile Tillaux fracture.

Common Soft Tissue Masses

The underlying diagnosis of some soft tissue masses can be suspected by clinical exam, such as lipomas (which are superficial & doughy by palpation) & ganglion cysts (which transilluminate & lie near a joint or tendon). Others warrant further evaluation by US &/or MR. US is excellent for characterizing the internal vascularity of a lesion & assessing any dynamic properties, such as compressibility & mobility. MR is particularly helpful in determining the deep extent of a lesion & recognizing characteristic features that may elude US (including the presence of fat, layering blood products, & surrounding muscle edema). Firm, round, solid masses are particularly concerning for malignancy & almost always require biopsy. Nonspecific but small & entirely superficial lesions on US may be considered for excision without MR.

The ganglion cyst is a homogeneously hyperintense round or lobulated mass with minimal peripheral enhancement on MR; it communicates with an adjacent tendon or joint space.

A lipoma follows fat signal on all MR sequences & has thin septations with no significant enhancement. Other fat-containing lesions in the 1st decade of life include lipoblastoma, fibrous hamartoma of infancy, involuted infantile hemangioma, & lipofibromatosis.

Vascular malformations are congenital anomalies that are present at birth but may not manifest until later in life. Slow-flow venous or lymphatic malformations are usually soft/compressible & may show layering fluid-fluid levels of stagnant blood products. Venous lesions will show gradual, patchy to diffuse enhancement (& may contain hard, painful phleboliths), while lymphatic malformations will only show rim or septal enhancement. Fast-flow arteriovenous malformations show a tangle of vascular flow voids with minimal soft tissue mass.

An infantile hemangioma is a benign neoplasm that is typically small or absent at birth with rapid growth over the 1st few months of life before involuting over months to years. On MR, this lobulated lesion is typically subcutaneous & shows hyperintense T2 signal, vascular flow voids, & intense contrast enhancement. On Doppler US, there are > 5 vessels/cm^2 in the lesion with numerous low-resistance arterial waveforms.

Fat-shearing injuries most commonly follow blunt trauma (though the patient may not remember the traumatic event) & typically manifest as a subcutaneous, elongated fluid collection with angular peripheral margins (± central fat globules).

Plexiform neurofibromas are found in NF1 & may show a target or bag-of-worms appearance. There is concern for a malignant peripheral nerve sheath tumor when the mass shows disproportionate enlargement, loses the target sign, invades the surrounding structures, or becomes painful.

Rhabdomyosarcoma (RMS) is the most common soft tissue sarcoma in children. Embryonal RMS accounts for 60-70% of childhood RMS & typically occurs in the GU tract & head/neck (but may occur in the extremities). Alveolar RMS occurs in adolescents, most commonly in the extremities, trunk, & perianal/perirectal area.

Synovial sarcoma is the 2nd most common soft tissue sarcoma of childhood. It most commonly presents at 15-35 years of age. There is Ca^{2+} in 1/3 of cases, & the lesion often occurs near a joint. The lesion may be small & indolent-appearing on MR, potentially mimicking a cyst.

Desmoid-type fibromatosis varies in appearance depending on the amount of intralesional collagen vs. cellularity. The mass may erode or scallop the adjacent bone. It is often infiltrating & slow growing with a high rate of local recurrence.

Focal Bone Lesions

In the evaluation of extremity bone tumors, begin the exam with T1 & STIR MR joint-to-joint imaging to exclude skip metastases of the marrow. Smaller field-of-view images targeted at the main tumor can then be obtained with dedicated surface coils.

Osteosarcoma is the most common malignant primary bone tumor in children & young adults. The bimodal age distribution is 10-30 years followed by > 60 years. It classically shows aggressive destruction + new osteoid formation with 55-80% occurring around the knee. It is typically metaphyseal (90%).

Ewing sarcoma is the 2nd most common primary bone malignancy in children. The typical age range is 5-25 years. It has an aggressive appearance that is permeative or moth eaten, though sclerosis (in the bone) may occur in up to 25%. Its aggressive periosteal reaction may include Codman triangles, a spiculated (i.e., sunburst or hair standing on end) appearance, or a lamellated onion-skin appearance. There is often a disproportionately larger soft tissue mass than the amount of bone destruction.

Langerhans cell histiocytosis has a variable radiographic appearance. It occurs between 0-30 years of age with a peak at 5-10 years. It is classically a lucent, round or geographic, punched-out lesion with a narrow zone of transition. Enhancing tissue usually fills the defect on MR but does not substantially extend beyond the bone.

Infection

The absence of radiographic findings early does not exclude osteomyelitis. It typically shows periosteal reaction &/or bony destruction with an aggressive look after 7-10 days. In subacute osteomyelitis, an intraosseous Brodie abscess may show the penumbra sign with a high T1 signal rim marginating a more hypointense center.

Selected References

1. Navarro OM: Pearls and pitfalls in the imaging of soft-tissue masses in children. Semin Ultrasound CT MR. 41(5):498-512, 2020
2. Kim HH et al: Pediatric elbow injuries. Semin Ultrasound CT MR. 39(4):384-96, 2018

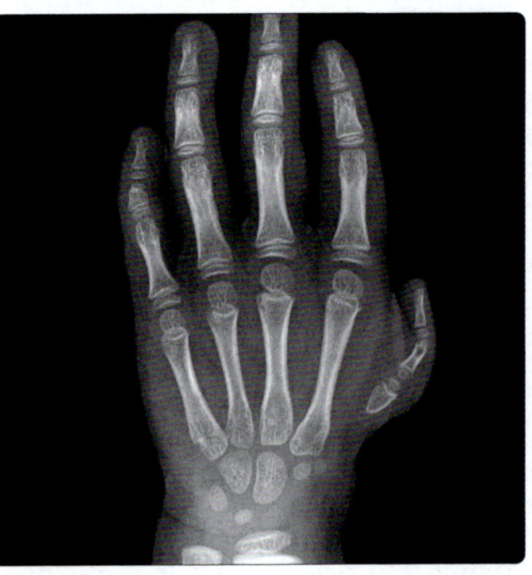

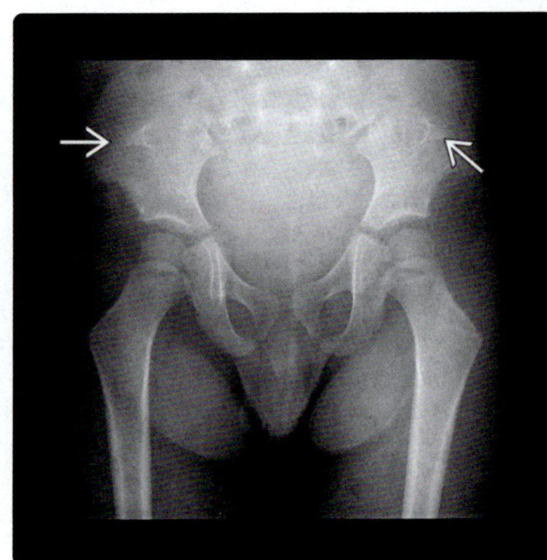

(Left) *PA radiograph in the left hand in a 4-year-old with Fanconi anemia shows a hypoplastic thumb with a truncated, triangular-shaped distal metacarpal & hypoplastic proximal & distal phalanges. Fanconi anemia is associated with radial ray dysplasia, which may be isolated to the thumb.* **(Right)** *AP radiograph in a 3-year-old shows bilateral posterior iliac horns ("Fong prongs") ➡ in a child with nail-patella syndrome or Fong disease. The iliac horns are considered pathognomonic for this syndrome.*

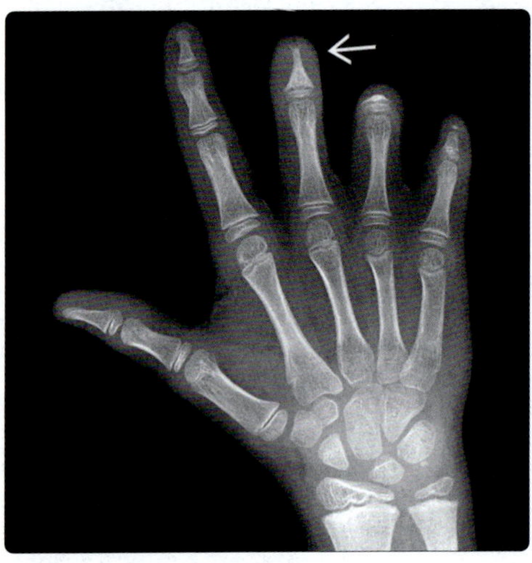

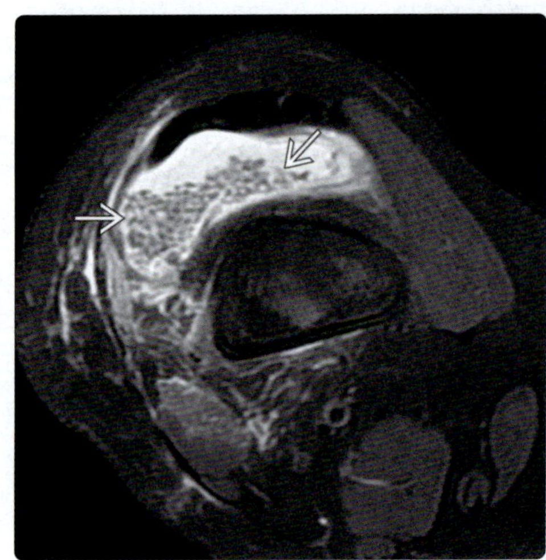

(Left) *PA radiograph in the hand in an 8-year-old with middle finger swelling shows loss of the distal portions of the 3rd-5th digits due to amniotic band syndrome. There is soft tissue swelling & irregularity of the tip of the middle finger ➡ in this child with cellulitis.* **(Right)** *Axial T2 FS MR in a child with juvenile idiopathic arthritis shows multiple, uniform hypointense rice bodies ➡ dependently within the knee joint.*

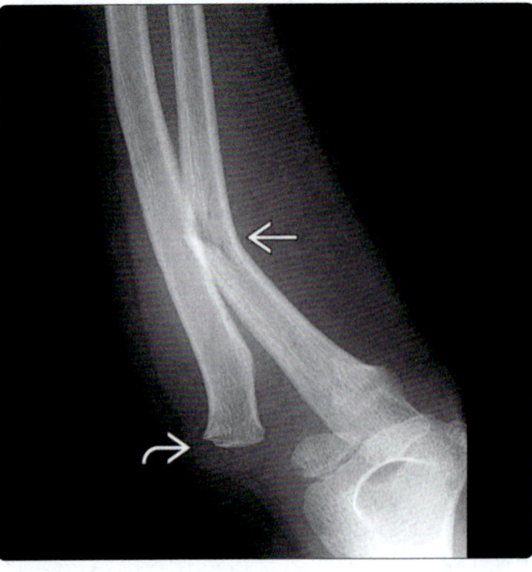

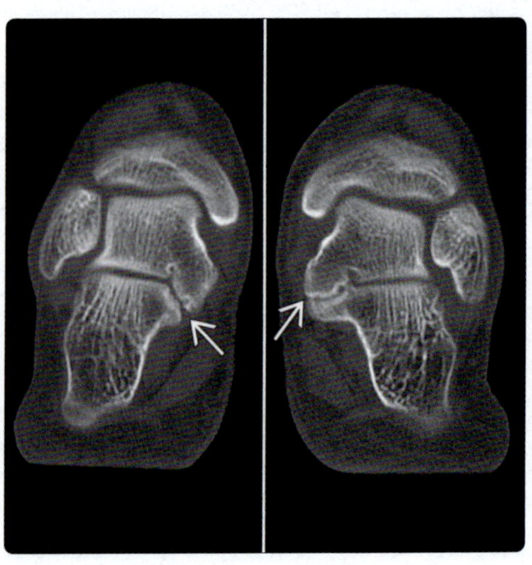

(Left) *AP radiograph in a child with a Monteggia fracture shows an angulated, incomplete proximal ulnar diaphyseal fracture ➡ with dislocation of the radial head ➡ laterally.* **(Right)** *Coronal bone CT in a 12-year-old with bilateral foot pain & flat feet shows bilateral middle facet, nonosseous talocalcaneal coalitions ➡, evidenced by narrowing & abnormal sloping of the articulations as well as irregularity of the apposed surfaces.*

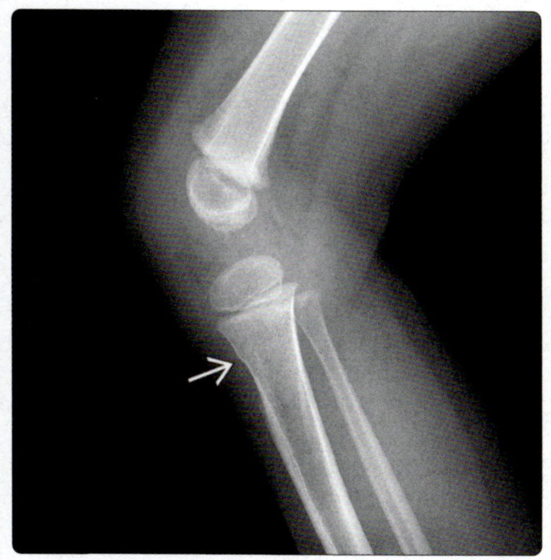

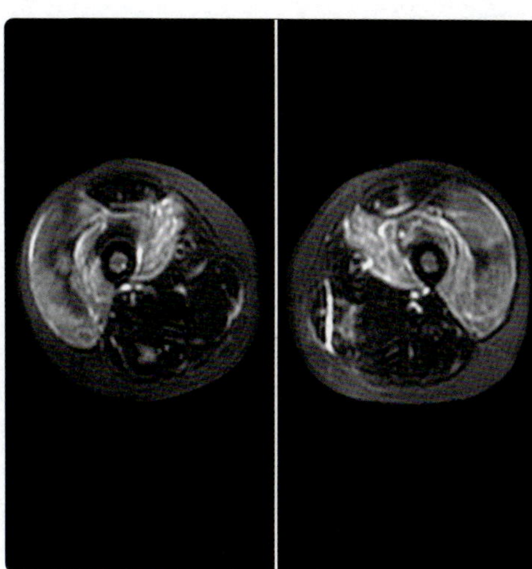

(Left) *Lateral radiograph in a 2.5-year-old after an injury on a trampoline shows a buckle fracture of the anterior tibia ➡.* **(Right)** *Axial T2 FS MR in an 8-year-old with weakness shows relatively symmetric, hyperintense signal within the anterior compartments of the thighs. Five major criteria for juvenile dermatomyositis include: Symmetric proximal muscle weakness, characteristic changes on muscle biopsy, ↑ muscle enzymes in the serum, EMG abnormality of myopathy & denervation, & a characteristic rash.*

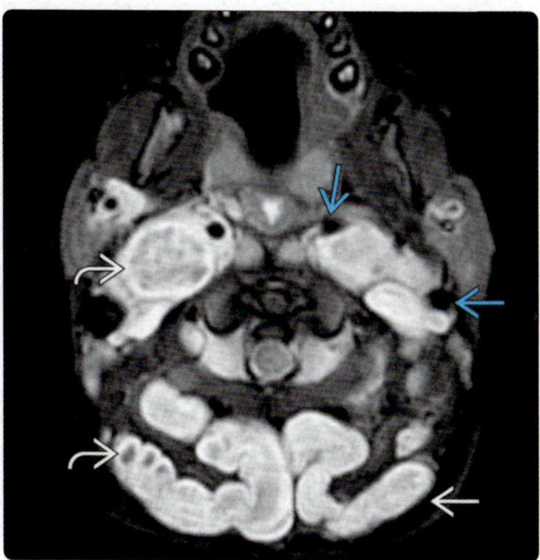

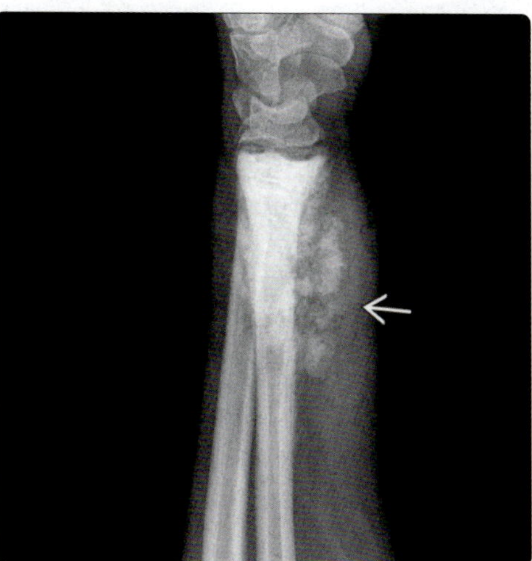

(Left) *Axial STIR MR shows the worm-like ➡ & target ➡ appearances of plexiform neurofibromas throughout the neck. These benign lesions can result in substantial mass effect on adjacent vessels ➡ & other vital structures (such as the airway).* **(Right)** *Lateral radiograph in a 13-year-old with osteosarcoma shows ↑ sclerosis of the distal radius with cloud-like Ca^{2+} (or osteoid) ➡ surrounding the bone.*

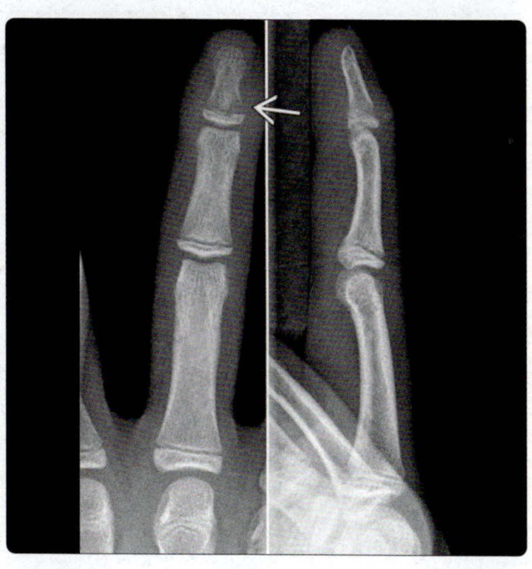

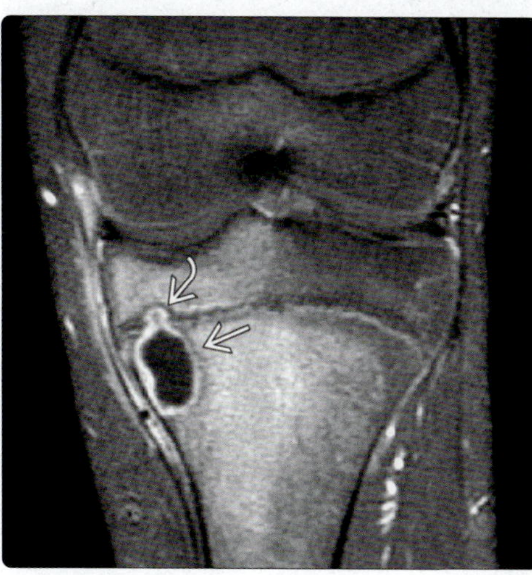

(Left) *Frontal & lateral radiographs of the middle finger in a 14-year-old after a basketball injury 2 weeks prior show ↑ lucency ➡ of the metaphysis of the distal phalanx. This is a "stubbed finger" fracture complicated by osteomyelitis.* **(Right)** *Coronal T1 C+ FS MR in a 14-year-old with proximal tibial pain shows a rim-enhancing intraosseous Brodie abscess ➡ with surrounding marrow edema. The abscess ends across the proximal tibial physis ➡.*

KEY FACTS

TERMINOLOGY

- Primary (1°) growth center = 1° ossification center
- Secondary (2°) growth center = 2° ossification center
- Endochondral ossification: Bone formation on preexisting cartilage model at 1° & 2° growth centers
- 1° growth centers: Where majority of ossification occurs
    - Predominately at long bone physes in childhood
- 2° growth centers: Ossification centers that do not significantly contribute to longitudinal growth
    - Surrounded by growth plate & unossified cartilage
    - Found at articulations of long bones (epiphyses) & epiphyseal equivalents (e.g., apophyses)

IMAGING

- Radiographs: Multiple &/or irregular growth centers are normal at some locations but can mimic pathology
    - Upper extremity: Trochlea, pisiform
    - Lower extremity: Femoral condyles, tibial tubercle, medial malleolus, calcaneal apophysis
- MR: Normal ossification centers do not show abnormal edema/fluid signal

TOP DIFFERENTIAL DIAGNOSES

- Osteochondroses
- Osteochondritis dissecans
- Osteomyelitis
- Osteonecrosis

CLINICAL ISSUES

- 1° & 2° growth centers are normally asymptomatic
- Pathology can occur at growth centers (e.g., acute/chronic trauma, infection, & osteonecrosis)

DIAGNOSTIC CHECKLIST

- Familiarity with normal sites of irregular or multiple ossification centers prevents mistaking them for pathology
- Comparison with contralateral side or prior studies of similar-aged children can be helpful
- MR is useful in difficult cases

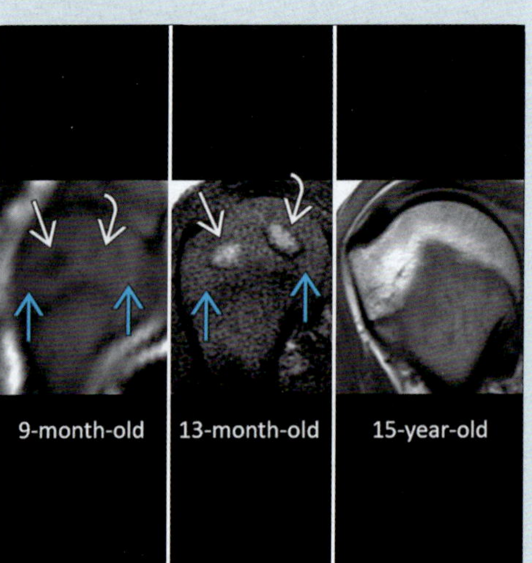

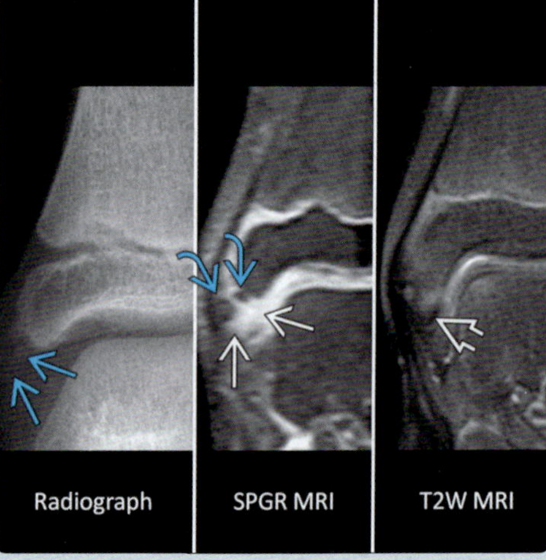

(Left) *Coronal T1 MR shows changes of the humerus at 3 ages. The 2° growth centers of the epiphysis* ➡ *& greater tuberosity* ➡ *are low to intermediate signal (red marrow) at 9 months & ↑ signal (yellow marrow) at 13 months. Epiphyseal cartilage* ➡ *surrounds these centers. The centers are fused in the 15 year old.* **(Right)** *Radiograph shows multiple medial malleolar ossification centers* ➡*. These are low signal* ➡ *on the SPGR MR within bright epiphyseal cartilage* ➡*. T2 MR shows no edema* ➡*.*

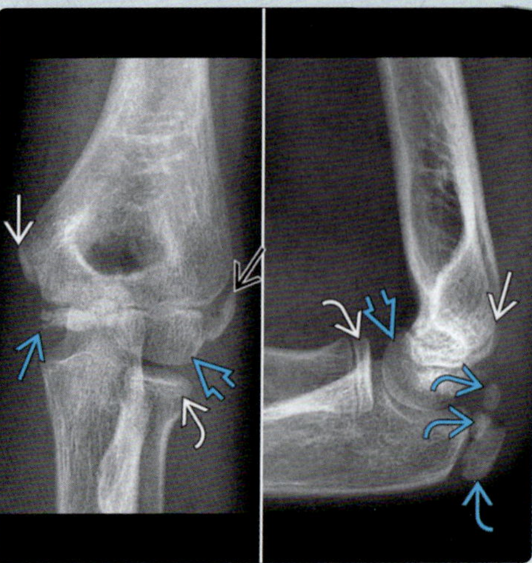

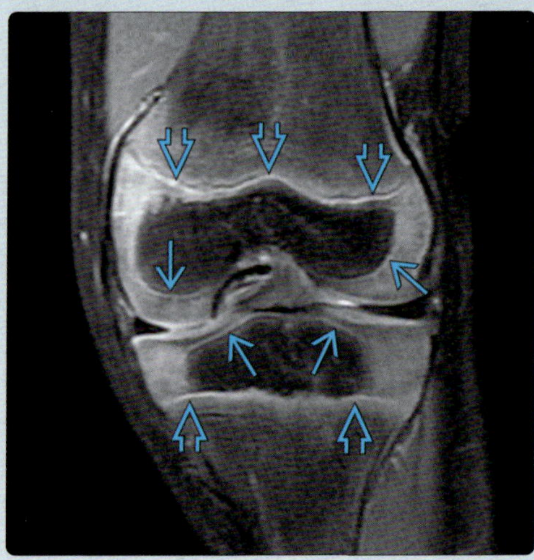

(Left) *Note the elbow 2° growth centers: Capitellum* ➡*, radial head* ➡*, internal (medial) epicondyle* ➡*, trochlea* ➡*, olecranon* ➡*, & external (lateral) epicondyle* ➡*. The trochlear irregular ossification & the multiple olecranon growth centers are normal findings.* **(Right)** *Coronal T2 FS MR in a 3 year old shows hyperintense lines along the metaphyses of the tibia & femur representing the 1° physes* ➡*. The hyperintense lines surrounding the 2° ossification centers represent the 2° physes* ➡*.*

TERMINOLOGY

Synonyms

- Primary (1°) growth (ossification) center
- Secondary (2°) growth (ossification) center

Definitions

- Endochondral ossification: Bone formation of preexisting cartilage model at 1° & 2° growth centers
  - Occurs at limbs, pelvis, vertebral column, & portions of clavicles, scapulae, skull base
- Intramembranous ossification: Bone formation from mesenchymal cells without prior cartilage model
  - Occurs at cranial vault, facial bones, & portions of clavicles, scapulae
- 1° growth centers: Provide majority of ossification
  - Form in central diaphyses of tubular bones in utero
    - Ossification proceeds outward (proximal & distal)
    - 1° growth plates (physes) form at leading edge(s) of expanding 1° ossification centers
  - Predominately found at tubular bone physes in childhood
  - Account for majority of longitudinal growth
- 2° growth centers: Do not significantly contribute to longitudinal growth
  - Surrounded by 2° growth plate & unossified cartilage
  - Found at articulations of long bones (epiphyses) & epiphyseal equivalents (e.g., apophyses)

IMAGING

General Features

- Location
  - Skull base: 1° growth centers develop ~ 12-17 weeks
  - Vertebrae: 1° growth centers are present at birth, 2° growth centers form in C2-L1 after birth
  - Elbow: Order of appearance of 2° growth centers is remembered by acronym **CRITOE**: **C**apitellum → **r**adial epiphysis → **i**nternal (medial) epicondyle → **t**rochlea → **o**lecranon → **e**xternal (lateral) epicondyle
  - Hand/wrist: Growth centers of carpals & 2° growth centers of phalanges form after birth
  - Pelvis: 2° growth centers form in teens, most fuse in 20s
  - Femur: 2° growth centers form in utero & in childhood
  - Tibia: 2° growth centers form at birth & in childhood
  - Fibula: 2° growth centers form throughout childhood
  - Foot: Growth centers of tarsals form before & after birth, 2° growth centers of phalanges form after birth
- Morphology
  - Multiple &/or irregular growth centers at some locations
  - Upper extremity
    - Trochlea of distal humerus: Irregular ossification
    - Pisiform: Irregular ossification
  - Lower extremity
    - Proximal femoral epiphyses: Mild irregularity < 3 years
    - Femoral condyles: Irregular ossification medially & posteriorly
      - Radiographically difficult to distinguish from osteochondritis dissecans (OCD)
      - Irregular ossification typically occurs in younger patients posteriorly & not in intercondylar region
    - Tibial tubercle: Multiple irregular centers
    - Medial malleolus: Multiple irregular centers
    - Calcaneal apophysis: Multiple irregular centers
    - Apophysis of 5th metatarsal base: Lateral & longitudinally oriented

Radiographic Findings

- Irregular growth centers can mimic pathology
- Unossified cartilage of 2° centers may mimic abnormal fluid on radiographs

MR Findings

- Helpful in difficult cases to distinguish irregular ossification & pathologic processes
- Normal development will show multiple &/or irregular dark ossification centers in normal bright surrounding cartilage without abnormal edema/fluid signal
  - Best for cartilage: PD FS or T2* GRE
  - Best for fluid: T2 FS or STIR

DIFFERENTIAL DIAGNOSIS

Osteochondroses

- Poorly defined group of painful growth disturbances (usually due to repetitive microtrauma &/or avascular necrosis) that occur at epiphyses & apophyses

Osteochondritis Dissecans

- Overuse injury in femoral condyles, talus, & capitellum

Osteomyelitis

- Can involve epiphysis: May be 1° site in infants vs. spread from metaphysis or joint in any child
- Typical signs & symptoms of infection

Osteonecrosis

- May see in sickle cell & steroid use or 1° idiopathic hip disease

CLINICAL ISSUES

Presentation

- Most common signs/symptoms
  - 1° & 2° growth centers are normal part of endochondral ossification & are asymptomatic
  - Growth center pathology can occur (e.g., acute/chronic trauma, infection, osteochondroses, & osteonecrosis)

DIAGNOSTIC CHECKLIST

Image Interpretation Pearls

- Familiarity with common sites of normal variant irregular ossification prevents mistaking multiple/irregular growth centers with pathology
- Comparison with contralateral side (in limited circumstances), prior studies of similar-aged children, & reference texts can be helpful
- MR may be useful in difficult cases

SELECTED REFERENCES

1. Walter WR et al: Pitfalls in MRI of the developing pediatric ankle. Radiographics. 41(1):210-23, 2021
2. Nguyen JC et al: Imaging of pediatric growth plate disturbances. Radiographics. 37(6):1791-812, 2017

Red to Yellow Marrow Conversion

KEY FACTS

IMAGING

- At birth, red marrow is present throughout entire skeleton
- Conversion of hematopoietic red to fatty yellow marrow begins shortly after birth & follows predictable pattern
  - Appendicular before axial skeleton
  - Distal before proximal extremities (e.g., phalanges of fingers begin conversion before humeri)
  - Within individual long bones
    - Epiphyses convert 1st: Within 6 months of appearance, epiphyseal ossification center should contain almost entirely yellow marrow
    - Central diaphyses next, spreading toward metaphyses
    - Metaphyseal red marrow often persists in adults
      - Typically flame-shaped or poorly defined
  - Conversion of red to yellow marrow is typically symmetric (i.e., similar appearance of R vs. L extremities)
- By 12-24 months, most appendicular marrow is approaching MR signal intensity of subcutaneous fat on spin-echo T1 (i.e., concordance of signal intensities)
  - Diffuse or multifocal discordance after this age (especially on spin-echo T1) implies pathology
- Variability exists among individuals as to exact timeframe
- Some degree of red marrow often persists in spine & pelvis
- On spin-echo T1 MR (best marrow sequence): Red marrow shows low to intermediate signal intensity
  - Typically iso- or slightly hyperintense as compared to muscle & intervertebral discs
- In- & opposed-phase T1 MR
  - Normal red marrow drops signal intensity on opposed-phase images compared to in-phase images
    - Due to water & fat protons in same voxel
  - Infiltrating processes (such as leukemia & metastases) generally do not drop signal on opposed-phase images
- Reconversion of yellow to red marrow (from variety of causes) occurs in reverse order from initial conversion

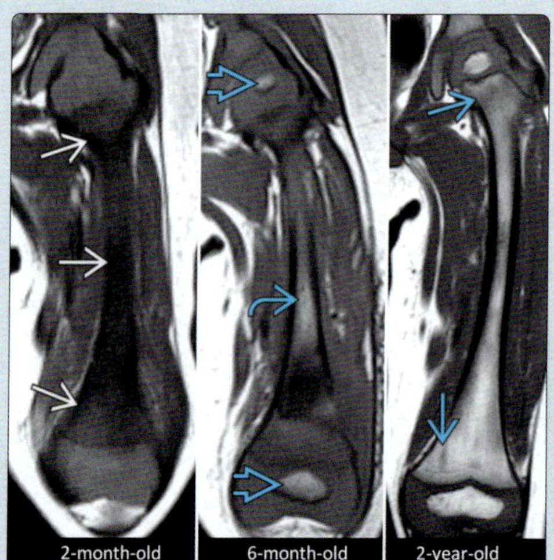

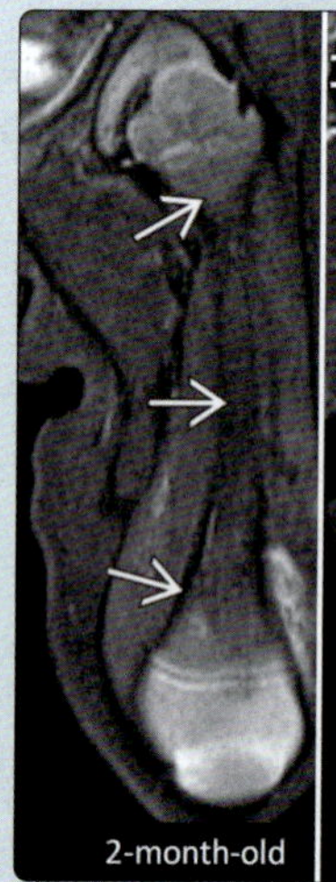

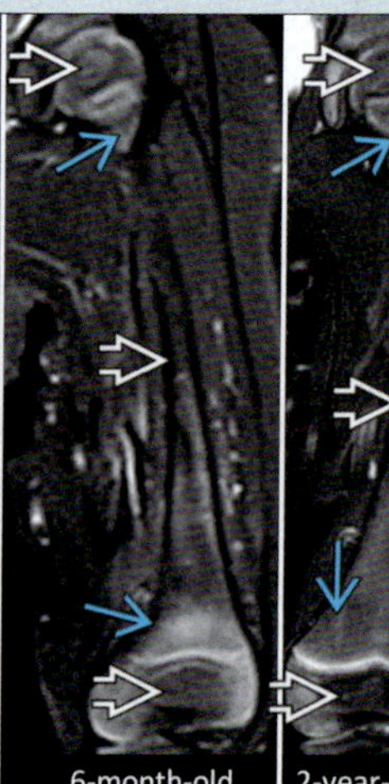

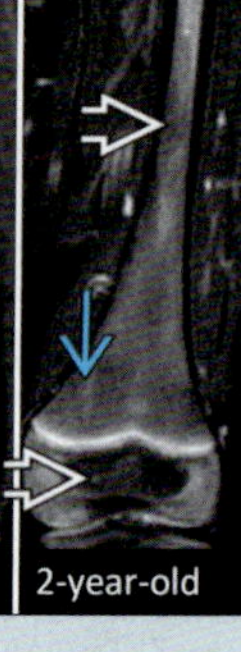

(Left) *Coronal T1 MR shows femurs in normal children of various ages. Initially, low signal intensity red marrow is seen diffusely. In infancy, yellow marrow appears 1st in the epiphyses & central diaphysis, progressing to the metaphyses, but metaphyseal foci of red marrow persist.* **(Right)** *Corresponding coronal STIR MRs show homogeneous low signal intensity early. Later, epiphyseal & diaphyseal yellow marrow are of lower signal intensity than metaphyseal red marrow.*

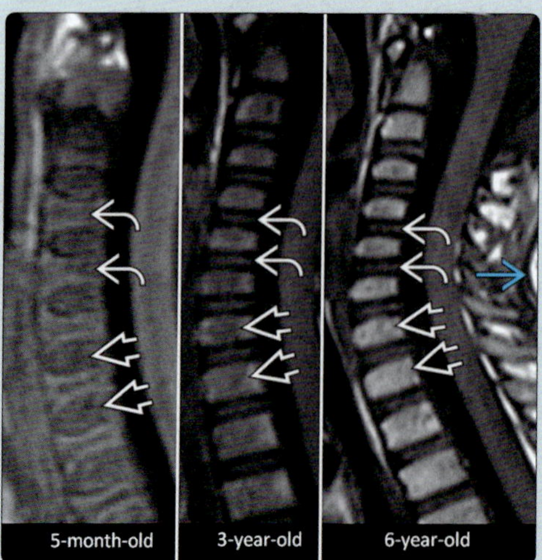

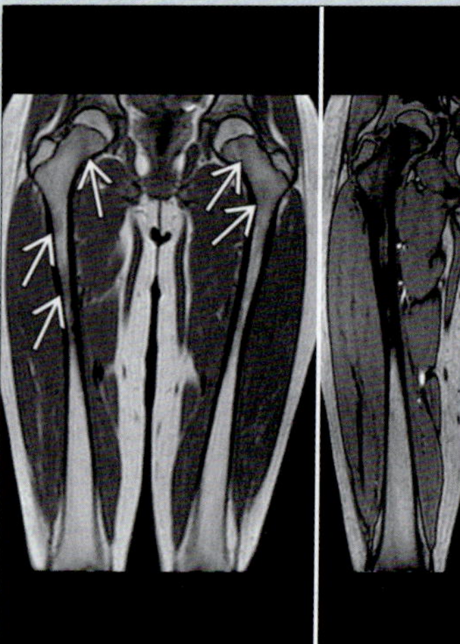

(Left) *Sagittal T1 MRs show the cervical spine at various ages. The signal intensity of vertebral body marrow, as compared to the intervertebral discs, is initially hypointense, gradually becoming iso- & hyperintense. In the 6 year old, the marrow signal is slightly < subcutaneous fat.* **(Right)** *Coronal T1 GRE MRs in a 9-year-old with residual red marrow show ill-defined foci of intermediate signal in the proximal femurs on the in-phase (L) image, which drop signal on the opposed-phase (R) image.*

TERMINOLOGY

Synonyms

- Red (hematopoietic) marrow, yellow (fatty) marrow

Definitions

- At birth, red marrow is present throughout entire skeleton
- Conversion to yellow marrow begins shortly after birth
- Reconversion from yellow to red marrow occurs secondary to variety of causes & must be distinguished from pathologic marrow infiltration

IMAGING

General Features

- Best diagnostic clue
  - In predictable pattern, appendicular skeleton converts from red to yellow marrow before axial skeleton
  - Conversion of red to yellow marrow is typically symmetric (i.e., R vs. L)
  - By 12-24 months, most appendicular marrow is generally approaching signal intensity of subcutaneous fat on T1-weighted spin-echo MR pulse sequences
    - On FS T2 or STIR MR, epiphyseal yellow marrow has greatest concordance with subcutaneous fat
  - Regions of red marrow often persist in spine, pelvis, & long bone metaphyses of normal adults
- Location
  - Appendicular skeleton conversion
    - Begins in bones of distal extremities (i.e., phalanges of fingers & toes) & progresses proximally
    - Within individual long bones
      - Epiphyses convert 1st: Within 6 months of appearance, epiphyseal ossification center should contain almost entirely yellow marrow
      - Central diaphyseal conversion occurs next, spreading proximally & distally toward metaphyses
      - Residual red marrow often persists in adult metaphyses, particularly proximal femurs & humeri
  - Spine: Marrow signal intensity of vertebral bodies changes on spin-echo T1-weighted MR by approximate ages
    - 0-1 year: Hypointense to intervertebral disc
    - 1-5 years: Iso- to mildly hyperintense to disc
    - > 5 years: Hyperintense to disc, hypointense to subcutaneous fat
  - Reconversion of yellow to red marrow generally occurs in reverse order as compared to initial conversion
    - Axial → appendicular skeleton
    - Proximal → distal extremities
    - Long bone metaphyses → diaphyses → epiphyses

MR Findings

- T1 MR (spin-echo)
  - Yellow marrow shows ↑ signal intensity
  - Red marrow shows ↓ to intermediate signal intensity
    - Mildly ↑ compared to muscle & intervertebral discs
    - Neonatal red marrow may be isointense or ↓ in signal intensity compared to muscle & discs
- T1 in-phase (IP) & opposed-phase (OP)
  - Red marrow drops signal on OP images due to water & fat protons in same voxel
  - Helps distinguish red marrow from infiltrating processes (such as leukemia & metastases), which generally do not drop signal on OP
  - Red marrow typically shows
    - ≥ 20% drop in signal on OP at 1.5T
    - ≥ 25% drop in signal on OP at 3T
- T2 FS & STIR
  - Yellow marrow shows ↓ signal intensity, most pronounced in epiphyses
  - Red marrow generally shows signal intensity similar to or mildly ↑ compared to skeletal muscle

DIFFERENTIAL DIAGNOSIS

Residual Red Marrow or Red Marrow Reconversion

- Iso- to mildly hyperintense on T1 MR compared to skeletal muscle & intervertebral discs
- Drops signal on OP MRs
- In long bones, normal residual red marrow is often flame-shaped in metaphyses

Systemic Marrow Infiltrating Processes

- Primarily leukemia or metastases
- Diffuse confluent or multifocal well-defined marrow lesions ± cortical destruction, periosteal reaction
- Iso- to hypointense to skeletal muscle & intervertebral discs on T1; usually hyperintense on T2 FS/STIR MR
- Typically drops < 20% of signal at 1.5T (< 25% at 3T) on OP

Marrow Deposition Diseases

- Gaucher disease: Most common lysosomal storage disease
  - Distribution & signal intensity can be similar to red marrow reconversion
  - Other imaging findings are typically present: Endosteal scalloping, Erlenmeyer flask deformities (undertubulation), bone infarcts, hepatosplenomegaly
- Iron deposition disease: ↓ signal intensity on all sequences

PATHOLOGY

General Features

- Differences in fat & water content account for imaging appearances of red & yellow marrow
- Red marrow ~ 40% adipocytes, 60% hematopoietic cells
- Yellow marrow ~ 95% adipocytes

CLINICAL ISSUES

Presentation

- Most common signs/symptoms
  - Conversion of red to yellow marrow is asymptomatic normal physiologic process
  - Physiologic stresses, disease processes, & medications may cause reconversion to red marrow

SELECTED REFERENCES

1. Chaturvedi A: Pediatric skeletal diffusion-weighted magnetic resonance imaging: part 1 - technical considerations and optimization strategies. Pediatr Radiol. 51(9):1562-74, 2021
2. van Vucht N et al: The Dixon technique for MRI of the bone marrow. Skeletal Radiol. 48(12):1861-74, 2019
3. Chan BY et al: MR Imaging of pediatric bone marrow. Radiographics. 36(6):1911-30, 2016

KEY FACTS

IMAGING

- Growing skeleton demonstrates range of normal age-related radiographic appearances due to
  - Abundant radiolucent growth cartilages
  - Gradual endochondral ossification of such cartilages
- Normal developmental variants have
  - Typical orientation, site, & patient age
  - No overlying swelling or point tenderness
    - May be clouded by isolated soft tissue injury
- MR is useful when source of symptoms is unclear (i.e., is fragmented growth center incidental normal variant or pathologic due to fracture, infarction, or infection)
  - Marrow edema on T2 FS/STIR MR favors pathology
  - ± soft tissue edema &/or joint effusion

TOP DIFFERENTIAL DIAGNOSES

- Physeal fractures
- Incomplete fractures
- Remote trauma
- Child abuse
- Ligamentous disruption
- Avascular necrosis

CLINICAL ISSUES

- Usually asymptomatic; come to attention incidentally by radiographs (often with history of regional trauma)

DIAGNOSTIC CHECKLIST

- If unclear whether or not bony appearance is abnormal vs. incidental normal developmental variant in regionally symptomatic child
  - Review prior radiographs
  - Discuss with referring clinician regarding exact site of symptoms (including point tenderness)
  - Consider
    - Contralateral radiographs of asymptomatic side
    - Splinting with follow-up radiographs in 10-14 days to assess for healing changes

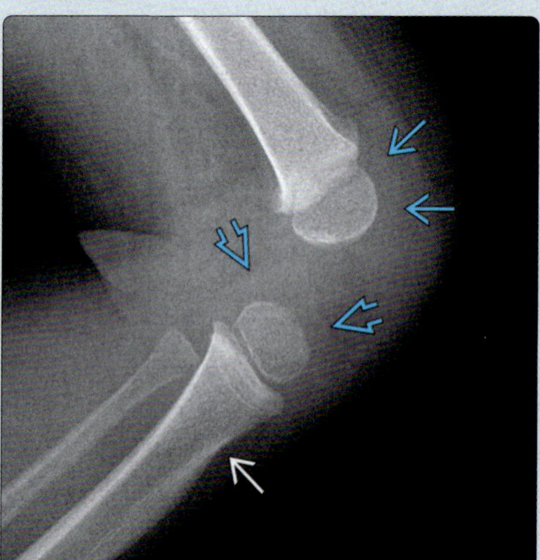

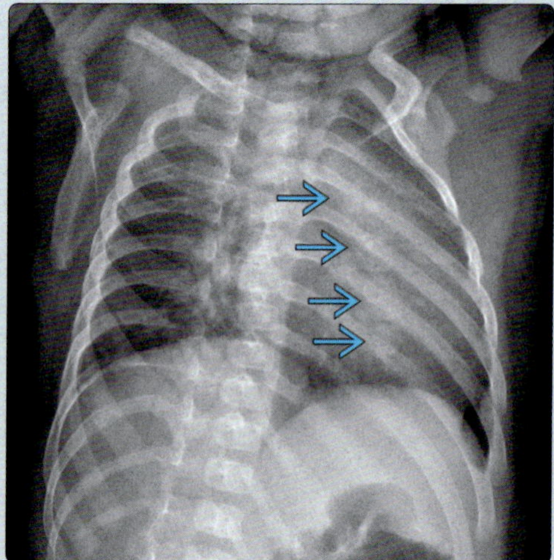

(Left) *Lateral knee radiograph in a 2-year-old shows a normal anterior tibial metadiaphyseal concavity ➡ at the site of the unossified tibial tubercle. Transversely oriented fractures may be seen at this level but show focal buckling or cortical interruption. Also note the unossified cartilages of the femoral ➡ & tibial ➡ epiphyses.* **(Right)** *Oblique rib radiograph from a skeletal survey in a 3-month-old shows multiple sternal ossification centers ➡ overlapping the left posterior ribs, which can mimic the bulbous callous of healing rib fractures.*

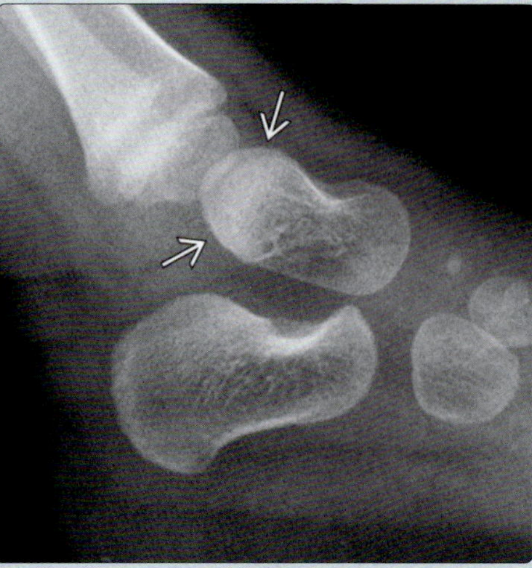

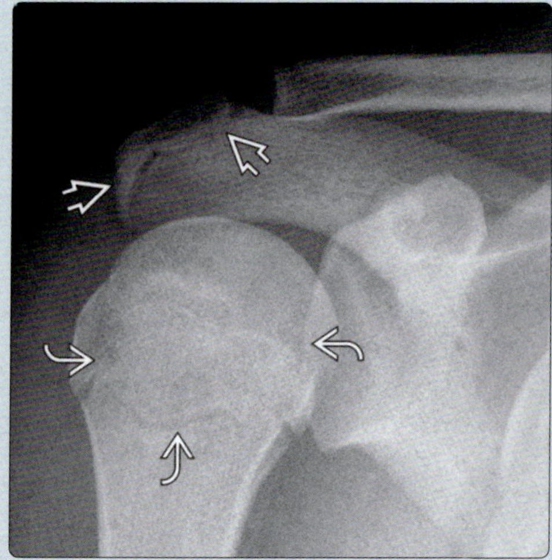

(Left) *Lateral radiograph in a 2-year-old girl shows poorly defined sclerosis in the posterior talus ➡, a commonly seen normal finding in this age. Linear sclerosis in the posterior calcaneus or cuboid (not present here) would suggest a fracture in this age group.* **(Right)** *AP internal rotation radiograph of the right shoulder in a 15-year-old boy shows an unfused acromion ossification center ➡. The sloped proximal humeral physis is viewed at different heights ➡ anteriorly & posteriorly (a common fracture mimic).*

TERMINOLOGY

Definitions

- Skeletally immature patients have numerous radiolucent growth centers composed of cartilage
  - Primary physis: Site of majority of longitudinal growth; lies between epiphysis & metaphysis
  - Secondary physis: Surrounds secondary ossification center (SOC) in epiphysis or equivalent bone
    - Interface where cartilaginous precursor is transformed into bone from central to peripheral
    - Process is uniform in some centers (capitellum, femoral head), nonuniform in others (fragmented trochlea, irregular medial femoral condyle)
  - Apophysis: Nonarticular SOC with muscle/tendon attachment (ischial & tibial tuberosities)
  - Zone of provisional calcification (ZPC): Thin, radiodense line at interface of physeal growth cartilage & newly mineralized bone
- Accessory ossification centers: Separate small rounded ossicles vs. SOCs in same unossified cartilage as adjacent epiphysis (or equivalent bone)
- Pseudoepiphysis: False appearance of growth centers at distal 1st & proximal 2nd-5th metatarsals & metacarpals
- Physiologic periosteal reaction (PPR): Smooth, solid, new bone being symmetrically & rapidly laid down along entire lengths of long bone diaphyses in infants

IMAGING

General Features

- Best diagnostic clue
  - No overlying swelling or point tenderness
    - May be clouded by isolated soft tissue injury
  - Orientation, site, & patient age are typical for specific variant
- Morphology
  - SOCs are widely spaced at carpals & tarsals before maturity (due to remaining unossified cartilage)
  - Some long bones (radius, ulna) have normal mild degrees of generalized curvature

Radiographic Findings

- Growth cartilages are normally lucent
- Bony metaphyseal & epiphyseal margins are often undulating; may be irregular in some instances
- Lack of interrupted cortex or ZPC
- No soft tissue edema (unless isolated soft tissue injury)
- PPR: Smooth, solid periosteal reaction along shafts of certain long bones (humeri, femurs, tibias)
  - Typical age: 1-6 months
  - Most commonly symmetric

MR Findings

- Useful when source of symptoms is unclear (i.e., is fragmented growth center incidental normal variant or pathologic, such as fractured, infarcted, or infected)
- Marrow edema on T2 FS/STIR MR favors pathology
  - ± soft tissue edema, joint effusion

DIFFERENTIAL DIAGNOSIS

Physeal Fractures

- Soft tissue edema ± physeal widening & displaced metaphyseal or epiphyseal fragment

Incomplete Fractures

- Buckle fractures: Abnormal focal cortical bump or angulation
- Plastic/bowing deformities: ↑ curvature

Remote Trauma

- Sclerotic margins; soft tissue edema is absent
- Differentiation from normal variant is not always possible

Child Abuse

- Subtle metaphyseal corner fracture in infant may lead to extensive periosteal reaction
- Typically unilateral/asymmetric

Ligamentous Disruption

- ↑ separation of bones with overlying soft tissue edema
- Stress views can be helpful

Avascular Necrosis

- Sclerosis, fragmentation, &/or collapse of SOC
- In otherwise healthy child, certain sites & ages are typical (such as Legg-Calvé-Perthes at hip)

CLINICAL ISSUES

Presentation

- Normal variants are usually asymptomatic; come to attention incidentally on imaging (often with history of regional trauma)

DIAGNOSTIC CHECKLIST

Image Interpretation Pearls

- If unclear whether or not bony appearance is abnormal vs. incidental normal developmental variant in regionally symptomatic child, then
  - Review prior radiographs
  - Discuss with referring clinician regarding exact site of symptoms (including point tenderness)
- Consider
  - Contralateral radiographs of asymptomatic side
  - Splinting + follow-up radiographs in 10-14 days to assess for healing changes

SELECTED REFERENCES

1. Kan JH et al: Embryology, anatomy, and normal findings. In: Caffey's Pediatric Diagnostic Imaging, 13th ed. Philadelphia: Elsevier Saunders. 1219-36, 2019
2. Lerisson H et al: Radiographic/MR imaging correlation of the pediatric knee growth. Magn Reson Imaging Clin N Am. 27(4):737-51, 2019
3. Woo TD et al: Radiographic morphology of normal ring apophyses in the immature cervical spine. Skeletal Radiol. 47(9):1221-8, 2018
4. Berko NS et al: Imaging appearances of musculoskeletal developmental variants in the pediatric population. Curr Probl Diagn Radiol. 44(1):88-104, 2015
5. Idriz S et al: CT of normal developmental and variant anatomy of the pediatric skull: distinguishing trauma from normality. Radiographics. 35(5):1585-601, 2015

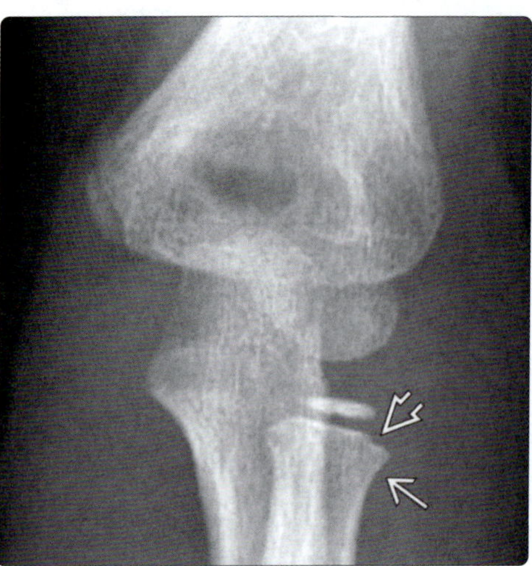

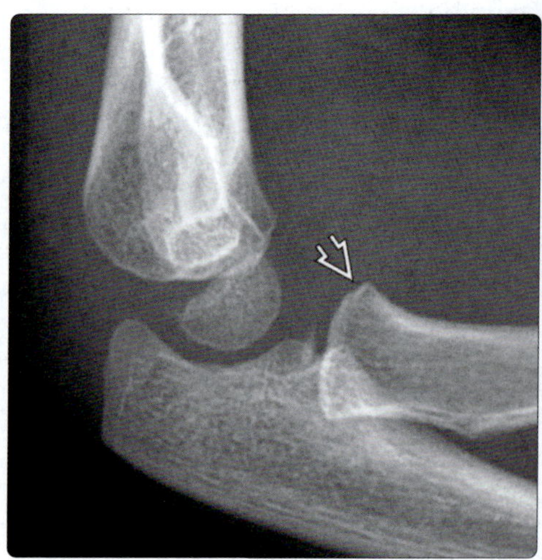

(Left) *AP radiograph of a 7-year-old patient shows a normal location for step-off at the lateral physeal margin of the proximal radial metaphysis ➲. Note the smooth radial metaphyseal neck laterally ➔ (which is a common site for Salter-Harris II injuries).* **(Right)** *Lateral elbow radiograph in a 4-year-old girl shows the commonly seen normal step-off at the anterior & lateral physeal margin of the proximal radial metaphysis ➲.*

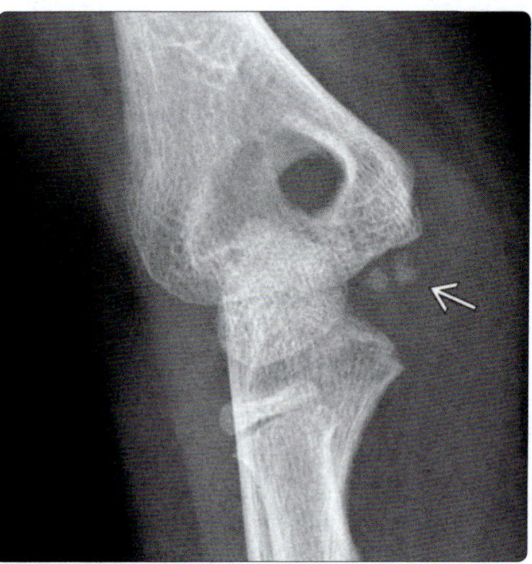

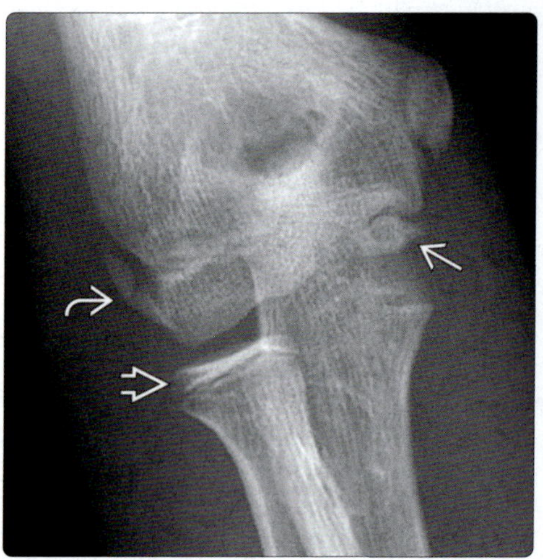

(Left) *Oblique radiograph of the elbow in an 8-year-old girl shows fragmentation of the trochlear ossification center ➔, a normal finding.* **(Right)** *AP radiograph in a 12-year-old patient shows the normal ossification centers about the elbow. The lateral or external epicondyle ➔ may be fragmented, the radial head ➲ may be sclerotic, & the trochlea ➔ may be irregular, sclerotic, &/or fragmented.*

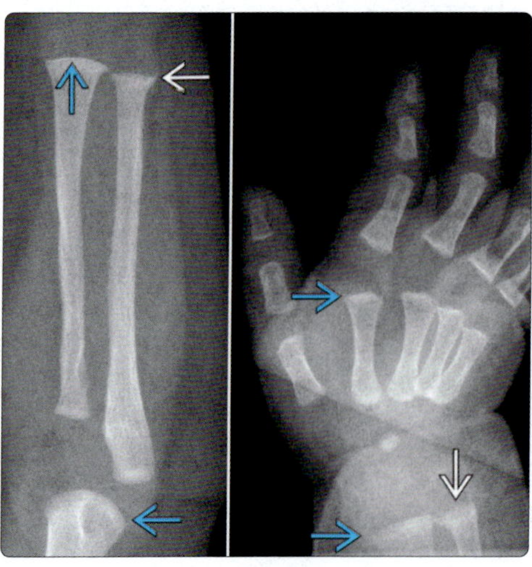

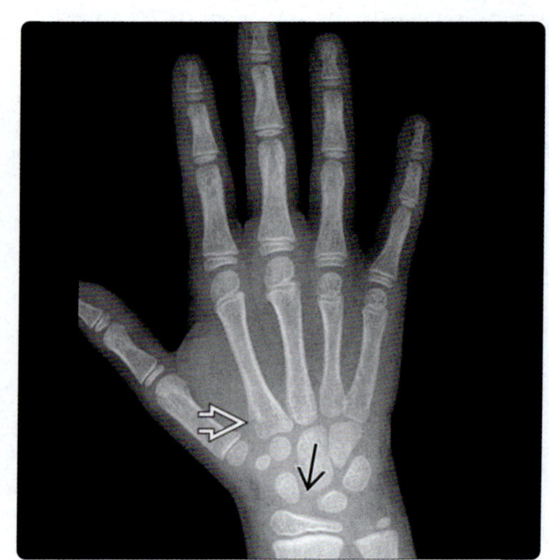

(Left) *AP left forearm & oblique right hand radiographs in a 3-month-old with a femur fracture show a normal variant appearance of the distal ulnar metaphyses ➔ mimicking "fraying & cupping." As the remaining growth centers show normal zones of provisional calcification ➔, underlying rickets is excluded.* **(Right)** *PA radiograph of a 7-year-old girl shows false widening of the scapholunate interval ➔ due to incomplete carpal ossification in this age. Note the pseudoepiphysis ➲ at the 2nd metacarpal.*

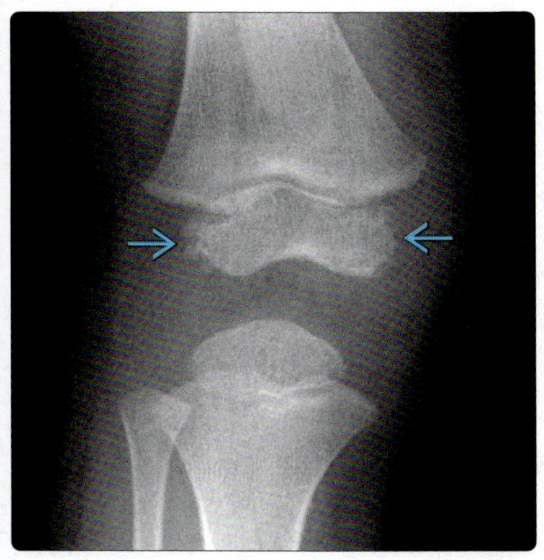

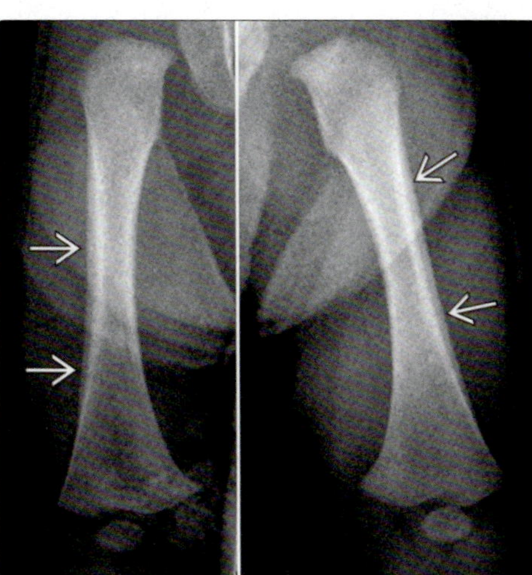

(Left) *AP radiograph in a 3-year-old with pain after a fall shows irregular peripheral margins ⇨ to the distal femoral secondary ossification center, a common normal variant in young children.* **(Right)** *AP femur radiographs in a 1-month-old patient show thin, smooth, solid periosteal reaction along the lateral aspects of the femoral diaphyses bilaterally ➡, typical of physiologic periosteal reaction.*

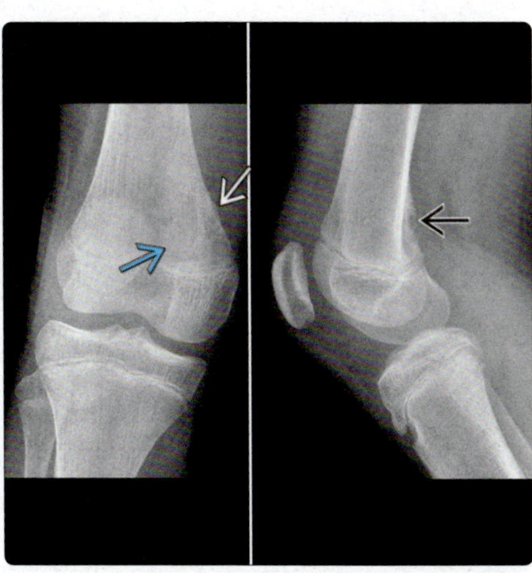

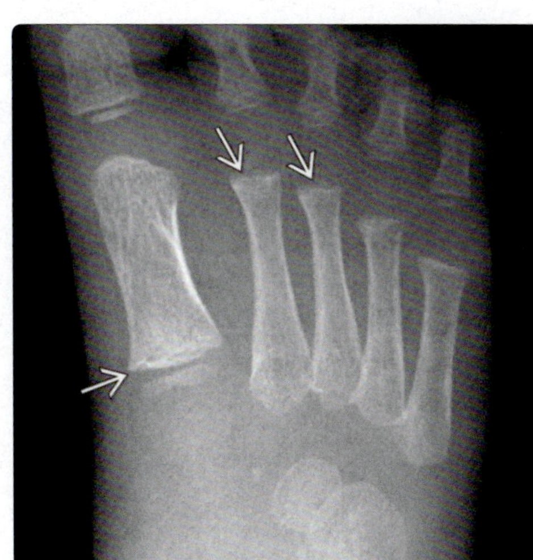

(Left) *AP (left) & lateral (right) radiographs show a typical location & configuration of avulsive irregularity of the posteromedial distal femur. A well-defined sclerotic margin ⇨ is often present with mild medial ➡ & posterior ⇨ irregularity being less frequent. Any lesion at this location appearing more aggressive than this should get further work-up.* **(Right)** *AP foot radiograph in a 2-year-old boy shows normal metaphyseal undulation ➡ at the base of the 1st metatarsal as well as the distal 2nd & 3rd metatarsals.*

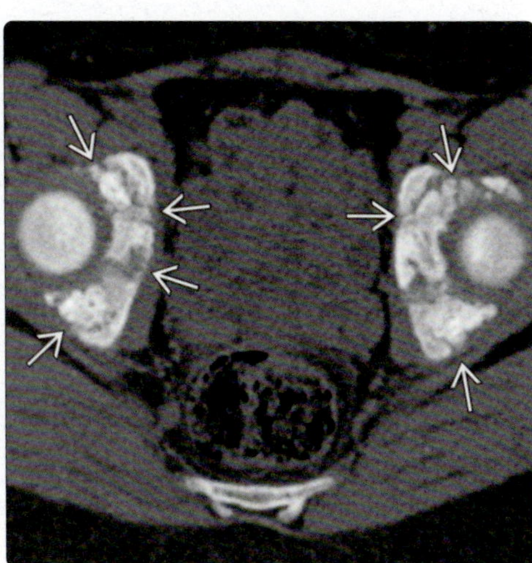

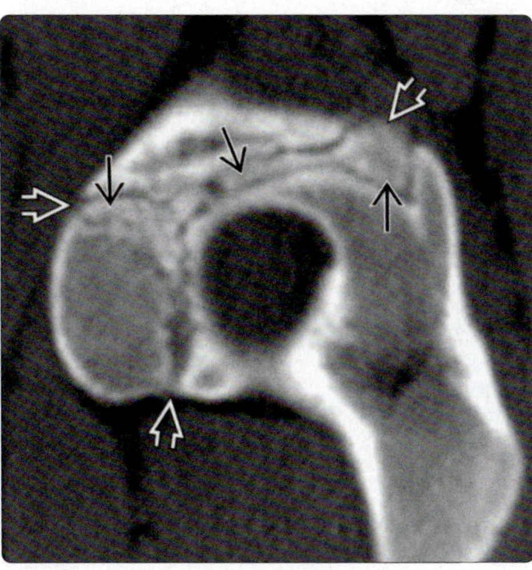

(Left) *Axial NECT in a 7-year-old patient shows multiple ossification centers within the triradiate cartilages of the medial acetabula bilaterally ➡.* **(Right)** *Sagittal NECT of the same patient more clearly displays the arrangement of the accessory ossification centers ⇨ within the triradiate cartilage ➡ of the medial acetabular wall.*

(Left) *Lateral radiograph in a 6-year-old patient with knee pain shows an irregular lucency in the posterior lateral femoral condyle ➙.* **(Right)** *Tunnel view of the same knee shows the irregularity/fragmentation ➙ of the posterior non-weight-bearing aspect of the lateral femoral condyle, a common location for developmental irregular ossification. This is in contrast to osteochondritis dissecans (OCD), which more classically affects the lateral & central aspects of the medial femoral condyle.*

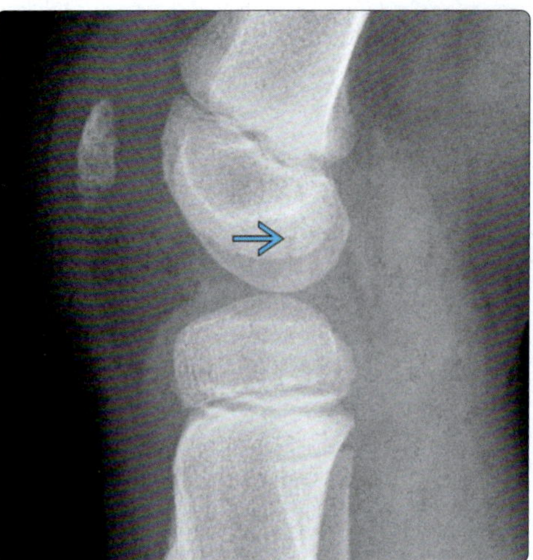

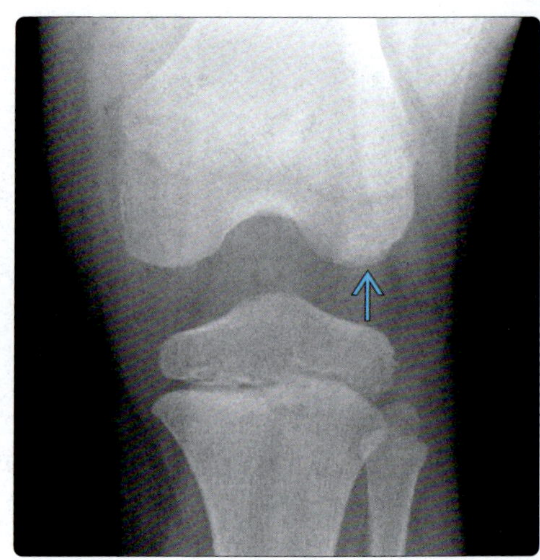

(Left) *Sagittal T2 FS MR in the same patient shows minimal ossific fragmentation posteriorly ➙ without adjacent marrow edema, cystic change, cartilage fissuring, or secondary growth plate interruption to suggest a true OCD lesion. Also note the normal dark signal of the weight-bearing unossified femoral condyle ➡ due to water displacement in the cartilage.* **(Right)** *Sagittal PD FS MR in the same patient shows the ossific "puzzle piece" fragmentation of the posterior lateral femoral condyle ➙, a normal variant.*

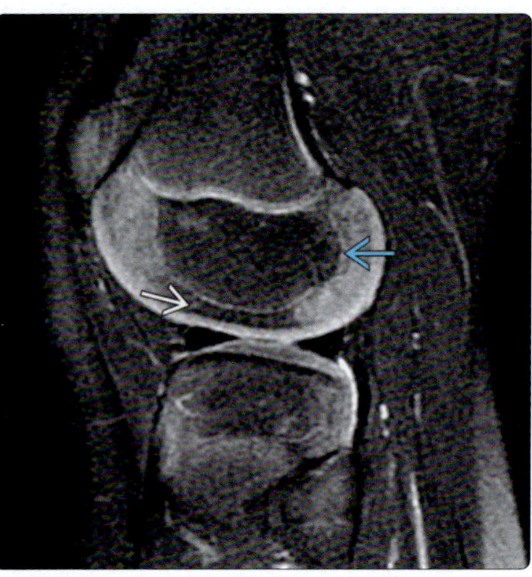

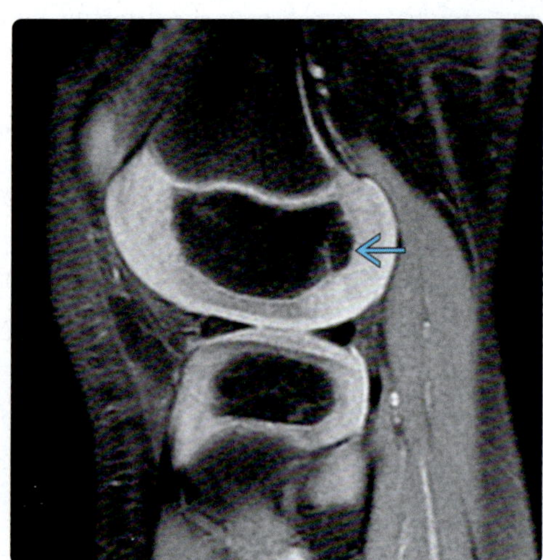

(Left) *AP ankle radiograph in a 9-year-old boy shows an ovoid ossification center with sclerotic margins at the medial malleolus ➡. This is a very common location for accessory ossification centers (which may be fragmented).* **(Right)** *Lateral radiograph of the calcaneus in a 10-year-old patient shows a normal fragmented & sclerotic appearance of the calcaneal apophysis ➡. Patients may have symptoms related to recurrent traction here (Sever disease), but this entity is not diagnosed by bony radiographic changes.*

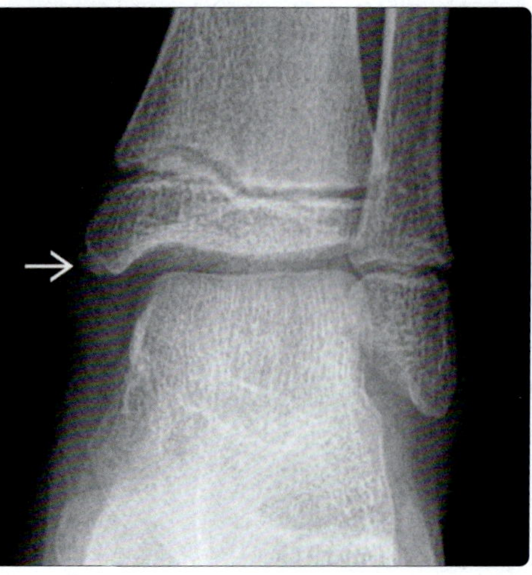

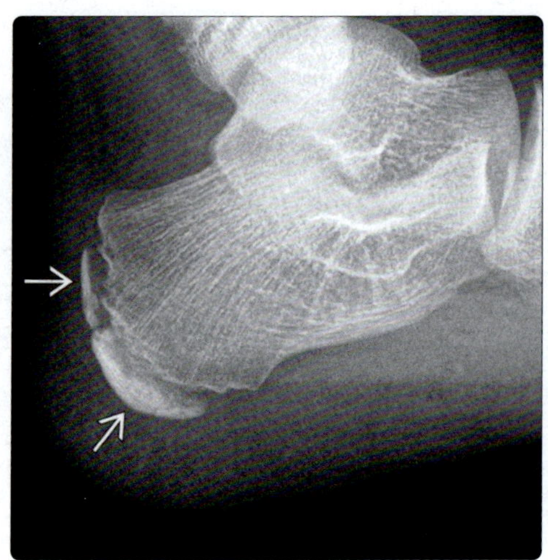

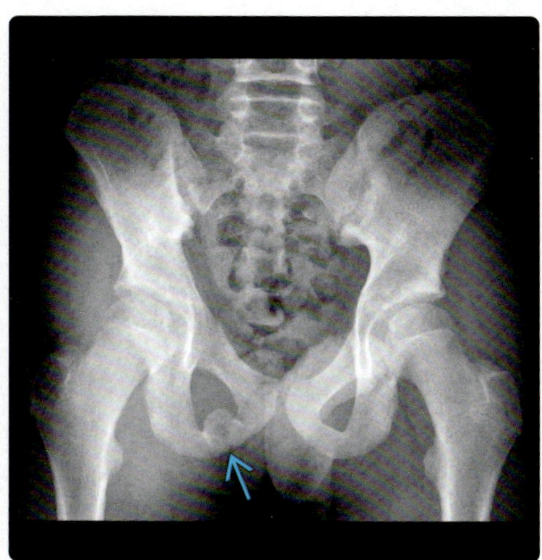

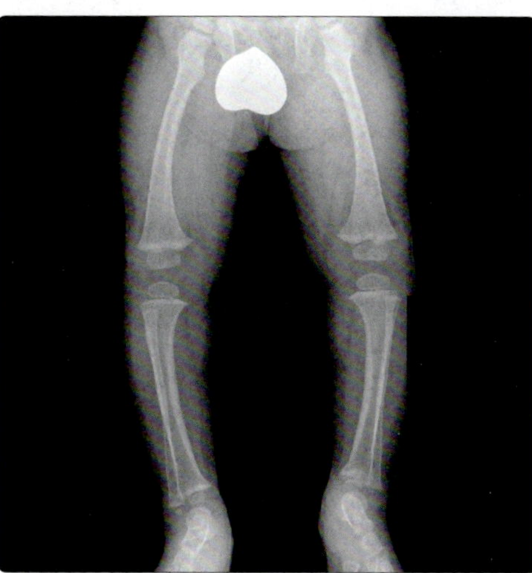

(Left) *AP radiograph of the pelvis in a 14-year-old boy with a coccygeal injury shows a mixed lucent & sclerotic expansile lesion at the right ischiopubic synchondrosis ➡. This is a recognized & typically asymptomatic normal variant occurring in some patients around puberty.* **(Right)** *AP radiograph of the lower extremities in a child with genu varum shows physiologic bowing of the tibias & femurs. Note that there is only mild medial downsloping of the proximal tibial metaphyses without fragmentation (in contrast to Blount disease).*

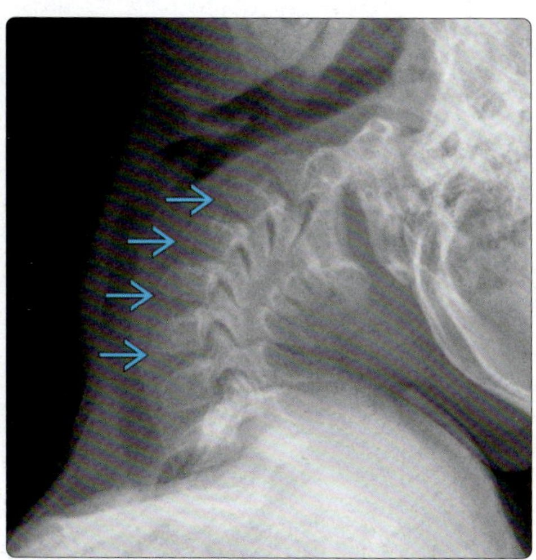

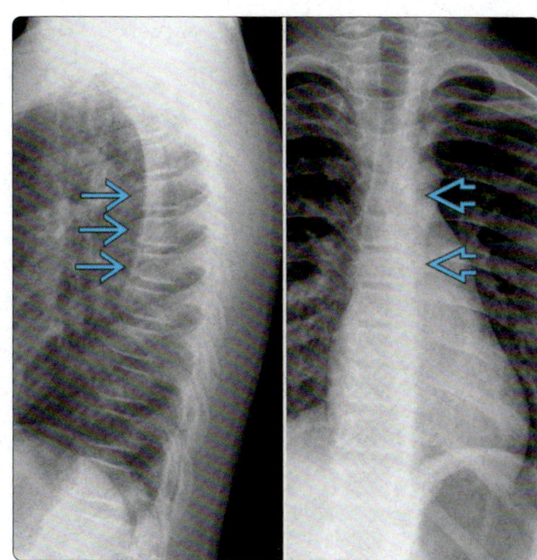

(Left) *Lateral cervical spine extension radiograph in a 6-year-old without trauma shows normal mild anterior wedging of vertebral bodies due to incomplete ossification. Note the small ring apophyses ➡.* **(Right)** *Chest radiographs in a 10-year-old with chest pain but no trauma show very mild gradual anterior wedging of several midthoracic vertebral bodies ➡ without focal concavity. The vertebral body heights are maintained from left to right ➡ on the AP view. This normal wedging can be difficult to separate from traumatic compression.*

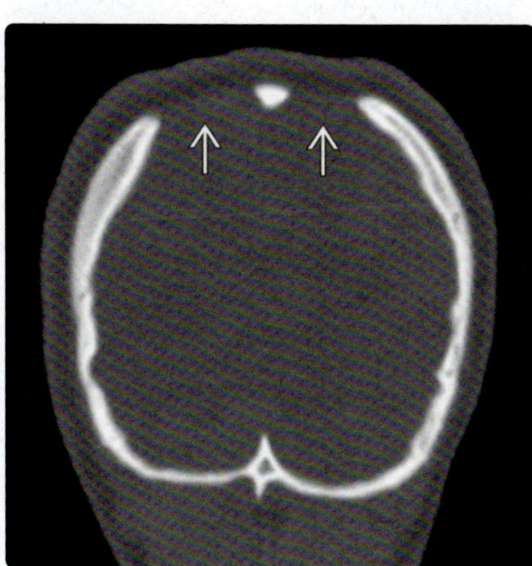

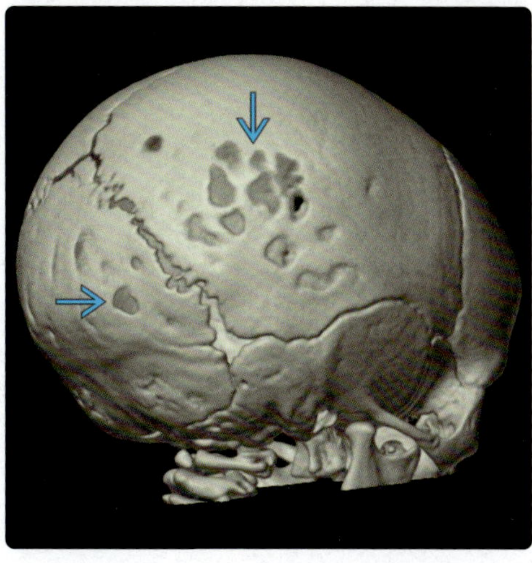

(Left) *Coronal NECT in an 11-year-old with a history of headaches shows a typical location & symmetric morphology of giant parietal foramina ➡, an appearance which was stable from a CT scan 2 years prior. Note the smoothly tapered bony margins without permeation or periosteal reaction.* **(Right)** *3D NECT shows apparent lytic skull lesions at sites of normal bone thinning ➡ (confirmed to be intact on source images) in the parietal & occipital bones, due to normal convolutional markings in an infant.*

Distal Femoral Avulsive Irregularity

KEY FACTS

TERMINOLOGY

- Common pediatric finding at posterior, medial distal femoral metaphysis: Cortical defect deep to medial gastrocnemius or adductor magnus attachments
  - Likely due to chronic avulsive forces
  - Typically incidental lesion; no treatment needed
- Synonyms
  - Avulsive cortical irregularity or tug lesion
  - Cortical desmoid: Misnomer as biology & histology differ from true desmoid tumors (which are locally aggressive benign neoplasms)

IMAGING

- Lucent focus of cortical interruption/irregularity at posterior, medial distal femoral metaphysis
- Deep margin is commonly concave ± sclerosis
- May have adjacent cortical thickening
- Frontal view may show well-defined round/ovoid lucent focus with sclerotic rim or mild medial cortical irregularity
- Bilateral: 25-100%

TOP DIFFERENTIAL DIAGNOSES

- Osteosarcoma
- Osteomyelitis
- Langerhans cell histiocytosis
- Fibroxanthoma
- Periosteal/juxtacortical chondroma
- Osteoid osteoma
- Metastases

PATHOLOGY

- Benign, self-limited reactive process (not neoplasm)
- Needle biopsy may lead to inappropriate treatment
  - "Do not touch" lesion

DIAGNOSTIC CHECKLIST

- Location of this entity is very typical
- More aggressive entities also occur here
  - Get MR or contralateral radiographs if unclear

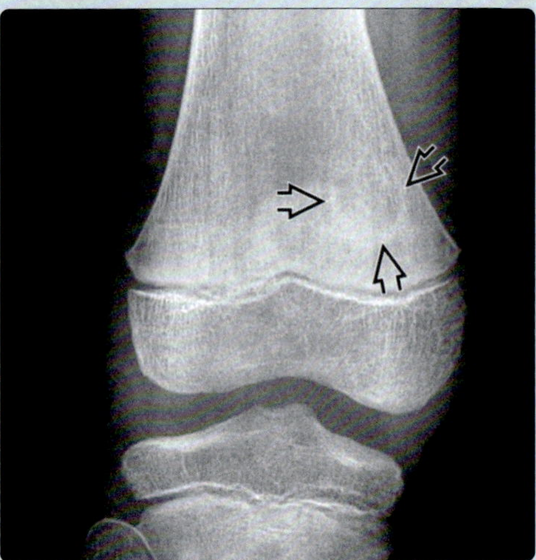

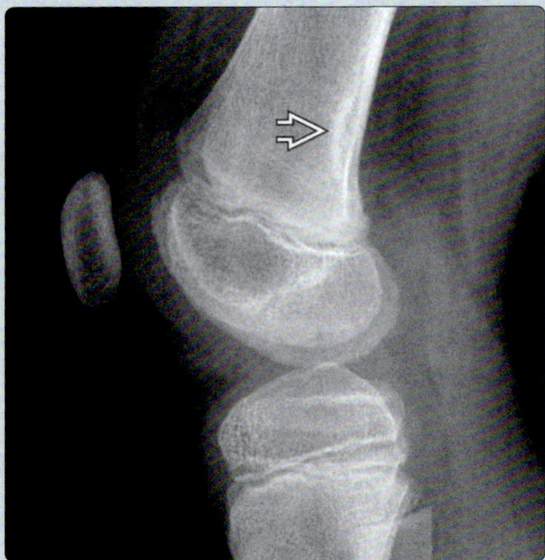

(Left) *AP radiograph from a 10-year-old boy shows a common appearance of distal femoral avulsive irregularity (DFAI) in the medial distal femoral metaphysis: it is well circumscribed, ovoid, & centrally lucent with mildly sclerotic margins ➩.* **(Right)** *Lateral radiograph in the same patient shows a scalloped appearance of the posterior distal femoral cortex ➨ at the site of the lesion. There is no periosteal reaction.*

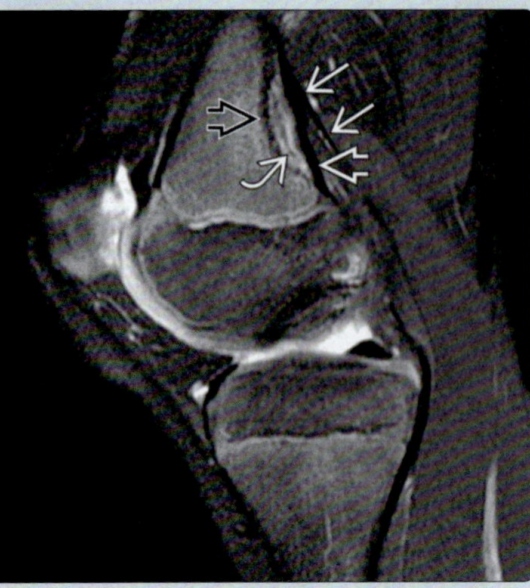

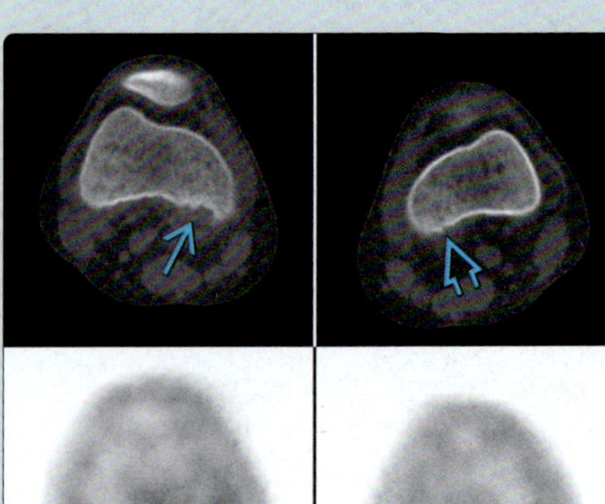

(Left) *Sagittal T2 FS MR through the same lesion shows heterogeneous signal intensity centrally ➨. There is typical, concave low signal intensity at the sclerotic deep margin ➩. The overlying periosteum (which is normally thickened at this level) is intact ➨ deep to the medial gastrocnemius muscle attachment ➨.* **(Right)** *Axial CT (top) & FDG PET (bottom) images in a teenager with a known chest wall Ewing sarcoma (not shown) demonstrate ↑ metabolic activity at bilateral foci of DFAI, R ➩ > L ➩.*

TERMINOLOGY

Synonyms

- Benign cortical irregularity of distal femur
- Avulsive cortical irregularity or tug lesion
- Cortical desmoid: Misnomer as biology & histology differ from true desmoid tumors (which are locally aggressive benign neoplasms)

Definitions

- Irregularity of posterior, medial distal femoral metaphyseal cortex deep to attachments of gastrocnemius muscle medial head or adductor magnus aponeurosis
- Benign self-limited lesion likely due to chronic avulsion

IMAGING

General Features

- Best diagnostic clue
  - Typically incidental radiographic finding at classic location without soft tissue mass or symptoms
- Location
  - Bilateral: 25-100%
  - Other chronic stress-related irregularities
    - Deltoid insertion on lateral humerus
    - Pectoralis major insertion on medial humerus
- Morphology
  - Round vs. elongated with femoral long axis
  - May appear as
    - Scalloped, concave, saucer-shaped cortical defect with well-defined border
    - Bulging, convex cortical lesion with irregular surface
    - Divergent lesion splitting cortex

Radiographic Findings

- Lateral view (key to visualization)
  - Lucent focus of cortical interruption/irregularity
    - Deep margin is commonly concave ± sclerosis
    - Solid periosteal reaction or cortical thickening may abut lesion
    - Lesion may contain bony spicules
- Frontal view may show round or ovoid lucent focus with sclerotic rim &/or subtle medial cortical irregularity
- Important negative findings
  - No associated soft tissue abnormality
  - No aggressive periosteal reaction

MR Findings

- Interruption of contiguous smooth cortex by intermediate T1/heterogeneous T2 signal intensity lesion
- Thin, concave, T1-/T2-hypointense deep rim
- Lesion may enhance on T1 C+ sequences
- Overlying periosteum is intact
- ± mild adjacent marrow edema (more likely if symptomatic)
- No overlying soft tissue mass

Nuclear Medicine Findings

- Bone scan
  - Healing lesions show mildly ↑ uptake
  - Inactive lesions show no uptake
- PET/CT
  - ↑ metabolic activity; accompanying CT is diagnostic

DIFFERENTIAL DIAGNOSIS

Osteosarcoma

- Destructive bone lesion most commonly arising from intramedullary distal femoral metadiaphysis
- Aggressive features are rule, not exception

Osteomyelitis

- Overlying soft tissue edema early
- Radiographic bone changes in 10-14 days
  - Lucent cortical destruction/permeation

Langerhans Cell Histiocytosis

- Flat bones > metaphyseal/diaphyseal long bones
- Classically: Geographic lytic lesion
- Sclerotic margins with healing

Fibroxanthoma/Nonossifying Fibroma

- Overlaps distal femoral avulsive irregularity in some cases
- Eccentric multilobulated lucent metaphyseal/metadiaphyseal lesion
- Thin sclerotic margin; narrow zone of transition

Periosteal/Juxtacortical Chondroma

- Uncommon benign surface lesion with scalloping & buttressing of cortex ± chondroid matrix

Bone Metastases

- Neuroblastoma & leukemia are most common < 10 years
- Lucent metaphyseal bands vs. poorly defined lesions with permeative destruction & aggressive periosteal reaction

Osteoid Osteoma

- Small lucent, highly vascular nidus ± central Ca^{2+}
- Adjacent periosteal reaction, cortical thickening, soft tissue & marrow edema

CLINICAL ISSUES

Presentation

- Most common signs/symptoms
  - Usually asymptomatic; local pain is uncommon

Demographics

- Age: 3-17 years; most common: 10-15 years
- Sex: M > F = 1.4-3:1

Treatment

- None if asymptomatic
- With localizing symptoms & no other etiologies, conservative therapy may relieve repetitive stress injury
- Avoid unnecessary biopsy

SELECTED REFERENCES

1. Lerisson H et al: Radiographic/MR imaging correlation of the pediatric knee growth. Magn Reson Imaging Clin N Am. 27(4):737-51, 2019
2. Kay M et al: Cortical desmoid of the humerus: radiographic and MRI correlation. Skeletal Radiol. 46(7):1011-5, 2017
3. Tscholl PM et al: Cortical desmoids in adolescent top-level athletes. Acta Radiol Open. 4(5):2058460115580878, 2015
4. Thapa MM et al: MRI of pediatric patients: part 2, normal variants and abnormalities of the knee. AJR Am J Roentgenol. 198(5):W456-65, 2012
5. Vieira RL et al: MRI features of cortical desmoid in acute knee trauma. AJR Am J Roentgenol. 196(2):424-8, 2011
6. Connolly SA et al: Avulsive cortical irregularity and F-18 FDG PET. Clin Nucl Med. 31(2):87-9, 2006

KEY FACTS

TERMINOLOGY

- Nonrandom association of anomalies involving multiple organ systems (except brain); causative gene is unknown
  - **V**ertebral/vascular
  - **A**nal atresia/auricular
  - **C**ardiac
  - **T**racheoesophageal fistula
  - **E**sophageal atresia
  - **R**enal/radial/rib
  - **L**imb
- VACTERL association is typically diagnosed when ≥ 3 malformations are present

IMAGING

- Actively seek other features of VACTERL association when 1-2 components are present
- Initial imaging in suspected cases: Radiographs & US
  - Radiographs: Spine & limbs (if limb anomaly is present on physical exam)
  - US: Head, spine, renal/bladder, echocardiography
- Further imaging depends on initial imaging & clinical exam findings

CLINICAL ISSUES

- Incidence of VACTERL association: 1/10,000 to 40,000 liveborn infants
- Children with VACTERL: 72% have 3 anomalies, 24% have 4 anomalies, 8% have 5 anomalies
- Frequency of anomalies in VACTERL
  - Cardiac: 40-80%
  - Renal: 50-80%
  - Anal: 55-90%
  - Tracheoesophageal: 50-80%
  - Vertebral: 60-80%
  - Limb: 40-50%

DIAGNOSTIC CHECKLIST

- Consider VACTERL in child with vertebral & other anomalies

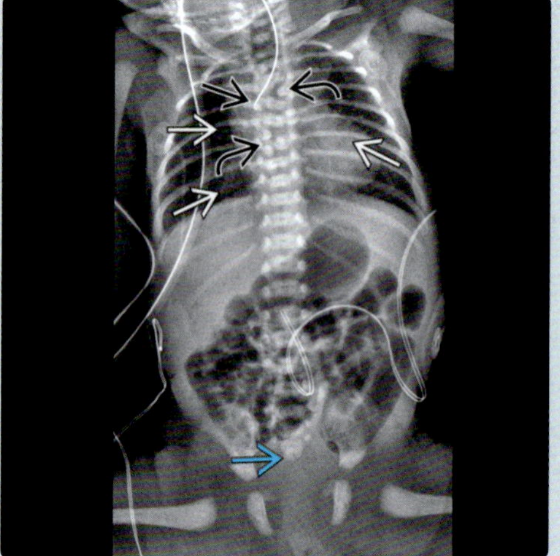

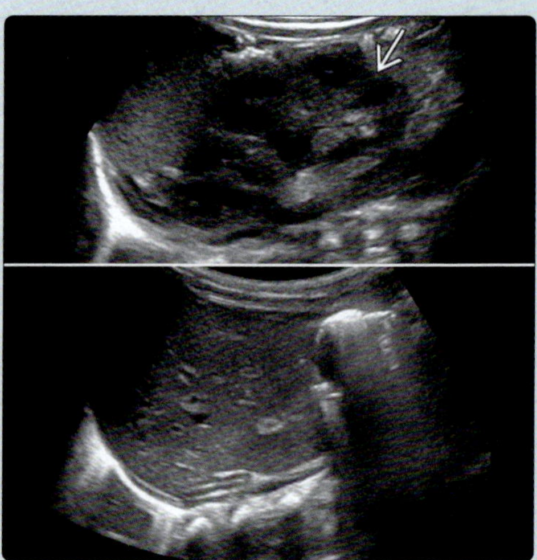

(Left) *AP radiograph in a newborn shows vertebral segmentation anomalies ⇨. The nasogastric tube (NGT) could not be advanced beyond the upper esophagus ⇨ due to esophageal atresia (EA) [with the bowel gas indicating an associated tracheoesophageal fistula (TEF)]. Mild central pulmonary vascular congestion ➡ is secondary to a VSD. There is partial sacral agenesis ⇨ in this child with an ARM.* **(Right)** *Longitudinal US of the left (top) & right (bottom) renal fossae in the same patient show a solitary left kidney ➡.*

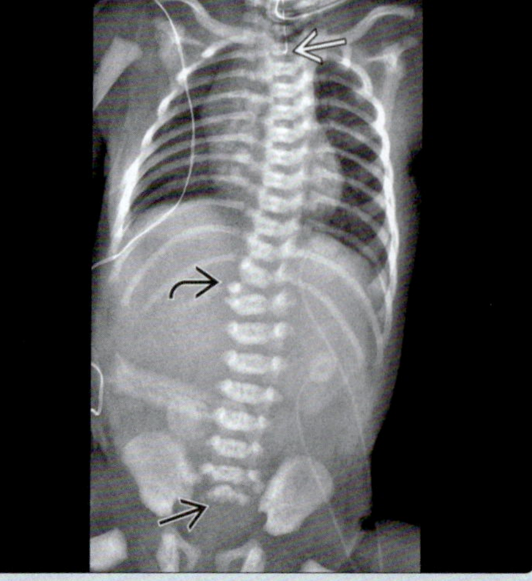

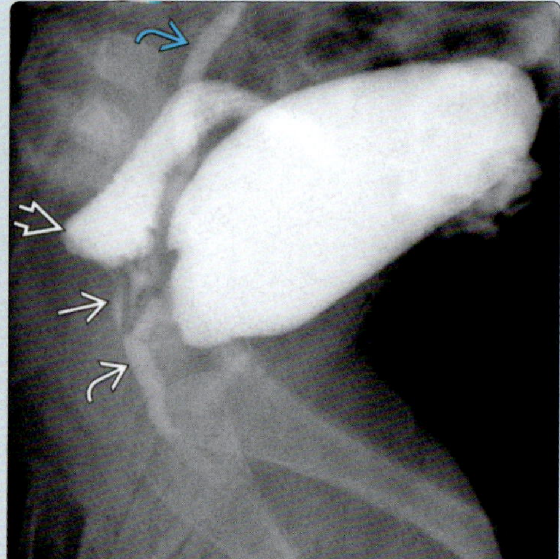

(Left) *AP radiograph in a newborn shows vertebral segmentation anomalies ⇨ & partial agenesis of the sacrum ⇨. The NGT could not be passed beyond the upper esophagus due to EA ➡ (with the lack of abdominal gas indicating the absence of a TEF).* **(Right)** *Lateral view from a VCUG in the same child shows a rectourethral fistula ➡ from the rectal pouch ➡ to the posterior urethra ➡. Left vesicoureteral reflux ⇨ is also seen in this child with an ARM.*

TERMINOLOGY

Synonyms

- VATER, VACTER, VACTEL association, TREACLE, ARTICLE, ARTICLE V, axial mesodermal dysplasia spectrum

Definitions

- Nonrandom association of anomalies involving multiple organ systems (except brain)
  - **V**ertebral/vascular
  - **A**nal atresia/auricular
  - **C**ardiac
  - **T**racheoesophageal fistula (TEF)
  - **E**sophageal atresia (EA)
  - **R**enal/radial/rib
  - **L**imb
- VACTERL association is typically diagnosed when ≥ 3 malformations are present
  - Clubfoot & hip dysplasia are excluded if no other limb anomalies are present
- No clinical or laboratory evidence of alternative diagnosis

IMAGING

General Features

- Best diagnostic clue
  - Vertebral anomalies in presence of other malformations

Radiographic Findings

- Radiography
  - Axial skeleton
    - Vertebral anomalies
      - Cleft, block, butterfly vertebrae; hemivertebrae; hypersegmentation; vertebral bars; caudal regression
      - Secondary scoliosis, kyphosis
    - Other spine issues: Cord tethering (8-78%)
    - Ribs: Fused, bifid, hypoplastic, supernumerary/cervical
  - Limbs or extremities
    - Radial ray: Dysplastic or absent radius, radioulnar synostosis, thumb hypoplasia, radial polydactyly, absent scaphoid, radial artery hypoplasia
    - Hands: Polydactyly (20%) is most common; syndactyly
    - Reduction deformities (34%): Aplasia/hypoplasia of humerus, radius, femur, tibia, or fibula
  - Head & neck
    - Choanal atresia, cleft lip/palate, auricular defects
  - Chest
    - Congenital heart disease: Ventricular septal defect (VSD) (30%); patent ductus arteriosus (PDA) (26%); atrial septal defect (ASD) (20%)
    - EA/TEF
    - Lung agenesis, horseshoe lung (posterior lung fusion), ectopic bronchus
  - Abdomen & pelvis
    - Imperforate anus ± fistula
    - Microgastria, duodenal atresia, malrotation, Meckel diverticulum

Ultrasonographic Findings

- Renal/bladder US to evaluate for renal/GU anomalies
  - Renal agenesis is most common (bilateral in ~ 13%); multicystic dysplasia, horseshoe kidney, ectopia, hydronephrosis
  - Persistent urachus; cryptorchidism
- Neonatal head US to evaluate for findings suggestive of other diagnoses (e.g., hydrocephalus)
- Spinal US to evaluate for tethered cord
- Prenatal detection rates of VACTERL anomalies
  - Renal malformations: 45%; TEF: 44%; cardiac malformations: 20%; vertebral: 13%; limb: 11%

Imaging Recommendations

- Actively seek other features of VACTERL when 1-2 components are present
- Multidisciplinary group suggests specific work-up for VACTERL in
  - All infants with 2 features of VACTERL association
  - All infants with TEF/EA
  - All infants with anorectal malformation (ARM)
- Radiographs & US are used initially for imaging in suspected cases
  - Radiographs: Spine & limbs (if limb anomaly is present on physical exam)
  - US: Head, spine, renal/bladder, echocardiography
  - Additional & advanced imaging depend on radiographic & clinical exam findings

DIFFERENTIAL DIAGNOSIS

Alagille Syndrome

- Butterfly vertebra & cardiac anomalies ± renal anomalies
- Differs from VACTERL: Bile duct paucity/cholestasis, ophthalmologic anomalies, neurologic anomalies, characteristic facies, *JAG1* mutations in > 90%

CHARGE Syndrome

- Cardiac malformations, GU anomalies ± TEF
- Differs from VACTERL: Coloboma, cranial nerve dysfunction, characteristic facial features, *CHD7* mutations in > 50%

Currarino Syndrome

- Partial sacral agenesis, presacral mass, & ARM
- Differs from VACTERL: Presacral mass, *MNX1* mutations

Fanconi Anemia

- Radial deficiency & many other features of VACTERL
- Differs from VACTERL: Pancytopenia, pigmentation anomalies

Holt-Oram Syndrome (Heart-Hand Syndrome)

- Cardiac conduction defect ± ASD/VSD; thumb, wrist, & forearm abnormalities
- Differs from VACTERL: Heterozygous mutations in *TBX5* gene

Oculoauriculovertebral Syndrome (Goldenhar Syndrome)

- Vertebral, cardiac, limb, & urogenital anomalies
- Differs from VACTERL: Ear anomalies, hemifacial microsomia

Thrombocytopenia/Absent Radius Syndrome

- Normal thumb

- Differs from VACTERL: Thrombocytopenia

VACTERL-H (VACTERL + Hydrocephalus)

- Severe intellectual disability; poor prognosis
- Differs from VACTERL: Hydrocephalus, various known mutations

22q11.2 Deletion Syndrome (DiGeorge/Velocardiofacial Syndrome)

- Cardiac malformations, renal anomalies
- Differs from VACTERL: Hypocalcemia, immune dysfunction, characteristic facial features, deletion of 1 copy of chromosome 22q11.2

PATHOLOGY

General Features

- Etiology
  - Classified as association due to no unifying causative gene identified
    - Association: Grouping of anomalies more frequently than expected by chance
  - Exact etiology unknown
  - Various overlapping theories for etiology of VACTERL
    - Malformations occur during blastogenesis → developmental field defect → polytopic anomalies affecting multiple organ systems
    - Undiscovered genetic & epigenetic causes
    - Nongenetic factors have been implicated in playing role in VACTERL (e.g., maternal diabetes mellitus, alcohol or antiepileptic use, assisted reproductive techniques, & in utero hypoxia)
- Genetics
  - *SHH* mutations are theorized based on animal models
    - Not established in humans
  - Associated with trisomies 13 & 18, cri du chat syndrome, Fanconi anemia
- Associated abnormalities
  - Cleft palate: 18%
  - Neural tube defect: 10%
  - Diaphragmatic hernia: 8%
  - Omphalocele: 6%
  - Exstrophy of cloaca
  - Congenital pulmonary airway malformation
  - Sirenomelia

Staging, Grading, & Classification

- No definitive consensus of criteria for VACTERL
  - Most require ≥ 3 components for diagnosis
- Some researchers/clinicians believe "core" features, such as TEF or ARMs, should be present for diagnosis
- Other etiologies in differential should be excluded based on clinical & laboratory work-up

CLINICAL ISSUES

Presentation

- Most common signs/symptoms
  - Neonatal: Depends on anomaly constellation
- Other signs/symptoms
  - Prenatal imaging
    - Polyhydramnios (EA), kyphoscoliosis, absent radius, cardiac &/or renal anomalies, single umbilical artery
  - Prematurity: ~ 1/3
  - Stillborn: 12%

Demographics

- Epidemiology
  - 1/10,000 to 40,000 liveborn infants
  - Frequency of anomalies in VACTERL
    - Cardiac: 40-80%
    - Renal: 50-80%
    - Anal: 55-90%
    - Tracheoesophageal: 50-80%
    - Vertebral: 60-80%
    - Limb: 40-50%
  - Concurrence of 2 specific VACTERL anomalies is 11x more frequent than expected by chance
    - Probably belongs to VACTERL continuum
  - Concurrence of ≥ 3 specific VACTERL anomalies is 95x more frequent than expected by chance
  - Children with VACTERL: 72% have 3 anomalies, 24% have 4 anomalies, 8% have 5 anomalies
    - Most common 3-anomaly combinations: Cardiac-renal-limb & cardiac-renal-anal
    - Most common 5-anomaly combination: Cardiac-renal-limb-anal-tracheoesophageal

Natural History & Prognosis

- Mortality (not due to any specific defect)
  - 28% neonatal mortality
  - 48% mortality in 1st year
- Intelligence is usually normal

Treatment

- If prenatal diagnosis: Delivery at tertiary care facility

DIAGNOSTIC CHECKLIST

Image Interpretation Pearls

- Consider VACTERL in child with vertebral & other anomalies

SELECTED REFERENCES

1. van de Putte R et al: Maternal risk factors for the VACTERL association: a EUROCAT case-control study. Birth Defects Res. 112(9):688-98, 2020
2. Lubinsky M: The VACTERL association: mosaic mitotic aneuploidy as a cause and a model. J Assist Reprod Genet. 36(8):1549-54, 2019
3. Solomon BD: The etiology of VACTERL association: current knowledge and hypotheses. Am J Med Genet C Semin Med Genet. 178(4):440-6, 2018
4. Debost-Legrand A et al: Prenatal diagnosis of the VACTERL association using routine ultrasound examination. Birth Defects Res A Clin Mol Teratol. 103(10):880-6, 2015
5. Solomon BD: VACTERL/VATER association. Orphanet J Rare Dis. 6:56, 2011
6. O'Neill BR et al: Prevalence of tethered spinal cord in infants with VACTERL. J Neurosurg Pediatr. 6(2):177-82, 2010
7. Castori M et al: Tibial developmental field defect is the most common lower limb malformation pattern in VACTERL association. Am J Med Genet A. 146A(10):1259-66, 2008

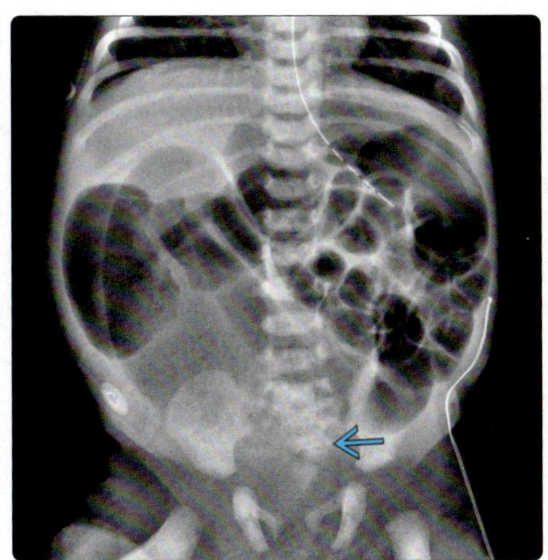

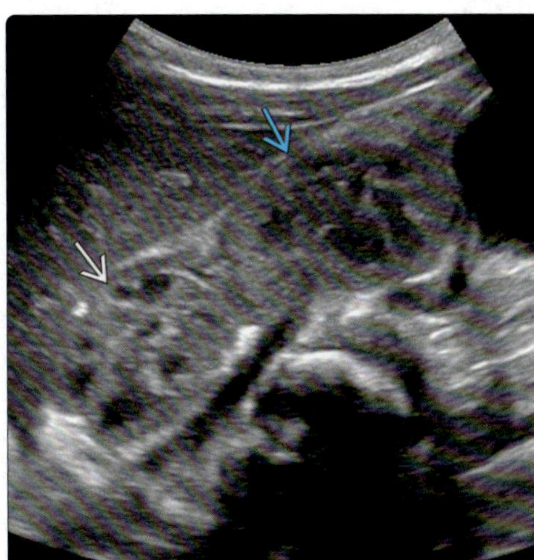

(Left) *AP abdominal radiograph in a newborn boy with an ARM shows diffusely dilated bowel loops, consistent with a distal bowel obstruction. The sacrum has an anomalous morphology ➡, nearly scimitar.* **(Right)** *Transverse US of the right renal fossa in the same patient shows a cross-fused ectopic left kidney ➡, which is inferior to & fused to the inferior pole of the normally positioned right kidney ➡.*

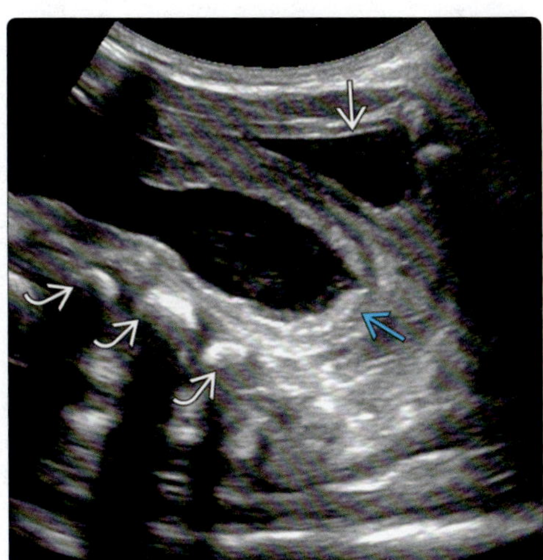

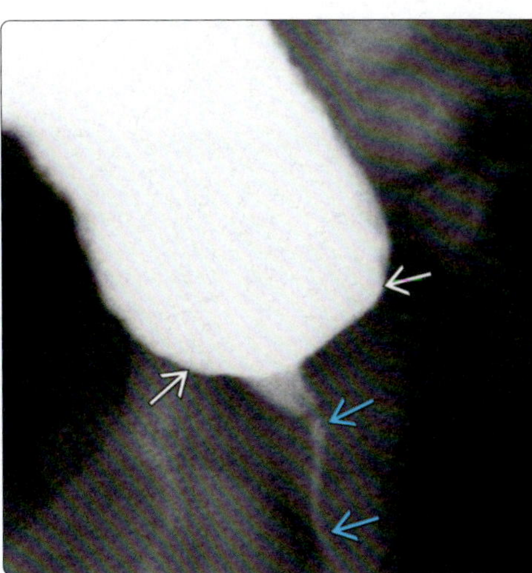

(Left) *Sagittal US of the pelvis in the same boy shows the blind-ending distal rectum ➡, consistent with an ARM. The urinary bladder ➡ is seen anteriorly & echogenic sacral vertebral bodies ➡ are seen posteriorly.* **(Right)** *Lateral fluoroscopy of the pelvis from a distal colostogram in the same boy with an ARM shows a long rectoperineal fistula ➡ extending from the distal rectal pouch ➡ to the perineum.*

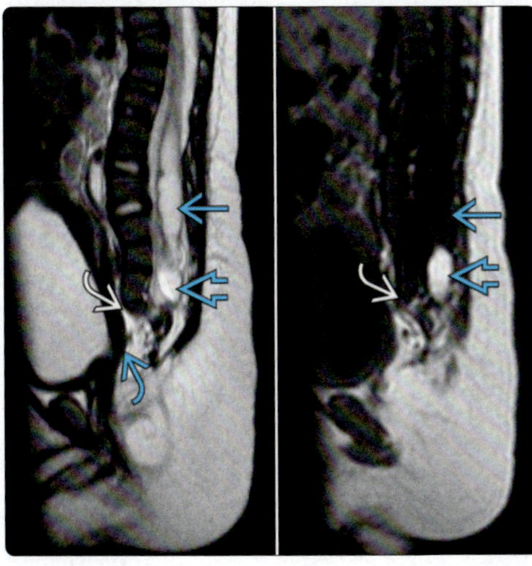

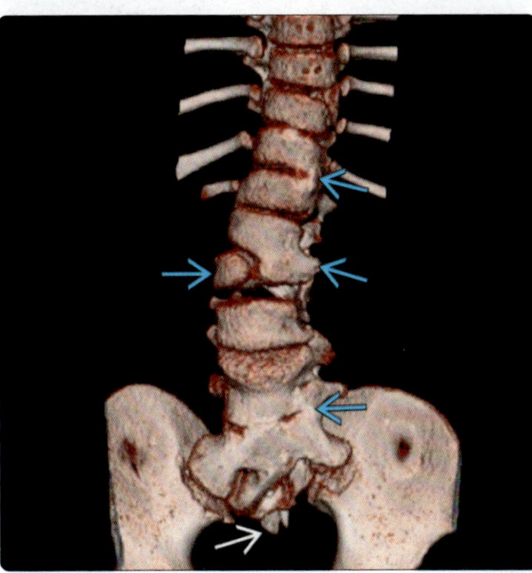

(Left) *Sagittal T2 (left) & T1 MR images in a 3-month-old boy with VACTERL show partial agenesis of the sacrum ➡. There is a low-lying conus with an associated syrinx ➡ & a terminal lipoma ➡. The decompressed blind-ending rectum ➡ does not extend to the perineum, consistent with this child's known ARM.* **(Right)** *3D surface-rendered CT in the same patient at 10 years of age shows multiple vertebral anomalies ➡ & partial sacral agenesis ➡.*

Polydactyly

KEY FACTS

TERMINOLOGY

- Polydactyly: Extra digits of hands or feet
  - Description of individual bones: Bifid (distal cleft) vs. duplication (complete distal to proximal cleft)
  - Preaxial: Radial side of hand, tibial side of foot
  - Post axial: Ulnar side of hand, fibular side of foot
  - Central (mesoaxial): Involves central digits
  - Mirror-image polydactyly: Central thumb/great toe-like digit with variable duplication of 2nd-5th digits
- Syndactyly: Fusion of digits
  - Simple (soft tissue fusion) vs. complex (osseous fusion)
  - Complete (entire digit) vs. incomplete (spares distal digit)
- Polysyndactyly: Polydactyly + syndactyly (soft tissue ± osseous fusion of digits)

IMAGING

- Radiographs of affected hand/foot are done primarily to detect skeletal elements within extra digit(s)
- Extra digit can range from small, entirely soft tissue skin tag → rudimentary digit with hypoplastic bones → fully developed extra digit
- Affected phalanges & metacarpals/metatarsals may be bifurcated or duplicated
- Skeletal survey is indicated if syndromic association is suspected

PATHOLOGY

- Most cases are sporadic & isolated
- However, ~ 300 syndromes are associated with polydactyly (e.g., trisomies, Meckel-Gruber, VACTERL, Ellis-van Creveld)

DIAGNOSTIC CHECKLIST

- If found on prenatal US/MR, search for other anomalies
- Description of each digital anomaly should include
  - Degree of bifurcation/duplication of each phalanx
  - Morphology of metacarpal/metatarsal (e.g., duplicated, bifurcated Y or T shape, broadening of head)
  - Any associated soft tissue (± osseous) syndactyly

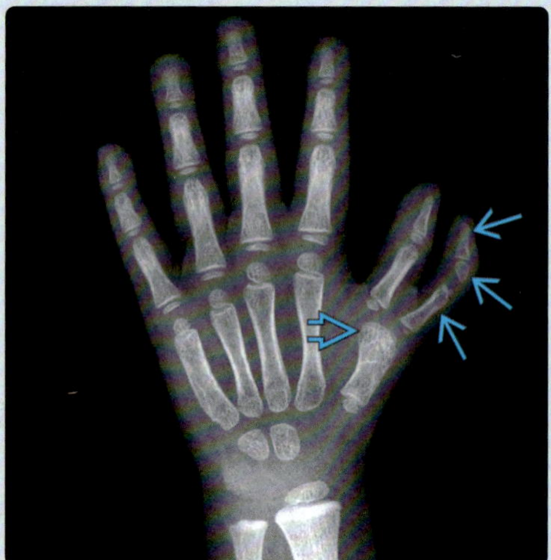

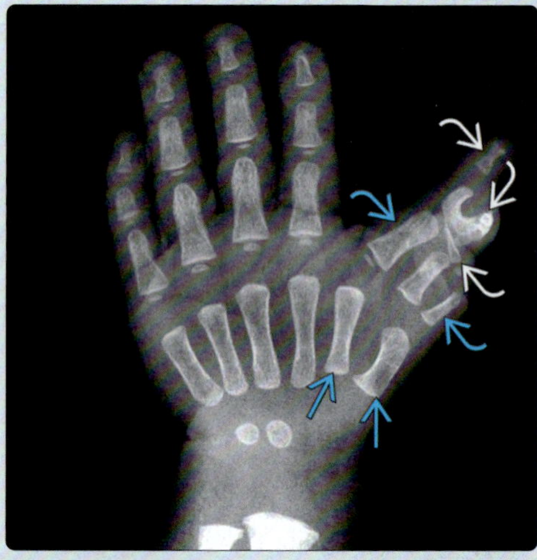

(Left) *PA radiograph shows the left hand in a 2-year-old girl with preaxial polydactyly. The duplicated thumb is triphalangeal ➡ (Wassel type VII). The distal end of the 1st metacarpal is broad ⇨ but not duplicated.* **(Right)** *PA radiograph of the left hand in a girl with multiple limb anomalies shows a complex, preaxial polydactyly with 2 metacarpals ➡, 3 proximal phalanges ↪, & a complex array of middle & distal phalanges ↪ with soft tissue & osseous fusion.*

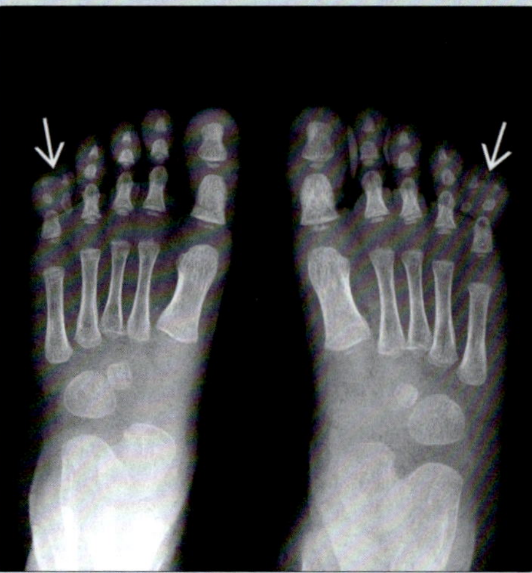

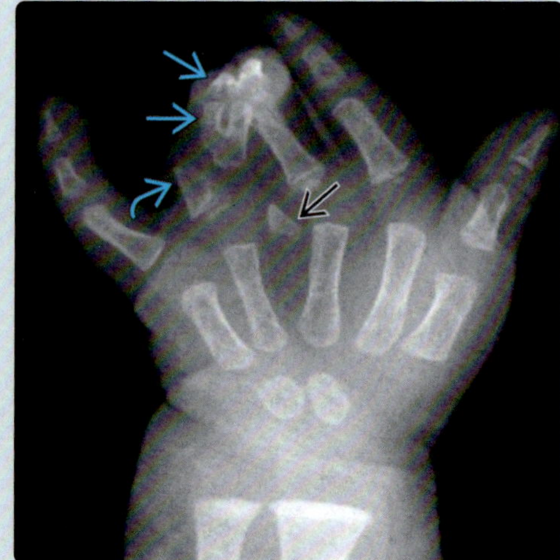

(Left) *AP radiograph of both feet in a 2-year-old girl shows bilateral, postaxial polydactyly (type B) with duplication of the 5th middle & distal phalanges ➡.* **(Right)** *PA radiograph in a 1-year-old with a complex, central polysyndactyly shows a ring finger proximal phalanx deformity/shortening ↪ with bifurcation of the middle & distal phalanges ➡. There is also ring/middle finger soft tissue syndactyly & a supernumerary bone ➡ between the 3rd & 4th metacarpals.*

KEY FACTS

TERMINOLOGY

- Hemimelia: Absence of all or portion of distal limb
  - Transverse hemimelia: Defects of both tibia & fibula
  - Paraxial hemimelia: Defect of only tibia (preaxial) or fibula (post axial)
  - Terminal hemimelia: Foot bones absent to some degree
  - Intercalary hemimelia: Foot spared

IMAGING

- Radiographs remain primary imaging modality for detection & characterization of hemimelia
- Both lower extremities should be imaged from hips to feet with AP & lateral views to characterize
  - Specific hemimelia defects
  - Associated limb shortening/limb length discrepancy
  - Other lower extremity bony anomalies
- US & MR more accurately define extent of
  - Cartilaginous anlage of unossified bone
  - Presence/absence of patella & quadriceps

DIAGNOSTIC CHECKLIST

- Differentiating fibular from tibial hemimelia
  - Fibular hemimelia associations
    - Tibial bowing (typically with anteromedial apex); tibia remains centered on femur
    - Absent lateral digits
    - Valgus foot deformity
  - Tibial hemimelia associations
    - ↑ fibular width; fibula overrides distal femur
    - Absent medial digits
    - Varus foot deformity
- Report details should include descriptions of
  - Complete vs. partial absence of each leg bone
    - Approximate fraction & position of affected segment
  - Specifics of foot involvement
    - Be aware of radiographically limited tarsal assessment in young children due to ossification timing
  - Associated lower extremity anomalies

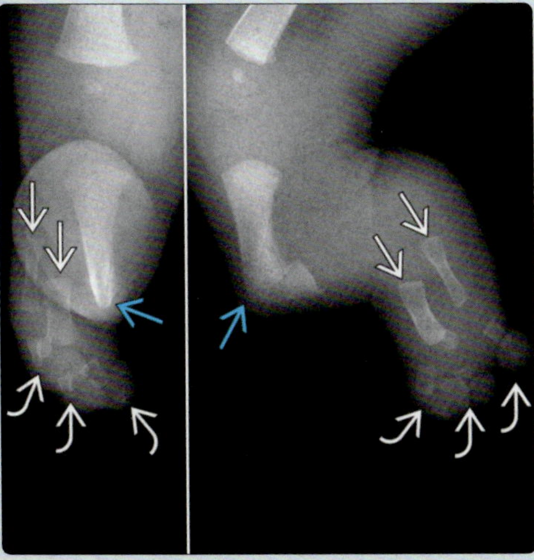

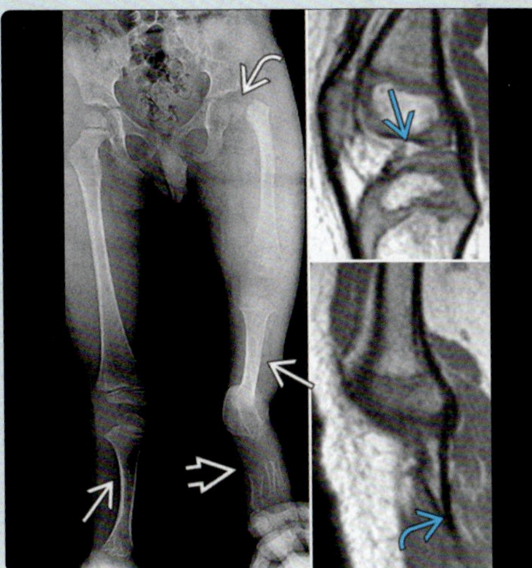

(Left) *Frontal (left) & lateral (right) radiographs in a 2-week-old show absence of the fibula with anteromedial tibial bowing ➡. Also note the foot deformity with only 2 metatarsals ➡ & 3 digits ➡.* **(Right)** *AP radiograph (left) in a 4-year-old shows bilateral fibular hemimelia ➡ with associated left proximal focal femoral deficiency ➡, shortening of the left lower extremity, & left foot anomalies ➡. Sagittal PD MR images of the left knee (right) show absence of the ACL ➡ & an elongated conjoined tendon ➡.*

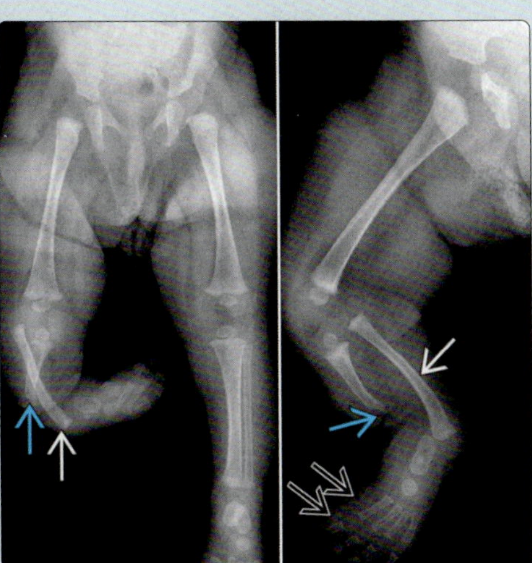

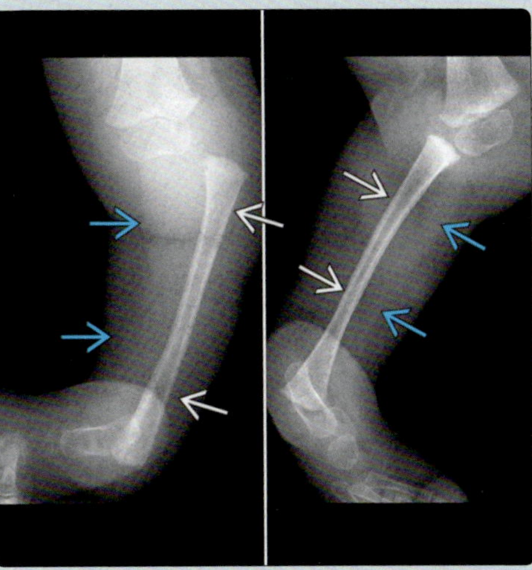

(Left) *Frontal (left) & lateral (right) radiographs in a 3-month-old with partial tibial hemimelia show absence of the distal right tibia ➡. The right fibula is thickened ➡. There is an associated preaxial foot anomaly with absence of a normal 1st metatarsal & great toe ➡.* **(Right)** *Frontal (left) & lateral (right) radiographs of the left leg in a 1-year-old with tibial hemimelia show complete absence of the tibia ➡. The left fibula is intact but thickened ➡. An associated foot anomaly is partially visualized.*

Tibial Bowing

KEY FACTS

TERMINOLOGY

- Tibial bowing: Typically unilateral, congenital or infantile diaphyseal deformity characterized by direction of apex
  - Posteromedial: Physiologic bowing frequently secondary to intrauterine positioning
  - Anteromedial: Associated with fibular hemimelia
  - Anterolateral: Associated with neurofibromatosis type 1
    - May develop fractures (secondary to osseous dysplasia) & pseudoarthrosis (secondary to abnormal cellular healing)

IMAGING

- Frontal & lateral leg radiographs are necessary to characterize apex of deformity
  - If tibial bowing is present, evaluate for
    - Cortical thickening or thinning
    - Fracture or pseudarthrosis
    - Underlying lesion or abnormal mineralization
    - Fibular hemimelia
    - Associated knee, ankle, & foot deformities
- Standing leg length radiograph
  - Characterizes limb length discrepancy
- Additional radiographs to evaluate for associated anomalies
  - Foot radiographs
    - Posteromedial bowing: Calcaneovalgus
    - Anteromedial bowing with fibular hemimelia: Absent rays, talipes equinovalgus, tarsal coalitions
- Advanced imaging may be used to evaluate associated conditions affecting management
  - Knee MR in fibular hemimelia may show congenital ligamentous & meniscal abnormalities

DIAGNOSTIC CHECKLIST

- Depending on apex direction/type, tibial bowing should prompt search for associated anomalies
  - Affects local diagnosis, prognosis, & therapy
  - May impart underlying systemic diagnosis

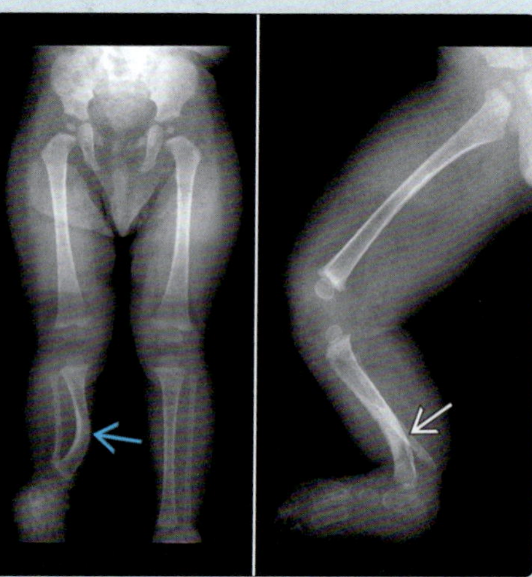

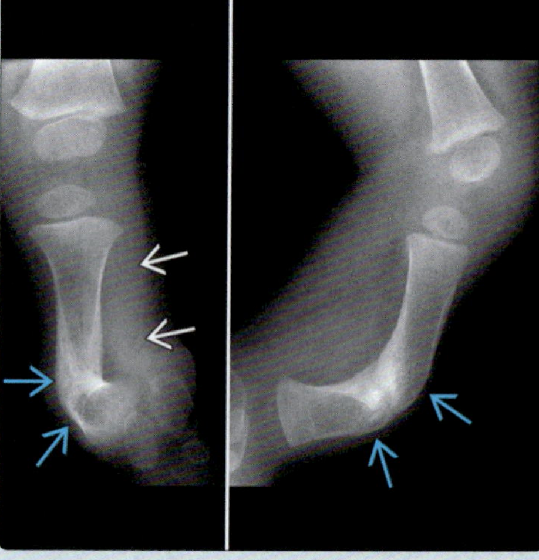

(Left) *Frontal radiograph (left) in a 1-year-old shows right medial tibial bowing ⇨ & shortening of the right tibia & fibula with a limb length discrepancy. The lateral radiograph (right) shows posterior tibial bowing ➡ & suggestion of a foot deformity (though weight-bearing views are required to adequately assess disorders of foot alignment).* **(Right)** *Frontal (left) & lateral (right) radiographs in an 8-month-old with fibular hemimelia show anteromedial tibial bowing ⇨ associated with absence of the fibula ➡.*

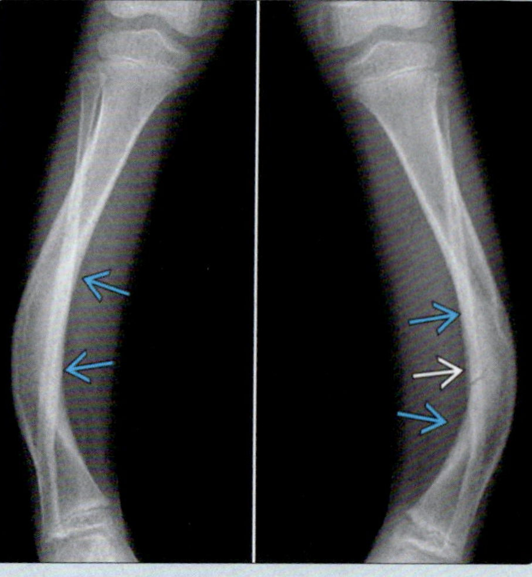

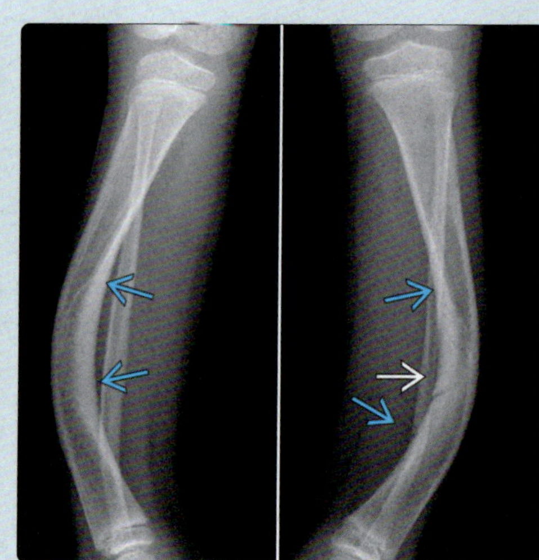

(Left) *AP radiographs in a 6-year-old girl with neurofibromatosis type 1 (NF1) show lateral bowing of the tibias ⇨. Additionally, an early, incomplete fracture line is present in the medial aspect of the mid to distal left tibial diaphysis ➡.* **(Right)** *Lateral radiographs of the legs in the same patient confirm bilateral anterolateral bowing ⇨, which is characteristic of NF1. The fracture ➡ is due to associated osseous dysplasia & may go on to form a pseudarthrosis because of abnormal cellular healing in NF1.*

Arthrogryposis

KEY FACTS

TERMINOLOGY

- Arthrogryposis multiplex congenita (AMC): Descriptive term for infant born with ≥ 2 joint contractures
  - **Not** specific diagnosis (> 300 underlying causes)

IMAGING

- Radiographs of affected limbs are typically performed
  - Static/fixed abnormal deviations/orientations of joints
    - Positioning for standard views is difficult
  - Gracile & osteoporotic bones with muscle wasting
  - Foot radiographs should simulate weight-bearing to accurately diagnose associated alignment disorders
- MR
  - Brain/spine evaluation if neurologic exam is abnormal
  - Extremities show ↓ muscle bulk with fatty replacement in many conditions
  - May aid in preoperative assessment of joints (e.g., soft tissue bands, abnormalities of unossified cartilage)

PATHOLOGY

- Broad categories of AMC etiologies
  - Neurologic (70-80%): Various CNS/PNS anomalies
    - Forebrain malformations, spinal muscular atrophy
  - Primary myopathies (~ 20%)
    - Amyoplasia (most common cause of AMC overall)
    - Distal arthrogryposis, congenital muscular dystrophies
  - Connective tissue disorders
    - Skeletal dysplasias, multiple pterygium syndromes
  - Maternal exposures: Teratogens, infections
  - Intrauterine compression: Oligohydramnios, multiple gestations, uterine anomalies

CLINICAL ISSUES

- Perinatal fractures are common in AMC
- Initial treatment of contractures is typically nonoperative: Passive manipulation & serial casting
- Operative treatments: Soft tissue release, tendon transfer, various osteotomies

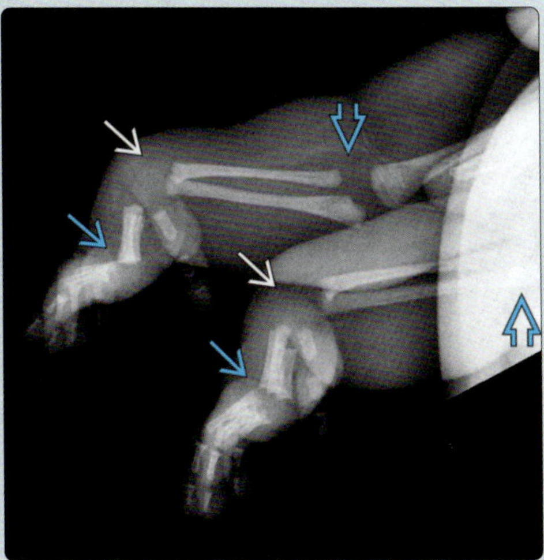

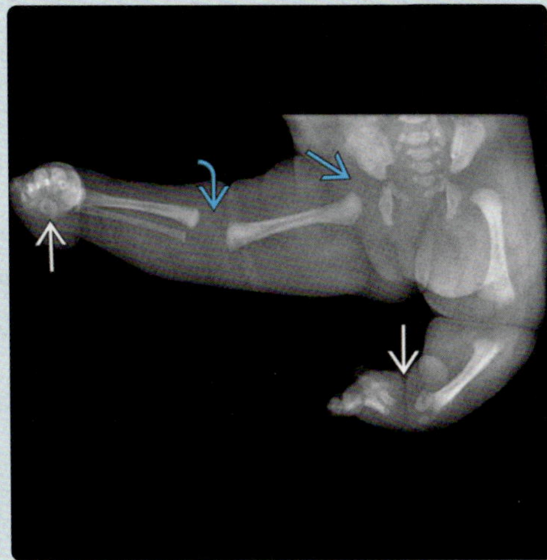

(Left) *Lateral radiograph of both arms in a newborn with arthrogryposis multiplex congenita (AMC) due to amyoplasia shows persistent extension at the elbows → with the forearms held straight out from the body. The wrists show hyperflexion → with hyperextension at the MCP joints →.* **(Right)** *Lower extremity radiograph in the same patient shows right hip flexion → & right knee hyperextension →. Bilateral talipes equinovarus deformities → are incompletely evaluated on this non-weight-bearing exam.*

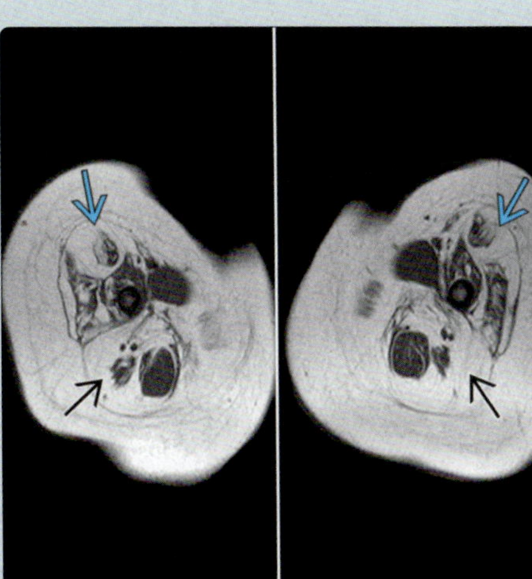

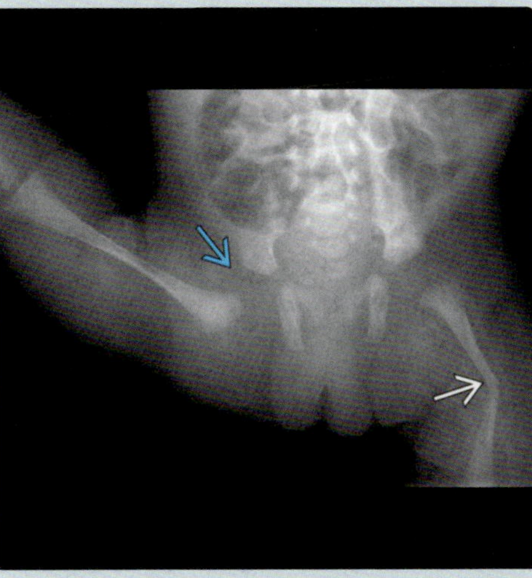

(Left) *Axial T1 MR in a 5-month-old with AMC due to amyoplasia shows severe loss of muscle bulk of the bilateral quadriceps → & hamstring → muscles with associated fatty replacement. Fatty & fibrous replacement of muscles is typical of amyoplasia.* **(Right)** *Frontal radiograph of the pelvis in a newborn with AMC shows right hip hyperflexion →. Both femurs are gracile (overtubulated) with muscle wasting of the bilateral thighs. There is a fracture of the left femoral diaphysis →. Perinatal fractures are common in infants with AMC.*

Clubfoot

KEY FACTS

TERMINOLOGY

- Synonym: Talipes equinovarus
- **C**avus, forefoot **a**dductus, hindfoot **v**arus & **e**quinus (CAVE)
- Plantarflexion of calcaneus relative to tibia (equinus) + hindfoot inversion (varus) + forefoot adduction (varus)

IMAGING

- Talus: Lateral rotation within ankle joint
  - Talus is point of reference for hindfoot
- Calcaneus: Relative medial rotation + equinus
- Navicular: Medial subluxation on talus
- Cuboid: Medial subluxation on calcaneus
- Metatarsals: Inverted, appears parallel on lateral view
- AP view: "Laterally pointing" hindfoot + adducted forefoot
  - Long axis of talus is very lateral to 1st metatarsal
  - Long axis of calcaneus is lateral to 5th metatarsal
- Measure on weight-bearing views (may be simulated)
  - ↑ tibiocalcaneal angle on lateral view (> 90° = calcaneal equinus)
  - ↓ talocalcaneal angle on lateral & AP views (hindfoot varus)
  - ↑ talus-1st metatarsal angle (forefoot varus)
- Frequently detected on 2nd-trimester ultrasound
- Prenatal MR performed for other abnormalities (e.g., myelomeningocele) may detect clubfoot

PATHOLOGY

- Isolated, idiopathic, & congenital form is most common
- Additional anomalies in 24-50%
  - Myelomeningocele, arthrogryposis, myotonic dystrophy
  - Various syndromes (trisomies 18, 21)
- Association with intrauterine "packing disorders" (e.g., oligohydramnios, twinning)

CLINICAL ISSUES

- 50% are bilateral
- Treatment is primarily conservative with manipulation & casting; selective use of surgery

(Left) *Oblique graphic shows a clubfoot deformity with equinus, inversion, & forefoot adduction.* **(Right)** *Sagittal US through the lower leg of a 27-weeks-gestational age fetus with amniotic band syndrome shows abnormal positioning of the foot relative to the foreleg with the tibia ➔, fibula ➔, & all metatarsals ➔ visible in their long axes on a single image. This finding is consistent with clubfoot.*

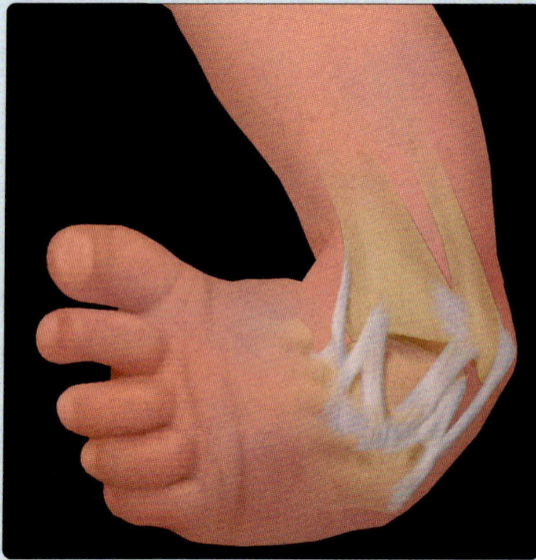

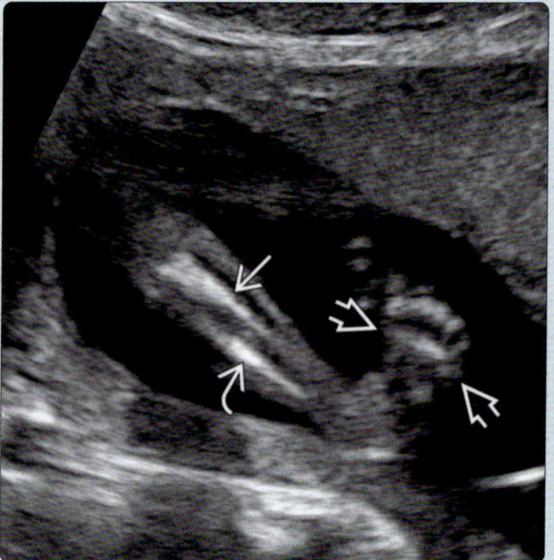

(Left) *AP radiograph in a 9-month-old with clubfoot shows hindfoot varus with a reduced talocalcaneal angle (black lines). There is varus angulation of the forefoot ➔ with the long axis of the talus ➔ far lateral to the 1st metatarsal & the long axis of the calcaneus ➔ lateral to the 5th metatarsal.* **(Right)** *Lateral view shows hindfoot varus with a reduced talocalcaneal angle (black lines). The angle between the long axes of the tibia ➔ & calcaneus ➔ is > 90° (hindfoot equinus). The inverted metatarsals ➔ appear parallel.*

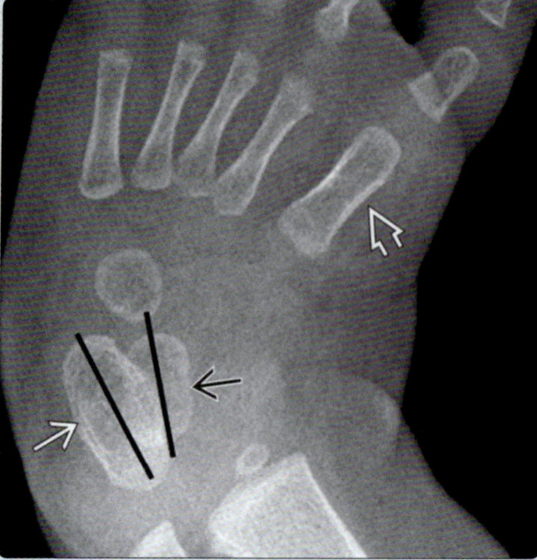

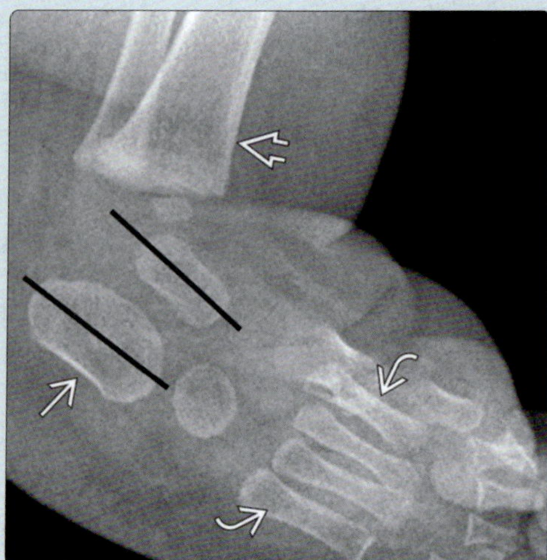

TERMINOLOGY

Abbreviations

- **C**avus, forefoot **a**dductus, hindfoot **v**arus, hindfoot **e**quinus (CAVE)

Synonyms

- Talipes equinovarus

Definitions

- Plantarflexion of calcaneus relative to tibia (equinus) + hindfoot inversion (varus) + forefoot adduction (varus)

IMAGING

General Features

- Best diagnostic clue
  - AP view: Hindfoot "points lateral" + adducted forefoot
    - Long axis of talus is very lateral to 1st metatarsal; long axis of calcaneus is lateral to 5th metatarsal

Radiographic Findings

- Measure on weight-bearing views (may be simulated)
- ↑ tibiocalcaneal angle (calcaneal equinus)
  - Lateral view: Normal 70-90°; > 90° in clubfoot
- ↓ talocalcaneal angle (hindfoot varus)
  - AP view: Normal 20-40°; ~ 0-10° in clubfoot
  - Lateral view: Normal 35-50°; ~ 10-20° in clubfoot
- ↑ talus-1st metatarsal angle (forefoot varus)
  - AP view: Normal 0-15°; ~ 20-40° in clubfoot
- Talus: Lateral rotation within ankle joint
  - Talus is point of reference for hindfoot
- Calcaneus: Relative medial rotation + equinus
- Navicular: Medial subluxation on talus
- Cuboid: Medial subluxation on calcaneus
- Metatarsals: Inverted, appearing parallel on lateral view

MR Findings

- Prenatal MR can detect clubfoot

Ultrasonographic Findings

- Prenatal
  - Affected foot is short, plantarflexed, bent medially
- Post natal
  - Dynamic visualization of unossified cartilage
  - Serial US to evaluate treatment response

DIFFERENTIAL DIAGNOSIS

Metatarsus Adductus

- Forefoot varus without other findings of clubfoot

Congenital Vertical Talus

- Talar plantarflexion with relative dorsal displacement of navicular + hindfoot equinus

Rocker-Bottom Foot

- Foot is foreshortened & convex ("Persian slipper")
- May be associated with clubfoot repair

Amniotic Band Syndrome

- Ranges from extremity ring constrictions (edema → fracture → amputation) to major craniofacial & visceral defects

Vertical Calcaneus in Myelodysplasia

- Imbalance of ankle/foot dorsi/plantar flexion → vertical calcaneal rotation

PATHOLOGY

General Features

- Etiology
  - Isolated: Idiopathic congenital is most common form
  - Additional anomalies: 24-50%
    - Neuromuscular etiologies: Myelomeningocele, arthrogryposis, myotonic dystrophy
    - Numerous syndromic associations
  - Intrauterine factors with ↑ risk: Intrauterine growth restriction, twinning, oligohydramnios, amniotic bands, 1st-trimester amniocentesis
  - Acquired/postnatal onset is seen in cerebral palsy (> 5 years)

CLINICAL ISSUES

Presentation

- Most common signs/symptoms
  - Hindfoot: Varus & equinus
  - Forefoot: Adduction
  - Stiffness: Ankle & foot
  - 50% are bilateral

Demographics

- Age: Most commonly congenital
- Sex: M:F = 2.5:1

Natural History & Prognosis

- Untreated → lateral weight-bearing → ↑ equinus & inversion → ↑ lateral column growth → ↑ deformity/stiffness

Treatment

- Goals: ↑ mobility, ↓ pain, ↓ stiffness
  - Nonsurgical: Birth to 12 months (better if earlier)
    - Ponseti method: Serial casting ± Achilles tenotomy
  - Surgery: Not primary therapy
    - Used in treatment-resistant cases & to correct posttreatment deformities

SELECTED REFERENCES

1. Brasseur-Daudruy M et al: Clubfoot versus positional foot deformities on prenatal ultrasound imaging. J Ultrasound Med. 39(3):615-23, 2020
2. Winfeld MJ et al: Management of pediatric foot deformities: an imaging review. Pediatr Radiol. 49(12):1678-90, 2019
3. Chawla S et al: Clinico-sonographical evaluation of idiopathic clubfoot and its correction by Ponseti method - A prospective study. Foot (Edinb). 33:7-13, 2017
4. Miron MC et al: Ultrasound evaluation of foot deformities in infants. Pediatr Radiol. 46(2):193-209; quiz 190-2, 2016
5. Faldini C et al: Congenital idiopathic talipes equinovarus before and after walking age: observations and strategy of treatment from a series of 88 cases. J Orthop Traumatol. 17(1):81-7, 2015
6. Moon DK et al: Soft-tissue abnormalities associated with treatment-resistant and treatment-responsive clubfoot: Findings of MRI Analysis. J Bone Joint Surg Am. 96(15):1249-56, 2014
7. Horn BD et al: Current treatment of clubfoot in infancy and childhood. Foot Ankle Clin. 15(2):235-43, 2010
8. Uglow MG et al: Residual clubfoot in children. Foot Ankle Clin. 15(2):245-64, 2010

Discoid Meniscus

KEY FACTS

IMAGING

- Modality of choice: MR
  - Sagittal images with confirmation on coronal data sets
    - Sagittal: Evaluate periphery
      - Complete "bow ties" on ≥ 3 consecutive images (with 4- to 5-mm slices) are suggestive
    - Coronal: Central images are key
      - > 50% coverage of unilateral tibial plateau
      - > 13- to 14-mm transverse width
      - ≥ 2 mm in height > medial meniscus
  - Frequent linear or amorphous ↑ intrameniscal signal (intermediate to hyperintense on PD, T2, or T2* GRE) in slab-like meniscus
    - Difficult to determine if intrameniscal signal indicates tear, vascularity, mucoid degeneration, or cyst

PATHOLOGY

- Watanabe classification
  - Complete discoid meniscus: Stable
    - Extends into intercondylar notch on coronal images
  - Incomplete: Stable
    - No extension into intercondylar notch
  - Wrisberg ligament type: Unstable, hypermobile
    - Lacks posterior meniscal attachments

CLINICAL ISSUES

- Most commonly asymptomatic in children
  - Symptoms may not develop until adolescence or later
  - Snapping knee syndrome: Wrisberg type
    - < 10 years old
    - Snaps in flexion & extension
  - Symptomatic in older children from tears or unstable variant: Locking, pain, clicking
- Treatment
  - Asymptomatic: Typically observe, no surgical treatment
  - Symptomatic: Saucerization & repair
    - Arthroscopic goal: Width of peripheral rim remaining at 5-8 mm

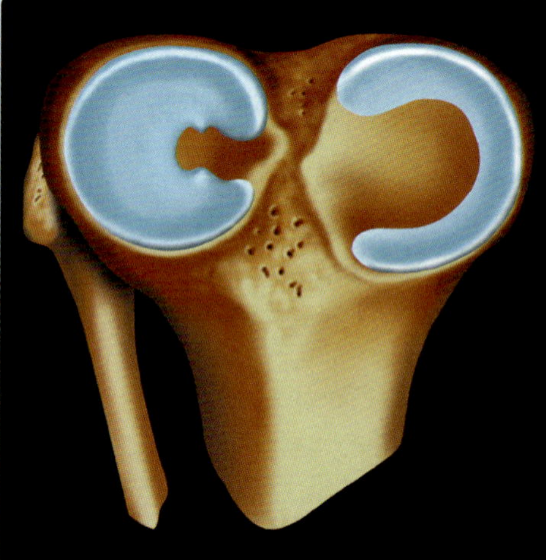

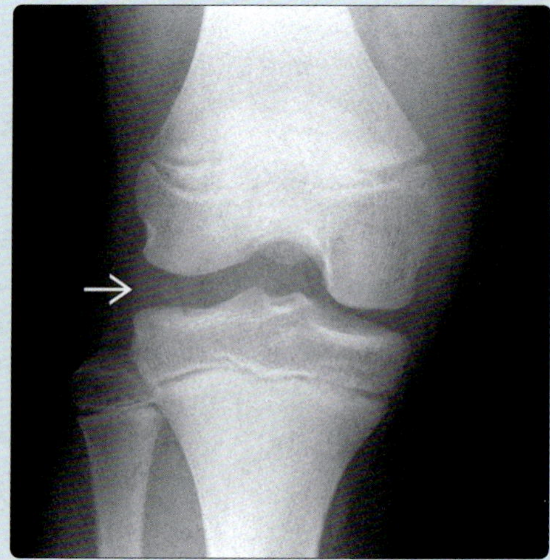

(Left) *Graphic shows a discoid lateral meniscus with minimal resorption of the central portion & > 50% coverage of the lateral tibial plateau surface.* **(Right)** *AP standing radiograph in a child with knee popping/clicking shows widening of the lateral joint compartment ➡. There is cupping of the lateral tibial plateau. This appearance proved to be a discoid lateral meniscus on MR & subsequent arthroscopy.*

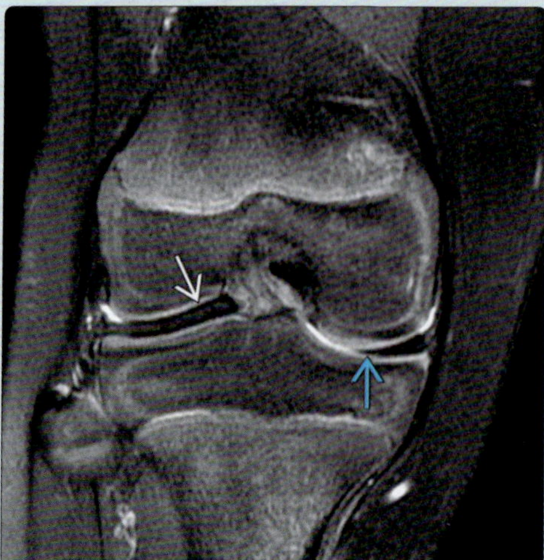

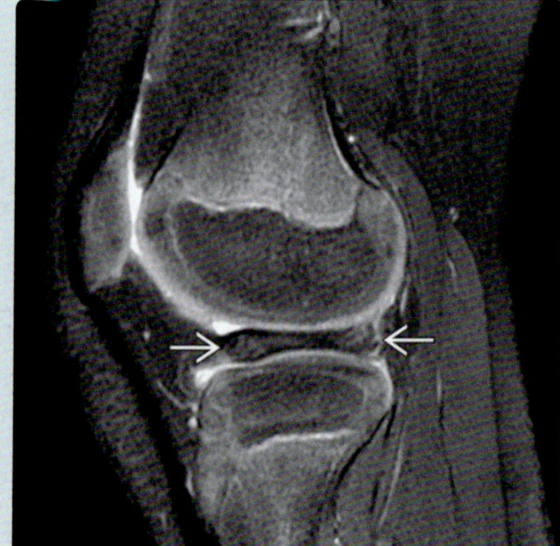

(Left) *Coronal T2 FS MR in an 8-year-old with knee pain & popping after playing basketball shows a complete discoid lateral meniscus ➡. Note the slab-like appearance with the lack of tapering of the inner margin of the lateral meniscus compared to the normal tapering of the medial meniscus ➡.* **(Right)** *Sagittal T2 FS MR in the same child shows the slab-like appearance of the discoid lateral meniscus ➡. Note the internally ↑ signal intensity in the meniscus on both images.*

TERMINOLOGY

Definitions

- Large, congenitally dysplastic meniscus with loss of normal semilunar shape

IMAGING

General Features

- Best diagnostic clue
  - Continuity of anterior & posterior horns on ≥ 3 consecutive MR sagittal images (with 4- to 5-mm slices)
    - Central meniscal portion covers > 50% of articular surface of lateral tibial plateau
    - Loss of normal semilunar morphology
- Location
  - Lateral > > medial discoid meniscus
  - Bilateral: 20-50%
- Size
  - ≥ 2 mm in craniocaudal height > medial meniscus
  - > 13-14 mm in transverse dimension on central coronal cross section (for both partial & complete discoid meniscus)
    - Normal: 5-13 mm from capsular margin to free edge on central coronal image
  - Ratio of minimal meniscal width to maximal tibial width of ≥ 20% on coronal image
- Morphology
  - Large slab/pancake-like complete discoid meniscus
  - Partial discoid meniscus tapers centrally

Radiographic Findings

- Discoid lateral meniscus
  - Normal radiographs in most
  - Widened lateral joint space (best on weight-bearing view)
  - High fibular head
  - Hypoplastic or squared femoral condyle
    - Condylar cutoff sign: ↓ prominence of lateral condyle adjacent to intercondylar notch on tunnel view (with complete discoid meniscus)
  - Hypoplastic lateral tibial spine
  - Cupping of lateral tibial plateau

MR Findings

- Continuous body with continuity of anterior & posterior horns ("bow ties") on ≥ 3 consecutive sagittal images (with 4- to 5-mm thick slices)
- Transverse meniscal dimension ("width") > 13-14 mm in cross section on central coronal image
  - Normal hypointense meniscus: 5-13 mm from capsular margin to free edge on central coronal image
- Complete discoid meniscus has pancake-like appearance (does not taper medially)
  - Hypointense, slab-like meniscus
  - Extending from intercondylar notch to periphery of compartment
- Partial discoid meniscus: Tapers centrally but too wide & tall peripherally
  - ≥ 2 mm in craniocaudal height > medial meniscus
- Frequent linear or amorphous ↑ intrameniscal signal (intermediate to hyperintense on PD, T2, or T2* GRE)
  - Difficult to determine if intrameniscal signal indicates tear, vascularity, mucoid degeneration, or cyst
    - Within substance of meniscus (intrameniscal tear) vs. extending to articular surface (tear)
      - Extensive signal abnormality may reflect tear
    - Discoid menisci are prone to more complex tears
- Prominent ligament of Wrisberg
- May see cord-like intermeniscal ligament
- MR arthrography may have role in distinguishing articular surface meniscal tear from intrameniscal tear
  - If contrast extends into meniscus: Articular surface tear
  - If contrast does not enter meniscus: Intrameniscal tear, cyst, or degeneration
- Advanced cartilage techniques (e.g., T2 mapping) can look at articular cartilage degeneration before/after discoid meniscus repair

Ultrasonographic Findings

- New literature supporting sonographic criteria for diagnosis of discoid meniscus
  - Anterior & posterior meniscus angles, meniscal body angle

Imaging Recommendations

- Best imaging tool
  - MR is modality of choice
  - MR sagittal images are suggestive with confirmation on coronal data sets
    - Coronal images are most accurate

DIFFERENTIAL DIAGNOSIS

Vacuum Phenomenon

- ↓ signal intensity in joint between weight-bearing surfaces
- Rarely homogeneous like discoid meniscus

Flipped Meniscus

- Abnormal morphology to "donor site" of torn meniscus
  - Portions of meniscus are missing, allowing distinction from discoid meniscus
  - < 2 "bow ties" on consecutive sagittal images (4- to 5-mm slices)
- Displaced meniscal fragment may be found in various locations
  - May lie along other portions of meniscus, creating abnormally thick/tall appearance focally

Bucket-Handle Tear

- Longitudinal vertical peripheral tear with displacement of meniscal fragment into intercondylar notch
  - Displaced fragment remains continuous with nondisplaced torn meniscus at anterior & posterior horns
- Double posterior cruciate ligament (PCL) sign
  - Displaced meniscal fragment anterior to PCL creates appearance of 2 PCLs
- Foreshortened, truncated, & abnormal-sized meniscus on sagittal images
  - < 2 "bow ties" on consecutive sagittal images (4- to 5-mm slices)

Osteochondritis Dissecans/Osteochondral Lesion

- Focal ovoid irregularity/defect of subchondral femoral condyle

- ± fissuring with fluid undercutting lesion, cystic change, surrounding marrow edema
- ± detached osteochondral fragment in joint space
- Most common at lateral aspect of medial femoral condyle
- May be due to acute trauma or repetitive microtrauma

PATHOLOGY

General Features

- Etiology
  - Failure of fetal discoid meniscal form to involute
    - Derived from mesenchyme that is initially disc-shaped then forms semilunar shape

Staging, Grading, & Classification

- Watanabe classification
  - Complete discoid meniscus (type 1)
    - Stable
    - Covers > 80% of unilateral tibial plateau on coronal image
    - Extending into intercondylar notch on coronal images (fills entire lateral compartment)
  - Incomplete (type 2)
    - Stable
    - Covers ≤ 80% of unilateral tibial plateau on coronal image
    - Does not extend into intercondylar notch on coronal images
  - Wrisberg type (type 3)
    - Unstable
    - Least common
    - Lacks posterior meniscal attachments
    - Hypermobile, can extend into intercondylar notch with knee extension

Gross Pathologic & Surgical Features

- Pancake-like or large, otherwise normal-appearing meniscus in lateral > > medial compartment
- Wrisberg-type discoid meniscus lacks posterior meniscotibial attachment
- More prone to tears
  - Due to meniscal thickness & mechanical relationships
  - Most common: Horizontal cleavage tear
- Peripheral rim instability patterns
  - 28% of discoid lateral meniscus patients at arthroscopy → requires repair
  - Most commonly involves anterior 1/3 of meniscus

CLINICAL ISSUES

Presentation

- Most common signs/symptoms
  - Often asymptomatic in children (most common), especially < 10 years of age
  - Snapping knee syndrome may be seen < 10 years
    - Snap in flexion & extension due to displacing meniscus
      - Wrisberg type
    - Virtually pathognomic for discoid lateral meniscus
  - Symptomatic in older children from tears or unstable variant
    - Patients often present with pain, clicking, & snapping
    - Locking is common in children
    - Recurrence of knee "giving way"
    - Lateral joint line tenderness
    - Effusion
- Other signs/symptoms
  - McMurray & Apley grinding test may have pain & audible snap or click

Treatment

- Asymptomatic: Debatable, but most observe without surgical treatment
- Symptomatic: Arthroscopic partial central meniscectomy (i.e., saucerization)
  - Stabilization to capsule if unstable
  - Repair tear if present
- Attempt to leave peripheral rim width of 5-8 mm
- Case reports of meniscal regrowth after repair

DIAGNOSTIC CHECKLIST

Consider

- Displaced meniscal tear may cause same symptoms

Image Interpretation Pearls

- Sagittal images: ≥ 3 consecutive images show "bow tie" configuration → think discoid meniscus
- Coronal images: Slab-like shape with meniscus not tapering centrally toward intercondylar notch
- Meniscus displacement & deformation → ↑ risk of tear
  - True tears of discoid meniscus may be difficult to diagnose on MR

SELECTED REFERENCES

1. Nishino K et al: Magnetic resonance imaging T2 relaxation times of articular cartilage before and after arthroscopic surgery for discoid lateral meniscus. Arthroscopy. 37(2):647-54, 2021
2. Tyler PA et al: Update on imaging of the discoid meniscus. Skeletal Radiol. ePub, 2021
3. Yang SJ et al: A reliable, ultrasound-based method for the diagnosis of discoid lateral meniscus. Arthroscopy. 37(3):882-90, 2021
4. Restrepo R et al: Discoid meniscus in the pediatric population: emphasis on MR imaging signs of instability. Magn Reson Imaging Clin N Am. 27(2):323-39, 2019
5. Park YB et al: Prediction models to improve the diagnostic value of plain radiographs in children with complete discoid lateral meniscus. Arthroscopy. 34(2):479-489.e3, 2018
6. Ha CW et al: The utility of the radiographic condylar cut-off sign in children and adolescents with complete discoid lateral meniscus. Knee Surg Sports Traumatol Arthrosc. 25(12):3862-8, 2017
7. Choi SH et al: Do the radiographic findings of symptomatic discoid lateral meniscus in children differ from normal control subjects? Knee Surg Sports Traumatol Arthrosc. 23(4):1128-34, 2015
8. Kushare I et al: Discoid meniscus: diagnosis and management. Orthop Clin North Am. 46(4):533-40, 2015
9. Song JG et al: Radiographic evaluation of complete and incomplete discoid lateral meniscus. Knee. 22(3):163-8, 2015
10. Yoo WJ et al: Meniscal morphologic changes on magnetic resonance imaging are associated with symptomatic discoid lateral meniscal tear in children. Arthroscopy. 28(3):330-6, 2012
11. Ha CW et al: The condylar cutoff sign: quantifying lateral femoral condylar hypoplasia in a complete discoid meniscus. Clin Orthop Relat Res. 467(5):1365-9, 2009
12. Yaniv M et al: The discoid meniscus. J Child Orthop. 1(2):89-96, 2007
13. Samoto N et al: Diagnosis of discoid lateral meniscus of the knee on MR imaging. Magn Reson Imaging. 20(1):59-64, 2002

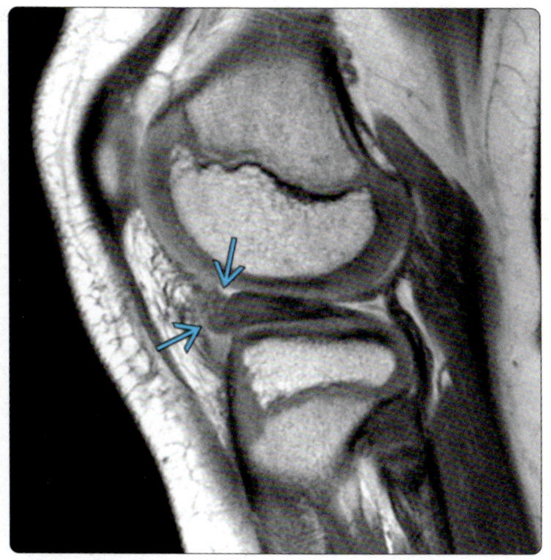

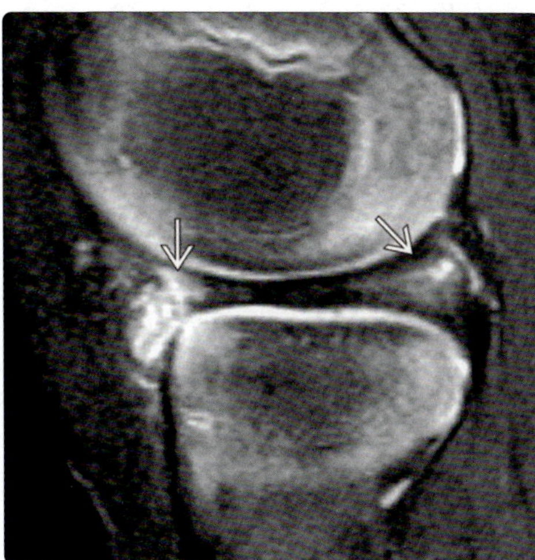

(Left) *Sagittal PD MR of the knee in a 9-year-old with a Wrisberg variant of a discoid meniscus shows anterior buckling of the meniscus ⇒. At arthroscopy, no posterior capsular attachment of the discoid lateral meniscus was found.* **(Right)** *Sagittal T2 FS MR shows hyperintense signal within the anterior & posterior horns of this discoid lateral meniscus ➡. The meniscus was found to be degenerated & torn at arthroscopy.*

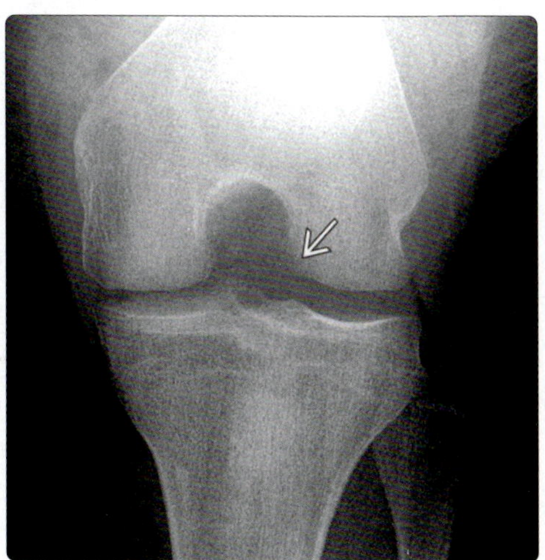

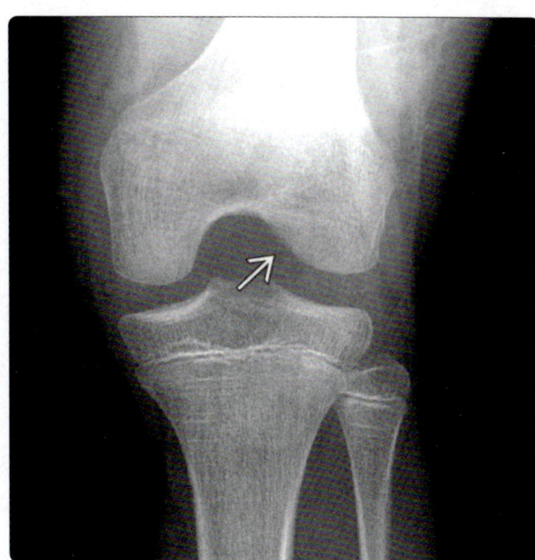

(Left) *Tunnel radiograph of the knee shows a normal prominence of the medial margin of the lateral femoral condyle ➡ adjacent to the intercondylar notch in a patient without a discoid meniscus.* **(Right)** *Tunnel radiograph in a 9-year-old with a discoid lateral meniscus shows ↓ prominence of the lateral femoral condyle, the positive cutoff sign ➡. This child had undergone a discoid lateral meniscus repair on the contralateral knee in the past.*

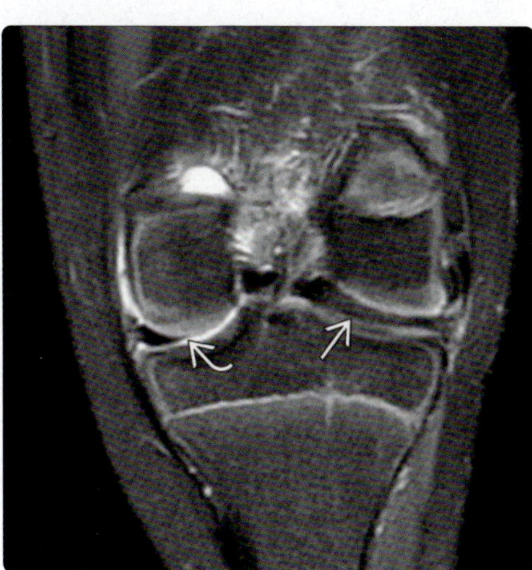

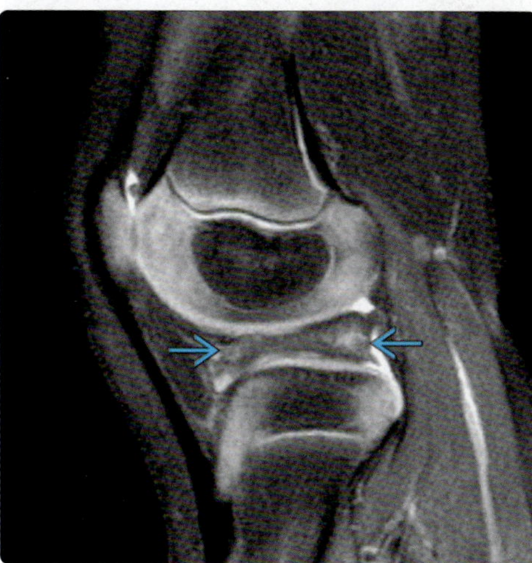

(Left) *Coronal T2 FS MR of the left knee in the same patient shows a complete discoid lateral meniscus ➡. Note the slab-like appearance of the meniscus covering the entire lateral tibial plateau with the lack of tapering of the meniscal inner margin (as compared to the normal tapering of the medial meniscus ➡).* **(Right)** *Sagittal T2 FS MR in a 3-year-old with pain, clicking, & popping shows enlargement of a discoid lateral meniscus with internal hyperintense signal ⇒. A radial tear was found at arthroscopy.*

Physeal Fractures

KEY FACTS

TERMINOLOGY

- Fracture of immature skeleton involving cartilaginous primary growth plate (physis)

IMAGING

- Most are detected & managed by radiographs alone
  - Widening or interruption of normally uniform, undulating lucent physis
  - Translation &/or angulation of bony fragment adjacent to physis with overlying soft tissue swelling
  - Persistent physeal widening > 3 mm post reduction suggests tissue entrapment requiring open reduction
- CT: Helps evaluate comminution, displacement, articular surface step-off, loose intraarticular fragment(s)
- MR: Can detect nondisplaced fractures, assess cartilaginous & soft tissue injury or entrapment

TOP DIFFERENTIAL DIAGNOSES

- Incomplete fracture
- Chronic physeal stress injury
- Rickets
- Osteomyelitis

CLINICAL ISSUES

- Peak age: 11-12 years
- 6-30% of childhood fractures involve physis
- Overall complication rate: ~ 14% (but varies by site)
  - Premature physeal closure with limb shortening or angulation
    - Growth disturbance risk is highest in distal femur, tibia
  - Joint incongruity due to intraarticular extension → degenerative arthritis
  - Osteomyelitis (particularly with nailbed injury)

DIAGNOSTIC CHECKLIST

- Always evaluate involved growth plate for premature closure on follow-up studies

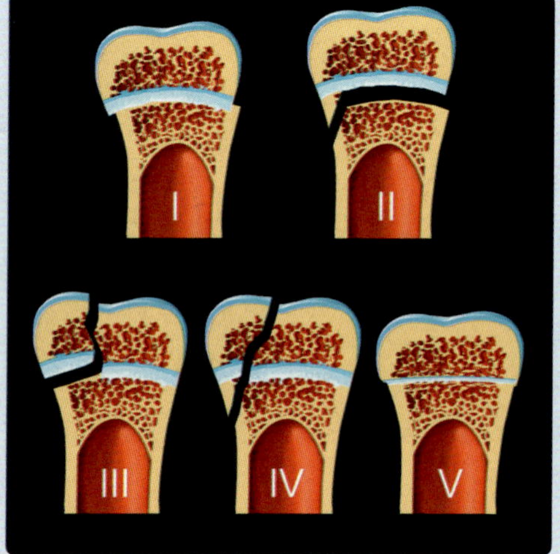

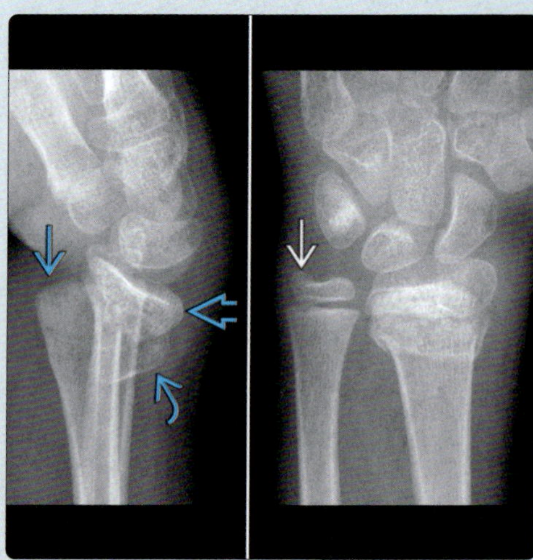

(Left) *Graphic shows the relationship of the epiphyseal, physeal, & metaphyseal components of the 5 classic Salter-Harris (SH) fractures. (SH V is a crush injury to the physis, quite uncommon.)* **(Right)** *Lateral (left) & PA (right) radiographs in a 9-year-old show an SH II fracture of the distal radius with ~ 60% dorsal translation of the epiphyseal ➔ & metaphyseal ➔ fracture fragments with ~ 45° apex volar angulation. Note the uncovering of the volar metaphysis ➔. Also note the nondisplaced ulnar styloid fracture ➔.*

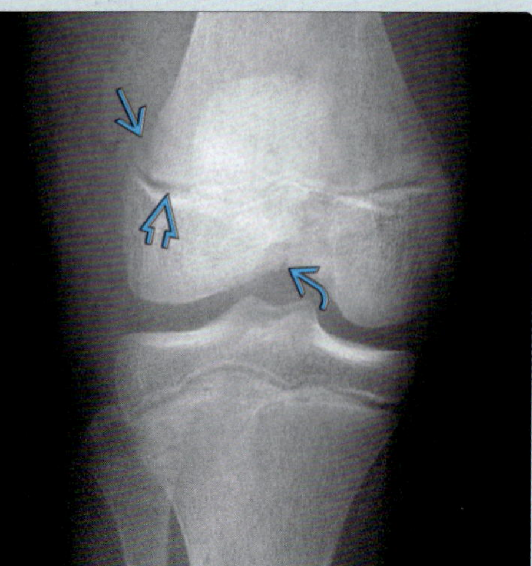

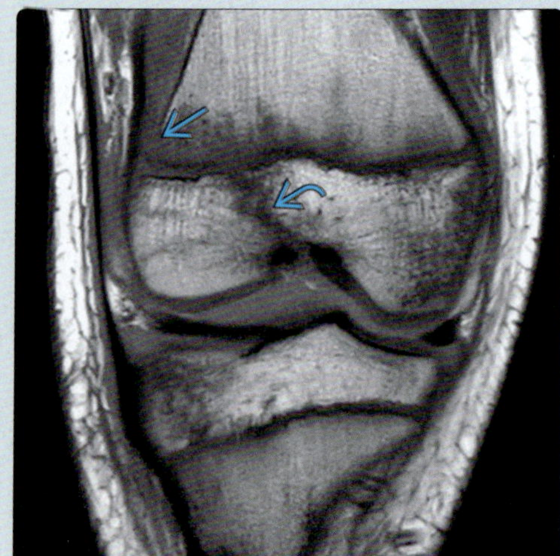

(Left) *Frontal radiograph of the right knee in a 13-year-old boy with a knee injury shows a very subtle SH IV fracture with a lateral metaphyseal component ➔, mild widening of the lateral physis ➔, & a more central fracture line extending through the epiphysis to the intercondylar notch ➔.* **(Right)** *Coronal T1 MR in the same child better shows the metaphyseal ➔ & epiphyseal ➔ components of the fracture.*

TERMINOLOGY

Synonyms

- Salter-Harris (SH) fractures 1-5 (I-V)

Definitions

- Fracture of immature skeleton involving cartilaginous primary growth plate (physis)

IMAGING

General Features

- Best diagnostic clue
  - Widening or interruption of normally uniform, undulating lucent physis
  - Translation/angulation of bony fragment adjacent to physis with overlying soft tissue swelling
- Location
  - Upper extremity
    - Distal radius: 28-50%
    - Phalanges: 26%
    - Distal humerus: 7-17%
    - Proximal radius: 5%
    - Distal ulna: 5%
    - Metacarpals: 4%
    - Proximal humerus: 2%
  - Lower extremity
    - Distal tibia: 9-11%
    - Phalanges: 7%
    - Distal fibula: 3%
    - Metatarsals: 1%
    - Proximal tibia: 1%
    - Distal femur: 1-5%

Radiographic Findings

- Upon presentation
  - Partial or complete physeal widening with metaphyseal &/or epiphyseal fracture lines
  - Varying degrees of translation &/or angulation of distal fragments
    - Thurstan Holland fragment: Metaphyseal fragment (often triangular) separated from parent bone by SH II or IV fractures
      - Remains attached to physis & travels with displaced epiphysis
      - Quite variable in size
  - Overlying soft tissue edema
- Immediately after reduction
  - Persistent physeal widening > 3 mm suggests entrapment requiring open reduction
    - Overlying periosteum is most common
    - Adjacent ligament or tendon
    - Bony fragment from comminution
- Long-term follow-up
  - Evaluate affected physis for premature closure

CT Findings

- Bone CT
  - Helps evaluate comminution, displacement, articular surface step-off, loose intraarticular fragment(s)
    - ≥ 2-mm articular surface gap or step-off generally requires open reduction + internal fixation

MR Findings

- T1WI
  - Low signal intensity fracture line
- T2WI FS
  - High signal intensity fracture line due to fluid
  - Surrounding marrow & soft tissue edema
  - Elevation of loose metadiaphyseal periosteum by subperiosteal hemorrhage
  - Low signal intensity periosteum, ligament, or tendon is rarely entrapped in fracture
- STIR
  - Similar to T2 FS (both are fluid-sensitive sequences)
- T2* GRE
  - Cartilage-sensitive sequence
  - Most useful in chronic setting to detect growth arrest (physeal bar/bridge) due to prior injury
- MR may alter clinical management in acute setting by
  - Detecting nondisplaced fractures
  - Visualizing fracture relationship to radiolucent cartilage (changing fracture classification)
  - Visualizing entrapped structures (requiring open reduction)
  - Visualizing adjacent neurovascular injury
- MR can alter clinical management of long-term complications by
  - Detecting & quantifying bone bridges
  - Detecting degenerative changes

Ultrasonographic Findings

- Useful in neonates/infants/toddlers with limited ossification of epiphyses
- May visualize displacement of cartilaginous epiphyses, physeal &/or cortical interruption, &/or subperiosteal fluid
- Sonographic comparison of contralateral side is helpful

Imaging Recommendations

- Best imaging tool
  - Typically detected & managed by radiographs alone
  - CT & MR have limited indications
- Protocol advice
  - Opposite side comparison radiographs may help (particularly for SH I)
  - Fluid-sensitive sequences are critical if MR is requested

DIFFERENTIAL DIAGNOSIS

Incomplete Fracture

- Cortical buckle deformity of metadiaphysis shows no fracture line extension to physis

Chronic Physeal Stress Injury

- Partially or completely widened physis mimics nondisplaced SH I fracture
  - Interruption of endochondral ossification results in persistence of growth cartilage without fracture
- Metaphyseal irregularity & sclerosis
- Chronic pain in adolescent high-level athletes

Epiphysiodesis

- Extremity may show physeal widening & irregularity after drilling

- Sometimes performed to halt growth in setting of growth arrest of contralateral long bone from remote insult (therefore preventing limb length discrepancy)

Rickets

- Variety of metabolic abnormalities can inhibit endochondral ossification with physeal widening
- Multiple physes are symmetrically involved
- Classic rickets has metaphyseal fraying, cupping, widening, & loss of zone of provisional calcification (ZPC)

Osteomyelitis

- Commonly affects metaphysis in children
- Soft tissue abnormalities precede bony radiographic findings
  - Permeative lytic bone destruction &/or periosteal reaction after 10 days
  - May cause physeal widening
- Pathologic fracture may result

PATHOLOGY

General Features

- Etiology
  - Structure of normal physis
    - Germinal zone (closest to epiphysis): Small active chondrocytes emerge from resting chondrocytes
    - Proliferative zone: Chondrocytes rapidly dividing; arranged in columns
    - Hypertrophic zone: Chondrocytes undergo hypertrophy; arranged in columns
    - ZPC (closest to metaphysis): Chondrocytes undergo apoptosis, cartilage matrix calcifies, osteoblasts form osteoid
- Associated abnormalities
  - ± injuries of neurovascular bundle, ligaments, cartilage, other bones
    - Depends on mechanism, fracture location, fracture type, & degree of displacement

Staging, Grading, & Classification

- Type I (~ 8.5%): Involves only physis
- Type II (~ 73%): Involves physis & metaphysis
- Type III (~ 6.5%): Involves physis & epiphysis
- Type IV (~ 12%): Involves physis, metaphysis, & epiphysis
- Type V (< 1%): Crush fracture involving physis
  - Usually recognized when cone epiphyses or partial physeal arrest becomes apparent later
- Types VI-IX, as described by Ogden 1981
  - Infrequently used classification

CLINICAL ISSUES

Presentation

- Most common signs/symptoms
  - Pain, swelling, point tenderness, limited range of motion, inability to bear weight

Demographics

- Peak age: 11-12 years
- Sex: Skeletal maturity occurs earlier in girls than in boys
  - Mean age of physeal injuries is 1-2 years earlier in girls
- Epidemiology: Up to 30% of childhood fractures involve physis; likely underestimated if based only on initial exam

Natural History & Prognosis

- Overall complication rate ~ 15%
  - Premature physeal closure with limb shortening or angulation
    - Much more common in lower than upper extremities (regardless of SH type)
      - 40-90% of distal femur, 25% of proximal tibia, 5-50% of distal tibia physeal fractures
      - 5-7% of distal radial physeal fractures
    - 2x as likely in displaced vs. nondisplaced fractures
  - Joint incongruity due to articular surface involvement → degenerative arthritis
    - Up to 29% of SH III or IV ankle injuries
  - Osteomyelitis with adjacent nailbed trauma ("stubbed toe osteomyelitis") or penetrating injury

Treatment

- Closed reduction & casting for low SH categories (unless unstable post reduction)
  - < 2-mm displacement → ↓ risk of growth arrest
  - Follow-up at 5-7 days to ensure stability
- Open reduction & internal fixation is often required with higher categories (due to articular surface involvement)
- Subsequent bone bridges → angular deformities or limb length discrepancies → bone bridge resection vs. contralateral epiphysiodesis

DIAGNOSTIC CHECKLIST

Consider

- Always evaluate involved growth plate for premature closure on follow-up studies
  - Follow-up of physeal injuries is prolonged due to risk of growth disturbances

Reporting Tips

- Include type, direction, & magnitude of displacement
  - Translation (including shortening & distraction), angulation, & rotation
- Presence of physeal &/or articular extension

SELECTED REFERENCES

1. Jalkanen J et al: Physeal fractures of distal tibia: a systematic review and meta-analysis. J Pediatr Orthop. ePub, 2021
2. Khan H et al: What are the risk factors and presenting features of premature physeal arrest of the distal radius? A systematic review. Eur J Orthop Surg Traumatol. 31(5):893-900, 2021
3. Nguyen JC et al: Imaging of pediatric growth plate disturbances. Radiographics. 37(6):1791-812, 2017
4. Chen J et al: Imaging appearance of entrapped periosteum within a distal femoral Salter-Harris II fracture. Skeletal Radiol. 44(10):1547-51, 2015
5. Mayer S et al: Pediatric knee dislocations and physeal fractures about the knee. J Am Acad Orthop Surg. 23(9):571-80, 2015
6. Abzug JM et al: Physeal arrest of the distal radius. J Am Acad Orthop Surg. 22(6):381-9, 2014
7. Little JT et al: Pediatric distal forearm and wrist injury: an imaging review. Radiographics. 34(2):472-90, 2014
8. Fassier A et al: Fractures in children younger than 18 months. Orthop Traumatol Surg Res. 99(1 Suppl):S160-70, 2013
9. Gufler H et al: MRI for occult physeal fracture detection in children and adolescents. Acta Radiol. 54(4):467-72, 2013
10. Laor T et al: Physeal widening in the knee due to stress injury in child athletes. AJR Am J Roentgenol. 186(5):1260-4, 2006

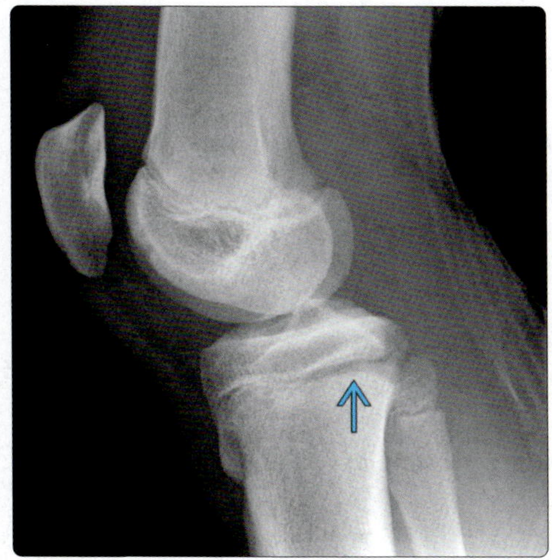

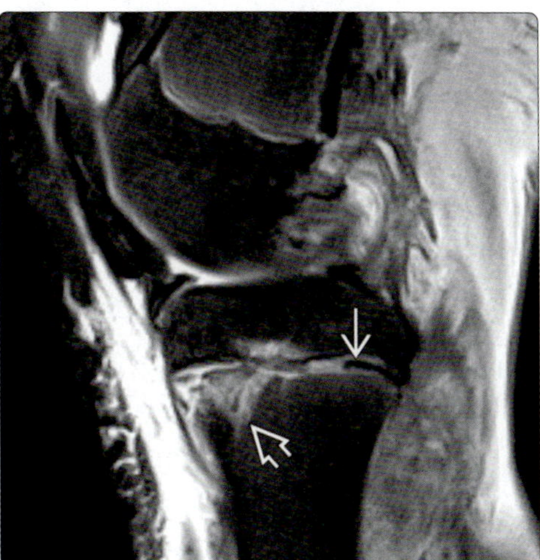

(Left) *Lateral radiograph in a 15-year-old with pain from a gymnastics injury shows widening of the posterior physis of the proximal tibia* ⇨. **(Right)** *Sagittal T2 FS MR in the same patient shows low signal intensity periosteum* ➡ *trapped in the widened physis. The metaphyseal components of an SH II fracture are present anteriorly* ➡*. Subsequent growth arrest is more likely when periosteal entrapment occurs.*

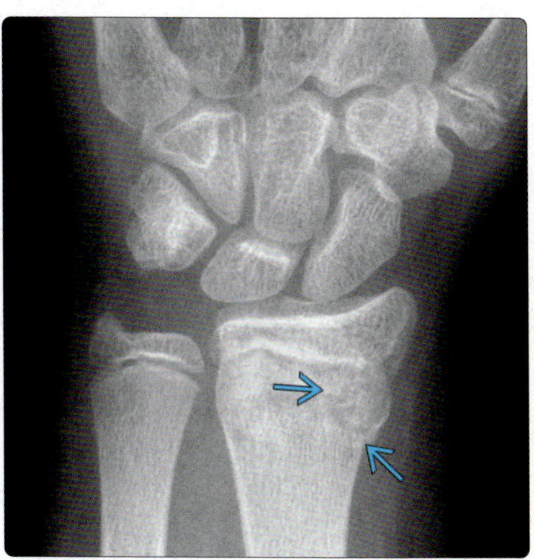

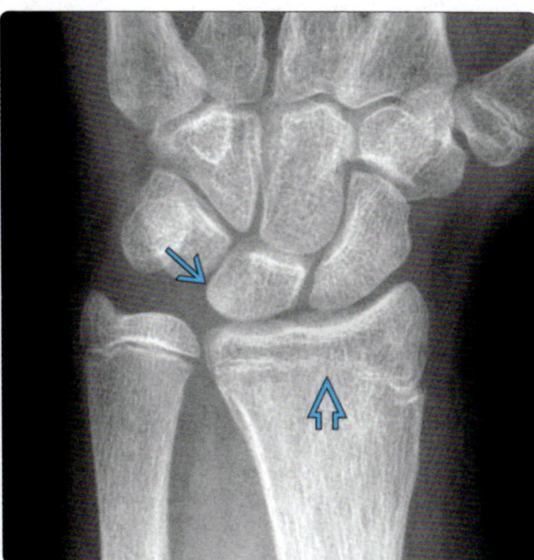

(Left) *Frontal radiograph in a 12-year-old girl with a right wrist injury shows an acute SH II fracture of the distal radius* ⇨. **(Right)** *Frontal radiograph in the same girl 2 years later shows the development of a distal radial physeal bridge* ⇨*. The growth arrest in the radius has lead to ulnar positive variance with associated ulnocarpal impaction, evidenced by the sclerosis in the proximal lunate* ⇨*. MR (not shown) confirmed lunate marrow edema with cartilage & TFCC injury.*

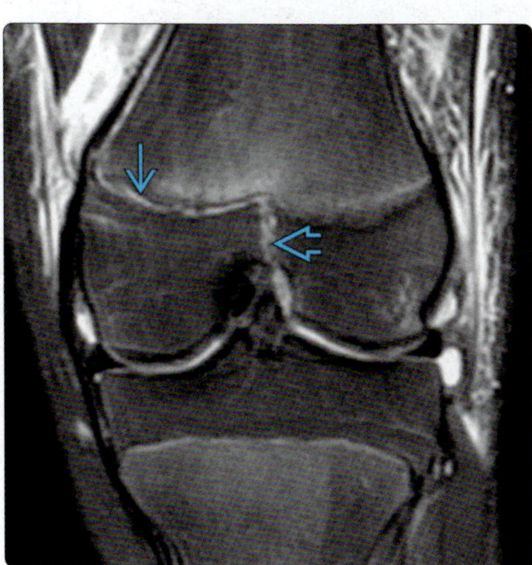

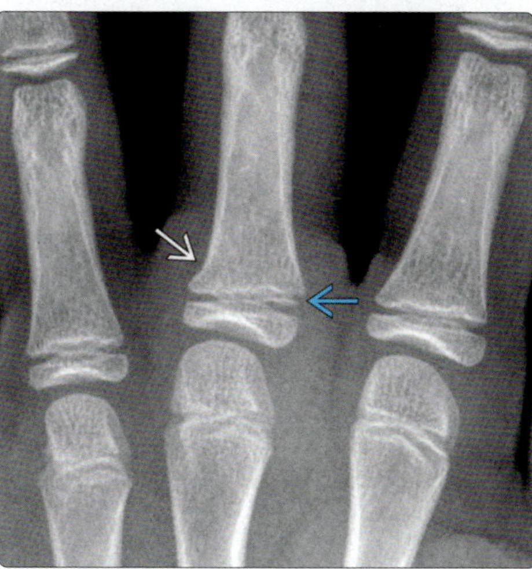

(Left) *Coronal T2 FS MR in a 12-year-old shows an SH III fracture of the distal femur with vertical intraarticular epiphyseal* ⇨ *& horizontal medial physeal* ⇨ *components. These fractures can be radiographically occult.* **(Right)** *PA radiograph of the hand in a 10-year-old shows slightly ↑ angulation of the ulnar-sided cortex* ➡ *of the middle finger proximal phalanx. A metaphyseal fragment* ⇨ *confirms an SH II fracture.*

Apophyseal Injuries

KEY FACTS

TERMINOLOGY

- Apophysis: Nonarticular secondary center of ossification that serves as attachment site for muscle or tendon
  - Considered epiphyseal equivalent
- Acute injury: Avulsion fracture of osseous &/or cartilaginous apophysis through subjacent physis
- Chronic injury: Repetitive submaximal tensile forces (avulsive microtrauma) exceed rate of repair, leading to local growth plate disturbance (± symptoms)

IMAGING

- Acute injury: Displaced apophyseal ossification center
- Chronic injury: Soft tissue swelling with ossific irregularity at tendon attachment site
- Radiographs are usually diagnostic of acute avulsion
- Further imaging may be required if fragment is nondisplaced, ossification center is not yet present, or chronic apophysitis is suspected
  - MR is more sensitive & specific than US

TOP DIFFERENTIAL DIAGNOSES

- Osteomyelitis
- Ewing sarcoma
- Muscle injury
- Stress injury of bone

CLINICAL ISSUES

- Acute injury: Sudden onset of pain with sensation of pop & instant ↓ in muscle function during athletic activity
- Chronic injury: Insidious onset of pain & swelling without specific event or associated bruising
- Majority of acute pelvic avulsions occur from ages 12-18 years; mean of 13.8-15.2 years
  - Most occur during kicking, sprinting, or jumping
  - AIIS, ASIS, ischial tuberosity > iliac crest, pubic symphysis
- Conservative (nonsurgical) therapy: Highly successful
  - Complications (nonunion, heterotopic ossification, chronic pain) are uncommon
- Surgical fixation is reserved for displacement > 1.5-2.0 cm

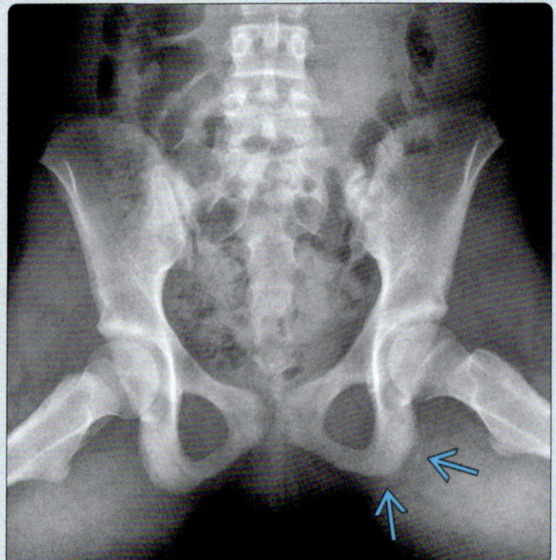

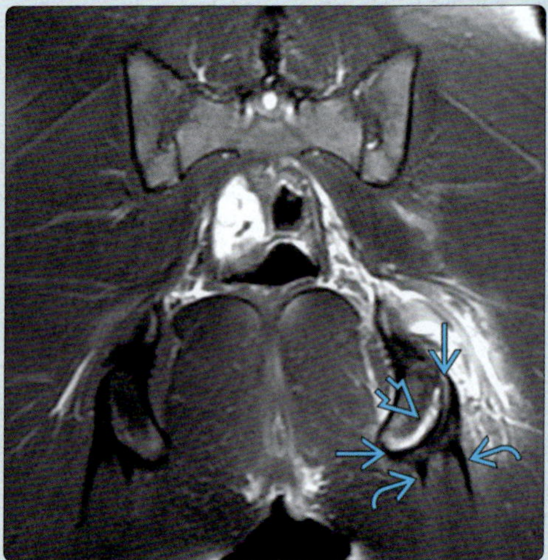

(Left) *Frog leg lateral radiograph in a 13-year-old girl with acute onset of left hip pain & sensation of a pop during cheerleading shows displaced bony fragments ➡ adjacent to the left ischial tuberosity.* **(Right)** *Coronal T2 FS MR in the same patient shows the attachments of the hamstring tendons ➡ to the displaced curvilinear osteocartilaginous apophysis ➡ at the ischial tuberosity. Fluid ➡ undercuts the displaced fragment, typical of an acute avulsion injury.*

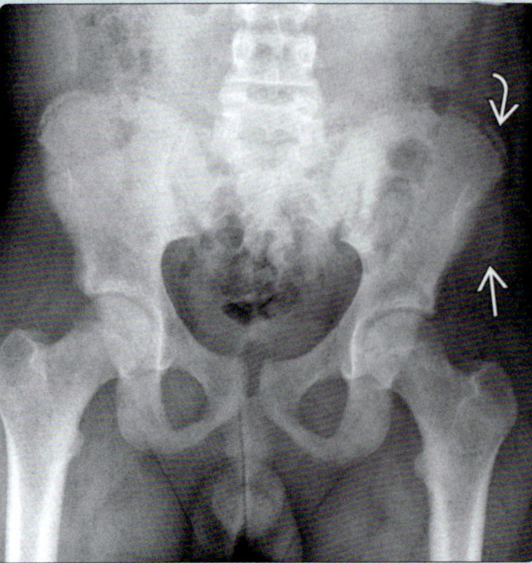

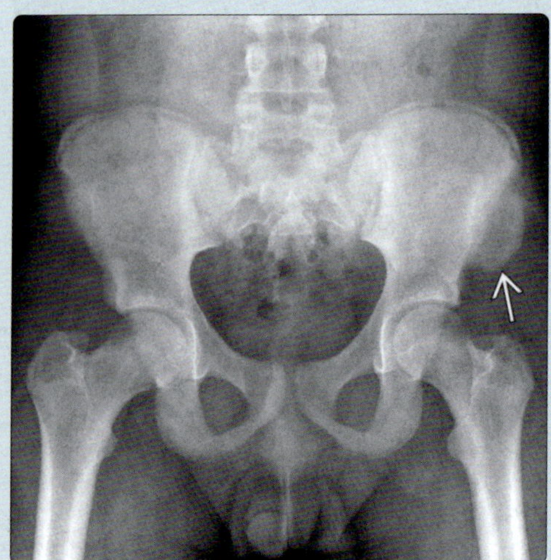

(Left) *AP radiograph in a 16-year-old boy with a history of pain & a pop while kicking a ball shows an inferiorly displaced bony fragment ➡ that was avulsed from the anterior superior iliac spine (ASIS). The lateral left iliac wing apophysis ➡ also shows fragmentation & growth plate widening, suggesting an additional avulsion component.* **(Right)** *AP radiograph in the same patient 3 months later shows progressive healing at the site of injury with callus now seen between the fragment & underlying iliac bone ➡.*

TERMINOLOGY

Synonyms

- Acute injury: Avulsion fracture
- Chronic injury: Apophysitis, physeal stress fracture, osteochondrosis, various eponyms specific to site

Definitions

- Apophysis: Nonarticular secondary center of ossification that serves as attachment site for muscle or tendon
  - Contributes to bony shape but not length
  - Considered epiphyseal equivalent
- Acute injury: Avulsion fracture of osseous &/or cartilaginous apophysis through subjacent physis
- Chronic injury: Repetitive submaximal tensile forces (avulsive microtrauma) exceed rate of repair, leading to local growth plate disturbance (± symptoms)

IMAGING

General Features

- Best diagnostic clue
  - Acute injury: Displaced apophyseal ossification center
  - Chronic injury: Soft tissue swelling with ossific irregularity at tendon attachment site
- Location
  - Acute avulsion injury
    - Pelvis/hips: High concentration of muscle attachments
      - Ischial tuberosity (hamstrings: Biceps femoris, semimembranosus, semitendinosus)
      - Anterior inferior iliac spine (AIIS) (rectus femoris)
      - Anterior superior iliac spine (ASIS) (sartorius)
      - Iliac crest (tensor fascia lata, abdominal wall muscles)
      - Pubic symphysis (adductors)
      - Greater trochanter (gluteus medius & minimus)
      - Lesser trochanter (iliopsoas)
    - Tibial tubercle (patellar tendon)
    - Medial epicondyle of humerus (flexor group & ulnar collateral ligament)
  - Chronic stress injury
    - Tibial tuberosity: Osgood-Schlatter disease
    - Humeral medial epicondyle: Little Leaguer's elbow
    - Iliac crest
    - Calcaneal apophysis: Sever disease

Radiographic Findings

- Acute avulsion injury
  - Displacement of apophyseal ossification center
    - Tangential view: Crescentic, triangular, or irregular bone fragment
    - En face view: Poorly defined or ovoid fragment
  - Moderate to marked soft tissue edema
    - May be only sign if ossification has not yet developed in apophysis
    - May be occult at pelvis due to overlapping structures
- Healed/remote acute avulsion fracture
  - Bony remodeling from prior injury that may result in apparent expansion/overgrowth
  - Heterotopic ossification of soft tissues may develop at site of prior injury
- Chronic stress injury
  - Ossific irregularity or fragmentation at site of tendon attachment
  - Underlying physeal widening (lengthening) without true fragment displacement
  - Mild overlying soft tissue swelling

MR Findings

- T1WI
  - Dark signal intensity of marrow & soft tissue edema
  - ± bright fatty marrow in avulsed bone
- T2WI FS
  - Long TE ↓ conspicuity of cartilage, especially unossified epiphyseal cartilage (appears dark)
  - Acute injury
    - Bright fluid deep to displaced apophysis
    - Dark tendon remains attached to osteocartilaginous fragment
    - Bright marrow edema of apophysis & adjacent metaphyseal equivalent donor site
    - Moderate/marked surrounding soft tissue edema
      - Fluid &/or hemorrhage at avulsion site
      - Muscle edema from strain ± laxity
  - Chronic injury
    - Mild edema of nondisplaced apophysis & metaphysis
    - Mild ↑ signal, widening (lengthening), & irregularity of physis without discrete fluid
- PD/intermediate FS
  - Bright cartilage fragment
    - Short TE improves cartilage visualization
- GRE FS
  - Bright cartilage fragment, dark bone fragment

Ultrasonographic Findings

- Grayscale ultrasound
  - Distortion of normal soft tissue planes & osteocartilaginous interfaces
    - Comparison to contralateral normal side is key
  - Acute injury: Displaced osteocartilaginous fragment attached to muscle/tendon
    - Hypoechoic cartilage surrounding hyperechoic, shadowing ossification center
    - Dynamic maneuvers can move fragment
  - Chronic: Soft tissue edema, tendon thickening, bony fragmentation

Imaging Recommendations

- Best imaging tool
  - Radiographs are usually diagnostic of acute avulsion
  - MR is useful in some settings
    - Acute injury: Nondisplaced fragment or purely cartilaginous fragment (prior to ossification)
    - Chronic apophysitis
- Protocol advice
  - T2 FS or STIR MR: Best for marrow & soft tissue edema
  - PD FS or GRE FS MR: Best for cartilaginous fragments

DIFFERENTIAL DIAGNOSIS

Osteomyelitis

- Pelvic bones adjacent to growth cartilages (i.e., metaphyseal equivalents) are frequently involved

- Marrow & soft tissue edema ± fluid collections

Ewing Sarcoma

- Often involves entire pelvic bone with permeation, expansion, aggressive periosteal reaction, & (sometimes large) soft tissue mass

Muscle Injury

- Musculotendinous junction becomes weak link of musculoskeletal system after physeal closure
- Edema, fluid, interruption of muscle fibers ± tendon; muscle retraction if tear is complete

Stress Injury of Bone

- Solid periosteal reaction ± linear sclerosis or lucency (often perpendicular to bone long axis)
- Dark T1 MR signal fracture line precedes radiographic findings
- Surrounding marrow & soft tissue edema on T2 FS MR

PATHOLOGY

General Features

- Etiology
    - Osteochondral junction: Weakest point of immature musculoskeletal system
    - ↑ muscle strength of adolescence causes ↑ forces on relatively weak sites of muscle/tendon attachments
    - Acute apophyseal avulsions: Essentially Salter-Harris growth plate fractures
    - Chronic injury (apophysitis): Repetitive submaximal tensile stresses exceed rate of bone repair
        - Physeal widening (lengthening) due to impaired endochondral ossification or chondrocyte hypertrophy
        - Chronic stress injury may weaken physis & predispose to acute avulsion

CLINICAL ISSUES

Presentation

- Most common signs/symptoms
    - Acute: Sudden onset of pain with sensation of pop & instant ↓ of muscle function during athletic activity
    - Chronic: Insidious onset of pain & swelling without specific event or associated bruising

Demographics

- Age
    - Acute pelvic avulsions: Majority occur from ages 12-18 years; mean of 13.8-15.2 years
        - Ossification centers about pelvis appear around ages 12-14 years, fuse by 25 years
        - Sites of radiographically diagnosed injuries correlate with timing of ossification center appearance
            - Older patients (Risser 4): Iliac crest, ASIS avulsions
            - Younger patients (Risser 0): AIIS, ischial tuberosity avulsions
    - Medial epicondyle avulsions: 9-14 years
    - Tibial tubercle avulsions: 13-16 years
- Sex
    - M:F = 3:1
- Epidemiology
    - Acute
        - Most pelvic avulsions occur with kicking or sprinting
            - Soccer, gymnastics, rugby, track & field
            - AIIS, ASIS, ischial tuberosity > iliac crest, pubic symphysis
            - Multiple fractures in 6% of cases
        - Tibial tubercle avulsions are common in basketball & American football
        - Medial epicondyle avulsions are common with throwing or dislocation
    - Chronic
        - Little Leaguer's elbow: Valgus stress of overhead throwing
        - Osgood-Schlatter disease: Repetitive traction of jumping
        - Sever disease: Traction by Achilles tendon

Natural History & Prognosis

- Complications are uncommon
    - Nonunion: Much more likely if displacement is > 2 cm
    - Chronic pain
        - Most common with AIIS avulsions
            - Concomitant or subsequent labral injury
            - Exuberant heterotopic ossification
        - Sciatic nerve irritation or entrapment from displaced ischial tuberosity avulsions
    - Not at risk for clinically significant growth arrest (unlike long bone physeal injuries)

Treatment

- Most therapy is conservative (nonsurgical) & highly successful
    - Initial rest followed by physical therapy
- Surgical fixation is reserved for higher grade injuries
    - More likely if displacement > 1.5-2.0 cm

DIAGNOSTIC CHECKLIST

Image Interpretation Pearls

- Check pelvic apophyses closely in teenager with acute hip pain & pop during activity
- Radiographs may be negative initially in younger patients who have not yet ossified their apophyses

SELECTED REFERENCES

1. Franz P et al: Tibial tubercle avulsion fractures in children. Curr Opin Pediatr. 32(1):86-92, 2020
2. Calderazzi F et al: Apophyseal avulsion fractures of the pelvis. A review. Acta Biomed. 89(4):470-6, 2018
3. Ghanem IB et al: Pediatric avulsion fractures of pelvis: current concepts. Curr Opin Pediatr. 30(1):78-83, 2018
4. Schiller J et al: Lower extremity avulsion fractures in the pediatric and adolescent athlete. J Am Acad Orthop Surg. 25(4):251-9, 2017
5. Schuett DJ et al: Pelvic apophyseal avulsion fractures: a retrospective review of 228 cases. J Pediatr Orthop. 35(6):617-23, 2015
6. Singer G et al: Diagnosis and treatment of apophyseal injuries of the pelvis in adolescents. Semin Musculoskelet Radiol. 18(5):498-504, 2014
7. Meyers AB et al: MRI of radiographically occult ischial apophyseal avulsions. Pediatr Radiol. 42(11):1357-63, 2012
8. McKinney BI et al: Apophyseal avulsion fractures of the hip and pelvis. Orthopedics. 32(1):42, 2009
9. Hébert KJ et al: MRI appearance of chronic stress injury of the iliac crest apophysis in adolescent athletes. AJR Am J Roentgenol. 190(6):1487-91, 2008

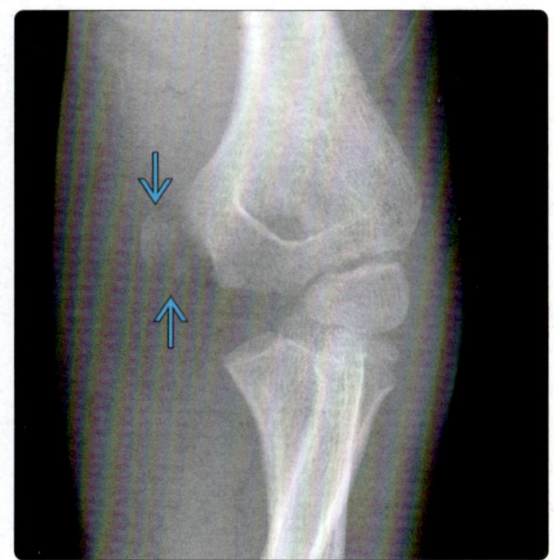

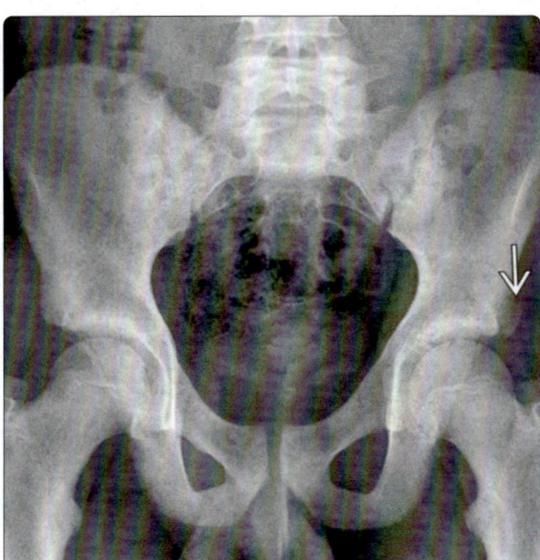

(Left) *Oblique radiograph in a 7-year-old boy after a fall shows medial translation & fragmentation of the medial epicondyle apophysis ➙ with marked overlying soft tissue swelling.* **(Right)** *AP radiograph of a 12-year-old patient with hip pain shows mild lateral displacement of an avulsed anterior inferior iliac spine (AIIS) ossification center ➙ at the attachment of the rectus femoris muscle.*

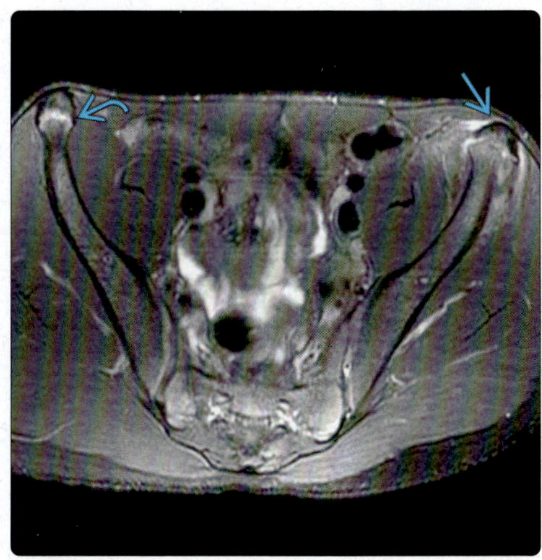

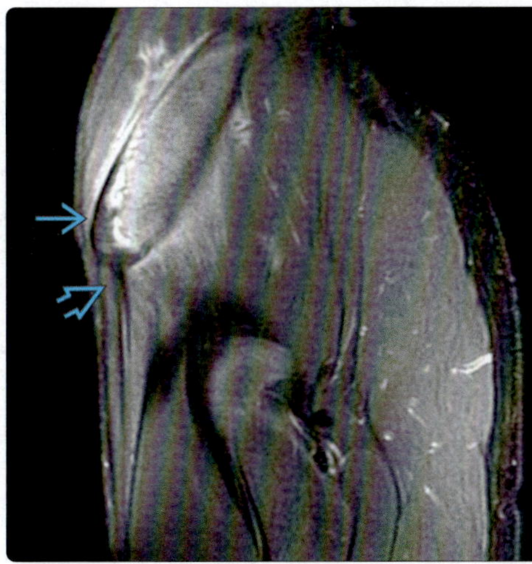

(Left) *Axial T2 FS MR in a 14-year-old boy who felt a pop while running shows a displaced apophyseal fragment ➙ due to sartorius avulsion of the left ASIS. The right ASIS shows chronic physeal stress injury with growth plate widening ➙.* **(Right)** *Sagittal T2 FS MR in the same patient shows cartilaginous apophyseal avulsion at the sartorius attachment ➙ to the left ASIS ➙. This fracture was radiographically occult.*

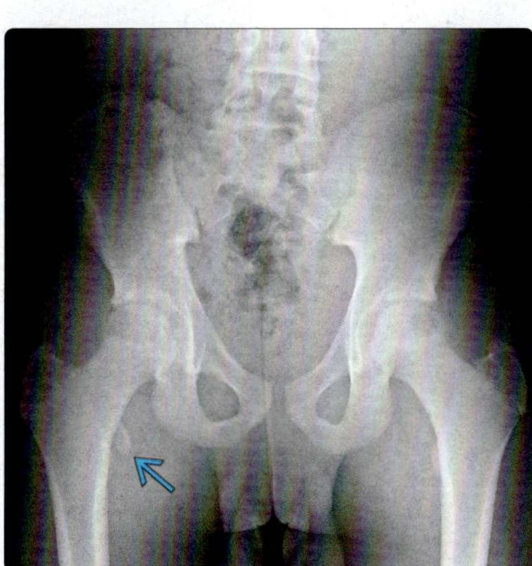

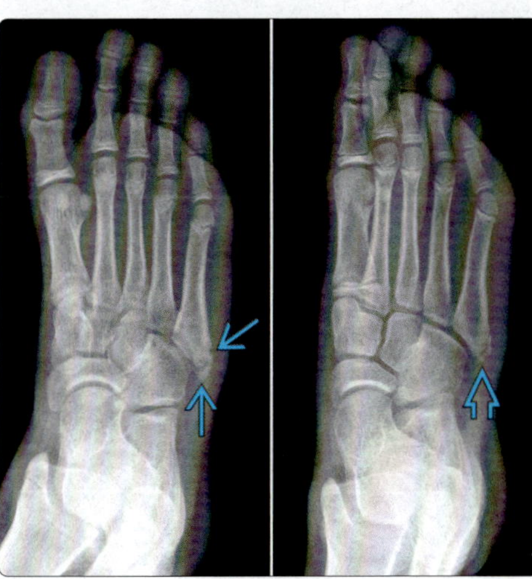

(Left) *AP radiograph in a 14-year-old patient who felt a pop while swimming shows avulsion of the unfused right lesser trochanter ➙. This fracture does not implicate underlying pathology in children.* **(Right)** *Oblique radiograph of the foot in a 13-year-old boy after a basketball injury (L) shows new proximal retraction of the 5th metatarsal base apophysis ➙ as compared to a normal appearance 5 months prior ➙ (R). Point tenderness at this level confirmed an acute avulsion fracture.*

Incomplete Fractures

KEY FACTS

TERMINOLOGY

- Incomplete fracture: Macroscopic fracture line does not traverse entire bony diameter
- Buckle fracture: Fracture on compression side
- Greenstick fracture: Fracture on tension side
- Plastic deformity: Smooth abnormal bending of diaphysis without visible fracture line

IMAGING

- 2 tangential views: At least 1 cortex disrupted & 1 intact
  - Exception: Smooth bowing of plastic deformity
- Contralateral comparison views may be helpful
  - Especially in plastic deformity
- Most commonly occurs in radial & ulnar diaphyses & metaphyses
  - Look for subtle fracture line extending distally to physis as Salter-Harris type II (SH II) fracture has different follow-up requirements

TOP DIFFERENTIAL DIAGNOSES

- Bowing due to underlying skeletal disease
- Normal developmental variants
- SH II fracture

PATHOLOGY

- Immature bone is more pliable with greater bending before breaking
- Fall on outstretched hand is most common mechanism

CLINICAL ISSUES

- Most common < 10 years of age
- Greenstick fracture is unstable: Refracture in 7-20%
- Reduction if needed + splint or cast immobilization
  - Acceptable displacement varies by age, location, type
- Greater remodeling potential in younger children
  - Will not correct rotational deformity
  - Limited remodeling potential in plastic deformity even when young

(Left) *PA & lateral wrist radiographs in an 11-year-old after a fall shows a buckle fracture of the distal radial diaphysis ➡ with minimal angulation. A focal contour protuberance of a nondisplaced ulnar buckle fracture ➡ is more subtle, best seen on the lateral view.* **(Right)** *AP & lateral radiographs of the forearm in a 5-year-old after a fall show incomplete fractures of the distal radial & ulnar diaphyses. Note the intact "bent but not broken" posterior cortex of each bone ➡, typical of greenstick fractures.*

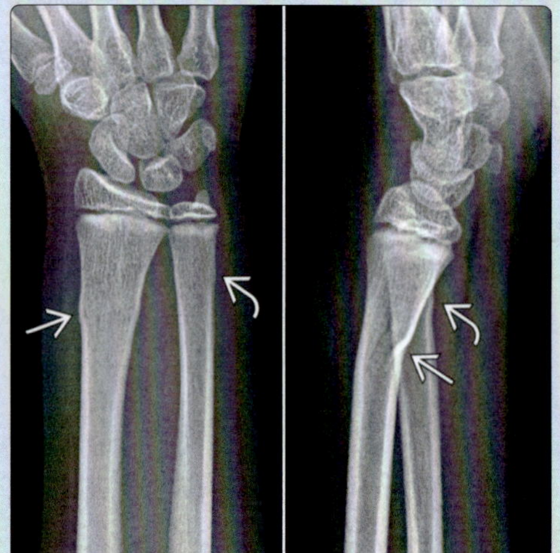

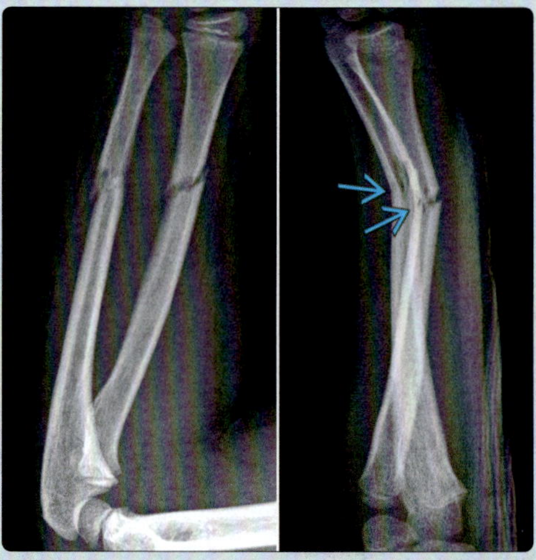

(Left) *AP radiograph of the forearm in a 5-year-old after a fall shows a plastic (bowing) deformity of the ulnar diaphysis ➡. The radial curvature is within normal limits. Note that the ulnar deformity is not readily visible on the lateral view.* **(Right)** *Axial T2 FS MR in the same patient 4 days later (performed for specific elbow complaints) shows marrow ➡, periosteal ➡, & soft tissue edema in/about the ulnar diaphysis with no cortical break. Subperiosteal hemorrhage ➡ is noted. The radius ➡ is normal.*

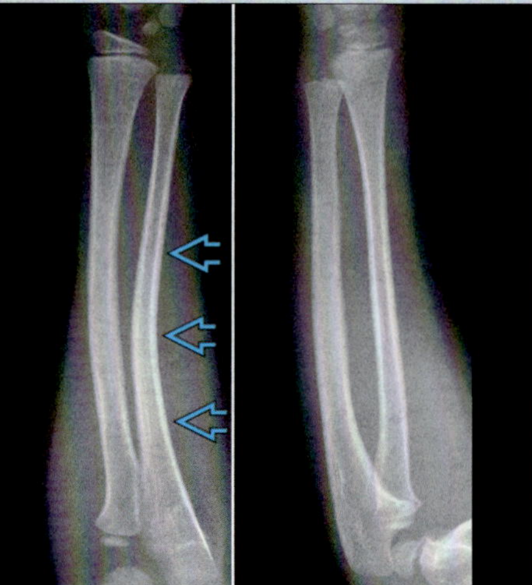

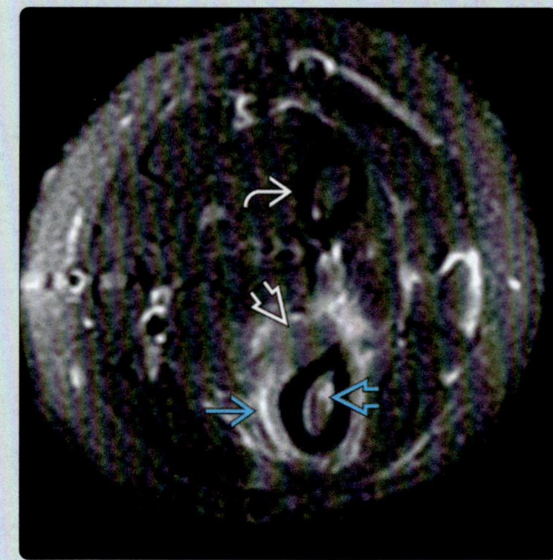

TERMINOLOGY

Definitions

- Incomplete fracture: Macroscopic fracture line does not traverse entire bony diameter
- Buckle fracture: Fracture on compression side
- Greenstick fracture: Fracture on tension side
- Plastic deformity: Smooth, abnormal bending of diaphysis without visible fracture line

IMAGING

General Features

- Best diagnostic clue
  - Cortical bump, break, or angulation at site of pain + overlying soft tissue swelling
- Most common locations
  - Buckle fracture: Distal radial & ulnar diaphysis or metadiaphysis, tibia, proximal 1st metatarsal
  - Greenstick fracture: Radial & ulnar diaphysis
  - Plastic deformity: Radial, ulnar, & fibular diaphysis

Radiographic Findings

- Obtain at least 2 tangential views
  - At least 1 cortex is intact
- Buckle fracture
  - Focal protuberance of cortex on compression side
  - May be very subtle; suspect with any disruption of smooth cortical contour
- Greenstick fracture
  - Cortical disruption on tension side
  - Usually angulated with fracture on convex margin
- Plastic deformity
  - ↑ curvature of long bone diaphysis without cortical disruption
  - Adjacent bone of forearm or lower leg is often fractured
    - May be different type or dislocation
    - Monteggia equivalent fracture: Plastic deformation of ulna with anterior dislocation of radial head

Ultrasonographic Findings

- Focal interruption/bulging of echogenic cortex ± subperiosteal hemorrhage, soft tissue edema

DIFFERENTIAL DIAGNOSIS

Bowing Due to Underlying Skeletal Disease

- Systemic or localized bony dysplasias
- Metabolic bone diseases

Normal Developmental Variants

- Few sites of normal cortical angulation/protuberance
- Comparison views of contralateral side may be helpful

Salter-Harris Type II (SHII) Fracture

- Fracture line extends to physis

PATHOLOGY

General Features

- Immature bone is softer, more pliable → greater bowing or bending before breaking
  - Thicker periosteum, ↑ porosity, ↓ mineralization
- Forearm is most common site
  - Fall on outstretched hand is most common mechanism
  - Rotational component is common with greenstick fracture & plastic deformity

CLINICAL ISSUES

Presentation

- Most common signs/symptoms
  - Pain, swelling, tenderness, disuse of limb, limp, or deformity

Demographics

- Most common < 10 years of age

Natural History & Prognosis

- Buckle fracture: Stable, typically heals without deformity
- Greenstick fracture: Unstable, at risk for refracture (7-20%)
- Plastic deformation: Limited remodeling potential, even in younger children

Treatment

- Nonsurgical reduction if needed + splint or cast immobilization
  - Fractured bones have greater remodeling potential in younger children (especially < 6 years)
    - Rotational deformity is not corrected with growth remodeling
  - Acceptable displacement, angulation, & malrotation varies by age, location, fracture type
- Buckle fracture
  - 3-week immobilization with splint
  - May not require follow-up imaging
- Greenstick fracture
  - May require closed reduction & casting
  - Some advocate completing fracture for improved alignment
  - Prolonged immobilization may reduce refractures
- Plastic deformation
  - May require closed reduction
    - Requires significant force over several minutes, adequate sedation

DIAGNOSTIC CHECKLIST

Image Interpretation Pearls

- Look carefully for metaphyseal fracture line extending to physis (implying SH II fracture)
  - Complications & follow-up are different from buckle

SELECTED REFERENCES

1. Laor T et al: Describing pediatric fractures in the era of ICD-10. Pediatr Radiol. 50(6):761-75, 2020
2. Iles BW et al: Differentiating stable buckle fractures from other distal radius fractures: the 1-cm rule. Pediatr Radiol. 49(3):358-64, 2019
3. Forestier-Zhang L et al: Bone strength in children: understanding basic bone biomechanics. Arch Dis Child Educ Pract Ed. 101(1):2-7, 2016
4. Herren C et al: Ultrasound-guided diagnosis of fractures of the distal forearm in children. Orthop Traumatol Surg Res. 101(4):501-5, 2015
5. Pountos I et al: Diagnosis and treatment of greenstick and torus fractures of the distal radius in children: a prospective randomised single blind study. J Child Orthop. 4(4):321-6, 2010

Child Abuse, Metaphyseal Fracture

KEY FACTS

TERMINOLOGY

- Classic metaphyseal lesion (CML) or metaphyseal corner fracture: Transverse fracture of subphyseal metaphysis that undercuts subperiosteal bone collar (SPBC) peripherally
  - Fracture of infants with high specificity for child abuse

IMAGING

- Most common at distal femur, proximal & distal tibia
- Radiographic appearance
  - Triangular fragment at metaphyseal corner when x-ray beam is perpendicular to bone long axis
  - Bucket-handle fragment adjacent to metaphysis when x-ray beam is angled caudal or cranial relative to physis
  - Healing fractures are more conspicuous
    - Extension of physeal lucency into metaphysis
    - May see sclerosis along fracture margin
    - Subperiosteal new bone formation & callus
- Tc-99m MDP bone scan & F-18 NaF PET are complementary to initial skeletal survey
  - Sensitivity is greater for most fractures except CML, skull, scapula, & remote

PATHOLOGY

- Planar fracture through junction of primary & secondary spongiosa at trabecular transition zone; fracture undercuts SPBC peripherally
- Due to tensile & torsional forces from twisting or pulling extremity or from acceleration/deceleration of shaking
- No established evidence that rickets or metabolic bone disease can cause CML

CLINICAL ISSUES

- Initial skeletal survey is obtained if
  - < 2 years old with suspicion of NAT
  - < 5 years old with suspicious fracture
  - Concern for NAT in any child unable to communicate
- Obtain follow-up skeletal survey in 2 weeks as healing ↑ fracture conspicuity
- 95% of cases with CML have ≥ 1 additional injury

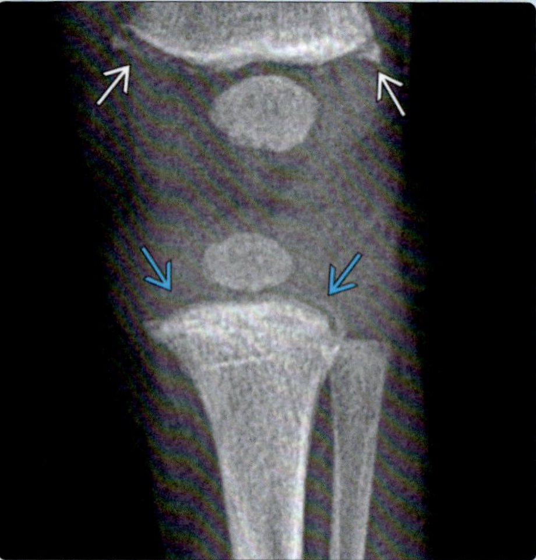
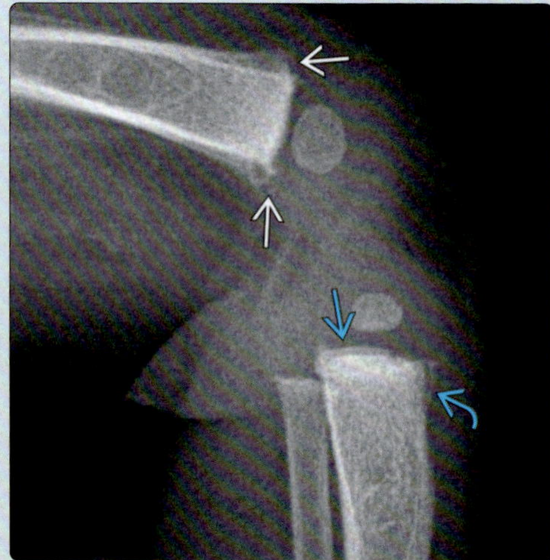

(Left) *AP radiograph of the left knee of a 9-month-old with lower extremity bruising shows the typical appearance of bucket-handle metaphyseal fractures [classic metaphyseal lesions (CMLs)] at the distal femur ➡ & proximal tibia ➡.* **(Right)** *Lateral radiograph of a 5-month-old's knee demonstrates CMLs of the distal femur ➡ & proximal tibia ➡. The tibial fracture extends anteriorly along the course of the unossified tibial tubercle ➡.*

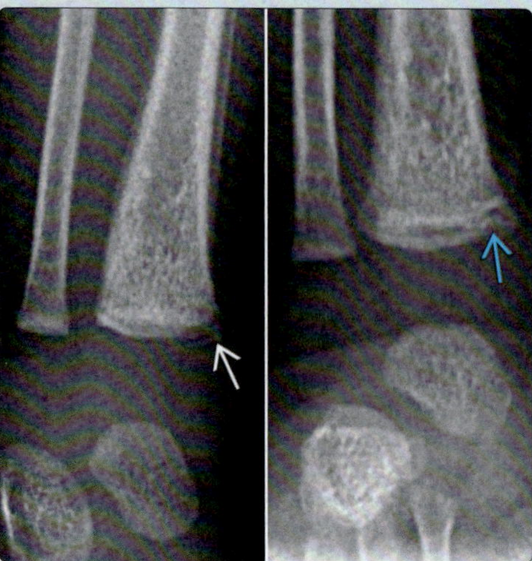
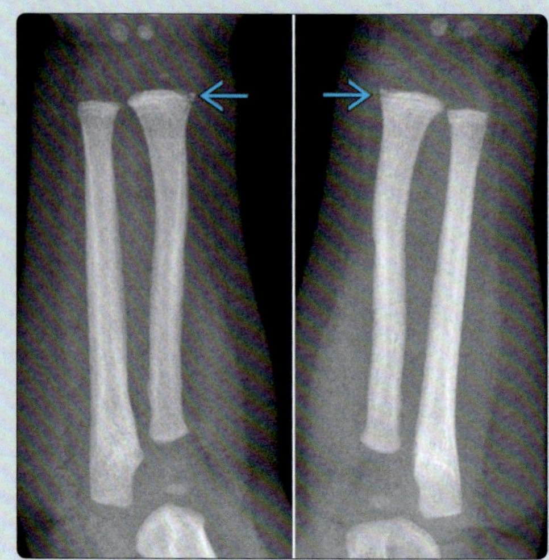

(Left) *AP radiograph of a 5-month-old with unexplained fractures at presentation (left) demonstrates a subtle metaphyseal fracture of the distal tibia ➡. A follow-up radiograph 3 weeks later (right) shows further healing changes with persistent subphyseal lucency ➡.* **(Right)** *AP radiographs in the same patient (at presentation) show bilateral metaphyseal corner fractures of the distal radial metaphyses ➡.*

TERMINOLOGY

Synonyms

- Nonaccidental trauma (NAT), battered child syndrome
- Metaphyseal corner fracture, classic metaphyseal lesion (CML), bucket-handle fracture

Definitions

- Fracture of infants that extends though subphyseal metaphysis & undercuts subperiosteal bone collar (SPBC) peripherally

IMAGING

General Features

- Best diagnostic clue
  - Triangular bone fragments at corners of metaphysis or bucket-handle, rim-like fragment of subphyseal metaphysis
- Location
  - Metaphyses of long bones, most commonly distal femur, proximal & distal tibia, proximal humerus

Radiographic Findings

- Acute fractures can be subtle & difficult to identify on initial skeletal survey
  - Transverse subphyseal lucency separates thin bone fragment from metaphysis & undercuts SPBC peripherally
    - May fully or partially extend across metaphysis
  - Appearance depends on radiographic projection
    - Triangular fragment lies at metaphyseal corner when x-ray beam is perpendicular to metaphysis long axis
    - Bucket-handle fragment lies along metaphysis when x-ray beam is angled caudal or cranial relative to physis
- Healing fractures are more conspicuous
  - Focal extension of physeal lucency into metaphysis due to persistent unossified cartilage
    - Most common at site of SPBC undercutting
    - May be broad with extensive fracture
  - Callus & subperiosteal new bone formation (SPNBF)
  - May see sclerosis along fracture margin
- Most common at distal femur, proximal & distal tibia
  - More commonly seen medially at these locations
  - Lateral & anterior fractures are always accompanied by medial fractures in series of cases
  - Proximal tibial fracture may extend anteriorly along tibial tubercle region, best seen in healing phase with sclerosis on lateral view
  - Distal tibial fracture vertical component undercutting SPBC is typically longer than in proximal tibia
- General comments on dating fractures
  - SPNBF appears after 7-10 days
  - SPNBF thickness ↑ with time
  - Callus develops by 15 days, not before 9 days
  - Callus thickness ↓ with age
  - Subphyseal lucency is late finding in healing
  - Up to 1/3 of distal tibial CML fails to demonstrate SPNBF
    - Normalization of metaphysis on follow-up does not exclude healed CML

CT Findings

- Not advocated for identification of fractures
- Evaluate proximal humeri & femurs on CT obtained to evaluate intrathoracic or intraabdominal injuries

MR Findings

- Whole-body MR shows very low sensitivity for signal abnormalities at sites of CML seen on skeletal survey: 31%
- May be complementary given ability to detect soft tissue abnormalities

Ultrasonographic Findings

- ↓ sensitivity (63%), ↑ specificity (97%)
  - Positive US may be helpful if radiographs are equivocal
- Metaphyseal collar fracture
- Metaphyseal collar thickening or deformity
- Irregularity of zone of provisional Ca^{2+}
- May see subtle edema in adjacent soft tissues

Nuclear Medicine Findings

- Tc-99m MDP skeletal scintigraphy or F-18 NaF PET is complementary to initial skeletal survey
  - Focal ↑ in radionuclide activity within 24 hours, normalizing within 6 months
  - Overall sensitivity of scintigraphy for detecting fractures > initial skeletal survey; exceptions include CML, skull & scapular fractures, remote injuries
    - ↓ sensitivity for CML due to physiologic uptake at physes
      - Tc-99m MDP bone scan 35%, F-18 NaF PET 67%
  - Scintigraphy specificity is lower than initial skeletal survey

Imaging Recommendations

- Initial skeletal survey
  - Indications
    - < 2 years old with suspicion of NAT
    - < 5 years old with suspicious fracture
    - Concern for NAT in any child unable to communicate
  - Images include: AP & lateral skull, lateral cervical & lumbar spine, AP & lateral & both obliques thorax (ribs), AP pelvis, AP humeri, AP forearms, shallow oblique hands, AP femurs, AP lower legs, AP feet
  - Additional views based on clinical & imaging findings
- Follow-up skeletal survey
  - Typically 2 weeks from initial evaluation
    - Minimum of 10 days
  - Indications
    - Concerning fractures on initial study
    - Normal initial study with persistent suspicion based on clinical or imaging findings
  - Used to confirm suspected fractures & identify additional fractures
  - In one study, clarified questionable fractures or identified new fractures in 48% of cases
    - Of 27 new fractures, 2 were CML
    - Of 29 questionable fractures, 6 were confirmed CML
- Tc-99m MDP skeletal scintigraphy or F-18 NaF PET as complementary or problem-solving tools
- CECT for suspected intrathoracic or intraabdominal injury

DIFFERENTIAL DIAGNOSIS

Osteogenesis Imperfecta

- Multiple fractures ± wormian bones, blue sclera
- ± osteoporosis

Metaphyseal Spur

- Distal extension of SPBC beyond chondroosseous junction, may be seen at lateral distal femur & other sites
- Typically lacks underlying lucency

Rickets

- Metaphyseal fraying, cupping, widening ± fractures
- Demineralization

Birth Trauma

- CML-like injuries are rarely reported with C-section

Leukemia

- Metaphyseal lucent bands ± fractures or more aggressive permeative lesions

Menkes Syndrome

- Osteoporosis, metaphyseal corner spurs, wormian bones, tortuous intracranial arteries, & brittle hair from abnormal copper metabolism

Spondylometaphyseal Dysplasia

- Metaphyseal irregularities resembling corner fractures due to abnormal endochondral ossification
- Scoliosis, platyspondyly, coxa vara, pectus carinatum

Metaphyseal Chondrodysplasia

- Early metaphyseal cupping → severe expansion → fragmentation or cystic changes
- Frontonasal hyperplasia, hypertelorism, proptosis, micrognathia, curved forearms & legs

PATHOLOGY

General Features

- Planar fracture through junction of primary & secondary spongiosa at trabecular transition zone; fracture undercuts SPBC peripherally
- Due to tensile & torsional forces from twisting or pulling extremity or from acceleration/deceleration of shaking
- No established evidence that rickets/metabolic bone disease can cause CML
- No established evidence that rickets/metabolic bone disease can cause fractures of any kind in absence of radiographic findings of underlying metabolic bone disturbance

CLINICAL ISSUES

Presentation

- Wide range of clinical presentations for NAT
  - Injury inconsistent with history or stage of development
  - Multiple injuries in various stages of healing
  - Bruising in nonmobile infant
  - Retinal hemorrhages
- CML
  - One study evaluating bruising as indicator for fracture
    - 25% had bruising at sites other than fracture site
    - Only 13% had bruising at/near fracture site
  - Another study found that 95% of cases with CML had at least 1 additional injury
    - 84% had additional non-CML fractures, most commonly long bone & rib
    - 43% had cutaneous injuries (bruising or burns)
    - 28% had traumatic brain injury

Demographics

- Epidemiology
  - ~ 702,000 child maltreatment victims in USA in 2014
    - Infants ≤ 1 year old are most at risk, account for 36.7%
    - Physical abuse in 41% of child maltreatment cases
  - CML has high specificity for NAT
    - Most common fracture in fatal NAT cases in one study
    - Present in 50% of infants at high risk for NAT compared to 0% in infants at low risk for NAT

Natural History & Prognosis

- ~ 1,580 fatalities from child maltreatment in USA in 2014
  - Death rate greatest in infants < 1 year old: 17.96/100,000 same-aged children in population
  - 71% of all deaths occurred in children < 3 years old
  - 79% of fatalities involved parent as perpetrator

Treatment

- Multidisciplinary investigation of maltreatment allegation
- Ensure at risk child & siblings are placed in safe environment

DIAGNOSTIC CHECKLIST

Reporting Tips

- Concern for child abuse raised by imaging must be discussed with referring clinician immediately
- Report represents legal document: Review carefully
- Provide clear, detailed description of each fracture, including location, fragments, & estimated age (i.e., acute, healing, healed/remote)

SELECTED REFERENCES

1. Karmazyn B et al: Accuracy of ultrasound in the diagnosis of classic metaphyseal lesions using radiographs as the gold standard. Pediatr Radiol. 50(8):1123-30, 2020
2. Karmazyn B et al: Establishing signs for acute and healing phases of distal tibial classic metaphyseal lesions. Pediatr Radiol. 50(5):715-25, 2020
3. Marine MB et al: Ultrasound findings in classic metaphyseal lesions: emphasis on the metaphyseal bone collar and zone of provisional calcification. Pediatr Radiol. 49(7):913-21, 2019
4. Tsai A et al: Subperiosteal new bone formation with the distal tibial classic metaphyseal lesion: prevalence on radiographic skeletal surveys. Pediatr Radiol. 49(4):551-8, 2019
5. Tsai A et al: The distal tibial classic metaphyseal lesion: medial versus lateral cortical injury. Pediatr Radiol. 48(7):973-8, 2018
6. Tsai A et al: Biomechanics of the classic metaphyseal lesion: finite element analysis. Pediatr Radiol. 47(12):1622-30, 2017
7. Servaes S et al: The etiology and significance of fractures in infants and young children: a critical multidisciplinary review. Pediatr Radiol. 46(5):591-600, 2016
8. Thackeray JD et al: The classic metaphyseal lesion and traumatic injury. Pediatr Radiol. 46(8):1128-33, 2016
9. Barber I et al: The yield of high-detail radiographic skeletal surveys in suspected infant abuse. Pediatr Radiol. 45(1):69-80, 2015
10. Kleinman, PK. Diagnostic imaging of child abuse, 3rd edition. Cambridge University Press, 2015
11. Perez-Rossello JM et al: Absence of rickets in infants with fatal abusive head trauma and classic metaphyseal lesions. Radiology. 275(3):810-21, 2015
12. Kleinman PK et al: Prevalence of the classic metaphyseal lesion in infants at low versus high risk for abuse. AJR Am J Roentgenol. 197(4):1005-8, 2011

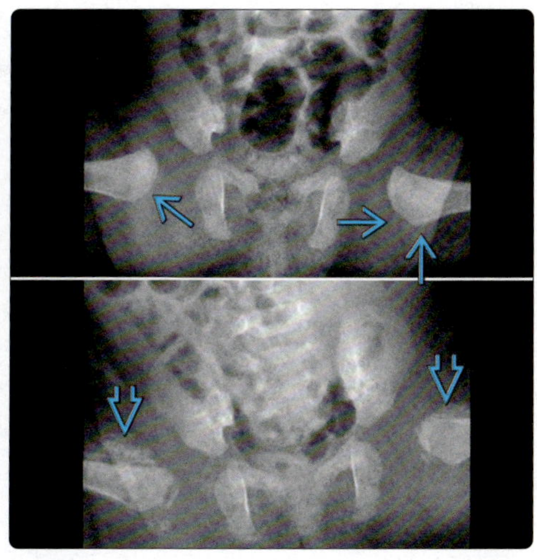

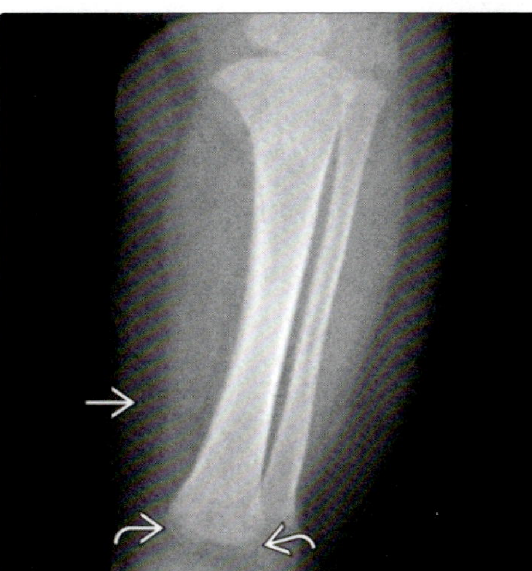

(Left) *Frog leg lateral radiograph in a 2-month-old with bruising (top) shows bilateral metaphyseal corner/bucket-handle fractures of the proximal femurs ⇨. MR (not shown) confirmed fractures traversing the primary spongiosa. Follow-up radiograph 2 weeks later (bottom) shows marked periosteal reaction ⇩.* **(Right)** *AP radiograph in a 3-month-old infant shows a bucket-handle fracture of the distal tibial metaphysis ↷ with overlying soft tissue swelling →.*

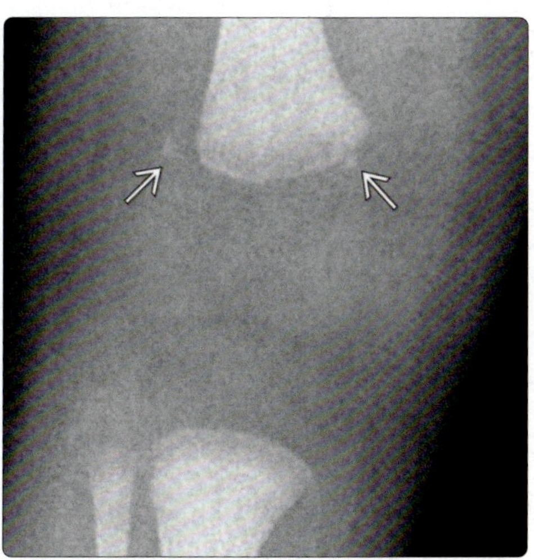

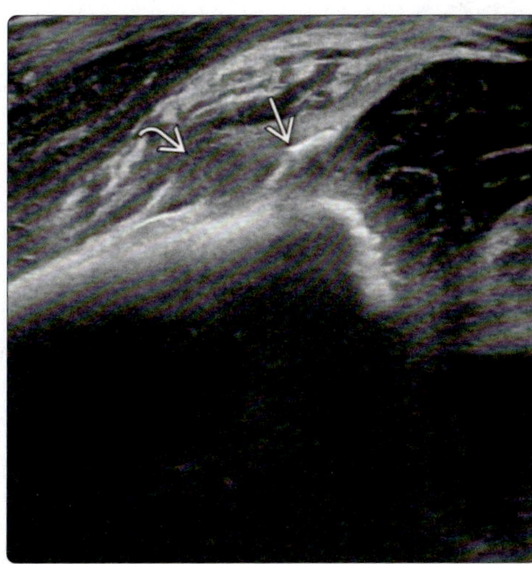

(Left) *AP radiograph of the right knee in a newborn who suffered birth trauma shows a CML-like fracture at the distal femur →. This is similar in appearance to metaphyseal fractures related to nonaccidental trauma (NAT).* **(Right)** *Longitudinal US from the same patient with birth trauma demonstrates the metaphyseal fracture → with associated hematoma ↷. There has been ↑ interest in using US to evaluate similar-appearing NAT-related CMLs, particularly when initial radiographs are unclear.*

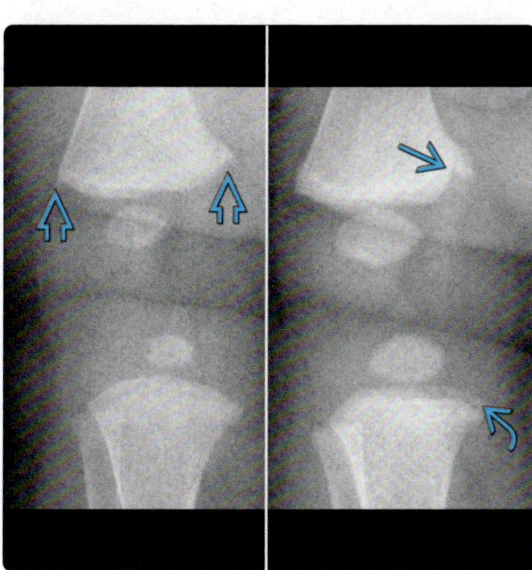

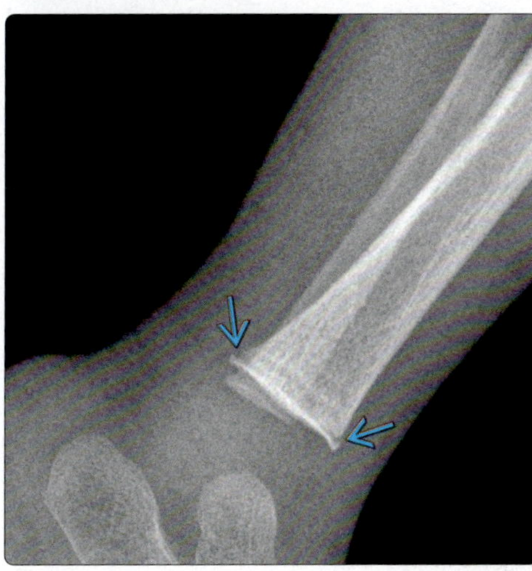

(Left) *AP radiographs of the right knee in a 3-month-old with a skull fracture (not shown) at presentation (left) & 7 weeks later (right) show evolution of a distal femoral metaphyseal corner fracture ⇧ with subphyseal lucency → on follow-up. A tibial CML is seen on the 2nd study ↷.* **(Right)** *Lateral view of the tibia in a 6-month-old with failure to thrive shows a metaphyseal fracture →. The periphery of the fracture undercuts the subperiosteal bone collar, which is thicker than the thin central component.*

Other Fractures of Child Abuse

KEY FACTS

IMAGING

- High specificity for child abuse
  - Classic metaphyseal lesions, posterior rib fractures
  - Scapular fractures
    - Transverse or oblique fractures of midacromion process are most common
    - Acromion tip fracture mimics ossification center
  - Sternal fractures
    - Linear lucency or buckling of anterior cortex
    - Widened sternal synchondrosis or malalignment of sternal segments
  - Spinous process fractures
    - Cartilage/bone avulsion at interspinous ligamentous attachment due to hyperflexion & shaking
    - Ossific density adjacent to spinous process may represent acute or remote injury
- Moderate specificity for child abuse
  - Vertebral body fractures
    - Compression deformity &/or anterosuperior endplate fracture
  - Vertebral fracture-dislocations
    - Neurocentral synchondrosis fracture extending through endplate apophyses with retropulsion of vertebral centrum
    - Facet dislocation ± fracture
  - Transphyseal fracture/distal humeral epiphyseal separation
    - Capitellar ossification center, radius, & ulna are displaced posteriorly & medially relative to distal humerus
    - Distal humeral cartilage maintains alignment with radius & ulna (not true dislocation)
  - Complex skull fractures, hand & foot fractures, pelvic fractures
- Low specificity for child abuse
  - Clavicle, long bone shaft, & linear skull fractures common but have low specificity for nonaccidental trauma

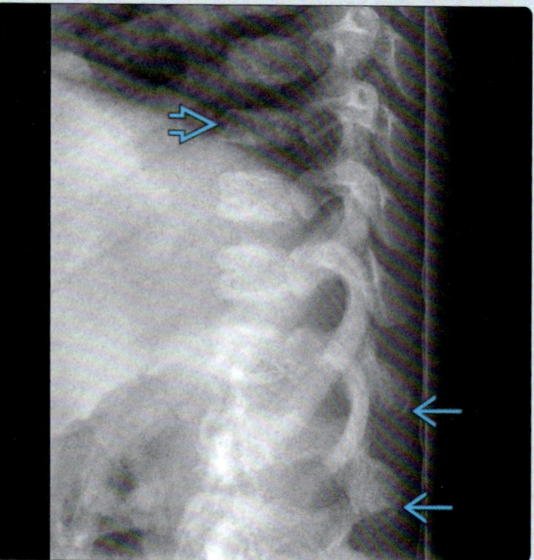

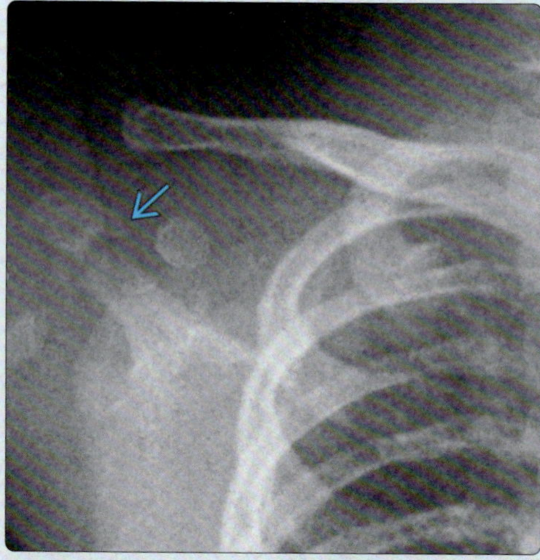

(Left) *Lateral radiograph of the spine in an 8-month-old with bruising & a subdural hematoma shows irregularity, lucency, & sclerosis of the T12 & L1 spinous processes ➡ as well as compression of the T9 vertebral body ⇨. Spinous process fractures are highly suggestive of child abuse.* **(Right)** *Frontal radiograph in an abused 6-week-old shows an acromial fracture ➡ with irregularity & elevation of the distal fragment. Follow-up images confirmed the presence of healing changes.*

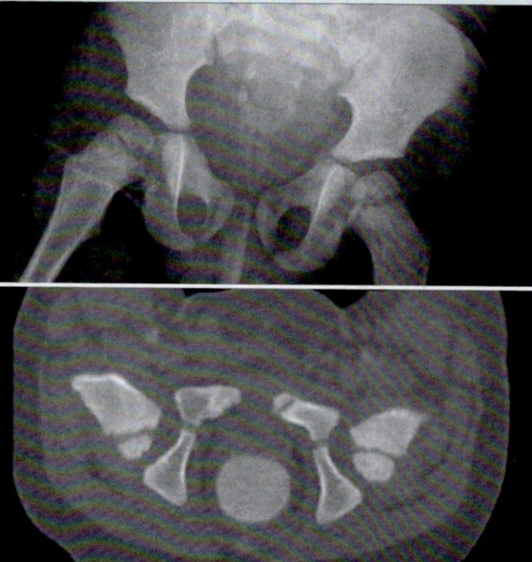

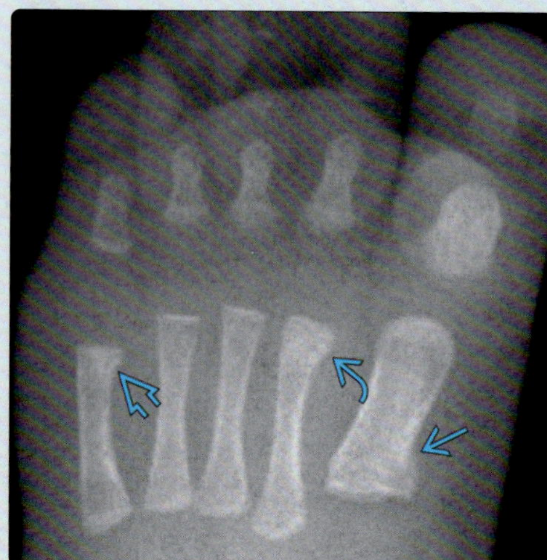

(Left) *AP radiograph (top) & axial CT (bottom) of an abused 2-year-old with numerous other high-specificity fractures (not shown) demonstrate sclerosis at the right superior pubic ramus ➡, compatible with healing fracture. Radiographic cortical irregularity at the left superior pubic ramus ➡ shows lucency on CT, also compatible with fracture.* **(Right)** *AP radiograph of the foot in the same patient shows healing fractures of the 1st ➡, 2nd ➡, & 5th ⇨ metatarsals.*

TERMINOLOGY

Synonyms

- Nonaccidental trauma (NAT), battered child syndrome

IMAGING

General Features

- Best diagnostic clue
  - Classic metaphyseal lesions (CMLs) & posterior rib fractures: High specificity for NAT
    - Other high-specificity injuries include scapular, spinous process, & sternal fractures
  - Multiple fractures, bilateral fractures, & fractures of varying ages: Moderate specificity for NAT
    - Other moderate-specificity injuries include epiphyseal separation, vertebral body, digital, complex skull, & pelvic fractures
  - Injury incompatible with age &/or history suspicious for NAT
- Distribution of fractures due to NAT
  - Skull 27%, ribs 18%, vertebra 2%, pelvis < 1%
  - Humerus 11%, forearm 7%, clavicle 4%, hand < 1%
  - Femur 18%, tibia & fibula & ankle 12%, tarsal & metatarsal < 1%

High-Specificity Fractures

- Scapular fractures
  - Acromion is most commonly involved
    - Transverse or oblique fractures of midprocess
    - Tip fractures are less common
    - Ossification centers can mimic fractures but are anterior/inferior & typically arise in 2nd decade
  - Coracoid & glenoid fractures are rare
  - Best evaluated on humerus & oblique rib views
  - CT or radionuclide exam for challenging cases
- Sternal fractures
  - Rare; result from direct force to sternum
  - Linear lucency or buckling of anterior cortex
  - Widened sternal synchondrosis or malalignment of sternal segments
  - Irregularity & sclerosis of synchondrosis osseous margins with healing
  - May require dedicated views or CT for evaluation
  - Likelihood of accidental cause ↑ > 1 year of age
- Spinous process fractures
  - Avulsion of cartilage &/or bone at interspinous ligamentous attachments due to shaking, hyperflexion
  - ± vertebral body compression deformity

Moderate-Specificity Fractures

- Vertebral body fractures
  - Compression &/or anterosuperior endplate fracture
  - Healing results in
    - Central vertebral body sclerosis
    - Anterosuperior endplate notching/lucency + marginal sclerosis with remote injuries
  - Findings may be subtle, underestimate injuries
    - MR & F-18 NaF PET are more sensitive
- Vertebral fracture-dislocations
  - Neurocentral synchondrosis injury
    - Fracture extends through superior & inferior endplate apophyses & neurocentral synchondrosis posteriorly due to hyperflexion
    - Extrusion of vertebral centrum, typically posteriorly
      - Retropulsion of vertebral body on lateral view
    - Widened interpediculate distance & disc space narrowing on AP view
    - ± vertebral body compression deformity
    - ± mass effect on thecal sac on MR
  - Facet dislocation ± fracture
    - Widened interspinous distance on AP & lateral views
    - Retrolisthesis on lateral view
    - Facet joint disruption/widening
    - ± compression deformity &/or fractures involving facets, posterior elements, endplates
  - Paraspinal Ca^{2+} with healing
- Epiphyseal separations (or transphyseal fractures)
  - Have also been described with birth trauma
  - US or MR can be very helpful for showing
    - Displacement of unossified epiphysis
    - Periosteal elevation along metaphysis acutely
  - Abundant periosteal new bone is typical of healing
  - Distal humeral epiphyseal separation
    - Largely unossified capitellar ossification center is translated posteriorly & (usually) medially relative to distal humerus but maintains alignment with radius
    - In absence of epiphyseal/capitellar ossification, posterior & medial translation of radius & ulna is suggested if
      - Radius aligns with central & medial humeral metaphysis with ulna medial to humerus
      - Dislocation is initially suspected: Rare in infants, & most dislocations occur laterally
    - ± metaphyseal fracture fragment
    - MR, US, or arthrogram is helpful to confirm diagnosis & evaluate degree of displacement
      - Discontinuity of distal humeral epiphyseal cartilage from bony metaphysis
      - Posterior & medial translation of epiphysis, which maintains alignment with radius & ulna
    - Up to 50% are due to NAT but can occur with birth or accidental trauma
  - Proximal humeral epiphyseal separation
    - Rare; classically seen with birth injuries
  - Proximal femoral epiphyseal separation
    - Proximal femoral diaphysis is translated laterally & proximally relative to ossified capital femoral epiphysis (or acetabulum if epiphysis is unossified)
    - If epiphysis is unossified, may simulate dislocation on radiograph
    - May develop coxa vara deformity
  - Distal femoral epiphyseal separation
    - Rare: Requires more force than CML
- Complex skull fractures
  - > 1 fracture line, stellate or branching, comminuted
- Digital fractures of hands & feet
  - Relatively uncommon, present in 4.9% of all positive skeletal surveys obtained for NAT
    - Buckle fractures of metatarsals, usually medial 1st metatarsal

- Buckle fractures of metacarpals & phalanges
- Likely result from twisting or bending forces

- Pelvic fractures
  - Subtle, typically involve superior pubic ramus in infants
  - ± association with sexual assault in older children
  - MR & F-18 NaF PET may be helpful

Low-Specificity Fractures

- Clavicle, long bone shaft, & linear skull fractures are common but have low specificity for NAT

Dating Fractures

- Soft tissue swelling only in first 1-2 days, ↓ by 7 days; seen again (less pronounced) from 15-35 days
- Subperiosteal new bone formation after 7-10 days, ↑ thickness until 25 days
- Soft callus usually by 15 days, ↓ by 35 days
- Bridging & remodeling by 14-21 days
- Hard callus by > 35 days

DIFFERENTIAL DIAGNOSIS

Accidental Trauma

- Age & clinical history are consistent with fracture

Osteogenesis Imperfecta

- Multiple fractures, wormian bones, diffuse osteoporosis, ± blue sclera

Birth Trauma

- Correlates with age, birth history, & typical location

Rickets

- Demineralization with metaphyseal fraying, cupping, widening; loss of normal zone of provisional Ca^{2+}

Metabolic Disorder-Related Bone Changes

- Mucopolysaccharidoses: Vertebral body beaking, oar-shaped ribs, short, thick metacarpals with proximal pointing
- Menkes disease: Metaphyseal spurs, brittle hair, tortuous intracranial arteries

Normal Variants Confused With Fractures

- Normal variant vertebral notching typically occurs at 1 level; no disc space narrowing or malalignment
- Minimal anterior sloping of midthoracic vertebrae

PATHOLOGY

General Features

- Hyperextension/hyperflexion with acceleration-deceleration forces from shaking account for many NAT-related fractures, including CMLs, posterior rib fractures, spinal fractures, & avulsion-type injuries of scapula
- Grabbing & twisting/torsional forces: Transphyseal & digital fractures
- Direct impact mechanism: Sternal, skull, & scapular body fractures

CLINICAL ISSUES

Presentation

- Wide range of clinical presentations for NAT
  - Injury inconsistent with history or stage of development
  - Multiple injuries in various stages of healing
  - Bruising in nonmobile infant
  - Burns, retinal hemorrhages
  - Seizures, altered mental status, acute life-threatening event
- Majority of spinal fractures are clinically inapparent
  - Severe & undiagnosed; may result in cord injury
  - Significant association with intracranial injury

Demographics

- Epidemiology
  - 678,000 child maltreatment victims in 2018 in USA
    - Infants ≤ 1 year old most at risk

Natural History & Prognosis

- 1,770 fatalities from child maltreatment in 2018
  - Death rate greatest in infants < 1 year old
  - 79% of fatalities involved parent as perpetrator

Treatment

- Multidisciplinary investigation of maltreatment allegations must involve physicians, social worker, Child Protective Services, legal authorities
- Ensure at risk child & siblings are given safe environment
  - May involve removal of child from home, temporary/protective custody

DIAGNOSTIC CHECKLIST

Consider

- Imaging findings & their specificity for NAT must be correlated with clinical history & physical exam findings

Reporting Tips

- Concern for child abuse raised by imaging must be discussed with referring clinician ASAP
- Report represents legal document; review carefully
- Provide clear, detailed description of each fracture, including location, fragments, & approximate age

SELECTED REFERENCES

1. Shalaby-Rana E et al: Proximal femoral physeal fractures in children: a rare abusive injury. Pediatr Radiol. 50(8):1115-22, 2020
2. Gunda D et al: Pediatric central nervous system imaging of nonaccidental trauma: beyond subdural hematomas. Radiographics. 39(1):213-28, 2019
3. Kleinman PK: Diagnostic Imaging of Child Abuse, 3rd edition. Cambridge University Press, 2015
4. Supakul N et al: Distal humeral epiphyseal separation in young children: an often-missed fracture-radiographic signs and ultrasound confirmatory diagnosis. AJR Am J Roentgenol. 204(2):W192-8, 2015
5. Bixby SD et al: Ischial apophyseal fracture in an abused infant. Pediatr Radiol. 44(9):1175-8, 2014
6. Walters MM et al: Healing patterns of clavicular birth injuries as a guide to fracture dating in cases of possible infant abuse. Pediatr Radiol. 44(10):1224-9, 2014
7. Barber I et al: Prevalence and relevance of pediatric spinal fractures in suspected child abuse. Pediatr Radiol. 43(11):1507-15, 2013
8. Kleinman PK et al: Yield of radiographic skeletal surveys for detection of hand, foot, and spine fractures in suspected child abuse. AJR Am J Roentgenol. 200(3):641-4, 2013
9. Prosser I et al: A timetable for the radiologic features of fracture healing in young children. AJR Am J Roentgenol. 198(5):1014-20, 2012
10. Hechter S et al: Sternal fractures as a manifestation of abusive injury in children. Pediatr Radiol. 32(12):902-6, 2002
11. Nimkin K et al: Distal humeral physeal injuries in child abuse: MR imaging and ultrasonography findings. Pediatr Radiol. 25(7):562-5, 1995

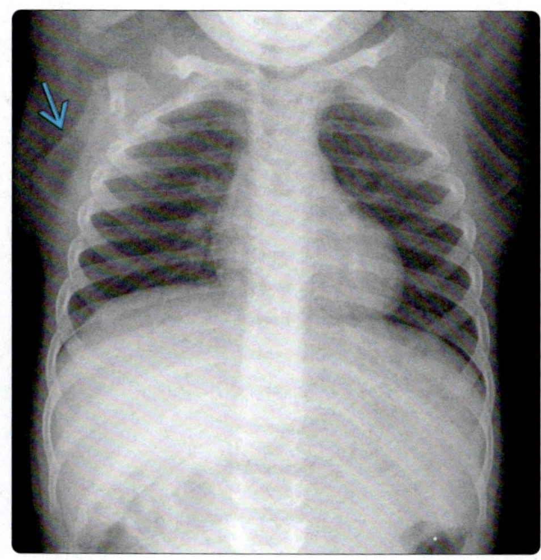

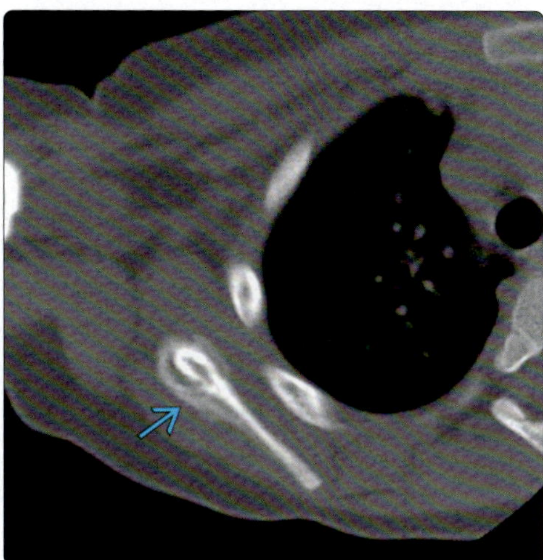

(Left) *AP chest radiograph in a 2-year-old with bruising shows a fracture of the right scapular body* ➡. **(Right)** *Axial bone CT in the same 2-year-old patient with bruising shows callus formation about the right scapular body fracture* ➡. *Scapular fractures in young children have a high specificity for child abuse, & those of the scapular body are typically the result of direct impact.*

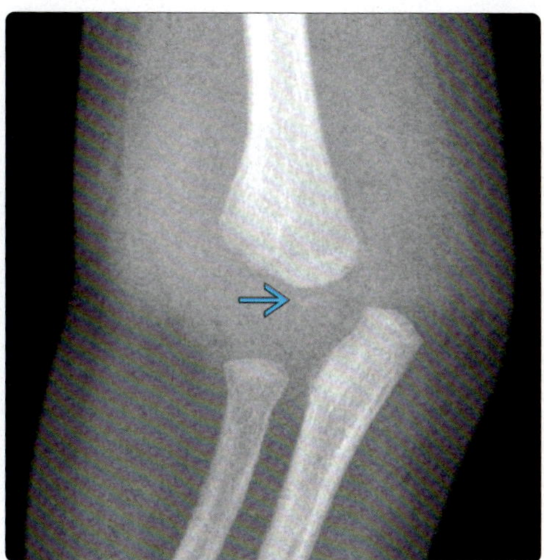

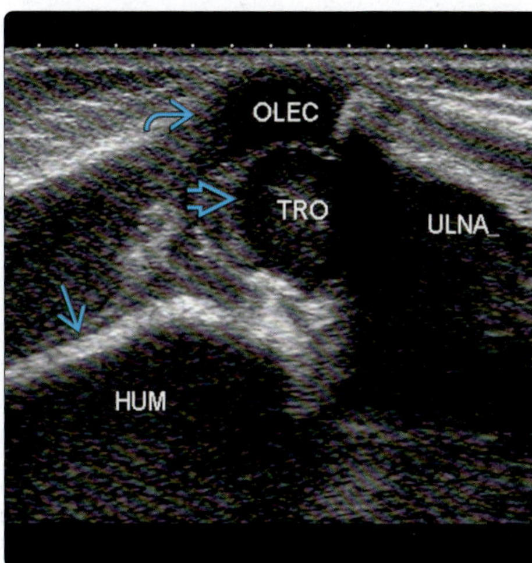

(Left) *External oblique radiograph in a 1-month-old not using his arm shows medial translation of the capitellar ossification center* ➡, *radius, & ulna relative to the distal humerus.* **(Right)** *Posterior longitudinal US of the elbow in the same patient shows posterior translation of the hypoechoic trochlear cartilage* ➡ *relative to the humerus* ➡. *The olecranon* ➡ *still articulates with the trochlea. These findings are consistent with a distal humeral epiphyseal separation fracture rather than an elbow dislocation.*

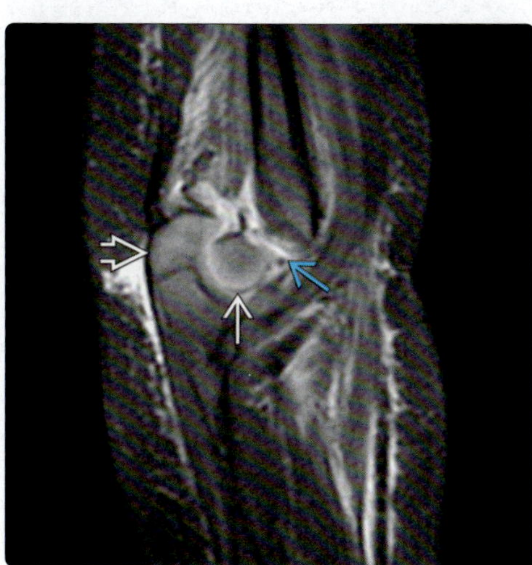

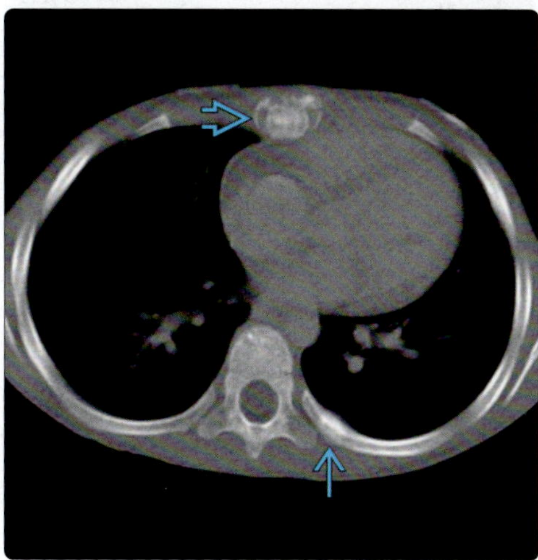

(Left) *Sagittal T2 FS MR in a 6-month-old after a reported fall shows a fracture through the distal humerus* ➡ *with posterior translation & angulation of the unossified trochlear cartilage* ➡ *& articulating olecranon cartilage* ➡. *These findings are consistent with a distal humeral epiphyseal separation.* **(Right)** *Axial CECT (in bone windows) in a young child with abdominal pain shows healing fractures of the sternum* ➡ *& a posterior left rib* ➡. *Both of these fractures are highly suggestive of child abuse.*

KEY FACTS

TERMINOLOGY

- Fatigue fracture: Fracture due to abnormal stresses applied (over time) to normal bone
- Insufficiency fracture: Fracture due to normal stresses applied to abnormal bone
- Stress response/reaction: Result of stresses upon bone prior to development of macroscopic fracture
- Chronic physeal stress injury: Repetitive stress to growth plate interrupts normal endochondral ossification

IMAGING

- Stress injury of formed bone
  - Periosteal new bone ± transversely oriented lucent cortical fracture or band of sclerosis on radiographs
  - Transverse linear focus of unicortical & medullary ↓ T1 & T2 signal (fracture line) + poorly defined surrounding ↑ T2 signal (edema) on MR = stress fracture
  - Limited marrow, periosteal, & soft tissue abnormalities without discrete fracture line = stress response
- Chronic physeal stress injury
  - Asymmetric lengthening (widening) of lucent growth plate with metaphyseal irregularity on radiographs
  - Broad metaphyseal extension of cartilaginous physeal signal intensity on MR (especially PD/T2 FS or T2* GRE)

CLINICAL ISSUES

- Fatigue fractures occur in
  - Athletes with recent changes in routine
  - Newly ambulating children
  - Children with malalignment or altered weight bearing
  - Preadolescent children without ↑ activity intensity
- Insufficiency fractures occur in children with focal or systemic processes leading to bone weakening
- Treatment includes cessation of stresses with adequate time for bone repair & recovery of normal ossification
  - Rest & immobilization to prevent completion of fracture or permanent growth disturbance from physeal injury

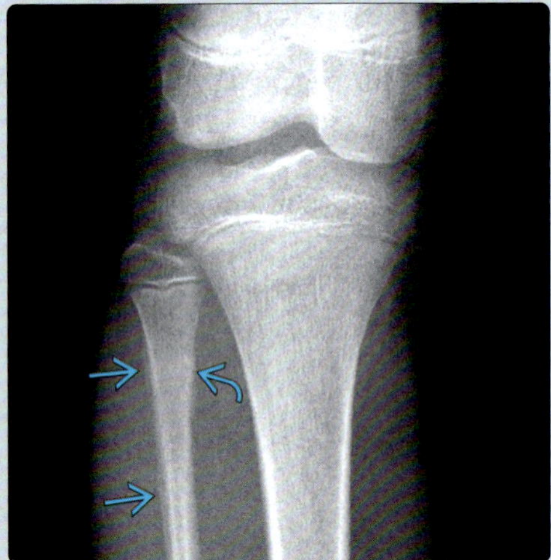

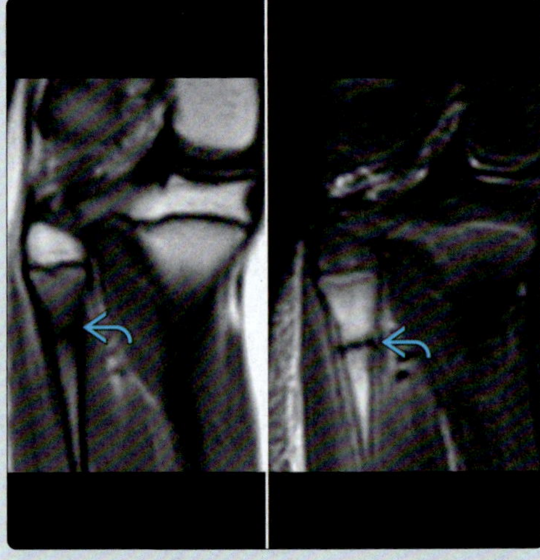

(Left) *Frontal radiograph of the right proximal leg in a 13-year-old girl with leg pain shows periosteal reaction along the proximal fibula* ➡. *A very subtle linear lucency is also seen* ➡, *suggesting a stress fracture that is poorly visualized on this study.* **(Right)** *Coronal T1 (left) & STIR (right) MR images of the proximal leg in the same child show a linear low signal intensity fracture line* ➡. *Adjacent periosteal & soft tissue edema are also seen on the STIR MR.*

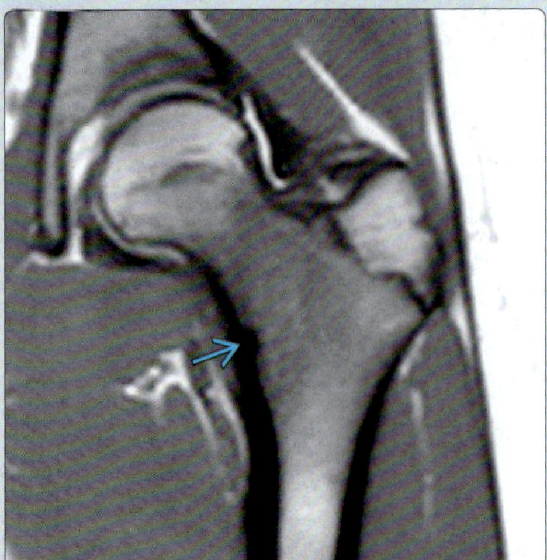

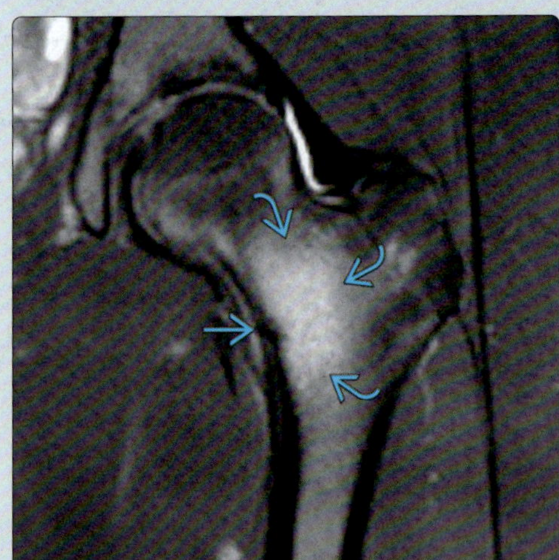

(Left) *Coronal PD MR in a 17-year-old female track athlete with left hip pain shows linear low signal intensity* ➡ *at the medial aspect of the left femoral neck.* **(Right)** *Coronal T2 FS MR in the same patient shows the low signal intensity fracture line* ➡ *with surrounding marrow edema* ➡. *This half-moon configuration of marrow edema in the femoral neck has been described with both osteoid osteoma & stress fractures.*

TERMINOLOGY

Definitions

- Fatigue fracture: Fracture due to abnormal stresses applied (over time) to normal bone
- Insufficiency fracture: Fracture due to normal stresses applied to abnormal bone
  - Demineralized or otherwise weakened bone from focal or systemic process
- Stress response/reaction: Result of stresses upon bone prior to development of macroscopic fracture
- Chronic physeal stress injury: Repetitive stress to metaphyseal vasculature & cartilaginous growth plate interrupts normal endochondral ossification

IMAGING

Radiographic Findings

- Stress fracture
  - Poor cortical definition with varying degrees of cortical thickening/periosteal new bone
  - ± transversely oriented findings, including
    - Hairline fracture lucency extending centrally from involved cortex
    - Sclerotic band of medullary cavity
- Chronic physeal stress injury
  - Broad or focal lengthening (widening) of lucent physis
  - Metaphyseal irregularity with loss of normal thin, radiodense zone of provisional calcification (ZPC)

CT Findings

- Hairline, transversely oriented, unicortical lucency extending centrally with adjacent solid, smooth periosteal reaction

MR Findings

- T1WI
  - Transverse hypointense stress fracture line extending from cortex into medullary cavity
  - Varying degrees of surrounding poorly defined hypointense marrow edema
- T2WI FS
  - Poorly defined hyperintense signal of marrow, periosteum, & soft tissues without discrete fracture line: Stress response
  - Transverse linear hypointense focus of medullary signal: Stress fracture
  - Metaphyseal extension of cartilaginous physeal signal intensity: Chronic physeal stress injury
    - Broad vs. small "tongue" of unossified cartilage
- T2* GRE
  - Cartilage-sensitive sequences nicely demonstrate abnormalities at interface of physis-metaphysis (i.e., chronic physeal stress injuries & rare secondary bony bridges)
- T1WI C+ FS
  - Enhancing marrow, periosteal, & soft tissue edema

Nuclear Medicine Findings

- Bone scan: Intense cortical uptake; sensitivity ~ 100%
- SPECT-CT: ↑ specificity for location & etiology
  - May help separate fracture from osteoid osteoma
  - Excellent for pars interarticularis stress fracture

DIFFERENTIAL DIAGNOSIS

Focal Periosteal Reaction, Marrow Edema

- Osteoid osteoma
- Osteomyelitis
- Bone malignancy
  - Ewing sarcoma, metastatic neuroblastoma, leukemia

Linear Sclerosis Within Bone

- Infarction

Lucent & Irregular Physes/Metaphyses

- Rickets
- Epiphysiodesis (drill type)
- Leukemia

CLINICAL ISSUES

Presentation

- Most common signs/symptoms
  - Stress fracture: Pain, swelling with appropriate history
  - Chronic physeal stress injury: Pain; rarely asymptomatic
  - Symptoms typically are present for weeks prior to presentation
- Clinical profile
  - Fatigue fractures in
    - Athletes with recent changes in routine
      - Medial tibial stress syndrome: Overuse or repetitive stress injury to shin area; may progress to fracture
    - Newly ambulating children
      - Young child with new refusal to bear weight
    - Children with malalignment or altered weight bearing
    - Preadolescent children with normal play activities & no elevation of activity intensity
  - Insufficiency fractures in
    - Children with focal or systemic processes leading to bone weakening
      - New stress reaction/insufficiency fracture in osteoporotic hindfoot due to ↑ ambulation after weeks of casting for preceding distal tibial fracture

Treatment

- Stress fracture
  - Prevention is paramount: Gradual ↑ in new activity intensity + prompt activity reduction when pain occurs
  - Combination of reduced activity, rest, immobilization, casting, & (rarely) internal fixation
- Chronic physeal stress injury: Rest & immobilization are typically sufficient for endochondral ossification to resume

SELECTED REFERENCES

1. Ditmars FS et al: MRI of tibial stress fractures: relationship between Fredericson classification and time to recovery in pediatric athletes. Pediatr Radiol. 50(12):1735-41, 2020
2. Sweeney E et al: Overuse knee pain in the pediatric and adolescent athlete. Curr Sports Med Rep. 19(11):479-85, 2020
3. Nguyen JC et al: Imaging of pediatric growth plate disturbances. Radiographics. 37(6):1791-812, 2017
4. Shelat NH et al: Pediatric stress fractures: a pictorial essay. Iowa Orthop J. 36:138-46, 2016
5. Bedoya MA et al: Overuse injuries in children. Top Magn Reson Imaging. 24(2):67-81, 2015

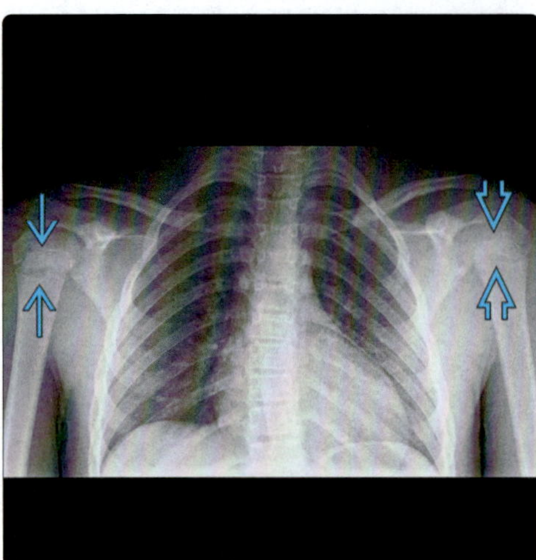

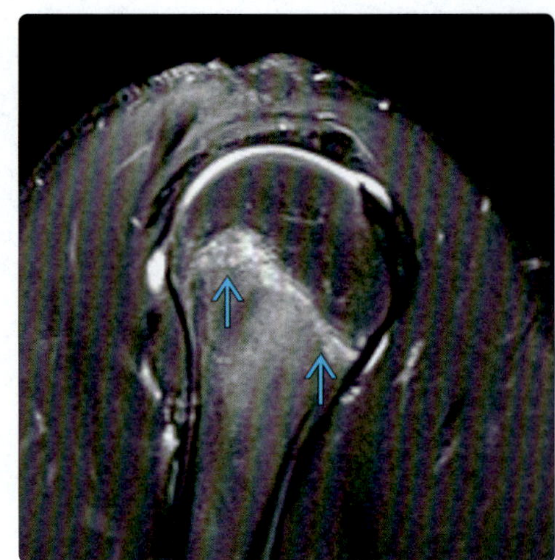

(Left) *AP radiograph of the shoulders in a 14-year-old pitcher with weeks of right shoulder pain shows lengthening of the proximal right humeral physis ➔ as compared to the normal left side ➔. Note the pseudofracture appearance of both proximal humeri due to the normal obliquity of the growth plates.* **(Right)** *Sagittal T2 FS MR in the same patient shows an abnormally long, irregular, & hyperintense physis ➔, typical of a chronic repetitive stress injury of the growth plate in this pitcher (Little Leaguer's shoulder).*

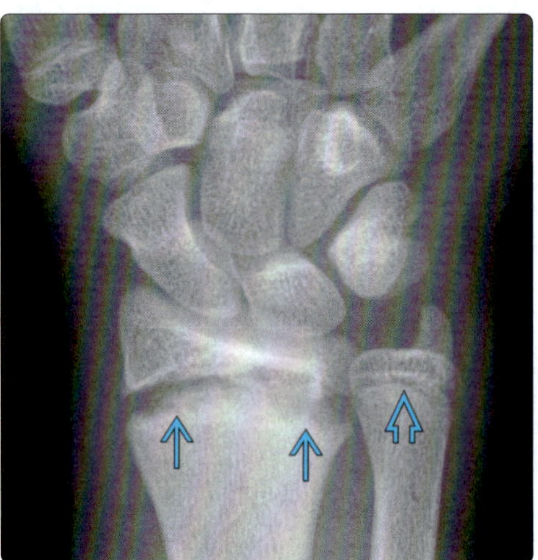

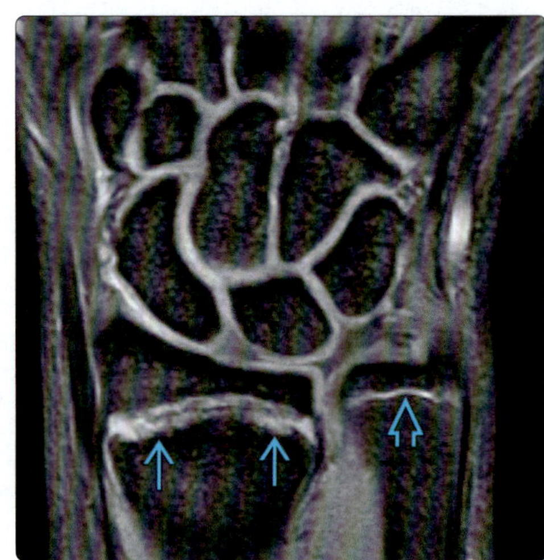

(Left) *PA wrist radiograph in a 13-year-old female gymnast with pain shows abnormal lengthening of the cartilaginous distal radial physis with metaphyseal irregularity ➔ & loss of the normal thin, dense zone of provisional Ca^{2+}. Note the normal distal ulnar physis ➔.* **(Right)** *Coronal T2* GRE MR in this patient confirms abnormal lengthening of the radial physis ➔ due to repetitive microtrauma (gymnast wrist). The ulnar physis is normal ➔ as it does not endure the same physical stresses as the radius.*

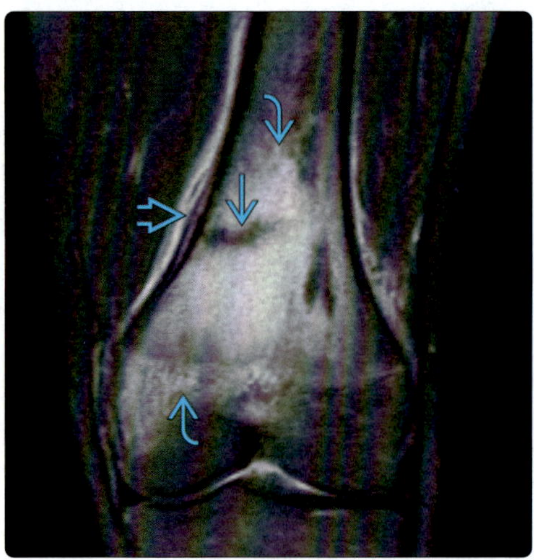

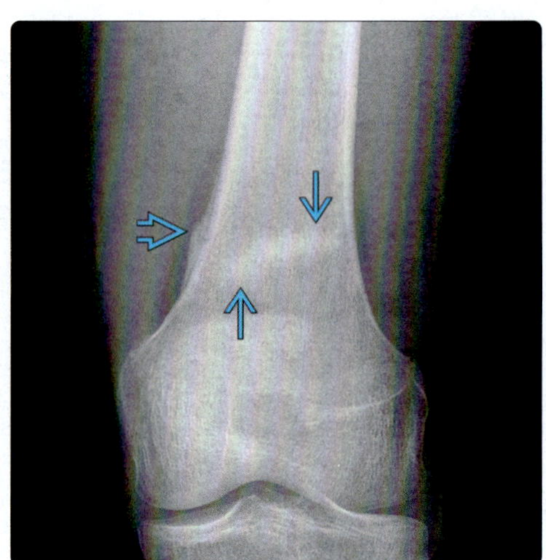

(Left) *Coronal T2 FS MR in a 16-year-old with knee pain shows a transverse band of low signal intensity ➔ in the distal femoral diaphysis, consistent with an incomplete stress fracture. There is surrounding marrow edema ➔ & overlying periosteal reaction ➔.* **(Right)** *Follow-up AP radiograph in the same patient 4 weeks later shows sclerosis of the healing stress fracture ➔ with focal solid periosteal reaction at this level ➔.*

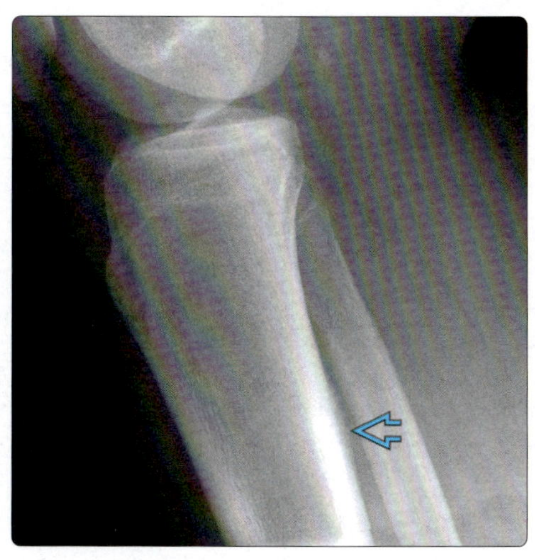

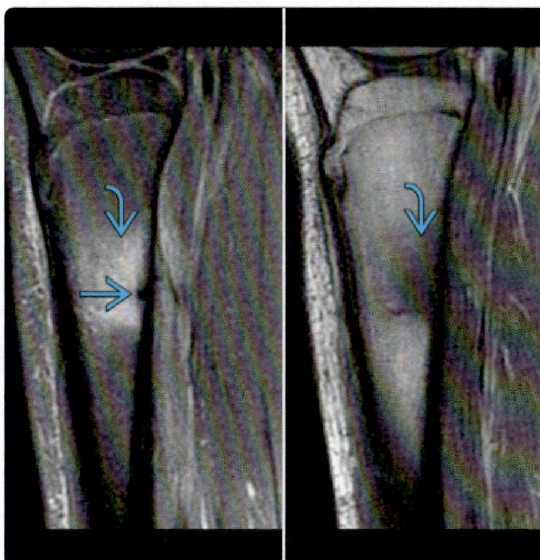

(Left) *Lateral radiograph in a 14-year-old with lower leg pain shows subtle solid periosteal reaction focally at the posterior proximal right tibial diaphysis* ➡. **(Right)** *Sagittal T2 FS (left) & T1 (right) MR images of the same patient show poorly defined marrow edema* ➡ *surrounding a small linear corticomedullary focus of low signal intensity* ➡, *consistent with a stress fracture.*

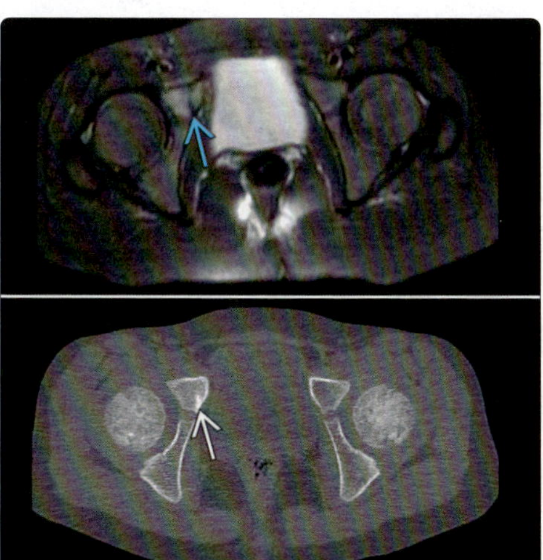

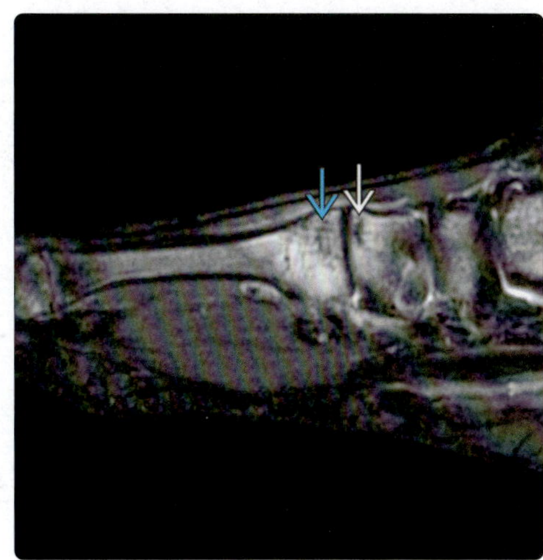

(Left) *Axial T2 FS MR (top) of the pelvis in a 6-year-old with pain shows a low signal intensity fracture line* ➡ *of the superior pubic ramus with surrounding marrow edema. Axial bone CT (bottom) shows sclerosis at this same level* ➡, *consistent with a healing stress fracture.* **(Right)** *Sagittal STIR MR in a 16-year-old cross country runner with pain shows linear low signal intensity foci in the 2nd metatarsal base* ➡ *& middle cuneiform* ➡ *with surrounding marrow edema, consistent with stress fractures.*

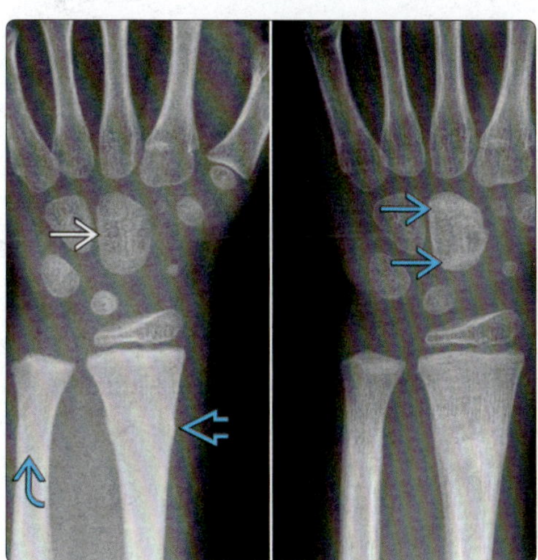

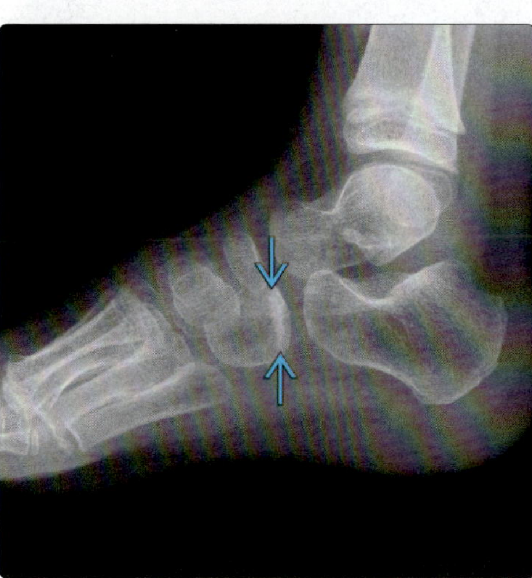

(Left) *PA wrist radiographs taken 6 weeks apart in a 6-year-old after a fall show incomplete fractures of the distal radius* ➡ *& ulna* ➡ *initially (left). The capitate is normal* ➡ *on the initial radiographs. Six weeks later (right), there is disuse osteoporosis distally with horizontal stress reaction* ➡ *of the capitate.* **(Right)** *Lateral radiograph of the foot in a 3-year-old shows a band of vertically oriented sclerosis in the posterior aspect of the cuboid* ➡, *a common location for a stress injury.*

Osteochondritis Dissecans

KEY FACTS

TERMINOLOGY

- Osteochondritis dissecans (OCD): Juvenile OCD (JOCD) when physes are open vs. adult OCD when physes are closed
- Focal joint disorder with progressive changes in subchondral bone & overlying articular cartilage that may lead to early joint degeneration

IMAGING

- Findings reported as specific for instability in JOCD
  - Fluid-filled osteochondral defect
  - High T2 signal intensity cartilage fracture line
  - Fluid signal intensity surrounding OCD
  - Multiple breaks in subchondral bone plate on T2 MR
  - Outer rim of T2 low signal intensity
  - Multiple cysts or single cyst > 5 mm
- Findings reported as specific for instability in adult OCD
  - Fluid-filled osteochondral defect
  - High T2 signal intensity rim
  - High T2 signal intensity cartilage fracture line
  - Cysts surrounding OCD

TOP DIFFERENTIAL DIAGNOSES

- Normal irregular distal femoral epiphyseal ossification
- Osteonecrosis
- Osteochondral impaction fracture
- Stress or insufficiency fracture

PATHOLOGY

- Etiology is likely multifactorial (traumatic, ischemic, genetic)
  - Favored mechanism: Repetitive microtrauma
  - JOCD may represent growth disturbance of secondary physis; little necrosis or inflammation on histology

CLINICAL ISSUES

- Most common in adolescent athletes
- Studies show high variability in MR accuracy for predicting instability compared to arthroscopy

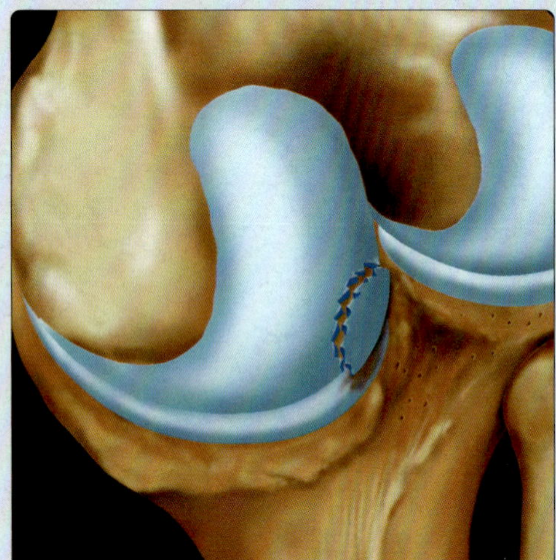

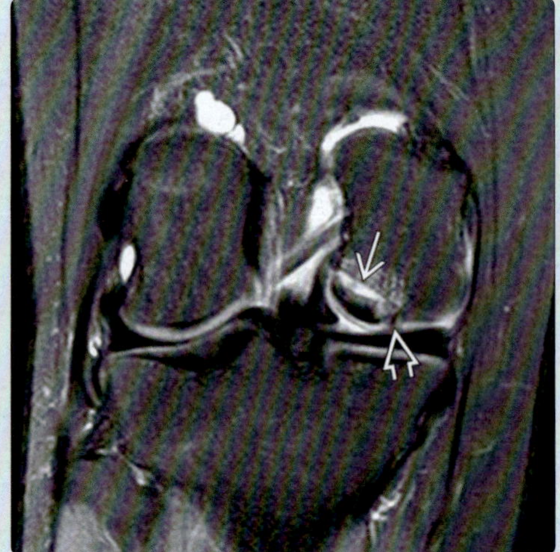

(Left) *Coronal oblique graphic shows circumferential fissuring of the articular cartilage of the posterolateral aspect of the medial femoral condyle.* **(Right)** *Coronal T2 FS MR in a 15-year-old girl shows the in situ portion of a complex osteochondral lesion of the medial femoral condyle. Fluid* ➔ *undercuts the fragment with an overlying T2-hypointense cartilage crack* ➔ *noted, which are MR findings consistent with an unstable lesion.*

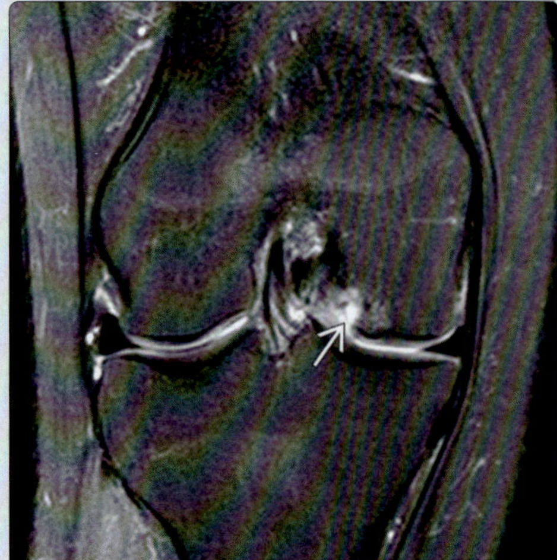

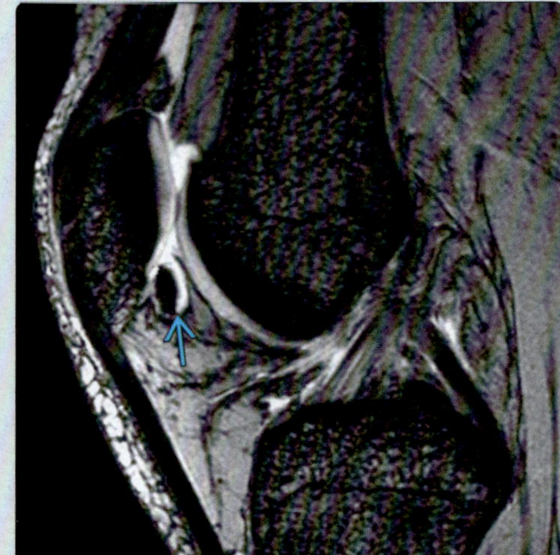

(Left) *Slightly more anterior T2 FS MR slice in the same patient shows fluid filling an osteochondral defect* ➔ *of the parent femoral condyle.* **(Right)** *Sagittal midline T2* GRE MR in the same patient shows the displaced osteochondral fragment* ➔ *along the inferior patellar articular surface. The fragment was shown to be loose (rather than synovialized & fixed) by interval changes in position on radiographs (not shown).*

TERMINOLOGY

Abbreviations

- Osteochondritis dissecans (OCD)

Synonyms

- Osteochondral lesion, juvenile OCD (JOCD), adult OCD

Definitions

- Focal joint disorder with progressive changes in subchondral bone & overlying articular cartilage that may lead to early joint degeneration
- JOCD is limited to skeletally immature patients (open physes)

IMAGING

General Features

- Best diagnostic clue
  - Osteochondral lesion at lateral aspect of medial femoral condyle ± loose fragment in young adolescent athlete
- Location
  - Large multicenter study of OCD: Knee is most common location
    - Medial femoral condyle: 77%
    - Lateral femoral condyle: 17%
    - Others at knee: Patella (7%), trochlea (1%), tibial plateau (0.2%)
    - Bilateral: ~ 15-30%
  - Less frequent in elbow, ankle, hip
- Morphology
  - Crescentic/ovoid osteochondral lesion contiguous with parent bone (in situ) vs. detached intraarticular fragment

Radiographic Findings

- Crescentic/ovoid lucent subchondral bone lesion surrounded by sclerotic margin
- ± in situ or displaced intraarticular osseous fragment
- Underestimates size, cannot assess cartilage integrity
- Radiographic findings of healing on follow-up exams
  - ↑ ossification within lesion
  - ↓ sclerotic halo between parent bone & lesion
  - Less defined lucency between parent bone & lesion
  - ↑ convexity of articular surface shape
  - ↓ overall volume of lesion

MR Findings

- T1WI
  - Hypointense fragment
  - ± hypointense subchondral marrow edema
  - ± hyperintense fibrovascular tissue on 3D T1 FS SPGR
- T2WI
  - Variable hyperintense signal in osteochondral fragment & adjacent marrow
  - Overlying fissures/defects in articular cartilage are best appreciated on PD/T2 ± FS
  - PD/T2 FS may demonstrate direct cartilaginous &/or bony extension of fluid
  - ± hyperintense cysts or fibrovascular tissue deep to lesion
  - ± hyperintense synovial thickening or joint fluid
  - Specifically in JOCD
    - Oreo cookie sign: Laminar T2 hyperintensity with deep & superficial margins of hypointensity
    - Disruption of thin, circumferential, hyperintense secondary physis overlying OCD lesion
    - Thickened overlying unossified epiphyseal cartilage
- T2* GRE
  - May help visualize displaced osteochondral fragment
    - Purely chondral fragments may be best seen on FSE FS images
- MR arthrography with gadolinium-based agent
  - Contrast between OCD fragment & parent bone = unstable fragment
- MR features for treatment planning (most studied in knee)
  - Findings reported as specific for instability in JOCD
    - Fluid-filled osteochondral defect
    - High T2 signal intensity cartilage fracture line
    - High T2 signal rim equal to fluid signal intensity surrounding OCD
    - Multiple breaks in subchondral bone plate on T2
    - Outer rim of T2 low signal intensity
    - Multiple cysts or single cyst > 5 mm
  - However, other studies have shown some JOCD with MR findings of instability to heal without surgery
  - Findings reported as specific for instability in adult OCD
    - Fluid-filled osteochondral defect
    - High T2 signal intensity rim
    - High T2 signal intensity cartilage fracture line
    - Cysts surrounding OCD
  - Predictors of stability
    - Fragment continuity with parent bone without linear fluid signal intensity interface, cyst, high T2 signal cartilage fracture line, or breaks in subchondral bone plate
  - MR accuracy for predicting stable vs. unstable OCD lesion as compared to arthroscopy: 30-92%
  - MR findings of healing after therapy
    - Variable osteochondral changes depending on type of intervention
    - In general, healing is indicated by
      - ↓ lesion size, cysts, marrow edema
      - ↑ bone filling OCD lesion bed
      - Improved morphology of articular cartilage surface

Imaging Recommendations

- Best imaging tool
  - MR or MR arthrography
- Protocol advice
  - PD/T2 FS MR sagittal, coronal ± axial sequences (depending on OCD site)
  - 3D GRE FS MR cartilage-sensitive sequence
  - MR arthrography with gadolinium-based contrast agent can aid instability assessment

DIFFERENTIAL DIAGNOSIS

Normal Irregular Distal Femoral Epiphyseal Ossification

- Asymptomatic younger patients
- Most commonly in posterior condyle
- Often has "puzzle piece" fragment-parent bone interface
- Deep rather than flat

- No adjacent bone marrow edema
- Overlying cartilage is intact, including thin, T2-hyperintense secondary physis

Osteonecrosis

- Serpentine sclerotic foci with characteristic double-line appearance on T2 MR
  - May lead to subchondral collapse
- History of steroid therapy, lupus, sickle cell disease, or other predisposing condition

Osteochondral Impaction Fracture

- Single traumatic event
- Different location than typical OCD lesion

Stress or Insufficiency Fracture

- Sclerotic band, often horizontal to bone long axis
- Not usually subchondral

PATHOLOGY

General Features

- Etiology
  - Favored mechanism: Repetitive microtrauma
    - Acute trauma, ischemia, &/or genetic predisposition may be contributory
  - JOCD may represent symptomatic growth disturbance of epiphyseal secondary physis
  - Adult OCD may be incompletely healed JOCD lesion

Staging, Grading, & Classification

- Arthroscopic grading: Multiple systems
  - Research in Osteochondritis of the Knee (ROCK)
    - Immobile lesions
      - Cue ball: No arthroscopic abnormality
      - Shadow: Cartilage intact but subtly demarcated
      - Wrinkle: Cartilage fissure, buckle &/or wrinkle
    - Mobile lesions
      - Locked door: Cartilage fissure, cannot hinge open
      - Trap door: Cartilage fissure, can hinge open
      - Crater: Exposed subchondral bone defect

Microscopic Features

- No substantial necrosis or inflammation in JOCD lesions
- Abundant fibrovascular tissue at osteochondral interface & in subchondral bone

CLINICAL ISSUES

Presentation

- Most common signs/symptoms
  - Pain aggravated by activity
  - Mechanical symptoms (clicking, catching, grinding, locking) raise concern for unstable OCD
- Other signs/symptoms
  - Can be asymptomatic

Demographics

- Age
  - Most present at 13-21 years of age
  - Mean age of JOCD is 11.3 years by one study
  - Symptoms often last > 1 year prior to diagnosis
- Sex
  - M:F = 2-4:1 (but ↑ in females with ↑ sports participation)
- Epidemiology
  - Incidence of JOCD = 2.3/100,000 to 31.6/100,000
  - Often seen in athletes

Natural History & Prognosis

- ↑ rate of spontaneous healing in JOCD vs. adult OCD
  - 50-67% of JOCD lesions heal in 6-18 months with conservative therapy only
    - Spontaneous healing: Stable > > unstable
- American Academy of Orthopaedic Surgeons (AAOS) practice guidelines state, "natural history of OCD of the knee remains unclear"

Treatment

- AAOS 2010 review of OCD evidence was largely inconclusive regarding diagnosis + treatment recommendations
- Stable lesions are generally treated with rest, casting, NSAIDs over 3-12 months
  - Failure to heal on conservative therapy → surgery
    - Drilling (transarticular or retroarticular) to create vascular channels
- Stable but symptomatic OCDs that fail nonoperative management may be treated with arthroscopic drilling
- Unstable lesions → surgery
  - Salvageable: Internal fixation of fragment
    - Metal screws; bioabsorbable pins, screws, or nails
    - ± bone autograft or allograft
  - Unsalvageable: Cartilage repair/restoration
    - Chondroplasty
    - Microfracture
    - Osteochondral autograft/allograft transfer system
    - Autologous chondrocyte implantation

DIAGNOSTIC CHECKLIST

Image Interpretation Pearls

- Careful evaluation for signs of instability ± loose body

SELECTED REFERENCES

1. Fabricant PD et al: Osteochondritis dissecans of the knee: an interrater reliability study of magnetic resonance imaging characteristics. Am J Sports Med. 48(9):2221-9, 2020
2. Masquijo J et al: Juvenile osteochondritis dissecans (JOCD) of the knee: current concepts review. EFORT Open Rev. 4(5):201-12, 2019
3. Haeri Hendy S et al: Juvenile osteochondritis dissecans of the knee: does magnetic resonance imaging instability correlate with the need for surgical intervention? Orthop J Sports Med. 5(11):2325967117738516, 2017
4. Wall EJ et al: The reliability of assessing radiographic healing of osteochondritis dissecans of the knee. Am J Sports Med. 45(6):1370-5, 2017
5. Carey JL et al: Novel arthroscopic classification of osteochondritis dissecans of the knee: a multicenter reliability study. Am J Sports Med. 44(7):1694-8, 2016
6. Roßbach BP et al: Discrepancy between morphological findings in juvenile osteochondritis dissecans (OCD): a comparison of magnetic resonance imaging (MRI) and arthroscopy. Knee Surg Sports Traumatol Arthrosc. 24(4):1259-64, 2016
7. Zbojniewicz AM et al: Juvenile osteochondritis dissecans: correlation between histopathology and MRI. AJR Am J Roentgenol. 205(1):W114-23, 2015
8. Laor T et al: Juvenile osteochondritis dissecans: is it a growth disturbance of the secondary physis of the epiphysis? AJR Am J Roentgenol. 199(5):1121-8, 2012

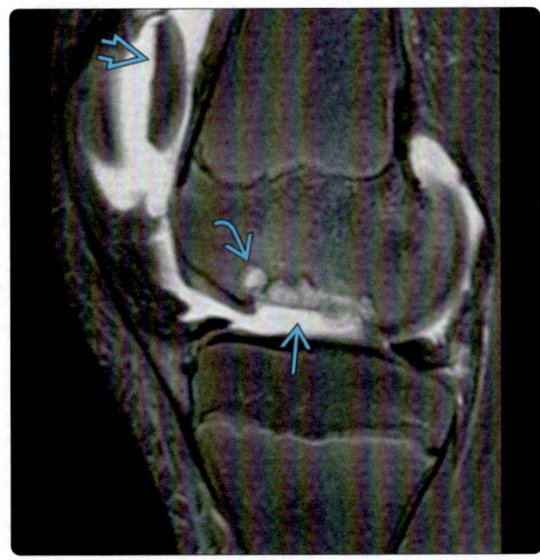

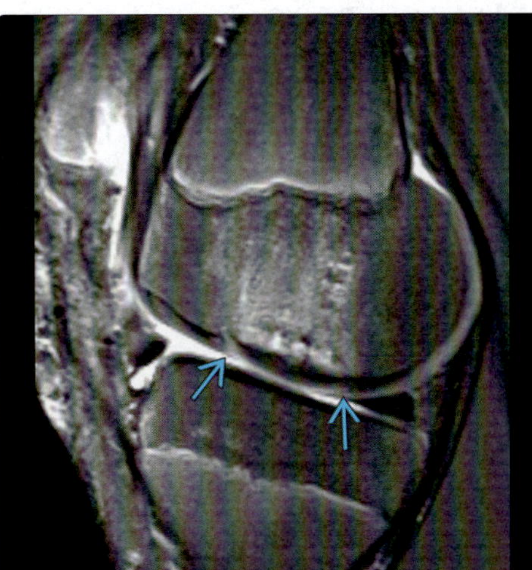

(Left) *Sagittal T2 FS MR in a 15-year-old with an unstable JOCD lesion shows a large, fluid-filled gap in the medial femoral condyle* ➡ *with multiple subjacent cysts* ➡ *in the parent bone. A large, displaced osteochondral fragment is noted* ➡. **(Right)** *Sagittal T2 FS MR in the same patient status post autologous bone graft to the donor site shows interval healing with early incorporation of the bone graft. The overlying articular cartilage is smooth & continuous* ➡ *with the adjacent native articular cartilage.*

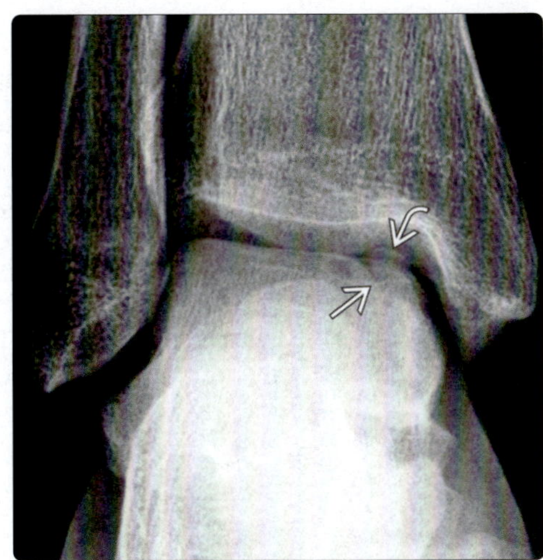

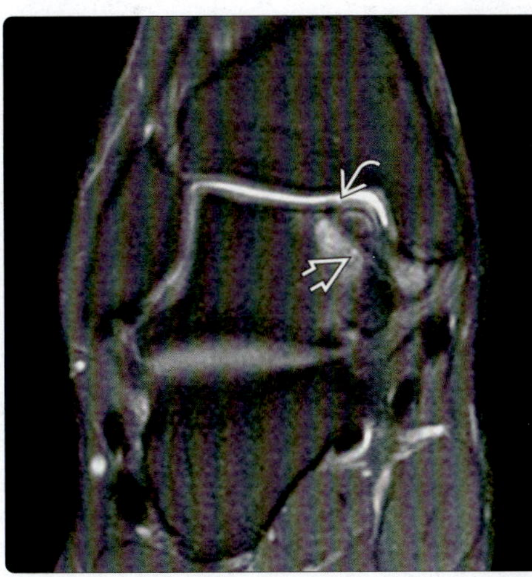

(Left) *AP ankle radiograph in a 16-year-old boy shows a crescentic lucent lesion in the medial talar dome* ➡ *with a bony fragment* ➡ *protruding into the joint space.* **(Right)** *Coronal T2 FS MR in the same patient confirms the OCD lesion of the medial talar dome with adjacent cartilage fissuring* ➡. *Cystic change* ➡ *& surrounding edema are noted in the parent bone. While no fluid is seen undercutting the fragment, the constellation of radiographic & MR findings remains suspicious for an unstable lesion.*

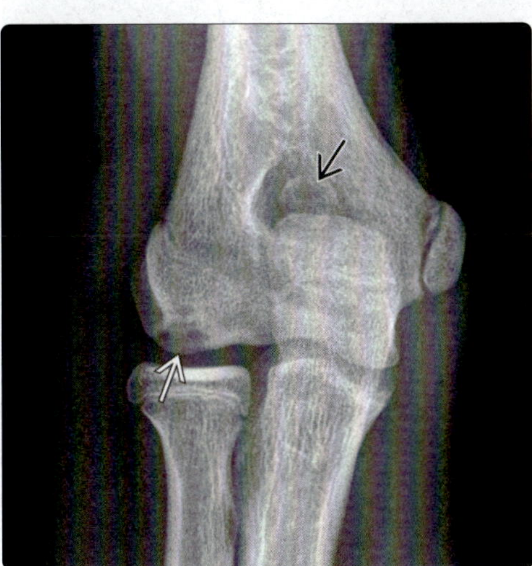

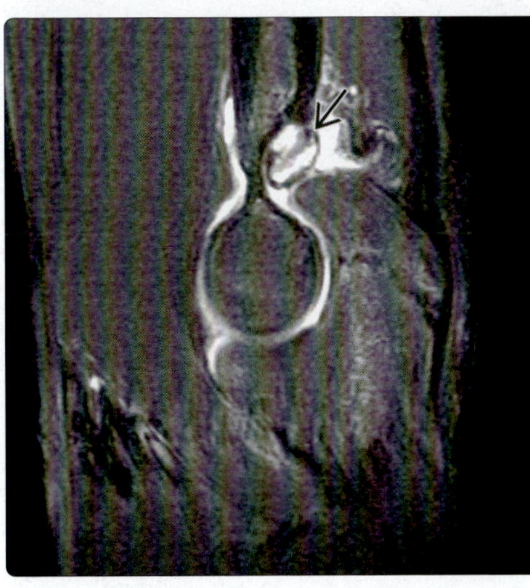

(Left) *AP elbow radiograph in a 13-year-old boy with pain & locking shows an irregular lucent defect* ➡ *with sclerotic margin in the humeral capitellum, typical of OCD. An ossific body* ➡ *projects over the olecranon fossa.* **(Right)** *Sagittal T2 FS MR in the same patient confirms an intraarticular osteochondral body in the olecranon fossa* ➡ *with high signal within the body. An associated elbow joint effusion & synovitis are also present.*

Fracture Complications

KEY FACTS

TERMINOLOGY

- Nonunion: Lack of progression to union > 6 months after injury with corresponding clinical signs & symptoms
- Malunion: Nonanatomic alignment of fracture fragments
- Premature physeal closure: Osseous physeal bridge (bar) formation across cartilaginous physis

IMAGING

- Nonunion: Sclerosis at fragment margins, absence of bridging trabecula, persistence of fracture line
- Premature physeal closure
  - Progressive focal narrowing or interruption of lucent physis ± discrete bone bridge/bar
  - Abnormal (obliquely oriented or asymmetric) growth arrest/growth recovery lines
    - Angulated toward & tethered by bridge
  - Peripheral bridge → angular deformity
  - Central bridge → longitudinal growth restriction
  - 3D SPGR or T2* GRE FS MR can generate physeal map
    - Assess percent of physis occupied by bridge
- Posttraumatic lipid inclusion cyst
  - Radiographs: Round or ovoid, lucent, eccentric, subperiosteal lesion, typically in distal radius or tibia
  - CT/MR: Fat characteristics
- Osteonecrosis: T1 C+ FS MR can help determine viability of proximal fragment in scaphoid nonunions

CLINICAL ISSUES

- Malunion is common in pediatric fractures (but there is high corrective potential due to remodeling in growing skeleton)
- Physeal bridges begin 1-2 months following injury but may not manifest until years later during adolescent growth

DIAGNOSTIC CHECKLIST

- Imaging findings of nonunion & malunion must be clinically correlated
  - From medicolegal standpoint, it may be best to be descriptive & discuss with orthopedist rather than use these terms in report

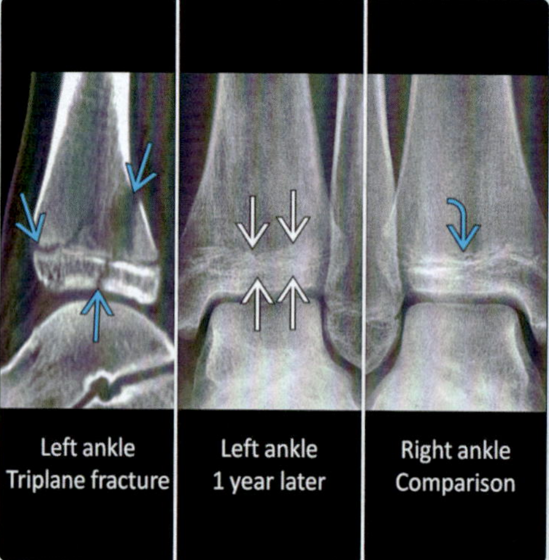

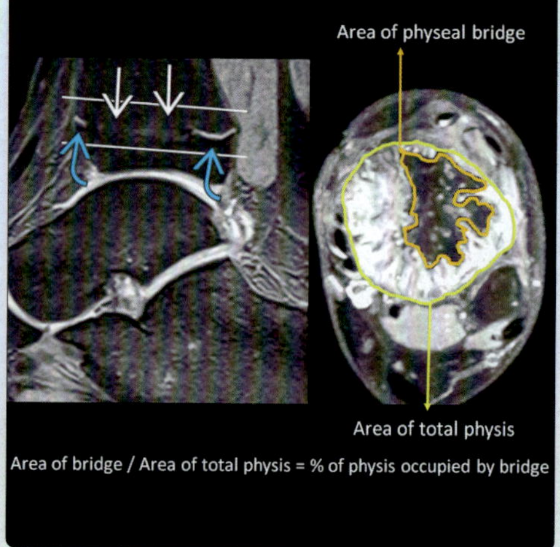

(Left) *Sagittal bone CT in a 13-year-old boy shows a triplane fracture ➔. Follow-up frontal radiographs show poor definition of the central physis ➔ due to a physeal bridge of the distal left tibia. Note the normal open distal right tibial physis ➔.* **(Right)** *Sagittal 3D SPGR FS MR (left) in the same patient shows a dark osseous bridge ➔ interrupting the bright cartilaginous physis ➔. The axial MIP of the physis (right) allows calculation of the areas of the osseous bridge (outlined in orange) & total physis (outlined in yellow).*

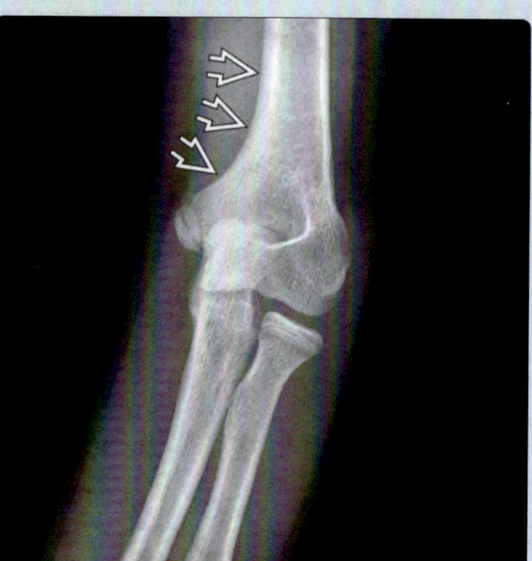

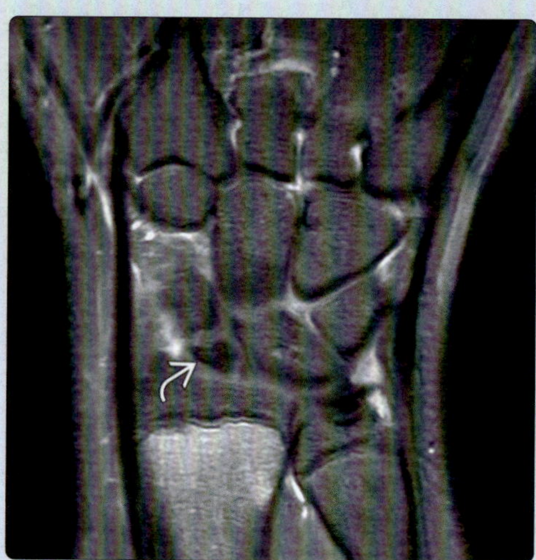

(Left) *AP radiograph in an 11-year-old girl with a deformity of the elbow (following a previously treated distal humeral supracondylar fracture) shows malunion with varus configuration to the distal humerus ➔ (cubitus varus).* **(Right)** *Coronal T1 FS C+ MR in a 14-year-old girl with a scaphoid fracture shows a diffuse lack of enhancement ➔ within the proximal pole of the scaphoid, which suggests nonviability.*

TERMINOLOGY

Complications Encountered

- Nonunion: Lack of bony union > 6 months after injury with corresponding clinical signs/symptoms
- Delayed union: Lack of union by 6 months but with imaging &/or clinical signs of healing; eventually heals
- Malunion: Healing with nonanatomic alignment of fracture fragments
- Premature physeal closure/growth arrest: Osseous physeal bridge (bar) forms across otherwise unfused cartilaginous physis
- Osteonecrosis: Disruption of blood supply to fracture fragment with resulting infarction
- Chondrolysis: Progressive destruction of articular cartilage; may lead to premature degenerative arthritis
- Posttraumatic lipid inclusion cyst: Subperiosteal focus of marrow fat entrapped in remodeled cortex (due to transposition of fatty marrow during prior fracture)
- Others: Infection, degenerative changes, refracture

IMAGING

General Features

- Nonunion
  - Radiographic findings
    - Absence of bridging trabecula with persistence of fracture lucency
    - Sclerosis of fragment margins along fracture
    - Lack of healing/callus progression on serial radiographs
      - Callus may not be seen normally with rigid fixation
  - Scaphoid nonunion
    - Humpback deformity
      - ↑ angulation between proximal & distal poles with settling/impaction of fragments & eventual dorsal bone formation
    - Carpal instability
    - Late complications
      - Scaphoid nonunion advanced collapse: Late development of arthritis
- Premature physeal closure
  - Peripheral bridge → angular deformity
    - Medial proximal femur → coxa vara
    - Anterior proximal tibia → genu recurvatum
    - Medial distal tibia → ankle varus
  - Central bridge → longitudinal growth restriction
    - Leg length discrepancy
    - Distal radial bridge → ulnar positive variance → ulnar abutment/impaction
  - Radiographs
    - May show bone bridge across physis; contralateral radiographs are helpful for comparison
      - Focal poor definition/frank interruption of lucent physis
    - Angled growth arrest/growth recovery line
      - Obliquely oriented or tethered growth recovery line extends to bony bridge at physis instead of paralleling physis
      - Asymmetry of transverse growth recovery line indicates focally diminished growth
    - Altered relative length of bone (as compared to adjacent long bone)
    - ↑ angulation of epiphysis
  - CT: Can depict bony physeal bridges but MR is preferred due to ability to evaluate residual cartilaginous physis
  - MR
    - Spin-echo T1 & PD/T2 FS sequences can demonstrate larger physeal bridges
    - 3D GRE FS sequences (with multiplanar reformatted images) detect even small bridges & can generate axial MIP physeal map
      - Cartilaginous physis is bright; bone bridge is dark
      - Area of bridge/area of total physis = % of physis occupied by bridge (used to determine therapy)
- Posttraumatic lipid inclusion cyst
  - Radiographs: Small, eccentric, round or ovoid lucent subperiosteal lesion, typically in distal radius or tibia
  - CT/MR: Fat characteristics
- Osteonecrosis
  - Scaphoid
    - Osteonecrosis in ~ 30% of midbody fractures & up to 100% of proximal pole fractures
    - Relative sclerosis of proximal pole on radiographs
    - STIR/T2 FS MR is not helpful in determining viability (i.e., lack of necrosis) of proximal pole
    - T1 MR may be of value with regard to assessing viability; literature is conflicting
    - T1 C+ FS MR is useful to assess viability of proximal fragment
      - Most studies report lack of contrast enhancement in proximal pole as being specific for osteonecrosis
      - However, enhancement of proximal pole can be seen in cases of osteonecrosis
    - T1 C+ FS MR is also helpful in guiding treatment & predicting surgical outcome
      - Higher rates of union when vascularized (vs. nonvascular) bone grafts are used when there is ↓ T1 signal or lack of enhancement on pretreatment MR
    - Dual-energy CECT: Early study shows promise for evaluating viability of proximal pole
  - Distal humerus: Fishtail deformity
    - Osteonecrosis of distal humerus predominantly involving radial aspect of trochlea
    - Reported after fractures of various types (e.g., supracondylar, lateral condylar)

CLINICAL ISSUES

Nonunion

- Rare complication in pediatrics
- Risk factors: Open fractures, infection, severe soft tissue loss, & insufficient fixation
- Types of nonunion
  - Reactive/hypertrophic: Callus formation without bridging
  - Nonreactive/atrophic: No callus at nonunion site
  - Infected: Due to acute or chronic osteomyelitis
- Most common in children: Diaphyseal long bone fractures & elbow (especially displaced lateral condyle) fractures
- Scaphoid nonunions are rare in children

- Nonunion typically results from delayed or missed diagnosis
- Treatment options: Debridement of nonunion site, bone grafting, electrical stimulation, & rigid internal fixation

Malunion

- Common in children but with high corrective potential due to ↑ chance for remodeling in growing skeleton
- Recommendations regarding maximum acceptable displacement at fracture sites in children are controversial & depend on age, location, & type of displacement
- Subsequent functional limitation & cosmetic deformity depend on site of fracture
  - Forearm shaft & distal radial fractures have great capacity for remodeling
  - Supracondylar fractures have less potential for remodeling
- Common sites of malunion
  - Supracondylar fracture
    - Cubitus varus deformity with medial angulation of distal fragment, not growth disturbance
    - Baumann (humerocapitellar) angle is used to predict final carrying angle following reduction of supracondylar fractures to attempt to avoid cubitus varus deformities
      - Angle formed by line along long axis of humeral shaft & line along physis of capitellum
      - Normal range: 64-81° (comparison to contralateral side is helpful)
  - Forearm fractures
    - May cause limited pronation/supination, refracture, cosmetic deformity, or distal radioulnar joint pain
    - Acceptable angulation is controversial
      - Some authors: > 10° in children > 8 years old = malunion
      - Other definitions: > 20° in children > 9 years old = malunion
  - Distal radius fracture
    - Usually remodels satisfactorily if < 11-12 years old
    - Malunion may result in functional limitation, pain, or cosmetic deformity
    - Features appear similar to adults prior to remodeling
      - ↓ radial inclination; abnormal dorsal tilt, radial shortening, articular incongruity
    - Adolescents & young adults can still develop significant distal radius malunion
      - One source suggests malunion if dorsal tilt ≥ 5°, radial inclination ≤ 10°, loss of radial height ≥ 5 mm
      - Normal values: Volar tilt (11°, range: 2-20°), radial inclination (21-25°), radial length (10-13 mm)
  - Femur fracture (definitions vary)
    - Some contend > 10° in coronal plane & > 15° in sagittal plane; others suggest > 5° & 10°, respectively
- Treatment may consist of osteotomy & epiphysiodesis

Premature Physeal Closure

- Secondary to fracture involving cartilaginous growth plate
- 15-30% of injuries to long bones in children involve physis
  - ~ 10% of physeal injuries are associated with significant growth disturbance
- Bridges start to form 1-2 months following injury but may not manifest until years later
  - Clinical follow-up to skeletal maturity is recommended in high-risk fractures due to possibility of delayed presentation during adolescent growth spurt
  - If caught early, only resection of bar may be necessary vs. correction of angular deformity
- Treatment
  - Indicated when deformity is present/developing & patient has 2 years or ≥ 2 cm of growth remaining
  - Bridge resection is considered if bridge occupies < 50% of physis
    - If resected, various interposition materials are placed to ↓ recurrence
  - Other treatments may include: Corrective osteotomy, completion epiphysiodesis, contralateral epiphysiodesis, bone lengthening

Posttraumatic Lipid Inclusion Cysts

- Seen at sites of prior fracture; thought to be due to extension of intramedullary fat through disrupted cortex with intact periosteum
- May mimic more aggressive process
- Distal radius is most common, followed by distal tibia

Degenerative Change

- Intraarticular fractures are at risk for posttraumatic arthrosis
- Fixation is typically necessary to reestablish articular congruence with articular surface disruption > 2 mm

Osteonecrosis

- Proximal pole of scaphoid: Sclerosis & humpback deformity
- Distal humerus: Fishtail deformity

DIAGNOSTIC CHECKLIST

Reporting Tips

- Describe residual deformity; however, radiographic appearance may not correlate with clinical outcome
  - Malunion may not be clinically relevant (e.g., patient with worrisome radiograph may have no functional limitation &/or may completely remodel over time)
- Lack of fracture healing may be suggestive of nonunion union if > 6 months but must be correlated with clinical findings
  - From medicolegal standpoint, best to describe & discuss with orthopedist, avoiding term "nonunion" in report
- Note changes in growth plate in setting of prior physeal fracture
  - Indicators of bridge: Focal poor definition of physis, new angulation, or tethered growth recovery line

SELECTED REFERENCES

1. Kim HHR et al: Uniquely pediatric upper extremity injuries. Clin Imaging. 80:249-61, 2021
2. Meyers AB: Physeal bridges: causes, diagnosis, characterization and post-treatment imaging. Pediatr Radiol. 49(12):1595-609, 2019
3. Nguyen JC et al: Imaging of pediatric growth plate disturbances. Radiographics. 37(6):1791-812, 2017
4. Larribe M et al: Usefulness of dynamic contrast-enhanced MRI in the evaluation of the viability of acute scaphoid fracture. Skeletal Radiol. 43(12):1697-703, 2014
5. Glotzbecker MP et al: Fishtail deformity of the distal humerus: a report of 15 cases. J Pediatr Orthop. 33(6):592-7, 2013
6. Bushnell BD et al: Malunion of the distal radius. J Am Acad Orthop Surg. 15(1):27-40, 2007

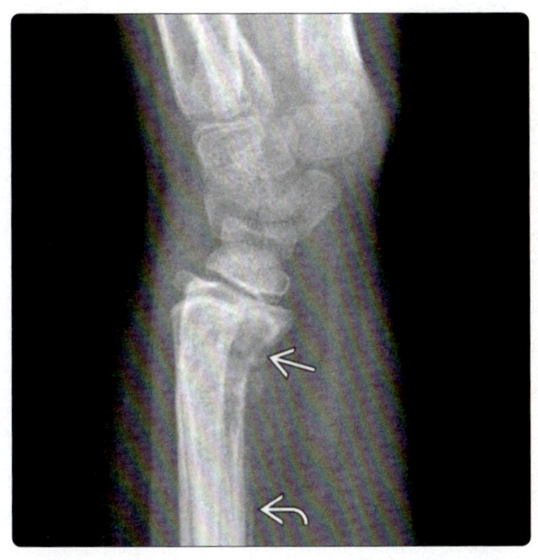

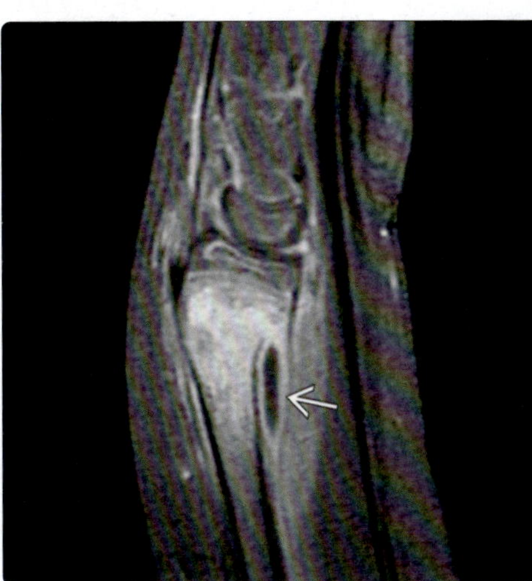

(Left) *Lateral wrist radiograph (obtained after cast removal) in a 6-year-old girl recently diagnosed with a Salter-Harris fracture shows an aggressive lytic process at the distal radius with cortical bone destruction ➡ & periosteal reaction ➡. These findings should raise concern for infection.* **(Right)** *Sagittal T1 C+ FS MR in the same patient shows a peripherally enhancing subperiosteal fluid collection ➡. Pus was found at surgery, & the patient was diagnosed with Staphylococcus aureus osteomyelitis.*

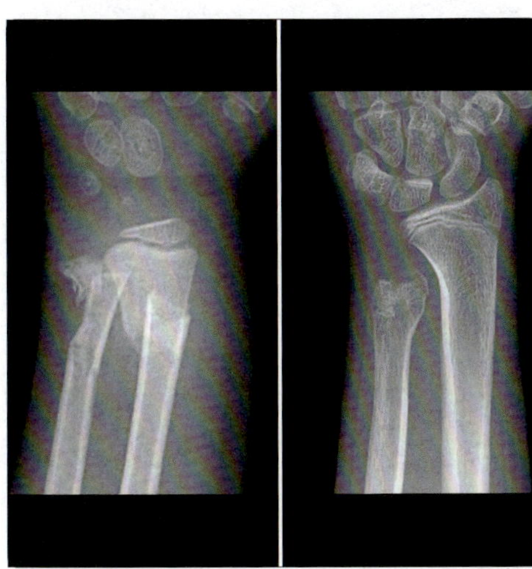

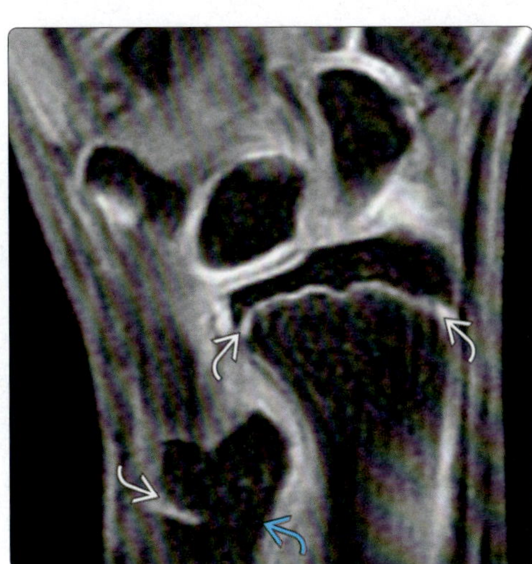

(Left) *Frontal radiograph of the distal forearm in a 4-year-old boy at presentation (left) shows a comminuted distal ulnar fracture & a distal radial metadiaphyseal fracture. A 6-year follow-up radiograph (right) shows marked negative ulnar variance & suggestion of a distal ulnar physeal bridge.* **(Right)** *Coronal 3D GRE MR in the same child shows osseous bridging across the lateral aspect of the distal ulnar physis ➡. The distal radial & medial distal ulnar physes remain open ➡.*

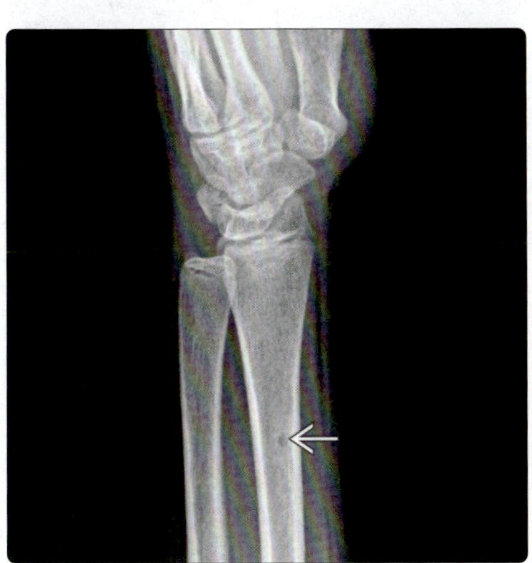

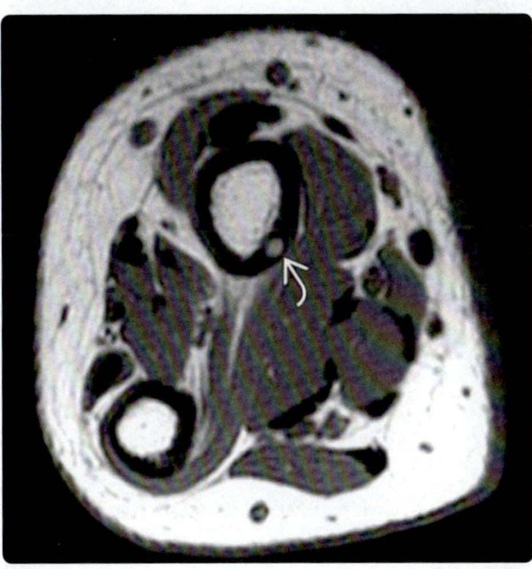

(Left) *Oblique radiograph of the distal forearm in a girl with a distal radial fracture 2 years prior shows a small, ovoid lucent lesion ➡. This is consistent with a lipid inclusion cyst.* **(Right)** *Axial T1 MR in the same patient shows an eccentrically located ovoid lesion in the volar distal radial cortex with ↑ T1 signal intensity ➡. This lesion followed the signal of fat on all sequences, compatible with a small lipid inclusion "cyst" related to the prior fracture.*

KEY FACTS

TERMINOLOGY

- Orthopedic hardware: Any of innumerable devices used for fracture fixation, realignment, ligament repair/reconstruction, arthroplasty, & other procedures

IMAGING

- External vs. internal fixation
- Goal of rigid fixation: Reduce motion
  - Look for endosteal rather than periosteal callus to indicate appropriate healing
    - Periosteal callus indicates motion at fracture site
- Radiographs remain primary evaluation of hardware
  - Malpositioning/migration or fracture of hardware
  - Fracture of bone at/adjacent to fixation site
  - Loosening or infection of hardware
  - Malunion, delayed union, or nonunion of fracture
- CT is more sensitive; used in select cases of clinical/imaging concern
- Comparing nuclear In-111 leukocyte & Tc-99m sulfur colloid exams is most specific evaluation of infected hardware
- MR for evaluation of ligament repair/reconstruction, soft tissue abscesses, & adverse local tissue reaction

CLINICAL ISSUES

- Goal of fracture treatment is to improve alignment & stabilize fracture to aid in healing & return function
- Numerous indications for orthopedic devices in children other than fracture fixation
  - Scoliosis, congenital deformity, growth disturbance, sports-related injuries

DIAGNOSTIC CHECKLIST

- Understanding purpose/function of orthopedic devices aids in evaluation of
  - Appropriate positioning of hardware
  - Hardware complications
  - Expected healing

(Left) *AP radiograph of a 12-year-old boy shows 2 fully threaded Steinmann pins ➡ transfixing a Salter-Harris II fracture ⮕.* **(Right)** *AP radiograph shows the same patient ~ 8 months later following a physeal bar resection. The bone block ➡ from the distal femoral window osteotomy is fixed with a single partially threaded cannulated screw ⮕. Steinman pins ➡ were placed to evaluate for subsequent growth. Cranioplasty material ➡ was placed across the physis to prevent new bar formation.*

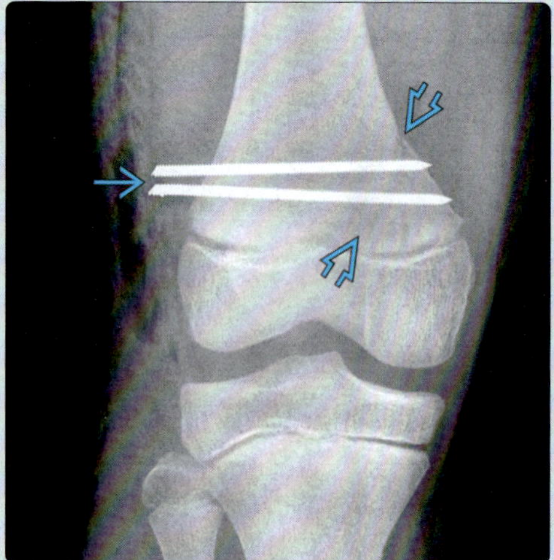

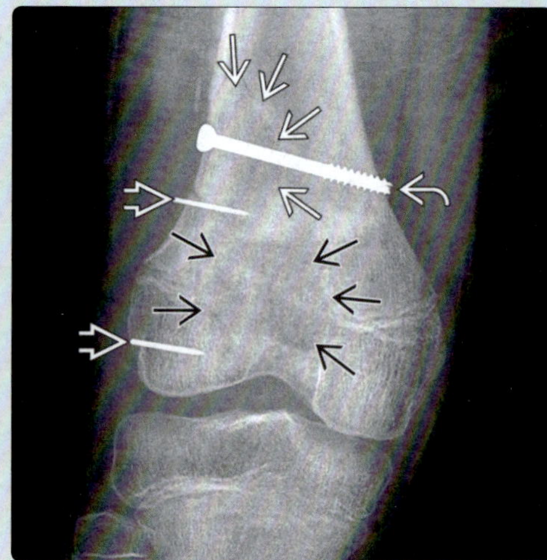

(Left) *Initial (L) & follow-up (R) frontal radiographs in a boy with neurofibromatosis type 1 & posterior spinal fusion for kyphoscoliosis show interval fractures of the hardware ➡. The patient had a fever at this time.* **(Right)** *Posterior images from In-111 leukocyte (L) & Tc-99m sulfur colloid (R) scans were obtained in the same patient. There is ↑ uptake in the left sacrum & iliac bones ➡ on the leukocyte scan with no corresponding ↑ uptake on the sulfur colloid scan. This discordance is consistent with infection.*

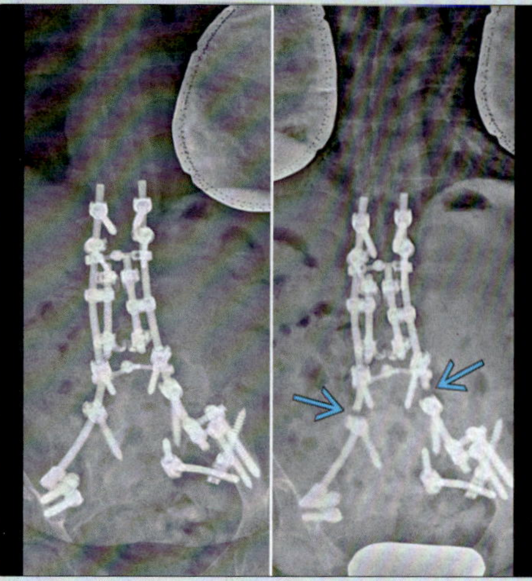

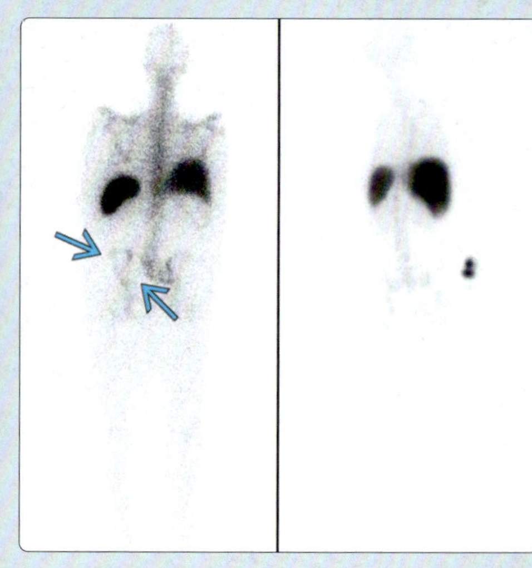

IMAGING

Radiographic Findings

- Radiographs: Primary modality for hardware assessment
- Evaluate for
  - Malpositioning/migration of hardware
  - Fracture of hardware components
  - Fracture of bone at or adjacent to fixation site
  - Loosening: Progressive lucency around hardware
  - Infection: Perihardware lucency, extensive periosteal reaction, erosions, subcutaneous emphysema, or ↑ edema
  - Malunion, delayed union, or nonunion of fracture
  - Osteonecrosis: Interruption of periosteal blood supply
  - Heterotopic bone formation

Fluoroscopic Findings

- Intraoperatively guides/confirms hardware placement

CT Findings

- More sensitive evaluation for hardware complications
- Modification of CT protocols to minimize artifacts
  - ↓ pitch setting, ↑ mAs, ↑ kVp (↑ radiation dose)
  - Dual-energy CT (no additional radiation)
  - Soft-tissue image reconstruction filters
- Must adjust window width/level for metal evaluation, not just bone

MR Findings

- MR is useful in certain postoperative situations
  - Ligament repair/reconstruction
  - Assessment of soft tissue abscesses
  - Adverse local tissue reaction (ALTR)
    - Various reactions to arthroplasty-related products (e.g., hypersensitivity reaction, metallosis)
    - Can lead to: Osteolysis, synovitis, soft tissue pseudotumors, soft tissue destruction
    - Most commonly described after hip arthroplasty
    - Recent studies have described metallosis with growing spinal rods in children
- Limited by metallic artifact; techniques to ↓ artifacts include

Ultrasonographic Findings

- Can be used to evaluate for fluid collections/abscesses
- May be helpful in evaluating nonmetallic hardware

Nuclear Medicine Findings

- Bone scan
  - Normal bone scan can exclude hardware infection
  - ↑ radiotracer activity may be due to infection or loosening
- Labeled leukocyte scintigraphy
  - ↑ radiotracer activity on leukocyte exam
    - Osteomyelitis
    - Marrow adjacent to fracture or hardware
  - Compare leukocyte & Tc-99m sulfur colloid exams
    - ↑ activity on labeled leukocyte exam but normal sulfur colloid exam = infection
    - Any other pattern is negative for infection

PATHOLOGY

General Features

- Fractures heal by primary or secondary mechanisms
  - Primary (direct) healing
    - Direct bone healing without callus formation
    - Occurs with rigid fracture fixation
  - Secondary (indirect) healing
    - Healing via callus formation
    - Occurs with flexible fracture fixation

CLINICAL ISSUES

Treatment

- Conservative treatment
  - Closed reduction with goal of restoring bone alignment
  - Stabilization via traction or external splinting
- Fracture fixation
  - External or internal fixation
  - Flexible vs. rigid fixation
    - Flexible: Allows interfragmentary movement under functional load
    - Rigid: Utilizes compression → ↑ stability; ↓ motion → primary healing without callus
      - Important at intraarticular sites where incongruity → osteoarthritis
- External or internal fixation is also used for nontraumatic purposes (i.e., leg lengthening, corrective osteotomy, etc.)
- External fixation advantages
  - Surgeon can control flexibility of fixation
  - ↓ injury to soft tissues, vasculature, & periosteum
- External fixation indications
  - Avoidance of physes in skeletally immature patients
  - Osteomyelitis (internal hardware must be avoided)
  - Substantial soft tissue injury requiring vascular procedures
  - Limb lengthening & other corrective osteotomies
- External fixation complications
  - Pin tract infection, breakage, or loosening
  - Delayed union, nonunion, malunion
- Internal fixation advantages
  - Potential for rapid return of function & rehabilitation
- Internal fixation indications & complications (categorized by different types of hardware)
  - Pin (K-wires & Steinman pins) indications
    - Temporary fixation of fragments during reduction
    - Attachment of skeletal traction devices
    - Guide accurate placement of larger cannulated screws
    - Occasionally used for definitive fracture treatment
    - Also used in setting of external fixation
  - Pin complications
    - Migration when used for definitive fracture treatment
  - Wire indications
    - Reattach osteotomized bone fragments
    - Tension banding (in combination with pins or screws, e.g., patella, olecranon fractures)
      - Converts tensile forces from adjacent tendon insertions into compressive forces across fracture
      - Aids with stability & fracture healing
    - Suture bone & soft tissue

- Cerclage wires (used with intramedullary fixation to stabilize long bone fragments)
- Wire complications
  - Breakage (insignificant if fragments maintain position)
  - Interruption of periosteal blood supply with subsequent osteonecrosis or fracture nonunion
- Screws: Types & indications
  - 2 basic types: Cortical & cancellous
    - Distance between threads = pitch
    - Screw diameter with threads = thread diameter
    - Core = diameter of screw without threads
  - Cortical screws
    - Designed for use in diaphysis
    - Typically fully threaded (threads along entire length) with smaller thread diameter & pitch
  - Cancellous screws
    - Can cross long segments of cancellous bone
    - Typically has deeper threads, larger thread diameter, greater pitch, partially threaded
  - Interfragmentary screw
    - Screw that crosses fracture line
    - Purpose: Act as lag screw providing compression of fragments → ↑ stability & healing
  - Cannulated screw
    - Possesses hollow shank, so can be placed over guide pin for ↑ accuracy
    - May be inserted percutaneously under fluoroscopy
  - Suture anchor
    - Anchor can be fixed into bone by screwing or lodging (e.g., press fit)
    - Used for capsular, ligamentous, or tendinous repair
  - Washer
    - Prevents screw head from sinking into bone
    - Enhances compressive area of screw in regions of thin cortex
    - Prevent fractures under screw
- Screw complications
  - Breakage, loosening, change in position
- Plates
  - Techniques for plating
    - Compression plating: Eccentric screw placement within sloped holes drives fragments into compression
    - Neutralization plating: Holds fracture fragments in place without compression; useful for severely comminuted fractures (bridging plate) & fractures with bone loss
    - Tension band plating: Placed along tension side of fracture; with loading, converts tensile to compressive force
    - Buttress plating: Often used in association with metaphyseal/epiphyseal shear or split fractures; prevents shear forces across fracture from displacing fragments
  - Dynamic compression plate: Can be used in compression, neutralization, tension band, or buttress
  - Additional plates
    - Tubular plate, reconstruction plate (malleable, used for pelvic fractures), less invasive stabilization system (LISS) plate, T-plate, blade plate, other special anatomically shaped plates
  - Locking plates may contain locking screws that contain threads at screw heads, allowing construct to better act as unit
- Plate complications
  - Plates have large contact area, may disrupt periosteal capillaries → compromise cortical perfusion
    - Low contact plates are available, reduce area of contact between plate & bone
  - Underlying bone resorption & old screw holes after plate removal may lead to fracture
  - Malposition, i.e., plate or screws violating articular surface or impinging upon joint motion
- Intramedullary nails or rods
  - Standard treatment for diaphyseal fractures of femur & tibia; may also be used in humerus
  - Rods are locked "statically" (proximal & distal interlocking screws) or "dynamically" (fixed at 1 end)
    - Dynamic locking ↑ compression across fracture site
    - Interlocking screws ↑ fixation stability & prevent rotation
  - Skeletally immature patients receive flexible intramedullary nails inserted through metaphysis
    - Typically 2 rods are placed through multiple insertion sites diverging at metaphyseal ends
    - Require additional external stabilization with cast
- Intramedullary nail or rod complications
  - Hardware fracture, loosening, or infection
  - Violation of joint by rods or screws
  - Intramedullary reaming is associated with ↑ infection rates (due to damage to internal cortical vasculature) & pulmonary fat embolism

- Antibiotic beads
  - Used for infected fractures
- Autogenous bone graft, allograft, or bone graft substitute
  - Treatment of bone defects

DIAGNOSTIC CHECKLIST

Image Interpretation Pearls

- On initial preoperative studies: Carefully evaluate fractured bone for any sign of underlying aggressive lesion
  - Placement of hardware may spread tumor cells
- On fluoroscopic intraoperative images: Carefully assess for hardware malposition or iatrogenic fracture
- On follow up postoperative studies: Carefully evaluate full complement of hardware (& adjacent bone) for interval change compared with prior studies

SELECTED REFERENCES

1. Fanelli D et al: Outcomes and complications following flexible intramedullary nailing for the treatment of tibial fractures in children: a meta-analysis. Arch Orthop Trauma Surg. ePub, 2021
2. Padgett DE et al: How useful is magnetic resonance imaging in evaluating adverse local tissue reaction? J Arthroplasty. 35(6S):S63-7, 2020
3. Teoh KH et al: Metallosis following implantation of magnetically controlled growing rods in the treatment of scoliosis: a case series. Bone Joint J. 98-B(12):1662-7, 2016
4. Coupal TM et al: Peering through the glare: using dual-energy CT to overcome the problem of metal artifacts in bone radiology. Skeletal Radiol. 43(5):567-75, 2014
5. Fayad LM et al: Value of 3D CT in defining skeletal complications of orthopedic hardware in the postoperative patient. AJR Am J Roentgenol. 193(4):1155-63, 2009

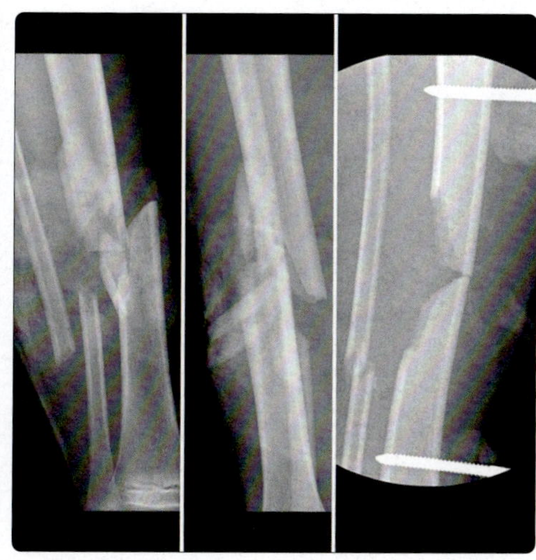

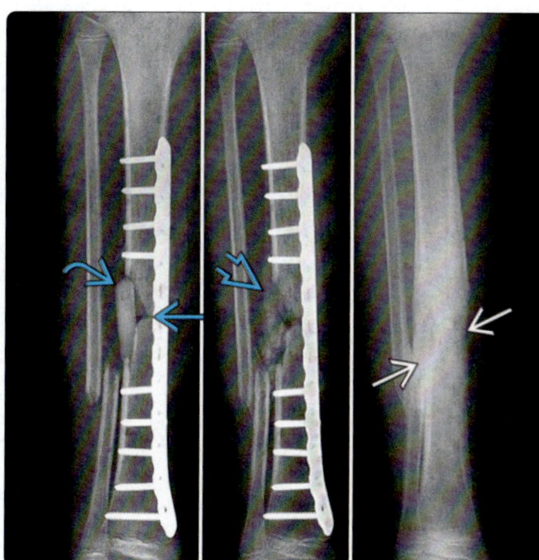

(Left) *Initial frontal (L) & lateral (M) radiographs in a boy show an open, comminuted tibial fracture. The initial treatment was with external fixation (R) due to the risk of infection.* **(Right)** *Radiograph in the same boy 7 months later (L) shows internal plate/screw fixation, placement of an antibiotic-impregnated spacer, & nonunion of the tibial fracture. Follow-up image (M) shows interval debridement & placement of bone graft with incorporation & bridging callus at the fracture 1 year later (R).*

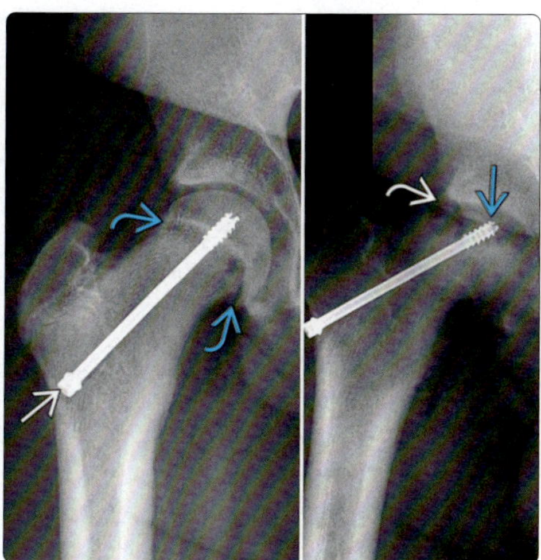

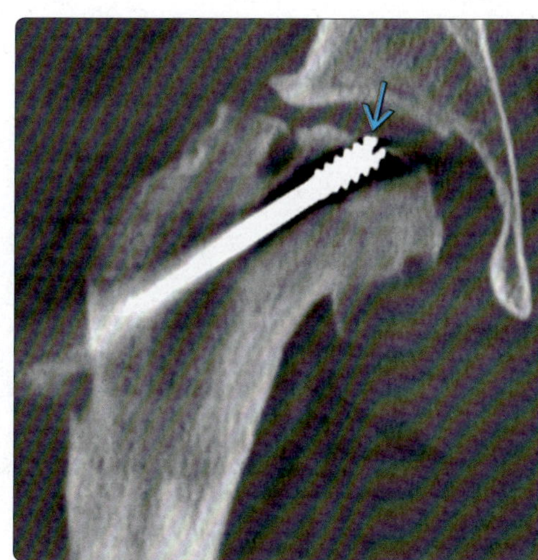

(Left) *Initial postoperative image (L) of a 12-year-old boy with a slipped capital femoral epiphysis (SCFE) shows fixation with a transphyseal partially threaded cannulated screw. Follow-up (R) shows collapse of the femoral head from osteonecrosis, a known complication of SCFE. The screw now extends beyond the articular surface.* **(Right)** *Coronal bone CT in the same patient confirms that the screw extends across the articular surface of the collapsed femoral head.*

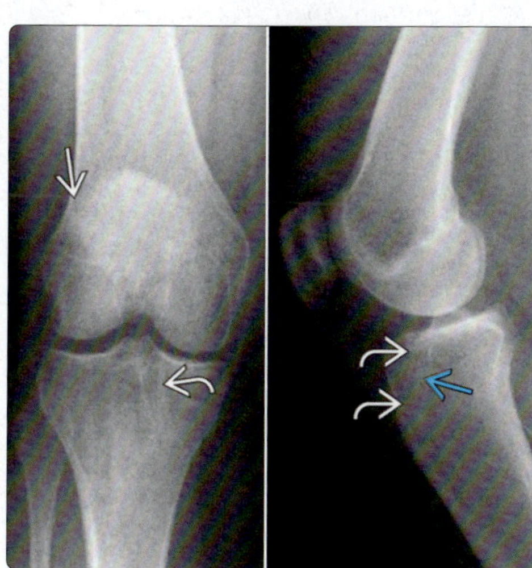

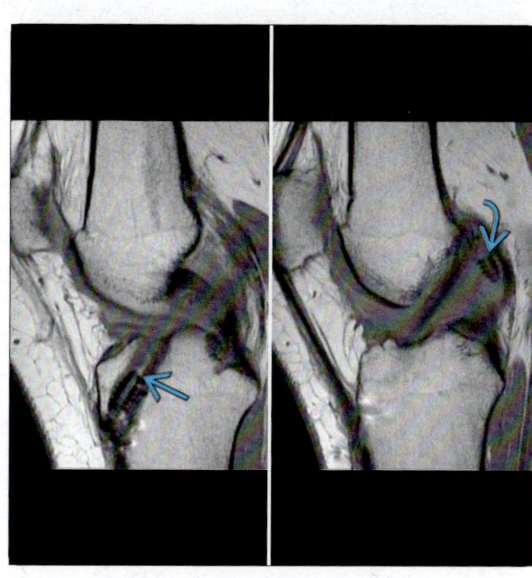

(Left) *AP (L) & lateral (R) radiographs in a reinjured 16-year-old boy with a history of an ACL tear & reconstruction 9 months prior show femoral & tibial tunnels with an interference screw faintly seen in the tibial tunnel.* **(Right)** *Sagittal PD MR images in the same boy show fracture of the interference screw in the tibial tunnel. A fractured portion of the screw has migrated into the posterior aspect of the joint.*

Soft Tissue Foreign Bodies, Acute and Chronic

KEY FACTS

TERMINOLOGY

- Penetrating injury → soft tissue foreign body (FB)
- Chronic FB → granulomatous reaction → soft tissue mass

IMAGING

- Most FBs are not radiopaque (e.g., wood splinters)
- Some FBs are radiopaque (e.g., metal, glass, bone)
- Radiographs assess radiopaque FBs & osseous changes
- US: Excellent detection of superficial FBs
  - Typically echogenic
  - ± posterior shadowing, depending on composition
  - Hypoechoic rim of edema/granulomatous reaction
- MR: FB is typically of low signal on all sequences
  - Nonanatomic, geographic shape (e.g., linear, triangular)
  - FB may be small or very subtle
  - GRE may show blooming if FB is metallic or Ca^{2+}
  - Adjacent edema or granulomatous reaction
  - Detects associated cellulitis, abscess, osteomyelitis

TOP DIFFERENTIAL DIAGNOSES

- Posttraumatic fat necrosis
- Soft tissue sarcoma
- Benign soft tissue tumors
- Venous malformation

PATHOLOGY

- Chronic FB → granulomatous reaction

CLINICAL ISSUES

- Acute: Sensation of FB under skin after injury
- Chronic: Firm, painless soft tissue mass
  - May occur long after injury that introduced FB
  - Often no specific trauma is recalled
- Treatment
  - Surgical or US-guided removal

DIAGNOSTIC CHECKLIST

- If radiolucent superficial FB is suspected → US

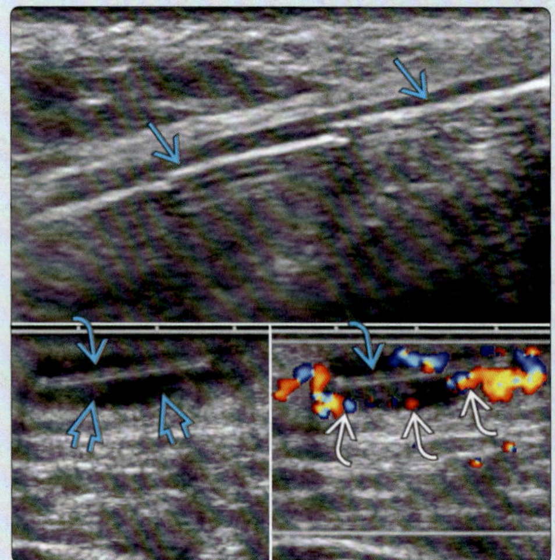

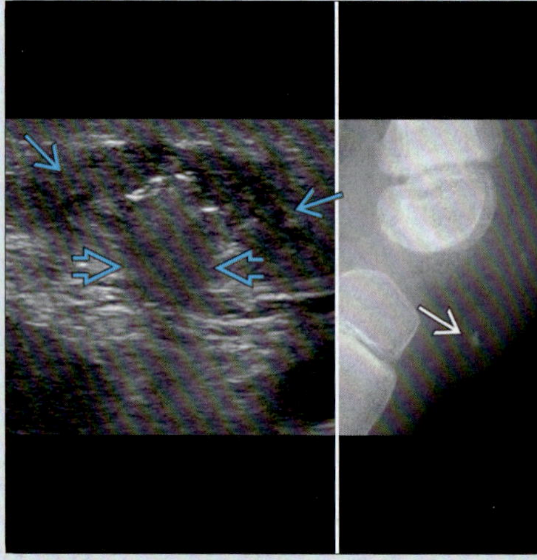

(Left) *US (top) of the left buttock in a 5-year-old who fell on a plastic toy shows a linear subcutaneous echogenic foreign body (FB) ➡. Removal was performed without imaging guidance. Repeat US 6 weeks later (bottom) shows a retained portion of the FB ➡ with adjacent hypoechoic ➡ but hypervascular ➡ granulation tissue.* **(Right)** *US in a 5-year-old patient with an anterior knee lump shows a heterogeneous mass ➡ with posterior shadowing ➡. Lateral radiograph confirms a glass FB ➡ at this site from a remote injury.*

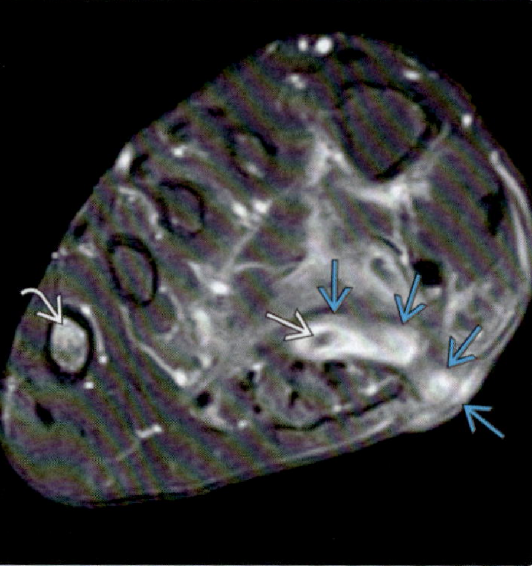

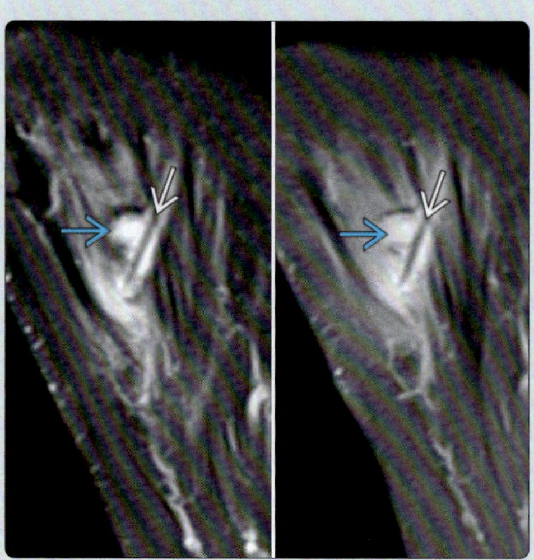

(Left) *Axial T2 FS MR in a 9-year-old girl who removed a toothpick from her foot 5 months prior shows a linear tract of ↑ signal ➡ extending from the plantar surface to a central focus of low signal ➡, concerning for a retained FB. There is adjacent soft tissue edema & distant marrow edema in the 5th metatarsal ➡ from infection vs. stress changes.* **(Right)** *Coronal T2 FS (left) & T1 C+ FS (right) MR images in the same patient show the linear low-signal retained toothpick ➡ surrounded by high-signal granulation tissue ➡.*

Soft Tissue Foreign Bodies, Acute and Chronic

TERMINOLOGY

Abbreviations

- Foreign body (FB)

Synonyms

- Chronic FB: FB granuloma, giant cell granulomatous reaction, fibrohistiocytic reaction

Definitions

- Penetrating injury → soft tissue FB deposition
  - Injury & retention of FB may not be recognized/recalled
- Chronic FB may lead to mass of granulomatous reaction

IMAGING

General Features

- Best diagnostic clue
  - Radiopaque FB identified on radiographs
  - Radiolucent FB may be identified on US, MR, or CT
- Location
  - Often confined to subcutaneous fat
  - Typically in areas prone to injury
    - Walking barefoot: Plantar aspect of feet
    - Areas commonly injured from fall: Anterior knee/shin, hands, elbows, buttocks

Radiographic Findings

- Radiodensity depends upon FB composition
- Conspicuity depends on size & degree of difference in radiodensity from surrounding soft tissues
- Most FBs are not radiopaque (e.g., wood splinters, thorns, plastic)
  - May only show nonspecific soft tissue fullness
- Some FBs are radiopaque (e.g., metal, glass, bone)
- ± findings of osteomyelitis in subacute/chronic setting

MR Findings

- FB: Typically low signal intensity on all sequences
  - Nonanatomic, geographic shape (e.g., linear or square)
  - Low signal intensity may be small or very subtle
  - GRE sequence can be helpful depending on composition
    - Blooming artifact if metal or bone
- Acute FB: Poorly defined edema in adjacent soft tissues
  - Reticular ↑ signal on T2 FS/STIR, ↓ signal on T1
  - Reticular enhancement on T1 C+ FS
- Chronic FB: May lead to granulomatous reaction
  - Mass-like ↑ signal on T2 FS/STIR, ↓ signal on T1
  - Diffuse enhancement on T1 C+ FS
- Associated findings
  - Linear tract of fluid signal extending from skin
  - Soft tissue abscess: Localized fluid collection with peripheral enhancement (vs. diffuse enhancement of FB granuloma)
  - Marrow edema/hyperenhancement of adjacent bone may be seen with osteomyelitis or stress changes (due to altered weight bearing in setting of pain)

Ultrasonographic Findings

- Excellent for identifying superficial acute & chronic FBs
- FBs are typically echogenic; often punctate or linear
- Variable posterior shadowing depending on composition
- Peripheral ↓ echogenicity from edema (acute) or granulomatous reaction (chronic)
- Exam may be confusing if US is only performed after attempted FB removal

Imaging Recommendations

- Best imaging tool
  - Radiography for radiopaque FBs (e.g., glass, metal, bone)
    - Also shows bone involvement by penetrating trauma
  - US for suspected superficial radiolucent FB

DIFFERENTIAL DIAGNOSIS

Posttraumatic Fat Necrosis

- Injury of subcutaneous fat with associated hematoma
- No central FB is seen at imaging

Soft Tissue Sarcomas

- More common in areas not prone to FBs (i.e., proximal to midextremities)
- No central FB is seen at imaging
- Typically well circumscribed without surrounding edema

Benign Soft Tissue Tumors

- Variety of nonmalignant soft tissue tumors occur in children
  - e.g., fibrous lesions (fibromatosis, nodular fasciitis), subcutaneous granuloma annulare
- No central FB is seen at imaging
- Can be well circumscribed or poorly defined & infiltrative

Venous Malformations

- Compressible serpentine tangle or mass of abnormal veins
- ↑ signal on T2 FS + gradual contrast enhancement
- ± phleboliths, fluid-fluid levels

CLINICAL ISSUES

Presentation

- Most common signs/symptoms
  - Acute: Sensation of FB under skin after injury
  - Chronic: Firm, painless soft tissue mass
    - May come to attention long after injury
    - Often no specific trauma is recalled
- Other signs/symptoms
  - Erythema, swelling, &/or induration of overlying skin
  - Sinus tract to skin surface may develop

Treatment

- Surgical removal: US or fluoroscopy can localize FB
- Alternatively, US-guided removal with needle or forceps
  - Hydrodissection technique may assist procedure

SELECTED REFERENCES

1. Mulholland D et al: The evaluation of palpable thigh nodularity in vaccination-age children - differentiating vaccination granulomas from other causes. J Med Ultrasound. 29(2):129-31, 2021
2. Javadrashid R et al: Visibility of different intraorbital foreign bodies using plain radiography, computed tomography, magnetic resonance imaging, and cone-beam computed tomography: an in vitro study. Can Assoc Radiol J. 68(2):194-201, 2017
3. Davis J et al: Diagnostic accuracy of ultrasonography in retained soft tissue foreign bodies: a systematic review and meta-analysis. Acad Emerg Med. 22(7):777-87, 2015
4. Jarraya M et al: Multimodality imaging of foreign bodies of the musculoskeletal system. AJR Am J Roentgenol. 203(1):W92-102, 2014

Morel-Lavallée Lesion

KEY FACTS

TERMINOLOGY

- Closed degloving injury of subcutaneous fat at interface with fascia, often overlying bony protuberance
- Results in chronic fluid collection (blood, lymph, fat)

IMAGING

- Classic Morel-Lavallée lesion occurs at hip/proximal thigh overlying greater trochanter
  - Other sites: Abdominal wall, lumbar spine, buttock, sacrum, thigh, knee, lower leg, scapula, scalp
- Mean size: 8 cm; range: 3-17 cm
- Appearance depends on timing of imaging & complications
  - Acute/subacute: Elongated with irregular margins & internal heterogeneity
  - Chronic: Elongated & smooth; ↓ heterogeneity
  - Angular margins of shear plane are suggestive
- MR: Collection ultimately follows fluid signal intensity internally except for fat nodules, blood products
  - Fibrous pseudocapsule is hypointense on all sequences
  - Nodular enhancement, typically peripheral, may be seen with granulation tissue, inflammation, or infection
- Ultrasound: Ultimately hypoechoic to anechoic internally (due to ↓ complexity over time)
  - Echogenic fat nodules are characteristic

PATHOLOGY

- Blunt trauma with compressive & shear forces creates potential space with disruption of vessels & nerves

CLINICAL ISSUES

- Fluctuant mass, bruising, ↑ skin mobility, ↓ skin sensation
  - Delayed presentation after injury in 1/3 of patients
- Variable course: Resolution, persistence, enlargement
  - Risk for infection: Up to 50%
- Treatment
  - Conservative: Compression wraps, rest, physical therapy
  - Intervention: Percutaneous drainage ± steroid injection or sclerodesis; surgical debridement or excision

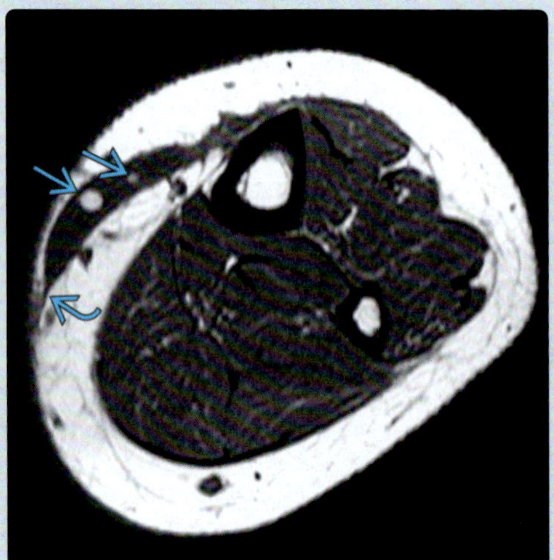

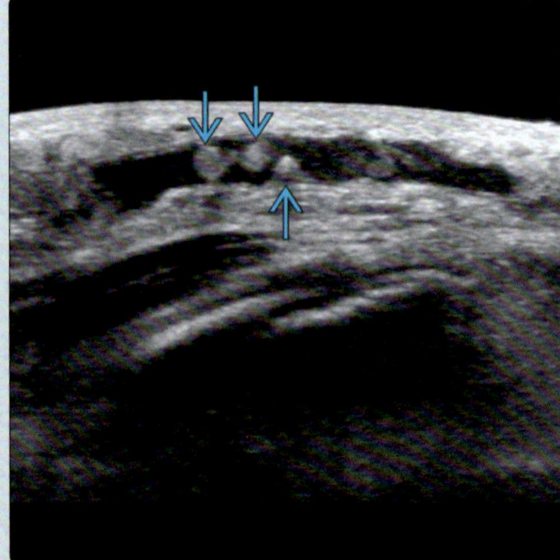

(Left) *Axial T1 MR of the lower leg in a 16-year-old soccer player shows an elongated collection containing nodules ➡ that followed fat signal on all sequences. A Morel-Lavallée-type injury was diagnosed. Note the acute angle at the margin of the shear plane ➡.* **(Right)** *Transverse ultrasound over the right iliac crest in a 15-year-old patient with a recent fall from a bicycle shows an elongated, hypoechoic subcutaneous collection containing echogenic fat nodules ➡, typical of a Morel-Lavallée lesion.*

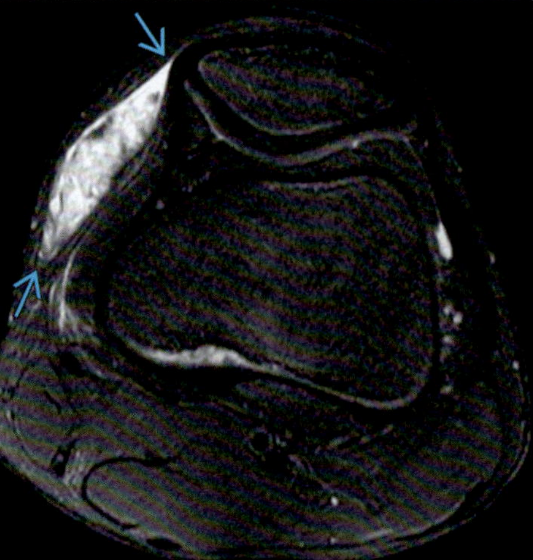

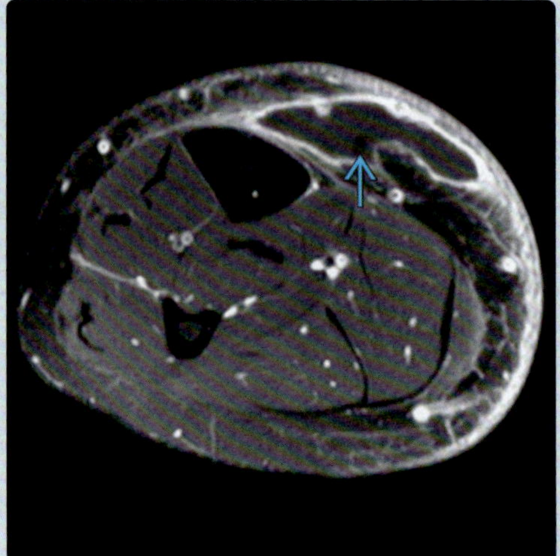

(Left) *Axial T2 FS MR in a 12-year-old patient after an American football injury shows an elongated collection in the medial soft tissues with internal heterogeneity. The collection lies in a single plane of shear injury in the subcutaneous fat & shows margins with acute angles ➡, typical of a Morel-Lavallée lesion.* **(Right)** *Axial T1 C+ FS MR in a 17-year-old with a history of leg hematoma 4 months prior & now presenting with new swelling & fever shows a superinfected Morel-Lavallée lesion containing a fat nodule ➡.*

Muscle Hernia

KEY FACTS

TERMINOLOGY

- Defect in fascia directly overlying muscle → focal muscle protrusion

IMAGING

- Lower > upper extremity
  - Most commonly affected muscle: Anterior tibialis
- MR: Bulging nodule should be isointense with muscle
  - Subtle defect of hypointense fascia may be only finding if hernia is reduced at time of static exam
- Ultrasound: Focal interruption of thin, linear hyperechoic fascia overlying hypoechoic, striated muscle
  - Focal bulge of hypoechoic muscle through fascial defect; may create mushroom cap appearance
    - Superficial broadening of herniated muscle directly overlying fascia with narrow waist of muscle in defect
  - Hernia accentuated by contraction or vigorous activity, reduced with relaxation or ↑ transducer pressure
    - Ankle dorsiflexion ↑ anterior tibialis muscle herniation
- Protocol advice (to optimize hernia visualization)
  - Use variety of provocative maneuvers
  - Reduce pressure applied by ultrasound transducer or MR skin marker (capsule) over site of clinical concern
  - Compare with contralateral extremity

TOP DIFFERENTIAL DIAGNOSES

- Vascular malformation
- Soft tissue malignancy
- Lipoma

PATHOLOGY

- Congenital or constitutional fascial hernia
- Acquired or traumatic fascial tear/rupture

CLINICAL ISSUES

- Asymptomatic vs. intermittent painless bulge/nodule vs. painful nodule appearing after vigorous exertion
- Surgery (fasciotomy favored over repair) for symptomatic cases not responding to conservative measures

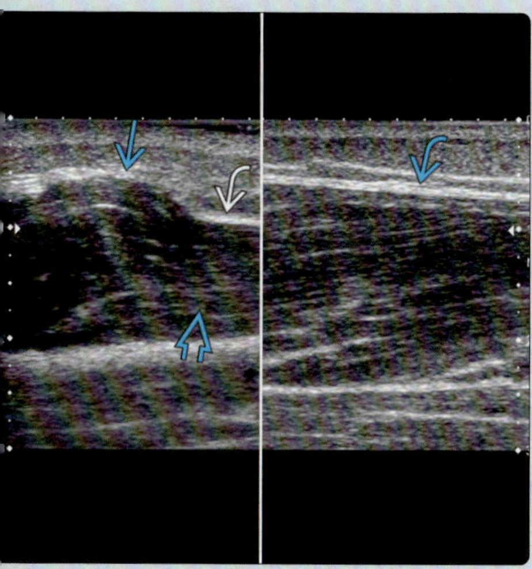

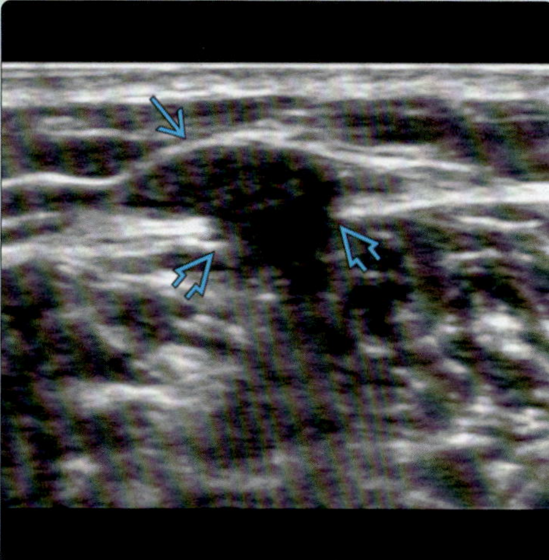

(Left) *Longitudinal ultrasound of the right lower leg in an 11-year-old girl with a palpable lump shows herniation of the anterior tibialis muscle through a fascial defect. Note the thin, linear, echogenic appearance of intact fascia distally on the right & in the contralateral left leg.* **(Right)** *Transverse ultrasound through the right lower leg in a 17-year-old girl shows herniation of muscle through a fascial defect, creating a mushroom cap appearance. The hernia intermittently reduced with relaxation.*

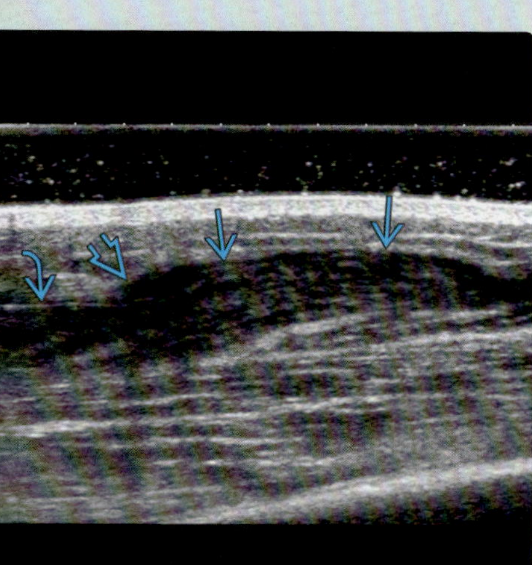

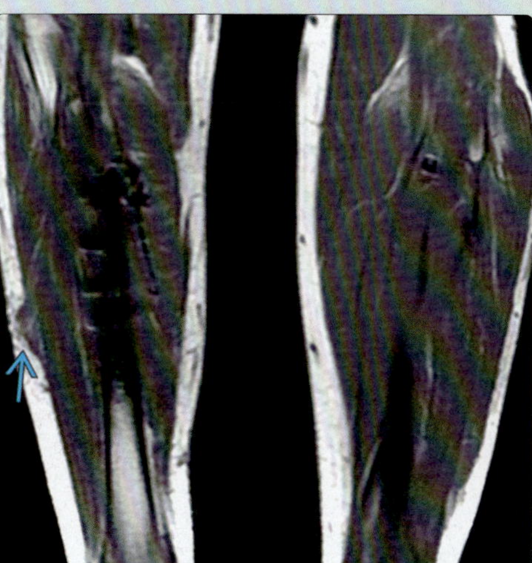

(Left) *Longitudinal ultrasound through the lower leg in a 16-year-old girl shows a focal muscle herniation through the overlying fascia. The convex superficial margin & overhanging edge of the herniated muscle are typical.* **(Right)** *Coronal T1 MR in an 18-year-old woman with a history of surgery for a right tibial osteosarcoma shows a focal herniation of peroneal muscle through a fascial defect.*

Clavicle Injuries

KEY FACTS

TERMINOLOGY

- Can be midshaft or medial or lateral ends
- Epiphyses are present at medial & lateral ends of clavicle
  - 2° ossification centers do not appear until teenage years
    - Fuse in late 2nd-3rd decades of life
  - Displaced fractures through unossified cartilage mimic acromioclavicular (AC) & sternoclavicular (SC) joint dislocations

IMAGING

- Lateral/medial fractures: Apparent AC or SC joint widening
- Apparent AC & SC dislocation on radiographs are typically Salter-Harris (SH)-type fractures in skeletally immature
  - Unossified epiphyses at ends of clavicle (not visible on radiographs) are areas of relative weakness
- CT in acute setting for suspected fracture/displacement of medial clavicle; compare alignment of bilateral medial clavicles on radiographs
  - CECT for posterior displacement → vascular injury

TOP DIFFERENTIAL DIAGNOSES

- Child abuse
  - Correlation with history is essential to distinguish accidental injury from abuse
  - Clavicle fractures have low specificity for abuse
- Congenital pseudoarthrosis
  - 2 separate portions of clavicle show smooth, intact cortices without callus
- AC & SC joint dislocations
  - Apparent AC or SC widening on radiographs is typically SH fracture in skeletally immature
- Normal unossified cartilage
  - Comparison contralateral view is helpful

DIAGNOSTIC CHECKLIST

- Infant fracture: Correlate age, radiographic findings, & clinical history to distinguish birth injury from abuse
- In skeletally immature, lateral & medial SH fractures can mimic AC & SC joint dislocations

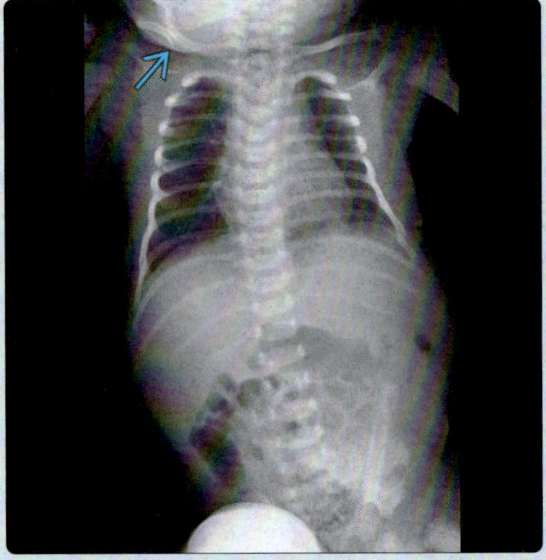

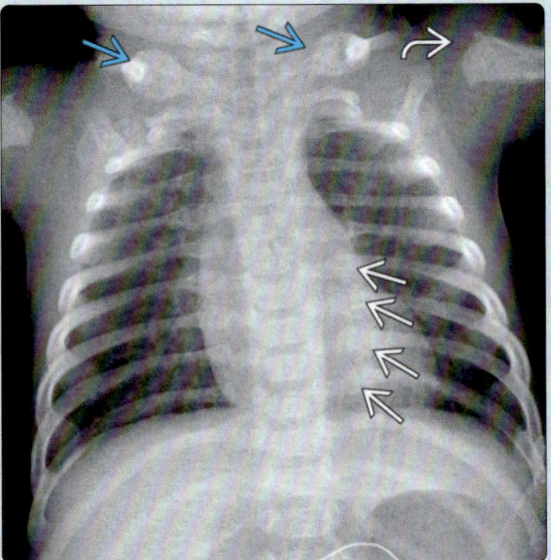

(Left) *Frontal radiograph of the chest & abdomen in a newborn taken while still in the hospital shows a right clavicle fracture ➔ secondary to birth injury. This was not apparent on clinical exam.* **(Right)** *AP chest radiograph in a 2-month-old boy with apnea shows healing bilateral clavicle fractures ➔. There are also multiple healing posterior left rib fractures ➔ & a healing left humeral metaphyseal corner fracture ↪. Subdural hematomas were found on a head CT, & abuse was clinically confirmed.*

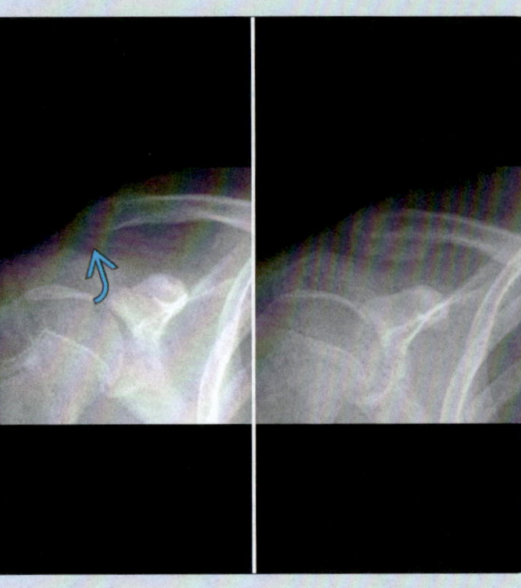

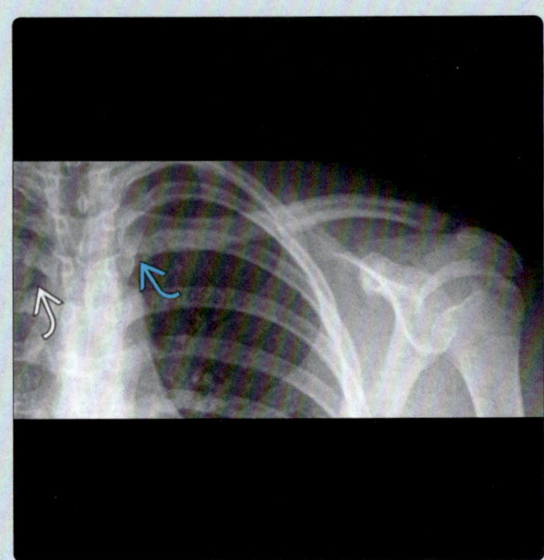

(Left) *Frontal radiographs at initial presentation (L) & 1 month (R) in a 13-year-old boy with an injury show a subtle fracture fragment ➔ aligned with the acromion with elevation of the more proximal clavicle. Callus at 1 month confirms that this was a healing fracture, not acromioclavicular joint dislocation.* **(Right)** *Frontal radiograph of the left clavicle in a 14-year-old boy with an acute injury shows elevation of medial left clavicle ➔ compared to right ➔. CT confirmed a Salter-Harris fracture of medial left clavicle.*

TERMINOLOGY

Definitions

- Occur at midshaft or at medial or lateral ends
- Growth plates & epiphyses are present at medial & lateral ends of clavicle
  - 2° ossification centers do not appear until 2nd decade of life & often do not fuse until 3rd decade
  - Displaced fractures through unossified cartilage mimic acromioclavicular (AC) & sternoclavicular (SC) joint dislocations

IMAGING

General Features

- Best diagnostic clue
  - Lateral/medial fractures: Apparent AC or SC widening
  - Midshaft fracture: Abnormal angulation
- Location
  - Fractures of clavicle are typically classified by location
    - Mid 1/3: 80-85% (most common)
    - Lateral 1/3: 15-20%
    - Medial 1/3: < 5%

Radiographic Findings

- Midclavicle fracture
  - Evolution of subperiosteal new bone & callus formation in birth trauma
    - No subperiosteal new bone < 7 days
    - Subperiosteal new bone is typically present by 10 days
    - Callus formation is typically not seen < 9 days but is often present by 15 days
- Apparent AC or SC dislocation on radiographs is typically Salter-Harris (SH)-type fracture in skeletally immature
  - Unossified epiphyses at ends of clavicle, not visible on radiographs, are areas of relative weakness
  - Distal clavicle SH fracture + periosteal avulsion
    - Periosteal sleeve avulsion allows superior displacement of clavicle relative to AC joint
    - Follow-up radiographs show callus formation
  - Medial clavicle fracture may be SH I or II
    - Clavicle may displace anterior, posterior, or superior
    - Can be very subtle on radiographs; compare to contralateral side

CT Findings

- CT in acute setting for suspected fracture/displacement of medial clavicle; CECT if concern for vascular injury
  - Posterior displacement may cause neurovascular, lung, tracheal, &/or esophageal injuries

MR Findings

- Allows visualization of cartilaginous epiphyses
- Allows delineation of associated soft tissue injuries in setting of distal clavicular fractures
- Can help differentiate posterior SC joint dislocation & medial clavicular physeal fracture

Imaging Recommendations

- Protocol advice
  - CT if concern for medial clavicle fracture or dislocation
    - CECT if concern for vascular injury

DIFFERENTIAL DIAGNOSIS

Child Abuse

- Correlation of radiographic findings & history is essential
- Clavicle fractures have low specificity for abuse
- Look closely for other fractures

Congenital Pseudoarthrosis

- Can be confused with fracture from birth trauma or abuse
- 2 separate portions of clavicle have smooth, intact cortices without callus

Acromioclavicular & Sternoclavicular Dislocations

- Apparent AC & SC widening on radiographs are typically SH fractures in skeletally immature children

Normal Unossified Cartilage

- AC joint often appears wide (by adult standards) prior to skeletal maturity
- Comparison view of contralateral side is helpful

CLINICAL ISSUES

Presentation

- Most common signs/symptoms
  - Birth-related clavicle fractures
    - Not moving extremity, tenderness, deformity
    - May go undetected if nondisplaced
  - Other presentations: Fall on outstretched arm, direct blow, child abuse
    - Tenderness, swelling, palpable deformity (if displaced)

Treatment

- Midclavicle fractures
  - Acute non-/minimally displaced fractures: Nonoperative management, immobilization
  - Open fractures & significant skin tenting/compromise: Open reduction internal fixation
- Medial & lateral clavicle fractures
  - Immobilization ± closed reduction
  - If fails → open reduction + various types of fixation

DIAGNOSTIC CHECKLIST

Consider

- Compare left & right medial clavicle positions for subtle malalignment of medial fracture/displacement
- CT in questionable cases (+ contrast if concern for posterior displacement & vascular injury)

Image Interpretation Pearls

- Infant clavicle fracture: Correlate age, radiographic findings, & clinical history to distinguish birth injury from abuse
- In skeletally immature, lateral & medial SH fractures can mimic AC & SC joint dislocations

SELECTED REFERENCES

1. Flores DV et al: Imaging of the acromioclavicular joint: anatomy, function, pathologic features, and treatment. Radiographics. 40(5):1355-82, 2020
2. Fadell M et al: Radiological features of healing in newborn clavicular fractures. Eur Radiol. 27(5):2180-7, 2017
3. Beckmann N et al: Posterior sternoclavicular Salter-Harris fracture-dislocation in a patient with unossified medial clavicle epiphysis. Skeletal Radiol. 45(8):1123-7, 2016

Supracondylar Fracture

KEY FACTS

IMAGING

- AP radiograph
  - Transverse fracture of distal humeral metadiaphyseal junction at level of coronoid & olecranon fossae
  - ± medial or lateral cortical buckling or angulation
- Lateral radiograph
  - Visible posterior fat pad due to joint effusion
    - May be only finding of nondisplaced fracture
  - Anterior humeral line fails to bisect capitellum due to apex volar angulation ± dorsal translation of distal fracture fragment
- Radiocapitellar alignment is generally maintained on all views (in contradistinction to true dislocation)

TOP DIFFERENTIAL DIAGNOSES

- Lateral condylar fracture
- Posterior dislocation
- Distal humeral epiphyseal separation/transphyseal fracture

PATHOLOGY

- Extension/FOOSH (fall on outstretched hand) mechanism (98%) vs. flexion injury with direct trauma (2%)
- Modified Gartland classification (I-IV) to direct treatment
  - Classified by degree of displacement, rotation, instability
  - Treatment ranges from casting to closed reduction with percutaneous fixation to open reduction internal fixation
- Neurovascular injury is much higher with completely displaced fractures (types III & IV)
  - Vascular injury requires urgent reduction + pinning at minimum; may need ORIF

CLINICAL ISSUES

- 60% of pediatric elbow fractures; peak age: 5-7 years

DIAGNOSTIC CHECKLIST

- Consider follow-up radiographs in 10-14 days to identify healing occult fracture if joint effusion is only finding initially (in setting of trauma)

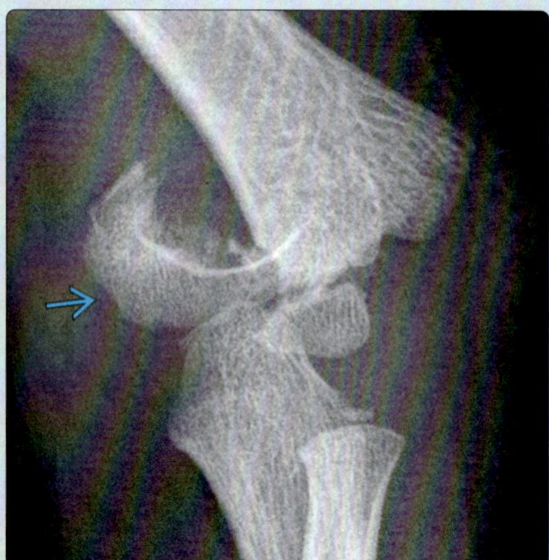

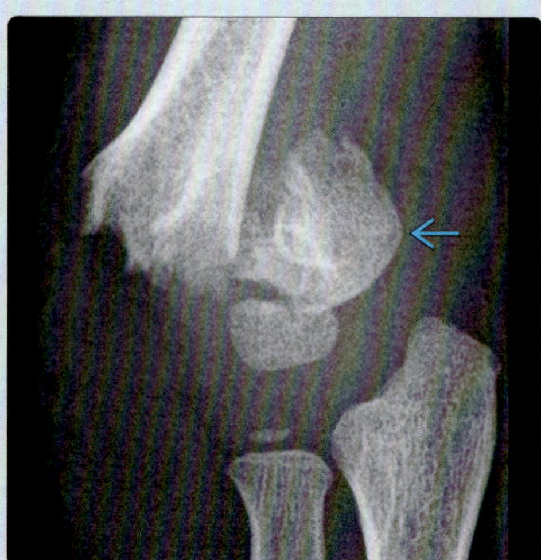

(Left) *AP radiograph in a 5-year-old after a fall shows a complete, transversely oriented distal humeral fracture through the olecranon & coronoid fossae with > 50% medial translation of the metaphysis* ➡. **(Right)** *Lateral radiograph in the same patient shows no cortical contact of the posteriorly translated distal fragment* ➡ *with the proximal fragment (a Gartland III or IV supracondylar fracture). The elbow articulations remain intact on both views.*

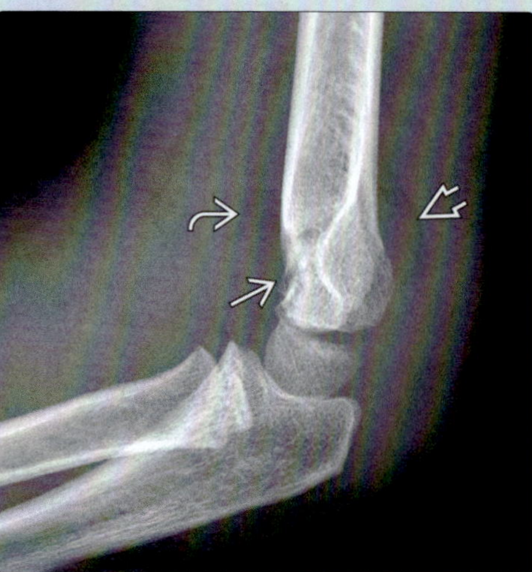

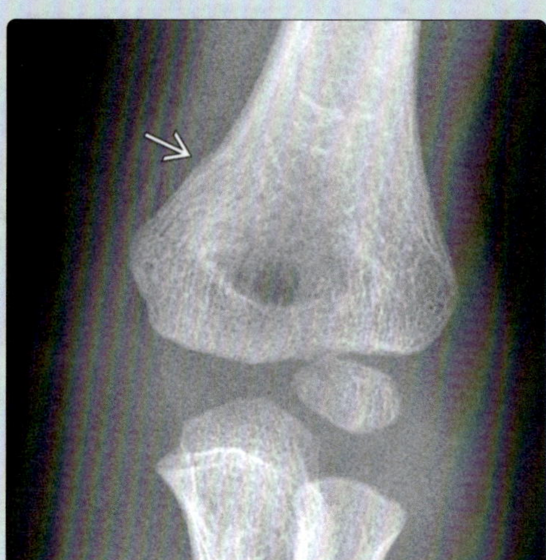

(Left) *Lateral radiograph after a fall shows anterior cortical disruption* ➡ *in the typical location of a supracondylar fracture. There is mild apex volar angulation (with hinged but intact posterior cortex), such that an anterior humeral line no longer bisects the capitellum (Gartland IIA). There is a large elbow joint effusion with elevation of the anterior* ➡ *& posterior* ➡ *fat pads.* **(Right)** *AP radiograph in the same child shows subtle medial cortical buckling* ➡ *of the supracondylar humerus.*

TERMINOLOGY

Synonyms

- Gartland fracture

Definitions

- Supracondylar fracture: Transverse fracture of distal humeral metadiaphyseal junction with varying degrees of displacement & comminution
- FOOSH injury: **F**all **o**n **o**ut**s**tretched **h**and
- Anterior humeral line: Vertical line drawn along anterior cortex of humeral diaphysis; normally bisects capitellum
  - Often courses through anterior 1/3 of capitellum in very young children
- Radiocapitellar (RC) line: Line drawn through long axis of radius; normally bisects capitellum on any view
  - Due to eccentric ossification of capitellum, RC line often does not bisect ossified capitellum < 10 years of age

IMAGING

General Features

- Best diagnostic clue
  - Lateral radiograph
    - Dorsal translation of distal humeral metaphysis/epiphysis with failure of anterior humeral line to bisect capitellum
      - Volar angulation of fracture apex
    - Displacement of anterior & posterior fat pads by joint effusion → may be only finding of nondisplaced fracture
  - AP radiograph
    - Transverse metadiaphyseal junction fracture lucency
- Location
  - Fracture occurs at thin distal humerus between olecranon (posterior) & coronoid (anterior) fossae
- Morphology
  - Various configurations depending on degree of angulation, translation, rotation, & comminution

Radiographic Findings

- Radiography
  - AP view
    - Transversely oriented linear lucency of distal humeral metadiaphyseal junction
    - Varying degrees of angulation, translation, & rotation of distal fragment
    - Fracture line may not be visible in up to 25%
    - Subtle buckling or angulation of medial or lateral cortex may be only finding on this view
  - Lateral view
    - Displacement of fat pads due to joint effusion
      - Posterior fat pad is not normally visible
    - Apex volar angulation ± dorsal translation of distal humeral fracture fragment
      - Anterior humeral line no longer bisects capitellum in majority
  - RC line is typically maintained
    - Disruption would indicate radial head subluxation/dislocation (or possibly patient < 10 years old if mild), which does not typically occur in this setting
  - Follow-up imaging
    - Baumann angle (shaft-capitellum angle) on AP view: Superolateral angle between humeral diaphyseal long axis & physis deep to capitellar ossification center
      - Normally 64-81° → mild valgus carrying angle
      - ↑ Baumann angle (> 5° vs. contralateral side): Cubitus varus (5-10%)
    - Fishtail deformity of central humeral epiphysis due to lateral trochlear avascular necrosis
      - Uncommon complication of distal humeral fractures (most frequently supracondylar)
      - May lead to proximal migration of ulna + radial head subluxation/dislocation

DIFFERENTIAL DIAGNOSIS

Lateral Condylar Fracture

- Fracture extends obliquely through lateral humeral metaphysis to central physis

Posterior Dislocation

- Ulna & radius are displaced posteriorly, laterally, & proximally
  - RC line no longer intersects capitellum
- No supracondylar metadiaphyseal fracture

Medial Epicondyle Avulsion

- Avulsion ± intraarticular entrapment of medial epicondyle
- Elbow dislocation in 50%

Distal Humeral Epiphyseal Separation (Transphyseal Fracture)

- Uncommon fracture of young children (< 2 years of age) through distal humeral physis
- May be difficult to recognize due to lack of radiographically visible ossification centers
- Capitellum, radius, & ulna translate medially
  - RC line is maintained (if capitellum visible)
- 25-50% are associated with child abuse

T-Condylar Fracture

- Generally considered variant of supracondylar fracture (with additional intraarticular extension) in skeletally immature patients

PATHOLOGY

General Features

- Etiology
  - Supracondylar humerus is susceptible to fracture due to thin bone between medial & lateral pillars at coronoid fossa anteriorly & olecranon fossa posteriorly
  - Mechanism: Hyperextension form (98%) in FOOSH injury vs. flexion type (2%) from fall onto posterior elbow with direct trauma to olecranon
- Associated abnormalities
  - Concomitant elbow & forearm fractures (11%)
    - Olecranon, medial epicondyle, distal radius
    - Floating elbow: Forearm fractures become unstable in setting of supracondylar fracture (5%)
      - ↑ risk of neurovascular injury & compartment syndrome
  - Nerve injuries (10-20%)

- Anterior interosseous/median, ulnar, &/or radial nerves
  - Ulnar nerve injury is more likely with flexion mechanism
  - Transection is uncommon, usually radial nerve
- Vascular injuries (3-14%)
  - Spasm, laceration, thrombus, rupture

Staging, Grading, & Classification

- Modified Gartland classification
  - Type I
    - Nondisplaced or minimally displaced (< 2 mm)
    - Intact anterior humeral line
    - Posterior fat pad sign may be only finding
  - Type IIA
    - Mildly displaced (> 2 mm) anterior cortex
    - Posterior cortex is intact but hinged
    - Anterior humeral line touches anterior capitellum but does not extend through middle 1/3
    - No rotational deformity on AP view
  - Type IIB
    - Mildly displaced + malrotation or lateral displacement with maintenance of cortical contact
  - Type III
    - Displaced fracture with no cortical contact
    - Periosteum is torn
    - Often with soft tissue & neurovascular injuries
  - Type IV
    - Multidirectional instability (determined intraoperatively)

CLINICAL ISSUES

Presentation

- Most common signs/symptoms
  - Pain, loss of function, swelling, discoloration
  - Varying degrees of deformity depending on displacement
- Other signs/symptoms
  - ↓ distal radial pulse, cool extremity
  - Open fracture in 3%

Demographics

- Age
  - Most common in children 5-7 years old
  - Suggestive of abuse in nonambulatory infants
- Epidemiology
  - 60% of pediatric elbow fractures
  - 3-16% of all pediatric fractures
  - Rare in adults (< 3%)
  - Common in nondominant side (1.5:1)

Natural History & Prognosis

- Return of function in > 90% regardless of Gartland type
- Return of range of motion may take 1 year
- In patients with cool, pulseless extremity, radial pulse often returns quickly (> 50%) after closed reduction
- Nerve dysfunction is typically transient; may require months

Treatment

- Conservative
  - Type I: Above elbow cast in 90° flexion for 3-4 weeks
- Surgical
  - Type II: Treatment controversial
    - Closed reduction & casting vs. pin fixation
  - Type III/IV: Percutaneous lateral pin fixation vs. open reduction internal fixation (ORIF)
  - Prompt reduction & pinning for vascular compromise or floating elbow
    - Delayed treatment of 8-24 hours is otherwise increasingly accepted
  - ORIF may be needed in up to 20%
    - Open fractures
    - Entrapped soft tissues preventing closed reduction
    - Worsening neurovascular compromise after closed treatment
- Complications
  - Neurovascular injury, compartment syndrome, infection, loss of reduction (even with pinning), malunion, restricted motion, hyperextension, cubitus varus or cubitus valgus, fishtail deformity

DIAGNOSTIC CHECKLIST

Image Interpretation Pearls

- Be sure to look for other elbow & forearm fractures
- Consider follow-up radiographs in 10-14 days to identify healing occult fracture if joint effusion is only finding initially (in setting of trauma)

SELECTED REFERENCES

1. Ducic S et al: T-condylar humerus fracture in children: treatment options and outcomes. Int Orthop. 45(4):1065-70, 2021
2. Hariharan AR et al: Transphyseal humeral separations: what can we learn? A retrospective, multicenter review of surgically treated patients over a 25-year period. J Pediatr Orthop. 40(6):e424-9, 2020
3. Farrow L et al: Early versus delayed surgery for paediatric supracondylar humeral fractures in the absence of vascular compromise: a systematic review and meta-analysis. Bone Joint J. 100-B(12):1535-41, 2018
4. Anari JB et al: Pediatric T-condylar humerus fractures: a systematic review. J Pediatr Orthop. 37(1):36-40, 2017
5. Usman R et al: Management of arterial injury in children with supracondylar fracture of the humerus and a pulseless hand. Ann Vasc Dis. 10(4):402-6, 2017
6. Emery KH et al: Pediatric elbow fractures: a new angle on an old topic. Pediatr Radiol. 46(1):61-6, 2016
7. Fader LM et al: Eccentric capitellar ossification limits the utility of the radiocapitellar line in young children. J Pediatr Orthop. 36(2):161-6, 2016
8. Hyatt BT et al: Complications of pediatric elbow fractures. Orthop Clin North Am. 47(2):377-85, 2016
9. Muchow RD et al: Neurological and vascular injury associated with supracondylar humerus fractures and ipsilateral forearm fractures in children. J Pediatr Orthop. 35(2):121-5, 2015
10. Zorrilla S de Neira J et al: Supracondylar humeral fractures in children: current concepts for management and prognosis. Int Orthop. 39(11):2287-96, 2015
11. Isa AD et al: Functional outcome of supracondylar elbow fractures in children: a 3- to 5-year follow-up. Can J Surg. 57(4):241-6, 2014
12. Little KJ: Elbow fractures and dislocations. Orthop Clin North Am. 45(3):327-40, 2014
13. Narayanan S et al: Fishtail deformity - a delayed complication of distal humeral fractures in children. Pediatr Radiol. 45(6):814-9, 2014
14. Pennock AT et al: Potential causes of loss of reduction in supracondylar humerus fractures. J Pediatr Orthop. 34(7):691-7, 2014
15. Valencia M et al: Long-term functional results of neurological complications of pediatric humeral supracondylar fractures. J Pediatr Orthop. 35(6):606-10, 2014
16. Wegmann H et al: The impact of arterial vessel injuries associated with pediatric supracondylar humeral fractures. J Trauma Acute Care Surg. 77(2):381-5, 2014
17. Glotzbecker MP et al: Fishtail deformity of the distal humerus: a report of 15 cases. J Pediatr Orthop. 33(6):592-7, 2013

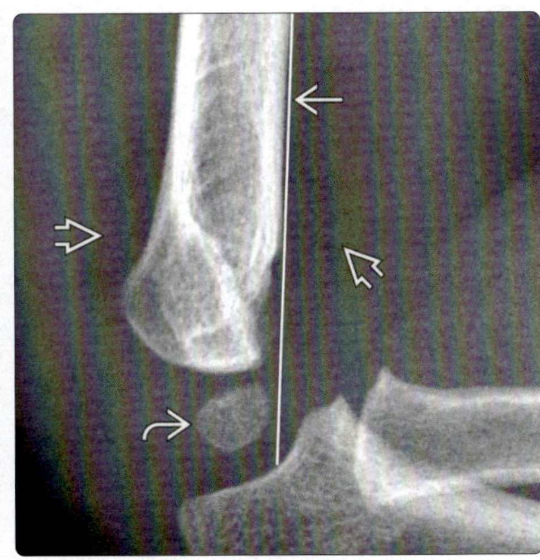

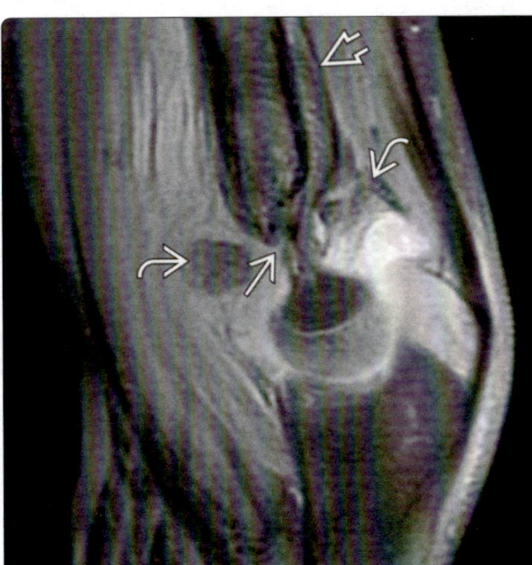

(Left) *Lateral radiograph shows that the anterior humeral line ➡ fails to intersect the capitellar ossification center ➡. This finding is consistent with a supracondylar fracture. Note the elevation of both the anterior & posterior fat pads ➡, indicating an elbow joint effusion.* **(Right)** *Sagittal PD FS MR in a 9-year-old with a healing supracondylar fracture shows anterior cortical disruption ➡ with displacement of the humeral fat pads ➡ by a joint effusion. Note the posterior humeral periosteal reaction ➡.*

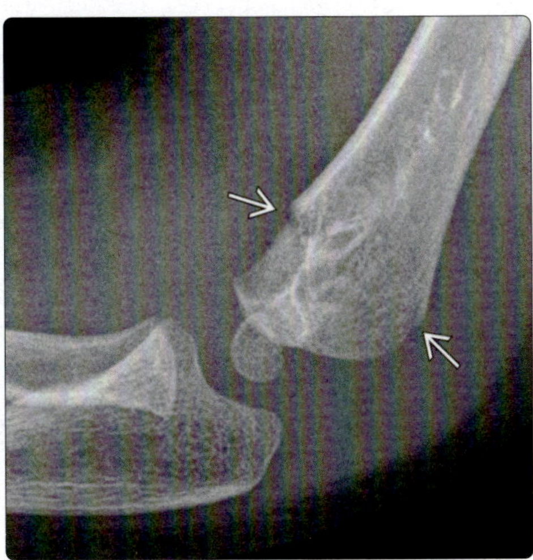

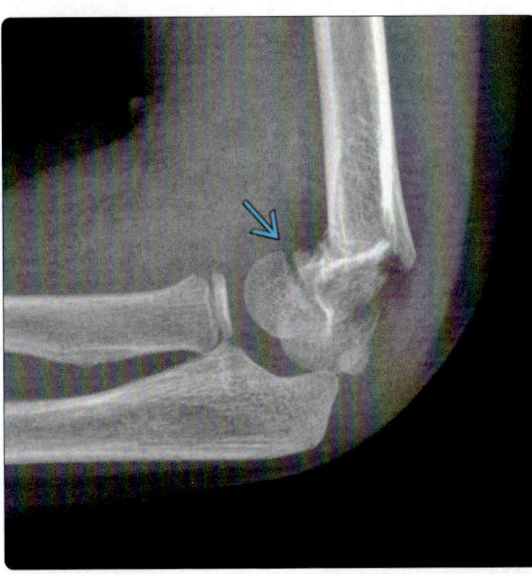

(Left) *Lateral radiograph in a patient after a fall shows a horizontally oriented fracture lucency ➡ through the supracondylar humerus with minimal apex volar angulation.* **(Right)** *Lateral radiograph in an 8-year-old girl after a fall shows an uncommon pattern of displacement for a supracondylar fracture with anterior translation ➡ & apex dorsal angulation. This pattern is associated with the less common (2%) mechanism of injury in supracondylar fractures (flexion injury with direct olecranon impact).*

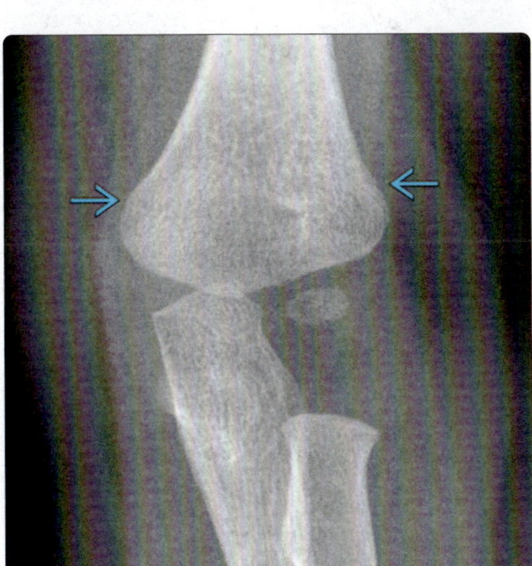

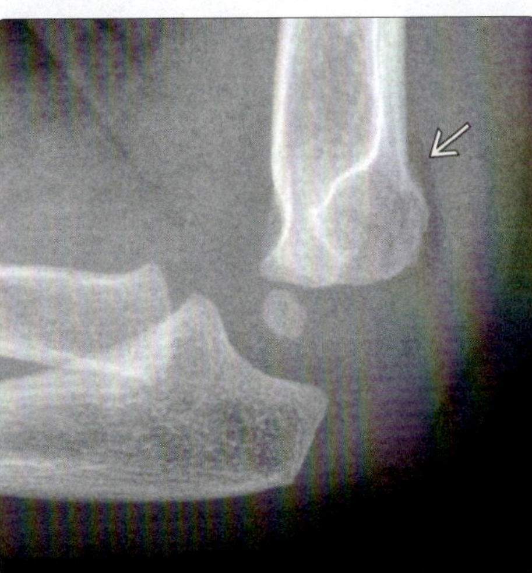

(Left) *AP radiograph in a 23-month-old patient shows slight cortical irregularity of the supracondylar humerus ➡ with overlying soft tissue swelling.* **(Right)** *Lateral radiograph in the same patient shows displacement of the posterior fat pad ➡ overlying a mildly angulated posterior humeral cortex. The anterior humeral line fails to bisect the capitellum.*

Lateral Condylar Fracture

KEY FACTS

TERMINOLOGY

- Posterior oblique fracture through lateral condyle of humeral metaphysis with distal extension through unossified epiphyseal cartilage (Salter-Harris IV)
  - Fracture line may dissipate within epiphyseal cartilage before reaching articular surface, leaving cartilaginous hinge/bridge

IMAGING

- AP view: Ranges from sliver of nondisplaced metaphyseal fracture fragment to marked translation & rotation of larger triangular metaphyseal fragment + capitellum
- Lateral view: Posterior oblique metaphyseal fracture plane; displacement of lucent anterior & posterior fat pads by joint effusion
- Internal oblique radiographs: More accurate for detecting fracture & determining displacement
- Distal cartilaginous extension is not radiographically visible but is implied by degree of bone fragment displacement
  - Lack of bone fragment displacement does not ensure cartilage integrity/fracture stability
  - Arthrography, MR, or US characterizes extent of cartilaginous articular surface injury

PATHOLOGY

- Jakob classification is used to determine therapy
  - Type I (≤ 2-mm displacement): Typically casted
  - Type II (> 2-mm displacement without rotation): Closed reduction with percutaneous pinning
  - Type III (> 2-mm displacement with rotation): Open reduction & fixation

CLINICAL ISSUES

- 10-20% of pediatric elbow fractures (2nd most common)
- Typically 5-10 years old; peak age: 6 years
- Complications include stiffness, late displacement, nonunion, delayed union, malunion, prominence or spurring of lateral condyle, capitellar osteonecrosis, tardy ulnar nerve palsy

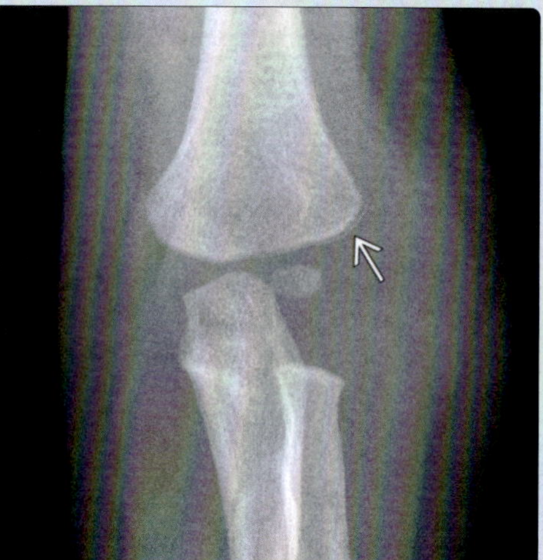

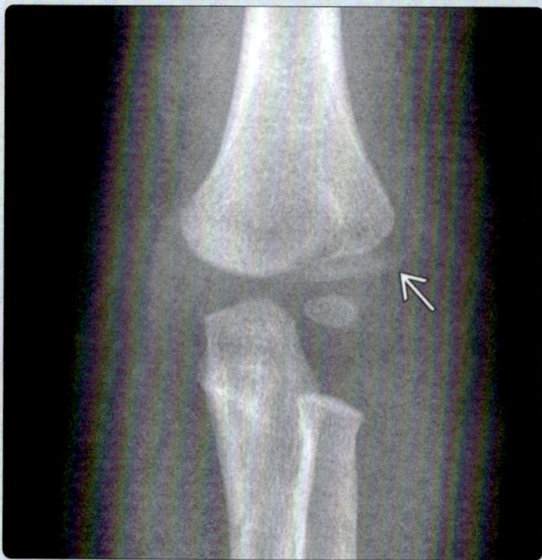

(Left) *AP radiograph in an 18-month-old after falling out of bed shows a subtle Jakob type I (≤ 2 mm of displacement) lateral condylar fracture* ➡ *of the distal humerus. Note the marked lateral soft tissue swelling.* **(Right)** *AP radiograph in the same child 1 week later shows ↑ displacement of the fracture* ➡ *despite immobilization. Delayed displacement is a known risk of nonoperative management in Jakob type I fractures.*

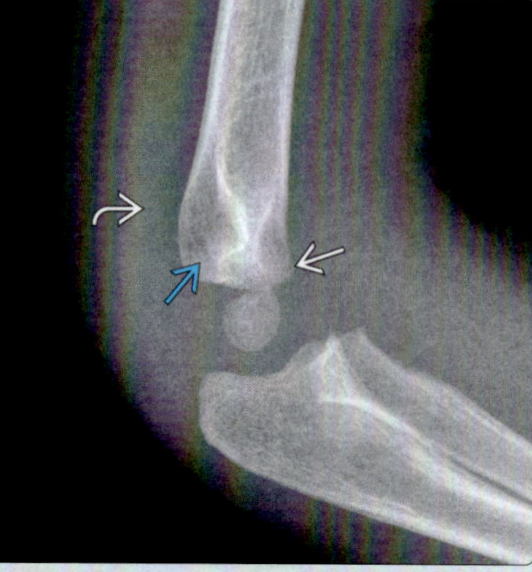

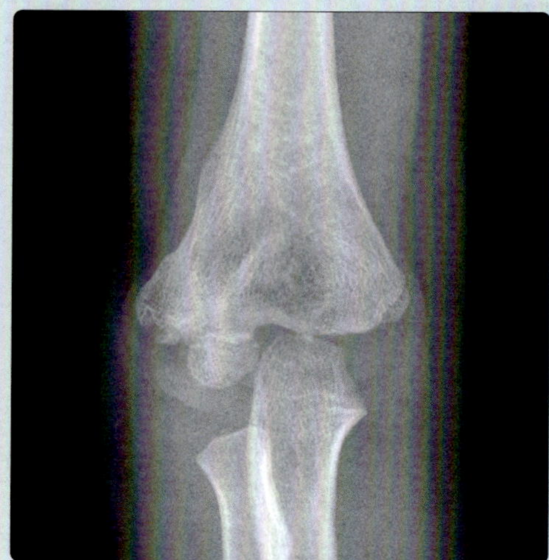

(Left) *Lateral radiograph in the same child shows an elbow joint effusion with elevation of the posterior* ➡ *fat pad. The fracture line* ➡ *has an oblique course posteriorly* ➡*, typical of lateral condylar fractures.* **(Right)** *AP radiograph in the same patient 8 months later shows a healed fracture with an enlarged lateral condyle & mild cubitus varus, both of which are recognized complications of lateral condylar fractures. This patient's fracture had been previously transfixed by 3 percutaneous K-wires.*

TERMINOLOGY

Definitions

- Posterior oblique fracture through lateral condyle of humeral metaphysis with distal extension through unossified epiphyseal cartilage
  - Fracture line may dissipate within epiphyseal cartilage before reaching articular surface

IMAGING

General Features

- Morphology
  - Metaphyseal fracture line parallels physis (or slightly steeper) on AP view
  - Salter-Harris IV fracture: Distal extension through unossified epiphyseal cartilage is not radiographically visible

Radiographic Findings

- AP view: Ranges from sliver of nondisplaced metaphyseal fracture fragment to marked translation & rotation of larger triangular metaphyseal fragment + capitellum
  - Nondisplaced fracture may be occult or easily missed
  - If missed &/or not treated appropriately, may lead to nonunion & joint incongruence
- Lateral view: Posterior oblique metaphyseal fracture plane; displacement of lucent anterior & posterior fat pads by joint effusion
- Internal oblique radiographs: More accurate for detecting fracture & determining displacement
  - May still underestimate true displacement
- External oblique views are rarely helpful
- Arthrography characterizes extent of cartilage/articular surface injury

CT Findings

- CT with reformation: Best assessment of displacement; also helpful for understanding complex fracture components to determine classification & treatment

MR Findings

- Horizontal to oblique linear high or low T1/T2 signal intensity fracture component in lateral metaphyseal humerus, ± surrounding marrow edema
- Vertical/oblique linear focus of fluid signal intensity through unossified distal humeral epiphyseal cartilage
- MR is also useful for follow-up of complications

Ultrasonographic Findings

- May be used to assess cartilage

Imaging Recommendations

- Protocol advice
  - Radiographs: AP & lateral views initially
    - Internal oblique view: Most sensitive for occult lateral condylar fractures & determining displacement
  - MR
    - Coronal & sagittal PD & T2 FS
    - Useful in assessing cartilage integrity/disruption
    - More expensive & often requires sedation in young child

DIFFERENTIAL DIAGNOSIS

Supracondylar Fracture

- Most common pediatric elbow fracture
- Transversely oriented fracture of distal humerus extending through level of olecranon fossa & coronoid fossa
  - Variable degrees of displacement
  - Disruption of anterior humeral line (normally bisects middle 1/3 of capitellum) on lateral view
  - May be occult, showing only elbow joint effusion

Olecranon Fracture

- Association with lateral condylar & other elbow fractures
- Must not confuse normal ossification center for fracture

Medial Epicondyle Avulsion

- ~ 10% of elbow fractures in pediatrics, usually in older children
- Distraction of medial epicondyle (ME) ossification center
  - Can become entrapped in elbow joint, simulating trochlear ossification center
- Unreliable fat pad displacement: ME tends to be extracapsular > 2 years old
- 50% are associated with elbow dislocations

Radial Neck Fracture

- 5% of elbow fractures in children
- Salter-Harris II fracture: 90%

Transphyseal Fracture

- Distal humeral epiphyseal separation, usually < 2 years old
- Displacement of largely unossified epiphyseal cartilage medially, resulting in malalignment between humeral metaphysis & radius (thereby suggesting elbow joint dislocation)
  - May be difficult to distinguish from dislocation when capitellum is not ossified
    - In true dislocation, radiocapitellar alignment is disrupted with radius displaced laterally & posteriorly
    - In transphyseal fracture, capitellum still aligns with radial head & radius/capitellum are usually shifted medially
- > 50% are associated with nonaccidental trauma

PATHOLOGY

General Features

- Etiology
  - Push-off: Fall on outstretched hand causing impaction of lateral condyle into radial head
  - Pull-off: Avulsion by lateral collateral ligamentous complex & common extensor tendons
  - Combination of push-off & pull-off

Staging, Grading, & Classification

- Distal extension of fracture through epiphysis (Salter-Harris IV) is much more common than extension through medial physis (Salter-Harris II)
- Jakob classification: Most common system used by surgeons; based on fragment displacement on internal oblique radiograph
  - Type I
    - Nondisplaced or ≤ 2 mm of displacement

- Fracture line is presumed not to extend to articular surface
- Type II
  - > 2 mm of displacement (typically < 4 mm)
  - Partial disruption of articular surface with intact hinge/bridge of cartilage
    - No rotation of lateral condylar fragment
- Type III
  - > 2 mm of displacement
  - Complete disruption of articular surface
    - Metaphyseal fragment & capitellum are rotated
    - Loss of radiocapitellar alignment → elbow instability
- Milch classification: Less commonly used due to high radiographic-surgical discordance
  - Type I
    - Fracture extends through capitellar ossification center lateral to trochlear groove
  - Type II
    - Fracture extends into trochlea rather than through capitellar ossification center

CLINICAL ISSUES

Presentation

- Lateral elbow swelling
- Lateral supracondylar ridge tenderness
- Absent pain over medial supracondylar ridge
- Ecchymosis

Demographics

- 10-20% of pediatric elbow fractures
  - 2nd in frequency after supracondylar fracture
  - Most common intraarticular pediatric elbow fracture
- Age: Typically 5-10 years old; peak: 6 years

Natural History & Prognosis

- Complications
  - Stiffness is most common
  - ↓ range of motion
  - Late fracture displacement 3 days to 3 weeks after nonoperative cast placement in ~ 11%
  - Nonunion
    - ↑ in intraarticular fractures
      - Bathed by synovial fluid, leading to ↓ healing
      - Pull of extensor muscles
      - Poor circulation to distal fracture fragment
    - ↑ in inadequately treated or displaced fractures
    - ↑ in missed or unrecognized fractures
  - Delayed union
    - > 6-8 weeks
  - Malunion
    - Fishtail deformity
      - Concavity with deepening of trochlear groove due to osteonecrosis
      - Rare; more common in supracondylar fractures
      - Usually minimal symptoms early; may have limited flexion & extension long term
    - Cubitus varus
      - More common than cubitus valgus
      - Most common with nondisplaced or minimally displaced fractures
    - Cubitus valgus
      - Fragment migration vs. lateral growth arrest
      - May lead to tardy ulnar nerve palsy
  - Tardy ulnar nerve palsy
    - Slow progressive paralysis of ulnar nerve
      - Atrophy of intrinsic hand muscles, sensory loss
      - Latency period of several months to many years
    - Treated by anterior transposition of ulnar nerve
  - Enlarged &/or spurred lateral condyle (nearly 50%)
    - Usually cosmetic without affecting function
  - Osteonecrosis of capitellum
    - Rare complication of extensive surgical dissection
  - Degenerative arthritis

Treatment

- Type I (≤ 2 mm of displacement)
  - Controversial: Some advocate surgical treatment
    - Occult extension to joint may occur without initial fracture displacement (thereby predisposing to late displacement if only casted initially)
  - Most commonly treated with long arm cast
    - Frequent follow-up radiographs every 7-10 days
      - Due to risk of late displacement
- Type II (> 2 mm of displacement without rotation)
  - Closed reduction with percutaneous pinning
    - Consider compression screws
  - Intraoperative arthrography is helpful in determining articular surface congruity
- Type III (> 2 mm of displacement with rotation)
  - Open reduction & fixation
    - K-wires &/or compression screws
- Cast is maintained for 4-6 weeks with operative or nonoperative treatment
- Removal of hardware after healing
- Physical therapy for stiffness

SELECTED REFERENCES

1. Wendling-Keim DS et al: Lateral condyle fracture of the humerus in children: Kirschner wire or screw fixation? Eur J Pediatr Surg. 31(4):374-9, 2021
2. Ganeshalingam R et al: Lateral condylar fractures of the humerus in children: does the type of fixation matter? Bone Joint J. 100-B(3):387-95, 2018
3. Salgueiro L et al: Rate and risk factors for delayed healing following surgical treatment of lateral condyle humerus fractures in children. J Pediatr Orthop. 37(1):1-6, 2017
4. Sinikumpu JJ et al: Paediatric lateral humeral condylar fracture outcomes at twelve years follow-up as compared with age and sex matched paired controls. Int Orthop. 41(7):1453-61, 2017
5. Bakarman KA et al: Humeral lateral condyle fractures in children: redefining the criteria for displacement. J Pediatr Orthop B. 25(5):429-33, 2016
6. Narayanan S et al: Fishtail deformity - a delayed complication of distal humeral fractures in children. Pediatr Radiol. 45(6):814-9, 2015
7. Little KJ: Elbow fractures and dislocations. Orthop Clin North Am. 45(3):327-40, 2014
8. Song KS et al: Lateral condylar humerus fractures: which ones should we fix? J Pediatr Orthop. 32 Suppl 1:S5-9, 2012
9. Marcheix PS et al: Distal humerus lateral condyle fracture in children: when is the conservative treatment a valid option? Orthop Traumatol Surg Res. 97(3):304-7, 2011
10. Tejwani N et al: Management of lateral humeral condylar fracture in children. J Am Acad Orthop Surg. 19(6):350-8, 2011
11. Song KS et al: Internal oblique radiographs for diagnosis of nondisplaced or minimally displaced lateral condylar fractures of the humerus in children. J Bone Joint Surg Am. 89(1):58-63, 2007

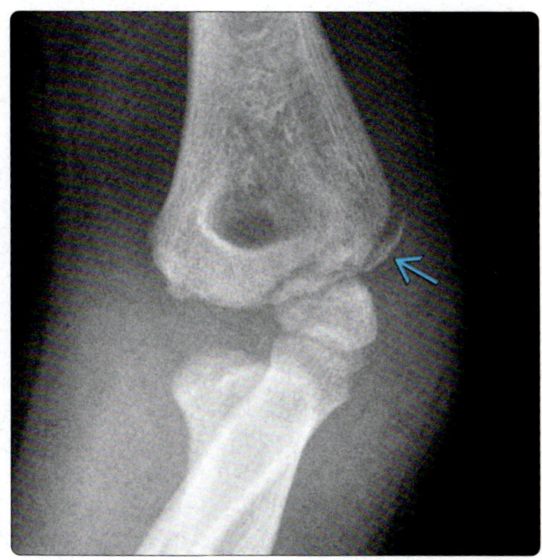

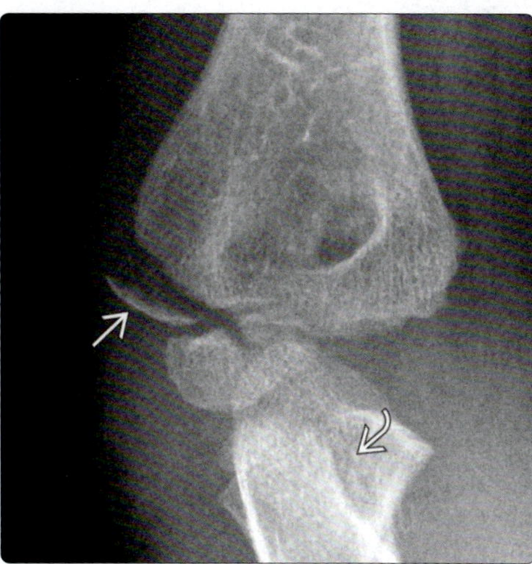

(Left) *Internal oblique radiograph in an 8-year-old after a fall shows a ≤ 2-mm displaced Jakob type I lateral condylar fracture* ➙ *with marked overlying soft tissue swelling.* **(Right)** *Oblique radiograph at 1 week of follow-up in a 5-year-old shows 4 mm of displacement to the lateral condylar fracture fragment* ➙*. On the initial images (not shown), the fracture was displaced ≤ 2 mm. There is also an olecranon process fracture* ➙*. Internal oblique radiographs are more accurate for fracture detection & displacement.*

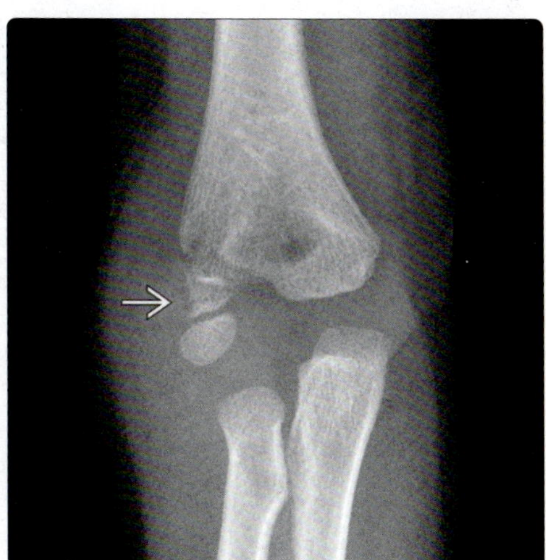

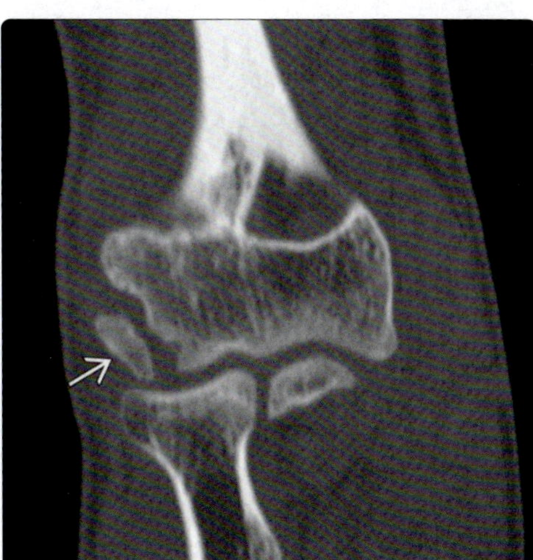

(Left) *AP radiograph in a 4-year-old who injured her elbow after falling off of a scooter shows a displaced & rotated Jakob type III lateral condylar fracture* ➙*.* **(Right)** *Coronal reformatted bone CT in a 15-year-old who sustained a lateral condylar fracture while playing football 3 years ago shows nonunion of a displaced fragment* ➙*. This complication is seen more often in children with inadequately treated or displaced fractures.*

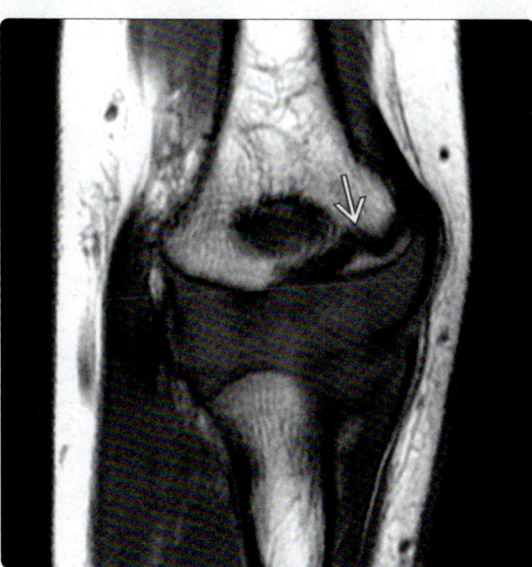

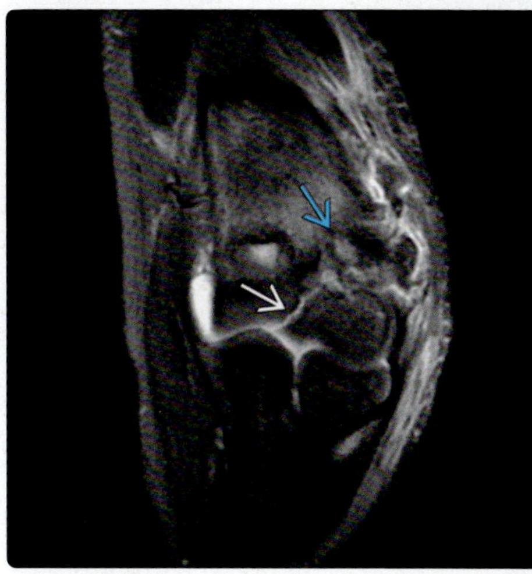

(Left) *Coronal T1 MR in a 5-year-old who sustained an elbow injury shows a hypointense oblique fracture line* ➙ *extending across the lateral condyle. No intraarticular extension of the fracture was identified.* **(Right)** *Coronal T2 FS MR in a patient after a fall shows an oblique hyperintense fracture line in the trochlear cartilage* ➙ *extending from the disrupted lateral condylar metaphysis* ➙ *to the articular surface.*

Medial Epicondyle Avulsion

KEY FACTS

TERMINOLOGY

- Acute injury: Avulsion fracture of medial epicondyle (ME) ossification center
- Chronic stress injury: Traction apophysitis, medial epicondylitis, Little Leaguer's elbow

IMAGING

- Acute injury: Distal & anterior translation of ME ossification center with moderate soft tissue swelling
  - May occur in setting of elbow dislocation
  - Remember CRITOE pattern of ossification at elbow
    - Should normally see ME in expected location on AP radiograph if trochlea is present
      - Avulsed, incarcerated ME can simulate trochlear ossification center
  - Unreliable fat pad sign: Joint effusion may be absent
- Chronic injury: Widening & irregularity of cartilaginous physis deep to ME
  - Less pronounced ME separation & soft tissue swelling
  - ± fragmentation & edema of ME on MR

PATHOLOGY

- Weakest link of immature musculoskeletal system: Osteocartilaginous interface
  - Acute tensile force → osteocartilaginous avulsion
    - Skeletally mature patients are more likely to injure ligaments, tendons, muscles
  - Chronic submaximal valgus forces (repetitive microtrauma) exceed healing capacity of system → irritation & disturbance of normal ossification

CLINICAL ISSUES

- Typical age for acute & chronic ME injuries: 8-14 years
- Acute avulsion fracture: Elbow dislocation in 50%, entrapped ME in 15-20%
- Chronic stress injury: Same valgus forces predispose to capitellar osteochondritis dissecans (OCD) & olecranon stress injuries
  - Typically overhead-throwing athletes (e.g., pitchers)

(Left) *AP radiograph in a 13-year-old girl after a fall shows an irregular defect ➡ at the expected site of the medial epicondyle (ME), which is entrapped in ➡ (& widening) the ulnohumeral articulation. Also note the impacted radial neck fracture ➡.* **(Right)** *Lateral radiograph in the same patient shows the donor site ➡ for the avulsed, incarcerated ME ➡ along the posterior aspect of the distal humerus. The impacted radial neck fracture ➡ is again noted.*

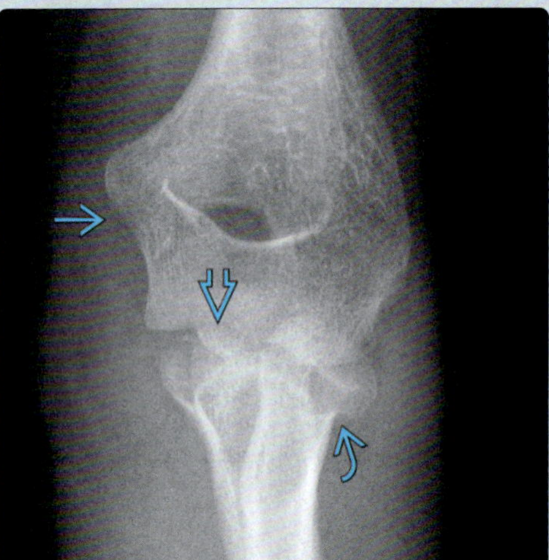

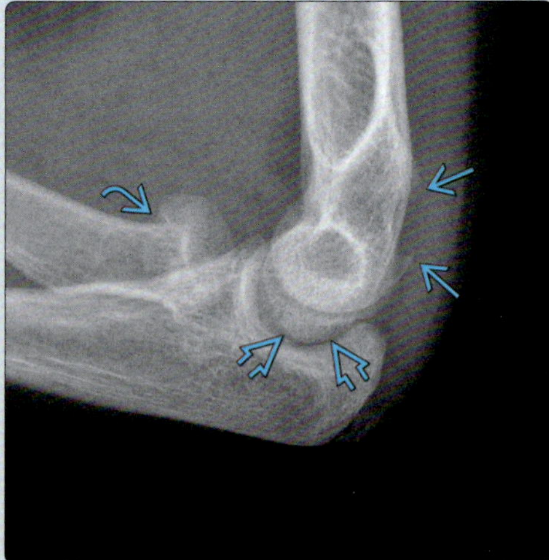

(Left) *AP radiograph shows an acute avulsion of the ME ossification center with mild rotation & distal translation of the fragment ➡.* **(Right)** *Coronal T2 FS MR in a 13-year-old pitcher with an acute injury shows a displaced ME ossification center ➡. Hyperintense fluid ➡ is interposed between the fragment & the medial humeral metaphysis, & there is moderate adjacent soft tissue edema. There is a low-grade tear of the ulnar collateral ligament ➡.*

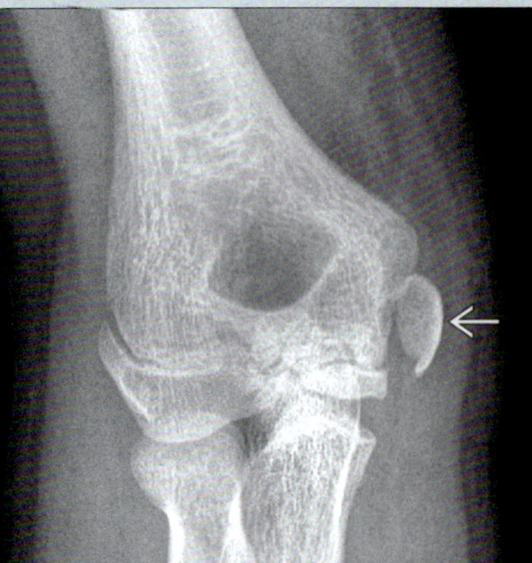

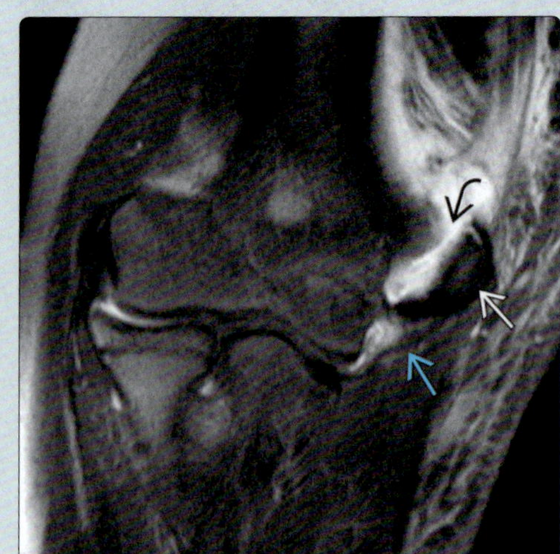

TERMINOLOGY

Synonyms

- Acute medial epicondyle (ME) injury: Avulsion fracture
- Chronic injury: Stress injury, medial epicondylitis, traction apophysitis, Little Leaguer's elbow

Definitions

- Acute injury: Avulsion of ME ossification center
- Chronic stress injury: Repetitive traction microtrauma exceeds healing capacity, causes inflammation, growth disturbance, degeneration
  - Skeletally immature: Apophysitis of ME
  - Skeletally mature: Partial tearing/degeneration of common flexor tendon, medial/ulnar collateral ligament

IMAGING

General Features

- Best diagnostic clue
  - Acute: Radiographic displacement of ME ossification center + overlying soft tissue swelling after injury
  - Chronic: MR fluid-sensitive sequence showing marrow & soft tissue edema at ME + widening, irregularity of physis
- Morphology
  - Should normally see ME in expected location on AP radiograph if trochlea is identified → excludes avulsed & entrapped ME, which can simulate trochlear ossification

Radiographic Findings

- Acute injury: Displacement of ME ossification center distally & anteriorly
  - Or laterally into joint (especially with lateral/posterior elbow dislocation) between olecranon & trochlea
  - ± joint effusion (therefore fat pad sign is unreliable)
- Chronic injury: Enlargement, sclerosis, fragmentation of ME with subjacent physeal widening & irregularity ± thickening of medial humeral cortex

MR Findings

- Acute: Separation of osteocartilaginous ME ossification center from humerus with interposed fluid signal
  - Moderate adjacent soft tissue edema ± marrow edema
- Chronic: Widening & irregularity of cartilaginous physis mimicking mild ME separation from humerus
  - Mild marrow & soft tissue edema, ± fragmentation of ME

DIFFERENTIAL DIAGNOSIS

Ulnar/Medial Collateral Ligament Injury

- More common with skeletal maturity
- Complete tear: Disruption of taut, linear/fan-shaped hypointense band
- Sprain: Thickened ligament with intermediate/high signal

Medial Condyle Avulsion

- Rare Salter-Harris type IV fracture with displaced sliver of bone along medial distal humeral metaphysis
  - Includes displacement of trochlea, which may be partially/completely unossified

Olecranon Stress Injury

- Olecranon fragmentation, edema, &/or physeal widening with appropriate history

Capitellar Osteochondritis Dissecans

- Repetitive impaction of radial head on capitellum with valgus stresses
- Lucent defect with flattening of anterior/midcapitellum
- Lateral pain & locking with loose intraarticular body

PATHOLOGY

General Features

- Etiology
  - ME serves as attachment for medial/ulnar collateral ligament & flexor-pronator muscle group of forearm
  - Osteocartilaginous interface is most likely site to fail under acute tensile stress in skeletally immature patients
    - Musculotendinous junction or ligament in adults
- Associated abnormalities
  - Elbow dislocation in 50% of acute avulsions
    - Ulnar nerve injury: 10-50%
    - ME trapped in elbow joint: 15-20%

CLINICAL ISSUES

Demographics

- Age: Similar ranges for acute ME avulsion fractures & chronic apophysitis: 8-14 years of age; peaks at 11-12 years of age
- Sex: M > F (4:1)
- Epidemiology: Acute avulsion is traditionally considered 3rd most common pediatric elbow fracture (10-20%)

Treatment

- Acute avulsion fracture treatment is controversial
  - Operative management
    - Absolute indications: Open fracture, incarcerated ME, entrapped ulnar nerve
    - Relative indications: Elbow instability, ME displacement, high-level athletes
      - Degree of displacement necessitating fixation is unclear: 2 vs. 5 vs. 10 mm
  - Nonoperative management
    - Good functional outcomes despite high nonunion rate
- Treatment of chronic stress injuries is largely conservative

SELECTED REFERENCES

1. García-Mata S et al: Prospective study of pediatric medial humeral epicondyle fractures nonoperatively treated. Clinical, radiologic, and functional evaluation at long term. J Pediatr Orthop B. 30(2):180-9, 2021
2. Fernandez FF et al: Medial humeral condyle fracture in childhood: a rare but often overlooked injury. Eur J Trauma Emerg Surg. 45(4):757-61, 2019
3. Griffith TB et al: Elbow injuries in the adolescent thrower. Curr Rev Musculoskelet Med. 11(1):35-47, 2018
4. Emery KH et al: Pediatric elbow fractures: a new angle on an old topic. Pediatr Radiol. 46(1):61-6, 2016
5. Pathy R et al: Medial epicondyle fractures in children. Curr Opin Pediatr. 27(1):58-66, 2015
6. Redler LH et al: Elbow trauma in the athlete. Hand Clin. 31(4):663-81, 2015

KEY FACTS

TERMINOLOGY

- Complete fracture: Macroscopic fracture line traverses entire bony diameter
  - Physeal (Salter-Harris): Fracture through cartilaginous growth plate, typically with adjacent bony involvement
- Incomplete fracture: Macroscopic fracture line does not traverse entire bony diameter
  - Buckle fracture, greenstick fracture, plastic deformity

IMAGING

- Focal abrupt cortical angulation, protuberance, &/or discrete fracture line with overlying soft tissue swelling
  - ± physeal extension with displacement of metaphyseal fragment & epiphysis
- Radius & ulna are often fractured together unless dislocated
  - Fractures may be of different types
- Distal radius: Buckle, complete transverse, or physeal
  - Up to 85% of pediatric forearm fractures
  - Distal ulnar injury is usually present: Styloid or incomplete metadiaphyseal fracture
- Radial & ulnar diaphyses: Complete, greenstick, or plastic deformity
- Proximal radius & ulna fractures are usually considered with elbow

PATHOLOGY

- Fall on outstretched hand > > direct blow
- Immature bone is more pliable → incomplete fractures (particularly < 10 years of age)

CLINICAL ISSUES

- Greater remodeling potential in younger children with remaining growth
- Usually managed with closed reduction as needed + cast/splint immobilization
- Risk of growth arrest with Salter-Harris fracture

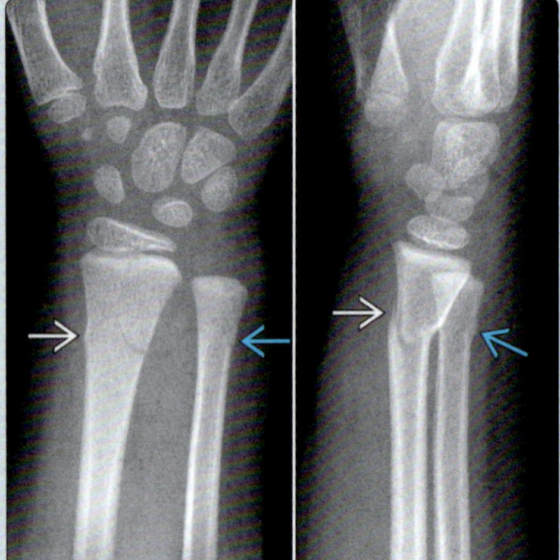

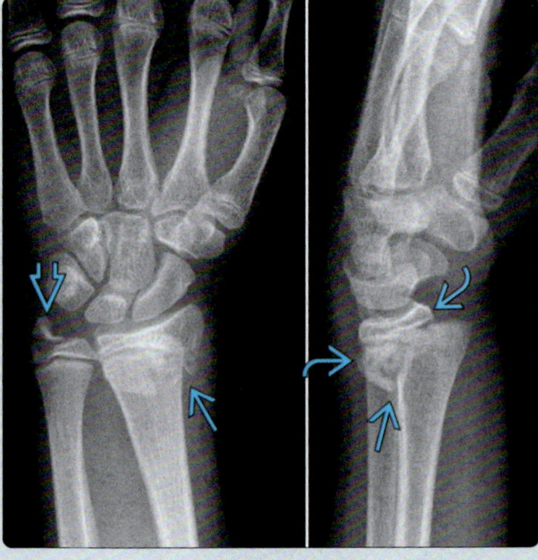

(Left) *PA & lateral radiographs of the wrist in a 5-year-old after a fall show a mildly angulated complete fracture of the distal radial metadiaphyseal junction ➡. A buckle fracture of the distal ulna ➡ is also noted. Ulnar fractures usually accompany distal radial fractures but may be subtle.* **(Right)** *PA & lateral views of the wrist in a 12-year-old show a comminuted Salter-Harris II (SHII) fracture ➡ of the distal radius with dorsal translation of the distal fracture fragment ➡. An ulnar styloid fracture ➡ is present.*

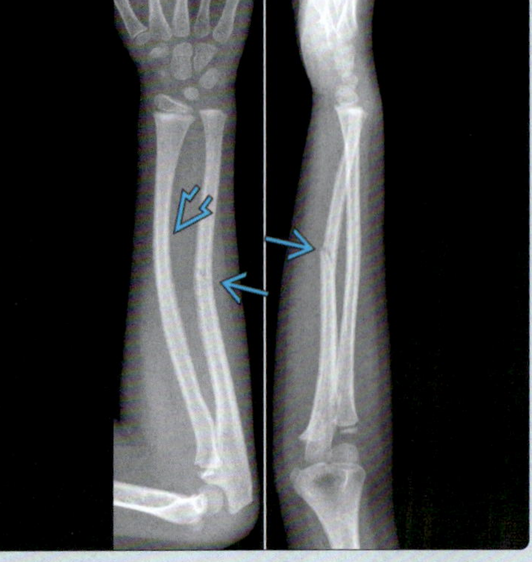

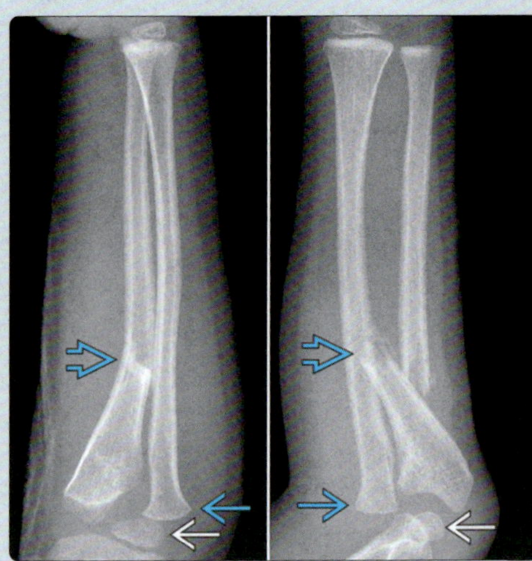

(Left) *AP & lateral forearm radiographs show 2 types of incomplete fractures with a greenstick fracture of the ulnar diaphysis ➡ (with cortical disruption on the tension or convex side) & a plastic deformity of the radial diaphysis ➡.* **(Right)** *AP & lateral forearm radiographs in a 4-year-old show a complete fracture of the proximal ulnar diaphysis ➡ & dislocation of the proximal radius ➡ relative to the capitellum ➡ (the Monteggia fracture-dislocation complex). The radial head has not yet ossified.*

TERMINOLOGY

Definitions

- Complete fracture: Macroscopic fracture line traverses entire bony diameter
  - Physeal (Salter-Harris): Fracture through cartilaginous growth plate, typically with adjacent bony involvement
  - Monteggia: Radial head dislocation + proximal ulnar shaft fracture
  - Galeazzi: Distal radial fracture + distal ulnar dislocation
- Incomplete fracture: Macroscopic fracture line does not traverse entire bony diameter
  - Buckle: Focal cortical deformity on compression side
    - Component of buckling often accompanies physeal fracture → look for subtle extension of lucency to growth plate
  - Greenstick: Cortical disruption on tension side
  - Plastic deformity: Smooth abnormal curvature of diaphysis without cortical interruption

IMAGING

General Features

- Best diagnostic clue
  - Abrupt angular deformity or frank interruption of normally smooth cortical contour
  - Radius & ulna are often both fractured ("both bone forearm fractures") unless dislocated
- Location
  - Distal radius: Buckle, complete transverse, or physeal
    - 25-43% of all pediatric fractures
    - 15% involve physis; almost all are Salter-Harris II (SHII)
    - Accompanying ulnar injury: Styloid or incomplete metadiaphyseal fracture is most common
      - Less commonly: Physeal injury or dislocation
  - Radial & ulnar diaphyses: Complete, greenstick, or plastic deformity
    - 10-30% of all pediatric fractures
  - Proximal radius & ulna fractures are typically considered as elbow fracture
    - Radial neck SHII & ulnar olecranon are most common

Radiographic Findings

- Focal abrupt cortical angulation, protuberance, &/or discrete fracture line with overlying soft tissue swelling
- ± physeal extension with displacement of metaphyseal & epiphyseal fragments
- May see displacement of pronator quadratus fat pad at volar radius

Ultrasonographic Findings

- Focal interruption/bulging of echogenic cortex ± subperiosteal hemorrhage, soft tissue edema

Imaging Recommendations

- Vast majority are diagnosed & managed by radiographs
- Obtain 2 tangential views as fracture may be subtle

DIFFERENTIAL DIAGNOSIS

Normal Developmental Variants

- Few sites of normally occurring mild cortical angulation/protuberance or bowing
- Contralateral comparison radiographs are helpful

Metabolic Bone Diseases

- Pathologically weakened bones ± multiple fractures, may show chronic bowing

Skeletal Dysplasias

- Bones of abnormal shapes & sizes, typically bilateral
- ± abnormal mineralization

PATHOLOGY

General Features

- Fall on outstretched hand > > direct blow
- Immature bone is softer, more pliable → greater bowing or bending before breaking → incomplete fractures
  - Particularly children < 10 years of age

CLINICAL ISSUES

Presentation

- Most common signs/symptoms
  - Pain, swelling, tenderness, ↓ use, deformity

Natural History & Prognosis

- Acceptable degree of displacement, angulation, & malrotation varies by fracture type, location, patient age
  - Greater remodeling potential in children (especially < 6-10 years of age)
    - Tolerate ↑ degrees of residual displacement of nonarticular fractures after closed reduction
  - 21-39% of reduced distal radial fractures will redisplace
    - Risk factors: Initial displacement ≥ 1 shaft width, "both bone" fractures, nonanatomic reduction
- Buckle fractures
  - 3-week immobilization with splint
  - Follow-up imaging is often not necessary
- Complete or incomplete diaphyseal fractures
  - > 90% are managed with closed reduction & casting
- Physeal injuries
  - < 5% develop subsequent symptomatic growth arrest at distal radius vs. ~ 50% growth arrest rate at distal ulna
- Ulnar styloid injuries
  - Vast majority are not treated; nonunion is common
  - Few patients will have long-term symptoms
- Forearm fracture patterns more likely to be managed operatively: Proximal 1/3, comminuted, Monteggia, older children/adolescents, & severe soft tissue injuries precluding cast placement

SELECTED REFERENCES

1. Laor T et al: Describing pediatric fractures in the era of ICD-10. Pediatr Radiol. 50(6):761-75, 2020
2. Sengab A et al: Risk factors for fracture redisplacement after reduction and cast immobilization of displaced distal radius fractures in children: a meta-analysis. Eur J Trauma Emerg Surg. 46(4):789-800, 2020
3. Iles BW et al: Differentiating stable buckle fractures from other distal radius fractures: the 1-cm rule. Pediatr Radiol. 49(3):358-64, 2019
4. Herren C et al: Ultrasound-guided diagnosis of fractures of the distal forearm in children. Orthop Traumatol Surg Res. 101(4):501-5, 2015
5. Little JT et al: Pediatric distal forearm and wrist injury: an imaging review. Radiographics. 34(2):472-90, 2014

ACL Injuries

KEY FACTS

TERMINOLOGY

- Intrasubstance anterior cruciate ligament (ACL) tears may be complete or partial; differentiation can be difficult
- Avulsion fractures of tibial eminence at distal ACL attachment are more frequent in skeletally immature patients
- Femoral avulsion fractures of ACL are rare

IMAGING

- Radiographs: Joint effusion is common but nonspecific
  - Less common but more specific secondary findings: Deep lateral condylar notch sign & Segond fracture
- MR: ↑ intrasubstance signal of ACL with disrupted fibers
  - Empty lateral intercondylar wall on coronal PD/T2 FS
  - "Kissing" contusions: Edema in lateral femoral & posterolateral tibial condyles
  - ACL tibial eminence avulsion
    - Meniscus or transverse ligament may be entrapped under avulsed tibial eminence fracture fragment

CLINICAL ISSUES

- Mid or proximal substance ACL tears are typical of athletic patients at or approaching skeletal maturity (F > M)
- Tibial eminence avulsion fractures are most common at 8-14 years of age (M > F); ACL is intact or partially torn

DIAGNOSTIC CHECKLIST

- Evaluate integrity of ACL in 3 standard planes
  - Oblique planes along course of ACL may improve detection of partial tears
- Important associated MR findings in setting of ACL tear
  - Meniscal tears
    - Posterior horn medial meniscus-capsular separation: "Ramp lesion"
      - May result in graft failure & joint degeneration
    - Posterior horn lateral meniscal tears are often missed
      - Closely inspect lateral meniscal-meniscofemoral ligament attachment
  - Posterolateral corner/medial collateral ligament injuries

(Left) *Lateral radiograph in a 17-year-old girl with a right knee injury during a soccer game shows a joint effusion & a deep lateral condylar notch that measures > 3 mm.* **(Right)** *Sagittal PD (left) & T2 FS (right) MR images (same patient) show a corresponding subchondral fracture of the lateral femoral condyle with underlying edema + complex tear of the lateral meniscus posterior horn. The more central PD image shows a complete midsubstance anterior cruciate ligament (ACL) tear.*

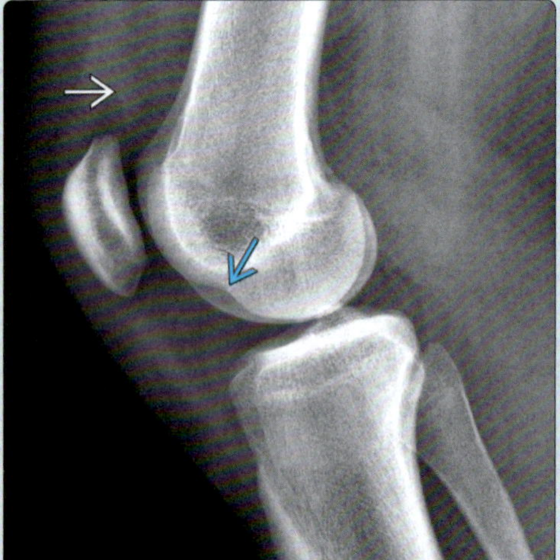

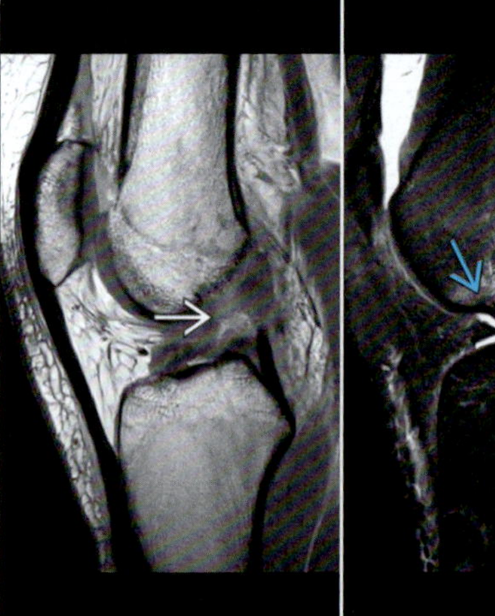

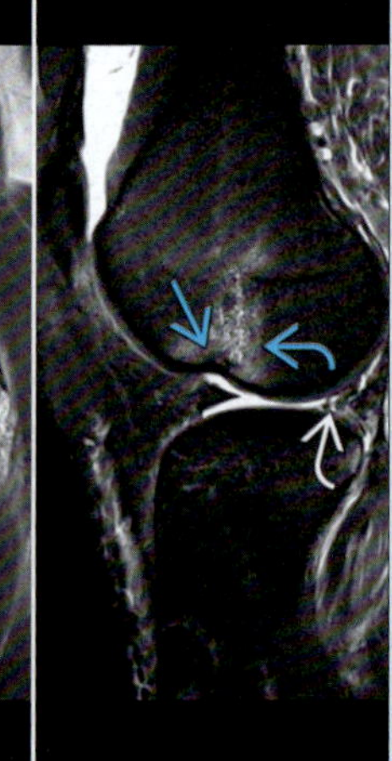

(Left) *Frontal (left) & lateral (right) radiographs in a boy with a right knee injury show a joint effusion & a Segond fracture. Segond fractures are nearly always associated with ACL tears.* **(Right)** *Sagittal T2 FS MR images from central (left) to lateral (right) in the same boy show a complete intrasubstance ACL tear, "kissing" contusions in the lateral femoral & posterolateral tibial condyles, & partial tearing of the popliteofibular ligament with edema in the fibular head.*

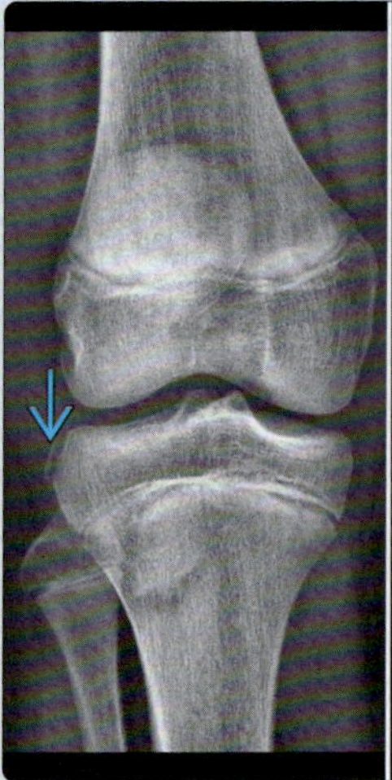

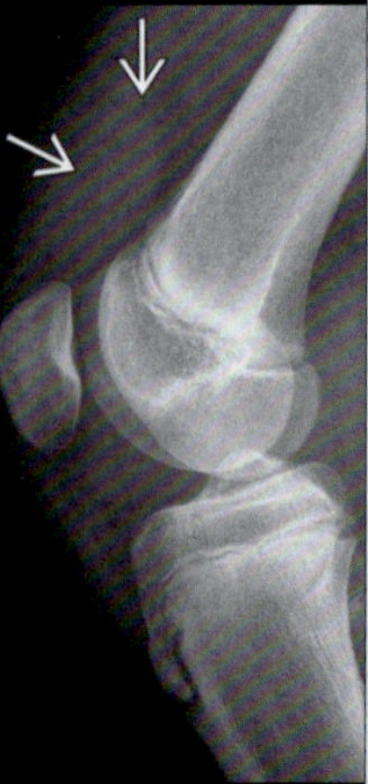

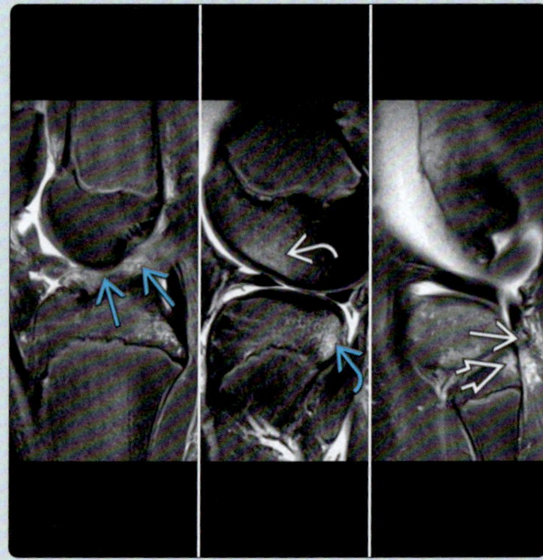

TERMINOLOGY

Abbreviations

- Anterior cruciate ligament (ACL)

Definitions

- ACL has anteromedial & posterolateral bundles
- ACL tears can be complete or partial

IMAGING

General Features

- Best diagnostic clue
  - Radiographs: Large joint effusion
    - Less common: Deep lateral condylar notch, Segond fracture
  - MR: ↑ intrasubstance T2 signal & disrupted fibers
    - Empty lateral intercondylar wall on coronal PD/T2 FS
    - "Kissing" contusions (lateral femoral & posterolateral tibial condyles)
- Location
  - Intrasubstance: Typically midsubstance or proximal
  - Tibial eminence avulsion fractures of ACL in younger (skeletally immature) children
  - Femoral avulsion fractures of ACL are rare but do occur

Radiographic Findings

- Intrasubstance ACL tears
  - Large joint effusion
    - Absence of joint effusion following acute injury virtually excludes ACL tear
  - Segond fracture: Vertically oriented avulsion from lateral proximal tibia
    - Associated ACL tear: 75-100%
    - Associated meniscal tear: 66-75%
  - Deep lateral femoral notch sign
    - Suggests ACL tear if > 1.5-2 mm
  - Fibular head avulsion fracture (arcuate sign)
    - Indicates injury to arcuate ligament complex
    - Associated with cruciate ligament [posterior cruciate ligament (PCL) > ACL] tears
- Tibial eminence fractures
  - Meyers & McKeever classification (modified)
    - Type I: Minimal displacement
    - Type II: "Trapdoor" configuration (elevation of anterior portion of fragment)
    - Type III: Completely displaced fragment
    - Type IV: Comminution of fragment
- Femoral avulsion fracture
  - Avulsion fracture at posteromedial aspect of lateral femoral condyle
  - May be radiographically occult if nondisplaced or predominantly cartilaginous

MR Findings

- T2 FS useful for marrow & soft tissue edema, ligamentous injuries
- PD useful to evaluate associated meniscal injuries
- Primary signs
  - ↑ intrasubstance signal, diffuse thickening, & clearly disrupted fibers
    - May be partial or complete: Can be difficult to distinguish, even at 3T
  - Empty lateral intercondylar wall on coronal images
    - Fluid signal at femoral attachment of ACL
  - Abnormal horizontal or bowed orientation of ligament relative to roof of intercondylar notch
- Secondary & associated signs
  - "Kissing" contusions: Edema in lateral femoral & posterolateral tibial condyles
  - Anterior tibial translation
  - Uncovered lateral meniscus sign
  - Laxity of PCL; posterolateral corner (PLC) injury
  - Medial collateral ligament (MCL) injury
  - Meniscal tears, including medial meniscus posterior horn meniscocapsular separation ("ramp lesion")
    - Posterior horn lateral meniscus tear: Most commonly missed tear associated with ACL injury
      - Often confused with "pseudotear" at lateral meniscal-meniscofemoral ligament attachment
      - Apparent ↑ lateral extension of this attachment site should raise suspicion for tear [≥ 4 images (on 3-mm slices) lateral to PCL = tear]
    - Lateral meniscus root tears with meniscal extrusion also associated with ACL tears
- Chronic ACL tears
  - Complete: Fatty signal in notch without ACL fibers
  - Chronic partial tears: Attenuated ACL
- Tibial eminence fracture
  - MR performed to assess for associated injuries
    - Partial intrasubstance ACL tears
    - Interposition of menisci or transverse ligament under avulsed fracture fragment
      - Up to 33% of type II & 65% of type III fractures
      - Can prevent reduction & healing
- Femoral avulsion fracture
  - MR may show radiographically occult femoral avulsion fracture & associated injuries
  - Avulsion fracture at posteromedial aspect of lateral femoral condyle at ACL femoral attachment

Imaging Recommendations

- Best imaging tool
  - Radiographs in acute setting
    - Evaluate for joint effusion, deep lateral condylar notch, Segond fracture, or tibial eminence avulsion
  - MR confirms ACL tear & evaluates associated injuries
    - Meniscal, MCL, PLC, & cartilaginous injuries
- Protocol advice
  - Evaluate ACL on all 3 standard planes (not just sagittal)

DIFFERENTIAL DIAGNOSIS

Congenital Absence of Anterior Cruciate Ligament

- Hypoplasia to complete absence of ACL
  - Could mimic chronic partial or complete ACL tears
- Small/absent intercondylar notch & dysplasia of tibial eminence

Anterior Cruciate Ligament Ganglion

- Lobular, septated fluid signal mass along or within ACL

Synovial Cleft of Anterior Cruciate Ligament
- Variant herniation of fluid-containing synovium into ACL

PATHOLOGY

Gross Pathologic & Surgical Features
- ACL is intraarticular but extrasynovial (i.e., encased by synovial lining such that joint fluid does not directly contact ACL)
- Tibial intercondylar eminence is divided into 4 regions
  - Medial & lateral intercondylar tubercles or spines
  - Anterior & posterior intercondylar area
- ACL footprint lies at anterior intercondylar area, between anterior attachments of medial & lateral menisci
- Due to this proximity, menisci &/or transverse ligament can become trapped under avulsed tibial eminence fragment → prevents fracture reduction & healing
- Strong association between ACL tears & meniscal tears

CLINICAL ISSUES

Presentation
- Most common signs/symptoms
  - Complete ACL tear
    - Acute swelling & pain with knee "giving out"
    - Sensation of &/or audible "pop" at time of injury
- Clinical profile
  - Complete ACL tears
    - Pivot shift injury
      - Noncontact injury seen commonly in American football players & skiers
      - Valgus stress is applied to flexed knee & external rotation of tibia or internal rotation of femur loads ACL → tear
      - ACL rupture → unrestrained anterior translation of tibia relative to femur → impaction of central lateral femoral & posterolateral tibial condyles
      - Various degrees of flexion may alter location of bone bruise in femoral condyle (i.e., ↑ flexion → more posterior, ↓ flexion → more anterior)
      - Can get contrecoup injury with bone contusion to posteromedial tibial condyle
  - Tibial eminence fractures
    - Typically hyperextension force ± valgus or rotational component
    - May occur from direct blow to femur with knee flexed
- Clinical examination
  - ACL injury
    - Lachman test: Anterior translation force applied to proximal tibia with knee mildly flexed
      - Lack of solid/firm endpoint = (+) test
    - Anterior drawer test: Anterior translational force applied to proximal tibia with knee flexed at ~ 80-90°
      - ↑ translation (vs. contralateral side) = (+) test

Demographics
- Epidemiology
  - ↑ frequency related to ↑ childhood athletic activities
  - Tibial eminence avulsion fractures are most common at 8-14 years of age (M > F)
  - Frequency of ACL tears in skeletally mature adolescents approaches that in adults (F > M)

Natural History & Prognosis
- Conservatively managed complete ACL tears in skeletally immature patients often have poor outcomes
  - Instability → degenerative change, meniscal tears, & chondral injury
  - Few patients return to preinjury sports level
- Partial ACL tears can progress to complete tears & symptomatic laxity within 1 year
- Tibial eminence fractures: May be associated with partial tear of ACL; contributes to residual sagittal laxity even following "anatomic" reduction & healing

Treatment
- Complete ACL tears need ligamentous reconstruction
  - May be complicated by presence of open growth plates
    - Various physeal-sparing approaches for children with substantial growth remaining
      - Intra- & extraarticular iliotibial band autograft
      - All epiphyseal approach: Uses epiphyseal tunnels & fixation
    - Transphyseal approach with metaphyseal fixation for children past peak growth
  - Adult reconstruction techniques in patients with closed or closing growth plates
- Tibial eminence fractures
  - Type I: Immobilization in long leg cast or fracture brace with knee flexed at ~ 10-20°
  - Type II: Optimal treatment is controversial
    - Closed reduction & casting
    - Surgical (typically arthroscopic) reduction & fixation
  - Type III-IV
    - Surgical (open or arthroscopic) reduction & fixation

DIAGNOSTIC CHECKLIST

Image Interpretation Pearls
- Important associated MR findings in setting of ACL tear
  - Posterior horn lateral meniscal tears are often missed
    - Closely inspect lateral meniscal-meniscofemoral ligament attachment
    - Apparent extension of attachment ≥ 4 images (with 3-mm slices) lateral to PCL indicates tear
  - Medial meniscus posterior horn ramp lesions
  - PLC & MCL injuries
  - Meniscus or transverse ligament trapped under avulsed tibial eminence fracture fragment

SELECTED REFERENCES

1. Kushare I et al: High Incidence of Intra-articular Injuries With Segond Fractures of the tibia in the pediatric and adolescent population. J Pediatr Orthop. 41(8):514-9, 2021
2. Adams AJ et al: Pediatric type II tibial spine fractures: addressing the treatment controversy with a mixed-effects model. Orthop J Sports Med. 7(8):2325967119866162, 2019
3. Dingel A et al: Pediatric ACL tears: natural history. J Pediatr Orthop. 39(Issue 6, Supplement 1 Suppl 1):S47-9, 2019
4. Green D et al: A new, MRI-based classification system for tibial spine fractures changes clinical treatment recommendations when compared to Myers and Mckeever. Knee Surg Sports Traumatol Arthrosc. 27(1):86-92, 2019
5. Beck NA et al: ACL tears in school-aged children and adolescents over 20 years. Pediatrics. 139(3), 2017
6. Dunn KL et al: Early operative versus delayed or nonoperative treatment of anterior cruciate ligament injuries in pediatric patients. J Athl Train. 51(5):425-7, 2016

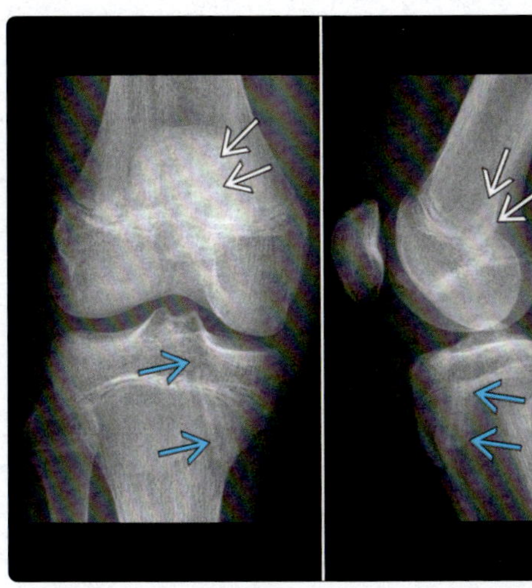

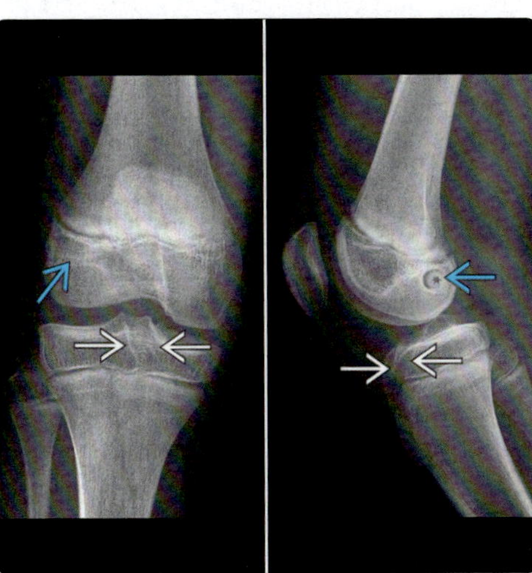

(Left) *Frontal (left) & lateral (right) radiographs after an ACL repair show that this boy was close enough to skeletal maturity to perform a transphyseal reconstruction. Note how the tibial tunnel & interference screw cross his tibial physis* → *. Two bioabsorbable pins* ➡ *fix the graft to the femur.* **(Right)** *Frontal (left) & lateral (right) radiographs in a 12-year-old with a physeal-sparing ACL reconstruction show that the femoral tunnel interference screw* → *& the tibial tunnel* ➡ *are completely epiphyseal & do not cross the physes.*

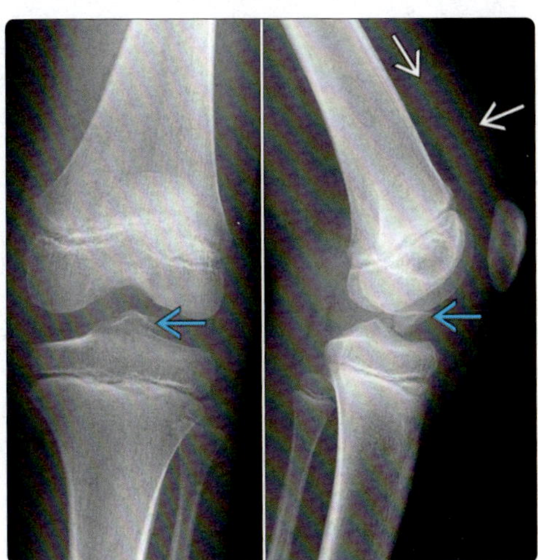

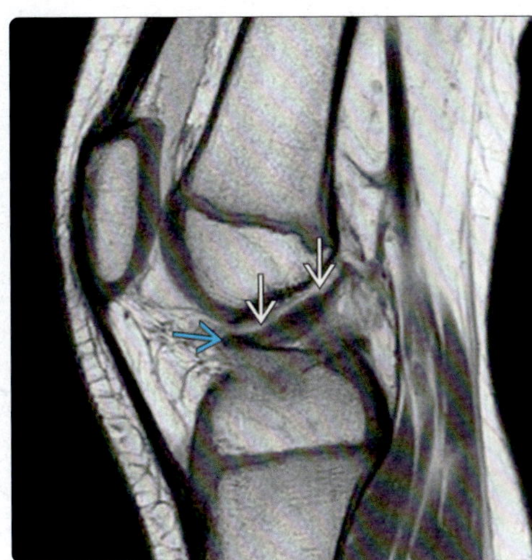

(Left) *Frontal (left) & lateral (right) radiographs in a 7-year-old boy with a left knee injury show an elevated tibial eminence avulsion fracture* → *with a joint effusion* ➡ *.* **(Right)** *Sagittal PD MR in the same boy shows that the intact ACL* ➡ *is attached to the avulsed tibial eminence fragment* → *, the anterior portion of which is elevated (consistent with a type II tibial eminence fracture). In this case, there is no meniscal tissue or transverse ligament trapped deep to the avulsed fragment.*

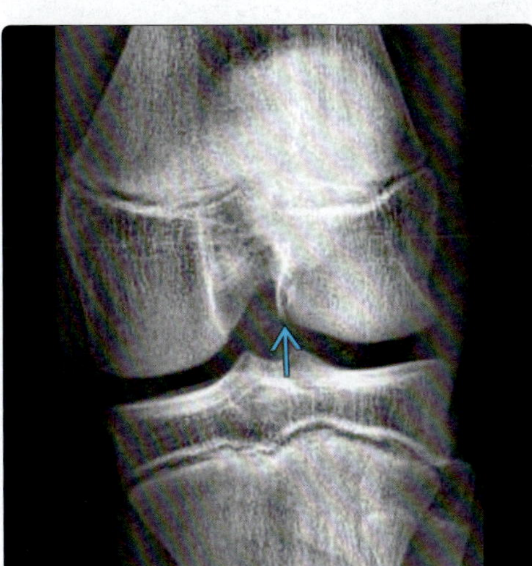

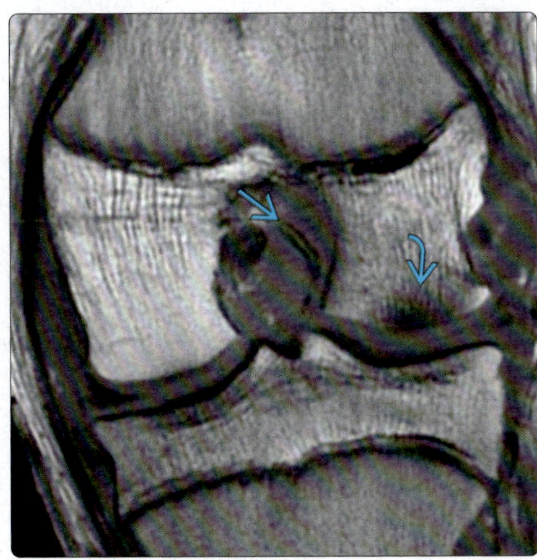

(Left) *AP radiograph in a 14-year-old boy with a left knee injury during a soccer game shows an avulsion fracture* → *along the central aspect of the lateral femoral condyle at the femoral attachment of the ACL.* **(Right)** *Coronal T1 MR in the same patient shows the avulsion fracture at the ACL femoral attachment site* → *on the posteromedial aspect of the lateral femoral condyle. A lateral condyle bone contusion* ⤷ *is also noted. Avulsion fractures at the ACL femoral attachment are rare & mostly occur in the skeletally immature.*

Patellar Dislocation

KEY FACTS

TERMINOLOGY

- Transient patellar dislocation (TPD): Lateral dislocation & relocation of patella from direct/indirect injury
  - Shearing, tensile, compressive forces → medial patella, lateral femur, & soft tissue injuries

IMAGING

- Radiographs
  - Large joint effusion after acute TPD
  - Osseous fragments (of patella & lateral femoral condyle)
- MR
  - Medial patella & lateral femoral condyle contusions
  - Chondral & osteochondral injuries
  - Medial patellofemoral ligament (MPFL) tears

PATHOLOGY

- MPFL = condensation of medial retinaculum
  - Extends from superomedial patella to medial femur (between adductor tubercle & medial epicondyle)
  - Strongest passive medial stabilizer of patella

CLINICAL ISSUES

- Predisposing factors may be congenital or acquired
  - Patella: Alta, lateral subluxation/tilt, dysplasia
  - Trochlear dysplasia
  - Lateralization of tibial tubercle
  - Deficient/absent soft tissue medial stabilizers
  - Generalized ligamentous laxity (e.g., Ehlers-Danlos or Marfan syndrome)

DIAGNOSTIC CHECKLIST

- Radiographic axial patellar view: Evaluate for small fragments & patellar articular surface integrity
- MR: Diagnosis (if unsuspected) + characterization of injuries
  - Patellar & lateral femoral condylar articular cartilage injuries ± osteochondral/chondral intraarticular bodies
  - MPFL tears (must evaluate entirety of MPFL)

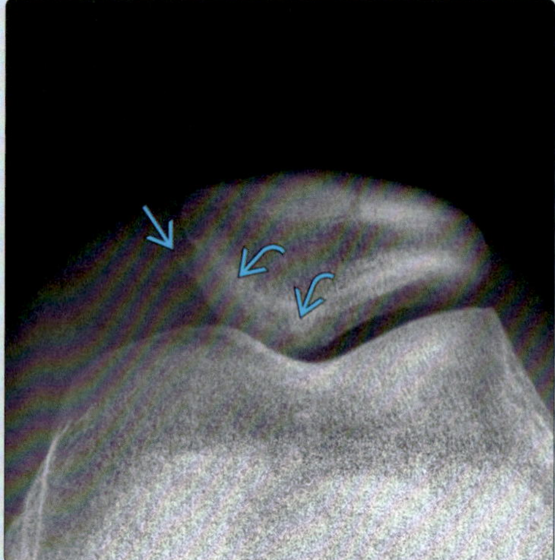
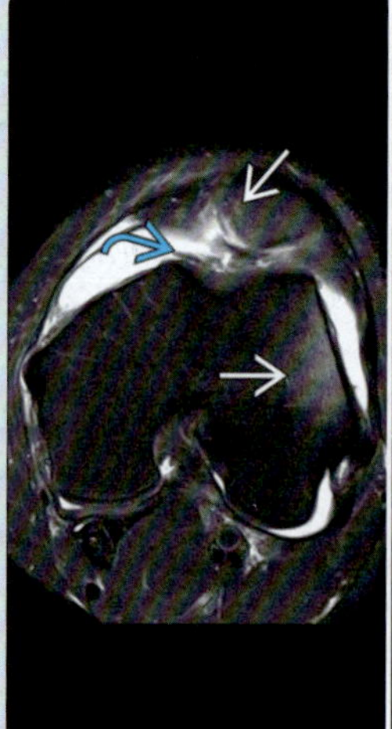
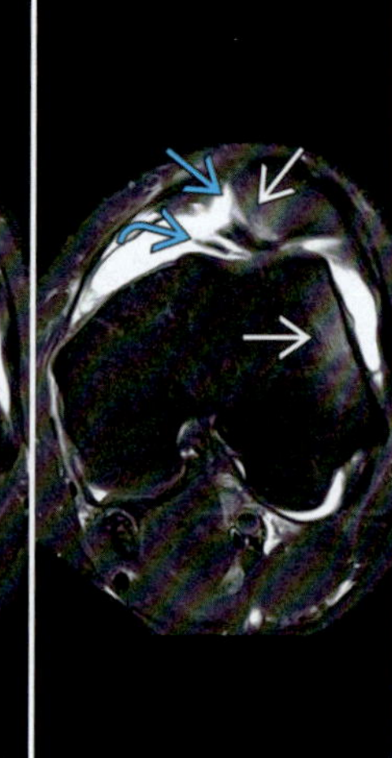

(Left) *Axial radiograph of the patella in a 16-year-old boy with a recent transient patellar dislocation (TPD) shows an osseous fragment ➡ adjacent to the medial patella with irregularity ➡ of the entire medial facet.* **(Right)** *Axial T2 FS MR (superior on the left, inferior on the right) in the same patient shows bone contusions ➡ of the lateral femoral condyle & medial patella. There is also full-thickness articular cartilage loss of the medial patellar facet ➡ with an associated intraarticular osteochondral body ➡.*

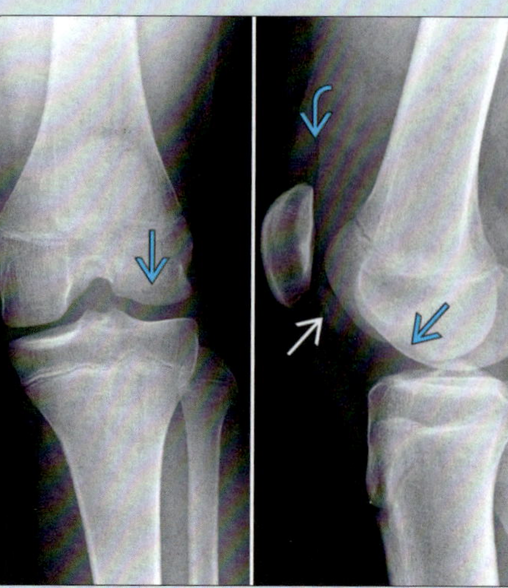
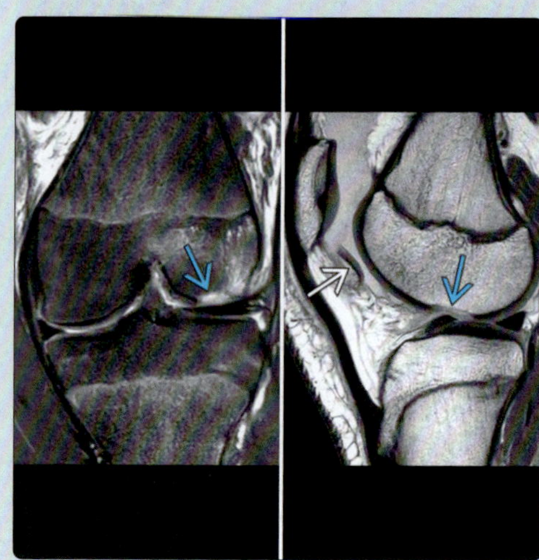

(Left) *Frontal & lateral radiographs in a 14-year-old boy with a recent TPD show a large osseous fragment in the anterior knee joint ➡ with an associated lucency in the lateral femoral condyle ➡. A lipohemarthrosis is also present ➡.* **(Right)** *Coronal T2 FS (left) & sagittal PD (right) MR images in the same boy confirm a displaced, rotated osteochondral fracture fragment ➡ in the anterior aspect of the joint with a donor site ➡ at the lateral femoral condyle.*

TERMINOLOGY

Abbreviations

- Transient patellar dislocation (TPD)

Definitions

- Lateral dislocation of patella from direct/indirect injury
- Dislocation/relocation → shearing, tensile, & compressive forces → injuries of medial patella, lateral femur, & soft tissues

IMAGING

General Features

- Best diagnostic clue
  - Radiographs
    - Large hemarthrosis
    - Patellar or femoral osseous/osteochondral fragments
  - MR
    - Medial patella & lateral femoral condyle contusions
    - Patellar & femoral osteochondral injuries
    - Medial patellofemoral ligament (MPFL) tear
- Morphology
  - Predisposing anatomic abnormalities of knee
    - Trochlear dysplasia, lateral patellar subluxation/tilt, patella alta, & tibial tubercle lateralization
  - MPFL is normally dark, linear, oblique band extending from medial distal femur to superior 2/3 of patella

Radiographic Findings

- Large joint effusion after acute TPD
- Osseous fragments
  - Medial patellar osseous avulsion (at MPFL attachment)
  - Patellar & femoral osteochondral fracture fragments from dislocation/relocation
- Importance of axial view of patella (e.g., Merchant, sunrise)
  - Avulsion & osteochondral fragments at medial patella
  - Patellar articular surface irregularities
  - Medial soft tissue swelling
- Patella typically relocates prior to radiographs

MR Findings

- T1WI
  - Bone contusions: Poorly defined ↓ marrow signal in medial patella & lateral femoral condyle
- T2WI FS
  - Bone contusions: Poorly defined ↑ marrow signal in medial patella & lateral femoral condyle
  - MPFL injury can occur at femoral or patellar attachments, midsubstance, or multiple sites
    - Grade 1/sprain: ↑ signal about ligament
    - Grade 2/partial tear: Intrasubstance ↑ signal, partial fiber discontinuity
    - Grade 3/complete tear: Complete fiber discontinuity
    - Chronic tears
      - Focal or diffuse attenuation of MPFL
  - Vastus medialis obliquus (VMO) muscle tears
  - Chondral abnormalities
    - Cartilage injury: Range from softening (↑ signal but normal morphology) to partial- or full-thickness defects
    - Osteochondral fractures
    - Displaced chondral & osteochondral fragments → intraarticular bodies
      - Often laminar in appearance from layered structure of cartilage & subchondral bone
  - Joint effusion
    - Hemarthrosis may be evident with hematocrit layer
    - Lipohemarthrosis is seen with osteochondral fractures
- Patella alta
  - Traditionally defined on radiographs
    - Insall-Salvati index = patellar tendon length (TL)/patella length (PL) → > 1.2 considered patella alta
  - Proposed MR criteria
    - Measured on single midsagittal image
    - Length of inner patellar tendon (TL)/anteroinferior to posterosuperior edge of patella (PL)
    - Ratios change during range of skeletal maturity
      - Values not definitively established in children
      - Some authors propose MR ratio > 1.3 in children
- Trochlear dysplasia
  - Lateral trochlear inclination (of femur)
    - Shallow lateral inclination predisposes to TPD
    - Angle between lines along subchondral bone of lateral trochlea & posterior aspect of femoral condyles on axial image
    - Inclination angle < 11° = trochlear dysplasia
  - Trochlear facet asymmetry (of femur)
    - On axial image 3 cm above tibiofemoral joint, ratio of length of medial facet:lateral facet x 100%
    - Facet ratio < 40% = trochlear dysplasia
  - Trochlear depth (of femur)
    - Measured on axial image 3 cm above knee joint
    - Reference line drawn along posterior femoral condyles
    - AP measurements are made perpendicular to posterior condylar line for largest AP dimensions of medial (A) & lateral (B) trochlear facets & deepest trochlear sulcus (C)
    - Trochlear depth = [(A+B)/2] - C
    - Trochlear depth ≤ 3 mm = trochlear dysplasia
- Tibial tubercle to trochlear groove (TT-TG) distance
  - Transverse distance from anterior-most osseous tibial tubercle to trochlear groove (deepest osseous portion)
    - Measurement of lateral offset of extensor mechanism
  - Mark anterior-most tibial tubercle on inferior image
  - Scroll to superior slice with deepest trochlea & mark position of tibial tubercle on this image
    - Posterior condylar line is drawn on this axial slice
  - Line perpendicular to posterior condylar line is drawn between marks for
    - Deepest portion of osseous trochlea
    - Position of tibial tubercle
  - Distance between these lines = TT-TG distance
  - TT-TG distance varies with age; general guideline
    - Normal < 15 mm, borderline 15-20 mm, abnormal > 20 mm
- Patellar tendon to trochlear groove (PT-TG) distance
  - Measurement of lateral offset of extensor mechanism developed specifically on MR, where soft tissue & cartilage landmarks can be seen
  - Similar but not equivalent to TT-TG distance

- Center of patellar tendon (PT) (on superior-most axial slice of tibial attachment) is used as distal landmark rather than tibial tubercle
- Deepest portion of cartilaginous (vs. osseous) trochlea is used as proximal landmark for TG location
- PT-TG vs. TT-TG distances may differ ≥ 4 mm in same individual
- PT-TG distance has better inter- & intraobserver reliability

- Postoperative: MPFL reconstructions
  - Normal graft: Low signal intensity with intact fibers
    - Continuous, taut, & oriented as native MPFL
  - Graft tear: Intrasubstance ↑ signal on T2 FS MR + partial or complete disruption of fibers

DIFFERENTIAL DIAGNOSIS

Dorsal Patellar Defect

- Well-defined lucent lesion in superolateral aspect of patella
- Location & appearance distinguish from fracture

Bipartite/Multipartite Patella

- Typical fragmentation at superolateral aspect of patella
- Location & appearance distinguish from fracture

PATHOLOGY

Gross Pathologic & Surgical Features

- Condensations of medial patellar retinaculum form complex of medial patellar retinacular ligaments
  - MPFL is most important
    - Strongest passive medial stabilizer of patella
      - Considerable variation in size & thickness of MPFL in normal individuals
    - Contributes up to 60% of medial restraining force on patella
    - Broader patellar attachment: Superomedial patella deep to fibers of VMO, creating bilaminar appearance on axial MR images
    - Narrower femoral attachment: Most often described between adductor tubercle & medial epicondyle on anatomic studies
  - Other condensations of medial patellar retinaculum include: Medial patellotibial ligament & medial patellomeniscal ligament
    - Growing realization of importance of medial patellotibial ligament for patellar tracking

CLINICAL ISSUES

Presentation

- Most common signs/symptoms
  - Knee giving way, swelling, tenderness along medial retinaculum, sensation of impending dislocation with manual pressure upon patella
  - Patellar dislocation is clinically occult in 45-73% of cases
    - Due to transient nature of process, patients are frequently unaware that patella has dislocated
- Clinical profile
  - May occur from direct or indirect injuries
  - Persons who dislocate with less forceful injuries typically have more predisposing factors
  - Predisposing factors may be congenital or acquired
    - Osseous factors
      - Patella: Alta, lateral subluxation/tilt, dysplasia
      - Trochlear dysplasia: ↓ depth, ↓ lateral inclination
      - Lateralization of tibial tubercle
    - Soft tissue factors
      - Deficiency/absence of medial retinacular complex
      - Hypoplasia of vastus medialis muscle
      - Tight lateral retinaculum
      - Generalized ligamentous laxity (e.g., Ehlers-Danlos or Marfan syndrome)
  - True congenital dislocation is rare & frequently associated with syndromes

Demographics

- Epidemiology
  - Overall incidence of 1st-time TPD = 5.8/100,000
  - In 10- to 17-year-olds, incidence ↑ to 29/100,000

Natural History & Prognosis

- After single episode of TPD
  - 50% of patients have persistent anterior knee pain
  - 15-40% have recurrent TPD (after conservative management of initial episode)
- After 2nd TPD, chance of recurrence ↑ to 50%
- Recurrent dislocations ↑ risk for persistent symptoms & degenerative changes

Treatment

- Treatment of acute TPD is controversial
- Conservative management is considered if
  - No osteochondral injury
  - Patella is stable on clinical exam
  - No more than partial injury to medial patellar stabilizers
- Conservative management
  - Patellar-stabilizing orthotic & early mobilization
  - Physical therapy to strengthen medial patellar stabilizers
- Surgical management is indicated for
  - 1st-time TPD with intraarticular bodies or major tear of medial stabilizers
  - Recurrent TPD
- Surgical procedures (performed alone or in combination)
  - Lateral retinacular release
  - MPFL repair or reconstruction
    - Reconstruction: Single or double graft fixed to medial distal femur & medial patella
  - Growing interest in medial patellotibial ligament reconstruction (with MPFL reconstruction)
  - Distal realignment procedure
    - Tibial tubercle repositioning medial &/or distal

SELECTED REFERENCES

1. Grantham WJ et al: Medial patellotibial ligament reconstruction improves patella tracking when combined with medial patellofemoral reconstruction: an in vitro kinematic study. Arthroscopy. 36(9):2501-9, 2020
2. Tanaka MJ et al: Recognition of evolving medial patellofemoral anatomy provides insight for reconstruction. Knee Surg Sports Traumatol Arthrosc. 27(8):2537-50, 2019
3. Zhang GY et al: Injury patterns of medial patellofemoral ligament after acute lateral patellar dislocation in children: correlation analysis with anatomical variants and articular cartilage lesion of the patella. Eur Radiol. 27(3):1322-30, 2017
4. Meyers AB et al: Imaging assessment of patellar instability and its treatment in children and adolescents. Pediatr Radiol. 46(5):618-36, 2016

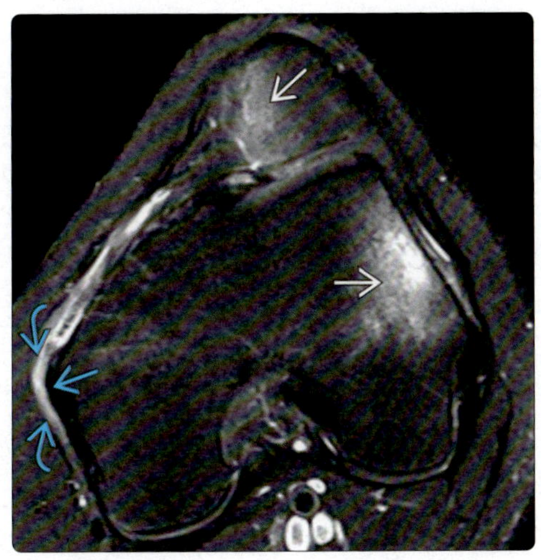

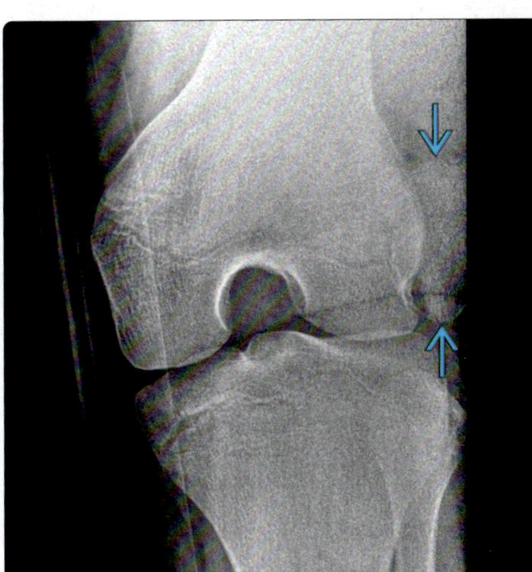

(Left) *Axial T2 FS MR in a 17-year-old boy with a recent TPD shows medial patella & lateral femoral condyle bone contusions ➡. There is ↑ signal at the MPFL femoral attachment ➡ with complete disruption of the fibers. Note the normal MCL attachment ➡ deep to the torn MPFL.* **(Right)** *Tunnel radiograph in a 12-year-old girl who was splinted immediately after a knee injury shows lateral dislocation of the patella ➡. Typically, the patella reduces spontaneously with knee extension prior to radiographic evaluation.*

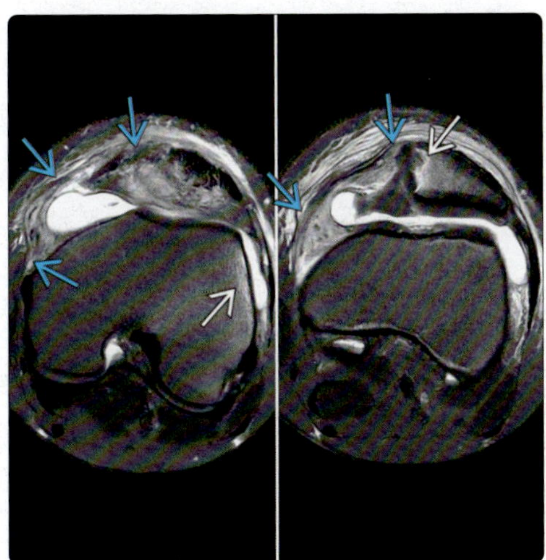

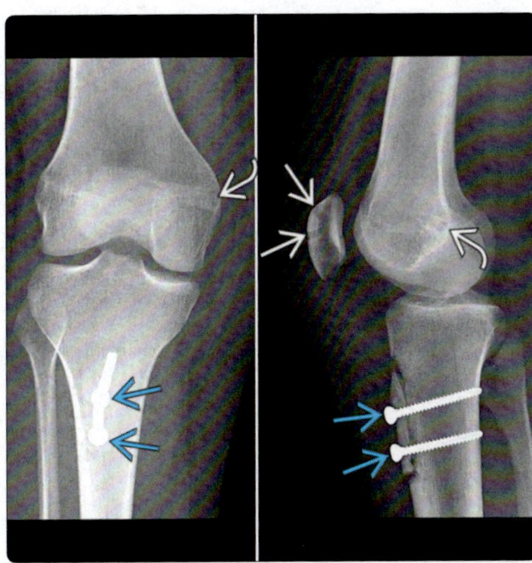

(Left) *Axial T2 FS MR (inferior on the left, superior on the right) in the same girl shows bone contusions ➡ in the lateral femoral condyle & medial patella with tearing of the MPFL throughout its course ➡.* **(Right)** *AP & lateral radiographs in a 15-year-old girl with prior patellar dislocations show findings of MPFL reconstruction & tibial tubercle repositioning. The MPFL graft loops through a patellar tunnel ➡ & is fixed to the medial femur with an interference screw ➡. Two screws ➡ fix the medially repositioned tibial tubercle.*

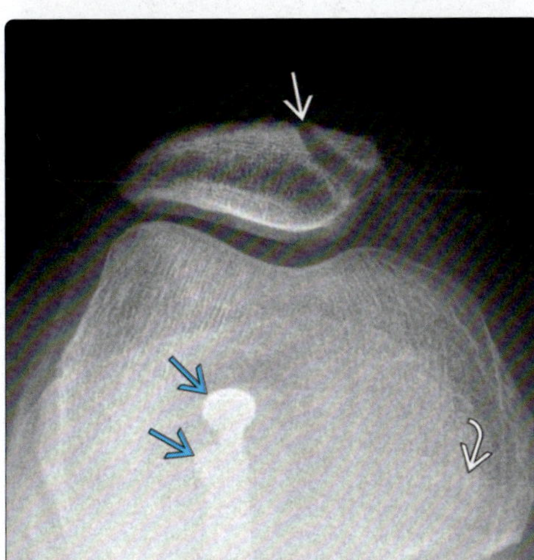

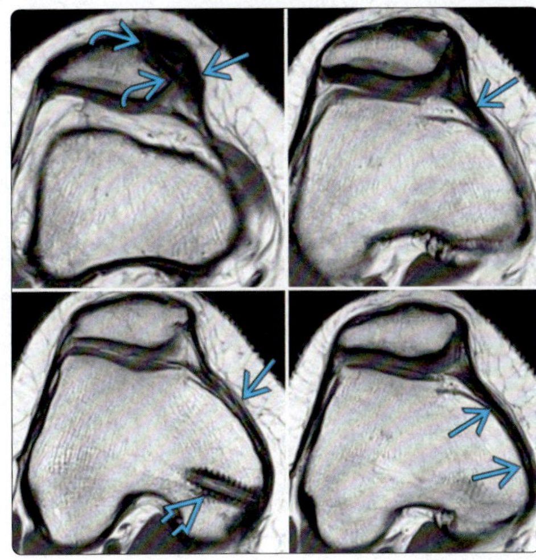

(Left) *Axial radiograph in the same girl shows the patellar tunnel ➡ through which the MPFL graft is looped. The femoral interference screw ➡ & tibial tubercle screws ➡ are also seen.* **(Right)** *Axial PD MR (clockwise superior to inferior from the upper left) in the same patient shows the MPFL graft within the patellar tunnel ➡ extending posteriorly ➡ in an oblique course (similar to the native MPFL). The graft has normal low signal intensity & is fixed in a femoral tunnel with an interference screw ➡.*

KEY FACTS

TERMINOLOGY

- Avulsion injury of patellar pole in skeletally immature
- Small bone fragment & larger sleeve of unossified "epiphyseal" cartilage are avulsed from patella at
  - Inferior pole by patellar tendon (more common)
  - Superior pole by quadriceps tendon (less common)
- **Not** periosteal sleeve avulsion (as patella has no periosteum)

IMAGING

- Radiographs
  - Inferior pole: Small, ossific fragment is displaced distally from irregular inferior pole, ± patella alta
  - Superior pole: Small, ossific fragment is retracted proximally from irregular superior pole, ± patella baja
  - Either site: Lax quadriceps &/or patellar tendons, soft tissue swelling, ± joint effusion
  - Extent of patellar injury & degree of fragment displacement are underestimated by radiographs alone
- Ultrasound & MR reveal larger sleeve of unossified cartilage surrounding displaced bony fragment
  - With minimal displacement, fluid signal intensity in fracture cleft stands out against darker unossified "epiphyseal" cartilage on fluid-sensitive MR sequences

TOP DIFFERENTIAL DIAGNOSES

- Normal variant ossification
- Sinding-Larsen-Johansson syndrome
- Tibial tubercle avulsion
- Isolated tendon rupture

CLINICAL ISSUES

- Peak incidence: 12-13 years; range: 8-16 years
- Sudden pain with "explosive force" (such as jumping) or fall
- Clinical findings: Swelling, extensor lag, palpable defect
- Treatment: Restore extensor mechanism function
  - Immobilization if minimally displaced (< 2-3 mm)
  - Open reduction, internal fixation is otherwise required

(Left) *Lateral radiograph in a 10-year-old girl after a fall shows ossific irregularity ➡ at the inferior pole of the high-riding patella (alta). The avulsed irregular ossific fragments ➡ remain attached to the proximal patellar tendon.* **(Right)** *Sagittal T2 FS MR in the same patient shows interruption of the low signal intensity unossified "epiphyseal" cartilage ➡ at the inferior pole of the superiorly retracted patella. An avulsed osteochondral sleeve ➡ remains attached to the patellar tendon ➡.*

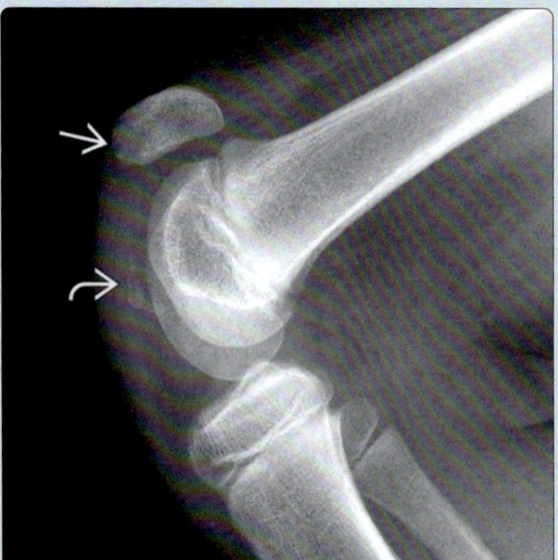

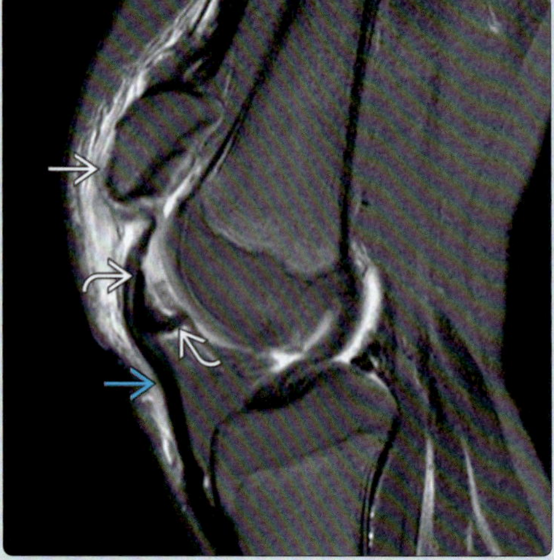

(Left) *Lateral radiograph of the right knee in a 10-year-old boy after a fall shows elevation of the patellar ossification center with irregularity of the inferior pole ➡. Several small, ossific fragments ➡ are retracted distally by the patellar tendon.* **(Right)** *Longitudinal ultrasound in the same patient confirms retraction of the osteocartilaginous fragments ➡ from the irregular inferior patellar pole ➡ by the patellar tendon ➡, consistent with a patellar sleeve avulsion fracture.*

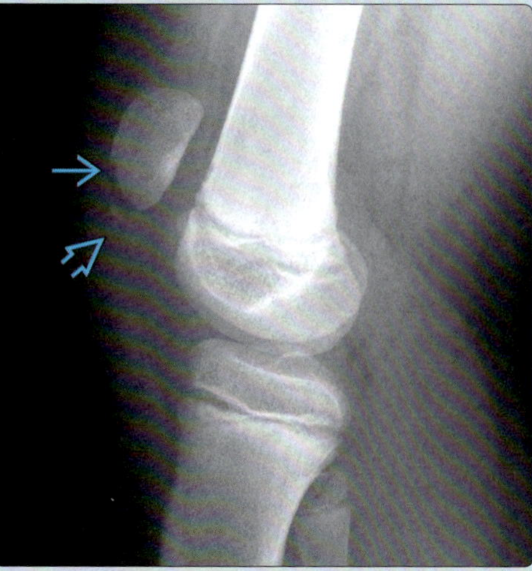

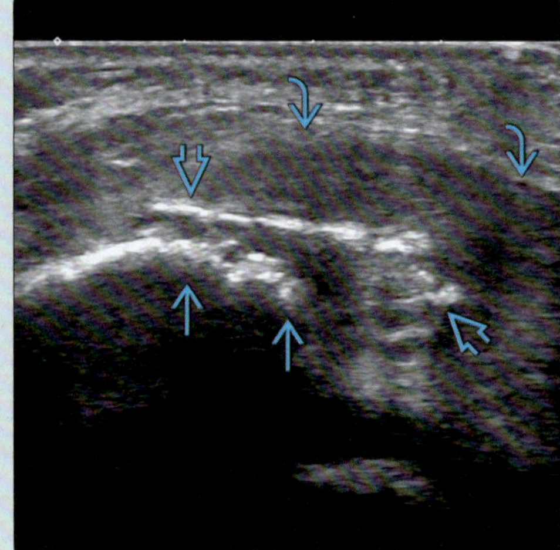

KEY FACTS

IMAGING

- Fragment of largely ossified but unfused anterior tibial tubercle is retracted proximally &/or rotated superiorly
- Many variables, including fragment size & shape, degree of comminution & displacement, pattern of extension
- Adjacent soft tissues may become entrapped

TOP DIFFERENTIAL DIAGNOSES

- Normal ossification variant
- Osgood-Schlatter disease
- Patellar sleeve avulsion fracture
- Patellar tendon rupture

PATHOLOGY

- Predisposing anatomy
  - Portion of physis deep to tibial tubercle ossification center is uniquely composed of strong fibrocartilage
  - As patient nears physeal closure, this growth plate converts to weaker hyaline cartilage
  - Timing coincides with ↑ muscle strength & athletic activity
- Prior Osgood-Schlatter disease in 25-31%
- Mechanisms include forceful quadriceps contraction with extension (i.e., jumping), passive knee flexion during quadriceps contraction (i.e., landing), or direct blow
- Associated injuries: Tears of patellar tendon, ACL, menisci
  - Anterior compartment syndrome in 2-20%

CLINICAL ISSUES

- Vast majority: Boys 11-17 years old
- Presentations include swelling, tenderness, knee held in flexion with inability to fully extend actively
- Nonoperative management for minimally displaced fractures limited to distal tibial tubercle
- Open reduction, internal fixation is otherwise required to
  - Restore extensor mechanism alignment
  - Establish congruence of articular surface of tibia

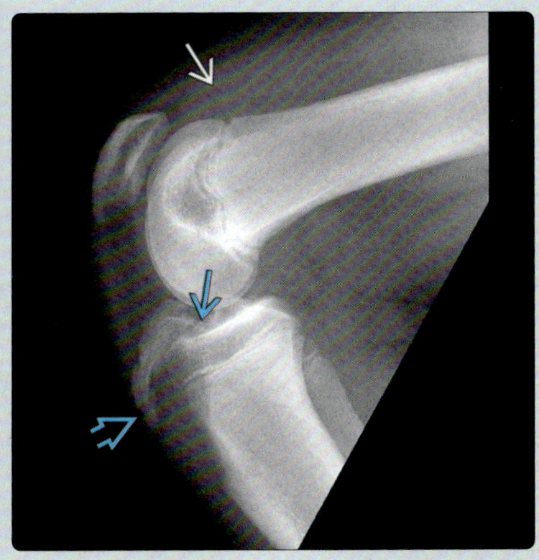

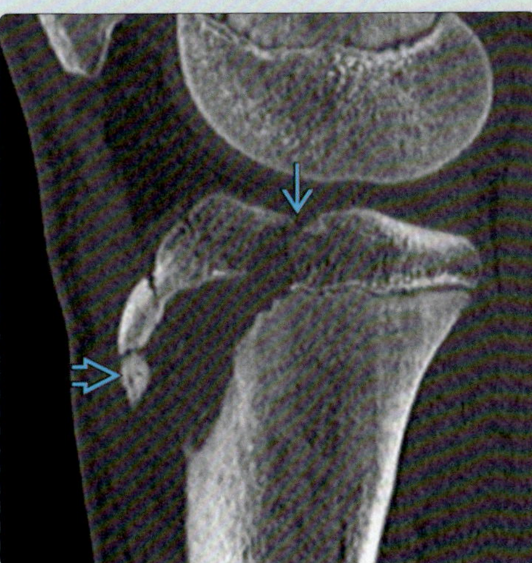

(Left) *Lateral radiograph in a 14-year-old boy after a jumping injury shows marked retraction & rotation of the avulsed tibial tubercle ⇨. There is intraarticular extension of the fracture plane ⇨ with a moderate joint effusion ➡. The findings are typical of an Ogden type III fracture.* **(Right)** *Sagittal bone CT in the same patient with a tibial tubercle avulsion ⇨ better demonstrates the degree of articular surface distraction ⇨ than radiographs.*

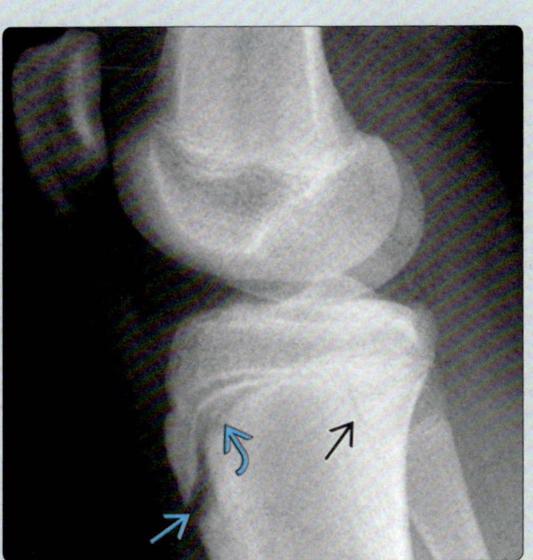

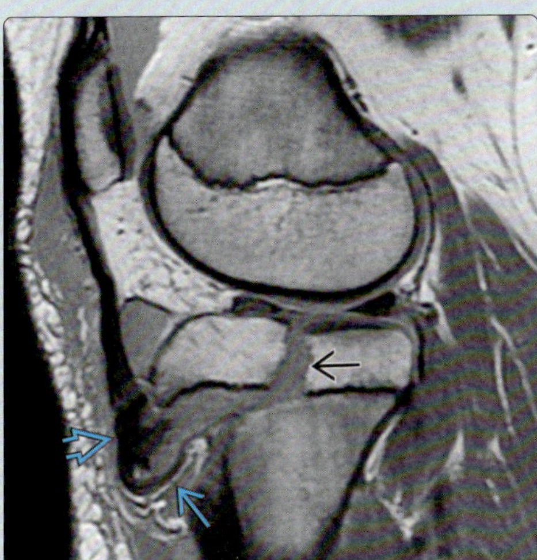

(Left) *Lateral knee radiograph in a 15-year-old boy after a fall shows mild widening & irregularity of the growth plate deep to the tibial tubercle ⇨ with posterior extension to the proximal tibial physis ⇨ & metaphysis ⇨ as a Salter-Harris II fracture (modified Ogden type IV).* **(Right)** *Sagittal PD MR in a 15-year-old boy after a fall shows avulsion of a tibial tubercle fragment ⇨. The fracture extends proximally with a Salter-Harris III configuration ⇨. Stripped distal periosteum ⇨ is entrapped in the fracture.*

Trampoline Fracture

KEY FACTS

TERMINOLOGY

- Proximal tibial impaction fracture seen in young children (2-5 years of age), incurred on bouncing surface

IMAGING

- Focal cortical buckling/convexity/disruption
  - More likely in younger child: Focal convexity is superimposed on normally smooth, concave proximal tibial metadiaphysis at site of unossified tibial tuberosity on lateral view
  - Exaggerates anterior tibial "scoop" (may be very subtle)
- Transverse/oblique fracture lucency may extend to physis
  - Salter-Harris II fracture in ~ 11%
  - More likely in older child
- Anterior tilt of proximal tibial physis
- May be initially occult → healing on follow-up in 7-10 days

PATHOLOGY

- Hyperextension injury & axial loading on bouncing surface
  - Often occurs when bouncing with larger individual
    - Recoil of mat as larger individual goes up, impacts foot of child coming down
  - ↑ risk with multiple bouncers
  - Surface: Trampoline >> inflatable bouncer > bed

CLINICAL ISSUES

- Beware of misleading history: Direct impact or fall is often reported, but fall typically occurs after fracture
- ↑ incidence in recent decades due to home trampolines & indoor trampoline parks
- Generally good outcomes with immobilization for 4-6 weeks
- Risk of late valgus deformity with proximal tibial fractures (Cozen phenomenon)
  - Valgus overgrowth over course of up to 18-24 months
  - Usually spontaneously resolves
  - Recent evidence suggests relatively low-impact, nondisplaced trampoline fracture may not be at risk

(Left) *Lateral radiograph of the knee in a 3-year-old with pain after jumping on a trampoline shows buckling of the anterior proximal tibia ➡, consistent with a nondisplaced trampoline fracture. The anterior proximal tibia normally has a smooth, concave contour at this age.* **(Right)** *Lateral knee radiograph in a 2-year-old after a trampoline injury demonstrates cortical buckling in the anterior proximal tibia ➡, exaggerating the normal anterior tibial "scoop" ⇨. There is also adjacent soft tissue swelling.*

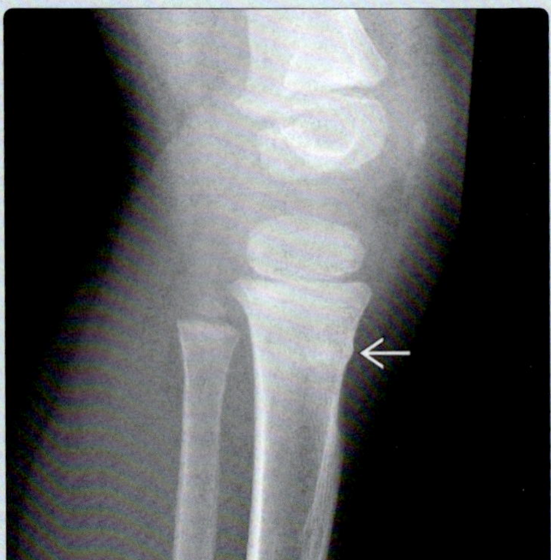

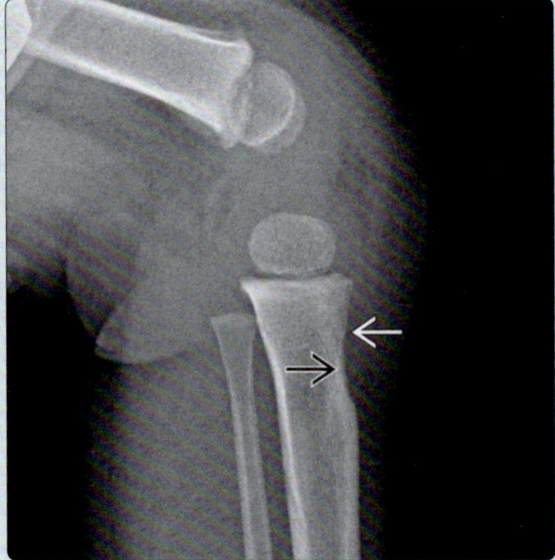

(Left) *AP & lateral radiographs of the knee in a 4-year-old with leg pain after jumping on a trampoline with their father show irregular contour of the anterior proximal tibia ➡. A subtle oblique fracture lucency ⇨ is also seen with extension toward the physis.* **(Right)** *Follow-up radiographs in the same patient 4 weeks after the injury demonstrate healing with sclerosis along the fracture plane ⇨. Extension to the physis is evident.*

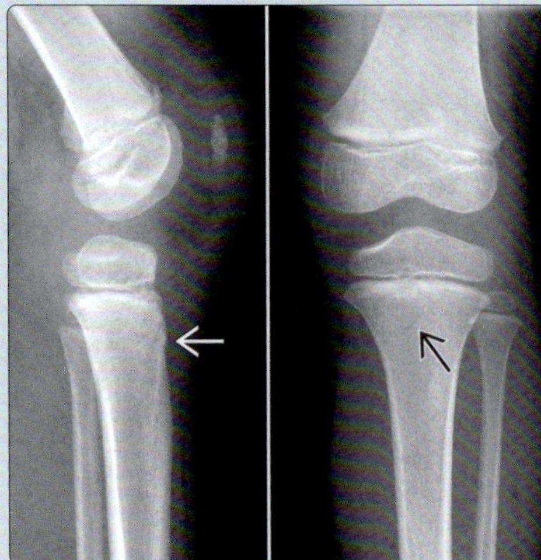

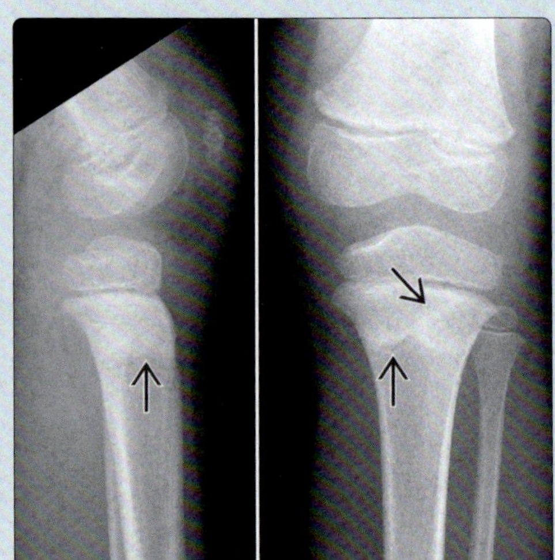

Toddler's Fracture

KEY FACTS

TERMINOLOGY

- Toddler's fracture: Nondisplaced spiral fracture of tibial diaphysis in newly ambulatory child
- Synonym: Childhood accidental spiral tibial (CAST) fracture
- "Toddler's fracture" is sometimes applied to other low-energy lower extremity fractures in young child (such as cuboid)

IMAGING

- Spiral or oblique fracture of mid/distal tibial diaphysis ± metaphysis
  - Fibula is intact
- Nondisplaced or minimally displaced
- May be best seen on oblique view
- Radiographically occult in up to 39%
  - Follow-up radiographs show healing change
- Ultrasound: Cortical disruption, hypoechoic subperiosteal hematoma

PATHOLOGY

- Axial loading &/or torsional forces
- Typically from low-energy injury, often goes unrecognized
  - Fall or twisting while walking
  - Also described with foot caught on slide, especially when riding on adult's lap

CLINICAL ISSUES

- Ambulatory child 9 months to 4 years of age
- Presentation: Refusal to bear weight, limp
- Isolated toddler's fracture in ambulatory child should not raise concern for child abuse
  - Lack of known injury is common
- Treatment: Immobilization with cast (short vs. long leg), walking boot, or long leg splint
  - Symptomatic follow-up without radiographs may be sufficient
  - Presumptive treatment is employed for high clinical suspicion despite negative radiographs

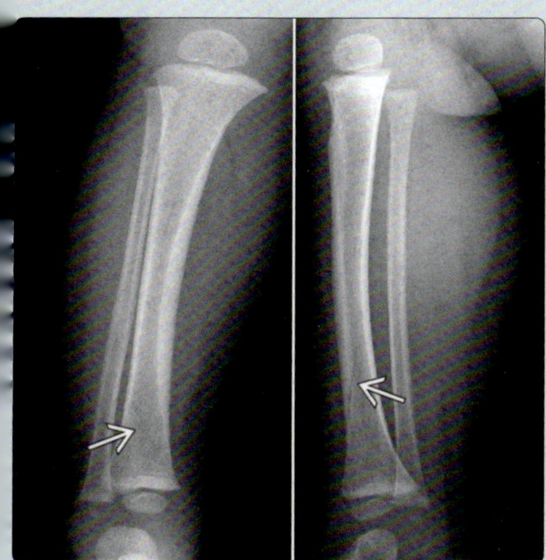

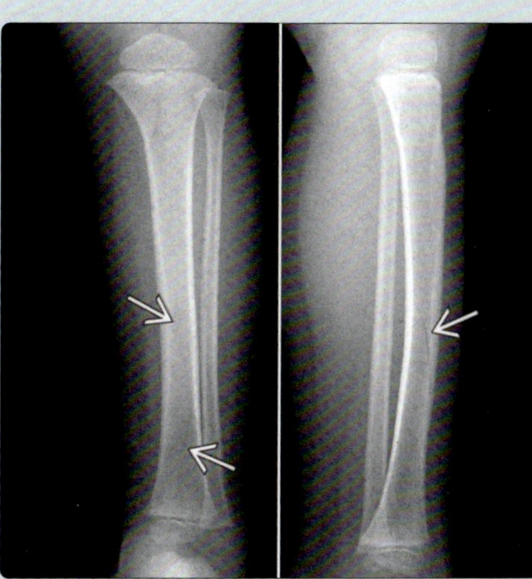

(Left) *AP & lateral radiographs of the tibia & fibula in a 20-month-old with pain after a fall while walking show a thin lucency ➡ in the distal tibial diaphysis, consistent with a nondisplaced spiral fracture. Mild overlying soft tissue swelling is seen in this child but is not reliably present.* **(Right)** *AP & lateral radiographs in a 2-year-old with pain after a twisting injury on a playground slide show a nondisplaced spiral fracture of the mid & distal tibial diaphysis ➡.*

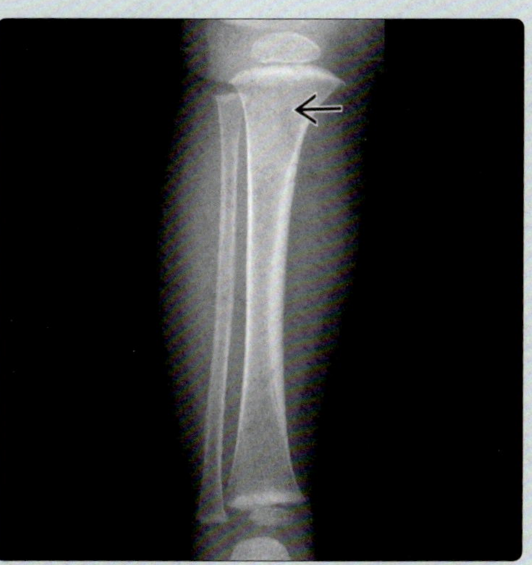

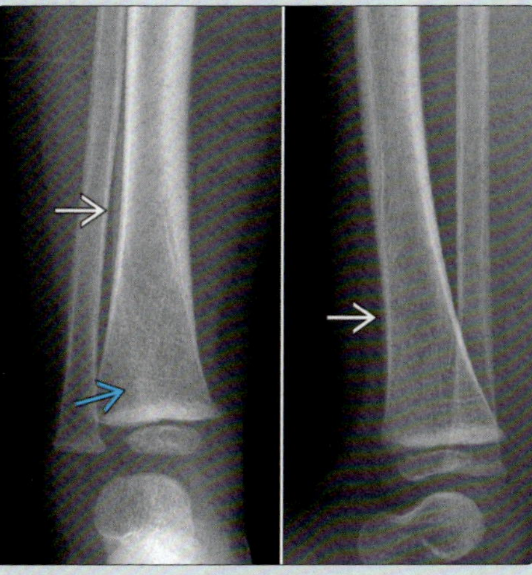

(Left) *Frontal radiograph in a 16-month-old after a fall does not demonstrate a visible fracture line. Normal structures that may mimic a fracture line include superimposed intermuscular fat planes ➡ & nutrient canals.* **(Right)** *Follow-up radiographs in the same patient 14 days later show healing with periosteal reaction ➡ & sclerosis ➡. Oblique views may be used to improve sensitivity if initial radiographs are negative in the setting of high clinical suspicion.*

Triplane Fracture

KEY FACTS

IMAGING

- Distal tibial fracture in 3 planes; may be true Salter-Harris IV (SH IV) or combinations of SH II & III
- Classic triplane fracture pattern
  - Oblique coronal fracture plane through posterior distal tibial metaphysis & diaphysis
  - Transverse fracture plane through physis (growth plate)
  - Sagittal fracture plane through epiphysis
    - Extension to tibial plafond (intraarticular) vs. medial malleolus (intra- or extraarticular)
- Oblique coronal plane of metaphysis/diaphysis may be hidden on lateral radiograph if nondisplaced & overlapping tibial-fibular interface
- CT is more accurate for determining course & comminution of fracture, amount of displacement, articular surface involvement, & presence of free intraarticular fragments

PATHOLOGY

- Triplane fracture occurs around time of earliest physeal closure, which has unique pattern in distal tibia
  - Earliest fusion at anteromedial tibial physis (Kump bump)
  - Affects planes of fracture extension
- Rapariz triplane fracture classification: Variations of 2-, 3-, or 4-part fractures for 6 possible subtypes

CLINICAL ISSUES

- 5-10% of pediatric intraarticular ankle fractures
- Typically affects adolescents within 18 months of tibial growth plate closure (12-15 years old)
- Nonoperative treatment
  - ≤ 2 mm of displacement
  - Extraarticular fractures
- Operative treatment
  - > 2 mm of articular step-off or distraction
- Complications: Growth arrest, pain, degenerative joint changes

(Left) *AP radiograph shows a triplane fracture ➡ with extension through the tibial epiphysis into the joint space & along the lateral physis. A tiny posterior metaphyseal fragment was also present (not shown).* **(Right)** *Sagittal bone CT in a 2-part triplane fracture shows a widened oblique coronal fracture plane along the posterior tibial metaphysis with extension across the anterior physis, creating a single posterolateral fragment ➡.*

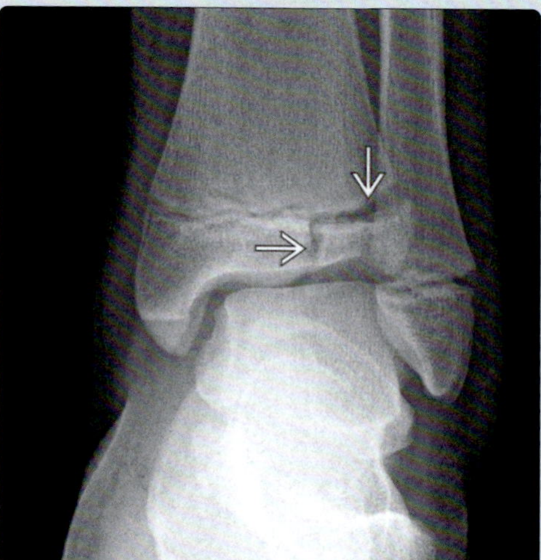

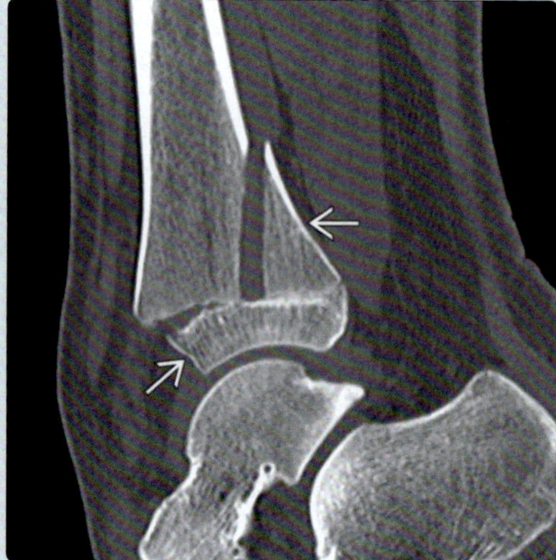

(Left) *Axial bone CT in a 15-year-old shows the predominantly sagittal fracture plane through the distal tibial epiphysis. In many cases, this plane allows the most accurate assessment of the articular surface distraction ➡, which is a key determinant for treating with a closed vs. open reduction.* **(Right)** *Coronal bone CT in a 13-year-old who sustained an ankle injury after falling from a scooter shows an extraarticular intramalleolar triplane fracture variant ➡.*

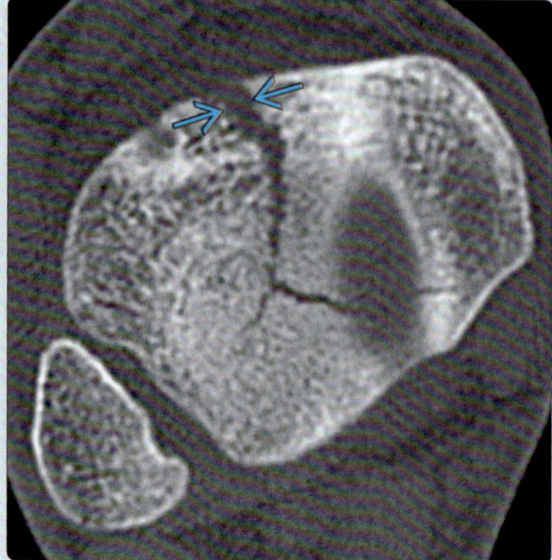

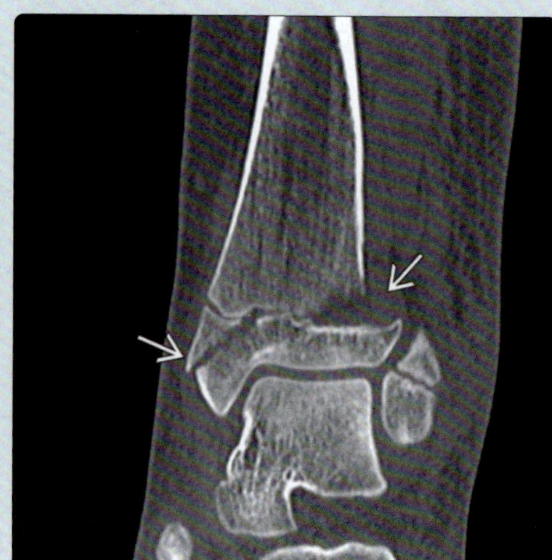

TERMINOLOGY

Synonyms

- Adolescent triplane fracture, transitional injury

IMAGING

General Features

- Best diagnostic clue
  - Complex fracture of adolescent distal tibia involving metaphysis, physis, & epiphysis
    - Fracture components in transverse, sagittal, & coronal planes
- Location
  - Classic triplane fracture pattern
    - Coronal fracture plane through posterior distal tibial metaphysis & diaphysis
    - Transverse fracture plane through physis (growth plate)
    - Sagittal fracture plane through epiphysis
      - Extension to tibial plafond (intraarticular) vs. medial malleolus (intra- or extraarticular)
- Morphology
  - Distal tibial growth plate closes in predictable unique pattern: Begins in anteromedial tibial physis at Kump bump
    - Injury at time of early closure affects planes of fracture extension

Radiographic Findings

- Distal tibial fracture in 3 planes; may be true Salter-Harris IV (SH IV) or combinations of SH II & III
  - Oblique coronal plane of metaphysis/diaphysis may be hidden on lateral view if it is nondisplaced & overlaps tibial-fibular interface
- Fibular fracture in 50%
- Soft tissue swelling & joint effusion

CT Findings

- Bone CT
  - Axial with sagittal & coronal reformations, ± 3D
  - More accurate than radiographs for determining course & comminution of fracture, amount of displacement, articular surface involvement, & presence of free intraarticular fragments
  - Axial fracture line may be helpful in determining optimal screw orientation for reduction

PATHOLOGY

General Features

- Mechanism: External rotation

Staging, Grading, & Classification

- Rapariz triplane fracture classification: Variations of 2-, 3-, or 4-part fractures for 6 possible subtypes
  - 2-part fracture: Most common
    - True SH IV fracture
    - Either medial or lateral
  - 3-part fracture: Combination of fractures: SH II (AP view) & SH III (lateral view)
    - ± separation at Kump bump
  - 4-part fracture: Combinations of above
- 2- or 3-part intramalleolar variant
  - Depending on fracture line extension, fracture may be intra- or extraarticular
    - Type I: Intraarticular at junction of medial malleolus & tibial plafond
    - Type II: Intraarticular outside weight-bearing zone of plafond
    - Type III: Extraarticular

CLINICAL ISSUES

Presentation

- Most common signs/symptoms
  - Pain
  - Swelling
  - Inability to bear weight
- Other signs/symptoms
  - Bruising
  - Associated fibular fracture in ~ 50% of patients

Demographics

- Age
  - Adolescent within 18 months of tibial growth plate closure
    - 12-15 years old
      - Males: 15-16 years old
      - Females: 13-14 years old
  - 2-part triplane fractures occur in younger children than 3-part triplane fractures
- Sex
  - M > F
- Epidemiology
  - 5-10% of pediatric intraarticular ankle fractures

Treatment

- Nonoperative treatment
  - ≤ 2 mm of displacement or extraarticular
  - Most 2-part fractures
  - Closed reduction with internal rotation of foot
    - Immobilization & long leg cast
- Operative treatment
  - > 2 mm of articular surface distraction or step-off
  - Most 3-part fractures
  - Internal fixation with screws, percutaneous K-wires

SELECTED REFERENCES

1. Gaudiani MA et al: Clinical outcomes of triplane fractures based on imaging modality utilization and management: a systematic review and meta-analysis. J Pediatr Orthop. 40(10):e936-41, 2020
2. Lurie B et al: Functional outcomes of Tillaux and triplane fractures with 2 to 5 millimeters of intra-articular gap. J Bone Joint Surg Am. 102(8):679-86, 2020
3. Mishra N et al: Comparison of K-wire versus screw fixation after open reduction of transitional (Tillaux and triplane) distal tibia fractures. J Pediatr Orthop B. 30(5):443-9, 2020
4. Hadad MJ et al: Surgically relevant patterns in triplane fractures: a mapping study. J Bone Joint Surg Am. 100(12):1039-46, 2018
5. Eismann EA et al: Pediatric triplane ankle fractures: impact of radiographs and computed tomography on fracture classification and treatment planning. J Bone Joint Surg Am. 97(12):995-1002, 2015
6. Choudhry IK et al: Functional outcome analysis of triplane and tillaux fractures after closed reduction and percutaneous fixation. J Pediatr Orthop. 34(2):139-43, 2014
7. Blackburn EW et al: Ankle fractures in children. J Bone Joint Surg Am. 94(13):1234-44, 2012
8. Kim JR et al: Treatment outcomes of triplane and Tillaux fractures of the ankle in adolescence. Clin Orthop Surg. 2(1):34-8, 2010

Juvenile Tillaux Fracture

KEY FACTS

IMAGING

- Salter-Harris III fracture of anterolateral distal tibial physis & epiphysis
  - Sagittal fracture component extending through epiphysis to tibiotalar joint
  - Widening of physis anterolaterally
- Occurs after fusion of central & medial physis but before anterolateral physis closes
  - Avulsion of anterolateral tibial epiphyseal fragment by anterior inferior tibiofibular ligament
  - Ligament usually remains intact
- Radiographs are typically diagnostic
  - Often best seen on mortise view
- CT is obtained to assess articular surface distraction (> 2 mm necessitates operative fixation)
  - Reformatted images in 3 planes are essential to fully characterize fracture

CLINICAL ISSUES

- 3-5% of pediatric ankle fractures
- Affects adolescents < 18 months from complete distal tibial growth plate closure
  - Age range: 12-15 years old
  - Median age: 12 years in females, 14 years in males
- Nonoperative treatment with fracture displacement < 2 mm
- Internal fixation with screws & K-wires for articular surface fracture displacement > 2 mm
  - Anatomic reduction at articular surface is required to restore joint function, prevent premature degeneration
- Subsequent growth disturbance is rare as majority of physis has already closed

DIAGNOSTIC CHECKLIST

- Differentiate from triplane fracture
  - Salter-Harris IV fracture with coronal metadiaphyseal fracture plane

(Left) *AP radiograph of the right ankle in a 13-year-old patient after a trampoline injury shows a Salter-Harris III fracture of the distal tibia. The fracture extends horizontally through the lateral physis ➩ & vertically through the epiphysis ➩ to the articular surface, typical of a juvenile Tillaux fracture.* **(Right)** *Coronal bone CT in the same patient demonstrates the physeal ➩ & epiphyseal ➩ fracture planes. The tibial articular surface gap is > 2 mm, requiring surgical fixation.*

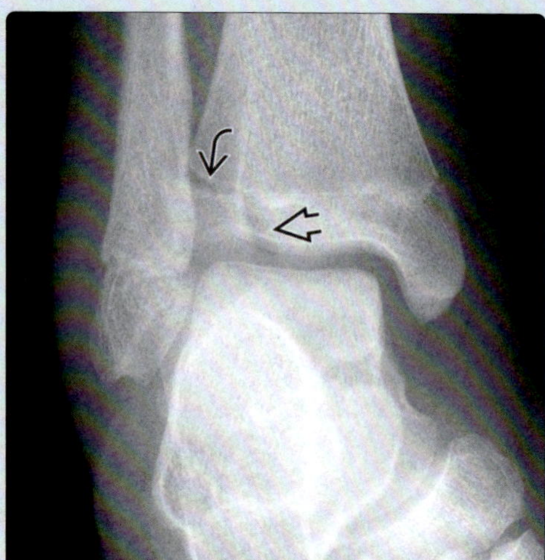

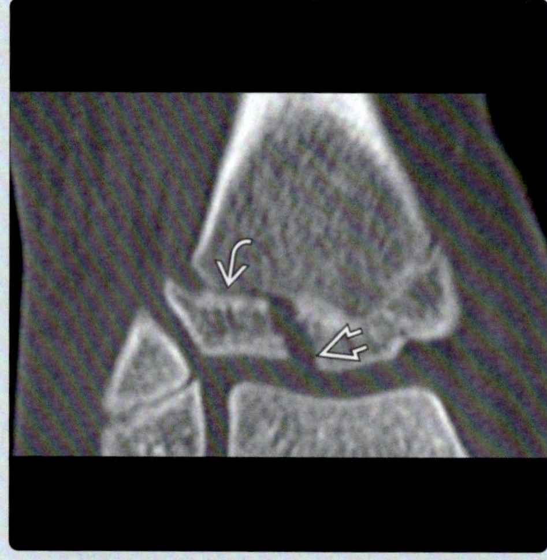

(Left) *Axial bone CT in the same patient shows distraction & rotation of the anterolateral epiphyseal fracture fragment ➩. This displacement is due to traction from the anterior inferior tibiofibular ligament.* **(Right)** *AP radiograph of the ankle in a 12-year-old girl after a fall shows the sagittal epiphyseal component ➩ of this juvenile Tillaux fracture. With only 1 mm of displacement at the articular surface, this fracture was successfully managed with closed reduction & casting.*

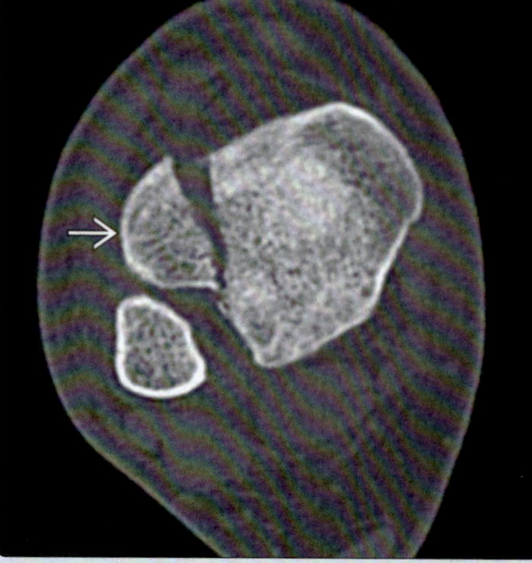

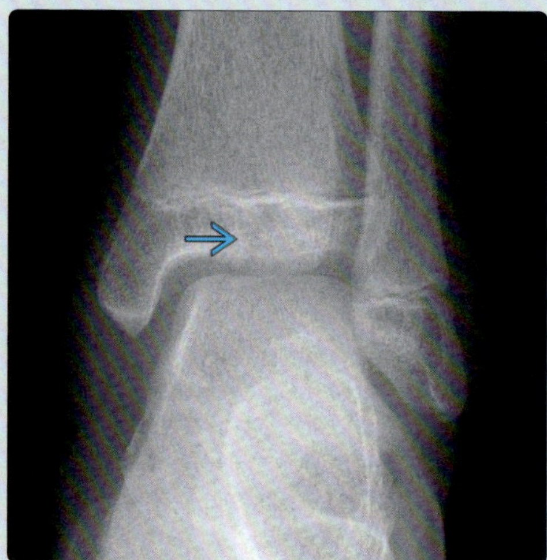

Juvenile Tillaux Fracture

TERMINOLOGY

Synonyms

- Tillaux fracture

IMAGING

General Features

- Best diagnostic clue
  - Sagittal fracture plane through distal tibial epiphysis with widening of lateral physis ± displacement of anterolateral epiphyseal fragment
- Location
  - Anterolateral aspect of distal tibial physis & epiphysis

Radiographic Findings

- Salter-Harris III fracture of anterolateral distal tibial epiphysis
- ± lateral displacement of epiphyseal fracture fragment
- Soft tissue swelling ± joint effusion
- Often best seen on mortise view, may be obscured by distal fibula on AP view

CT Findings

- Obtained to assess articular surface distraction
  - > 2 mm necessitates operative fixation
- Reformatted images in 3 planes are essential to fully characterize fracture
  - Width & location of greatest distraction
  - Degree of vertical step-off
  - Presence of loose intraarticular fragments
  - May reveal radiographically obscured metaphyseal fracture in coronal plane → triplane fracture

Imaging Recommendations

- Best imaging tool
  - AP, lateral, & mortise/oblique radiographic views
  - Bone CT to determine articular surface distraction

PATHOLOGY

General Features

- Salter-Harris III fracture of distal tibia extending through open lateral aspect of partially closed physis
  - Distal tibial physeal closure: Central → medial → lateral
  - Transitional fractures = fractures that occur in partially closed physis
    - Juvenile Tillaux & triplane fractures
- Avulsion of anterolateral tibial epiphyseal fragment by anterior inferior tibiofibular ligament
  - Ligament usually remains intact
- Mechanisms of injury
  - External rotation & supination of foot
  - Medial rotation of leg on fixed foot

CLINICAL ISSUES

Presentation

- Most common signs/symptoms
  - Anterior &/or lateral ankle pain, tenderness
  - Lateral swelling, bruising
  - Inability to bear weight
- Other signs/symptoms
  - Limp, external rotation of foot

Demographics

- Age
  - Adolescents < 18 months prior to complete distal tibial growth plate closure
    - Most common 12-15 years
    - Median age: 12 years in females, 14 years in males
    - After closure of central & medial physis, but before lateral physis
- Sex
  - More common in girls (F:M = 4:1)
- Epidemiology
  - 3-5% of pediatric ankle fractures

Natural History & Prognosis

- Risk for premature degeneration with residual articular surface irregularity
- Subsequent growth disturbance is rare as majority of physis has already closed

Treatment

- Displacement < 2 mm at articular surface: Closed reduction + immobilization
- Displacement > 2 mm: Operative management
  - Internal fixation with screws & K-wires
    - Anatomic reduction at articular surface is required to restore joint function, prevent premature degeneration
  - Alternatively, percutaneous pinning ± arthroscopic assistance may be considered

DIAGNOSTIC CHECKLIST

Consider

- Differentiate from triplane fracture
  - Salter-Harris IV fracture with coronal metadiaphyseal fracture plane

SELECTED REFERENCES

1. Ali Al-Ashhab ME et al: Treatment for displaced Tillaux fractures in adolescent age group. Foot Ankle Surg. 26(3):295-8, 2020
2. Lurie B et al: Functional outcomes of Tillaux and triplane fractures with 2 to 5 millimeters of intra-articular gap. J Bone Joint Surg Am. 102(8):679-86, 2020
3. Nenopoulos A et al: The role of CT in diagnosis and treatment of distal tibial fractures with intra-articular involvement in children. Injury. 46(11):2177-80, 2015
4. Wuerz TH et al: Pediatric physeal ankle fracture. J Am Acad Orthop Surg. 21(4):234-44, 2013
5. Crawford AH: Triplane and Tillaux fractures: is a 2 mm residual gap acceptable? J Pediatr Orthop. 32 Suppl 1:S69-73, 2012
6. Liporace FA et al: Does adding computed tomography change the diagnosis and treatment of Tillaux and triplane pediatric ankle fractures? Orthopedics. 35(2):e208-12, 2012
7. Rosenbaum AJ et al: Review of distal tibial epiphyseal transitional fractures. Orthopedics. 35(12):1046-9, 2012
8. Ayyagari S et al: Radiologic case study. Diagnosis: juvenile tillaux fracture. Orthopedics. 33(3):134, 2010
9. Kim JR et al: Treatment outcomes of triplane and Tillaux fractures of the ankle in adolescence. Clin Orthop Surg. 2(1):34-8, 2010
10. Kaya A et al: Open reduction and internal fixation in displaced juvenile Tillaux fractures. Injury. 38(2):201-5, 2007
11. Horn BD et al: Radiologic evaluation of juvenile tillaux fractures of the distal tibia. J Pediatr Orthop. 21(2):162-4, 2001

KEY FACTS

IMAGING

- Long bone metaphyses 70% (femur > tibia > humerus), short bones 6%, pelvis 5%, spine 2%
  - Metaphysis or equivalent > epiphysis, diaphysis
  - Multifocal in 10% overall but 22-55% in neonates
- Absence of radiographic bone findings does not exclude early osteomyelitis
  - Earliest finding: Soft tissue swelling next to bone
  - Bone destruction, periosteal reaction by 7-14 days
- MR: Best advanced imaging choice if diagnosis is unclear with localized symptoms or concern for complications
  - T1: Poorly defined metaphyseal marrow abnormality
  - T2 FS/STIR: Bright marrow, periosteal, & soft tissue edema; ± adjacent joint effusion
  - T1 C+ FS: Rim-enhancing abscesses (soft tissue, subperiosteal, intraosseous); ↓ enhancement of otherwise occult, unossified epiphyseal cartilage lesions in infants

TOP DIFFERENTIAL DIAGNOSES

- Ewing sarcoma
- Neuroblastoma metastases
- Langerhans cell histiocytosis
- Septic arthritis
- Bone infarct
- Leukemia
- Chronic recurrent multifocal osteomyelitis

PATHOLOGY

- Hematogenous source is most common
- *Staphylococcus aureus* > 80-90% of cases
  - Identification of infectious agent often fails despite blood cultures & site sampling

CLINICAL ISSUES

- Fever, pain, limp, tenderness, swelling
- Presentation is often nonspecific, may delay diagnosis
- Treat with IV then PO antibiotics + abscess drainage

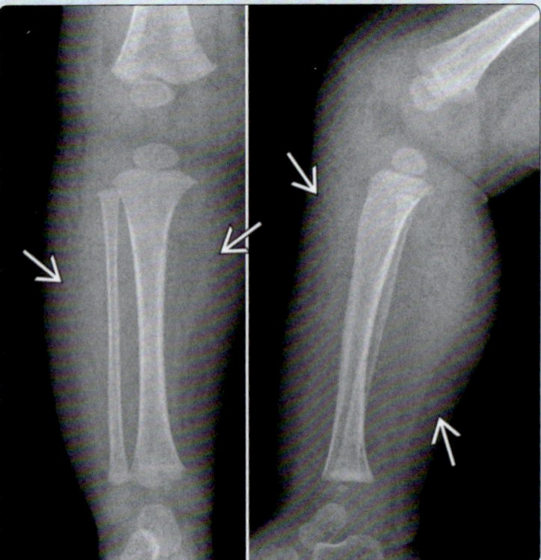

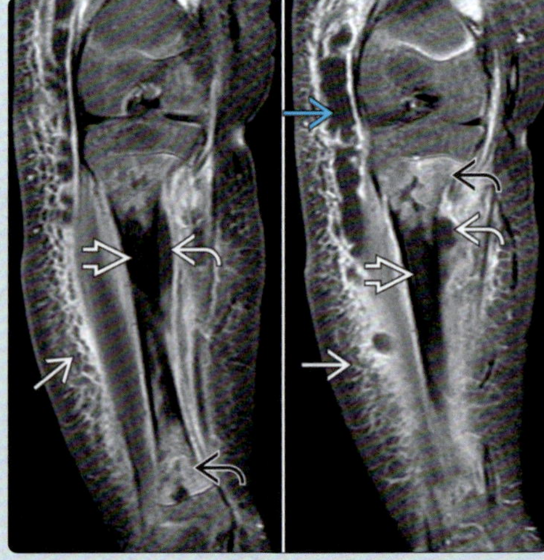

(Left) *AP (left) & lateral (right) radiographs in a 9-month-old infant show extensive, subcutaneous edema of the lower leg with blurring of soft tissue planes ➡ but no discrete bony abnormality.* **(Right)** *Coronal T1 C+ FS MR images in the same patient show foci of marrow necrosis ➡ with adjacent ↑ enhancement ↪ from infected or reactive viable marrow. Subperiosteal ➡ & soft tissue ➡ fluid collections & overlying fat edema ➡ are noted in this patient with MRSA osteomyelitis.*

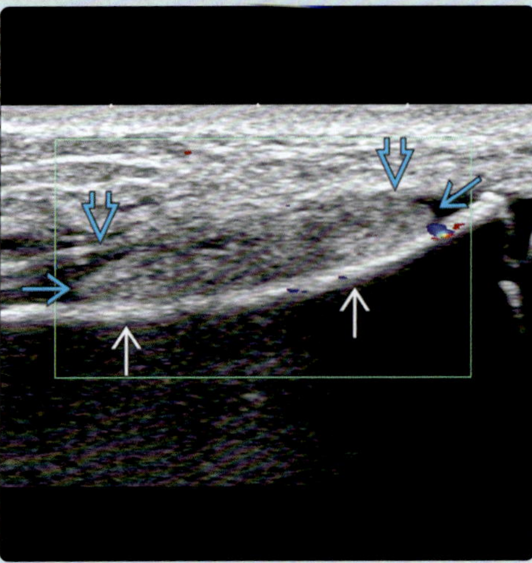

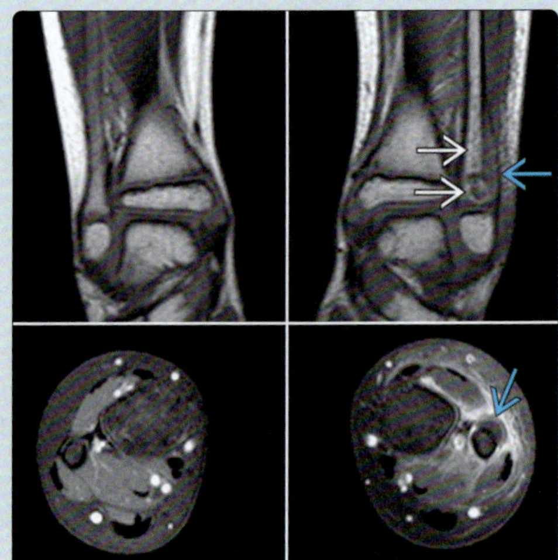

(Left) *Longitudinal color Doppler ultrasound in a 6-year-old with fever & lower extremity swelling shows an echogenic, avascular collection ➡ that is lifting the periosteum ➡ off of the cortex ➡.* **(Right)** *Coronal T1 (top) & axial T1 C+ FS (bottom) MR images in the same patient show heterogeneous marrow of the distal left fibula ➡ with a rim-enhancing subperiosteal abscess ➡. Surrounding soft tissue edema is also noted in this patient with MSSA osteomyelitis.*

TERMINOLOGY

Definitions

- Osteomyelitis: Bone infection, most commonly bacterial
- Osteoarticular infection: Osteomyelitis &/or septic arthritis

IMAGING

General Features

- Best diagnostic clue
  - Radiographs: Nonspecific soft tissue edema in setting of limp, pain, swelling, &/or fever (< 7-10 days)
  - MR: Heterogeneous, poorly defined metaphyseal or metadiaphyseal marrow signal abnormalities + subperiosteal fluid & soft tissue edema
- Location
  - Long bone metaphyses 70% (femur > tibia > humerus), short bones 6%, pelvis 5%, spine 2%
    - Metaphysis or equivalent > epiphysis, diaphysis
      - Bone adjacent to growth cartilage (e.g., synchondrosis or apophysis) is considered metaphyseal equivalent
  - Multifocal in 10% overall but 22-55% in neonates

Radiographic Findings

- Absence of findings does not exclude early osteomyelitis
- Earliest finding: Soft tissue swelling next to bone
  - Displacement or obliteration of fat planes
  - Reticulation of subcutaneous fat
- Lytic bone lesion in 7-14 days (or longer) after onset
  - Vague lucency → permeation → destruction
- Periosteal reaction is seen by 7-14 days
- Epiphyseal displacement/separation may occur in infants
- Healing changes on follow-up may look bizarre due to extensive bone involvement &/or superimposed pathologic fracture (due to ↑ activity on weak bone)
- Subacute: Lucent lesion + sclerotic rim (Brodie abscess)
- Chronic: Sclerosis or mixed sclerotic/lucent foci
  - ± cloaca (lucent drainage tract through cortex)
  - ± sequestrum (radiodense necrotic bone)
  - Garré sclerosing osteomyelitis (thick cortex)

Ultrasonographic Findings

- Sensitive for drainable fluid collections
  - Joint effusions; soft tissue &/or subperiosteal fluid
- Cortical bone changes are rarely seen

MR Findings

- T1WI
  - Poorly defined, heterogeneous dark marrow (due to loss of normal fatty marrow signal)
  - Subperiosteal foci of bright fat (from cortical disruption & marrow lipocyte necrosis)
  - Penumbra sign (in subacute Brodie abscess): ↑ T1 signal rim of granulation tissue
- T2WI FS/STIR
  - Bright marrow + soft tissue edema
    - Soft tissue changes are usually moderate to marked
  - Discrete soft tissue & subperiosteal fluid collections
    - Elevated thin, dark periosteum
    - Disrupted dark cortex
  - ± adjacent joint effusion
    - Concomitant septic arthritis in up to 55%
      - Spread of infection to joint ↓ > 1-2 years of age
  - Chronic: Dark signal sclerotic sequestrum & involucrum
- T1WI C+ FS
  - ↑ marrow enhancement: Hyperemia/edema
  - ↓ marrow enhancement: Pressure necrosis, vessel thrombosis, pus
  - Rim-enhancing soft tissue & subperiosteal abscesses
  - Brodie abscess: Central nonenhancement (pus), inner rim of ↑ enhancement (granulation tissue), outer low signal rim (sclerosis)

Nuclear Medicine Findings

- Bone scan: ↑ uptake in angiographic, blood pool, & delayed phases: 80-94% sensitive
  - Positive in 24-72 hours; can demonstrate multiple sites
  - Central photopenia with bone infarct or abscess

Imaging Recommendations

- Best imaging tool
  - MR is most sensitive & specific modality for early infection with localized symptoms
    - Confirms diagnosis or delineates alternative processes
    - Shows drainable abscesses & intraspinal extension
  - Bone scintigraphy can be helpful if site & diagnosis are unclear (as less likely to require sedation than MR)
  - Whole-body MR is helpful for localizing multifocal, drainable collections in ill patient
- Protocol advice
  - T2 FS or STIR MR is crucial for edema/fluid detection
  - T1 C+ FS MR delineates drainable fluid & otherwise occult foci of epiphyseal cartilage involvement in infancy
    - Contrast is of questionable utility with otherwise normal study beyond 18 months of age

DIFFERENTIAL DIAGNOSIS

Ewing Sarcoma

- Aggressive lytic diaphyseal/metadiaphyseal lesion, most common in patients > 5 years old
- Sharply marginated interface of intramedullary tumor with normal fatty marrow on T1 MR; large, heterogeneously enhancing soft tissue mass with contrast

Neuroblastoma Metastases

- Aggressive but frequently subtle lytic lesions, most common in patients < 5 years old
- Calcified primary suprarenal/paraspinal tumor

Langerhans Cell Histiocytosis

- Punched-out, well-defined lytic lesions + enhancing mass
- Flat bones & spine are frequently involved

Septic Arthritis

- Effusion + enhancing, mildly thickened synovium
- Adjacent marrow & soft tissue edema favor infected joint

Bone Infarct

- Acute: Focal, poorly defined marrow edema with nonenhancement & mild, adjacent soft tissue changes
- Chronic: Serpentine medullary sclerosis on radiographs; MR shows characteristic double line sign (low/high T2 signal)

Leukemia

- Metaphyseal lucent bands &/or permeative lytic lesions in patients < 10 years old
- Diffuse marrow replacement on T1 MR is classic

Chronic Recurrent Multifocal Osteomyelitis

- Noninfectious, episodic bone inflammation
- Mixed bubbly, lucent, & sclerotic periphyseal lesions of femur, tibia; spine, pelvis, clavicle, & mandible also typical
- Multifocal, often symmetric sites of MR marrow edema on either side of physis, ± physeal widening

PATHOLOGY

General Features

- Pathophysiology
  - Hematogenous seeding >> penetrating injury or contiguous spread
    - After infancy, transphyseal vessels resolve
      - Avascular physis maintains relative barrier between epiphysis & metaphysis, making continuous epiphyseal & intraarticular spread less likely
      - Barrier is nonexistent in infants or after skeletal maturity → ↑ rates of septic arthritis
    - Slow flow through looping metaphyseal venules
      - Primary sites for bacterial lodging
    - Intramedullary infection → edema, vascular congestion → ↑ pressure → transcortical spread
    - Periosteal attachment is tight at physis, loose at metaphysis/diaphysis in children
      - Marked elevation by pus or tumor is possible
- Organisms
  - Identified in only 35-66% of needle aspirates, 36-55% of blood cultures
  - *Staphylococcus aureus* > 80-90% of cases (> 55% due to methicillin-resistant strains)
    - Panton-Valentine leukocidin: Necrotizing toxin secreted by some strains of MRSA or MSSA → more invasive infections
      - Persistent bacteremia despite IV antibiotics
      - ↑ rates of shock, septic emboli, deep venous thrombosis, & fluid collections requiring drainage
  - Streptococcus in ~ 10%: Group A β hemolytic, *S. pyogenes*, *S. pneumoniae*
  - Children 6 months to 4 years of age: *Kingella kingae*
    - Relatively ↓ bone & soft tissue reaction & ↑ epiphyseal cartilage lesions vs. other organisms
    - PCR is much more sensitive than culture
  - Neonates: MSSA (premature infants with multifocal infection), group B *Streptococcus* (term infants with single-site disease)
  - Sickle cell disease: *Salmonella* in children; *S. aureus* also reported in adults
  - Immunocompromised: *Streptococcus pneumoniae*, tuberculosis
  - Penetrating foot trauma: *Pseudomonas aeruginosa*
  - Purpuric rash, shock: Meningococcemia (severe infarctions → amputation; less severe → growth arrest)
  - Kitten exposure (cat-scratch disease): *Bartonella henselae*

CLINICAL ISSUES

Presentation

- Most common signs/symptoms
  - Pain, ↓ range of motion, ↓ weight bearing, tenderness, swelling, fever
  - Minor trauma history in 1/3 of patients
- Labs: ↑ ESR, CRP > ↑ WBC
  - Higher inflammatory markers are more likely with disseminated than localized infection

Demographics

- Age
  - Primarily disease of infants & young children
    - 1/2 of cases occur before 5 years of age
- Epidemiology
  - Incidence has nearly tripled in USA in last several decades

Natural History & Prognosis

- Complications include septic arthritis, deep venous thrombosis, fracture, septic emboli, multisystem failure, growth disturbance
  - More likely with treatment delay of > 4 days

Treatment

- Identify infectious agent: Image-guided needle aspiration or open surgical biopsy + blood culture
- Antibiotics (IV followed by PO), pain management
  - Longer antibiotic therapy is required for multifocality
- Surgery/intervention: Abscess (intraosseous, subperiosteal, soft tissue) drainage, sequestrectomy, management of sinus tracts & pathologic fractures

DIAGNOSTIC CHECKLIST

Consider

- Immediate preoperative MR will require concurrent interpretation to facilitate single sedation (for imaging & surgery) in young children
- Imaging after treatment: Uncomplicated osteomyelitis may require 6 months for MR normalization
  - Nonspecific for ongoing bone infection vs. resolving inflammation/healing
  - Drainable collections can be sampled to guide therapy

SELECTED REFERENCES

1. Weisman JK et al: Characteristics and outcomes of osteomyelitis in children with sickle cell disease: a 10-year single-center experience. Pediatr Blood Cancer. 67(5):e28225, 2020
2. Wyers MR et al: Physeal separation in pediatric osteomyelitis. Pediatr Radiol. 49(9):1229-33, 2019
3. Greer MC: Whole-body magnetic resonance imaging: techniques and non-oncologic indications. Pediatr Radiol. 48(9):1348-63, 2018
4. Manz N et al: Evaluation of the current use of imaging modalities and pathogen detection in children with acute osteomyelitis and septic arthritis. Eur J Pediatr. 177(7):1071-80, 2018
5. Mignemi ME et al: A novel classification system based on dissemination of musculoskeletal infection is predictive of hospital outcomes. J Pediatr Orthop. 38(5):279-86, 2018
6. Jaramillo D et al: Hematogenous osteomyelitis in infants and children: imaging of a changing disease. Radiology. 283(3):629-43, 2017
7. Chan BY et al: MR Imaging of pediatric bone marrow. Radiographics. 36(6):1911-30, 2016
8. Browne LP et al: Community-acquired staphylococcal musculoskeletal infection in infants and young children: necessity of contrast-enhanced MRI for the diagnosis of growth cartilage involvement. AJR Am J Roentgenol. 198(1):194-9, 2012

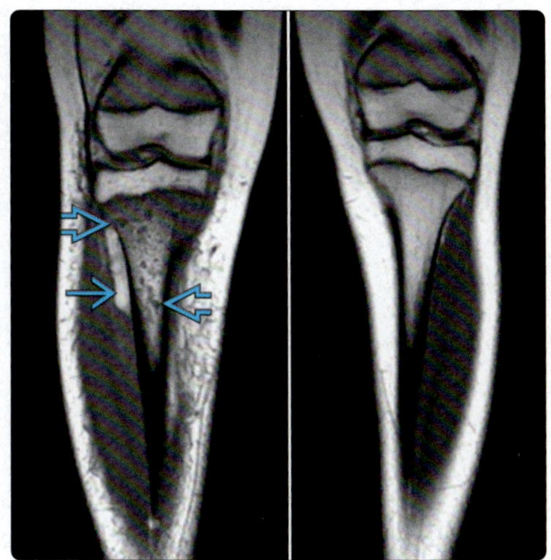

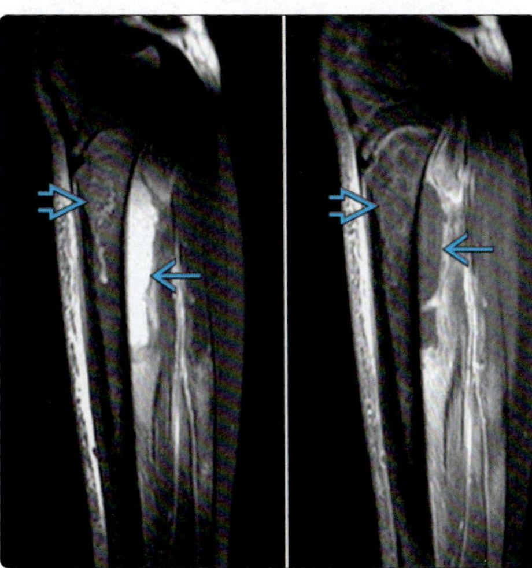

(Left) *Coronal T1 MR in an 11-year-old with 5 days of fever & leg swelling shows heterogeneous, "speckled" signal abnormalities in the proximal right tibia ⇨. Fat within an overlying subperiosteal collection ➙ is due to marrow lipocyte necrosis by PVL, an enzyme often associated with aggressive MRSA infections.* **(Right)** *Sagittal T2 FS (L) & T1 C+ FS (R) MR images in the same patient show the heterogeneous proximal tibial marrow ⇨ & large subperiosteal abscess ➙. MRSA was cultured at surgery.*

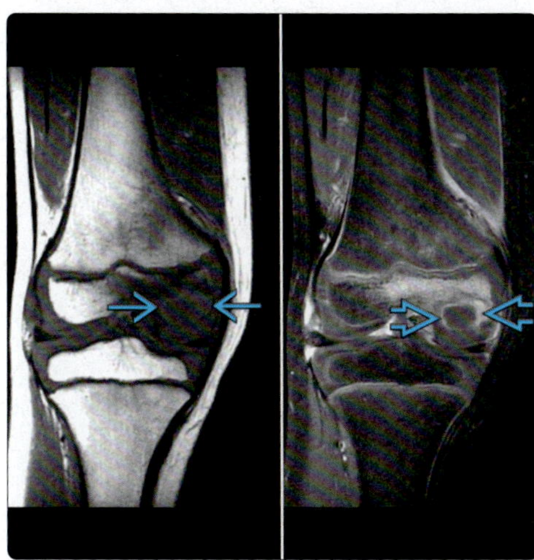

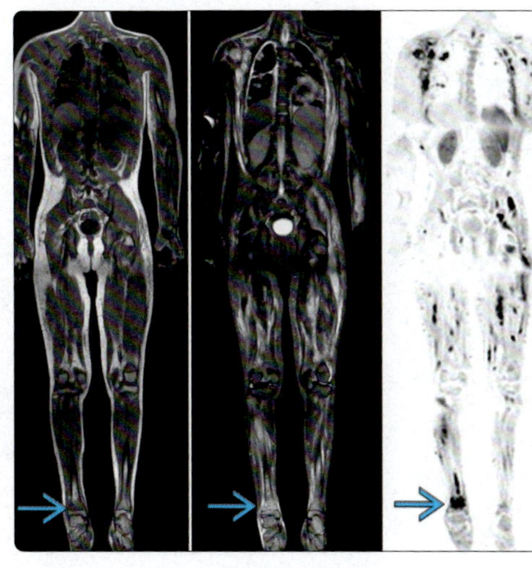

(Left) *Coronal T1 (L) & T1 C+ FS (R) MR images in a 5-year-old with 3 weeks of pain after an injury show a Brodie abscess of the medial femoral condyle with high T1 signal of granulation tissue along the abscess rim ➙ (the penumbra sign) that enhances after contrast ⇨.* **(Right)** *Coronal T1 (L), STIR (middle), & DWIBS (R) MR images in a 9-year-old with MRSA bacteremia & septic emboli show right distal tibial osteomyelitis ➙, pulmonary nodules, & numerous foci of myositis & fasciitis with muscular abscesses.*

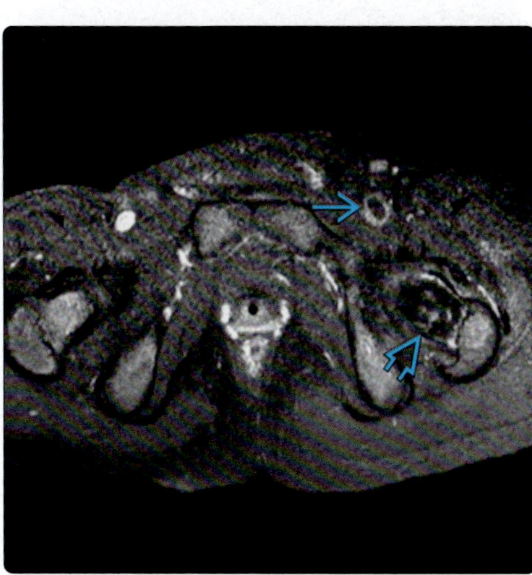

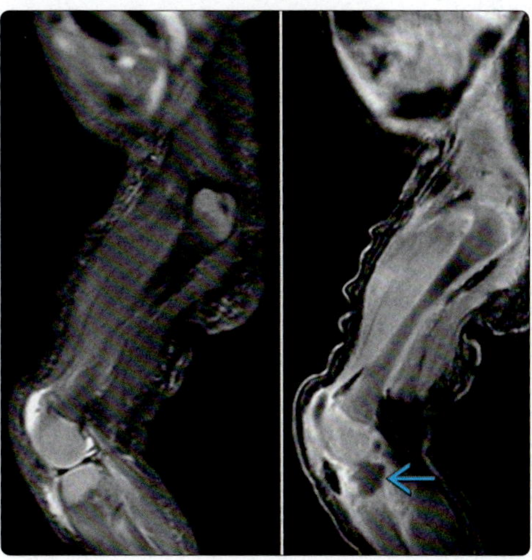

(Left) *Axial T1 C+ FS MR in a 7-year-old with septic emboli shows osteomyelitis of the left femoral neck ⇨ & thrombus of the left common femoral vein ➙. MSSA was grown from blood cultures in this patient.* **(Right)** *Sagittal STIR (L) & T1 C+ FS (R) MR images in a 19-day-old with MRSA septic emboli & known pelvic abscesses show diminished enhancement of the unossified proximal tibial epiphyseal cartilage ➙ due to infection. Note the lack of signal abnormality at this level on the STIR image.*

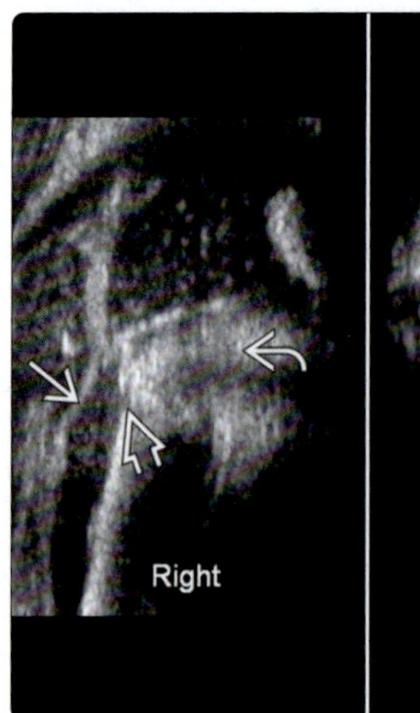

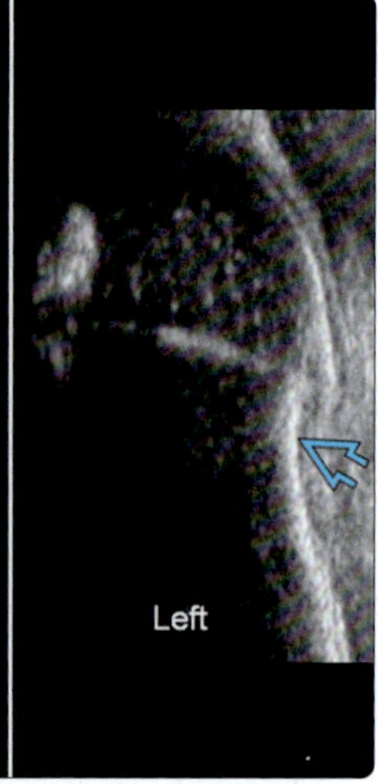

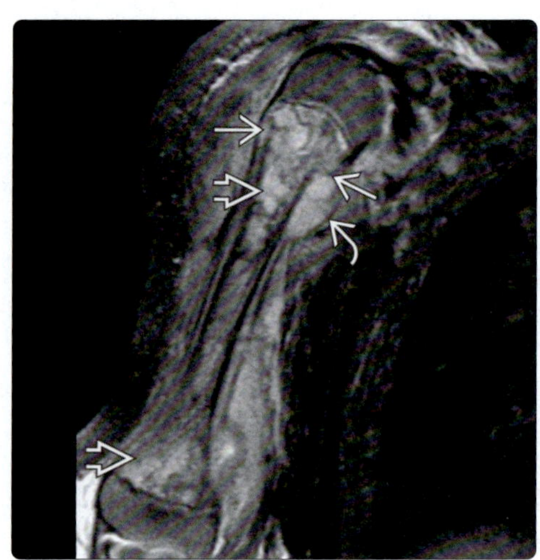

(Left) *Coronal ultrasound of the proximal right humerus in a 5-month-old boy shows a subperiosteal fluid collection ➡ with disruption of the metaphyseal cortex ➡ & disturbed underlying medullary echotexture ➡. Compare the normal left humeral sonographic architecture ➡.* **(Right)** *Coronal STIR MR of the same patient with osteomyelitis shows abnormal fluid signal throughout the right humerus ➡ + a nondisplaced, pathologic metaphyseal fracture ➡. A subperiosteal fluid collection ➡ is noted.*

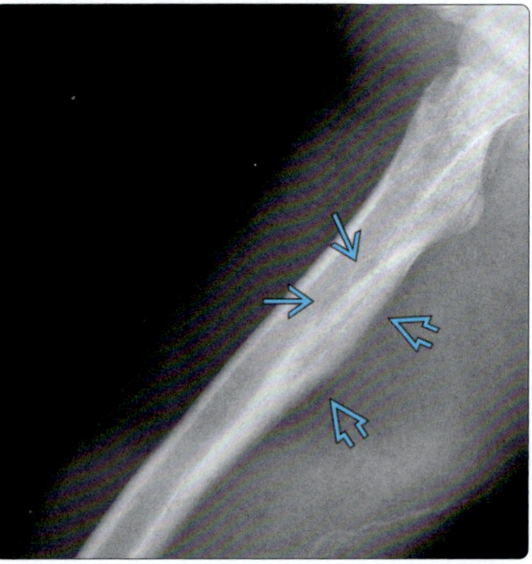
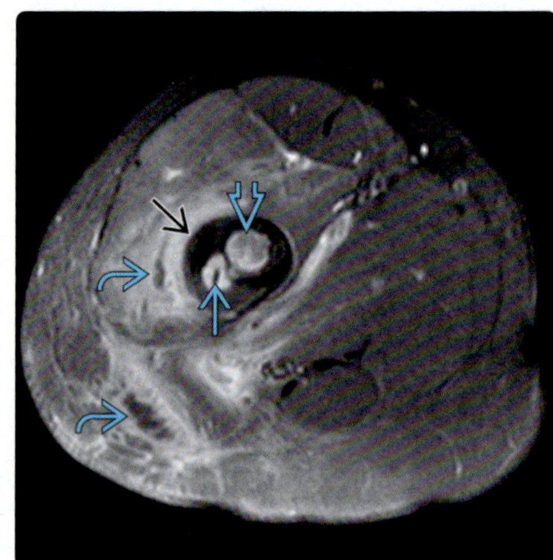

(Left) *Lateral radiograph in an 11-year-old with 3 weeks of thigh pain & swelling shows eccentric intramedullary lucencies ➡ with overlying cortical thickening & subtle aggressive periosteal reaction ➡.* **(Right)** *Axial T1 C+ FS MR in the same patient shows a sequestrum ➡ with surrounding involucrum ➡ & marrow signal abnormalities ➡. A cloaca was visible superior to this level (not shown). Note the overlying soft tissue abscesses ➡. MSSA grew from cultures in this case of chronic osteomyelitis.*

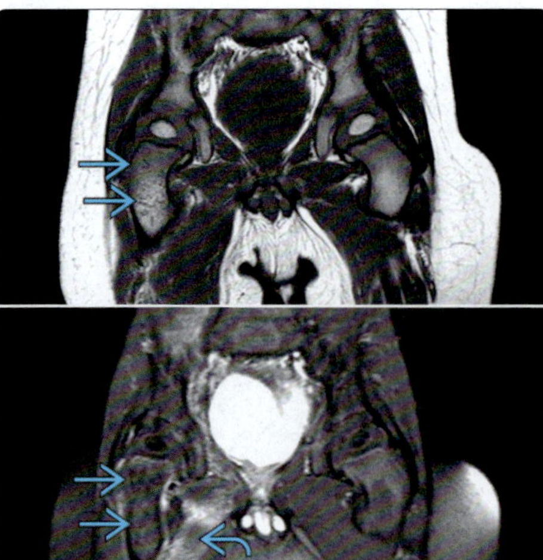
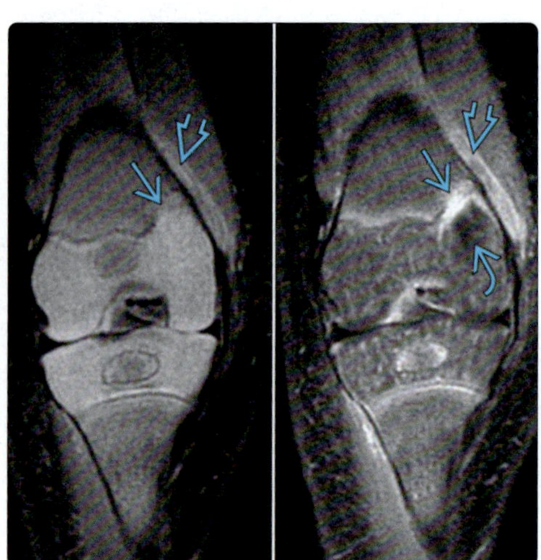

(Left) *Coronal T1 (top) & T1 C+ FS (bottom) MR images in a 1-year-old with fever & a limp show abnormal, poorly defined marrow heterogeneity of the proximal right femur ➡ with surrounding soft tissue edema ➡, typical of osteomyelitis.* **(Right)** *Coronal PD FS (L) & T1 C+ FS (R) MR images in a neonate with femoral osteomyelitis show focal loss of normal low-signal zone of provisional calcification (ZPC) ➡ with poor enhancement of unossified epiphyseal cartilage ➡ & overlying soft tissue edema ➡.*

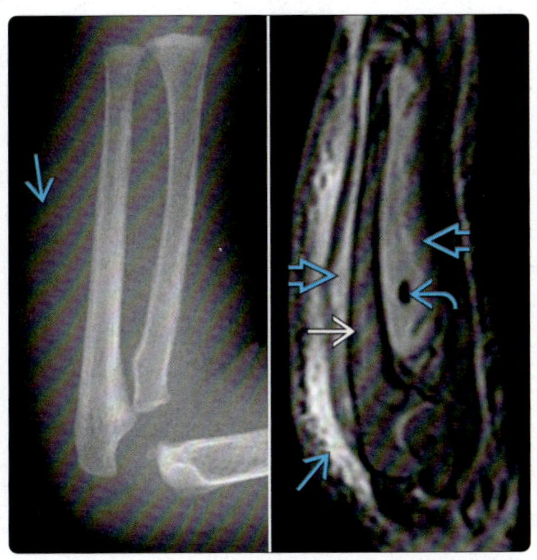

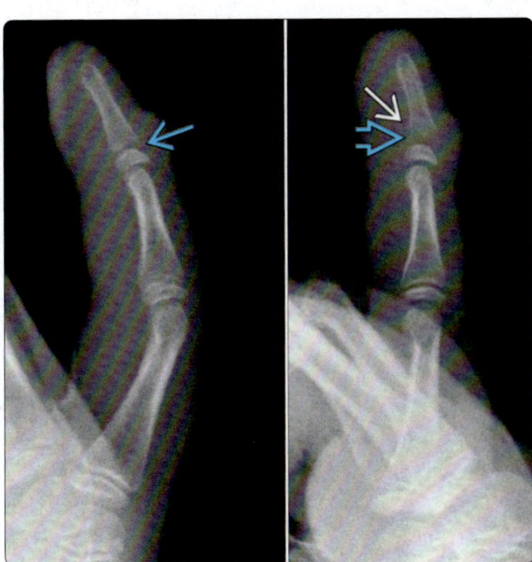

(Left) *Lateral radiograph (L) & sagittal STIR MR (R) images in an infant with ulnar osteomyelitis show soft tissue edema, a large subperiosteal abscess, & marrow heterogeneity. A small, subperiosteal globule followed fat signal on all sequences, consistent with marrow lipocyte necrosis.* **(Right)** *Lateral radiographs 1 (L) & 3 (R) weeks after a nailbed injury in an 11-year-old show a subtle Salter-Harris 2 fracture with subsequent metaphyseal bone loss & periosteal reaction due to osteomyelitis.*

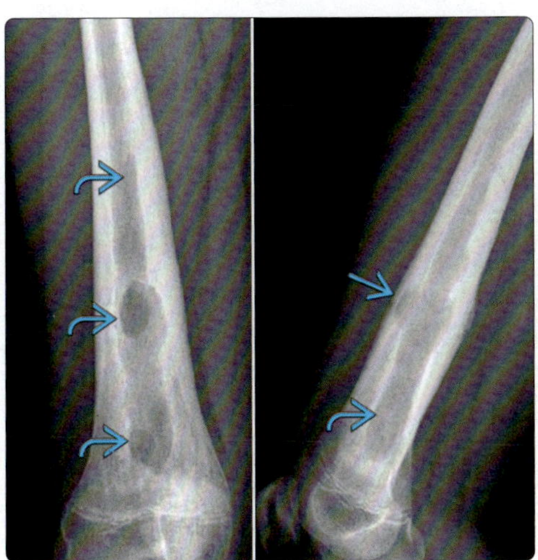

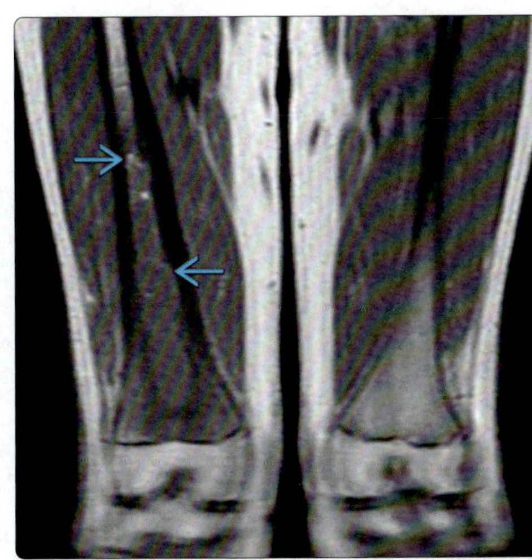

(Left) *AP (L) & lateral (R) radiographs of the distal femur in a teenager with months of pain show central, elongated lucent lesions, some of which have narrow zones of transition. There is mild expansile remodeling with foci of endosteal scalloping intermixed with cortical thickening.* **(Right)** *Coronal T1 MR in the same patient shows a high-signal rim to the central medullary lesion, the typical penumbra sign of granulation tissue in a subacute to chronic Brodie abscess.*

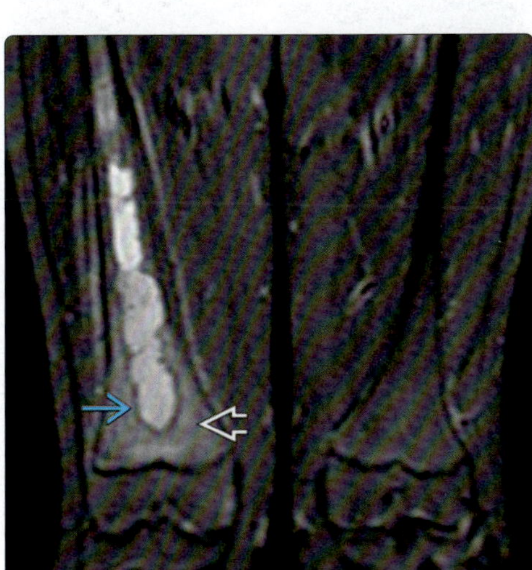

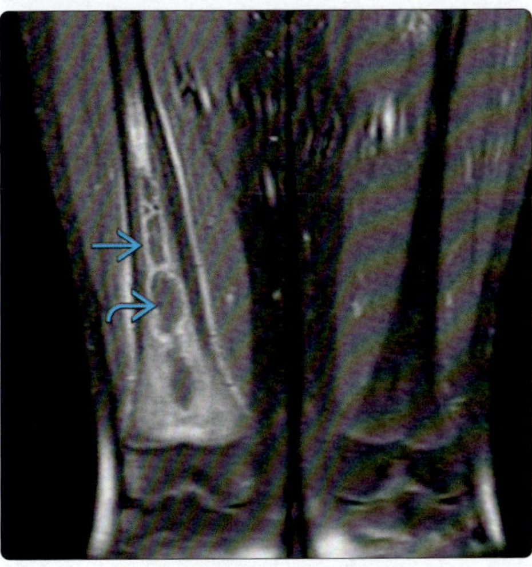

(Left) *Coronal STIR MR in the same patient shows that the high signal intensity intramedullary collection is surrounded by a hypointense outer rim of fibrosis &/or sclerosis, a feature not seen with acute infections. There is surrounding poorly defined marrow edema.* **(Right)** *Coronal T1 C+ FS MR in the same patient shows intense rim enhancement of the medullary abscess. The periosteal & soft tissue edema in this case of subacute to chronic osteomyelitis is less pronounced than is typically seen with acute infection.*

Syphilis

KEY FACTS

TERMINOLOGY

- Congenital syphilis (CS): Transmission of *Treponema pallidum* to fetus from infected mother
  - Early-onset CS: Clinically manifests < 2 years of age
  - Late-onset CS: Clinically manifests > 2 years of age

IMAGING

- Usually widespread, symmetric
  - Can be asymmetric or solitary
- Periosteal reaction is most common finding
- Metaphyseal lesions
  - Nonspecific lucent bands with intact zone of provisional calcification (ZPC) are typical
    - Can have serrated/sawtooth metaphyses
  - Wimberger corner sign: Destruction of proximal medial tibias with sparing of 1st few mm of new bone
- Saber shins: Anterior tibial cortical thickening & bowing (in older children)
- Pathologic fractures, usually metaphyseal

TOP DIFFERENTIAL DIAGNOSES

- Bacterial osteomyelitis
- Neuroblastoma or leukemia
- Physiologic periosteal reaction
- Infantile myofibromatosis
- Child abuse

CLINICAL ISSUES

- Fetal/perinatal demise in 40% of infants with CS
- 2/3 of infants with CS are asymptomatic at birth
  - Prenatal screening is important for early treatment
- Symptoms: Hepatosplenomegaly, rhinitis ("snuffles"), rash
  - Parrot pseudoparalysis: Not moving painful extremity
- Prevention of CS: Treatment of seropositive mothers
- Treatment of CS: IV penicillin for infants

DIAGNOSTIC CHECKLIST

- Consider CS in infant with widespread polyostotic findings
- Infant with CS & multiple fractures may mimic abuse

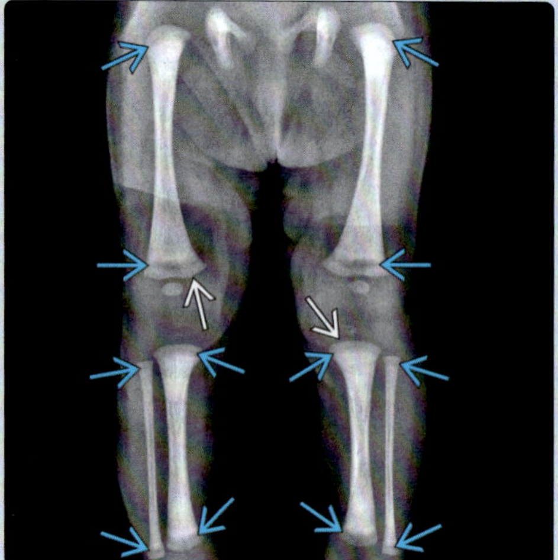

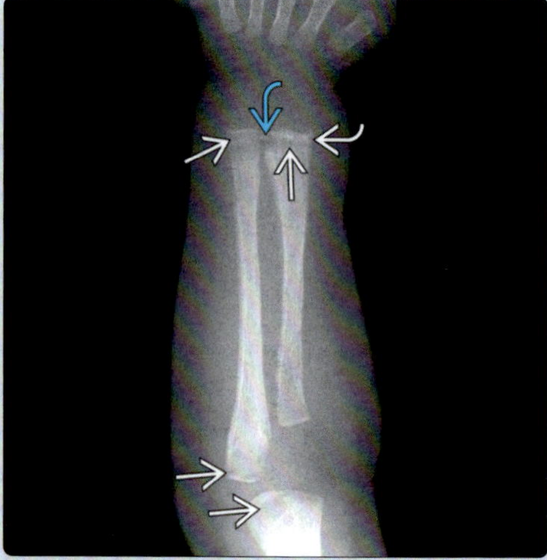

(Left) *Frontal radiograph of the lower extremities in a 3-week-old girl with acute congenital syphilis (CS) shows metaphyseal lucent bands in all of the long bones ➡, though the ZPCs are intact ➡. This finding is nonspecific as systemic stress, neuroblastoma, & leukemia can cause a similar appearance.* **(Right)** *AP radiograph shows metaphyseal lucent bands ➡ in the radius, ulna, & humerus. Periosteal reaction ➡ & a destructive metaphyseal lesion ➡ are also seen in the distal radius.*

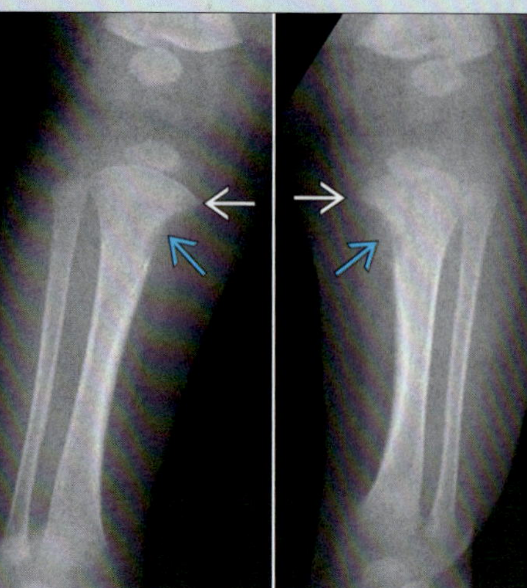

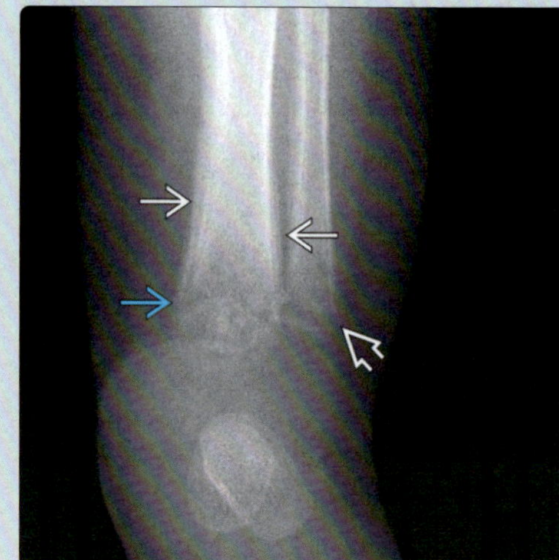

(Left) *AP radiographs in a 2-month-old girl with known CS show destructive lytic lesions in the bilateral medial tibial metaphyses ➡ with sparing of the proximal few mm of bone ➡. This is the Wimberger corner sign, which is highly suggestive of (but not specific for) CS.* **(Right)** *Newborn ankle radiograph of CS shows a fracture ➡ through a lucent band in the distal fibula. Periostitis ➡ & permeation ➡ are seen in the distal tibia. Fractures in CS can be confused with abuse.*

TERMINOLOGY

Definitions

- Congenital syphilis (CS): Transmission of *Treponema pallidum* to fetus from infected mother
  - Early-onset CS: Clinically manifests < 2 years of age
  - Late-onset CS: Clinically manifests > 2 years of age
- "Great imitator" (coined by Sir William Osler)

IMAGING

General Features

- Best diagnostic clue
  - Infant with widespread metaphyseal findings
  - Wimberger corner sign: Bilateral destruction of proximal medial tibias
    - Spares 1st few mm of newly formed bone
    - Highly suggestive but not specific for CS
- Location
  - Often widespread but can involve single bone

Radiographic Findings

- Periosteal reaction is most common finding
  - Typically symmetric
- Long bones
  - Metaphyses: Typically 1st area of involvement
    - Nonspecific horizontal lucent bands, classically sparing thin radiodense periphyseal zone of provisional calcification (ZPC)
      - Can see metaphyseal irregularity (serrated, sawtooth)
    - Destructive lucent lesion
      - Tibia > femur > humerus
      - Wimberger corner sign: Upper medial tibias
  - Diaphyses
    - Cortical thickening ± destructive lesions
      - Saber shin: Anterior tibial cortical thickening/bowing (late childhood)
- Pathologic fractures, frequently multiple
  - Most common at metaphysis
  - May mimic nonaccidental trauma
- Skull: Multiple lytic calvarial lesions
- Chest: Diffuse pulmonary opacities

DIFFERENTIAL DIAGNOSIS

Bacterial Osteomyelitis

- Usually monostotic with edema ± fluid collections

Leukemia

- Symmetric, metaphyseal lucent bands

Neuroblastoma

- Diffuse bone metastases (asymmetric)

Systemic Stress

- May cause metaphyseal lucent bands with intact ZPC
- Common in 1st month of life

Rickets

- Metaphyseal cupping, fraying, & splaying
- Loss of ZPC

Physiologic Periosteal Reaction

- Symmetric & smooth along entire diaphysis
- Most commonly of humeri, femurs, & tibias
- Appears > 1 month, peaks ~ 6 months

Infantile Myofibromatosis

- Relatively symmetric, bubbly, metadiaphyseal lucent lesions of infant, often with ≥ 1 soft tissue myofibroma

Child Abuse

- Healing classic metaphyseal lesion can mimic CS

PATHOLOGY

General Features

- Typically due to transplacental transmission

Microscopic Features

- Focal erosions are due to syphilitic granulation tissue
- Metaphyseal lucent bands may be secondary to
  - Stress response from systemic disease
  - Syphilitic granulation tissue

CLINICAL ISSUES

Presentation

- Most common signs/symptoms
  - Hepatosplenomegaly, rhinitis ("snuffles"), rash
  - 2/3 of infants with CS are asymptomatic at birth
    - Prenatal screening is important for early treatment
    - Adequately treated maternal syphilis 30 days before delivery prevents up to 98% of CS
    - Untreated CS typically shows symptoms by 5 weeks
- Other signs/symptoms
  - Early-onset (0-2 years) CS
    - Parrot pseudoparalysis: Immobile limb due to pain
      - Radiograph of limb shows destructive lesion
  - Late-onset (2 to ~ 30 years) CS
    - Bone changes: Frontal bossing, saddle nose, maxillary hypoplasia, saber tibia, gummatous periostitis

Natural History & Prognosis

- Fetal/perinatal demise in 40% of infants with CS
- Early CS bone lesions usually resolve with treatment

Treatment

- Prevention of CS: Treatment of seropositive mothers
- IV penicillin for infected infants

DIAGNOSTIC CHECKLIST

Image Interpretation Pearls

- Consider CS in infant with widespread polyostotic findings
- Infant with CS & multiple fractures may mimic abuse

SELECTED REFERENCES

1. Kimball A et al: Congenital syphilis diagnosed beyond the neonatal period in the United States: 2014-2018. Pediatrics. 148(3), 2021
2. Medoro AK et al: Syphilis in neonates and infants. Clin Perinatol. 48(2):293-309, 2021
3. Jacobs K et al: Congenital syphilis misdiagnosed as suspected nonaccidental trauma. Pediatrics. 144(4), 2019
4. Kan JH et al: Musculoskeletal infections. Caffey's pediatric diagnostic imaging. 13th ed. Elsevier. 1349-64, 2019

Septic Arthritis

KEY FACTS

TERMINOLOGY

- Septic arthritis: Microbial (typically bacterial) invasion of joint leading to inflammation & purulence

IMAGING

- Best clue: Joint effusion in non-weight-bearing child with fever > 38.5°C + ↑ serum inflammatory markers
- Radiographs: Displacement of fat pads ± widened joint
- US: Highly sensitive for fluid distending joint capsule
  - Complexity & volume do not predict/exclude infection
- MR: Nonspecific joint fluid with synovial thickening & enhancement
  - Findings favoring septic arthritis over transient synovitis
    - Presence of marrow &/or soft tissue edema
    - ↓ early enhancement/perfusion of articular epiphysis

TOP DIFFERENTIAL DIAGNOSES

- Transient synovitis
- Juvenile idiopathic arthritis
- Trauma
- Reactive effusion due to adjacent bone pathology

PATHOLOGY

- Mechanism: Hematogenous spread vs. direct spread from adjacent osteomyelitis or puncture wound
- Most common organisms overall: *Staphylococcus aureus* > streptococcal species
  - Neonates: Group B streptococci, gram-negative rods, *Neisseria gonorrhoeae*
  - < 4 years of age: *Kingella kingae* most common

CLINICAL ISSUES

- Treatment: Emergent arthroscopy/arthrotomy with joint irrigation + IV antibiotics to prevent long-term sequelae

DIAGNOSTIC CHECKLIST

- Synovitis has many etiologies; always consider infection
  - Imaging alone cannot exclude infection of joint fluid
  - Joint aspiration required for 100% confidence

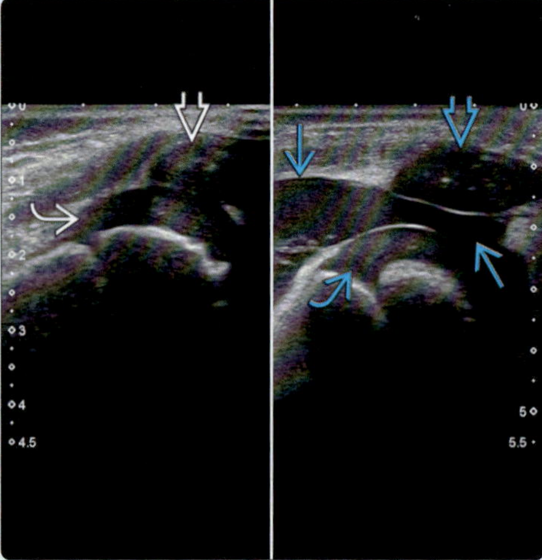

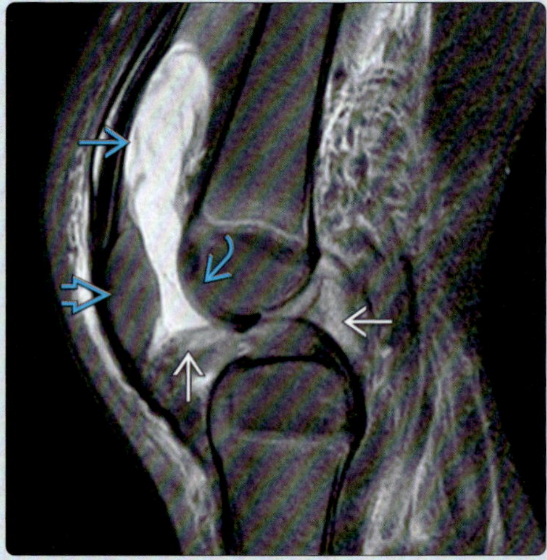

(Left) *Sagittal US in a 2-year-old with Staphylococcus aureus septic arthritis shows a large joint effusion ➡ of the left knee displacing the unossified patellar cartilage ➡ from the femoral condylar cartilage ➡. There is no fluid separating the right knee patellar ➡ & femoral ➡ cartilages.* **(Right)** *Sagittal T2 FS MR in the same child shows the large effusion ➡ separating the patellar ➡ & femoral ➡ cartilages. The inflamed synovium ➡ is of intermediate signal intensity. Note the surrounding soft tissue edema.*

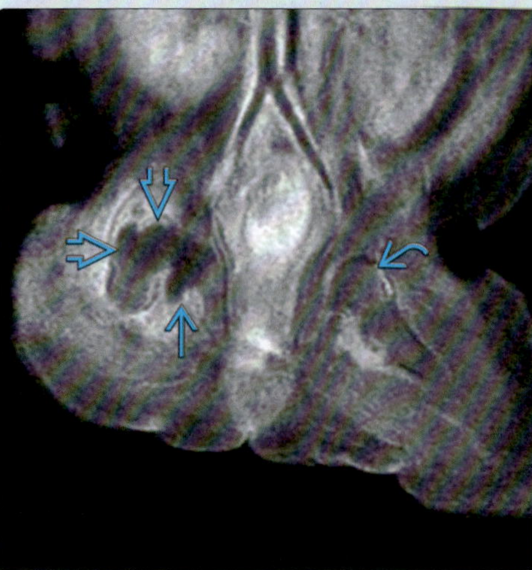

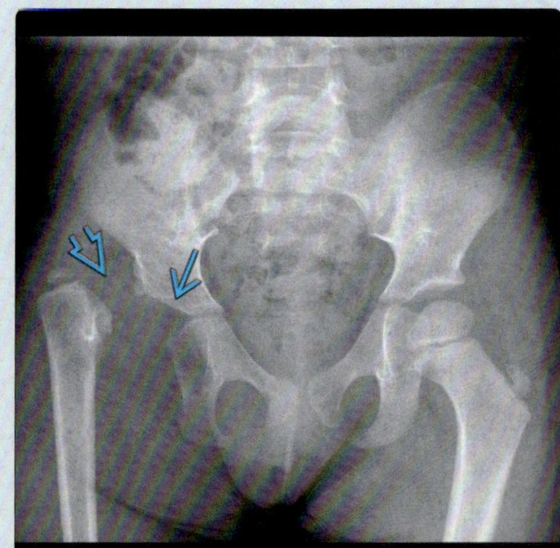

(Left) *Coronal T1 C+ FS MR in a 1-month-old with S. aureus bacteremia shows nonenhancing fluid ➡ of the right hip joint displacing & eroding a necrotic right femoral head ➡. Note the surrounding inflammation. The left femoral head ➡ is normal without joint effusion.* **(Right)** *AP radiograph in the same patient 4 years later shows no discernible right femoral head or neck ➡ with displacement of the femur from an abnormal acetabulum ➡. Hip destruction is a feared complication of septic arthritis.*

TERMINOLOGY

Definitions

- Septic arthritis: Microbial (typically bacterial) invasion of joint leading to inflammation & purulence

IMAGING

General Features

- Location
  - Affects lower extremity joints in ≥ 75% of cases
  - Multiple joints in ~ 10-15%

Radiographic Findings

- Displacement of fat pads ± widening of joint space, soft tissue edema with blurred fat-muscle interfaces
- Sensitivity for fluid distending joint capsule varies on location: Knee, ankle, elbow > > hip, shoulder
  - Only 20-73% sensitive at hip

Ultrasonographic Findings

- Anechoic to complex fluid distending joint capsule; complexity & volume do not predict sterile vs. infected fluid
  - Septic joint is unlikely if fluid is absent (but must know where to look)
- Synovial thickening, ± hyperemia

MR Findings

- Nonspecific synovitis (as with many etiologies)
  - Bright T2/STIR fluid in joint
    - ± debris, fluid-fluid level
  - Synovial thickening & enhancement
- Findings favoring septic arthritis over transient synovitis
  - Presence of marrow &/or soft tissue edema
  - ↓ early enhancement/perfusion of articular epiphysis, especially in tight joint (e.g., femoral head at hip)
- Findings favoring septic arthritis over reactive fluid secondary to adjacent metaphyseal osteomyelitis
  - Epiphyseal marrow edema, surrounding soft tissue edema, epiphyseal nonenhancement

Imaging Recommendations

- Best imaging tool
  - US: Highly sensitive for joint fluid; ~ 5% false-negative rate in first 24 hours
  - MR ± contrast
    - Best tool for detecting adjacent bone & soft tissue infections/collections
    - Can detect other diagnoses

DIFFERENTIAL DIAGNOSIS

Transient Synovitis

- Typically occurs at hip, leading to limp
- Usually without fever or ↑ serum inflammatory markers
- Nonspecific MR appearance of synovitis
  - Joint fluid + mild synovial thickening & enhancement
  - Lacks surrounding marrow or soft tissue edema

Juvenile Idiopathic Arthritis

- ± rice bodies: Numerous, tiny low T2 signal intensity bodies of uniform size throughout joint fluid

Trauma

- ± marrow & soft tissue edema, ligament & cartilage injuries

Reactive Effusion Due to Adjacent Bone Pathology

- Osteomyelitis, bone tumor, Legg-Calvé-Perthes

PATHOLOGY

General Features

- Mechanisms of joint seeding
  - Hematogenous spread: Vascularized synovium lacking basement membrane allows bacterial entry
  - Direct spread: Adjacent osteomyelitis, puncture wound
    - Epiphyseal osteomyelitis leading to septic arthritis is common in neonates
- Causative organisms
  - *Staphylococcus aureus* > streptococcal species overall
  - Neonates: Group B streptococci, gram-negative rods, *Neisseria gonorrhoeae, S. aureus*
  - 3 months to 4 years of age: Gram-negative bacteria, streptococcal species, *Kingella kingae*
    - *K. kingae* often lacks systemic markers of inflammation
- Osteocartilaginous destruction caused by
  - Neutrophil & bacterial proteolytic enzymes → articular & unossified epiphyseal cartilage damage
  - ↑ joint pressure by pus → ↓ perfusion of articular epiphysis → ischemic injury

CLINICAL ISSUES

Presentation

- Fever, pain, swelling, ↓ motion, non-weight-bearing
- Kocher criteria: ↑ likelihood for hip septic arthritis over transient synovitis with ↑ number of predictors
  - Fever > 38.5°C (101.3°F) , non-weight-bearing, WBC > 12,000 cells/mm³, ESR ≥ 40 mm/hour; later addition to original criteria: CRP > 20 mg/L
    - If all are present, specificity is ~ 60-99%

Demographics

- Peak age: ~ 2-3 years
- Coexistent osteomyelitis in 15-68%

Natural History & Prognosis

- Long-term sequelae in 10-50%
  - Limited motion, dislocation, degeneration, ankylosis, limb length discrepancy, avascular necrosis

Treatment

- Emergent arthroscopy or arthrotomy + joint irrigation
  - Serial joint aspiration + lavage may be acceptable in certain scenarios
- IV antibiotics for 2-4 days followed by oral antibiotics for 10 days; longer course for concomitant osteomyelitis

SELECTED REFERENCES

1. Erkilinc M et al: Current concepts in pediatric septic arthritis. J Am Acad Orthop Surg. 29(5):196-206, 2021
2. Royle LN et al: Inflammatory conditions of the pediatric hand and non-inflammatory mimics. Pediatr Radiol. ePub, 2021
3. Nguyen JC et al: US evaluation of juvenile idiopathic arthritis and osteoarticular infection. Radiographics. 37(4):1181-201, 2017

Transient Synovitis

KEY FACTS

TERMINOLOGY

- Idiopathic, self-limited inflammation of pediatric hip
- Synonyms: Toxic synovitis

IMAGING

- Radiographs: Low sensitivity for hip joint effusion; look for convex gluteal fat pad & medial joint space widening
- US: Highly sensitive for joint fluid
  - Distention of joint capsule by anechoic or hypoechoic fluid
  - ± synovial thickening, hyperemia
- MR: Nonspecific fluid + synovial enhancement
  - Findings favoring transient synovitis over septic arthritis
    - Absence of adjacent marrow or soft tissue edema
    - Normal enhancement/perfusion of femoral head

TOP DIFFERENTIAL DIAGNOSES

- Septic arthritis
- Lyme arthritis
- Juvenile idiopathic arthritis
- Trauma
- Reactive effusion due to adjacent bone pathology

PATHOLOGY

- Viral etiology is considered most likely

CLINICAL ISSUES

- 3-8 years of age; mean: 4.7-5.5 years
- Limping ± pain; fever is typically absent or low
- Kocher criteria: ↑ likelihood for septic arthritis over transient synovitis with ↑ number of positive parameters
  - Fever > 38.5°C (101.3°F), non-weight-bearing, ↑ WBC, ↑ ESR; ↑ CRP is also predictive
- Transient synovitis is self-limited, lasting 7-10 days
- Conservative management with bed rest + NSAIDs
  - Hip aspiration expedites clinical improvement

DIAGNOSTIC CHECKLIST

- Imaging alone cannot exclude infection of fluid

(Left) *AP radiograph of the pelvis in an afebrile 5-year-old with the new onset of a limp & left hip pain shows bowing of the left gluteal fat pad* ➡ *as compared to the normal right side* ➡*, suggesting a left hip joint effusion.* **(Right)** *Sagittal US of the left hip in the same patient shows convex bowing of the joint capsule* ➡ *by hypoechoic fluid that distends the joint at the femoral neck* ➡*. The patient had normal laboratory markers & was successfully treated conservatively for transient synovitis.*

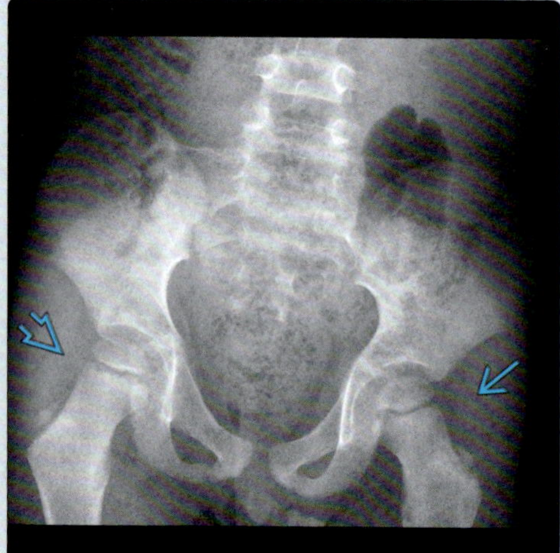

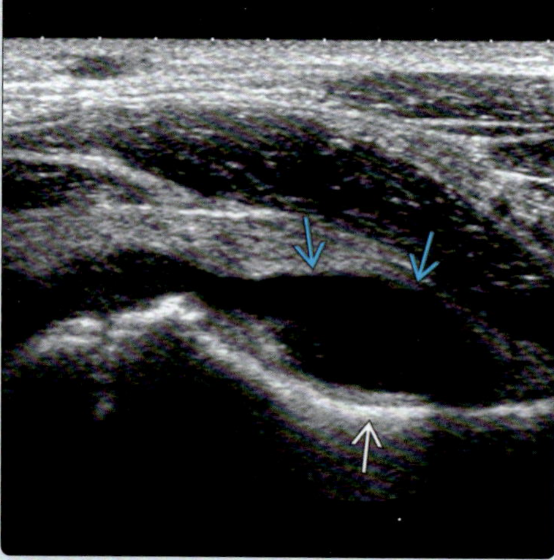

(Left) *Coronal T2 FS MR in a 4-year-old with several days of left thigh pain & limping shows a small left hip joint effusion* ➡ *with no adjacent marrow or soft tissue edema.* **(Right)** *Axial T1 C+ FS MR in the same patient shows mildly ↑ synovial enhancement of the left hip joint* ➡ *as compared to the right. The patient was successfully treated conservatively for transient synovitis given the combination of clinical & imaging features.*

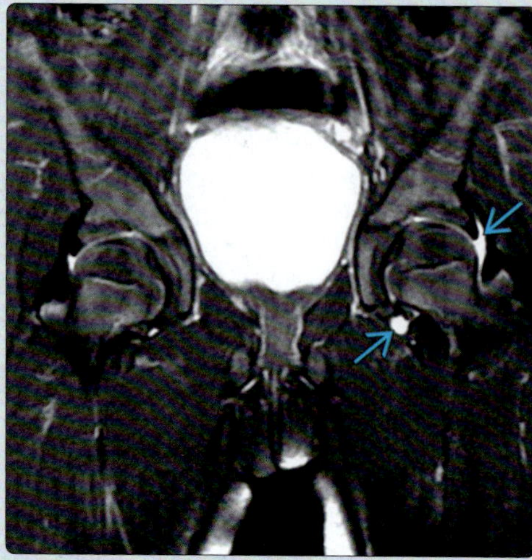

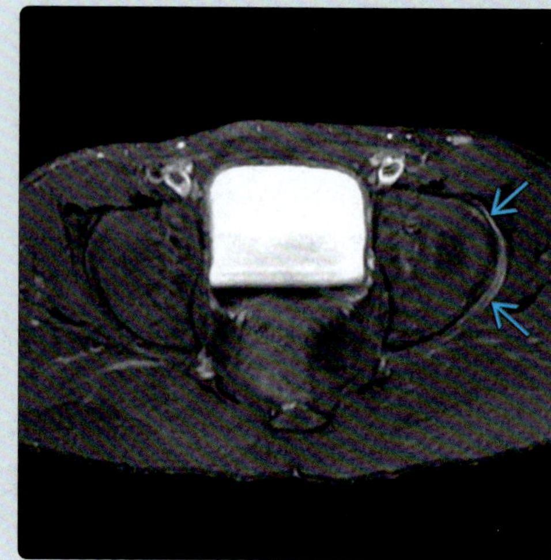

TERMINOLOGY

Synonyms

- Toxic synovitis

Definitions

- Idiopathic, self-limited inflammation of pediatric hip

IMAGING

General Features

- Best diagnostic clue
  - Hip effusion & limp in child with absent to mild systemic findings of inflammation (i.e., fever & elevated serum markers)
- Location
  - Bilateral in ~ 5%

Radiographic Findings

- Low sensitivity for hip joint effusion
- ± convex gluteal fat pad & medial joint space widening

Ultrasonographic Findings

- Distention of joint capsule by fluid
  - Anterior joint capsule demonstrates convex bulge (rather than normal concavity) over femoral neck
- ± synovial thickening, hyperemia

MR Findings

- Features of nonspecific synovitis (with many etiologies)
  - Homogeneously bright T2/STIR fluid in hip joint
  - Mild synovial thickening & enhancement
- Findings favoring transient synovitis over septic arthritis
  - Absence of adjacent marrow or soft tissue edema
  - Normal enhancement/perfusion of femoral head

Imaging Recommendations

- Best imaging tool
  - US: Highly sensitive for hip joint fluid
    - Not specific for sterile vs. infected fluid (regardless of size or complexity)
- Protocol advice
  - US: Patient lies supine with hip in neutral position
    - Anterior oblique approach with transducer oriented along femoral neck long axis
    - Obtain comparison images of contralateral hip
  - MR: Coronal plane is key to compare femoral heads
    - T1, T2 FS/STIR, T1 C+ FS

DIFFERENTIAL DIAGNOSIS

Septic Arthritis

- Favored over transient synovitis with
  - High number of clinical/laboratory Kocher criteria
  - MR showing adjacent marrow & soft tissue edema &/or ↓ enhancement/perfusion of femoral head

Juvenile Idiopathic Arthritis

- ± rice bodies: Numerous, tiny low T2 signal intensity bodies of uniform size throughout joint fluid

Lyme Arthritis

- Presentation tends to be less acute
- Traditionally limited to certain geographic regions

Trauma

- ± marrow & soft tissue edema, ligament & cartilage injuries

Reactive Effusion Due to Adjacent Bone Pathology

- Osteomyelitis, bone tumor, Legg-Calvé-Perthes

PATHOLOGY

General Features

- Viral etiology is more likely than trauma or allergy

CLINICAL ISSUES

Presentation

- Most common signs/symptoms
  - Acute pain + limping; afebrile (> 90%)
    - Pain at groin, thigh, or medial knee
- Clinical profile
  - Kocher criteria must be considered to differentiate from septic arthritis: Fever > 38.5°C (101.3°F), non-weight-bearing, WBC > 12,000 cells/mm^3, ESR ≥ 40 mm/hour
    - ↑ likelihood for septic arthritis with ↑ number of positive parameters
      - CRP > 20 mg/L also suggests septic joint

Demographics

- Typically 3-8 years of age; mean: 4.7-5.5 years
- M:F = 2-3:1

Natural History & Prognosis

- Self-limited; lasts 7-10 days

Treatment

- Conservative management with bed rest + NSAIDs
- Hip aspiration expedites clinical improvement
  - Also allows confident exclusion of septic joint

DIAGNOSTIC CHECKLIST

Consider

- Primary concern: Missing septic joint that needs emergent drainage & IV antibiotics to prevent long-term damage
- Imaging alone cannot exclude infection of fluid
  - Combination of certain clinical & imaging parameters can raise or lower likelihood
  - Joint aspiration is required for 100% confidence

Image Interpretation Pearls

- Synovitis has many etiologies; always consider infection

SELECTED REFERENCES

1. Clever D et al: Pilot study analysis of serum cytokines to differentiate pediatric septic arthritis and transient synovitis. J Pediatr Orthop. 41(10):610-6., 2021
2. Kang MS et al: Differential MRI findings of transient synovitis of the hip in children when septic arthritis is suspected according to symptom duration. J Pediatr Orthop B. 29(3):297-303, 2019
3. Cruz AI Jr et al: Distinguishing pediatric Lyme arthritis of the hip from transient synovitis and acute bacterial septic arthritis: a systematic review and meta-analysis. Cureus. 10(1):e2112, 2018
4. Nouri A et al: Transient synovitis of the hip: a comprehensive review. J Pediatr Orthop B. 23(1):32-6, 2014
5. Kim EY et al: Usefulness of dynamic contrast-enhanced MRI in differentiating between septic arthritis and transient synovitis in the hip joint. AJR Am J Roentgenol. 198(2):428-33, 2012

Soft Tissue Abscess

KEY FACTS

TERMINOLOGY

- Abscess: Walled-off, liquefied collection of necrotic tissue, inflammatory cells, & bacteria

IMAGING

- Most commonly affects single site: Expected lymph node location vs. other subcutaneous or intramuscular focus
  - Septic emboli can cause multifocal collections
- US: Excellent for detecting superficial collections & defining drainability
  - Thick-walled, centrally avascular collection with surrounding edema ± hyperemia
  - Swirling internal debris upon compression
- MR: Clearly defines deep extent, evaluates adjacent bone/joint, & helps exclude other diagnoses
  - Centrally nonenhancing fluid collection with thick, enhancing wall & peripheral, poorly defined edema
  - Restricted diffusion centrally

TOP DIFFERENTIAL DIAGNOSES

- Soft tissue sarcoma
- Lymphatic malformation
- Hematoma
- Myositis ossificans
- Morel-Lavalleé lesion

PATHOLOGY

- *Staphylococcus aureus* > > streptococcal species
- *Bartonella henselae*: Regional lymphadenitis ± suppuration in cat-scratch disease

CLINICAL ISSUES

- Presentation: Swelling, erythema, tenderness, limited motion, fever; ± fluctuance, sepsis
- Treatment: Drainage procedure + IV antibiotics
  - Whole-body MR may be useful to screen large territories for drainable collections in setting of systemic infection

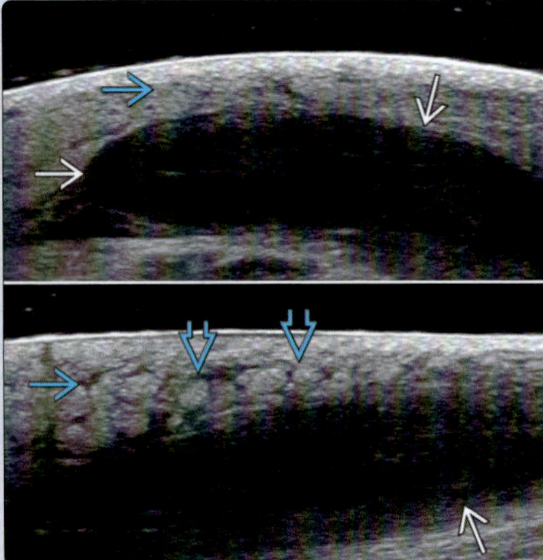

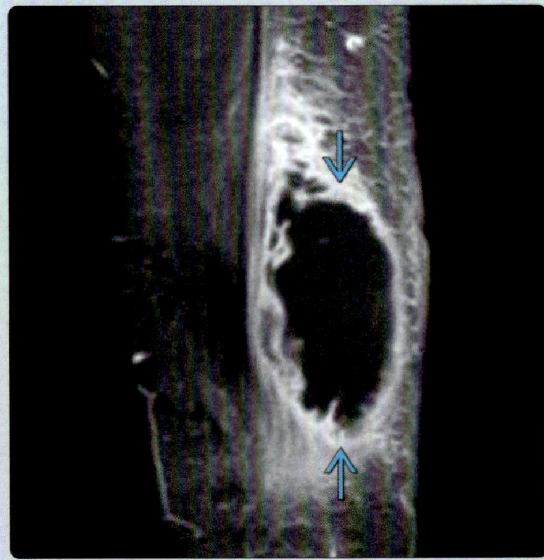

(Left) *Longitudinal US images in an 11-year-old with thigh swelling & tenderness show thickening & reticular edema of the subcutaneous fat ⇨ overlying a heterogeneously hypoechoic, ovoid collection ➡. The more inferior image demonstrates the typical cobblestone appearance of the fat ⇨ that can imply purulence.* **(Right)** *Sagittal T1 C+ FS MR in the same patient shows thick, irregular rim enhancement of the fluid collection ⇨, typical of an abscess. Pus was encountered upon surgical drainage.*

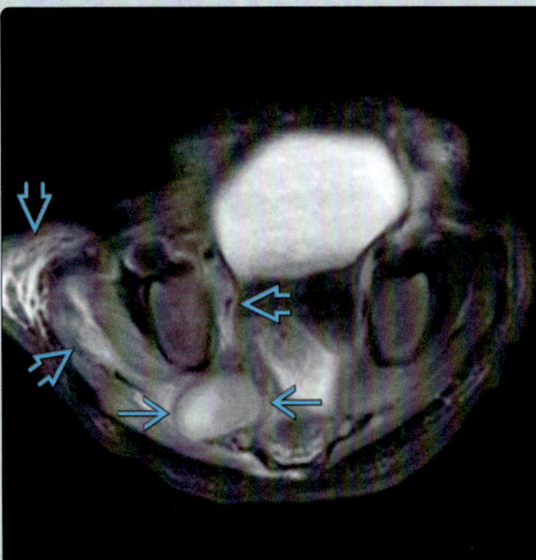

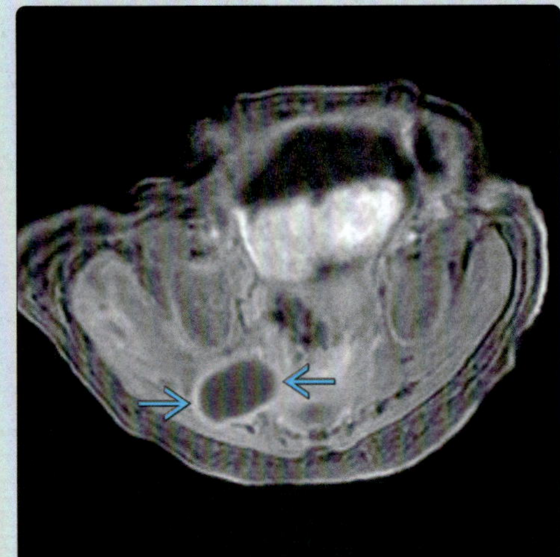

(Left) *Axial T2 FS MR in a 20-day-old with Staphylococcus aureus bacteremia shows a well-defined collection ⇨ traversing the right greater sciatic notch with a low-signal rim & high-signal center. Note the adjacent soft tissue edema ⇨.* **(Right)** *Axial T1 C+ FS MR in the same patient shows only rim enhancement of the collection ⇨, typical of an abscess. This collection was percutaneously drained.*

TERMINOLOGY

Definitions

- Suppurative or purulent: Pus forming/pus containing
- Abscess: Walled-off, liquefied collection of necrotic tissue, inflammatory cells, & bacteria
- Phlegmon: Poorly defined focus of necrotic & inflammatory tissue ± components of liquefaction
- Cellulitis: Poorly defined changes of superficial (i.e., skin & subcutaneous fat) soft tissue infections
- Fasciitis: Inflammation in & along superficial & deep fascial planes investing muscles
- Pyomyositis: Deep muscle infection
- Skin & soft tissue infections (SSTI): Any of above

IMAGING

General Features

- Best diagnostic clue
  - US: Focal, thick-walled, avascular collection with swirling internal echoes (upon compressions) & overlying edema
  - MR: Centrally nonenhancing fluid collection with thick, enhancing wall & peripheral, poorly defined edema

Radiographic Findings

- Edema: Subcutaneous reticulation with blurring of normally sharp fat-muscle interfaces
- ± focal bulge at site of collection
- ± retained foreign body, gas

Ultrasonographic Findings

- Grayscale ultrasound
  - Well-defined collection with thick, irregular wall
  - Contents range from anechoic to isoechoic
    - Internal debris swirls with dynamic compression
  - Branching interstitial fluid throughout edematous & lobulated subcutaneous fat ("cobblestoning")
    - May also be purulent; overlaps with classic description of nonpurulent cellulitis
  - May detect retained foreign body
- Color Doppler
  - No internal vascularity; ± ↑ peripheral vascularity

MR Findings

- T2 FS/STIR
  - Collection of hyperintense fluid centrally
  - Wall may show hypointense inner rim (minerals, hemorrhage, fibrous tissue) & hyperintense outer rim (granulation tissue)
  - Surrounding edema
- T1 C+ FS: Mildly thickened, irregular, enhancing rim after contrast without substantial nodularity
- DWI: Restricted diffusion centrally

Imaging Recommendations

- Best imaging tool
  - US is excellent for detecting superficial collections & defining drainability
  - MR more clearly defines collection deep extent & relationships to vital structures, evaluates adjacent bone & cartilage, & helps exclude other diagnoses

DIFFERENTIAL DIAGNOSIS

Soft Tissue Sarcoma

- Typically solid, well-circumscribed mass with little (if any) surrounding edema

Lymphatic Malformation

- Multicystic mass crossing soft tissue compartments
- Fluid-fluid levels due to internal hemorrhage

Myositis Ossificans

- Heterogeneous, intramuscular mass with marked surrounding edema
- Peripheral Ca^{2+} within weeks is diagnostic

Morel-Lavalleé Lesion

- Closed degloving injury of subcutaneous fat, usually over bony protuberance
- Typically elongated with angular margins
- Often contains foci of fat in collection

PATHOLOGY

General Features

- Most common organisms
  - *Staphylococcus aureus* > > streptococcal species
    - ↑ incidence of methicillin-resistant *S. aureus* (MRSA) → ↑ number of SSTIs in last 20 years
  - *Bartonella henselae*: Regional lymphadenitis ± suppuration in cat-scratch disease
    - Axillary, epitrochlear > head/neck or inguinal nodes

CLINICAL ISSUES

Presentation

- Swelling, erythema, tenderness, limited motion, fever; ± fluctuance, septic shock

Treatment

- Drainage procedure + IV antibiotics
  - Drainage may not be necessary if collection is < 2 cm in noncritical location

DIAGNOSTIC CHECKLIST

Image Interpretation Pearls

- US cine clips with dynamic compression can help confirm drainable fluid within collection
- Make sure US visualizes entirety of soft tissues down to bone → prevents missing deep collection
  - Cortical irregularity & subperiosteal collections can provide clue about site of origin (i.e., osteomyelitis)

SELECTED REFERENCES

1. Altmayer S et al: Imaging musculoskeletal soft tissue infections. Semin Ultrasound CT MR. 41(1):85-98, 2020
2. Nelson CE et al: Ultrasound features of purulent skin and soft tissue infection without abscess. Emerg Radiol. 25(5):505-11, 2018
3. Chang CD et al: Imaging of musculoskeletal soft tissue infection. Semin Roentgenol. 52(1):55-62, 2017
4. Pattamapaspong N et al: Pitfalls in imaging of musculoskeletal infections. Semin Musculoskelet Radiol. 18(1):86-100, 2014

Juvenile Idiopathic Arthritis

KEY FACTS

TERMINOLOGY

- Synovial inflammation of unknown cause
- Diagnostic criteria
  - Arthritis begins < 16 years of age
  - ≥ 6 weeks of symptoms
  - Other conditions have been excluded
- International League of Associations for Rheumatology (ILAR) classification of juvenile idiopathic arthritis (JIA)
  - Systemic arthritis: Arthritis of ≥ 1 joint + daily spiking fever for ≥ 3 consecutive days
    - Accompanied by ≥ 1 of following: Evanescent rash, hepatomegaly &/or splenomegaly, serositis
  - Oligoarticular arthritis: Arthritis of < 5 joints in first 6 months of disease
  - Polyarticular arthritis: Arthritis of ≥ 5 joints in first 6 months of disease; RF positive or negative
  - Psoriatic arthritis
  - Enthesitis-related arthritis
  - Undifferentiated or unclassified arthritis

IMAGING

- Radiographs: Classic findings are seen late in disease
  - Early to intermediate: Osteoporosis, periarticular soft tissue swelling, joint capsule distention (by effusion &/or thickened synovium/pannus), marginal erosions
  - Late: Joint space loss with gradual ankylosis, growth disturbances (e.g., hypoplasia vs. overgrowth)
- MR: Joint effusion with synovial thickening & enhancement, bone marrow edema, cartilage loss ± bone erosions
  - Hypointense rice bodies in joint fluid
- US: Compressible hypoechoic joint fluid vs. noncompressible synovial pannus
  - Color/power Doppler for active vs. inactive synovitis

CLINICAL ISSUES

- Presents with joint swelling/effusion, stiffness, pain & tenderness, ↑ warmth
- 1-3 years of age (largest peak); 8-10 years (smaller peak)

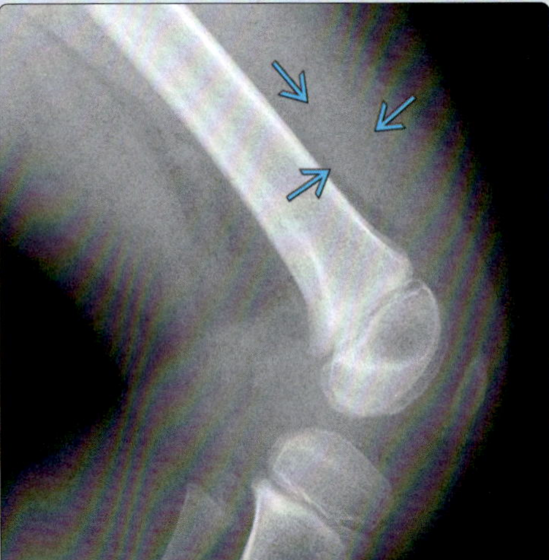

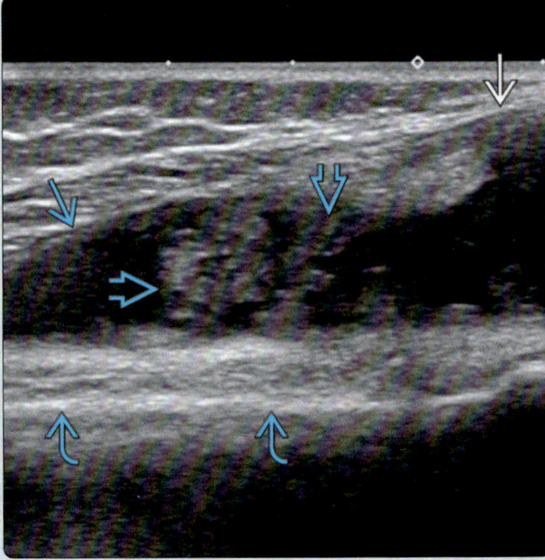

(Left) *Lateral radiograph in a 5-year-old with weeks of knee pain & swelling shows a moderate joint effusion distending the suprapatellar pouch.* **(Right)** *Longitudinal US of the knee in the same patient shows hypoechoic fluid distending the suprapatellar pouch. There is moderate internal debris with regions of synovial thickening due to juvenile idiopathic arthritis (JIA). The patella & femur are noted for reference.*

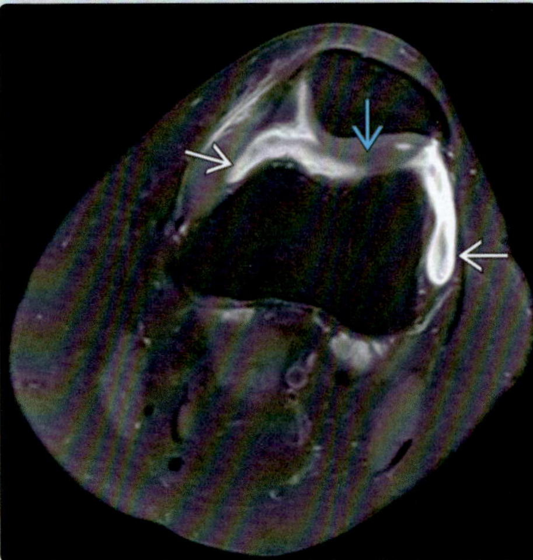

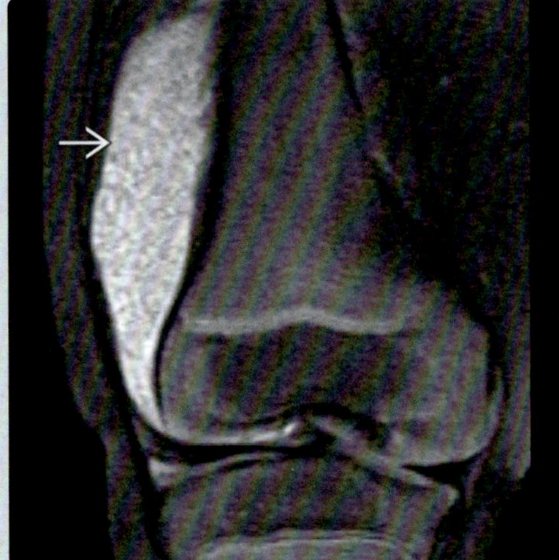

(Left) *Axial T1 C+ FS MR in an 18-year-old with a history of JIA shows moderate diffuse synovial thickening & enhancement (synovitis) of the knee. Only a small joint effusion is present.* **(Right)** *Coronal T2 FS MR in a toddler with JIA shows a large knee joint effusion containing numerous small (& uniform in size) hypointense rice bodies.*

TERMINOLOGY

Synonyms

- Juvenile rheumatoid arthritis (JRA), juvenile chronic arthritis

Definitions

- Juvenile idiopathic arthritis (JIA): Synovial inflammation of unknown cause
- Diagnostic criteria: Arthritis begins < 16 years of age, ≥ 6 weeks of symptoms, & other conditions excluded (diagnosis of exclusion)
- Most widely used classification developed by International League of Associations for Rheumatology (ILAR)
  - Systemic arthritis (sJIA), previously known as Still disease: 10-20%
    - Arthritis of ≥ 1 joint + fever of ≥ 2-weeks duration with daily (quotidian) fever for at least 3 consecutive days
    - Accompanied by ≥ 1 of following: Evanescent rash, hepatomegaly &/or splenomegaly, serositis (pericarditis, pleuritis, peritonitis), generalized lymphadenopathy
    - Can be associated with interstitial lung disease, macrophage activation syndrome, amyloidosis
  - Oligoarticular arthritis: Most common form of JIA (50%)
    - Arthritis of < 5 joints in first 6 months of disease
      - Persistent: < 5 joints affected during entire disease
      - Extended: ≥ 5 joints affected after first 6 months
    - Young girls
    - Large joints: Knee, ankle, elbow
    - Iridocyclitis in up to 30%
  - Polyarticular rheumatoid factor (RF)-positive arthritis
    - Arthritis of ≥ 5 joints in first 6 months of disease
    - ≥ 2 positive tests for RF at least 3 months apart within first 6 months of disease
    - More commonly adolescent girls
    - Typical: Symmetric, small joints of hands
  - Polyarticular RF-negative arthritis
    - Arthritis of ≥ 5 joints in first 6 months of disease
    - No characteristic pattern
    - Any age throughout childhood
  - Psoriatic arthritis (< 15%)
    - Arthritis & psoriasis or arthritis & ≥ 2 of following: Dactylitis ("sausage digit"), nail pitting or onycholysis, psoriasis in 1st-degree relative
  - Enthesitis-related arthritis (< 7%)
    - Arthritis & enthesitis, or
    - Arthritis or enthesitis with ≥ 2 of following
      - Sacroiliac joint tenderness &/or inflammatory lumbosacral pain
      - Positive HLA-B27 antigen test
      - Onset of arthritis in male ≥ 6 years old
      - Symptomatic anterior uveitis
      - Presence of 1st-degree relative with ankylosing spondylitis, enthesitis-related arthritis, inflammatory bowel disease with sacroiliitis, Reiter syndrome, or acute anterior uveitis
    - Enthesitis is most commonly at Achilles, plantar fascia
  - Undifferentiated arthritis
    - Does not fulfill criteria for any category or fulfills criteria for multiple categories

IMAGING

General Features

- Best diagnostic clue
  - Joint effusion with synovial thickening & enhancement in patient with symptoms suggestive of JIA
- Location
  - Any joint; large joints are most common
    - Polyarticular also involves small joints (hands & feet)
    - Cervical spine apophyseal joints are rare at presentation but > 50% eventually develop involvement

Radiographic Findings

- Classic findings are seen late in disease
- General
  - Early to intermediate: Osteoporosis, periarticular soft tissue swelling, joint capsule distention (by effusion &/or pannus/thickened synovium), marginal erosions
  - Late: Joint space loss with gradual ankylosis, subluxation, adjacent periosteal reaction, growth disturbances (including shortening/hypoplasia due to premature growth plate closure, enlarged overgrown epiphyses, limb length discrepancy)
- Mandible
  - Micrognathia or unilateral hypoplasia
  - Antegonial notching of mandible (concave undersurface)
- Wrist
  - Squared or angular carpal bones
  - Carpal erosions (which overlap normal indentations)
  - Accelerated maturation
- Hip
  - Coxa valga, coxa magna, protrusio acetabuli
  - Overgrowth of femoral capital epiphysis
  - Abnormal growth of femoral neck
- Knee
  - Squared inferior margin of patella
  - Widened intercondylar notch
- Cervical spine
  - Atlantoaxial subluxation
  - ↓ disc space with narrowed vertebral body height, ankylosis

MR Findings

- Only modality for marrow edema (preerosive finding)
- Most sensitive technique for detecting active inflammation (synovitis & marrow edema)
- T2 FS/STIR
  - Intermediate to hyperintense pannus & hyperintense joint effusion
    - Small, hypointense rice bodies (generally of uniform size): Detached fragments of necrotic synovium
  - Patchy, hyperintense marrow edema
  - Cartilage loss ± bone erosions
  - Hyperintense tenosynovitis: Most common at extensor tendons of hand & feet, peroneal & posterior tibialis tendons of ankle
  - Hypoplastic menisci & cruciate ligaments
  - Regional lymphadenopathy
- T1 C+ FS

- Early scanning after contrast administration (< 5 minutes) is most sensitive & specific for abnormal synovium
  - Contrast gradually leaks into joint fluid
- Actively inflamed enhancing synovium largely outlines (except where synovium is routinely lacking) nonenhancing joint effusion &/or fibrotic/necrotic pannus
  - Early dynamic synovial enhancement correlates with active disease & better reflects treatment response than synovial volumes
- T2* GRE
  - Marginal erosions
- Advanced techniques
  - T2 mapping, DTI, perfusion,T1 rho, dGEMRIC: May reveal microstructural cartilage changes prior to conventional sequences

Ultrasonographic Findings

- More sensitive for synovitis than clinical exam
- Distinguishes articular vs. tenosynovial disease
- Compressible hypoechoic joint fluid vs. noncompressible, synovial pannus
- Color/power Doppler is helpful for active vs. inactive synovitis
  - Developing role for CEUS
- Can visualize some erosions, evaluate cartilage thickness
- Guides injections & biopsies

DIFFERENTIAL DIAGNOSIS

Septic Arthritis

- Majority are monoarticular, often from adjacent osteomyelitis
  - *Staphylococcus aureus* is most common
- Rapid presentation with adjacent marrow & soft tissue edema favor infection
  - Synovial thickening is typically less severe in acute pyogenic infections as compared to JIA
- Kocher criteria: If specific thresholds are met for fever, non-weight-bearing, leukocytosis, ESR, & CRP → strongly favor infected joint
  - Urgent washout is required to prevent long-term damage

Transient Synovitis

- Self-limited, typically at hip of children 3-6 years of age
- Diagnosis of exclusion: Absence of Kocher criteria

Recent Trauma

- Nonspecific effusion ± synovitis with trauma history

Leukemia

- Can present with arthritis symptoms
- ± lucent metaphyseal bands, permeative lesions, osteoporosis

Synovial Venous Malformation

- Septated, fluid-filled channels/cysts infiltrating synovium → hemarthrosis → eventual joint degeneration
- ± phleboliths, fluid-fluid levels, delayed patchy enhancement

Lyme Disease

- Characteristic rash + history of tick bite

Hemophilic Arthropathy

- Relevant clinical history is usually apparent
- Repetitive hemorrhage into joints with hemosiderin deposition & eventual joint degeneration

Pigmented Villonodular Synovitis

- Monoarticular with hemosiderin deposition

CLINICAL ISSUES

Presentation

- Most common signs/symptoms
  - Arthritis (≥ 1 joints): Swelling/effusion, stiffness, pain & tenderness, ↑ warmth
- Other signs/symptoms
  - Fatigue, fevers, weight loss, rash, growth failure
  - TMJs are often involved but often asymptomatic

Demographics

- Age
  - 1-3 years (largest peak); 8-10 years (smaller peak)
- Sex
  - M < F overall; systemic form: M = F

Treatment

- NSAIDs, systemic/local corticosteroids, disease-modifying agents (e.g., methotrexate), biologic agents (monoclonal antibodies or soluble receptors), anti-TNF
- Interleukin-1 & interleukin-6 inhibitors
- Stem cell transplant in very rare cases

DIAGNOSTIC CHECKLIST

Consider

- Whole-body MR may have prognostic & therapeutic implications, as active synovitis may be detected in clinically asymptomatic joints

Image Interpretation Pearls

- Synovitis has many causes; use clinical & imaging clues to narrow differential diagnosis
  - Do not overlook septic arthritis
- Difficult to distinguish ongoing active inflammation vs. reactive & degenerative changes in longstanding JIA

SELECTED REFERENCES

1. Pracoń G et al: Conventional radiography and ultrasound imaging of rheumatic diseases affecting the pediatric population. Semin Musculoskelet Radiol. 25(1):68-81, 2021
2. Schiettecatte E et al: MR imaging of rheumatic diseases affecting the pediatric population. Semin Musculoskelet Radiol. 25(1):82-93, 2021
3. Lee JJY et al: Systemic juvenile idiopathic arthritis. Pediatr Clin North Am. 65(4):691-709, 2018
4. Hemke R et al: Magnetic resonance imaging (MRI) of the knee as an outcome measure in juvenile idiopathic arthritis: an OMERACT reliability study on MRI scales. J Rheumatol. 44(8):1224-30, 2017
5. Nguyen JC et al: US evaluation of juvenile idiopathic arthritis and osteoarticular infection. Radiographics. 37(4):1181-201, 2017
6. Avenarius DF et al: Erosion or normal variant? 4-year MRI follow-up of the wrists in healthy children. Pediatr Radiol. 46(3):322-30, 2016
7. Sheybani EF et al: Imaging of juvenile idiopathic arthritis: a multimodality approach. Radiographics. 33(5):1253-73, 2013

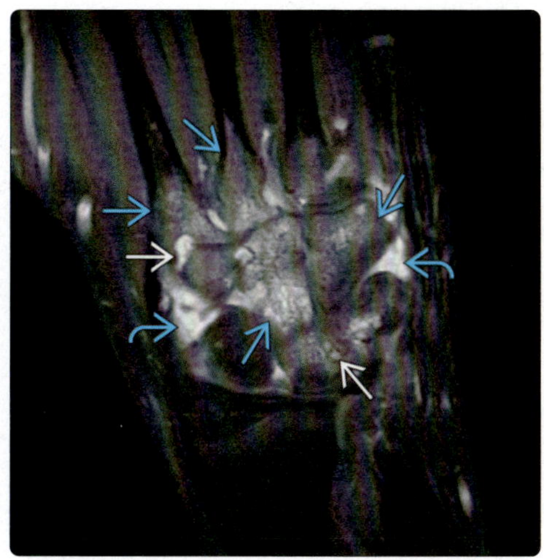

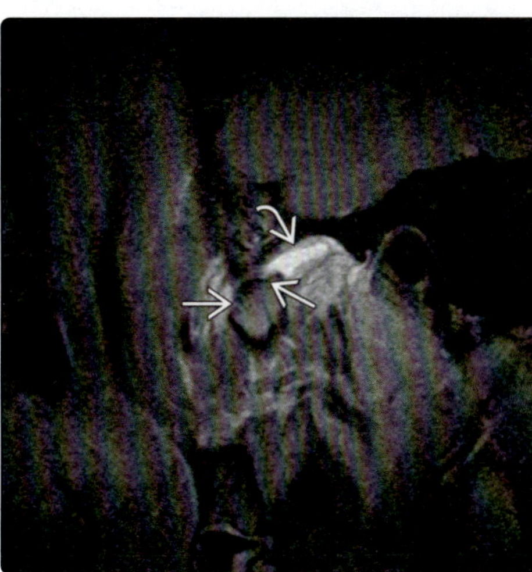

(Left) *Coronal T1 C+ FS MR in a teenager shows multiple wrist erosions ➡ & moderate synovial enhancement (or synovitis) ➡. The marrow edema ➡ is much more extensive than seen on the precontrast T1 sequence (not shown).* **(Right)** *Open-mouth sagittal T1 C+ FS MR of the TMJ shows erosions & flattening of the mandibular condyle ➡ with synovial thickening & enhancement ➡. The normally visible articular disc is unrecognizable, & is likely degenerated & torn.*

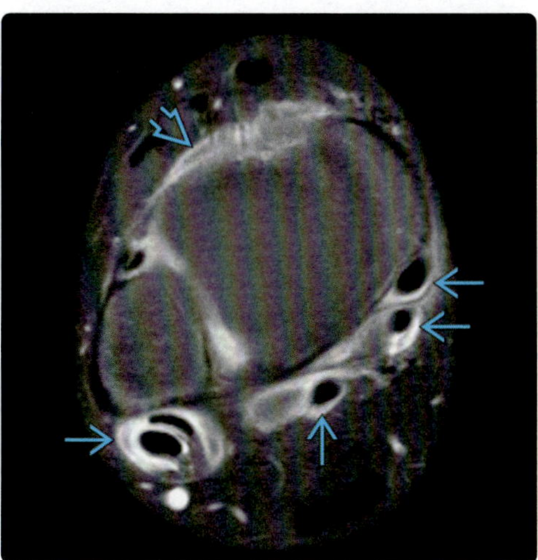

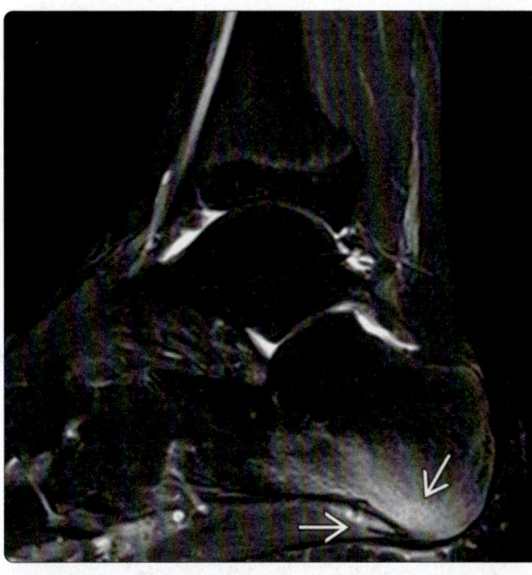

(Left) *Axial T1 C+ FS MR of the ankle ➡ shows marked synovial enhancement (or tenosynovitis) surrounding the posterior tibial, flexor digitorum longus, flexor hallucis longus, & peroneal tendons. Diffuse ankle joint synovitis ➡ was also present.* **(Right)** *Sagittal T2 FS MR in a 17-year-old with a history of JIA shows plantar fascial enthesitis with edema ➡ of the calcaneal bone marrow & adjacent soft tissues at & surrounding the attachment of the plantar fascia.*

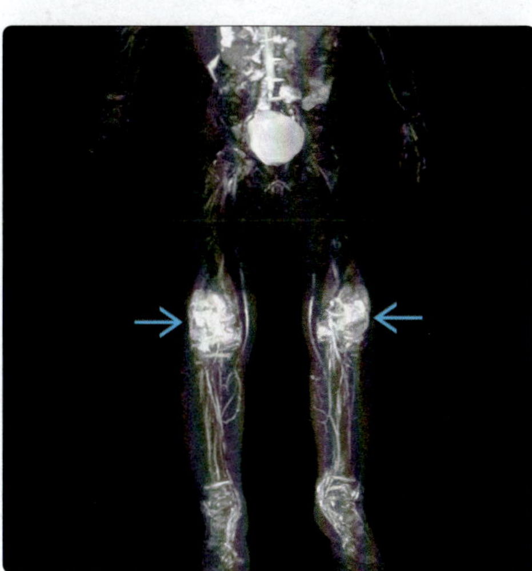

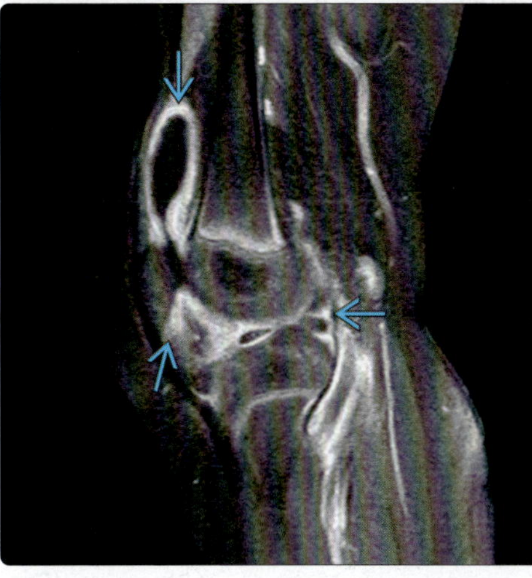

(Left) *Coronal STIR MR MIP in a 15-month-old girl with refusal to bear weight for days shows synovial proliferation at multiple joints but is most pronounced at the knees ➡. The patient had ↑ inflammatory markers & was ultimately diagnosed with polyarticular JIA.* **(Right)** *Sagittal T1 C+ FS MR of the right knee in the same patient shows moderate synovial thickening ➡ with a moderate joint effusion. The degree of synovial thickening is > typically seen with septic arthritis.*

KEY FACTS

TERMINOLOGY

- Juvenile dermatomyositis (JDM): Diffuse, nonsuppurative inflammation of striated muscle, subcutaneous fat, & skin
- Most common (85%) of juvenile idiopathic inflammatory myopathies

IMAGING

- Patchy to diffusely infiltrative ↑ fluid signal intensity of muscles on STIR or T2 FS MR
  - Symmetric involvement of proximal musculature
    - Thighs > pelvis > shoulders
      - Vastus lateralis & intermedius are most common
  - ± fatty muscle infiltration & atrophy chronically; not prominent feature early
- Subcutaneous fat involvement: High specificity (but low sensitivity) for predicting progression to chronic forms
- Soft tissue Ca^{2+} (30-70%)
  - Develops months to years after disease onset; usually periarticular

CLINICAL ISSUES

- Median age of onset of JDM: 7-11 years
- Most common symptoms
  - Proximal muscle weakness ± tenderness, easily fatigued
  - Rash (heliotrope eyelid rash & Gottron papules)
- Other manifestations: Arthritis, pericarditis, pulmonary fibrosis, gastrointestinal symptoms, including dysphagia & ulceration, fever, weight loss
- JDM diagnosis is classically made by characteristic skin rash + 3 of following
  - Symmetric proximal muscle weakness
  - ↑ muscle enzymes in serum
  - Characteristic electromyography
  - Characteristic changes on muscle biopsy
- Diagnosis confirmation now more commonly employs characteristic MR findings & autoantibody profiles
- Variable disease course: Up to 73% with active disease > 10 years after diagnosis; 3% mortality

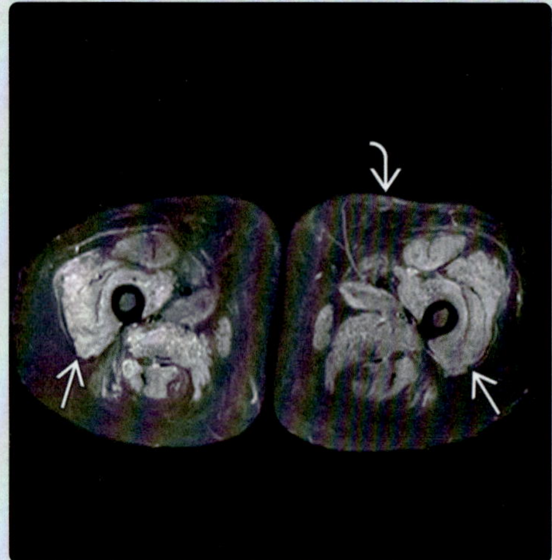

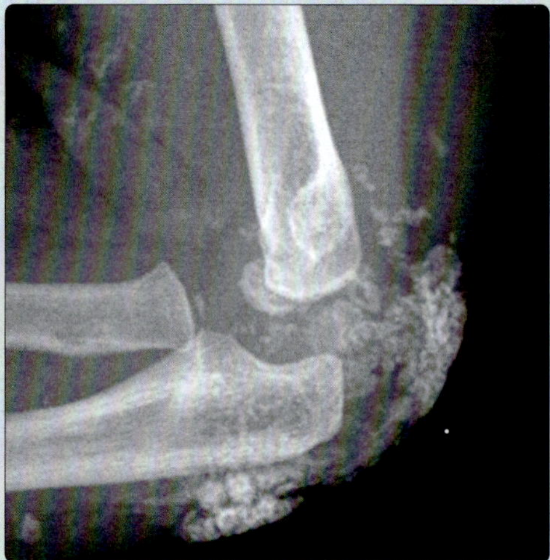

(Left) *Axial STIR MR in a 12-year-old patient with proximal muscle weakness, myalgias, & a malar heliotrope rash shows diffuse symmetric muscle abnormalities of the bilateral thighs, including ↓ muscle bulk & muscle edema ➡. Hyperintense signal within the subcutaneous fat ➡ has a significant association with a more aggressive course of juvenile dermatomyositis (JDM).* **(Right)** *Lateral elbow radiograph shows diffuse, periarticular Ca^{2+} in this young patient several years after the initial presentation of JDM.*

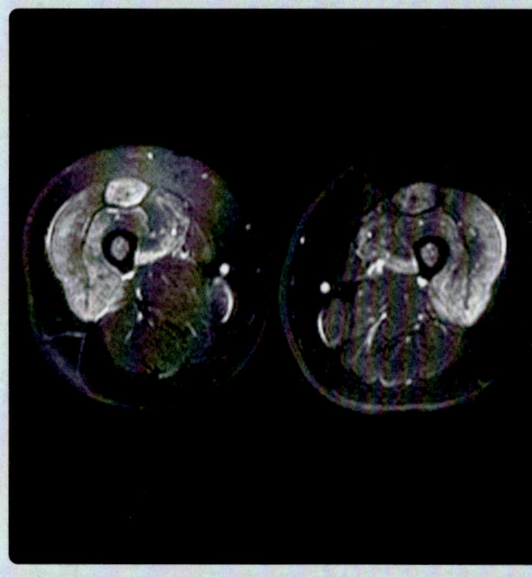

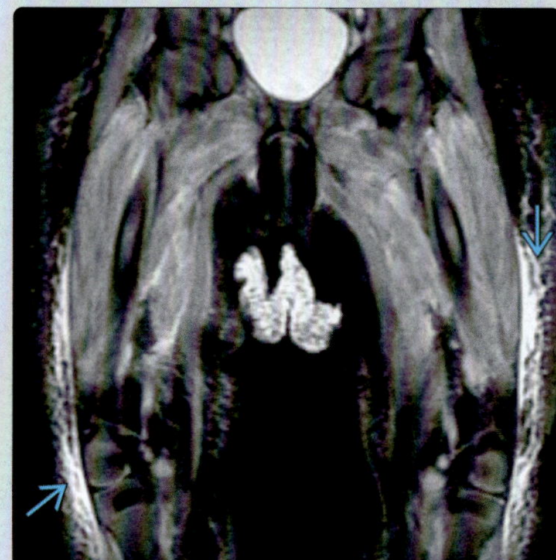

(Left) *Axial T2 FS MR in an 8-year-old girl with suspected JDM shows abnormal hyperintense signal of muscles within the anterior compartments of both thighs. The study was performed to help localize a biopsy target.* **(Right)** *Coronal STIR MR in a patient with JDM shows diffusely infiltrating, hyperintense signal abnormalities in all visible pelvic & thigh musculature. Extensive reticular signal abnormalities of the subcutaneous fat ➡ are also noted.*

TERMINOLOGY

Definitions

- Juvenile dermatomyositis (JDM): Diffuse, nonsuppurative inflammation of striated muscle, subcutaneous fat, & skin
- Most common (85%) of juvenile idiopathic inflammatory myopathies

IMAGING

General Features

- Best diagnostic clue
  - Patchy to diffusely infiltrative ↑ fluid signal intensity of muscles on MR, symmetric in anterior thighs & pelvis
- Location
  - Proximal musculature: Thighs > pelvis > shoulders
    - Most common: Vastus lateralis & vastus intermedius
  - ± pharyngeal striated muscles → dysphagia

Radiographic Findings

- Soft tissue Ca^{2+} (30-70% of JDM patients)
  - Develops from months to years after disease onset
  - Amorphous, globular, or sheet-like; usually periarticular

CT Findings

- High-resolution NECT of lung
  - Interstitial lung disease, chest wall Ca^{2+}, airway disease
  - ≥ 50% of JDM patients have abnormal pulmonary function tests

MR Findings

- Streaky or infiltrative ↑ fluid signal intensity (edema) of affected muscles, most conspicuous on T2 FS or STIR
- ± elongated, crescentic, & reticular foci of fluid signal intensity along fascial planes & in subcutaneous fat
  - Subcutaneous fat involvement: High specificity (but low sensitivity) for predicting progression to chronic forms
    - May lead to calcinosis or lipodystrophy (focal or generalized subcutaneous fat loss)
- ± chronic fatty muscle atrophy (not predominant feature)
- Whole-body STIR MR: Potential screening for disease extent &/or therapy-induced osteonecrosis (ON)

PATHOLOGY

General Features

- Etiology
  - Common reports of preceding illness or ultraviolet exposure
  - Multiple autoantibodies have been identified
    - Profiles/panels are helpful in distinguishing subtypes of myopathy & myositis overlap syndromes

Staging, Grading, & Classification

- Classifications of JDM disease patterns include
  - Limited, chronic nonulcerative, chronic ulcerative (involves skin & gastrointestinal tract)
  - Monocyclic, polycyclic, chronic continuous

CLINICAL ISSUES

Presentation

- Most common signs/symptoms
  - Symmetric proximal muscle weakness ± tenderness; easily fatigued
- Other signs/symptoms
  - Heliotrope rash & Gottron papules are classic; may occur prior to, during, or after muscle weakness symptoms
    - Heliotrope rash: Purplish or violet rash of upper > lower eyelids
    - Gottron papules: Elevated violaceous papules on extensor surfaces of metacarpophalangeal, proximal interphalangeal, or distal interphalangeal joints of hands; elbows & knees are also affected
  - Other cutaneous manifestations
    - Periungual telangiectasis, scaly alopecia, ulcers
    - Photosensitive rash
    - Shawl sign: Poikilodermatous rash on upper chest or V-shaped rash on upper back
  - Subcutaneous & periorbital edema
  - Other manifestations: Arthritis, pericarditis, pulmonary fibrosis, gastrointestinal symptoms, including dysphagia & ulceration, fever, weight loss
- JDM diagnosis is classically made by characteristic skin rash + 3 of following
  - Symmetric proximal muscle weakness
  - ↑ muscle enzymes in serum
    - Creatine kinase (CK), aldolase, aspartate aminotransferase (AST), lactate dehydrogenase (LDH)
  - Characteristic electromyography
  - Characteristic changes on muscle biopsy
- Diagnosis confirmation now more commonly employs combination of characteristic MR findings & autoantibody profiles in correct clinical setting

Demographics

- Age
  - Median age of onset of JDM: 7-11 years
  - Bimodal distribution of dermatomyositis overall
    - 5-14 years is less common than 40s-50s
- Epidemiology
  - 3-5/1,000,000

Natural History & Prognosis

- Variable course of disease
  - Up to 73% with active disease > 10 years after diagnosis
- Complications: Calcinosis, contractures, ON (steroids)
- Mortality up to 3%

SELECTED REFERENCES

1. Zadig P et al: Whole-body magnetic resonance imaging in children - how and why? A systematic review. Pediatr Radiol. 51(1):14-24, 2021
2. Sag E et al: Clinical features, muscle biopsy scores, myositis specific antibody profiles and outcome in juvenile dermatomyositis. Semin Arthritis Rheum. 51(1):95-100, 2020
3. Sudoł-Szopińska I et al: Imaging in dermatomyositis in adults and children. J Ultrason. 20(80):e36-42, 2020
4. Pachman LM et al: Advances in juvenile dermatomyositis: myositis specific antibodies aid in understanding disease heterogeneity. J Pediatr. 195:16-27, 2018
5. Bellutti Enders F et al: Consensus-based recommendations for the management of juvenile dermatomyositis. Ann Rheum Dis. 76(2):329-40, 2017
6. Damasio MB et al: Whole-body MRI: non-oncological applications in paediatrics. Radiol Med. 121(5): 454-61, 2016
7. Deakin CT et al: Muscle biopsy findings in combination with myositis-specific autoantibodies aid prediction of outcomes in juvenile dermatomyositis. Arthritis Rheumatol. 68(11):2806-16, 2016

Chronic Recurrent Multifocal Osteomyelitis

KEY FACTS

TERMINOLOGY

- Idiopathic disorder with nonpyogenic inflammatory bone lesions, typically multifocal with relapsing/remitting course
- Associated with other inflammatory conditions (e.g., psoriasis, inflammatory bowel disease)

IMAGING

- Multiple sites involved over course of disease: > 80%
  - Can be bilateral with relatively symmetric distribution
- Most commonly at periphyseal long bone metaphyses or metaphyseal-equivalent regions
- Most common sites: Tibia, femur, clavicle, spine, pelvis
  - Most common disease to involve medial clavicle
- Radiographs: Features may be mixed at presentation
  - Acute: Lytic lesion (usually in metaphysis near physis)
  - Late: Progressive adjacent sclerosis
  - Recurrence: New lytic areas or periosteal reaction
- MR with contrast
  - Edema & enhancement of lesion & surrounding marrow
  - ± soft tissue & periosteal inflammation but no abscess
  - ± mild reactive adjacent joint effusion/synovitis

TOP DIFFERENTIAL DIAGNOSES

- Bacterial osteomyelitis
- Ewing sarcoma
- Langerhans cell histiocytosis
- Leukemia
- Scurvy

CLINICAL ISSUES

- Most common age: 9-14 years
- Typically presents with symptoms at 1 site
  - Most (not all) develop other symptomatic sites

DIAGNOSTIC CHECKLIST

- Whole-body MR or bone scan to screen asymptomatic sites
- Report physeal involvement (due to risk of premature physeal closure)

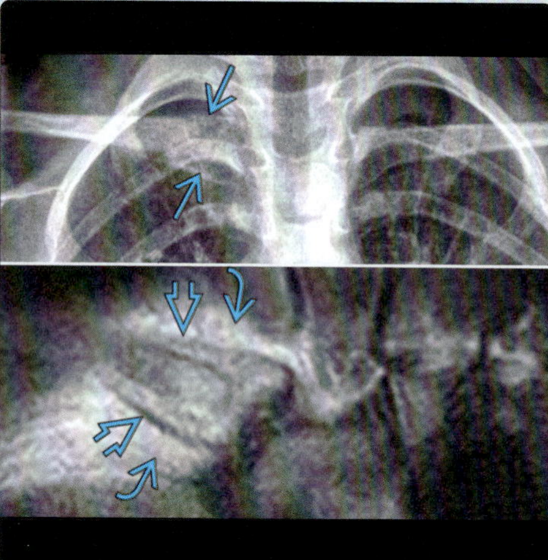

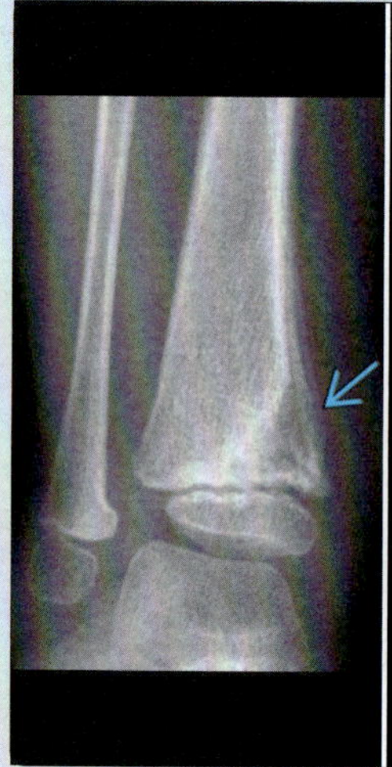

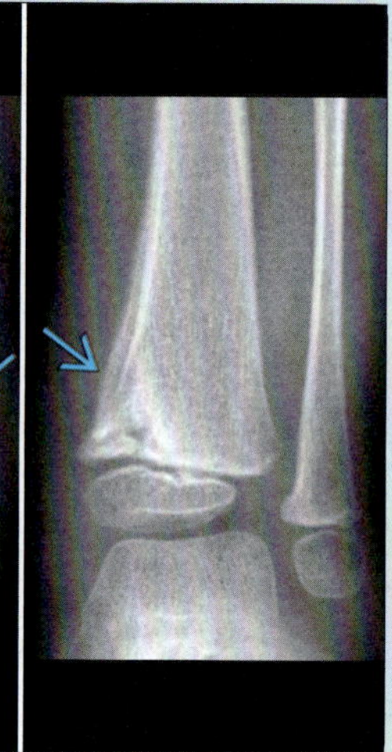

(Left) *AP radiograph (top) in a 4-year-old girl with right clavicle & bilateral ankle pain shows expansion & permeation of the right medial clavicle ➔. On the coronal STIR MR (bottom), there is ↑ signal within & periosteal reaction along the right clavicle ➔ with adjacent soft tissue inflammation ➔.* **(Right)** *Frontal ankle radiographs in the same child with chronic recurrent multifocal osteomyelitis (CRMO) show lucent lesions in the distal tibial metaphyses with cortical thinning & layered periosteal reaction ➔.*

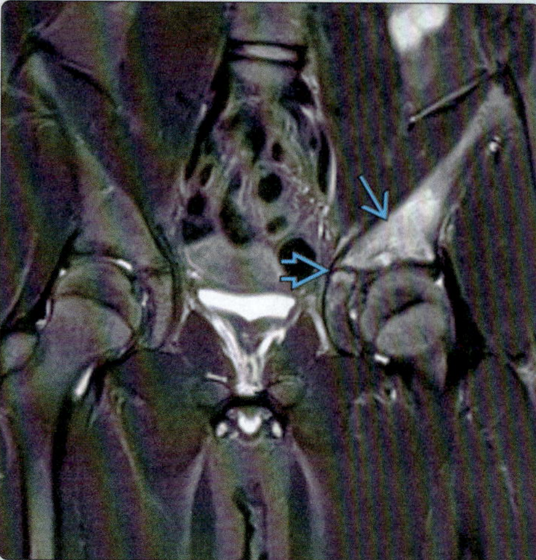

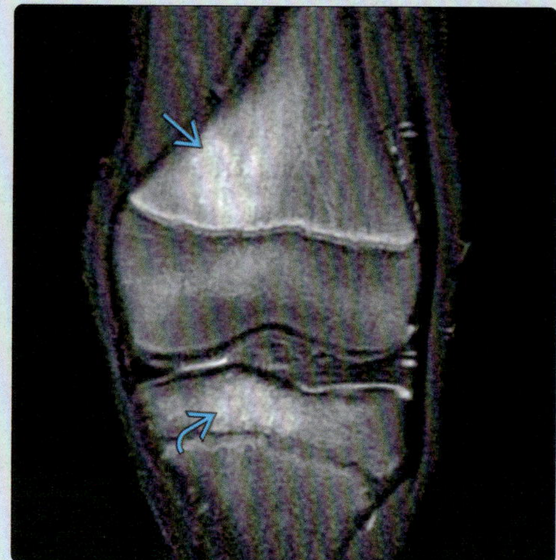

(Left) *Coronal T2 FS MR of the pelvis in a 12-year-old boy with left hip & knee pain shows poorly defined, hyperintense signal within the left iliac bone ➔. This region of the iliac bone is considered a metaphyseal equivalent due to its proximity to the triradiate growth cartilage ➔.* **(Right)** *Coronal T2 FS MR of the left knee in the same patient shows poorly defined signal abnormalities within the distal femoral metaphysis ➔ & proximal tibial epiphysis ➔. The patient was ultimately diagnosed with CRMO.*

TERMINOLOGY

Abbreviations

- Chronic recurrent multifocal osteomyelitis (CRMO)

Synonyms

- Chronic nonbacterial osteomyelitis (CNO)
  - Newer term proposed as process may be unifocal

Definitions

- Idiopathic disorder with multifocal, nonpyogenic inflammatory bone lesions & relapsing/remitting course

Associated Syndromes

- May be in spectrum of diseases with SAPHO (**s**ynovitis, **a**cne, **p**ustulosis, **h**yperostosis, **o**steitis)
- Associated with other inflammatory conditions [e.g., psoriasis, inflammatory bowel disease (IBD)]

IMAGING

General Features

- Best diagnostic clue
  - Multifocal lytic & sclerotic lesions of periphyseal metaphyses/metaphyseal equivalents or medial clavicle
- Location
  - Multiple sites over course of disease: > 80%
    - Can be bilateral with relatively symmetric distribution
  - Most common location: Long bone metaphyses (periphyseal)
    - Lower extremity > upper extremity (3:1)
  - Most commonly involved bones
    - Tibia, femur, clavicle (especially medial), spine, pelvis
  - Additional locations
    - Metaphyseal equivalent bones (next to growth cartilage)
    - Fibula, ribs, mandible, sternum, scapula, hands, & feet

Radiographic Findings

- Early: Lytic lesion (usually metaphyseal)
- Late: Progressive adjacent sclerosis
  - Chronic lesions may be mixed lytic/sclerotic or purely sclerotic
  - Hyperostosis with cortical thickening
- Recurrence
  - New lytic area &/or periosteal reaction

MR Findings

- T1WI
  - ↓ signal within metaphysis adjacent to growth plate
- T2WI FS/STIR
  - Focal, well-circumscribed, periphyseal metaphyseal lesion of ↑ signal
    - ± breach of physis (which can lead to subsequent growth arrest)
  - Less pronounced, poorly defined ↑ signal of bone marrow in adjacent metadiaphysis & epiphysis
    - Epiphyseal signal may be out of proportion to physeal involvement
  - ± periosteal/soft tissue edema/inflammation
  - ± small reactive adjacent joint effusion
- T1WI C+ FS
  - Diffuse enhancement of bone & soft tissue abnormalities
    - No drainable soft tissue or subperiosteal collection
  - ± small foci of peripheral enhancement in bone (due to sterile intraosseous abscess or necrosis)
  - ± mild synovial thickening & enhancement in adjacent joints
- Whole-body MR
  - Techniques differ but typically include coronal STIR ± T1, DWI; ± sagittal STIR for vertebral involvement
  - Detects clinically asymptomatic lesions
  - At long-term follow-up (≥ 10 years), clinically asymptomatic patients may still have lesions

Nuclear Medicine Findings

- Bone scan
  - Tc-99m whole-body bone scan can also evaluate for asymptomatic lesions: ↑ radiotracer uptake

Imaging Recommendations

- Best imaging tool
  - Imaging work-up should begin with radiographs
  - Targeted MR helps confirm diagnosis & define extent of symptomatic disease
  - Whole-body imaging (MR or bone scan) to evaluate for additional asymptomatic sites
    - May play role in long-term follow-up

DIFFERENTIAL DIAGNOSIS

Osteomyelitis

- Single site is most common; medial clavicle is rare
- Typically presents before lytic lesions occur
- Soft tissue &/or subperiosteal abscesses are common

Ewing Sarcoma

- Permeative bone tumor with aggressive periosteal reaction
- Sharp interface between tumor & normal marrow on T1 MR
- Relatively large soft tissue mass is common

Langerhans Cell Histiocytosis

- Punched-out lytic lesion is classic
- Homogeneously enhancing soft tissue mass fills defect & emanates from bone
- Marked surrounding marrow edema with less pronounced soft tissue findings
- Peak age: 5-10 years

Leukemia

- Osteoporosis, lucent metaphyseal bands ± subtle permeative lytic lesions & aggressive periosteal reaction
- Diffuse replacement of fatty marrow on T1 MR
- Peak age: 2-10 years

Scurvy

- Rare, but seen in patients with restrictive diets (e.g., autism)
- Lucent metaphyseal bands
- Multifocal metaphyseal ↑ T2 signal
  - ± periosteal edema/hyperenhancement
  - May develop subperiosteal hemorrhages

PATHOLOGY

General Features

- Etiology
  - Unknown; genetic & autoinflammatory causes have been suggested
  - Diagnosis of exclusion
- Genetics
  - Susceptibility locus identified at 18q21.3-22
- Associated abnormalities
  - Dermatologic disorders
    - Palmoplantar pustulosis
    - Psoriasis
  - Autoinflammatory disorders
    - Takayasu arteritis
    - Wegener granulomatosis
  - Gastrointestinal disorders
    - IBD: Crohn disease & ulcerative colitis
  - Genetic disorders
    - Majeed syndrome
  - Others
    - Enthesis-related arthritis
    - SAPHO syndrome
      - Thought to be adult equivalent of CRMO but with some distinct differences
      - Etiology unknown (genetic, immunologic, & bacterial mechanisms are proposed)
      - Mean age: 28 years
      - Chest wall & pelvic disease predominates (especially at sternoclavicular & 1st sternocostal joints)
      - Arthritis of peripheral joints
      - Associated dermatologic disorders are more common

Gross Pathologic & Surgical Features

- Microscopic features
  - Nonspecific inflammatory changes with granulocytic infiltration
  - Acute: Polymorphonuclear leukocytes, osteoclastic bone resorption, ± multinucleated giant cells
  - Chronic: Lymphocytes, plasma cells, histiocytes with occasional granulomas, ↑ osteoblastic activity
  - Acute to chronic findings may be found in single lesion
  - Appearance of biopsy specimen may not correlate with clinical time course of disease
- Cultures are negative for organisms

Laboratory Tests

- Nonspecific laboratory markers
  - Mildly elevated C-reactive protein (CRP) & erythrocyte sedimentation rate
  - Normal WBC count

CLINICAL ISSUES

Presentation

- Most common signs/symptoms
  - Typically starts with 1 symptomatic site: Pain, tenderness, swelling, limited range of motion
    - Most (not all) develop other symptomatic sites
  - May be symptomatic days to years prior to presentation
    - Often insidious with vague, nonspecific symptoms
- Other signs/symptoms
  - Systemic signs may be present but are uncommon
    - Fever, weight loss, lethargy
  - Associated with dermatologic disorders & IBD

Demographics

- Age: Most commonly 9-14 years old
  - Reported as young as 6 months & as old as 55 years
- Sex: Female predominance
  - M:F = 1:2.1

Natural History & Prognosis

- Most patients undergo spontaneous resolution over months to years
  - Symptoms up to 25 years following initial diagnosis

Treatment

- 1st-line treatment: NSAIDs
- 2nd-line treatment: Methotrexate, TNF inhibitors, bisphosphonates

DIAGNOSTIC CHECKLIST

Consider

- Lack of improvement on antibiotics & presence of associated inflammatory disorder lend support to imaging findings suggestive of CRMO
- Whole-body MR or bone scan to evaluate multifocality
- Medial clavicular involvement strongly suggests CRMO

Image Interpretation Pearls

- Carefully inspect metaphyses on radiographs in patients with extremity pain
- ± soft tissue inflammation & joint effusion/synovitis
- ± small, intraosseous fluid collections or necrotic bone
  - Soft tissue abscess, sequestra, or presence of fistula suggests bacterial osteomyelitis

Reporting Tips

- Suggest diagnosis along with appropriate differential considerations if imaging appearance is characteristic
- Include presence/absence of transphyseal involvement
  - ↑ risk of growth disturbance

SELECTED REFERENCES

1. Sato TS et al: Imaging mimics of chronic recurrent multifocal osteomyelitis: avoiding pitfalls in a diagnosis of exclusion. Pediatr Radiol. 50(1):124-36, 2020
2. Andronikou S et al: Radiological diagnosis of chronic recurrent multifocal osteomyelitis using whole-body MRI-based lesion distribution patterns. Clin Radiol. 74(9):737.e3-e15, 2019
3. Zhao Y et al: Chronic nonbacterial osteomyelitis and chronic recurrent multifocal osteomyelitis in children. Pediatr Clin North Am. 65(4):783-800, 2018
4. Leclair N et al: Whole-body diffusion-weighted imaging in chronic recurrent multifocal osteomyelitis in children. PLoS One. 11(1):e0147523, 2016
5. Voit AM et al: Whole-body magnetic resonance imaging in chronic recurrent multifocal osteomyelitis: clinical longterm assessment may underestimate activity. J Rheumatol. 42(8):1455-62, 2015
6. Falip C et al: Chronic recurrent multifocal osteomyelitis (CRMO): a longitudinal case series review. Pediatr Radiol. 43(3):355-75, 2013
7. Iyer RS et al: Chronic recurrent multifocal osteomyelitis: review. AJR Am J Roentgenol. 196(6 Suppl):S87-91, 2011

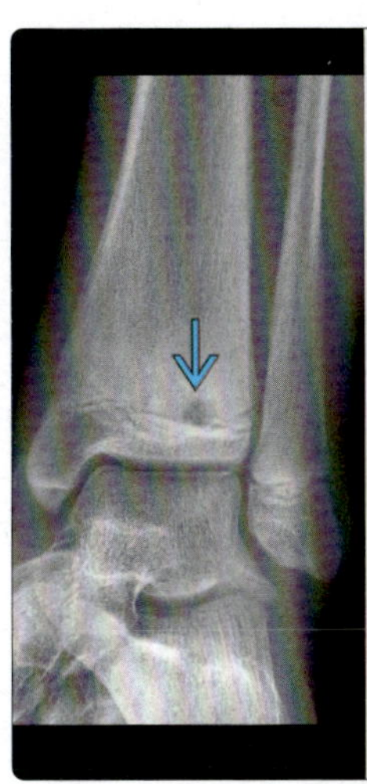
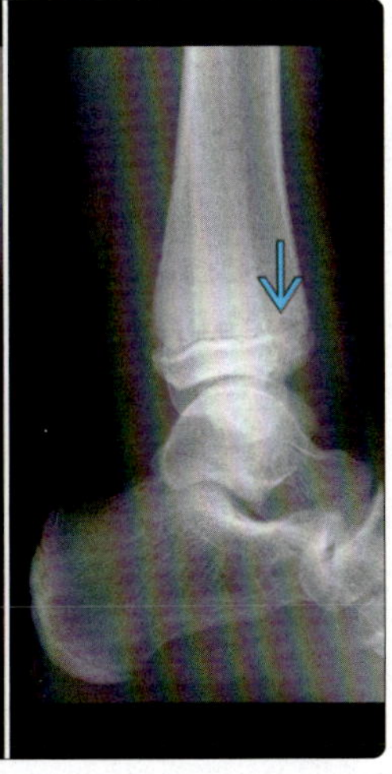
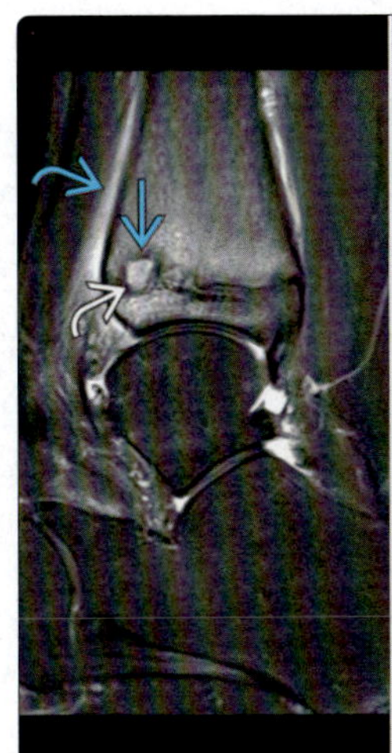
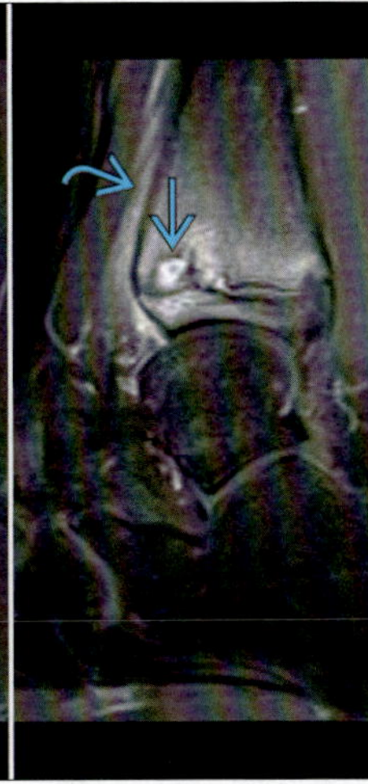

(Left) *Frontal (left) & lateral (right) ankle radiographs in a 12-year-old girl with left ankle & knee pain show a lytic lesion in the distal tibial metaphysis* ➡ *with mild adjacent sclerosis.* **(Right)** *Sagittal T2 FS (left) & T1 C+ FS (right) MR images in the same girl show a focal metaphyseal lesion* ➡ *with ↑ T2 signal & enhancement. There is physeal extension* ➡ *with adjacent metaphyseal, epiphyseal, & periosteal* ➡ *edema.*

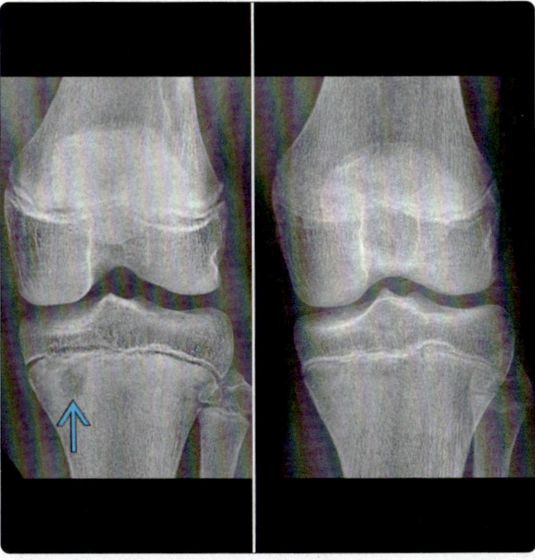
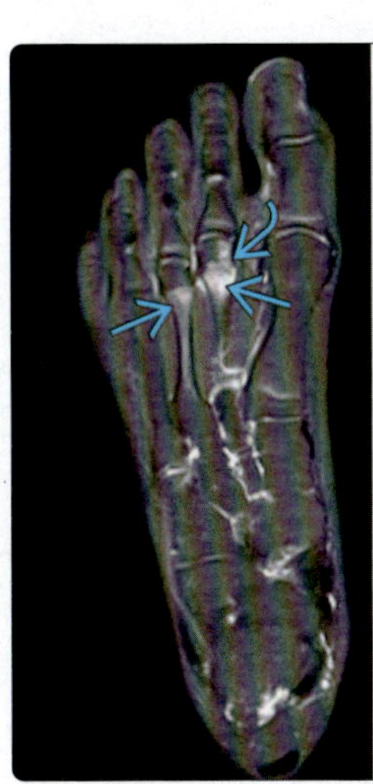
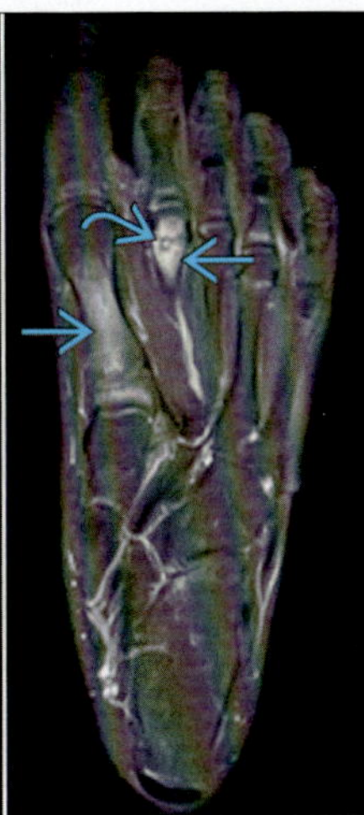

(Left) *AP knee radiograph in the same girl at presentation (left) shows a focal lytic lesion in the proximal left tibial metaphysis* ➡*. Biopsy with culture grew no organisms. After treatment with a TNF-a antagonist, her symptoms & tibial lesion resolved (right), typical of CRMO.* **(Right)** *Long-axis T2 FS MR images of the feet in a 13-year-old girl with bilateral foot & ankle pain show edema of several metatarsals* ➡*. Note the transphyseal extension in both 2nd metatarsals* ➡*. Biopsy & culture revealed no organism, typical of CRMO.*

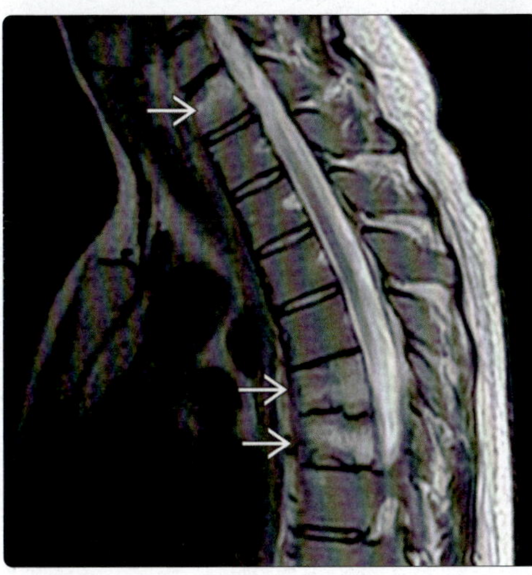
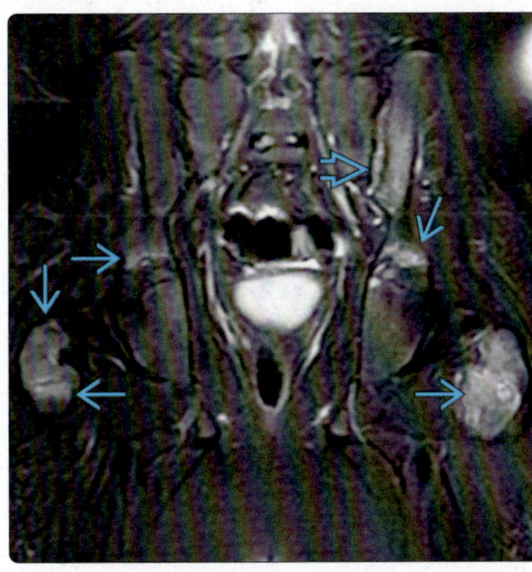

(Left) *Sagittal T2 MR in a patient with Crohn disease & rashes shows ↑ signal within the T1, T6, & T7 vertebral bodies* ➡ *with height loss at T6 & T7. The patient was ultimately diagnosed with CRMO.* **(Right)** *Coronal T2 FS MR in a 13-year-old patient with CRMO shows relatively symmetric foci of ↑ signal* ➡ *in the pelvis & proximal femurs adjacent to growth cartilages. There is also left sacroiliitis* ➡*.*

Infantile Hemangioma

KEY FACTS

TERMINOLOGY

- Widespread misuse of term "hemangioma" in literature
  - True hemangioma: Benign vascular neoplasm
- Infantile hemangioma (IH)
  - Most common soft tissue tumor of childhood
  - Predictable life cycle: Usually absent at birth, rapid growth over 1st few weeks/months of life (proliferating phase), spontaneous regression over subsequent months to years (involuting phase)

IMAGING

- Soft/"squishy," elongated, lobulated, well-defined, highly vascular, solitary or multifocal superficial soft tissue mass
- Grayscale US shows moderately compressible subcutaneous mass with variable internal echogenicity & few discrete vessels
- Doppler US should clearly document characteristic internal vascularity (i.e., high vessel density with many low-resistance arterial waveforms) throughout proliferating IH
- MR shows diffusely high T2 signal with scattered flow voids, relatively high ADC values, & diffuse enhancement
- Imaging features change with involution

TOP DIFFERENTIAL DIAGNOSES

- Other vascular neoplasms: Congenital hemangioma, kaposiform hemangioendothelioma
- Vascular malformations: Venous, lymphatic, arteriovenous
- Soft tissue sarcomas

CLINICAL ISSUES

- Most follow benign course without requiring therapy
- Complications &/or associated anomalies are more likely if IH is large, segmental, facial, or multifocal
  - 1st-line therapy: Propranolol (β-blocker)

DIAGNOSTIC CHECKLIST

- If imaging appearance, timeline, or physical exam findings are atypical for IH, exclude other lesions by biopsy

(Left) *Photograph of a 4-month-old patient shows a well-defined, raised strawberry lesion on the neck that appeared after birth, typical of a proliferating infantile hemangioma (IH).* **(Right)** *Longitudinal US images in a 3-month-old with a soft, growing palpable mass of the back show a well-circumscribed elongated mass ➙ that lies within the subcutaneous fat ➙ & does not extend deeper into muscle ➙. The mass is somewhat lobulated & mildly heterogeneous in echogenicity.*

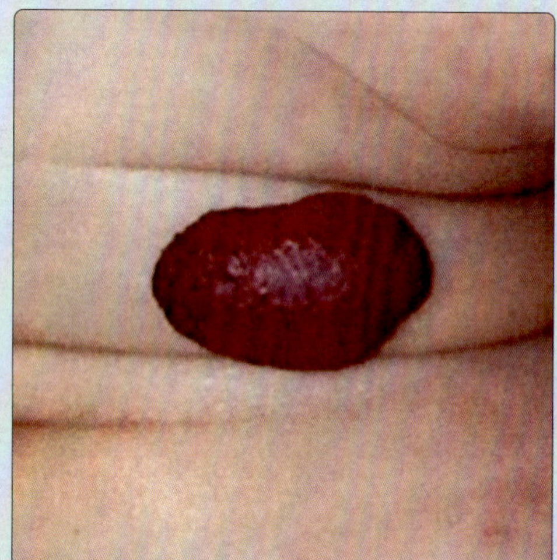

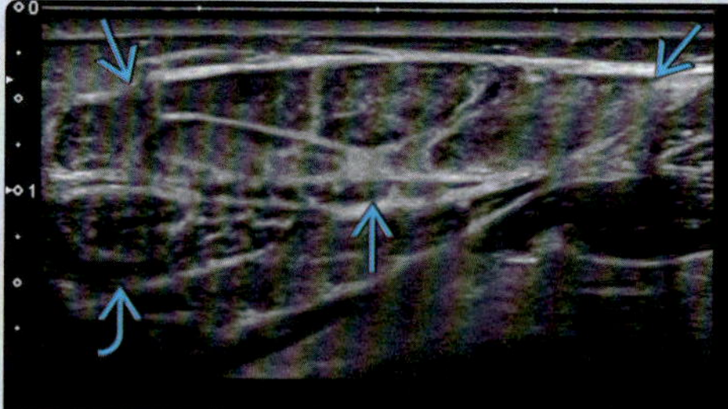

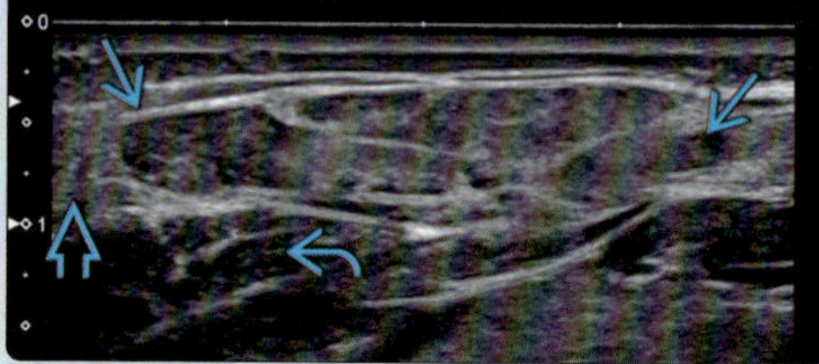

(Left) *Transverse Doppler US of the same mass shows a high vessel density with many low-resistance arterial waveforms. The overall findings are very typical of an IH.* **(Right)** *Axial STIR (left) & T1 C+ FS (right) MR images in an infant with facial IHs & aortic coarctation show numerous lobulated lesions of the superficial & deep neck with bright (nearly fluid) signal ➙ & diffuse enhancement ➙. The findings are consistent with IHs, though deeper extension is typically seen only with an associated syndrome (such as PHACE in this patient).*

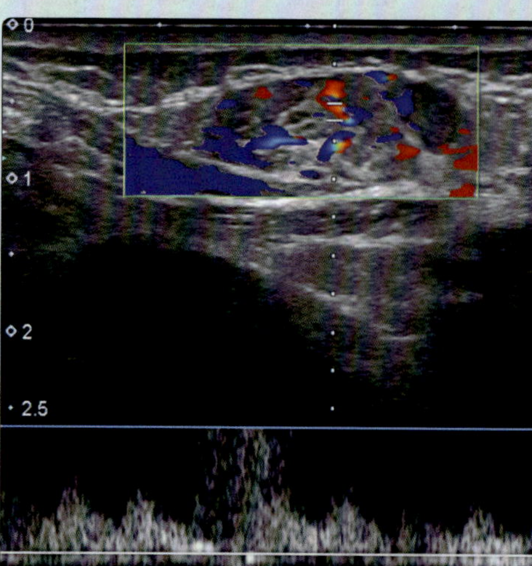

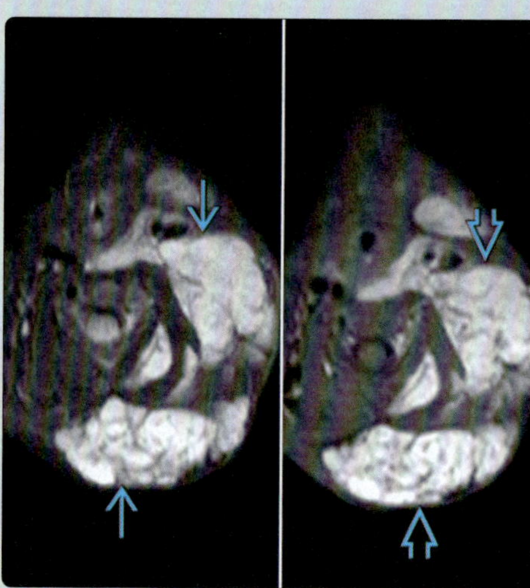

TERMINOLOGY

Synonyms

- Capillary hemangioma, strawberry hemangioma
- Not cavernous hemangioma (actually venous malformation)
- Not synovial hemangioma (actually venous malformation)
- Not hemangioendothelioma (actually intermediate-grade vascular tumor)

Definitions

- 2018 revised classification by International Society for Study of Vascular Anomalies (ISSVA) retains 2 main categories
  - Vascular tumors (true neoplasms with cellular proliferation that generally grow out of proportion to patient)
  - Vascular malformations (congenital errors of vessel development that generally grow commensurate with patient)
- Hemangioma: Benign vascular neoplasm with predictable life cycle
  - Infantile hemangioma (IH)
    - Most common soft tissue tumor of childhood
    - Usually absent at birth with rapid growth over 1st few weeks/months of life (proliferating phase) followed by spontaneous regression over subsequent months to years (involuting phase)
  - Congenital hemangioma (CH)
    - Fully developed at birth
    - Rapidly involuting (RICH) vs. noninvoluting (NICH) vs. partially involuting (PICH)
      - RICH is mostly involuted by 14 months

IMAGING

General Features

- Best diagnostic clue
  - Lobular, well-defined, highly vascular solitary or multifocal superficial soft tissue masses appearing in 1st few weeks of life
    - Common cutaneous lesions are not usually imaged due to typical appearance & timeline
    - Deeper subcutaneous lesions without typical skin findings are likely to be imaged, as diagnosis is less clear to clinician
- Location
  - Head & neck (60%), trunk (25%), extremities (15%)
  - Typically confined to cutaneous or subcutaneous tissues
    - Deeper lesions are typically only seen in syndromic cases or with multifocal cutaneous lesions
- Morphology
  - Frequently ovoid or elongated rather than round
- Other imaging characteristics
  - Depends on timing of imaging
    - Proliferating phase: Homogeneous & diffuse enhancement; high-flow vessels in/adjacent to mass
    - Involuting phase: Heterogeneous with varying fatty infiltration; ↓ flow/enhancement of mass

Radiographic Findings

- Soft tissue mass without Ca^{2+}
  - Phleboliths are found in venous malformations, not IH

Ultrasonographic Findings

- Grayscale ultrasound
  - Lobular mass with variable echogenicity & few macroscopic vessels
    - Relative to subcutaneous fat: ~ 30% hypoechoic, 30% hyperechoic, 40% mixed echogenicity
  - Soft "squishy" mass: Moderately compressible with relatively high elasticity/strain
- Color Doppler
  - "Lights up" during proliferating phase
    - High vessel density on color Doppler (> 5 vessels/cm^2)
    - High systolic Doppler shift (> 2 kHz): Many arterial tracings with low resistive index but no arterialized veins to suggest shunting
  - With involution/treatment: ↓ vessel density & size, ↓ flow velocity, ↑ resistive index

MR Findings

- Proliferating phase
  - Largely homogeneous except for occasional flow voids & intervening thin septa
  - T1: Intermediate signal intensity
  - T2 FS/STIR: High signal intensity
    - May not be as bright as fluid
    - Many internal low signal flow voids are often present
  - T1 C+ FS: Diffuse early homogeneous enhancement
  - DWI: ADC values are higher in IHs vs. pediatric soft tissue malignancies
    - IHs: ~ 1.3-1.6 x 10^{-3} mm^2/s
    - Sarcomas: ~ 0.6-1.1 x 10^{-3} mm^2/s
- Involuting phase
  - Varying degrees of fatty infiltration with ↓ flow/enhancement

Imaging Recommendations

- Best imaging tool
  - Cutaneous IH (majority) can be diagnosed by physical appearance & temporal growth history without imaging
  - For deeper lesions, US with Doppler can be highly suggestive of IH in right age range
  - Imaging may also be employed when location/number of cutaneous lesions implicate associated anomalies &/or complications
    - IH over lower midline back: Spine anomalies
    - Perineal IH: PELVIS/LUMBAR syndrome
    - Segmental or bearded facial IH: PHACE(S), airway involvement
    - Periocular IH: ± intraorbital components, various ophthalmologic complications
    - ≥ 5 cutaneous IHs: ↑ likelihood of visceral involvement, especially liver
      - Numerous liver lesions can lead to hepatic & heart failure, abdominal compartment syndrome, &/or hypothyroidism

DIFFERENTIAL DIAGNOSIS

Venous Malformation

- Multiple serpentine channels &/or lobular soft tissue mass(es) infiltrating various compartments
- Fluid signal intensity mass ± fluid-fluid levels

- Delayed/gradual patchy enhancement (except for thrombi)
- Phleboliths are virtually diagnostic in children

Lymphatic Malformation

- Multicystic mass crossing soft tissue planes
- May contain fluid-fluid levels, debris
- Rim/septal enhancement
  - Microcystic components may appear more solid

Arteriovenous Malformation

- Tangle of high-flow vessels with shunting
- ± other soft tissue components

Congenital Hemangioma

- Solid, heterogeneous, less well-defined mass ± Ca^{2+}, hemorrhage, necrosis, & larger vessels
- Fully developed at birth; different cutaneous features vs. IH

Kaposiform Hemangioendothelioma

- Usually poorly defined, infiltrating, solid enhancing mass presenting in infant with Kasabach-Merritt phenomenon
- ± marked surrounding edema: Difficult to discern from lesion margins

Soft Tissue Sarcomas

- Usually firm, solid, round mass with heterogeneous enhancement & intermediate to low vascularity
- Relatively uncommon in 1st few months of life
- Restricted diffusion (with lower ADC values)

PATHOLOGY

Microscopic Features

- Proliferating phase: Masses of plump endothelial cells forming small vascular channels
- Involuting phase: Flat endothelial cells + fibrofatty replacement

Immunohistochemical Features

- GLUT1(+) during all phases
  - CH: GLUT1(-)

CLINICAL ISSUES

Presentation

- Most common signs/symptoms
  - Usually presents during infancy as asymptomatic soft mass
    - With cutaneous involvement (most common): Lobular bright red or pink lesion
      - Localized: Nodule, papule
      - Segmental: Plaque-like over region
    - With deeper subcutaneous lesions: Bluish hue to skin
- Other signs/symptoms
  - During proliferation, high flow may cause bruit, warmth
  - May present with complication
    - Compression of vital structures, liver failure, etc.

Demographics

- Age
  - At birth: Typically absent
    - 30% have precursor lesion (pallor, ecchymosis, telangiectasia)
  - 0-2 months: Almost all double in size
  - 3-5 months: 80% of maximum size
  - 9-12 months: Peak size reached in almost all lesions
  - 12-48 months: Most rapid phase of involution
  - By 84-108 months: Involution usually complete
    - 20-50% with cutaneous residua
- Sex
  - Female predominance (F:M = 1.5-4.0:1.0)
- Ethnicity
  - White > > Black, Hispanic, Asian patients
- Epidemiology
  - Multiple lesions in 15-30% of patients
  - Up to 10% of premature infants affected vs. 5% overall

Natural History & Prognosis

- Most follow benign course
- Complications are more likely if IH is large, segmental, multifocal, or on face
  - Ulceration (most likely with intertriginous & perioral lesions), bleeding
  - Compression of vital structures (airway, orbit)
  - Heart failure, liver failure, hypothyroidism, &/or compartment syndrome with high liver lesion burden
  - Psychologic issues (especially with facial lesions)
  - Coagulopathy is not associated with IH

Treatment

- Most IHs require no imaging or therapy
- Therapy is reserved for large or complicated lesions or for significant residua (such as fibrofatty tissue or cutaneous telangiectasias) following involution
- 1st-line treatment is medical
  - Propranolol (β-blocker) has replaced oral steroids as primary therapy due to low side effect profile
- Other therapies: Intralesional steroids, embolization, surgical removal, pulsed-dye laser

DIAGNOSTIC CHECKLIST

Consider

- If imaging appearance, timeline, or physical exam findings are atypical for IH, exclude other lesions by biopsy
- IH patients with cutaneous segmental lesions, certain facial lesions, or ≥ 5 lesions otherwise require further directed imaging due to associated anomalies/complications

SELECTED REFERENCES

1. Abu Ata N et al: Neonatal vascular anomalies manifesting as soft-tissue masses. Pediatr Radiol. ePub, 2021
2. Abu Ata N et al: Imaging of vascular anomalies in the pediatric musculoskeletal system. Semin Roentgenol. 56(3):288-306, 2021
3. Gong X et al: Conventional ultrasonography and elastography for the diagnosis of congenital and infantile hemangiomas. J Dermatol. 47(5):527-33, 2020
4. Peterman CM et al: Clinical and radiological characteristics of patients with retroperitoneal infantile hemangiomas. Pediatr Dermatol. 36(6):823-9, 2019
5. Saito M et al: Usefulness of diffusion-weighted magnetic resonance imaging using apparent diffusion coefficient values for diagnosis of infantile hemangioma. J Comput Assist Tomogr. 43(4):563-7, 2019
6. Johnson CM et al: Clinical and sonographic features of pediatric soft-tissue vascular anomalies part 1: classification, sonographic approach and vascular tumors. Pediatr Radiol. 47(9):1184-95, 2017
7. Merrow AC et al: 2014 Revised classification of vascular lesions from the International Society for the Study of Vascular Anomalies: radiologic-pathologic update. Radiographics. 36(5):1494-516, 2016
8. Blei F et al: Current workup and therapy of infantile hemangiomas. Clin Dermatol. 32(4):459-70, 2014

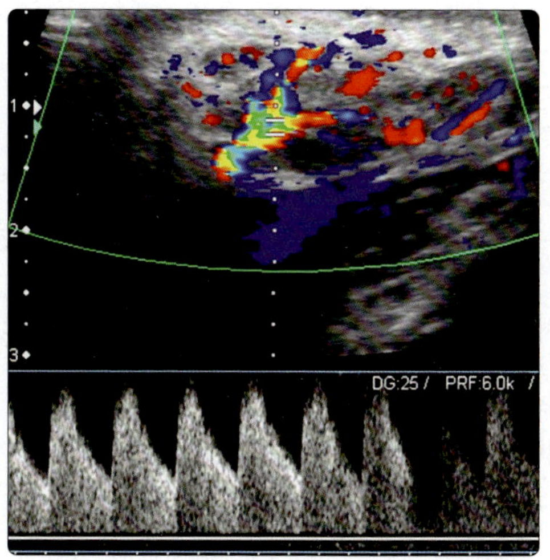

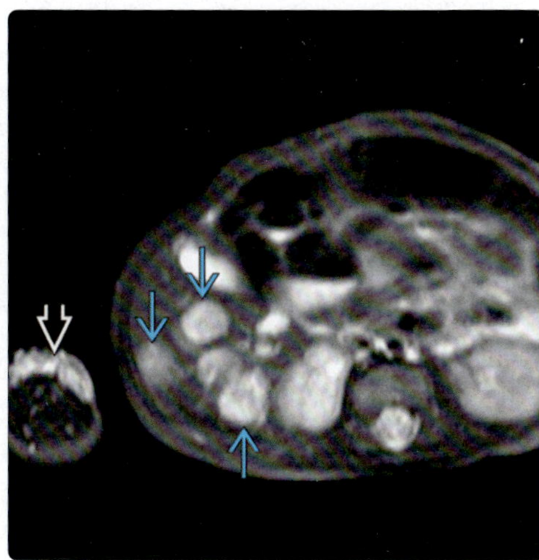

(Left) *Transverse color Doppler US in a 2-month-old at the level of a growing soft tissue mass of the back (which was not present at birth) shows a heterogeneously echogenic mass of the subcutaneous fat. There is a high vessel density with low-resistance arterial waveforms, typical of IH.* **(Right)** *Axial T2 FS MR in a 3-month-old with a known forearm IH shows multiple round, hyperintense hepatic lesions. Having ≥ 5 skin IHs ↑ the risk of visceral lesions with the liver being the most frequently affected organ.*

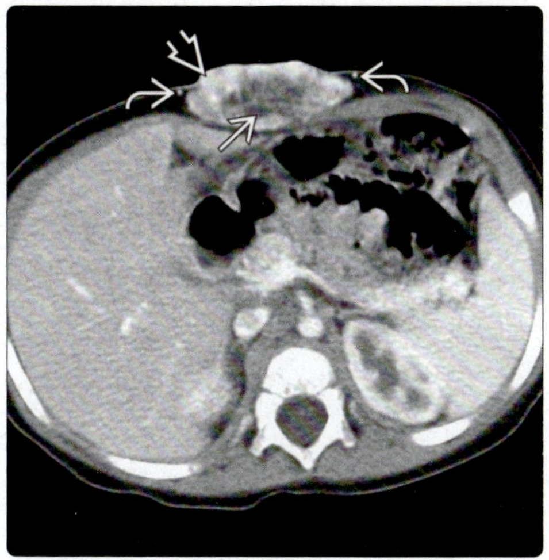

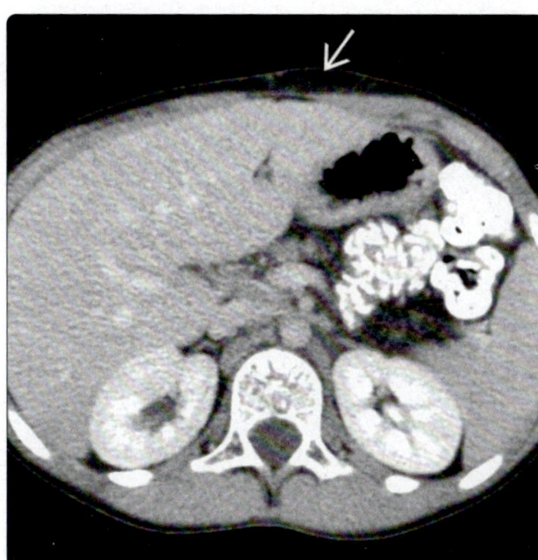

(Left) *Axial abdominal CECT in a 12-month-old girl with a known superficial IH shows an elongated, well-defined, lobular mass with peripheral enhancement & central fatty infiltration. Note the prominent vessels along the lesion margins. These findings are typical of an IH during early involution.* **(Right)** *Axial CECT in the same patient 7 years later shows minimal residual prominence of fat at the site of the previously visualized lesion, consistent with an involuted IH.*

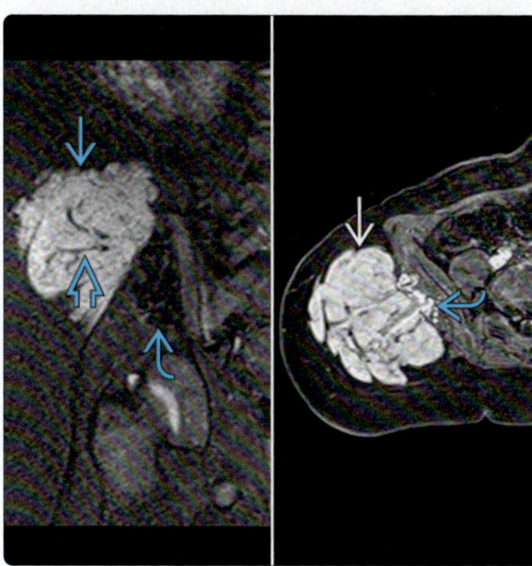

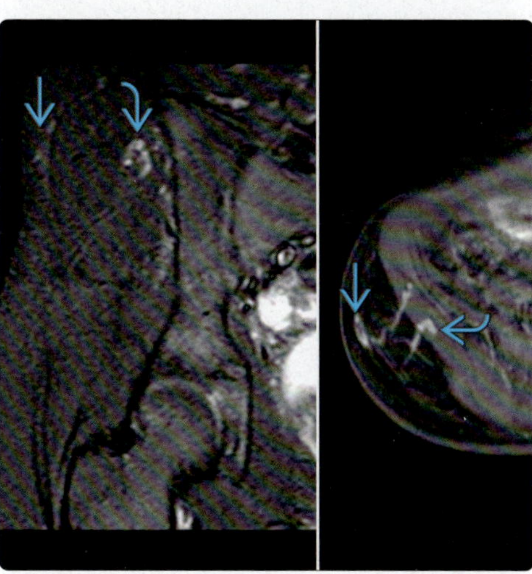

(Left) *Coronal STIR (left) & axial T1 C+ FS (right) MR images in a 9-month-old show a large, lobulated hyperintense & diffusely enhancing subcutaneous mass with internal flow voids. Numerous large feeding & draining vessels are seen deep to the lesion in the gluteal musculature. Biopsy confirmed an IH.* **(Right)** *Coronal STIR (left) & axial T1 C+ FS (right) MR images in the same patient 10 years later show involution of the IH with minimal residual lesion & substantial ↓ in the subjacent gluteal vessels.*

KEY FACTS

TERMINOLOGY

- KHE: Aggressive, locally invasive vascular neoplasm of spindled endothelial cells & abnormal lymphatics

IMAGING

- Best clue: Poorly defined, diffusely enhancing soft tissue mass infiltrating multiple tissue planes/compartments in infant with coagulopathy
  - ~ 80-90% have continuous cutaneous lesions & deep components
- Most common locations: Extremity > trunk > head & neck; regional lymph node involvement is common

CLINICAL ISSUES

- Characteristic cutaneous vascular lesion ~ 90%: Indurated, ill-defined, red-purple mass or plaque
- Profound, sustained consumptive coagulopathy: Kasabach-Merritt phenomenon (KMP) in 33-70%
  - ↓ platelets, fibrinogen, hematocrit; ↑ D-dimer
  - KHE lesions at risk for KMP include those with
    - Deeper > superficial components (78% vs. 36%)
    - Retroperitoneal & thoracic involvement
    - Cutaneous lesion > 8 cm
- > 90% present in infancy; median age: 2-5 months
- Mortality ranges from 12-30%
- Treated lesions do not fully regress & may recur
- Treatment in setting of KMP includes steroids + sirolimus &/or vincristine
  - Limited role for platelet transfusions
  - Complete surgical excision curative but rarely option due to infiltrative nature of KHE with extension into vital regions

DIAGNOSTIC CHECKLIST

- Enhancing poorly defined soft tissue mass in infant with thrombocytopenia should raise concern for KHE
- In conjunction with characteristic cutaneous lesion, these features may obviate biopsy

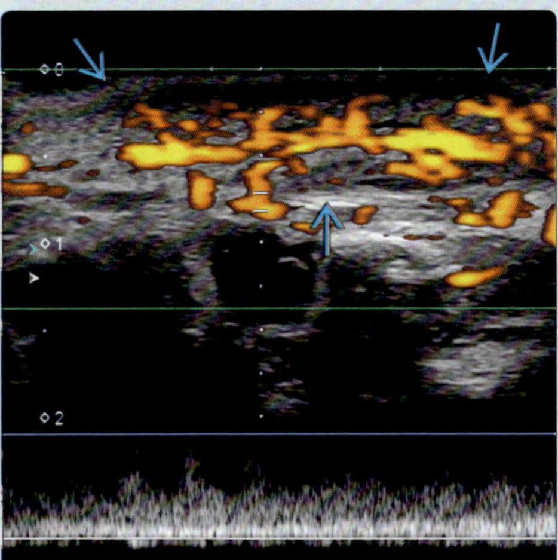

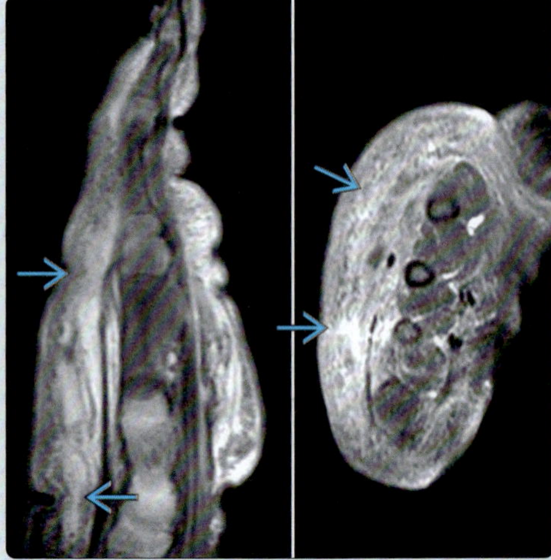

(Left) *Sagittal power Doppler ultrasound shows an infiltrative, poorly defined, hypervascular mass ➙ expanding the right hand dorsal soft tissues of a 3 week old with redness & swelling since birth.* **(Right)** *Sagittal T2 FS (L) & axial T1 C+ FS (R) MR in the same infant 1 week later show heterogeneous enhancement of the infiltrating lesion ➙. The margins are inseparable from surrounding edema. A typical coagulopathy of Kasabach-Merritt phenomenon confirmed kaposiform hemangioendothelioma (KHE).*

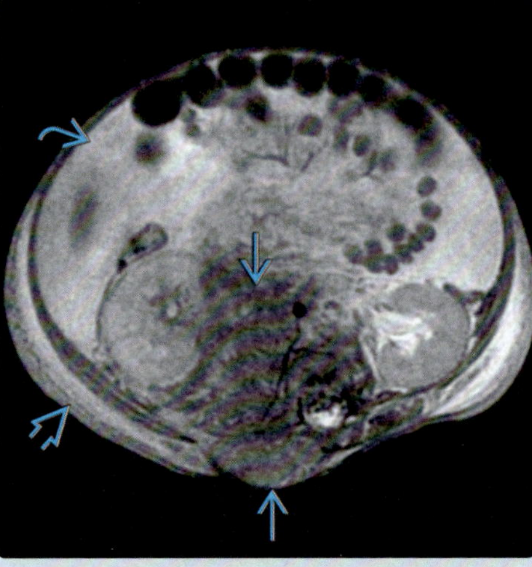

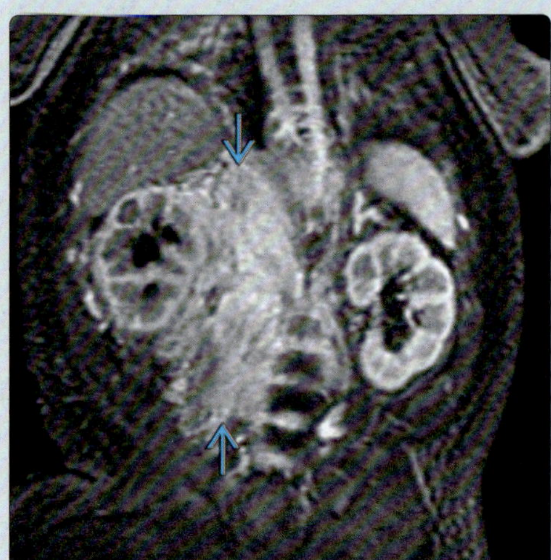

(Left) *Axial FS T2 MR in a 3-week-old with consumptive coagulopathy & abdominal distention shows a large, poorly defined intermediate T2 signal intensity mass ➙ extending from the skin into the retroperitoneum. There is diffuse body wall edema ➙ & a large volume of ascites ➙.* **(Right)** *Coronal T1 C+ FS MR in the same patient shows early, diffuse enhancement of the infiltrative mass ➙, confirmed to be a KHE.*

TERMINOLOGY

Definitions

- Kaposiform hemangioendothelioma (KHE): Aggressive, locally invasive vascular neoplasm of spindled endothelial cells & abnormal lymphatics
  - **Not** equivalent to hemangioma

IMAGING

General Features

- Best diagnostic clue
  - Poorly defined soft tissue mass infiltrating across tissue planes in infant with coagulopathy
- Location
  - Extremity > trunk > head & neck
    - ~ 26% have continuous extension into > 1 region
  - Most have superficial & deep involvement, extending from skin through subcutaneous fat into muscle
  - Regional lymph node involvement is common
  - Visceral & bony involvement are uncommon
  - Very rare reports of multifocality vs. distant metastases
    - May actually represent distinct entity: Kaposiform lymphangiomatosis
- CT/MR/US
  - Classic appearance: Infiltrating, poorly defined mass
    - Thickening/expansion of involved soft tissues
    - Variable degree of reticular foci or stranding extending from mass into surrounding tissues
      - Difficult to distinguish surrounding edema from true tumor margins
  - Less common: Well-defined lesion
  - Often heterogeneous internally: May have foci of hemorrhage & fibrosis
    - Intermediate to dark T2 components amidst otherwise T2 bright lesion on MR
    - Variable enhancement; can be strikingly vigorous & diffuse (particularly on CECT)
  - Moderately ↑ vascularity
    - ± prominent feeding/draining vessels
    - No large tangles of vessels or significant shunting

DIFFERENTIAL DIAGNOSIS

Soft Tissue Infection (Cellulitis/Fasciitis/Myositis)

- Redness, swelling, pain, ↑ inflammatory markers
- Indurated soft tissues with serpiginous hypoechoic fluid

Microcystic Lymphatic Malformation

- Longstanding tissue thickening ± cutaneous blebs

Hemangioma, Infantile vs. Congenital

- Typically well-defined, high-flow cutaneous/subcutaneous mass of infancy without muscular involvement

Infantile Myofibroma

- Solid soft tissue mass of infants with variable heterogeneity, Ca^{2+}, tissue infiltration, bone involvement

Rhabdomyosarcoma

- Well-defined, solid soft tissue mass of children (usually not neonates) with variable vascularity

PATHOLOGY

General Features

- Histologic & clinical overlap with more limited superficial lesion of tufted angioma (TA)

Microscopic Features

- Coalescing nodules of spindled endothelial cells surrounded by abnormal lymphatic channels
  - Intermixed platelet microthrombi, extravasated RBCs, hemosiderin

CLINICAL ISSUES

Presentation

- Most common signs/symptoms
  - Characteristic cutaneous vascular lesion ~ 90%
    - Indurated, ill-defined, red-purple mass or plaque
  - Profound, sustained consumptive coagulopathy with microangiopathic hemolytic anemia: Kasabach-Merritt phenomenon (KMP) in 33-70%
    - ↓ platelets, ↓ fibrinogen, ↓ hematocrit, ↑ D-dimer
    - KHE lesions at risk for KMP include those with
      - Deeper > superficial components (78% vs. 36%)
      - Retroperitoneal & thoracic involvement
      - Cutaneous lesion > 8 cm
- Other signs/symptoms
  - Musculoskeletal symptoms: Pain, ↓ range of motion
  - Clinically inert soft tissue mass

Demographics

- > 90% present in infancy; median age: 2-5 months
  - Patients with KMP present earlier than those without

Natural History & Prognosis

- Mortality ranges from 12-30%
- Treated lesions do not fully regress & may recur

Treatment

- KHE with KMP
  - Steroids, sirolimus (m-TOR inhibitor), &/or vincristine
  - Limited role for platelet transfusions (only prior to surgery or for active bleeding)
  - Complete surgical excision is curative but rarely option due to infiltration & extension into vital regions
  - Embolization can be temporizing
- KHE without KMP
  - Oral steroids alone may be used for growing lesions

SELECTED REFERENCES

1. Abu Ata N et al: Imaging of vascular anomalies in the pediatric musculoskeletal system. Semin Roentgenol. 56(3):288-306, 2021
2. Peng S et al: Kaposiform haemangioendothelioma: magnetic resonance imaging features in 64 cases. BMC Pediatr. 21(1):107, 2021
3. Gong X et al: Ultrasonography and magnetic resonance imaging features of kaposiform hemangioendothelioma and tufted angioma. J Dermatol. 46(10):835-42, 2019
4. Hu PA et al: Clinical and imaging features of kaposiform hemangioendothelioma. Br J Radiol. 91(1086):20170798, 2018
5. Ryu YJ et al: Imaging findings of kaposiform hemangioendothelioma in children. Eur J Radiol. 86:198-205, 2017
6. Croteau SE et al: Kaposiform hemangioendothelioma: atypical features and risks of Kasabach-Merritt phenomenon in 107 referrals. J Pediatr. 162(1):142-7, 2013

KEY FACTS

TERMINOLOGY

- Subtype of congenital slow- or low-flow vascular malformation due to error in vein formation; not neoplastic
  - **Not** hemangioma (benign vascular neoplasm of capillaries) or arteriovenous malformation (high flow)

IMAGING

- Locations
  - Most commonly subcutaneous &/or intramuscular but may involve bone, synovium, viscera
  - Focal, multifocal, or diffuse throughout region
- Morphology
  - Well-circumscribed, lobulated mass vs. extensive confluent, infiltrative lesion
  - ± discrete serpentine venous channels of abnormal number, size, shape, & location
- Radiography: Phleboliths in mass are essentially diagnostic
- MR: High fluid signal intensity ± layering fluid-fluid levels
  - Phleboliths are typically small, round, & dark
  - Diffuse or patchy delayed enhancement of mass; discrete venous channels will diffusely enhance
- US: Mass of heterogeneous echotexture
  - Hypoechoic/anechoic tubular channels in clusters
    - Compressible; will slowly refill
  - Phleboliths: Round echogenic foci with posterior acoustic shadowing & twinkling artifact
  - Detectable venous waveforms are often sparse

CLINICAL ISSUES

- Soft, compressible mass without thrill
  - Enlarges with Valsalva/crying/dependent positioning
  - Bluish skin discoloration with superficial lesions
  - Episodic pain &/or swelling
- Grow proportional to child but may enlarge suddenly due to hemorrhage, thrombosis, or hormonal changes
- Treatments include conservative therapy (compression garments, antiinflammatory medications), percutaneous procedures (sclerotherapy, laser), surgical resection

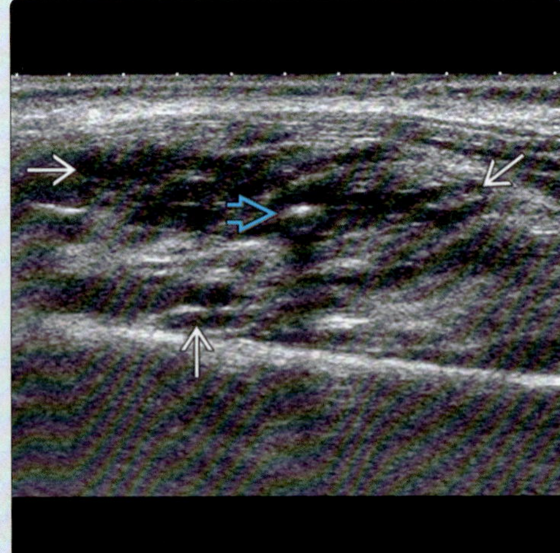

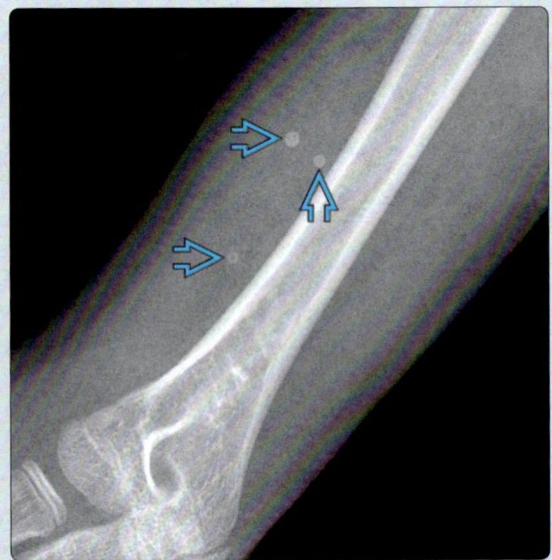

(Left) *Longitudinal US of the upper arm in a 9-year-old girl with new pain & swelling shows a multilobulated collection of hypoechoic channels ➡ within the biceps muscle. There is an echogenic focus ➡ in the mass with posterior acoustic shadowing.* **(Right)** *AP radiograph of the humerus in the same patient confirms numerous round, intralesional Ca^{2+} with lucent centers ➡, typical of phleboliths in a venous malformation (VM).*

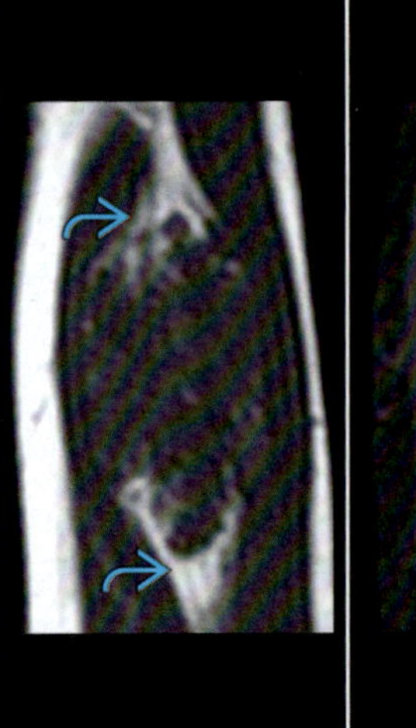

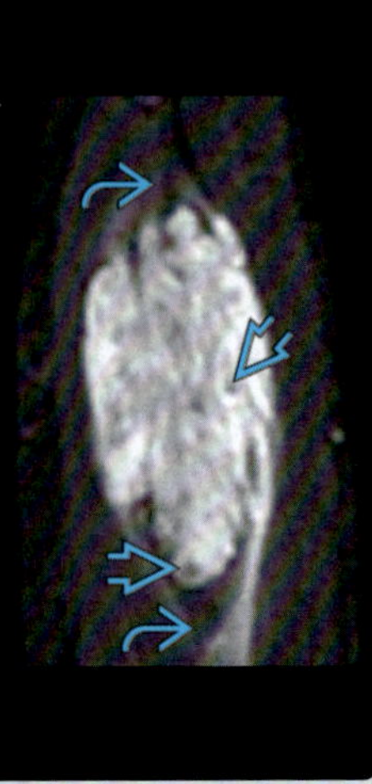

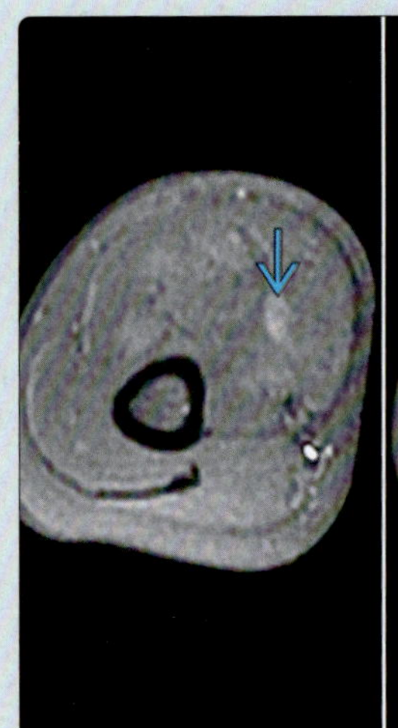

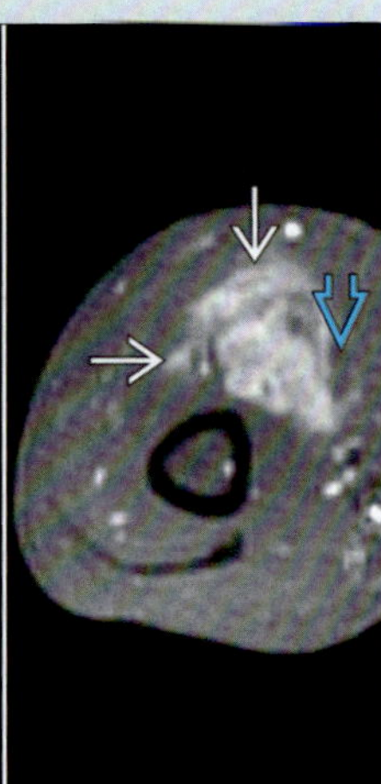

(Left) *Coronal T1 (left) & STIR (right) MR images of the same VM show the lobulated soft tissue mass following fluid signal intensity except for the thin septations & phleboliths ➡. Note the associated fat ➡ along the margins & septations.* **(Right)** *Axial T1 FS pre- (left) & postcontrast (right) MR images through the same mass show that the lesion is largely isointense to muscle before contrast with subsequent heterogeneous enhancement ➡. A focal thrombus shows T1 shortening before contrast ➡ but no enhancement ➡.*

TERMINOLOGY

Synonyms

- Venous anomaly, common venous malformation (VM)
- **Not** hemangioma (benign vascular neoplasm of capillaries) or arteriovenous malformation (high-flow lesion)

Definitions

- Subtype of congenital slow- or low-flow vascular malformation due to error in vein formation; not neoplastic

IMAGING

General Features

- Location
  - Head/neck (40%), extremities (40%), trunk (20%)
  - Focal, multifocal, or diffuse throughout region
  - Most commonly subcutaneous &/or intramuscular but may involve bone, synovium, &/or viscera
    - Often cross soft tissue planes/compartments
- Morphology
  - Well-circumscribed, lobulated (spongiform) mass vs. extensive confluent, infiltrative lesion
  - ± discrete serpentine venous channels of abnormal number, size, shape, & location (phlebectasia)

Radiographic Findings

- Lobulated soft tissue mass ± calcified phleboliths (30%)

MR Findings

- T1WI
  - Largely isointense to muscle
    - Layering stagnant blood &/or thrombi may have ↑ signal intensity
    - Bright fat may be interspersed within & around lesion, particularly intramuscular components
- T2WI FS
  - Serpentine venous channels of high (fluid) signal intensity
    - Tightly clustered masses of abnormal channels show thin, dark, intervening septations
    - Large varicosities may show low signal internally due to disturbed flow; can mimic clot
  - Layering fluid-fluid levels are often present due to settling of blood products
    - Dependent sediment is of intermediate signal intensity vs. bright plasma
  - Absence of flow voids
  - Phleboliths are typically small, round, & dark
- T2* GRE
  - Useful to show chronic joint complications of hemarthroses from synovial VM
    - Blooming (exaggerated signal loss) of synovium from hemosiderin deposits; focal or diffuse cartilage loss
- T1WI C+ FS
  - Discrete ectatic venous channels diffusely enhance
  - Diffuse or patchy enhancement in lobulated mass-like components; thrombi & intermixed lymphatic components will not enhance
    - Dynamic imaging shows gradual contrast filling + absence of large arteries or arteriovenous shunting
- MRV
  - Useful to exclude intralesional high-flow vessels & confirm patency of deep venous system & varicosities
    - Slow-flow or in-plane flow can lose signal & mimic clot

Ultrasonographic Findings

- Grayscale ultrasound
  - Mass of heterogeneous echotexture
    - Hypoechoic/anechoic tubular channels in clusters with ↑ through transmission
      - Often compressible; will slowly refill
    - Intermixed & peripheral patchy foci of ↑ echogenicity due to fat, particularly in atrophied muscle
    - Phleboliths: Round echogenic foci with posterior acoustic shadowing & twinkle artifact
  - ± discrete venous channels of abnormal number, size, shape, & location in surrounding tissues
- Pulsed Doppler
  - Lack of arterial waveforms or arterialized draining veins
    - However, 1-2 normal arteries can be encased by VM
  - Detectable venous waveforms are often sparse
- Color Doppler
  - Majority show little internal vascular flow due to slow flow through dysplastic venous channels
    - Valsalva or compression/release will ↑ flow

Imaging Recommendations

- Best imaging tool
  - US (& potentially radiographs) can be diagnostic of VM
  - MR will show confirmatory features & clarify extent
- Protocol advice
  - US: Assess lesion response to compression
  - MR: Rapid T1 C+ FS 3D GRE sequence (FSPGR or Dixon) can confirm deep venous system or varicosity patency (as noncontrast MRV may be confounded by slow flow)

DIFFERENTIAL DIAGNOSIS

Infantile Hemangioma

- Characteristic life cycle: Small or absent at birth, rapid growth during early infancy, gradual involution over years
- Solid ovoid vs. lobular, elongated soft tissue mass, typically in cutaneous &/or subcutaneous tissues
- Variable sonographic echogenicity due to mix of proliferating & involuting components; no phleboliths
  - Soft & mildly compressible; not firm
- Highly vascular by Doppler US with many low-resistance arterial waveforms
- Bright (but not fluid) T2 signal intensity with diffuse early enhancement on MR

Arteriovenous Malformation

- Tangle of enlarged tortuous arteries & veins with variable soft tissue components
- High flow with shunting by US, MRA/MRV

Lymphatic Malformation

- Another common slow-flow lesion
- Compressible, fluid-filled macrocystic soft tissue mass
  - Thin, enhancing internal septations, internal debris/fluid-fluid levels, no internal vascularity
- Microcystic lesion is more solid-appearing, infiltrative

Soft Tissue Sarcoma

- Typically firm, well-defined, round or ovoid hypovascular solid soft tissue mass with variable enhancement
- ± cystic foci, but solid components are typically visible

Plexiform Neurofibroma

- Elongated lobular masses along courses of nerves
  - In multiple adjacent nerves: Bag of worms appearance
- Cross section of lesion shows target sign on MR
  - Bright peripherally, dark centrally on T2/STIR
  - Dark peripherally, bright centrally on T1 C+ FS

Fibroadipose Vascular Anomaly

- Uncommon solid lesion of extremity musculature
- Contains abnormal veins + dense fibrous & fatty tissue
- Constant pain + contracture

PATHOLOGY

General Features

- Genetics
  - Mutations in *TEK* (*TIE2*) or *PIK3CA*
- Associated abnormalities
  - Klippel-Trenaunay syndrome
    - Capillary-lymphatic-venous malformation of extremity (usually lower) + lipomatous & osseous overgrowth
    - Port-wine capillary stain on lateral extremity with lymphatic vesicles
    - Varicosities of superficial veins
      - Marginal primitive venous system may dominate over diminutive or absent deep venous system
  - Maffucci syndrome
    - Vascular soft tissue masses + enchondromatosis
      - Soft tissue masses likely represent spindle cell hemangiomas rather than true VM

Staging, Grading, & Classification

- 2018 revised classification of VMs by International Society for Study of Vascular Anomalies
  - Common VM (94%)
  - Familial VM cutaneomucosal
    - Multifocal lesions of lips, tongue
    - Dilated neck, upper extremity veins
  - Blue rubber bleb nevus syndrome
    - Multifocal cutaneous, muscular, gastrointestinal VMs
      - Intestinal VMs lead to chronic bleeding, anemia
  - Glomuvenous malformation
    - Presence of glomus cells in VM
    - Darker, less compressible superficial lesions
  - Cerebral cavernous malformation
  - Familial intraosseous vascular malformation
  - Verrucous VM
- Morphologic/drainage classification based on direct injection (Dubois & Puig)
  - Type I: Well circumscribed, isolated without venous drainage
  - Type II: Drainage into normal veins
  - Type III: Drainage into dysplastic ectatic veins
  - Type IV: Composed of ectatic veins

Microscopic Features

- Irregular, variably sized channels of flattened endothelium with variable smooth muscle & no internal elastic lamina
- Intraluminal thrombi are common
- May contain intermixed lymphatic components

CLINICAL ISSUES

Presentation

- Most common signs/symptoms
  - Soft, compressible mass without thrill
    - ± small internal firm thrombi/hard phleboliths
    - Enlarges with Valsalva/crying/dependent positioning
  - Bluish skin discoloration with superficial lesions
  - Episodic pain &/or swelling, which may be due to
    - Engorgement from stasis
    - Intralesional thrombosis
    - Hemorrhage into adjacent tissues, joints
    - Local compression of adjacent tissues
    - Local muscular dysfunction
- Other signs/symptoms
  - Grow proportional to child but may enlarge suddenly due to hemorrhage, thrombosis, or hormonal changes
  - Large varicosities can lead to thromboembolism

Natural History & Prognosis

- Prognosis depends on lesion size, extent, & location
- Larger, more extensive lesions may cause lifelong morbidity

Treatment

- Conservative therapy
  - Compression garments; antiinflammatory medication
  - Low molecular weight heparin if thrombosis risk is ↑
- Percutaneous procedures
  - Direct injection with sclerosing agent under fluoroscopic/US guidance
    - Multiple procedures may be required
  - Laser ablation (Nd:YAG laser) of superficial VM
  - Endovenous ablation of varicosities
    - Radiofrequency vs. laser
- Surgical resection of focal lesions
  - ± percutaneous sclerosis for more extensive VM

SELECTED REFERENCES

1. Abu Ata N et al: Imaging of vascular anomalies in the pediatric musculoskeletal system. Semin Roentgenol. 56(3):288-306, 2021
2. Mattila KA et al: Intra-articular venous malformation of the knee in children: magnetic resonance imaging findings and significance of synovial involvement. Pediatr Radiol. 50(4):509-15, 2020
3. Restrepo R et al: Three distinct vascular anomalies involving skeletal muscle: simplifying the approach for the general radiologist. Radiol Clin North Am. 58(3):603-18, 2020
4. Bertino F et al: Congenital limb overgrowth syndromes associated with vascular anomalies. Radiographics. 39(2):491-515, 2019
5. ISSVA Classification of Vascular Anomalies. Published April 2014. Updated May 2018. Accessed April 27, 2020. https://www.issva.org/UserFiles/file/ISSVA-Classification-2018.pdf
6. Merrow AC et al: 2014 Revised classification of vascular lesions from the International Society for the Study of Vascular Anomalies: radiologic-pathologic update. Radiographics. 36(5):1494-516, 2016
7. Olivieri B et al: Low-flow vascular malformation pitfalls: from clinical examination to practical imaging evaluation–part 2, venous malformation mimickers. AJR Am J Roentgenol. 206(5):952-62, 2016
8. Dasgupta R et al: Venous malformations. Semin Pediatr Surg. 23(4):198-202, 2014

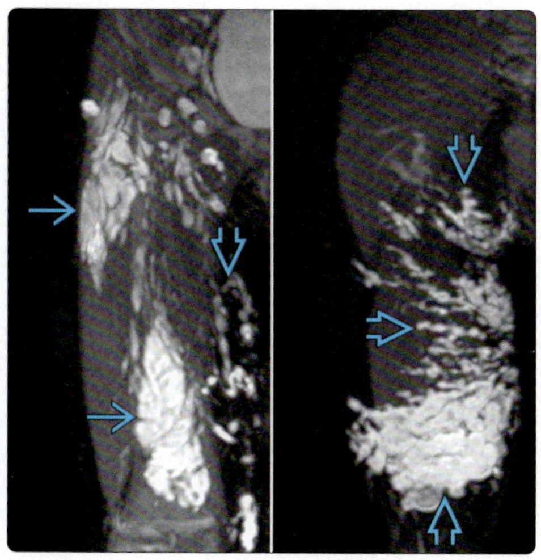

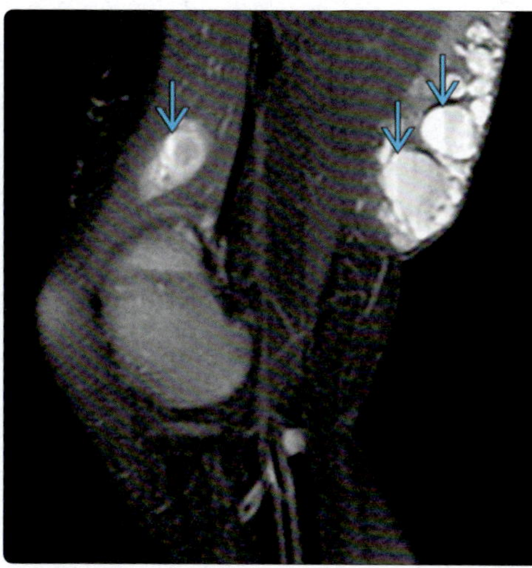

(Left) *Coronal STIR MR MIP images in a 2-year-old show mass-like clusters of malformed intramuscular veins* ➔ *as well variably sized abnormal subcutaneous veins* ➔. **(Right)** *Sagittal T2 FS MR in the same patient using a dedicated knee coil shows higher detail of the malformed veins with fluid-fluid levels seen in multiple channels* ➔ *(due to layering stagnant blood products). Note that the darker sediment lies dependently vs. the higher signal intensity plasma.*

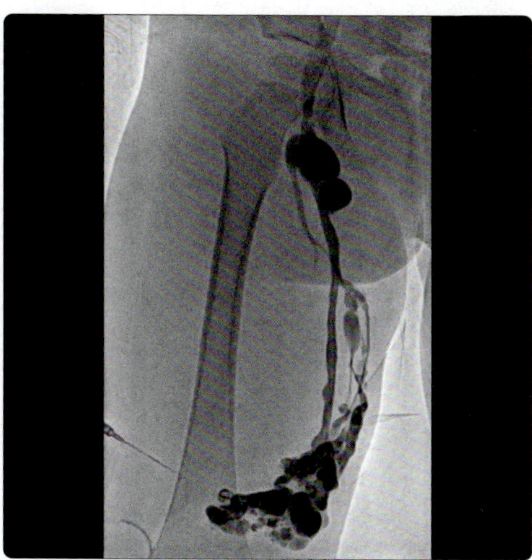

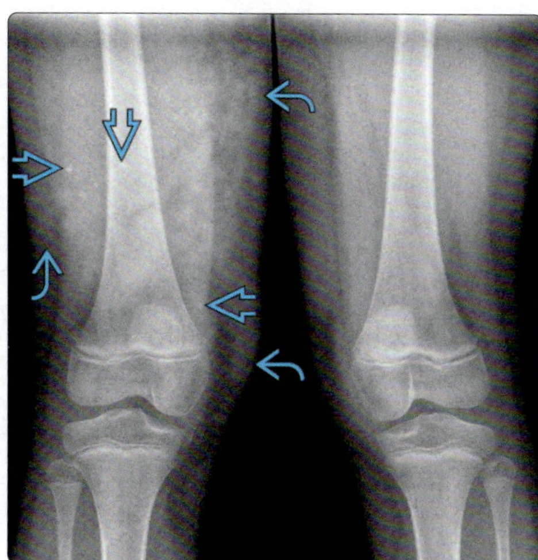

(Left) *Frontal fluoroscopic image during a presclerotherapy diagnostic injection of the same right thigh VM shows continuity of the mass-like clusters of abnormal veins by elongated, smaller caliber abnormal venous channels.* **(Right)** *Frontal radiograph in the same patient 5 years later shows multiple small phleboliths* ➔ *amidst residual lobulated soft tissue masses* ➔*, an essentially pathognomonic x-ray appearance of VMs.*

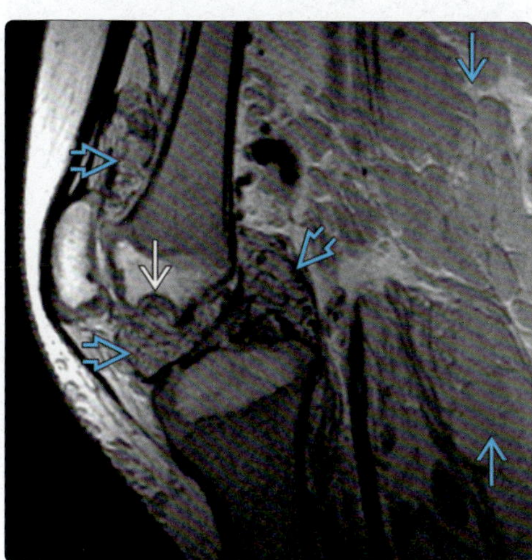

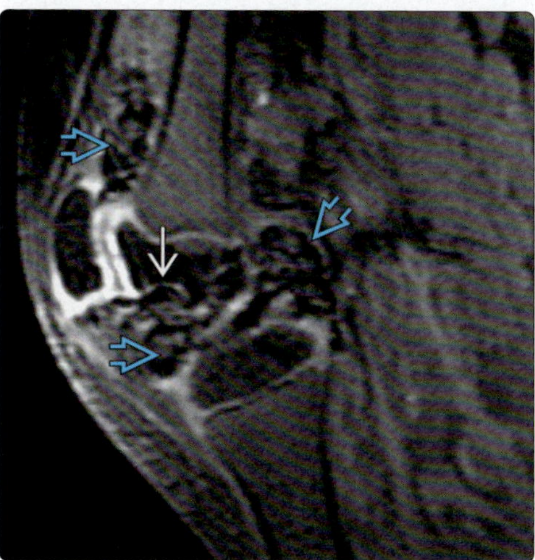

(Left) *Sagittal PD MR in a 9-year-old with an extensive lower extremity VM shows the masses infiltrating all visible muscles* ➔ *& extending into the knee joint* ➔*. There is marked cartilage loss with a large distal femoral erosion* ➔. **(Right)** *Sagittal T2* GRE MR in the same patient shows blooming of hemosiderin within the joint* ➔ *due to recurrent hemarthrosis from the synovial VM. Severe cartilage loss & a large femoral erosion* ➔ *are again noted.*

KEY FACTS

TERMINOLOGY

- Subtype of congenital slow-/low-flow vascular malformation due to error in lymphatic vessel formation
- Results in well-defined, cyst-like (macrocystic) &/or infiltrative, solid-appearing (microcystic) mass of abnormal lymphatic channels
  - Individual cyst size: Macrocyst > 1 cm, microcyst < 1 cm

IMAGING

- Macrocystic lymphatic malformation (LM): Lobulated, well-defined cystic lesion with numerous thin internal septations
  - ± multiple fluid-fluid levels, typically due to hemorrhage
  - Soft & compressible by US with internal swirling debris
  - Protein, blood products, chyle/fat may cause bright T1 signal intensity on MR
  - Enhancement is limited to rim, septations
- Microcystic LM: More poorly defined & solid-appearing
  - ± diffuse enhancement
- Locations: Face, neck, chest, axilla > > abdomen, pelvis, extremities
  - Frequently extend across tissue planes/compartments

TOP DIFFERENTIAL DIAGNOSES

- Venous malformation
- Soft tissue sarcoma
- Soft tissue infection

CLINICAL ISSUES

- Soft & pliable mass, often apparent at birth
  - Can compress airway or other vital structures
  - May present later with pain & rapid enlargement due to hemorrhage, inflammation, or hormonal stimulation
- Primary treatment: Surgical resection &/or percutaneous sclerotherapy
  - Reports of successful medical therapy with sirolimus

(Left) *Transverse ultrasound of the left buttock in a 2-day-old with a clinically apparent capillary lymphaticovenous malformation shows a predominantly anechoic mass with thin septations in the subcutaneous soft tissues ➡, typical of a macrocystic lymphatic malformation.* **(Right)** *Longitudinal color Doppler ultrasound in the same patient shows no significant internal vascular flow within the cysts.*

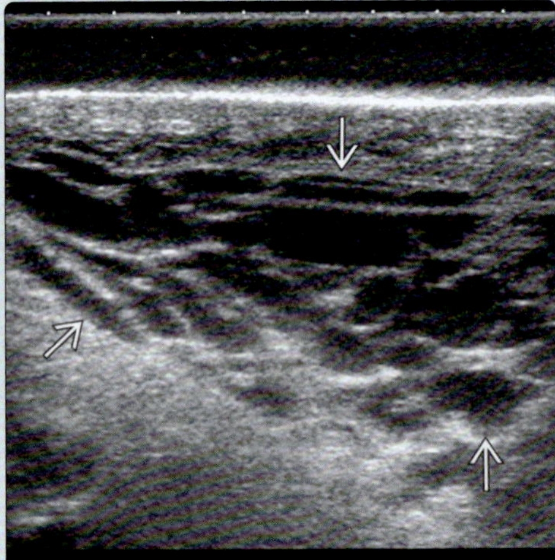

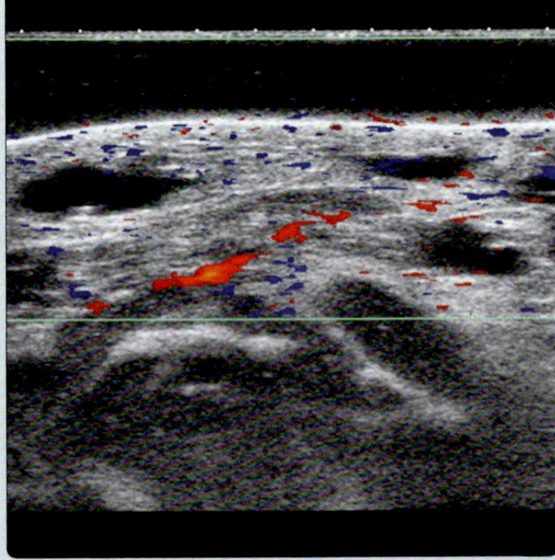

(Left) *Axial T2 FS MR in the same patient shows contiguous cystic foci with internal septations ➡, typical of macrocystic components. The lesion is poorly defined & infiltrative superficially with slightly lower signal intensity ➡, typical of microcystic components. The mildly thickened septations were likely due to interval infection.* **(Right)** *Axial T1 C+ FS MR in the same patient shows mild septal enhancement of the macrocystic components ➡ with more confluent enhancement of the microcystic components ➡.*

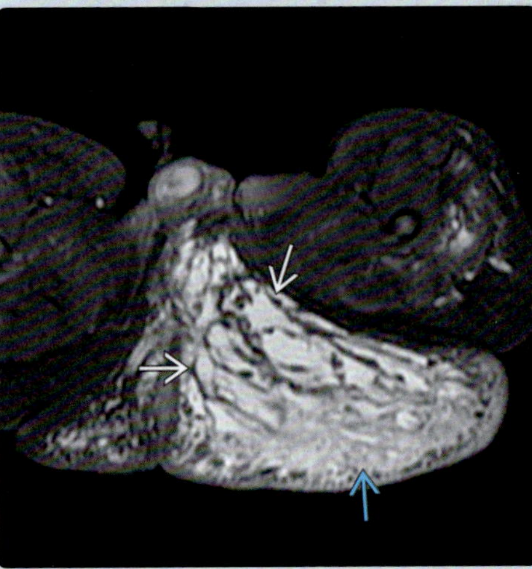

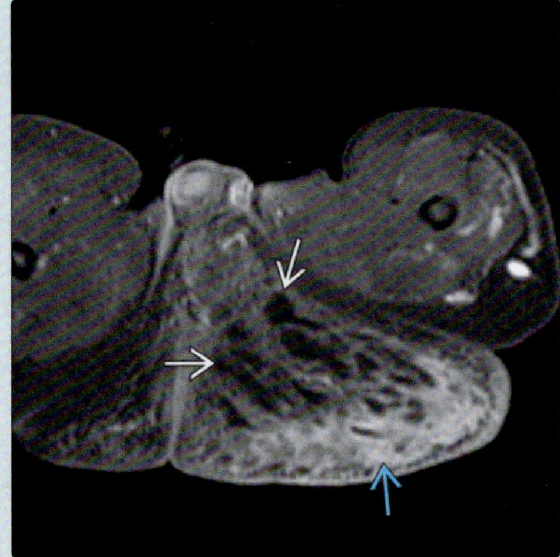

TERMINOLOGY

Abbreviations

- Lymphatic malformation (LM)

Synonyms

- Common (cystic) LM, lymphatic anomaly
- Avoid incorrect & confusing terminology
  - Cystic hygroma is reserved for abnormal midline posterior nuchal translucency on early fetal US
    - Different than anterolateral neck LM, which does not necessarily implicate chromosomal anomalies
  - Lymphangioma implies neoplasm
    - LM is not neoplastic

Definitions

- Subtype of congenital slow-/low-flow vascular malformation due to error in lymphatic vessel formation
  - Results in well-defined, cyst-like (macrocystic) &/or infiltrative, solid-appearing (microcystic) mass of abnormal lymphatic channels
    - Individual cyst size: Macrocyst > 1 cm, microcyst < 1 cm
  - Mass lacks communication with normal lymphatics

IMAGING

General Features

- Location
  - Face, neck, chest, axilla > > abdomen, pelvis, extremities
  - Focal > > multifocal
  - Soft tissue > > bone
  - Frequently extend across tissue planes/compartments
- Size
  - Highly variable
  - May enlarge rapidly with hemorrhage, infection, or hormonal stimulation (puberty, pregnancy)
- Morphology
  - Macrocystic: Lobulated, well-defined cystic lesion with numerous thin internal septations
  - Microcystic: More poorly defined, infiltrative, & solid-appearing
  - Components of both may be present

Ultrasonographic Findings

- Grayscale ultrasound
  - Macrocystic LM: Anechoic cystic mass, usually with thin internal septations
    - ± ↑ echogenicity related to hemorrhage or proteinaceous fluid
    - Soft, compressible with swirling debris internally
  - Microcystic LM: Poorly defined region of subcutaneous soft tissue thickening
    - Mildly hypo- or hyperechoic
- Color Doppler
  - No vascular flow identified in cysts
  - Flow may be identified in septations, typically from encased normal vessels

MR Findings

- **T2 FS/STIR**: Largely fluid signal intensity mass
  - Intervening hypointense septa
  - Fluid-fluid levels due to hemorrhage within some cysts
    - Less frequently seen on other sequences
- **T1**: Hemorrhage, protein, fat/chyle within cysts may cause bright signal intensity; otherwise follows fluid signal
  - Patchy multifocal ↑ fat deposition may be seen in vertebrae in systemic lymphatic disorders
- **T1 C+ FS**
  - Macrocystic LM: Thin rim/septal enhancement of cysts
    - Septations may be thicker from recent inflammation or hemorrhage
  - Microcystic LM: ± confluent enhancement of infiltrating tissue
- **DWI/ADC**: Internal blood products may restrict diffusion, but mean ADC values are typically > 1.9 x 10^{-3} mm²/s
- **MRA/MRV**: No high-flow vessels intrinsic to lesion
  - Nearby normal vessels may be encased by infiltrating LM
- **MR lymphangiogram**: Injection of contrast into lymph nodes with passage followed on dynamic 3D T1 FS sequences
  - More commonly used in setting of lymphedema or chylous ascites/effusions

Imaging Recommendations

- Best imaging tool
  - US is often diagnostic for macrocystic LM, though deep extent & relationship to vital structures may be unclear
  - MR will typically confirm diagnosis & extent of disease
- Protocol advice
  - US: For any soft tissue mass include
    - Compression cine to evaluate internal contents
    - Doppler assessment for presence & types of vascularity
  - MR: For any soft tissue mass include
    - Subtracted (pre- from post-) contrast-enhanced FS T1
      - Particularly relevant in LM as intrinsic T1 shortening from hemorrhage/protein may confound postcontrast images

DIFFERENTIAL DIAGNOSIS

Venous Malformation

- Focal mass vs. conglomeration of abnormal tubular slow-flow channels
- Phleboliths in soft tissue mass are essentially pathognomonic
- Bright (fluid) T2 signal intensity ± fluid-fluid levels on MR
- May have fat along margins or septa
- Gradual patchy enhancement after contrast

Soft Tissue Sarcoma

- Typically firm, well-defined round or ovoid hypovascular solid soft tissue mass with variable enhancement
- May have cystic components, but solid components with internal vascularity are usually visible
- Mean MR ADC values are typically < 1.1 x 10^{-3} mm²/s

Soft Tissue Infection

- Cellulitis: Poorly defined soft tissue thickening with irregular serpentine pockets of fluid
- Abscess: Well-defined hypoechoic collection with mobile debris, thick & irregular walls

PATHOLOGY

General Features

- Associated abnormalities
  - Klippel-Trenaunay syndrome
    - Capillary lymphaticovenous malformation malformation of extremity (usually lower) + lipomatous & osseous overgrowth
    - Port-wine capillary stain on lateral extremity with lymphatic vesicles
    - Varicosities of superficial veins
      - Marginal venous system may dominate over diminutive or absent deep venous system
  - Congenital lipomatous overgrowth with vascular malformations, epidermal nevi, & skeletal anomalies (CLOVES)
    - Truncal lipomatous masses ± LM
    - Other vascular malformations are often present
  - LM may be associated with trisomies 13, 18, 21, or Turner syndrome

Staging, Grading, & Classification

- 2014 revised classification by International Society for Study of Vascular Anomalies (updated 2018)
  - Common (cystic) LM: Macrocystic, microcystic, mixed
  - Generalized lymphatic anomaly (GLA)
    - Multifocal cystic lesions commonly involving pleura, spleen, bones (axial & appendicular skeleton)
      - Progressive cortical destruction is not seen in GLA
    - Macrocystic LM is often present
  - Kaposiform lymphangiomatosis (KLA)
    - May be subtype of GLA
    - Extensive lymphangiectasia of lungs & mediastinum + coagulopathy
  - Gorham-Stout disease (GSD) ("vanishing bone disease")
    - Overlap with GLA but with less extensive disease
    - Favors axial skeleton
    - Progressive regional osteolysis (hallmark of disease) due to focal microcystic LM
      - Multiple adjacent bones are typically involved
  - Channel-type (or "central conducting-type") LM
    - May see dilated central lymphatics &/or secondary manifestations
      - Intestinal lymphangiectasia with bowel wall thickening & abnormal mesentery causing protein-losing enteropathy
      - Chylous pleural effusions & ascites
      - Extremity edema
  - Primary lymphedema

Immunohistochemical Features

- Endothelium stains positive for lymphatic markers
  - PROX1 & VEGFR-3 most sensitive, specific
  - D2-40 & LYVE-1 less sensitive in large channel LM

CLINICAL ISSUES

Presentation

- Most common signs/symptoms
  - Soft & pliable mass without pain
- Other signs/symptoms
  - Pain &/or rapid enlargement due to hemorrhage, inflammation, or hormonal stimulation
  - Cutaneous vesicles suggest LM, though overlying skin is often normal
  - Compression of airway or other vital structures
  - Diffuse limb enlargement

Demographics

- Age
  - Identified at birth or prenatally in majority of cases

Natural History & Prognosis

- LMs generally grow commensurate with patient
  - May enlarge rapidly due to hemorrhage, inflammation, or hormonal stimulation
- Prognosis is better for small focal lesions
  - Difficult to treat entirety of large, infiltrating lesion with surgery or sclerotherapy, leading to recurrence

Treatment

- Compression garments
- Surgical resection &/or percutaneous sclerotherapy
  - Combination is often required for larger infiltrating lesions
  - Sclerotherapy for macrocystic > microcystic disease
    - Direct injection of sclerosing agent into LM under sonographic/fluoroscopic guidance
      - Doxycycline, bleomycin, OK-432, ethanol
      - Utility of bleomycin is also reported in microcystic LM
    - Major complications (skin necrosis, nerve damage, extremity swelling, muscle atrophy, disseminated intravascular coagulation) are uncommon
    - Full results of sclerosis can take months to manifest
      - May take multiple staged procedures to treat lesion
- Medical therapy with sirolimus (mTOR inhibitor) is gaining favor

SELECTED REFERENCES

1. Abu Ata N et al: Imaging of vascular anomalies in the pediatric musculoskeletal system. Semin Roentgenol. 56(3):288-306, 2021
2. Kronfli AP et al: Lymphatic malformations: a 20-year single institution experience. Pediatr Surg Int. 37(6):783-90, 2021
3. Ramirez-Suarez KI et al: Dynamic contrast-enhanced magnetic resonance lymphangiography. Pediatr Radiol. ePub, 2021
4. Zobel MJ et al: Management of cervicofacial lymphatic malformations requires a multidisciplinary approach. J Pediatr Surg. 56(5):1062-7, 2021
5. Bertino F et al: Congenital limb overgrowth syndromes associated with vascular anomalies. Radiographics. 39(2):491-515, 2019
6. ISSVA Classification of Vascular Anomalies. Published April 2014. Updated May 2018. Accessed April 29, 2020. https://www.issva.org/UserFiles/file/ISSVA-Classification-2018.pdf
7. Johnson CM et al: Clinical and sonographic features of pediatric soft-tissue vascular anomalies part 2: vascular malformations. Pediatr Radiol. 47(9):1196-208, 2017
8. Kim SH et al: Clinical features of mesenteric lymphatic malformation in children. J Pediatr Surg. 51(4):582-7, 2016
9. Merrow AC et al: 2014 Revised classification of vascular lesions from the International Society for the Study of Vascular Anomalies: radiologic-pathologic update. Radiographics. 36(5):1494-516, 2016
10. Wassef M et al: Vascular anomalies classification: recommendations from the International Society for the Study of Vascular Anomalies. Pediatrics. 136(1):e203-14, 2015
11. Lala S et al: Gorham-Stout disease and generalized lymphatic anomaly–clinical, radiologic, and histologic differentiation. Skeletal Radiol. 42(7):917-24, 2013

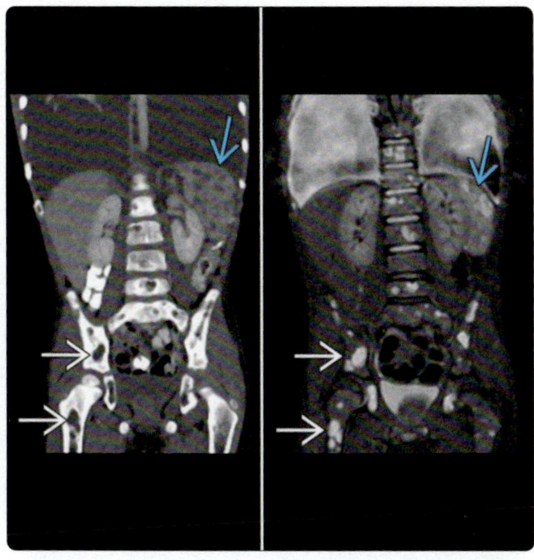

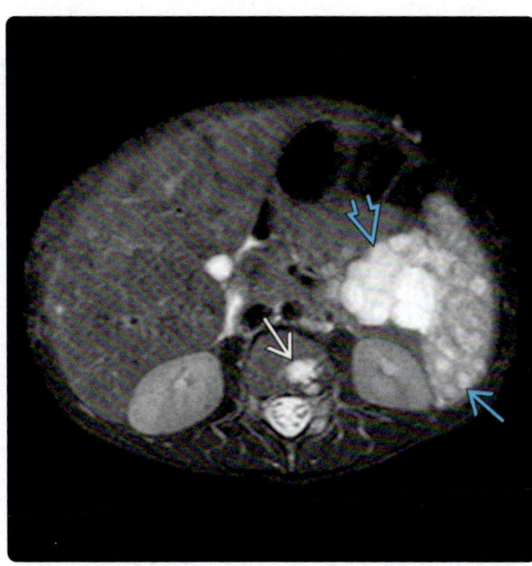

(Left) *Coronal CECT (left) & STIR MR (right) images of the abdomen in a 5-year-old patient with shortness of breath show large, bilateral pleural effusions, numerous well-defined lucent (CT) & fluid signal intensity (MR) bone lesions without cortical destruction ➡, + multiple splenic lesions ➡.* **(Right)** *Axial T2 FS MR in the same patient shows the bone ➡ & splenic lesions ➡ as well as a lobulated macrocystic mass ➡ in the splenic hilum. The constellation of findings in this case is typical of generalized lymphatic anomaly.*

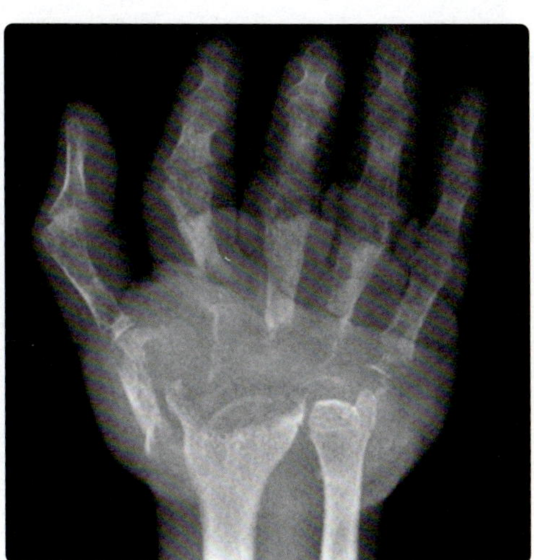

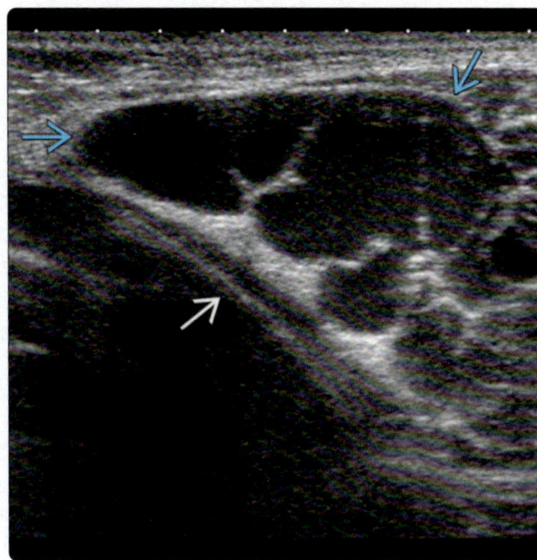

(Left) *PA radiograph in a 14-year-old patient with years of pain shows severe osteolysis of the wrist & hand, typical of Gorham-Stout disease. The bone resorption had progressed severely over 3 years compared to a prior radiograph (not shown).* **(Right)** *Ultrasound of the axillary soft tissues in a 2-year-old patient with a soft, pliable mass shows a well-defined, lobulated, multicystic lesion ➡ with thin internal septations, typical of a macrocystic lymphatic malformation. Note the intact underlying rib ➡.*

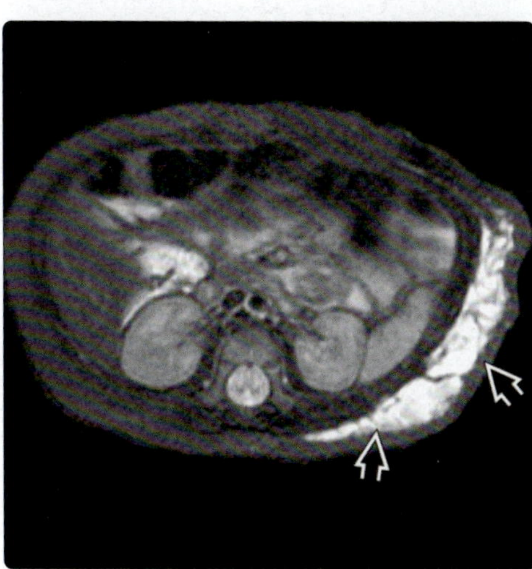

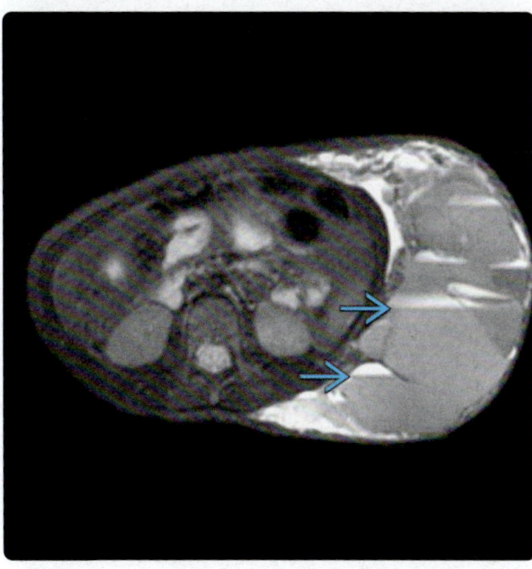

(Left) *Axial T2 FS MR shows an elongated, septated fluid signal intensity mass of the subcutaneous left flank ➡, typical of a lymphatic malformation.* **(Right)** *Axial T2 FS MR obtained 1 month later in the same patient shows marked interval enlargement of the mass. Numerous fluid-fluid levels ➡ are now seen in the mass, typical of layering blood products due to interval hemorrhage.*

Arteriovenous Malformation (Musculoskeletal)

KEY FACTS

TERMINOLOGY

- Congenital high-flow vascular lesion with abnormal direct connections between arteries & veins (with no intervening capillary bed)

IMAGING

- Tangle of abnormal high-flow vessels with variable (often minimal) soft tissue mass
- Draining veins are enlarged > tortuous feeding arteries
- Grayscale US: Clustered, anechoic tubular channels
- Color Doppler US: Channels all fill with color; artifactual flow in surrounding soft tissues due to vibration
- Pulsed Doppler US: Numerous low-resistance (high diastolic flow) arterial waveforms & arterialized venous waveforms; spectral broadening
- MR spin-echo: Tangle of flow voids in lesion (before & after contrast); phase-encoding pulsation artifact at nidus; ± surrounding edema or soft tissue components
- CTA/MRA: Rapid contrast enhancement of nidus; early enhancement of draining veins due to shunting

TOP DIFFERENTIAL DIAGNOSES

- Infantile hemangioma
- Venous malformation
- Arteriovenous fistula
- Soft tissue sarcoma
- *PTEN* hamartoma

CLINICAL ISSUES

- Presentation: Warm, pulsatile mass with thrill/bruit, pain, congestive heart failure (< 2%), steal phenomenon, skin discoloration, ulceration, prolonged bleeding
- Treatment generally consists of transarterial embolization without, or in conjunction with, surgical resection
- ~ 80% of superficial AVMs present in childhood
  - Hormonal stimulation of puberty or pregnancy → ↑ AVM size & symptoms in 2nd/3rd decades of life

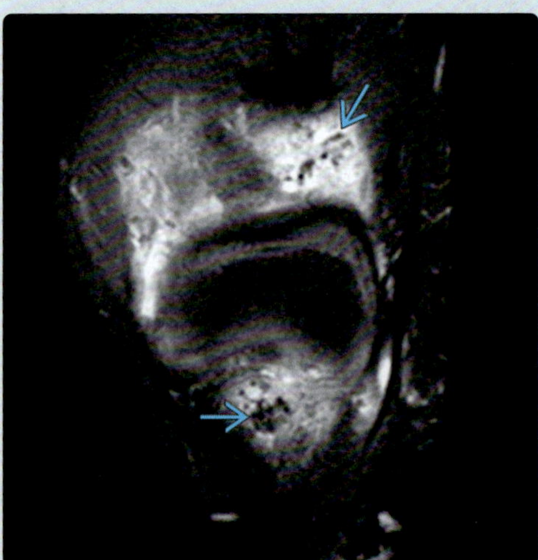

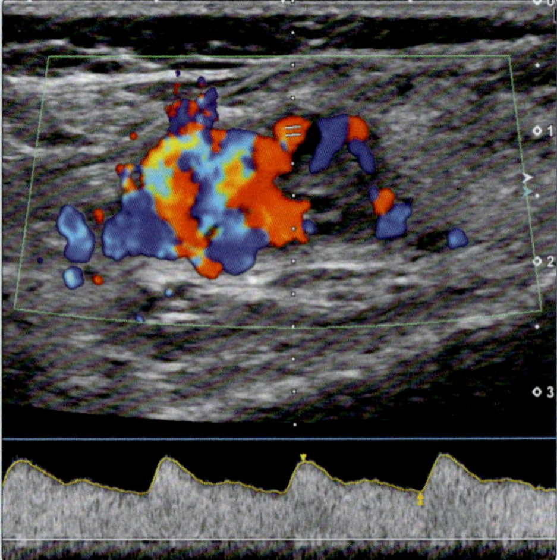

(Left) *Coronal T2 FS MR in a 5-year-old with a longstanding mass & worsening knee pain shows clusters of small flow voids* → *(due to high-flow vessels) within surrounding poorly defined hyperintense tissue about the patella.* **(Right)** *Longitudinal spectral Doppler US in the same patient shows abnormally low-resistance arteries within one of the clusters of vessels, typical of an arteriovenous malformation (AVM).*

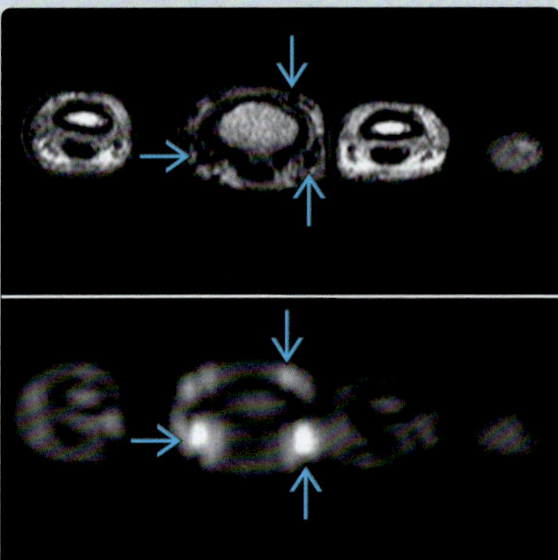

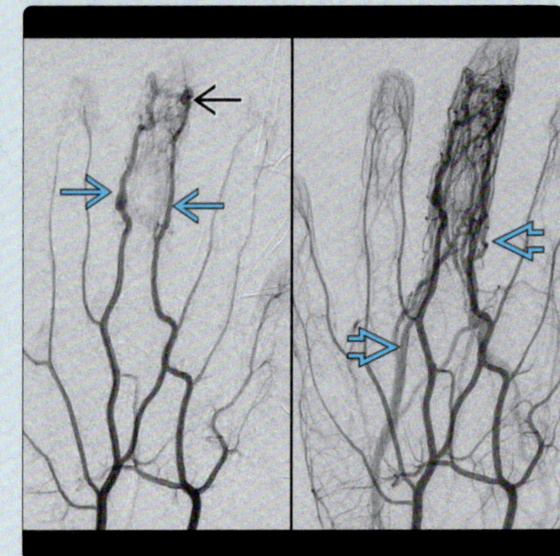

(Left) *Axial PD (top) & 2D TOF (bottom) MR images in a 9-year-old with a painful blue finger show numerous enlarged vessels (flow voids on PD & flow-enhancement on TOF)* → *throughout the visualized digit.* **(Right)** *Arterial- (left) & early venous- (right) phase DSA images of the hand in the same patient show a nidus of abnormal tangled arteries* → *in the distal middle finger with enlargement of the supplying digital arteries* →*. There is early visualization of enlarged draining veins* ⇨*, consistent with shunting in this AVM.*

TERMINOLOGY

Definitions

- Arteriovenous malformation (AVM): Congenital high-flow vascular lesion with abnormal direct connections between arteries & veins (i.e., no intervening capillary bed)

IMAGING

General Features

- Morphology: Cluster of abnormal high-flow vessels; variable (but often minimal) associated soft tissue mass; draining veins are enlarged > tortuous feeding arteries
- Location: Essentially anywhere; often transspatial
  - Up to 20% of extremity AVMs have bone involvement
- **Radiographs**: ± mass-like density of soft tissues without phleboliths, limb/bone overgrowth; rare bone destruction
- **US:** Often used for initial investigation of mass
  - Grayscale: Clustered anechoic tubular channels (high vessel density) ± adjacent soft tissue edema/distortion (but classically without well-defined mass)
  - Color Doppler: Channels all fill with color flow; artifactual flow in surrounding soft tissues due to vibration
  - Pulsed Doppler: Numerous low-resistance (high diastolic flow) arterial waveforms with spectral broadening; arterialized venous waveforms
- **MR**
  - Spin-echo: Tangle(s) of flow voids in lesion due to high flow; phase-encoding pulsation artifact of nidus; ± surrounding edema or soft tissue components (in up to 50%, especially multicompartmental AVMs)
  - Gradient-echo: High-flow vessels are typically bright before & after contrast
- **CTA/MRA**: Useful for characterizing lesion, determining involvement of adjacent tissues, & planning embolization or surgery through measurement & mapping of vessels
  - Rapid contrast enhancement of nidus
    - Time-resolved/dynamic MRA: "Contrast rise time" < 20 seconds is highly specific for high-flow lesions
  - Early enhancement of draining veins due to shunting
  - Enlargement of otherwise normal vessels supplying/draining lesion

DIFFERENTIAL DIAGNOSIS

Infantile Hemangioma

- Discrete, heterogeneous, typically subcutaneous, high-flow, benign soft tissue neoplasm in infant
- US shows patchy regions of ↑ & ↓ echogenicity
  - High vessel density by color Doppler (not grayscale)
  - Low-resistance arterial waveforms during proliferation (but no shunting)

Venous Malformation

- Discrete or infiltrating low-flow mass, often intramuscular
  - Multiple high-signal serpentine channels on T2 FS MR
  - ± fluid-fluid levels in stagnant channels
- Phleboliths in pediatric mass are virtually diagnostic

Arteriovenous Fistula

- Direct high-flow communication between artery & vein without surrounding tangle of abnormal vessels

Soft Tissue Sarcomas

- Typically well-circumscribed, firm, solid mass
- Most have low to intermediate levels of vascularity

PTEN Hamartoma of Soft Tissue

- Heterogeneous mass with variable soft tissue components, including myxomatous & fatty elements
- High-flow vessels are typical
- Phenotype of *PTEN* mutation: Macrocrania, skin lesions

CLINICAL ISSUES

Presentation

- Most common signs/symptoms
  - Warm, pulsatile mass with thrill/bruit, pain
- Other signs/symptoms
  - Congestive heart failure (< 2%), steal phenomenon, skin discoloration, ulceration, prolonged bleeding
  - Limb length discrepancy: Bone overgrowth
  - Associated capillary stains (CM-AVM) are often multifocal & surrounded by characteristic pale halo
    - Number ↑ with age
  - May rarely present in utero with hydrops

Demographics

- ~ 80% of superficial AVMs present in childhood
  - Large shunting lesions may present soon after birth
  - Hormonal stimulation of puberty or pregnancy → ↑ AVM size & symptoms in 2nd/3rd decades of life

Natural History & Prognosis

- Schobinger classification: Outlines progressive clinical course of untreated AVMs
  - Stage 1 (quiescence)
    - All progress with > 80% doing so before adulthood
  - Stage 2 (expansion): ↑ pulse & thrill
  - Stage 3 (destruction): Local destruction with pain, ischemia, necrosis
  - Stage 4 (decompensation): High-output cardiac failure

Treatment

- Cure is rarely achievable; main goal is clinical improvement
- Conservative management: Compression garments
- Transarterial embolization
  - 75% volume devascularization rates are reported in 47-94%
- Surgical excision
  - Resection is best < 24 hours after embolization
- Recurrence rate: > 80-90%

SELECTED REFERENCES

1. Hawkins CM et al: Diagnosis and management of extracranial vascular malformations in children: arteriovenous malformations, venous malformations, and lymphatic malformations. Semin Roentgenol. 54(4):337-48, 2019
2. Sibley CD et al: Capillary malformation-arteriovenous malformation syndrome. JAMA Dermatol. 155(6):733, 2019
3. Do YS et al: Special consideration for intraosseous arteriovenous malformations. Semin Intervent Radiol. 34(3):272-9, 2017
4. Johnson CM et al: Clinical and sonographic features of pediatric soft-tissue vascular anomalies part 2: vascular malformations. Pediatr Radiol. 47(9):1196-208, 2017
5. Dunham GM et al: Finding the nidus: detection and workup of non-central nervous system arteriovenous malformations. Radiographics. 36(3):891-903, 2016

KEY FACTS

TERMINOLOGY

- Synonyms: Desmoid-type fibromatosis, aggressive fibromatosis, extraabdominal desmoid tumor, musculoaponeurotic fibromatosis
- Most common of fibrous tumors in children (60%)
- Locally aggressive with tendency to slowly infiltrate adjacent tissues
- Frequently recurs but lacks metastatic disease

IMAGING

- Homogeneous or heterogeneous with low T1 & T2 signal
  - Cellular components: T2 hyperintense/enhancing
  - Collagenous components: T2 hypointense/nonenhancing
- May be well defined or infiltrative
- Often in/adjacent to muscle; often multicompartmental
- Can remodel adjacent bone
- May arise at site of prior surgery or from preexisting Gardner fibroma
  - Gardner fibromas are typically plaque-like

PATHOLOGY

- Most are due to sporadic mutations activating β-catenin signaling pathway
- *APC* gene mutation (long arm of chromosome 5q21-22): Gardner syndrome

CLINICAL ISSUES

- Wait & see in some cases: May regress or stop growing
- Complete excision is often difficult due to infiltration
- Frequent local recurrence: 25-88%
  - Involvement of neurovascular bundle on baseline MR is greatest predictor for residual or recurrent disease

DIAGNOSTIC CHECKLIST

- Can mimic soft tissue sarcomas
- Due to slow growth, comparison to multiple prior exams is recommended to appreciate interval change

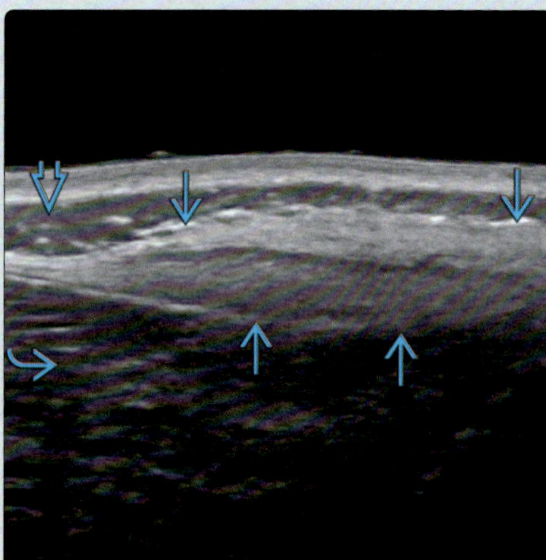

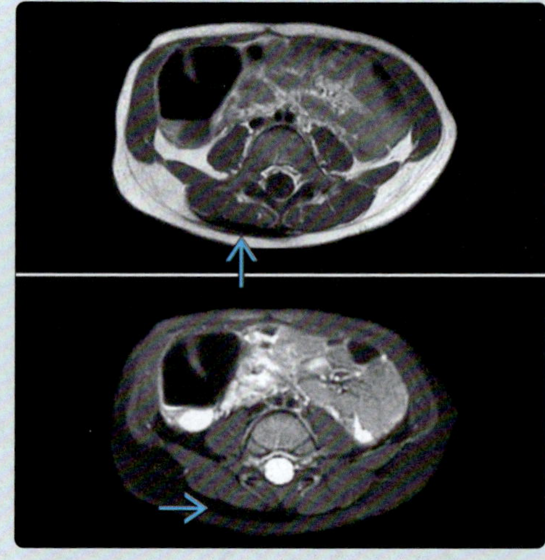

(Left) *Transverse ultrasound of the back in a 2-year-old with a palpable firm mass shows elongated echogenic tissue ➡ at the interface of the subcutaneous fat ➡ & muscle ➡.* **(Right)** *Axial T1 (top) & T2 FS (bottom) MR images in the same patient show diffusely hypointense signal throughout the plaque-like mass ➡, proven to be a Gardner fibroma in a patient with an APC mutation.*

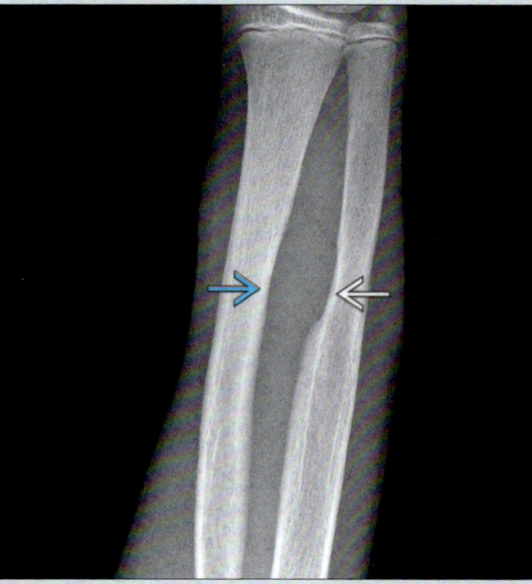

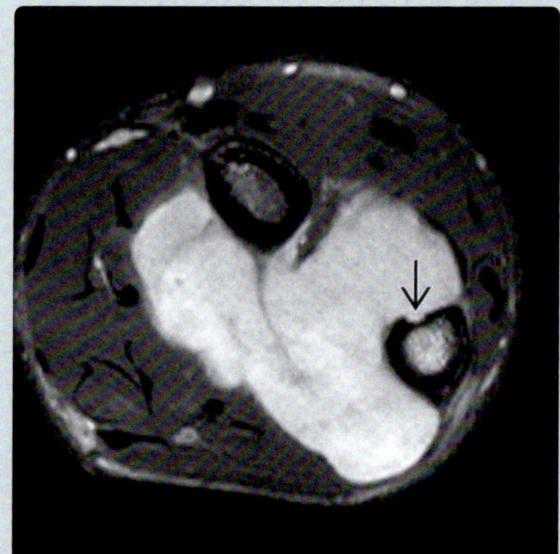

(Left) *AP radiograph in a 14-year-old boy who injured his forearm 2 weeks prior shows subtle remodeling of the radius ➡ & ulna ➡ with cortical scalloping.* **(Right)** *Axial T2 FS MR in the same teenager shows a lobulated hyperintense mass along the interosseous membrane between the radius & ulna. Note the cortical remodeling of the volar margin of the ulna ➡ by this desmoid-type fibromatosis. With chemotherapy, increasing streaks of ↓ signal were noted in the lesion over time.*

TERMINOLOGY

Synonyms

- Desmoid-type fibromatosis, aggressive fibromatosis, extraabdominal desmoid tumor, musculoaponeurotic fibromatosis

Definitions

- Most common of fibrous tumors in children (60%)
- Locally aggressive with tendency to slowly infiltrate adjacent tissues
- Frequently recurs but lacks metastatic disease

IMAGING

General Features

- Location
  - Often in/adjacent to muscle; often multicompartmental
  - May arise at site of prior surgery or from preexisting Gardner fibroma
- Size
  - Varies widely; may be up to 20 cm (especially in Gardner syndrome)
- Morphology
  - Abdominal wall lesions tend to be more round/ovoid & well defined
  - Extremity lesions tend to be more elongated with nodular or tendril-like extensions
- **Desmoid-type fibromatosis (aggressive fibromatosis)**
  - 1st peak: 4-5 years old; 2nd peak: 25-35 years
  - F > M in younger patients
  - Erosions, scalloping, or bowing of bones
  - Nodular (more common in adults) or infiltrative (children) patterns
  - High potential for recurrence, locally aggressive
  - May spontaneously regress
- **Abdominal wall fibromatosis**
  - Most commonly in rectus abdominis muscles & adjacent fascia
  - Often related to recent pregnancy (in past year)
- **Gardner fibroma**
  - Mostly occur in 1st decade of life
  - Detection may be sentinel event leading to diagnosis of Gardner syndrome
  - Strong association with desmoid fibromatosis & Gardner syndrome
  - Plaque-like mass, typically hypointense T1 & T2 on MR with variable contrast enhancement
  - Common in trunk, paraspinal, head/neck, & extremities

Radiographic Findings

- Nondescript soft tissue mass
- ± periosteal reaction, scalloping, or erosions

CT Findings

- CECT
  - Soft tissue mass hyperdense to muscle
  - ± adjacent osseous changes, typically sparing medullary space

Ultrasonographic Findings

- Common 1st-line imaging modality for palpable mass
- Nonspecific soft tissue mass with variable echogenicity; may be well circumscribed or infiltrative & poorly defined

MR Findings

- T1WI
  - Typically hypointense to muscle; can be isointense
  - Frequently centered in intermuscular location with rim of surrounding fat (split fat sign)
- T2WI
  - Hyperintense or heterogeneous with bands of hypointense signal (fibrous components)
    - Depends on cellular compared (high signal) to collagen (low signal) components
  - Wide variability from diffusely low signal to diffusely high signal intensity
    - Significant portion of very hypointense signal is typical
    - Lesions with high signal at baseline are more likely to progress on therapy
  - Often insinuates slowly along fascial planes (fascial tail sign); may extend distance from main lesion
- DWI
  - Mean ADC value is higher than malignant soft tissue tumors
- T1WI C+
  - Variable enhancement depending on lesion activity

Nuclear Medicine Findings

- PET
  - Mild F-18 FDG uptake (with mean SUV of 3.1 in one study)

DIFFERENTIAL DIAGNOSIS

Infantile Myofibromatosis

- Most common in infancy but may occur in adults
- 90% in first 2 years of life, 50% in newborns
- ↑ in size & number to 1 year of age, then can regress
- 3 types: Solitary or multicentric involvement of soft tissues & bone, ± visceral involvement
  - Sharply defined bubbly lucent lesions of bone (metaphyseal > diaphyseal), often relatively symmetric
- MR: May have target appearance with nonenhancing center
  - ± Ca^{2+}

Congenital or Infantile Fibrosarcoma

- Typically presents < 2 years of age, commonly neonatal or congenital
- Can erode adjacent bone, rarely metastasize
- US: May be hypervascular with solid & cystic/hemorrhagic components
- MR: Heterogeneous enhancement, may be cystic
- Better prognosis than adults

Rhabdomyosarcoma

- Well-circumscribed solid soft tissue mass ± necrotic or hemorrhagic foci
- MR: Intermediate to high T2 signal, variable enhancement

Synovial Sarcoma

- Well-circumscribed soft tissue mass in close proximity to joint
- Amorphous Ca^{2+}

- MR: May be small & cystic-appearing before contrast

Venous Malformation

- Low-flow lesion with lobulated &/or tubular clusters
- MR: Fluid signal intensity ± phleboliths &/or thrombi, fluid-fluid levels, & patchy or diffuse enhancement

Plexiform Neurofibromas

- Clinical diagnosis of neurofibromatosis type 1 has often been established prior to imaging, but not always
- Elongated lobulated soft tissue lesions following course of nerve/nerves
  - With clustering of numerous lesions, may infiltrate/distort tissue planes & create bag of worms appearance
- MR: Typically T2 hyperintense; in cross section, individual lobules often have target appearance with central hypointensity

Fibrous Hamartoma of Infancy

- Neonates → young children (typically first 2 years of life, 1/4 are congenital)
- Subcutaneous or reticular dermis, 0.5 → 4 cm
- Axilla, shoulders, inguinal region, & chest wall are most common locations
- Excision is usually curative, excellent prognosis
- MR: Varying amounts of fibrous & fatty tissue
  - May have streaks of fat

Inflammatory Myofibroblastic Tumor

- Median age: 9 years old
- Most common in lung, mesentery, omentum
- May have inflammatory syndrome with fever, weight loss, abnormal lab values
- MR: Variable signal intensity depending on fibrous components

PATHOLOGY

General Features

- Etiology
  - β-catenin signaling pathway activation
- Genetics
  - Most are sporadic mutations
  - *APC* gene mutation (long arm of chromosome 5q21-22): Gardner syndrome
- Associated abnormalities
  - Familial adenomatosis fibromatosis (FAP) in 5% of Gardner syndrome patients
    - 1,000x greater risk of developing fibromatosis due to *APC* gene
    - Fibromatosis in 10-20% of FAP patients
  - Trisomies 7, 8, 14, 20

CLINICAL ISSUES

Presentation

- Most common signs/symptoms
  - Palpable mass
  - Firm, poorly circumscribed, slowly growing mass
  - Tends to extend beyond palpable limits
  - Flexion contractures
  - ± tenderness (related to nerve compression or infiltration)

Demographics

- Ethnicity
  - More common in White patients
- Epidemiology
  - 2-4/1 million per year

Natural History & Prognosis

- Recurrence: 25-88% locally
  - Involvement of neurovascular bundle on baseline MR is greatest predictor for residual or recurrent disease
  - Larger lesions, < 30 years old, female predominance, location
  - Controversy over positive resection margin

Treatment

- With tissue confirmation: Wait & see; some lesions regress
- Surgical excision with wide margins; recurrence in 33-88%
  - For abdominal wall, symptomatic lesions, & progressive disease
  - Often wide excision is not feasible due to loss of function
- Chemotherapy, radiation therapy

DIAGNOSTIC CHECKLIST

Consider

- Can mimic soft tissue sarcomas

Image Interpretation Pearls

- Often contains regions of ↓ signal on T2 FS & T1 C+ FS MR
  - Inactive fibrous rather than active cellular components
- Due to slow growth, comparison to multiple prior exams is recommended to appreciate interval change

SELECTED REFERENCES

1. Zanchetta E et al: Magnetic resonance imaging patterns of tumor response to chemotherapy in desmoid-type fibromatosis. Cancer Med. 10(13):4356-65, 2021
2. Davis JL et al: Pediatric and infantile fibroblastic/myofibroblastic tumors in the molecular era. Surg Pathol Clin. 13(4):739-62, 2020
3. Garcia-Ortega DY et al: Desmoid-type fibromatosis. Cancers (Basel). 12(7), 2020
4. Navarro OM: Pearls and pitfalls in the imaging of soft-tissue masses in children. Semin Ultrasound CT MR. 41(5):498-512, 2020
5. Caro-Domínguez P et al: Imaging appearances of soft-tissue tumors of the pediatric foot: review of a 15-year experience at a tertiary pediatric hospital. Pediatr Radiol. 47(12):1555-71, 2017
6. Sargar KM et al: Pediatric fibroblastic and myofibroblastic tumors: a pictorial review. Radiographics. 36(4):1195-214, 2016
7. He XD et al: Prognostic factors for the recurrence of sporadic desmoid-type fibromatosis after macroscopically complete resection: analysis of 114 patients at a single institution. Eur J Surg Oncol. 41(8):1013-9, 2015
8. Xu H et al: Desmoid-type fibromatosis of the thorax: CT, MRI, and FDG PET characteristics in a large series from a tertiary referral center. Medicine (Baltimore). 94(38):e1547, 2015
9. Murphey MD et al: From the archives of the AFIP: musculoskeletal fibromatoses: radiologic-pathologic correlation. Radiographics. 29(7):2143-73, 2009

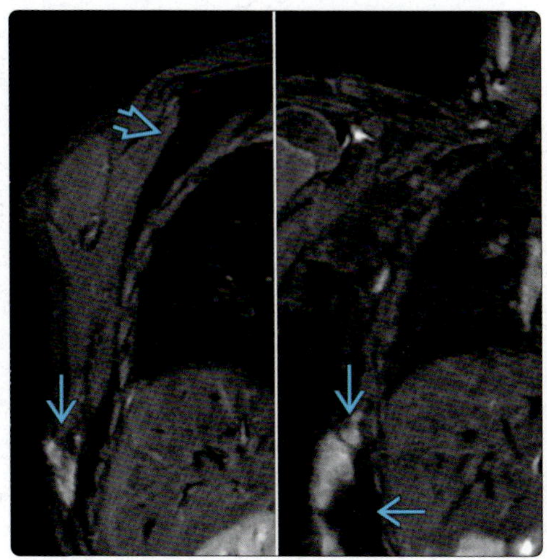

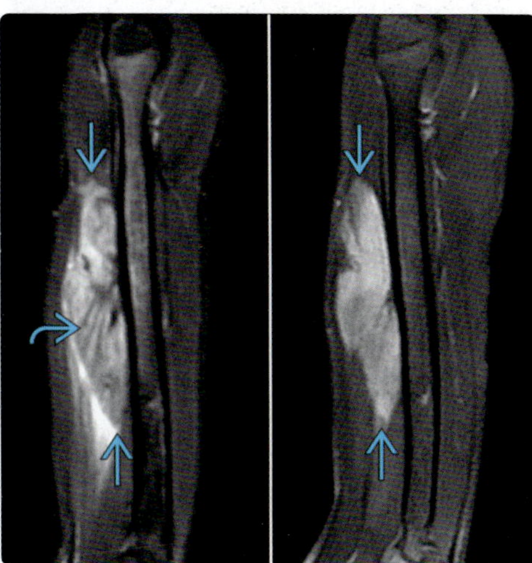

(Left) *Coronal STIR MR images in a 3-year-old with APC mutation-confirmed Gardner fibromatosis show 2 lesions: A stable, homogeneously low signal, plaque-like mass of the chest wall ⇨ & a heterogeneous lobulated growing mass of the flank ⇨.* **(Right)** *Sagittal STIR (left) & T1 C+ FS (right) MR images in a 9-year-old show an elongated heterogeneous intramuscular mass ⇨ proven to be desmoid fibromatosis. Note streaks of internal hypointensity ⇨. Due to progressive growth toward the chest, amputation was ultimately performed.*

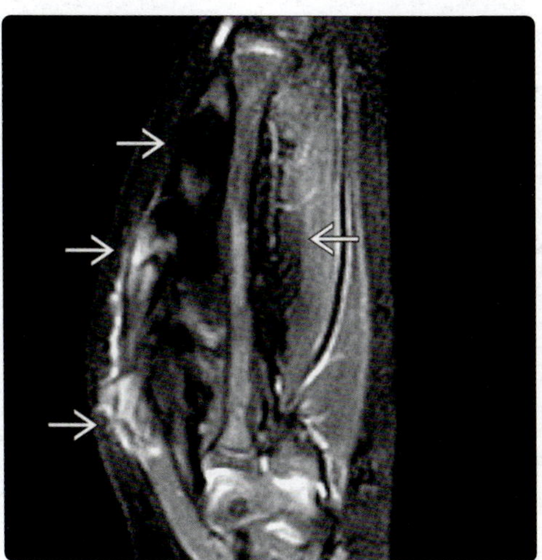

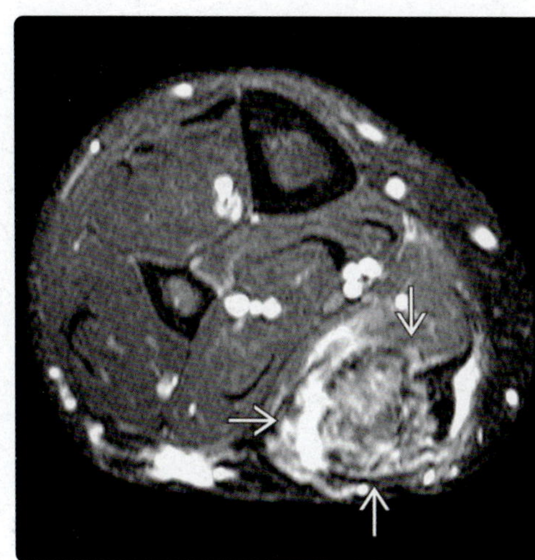

(Left) *Coronal STIR MR of the forearm in a child just under 2 years of age shows a heterogeneous but predominantly hypointense ill-defined & infiltrative soft tissue mass ➡. This was biopsied & proven to be desmoid-type fibromatosis.* **(Right)** *Axial T2 FS MR shows a heterogeneous, ill-defined soft tissue mass ➡ in the posterior right calf of a 16-year-old patient who had recurrent desmoid-type fibromatosis.*

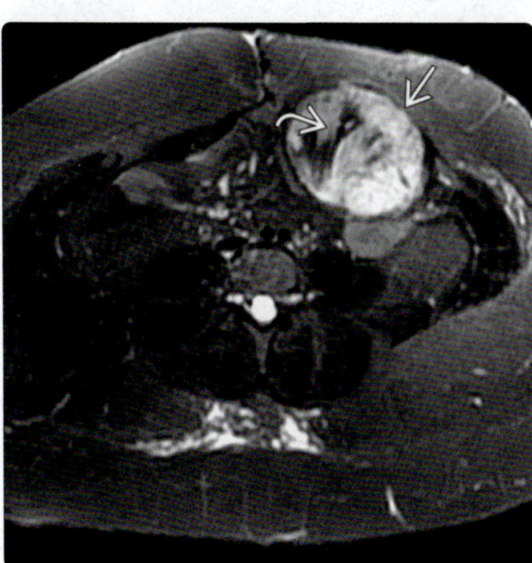

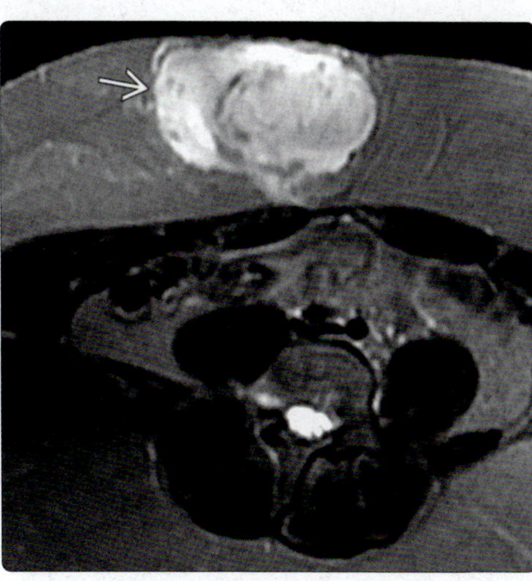

(Left) *Axial T2 FS MR shows a heterogeneous mass ➡ within the left rectus abdominis muscle of a 25-year-old with Down syndrome & a history of multiple abdominal surgeries. Note the hypointense bands ➡ within this desmoid fibromatosis.* **(Right)** *Axial T2 FS MR shows a hyperintense subcutaneous mass ➡ extending to the anterior margin of the right rectus abdominis muscle in a 17-year-old boy. The mass was intensely enhancing (not shown) & proved to be a desmoid fibromatosis.*

Infantile Myofibroma/Myofibromatosis

KEY FACTS

TERMINOLOGY

- Infantile myofibroma: Solitary, benign fibrous tumor of young children with high rate of spontaneous regression
- Myofibromatosis: Multicentric disease with soft tissue & bone lesions ± visceral involvement
  - Poorer prognosis with visceral lesions

IMAGING

- Myofibroma: Solitary, solid soft tissue mass in infant
  - ± internal Ca^{2+}, bizarre adjacent bone remodeling
  - Hypovascular internally by Doppler
  - T2 FS MR: Variable internal signal intensity
  - T1 C+ FS MR: Peripheral/rim enhancement
  - Typical locations
    - Cutaneous, subcutaneous, muscular: 86%
    - Head & neck (50%) > trunk > extremities
- Myofibromatosis (25-55% of myofibroma cases)
  - Soft tissue masses
  - Relatively symmetric bony metaphyseal/metadiaphyseal lucent lesions ± remodeling, cortical loss
  - Visceral involvement in 25-37% of multicentric cases
    - Lungs > gastrointestinal tract > heart > liver

PATHOLOGY

- Peripheral clusters of spindled myofibroblastic cells
- Central cellularity & vascularity similar to hemangiopericytoma

CLINICAL ISSUES

- Presentations: Soft tissue mass ± red-purple skin nodules
  - Perinatal in 50%; 90% diagnosed by age 2
- Solitary/multicentric without visceral involvement: High rate of spontaneous regression over 1-2 years; 1% mortality
  - Observation vs. surgical resection
- Multicentric with visceral involvement: 48-75% mortality historically due to obstruction, organ failure
  - Favorable outcomes with low-dose chemotherapy

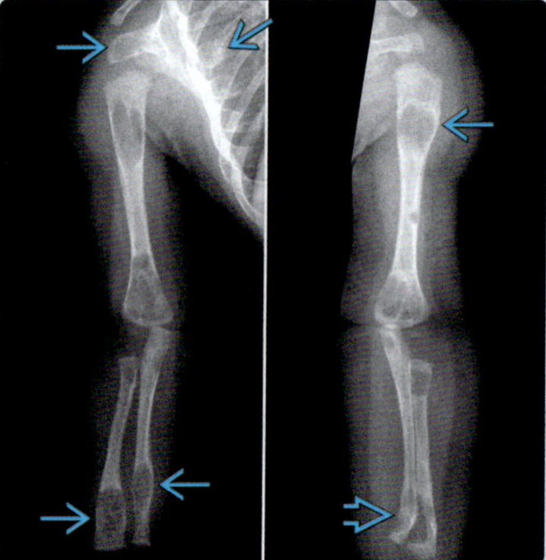

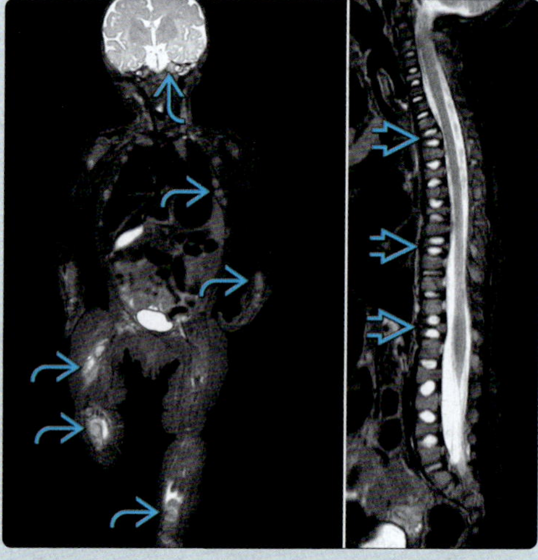

(Left) *AP radiographs of upper extremities in a 4-month-old with myofibromatosis show relatively symmetric, well-circumscribed lucent lesions of all visualized metadiaphyses. Many lesions demonstrate remodeling with expansion or bowing.* **(Right)** *Coronal (left) & sagittal (right) STIR MR images in the same patient show mild to moderate hyperintensity of the numerous skeletal lesions. There is deformity of many involved vertebral bodies, including several levels of vertebra plana. No visceral lesions were identified.*

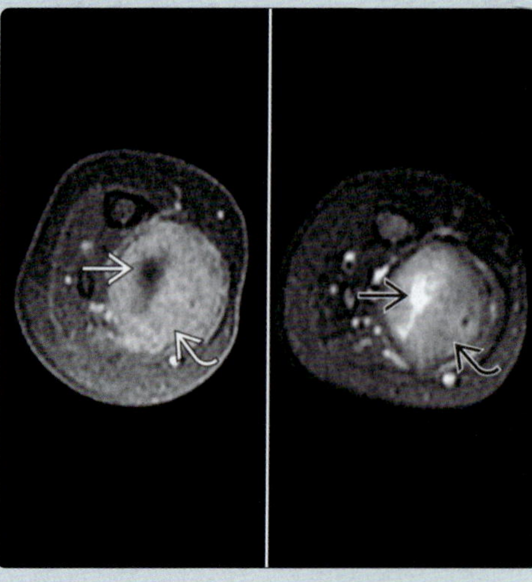

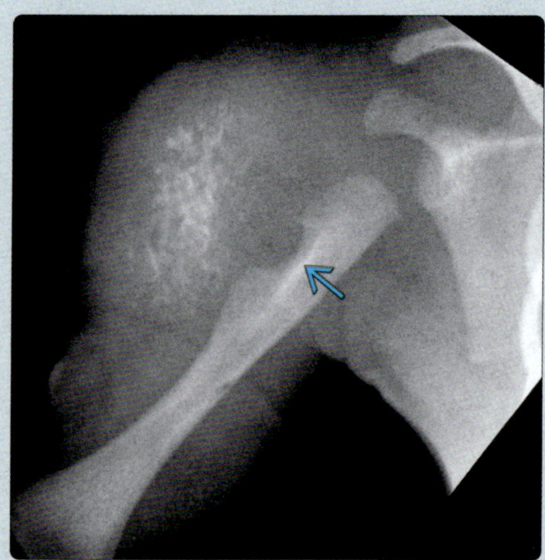

(Left) *Axial T1 C+ FS (left) & axial T2 FS (right) MR images in a 4-month-old with multiple soft tissue masses show peripheral enhancement & T2 hypointensity with central nonenhancement & T2 hyperintensity of an infantile myofibroma.* **(Right)** *AP radiograph in a newborn with a large shoulder mass shows clustered speckled Ca^{2+} in the central necrotic portion of the mass. There is unusual remodeling of the adjacent humerus with expansion & focal surface scalloping. Myofibroma was confirmed on biopsy.*

TERMINOLOGY

Definitions

- Infantile myofibroma: Solitary, benign fibrous tumor of young children with high rate of spontaneous regression
- Myofibromatosis: Multifocal disease
  - Multicentric without visceral involvement: Soft tissue &/or bone lesions
  - Multicentric with visceral involvement (or generalized): Additional organ systems are involved with poorer prognosis

IMAGING

General Features

- Best diagnostic clue
  - Myofibroma: Solitary, solid, centrally nonenhancing soft tissue mass in newborn
    - Typically in skin & subcutaneous tissues
  - Myofibromatosis: Numerous, relatively symmetric, well-defined metaphyseal/metadiaphyseal lucent lesions ± remodeling, cortical loss
- Location
  - Cutaneous, subcutaneous, muscular: 86%
  - Solitary lesions: Head & neck (50%) > trunk > extremities
  - Multicentric disease in 25-55%
    - Visceral involvement in 25-37% of multicentric cases
      - Lungs > gastrointestinal tract > heart > liver
    - Uncommon forms
      - Large, extensive retroperitoneal/paraspinal lesions
      - Intracranial involvement, intra- or extraaxial

Radiographic Findings

- Soft tissue mass ± internal Ca^{2+}, bizarre adjacent bone remodeling
- Multifocal extensive, well-circumscribed, lucent metaphyseal & metadiaphyseal lesions of bone
  - Relatively symmetric distribution
  - ± cortical loss, expansile remodeling
  - Periosteal reaction is usually absent or solid
  - Can cause vertebra plana
  - Sclerosis may represent early healing

MR Findings

- T2 FS/STIR: Variable internal signal intensity
- T1 C+ FS: Peripheral/rim enhancement
  - Diffuse enhancement is less common
- DWI: Often restrict diffusion

Ultrasonographic Findings

- Heterogeneous, may be hypo- or isoechoic
- Hypovascular internally by Doppler

Nuclear Medicine Findings

- Bone scan: Lacks sensitivity
- PET/CT: Highly sensitive

DIFFERENTIAL DIAGNOSIS

Solitary Congenital/Neonatal Soft Tissue Mass

- Other fibrous lesions
  - Fibrosarcoma
  - Fibrous hamartoma of infancy
- Vascular anomalies
  - Neoplasm
    - Hemangioma, infantile or congenital
    - Kaposiform hemangioendothelioma
  - Malformation
    - Venous
    - Lymphatic
- Teratoma
- Neuroblastoma

Multifocal Infantile Lesions

- Langerhans cell histiocytosis
- Metastatic neuroblastoma
- Multifocal vascular anomalies
- Disseminated infection

PATHOLOGY

Microscopic Features

- Peripheral clusters of spindled myofibroblastic cells
- Central cellularity & vascularity are similar to hemangiopericytoma

CLINICAL ISSUES

Presentation

- Most common signs/symptoms
  - Soft tissue mass ± red-purple skin nodules

Demographics

- Age: Perinatal in 50%; 90% diagnosed by age 2

Natural History & Prognosis

- Solitary/multicentric without visceral involvement: High rate of spontaneous regression over 1-2 years
  - May ↑ in size & number prior to regression
  - Overall 1% mortality
- Multicentric with visceral involvement: 48-75% mortality historically due to obstruction, organ failure

Treatment

- Solitary: Observation or surgical resection
  - 7-10% recurrence
- Multicentric with visceral involvement: Favorable outcomes with low-dose chemotherapy

SELECTED REFERENCES

1. Manisterski M et al: Diverse presentation and tailored treatment of infantile myofibromatosis: a single-center experience. Pediatr Blood Cancer. 68(2):e28769, 2021
2. Naffaa L et al: Infantile myofibromatosis: review of imaging findings and emphasis on correlation between MRI and histopathological findings. Clin Imaging. 54:40-7, 2019
3. Rekawek P et al: Prenatal sonography of multicentric infantile myofibromatosis: case report and review of the literature. J Clin Ultrasound. 47(8):490-3, 2019
4. Tang ER et al: Utility of 18F-FDG PET/CT in infantile myofibromatosis. Clin Nucl Med. 44(8):676-9, 2019
5. Ushida T et al: A large mediastinal tumour invading into the liver with foetal hydrops: a rare case of infantile myofibromatosis. J Obstet Gynaecol. 37(6):821-3, 2017
6. Salerno S et al: Whole-body magnetic resonance imaging in the diagnosis and follow-up of multicentric infantile myofibromatosis: a case report. Mol Clin Oncol. 6(4):579-82, 2017
7. Sargar KM et al: Pediatric fibroblastic and myofibroblastic tumors: a pictorial review. Radiographics. 36(4):1195-214, 2016

Plexiform Neurofibroma

KEY FACTS

TERMINOLOGY

- Neurofibroma: Type of benign peripheral nerve sheath tumor with 3 subtypes (localized, diffuse, plexiform)
  - Plexiform subtype occurs almost exclusively in neurofibromatosis type 1 (NF1)
  - Extensive plexiform neurofibromas → massive enlargement of body part (elephantiasis neuromatosa)
- Malignant peripheral nerve sheath tumor (MPNST)
  - Plexiform neurofibromas are at ↑ risk → MPNST

IMAGING

- Plexiform neurofibroma: Tortuous, lobulated expansion of long segments of nerves & branches ("bag of worms")
- Radiographs: Nonspecific soft tissue mass without Ca^{2+}; bony remodeling/erosions or mass effect on vital structures may occur from numerous adjacent neurofibromas
- T1 MR: Hypo- to isointense to skeletal muscle
  - Split fat sign: Rim of fat surrounding surrounding mass
- T2/STIR MR: Hyperintense lobules along nerve
  - Target sign: ↑ peripheral & ↓ central signal intensity
- T1 C+ MR: Heterogeneous or central enhancement
- MR features suggesting MPNST: ↑ size, cysts, peripheral enhancement, perilesional edema, heterogeneity on T1 (specific to NF1), ↓ ADC values
- FDG PET: SUVmax ≥ 3.5 is sensitive but not specific for MPNST

TOP DIFFERENTIAL DIAGNOSES

- Venous malformation, soft tissue sarcoma, MPNST, polyneuropathy

CLINICAL ISSUES

- Symptoms include pain, neurologic deficit, mass effect
- Treatment of plexiform neurofibroma is typically conservative due to inseparability of lesion & involved nerve
  - Surgery: For debulking symptomatic lesions & foci concerning for MPNST
  - Some chemotherapeutics shown to ↓ tumor bulk & symptoms

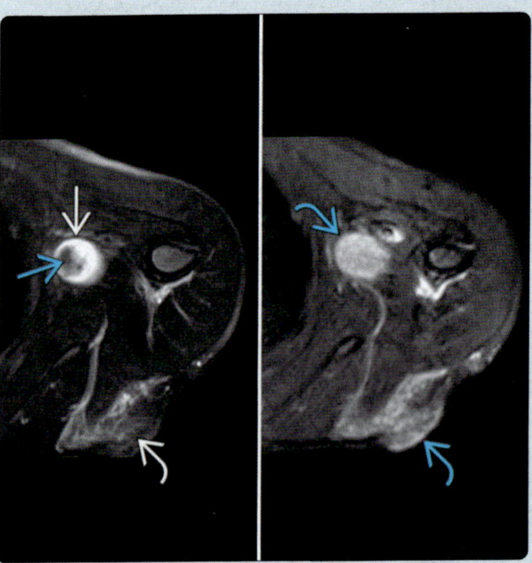

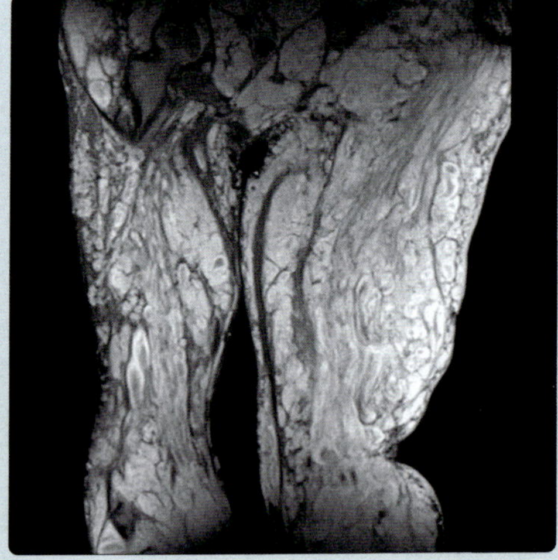

(Left) *Axial T2 FS MR (left) in a 14-year-old with neurofibromatosis type 1 (NF1) shows a localized neurofibroma in the left axilla with a target sign (high peripheral ➡ & low central ⇨ signal). There is a poorly defined diffuse neurofibroma posteriorly ↷. Axial T1 C+ FS MR (right) shows variable enhancement of the lesions ↷.* **(Right)** *Coronal STIR MR in a 15-year-old with NF1 shows extensive plexiform neurofibromas with massive enlargement of both thighs (elephantiasis neuromatosa).*

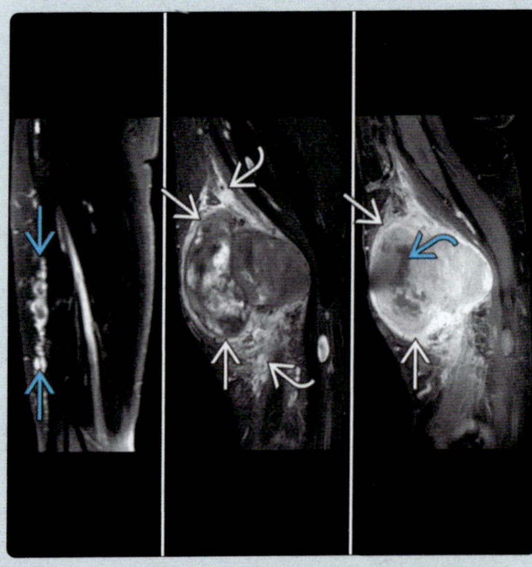

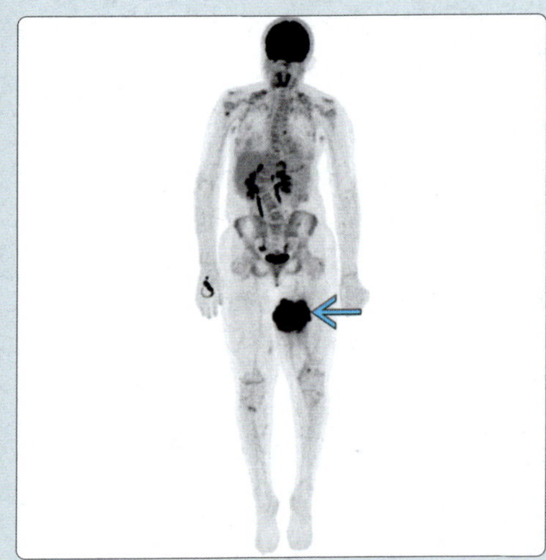

(Left) *Initial sagittal T2 FS MR (left) in an NF1 patient shows a thin, elongated plexiform neurofibroma in the anterior thigh ⇨. Seven years later, this mass had rapidly enlarged with sagittal T2 FS (middle) & T1 C+ FS (right) MR images showing marked enlargement & heterogeneity of the mass ➡ with central nonenhancement ↷ from necrosis. Perilesional edema ↷ is also present.* **(Right)** *Coronal FDG PET in the same patient shows ↑ uptake ⇨ (SUVmax of 13.7) within the mass. Pathology confirmed an MPNST.*

TERMINOLOGY

Definitions

- Neurofibroma: Type of benign peripheral nerve sheath tumor (BPNST)
  - 3 neurofibroma subtypes: Localized, diffuse, plexiform
- Malignant peripheral nerve sheath tumor (MPNST): Spindle cell sarcoma arising from nerve or BPNST
  - Plexiform neurofibromas have ↑ risk of MPNST

IMAGING

General Features

- Morphology
  - Plexiform type: Tortuous expansion of nerve(s) & branches by elongated lobules of varying size
    - May be relatively limited to courses of nerves vs. massive lobular proliferations engulfing & compressing adjacent tissues
      - Bag of worms appearance
      - Massive, disfiguring enlargement of body part (elephantiasis neuromatosa)
  - MPNST: ↑ heterogeneity with indistinct margins

Radiographic Findings

- Nonspecific soft tissue swelling without Ca^{2+}
- Large plexiform neurofibromas → bony remodeling from pressure erosions & mass effect on vital structures

Ultrasonographic Findings

- Predominantly hypoechoic lobular mass(es) along nerve(s)
  - May show ↑ echogenicity centrally

MR Findings

- T1WI
  - Hypo- to isointense to skeletal muscle
  - Split fat sign: Rim of fat surrounding tumor
- T2 FS or STIR
  - Predominately ↑ signal intensity
  - Target sign: ↑ peripheral, ↓ central signal intensity of lesion in cross section
- T1WI C+
  - Variable: Often heterogeneous & diffuse
- Whole-body MR
  - Used to evaluate neurofibromatosis type 1 (NF1) tumor burden, characterization, & treatment response

Nuclear Medicine Findings

- FDG PET/CT
  - SUVmax ≥ 3.5: Concerning for MPNST

Imaging Recommendations

- Best imaging tool
  - MR to characterize neurofibromas & evaluate depth & relationship to vital structures
  - FDG PET/CT is useful in differentiating MPNST vs. BPNST

DIFFERENTIAL DIAGNOSIS

Venous Malformation

- Low-flow vascular anomaly (localized or extensive)
- Numerous thin, low-signal septa in fluid-filled mass
  - ± fluid-fluid levels of stagnant blood
- Round, lucent-centered Ca^{2+} (phleboliths) are confirmatory
- Gradual patchy enhancement (often peripheral > central)

Soft Tissue Sarcoma

- Well-defined, solid, firm mass without entering/exiting nerve; no target sign or split fat sign
- Typically intermediate to high signal on T2/STIR MR; variable enhancement

Malignant Peripheral Nerve Sheath Tumor

- MR features favoring MPNST over plexiform neurofibroma (≥ 2: Specificity 90%, sensitivity 61%)
  - > 5 cm, cystic foci, peripheral enhancement, perilesional edema, heterogeneity on T1 (in NF1)
  - Also consider with preferential growth loss of target sign (if previously present), &/or ↓ ADC values

Polyneuropathy

- Various acute & chronic polyneuropathies cause diffuse enlargement of multiple adjacent nerves ± ↑ enhancement
- Nerve architecture is maintained without "target" lobules

CLINICAL ISSUES

Presentation

- Most common signs/symptoms
  - Plexiform type: Symptoms depend on location/extent
    - Pain & neurologic deficit vary with nerve involved
    - Symptoms from compression of adjacent structures
  - MPNST: ↑ pain, ↑ neurologic defect, & rapid growth

Natural History & Prognosis

- Neurofibromas (of all types) typically grow slowly
- Transformation of neurofibroma to MPNST
  - Lifetime risk of MPNST in patients with NF1: 8-13%
  - MPNST has poor prognosis with 5-year survival: 23-44%

Treatment

- Plexiform neurofibromas
  - Typically conservative management (as total resection → extensive neurologic deficit)
  - Surgery reserved for debulking of symptomatic lesions & masses concerning for MPNST
  - Some chemotherapeutics (e.g., tyrosine kinase inhibitors) ↓ tumor bulk & symptoms
- MPNST: Wide surgical excision + chemotherapy & radiation

SELECTED REFERENCES

1. Koike H et al: Diffusion-weighted magnetic resonance imaging improves the accuracy of differentiation of benign from malignant peripheral nerve sheath tumors. World Neurosurg. ePub, 2021
2. Liu Y et al: Correlation between NF1 genotype and imaging phenotype on whole-body MRI: NF1 radiogenomics. Neurology. 94(24):e2521-31, 2020
3. Markham A et al: Selumetinib: first approval. Drugs. 80(9):931-7, 2020
4. Ahlawat S et al: Current whole-body MRI applications in the neurofibromatoses: NF1, NF2, and schwannomatosis. Neurology. 87(7 Suppl 1):S31-9, 2016
5. Tovmassian D et al: The role of [18F]FDG-PET/CT in predicting malignant transformation of plexiform neurofibromas in neurofibromatosis-1. Int J Surg Oncol. 2016:6162182, 2016
6. Sabatini C et al: Treatment of neurofibromatosis type 1. Curr Treat Options Neurol. 17(6):355, 2015
7. Kransdorf MJ et al: Neurogenic lesions. In Kransdorf MJ et al: Imaging of Soft Tissue Tumors. 3rd ed. Lippincott, Williams & Wilkins. 395-460, 2014

Lipoblastoma

KEY FACTS

TERMINOLOGY

- Benign neoplasm of mature & immature adipocytes + myxoid stroma occurring in young children
- Termed lipoblastomatosis if lesion is poorly circumscribed or infiltrative

IMAGING

- Occurs at any soft tissue location: Extremities, trunk > head/neck; retroperitoneum in up to 5%
- Variable in size: 3-25 cm
- Imaging characteristic depend on percentage of fatty vs. myxoid components
  - Most commonly homogeneous & hyperechoic to muscle on ultrasound

TOP DIFFERENTIAL DIAGNOSES

- Lipoma: Well-circumscribed soft lesion of only fat ± few thin internal septations
- Involuting infantile hemangioma: Gradually increasing fat content with decreasing size, vascularity, & enhancing soft tissue relative to proliferating phase
- Fibrous hamartoma of infancy: Streaks of fat in solid mass
- Liposarcoma: Not reported < 5 years of age
- Hibernoma: Rare tumor of brown fat
- Teratoma: Abundant soft tissue & cystic components ± fat & Ca^{2+}; occurs in characteristic locations
- *PTEN* hamartoma: Abundant fatty, solid, & high-flow vascular elements in hamartoma-forming syndrome due to *PTEN* mutation
- Angiolipoma: Tender subcutaneous lesion of teenagers

CLINICAL ISSUES

- Often asymptomatic palpable mass; may grow rapidly &/or exert mass effect on critical structures
- 90% occur < 3 years of age; mean of 16-17 months
- Resection is curative; recurrence in up to 25%

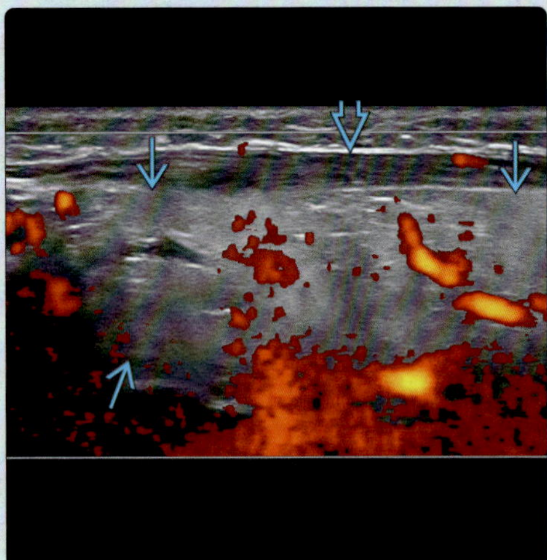

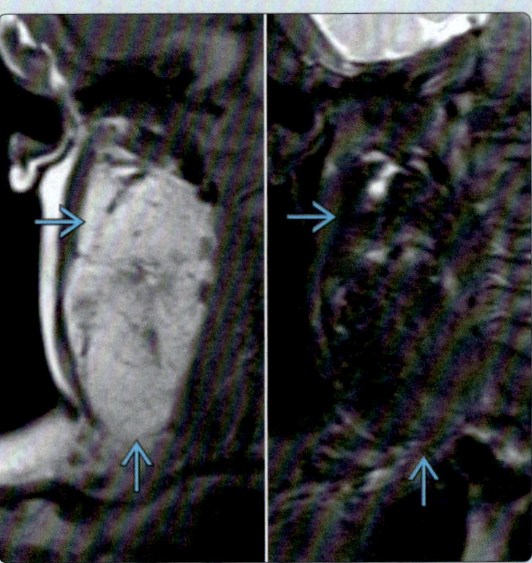

(Left) *Longitudinal power Doppler ultrasound in a 6-month-old with a neck mass shows an elongated, mildly lobulated echogenic mass → deep to the sternocleidomastoid muscle ⇨ with scattered internal vascularity.* **(Right)** *Coronal T1 & STIR MR images of the same patient show that the mass is predominantly of fat signal intensity → with scattered internal vessels & patchy solid components that enhanced (not shown). Lipoblastoma was confirmed upon resection.*

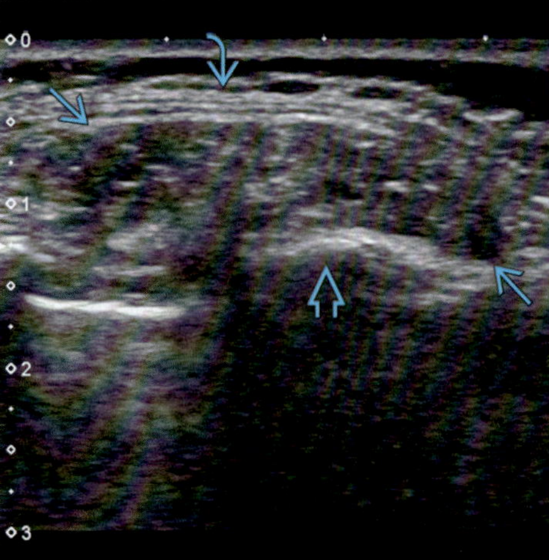

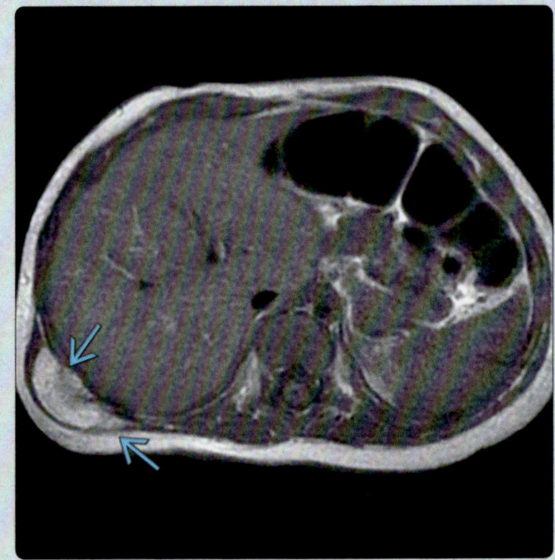

(Left) *Transverse ultrasound of the chest wall in a 9-month-old shows an elongated, mildly heterogeneous hypoechoic mass → overlying the ribs ⇨ & displacing adjacent musculature ↷.* **(Right)** *Axial T1 MR in the same patient shows a well-circumscribed, mildly heterogeneous but predominantly fatty mass → of the right chest wall musculature. Lipoblastoma was confirmed at resection.*

KEY FACTS

TERMINOLOGY

- Benign soft tissue neoplasm of hair follicle matrix cells
- a.k.a. pilomatricoma, calcifying epithelioma of Malherbe

IMAGING

- Occurs in subcutaneous fat at junction with dermis
  - Head & neck > extremities & trunk
    - Midface & periauricular regions are most common
  - Multiple lesions in 2-10%
- Mean of 0.8 cm; rarely "giant" (> 5 cm)
- Ultrasound: Well-circumscribed subcutaneous nodule with hypoechoic rim & internal heterogeneity
  - Nodule may be predominantly hyper-, iso-, or hypoechoic
  - Most show internal Ca^{2+} as echogenic foci in patterns of arcs, clumps, or dots
    - ± posterior acoustic shadowing
  - Less commonly show cystic degeneration
  - ± ↑ peritumoral echogenicity (due to inflammation)
  - Color Doppler flow is more likely peripheral than central
- Radiographs: Ca^{2+} in up to 55%, of various morphologies
- CT: Nonspecific soft tissue nodule; Ca^{2+} in up to 81%, ranging from punctate/scattered to diffuse/complete
- MR: T2: Heterogeneously isointense to muscle with patchy & reticulated foci of ↑ signal; ± surrounding fat stranding
  - T1 C+ FS: Rim, patchy, or reticular enhancement

CLINICAL ISSUES

- Asymptomatic, mobile, firm nodule; often with reddish/blue skin discoloration
- Mean age at diagnosis: 16 years; range: 5 months to 97 years
- Various underlying syndromes have been reported (though most occur without syndrome)
- Rare recurrence status post excision
- Malignant degeneration rarely occurs in adults

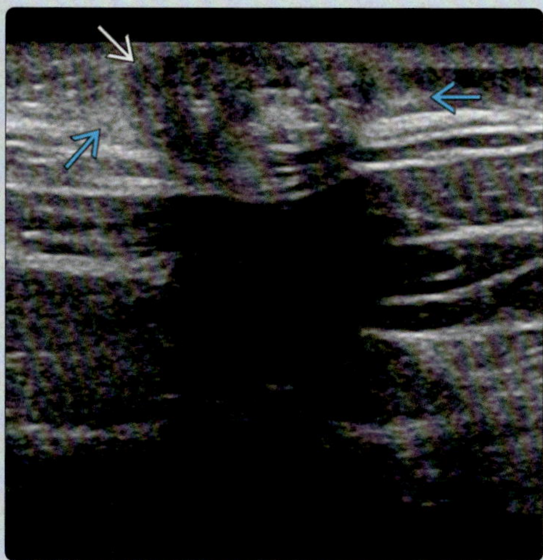

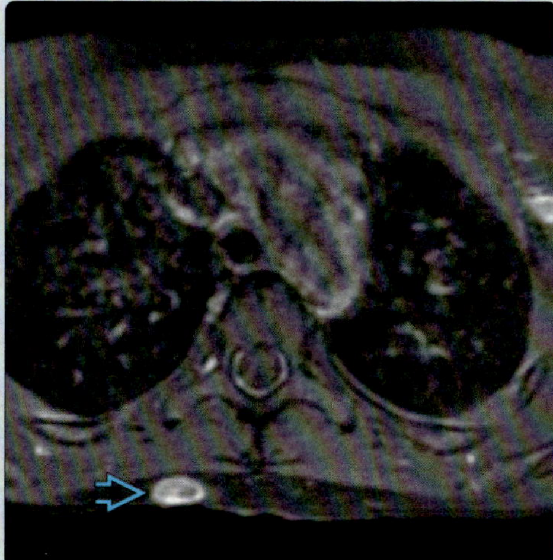

(Left) *Longitudinal ultrasound of the back soft tissues in a 12-year-old shows a well-circumscribed ovoid lesion ➡ of the subcutaneous fat with internal heterogeneity, posterior acoustic shadowing, & ↑ peritumoral echogenicity ⇨.* **(Right)** *Axial T1 C+ FS MR in the same patient shows predominantly peripheral enhancement of the lesion ⇨. Central low & peripheral high T2 signal intensity was also seen (not shown). Pilomatrixoma was confirmed upon resection.*

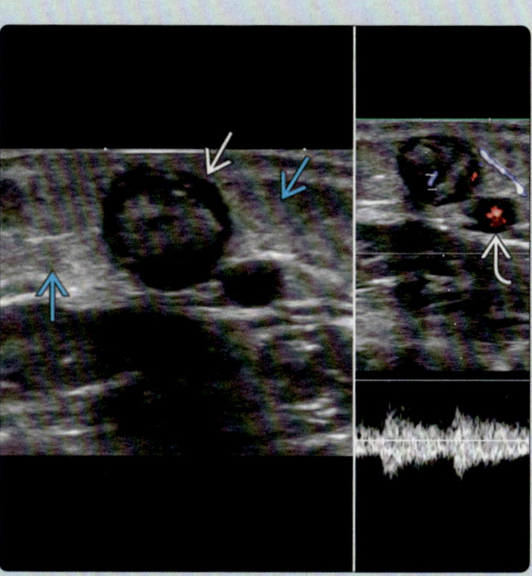

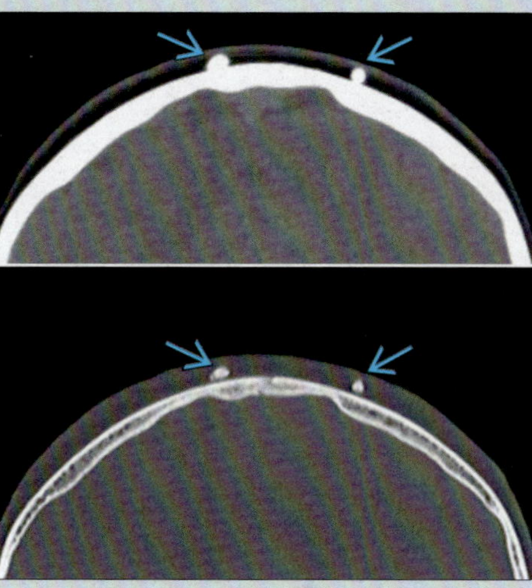

(Left) *Transverse grayscale & pulsed Doppler images of a 1-cm forearm mass in a 9-year-old show a round, well-circumscribed subcutaneous lesion with a peripheral hypoechoic rim ➡ & ↑ peritumoral echogenicity ⇨. A small amount of internal arterial flow is noted (as compared to the normal adjacent vein ➡).* *Pilomatrixoma was confirmed at surgery.* **(Right)** *Axial NECT images in an 8-year-old show 2 heavily calcified pilomatrixomas ⇨. Note the normal underlying calvarium.*

KEY FACTS

TERMINOLOGY

- Arises from rhabdomyoblasts (primitive muscle cells); lacks normal differentiation into skeletal muscle
  - Embryonal rhabdomyosarcoma (RMS): 60-70% of childhood RMS
    - Most common type in patients < 15 years old
    - Most commonly GU, head & neck, retroperitoneum
  - Alveolar RMS: 20% of RMS
    - Average age: 15 years old
    - Most commonly extremity, trunk, & perianal/perirectal
  - Undifferentiated RMS
    - 30-50 year olds; rarely in children

IMAGING

- Best clue: Solid, firm, mildly heterogeneous, intramuscular mass without significant surrounding soft tissue edema
- Usually round with well-circumscribed, lobular margins
  - May have tail of tumor extending proximal/distal
- Radiographs: Ca^{2+} is not typical
- US: Variable internal vascularity; not compressible
- MR: Moderately to markedly hyperintense (T2 FS/STIR) to skeletal muscle, ± heterogeneity (necrosis & hemorrhage)
  - Variable enhancement, ranging from minimal to diffuse, heterogeneous to homogeneous
  - Typically restricts diffusion
- US & MR features can strongly suggest sarcoma
- MR is better at defining deep extent & relationship to critical structures (e.g., neurovascular bundle, joints, etc.)
- PET is best for staging

CLINICAL ISSUES

- Most common soft tissue sarcoma in children
- Typically presents as enlarging, firm, painless mass
- 2 age peaks: 2-6 years, 14-18 years
- Prognosis is worse with alveolar subtype, tumor > 5 cm, metastatic disease at presentation (lung, bone marrow, & lymph nodes are most common)

(Left) *Longitudinal color Doppler US in a 12-month-old with weeks of arm swelling shows a heterogeneous, ovoid, intramuscular soft tissue mass → with moderate internal vascularity. The mass showed no significant deformation upon compression by the transducer.* **(Right)** *Coronal STIR MR in the same infant shows mild internal heterogeneity of the predominantly hyperintense mass →, which involved the brachioradialis & extensor carpi radialis muscles.*

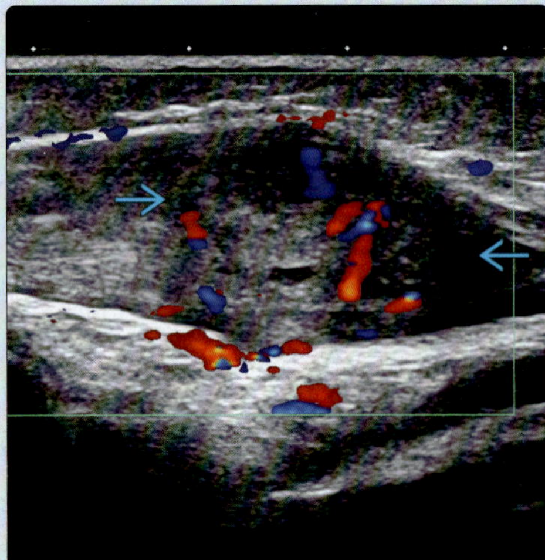

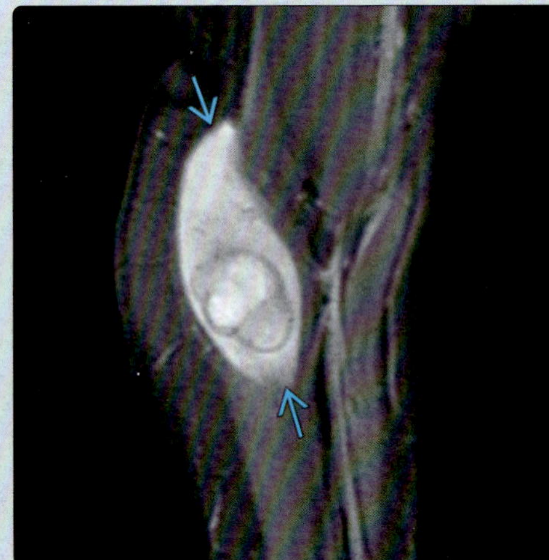

(Left) *Axial T1 C+ FS MR in the same infant shows nearly uniform enhancement of the forearm rhabdomyosarcoma (RMS) → with a central region of necrosis &/or hemorrhage →. Diffusion restriction (not shown) was variable in the mass with ADC values ranging from 0.8-1.2 x 10^{-3} mm/s^2.* **(Right)** *Coronal CECT in a 21-month-old with an enlarging chest wall mass shows deep extension of the predominantly superficial mass → into the diaphragm → & liver →. RMS was proven at biopsy.*

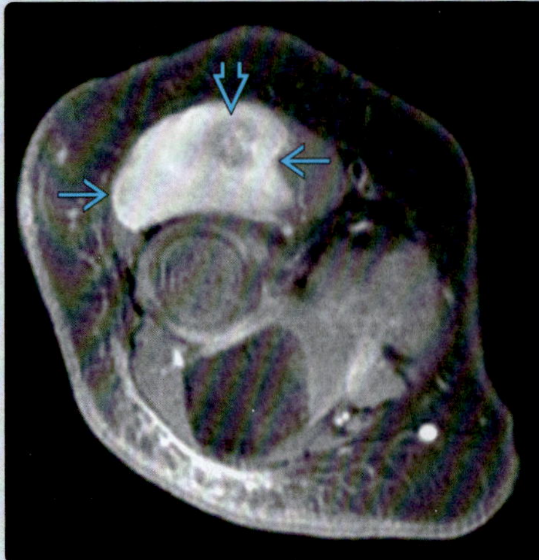

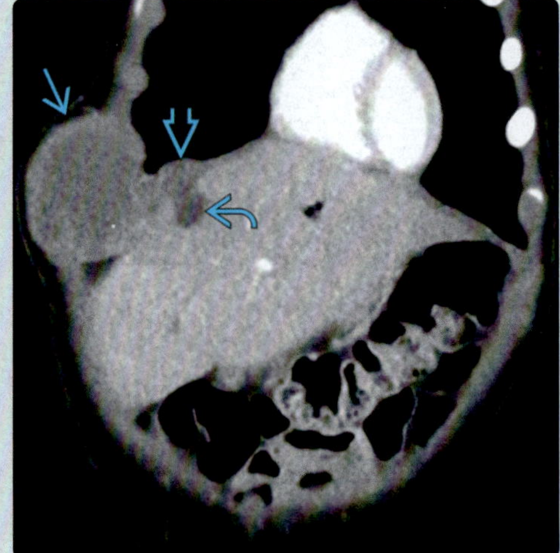

TERMINOLOGY

Definitions

- Mesenchymal sarcoma arising from rhabdomyoblasts (primitive muscle cells); lacks normal differentiation into skeletal muscle
  - Embryonal rhabdomyosarcoma (RMS): 60-70% of childhood RMS
    - Resembles skeletal muscle of 6- to 8-week fetus
    - Most common type in patients < 15 years old
    - Most common locations: GU, head & neck, retroperitoneum
    - Botryoid subtype (sarcoma botryoides): 10% of RMS
      - Grape-like polyploid masses or clusters protruding into lumen of vagina, bladder, biliary tree, or nasopharynx
  - Alveolar RMS: 20% of RMS
    - Resembles skeletal muscle of 10-week fetus
    - Average age: 15 years
    - Most common locations: Extremity, trunk, & perianal/perirectal
  - Undifferentiated RMS
    - 30- to 50-year-olds; rarely in children

IMAGING

General Features

- Best diagnostic clue
  - Well-circumscribed, solid, mildly heterogeneous intramuscular mass without significant surrounding soft tissue edema
- Location
  - Head & neck (28-40%)
    - Nasopharynx, sinuses, orbit, soft tissues (7%)
  - GU (20%)
    - Prostate, bladder, vagina, paratesticular
  - Extremities (15-20%)
    - Typically intramuscular
  - Truncal/retroperitoneal (11-17%)
- Size
  - Quite variable
- Morphology
  - Usually round with well-circumscribed, lobular margins
  - May have tail of tumor extending proximal/distal

Radiographic Findings

- Soft tissue fullness similar to muscle density on radiographs
- Rarely shows adjacent bone involvement
- Ca^{2+} is not typical

CT Findings

- Not used for primary mass investigation
- Lung CT for metastatic work-up

Ultrasonographic Findings

- Solid, firm, mildly heterogeneous soft tissue mass with variable amounts of internal vascularity
- Often round & well-circumscribed, though deeper infiltration is possible

MR Findings

- T1WI
  - Similar signal to skeletal muscle
- T2 FS/STIR
  - Moderately to markedly hyperintense to skeletal muscle
    - Not typically cystic
  - Can be heterogeneous with necrosis & hemorrhage
  - Typically minimal (if any) surrounding edema
- T1WI C+ FS
  - Variable enhancement, ranging from minimal to diffuse, heterogeneous to homogeneous
- DWI
  - Typically restricts diffusion; can ↑ conspicuity of primary & metastatic lesions
    - Mean ADC values reported from 0.7-1.2 x 10^{-3} mm/s^2
- MRA/MRV
  - May be helpful to determine relationship of mass to neurovascular bundle

Nuclear Medicine Findings

- PET
  - Intense FDG uptake by soft tissue tumor
  - Better than conventional imaging in staging disease (except for very small lung lesions)
  - May not predict event-free survival in intermediate- or high-risk RMS

Imaging Recommendations

- Best imaging tool
  - US & MR features can strongly suggests sarcoma
  - MR is better at defining deep extent & relationship to critical structures (e.g., neurovascular bundle, joints, etc.)
  - Extremity RMS: Important to image entire extremity, including lymph node drainage basins
- Protocol advice
  - Consider subtraction MR images of pre- from postcontrast T1 FS
    - Avoids pseudoenhancement postcontrast due to preexisting hemorrhage, protein, etc.

DIFFERENTIAL DIAGNOSIS

Other Soft Tissue Sarcomas

- Synovial sarcoma
  - Ca^{2+} in 1/3, may be small & cystic-appearing
  - Usually not intraarticular but near joint; often abuts bone
- Extraosseous Ewing sarcoma
  - Similar in appearance to RMS, usually 2nd-3rd decades
- Fibrosarcoma
  - Typically infantile in children
  - May be highly cystic or solid & highly vascular
  - Frequently infiltrative

Plexiform Neurofibroma

- Most common in neurofibromatosis type 1 (NF1)
- Lobular masses following course of nerve
- Classic target appearance in cross section on T2/STIR MR
  - Bright periphery, intermediate/dark center
- Loss of target appearance & disproportionate growth suggest malignant degeneration

Venous Malformation

- Patchy enhancement, fluid-fluid levels, ± phleboliths

Infantile Hemangioma

- Solid but soft subcutaneous mass of infants with mild lobulations, variable echogenicity
- Highly vascular on color Doppler US with > 5 vessels/cm²
  - Low-resistance arterial waveforms during proliferation

Myositis Ossificans

- Heterogeneous intramuscular mass in older children with prior acute trauma (2/3) or microtrauma history
- Marked inflammatory reaction of surrounding muscle
- Calcifies peripheral to central over weeks/months

Abscess

- Heterogeneous collection with thick, irregular wall & septations; swirling internal debris with compression
- Peripheral hyperemia/enhancement
- Moderate to marked surrounding edema

PATHOLOGY

General Features

- Genetics
  - Embryonal: Loss of chromosome 11 genomic material
  - Alveolar: Translocation of chromosomes 1 or 2 & 13
    - Translocation t(2;13) (q35;q14), results in *PAX3-FKHR* fusion gene (55%)
    - Translocation t(1;13) (p36;q14), results in *PAX7-FKHR* fusion gene (22%)
    - Better prognosis in *PAX7-FKHR* than *PAX3-FKHR* (more invasive)
- Associated abnormalities
  - Syndromes: NF1, Li-Fraumeni, Costello, Noonan, *DICER1*

Microscopic Features

- Embryonal RMS: Primitive with dense, spindle-shaped cells with hyperchromatic nuclei & cytoplasmic processes, strap cell appearance
- Alveolar RMS: Large oval cells separated into nests of "alveoli" separated by fibrous septa
- Central cells are necrotic & loosely arranged with peripheral cells arranged into well-organized picket fence appearance
- Immunohistochemical staining: MyoD1, myoglobin, myogenin, actin, & desmin

CLINICAL ISSUES

Presentation

- Most common signs/symptoms
  - Enlarging, firm soft tissue mass
- Other signs/symptoms
  - < 1/2 experience pain; symptoms depend on location

Demographics

- Age
  - 65% present < 6 years old
  - 2 age peaks: 2-6 & 14-18 years of age
    - Embryonal: < 15 years old; head & neck, GU
      - 46% occur in patients < 5 years old
    - Alveolar: Typically adolescents & young adults (extremity, paratesticular, & truncal)
      - Occurs at all ages
- Sex
  - Overall M > F (1.5:1), extremity: M < F (0.8:1), GU: M > F (3:1)
- Epidemiology
  - 5-10% of childhood malignant solid tumors overall
    - 4-6 cases/1 million per year
  - Most common soft tissue sarcoma in children

Natural History & Prognosis

- Prognosis depends on
  - Site of tumor
    - Orbit & nonparameningeal sites: More favorable
    - Extremity: Poorer prognosis, ↑ incidence of alveolar RMS, often lymph node (+), ↑ metastases at presentation
    - Chest: Poorer prognosis with 45% 5-year survival, tends to be alveolar RMS, ↑ metastases at presentation, location difficult for resection & radiation
  - Size: < 5 cm more favorable
  - Age: Alveolar ↓ prognosis < 1 year old & > 10 years old
  - Histiologic type: Embryonal is better than alveolar RMS
  - DNA component: Hyperdiploid (embryonal RMS) is better than diploid or tetraploid (alveolar RMS)
  - Tumor expression of p-glycoprotein gene: More likely multidrug resistant
  - Metastatic disease at presentation has much poorer prognosis: Lung, bone marrow, lymph nodes are most common

Treatment

- Neoadjuvant & adjuvant chemotherapy, surgery, radiation

SELECTED REFERENCES

1. Harrison DJ et al: Metabolic response as assessed by 18 F-fluorodeoxyglucose positron emission tomography-computed tomography does not predict outcome in patients with intermediate- or high-risk rhabdomyosarcoma: a report from the Children's Oncology Group Soft Tissue Sarcoma Committee. Cancer Med. 10(3):857-66, 2021
2. Li H et al: Germline cancer-predisposition variants in pediatric rhabdomyosarcoma: a report from the Children's Oncology Group. J Natl Cancer Inst. 113(7):875-83, 2021
3. Maldonado FR et al: Quantitative characterization of extraocular orbital lesions in children using diffusion-weighted imaging. Pediatr Radiol. 51(1):119-27, 2021
4. Rogers TN et al: Management of rhabdomyosarcoma in pediatric patients. Surg Oncol Clin N Am. 30(2):339-53, 2021
5. Morris CD et al: Surgical management of extremity rhabdomyosarcoma: a consensus opinion from the Children's Oncology Group, the European Pediatric Soft-Tissue Sarcoma Study Group, and the Cooperative Weichteilsarkom Studiengruppe. Pediatr Blood Cancer. ePub, 2020
6. Navarro OM: Pearls and pitfalls in the imaging of soft-tissue masses in children. Semin Ultrasound CT MR. 41(5):498-512, 2020
7. Harrison DJ et al: The role of 18F-FDG-PET/CT in pediatric sarcoma. Semin Nucl Med. 47(3):229-41, 2017
8. Norman G et al: An emerging evidence base for PET-CT in the management of childhood rhabdomyosarcoma: systematic review. BMJ Open. 5(1):e006030, 2015
9. Thacker MM: Malignant soft tissue tumors in children. Orthop Clin North Am. 44(4):657-67, 2013
10. Navarro OM: Soft tissue masses in children. Radiol Clin North Am. 49(6):1235-59, vi-vii, 2011
11. Stegmaier S et al: Prognostic value of PAX-FKHR fusion status in alveolar rhabdomyosarcoma: a report from the cooperative soft tissue sarcoma study group (CWS). Pediatr Blood Cancer. 57(3):406-14, 2011

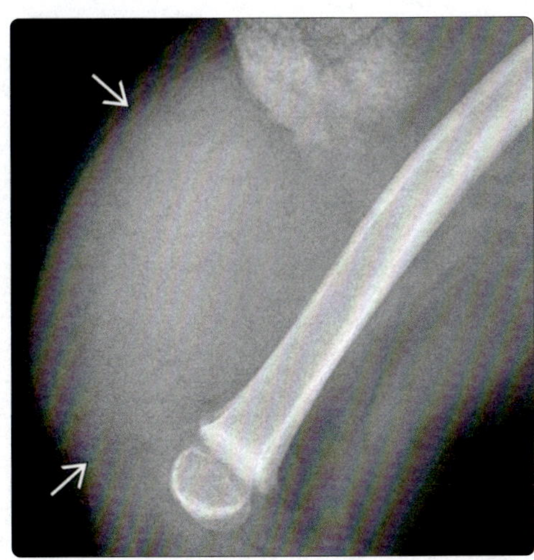

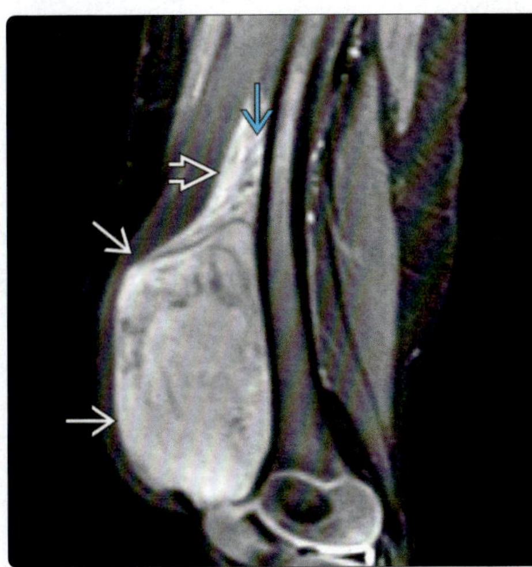

(Left) *Lateral radiograph in 2-year-old patient shows a large soft tissue mass in the mid- & lower anterior thigh ➡ with mild saucerization of the outer anterior femoral cortex.* **(Right)** *Sagittal STIR MR in the same patient shows a heterogeneously hyperintense soft tissue mass ➡ within the thigh anteriorly. There is tumor ➡ & edema ➡ extending proximally in this embryonal RMS.*

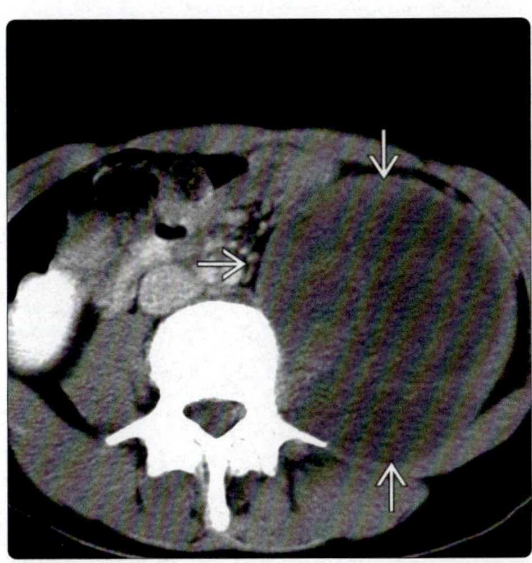

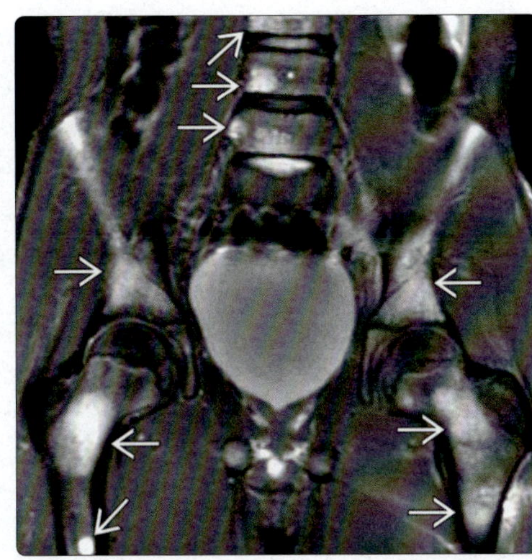

(Left) *Axial CECT shows massive enlargement & replacement of the left psoas muscle by a hypodense RMS ➡.* **(Right)** *Coronal STIR MR in a 10-year-old with an intramuscular gluteal mass (not shown) demonstrates numerous hyperintense osseous metastatic foci ➡ within the lower lumbar spine, pelvis, & femurs. Biopsy of the mass showed alveolar RMS.*

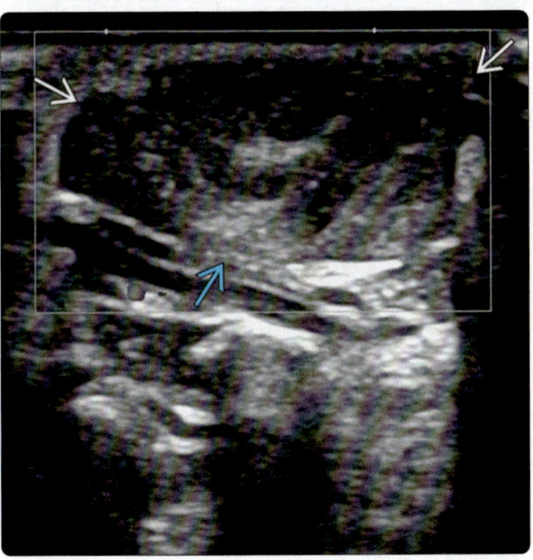

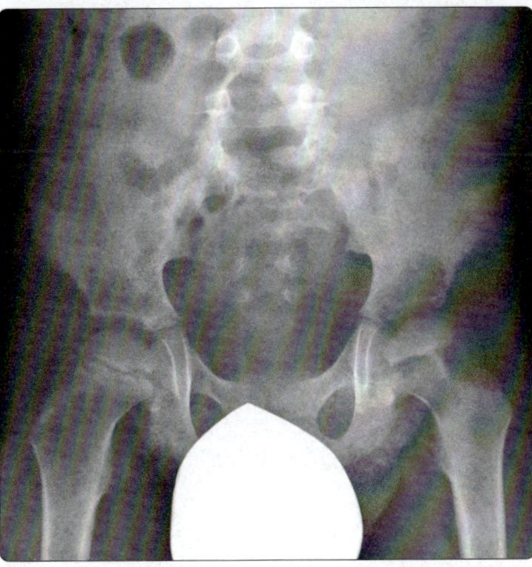

(Left) *Color Doppler US in a 6-month-old with a firm hand mass shows a mildly heterogeneous palmar soft tissue lesion ➡. Features that lead away from considering an infantile hemangioma include the lack of significant internal vascularity, the presence of deep extension ➡, & firmness. Biopsy confirmed an RMS.* **(Right)** *AP radiograph in a 4-year-old with left knee pain shows multifocal lytic lesions throughout the pelvis & proximal femurs. This was biopsy-proven metastatic embryonal RMS of prostate origin.*

KEY FACTS

TERMINOLOGY

- Heterogenous group of malignant mesenchymal tumors
- Pediatric soft tissue sarcomas: ~ 40% are rhabdomyosarcoma, ~ 60% are nonrhabdomyosarcoma soft tissue sarcomas (NRSTS)

IMAGING

- Best clue: Well-circumscribed, round or ovoid, predominantly solid (firm) soft tissue mass without substantial surrounding edema
  - Overlaps many benign pediatric soft tissue masses
- Variable internal heterogeneity
  - Solid tumor components show variable enhancement
  - Intermixed nonenhancing foci: Hemorrhage, necrosis, Ca^{2+}
    - Some sarcomas may appear partially or entirely cystic until contrast is administered
- MR with IV contrast: Best study to characterize mass, determine local extent, & follow local therapy response

TOP DIFFERENTIAL DIAGNOSES

- Vascular anomalies
- Periarticular cysts or cyst-like lesions
- Myositis ossificans
- Benign fibrous or neurogenic tumors
- Abscess

CLINICAL ISSUES

- Most common signs/symptoms: Palpable, firm mass

DIAGNOSTIC CHECKLIST

- Benign & malignant soft tissue masses overlap in appearances
- Without specific clinical & imaging features of benign process → biopsy required
- If specific features strongly suggest benign, self-limited or medically treatable process → close clinical & imaging follow-up
- Smaller focal lesions are frequently excised regardless

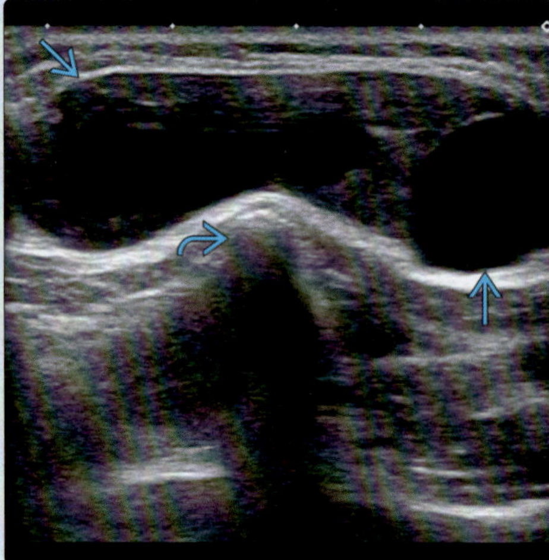

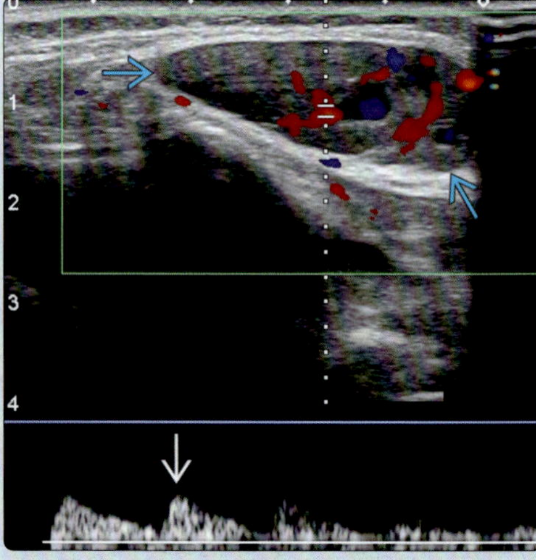

(Left) *Longitudinal ultrasound through a firm mass in the posterior right shoulder of a 5-year-old shows a mixed cystic & solid lesion* ⇨ *overlying the scapula* ⇨. **(Right)** *Transverse pulsed Doppler ultrasound in the same patient shows a moderate amount of internal vascularity throughout the solid portions of the lesion* ⇨, *including several arterial waveforms* ➡. *Spectral tracings (at several locations) are critical for characterizing flow within a lesion.*

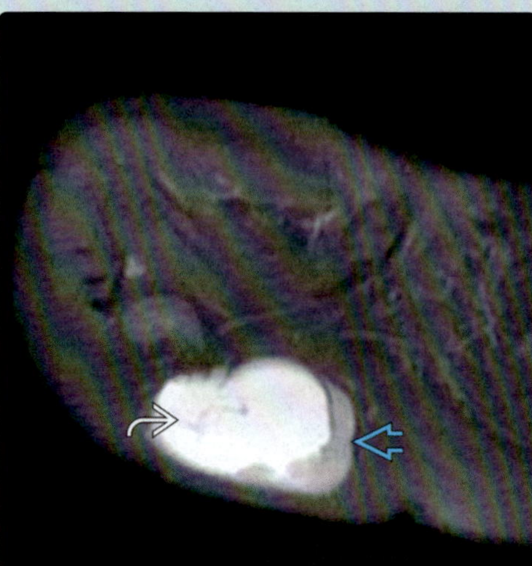

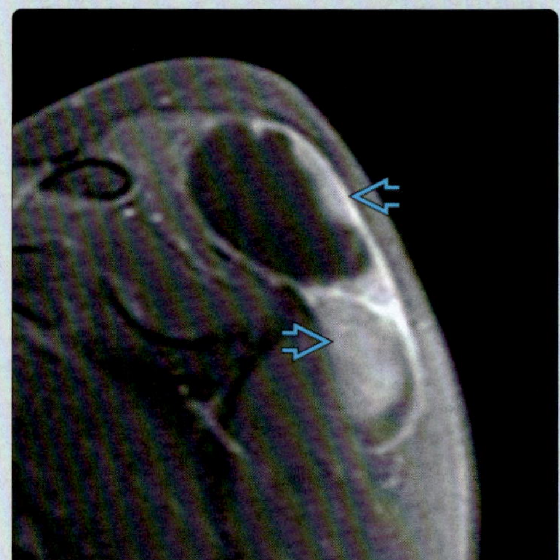

(Left) *Axial T2 FS MR in the same patient shows nodular intermediate signal intensity components along the wall of the mass* ⇨. *Some of the cystic portions* ➡ *show thin internal septations.* **(Right)** *Sagittal T1 C+ FS MR in the same patient shows enhancement of the solid components* ⇨ *of the mass. While some of the cystic features could be seen in a lymphatic malformation, the enhancing, solid components are concerning for malignancy. An extraskeletal Ewing sarcoma was confirmed with biopsy.*

TERMINOLOGY

Abbreviations

- Nonrhabdomyosarcoma soft tissue sarcomas (NRSTS)

Definitions

- Soft tissue sarcomas: Heterogenous group of malignancies arising in extraskeletal mesenchymal tissues
- In children: ~ 40% are rhabdomyosarcoma, ~ 60% are NRSTS
- > 40 subtypes of NRSTS (e.g., synovial sarcoma, infantile fibrosarcoma, malignant peripheral nerve sheath tumor, undifferentiated sarcoma, extraskeletal Ewing sarcoma, etc.)

IMAGING

General Features

- Best diagnostic clue
  - Well-circumscribed, round or ovoid, predominantly solid (firm) soft tissue mass without surrounding edema
    - Overlaps many benign pediatric soft tissue masses

MR Findings

- T1: Typically similar to muscle signal intensity ± bright foci of hemorrhage
- T2 FS/STIR: Relatively uniform intermediate to bright signal intensity of solid tissue
  - ± cystic/necrotic foci of very bright signal; purely cystic appearance is uncommon (but still requires contrast)
  - Typically lacks significant surrounding muscle edema
- T1 C+ FS: Wide range of enhancement patterns
  - Often intermediate- to low-level enhancement
    - ± nonenhancing foci of necrosis or hemorrhage
- DWI: Highly cellular tumors show restricted diffusion, typically with ADC values < 1.0×10^{-3} mm/s^2

Ultrasonographic Findings

- Grayscale ultrasound
  - Firm mass of variable internal echogenicity
    - Typically of intermediate- or low-level echoes
  - Rarely anechoic with posterior acoustic enhancement & compressibility → favors benign, fluid-filled process
    - Must look closely for solid nodular components
- Color Doppler
  - Variable internal vascularity
    - Frequently only mild to intermediate
    - Check for spectral waveforms to confirm true flow

Imaging Recommendations

- Best imaging tool
  - MR ± IV contrast: Best study to characterize mass, determine local extent, & follow local response during/after therapy
- Protocol advice
  - MR technique
    - T1 sequence in at least 1 plane
      - ▫ Axial images show relationship of mass to neurovascular bundle (normally encased by fat)
      - ▫ Additional T1 FS sequence may help evaluate etiologies of bright signal in mass & determine true enhancement after contrast administration
    - Multiplanar fluid-sensitive T2 FS or STIR sequences to highlight most pathologies
    - Contrast is critical for showing solid vs. necrotic foci
      - ▫ Subtraction of precontrast images is most accurate

DIFFERENTIAL DIAGNOSIS

Vascular Anomalies

- Infantile hemangioma
- Venous malformation
- Lymphatic malformation

Benign Fibrous/Fibrohistiocytic Tumors

- Fibrous hamartoma of infancy
- Myofibroma/myofibromatosis
- Nodular fasciitis
- Fibromatosis

Neurogenic Tumors

- Plexiform, localized, or diffuse neurofibroma
- Schwannoma

Fat-Containing Neoplasms

- Lipoma
- Lipoblastoma
- Hibernoma

Periarticular Cysts

- Ganglion vs. synovial or parameniscal cysts

Infectious/Inflammatory Masses

- Granuloma annulare
- Abscess

Posttraumatic Lesions

- Myositis ossificans
- Fat trauma/necrosis
- Hematoma

CLINICAL ISSUES

Presentation

- Most common signs/symptoms: Palpable, painless, firm mass

Natural History & Prognosis

- Prognosis varies greatly based on subtype, staging, grade

Treatment

- Combination of surgery, chemotherapy, &/or radiation

DIAGNOSTIC CHECKLIST

Consider

- Benign & malignant soft tissue masses overlap in appearances; biopsy is often required
- Correlation with clinical history is important
  - Inflammatory & posttraumatic etiologies should be considered when pain & surrounding edema are present
  - Firm & painless or mildly tender mass is more concerning
  - Indolent growth does not exclude malignancy

Image Interpretation Pearls

- Soft tissue sarcomas often show well-defined margins

Pediatric Soft Tissue Malignancies

Tumor	Characteristic Imaging Features	Clinical Features	Prognosis
Rhabdomyosarcoma	Typical soft tissue sarcoma without specific features: Well-circumscribed, round/ovoid solid mass of intermediate/high T2 MR signal intensity with diffusion restriction & variable enhancement	Peak incidence overall: 2-6 years old; head/neck & genitourinary sites are more common than extremities; metastases in 15-20% at presentation	Overall 5-year survival: ~70%
Synovial sarcoma	30% show Ca^{2+}; often cystic-appearing; enhances with IV contrast; T2 MR triple sign (of intensities) is not specific; fluid-fluid levels in up to 25%; contiguity with bone is more common than remodeling or invasion	30% < 20 years old with median of 13-14 years in children; lower extremity is most common, often near joint (rarely in joint); slow growth is common	5-year survival: 36-76%; late recurrence is common
Extraskeletal Ewing sarcoma/PNET	No specific features overall; aggressive chest wall mass (Askin tumor) with pleural effusion & rib destruction is very suggestive	10-30 years old; most common in White patients; extraskeletal is less common than skeletal	Overall 5-year survival: ~ 61%
Infantile fibrosarcoma	Frequently infiltrative; often contains prominent cystic spaces; may be highly vascular	0-2 years old; 30-80% detected by/at birth; rapidly growing; skin involvement mimics vascular lesion; distal extremities are most common	5-year survival: 80% (better than adolescent/adult fibrosarcoma)
Undifferentiated sarcoma	No specific features	Multiple subtypes within this group	Varies by type, grade, stage
Extrarenal malignant rhabdoid tumor	No specific features overall; reported in virtually all anatomic sites (head/neck, trunk/viscera, limbs)	Older than renal rhabdoid patients with median < 4 years; ± concomitant CNS or renal rhabdoid tumors	5-year survival: 25-50%
MPNST	Features that can help distinguish from PN: Enlarging mass (> 5 cm) amidst stable PNs, loss of target sign on MR, ↑ activity on PET	~ 50% in neurofibromatosis type 1: 8-13% lifetime risk of MPNST	5-year survival: 23-69%
Dermatofibrosarcoma protuberans	Nodular, superficial mass with cutaneous elongation ± satellite nodules	Slow-growing, discolored skin mass	5-year survival: > 99%
Granulocytic/myeloid sarcoma (chloroma)	Background of diffuse marrow abnormalities	Acute myelogenous leukemia	5-year survival: 20-25%
Neuroblastoma	Typically small cutaneous & subcutaneous masses; ± discrete paraspinal primary mass; ± extensive marrow abnormalities	Wide range of clinical presentations; soft tissue metastases are most common < 18 months of age	Excellent in infant with metastases limited to liver, skin, & bone marrow; otherwise variable
Alveolar soft part sarcoma	Often brighter than muscle on T1 MR; typically shows prominent intra- & peritumoral vascularity, central necrosis, & infiltration	Head/neck is most common in children	5-year survival: 56-70%
Epithelioid sarcoma	Ca^{2+} in 20-30%; may have moderate surrounding edema with extension along fascia & tendon sheaths (uncommon for other sarcomas)	75% are 10-39 years old; distal upper extremity is most common, slow growth is frequent; proximal type is more aggressive	5-year survival: 50-70%
Angiosarcoma	Evidence of prior hemorrhage; tangles of high-flow vessels are uncommon	Typically de novo; rarely arise from preexisting vascular malformation	5-year survival: As low as 15%
Liposarcoma	Fat-poor myxoid subtype in 2nd decade of life	Extremely uncommon < 8-10 years old	Better than adult types

PNET = primitive neuroectodermal tumor; PN = plexiform neurofibroma; MPNST = malignant peripheral nerve sheath tumor.

- Significant surrounding edema favors (but does not confirm) infectious/inflammatory or posttraumatic etiology; consider close follow-up before biopsy

SELECTED REFERENCES

1. Milgrom SA et al: Non-rhabdomyosarcoma soft-tissue sarcoma. Pediatr Blood Cancer. 68 Suppl 2:e28279, 2021
2. Renzi S et al: Non-rhabdomyosarcoma soft tissue sarcomas diagnosed in patients at a young age. An overview of clinical, pathological, and molecular findings. Pediatr Blood Cancer. e29022, 2021
3. Cheng H et al: Clinical and prognostic characteristics of 53 cases of extracranial malignant rhabdoid tumor in children. a single-institute experience from 2007 to 2017. Oncologist. 24(7):e551-8, 2019
4. Kao SC: Overview of the clinical and imaging features of the most common non-rhabdomyosarcoma soft-tissue sarcomas. Pediatr Radiol. 49(11):1524-33, 2019
5. Tinkle CL et al: Nonrhabdomyosarcoma soft tissue sarcoma (NRSTS) in pediatric and young adult patients: results from a prospective study using limited-margin radiotherapy. Cancer. 123(22):4419-29, 2017
6. Kransdorf MJ et al: Imaging of Soft Tissue Tumors. 3rd ed. Lippincott Williams & Wilkins, 2014

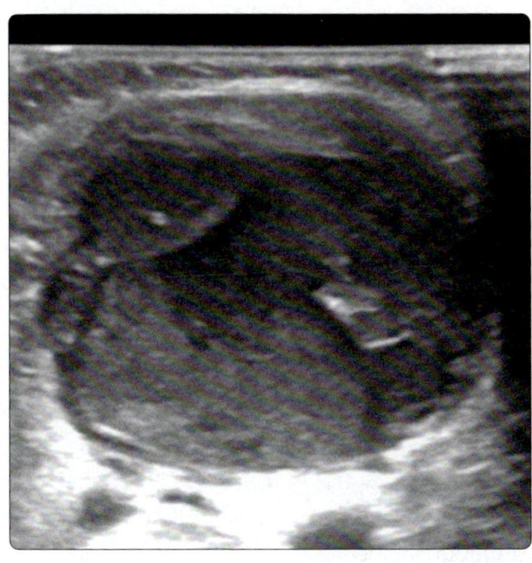

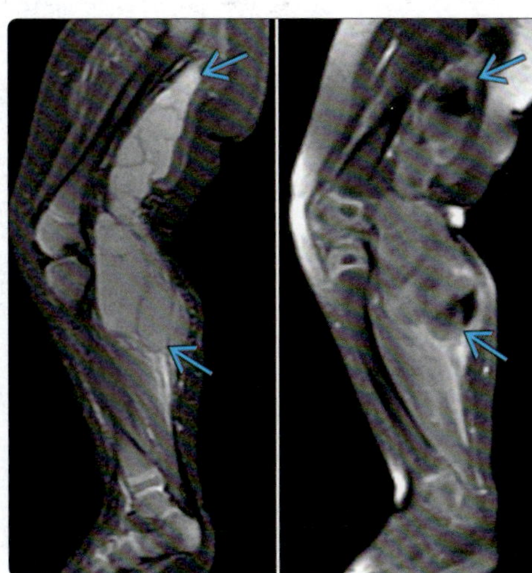

(Left) *Transverse ultrasound of the posterior calf in a 2-year-old girl with a palpable mass shows a well-circumscribed, heterogeneous, solid mass that was noncompressible. Internal vascularity was seen on Doppler (not shown).* **(Right)** *Sagittal T2 FS (left) & T1 C+ FS (right) MR images in the same patient demonstrate the full extent of the soft tissue mass → extending from the posterior upper thigh to the midleg. Biopsy showed an undifferentiated round cell sarcoma.*

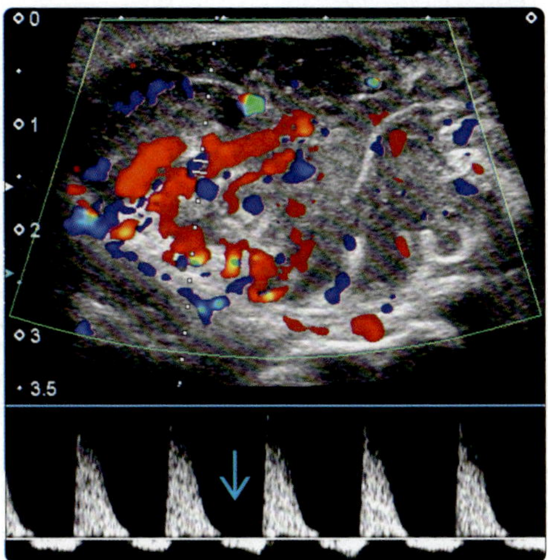

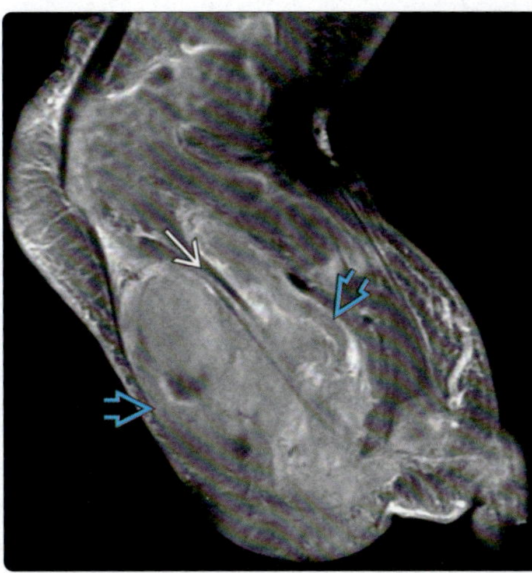

(Left) *Transverse color Doppler ultrasound through a growing plantar soft tissue mass of the foot in a young infant shows a heterogeneous & highly vascularized lesion. The high-resistance waveforms (with reversed diastolic flow →) & deep extent would be atypical for an infantile hemangioma.* **(Right)** *Sagittal T1 C+ FS MR in the same patient shows heterogeneous enhancement of the deep & infiltrative mass → that encases the flexor tendons →. An infantile fibrosarcoma was found upon biopsy.*

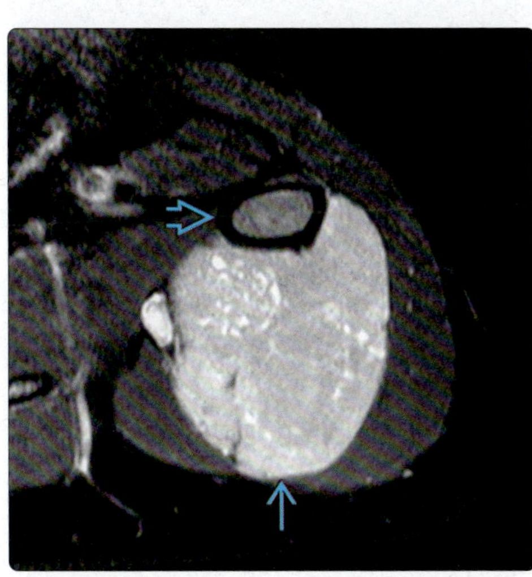

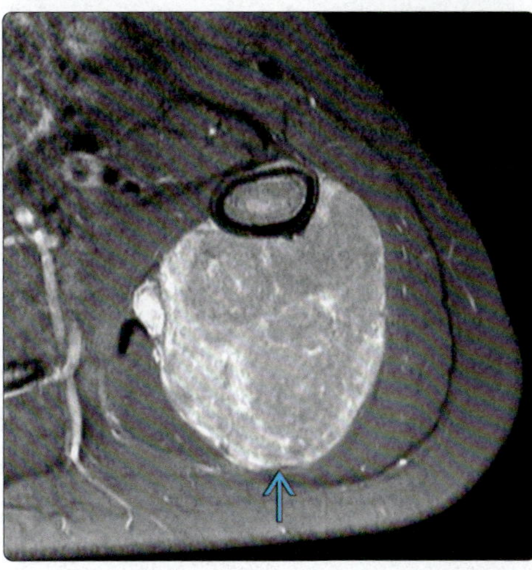

(Left) *Axial T2 FS MR in a 4-year-old with a firm mass shows a well-circumscribed, round, mildly heterogeneous, intermediate to bright intramuscular mass → directly abutting the posterior left humerus →. Note the lack of surrounding edema.* **(Right)** *Axial T1 C+ FS MR in the same patient shows moderate heterogeneous enhancement throughout the mass →. The overall appearance as a "solid soft tissue ball" is highly suggestive of a soft tissue malignancy. Biopsy confirmed a synovial sarcoma.*

Granuloma Annulare

KEY FACTS

TERMINOLOGY

- Benign, inflammatory lesion of superficial soft tissues
- Cutaneous form is very familiar to dermatologists
- Subcutaneous granuloma annulare (SGA) is type most frequently encountered by radiologists due to
  - Deeper location
  - Nonspecific clinical appearance

IMAGING

- Subcutaneous lesion(s) of extensor surfaces of lower leg (pretibial), foot, & forearm/elbow or scalp
- Elongated, nodular, & poorly defined
- Radiography: Swelling without Ca^{2+} or bone involvement
- Ultrasound: Hypoechoic, mildly heterogeneous, infiltrating superficial lesion
- T2 FS MR: Heterogeneous with regions of ↓ & ↑ signal
  - Indistinct margins with surrounding edema is common
- T1 C+ FS MR: Homogeneous to mildly heterogeneous

TOP DIFFERENTIAL DIAGNOSES

- Trauma (contusion or fat necrosis)
- Chronic foreign body
- Microcystic lymphatic malformation
- Cellulitis
- Fibromatosis

PATHOLOGY

- Fine-needle aspiration is not adequate for diagnosis
  - May lead to mistaken diagnosis of malignancy
- Mucin staining is characteristic

CLINICAL ISSUES

- Typical presentation: Firm, painless, subcutaneous nodule in otherwise healthy young child
- Natural history: Spontaneous involution
- Lesions with characteristic history, location, & imaging: Consider observation vs. incisional biopsy for diagnosis
- May recur even after excisional biopsy

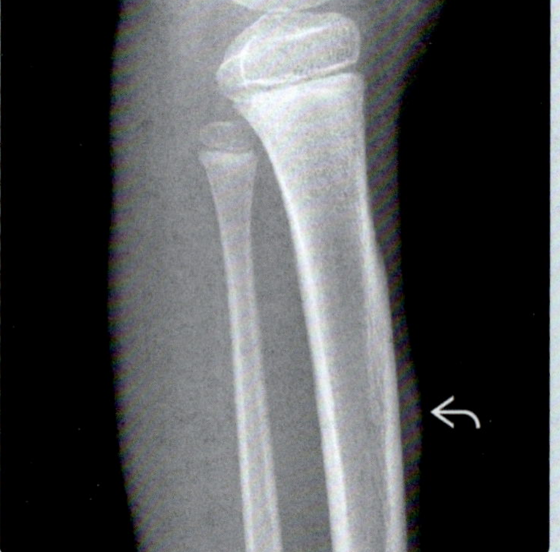
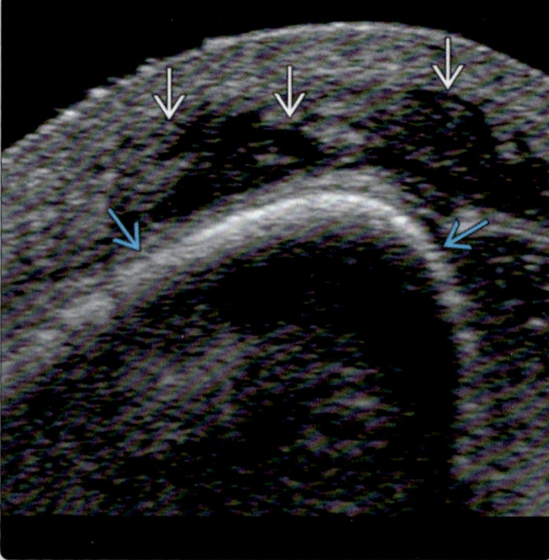

(Left) *Lateral radiograph of a 6-year-old girl presenting with a painless, firm bump at the anterior tibia shows a soft tissue mass ➡ without Ca^{2+} or underlying bony abnormality. A similar but smaller mass was present on the contralateral side (not shown).* **(Right)** *Transverse ultrasound in the same patient shows an elongated & lobulated hypoechoic mass ➡ with indistinct margins in the subcutaneous fat anterior to the tibial diaphysis ➡. The mass proved to be subcutaneous granuloma annulare (SGA) on biopsy.*

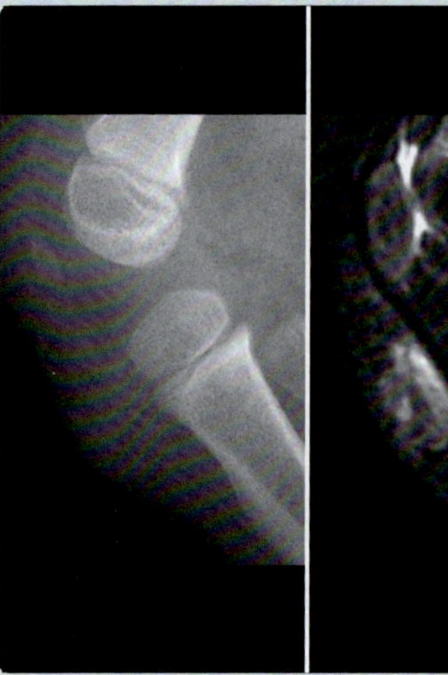
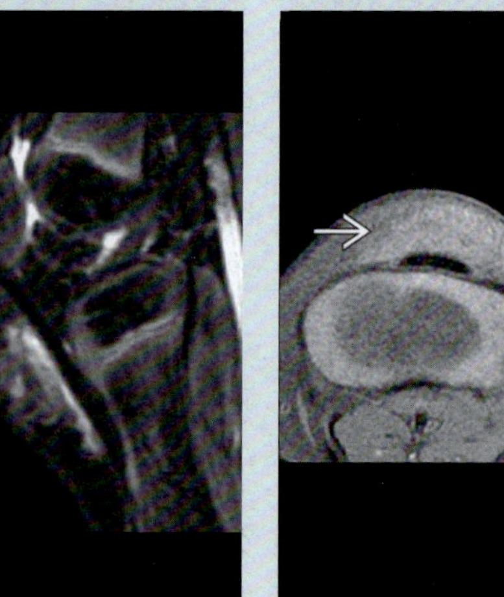
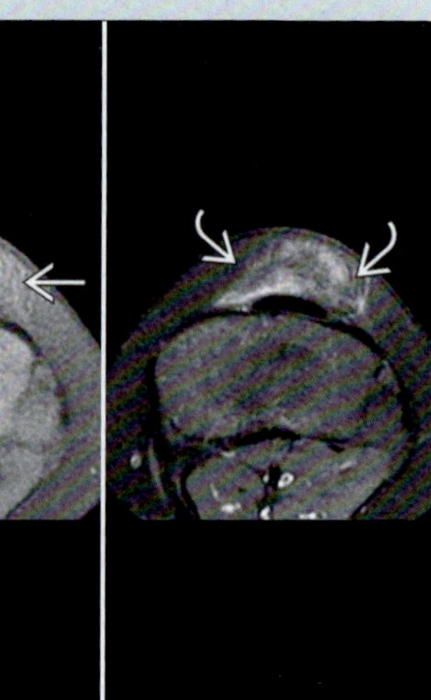

(Left) *Knee radiograph (left) in a 3-year-old girl shows nonspecific soft tissue swelling ➡ anterior to the patellar tendon. On the sagittal T2 FS MR (right), the mass is poorly defined ➡ with areas of intermediate & high signal intensity.* **(Right)** *Axial T1 FS MR images were performed before (left) & after (right) contrast in the same patient. The mass is isointense to slightly hyperintense ➡ to skeletal muscle before contrast with heterogeneous enhancement ➡ after contrast. Biopsy confirmed SGA.*

TERMINOLOGY

Abbreviations

- Subcutaneous granuloma annulare (SGA)

Synonyms

- Benign rheumatoid nodule, pseudorheumatoid nodule, deep granuloma annulare, subcutaneous palisading granuloma, palisading granuloma nodosum, isolated subcutaneous nodule, isolated subcutaneous granuloma, necrobiotic granuloma

Definitions

- Benign inflammatory skin lesion of unknown etiology
- 4 clinically distinct subtypes
  - Localized
  - Generalized
  - Perforating
  - Subcutaneous: Subtype of concern to radiologists

IMAGING

General Features

- Location
  - Extension up to (but not deep to) investing fascia
    - Abnormal muscle signal is highly atypical
  - Distributed within feet, lower legs, fingers, hands, forearms, & scalp; can be multifocal & bilateral
    - Primarily affects extensor surfaces of extremities
    - Classic location: Pretibial (19-65%)
- Morphology
  - Elongated, mildly nodular mass with indistinct margins

Radiographic Findings

- Superficial soft tissue mass
  - No Ca^{2+} or bone involvement

Ultrasonographic Findings

- Hypoechoic, mildly heterogeneous nodular lesion

MR Findings

- T1WI
  - Iso- to slightly hyperintense to skeletal muscle
- T2WI FS
  - Heterogeneous with areas of ↓ & ↑ signal intensity
  - Reticular ↑ signal in surrounding subcutaneous fat
- T1WI C+ FS
  - Homogeneous to mildly heterogeneous enhancement

DIFFERENTIAL DIAGNOSIS

Trauma (Contusion or Fat Necrosis)

- Focally edematous soft tissue after trauma, often overlying bony protuberance
- May ultimately lead to focal fat thinning

Chronic Foreign Body

- Hyperechoic foreign body surrounded by poorly defined hypoechoic tissue or fluid

Microcystic Lymphatic Malformation

- Longstanding, poorly defined infiltrative lesion
- ± macrocysts (> 1 cm)
- Often has characteristic cutaneous blebs

Cellulitis

- Poorly defined, serpentine foci of fluid tracking through indurated fat
- Erythema & tenderness are typical

Nodular Fasciitis

- Benign rapidly growing lesion, often painful
- Frequently at subcutaneous fat-fascial interface

Muscle Hernia

- Superficial fascial defect with dynamic muscle protrusion

Fibromatosis

- Typically deeper & infiltrative but benign locally aggressive lesion
- Often has foci of ↓ & ↑ T2 signal intensity

PATHOLOGY

Microscopic Features

- Degenerating collagen with peripheral palisading histiocytes & surrounding reactive inflammatory cells
- Mucin staining is characteristic
- Fine-needle aspiration is suboptimal
  - May cause lesion to look aggressive (like malignancy)

CLINICAL ISSUES

Presentation

- Most common signs/symptoms
  - Painless, firm subcutaneous nodules in extremities or scalp

Demographics

- Age
  - Subcutaneous form is almost exclusively seen in children
  - Classic range: 2-5 years; mean age: 4.3 years

Natural History & Prognosis

- Spontaneous involution is typical (over months to years)
- Recurrence in 19-75% of cases
  - May occur following incisional or excisional biopsy

Treatment

- Observation with typical clinical & imaging findings
- No proven efficacious medical treatment
- Incisional or excisional biopsy is diagnostic but not necessarily curative

SELECTED REFERENCES

1. Joshi TP et al: Granuloma annulare: an updated review of epidemiology, pathogenesis, and treatment options. Am J Clin Dermatol. 8;1-14, 2021
2. Rodríguez-Garijo N et al: Granuloma annulare subtypes: sonographic features and clinicopathological correlation. J Ultrasound. ePub, 2021
3. Vázquez-Osorio I et al: Usefulness of ultrasonography in the diagnosis of subcutaneous granuloma annulare. Pediatr Dermatol. 35(3):e200-1, 2018
4. Fathi K et al: Subcutaneous granuloma annulare of the penis associated with a urethral anomaly: case report and review of the literature. Pediatr Dermatol. 31(4):e100-3, 2014
5. Agrawal AK et al: An unusual presentation of subcutaneous granuloma annulare in association with juvenile-onset diabetes: case report and literature review. Pediatr Dermatol. 29(2):202-5, 2012
6. Navarro OM: Soft tissue masses in children. Radiol Clin North Am. 49(6):1235-59, vi-vii, 2011

KEY FACTS

TERMINOLOGY

- Myositis ossificans (MO): Benign reactive ossifying soft tissue mass; clear history of trauma in 60-75%

IMAGING

- Best diagnostic clue: Heterogeneous intramuscular mass occurring after trauma with evolving imaging appearance
- Radiographic findings
  - 0-2 weeks: Nonspecific soft tissue swelling/mass
  - 2-6 weeks: Faint but increasing peripheral Ca^{2+}
  - 6-8 weeks: Sharply circumscribed osseous mass
  - 5-6 months: Ossified mass with ↑ maturity, ↓ size
- CT: Rim of mineralization by 4 weeks; cortical & trabecular bone ± fatty marrow within months
- MR appearance also varies with age of lesion
  - Early: T2 heterogeneity internally with mild peripheral mineralization + marked surrounding edema
    - Active areas show intense enhancement
  - Late (mature): Well-circumscribed mass with rim of low signal cortex & little surrounding edema
    - Internal foci of fatty yellow marrow on all sequences
  - GRE: Sensitive for mineralization (blooming artifact)

TOP DIFFERENTIAL DIAGNOSES

- Soft tissue sarcoma
- Hematoma
- Abscess
- Surface osteosarcoma

DIAGNOSTIC CHECKLIST

- Short-term radiographic follow-up or CT to demonstrate zonal ossification
- MR of early MO can mimic malignant soft tissue tumors
  - Marked surrounding edema is atypical in sarcomas
- Indeterminate lesions should undergo adequate biopsy
  - Pathologist to be aware if MO is being considered, as early MO may mimic malignancy under microscope

(Left) *Serial lateral radiographs in a 14-year-old dancer with a popliteal mass show an evolving lesion with only soft tissue edema present initially (left) ➡. A 6-week follow-up (middle) shows peripheral ossification ➡ with progressive maturation at 6 months (right) ➡.* **(Right)** *Initial sagittal MR in the same patient shows a mass that is isointense on PD (left) ➡, hyperintense on T2 FS (middle) ➡, & diffusely enhancing on T1 C+ FS (right) ➡. Small peripheral hypointense foci ➡ represent early ossification. Note adjacent edema ➡.*

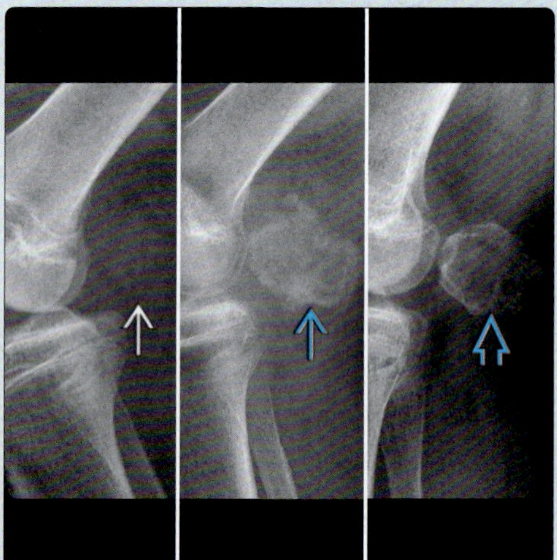

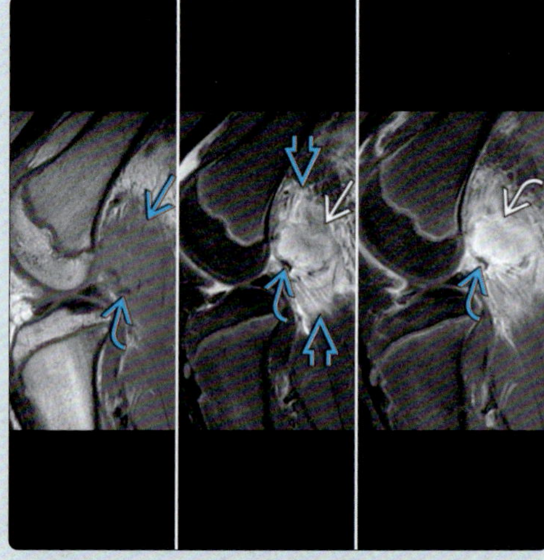

(Left) *Sagittal T2 FS (left) & GRE (right) MR images in the same patient 6 weeks later show heterogeneous internal signal in the mass ➡ with a peripheral hypointense rim ➡ that blooms on the GRE sequences. There is continued surrounding edema ➡.* **(Right)** *Coronal T1 MR in the same patient at 6 weeks (left) & 1 year (right) of follow-up shows progressive maturation of the mass ➡ to an ossified lesion of fatty yellow marrow with no surrounding edema. The mass was then resected.*

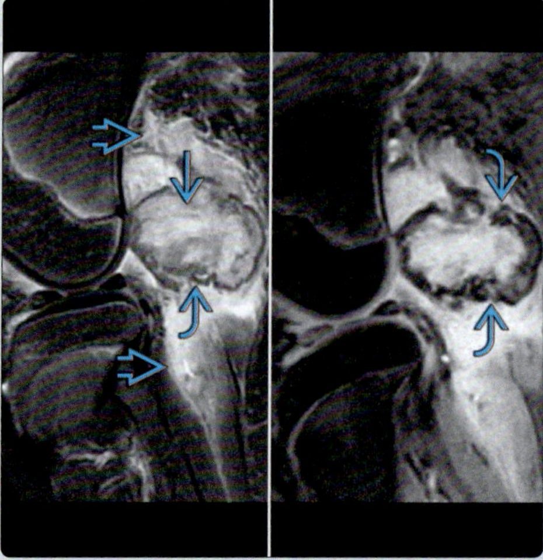

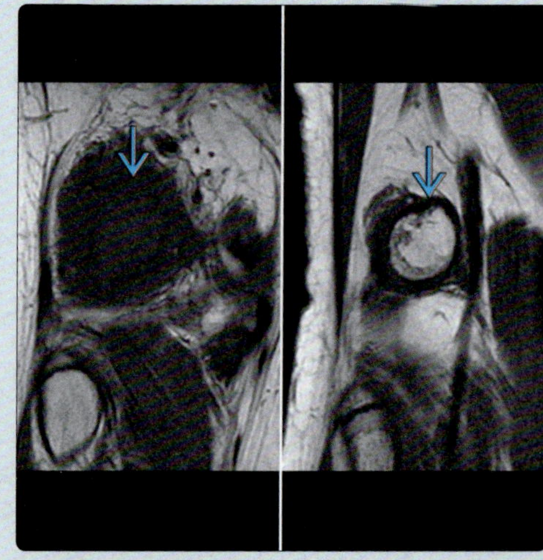

Myositis Ossificans

TERMINOLOGY

Abbreviations

- Myositis ossificans (MO)

Definitions

- Benign ossifying soft tissue mass; reactive lesion typically occurring after muscle insult
  - Clear history of trauma in 60-75% of cases
  - Others: Repetitive microtrauma, inflammation, ischemia

IMAGING

General Features

- Best diagnostic clue
  - Heterogeneous intramuscular mass with peripheral mineralization developing within weeks
    - Appearance changes over time as lesion matures

Radiographic Findings

- 0-2 weeks: Nonspecific soft tissue swelling/mass
- 2-6 weeks: Faint Ca^{2+}, largely peripheral
- 6-8 weeks: Sharply circumscribed peripheral Ca^{2+}
- 5-6 months: More mature ossified mass with ↓ size

Ultrasonographic Findings

- Early: Heterogeneous lesion with ↓ central & ↑ peripheral echogenic zones
- Late: Peripheral zone shows posterior shadowing

CT Findings

- NECT
  - Low-attenuation mass without mineralization early
  - Rim of mineralization usually seen by 4 weeks
  - Gradual maturing ossification demonstrates cortical & trabecular bone ± fat attenuation of yellow marrow

MR Findings

- Early: Round, elongated, or poorly defined intramuscular mass + intense surrounding edema
  - T2 FS/STIR: Heterogeneous signal intensity
  - T1: Isointense to skeletal muscle
  - ± small areas of ↓ peripheral signal (mineralization)
- Intermediate: ↓ peripheral signal is more apparent
  - ± central areas of irregular low signal; ± fluid/fluid levels from hemorrhage
- Late (mature): Well-defined mass of variable heterogeneity with minimal, if any, surrounding edema
  - Internal foci that are isointense to fat (yellow marrow) on all sequences; confluent peripheral rim of low signal intensity
- GRE: Most sensitive for mineralization; exaggerated signal loss or blooming artifact
- T1 C+ FS: Heterogeneous to intense enhancement if active

Imaging Recommendations

- Best imaging tool
  - Radiographs: Short interval follow-up in 3-4 weeks (when MO is suspected) → new peripheral mineralization
  - CT: Earliest detection of zonal pattern of mineralization

DIFFERENTIAL DIAGNOSIS

Soft Tissue Sarcoma

- Typically well-circumscribed with little surrounding edema
- May contain disorganized Ca^{2+}

Hematoma

- Heterogeneous mass after trauma or with coagulopathy
- Subacute/chronic hematomas may develop Ca^{2+}

Venous Malformation

- Large phleboliths may occur in extensive lesions

Soft Tissue Abscess

- Clinical symptoms typically suggest infection
- Mass with thick, irregular enhancing wall & central nonenhancing fluid

Surface Osteosarcoma

- Underlying bone shows cortical scalloping, periosteal reaction

PATHOLOGY

Microscopic Features

- Early: Immature, highly cellular fibroblastic lesion
  - Differentiation from sarcoma may be difficult
- Late (mature): Distinct zonal pattern of ossification
  - Peripheral: Rim of mature lamellar bone

CLINICAL ISSUES

Presentation

- Most common signs/symptoms
  - Firm/hard soft tissue mass ± pain, tenderness
  - Clear history of traumatic event is absent in up to 40%

Treatment

- Surgical excision of symptomatic lesions

DIAGNOSTIC CHECKLIST

Consider

- Heterogeneous, solid, intramuscular mass in teenager/young adult with marked surrounding muscle edema → strongly consider MO, especially after trauma
  - Recommend short-term follow-up radiographs or CT rather than immediate biopsy
- If biopsy is required for indeterminate lesion → obtain core, incisional, or excisional biopsy; FNA may be inconclusive

Image Interpretation Pearls

- Earliest MR findings of MO: Mass with small peripheral areas of ↓ signal + marked surrounding edema
  - Recent study found that perilesional edema on MR > 2x size of central lesion favors early/intermediate MO vs. malignant soft tissue mass

SELECTED REFERENCES

1. Zubler V et al: Diagnostic utility of perilesional muscle edema in myositis ossificans. Skeletal Radiol. 49(6):929-36, 2020
2. Meyers C et al: Heterotopic ossification: a comprehensive review. JBMR Plus. 3(4):e10172, 2019
3. Tyler P et al: The imaging of myositis ossificans. Semin Musculoskelet Radiol. 14(2):201-16, 2010

KEY FACTS

TERMINOLOGY

- Ewing sarcoma family of tumors: Ewing sarcoma, primitive neuroectodermal tumor, Askin tumor, extraosseous Ewing sarcoma
- Aggressive small round blue cell tumor that typically arises in bone

IMAGING

- Highly aggressive appearance
  - Lucent, ill-defined, intramedullary lesion; poorly marginated; can show mild expansile remodeling
    - Sclerosis in up to 25% of cases (not beyond bone)
  - Permeative or moth-eaten cortical destruction
  - Aggressive periosteal reaction: Spiculated, sunburst, lamellated onion skin appearance, &/or Codman triangle
  - Associated soft tissue mass
    - Disproportionately larger than amount of bone destruction
- Greater propensity for flat bones (scapula, pelvis) than other primary bone malignancies
- Diaphyseal involvement is more common than with other bone malignancies
- MR for local evaluation: Intraosseous & soft tissue extent, relationship to joint & neurovascular bundle
  - Coronal/sagittal T1 MR best shows true tumor margin in bone: Sharp demarcation vs. adjacent fatty marrow
  - Early joint-to joint marrow sequence (coronal T1 &/or STIR) to look for intraosseous skip metastases before smaller field-of-view high-detail assessment
- Chest CT, PET/CT for staging

CLINICAL ISSUES

- 2nd most common primary bone malignancy in children after osteosarcoma
- Most common during 2nd decade of life

(Left) *AP radiograph in a 5-year-old with shoulder pain shows abnormal lucency, permeation, & expansion of the entire right scapula* ➔. **(Right)** *Axial T2 FS MR in the same patient shows that the entire scapula has been replaced by a solid mass* ➔ *that extends into the surrounding soft tissues. A thin, low-signal rim of expanded & permeated cortex remains* ➔. *Note the residual glenoid articular cartilage & labrum* ➔. *Biopsy of the mass confirmed Ewing sarcoma.*

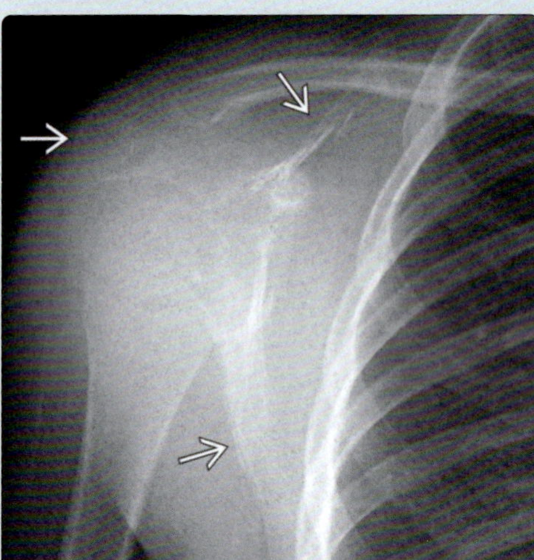

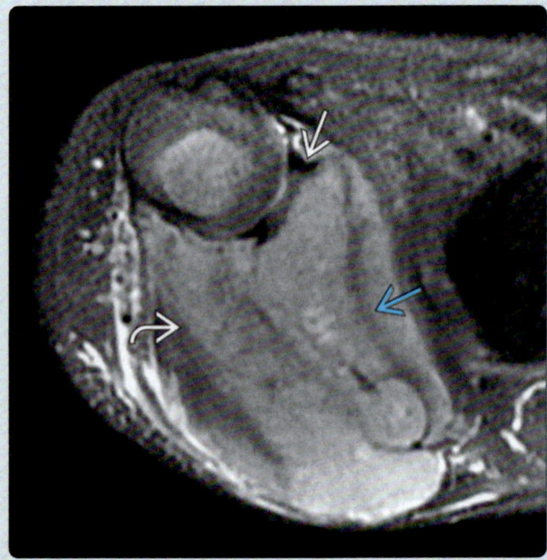

(Left) *Lateral radiograph in a 10-year-old with weeks of knee pain shows poorly circumscribed lucency & permeation of the mid to lower patella.* **(Right)** *Coronal T1 MR (left) in the same patient show a relatively sharp interface* ➔ *between the lesion & yellow marrow. Coronal T1 C+ FS MR (right) shows heterogeneous enhancement of the lesion with adjacent marrow & soft tissue signal abnormality. Ewing sarcoma was proven at biopsy.*

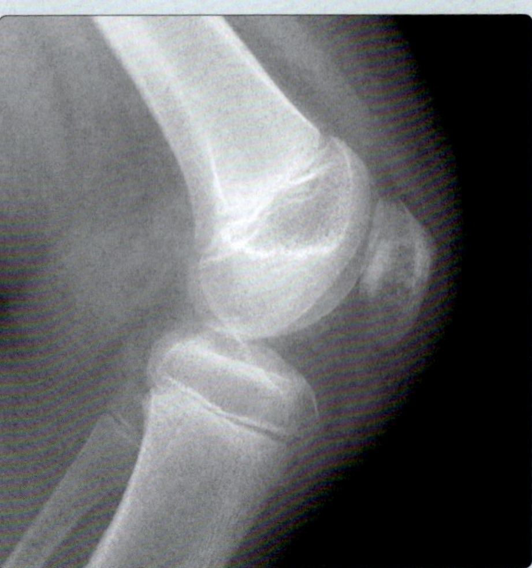

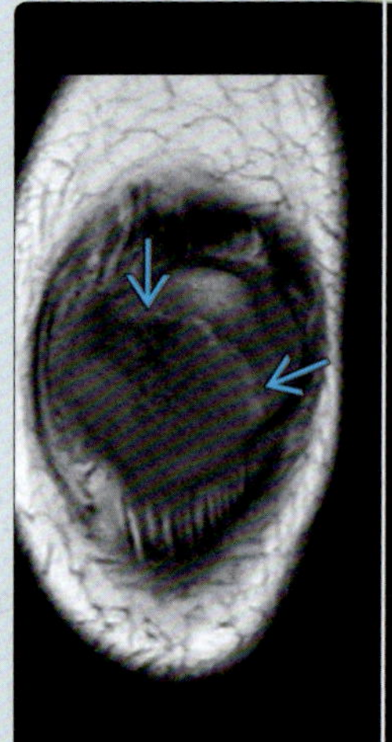

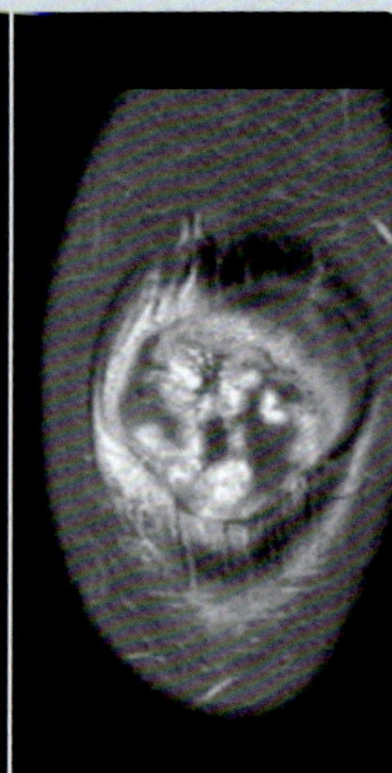

TERMINOLOGY

Synonyms

- Malignant primary bone tumor
- Ewing sarcoma (EWS) family of tumors: Ewing, primitive neuroectodermal tumor (PNET), Askin tumor, extraosseous Ewing

Definitions

- Aggressive small round blue cell tumor that typically arises in bone

IMAGING

General Features

- Best diagnostic clue
  - Central, diaphyseal, permeative lytic lesion with lamellated "onion skin" periosteal reaction
- Location
  - Can occur in any bone & soft tissue
    - Metaphyseal & diaphyseal: 94%
      - Diaphyseal involvement is more common than with other bone malignancies, tends to be central
      - Metaphyseal involvement tends to be eccentric
    - Greater propensity for flat bones (scapula, pelvis) than other primary bone malignancies
  - Lower extremity: 41%
  - Pelvis: 26%
  - Chest wall: 16%
  - Extraosseous: Chest wall & retroperitoneum or paravertebral are most common
  - Metastatic disease
    - Most commonly lungs, bones
- Morphology
  - Bone lesions classically (but not always) have large soft tissue mass relative to degree of bone change
  - Extraosseous EWS arises from soft tissues, not bone
    - Typically adjacent to or involving neurovascular bundles
    - Appears as nonspecific, well-circumscribed soft tissue mass

Radiographic Findings

- Radiography
  - Highly aggressive appearance overall
    - May sometimes show expansile remodeling but not without other more aggressive features
  - Ill-defined (wide zone of transition) intramedullary lesion
  - Mixed lytic & sclerotic intraosseous components
  - Permeative or moth-eaten appearance of cortical destruction
    - Infiltration of tumor through haversian canals of cortical bone
  - Cortical thickening, violation, or rarely, saucerization
  - Aggressive periosteal reaction, often interrupted
    - Spiculated
    - Lamellated onion skin appearance
    - Sunburst or hair standing on end patterns: Periosteal reaction laid down along Sharpey fibers (which attach periosteum to underlying cortical bone) in attempt to wall off tumor
    - Codman triangle: Interrupted elevation of periosteal new bone along margin of tumor
  - No ossified tumor matrix (i.e., no soft tissue osteoid) but can be sclerotic in flat bones
    - Bone necrosis, reactive sclerosis
  - Associated soft tissue mass, often disproportionately larger than amount of bone destruction
  - ± pathologic fracture

CT Findings

- NECT
  - Depicts aggressive periosteal reaction & bone destruction
  - May be helpful in complex anatomic areas (pelvis, spine, skull base)
  - Chest CT for pulmonary metastasis

MR Findings

- T1WI
  - Coronal/sagittal best shows true tumor margin in bone: Sharp demarcation vs. adjacent normal fatty marrow
  - Axial may be helpful for relationship of tumor to neurovascular bundle
- T2 FS/STIR
  - Heterogeneous mass of intermediate to high signal intensity
  - Surrounding marrow, periosteal, & soft tissue edema
- DWI
  - Typically restricts diffusion in cellular areas
  - ADC values are lower than osteosarcoma
  - ADC value may help in monitoring response to therapy
- T1WI C+ FS
  - Heterogeneous enhancement
  - Baseline for postchemotherapy response assessment

Nuclear Medicine Findings

- Bone scan
  - Intense uptake
  - Traditionally used for evaluation of metastatic bone disease
- PET
  - Lesions demonstrate F-18 FDG avidity
  - Useful in staging & monitoring response to therapy
    - More likely to detect osseous metastases than bone scan
  - Possible predictor of outcome

Imaging Recommendations

- Best imaging tool
  - MR for local evaluation: Intraosseous & soft tissue extent, relationship to joint & neurovascular bundle
- Protocol advice
  - Early joint-to-joint marrow sequence (coronal T1 &/or STIR) to look for intraosseous skip metastases
  - Then smaller field-of-view pre- & postcontrast sequences for high detail

DIFFERENTIAL DIAGNOSIS

Osteomyelitis

- May be difficult to differentiate from EWS as both can have very aggressive imaging appearances

- Typically has less enhancing soft tissue & more nonenhancing fluid pockets & surrounding inflammation than EWS
- More common in children < 5 years of age
- More rapid presentation of symptoms

Osteosarcoma

- Osteoid tumor matrix in 90%
- More commonly involves long bone metaphysis than diaphysis or axial skeleton

Metastatic Neuroblastoma

- More common in children < 3 years of age
- Multifocal permeative lucent lesions
- Calcified abdominopelvic mass

Langerhans Cell Histiocytosis

- Lytic bone lesion, often with sharp, punched-out margins & minimal to no periosteal reaction
- Homogeneously enhancing soft tissue mass in bone defect
- ± T2 MR hypointense rim, surrounding marrow edema > soft tissue edema

PATHOLOGY

General Features

- Genetics
  - EWS family of tumors: t(11;22)(q24;q12) (85%)

Microscopic Features

- Highly cellular with sheets of cells, little stroma
- Small round blue cell tumor

CLINICAL ISSUES

Presentation

- Most common signs/symptoms
  - Presents with pain & swelling
  - Tenderness/palpable mass
- Other signs/symptoms
  - May be associated with systemic symptoms/signs: Leukocytosis, fever, anemia, elevated sedimentation rate
    - Mimics osteomyelitis
  - Pathologic fracture (up to 15%)
    - Not considered adverse prognostic sign

Demographics

- Age
  - 2nd most common primary bone malignancy in children after osteosarcoma
  - Median age: 15 years
  - 80% are < 20 years old
  - Rare before 5 years of age
  - Extraosseous EWS is typically slightly older age group
- Sex
  - M > F (1.5-2:1)
- Ethnicity
  - White patients are 9x more common than Black patients

Natural History & Prognosis

- Poorer prognosis in
  - Boys
  - Patients 15-18 years & older
  - Metastatic disease
  - Larger tumor volume
  - Pelvic location
  - Higher serum lactate dehydrogenase levels prior to treatment
  - Previous treatment of malignancy: EWS as 2nd malignancy
- Survival is better for lesions of extremities than those of axial skeleton
  - Pelvic lesions tend to be larger at presentation
- ↑ incidence of developing other future solid neoplasms
  - Treatment-related acute myeloid leukemia & myelodysplastic syndrome in 1-2% of patients
- Overall survival rate: 41%

Treatment

- Neoadjuvant & adjuvant chemotherapy
  - Vincristine, cyclophosphamide, doxorubicin, or actinomycin D
- Radiation therapy
- Resection of primary tumor
- Limb salvage procedures
- IGF-1R antibody
- Investigational: High-dose therapy followed by stem cell transplant for metastatic disease at presentation & patients with poor response to initial chemotherapy

DIAGNOSTIC CHECKLIST

Consider

- F-18 FDG PET in determining active residual/recurrent tumor from therapeutic changes

Image Interpretation Pearls

- May mimic osteomyelitis clinically or in laboratory findings

SELECTED REFERENCES

1. Murphey MD et al: Staging and classification of primary musculoskeletal bone and soft tissue tumors based on the 2020 WHO update, from the AJR special series on cancer staging. AJR Am J Roentgenol. ePub, 2021
2. Parlak Ş et al: Diffusion-weighted imaging for the differentiation of Ewing sarcoma from osteosarcoma. Skeletal Radiol. 50(10):2023-30, 2021
3. Harrison DJ et al: PET with 18F-Fluorodeoxyglucose/computed tomography in the management of pediatric sarcoma. PET Clin. 15(3):333-47, 2020
4. Saleh MM et al: Multiparametric MRI with diffusion-weighted imaging in predicting response to chemotherapy in cases of osteosarcoma and Ewing's sarcoma. Br J Radiol. 93(1115):20200257, 2020
5. Tal AL et al: The utility of 18FDG PET/CT versus bone scan for identification of bone metastases in a pediatric sarcoma population and a review of the literature. J Pediatr Hematol Oncol. 43(2):52-8, 2020
6. Veselis CA et al: Bone tumors occurring in the soft tissues: a review of the clinical, imaging, and histopathologic findings. Curr Probl Diagn Radiol. 50(3):419-29, 2020
7. McCarville MB et al: Distinguishing osteomyelitis from Ewing sarcoma on radiography and MRI. AJR Am J Roentgenol. 205(3):640-50; quiz 651, 2015
8. Orr WS et al: Analysis of prognostic factors in extraosseous Ewing sarcoma family of tumors: review of St. Jude Children's Research Hospital experience. Ann Surg Oncol. 19(12):3816-22, 2012
9. Mody RJ et al: FDG PET imaging of childhood sarcomas. Pediatr Blood Cancer. 54(2):222-7, 2010
10. Peersman B et al: Ewing's sarcoma: imaging features. JBR-BTR. 90(5):368-76, 2007
11. Hayashida Y et al: Monitoring therapeutic responses of primary bone tumors by diffusion-weighted image: Initial results. Eur Radiol. 16(12):2637-43, 2006
12. Ewing Sarcoma Treatment (PDQ®)–Health Professional Version

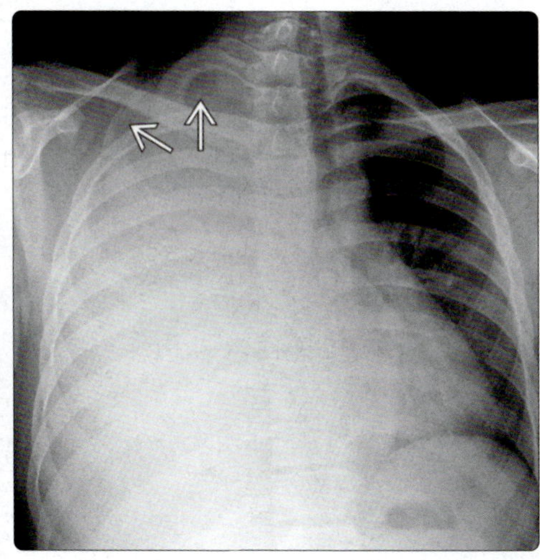

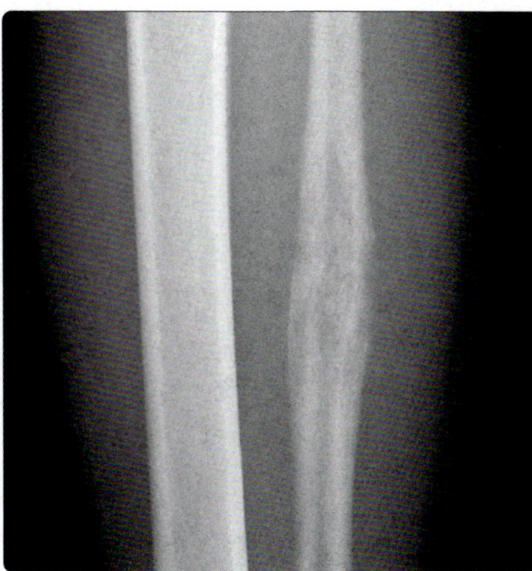

(Left) *Frontal radiograph in a 15-year-old boy shows a large mass & effusion filling the entire right hemithorax. Note the destructive right 2nd rib lesion ➡ due to Ewing sarcoma.* **(Right)** *AP radiograph in a 10-year-old with leg pain shows an aggressive-appearing lucent lesion of the midfibular diaphysis with permeation, wide zone of transition, & expansile remodeling. Biopsy confirmed Ewing sarcoma.*

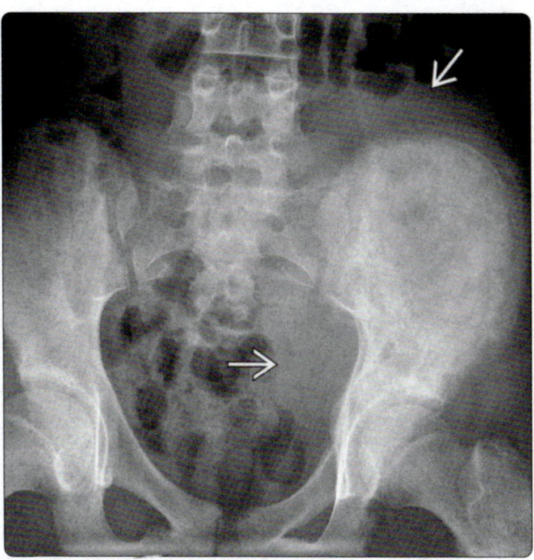

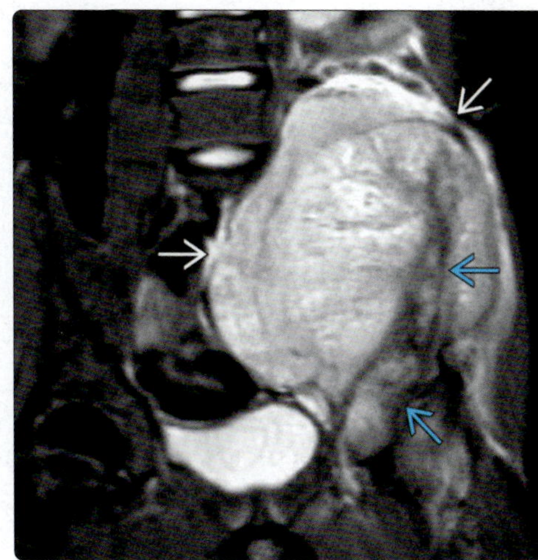

(Left) *AP radiograph shows a large soft tissue mass ➡ displacing bowel from a permeated, mottled, & expanded left iliac bone with overlying periosteal reaction. Ewing sarcoma was proven on biopsy.* **(Right)** *Coronal STIR MR in the same patient confirms the large soft tissue component ➡ of the Ewing sarcoma emanating from an expanded & permeated iliac bone ➡. This patient had innumerable lung metastases (not included).*

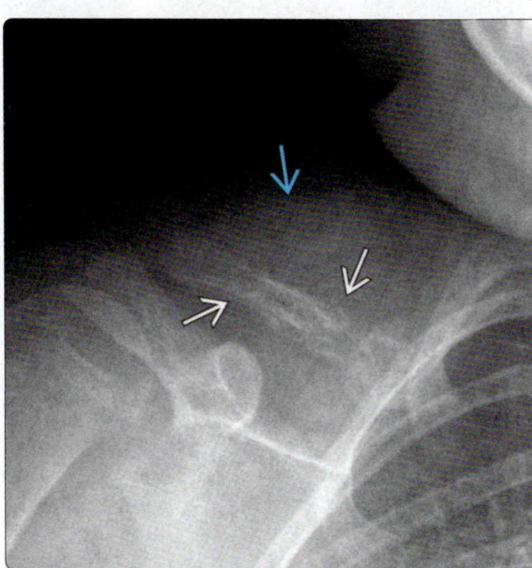

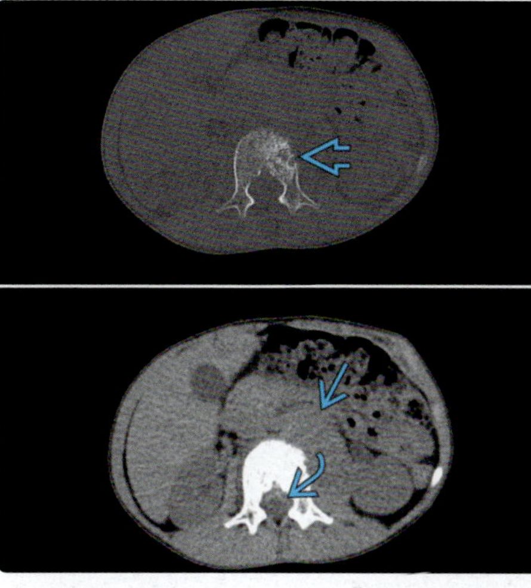

(Left) *AP radiograph in a 7-year-old who presented with soft tissue swelling shows an expanded & permeated lucent clavicle ➡ with aggressive periosteal reaction & a soft tissue mass ➡ from Ewing sarcoma.* **(Right)** *Axial NECT in bone (top) & soft tissue (bottom) windows from an 11-year-old with back pain shows L2 vertebral body permeation by a Ewing sarcoma ⇨. Note the overlying soft tissue expansion ➡ & epidural space infiltration ↗.*

Osteosarcoma

KEY FACTS

TERMINOLOGY

- Conventional high-grade intramedullary osteosarcoma (OS): 75-85%
- Less common OS subtypes (5% or less each): Telangiectatic, low-grade intramedullary, surface (low to high grade), multicentric, extraskeletal, secondary

IMAGING

- Aggressive metaphyseal/metadiaphyseal lesion with variable mix of bone destruction & bone production (cloud-like osteoid)
  - 55-80% around knee; axial skeleton < 20%
- Radiographs are often diagnostic or highly suggestive
- MR to characterize tumor + intra- & extraosseous extent
  - Large field of view joint-to-joint imaging
    - Look for skip metastases
    - T1 is best sequence for intraosseous tumor margin
  - High-detail focused imaging with surface coils
    - Heterogeneous signal intensity on all sequences
      - ◻ Mineralized tumor: Dark T2
      - ◻ Nonmineralized tumor: Intermediate to bright T2
      - ◻ Necrosis: Bright T2; extensive fluid-fluid levels (layering blood products) in telangiectatic subtype
    - Evaluate relationship to physis, joint, neurovascular bundle
- PET for distant metastases; chest CT for small nodules

CLINICAL ISSUES

- Most common malignant primary bone tumor in children/young adults
- Bimodal age distribution: 10-30 years, > 60 years
- Presentations: Pain, mass, recent trauma
- Treatment
  - Neoadjuvant chemotherapy → surgical resection → adjuvant chemotherapy
    - Improved survival if necrosis > 90% at resection
  - Lung nodule metastasectomy (if low-volume disease)

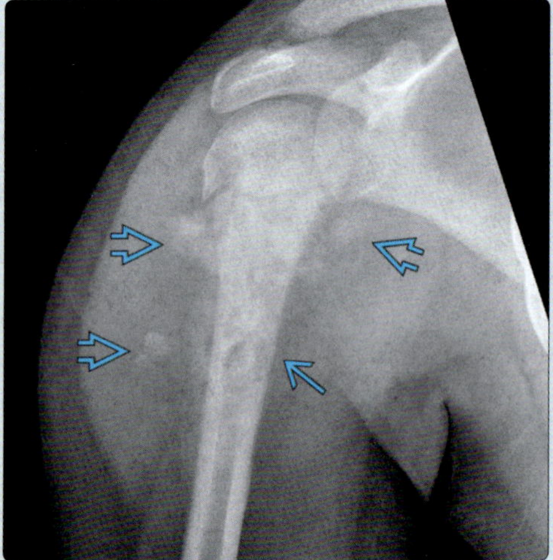

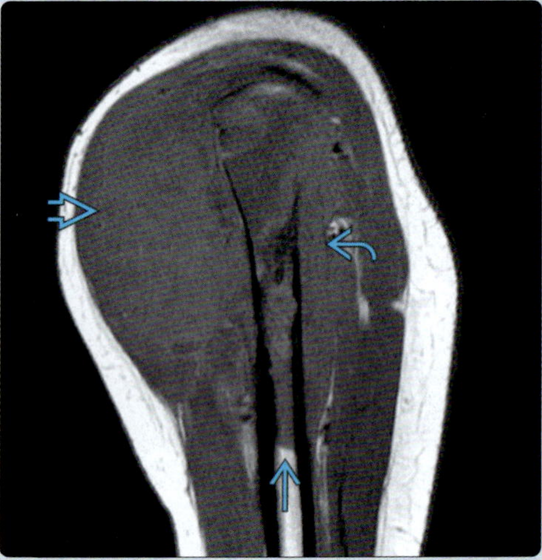

(Left) *Internal rotation radiograph in a 13-year-old with pain shows a mixed lucent & sclerotic lesion of the proximal humerus with many aggressive features, including a wide zone of transition & a Codman triangle ➾ of periosteal reaction. The cloud-like osteoid in the overlying soft tissues ➾ is diagnostic of osteosarcoma (OS).* **(Right)** *Sagittal T1 MR in the same patient shows the typical sharp margin ➾ of bone tumors on T1 against normal yellow marrow. Note the large soft tissue ➾ & subperiosteal ➾ components.*

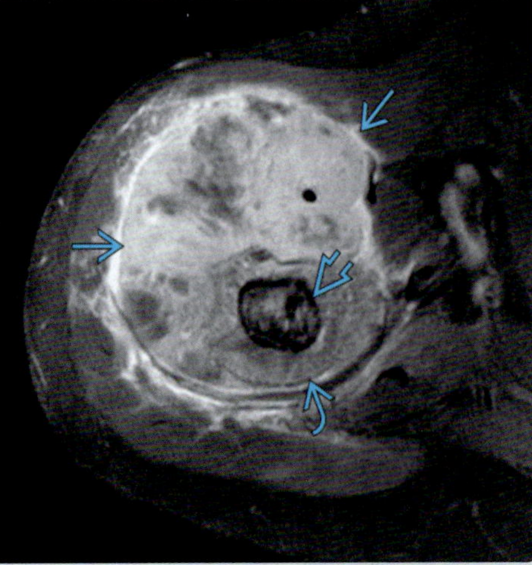

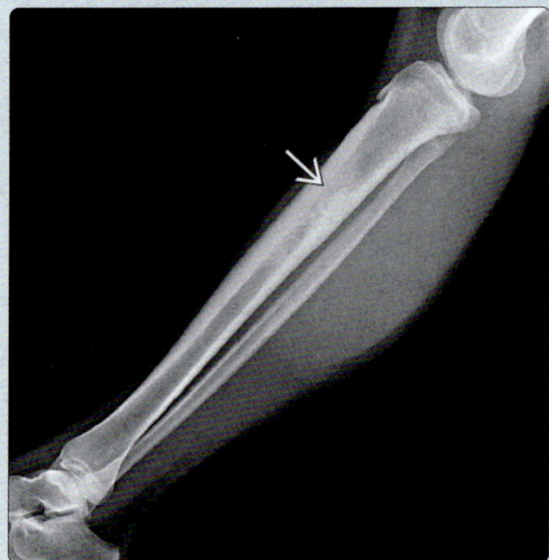

(Left) *Axial T1 C+ FS MR in the same patient shows cortical permeation ➾ & periosteal elevation ➾ by the OS with heterogeneous enhancement of the large soft tissue mass ➾. Though not shown in this case, axial T1 without contrast or FS is particularly helpful for evaluating the relationship of the tumor to the neurovascular bundle.* **(Right)** *Lateral radiograph shows a poorly defined intramedullary sclerotic lesion ➡ within the right tibial diaphysis. There is no visible periosteal reaction or soft tissue mass in this osteoblastic OS.*

TERMINOLOGY

Definitions

- Osteosarcoma (OS): Malignant tumor with ability to produce osteoid directly from neoplastic cells

IMAGING

General Features

- Best diagnostic clue
  - Aggressive metaphyseal/metadiaphyseal lesion with mix of bone destruction & new bone formation
    - Sclerotic (cloud-like) osteoid density extending beyond margins of underlying bone is classic

Radiographic Findings

- Radiography
  - Conventional OS (75-85%)
    - Poorly defined, intramedullary mass
    - Extends through cortex: Frank lysis &/or moth-eaten destruction
    - Aggressive periosteal reaction: Codman triangle, sunburst appearance
    - Soft tissue mass with cloud-like osteoid matrix (90%)
  - Telangiectatic OS (< 5%)
    - Purely lytic geographic lesion; blown-out appearance
    - Cystic cavities filled with blood/necrosis
      - Fluid-fluid levels in 90% (may mimic aneurysmal bone cyst)
    - Enhancing nodular components
    - Pathologic fracture in 25%
  - Parosteal OS (3%)
    - Low-grade surface OS; better prognosis than conventional OS
      - > 90% 5-year survival
    - Age: 20-50 years (older than conventional OS)
    - Classically at distal posterior femoral metaphysis
    - Invasion of marrow in 25%
  - Periosteal OS (1%)
    - Intermediate- to high-grade surface OS
      - Metastatic disease in 15%
      - Recurrence rate as high as 70%
    - Attached to underlying cortex with thickening, scalloping, &/or saucerization of cortex
    - Usually diaphyseal with no medullary involvement
      - Medullary involvement may have poorer prognosis
    - Femur + tibia (85-95%); ulna + humerus (5-10%)
  - High-grade surface OS (1%)
    - Peak incidence in 2nd decade of life
    - Partially mineralized mass
    - Underlying cortex is often partially destroyed
    - Periosteal new bone along margins of lesion
    - May have minimal medullary involvement
  - Multicentric OS (1%)
    - Synchronous osteoblastic osteosarcomas at multiple sites (usually symmetric)
    - Exclusively in children (5-10 years)
    - Extremely poor prognosis
  - Secondary OS (5%)
    - Association with preexisting bone lesion: Paget disease, prior radiation, bone infarct

CT Findings

- Critical for detecting lung metastases

MR Findings

- T1WI
  - Very low signal: Mineralized tumor
  - Low/intermediate signal: Solid, nonmineralized tumor
  - High signal: Hemorrhage
  - Best sequence for determining true tumor margin
- T2 FS/STIR
  - Very low signal: Mineralized tumor
  - Intermediate/high signal: Nonmineralized tumor
  - High signal: Necrosis
    - Fluid-fluid levels with hemorrhagic components, especially telangiectatic OS
  - Tumor margin may blend with surrounding edema
- DWI
  - Highly cellular components restrict diffusion
    - Hemorrhage may also restrict diffusion
  - ADC values may help evaluate treatment response & help differentiate OS from Ewing sarcoma
- T1WI C+ FS
  - Heterogeneous, variable enhancement
    - Subtracted postminus precontrast images are helpful to determine true enhancement vs. T1 shortening due to hemorrhage
  - Changes in dynamic enhancement parameters reflect therapy response better than tumor volume changes

Nuclear Medicine Findings

- Bone scan
  - Much less sensitive for metastatic OS than PET
- PET
  - Intense metabolic activity in viable tumor
    - Differentiates from necrosis/posttherapeutic change
    - May help stage & predict/evaluate treatment response

Imaging Recommendations

- Best imaging tool
  - Radiograph: Primary investigative tool for bone pain
    - Often diagnostic in OS
  - MR to further characterize lesion, including extent in marrow, physis, joint, & soft tissues, including relationship to neurovascular (NV) bundle
  - CT of chest for pulmonary metastatic disease
- Protocol advice
  - Joint-to-joint T1 & STIR MR imaging to determine marrow extent & look for skip metastases
  - Targeted high-detail imaging of lesion to determine relationship to physis, joint, NV bundle

DIFFERENTIAL DIAGNOSIS

Ewing Sarcoma

- Aggressive long bone diaphyseal or flat bone lesion
- Often shows permeation, mild remodeled expansion, large soft tissue mass
- No osteoid production

Stress Fracture

- Linear sclerosis without bone destruction

- Often perpendicular to bone long axis
- Subtle, solid periosteal reaction or cortical thickening

Aneurysmal Bone Cyst

- Numerous fluid-fluid levels with septal enhancement
- No soft tissue mass, nodular enhancement, or sclerosis
- Bony expansion is more frequent than cortical disruption

Osteomyelitis

- Acute (most common): Typically presents prior to development of aggressive radiographic change
  - MR shows poorly defined marrow abnormalities ± subperiosteal & soft tissue fluid collections
- Chronic: Can show mixed sclerotic & lucent foci

Myositis Ossificans

- Reactive lesion, typically to muscle injury
- Marked edema often surrounds intramuscular mass
- Ca^{2+} is first seen at periphery of lesion within weeks

Bone Infarction

- Acute: May show only periosteal reaction & marrow edema
- Chronic: Classic serpentine/geographic sclerotic foci

PATHOLOGY

General Features

- Genetics
  - Most cases are sporadic
  - Predisposing syndromes
    - Li-Fraumeni (*TP53* mutation)
    - Hereditary retinoblastoma (*RB1* mutation)
    - Rothmund-Thomson (*RECQL4* mutation)

Microscopic Features

- Highly pleomorphic, spindle-shaped tumor cells producing different forms of osteoid
- 3 main histologic subtypes depending on sarcomatous component: Osteoblastic (50%), chondroblastic (25%), fibroblastic (25%)

CLINICAL ISSUES

Presentation

- Most common signs/symptoms
  - Pain, soft tissue swelling/mass
- Clinical profile
  - Pathologic fracture: 5-10% in conventional OS
  - Pulmonary metastases can cause pneumothorax (calcifying)
  - Less common metastases: Bone, lymph nodes, liver, brain

Demographics

- Age
  - Bimodal distribution: 10-30 years; over 60 years
- Sex
  - M ≥ F, 3:2 to 2:1
- Epidemiology
  - Most common malignant primary bone tumor in children/young adults
  - Incidence: 5/1 million children ≤ 19 years old

Natural History & Prognosis

- Prognosis depends on
  - Age, sex, extent of disease at diagnosis, time to 1st relapse, location, & stage
    - Better prognosis for extremity vs. axial tumors
    - 15-20% have metastatic disease at diagnosis
      - 80-85% to lungs; bone is 2nd most common
  - Best predictor: Degree of necrosis following neoadjuvant chemotherapy
    - Improved survival with > 90% necrosis
  - OS has ↑ incidence of secondary malignancies
- 5-year survival
  - Without metastases: 70-80%
  - With metastases at presentation: 20-30%
    - Pulmonary is more favorable than bone or other sites
  - With metastases > 2 years after chemotherapy: 40%

Treatment

- Neoadjuvant chemotherapy → surgical resection → adjuvant chemotherapy
- Limb salvage procedures (> 80% of cases)
- Pulmonary nodule metastasectomy in isolated or low-volume metastatic disease (can be curative)

DIAGNOSTIC CHECKLIST

Image Interpretation Pearls

- Bone MR
  - Do not miss distinct skip or other metastatic lesions
    - Requires joint-to-joint imaging
  - Evaluate relationship to physis, joint, & NV bundle
    - Requires focused high-detail imaging
- Chest CT: Calcified & noncalcified pulmonary nodules must be presumed as metastatic until proven otherwise
  - Even in geographic locations with endemic granulomatous diseases (such as histoplasmosis)

SELECTED REFERENCES

1. Habre C et al: Diffusion-weighted imaging in differentiating mid-course responders to chemotherapy for long-bone osteosarcoma compared to the histologic response: an update. Pediatr Radiol. 51(9):1714-23, 2021
2. Parlak Ş et al: Diffusion-weighted imaging for the differentiation of Ewing sarcoma from osteosarcoma. Skeletal Radiol. 50(10):2023-30, 2021
3. Tal AL et al: The utility of 18FDG PET/CT versus bone scan for identification of bone metastases in a pediatric sarcoma population and a review of the literature. J Pediatr Hematol Oncol. 43(2):52-8, 2021
4. Liu F et al: Effectiveness of 18F-FDG PET/CT in the diagnosis and staging of osteosarcoma: a meta-analysis of 26 studies. BMC Cancer. 19(1):323, 2019
5. Spraker-Perlman HL et al: Factors influencing survival after recurrence in osteosarcoma: a report from the Children's Oncology Group. Pediatr Blood Cancer. 66(1):e27444, 2019
6. Takeuchi A et al: Joint-preservation surgery for pediatric osteosarcoma of the knee joint. Cancer Metastasis Rev. 38(4):709-22, 2019
7. Harrison DJ et al: Current and future therapeutic approaches for osteosarcoma. Expert Rev Anticancer Ther. 18(1):39-50, 2018
8. Anderson ME: Update on survival in osteosarcoma. Orthop Clin North Am. 47(1):283-92, 2016
9. Salah S et al: Factors predicting survival following complete surgical remission of pulmonary metastasis in osteosarcoma. Mol Clin Oncol. 3(1):157-62, 2015
10. Lee JS et al: Secondary malignant neoplasms among children, adolescents, and young adults with osteosarcoma. Cancer. 120(24):3987-93, 2014
11. Guo J et al: Dynamic contrast-enhanced magnetic resonance imaging as a prognostic factor in predicting event-free and overall survival in pediatric patients with osteosarcoma. Cancer. 118(15):3776-85, 2012

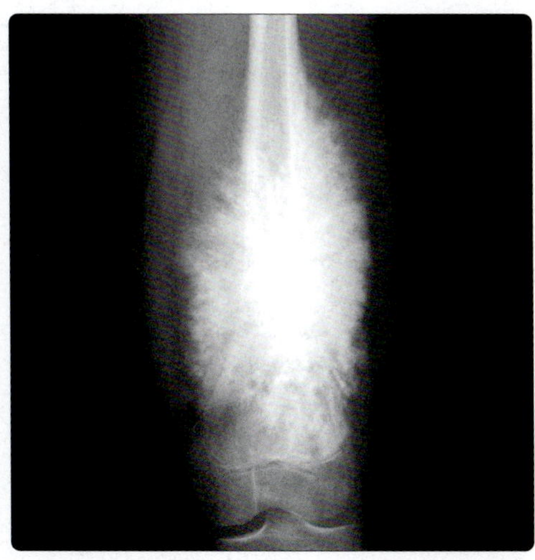

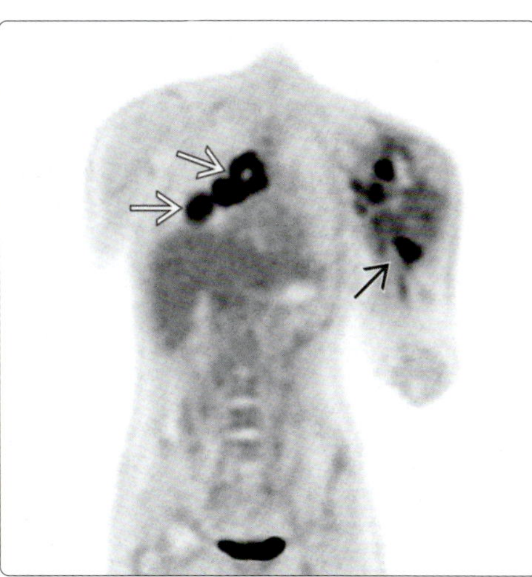

(Left) *AP radiograph of a 12-year-old with leg swelling for 2 weeks shows an aggressive sunburst periosteal reaction within this distal femoral osteoblastic OS.* **(Right)** *Coronal PET/CT in a teenager with a left humeral OS shows ↑ metabolic activity in the primary mass ⇨ with an SUVmax of 8.7. Intense FDG accumulation is also seen within the right subcarinal/hilar & lung metastases ➡ with an SUVmax of 11.3. Metastatic lesions were also found in the brain & right adrenal gland (not shown).*

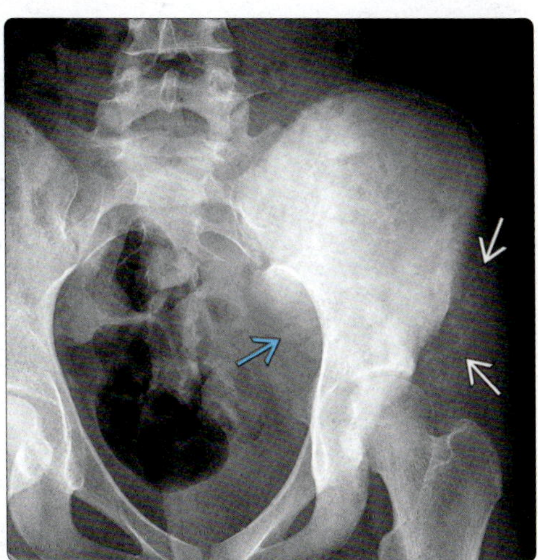

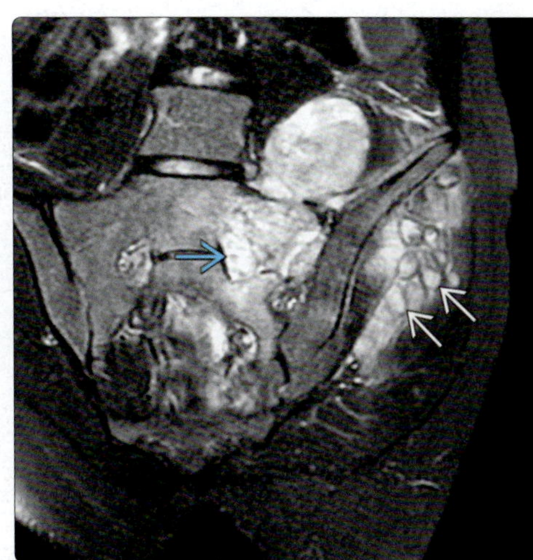

(Left) *AP radiograph in a 16-year-old presenting with back & leg pain shows sclerosis of the left iliac wing with aggressive sunburst periosteal reaction ⇨. Ring & arc chondroid Ca^{2+} ➡ are seen within the lateral soft tissues in this chondroblastic OS.* **(Right)** *Coronal oblique T2 FS MR in the same patient shows heterogeneity of the sacrum & left ilium due to tumor. Soft tissue components of the mass extend into multiple left neural foramina ⇨. Note the multiple tumor cartilage lobules ➡ in this chondroblastic OS.*

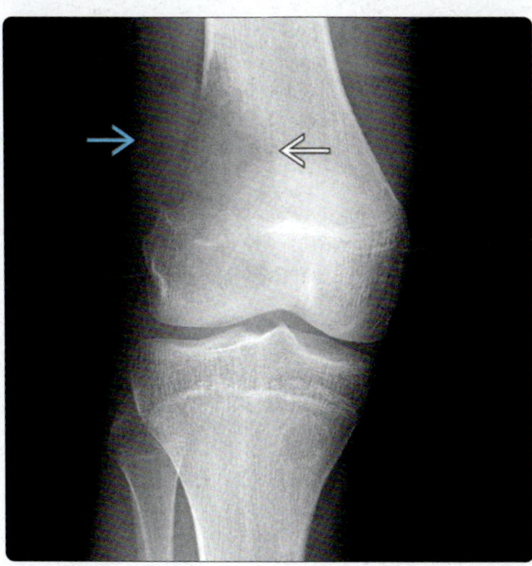

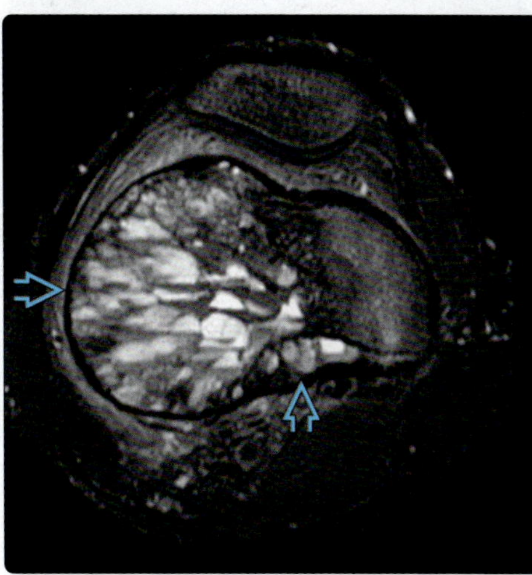

(Left) *AP radiograph of the knee in a 15-year-old with pain shows a lytic metaphyseal OS with a wide zone of transition ➡, overlying soft tissue mass ⇨, & no substantial osteoid production.* **(Right)** *Axial T2 FS MR in the same patient shows numerous fluid-fluid levels throughout the lesion, typical of layering blood products. The lateral cortex is completely absent with ballooning of the periosteum by tumor ⇨. A telangiectatic OS was confirmed histologically.*

Leukemia

KEY FACTS

TERMINOLOGY

- Leukemia: Malignancy of hematopoietic stem cells diffusely infiltrating or replacing normal bone marrow
- Granulocytic sarcoma or chloroma: Soft tissue mass of leukemic cells typically found with AML

IMAGING

- Radiographs are often normal or have subtle findings
  - Diffuse osteoporosis
  - Leukemic lines
    - Radiolucent metaphyseal bands; zone of provisional calcification (ZPC) is often intact
  - Focal bone destruction
    - Poorly defined, metaphyseal osteolytic lesions with moth-eaten or permeative appearance
  - Aggressive periosteal reaction (lamellated, spiculated, interrupted), even if some components appear smooth
  - Pathologic fracture
  - Chloroma (granulocytic sarcoma)
  - ± chronic bone infarcts in treated patients
    - Osteonecrosis with subchondral collapse
- MR: Leukemia may completely replace normal fatty marrow
  - Discordance of signal between abnormal, infiltrated marrow & subcutaneous fat
  - ± superimposed acute infarction, fracture, or osteomyelitis causing focal symptoms

CLINICAL ISSUES

- Leukemia is most common childhood malignancy
  - Subtypes: ALL > 75%, AML 15-20%, CML < 5%
- Most common presentations
  - Bone or joint pain, limp, swelling
  - Fatigue (anemia), fever ± infection, petechiae, bleeding
  - Hepatosplenomegaly, lymphadenopathy > 60%
- ALL: 5-year survival > 85%; 60-80% for others
- Treatment: Chemotherapy with steroids ± radiation, GCSF (→ ↑ red marrow content), stem cell transplant

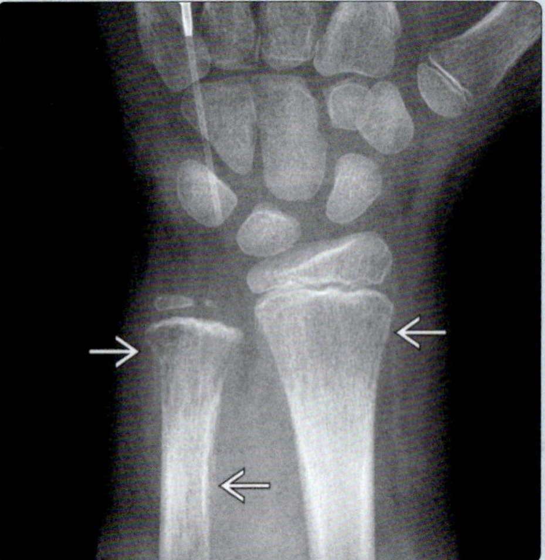

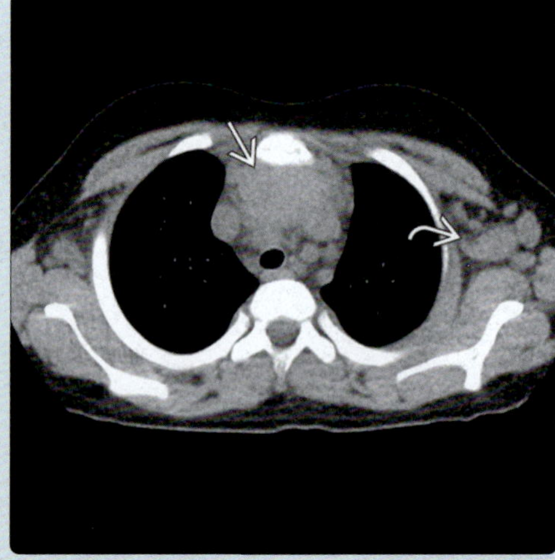

(Left) *PA radiograph of the wrist in a 9-year-old with acute lymphoblastic leukemia (ALL) presenting with bone pain for 1 month & periorbital ecchymosis shows permeative osteolytic changes of the distal radius & ulna ➡.* **(Right)** *Axial NECT in the same patient shows lobular thymic infiltration/expansion ➡ & bilateral axillary lymphadenopathy ➡. The largest axillary nodes on more superior images measured up to 2 cm in short axis. The spleen was also enlarged (not shown).*

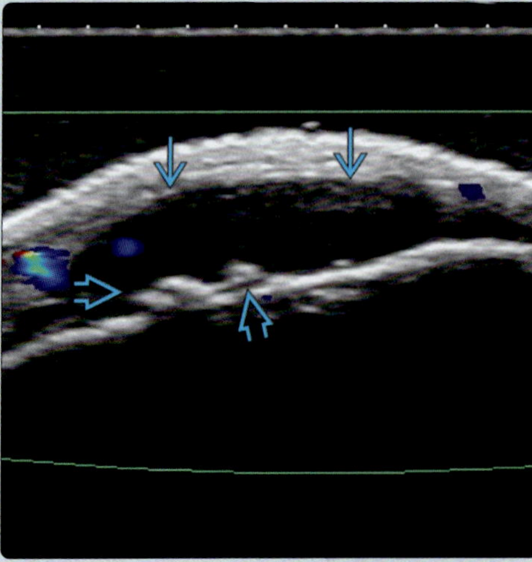

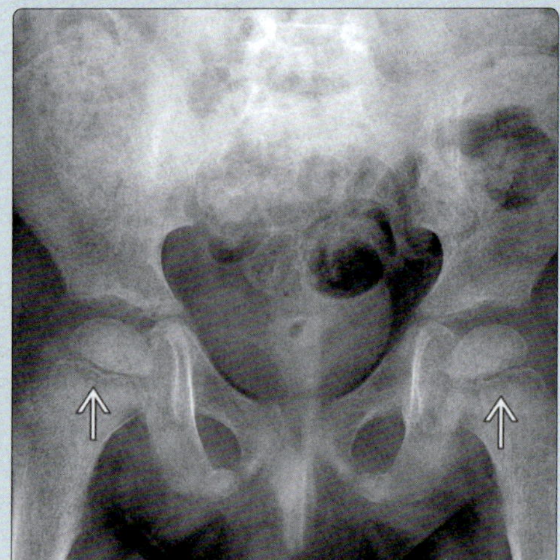

(Left) *Transverse Doppler US shows a left temporal soft tissue mass ➡ with calvarial permeation & irregular periosteal reaction ➡ due to a granulocytic sarcoma in acute myelogenous leukemia (AML).* **(Right)** *AP radiograph in an anemic patient with cardiomegaly & splenomegaly shows transverse radiolucent lines ➡ in the femurs due to leukemia. Note the intact thin sclerotic zones of provisional Ca^{2+} abutting the physes (just proximal to the lucent lines), which help differentiate leukemia from rickets.*

TERMINOLOGY

Synonyms

- Acute lymphocytic (or lymphoblastic) leukemia (ALL), acute myelogenous leukemia (AML), myeloblastoma, chronic myelogenous leukemia (CML), chronic lymphocytic leukemia (CLL), juvenile chronic myeloid leukemia (JCML)

Definitions

- Leukemia: Malignancy of hematopoietic stem cells diffusely infiltrating or replacing normal bone marrow
- Granulocytic sarcoma or chloroma: Soft tissue mass of leukemic cells typically found with AML
- Extramedullary sanctuary sites: Sites of leukemia with barriers to systemic therapy (CNS & reproductive organs)

IMAGING

Radiographic Findings

- Radiography
  - Often normal or with very subtle metaphyseal findings
    - Only 40% have radiographic findings
  - Diffuse osteoporosis
    - Coarse trabeculae with abnormally well-visualized sclerotic rim due to intact zone of provisional calcification (ZPC) or subchondral bone
    - Multiple flattened, collapsed, or biconcave vertebrae
  - Leukemic lines
    - Radiolucent metaphyseal bands; ZPC is often intact
      - Stress of disease or leukemic infiltration
    - ± dense metaphyseal bands post therapy
  - Focal bone destruction
    - Poorly defined osteolytic lesions with moth-eaten or permeative bone destruction
  - Periosteal reaction
    - Usually has some aggressive features (lamellated, spiculated, interrupted) even if some components appear smooth
      - Subperiosteal infiltration by malignant cells through haversian canals
      - Subperiosteal hemorrhage is less common
  - Sclerotic foci
    - Typically in myelogenous leukemia
    - ± chronic bone infarcts in treated patients
  - Pathologic fracture
    - Usually metaphyseal
    - Can simulate nonaccidental trauma
  - Chloroma (granulocytic sarcoma)
    - Nonspecific soft tissue mass
    - Most commonly in head & neck, musculoskeletal soft tissues, GI system, lymph nodes, peritoneum, or bony mass
      - Can simulate meningioma or epidural hematoma
    - Poor prognosis
  - Late findings
    - Osteonecrosis (ON) with subchondral collapse
    - Endochondral ossification is rarely interrupted with persistence of unossified cartilage in metaphysis
  - Other organs: Splenomegaly, cardiomegaly, thymic infiltration

CT Findings

- Bone CT
  - Permeative bone destruction, periosteal reaction
  - ± soft tissue mass of chloroma
  - Sclerotic foci of ON

MR Findings

- T1: Confluent dark leukemic infiltrate replacing normal high-signal fatty yellow marrow
  - Marrow signal abnormally is abnormally discordant from signal of bright subcutaneous fat
    - Must be interpreted in light of normal red to yellow marrow conversion patterns in children
- T2 FS/STIR: Poorly defined patchy or diffusely bright marrow signal of visualized bones
  - Marrow signal is abnormally discordant from signal of dark subcutaneous fat
- T1 C+ FS: Intermediate to mildly bright enhancement of leukemic marrow diffusely
- DWI: May show restricted diffusion
- Special circumstances
  - Acute infarction or osteomyelitis
    - May present before, during, or after treatment
    - Focal regions of superimposed marrow heterogeneity with ↓ enhancement & overlying periosteal & soft tissue edema
  - Chloroma
    - Intermediate to bright T2 FS/STIR signal soft tissue mass with heterogenous or uniform enhancement
  - Recovery of normal marrow signal after treatment
    - Gradual process in setting of effective therapy
      - ↑ fat fraction, T1 shortening
  - Relapse after stem cell transplant
    - Numerous, round, well-circumscribed "dots" of leukemic infiltrate
    - T1 dark, T2 FS/STIR bright; enhance with contrast
    - May require targeted biopsy rather than blind iliac marrow aspiration to confirm recurrence

Nuclear Medicine Findings

- Bone scan
  - ↑ radiotracer uptake in tumor
    - May underestimate disease
- PET
  - Helpful to identify extramedullary disease with ↑ metabolic activity

Imaging Recommendations

- Best imaging tool
  - MR: T1, T2 FS/STIR, T1 C+ FS
    - Musculoskeletal symptoms with normal radiographs
    - Whole-body MR can screen for ON

DIFFERENTIAL DIAGNOSIS

Metastatic Neuroblastoma

- Bone involvement is similar to leukemia
  - Metaphyseal lucent bands
  - "Moth-eaten" bone destruction
  - Circumscribed or diffuse marrow replacement
  - Spiculated periosteal reaction of skull

- Look for primary retroperitoneal/suprarenal mass

Langerhans Cell Histiocytosis

- Focal/multifocal, punched-out lytic lesion(s)
- Intense marrow edema + homogeneous small soft tissue mass
- ± periosteal reaction, soft tissue edema

Osteomyelitis

- Symptoms similar to leukemia
- Adjacent, poorly defined soft tissue abnormalities
- Poorly defined metaphyseal-centric marrow process
  - ± drainable fluid collections

Congenital Syphilis

- Metaphyseal lucent bands
- Hepatosplenomegaly, lymphadenopathy, anemia, skin rash
- Wimberger corner sign: Focal destruction of medial proximal tibial metaphysis

Lymphoma

- Typically solitary, often sclerotic focus
- Older age group

Ewing Sarcoma

- Diaphyseal or flat bone lesion with aggressive periosteal reaction & permeative bone destruction
- Sharply circumscribed marrow interface on T1 MR
- Large soft tissue mass

Rickets

- Physeal lengthening/widening with loss of ZPC
- Metaphyseal fraying, cupping, & splaying

Physeal Stress Injuries

- Physeal lengthening/widening with loss of ZPC
- Isolated to painful extremity

PATHOLOGY

General Features

- Etiology
  - Arises from primitive stem cells either de novo or from preleukemic state
- Genetics
  - ↑ ALL risk in Down syndrome, Li-Fraumeni syndrome, Fanconi anemia, immunodeficiencies
  - CML translocation chromosome 9 & 22 is classic (Philadelphia chromosome)
- Associated abnormalities
  - Myelodysplastic syndrome (1/3 develop AML)
  - Long-term risk from low medical levels of diagnostic imaging ionizing radiation is debated
- Classified
  - Basis of cell maturity: Acute (blasts) or chronic (more mature cells)
  - Basis of cell type: Lymphocytic or myelogenous form

Microscopic Features

- Acute: Infiltration of bone marrow by poorly differentiated blast cells
  - ALL: Patternless sheets of small blue cells
  - AML: Wright stain or Giemsa preparation with lysosomal cytoplasmic structure (Auer rods)
- Chronic: Mature leukocyte infiltration
  - CML: Mature granulocyte with normal lymphocyte count, Philadelphia chromosome
  - CLL: Mature lymphocytes

CLINICAL ISSUES

Presentation

- Most common signs/symptoms
  - Bone or joint pain, limp, swelling
    - Sharp, localized, recurrent arthralgias (75%)
  - Fatigue (anemia), fever ± infection, petechiae, bleeding
  - Hepatosplenomegaly, lymphadenopathy > 60%
- Other signs/symptoms
  - Chest radiographs are often obtained prior to sedated procedures
    - Mediastinal mass, tracheal deviation, lung opacities, cardiomegaly, humeral metaphyseal lucent bands
  - SVC syndrome, tachypnea, respiratory distress
  - ↑ ESR, thrombocytopenia, neutropenia

Demographics

- Age
  - ALL: Peak 2-10 years
  - AML: Peak > 65 years but accounts for 15-20% of childhood leukemias
  - CML: Peak 30-50 years
  - CLL: Median 60 years
- Epidemiology
  - Most common pediatric malignancy
    - ALL is most common form in children
      - ALL > 75%, AML 15-20%, CML < 5%

Natural History & Prognosis

- ALL: 5-year survival > 85%
- AML: 5-year survival ~ 60-70%
- CML: 5-year survival ~ 60-80%

Treatment

- Chemotherapy with steroids ± radiation
- Intrathecal chemotherapy for CNS disease
- CD19-directed chimeric antigen receptor (CAR) T cells for relapsed or refractory disease in ALL
- Granulocyte colony-stimulating factor (GCSF)
- Stem cell transplant

SELECTED REFERENCES

1. Inaba H et al: Whole-joint magnetic resonance imaging to assess osteonecrosis in pediatric patients with acute lymphoblastic lymphoma. Pediatr Blood Cancer. 67(8):e28336, 2020
2. Smith WT et al: Evaluation of chest radiographs of children with newly diagnosed acute lymphoblastic leukemia. J Pediatr. 223:120-7.e3, 2020
3. Chambers G et al: 18F-FDG PET-CT in paediatric oncology: established and emerging applications. Br J Radiol. 92(1094):20180584, 2019
4. Pehlivan KC et al: CAR-T cell therapy for acute lymphoblastic leukemia: transforming the treatment of relapsed and refractory disease. Curr Hematol Malig Rep. 13(5):396-406, 2018
5. Cunningham I et al: (18) FDG-PET/CT: 21st century approach to leukemic tumors in 124 cases. Am J Hematol. 91(4):379-84, 2016
6. Guillerman RP: Marrow: red, yellow and bad. Pediatr Radiol. 43 Suppl 1:S181-92, 2013
7. Sinigaglia R et al: Musculoskeletal manifestations in pediatric acute leukemia. J Pediatr Orthop. 28(1):20-8, 2008

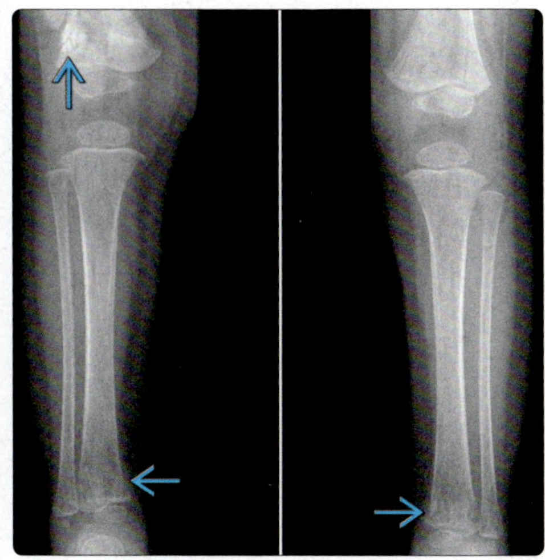

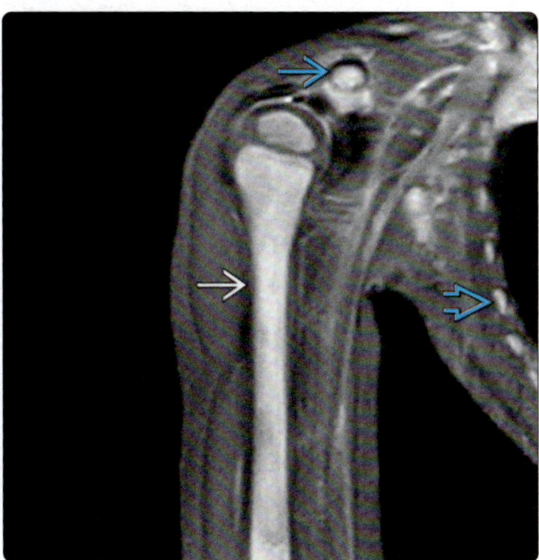

(Left) *AP radiograph in an 11-month-old shows pathologic fractures of the femoral, tibial, & fibular metaphyses* ➔ *at sites of underlying permeative osteolytic change. The patient was ultimately diagnosed with leukemia.* **(Right)** *Coronal STIR MR in a 3-year-old with arm pain & fever shows diffuse hyperintense marrow throughout the humerus* ➔, *coracoid process* ➔, *& ribs* ➔. *The marrow was diffusely dark on T1 MR (not shown). The patient was eventually diagnosed with B-cell ALL.*

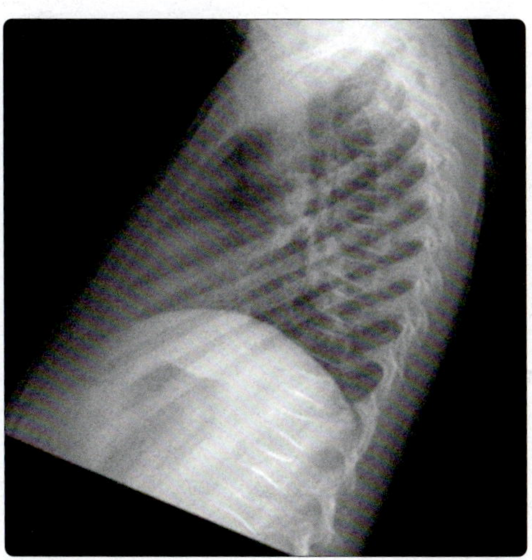

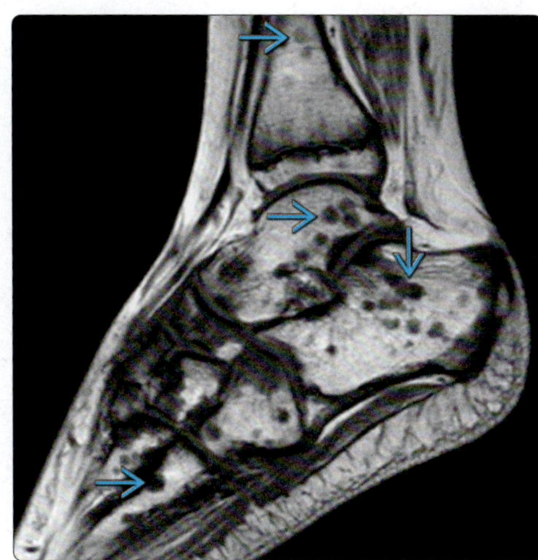

(Left) *Lateral chest radiograph in a 5-year-old with newly diagnosed ALL who had lucent metaphyseal bands on hip radiographs (not shown) demonstrates osteoporosis & compression fractures throughout the spine.* **(Right)** *Sagittal T1 MR in a 14-year-old with a history of ankle pain 2 years after a bone marrow transplant for ALL shows numerous round lesions* ➔ *in a background of normal yellow marrow. Recurrent leukemia was confirmed by biopsy.*

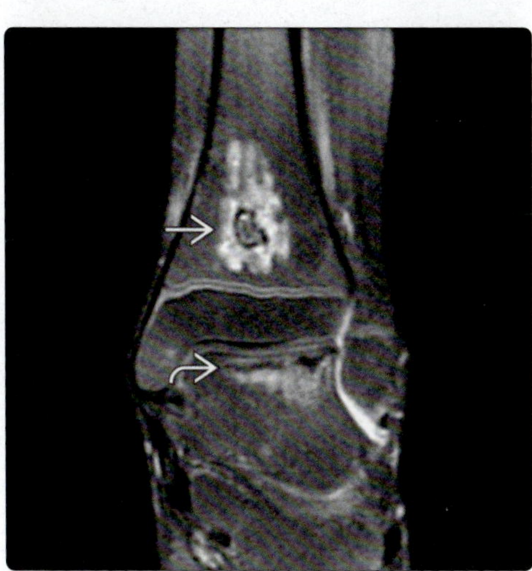

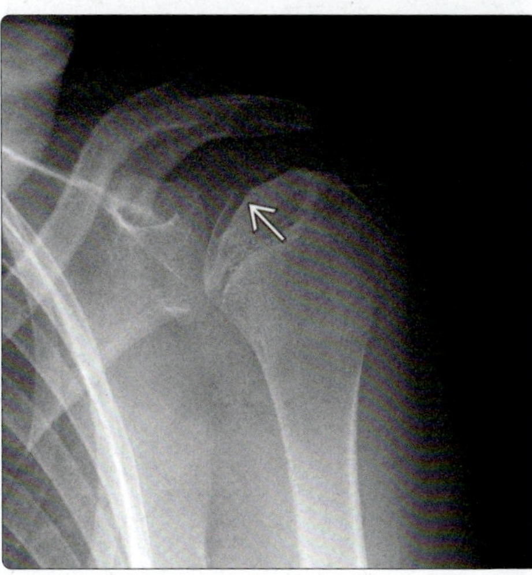

(Left) *Coronal T2 FS MR in a 10-year-old with history of T-cell ALL shows a bone infarct* ➔ *within the distal tibia as well as talar dome osteonecrosis with a hypointense subchondral fracture* ➔. *Subchondral collapse of the talar dome was visible on 1-year follow-up radiographs (not shown).* **(Right)** *AP radiograph in a 12-year-old with relapsed ALL & bilateral shoulder pain shows humeral head osteonecrosis with a lucent subchondral fracture* ➔ *due to steroid therapy.*

Langerhans Cell Histiocytosis

KEY FACTS

TERMINOLOGY

- Langerhans cell histiocytosis (LCH): Spectrum of disease caused by neoplastic clonal proliferations of CD1a, CD207, & S100 protein (+) dendritic cells
- Single system (SS) (unifocal or multifocal) vs. multisystem (MS) disease
  - Most frequently involved: Bone (80-90%) & skin (40-50%)
  - Risk organ (RO) involvement: Liver, spleen, marrow; confers worse prognosis (high risk)
  - Others: Lymph nodes, lung, pituitary, thymus, GI tract

IMAGING

- Best clue: Well-defined, round or lobulated lytic punched-out skull lesion(s) without sclerotic rim
- Monostotic vs. multifocal involvement: 50-75% vs. 10-20%
- Affected sites: Flat bones (50%) vs. long bones (30%)
  - Skull > ribs > femur > pelvis > spine
  - Classic cause of vertebra plana & "floating tooth"
  - Typically lacks large soft tissue mass
- Sensitivity for LCH: FDG PET & whole-body MR > > radiographs > bone scan
  - FDG PET is better for active vs. healing disease

CLINICAL ISSUES

- Age: 90% of LCH cases are < 15 years at presentation
  - SS, unifocal (70% of cases); peak age: 5-15 years
  - SS, multifocal (20% of cases); peak age: 1-5 years
  - MS RO(+) disease (10% of cases); peak age: 0-2 years
- Spontaneous regression of unifocal bone disease is common; chemotherapy & steroids are used otherwise
- Mortality: SS or MS RO(-) disease < 5%; MS RO(+) disease 10-50%
- Disease reactivation &/or long-term sequelae in 25-75% (MS > SS)

DIAGNOSTIC CHECKLIST

- LCH should be considered for most lytic pediatric bone lesions due to variable appearances

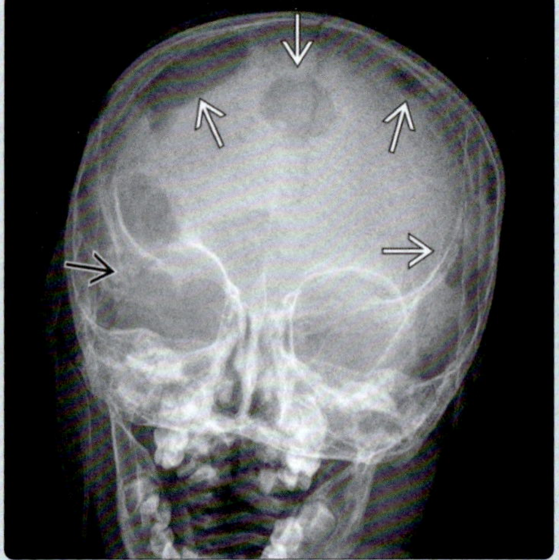

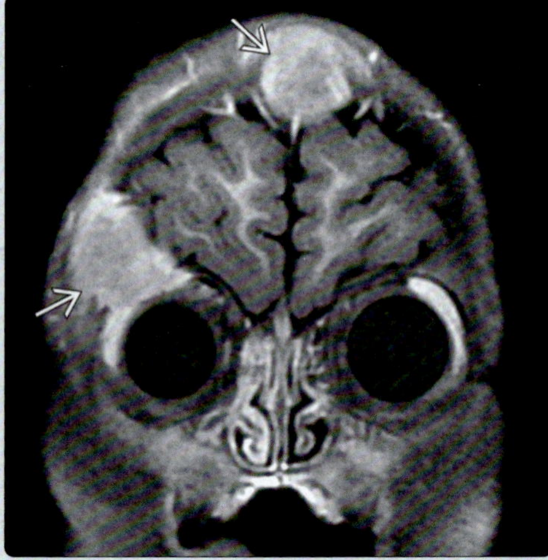

(Left) *AP radiograph of the skull in a 1-year-old girl with palpable masses shows multiple punched-out lytic lesions of the calvarium ➡. The superior & lateral walls of the right orbit are destroyed ➡. An ultrasound performed at the same time (not shown) demonstrated hypovascular soft tissue filling these sites of complete bone absence (rather than bone permeation or spiculation).* **(Right)** *Coronal T1 C+ FS MR in the same patient shows enhancing soft tissue masses ➡ at the sites of the lytic bone lesions. LCH was confirmed at biopsy.*

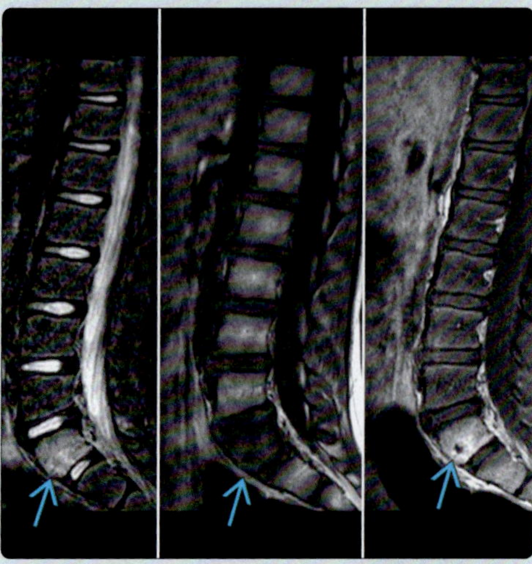

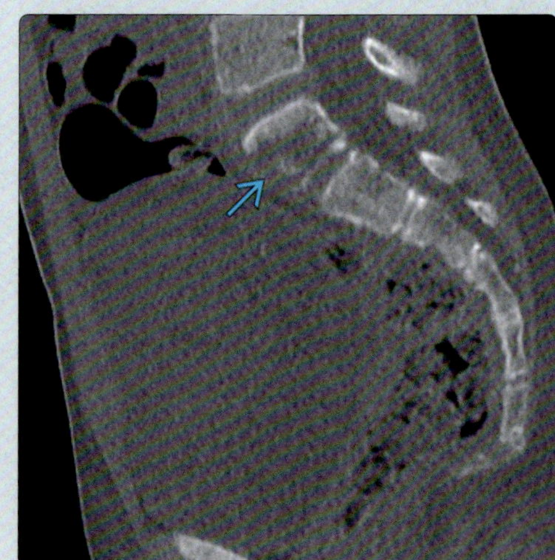

(Left) *Sagittal (from left to right) STIR, T1, & T1 C+ FS MR images in an 8-year-old patient with 1 month of back pain show a heterogeneous poorly defined lesion of the S1 vertebral marrow ➡. No soft tissue mass is seen.* **(Right)** *Sagittal bone CT in the same patient shows a lytic lesion ➡ of S1 with destruction of the anterior cortex. LCH was found at biopsy. A subsequent PET/CT (not shown) demonstrated no other foci of involvement.*

TERMINOLOGY

Definitions

- Langerhans cell histiocytosis (LCH): Spectrum of disorders caused by neoplastic clonal proliferations of CD1a, CD207, & S100 protein (+) dendritic cells
- Single system (SS) (unifocal or multifocal) vs. multisystem (MS) disease
  - Bone (80-90%) & skin (40-50%) are most frequently involved
    - Lung is most common SS site in adults
  - Risk organ (RO) involvement: Liver, spleen, marrow; confers worse prognosis (high risk)
    - Lung is no longer considered RO
  - Other organs: Lymph nodes, pituitary, thymus, GI tract
  - CNS-risk lesion: Skull base & many facial lesions
    - Diabetes insipidus (25% overall, 50% with MS disease), growth hormone deficiency (10%), parenchymal mass lesions (1%), & delayed neurodegenerative changes

IMAGING

General Features

- Best diagnostic clue
  - Well-defined, round or lobulated lytic punched-out skull lesion(s) without sclerotic rim
- Location
  - Monostotic involvement (unifocal SS): 50-75%
  - Multifocal SS involvement: 10-20%
  - Predilection for flat bones (> 50% of cases): Skull, ribs, pelvis, scapula
  - Long bones affected ~ 30% of cases
    - Metaphysis, diaphysis > epiphysis
  - Decreasing order of frequency: Skull, ribs, femur, pelvis, spine
- Morphology
  - Variable radiographic appearance of skeletal lesions depending on phase of disease ± therapy
    - Lucent/lytic > > sclerotic; well-defined vs. poorly defined borders; aggressive vs. nonaggressive vs. absent periosteal reaction

Radiographic Findings

- Radiography
  - Skull (50%)
    - Well-defined lytic lesion, most commonly solitary, without sclerotic rim
      - Sclerotic rim develops during healing phase (which may occur before therapy)
      - Coalescence of lesions: Geographic skull
    - Periosteal reaction is often absent in skull LCH
      - Does not produce radiating spicules of new bone as seen with metastases
    - ± beveled edge: Asymmetric involvement of inner vs. outer table of skull
    - ± button sequestrum: Sclerotic focus within lytic lesion
    - Small soft tissue mass may extend from lytic lesion
    - Floating tooth sign: Lesion in alveolar mandible → loss of dense lamina dura
  - Appendicular skeleton: Variable appearance
    - Lesions generally respect joint space & growth plate
  - Spine: Variable loss of height
    - Classic vertebra plana: Complete collapse of vertebral body ("wafer thin")
    - Height recovers to some degree over years

MR Findings

- T1WI
  - Intermediate- to low-signal lesion replacing marrow fat
- T2WI FS
  - Intermediate to high signal within focal lesion
    - ± hypointense lesion rim
    - Surrounded by ill-defined hyperintense marrow > soft tissue edema
    - Hyperintense signal deep to or overlying periosteum
  - Purely medullary lesion vs. cortical destruction with relatively small soft tissue mass extending beyond bone
  - Findings may change with phase of disease
- STIR
  - Whole-body STIR to assess for multifocal disease
    - Much more sensitive for skeletal & extraskeletal LCH than radiographs or bone scan
    - Limited ability to distinguish active vs. residual disease
- T1WI C+ FS
  - Diffuse enhancement of lesion & adjacent edema is typical

Nuclear Medicine Findings

- Bone scan
  - Lower sensitivity than radiographic survey or whole-body MR
- PET/CT
  - FDG PET is highly sensitive for active LCH (FDG avid)
    - Less sensitive than MR in vertebral disease
  - Also demonstrates healing before other modalities
  - Higher radiation dose than other modalities; radiation dose reduction can be achieved with
    - Low-dose lesion-selective CT technique
    - PET/MR fusion

Imaging Recommendations

- Best imaging tool
  - PET/CT vs. whole-body STIR MR

DIFFERENTIAL DIAGNOSIS

Osteomyelitis

- Cortical & marrow abnormalities are less well defined
- Moderate to marked soft tissue inflammation
- Rim-enhancing fluid collections are often present

Metastatic Neuroblastoma

- Lucent metaphyseal bands &/or lytic permeative metaphyseal lesions
- Radiating spicules of periosteal new bone formation are typical in permeative skull lesions
  - May also cause mild expansile remodeling

Leukemia

- Lucent metaphyseal bands &/or lytic permeative metaphyseal lesions
- ± diffusely abnormal background marrow

Ewing Sarcoma

- Permeative bone destruction, wide zone of transition, aggressive periosteal reaction; often with large soft tissue mass
- ± remodeling with expansion, saucerization
- May involve entire flat bone, but calvarium is uncommon

Congenital Syphilis

- Hepatosplenomegaly, lymphadenopathy, rash, lucent metaphyseal bands
- Wimberger sign: Lytic lesion of proximal medial tibia

Infantile Myofibromatosis

- Single or multifocal bone &/or soft tissue lesions
- Expansile bubbly lucent metadiaphyseal lesions, often relatively symmetric

PATHOLOGY

General Features

- Historic categorization
  - Letterer-Siwe (acute disseminated form): < 10%
  - Hand-Schüller-Christian (chronic disseminated form): 15-30%
  - Eosinophilic granuloma (isolated bone or lung involvement): 60-80%

Microscopic Features

- Active lesion: Granuloma of dendritic Langerhans cells > inflammatory cells
- Later stages: Macrophages > Langerhans cells + fibrotic & xanthomatous changes
- Birbeck granule: Classic "tennis racquet" organelle found by electron microscopy in up to 40% of Langerhans cells
  - Diagnostic importance is now diminished due to immunostaining of specific markers

CLINICAL ISSUES

Presentation

- Most common signs/symptoms
  - Localized bone pain, tenderness
  - Soft tissue swelling or mass
- Other signs/symptoms
  - Rash, limping, exophthalmos, hepatosplenomegaly, lymphadenopathy, otitis externa, mastoiditis, gingivitis
  - Fever, ↑ erythrocyte sedimentation rate, & leukocytosis may occur

Demographics

- Age
  - 90% of cases are < 15 years at presentation; median is 3 years of age at diagnosis
  - SS, unifocal (70% of cases); peak age: 5-15 years
  - SS, multifocal (20% of cases); peak age: 1-5 years
  - MS RO(+) (10% of cases); peak age: 0-2 years
- Sex
  - M:F = 1.2-3:1

Natural History & Prognosis

- Mortality
  - SS or no RO [MS RO(-)] disease: < 5%
    - Spontaneous regression of unifocal bone disease is common
  - MS disease + RO involvement [MS RO(+)]: 10-50%
    - Progressive disease on multiagent chemotherapy at 6 weeks: 40-80% mortality
  - Lung disease in adults: 25% at 5 years
    - Regresses with smoking cessation
- Disease reactivation
  - Unpredictable timeframe, number of episodes
  - Up to 25% in multifocal SS (bone) disease
  - 50-75% in MS disease
  - Bone is most frequent site of reactivation
- Long-term sequelae
  - 70% in MS disease, 25% in SS disease
  - Often related to destructive/fibrotic changes at site(s) of initial disease
  - Diabetes insipidus & CNS degeneration (which may be paraneoplastic) are most serious

Treatment

- SS disease
  - Unifocal bone disease: Watchful waiting vs. curettage & local steroid injection
  - Multifocal bone disease or CNS-risk lesion: Chemotherapy & steroids x 6-12 months
- MS disease (± RO): Multiagent chemotherapy x 12 months

DIAGNOSTIC CHECKLIST

Consider

- LCH should be considered in differential diagnosis for most pediatric bone lesions due to variable appearances
- If favoring LCH on initial targeted radiographs, consider whole-body survey (MR vs. PET) to help direct biopsy & determine disease extent

SELECTED REFERENCES

1. Jessop S et al: FDG PET-CT in pediatric Langerhans cell histiocytosis. Pediatr Blood Cancer. 67(1):e28034, 2020
2. Kim JR et al: Comparison of whole-body MRI, bone scan, and radiographic skeletal survey for lesion detection and risk stratification of Langerhans cell histiocytosis. Sci Rep. 9(1):317, 2019
3. Krooks J et al: Langerhans cell histiocytosis in children: history, classification, pathobiology, clinical manifestations, and prognosis. J Am Acad Dermatol. 78(6):1035-44, 2018
4. Lee SW et al: Long-term clinical outcome of spinal Langerhans cell histiocytosis in children. Int J Hematol. 106(3):441-9, 2017
5. Sher AC et al: PET/MR in the assessment of pediatric histiocytoses: a comparison to PET/CT. Clin Nucl Med. 42(8):582-8, 2017
6. Emile JF et al: Revised classification of histiocytoses and neoplasms of the macrophage-dendritic cell lineages. Blood. 127(22):2672-81, 2016
7. Samet J et al: MRI and clinical features of Langerhans cell histiocytosis (LCH) in the pelvis and extremities: can LCH really look like anything? Skeletal Radiol. 45(5):607-13, 2016
8. Allen CE et al: How I treat Langerhans cell histiocytosis. Blood. 126(1):26-35, 2015
9. Gelfand MJ et al: Selective CT for PET/CT: dose reduction in Langerhans cell histiocytosis. Pediatr Radiol. 45(1):81-5, 2015
10. Monsereenusorn C et al: Clinical characteristics and treatment of Langerhans cell histiocytosis. Hematol Oncol Clin North Am. 29(5):853-73, 2015
11. Lee JW et al: Clinical characteristics and treatment outcome of Langerhans cell histiocytosis: 22 years' experience of 154 patients at a single center. Pediatr Hematol Oncol. 31(3):293-302, 2014
12. Zaveri J et al: More than just Langerhans cell histiocytosis: a radiologic review of histiocytic disorders. Radiographics. 34(7):2008-24, 2014

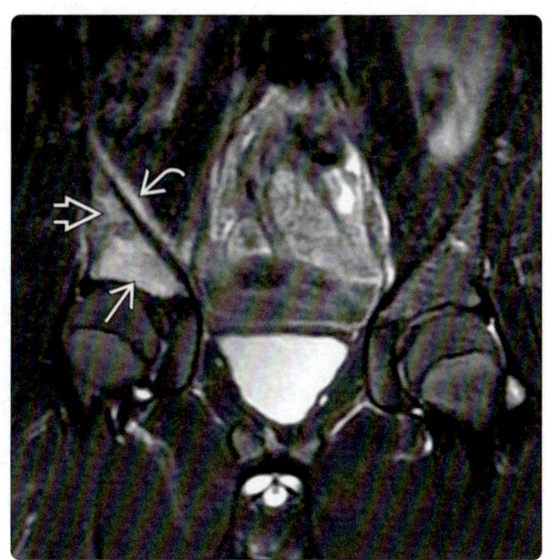

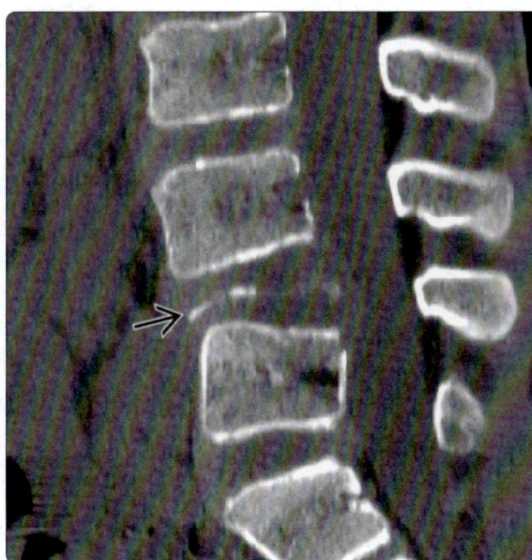

(Left) *Coronal T2 FS MR in a 10-year-old patient with right hip pain shows a homogeneously hyperintense lesion ➡ of the right iliac marrow without adjacent bone destruction. There is surrounding marrow ➡ & juxtacortical ➡ edema. LCH was confirmed with biopsy.* **(Right)** *Sagittal bone CT in a 12-year-old patient undergoing evaluation for a spinal deformity shows a wafer-like L4 vertebral body (vertebra plana) ➡, ultimately proven to be secondary to LCH.*

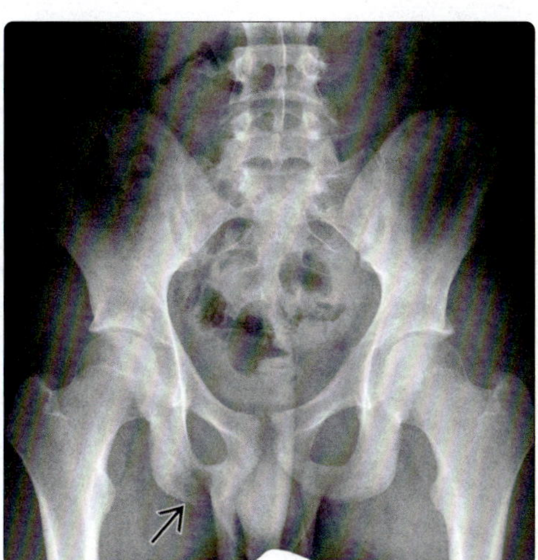

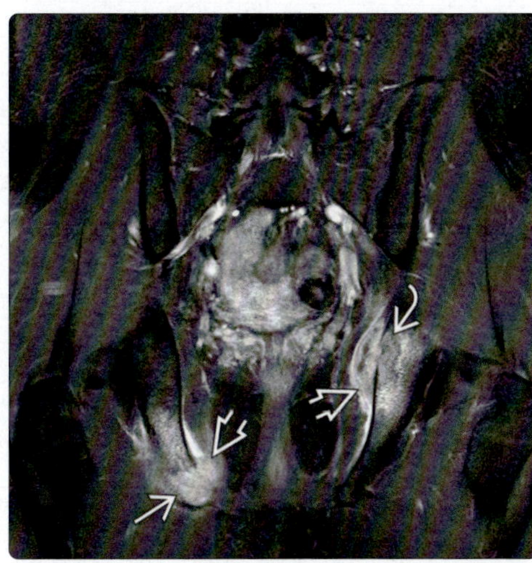

(Left) *AP radiograph in a 15-year-old boy with weeks of pelvic pain shows a lucent lesion ➡ with intermediate zone of transition in the right ischium.* **(Right)** *Coronal T1 C+ FS MR in the same patient shows enhancing bone lesions arising from the right ischial tuberosity ➡ & left posterior acetabular wall ➡. Contiguous enhancing soft tissue masses ➡ overlie foci of cortical destruction, & there is adjacent soft tissue & marrow edema at each site.*

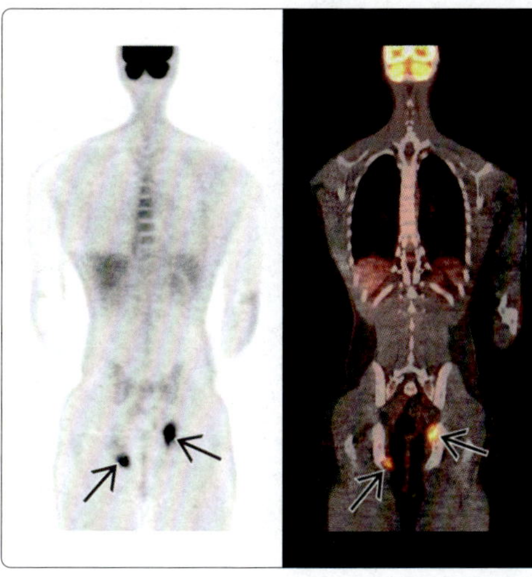

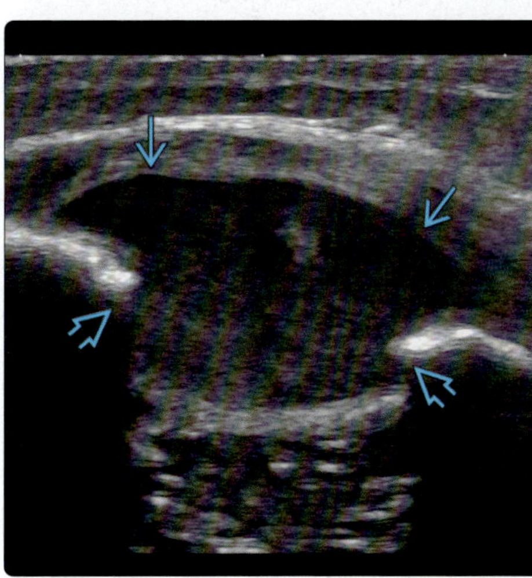

(Left) *Coronal FDG PET/CT in the same patient shows FDG avidity (or ↑ metabolic activity) in the lesions ➡, typical of LCH. No other lesions were identified.* **(Right)** *Longitudinal ultrasound of the occipital calvarium in a 6-month-old patient with a palpable mass shows complete interruption of the bone ➡ by a mildly heterogeneous ovoid mass ➡, confirmed as LCH on biopsy.*

Nonossifying Fibroma

KEY FACTS

TERMINOLOGY

- Very common benign fibrous lesion of pediatric bone
- Terms fibroxanthoma & metaphyseal fibrous defect include
  - Nonossifying fibroma (NOF)
    - > 2- or 3-cm length; encroachment on medullary cavity
  - Fibrous cortical defect (FCD)
    - < 2- or 3-cm length
    - Essentially isolated to cortex

IMAGING

- Eccentric, elongated, & bubbly lucent lesion in long bone metaphysis/diaphysis with narrow zone of transition, lobular or smooth sclerotic margin, & no periosteal reaction
- Expected involution/healing → gradual sclerosis, resolution
- Typical locations
  - Metaphysis of long bone: Up to 93%
    - Distance from physis ↑ with age
  - Located around knee: 55-89%
- Radiographs are usually diagnostic
  - Atypical features should suggest other lesion or superimposed complication (such as pathologic fracture)

CLINICAL ISSUES

- May be developmental defect rather than neoplasm
- Usually asymptomatic & incidentally discovered
- Occurs in up to 35% of children
  - Peak age: 10-15 years (75% in 2nd decade)
- May develop symptoms (uncommon)
  - Acute pain with pathologic fracture
    - Classic predictors: > 50% of cortical thickness involved or > 3.3 cm in size in weight-bearing bone
  - Gradual pain with stress fracture of adjacent bone (very rare)
  - Paraneoplastic rickets/osteomalacia (extremely rare)
- Gradual healing with spontaneous regression of most cases in late adolescence
- Treatment is only required if patient is at high risk for pathologic fracture

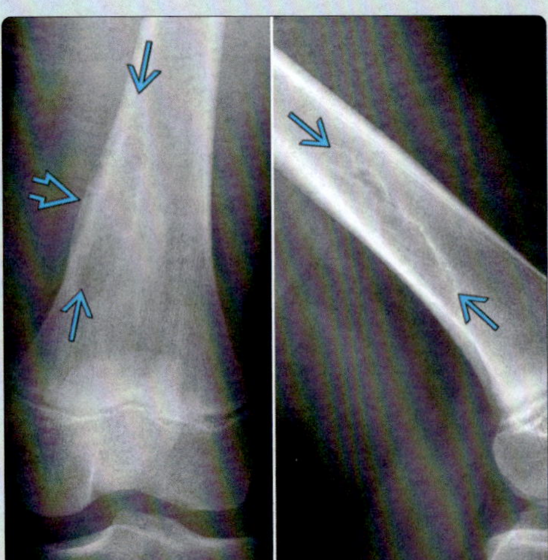

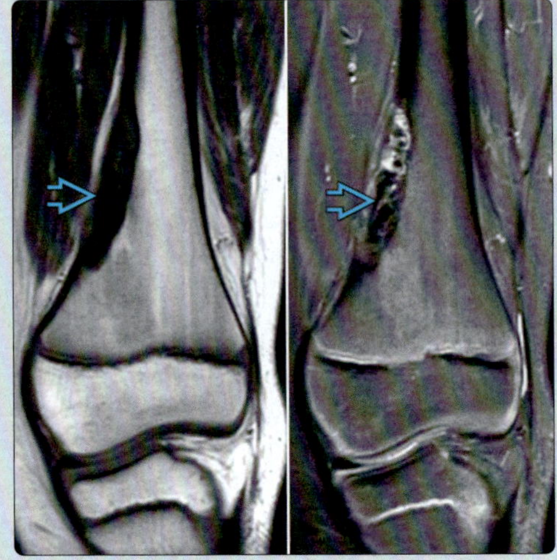

(Left) *AP (left) & lateral (right) radiographs in a 9-year-old after an injury show a well-circumscribed, elongated, lucent & bubbly, eccentric lesion ➡ of the distal femoral diaphysis with mild expansile remodeling ➡.* **(Right)** *Coronal T1 (left) & STIR (right) MR images in the same patient show heterogeneous but predominantly low signal intensity ➡ throughout the 6-cm lesion. Note the lack of adjacent marrow & soft tissue edema or periosteal reaction. The features are typical of a nonossifying fibroma (NOF).*

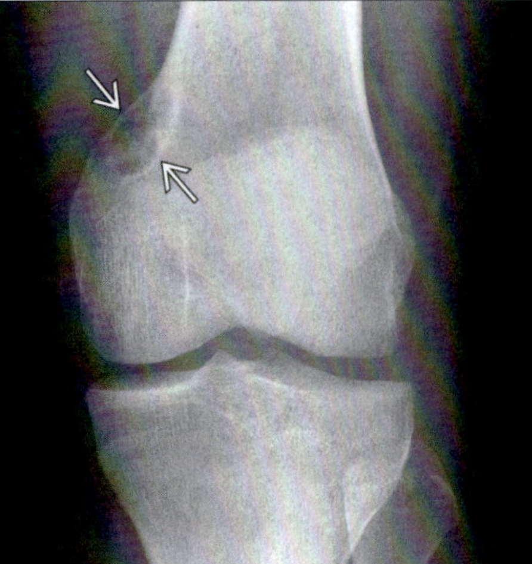

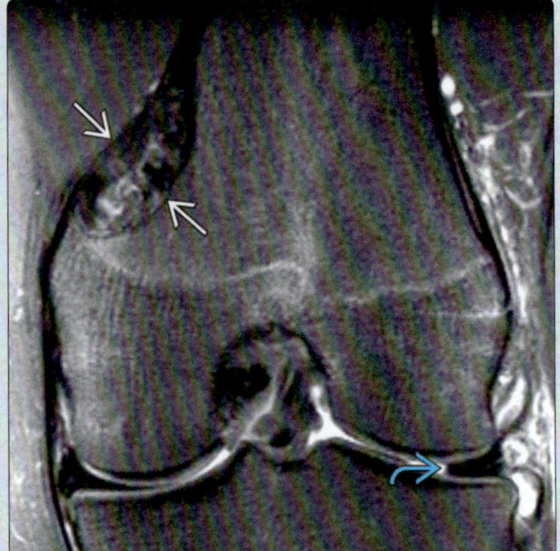

(Left) *AP radiograph in a 14-year-old after an injury shows an incidental, elongated, lucent & bubbly, eccentric lesion ➡ in the medial femoral metaphysis with a narrow zone of transition & sclerotic border, typical of an NOF or fibroxanthoma. There is mild expansile remodeling & endosteal scalloping without periosteal reaction.* **(Right)** *Coronal T2 FS MR in the same patient shows heterogeneous but largely hypointense signal of the lesion ➡ with normal adjacent marrow & soft tissues. (Note the torn lateral meniscus ➡.)*

TERMINOLOGY

Abbreviations

- Nonossifying fibroma (NOF)

Synonyms

- Non-ossifying fibroma, fibrous cortical defect (FCD), metaphyseal fibrous defect, fibroxanthoma

Definitions

- Very common benign fibrous lesion of pediatric bone, usually asymptomatic
- Terms fibroxanthoma & metaphyseal fibrous defect include
  - NOF
    - > 2- or 3-cm length
    - Encroachment on medullary cavity
  - FCD
    - < 2- or 3-cm length
    - Essentially isolated to cortex

IMAGING

General Features

- Best diagnostic clue
  - Eccentric, elongated, & bubbly lucent lesion in long bone metaphysis/diaphysis with narrow zone of transition, sclerotic margin, & no periosteal reaction
- Location
  - Metaphysis of long bone involved in up to 93%
    - Distance from physis ↑ with age
  - Tibia (43%), femur (38%), fibula (8%)
    - Around knee: 55-89%
  - Less common in upper extremity: 8%
    - Humerus: 5%
  - Usually solitary in absence of syndrome
- Size
  - 0.5-7.0 cm
- Morphology
  - Elongated, lobular, eccentric lesion

Radiographic Findings

- Radiography
  - Eccentric, cortically based, lucent lesion
  - Lesion long axis parallels bone long axis
  - Narrow zone of transition
  - Scalloped, lobular, or smooth deep sclerotic margin
  - ± mild expansile remodeling of overlying cortex &/or endosteal scalloping
    - Cortex thinned but usually intact (not always)
  - No matrix Ca^{2+}
  - ± septation/trabeculation
  - No periosteal reaction without fracture or other complication
  - ↑ mineralization in healing stages

CT Findings

- Bone CT
  - Parallels radiographic findings
  - Attenuation of lesion matrix is slightly > bone marrow

MR Findings

- T1WI
  - Intermediate to low signal intensity centrally
  - Peripheral hypointense rim (reactive sclerosis)
- T2WI
  - Variable signal intensity centrally, most commonly low
    - T2-hypointense components are due to fibrous tissue ± hemosiderin
  - Visible internal septa
  - Peripheral hypointense rim (reactive sclerosis)
  - No overlying soft tissue mass
  - No adjacent marrow, periosteal, or soft tissue edema without superimposed complication
- T1WI C+
  - Variable enhancement centrally, may be avid

Ultrasonographic Findings

- Grayscale ultrasound
  - Expanded, thinned, or scalloped cortex filled with hypoechoic tissue
  - ↓ size, ↑ echogenic foci with healing
- Color Doppler
  - May show prominent internal blood flow

Nuclear Medicine Findings

- Bone scan
  - Almost all lesions show some degree of uptake
    - Mild to intense uptake in healing lesions
    - Faint to absent uptake in inactive or fully healed lesions
- PET/CT
  - Mildly to intensely ↑ metabolic activity (may mimic malignancy)
    - ↓ activity with healing, though FDG avidity of these lesions often differs from Tc-99m bone scan uptake
    - Correlation with CT appearance is critical (or radiographs if PET performed without CT)

Imaging Recommendations

- Best imaging tool
  - Radiographs are diagnostic in most cases
  - Usually no other imaging needed unless
    - Complications are suspected by clinical or radiographic features
    - Larger lesion is identified
      - ☐ May be less pathognomonic
      - ☐ Follow-up to evaluate growth & fracture risk
  - CT/MR is helpful in confirming underlying fibroxanthoma in atypical or complicated lesion or with unusual clinical symptoms

DIFFERENTIAL DIAGNOSIS

Distal Femoral Metaphyseal Irregularity

- Cortical undulation/irregularity/interruption by lucent lesion with concave sclerotic deep margin
- Always at posterior, medial distal femur near medial gastrocnemius or adductor magnus attachments
- Overlaps fibroxanthoma imaging & histology despite poorly applied term "cortical desmoid"

Aneurysmal Bone Cyst

- Lucent metadiaphyseal lesion with marked expansile remodeling of cortex ± internal septations

- CT/MR: Fluid-fluid levels + thin septal enhancement

Unicameral Bone Cyst

- Centrally located, well-defined metadiaphyseal lucent lesion without profound expansion or septations
- Fallen fragment sign is pathognomonic in cases of fracture
- Classic location: Proximal humerus

Fibrous Dysplasia

- Mildly expansile, medullary diaphyseal lesion
- Ground-glass (think frosted or smudged glass) appearance of matrix

Chondromyxoid Fibroma

- Eccentric, bubbly, lucent metadiaphyseal lesion
- ~ 90% are expansile
- Much less common than fibroxanthoma

Enchondroma

- Central diaphyseal bubbly lucent lesion with endosteal scalloping & mild expansile remodeling
- ± ring & arc chondroid matrix
- Most commonly found in hands & feet

PATHOLOGY

General Features

- Genetics
  - Vast majority of these lesions are sporadic
  - Multiple lesions are seen in
    - Neurofibromatosis type 1 (NF1)
    - Jaffe-Campanacci syndrome (may be NF1 subset)
      - Multifocal fibroxanthomas with extraskeletal manifestations in children
      - Café au lait spots, mental restrictions, hypogonadism, & cryptorchidism + cardiovascular, renal, & ocular abnormalities

Microscopic Features

- NOF & FCD are histologically identical
- Bundles of spindle-shaped fibroblasts, scattered multinucleated giant cells, & foamy histiocytes
- Arranged in storiform pattern

CLINICAL ISSUES

Presentation

- Most common signs/symptoms
  - Usually asymptomatic & identified incidentally
- Other signs/symptoms
  - Acute pain with pathologic fracture
    - Risk greatest if lesion is > 3.3 cm in size or causing loss of > 50% cortical thickness in weight-bearing bone
    - Recent literature touts 4 point scale for assessment of fracture risk by CT: Risk ↑ with more positive factors
      - > 50% width in sagittal plane
      - > 50% width in coronal plane
      - Breach of cortex
      - Lack of "neocortex" (i.e., sclerotic deep margin that is similar in thickness to true cortex)
  - Adjacent stress fractures are reported rarely with gradual pain onset
  - Rarely complicated by other processes (such as infection)
  - Oncogenic osteomalacia is extremely rare
    - Paraneoplastic syndrome where benign bone tumor releases factors, resulting in renal phosphate wasting with subsequent rickets/osteomalacia
    - Usually in adults (mean age: 35-40 years)

Demographics

- Age
  - 2-20 years; peak: 10-15 years
    - 75% are found in 2nd decade of life
    - Usually not seen after age 30
- Sex
  - M:F = 2:1
- Epidemiology
  - Most common fibrous lesion of bone
  - Occurs in up to 35% of children

Natural History & Prognosis

- Benign lesion; no malignant transformation risk
  - More likely to be developmental defect than neoplasm
- Presents during childhood, usually disappears in late adolescence
  - Involution over 2-4 years
- Rarely grows rather than involutes

Treatment

- Usually not required
- Curettage with bone grafting of larger lesions at risk for fracture
- Conventional casting or internal fixation if fracture occurs
  - Lesion may heal after fracture

DIAGNOSTIC CHECKLIST

Consider

- No need to biopsy or treat if appearance is typical & fracture risk is low ("do not touch")
- MR to assess any atypical radiographic features

SELECTED REFERENCES

1. Goldin AN et al: Nonossifying fibromas: a computed tomography-based criteria to predict fracture risk. J Pediatr Orthop. 40(2):e149-54, 2020
2. Shah JN et al: Pediatric benign bone tumors: what does the radiologist need to know? Pediatric Imaging. Radiographics. 37(3):1001-2, 2017
3. Wodajo FM: Top five lesions that do not need referral to orthopedic oncology. Orthop Clin North Am. 46(2):303-14, 2015
4. Jagtap VS et al: Tumor-induced osteomalacia: a single center experience. Endocr Pract. 17(2):177-84, 2011
5. Shimal A et al: Fatigue-type stress fractures of the lower limb associated with fibrous cortical defects/non-ossifying fibromas in the skeletally immature. Clin Radiol. 65(5):382-6, 2010
6. Wootton-Gorges SL: MR imaging of primary bone tumors and tumor-like conditions in children. Magn Reson Imaging Clin N Am. 17(3):469-87, vi, 2009
7. Hetts SW et al: Case 110: Nonossifying fibroma. Radiology. 243(1):288-92, 2007
8. Hod N et al: Scintigraphic characteristics of non-ossifying fibroma in military recruits undergoing bone scintigraphy for suspected stress fractures and lower limb pains. Nucl Med Commun. 28(1):25-33, 2007
9. Goodin GS et al: PET/CT characterization of fibroosseous defects in children: 18F-FDG uptake can mimic metastatic disease. AJR Am J Roentgenol. 2006 Oct;187(4):1124-8. Erratum in: AJR Am J Roentgenol. 187(5):1146, 2006
10. Levine SM et al: Cortical lesions of the tibia: characteristic appearances at conventional radiography. Radiographics. 23(1):157-77, 2003
11. Smith SE et al: Primary musculoskeletal tumors of fibrous origin. Semin Musculoskelet Radiol. 4(1):73-88, 2000

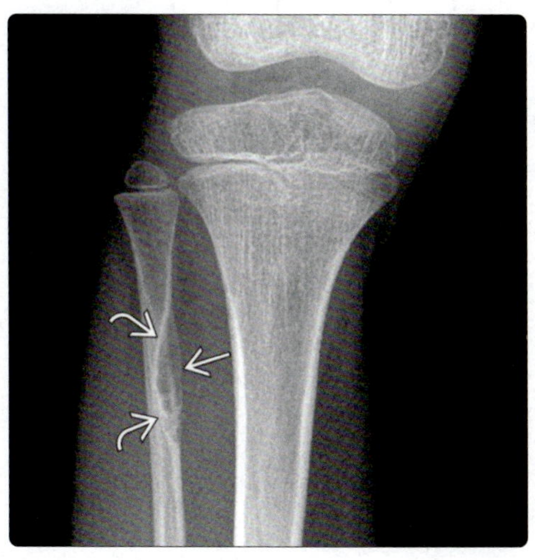

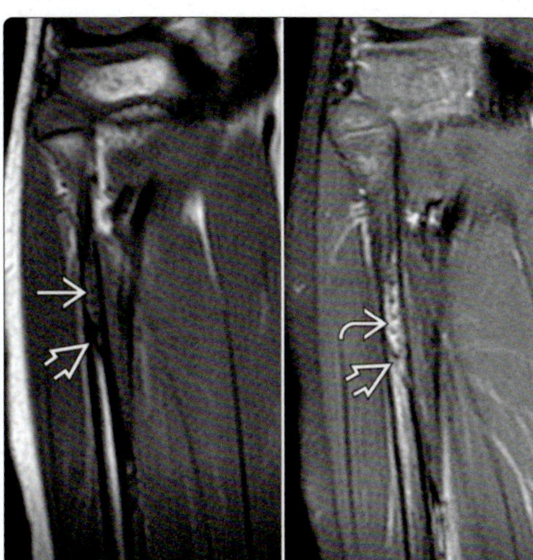

(Left) *AP radiograph shows a well-circumscribed, bubbly, lucent lesion eccentrically located in the proximal fibular diaphysis with a deep margin of sclerosis ➡ & mild expansile remodeling of the overlying cortex ➡, typical of an NOF.* **(Right)** *Coronal T1 (left) & T1 C+ FS (right) MR images in the same patient show the low signal intensity rim ➡ of the lesion. The lesion shows intermediate signal intensity internally ➡ prior to contrast administration with heterogeneous enhancement ➡ after contrast.*

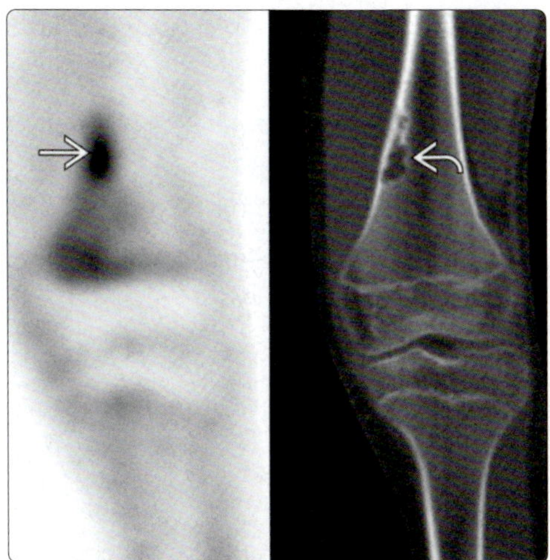

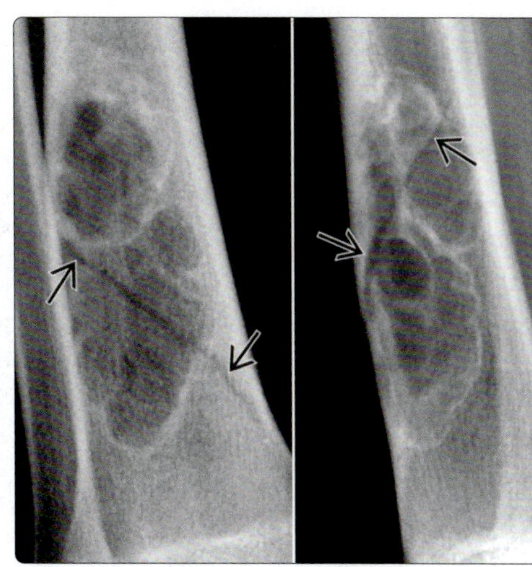

(Left) *Coronal FDG PET/CT in a teenager with nasopharyngeal carcinoma shows ↑ metabolic activity ➡ in an eccentric distal femoral lesion that has typical CT characteristics ➡ of an NOF.* **(Right)** *AP (left) & lateral (right) radiographs show an obliquely oriented pathologic fracture ➡ through a relatively large NOF in the distal tibia of this teenage patient who fell from a height of 12 feet.*

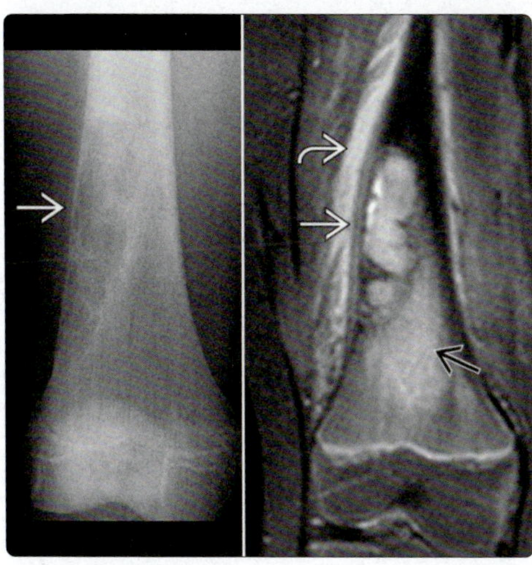

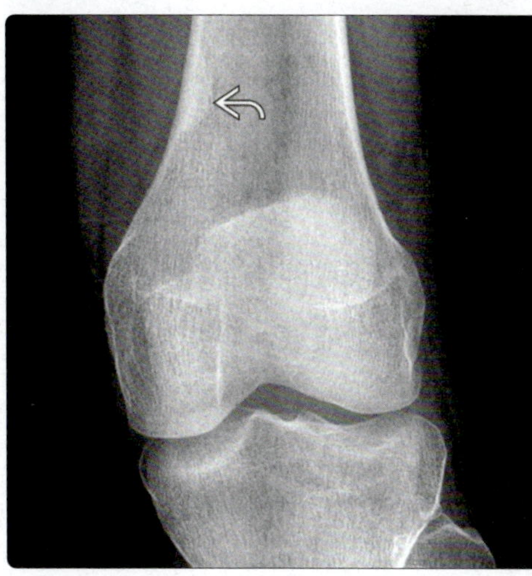

(Left) *AP radiograph (left) & coronal T2 FS MR (right) in a 10-year-old boy with knee pain show a large NOF with atypical periosteal reaction ➡ & edema of the surrounding soft tissues ➡ & marrow ➡. No fracture was identified. Biopsy confirmed an NOF with superimposed osteomyelitis.* **(Right)** *AP radiograph of the knee in a 16-year-old girl shows a well-defined, crescentic, sclerotic lesion in the medial aspect of the distal femoral metadiaphysis ➡, typical of a nearly healed fibroxanthoma/NOF.*

KEY FACTS

TERMINOLOGY

- Benign osteoblastic lesion characterized by < 2-cm nidus of osteoid/woven bone in fibrovascular stroma

IMAGING

- Best clue: Well-defined, small, lucent lesion in tubular bone cortex with surrounding sclerosis & edema
- Locations
  - Cortical: 70-80%
    - Diaphyses > metaphyses of tubular bones
  - Medullary: 20-30%
    - Epiphyses or equivalents (intraarticular in 10%)
    - Spine posterior elements
- Radiographs/CT
  - Small, round, or ovoid lucent nidus ± central Ca^{2+}
  - Surrounding cortical thickening, solid periosteal reaction
  - Prominent cortical vessels near nidus
- MR
  - Variable nidus signal on T2 FS MR; may be "target"
  - Surrounding marrow, periosteal, & soft tissue edema
    - Joint effusion/synovitis if osteoid osteoma is intraarticular
  - Hyperenhancing nidus on early dynamic T1 C+ FS MR
- NM bone scan: Double density sign

TOP DIFFERENTIAL DIAGNOSES

- Osteomyelitis, Langerhans cell histiocytosis, stress injury, osteoblastoma, osteosarcoma

CLINICAL ISSUES

- Insidious pain, classically worse at night & relieved by NSAIDs
- Gradual spontaneous regression is accelerated by NSAIDs
- Surgery is curative if nidus is completely resected
- Image-guided percutaneous interventions are highly effective due to nidus visualization

(Left) *AP & lateral views in an 8-year-old with months of left hip pain show cortical thickening ⇨ & medullary sclerosis ➡ at the medial & anterior proximal femur surrounding a subtle lucent focus ⇨.* **(Right)** *Coronal STIR MR in the same patient shows well-circumscribed edema ➡ (a.k.a. the half-moon sign) surrounding the subtle cortical lesion ⇨. Note the edema ↗ overlying the periosteum.*

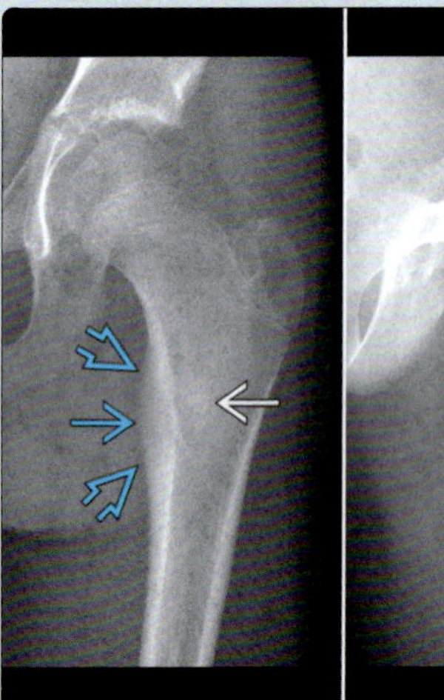

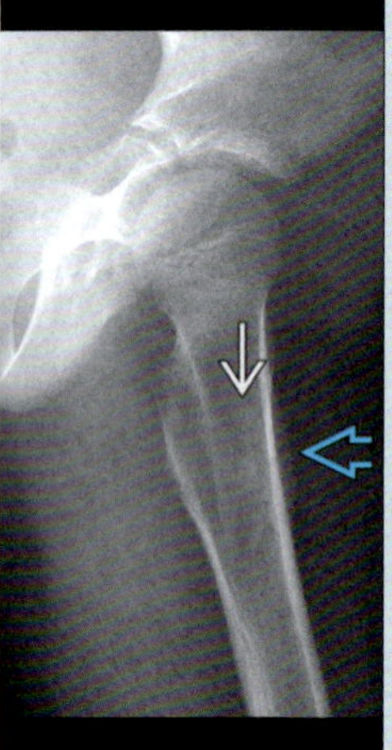

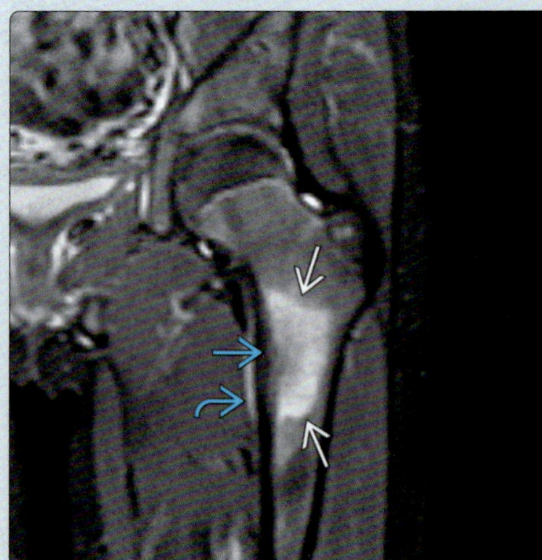

(Left) *Axial T2 FS MR in the same patient shows hyperintense signal at the osteoid osteoma nidus ⇨ with overlying soft tissue & periosteal edema ↗ + subjacent medullary edema ➡.* **(Right)** *Axial NECT in the same patient at the time of radiofrequency ablation shows a tiny focus of calcification in the lucent nidus ⇨ of this osteoid osteoma (OO). The characteristic adjacent cortical thickening ⇨ & medullary sclerosis ➡ are again noted.*

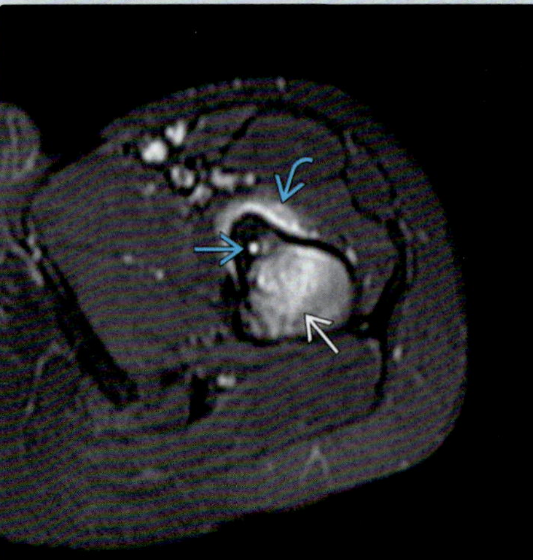

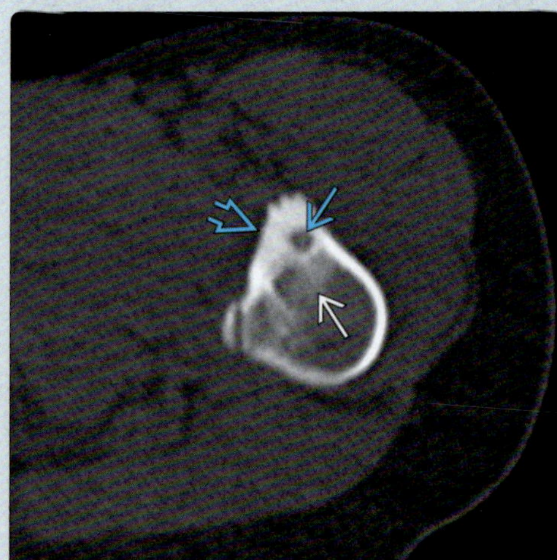

TERMINOLOGY

Abbreviations

- Osteoid osteoma (OO)

Definitions

- Benign osteoblastic lesion characterized by < 2-cm nidus of osteoid/woven bone in fibrovascular tissue

IMAGING

General Features

- Best diagnostic clue
  - Small, well-defined, cortically-based lucent lesion of tubular bone with surrounding sclerosis & edema
- Location
  - Distribution in body
    - Femur, tibia: 53-60%
    - Hands & feet: 15-25%
    - Spine: 9-20%
      - Posterior elements: 90%
      - Vertebral body: 10%
      - Lumbar > cervical > thoracic > sacral
  - Distribution in bone
    - Cortical: 70-80%
      - Diaphyses > metaphyses of tubular bones
    - Medullary: 20-30%
      - Epiphyses or equivalents (10% are intraarticular)
      - Posterior vertebral elements
    - Subperiosteal

Radiographic Findings

- Radiolucent central nidus is usually < 1 cm
  - Nidus is often partly calcified
- Adjacent cortical thickening & medullary sclerosis are common
  - Less frequent with medullary/intraarticular OO
- Periosteal reaction: Solid > lamellated
  - Often distant from intraarticular OO
- Focal cortical bulge or scalloping may be present
- Joint effusion & synovitis with intraarticular OO
- ± osteoporosis, muscle atrophy distally

CT Findings

- Small, well-defined, round or ovoid hypoattenuating nidus surrounded by thickened cortex & medullary sclerosis
  - Elongated/eccentric nidus is more likely to have treatment failure
- Central Ca^{2+} of nidus is often present, may have target appearance
- Overlying nonaggressive periosteal reaction
- Prominent cortical vascular channels extending toward nidus

MR Findings

- T1WI
  - Low- to intermediate-signal nidus
  - ± adjacent muscle atrophy
- T2WI FS/STIR
  - Unmineralized nidus shows intermediate to high signal; mineralized nidus shows low signal
  - ± target appearance of nidus
    - Low signal centrally from nidus Ca^{2+}
    - Surrounding high signal of unmineralized nidus
    - Outer low-signal rim of sclerosis
  - Adjacent abnormal fluid signal
    - Marrow, periosteal, & soft tissue edema
      - Extensive marrow edema can obscure small nidus
      - Half-moon sign (or half-circle) of marrow edema may be suggestive of femoral neck OO (but is also seen with stress injuries)
      - "Pseudotumor" of surrounding soft tissue inflammation is reported at phalangeal OO
    - Joint effusion/synovitis if OO is intra/periarticular
- T1WI C+ FS
  - Dynamic imaging: Peak enhancement of nidus occurs during early arterial phase with subsequent partial washout
    - Slower enhancement of adjacent marrow edema
  - Reactive synovitis with intra/periarticular OO
- Post ablation (by radiofrequency)
  - ↓ nidus volume
  - T2 hypointense center with hyperintense band
  - ↑ ADC values of nidus
  - No dynamic enhancement

Ultrasonographic Findings

- Color Doppler
  - ↑ vascularity of superficial nidus
    - May be obscured by overlying thickened cortex
  - Can be used to localize lesion for biopsy

Nuclear Medicine Findings

- Bone scan
  - ↑ radiotracer uptake
    - Double density sign: Small focus of intensely ↑ activity (nidus) surrounded by larger area of less intensely ↑ activity (reactive sclerosis)
  - SPECT: ↑ sensitivity for subtle spine OO
    - Fusion with targeted CT at site of abnormal uptake provides optimal localization

Imaging Recommendations

- Best imaging tool
  - SPECT-CT (if OO suspected)
- Protocol advice
  - CT: Limit coverage to region of abnormality based on preceding imaging studies
  - MR: Dynamic postcontrast sequence is most helpful for localizing nidus

DIFFERENTIAL DIAGNOSIS

Osteomyelitis

- Chronic infection with Brodie abscess
  - Sclerosis & periosteal reaction ± lucent abscess cavity, necrotic bone sequestrum
    - Margins of abscess & sequestrum are more likely to be irregular
      - Peripheral enhancement of abscess
      - Penumbra sign of subacute/chronic intraosseous abscess: High T1 signal rim (precontrast) of granulation tissue lining sclerotic margin
    - Cloaca drainage tract may be present

- Acute infection
  - Poorly defined marrow edema, periosteal reaction
    - Intramedullary OO may be confused for early infection by MR if nidus not clearly seen
  - More likely to have osteolysis & fluid collections than OO

Langerhans Cell Histiocytosis

- Lytic lesion with well-defined or permeative margins ± lamellated periosteal reaction
- Sclerotic rim with healing

Stress Injury

- Radiolucency & sclerosis are more linear & perpendicular to cortex (rather than parallel)

Osteoblastoma

- Histologically similar but larger than OO (> 2-2.5 cm)
- More frequently involves spine
- Constellation of symptoms is less classic than OO
- Reactive bone formation is uncommon

Osteosarcoma

- Intramedullary location is most common
- Combination of aggressive bony destructive features & cloud-like osteoid matrix

PATHOLOGY

General Features

- Benign tumor consisting of osteoblastic mass (nidus) surrounded by zone of reactive sclerosis
  - Zone of sclerosis is not integral part of tumor: Represents reversible reactive change; not always present
  - Nidus has limited growth potential
- Prostaglandin E2 is elevated 100-1000x within nidus
  - May be cause of pain & vasodilation

Microscopic Features

- Nidus is composed of osteoid tissue or mineralized, immature bone surrounded by fibrovascular stroma
  - Variable amounts of osteoblasts & giant cells resembling osteoclasts
  - Unmyelinated nerve fibers are present
- Sclerosis surrounding nidus is composed of dense bone

CLINICAL ISSUES

Presentation

- Most common signs/symptoms
  - Local pain, worse at night; ↓ by aspirin/NSAIDs in < 30 minutes (75%)
    - Up to 5% of patients present without pain
- Other signs/symptoms
  - Local swelling, erythema, point tenderness
  - Symptoms may last weeks to years before presentation
  - Spinal involvement: Painful scoliosis with concavity of curvature toward side of lesion
    - Scoliosis improves/resolves if nidus is resected within 15 months of diagnosis
  - Intraarticular lesion
    - Pain, limp, ↓ range of motion, swelling
    - Some literature reports that intraarticular OO takes up to 3x as long as extraarticular OO due to variety of other joint pathologies considered in work-up
  - ↑ urinary excretion of major prostacyclin metabolite (6-keto-PGF1α)
    - Returns to normal after removal of nidus

Demographics

- Age
  - 5-35 years old; 50% between ages 10-20 years
- Sex
  - M:F = 2-4:1
- Epidemiology
  - 4% of primary bone tumors
  - 11-14% of benign bone tumors

Natural History & Prognosis

- No malignant potential
- No growth progression
- Without treatment, lesion ultimately regresses in 6-15 years with symptom resolution
- Long-term bone growth disturbances can result from hyperemia of OO
  - Overgrowth, angular deformities

Treatment

- Medical: NSAIDs
  - Can expedite lesion healing/regression to < 3 years
- Surgical resection is curative if nidus is completely removed
  - Tetracycline with fluorescence or radionuclide labeling was used historically for lesion localization at surgery
- CT-guided percutaneous interventions
  - Radiofrequency ablation, laser photocoagulation, cryoablation, trephine/drill excision
- MR-guided high intensity focused ultrasound or other percutaneous interventions

DIAGNOSTIC CHECKLIST

Consider

- Image-guided therapy is often more successful than surgical resection due to nidus visualization

SELECTED REFERENCES

1. French J et al: MR imaging of osteoid osteoma: pearls and pitfalls. Semin Ultrasound CT MR. 41(5):488-97, 2020
2. Malghem J et al: Osteoid osteoma of the hip: imaging features. Skeletal Radiol. 49(11):1709-18, 2020
3. Arrigoni F et al: Magnetic-resonance-guided focused ultrasound treatment of non-spinal osteoid osteoma in children: multicentre experience. Pediatr Radiol. 49(9):1209-16, 2019
4. Baal JD et al: Factors associated with osteoid osteoma recurrence after CT-guided radiofrequency ablation. J Vasc Interv Radiol. 30(5):744-51, 2019
5. Bhure U et al: Osteoid osteoma: multimodality imaging with focus on hybrid imaging. Eur J Nucl Med Mol Imaging. 46(4):1019-36, 2019
6. Erbaş G et al: Treatment-related alterations of imaging findings in osteoid osteoma after percutaneous radiofrequency ablation. Skeletal Radiol. 48(11):1697-703, 2019
7. Pottecher P et al: Dynamic contrast-enhanced MR imaging in osteoid osteoma: relationships with clinical and CT characteristics. Skeletal Radiol. 46(7):935-48, 2017
8. Carra BJ et al: The half-moon sign of the femoral neck is nonspecific for the diagnosis of osteoid osteoma. AJR Am J Roentgenol. 206(3):W54, 2016
9. Rheinheimer S et al: Diffusion weighted MRI of osteoid osteomas: higher ADC values after radiofrequency ablation. Eur J Radiol. 85(7):1284-8, 2016

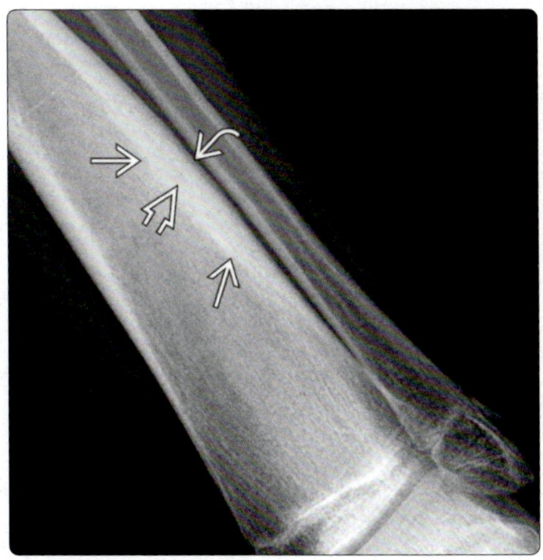

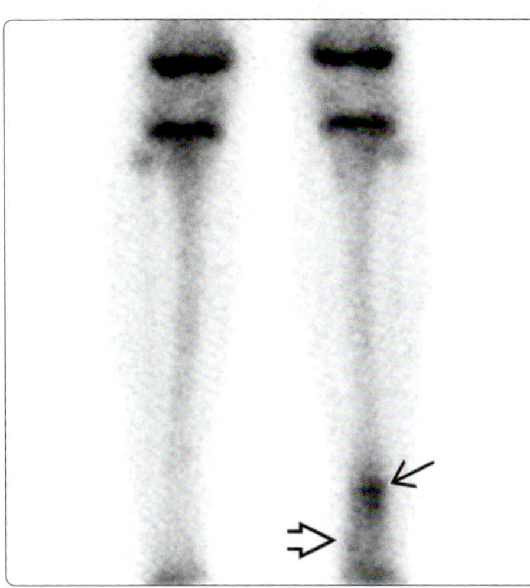

(Left) *AP radiograph of the left tibia in a 15-year-old girl with 1 year of lower leg pain shows a region of diaphyseal cortical thickening laterally* → *with mild overlying solid periosteal reaction* → *& a subtle lucent focus centrally* →. **(Right)** *Anterior Tc-99m nuclear medicine bone scan in the same patient shows focally ↑ uptake at the level of the nidus* →. *This "hot" focus is superimposed on a background of mildly ↑ radiotracer activity in the distal tibia* → *(the double density sign, typical of OO).*

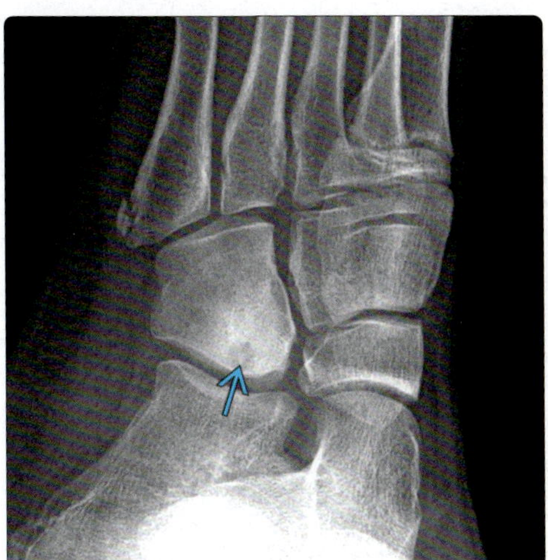

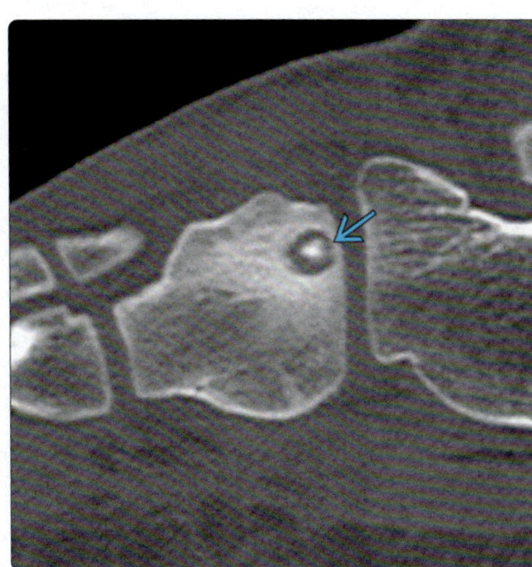

(Left) *Oblique radiograph in a 13-year-old boy with lateral foot pain shows a centrally calcified lucent focus* → *in the posterior cuboid. Note the medullary sclerosis surrounding the lesion.* **(Right)** *Sagittal bone CT in the same patient shows the hypoattenuating round nidus* → *of the cuboid OO with central* Ca^{2-} *& surrounding sclerosis.*

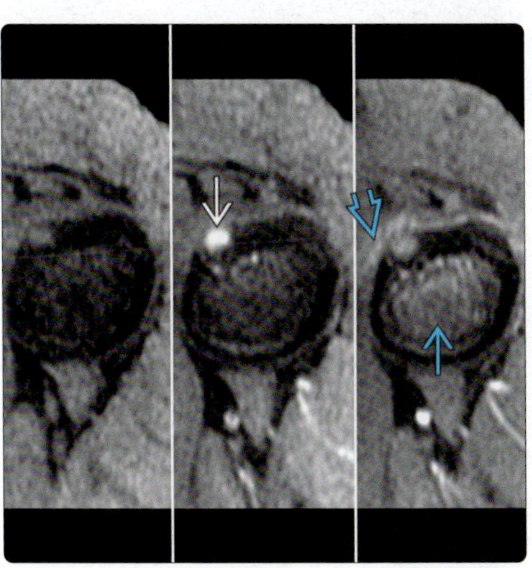

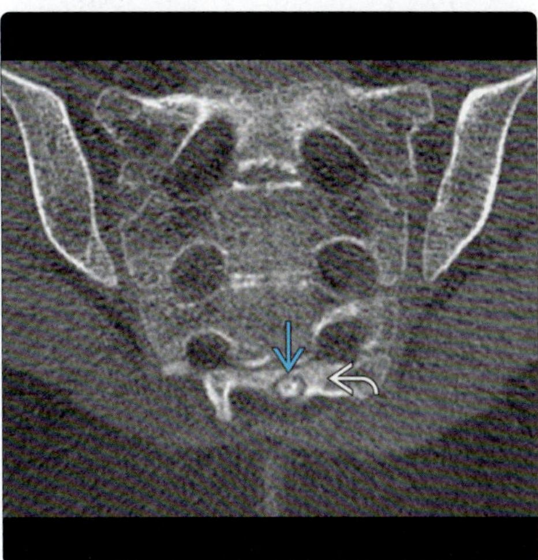

(Left) *Axial dynamic T1 FS MR images before (left), 1 minute after (middle), & 8 minutes after (right) contrast administration in an 11-year-old patient with an OO of the humeral cortex show early intense enhancement of the nidus* → *with gradual vague enhancement of the adjacent marrow* → *& overlying tissues* →. **(Right)** *Coronal oblique bone CT of the sacrum in an 8-year-old girl with pain shows a round, hypoattenuating nidus with central* Ca^{2+} → *& adjacent sclerosis* →, *consistent with an OO.*

Chondroblastoma

KEY FACTS

TERMINOLOGY

- Benign to intermediate-grade bone tumor with immature cartilage cells (chondroblasts) in heterogeneous matrix

IMAGING

- Vast majority originate in epiphysis (85%), apophysis (12%), or other epiphyseal equivalent (tarsals, carpals, patella)
  - Up to 55% extend to adjacent metaphysis
  - Pure metaphyseal/diaphyseal location is uncommon
- Tubular bones are affected most frequently
  - Long bones in 75-80%
- Radiographs
  - Well-circumscribed, lucent epiphyseal lesion
  - Chondroid ring & arc Ca^{2+} in 30-50%
  - Solid periosteal reaction of adjacent metaphysis in 50-60%
- T2 FS MR
  - Heterogeneous internally with foci of low or intermediate T2 signal intensity
    - Distinct from most other cartilage tumors
  - Low signal intensity rim
  - Surrounding marrow, periosteal, & soft tissue edema
  - Reactive joint effusion in up to 50%
  - Secondary aneurysmal bone cyst in 23-33%

TOP DIFFERENTIAL DIAGNOSES

- Osteoid osteoma
- Osteomyelitis
- Langerhans cell histiocytosis
- Metastatic disease
- Giant cell tumor

CLINICAL ISSUES

- Presentations: Pain, tenderness, stiffness, swelling, limping
- Peak age: 15-20 years
- Treatment: Surgical curettage ± bone grafting vs. RFA; must consider risks to adjacent growth plate
  - Recurrence in 5-35%; rare lung metastases

(Left) *AP radiograph in a 14-year-old girl with right shoulder pain shows a well-circumscribed, round, lucent lesion of the humeral head. The adjacent growth plate appears intact.* **(Right)** *Axial STIR MR in the same patient shows nearly homogeneous low signal intensity throughout the round lesion with an even lower signal rim of sclerosis. Note the marked edema of the surrounding marrow of the humeral head (as compared to the normal scapular marrow), typical of a chondroblastoma.*

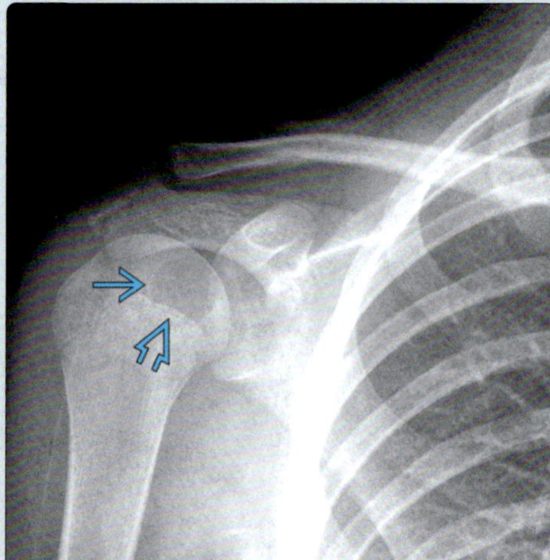

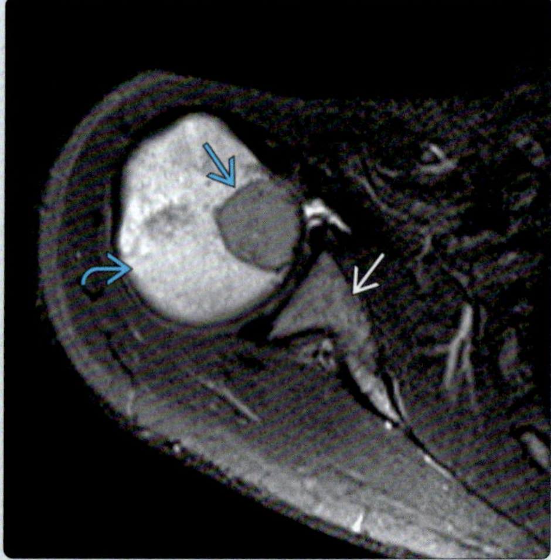

(Left) *Lateral knee radiograph in a 13-year-old girl with 1 year of pain shows a lobular, lucent lesion in the posterior tibial epiphysis. There is fullness & poor definition of the surrounding soft tissues, suggesting edema.* **(Right)** *Sagittal T2 FS MR in the same patient shows heterogeneous low signal intensity in the lesion with metaphyseal extension & cortical breach. There is surrounding marrow & soft tissue edema as well as a joint effusion. Chondroblastoma was confirmed at surgery.*

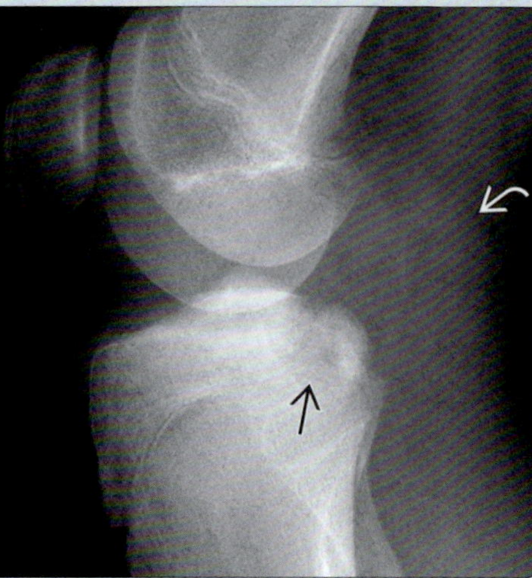

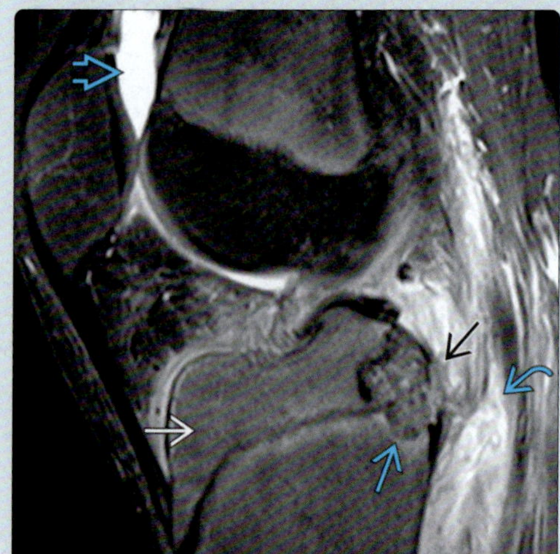

TERMINOLOGY

Definitions

- Benign to intermediate-grade bone tumor with immature cartilage cells (chondroblasts) in heterogeneous matrix

IMAGING

General Features

- Best diagnostic clue
  - Well-circumscribed, lucent epiphyseal lesion in teenager
- Location
  - Majority originate in epiphysis (85%), apophysis (12%), or other epiphyseal equivalent (tarsals, carpals, patella)
    - Up to 55% extend to metaphysis
    - Pure metaphyseal/diaphyseal location is rare
  - Tubular bones are affected most frequently
    - Long bones in 75-80%
      - Proximal tibia, distal & proximal femur, & proximal humerus are most frequent
    - Foot involved in 5-16%
      - Talus, calcaneus: ~ 40% each
  - Rare cortical disruption with extraosseous or intraarticular extension

Radiographic Findings

- Well-circumscribed, lucent epiphyseal lesion
- Mildly lobulated with sclerotic rim
- Chondroid ring & arc Ca^{2+} in 30-50%
- Solid periosteal reaction of adjacent metaphysis in 60%
- Bubbly expansile remodeling if aneurysmal bone cyst (ABC) develops

CT Findings

- ± chondroid Ca^{2+} (~ 44%)
- Cortical disruption (19%)
- Periosteal reaction of adjacent metaphysis

MR Findings

- T2WI FS
  - Heterogeneous internally with foci of low or intermediate T2 signal intensity
    - Ca^{2+} vs. hemosiderin vs. cellular regions
    - Distinct from most other high T2 signal intensity cartilage tumors
  - Low signal intensity rim
  - Surrounding marrow, periosteal, & soft tissue edema
  - Reactive joint effusion in up to 50%
  - Multiloculated component containing fluid-fluid levels due to secondary ABC (15-33%)
- T1WI C+ FS
  - Variable enhancement of lesion internally
  - Enhancement of edematous marrow & soft tissues

DIFFERENTIAL DIAGNOSIS

Osteoid Osteoma

- Cortical metaphysis/diaphysis is most common location (but can be epiphyseal)
- Adjacent edema & cortical thickening
- Lucent nidus is usually small
  - Enhances early on dynamic MR imaging

Osteomyelitis

- Metaphyseal origin is most common
- Typically presents early, often with only soft tissue edema on radiographs
- Abundant marrow & soft tissue edema on MR, usually without well-defined lesion
- Fluid collections are often present

Langerhans Cell Histiocytosis

- Cortical destruction with soft tissue mass
  - Typically well circumscribed
  - Often has uniform high T2 signal & enhancement
  - May have low T2 signal intensity rim
- Favors metadiaphysis or flat bones

Metastatic Disease

- Often multifocal with aggressive features & enhancement

Giant Cell Tumor

- Subchondral epiphyseal lesion without sclerotic rim
- Uncommon in skeletally immature patients but more likely to involve metaphysis

PATHOLOGY

General Features

- Closely packed immature cartilage cells (chondroblasts) with scattered mature cartilage & giant cells
- Intercellular Ca^{2+} (chicken wire) in 60%
- Frequency of secondary ABC depends on definition
  - "ABC-rich" form: 23-33%
  - Microcysts + hemorrhage: Up to 83%

CLINICAL ISSUES

Presentation

- Most common signs/symptoms
  - Pain, tenderness, stiffness, swelling, limping

Demographics

- 1% of primary bone tumors
- Peak age: 15-20 years; range: 3-85 years
- M:F = 1.6-3.5:1.0

Natural History & Prognosis

- Rare lung metastases

Treatment

- Surgical curettage ± bone grafting preferred over resection due to adjacent growth plate
  - Recurrence in 5-35%
    - More likely with skeletal immaturity
- Radiofrequency ablation (RFA) in some cases

SELECTED REFERENCES

1. Arkader A et al: Pediatric chondroblastoma and the need for lung staging at presentation. J Pediatr Orthop. 40(9):e894-7, 2020
2. John I et al: Chondroblastomas presenting in adulthood: a study of 39 patients with emphasis on histologic features and skeletal distribution. Histopathology. ePub, 2019
3. Laitinen MK et al: Chondroblastoma in pelvis and extremities- a single centre study of 177 cases. J Bone Oncol. 17:100248, 2019
4. Douis H et al: The imaging of cartilaginous bone tumours. I. Benign lesions. Skeletal Radiol. 41(10):1195-212, 2012

Osteochondroma

KEY FACTS

TERMINOLOGY

- Common benign, developmental bony surface lesion resulting from displaced growth cartilage; not neoplastic

IMAGING

- Lobulated, sessile or pedunculated bony protuberance
    - Demonstrates flowing corticomedullary continuity with underlying (parent) bone
    - Covered by cap of hyaline cartilage
- Radiographs are usually diagnostic
- MR is typically reserved for pain/complications or if diagnosis is unclear
    - Fracture (± radiographic visibility) may occur at stalk
    - Mass effect may lead to
        - Friction/irritation of overlying soft tissues ± bursa formation
        - Compression neuritis leading to denervation
        - Vascular compression or rarely occlusion, pseudoaneurysm

TOP DIFFERENTIAL DIAGNOSES

- Osteosarcoma (parosteal)
- Myositis ossificans
- Periosteal chondroma

PATHOLOGY

- Solitary > > multiple
    - Hereditary multiple exostoses (HME) patients
        - Develop characteristic growth disturbances
        - Have 5-11% lifetime risk of malignant degeneration vs. < 1% risk for solitary osteochondroma (OC)
            - OC cartilage cap thickness > 2 cm in skeletally mature patient is more likely to harbor malignancy

CLINICAL ISSUES

- Most commonly found in ages 10-35 years
- Typically presents as painless hard mass
- Lesion growth should cease at skeletal maturity
    - Further ↑ suggests malignant degeneration

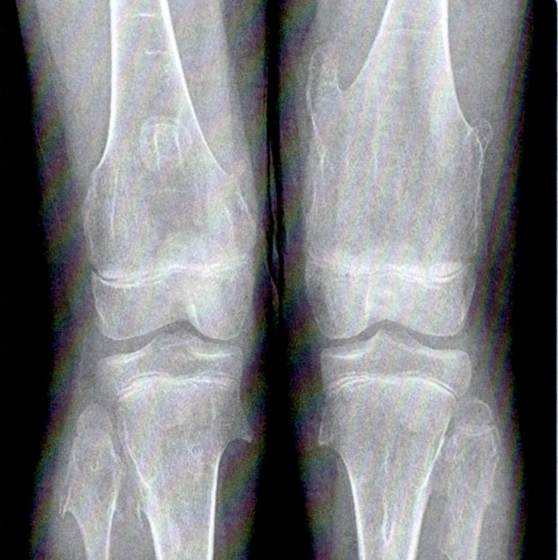

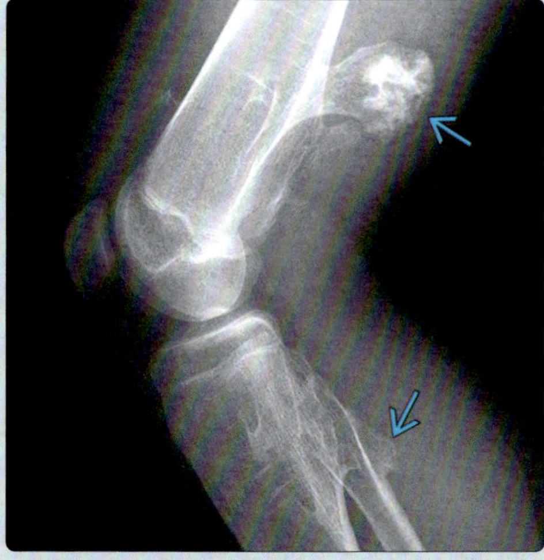

(Left) *AP radiograph of the lower extremities in a 13-year-old with hereditary multiple exostoses (HME) shows numerous osteochondromas (OCs) about the knees, ranging in morphology from pedunculated to sessile. Note the broadened metadiaphyses typical of HME.* **(Right)** *Subsequent lateral radiograph of the right knee in the same patient shows that the pedunculated OCs → point away from the joint. Note the characteristic corticomedullary continuity of the OCs with the underlying bones.*

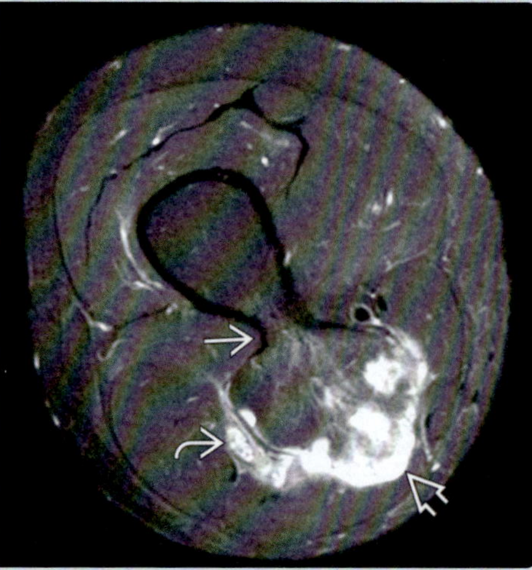

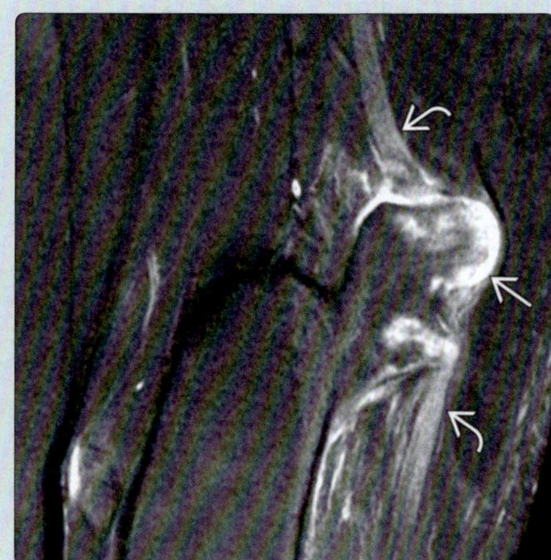

(Left) *Axial T2 FS MR of the right thigh in a 14-year-old girl shows a pedunculated OC with a thin stalk → arising from the posteromedial femur. A thin high-signal cartilage cap is noted →. The sciatic nerve is displaced laterally → & shows abnormal high T2 signal internally.* **(Right)** *Sagittal T2 FS MR in the same patient shows displacement & abnormal fluid signal of the sciatic nerve → due to mass effect from the adjacent OC →.*

TERMINOLOGY

Definitions

- Osteochondroma (OC): Benign, developmental bony surface lesion arising from displaced growth cartilage
  - Not true neoplasm
  - Generally synonymous with exostosis
- Maintains corticomedullary continuity with underlying bone
- Covered by hyaline cartilage cap

IMAGING

General Features

- Best diagnostic clue
  - Lobulated, sessile or pedunculated bony protuberance demonstrating flowing corticomedullary continuity with underlying bone (parent bone)
- Location
  - Any bone that develops by endochondral ossification
    - Distal femur > proximal femur, proximal tibia, humerus
      - Metaphysis/metadiaphysis > diaphysis > epiphysis
    - Hands, feet, scapula, spine, pelvis, skull base < 10% each; cervical > thoracic > lumbar
      - C2 is most common spine site
  - > 80% solitary, < 20% multiple
- Morphology
  - Spectrum between extremes
    - Sessile: Broad base with underlying bone
    - Pedunculated: Narrow or bulbous mass with thin stalk of attachment to bone
      - Usually points away from joint due to traction

Radiographic Findings

- Sessile or pedunculated bony lesion arising from bone surface
- Corticomedullary continuity with underlying bone
- Chondroid Ca^{2+} may be seen in cartilage cap
- U-shaped rim of sclerosis if viewed en face

CT Findings

- CTA is useful for assessing vascular complications
  - Vessel compression, occlusion, arteriovenous fistula, or pseudoaneurysm (PSA) may result from mass effect by adjacent OC

MR Findings

- T1WI
  - Continuity of dark cortex & bright fatty marrow signal between lesion & underlying bone
- T2WI FS
  - Marrow & cortex signal similar to parent bone
    - Marrow edema due to contusion or fracture
  - Bright cartilage cap overlying ossified lesion
    - Cartilage cap thickness > 2 cm after skeletal maturity → ↑ ↑ likelihood of malignant transformation
    - Size of cartilage cap may be irrelevant prior to skeletal maturity, though some report risk if > 3 cm
  - Very sensitive for soft tissue complications
    - Friction/compression of overlying muscle & fat ± bursa formation
    - Nerve compression
    - Vascular compression & PSA formation
      - PSAs are very heterogeneous due to turbulent internal flow & layers of thrombus; pulsation artifact in phase-encoding direction
      - Popliteal artery is most common PSA location due to OC
    - Edema from fracture through stalk
- T1WI C+ FS
  - Enhancement of growth plate at osteocartilaginous junction
  - Variable enhancement of remaining cartilage cap
    - May show lobular septal & rim enhancement

Ultrasonographic Findings

- Can confirm cortical continuity, cartilage cap
- May be useful to evaluate surrounding soft tissues
  - Relationship of OC to nerve or vessel
    - Color Doppler to look for vascular complication
  - Bursa formation

Nuclear Medicine Findings

- Bone scan
  - ↑ activity at growth plate of cartilage cap
  - ↓ activity with skeletal maturity
  - ↑ activity beyond skeletal maturity: Concerning for malignancy
- PET/CT
  - FDG PET can help identify malignant change

Imaging Recommendations

- Best imaging tool
  - Radiographs are usually diagnostic
  - MR is excellent for soft tissue complications
- Protocol advice
  - T2 FS/STIR most sensitive MR sequence for complications
  - Contrast-enhanced MR is rarely needed

DIFFERENTIAL DIAGNOSIS

Osteosarcoma (Parosteal)

- Most common surface osteosarcoma
- Ossified soft tissue mass arising from outer periosteum
- May have broad base vs. cleavage plane with bone
  - Lacks "flowing" corticomedullary continuity of OC
- Most common at posterior distal femoral metaphysis
- Peak incidence: 20-40 years of age

Myositis Ossificans

- Initially, noncalcified soft tissue mass overlying bone
- Typically shows marked surrounding muscular edema by MR
- Develops peripheral Ca^{2+} within weeks, progressing to center
- Trauma history is often (but not always) present

Periosteal/Juxtacortical Chondroma

- Uncommon cartilaginous surface lesion
- Partially interrupted & layered or scalloped cortex deep to cartilage focus (rather than corticomedullary continuity)

PATHOLOGY

General Features

- Etiology
  - Displaced physeal cartilage herniates through periosteal bone cuff
  - Endochondral ossification of this cartilage yields growing bony protuberance
  - Growth of OC is expected to cease at skeletal maturity
    - Continued growth or pain is concerning for malignant transformation
  - ↑ OC incidence with prior radiation (up to 24% develop exostoses)
    - Mean latency of 5-12 years
- Associated abnormalities
  - Hereditary multiple exostoses (HME)
    - Numerous OCs with resulting growth disturbances
      - Valgus tibiotalar tilt, limb length discrepancy, pseudo-Madelung deformity, coxa valga
    - Autosomal dominant with incomplete penetrance
      - Mutations of exostosin tumor suppressor genes on chromosomes 8 (*EXT1*), 11 (*EXT2*), & 19 (*EXT3*)
    - ↑ likelihood of malignant transformation to chondrosarcoma
      - 5-11%; typically after skeletal maturity
  - Dysplasia epiphysealis hemimelica (Trevor disease)
    - Classically considered to be epiphyseal (or equivalent) OCs
      - Now seen as epiphyseal cartilage overgrowth
    - Multiple bones of single extremity are often involved on either medial or lateral side (not both)
    - Lower extremity (particularly foot/ankle) is much more commonly affected than upper
    - Mechanical symptoms & limb deformities are common
  - Metachondromatosis
    - Very rare disease of multiple OCs & enchondromas
  - Subungual exostosis
    - Lesion deep to nailbed
  - Bizarre parosteal osteochondromatous proliferation (BPOP or Nora lesion)
    - Phalanges involved in 70% of cases
      - Middle phalanx is most common
      - Hands > > feet
    - Ossified pedunculated lesion attached to (but not flowing from) cortex
    - Most common in 20-30 year olds
    - May grow rapidly

Gross Pathologic & Surgical Features

- Lobulated cartilage cap with shiny bluish-gray surface
  - Thickness is typically on order of several mm but up to 2 cm is acceptable
    - > 2 cm in skeletally mature patient is more likely to harbor malignancy

CLINICAL ISSUES

Presentation

- Most common signs/symptoms
  - Hard painless mass with deformity
- Other signs/symptoms
  - Pain secondary to
    - Soft tissue friction or bursitis
    - Nerve or vessel compression
    - Fracture of exostosis stalk
    - Malignant transformation (uncommon in pediatrics)
      - Chondrosarcoma is most likely
  - Spinal cord compression from vertebral lesion
  - Hemo-/pneumothorax from rib lesion
  - Hip pain in HME can also be from labral or chondral injury or ischiofemoral impingement

Demographics

- Age
  - 10-35 years of age for solitary lesion
  - Most HME patients are diagnosed by age 10
- Epidemiology
  - Most common bone "tumor"
    - Solitary OC in 1-2% of population
    - Up to 15% of all bone tumors
    - Up to 50% of benign bone tumors

Natural History & Prognosis

- Lesion growth should cease at skeletal maturity
  - Spontaneous regression has been reported
- Continued growth suggests malignant transformation
  - Extremely rare in skeletally immature
  - Solitary exostosis lifetime risk: < 1%
  - HME lifetime risk: 5-11%

Treatment

- Surgical resection for symptomatic lesions or lesions growing beyond skeletal maturity
  - Entire cartilage cap & perichondrium must be removed to prevent recurrence
- Additional procedures are often required in HME to correct deformities

SELECTED REFERENCES

1. Iqbal A et al: Osteochondroma-induced pseudoaneurysms of the extremities mimicking sarcoma: a report of seven contemporary and one historical case. Clin Radiol. 75(8):642.e9-13, 2020
2. Jurik AG et al: Whole-body MRI in assessing malignant transformation in multiple hereditary exostoses and enchondromatosis: audit results and literature review. Skeletal Radiol. 49(1):115-24, 2020
3. Jackson TJ et al: Is Routine spine MRI necessary in skeletally immature patients with MHE? Identifying patients at risk for spinal osteochondromas. J Pediatr Orthop. 39(2):e147-52, 2019
4. Tsuda Y et al: Secondary chondrosarcoma arising from osteochondroma: outcomes and prognostic factors. Bone Joint J. 101-B(10):1313-20, 2019
5. Aiba H et al: Spontaneous shrinkage of solitary osteochondromas. Skeletal Radiol. 47(1):61-8, 2018
6. Degnan AJ et al: More than epiphyseal osteochondromas: updated understanding of imaging findings in dysplasia epiphysealis hemimelica (Trevor Disease). AJR Am J Roentgenol. 211(4):910-9, 2018
7. Duque Orozco MDP et al: Magnetic resonance imaging in symptomatic children with hereditary multiple exostoses of the hip. J Pediatr Orthop. 38(2):116-21, 2018
8. Kim HK et al: T2 relaxation time mapping of the cartilage cap of osteochondromas. Korean J Radiol. 17(1):159-65, 2016
9. Douis H et al: The imaging of cartilaginous bone tumours. I. Benign lesions. Skeletal Radiol. 41(10):1195-212, 2012
10. Murphey MD et al: Imaging of osteochondroma: variants and complications with radiologic-pathologic correlation. Radiographics. 20(5):1407-34, 2000

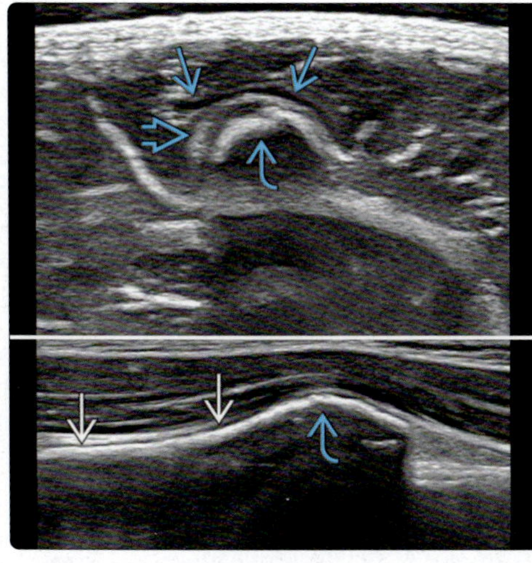

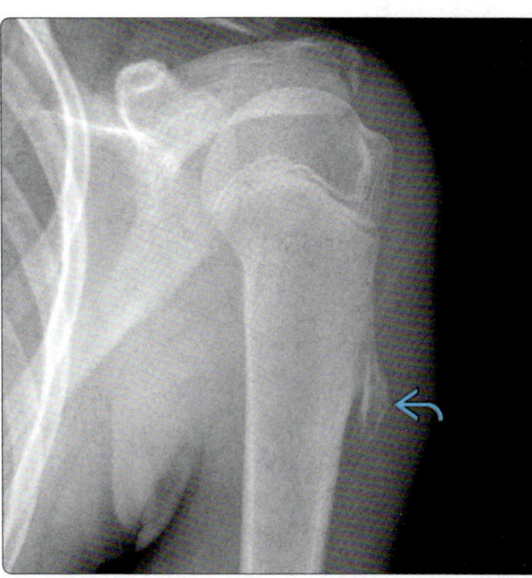

(Left) *Transverse (top) & longitudinal (bottom) ultrasounds in a 14-year-old with a hard bump for 3 years along the upper arm show flowing cortical continuity of the humerus ➡ to the osseous excrescence ➡. Note the overlying cartilage cap ➡ & small bursa ➡.* **(Right)** *External rotation radiograph in the same patient confirms the typical OC ➡ pointing away from the joint & demonstrating flowing corticomedullary continuity with the underlying bone.*

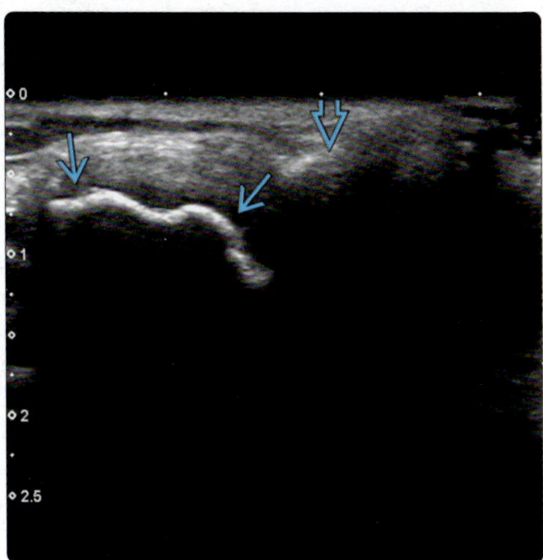

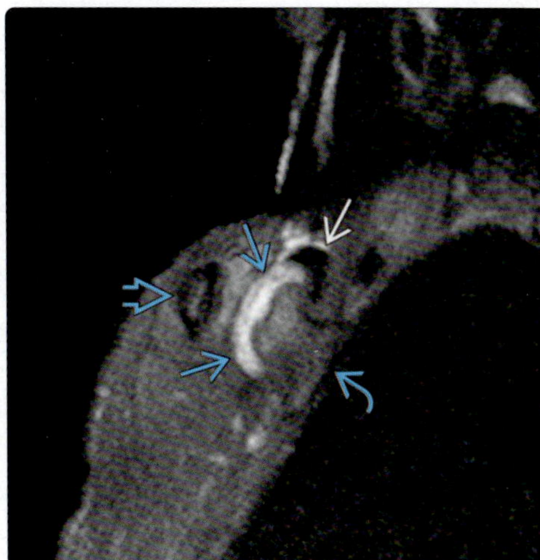

(Left) *Longitudinal ultrasound of the upper chest in a 10-year-old with a newly noted palpable mass shows a lobulated bony protuberance ➡ at the superior margin of the left clavicle ➡.* **(Right)** *Sagittal T2 FS MR in the same patient shows an OC protruding from the anterior 1st rib ➡ deep to the clavicle ➡. Note the hyperintense cartilage cap ➡ & deformation of the adjacent subclavian vein ➡.*

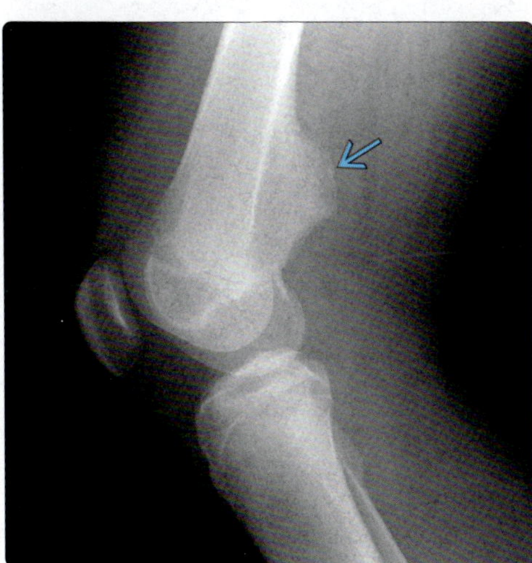

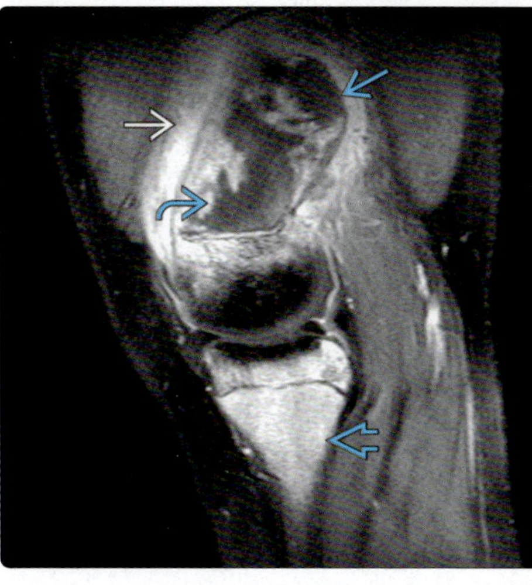

(Left) *Lateral radiograph of the right knee in a patient with recently diagnosed leukemia & subsequent onset of acute knee pain shows a sessile OC ➡ of the distal femur.* **(Right)** *Sagittal T1 C+ FS MR in the same patient shows homogeneous, diffusely abnormal marrow enhancement of the proximal tibia ➡ due to leukemic infiltration. Heterogeneous enhancement of the distal femoral marrow ➡ (with overlying soft tissue edema ➡) was due to superimposed acute infarction with extension into the OC ➡.*

Developmental Hip Dysplasia

KEY FACTS

TERMINOLOGY

- Developmental dysplasia of hip (DDH): Spectrum of hip abnormalities, including dysplastic acetabulum & femoral head malpositioning
- Risk factors: Female, 1st-born infant, breech positioning, oligohydramnios, White patients, family history, swaddling
- Ligamentous laxity contributes to DDH

IMAGING

- US is modality of choice for infants 1-4 months old
- Radiographs necessary after 4-5 months
  - Proximal femoral epiphysis ossifies, blocks ultrasound beam, limits evaluation

PATHOLOGY

- Normal
  - α angle ≥ 60°, coverage ≥ 50%, no instability
- Immature hip (applies only to infants < 3 months of age)
  - α angle 50-59°, coverage 45-50%, no instability
  - Small risk of delayed DDH; follow-up recommended to confirm normal development
- Mild hip dysplasia
  - α angle 50-59°, coverage 40-50%
  - May observe, repeat US in 1 month, especially if ≤ 2 months; older infants usually treated with harness
- Moderate hip dysplasia
  - α angle ≤ 50°, coverage ≤ 40%, any instability
  - Treated with harness; repeat US q4 weeks until normal
- Severe hip dysplasia
  - Grossly dysplastic acetabulum, dislocated hip
  - No improvement in harness by 4 weeks → operative management

CLINICAL ISSUES

- Treat with Pavlik harness to flex, abduct, & externally rotate hips
- Frequently repeat US to evaluate progression
- Occasionally surgical hip reduction & casting are required

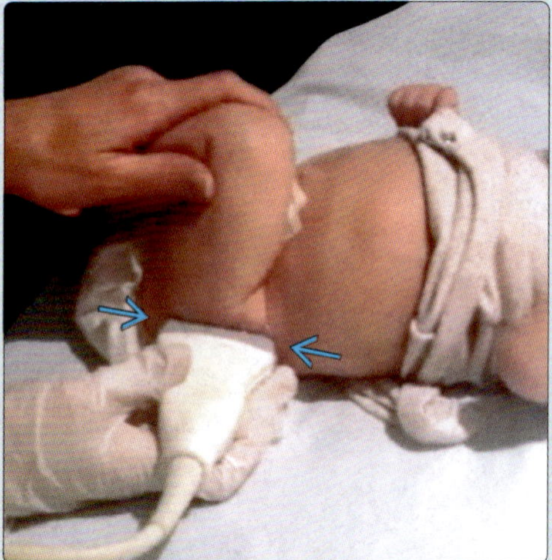

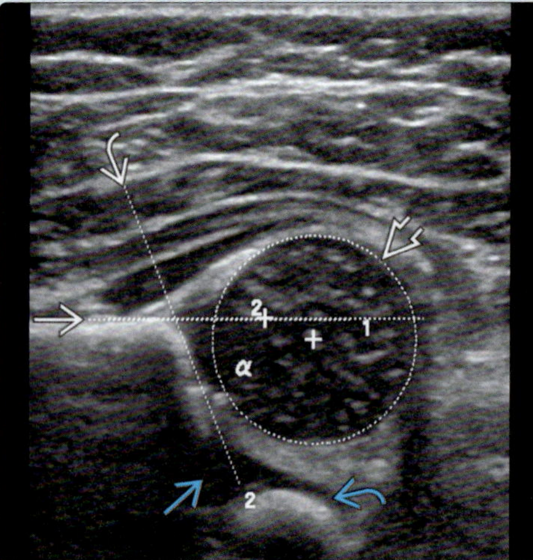

(Left) *The US transducer is placed over the lateral hip with slight posterior obliquity to obtain a coronal flexed image. Note the use of 2 hands (& the foot pedal to save images).* **(Right)** *Coronal flexed US in the same patient shows the unossified femoral head, the straight segment of the iliac bone, & a line drawn along the acetabular roof. The α angle is measured between these lines & should be ≥ 60°. The iliac line should cover the femoral head by ≥ 50%. Note the triradiate cartilage & ischium.*

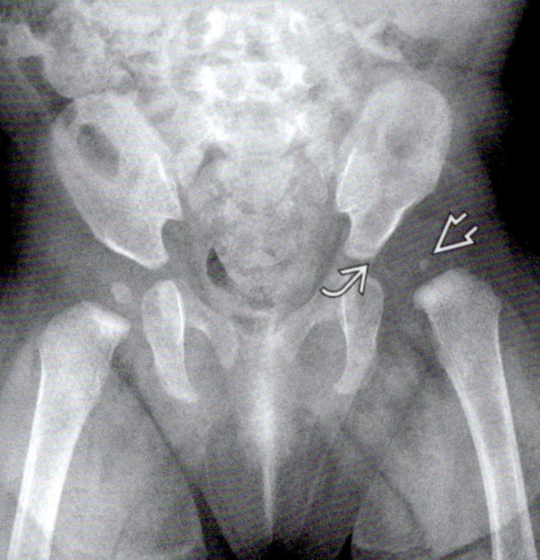

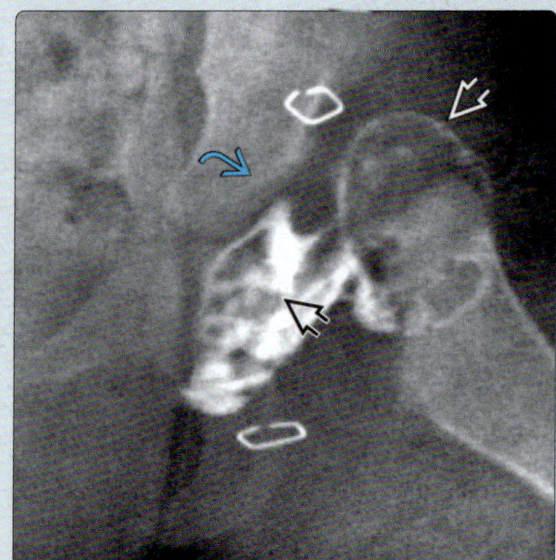

(Left) *Frontal radiograph in a 6-month-old boy with a left hip clunk reveals severe left developmental dysplasia of the hip. The acetabular roof is quite steep, & the ossified femoral head is small with superolateral dislocation.* **(Right)** *An intraoperative arthrogram shows contrast outlining a dysplastic, mostly unossified left femoral head. Note that the acetabular roof is quite steep. The femur is dislocated from the severely dysplastic & shallow joint space. This child required an osteotomy.*

TERMINOLOGY

Synonyms

- Congenital dislocation of hip (archaic)

Definitions

- Developmental dysplasia of hip (DDH): Spectrum of progressive hip abnormalities developing during infancy & resulting in acetabular dysplasia with femoral head malpositioning
  - Ranges from mild subluxation → dislocatable hip → fixed hip dislocation

IMAGING

General Features

- Best diagnostic clue
  - Abnormal position & delayed ossification of femoral head with abnormally steep & shallow acetabulum

Ultrasonographic Findings

- Grayscale ultrasound
  - Sonography directly visualizes cartilaginous & osseous components of hip
  - Static (anatomic) & stress (dynamic) imaging evaluates
    - Acetabular morphology
    - α angle (normal ≥ 60°)
    - Coverage of femoral head (normal ≥ 50%)
    - Dynamic subluxation during stress maneuvers
- Color Doppler
  - May be helpful in assessing femoral head perfusion, especially in patients abducted in Pavlik harness

Radiographic Findings

- Radiography
  - Hilgenreiner (horizontal) line
    - Drawn through bilateral triradiate cartilages
  - Perkin (perpendicular) line
    - Drawn from superolateral rim of acetabulum through line of Hilgenreiner
    - Should intersect lateral femoral metaphysis with femoral head mostly medial to line
      - Femoral head begins ossification by 3-6 months
  - Acetabular angle
    - Angle between line drawn along acetabular roof & Hilgenreiner line
      - Mathematically complementary to α angle of US
    - ↓ as hip matures
      - Normal < 30° in 1st year of life
      - Normal < 24° in 2nd year of life
  - Shenton line
    - Drawn along superior aspect of obturator foramen & medial femoral neck
    - Normally represents contiguous arc
    - If noncontiguous, suggests hip subluxation (DDH)

CT Findings

- NECT
  - Limited CT scans are sometimes performed to confirm hip position after open surgical reduction & spica casting

MR Findings

- Used only in difficult cases & casted/postoperative patients
  - Contrast may be used to look for ↓ femoral head perfusion

Nonvascular Interventions

- Arthrogram
  - Occasionally performed intraoperatively

Imaging Recommendations

- Best imaging tool
  - US is modality of choice for infants 1-4 months of age
    - Screening hip US is not recommended < 4 weeks of age due to presence of physiologic laxity
    - However, US should be performed early if clinical exam suggests dislocation or significant instability
  - Radiographs are necessary after 4-5 months
    - Proximal femoral epiphysis ossifies, blocks ultrasound beam, limits evaluation
- Protocol advice
  - Important to examine both hips
  - Careful US technique is mandatory; use high-frequency transducer (7-9 MHz), MSK settings, foot pedal
  - Coronal view
    - Infant at rest, in supine or lateral decubitus position
    - Transducer is parallel to lateral aspect of hip; may need to angle transducer 10-15° posteriorly into oblique coronal plane
    - Normal: α angle ≥ 60°, ≥ 50% femoral head coverage
    - Image should show
      - Straight segment of iliac wing
      - Center of femoral head (maximal diameter)
      - Deepest part of acetabulum (should see triradiate cartilage & ischium posteriorly)
  - Transverse flexion view
    - Infant's hip is held in 90° flexion
    - Place transducer over posterolateral hip in anatomic transverse plane
    - Image should show
      - Femoral metaphysis, femoral head, ischium (posterior acetabulum)
      - Femoral head should rest on ischium
    - Considered unstable if head slips or pistons beyond ischium on stress maneuvers
  - Posterior lip view
    - Stay in coronal flexed position, slide transducer posteriorly, remove 10-15° obliquity
    - Image should show
      - Ilium, ischium, & intervening triradiate cartilage: Posterior acetabular lip
      - Should **not** see femoral head
    - If normal, gently push thigh posterior to check stability
    - If subluxed, gently pull to determine if head can be easily reduced

DIFFERENTIAL DIAGNOSIS

Cerebral Palsy, Congenital Coxa Valga, Neuromuscular Disease

- Abnormal muscular tension causes subluxation/abnormal alignment

- Other radiographic findings of neuromuscular disease are often present
  - Gracile long bones, muscle wasting, coxa valga, "windswept pelvis"

Septic Arthritis

- Acute: Joint fluid may displace femoral head
  - Clinical/laboratory findings of infection are present
- Chronic: Abnormally small & misshapen femoral head & acetabulum

Proximal Focal Femoral Deficiency

- Rare congenital anomaly characterized by varying degrees of proximal femoral hypoplasia/aplasia; acetabulum may be normal

PATHOLOGY

General Features

- Etiology
  - Cartilaginous components on both sides of hip joint must be closely apposed to develop properly
  - DDH is likely multifactorial, includes ligamentous laxity
    - Effect of maternal hormones (especially relaxin)
    - Intrinsic acetabular/femoral head deficiency
    - Reduced in utero space
      - Breech position (extreme hip flexion, knee extension)
      - Oligohydramnios
      - 1st-born child or multiple gestation pregnancy
      - Large for gestational age, twins

Staging, Grading, & Classification

- Graf staging is based on single, static coronal image
- Most recommendations now include description of femoral head coverage & require stress imaging
- Simpler US classification includes normal, immature, & abnormal (with mild, moderate, severe modifier)
- Normal
  - Sometimes called Graf type 1
  - α angle ≥ 60°, coverage ≥ 50%
  - Requires no treatment
- Immature hip
  - Sometimes called Graf type 2a
  - Applies only to infants < 3 months of age
  - α angle 50-59°, coverage 45-50%
  - Small risk of delayed DDH
    - Recommend follow-up to confirm normal development
    - Requires no treatment
- Mild hip dysplasia
  - α angle 50-59°, coverage 40-50%
  - May be observed by orthopedists with repeat US in 1 month, especially if < 2 months of age
  - Older infants usually treated with harness
- Moderate hip dysplasia
  - α angle ≤ 50°, coverage ≤ 40%
  - Unstable on stress imaging or clinical exam
  - Treated with Pavlik harness with repeat US every 4 weeks until normal
- Severe hip dysplasia
  - Grossly dysplastic acetabulum with dislocated hip
  - Can treat with Pavlik harness for no more than 4 weeks
    - If no improvement in Pavlik harness by 4 weeks, continue to operative management

CLINICAL ISSUES

Presentation

- Most common signs/symptoms
  - Asymmetric skin or gluteal folds
  - Leg length discrepancy
  - Palpable click or clunk during stress maneuvers: Ortolani & Barlow
- Other signs/symptoms
  - Delayed ambulation or limp in toddlers

Demographics

- Sex
  - M:F = 1:5-8
- Epidemiology
  - Incidence: 2-20 per 1,000 births

Natural History & Prognosis

- Mild hip dysplasia may resolve spontaneously & never cause clinical problems
  - 60-80% of abnormalities found by clinical exam resolve spontaneously
  - 90% of abnormalities found by US resolve spontaneously
- Moderate or severe dysplasia can cause long-term disability, limb shortening, ↓ range of motion, degenerative change, avascular necrosis
  - Some patients may eventually require hip replacement
- Excellent prognosis when diagnosed & treated early with Pavlik harness
- Some authors recommend follow-up radiographs at 6 months for breech presentation, even after normal screening US
- Delayed diagnosis or treatment can result in irreversible dysplasia requiring iliac osteotomy/shelving procedure

Treatment

- Pavlik harness to flex, abduct, & externally rotate hips
  - Increases femoral head engagement with acetabulum
  - Overabduction can cause femoral head ischemia
- Occasionally, surgical hip reduction & casting are required
  - Salter osteotomy, Steele triple osteotomy, Pemberton or Chiari procedure, femoral osteotomy

SELECTED REFERENCES

1. Nguyen JC et al: Developmental dysplasia of the hip: can contrast-enhanced MRI predict the development of avascular necrosis following surgery? Skeletal Radiol. 50(2):389-97, 2021
2. Harsanyi S et al: Developmental dysplasia of the hip: a review of etiopathogenesis, risk factors, and genetic aspects. Medicina (Kaunas). 56(4), 2020
3. Barrera CA et al: Imaging of developmental dysplasia of the hip: ultrasound, radiography and magnetic resonance imaging. Pediatr Radiol. 49(12):1652-68, 2019
4. Gkiatas I et al: Developmental dysplasia of the hip: a systematic literature review of the genes related with its occurrence. EFORT Open Rev. 4(10):595-601, 2019
5. Louer CR et al: Should paediatricians initiate orthopaedic hip dysplasia referrals for infants with isolated asymmetric skin folds? J Child Orthop. 13(6):593-9, 2019
6. Vaquero-Picado A et al: Developmental dysplasia of the hip: update of management. EFORT Open Rev. 4(9):548-56, 2019

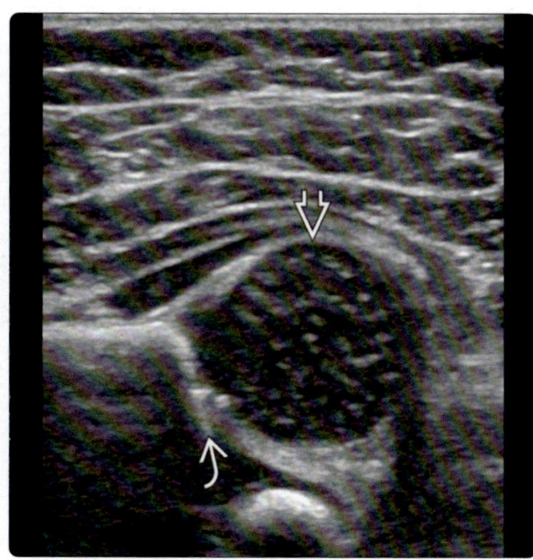

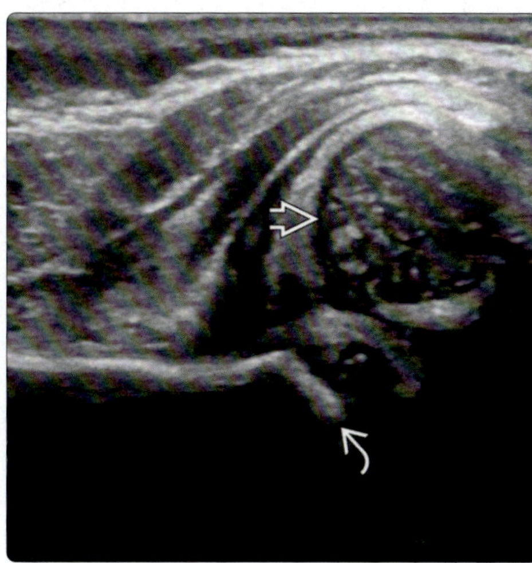

(Left) *Coronal flexed US of a normal right hip shows ≥ 50% coverage of the unossified femoral head ➡. The acetabular roof ➡ is normal with an a angle ≥ 60° (measurement not shown).* **(Right)** *Similar image of the left hip in the same patient shows dislocation of the femoral head ➡ & a steep acetabular roof ➡ (with an a angle of 40°). As is customary, the image is rotated 90° counterclockwise from the anatomic position, so a radiographically steep acetabular roof appears as a "shallow" angle on US.*

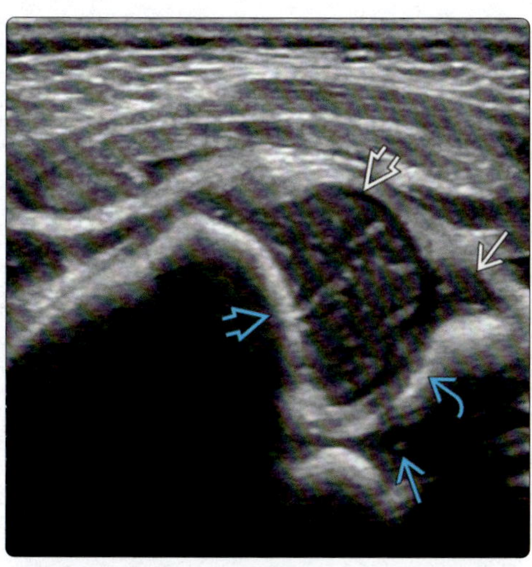

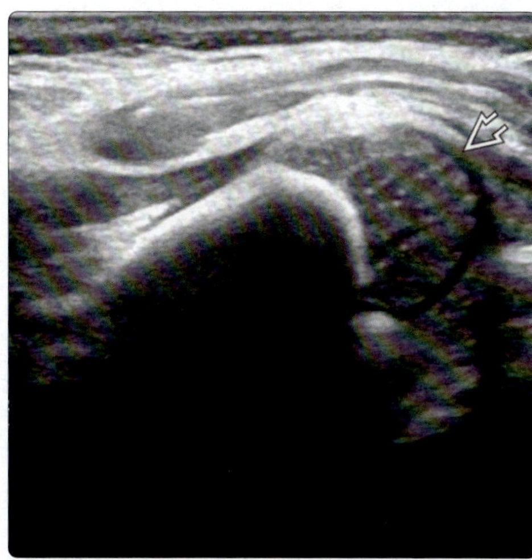

(Left) *Transverse flexed stress view shows a normal, stable right hip. Note how the femoral metaphysis ➡, triradiate cartilage ➡, & ischium ➡ form a U-shaped concavity in which the unossified femoral head ➡ rests. Even with stress, a stable hip will remain resting against the ischium & posterior labrum ➡.* **(Right)** *In contradistinction, the unstable left hip (in the same patient) is dislocated on this transverse flexed stress view. The femoral head ➡ lies posterior & lateral, no longer resting in a U-shaped concavity.*

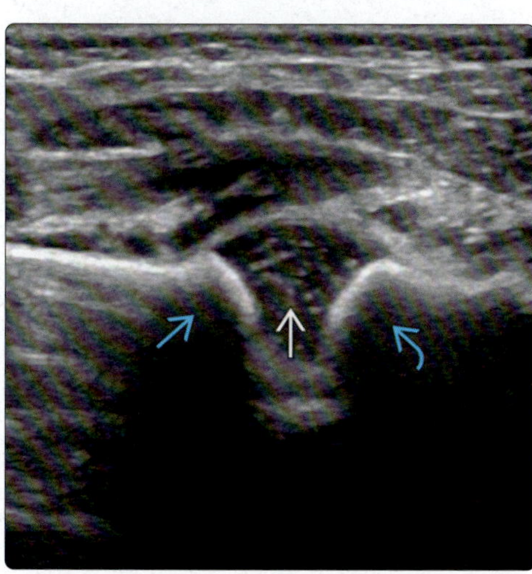

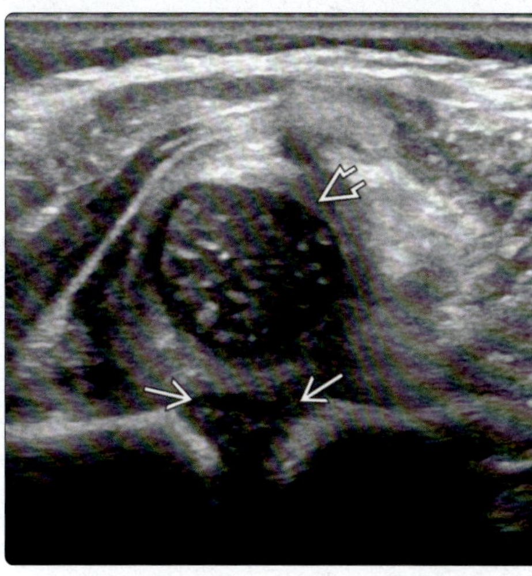

(Left) *The posterior lip US view is useful to determine stability but is often misunderstood. The unossified cartilage ➡ between the iliac bone ➡ & ischium ➡ is actually the posterior lip of the acetabulum, not the femoral head. If a hip is unstable, the femoral head will be seen rising over the convex margin of the acetabular cartilage with stress.* **(Right)** *In this already dislocated hip, the femoral head ➡ is seen just above (posterior & lateral) the posterior lip of the acetabulum ➡.*

Proximal Focal Femoral Deficiency

KEY FACTS

TERMINOLOGY

- Proximal femoral focal deficiency: Malformation in which complete growth & development of upper femur fails to occur

IMAGING

- Often difficult to classify with radiographs at early age (due to delayed ossification)
- Can classify earlier with MR

PATHOLOGY

- Aitken classification
  - Class A (38%)
    - Femoral head is present, & acetabulum is normal
    - All parts of femur are connected by bone
    - Subtrochanteric varus is common
  - Class B (32%)
    - Femoral head is present within acetabulum; acetabulum is adequate or moderately dysplastic
    - Bone does not connect femoral head & shaft
    - Pseudoarthrosis is often present but does not heal at skeletal maturity
  - Class C (17%)
    - Femoral head is absent or represented by ossicle
    - Femur tapers proximally
    - Acetabulum is severely dysplastic
  - Class D (13%)
    - Both femoral head & acetabulum are absent
    - Distal femoral segment is shortened & deformed
    - Obturator foramen of pelvis is enlarged
- Associations: Ipsilateral fibular hemimelia in ~ 50%, unstable knee, tarsal coalition, ↓ number of foot rays; abnormal contralateral extremity in 26%

CLINICAL ISSUES

- 4 major biomechanical problems: Hip instability, malrotation of thigh with flexed knee, deficient proximal musculature, & leg length discrepancy

(Left) *AP radiograph in a 6-month-old shows bilateral (right worse than left) proximal femoral focal deficiency (PFFD). Note the right-sided fibular hemimelia, anterior tibial bowing, 4 rays of the right foot, & severely dysplastic acetabulum.* **(Right)** *AP radiograph in a 2-year-old shows a short right femur with small right femoral head ossification center ➡ & developing proximal femoral pseudoarthrosis ➡. This is best classified as Aitken class B.*

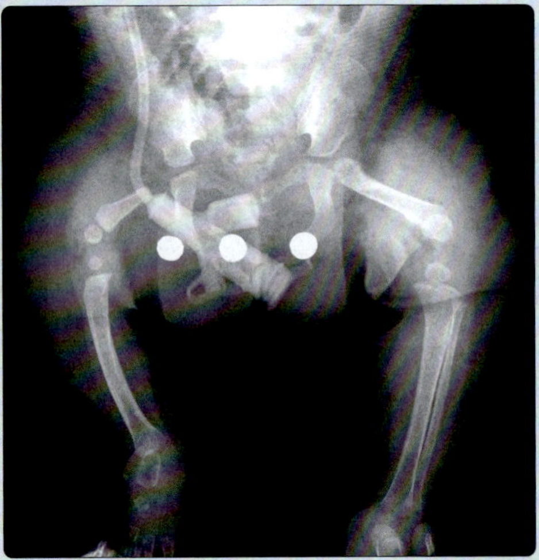

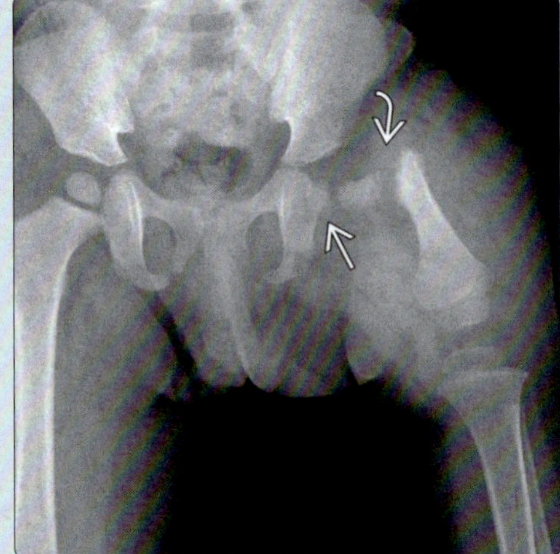

(Left) *AP radiograph in a 4-month-old shows bilateral tiny femoral head ossification centers ➡ with left worse than right PFFD changes.* **(Right)** *Coronal T2 FS MR in the same child at 20 months of age shows no connection of the right femoral head ➡ to the remainder of the femur. There is continuity of the left femoral head & neck, which eventually developed pseudoarthrosis 1 year later (not shown), effectively making this bilateral Aitken class B.*

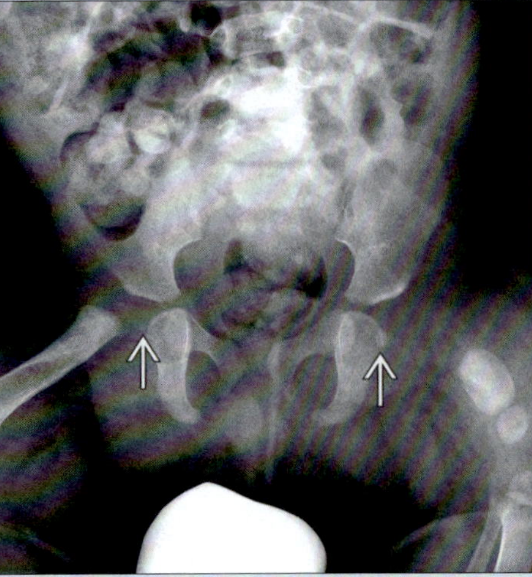

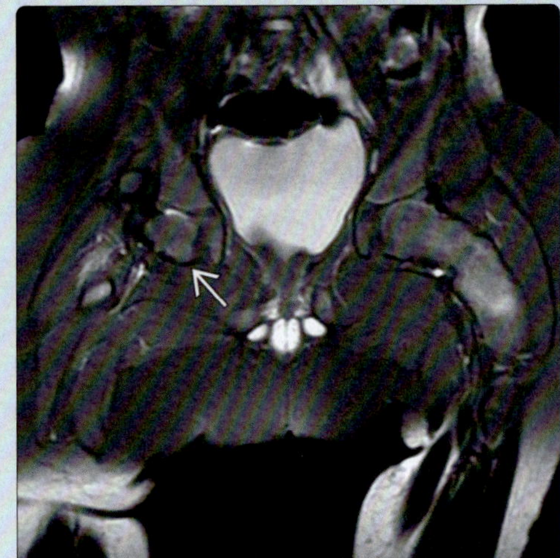

TERMINOLOGY

Abbreviations

- Proximal femoral focal deficiency (PFFD)

Definitions

- Malformation in which complete growth & development of upper femur fails to occur
- Spectrum ranging from mild shortening & varus deformity of otherwise normal femur to absence of all but distal femur
- Accompanied by varying degrees of acetabular dysplasia, thigh muscular hypoplasia, fibular & foot maldevelopment, & shortened lower extremity length

IMAGING

Radiographic Findings

- At 2 years of age, radiographs are more accurate in classifying Aitken type
- Pelvis
  - Obturator foramen: Enlarged
  - Acetabulum: Supraacetabular bump of Court, horizontal or small/shallow/dysplastic roof
  - If detached femoral head is fixed in acetabulum, then supraacetabular bump, enlarged obturator foramen, horizontal acetabular roof, & pencil-pointing of upper end of detached distal femur are common
- Femur
  - Short femur; delayed appearance or nonappearance of femoral capital ossification center
    - Average age of appearance in PFFD is 25 months vs. 3-6 months in normal patients
  - Misshapen femoral head & neck, coxa vara
  - Upper end of disconnected distal femur: Either bulbous or pencil-pointed

MR Findings

- Shows cartilage structure of acetabulum & upper femur in infants to assist prognosis & treatment planning
  - More accurate than radiographic evaluation for classification of PFFD
    - Radiographs tend to overestimate degree of deficiency prior to complete ossification of cartilaginous femur
- Presence or absence of unossified femoral head & neck & their degree of connection to shaft can be identified
- Hip joint poorly forms when femoral head is fixed in acetabulum
- Sartorius muscle is enlarged, which may explain flexion, abduction, & external rotation of hip

PATHOLOGY

General Features

- Etiology
  - Embryology
    - Developmental insult: PFFD occurs at 4-6 weeks during limb bud formation, growth, & differentiation
    - Acetabulum & proximal femur develop from common anlage in embryo
- Associated abnormalities
  - Ipsilateral fibular hemimelia (absence) in ~ 50%
  - Knee is often unstable & may dislocate
    - Absent or hypoplastic cruciate ligaments & menisci
  - Ball-&-socket ankle, clubfoot, tarsal coalition, ↓ number of foot rays
  - Abnormal contralateral extremity in 26%

Staging, Grading, & Classification

- Goals: Predict limb function & treatment planning
- Aitken classification (1968)
  - Class A (38%): Femoral head is present, & acetabulum is normal; short femur with all parts of femur connected by bone; subtrochanteric varus is common
  - Class B (32%): Femoral head is present within acetabulum, & acetabulum is adequate or moderately dysplastic; bone does not connect femoral head & shaft
  - Class C (17%): Femoral head is absent or represented by ossicle; acetabulum is severely dysplastic
  - Class D (13%): Both femoral head & acetabulum are absent; distal femoral segment is shortened & deformed; obturator foramen of pelvis is enlarged

CLINICAL ISSUES

Demographics

- Epidemiology
  - Incidence: 1.1-2 per 100,000 live births
  - Bilateral PFFD in 10-15%, often Aitken class D

Treatment

- 4 major biomechanical problems
  - Hip instability, malrotation of thigh with flexed knee, poor development of proximal musculature, & leg length discrepancy
- Treatment is highly individualized; options include (when PFFD is unilateral): Prosthesis, limb lengthening, hip reconstruction, Van Ness rotationplasty, & Syme amputation
- Bilateral PFFD: Most ambulate well on shortened legs
  - Usually not treated surgically without severe foot deformities
  - Children ambulate at home without prostheses; prostheses may be used in social settings to achieve stature closer to that of peers

DIAGNOSTIC CHECKLIST

Image Interpretation Pearls

- If radiographs show normal acetabulum at birth, normal cartilaginous femoral head is likely

SELECTED REFERENCES

1. Uduma FU et al: Proximal femoral focal deficiency - a rare congenital entity: two case reports and a review of the literature. J Med Case Rep. 14(1):27, 2020
2. D'Ambrosio V et al: Prenatal diagnosis of proximal focal femoral deficiency: literature review of prenatal sonographic findings. J Clin Ultrasound. 44(4):252-9, 2016
3. Bedoya MA et al: Common patterns of congenital lower extremity shortening: diagnosis, classification, and follow-up. Radiographics. 35(4):1191-207, 2015
4. Bergère A et al: Imaging features of lower limb malformations above the foot. Diagn Interv Imaging. 96(9):901-14, 2015
5. Biko DM et al: Proximal focal femoral deficiency: evaluation by MR imaging. Pediatr Radiol. 42(1):50-6, 2012

Legg-Calvé-Perthes Disease

KEY FACTS

TERMINOLOGY

- Symptomatic growth disturbance of capital femoral epiphysis due to idiopathic osteonecrosis

IMAGING

- Radiographic flattening & fragmentation of sclerotic capital femoral epiphysis ± "cystic" metaphyseal changes
- ↓ perfusion of femoral head acutely
  - Photopenia on nuclear medicine bone scan
  - ↓ enhancement on MR: Sagittal plane detects early anterior involvement
- Gradual coxa magna, coxa plana, & coxa brevis with femoral head extrusion, femoroacetabular impingement, labral tears, joint degeneration

TOP DIFFERENTIAL DIAGNOSES

- Septic arthritis
- Transient synovitis
- Juvenile idiopathic arthritis
- Slipped capital femoral epiphysis
- Epiphyseal dysplasias

CLINICAL ISSUES

- Limp due to groin, thigh, or referred knee pain
- Age: 4-12 years; peak: 4-8 years
- 10-20% bilateral, usually asynchronous
- Worse prognosis: > 8 years old at onset, greater femoral head + lateral pillar involvement, subchondral fracture, metaphyseal changes, physeal arrest, aspherical femoral head with joint incongruence
- Surgical interventions: Femoral head containment with joint congruence is key to maintaining femoral head shape & preventing accelerated joint degeneration

DIAGNOSTIC CHECKLIST

- Anterior femoral head is most frequently affected: Include sagittal MR plane
- Subtracted pre- from postcontrast T1 FS: Most sensitive MR sequence for acute ischemia & revascularization

(Left) *AP radiograph in a 10-year-old boy with left hip pain shows flattening, broadening, & sclerosis of the left femoral head ➡. The left hip joint is widened, & the acetabular roof is flattened. The femoral neck is short & broad with a lateral metaphyseal lucency ⮫.* **(Right)** *Frog leg lateral radiograph in the same patient shows similar left hip findings with better definition of the cystic-appearing femoral neck lucency ⮫. The constellation of findings is typical for Legg-Calvé-Perthes (LCP) disease.*

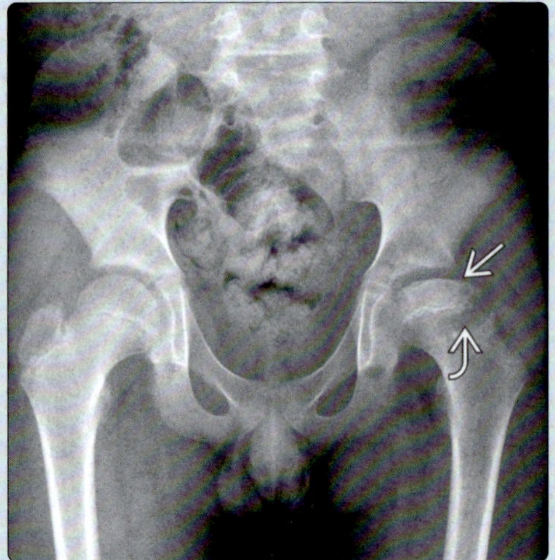

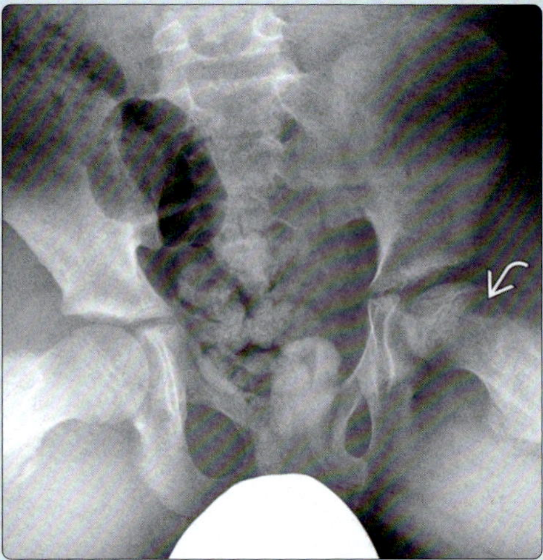

(Left) *Coronal T2 FS MR in the same patient shows fluid ➡ within a subchondral fracture of the flattened & hypointense left femoral head. There is hyperintense marrow edema ➡ in the femoral neck with an adjacent joint effusion ⮫.* **(Right)** *Subtracted T1 C+ FS MR in the same patient shows no enhancement of ~ 80% of the left femoral head ➡ (as compared to the normal right) with the medial ~ 20% showing hyperenhancement ➡. Adjacent reactive synovitis ⮫ is noted.*

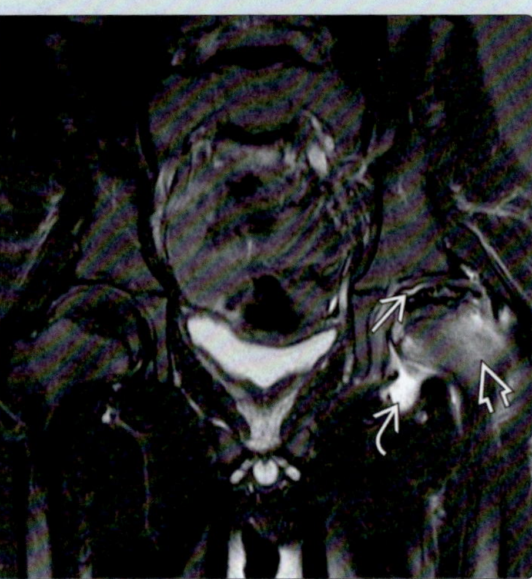

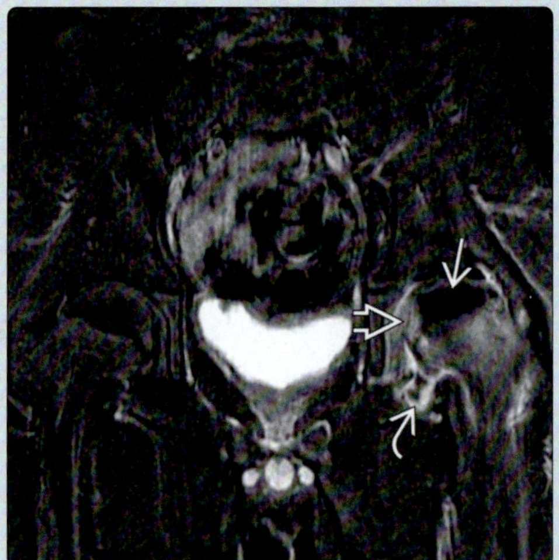

TERMINOLOGY

Abbreviations

- Legg-Calvé-Perthes (LCP) disease

Synonyms

- Legg-Perthes or Perthes disease
- Juvenile idiopathic osteonecrosis

Definitions

- Idiopathic osteonecrosis of femoral head in children

IMAGING

General Features

- Best diagnostic clue
  - Sclerosis, fragmentation, & flattening of capital femoral epiphysis in child 4-8 years old
  - ↓ perfusion of femoral head (earliest stage) in otherwise healthy child with pain
    - Photopenia on Tc-99m nuclear medicine bone scan
    - ↓ enhancement on MR
- Morphology
  - Proximal femoral configuration depends on extent & severity of involvement & timing of imaging

Radiographic Findings

- Radiography
  - Does not depict earliest stages of insult or repair
  - Active early: Sclerosis, subchondral fracture (lucency), early fragmentation of femoral head
  - Active late: Late fragmentation (± reossification) with flattening (asphericity), extrusion of femoral head, metaphyseal irregularity or "cystic" change
    - Hinge abduction: Medial joint space widening with abnormal lateral femoral head rotating on superolateral acetabular rim
  - Healed: Reossification completed with absence of sclerotic avascular bone
    - Coxa magna (enlarged femoral head), coxa plana (flattened), coxa irregularis (irregular), coxa brevis (short neck, greater trochanter overgrowth), hip joint incongruence
  - Waldenström classification: Radiographic reflection of LCP natural evolution; developed in 1922
    - Initial/necrotic stage (lasts 6 months to 1 year)
    - Fragmentation stage (lasts 2-3 years)
    - Reparative/healing/reossification stage (lasts 1-2 years)
    - Growing/remodeling stage (changes up to skeletal maturity)
    - Definite stage (final shape with congruent or incongruent joint)

MR Findings

- T1WI
  - Patchy hypointensity replacing fatty marrow signal due to necrosis
  - Returning fatty marrow signal intensity with revascularization
- T2WI FS
  - Patchy femoral head ↑ signal (edema) or ↓ signal (sclerosis)
  - Hyperintense joint effusion & synovitis
- T2* GRE
  - Cartilage & osteochondral disturbances: Epiphyseal thickening, metaphyseal abnormalities, physeal bone bridge, articular surface degeneration
- DWI
  - Restricted diffusion immediately after ischemic event
  - Days to hours after event: ↑ diffusion & ADC values
- T1WI C+ FS
  - Acute ischemia: ↓ enhancement
    - Subtraction of unenhanced T1 FS from T1 C+ FS (perfusion): Earliest detection/extent assessment
    - Sagittal images show early anterior involvement
  - Adjacent marrow edema, synovitis: ↑ enhancement
  - Revascularized bone: ↑ enhancement
    - Improved prognosis with lateral pillar perfusion; may predict radiographic maintenance of lateral pillar
- MR arthrogram
  - Long-term sequelae include joint degeneration & femoroacetabular impingement with labral tears
- Advanced techniques
  - Delayed gadolinium enhancement, T1rho, & T2 mapping detect cartilage degeneration prior to conventional sequences

Ultrasonographic Findings

- Some studies propose using ultrasound to evaluate femoral head lateral containment

Nuclear Medicine Findings

- Bone scintigraphy
  - Photopenia from ischemia
    - In correct clinical setting, associated joint effusion must be sampled to exclude septic arthritis
  - ↑ uptake with revascularization

Imaging Recommendations

- Best imaging tool
  - MR or nuclear medicine bone scan for early changes of ischemia & revascularization
    - MR better delineates location of involvement
- Protocol advice
  - MR: FS postcontrast images are key
    - Subtraction is most helpful (perfusion)
    - Sagittal plane is most sensitive for early changes
    - Specific thresholds of ↓ enhancement & ↑ ADC values may predict worse outcomes
  - Nuclear medicine bone scan: Pinhole hip images

DIFFERENTIAL DIAGNOSIS

Septic Arthritis

- Fever, leukocytosis, ↑ erythrocyte sedimentation rate
- Hip held in flexion, abduction, external rotation
- Joint effusion ± marrow edema
  - Reduced perfusion of femoral head due to large effusion
- May yield long-term ossific abnormalities or joint destruction

Transient Synovitis

- Self-limited acute synovitis in ages 3-10 years
- Significant effusion & capsular distention

- No long-term femoral head changes

Juvenile Idiopathic Arthritis

- Synovitis predominates over bone findings early
- ± rice bodies in joint fluid

Slipped Capital Femoral Epiphysis

- Posterior, medial displacement of femoral head
- Older patients (age 10-15 years), often obese

Osteoid Osteoma

- Local pain worse at night, ↓ by salicylates
- Uncommonly epiphyseal; more commonly in femoral neck
- May have sclerosis, marrow/soft tissue edema, effusion

Juvenile Osteonecrosis

- Osteonecrosis due to known cause: Sickle cell anemia, steroids, Gaucher, after hip dislocation

Epiphyseal Dysplasias

- Multifocal: Spondyloepiphyseal & multiple epiphyseal dysplasias
- Limited to hips: Meyer dysplasia
  - Age 2-4 years, bilateral in 60%, asymptomatic

Juvenile Idiopathic Chondrolysis

- Band area of ↑ T2 signal/enhancement in central femoral head
- Often has adjacent ill-defined acetabular marrow edema
- ± mild synovitis & minimal effusion

PATHOLOGY

Staging, Grading, & Classification

- Prognostic staging during radiographic evolution
  - Catterall classification (originated in 1971; 1st widely used system): Based on extent of epiphyseal involvement
  - Salter-Thompson scheme (originated in 1984): Based on extent of subchondral fracture
  - Herring system (originated in 1992): Based on lateral pillar (lateral 1/3 of femoral head) involvement by AP view
    - Most reliable, reproducible
- Prognostic staging of final morphology at maturity
  - Stulberg classification based on shape & congruency of femoral head
- Radiographic systems may miss window of opportunity for intervention while waiting to predict outcomes at (or beyond) midfragmentation stage; perfusion MR allows assessment during initial stage

CLINICAL ISSUES

Presentation

- Most common signs/symptoms
  - Limping with groin, thigh, or referred knee pain
- Clinical profile
  - No specific history of trauma
  - ↓ range of motion with loss of abduction & internal rotation

Demographics

- Age
  - 4-12 years; peak: 4-8 years
- Sex
  - M:F = 4-5:1
- Epidemiology
  - Prevalence: 0.4 to 29/100,000 in children < 15 years old
  - 10-20% bilateral, usually asynchronous

Natural History & Prognosis

- Worse prognosis
  - > 8 years old at onset
  - Greater extent of femoral head involvement
  - Necrosis/height loss of lateral pillar
  - Subchondral fracture
  - Metaphyseal changes
  - Premature physeal closure
  - Aspherical femoral head
  - Lateral subluxation with joint incongruence
- 21-77% with premature physeal closure at hip
  - 3.5 years earlier than unaffected side
  - High percentage develop limb length discrepancy > 1 cm

Treatment

- Conservative
  - Bed rest, abduction stretching, bracing
  - Best nonoperative outcomes in patients < 6 years old
- Surgical
  - Femoral/pelvic osteotomies, shelf acetabuloplasty
    - Femoral head containment with joint congruence is key to maintaining femoral head shape & preventing accelerated joint degeneration
  - Greater trochanter epiphysiodesis to prevent overgrowth with abnormal gait & instability

DIAGNOSTIC CHECKLIST

Consider

- MR & nuclear medicine bone scan detect early ischemia & revascularization
- Anterior femoral head is most frequently affected → include sagittal MR plane

SELECTED REFERENCES

1. Chong DY et al: Reliability and validity of visual estimation of femoral head hypoperfusion on perfusion MRI in Legg-Calve-Perthes disease. J Pediatr Orthop. 41(9):e780-6, 2021
2. Jones CE et al: T1ρ and T2 MRI show hip cartilage damage in adolescents with healed Legg-Calvé-Perthes disease. J Pediatr Orthop B. ePub, 2021
3. Tis JE et al: Reproducibility of radiographic measurements made in the active stages of Legg-Calvé-Perthes disease: evaluation of a prognostic indicator and an interim outcome measure. J Pediatr Orthop. 41(2):93-8, 2021
4. Pavone V et al: Aetiology of Legg-Calvé-Perthes disease: a systematic review. World J Orthop. 10(3):145-65, 2019
5. Jandl NM et al: MRI and sonography in Legg-Calvé-Perthes disease: clinical relevance of containment and influence on treatment. J Child Orthop. 12(5):472-9, 2018
6. Yoo WJ et al: Risk factors for femoral head deformity in the early stage of Legg-Calvé-Perthes disease: MR contrast enhancement and diffusion indexes. Radiology. 279(2):562-70, 2016
7. Heesakkers N et al: The long-term prognosis of Legg-Calvé-Perthes disease: a historical prospective study with a median follow-up of forty one years. Int Orthop. 39(5):859-63, 2015
8. Accadbled F et al: "Femoroacetabular impingement". Legg-Calve-Perthes disease: from childhood to adulthood. Orthop Traumatol Surg Res. 100(6):647-9, 2014
9. Mazloumi SM et al: Evolution in diagnosis and treatment of Legg-Calve-Perthes disease. Arch Bone Jt Surg. 2(2):86-92, 2014

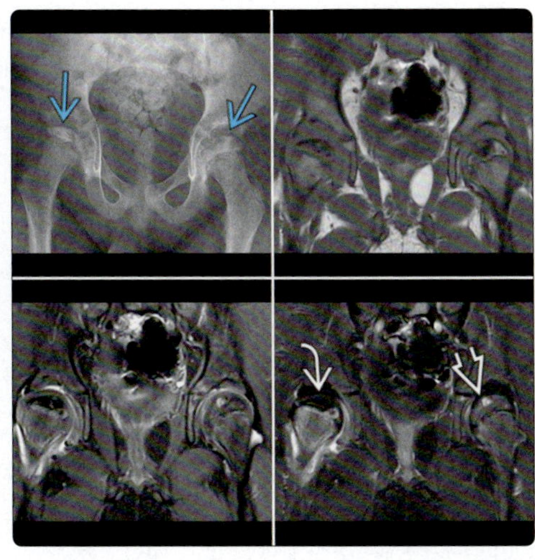

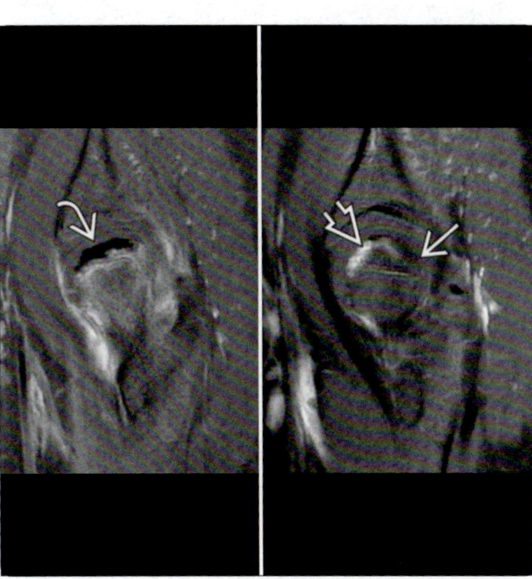

(Left) *Images (clockwise from upper left: AP radiograph, coronal T1, subtracted T1 C+ FS, & T2 FS MR) in an 8-year-old boy show bilateral LCP with regions of bilateral femoral head sclerosis ➡. Most of the right femoral head is of low signal intensity on all sequences & is nonenhancing ➡. Note the focal hyperenhancement ➡ of the left femoral head.* **(Right)** *Sagittal T1 C+ FS MR from the same exam shows the nonenhancement (necrosis) of the right femoral head ➡ vs. left hyper-(revascularization) ➡ & normal ➡ enhancement.*

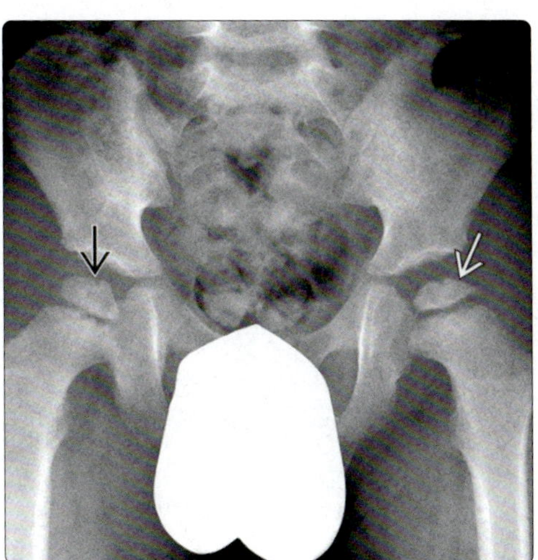

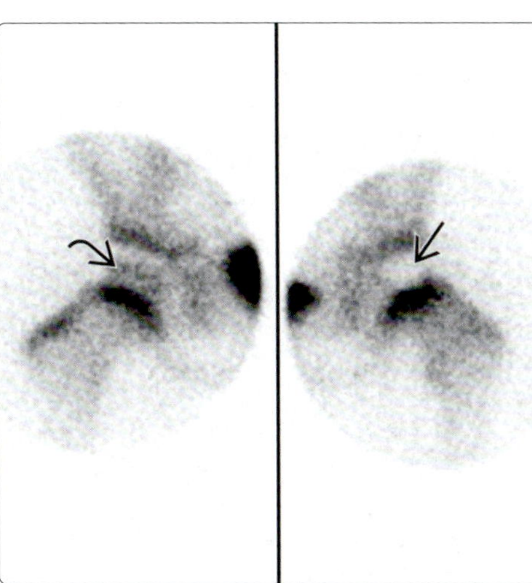

(Left) *AP radiograph in a 4-year-old boy with left hip pain shows left femoral head flattening & sclerosis ➡, consistent with LCP. Note the central femoral notch ➡ in the otherwise normal right femoral head, a normal variant.* **(Right)** *Pinhole images from a Tc-99m MDP bone scan show ↓ radiotracer uptake in the left femoral head ➡ as compared to the normal right side ➡, consistent with ischemia.*

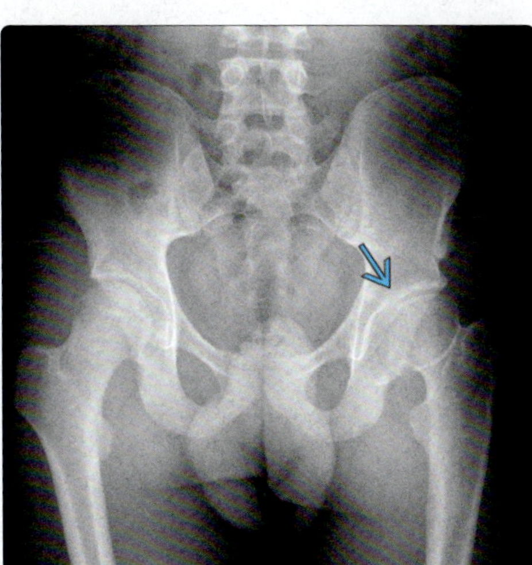

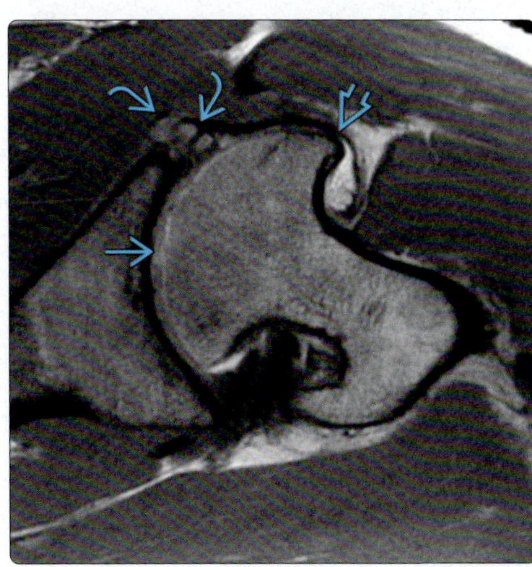

(Left) *AP radiograph in an 18-year-old with a history of left hip LCP & chronic pain shows a dysplastic left acetabulum ➡ with coxa magna, plana, & breva of the proximal femur.* **(Right)** *Axial oblique PD MR arthrogram in the same patient shows chronic LCP findings of coxa magna, plana, & breva with an anterior femoral head protuberance ➡ that is causing femoroacetabular impingement. The anterior superior labrum is torn & replaced by para- & intralabral cysts ➡. Articular cartilage degeneration is noted ➡.*

Slipped Capital Femoral Epiphysis

KEY FACTS

TERMINOLOGY

- SCFE: Salter-Harris I fracture of subcapital femoral physis due to chronic stress of weight bearing
  - Femoral head slips posterior & medial to metaphysis

IMAGING

- AP view: Subcapital femoral physis is abnormally smooth, lucent, & elongated ("wide")
  - Visible before medial femoral head displacement
- Frog leg lateral view (essential for diagnosis): Posterior displacement of femoral head relative to metaphysis
  - Femoral head-neck angle for severity assessment
- CT/MR more accurately determine severity of slip
- MR is more sensitive than radiographs for diagnosis & complications
  - "Preslip" physeal elongation ("widening") on T1
  - ± marrow edema, synovitis with slip on T2 FS/STIR
  - Long term: Femoroacetabular impingement, labral tear, articular cartilage damage, osteonecrosis (ON)
- Incidence of bilateral SCFE varies widely: 18-80%
  - At initial presentation: 9-22%
  - Contralateral slip usually occurs in 18 months

CLINICAL ISSUES

- Limp, pain, limited motion; symptoms are often mild for weeks with acute worsening
  - Pain in hip, groin, or proximal thigh in 85%
  - Distal thigh or knee pain in 15%
- Girls average 11-12 years, boys average 13-14 years
- Major predisposing factor: Obesity
- Prognosis is poorer for unstable (unable to bear weight) SCFE: ↑ ON risk
- Most common treatments
  - Percutaneous single screw in situ fixation without femoral head manipulation (stable & mild unstable SCFE)
  - Open surgical hip dislocation with capital realignment (↑ use in moderate & severe unstable SCFE)
  - Prophylactic contralateral fixation is controversial

(Left) *AP radiograph in an obese 10-year-old girl with left hip pain shows intersection of the lateral right femoral head ➡ by the line of Klein (normal). Such a line would not intersect the slipped left femoral head ➡. A normal continuous Shenton arc can be drawn on the right ➡ but not the left ➡.* **(Right)** *Axial (top left) & coronal (bottom left) 2D & posterior (bottom right) & anterior (top right) 3D surface-rendered CT images in a 12-year-old show a chronic SCFE with a posteromedial slip of the right femoral head ➡ relative to the neck ➡.*

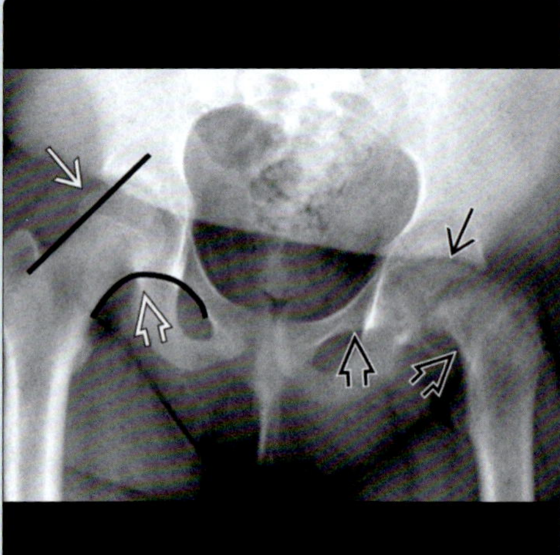

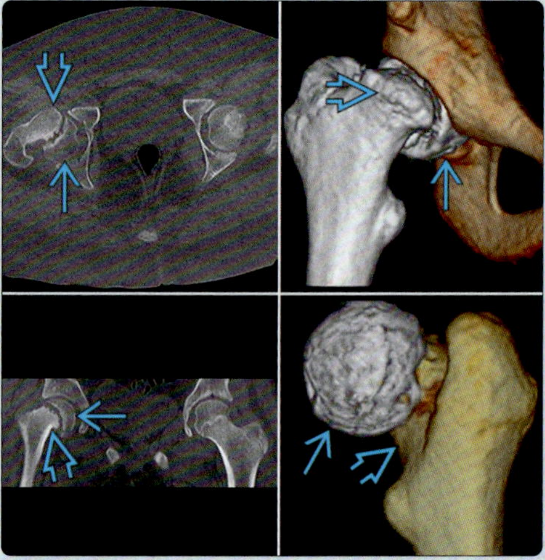

(Left) *AP (top) & frog leg lateral (bottom) radiographs in an obese 12-year-old patient with right hip pain show an abnormally smooth & lucent right subcapital physis ➡ with offset of the femoral head-neck junction ➡, consistent with a SCFE.* **(Right)** *Follow-up radiographs 1 month later in the same patient status post right SCFE pinning demonstrate interval development of an abnormally smooth & lucent left subcapital physis ➡ with mild head-neck offset on the frog leg lateral view ➡, consistent with a left SCFE.*

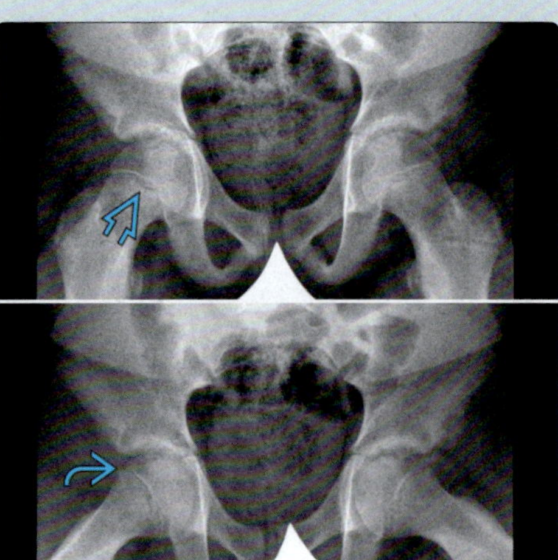

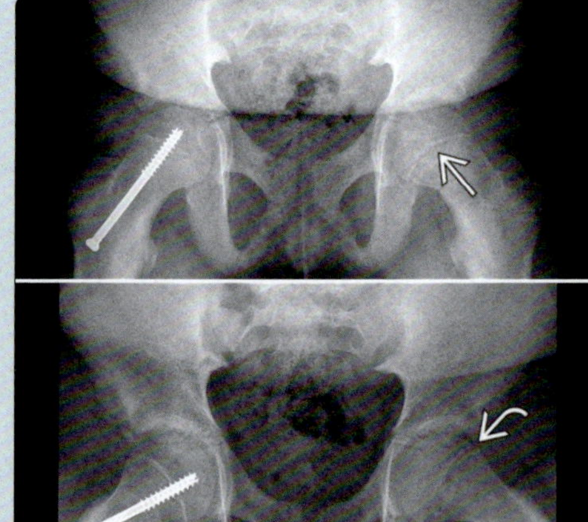

TERMINOLOGY

Abbreviations

- Slipped capital femoral epiphysis (SCFE)

Definitions

- Salter-Harris I fracture of subcapital femoral physis due to chronic stress of weight bearing
  - SCFE term is not used for acute trauma
- Capital femoral epiphysis = femoral head
- Subcapital physis = proximal femoral growth plate

IMAGING

General Features

- Best diagnostic clue
  - Posterior displacement of femoral capital epiphysis relative to femoral neck on frog leg lateral view
- Location
  - Rates of bilateral SCFE vary widely: 18-80%
    - At initial presentation: 9-22%
    - 88% of contralateral SCFE occurs within 18 months
- Morphology
  - Femoral head slips posterior, inferior, & medial relative to metaphysis

Radiographic Findings

- Wide (elongated), smooth, & lucent subcapital femoral physis
  - May occur before visible femoral head displacement
- AP view: Medial displacement of femoral head relative to metaphysis
  - Klein line: Straight line drawn along lateral femoral neck normally intersects outer 15-20% of femoral head
    - Slipped femoral head lies medial to Klein line
    - ↑ sensitivity if > 2-mm difference in amount of femoral head lateral to line vs. contralateral side
  - Shenton arc: Normally continuous smooth curve drawn along undersurface of superior pubic ramus & medial femoral neck
    - SCFE disrupts arc as slipped femoral head displaces femoral neck laterally & superiorly
  - Dense medial femoral metaphysis due to normal overlap with ischium
    - Lost in SCFE due to lateral & superior displacement of femoral neck
- Frog leg lateral view: Posterior displacement of femoral head relative to metaphysis
  - Appears medial relative to acetabulum, pelvis
  - More sensitive for slip than AP view
  - Staging on frog leg lateral view
    - Percentage of epiphyseal displacement: Mild 0-33%, moderate 34-49%, severe > 50%
- Metaphysis: Scalloping, irregularity, sclerosis, & posterior beaking if chronic
- Valgus SCFE (lateral & superior slip of epiphysis) is very uncommon
  - Typically has posterior component revealed on lateral view (as Klein line is insensitive)

CT Findings

- Axial oblique & sagittal planes best reveal maximum displacement
- Osteoporosis & ↓ muscle bulk if chronic

MR Findings

- Physeal elongation ("widening") of "preslip" is best seen on coronal T1
- ± marrow edema, synovitis with slip on T2 FS/STIR
- Severity of slip angle is more accurate than radiographs
- Periosteal disruption confirms instability
- Chronicity is suggested with remodeling, osteoporosis, ↓ muscle bulk
- Long term: Femoroacetabular impingement (FAI), labral tear, & articular cartilage damage are likely ↑ with greater degree of slip & residual head-neck offset

Nuclear Medicine Findings

- Bone scan
  - Acute SCFE: ↑ uptake at physis (fracture)
  - Chondrolysis: ↑ uptake on acetabular & femoral sides of joint (synovitis)
  - Osteonecrosis (ON): ↓ uptake in femoral epiphysis (infarct)

Imaging Recommendations

- Best imaging tool
  - AP & frog leg lateral radiographs of both hips
    - Frog leg view: Abducted, externally rotated femurs
    - Do not use force to secure frog leg lateral position (may worsen slip)
- Protocol advice
  - SCFE may be subtle on radiographs; consider urgent MR to include coronal T1 if any doubt exists

DIFFERENTIAL DIAGNOSIS

Legg-Calvé-Perthes Disease

- Idiopathic ON of hip, classically 5-8 years old
- Marrow edema, synovitis/effusion, ↓ femoral head enhancement early on MR
- Subsequent radiographic sclerosis & collapse of femoral head ossification center, coxa magna

Juvenile Idiopathic Arthritis

- Nonspecific joint effusion & synovitis, often insidious
- ± multiple joints, characteristic rash, systemic symptoms

Renal Osteodystrophy

- Generalized bony sclerosis with "fuzzy" margins
- Subperiosteal & subsymphyseal resorption
- Multifocal physeal elongation ("widening"): ↑ SCFE risk

Traumatic Salter-Harris I Fracture

- Unequivocal history of acute trauma in adolescence
- Rarely in newborns with difficult delivery

Septic Arthritis

- ↑ WBC, ESR, fever, & failure to bear weight
- Marrow & soft tissue edema often surround effusion

Transient Synovitis

- Limp & pain without systemic findings

- Lack of marrow & soft tissue edema surrounding effusion

Idiopathic Chondrolysis

- Accelerated hip joint cartilage destruction in preadolescent without clear etiology
- Early: Geographic ↑ T2 signal & enhancement centrally in femoral head ± synovitis
- Late: Joint space loss & degenerative change

PATHOLOGY

General Features

- Associated abnormalities
  - ON may be due to
    - Vessel injury acutely at time of slip
    - Vascular compression from operative reduction
    - ↑ intracapsular pressure by effusion reducing flow
  - Residual head-neck offset post therapy can result in cam-type FAI & premature joint degeneration

Microscopic Features

- Physeal architectural distortion before fracture
- Fracture occurs in zone of hypertrophic chondrocytes

CLINICAL ISSUES

Presentation

- Most common signs/symptoms
  - Limp, pain, limited motion
    - Pain in hip, groin, or proximal thigh in 85%
    - Distal thigh or knee pain in 15%
- Other signs/symptoms
  - Clinical staging
    - Stable: Able to bear weight (even with crutches)
      - More likely to have delayed presentation
    - Unstable: Unable to bear weight
    - Timing of symptoms: Acute < 3 weeks, chronic > 3 weeks
      - Acute on chronic: Gradual onset, suddenly worse (most common)

Demographics

- Age
  - Girls: Range 8-15 years, average 11-12 years
  - Boys: Range 10-17 years, average 13-14 years
  - Can see at younger age with endocrine/metabolic disorder
- Sex
  - M:F = 2.5:1:0
- Ethnicity
  - Nearly 4:1 = Black patients:White patients
- Epidemiology
  - Most common hip disorder in adolescents
  - Incidence: 0.7-10.8 per 100,000
- Predisposing factors
  - Obesity is most significant factor
  - Adolescent growth spurt
  - Endocrine: Primary hypothyroidism, hypogonadism
  - Renal rickets, radiation therapy, chemotherapy

Natural History & Prognosis

- Prognosis is poorer for unstable SCFE → 10-60% develop ON
  - ↑ risk with slip severity, younger age, manual reduction, ↑ intracapsular pressure
    - Some advocate surgery within 24 hours to ↓ risk
- Chondrolysis from SCFE is most frequently due to persistent (not transient) joint penetration by pin
- Joint degeneration secondary to incongruity, residual head-neck offset → cam-type FAI

Treatment

- Percutaneous screw/pin fixation of epiphysis to femoral neck through physis
  - In situ fixation (no attempted reduction due to ↑ risk of ON with manual reduction)
    - Placement of threaded screw across physis
      - Traditional placement promotes growth arrest (growth-restricting method) → ↑ stabilization
      - Also promotes continued deformity of femoral-head neck junction → FAI & joint degeneration
      - Up to 45% of patients with SCFE need total hip replacement 50 years after slip
    - Newer (growth-sparing) techniques
      - Use nonthreaded fixation or gliding/telescoping screw techniques
      - Allow for continued growth & remodeling (improvement of α angle)
      - Goal: ↓ late complications of FAI & degenerative joint disease
- Surgical hip dislocation (open reduction + internal fixation)
  - Used for unstable severe slip & chronic slip
    - Capsulotomy advocated to ↓ risk of ON
    - Modified Dunn procedure with capital realignment ± osteochondroplasty
      - ↓ FAI & ON
- Prophylactic contralateral fixation is controversial; strongly considered in
  - Predisposing disease
  - Girls < 10 years old, boys < 12 years old

DIAGNOSTIC CHECKLIST

Image Interpretation Pearls

- Frog leg lateral view is essential
- Beware comparison to contralateral side
  - Up to 22% have contralateral SCFE at presentation
- Bilateral SCFE below typical age range should raise suspicion for underlying disorder

SELECTED REFERENCES

1. Samelis PV et al: Factors affecting outcomes of slipped capital femoral epiphysis. Cureus. 12(2):e6883, 2020
2. Balch Samora J et al: MRI in idiopathic, stable, slipped capital femoral epiphysis: evaluation of contralateral pre-slip. J Child Orthop. 12(5):454-60, 2018
3. Hesper T et al: Imaging modalities in patients with slipped capital femoral epiphysis. J Child Orthop. 11(2):99-106, 2017
4. Boyle MJ et al: The alpha angle as a predictor of contralateral slipped capital femoral epiphysis. J Child Orthop. 10(3):201-7, 2016
5. Roaten J et al: Complications related to the treatment of slipped capital femoral epiphysis. Orthop Clin North Am. 47(2):405-13, 2016
6. Thawrani DP et al: Current practice in the management of slipped capital femoral epiphysis. J Pediatr Orthop. 36(3):27-37, 2016

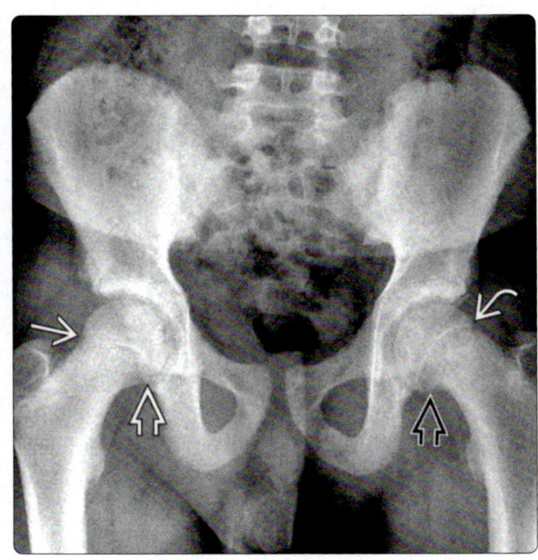

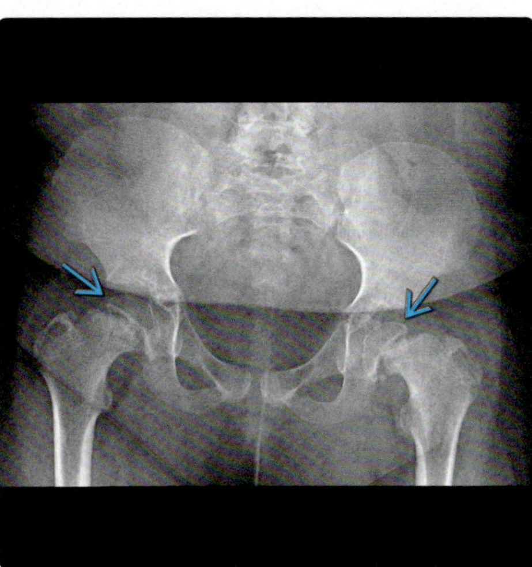

(Left) *AP radiograph in an obese 15-year-old boy shows slight posterior slippage of the left femoral head with an abnormally smooth, widened, & lucent physis ➨. The left medial femoral metaphyseal corner ➨ does not overlap the ischium. Note the normal undulating right physis ➨ & normal metaphyseal/ischium relationship ➨.* **(Right)** *AP radiograph in an obese 13-year-old girl with hip pain & hypothyroidism shows bilateral SCFE ➨ with widened physes & metaphyseal irregularities.*

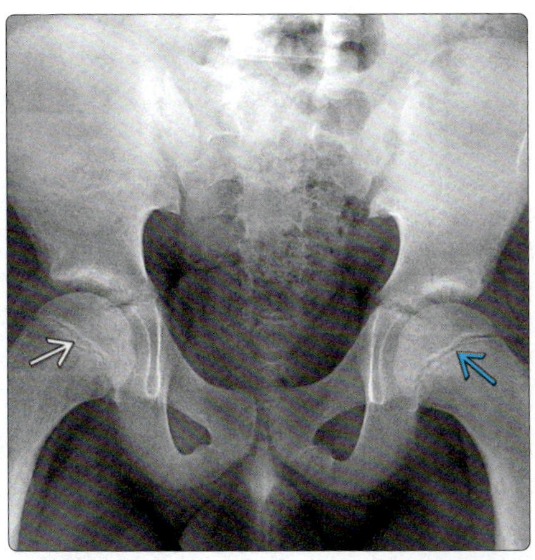

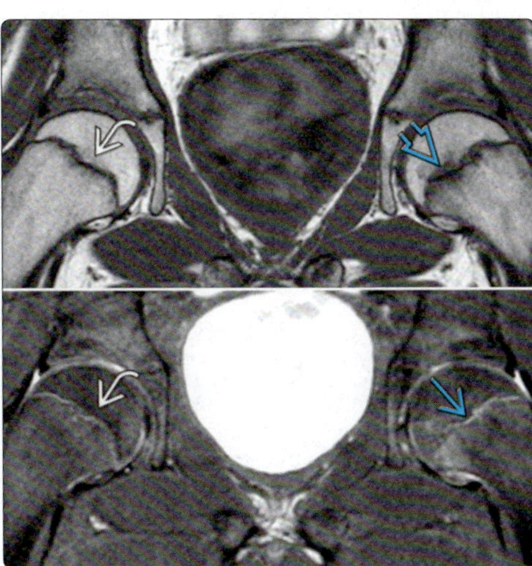

(Left) *AP radiograph in a 14-year-old boy with left hip pain shows slightly ↑ smoothness & lucency to the left femoral physis ➨ relative to the right ➨.* **(Right)** *Coronal T1 MR (top) of the same patient shows periphyseal foci of fatty marrow signal loss with poor definition of the subcapital femoral physis, suggesting a "preslip" ➨. No physeal abnormality can be seen on the corresponding T2 FS MR (bottom) ➨. Note the normal right side ➨.*

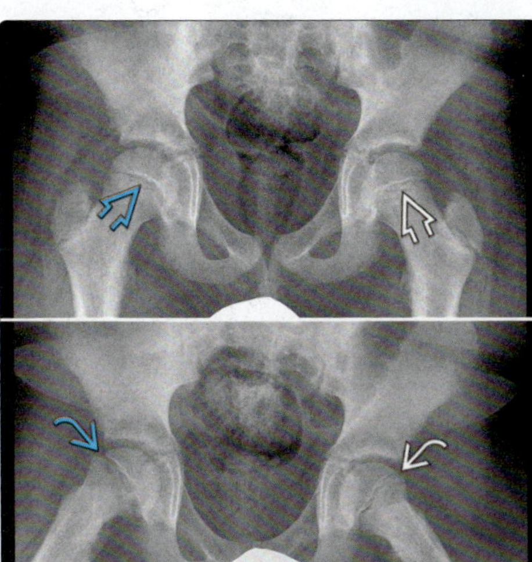

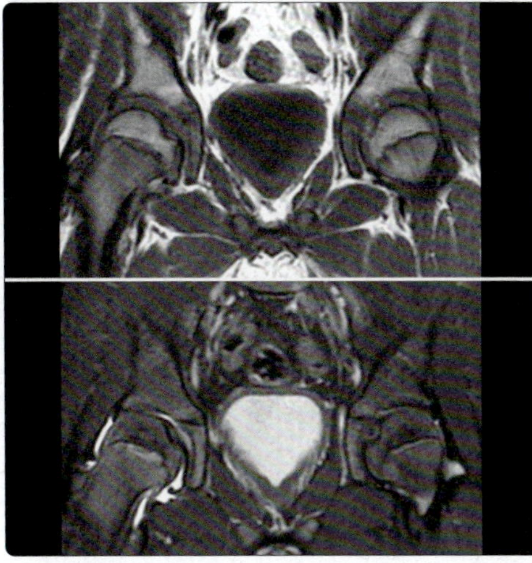

(Left) *AP (top) & frog leg lateral (bottom) radiographs in an 11-year-old with hip pain show an abnormally smooth & wide right subcapital physis ➨ with femoral head-neck offset ➨, consistent with SCFE. The left subcapital physis appears normal ➨ with questionable head-neck offset ➨.* **(Right)** *Coronal T1 (top) & T2 FS (bottom) MR images of the same patient show an abnormal right subcapital physis & associated joint effusion from SCFE. However, the left subcapital physis is normal.*

Achondroplasia

KEY FACTS

TERMINOLOGY

- Most common nonlethal skeletal dysplasia

IMAGING

- Symmetric shortening of all long bones
  - Proximal are most affected (rhizomelic)
- Upper extremity shortening
  - Humerus is barely longer than ulna
  - Short metacarpals & phalanges with trident hand configuration: 3 forks = thumb, digits 2 & 3, digits 4 & 5
- Lower extremity shortening
  - Femur is barely longer than tibia
  - Ice cream scoop shape of proximal femurs in infants
  - Lower femoral & proximal tibial epiphyses/metaphyses have cone or chevron shapes
  - Relatively elongated fibulae
- Pelvis: Squared iliac wings, narrowed sacrosciatic notches, horizontal acetabular roofs, overall coupe-type champagne glass configuration
- Spine: Gibbus deformity of thoracolumbar junction, anterior vertebral body beaking or wedging (bullet-shaped), posterior vertebral body scalloping, progressive narrowing of interpediculate distances from L1-L5
- Skull base: Keyhole foramen magnum, narrow jugular foramina → venous hypertension → ventriculomegaly

PATHOLOGY

- Autosomal dominant; 80% are sporadic
- Mutation at chromosome 4p16.3: Fibroblast growth factor receptor-3 gene (*FGFR3*)
  - Other mutations of same gene cause mild hypochondroplasia or lethal thanatophoric dysplasia
- Fetal cell-free DNA from maternal plasma is replacing amniocentesis for prenatal diagnosis

CLINICAL ISSUES

- ↑ risk of sudden death from cervicomedullary compression
- Otherwise, lifespan is near normal

(Left) *Sagittal T2 MR in a 2-month-old with achondroplasia shows narrowing of the craniocervical junction with cervicomedullary compression ➔. Note the enlarged lateral ventricles & subarachnoid spaces (due to jugular foramen stenosis with venous hypertension & impaired CSF resorption).* **(Right)** *Sagittal T2 MR in a 4-year-old shows lumbar spinal canal stenosis with scalloping of the posterior vertebral bodies. A bullet configuration with anterior vertebral body wedging is seen at T12-L2.*

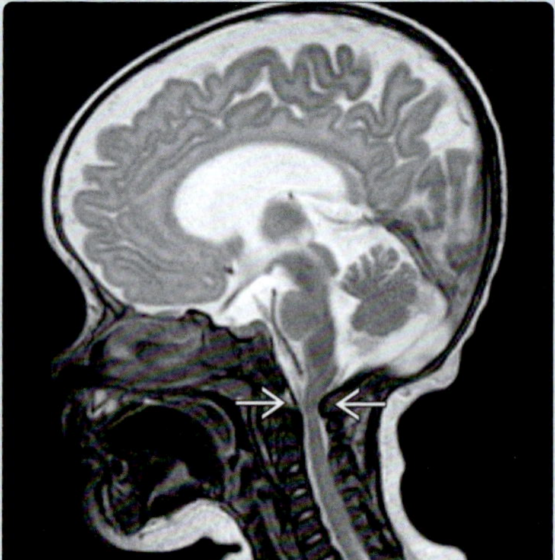

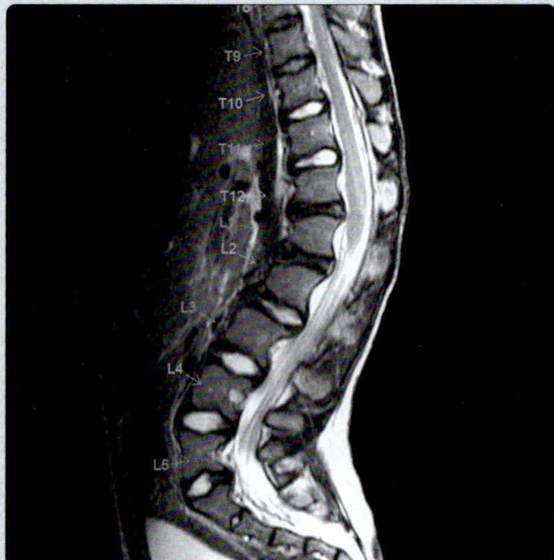

(Left) *AP radiograph shows inferiorly decreasing interpediculate distances of the lower lumbar spine, squared iliac wings, narrow sciatic notches, & horizontal acetabular roofs characteristic of achondroplasia.* **(Right)** *PA radiograph shows a trident hand configuration in a newborn with achondroplasia. The fingers are of approximately equal length & diverge from one another in 2 pairs + the thumb (i.e., there is splaying of the middle & ring fingers). The metacarpals & phalanges are short & broad.*

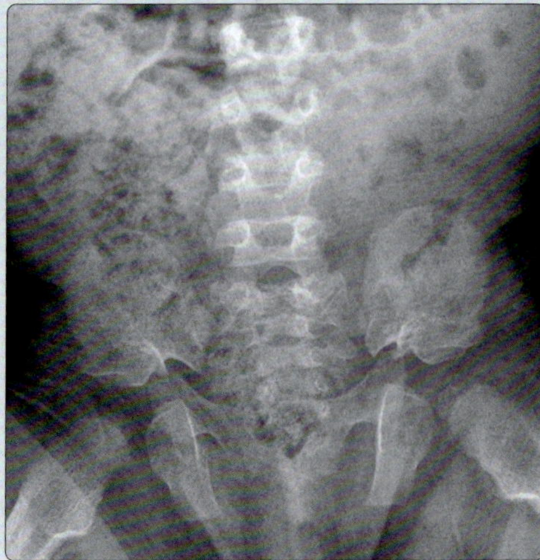

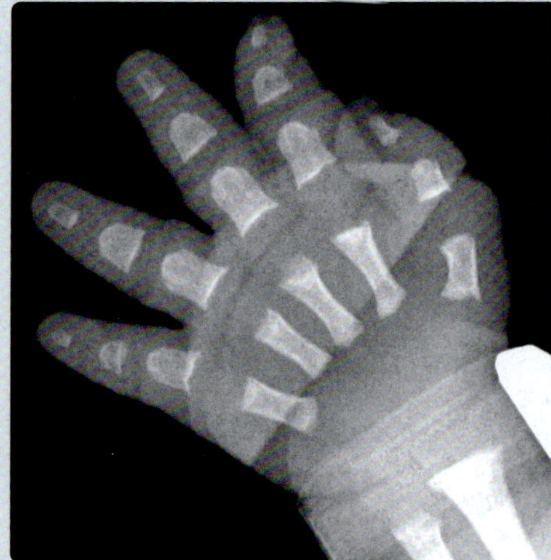

TERMINOLOGY

Definitions

- Mutations of fibroblast growth factor receptor-3 gene (*FGFR3*) at chromosome location 4p16.3 underlie achondroplasia & related dysplasias (FGFR3 group)
  - Achondroplasia (ACH)
    - Most common nonlethal skeletal dysplasia
    - Large cranium; small face & chest; short limbs
  - Hypochondroplasia
    - Milder skeletal dysplasia affecting similar sites
      - Usually not recognized until child is > 2 years old
      - Severe forms overlap with achondroplasia
    - Milder changes of hands & spine
    - Fibular overgrowth
  - Thanatophoric dysplasia
    - Most common lethal bone dysplasia
    - Lungs cannot fully develop/ventilate due to short ribs; micromelia

IMAGING

Radiographic Findings

- Radiologic evaluation begins with skeletal survey
- Skull, face, & brain
  - Calvarium is enlarged with frontal bossing, megalencephaly
  - Flat nasal bridge
  - Skull base is small with narrow foramen magnum
    - Concern for brainstem compression
  - Petrous pyramids are closer to midline than normal
  - Basal angle is low: 85-120°; steep clivus
  - Basilar impression
  - Narrow jugular foramina may cause ventriculomegaly via venous hypertension
  - Short petrous carotid canals
  - Mastoids are underpneumatized
  - Midface hypoplasia, dental crowding
  - Choanal atresia: Occasional
- Spine
  - Spinal canal stenosis is seen as short pedicles on lateral view with ↓ interpediculate distances on AP view
    - Interpediculate distances become progressively smaller lower in lumbar spine (opposite of normal)
  - Vertebral bodies: Short, bullet-shaped in early life; concave posterior surfaces (scalloping)
    - Vertebral heights are normal
  - Transverse processes are short
  - Thoracolumbar gibbus or kyphosis in infancy
  - ↑ lumbar lordosis after infancy with horizontal sacrum
  - Cervical instability
- Chest
  - Short ribs & sternum
  - Cup-shaped anterior rib ends
  - Clavicles: Musk ox horn shape, relatively long
- Pelvis
  - Champagne glass shape (coupe type of glass, not tulip or flute) of inner margin
    - Pelvic cavity broad & short
  - Small, squared iliac wings with horizontal acetabular roofs & rounded iliac crests (tombstone or elephant ear appearance)
  - Narrowed sacrosciatic notches
- Lower extremity
  - Rhizomelic shortening: Femur is barely longer than tibia
  - Femoral necks are short with coxa vara
  - Hemispheric femoral head
  - Ice cream scoop shape of proximal femurs in infants
  - Flared (widened) metaphyses capped by large epiphyses
  - Diaphyseal widths are normal but appear broadened due to shortening
  - Distal femoral & proximal tibial metaphyses/epiphyses are cone or chevron in shape
  - Bowlegs: Genu varum (> 90%)
  - Delayed ossification of tibial epiphysis
  - Fibula is longer than tibia
  - Posteroinferior calcaneal pseudospurs before ossification of calcaneal apophysis
  - Joint laxity
- Upper extremity
  - Rhizomelic shortening: Humerus is barely longer than ulna
  - Outward lateral bulging of humerus at deltoid insertion
  - Concave medial distal radial metaphysis
  - Hand: Delayed bone age
  - Metacarpals & phalanges are short & broad
  - "Trident hand" with 3 forks: Thumb, digits 2 & 3, digits 4 & 5
    - Splaying of middle & ring fingers

Ultrasonographic Findings

- Prenatal studies may be normal on early scan with long bone shortening not detected until 22- to 24-weeks gestation
  - Foreshortening of limbs (< 3rd percentile)
  - ↑ biparietal diameter (> 95th percentile)
  - Flat nasal bridge
  - Collar hoop sign: Overgrowth of periosteum with small, echogenic hook at proximal femoral metaphyseal-epiphyseal junction
  - Rounded metaphyseal-epiphyseal interface
  - Possible temporal lobe abnormalities

Other Modality Findings

- MR: Herniated nucleus pulposus
- CT/MR: Narrowed foramen magnum, enlargement of convexity subarachnoid CSF spaces & ventricles

DIFFERENTIAL DIAGNOSIS

Hypochondroplasia

- Milder short-limbed dwarfism with similarly affected sites
  - Hands & feet are short & broad
  - Midface hypoplasia
  - Foramen magnum is small
  - Lumbar spine: ↓ interpediculate distance
  - Vertebral bodies: Posterior scalloping
- Often not clinically apparent until 2 years of age

Pseudoachondroplasia

- Normal skull; severe epiphyseal findings

Metatropic Dysplasia

- Dumbbell-shaped femurs
- Kyphoscoliosis, caudal appendage (tail)

Other Conditions With Endochondral Growth Slowing

- Homozygous achondroplasia (lethal), Ellis van Creveld syndrome, thanatophoric dysplasia (lethal), Morquio disease

PATHOLOGY

General Features

- Etiology
  - ↓ rate of endochondral ossification
- Genetics
  - Defect on chromosome 4p16.3
    - Fibroblast growth factor receptor-3 (*FGFR3*) gene
      - > 98% are due to G1138A (glycine to arginine substitution at nucleotide 1138)
    - Prenatal diagnosis by next-generation sequencing of cell-free fetal DNA from maternal plasma
      - Traditional methods: Amniocentesis or chorionic villus sampling
  - Autosomal dominant
    - 80% of cases are new (de novo) mutations
    - Heterozygous: Common
    - Homozygous: Rare, lethal

Microscopic Features

- Histology of epiphyseal & physeal growth cartilage is normal

CLINICAL ISSUES

Presentation

- Most common signs/symptoms
  - Characteristic face with midface hypoplasia, saddle nose, & macrocephaly with frontal bossing
  - Rhizomelic limb shortening
  - Limited elbow extension
  - Trident hand
  - Thoracolumbar gibbus or kyphosis
  - Lumbar lordosis is exaggerated
    - Buttocks prominent & abdomen protuberant after walking begins
  - Hypermobility of joints, especially knees
  - Hypotonia
- Clinical profile
  - At birth, physical appearance commonly makes the diagnosis

Demographics

- Epidemiology
  - Heterozygous achondroplasia
  - Incidence: 1:10,000-40,000 live births
  - Increasing incidence with advancing paternal age

Natural History & Prognosis

- 2-5% risk of sudden death due to cervicomedullary compression
  - Suspect with central hypopnea, ↓ arousal state, small foramen magnum, hypotonia, hyperreflexia
- Lifespan is near normal without craniocervical junction stenosis
- Obesity is common
- ↑ incidence of orthopedic & neurologic complications
  - Cervical instability in infancy
  - Basilar impression, Chiari 1, syringomyelia
  - Lumbosacral stenosis
  - Tibial bowing in 42%
    - Tibial osteotomy is required in 22%
- Upper airway obstruction/obstructive sleep apnea
- Otitis media in 60% of infants & 93% of toddlers
  - Myringotomy tubes in 80% over lifespan
  - Conductive hearing loss in 40%
- Normal intelligence but delayed motor & speech development
- Average adult height is 4 feet

Treatment

- Available for most complications
  - Cervicomedullary decompression surgery in 17%
    - Potentially urgent to prevent sudden death
  - Cardiorespiratory & sleep dysfunction
    - Mild midface hypoplasia & relative adenotonsillar hypertrophy: Treat with tonsillectomy & adenoidectomy
    - Upper airway obstruction: Nocturnal, continuous positive airway pressure
    - Upper airway obstruction associated with hypoglossal canal stenosis: Various options, including foramen magnum decompression
    - Ventriculomegaly from jugular foramen stenosis: Treat with shunt as needed clinically
- Limb lengthening: Controversial
  - Ilizarov procedure with average length gain of 20.5 cm
    - High complication rate includes fracture, infection, joint stiffness, contractures
  - Magnetically driven intramedullary nail

SELECTED REFERENCES

1. Khalid K et al: Pictorial review: imaging of the spinal manifestations of achondroplasia. Br J Radiol. 94(1123):20210223, 2021
2. Sarioglu FC et al: Neuroimaging and calvarial findings in achondroplasia. Pediatr Radiol. 50(12):1669-79, 2020
3. Pauli RM: Achondroplasia: a comprehensive clinical review. Orphanet J Rare Dis. 14(1):1, 2019
4. Manikkam SA et al: Temporal lobe malformations in achondroplasia: expanding the brain imaging phenotype associated with FGFR3-related skeletal dysplasias. AJNR Am J Neuroradiol. 39(2):380-4, 2018
5. Daugherty A: Achondroplasia: etiology, clinical presentation, and management. Neonatal Netw. 36(6):337-42, 2017
6. Ornitz DM et al: Achondroplasia: development, pathogenesis, and therapy. Dev Dyn. 246(4):291-309, 2017
7. Sargar KM et al: Imaging of skeletal disorders caused by fibroblast growth factor receptor gene mutations. Radiographics. 37(6):1813-30, 2017
8. Gajarajulu V et al: The radiograph of the pelvis as a window to skeletal dysplasias. Indian J Pediatr. 83(6):543-52, 2016
9. Donaldson J et al: Achondroplasia and limb lengthening: Results in a UK cohort and review of the literature. J Orthop. 12(1):31-4, 2015
10. Panda A et al: Skeletal dysplasias: A radiographic approach and review of common non-lethal skeletal dysplasias. World J Radiol. 6(10):808-25, 2014
11. Boulet S et al: Prenatal diagnosis of achondroplasia: new specific signs. Prenat Diagn. 29(7):697-702, 2009
12. King JA et al: Neurosurgical implications of achondroplasia. J Neurosurg Pediatr. 4(4):297-306, 2009

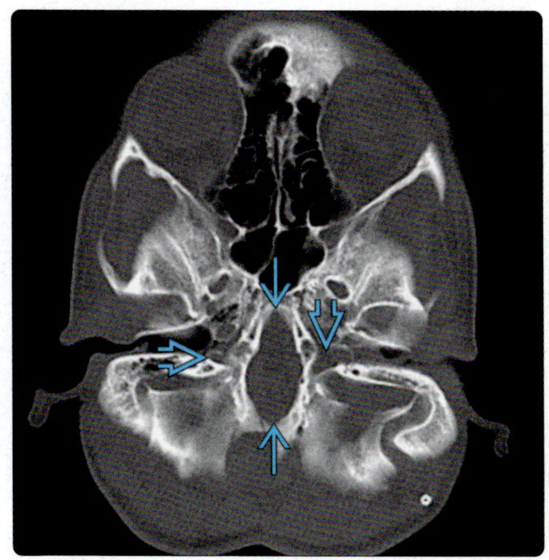

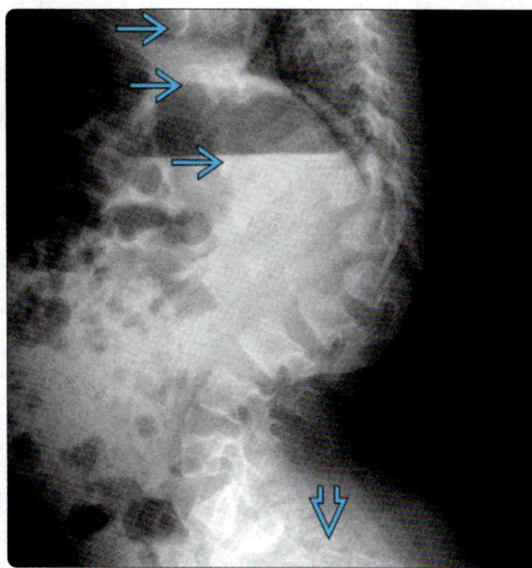

(Left) *Axial bone CT in a teenager with achondroplasia & shunted hydrocephalus shows a typical keyhole foramen magnum ➔ with jugular foramen hypoplasia ➔.* **(Right)** *Lateral radiograph in a 5-year-old shows thoracolumbar kyphosis (or gibbus deformity) with multilevel anterior wedging & an exaggerated lumbar lordosis. There is ↑ concavity of the posterior vertebral bodies. Note the nearly horizontal sacrum ➔ & rib shortening with anterior flaring ➔.*

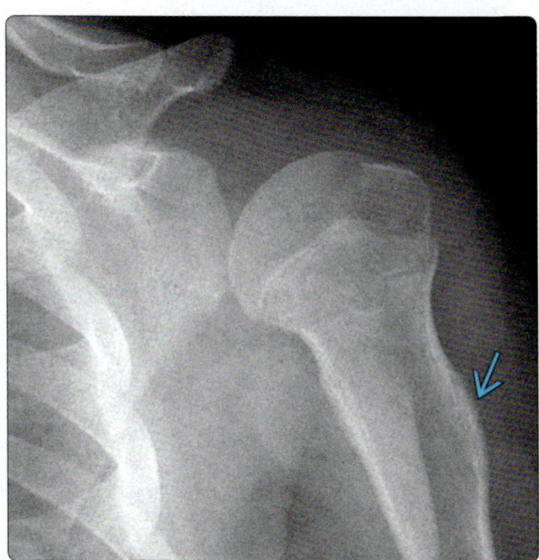

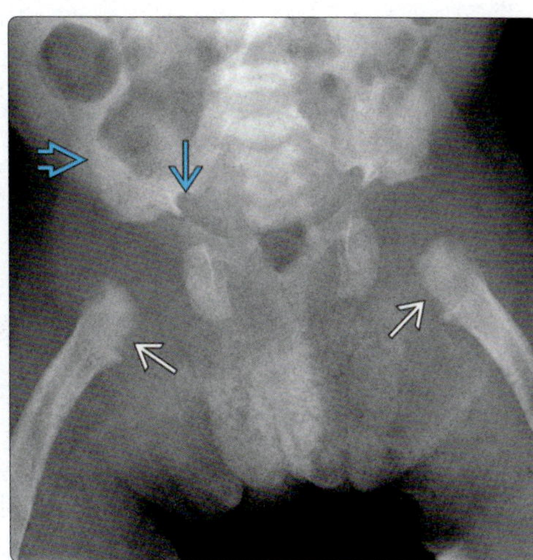

(Left) *External rotation radiograph in a child with achondroplasia shows a prominent deltoid insertional irregularity ➔ of the proximal humerus.* **(Right)** *AP radiograph shows ice cream scoop configurations ➔ of the proximal femurs in this infant with achondroplasia. Also note the elephant ear configurations of the iliac wings ➔ with small sciatic notches ➔.*

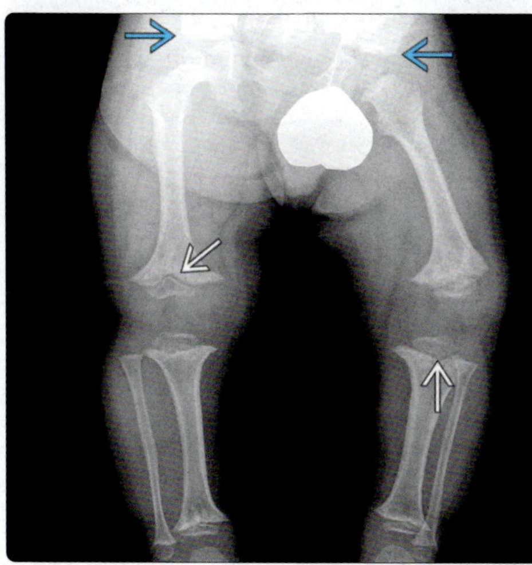

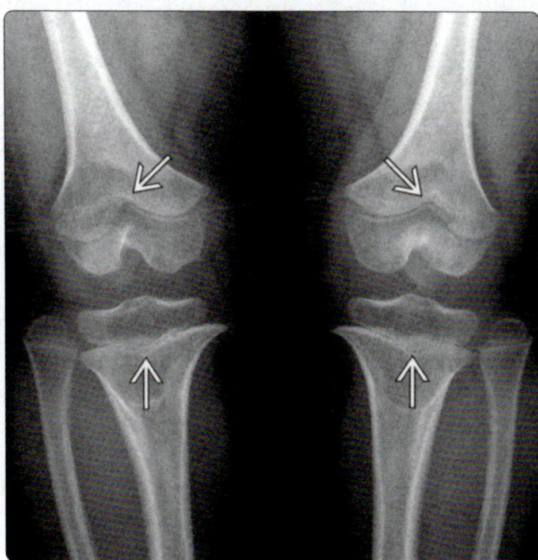

(Left) *AP radiograph in an infant with achondroplasia shows horizontal acetabular roofs ➔, metaphyseal flaring, & chevron or upside-down chevron deformities of the knees ➔ with long fibulae.* **(Right)** *AP radiograph in a 7-year-old with knee pain & achondroplasia shows metaphyseal flaring with chevron or upside-down chevron deformities of the distal femoral & proximal tibial epiphyses bilaterally ➔. The fibulae are elongated.*

Mucopolysaccharidoses

KEY FACTS

TERMINOLOGY

- Heterogeneous group of lysosomal storage diseases due to deficiency of enzymes that degrade glycosaminoglycans (GAGs)
- Dysostosis multiplex: Constellation of bone dysplasia features seen variably in mucopolysaccharidoses (MPS)

IMAGING

- Thoracolumbar gibbus (sharply angled kyphosis) with anteriorly beaked vertebral bodies
- Oar-shaped ribs (thin proximally, wide distally)
- Short, thick clavicles
- Pelvis: Ilia small & tapered inferiorly, steep acetabular roofs, hip subluxation, coxa valga, ± femoral head avascular necrosis
- Pointed proximal 2nd-5th metacarpals
- Diaphyseal widening of tubular bones
- Odontoid hypoplasia & other C1/C2 abnormalities → atlantoaxial subluxation → cord compression

TOP DIFFERENTIAL DIAGNOSES

- Legg-Calvé-Perthes disease
- Sickle cell disease
- Gaucher disease
- Spondyloepiphyseal dysplasia
- Multiple epiphyseal dysplasia
- Spondylometaphyseal dysplasia

PATHOLOGY

- GAGs are ubiquitous in connective tissues throughout body
- GAGs accumulate in lysosomes in bone marrow & multiple viscera → dysfunction

CLINICAL ISSUES

- Stem cell transplantation by unrelated donor umbilical cord blood: MPS I-H, VI
  - Best done when < 2 years old, no CNS disease
- Enzyme replacement therapy: MPS I, II, VI

(Left) *Frontal (left) & lateral (right) radiographs in a 6-year-old girl with MPS IV show thoracolumbar kyphosis, small irregular vertebrae, beaked vertebrae, wide ribs, hepatomegaly, coxa valga deformities, steep acetabula, & rounded iliac wings with inferiorly tapered ilia.* **(Right)** *Frontal radiographs of the hands in the same child show short, wide 2nd-5th metacarpals with pointed proximal ends, small, irregular carpal bones, & irregular, centrally-sloped metaphyses of the distal radius & ulna.*

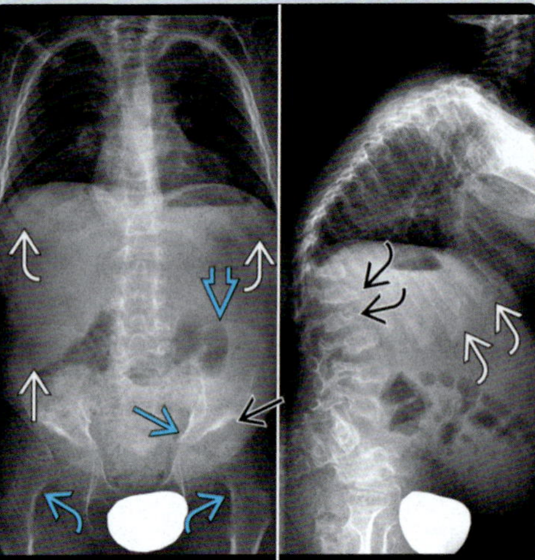

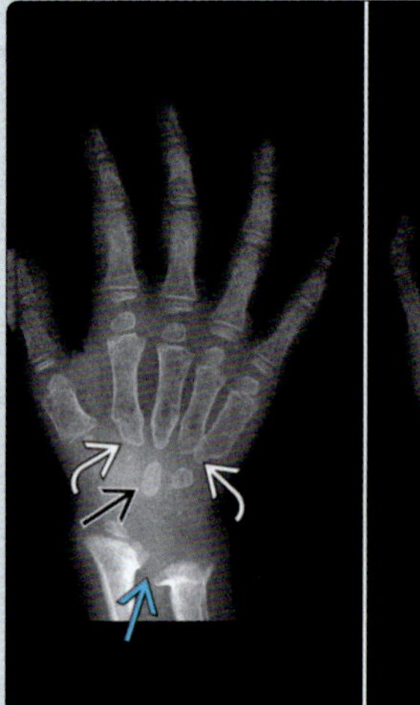

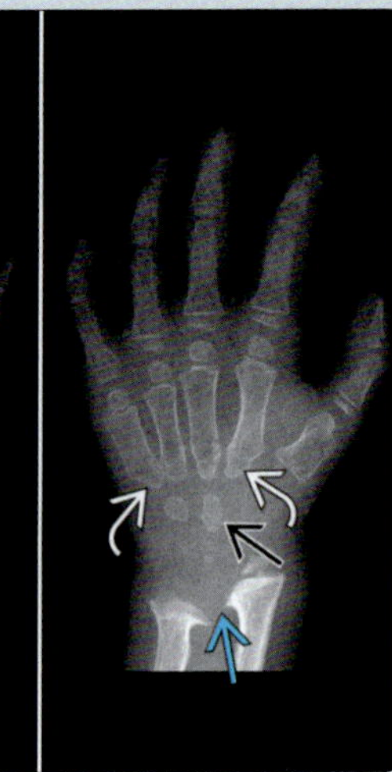

(Left) *Sagittal CT (left) & T2 MR (right) images show the C-spine in the same child. The odontoid is hypoplastic with dark soft tissue filling the expected location of odontoid. There is also narrowing of the spinal canal at the craniocervical junction with cord compression.* **(Right)** *Lateral radiograph shows the same child after craniocervical junction decompression & fusion from the occiput to the C2 level. Cord compression in MPS can lead to cervical/brainstem myelopathy & respiratory failure.*

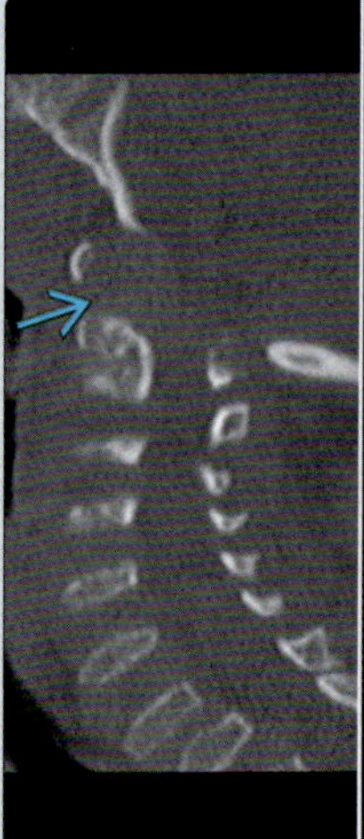

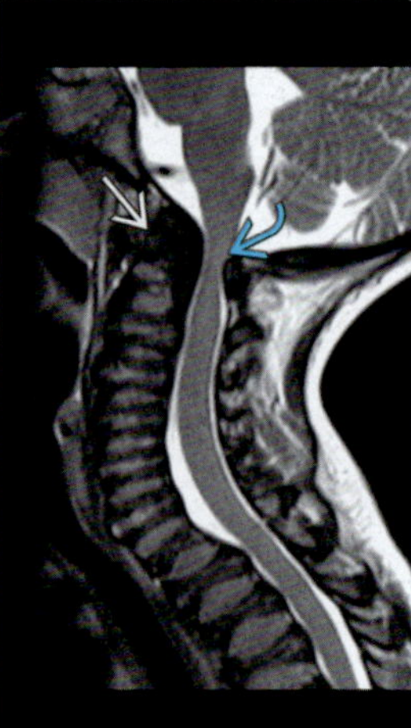

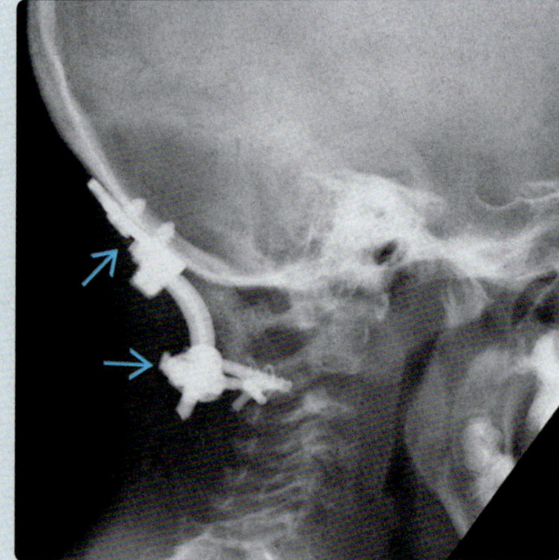

TERMINOLOGY

Abbreviations

- Mucopolysaccharidosis/mucopolysaccharidoses: MPS
- MPS I-H: Hurler syndrome
- MPS I-S: Scheie syndrome
- MPS I-H/S: Hurler-Scheie syndrome
- MPS II: Hunter syndrome
- MPS III: Sanfilippo syndrome
- MPS IV: Morquio syndrome
- MPS V: Nonexistent, now classified as MPS I-S
- MPS VI: Maroteaux-Lamy syndrome
- MPS VII: Sly syndrome or β-glucuronidase deficiency
- MPS VIII: Nonexistent
- MPS IX: Natowicz syndrome or Hyaluronidase deficiency

Definitions

- Heterogeneous group of lysosomal storage diseases due to deficiency of glycosaminoglycan (GAG)-degrading enzymes
  - GAGs were formerly called mucopolysaccharides
- Dysostosis multiplex (DM): Constellation of bone dysplasia features seen variably in MPS
- DM group: Includes all storage diseases that lead to skeletal dysplasia
  - MPS, mucolipidoses, others (Gaucher, Niemann-Pick, gangliosidosis, fucosidosis, mannosidosis, sialidosis)

IMAGING

Radiographic Findings

- Key features
  - Thoracolumbar gibbus (sharply angled kyphosis) with anteriorly beaked vertebral bodies
  - Oar-shaped ribs (thin proximally, wide distally)
  - Short, thick clavicles
  - Pelvis: Ilia are small & tapered inferiorly with steep & poorly formed acetabular roof, hip subluxation, coxa valga, femoral head deformities ± avascular necrosis (AVN)
  - Pointed proximal 2nd-5th metacarpals
  - Diaphyseal widening of small tubular bones

Other Modality Findings

- MPS I-H typifies DM features seen in other MPS types
- MPS I-H, Hurler syndrome: Severe DM
  - Brain: Abnormal white matter; delayed myelination; ↑ size of perivascular spaces, sulci, ventricles
  - Neurocranium: Enlarged; early closure of sagittal & lambdoid sutures; thickened skull base; J-shaped (elongated) sella
  - Face: Mandibular condyles flat/concave ± TMJ ankylosis; underpneumatized mastoids
  - Craniocervical junction: Spinal cord compression
  - Spine: Hypoplastic dens with C1/C2 subluxation; C3/C4 subluxation; thoracolumbar gibbus; anterior mid to inferior vertebral beak
    - May lead to spinal canal stenosis ± syringohydromyelia
  - Chest & shoulders: Trachea narrow; ribs wide & oar-shaped; clavicles short & thick; scapulae elevated with dysmorphic glenoid fossae
  - Pelvis & hips: Ilia small & taper inferiorly; steep, poorly formed acetabula; femoral head subluxation & developmental deformity ± AVN; coxa valga
  - Knees: Genu valgum
  - Arms: Humeral neck varus (hatchet-shaped humerus); wide humeral midshaft; distal radial & ulnar physes tilt toward each other
  - Wrists: Carpals small & irregular
  - Hands: Wide & short metacarpals with proximal pointed ends at 2-5; wide proximal & middle phalanges; synovitis & claw deformity, trigger finger
  - Cardiovascular: Cardiomyopathy; arterial narrowing; mitral/aortic stenosis
- MPS I-S: Scheie syndrome
  - Mild DM
- MPS II: Hunter syndrome
  - Mild to severe DM
- MPS I-H/S: Hurler-Scheie syndrome
  - Mild to moderate DM
- MPS IIIA-D: Sanfilippo syndrome
  - Mild or absent DM
  - Attenuated (mild) form: Intellectual disability, no DM
- MPS IVA-B: Morquio syndrome
  - Type A: Severe DM
    - Cord compression at C1/C2 level due to ≥ 1 of following
      - Transverse ligament laxity
      - Dural thickening from deposition of GAGs
      - Odontoid hypoplasia ± anterior soft tissue mass of unossified fibrocartilage & reactive changes
      - Indentation of posterior arch of C1
      - Chronic subluxation at C1/C2 → ligamentous hypertrophy → further narrowing at craniocervical junction → additional cord compression
      - Cervical cord compression can lead to myelopathy & respiratory failure
    - Cord compression at thoracic/thoracolumbar level from gibbous formation due to vertebral malformations; generalized platyspondyly; anterior vertebral beak (typically midportion)
    - Narrow; soft trachea collapses during neck flexion
    - Pectus carinatum
    - AVN of femoral heads
    - Ribs wide but not oar-shaped
  - Type B: Moderate DM
- MPS VI: Maroteaux-Lamy syndrome
  - Mild to severe DM
  - Severe form may have cervical & thoracic cord compression similar to type IV
- MPS VII: Sly syndrome
  - Mild to severe DM
    - Femoral head: AVN
- MPS IX: Hyaluronidase deficiency
  - Mild DM: Extremely rare

Imaging Recommendations

- Best imaging tool
  - Most findings are made on radiographs
    - Brain & spine MR may be needed

DIFFERENTIAL DIAGNOSIS

Legg-Calvé-Perthes Disease

- Idiopathic AVN of femoral head
- Isolated to hip without other MPS/DM features

Sickle Cell Disease

- Hemoglobinopathy
- Widespread marrow hyperplasia & osteonecrosis with H-shaped vertebral bodies

Gaucher Disease

- Storage disorder (not MPS) under DM group
- Osteoporosis with medullary expansion, undertubulation
- Osteonecrosis, H-shaped vertebral bodies

Spondyloepiphyseal Dysplasia

- No clinical or lab features of MPS
- Platyspondyly & abnormal epiphyses

Multiple Epiphyseal Dysplasia

- No clinical or lab features of MPS
- Findings at multiple epiphyses

Spondylometaphyseal Dysplasia

- No clinical or lab features of MPS
- Findings in spine & metaphyses

PATHOLOGY

General Features

- Etiology
  - Enzymatic deficiencies prevent GAG degradation
  - GAGs accumulate in lysosomes in bone marrow & multiple viscera → dysfunction
- Genetics
  - All MPS have autosomal recessive genetic abnormality (except MPS II: X-linked recessive)
    - MPS I-H, I-S, & I-H/S have same biochemical defect with spectrum of phenotypic severity
  - MPS I-H/S: > 110 gene mutations reported

CLINICAL ISSUES

Presentation

- Most common signs/symptoms
  - Many USA states are now screening newborns for MPS I
  - Spectrum of phenotypes (mild to severe)
    - Most common: Organomegaly, DM, intellectual disability/developmental delay
  - Brain: Regression of speech & learning skills → intellectual disability (not in MPS IV & VI)
  - Head/face: Large head, coarse hair & facial features, proptosis, corneal opacification, recurrent otitis media, flared nostrils, protruding tongue, ↓ hearing
  - Neck: Adenotonsillar enlargement, snoring, sleep apnea, tracheobronchomalacia
  - Spine & chest: Thoracolumbar gibbus (age 6-14 months in MPS I-H), scoliosis, spondylolisthesis in adults with MPS III, pectus carinatum
  - Respiratory: Frequent pneumonia
  - Cardiovascular: Valvular thickening, stenosis, insufficiency; cardiomyopathy, heart failure
  - Abdomen: Protuberant due to hepatosplenomegaly, umbilical/inguinal hernia, intestinal pseudoobstruction, idiopathic diarrhea
  - General: Short (except MPS I-S), claw hand, trigger finger, thick skin, carpal tunnel syndrome, ↓ joint mobility
  - Hydrops fetalis: MPS IV, VII
  - General anesthesia: ↑ risk due to redundant supraglottic tissue, ↓ airway size & stability, unstable C1/C2 joints in MPS I, II, IV, VI, & VII

Demographics

- Age
  - Clinical onset usually < 6 years old
  - Radiographic onset: May be at birth
- Epidemiology
  - Overall incidence of all types of MPS ~ 1 in 20,000 live births

Natural History & Prognosis

- Varies depending on type & severity
- Life span without treatment: MPS I-H < 10 years, MPS II roughly 15 years
- Near-normal lifespan: MPS I-S

Treatment

- Prevention of CNS damage: Perinatal screening → earliest possible treatment
- Stem cell transplantation using unrelated donor umbilical cord blood
  - Replacing conventional bone marrow transplant
  - Most primitive stem cells in cord blood have proliferative advantage & ↓ frequency & severity of graft-vs.-host disease (GVHD)
  - Early transplant is beneficial: MPS I-H (but does not arrest bone dysplasia), MPS VI
    - Best if performed when < 2 years old & no CNS disease
  - Transplant is not beneficial: MPS II, MPS III
    - Fails to arrest encephalopathy
- Enzyme replacement therapy: MPS I, II, VI
- Surgery
  - Hydrocephalus: Ventriculoperitoneal shunt (fewer complications prior to stem cell transplant)
  - Corneal opacity: Corneal transplant
  - Spine: C1/C2 stabilization, craniocervical junction decompression, fusion of progressive kyphosis
  - Airway obstruction or eustachian tube obstruction: Tonsillectomy & adenoidectomy
  - Valvular heart disease: Valve replacement
  - Carpal tunnel decompression
  - Hernia repair

SELECTED REFERENCES

1. Kubaski F et al: Mucopolysaccharidosis type I. Diagnostics (Basel). 10(3), 2020
2. Reichert R et al: Neuroimaging findings in patients with mucopolysaccharidosis: what you really need to know. Radiographics. 36(5):1448-62, 2016
3. Palmucci S et al: Imaging findings of mucopolysaccharidoses: a pictorial review. Insights Imaging. 4(4):443-59, 2013
4. Muenzer J: Overview of the mucopolysaccharidoses. Rheumatology (Oxford). 50 Suppl 5:v4-12, 2011
5. Rasalkar DD et al: Pictorial review of mucopolysaccharidosis with emphasis on MRI features of brain and spine. Br J Radiol. 84(1001):469-77, 2011

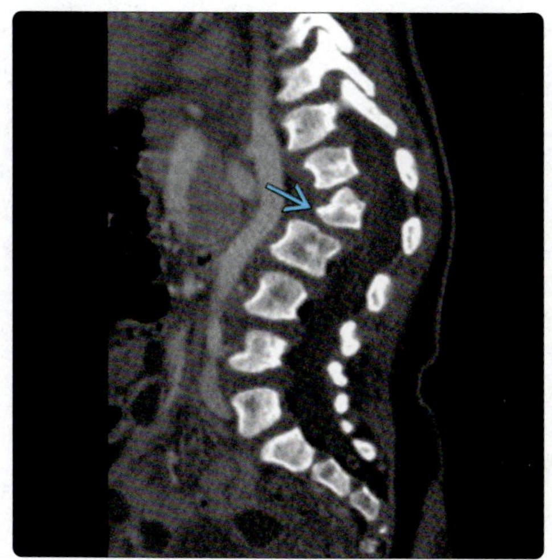

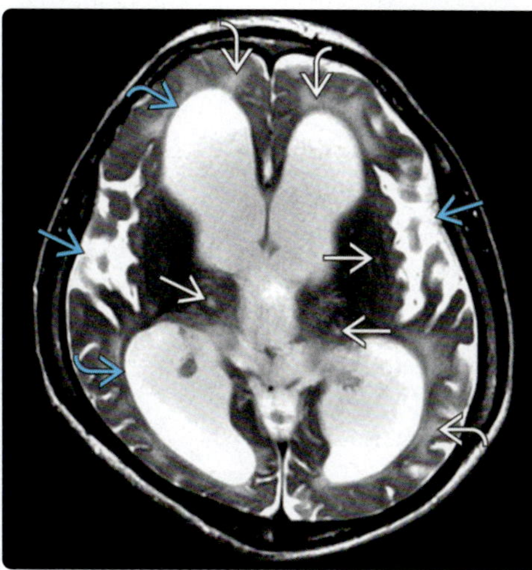

(Left) *Sagittal NECT shows the thoracolumbar spine in a 9-year-old girl with MPS II (Hunter syndrome). There is gibbus deformity with anterior beaking of the L1 vertebral body ⇒.* **(Right)** *Axial T2 brain MR in the same patient shows enlarged ventricles ⇒ & sulci ⇒. There is also ↑ signal within the periventricular white matter ⇒ with a few enlarged perivascular spaces ⇒.*

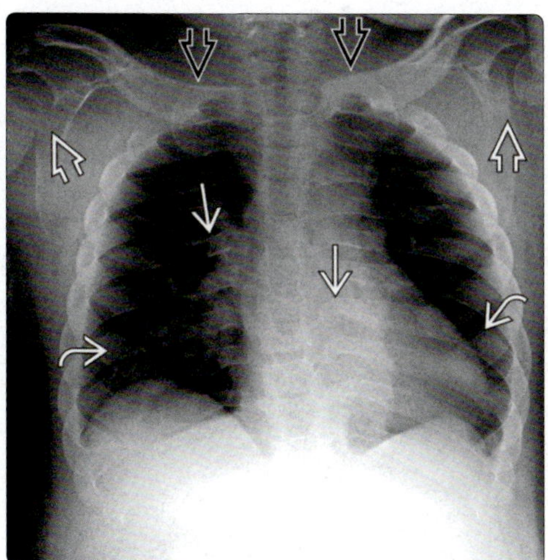

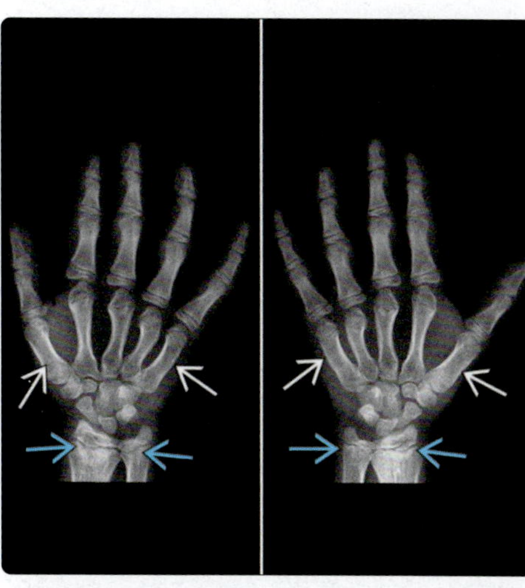

(Left) *AP radiograph in a 10-year-old girl with MPS II (Hunter syndrome) shows thickened clavicles bilaterally ⇒. The ribs have a characteristic oar shape with narrowing medially ⇒ but progressive broadening anterolaterally ⇒. Note the poorly formed glenoid fossae bilaterally ⇒.* **(Right)** *Bilateral frontal radiographs of the hands in a girl with MPS VI show short, wide metacarpals ⇒. There is also irregularity of the metaphyses of the distal radius & ulna ⇒ & slight irregularity of the distal radial epiphyses.*

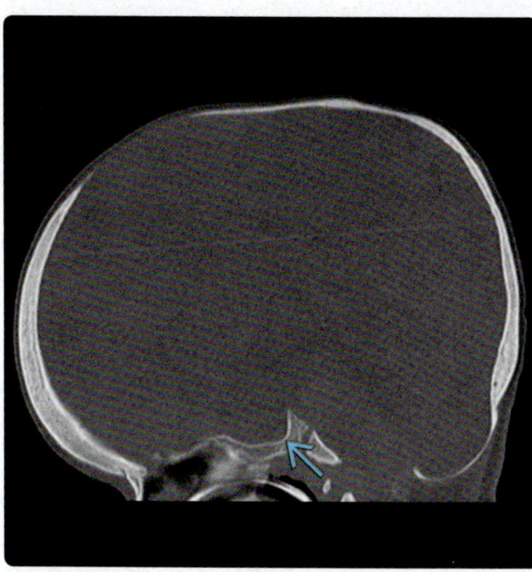

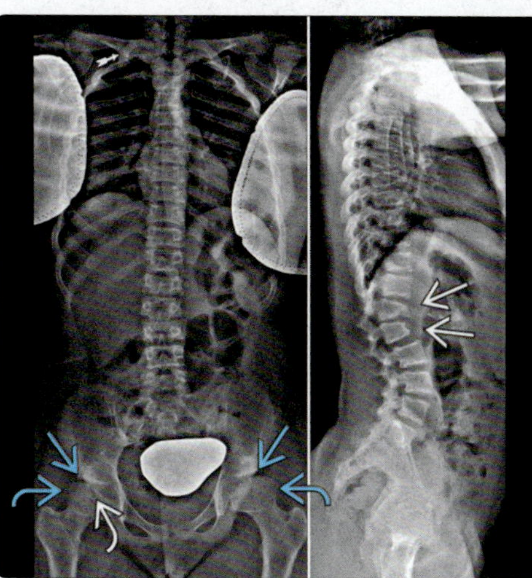

(Left) *Sagittal bone CT in a 5-year-old boy with Hurler's syndrome (MPSI-H) shows macrocephaly with an elongated, J-shaped sella turcica ⇒.* **(Right)** *Frontal (left) & lateral (right) radiographs of the spine in a 15-year-old girl with MPS VI show focal kyphosis with anterior beaking of the L1 & L2 vertebrae ⇒. There is underdevelopment of the acetabula ⇒. The femoral heads are broad with lateral uncovering ⇒. Lucency & sclerosis in the right femoral head suggests avascular necrosis (AVN) ⇒.*

Osteogenesis Imperfecta

KEY FACTS

TERMINOLOGY

- Osteogenesis imperfecta (OI): Group of clinically heterogeneous genetic disorders, most often caused by type I collagen alterations
- ↑ bone fragility → frequent fractures → malunion & bowing
  - ↑ likelihood of subsequent fractures

IMAGING

- Numerous in utero or perinatal fractures of short, poorly mineralized bones (OI type II)
- Other OI types: Multiple fractures in thin, overtubulated long bones + vertebral fractures + osteoporosis
- Radiographs are generally sufficient to suggest diagnosis
- CT or MR for axial skeleton complications

PATHOLOGY

- Nosology & Classification of Genetic Skeletal Disorders (2019) identifies 5 clinical forms
  - Type I: Nondeforming with persistently blue sclera
  - Type II: Perinatal lethal form
  - Type III: Progressively deforming type; most severe form that survives infancy
  - Type IV: Moderate form
  - Type V: Similar to type IV + interosseous membrane Ca^{2+} &/or hypertrophic callus
- Currently 20 genetic types of OI

CLINICAL ISSUES

- Severity of OI (mild → severe)
  - Type I < IV < III < II
- Type II: Lethal in perinatal period
- Type III: Premature death
- Treatment: Intravenous bisphosphonates, surgery

DIAGNOSTIC CHECKLIST

- Wide range of radiographic features across OI types
- Radiographic appearance alone does not classify OI

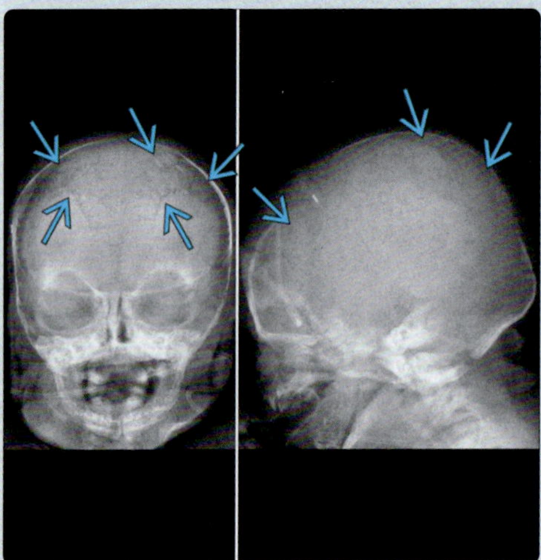

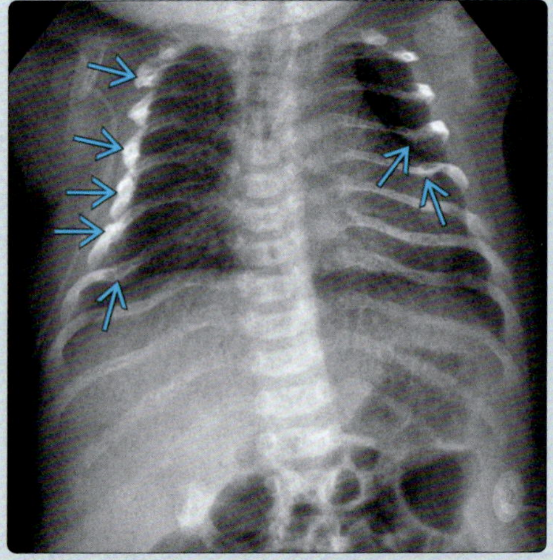

(Left) *Frontal & lateral radiographs of the skull in a 1-day-old girl with multiple fractures seen on fetal ultrasound shows numerous (> 10) wormian bones* ➔ *throughout the skull. The patient was subsequently diagnosed with type III osteogenesis imperfecta (OI).* **(Right)** *Frontal radiograph of the chest in the same patient shows deformities & healing fractures of multiple bilateral ribs* ➔*. Intrauterine fractures can be seen in OI, particularly in types II & III.*

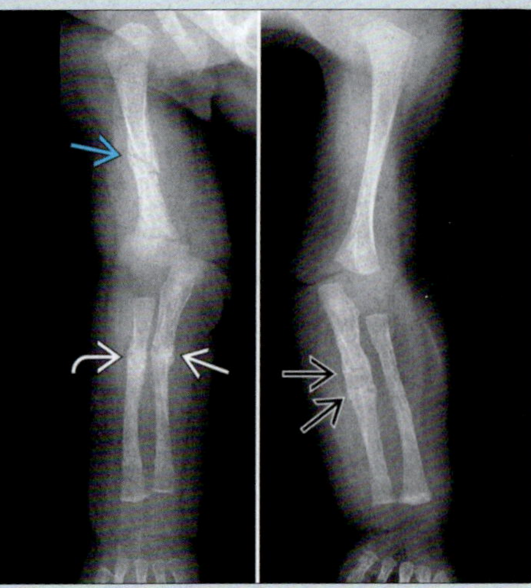

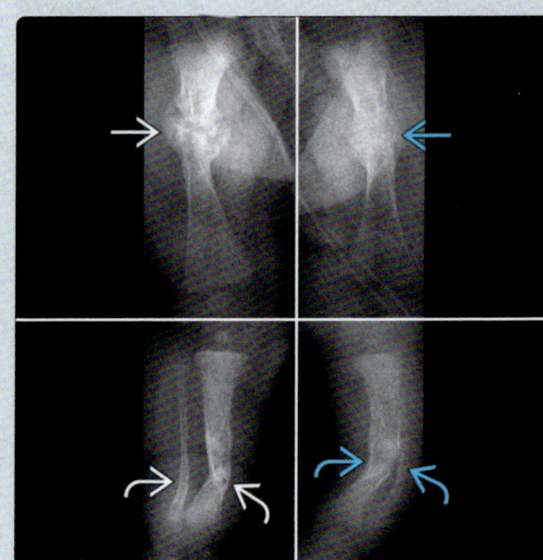

(Left) *Frontal radiographs show the right & left upper extremities in the same patient. There are healing fractures of the right humerus* ➔*, right radius* ➔*, & right ulna* ➔*, as well as multiple healing fractures of the left ulna* ➔*.* **(Right)** *Frontal radiographs show the right & left lower extremities in the same patient with OI type III. There are healing fractures of the right* ➔ *& left* ➔ *femurs. Bowing deformities of both the right* ➔ *& left* ➔ *tibias/fibulae (secondary to healing fractures) are also noted.*

TERMINOLOGY

Abbreviations

- Osteogenesis imperfecta (OI)

Definitions

- Group of clinically heterogeneous genetic disorders most often caused by type I collagen alterations
- ↑ bone fragility → frequent fractures → malunion & bowing
  - Further ↑ likelihood of subsequent fractures
- Dentinogenesis imperfecta: Soft, cracked, discolored teeth

IMAGING

General Features

- Best diagnostic clue
  - Multiple in utero/perinatal fractures of short, poorly mineralized bones (OI type II)
  - Other OI types: Multiple fractures in thin, overtubulated long bones + vertebral fractures + osteoporosis

Radiographic Findings

- Radiography
  - Skull
    - Macrocranium
    - Frontal bossing, wide fontanelles, & sutures
    - Multiple wormian bones (≥ 10)
    - Platybasia & basilar impression/invagination
  - Spine
    - Kyphoscoliosis, biconcave or flattened vertebral bodies (platyspondyly), compression fractures
      - High rates of scoliosis progression in types III, IV, & V
      - Lower rate of progression in type I
    - Spondylolisthesis due to pedicle elongation
  - Chest
    - Thorax deformity → respiratory insufficiency
    - Sternum/manubrium bowing (convex outward)
    - Cardiac anomalies
  - Pelvis & hips
    - Coxa vara, protrusio acetabuli
  - Long bones
    - Diaphyseal overtubulation (thin, gracile)
    - Thin cortex
    - Bowing
    - "Popcorn Ca^{2+}" in epiphyses, metaphyses
      - Most common with type III
      - Especially knee & ankle
      - Typically resolves with physeal closure
    - Hyperplastic callus formation &/or interosseous membrane Ca^{2+} (type V)
      - Radioulnar interosseous membrane Ca^{2+} → radial head dislocation
      - Tibiofibular interosseous membrane Ca^{2+} (less common)
    - Zebra sign with bisphosphonate therapy
      - Sclerotic metaphyseal bands paralleling growth plates
      - Number of bands = number of treatments
  - Feet
    - Flatfoot & skewfoot (forefoot adduction, heel valgus, navicular abduction on talus)

Ultrasonographic Findings

- Fetal US may detect more severe types (II & III)
  - ↓ echogenicity of skull, spine, & long bones
    - Unusually well-visualized brain
  - Small thorax ± rib fractures
  - Long bones: Short, bowed multiple fractures ± callus
    - "Crinkled" or "crumpled" or "accordion" long bones

CT Findings

- Bone CT
  - Can help evaluate complications in axial skeleton
    - Cervical spine: Basilar invagination
    - Temporal bone: Otic capsule abnormalities resembling otospongiosis; stapes crura fractures & footplate fixation
    - Lumbar spine: Pedicle elongation + spondylolisthesis
  - Fetal CT done at some institutions if type II OI suspected
    - ↓ skull ossification, ↓ thorax size, bowed long bones with multiple fractures
- CTA
  - Rare: Aortic & carotid or vertebral artery dissection

MR Findings

- T2WI
  - Assess brainstem & spinal cord in basilar invagination

Nuclear Medicine Findings

- Bone scan
  - ↑ uptake with fractures

Imaging Recommendations

- Best imaging tool
  - Radiographs are usually sufficient to suggest diagnosis
  - CT or MR for axial skeleton complications

DIFFERENTIAL DIAGNOSIS

Child Abuse

- Fractures, retinal hemorrhages, intracranial injury, bruises
- No wormian bones, osteoporosis, or blue sclera

Diseases That Cause Bone Bowing

- Neurofibromatosis type 1
- Fibrous dysplasia
- Hyperparathyroidism
- Rickets
- Many bone dysplasias

Diseases With Fragile Bones

- Bruck syndrome
  - Fragile bones with congenital joint contractures
- Osteoporosis-pseudoglioma syndrome
  - Fragile bones with congenital blindness
- Cole-Carpenter syndrome
  - Fragile bones with craniosynostosis & ocular proptosis
- Idiopathic juvenile osteoporosis
  - No extraskeletal abnormalities

Hyperplastic Bone Formation

- Stress injury
- Myositis ossificans/heterotopic ossification
- Osteosarcoma

- Chronic osteomyelitis

Increased Wormian Bones

- Cleidocranial dysplasia
- Hypophosphatasia
- Hypothyroidism
- Pyknodysostosis
- Menkes syndrome

PATHOLOGY

General Features

- Genetics
  - Type I collagen is composed of triple helix
    - 2 α-1 chains (*COL1A1* gene)
    - 1 α-2 chain (*COL1A2* gene)
  - > 800 type I collagen mutations are known
  - 20 genetic types of OI are currently recognized
  - OI types I-IV: Mutations in *COL1A1* or *COL1A2*
    - OI type I: ↓ amount of type I collagen
    - OI types II-IV: Type I collagen folding, secretion, &/or mineralization abnormality
  - OI types V-XX involve mutations other than *COL1A1* or *COL1A2*
  - Screening for OI biochemical abnormalities
    - DNA sequencing is most sensitive
    - Cultured skin fibroblast test is rarely used now
- Associated abnormalities
  - Hearing loss (usually as adults), thin skin with subcutaneous hemorrhages, cardiac disease, hernias

Staging, Grading, & Classification

- Original Sillence classification (1979) included types I-IV
  - Based on clinical & radiologic manifestations & inheritance
  - Subsequent types were based on mutations outside type I collagen ± different phenotypes, inheritance
- OI type I: Mild, not deforming
  - Sclerae: Blue in most
  - Fractures: Spectrum of none (in 10%) → numerous; less common after puberty
  - Stature: Often normal, 20% with mild kyphoscoliosis in adults
  - Dentinogenesis imperfecta: Usually not present
- OI type II (subtypes A-C): Perinatal lethal
  - Sclerae: Blue
  - Beaded ribs, "accordion" femurs
  - Myriad of prenatal fractures
  - Poor to no ossification of skull
  - Intracranial hemorrhage, lung hypoplasia → death
- OI type III: Deformation severe
  - Triangular face due to underdeveloped facial bones
  - Sclerae: Gray
  - Kyphoscoliosis, chest deformity, bowed bones
  - Stature: Short
  - Usually wheelchair bound
- OI type IV: Deformation moderate
  - Sclerae: White
  - Bowing of long bones, vertebral fractures
  - Dentinogenesis imperfecta: In some but not all
  - Stature: Short
  - Walk with braces or crutches
- OI type V: Deformation moderate
  - Similar to type IV + interosseous membrane Ca^{2+} &/or hypertrophic callus
  - Dentinogenesis imperfecta: Absent
- OI type VI: Deformation moderate to severe
  - Sclerae: White or faintly blue
  - Stature: Moderately short
  - Vertebral compression fractures
  - Distinct histologic features
- Nosology & Classification of Genetic Skeletal Disorders (2019) identifies 5 clinical forms
  - Type I: Nondeforming with persistently blue sclera
    - Mildest form
  - Type II: Perinatal lethal
  - Type III: Progressively deforming
    - Most severely affected patients that survive infancy
  - Type IV: Moderate form
  - Type V: Similar phenotype to type IV + intramembranous ossification &/or hypertrophic callus

CLINICAL ISSUES

Demographics

- Epidemiology
  - All types: Incidence 1:10,000-20,000
  - OI type I: Incidence ~ 1:30,000
  - OI type II: Incidence ~ 1:60,000
  - Other types are rarer

Natural History & Prognosis

- Severity of OI (mild → severe)
  - Type I < IV < III < II
- Type II: Lethal in perinatal period
- Type III: Premature death

Treatment

- Intravenous bisphosphonates
  - Inhibit osteoclasts, ↑ bone mass/mineralization
  - ↓ bone pain & fractures
  - ↓ rate of scoliosis progression in type III if started < 6 years
  - Jaw osteonecrosis is not reported in this population
- Physical therapy, orthopedic surgery

DIAGNOSTIC CHECKLIST

Image Interpretation Pearls

- Wide range of radiographic features across OI types
- Radiographic appearance alone does not classify OI
  - Family history, clinical features, histology, & genetic screening all contribute

SELECTED REFERENCES

1. Marom R et al: Osteogenesis imperfecta: an update on clinical features and therapies. Eur J Endocrinol. 183(4):R95-106, 2020
2. Mortier GR et al: Nosology and classification of genetic skeletal disorders: 2019 revision. Am J Med Genet A. 179(12):2393-419, 2019
3. Pereira EM: Clinical perspectives on osteogenesis imperfecta versus non-accidental injury. Am J Med Genet C Semin Med Genet. 169(4):302-6, 2015
4. Renaud A et al: Radiographic features of osteogenesis imperfecta. Insights Imaging. 4(4):417-29, 2013

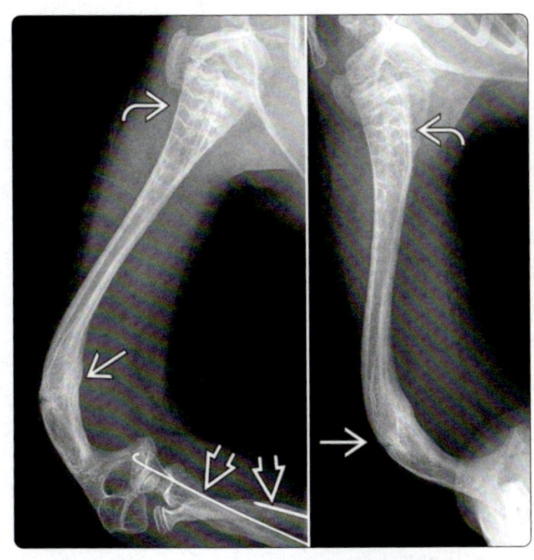

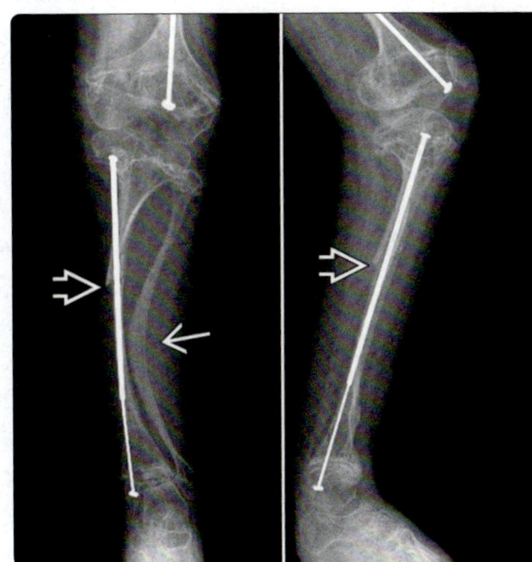

(Left) *AP (left) & lateral (right) radiographs in an 11-year-old OI patient show a gracile, bowed appearance of the right humerus with the apex at the site of a prior fracture. Sclerotic metaphyseal lines are seen in the proximal humerus secondary to episodes of bisphosphonate therapy. Rods are seen in the radius & ulna.* **(Right)** *AP (left) & lateral (right) radiographs of the lower leg in the same patient show osteoporotic, gracile, & bowed bones with a prior fracture & hardware.*

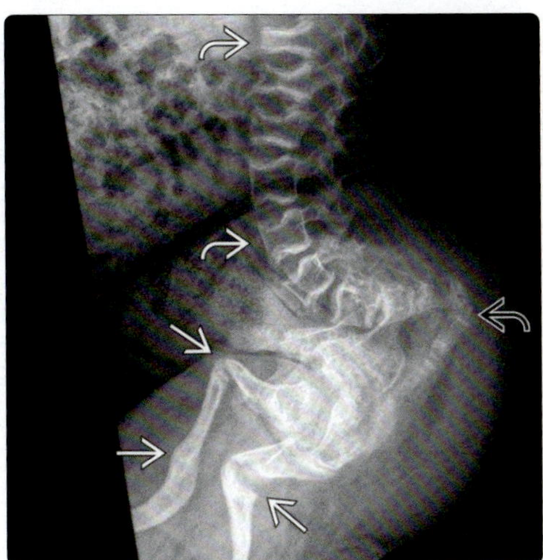

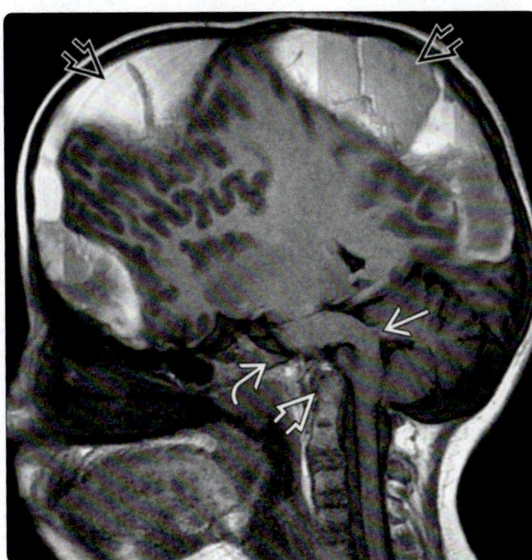

(Left) *Lateral lumbar radiograph in a 16-year-old with OI shows diffuse demineralization, biconcave/flattened vertebral bodies, severe sacral kyphosis, & bilateral femur fractures with malunion & bowing.* **(Right)** *Sagittal T1 brain MR in a child with OI shows the dens protruding into the foramen magnum with a horizontal clivus & brainstem angulation. Large subdural hematomas are present. Patients with OI are predisposed to intracranial hemorrhages after minor trauma.*

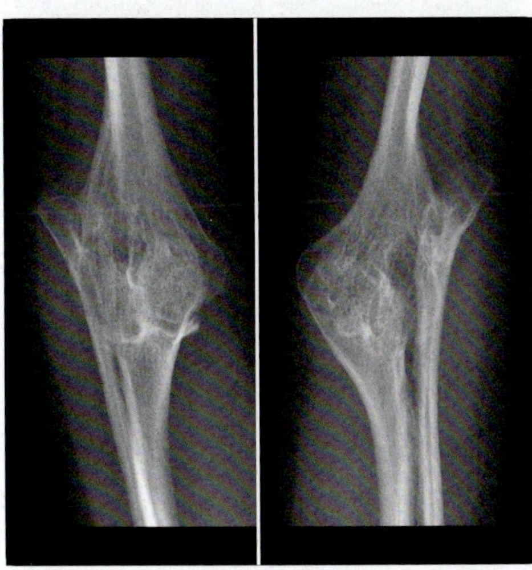

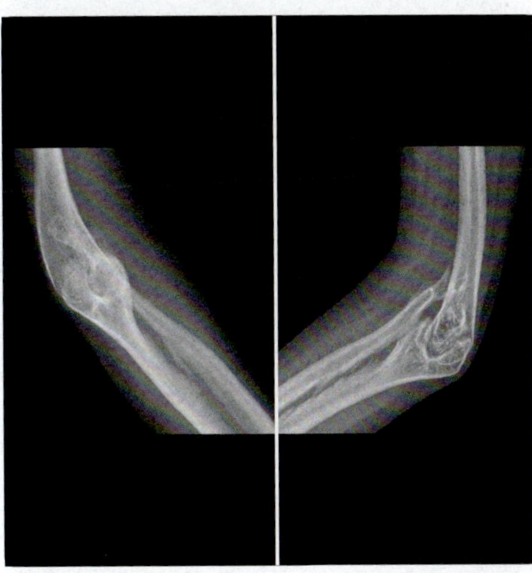

(Left) *Frontal radiographs of the right (left) & left (right) elbows in a 14-year-old girl with OI type V show a gracile appearance of the long bones & chronic bilateral radial head dislocations.* **(Right)** *Lateral radiographs of the right (left) & left (right) elbows in the same patient shows bilateral, volar radial head dislocations & ossification of the interosseous membranes. OI type V can have features of intramembranous ossification &/or hypertrophic callus formation.*

KEY FACTS

TERMINOLOGY

- Heterogeneous group of genetic disorders with ↑ bone density due to impaired bone resorption by osteoclasts
  - Osteopetrosis, autosomal recessive (ARO)
    - > 50% due to mutation of *TCIRG1* → infantile malignant osteopetrosis (IMO)
      - Typically presents in 1st year of life with macrocephaly, progressive blindness > deafness, hepatosplenomegaly, recurrent infections, severe anemia, fractures
      - Uniformly fatal without stem cell transplant
    - Other forms of ARO range from mild to severe
  - Osteopetrosis, autosomal dominant type 1
    - Not true osteopetrosis (unrelated to osteoclasts)
  - Osteopetrosis, autosomal dominant type 2
    - Most common form of osteopetrosis
    - More likely to present incidentally or due to pathologic fracture later in life

IMAGING

- Generalized osteosclerosis ± alternating radiolucent bands in metaphyses
  - Loss of corticomedullary definition
  - Undertubulated Erlenmeyer flask deformity of metaphyses, especially distal femurs
  - Bone-in-bone appearance of flat or small bones
  - ± pathologic fractures
- Thick, dense skull base &/or calvarium
- Well-defined sclerotic borders at vertebral endplates (sandwich vertebrae) vs. diffuse sclerosis

PATHOLOGY

- Defective bone remodeling results in effacement of marrow cavity & abnormal bone structure, impairing
  - Hematopoiesis → anemia, recurrent infections
  - Foraminal development → cranial nerve compression
  - Bone strength → pathologic fractures

(Left) *Bilateral lower extremity radiographs in a 6-month-old with fever show ↑ sclerosis of all visualized bones. The distal femurs show undertubulation (Erlenmeyer flask deformity) with loss of normal corticomedullary interfaces. Genetic testing confirmed autosomal recessive osteopetrosis (ARO).* **(Right)** *Lateral skull radiographs in an ARO patient taken at 6 months of age (left) & 2 years after bone marrow transplant (right) show interval restoration of normal bony mineralization.*

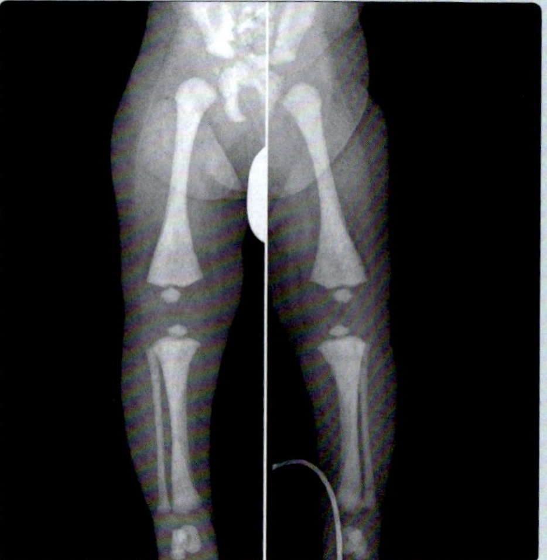

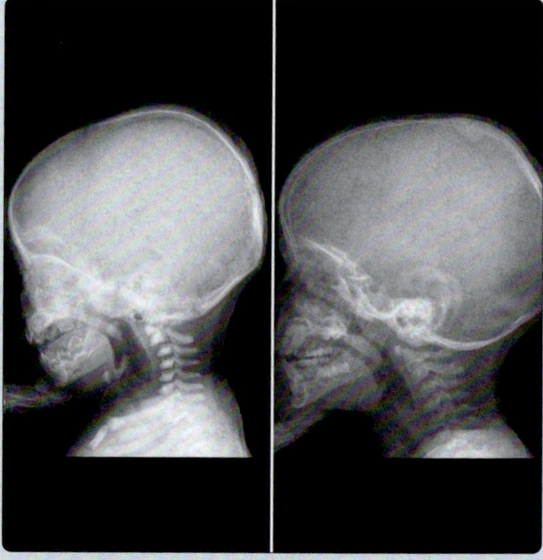

(Left) *AP radiograph in a 4-month-old with optic nerve atrophy, anemia, & thrombocytopenia shows diffusely ↑ bone density with marked splenomegaly ➙. Genetic testing confirmed ARO. Note the irregular metaphyses ➙ with fraying & cupping due to superimposed rickets ("osteopetrorickets").* **(Right)** *Axial NECT in the same patient with ARO shows diffusely ↑ density & thickening of the skull with severely narrowed optic foramina ➙.*

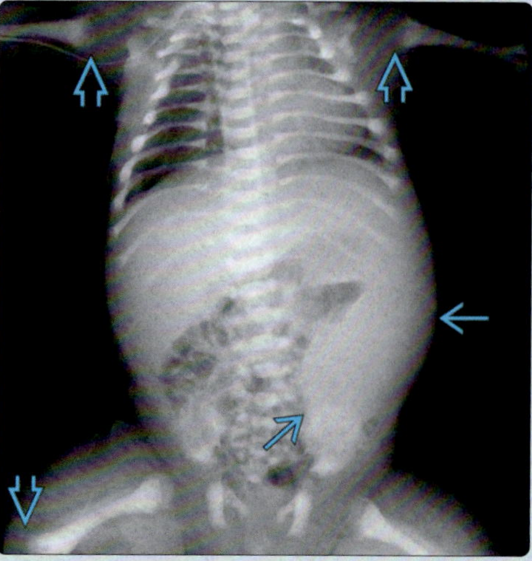

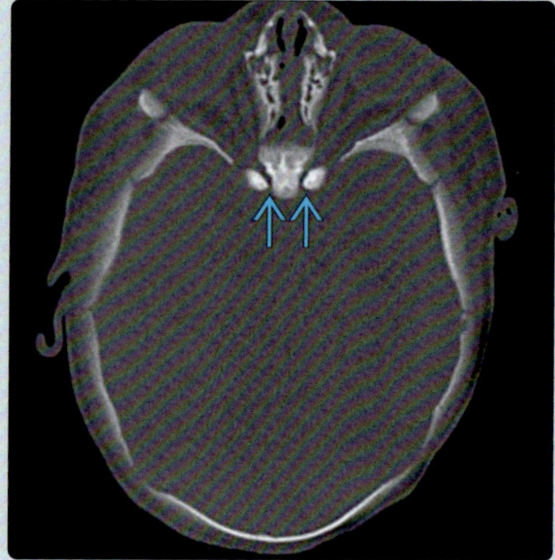

TERMINOLOGY

Definitions

- Heterogeneous group of genetic disorders characterized by ↑ bone density due to impaired bone resorption by dysfunctional osteoclasts
  - Osteopetrosis, autosomal recessive (ARO)
    - > 50% due to mutations of *TCIRG1* → infantile malignant osteopetrosis (IMO)
      - Severe anemia, hepatosplenomegaly, recurrent infections, fractures, macrocephaly, progressive blindness > deafness, ± hydrocephalus, coxa vara
    - Other forms of ARO range from mild to severe
  - Osteopetrosis, autosomal dominant type 1 (ADO1)
    - Not true osteopetrosis
      - *LRP5* mutation → enhanced osteoblast activity → high bone mass
  - Osteopetrosis, autosomal dominant type 2 (ADO2)
    - Albers-Schönberg disease, osteoclast rich
    - Most common form of osteopetrosis
    - *CLCN7* mutation in most → ↓ of chloride channel 7
      - Variable penetrance & expressivity; 20-40% are asymptomatic
  - Osteopetrosis, X-linked recessive (very rare)
    - *IKBKG* mutation → osteopetrosis, lymphedema, anhidrotic ectodermal dysplasia, immunodeficiency (OL-EDA-ID)

IMAGING

General Features

- Location
  - Skull, brain, face
    - Thick, dense skull base &/or calvarium
    - Macrocrania with frontal bossing
    - Neural: Narrowed foramina, including foramen magnum
    - Mandible: Frequent site of osteomyelitis
  - Axial skeleton
    - Vertebrae: Well-defined sclerotic borders at endplates (sandwich vertebrae) in ADO are classic; however, uniform sclerosis may be present
      - Bone-in-bone appearance
      - Osteomyelitis, scoliosis, fractures
    - Pelvis: Bone-in-bone appearance
  - Appendicular skeleton
    - Dense skeleton: Generalized sclerosis vs. radiolucent bands in metaphyses
      - Loss of corticomedullary definition
      - Bone-in-bone (endobone) appearance
    - Metaphyseal widening/flaring caused by defective tubular remodeling
      - Erlenmeyer flask deformity of distal femur, proximal humerus & tibia
    - Pathologic fractures
    - Coxa vara
    - ± osteopetrorickets (in ARO)
      - ↓ gastric acidity → ↓ calcium absorption; most commonly in *TCIRG1* mutation
      - Metaphyseal widening, cupping, & fraying superimposed over findings of osteopetrosis

PATHOLOGY

General Features

- Genetics
  - Different mutations affect osteoclasts in various ways
    - Osteoclast poor forms: ↓ number
    - Osteoclast rich forms: ↓ functionality
  - Mutations found in > 90% of cases

Microscopic Features

- Primary spongiosa persists & fills medullary cavity (rather than being removed during normal growth)
  - Leaves no room for hematopoietic marrow
  - Prevents development of normal mature trabeculae that provide strength to bone

CLINICAL ISSUES

Presentation

- Most common signs/symptoms
  - ARO/IMO: Impaired hematopoiesis → thrombocytopenia, anemia, infection, & extramedullary hematopoiesis; cranial nerve compression → impaired vision, sensorineural hearing loss
  - ADO: Nontraumatic fractures, cranial nerve palsy, osteoarthritis of hip, mandibular osteomyelitis

Demographics

- Age
  - ARO/IMO typically presents < 1 year old
  - ADO2 typically presents in late childhood or adolescence

Natural History & Prognosis

- IMO: Uniformly fatal if untreated
- ADO: Can be completely asymptomatic

Treatment

- Hematopoietic stem cell transplant: Only cure for ARO
  - Addresses bone marrow failure & underlying bone resorption abnormality
    - Successful engraftment is indicated by changes in
      - Platelet & neutrophil counts
      - Calcium & phosphate levels
      - Bone morphology & mineralization (improving by 3-12 months)
- Fracture fixation: Unique problems are encountered due to abnormal bone density & fragility, lack of medullary canal, & ↓ vascularity with impaired healing & infection risks

SELECTED REFERENCES

1. Shapiro G et al: Skeletal changes following hematopoietic stem cell transplantation in osteopetrosis. J Bone Miner Res.35(9):1645-51, 2020
2. Chawla A et al: Fractures in patients with osteopetrosis, insights from a single institution. Int Orthop. 43(6):1297-302, 2019
3. Vomero A et al: Malignant Infantile osteopetrosis. Rev Chil Pediatr. 90(4):443-7, 2019
4. Palagano E et al: Genetics of osteopetrosis. Curr Osteoporos Rep. 16(1):13-25, 2018
5. Simanovsky N et al: Extending the spectrum of radiological findings in patients with severe osteopetrosis and different genetic backgrounds. Pediatr Blood Cancer. 63(7):1222-6, 2016
6. Orchard PJ et al: Hematopoietic stem cell transplantation for infantile osteopetrosis. Blood. 126(2):270-6, 2015
7. Gonen KA et al: Infantile osteopetrosis with superimposed rickets. Pediatr Radiol. 43(2):189-95, 2013

KEY FACTS

TERMINOLOGY

- Collection of poorly understood "disorders" of immature skeleton
  - > 70 entities, many with eponyms
- Many are symptomatic growth disturbances with elements of idiopathic osteonecrosis &/or overuse injury
- Symptoms vary: Asymptomatic → pain → long-term growth disturbances
- Outcomes vary: Resolution of self-limited process → permanent deformity if untreated

IMAGING

- Affect certain sites where bone growth occurs by endochondral ossification (epiphyses, apophyses > metaphyses)
- Radiographs: Fragmentation, sclerosis, flattening
  - Depending on location, symptoms, & patient age, such findings do not necessarily indicate disease
  - Normal variants of irregular epiphyseal ossification can occur at certain locations
- MR: Marrow & soft tissue edema typically correlate with symptoms
  - Subtracted pre-/postcontrast T1 FS images may show ↓ enhancement in setting of ischemia/necrosis
  - DWI/ADC may also reflect ischemia

CLINICAL ISSUES

- Conservative therapy with rest is effective for many
- Certain entities (e.g., Blount, Legg-Calvé-Perthes) often require surgical intervention to preserve long-term function

DIAGNOSTIC CHECKLIST

- Not every irregular ossification center is abnormal
  - Correlate with site, patient age, & symptoms
    - Helpful to know locations where irregular ossification normally occurs vs. never occurs
  - MR is useful adjunct for determining source of pain

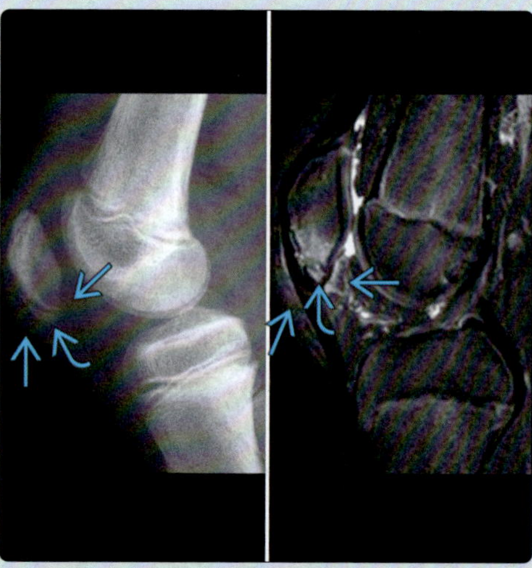

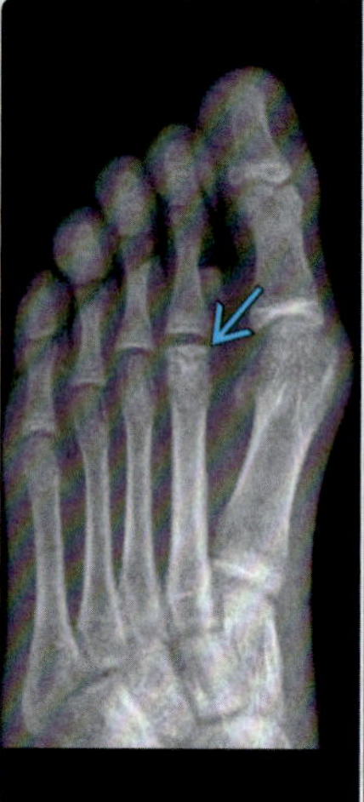

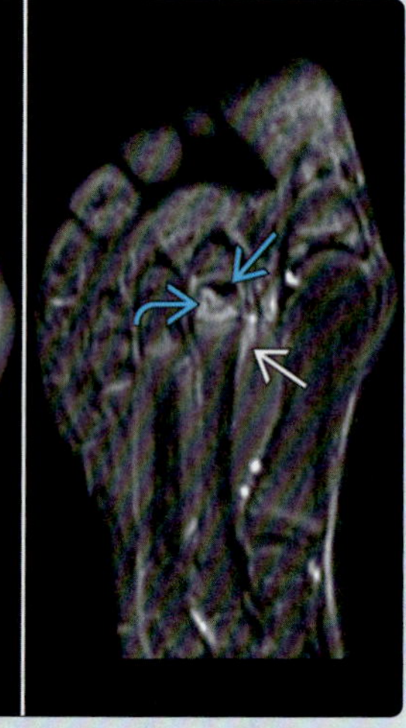

(Left) *Lateral radiograph (left) & sagittal T2 FS MR (right) of a 12-year-old boy with anterior knee pain show fragmentation of the inferior pole of the patella ➡ with adjacent soft tissue swelling ➡. The findings are consistent with Sinding-Larsen-Johansson syndrome.* **(Right)** *Oblique radiograph (left) & T2 FS MR (right) of the left foot in a 13-year-old girl with Freiberg disease show flattening & sclerosis of the 2nd metatarsal head ➡. Additionally, the MR shows adjacent marrow ➡ & soft tissue ➡ edema.*

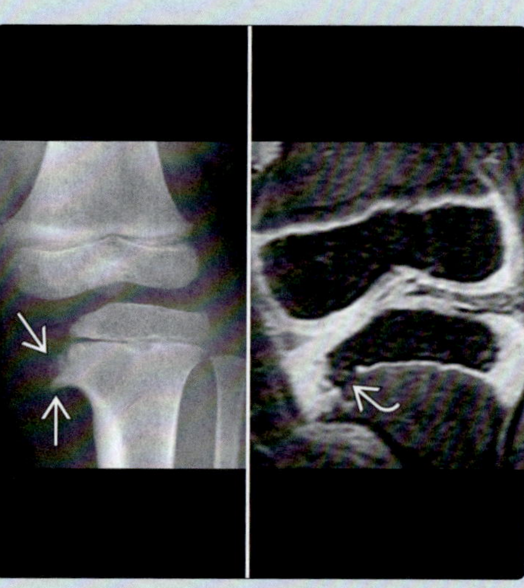

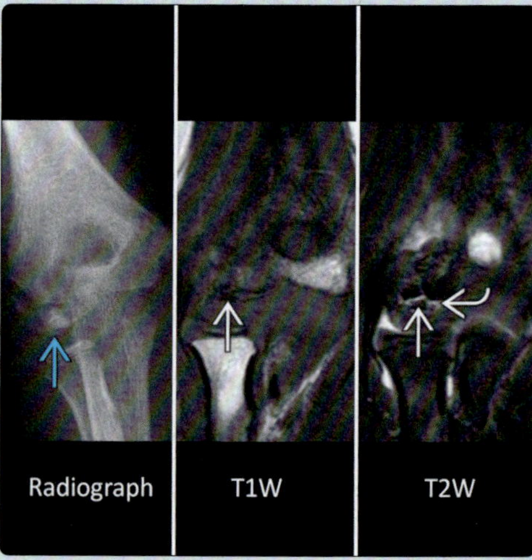

(Left) *AP radiograph (left) shows downsloping, beaking, & irregularity of the medial tibial metaphysis ➡ (Blount disease). Coronal GRE MR (right) shows abnormal ossification of the medial tibial epiphysis & metaphysis with an osseous bridge ➡ crossing the physis.* **(Right)** *AP radiograph (left) of an 8-year-old girl with Panner disease shows fragmentation & sclerosis of the capitellum ➡. There is associated low signal intensity at this level on the T1 (middle) & T2 FS (right) MR images ➡ with interspersed ↑ signal intensity ➡.*

TERMINOLOGY

Synonyms

- > 70 entities, many with eponyms

Definitions

- Collection of poorly understood "disorders" of immature skeleton
- Many entities reflect symptomatic growth disturbances with elements of idiopathic osteonecrosis &/or overuse
- Symptoms range from asymptomatic → pain → chronic manifestations of growth disturbances
- Outcomes range from resolution of self-limited process → permanent deformity if untreated

IMAGING

General Features

- Best diagnostic clue
  - Radiographic fragmentation, sclerosis, flattening
    - Depending on location, symptoms, & patient age, such findings do not necessarily indicate disease
    - Normal variants of irregular epiphyseal ossification can occur at certain locations
  - Bone marrow & soft tissue edema by MR
    - Typically correlate with symptoms
- Location
  - Affect certain sites where bone growth occurs by endochondral ossification (epiphyses, apophyses > metaphyses)
  - > 1 osteochondrosis can occur at some locations with differing clinical implications
  - Most frequent sites
    - Thoracic spine: Scheuermann disease
    - Capitellum: Panner disease, osteochondritis dissecans (OCD)
    - Lunate: Kienbock disease
    - Hip: Legg-Calvé-Perthes (LCP), Meyer dysplasia
    - Inferior patella: Sinding-Larsen-Johansson syndrome
    - Proximal, medial tibia: Blount disease
    - Tibial tubercle: Osgood-Schlatter disease
    - Calcaneal apophysis: Sever disease
    - Tarsal navicular: Köhler disease
    - 2nd or 3rd metatarsal head: Freiberg disease

Radiographic Findings

- Irregularity, fragmentation, sclerosis, flattening at site of endochondral ossification
  - Chronic changes may lead to deformity (e.g., LCP) &/or osteoarthritis (e.g., Freiberg)
- Bony bridges may rarely form across physes in this setting, leading to angular deformities or limb length discrepancy (e.g., Blount)
- ± adjacent soft tissue edema

MR Findings

- Abnormal sclerosis: Low T1 & T2 signal
- Marrow & soft tissue edema: Poorly defined high T2 signal
- Fragmentation/collapse: Discrete linear fluid signal intensity
- Osteonecrosis: Variable depending on stages
  - Subtracted pre-/postcontrast T1 FS images show earliest findings of ischemia & necrosis (↓ enhancement) & subsequent revascularization (↑ enhancement)
  - DWI can show early ischemia

Imaging Recommendations

- Best imaging tool
  - Radiographs correlated with specific symptoms
  - MR is useful adjunct if clinically uncertain

DIFFERENTIAL DIAGNOSIS

Normal Developmental Variants

- Asymptomatic
- Radiographic findings only with essentially normal MR
  - No marrow edema
- Characteristic locations (e.g., humeral trochlea)

Osteonecrosis of Systemic Disorders

- Sclerosis, fragmentation, collapse of epiphyses
- Often widespread with predisposing conditions

Spondyloepiphyseal Dysplasia

- Epiphyseal dysplasias may or may not involve spine
- Epiphyses are affected throughout body

Septic Arthritis

- Joint effusion, synovitis, marrow & soft tissue edema
- Fever, leukocytosis, & altered weight bearing

Juvenile Idiopathic Arthritis

- Swelling, pain, joint effusion, synovitis acutely
- Epiphyseal overgrowth, erosions, joint space loss chronically

CLINICAL ISSUES

Presentation

- Site dependent: Pain, limp, or limb deformity possible

Treatment

- Conservative therapy with rest is effective for many
- Certain entities (e.g., Blount, LCP) often require surgical intervention to preserve long-term function

DIAGNOSTIC CHECKLIST

Image Interpretation Pearls

- Not every irregular ossification center is abnormal
- Helpful to know locations where irregular ossification
  - Occurs normally (e.g., trochlea of humerus)
  - May occur normally without symptoms or with symptomatic osteochondrosis (e.g., calcaneal apophysis: Sever disease)
  - Does not normally occur (e.g., capitellum of elbow)
- MR is useful adjunct for determining source of pain

SELECTED REFERENCES

1. Ahuja K et al: Osteochondroses of the bilateral metacarpal heads: Dieterich disease. A case report with review of the literature. Clin Imaging. 67:7-10, 2020
2. West EY et al: Imaging of osteochondrosis. Pediatr Radiol. 49(12):1610-6, 2019
3. Launay F: Sports-related overuse injuries in children. Orthop Traumatol Surg Res. 101(1 Suppl):S139-47, 2015

Rickets

KEY FACTS

TERMINOLOGY

- Failure to mineralize cartilage & osteoid at growth plates (physes) of immature skeleton in setting of low ion concentrations (calcium or phosphorous)
  - Lack of phosphate (ultimate problem in all rickets) → failure of chondrocyte apoptosis → disruption of endochondral ossification
- Most common cause: Nutritional vitamin D deficiency

IMAGING

- Loss of normally thin, dense, well-defined zone of provisional Ca^{2+} at interface of physis & metaphysis
- Metaphyseal cupping, splaying, & fraying with lengthening ("widening") of adjacent radiolucent physis
- All sites of endochondral bone formation are affected
  - Most pronounced at long bone metaphyses with greatest linear growth
- Sites of membranous bone growth are less affected

TOP DIFFERENTIAL DIAGNOSES

- Newborn stress demineralization
- Leukemia or metastatic neuroblastoma
- Congenital syphilis
- Metaphyseal fracture of child abuse
- Physeal stress injury
- Physeal fracture
- Metaphyseal chondrodysplasias
- Hypophosphatasia

CLINICAL ISSUES

- Peak age for dietary rickets: 3 months to 2 years
- Most rickets responds to vitamin D therapy ± calcium

DIAGNOSTIC CHECKLIST

- Unexplained physeal widening at 1 site (i.e., without acute or chronic trauma) merits survey at other sites of rapidly growing long bones (knees, wrists)
  - Multisite physeal widening → get metabolic work-up

(Left) *AP radiograph in a young child with rickets shows fraying, cupping, & splaying of the proximal tibial ➔ & fibular ➔ metaphyses. There is loss of the normally dense, well-defined zones of provisional Ca^{2+} (ZPC) that should be seen at the metaphyseal-physeal junctions. The radiolucent tibial physis is lengthened ➔. The epiphyseal ZPC is also lost ➔ with poor bony margin definition.* **(Right)** *AP knee radiograph in a 3-year-old with rickets shows typical metaphyseal fraying, cupping, & splaying ➔, as well as physeal lengthening ➔.*

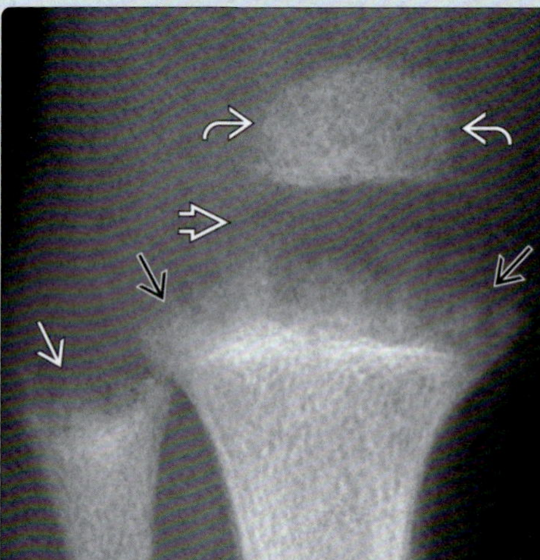

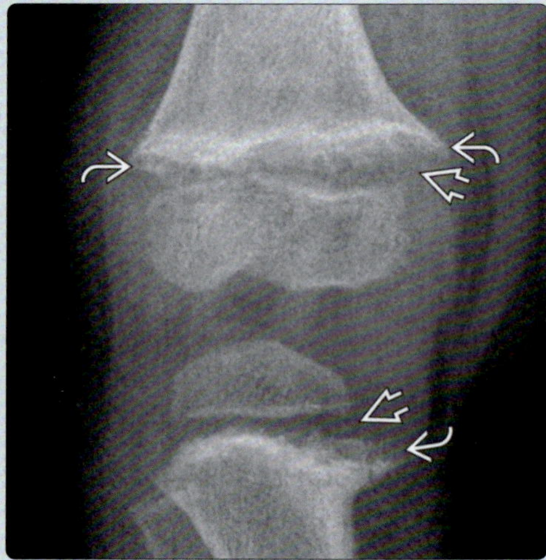

(Left) *PA wrist radiograph in this young child with rickets shows fraying, cupping, & splaying of every visualized metaphysis ➔. The normal ZPCs are lost.* **(Right)** *PA radiograph in the same child 9 weeks after initiation of therapy shows that endochondral ossification has resumed with improved bone formation at all the growth centers. The visualized metaphyses ➔ are normalizing in shape & density as compared to the prior study.*

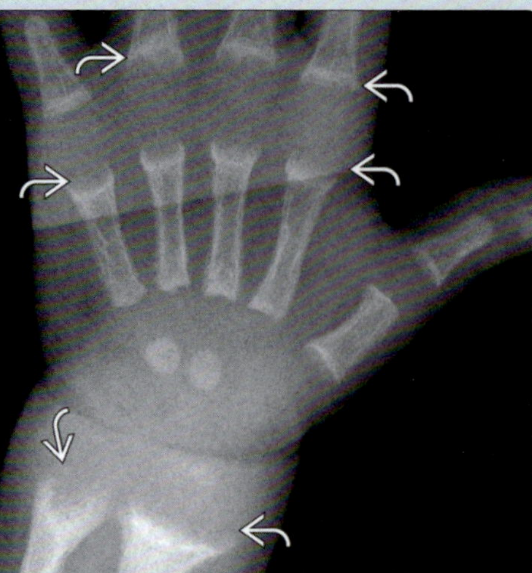

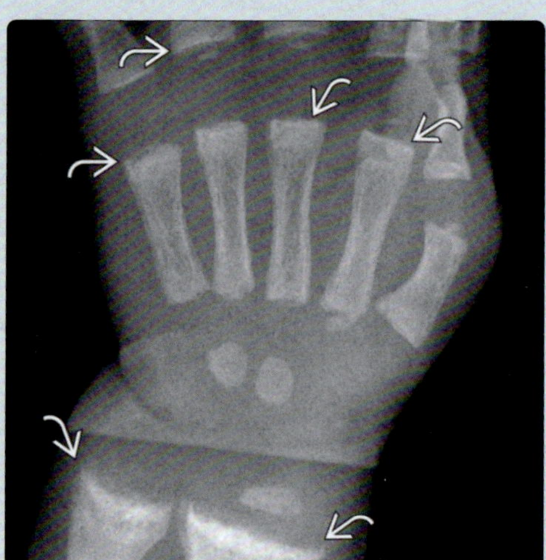

TERMINOLOGY

Definitions

- Failure to mineralize cartilage & osteoid at growth plates (physes) of immature skeleton in setting of low ion concentrations
  - Initial deficiency may be considered as calcipenic or phosphopenic
  - Lack of phosphate becomes ultimate problem
    - Underlying factor in all rickets: Failed apoptosis of hypertrophic chondrocytes
      - Key enzyme (caspase-9) is dependent on phosphorylation
      - Failure of apoptosis disrupts endochondral ossification
- Most common cause: Nutritional vitamin D deficiency
  - ↓ dietary vitamin D &/or ↓ exposure to sunlight
  - Primary calcium deficiency is uncommon
- Many other causes, including
  - Prematurity
    - < 28-weeks gestational age, birth weight < 1,000 g
    - 80% of fetal bone mineralization occurs in 3rd trimester
      - Typical neonatal nutrition is not sufficient
      - Exacerbated by medications used for chronic lung disease of prematurity, including steroids & calcium-excreting diuretics
  - Prenatal factors
    - Maternal medical problems → severe vitamin D deficiency
  - Malabsorption: Binding with malabsorbed fatty acids → ↓ calcium & vitamin D absorption
  - Liver disease: ↓ formation of 25-hydroxy vitamin D; unconjugated bilirubin interferes with osteoblasts
    - Chronic liver disease
    - Anticonvulsant therapy
  - Vitamin D-dependent types 1A, 1B, 2A, 2B
    - Various genetic disorders of vitamin D metabolism
  - Hypophosphatemic rickets: Renal loss of phosphates
    - > 10 phenotypes with FGF-23-dependent & -independent forms, including
      - X-linked, autosomal dominant & recessive forms
      - Syndromes, including neurofibromatosis type 1, McCune-Albright
    - Chemotherapy: Ifosfamide renal-tubule toxicity
  - Oncogenic rickets: Rare paraneoplastic syndrome caused by ↑ production of FGF-23
    - Phosphaturic mesenchymal tumor
    - Nonossifying fibroma
    - Hemangiopericytoma
    - Osteoblastoma
    - Linear sebaceous nevus syndrome
  - Chronic renal disease: Renal osteodystrophy with secondary hyperparathyroidism
    - ↓ glomerular function → phosphorus retention → hypocalcemia
    - Tubular dysfunction → ↓ synthesis of 1,25-dihydroxy vitamin D → hypocalcemia
    - Hypocalcemia → hyperparathyroidism

IMAGING

General Features

- Best diagnostic clue
  - Loss of normally thin, dense, well-defined zone of provisional Ca^{2+} (ZPC) at interface of physis & metaphysis
  - Metaphyseal cupping, splaying, & fraying with lengthening ("widening") of adjacent physis
- Location
  - All sites of endochondral bone formation are affected
    - Most pronounced at long bone metaphyses with greatest linear growth
      - Distal femur, proximal tibia, proximal humerus, distal radius
  - Sites of membranous bone growth are less affected

Radiographic Findings

- Axial skeleton
  - Costochondral junctions: Cupping, widening of anterior rib ends ("rachitic rosary")
  - Spine: Scoliosis, biconcave vertebral bodies
  - Skull, face (largely membranous growth, except skull base)
    - Widened sutures, delayed sutural & fontanel closure
    - Postural molding, frontal bossing, platybasia
    - Delayed eruption of teeth, enamel hypoplasia
- Appendicular skeleton
  - Epiphyses: Loss of dense outline (ZPC) of secondary ossification centers → irregular margins
  - Physes: Lengthening (longitudinal "widening") of radiolucent growth plates (due to ↑ unossified cartilage)
  - Metaphyses: Fraying, splaying/transverse widening, & cupping with loss of normal dense ZPC
    - Loss of metaphyseal collar of Laval-Jeantet
  - Diaphyses: Bowing, osteoporosis, tunneling, fractures
    - Looser zones: Transversely oriented lucencies of insufficiency fractures in severe cases
  - Pelvis: Inward migration of sacrum, acetabula → triradiate appearance; causes dystocia in adulthood
  - Hip: Coxa vara, protrusio acetabuli
  - Knees: Genu valgum or varum
  - Periosteal reaction: Occult fracture or subperiosteal accumulation of unmineralized osteoid
- Renal osteodystrophy with secondary hyperparathyroidism
  - Subperiosteal bone resorption
    - Distal clavicle, distal radius + ulna, middle phalanges of hands, medial femoral neck, medial proximal tibia
    - Lamina dura of teeth
  - Resorption at phalangeal tufts, pubic symphysis
  - Subchondral, subtendinous, subligamentous resorption
  - Endosteal bone resorption → lacy pattern of inner cortex (cortical tunneling)
  - Lengthened ("widened") physes (subphyseal resorption, fibrous tissue deposition)
    - ↑ risk for slipped capital femoral epiphysis
  - Bone margins unsharp, hazy
  - Sclerosis with "smudged" trabeculae
  - Soft tissue Ca^{2+}
- Healing rickets after vitamin D therapy
  - ↑ density at ZPC after treatment in 2-3 weeks with nutritional rickets, 2-3 months with renal rickets

MR Findings

- Elongated cartilaginous physes with ↑ PD/T2 signal
- Absence of normal thin, low signal intensity ZPC

DIFFERENTIAL DIAGNOSIS

Newborn Stress Demineralization

- Metaphyseal lucent bands with intact ZPC in first 2 months after delivery

Leukemia or Metastatic Neuroblastoma

- Metaphyseal lucent bands with intact ZPC
- ± osteoporosis, permeative lesions, periosteal reaction

Congenital Syphilis

- Serrated lucent metaphyses
- Focal destruction of upper medial tibial metaphyseal cortex (Wimberger corner sign)

Metaphyseal Fracture of Child Abuse

- Classic metaphyseal corner injury (or bucket-handle fracture) due to fracture through primary spongiosa
- Only at sites of injury (not diffuse)
- ZPC & bony mineralization are normal

Physeal Stress Injury

- Repetitive microtrauma to growth plate causes focal or diffuse longitudinal physeal widening & irregularity without transverse metaphyseal widening or cupping
  - Likely due to chronic metaphyseal vasculature injury impairing endochondral ossification in high-level athletes
- Single site is usually affected (e.g., distal radius of "gymnast wrist" or proximal humerus of "Little Leaguer shoulder")
- Non-weight-bearing long bones (e.g., fibula, ulna) are typically spared

Physeal Fracture

- Acute growth plate widening in Salter-Harris injuries
  - ± displacement of epiphysis + metaphyseal fragment
- Overlying soft tissue swelling
- Clear history of trauma is usually present

Metaphyseal Chondrodysplasias

- Widespread abnormal metaphyseal configurations
- Varying etiologies & associated anomalies

Hypophosphatasia

- Wide spectrum of disease severity; due to inactive enzyme despite normal mineral concentrations
- In milder forms, metaphyseal disturbances may be focal rather than uniform
- Bowdler spurs are characteristic

PATHOLOGY

General Features

- Etiology
  - Normal bone development requires adequate calcium + phosphorus (facilitated by vitamin D)
    - Essential for formation of hydroxyapatite crystals
    - Rickets is due to ↓ availability of these substances
      - Also need adequate blood supply & cartilage for endochondral ossification
  - Vitamin D
    - ↑ absorption of calcium from intestine
    - ↑ calcium resorption in renal proximal tubules
    - Regulates apoptosis of chondrocytes, cartilage matrix mineralization, & metaphyseal angiogenesis
- Associated abnormalities
  - Fractures due to vitamin D deficiency do occur in mobile patients with radiologic manifestations of rickets
  - Findings **not** attributable to rickets that must prompt child abuse evaluation
    - Fractures in nonmobile infants
    - Fractures otherwise typical of child abuse (e.g., classic metaphyseal lesion or corner fracture, etc.)
    - Subdural hematoma or retinal hemorrhage

Microscopic Features

- Normal physis consists of 4 zones of cartilage
  - Germinal/resting cartilage cells (near epiphysis)
  - Proliferating cartilage cells
  - Hypertrophic columns of cartilage cells
  - Provisional Ca^{2+} of cartilage (ZPC)
    - First 3 zones: Radiolucent
    - ZPC: Thin, dense, undulating line at metaphyseal edge
- Metaphyseal spongiosa adjacent to ZPC: Cartilage matrix replaced by osteoid with remodeling & Ca^{2+} leading to spongy bone occupying marrow cavity
  - Rickets: Ca^{2+} of cartilage & osteoid does not occur → physeal/metaphyseal abnormalities

CLINICAL ISSUES

Demographics

- Peak age for dietary rickets: 3 months to 2 years

Treatment

- Most rickets responds to vitamin D therapy ± calcium

DIAGNOSTIC CHECKLIST

Consider

- Unexplained physeal widening at 1 site (i.e., without acute or chronic trauma) merits survey at other sites of rapidly growing long bones (knees, wrists)
  - If widening is present at multiple sites, including non-weight-bearing long bones, suspect metabolic disease

Image Interpretation Pearls

- Be sure to look at growth centers of proximal humeri & femurs on neonatal chest & abdominal radiographs

SELECTED REFERENCES

1. Aldana Sierra MC et al: Vitamin D, rickets and child abuse: controversies and evidence. Pediatr Radiol. 51(6):1014-22, 2021
2. Servaes S et al: Rachitic change and vitamin D status in young children with fractures. Skeletal Radiol. 49(1):85-91, 2020
3. Ma GM et al: Review of paraneoplastic syndromes in children. Pediatr Radiol. 49(4):534-50, 2019
4. Michałus I et al: Rare, genetically conditioned forms of rickets: differential diagnosis and advances in diagnostics and treatment. Clin Genet. 94(1):103-14, 2018
5. Chang CY et al: Imaging findings of metabolic bone disease. Radiographics. 36(6):1871-87, 2016
6. Servaes S et al: The etiology and significance of fractures in infants and young children: a critical multidisciplinary review. Pediatr Radiol. 46(5):591-600, 2016
7. Shore RM et al: Rickets: part I. Pediatr Radiol. 43(2):140-51, 2013
8. Shore RM et al: Rickets: part II. Pediatr Radiol. 43(2):152-72, 2013

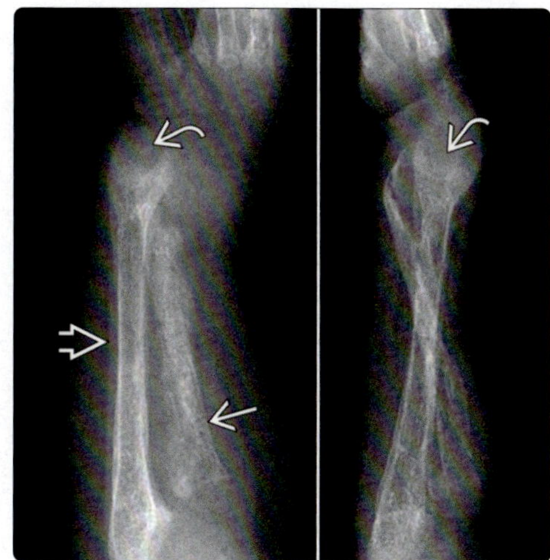

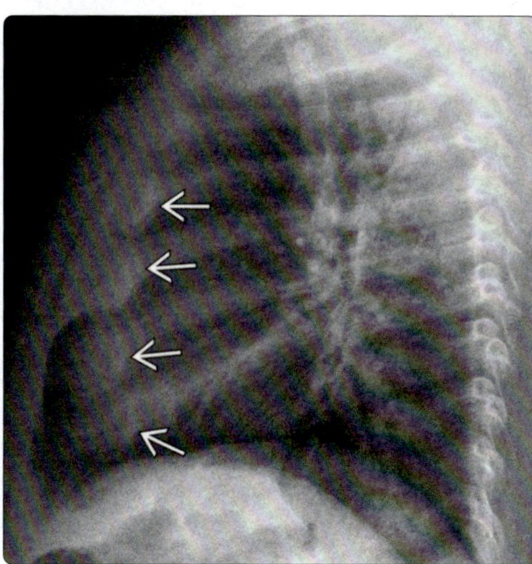

(Left) *Lateral radiographs of the forearm in a 2-year-old child with linear nevus sebaceous syndrome & associated paraneoplastic hypophosphatemic rickets show severe demineralization with periosteal reaction ➡, cortical tunneling ➡, & cupped, frayed metaphyses ➡.* **(Right)** *Lateral radiograph in a 7-month-old boy with failure to thrive shows the widened & cupped anterior ribs ➡ typical of the "rachitic rosary."*

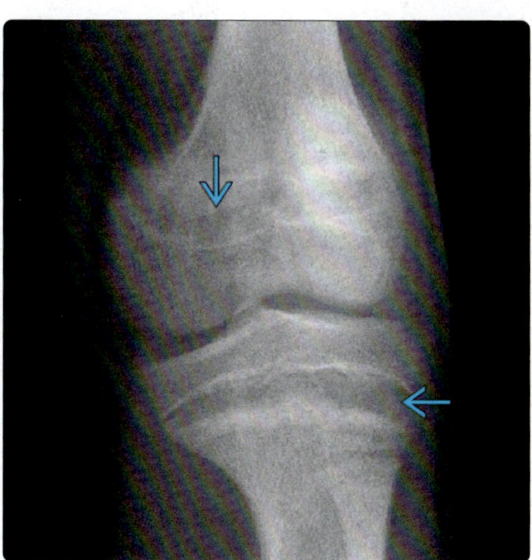

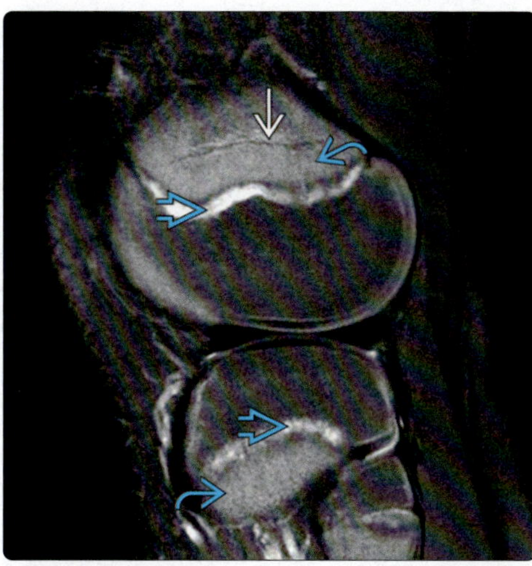

(Left) *AP radiograph of a 15-year-old with knee pain shows loss of the normal dense ZPCs with partial mineralization of hypertrophied physeal cartilage ➡. The metaphyses appear mildly frayed & cupped.* **(Right)** *Sagittal T2 FS MR in the same patient shows mild physeal lengthening ("widening") ➡ with abnormally hyperintense metaphyses that are partially mineralized ➡. The thin, low-signal line ➡ represents an aberrant ZPC in this patient with nutritional rickets.*

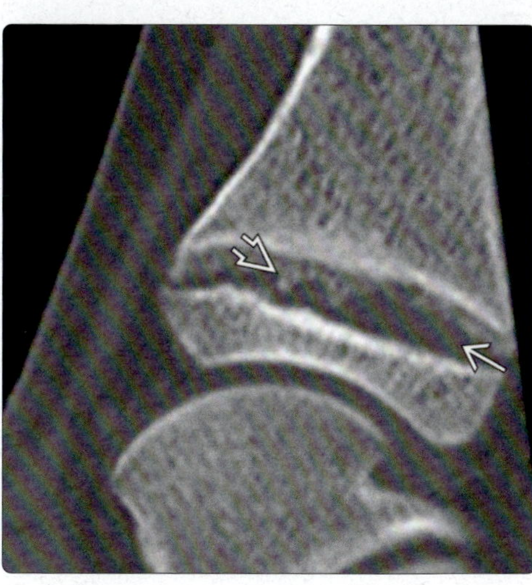

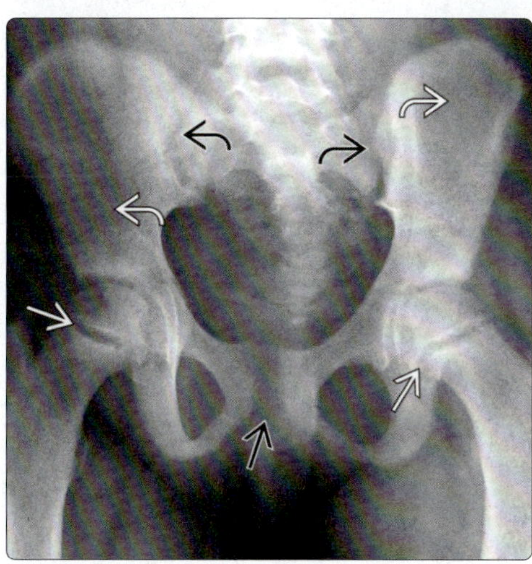

(Left) *Sagittal CT reconstruction in a 12-year-old boy with ankle pain shows a lengthened ("widened") distal tibial physis ➡ with metaphyseal cupping & irregularity ➡. This finding was present bilaterally at the tibias & fibulas.* **(Right)** *AP radiograph in the same patient, who was found to be in renal failure, shows typical changes of renal osteodystrophy & renal rickets with proximal femoral physeal lengthening ➡, widened & irregular pubic symphysis ➡ & sacroiliac joints ➡, & diffuse "smudging" of trabeculae ➡.*

Sickle Cell Disease

KEY FACTS

IMAGING

- Vertebrae
  - Infarctions: Central endplate depressions (H-shape or Lincoln log morphology)
  - Marrow hyperplasia with bone softening: Biconcave endplates (fish mouth)
- Ribs: Infarction is part of acute chest syndrome (chest pain, dyspnea, cough + pulmonary consolidation)
- Long bone infarctions
  - Acute/subacute: Poorly defined marrow, soft tissue, & periosteal edema ± fluid collections
    - Not easily distinguished from osteomyelitis
    - Dactylitis (hand-foot syndrome): Hand & foot small tubular bone infarcts, usually at age 6-24 months
  - Chronic: Lucent or sclerotic medullary cavity
    - Diaphysis, metaphysis
    - Epiphyseal infarction is most common in humeral & femoral heads: Sclerosis, subchondral collapse

PATHOLOGY

- Bony manifestations result from
  - Chronic anemia → red marrow hyperplasia
  - Immunocompromise & altered blood flow → osteomyelitis
  - Vasoocclusion → medullary infarction

CLINICAL ISSUES

- Typical presentation: Pain due to vasoocclusive crisis involving any organ, most commonly bone
- Patients of African descent are most commonly affected
- Mean survival: 42 years

DIAGNOSTIC CHECKLIST

- Differentiation of acute bone infarct vs. osteomyelitis in SCD is very difficult
  - Episodes of vasoocclusion > > osteomyelitis in SCD
  - Cortical disruption & fluid collections (especially larger) favor osteomyelitis

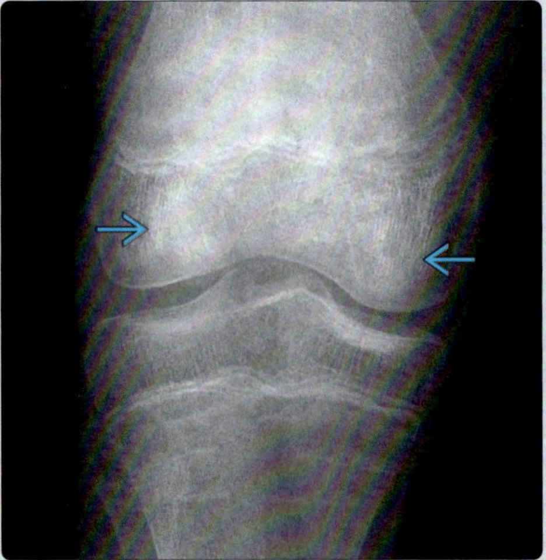

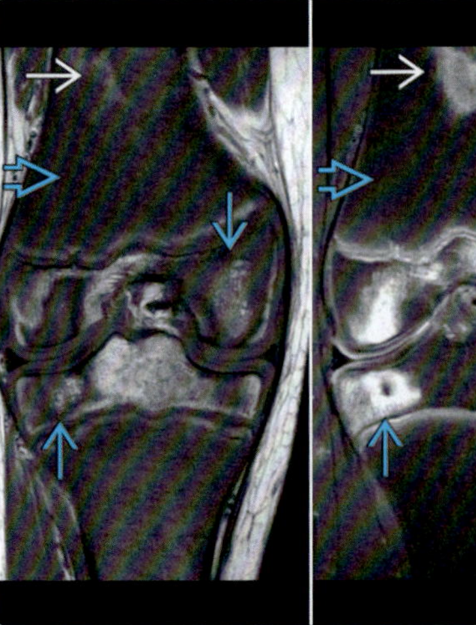

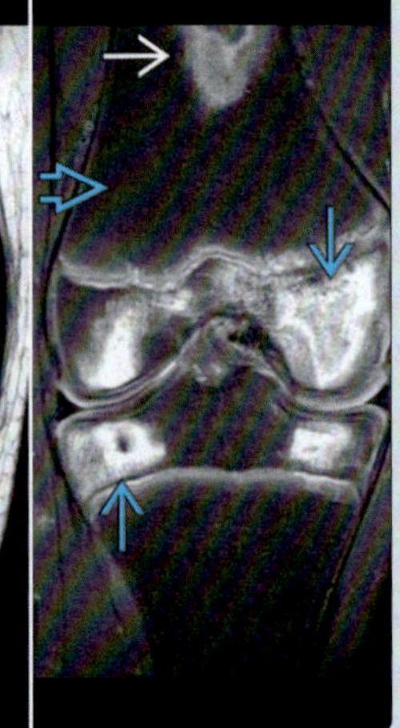

(Left) *AP radiograph of the right knee in a patient with sickle cell disease (SCD) & pain shows patchy sclerosis ⇨ of the femoral condyles, suggesting bone infarcts.* **(Right)** *Coronal T1 (L) & T2 FS (R) MR images in the same patient show heterogeneous, geographic foci with serpiginous margins in the femoral & tibial epiphyses ⇨ & femoral diaphysis ➡, typical of bone infarcts. The abnormally low T1 & T2 signal intensity of the visualized metadiaphyses ⇨ is due to ↑ red marrow & iron overload.*

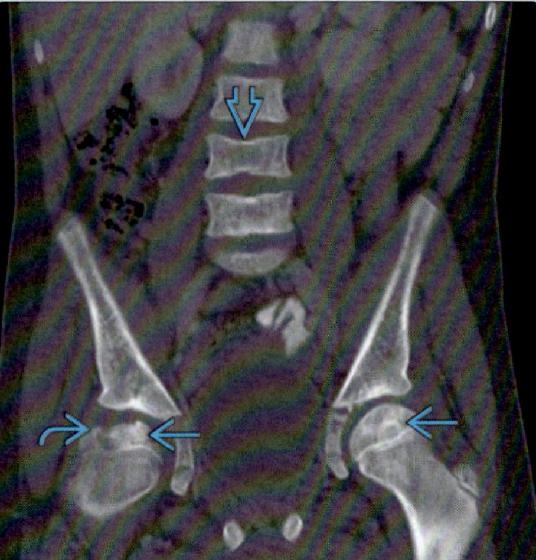

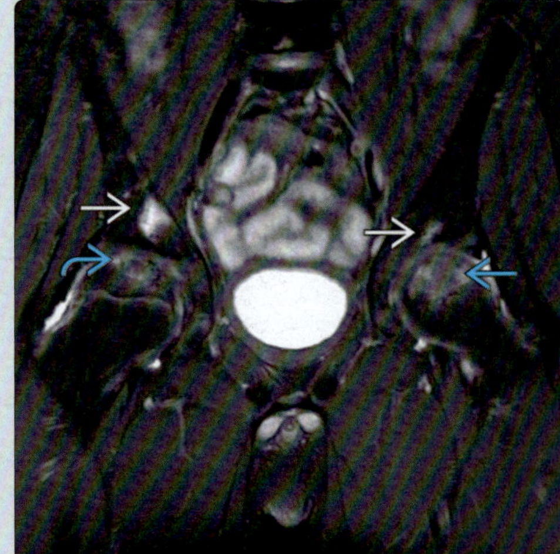

(Left) *Coronal CECT in the same patient shows heterogeneous sclerosis of the femoral heads ⇨, consistent with avascular necrosis (AVN). There is subchondral collapse & fragmentation on the right ⇨ with associated acetabular dysplasia. Central depressions are seen at several vertebral body endplates ⇨.* **(Right)** *Coronal T2 FS MR in the same patient shows articular cartilage loss on the right at the site of fragmentation ⇨. Infarcts are also seen in the left femoral head ⇨ & bilateral iliac bones ➡.*

TERMINOLOGY

Abbreviations

- Sickle cell disease (SCD); hemoglobin SS (Hb SS, Hgb SS)

Definitions

- SCD: Hb SS (homozygous) → severe anemia
- Sickle cell-hemoglobin C disease: Hb SC → mild anemia
- Sickle cell-α thalassemia: Hb S-α thal → severe anemia
- Sickle cell-β thalassemia: Hb S-β thal → mild to severe anemia
- Sickle cell trait: Hb SA (heterozygous gene carrier)
- Normal: Hb AA

IMAGING

General Features

- Best diagnostic clue
  - H-shaped vertebrae
  - Bone marrow infarctions with sclerosis
- Location
  - Percentage of all bone infarcts found in individual bones: Femur 16%, tibia 15%, humerus 13%, spine 11%, radius 10%, ulna 8%, pelvis 8%, others 19%

Radiographic Findings

- Skull
  - Expanded diploic space; hair-on-end appearance is rare
  - Extramedullary hematopoiesis (EMH): Middle ear, paranasal sinuses
  - Mandible: Coarse trabeculae; condyle infarction
  - Orbital wall infarction → subperiosteal hemorrhage → proptosis (orbital compression syndrome)
- Spine
  - Vertebral infarctions
    - Central endplate depression (superior + inferior endplate → H-shape or Lincoln log morphology)
    - ± compensatory enlargement of adjacent vertebra (tower vertebra)
    - ↓ height → kyphosis, lordosis
  - Smooth endplate concavities from marrow hyperplasia → osteoporosis with bone softening → insufficiency fractures (fish mouth appearance formed by adjacent inferior & superior endplates)
  - EMH: Paraspinal/intraspinal masses
- Chest
  - Rib & sternal infarction: Part of acute chest syndrome (chest pain, dyspnea, cough + pulmonary consolidation)
    - Bone infarctions → lucent or sclerotic foci
  - EMH: Posterior mediastinal masses
  - Soft tissue findings provide useful clues
    - Enlarged heart (chronic anemia)
    - Absent splenic shadow (infarction)
    - Cholecystectomy clips (pigment gallstones)
- Pelvis
  - Osteomyelitis, protrusio acetabuli, infarction
- Extremities
  - Diametaphyseal infarction: Lucent or sclerotic serpiginous/geographic foci with healing (months)
  - Epiphyseal infarctions (avascular necrosis) are most common in humeral & femoral heads
    - Sclerosis, subchondral fracture, coxa magna
  - Dactylitis (hand-foot syndrome): Hand & foot small tubular bone infarcts, usually at age 6-24 months
    - Soft tissue edema, solid periosteal reaction, cortical mottling, sclerosis
  - Infarctions up to physis → growth disturbances
    - Cone-shaped epiphyses of metacarpals, phalanges
    - Premature physeal fusion
  - Osteomyelitis: Femur, tibia, & humerus are most common
  - Marrow hyperplasia: Osteoporosis, thinned cortex, widened medullary spaces, coarsened trabeculae

MR Findings

- T1WI
  - Marrow hyperplasia: Bright yellow marrow replaced by darker red marrow (↓ fat, ↑ water content)
  - Variable appearance of infarctions
    - Serpiginous low signal intensity foci if chronic
- T1WI FS
  - Bright, patchy foci can favor infarction but not reliable for differentiating from infection
- T2WI FS
  - Poorly defined bright marrow, periosteal, & soft tissue edema from acute infarction or osteomyelitis
  - Soft tissue or subperiosteal collections or joint fluid seen in either process
    - Larger collections favor infection
  - Interrupted dark signal cortex favors infection
  - Double-line sign: Alternating bright + dark T2 serpiginous foci of chronic infarctions throughout medullary cavities & epiphyses
  - ↓ marrow signal of iron overload from numerous transfusions
- T1WI C+ FS
  - Enhancement in infarction & infection is variable
    - ↓ marrow enhancement (± fluid) in regions of acute infarction or ↑ pressure from infection/abscess
      - Thin rim enhancement favors infarct
      - Thick rim enhancement favors infection
  - Extensive geographic regions of ↓ marrow enhancement: Bone marrow necrosis
    - Preservation of trabeculae

Ultrasonographic Findings

- Fluid collections (especially larger) favor osteomyelitis
- Imaging guidance is useful for sampling fluid for culture

Nuclear Medicine Findings

- Bone scan
  - Symmetric expansion of hematopoietic marrow involving femur, calvaria, small bones of hands/feet
  - Bone marrow infarction: Photopenic defect initially; may show ↑ activity with healing & revascularization
  - Bone infarction vs. osteomyelitis
    - Infarction: Tc-99m MDP bone scan shows ↑ activity; Tc-99m sulfur colloid marrow scan shows ↓ activity
    - Osteomyelitis: Bone scan shows ↑ activity; sulfur colloid marrow scan shows normal activity
- Tc-99m sulfur colloid
  - Can confirm masses as EMH

DIFFERENTIAL DIAGNOSIS

Langerhans Cell Histiocytosis

- Vertebra plana (flat vertebral body)
- Punched-out lytic bone lesions

Leukemia

- Osteoporosis, metaphyseal lucent bands, pathologic fractures
- May have more aggressive bone lesions & periosteal reaction

Thalassemia

- Changes of bone marrow expansion are similar to SCD but exaggerated
  - H-shaped vertebra
  - Hair-on-end appearance of skull diploic space
  - Avascular necrosis is less common than SCD
  - Paravertebral masses: EMH

PATHOLOGY

General Features

- Etiology
  - Normal human hemoglobin A contains 4 globin chains: 2 α + 2 β chains
    - Hb SS: Abnormal β chains twist (polymerization) → RBC distortion
    - RBC distortion is exaggerated with deoxygenation → irreversible sickling (banana-shaped RBCs)
      - Sickled RBCs occlude vessels → infarction
      - Sickled RBCs are quickly removed → anemia
  - Bony manifestations result from
    - Chronic anemia → red marrow hyperplasia → medullary cavity expansion, bone softening
    - Immunocompromise + abnormal blood flow → osteomyelitis
      - Osteomyelitis 2:1 *Salmonella:Staphylococcus*
    - Vasoocclusion → medullary infarction
- Genetics
  - Abnormal β globin gene on short arm of chromosome 11 → valine substituted for glutamic acid at β globin position 6 → Hb S

Microscopic Features

- Normally, red/cellular marrow of appendicular skeleton converts to yellow/fatty marrow during childhood
  - Begins in epiphyses & central diaphyses, gradually spreading toward metaphyses
  - Red marrow persists in normal adult axial skeleton
- Expansion of red marrow throughout skeleton in SCD

CLINICAL ISSUES

Presentation

- Most common signs/symptoms
  - Pain due to vasoocclusive crisis involving any organ, most commonly bone
    - Infarction dactylitis is often 1st manifestation
    - Painful chest/abdominal crises begin at age 2-3 years
  - Skeletal pain due to marrow infarction > > osteomyelitis
    - Fever, pain, swelling, ↓ motion, leukocytosis, ↑ inflammatory markers in either diagnosis
      - C-reactive protein tends to be much higher in osteomyelitis
    - Osteomyelitis is 10-50x less common than bone infarction in SCD
  - Splenomegaly initially, then splenic atrophy
    - Autosplenectomy by progressive infarction
  - Hemolytic anemia: Jaundice, gallstones
    - 50-70% have gallstones by adulthood
  - Marrow, liver, pancreas hemosiderosis (transfusions)
  - Stroke in 11% before 20 years old

Demographics

- Age
  - Typically detected on newborn genetic screening
  - Painful crisis of bone in 50% by age 5
    - Most common cause of hospitalization
      - Acute chest syndrome is 2nd most common
- Epidemiology
  - Incidence: 1 in 375-650 Black Americans have SCD
    - 8% of Black Americans carry *HbS* gene
      - Up to 40% in some African tribes
  - Incidence: 1 in 2,000 Hispanic individuals from Caribbean, Central America, South America

Natural History & Prognosis

- Mean survival: 42 years
- Acute chest syndrome: Most common cause of death
- Frequency of vasoocclusive crises may predict presence of bone infarcts on imaging

Treatment

- Sickle cell crisis: Oxygen, hydration, pain management, blood transfusion
- Hydroxyurea to prevent vasoocclusive crises
- Autologous stem cell implantation at site of osteonecrosis may improve symptoms & prevent joint degeneration
- Prophylactic penicillin + pneumococcal & *Haemophilus influenzae* vaccines to prevent infection

DIAGNOSTIC CHECKLIST

Consider

- Differentiation of acute bone infarcts vs. osteomyelitis in SCD is very difficult clinically & radiologically
- Episodes of vasoocclusion > > osteomyelitis (up to 50:1)

Image Interpretation Pearls

- Cortical disruption &/or fluid collections favor osteomyelitis

SELECTED REFERENCES

1. Kao CM et al: Microbiology and radiographic features of osteomyelitis in children and adolescents with sickle cell disease. Pediatr Blood Cancer. 67(10):e28517, 2020
2. Fontalis A et al: The challenge of differentiating vaso-occlusive crises from osteomyelitis in children with sickle cell disease and bone pain: a 15-year retrospective review. J Child Orthop. 13(1):33-9, 2019
3. Daltro G et al: Use of autologous bone marrow stem cell implantation for osteonecrosis of the knee in sickle cell disease: a preliminary report. BMC Musculoskelet Disord. 19(1):158, 2018
4. Kosaraju V et al: Imaging of musculoskeletal manifestations in sickle cell disease patients. Br J Radiol. 90(1073):20160130, 2017
5. Sundu C et al: Bilateral subperiosteal hematoma and orbital compression syndrome in sickle cell disease. J Craniofac Surg. 28(8):e775-6, 2017

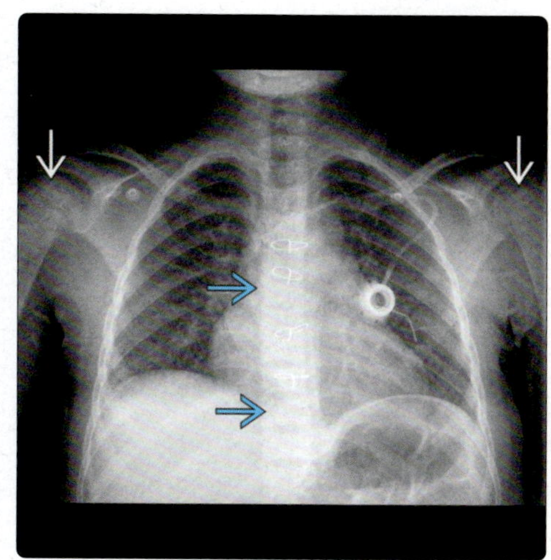

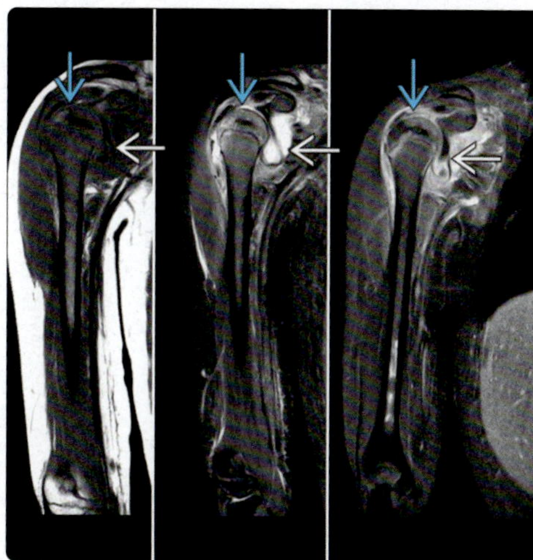

(Left) *AP chest radiograph in a 7-year-old with SCD shows sclerosis of the humeral heads, consistent with AVN. Vertebral endplate concavities & central depressions are noted at multiple levels.* **(Right)** *Coronal T1 (L), STIR (M), & T1 C+ FS (R) MR images in the same patient show heterogeneous epiphyseal marrow, a moderate joint effusion, & surrounding soft tissue edema. These findings can be seen with acute bone infarction or osteomyelitis in SCD.*

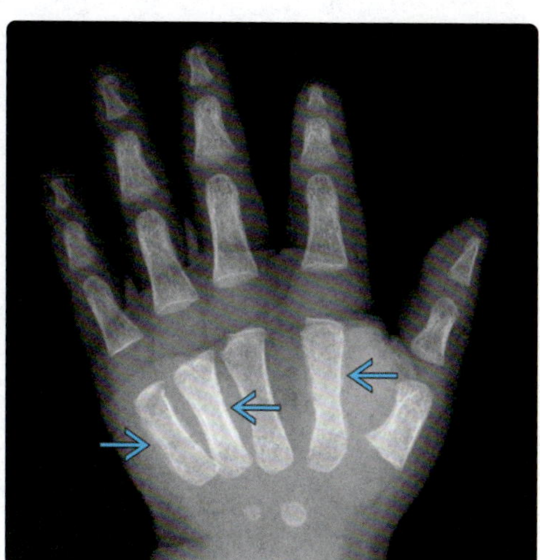

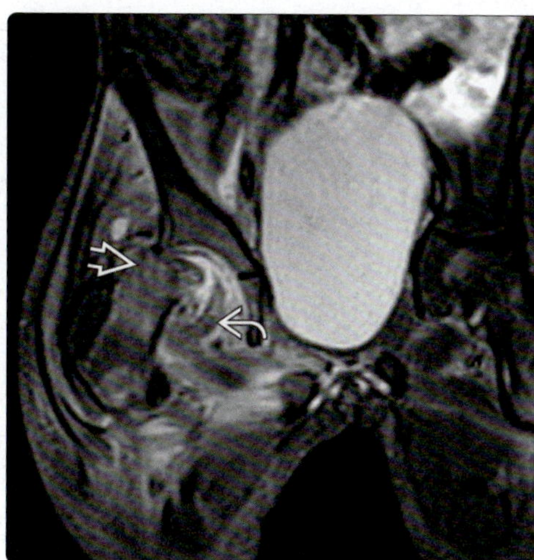

(Left) *PA radiograph of the hand in an 11-month-old SCD patient with swelling shows medullary sclerosis & periosteal reaction of the 2nd, 4th, & 5th metacarpals, typical of dactylitis.* **(Right)** *Coronal T1 C+ FS MR in an SCD patient with recently diagnosed pelvic osteomyelitis, septic arthritis, & soft tissue abscesses shows an unusual complication: Complete slip of the capital femoral epiphysis from the femoral neck.*

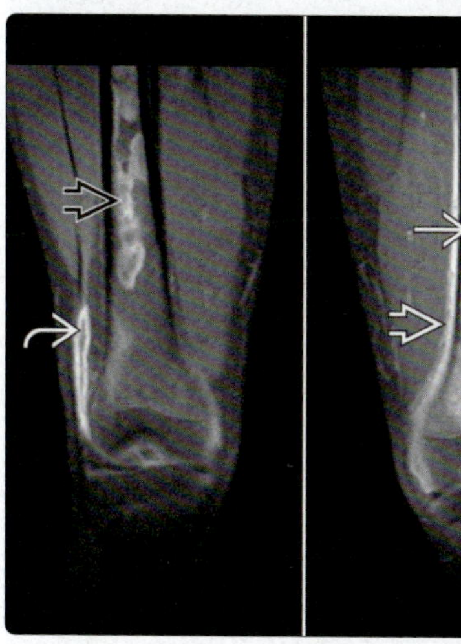

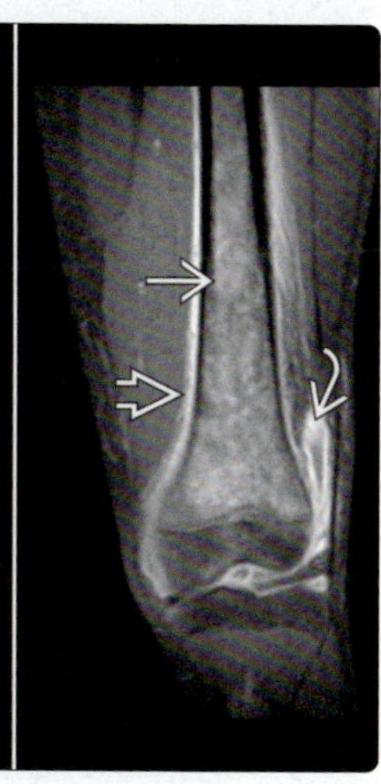

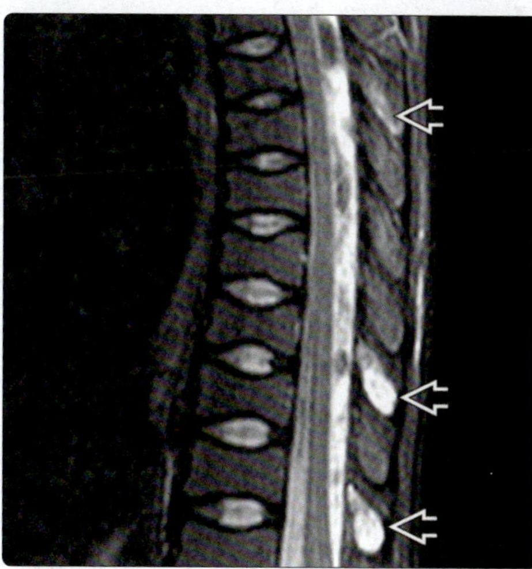

(Left) *Coronal T1 C+ FS MR in a 14-year-old boy with SCD shows heterogeneous enhancement of the distal left femur with periosteal edema (due to infection vs. acute infarction). The bilateral knee synovitis could be reactive from either process or from septic arthritis. Subacute infarction is seen in the right femoral shaft.* **(Right)** *Sagittal STIR MR shows biconcave vertebral bodies at each level, typical of bone softening. There is also high signal intensity in multiple spinous processes from recent infarctions.*

KEY FACTS

TERMINOLOGY

- Lateral curvature(s) of spine with Cobb angle of ≥ 10°
- Flexible: Nonstructural; corrects with ipsilateral bending
  - Usually does not progress; need not be included in fusion
- Rigid: Structural; does not correct with ipsilateral bending
  - Cobb angle remains ≥ 25° on ipsilateral bending
  - Included in spinal fusion
- Curve etiologies
  - Some diagnoses span categories
  - Idiopathic: Most common; 70-85% of all scoliosis
    - Classified according to time of onset
    - Infantile: < 3 years of age
      - Mostly develops during first 6 months of life
      - Typical: Convex left thoracic curve (70%)
      - M > F
    - Juvenile: 4-9 years
      - Typical: Convex right thoracic curve
      - Most likely to progress
    - Adolescent: > 10 years
      - Most common type: Convex right thoracic curve
      - M < < F
  - Congenital: 10%
    - Osteogenic: Segmentation anomaly
    - Neuropathic: Syrinx, tethered cord, diastematomyelia
  - Neuromuscular (neuropathic or myopathic)
    - Single long curve
    - Neuropathic: Chiari 1, cerebral palsy
    - Myopathic: Muscular dystrophies, spinal muscular atrophy
  - Developmental (skeletal dysplasia or dysostosis)
  - Tumor associated
    - Osteoid osteoma, cord neoplasm, neurofibromas

CLINICAL ISSUES

- Younger patients presenting with severe curves are more likely to progress than older children with less severe curves
- Progression is most likely during adolescent growth spurt

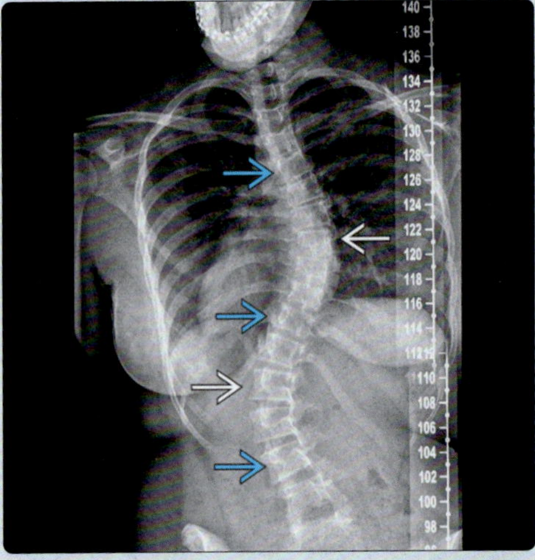

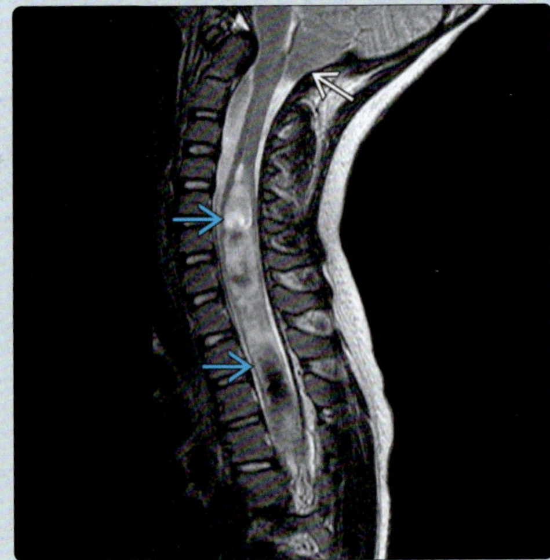

(Left) *PA radiograph of a 13-year-old during follow-up for adolescent idiopathic scoliosis shows 47° convex right thoracic & 47° convex left thoracolumbar curvatures. The terminal ⇨ & apical ➡ vertebrae for each curve are noted. The image is displayed from the perspective of the examining/operating orthopedist.* **(Right)** *Sagittal T2 MR shows a large syrinx ⇨, which extended to T10 (not shown). Note the Chiari 1 configuration of the cerebellar tonsils ➡. The patient was imaged due to a rapidly progressive curve.*

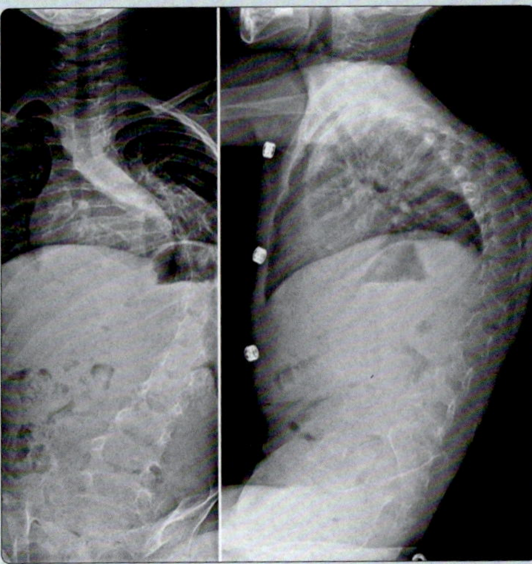

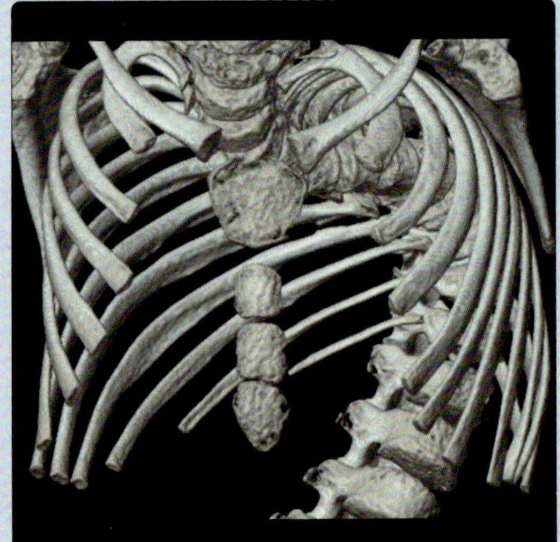

(Left) *Frontal (L) & lateral (R) radiographs of the spine in a 4-year-old with an uncommon form of muscular dystrophy show a severe apex left curve of the thoracolumbar spine with marked kyphosis.* **(Right)** *Anterior 3D bone CT in the same patient shows the severe thoracic deformity from the rotary as well as the sagittal & coronal components of the curvature.*

TERMINOLOGY

Definitions

- Presence of lateral curvature(s) of spine with Cobb angle of ≥ 10°, often associated with vertebral rotation
- 2 types
  - Flexible: Nonstructural, corrects with ipsilateral bending, usually does not progress
  - Structural: Rigid, does not demonstrate correction with ipsilateral bending
    - Cobb angle remains ≥ 25° on ipsilateral bending

IMAGING

General Features

- Idiopathic: No clear cause by clinical exam or radiographs
  - Most common: 70-85% of all scoliosis
  - Classified according to time of onset
    - Infantile: ≤ 3 years of age
      - Most develop during first 6 months of life; M > F
      - 1/4 are associated with hip dysplasia
      - Typical: Convex left thoracic curve (70%)
    - Juvenile: 4-10 years
      - Typical: Convex right thoracic curve, progressive
    - Adolescent idiopathic scoliosis (AIS): > 10 years
      - Most common type: Convex right S-shaped thoracic
      - Compensatory left convex lumbar; ↑ rapidly with growth spurts; M < < F
    - Adult: Curve begins after maturation
  - Note that other categories may cause similar curves
- Congenital: 10%
  - Result of vertebral anomalies: Hemivertebrae (45%), occult spinal abnormality (15-40%)
  - Typical: Thoracic or thoracolumbar curve
  - Progressive scoliosis (3/4)
  - If curve is progressive or surgery is planned, image with MR; fine osseous detail may be better seen on CT
  - Associated with
    - Spinal dysraphism: Lipoma, diastematomyelia, syringohydromyelia, tethered cord
    - Genitourinary anomalies (6%), cardiac anomalies (15%), rib anomalies
- Neuromuscular (neuropathic or myopathic)
  - Chiari 1
  - Cerebral palsy, muscular dystrophy, spinal muscular atrophy, poliomyelitis
- Developmental (skeletal dysplasia or dysostosis)
  - Neurofibromatosis, achondroplasia, osteogenesis imperfecta
- Tumor associated: Osteoid osteoma, cord neoplasm, neurofibroma

Radiographic Findings

- Imaging evaluation depends on cause of scoliosis
  - Initial erect anteroposterior view from chin to greater trochanter
    - Posteroanterior on follow-up (less breast radiation)
  - Lateral for clinical concern of excessive kyphosis or lordosis
  - Cobb method of measuring scoliosis angle
    - Parallel lines to superior terminal vertebra superior endplate & inferior terminal vertebra inferior endplate
      - If endplates are not seen, use pedicles
    - Perpendicular intersecting lines then yield Cobb angle
    - Same vertebral bodies are used for follow-up measurements
    - Curve progression is present when > 5° between studies
- Lateral bending films to assess flexibility prior to surgery
- Skeletal maturity assessment (to determine potential curvature progression & timing of surgery)
  - Iliac crest apophysis ossification center appearance/fusion on scoliosis study
    - Iliac crest is divided into 4 quadrants; Risser grade is given according to ossification of iliac apophysis
    - Risser 0: No ossification; Risser 1: Only lateral 1/4 is ossified; Risser 4: All 4 quadrants are ossified; Risser 5: Fused iliac apophysis
    - At skeletal maturity, scoliosis unlikely to progress if < 30°
  - Posteroanterior view of left hand/wrist for bone age
- Assessment of balance
  - Central sacral vertical line (CSVL): Vertical line drawn on frontal view perpendicular to imaginary tangential line across top of iliac crests, bisects sacrum
  - Plumb line: Center of C7 parallel to radiographic edges extending distally
  - Coronal balance on standing frontal image: Distance between CSVL & plumb line: > 2 cm is abnormal
  - Sagittal balance: Distance between posterosuperior aspect of S1 vertebral body & plumb line: > 2 cm is abnormal
- Vertebral rotation
  - Nash-Moe method: Percentage of pedicle on convex side of curve displaced in respect to vertebral body width
- **Findings by curve types**
  - Idiopathic
    - Prevalence of typical curvature: Convex right thoracic curve > right thoracic & left lumbar > right thoracolumbar > right lumbar
    - Vertebral rotation is often present; lower lumbar spondylolysis may be present
  - Congenital
    - Failure of vertebral formation (wedge vertebra, hemivertebra)
    - Failure of segmentation (pedicle bar, block vertebra)
  - Tumor associated
    - Look for osseous remodeling or destruction
  - Neurofibromatosis
    - Many lack distinctive diagnostic features
    - Classic: High thoracic acute curvature, kyphosis, rib & pedicle anomalies, posterior vertebral scalloping, ± paraspinal mass
  - Neuromuscular
    - Tethered cord, syrinx, Chiari 1
    - Single long curve
- EOS system: Biplanar x-ray imaging
  - Several times ↓ radiation dose compared to conventional radiographs
  - ↑ artifacts

CT Findings

- NECT
  - Coronal, sagittal, & 3D reconstruction for surgical planning
  - Evaluates congenital vertebral anomalies
  - May be used to size pedicles for screws
  - Assess for pseudoarthrosis following spinal fusion

MR Findings

- Indications for MR
  - Congenital scoliosis
  - Neuropathic cause
  - Juvenile onset: 4-10 years
  - Suspected adolescent idiopathic but with atypical feature
    - Rapid progression of curve
    - Unusual curves: Convex left thoracic, long right thoracolumbar curve, double thoracic
    - Widened spinal canal or foramina, osseous lesion, foot deformity
    - Pain, headache, neck pain, neurologic deterioration
    - Debatable utility of MR without other indications; some literature reports 1/7 will have neuraxis abnormality

Ultrasonographic Findings

- Several papers report curve measurements by US
- 3D imaging for measuring vertebral rotation
- Measuring lengthening in magnetically controlled rods

Nuclear Medicine Findings

- Bone scan
  - SPECT imaging for pseudoarthrosis following spinal fusion surgery

DIFFERENTIAL DIAGNOSIS

Other Causes for Scoliosis

- Differentiated by clinical history, radiographic findings, & MR
  - Osteoid osteoma
  - Paraspinal tumor
  - Inflammation, infection
    - Many etiologies
  - Limb length discrepancy

CLINICAL ISSUES

Presentation

- Most common signs/symptoms
  - Usually asymptomatic
    - Idiopathic scoliosis usually detected during physical exam
  - Pain from progressive curvature or degenerative disc & facet disease

Demographics

- Epidemiology
  - 0.2-0.5% of population in USA
- Sex: AIS: Female predilection
  - Girls tend to progress more than boys in idiopathic scoliosis

Natural History & Prognosis

- Worsening curve in 10-25% of cases
  - During adolescent growth spurts
    - Younger patients with more severe curves at presentation are much more likely to progress than older children with less severe curves
  - Curves > 40-50° after skeletal maturity
  - Cardiopulmonary complications from severe scoliosis

Treatment

- Mehta casting for infantile scoliosis
- Idiopathic
  - Observe if < 20° in adolescent or < 30° in skeletally mature at presentation
  - Brace (orthotics)
    - ≥ 10 years
    - 25-45° at presentation (Risser 0-2)
    - > 25° with progression
  - Surgical
    - Curves > 45°
    - Progressive curves that fail bracing
    - Posterior spinal fusion with engagement of all 3 spinal columns (as by pedicle screw)
- Congenital
  - Observation
  - Surgical: With progressive curve
    - In situ fusion, anterior & posterior epiphysiodesis, hemivertebrae resection, reconstructive osteotomies
- Neuromuscular
  - Typical: Anterior & posterior spinal fusion
- Complications of surgery
  - Rod, screw, or wire breakage; slippage of hook; infection; spondylolysis; neurologic injury; superior mesenteric artery syndrome; pseudoarthrosis

DIAGNOSTIC CHECKLIST

Consider

- Atypical/painful scoliosis: MR to exclude spinal pathology

SELECTED REFERENCES

1. de Oliveira RG et al: Magnetic resonance imaging effectiveness in adolescent idiopathic scoliosis. Spine Deform. 9(1):67-73, 2021
2. Guglielmi R et al: Preoperative and postoperative imaging in idiopathic scoliosis: what the surgeon wants to know. Semin Musculoskelet Radiol. 25(1):155-66, 2021
3. Jarrett DY et al: EOS imaging of scoliosis, leg length discrepancy and alignment. Semin Roentgenol. 56(3):228-44, 2021
4. Lee TT et al: 3D ultrasound imaging provides reliable angle measurement with validity comparable to x-ray in patients with adolescent idiopathic scoliosis. J Orthop Translat. 29:51-9, 2021
5. Chen J et al: Risk factors for neurological complications in severe and rigid spinal deformity correction of 177 cases. BMC Neurol. 20(1):433, 2020
6. Girdler S et al: Emerging techniques in diagnostic imaging for idiopathic scoliosis in children and adolescents: a review of the literature. World Neurosurg. 136:128-35, 2020
7. Mackel CE et al: A comprehensive review of the diagnosis and management of congenital scoliosis. Childs Nerv Syst. 34(11):2155-71, 2018
8. Tully PA et al: Should all paediatric patients with presumed idiopathic scoliosis undergo MRI screening for neuro-axial disease? Childs Nerv Syst. 34(11):2173-8, 2018
9. Cheung JP et al: Clinical utility of ultrasound to prospectively monitor distraction of magnetically controlled growing rods. Spine J. 16(2):204-9, 2016
10. Wang Q et al: Validity study of vertebral rotation measurement using 3-D ultrasound in adolescent idiopathic scoliosis. Ultrasound Med Biol. 42(7):1473-81, 2016

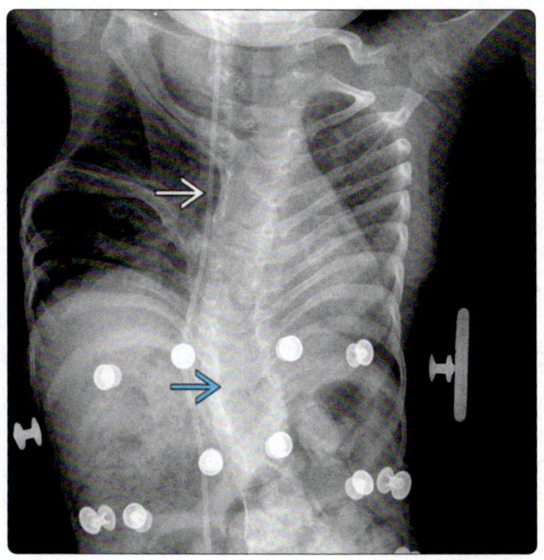

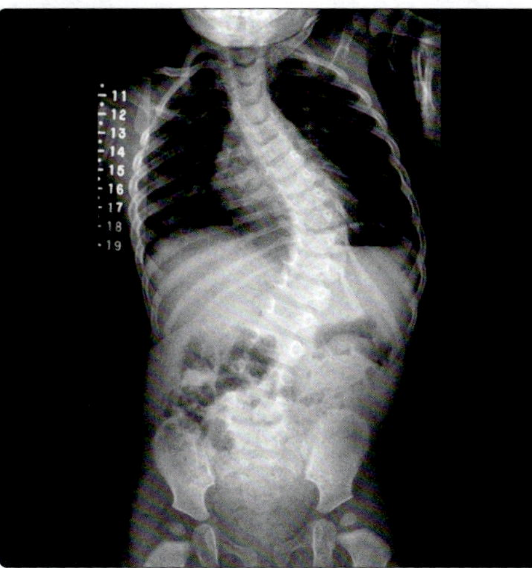

(Left) *AP radiograph shows numerous vertebral & rib anomalies throughout the spine. In addition to segmentation anomalies, there are multiple thoracolumbar levels with dysraphic bony elements + a ventriculoperitoneal shunt, suggesting a neurologic component to the curve as well.* **(Right)** *Frontal radiograph shows ~ 60° of convex leftward scoliosis of the spine from T7 to L2. This is a 1-year-old with the infantile type of idiopathic scoliosis.*

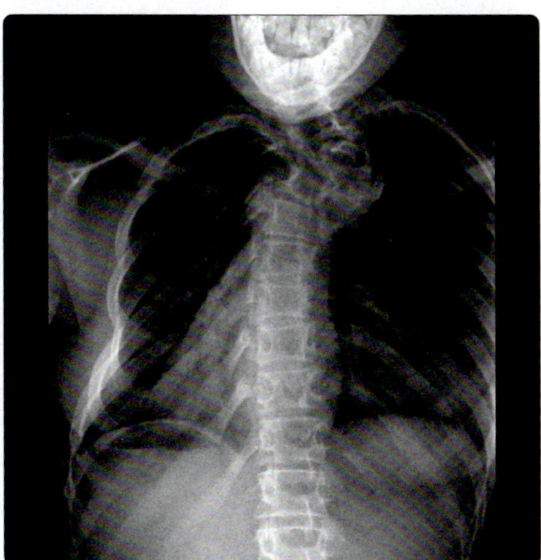

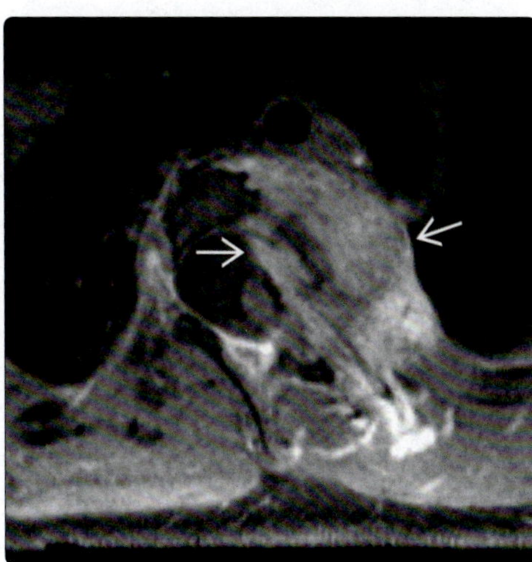

(Left) *Frontal radiograph (displayed from the orthopedic perspective) in a 12-year-old with back pain, café au lait spots, & neurofibromatosis type 1 (NF1) shows a short-segment, convex, right upper thoracic curvature. This dystrophic curvature is frequently associated with paraspinal plexiform neurofibromas.* **(Right)** *Axial T1 C+ FS MR in the same patient with NF1 shows lobular, enhancing paraspinal & intraspinal infiltrative lesions of plexiform neurofibromas.*

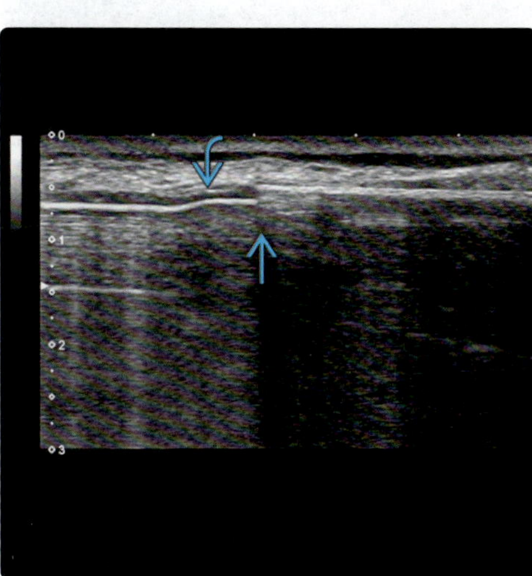

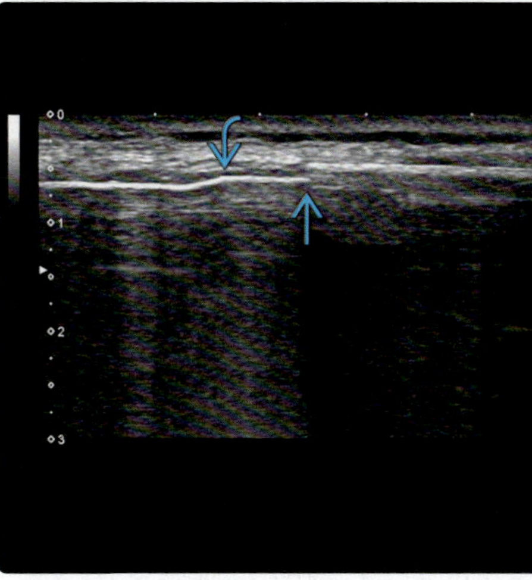

(Left) *Longitudinal US in a 4-year-old with infantile idiopathic scoliosis & magnetically controlled growing rod shows a 5-mm distance between the housing unit & the neck of the extended part. This was performed in ultrasound prior to lengthening.* **(Right)** *Longitudinal US in the same child performed 5 minutes later (status post 3 mm of lengthening) shows that the distance between the housing & neck of the extending part now measures 8 mm, confirming success of the manipulation by the magnet.*

Tarsal Coalition

KEY FACTS

TERMINOLOGY

- Congenital or acquired abnormal fusion of ≥ 2 tarsal bones; fusion may be osseous, cartilaginous, or fibrous

IMAGING

- Tarsal coalitions
  - Calcaneonavicular (CN)
  - Talocalcaneal (TC)
  - Uncommon: Talonavicular, calcaneocuboid, cubonavicular
- CN coalition
  - 45° internal oblique foot radiograph view (Slomann view)
  - Anteater nose sign = elongation of anterosuperior calcaneus on lateral view
  - ± hypoplastic talar head
- TC coalition
  - Most common: Middle facet in up to 70%; posteromedial (posterior to middle facet) in up to 1/3; less common involvement of anterior or posterior facets
    - Extraarticular posteromedial TC coalitions lack classic indirect radiographic findings
  - Harris-Beath (axial) & lateral radiographic views are best
    - Difficult to see actual coalition, CT is often needed; many indirect signs
      - Talar beak
      - C sign: Continuous uninterrupted sclerotic line formed posteriorly by talar dome & sustentaculum tali on lateral view
      - Rounding of lateral talar process
      - Narrowing of posterior subtalar joint
      - "Ball-&-socket" ankle joint

CLINICAL ISSUES

- Recurrent sprains, midfoot pain, limited subtalar motion, peroneal spastic flatfoot
- 90% of all coalitions: TC or CN
- Up to 50% are bilateral
- Look for > 1 coalition in same foot (rare)

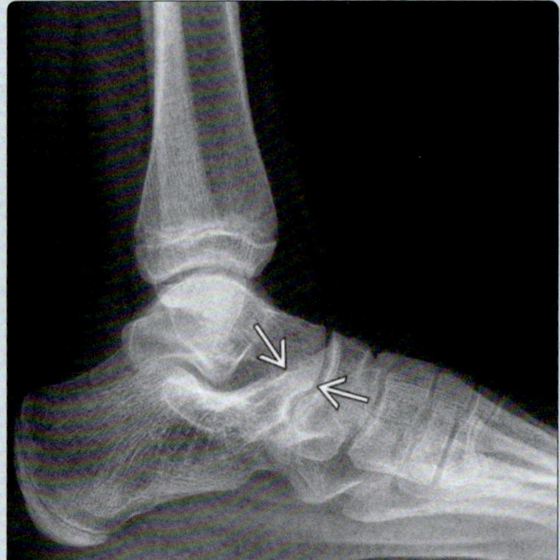

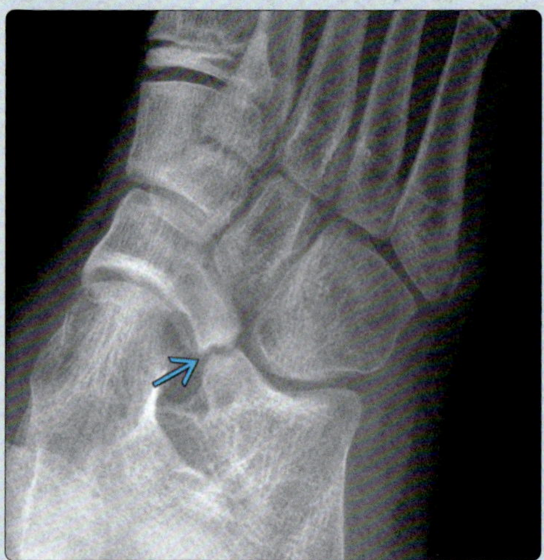

(Left) *Lateral radiograph in a 10-year-old girl with foot pain for 1 year shows elongation of the anterior process of the calcaneus (anteater nose sign) ➔. The oblique view (not shown) confirmed a calcaneonavicular (CN) coalition.* **(Right)** *Oblique foot radiograph in a 10-year-old shows narrowing of the CN articulation ➔ with sclerosis & irregularity of the apposed navicular & calcaneus, consistent with a nonosseous coalition.*

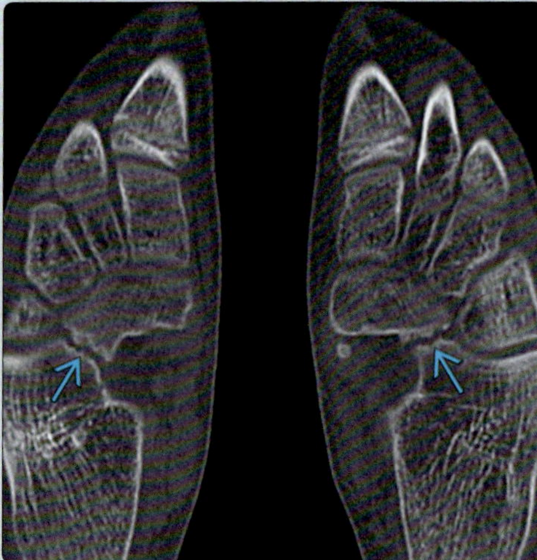

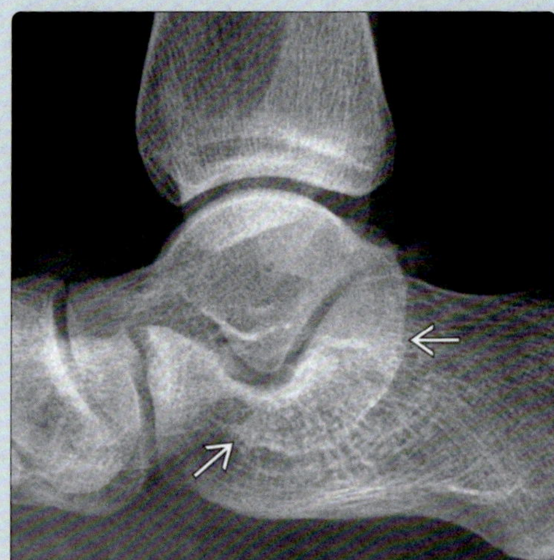

(Left) *Coronal oblique bone CT images in the same patient confirm bilateral nonosseous CN coalitions with narrowing, irregularity, & sclerosis at the CN articulations ➔.* **(Right)** *Lateral radiograph in a 15-year-old that presented with limited talar motion on physical examination shows a continuous C sign ➔ of a talocalcaneal coalition. The C-shaped line is formed superiorly by the medial talar dome & outline of the sustentaculum tali inferiorly.*

TERMINOLOGY

Synonyms

- Tarsal fusion

Definitions

- Congenital or acquired abnormal fusion of ≥ 2 tarsal bones
  - Union may be osseous, cartilaginous, or fibrous

IMAGING

General Features

- Best diagnostic clue
  - Close apposition or fusion of tarsal bones at/posterior to middle facet of talocalcaneal (TC) joint or calcaneonavicular (CN) joint at anterior process of calcaneus to navicular
- Location
  - Most common: CN, TC
    - Up to 1/3 of subtalar coalitions are at extraarticular posteromedial location (posterior to middle facet)
  - Uncommon: Talonavicular, calcaneocuboid, or cubonavicular
- Morphology
  - Synostosis = ossific bar
  - Synchondrosis = cartilaginous bar
  - Syndesmosis = fibrous union

Radiographic Findings

- Radiography
  - CN coalition
    - 45° internal oblique view (Slomann view) of foot
      - Ossific bar connects anterior process of calcaneus to dorsolateral navicular
      - Irregularity, sclerosis, or narrowing of CN space (fibrous or cartilaginous coalition)
    - Anteater nose sign: Elongation of anterosuperior calcaneus on lateral view
    - Broadening of medial aspect of anterosuperior calcaneus in close apposition to navicular
    - ± hypoplastic talar head
    - Radiography is typically diagnostic; other imaging may not be needed
  - TC coalition
    - Harris-Beath (axial) & lateral views
    - Difficult to see; CT is often needed
    - Most commonly at middle facet, though posteromedial extraarticular location may represent 1/3 of subtalar cases; less common involvement of anterior or posterior facets
    - Talar beak: Impaired subtalar motion → elevation stress at insertion of TC ligament → cycles of osseous repair → beak immediately adjacent to dorsal aspect of talonavicular joint (not specific for coalition)
    - Rounding or blunting of lateral talar process
    - C sign: Continuous uninterrupted sclerotic line formed by medial talar dome & sustentaculum tali on lateral view (50%)
      - False positive in some due to pes planus & abnormal positioning
    - Absent middle facet sign: Middle facet may be inapparent on lateral view
    - "Ball-&-socket" ankle joint: Concave surfaces of tibia & fibula, domed talus (convex proximal margin); uncommon & nonspecific
    - Narrowing of posterior subtalar joint
    - Normal middle & posterior facets are parallel to each other on Harris-Beath view; middle facet slants inferomedially in fibrous or cartilaginous coalition (bar in ossific coalition)
    - Extraarticular posteromedial TC can not be diagnosed by classic indirect radiographic signs
      - Prominence of posterior subtalar joint
- CT findings
  - Axial, coronal, & sagittal reformats
  - CN coalition
    - Joint space narrowing or reactive sclerosis
    - Widening of medial aspect of anterosuperior calcaneus
    - ± bony bridge
    - Best seen on axial or sagittal planes
  - TC coalition
    - Ossific bar (best on coronal images)
    - Downward (may be horizontal) orientation/sloping of sustentaculum along middle facet (normally slopes upward medially)
    - Reactive subchondral sclerosis & narrowing with cystic & hypertrophic changes of TC joint (especially middle facet)
    - ± broadening or hypoplasia of sustentaculum
      - Middle facet is shorter in posteromedial coalition

MR Findings

- T1WI
  - CN coalition
    - Sagittal & axial images are best for detecting coalition
    - Hypointense reactive changes
  - TC coalition
    - Most commonly at middle facet
    - Coronal image is best for detecting coalition
    - Osseous: Bar with marrow signal connection
    - Fibrous & cartilaginous: Hypointense signal connection with hypointense subchondral marrow changes
- T2WI
  - Ossific: Bone marrow contiguity across either TC or CN coalition
  - Cartilaginous: Hyperintense fluid signal connection with reactive, hyperintense subchondral bone marrow edema
  - Fibrous: Intermediate-signal connection with reactive, hyperintense subchondral bone marrow edema
  - Cartilaginous & fibrous: ↓ joint space

Imaging Recommendations

- Best imaging tool
  - Bone CT or 3-plane MR: TC coalition
  - 45° oblique radiograph: CN coalition

DIFFERENTIAL DIAGNOSIS

Subtalar Fractures

- Talar fractures
- Calcaneal fractures

Osteomyelitis

- Poorly defined marrow hyperintensity ± erosion or sinus tract
- Pain, fever, erythema; ↑ C-reactive protein, sedimentation rate, leukocytosis

Osteochondritis Dissecans

- Osteocartilaginous change at medial talar dome ± cysts, edema, sclerosis, fissuring, detached fragment
- Mostly adolescents, M > F

Juvenile Idiopathic Arthritis

- Synovitis with effusions, ± cartilage or bone erosions
  - Can eventually lead to ankylosis
- Reactive marrow edema
- ± tenosynovitis

PATHOLOGY

General Features

- Etiology
  - Congenital failure of segmentation & differentiation of primitive mesenchyme
  - Acquired: Trauma, infection, arthritis, or surgery
- Genetics
  - Autosomal dominance with high penetrance
- Associated abnormalities
  - Apert
  - Hand-foot-uterus syndrome
  - Proximal focal femoral deficiency
  - Hereditary symphalangism
  - Nievergelt syndrome

Staging, Grading, & Classification

- TC coalition classification scheme is based on 3D CT reconstruction (Rozansky et al.)
  - Type I: Linear coalition
  - Type II: Linear coalition with posterior hook
  - Type III: Shingled coalition
  - Type IV: Complete osseous coalition
  - Type V: Posterior coalition

Gross Pathologic & Surgical Features

- Osseous, fibrous, or cartilaginous connection

CLINICAL ISSUES

Presentation

- Most common signs/symptoms
  - Often asymptomatic in 1st decade of life
  - May lead to recurrent sprains, chronic midfoot pain, limited subtalar motion
- Other signs/symptoms
  - Commonly asymptomatic, discovered after imaging for trauma
  - Pes planus + heel valgus
  - Flattening of medial arch
  - Pain with activity
  - Peroneal spastic flatfoot
    - Rigid valgus deformity, pain, & peroneal muscle spasm
    - Tarsal coalition most common cause
    - Other causes: Fracture, arthritis, & some tumors
  - TC: Limited subtalar motion & prominence inferior to medial malleolus (double medial malleolus sign)

Demographics

- Age
  - Symptoms occur as coalition ossifies
    - Talonavicular (3-5 years)
    - CN (8-12 years)
    - TC (12-16 years)
- Sex
  - M > F
- Epidemiology
  - 1% incidence
  - 90% of all coalitions are TC or CN
  - Bilateral: 25-50%
  - Other tarsal coalitions are uncommon

Natural History & Prognosis

- Coalitions at birth may be fibrous or cartilaginous & later ossify
- Symptoms are more severe when coalition ossifies
- ↓ hindfoot motion makes child prone to ankle sprains
- Commonly discovered after imaging for ankle injuries

Treatment

- Initially conservative
  - Nonsteroidal antiinflammatory medication, arch supports, steroids, trial of casting, orthotics, & physical therapy
- Open surgical or arthroscopic resection
  - CN: Resection of bony bridge or arthrodesis
    - Fat autograft interposition, extensor digitorum brevis interposition
  - TC: Resection of middle facet bony bridge with fat interposition
  - If excision fails or if there is severe degenerative disease: Fusion or triple arthrodesis

DIAGNOSTIC CHECKLIST

Consider

- TC coalition: Coronal NECT or MR
- CN coalition: 45° internal oblique radiograph

Reporting Tips

- CT: Location & size of coalition; presence of other coalitions (bilateral or in same foot) or degenerative changes

SELECTED REFERENCES

1. King A et al: Endoscopic resection of tarsal coalitions. Foot Ankle Clin. 25(3):493-503, 2020
2. Phyo N et al: The radiological diagnosis of extra-articular posteromedial talocalcaneal coalition. Skeletal Radiol. 49(9):1413-22, 2020
3. Docquier PL et al: Tarsal coalition in paediatric patients. Orthop Traumatol Surg Res. 105(1S):S123-31, 2019
4. Steinborn M et al: Normal variations and pathologic disorders of chondrification and ossification of the foot and related diseases. Semin Musculoskelet Radiol. 23(5):497-510, 2019
5. Bixby SD et al: Posteromedial subtalar coalitions: prevalence and associated morphological alterations of the sustentaculum tali. Pediatr Radiol. 46(8):1142-9, 2016
6. Murphy JS et al: Talocalcaneal coalitions. Foot Ankle Clin. 20(4):681-91, 2015

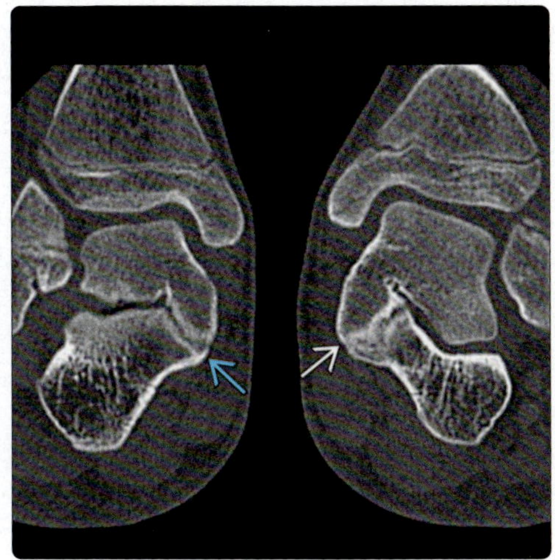

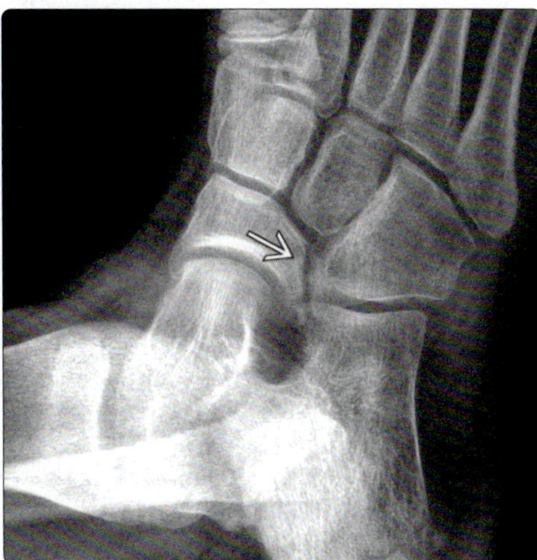

(Left) *Coronal bone CT in a 12-year-old with bilateral ankle pain shows partial osseous bridging on the left ➔ & close apposition on the right ➔ at the posteromedial aspects of the middle facets with broadening & downsloping of each sustentaculum tali.* **(Right)** *Oblique radiograph of the foot shows an uncommon nonosseous coalition between the cuboid & navicular, evident by sclerosis, irregularity, & joint space narrowing ➔.*

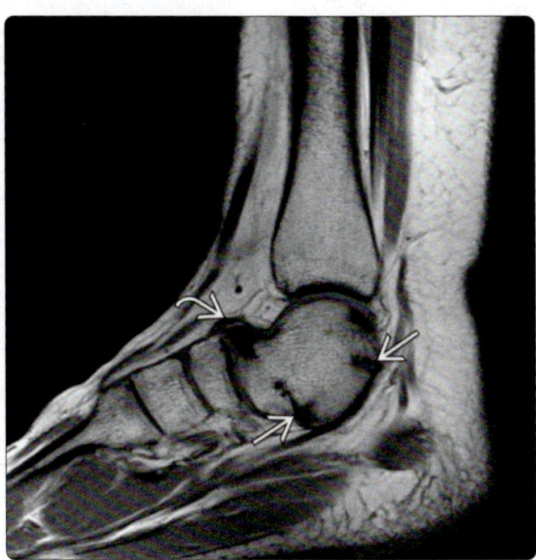

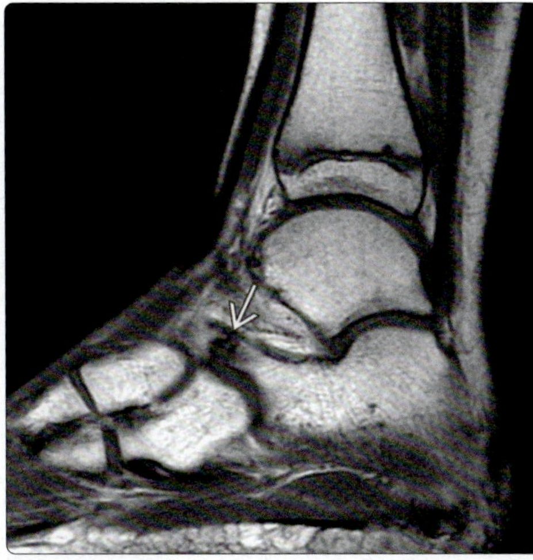

(Left) *Sagittal T1 MR in a 16-year-old with ankle pain shows a large osseous TC coalition ➔ of the middle facet. Note the talar beaking ➔, a common secondary finding that is the result of impaired talar motion.* **(Right)** *Sagittal T1 MR in an 11-year-old with acute-on-chronic ankle pain shows irregularity & narrowing of the CN joint ➔, indicating a nonosseous coalition. No other coalitions were found.*

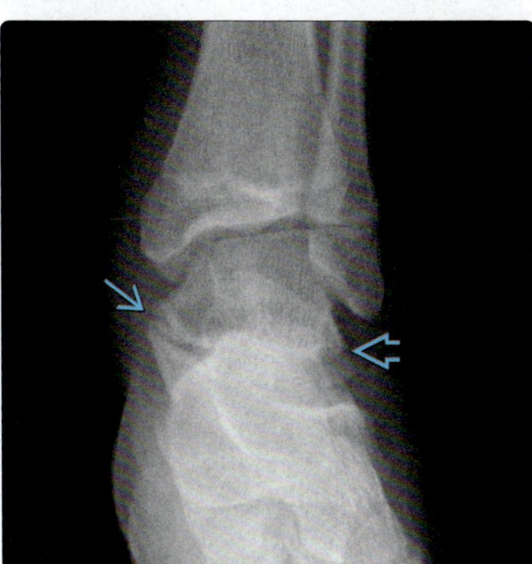

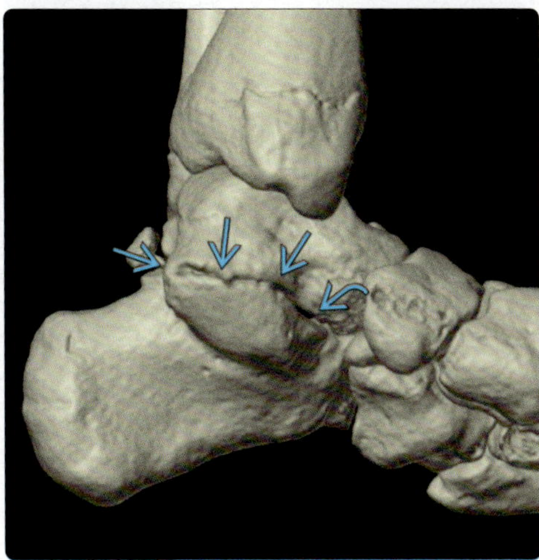

(Left) *AP radiograph of the ankle in a 15-year-old after a football injury shows a lateral process fracture of the talus ➔. Additionally, there is abnormal enlargement & orientation at the middle subtalar facet ➔.* **(Right)** *Medial view of a 3D bone CT in the same patient shows the large posteromedial coalition ➔ with a largely intact middle facet ➔.*

KEY FACTS

TERMINOLOGY

- Brachial plexopathy: Injury to ≥ 1 brachial plexus nerve roots, trunks, or cords → upper extremity contracture
- Glenohumeral dysplasia: Sequelae of brachial plexopathy on developing glenoid & humeral head

IMAGING

- Affected & unaffected shoulders imaged for comparison
- Radiographs
  - Dysplastic glenoid, winged scapula, hooked coracoid
  - Humeral head is small & ovoid
- Ultrasound
  - Uses posterior axial approach to glenohumeral joint
  - Can assess humeral head prior to ossification
  - α angle = angle between posterior scapular margin & tangent to humeral head from posterior edge of glenoid (normal ≤ 30°)
  - Percentage of humeral head posterior to scapular margin; humeral head ossification center should lie anterior to posterior scapular margin
- MR
  - Cartilage-sensitive GRE & PD FS sequences show unossified & ossified portions of glenoid & humeral head
    - Angle of glenoid version
      - ↑ retroversion with ↑ glenohumeral dysplasia
      - > 5° difference to unaffected side is abnormal
    - Percentage of humeral head anterior to scapular line
      - ~ 50% normally; ↓ with ↑ glenohumeral dysplasia
  - T1 shows fatty atrophy of shoulder musculature

CLINICAL ISSUES

- Shoulder traction at delivery → nerve injury → muscle imbalance → unopposed internal rotation → posterior glenoid/anterior humeral head cartilage loading → glenohumeral dysplasia → posterior subluxation
- Most deficits recover by 3 months; 20-30% are permanent

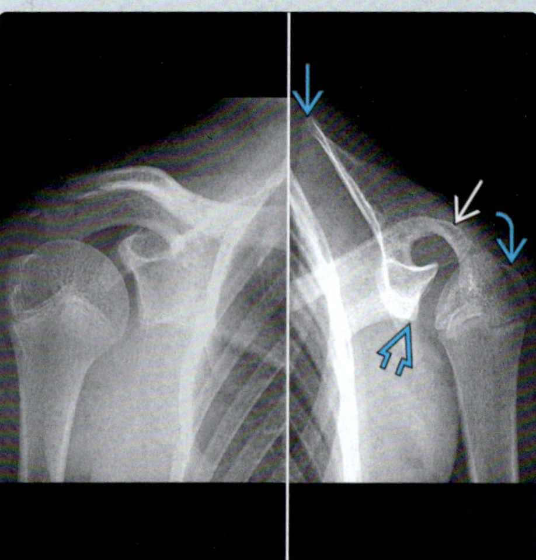

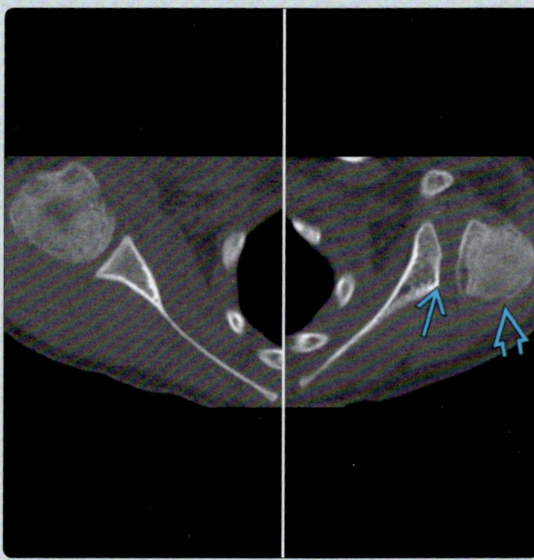

(Left) *Frontal radiographs of the normal right shoulder (left) & abnormal left shoulder (right) in a 12-year-old with glenohumeral dysplasia secondary to a left brachial plexopathy show a small, ovoid left humeral head ➢, winging of the left scapula ➢, a hooked coracoid ➡, & a dysplastic left glenoid ➢.* **(Right)** *Axial NECT images of the right (left) & left (right) shoulders in the same girl show that the small left humeral head is posteriorly displaced ➢, articulating with a false glenoid ➢.*

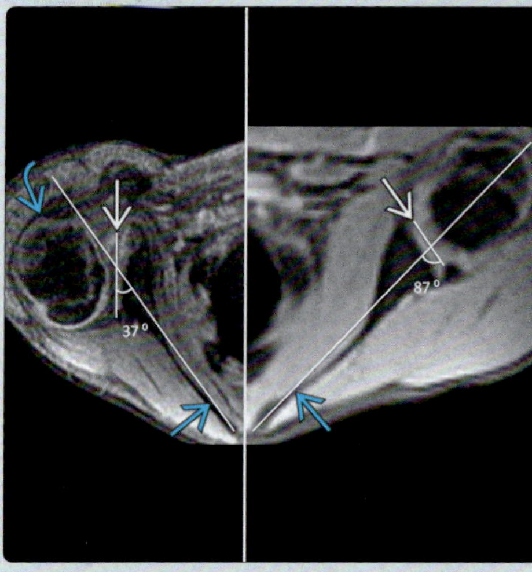

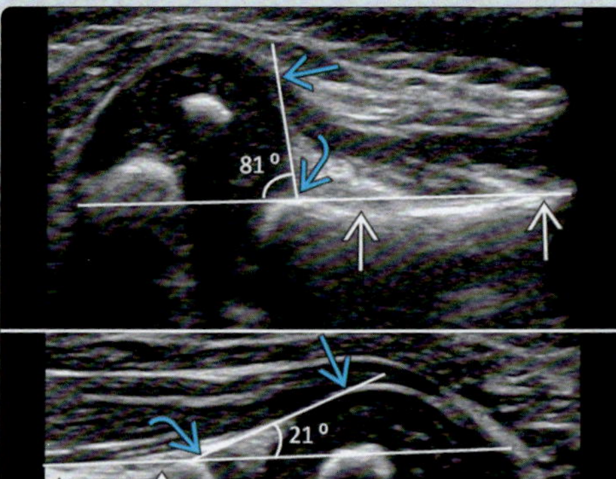

(Left) *Axial GRE MR of abnormal right (left) & normal left (right) shoulders shows a low right glenoscapular angle (between the scapular ➢ & glenoid ➡ lines) with the humeral head ➢ posterior to the scapular line.* **(Right)** *Posterior axial US of the left shoulder (top) in an infant with left brachial plexopathy shows a high α angle (between the posterior scapular margin ➡ & a tangent to the humeral head ➢ from the posterior glenoid ➢), indicating posterior subluxation. The right α angle (bottom) is normal.*

TERMINOLOGY

Synonyms

- Neonatal/perinatal brachial plexus palsy, birth palsy, brachial plexus birth injury (BPBI), shoulder contracture

Definitions

- Brachial plexopathy: Injury to ≥ 1 brachial plexus nerve roots, trunks, or cords → upper extremity contracture
- Glenohumeral dysplasia: Sequelae of brachial plexopathy on developing glenoid & humeral head

IMAGING

General Features

- Best diagnostic clue
  - Retroverted glenoid + posteriorly displaced humeral head

Radiographic Findings

- Small & ovoid humeral head
- Dysplastic glenoid, winged scapula, hooked coracoid

Ultrasonographic Findings

- Assesses humeral head prior to ossification
- Uses posterior axial approach to glenohumeral joint
- Measurements made with neutral, internal, & external rotation of humerus
- α angle: Angle between posterior scapular margin & tangent to humeral head from posterior edge of glenoid
  - Normal ≤ 30°
- Percentage of humeral head posterior to posterior scapular margin
  - Humeral head ossification center normally lies anterior to posterior scapular margin
    - Posterior position indicates posterior subluxation

MR Findings

- GRE & PD FS: Cartilage-sensitive sequences show unossified & ossified portions of glenoid & humeral head
- T1: Shows fatty atrophy of shoulder musculature
- Measurements on axial images
  - Glenoscapular angle (GSA): Posterior angle between scapular & glenoid lines
    - Scapular line: Line connecting medial most scapula & midglenoid cartilage
    - Glenoid line: Line parallels glenoid articular cartilage
  - Glenoid version angle = GSA -90°
    - Negative number = glenoid retroversion
    - > 5° more retroversion vs. unaffected side indicates glenoid dysplasia
  - Percentage of humeral head anterior to scapular line (PHHA)
    - Normal ~ 50%; ↓ with ↑ glenohumeral dysplasia
- Recent papers show abnormal scapular position of affected shoulder → inaccurate measurement of GSA & PHHA
  - Corrected by measuring on reconstructed images truly axial to scapula (from 3D data set)
  - Another study found "modified Friedman method" to give similar values to 3D reformatted method

Imaging Recommendations

- Best imaging tool
  - MR provides best overall articular & soft tissue evaluation
- Protocol advice
  - Compare affected vs. unaffected shoulders

DIFFERENTIAL DIAGNOSIS

Pseudoparesis of Upper Extremity

- Due to birth trauma → clavicular or humeral fracture

Arthrogryposis

- Infant born with ≥ 2 joint contractures

Cervical Spinal Cord Injury

- Affects bilateral extremities + bladder & bowel function

PATHOLOGY

General Features

- Etiology
  - Shoulder traction at delivery → nerve injury → muscle imbalance → internal rotation → posterior glenoid/anterior humeral head cartilage loading → glenohumeral dysplasia → posterior subluxation
    - Subluxation develops gradually in 1st year of life in infants with more severe birth injuries

Staging, Grading, & Classification

- Birch glenoid classification: Concave-flat, convex, biconcave
- Waters classification system: Glenoid version, humeral head coverage/position, ± pseudoglenoid

CLINICAL ISSUES

Presentation

- Most common signs/symptoms
  - Depends on level of injured nerves (C5-T1)

Demographics

- Epidemiology: 1-3 per 1,000 live births in USA

Natural History & Prognosis

- Most BPBI patients have temporary injuries & recover by 1-3 months of age; persistence depends on
  - Type of nerve injury
  - Number of roots involved
- 20-30% have residual neurologic deficits at 3 years
  - Posterior humeral head subluxation in up to 33% of permanent BPBI

Treatment

- Conservative: Physical therapy, Botox injections, & closed reduction
- Surgical: Anterior soft tissue release ± tendon transfers

SELECTED REFERENCES

1. Kim HHR et al: Contemporary imaging of the pediatric shoulder: pearls and pitfalls. Pediatr Radiol. 51(3):338-52, 2021
2. Ditzler MG et al: Modified Friedman technique: a new proposed method of measuring glenoid version in the setting of glenohumeral dysplasia. Pediatr Radiol. 48(12):1779-85, 2018
3. Donohue KW et al: Comparison of ultrasound and MRI for the diagnosis of glenohumeral dysplasia in brachial plexus birth palsy. J Bone Joint Surg Am. 99(2):123-32, 2017
4. van de Bunt F et al: Analysis of normal and dysplastic glenohumeral morphology at magnetic resonance imaging in children with neonatal brachial plexus palsy. Pediatr Radiol. 47(10):1337-44, 2017

Hemophilia

KEY FACTS

TERMINOLOGY

- X-linked recessive bleeding disorder resulting from clotting factor deficiencies
  - Hemophilia A (> 80% of cases): Factor VIII deficiency
  - Hemophilia B (< 15% of cases): Factor IX deficiency
- Hemophilic arthropathy: Progressive joint destruction due to recurrent hemarthrosis, synovitis, & erosions

IMAGING

- Location of arthropathy: Ankle > knee, elbow > shoulder
- Radiographs
  - Distention of joint capsule by effusion & synovitis with eventual cartilage damage, erosions, & subchondral cysts
- MR
  - Variable signal intensity & heterogeneity of effusions due to blood products of different ages
  - Chronic hemosiderin deposits line synovium
    - Low signal intensity on all sequences with characteristic blooming of signal loss on T2* GRE
  - Eventual development of osteocartilaginous erosions
- US
  - Effusion of variable echogenicity/complexity
  - Synovial thickening with hyperemia by Doppler
  - Thinning, irregularity of hypoechoic cartilage

TOP DIFFERENTIAL DIAGNOSES

- Synovial venous malformation
- Pigmented villonodular synovitis
- Juvenile idiopathic arthritis

CLINICAL ISSUES

- Prevention: Early initiation of aggressive prophylaxis regimen with clotting factors
  - Significantly ↓ joint bleeds & chronic degeneration
- Acute hemarthrosis: Factor replacement + joint aspiration
- Chronic hemarthrosis: Synovectomy (surgical or radiosynovectomy); arthroplasty

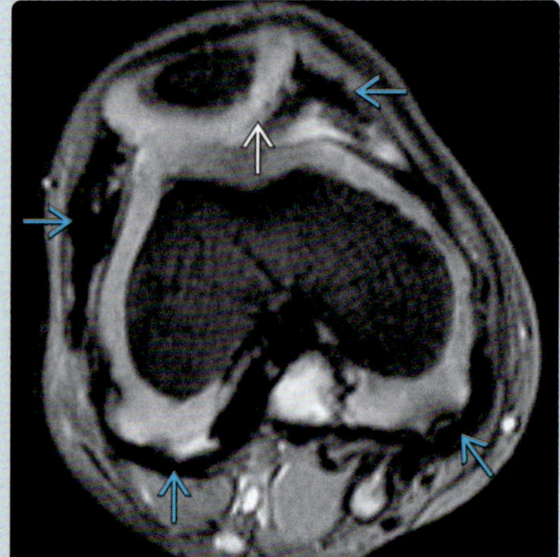

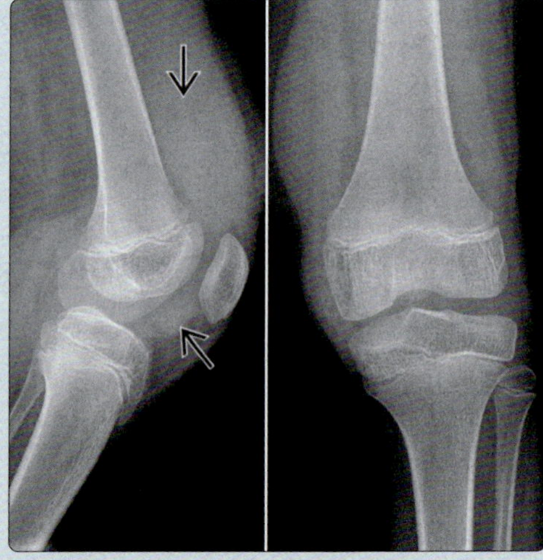

(Left) *Axial T2* GRE MR of the knee in a 7-year-old with hemophilia A shows extensive blooming (exaggerated signal loss) along the joint capsule ➔ due to prior episodes of hemarthrosis. Early cartilage irregularity is seen at the patellar medial facet ➔.* **(Right)** *Lateral & AP knee radiographs in the same patient 6 years later at a time of swelling show a large dense joint effusion ➔. The epiphyses are mildly large & irregular due to repeated hemarthroses & synovitis causing local hyperemia & cartilage damage.*

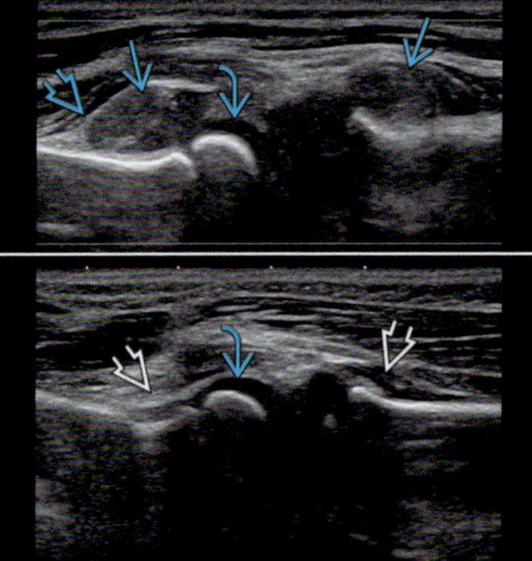

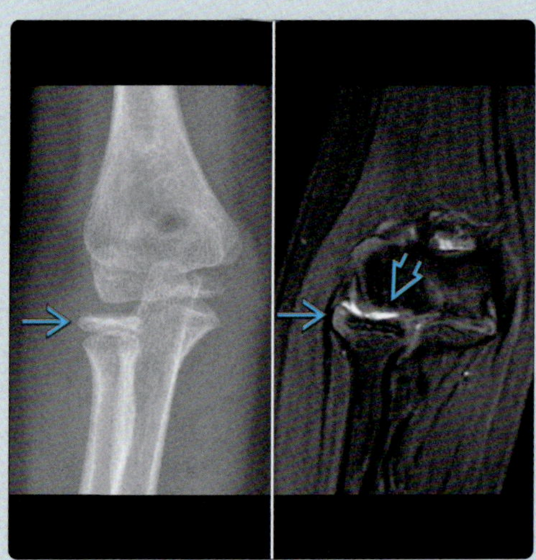

(Left) *Sagittal US of the right (top) & left (bottom) elbows in a child with hemophilia A & right arm swelling shows a complex effusion ➔ anterior to the distal right humerus & radial neck. There is anterior fat pad displacement ➔. No effusion is seen on the left ➔. Normal hypoechoic humeral capitellar cartilage is seen bilaterally ➔.* **(Right)** *AP radiograph (left) & T2 FS MR (right) in the same patient 3 years later show overgrowth & irregularity of the radial head ➔ with associated cartilage loss at the radiocapitellar articulation ➔.*

TERMINOLOGY

Synonyms

- Hemophilia A: Factor VIII deficiency
- Hemophilia B: Factor IX deficiency, Christmas disease

Definitions

- Hemophilia: X-linked recessive bleeding disorder due to clotting factor deficiencies
- Hemophilic arthropathy: Spontaneous bleeding into joint → inflamed & friable synovium → recurrent bleeding → pain & loss of function with accelerated joint degeneration
- Hemophilic pseudotumor: Nonneoplastic mass from focally recurrent intraosseous, subperiosteal, or soft tissue bleeds

IMAGING

Radiographic Findings

- Hemophilic arthropathy: Historically common; substantially ↓ now due to aggressive factor replacement regimens
  - Distention of joint capsule by effusion & synovitis
  - Hyperemia leads to
    - Overgrowth (ballooning) of epiphyses
    - Premature physeal fusion → limb shortening
  - Inflammatory synovitis → cartilage destruction, erosions, subchondral cysts, recurrent bleeds
- Hemophilic pseudotumor (very uncommon)
  - Intraosseous: Large expansile or lytic bubbly lesion with mass effect on adjacent tissues
  - Subperiosteal or soft tissue: Extrinsic scalloping of bone

Ultrasonographic Findings

- Effusion (hemorrhage) showing variable complexity
  - Simple fluid & hemorrhagic fluid are not reliably differentiated by US
- Synovial thickening with hyperemia by Doppler
  - ↑ power Doppler signal of synovium → ↑ bleeding risk
- Thinning & irregularity of hypoechoic cartilage ± bone erosions at margins of joints
  - US is limited at central articular surfaces

MR Findings

- Hemophilic arthropathy
  - Variable signal intensity & heterogeneity of effusions due to blood products of different ages
  - Chronic hemosiderin lines synovium
    - Low signal intensity on all sequences with characteristic blooming of signal loss on T2* GRE
    - Hypertrophied enhancing synovium
  - Eventual development of osteocartilaginous erosions

Imaging Recommendations

- US for acute hemarthrosis
- MR provides superior assessment of entire joint

DIFFERENTIAL DIAGNOSIS

Pediatric Arthropathies

- Synovial venous malformation
  - Blood-filled intraarticular mass → hemarthrosis, synovitis, erosions, degeneration
  - Infiltrating or discrete lobular &/or tubular fluid signal intensity masses with septations
    - ± fluid-fluid levels, thrombi
- Pigmented villonodular synovitis
  - Diffuse intraarticular form: Intermixed hemosiderin deposits & enhancing proliferative synovium often have radiating frond-like appearance
- Juvenile idiopathic arthritis
  - Joint effusion ± rice bodies; blood products are rare
  - Synovitis → erosions & growth disturbances
    - Similar chronic radiographic appearance to hemophilia

PATHOLOGY

General Features

- Etiology
  - Sites of bleeds depend on clotting factor levels
    - Musculoskeletal system (exposed to repetitive mild trauma) accounts for up to 90% of sites
      - Joints: 70-80%; muscles: 10-20%

CLINICAL ISSUES

Presentation

- Most common signs/symptoms
  - Acute hemarthrosis: Tense, swollen, red, painful joint occurring spontaneously or with minor trauma
  - Subacute or chronic hemarthrosis: Degenerative arthrosis, ↓ range of motion, contractures

Demographics

- Age
  - 1st episode of joint hemorrhage by 2-3 years of age
- Epidemiology
  - Hemophilia A (> 80% of cases): 1 in 5,000 male patients
  - Hemophilia B: 1 in 30,000 male patients

Natural History & Prognosis

- Hemarthrosis classically occurs in 70-90% of cases
  - Substantial reduction in modern era by early initiation of aggressive prophylactic replacement of synthetic clotting factors
    - Patients may develop antibodies (inhibitors) to replacement clotting factors: Up to 30% of severe A vs. 2% of B

Treatment

- Hemophilic arthropathy
  - Acute bleed: Clotting factor, joint aspiration
  - Chronic: Synovectomy (surgical vs. radiosynovectomy); intraarticular hyaluronic acid; if end stage → arthroplasty

SELECTED REFERENCES

1. Kizilocak H et al: Diagnosis and treatment of hemophilia. Clin Adv Hematol Oncol. 17(6):344-51, 2019
2. Rodríguez-Merchán EC: The role of orthopaedic surgery in haemophilia: current rationale, indications and results. EFORT Open Rev. 4(5):165-73, 2019
3. Ligocki CC et al: A systematic review of ultrasound imaging as a tool for evaluating haemophilic arthropathy in children and adults. Haemophilia. 23(4):598-612, 2017
4. Soliman M et al: Imaging of haemophilic arthropathy in growing joints: pitfalls in ultrasound and MRI. Haemophilia. 23(5):660-72, 2017
5. Doria AS et al: Diagnostic accuracy of ultrasound for assessment of hemophilic arthropathy: MRI correlation. AJR Am J Roentgenol. 204(3):W336-47, 2015
6. Keshava SN et al: Imaging evaluation of hemophilia: musculoskeletal approach. Semin Thromb Hemost. 41(8):880-93, 2015

SECTION 7
Brain

Overview

This 4th edition of *Diagnostic Imaging: Pediatrics* presents another great opportunity to expand & update the neuroradiology sections. As in the 3rd edition, we continue to add new diagnoses to the book. Length constraints mean that many diagnoses are only 1 or 2 pages long. We hope readers will see the increased number of diagnoses as outweighing the decreased in length & will explore the additional material in the Elsevier eBook & Expert Consult, where they will find expanded descriptions, case examples, & selected references to support the printed text.

The most difficult task in organizing the Brain section is deciding what to include & what to leave out. The brain section is divided into 6 subsections: Normal Developmental Variation, Congenital Malformations, Phakomatoses, Cysts & Neoplasms, Traumatic & Vascular Lesions, & Metabolic, Infectious, & Inflammatory Disorders. The included diagnoses are not meant to be all-encompassing but were selected to be the most helpful to the pediatric radiology practitioner. Some topics, such as pineal cyst & enlarged perivascular spaces, are included because they are so common. Conversely, metabolic brain diseases are rarely encountered but are complex entities that may be overwhelming to approach without a resource to provide direction. Some diagnoses that are not exclusively pediatric, such as cerebral venous sinus thrombosis, often get overlooked in specialty texts but have been included here because they constitute an important pathology for which we can provide a unique pediatric perspective.

As in the transition from the 2nd edition to the 3rd edition, there have been a number of changes to the neoplasm diagnoses in this edition. With an increasingly rapid evolution of our understanding of the molecular & genetic underpinnings of pediatric CNS tumors, we have seen previous diagnoses (e.g., CNS PNET) disappear from the WHO tumor classification lexicon, while others (e.g., embryonal tumor with multilayered rosettes) have grown up in their place. Not unexpectedly, the new 2021 WHO CNS classification increasingly relies on the molecular & genetic profile of tumors with a trend towards subgrouping of tumors, which previously represented a single diagnosis. Some tumors, which were once considered to be similar because they looked similar under the microscope, are now understood to represent remarkably unique tumors molecularly & genetically. Possibly the best example of this is ependymoma, which was previously addressed in the 3rd edition as a single chapter but is now split into posterior fossa ependymoma & supratentorial ependymoma. This change reflects the recent advances that show these tumors to be distinct entities based upon their genetic & molecular profiles. Posterior fossa ependymomas are subdivided into PFE-A & PFE-B with unique clinical & prognostic profiles. Supratentorial ependymomas are divided into those with *RELA* fusion & those without (e.g., *YAP1* fusion). The trend towards increased molecular subtyping of CNS tumors has driven forward remarkably targeted therapies. A great example of this is the targeting of the RAS-MAPK pathway in low-grade glial tumors with *BRAF* mutations. As radiologists, we have come to discover a number of important imaging markers that correlate well with molecular subtypes in pediatric CNS tumors, including both medulloblastoma & ependymoma. It is expected that radiogenomics, or the correlation of imaging & molecular data, will be a major area of research & clinical interest in the coming years.

Terminology

There is a constant process in science & medicine of renaming entities to more accurately reflect new knowledge gained. This can make understanding, teaching, & researching these disease processes difficult. When a disease has many names, a comprehensive literature search becomes significantly more difficult to confidently perform. For this reason, we have made every effort to be comprehensive in listing the synonyms used both in the past & present to describe certain disease processes. We have also updated the titles of certain diagnoses (e.g., white matter injury of prematurity rather than periventricular leukomalacia, & hypoxic-ischemic encephalopathy rather than perinatal asphyxia) to reflect evolving descriptions found in recent medical literature.

Normal Development

One of the great challenges in pediatric neuroimaging is understanding the dynamic development of the human brain from the fetus to the adult. Understanding this normal development allows for accurate identification of normal vs. abnormal & gives the imaging professional a conceptual framework to understand many CNS diagnoses, especially the congenital malformations. For instance, when evaluating a fetal MR of the brain, it is critical to know the expected sulcation pattern for a given gestational age in order to identify possible malformations of cortical development. A delayed sulcation pattern may suggest a malformation of cortical development on the spectrum of lissencephaly or gyral simplification, whereas the presence of too many sulci for gestational age may suggest polymicrogyria.

During the first 2 years of life, an understanding of the normal myelination pattern allows for accurate identification of conditions associated with delayed myelination (e.g., Pelizaeus-Merzbacher disease). Because understanding normal myelination is so critical, this edition includes a 4-page chapter dedicated to the topic. Another important point regarding myelination is that certain diseases have very different imaging characteristics during the 1st year of life compared with later years. A prime example of this can be seen in tuberous sclerosis in which cortical tubers & radial migration lines are T1 hyperintense & T2 isointense prior to myelination & exactly the opposite (T1 hypointense & T2 hyperintense) following myelination. Tuberous sclerosis is just one of many diagnoses with such dynamic imaging characteristics over time.

One final example of the importance of understanding normal CNS development can be found in the pituitary, which undergoes both age- & sex-specific changes in size & signal characteristics with time. The anterior pituitary in the newborn is very T1 hyperintense, often equal to that of the posterior pituitary. This is normal & should not be mistaken for hemorrhage or other pathology. This hyperintensity is presumed to be related to maternal hormones, as the same finding is not seen in early premature infants when imaged at term-equivalent age. The anterior pituitary slowly decreases in T1 signal intensity & becomes isointense to the pons after the 1st few months of life. Regarding pituitary size, the normal pituitary often has a convex superior margin at birth, slowly becoming flat or concave over the ensuing weeks, an appearance that is typically maintained in male patients throughout life & in female patients until puberty. The imaging professional should not be alarmed to see an enlarged pituitary with a convex superior border in a teenage girl. This is a normal appearance in this age & sex should not in & of itself raise suspicion for a pituitary lesion.

Hydrocephalus

Hydrocephalus is a distressingly common entity in pediatrics, the consequence of a multitude of primary pathologies that result in alterations in the production, distribution, & resorption of CSF. Traditional views of intracranial fluid management as related to the choroid plexus, ventricles, subarachnoid space (SAS), arachnoid granulations, pia, arachnoid, & dural sinuses to manage the flow & distribution of interstitial fluid (ISF) have recently expanded to include the glymphatic system, which is a network of perivascular channels involved in fluid, nutrient, & metabolite exchange between the CSF & ISF.

Obstruction within the ventricular system will prevent egress of intraventricular CSF into the SAS, & increased pressure within the ventricles will cause ISF to accumulate in the periventricular white matter (transependymal edema). Elevated pressure in the dural sinuses will prevent the transmission of CSF from the SAS into the sinuses, as will alteration in arachnoid granulation function caused by inflammation or metabolic disorders (communicating hydrocephalus).

Cerebral Edema

A common & important neuroimaging finding is the development of brain edema, of which 4 basic types are recognized. Vasogenic edema reflects expansion of the ISF compartment in response to an irritating stimulus, such as tumor or inflammation. Cytotoxic edema is due to expansion of the intracellular fluid compartment secondary to failure of the sodium-potassium pump regulation of the cell membrane. In transependymal edema, increased hydrostatic pressure in the ventricular system prevents the normal progression of ISF into the ventricles & causes congestion in the periventricular white matter. Perhaps the least understood is posttraumatic edema, in which diffuse brain swelling is caused by a combination of cytotoxic & vasogenic edema resulting from a cascade of events that include sodium-potassium pump failure, diminished cerebral perfusion & autoregulation, & loss of integrity of the blood-brain barrier. Posttraumatic cerebral edema typically sets in several hours after the initial injury & can lead to rapid increase in intracranial pressure & death. Clinical management of traumatic brain injury usually includes imaging reassessment within the first 12 hours after presentation to look for progression of initially identified injuries, such as contusions & intracranial hemorrhage. The radiologist must be diligent in looking for signs of increased brain swelling at this time also; such signs include effacement of previously identifiable sulci at the vertex & decrease in size of basal cisterns. The presence of these signs should lead to more aggressive monitoring & management of intracranial pressure. Waiting until clinical signs develop is too late to effectively combat the cycle of reduced cerebral perfusion & progressive cellular injury. Diffuse cerebral edema is the leading cause of death from cases of child abuse, & the traumatic nature of the insult may not be readily apparent at first presentation. Nontraumatic insults, such as acute encephalitis & status epilepticus, can also lead to this potentially fatal complication.

Imaging Protocols

The development & use of high-quality indication-specific imaging protocols are essential to the practice of pediatric neuroradiology. For CT imaging in the age of the Image Gently campaign, much of the focus has been appropriately on the reduction of radiation exposure to the patient. When an indicated CT exam is performed, it is imperative that we extract the maximum information from this study. One of the best ways to do so is to perform multiplanar reconstructions (MPR) in coronal & sagittal planes. MPRs have been shown to ↑ the detection of small intracranial hemorrhages & reduce the number of false-positives by accurately characterizing some findings as artifactual. The same can be said for the detection of skull fractures, which is improved with MPR as well as 3D surface rendering.

Brain MR protocols for the neonate should be adjusted to confidently identify perinatal injuries, congenital malformations, & metabolic derangements. For the infant younger than 3 years, a focus on myelin maturation is key with T1 included in all protocols. Conversely, FLAIR sequences are typically avoided in the child under 24 months, as these may cause confusion in the incompletely myelinated brain. For the child over 24 months, adult-type sequences can be employed but should be specifically tailored to answer the clinical question at hand.

Volumetric MR is becoming increasingly important in pediatric imaging with most weightings (e.g., T1, T2, PD, FLAIR, & SSFP) now available on most platforms. Volumetric imaging is optimal for tumor follow-up, giving the imaging professional confidence in tumor size measurements from one exam to the next. Volumetric FLAIR has become a critical sequence in seizure protocols to increase sensitivity for the often subtle findings of focal cortical dysplasia. 3D SSFP (e.g., FIESTA, CISS) images remove CSF flow artifact & provide high spatial resolution for the optimal evaluation of masses with a CSF interface. Finally, volumetric imaging is helpful because it allows reconstruction in multiple planes with no penalty in exam length.

Pediatric radiologists should be eager to employ advanced MR techniques, such as diffusion tensor imaging (DTI), susceptibility weighted imaging (SWI), arterial spin labeling (ASL), & vessel wall imaging. DTI provides high-quality DWI & ADC derivatives, & the ability to perform tractography is very helpful in preoperative tumor & epilepsy planning. SWI provides highly sensitive detection of hemorrhagic foci in the brain parenchyma & important insight into the vascular supply to tumors & malformations. ASL provides the opportunity to acquire brain perfusion information without the need for contrast administration, opening the door for perfusion imaging in the routine setting. Finally, vessel wall imaging is becoming an increasingly important technique for identifying inflammatory arteriopathies in children.

Selected References

1. Taoka T et al: Neurofluid dynamics and the glymphatic system: a neuroimaging perspective. Korean J Radiol. 21(11):1199-209, 2020
2. Ho ML et al: Pediatric brain MRI, part 2: advanced techniques. Pediatr Radiol. 47(5):544-55, 2017
3. Louis DN et al: The 2016 World Health Organization Classification of Tumors of the Central Nervous System: a summary. Acta Neuropathol. 131(6):803-20, 2016

(Left) *Sagittal T1 MR images in a 7-day-old infant (top) & a 2-month-old infant (bottom) show the typical imaging evolution of the neonatal anterior pituitary, which is often very hyperintense (sometimes equal to the posterior pituitary) early with a superior convex border ➲. This signal & morphology are presumably related to maternal hormones, as early premature infants imaged at term-equivalent ages do not have this appearance. Over the 1st few weeks of life, the anterior pituitary becomes isointense to the pons with a flat or concave superior border ➙.* **(Right)** *Sagittal T1 MR images in a 6-year-old girl (top) & a 17-year-old girl (bottom) show typical appearances of the anterior pituitary at these ages. An enlarged (up to 9-mm vertical) anterior pituitary with a convex, superior border in a teenage girl should not raise concern.*

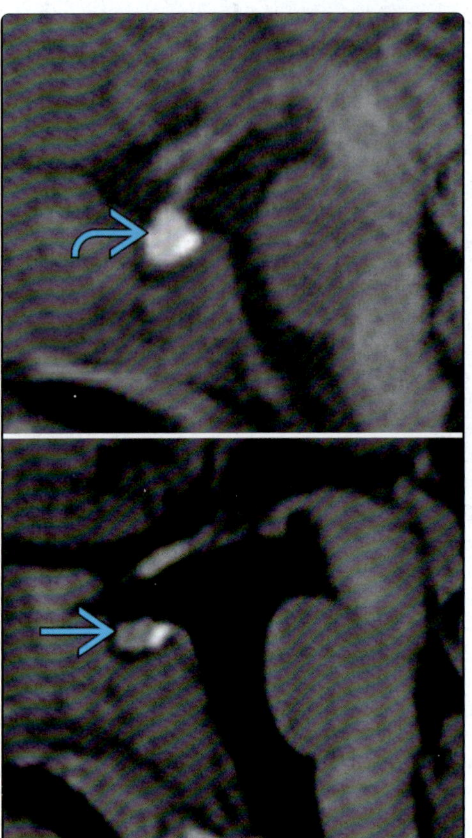

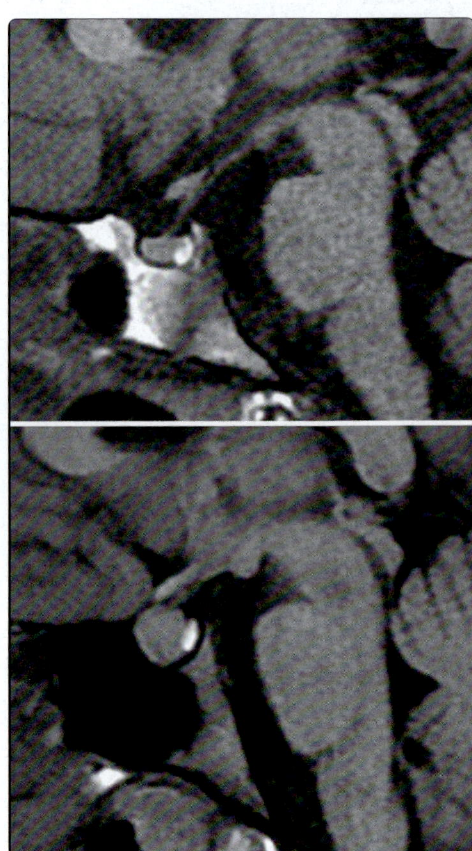

(Left) *Sagittal T1 MR images at 2, 4, 7, & 10 months (top to bottom, respectively) show development of the corpus callosum during the 1st year of life. Progressive myelination & thickening of the corpus callosum begin with the posterior body & splenium. The posterior 1/2 of the corpus callosum continues to thicken as the anterior body, genu, & rostrum begin to myelinate at 4 months. By the end of the 1st year of life, the corpus callosum is completely myelinated with uniform signal intensity.* **(Right)** *Axial T1 MR images in a patient with tuberous sclerosis complex at 3 months (top) & 10 months (bottom) show that, prior to significant myelination, the cortical tubers & radial migration lines are hyperintense ➙. Following myelination, these lesions show varying degrees of hypointensity ➙ compared with adjacent white matter.*

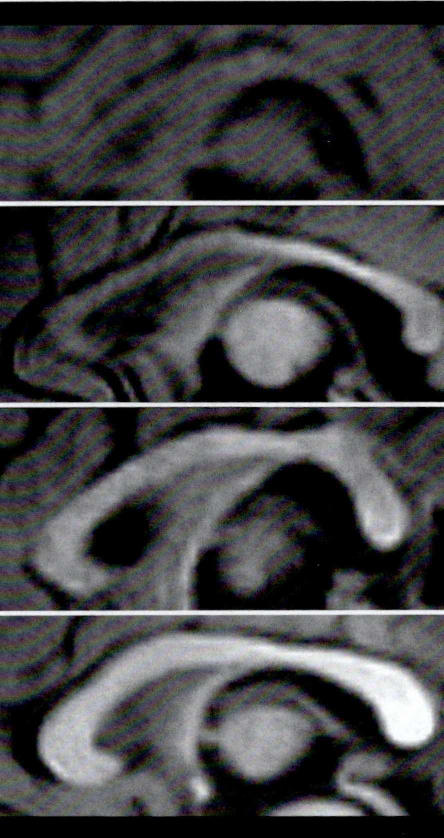

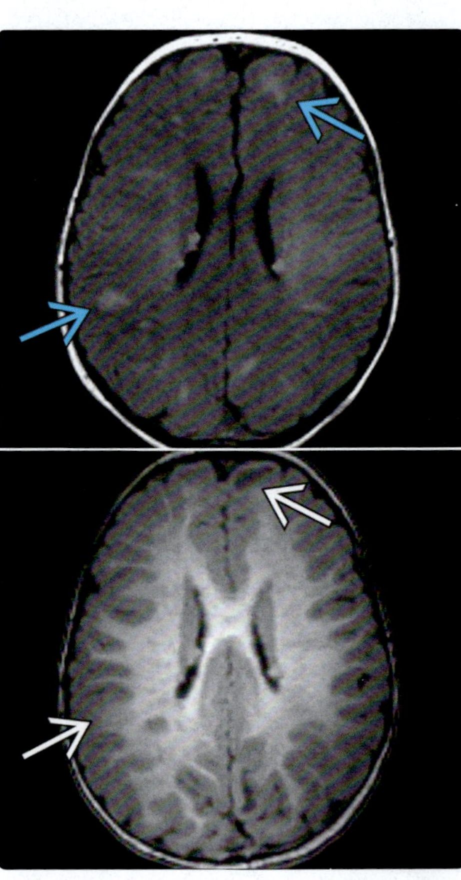

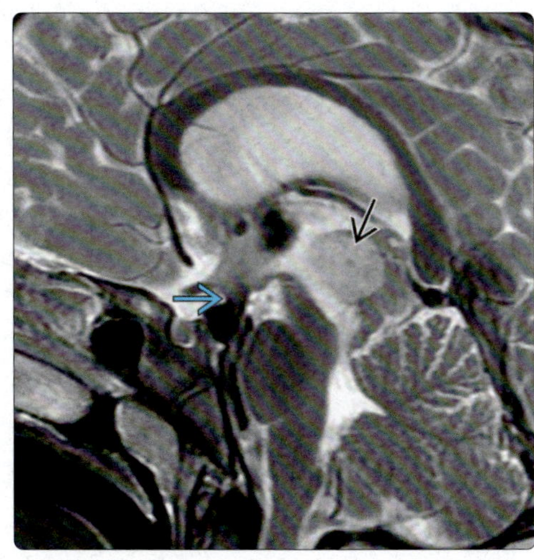

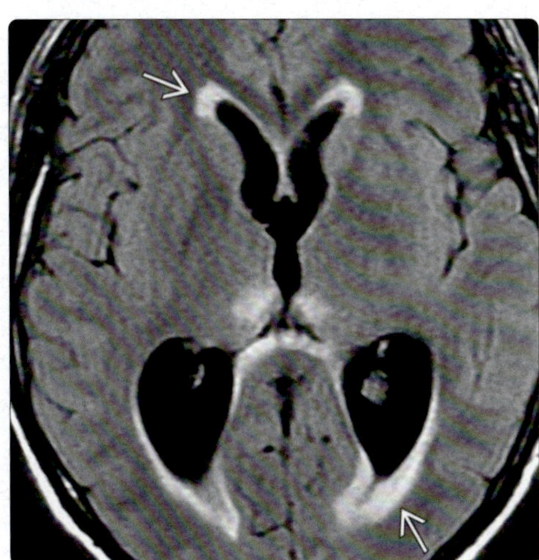

(Left) *Midline sagittal T2 MR in a 6-year-old child with a tectal mass* ⇒ *shows obstruction of the cerebral aqueduct with mass effect on the midbrain. Treatment is an endoscopic 3rd ventriculostomy, which appears patent as evidenced by the dark flow artifact* ⇒ *across the floor of the 3rd ventricle.* **(Right)** *Axial FLAIR MR in a 19-year-old man with a pineal germinoma shows ventriculomegaly with transependymal edema* ➡ *in the frontal & occipital regions (where hydrostatic pressure of interstitial fluid is highest).*

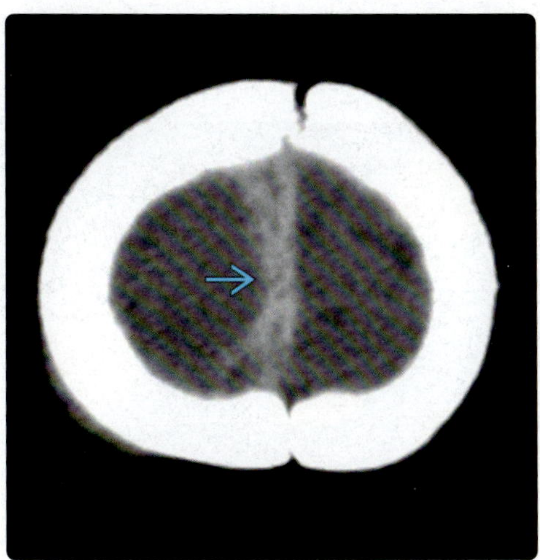

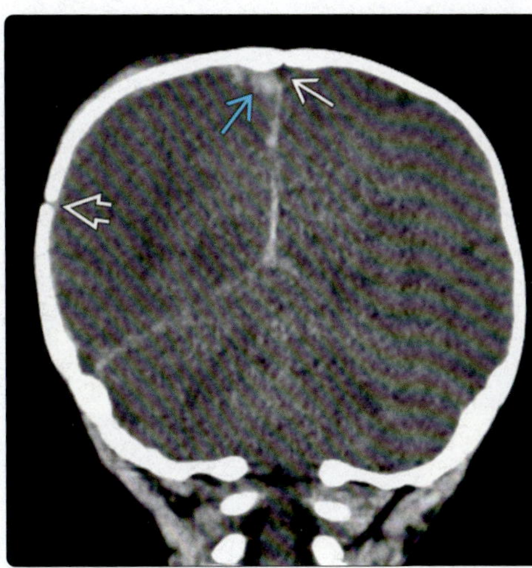

(Left) *Axial NECT in a 6-month-old infant with nonaccidental trauma shows hyperdensity* ⇒ *in the region of the superior sagittal sinus. With axial images alone, it can be difficult to distinguish subdural hemorrhage from venous sinus thrombosis.* **(Right)** *Coronal NECT in the same patient clearly delineates the superior sagittal sinus* ➡ *from the adjacent subdural hemorrhage* ⇒*. Also note the axially oriented right parietal bone fracture* ➡*, which was difficult to see on axial images.*

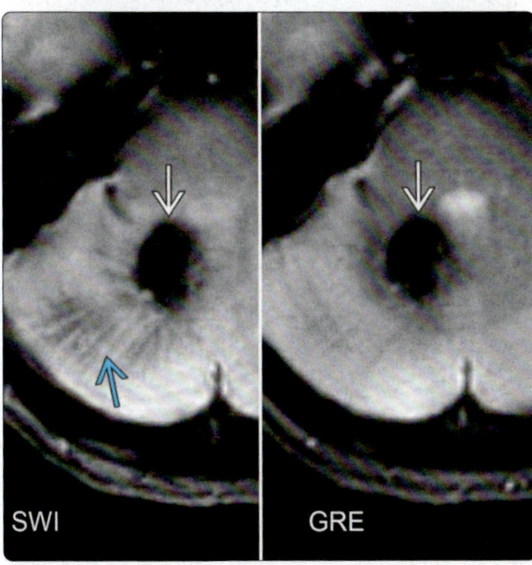

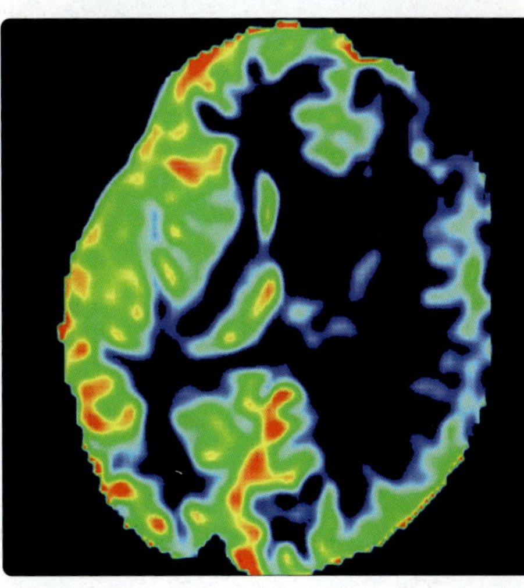

(Left) *Axial SWI (L) & T2* GRE (R) MRs in a patient with a cavernous malformation* ➡ *show the ↑ conspicuity of the associated developmental venous anomaly* ⇒ *on SWI compared with GRE.* **(Right)** *Axial ASL in a 10-year-old boy with Sturge-Weber syndrome shows substantially ↓ perfusion within the left frontal lobe (which was severely affected with pial angiomatosis & parenchymal atrophy). ASL is a perfusion technique that does not require contrast administration.*

Normal Myelination

KEY FACTS

IMAGING

- T1 is key sequence in assessing myelination < 1 year
  - Bright signal reflects presence of proteolipid protein (PLP)
  - Extent of bright signal on T1 reflects distribution of myelinating oligodendrocytes in infant brain
- T2 is key sequence in assessing myelination in children 1-2 years of age
  - As myelin sheaths thicken, surrounding interstitial (extraaxonal) water is displaced
  - Less interstitial water → darker signal on T2
  - Drop in T2 signal lags considerably behind presence of bright T1 signal
- PD/intermediate echo images are especially valuable < 24 months
  - Very helpful in distinguishing gliosis from lack of myelination
  - Gliosis is brighter than terminal zones
- Difficult to distinguish pathology from normal in infant on FLAIR
- Presence of myelin has significant effect on ability of water to diffuse
  - Fractional anisotropy (FA) ↑ with brain maturation

DIAGNOSTIC CHECKLIST

- MR demonstration of normal myelination closely parallels developmental functional milestones
  - Assessment of myelination is essential aspect of interpreting MR in children
    - Analogous to documentation of developmental milestones by pediatrician
- Know gestational age before assigning myelination stage
  - Normal myelination milestones are based upon postconception age, regardless of degree of maturity at delivery

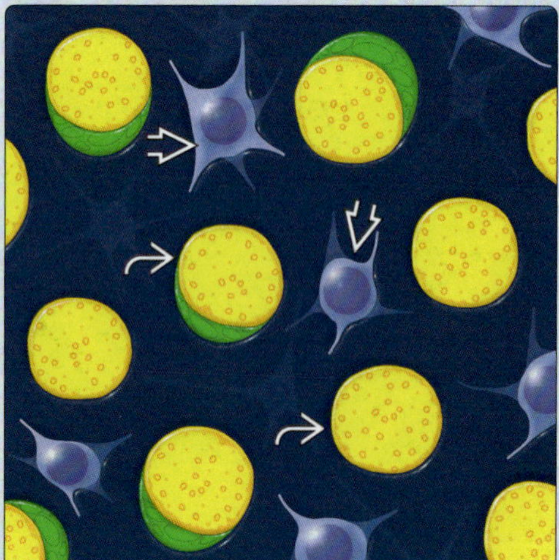
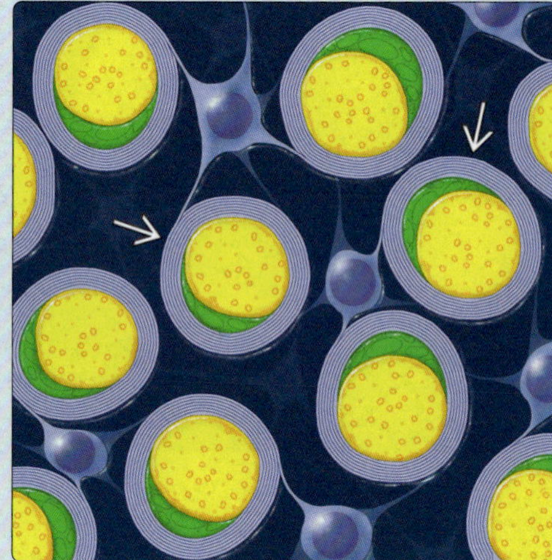

(Left) *Oligodendrocytes ➡ lie in proximity to axons ➡ after migration. The presence of proteolipid protein in the oligodendrocytes results in T1 shortening (T1 bright signal) on MR, but the large amount of interstitial water (dark blue background) results in T2 prolongation (T2 bright signal) on MR.* **(Right)** *With time, the oligodendrocytes lay down multiple layers of myelin ➡ around each axon. As it thickens, the hydrophobic myelin drives out the interstitial water, causing reduced T2 signal (or T2 shortening) on MR.*

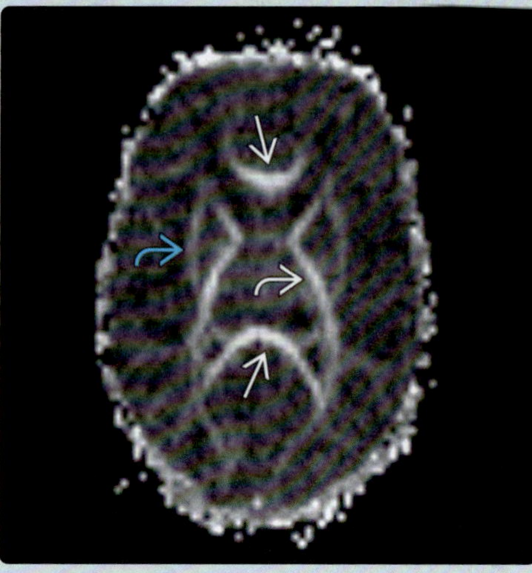
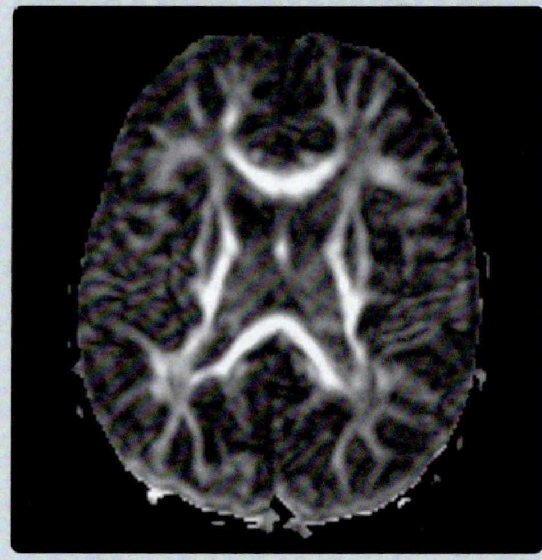

(Left) *Axial fractional anisotropy (FA) map in a newborn shows bright signal in the corpus callosum ➡ & internal ➡ & external ➡ capsules, reflecting the relatively dense axonal population & early myelination in these regions. FA maps can demonstrate white matter tracts prior to their delineation on conventional MR sequences.* **(Right)** *Axial FA map in a 9-month-old shows extension of bright signal throughout the brain, reflecting the greater structural organization resulting from myelination.*

TERMINOLOGY

Synonyms

- Myelin maturation, white matter (WM) development

Definitions

- Process of myelin sheath development around axons throughout CNS
  - Begins in 5th fetal month & continues throughout life

IMAGING

General Features

- Best diagnostic clue
  - Appearance of myelination on imaging reflects presence of proteolipid & its effect on interstitial water
  - Myelin development correlates with functional milestones
- Location
  - In general, myelin maturation proceeds caudal to rostral, central to peripheral, dorsal to ventral
- Size
  - WM tracts, especially corpus callosum, ↑ in size with myelin formation
- Morphology
  - Diffusion tractography can demonstrate morphology & integrity of developing tracts

CT Findings

- NECT
  - Gray matter (GM)-WM differentiation is accentuated in neonate due to high water content of WM
    - Unmyelinated WM is hypodense relative to GM & to myelinated WM
      - Reflects high ratio of interstitial water:axons
  - Density ↑ with myelination is relatively subtle, making CT insensitive to detecting delays in myelination

MR Findings

- T1WI
  - Key sequence in assessing myelination < 1 year
  - Bright signal reflects presence of proteolipid protein (PLP)
    - PLP is expressed by mature (myelinating) oligodendrocytes as they start laying down myelin sheath
    - Extent of bright signal on T1 reflects distribution of myelinating oligodendrocytes in infant brain
  - Detection of myelination (represented by hyperintense signal) progresses in predictable fashion
    - By term
      - Dorsal brainstem
      - Dentate nucleus
      - Optic tracts
      - Anterior commissure
      - Posterior limb of internal capsule
      - Rolandic & perirolandic gyri
      - Pyramidal tracts
    - By 2 months
      - Splenium of corpus callosum
      - Anterior limb internal capsule
      - Early optic radiations
    - By 4 months
      - Genu of corpus callosum
      - Optic radiations become more apparent
      - Peripheral rami in pyramidal tracts (perirolandic gyri)
    - By 6 months
      - Genu & splenium are equally hyperintense
      - Peripheral rami in parietal & occipital lobes become hyperintense
    - By 8 months
      - All but most peripheral rami of frontal gyri are hyperintense
    - By 10-12 months
      - Adult appearance of myelin is achieved on T1
- T2WI
  - Key sequence in assessing myelination in children 1-2 years of age
  - As myelin sheaths thicken, surrounding interstitial (extraaxonal) water is displaced
    - PLP is hydrophobic
    - Less interstitial water → darker signal on T2
  - Drop in T2 signal lags considerably behind presence of bright T1 signal
    - Process starts immediately after oligodendrocytes begin laying down myelin sheath
    - Sheath has to thicken considerably before enough water is displaced to reduce signal
  - Detection of myelination (represented by hypointense signal) progresses in predictable fashion
    - By term
      - Dorsal brainstem
      - Part of posterior limb of internal capsule
      - Perirolandic gyri
    - By 4 months
      - More hypointense signal in rolandic & perirolandic gyri
      - Splenium of corpus callosum
      - More anterior extension in internal capsule
    - By 8 months
      - Genu & splenium of corpus callosum
      - Anterior limb of internal capsule
      - ↓ signal in centrum semiovale & optic radiations
      - ↓ signal in basal ganglia & thalamus
    - By 12 months
      - External capsule hypointense signal becomes apparent
      - Expansion of centrum semiovale hypointensity
      - Clearly defined peripheral rami around central sulcus & in occipital poles
    - By 16 months
      - Better definition of deep nuclei in brainstem & basal ganglia
      - Peripheral rami in parietal lobes become hypointense
    - By 18 months
      - All but most peripheral frontal WM rami are now hypointense

- Some residual hyperintense signal around trigones of lateral ventricles (terminal zones) due to greater hydrostatic pressure in this region from confluence of WM tracts
  - By 36 months
    - Adult appearance of myelin achieved on T2
- PD/intermediate
  - Very helpful in distinguishing gliosis from lack of myelination
    - Gliosis is brighter than terminal zones
- FLAIR
  - Relatively "flat" images in immature brains
  - Signal changes associated with myelination (hyperintense to hypointense) are similar to T2
    - Tend to occur 2-3 months after changes visible on T2
      - Smaller amounts of interaxonal water may exert greater influence on FLAIR sequences
  - Difficult to distinguish pathology from normal in infant
- DWI
  - ADC values predate T1/T2 signal changes
  - Presence of myelin has significant effect on ability of water to diffuse
    - Fractional anisotropy (FA) ↑ with brain maturation
    - Diffusion perpendicular to myelin sheaths is restricted with ↓ in extraaxonal water
    - Diffusivity along axon ↑
  - Diffusion tractography (DTI) can elucidate fiber tracts as they become myelinated
    - Correlates with functional milestones
    - May allow more specific identification of developing functional tracts
    - Mean diffusivity & FA measurements can be used to assess integrity of tracts
- MRS
  - Changes in relative metabolite concentrations in first 2 years of life may reflect myelination
  - Myoinositol & choline are high in neonate
    - Choline ↓ with myelination
  - NAA ↑ with myelination in 1st year of life

Imaging Recommendations

- Best imaging tool
  - Use both T1 & T2 to assess myelination
    - T1 < 12 months
    - T2 from 12-24 months
- Protocol advice
  - IR may ↑ sensitivity to T1 shortening
  - FSE sequences may minimize appearance of abnormal hyperintensity
  - Conventional double spin-echo sequences are preferred for T2
    - PD/intermediate echo images are especially valuable < 24 months

PATHOLOGY

General Features

- Etiology
  - Oligodendrocyte precursors proliferate in germinal matrix
  - Immature oligodendrocytes (prooligodendrocytes) migrate throughout brain
    - Follow distribution of neurons
    - Mature to myelinating oligodendrocytes after reaching destination
    - Neuron induces myelinization by electrical impulse
- Genetics
  - 2 major structural proteins of myelin: Myelin basic protein (MBP) & PLP
    - *MBP* gene encoded on chromosome 18q
    - *PDXP* gene encoded on chromosome Xq21-q22
- General path comments
  - Oligodendrocytes form & maintain axon myelin sheath
  - 1 oligodendrocyte may invest up to 50 axons

Staging, Grading, & Classification

- Myelination is assessed as "appropriate" for age or delayed
- Delay in myelination should prompt investigation for possible causes

Gross Pathologic & Surgical Features

- Premyelinated brain is "soft" due to high water content
  - Presence of myelin is required for fixation

Microscopic Features

- Myelin sheath is formed of multiple layers wrapped around axon
  - Forms protein-lipid-protein-lipid-protein stack

CLINICAL ISSUES

Demographics

- Age
  - All children should achieve adult appearance of WM by 36-40 months
- Sex
  - No significant male/female difference

DIAGNOSTIC CHECKLIST

Consider

- MR demonstration of normal myelination closely parallels developmental functional milestones
- Assessment of myelination is essential aspect of interpreting MR in children
- Know gestational age before assigning myelination stage
  - Normal myelination milestones are based upon postconception age, regardless of degree of maturity at delivery

Image Interpretation Pearls

- Use IR for T1 < 10 months
- Use conventional double spin-echo sequences for T2

SELECTED REFERENCES

1. Bhatia V et al: MRI in normal myelination: a pictorial review. Curr Pediatr Rev. ePub, 2021
2. Barkovich MJ et al: MR imaging of normal brain development. Neuroimaging Clin N Am. 29(3):325-37, 2019
3. Uda S et al: Normal development of human brain white matter from infancy to early adulthood: a diffusion tensor imaging study. Dev Neurosci. 37(2):182-94, 2015
4. Branson HM: Normal myelination: a practical pictorial review. Neuroimaging Clin N Am. 23(2):183-95, 2013

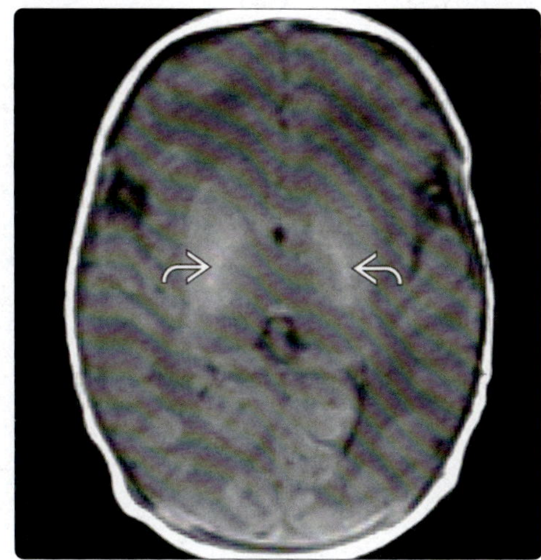

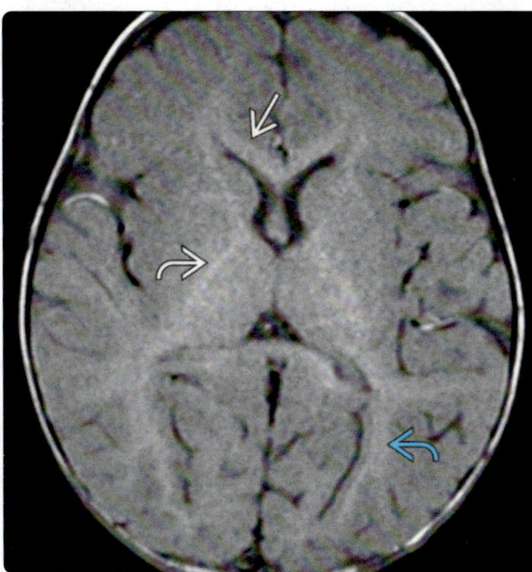

(Left) *Axial T1 MR in a term newborn shows faint bright signal in the posterior limbs of the internal capsules, indicating the presence of mature oligodendrocytes that are producing myelin in these regions. This process begins in the 2nd trimester of gestation.* **(Right)** *Axial T1 MR in a normal 6-month-old shows faint bright signal in the internal capsules, corpus callosum, & optic radiations well before any hypointense signal will be obvious in these structures on T2.*

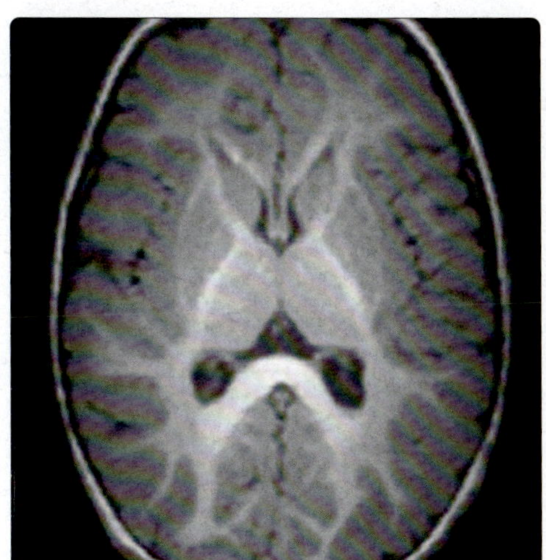

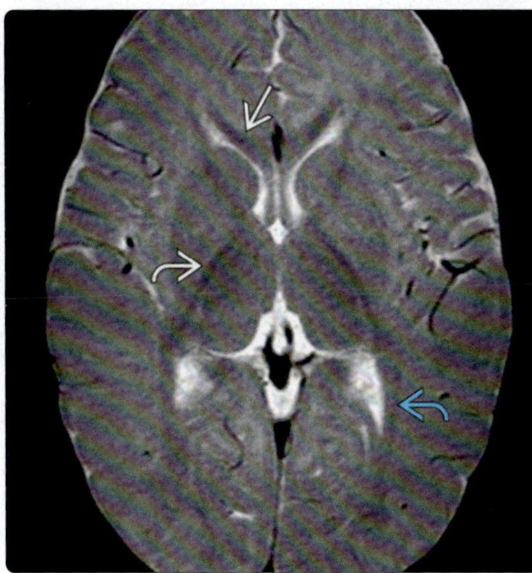

(Left) *Axial T1 MR in a 9-month-old shows bright signal throughout the white matter. Myelination is far from complete at this stage, but the T1 confirms the presence of mature oligodendrocytes throughout the brain.* **(Right)** *Axial T2 MR in another 9-month-old shows hypointensity in the internal capsules, corpus callosum, & optic radiations, areas that appear fully mature on T1. The displacement of interstitial water by the thickening myelin sheath lags far behind the signal changes on T1.*

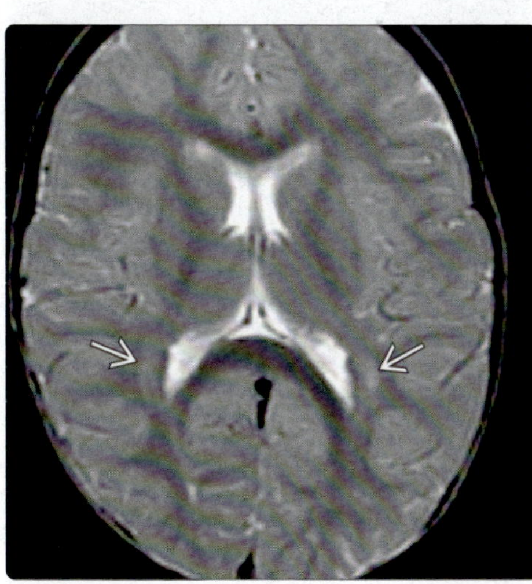

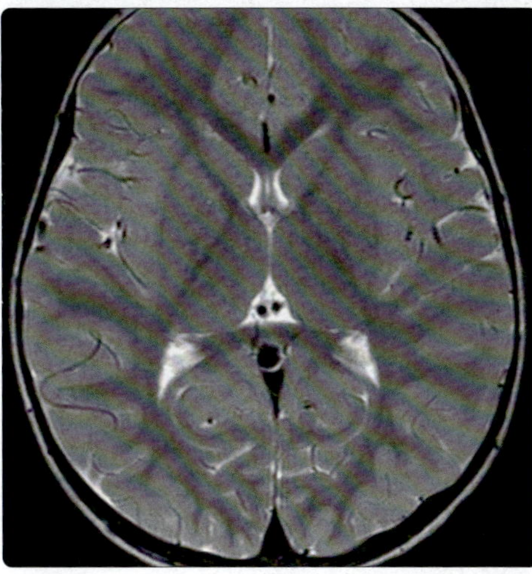

(Left) *Axial T2 MR at 18 months of age shows some residual bright signal in the periventricular white matter of the parietal lobes. Displacement of interstitial water may lag in these regions due to the large volume of parenchyma contributing to centripetal CSF flow.* **(Right)** *Axial T2 MR in a 2-year-old shows an adult pattern of myelination. Progressive myelination beyond this stage is not detectable by standard MR techniques.*

Enlarged Subarachnoid Spaces

KEY FACTS

TERMINOLOGY

- Idiopathic enlargement of subarachnoid spaces (SAS) during infancy

IMAGING

- Primary imaging modality: US
    - CT/MR is used if fontanelle is closing or to further investigate atypical clinical/US findings
- Best clue: Enlarged SAS & ↑ head circumference (> 95th percentile)
    - Ventricles may be mildly enlarged
- Symmetric bifrontal & bitemporal SAS
- All modalities show veins coursing through SAS
- SAS follow CSF appearance on all modalities
- No compression of veins or gyri
- No inward displacement of arachnoid membrane by subdural fluid
    - Small, nonhemorrhagic subdural collections are seen in ~ 4% of patients with enlarged SAS

TOP DIFFERENTIAL DIAGNOSES

- Brain volume loss
- Nonaccidental trauma (NAT)
- Communicating hydrocephalus

PATHOLOGY

- Immature CSF drainage pathways are likely cause
- Family history of macrocephaly in > 80%

CLINICAL ISSUES

- Mild developmental delay alone should not prompt further imaging or subspecialty evaluation
    - Further evaluation is required only in setting of focal neurologic signs &/or developmental regression
- Consider NAT if enlarged extraaxial spaces are atypical
    - Moderate/large/complex subdural collection → NAT work-up
- SAS enlargement & developmental delay typically resolve without therapy by 2 years of age

(Left) *Coronal US in a 7-month-old boy with macrocrania shows enlarged subarachnoid spaces (SAS) ⇨ & normal ventricular size ⇨. Note the normal size of the sulci. This is a typical clinical history & imaging appearance for benign enlargement of the SAS (BESS). US is the initial exam of choice for infants with macrocrania.* **(Right)** *Coronal color Doppler US in a 4-month-old girl shows vessels ➡ traversing the enlarged SAS ⇨. Doppler US is often helpful to exclude subdural collections by demonstrating normal veins in the SAS.*

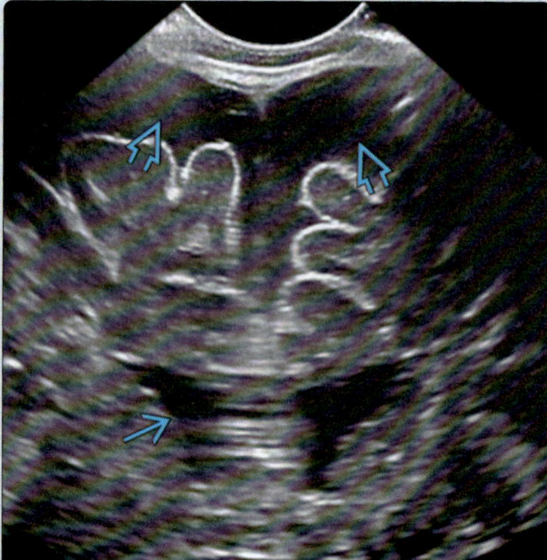

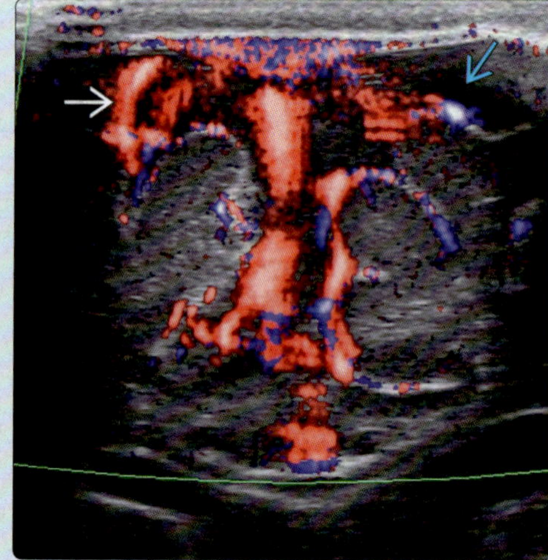

(Left) *Coronal T2 MR at 13 months (left) & NECT at 5 years (right) of age show expected resolution of the enlarged SAS ⇨ over a 4-year period. Enlarged SAS typically resolve by 24 months of age.* **(Right)** *Axial PD MR in a 4-month-old girl with macrocrania shows enlarged SAS ⇨, which are isointense to the brain. Also note the small, bilateral, hyperintense subdural fluid collections ➡. GRE/SWI (not shown) showed no hemorrhage. Small, nonhemorrhagic subdural collections can be seen in ~ 4% of patients with enlarged SAS.*

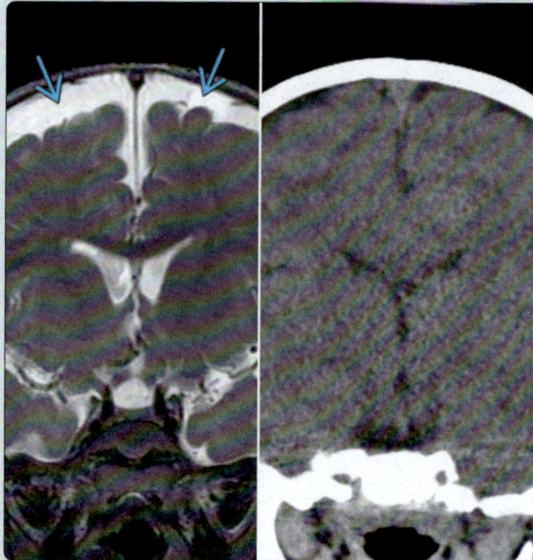

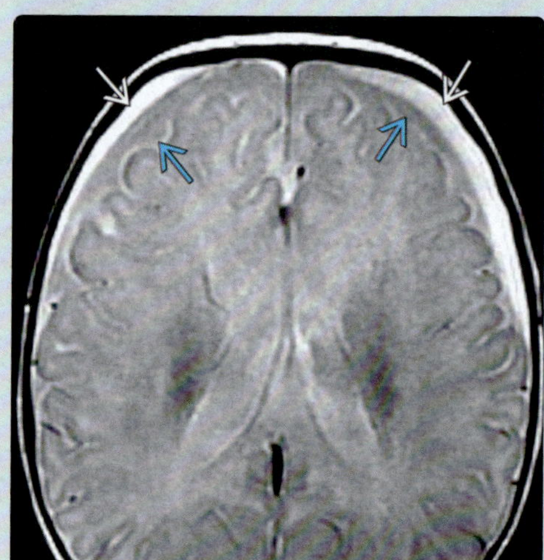

TERMINOLOGY

Abbreviations

- Subarachnoid spaces (SAS)

Definitions

- Enlarged SAS in patient < 1 year of age with macrocrania [head circumference (HC) > 95%]

IMAGING

General Features

- Enlarged SAS in infant with macrocrania
  - Symmetric at bifrontal & bitemporal SAS
  - Normal SAS values differ significantly between studies
    - Interhemispheric width: 95th percentile ~ 8 mm
    - Craniocortical width: 95th percentile ~ 10 mm
    - Sinocortical width: 95th percentile ~ 7 mm
- Ultrasound: Primary modality used whenever possible
  - Numerous cortical veins traverse singular fluid space on grayscale & Doppler
    - No mass effect displacing veins against pia
    - No inward displacement of arachnoid membrane by subdural fluid (which lack traversing veins)
  - ± mild ventricular enlargement
- CT/MR: Used for screening when no acoustic window is available for US (due to fontanelle closure) or if other neurologic signs/symptoms are present
  - NECT: Enlarged, homogeneous SAS (isodense to ventricular CSF) with normal sulci; no hemorrhage
    - Enlarged cisterns (especially suprasellar/chiasmatic)
  - CECT: Easily demonstrates veins traversing SAS
    - No abnormal meningeal enhancement
  - MR: Normal brain parenchyma without edema
    - SAS fluid follows CSF signal on all sequences
    - Small, nonhemorrhagic subdural collections in ~ 4%

Imaging Recommendations

- Protocol advice
  - After diagnosis, best follow-up: Clinical monitoring of HC & development of any neurologic findings
  - Follow-up with MR/CT is typically not necessary, unless
    - Focal neurologic signs/symptoms develop
    - Subdural collection is suspected on US

DIFFERENTIAL DIAGNOSIS

Brain Volume Loss

- Small HC; sulcal prominence is out of proportion

Nonaccidental Trauma

- Moderate/large or hemorrhagic subdural collections or unusual clinical findings should raise concern

Incidental Bilateral Subdural Fluid Collections

- Subdural fluid is not normally visualized
  - Small, nonhemorrhagic subdural collections are seen in 4% of benign macrocrania patients
  - Characterized by crescentic fluid collection separating dura from arachnoid
    - No cortical veins traverse subdural space
    - Discrete arachnoid membrane is displaced toward cortex & may be compressing SAS veins
    - May have different signal intensity on MR vs. CSF
  - Discuss need for further work-up with referring clinician
    - Close clinical follow-up at minimum; work-up for nonaccidental trauma (NAT) at discretion of clinician

Glutaric Aciduria Type 1

- Enlarged sylvian fissures with delayed myelination
- Subdural collections may be present
- T2-hyperintense basal ganglia

Elevated Venous Pressures

- Causes: Cardiac disease, internal jugular vein sacrifice for ECMO, arteriovenous fistula, or sinus venous thrombosis

Communicating Hydrocephalus

- Often posthemorrhagic/postinflammatory/neoplastic

PATHOLOGY

General Features

- Etiology
  - Immature CSF drainage pathways: Most accepted theory
  - Family history of macrocephaly > 80%
- Associated abnormalities
  - Predisposition to bleed with minor trauma: Controversial
    - Possibility of ↑ risk for bridging vein injury & subdural collection/hematoma in absence of major trauma

CLINICAL ISSUES

Presentation

- Most common signs/symptoms
  - Macrocrania: HC > 95th percentile
  - Danger signs: Persistent or rapid deviation of HC from normal curve; developmental regression, focal neurologic signs, vomiting, bruising
- Other signs/symptoms
  - Mild developmental delay is common (20-50%) & usually resolves over time

Natural History & Prognosis

- Self-limited; resolves without therapy by 12-24 months

DIAGNOSTIC CHECKLIST

Image Interpretation Pearls

- Crucial to know HC
- Further evaluation with brain MR or CT if US is atypical
  - Moderate/large/complex subdural collection → NAT work-up
  - Even small/simple subdural collections should be discussed with referring clinician to identify any concerns for NAT that merit further work-up

SELECTED REFERENCES

1. Caré MM: Macrocephaly and subdural collections. Pediatr Radiol. 51(6):891-7, 2021
2. Zahl SM et al: Clinical, radiological, and demographic details of benign external hydrocephalus: a population-based study. Pediatr Neurol. 96:53-7, 2019
3. Haws ME et al: A retrospective analysis of the utility of head computed tomography and/or magnetic resonance imaging in the management of benign macrocrania. J Pediatr. 182:283-9.e1, 2017

Cavum Septum Pellucidum

KEY FACTS

TERMINOLOGY

- Cavum septi pellucidi (CSP)
  - ± cavum vergae (CV)

IMAGING

- Visible CSF space between leaves of CSP
- Normally ≤ 1 cm in width
- ± CV = posterior continuation of CSP
  - CSP & CV are divided by arbitrary vertical plane formed by forniceal columns
  - CV is usually seen with CSP but can be seen in isolation
- CSP is normal structure in fetal life & should be present on 2nd-trimester screening US
- Usually begins to close from back to front at 6 months gestation, forming septum pellucidum
  - CSP is present in 100% of premature & 85% of term infants
  - CSP is seen in up to 15-20% of adults

TOP DIFFERENTIAL DIAGNOSES

- Cyst of CSP
- Interhemispheric cyst
- Acquired intracranial cyst
- Dermoid/epidermoid cyst
- Pilocytic astrocytoma

CLINICAL ISSUES

- Almost always incidental finding
- Link to various pathologic conditions is unclear given how commonly this is seen in normal patients
- Rare reports of CSP cyst requiring surgical drainage
  - Look for outward bowing of CSP leaves; likely still incidental unless causing hydrocephalus

DIAGNOSTIC CHECKLIST

- CSP > 10 mm is considered enlarged, particularly in fetus; usually still incidental

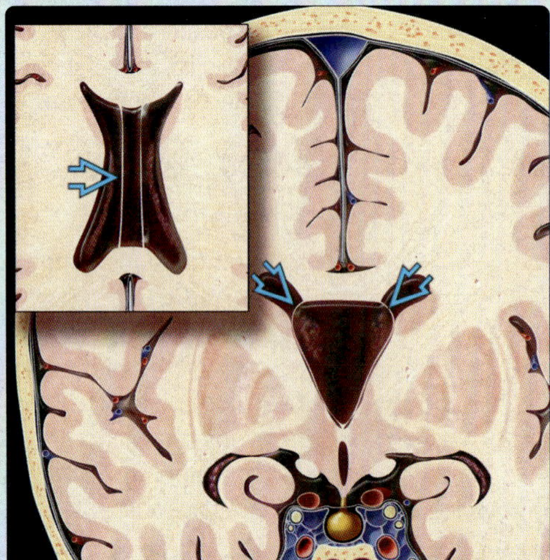

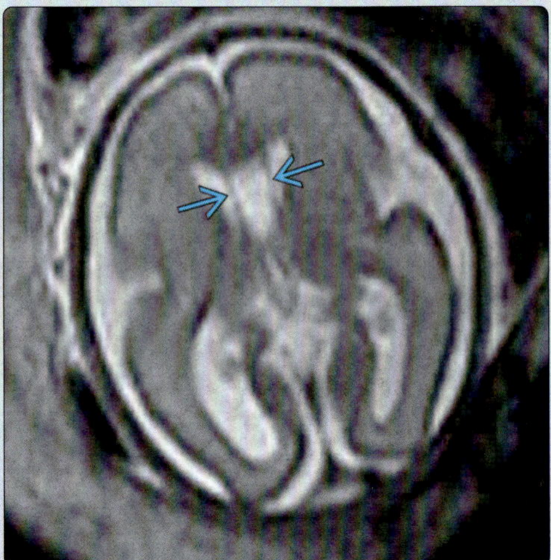

(Left) *Coronal graphic with axial insert shows a classic cavum septi pellucidi (CSP) with cavum vergae (CV). Note the CSF space between the leaves of the CSP ⇨ that is bordered by the medial walls of the lateral ventricles.* **(Right)** *Axial T2 SSFSE MR of a 26-weeks-gestation fetus imaged for an umbilical cord cyst shows a normal brain with a normal CSP ⇨, which should be visible in a 2nd-trimester fetus.*

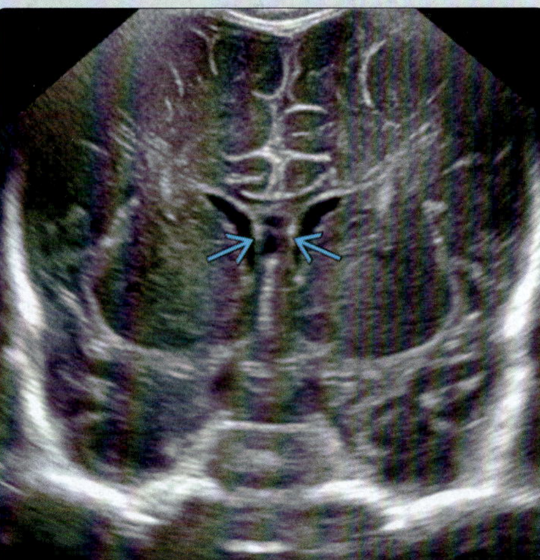

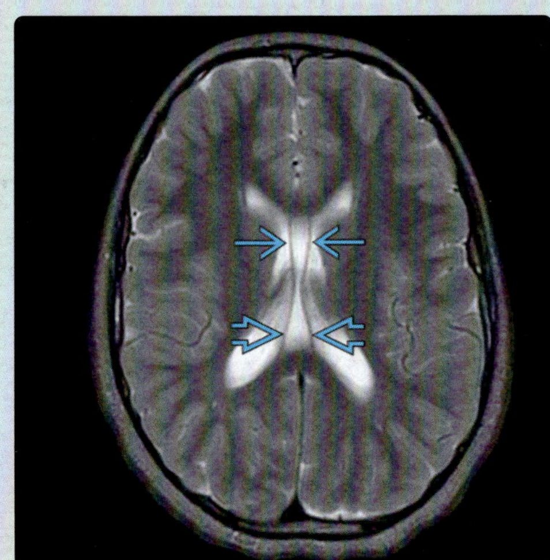

(Left) *Coronal ultrasound in a 22-day-old term infant with cholestasis of unknown etiology shows a normal brain & a normal appearance of the CSP ⇨.* **(Right)** *Axial T2 MR in a 7-year-old boy with generalized tonic clonic seizures shows an incidental CSP ⇨ with cavum vergae ⇨. No abnormalities were identified in the brain. Note the normal ventricular size & lack of periventricular edema.*

KEY FACTS

TERMINOLOGY

- Cavum veli interpositi (CVI); cyst of velum interpositum

IMAGING

- Triangular CSF space
  - Between lateral ventricles & posterior thalami
  - Apex points toward foramina of Monro
  - Elevates & laterally displaces forniceal body & columns
  - Displaces internal cerebral veins inferolaterally
  - Anterior to splenium of corpus callosum, above pineal gland
- Size varies from slit-like/linear to triangular to round/ovoid CSF collection (CVI cyst)
- Isodense/isointense with CSF; on MR
  - Suppresses completely on FLAIR
  - Does not restrict on DWI
  - Does not enhance
- Infant head US can be diagnostic: Typical morphology & location with lack of internal echoes or Doppler signal

TOP DIFFERENTIAL DIAGNOSES

- Pineal cyst
- Arachnoid cyst
- Epidermoid cyst

CLINICAL ISSUES

- Can be found at any age
  - Common in infants, less common in adults
- Symptoms
  - Usually asymptomatic, found incidentally
  - Headache (but relationship to cyst is unclear)
  - CVI cyst can obstruct normal CSF flow though rare → may require neurosurgical drainage

DIAGNOSTIC CHECKLIST

- Considered normal variant but can be associated with cyst
  - Look for signs of ventricular obstruction (rare)

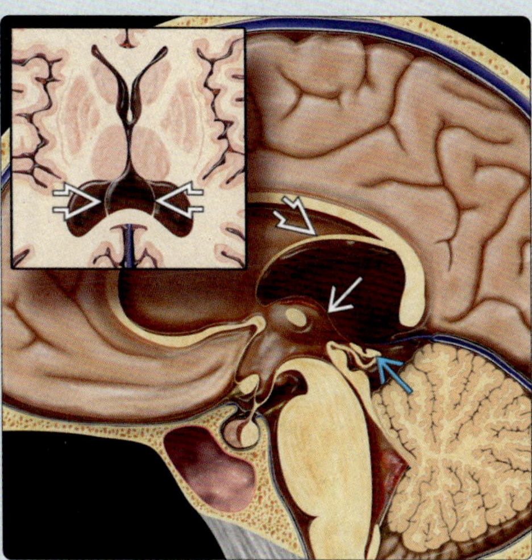

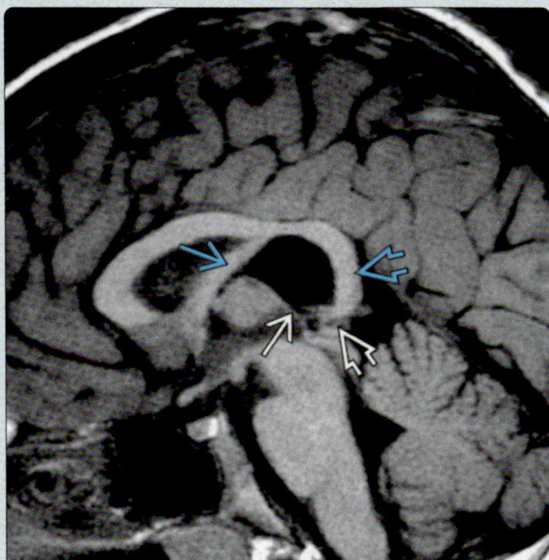

(Left) *Sagittal graphic with axial insert shows a cavum veli interpositi (CVI) with elevation & lateral displacement of the fornices ➡. Also note the inferior displacement of the internal cerebral veins ➡ & pineal gland ➡.* **(Right)** *Sagittal T1 MR of a 7-year-old patient with precocious puberty shows an incidentally noted CVI posterior to the forniceal body/columns ➡, anterior to the corpus callosum splenium ➡, & superior to the tela choroidea ➡ of the 3rd ventricular roof. The pineal gland ➡ is displaced inferiorly.*

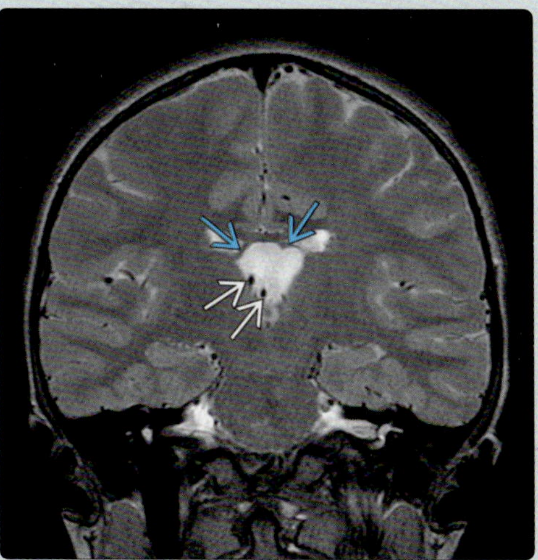

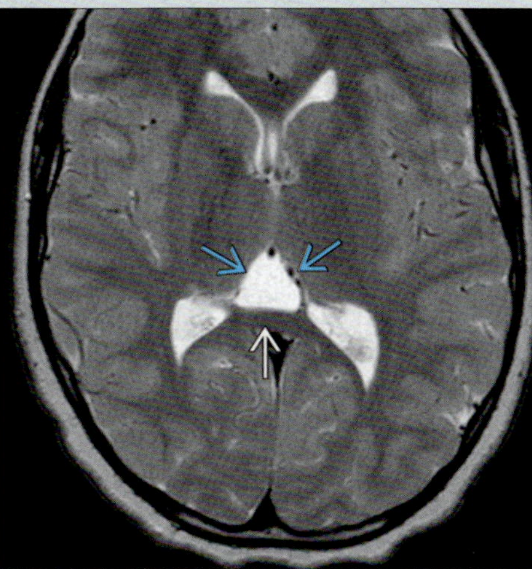

(Left) *Coronal T2 MR in the same patient demonstrates mild mass effect on the forniceal columns ➡ & internal cerebral veins ➡, suggesting a cyst of the CVI, (which is usually incidental).* **(Right)** *Axial T2 MR in the same patient shows a characteristic triangular morphology of the CVI ➡ between the posterior thalami & anterior to the corpus callosum splenium ➡. There is no associated ventriculomegaly.*

KEY FACTS

TERMINOLOGY

- Dandy-Walker continuum is clinically & radiologically heterogeneous group of posterior fossa (PF) malformations
  - Classic Dandy-Walker malformation (DWM)
  - Vermian hypoplasia (VH)
  - Blake pouch (BP) remnant/cyst
  - Mega cisterna magna (MCM)

IMAGING

- Most severe to mildest: Classic DWM → VH → BP → MCM
- Classic DWM
  - Triad of vermian agenesis/hypogenesis, 4th ventricle cystic dilation, & enlarged PF with elevation of torcular Herophili (torcular-lambdoid inversion)
  - ± hydrocephalus
- VH
  - Variable VH ± superior rotation/elevation of vermis
  - No upward sloping of tentorium or torcular-lambdoid inversion
- BP remnant
  - Elevated tegmentovermian angle
  - Normal size & morphology of vermis
- MCM
  - Enlarged retrocerebellar CSF cistern (≥ 10 mm)

TOP DIFFERENTIAL DIAGNOSES

- PF arachnoid cyst
- Joubert syndrome & related disorders
- Dystroglycanopathies
- Cerebellar hypoplasia

CLINICAL ISSUES

- Conflicting terminology, not universally agreed upon
- Wide range of clinical severity
- Classic DWM & VH may be difficult to distinguish; anatomic descriptions may be most useful clinically

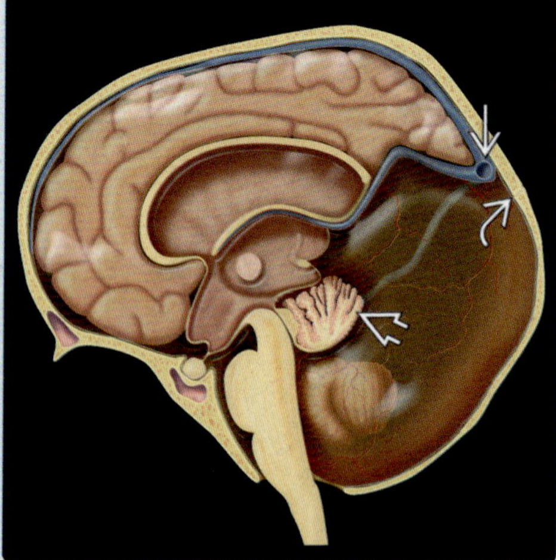

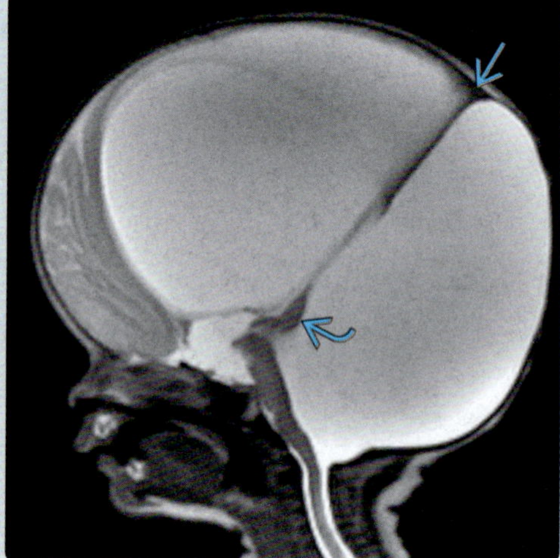

(Left) *Graphic of the classic Dandy-Walker malformation (DWM) shows an enlarged posterior fossa, elevated torcular Herophili ➡ (above the lambdoid suture ➡), superior rotation of a hypoplastic cerebellar vermis ➡, & posterior cystic expansion of the 4th ventricle.* **(Right)** *Sagittal T2 MR of a 2-day-old girl with prenatally diagnosed classic DWM shows the hypoplastic rotated vermis ➡, upward slanting tentorium with elevated torcular Herophili ➡, & obstructive hydrocephalus.*

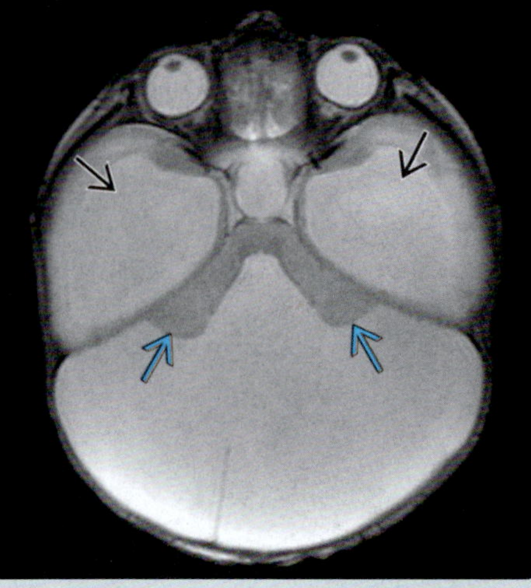

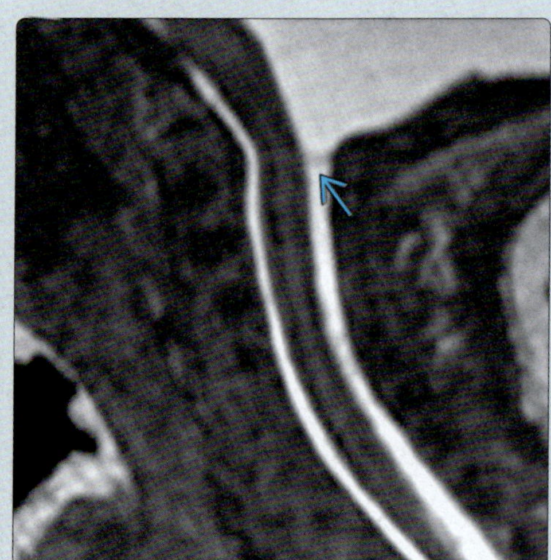

(Left) *Axial T2 MR in the same patient with classic DWM shows lateral displacement of the cerebellar hemispheres ➡ & obstructive hydrocephalus with dilated lateral ventricular temporal horns ➡. The presence of hydrocephalus & other associated brain malformations are critical in helping to establish prognosis.* **(Right)** *Sagittal 3D FIESTA MR of the craniocervical junction in the same patient demonstrates the Blake pouch remnant ➡ obstructing the 4th ventricular outflow tracts.*

TERMINOLOGY

Abbreviations

- Classic Dandy-Walker malformation (DWM)

Synonyms

- Terms DW spectrum, DW variant, & DW complex have complicated clinical & imaging implications in literature

Definitions

- DW continuum represents clinically & radiologically heterogeneous group of posterior fossa (PF) malformations
- Referred to as continuum by some based on belief that DWM, vermian hypoplasia (VH), Blake pouch (BP) remnant/cyst, & mega cisterna magna (MCM) are spectrum of developmental anomalies of rhombencephalic vesicle roof
  - Terminology is controversial & not uniformly accepted
  - Clinical severity ranges widely in this group

IMAGING

General Features

- Best diagnostic clue
  - Classic DWM triad: Vermian agenesis/hypogenesis, 4th ventricle cystic dilation, & enlarged PF with elevation of torcular Herophili (torcular-lambdoid inversion)
  - VH: Vermis is small & usually rotated, may be dysplastic; no torcular-lambdoid inversion
  - BP: Vermis is normal in size & morphology with rotation marked by elevated tegmentovermian angle (≥ 18°)
  - MCM: Enlarged retrocerebellar CSF space (≥ 10 mm) with normal size & orientation of vermis (normal tegmentovermian angle)
- Morphology
  - DW continuum (from most to least severe)
    - DWM classic triad
      - ▫ Complete or partial agenesis of vermis
      - ▫ Cystic dilation of 4th ventricle → rotation of hypoplastic vermis
      - ▫ Enlarged PF with upward displacement of tentorium & torcular Herophili (torcular-lambdoid inversion)
      - ▫ Obstructive hydrocephalus: 70-90%, callosal anomalies: 20%, polymicrogyria or gray matter heterotopia: 5-10%
    - VH
      - ▫ Variable degree of VH ± rotation
      - ▫ ± abnormal vermian foliation/dysplasia
      - ▫ No upward slanting tentorium, no torcular-lambdoid inversion
      - ▫ May be difficult to distinguish from DWM
    - BP remnant (a.k.a. BP "cyst")
      - ▫ Elevated tegmentovermian angle (a.k.a. "open" 4th ventricle)
      - ▫ Normal size & morphology of vermis
    - MCM
      - ▫ Enlarged retrocerebellar cistern (≥ 10 mm) without mass effect on hindbrain
      - ▫ Normal vermis, 4th ventricle, & tegmentovermian angle
      - ▫ In isolation, incidental finding

CT Findings

- NECT
  - DWM: Large PF
    - Torcular-lambdoid inversion (torcular above lambdoid sutures)
  - Scalloped occipital bone, remodeled in all types of DW continuum

MR Findings

- T1, T2, FLAIR
  - DWM
    - Vermian agenesis/hypogenesis, hypoplastic vermis with superior rotation/elevation
    - Variable cerebellar hemisphere & brainstem hypoplasia &/or compression
    - Enlarged 4th ventricle communicating with retrocerebellar cystic space
    - Elevated torcular Herophili with upward-slanting tentorium
    - Hydrocephalus is common, though not originally described as part of DWM
  - VH
    - Varying degrees of vermian tissue are present
    - Vertical height of vermis does not reach level of obex
    - ± rotation of vermis
      - ▫ Normal tegmentovermian angle is usually close to 0°; however, < 18° has been reported as normal
      - ▫ Angle as large as 30° may be normal before 20-weeks gestation on fetal MR
    - ± abnormal foliation/dysplasia
    - May be difficult to distinguish from DWM, particularly in fetus in which there are no reliable landmarks to identify lambdoid sutures
  - BP remnant
    - Rotated but normal-appearing vermis
    - 4th ventricle communicates inferiorly with retrocerebellar CSF cystic space
    - Cyst wall is variably present, often imperceptible on MR
    - Choroid plexus may be seen along inferior surface of vermis (superior margin of cyst wall)
  - MCM
    - Enlarged retrocerebellar CSF space
    - Normal vermis (not rotated, dysplastic, or hypoplastic)
  - ± callosal anomalies, polymicrogyria, gray matter heterotopia, occipital cephalocele, myelination delay

Imaging Recommendations

- Protocol advice
  - Routine MR with thin-section sagittal 3D true FISP/FIESTA to look for cyst wall

DIFFERENTIAL DIAGNOSIS

Posterior Fossa Arachnoid Cyst

- True cyst that does not communicate with 4th ventricle
- ± mass effect on adjacent structures
- May be impossible to distinguish from MCM without CT cisternography

- Distinguishing small AC from MCM is not typically clinically significant

Joubert Syndrome & Related Disorders

- Hypoplastic/dysplastic vermis, "bat wing" 4th ventricle on axial images, thickened & horizontal superior cerebellar peduncles with midbrain cleft → molar tooth appearance on axial images

Dystroglycanopathies

- VH with cobblestone cortex & Z-shaped brainstem (Walker-Warburg phenotype)

Cerebellar Hypoplasia

- ± brainstem hypoplasia (pontocerebellar hypoplasia)

PATHOLOGY

General Features

- Etiology
  - DW continuum is result of abnormal development of posterior fossa mesenchyme
  - Rhombencephalic vesicle roof divides into cranial [anterior membranous area (AMA)] & caudal [posterior membranous area (PMA)] segments
    - AMA invaded by neural cells → cerebellum
    - PMA expands then disappears to form outlet foramina of 4th ventricle
  - Hindbrain development arrest
    - Defective AMA & PMA → DWM & VH
    - Defective PMA only → BP (incomplete/nonperforation of foramen of Magendie) & MCM (delayed perforation)
- Genetics
  - Multiple causative genes identified
    - *FOXC1* (chromosome 6p25.3)
    - Deletion of 3q24 (includes *ZIC1* & *ZIC4* genes)
    - *FGF17*, *LAMC1*, *NID1*
  - DWM can be in isolation or in well-defined syndrome
    - Ritscher-Schinzel syndrome
    - Cranio-cerebello-cardiac syndrome
- Associated abnormalities
  - 2/3 of DWM & related disorders have associated CNS &/or extracranial anomalies
    - Midline anomalies, neurocutaneous melanosis, PHACE(S) syndrome
    - Craniofacial, cardiac, urinary tract, & orthopedic anomalies
    - Trisomy 18 > other trisomies
- Embryology
  - Common association of DWM/VH with facial & cardiovascular anomalies suggests onset between formation & migration of neural crest cells

Gross Pathologic & Surgical Features

- DWM: Large PF with cystic dilation of 4th ventricle
  - Roof of 4th ventricle is in continuity with cyst wall that attaches to hypoplastic vermis anteriorly, cerebellar hemispheres laterally, & medulla caudally
- BP can have variable degrees of perforation & is not true cyst; rather, remnant of PMA

CLINICAL ISSUES

Presentation

- Most common signs/symptoms
  - DWM: Macrocephaly, bulging fontanel (obstructive hydrocephalus)
  - MCM: Incidental finding
- Clinical profile
  - Motor developmental delay, spastic paraplegia, seizures, variable intellectual disability
    - Marked heterogeneity in clinical findings, even in families with same genetic mutations

Demographics

- Age
  - DWM: 80% diagnosed by 1 year of age
    - Age of diagnosis depends on degree of hydrocephalus, supratentorial anomalies, & cerebellar dysfunction
- Epidemiology
  - 1:25,000-30,000 births

Natural History & Prognosis

- Cognitive outcome depends on associated syndromes, supratentorial anomalies, & hydrocephalus
- Classic DWM: Poor prognosis overall
  - Though developmental delay was previously reported in 40-60%, recent literature suggests much higher incidence in true DWM
  - 70-90% with hydrocephalus
  - Seizures, hearing &/or visual difficulties, systemic abnormalities
- VH: Highly variable
  - Cognitive abnormalities in 40-50%, though normal neurodevelopment has been reported in isolated VH
- BP: Favorable outcome in isolation; however, significant proportion are associated with other anomalies
- MCM: Normal neurodevelopmental outcome in isolation

Treatment

- CSF diversion for hydrocephalus: Ventriculoperitoneal shunt ± cyst shunt or marsupialization

DIAGNOSTIC CHECKLIST

Reporting Tips

- Terms, such as DW spectrum, variant, & continuum, can be confusing
  - Use clear description & best categorization of abnormal PF findings when possible (may not always be clear cut)
  - Note hydrocephalus & supratentorial anomalies

SELECTED REFERENCES

1. Nagaraj UD et al: evaluation of posterior fossa biometric measurements on fetal MRI in the evaluation of Dandy-Walker continuum. AJNR Am J Neuroradiol. 42(9):1716-21, 2021
2. Aldinger KA et al: Redefining the etiologic landscape of cerebellar malformations. Am J Hum Genet. 105(3):606-15, 2019
3. Bosemani T et al: Congenital abnormalities of the posterior fossa. Radiographics. 35(1):200-20, 2015
4. Robinson AJ: Inferior vermian hypoplasia–preconception, misconception. Ultrasound Obstet Gynecol. 43(2):123-36, 2014

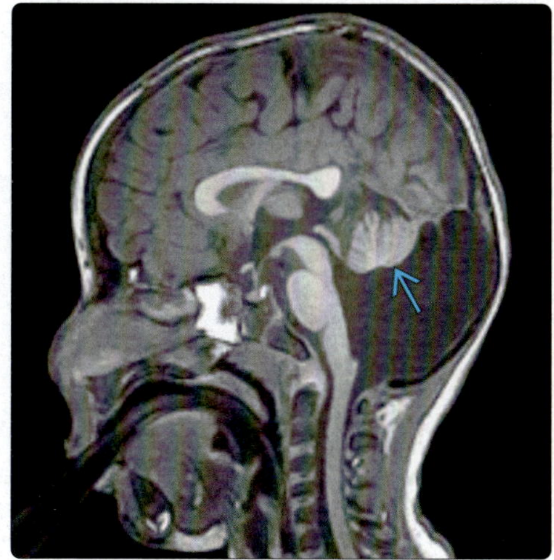

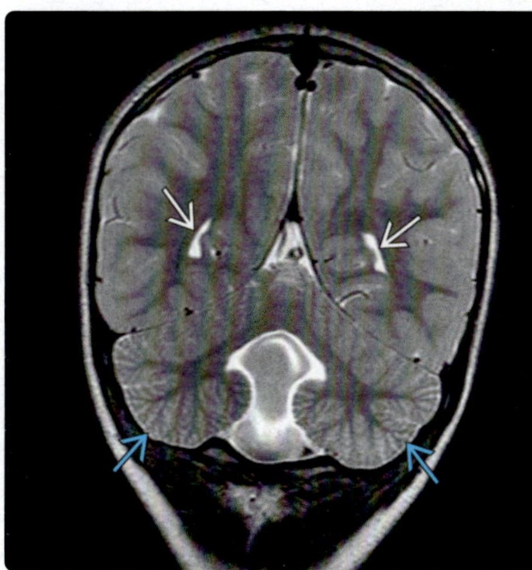

(Left) *Sagittal T1 MR in a 4-year-old with vermian hypoplasia shows a small & rotated vermis ➲ with no significant torcular-lambdoid inversion (though the lambdoid suture is difficult to see on this image).* **(Right)** *Coronal T2 MR in the same patient demonstrates mild separation of the cerebellar hemispheres ➲. The supratentorial ventricles are normal in size ➔, & there is no evidence of ventricular obstruction.*

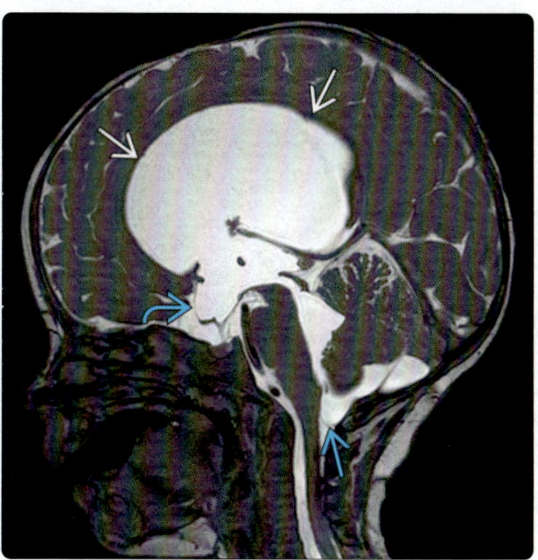

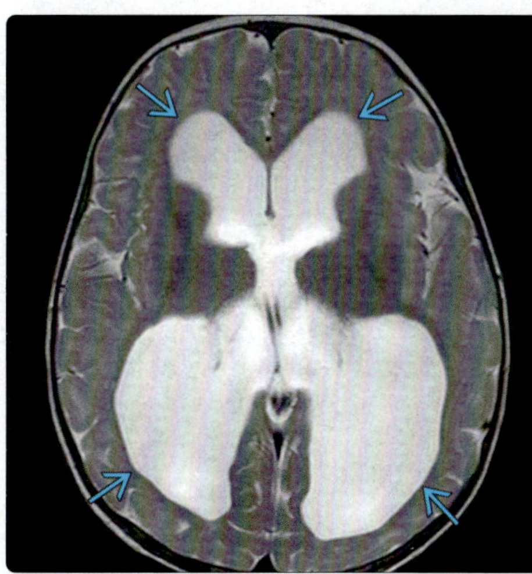

(Left) *Sagittal 3D FIESTA MR of a 9-month-old with a Blake pouch remnant ➲ shows ventricular obstruction with upward stretching of the corpus callosum ➔ & anterior bowing of the lamina terminalis ➲. The vermis is normal in size.* **(Right)** *Axial T2 MR in the same patient demonstrates ventriculomegaly of the lateral ➲ & 3rd ventricles. However, there is evidence of chronic compensation, as there is no periventricular edema or sulcal effacement.*

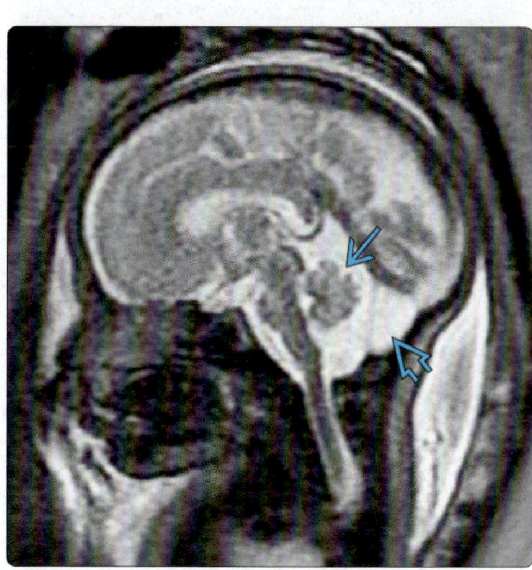

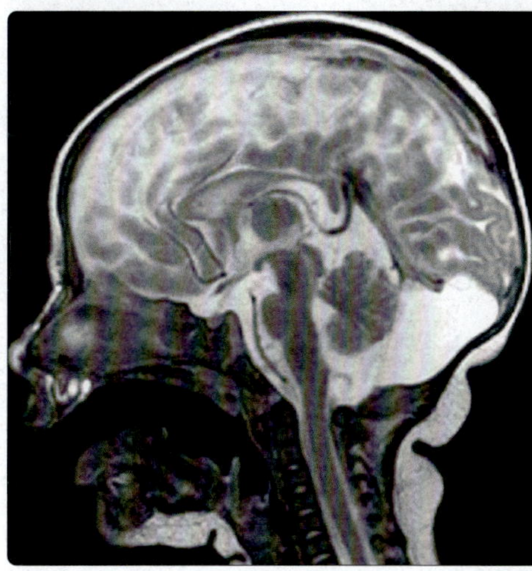

(Left) *Sagittal T2 SSFSE fetal MR at 33-weeks gestation shows a mega cisterna magna. In this patient, the cisterna magna ➲ is enlarged, measuring 15 mm in AP dimension. The vermis ➲ is normal in size, morphology, & orientation.* **(Right)** *Postnatal sagittal T2 MR of the same patient at 6 weeks of age shows that the cisterna magna remains enlarged with a normal vermis. Note the lack of mass effect on the cerebellum & brainstem. In isolation, this is an incidental finding.*

KEY FACTS

TERMINOLOGY

- Rhombencephalosynapsis (RS)
- Lhermitte-Duclos disease (LDD) (dysplastic cerebellar gangliocytoma, Cowden syndrome)
- Joubert syndrome & related disorders (JSRD) (molar tooth malformation)

IMAGING

- RS: Incomplete separation of cerebellar hemispheres
  - Partial or complete absence of cerebellar vermis with folia continuous across midline
  - ~ 65% have coexisting aqueductal stenosis & hydrocephalus
- LDD: Well-circumscribed ↑ T2, ↓ T1 expansile lesion with enlarged & dysplastic cerebellar folia
  - Characteristic tiger stripe or corduroy striated pattern
- JSRD: Molar tooth configuration of brainstem is marked by absent decussation of superior cerebellar peduncles
  - Thickened & horizontally oriented superior cerebellar peduncles, deep & broad interpeduncular fossa, deformed 4th ventricle, hypoplastic vermis

TOP DIFFERENTIAL DIAGNOSES

- Hypoplastic cerebellum: Dandy-Walker continuum, congenital muscular dystrophy, isolated cerebellar hypoplasia, pontocerebellar hypoplasia
- Expanded cerebellar hemisphere: Infarct, cerebellitis, tumor

CLINICAL ISSUES

- RS: Widely varied depending on degree of associated anomalies
- LDD: Diagnosis of exclusion; continued imaging follow-up is warranted
- JSRD: Clinically heterogeneous; molar tooth sign must be correlated with clinical presentation & genetic testing (ciliopathy)

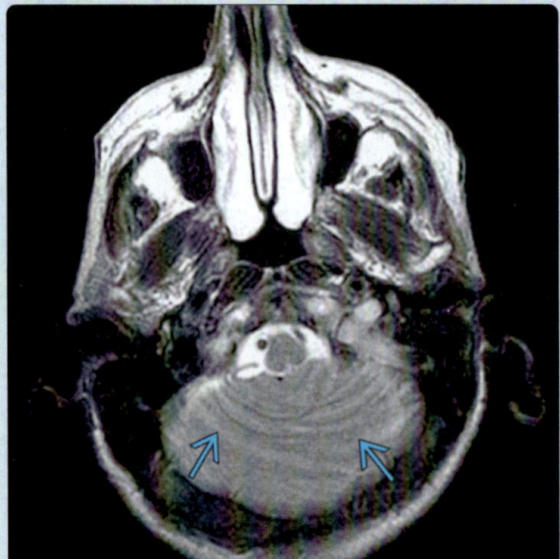

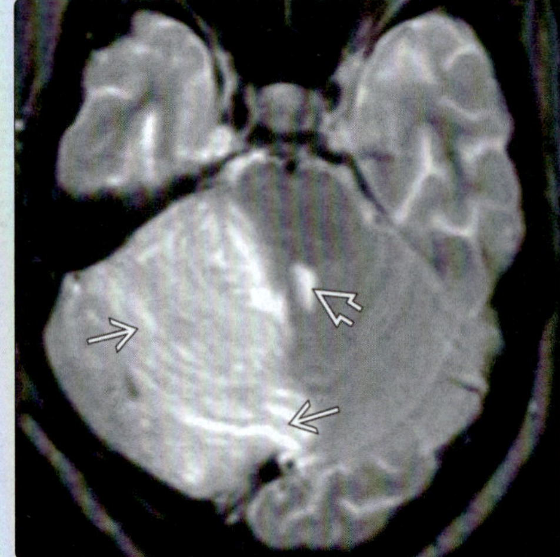

(Left) *Axial T2 MR in a patient with rhombencephalosynapsis (RS) shows lack of separation of the cerebellar hemispheres with transversely oriented folia* ➡ *that are continuous across the midline. No discrete vermis is seen. Look carefully for associated aqueductal stenosis in the setting of RS (& vice versa).* **(Right)** *Axial T2 MR shows an expanded, striated, hyperintense right cerebellar hemisphere* ➡ *characteristic of Lhermitte-Duclos disease (LDD). Note the 4th ventricular compression* ➡*.*

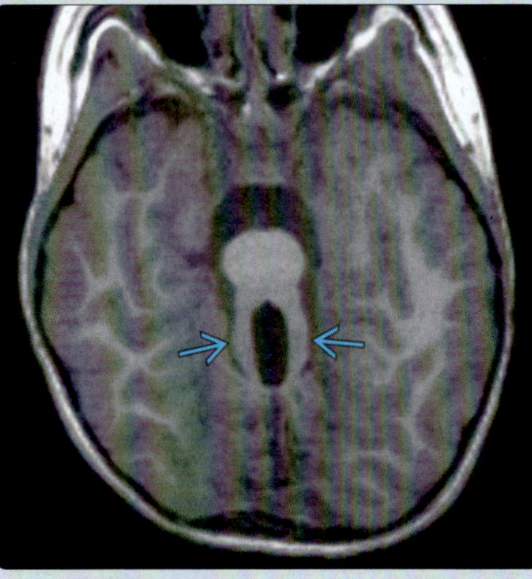

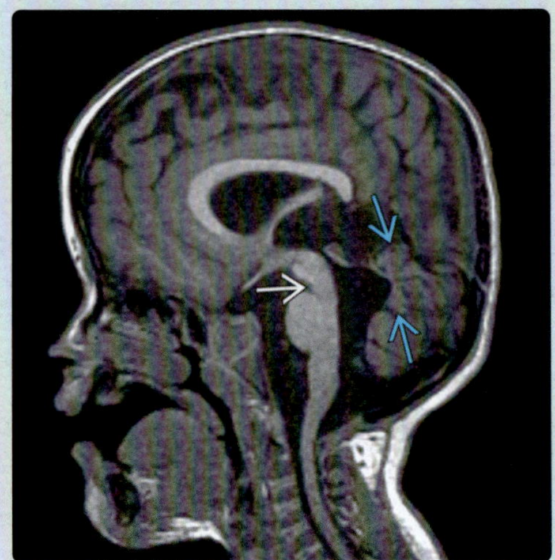

(Left) *Axial T1 MR in a 4-year-old patient shows a classic molar tooth configuration of the midbrain, consistent with Joubert syndrome & related disorders (JSRD). There is characteristic thickening & elongation of the superior cerebellar peduncles* ➡*.* **(Right)** *Sagittal T1 MR in the same patient with JSRD demonstrates marked cerebellar vermian hypoplasia* ➡ *& flattening of the dysplastic fastigial recess. There is also narrowing of the midbrain at the pontomesencephalic junction* ➡*.*

TERMINOLOGY

Abbreviations

- Rhombencephalosynapsis (RS)
- Lhermitte-Duclos disease (LDD)
- Joubert syndrome & related disorders (JSRD)

Synonyms

- LDD: Cowden syndrome, dysplastic cerebellar gangliocytoma, diffuse hypertrophy of cerebellar cortex
- JSRD: Molar tooth malformation

Definitions

- RS: Incomplete separation of cerebellar hemispheres with complete or partial absence of vermis
- LDD: Focal enlargement of cerebellar cortex
  - Low-grade tumor vs. dysplasia: Molecular subtype (usually *PTEN* mutation) & location are distinct from gangliocytomas (WHO grade 1) in other locations
- JSRD: Absence of decussation of superior cerebellar peduncles leading to molar tooth sign
  - Ciliopathy: Caused by mutation of genes encoding ciliary proteins

IMAGING

General Features

- Best diagnostic clue
  - RS: Midline continuation of cerebellar hemispheres (a.k.a. fusion) with at least partial absence of vermis
  - LDD: Sharply marginated region of enlarged & dysplastic cerebellar cortex with characteristic striated (a.k.a. tiger stripe) folial pattern on MR
  - JSRD: Molar tooth sign of midbrain with absence of decussation of superior cerebellar peduncles on DTI + small, malformed vermis

MR Findings

- RS
  - Incomplete separation of cerebellar hemispheres: Diamond-shaped 4th ventricle on axial images, flattened fastigial recess, transversely oriented continuous folia, flat-based cerebellum
  - ± aqueductal stenosis with ventriculomegaly (~ 65%)
  - ± supratentorial anomalies of midline development: Deficiency/absence of septum pellucidum, corpus callosum hypogenesis/dysgenesis, absent anterior commissure, united fornices, incompletely separated thalami, holoprosencephaly, pituitary abnormalities
- LDD
  - Well-circumscribed, nonenhancing ↓ T1, ↑ T2 expansile cerebellar mass
  - Enlargement of dysplastic cerebellar folia creating striated pattern
  - Mass effect can cause obstructive hydrocephalus
  - DWI: Intermediate diffusion (similar to cerebellar cortex)
- JSRD
  - Molar tooth sign: Deep & broad posterior interpeduncular fossa + thick, elongated superior cerebellar peduncles
  - Hypoplastic & dysplastic cerebellar vermis, high position of fastigium, superior midline vermian cleft on coronal images, enlarged posterior fossa
  - Deformed 4th ventricle: Triangular-shaped in midportion & batwing-shaped in superior portion on axial images
  - Hypoplasia of middle cerebellar peduncles, hypoplastic brainstem at pontomesencephalic junction, hypoplastic/dysplastic cerebellar hemispheres
  - ± supratentorial anomalies: Ventriculomegaly, ↓ cerebral volume, hypomyelination, corpus callosum dysgenesis

DIFFERENTIAL DIAGNOSIS

Dandy-Walker Continuum

- Absence or hypoplasia of vermis, communication of 4th ventricle with posterior cyst, enlargement of posterior fossa

Congenital Muscular Dystrophy

- Cerebellar hypoplasia, Z-shaped brainstem
- Extensive cortical abnormalities, eye anomalies

Isolated Cerebellar Hypoplasia

- TORCH infections, trisomy 21, many other causes

Pontocerebellar Hypoplasia

- Numerous syndromic forms

CLINICAL ISSUES

Presentation

- Most common signs/symptoms
  - RS: Widely varied depending on degree of associated anomalies; isolated cases may have subclinical symptomatology
  - LDD: Longstanding history of poorly localized neurological symptoms
  - JSRD: Clinically heterogeneous, including neonatal hyperpnea intermixed with central apnea, oculomotor apraxia, developmental delay, hypotonia/ataxia

DIAGNOSTIC CHECKLIST

Image Interpretation Pearls

- RS: Can be partial or complete; isolated partial can be difficult to diagnose → midline sagittal image is necessary to identify all parts of vermis
- LDD: Classic striated pattern, but LDD is diagnosis of exclusion → continued imaging follow-up is warranted to exclude other etiologies (infarct, cerebellitis, tumor)
- JSRD: Molar tooth sign is classic, though must be correlated with clinical presentation & genetic work-up (ciliopathy)

SELECTED REFERENCES

1. Surisetti BK et al: Clinical and imaging profile of patients with Joubert syndrome. J Mov Disord. 14(3):231-5, 2021
2. Dhamija R et al: Imaging of PTEN-related abnormalities in the central nervous system. Clin Imaging. 60(2):180-5, 2020
3. Parisi MA: The molecular genetics of Joubert syndrome and related ciliopathies: the challenges of genetic and phenotypic heterogeneity. Transl Sci Rare Dis. 4(1-2):25-49, 2019
4. Bosemani T et al: Congenital abnormalities of the posterior fossa. Radiographics. 35(1):200-20, 2015
5. Whitehead MT et al: Rhombencephalosynapsis as a cause of aqueductal stenosis: an under-recognized association in hydrocephalic children. Pediatr Radiol. 44(7):849-56, 2014

Cephalocele

KEY FACTS

TERMINOLOGY

- Extracranial extension of intracranial contents through defect in skull
  - Contents
    - Meningocele: Meninges & CSF
    - Encephalocele: Brain tissue, meninges, CSF
  - Locations
    - Occipital (most common)
    - Frontoethmoidal/sincipital
    - Parietal (usually atretic)
    - Basal/nasopharyngeal
    - Remaining cranial vault, including calvarium, mastoid & petrous temporal bones, cavum trigeminale

IMAGING

- Meninges & CSF ± brain tissue protrude through defect
  - Herniated brain tissue is often dysplastic
- MR + MRV to assess cephalocele contents & abnormal venous sinuses; CT to assess bone defect

TOP DIFFERENTIAL DIAGNOSES

- Dermoid/epidermoid cyst
- Nasal glial heterotopia ("nasal glioma")
- Sinus pericranii
- Assorted vascular anomalies (neoplasms & malformations)
- Cutis aplasia congenita
- Giant parietal foramina

CLINICAL ISSUES

- Congenital is more common than acquired
- Most cephaloceles (occipital) are clinically obvious at birth
- Basal/nasopharyngeal cephaloceles may not manifest until end of 1st decade
- Prognosis & surgical options depend on cephalocele size, location, contents, & associated anomalies

DIAGNOSTIC CHECKLIST

- Normal cartilaginous nasofrontal region in infants can mimic defect on CT; correlate with MR

(Left) *Sagittal T1 MR of a 2-year-old patient shows a giant occipital encephalocele containing a portion of the cerebrum ➡, cerebellum ➡, & dilated lateral ventricle ➡. There is no associated cervical spinal dysraphism (which would suggest a Chiari 3 malformation).* **(Right)** *Sagittal T2 MR of a 5-day-old patient shows a parietal cephalocele containing CSF & fibrous tissue ➡. Note the persistent falcine sinus ➡. Special attention to vascular involvement is critical in cephalocele evaluation.*

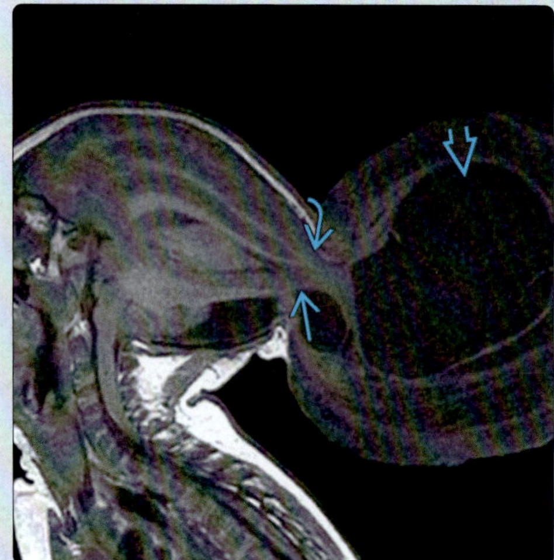

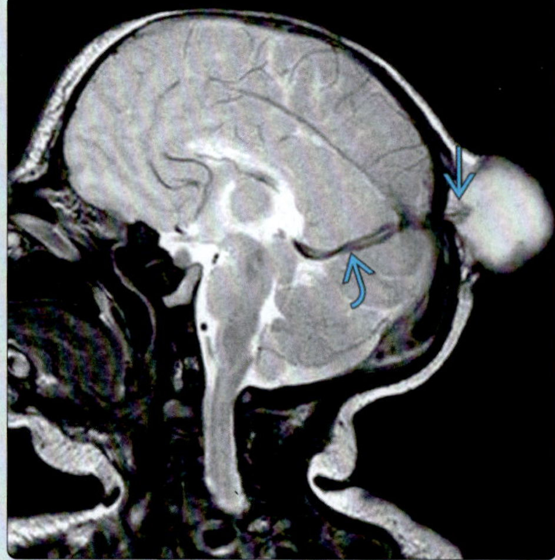

(Left) *Sagittal T2 MR of a 1-month-old patient shows a frontonasal encephalocele ➡. There is associated microcephaly & lateral ventriculomegaly ➡.* **(Right)** *Sagittal T2 SSFSE MR of a 32-week fetus demonstrates a large basal cephalocele ➡ due to Sakoda complex. Agenesis of the corpus callosum is present ➡, & there is an associated midline cleft lip/palate. This patient required an EXIT-to-airway procedure at delivery.*

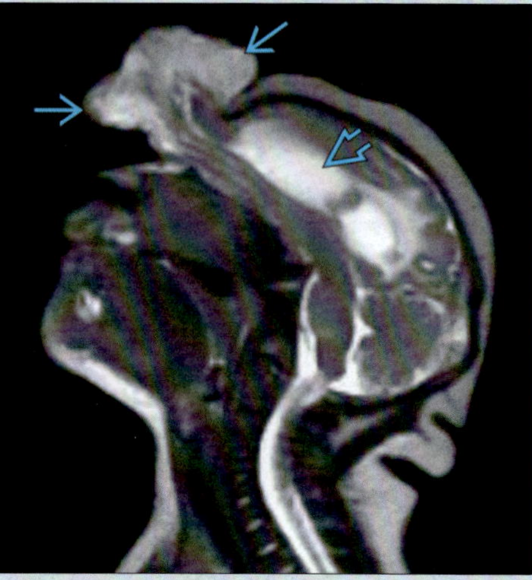

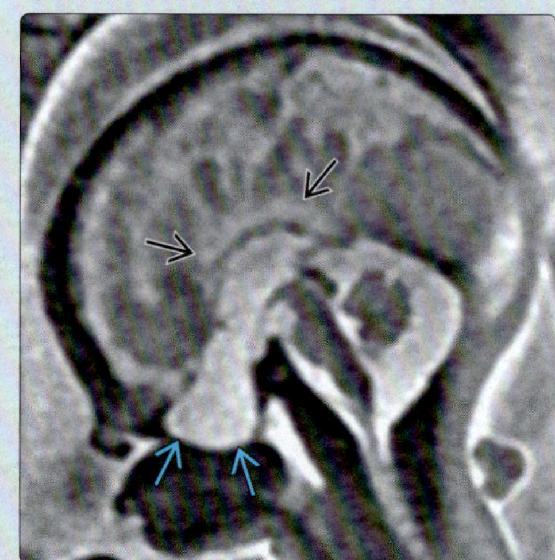

TERMINOLOGY

Definitions

- Extracranial extension of intracranial contents through defect in skull; categorized by contents & location
  - Congenital is more common than acquired
- Contents
  - Cephalocele: Broad term for any focal extracranial extension of intracranial contents
  - Meningocele: Meninges & CSF only
  - Encephalocele: Brain, meninges, CSF
    - a.k.a. meningoencephalocele
  - Meningoencephalocystocele: Ventricle, brain, meninges, CSF
  - Atretic cephalocele: Meningeal & neuroglial elements retain fibrous connection to intracranial compartment, often without significant protrusion through defect
- Locations
  - Occipital: Most common location, up to 80% of cases
    - Supra- &/or infratentorial structures in cephalocele, including tentorium cerebelli & dural venous sinuses
    - Occipitocervical form (Chiari 3): Very rare
  - Frontoethmoidal/sincipital/anterior: 15% (↑ in Southeast Asia)
  - Parietal: 10% (↑ in Japan at 38%)
    - Atretic parietal cephalocele is most common
      - Majority have benign clinical course
  - Basal/nasopharyngeal: Up to 10% of cases
  - Remaining calvarium: Rare
  - Mastoid &/or petrous temporal bone: Rare
  - Cavum trigeminale: Rare

IMAGING

General Features

- Best diagnostic clue
  - Meninges & CSF ± brain tissue protruding through skull defect

CT Findings

- Best for delineation of osseous defect

MR Findings

- T1, T2, FLAIR
  - Heterogeneous signal intensity of cephalocele contents reflecting brain parenchyma & CSF
    - Neural tissue may be dysplastic/gliotic
- MRV
  - Helps to characterize venous relationships to cephaloceles, particularly occipital
  - Venous anomalies occur in most atretic parietal cephaloceles
    - Persistent falcine sinus (± absent vein of Galen, straight sinus)
    - Superior sagittal sinus fenestration/duplication

Ultrasonographic Findings

- Prenatal: Cephaloceles (mainly occipital) can be detected in utero
- Postnatal: Small superficial bumps over calvarium may receive ultrasound request first (particularly for small nasofrontal or atretic parietal cephaloceles)
  - May visualize calvarial defect, altered venous anatomy

DIFFERENTIAL DIAGNOSIS

Dermoid/Epidermoid Cyst

- ± T1-hyperintense fat, diffusion restriction
- Commonly seen near suture lines (scalp, orbit)
- ± nasal pit in association with nasal dermal sinus

Nasal Glial Heterotopia

- Dysplastic neural tissue (a.k.a. "nasal glioma" but not true glioma)
- No communication with subarachnoid space

Sinus Pericranii

- Anomalous connection of intracranial & extracranial veins
- Compressible; engorge with Valsalva/crying

Vascular Anomaly

- Variety of solid & cystic lesions found in neonatal period
- Other than sinus pericranii, rarely have communication through calvarium

Cutis Aplasia Congenita

- Skin defect ± calvarial defect, typically off midline

Giant Parietal Foramina

- Symmetric round/ovoid calvarial defects of paramidline parietal bones
- Can be single midline defect early

CLINICAL ISSUES

Presentation

- Most common signs/symptoms
  - Majority (occipital) are clinically obvious
  - Smaller lesions: Soft & bluish mass if skin covered (majority) or moist & red if lacking skin covering (rare)
- Other signs/symptoms
  - Occipital: Microcephaly, hydrocephalus
  - Basal/nasopharyngeal: Occult mass in oro-/nasopharynx → changes in size with Valsalva + upper airway obstruction, nasal stuffiness/mouth breathing
  - Frontoethmoidal: Hypertelorism, broad nasal bridge, CSF rhinorrhea → meningitis

Treatment

- Depends on cephalocele location, contents, size, & associated anomalies
- Goals of surgery: Prevent CSF leak & meningitis, improve functional & cosmetic deformities

DIAGNOSTIC CHECKLIST

Image Interpretation Pearls

- Always consider cephalocele when encountering cystic skull base lesion

SELECTED REFERENCES

1. Khodarahmi I et al: Imaging spectrum of calvarial abnormalities. Radiographics. 41(4):1144-63, 2021
2. Nagaraj UD et al: Prenatal evaluation of the Sakoda complex. Pediatr Radiol. 49(13):1843-7, 2019
3. Yucetas SC et al: A retrospective analysis of neonatal encephalocele predisposing factors and outcomes. Pediatr Neurosurg. 52(2):73-6, 2017

KEY FACTS

TERMINOLOGY

- Holoprosencephaly (HPE): Spectrum of congenital forebrain malformations characterized by failure of differentiation & midline cleavage of prosencephalon
- Traditionally divided (from most to least severe) into alobar, semilobar, & lobar subtypes
- Middle interhemispheric variant (MIH) or syntelencephaly is generally accepted as subtype of HPE

IMAGING

- Abnormal midline communications of gray & white matter
- Categories represent continuum of forebrain malformations without clear distinction between subtypes
- Alobar HPE: Complete absence of cleavage with "pancake" of anterior cerebral tissue, crescent-shaped anterior monoventricle communicating with large dorsal cyst, fused thalami
- Semilobar HPE: Interhemispheric fissure & falx cerebri are formed posteriorly with absence of frontal lobe separation & varying degrees of failed diencephalon cleavage
- Lobar HPE: 3rd ventricle is fully formed (diencephalon separation), interhemispheric fissure & falx are mostly formed with absent cleavage in inferior frontal lobes
- MIH: Lack of posterior frontal & parietal midline separation with cleavage of anterior frontal & occipital lobes

TOP DIFFERENTIAL DIAGNOSES

- Aqueductal stenosis
- Hydranencephaly
- Callosal agenesis with interhemispheric cyst
- Open-lip schizencephaly
- Hypoplastic optic nerve syndrome (a.k.a. septooptic dysplasia)

CLINICAL ISSUES

- Presentation varies widely depending on severity of malformation

(Left) *Axial T1 MR of a 4-day-old with alobar holoprosencephaly shows a monoventricle ➡ & a dorsal cyst that displaces the brain anteriorly ➡ in a pancake configuration. Note the normal lack of myelination of the cerebral white matter at this age.* **(Right)** *Axial T1 MR in a 6-year-old with semilobar holoprosencephaly shows nonseparation of the frontal lobes ➡ & anterior caudate nuclei ➡. However, there is separation of the parietal & occipital lobes with the falx cerebri ➡ identified posteriorly.*

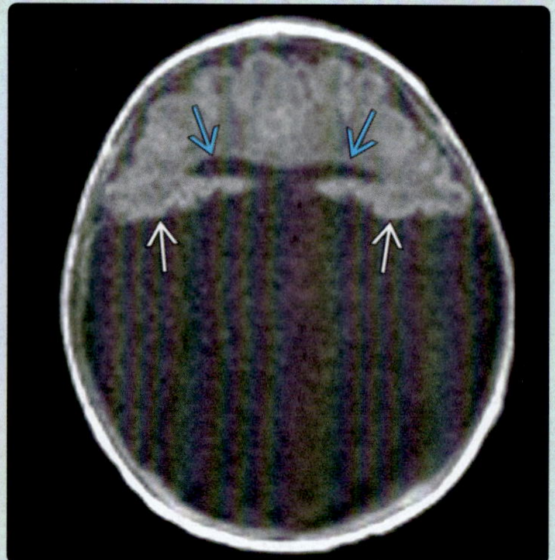

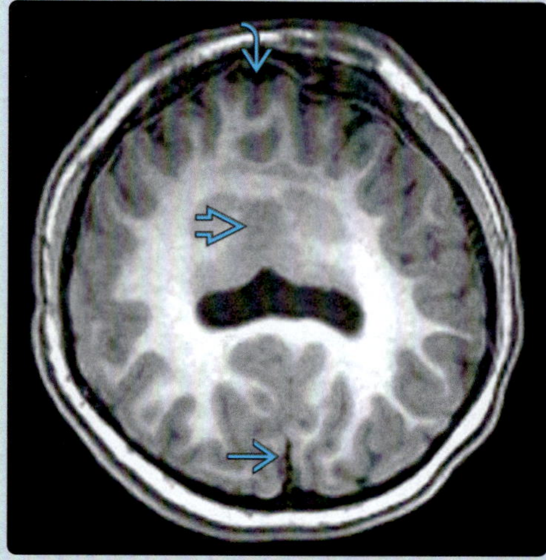

(Left) *Axial T1 MR in a 2-year-old with lobar holoprosencephaly shows failed separation of the anterior inferior frontal lobes with a small amount of gray matter ➡ crossing the midline. Note the characteristic azygous anterior cerebral artery ➡. The 3rd ventricle ➡ is not hypoplastic.* **(Right)** *Axial T1 MR in a 13-year-old with seizures shows the middle interhemispheric variant of holoprosencephaly marked by focal incomplete separation of the posterior frontal & anterior parietal regions ➡.*

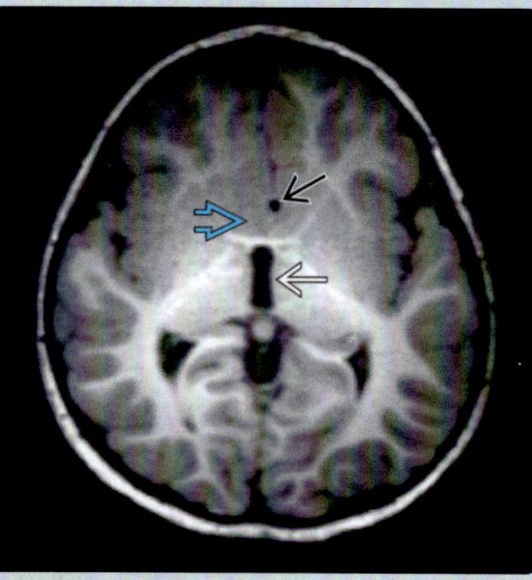

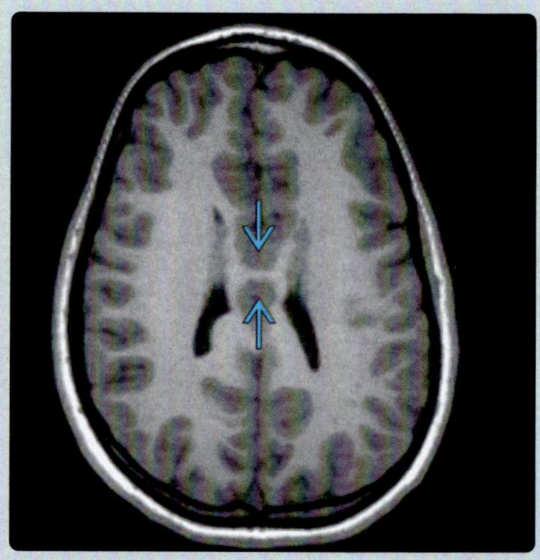

TERMINOLOGY

Abbreviations

- Holoprosencephaly (HPE)

Definitions

- Spectrum of congenital forebrain malformations characterized by failure of differentiation & midline cleavage of prosencephalon
- Traditionally, classic HPE is divided into alobar, semilobar, & lobar subtypes
- Middle interhemispheric variant (MIH) (a.k.a. syntelencephaly) is generally accepted as subtype of HPE
- Subtypes represent continuum of forebrain malformations without clear distinction between different subtypes

IMAGING

General Features

- Best diagnostic clue
  - Alobar HPE: Complete absence of cleavage with "pancake" of anterior cerebral tissue, crescent-shaped anterior monoventricle communicating with large dorsal cyst, fused thalami
  - Semilobar HPE: Absent frontal lobe cleavage with parietooccipital lobe separation
  - Lobar HPE: Interhemispheric fissure & falx are mostly formed with partial nonseparation of frontal lobes
  - MIH: Hemispheres are not separated in posterior frontal & anterior parietal regions

MR Findings

- T1, T2, FLAIR
  - Alobar: Anterior monoventricle ± communication with dorsal cyst
    - Cerebral tissue is flattened anteriorly like pancake
    - Absent corpus callosum, falx, interhemispheric fissure
  - Semilobar: Frontal lobes are largely continuous across midline
    - Varying degrees of diencephalon separation (absent/small 3rd ventricle)
    - Posterior corpus callosum (splenium) is present
  - Lobar: Interhemispheric fissure is present along nearly entire midline
    - Rudimentary frontal horns are typical, inferior portions of frontal lobes are uncleaved
    - 3rd ventricle is fully formed
    - Absence of genu & rostrum of corpus callosum
  - MIH: Lack of midline separation in posterior frontal & anterior parietal regions with normal cleavage of polar areas of cerebrum
    - Genu & splenium are present with absent body of corpus callosum
    - Normal basal ganglia
  - Absent septum pellucidum is typical though it can be seen in milder subtypes
  - No precise distinction between lobar & semilobar HPE
- Variable findings
  - Brainstem & cerebellar anomalies, such as rhombencephalosynapsis
  - Gray matter heterotopia: MIH > classic HPE
  - Azygous anterior cerebral artery

DIFFERENTIAL DIAGNOSIS

Aqueductal Stenosis

- Macrocephalic with moderate to severe enlargement of ventricles; small rind of cerebral tissue in maximal cases
- Falx may be disrupted

Hydranencephaly

- Absence of anterior circulation cerebrum with fluid-filled cranial vault
- Preservation of falx

Hypoplastic Optic Nerve Syndrome (a.k.a. Septooptic Dysplasia)

- Optic nerve hypoplasia ± absent/deficient septum pellucidum, hypothalamic-pituitary axis abnormalities, schizencephaly

PATHOLOGY

General Features

- Etiology
  - Teratogen exposure
    - Ethanol, diabetes, cigarette smoking, retinoic acid
  - Many genetic/syndromic etiologies
    - Smith-Lemli-Opitz, Stromme, Steinfeld, Hartsfield, Kallman syndrome 2
- Genetics
  - Standard karyotyping is abnormal in 40-60% of HPE
    - Classically trisomy 13 (Patau syndrome)
      - Arrhinencephaly is seen in ~70%
  - 18-25% have pathogenic variant in single gene
    - > 20 known HPE-associated genes
- Associated abnormalities
  - Facial anomalies → hypotelorism/cyclopia, ethmocephaly (proboscis), cebocephaly (single naris), arrhinia, central incisor, midline or bilateral cleft lip/palate

Staging, Grading, & Classification

- Alobar, semilobar, lobar classification of DeMyer
- MIH described as HPE variant by Barkovich in 1993
- Milder subtypes may be often observed in clinical practice, such as preseptooptic subtype

DIAGNOSTIC CHECKLIST

Image Interpretation Pearls

- HPE represents continuum of forebrain malformations
  - No clear distinction amongst different categories → provide clear anatomic descriptions in reports
  - Less severe lack of separation is described at many different locations in telencephalon & considered as midline anomalies vs. forme fruste of HPE

SELECTED REFERENCES

1. Riddle A et al: Fetal magnetic resonance imaging (MRI) in holoprosencephaly and associations with clinical outcome: implications for fetal counseling. J Child Neurol. 36(5):357-64, 2021
2. Choi JJ et al: Fetal magnetic resonance imaging: supratentorial brain malformations. Pediatr Radiol. 50(13):1934-47, 2020
3. Kousa YA et al: Prenatal diagnosis of holoprosencephaly. Am J Med Genet C Semin Med Genet. 178(2):206-13, 2018
4. Winter TC et al: Holoprosencephaly: a survey of the entity, with embryology and fetal imaging. Radiographics. 35(1):275-90, 2015

KEY FACTS

TERMINOLOGY

- Agenesis (absence) of corpus callosum (ACC)
- Dysgenesis of CC
  - Hypogenesis of CC (partial agenesis)
  - Hypoplasia of CC

IMAGING

- Axial: Parallel configuration of lateral ventricles with colpocephaly (dilation of trigones/posterior horns of lateral ventricles)
  - Probst bundles: Densely packed heterotopic white matter (WM) tracts parallel to interhemispheric fissure
- Sagittal: Absent or abnormal CC
  - Absent cingulate sulcus
  - Interhemispheric sulci radiate to 3rd ventricular margin
- Coronal images: No band of WM bridging cerebral hemispheres over 3rd ventricle
  - Upturned anterior horns of lateral ventricles & high-riding 3rd ventricle
- ± interhemispheric cyst or lipoma

TOP DIFFERENTIAL DIAGNOSES

- Destruction, attenuation, or immaturity of CC
- Failure of forebrain cleavage (holoprosencephaly spectrum)

PATHOLOGY

- Associated with hundreds of described genetic abnormalities & nongenetic syndromes
- Can be seen in isolation in minority of cases

CLINICAL ISSUES

- Typical manifestations include seizures, developmental delay, anomalies of hypothalamic-pituitary axis

DIAGNOSTIC CHECKLIST

- When CC is absent, evaluate presence & morphology of other forebrain commissures
- Description of other brain anomalies is important in prognosis

(Left) *Coronal graphic shows agenesis of the corpus callosum (ACC) with bundles of Probst ➡ & everted cingulate gyri. The 3rd ventricle is high riding ➡ with upturned lateral ventricles ➡ in a trident configuration. The hippocampi are underrotated with vertical orientation ➡.* **(Right)** *Sagittal SSFP MR in a 31-weeks-gestational age female fetus with ACC shows that the cingulate sulcus is absent, & the interhemispheric sulci reach the 3rd ventricle margin. The anterior commissure ➡ is present.*

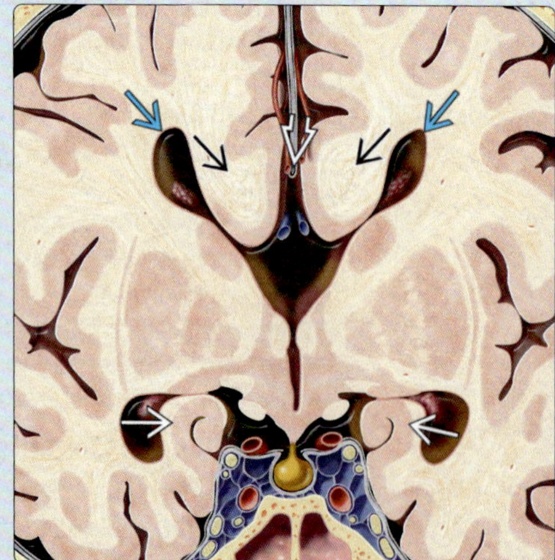

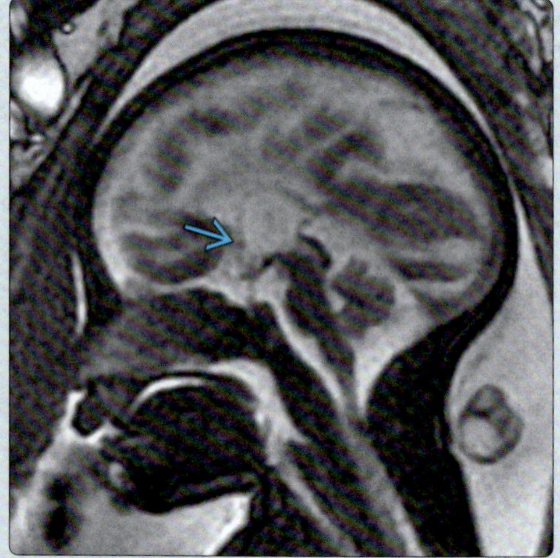

(Left) *Axial T2 SSFSE MR in the same fetus shows a parallel configuration of the lateral ventricles with colpocephaly characterized by selective dilation ➡ of the atria & occipital horns of lateral ventricles.* **(Right)** *Coronal T2 MR in a 4-year-old patient shows ACC ➡ with upturned lateral ventricular frontal horns ➡ in a trident configuration. Note the foci of associated subependymal gray matter heterotopia ➡. MR is the most sensitive examination for the detection of associated anomalies in ACC.*

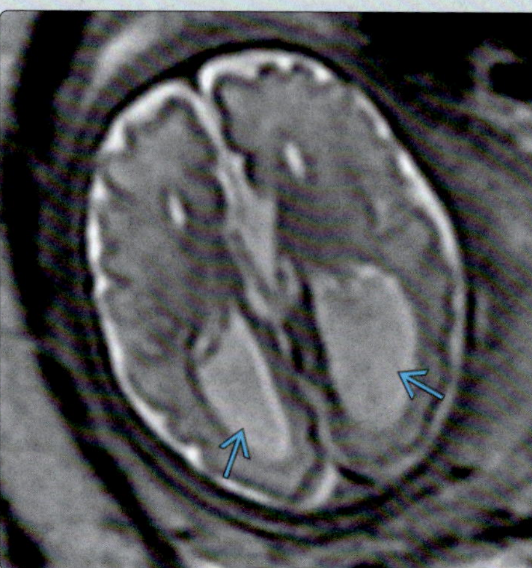

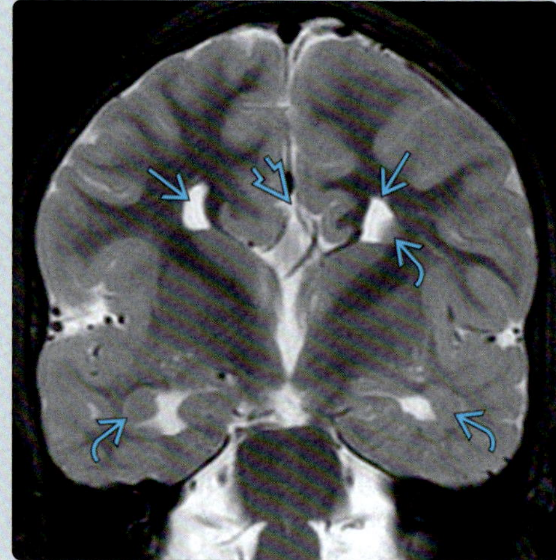

TERMINOLOGY

Definitions

- Heterogeneous condition of congenital hypoplasia/dysplasia or absence of corpus callosum
- Complete agenesis of corpus callosum (ACC)
  - Agenesis of CC & hippocampal commissure with presence of anterior commissure: Most common
  - ACC with presence of anterior & hippocampal commissures
  - Tricommissural agenesis: Complete absence of CC, anterior commissure, & hippocampal commissure
- Dysgenesis of corpus callosum
  - Hypogenesis of corpus callosum (partial agenesis of corpus callosum)
    - All 5 parts of CC are not present → shortening of CC in AP dimension
  - Hypoplasia of corpus callosum
    - Diffusely thin CC with normal AP length & all parts present

IMAGING

General Features

- Best diagnostic clue
  - Axial: Parallel configuration of lateral ventricles with colpocephaly
  - Sagittal: Absent cingulate sulcus with interhemispheric sulci radiating to margin of 3rd ventricle
  - Coronal: High-riding 3rd ventricle with upturned lateral ventricles in trident morphology
  - Absent septum pellucidi
  - Associated interhemispheric lipoma or cyst
    - Interhemispheric cyst of ACC may be communicating (type I) or noncommunicating (type II) with ventricle
  - Anterior cerebral arteries & branches do not conform to expected normal CC shape

Imaging Recommendations

- Best imaging tool
  - MR is most sensitive examination for detection of associated anomalies

DIFFERENTIAL DIAGNOSIS

Destruction of Corpus Callosum

- Surgery (callosotomy), trauma
- WM injury of prematurity
- Cerebral infarcts → focal thinning of CC

Attenuation of Corpus Callosum

- Hydrocephalus stretches/deforms CC, flattens fiber tracts
- CC often looks "dysplastic" in severe hydrocephalus s/p shunting

Immaturity of Corpus Callosum

- CC is relatively thin & unmyelinated in normal neonates

Failure of Forebrain Cleavage

- Varying degrees of CC absence depending on type of holoprosencephaly

PATHOLOGY

General Features

- Associated abnormalities
  - Additional CNS malformations may be present
  - Associated with hundreds of described genetic abnormalities & nongenetic syndromes
    - Aicardi: ACC in female patient with polymicrogyria, interhemispheric cyst, & gray matter heterotopias
    - Genetic Syndromes: Rubinstein-Taybi, Apert, Smith-Lemli-Opitz syndrome
    - Ciliopathies: Joubert, acrocallosal, Meckel syndrome
- Embryology
  - Cells destined for CC begin forming at 6-weeks gestation
  - Glial sling connecting anterior & hippocampal commissure begins to form at 12 weeks
  - Developing anterior & posterior parts fuse to form single structure with all parts of CC present by 15 weeks

Staging, Grading, & Classification

- Complete ACC
  - Classification of ACC based on evaluation of 3 main forebrain commissures: Corpus callosum, anterior commissure, & hippocampal commissure
  - Only anterior commissure is present (most common)
    - Anterior commissure may be small or thickened
  - Both anterior & hippocampal commissures are present
    - Hippocampal commissure can be difficult to differentiate from hypogenetic CC
    - Hippocampal commissure connects forniceal crura while CC connects cerebral hemispheres
  - Tricommissural agenesis: Complete absence of all 3 commissures (least common)

CLINICAL ISSUES

Presentation

- Most common signs/symptoms
  - Seizures, developmental delay
  - Anomalies of hypothalamic-pituitary axis
- Other signs/symptoms
  - Widely variable depending on type of CC anomaly, associated CNS malformations, genetic syndromes
  - In isolated ACC, patients may be asymptomatic

DIAGNOSTIC CHECKLIST

Consider

- Anterior commissure is usually present in complete ACC & should be described

Image Interpretation Pearls

- Look for additional CNS malformations

SELECTED REFERENCES

1. Sileo FG et al: Role of prenatal magnetic resonance imaging in fetuses with isolated agenesis of corpus callosum in the era of fetal neurosonography: a systematic review and meta-analysis. Acta Obstet Gynecol Scand. 100(1):7-16, 2021
2. Cesaretti C et al: Variability of forebrain commissures in callosal agenesis: a prenatal MR imaging study. AJNR Am J Neuroradiol. 37(3):521-7, 2016

Hemimegalencephaly

KEY FACTS

TERMINOLOGY

- Hemimegalencephaly (HMEG): Overgrowth & malformation of part vs. entire hemisphere
- Due to defects in neuronal proliferation, migration, & organization

IMAGING

- Large cerebral hemisphere & hemicranium
  - Displaced posterior falx & occipital pole extending to contralateral side
  - Enlarged ipsilateral ventricle with abnormally shaped frontal horn (often pointed)
- Associated cortical malformations include pachygyria, polymicrogyria, & heterotopias
- White matter (WM) abnormalities
  - ↑ volume, abnormal T2 signal intensity
    - Often dark prior to typical myelination timeframe
- Size & signal intensity of HMEG can change over time
  - May atrophy with chronic seizure activity

PATHOLOGY

- Classified as cortical dysgenesis with abnormal cell proliferation but without neoplasia
- Same pathologic & genetic spectrum as focal cortical dysplasia type II & tuberous sclerosis complex

CLINICAL ISSUES

- Most common presentations: Seizures, hemiparesis, developmental delay
  - 50% have associated skin lesions, truncal/extremity overgrowth, &/or vascular malformations
    - Seen in *PIK3CA*-related overgrowth spectrum (PROS)
- Functional hemispherectomy is used for seizure control (as anticonvulsants are usually ineffective)

DIAGNOSTIC CHECKLIST

- Must exclude contralateral abnormalities for successful epilepsy surgery

(Left) *Coronal SSFSE T2 fetal MR at 20-weeks gestational age shows left hemimegalencephaly (HMEG). The left germinal matrix ➡ is asymmetrically larger than the right, compatible with ↑ neuronal proliferation.* **(Right)** *Coronal T2 MR in the same patient after delivery shows extensive associated left polymicrogyria ➡, consistent with abnormal neuronal organization. There is also callosal hypogenesis ➡ & right perisylvian polymicrogyria ➡, making this patient a poor surgical candidate.*

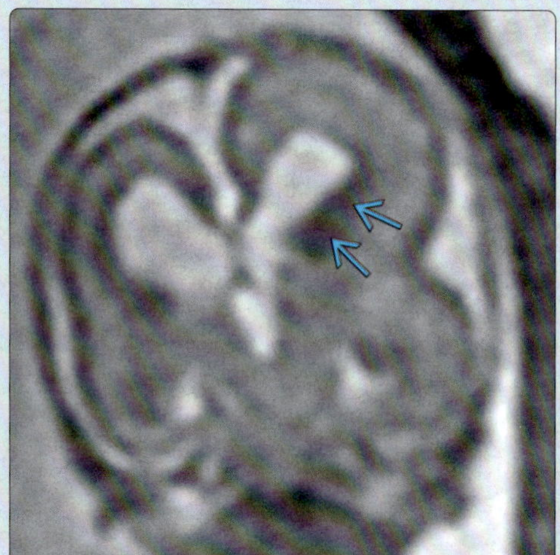

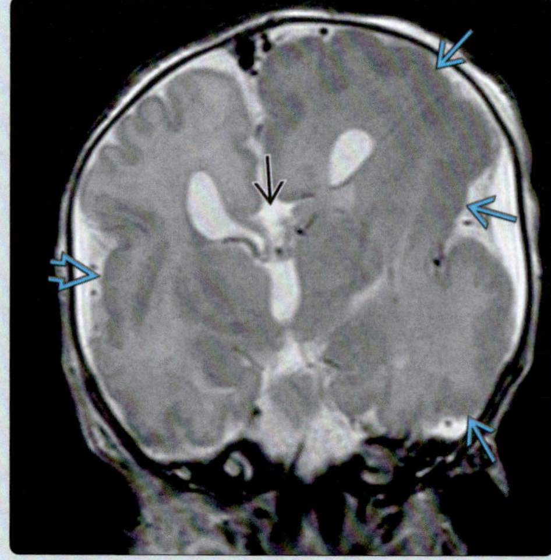

(Left) *Axial T2 MR in the same newborn with left HMEG shows asymmetric relative T2 hypointensity of the white matter in the left cerebral hemisphere, compatible with abnormal neuronal migration. Extensive left polymicrogyria ➡ is again seen.* **(Right)** *Axial T1 MR in the same patient with HMEG shows characteristic asymmetric enlargement of the lateral ventricle on the affected side ➡ with the occipital lobe crossing midline posteriorly ➡. Note the abnormal gray matter-white matter differentiation on the left.*

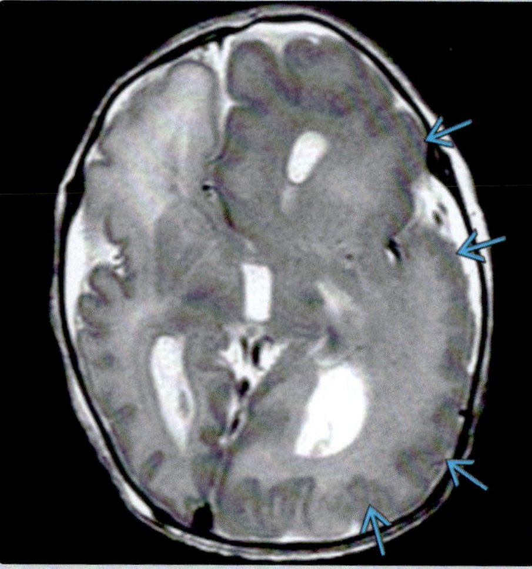

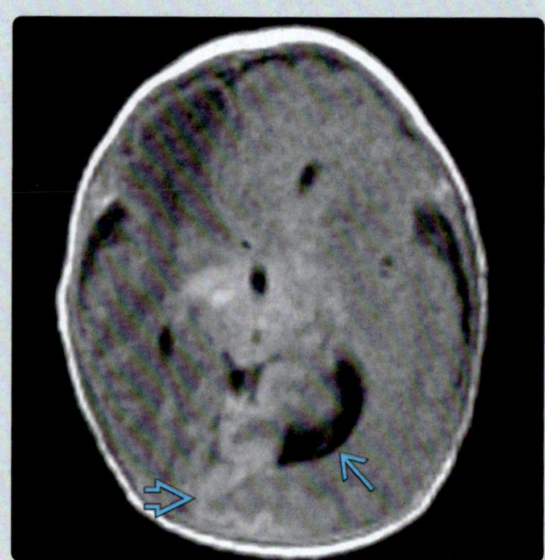

TERMINOLOGY

Definitions

- Hemimegalencephaly (HMEG): Nonneoplastic overgrowth of part or entire hemisphere
  - Classic HMEG (or unilateral megalencephaly): Holohemispheric involvement
  - Partial HMEG (or focal megalencephaly): Portion of hemisphere involved
- Dysplastic megalencephaly (DMEG): Macrocephaly with significant portions of both hemispheres involved
- Same pathologic & genetic spectrum as focal cortical dysplasia type II & tuberous sclerosis complex (TSC)

IMAGING

General Features

- Best diagnostic clue
  - Enlarged dysplastic cerebral hemisphere (or portion of hemisphere) with enlarged ipsilateral lateral ventricle
    - Abnormal gray matter (GM) & white matter (WM)
  - Displaced posterior falx with enlarged occipital lobe crossing midline

MR Findings

- T1, T2, FLAIR
  - Abnormal GM: Pachygyria, polymicrogyria, heterotopia
  - Abnormal WM: ↑ volume, ↓ T2 signal intensity prior to expected myelination timeframe, variable T2 signal intensity after myelination is complete
  - Blurring of GM-WM junction
  - Enlarged ipsilateral ventricle, pointed frontal horn
  - ± cerebellar, brainstem ipsilateral overgrowth
  - Size & signal intensity of HMEG can change over time
- T2* GRE
  - Signal loss from dystrophic Ca^{2+}
- Fetal MR, 2nd trimester
  - Disruption of normal cerebral mantle lamination (described on SSFSE T2) secondary to abnormal neuronal migration & proliferation
  - Mass-like low T2 signal proliferation of germinal matrix/ventricular zone mimics hemorrhage

DIFFERENTIAL DIAGNOSIS

Rasmussen Encephalitis

- Unilateral encephalitis with progressive atrophy

Gliomatosis Cerebri

- Diffusely infiltrating glioma effaces ipsilateral ventricle (rather than enlarging it)

Unilateral Cerebral Edema

- May be seen with trauma, infarction, or infection
- Effaces ipsilateral ventricle

PATHOLOGY

General Features

- Etiology
  - Defect in neuronal proliferation, migration, & organization
- Genetics
  - Classified as cortical dysgenesis with abnormal cell proliferation but without neoplasia
    - 3 subtypes: Isolated, associated with TSC, & associated with other neurocutaneous syndromes
      - TSC is given its own subcategory based on differences in etiology & treatment (i.e., mTOR inhibitors)
    - Abnormal cellular proliferation, migration, & differentiation
  - Currently believed to be result of gene mutations coding PI3K-AKT-mTOR pathway proteins → *PIK3CA*-related overgrowth spectrum (PROS)

Microscopic Features

- Dyslamination, dysplastic neurons, immature neurons, astrogliosis
- ± hypercellularity, balloon cells, dystrophic Ca^{2+}

CLINICAL ISSUES

Presentation

- Most common signs/symptoms
  - Macrocephaly
  - Seizures, hemiparesis, developmental delay
- Other signs/symptoms
  - 50% of patients have associated abnormalities
    - Cutaneous lesions, hemihypertrophy

Demographics

- Usually diagnosed during 1st year of life

Natural History & Prognosis

- Intractable seizures with progressive hemiparesis
- Best seizure control is offered by functional hemispherectomy, though motor deficits/hemiparesis frequently persist
- Some infants develop obstructive hydrocephalus requiring CSF diversion

Treatment

- Anticonvulsants are usually ineffective
- Functional hemispherectomy or hemispherotomy
  - Earlier surgical intervention yields better outcomes
  - Must first confirm normal contralateral hemisphere

DIAGNOSTIC CHECKLIST

Reporting Tips

- Define extent of HMEG + contralateral abnormalities

SELECTED REFERENCES

1. Reghunath A et al: A journey through formation and malformations of the neo-cortex. Childs Nerv Syst. 36(1):27-38, 2020
2. Barkovich AJ et al: Pediatric Neuroimaging. 6th ed. Wolters Kluwer. 448-51, 2019
3. Shrot S et al: Dysplasia and overgrowth: magnetic resonance imaging of pediatric brain abnormalities secondary to alterations in the mechanistic target of rapamycin pathway. Neuroradiology. 60(2):137-50, 2018
4. Keppler-Noreuil KM et al: PIK3CA-related overgrowth spectrum (PROS): diagnostic and testing eligibility criteria, differential diagnosis, and evaluation. Am J Med Genet A. 167A(2):287-95, 2015
5. Sarnat HB et al: Infantile tauopathies: hemimegalencephaly; tuberous sclerosis complex; focal cortical dysplasia 2; ganglioglioma. Brain Dev. 37(6):553-62, 2015

Lissencephaly

KEY FACTS

TERMINOLOGY

- Extensive cortical malformation caused by ↓ transmantle neuronal migration
  - Results in thick cortex & ↓ sulcation
- Spectrum of agyria, pachygyria, & band heterotopia

IMAGING

- Classic lissencephaly: Most common, considered subtype of tubulinopathies
  - Spectrum of ↓ number & depth of sulci + broad gyri
    - Graded based on anteroposterior predominance ± band heterotopia
  - Hourglass or figure 8 cerebral hemispheres in agyria
  - Few other major brain abnormalities; no severe congenital microcephaly
- Variant lissencephaly
  - Thick cortex, though not as thick as classic lissencephaly; no cell-sparse zone
  - Additional anomalies: Marked callosal dysgenesis, dysmorphic basal ganglia, cerebellar hypoplasia
- Microcephaly & additional anomalies with tubulinopathies from TUBA & TUBB mutations
- Deep white matter: Volume loss, ↓ arborization
- Ventriculomegaly

TOP DIFFERENTIAL DIAGNOSES

- Microcephaly with simplified gyral pattern
- Congenital muscular dystrophies: Dystroglycanopathies
- Expected immature sulcation pattern of prematurity
- Polymicrogyria

PATHOLOGY

- Many genetic mutations → spectrum of phenotypes
- Genetically based classification divides into tubulinopathies & variant lissencephalies
- Classic lissencephaly is most common, subtype of tubulinopathies

(Left) *Axial T2 MR in a 10-year-old girl with a LIS1 gene mutation shows posterior predominant agyria & bifrontal pachygyria. There is diffuse cortical thickening & vertically oriented sylvian fissures ➡, consistent with classic lissencephaly. Posterior predominant ventriculomegaly ➡ is seen as well as right frontal gray matter heterotopia ➡.* **(Right)** *Axial T1 MR in the same patient shows similar findings. The T1-hyperintense cell-sparse zone ➡ can be faintly seen posteriorly.*

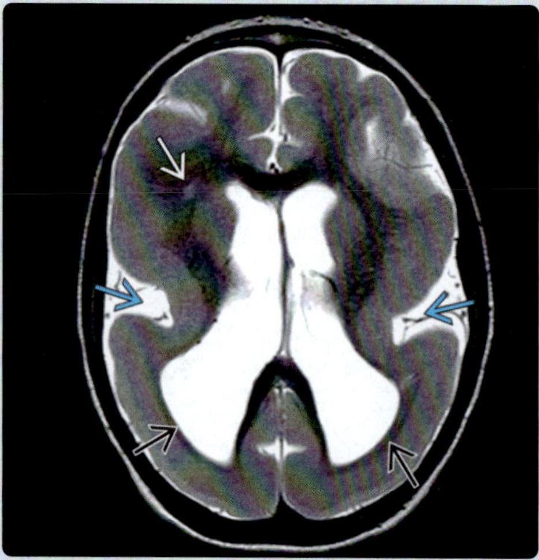

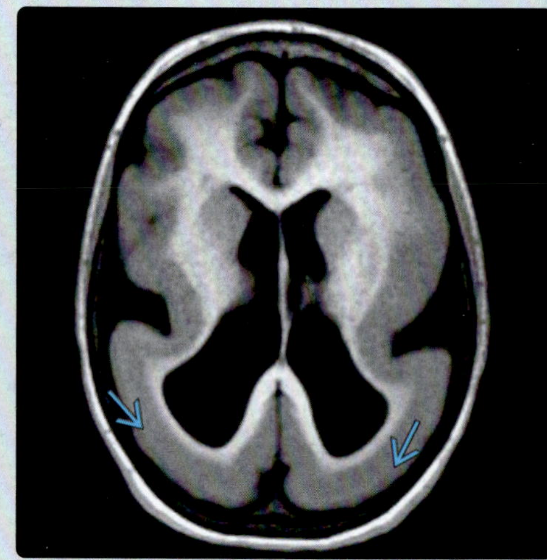

(Left) *Axial T1 MR in an 8-year-old girl with a DCX mutation & generalized seizures shows diffuse subcortical band heterotopia ➡, which is in the classic lissencephaly spectrum.* **(Right)** *Axial T2 MR in the same patient shows bilateral hemispheric band heterotopia ➡. The overlying gyral-sulcal pattern is normal with normal cortical thickness. Band heterotopia can be diffuse (as in this case), but in some cases may only involve the frontal or parietooccipital regions.*

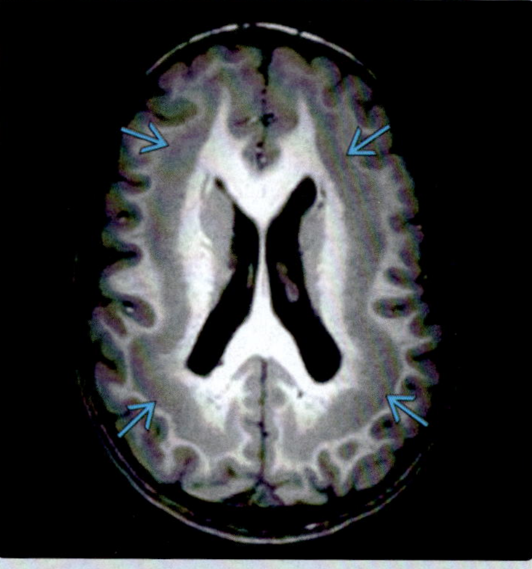

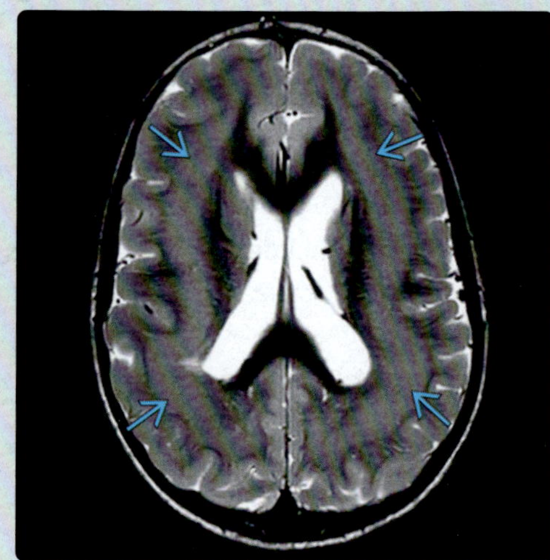

TERMINOLOGY

Definitions

- Spectrum of cortical malformation caused by arrested or ↓ transmantle neuronal migration
  - Agyria, pachygyria, & subcortical band heterotopia
- Most updated classification is based on combination of involved stage of neuronal migration & genetic information
- Abnormalities of neuronal proliferation (microlissencephaly, microcephaly with simplified gyral pattern, megalencephalies) & dystroglycanopathies (cobblestone malformations, previously type II lissencephaly) are described in separate categories
  - However, there is phenotypic & genetic overlap with congenital microcephaly & tubulinopathies

IMAGING

General Features

- Best diagnostic clue
  - Thick cortex with absence (agyria) or ↓ (pachygyria) number of sulci
  - Hourglass or figure 8 shape of cerebral hemispheres on axial images
- Location
  - Gradients of anterior to posterior cerebral hemispheric involvement are described in classic lissencephalies

MR Findings

- Smooth cortical surface
  - Spectrum of ↓ number & depth of sulci with large, broad gyri
- Thick, abnormal cortex
  - Classic lissencephaly: Thick cortex
    - 4-layer pattern described with cell-sparse zone deep to thin outer cortical layer & superficial to thick deeper cortical layer
      - Not always seen on MR; can be difficult to distinguish from band heterotopia in certain cases
  - Variant lissencephaly: Thick cortex, not as thick as classic lissencephaly (5-7 mm)
    - No cell-sparse zone
- Deep white matter abnormalities
  - ↓ volume with ↓ arborization
- Enlarged lateral ventricles
- Common associated findings
  - Callosal dysgenesis/agenesis
  - Pontocerebellar hypoplasia
  - Hippocampal anomalies

DIFFERENTIAL DIAGNOSIS

Microcephaly With Simplified Gyral Pattern

- Head circumference > 3 standard deviations below normal
- Broad gyri, ↓ number of sulci without cortical thickening

Congenital Muscular Dystrophies: Dystroglycanopathies

- Cobblestone cortex (formerly type II lissencephaly)
- Z-shaped hypoplastic brainstem on sagittal images
- Walker-Warburg, Fukuyama, muscle-eye-brain disease

Delayed Gyral-Sulcal Pattern

- Seen in preterm infants, infants with prenatal/neonatal systemic stressors, or genetic abnormalities/syndromes

Polymicrogyria

- Irregular pial surface ("lumpy-bumpy") & gray matter-white matter junction, shallow sulci + abnormal gyri

PATHOLOGY

General Features

- Genetics
  - Many identified mutations → spectrum of phenotypes
    - Tubulinopathies
      - Microtubules are essential in neuronal proliferation, migration, & axonal pathfinding
      - Mutations of genes encoding microtubule-associated proteins (MAPs: *LIS1*, *DCX*, *KIF5C*, *KIF2A*, & *DYNC1H1*), α-tubulin (TUBA genes, mainly *TUBA1A*), & β-tubulin (TUBB genes, mainly *TUBB2B* & *TUBB3*)
      - Classic lissencephalies fall under this category, most caused by MAP mutations (50% *LIS1*, 10% *DCX*), but up to 7% are from tubulin mutations
      - *DCX* mutations: Classic lissencephaly in male patients, band heterotopia in female patients
    - Variant lissencephalies
      - Primarily consists of *ARX* mutations & mutations of Reelin signaling pathway

CLINICAL ISSUES

Presentation

- Clinical profile depends on severity of malformation & associated anomalies
  - Complete agyric lissencephaly: Neonatal hypotonia, gradual spasticity, severe epilepsy
  - Isolated band heterotopia (BH): Intellectual disability, seizures

DIAGNOSTIC CHECKLIST

Consider

- Patterns of gyral abnormalities may provide insight into underlying genetic defect

Image Interpretation Pearls

- If lissencephaly is suspected in fetus or neonate, verify gestational age

Reporting Tips

- Describe regions & types of involvement ± associated abnormalities to help in classification

SELECTED REFERENCES

1. Kolbjer S et al: Lissencephaly in an epilepsy cohort: molecular, radiological and clinical aspects. Eur J Paediatr Neurol. 30:71-81, 2021
2. Lerman-Sagie T et al: A practical approach to prenatal diagnosis of malformations of cortical development. Eur J Paediatr Neurol. 34:50-61, 2021
3. Di Donato N et al: Lissencephaly: expanded imaging and clinical classification. Am J Med Genet A. 173(6):1473-88, 2017
4. Barkovich AJ et al: Malformations of cortical development and epilepsy. Cold Spring Harb Perspect Med. 5(5):a022392, 2015

Heterotopic Gray Matter

KEY FACTS

TERMINOLOGY

- Heterotopia (HTP): Abnormally located gray matter (GM) due to foreshortened or prolonged neuronal migration
  - Anywhere from periventricular germinal zone to pia

IMAGING

- Ectopic nodular or ribbon-like foci following GM signal intensity on every MR sequence
- Locations: Periventricular, subcortical, pial
  - Periventricular nodular HTP (most common)
  - Band HTP ≈ laminar HTP, double cortex
  - Subcortical nodular HTP (focal or multinodular)
  - Pial: Cobblestone cortex
- Best MR sequences (with multiplanar reformats)
  - Myelinated brain: 3D T1-spoiled GRE (e.g., SPGR)
  - Unmyelinated brain: 3D T2 FSE (e.g., Cube/VISTA/SPACE)

TOP DIFFERENTIAL DIAGNOSES

- Tuberous sclerosis
- Closed-lip schizencephaly
- Ependymal spread of tumor
- Congenital cytomegalovirus

PATHOLOGY

- Genetic & acquired etiologies cause disturbed neuronal migration resulting in ectopic rests of GM
  - At germinal zone → periventricular HTP
  - Before reaching cortex → subcortical & band HTP
  - At pia → cobblestone brain

CLINICAL ISSUES

- Symptoms: Developmental delay, motor dysfunction, seizures (40% of intractable epilepsy cases)
- Palliative surgery is reserved for intractable seizures

DIAGNOSTIC CHECKLIST

- Look closely for associated anomalies of adjacent cortex

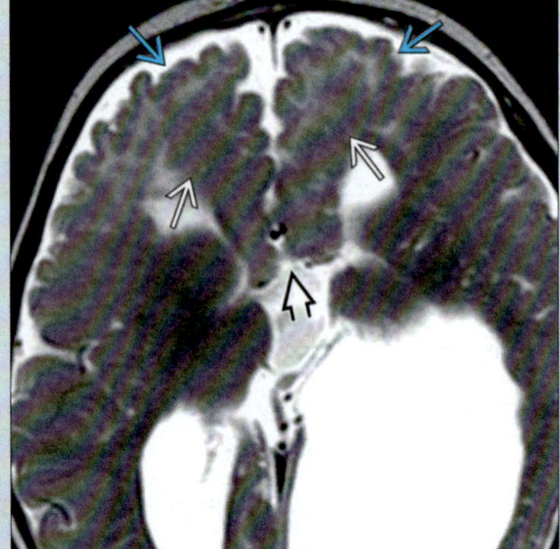

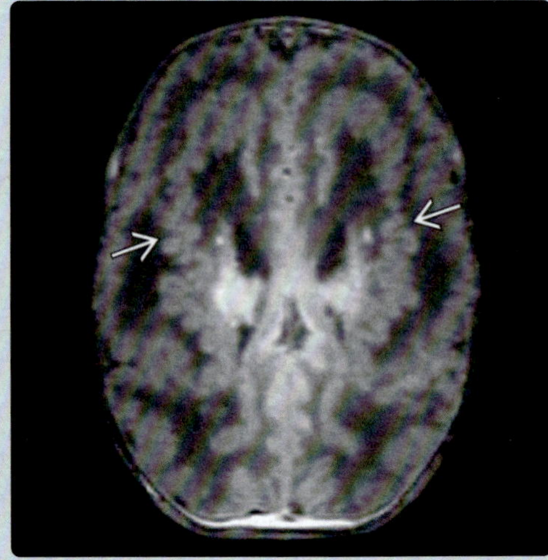

(Left) *Axial T2 MR in an 18-month-old girl with Aicardi syndrome & seizures shows extensive bifrontal periventricular & subcortical gray matter heterotopia ➡. Note the thin, irregular cortex ➡ overlying the foci of heterotopia. The corpus callosum is absent ⇨.* **(Right)** *Axial T1 MR in a 2-month-old with seizures shows extensive, symmetric heterotopic gray matter ➡ with a brain-in-brain appearance. The more superficial cortex is thinner than usual with poor sulcation.*

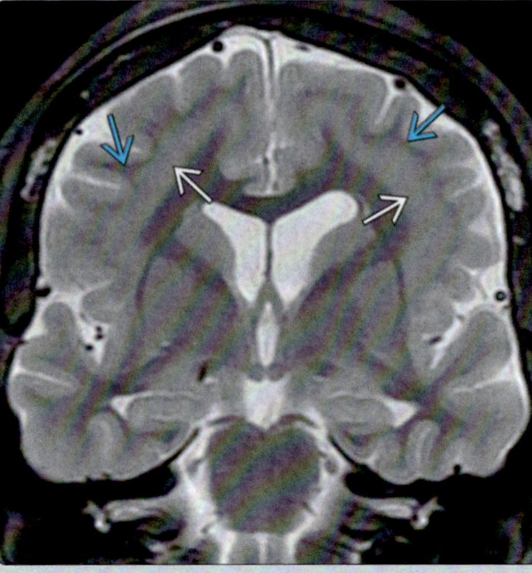

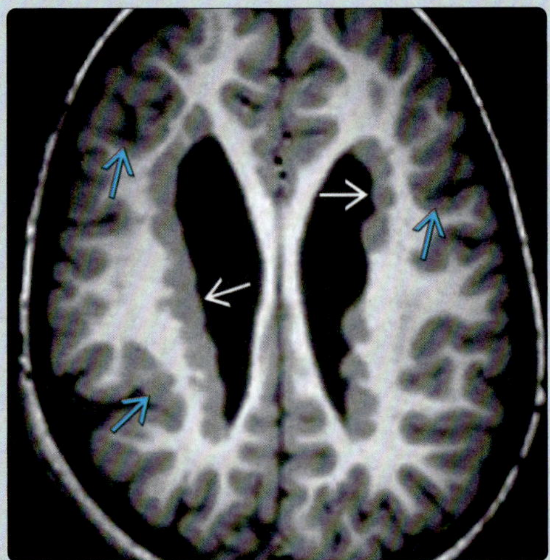

(Left) *Coronal T2 MR in a 15-year-old girl with seizures demonstrates a band of gray matter of variable thickness ➡ within the deep & subcortical white matter, consistent with band heterotopia. Note the thin layer of intervening white matter ➡ between the band of heterotopic gray matter & cortex.* **(Right)** *Axial T1 MR in a 9-year-old boy with epilepsy shows the diffuse form of periventricular nodular heterotopia ➡. Note the abnormal overlying cortex ➡ in multiple areas.*

Heterotopic Gray Matter

TERMINOLOGY

Synonyms

- Gray matter (GM) heterotopia (HTP)
- Double cortex ≈ band HTP

Definitions

- Abnormally located GM due to foreshortened or prolonged migration of neuronal groups
  - Occurs anywhere from periventricular germinal zone (GZ) to pia

IMAGING

General Features

- Best diagnostic clue
  - Nodules or ribbons of ectopic tissue that follow GM on all MR sequences
- Location
  - Periventricular, subcortical/transcerebral, pial

CT Findings

- NECT**:** Isodense with GM; rare dysplastic Ca^{2+}

MR Findings

- T1: Isointense to GM; well marginated
- T2: Isointense to GM
- FLAIR: Isointense to minimally hyperintense to GM
- DWI: Isointense to GM
- T1 C+: No enhancement
- Fetal MR: Nodular, irregular ventricular lining ± abnormal sulcation

Ultrasonographic Findings

- Nodular periventricular HTP may be evident as irregular/lobulated ventricular margin

Imaging Recommendations

- Protocol advice
  - Multiplanar reconstructions of
    - Volumetric 3D T1 spoiled GRE MR (e.g., SPGR) in myelinated brain
    - Volumetric 3D T2 FSE MR (e.g., Cube/VISTA/SPACE) in unmyelinated brain

DIFFERENTIAL DIAGNOSIS

Tuberous Sclerosis

- Subependymal nodules in regions of fetal germinal matrix
- Often calcify; may enhance
- Associated with cortical/subcortical tubers

Closed-Lip Schizencephaly

- Polymicrogyric GM lines apposed walls of pial-ependymal cleft with funnel-shaped outpouching (dimple) of ventricular wall

Ependymal Spread of Tumor

- Nodular or crescentic foci along ventricular lining
- Usually enhance, may restrict diffusion

Congenital Cytomegalovirus

- Periventricular Ca^{2+} without protrusion into ventricle
- ± white matter injury, polymicrogyria, schizencephaly, cerebellar hypoplasia, microcephaly

PATHOLOGY

General Features

- Etiology
  - Genetic: Mutations alter molecular interactions at multiple migration points → migration arrest → HTP
  - Acquired: Fetal insult (ischemia, infection, etc.) → disturbed neuronal migration/cortical positioning
- Genetics
  - Diffuse periventricular nodular HTP is often genetic
    - *FLNA* (Xq28), *ARFGEF2* (20q13.13), 5p15
  - Band HTP: Mild form of classic lissencephaly (agyria/pachygyria/double cortex)
    - *LIS1* (17p13.3), *DCX* (Xq22.3-q23), tubulin genes
- Associated abnormalities
  - Focal periventricular nodular HTP in 30% of Chiari 2
- Embryology
  - Landing zones with abnormal neuronal migration
    - At GZ → periventricular HTP
    - Before reaching cortex → subcortical & band HTP
    - At pia → cobblestone brain

Microscopic Features

- Multiple types of immature/dysplastic cells
  - Excitatory exceed inhibitory

CLINICAL ISSUES

Presentation

- Most common signs/symptoms
  - Developmental delay, seizures, motor dysfunction
  - Age of onset & severity of symptoms depend on location & extent of abnormalities

Demographics

- Epidemiology
  - Found in up to 40% of patients with intractable epilepsy

Natural History & Prognosis

- Prognosis depends on location & extent of HTP, associated malformations, & seizure severity
- Focal HTP can be incidental on imaging/autopsy

Treatment

- Palliative surgery is reserved for intractable seizures

DIAGNOSTIC CHECKLIST

Image Interpretation Pearls

- HTP is commonly associated with other anomalies
  - Look closely for overlying cortical abnormalities

SELECTED REFERENCES

1. Deleo F et al: Whole-brain multimodal MRI phenotyping of periventricular nodular heterotopia. Neurology. 95(17):e2418-26, 2020
2. Oegema R et al: Subcortical heterotopic gray matter brain malformations: classification study of 107 individuals. Neurology. 93(14):e1360-73, 2019
3. Watrin F et al: Causes and consequences of gray matter heterotopia. CNS Neurosci Ther. 21(2):112-22, 2015
4. Barkovich AJ et al: A developmental and genetic classification for malformations of cortical development: update 2012. Brain. 135(Pt 5):1348-69, 2012

Schizencephaly

KEY FACTS

IMAGING

- Transmantle cleft lined by gray matter (GM) extending from cortical surface to ventricle
  - Closed-lip defect: Cleft walls are closely apposed
    - Dimple along ependymal surface of lateral ventricle
    - CSF cleft should be present but may be subtle
  - Open-lip defect: Cleft walls are clearly separated by CSF; widths & shapes of clefts are variable
- GM lining cleft is inherently abnormal
  - Polymicrogyria, heterotopia
- May occur anywhere but most often perisylvian
- Bilateral in up to 1/2 of patients
  - Unilateral often shows contralateral polymicrogyria
- ± hemosiderin staining of cleft, ventricles
- Associated with absence of cavum septum pellucidum ± optic nerve hypoplasia (a.k.a. septo-optic dysplasia)
  - Anomalies of hypothalamic-pituitary axis
  - Callosal hypogenesis other midline anomalies

TOP DIFFERENTIAL DIAGNOSES

- Encephaloclastic porencephaly
- Transmantle heterotopia
- Ventricular rupture
- Hydranencephaly

PATHOLOGY

- In utero insult affecting neuronal organization
- Considered to be extreme spectrum of polymicrogyria
- Etiologies include: Vascular insult, infection (CMV, HSV), maternal trauma, toxins; rare genetic etiologies

CLINICAL ISSUES

- Seizures, motor abnormalities, developmental delay
- Type & severity of clinical impairment is determined by
  - Number, size, & location of clefts
    - Worse prognosis for bilateral open clefts vs. unilateral closed defect
  - Presence of associated malformations

(Left) *Coronal graphic shows bilateral schizencephalic clefts, closed lip on the right ➔ & open lip on the left ➩. Both clefts are lined by dysplastic gray matter. Note the absence of the septum pellucidum ➨.* **(Right)** *Axial T2 MR of a 4-month-old girl with a left open-lip schizencephaly shows mild overlying calvarial thinning/expansion ➔ secondary to CSF pulsation. There is polymicrogyria ➔ of gray matter lining the cleft. The septum pellucidum is absent ➩.*

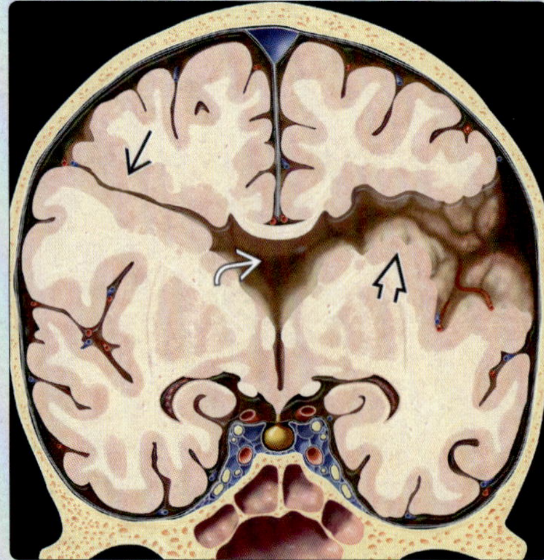

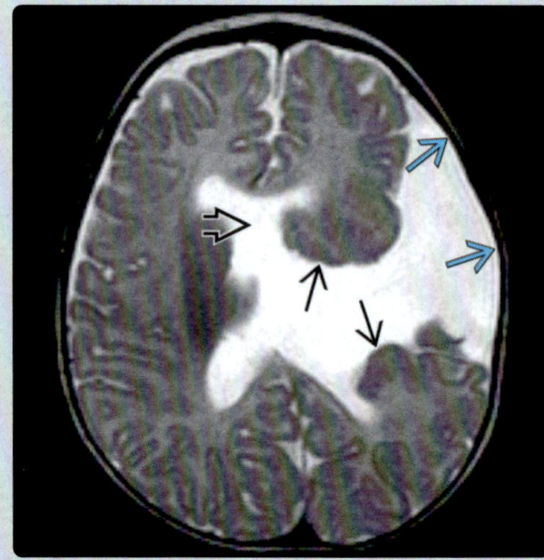

(Left) *Coronal T2 MR in a 13-year-old boy with a right closed-lip schizencephaly shows buckling of the inner ependymal margin on the right ➔. There is also left polymicrogyria with transmantle heterotopia ➨.* **(Right)** *Coronal T2 MR in an 11-month-old with septo-optic dysplasia (SOD) shows left closed-lip schizencephaly ➔, absence of the septum pellucidum ➔, & contralateral right polymicrogyria ➩. Schizencephaly & polymicrogyria are commonly associated with SOD.*

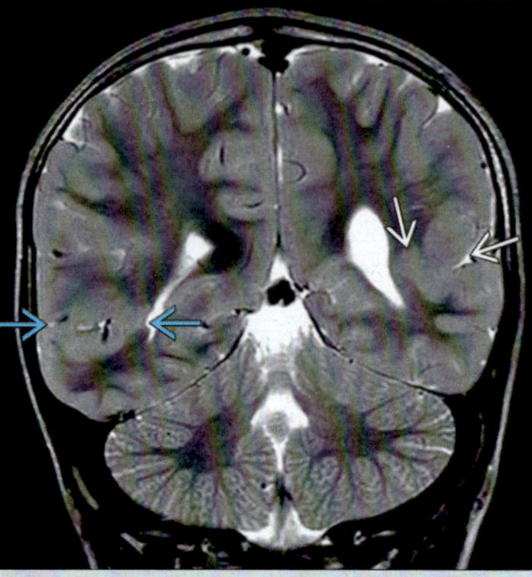

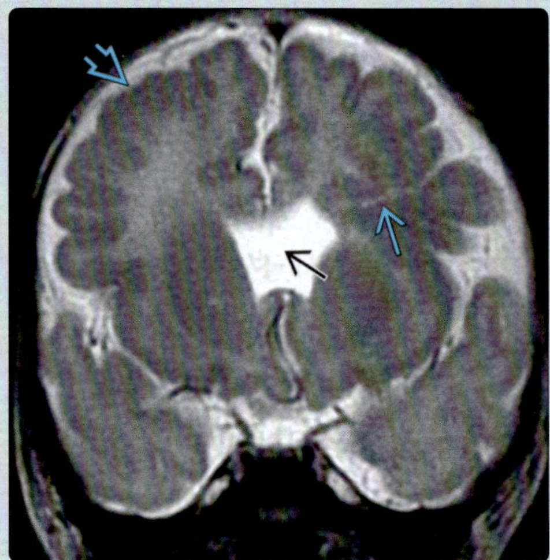

TERMINOLOGY

Definitions

- Transmantle cleft in brain parenchyma extending from cortical surface to ventricle (i.e., pia to ependyma)
  - Lined by dysplastic gray matter (GM)

IMAGING

General Features

- Best diagnostic clue
  - Full-thickness transmantle, GM-lined cleft extending from pial to ependymal surfaces
    - Closed lip (type I): Walls of cleft are in direct contact
    - Open lip (type II): CSF throughout cleft
      - Variable cleft widths
  - Up to 50% are bilateral

CT Findings

- NECT
  - Cerebral cleft of CSF density (in open-lip type)
  - Thinned, expanded calvarium with large open-lip clefts
    - Calvarial remodeling from CSF pulsations through cleft or expansion of diverticulum associated with cleft (roofing membrane)

MR Findings

- T1, T2, FLAIR
  - Closed type may appear as irregular tract of GM from cortical surface to ventricle (fused cleft)
    - Look for dimple in wall of lateral ventricle
  - Open type can be wide & wedge-shaped or have nearly parallel walls
  - Abnormal GM lining cleft: Polymicrogyria or heterotopia
  - ± thin overlying membrane of pia or ependyma (a.k.a. roofing membrane)
- T2* GRE
  - ± hemosiderin staining of ventricles &/or cleft from prenatal insult

Imaging Recommendations

- Protocol advice
  - Multiplanar sequences (± volumetric acquisition) are particularly important for closed-lip type

DIFFERENTIAL DIAGNOSIS

Encephaloclastic Porencephaly

- Parenchymal cavity due to insult after cortical organization is complete
- Lined by gliotic white matter, not dysplastic GM

Transmantle Heterotopia

- No cleft; can be difficult to differentiate from closed-lip schizencephaly (lies along same pathologic spectrum)

Ventricular Rupture

- Due to severe congenital hydrocephalus (e.g., aqueductal stenosis), most often in medial parietal region

Hydranencephaly

- Destruction of middle & anterior cerebral artery territories
- May mimic severe bilateral open-lip schizencephaly

PATHOLOGY

General Features

- Etiology
  - In utero injury to developing brain prior to completion of neuronal organization
    - Often considered to be extreme spectrum of polymicrogyria
  - Etiologies may be hypoxic-ischemic, vascular, teratogenic (alcohol, warfarin, & cocaine), infectious (CMV, HSV)
- Genetics
  - Genetic cause is uncommon
  - Single gene mutations
    - Mutations of *COL4A1*, *EMX2*
- Associated abnormalities
  - GM heterotopia is often seen adjacent to cleft
  - Contralateral polymicrogyria is common
  - Septum pellucidum is absent in large percentage of schizencephaly cases, especially bilateral clefts
  - Hypoplastic optic nerve syndrome [a.k.a. septo-optic dysplasia (SOD)]
    - Optic nerve hypoplasia: Key to diagnosis (& best determined by ophthalmologic exam) ± other commonly associated findings
      - Absence of septum pellucidum
      - Abnormalities of hypothalamic-pituitary axis
      - Corpus callosum dysgenesis
    - Schizencephaly in 30-50% of SOD patients

CLINICAL ISSUES

Presentation

- Most common signs/symptoms
  - Seizures, hemiparesis, developmental delay
  - Bilateral clefts: Tetraparesis, blindness, more severe cognitive impairment

Demographics

- Epidemiology
  - Incidence: 1.5/100,000 births
  - 1 in 3 children have non-CNS abnormalities
    - > 50% likely due to vascular disruption
      - Gastroschisis, bowel atresias, & amniotic band disruption sequence
  - Associated with ↓ maternal age, lack of prenatal care, ethanol abuse
  - Other risk factors: Prenatal infection, thrombophilia, disorders of blood vessel wall integrity

Treatment

- Surgery for medically intractable epilepsy
- CSF diversion/shunting in cases of ↑ intracranial pressure
  - Abnormal CSF dynamics associated with cleft

SELECTED REFERENCES

1. Park KB et al: The spectrum of brain malformations and disruptions in twins. Am J Med Genet A. 185(9):2690-718, 2021
2. Braga VL et al: Schizencephaly: a review of 734 patients. Pediatr Neurol. 87:23-9, 2018
3. Kutuk MS et al: Prenatal diagnosis and postnatal outcome of schizencephaly. J Child Neurol. 30(10):1388-94, 2014
4. Nabavizadeh SA et al: Correlation of prenatal and postnatal MRI findings in schizencephaly. AJNR Am JNeuroradiol. 35(7):1418-24, 2014

KEY FACTS

TERMINOLOGY

- Polymicrogyria (PMG)
- Traditionally considered malformation of late neuronal migration & cortical organization resulting in abnormal distribution of neurons; disputed by some literature

IMAGING

- Excessively small & disorganized gyral convolutions with shallow sulci, creating appearance of nodular cortex
- Commonly perisylvian; may be unilateral or bilateral
- Imaging findings depend on patient age
  - Fetal: Premature appearance of sulci
  - 1-2 years: Abnormal sulcation pattern
  - > 2 years: Abnormally thick, irregular cortex
- Optimal MR sequence depends on brain maturation
  - Incomplete myelination (< 1 year): Thin-section T2 MR
  - Complete myelination (> 1-2 years): 3D SPGR T1 MR
- Look for additional findings to suggest underlying CMV or metabolic/syndromic diagnosis
  - NECT or SWI/GRE MR may detect Ca^{2+} in CMV

TOP DIFFERENTIAL DIAGNOSES

- Microcephaly with simplified gyral pattern
- Hemimegalencephaly
- Pachygyria
- Cobblestone malformations

PATHOLOGY

- Causes: Fetal infection, ischemia, or genetic/syndromic
- Associated syndromes: Aicardi, Zellweger, DiGeorge, Warburg microsyndromes
- PMG lines clefts of schizencephaly

CLINICAL ISSUES

- Most common presentation: Seizures, developmental delay, spasticity; varies with extent/location of PMG
  - Neonatal (in severe) vs. adolescence (in mild, focal)

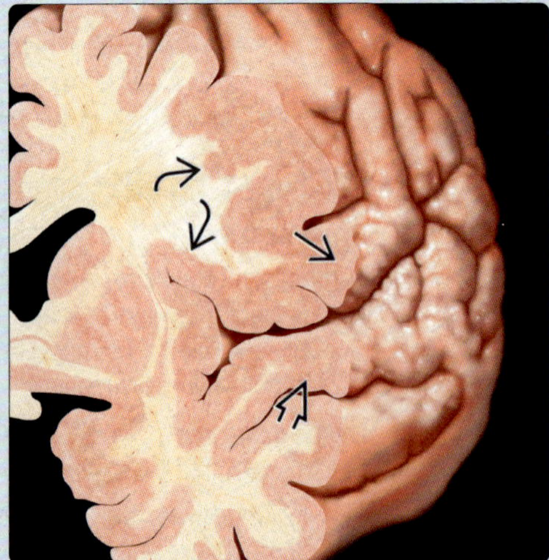

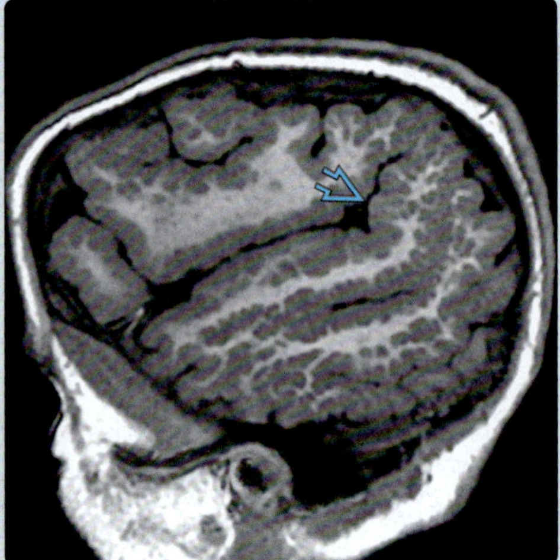

(Left) *Coronal oblique graphic shows thickened "pebbly" or nodular gyri of polymicrogyria (PMG) involving the frontal ➡ & temporal ➡ opercula. Note the abnormal sulcation & irregular gray matter-white matter (GM-WM) junctions ➡ in the affected regions.* **(Right)** *Sagittal T1 MR in a 17-year-old with extensive PMG shows diffuse nodularity along the surface of the cortex & at the GM-WM junction. Note the continuation of the sylvian fissure into the superior parietal lobule ➡, a characteristic appearance for PMG.*

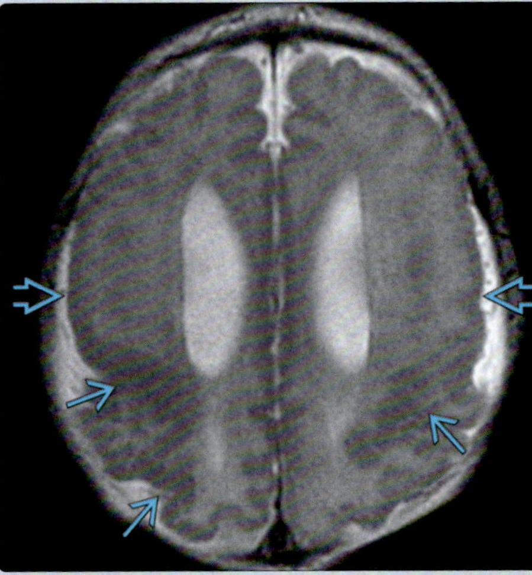

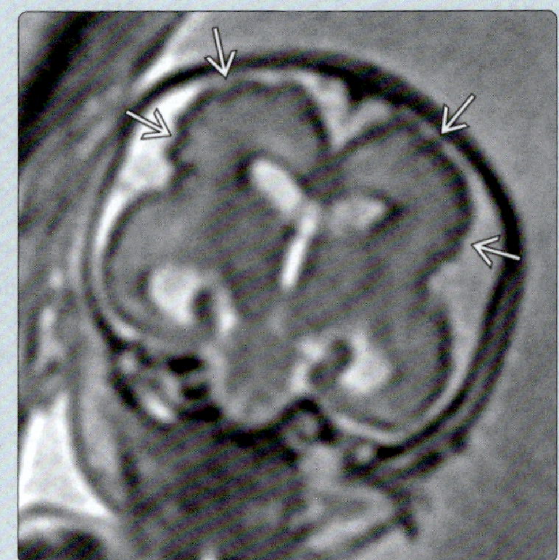

(Left) *Axial T2 MR in a 3-month-old with congenital CMV shows a nearly symmetric appearance of abnormally thick & irregular/nodular cortex ➡ in a perisylvian distribution, consistent with PMG. A paucity of gyri & sulci is seen more anteriorly ➡.* **(Right)** *Coronal SSFSE T2 MR in a 25-weeks-gestation fetus shows bilateral foci of irregular cortex ➡, consistent with extensive PMG. The cortex in these regions should appear smooth at this time in gestation.*

TERMINOLOGY

Abbreviations

- Polymicrogyria (PMG)

Definitions

- Traditionally considered malformation of late neuronal migration & cortical organization resulting in abnormal distribution of neurons; disputed by some literature
  - Regardless, macroscopic result is nodular cortex with disorganized small, undulating gyri & shallow sulci

IMAGING

General Features

- Best diagnostic clue
  - Excessively small & numerous gyri
- Location
  - Can be unilateral, bilateral, multifocal
  - Most common in perisylvian regions (60-70%)
- Size
  - Ranges from single gyrus to entire cerebrum
- Morphology
  - Small, irregular gyri
  - Thick nodular cortex with irregular gray matter-white matter (GM-WM) junctions
  - May appear as deep infolding of thick cortex
  - Schizencephalic clefts are lined by PMG
  - Sylvian fissure may extend into parietal lobe

CT Findings

- Look for altered sulcation pattern (suggests PMG)
- Periventricular Ca^{2+} in CMV

MR Findings

- **T1**: Irregular cortical surface; thick-appearing cortex; deep infolding of irregular cortex
- **T2**: 2 imaging patterns depending on patient age
  - < 12 months: Undulating cortex of normal thickness
  - > 18 months: Thick, bumpy cortex (6-8 mm)

Nuclear Medicine Findings

- **PET**: Ictal hypermetabolism & interictal hypometabolism

Imaging Recommendations

- Protocol advice
  - Volumetric 3D SPGR (T1) MR in mature brain
  - Thin-section T2 MR if unmyelinated

DIFFERENTIAL DIAGNOSIS

Microcephaly With Simplified Gyral Pattern

- Normal cortex with primary & secondary sulci but absent tertiary sulci

Hemimegalencephaly

- ↑ size of involved hemisphere (vs. ↓ in PMG)

Pachygyria

- Thick cortex (8-10 mm), smooth GM-WM junction

Cobblestone Malformations

- Hypomyelination, cerebellar dysgenesis, pontine hypoplasia
- Often associated with congenital muscular dystrophy

PATHOLOGY

General Features

- Etiology
  - Intrauterine infection, ischemia, or gene mutations
- Genetics
  - Most common: 1p36.3 & 22q11.2 microdeletions
- Associated abnormalities
  - Aicardi, Zellweger, Warburg microsyndromes
  - Congenital bilateral perisylvian syndrome (Foix-Chavany-Marie)
  - Corpus callosum dysgenesis, periventricular nodular heterotopia, & subcortical heterotopia
  - Microcephaly (~ 50%); more common in generalized forms of PMG

Gross Pathologic & Surgical Features

- Multiple small gyri lie in haphazard orientation

Microscopic Features

- Derangements of normal 6-layered cortex
  - Reduced numbers of neurons
  - Areas of 2-, 4-, & 6-layered cortex are described, even in different regions of same brain
    - Normal vs. abnormal laminar arrangement is disputed

CLINICAL ISSUES

Presentation

- Most common signs/symptoms
  - Seizures, developmental delay, spasticity

Demographics

- Age
  - Symptom onset varies with extent/location of malformation
    - Neonatal manifestations in severely affected vs. 2nd decade of life for focal unilateral PMG
- Epidemiology
  - Malformations of cortical development are found in ~ 40% of children with intractable epilepsy

Treatment

- Surgical options with medically refractory seizures
  - Focal PMG may be resected
  - Corpus callosotomy if bilateral or unresectable lesions

DIAGNOSTIC CHECKLIST

Image Interpretation Pearls

- Look for PMG in congenital hemiplegia with epilepsy
  - Schizencephaly is always lined by PMG
  - Open sylvian fissures with thick cortex suggest PMG
- Look for secondary findings of CMV or syndrome

SELECTED REFERENCES

1. Arrigoni F et al: Characterizing white matter tract organization in polymicrogyria and lissencephaly: a multifiber diffusion mri modeling and tractography study. AJNR Am J Neuroradiol. 41(8):1495-502, 2020
2. Jansen AC et al: The histopathology of polymicrogyria: a series of 71 brain autopsy studies. Dev Med Child Neurol. 58(1):39-48, 2016

KEY FACTS

TERMINOLOGY

- Cortical disorganization & abnormal laminar architecture

IMAGING

- Focal cortical dysplasia (FCD) type 1
  - MR imaging findings are present in 22-64%, may be lower in children
    - White matter (WM) volume loss
    - Ill-defined WM ↑ signal
    - Blurring of gray matter-WM junction
    - Cortical signal change
    - Abnormal sulcal & gyral pattern
- FCD type 2
  - MR imaging findings are more commonly present (60-100%)
    - Focal signal abnormality in subcortical WM
    - Blurring of gray matter-WM junction
    - Cortical thickening & signal change
    - Abnormal sulcal & gyral pattern

PATHOLOGY

- FCD type 1
  - Abnormal lamination of cortex without dysmorphic neurons
- FCD type 2
  - Abnormal lamination of cortex with dysmorphic neurons, ± balloon cells
- FCD type 3
  - FCD associated with other structural lesions

CLINICAL ISSUES

- FCD is most common pathology seen in pediatric patients with surgically treated epilepsy
  - Type 1 dysplasias are more commonly seen in adults
- Epilepsy surgery effectiveness is dependent on type of underlying pathology
  - Type 1 FCD: 13-21% seizure free
  - Type 2 FCD: 52-91% seizure free

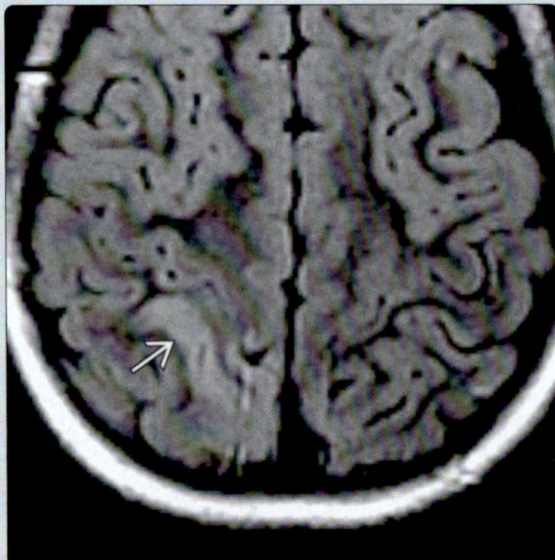

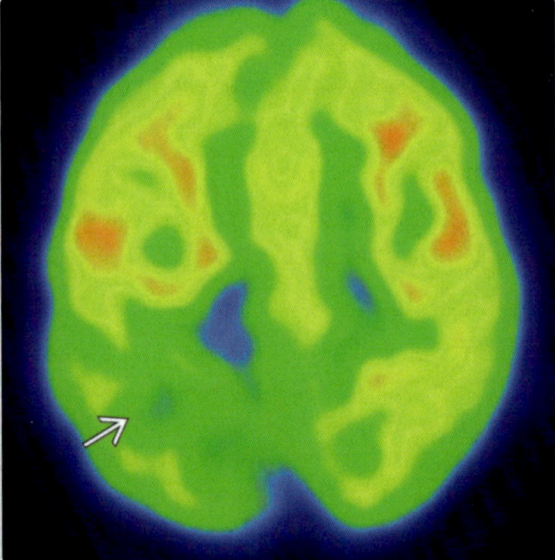

(Left) *Axial FLAIR MR in an 8-year-old girl shows hyperintense signal ➡ in the right parietal cortex, a common finding in focal cortical dysplasia (FCD). Pathology demonstrated FCD type 2B, which is usually visible on imaging.* **(Right)** *Axial color-coded FDG PET in the same patient shows focally ↓ metabolism ➡ in the area of MR signal abnormality. FDG PET is particularly helpful in identifying FCD lesions that are not visible or very subtle on conventional MR imaging.*

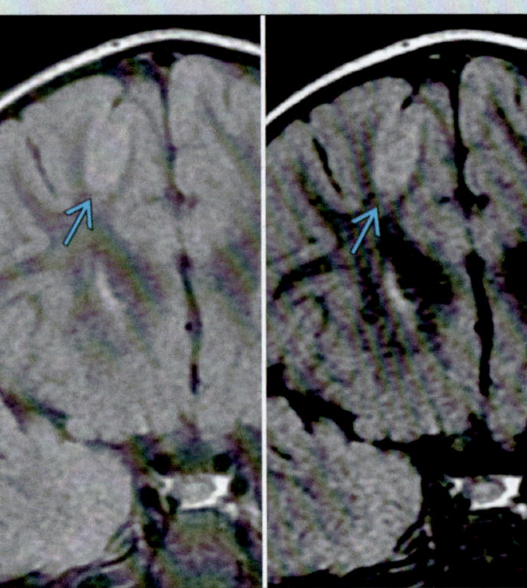

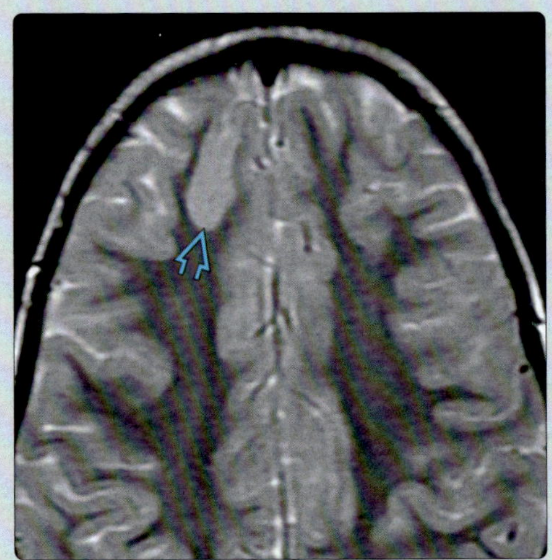

(Left) *Coronal FLAIR MR images in a 3-year-old with FCD type 2B ➡ with varying contrast windowing are shown. Note how FCD is much more conspicuous in the image on the right with windowing emphasizing greater contrast. Windowing is an important means to increasing detection of subtle FCD lesions.* **(Right)** *Axial T2 MR in the same patient shows an abnormally deep sulcus ➡ with cortex that is both thickened & slightly ↑ in signal intensity compared to adjacent normal cortex, typical findings in FCD.*

TERMINOLOGY

Definitions

- Focal cortical dysplasia (FCD)
  - Cortical disorganization & abnormal laminar architecture

IMAGING

General Features

- FCD type 1
  - Only 22-64% have imaging findings, may be lower in children (12%)
  - When present, MR findings are often subtle
    - White matter (WM) volume loss
    - Ill-defined WM ↑ signal
    - Blurring of gray matter-WM junction
    - Cortical signal change
    - Abnormal gyral & sulcal pattern
- FCD type 2
  - 60-100% have identifiable abnormalities on MR
    - Focal signal abnormality in subcortical WM
    - Blurring of gray-WM junction
    - ↑ cortical thickness
    - Cortical signal change
    - Abnormal gyral & sulcal pattern
  - MR findings highly suggestive of type 2
    - Transmantle sign: WM signal tapering from subcortical region to ventricular margin
    - Depth of sulcus morphology: ↑ signal at depth of abnormal sulcus ± transmantle sign

Nuclear Medicine Findings

- PET
  - ↓ interictal vs. ↑ ictal metabolic activity
- Perfusion SPECT
  - Comparative ictal & interictal scans with Tc-99m HMPAO or Tc-99m ECD
    - ↑ ictal vs. ↓ interictal perfusion

Imaging Recommendations

- Protocol advice
  - Higher field strength (3T) is preferred
  - 3D isotropic MR techniques (T1 & FLAIR) allow multiplanar reconstruction, PET/SPECT/MEG fusion, & intraoperative guidance

DIFFERENTIAL DIAGNOSIS

Tuberous Sclerosis

- Radial migration lines & cortical tubers share many imaging features with FCD, especially FCD type 2B
- Tubers & FCD type 2B share similar histopathology

Cortical Neoplasm

- Especially DNET, ganglioglioma, or other low-grade glioma
- Abnormal enhancement excludes FCD

Incomplete or Delayed Myelination

- Focal incomplete myelination may mimic FCD
- Follow-up imaging after myelin maturation is helpful

PATHOLOGY

General Features

- Etiology
  - FCD type 1: Disturbance of cortical organization
  - FCD type 2: Disturbance of cellular proliferation

Staging, Grading, & Classification

- FCD type 1
  - Isolated alterations in cortical organization & lamination
    - 1A: Abnormal radial cortical lamination
    - 1B: Abnormal tangential cortical lamination
    - 1C: Abnormal radial & tangential cortical lamination
- FCD type 2
  - Isolated alterations in cortical organization & lamination with dysmorphic neurons
    - 2A: Presence of dysmorphic neurons
    - 2B: Dysmorphic neurons & balloon cells
- FCD type 3
  - FCD associated with another principal (non-FCD) lesion
    - 3A: FCD associated with hippocampal sclerosis
    - 3B: FCD associated with glial or glioneuronal tumor
    - 3C: FCD associated with vascular malformation
    - 3D: FCD associated with early-acquired encephaloclastic lesion

CLINICAL ISSUES

Presentation

- 10% of all epilepsy patients
- 50% of children undergoing surgery for intractable epilepsy

Natural History & Prognosis

- Seizure-free outcome following surgery is much better in FCD type 2 (52-91%) compared to FCD type 1 (21%)

Treatment

- Focal resection ± preceding subdural EEG grid localization

DIAGNOSTIC CHECKLIST

Consider

- Review localizing EEG findings during image interpretation if available

Image Interpretation Pearls

- Consideration of seizure semiology, localizing EEG findings, & NM imaging to help localize MR abnormalities
- ~ 1/3 of cases are initially missed because findings are subtle
- Proper MR imaging technique improves lesion detection
- Windowing to ↑ contrast on T2 & FLAIR imaging is helpful to improve subtle FCD detection.

SELECTED REFERENCES

1. Tahta A et al: Focal cortical dysplasia: etiology, epileptogenesis, classification, clinical presentation, imaging, and management. Childs Nerv Syst. 36(12):2939-47, 2020
2. Jayalakshmi S et al: Focal cortical dysplasia and refractory epilepsy: role of multimodality imaging and outcome of surgery. AJNR Am J Neuroradiol. 40(5):892-8, 2019

Chiari 1

KEY FACTS

TERMINOLOGY

- Chiari 1 malformation (CM1); synonyms: Chiari type 1, Chiari 1 deformity, cerebellar tonsillar ectopia

IMAGING

- Pointed cerebellar tonsils extending ≥ 5 mm below foramen magnum (basion-opisthion/McRae line) with effacement of CSF spaces
- ± retroflexed odontoid, horizontal shortened clivus, basilar invagination, atlantooccipital assimilation
- ± caudal descent of brainstem, brainstem compression, medullary bump
- ± syringohydromyelia, scoliosis

TOP DIFFERENTIAL DIAGNOSES

- Normal low-lying cerebellar tonsils
- Chiari 2 malformation
- Tonsillar herniation due to ↑ intracranial pressure
- Intracranial hypotension

PATHOLOGY

- Most common cause is believed to be small/underdeveloped posterior fossa; no association with open spinal dysraphism
- Can result from premature closure of sutures
  - Causes include shunted infantile hydrocephalus, bone dysplasias, genetic syndromes

CLINICAL ISSUES

- Most common presenting symptom: Occipital headache
  - Up to 30% of patients are asymptomatic
- Goal of surgery in symptomatic patients: Restore normal CSF flow at foramen magnum
  - Suboccipital decompression, resection of C1 posterior arch ± duraplasty, cerebellar tonsil cautery

DIAGNOSTIC CHECKLIST

- Look for presence of syrinx → usually requires surgical treatment of Chiari 1

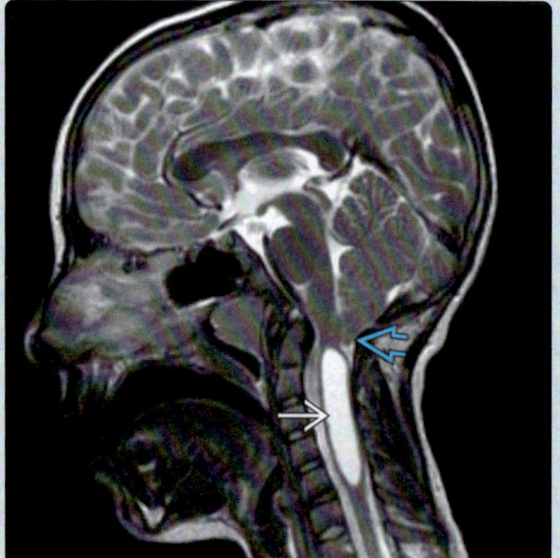

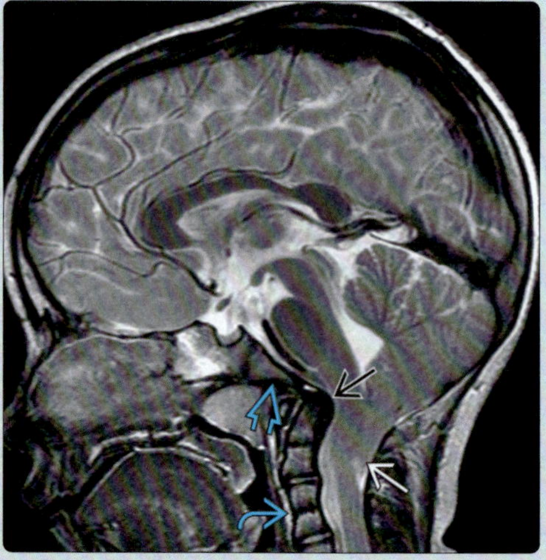

(Left) *Sagittal T2 MR shows the low-lying, pointed cerebellar tonsils* ⇨ *typical of a Chiari 1 malformation. Note the expansion of the cervical spinal cord by a large syrinx* ➡. **(Right)** *Sagittal T2 MR in a 5-year-old with occipital headaches demonstrates pointed, low-lying cerebellar tonsils* ➡ *with associated effacement of CSF spaces. Note the short horizontal clivus* ⇨, *retroverted dens* ⇨, *impression upon the medulla, & segmentation anomaly at the C3-C4 levels* ⇨, *consistent with a complex Chiari 1 malformation.*

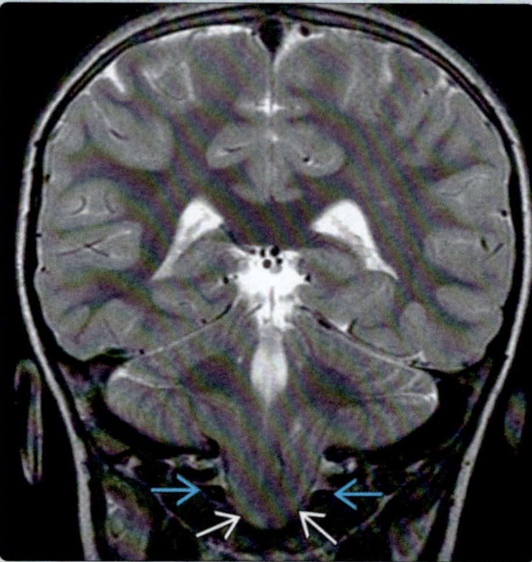

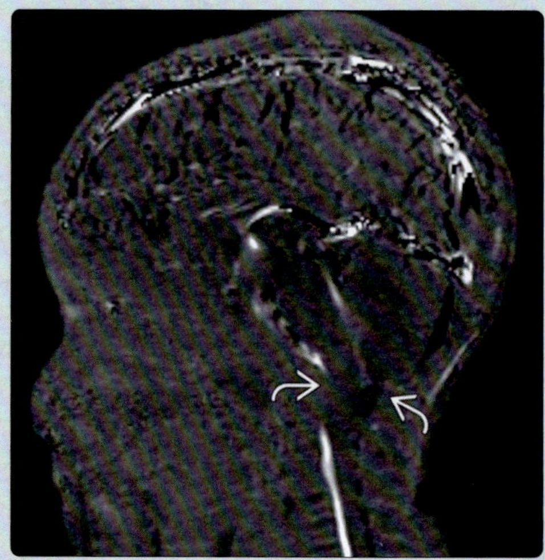

(Left) *Coronal T2 MR in the same patient demonstrates pointed, low-lying cerebellar tonsils* ➡ *extending below the C1 ring* ⇨, *typical of a Chiari 1 malformation.* **(Right)** *Sagittal image from a phase-contrast cine MR (with hyperintense signal at sites of active CSF or venous flow) in the same patient shows absence of CSF flow at the craniocervical junction* ➡ *due to the Chiari 1 malformation.*

TERMINOLOGY

Definitions

- Compressed & pointed cerebellar tonsils extending below foramen magnum with effacement of CSF spaces

IMAGING

General Features

- Best diagnostic clue
  - Pointed cerebellar tonsils (unilateral or bilateral) extending ≥ 5 mm below foramen magnum (basion-opisthion line)
    - No consensus statement on exact definition

CT Findings

- Crowding of foramen magnum on axial CT images
  - Sagittal reconstructed images are very helpful
  - Beware that streak artifact from skull base can falsely simulate Chiari 1 malformation
- Superior aspect of syrinx may be imaged on head CT
- Associated osseous anomalies may include small posterior fossa, short horizontal clivus, retroverted dens, basilar invagination, platybasia, hypoplastic occipital condyles, segmentation anomalies (such as atlantooccipital assimilation), scoliosis

MR Findings

- T1, T2, FLAIR
  - Pointed (not rounded) cerebellar tonsils extending ≥ 5 mm below foramen magnum
  - Crowded foramen magnum with small/effaced cisterns ± brainstem compression
  - ± small posterior fossa, elongated 4th ventricle
  - ± syringohydromyelia/syrinx, scoliosis
  - ± dorsal cervicomedullary "bump"
  - Other descriptions are usually considered subtypes
    - Chiari 1.5: Brainstem herniation
    - Complex Chiari: Retroflexed odontoid causes medullary bump, abnormally acute clival-cervical angle; ± atlantooccipital assimilation, ± basilar invagination, ± platybasia
- MR cine
  - Restricted CSF flow through foramen magnum ± ↑ brainstem/cerebellar tonsil motion (pistoning)

DIFFERENTIAL DIAGNOSIS

Normal Variation of Cerebellar Tonsil Position

- Tonsils may normally lie below foramen magnum
  - May be accentuated by certain head positions
- Rounded tonsils but no crowding at foramen magnum

Chiari 2 Malformation

- Very small posterior fossa with hindbrain herniation in setting of open spinal dysraphism at birth
- ± hydrocephalus, tectal beaking, & other findings

Tonsillar Herniation Due to ↑ Intracranial Pressure

- Neoplasm, hemorrhage, hydrocephalus, infarct

Intracranial Hypotension

- Sagging brain with dural thickening/enhancement, distended dural sinuses

PATHOLOGY

General Features

- Etiology
  - Primary congenital malformation vs. secondarily acquired morphologic changes
  - Primary: Posterior fossa underdevelopment theory is most common
  - Secondary: Premature closure of cranial sutures &/or generalized abnormal bone formation
    - Shunted infantile hydrocephalus
    - Calvarial thickening of bone dysplasias or thalassemia
    - Genetic syndromes
  - Seen in 2-10% of patients with idiopathic intracranial hypertension (a.k.a. pseudotumor cerebri)

CLINICAL ISSUES

Presentation

- Most common signs/symptoms
  - Occipital headache
    - Exacerbated by cough, Valsalva, neck extension, or physical exertion
  - Less common: Cerebellar, brainstem, bulbar, cord motor/sensory symptoms

Demographics

- True prevalence is unknown given how frequently Chiari 1 is picked up incidentally

Treatment

- Posterior fossa decompression (PFD): Suboccipital craniectomy with C1 laminectomy ± duraplasty, arachnoid opening/dissection, cerebellar tonsillar reduction/cautery
- Complex Chiari 1 may also require odontoid resection &/or craniocervical junction fusion
- Operative complications depend upon surgery
  - PFD: ~ 2% have CSF-related complications with ↑ reoperation rate
  - PFD + duraplasty: ~ 18% have CSF-related complications but ↓ reoperation rate
  - Most common: CSF leak, pseudomeningocele, infection
- Conservative management for asymptomatic or minimally symptomatic children without syrinx

DIAGNOSTIC CHECKLIST

Consider

- Degree of tonsillar descent does not always correlate with symptoms: Chiari 1 is frequently picked up incidentally

SELECTED REFERENCES

1. Alford EN et al: Imaging characteristics associated with surgery in Chiari malformation type I. J Neurosurg Pediatr. 1-9, 2021
2. Hiremath SB et al: The perplexity surrounding Chiari malformations - are we any wiser now? AJNR Am J Neuroradiol. 41(11):1975-81, 2020
3. Dangouloff-Ros V et al: Incidental brain MRI findings in children: a systematic review and meta-analysis. AJNR Am J Neuroradiol. 40(11):1818-23, 2019

KEY FACTS

TERMINOLOGY

- Constellation of intracranial findings, mainly hindbrain herniation, due to open spinal dysraphism [either myelomeningocele (MMC) or myelocele]

IMAGING

- Small posterior fossa: Cerebellum herniates downward through foramen magnum & upward through incisura
- Caudal brainstem herniation with cervicomedullary kink, tectal beaking
- ± ventriculomegaly
- Falx insufficiency, thickened massa intermedia, callosal dysgenesis, ↓ white matter volume
- ± subependymal gray matter heterotopias
- Lacunar skull (lückenschädel)

TOP DIFFERENTIAL DIAGNOSES

- Chiari 1 malformation
- Chiari 3 malformation
- Intracranial hypotension
- Severe, chronic shunted hydrocephalus

PATHOLOGY

- Secondary to sequelae of chronic in utero CSF leakage through open spinal dysraphism (4th fetal week)

CLINICAL ISSUES

- Lower extremity paresis/spasticity, bowel/bladder dysfunction, symptoms of brainstem compression (swallowing difficulties, stridor, apnea), epilepsy
- In utero repair of MMC ↓ need for postnatal CSF diversion (shunting) & may improve neurologic outcomes in some patients

DIAGNOSTIC CHECKLIST

- Confirm history of open spinal dysraphism before assigning Chiari 2 malformation
- Fetal surgery results in milder Chiari 2 phenotype with less hindbrain herniation

(Left) *Sagittal SSFP FIESTA MR of a 23-weeks-gestation fetus shows hindbrain herniation ➡ in the setting of an open sacral spinal dysraphism ➡, consistent with Chiari 2 malformation. Effacement of the 4th ventricle & cisterna magna is consistent with grade 3 Chiari 2 malformation based on fetal grading system.* **(Right)** *Axial SSFSE T2 MR in the same fetus demonstrates classic bifrontal concavity ➡ of the calvarium (a.k.a. lemon sign) & associated lateral ventriculomegaly. Note the effacement of subarachnoid CSF spaces.*

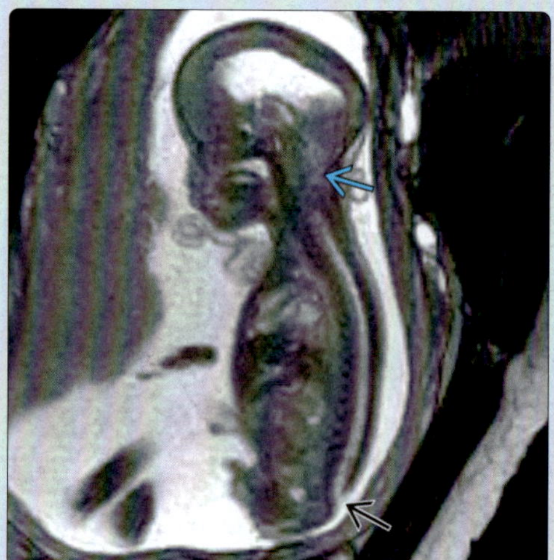

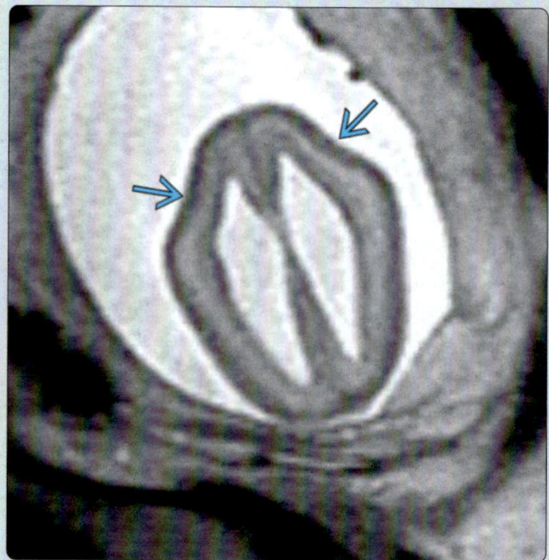

(Left) *Sagittal T2 MR in a 1-year-old after postnatal repair of a myelomeningocele (MMC) shows typical findings of Chiari 2 malformation, including cerebellar herniation ➡, elongated & effaced 4th ventricle ➡, tectal beaking ➡, enlarged massa intermedia ➡, & callosal hypogenesis ➡.* **(Right)** *Sagittal T1 MR in a 1-month-old status post prenatal repair of a MMC shows no hindbrain herniation. Other findings of Chiari 2 are present, including callosal hypogenesis ➡, large massa intermedia ➡, & tectal beaking ➡.*

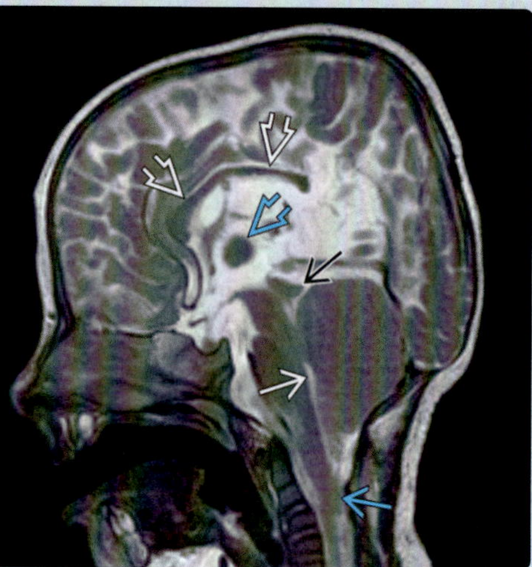

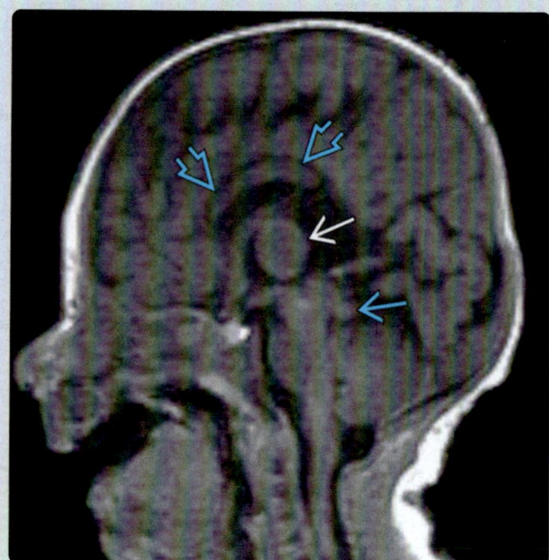

TERMINOLOGY

Definitions

- Constellation of intracranial anomalies, mainly hindbrain herniation, due to open spinal dysraphism [either myelomeningocele (MMC) or myelocele]

IMAGING

General Features

- Best diagnostic clue
  - Small posterior fossa (PF) with inferior cerebellar & brainstem herniation in presence of open spinal dysraphism

Radiographic Findings

- Radiography
  - Lacunar skull (lückenschädel) → numerous undulations of inner calvarium with focal thinning

MR Findings

- Infratentorial
  - Small PF with downward sloping tentorium, low torcular Herophili
  - Hindbrain herniation (postnatal repair)
    - Caudal descent of pointed cerebellar tonsils/vermis
    - Towering appearance of cerebellum with upward herniation through widened incisura
    - Elongated, effaced, inferiorly displaced 4th ventricle with flattened fastigium
    - Cerebellar hemispheres wrap around brainstem on axial images
  - Significant hindbrain herniation is unusual after prenatal repair
  - Tectal beaking, brainstem caudal displacement ± cervicomedullary kink
- Supratentorial
  - ± ventriculomegaly
  - Midline anomalies: Large massa intermedia, callosal hypogenesis/dysgenesis, absent septum pellucidum
  - ± neuronal migrational anomalies: Subependymal gray matter (GM) heterotopia (~ 25%), polymicrogyria (rare)
  - Falx insufficiency with interdigitation of hemispheric gyri
  - Stenogyria (elongated, compact gyri) after shunting (differs from polymicrogyria)

Ultrasonographic Findings

- Grayscale ultrasound
  - Prenatal US is key for early diagnosis
    - Lemon sign: Bifrontal concavity of calvarium
    - Banana sign: Cerebellum wraps around brainstem with effacement of cisterna magna

DIFFERENTIAL DIAGNOSIS

Chiari 1 Malformation

- Low pointed cerebellar tonsils effacing CSF at foramen magnum
- Absence of associated open spinal dysraphism
- None of associated supratentorial findings seen in Chiari 2

Chiari 3 Malformation

- PF contents herniate through suboccipital encephalocele + high cervical spinal dysraphism

Intracranial Hypotension

- Dural enhancement, venous sinus engorgement, ± subdural collections
- Typically in setting of CSF leak with postural headaches

Severe Chronically Shunted Hydrocephalus

- May cause collapsed & dysmorphic brain with upward cerebellar herniation

PATHOLOGY

General Features

- Etiology
  - Folate deficiency during pregnancy is leading preventable risk factor

Staging, Grading, & Classification

- Grading system for Chari 2 malformation on fetal MR is based on PF morphology
  - Grade 1: 4th ventricle & cisterna magna are patent
  - Grade 2: 4th ventricle is effaced, cisterna magna is patent
  - Grade 3: 4th ventricle & cisterna magna are effaced

CLINICAL ISSUES

Presentation

- Most common signs/symptoms
  - 80-90% develop hydrocephalus requiring shunting, though incidence is lower in those who undergo prenatal repair of open spinal dysraphism
  - Varying degrees of lower extremity paresis/spasticity, clubfoot, bowel/bladder dysfunction
  - ± epilepsy, symptoms from brainstem compression (swallowing difficulties, stridor, apnea)

Treatment

- Surgical management
  - MMC is classically repaired in first 48 hours after delivery
  - CSF diversion/shunting is classically required in 80-90%
  - PF decompression in those who do not improve with shunting
  - Fetal MMC repair in select patients
    - Must have hindbrain herniation & upper level of spinal defect T1-S1
    - Reduces need for shunting; may improve neurologic outcomes in some patients
    - Improved neurologic outcomes must be balanced with potential surgical risks (e.g., premature birth)

SELECTED REFERENCES

1. Khalaveh F et al: Myelomeningocele-Chiari II malformation-neurological predictability based on fetal and postnatal magnetic resonance imaging. Prenat Diagn. 41(8):922-32, 2021
2. Miller JL et al: Spinal dysraphia, Chiari 2 malformation, unified theory, and advances in fetoscopic repair. Neuroimaging Clin N Am. 29(3):357-66, 2019
3. Kim I et al: Decompression for Chiari malformation type II in individuals with myelomeningocele in the National Spina Bifida Patient Registry. J Neurosurg Pediatr. 22(6):652-8, 2018
4. Nagaraj UD et al: Hindbrain herniation in Chiari II malformation on fetal and postnatal MRI. AJNR Am J Neuroradiol. 38(5):1031-6, 2017

Aqueductal Stenosis

KEY FACTS

TERMINOLOGY

- Aqueductal stenosis (AS)

IMAGING

- Lateral & 3rd ventriculomegaly with normal 4th ventricle
- Obstruction of cerebral aqueduct ± tectal thickening
- Funnel-shaped enlargement of proximal cerebral aqueduct or diffuse ↓ caliber of entire aqueduct
- Absent CSF flow void in cerebral aqueduct in most cases
- Macrocephaly in fetus & infant
- Best imaging tool: MR with sagittal 3D SSFP/FISP/BTFE sequence to evaluate aqueduct

TOP DIFFERENTIAL DIAGNOSES

- Posthemorrhagic hydrocephalus
- Secondary obstructive hydrocephalus
- Supratentorial volume loss
- Communicating hydrocephalus

PATHOLOGY

- Congenital AS is common cause of fetal hydrocephalus
- Can be isolated or associated with genetic disorder
- Subsets include stenosis from tectal thickening, obstructing web/gliotic tissue, or forking

CLINICAL ISSUES

- May present at any time from birth to adulthood; bimodal distribution: 1st year of life vs. adolescence
- Fetus/infant: Macrocephaly, bulging fontanelle
- Older children: Headache, papilledema, 6th nerve palsy
- C-section may be required for prenatally diagnosed cases due to macrocephaly
- Preferred treatment → endoscopic 3rd ventriculostomy

DIAGNOSTIC CHECKLIST

- Identify associated brain anomalies, such as rhombencephalosynapsis
  - Important for prognosis

(Left) *Sagittal graphic shows obstructive hydrocephalus with a stretched (thinned) corpus callosum ➔ & a funnel-shaped cerebral aqueduct ➔ related to obstruction at its inferior aspect. This site of obstruction allows for a normal 4th ventricle but a depressed floor of the enlarged 3rd ventricle ➔.* **(Right)** *Sagittal SSFSE T2 MR of a fetus at 25-weeks gestation shows macrocephaly from aqueductal stenosis causing lateral & 3rd ventriculomegaly. There is no CSF in the cerebral aqueduct ➔.*

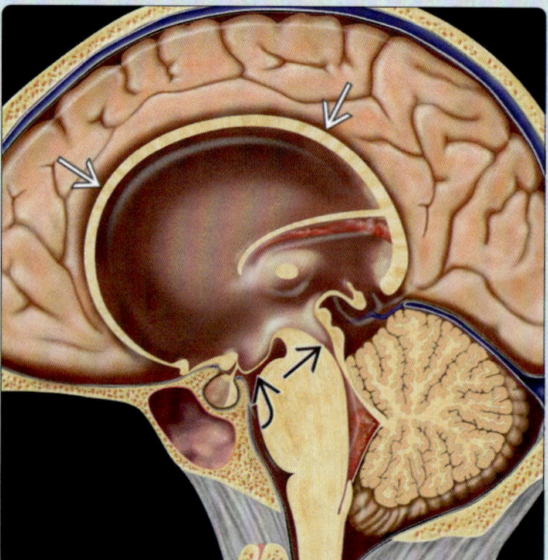

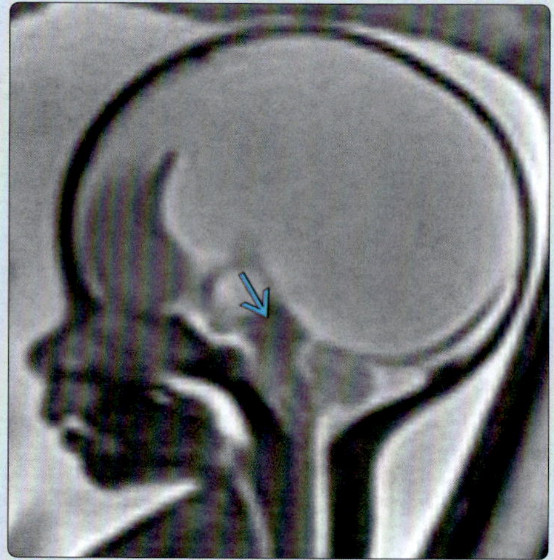

(Left) *Sagittal 3D SSFP MR in a 15-year-old girl with a several-year history of headaches & new generalized seizures shows aqueductal stenosis with an obstructing web ➔ at the inferior margin of the aqueduct.* **(Right)** *Axial T2 MR in the same patient shows ventriculomegaly of the lateral ➔ & 3rd ➔ ventricles. There is no periventricular edema as late-presentation cases are often offset by alternative microscopic pathways of CSF drainage.*

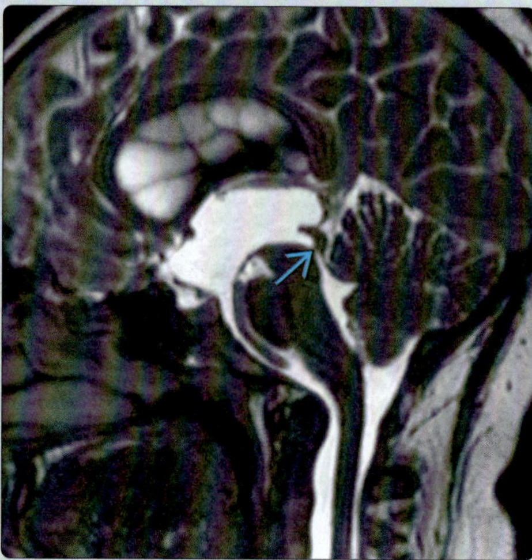

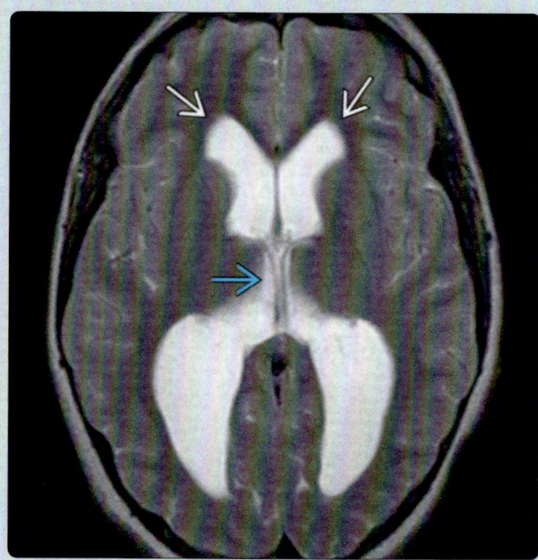

TERMINOLOGY

Definitions

- Aqueductal stenosis (AS): Lateral & 3rd ventriculomegaly due to complete or partial obstruction of CSF flow through cerebral aqueduct

IMAGING

General Features

- Best diagnostic clue
  - Lateral & 3rd ventriculomegaly with normal 4th ventricle

MR Findings

- T1WI
  - Enlargement of lateral & 3rd ventricles
    - Corpus callosum (CC) is thinned & stretched upward
    - ± lateral ventricular diverticulum (a.k.a. ventricular rupture or dehiscence)
    - Extraaxial CSF effacement
      - Limits ability to evaluate gyral-sulcal pattern
- T2WI
  - Funnel-shaped enlargement of proximal cerebral aqueduct or diffuse ↓ caliber of entire aqueduct
  - Typical CSF flow void in cerebral aqueduct is usually absent
  - ± tectal plate thickening
  - Septum pellucidum is often absent due to perforation
- MR cine
  - Phase-contrast imaging may demonstrate absent or diminished CSF flow in aqueduct
  - Useful in posttreatment setting to confirm patency of endoscopic 3rd ventriculostomy
- 3D SSFP/FISP/BTFE: Sagittal plane may demonstrate membrane/web or narrowed aqueduct

Ultrasonographic Findings

- Grayscale ultrasound
  - Lateral & 3rd ventriculomegaly in newborn with macrocephaly
  - Obstetrical ultrasound may permit prenatal diagnosis
    - Usually severe lateral ventriculomegaly (> 15 mm)

Imaging Recommendations

- Best imaging tool
  - Multiplanar MR with sagittal 3D SSFP/FISP/BTFE (i.e., FIESTA, CISS, etc.) to evaluate aqueduct

DIFFERENTIAL DIAGNOSIS

Posthemorrhagic Hydrocephalus

- Most common cause of acquired hydrocephalus in infancy
- Look for blood products in ventricles & cerebral aqueduct

Secondary Obstructive Hydrocephalus

- Cause of obstruction extrinsic to aqueduct: Tumor, vascular lesion, etc.

Supratentorial Volume Loss

- Normal or ↓ head circumference
- Extraaxial CSF spaces should not be effaced

Communicating Hydrocephalus

- Secondary to impaired absorption of CSF in subarachnoid spaces rather than anatomic obstruction
- Causes include meningitis, leptomeningeal metastatic disease, venous hypertension

PATHOLOGY

General Features

- Etiology
  - AS pathologically obstructs CSF flow into 4th ventricle
    - CSF production in choroid plexus continues → ↑ CSF pressure → lateral & 3rd ventriculomegaly
- Genetics
  - X-linked hydrocephalus
    - One of most common inherited causes of AS
- Associated abnormalities
  - Rhombencephalosynapsis
    - Up to 65% have coexisting AS

CLINICAL ISSUES

Presentation

- Most common signs/symptoms
  - Symptoms depend on patient age at time of diagnosis
  - Onset can be insidious in older patients
- Other signs/symptoms
  - Fetus/infants: Macrocrania
  - Older patients: Headache, papilledema, 6th nerve palsy

Demographics

- Age
  - 2 peaks: 1st year of life (more common) vs. adolescence
- Epidemiology
  - AS is responsible for ~ 20% of congenital hydrocephalus

Natural History & Prognosis

- Hydrocephalus is usually progressive unless treated
  - May stabilize as compensated hydrocephalus
- Isolated congenital AS has much better prognosis than AS with genetic disorder or other brain anomalies

Treatment

- Endoscopic 3rd ventriculostomy (preferred) vs. CSF diversion by shunt
- Fetal cases may require C-section due to macrocephaly

DIAGNOSTIC CHECKLIST

Consider

- Look for coexisting brain anomalies that affect prognosis

SELECTED REFERENCES

1. Mirsky DM et al: Imaging of fetal ventriculomegaly. Pediatr Radiol. 50(13):1948-58, 2020
2. Heaphy-Henault KJ et al: Congenital aqueductal stenosis: findings at fetal mri that accurately predict a postnatal diagnosis. AJNR Am J Neuroradiol. 39(5):942-8, 2018
3. Kline-Fath BM et al: Congenital aqueduct stenosis: progressive brain findings in utero to birth in the presence of severe hydrocephalus. Prenat Diagn. 38(9):706-12, 2018

Neurofibromatosis Type 1

KEY FACTS

IMAGING

- Nonenhancing T2/FLAIR MR hyperintense lesions
  - 60-85% of children with neurofibromatosis type 1 (NF1)
  - Characteristic sites: Globus pallidus, cerebellar WM
  - Little/no mass effect, no enhancement
  - Higher lesion burden may ↓ cognitive functioning
  - ↓ with puberty, resolved by adulthood
- Optic pathway glioma (OPG)
  - 15-20% of children with NF1
  - Anywhere from optic nerve (ON) through optic radiations
  - Fusiform to lobular in shape, ± ON tortuosity
  - ± contrast enhancement
- Plexiform neurofibromas (PNF)
  - Lobular infiltrating soft tissue masses
  - Target appearance in cross section on T2 MR
  - Orbital PNFs are associated with sphenoid wing defects
- Vascular dysplasia (moyamoya arteriopathy)
  - 3-7% of children with NF1
  - Vessel narrowing (especially distal ICA) with collaterals

PATHOLOGY

- *NF1* gene locus on long arm of chromosome 17
- Autosomal dominant; 50% are new mutations
- Variable expression, virtually 100% penetrance

CLINICAL ISSUES

- 1:3,000-5,000 people have NF1
- NF1-related learning disability in 30-60%
- OPG & brainstem gliomas have more indolent behavior in NF1 compared to non-NF1 patients
  - OPG is typically not progressive; treatment in ~ 15%
- Phenotype is quite variable: Can be dominated by peripheral, paraspinal, or intracranial lesions

DIAGNOSTIC CHECKLIST

- Include dedicated imaging of orbits with all brain MR scans
- Look closely for vascular dysplasia

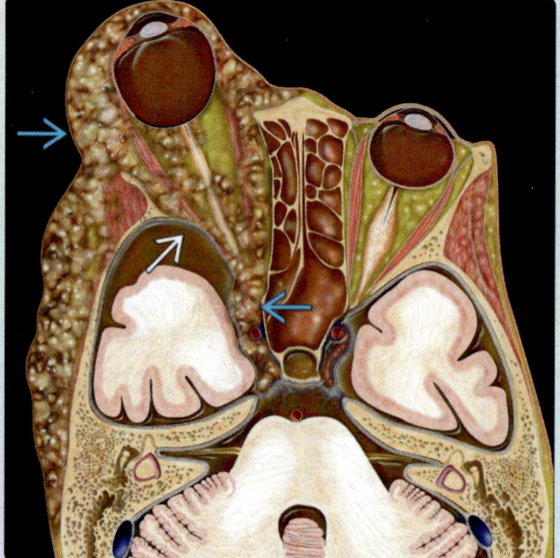

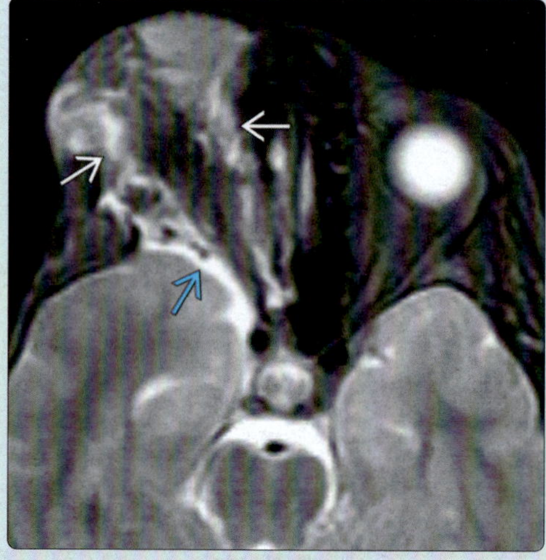

(Left) *Axial graphic of the orbits shows an infiltrating plexiform neurofibroma (PNF) extending from the cavernous sinus through the orbit with associated "dysplasia" of the sphenoid wing.* **(Right)** *Axial T2 FS MR in a 12-year-old girl with NF1 shows a large infiltrating hyperintense lesion in the right orbit, consistent with a PFN. Note the absence of the greater sphenoid wing, consistent with sphenoid wing dysplasia. Such osseous changes in the sphenoid occur almost exclusively in the setting of a PFN.*

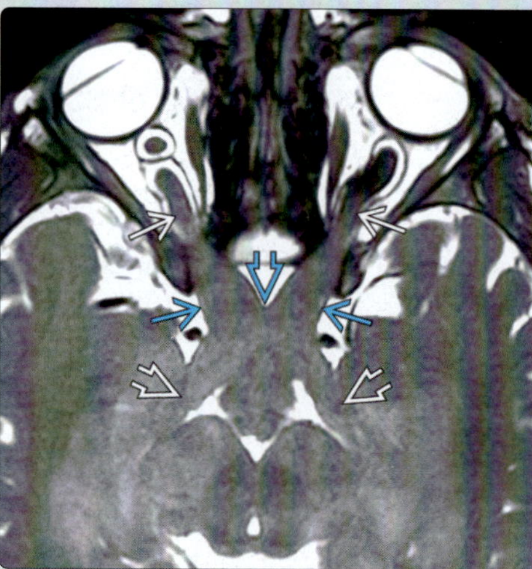

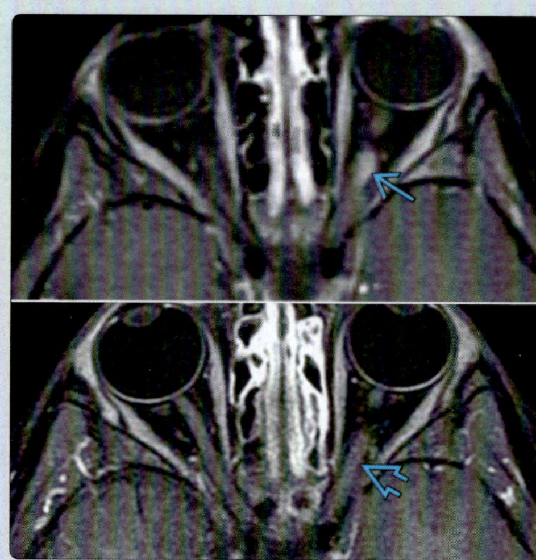

(Left) *Axial MIP of a 3D CISS MR in a 3-year-old with NF1 shows enlargement & tortuosity of the orbital & prechiasmatic optic nerves, optic chiasm, & optic tracts, consistent with an OPG.* **(Right)** *Axial T1 C+ FS MRs show a patient with NF1 at 3 years (top) & 6 years (bottom) of age. The initial image shows mild enlargement & marked enhancement of the left orbital optic nerve, consistent with an OPG. Without any therapy, the lesion has resolved spontaneously over a 3-year period.*

TERMINOLOGY

Abbreviations

- Neurofibromatosis type 1 (NF1)

Synonyms

- von Recklinghausen disease

Definitions

- Neurocutaneous disorder (phakomatosis) characterized by
  - Nonenhancing T2/FLAIR MR signal abnormalities at characteristic brain locations
    - Unidentified bright objects (UBOs) or focal abnormal signal intensities (FASI)
  - Plexiform neurofibromas (PNF) of soft tissues
    - Differ from diffuse & localized neurofibromas (NF)
  - Astrocytomas, primarily optic pathway glioma (OPG)
  - Vascular dysplasias (moyamoya arteriopathy)
  - Skeletal dysplastic lesions
  - Café au lait spots of skin

IMAGING

General Features

- **Nonenhancing T2/FLAIR MR hyperintense lesions**
  - 60-85% of children with NF1
  - Commonly found in deep gray matter (especially globus pallidus & thalamus), hippocampus, brainstem, cerebellar white matter (WM)
  - Hyperintense on T2/FLAIR, little/no mass effect
  - Often inapparent on T1 & CT
  - No enhancement
  - Characteristic time course
    - Not present in first 1-2 years of life
    - ↑ in number/size in younger children
    - ↓ in teenage years; usually resolved by adulthood
- **Increased WM volume**
  - Macrocephaly &/or thickened corpus callosum
- **OPG**
  - Occur in ~ 15-20% of children with NF1
  - Anywhere from optic nerves through optic radiations
  - Fusiform enlargement ± enhancement
    - Tortuosity in orbit: Dotted i sign on axial images
- **Plexiform neurofibroma**
  - Infiltrating soft tissue lobules along peripheral nerves
  - Hyperintense on T2/STIR MR
    - Target sign in cross section (central hypointensity)
  - Variable enhancement, classically central
- **Sphenoid wing dysplasia**
  - Almost always associated with orbital PNF
  - Distortion/absence of lateral orbital wall with anterior expansion of middle cranial fossa
- **Lambdoid defect**
  - Absence of bone along lambdoid suture
- **Vascular dysplasia (moyamoya arteriopathy)**
  - Occurs in 3-7% of children with NF1
  - Vessel narrowing (especially distal internal carotid artery) with collateral formation

CT Findings

- NECT
  - Bone defects of sphenoid wing & lambdoid suture
  - Enlargement of ON, chiasm, superior orbital fissure
- CECT
  - ± enhancement in OPG
  - PNFs typically have little enhancement
- CTA
  - May be best test to determine degree of stenosis in moyamoya arteriopathy

MR Findings

- T1WI
  - Thick corpus callosum on sagittal images
  - OPG: Enlargement of optic nerve & chiasm
  - PNF: Isointense to brain/cord
  - May see hyperintense globus pallidus & dentate nuclei in older patients who have had multiple gadolinium administrations from prior screening MRs
    - Pathologically proven to represent gadolinium deposition
- T2WI
  - Poorly defined, round, or ovoid hyperintense WM lesions in characteristic locations
- T2WI FS
  - OPG may have hyperintense signal
- STIR
  - Helpful to identify soft tissue PNFs
- FLAIR
  - Best sequence to identify nonenhancing parenchymal signal abnormalities
- DWI
  - ↑ ADC values in nonenhancing signal abnormalities
- T1WI C+
  - PNF & OPG have variable enhancement patterns that often change over time
  - Parenchymal signal abnormalities should not enhance (which would suggest gliomatous degeneration)
- MRA
  - Major cerebral artery narrowing (especially carotid terminus) in moyamoya arteriopathy
- MRS
  - Can help distinguish nonenhancing signal abnormalities from glioma
    - Nonenhancing signal abnormalities → ↑ myoinositol (mI), preserved NAA
    - Glioma → ↑ choline, ↓ NAA

Angiographic Findings

- Typically reserved for cases of moyamoya arteriopathy where revascularization is contemplated

Imaging Recommendations

- Best imaging tool
  - Brain/orbits MR C+
- Protocol advice
  - Dedicated orbital protocol to include T1 C+ FS MR for optimal detection of OPG & orbital PNF
  - Thin-section T2 or MRA for vascular dysplasia
  - 3D volumetric analysis is helpful for treatment surveillance

DIFFERENTIAL DIAGNOSIS

Neurocutaneous Syndromes: Phakomatoses

- **Tuberous sclerosis complex (TSC)**
  - Dysplasias (a.k.a. tubers) + subependymal nodules
- **Sturge-Weber syndrome (SWS)**
  - Retinal & pial angiomatosis with focal/lobar cerebral atrophy due to abnormal cerebral venous drainage
- **Neurofibromatosis type 2 (NF2)**
  - Multiple schwannomas, meningiomas, & ependymomas
- **PHACE(S)**
  - **P**osterior fossa malformations, infantile **h**emangiomas, **a**rterial anomalies, **c**ardiac anomalies, **e**ye anomalies, & **s**ternal clefting
- **von Hippel-Lindau disease (VHL)**
  - Hemangioblastomas, retinal angiomas, renal cysts & carcinomas, pancreatic cysts & tumors
- **Other phakomatoses**
  - Multiple others, including ataxia-telangiectasia, neurocutaneous melanosis, incontinentia pigmenti, basal cell nevus syndrome

PATHOLOGY

General Features

- Genetics
  - *NF1* gene locus lies on long arm of chromosome 17
    - Neurofibromin, inactivated in NF1 → allows cellular proliferation & tumor development
      - Neurofibromin: RAS GTPase-activating protein responsible for tumor suppression
    - Oligodendrocyte myelin glycoprotein lies within *NF1* gene
      - May cause myelin dysplasia UBOs & FASIs
  - Autosomal dominant; 50% are new mutations
  - Variable expression; virtually 100% penetrance
- Associated abnormalities
  - Pheochromocytomas, malignant peripheral nerve sheath tumors (MPNST)

Staging, Grading, & Classification

- NF1 if ≥ 2 of following
  - ≥ 6 skin café au lait spots, > 5 mm
  - ≥ 2 NF or 1 PNF
  - Axillary/inguinal freckling
  - Optic nerve glioma
  - Distinctive bone lesion
  - Primary relative with NF1

Gross Pathologic & Surgical Features

- Visual pathway glioma is usually low grade
  - Can extend to geniculate bodies & optic radiations
  - Perichiasmatic infiltration → more likely to be aggressive, ↑ frequency of precocious puberty
- Lisch nodules (iris hamartomas) in 85% > 10 years old
- Buphthalmos (globe)

Microscopic Features

- Nonenhancing T2/FLAIR MR hyperintense lesions: Foci of "myelin vacuolization"; no inflammation/demyelination
- PNF: Schwann cells, perineural fibroblasts, growth along nerve fascicles

CLINICAL ISSUES

Presentation

- Most common signs/symptoms
  - > 95% have skin lesions
  - > 95% have Lisch nodules (adults)
  - ~ 50% have macrocephaly → ↑ WM volume
  - > 30% have learning disabilities
  - ~ 15% have scoliosis
  - ~ 15% have OPG
- Phenotype is quite variable: Can be dominated by peripheral, paraspinal, or intracranial lesions

Demographics

- Age
  - Café au lait spots appear in 1st year of life
  - OPG usually occurs in 1st few years
    - Median age at diagnosis: 3 years
    - If no OPG is identified before 15 months, patient is unlikely to develop symptomatic OPG
- Epidemiology
  - Most common autosomal dominant disorder
  - 1:3,000-5,000 people have NF1

Natural History & Prognosis

- NF1-related learning disability in 30-60%
  - May be associated with ↑ number of characteristic T2/FLAIR MR parenchymal lesions
- 1-3% risk of other CNS glial tumors
  - Typically low grade in children, higher grade in adults
- 8-13% lifetime risk of MPNST
- Vascular dysplasia: If progressive, may cause ischemic injury
- OPG typically has indolent course with observation being sufficient in most cases
  - Chiasmatic & postchiasmatic are more likely to progress than prechiasmatic
  - Small percentage resolve spontaneously

Treatment

- Observation/surveillance is sufficient unless symptoms arise
- PNF: Debulking surgery if symptomatic, though not preferable, as tumor cannot be separated from nerves
  - MEK inhibitors (e.g., selumetinib) for inoperable lesions
- OPG: ~ 15% require chemotherapy for progression
  - Decision to treat is based on combination of clinical & radiologic findings
- Moyamoya arteriopathy: Surgical revascularization

DIAGNOSTIC CHECKLIST

Image Interpretation Pearls

- Remember to look for vascular lesions
- Signal abnormalities with mass effect, enhancement, or atypical location should be viewed with suspicion

SELECTED REFERENCES

1. Batchala PP et al: Imaging of tumor syndromes. Radiol Clin North Am. 59(3):471-500, 2021
2. de Blank PMK et al: Optic pathway gliomas in neurofibromatosis type 1: an update: surveillance, treatment indications, and biomarkers of vision. J Neuroophthalmol. 37 Suppl 1:S23-32, 2017

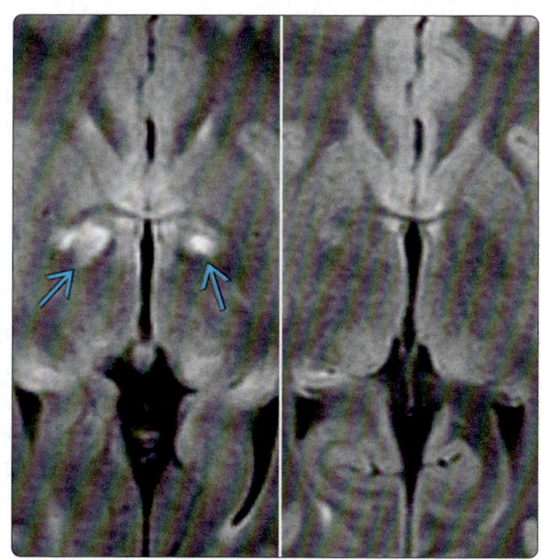

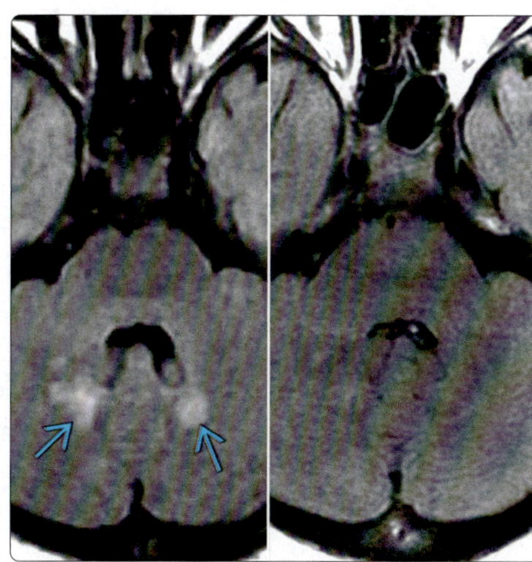

(Left) *Axial FLAIR MRs in a patient with NF1 at 10 (L) & 15 (R) years of age show interval near-complete resolution of the characteristic nonenhancing signal abnormalities ➔ within the globus pallidus nuclei.* **(Right)** *Axial FLAIR MRs in a patient with NF1 at 10 (L) & 15 (R) years of age show interval near-complete resolution of the nonenhancing signal abnormalities ➔ within the cerebellar white matter & dentate nuclei. These signal abnormalities typically resolve in the late teenage years.*

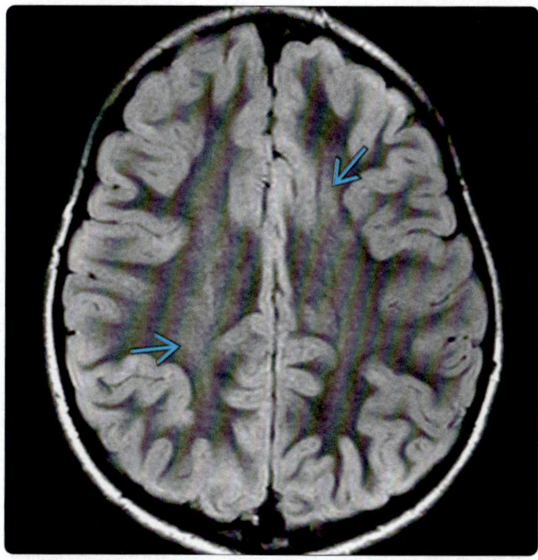

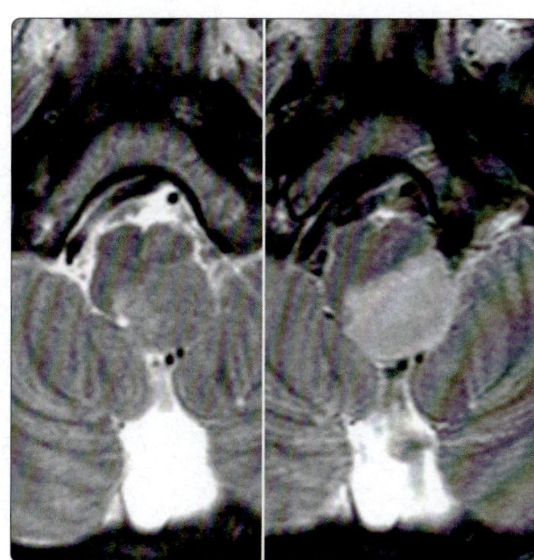

(Left) *Axial FLAIR MR in an 8-year-old with NF1 shows nearly symmetric ↑ signal intensity within the centrum semiovale ➔ without volume loss. This degree of delayed/abnormal myelination is uncommon, though mildly delayed myelination is frequently seen in younger NF1 patients.* **(Right)** *Axial T2 MRs in a patient with NF1 at 6 (L) & 9 (R) years of age show minimal change in the lesion size over time. Brainstem masses in NF1 typically have a more indolent behavior than brainstem masses seen in otherwise healthy individuals.*

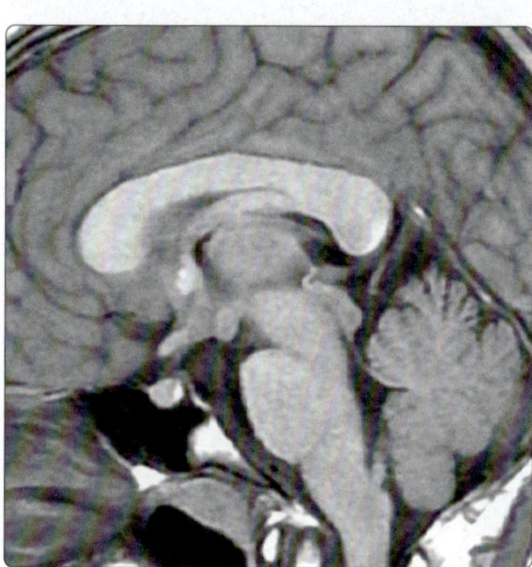

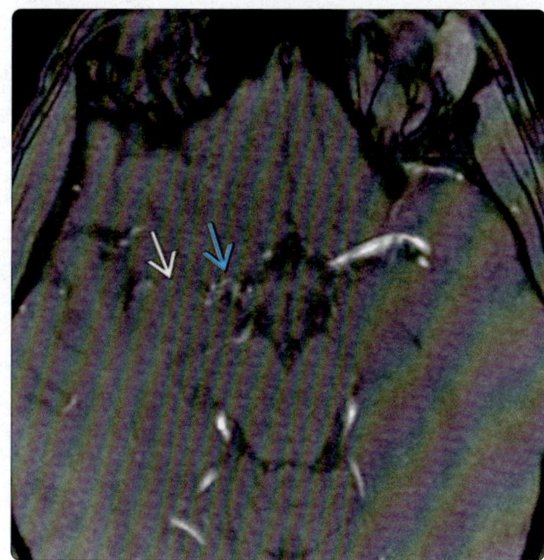

(Left) *Sagittal T1 MR in a 15-year-old with NF1 shows a diffusely thickened corpus callosum with normal signal. On average, NF1 patients have higher corpus callosum volumes compared to normal subjects.* **(Right)** *Axial 3D TOF MRA in a 14-year-old with NF1 shows a complete lack of flow-related signal in the right middle cerebral artery ➔ with multiple small collateral vessels ➔ in the expected region of the M1 segment, consistent with moyamoya arteriopathy. Moyamoya arteriopathy is seen in 3-7% of patients with NF1.*

Tuberous Sclerosis

KEY FACTS

TERMINOLOGY

- Tuberous sclerosis complex (TSC): Hamartomas of multiple organs → CNS, skin, kidney, bone

IMAGING

- Cerebral tubers
  - Cortical/subcortical lesion expanding overlying gyrus
  - T2/FLAIR hyperintense, T1 hypointense after myelination
    - T1 hyperintense prior to myelination
- Cerebellar tubers
  - Wedge-shaped foci of volume loss
  - More likely to enhance & calcify
- Subependymal nodules (SENs)
  - Elongated nodules in locations of fetal germinal matrix
  - ↑ Ca^{2+} over time
  - 30-80% enhance
- Subependymal giant cell astrocytoma (SEGA)
  - Growing nodule at caudothalamic groove
  - WHO grade 1 neoplasm

TOP DIFFERENTIAL DIAGNOSES

- Focal cortical dysplasia
- Dysembryoplastic neuroepithelial tumor
- Ganglioglioma
- TORCH infections that cause periventricular Ca^{2+}
- X-linked subependymal heterotopia

PATHOLOGY

- 2 distinct gene loci
  - *TSC1* (9q34) encodes hamartin
  - *TSC2* (16p13) encodes tuberin → more severe

CLINICAL ISSUES

- Medical antiseizure therapy, resection of seizure focus
- mTOR inhibitors are now 1st-line therapy for SEGA

DIAGNOSTIC CHECKLIST

- Tubers + SEN → pathognomonic for TSC
- Surveillance imaging is performed to detect SEGA

(Left) *Axial FLAIR MR of a 6-year-old girl with tuberous sclerosis complex (TSC) shows a moderate to severe burden of cerebral tubers ➔. Tubers are dysplastic lesions that are present in nearly all patients with TSC. After the brain is myelinated, FLAIR is the most sensitive sequence for tuber detection.* **(Right)** *Axial T1 C+ MR in the same patient shows a wedge-shaped, enhancing right cerebellar tuber ➔. Cerebellar tubers differ from cerebral tubers in that volume loss, Ca^{2+}, & enhancement are very common.*

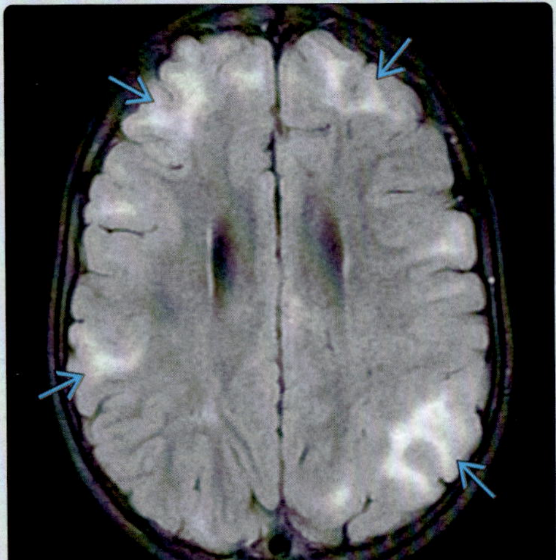

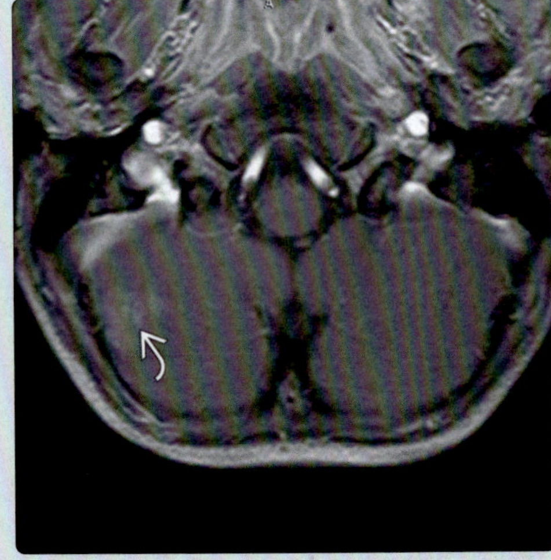

(Left) *Axial T1 C+ MR in a 4-year-old boy with TSC shows a lobular, homogeneously enhancing mass ➔ in the right caudothalamic groove, consistent with a subependymal giant cell astrocytoma (SEGA).* **(Right)** *Axial NECT in the same patient 1 year after resection of the SEGA (note the surgical tract ➔) shows multiple calcified subependymal nodules ➔. The location of the subependymal nodules adheres to the anatomic distribution of fetal germinal matrix with a preponderance in the caudothalamic grooves.*

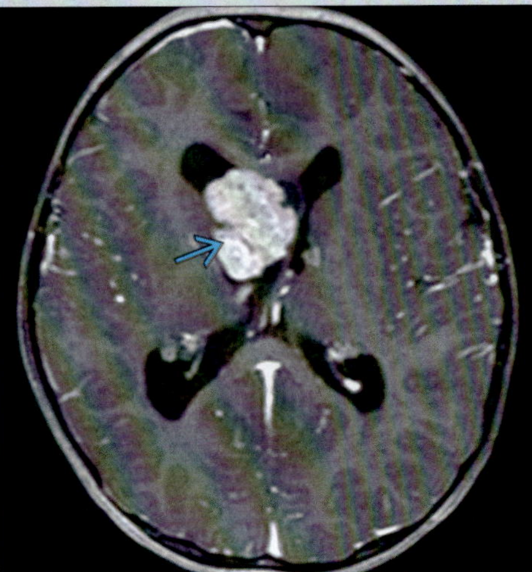

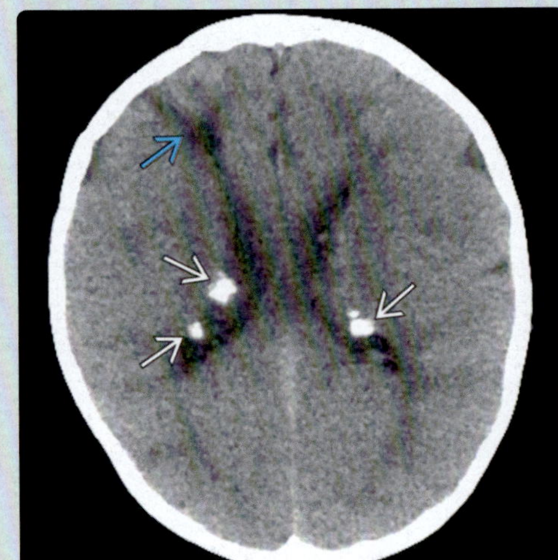

TERMINOLOGY

Synonyms

- Tuberous sclerosis complex (TSC), Bourneville syndrome, Pringle disease

Definitions

- Neurocutaneous syndrome: Hamartomatosis
  - Hamartomas of multiple organs → CNS, skin, kidney, bone

IMAGING

General Features

- Best diagnostic clue
  - Cerebral & cerebellar "tubers"
  - Subependymal nodules (SENs)
  - Subependymal giant cell astrocytoma (SEGA)

Tubers

- Cerebral
  - Cortical/subcortical tubers expand overlying gyri
  - Hyperintense on T2/FLAIR, hypointense on T1 MR
    - T1 hyperintense prior to myelination
  - Typically hypoattenuating on CT
  - Subcortical cystic degeneration in tubers → "empty gyrus"
  - Often associated with radial migration lines extending toward lateral ventricles
  - 3-4% enhance; 50% calcify (by age 10)
- Cerebellar
  - Typically wedge-shaped with volume loss & folia distortion
  - Many show enhancement (33-92%)
  - Many calcify (29%)

SEN

- Located in areas of fetal germinal matrix with preponderance in caudothalamic grooves
- Caudothalamic groove > body/atrium > temporal horn
- ↑ Ca^{2+} over time; 30-80% enhance

SEGA

- Growing nodule at caudothalamic groove
  - NAA ↓, choline ↑ compared to SEN
  - WHO grade 1 neoplasm
- Irregular & diffuse enhancement
- Can cause obstructive hydrocephalus

Other Lesions

- Cerebral aneurysms (0.78%) & dolichoectasia
- Retinal hamartoma
- Renal angiomyolipoma (AML)
- Lymphangioleiomyomatosis (LAM)
- Cardiac rhabdomyoma

Imaging Recommendations

- Best imaging tool
  - Traditionally: MR with contrast
    - Recent studies suggest contrast is likely not necessary for detection of SEGAs

DIFFERENTIAL DIAGNOSIS

Infection

- TORCH infections that cause periventricular Ca^{2+}
  - Cytomegalovirus (CMV), toxoplasmosis
  - Periventricular, not subependymal

Neoplasms

- Superficial tumors that can resemble tubers
- Intraventricular tumors

Cortical Dysplasia

- Focal cortical dysplasia, especially type II

X-Linked Subependymal Heterotopia

- Gray matter heterotopia along lateral ventricle margins
- No Ca^{2+} or enhancement

PATHOLOGY

General Features

- Etiology
  - Tuberin & hamartin combine to form complex in vivo
    - Act together to regulate mTOR pathway
      - **M**ammalian **t**arget **o**f **r**apamycin
    - Regulate cell growth & proliferation
  - Mutations prevent them from downregulating mTOR
  - Affects germinal matrix → disordered neuronal migration & growth
- Genetics
  - 2 distinct gene loci
    - *TSC1* (9q34) encodes hamartin
    - *TSC2* (16p13) encodes tuberin
    - *TSC2* is most common with severe phenotype
      - More likely to have complex partial seizures, infantile spasms, SEGAs, & intellectual disability

Staging, Grading, & Classification

- Diagnostic criteria: 2 major (definite) or 1 major + 1 minor (probable)
  - Major: Tuber, SEN, SEGA, cardiac rhabdomyoma, renal AML, LAM, adenoma sebaceum, sub-/periungual fibroma, hypomelanotic macules, shagreen patch, retinal hamartoma
  - Minor: WM lesions, dental pits, gingival fibromas, rectal polyps, bone cysts, nonrenal hamartoma, retinal achromic patch, confetti skin lesions, multiple renal cysts

CLINICAL ISSUES

Treatment

- Medical antiseizure therapy, resection of seizure focus
- mTOR inhibitors are now 1st-line therapy for SEGA

SELECTED REFERENCES

1. Gaillard AL et al: Magnetic resonance imaging diagnosis of subependymal giant cell astrocytomas in follow-up of children with tuberous sclerosis complex: should we always use contrast enhancement? Pediatr Radiol. 50(10):1397-408, 2020
2. Gül Mert G et al: Factors affecting epilepsy prognosis in patients with tuberous sclerosis. Childs Nerv Syst. 35(3):463-8, 2019
3. Curatolo P et al: Management of epilepsy associated with tuberous sclerosis complex: updated clinical recommendations. Eur J Paediatr Neurol. 22(5):738-48, 2018

Sturge-Weber Syndrome

KEY FACTS

TERMINOLOGY

- Syndrome of abnormal cortical venous development
- Imaging features result from progressive venous occlusion, recruitment of alternate drainage pathways, & chronic venous ischemia

IMAGING

- **CT**: Gyral/subcortical Ca^{2+} → tram-track appearance
    - ± calvarial thickening & sinus hyperpneumatization
- **MR**: Regions of atrophy ± abnormal myelination
    - **T2**: Flow voids in enlarged deep/transcerebral veins
    - **FLAIR**: Atrophied lobe(s) ± bright sulcal signal of leptomeningeal angiomatosis
    - **SWI/T2* GRE**: ↓ cortical/subcortical signal from Ca^{2+}
    - **T1 C+**: Enhancing leptomeningeal angiomatosis
        - Abundant medullary & deep draining veins
        - Choroidal globe enhancement of angioma
    - **MRV**: Absent normal cortical veins in affected region
    - **PWI**: ↑ perfusion early, ↓ perfusion late
- **FDG PET**: Progressive ↓ metabolism in affected brain

TOP DIFFERENTIAL DIAGNOSES

- Acquired meningeal processes
- PHACE(S) syndrome
- Blue rubber bleb nevus syndrome
- Meningioangiomatosis

CLINICAL ISSUES

- Seizures (75-90%), hemiparesis (30-66%)
    - Holohemispheric/bilateral angiomatosis (10-20%) → worse than focal involvement
- Forehead cutaneous capillary malformation (port-wine stain) in ~ 95%
- Choroidal angioma in 70% → glaucoma
- Treatment: Aggressive seizure control, resection/hemispherectomy for intractable epilepsy
- MR in early infancy may be normal: Recommend follow-up if patient is at risk for Sturge-Weber syndrome clinically

(Left) *Axial NECT in an 11-year-old girl with intractable epilepsy shows bilateral (right > left) subcortical Ca^{2+} →, characteristic of Sturge-Weber syndrome.* **(Right)** *Axial T1 C+ FS MR in the same patient shows bilateral leptomeningeal enhancement → & enlargement of the right choroid plexus →. Note the low signal within the subcortical white matter at the depth of sulci →, consistent with Ca^{2+}. There is mildly ↑ right calvarial thickness → secondary to underlying brain parenchymal volume loss.*

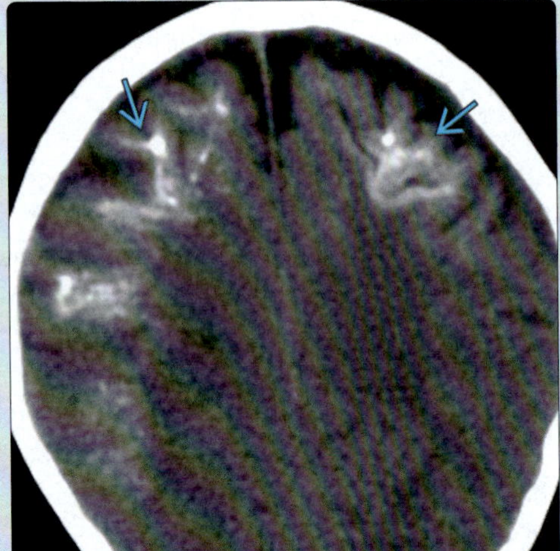

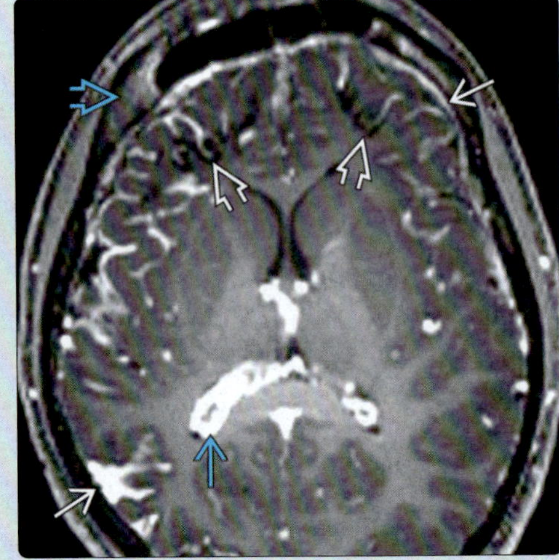

(Left) *Axial T2 MR in a 10-year-old boy with right-sided hemiplegia & seizures shows marked parenchymal volume loss & low signal → corresponding to an area of cortical/subcortical Ca^{2+} seen on CT. Also note the ipsilateral enlarged deep draining vein →.* **(Right)** *Axial T1 C+ MR in the same patient shows extensive left cerebral leptomeningeal enhancement → with multiple prominent medullary veins → & a large subependymal draining vein →. The enlargement of the left lateral ventricle is due to left cerebral volume loss.*

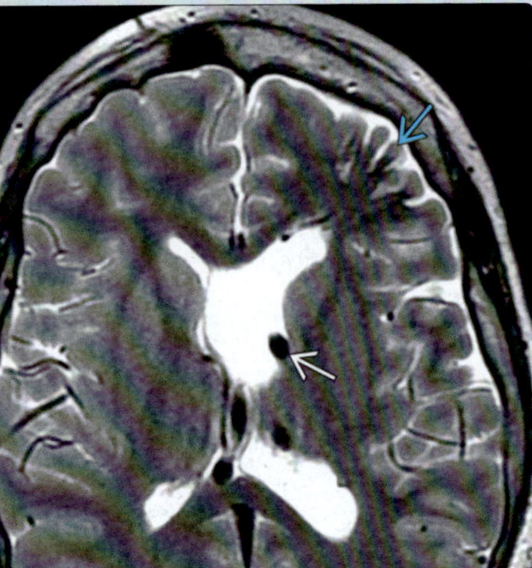

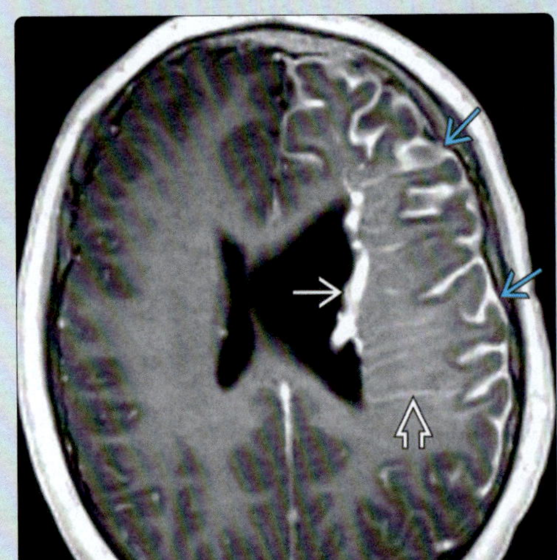

TERMINOLOGY

Abbreviations

- Sturge-Weber syndrome (SWS)

Definitions

- Congenital (but not inherited) syndrome in which cortical veins fail to develop normally, leading to numerous long-term intracranial manifestations of chronic ischemia & expanded alternate routes of venous drainage

IMAGING

General Features

- Best diagnostic clue
  - Cerebral lobar atrophy with cortical/subcortical Ca^{2+}, leptomeningeal enhancement, & enlarged ipsilateral choroid plexus in patient with V1 port-wine stain
- Location
  - Leptomeningeal angiomatosis is unilateral in 80-90%, bilateral in 10-20%

CT Findings

- NECT
  - Gyral/subcortical Ca^{2+} (may have tram-track appearance)
    - Progressive process, usually not present in very young
  - Calvarial thickening & hyperpneumatization of sinuses

MR Findings

- **T1**: Altered ("accelerated") white matter (WM) myelination in young patients
- **T2**: Hypointense subcortical signal of Ca^{2+} at depth of sulci; ↓ WM signal of accelerated myelination &/or low oxygen tension; enlarged deep vein flow voids
- **FLAIR**: Gliosis is often seen late in affected regions
- **SWI/T2* GRE**: ↓ cortical/subcortical signal (Ca^{2+})
  - SWI: Most sensitive to transcerebral medullary collaterals
- **T1 C+**: Leptomeningeal enhancement (angiomatosis)
  - Late stage: ↓ leptomeningeal enhancement, atrophy
  - Choroidal globe enhancement (choroidal angioma)
- **MRA**: Normal early but ↓ artery size in affected areas later
- **MRV**: Absent cortical veins in affected region
  - ↑ size of medullary & deep draining veins
- **Perfusion imaging (arterial spin labeling & contrast perfusion)**
  - Early: ↑ perfusion in affected regions
  - Late: ↓ perfusion in affected regions
    - ↓ perfusion associated with frequent seizures, ↑ duration of epilepsy, & brain atrophy

Nuclear Medicine Findings

- **FDG PET**: Progressive hypometabolism in affected regions
- **SPECT**: Hyperperfusion (early), hypoperfusion (late) on interictal scans
- Note that ictal scans (which may be intentional on SPECT or unintentional on FDG PET) will show ↑ activity

Imaging Recommendations

- Protocol advice
  - MR C+: May be normal at early age; consider follow-up
    - FLAIR C+ improves detection of leptomeningeal angiomatosis
    - Perfusion may predict progression

DIFFERENTIAL DIAGNOSIS

Acquired Meningeal Processes

- Meningitis, tumor spread, hemorrhage, high inspired oxygen content of CSF (usually with anesthesia)

PHACE(S) Syndrome

- **P**osterior fossa malformations, infantile **h**emangiomas, **a**rterial anomalies, **c**oarctation of aorta, **c**ardiac, **e**ye, & **e**ternal anomalies
- Segmental hemangioma of face is not fully present at birth

Blue Rubber Bleb Nevus Syndrome

- Multiple small soft tissue venous malformations + intracranial developmental venous anomalies

Klippel-Trenaunay Syndrome

- Extremity overgrowth with extensive capillary-venous-lymphatic malformations & abnormal deep venous system

Meningioangiomatosis

- Rare meningovascular hamartomatous plaque-like mass ± Ca^{2+} & cyst formation

PATHOLOGY

General Features

- Sporadic: Mosaic somatic mutation in gene *GNAQ* (9q21)

CLINICAL ISSUES

Presentation

- Most common signs/symptoms
  - Seizures (75-90%), hemiparesis (30-66%)
  - Stroke-like episodes, neurological deficit, headaches, & intellectual disability
  - Facial capillary malformation (port-wine stain) in ~ 95%
    - V1 distribution is classic
  - Choroidal angioma (70%), especially with eyelid stain
    - ↑ intraocular pressure/congenital glaucoma → buphthalmos in young

Demographics

- Rare: 1:20,000-50,000
- Seizures typically develop in 1st year of life

Natural History & Prognosis

- Seizures exacerbate vascular compromise to affected brain → progressive brain injury
- Holohemispheric &/or bilateral involvement is worse compared with focal involvement

Treatment

- Presymptomatic: Some recommend low-dose aspirin ± anticonvulsant
- Symptomatic: Aggressive medical management of seizures
- Symptomatic & medically refractory: Consider surgical resection/hemispherectomy

SELECTED REFERENCES

1. Sabeti S et al: Consensus statement for the management and treatment of sturge-weber syndrome: neurology, neuroimaging, and ophthalmology recommendations. Pediatr Neurol. 121:59-66, 2021
2. Brinjikji W et al: Cerebrofacial venous metameric syndrome-spectrum of imaging findings. Neuroradiology. 62(4):417-25, 2020

KEY FACTS

TERMINOLOGY

- **PHACE(S)**: Association of segmental craniofacial infantile hemangioma (IH) & 1 or more other features listed in acronym
  - **P**osterior fossa malformations
  - **H**emangioma
  - **A**rterial lesions
  - **C**ardiac abnormalities/aortic coarctation
  - **E**ye abnormalities
  - **S**ternal defects or supraumbilical raphe
    - Deemphasized in recent literature

IMAGING

- Proliferating regional or midline cervicofacial IH: Lobulated or plaque-like, prominent vascularity
- Unilateral cerebellar hypoplasia & prominent retrocerebellar CSF space
- Widened internal auditory canal ± IH ± persistent stapedial artery
- Hypoplasia, aplasia, aberrancy, ectasia, tortuosity, &/or stenoocclusive changes of major craniocervical arteries
- ± reduced perfusion (or infarction) in affected arterial territory

TOP DIFFERENTIAL DIAGNOSES

- Sturge-Weber syndrome
- Vestibular schwannoma
- Loeys-Dietz syndrome

CLINICAL ISSUES

- Cutaneous: Large regional or midline craniofacial IH → 20% have PHACE
  - IH appears in early neonatal period
- Sex: 80-90% female

DIAGNOSTIC CHECKLIST

- Look for ipsilateral cerebellar hemisphere anomaly of PHACE in patient clinically mistaken for Sturge-Weber syndrome with port-wine stain

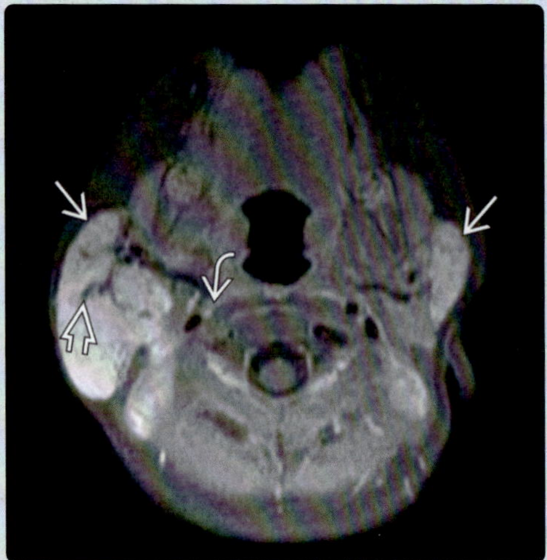

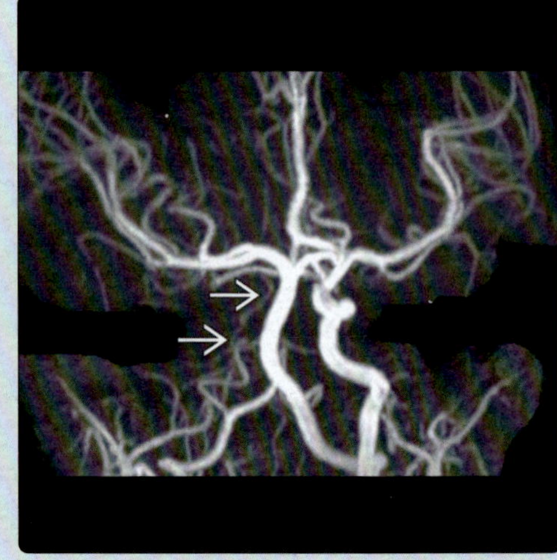

(Left) *Axial T1 C+ FS MR in an 8-month-old with PHACE syndrome shows R > L parotid/periparotid infantile hemangiomas (IHs)* ➡ *with typical intense enhancement, well-defined margins, & intralesional flow voids* ➡*. Also note the absence of a normal flow void in the expected location of the right internal carotid artery (ICA)* ➡*.* **(Right)** *Anterior 3D time-of-flight (TOF) MRA in the same child shows marked hypoplasia of the right ICA* ➡*. The patient also had IHs in a bearded distribution as well as in the floor of mouth & airway.*

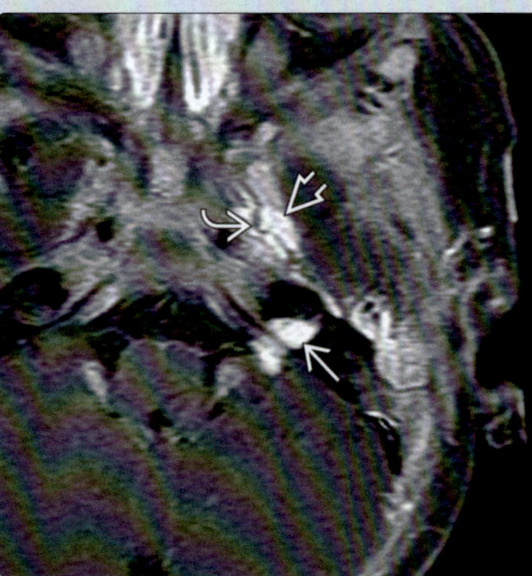

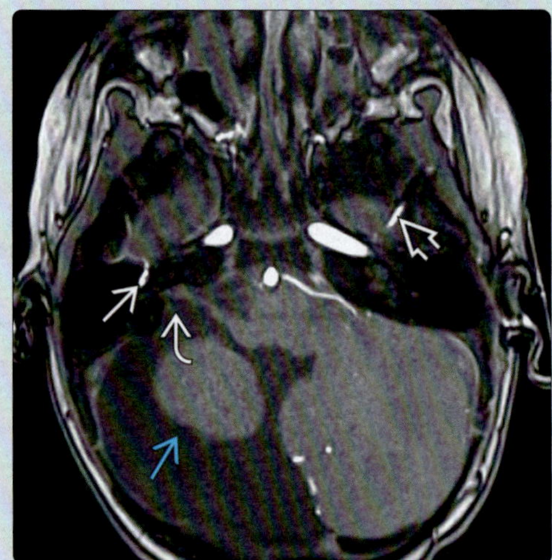

(Left) *Axial T1 C+ FS MR in a 3-week-old boy with left facial palsy shows avidly enhancing masses within the left internal auditory canal (IAC)* ➡ *& cavernous sinus* ➡ *with a prominent flow void* ➡ *in the left cavernous sinus mass. The IAC mass mimics a schwannoma. These IHs involuted after the 1st year of life.* **(Right)** *Axial 3D TOF MRA of an infant girl with PHACE & right cerebellar hypoplasia* ➡ *shows a right persistent stapedial artery* ➡*. Note the normal left middle meningeal artery* ➡*. The right IAC* ➡ *is widened.*

KEY FACTS

TERMINOLOGY

- Congenital phakomatosis characterized by giant or multiple cutaneous melanocytic nevi (CMN) + benign & malignant melanotic lesions of CNS
  - Parenchymal melanosis (Ms): Nonmalignant intraparenchymal foci
  - Leptomeningeal melanosis (LMs): Excess of benign melanotic cells in leptomeninges
  - Leptomeningeal melanoma (LM): Malignant melanoma of leptomeninges
  - Primary CNS malignant melanoma (MM): Focal malignant melanoma of CNS

IMAGING

- Parenchymal melanosis: CMN + foci of intraaxial T1 MR hyperintensity (hyperdense on CT, echogenic on US)
  - Medial temporal lobe, cerebellum, pons, thalami, base of frontal lobes
- LMs & LM: CMN + diffuse leptomeningeal enhancement
  - Typically develop communicating hydrocephalus
- MM: Focal intraparenchymal enhancing mass

PATHOLOGY

- Focal or diffuse proliferation of melanin-producing cells in both skin & leptomeninges
- Associated cerebellar hypoplasia ~ 10%

CLINICAL ISSUES

- Only ~ 10-15% of CMN patients have NCM
  - ~ 80-90% of have parenchymal Ms
  - ~ 10% have LMs or LM
  - ~ 1-5% have MM
- Screening is recommended for CMN patients < 6 months
- Poor prognosis with LMs, LM, or MM

DIAGNOSTIC CHECKLIST

- Normal MR does not exclude diagnosis of NCM
- LMs cannot be distinguished from LM by imaging

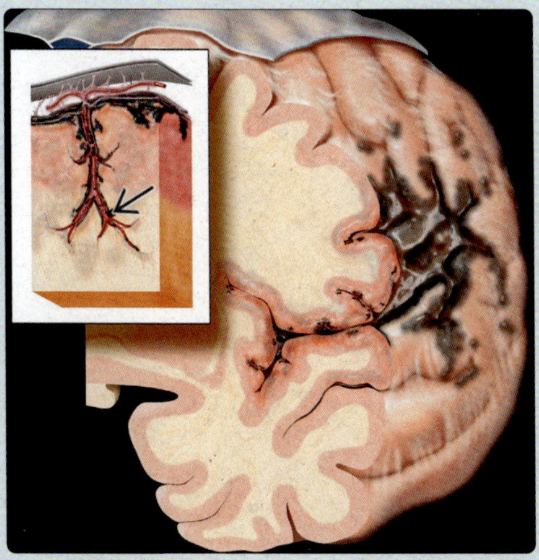

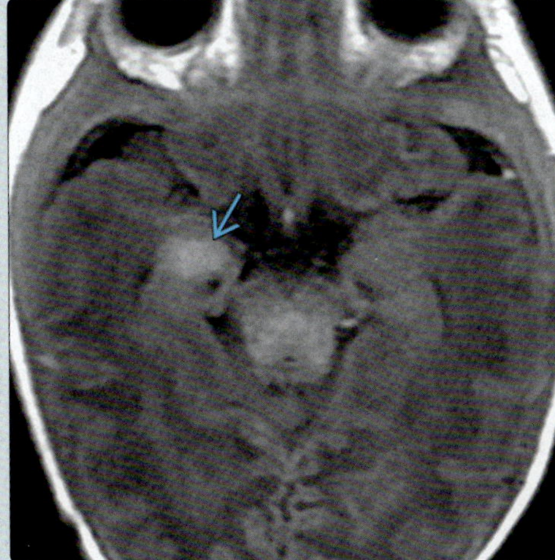

(Left) *Graphic shows localized dark (melanotic) pigmentation of the leptomeninges. Inset demonstrates extension of melanosis into the brain substance along the Virchow-Robin spaces* ➜. **(Right)** *Axial T1 MR in a 4-day-old patient with a giant congenital melanocytic nevus on the buttock shows a hyperintense lesion* ➜ *in the medial right temporal lobe. A solitary focus of T1 hyperintensity in the medial temporal lobe is the most common appearance of neurocutaneous melanosis (NCM).*

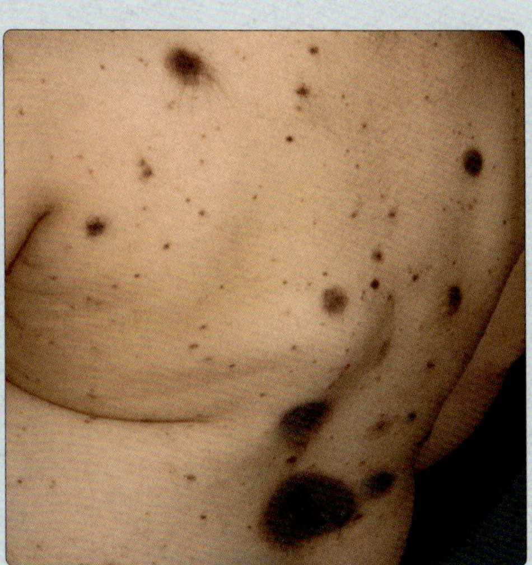

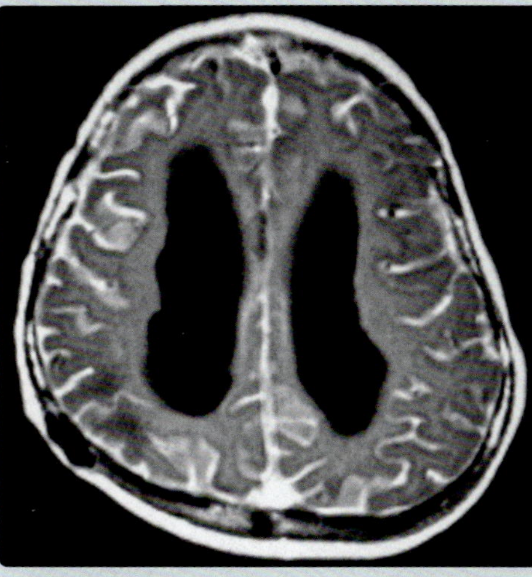

(Left) *Clinical photograph of the back of a young child with NCM shows numerous cutaneous melanocytic nevi, many of which are several centimeters in size, qualifying for the distinction of "giant" nevi.* **(Right)** *Axial T1 C+ MR in a 6-year-old patient shows diffuse leptomeningeal NCM. The pial melanosis involves virtually the entire surface of the brain, enhancing strongly & uniformly. There is moderate ventriculomegaly from associated communicating hydrocephalus.*

KEY FACTS

TERMINOLOGY

- Benign epithelial-lined cyst of anterior 3rd ventricle

IMAGING

- Best clue: Round, homogeneous midline mass at foramen of Monro with lateral ventricular enlargement
- Mean size: Asymptomatic = 0.8 cm, symptomatic = 1.4 cm
- CT: Hyperdense (70-80%); iso-/hypodense (20-30%)
- MR: Variable signal characteristics
  - T1 hyperintense (40-60%)
  - T2 hypointense (50-60%)
  - No FLAIR suppression
  - No restricted diffusion
  - No enhancement; rarely, thin rim enhancement
- Pillars of fornix straddle anterior aspect of cyst

TOP DIFFERENTIAL DIAGNOSES

- CSF flow artifact (MR pseudocyst)
- Subependymal giant cell astrocytoma (SEGA)
- Arachnoid cyst
- Neurocysticercosis

PATHOLOGY

- Derived from embryonic endoderm
  - Outer wall: Thin fibrous capsule
  - Inner lining: Columnar epithelium
  - Cyst contents: Proteinaceous material, exfoliated cells

CLINICAL ISSUES

- 40-50% are asymptomatic & discovered incidentally
- ~ 90% stable over time
- Most common treatment: Complete surgical resection
  - Recurrence rare if resection is complete
- Asymptomatic patients may be treated conservatively with clinical & imaging follow-up

DIAGNOSTIC CHECKLIST

- NECT & T1 MR are often more sensitive than T2, FLAIR, or DWI MR

(Left) *Axial NECT in a 14-year-old boy with headaches shows a hyperattenuating lesion ➡ at the foramen of Monro, which is causing mild enlargement of the lateral ventricles ➡. The finding of ventricular enlargement suggests that the cyst is likely symptomatic. The lesion was endoscopically resected, & pathology confirmed a colloid cyst.* **(Right)** *Follow-up axial 3D SSFP MR in the same patient shows recurrence of the colloid cyst ➡, an uncommon occurrence. Note the small focus of hemosiderin ➡ from the prior resection.*

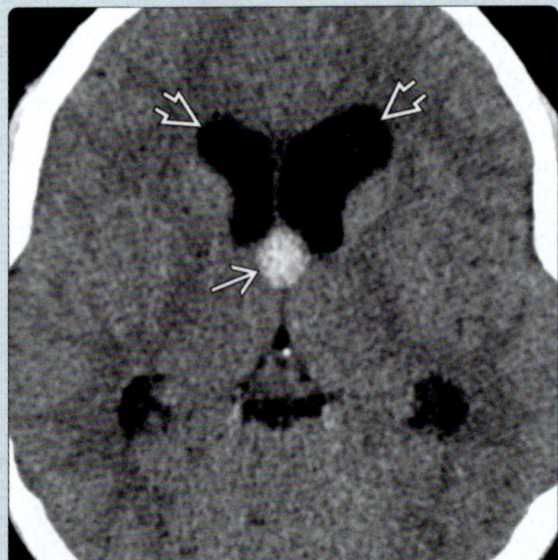

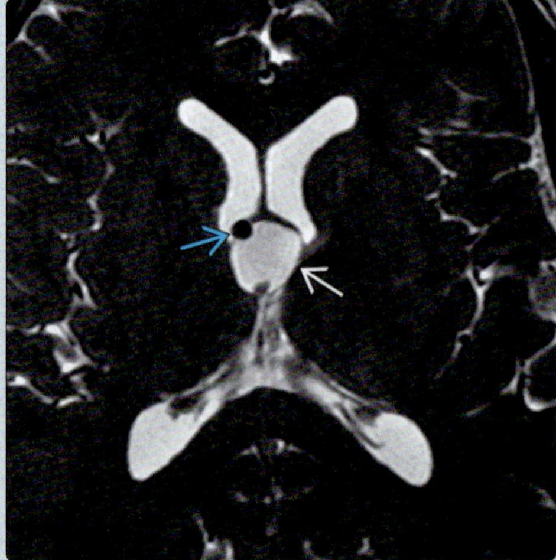

(Left) *Sagittal T1 MR images in an asymptomatic boy at 10 (left) & 15 (right) years of age show an interval ↑ in the size of the colloid cyst ➡ in the anterior superior 3rd ventricle. Most colloid cysts are stable over years but some will ↑.* **(Right)** *Axial T2 MR in the same patient shows a foramen of Monro mass ➡ with contents that are isointense to gray matter. The majority of colloid cysts are hypo- or isointense to gray matter on T2 MR, as ↓ T2 signal correlates with ↑ cholesterol content & viscosity.*

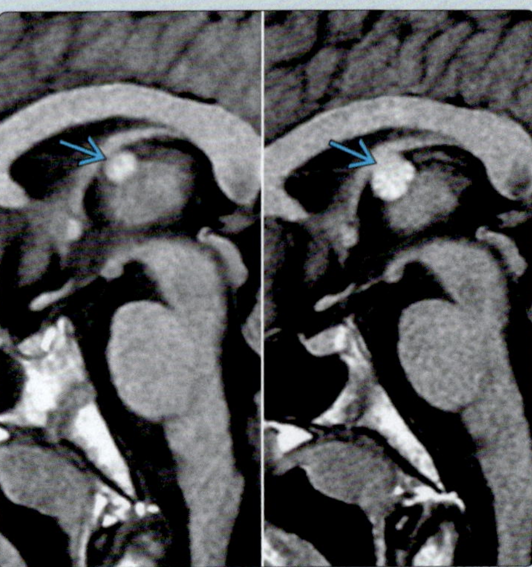

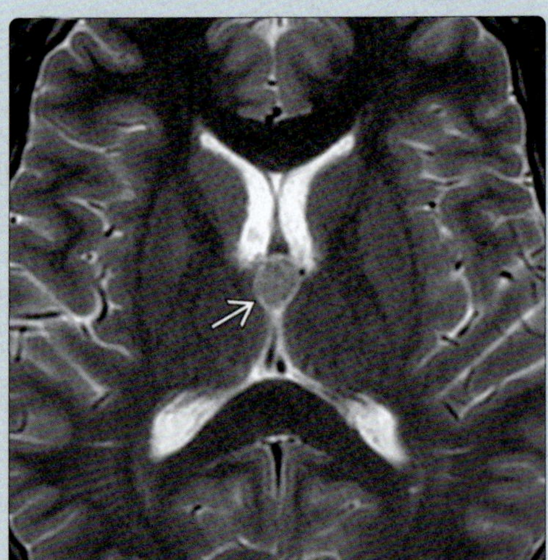

TERMINOLOGY

Definitions

- Benign epithelial-lined, mucin-containing cyst; almost exclusively located in anterior superior 3rd ventricle

IMAGING

General Features

- Best diagnostic clue
  - Hyperdense midline foramen of Monro mass on NECT
- Location
  - 99% in anterior superior 3rd ventricle
    - Anterior to interthalamic adhesion
    - Posterior to fornices
    - Posteromedial but bulging into foramen of Monro
- Size
  - Few millimeters to 3 cm
    - Symptomatic mean size: 1.4 cm
    - Asymptomatic mean size: 0.8 cm
- Morphology
  - Usually spherical or ovoid

CT Findings

- NECT
  - Usually hyperdense (70-80%)
    - ↑ density correlates with ↑ T1 & ↓ T2 signal on MR
  - Minority are iso-/hypodense (20-30%)
  - ± hydrocephalus

MR Findings

- **T1**: Hyper- (40-60%), isointense (~ 20%); hypointense (~ 20%)
- **T2**: Hypointense (50-60%); iso-/hyperintense (~ 40%)
- **FLAIR**: Does not suppress like CSF; usually iso-/hyperintense
- **DWI**: No diffusion restriction
- **T1 C+**: Nonenhancing or rare peripheral (rim) enhancement

DIFFERENTIAL DIAGNOSIS

CSF Flow Artifact (MR Pseudocyst)

- Most pronounced on FLAIR MR
- Multiple different sequences & planes confirm artifact

Subependymal Giant Cell Astrocytoma

- Off-midline solid, lobulated, enhancing mass at foramen of Monro in child with tuberous sclerosis

Arachnoid Cyst

- Rare in ventricle; usually arises from suprasellar cistern
- Follows CSF signal intensity on all sequences

Craniopharyngioma

- Suprasellar location is much more common than 3rd ventricle
- Often multilobulated with Ca^{2+} & rim/nodular enhancement

Metastases

- Dissemination of tumor in CSF, most commonly of primary CNS origin in children

Neurocysticercosis

- Single or multiple lesions within parenchyma & cisterns
  - Look for scolex along margin of cyst
- Ca^{2+} is frequent

PATHOLOGY

General Features

- Outer wall: Thin fibrous capsule
- Inner lining
  - Pseudostratified epithelium with ciliated & goblet cells
  - Individual cells are positive for cytokeratin & EMA
- Cyst contents
  - Amorphous proteinaceous ("colloid") material
  - Scattered exfoliated cells

CLINICAL ISSUES

Presentation

- Most common signs/symptoms
  - Headache (~ 75%), nausea & vomiting, visual symptoms
  - 40-50% are asymptomatic & discovered incidentally
    - 3-, 5-, 10-year incidence of developing cyst-related symptoms: 0%, 0%, 8%, respectively
- Other signs/symptoms
  - Acute foramen of Monro obstruction may rarely lead to acute hydrocephalus, herniation, death (usually with cysts > 1 cm)

Demographics

- Age
  - Mean: 30-40 years; 8% < 15 years at diagnosis

Natural History & Prognosis

- Factors associated with symptomatic cysts
  - Younger age
  - Ventricular dilation
  - Larger cyst size
  - ↑ signal intensity on T2/FLAIR MR
  - Location immediately adjacent to foramen of Monro
- Rare cases of sudden death are reported in literature

Treatment

- Symptomatic patients
  - Complete resection: Endoscopic vs. microsurgical
  - Recurrence is rare, especially with complete resection
- Asymptomatic (incidental) patients
  - Conservative management: Clinical & imaging follow-up
  - However, with relatively low morbidity, surgery is also considered for asymptomatic patients

DIAGNOSTIC CHECKLIST

Image Interpretation Pearls

- NECT & T1 MR are often more obvious than pathology-weighted sequences (T2, FLAIR, or DWI)

SELECTED REFERENCES

1. Alford EN et al: Independent validation of the colloid cyst risk score to predict symptoms and hydrocephalus in patients with colloid cysts of the third ventricle. World Neurosurg. 134:e747-53, 2020
2. O'Neill AH et al: Natural history of incidental colloid cysts of the third ventricle: a systematic review. J Clin Neurosci. 53:122-6, 2018

Arachnoid Cyst

KEY FACTS

TERMINOLOGY

- Focal extraaxial CSF collection lined by arachnoid

IMAGING

- Location
  - Middle cranial fossa: 50-70%
  - Retrocerebellar: 15-20%
  - Less common: Basilar cisterns, interhemispheric fissure, cerebral convexities
  - Rare: Intraventricular
- Displaces adjacent vessels & nerves
- Typically shows less mass effect than expected
  - Adjacent brain accommodates cyst
- Calvarial remodeling: Thinning/scalloping ± bulging
- **US**: Anechoic; no internal vascularity
- **NECT**: Isodense to CSF, unless hemorrhage occurs (rare)
- **MR**: Follows CSF signal intensity on all sequences
  - Fluid signal suppression on FLAIR
  - DWI/ADC signal equal to CSF

TOP DIFFERENTIAL DIAGNOSES

- Epidermoid cyst
- Chronic subdural hematoma
- Subdural hygroma
- Mega cisterna magna

PATHOLOGY

- Wall consists of flattened but normal arachnoid cells

CLINICAL ISSUES

- Asymptomatic in vast majority (typically found incidentally)
- More likely to grow in younger patients (< 4 years of age)
- In young children: 80% stable, 10% enlarge, 10% ↓
- Surgery is only indicated if symptoms are directly attributable to arachnoid cyst

DIAGNOSTIC CHECKLIST

- FLAIR & DWI are best MR sequences for distinguishing cystic-appearing intracranial masses

(Left) *Axial NECT in a 6-year-old boy shows a right retrocerebellar cystic collection ➡. Note the characteristic imaging features of an arachnoid cyst (AC): Isoattenuating to CSF, bulging & thinning of the overlying calvarium ➡, & relatively mild mass effect on the 4th ventricle ➡.* **(Right)** *Axial FLAIR MR in a 14-year-old girl with headaches shows fluid signal suppression within the right middle cranial fossa arachnoid cyst ➡.*

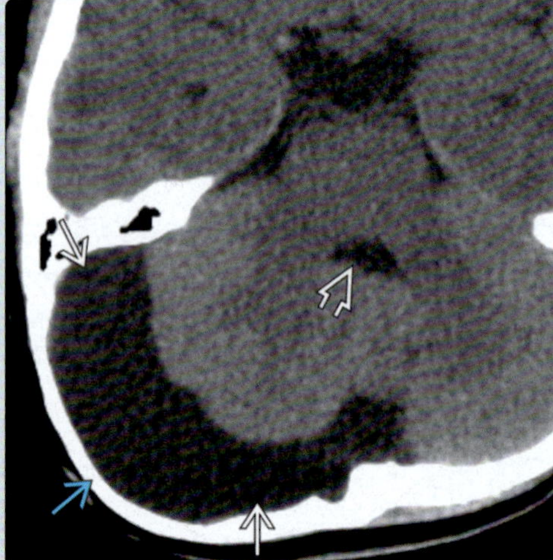

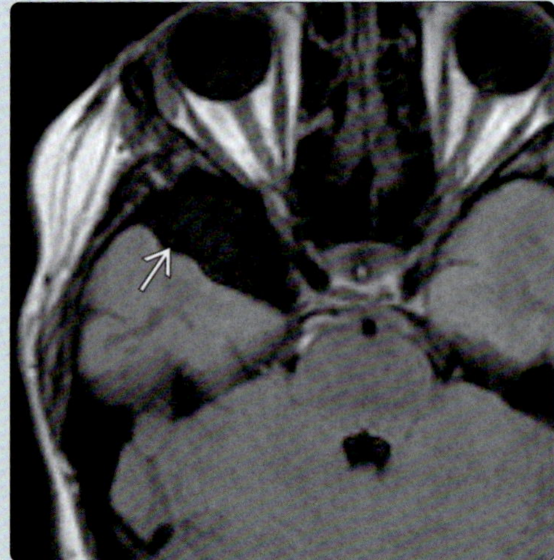

(Left) *Axial T2 MR in a 10-year-old with a head deformity shows a moderate left frontal AC ➡. Note the expansion & remodeling of the overlying calvarium ➡ & minimal mass effect on the brain relative to the size of the cyst.* **(Right)** *Sagittal 3D FIESTA MR in an infant with macrocephaly shows a large posterior fossa AC ➡. Note the mass effect on the cerebellum ➡ & associated ventriculomegaly ➡. While most ACs are incidental, larger cysts in the posterior fossa & basilar cisterns may cause significant mass effect & symptoms.*

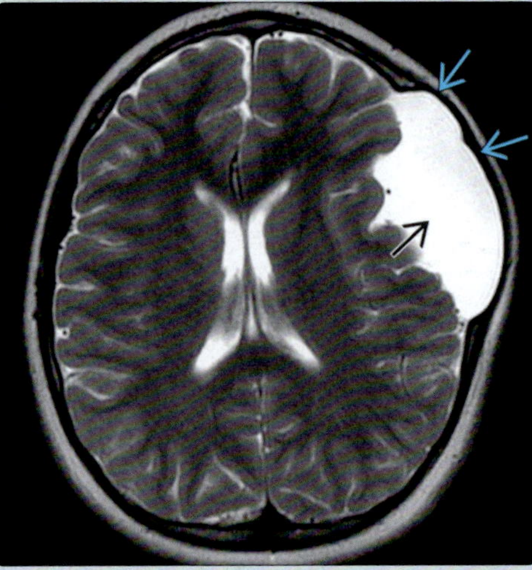

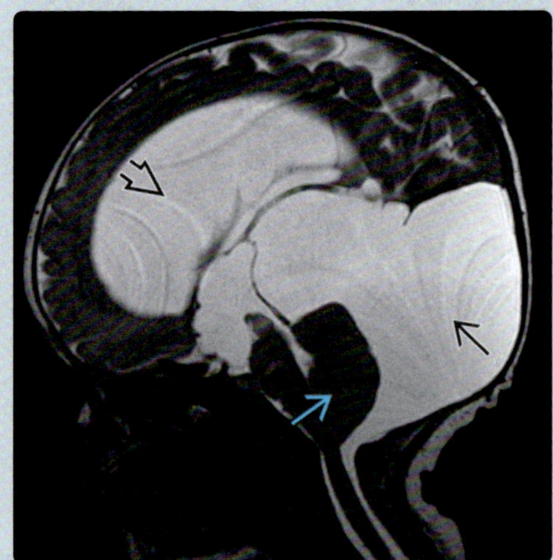

TERMINOLOGY

Abbreviations

- Arachnoid cyst (AC)

Definitions

- Focal extraaxial CSF collection lined by arachnoid; generally lacks free communication with ventricles or subarachnoid space

IMAGING

General Features

- Location
  - Middle cranial fossa (MCF): 50-70%
  - Retrocerebellar: 15-20%
  - Less common locations: Cerebral convexities or interhemispheric fissure (5-10%), cerebellopontine angle (5-10%), quadrigeminal plate (1-5%), suprasellar (1-5%)
- Size
  - Mean diameter: 3 cm; ~ 20% > 5 cm
- Morphology
  - Sharply marginated extraaxial fluid collection
    - Lentiform, crescentic, ovoid, or lobular
    - Thin, nearly imperceptible wall
  - Less than expected mass effect
    - Adjacent brain accommodates cyst; parenchyma may be mildly hypoplastic
  - Thinning/scalloping ± bulging of overlying calvarium

CT Findings

- **NECT**: Isodense to CSF
- **CECT**: Nonenhancing cystic mass displaces vessels
- **CT cisternogram**: AC shows absent or delayed opacification relative to subarachnoid spaces

MR Findings

- **T1**: Isointense to CSF
- **T2**: Isointense to CSF
  - Displaces vascular flow voids; mild deformation of adjacent cortex
- **DWI**: Follows CSF signal
- **FLAIR**: Suppresses completely, similar to CSF
  - No edema in adjacent brain parenchyma
- **T1 C+**: No cyst enhancement
- **Phase-contrast cine**: Reduced/absent CSF flow compared to subarachnoid spaces (e.g., mega cisterna magna)

Ultrasonographic Findings

- Only useful in young infants with open fontanelle
- **Grayscale**: Anechoic with ↑ posterior acoustic shadowing
- **Color Doppler**: No internal vascularity

DIFFERENTIAL DIAGNOSIS

Epidermoid Cyst

- Does not follow CSF on all modalities/sequences
  - Markedly restricted diffusion on MR
- Engulfs (rather than displaces) vessels & nerves

Chronic Subdural Hematoma

- Crescentic collection differing from CSF appearance
  - Hyperdense on CT & hyperintense on FLAIR, PD, & T1 MR relative to CSF (difference may only be mild)

Subdural Hygroma

- CSF leak from subarachnoid space into subdural space
  - 2-7 days after trauma

Mega Cisterna Magna

- Communicates freely with subarachnoid space

Porencephalic Cyst

- Result of remote trauma or ischemic injury
- Surrounded by injured, chronically abnormal brain

Neuroepithelial Cyst

- Periventricular, intraventricular, or choroidal fissure cyst

Epidural Abscess

- Collection with enhancing wall & restricted diffusion
- Typically with relevant causative findings (e.g., sinusitis, penetrating injury)

PATHOLOGY

Microscopic Features

- Wall consists of flattened but normal arachnoid cells
- No inflammation or neoplastic changes

CLINICAL ISSUES

Presentation

- Most common signs/symptoms
  - Vast majority are asymptomatic & found incidentally
  - Associated symptoms vary with size & location of cyst

Demographics

- Age: Most symptomatic ACs are diagnosed in infants & young children; cysts in older children & adults are usually incidental

Natural History & Prognosis

- More likely to enlarge in younger patients (< 4 years old)
  - In young children: 80% stable, 10% ↑, 10% ↓

Treatment

- Typically none
- Treatment only if symptoms are directly attributable to AC & potential benefits of surgery outweigh risks
- Surgical options
  - Long-term outcomes are similar among different options
    - Endoscopic cyst fenestration; open microsurgical cyst resection/fenestration; cystoperitoneal shunt

DIAGNOSTIC CHECKLIST

Image Interpretation Pearls

- FLAIR & DWI are best MR sequences for distinguishing cystic-appearing intracranial masses

SELECTED REFERENCES

1. Beresford C et al: Prenatal diagnosis of arachnoid cysts: a case series and systematic review. Childs Nerv Syst. 36(4):729-41, 2020
2. Yahal O et al: Prenatal diagnosis of arachnoid cysts: MRI features and neurodevelopmental outcome. Eur J Radiol. 113:232-7, 2019
3. Al-Holou WN et al: Prevalence and natural history of arachnoid cysts in children. J Neurosurg Pediatr. 5(6):578-85, 2010

Dermoid and Epidermoid Cysts

KEY FACTS

TERMINOLOGY

- Intracranial inclusion cysts containing ectodermal tissue
  - Dermoids contain squamous epithelium & associated dermal appendages
  - Epidermoids consist of squamous epithelium

IMAGING

- Dermoid: Fatty mass with layered septations
  - NECT: Fat density may mimic gas; Ca^{2+} in 20%
  - MR: Striated/layered appearance, nonenhancing
    - T1: Iso-/hyperintense to brain
      - Incomplete fat suppression
    - T2: Heterogeneous signal
- Epidermoid: Nonenhancing, T2-hyperintense (~ CSF) mass
  - NECT: Iso- to slightly hyperdense to CSF
  - MR: Well-defined mass, lobulations on 3D SSFP images
    - T1: Iso-/hyperintense to CSF on T1
    - T2: Isointense to CSF but no FLAIR suppression
    - DWI: Marked diffusion restriction

TOP DIFFERENTIAL DIAGNOSES

- Craniopharyngioma
- Arachnoid cyst
- Lipoma
- Teratoma

PATHOLOGY

- Dermoids: Mixture of greasy lipid, cholesterol debris
- Epidermoids: Lobular mass with shiny (pearl-like) surface

CLINICAL ISSUES

- Dermoid rupture → acute severe headache, collapse
- Dermoids are rare: < 0.5% of primary intracranial tumors
- Epidermoids 5-10x more common

DIAGNOSTIC CHECKLIST

- Fat suppression of dermoid is much less "clean" than lipoma
- IV contrast helps distinguish dermoid from craniopharyngioma

(Left) *Axial T2 MR in a 7-year-old child shows an epidermoid cyst ➡ in the left cerebellopontine angle. The T2 signal is essentially isointense to CSF. Without the associated mass effect on the brainstem & cerebellum, this lesion would not be visible on this sequence.* **(Right)** *Axial DWI MR in the same patient shows "light bulb" hyperintense signal within the mass ➡, consistent with diffusion restriction. This is a characteristic feature of an epidermoid cyst, which was confirmed at surgery.*

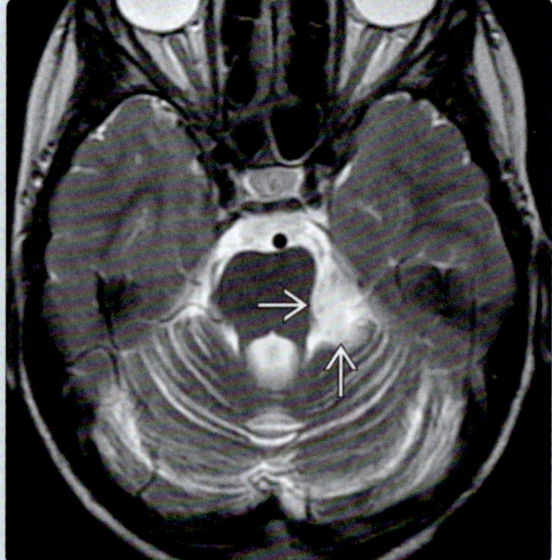

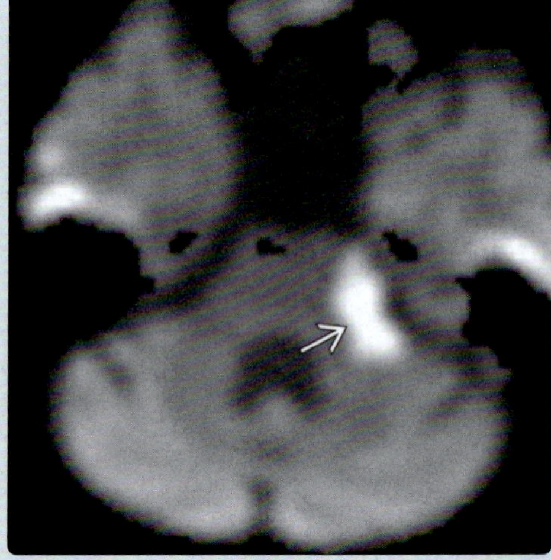

(Left) *Axial T1 MR images in a patient at 1 year (right) & 15 years (left) show a hyperintense parasellar mass ➡ that has ↑ in size. It can be difficult to distinguish a lipoma from a dermoid cyst, but growth over time favors the latter.* **(Right)** *Axial NECT (left) in a 14-year-old shows a very low-density mass ➡ in the right sylvian fissure. Axial T2 MR (right) shows the mass to be CSF isointense ➡ with many dark striations. DWI (not shown) demonstrated diffusion restriction. Pathology confirmed an epidermoid cyst.*

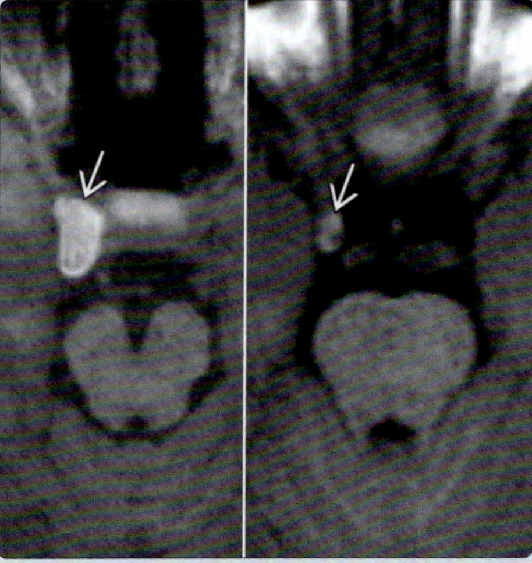

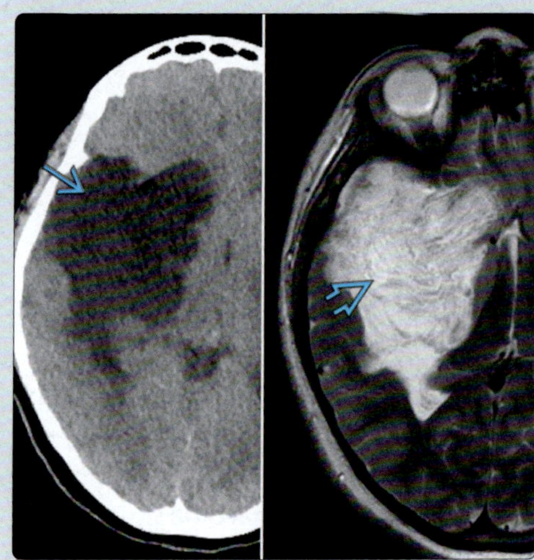

TERMINOLOGY

Definitions

- Intracranial inclusions of ectodermal tissue
- Dermoids contain squamous epithelium & associated dermal appendages
  - Sebaceous glands, dental enamel, hair follicles
- Epidermoids consist of squamous epithelium

IMAGING

General Features

- Best diagnostic clue
  - Dermoids: Fatty, nonenhancing mass with layered septations
  - Epidermoids: T2-hyperintense (~ CSF intensity), nonenhancing, diffusion-restricting mass
- Location
  - Dermoids: Usually midline, common in parasellar & frontonasal regions
  - Epidermoids: Most commonly in cerebellopontine angle & near 4th ventricle
    - Peripheral epidermoids are typically located adjacent to cranial sutures

CT Findings

- NECT
  - Dermoids: Often have fat density; Ca^{2+} in 20%
    - Rupture → fat droplets within cisterns & sulci, fat/fluid levels in ventricles
  - Epidermoids: Usually iso- to hyperdense to CSF

MR Findings

- Dermoids: Striated or layered internal appearance
  - **T1:** Iso- to hyperintense to brain
    - Not as uniformly bright as lipomas
    - Suppress with fat saturation but not as uniformly as lipoma
  - **T2:** Heterogeneous signal
  - **DWI:** Variable but diffusion restriction is typically < epidermoids
  - **T1 C+:** No internal contrast enhancement
    - Rupture → chemical ventriculitis & ependymal enhancement
- Epidermoids: Small septations or lobules may be visible, especially on 3D SSFP imaging
  - **T1:** Iso- to slightly hyperintense to CSF
  - **T2:** Isointense to CSF (may mimic arachnoid cyst)
  - **FLAIR:** Does not suppress like CSF
  - **DWI:** Marked diffusion restriction ("light bulb bright")
  - **T1 C+:** No internal contrast enhancement
  - "Atypical" epidermoids (< 5%)
    - T1 hyperintense & T2 hypointense
    - Atypical signal corresponds to hemorrhage

Imaging Recommendations

- Best imaging tool
  - MR with contrast
- Protocol advice
  - Use fat suppression, DWI, & FLAIR
  - Use MRA to assess vascular narrowing/encasement
  - Look for chemical shift artifact, especially with rupture

DIFFERENTIAL DIAGNOSIS

Craniopharyngioma

- T1-hyperintense foci do not change with fat suppression
- Enhancement in > 90%

Arachnoid Cyst

- Similar to epidermoids on NECT & T2 MR
- Suppresses on FLAIR MR; does not restrict diffusion

Lipoma

- Fatty signal/attenuation is more homogeneous

Teratoma

- Germ cell tumor that contains ≥ 2 embryologic layers
- Usually has enhancing components

PATHOLOGY

General Features

- Etiology
  - Congenital: Inclusion of cutaneous ectoderm during neural tube closure
  - Acquired: Displacement of epithelium into CNS during lumbar puncture, trauma, surgery

Gross Pathologic & Surgical Features

- Dermoids: Mixture of greasy lipid, cholesterol debris
  - Often contain hair, may contain enamel
- Epidermoids: Lobular mass with shiny (pearl-like) surface
  - Cyst contents: Soft, waxy, flaky material

CLINICAL ISSUES

Demographics

- Epidemiology
  - Dermoids are rare: < 0.5% of primary intracranial tumors
  - Epidermoids are 5-10x more common

Natural History & Prognosis

- Slowly growing, often asymptomatic
- Dermoid rupture can cause significant morbidity/mortality

Treatment

- Complete microsurgical excision
  - Residual capsule may lead to recurrence
  - Subarachnoid dissemination of contents may occur

DIAGNOSTIC CHECKLIST

Image Interpretation Pearls

- Use contrast to distinguish suprasellar dermoid from craniopharyngioma
- Fat suppression of dermoid is less "clean" than lipoma
- Epidermoids are easily distinguished from arachnoid cysts with appropriate MR sequences; FLAIR, DWI, & 3D SSFP (FIESTA, CISS, etc.)

SELECTED REFERENCES

1. Lundy P et al: A rare case of a pediatric white epidermoid cyst. Childs Nerv Syst.36(8):1795-8, 2020
2. Shashidhar A et al: Ruptured intracranial dermoid cysts: a retrospective institutional review. J Clin Neurosci. 67:172-7, 2019
3. Kannan S et al: A rare case of pediatric intraparenchymal epidermoid cyst: case report and review of literature. J Pediatr Neurosci. 13(1):96-9, 2018

Pineal Cyst

KEY FACTS

TERMINOLOGY

- Nonneoplastic, intrapineal, glial-lined cyst

IMAGING

- Most common appearance: Single, round/ovoid cyst < 1 cm
- Lobulations & internal septations are common
- CT
  - Low-attenuation focus in pineal region
    - May be difficult to identify thin walls on CT
  - 25% show Ca^{2+} in cyst wall; more common with ↑ age
- MR
  - Cyst contents are typically similar to CSF on T1, T2
  - Cyst contents do not suppress on FLAIR
  - Cyst contents do not restrict diffusion
  - ~ 90% show wall enhancement
    - Most common pattern: Thin rim (≤ 2 mm)

TOP DIFFERENTIAL DIAGNOSES

- Arachnoid cyst
- Epidermoid cyst
- Velum interpositum cyst
- Pineocytoma

CLINICAL ISSUES

- Very common: > 50% prevalence with high-resolution MR
- Occur at all ages but prevalence ↓ in older adults
- Most commonly incidental
- Large cysts (> 1 cm) may become symptomatic
  - Headache (aqueduct compression → hydrocephalus)
  - Parinaud syndrome (due to tectal plate compression)
  - In absence of hydrocephalus & visual changes, symptoms are unlikely to be related to cyst

DIAGNOSTIC CHECKLIST

- Development of pineal gland cyst is considered normal
- Imaging follow-up is typically not necessary in children
  - Unless size or degree of enhancement are unusual
- Pineocytoma appearance overlaps (but rare in children)

(Left) *Sagittal T2 MR in a 17-year-old girl with headaches shows a simple pineal cyst ➡. The lesion is well defined, isointense to CSF, & contains no septations. There is mild mass effect on the tectum & cerebral aqueduct ➡. Given the lack of associated hydrocephalus, this finding is likely incidental.* **(Right)** *Axial FLAIR MR in the same patient shows that the cyst ➡ does not suppress like CSF, typical of pineal cysts.*

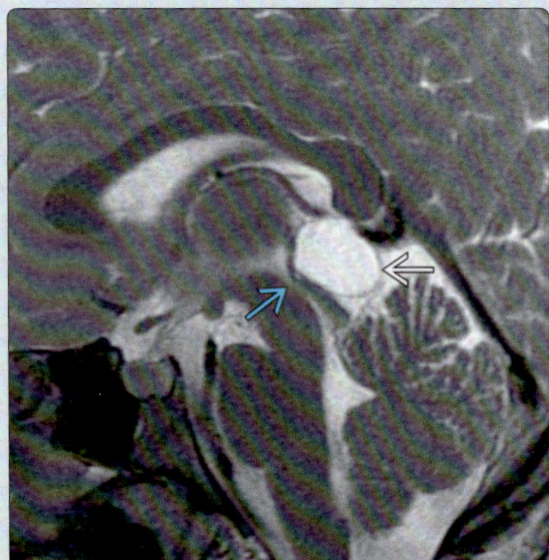

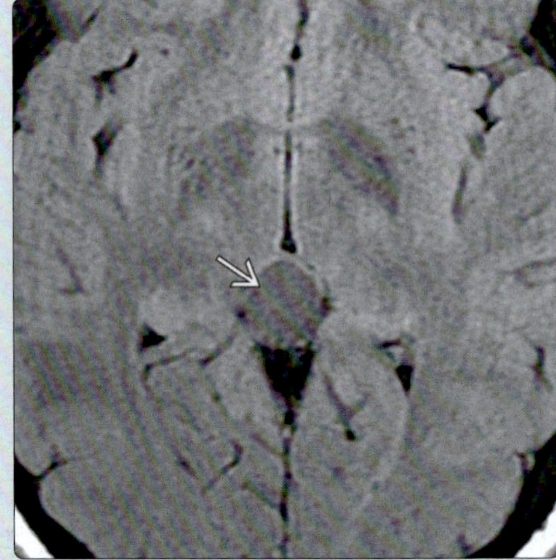

(Left) *Axial NECT in a 9-year-old with headaches shows a hypodense (but slightly hyperdense to CSF) lesion ➡ in the pineal region. It is difficult to clearly delineate the borders of the cyst on CT. Note the lack of ventriculomegaly.* **(Right)** *Sagittal T2 MR in a 6-year-old with seizures shows a pineal cyst, either containing a septation ➡ or representing 2 adjacent cysts. Septations are a common finding, seen in ≥ 25% of pineal cysts, & are especially evident when using high spatial resolution MR imaging.*

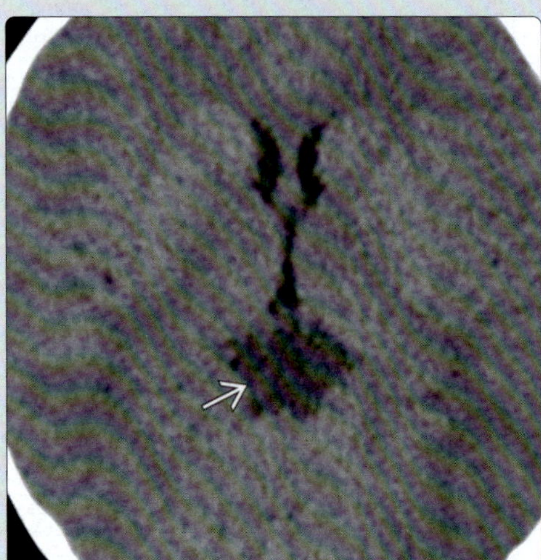

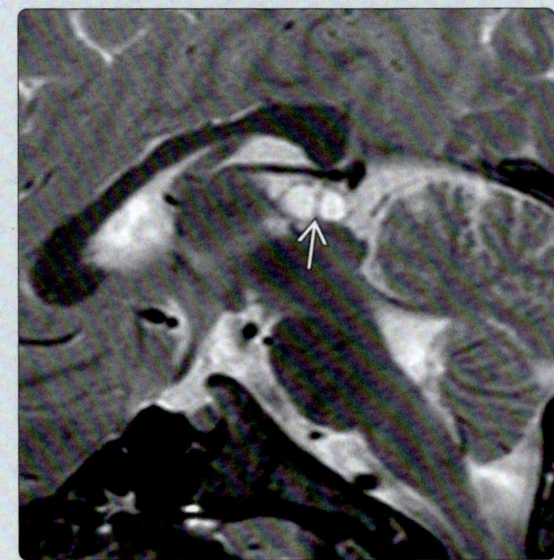

KEY FACTS

TERMINOLOGY

- Fluid-filled channels in subpial space that accompany penetrating arteries into brain

IMAGING

- Round/oval in basal ganglia; tubular in white matter
- Found in virtually all locations; conspicuity ↑ at 3T MR
  - Inferior basal ganglia > cerebral white matter
- **NECT**: Well-defined low-attenuation lesion (~ CSF)
- **MR**: PVS contents follow CSF signal on all sequences
  - May see penetrating vessels within PVS
  - No significant adjacent parenchymal signal abnormality
- ↑ size & number with ↑ age
- "Giant" or "tumefactive" clusters of PVSs are most often located in midbrain; may have associated mass effect

TOP DIFFERENTIAL DIAGNOSES

- Mucopolysaccharidoses
- Cystic neoplasms (e.g., DNET)
- Multiple sclerosis
- Cystic encephalomalacia
- Neurocysticercosis & other cyst-forming parasites
- Lacunar infarcts (typically in older patients)

PATHOLOGY

- Actually contain interstitial fluid, not CSF
- Single or double layer of invaginated pia

CLINICAL ISSUES

- Most common history: Incidentally identified focus of low attenuation on CT
- "Leave alone" lesion; MR ± contrast can typically distinguish from more serious considerations
  - PVSs are usually stable in otherwise normal patients
- "Giant" or "tumefactive" PVSs are very uncommon in children, consider mucopolysaccharidosis
- Recent studies in adults have shown PVSs to be imaging markers of cerebral small vessel disease

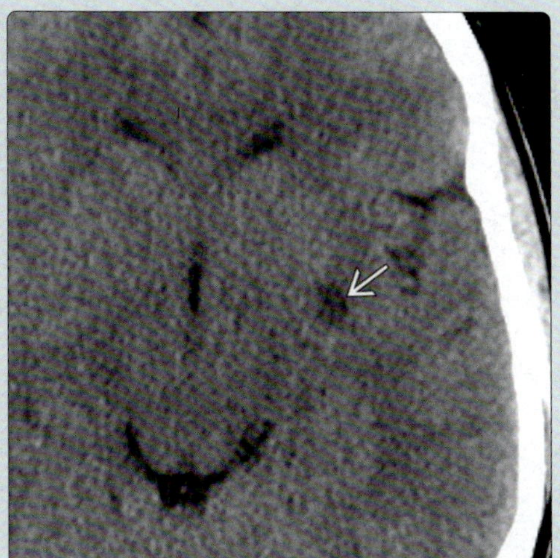

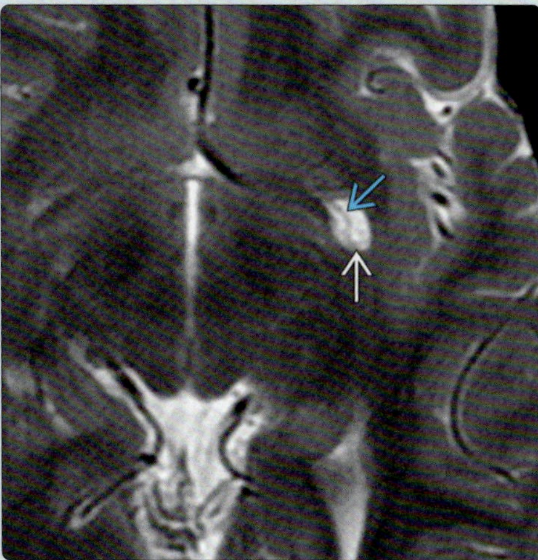

(Left) *Axial NECT in a 15-year-old girl with headache shows a focus of low attenuation ➡ in the left basal ganglia. While statistically this most likely represents an enlarged perivascular space (PVS), the finding is nonspecific on CT & warrants MR.* **(Right)** *Axial T2 MR in the same patient further characterizes the lesion seen on CT as an ovoid focus ➡ isointense to CSF & centered around a vessel ➡, consistent with an incidental PVS. The inferior basal ganglia are the most common locations for PVSs.*

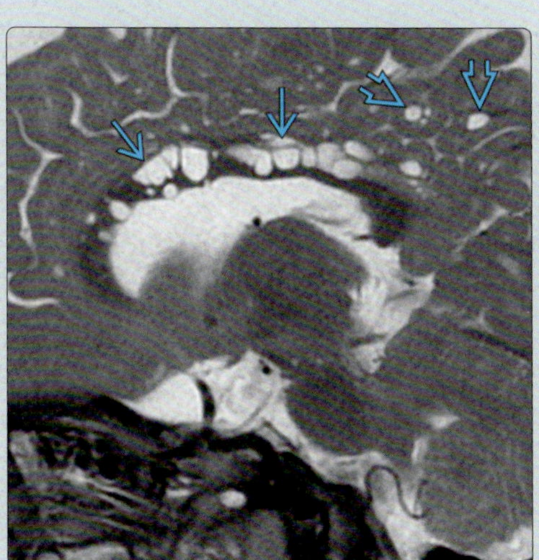

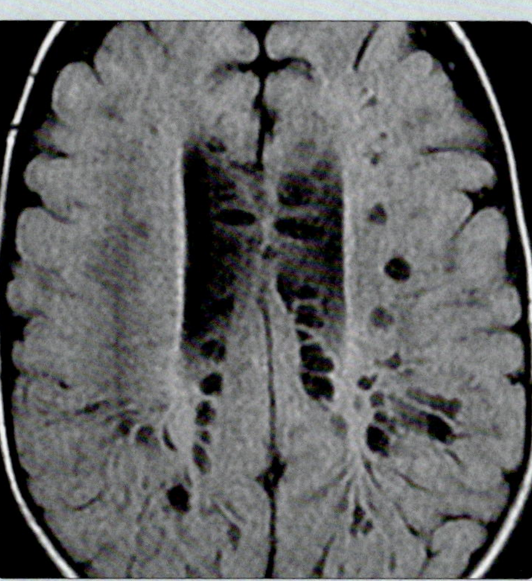

(Left) *Sagittal T2 MR in a 17-month-old patient with Hurler syndrome shows extensive cystic spaces within the corpus callosum ➡ & more peripheral subcortical white matter ➡.* **(Right)** *Axial FLAIR MR in the same patient shows signal suppression of the cysts. This extent of PVSs in a child is rare & should prompt consideration of an underlying mucopolysaccharidosis (MPS). Solitary, small PVSs are common in children, but extensive PVSs are extremely rare outside of MPS & a few other rare syndromes.*

Pilocytic Astrocytoma

KEY FACTS

TERMINOLOGY

- Pilocytic astrocytoma (PA)
  - WHO grade 1 astrocytic tumor
  - Most common primary brain tumor of children

IMAGING

- Location
  - Without neurofibromatosis type 1 (NF1): Cerebellum (midline or off midline) > hypothalamus, brainstem, cerebral hemispheres > optic pathway (OP)
  - With NF1: OP is most common
- Size: Cerebellar & cerebral lesions are often > 5 cm
- > 95% enhance (patterns vary)
  - Nonenhancing cyst with enhancing mural nodule: 50%
  - Heterogeneous enhancement with smaller cysts: 40%
  - Solid, (typically) avid enhancement: 10%
- Ca^{2+} in 20%; hemorrhage is uncommon
- May show little surrounding vasogenic edema
- Often causes obstructive hydrocephalus
- ↑ diffusivity is typical (unlike highly cellular tumors)
- Paradoxical aggressive-appearing MR spectroscopy
  - High choline, low NAA, ± lactate

TOP DIFFERENTIAL DIAGNOSES

- Posterior fossa: Medulloblastoma, ependymoma
- Hypothalamus/OP: Pilomyxoid astrocytoma, optic neuritis

PATHOLOGY

- Sporadic > syndromic
  - 15% of NF1 patients develop PAs: OP > brainstem
    - 50-60% of patients with OP PAs have NF1

CLINICAL ISSUES

- Location determines presentation, treatment, prognosis
  - Headaches, nausea/vomiting, cerebellar signs, visual loss
  - Cerebellar & cerebral lesions: Cured with total resection
  - OP lesions (especially NF1) may be observed for growth or visual loss prior to chemotherapy or radiation
- 10-year survival > 90%

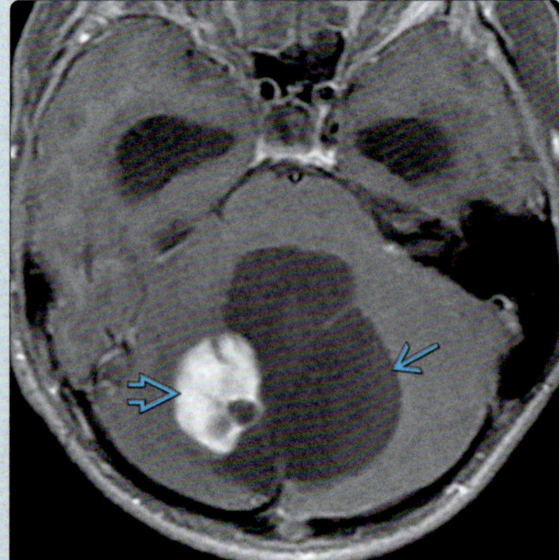

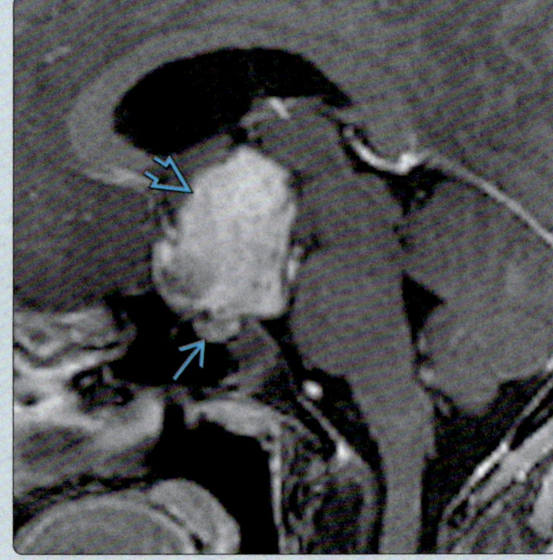

(Left) *Axial T1 C+ MR in a 13-year-old with a pilocytic astrocytoma (PA) shows a large, cystic mass ➾ with an enhancing mural nodule ➾ centered in the midline cerebellum. This is the classic appearance for a PA.* **(Right)** *Sagittal T1 C+ MR in a 10-year-old with PA shows an avidly enhancing mass ➾ centered in the hypothalamus. Note the normal pituitary ➾, which excludes a pituitary tumor. The hypothalamus/optic chiasm is a common location for PA.*

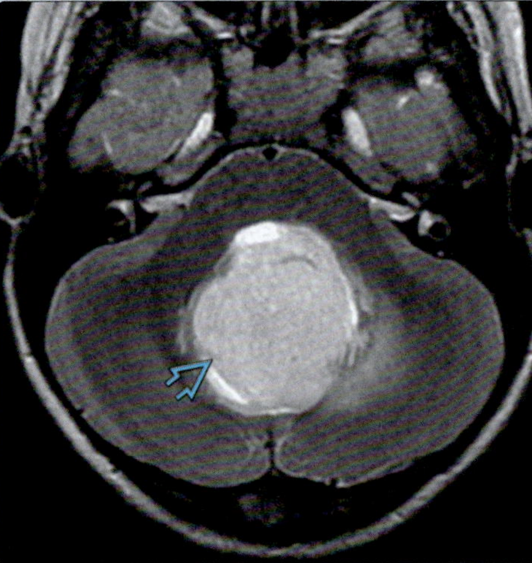

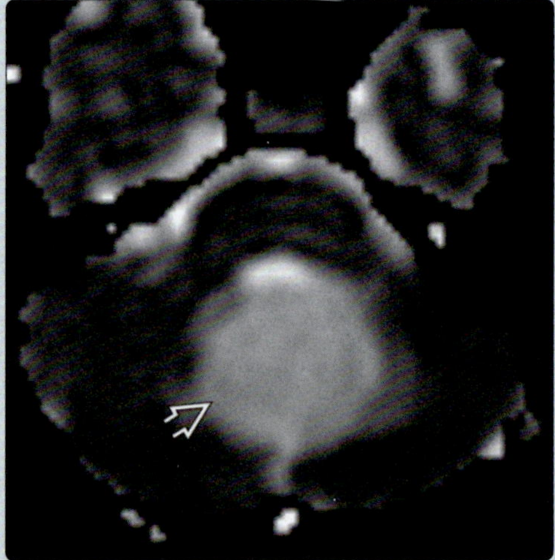

(Left) *Axial T2 MR in a 9-year-old girl with headaches shows a solid-appearing midline mass ➾ with ↑ signal intensity that is slightly lower than CSF, typical for PA.* **(Right)** *Axial ADC map MR in the same patient shows signal intensity in the mass ➾ that is much > the adjacent brain parenchyma. This ↑ diffusivity is typical of a PA. Diffusion characteristics can be helpful in distinguishing PA from medulloblastoma, especially with midline tumors extending into the 4th ventricle.*

TERMINOLOGY

Abbreviations

- Pilocytic astrocytoma (PA)

IMAGING

General Features

- Location
  - In patients without neurofibromatosis type 1 (NF1): Cerebellum > hypothalamus, brainstem, cerebral hemispheres > optic pathway (OP)
  - With NF1: OP is most common

CT Findings

- Mixed cystic/solid mass
  - Solid component: Iso- or hypoattenuating to white matter (WM)
  - Cystic component: Similar attenuation to CSF
- Ca^{2+} in 20%; hemorrhage is rare
- Frequently cause obstructive hydrocephalus

MR Findings

- T1WI
  - Cyst contents: Iso- to slightly hyperintense to CSF
- T2WI
  - Solid portions: Hyperintense to gray matter (GM)
- FLAIR
  - Solid portions are hyperintense to GM
  - Cyst contents are iso- to hyperintense to nulled CSF
    - Can help determine relationship to 4th ventricle
  - May cause only mild surrounding vasogenic edema
- DWI
  - Variable, but classically bright on ADC (not DWI)
    - ↑ diffusivity is typical in PA
- T1WI C+
  - > 95% enhance (with exception of OP glioma)
    - 50% with large cyst & enhancing mural nodule
      - ± cyst wall enhancement
    - 40% with heterogeneous enhancement
    - 10% with solid homogeneous enhancement
  - Leptomeningeal spread of tumor is very uncommon
- MRS
  - Paradoxical aggressive-appearing pattern
    - High Cho, low NAA ± lactate

DIFFERENTIAL DIAGNOSIS

Medulloblastoma

- Midline posterior fossa mass with hyperattenuation (CT) & diffusion restriction (MR)
- Younger patient age (median: 6 years)

Ependymoma

- "Plastic" tumor: Extends out 4th ventricular foramina
- Ca^{2+}, cysts, & hemorrhage are common

Pilomyxoid Astrocytoma

- More aggressive, less common tumor; usually suprasellar
- Hemorrhage & ↑ arterial spin labeling perfusion are suggestive

PATHOLOGY

General Features

- WHO grade 1, localized astrocytic neoplasm
  - Progression to higher grades is uncommon
- Genetics
  - Sporadic (majority): *BRAF* gene (at chromosome 7q34) mutations are most common → activation of RAS/ERK/MAPK pathways
  - Syndromic: Loss of neurofibromin protein (*NF1* gene at 17q11.2) activates RAS pathway
    - 15-21% of NF1 patients develop PAs, usually of OP
      - 50-60% of OP PAs occur in NF1

Microscopic Features

- Typically biphasic histologic pattern
  - Dense fibrillar piloid with Rosenthal fibers
  - Hypofibrillar spongy tissue

CLINICAL ISSUES

Presentation

- Most common signs/symptoms
  - ↑ intracranial pressure: Headaches, nausea, vomiting
  - Cerebellar lesions: Ataxia, dysdiadochokinesia
  - OP lesions: Visual loss
- Clinical profile
  - Most common primary CNS tumor in children
  - Most common posterior fossa tumor in ages 5-19 years

Natural History & Prognosis

- > 90% survival at 10 years
- Poorer prognosis: Solid lesions, brainstem extension, hypothalamic location, leptomeningeal spread, anaplasia
  - Pathology still demonstrates WHO grade 1 tumor

Treatment

- Cerebellar or cerebral locations: Surgical
  - Prognosis is related to success of total resection
    - Complete resection is curative
  - Adjuvant chemotherapy or radiation only with residual progressive unresectable tumor
  - Recent major advances in targeted molecular therapy for unresectable low-grade tumors
    - Biopsy & molecular characterization is critical
- OP: Often none, especially in NF1
  - Decision to treat is driven by vision loss & tumor growth
  - Radiation or chemotherapy for progressive disease

SELECTED REFERENCES

1. Campion T et al: Surveillance imaging of grade 1 astrocytomas in children: can duration and frequency of follow-up imaging and the use of contrast agents be reduced? Neuroradiology. 63(6):953-8, 2021
2. Sathyakumar K et al: Neuroimaging of pediatric infratentorial tumors and the value of diffusion-weighted imaging (DWI) in determining tumor grade. Acta Radiol. 62(4):533-40, 2021
3. McAuley E et al: The benefit of surveillance imaging for paediatric cerebellar pilocytic astrocytoma. Childs Nerv Syst. 35(5):801-5, 2019
4. Gaudino S et al: MR imaging of brain pilocytic astrocytoma: beyond the stereotype of benign astrocytoma. Childs Nerv Syst. 33(1):35-54, 2017
5. Alkonyi B et al: Differential imaging characteristics and dissemination potential of pilomyxoid astrocytomas versus pilocytic astrocytomas. Neuroradiology. 57(6):625-38, 2015
6. Collins VP et al: Pilocytic astrocytoma: pathology, molecular mechanisms and markers. Acta Neuropathol. 129(6):775-88, 2015

Medulloblastoma

KEY FACTS

TERMINOLOGY

- Malignant (WHO grade 4), invasive, highly cellular embryonal tumor

IMAGING

- Round midline 4th ventricular mass
  - If hemispheric → SHH subtype
- Obstructive hydrocephalus in 95%
- CT: 90% hyperattenuating (due to ↑ cellularity)
- CT: Ca^{2+} in up to 20%; hemorrhage is rare
- MR: Restricted diffusion reflects ↑ cellularity
- Complete neuraxis C+ MR to detect CSF spread
- 33% have subarachnoid metastatic disease at diagnosis
- 5% develop bone metastases, usually sclerotic

TOP DIFFERENTIAL DIAGNOSES

- Atypical teratoid/rhabdoid tumor (AT/RT)
- Ependymoma
- Pilocytic astrocytoma

PATHOLOGY

- 4 major molecular subgroups
  - Wnt-wingless (favorable prognosis)
  - SHH-Sonic hedgehog (intermediate prognosis)
  - Group 3 (poor prognosis)
  - Group 4 (intermediate prognosis)
- Histology is still important in treatment decisions
  - Classic, desmoplastic/nodular, & large cell/anaplastic

CLINICAL ISSUES

- Most common posterior fossa tumor in ages 0-4 years
  - 15-20% of all pediatric brain tumors
- Prognosis depends on residual tumor status post resection & presence of metastatic disease

DIAGNOSTIC CHECKLIST

- 4th ventricular tumor arising from roof: Medulloblastoma
- 4th ventricular tumor arising from floor: Ependymoma
- Consider AT/RT in patients < 3 years of age

(Left) *Sagittal NECT in a 3-year-old boy with intractable vomiting shows a predominantly solid hyperdense mass ➔ centered in the midline posterior fossa. The ↑ attenuation is consistent with high cellularity & should suggest medulloblastoma (MB).* **(Right)** *Axial DWI MR in the same patient shows diffusion restriction throughout most of the midline mass ➔, consistent with a highly cellular tumor.*

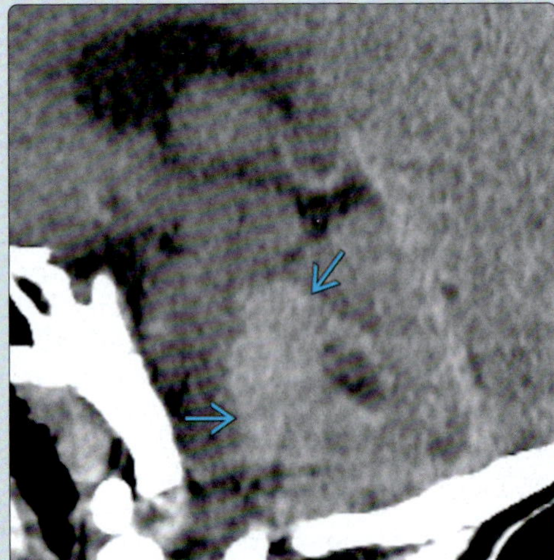

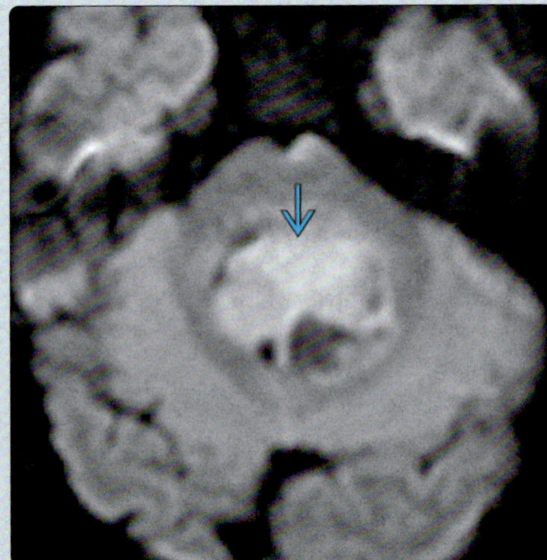

(Left) *Sagittal T1 C+ MR in a 14-year-old patient with Rubenstein-Taybi syndrome shows mild patchy enhancement of a midline posterior fossa mass ➔. Note the indistinct interface with the posterior 4th ventricle (roof) ➲, typical of MB.* **(Right)** *Axial DWI MR in a 13-year-old with MB status post gross total resection 3 years ago shows CSF dissemination of recurrent multifocal tumor ➔ along ventricular margins. DWI is helpful in surveillance imaging & is often the most sensitive sequence for detecting recurrent disease.*

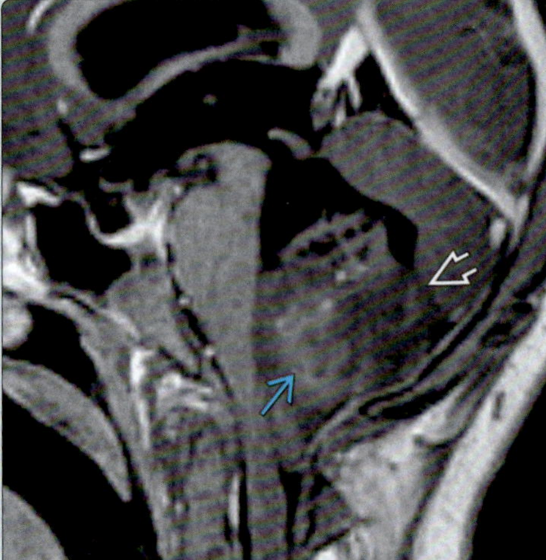

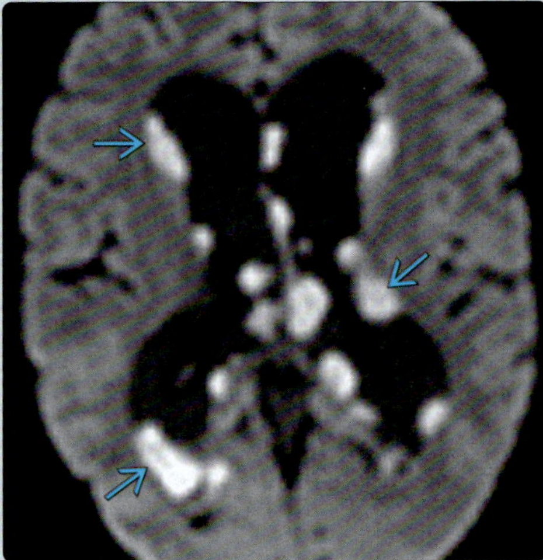

TERMINOLOGY

Abbreviations

- Medulloblastoma (MB)

Definitions

- Malignant (WHO grade 4), invasive, highly cellular embryonal tumor

IMAGING

General Features

- Best diagnostic clue
  - Midline 4th ventricular mass in 1st decade of life
  - Hyperattenuating (CT), diffusion restricting (MR)
- Location
  - 75-90% occur in midline
    - 4th ventricular mass arising from roof (dorsal 4th ventricle)
    - Cerebellar hemisphere is more frequent location in older children & adults
  - ~ 33% have subarachnoid metastatic disease at diagnosis
  - Bony metastases may occur in ~ 5%; usually sclerotic

CT Findings

- Hyperattenuation (90%) reflects high cellularity
- Ca^{2+} in up to 20%; hemorrhage is rare
- Obstructive hydrocephalus in up to 95%

MR Findings

- **T1**: Hypointense to gray matter (GM)
- **T2**: Iso- to hyperintense to GM
- **FLAIR**: Hyperintense to brain
- **DWI**: Hyperintense on DWI; hypointense on ADC
  - Reflects high cellularity
  - Excellent detection of recurrent nonenhancing MB
- **MRS**: Taurine peak may be detected at 3.4 ppm
- **T1 C+**: Variable enhancement of primary tumor
  - Contrast improves detection of CSF dissemination

Imaging Recommendations

- Best imaging tool
  - MR with DWI & postcontrast sequences
- Protocol advice
  - Sagittal images pre- & postcontrast often show site of origin (roof vs. floor of 4th ventricle)
  - Appropriate staging requires total spine imaging

DIFFERENTIAL DIAGNOSIS

Atypical Teratoid/Rhabdoid Tumor

- No differentiating imaging features; often more heterogeneous than MB
- Younger children (usually < 3 years of age)

Ependymoma

- Punctate Ca^2 & hemorrhage are more common than MB
- Extension through 4th ventricle foramina: "Plastic" tumor

Pilocytic Astrocytoma

- Cerebellar hemispheric lesion; often cystic
- Solid portion: ↑ ADC signal (↑ diffusivity, not ↓)

Choroid Plexus Papilloma

- 4th ventricle location is less common
- Vigorous enhancement is typical
- No diffusion restriction unless higher grade (carcinoma)

PATHOLOGY

General Features

- Most common posterior fossa tumor in ages 0-4 years
- Associated with many familial cancer syndromes

Staging, Grading, & Classification

- Molecular subgroups are increasingly important
  - Wnt-wingless (least common): Favorable prognosis
    - Often located in cerebellopontine angle
  - SHH-Sonic hedgehog: Intermediate prognosis, except infants → good prognosis
    - 50% located in cerebellar hemisphere
  - Group 3: Poor prognosis
    - *MYC* amplification is common
    - Located in midline/4th ventricle
  - Group 4 (most common): Intermediate prognosis
    - i17q mutation is common
    - Located in midline/4th ventricle

Microscopic Features

- Densely packed hyperchromatic cells with scant cytoplasm
- Histologic subtypes (still important in treatment decisions)
  - Classic (~ 70%)
  - Nodular/desmoplastic (~ 20%)
  - Anaplastic/large cell (~ 10%)

CLINICAL ISSUES

Presentation

- Ataxia, signs of ↑ intracranial pressure

Demographics

- M > F = 2-4:1
- 75% < 10 years of age

Treatment

- Surgical excision, adjuvant chemotherapy
- Craniospinal irradiation if > 3 years of age
- 5-year survival rate
  - No metastases or gross residual tumor status post resection: 60-100%
  - Presence of gross residual tumor after surgery or metastatic disease: 20%

SELECTED REFERENCES

1. Zhang M et al: Radiomic phenotypes distinguish atypical teratoid/rhabdoid tumors from medulloblastoma. AJNR Am J Neuroradiol. 42(9):1702-8, 2021
2. Iv M et al: MR imaging-based radiomic signatures of distinct molecular subgroups of medulloblastoma. AJNR Am J Neuroradiol. 40(1):154-61, 2019
3. Aboian MS et al: Early detection of recurrent medulloblastoma: the critical role of diffusion-weighted imaging. Neurooncol Pract. 5(4):234-40, 2018
4. Shih RY et al: Embryonal tumors of the central nervous system: from the radiologic pathology archives. Radiographics. 38(2):525-41, 2018
5. Perreault S et al: MRI surrogates for molecular subgroups of medulloblastoma. AJNR Am J Neuroradiol. 35(7):1263-9, 2014
6. Pierce T et al: Use of apparent diffusion coefficient values for diagnosis of pediatric posterior fossa tumors. Neuroradiol J. 27(2):233-44, 2014

Posterior Fossa Ependymoma

KEY FACTS

TERMINOLOGY

- Posterior fossa ependymoma (PF-EPN)

IMAGING

- Posterior fossa (2/3 of all CNS ependymomas)
  - Lobulated mass in body/inferior 4th ventricle
    - Soft or "plastic" tumor
      - Accommodates to shape of ventricle
      - Squeezes through foramen of Magendie into cisterna magna
      - ± extension through foramina of Luschka into CPA cisterns
- NECT
  - Fine, stippled Ca^{2+} is common (50%)
  - ± cysts, hemorrhage
  - Obstructive hydrocephalus is common
- MR
  - Variable enhancement
  - Iso- to hyperintense on ADC compared to brain

TOP DIFFERENTIAL DIAGNOSES

- Medulloblastoma (MB)
- Pilocytic astrocytoma (PA)
- Choroid plexus papilloma
- Atypical teratoid/rhabdoid tumor

PATHOLOGY

- PF-EPN subtype A (PF-EPN-A)
  - Most common (~ 80% of PF-EPNs)
  - Predominately infants & young children
  - Poor prognosis
- PF-EPN subtype B (PF-EPN-B)
  - Less common (~ 10-20% of PF-EPNs)
  - Predominantly older children & adults
  - Better prognosis
- 3-17% have CSF dissemination

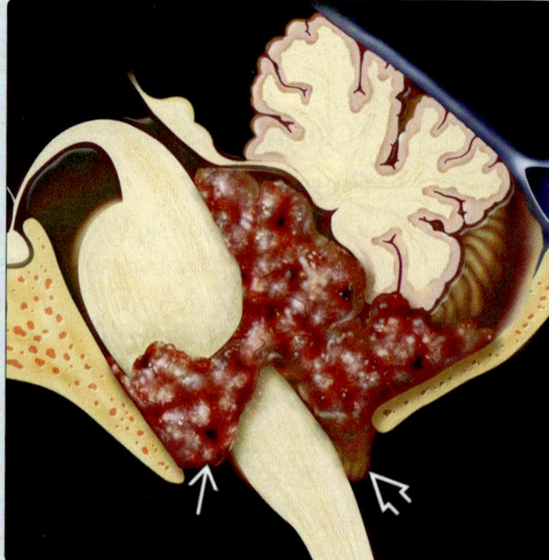

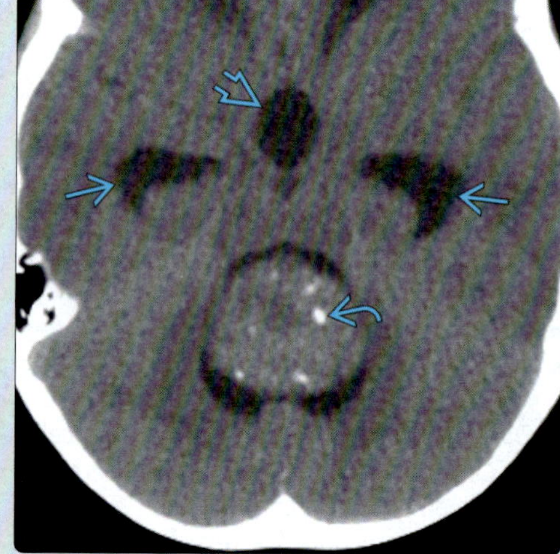

(Left) *Sagittal graphic shows a posterior fossa ependymoma (PF-EPN) extending through the 4th ventricular outlets into the cisterna magna ➡ & cerebellopontine angle (CPA) cistern ➡. This plastic pattern of growth is typical of EPN.* **(Right)** *Axial NECT in a 2-year-old girl shows a mass centered in the 4th ventricle containing scattered fine, stippled Ca^{2+} ↩, which are seen in ~ 50% of PF-EPNs. Note the enlargement of the temporal horns ➡ & 3rd ventricle ➡, consistent with obstructive hydrocephalus.*

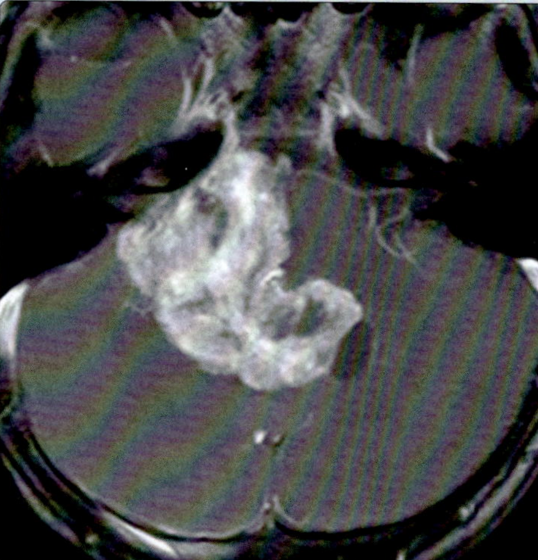

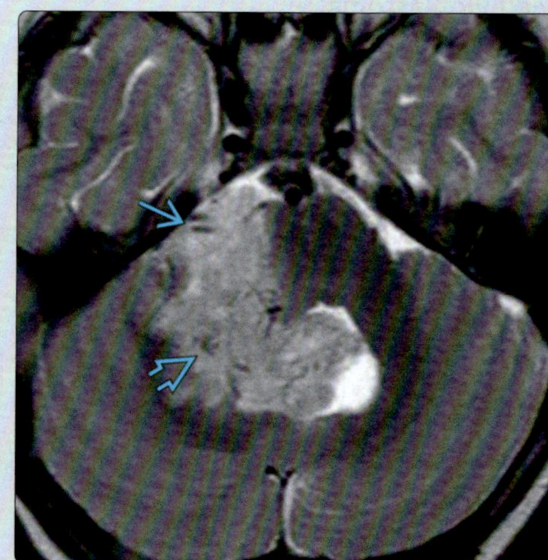

(Left) *Axial T1 C+ MR in a 2-year-old girl shows a heterogeneously enhancing mass centered in the right foramen of Luschka with extension to the 4th ventricle & CPA.* **(Right)** *Axial T2 MR in the same patient shows a heterogeneously hyperintense tumor ➡. This tumor likely corresponds to the PF-EPN molecular subtype A given the lateral location & patient age. Note flow voids ➡ encased by tumor. Involvement of the CPA & cranial nerves & vessels that course through it often makes complete resection difficult.*

TERMINOLOGY

Definitions

- Posterior fossa ependymoma (PF-EPN)
  - Slow-growing tumor of ependymal cells

IMAGING

General Features

- Best diagnostic clue
  - Soft "plastic" tumor squeezes out through 4th ventricle foramina into cisterns
- Location
  - Posterior fossa (typically in 4th ventricle)
    - Usually arises from inferior 1/2 of 4th ventricle
      - Much less commonly arises from cerebellopontine angle (CPA)
    - Anterolateral extension through foramina of Luschka into CPA cistern
    - Posteroinferior extension through foramen of Magendie into cisterna magna

CT Findings

- NECT
  - Fine, stippled Ca^{2+} is common (50%); ± cysts, hemorrhage

MR Findings

- T1: Heterogeneous; hyperintense Ca^{2+} & hemorrhage
- T2: Hyperintense cystic foci; hypointense Ca^{2+}
- FLAIR: Tumor cysts are hyperintense to CSF
- DWI: ADC usually iso- to hyperintense to gray matter
  - Diffusion restriction depends on tumor grade
- GRE/SWI: Hypointense blooming of Ca^{2+} & blood products
- T1 C+: Variable, heterogeneous enhancement
- MRS: ↓ NAA; ↑ Cho, lipid/lactate peaks

Imaging Recommendations

- Best imaging tool
  - MR of brain & spine with contrast
    - Spine imaging is necessary for complete staging
- Protocol advice
  - Sagittal imaging may distinguish point of origin as floor vs. roof of 4th ventricle
  - High-resolution 3D SSFP MR can visualize cranial nerve involvement by tumor extending into cisterns
  - MR angiography can delineate involvement of posterior fossa vessels by tumor extending into cisterns

DIFFERENTIAL DIAGNOSIS

Medulloblastoma

- Hyperdense on NECT; diffusion restriction (↑ DWI, ↓ ADC)
- Arises from roof of 4th ventricle with 90% in midline

Cerebellar Pilocytic Astrocytoma

- Arises from cerebellar parenchyma
- 90% are off midline
- Most have cystic component
- Enhancing portion enhances vigorously in > 90%

Choroid Plexus Papilloma

- Vigorously enhancing, intraventricular tumor
- 4th ventricle location is more common in adults
- Look for lobulated, frond-like border

Atypical Teratoid/Rhabdoid Tumor

- Cellular mass with diffusion restriction (↑ DWI, ↓ ADC)
- More likely to be off midline compared to medulloblastoma (MB)
- More likely to have cysts & hemorrhage compared to MB
- Most common in very young children

PATHOLOGY

General Features

- Genetics
  - Supratentorial, posterior fossa, & spinal ependymomas are genetically distinct
  - 3 PF-EPN subgroups
    - Subependymoma (PF-SE)
    - PF-EPN subtype A (PF-EPN-A)
      - ~ 80% of posterior fossa EPN
      - Location: Foramen of Luschka & CPA are common
      - More common in younger children; M:F = 2:1
      - Worse prognosis
    - PF-EPN subtype B (PF-EPN-B)
      - ~ 10-20% of all cases
      - Location: Midline 4th ventricle
      - Older children, adults; M:F = 1:1
      - Better prognosis

CLINICAL ISSUES

Presentation

- Most common signs/symptoms
  - ↑ intracranial pressure: Headache, nausea, vomiting
- Less common: Ataxia, hemiparesis, visual disturbances, neck pain, torticollis, dizziness

Demographics

- Epidemiology
  - 3-5% of all intracranial tumors
  - 15% of posterior fossa tumors in children

Natural History & Prognosis

- Prognosis is highly variable
  - PF-EPN-A: 50-60% 5-year survival
  - PF-EPN-B: 90-95% 5-year survival
- 3-17% have CSF dissemination
- 15% 5-year survival after recurrence

Treatment

- Maximal safe surgical resection, then XRT
- Chemotherapy has limited role, if any

SELECTED REFERENCES

1. Dong J et al: Differentiation between ependymoma and medulloblastoma in children with radiomics approach. Acad Radiol. 28(3):318-27, 2020
2. Takeishi Y et al: Advantage of high b value diffusion-weighted imaging for differentiation of common pediatric brain tumors in posterior fossa. Eur J Radiol. 128:108983, 2020
3. Ma SC et al: Clinical characteristics and prognostic factors of treatment in pediatric posterior cranial fossa ependymoma. Pediatr Neurosurg. 54(2):98-107, 2019

Supratentorial Ependymoma

KEY FACTS

TERMINOLOGY

- Genetically & molecularly distinct entity from posterior fossa & spinal cord ependymomas

IMAGING

- Imaging features
  - Large, complex-appearing, mixed solid/cystic mass ± Ca^{2+} & hemorrhage
  - Common locations of supratentorial ependymoma (ST-EPN): Cerebral hemisphere > 3rd ventricle > lateral ventricle
  - CT: Heterogeneous, cystic & solid mass ± Ca^{2+}
  - MR: Complex, mixed solid & cystic mass
    - SWI/GRE: Foci of ↓ signal → hemorrhage or Ca^{2+}
    - DWI: Often shows ↑ DWI, ↓ ADC in solid portions
    - Variable enhancement, usually moderately heterogeneous
    - Surrounding vasogenic edema is typical

TOP DIFFERENTIAL DIAGNOSES

- Glioblastoma
- Embryonal tumor with multilayered rosettes
- Atypical teratoid/rhabdoid tumor
- Ganglioglioma
- Astrocytoma (other)

PATHOLOGY

- Most ST-EPNs are WHO grade 3 tumors (anaplastic ependymoma)
- *RELA* fusion is present in ~ 70% of ST-EPNs
  - Associated with worse prognosis

CLINICAL ISSUES

- Most important prognostic factor: Location
- Children < 3 years have poor outcome

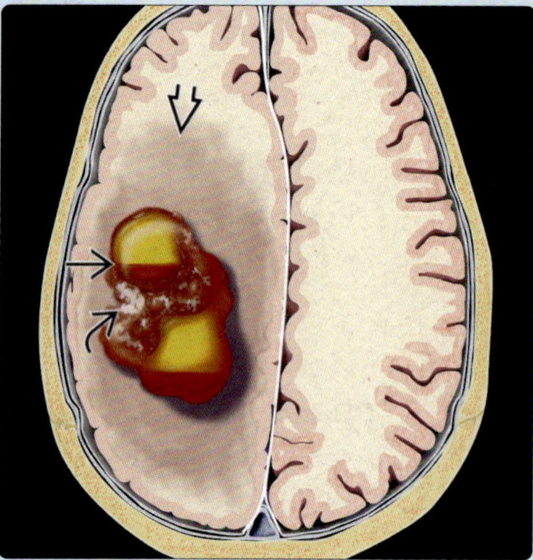

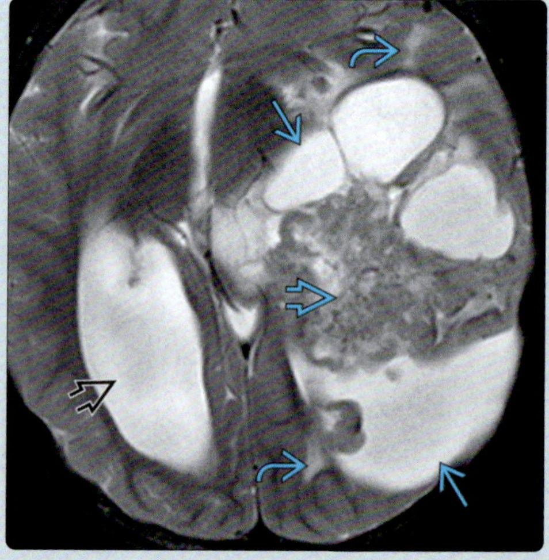

(Left) *Graphic depicts supratentorial ependymoma (ST-EPN) as a large, hemorrhagic, hemispheric mass with multiple cysts, fluid-fluid levels ➡, Ca^{2+} ➡, mass effect, & peritumoral edema ➡.* **(Right)** *Axial T2 MR in a 2-year-old patient demonstrates a large, mixed cystic ➡ & solid ➡ mass with peritumoral edema ➡. The large size, heterogeneous solid component, & cysts are typical of a ST-EPN. When large, entrapment of the contralateral lateral ventricle ➡ is common.*

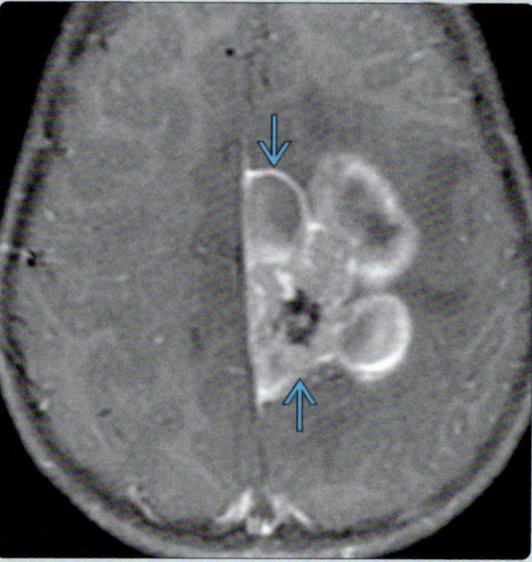

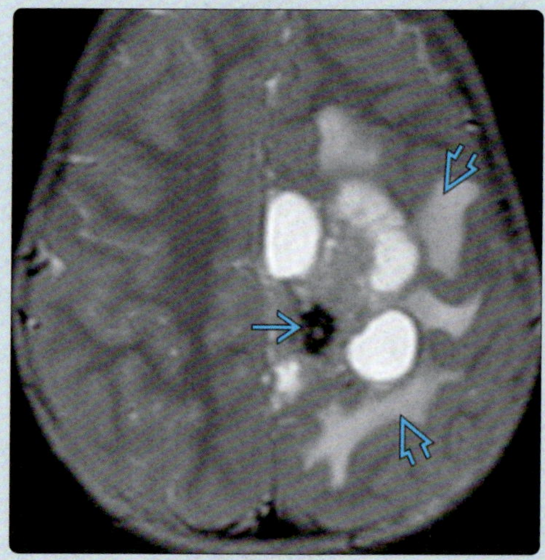

(Left) *Axial T1 C+ FS MR in a 5-year-old with ataxia & double vision shows a lobulated, multicystic mass ➡ in the periphery of the left frontoparietal region.* **(Right)** *Axial T2 MR in the same patient shows the mixed solid & cystic nature of the lesion. Note the focal ↓ signal ➡, consistent with Ca^{2+}, a common finding in ST-EPN. Also note the peritumoral edema ➡. Any time a large, heterogeneous supratentorial lesion is encountered, ST-EPN should be considered.*

KEY FACTS

TERMINOLOGY

- Rapidly enlarging, malignant WHO grade 4 astrocytic tumor characterized by necrosis & neovascularity

IMAGING

- Best imaging clue: Thick, irregularly enhancing rind of neoplastic tissue surrounding necrotic core
- Heterogeneous, hyperintense mass with adjacent tumor infiltration/vasogenic edema
- Necrosis, cysts, hemorrhage, fluid/debris levels, & flow voids (neovascularity) may be seen
- Supratentorial white matter is most common location
  - Cerebral hemispheres > brainstem > cerebellum
- Viable tumor often extends far beyond signal changes

TOP DIFFERENTIAL DIAGNOSES

- Abscess
- Anaplastic astrocytoma
- Supratentorial ependymoma
- Atypical teratoid/rhabdoid tumor
- Ganglioglioma
- Embryonal tumor with multilayered rosettes
- Tumefactive demyelination
- Subacute ischemia

PATHOLOGY

- 2 types: Primary (de novo) & secondary (degeneration from lower grade astrocytoma)
- Necrosis & microvascular proliferation are hallmarks

CLINICAL ISSUES

- Symptoms vary with location: Seizures & focal neurologic deficits are common
- Much less common in children (~ 5% of pediatric CNS neoplasms)
- Prognosis is poor but better in children than adults

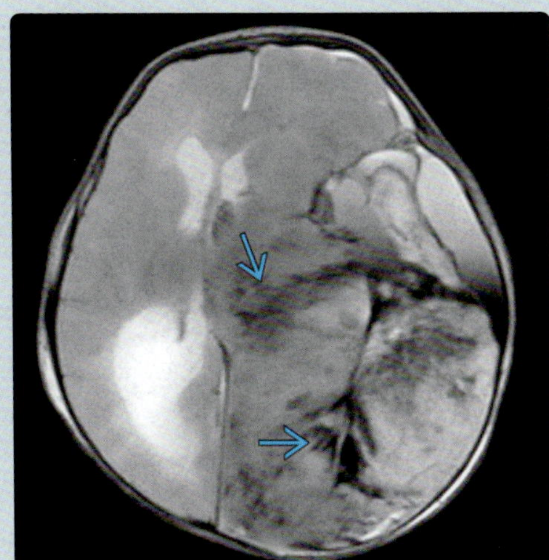

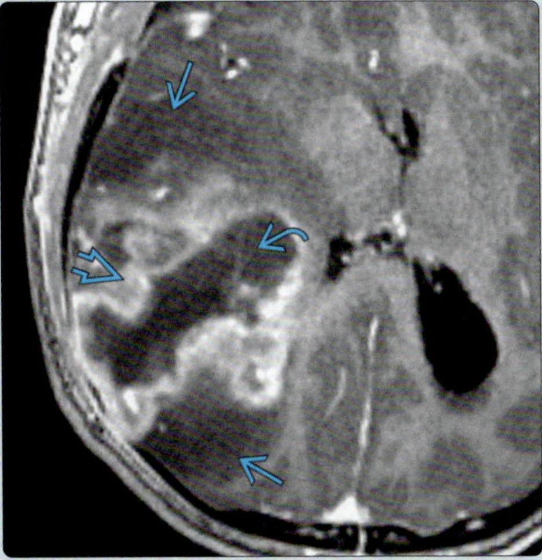

(Left) *Axial PD MR in a neonate shows a large mass of the posterior left cerebral hemisphere with numerous low signal intensity foci → due to hemorrhage. Glioblastomas in neonates & infants are often large & hemorrhagic at presentation.* **(Right)** *Axial T1 C+ MR in a 17-year-old with Lynch syndrome shows a heterogeneously enhancing glioblastoma → with central necrosis →, a typical finding in glioblastoma. Also note the extensive peritumoral signal changes →.*

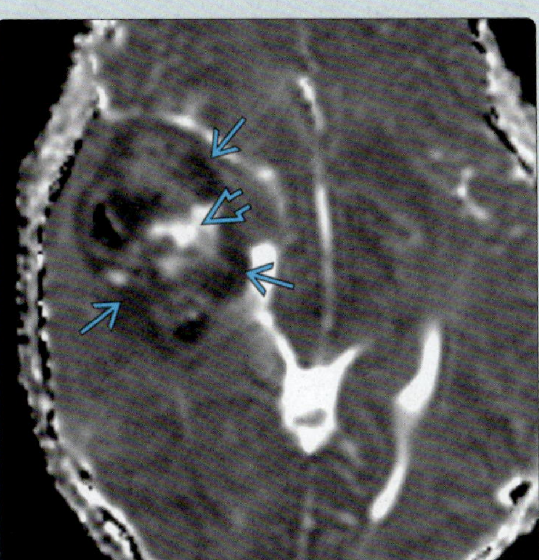

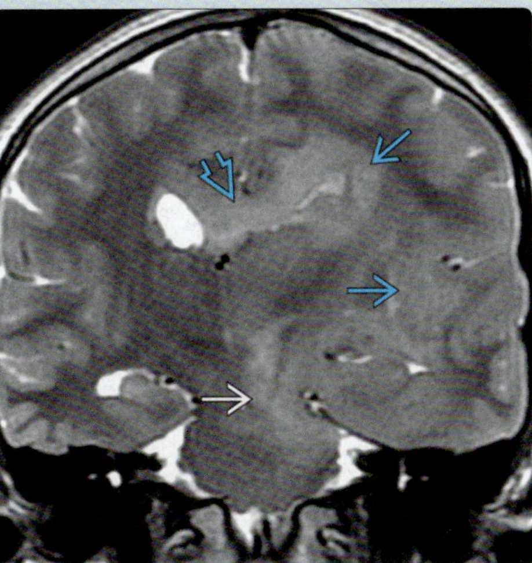

(Left) *Axial ADC map in an 8-year-old with right temporal glioblastoma shows markedly ↓ signal in the solid periphery of the lesion →, consistent with high cellularity. The area of central hyperintensity → corresponds to necrosis.* **(Right)** *Coronal T2 MR in a 10-year-old with glioblastoma shows extensive infiltrative signal throughout the left cerebral white matter →, crossing the corpus callosum → & involving the brainstem →.*

Brainstem Tumors

KEY FACTS

TERMINOLOGY

- Brainstem tumors (BSTs) are distinguished by location, imaging appearance, & histology
  - Medullary, pontine, mesencephalic, or tectal
  - Diffuse or focal

IMAGING

- Diffuse intrinsic pontine glioma (DIPG): Expansile diffuse midline glioma (DMG) in pons with poorly defined margins, effacing CSF cisterns & 4th ventricle; often encases basilar artery
  - Fibrillary tumors: Little or no enhancement
  - High grade: Focal enhancement with central necrosis
  - Foci of diffusion restriction in up to 63%, though, classically, DIPG does not restrict
- PA: Exophytic, enhancing tumor anywhere in brainstem
- Tectal plate glioma: Nonenhancing mass in tectum
- Midbrain tumors: Heterogeneous group

TOP DIFFERENTIAL DIAGNOSES

- Acute disseminated encephalomyelitis, brainstem abscess, neurofibromatosis type 1, osmotic demyelination syndrome, cavernous malformation

PATHOLOGY

- BSTs: 10-15% of pediatric brain tumors
  - Astrocytomas (WHO grades 1-4) > > embryonal tumor, ganglioglioma, atypical teratoid rhabdoid tumor
    - 80% of BSTs are pontine DMG (DIPG)

CLINICAL ISSUES

- Presentation: Cranial nerve palsies, hemiparesis, gait disturbance, ataxia, headache, nausea, vomiting
- Prognosis depends on location & histology
  - Pons: Poor prognosis (unresectable)
    - DIPG/DMG: Median survival ~ 1 year
  - Medulla or midbrain: Variable prognosis
  - Tectum: Good prognosis (only requires CSF diversion)

(Left) *Axial NECT in an 8-year-old patient with a diffuse intrinsic pontine glioma (DIPG)/pontine diffuse midline glioma (DMG), H3 K27M mutant, shows enlargement of the pons with effacement of the cisterns ➡ & near-complete effacement of the 4th ventricle ➡. Mass effect on the cisterns & 4th ventricle may be the only clue to DIPG on CT.* **(Right)** *Axial T2 MR in the same patient shows the pontine mass extending into the left cerebellum with indistinct margins ➡. Note partial encasement of basilar artery ➡, typical of DIPG.*

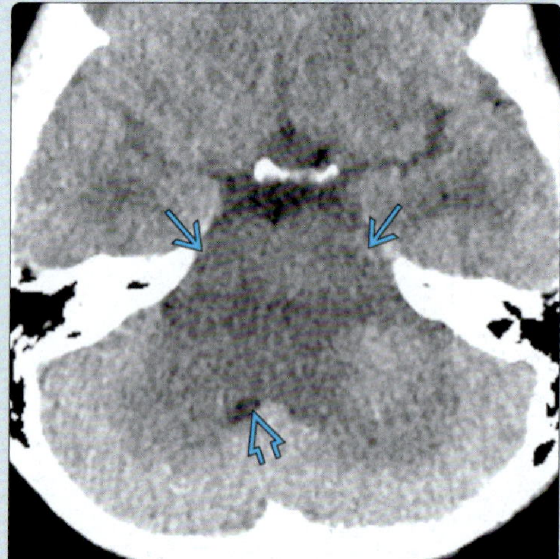

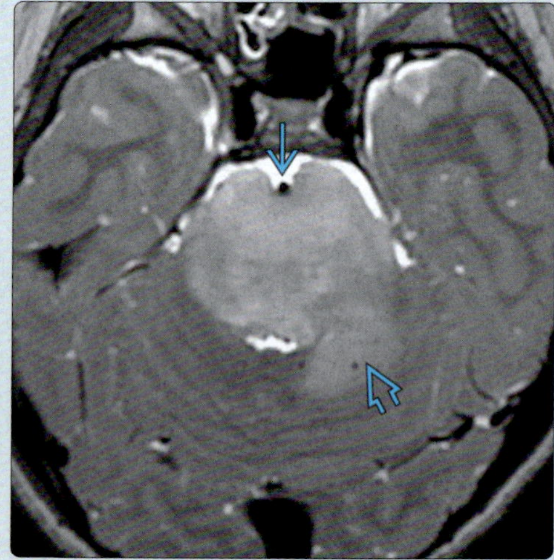

(Left) *Axial T1 C+ MR in a 9-year-old patient with a DIPG/DMG shows focal areas of enhancement with central nonenhancement ➡, suggesting necrosis. Enhancement has been shown to be associated with shorter survival time in midline glioma.* **(Right)** *Coronal FLAIR MR in the same patient with DIPG/DMG ➡ shows extension of abnormal signal into the bilateral thalami ➡ & medulla ➡. Such distant extension of signal abnormality typically suggests an infiltrative, higher grade tumor.*

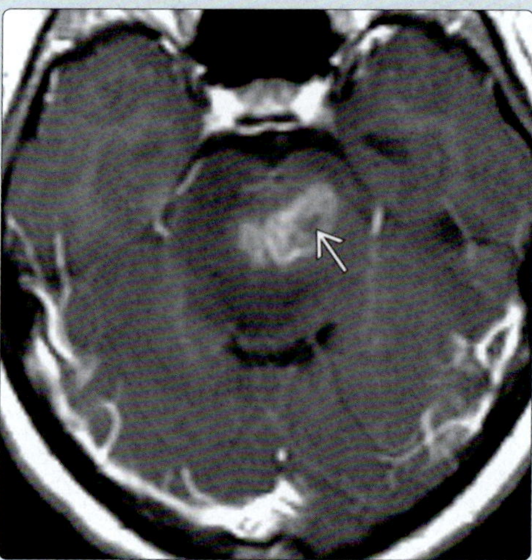

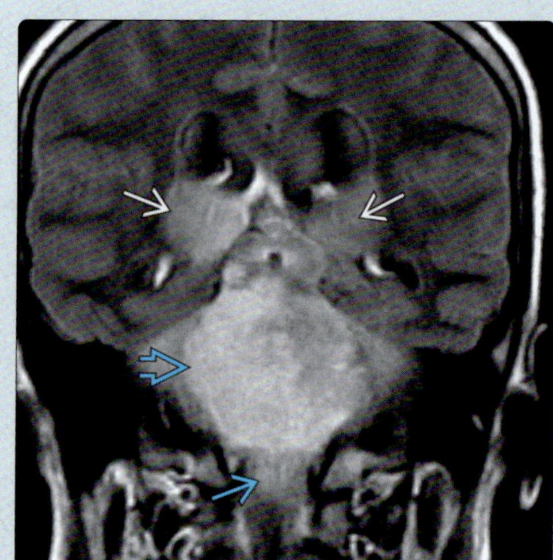

TERMINOLOGY

Abbreviations

- Brainstem tumors (BSTs)
- Diffuse intrinsic pontine glioma (DIPG): Diffuse midline glioma (DMG) in pons
  - Most common form of DMG in children

Synonyms

- Pontine glioma, midbrain glioma, medullary glioma, dorsally exophytic medullary glioma

Definitions

- BSTs are distinguished by location & imaging/histologic characteristics of tumor
  - DMG in pons (classically referred to as DIPG)
    - Glial tumor centered in pons (WHO grades 2-4)
    - 80% of pediatric BSTs
    - Expansile, often poorly marginated, often lacks enhancement
    - 70-80% harbor H3 K27M mutation → poor prognosis
  - Focal pontine tumors: Embryonal tumor with multilayered rosettes (ETMR), ganglioglioma
    - Much less common than DIPG/DMG
  - Tectal gliomas
    - Present with hydrocephalus in 6- to 10-year-olds
    - Rarely progressive
    - CSF diversion is often only treatment required
  - Midbrain or mesencephalic tumors
    - All histologies occur (including embryonal tumors & atypical teratoid/rhabdoid tumors)
  - Medullary tumors
    - Pilocytic astrocytoma (PA) is most likely histology
    - Usually dorsally exophytic & solidly enhancing
  - BSTs associated with neurofibromatosis type 1 (NF1)
    - Typically PA
    - Rarely enlarge, often asymptomatic

IMAGING

General Features

- Best diagnostic clue
  - DIPG/DMG: Expansile lesion in pons
  - PA: Exophytic enhancing lesion anywhere in brainstem
  - Tectal plate glioma: Nonenhancing lesion in tectum
- Location
  - Cervicomedullary junction to cerebral peduncles
    - Medullary, pontine, midbrain, tectal
  - DIPG/DMG: Typically centered in pons
    - Extends out of pons in 86%
      - Extension into cerebellar peduncles, midbrain, or medulla → higher grade
    - CSF dissemination in 3-7%
- Size
  - Varies greatly, partly related to location
    - DIPG is often large at presentation
    - Tectal plate gliomas are often small
- Morphology
  - Depends on histology; focal vs. large/infiltrative
    - Sometimes exophytic

CT Findings

- NECT
  - Brainstem enlargement with ↓ attenuation & effacement of adjacent CSF cisterns
    - Streak artifact from skull base can mimic tumor
  - Pontine tumors → flattening of anterior 4th ventricle
- CECT
  - Variable enhancement
    - PA in any region of brainstem usually enhances

MR Findings

- T1WI
  - Mild to moderate hypointensity
  - Central areas of preserved signal may represent relatively preserved white matter (WM) tracts
- T2WI
  - Hyperintense mass (homogeneous to heterogeneous) & margins (edema vs. infiltrating tumor)
    - Treatment often results in ↑ heterogeneity
  - Basilar artery flow void is often engulfed by DIPG
- FLAIR
  - Hyperintense mass, ± better definition than on T2
- T2* GRE
  - Areas of signal loss usually represent intratumoral hemorrhage
    - Mineralization is uncommon in BST
- DWI
  - DIPG/DMG shows foci of restricted diffusion in up to 63%, though lack of restricted diffusion is classic
    - ↓ ADC values are associated with shorter survival time & higher grade tumor
  - ETMR shows marked diffusion restriction
  - Diffusion tractography (DTI) can show displacement of WM tracts by tumor
    - WM tracts are typically infiltrated or displaced by DIPG (but not interrupted)
- T1WI C+
  - Fibrillary tumors: Variable enhancement, usually minimal
  - High-grade DIPG: Foci of enhancement in 70% ± central necrosis/rim enhancement
    - Changes from treatment are of unclear etiology
      - May reflect steroid effect on blood-brain barrier, not necessarily change in tumor
  - PA: Solid portion enhances
    - ± solid, cystic with nodule, or rim enhancing; most often located dorsally with exophytic component
  - Metastatic disease is more common than initially reported
    - Especially late in disease or post bevacizumab therapy
- MRS
  - ↑ Cho:NAA ratio is associated with shorter survival
  - Lactate implies necrosis & poor prognosis in some studies

Nuclear Medicine Findings

- PET/CT: FDG uptake in ≥ 50% of tumor → shorter survival
  - Hypermetabolic tumors are likely to be higher grade

Imaging Recommendations

- Best imaging tool
  - MR with contrast

- Protocol advice
  - DTI, PWI, & MRS may have prognostic significance in DIPG & can help distinguish high- vs. low-grade tumors

DIFFERENTIAL DIAGNOSIS

Acute Disseminated Encephalomyelitis/Other Autoimmune Inflammation

- Supratentorial & spinal sites are often affected as well
- Delayed onset after viral prodrome or vaccination

Brainstem Abscess

- *Listeria monocytogenes* is often implicated
  - Viral agents: West Nile virus, adenovirus, EBV, HSV
- More acute clinical course; often febrile

Neurofibromatosis Type 1

- Asymptomatic, poorly defined, T2-hyperintense foci in brainstem, cerebellum, globus pallidus
  - Develop in early childhood, diminish with age
- Cerebellar WM involvement is more common than pons
  - Look for additional findings of NF1

Osmotic Demyelination Syndrome

- Central pontine T2 hyperintensity with sparing of periphery
- Classic clinical setting: Rapid correction of hyponatremia

Cavernous Malformation

- Low-flow vascular malformation with locules containing fluid-fluid levels
- SWI/T2* GRE hypointensity is classic
- Often associated with DVA

PATHOLOGY

General Features

- Genetics
  - DIPG/DMG: H3 K27M mutants carry worse prognosis, regardless of histologic grade
- Associated abnormalities
  - Better prognosis of BST if associated with NF1
    - Medulla is most common site in NF1

Staging, Grading, & Classification

- DMG: Astrocytomas of varying grade (WHO grades 2-4)
  - Biopsy of presumed DIPG is becoming more common
    - Molecular subtyping allows improved prognostication & potential targeted therapy
- PA, ganglioglioma, embryonal tumors
  - If suspected based on imaging, recommend biopsy

Gross Pathologic & Surgical Features

- Pontine swelling in DIPG/DMG
  - Diffuse tumor infiltration; craniocaudal extension along fiber tracts

Microscopic Features

- Variable cellularity & mitoses with pleomorphism & nuclear atypia, necrosis, & endothelial proliferation

CLINICAL ISSUES

Presentation

- Most common signs/symptoms
  - Cranial nerve palsies with long tract signs
  - Hemiparesis, ataxia, gait disturbance
  - Headache, nausea, vomiting

Demographics

- Age
  - Peak incidence ~ 3-10 years of age
- Epidemiology
  - ~ 10-15% of pediatric brain tumors
  - 20-30% of pediatric posterior fossa tumors

Natural History & Prognosis

- DIPG/DMG: Very poor prognosis
  - CSF dissemination in 50% prior to death
  - Median survival ~ 1 year
  - 20% survival at 2 years
  - Worse prognosis: Enhancement, necrosis, low ADC, dissemination
- PA (dorsally exophytic): Fair to good prognosis, especially in setting of NF1
- Tectal plate gliomas: Good prognosis

Treatment

- DIPG/DMG: Radiation therapy if > 3 years old
  - Chemotherapy, though not particularly effective
- PA: Consider surgical resection based upon location
- Tectal plate glioma: Often only requires 3rd ventriculostomy followed by observation

DIAGNOSTIC CHECKLIST

Consider

- Rapid onset of symptoms: Abscess
- Blood products: Cavernous malformation (look for associated DVA)
- Lesions in other locations: Infection or demyelination
- Atypical appearance → consider biopsy

Image Interpretation Pearls

- Sagittal T2/FLAIR is helpful to show extent of lesion
- Hydrocephalus is usually late finding

Reporting Tips

- Pontine tumor signal extending to cerebellum, midbrain, or medulla suggests higher grade
- Solid exophytic enhancement is most common in PA; may suggest better prognosis

SELECTED REFERENCES

1. Sarma A et al: Magnetic resonance imaging of the brainstem in children, part 2: acquired pathology of the pediatric brainstem. Pediatr Radiol. 51(2):189-204, 2021
2. Cooney TM et al: Response assessment in diffuse intrinsic pontine glioma: recommendations from the Response Assessment in Pediatric Neuro-Oncology (RAPNO) working group. Lancet Oncol. 21(6):e330-6, 2020
3. Leach JL et al: MR imaging features of diffuse intrinsic pontine glioma and relationship to overall survival: report from the International DIPG Registry. Neuro Oncol. 22(11):1647-57, 2020
4. Pfaff E et al: Brainstem biopsy in pediatric diffuse intrinsic pontine glioma in the era of precision medicine: the INFORM study experience. Eur J Cancer. 114:27-35, 2019
5. Hoffman LM et al: Clinical, radiologic, pathologic, and molecular characteristics of long-term survivors of diffuse intrinsic pontine glioma (DIPG): a collaborative report from the International and European Society for Pediatric Oncology DIPG Registries. J Clin Oncol. 36(19):1963-72, 2018

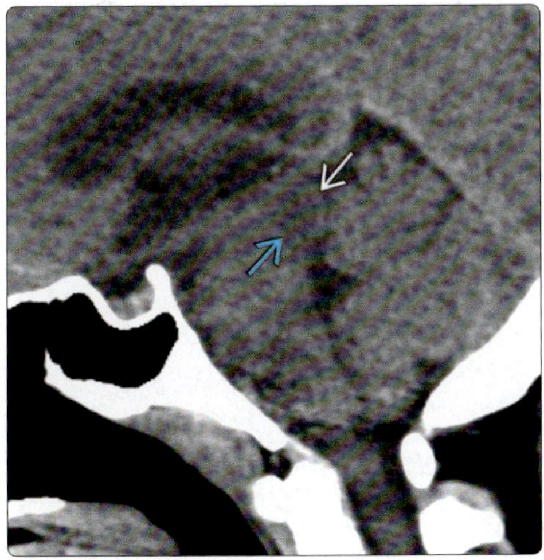

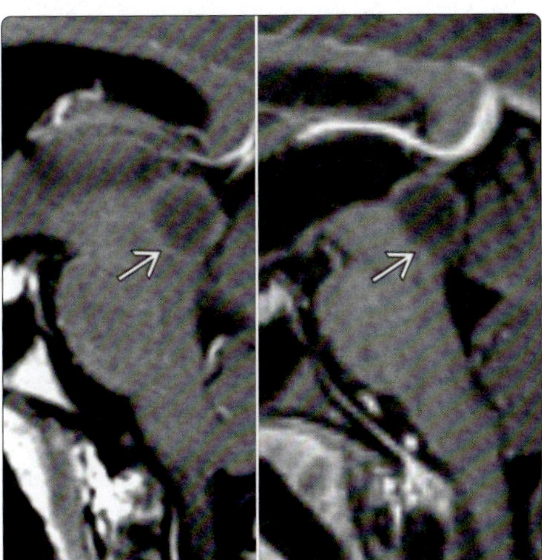

(Left) *Midline sagittal NECT in a 16-year-old girl involved in a motor vehicle accident shows a low-attenuation, expansile mass centered in the tectum ➡ with obliteration of the cerebral aqueduct ➡.* **(Right)** *Midline sagittal T1 C+ MR in the same patient at diagnosis (left) & 16 months later (right) shows a nonenhancing, expansile mass centered in the tectum ➡. The lack of enhancement & lack of interval growth (or very slow growth over time) is typical for a tectal plate glioma.*

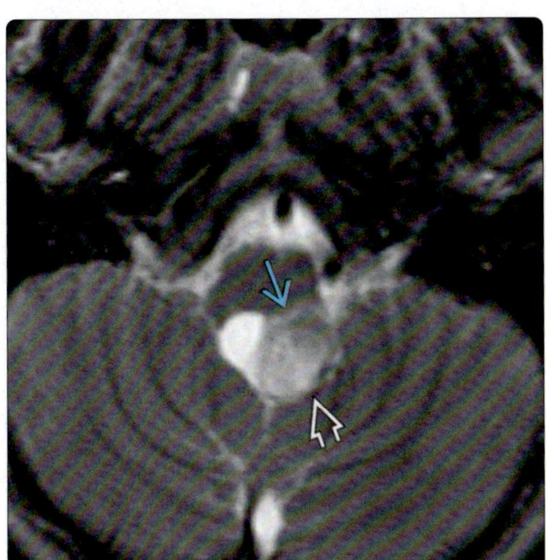

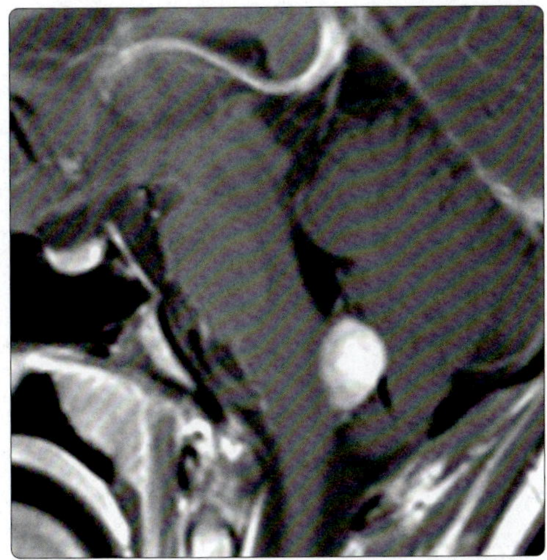

(Left) *Axial T2 MR in an 11-year-old patient with a heterogeneously hyperintense mass at the inferior 4th ventricle shows an indistinct border ➡ of the mass with the medulla, but a distinct border ➡ with the cerebellum, suggesting an exophytic origin from the dorsal medulla.* **(Right)** *Sagittal T1 C+ MR in the same patient shows homogeneous enhancement of the mass arising from the dorsal medulla, a typical pattern of enhancement for a pilocytic astrocytoma (confirmed histologically).*

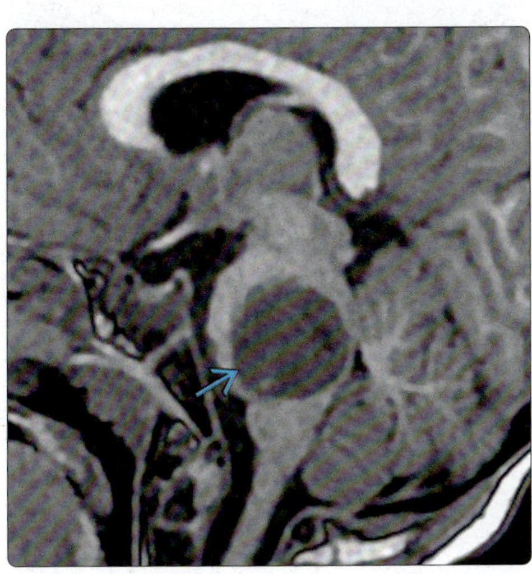

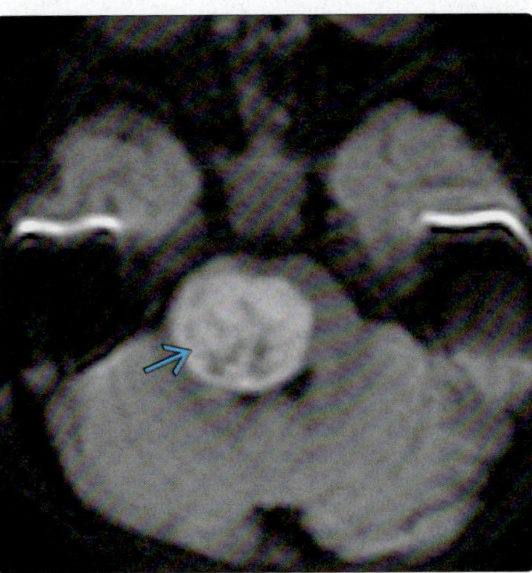

(Left) *Sagittal T1 MR in a 3-year-old patient with poor tracking shows a well-defined, hypointense mass ➡ centered in the pons. Note the sharp margins of the mass, atypical for DIPG/DMG.* **(Right)** *Axial DWI MR in the same patient shows diffusely ↑ signal ➡ (↓ ADC not shown), consistent with a highly cellular tumor. Pathology showed an embryonal tumor with multilayered rosettes (ETMR). While uncommon in the brainstem, embryonal tumors should be considered in any highly cellular focal brainstem tumor.*

KEY FACTS

TERMINOLOGY

- Dysembryoplastic neuroepithelial tumor (DNET)
  - Benign mixed glial-neuronal neoplasm
  - Adjacent cortical dysplasia is frequently present

IMAGING

- May occur in any region of supratentorial cortex
  - Medial temporal lobe is most common
- Typically sharply demarcated, often wedge-shaped
  - Often cystic ("bubbly")
  - Minimal or no mass effect
  - No peritumoral edema
- Some DNETs have less distinct margins
  - Associated cortical dysplasia is more likely in these cases
- Faint focal punctate or ring enhancement in 20-30%
- Ca^{2+} in 6-36%
- Slow or no growth over years
- Remodel overlying bone in 20-44%

TOP DIFFERENTIAL DIAGNOSES

- Ganglioglioma
- Focal cortical dysplasia
- Neuroepithelial cyst
- Pleomorphic xanthoastrocytoma
- Angiocentric glioma

PATHOLOGY

- WHO grade 1
- Pathologic hallmark: Specific glioneuronal element
- Histologic subtypes: Simple, complex, & nonspecific
  - Complex: Associated cortical dysplasia is present

CLINICAL ISSUES

- Typical history: Child or young adult with seizures
- Gross total resection (including adjacent dysplasia) is usually curative & is most important factor for seizure freedom
- Histology usually remains benign even with enhancing tumor recurrence

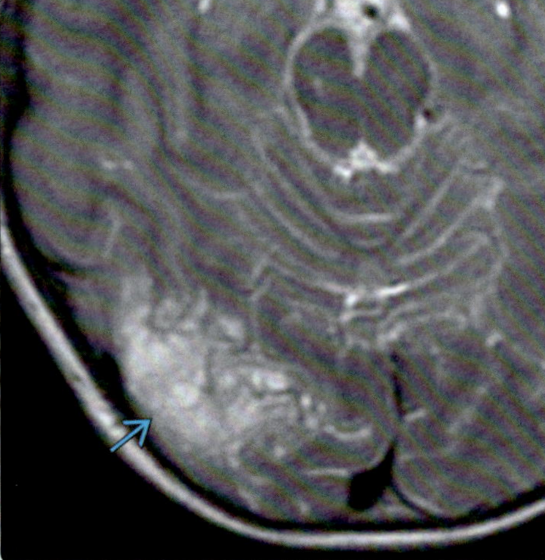

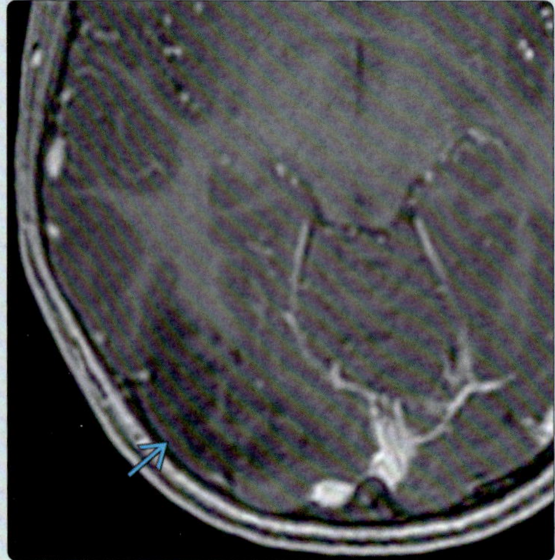

(Left) *Axial T2 MR in a 12-year-old patient with seizure shows a bubbly, microcystic lesion ➡ in right occipital lobe with no significant mass effect. This bubbly replacement of normal brain parenchyma is the most specific appearance for dysembryoplastic neuroepithelial tumor (DNET).* **(Right)** *Axial T1 C+ MR in the same patient shows hypointensity & no associated enhancement within the lesion ➡. The vast majority of DNETs do not enhance, particularly those with the microcystic bubbly appearance.*

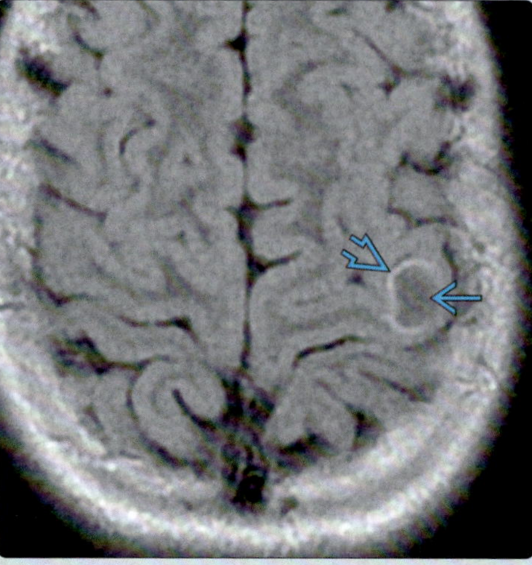

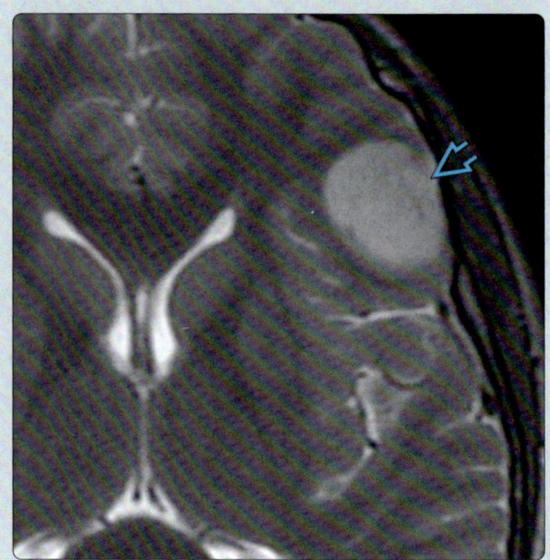

(Left) *Axial FLAIR MR in a 10-year-old patient with seizures shows a unilocular lesion with central hypointensity ➡ & a hyperintense rim ⇨, recently described as the T2-FLAIR mismatch sign. Even in multicystic lesions, the central portions often suppress on FLAIR, while the margins are typically hyperintense.* **(Right)** *Axial T2 MR in a 14-year-old patient with epilepsy shows the less common solid-appearing cortical DNET ⇨ with homogenous hyperintensity. T1 C+ MR (not shown) demonstrated no enhancement.*

KEY FACTS

TERMINOLOGY

- Well-differentiated, slowly growing neuroepithelial tumor composed of neoplastic ganglion & glial cells

IMAGING

- Best imaging clue: Partially cystic, partially enhancing, cortically based mass in child/young adult with temporal lobe epilepsy
- Supratentorial: 85-90%; infratentorial: 10-15%
- Most commonly involves cerebral cortex, especially temporal lobe (~ 50%)
- Ca^{2+} in up to 50%
- Enhancement in ~ 50%
- Superficial lesions may remodel overlying calvarium
- Ill-defined, adjacent, cortical signal abnormality suggests associated focal cortical dysplasia (FCD)

TOP DIFFERENTIAL DIAGNOSES

- Dysembryoplastic neuroepithelial tumor (DNET)
- FCD
- Pleomorphic xanthoastrocytoma
- Pilocytic astrocytoma
- Diffuse astrocytoma (grade 2)
- Oligodendroglioma

PATHOLOGY

- WHO grade 1 (80%) or 2
- Uncommon: Anaplastic ganglioglioma (WHO grade 3)
- Rare: Malignant with glioblastoma multiforme-like glial component (WHO grade 4)

CLINICAL ISSUES

- Occurs at all ages; peak: 10-20 years
- 1-4% of all pediatric CNS neoplasms
- Most common glioneuronal tumor
- Most common neoplastic cause of temporal lobe epilepsy
- Excellent prognosis with complete resection
- Seizure freedom is improved by early surgical intervention

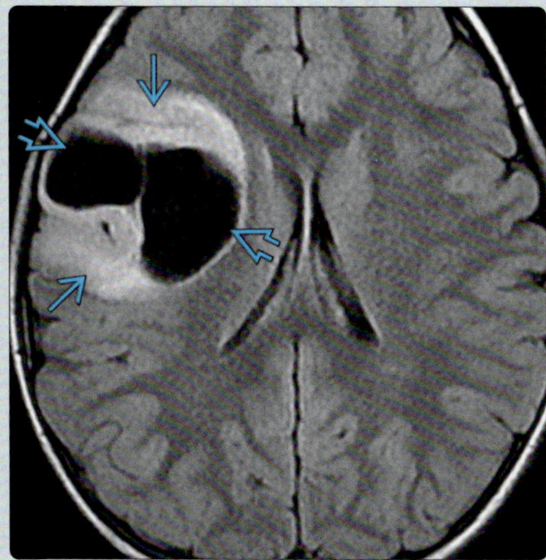

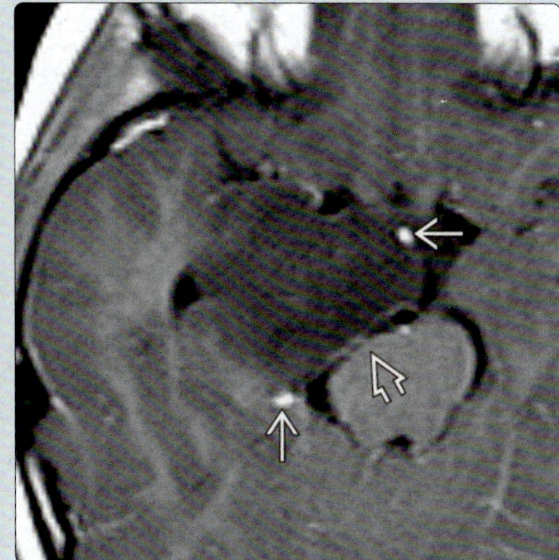

(Left) *Axial FLAIR MR in a 6-year-old with a ganglioglioma (GG) shows a mixed solid ➙ & cystic ➙ lesion involving the frontal cortex with extension to the underlying white matter. Approximately 25-50% of GGs will have a cystic component.* **(Right)** *Axial T1 C+ MR in a 5-year-old boy with episodes of eyelid fluttering & left arm dystonia shows a nonenhancing expansile mass in the right mesial temporal lobe. There is mass effect upon the adjacent vessels ➙ & brainstem ➙. Approximately 50% of GGs will demonstrate no enhancement.*

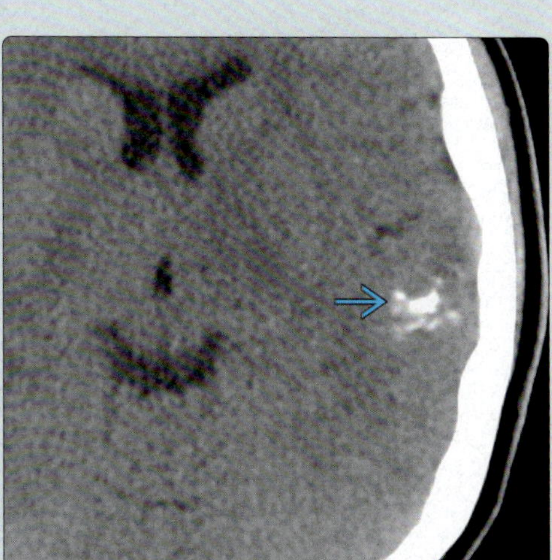

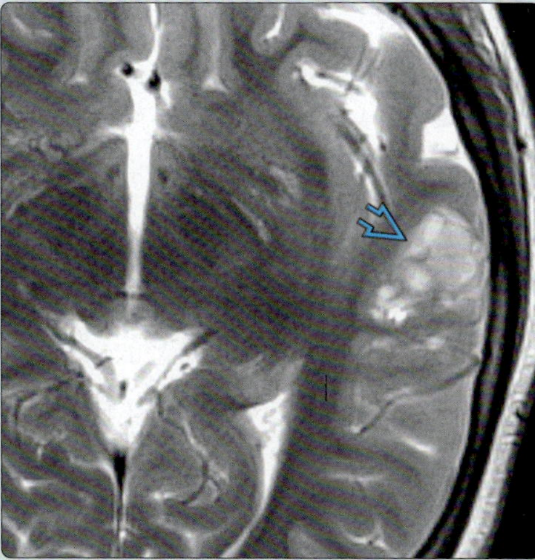

(Left) *Axial NECT in a 14-year-old patient with seizures shows a partially calcified GG ➙ in the left temporal lobe. Ca^{2+} is common in GG, seen in ~ 50% of tumors.* **(Right)** *Axial T2 MR in the same patient with a GG shows a cortically based, hyperintense lesion ➙ in the left temporal lobe, which is the most common location for GG. The lesion shows relatively little mass effect, another common finding. The associated Ca^{2+} & enhancement (not shown) in this lesion are strongly suggestive of GG.*

KEY FACTS

TERMINOLOGY

- Large, cystic tumors of infants involving superficial cerebral cortex & leptomeninges
- Desmoplastic infantile ganglioglioma (DIG)
  - Prominent desmoplastic stroma + neoplastic astrocytes & variable neuronal component
- Desmoplastic infantile astrocytoma (DIA)
  - Desmoplastic stroma + neoplastic astrocytes

IMAGING

- Peripheral, supratentorial tumor with large cyst(s) & cortically-based, solid nodule/plaque in child < 2 years of age
- Variable T2 signal of solid component, often markedly ↓
  - Peritumoral edema may be vasogenic or interstitial from obstructive hydrocephalus
- May have diffusion restriction despite low histologic grade
- Peripheral, solid component often avidly enhances
- Broad dural base + enhancement of adjacent meninges
- Hemorrhage & Ca^{2+} are uncommon

TOP DIFFERENTIAL DIAGNOSES

- Embryonal tumor with multilayered rosettes (ETMR)
- Infantile glioblastoma
- Atypical teratoid/rhabdoid tumor
- Supratentorial ependymoma
- Pleomorphic xanthoastrocytoma
- Pilocytic astrocytoma

PATHOLOGY

- WHO grade 1; areas of cellular proliferation, mitoses, & necrosis may cause misdiagnosis as higher grade tumor

CLINICAL ISSUES

- Most are found at 1-24 months of age (peak: 3-6 months)
- 16% of intracranial tumors in 1st year of life
- Median survival rate > 75% at 15 years
- Complete surgical resection is typically curative
  - 40% require additional therapy beyond surgery

(Left) *Coronal 3D SSFP MR in a 5-month-old girl with increasing head circumference shows a large mass with a peripheral, hyperintense, solid component ➡ & more central cystic component ➡. Note also the peritumoral edema ➡.* **(Right)** *Axial T1 C+ MR in the same patient shows homogeneous enhancement of the peripheral solid component ➡ & no significant enhancement along the margins of the central cystic component ➡. Note the broad-based dural attachment ➡ of this desmoplastic infantile ganglioglioma (DIG).*

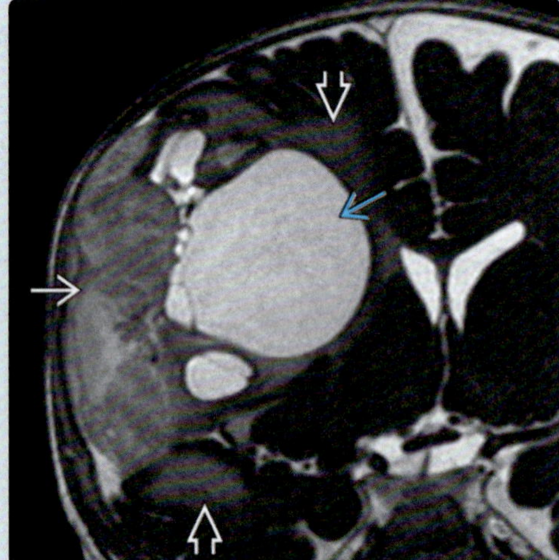

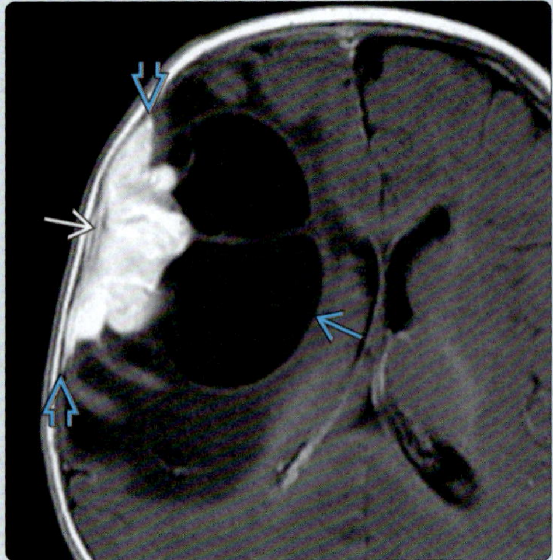

(Left) *Axial T2 MR in a 20-month-old with DIG shows a heterogeneous right temporal lobe mass with multiple cystic components ➡. The 2 most common appearances of DIG/DIA include a single large cyst with a solid, peripheral, enhancing component or a mixed solid & cystic mass with multiple prominent cysts.* **(Right)** *Axial T2 MR in a 1-year-old with a DIG shows a solid mass ➡ centered in the left thalamus with associated obstructive hydrocephalus. A solid lesion is the least common appearance of DIG/DIA.*

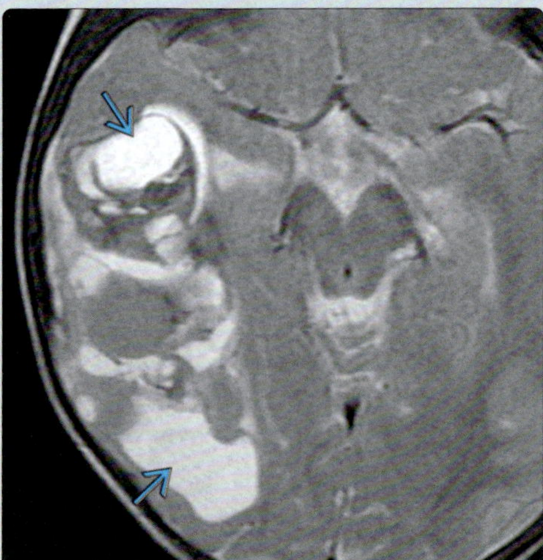

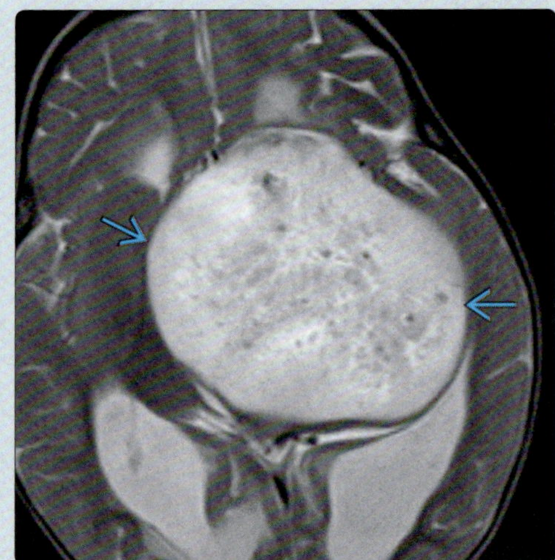

KEY FACTS

TERMINOLOGY

- Embryonal tumor with multilayered rosettes (ETMR)
- Includes former histologic diagnoses: Ependymal tumor with abundant neuropil & true rosettes (ETANTR) & ependymoblastoma
- Now molecularly & genetically distinct entities considered under embryonal tumors (all WHO grade 4) include
  - ETMR, C19MC altered
  - CNS embryonal tumor, not otherwise specified (NOS)
    - Medulloepithelioma
    - CNS neuroblastoma
  - Medulloblastoma
  - Atypical teratoid/rhabdoid tumor

IMAGING

- Large (mean: 5 cm), complex-appearing, hemispheric mass in infant/young child
- ~ 50% are well defined with minimal peritumoral edema
- Ca^{2+} in 50-70%; hemorrhage is common
- Variable enhancement
- Restricted diffusion of solid highly cellular components
- Subarachnoid spread is common at presentation

TOP DIFFERENTIAL DIAGNOSES

- Glioblastoma
- Supratentorial ependymoma
- Atypical teratoid/rhabdoid tumor
- Desmoplastic infantile ganglioglioma/astrocytoma
- Choroid plexus carcinoma
- Giant cavernoma

PATHOLOGY

- Defined by genetic alteration at 19q13.42 (*C19MC* amplification), regardless of histology

CLINICAL ISSUES

- Most common in younger children
- Treatment: Aggressive surgical resection, chemotherapy, craniospinal radiation (if of tolerable age)

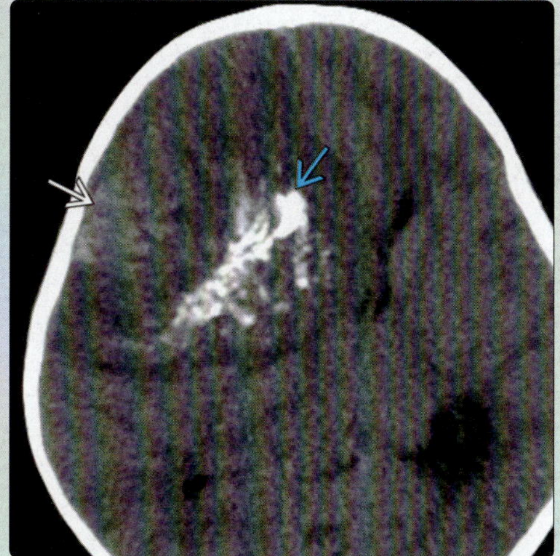

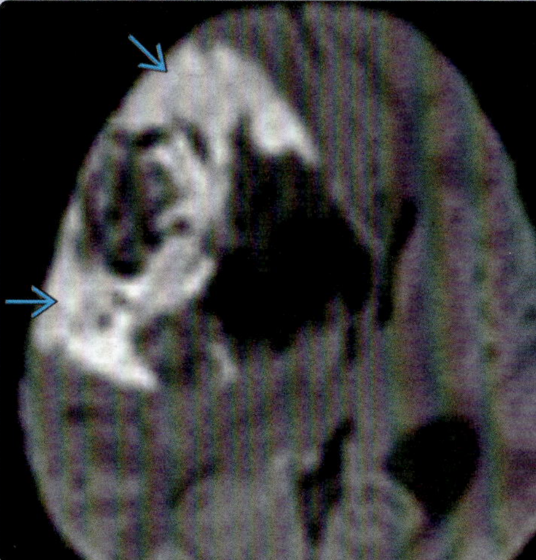

(Left) *Axial NECT in a 2-year-old child with altered mental status shows a large, heterogeneous, intraaxial mass. Areas of ↑ attenuation ➡ correspond to cellular or hemorrhagic areas foci. Calcification ➡ is present in ~ 50% of embryonal tumor with multilayered rosettes (ETMR).* **(Right)** *Axial DWI MR in the same patient shows restricted diffusion ➡ in the solid portions of the mass, consistent with high cellularity. ETMR should be considered in any cellular hemispheric tumor, especially in young children.*

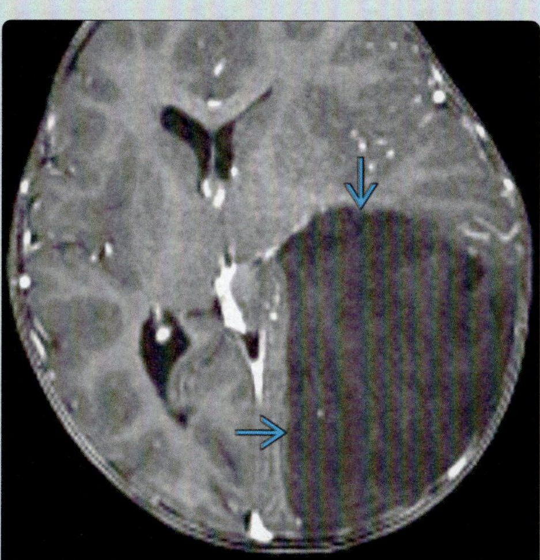

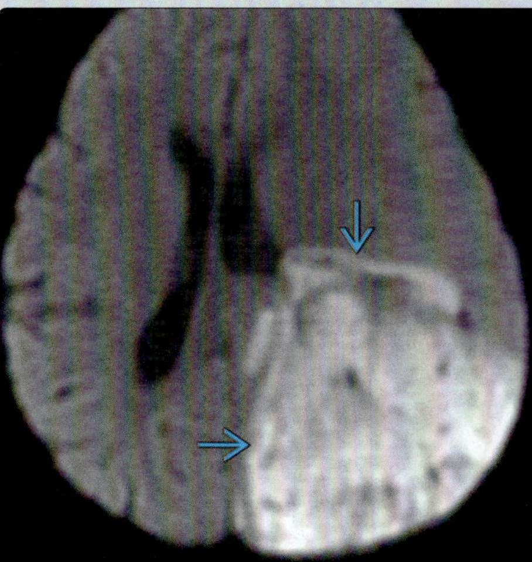

(Left) *Axial T1 C+ FS MR in a 1-year-old shows a well-demarcated tumor ➡ in the left parietooccipital region with no significant enhancement. The enhancement of ETMR is highly variable, ranging from avid to no enhancement. Note the lack of peritumoral edema, typical of ETMR.* **(Right)** *Axial DWI MR in the same patient shows marked diffusion restriction ➡ (↓ ADC not shown), consistent with a highly cellular tumor. Pathology revealed an ETMR, C19MC altered.*

KEY FACTS

IMAGING

- Best clue: Complex suprasellar cystic mass with Ca^{2+} & wall enhancement
- Location: Suprasellar 75%, suprasellar + intrasellar 21%
  - Larger tumors can extend into multiple cranial fossae
- "90% rule"
  - 90% cystic: MR signal intensity is highly variable
    - Cystic components are frequently T1 hyperintense
  - 90% calcified: SWI/T2* GRE MR are helpful to identify Ca^{2+}
  - 90% enhance (wall & solid portions)
- Often develop obstructive hydrocephalus
- Optic chiasm, hypothalamus, & vessels are often involved
  - Thin sagittal T2 or 3D SSFP MR sequences to assess

TOP DIFFERENTIAL DIAGNOSES

- Rathke cleft cyst
- Pituitary adenoma
- Germinoma
- Hypothalamic-chiasmatic glioma

PATHOLOGY

- 2 clinically & pathologically distinct subtypes
  - Adamantinomatous: Cystic & solid, mostly in children
  - Squamous-papillary: Mostly solid tumor found in adults

CLINICAL ISSUES

- 6-9% of all pediatric intracranial tumors
- Symptoms: Visual changes, endocrine related, academic decline, headache/vomiting (obstructive hydrocephalus)
  - ~ 1/3 of patients have endocrine symptoms (↓ growth hormone, ↓ thyroid function, diabetes insipidus)
- Benign tumor with high rate of recurrence
- Poor prognostic factors: Hypothalamic involvement, ↑ tumor size

DIAGNOSTIC CHECKLIST

- Must identify relationship of tumor to optic chiasm, hypothalamus, & vessels

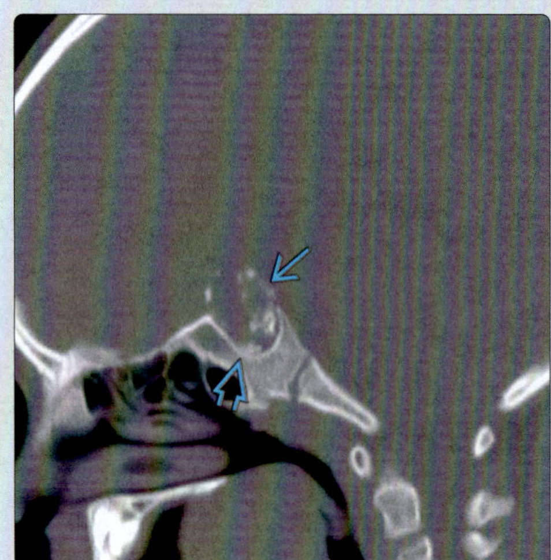

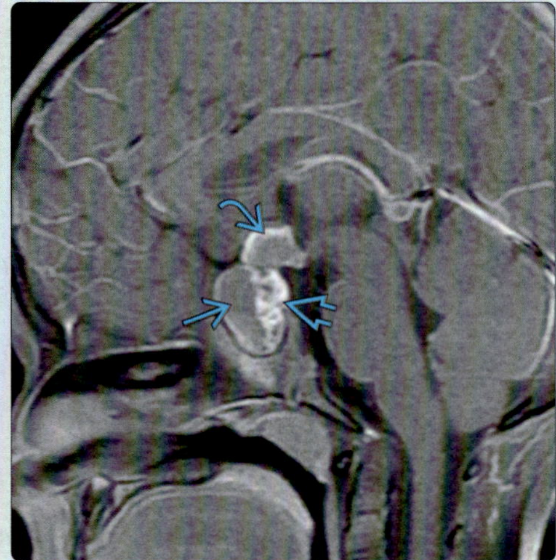

(Left) *Sagittal NECT in a 7-year-old patient with diabetes insipidus shows smooth remodeling of the sella turcica ⇨ by a partially calcified mass ⇨, highly suggestive of craniopharyngioma.* **(Right)** *Sagittal T1 C+ MR in the same patient shows a nonenhancing cystic component ⇨ & a nodular enhancing component ⇨. A rim-enhancing lobular component ⇨ protrudes superiorly. This case represents a typical craniopharyngioma with Ca^{2+}, cysts, & solid, enhancing tissue.*

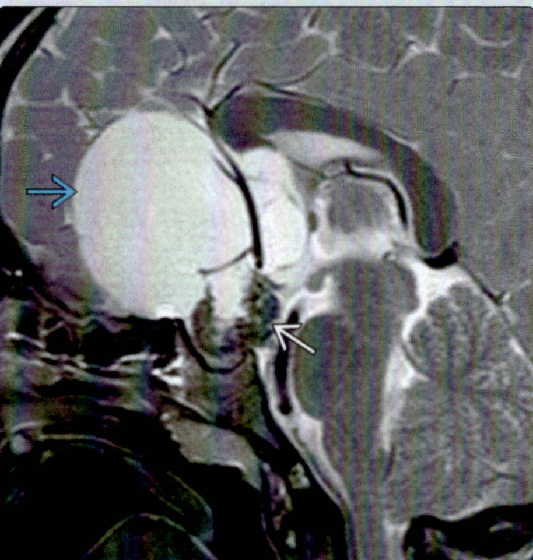

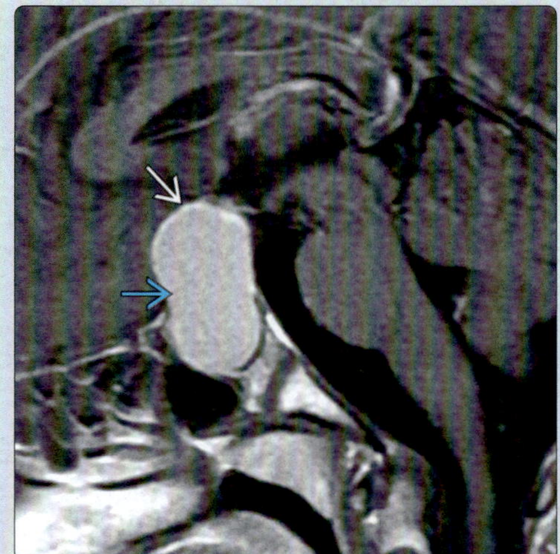

(Left) *Sagittal T2 MR in a 3-year-old patient shows hypointense signal in the posterior components ➡ of a suprasellar mass, corresponding to Ca^{2+}. Frontal extension of the large cystic components ⇨ is typical of a prechiasmatic location.* **(Right)** *Sagittal T1 C+ MR in a 10-year-old boy with increasing headaches shows a predominantly cystic mass with a very thin rim of enhancement ➡. The majority of the mass showed intrinsic T1 shortening ⇨ before contrast, a common finding in craniopharyngioma.*

TERMINOLOGY

Definitions

- Craniopharyngioma (CP): Histologically benign epithelial tumor arising from squamous rests along involuted hypophyseal-Rathke duct

IMAGING

General Features

- Best diagnostic clue
  - Cystic suprasellar mass with Ca^{2+} & enhancing wall or mural nodule
- Location
  - Suprasellar: 75%; mixed suprasellar + intrasellar: 21%; intrasellar: 4%
  - Retrochiasmatic vs. prechiasmatic configuration is key determinant for surgical approach
  - Larger tumors can extend into multiple cranial fossae
- Often large at presentation (> 5 cm)
  - Cyst is typically largest component

CT Findings

- "90% rule": 90% cystic, 90% calcified, 90% enhance (wall & solid portions)
- May present with obstructive hydrocephalus from compression on 3rd ventricle & foramen of Monro

MR Findings

- T1: Cysts are often very hyperintense, reflecting protein, cholesterol, &/or blood products in fluid
- T2: Heterogeneous, solid tumor: Hypointense foci of Ca^{2+}, variable signal intensity of cysts
- FLAIR: Cysts typically do not suppress like CSF
- SWI/T2* GRE: Areas of signal loss correspond to Ca^{2+}
- DWI: Variable cystic signal, typically closer to CSF than brain
- T1 C+: Solid portions enhance heterogeneously; cyst wall may show smooth or irregular enhancement

Imaging Recommendations

- Protocol advice
  - Volumetric T1 ± contrast; SWI/GRE for Ca^{2+}
  - Thin 3D sagittal T2 or SSFP sequences help define relationship of tumor to adjacent structures
  - MRA for preoperative identification of arterial involvement

DIFFERENTIAL DIAGNOSIS

Rathke Cleft Cyst

- Ca^{2+} uncommon; no nodular/solid component
- Cyst is more homogeneous, although small, T2-hypointense, intracystic nodules may be present

Germinoma

- Predominantly solid & lobular
- Ca^{2+} is very rare in suprasellar germinoma
- Strong association with diabetes insipidus

Pituitary Adenoma

- Solid tumor arising from adenohypophysis
- Diffuse & homogeneous enhancement

Hypothalamic-Chiasmatic Glioma

- More solid & homogeneous
- Extension into prechiasmatic optic nerves/tracts

Arachnoid Cyst

- Thin/imperceptible nonenhancing wall
- Cyst contents follow CSF

Dermoid & Epidermoid Cysts

- Epidermoids are solid but mimic cysts
- Suprasellar locations rare in children
- Minimal enhancement; marked diffusion restriction

PATHOLOGY

General Features

- 2 clinically & pathologically distinct subtypes
  - Adamantinomatous (~ 90%): Classic calcified cyst with mural nodule, seen in children
  - Papillary (~ 10%): Mostly solid tumor almost exclusively found in adults
  - Adamantinomatous & papillary: WHO grade 1
- Genetics
  - Targetable mutations present in subset of tumors
    - *BRAF* (V600E) in many papillary CPs
    - *CTNNB1* in many adamantinomatous CPs

CLINICAL ISSUES

Presentation

- Headache, vomiting, hydrocephalus, papilledema
- Visual disturbance, decline in school performance
- Endocrine symptoms in at least 1/3 of cases due to mass effect on pituitary/hypothalamus
  - Growth hormone deficiency, hypothyroidism, diabetes insipidus

Demographics

- Epidemiology
  - Most common nonglial pediatric intracranial tumor
    - > 50% of all pediatric suprasellar region tumors

Natural History & Prognosis

- 88% overall survival at 20 years
- Hypothalamic involvement: ↓ overall survival, quality of life
- Factors affecting recurrence
  - Gross total vs. partial resection
  - Radiation therapy (for residual tumor) ↓ recurrence
  - Tumor size (↑ recurrence in larger tumors)

Treatment

- Surgical: Complete resection is ideal but must be weighed against high morbidity associated with extensive resection in suprasellar/hypothalamic region
- Radiation therapy for incomplete resection

SELECTED REFERENCES

1. Chen X et al: Noninvasive molecular diagnosis of craniopharyngioma with MRI-based radiomics approach. BMC Neurol. 19(1):6, 2019
2. Plaza MJ et al: Conventional and advanced MRI features of pediatric intracranial tumors: posterior fossa and suprasellar tumors. AJR Am J Roentgenol. 200(5):1115-24, 2013

KEY FACTS

TERMINOLOGY

- Tumor of primordial germ cells, histologically identical to gonadal & nongonadal seminoma or dysgerminoma

IMAGING

- CT: Hyperattenuating, solid components
  - Pineal region: Localized "engulfed" Ca^{2+}
  - Other sites: Ca^{2+} rare, but hemorrhage may occur
- MR: Mass in suprasellar, pineal, or basal ganglia regions
  - T2: Multiple small cysts are not unusual (~ 25%)
  - DWI: Diffusion restriction in solid components
  - T1 C+: Avid enhancement, often "speckled"
  - Pineal: Bithalamic extension, peritumoral edema
  - Suprasellar: Absent T1 posterior pituitary bright spot
  - Metastatic CSF dissemination is common (25-40%)

TOP DIFFERENTIAL DIAGNOSES

- Pineal region
  - Pineoblastoma
  - Nongerminomatous germ cell tumors (teratoma, etc.)
  - Tectal plate glioma
- Suprasellar
  - Craniopharyngioma
  - Hypothalamic/chiasmatic astrocytoma
  - Langerhans cell histiocytosis

CLINICAL ISSUES

- M > F, especially in pineal region
- Mean age: 10-15 years
- Pineal: Headache, paralysis of upward gaze
- Suprasellar: Diabetes insipidus (DI), vision changes
- ± ↑ serum & CSF human chorionic gonadotropin
- Favorable prognosis (5-year survival > 90%)

DIAGNOSTIC CHECKLIST

- Image entire neuraxis to detect CSF dissemination
- Occult germinoma is possible in child with DI & normal MR
  - Repeat MR in 3-6 months to assess for growing mass

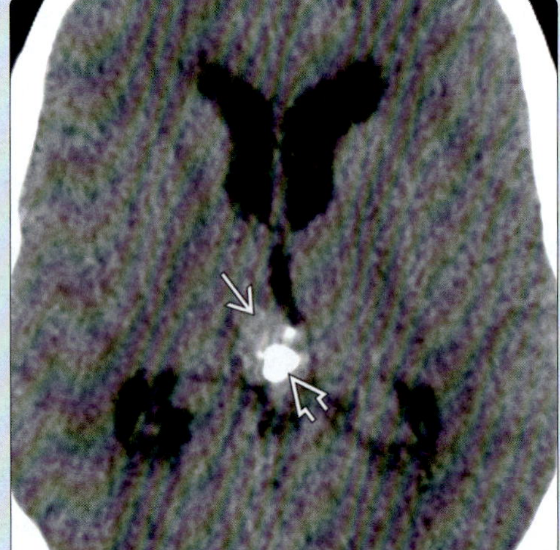

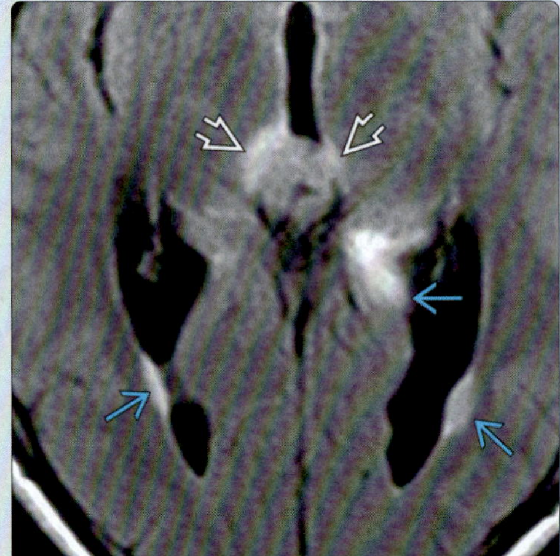

(Left) *Axial NECT in a 14-year-old boy with worsening headaches shows a hyperattenuating mass ➡ with localized Ca^{2+} ➡. Calcifications are common in pineal germinoma & are thought to represent pineal Ca^{2+} "engulfed" by tumor.* **(Right)** *Axial FLAIR MR in the same patient shows tumor extension into the right thalamus, parenchymal edema ➡ in the thalami (R > L), & CSF spread of tumor ➡. Peritumoral edema & thalamic extension are common findings in pineal germinoma, as is CSF spread of tumor.*

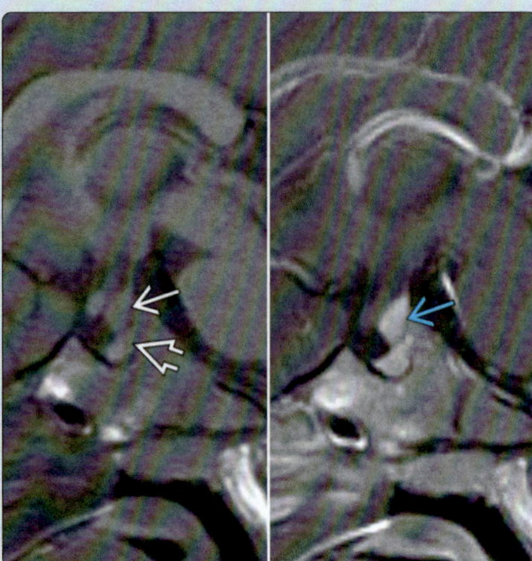

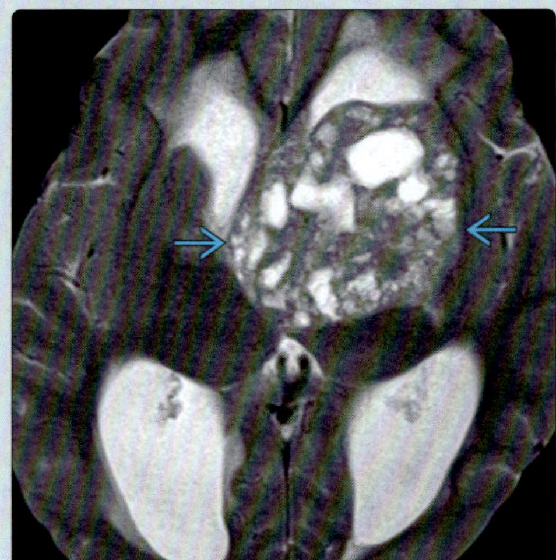

(Left) *Sagittal T1 C+ MR (left) in a 4-year-old boy with central diabetes insipidus (DI) shows an infundibular mass ➡ & absence of the posterior pituitary bright spot ➡. After contrast (right), the infundibular mass enhances homogeneously ➡, typical of germinoma.* **(Right)** *Axial T2 MR in a 10-year-old girl with fatigue, headaches, & vomiting shows a large solid, cystic mass ➡ centered in the left basal ganglia. The basal ganglia are a less common (~ 15%) location for germinoma (though these tumors are often large).*

TERMINOLOGY

Definitions

- Tumor of primordial germ cells, essentially identical to gonadal or extragonadal seminoma & dysgerminoma

IMAGING

General Features

- Best diagnostic clue
  - Pineal mass with localized Ca^{2+} & bithalamic extension
  - Suprasellar mass with diabetes insipidus (DI)
- Location
  - CNS germinomas typically occur in midline near 3rd ventricle
    - Pineal region (40-50%)
    - Suprasellar (30-40%)
    - Basal ganglia (BG) tumors are less common (5-15%)
  - CSF spread of metastases is common (25-40%)
- Size
  - Typically small (1-3 cm)
  - Tiny or inapparent suprasellar germinoma may cause DI

CT Findings

- Sharply circumscribed, heterogeneously hyperdense mass
- Localized ("engulfed") Ca^{2+} is common in pineal tumors
- Ca^{2+} is rare in suprasellar tumors
- Primary tumors & metastases usually enhance avidly

MR Findings

- T1: Isointense to hypointense
- T2: Hyperintense cystic components
- FLAIR: Sensitive for peritumoral edema
- DWI: Solid components typically show diffusion restriction
- GRE/SWI: Hypointense signal may represent Ca^{2+} (pineal) or hemorrhage (suprasellar & BG)
- T1 C+: Most tumors show marked enhancement
  - Speckled pattern in tumors with small cysts
  - Most sensitive sequence for CSF metastases

DIFFERENTIAL DIAGNOSIS

Pineal Region Masses

- Pineoblastoma
  - Highly cellular pineal mass in young child
  - Scattered ("exploded") Ca^{2+} rather than localized ("engulfed") Ca^{2+} in germinoma
  - Less common than germinoma & typically younger age
- Tectal plate glioma
  - Little or no enhancement
  - High ADC signal (no diffusion restriction)

Sellar/Suprasellar Masses

- Craniopharyngioma
  - Dominant cystic components ± T1 shortening, Ca^{2+}
  - DI is less common until after surgery
- Hypothalamic/chiasmatic astrocytoma
  - No diffusion restriction
  - Rarely associated with DI
- Langerhans cell histiocytosis (LCH)
  - Thickened infundibulum; look for osseus lesions

PATHOLOGY

General Features

- Etiology
  - Germ cell tumors (GCTs) are found in gonads, mediastinum, & intracranial (parasellar & pineal) locations
- Associated abnormalities
  - ± ↑ serum & CSF human chorionic gonadotropin

CLINICAL ISSUES

Presentation

- Most common signs/symptoms
  - Pineal region germinoma
    - Headache secondary to aqueduct obstruction & hydrocephalus
    - Parinaud syndrome (paralysis of upward gaze)
    - Precocious puberty
  - Suprasellar germinoma
    - DI
    - Hypothalamic-pituitary dysfunction (↓ growth, precocious puberty)
    - Visual symptoms

Demographics

- Age
  - Mean age in most studies: 10-15 years
- Sex
  - M > F, especially in pineal region

Natural History & Prognosis

- Pure germinoma has favorable prognosis
- Treatment with radiotherapy ± adjuvant chemotherapy
  - 5-year survival > 90%

DIAGNOSTIC CHECKLIST

Image Interpretation Pearls

- Child or adolescent with DI
  - Expect absence of posterior pituitary bright spot
  - Lobular enhancing suprasellar mass = germinoma
  - Thick, enhancing infundibulum = LCH or germinoma
  - No enhancing lesion = could be occult germinoma
- Adolescent with pineal mass = germinoma or nongerminomatous GCT (NGGCT)
- Child with pineal mass
  - Complex, cystic = also consider NGGCT
  - Homogeneous with restricted diffusion = germinoma vs. pineoblastoma

SELECTED REFERENCES

1. Hirata K et al: Time to diagnosis and clinical characteristics in pediatric brain tumor patients. Childs Nerv Syst. 36(9):2047-54, 2020
2. Juliano J et al: Imaging features predictive of recurrence in pediatric intracranial germ-cell tumors. Pediatr Neurosurg. 1-8, 2019
3. Wu CC et al: MRI features of pediatric intracranial germ cell tumor subtypes. J Neurooncol. 134(1):221-30, 2017
4. Awa R et al: Neuroimaging diagnosis of pineal region tumors-quest for pathognomonic finding of germinoma. Neuroradiology. 56(7):525-34, 2014
5. Kakigi T et al: Quantitative imaging values of CT, MR, and FDG-PET to differentiate pineal parenchymal tumors and germinomas: are they useful? Neuroradiology. 56(4):297-303, 2014
6. Wang Y et al: Intracranial germinoma: clinical and MRI findings in 56 patients. Childs Nerv Syst. 26(12):1773-7, 2010

KEY FACTS

TERMINOLOGY

- Choroid plexus tumor (CPT)
  - Choroid plexus papilloma (CPP): WHO grade 1
  - Atypical choroid plexus papilloma (aCPP): WHO grade 2
  - Choroid plexus carcinoma (CPCa): WHO grade 3

IMAGING

- Strongly enhancing, lobulated intraventricular mass
  - 60-70%: Lateral ventricles (most commonly atrium)
  - 20-30%: 4th ventricle (most common site in adults)
  - < 10%: 3rd ventricle, cerebellomedullary cistern
- Ventriculomegaly from obstruction or ↑ CSF production
- **CT**: Ca^{2+} in 25%
- **MR**: Iso- to hyperintense on T2; internal flow voids
- CPCa are more likely than CPP to show heterogeneous enhancement, necrosis, brain invasion, & CSF spread

TOP DIFFERENTIAL DIAGNOSES

- Intraventricular hemorrhage
- Atypical teratoid/rhabdoid tumor
- Medulloblastoma
- Ependymoma

PATHOLOGY

- ↓ ADC & ↑ tumor volume → ↑ grade & poorer prognosis
- ↑ *TP53* mutations in tumor correlate with poor prognosis
- Molecular subtype may be more prognostic than histology
  - Cluster 1: Pediatric, supratentorial, good prognosis
  - Cluster 2: Adult, infratentorial, good prognosis
  - Cluster 3: Pediatric, supratentorial, poor prognosis
- Associated with Li-Fraumeni & Aicardi syndromes

CLINICAL ISSUES

- ~ 25-33% present < 1 year of age; ~ 49-75% present < 5 years of age

DIAGNOSTIC CHECKLIST

- T1 C+ MR of entire neuraxis before surgery
- Imaging is not reliable for distinguishing CPP from CPCa

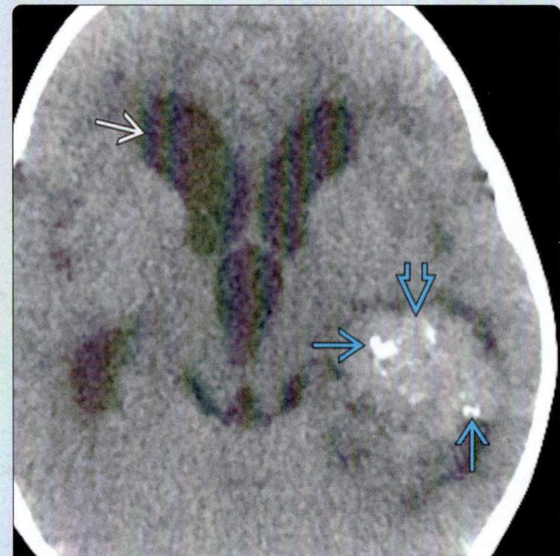

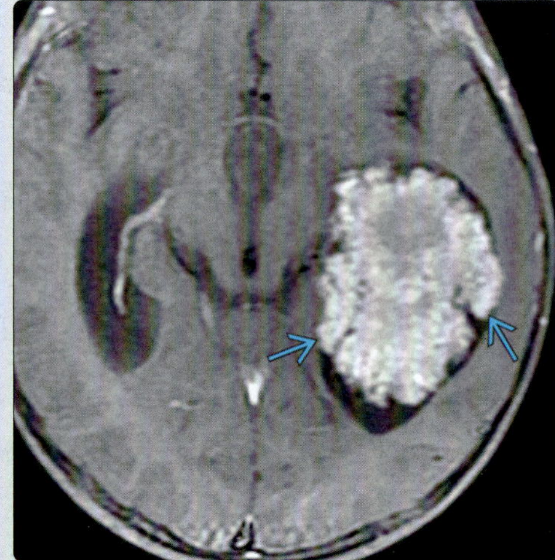

(Left) *Axial NECT in a 22-month-old with macrocephaly shows a large mass ⇨ centered in the atrium of the left lateral ventricle with scattered foci of Ca^{2+} ⇨. Note the lateral & 3rd ventricular enlargement ➡ without evidence of obstruction, consistent with hydrocephalus due to overproduction of CSF by this choroid plexus papilloma (CPP).* **(Right)** *Axial T1 C+ MR in the same patient shows avid enhancement of the mass & frond-like margins ⇨ of the tumor. These features are very common in CPP.*

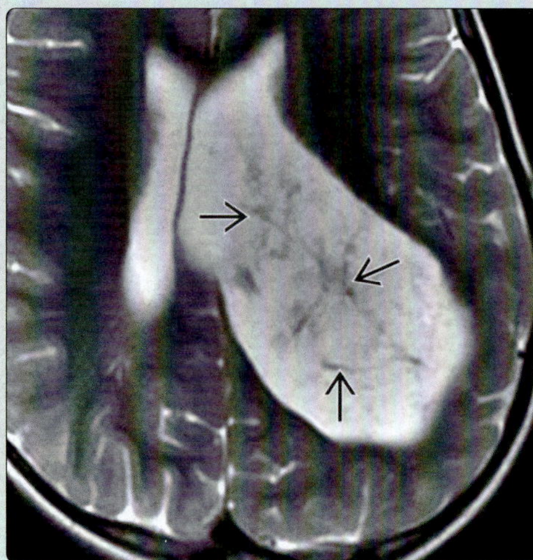

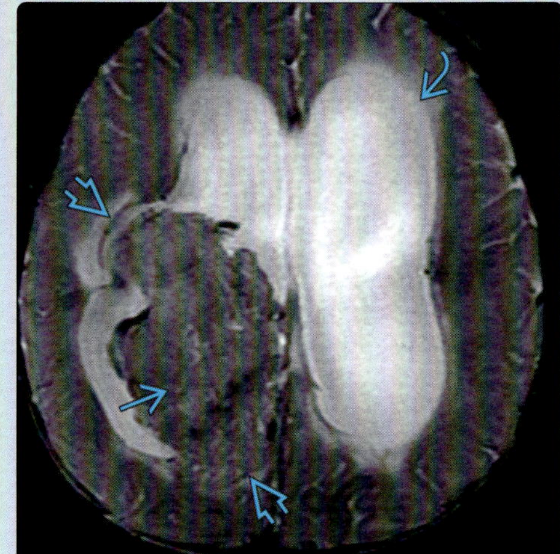

(Left) *Axial T2 MR in a 3-year-old girl shows predominantly hyperintense signal (equal to CSF) throughout a large mass that expands the lateral ventricle. A few branching, hypointense foci ➡ within the lesion represent high-flow vessels. CPP was proven upon resection.* **(Right)** *Axial T2 MR in a 9-month-old with macrocephaly shows a heterogeneous choroid plexus carcinoma (CPCa) ⇨ centered in the right atrium with right frontal & parietal lobe invasion ⇨. Also note the hydrocephalus ⇨.*

TERMINOLOGY

Abbreviations

- Choroid plexus tumor (CPT)
  - Choroid plexus papilloma (CPP): WHO grade 1
  - Atypical choroid plexus papilloma (aCPP): WHO grade 2
  - Choroid plexus carcinoma (CPCa): WHO grade 3

Definitions

- Intraventricular, papillary neoplasm of CP epithelium

IMAGING

General Features

- Best diagnostic clue
  - Strongly enhancing, lobulated intraventricular mass
  - Associated hydrocephalus may be obstructive or related to overproduction of CSF by tumor
- Location
  - 60-70%: Lateral ventricle (most commonly atrium)
  - 20-30%: 4th ventricle (most common site of origin in adults)
  - < 10%: 3rd ventricle, cerebellomedullary cistern

CT Findings

- Iso- or hyperattenuating in 75%; Ca^{2+} in 25%

MR Findings

- **T1**: Well-delineated, iso- to hypointense mass
- **T2**: Iso- to hyperintense mass
  - Internal dark signal: Ca^{2+} (nodular or irregular) vs. vascular flow voids (linear & branching)
- **FLAIR**: ↑ generalized periventricular signal → transependymal edema due to ventricular obstruction
  - Brain invasion causing focally abnormal signal is more common in CPCa
- **SWI/T2* GRE**: ± foci of low signal → Ca^{2+} or hemorrhage
- **DWI**: Iso- to hyperintense on ADC
  - ↓ ADC correlates with higher grade tumors
- **T1 C+**: Robust enhancement; frond-like margins
  - Heterogeneity with necrosis suggests CPCa
  - CPCa often shows enhancing CSF dissemination
- **Perfusion**: Typically elevated CBF & CBV

Ultrasonographic Findings

- Hyperechoic mass with frond-like projections
- Echogenicity is similar to normal choroid plexus
- ↑ central vascularity on color Doppler

Imaging Recommendations

- Best imaging tool
  - MR with contrast of entire neuraxis prior to surgery
  - US may be obtained 1st in young infant with open fontanelle & macrocephaly

DIFFERENTIAL DIAGNOSIS

Intraventricular Hemorrhage

- Originates from germinal matrix in premature neonate
- Clot adherent to choroid can be echogenic & mass-like but lacks internal vascularity/enhancement

Atypical Teratoid/Rhabdoid Tumor

- May be intraventricular & lobulated
- Shows less enhancement, more diffusion restriction

Medulloblastoma

- Most common 4th ventricular neoplasm in children
- Shows less enhancement, more diffusion restriction

Ependymoma

- Ependymoma is typically intraaxial when supratentorial
- 4th ventricular ependymoma is similar to CPT

PATHOLOGY

General Features

- Genetics
  - 3 molecular subtypes by methylation pattern (which may be more predictive of prognosis than histology)
    - Cluster 1: Pediatric, supratentorial, good prognosis
      - CPP = aCPP histologically
    - Cluster 2: Adult, infratentorial, good prognosis
      - CPP > aCPP histologically
    - Cluster 3: Pediatric, supratentorial, poor prognosis
      - CPCa > aCPP > CPP histologically
  - Associated with Li-Fraumeni & Aicardi syndromes

CLINICAL ISSUES

Presentation

- Young child with signs & symptoms of ↑ intracranial pressure: Macrocrania, bulging fontanelle, vomiting, headache, ataxia, seizure

Demographics

- Age: CPP: 49% < 5 years, 26% < 1 year
  - CPCa: 75% < 5 years, 33% < 1 year

Natural History & Prognosis

- CPP is benign, slowly growing; 5-year survival ~ 100%
- CPCa is usually large & invasive; 5-year survival ~ 60%
- Either may seed CSF pathways

Treatment

- Gross total resection (GTR)

DIAGNOSTIC CHECKLIST

Consider

- Imaging alone is not reliable for distinguishing CPP vs. CPCa
  - ↓ ADC & ↑ tumor volume → higher grade & poorer prognosis
- 4th ventricular CPT is less common than other pediatric posterior fossa tumors

SELECTED REFERENCES

1. Trybula SJ et al: Infratentorial choroid plexus tumors in children. Childs Nerv Syst. 36(8):1761-6, 2020
2. Crawford JR et al: Perinatal (fetal and neonatal) choroid plexus tumors: a review. Childs Nerv Syst. 35(6):937-44, 2019
3. Dash C et al: Management of choroid plexus tumors in infants and young children up to 4 years of age: an institutional experience. World Neurosurg. 121:e237-45, 2019
4. Sasaki T et al: Roles of the apparent diffusion coefficient and tumor volume in predicting tumor grade in patients with choroid plexus tumors. Neuroradiology. 60(5):479-86, 2018

KEY FACTS

IMAGING

- Scalp hematomas
  - Caput succedaneum: In superficial soft tissues; crosses sutures & midline
  - Subgaleal hematoma: Deep to epicranial aponeurosis; crosses sutures & midline
  - Cephalohematoma: Subperiosteal; limited by sutures; ↓ & calcifies over time
- Calvarial fractures
  - Usually nondisplaced
  - Depressed fractures often have smooth margins ("ping pong fracture")
- Intracranial hemorrhages
  - Subdural hematomas are most common: Usually small (< 3-mm thickness) without associated mass effect
  - Epidural hematomas are rare & usually associated with skull fracture
- Hypoxic-ischemic injury: Considered separately

TOP DIFFERENTIAL DIAGNOSES

- Coagulopathy
- Abusive head trauma
- Accidental postnatal head injury
- Venous sinus thrombosis

CLINICAL ISSUES

- Subdural hematomas, typically small, are seen in 26-63% of uncomplicated vaginal deliveries
- Cephalohematomas occur in 1% of all births; ↑ incidence in forceps &/or vacuum assisted deliveries
- Usually of no clinical significance & managed conservatively
  - However, subgaleal hematoma may lead to significant blood loss & shock

DIAGNOSTIC CHECKLIST

- US or CT can exclude need for surgical intervention
- Parenchymal injury not typical; MR study of choice to evaluate for suspected hypoxic-ischemic injury

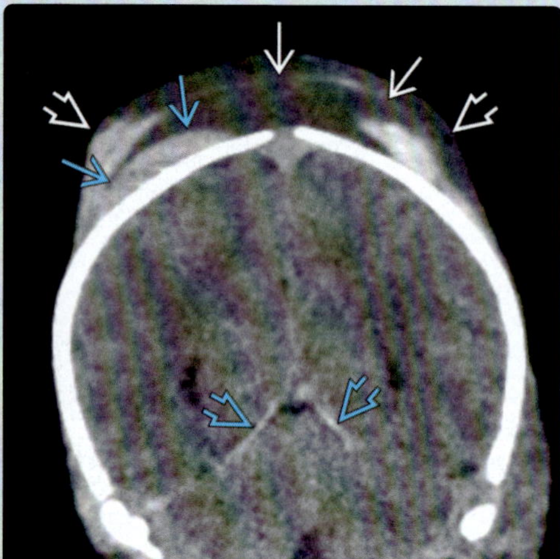

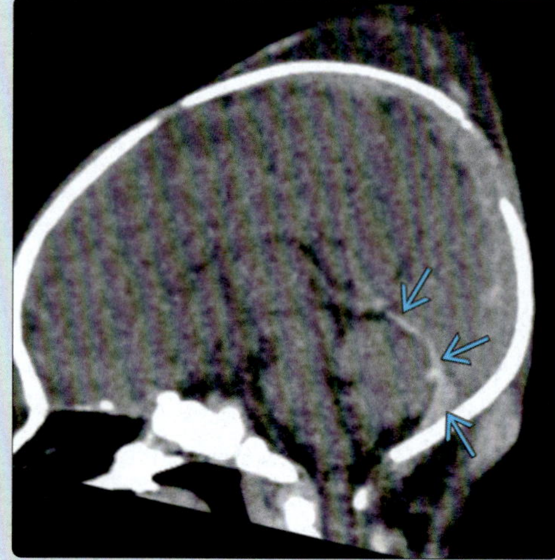

(Left) *Coronal NECT in a 1-day-old infant status post vaginal delivery with vacuum & forceps assist shows marked scalp swelling. There is subperiosteal cephalohematoma ⇨, subgaleal hematoma deep to the epicranial aponeurosis ➡, & diffuse overlying caput succedaneum ➡. Also note the small subdural hemorrhages along the tentorial leaflets ⇨.* **(Right)** *Sagittal NECT in the same patient demonstrates subdural hemorrhage ⇨ along the tentorium & in the posterior fossa.*

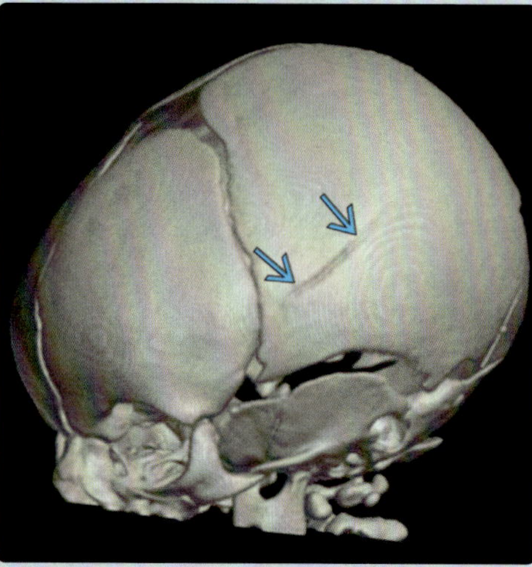

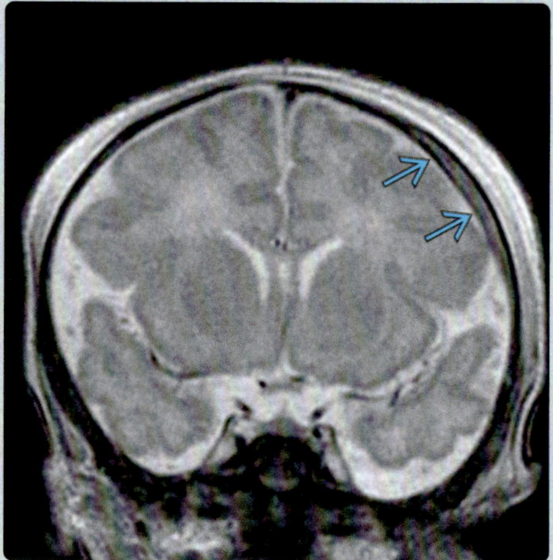

(Left) *Left lateral view of a NECT 3D reformat in the same patient demonstrates an obliquely oriented nondisplaced fracture ⇨ of the left parietal bone.* **(Right)** *Coronal T2 MR in the same patient shows a small, left-sided epidural hematoma ⇨ in association with the skull fracture. No brain parenchymal abnormality was seen. This was managed conservatively given the small size & lack of mass effect.*

IMAGING

General Features

- Location
  - Scalp injury
    - Caput succedaneum: Hemorrhage & edema in subcutaneous tissues; extends across suture lines, crosses midline, & extends into facial soft tissues
    - Subgaleal hematoma: Deep to aponeurosis of scalp, beneath occipitofrontalis muscle
    - Cephalohematoma: Subperiosteal hematoma; confined by sutures
  - Calvarial fractures
    - Frontal & parietal bones are most common
    - Most are nondisplaced
    - Due to ↑ plasticity of infant skull, depressed fractures tend to be of concave morphology rather than angulated
      - a.k.a. "ping pong fracture"
  - Subdural hematoma
    - Usually posterior in location (dependent)

Imaging Recommendations

- Best imaging tool
  - Ultrasound vs. CT: Initial study to exclude large intracranial hemorrhages requiring surgical intervention
  - MR: Used to exclude hypoxic-ischemic injury (if there is clinical concern)
- Protocol advice
  - MR: SWI most sensitive for intraparenchymal hemorrhage; DWI most sensitive for acute infarct

DIFFERENTIAL DIAGNOSIS

Coagulopathy

- Such as neonatal alloimmune thrombocytopenia

Abusive Head Trauma

- Usually not considered if patient has not yet left hospital
- Look for atypical patterns of fracture & hemorrhage

Accidental Postnatal Head Trauma

- Appropriate history for degree of injury

Venous Sinus Thrombosis

- Common cause of newborn intraparenchymal hemorrhage

PATHOLOGY

General Features

- Subdural hematoma
  - Typically < 3 mm in thickness
  - Supratentorial: Caused by lacerations of falx or subdural veins (near falcotentorial junction) from molding of head
  - Posterior fossa: Caused by tentorial lacerations or occipital osteodiastasis (at posterior occipital or supraoccipital-exoccipital synchondrosis)
- Subarachnoid hemorrhage
  - Germinal matrix origin in preterm neonate; usually associated with subdural hematoma in term neonate
- Epidural hematoma
  - Usually associated with cephalohematoma & fracture
- Intraventricular hemorrhage common in premature neonates but presumed to be germinal matrix in origin
- Intraparenchymal hemorrhage
  - Thought to be related to venous obstruction or injury, though may be contusional
  - Parenchymal brain injury not typical of birth trauma, though small parenchymal hemorrhages can be seen

CLINICAL ISSUES

Demographics

- Epidemiology
  - Subdural hematomas are seen in 26-63% of uncomplicated vaginal deliveries
  - Cephalohematomas occur in 1% of all births; ↑ incidence with forceps &/or vacuum-assisted deliveries
  - Epidural hematomas are rare

Natural History & Prognosis

- Scalp hematomas
  - Caput succedaneum: Steadily ↓ 1-2 days after birth
  - Subgaleal hematoma: ↑ in size after birth; resolves over 2-3 weeks
    - May lead to significant blood loss & shock
  - Cephalohematoma: Eventually calcifies, resolving over weeks to months
- Intracranial hemorrhage
  - Subdural hematoma: Most resolve by 1 month; nearly all resolve by 3 months
  - Subarachnoid hemorrhage: Usually of no clinical significance unless large (possibly leading to communicating hydrocephalus)

Treatment

- Depressed skull fractures can be treated neurosurgically, though vacuum/breastpump reduction & spontaneous resolution have been described

DIAGNOSTIC CHECKLIST

Image Interpretation Pearls

- On CT, dural venous sinuses are diffusely hyperdense in normal neonates, which can be confused for dural venous sinus thrombosis or subdural hemorrhage

Reporting Tips

- Important to communicate significance of findings
  - Small subdural hematomas & trace amounts of subarachnoid hemorrhage are not unexpected in neonates & are of no clinical significance
  - Scalp hematomas are not unexpected in neonatal period & typically do not need to be imaged

SELECTED REFERENCES

1. Gupta R et al: Neonatal birth trauma: analysis of yearly trends, risk factors, and outcomes. J Pediatr. ePub, 2021
2. Nikam RM et al: Birth-related subdural hemorrhage: prevalence and imaging morphology. Pediatr Radiol. 51(6):939-46, 2021
3. Bansal AG et al: US of pediatric superficial masses of the head and neck. Radiographics. 38(4):1239-63, 2018
4. Chaturvedi A et al: Mechanical birth-related trauma to the neonate: an imaging perspective. Insights Imaging. 9(1):103-18, 2018
5. Tan AP et al: Intracranial hemorrhage in neonates: a review of etiologies, patterns and predicted clinical outcomes. Eur J Paediatr Neurol. 22(4):690-717, 2018

Abusive Head Trauma

KEY FACTS

TERMINOLOGY

- Nonaccidental trauma (NAT), abusive head trauma (AHT)
- Traumatic injury inflicted on infants & children by adults

IMAGING

- Direct impact injury: Direct blow to cranium or impact of skull on object
    - Calvarial (often complex) & skull base fractures
    - Focal brain injury deep to impact
- Shaking injury: Result of violent to-&-fro motion of head
    - Subdural hematomas (SDHs) in 90-98%
    - Generalized parenchymal injuries (cytotoxic edema, lacerations, axonal injury)
    - Bridging vein injury & thrombosis are common
- NECT is primary imaging tool in initial evaluation of AHT
    - Multiplanar reconstructions improve detection of
        - Small intracranial hemorrhages (ICHs)
        - Fractures (with bone algorithm & 3D reformats)
- MR is best for determining full extent of injury
    - DWI is paramount for parenchymal injury
    - PD & SWI/T2* GRE for hemorrhage
    - T1 C+ for chronic SDH membranes

TOP DIFFERENTIAL DIAGNOSES

- Accidental trauma
- Benign macrocrania of infancy
- Mitochondrial encephalopathies
- Bleeding disorders

CLINICAL ISSUES

- Discordance between stated history & degree of injury
    - "Killer couch": Injuries blamed on infant rolling off couch
- Retinal hemorrhages in ~ 75%
- Most common cause of brain injury death in children < 2 years of age
    - 17-25:100,000 annual incidence
    - Cause of death in 80% of fatalities is brain swelling

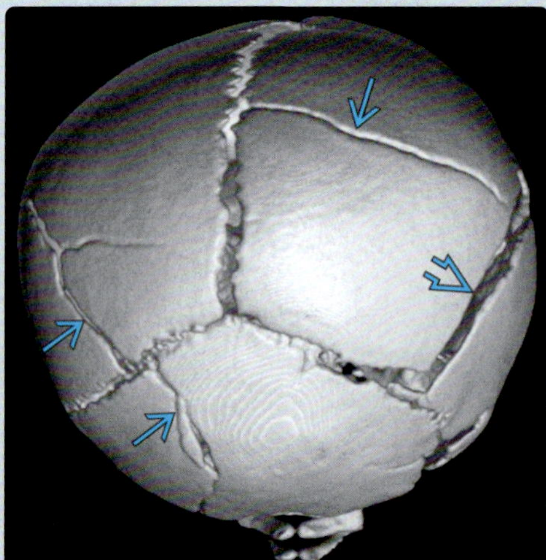

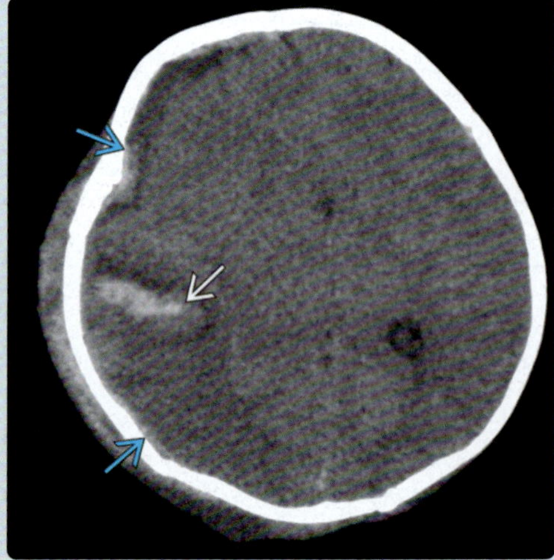

(Left) *Posterior oblique view of a 3D NECT in a 9-week-old who "fell off the couch" shows multiple complex skull fractures ⇨, including a displaced right parietal fracture ⇨. 3D renderings are helpful in improving the detection & characterization of skull fractures.* **(Right)** *Axial NECT in the same patient shows a right subdural hematoma (SDH) ⇨ & right opercular parenchymal laceration ➡ with significant midline shift & sulcal effacement. Parenchymal lacerations are seen in 10-15% of abusive head trauma (AHT).*

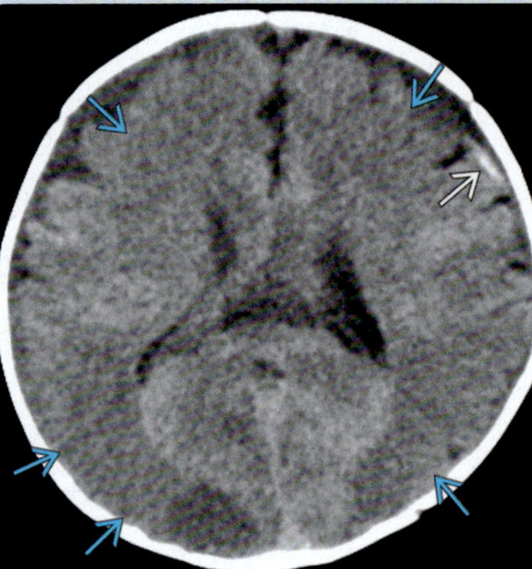

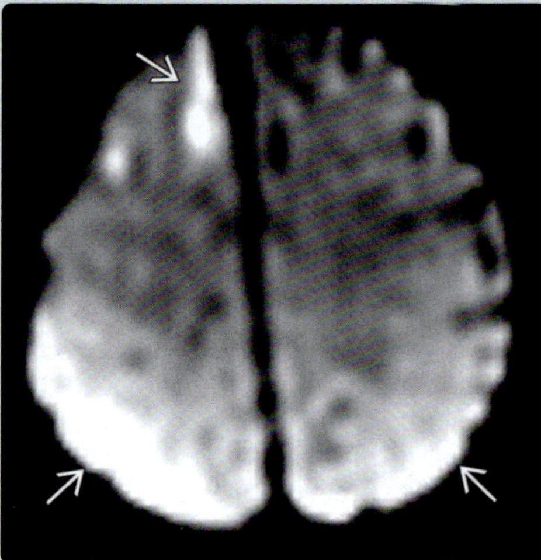

(Left) *Axial NECT in a 4-month-old boy with seizure activity shows multiple bilateral foci of low attenuation with loss of cortical differentiation ⇨ as well as a left frontal SDH ➡. There was no fracture, making these findings highly concerning for the shaking type of AHT.* **(Right)** *Axial DWI MR in a 2-month-old boy with AHT shows areas of diffusion restriction ➡ in the right frontal lobe & bilateral parietal lobes, consistent with parenchymal injury. MR is the most sensitive examination for parenchymal injury.*

TERMINOLOGY

Abbreviations

- Nonaccidental trauma (NAT), abusive head trauma (AHT)

Definitions

- Traumatic injury inflicted on infants & children by adults

IMAGING

General Features

- Multiple brain injuries disproportionately severe relative to offered history
- 2 major groupings of injuries (but can occur together)
  - Direct impact injury: Result of direct blow to cranium or impact of skull on object
  - Shaking injury: Result of violent to-&-fro head motion
- Direct impact injury is typified by skull fractures & injury to immediate subjacent brain
  - Scalp laceration, hematoma, & swelling are strongly associated
  - High association with injuries to other organs
- Shaking injury is typified by subdural hematoma (SDH), generalized parenchymal injury, & absence of fracture(s)
  - Cytotoxic injury not conforming to arterial territories
    - Exact etiology of injury is uncertain but usually permanent
      - Hypoxic-ischemic vs. direct traumatic brain injury
  - May see bridging vein injury ± thrombosis
  - Imaging findings may suggest injuries of differing ages

Radiographic Findings

- Sensitive in detection of linear skull fractures
  - Fracture detection is key component in forensic evaluation of suspected NAT
- Some fractures are considered more suspicious for NAT but evidence does not support this
  - Multiple compound, diastatic fractures, & fractures crossing sutures imply significant trauma but are not specific for NAT
  - Discordance with provided history is best indicator

CT Findings

- NECT: Primary imaging tool for initial evaluation of AHT
- Intracranial hemorrhage (ICH)
  - SDH: 90-98% (dominant feature of shaking injury)
    - Overlie cerebral convexities, extend into interhemispheric fissure, overlie tentorium
    - Normal density of subarachnoid space (SAS) stands out next to ↑ density of SDH
    - Acute SDHs are usually hyperdense but often have associated low-attenuation subdural hygromas (SDHys)
      - Blood density based upon multiple factors: CSF dilution, hematocrit, coagulation status
  - Subarachnoid hemorrhage: > 50%
  - Epidural hemorrhage (EDH) is uncommon but may occur
    - More characteristic of accidental trauma
- SDHy may develop after injury
  - CSF density subdural collection due to arachnoid membrane tear with CSF leakage from SAS
  - Usually develops ~ 12-24 hours after injury
  - Typically resolves without direct treatment
- Bridging vein injury ± thrombosis: 40-50%
  - Areas of ↑ density in paramedian high convexities
    - Pollywog & lollipop signs: Small round focus of clot adjacent to small segment of thrombosed injured vein
      - Fairly specific signs for AHT
- Extensive parenchymal ischemic injury is often seen in shaking injuries
  - Areas of ↓ density (with loss of gray-white differentiation) & sulcal effacement not confined to arterial territories; may be diffuse
  - ↓ density of cerebrum vs. cerebellum: "Bright cerebellum"
- Subcortical laceration or contusional tear: ~ 15%
  - More commonly seen in AHT vs. accidental injury
- Shear injury (axonal injury): ~ 15%
- Retinal hemorrhages are uncommonly visualized on CT
- CECT: Enhancing membranes are best sign of chronic SDHs

MR Findings

- DWI: Key sequence for parenchymal injury
- T1: Bright foci of hemorrhage or evolving cortical injury
- T2: Loss of normal lower signal intensity cortical ribbon & deep nuclei in neonates
- PD/intermediate echo sequences: Very sensitive for detection of small subdural collections
- SWI/T2* GRE: Detects small ICHs ± retinal hemorrhages
  - SWI is ~ 50% sensitive & 100% specific for retinal hemorrhage
- T1 C+: Enhancing membranes are best sign of chronic SDH
- MRA: Proximal vascular correlate (e.g., dissection, spasm) is rarely shown in association with parenchymal injury
- MRS: ↓ NAA, ↑ lactate in regions of parenchymal injury
  - May detect injury in normal-appearing regions

Ultrasonographic Findings

- Not used primarily for suspected AHT
- May be ordered in infant for other indications (e.g., macrocrania, scalp swelling) with incidental detection of NAT findings
  - Subdural collections: Displacement of discrete arachnoid membrane & subjacent vessels toward pial surface
  - Skull fracture: Linear interruption of bone not corresponding to predictable & symmetric suture

Imaging Recommendations

- Best imaging tool
  - NECT (with 3D bone reconstructions): Gold standard exam for acute evaluation of suspected AHT
    - Best for detection & characterization of fractures
    - Very sensitive in detection & characterization of ICH
  - ↑ interest in using limited SSFSE MR as initial screening tool
  - Complete MR after 2-4 days: Most sensitive to define full extent of brain injury
- Protocol advice
  - NECT: Multiplanar reconstructions improve detection of
    - Small ICHs
    - Skull fractures (especially with bone algorithm & 3Ds)
    - Craniocervical junction/upper cervical spine injuries (so cover through C2)

- MR: DWI to assess parenchymal injury; PD/SWI sequence to detect subtle SDH/SDHy
- Perform spine imaging (as spine injury seen in ~ 50%)
  - NAT in spine: SDH > EDH > osseous > cord

DIFFERENTIAL DIAGNOSIS

Accidental Trauma

- Appropriate history for degree of injury

Benign Macrocrania of Infancy

- Self-limited communicating hydrocephalus
- Symmetric enlargement of bifrontal SASs that are isodense to CSF & contain numerous tiny cortical vessels

Mitochondrial Encephalopathies

- May cause atrophy with subdural collections
  - Glutaric acidurias (types I & II), Menkes syndrome
  - Rare diseases with preexisting neurologic symptoms

Overshunting

- "Passive" subdurals can develop from ↓ volume associated with CSF shunting

Subdural Empyema

- Febrile, sinusitis, meningitis

Bleeding Disorders

- von Willebrand, thrombocytopenia
- Intracranial bleeding with minor trauma

PATHOLOGY

General Features

- ↑ vulnerability in infants due to
  - Large head:body ratio + weak neck muscles
  - Developing brain has less structural integrity prior to myelination → greater susceptibility to injury
- 85% of fatal child abuse victims have evidence of impact head injury at postmortem examination
- Retinal hemorrhages in ~ 75% (50-100% in literature)
  - Much less common in accidental head trauma (~ 6%)
- Retroclival collections can be seen in ~ 30% of AHT victims

CLINICAL ISSUES

Presentation

- Most common signs/symptoms
  - Discordance between stated history & degree of injury
    - Attempt by perpetrator to minimize suspicion
    - "Killer couch": Severe injuries are blamed on infant rolling off of couch onto floor
      - Infants are frequently too young to roll over at all
  - Unprovoked seizures & apnea raise suspicion for AHT
- Other signs/symptoms
  - Poor feeding, vomiting, irritability, seizures, lethargy, coma, apnea
  - Retinal hemorrhages (detected on eye exam)
    - Can be missed on cursory evaluation
  - Cause of death in 80% of fatalities is brain swelling
    - Severe hypoxic-ischemic encephalopathy > diffuse axonal injury
- Clinical profile
  - Perpetrators are most often direct caretakers: Parents, babysitters, mother's boyfriend
  - Developmentally delayed & "colicky," premature or low-birth-weight infants at higher risk
  - Psychosocial stressors & poor coping mechanisms are often present in family environment

Demographics

- Most common from 1-6 months of age
- 17-25:100,000 annual incidence
  - Almost certainly underreported
  - Leading cause of brain injury death in children < 2 years of age

Natural History & Prognosis

- Mortality rate: 20-25%
- High rates of impairment for survivors
  - Psychomotor delay, epilepsy, visual impairment, cognitive/behavioral disorders

Treatment

- Multidisciplinary child abuse & neglect team intervention
- Notification of local Child Protection Agency

DIAGNOSTIC CHECKLIST

Image Interpretation Pearls

- Avoid temptation to precisely time ICH
  - Impossible to precisely state age of bleeding in absence of "before & after" imaging
    - Mixed-density hematohygromas are most commonly caused by single acute injury with mixing of blood & CSF
      - **Should not** be mistaken for acute-on-chronic SDHs
  - Reasonable estimates & conclusions are more defensible in court

Reporting Tips

- Carefully proofread, as report may become legal document
- Avoid use of vague, oblique, obscuring language
  - Can hamper care of child & legal investigation
  - May ↑ likelihood of interpretation being challenged in legal proceedings
- Avoid speculation regarding source of injury
  - Report for identification & evaluation of injuries
  - May be appropriate to note discordance between reported mechanism & extent of injury

SELECTED REFERENCES

1. Orman G et al: MRI findings in pediatric abusive head trauma: a review. J Neuroimaging. 30(1):15-27, 2020
2. Rabbitt AL et al: Characteristics associated with spine injury on magnetic resonance imaging in children evaluated for abusive head trauma. Pediatr Radiol. 50(1):83-97, 2020
3. Mankad K et al: The neuroimaging mimics of abusive head trauma. Eur J Paediatr Neurol. 23(1):19-30, 2019
4. Thamburaj K et al: Susceptibility-weighted imaging of retinal hemorrhages in abusive head trauma. Pediatr Radiol. 49(2):210-6, 2019
5. Wittschieber D et al: Understanding subdural collections in pediatric abusive head trauma. AJNR Am J Neuroradiol. 40(3):388-95, 2019
6. Choudhary AK et al: Consensus statement on abusive head trauma in infants and young children. Pediatr Radiol. 48(8):1048-65, 2018

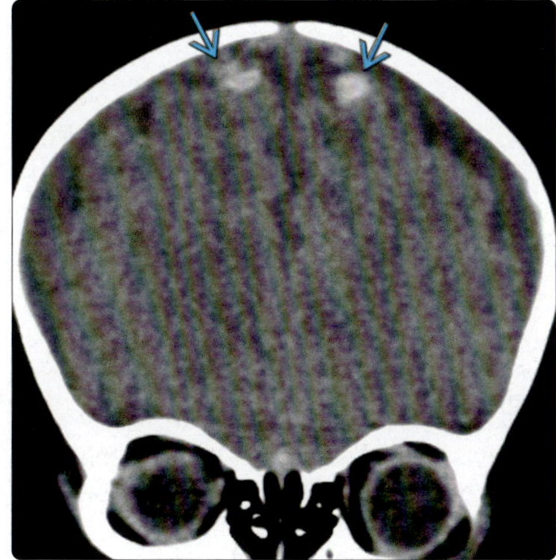

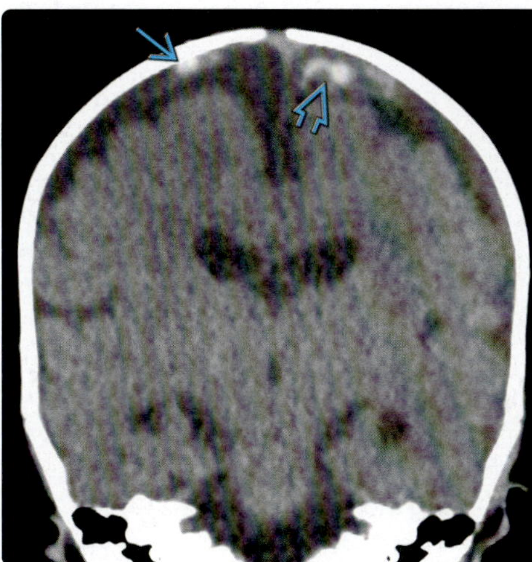

(Left) *Coronal NECT in a 1-month-old patient with AHT shows bilateral paramedian extraaxial hemorrhages ➡, a characteristic finding in AHT attributed to bridging vein injury & thrombosis. In all, 40-50% of AHT cases show evidence of bridging vein injury.* **(Right)** *Coronal NECT in a 3-month-old patient with AHT shows focal areas of parasagittal hemorrhage ➡. The lesion on the left has a lollipop or pollywog appearance ➡, typical for cortical vein avulsion, a finding that is fairly specific for AHT.*

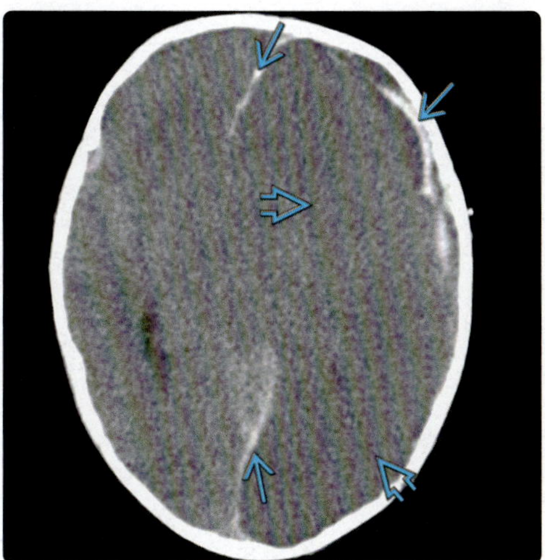

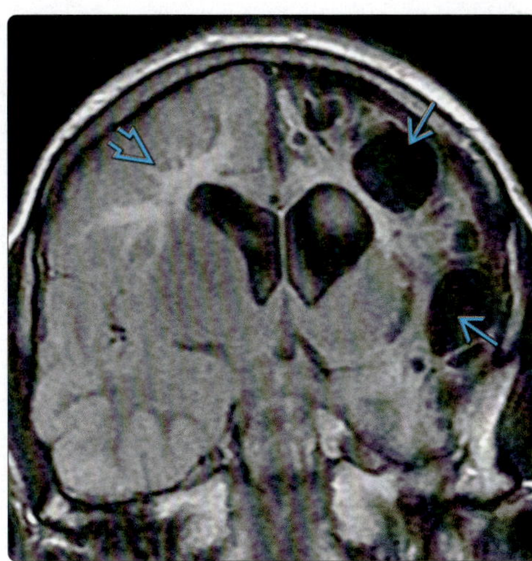

(Left) *Axial NECT in a 2-month-old patient with AHT shows subdural hemorrhage ➡ over the left frontal lobe & along the falx. Note the extensive left cerebral ↓ attenuation ➡ with loss of gray-white differentiation & significant left-to-right midline shift.* **(Right)** *Coronal FLAIR MR in the same patient 7 years later shows extensive cystic ➡ & noncystic ➡ encephalomalacia affecting the left > right cerebral hemispheres. There is associated ex vacuo ventriculomegaly.*

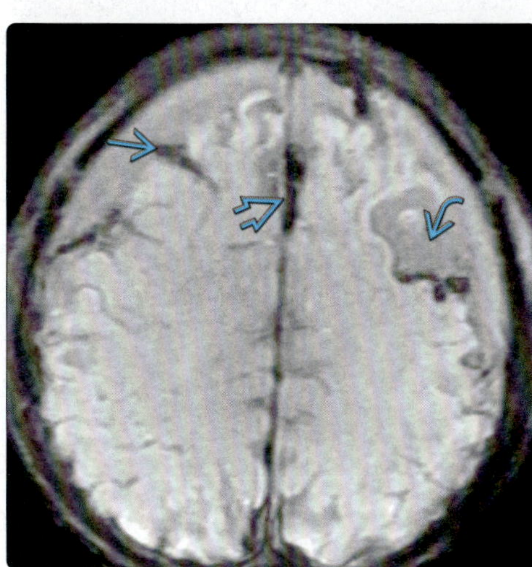

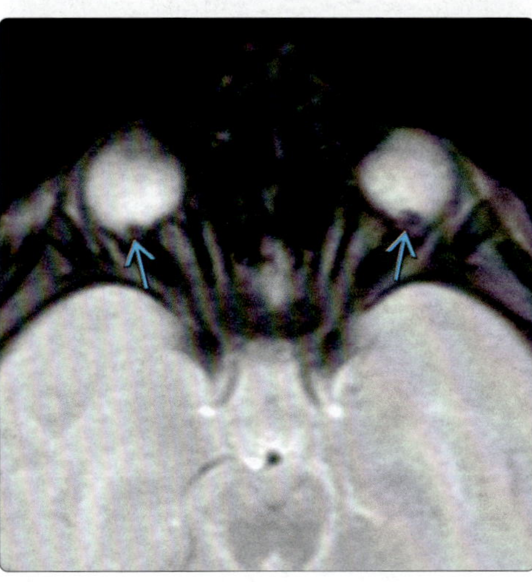

(Left) *Axial SWI MR in a 6-week-old shows subdural ➡ & subarachnoid ➡ hemorrhages as well as an evolving left frontal lobe laceration ➡ containing a hemorrhage level, a constellation of findings very suspicious for AHT.* **(Right)** *Axial SWI MR in a 4-month-old with AHT shows bilateral retinal hemorrhages ➡. Although SWI is the most sensitive imaging sequence for retinal hemorrhages, it is insensitive relative to a funduscopic exam. Note that a normal MR appearance of the globes does not exclude retinal hemorrhages.*

KEY FACTS

TERMINOLOGY

- Hemorrhage that occurs in richly vascular, but fragile, germinal matrix in premature infants

IMAGING

- Can occur anywhere along germinal matrix
  - Most commonly at caudothalamic groove
- Look for intraventricular extension, ventriculomegaly, & secondary intraparenchymal hemorrhage
- US: Globular echogenic focus in caudothalamic groove
  - Acute blood is echogenic; clot later retracts & becomes iso- to hypoechoic
  - May appear as abnormally thick choroid plexus but of slightly different echogenicity & lacking vascularity
  - Fluid-debris levels may be visible in dependent ventricles
  - Coronal & sagittal cine clips sweeping though ventricles help differentiate hemorrhage from normal choroid
- MR: Sensitive for detection of germinal matrix hemorrhage (GMH) & intraventricular hemorrhage (IVH)
  - ↑ T1 signal; ↓ SWI/T2* GRE
  - Best imaging modality for detection of associated parenchymal abnormalities

PATHOLOGY

- Germinal matrix is transiently present as region of fragile, thin-walled vessels & migrating neuronal components
  - Involutes by 34 weeks of gestation
- In premature infants, perinatal stresses + poor cerebral autoregulation + germinal matrix → hemorrhage
- GMH-IVH grading system
  - Grade 1: GMH only
  - Grade 2: GMH + IVH, normal ventricle size
  - Grade 3: GMH + IVH + ventricular expansion
  - Grade 4: GMH-IVH + intraparenchymal hemorrhage
    - Venous compression leads to venous infarction

CLINICAL ISSUES

- Most common < 32 weeks of gestation & < 1,500 grams

(Left) *Axial graphic shows germinal matrix hemorrhages (GMHs) grades 1 (top left) to 4 (bottom right) with ventricular dilation seen above grade 2 & parenchymal involvement (from hemorrhagic venous infarction) in grade 4.* **(Right)** *Coronal head US in a former 29-weeks-gestation male fetus 1 day after delivery shows an asymmetric globular echogenic focus in the right caudothalamic groove ➞, consistent with a GMH. The lack of intraventricular hemorrhage (IVH) makes this a grade 1 hemorrhage.*

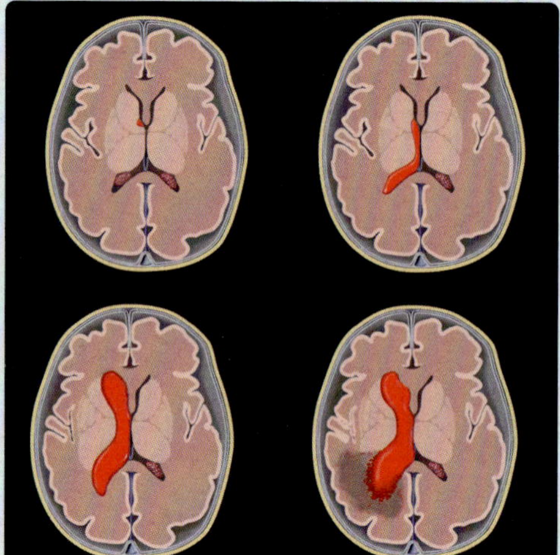

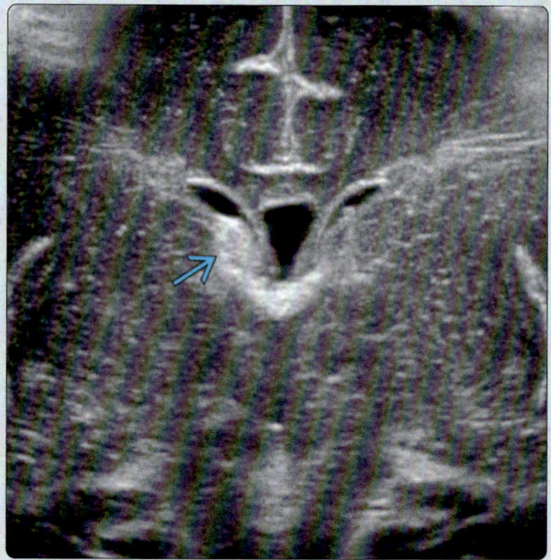

(Left) *Coronal US in a 1-day-old neonate born at 25-weeks gestation shows a heterogeneously echogenic IVH ➞ that expands the left lateral ventricle, consistent with a grade 3 IVH. Note the ↓ parenchymal sulcation, reflective of prematurity.* **(Right)** *Coronal US in a 3-day-old neonate born at 24-weeks gestation shows a large right IVH ➞ with a fan-shaped area of hyperechogenicity ➩ in the adjacent white matter, consistent with hemorrhagic venous infarction (grade 4 IVH).*

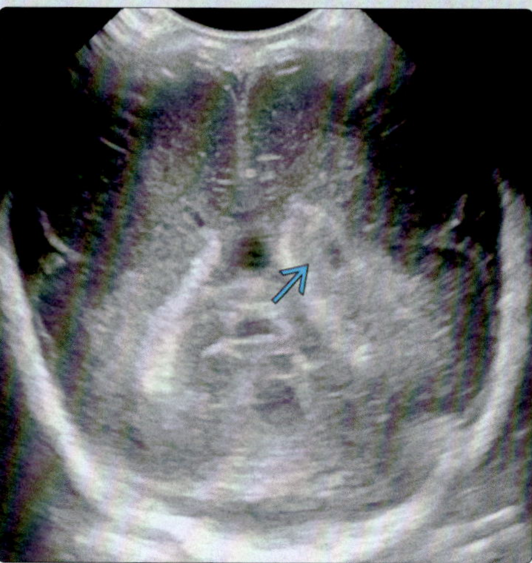

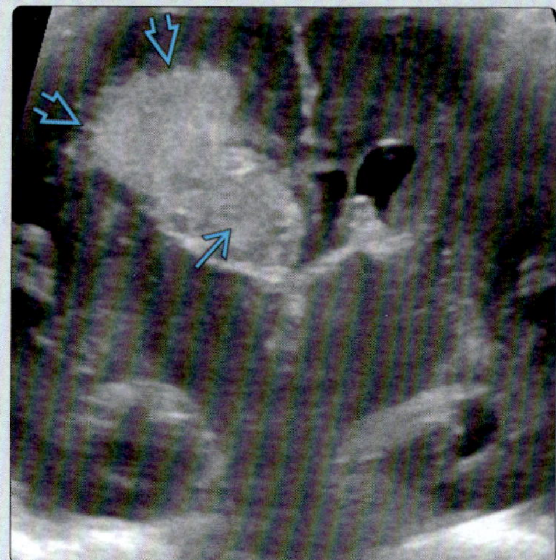

TERMINOLOGY

Abbreviations

- Germinal matrix hemorrhage (GMH), intraventricular hemorrhage (IVH)

Synonyms

- Germinal matrix bleed, preterm caudothalamic hemorrhage, GMH-IVH

Definitions

- Hemorrhage that occurs in very specific, richly vascular, stress-sensitive areas of premature brain
- Germinal matrix has developed more sturdy blood vessels by 34 weeks of gestation

IMAGING

General Features

- Best diagnostic clue
  - Globular echogenic focus in caudothalamic groove
    - Clearly asymmetric from contralateral normal choroid plexus
- Location
  - Within distribution of fetal germinal matrix
    - Most commonly caudothalamic groove
  - May extend into ventricular system
    - Adherent to choroid plexus or layering in occipital horns
- Size
  - Variable
- Morphology
  - Globular & rounded when limited to caudothalamic groove (grade 1)
  - Lobulated or amorphous with posterior intraventricular extension (grade 2)

Ultrasonographic Findings

- Grayscale ultrasound
  - Hyperechoic acute hemorrhage
    - Evolving clot retracts & becomes iso- to hypoechoic
  - IVH is often adherent to choroid plexus
    - Fluid-debris levels may be visible in dependent ventricular occipital horns
    - Chemical ventriculitis in 2-3 days after IVH
      - Ependymal lining becomes thick & echogenic
  - Larger IVH will expand ventricle(s) (grade 3)
    - Posthemorrhagic hydrocephalus often develops
  - Fan-shaped echogenic parenchymal focus due to hemorrhagic venous infarction (grade 4)
  - Examine remainder of brain for
    - Associated white matter injury
    - Lack of congenital anomalies
- Color Doppler
  - Useful to differentiate avascular hemorrhage from vascular choroid plexus

MR Findings

- Variable signal intensity based on age of blood
  - **T1**: ↑ in subacute blood, ↓ in chronic hemosiderin
  - **T2**: ↓ in most phases of hemorrhage evolution
  - **SWI**: Most sensitive for small or remote GMH-IVH
- Helpful to identify brain injury often associated with GMH-IVH
  - White matter injury of prematurity
  - Cerebellar microhemorrhage
- Also useful to detect underlying congenital anomalies

CT Findings

- Not typically used in premature neonate due to availability of US & superior soft tissue contrast of MR
- Excellent for detection of intracranial hemorrhage elsewhere: Parenchymal, subdural, subarachnoid

Imaging Recommendations

- Best imaging tool
  - US is primary imaging modality
    - Portability allows US to go to patient in NICU
    - Available sonographic windows of anterior & mastoid fontanelles
    - Lack of ionizing radiation
    - High sensitivity & specificity for GMH-IVH
  - MR is useful adjunctive imaging modality
    - More sensitive, specific, & reproducible than US but not usually practical in critically ill premature infants
    - MR is rarely performed acutely; usually performed later to evaluate extent of parenchymal injury
- Protocol advice
  - US: Use small-footprint, high-frequency linear transducer with multiple focal zones
    - Coronal & sagittal cine clips are helpful in distinguishing hemorrhage from normal choroid plexus
  - MR: Include SWI or T2* GRE to identify hemorrhage

DIFFERENTIAL DIAGNOSIS

Hypoxic-Ischemic Encephalopathy

- Deep or peripheral patterns of parenchymal injury due to perinatal insult to preterm or term infant
- Abnormal ↑ echogenicity of white matter ± deep gray nuclei
- Usually fairly symmetric

Hemorrhagic Infarction From Venous Thrombosis

- Superficial or deep venous thrombosis may lead to echogenic parenchyma ± discrete hematoma in neonate
  - Can liquefy & mimic abscess
- Isolated or secondary to infection or systemic processes

Choroid Plexus Cysts or Hematoma

- Small cysts &/or hemorrhage may occur in choroid plexus
- Often without consequence

Ventriculitis

- Echogenic ependyma & infectious debris may mimic IVH
- May lead to communicating hydrocephalus

Periventricular Calcifications

- Not typically seen in caudothalamic groove
- Related to TORCH infections most commonly

Periventricular Gray Matter Heterotopia

- Nodular heterotopic foci are less echogenic than blood
- Follow gray matter on all MR sequences

Tuberous Sclerosis

- Echogenic nodular periventricular foci
- Echogenic cortical/subcortical tubers

PATHOLOGY

General Features

- Etiology
  - Germinal matrix is transiently present as vascular-rich area of neuronal precursors
    - Involutes gradually → hemorrhage is less likely with ↑ gestational age
    - Most GMHs occur in 1st week of life
  - Germinal matrix is prone to hemorrhage in prematurity
    - High density of fragile vascularized tissue
    - Poor cerebral autoregulation in premature infants
  - Hemorrhage occurs secondary to perinatal stresses: Labile blood pressure, hypoxia, hypercarbia, etc.

Staging, Grading, & Classification

- Germinal matrix grading system created by Burstein et al in 1979
  - Performed on initial head US within days of delivery
  - Grading is not changed on follow-up exams (even with progression)
- Grade 1: GMH only
- Grade 2: GMH, IVH, normal ventricle size
- Grade 3: GMH, IVH, & ventricular expansion from IVH
  - Secondary hydrocephalus occurring several days after grade 2 IVH should not be mislabeled as grade 3 IVH
- Grade 4: IVH + intraparenchymal hemorrhage
  - Intraparenchymal hemorrhage represents hemorrhagic venous infarction, not direct extension of GMH or IVH
    - Deep draining vein compression → venous congestion → venous infarction → hemorrhagic infarction
    - Debated whether or not ventricular dilation is necessary
      - Is periventricular hemorrhagic infarction of premature infant with grade 1 or 2 GMH actually due to GMH vs. discrete focus of hypoxic-ischemic injury or venous thrombosis
  - Grade 4 may be called posthemorrhagic venous infarction

Gross Pathologic & Surgical Features

- Areas of hemorrhagic necrosis, liquefaction, & gliosis

CLINICAL ISSUES

Presentation

- Most common signs/symptoms
  - Variable: Hypotonia, seizures, hyperreflexia, falling hematocrit, irritability, failure to thrive, paresis, acidosis, feeding difficulties
- Other signs/symptoms
  - GMH may occur in utero & follow same pathway of evolution & complications

Demographics

- Age
  - Premature infants in 1st week of life
  - 1/3-1/2 of all GMHs occur on 1st day of life
- Sex
  - M:F = 1:1
- Ethnicity
  - No predisposition
- Epidemiology
  - Most common in infants < 32 weeks of gestation & < 1,500 grams
  - Higher risk of GMH in premature infants with congenital heart disease, surgical procedures, severe respiratory distress
  - Incidence of GMH-IVH: 50% from 1975 to 1980 & then ↓ to ~ 15% after 2005
    - Improved modern outcomes attributed to prenatal steroids & surfactant, among other therapies

Natural History & Prognosis

- GMHs may progress or rebleed
- In general, clot retracts, lyses, & becomes hypoechoic, leaving behind cyst or area of porencephaly
- Prognosis
  - Grades 1 & 2 bleeds generally have good prognosis
  - Grades 3 & 4 bleeds have variable long-term deficits
    - Spastic diplegia, seizures, neurocognitive impairment
    - Up to 44% mortality
- Posthemorrhagic hydrocephalus develops in 60% of grade 3-4 IVHs
  - Classically due to blood products, fibrosis, &/or gliosis obstructing ventricular outlets & arachnoid granulations
  - May also impair CSF dynamics at levels of microvasculature & ependyma

Treatment

- Prenatal
  - Prevent preterm delivery
  - Prenatal steroids
- Postnatal
  - Optimize neonatal resuscitation
  - Reduce fluctuations in cerebral blood flow
    - Minimize handling, gentle/synchronized ventilation, prompt treatment of patent ductus arteriosus, maintain normal oxygenation
- Posthemorrhagic hydrocephalus often requires CSF shunting (20-25% of grades 3-4 IVH)

SELECTED REFERENCES

1. Guillot M et al: Routine imaging of the preterm neonatal brain. Paediatr Child Health. 25(4):249-62, 2020
2. Parodi A et al: Cranial ultrasound findings in preterm germinal matrix haemorrhage, sequelae and outcome. Pediatr Res. 87(Suppl 1):13-24, 2020
3. Klebe D et al: Posthemorrhagic hydrocephalus development after germinal matrix hemorrhage: established mechanisms and proposed pathways. J Neurosci Res. 98(1):105-20, 2019
4. Coskun Y et al: A clinical scoring system to predict the development of intraventricular hemorrhage (IVH) in premature infants. Childs Nerv Syst. 34(1):129-36, 2018
5. Hinojosa-Rodríguez M et al: Clinical neuroimaging in the preterm infant: diagnosis and prognosis. Neuroimage Clin. 16:355-68, 2017
6. Raets MM et al: Neonatal disorders of germinal matrix. J Matern Fetal Neonatal Med. 28 Suppl 1:2286-90, 2015
7. Ballabh P: Pathogenesis and prevention of intraventricular hemorrhage. Clin Perinatol. 41(1):47-67, 2014
8. Intrapiromkul J et al: Accuracy of head ultrasound for the detection of intracranial hemorrhage in preterm neonates: comparison with brain MRI and susceptibility-weighted imaging. J Neuroradiol. 40(2):81-8, 2013

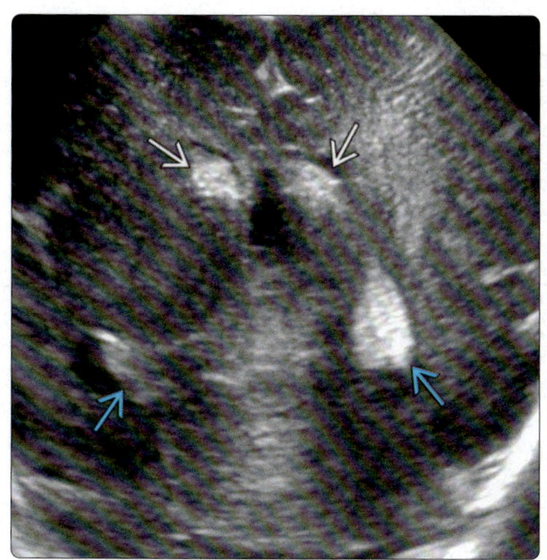

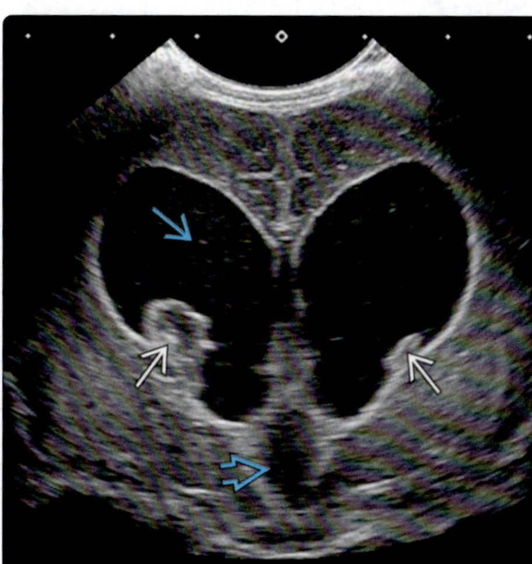

(Left) *Coronal head US in a former 30-weeks-gestation premature infant < 24 hours after delivery shows bilateral GMHs ➡ & IVHs ➡ without ventriculomegaly, consistent with grade 2 IVH. Cine clips are the easiest way to distinguish GMH/IVH from normal choroid plexus (which is not easily done on this static image).* **(Right)** *Coronal head US in the same patient 3 weeks later shows evolution of the IVHs ➡ with interval enlargement of the lateral ➡ & 3rd ➡ ventricles, consistent with posthemorrhagic hydrocephalus.*

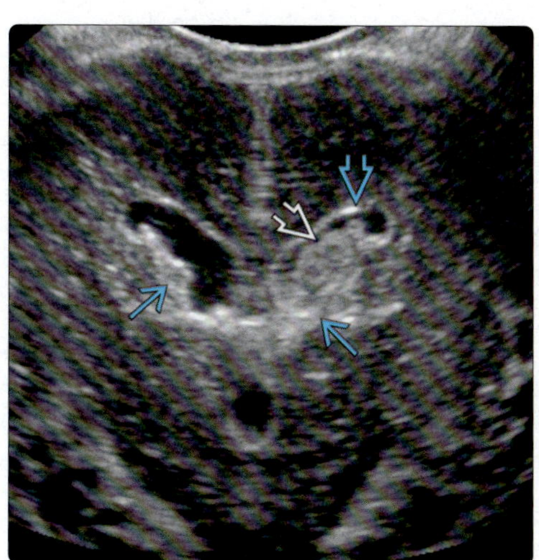

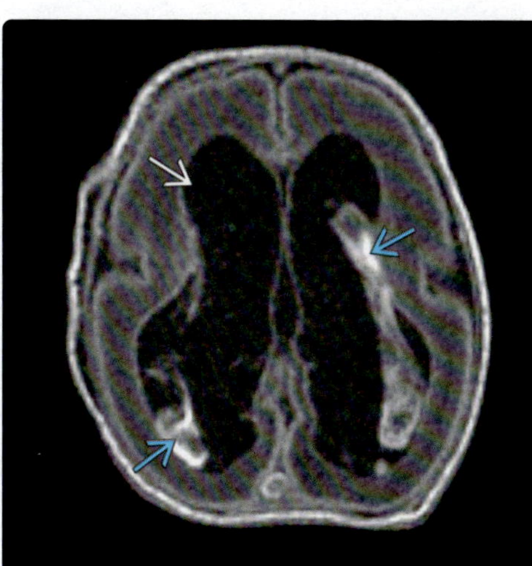

(Left) *Coronal head US in a former 24-weeks-gestation premature infant (now 6 days old) shows bilateral GMHs ➡. There is left intraventricular extension of the hemorrhage ➡ with expansion of the left frontal horn ➡, consistent with a grade 3 IVH. A grade 2 IVH was seen on the right.* **(Right)** *Axial T1 MR 3 weeks later in the same patient shows foci of T1 shortening from the prior IVHs ➡. Further ventriculomegaly ➡ has developed, consistent with posthemorrhagic hydrocephalus.*

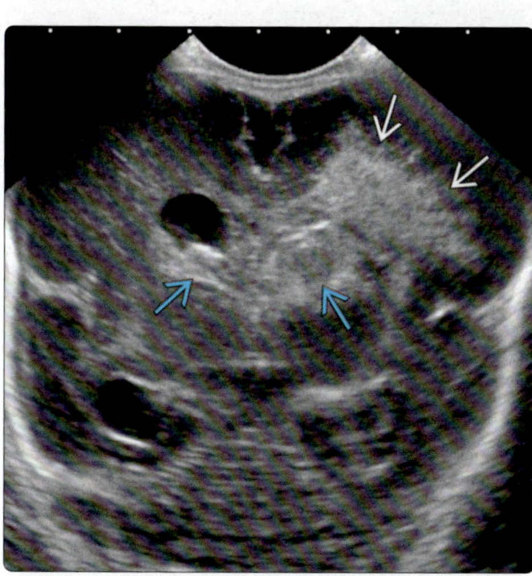

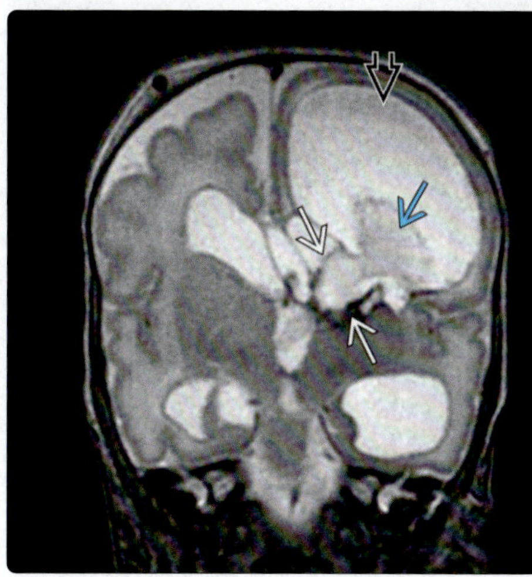

(Left) *Coronal US in a 28-weeks-gestational age premature infant at 2 days of life shows bilateral germinal matrix hemorrhage (GMH) ➡ (L > R) & fan-shaped echogenic hemorrhagic infarction ➡ in the left centrum semiovale, consistent with grade 4 IVH.* **(Right)** *Coronal T2 MR in the same infant 6 weeks later shows residua of the left-sided IVH ➡ & intraparenchymal hemorrhage ➡ with the development of cystic encephalomalacia ➡, an expected evolution of grade 4 IVH.*

White Matter Injury of Prematurity

KEY FACTS

TERMINOLOGY

- White matter (WM) injury of prematurity
- Brain injury occurring before 34-weeks gestation, resulting in loss of periventricular WM

IMAGING

- Ultrasound: Reliable for more severe or late disease; less reliable for mild/moderate or early disease
  - Acute findings
    - Patchy, globular foci of ↑ echogenicity in periventricular/deep WM
  - Subacute/chronic findings
    - Clusters of periventricular cysts
- MR: Reliable for entire spectrum of disease
  - Acute findings
    - T1-hyperintense, T2-hypointense foci
    - Hypointense SWI/GRE foci with hemorrhage
    - ↓ ADC (may miss if imaging < 24 hours or > 5 days)
    - MRS: Lactate peak or ↑ excitatory neurotransmitters
  - Subacute findings
    - Periventricular cysts
  - Chronic finding
    - Periventricular/deep WM volume loss
    - Typically minimal associated gliosis

TOP DIFFERENTIAL DIAGNOSES

- Normal periventricular halo on ultrasound
- Infection
- Shunted hydrocephalus

PATHOLOGY

- Preceding inflammation (e.g., chorioamnionitis) + ischemia superimposed on vulnerable premature brain
- Characteristic pattern of injury reflects distribution of immature oligodendrocytes during vulnerable period
  - Selective injury to immature oligodendrocytes dramatically reduces WM volume in affected areas
- Some WM injury is due to deep medullary vein thrombosis

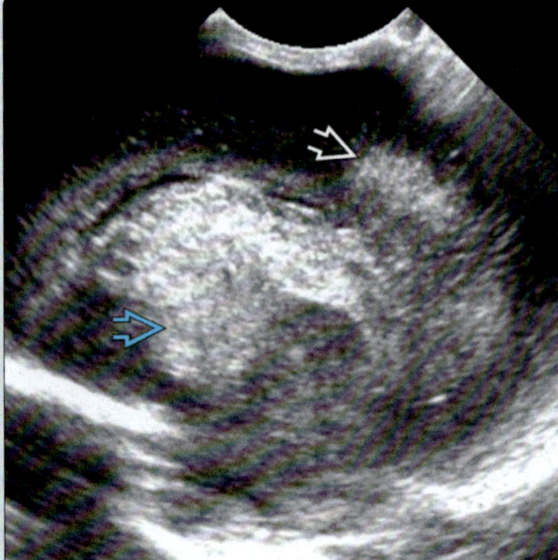

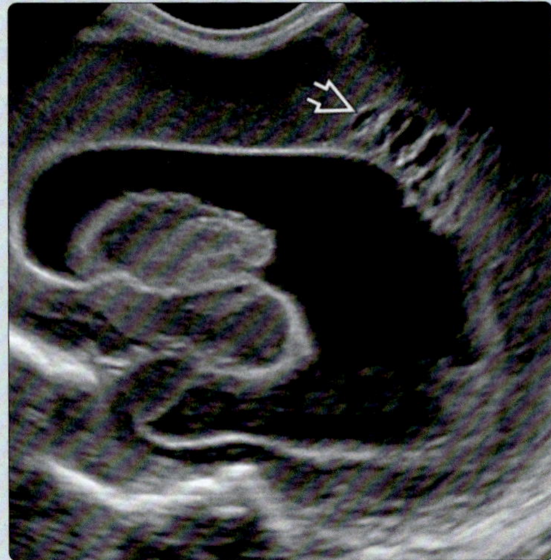

(Left) *Sagittal head ultrasound in a 5-day-old, former 27-weeks-gestational age (GA) infant shows globular ↑ echogenicity* ➡ *in the periventricular white matter (WM), consistent with ischemic injury. Intraventricular hemorrhage & deep gray nuclei insult* ➡ *were also noted.* **(Right)** *Sagittal head ultrasound 1 month later shows that the previously seen focus of ↑ echogenicity has now evolved into cystic encephalomalacia* ➡*. The new ventriculomegaly is likely due to volume loss & obstruction by blood products.*

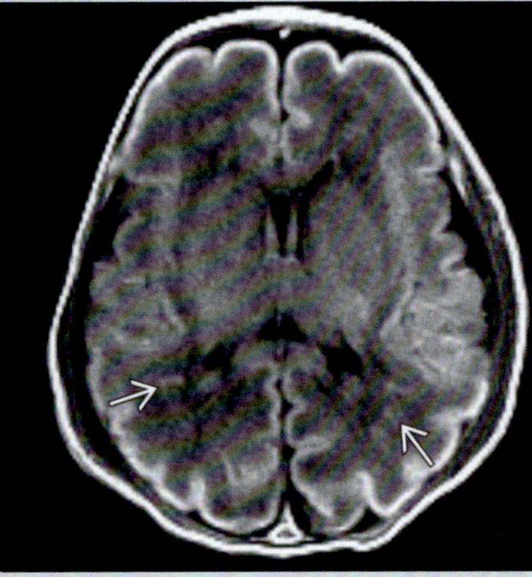

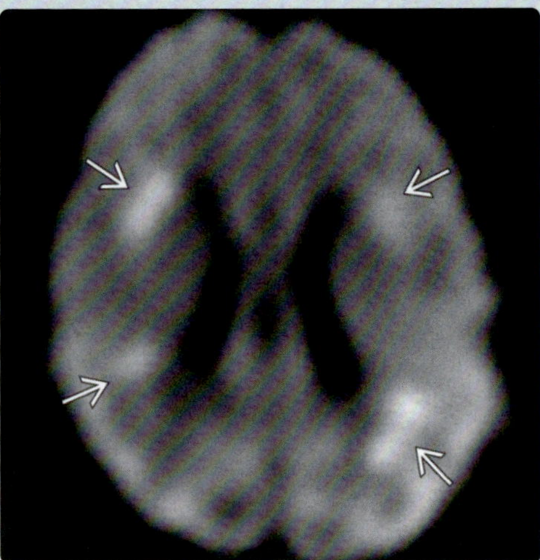

(Left) *Axial T1 MR in an 18-day-old, former 33-weeks-GA neonate with tricuspid atresia demonstrates patchy foci of hyperintense signal* ➡ *in the bilateral parietooccipital periventricular WM.* **(Right)** *Axial DWI MR in the same patient shows corresponding foci of restricted diffusion* ➡ *(↓ signal on the ADC map, not shown) in the bilateral periventricular WM, consistent with acute injury. MR is the most sensitive test for WM injury in neonates that can safely tolerate the exam.*

TERMINOLOGY

Synonyms

- White matter (WM) injury of prematurity, perinatal WM damage, punctate WM lesions, periventricular leukomalacia (PVL)

Definitions

- Perinatal WM injury occurring before 34-weeks gestation

IMAGING

Ultrasonographic Findings

- Reliable for more severe or late disease; less reliable for mild/moderate or early injury
- Acute findings
  - Patchy, globular foci of ↑ echogenicity in periventricular/deep WM
  - Loss of normal WM echotexture
- Subacute findings
  - Periventricular cystic foci

CT Findings

- Reliable for more severe or late disease; less reliable for mild/moderate or early injury
  - Due to high water content of normal newborn brain

MR Findings

- T1WI
  - Acute: Areas of T1 hyperintensity
  - Chronic: WM volume loss, callosal thinning
- T2WI
  - Acute: Areas of T2 hypointensity
  - Subacute: Cystic changes in periventricular WM
  - Chronic: WM volume loss, ventriculomegaly
    - Cortical ribbon extending down to ventricular margin
    - Angular ventricles with "squared-off" trigones
- FLAIR
  - Not usually performed in newborn due to high water content & lack of myelination in normal neonatal brain
  - Chronic: Hyperintense signal in periventricular/deep WM
- T2* GRE
  - Hypointense SWI/GRE foci in areas of hemorrhage
- DWI
  - Restricted diffusion often precedes other abnormalities
  - May miss or underestimate WM injury if DWI is performed < 24 hours or > 5 days after injury
    - ADC values may "normalize" after 5 days
  - Always review ADC maps as DWI may be falsely negative due to normally long T2 values in neonatal brain
- MRS
  - Lactate peak, ↓ NAA, ↑ excitatory neurotransmitters; alterations may antedate MR image abnormalities

Imaging Recommendations

- Best imaging tool
  - Ultrasound in perinatal period
    - Convenient & well tolerated by neonates
    - Poor sensitivity/specificity for WM injury, especially for mild, early, or noncavitary lesions
  - MR (including DWI & MRS)
    - Best performed 1-5 days after suspected injury

DIFFERENTIAL DIAGNOSIS

Normal Periventricular Halo

- Specular reflections of normal perpendicular WM tracts
- Most prominent in posterior periventricular WM but less echogenic than choroid plexus
- Usually linear & symmetric, not heterogeneous & globular

Infection

- CMV: Microcephaly, periventricular Ca^{2+}, ± periventricular WM abnormalities, ± polymicrogyria

Shunted Hydrocephalus

- Ventricular distortion ± abnormal WM after shunting

PATHOLOGY

General Features

- Etiology
  - Predisposing factors of premature brain: Unique cellular vulnerability, impaired cerebrovascular autoregulation, periventricular arterial end zones
  - Superimposed insult
    - Chorioamnionitis → vasculitis of chorionic plate → ↑ inflammatory cytokines
    - With pre-/perinatal hypoxia → WM damage via inflammatory response, oxidative stress linked to reoxygenation during perinatal period
  - Subset of WM injury is due to deep medullary vein thrombosis
    - More common in late preterm (> 32-weeks) & term (> 37-weeks) infants

CLINICAL ISSUES

Presentation

- Most common signs/symptoms
  - May be clinically silent initially ± EEG findings
  - Spastic diplegia, visual & cognitive impairment
- Clinical profile
  - Risk factors for WM injury of prematurity
    - Pregnancy: Low gestational age/weight, previous preterm birth, spontaneous preterm labor
    - Intrapartum: Preeclampsia, premature rupture of membranes, chorioamnionitis, group B *Streptococcus* infection
    - Perinatal: Respiratory distress, patent ductus arteriosus, ↓ PaCO2, sepsis, anemia, apnea, bradycardia, cardiac arrest

SELECTED REFERENCES

1. Guillot M et al: Comparative performance of head ultrasound and MRI in detecting preterm brain injury and predicting outcomes: a systematic review. Acta Paediatr. 110(5):1425-32, 2021
2. Jansen L et al: Associations between neonatal magnetic resonance imaging and short- and long-term neurodevelopmental outcomes in a longitudinal cohort of very preterm children. J Pediatr. 234:46-53.e2, 2021
3. Neil JJ et al: Diffusion magnetic resonance imaging of infants. Magn Reson Imaging Clin N Am. 29(2):185-93, 2021
4. Agut T et al: Preterm white matter injury: ultrasound diagnosis and classification. Pediatr Res. 87(Suppl 1):37-49, 2020
5. Benninger KL et al: MR imaging scoring system for white matter injury after deep medullary vein thrombosis and infarction in neonates. AJNR Am J Neuroradiol. 40(2):347-52, 2019

Hypoxic-Ischemic Encephalopathy

KEY FACTS

TERMINOLOGY

- Brain injury in neonate caused by hypoxic-ischemic insult

IMAGING

- Deep or central pattern of injury
  - Basal ganglia, thalamus, ± brainstem
- Peripheral pattern of injury
  - Injury to watershed zones of hemispheres
- Mixed (deep gray + cortex) pattern is often encountered
- US may be used for screening, particularly in acute setting or with concern for hemorrhage
  - Less sensitive for early injury or certain patterns
- MR is best imaging test for parenchymal injury
  - T1 & T2: Usually normal in 1st few days
    - T1: ↑ signal in affected regions
    - T2: ↑ or ↓ signal in affected regions
  - DWI: Best sequence to define extent of injury
    - ↑ DWI, ↓ ADC in affected regions from 1-10 days
  - MRS: ↓ NAA & ↑ lactate in affected areas

PATHOLOGY

- Central pattern is due to severe hypoxia of relatively brief (10-25 minutes) duration
  - Injury to regions of greatest metabolic demand
- Peripheral pattern is due to less severe hypoxia over longer period of time
  - Regions of greatest metabolic demand are protected
- Preterm infants are more susceptible to equivalent ischemic injury compared to term infants
- Preterm neonates are more likely to have associated white matter injury & hemorrhage

CLINICAL ISSUES

- Deep pattern is associated with dyskinetic cerebral palsy
- Peripheral pattern is associated with spastic cerebral palsy

DIAGNOSTIC CHECKLIST

- Findings may be inapparent/subtle in first 24 hours
- Image at 3-7 days for best MR evaluation of injury extent

(Left) *Axial DWI MR in a 5-day-old term neonate with HIE from meconium aspiration shows symmetric diffusion restriction in the watershed cortex & white matter. The involvement of cerebral cortex with sparing of the deep gray nuclei is consistent with a partial prolonged pattern of asphyxia.* **(Right)** *Axial T2 MR in a 7-day-old term neonate with HIE from placental abruption shows symmetric T2 signal hypointensity in the posterior putamina ➔ & anterolateral thalami ➔, typical of an acute profound pattern of asphyxia.*

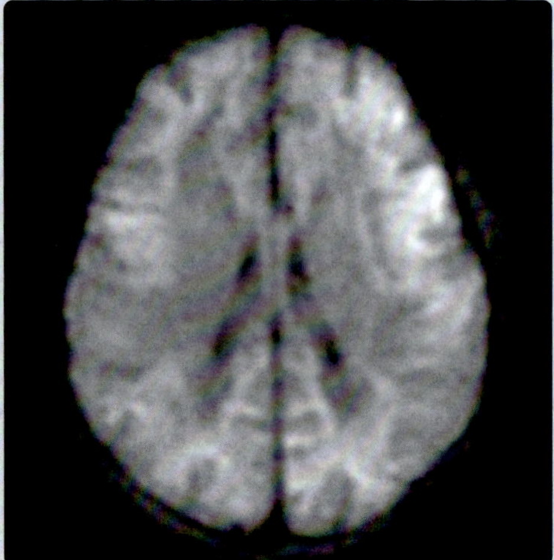

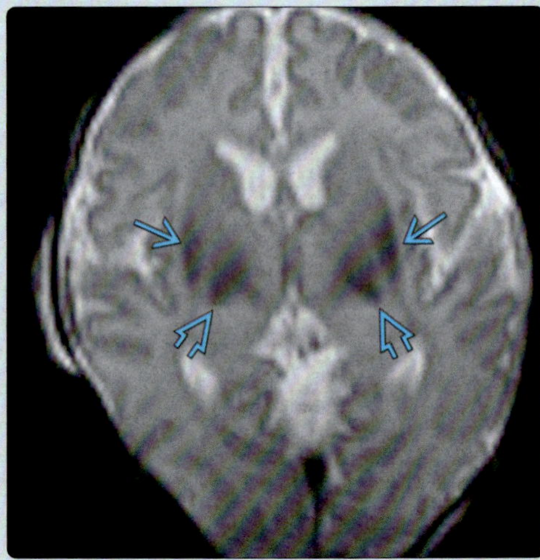

(Left) *Axial DWI MR in a 4-day-old term neonate with severe HIE shows a "superscan" with marked diffusion restriction throughout the brain. With the symmetry of severe findings, this is sometimes interpreted as normal. Comparing it to usually normal cerebellum is helpful.* **(Right)** *Axial T1 MR in a 31-week premature infant 11 days following placental abruption shows irregular hyperintense signal ➔ in the bilateral thalami & nuclei of the globus pallidus. Also note the GMH ➔ & small layering IVH ➔, findings often seen in this setting.*

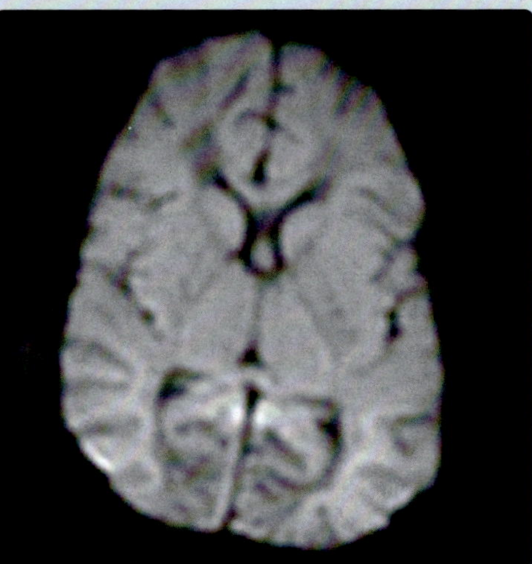

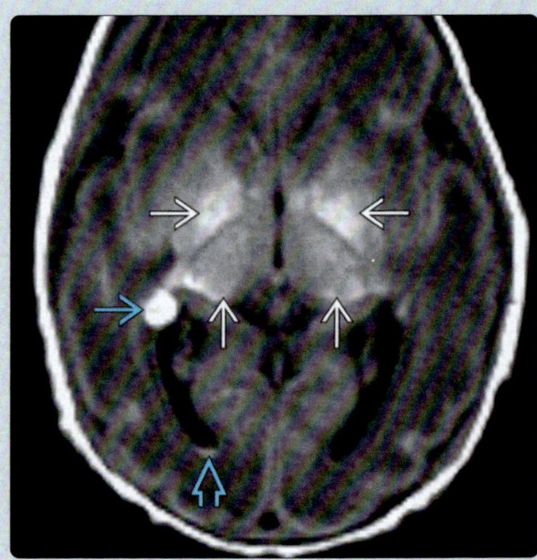

TERMINOLOGY

Definitions

- Hypoxic-ischemic encephalopathy (HIE): Neonatal brain injury caused by perinatal hypoxic-ischemic insult

IMAGING

General Features

- 2 patterns of injury have been described
  - Deep or central pattern
    - Injury to basal ganglia, thalami, ± perirolandic cortex
    - Profound hypoxic-ischemic injury (e.g., placental abruption)
    - More severe motor/cognitive outcomes
  - Peripheral pattern
    - Injury to watershed zones of cerebral hemispheres
    - Prolonged partial ischemia (e.g., fetal bradycardia)
    - Less severe motor/cognitive outcomes
  - Often have mixed pattern
    - Involving deep gray nuclei & cortex
  - Late findings: Atrophy, gliosis/encephalomalacia

Ultrasonographic Findings

- Insensitive compared to MR, especially early & for certain injury patterns
- Patchy or extensive hyperechoic foci in white matter (WM) & deep gray nuclei
  - May accentuate gray matter (GM)-WM differentiation at cortical/subcortical level
- Slit-like lateral ventricles & sulcal effacement
  - Common normally in newborns due to compression during labor &/or hypovolemia

MR Findings

- T1: Usually normal during 1st few days
  - ↑ signal in affected areas beginning at ~ 2-3 days
  - Loss of normal bright T1 signal in posterior limb of internal capsule
- T2: Usually normal during 1st few days
  - Indistinct deep gray nuclei & loss of cortical ribbon
  - ↑ or ↓ signal in affected areas after ~ 2-3 days
- SWI: Germinal matrix & intraventricular hemorrhages are often seen in preterm, less commonly in term neonates
- DWI: Most important sequence
  - Restricted diffusion is seen ~ 1-10 days after injury
  - Pseudonormalization occurs at ~ 7-10 days
  - Primary injury is apparent early; secondary injury (e.g., corpus callosum) develops days later
- MRS: ↓ NAA & ↑ lactate in affected areas
  - ↑ Lac:NAA ratio correlates with more severe injury
- Perfusion: ↑ ASL in affected deep gray nuclei during 1st week

Imaging Recommendations

- Best imaging tool
  - MR with DWI & MRS
- Protocol advice
  - Findings may be inapparent/subtle in first 24 hours
  - Image at 3-7 days for best MR evaluation of injury extent
    - ADC changes peak at ~ 5 days

DIFFERENTIAL DIAGNOSIS

Urea Cycle Disorders

- Elevated ammonia, present at 24-28 hours
- Diffuse cerebral edema

Maple Syrup Urine Disease

- Edema in myelinated areas
- Brainstem, perirolandic & cerebellar WM

Hypoglycemia

- Characteristic occipital cortex injury

Arterial Ischemic Stroke

- Focal arterial territory injury without hypoxic event

Venous Injury

- Edema, hemorrhage, &/or ischemia in venous distribution

TORCH Infections

- Microcephaly, migration anomalies, Ca^{2+}

PATHOLOGY

General Features

- Etiology
  - Central pattern is associated with severe hypoxia of relatively brief (10-25 minutes) duration
    - Causative (sentinel) event is usually identifiable
    - Injury to regions of greatest metabolic demand
  - Peripheral pattern is associated with less severe hypoxia over longer period
    - Causative event is sometimes cryptic
    - Regions of greatest metabolic demand are protected
    - Watershed regions are susceptible
  - Preterm infants are more susceptible to equivalent ischemic injury as compared to term infants
    - Preterm neonates more likely to have associated WM injury & hemorrhage
- Associated abnormalities
  - Maternal: Infection, preeclampsia, diabetes, cocaine

Staging, Grading, & Classification

- Sarnat stage (based on clinical & EEG findings)
  - I (mild): Hyperalert/irritable, mydriasis, ↑ heart rate, EEG is normal
  - II (moderate): Lethargy, hypotonia, miosis, ↓ heart rate
  - III (severe): Stupor, flaccid, reflexes absent, seizures

CLINICAL ISSUES

Natural History & Prognosis

- Deep pattern is associated with dyskinetic cerebral palsy
- Peripheral pattern is associated with spastic cerebral palsy

SELECTED REFERENCES

1. O'Kane A et al: Early versus late brain magnetic resonance imaging after neonatal hypoxic ischemic encephalopathy treated with therapeutic hypothermia. J Pediatr. 232:73-79.e2, 2021
2. Misser SK et al: A pictorial review of the pathophysiology and classification of the magnetic resonance imaging patterns of perinatal term hypoxic ischemic brain injury - what the radiologist needs to know.... SA J Radiol. 24(1):1915, 2020

KEY FACTS

TERMINOLOGY

- Acute alteration of neurologic function due to loss of vascular integrity

IMAGING

- NECT: ↓ attenuation of affected gray matter
  - Insular ribbon sign → loss of distinct insular cortex
  - Hyperdense middle cerebral artery (MCA) sign → thrombosed MCA
- MR: ↓ diffusion within ~ 30 minutes of arterial occlusion
  - Cytotoxic edema is evident in affected territory on FLAIR/T2 by 4-6 hours after arterial occlusion
  - Enhancement of infarct typically occurs after 5-7 days
- CTA/MRA: Critical for early evaluation & identification of possible etiology (e.g., dissection, arteriopathy)
- MR perfusion imaging can provide valuable information regarding region at risk in setting of acute stroke
- MR vessel wall imaging is helpful to identify inflammatory arteriopathy

TOP DIFFERENTIAL DIAGNOSES

- Complex migraine
- Seizure-related injury
- Acute encephalitis
- Mitochondrial encephalopathies
- Posterior reversible encephalopathy syndrome

PATHOLOGY

- Major causes: Cardiac disease (~ 25%), moyamoya-type arteriopathy, dissection, vasculitis, hematologic/metabolic
- No underlying cause discovered in ~ 25% of cases

CLINICAL ISSUES

- Incidence: 2-3/100,000 per year in USA
  - Mortality: 0.6/100,000
- Children typically present later than adults (> 24 hours)
- Focal deficit may be masked by lethargy, coma, irritability
- Treatment in pediatric acute stroke is often conservative
- Capacity for recovery in children much better than adults

(Left) *Axial DWI MR in a 4-day-old term neonate presenting with seizures shows diffusion restriction ➡ throughout the left middle cerebral artery (MCA) territory, consistent with a perinatal arterial ischemic stroke (PAIS).* **(Right)** *Axial T2 MR in the same patient 2 years later shows cystic encephalomalacia ➡ throughout left MCA territory & passive enlargement of the left lateral ventricle ➡. Patients with PAIS who do not present near birth with seizures may later present with early hand preference or extremity weakness.*

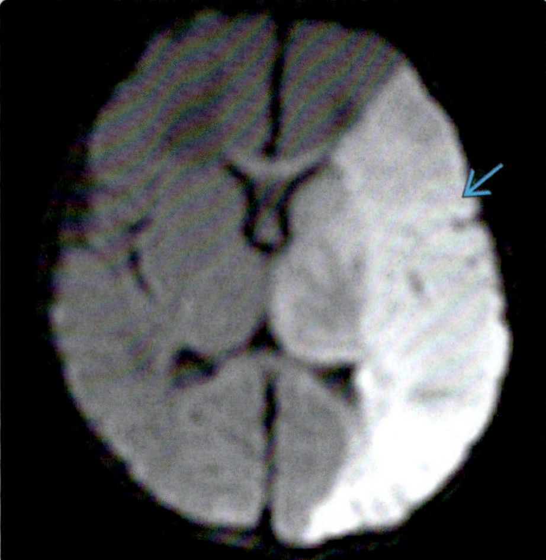

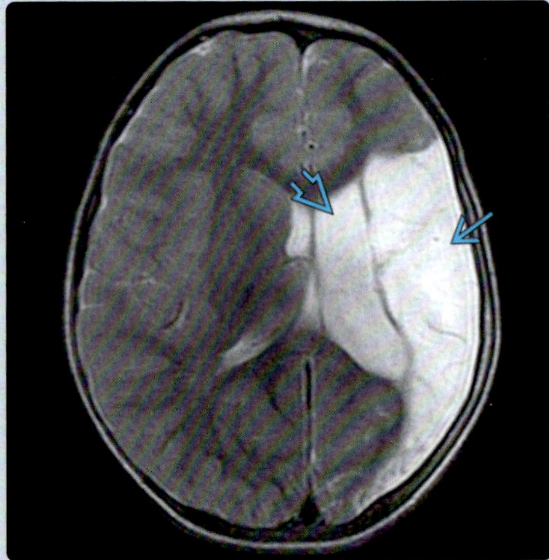

(Left) *Axial FLAIR MR in a 2-year-old girl shows multiple areas of cytotoxic edema ➡ in both cerebral hemispheres in this patient with moyamoya-type vasculopathy.* **(Right)** *Axial DWI MR in the same patient with moyamoya-type vasculopathy shows diffusion restriction in the right frontoparietal foci of signal abnormality ➡, suggesting an acute/subacute infarct. However, there is no diffusion restriction in the left parietal region ➡, suggesting this infarct is of an older age. Acute stroke should prompt careful arterial evaluation.*

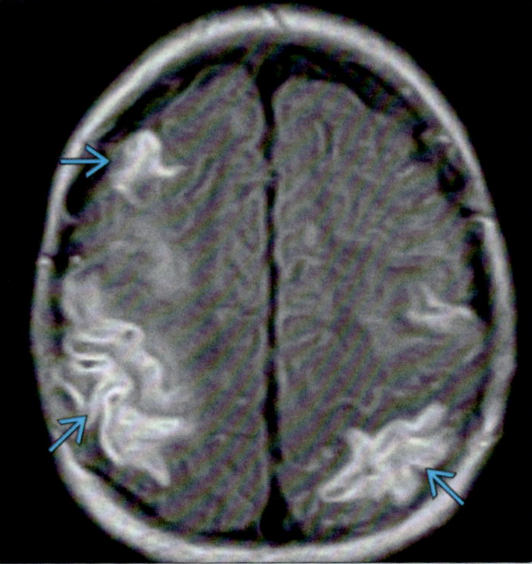

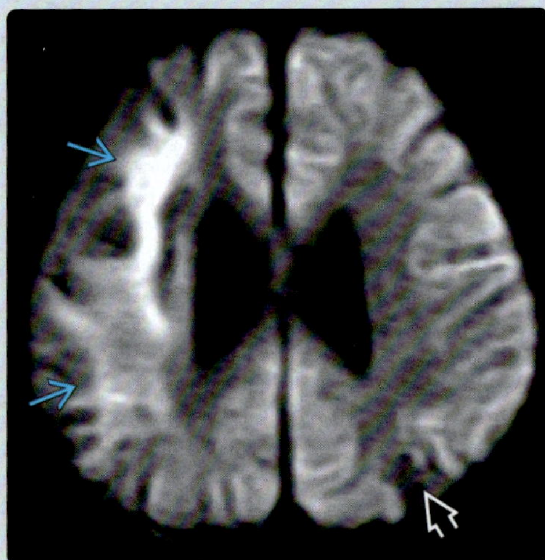

IMAGING

CT Findings

- NECT
  - ↓ attenuation of affected gray matter (GM) with loss of normal GM-white matter (WM) differentiation
    - ↓ in WM attenuation is less pronounced
    - Often wedge-shaped & localized to 1 arterial territory
  - Insular ribbon sign → loss of distinct insular cortex
  - Hyperdense middle cerebral artery (MCA) sign → ↑ density of acutely thrombosed MCA
  - Hemorrhagic transformation (HT)
    - Symptomatic HT in 3%; asymptomatic HT in 30%
- CTA
  - Invaluable for demonstrating focal vascular abnormalities in acute setting
    - Intimal flap in acutely dissected vessel
    - Major arterial occlusion may prompt thrombolysis or mechanical thrombectomy in appropriate setting

MR Findings

- **T1**: Acute: ↓ signal with gyral swelling
  - Chronic: ± ↑ signal in cortical laminar necrosis
- **T2**: Loss of flow void in thrombosed vessel
- **FLAIR**: ↑ signal with gyral swelling (within 4-6 hours)
  - Abnormal sulcal ↑ signal (climbing ivy sign) of chronic slow flow collaterals in setting of longstanding proximal vascular occlusion
- **DWI**: Most sensitive for early detection of ischemia
  - Acute: Restricted diffusion (↑ DWI, ↓ ADC signal) ≤ 30 minutes after ischemic insult
  - Subacute (7-14 days): Pseudonormalization of signal
  - Chronic: Facilitated diffusion in gliotic brain
- **T1 C+**: Cortical & leptomeningeal enhancement is seen after 5-7 days following acute infarct
  - Enhancing climbing ivy sign
- **MRA**: Can detect arterial occlusion & stenosis in large- & medium-sized cerebral vessels
- **PWI**: Provides valuable information about affected brain
  - Ischemic penumbra: ↓ perfusion, no DWI change (PWI-DWI mismatch)
- **MRS**: ↑ lactate is hallmark of ischemia/infarct
- **Vessel wall imaging**: Vessel wall enhancement suggests inflammatory arteriopathy

DIFFERENTIAL DIAGNOSIS

Complex Migraine

- ↓ (early) or ↑ (late) perfusion with normal DWI
- Engorgement of vessels on SWI

Seizure-Related Injury

- Swelling & restricted diffusion secondary to persistent seizure activity
- Differentiation by clinical presentation & EEG

Acute Encephalitis

- Acute parenchymal inflammation secondary to infectious agents, typically viral
- Slower onset with encephalopathy

Mitochondrial Encephalopathies

- Symmetric basal ganglia involvement is common
- Usually have manifestations beyond CNS

Posterior Reversible Encephalopathy Syndrome

- Patchy cortical/subcortical edema is most common in parietal & occipital lobes, typically in setting of hypertension
- Diffusion restriction is uncommon

PATHOLOGY

General Features

- 6 major causes of arterial stroke in children
  - Cardiac disease (~ 25%)
  - Moyamoya-type arteriopathy
  - Arterial dissection (e.g., trauma)
  - CNS vasculitis
  - Hematologic/metabolic (e.g., coagulopathy)
  - Idiopathic (~ 25%)

CLINICAL ISSUES

Presentation

- Most common signs/symptoms
  - Depends on patient age, etiology, & involved artery
    - < 1 year: Seizures, encephalopathy > focal neurologic
    - > 1 year: Usually focal neurologic (e.g., hemiplegia)
    - Speech difficulties, gait abnormality, seizure
    - Embolic cause: Sudden onset of symptoms
    - Stenoocclusive cause: Gradual/intermittent (e.g., TIA)
  - Focal deficit may be masked by lethargy, coma, irritability
- Children typically present later than adults (> 24 hours)

Demographics

- Epidemiology
  - Incidence: 2-3/100,000 per year in USA
    - Mortality: 0.6/100,000
  - Underrecognized as significant source of morbidity in pediatric population

Natural History & Prognosis

- Capacity for recovery is better than in adults, due to
  - Better compensatory mechanisms, collateral recruitment, neuronal plasticity
  - Fewer concomitant risk factors

Treatment

- Clinical window of opportunity/benefit is not as well understood in children as compared to adults
- Mainstay of chronic therapy for fixed vascular lesions & vasculopathies: Aspirin
- Transfusion therapy for at-risk children with sickle cell disease

SELECTED REFERENCES

1. van Es ACGM et al: Endovascular treatment for acute ischemic stroke in children: experience from the MR CLEAN Registry. Stroke. 52(3):781-8, 2021
2. Visser MJ et al: Automated perfusion-diffusion magnetic resonance imaging in childhood arterial ischemic stroke. Stroke. 52(10):3296-304, 2021
3. Donahue MJ et al: Neuroimaging advances in pediatric stroke. Stroke. 50(2):240-8, 2019
4. Khalaf A et al: Pediatric stroke imaging. Pediatr Neurol. 86:5-18, 2018

Moyamoya

KEY FACTS

TERMINOLOGY

- Progressive narrowing of distal internal carotid artery (ICA) & proximal circle of Willis (COW) vessels → characteristic adjacent clusters of collateral flow appearing as puff of smoke on real-time angiography
- Moyamoya disease = primary (idiopathic) moyamoya
- Moyamoya arteriopathy (a.k.a. moyamoya syndrome or secondary moyamoya) is due to other disorders

IMAGING

- Absent or narrowed distal ICA & abnormal COW
- Excessive tiny collaterals in basal ganglia & cisterns
  - "Puff of smoke" ("moyamoya" in Japanese) of lenticulostriate & thalamoperforator collaterals
- Prominent collaterals in sulci
  - Ivy sign on FLAIR & T1 C+ MR
- Acute & chronic infarcts
- CT/CTA: Acute use for ischemia or hemorrhage
- MR C+/MRA: Vascular protocol with DWI & perfusion
  - DWI: Helpful to identify acute-on-chronic injury

PATHOLOGY

- Moyamoya disease: Inherited idiopathic disorder
- Moyamoya arteriopathy: Secondary process
  - Sickle cell disease, neurofibromatosis type 1, radiation therapy, trisomy 21, Alagille syndrome, morning glory syndrome, TB meningitis, among others

CLINICAL ISSUES

- Bimodal age peaks: 6 & 35 years
- Most frequent cause of stroke in Asian children
- Presentation (children): Transient ischemic attacks (TIAs), alternating hemiplegia (exacerbated by crying), headache
- Presentation (adults): TIAs, hemorrhage (~ 30%), & cerebral infarct
- Prognosis depends on etiology, ability to form collaterals, age/stage at diagnosis
- Treatment: Indirect (more common in children) or direct (more common in adults) vascular bypass

(Left) *Axial DWI MR in a 13-month-old with increasing seizures shows left MCA distribution ischemia as well as a remote infarct in right MCA territory. This is a typical acute-on-chronic ischemic pattern of moyamoya.* **(Right)** *Anterior 3D TOF MRA in the same patient at 8 years of age shows occlusions of the small terminal ICAs →, absence of the MCAs, & numerous lenticulostriate collaterals ➡, forming a "puff of smoke." The PCAs are also occluded. Note the enlarged ECA collaterals ⇨ status post synangiosis & dural inversion.*

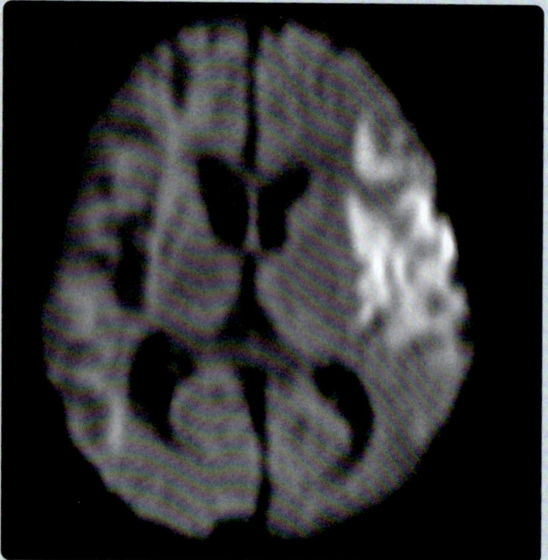

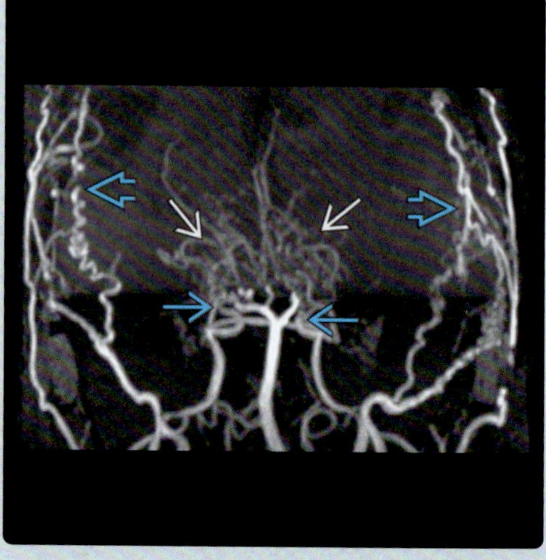

(Left) *Axial 3D TOF MRA in a 5-year-old with idiopathic moyamoya arteriopathy shows multiple small collateral vessels → where one would expect to see the proximal MCAs.* **(Right)** *Axial FLAIR MR in the same patient shows areas of gliosis ⇨ from vascular insufficiency, multiple linear hyperintensities representing deep medullary collateral vessels →, & hyperintensities conforming to the surface of the gyri & sulci representing pial collaterals ➡ (the leptomeningeal ivy sign).*

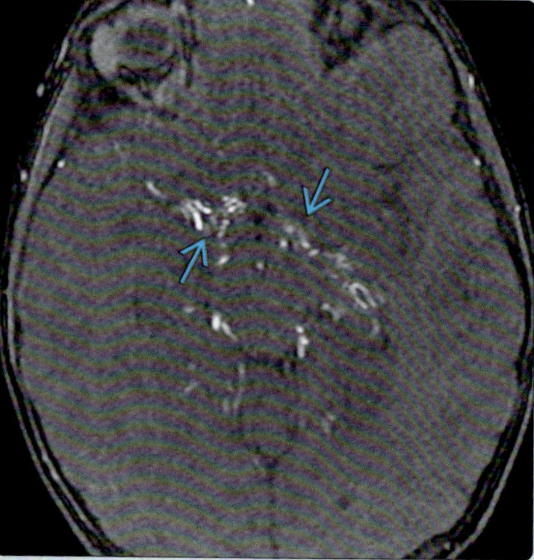

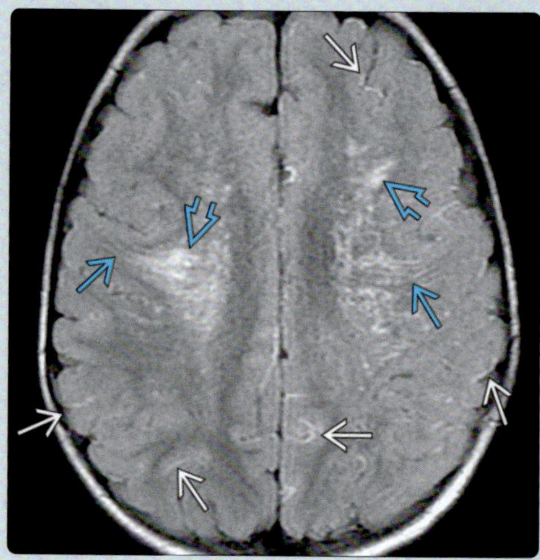

TERMINOLOGY

Definitions

- Progressive narrowing of distal internal carotid artery (ICA) & proximal circle of Willis (COW) vessels → characteristic adjacent clusters of collateral flow appearing as puff of smoke on real-time angiography
- Moyamoya disease: Primary (idiopathic) moyamoya
- Moyamoya arteriopathy (a.k.a. moyamoya syndrome or secondary moyamoya) occurs in association with other disorders or after radiation treatment

IMAGING

General Features

- Best diagnostic clue: Multiple enhancing punctate dots (CECT) & flow voids (MR) in basal ganglia & cisterns
- Arterial occlusions: Distal ICA, COW, branches
  - Anterior > posterior circulation
- Leads to prominent clusters of nearby collaterals
  - Cloud-like lenticulostriate & thalamoperforator collaterals on angiography: "Puff of smoke" ("moyamoya" in Japanese)
- Also leads to prominent sulcal collaterals distally

CT Findings

- NECT
  - Children: Acute ischemia ± old infarcts
  - Older children/adults: Usually ischemia but may present with intracranial hemorrhage
- CTA: Abnormal COW + basilar net-like collaterals

MR Findings

- **T2**: ↑ signal in gliotic areas from prior infarcts
  - Collateral vessels: Net-like cisternal flow voids
- **FLAIR**: Bright sulci = leptomeningeal ivy sign
  - Slow-flowing engorged pial collateral vessels, thickened arachnoid membranes
  - Correlates with ↓ cerebral vascular reserve
- **SWI/T2* GRE**: Hemosiderin if prior hemorrhage
- **DWI**: Very useful for acute-on-chronic infarcts
- **T1 C+**: Lenticulostriate collaterals → enhancing "dots" in basal ganglia & net-like thin vessels in cisterns
  - Leptomeningeal enhancement (ivy sign)
  - Vessel wall (spin-echo-based) imaging shows concentric enhancement of larger vessels
- **MRA**: Narrowed/occluded distal ICA & COW vessels
- **PWI**: ↓ perfusion in affected territories
  - May be used to measure response to revascularization

Angiographic Findings

- Predominantly (not exclusively) anterior circulation
  - Narrow proximal COW & ICA (early phase)
  - Lenticulostriate & thalamoperforator collaterals (intermediate phase)
  - Transdural/transosseous external carotid artery (ECA)-ICA collaterals (late phase)

Imaging Recommendations

- Best imaging tool: MR C+/MRA
- Catheter angiography defines anatomy prior to bypass

DIFFERENTIAL DIAGNOSIS

Ivy Sign

- Leptomeningeal metastases; subarachnoid hemorrhage; meningitis; ↑ inspired oxygen; collateral veins of Sturge-Weber or other chronic venous occlusion

Large Vessel Narrowing

- Vasculitis: Postvaricella vasculitis, lupus, & others; focal cerebral arteriopathy; arterial dissection; subarachnoid hemorrhage (spasm); meningitis; tumor encasement

PATHOLOGY

General Features

- Etiology
  - Moyamoya disease
    - Inherited polygenic or autosomal dominant
  - Moyamoya arteriopathy (a.k.a. moyamoya syndrome or secondary moyamoya)
    - Sickle cell disease, neurofibromatosis type 1, radiation therapy, trisomy 21, Alagille syndrome, morning glory syndrome, tuberculous meningitis, many others

Staging, Grading, & Classification

- Staging criteria (Suzuki)
  - Stage 1: Narrowing of ICA bifurcation
  - Stage 2: Anterior cerebral artery (ACA), middle cerebral artery (MCA), posterior cerebral artery (PCA) are dilated
  - Stage 3: Maximal basal collaterals; small ACA/MCA
  - Stage 4: Fewer collaterals (vessels); small PCA
  - Stage 5: Further ↓ in collaterals; absent ACA/MCA/PCA
  - Stage 6: Extensive ECA-pial collaterals

CLINICAL ISSUES

Presentation

- Most common signs/symptoms
  - Children: Transient ischemic attacks (TIAs), alternating hemiplegia (exacerbated by crying), headache
  - Adults: TIAs, hemorrhage (~ 30%), cerebral infarct

Natural History & Prognosis

- Pediatric cases usually advance to stage 5 in < 10 years
- Hemorrhagic moyamoya is more common in older patients

Treatment

- Aspirin therapy
- Direct bypass: Superficial temporal artery (STA)-MCA is more common in adults
- Indirect bypass
  - Pial synangiosis & encephaloduroarteriosynangiosis with STA is more common in children
  - Dural inversion with middle meningeal artery

SELECTED REFERENCES

1. Kaseka ML et al: Distinct clinical and radiographic phenotypes in pediatric patients with moyamoya. Pediatr Neurol. 120:18-26, 2021
2. Wang LX et al: Ivy sign in moyamoya disease: a comparative study of the FLAIR vascular hyperintensity sign against contrast-enhanced MRI. AJNR Am J Neuroradiol. 42(4):694-700, 2021
3. Lee S et al: Monitoring cerebral perfusion changes after revascularization in patients with moyamoya disease by using arterial spin-labeling MR imaging. Radiology. 288(2):565-72, 2018

Cerebral Venous Sinus Thrombosis

KEY FACTS

TERMINOLOGY

- Pathologic clot formation in cerebral veins & sinuses

IMAGING

- NECT: Acute thrombus is usually hyperdense (> 58 HU)
  - HU:hCT ratio > 1.4 ↑ sensitivity
  - Look for associated edema ± hemorrhage
- CTV: Filling defects or lack of opacification within sinus/vein
- MR: Be wary of artifacts [e.g., slow flow on spin-echo sequences, in-plane flow on time of flight (TOF)]
  - T2: Lack of flow void in affected vessels
  - FLAIR: May show edema within parenchyma
  - T2*/SWI: Blooming in areas of thrombosis
  - DWI: Look for areas of "venous infarct" within brain
  - 3D T1 GRE C+: Filling defects or nonopacification within sinus/vein, ± dural & leptomeningeal enhancement
  - PWI: ± altered areas of perfusion
  - MRV: Lack of flow-related signal in affected vessels
    - Helpful for chronic thrombus vs. recanalized vessel

TOP DIFFERENTIAL DIAGNOSES

- Subdural hemorrhage
- Arachnoid granulation
- Normal asymmetry/hypoplasia of transverse sinuses
- Idiopathic intracranial hypertension
- Hemoconcentration

PATHOLOGY

- Virchow triad: (1) Stasis, (2) vessel injury, (3) ↑ coagulability
- Occlusive thrombus → inadequate collaterals → edema, ischemia, & hemorrhage

CLINICAL ISSUES

- Risk factors: Infection, acute systemic illness, thrombophilia, cancer, trauma, & medications
- Common symptoms: Headache, nausea/vomiting, seizures, visual disturbances

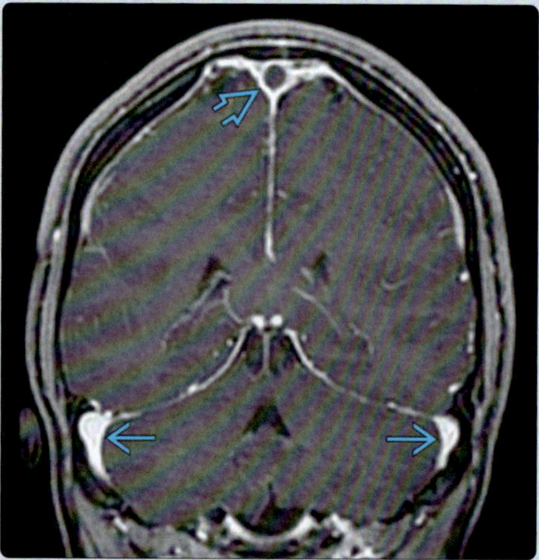
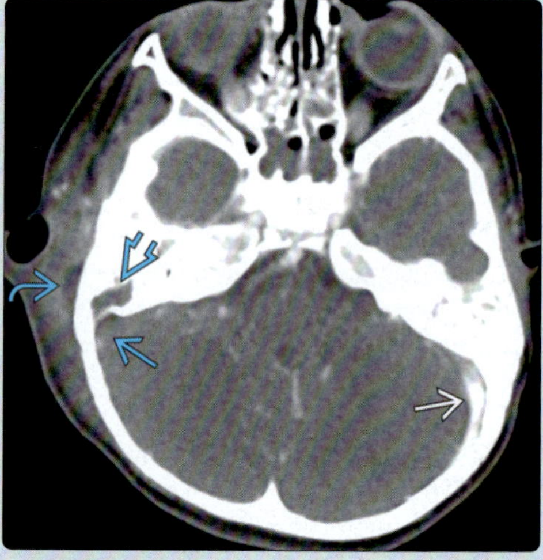

(Left) *Coronal 3D T1 C+ FS MR in a 17-year-old girl on oral contraceptives shows a lack of enhancement in the superior sagittal sinus ➡ (the empty delta sign), consistent with sinus thrombosis. Note the normal opacification of the sigmoid sinuses ➡.* **(Right)** *Axial CECT in a 2-year-old with mastoiditis shows opacification of the right mastoid ➡ & a subperiosteal abscess ➡. There is no contrast in the right sigmoid sinus ➡, consistent with thrombosis. Compare to the normal left sigmoid sinus ➡.*

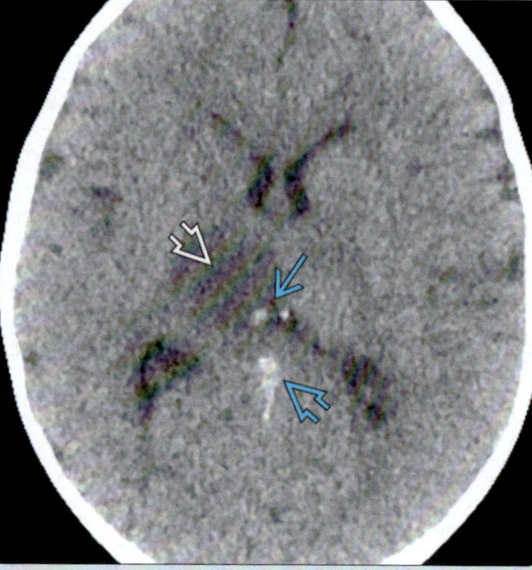
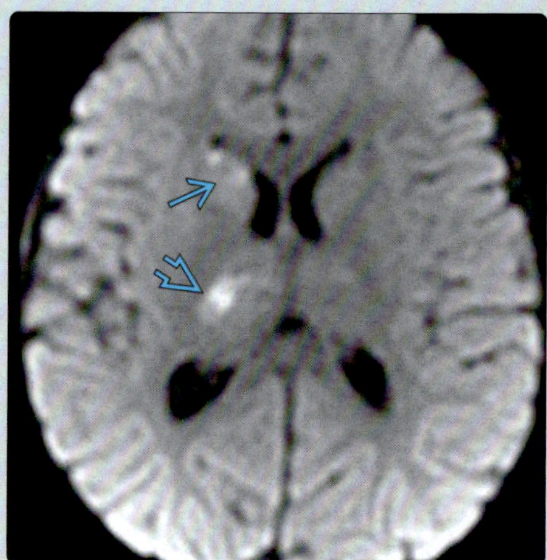

(Left) *Axial NECT in a 1-year-old with left facial droop shows hyperattenuation in the bilateral internal cerebral veins ➡ & vein of Galen ➡. Also note the ↓ attenuation & swelling of the right thalamus ➡.* **(Right)** *Axial DWI MR in the same patient shows an enlarged right thalamus ➡ & caudate head ➡ with areas of diffusion restriction, often referred to as venous infarctions. This term should be used with caution, however, as the diffusion restriction can resolve without imaging sequelae.*

TERMINOLOGY

Definitions

- Pathologic clot formation in cerebral veins & sinuses

IMAGING

General Features

- Best diagnostic clue
  - Lack of flow or enhancement in cerebral veins & sinuses
- Location
  - Dural venous sinuses & cerebral veins
    - Transverse sinus (86%), superior sagittal sinus (62%), straight sinus (18%), cortical veins (17%), jugular veins (12%), & internal cerebral veins (11%)

CT Findings

- NECT
  - Acute thrombus is usually hyperdense; in cortical vein → dense cord sign
    - Acute thrombus detection: NECT is > 70% sensitive
      - Typically > 60 HU; suggested cutoff values range from 58-62
    - HU:hCT ratio of > 1.4 is advocated for higher sensitivity/specificity
  - Chronic thrombus is usually iso- or hypodense
- CT venography: Filling defects or lack of opacification within sinus/vein; empty delta sign in sagittal & transverse sinuses

MR Findings

- T1: Variable signal based on age of thrombus
- T2: Lack of flow void within affected sinus/vein
- FLAIR: May show edema within parenchyma
- T2*/SWI: Blooming in areas of thrombosis
  - Excellent for detection of cortical vein thrombus
- DWI: Diffusion restriction in areas of "venous infarct"
  - Changes may be reversible without permanent injury
- 3D GRE T1 C+: Filling defects within sinus/vein
  - Empty delta sign in sagittal & transverse sinuses
  - Chronic thrombus may enhance despite lack of flow
  - ± dural & leptomeningeal enhancement
- PWI: ± altered areas of perfusion due to venous congestion
- MRV: Lack of flow-related signal on time of flight (TOF) & PC sequences; T1 shortening in clot may mimic flow on TOF

Ultrasonographic Findings

- May use to evaluate sagittal & transverse sinuses in infants

Imaging Recommendations

- Best imaging tool
  - NECT + CTV: Excellent for detection of thrombus & gross parenchymal hemorrhage
  - MR + MRV: Superior to CTV in detection of parenchymal edema, infarct, & microhemorrhage
- Protocol advice
  - Use both flow-related venography (e.g., TOF or phase contrast) to distinguish chronic thrombus from patent recanalized vessel (both enhance on T1 C+)
  - 3D GRE-based T1 (e.g., BRAVO, MP-RAGE, SPGR) is best to avoid flow artifacts

DIFFERENTIAL DIAGNOSIS

Subdural Hemorrhage

- Subdural hemorrhage (SDH) along tentorium & falx may mimic thrombus
- Dense (CT) & T1 bright (MR) blood may mimic thrombus
- Multiplanar reconstructions help distinguish SDH vs. clot

Arachnoid Granulation

- Focal filling defects on CTV & MRV
- Most often occur in transverse & sagittal sinuses
- Follow CSF on MR ± small vessel within arachnoid granulation

Asymmetric or Hypoplastic Transverse Sinus

- Normal for transverse sinuses to be asymmetric in size
- If little/no flow on MRV, confirm hypoplasia with T1 C+ & T2

Idiopathic Intracranial Hypertension

- Identical symptoms of ↑ intracranial pressure (ICP)
- Look for flattening of lateral transverse sinuses

Hemoconcentration

- ↑ hCT→ ↑ blood density; may mimic thrombus
- Dense vessels throughout, including arteries
- Usually < 58 HU; HU:hCT ratio < 1.4; common in newborns

PATHOLOGY

General Features

- Virchow triad: (1) Stasis, (2) vessel injury, (3) ↑ coagulability
- ↓ venous outflow → ↑ venous pressure → ↑ ICP
- Inadequate collaterals → edema, infarction, & hemorrhage
- Chronic: Conversion of thrombus into fibrotic mass with multiple endothelial-lined channels

CLINICAL ISSUES

Presentation

- ↑ ICP: Headache, nausea/vomiting, visual symptoms, altered mental status;
- Parenchymal injury: Seizure, focal neurologic deficits

Demographics

- Risk factors: Infection (e.g., meningitis), acute illness (e.g., dehydration), thrombophilia, cancer, trauma, & medications

Natural History & Prognosis

- Neonates in general have poorer outcomes; vast majority have full recovery with appropriate therapy
- Permanent symptoms due to brain injury (e.g., hemorrhage)

Treatment

- Anticoagulation (heparin & low molecular weight heparin)

SELECTED REFERENCES

1. Bonatti M et al: Accuracy of unenhanced CT in the diagnosis of cerebral venous sinus thrombosis. Radiol Med. 126(3):399-404, 2021
2. Pai V et al: Pearls and pitfalls in the magnetic resonance diagnosis of dural sinus thrombosis: a comprehensive guide for the trainee radiologist. J Clin Imaging Sci. 10:77, 2020

KEY FACTS

TERMINOLOGY

- Vein of Galen aneurysmal malformation (VGAM): High-flow arteriovenous fistula (AV) between deep choroidal arteries & median prosencephalic vein (MPV) of Markowski
- Not actually aneurysm of true vein of Galen, which fails to form because of fistula

IMAGING

- 2 major goals of imaging
  - Assess degree of brain injury
  - Define VGAM architecture to help plan embolization
- Some degree of ventriculomegaly is typical
  - ↓ CSF resorption due to venous hypertension
  - Chronic volume loss
    - Due to venous hypertension & arterial steal
  - Obstruction from compression of tectum
- Venous outflow stenosis affects end-organ damage
  - Sigmoid/jugular stenoses protect heart, injure brain
- Classification system for VGAMs (Lasjunias)
  - Choroidal type: Multiple primitive choroidal arteries pass through nidus before entering MPV
  - Mural type: 1 or more (usually multiple) direct AV fistulas within wall of MPV

CLINICAL ISSUES

- Most common extracardiac cause of high-output heart failure in newborn
- Preferred treatment: Transcatheter embolization at 4-6 months with occlusion of fistula, ideally from arterial side
  - May require staged embolizations
- Bicêtre neonatal evaluation score guides therapy
  - Assesses end-organ damage
- Prognosis is related to volume of shunt & timing/success of treatment
  - High-volume shunts requiring treatment in newborn period have worse prognosis
  - Ability to delay treatment until 4-6 months is associated with better outcome

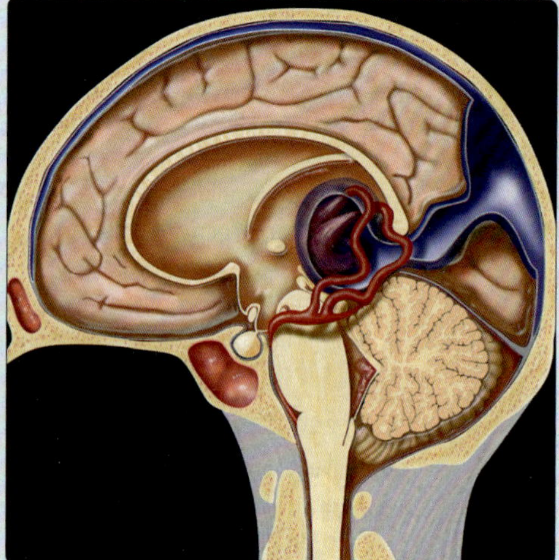

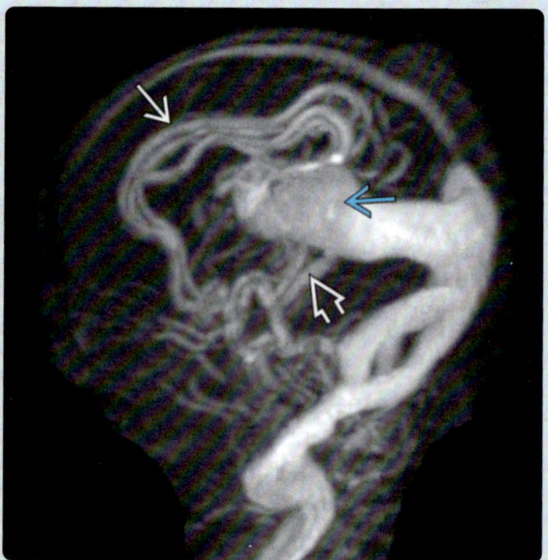

(Left) *Sagittal graphic shows medial & lateral posterior choroidal arteries with a fistulous connection to an enlarged midline vein [median prosencephalic vein (MPV)], which drains through a persistent falcine sinus to the superior sagittal sinus. This would be a mural-type vein of Galen aneurysmal malformation (VGAM).* **(Right)** *Lateral 3D MRA with contrast in a newborn with high-output cardiac failure shows enlarged choroidal ➡ & pericallosal ➡ arteries feeding a large MPV ➡ & straight sinus. No venous outflow stenosis is identified.*

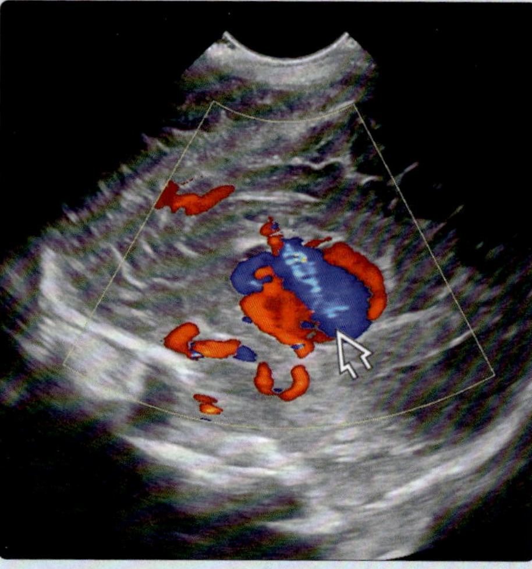

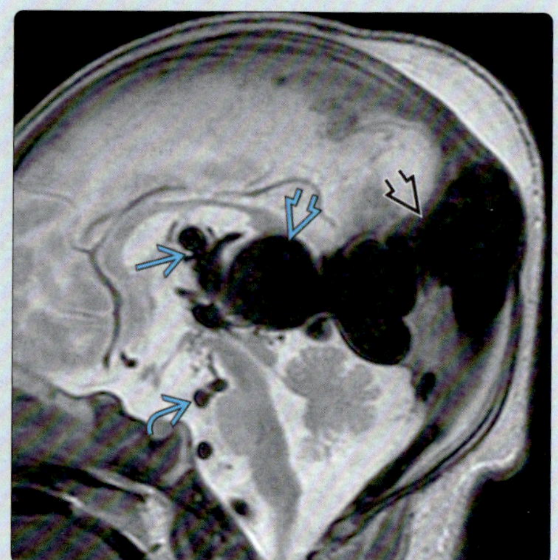

(Left) *Sagittal color Doppler US in a neonate with heart failure shows a large ovoid vascular lesion ➡ with turbulent flow located in the region of the MPV, characteristic for a VGAM.* **(Right)** *Sagittal T2 MR in the same patient shows a markedly dilated MPV ➡ & persistent falcine sinus ➡ with enlarged feeding arteries ➡, including the basilar ➡ & internal carotid arteries (not shown). In this case, multiple feeding arteries fistulize directly into the wall of the MPV, consistent with a mural-type VGAM.*

Vein of Galen Aneurysmal Malformation

TERMINOLOGY

Synonyms

- Vein of Galen aneurysmal malformation (VGAM), galenic varix

Definitions

- High-flow arteriovenous (AV) fistula between deep choroidal arteries & median prosencephalic vein (MPV) of Markowski
  - Not actually aneurysm of true vein of Galen, which fails to form because of fistula

IMAGING

General Features

- 2 major goals of imaging
  - Assess brain injury to determine if treatment is warranted
  - Delineate malformation architecture for embolization

CT Findings

- NECT
  - Hydrocephalus
  - Various stages of parenchymal injury, including cytoxic edema, volume loss, & white matter Ca^{2+} from chronic venous ischemia
- CTA
  - Excellent preangiography delineation of vessels

MR Findings

- Large flow void of varix
- Phase-encoding pulsation artifact from varix
- Prominent flow voids of feeding arteries around varix
- Some degree of ventriculomegaly is typical; ± ↑ T2 signal of white matter
  - ↓ CSF resorption due to venous hypertension
  - Obstruction from compression of tectum
  - Chronic volume loss
- Restricted diffusion in areas of acute ischemia/infarction
  - Due to venous hypertension & arterial steal phenomenon
  - ± focal or extensive loss of cortical ribbon on T2
- MRV: High flow through veins → venous stenoses
  - Affects end-organ damage
    - Venous stenosis protects heart at expense of brain
    - Jugular stenosis/atresia is associated with poor outcome
- MRA: Key to define architecture of lesion
  - Major arterial feeders: Targets for embolization
  - Unaffected by embolics (ideal for posttreatment evaluation)
- Perfusion: Arterial spin labeling can assess AV shunt reduction following embolization
- Fetal MR can identify malformation in 2nd & 3rd trimester & provide information about end-organ injury
  - Diameter of fetal or neonatal falcine or straight sinus may predict outcome

Angiographic Findings

- Choroidal or mural classification (Lasjunias) based on angioarchitecture of VGAM
  - Choroidal type: Primitive vessel morphology with multiple choroidal feeding arteries passing through nidus network before draining into MPV
  - Mural type: 1 or more (usually multiple) direct AV fistulas within wall of MPV
- Frequent venous abnormalities
  - Embryonic falcine sinus drains MPV in ~ 50%
  - Stenoses at sigmoid-jugular junction

PATHOLOGY

General Features

- Embryology
  - Abnormal connection of choroidal arteries to MPV occurs at 6- to 11-weeks gestation
  - Flow through fistula prevents normal regression of MPV

CLINICAL ISSUES

Presentation

- Most common signs/symptoms
  - Neonate: High-output CHF, cranial bruit
  - Infant: Macrocrania (hydrocephalus), seizures, or neurocognitive delay
  - Older children/adults: Usually compensated; may present with hemorrhage

Natural History & Prognosis

- Prognosis is related to volume of shunt & timing/success of treatment
  - High-volume shunts requiring treatment in newborn period have worse prognosis
- Severe cases → ischemia & cerebral atrophy: "Melting brain"
  - Due to venous insufficiency & arterial steal

Treatment

- Treatment in neonatal period is based upon Bicêtre neonatal evaluation score
  - 21-point system based upon cardiac (5), cerebral (5), respiratory (5), hepatic (3), & renal (3) function
  - High score: Good function; low score: Poor function
    - < 8: No treatment
    - 8-12: Emergent embolization
    - > 12: Medical management initially followed by delayed embolization at 4-6 months
- Transcatheter embolization
  - Permanent occlusion of fistula, ideally from arterial side
    - Liquid agents or coils
  - Outcome following embolization: 75% normal; 15% moderate impairment; 10% severe impairment

SELECTED REFERENCES

1. D'Amico A et al: Outcome of fetal vein Galen aneurysmal malformations: a systematic review and meta-analysis. J Matern Fetal Neonatal Med. 1-6, 2021
2. Arko L et al: Fetal and neonatal MRI predictors of aggressive early clinical course in vein of Galen malformation. AJNR Am J Neuroradiol. 41(6):1105-11, 2020
3. Li TG et al: Diagnosis of foetal vein of galen aneurysmal malformation by ultrasound combined with magnetic resonance imaging: a case series. BMC Med Imaging. 20(1):63, 2020
4. Berenstein A et al: Vein of Galen aneurysmal malformation: advances in management and endovascular treatment. Neurosurgery. 84(2):469-78, 2019

Arteriovenous Malformation

KEY FACTS

TERMINOLOGY

- High-flow vascular malformation with arteriovenous shunting through complex nidus of arterioles & venules (without intervening capillary bed)

IMAGING

- NECT: Parenchymal hematoma is most common
  - Small, unruptured AVMs are often not visible
- CTA: Enhancing feeding arteries, nidus, & draining veins
  - May be negative if AVM is compressed by hematoma
- MR
  - T1: Bright hemorrhage
  - T2: Prominent dark flow voids
  - T1 C+ (volumetric gradient): Enhancing abnormal vessels
- MRA: Gross depiction of AVM components
  - 3D TOF flow-related signal in draining veins from shunt
- Advanced MR
  - ASL: High signal in nidus & draining veins
  - SWI: High (arterial) signal in draining veins
- Digital subtraction catheter angiography
  - Best identifies all 3 components of AVM
    - Multiple arterial feeding vessels (internal-external carotid, vertebrobasilar)
    - Deep vs. superficial venous drainage
    - Associated arterial/nidus aneurysms, venous stenoses

PATHOLOGY

- Most AVMs are sporadic; micro-AVMs are typical in hereditary hemorrhagic telangiectasia (HHT)
- Spetzler-Martin surgical risk grading system (1-5 points)
  - Size: < 3 cm (1 point), 3-6 cm (2), > 6 cm (3)
  - Location: Eloquent (1) vs. noneloquent (0)
  - Venous drainage: Deep (1) vs. superficial (0)

CLINICAL ISSUES

- Spontaneous parenchymal hemorrhage in child should be considered AVM until proven otherwise
- Annual bleeding risk: 2-4%

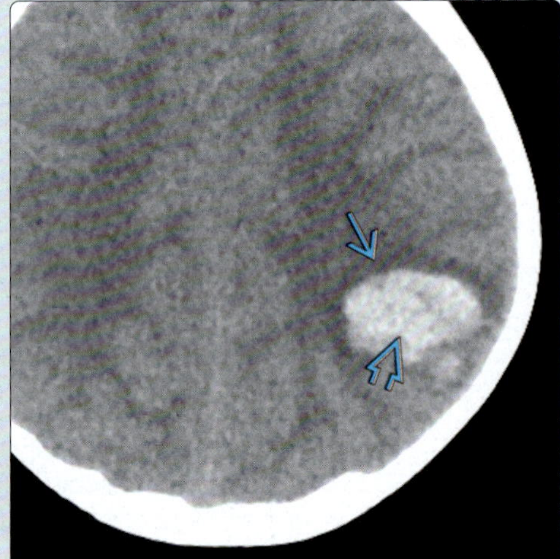

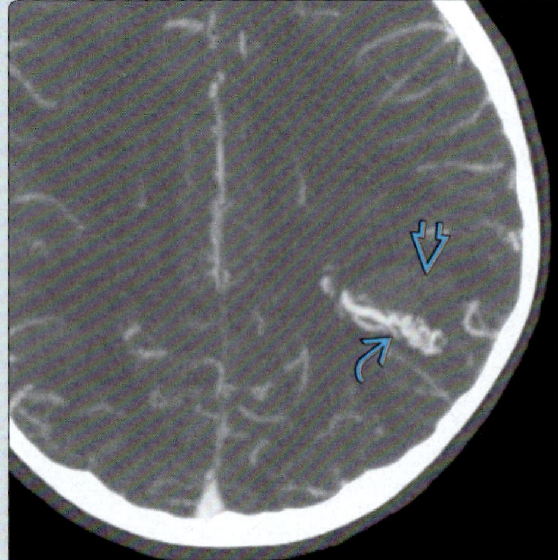

(Left) *Axial NECT in a 5-year-old with new-onset seizures shows intraparenchymal hemorrhage in the left parietal lobe with surrounding low-attenuation vasogenic edema. Such a finding should prompt immediate evaluation with CTA to detect an AVM, which is the most likely underlying cause of spontaneous hemorrhage in children.* **(Right)** *Axial CTA MIP in the same patient shows a nidus of abnormal vessels along the posterior margin of the intraparenchymal hemorrhage, consistent with an AVM.*

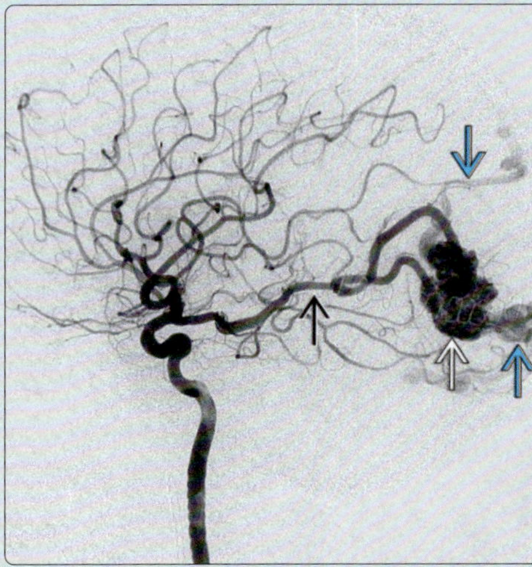

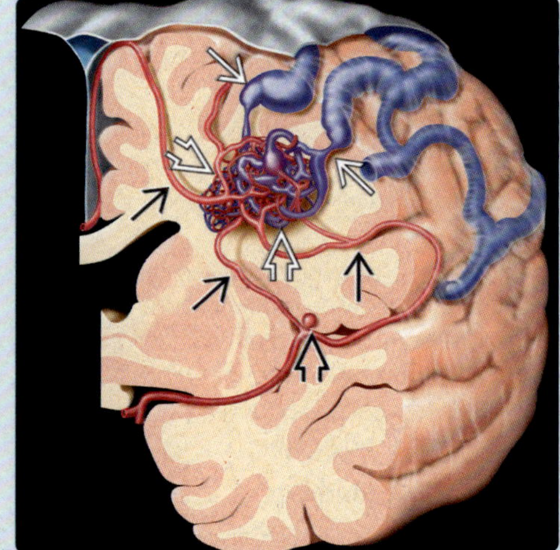

(Left) *Lateral DSA (right ICA injection) in a 15-year-old girl shows an enlarged arterial feeder arising from the right ICA via the PCOM artery. The tightly packed nidus is well defined. Note the 2 enlarged superficial draining veins that opacify early during the arterial phase, typical of an AVM.* **(Right)** *Graphic shows a cerebral AVM with a centrum semiovale nidus fed from cortical & central arteries (with a proximal flow-related aneurysm) & drained by enlarged cortical veins.*

TERMINOLOGY

Definitions

- Arteriovenous malformation (AVM): High-flow vascular malformation with AV shunting through complex nidus of arterioles & venules (without intervening capillary bed)

IMAGING

CT Findings

- NECT: Unruptured AVM is often occult, unless large; ± Ca^{2+}
  - Ruptured AVM: Spontaneous parenchymal hemorrhage ± intraventricular extension
- CTA: Enlarged feeding arteries, nidus, draining veins
  - Nidus may be compressed by hematoma

MR Findings

- T1: Hematoma in ruptured AVM is typically of ↑ signal
- T2: Flow voids of arterial feeder, nidus, & draining veins
- FLAIR: May see adjacent gliosis, especially with prior bleed
- SWI/T2* GRE: Blooming with hemorrhagic blood products
  - Hyperintense (arterial) SWI signal in draining veins
- DWI: Usually normal on initial imaging studies
  - ± ischemic complications following intervention
- T1 C+: Avid enhancement of nidus & draining veins with GRE T1 (not spin echo)
  - Important for micro-AVMs as found in hereditary hemorrhagic telangiectasia (HHT)
- MRA/MRV: Gross depiction of AVM components
  - Flow-related signal in draining veins on 3D TOF MRA reflects AV shunt
- ASL: High signal in AVM nidus & draining veins
  - Sensitive sequence for detection of micro-AVMs

Angiographic Findings

- DSA provides high spatial & temporal resolution
  - Arterial feeders
    - Enlarged; often from multiple arteries (internal-external carotid, vertebrobasilar)
    - Feeding artery aneurysms in 10-15%
  - AVM nidus
    - Central tangle of vessels where AV shunting occurs
    - Small aneurysms within nidus (~ 50%)
  - Venous drainage
    - Must identify drainage as deep &/or superficial
    - ± venous varix, which suggests distal stenosis
    - Unbalanced inflow vs. outflow
      - Fast AV shunt + small outflow vein

Imaging Recommendations

- Best imaging tool
  - CTA for atraumatic intracranial hemorrhage on NECT
    - If initially negative, repeat when hematoma resolves as small AVM may be compressed by initial hematoma

DIFFERENTIAL DIAGNOSIS

Cavernous Malformation

- "Angiographically occult" lesion
- Popcorn appearance on MR with fluid-fluid levels, hemosiderin staining, ± Ca^{2+}

Arterial Aneurysm

- No nidus or enlarged draining veins
- Subarachnoid blood is common

Hemorrhagic Tumor

- Often enhances on MR; tumor blush on DSA
- No enlarged draining veins

Arteriovenous Fistula

- Direct AV shunting without nidus

PATHOLOGY

General Features

- Associated abnormalities
  - Syndromic AVMs (2% of cases)
    - HHT: 40-50% have micro-AVMs of brain
      - Additional lung & hepatic AVMs; cutaneous & mucosal telangiectasias

Staging, Grading, & Classification

- Spetzler-Martin scale predicts surgical morbidity: ↑ score = ↑ risk of open surgery
  - Size: < 3 cm (1 point), 3-6 cm (2), > 6 cm (3)
  - Location: Noneloquent (0) or eloquent (1)
  - Drainage: Superficial (0) or deep (1)

CLINICAL ISSUES

Presentation

- ~ 50% have acute hemorrhage (headache, ↓ consciousness), ~ 25% seizure, ~ 15% focal neurologic findings, ~ 10% incidental
  - Spontaneous parenchymal hemorrhage in child should be considered AVM until proven otherwise

Natural History & Prognosis

- Annual bleeding risk: 2-4%
- Factors that ↑ annual bleeding risk
  - Prior AVM rupture, exclusively deep venous drainage, small size (< 3 cm), single feeder, single outflow vein
- Possible factors that ↑ annual bleeding risk
  - Arterial or intranidal aneurysms
  - Unbalanced inflow vs. outflow
  - Size of outflow veins (controversial)

Treatment

- Acute surgical decompression may be required for mass effect from hematoma
- Optimal treatment for underlying AVM is based on variety of factors; options include
  - Microsurgical resection
  - Endovascular embolization
  - Stereotactic radiosurgery

SELECTED REFERENCES

1. Hong S et al: Long-term outcomes in pediatric unruptured brain arteriovenous malformation treated by nonconservative management: a single center analysis. Childs Nerv Syst. 35(8):1363-9, 2019
2. Ai X et al: The factors associated with hemorrhagic presentation in children with untreated brain arteriovenous malformation: a meta-analysis. J Neurosurg Pediatr. 23(3):343-54, 2018
3. Hodel J et al: Intracranial arteriovenous shunting: detection with arterial spin-labeling and susceptibility-weighted imaging combined. AJNR Am J Neuroradiol. 38(1):71-6, 2017

Cavernous Malformation

KEY FACTS

TERMINOLOGY

- Benign vascular lesion with dilated sinusoids lined by thin, immature walls & containing blood products of various ages

IMAGING

- Supratentorial > infratentorial > spinal cord
- Vary in size from microscopic to giant (> 6 cm)
- **CT**: Hyperdense lesion ± Ca^{2+}; 50% are not visible
- **MR**: Heterogeneous core with T2-hypointense rim
  - Popcorn ball appearance with internal fluid-fluid levels
  - Adjacent ↑ FLAIR signal suggests recent hemorrhage
  - SWI/T2* GRE is most sensitive for small lesions
  - Absent or minimal enhancement, except for associated developmental venous anomaly (DVA)

TOP DIFFERENTIAL DIAGNOSES

- Diffuse axonal injury
- Intracerebral hematoma
- Neoplasm

PATHOLOGY

- Etiology: Initial parenchymal microhemorrhage is followed by neoangiogenesis & recurrent hemorrhage
  - ↑ in size from recurring intralesional hemorrhages
- Multiple (familial) cavernous malformation syndrome: Autosomal dominant
  - *KRIT1* (CCM1), *CCM2, PDCD10* (CCM3) genes; variable penetrance
- 25% of CMs are associated with DVAs

CLINICAL ISSUES

- 0.6% incidence in children undergoing brain MR
- 50% incidental, 25% seizures, 25% neurologic deficits
- 70% solitary, 30% multiple (if familial or prior radiation)
- Factors that ↑ annual risk of hemorrhage are
  - Zabramski MR classification (I & II > III, IV)
  - Prior hemorrhage; brainstem location; associated DVA
- Treatment: Total surgical excision, sparing DVA

(Left) *Axial NECT in a 1-year-old patient with focal facial seizures shows heterogeneous high attenuation ➔ in the right frontal lobe with low attenuation (edema) ➔ deep to the lesion.* **(Right)** *Axial T1 (left) & T1 C+ (right) MR images in the same patient demonstrate intrinsically high signal ➔ (Zabramski type I) in the lesion. There are multiple small vessels ➔ along the medial margin coalescing into a draining vein ➔, consistent with a developmental venous anomaly (DVA). DVAs are found in ~ 25% of cavernous malformations (CMs).*

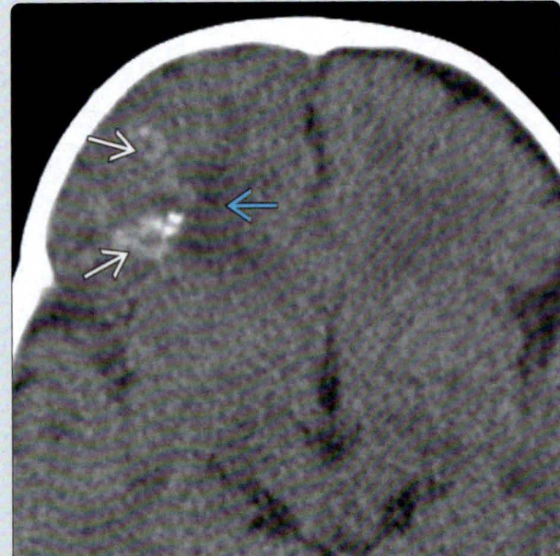

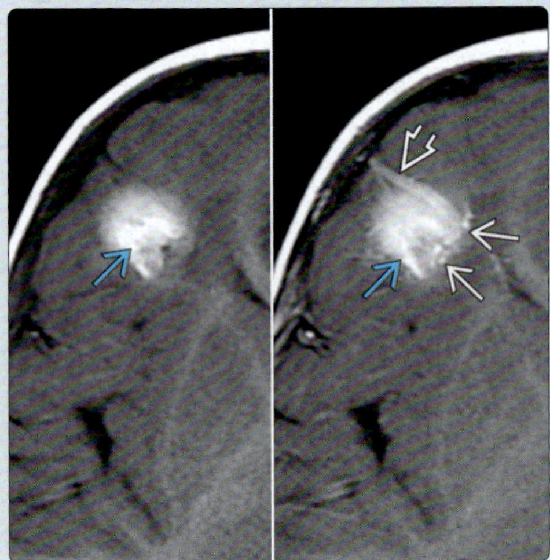

(Left) *Axial T2 MR in a 16-year-old patient shows a characteristic CM with a hypointense rim ➔ & fluid level ➔. The adjacent vasogenic edema ➔ suggests recent hemorrhage of the CM.* **(Right)** *Axial SWI MR in a 15-year-old patient with multiple familial CM syndrome shows 2 larger lesions ➔ in the left basal ganglia & right occipital lobe + a smaller lesion ➔ (Zabramski IV) in the right frontal lobe. The 2 larger lesions were visible on T2, but the smaller lesion was only visible on the more sensitive SWI sequence.*

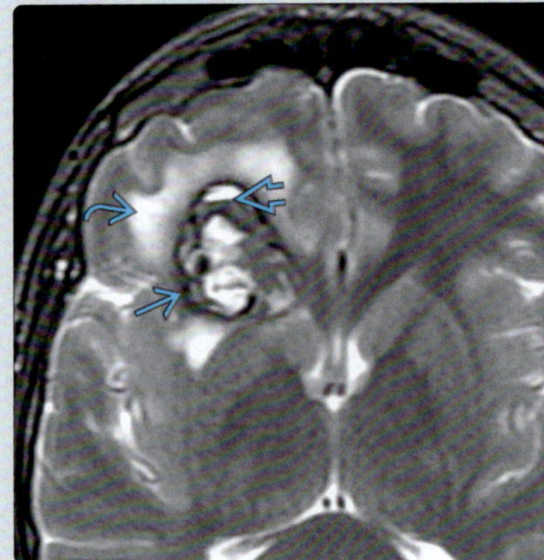

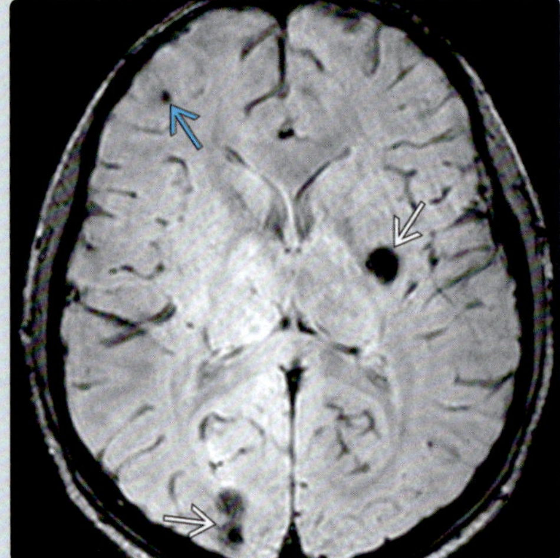

TERMINOLOGY

Definitions

- Cavernous malformation (CM): Benign vascular lesion arising in CNS
- Consists of dilated sinusoids containing blood products of various ages & lined by thin, immature walls

IMAGING

General Features

- Location: Can be found throughout CNS
  - Supratentorial: ~ 80%
  - Infratentorial: ~ 20%
  - Rarely in spinal cord, except in multiple CMs
- Vary in size from microscopic to giant (> 6 cm)

CT Findings

- **NECT**: Round or irregular hyperdense lesion
  - ± hemorrhage & associated perilesional edema
  - Often shows small areas of Ca^{2+}
  - CT is negative in up to 50%, especially for small lesions
- **CECT**: No enhancement of actual lesion
  - ± associated developmental venous anomaly (DVA)

MR Findings

- **T1**: Heterogeneous with blood of varied ages & Ca^{2+}
- **T2**: Mixed signal core with complete hypointense rim corresponding to hemosiderin
  - Numerous septations or locules
  - ± fluid-fluid levels of layering blood products
  - Small lesions may appear as focal hypointensities
- **FLAIR**: Surrounding edema suggests recent hemorrhage
- **SWI/T2* GRE**: Exaggerated signal loss (blooming)
  - Most sensitive for detection of small CMs
    - Numerous punctate hypointense foci (black dots)
- **DWI**: Usually normal; may show susceptibility effect
- **T1 C+**: Minimal or no enhancement
  - Associated enhancing DVA in ~ 25% of cases
- **MRA**: Normal
  - CMs are "angiographically occult"

DIFFERENTIAL DIAGNOSIS

Diffuse Axonal Injury

- Multiple small foci of hemosiderin deposition
- History of prior trauma with severe neurologic impairment

Venous Infarction

- More often hemorrhagic compared to arterial infarction
- Less complex-appearing without hemosiderin rim if acute

Intracerebral Hematoma

- Usually more simple-appearing
- No hemosiderin at acute presentation

Neoplasm

- Hemorrhage or Ca^{2+} in primary brain tumor
- Often has enhancing soft tissue component

Neurocysticercosis

- May mimic familial CM with many small CNS Ca^{2+}

Capillary Telangiectasia

- Subtle enhancement following contrast administration

PATHOLOGY

General Features

- Etiology
  - Initial microhemorrhage from variety of conditions followed by neoangiogenesis & recurrent hemorrhage
    - ↑ vascular permeability (familial CMs); ↑ venous flow/pressure (CMs associated with DVAs); small vessel injury (CMs associated with radiation)
- Genetics
  - Multiple (familial) CM syndrome: Autosomal dominant
    - 3 separate loci implicated: *KRIT1* (CCM1), *CCM2*, *PDCD10* (CCM3)
- Associated abnormalities
  - DVA: 25% of CMs have associated DVA; < 5% of DVAs have associated CM

Staging, Grading, & Classification

- Zabramski classification of CMs
  - Type I: Subacute hemorrhage (↑ T1; ↑ or ↓ T2)
  - Type II: Reticulated mixed T1 & T2 with ↓ T2 rim
  - Type III: Chronic hemorrhage (iso/↓ T1; ↓ T2)
  - Type IV: Tiny microhemorrhages only seen on SWI/T2*

CLINICAL ISSUES

Presentation

- Most common signs/symptoms
  - Identified incidentally (40-50%)
  - Seizures (20-25%)
  - Neurologic deficit from hemorrhage (20-25%)

Demographics

- ~ 0.6% prevalence in all children undergoing brain MR
- ~ 70% solitary, 30% multiple

Natural History & Prognosis

- Factors that ↑ risk of symptomatic hemorrhage in children
  - Prior hemorrhage: 11.3% annually
  - Brainstem or spine location: 16.7% & 8.2% annually
  - Associated DVA: 9.7% annually
- Annual risk of hemorrhage also predicted by MR imaging
  - Zabramski I & II: 23.4% (5-60% in literature)
  - Zabramski III: 3.4% (0-6% in literature)
  - Zabramski IV: 1.3%

Treatment

- Total removal via microsurgical resection
- If DVA is present, venous drainage should be preserved
  - DVA removal → venous injury & venous infarct

SELECTED REFERENCES

1. Ren J et al: Characteristics and long-term outcome of 20 children with intramedullary spinal cord cavernous malformations. Neurosurgery. 86(6):817-24, 2020
2. Young A et al: Sensitivity of susceptibility-weighted imaging in detecting developmental venous anomalies and associated cavernomas and microhemorrhages in children. Neuroradiology. 59(8):797-802, 2017
3. Gross BA et al: The natural history of cerebral cavernous malformations in children. J Neurosurg Pediatr. 1-6, 2015

KEY FACTS

TERMINOLOGY

- Peroxisomal biogenesis disorders (PBD)
  - Zellweger syndrome (ZS)
- Mucopolysaccharidoses (MPS)
- Organic & aminoacidopathies
  - Molybdenum cofactor deficiency (MoCD)
  - Nonketotic hyperglycinemia (NKH)
- Urea cycle disorders
- Fatty acid oxidation disorders
  - Short-, medium-, & long-chain acyl-CoA dehydrogenase deficiency (SCAD, MCAD, LCAD)

IMAGING

- ZS: Polymicrogyria is most severe in perisylvian region
- MPS: Enlarged perivascular spaces, confluent WM lesions
- MoCD: Hypoxic ischemic encephalopathy mimic
- NKH: Causes vacuolating myelinopathy, affecting structures that are myelinated at birth

TOP DIFFERENTIAL DIAGNOSES

- Hypoxic ischemic encephalopathy
  - Many metabolic disorders are thought to represent perinatal asphyxia at 1st presentation
- Traumatic brain injury
- Mitochondrial encephalopathies
  - May present with encephalopathy or stroke-like symptoms
- Leukodystrophies
  - Do not have migrational abnormalities like PBD

DIAGNOSTIC CHECKLIST

- Remember to consider metabolic diseases when encountering acutely ill neonate
- Characteristic laboratory abnormalities may provide clue
  - Hyperammonemia → urea cycle disorder
  - Severe hypoglycemia → MCAD deficiency

(Left) *Sagittal T2 MR in a 12-year-old with Hurler syndrome shows dilated perivascular spaces ➡, flattening of the anterior clinoids ➡, & hypertrophy of the tectorial membrane ➡.* **(Right)** *Coronal T2 MR shows confluent white matter (WM) lesions ➡ & dilated perivascular spaces ➡ in the corpus callosum & basal ganglia in this 5-year-old with Hunter syndrome (MPS 2). Perivascular space dilation is most pronounced in MPS 1 & 2 with WM lesions more common in 1, 2, 3, & 7.*

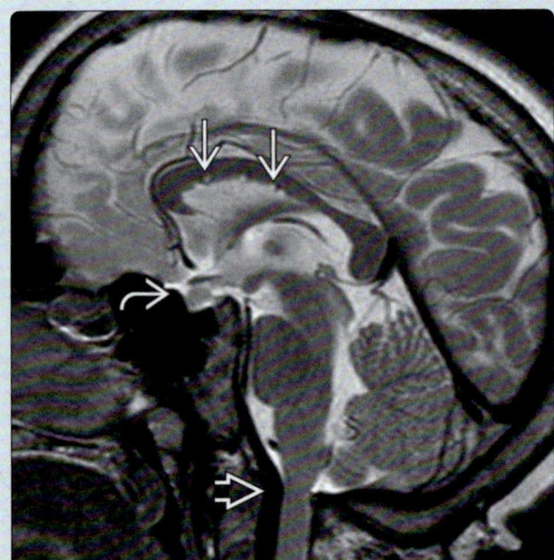

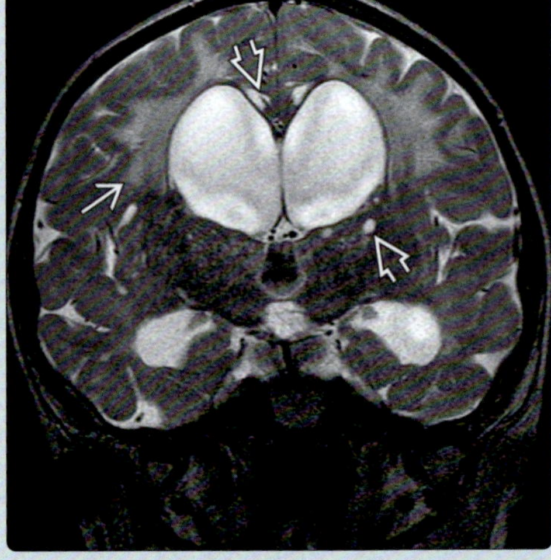

(Left) *Axial T2 MR in a 4-month-old with failure to thrive, hypotonia, & elevated liver enzymes shows polymicrogyria ➡ lining the sylvian fissure in each hemisphere. In combination with liver dysfunction, this is indicative of Zellweger syndrome.* **(Right)** *Axial T1 MR shows perisylvian polymicrogyria ➡ & germinolytic cysts ➡ in this 2-week-old with neonatal adrenoleukodystrophy, a peroxisomal biogenesis disorder with less severe enzymatic deficiencies than Zellweger syndrome.*

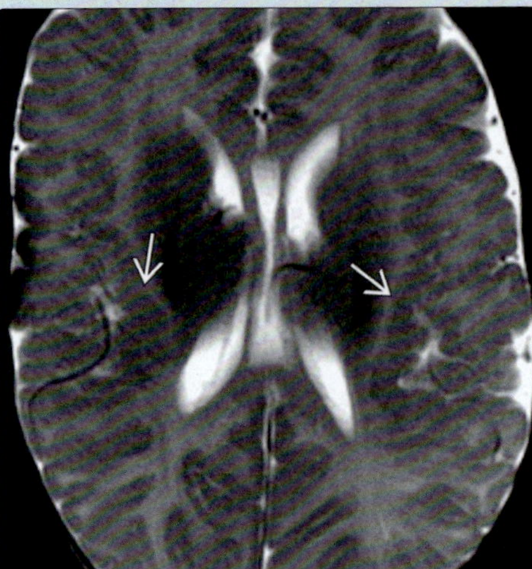

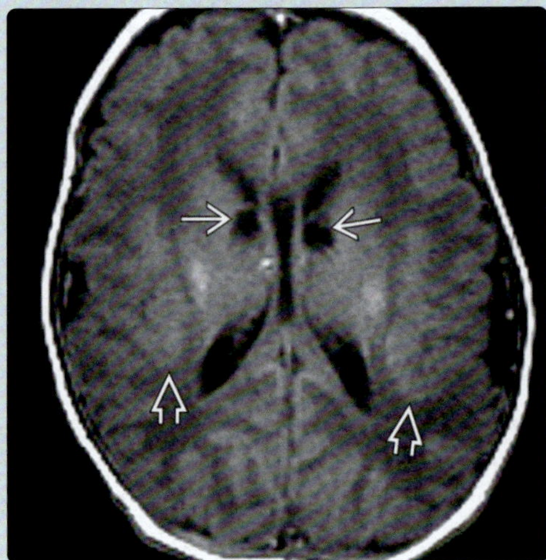

TERMINOLOGY

Definitions

- Inborn errors of metabolism affecting brain
  - Exclusive of mitochondrial encephalopathies & leukodystrophies
- Peroxisomal biogenesis disorders (PBD)
  - Severe: Zellweger syndrome (ZS)
  - Moderate: Neonatal adrenoleukodystrophy (NALD)
  - Mild: Infantile Refsum disease
- Mucopolysaccharidoses (MPS)
  - Lysosomal storage disease
  - Hunter, Hurler, Sanfilippo, Morquio, Maroteaux-Lamy, Sly, Natowicz syndromes
- Organic & aminoacidopathies
  - Molybdenum cofactor deficiency (MoCD)
  - Maple syrup urine disease (MSUD)
  - Phenylketonuria (PKU)
  - Nonketotic hyperglycinemia (NKH)
- Urea cycle disorders
  - Deficiency of enzymes in urea cycle
- Fatty acid oxidation disorders
  - Short-chain acyl-CoA dehydrogenase deficiency (SCAD)
  - Medium-chain acyl-CoA dehydrogenase deficiency (MCAD)
  - Long-chain acyl-CoA dehydrogenase deficiency (LCAD, VLCAD)
  - Carnitine palmitoyl transferase deficiencies (CPT1, CPT2)

IMAGING

Key Imaging Findings

- ZS
  - Leukoencephalopathy with abnormal myelin in corticospinal tracts & dentate nuclei
  - Polymicrogyria is most severe in perisylvian region
  - Germinolytic cysts near foramen of Monro
  - May see T1 shortening in globus pallidus from hyperbilirubinemia
  - May see enhancement of corticospinal tracts in brainstem
- MPS
  - CNS imaging abnormalities due to accumulated glycosaminoglycan (GAG)
  - Enlarged perivascular spaces
    - Pronounced in MPS 1 & 2
    - Not seen in MPS 4, 7, 9
  - Confluent WM lesions
    - Hypointense T1, hyperintense T2/FLAIR
    - Pronounced in MPS 1, 2, 3, & 7
  - Hydrocephalus & cortical atrophy
- MSUD
  - Edema prominently involving brainstem & cerebellar WM
  - Hypointense on T1, hyperintense on T2, hypodense on CT
  - Cytotoxic edema → markedly restricted diffusion
- MoCD
  - Diffuse cerebral edema/infarction
  - Diffusion restriction in globus pallidi & upper brainstem
  - Hypoxic-ischemic encephalopathy (HIE) mimic
- PKU
  - ↑ signal on T2 in periventricular WM
- NKH
  - Restricted diffusion & abnormal signal in posterior limb of internal capsule, dorsal midbrain, cerebellar WM in neonate
    - Causes vacuolating myelinopathy, affecting structures that are myelinated at birth
- Urea cycle disorders
  - Diffuse brain edema, not sparing basal ganglia or thalami
- MCAD deficiency
  - Cerebral cortical edema

DIFFERENTIAL DIAGNOSIS

Hypoxic Ischemic Encephalopathy

- Many metabolic disorders are thought to represent perinatal asphyxia at 1st presentation
- Atypical response to treatment raises concerns for metabolic disease

Traumatic Brain Injury

- May present with diffuse edema
- Close evaluation for signs of trauma is essential in obtunded neonate

Mitochondrial Encephalopathies

- May present with encephalopathy or stroke-like symptoms

Leukodystrophies

- Do not have migrational abnormalities like PBD

PATHOLOGY

PBD

- Defective transport of proteins into peroxisomal matrix → accumulation of very long chain fatty acids (VLCFA)
- ↓ peroxisomal function
  - Elevated plasma levels of sphingomyelin, VLCFA, pristanic acid, phytanic acid, pipecolic acid
- Caused by mutations in 1 of 14 known *PEX* genes
  - 70% associated with *PEX1* mutations
  - 15-20% associated with *PEX6* mutations

MPS

- Deficiencies of various enzymes required to break down GAG → accumulation of GAG in multiple organs, including brain & connective tissues
  - MPS 1 (Hurler): α-L-iduronidase
    - *IDUA* gene on chromosome 4
  - MPS 2 (Hunter): Iduronate 2-sulfatase
    - *IDS* gene on X chromosome
  - MPS 3 (Sanfilippo): Heparan sulfamidase
    - *SGSH* gene on chromosome 17
    - *NAGLU* gene on chromosome 17
    - *HGSNAT* gene on chromosome 8
    - *GNS* gene on chromosome 12
  - MPS 4 (Morquio): Galactose 6-sulfatase
    - *GALNS* gene on chromosome 16
    - *GLB1* gene on chromosome 3
  - MPS 6 (Maroteaux-Lamy): Arylsulfatase B
    - *ARSB* gene on chromosome 5

- MPS 7 (Sly): β-glucuronidase
  - *GUSB* gene on chromosome VII
- MPS 9 (Natowicz): Hyaluronidase
  - *HYAL1* gene on chromosome 3

Organic & Aminoacidopathies

- MoCD: Mutations in either *MOCS1*, *MOCS2*, or *GPHN* → inability to synthesize molybdopterin → deficiency of sulfite oxidase, xanthine dehydrogenase, aldehyde oxidase, & mitochondrial amidoxime reducing component
  - Enzyme deficiencies result in accumulation of sulfite, taurine, S-sulfocysteine, & thiosulfate
- MSUD: ↓ activity of branched chain α-keto acid dehydrogenase complex → accumulation of branched chain amino acids, particularly L-leucine
- PKU: ↓ phenylalanine dehydroxylase → accumulation of phenylalanine in brain (toxic to developing brain)
- NKH: Defect in 1 of 4 protein components (usually P-protein) of glycine cleavage system → accumulation of glycine (toxic to developing brain)

Urea Cycle Disorders

- Deficiencies of specific urea cycle enzymes
  - Ornithine transcarbamylase
  - Carbamoyl phosphate synthetase 1
  - Argininosuccinate synthetase (citrullinemia)
  - Arginase (argininemia)
  - N-acetylglutamate synthetase
  - Ornithine translocase (ORNT1 deficiency, hyperornithinemia-hyperammonemia-homocitrullinuria syndrome)
  - Citrin deficiency
- Enzyme deficiencies prevent conversion of ammonia into urea → hyperammonemia, neurotoxicity

Fatty Acid Oxidation Disorders

- MCAD deficiency: Enzyme deficiency prevents oxidization of medium-chain fatty acids → hypoketotic hypoglycemia when fatty acid oxidation is required to supplement cellular energy stores

CLINICAL ISSUES

PBD

- Severe hypotonia, seizures, poor sucking
- Elevated liver enzymes, hepatomegaly
- Characteristic facies in ZS: High forehead, broad nasal bridge, hypertelorism
- Renal cortical cysts

MPS

- Progressive coarsening of features, developmental delay
- Skeletal dysplasia: Dysostosis multiplex (**not** in MPS 3 or 9)
  - Flattening of anterior clinoid processes (J-shaped sella)
  - Inferior vertebral beaking (superior notch)
    - Middle of vertebral body in MPS 4
  - Rounded iliac wings
  - Thick diaphyses & metacarpals
  - Oar-shaped ribs
- Atlantoaxial instability
  - Result of odontoid hypoplasia & ligamentous laxity
  - Compensatory ligamentous hyperplasia contributes to craniocervical junction stenosis

Organic & Aminoacidopathies

- Catastrophic illness in neonatal period
- MoCD: Unremitting seizure activity
  - Type A, caused by mutations in *MOCS1*, amenable to treatment with *E. coli* derived cyclic PMP

Urea Cycle Disorders

- Hyperammonemia & coma in neonatal period

Fatty Acid Oxidation Disorders

- Severe hypoglycemia in response to illness or fasting

DIAGNOSTIC CHECKLIST

Consider

- Remember to consider metabolic diseases when encountering acutely ill neonate

Image Interpretation Pearls

- Characteristic laboratory abnormalities may provide clue
  - Hyperammonemia → urea cycle disorder
  - Severe hypoglycemia → MCAD deficiency

SELECTED REFERENCES

1. Lim YT et al: Neuroimaging spectrum of inherited neurotransmitter disorders. Neuropediatrics. 51(1):6-21, 2020
2. Reddy N et al: Neuroimaging findings of organic acidemias and aminoacidopathies. Radiographics. 38(3):912-31, 2018
3. Tan AP et al: Clinical and neuroimaging spectrum of peroxisomal disorders. Top Magn Reson Imaging. 27(4):241-57, 2018
4. Atwal PS et al: Molybdenum cofactor deficiency. Mol Genet Metab. 117(1):1-4, 2016
5. Braverman NE et al: Peroxisome biogenesis disorders in the Zellweger spectrum: An overview of current diagnosis, clinical manifestations, and treatment guidelines. Mol Genet Metab. 117(3):313-21, 2016
6. Reichert R et al: Neuroimaging findings in patients with mucopolysaccharidosis: what you really need to know. Radiographics. 36(5):1448-62, 2016
7. Alqahtani E et al: Mucopolysaccharidoses type I and II: new neuroimaging findings in the cerebellum. Eur J Paediatr Neurol. 18(2):211-7, 2014
8. Ruder J et al: Neonatal citrullinemia: novel, reversible neuroimaging findings correlated with ammonia level changes. Pediatr Neurol. 51(4):553-6, 2014
9. Das S et al: Rare magnetic resonance imaging findings in medium-chain acyl-coenzyme A dehydrogenase deficiency. Pediatr Neurol. 45(3):203-5, 2011
10. Gropman A: Brain imaging in urea cycle disorders. Mol Genet Metab. 100 Suppl 1:S20-30, 2010
11. Oldham MS et al: Diffusion tensor imaging in arginase deficiency reveals damage to corticospinal tracts. Pediatr Neurol. 42(1):49-52, 2010
12. Bindu PS et al: Cranial MRI in acute hyperammonemic encephalopathy. Pediatr Neurol. 41(2):139-42, 2009
13. Mourmans J et al: Sequential MR imaging changes in nonketotic hyperglycinemia. AJNR Am J Neuroradiol. 27(1):208-11, 2006

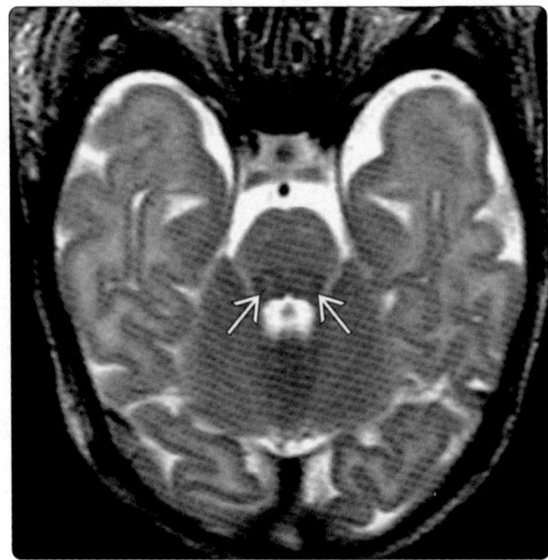

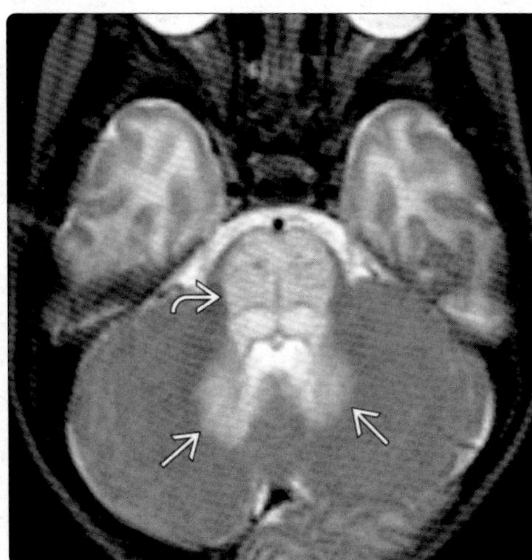

(Left) *Axial T2 MR in a 3-day-old with nonketotic hyperglycinemia (NKH) shows the characteristic "owl's eye" paired signal abnormalities in the central tegmental tracts of the brainstem* ➡*. Although this finding is not specific for NKH, it should raise the possibility of the diagnosis in the appropriate clinical setting.* **(Right)** *Axial T2 MR in an infant with maple syrup urine disease shows striking edema in the pons* ↪ *& cerebellar WM* ➡*. This degree of brainstem edema should raise concern for metabolic brain disease.*

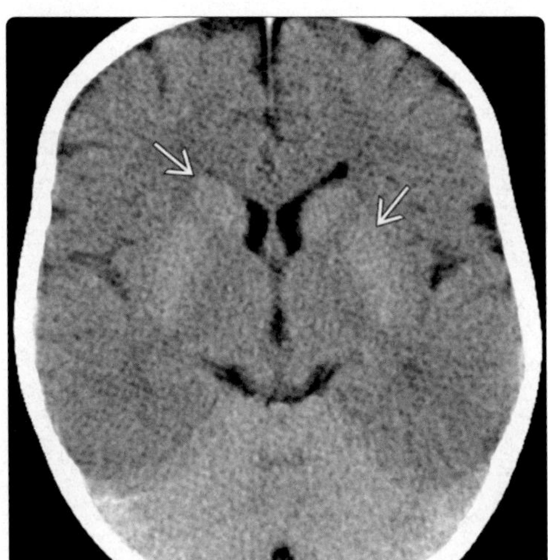

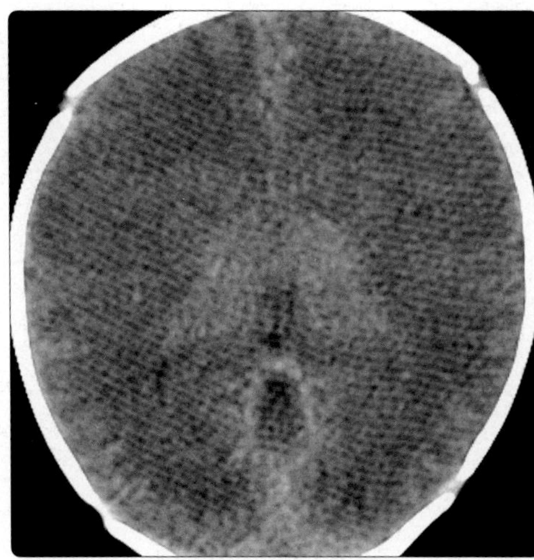

(Left) *Axial NECT in a 2-year-old presenting with severe hypoglycemia & seizures due to a medium-chain acyl-CoA dehydrogenase deficiency shows ↓ attenuation of the cerebrum with preservation of the basal ganglia* ➡*.* **(Right)** *Axial NECT in a neonate with an inborn deficiency of ornithine transcarbamylase (a urea cycle enzyme) shows diffuse cerebral & basal ganglia low attenuation with loss of gray matter-white matter differentiation from cytotoxic edema brought on by hyperammonemia.*

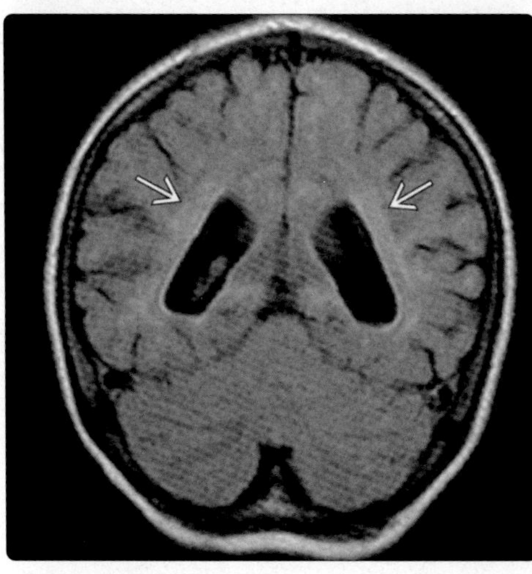

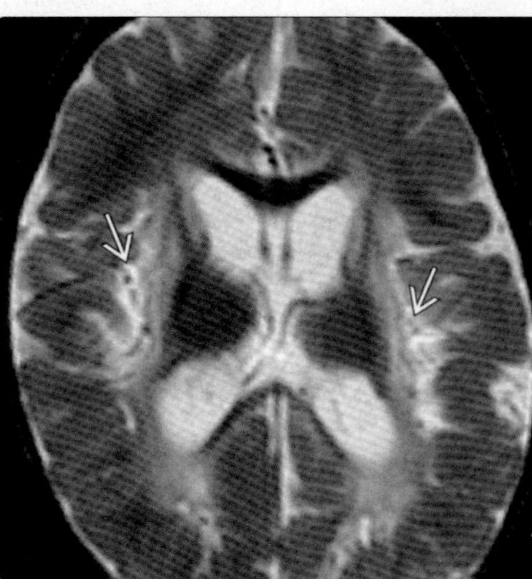

(Left) *Coronal FLAIR MR shows ill-defined, abnormal hyperintensity* ➡ *in the periventricular WM of this teenager with Sanfilippo syndrome (MPS 3).* **(Right)** *Axial T2 MR shows bilateral & symmetric volume loss & gliosis in the insular cortex* ➡ *& periventricular WM as a consequence of prior hyperammonemia in this 20-month-old with citrullinemia, a urea cycle disorder caused by deficiency of argininosuccinate synthetase.*

Mitochondrial Encephalopathies

KEY FACTS

TERMINOLOGY

- Genetically based disorders of mitochondrial function resulting in progressive or intermittent brain injury
  - Leigh syndrome (LS)
  - Myopathy, encephalopathy, lactic acidosis, & stroke-like episodes (MELAS)
  - Kearns-Sayre syndrome (KSS)
  - DNA polymerase γ-related disorders (POLG-RD)
  - Disorders of pyruvate metabolism
    - Pyruvate dehydrogenase (PDH) deficiency
  - Mitochondrial aminoacyl tRNA synthetase deficiencies
    - Leukoencephalopathy with brainstem & spinal cord involvement & high lactate (LBSL)
- Mitochondrial dysfunction has been associated with myriad clinical pathologies, ranging from autism to Alzheimer dementia to normal aging

IMAGING

- Broad range of imaging appearances, characterized by regions of edema, brain destruction, volume loss, &/or mineralization
- Typically hyperintense lesions on T2 & FLAIR
  - LS typically causes speckled pattern in deep nuclei
- MRS can be helpful although often nonspecific
  - ↑ lactate & restricted diffusion can be clue to true etiology
    - Especially if found in normal-appearing regions
- Cerebellar atrophy is common feature

PATHOLOGY

- LS → associated with mutations in > 60 genes, both mitochondrial (mtDNA) & nuclear (nDNA)
  - As specific mutations affecting specific metabolic pathways are determined, enzymatic deficiencies resulting in LS are now diagnosed as separate entities

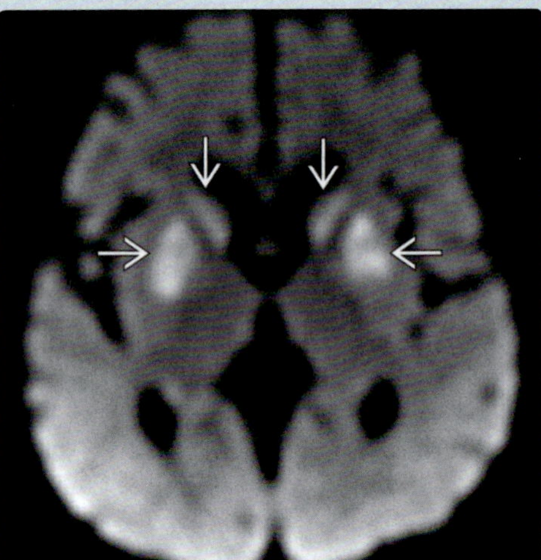

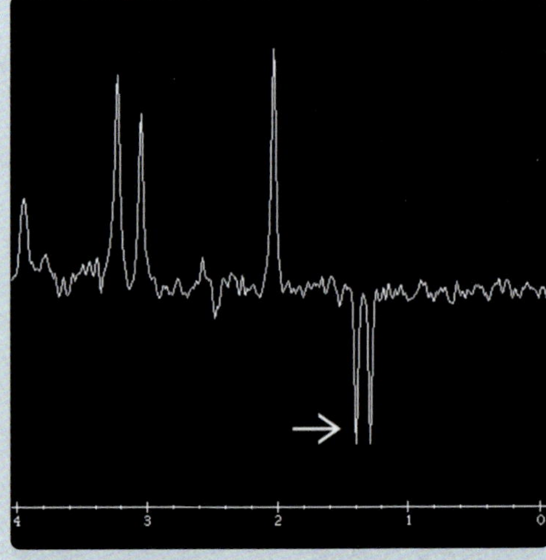

(Left) *Axial DWI MR in a 10-month-old with hypotonia & developmental delay shows restricting lesions in the basal ganglia that are bilateral & relatively symmetric ➡, characteristic of mitochondrial encephalopathy.* **(Right)** *Intermediate (144 msec) echo proton MR spectroscopy acquired in one of the lesions in this patient shows a characteristic inverted doublet at 1.3 ppm ➡, indicating elevated lactate. This child has Leigh disease caused by a mitochondrial DNA mutation.*

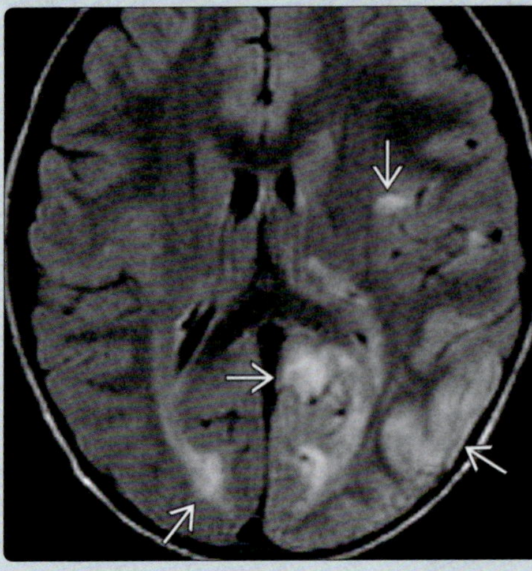

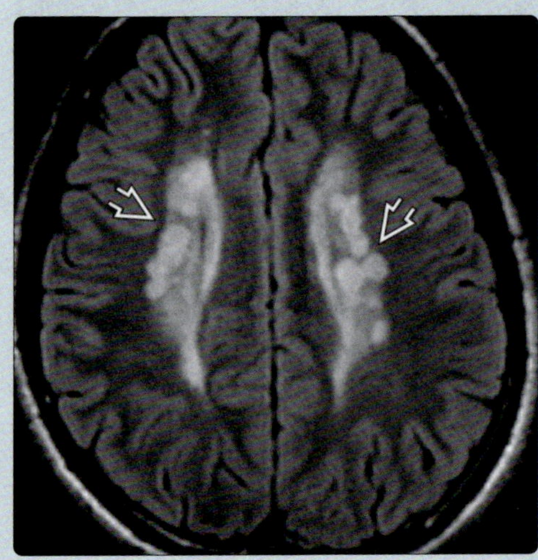

(Left) *Axial FLAIR MR in a 7-year-old with seizures shows numerous stroke-like lesions in both hemispheres ➡, not correlating with arterial territories. A diagnosis of myopathy, encephalopathy, lactic acidosis, & stroke-like episodes (MELAS) was confirmed.* **(Right)** *Axial FLAIR MR in a teenager with LBSL shows extensive bilateral signal abnormalities in the corona radiata ⇨. The patient's only symptoms were transient paresthesias (tingling) in the lower extremities.*

TERMINOLOGY

Abbreviations

- Mitochondrial encephalopathies (MEs)

Definitions

- Genetically based disorders of mitochondrial function resulting in progressive or intermittent brain injury
  - Leigh syndrome (LS)
  - Myopathy, encephalopathy, lactic acidosis, & stroke-like episodes (MELAS)
  - Kearns-Sayre syndrome (KSS)
  - DNA polymerase γ-related disorders (POLG-RD)
  - Disorders of pyruvate metabolism
    - Pyruvate dehydrogenase (PDH) deficiency
  - Mitochondrial aminoacyl tRNA synthetase deficiencies
    - Leukoencephalopathy with brainstem & spinal cord involvement & high lactate (LBSL)
- Mitochondrial dysfunction has been associated with myriad clinical pathologies, ranging from autism to Alzheimer dementia to normal aging

IMAGING

General Features

- Best diagnostic clue
  - Broad range of imaging appearances, characterized by regions of edema, brain destruction, volume loss, &/or mineralization
    - LS, PDH deficiency: Symmetric speckled lesions in basal ganglia (BG)
    - MELAS: Peripheral, stroke-like lesions
    - KSS: Cerebellar atrophy, ↑ T2 in subcortical white matter (WM)
    - POLG-RD: Volume loss, asymmetric thalamic lesions with restricted diffusion
    - LBSL: ↑ T2 in WM, posterior limbs of internal capsules, dorsal columns of spinal cord
- Location
  - Variable: Most common in BG, brainstem, thalami, dentate nuclei

Imaging Recommendations

- Protocol advice
  - MRS can be helpful but is often nonspecific
  - ↑ lactate & restricted diffusion can be clue to true etiology, especially if found in normal-appearing brain

DIFFERENTIAL DIAGNOSIS

Hypoxic Ischemic Encephalopathy

- Central pattern of injury → ventrolateral thalamus & BG

Near Drowning

- History is generally definitive

Neurofibromatosis Type 1

- Signal abnormalities in globus pallidus (GP) are most common brain manifestation in children

Encephalitis

- Viral encephalitides can cause symmetric ↑ T2 of BG
- Acute disseminated encephalomyelitis can affect BG, mimic MELAS/myoclonic epilepsy with ragged red fibers (MERRF)

PATHOLOGY

General Features

- Genetics
  - Syndromes attributed to mutations in mtDNA
    - MELAS
    - KSS
    - LHON
    - MERRF
  - Syndromes attributed to mutations in nDNA
    - POLG-RD
      - Alpers-Huttenlocher syndrome
      - Myoclonic epilepsy, myopathy, sensory ataxia (MEMSA)
      - Ataxia neuropathy spectrum (ANS)
    - Mitochondrial neurogastrointestinal encephalomyopathy (MNGIE)
    - Coenzyme Q10 (CoQ10) deficiency
  - LS → associated with mutations in > 60 genes, both mtDNA & nDNA
- Associated abnormalities
  - KSS → ophthalmoplegia, heart block, retinitis pigmentosa
  - Alpers → micronodular cirrhosis
- Broad phenotypic presentations are due to varied distribution of mitochondria throughout various cell types

CLINICAL ISSUES

Presentation

- Most common signs/symptoms
  - Psychomotor delay/regression, hypotonia
  - Stroke-like episodes, episodic paresis
  - Metabolic stressors (e.g., infection) may unmask disease or cause deterioration

Demographics

- Age: Majority have clinical symptoms in infancy
  - MELAS usually presents in teenagers
  - Age at onset & severity correlates with degree of enzyme deficit

DIAGNOSTIC CHECKLIST

Image Interpretation Pearls

- Think of MEs when encountering atypical presentation of stroke, severe encephalitis, or seizure
- Bilateral, speckled, hyperintense lesions on T2 & FLAIR MR = LS or PDH deficiency
- Bilateral GP lesions = toxin exposure, hypoxic-ischemic injury (HIE), or mitochondrial dysfunction
- Cerebellar atrophy is common feature in MEs

SELECTED REFERENCES

1. Gonçalves FG et al: Primary mitochondrial disorders of the pediatric central nervous system: neuroimaging findings. Radiographics. 40(7):2042-67, 2020
2. Alves CAPF et al: Neuroimaging of mitochondrial cytopathies. Top Magn Reson Imaging. 27(4):219-40, 2018
3. Finsterer J et al: Cerebral imaging in paediatric mitochondrial disorders. Neuroradiol J. 31(6):596-608, 2018

KEY FACTS

TERMINOLOGY

- Heritable disorders primarily impacting structure & function of white matter (WM) in CNS
- Recent classification is based upon component of WM that is impacted
  - Myelin & oligodendrocytes
    - Metachromatic leukodystrophy (MLD), X-linked adrenoleukodystrophy (ALD), Canavan disease
  - Astrocytes
    - Alexander disease (AD), megalencephalic leukodystrophy with subcortical cysts (MLC), vanishing WM (VWM), globoid cell leukodystrophy (GLD, Krabbe disease)
  - Neurons & axons
    - POLR3-related leukodystrophies, hypomyelination with atrophy of basal ganglia & cerebellum (H-ABC)

IMAGING

- ALD
  - Characteristic early involvement of parietal periventricular WM
  - Enhancement of zone of active inflammation
- MLD
  - Early sparing of subcortical U fibers & perivascular WM → tigroid appearance
- GLD
  - ↑ density on CT in basal ganglia
- AD
  - Enhancement of ventricular lining, periventricular rim, frontal WM, & more
- Canavan disease
  - Megalencephaly with ↑ signal in occipital WM early, progressing to entire brain
  - ↑ NAA on MRS
- MLC
  - Subcortical cysts in anterior temporal &/or frontal WM

(Left) *Axial T2 MR in a 3-year-old with Alexander disease shows bilateral & symmetric abnormal signal in the cerebral white matter (WM). The frontal predominance is characteristic of this leukodystrophy caused by accumulation of GFAP.* **(Right)** *Coronal T2 MR in a 9-year-old with metachromatic leukodystrophy shows abnormal hyperintense cerebral WM signal interrupted by speckled/linear regions of preserved signal ➡. The linear streaks of normal signal give rise to the phrase "tigroid demyelination."*

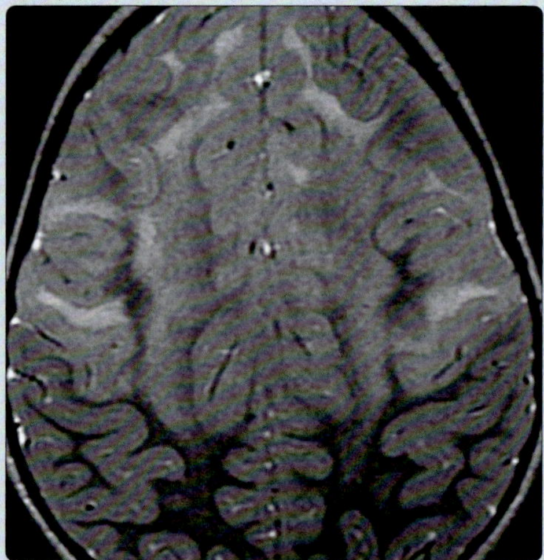

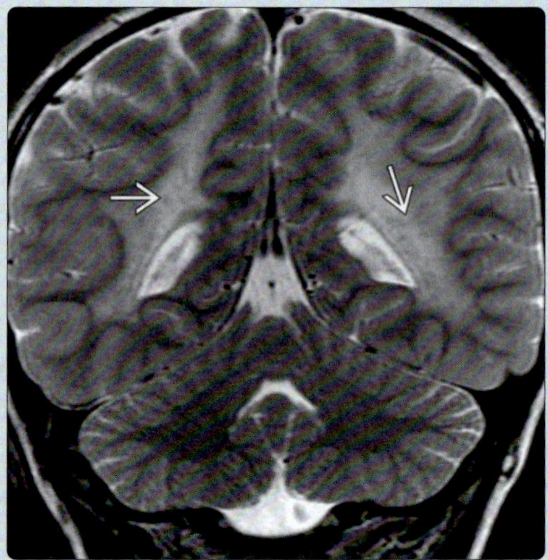

(Left) *Axial T2 MR in a 20-month-old with macrocephaly shows normal WM signal both proximal ➡ & distal ➡ to regions of myelin edema, confirming that this signal does not represent hypomyelination. This is MLC2B, a more benign phenotype of megalencephalic leukoencephalopathy caused by dominant mutations in the GLIALCAM gene.* **(Right)** *Axial NECT in a 9-year-old with vanishing WM shows marked hypoattenuation throughout the cerebral WM, caused by extensive myelin vacuolization & edema.*

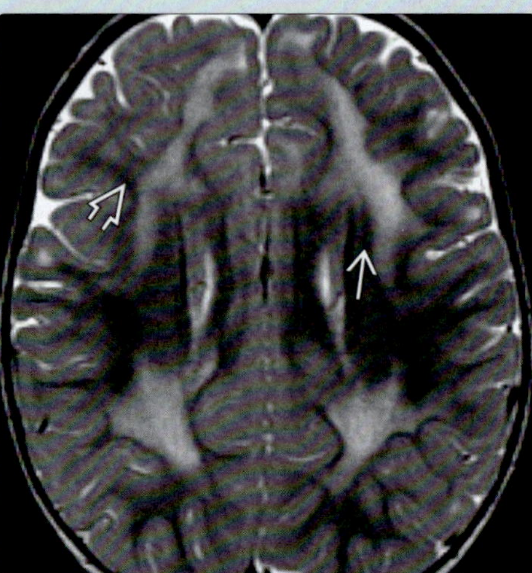

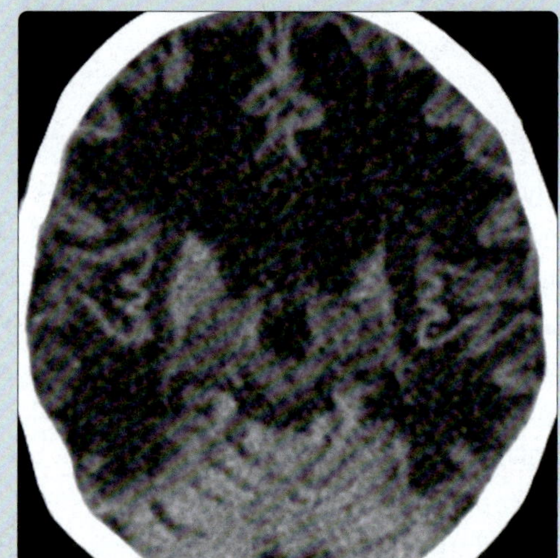

TERMINOLOGY

Definitions

- Heritable disorders primarily impacting structure & function of white matter (WM) in CNS

Classification

- Multiple classification schemes have been proposed
  - Based on clinical phenotype, imaging phenotype, pathologic phenotype, &/or cellular organelle affected
- Recent classification is based upon component of WM impacted
  - Myelin & oligodendrocytes
    - Metachromatic leukodystrophy (MLD), X-linked adrenoleukodystrophy (ALD), Canavan disease
  - Astrocytes
    - Alexander disease (AD), megalencephalic leukodystrophy with subcortical cysts (MLC), vanishing WM (VWM), globoid cell leukodystrophy (GLD, Krabbe disease)
  - Neurons & axons
    - POLR3-related leukodystrophies, hypomyelination with atrophy of basal ganglia & cerebellum (H-ABC)

IMAGING

General Features

- Location
  - Some leukodystrophies have characteristic distributions, especially early in disease course
- ALD
  - Characteristic early involvement of parietal periventricular WM
  - Enhancement of zone of active inflammation
- MLD
  - ↑ signal in hemispheric WM on T2
  - Early sparing of subcortical U-fibers & perivascular WM
- GLD
  - ↑ density on CT in basal ganglia
- AD
  - Megalencephaly with ↑ signal in frontal WM, thalami, & brainstem structures on T2
  - Enhancement of ventricular lining, periventricular rim, frontal WM, & more
- Canavan disease
  - Megalencephaly with ↑ signal in occipital WM early, progressing to entire brain
  - ↑ NAA on MRS
- VWM
  - Diffuse ↑ WM signal on T2, ↓ on T1
- MLC
  - Megalencephaly with swelling & ↑ signal in cerebral > cerebellar WM
  - Subcortical cysts in anterior temporal &/or frontal WM
- POLR3
  - Hypomyelination & cerebellar atrophy

DIFFERENTIAL DIAGNOSIS

Periventricular Leukomalacia

- Static injury to periventricular WM in immature brain

Multiple Sclerosis

- Autoimmune demyelination

Anti-MOG Antibody Disease

- Autoimmune myelin inflammation & injury

PATHOLOGY

General Features

- Etiology
  - ALD: Absent/deficient peroxisomal enzyme acyl-CoA synthetase → accumulation of very long-chain fatty acids (VLCFA)
    - Mechanism by which VLCFA induces demyelination is still undetermined
  - MLD: Absent/deficient lysosomal enzyme arylsulfatase A → accumulation of sulfatide
    - Sulfatide accumulation triggers inflammation & demyelination
  - Canavan: Absence/deficiency of aspartoacylase → accumulation of NAA
  - Alexander: Mutations in gene for glial fibrillary acidic protein → excess GFAP
    - GFAP aggregates in Rosenthal fibers in astrocytes, prevent myelination
  - MLC: Mutations in genes encoding for astrocytic proteins *MLC1* or *GLIALCAM* genes
    - Normal myelin volumes with excessive vacuolization
  - GLD: Absent/deficient lysosomal enzyme galactosylceramidase I → accumulation of psychosine & cerebroside
    - Psychosine induces astrocytic apoptosis, secondarily causing demyelination
  - VWM: Defects in eukaryotic initiation factor 2B (eIF2B) → episodic WM cavitation after febrile infections or minor head trauma
    - Global protein synthesis regulated by eIF2B → abnormal cellular stress response
  - POLR3: Mutations in genes *POLR3A*, *POLR3B*, &/or *POLR1C* encoding for components of RNA polymerase III
    - Impacts function of oligodendrocyte, astrocyte, neuron, & microglia

SELECTED REFERENCES

1. Mallack EJ et al: MRI surveillance of boys with X-linked adrenoleukodystrophy identified by newborn screening: meta-analysis and consensus guidelines. J Inherit Metab Dis. 44(3):728-39, 2021
2. Yazbeck E et al: Progressive leukodystrophy-like demyelinating syndromes with MOG-antibodies in children: a rare under-recognized phenotype. Neuropediatrics. 52(4):337-40, 2021
3. Perrier S et al: Expanding the phenotypic and molecular spectrum of RNA polymerase III-related leukodystrophy. Neurol Genet. 6(3):e425, 2020
4. Soderholm HE et al: Elevated leukodystrophy incidence predicted from genomics databases. Pediatr Neurol. 111:66-9, 2020
5. van der Knaap MS et al: Diagnosis, prognosis, and treatment of leukodystrophies. Lancet Neurol. 18(10):962-72, 2019
6. van der Knaap MS et al: Leukodystrophies: a proposed classification system based on pathological changes and pathogenetic mechanisms. Acta Neuropathol. 134(3):351-82, 2017
7. Bugiani M et al: Defective glial maturation in vanishing white matter disease. J Neuropathol Exp Neurol. 70(1):69-82, 2011

KEY FACTS

TERMINOLOGY

- TORCH/TORCHES: Acronym for congenital infections caused by transplacental transmission of pathogens
  - **T**oxoplasmosis (toxo) → *Toxoplasma gondii*
  - **O**ther (Zika → Zika virus)
  - **R**ubella → rubella virus
  - **C**ytomegalovirus (CMV) → most common TORCH infection
  - **He**rpes → herpes simplex virus 2 (HSV-2)
  - Human immunodeficiency virus (HIV)
  - **S**yphilis → *Treponema pallidum*

IMAGING

- Toxo, CMV, HIV, Zika, & rubella all cause parenchymal Ca^{2+}
- CMV causes migrational defects, white matter gliosis/hypomyelination, & cystic foci in temporal poles
- Rubella, Zika, & HSV cause lobar destruction/encephalomalacia
- ± microcephaly (not unique to Zika virus)

PATHOLOGY

- CMV
  - Ubiquitous DNA virus of herpesvirus family
- Zika
  - Arbovirus of flavivirus family
- Herpes encephalitis
  - 75-90% of congenital herpes encephalitis
  - Most commonly from transmission during delivery
  - Transplacental infection can be from HSV-1 or HSV-2
- Toxoplasmosis
  - Active infection in pregnancy → 20-50% congenital infection
- HIV
  - 30% of pregnancies in HIV(+) women will result in transmission unless preventative measures are taken

DIAGNOSTIC CHECKLIST

- CMV is most frequently encountered TORCH infection in USA

(Left) *Axial NECT shows extensive periventricular Ca^{2+} in this 2-day-old, 32-weeks-premature infant with microcephaly, caused by in utero CMV infection.* **(Right)** *Axial T2 MR in a 14-year-old with seizures & developmental delay shows subcortical temporal lobe cysts ➡. In combination with gliotic white matter lesions, such cysts are highly suggestive of congenital CMV.*

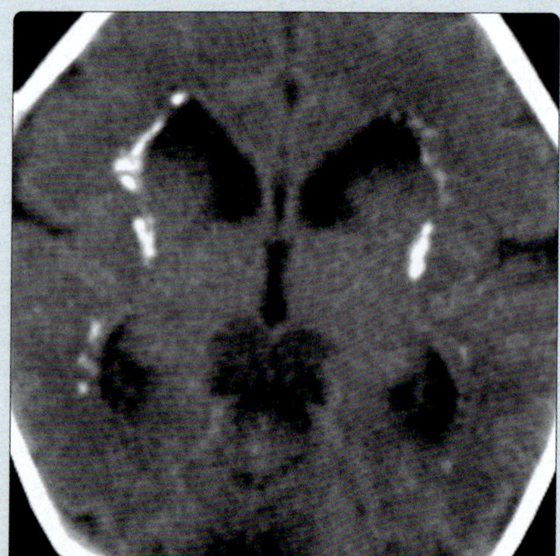

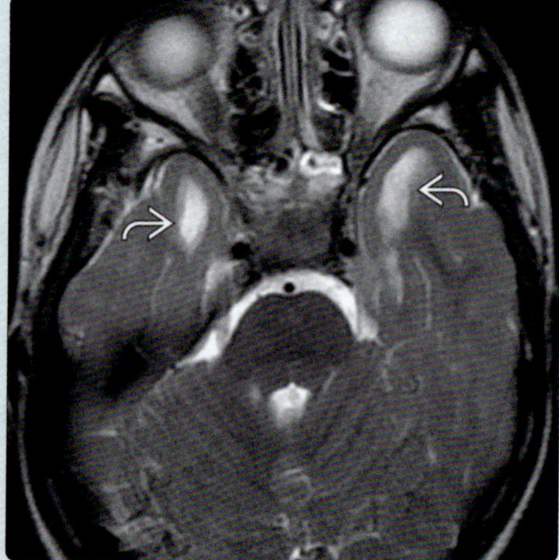

(Left) *Axial NECT in an infant with in utero Zika virus infection shows periventricular & subcortical Ca^{2+} with marked volume loss, resulting in microcephaly (despite the presence of ventriculomegaly). (Courtesy T. Fazecas, MD.)* **(Right)** *Axial NECT shows a focal parenchymal hemorrhage ➡ in a region of occipital pole cerebritis in this 3-week-old with disseminated herpes simplex virus (HSV) & lethargy. HSV acquired during delivery typically presents at 3-15 days.*

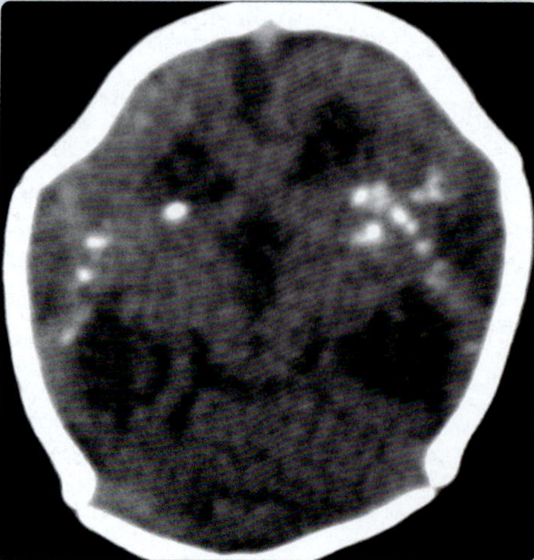

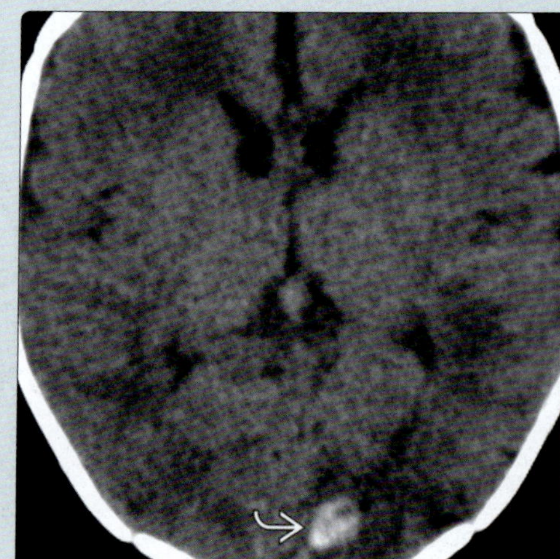

TERMINOLOGY

Synonyms

- Congenital infections, intrauterine infection, TORCHES

Definitions

- Acronym for congenital infections caused by transplacental transmission of pathogens
  - **T**oxoplasmosis (toxo) → *Toxoplasma gondii*
  - **O**ther (Zika → Zika virus)
  - **R**ubella → rubella virus
  - **C**ytomegalovirus (CMV) → most common TORCH infection
  - **He**rpes → herpes simplex virus 2 (HSV-2)
  - Human immunodeficiency virus (HIV)
  - **S**yphilis → *Treponema pallidum*

IMAGING

General Features

- Toxo, CMV, HIV, Zika, & rubella all cause parenchymal Ca^{2+}
  - Toxo Ca^{2+} is typically less extensive than CMV
  - HIV causes basal ganglia & frontal subcortical Ca^{2+}
- CMV causes migrational defects, white matter (WM) gliosis/hypomyelination, & cystic foci in temporal poles
- Rubella, Zika, & HSV cause lobar destruction/encephalomalacia; HSV is often hemorrhagic
- Syphilis causes basilar meningitis
- Unless complicated by hydrocephalus, volume loss caused by TORCH infections typically results in microcephaly
  - Zika is not unique in this regard
- Zika is also associated with macular atrophy

Imaging Recommendations

- Best imaging tool
  - MR brain to completely characterize abnormalities
  - CT is of benefit in confirming Ca^{2+}

DIFFERENTIAL DIAGNOSIS

Tuberous Sclerosis

- Subependymal Ca^{2+} is characteristic

Neurocysticercosis

- Most common cause of cerebral Ca^{2+} < 30 years of age

Chronic Venous Ischemia

- From arteriovenous fistula or venous malformation
- Subcortical Ca^{2+} with volume loss

Congenital Lymphocytic Choriomeningitis

- Produces necrotizing ependymitis, leading to aqueductal obstruction; macrocephaly (43%) > microcephaly (13%)
- NECT may perfectly mimic CMV

Pseudo-TORCH Syndromes

- Baraister-Reardon, Aicardi-Goutieres (CSF pleocytosis, ↑ CSF α-interferon)
  - Basal ganglia Ca^{2+}, ± periventricular Ca^{2+}

Megalencephalic Leukoencephalopathy With Subcortical Cysts

- Leukodystrophy with subcortical cysts in temporal lobes is similar to those seen in CMV

PATHOLOGY

General Features

- Etiology
  - CMV
    - Ubiquitous DNA virus of herpesvirus family
    - CMV is most common cause of intrauterine infection
  - Zika
    - Arbovirus of flavivirus family
    - Most commonly spread by *Aedes aegypti* mosquito
  - Herpes encephalitis
    - Active HSV-2 genital infection during delivery can pass directly to child
      - 75-90% of congenital herpes encephalitis
    - Transplacental infection can be from HSV-1 or HSV-2
  - Rubella
    - Togaviridae family of viruses
  - Toxoplasmosis
    - Active infection in pregnancy → 20-50% risk of congenital infection
  - HIV
    - 30% of pregnancies in HIV(+) women will result in transmission unless preventative measures are taken
  - Syphilis
    - Transplacental transmission from mother with primary or secondary syphilis

CLINICAL ISSUES

Presentation

- Most common signs/symptoms
  - CMV can present at birth (10%) with microcephaly, hepatosplenomegaly, petechial rash
    - 55% with systemic disease have CNS involvement
  - Congenital toxoplasmosis is usually inapparent at birth, presenting at 2-3 months
  - HSV acquired during delivery typically presents at 3-15 days with seizures, lethargy
    - HSV acquired in utero (5%) typically presents at birth
  - Zika is typically apparent at birth due to microcephaly

DIAGNOSTIC CHECKLIST

Image Interpretation Pearls

- Consider congenital CMV encephalitis when MR shows
  - Microcephaly & cerebellar hypoplasia
  - Cortical gyral abnormalities or schizencephaly with Ca^{2+}
  - WM gliosis & subcortical temporal cysts
- Zika virus causes brain destruction & dysmorphism in addition to microcephaly with Ca^{2+}

SELECTED REFERENCES

1. Buca D et al: Outcome of fetuses with congenital cytomegalovirus infection and normal ultrasound at diagnosis: systematic review and meta-analysis. Ultrasound Obstet Gynecol. 57(4):551-9, 2021
2. Levine D et al: How does imaging of congenital Zika compare with imaging of other TORCH infections? Radiology. 285(3):744-61, 2017

Brain Abscess

KEY FACTS

TERMINOLOGY

- Focal pyogenic infection of brain parenchyma

IMAGING

- Varies with stage of abscess development
- Early cerebritis: Ill-defined, hypodense (CT)/hyperintense (T2 MR) subcortical lesion with mass effect & patchy enhancement
- Late cerebritis: T2-hypointense rim (MR) with irregular, peripheral rim enhancement (CT/MR)
- Early capsule: T2-hypointense rim (MR) with well-defined, thin, enhancing wall (CT/MR)
- Late capsule: Cavity shrinks, edema & mass effect diminish, capsule thickens (CT/MR)
- DWI MR: Restricted diffusion in cerebritis & abscess

TOP DIFFERENTIAL DIAGNOSES

- Resolving hematoma
- Pilocytic astrocytoma
- Demyelinating disease

PATHOLOGY

- Early cerebritis (3-5 days)
  - Unencapsulated mass of leukocytes & edema
- Late cerebritis (4-5 days up to 2 weeks)
  - Necrotic foci coalesce
- Early capsule (begins ~ 2 weeks)
  - Well-delineated, collagenous capsule
- Late capsule (weeks to months)
  - Central cavity shrinks

CLINICAL ISSUES

- 25% occur in patients < 15 years
- Headache is most common symptom (up to 90%)
  - Fever in only 50%

DIAGNOSTIC CHECKLIST

- Search for local cause, such as sinusitis, mastoiditis

(Left) *Axial MR DWI in a teenager with a headache shows characteristic diffusion restriction in multiple intraparenchymal abscesses. Diffusion restriction layering in the left occipital horn ➡ reflects ventriculitis due to the intraventricular extension of a periventricular abscess, substantially increasing morbidity.* **(Right)** *Axial MR SWI in the same patient shows hemorrhage into an abscess in the left globus pallidus. Hemorrhagic changes in the walls of pyogenic abscesses are more frequently seen with SWI.*

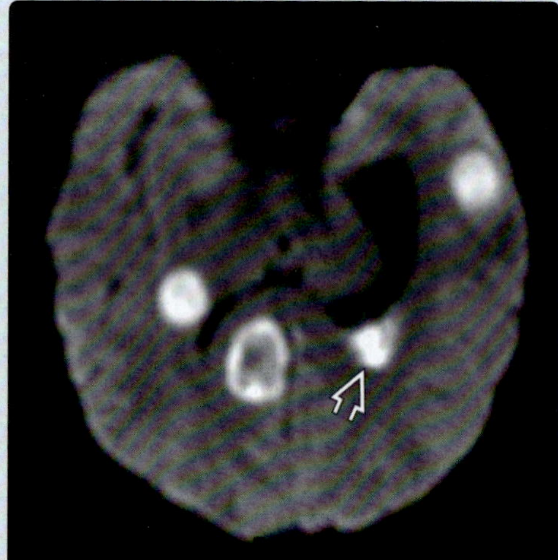

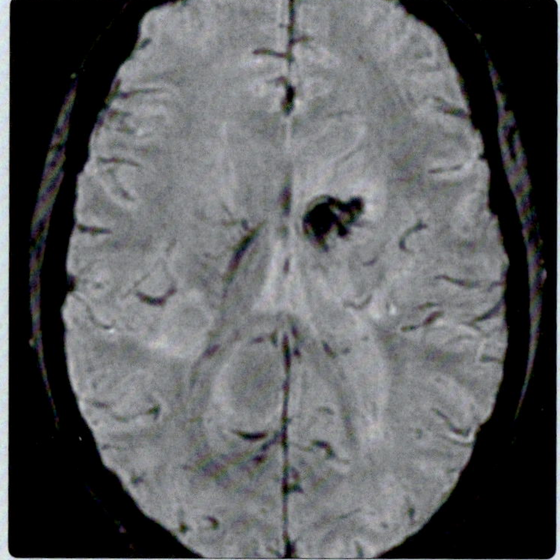

(Left) *Axial CECT in a 5-year-old with fever & COVID-19 positive serology who developed right-sided weakness shows a large left subdural empyema ➡ & right frontal lobe abscess ➡ as a complication of bacterial sinusitis.* **(Right)** *Axial T2 MR in a previously healthy teenager with fever & altered mental status shows multiple clusters of abscesses in the frontal & occipital lobes + the splenium of the corpus callosum. The dark signal in the abscess walls ➡ is thought to reflect the presence of free radicals.*

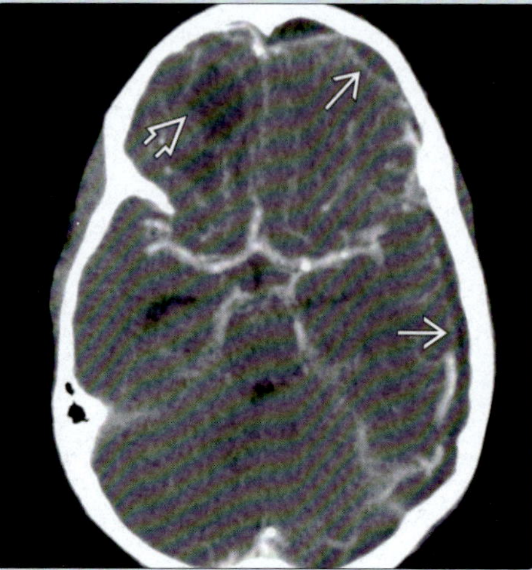

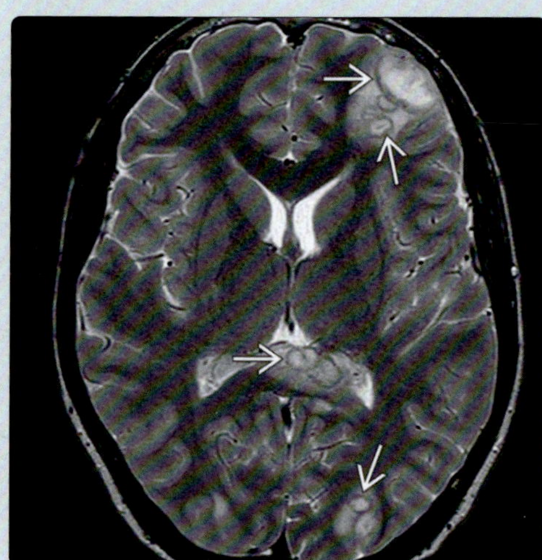

TERMINOLOGY

Definitions

- Focal pyogenic infection of brain parenchyma
  - Typically bacterial; fungal or parasitic is less common

IMAGING

General Features

- Best diagnostic clue
  - Ring-enhancing lesion
  - T2-hypointense rim on MR with surrounding edema
  - High signal (restricted diffusion) on DWI MR with low ADC
- Location
  - Supratentorial > > infratentorial
    - Frontal & parietal lobes are most common

CT Findings

- Early cerebritis: Ill-defined, hypodense subcortical lesion with mass effect
- Late cerebritis: Irregular, peripheral rim enhancement
- Early capsule: Thin, distinct, enhancing capsule
  - Capsule is thickest near cortex
- Late capsule: Cavity shrinks, capsule thickens

MR Findings

- Early cerebritis: Ill-defined, T2-hyperintense mass with patchy enhancement
- Late cerebritis: Hypointense rim on T2; intense but irregular rim enhancement
- Early capsule: Hypointense rim on T2; well-defined, enhancing, thin wall
- Late capsule: Edema & mass effect ↓; ↑ of thick wall
- Restricted diffusion in cerebritis & abscess
  - Markedly ↓ signal centrally on ADC map
- Central necrotic area may show presence of acetate, lactate, alanine, succinate, pyruvate on MRS

Imaging Recommendations

- Best imaging tool
  - Contrast-enhanced MR + DWI

DIFFERENTIAL DIAGNOSIS

Resolving Hematoma

- Rim enhancement starts ~ 7 days after event

Pilocytic Astrocytoma

- Cyst with enhancing mural nodule
- Low signal of cyst contents on DWI

Demyelinating Disease

- Multiple sclerosis, acute disseminated encephalomyelopathy
- May have incomplete rim enhancement
- Characteristic lesions elsewhere in brain

Aging Infarction

- Enhancement at periphery of subacute to chronic infarction may mimic abscess

PATHOLOGY

General Features

- Etiology
  - Hematogenous from extracranial location
  - Extension from sinus infection via valveless emissary veins
  - Direct extension from calvarial or meningeal infection
  - Right-to-left shunts (congenital cardiac malformations, pulmonary arteriovenous fistulas)
  - 20-30% have no identifiable source → cryptogenic
  - Often polymicrobial → streptococci, staphylococci, anaerobes

Staging, Grading, & Classification

- Early cerebritis (3-5 days)
  - Unencapsulated mass of leukocytes & edema
- Late cerebritis (4-5 days up to 2 weeks)
  - Necrotic foci coalesce
- Early capsule (begins at ~ 2 weeks)
  - Well-delineated, collagenous capsule
  - Liquefied necrotic core
- Late capsule (weeks to months)
  - Central cavity shrinks

CLINICAL ISSUES

Presentation

- Headache is most common symptom (up to 90%)
  - Fever in only 50%

Demographics

- 25% occur in patients < 15 years

Natural History & Prognosis

- Complications of inadequately or untreated abscesses
  - Intraventricular rupture, ventriculitis (may be fatal)
  - Meningitis, daughter lesions
  - Mass effect, herniation
- Mortality is variable, 0-30%

Treatment

- Antibiotics only, if small (< 2.5 cm) or early cerebritis
- Steroids to treat edema & mass effect
- Surgical drainage or excision may be required
- Drainage of adjacent source (e.g., infected paranasal sinuses, mastoids)

DIAGNOSTIC CHECKLIST

Image Interpretation Pearls

- Search for local cause, such as sinusitis, mastoiditis
- T2-hypointense abscess rim resolves before enhancement in successfully treated patients

SELECTED REFERENCES

1. Antkowiak Ł et al: Clinical features, microbiology, and management of pediatric brainstem abscess. Childs Nerv Syst. 36(12):2919-26, 2020
2. Lai PH et al: Susceptibility-weighted imaging provides complementary value to diffusion-weighted imaging in the differentiation between pyogenic brain abscesses, necrotic glioblastomas, and necrotic metastatic brain tumors. Eur J Radiol. 117:56-61, 2019
3. Mameli C et al: Brain abscess in pediatric age: a review. Childs Nerv Syst. 35(7):1117-28, 2019

Acute Encephalitis

KEY FACTS

TERMINOLOGY

- Acute brain inflammation caused by infectious agents, most commonly viruses
- Noninfectious (autoimmune) brain inflammation

IMAGING

- Most viral encephalitides have wide ranging, nonspecific imaging findings
  - Poorly defined white matter signal abnormalities
  - Bilateral, symmetric basal ganglia &/or thalamic signal abnormalities
  - Minimal leptomeningeal enhancement
- Focal splenium signal abnormality
  - Influenza & other viral encephalitides
- Symmetric thalamic & basal ganglia necrosis
  - Acute necrotizing encephalitis of childhood (ANEC)
- Abnormal cranial nerve enhancement (neuritis)
  - COVID-19

TOP DIFFERENTIAL DIAGNOSES

- Acute ischemia
- Gliomatosis cerebri
- Status epilepticus
- Mitochondrial encephalopathy

PATHOLOGY

- Herpesviruses include HSV1, HSV2, CMV, EBV, VZV, B virus, HSV6, HSV7
- Arboviruses transmitted by mosquitoes & ticks
  - Include Eastern & Western equine encephalitis, West Nile, Zika, St. Louis encephalitis, Lacrosse encephalitis, California encephalitis

CLINICAL ISSUES

- Presentation varies widely: Slight meningeal to severe encephalitic symptoms, ± fever, prodrome
- Rapid diagnosis & early treatment with antiviral or antibacterial agents can ↓ mortality, may improve outcome

(Left) *Axial T1 C+ FS MR in 9-year-old with left-sided weakness shows a right cerebral lesion with cortical enhancement ➔ & hemorrhagic necrosis due to COVID-19-associated vasculitis & infarction.* **(Right)** *Axial DWI MR in a 12-year-old with seizures shows abnormal signal & swelling of the right insular cortex ➔ due to GAD65 autoimmune encephalitis. GAD65 antibody is a biomarker of CNS & nonneurological autoimmune diseases.*

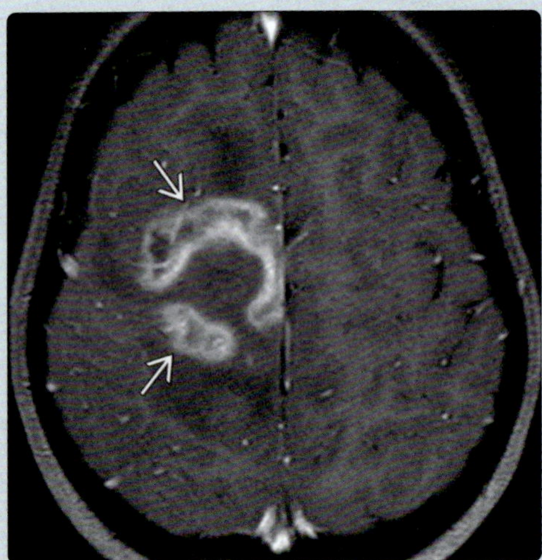

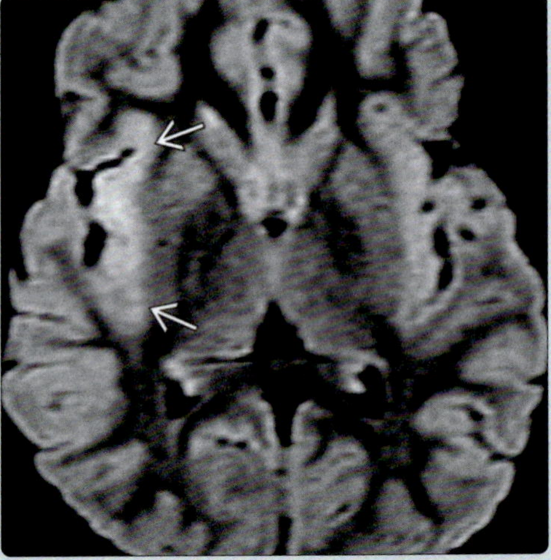

(Left) *Axial T1 C+ FS MR in a teenager presenting with nausea, headache, fever, & somnolence shows abnormal leptomeningeal enhancement in the frontal & parietal sulci ➔. Serology was positive for West Nile virus.* **(Right)** *Axial DWI MR in a 14-year-old with seizures after 1 week of cough & fever shows restricted diffusion in the splenium of the corpus callosum ➔ due to influenza encephalitis.*

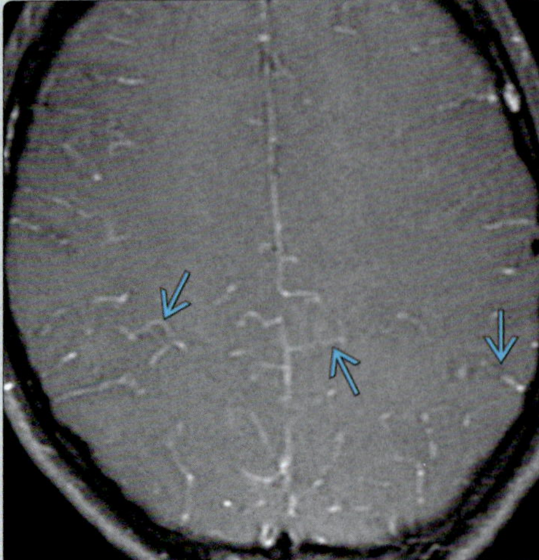

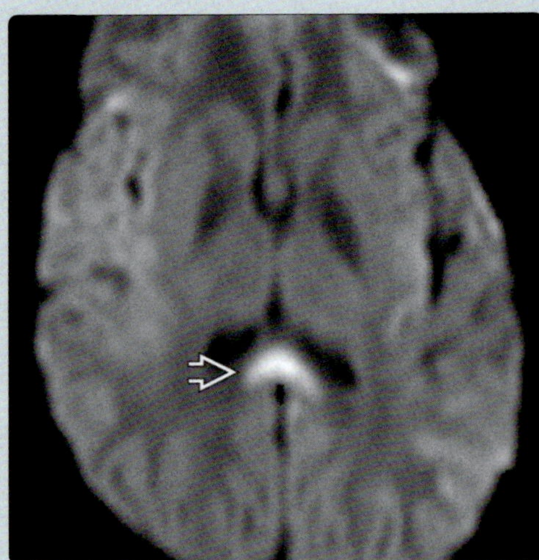

TERMINOLOGY

Definitions

- Acute brain inflammation caused by infectious agents, most commonly viruses
- Noninfectious (autoimmune) brain inflammation

IMAGING

General Features

- Most viral encephalitides have wide ranging, nonspecific imaging findings
  - West Nile, St. Louis, LaCrosse, California, Eastern equine
    - Poorly defined signal abnormalities in white matter
    - Bilateral, symmetric basal ganglia or thalamic signal abnormalities
      - ± diffusion restriction
    - Little or no parenchymal enhancement
    - Minimal leptomeningeal enhancement
- Some pathogens have characteristic imaging features
  - COVID-19
    - Abnormal cranial nerve enhancement (neuritis)
    - Vasculitic/thrombotic pattern with ischemic lesions
  - Herpetic encephalitis (HSV1) reactivation pattern
    - Temporal & subfrontal involvement, typically spares basal ganglia with early hemorrhagic conversion
      - Characteristic in adults
    - Majority of children with HSV1 encephalitis do not follow this pattern but have multilobar distribution instead
  - Rocky Mountain spotted fever (RMSF)
    - Multiple punctate foci of diffusion restriction in cerebral white matter
    - Minimal or no enhancement
  - Some features are associated with variety of pathogens
    - Focal splenium signal abnormality
      - Ovoid focus of diffusion restriction in splenium of corpus callosum
      - Associated with influenza & other viral encephalitides
      - Reported in COVID-19 infection
    - Acute necrotizing encephalitis of childhood (ANEC)
      - Symmetric thalamic & basal ganglia necrosis

Imaging Recommendations

- Best imaging tool
  - MR with FLAIR, DWI, & contrast is most sensitive
    - SWI or GRE to detect hemorrhage

DIFFERENTIAL DIAGNOSIS

Acute Ischemia

- Cytotoxic edema in typical vascular distribution; DWI positive

Gliomatosis Cerebri

- Lobar or hemispheric infiltration & expansion with subacute onset

Status Epilepticus

- Hyperintense on T2/FLAIR MR ± diffusion restriction

Mitochondrial Encephalopathy

- Symmetric basal ganglia or thalamic involvement common

PATHOLOGY

General Features

- Etiology
  - Herpesviruses include HSV1, HSV2, CMV, EBV, VZV, B virus, HSV6, HSV7
    - HSV2 is major cause of neonatal encephalitis
  - Arboviruses are transmitted by mosquitoes & ticks
    - Include Eastern & Western equine encephalitis, West Nile, Zika, St. Louis encephalitis, Lacrosse encephalitis, California encephalitis
  - Enteroviruses include Coxsackie viruses A & B, poliovirus, echoviruses, enteroviruses 68 to 71

Microscopic Features

- Infiltration by polymorphonuclear cells, lymphocytes, plasma cells, & mononuclear cells
- May see inclusion bodies (i.e., Negri bodies in rabies)

CLINICAL ISSUES

Presentation

- Most common signs/symptoms
  - Varies widely: Slight meningeal to severe encephalitic symptoms; ± fever, prodrome
  - Varicella & herpes zoster: Different clinical manifestations of infection by same virus (VZV)
    - Varicella encephalitis: Fever, headache, vomiting, seizures, altered mental status days to weeks after onset of (chicken pox) rash
    - Zoster: Immunocompetent patient with cranial nerve & peripheral nerve palsies in dermatomes involved by skin lesions
  - EV71
    - Hand, foot, & mouth disease: Fever, vesicles on hands, feet, elbows, knees, lips

Demographics

- Epidemiology
  - Herpes: Most common cause of sporadic (nonepidemic) viral encephalitis
  - Japanese encephalitis: Most common endemic encephalitis in Asia

Natural History & Prognosis

- Many encephalitides have high morbidity, mortality
- Rapid diagnosis & early treatment with antiviral or antibacterial agents can ↓ mortality, may improve outcome

SELECTED REFERENCES

1. Lindan CE et al: Neuroimaging manifestations in children with SARS-CoV-2 infection: a multinational, multicentre collaborative study. Lancet Child Adolesc Health. 5(3):167-77, 2020
2. Starkey J et al: Cytotoxic lesions of the corpus callosum that show restricted diffusion: mechanisms, causes, and manifestations. Radiographics. 37(2):562-76, 2017
3. Gagnon MM et al: Limbic encephalitis associated with GAD65 antibodies: brief review of the relevant literature. Can J Neurol Sci. 43(4):486-93, 2016
4. Bajaj M et al: Clinical and neuroimaging findings in neonatal herpes simplex virus infection. J Pediatr. 165(2):404-7.e1, 2014
5. Crapp S et al: Rocky Mountain spotted fever: 'starry sky' appearance with diffusion-weighted imaging in a child. Pediatr Radiol. 42(4):499-502, 2011

KEY FACTS

DIAGNOSTIC CHECKLIST

- Multiple sclerosis (MS)
  - Demyelinating disease characterized by multiple lesions disseminated in time & space
  - Brain lesions: Multiple T2- & FLAIR MR hyperintense foci, typically small (5-10 mm), ovoid, discrete, periventricular, & perpendicular to ventricular margins
  - Optic neuritis (ON): Unilateral, short segment, intraorbital; myelitis: < 2 vertebrae in length, < 50% of cross-sectional area, typically peripheral
- Acute disseminated encephalomyelitis (ADEM)
  - Acute demyelinating disease with encephalopathy, without NMOSD or anti-MOG associated antibodies
  - Characteristically arises subsequent to infection (viral respiratory) or vaccination
  - Brain: Ill-defined, larger T2-/FLAIR hyperintense lesions
- Neuromyelitis optica spectrum disorders (NMOSD)
  - Inflammatory CNS disease caused by antibodies to aquaporin-4 (AQP-4) on astrocytic end feet
  - ON & transverse myelitis predominate clinically
  - Brain: Commonly periventricular but parallel to ependymal lining; area postrema involvement is classic
  - ON: Bilateral, posterior predominant (including chiasm)
  - Myelitis: Longitudinally extensive transverse myelitis (LETM) (> 3 vertebrae), > 50% of cord cross section, central
- Anti-MOG syndromes
  - Acute demyelinating disease caused by antibodies to myelin oligodendrocyte glycoprotein (MOG)
  - Extensive clinical overlap with ADEM & NMOSD; encephalopathy in younger patients, ON in older
  - Brain: Similar to ADEM
  - ON: Bilateral anterior predominant (including optic disc) with perineural enhancement
  - Myelitis: LETM vs. short segment; conus involvement
- Lyme disease
  - May be accompanied by ON or other CN inflammation

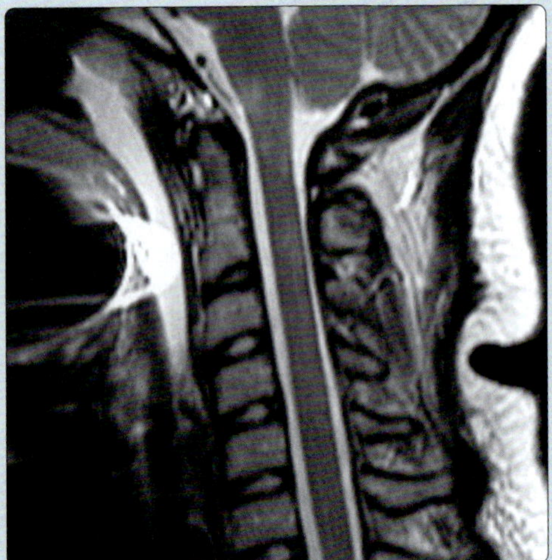

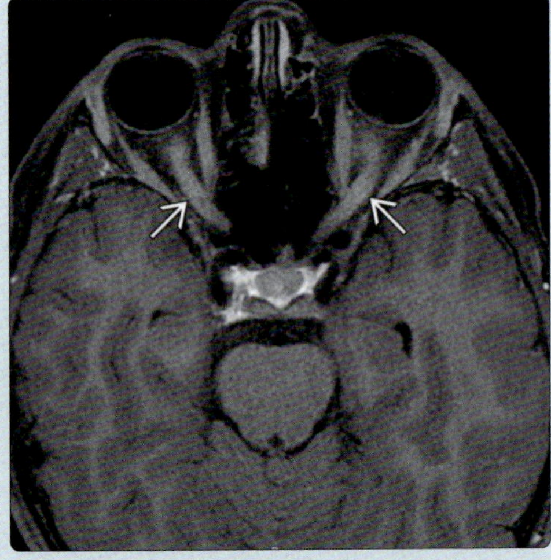

(Left) *Sagittal T2 MR in a 9-year-old with optic neuritis shows multiple ill-defined hyperintensities in the medulla & cervical cord. Subsequent serum testing revealed antibodies to aquaporin 4, confirming a diagnosis of neuromyelitis optica spectrum disorders (NMOSD).* **(Right)** *Axial T1 C+ FS MR through the orbits shows diffuse bilateral optic nerve enhancement ➡ in this 9-year-old with vision loss. Clinical features were suggestive of NMOSD, but CSF analysis confirmed anti-myelin oligodendrocyte glycoprotein (MOG) disease.*

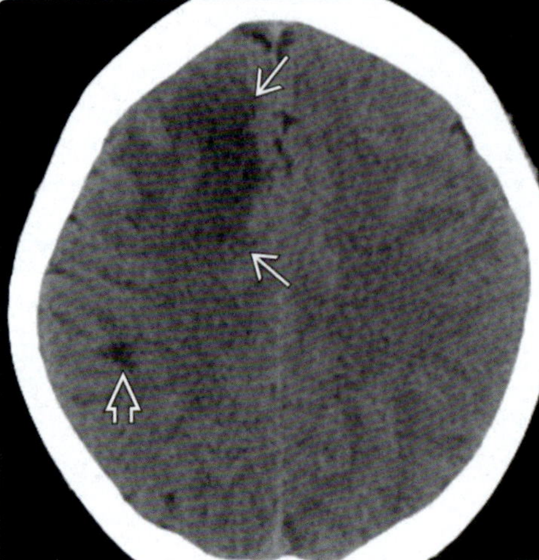

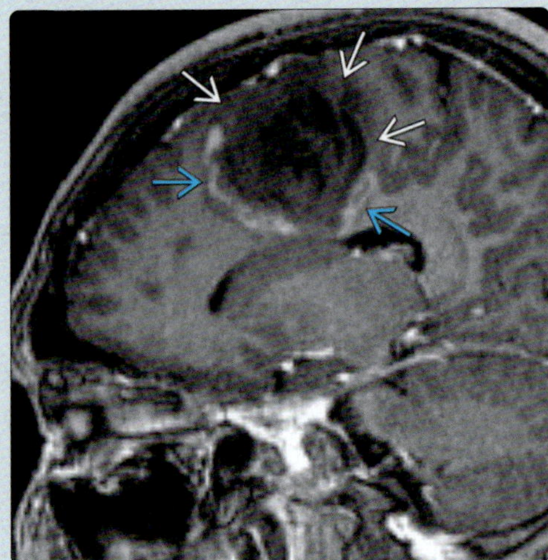

(Left) *Axial NECT in a 16-year-old with progressive left-sided weakness after minor trauma shows a large, low-attenuation white matter lesion in the anterior right frontal lobe ➡ & a smaller one near the right motor strip ➡.* **(Right)** *Sagittal T1 C+ MR in the same patient shows the borders of the large lesion nearest to the cortex to be nonenhancing ➡ as compared to the other margins ➡. This open ring appearance can help distinguish tumefactive MS from abscess or neoplasm (which more typically have complete ring enhancement).*

TERMINOLOGY

Definitions

- Acquired demyelinating processes characterized by inflammation
  - Multiple sclerosis (MS)
    - Demyelinating disease characterized by multiple lesions disseminated in time & space
  - Acute disseminated encephalomyelitis (ADEM)
    - Acute demyelinating disease with encephalopathy, without NMOSD or anti-MOG-associated antibodies
  - Neuromyelitis optica spectrum disorders (NMOSD)
    - Inflammatory CNS disease caused by antibodies to aquaporin-4 (AQP-4) on astrocytic end feet
    - Clinically characterized by optic neuritis & transverse myelitis
  - Antimyelin oligodendrocyte glycoprotein (MOG) syndromes
    - Acute demyelinating disease caused by antibodies to MOG
    - Extensive clinical overlap with ADEM & NMOSD
  - Lyme disease
    - CNS inflammation associated with *Borrelia burgdorferi* infection

IMAGING

General Features

- MS
  - Brain: Multiple T2- & FLAIR MR hyperintense lesions, typically small (5-10 mm), ovoid, discrete
    - > 85% are periventricular: Callosal involvement, hemispheric white matter; perpendicular to ventricle margin in perivenular distribution
    - Variable enhancement: Presumed to reflect active demyelination
      - Can be mass-like: Tumefactive MS
    - "Black holes" (due to axonal destruction) on T1 are much more likely to be seen in MS than ADEM
  - Optic neuritis (ON): Unilateral, short length, intraorbital
  - Myelitis: < 2 vertebral lengths, < 50% of cord cross section, cervical > thoracic
- ADEM
  - Brain: Ill-defined larger T2-/FLAIR hyperintense lesions
    - Lesions are more likely to be diffuse & bilateral
    - Frequent brainstem & thalamic involvement
  - ON: Less common; myelitis: Less common
- NMOSD
  - Brain: May have extensive lesions
    - Commonly periventricular but parallel
    - Dorsal brainstem (especially area postrema)
  - ON: Bilateral long segment
    - Posterior predominant, including chiasm
  - Myelitis: Longitudinally extensive transverse myelitis (LETM) (> 3 segments), typically central & > 50% circumference
- Anti-MOG syndromes
  - Brain: Similar in appearance to ADEM
    - Much less likely to involve corpus callosum
  - ON: Bilateral long length with perineural enhancement
    - Anterior predominant, including optic disc
  - Myelitis: LETM vs. short segment; conus often affected
- Lyme disease
  - May be accompanied by ON or other cranial nerve inflammation; Bell palsy is characteristic

DIFFERENTIAL DIAGNOSIS

Posterior Reversible Encephalopathy Syndrome

- Subcortical vasogenic edema associated with hypertension

Viral Encephalitis

- Widely variable, but often affects white matter & deep gray nuclei

Autoimmune-Mediated Vasculitis

- Reported in COVID-19 infection

Leukodystrophies

- Patterns vary by metabolic defect

Toxin-Induced Brain Injury

- Carbon monoxide or methanol poisoning

PATHOLOGY

General Features

- Etiology
  - MS
    - Activated T cells attack myelinated axons
    - B cells, antibodies, macrophages, & microglia all contribute to lesions
  - ADEM
    - Characteristically arises subsequent to infection (viral respiratory) or vaccination
  - NMOSD
    - Antibodies to aquaporin-4 (AQP-4) channels on astrocytic end feet
    - AQP-4 is dispersed throughout CNS
      - Highly expressed in optic nerves & spinal cord
  - Anti-MOG syndromes: Antibodies to MOG

CLINICAL ISSUES

Natural History & Prognosis

- MS: 45% of MS patients are not severely affected & are nearly normal
  - > 80% with "probable" MS & positive MR progress to clinically definite MS
- ADEM: Characteristically monophasic
  - Recurrence suggests anti-MOG
- Anti-MOG syndromes are more frequently seen in young
  - Encephalopathy is more common in younger patients, ON in older
- > 90% of NMOSD in pediatrics have relapsing disease
- Lyme disease: 11% develop neurologic manifestations

SELECTED REFERENCES

1. Chhabda S et al: Relapsing demyelinating syndromes in children: a practical review of neuroradiological mimics. Front Neurol. 11:627, 2020
2. Padilha IG et al: Pediatric multiple sclerosis: from clinical basis to imaging spectrum and differential diagnosis. Pediatr Radiol. 50(6):776-92, 2020
3. Bulut E et al: Brain MRI findings in pediatric-onset neuromyelitis optica spectrum disorder: challenges in differentiation from acute disseminated encephalomyelitis. AJNR Am J Neuroradiol. 40(4):726-31, 2019

Craniosynostoses

KEY FACTS

TERMINOLOGY

- Premature fusion of 1 or more cranial sutures, often resulting in abnormal cranial morphology &/or size
- Synonyms: Craniosynostosis, craniostenosis, sutural synostosis, premature sutural fusion

IMAGING

- Fibrous or osseous "bridging" ± ridging along suture
- Patterns of calvarial (& facial) dysmorphology depend on which suture(s) involved
  - Dolichocephaly: ↑ AP elongation, ↓ transverse dimension → sagittal synostosis
  - Trigonocephaly: Anterior pointing of frontal bone → metopic synostosis
  - Plagiocephaly: Calvarial asymmetry → unilateral coronal or lambdoid synostosis
  - Brachycephaly: ↑ transverse dimension, ↓ AP → bicoronal synostosis
  - Kleeblattschädel: Cloverleaf skull → sagittal & bilateral coronal ± bilateral lambdoid synostosis
  - Turricephaly (oxycephaly, acrocephaly): Towering skull → bilateral coronal, bilateral lambdoid, & sagittal synostosis
- Can be primary (nonsyndromic or syndromic) or secondary (e.g., shunt related, abnormally ↓ brain growth)

TOP DIFFERENTIAL DIAGNOSES

- Positional plagiocephaly or molding

CLINICAL ISSUES

- Nonsyndromic craniosynostosis: Most common, 1 or 2 sutures involved, typically normal outcomes
- Syndromic craniosynostosis: ↓ head growth, extremity anomalies, developmental delay
- Treatment with surgical cranial vault reconstruction or cranial vault distraction osteogenesis

DIAGNOSTIC CHECKLIST

- Low-dose head CT with 3D skull reformats is study of choice

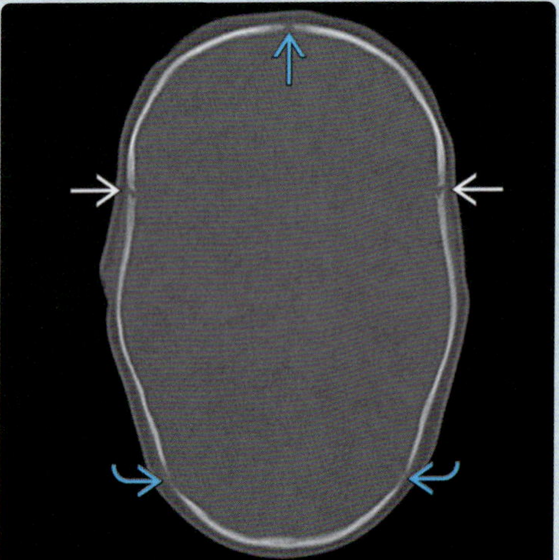

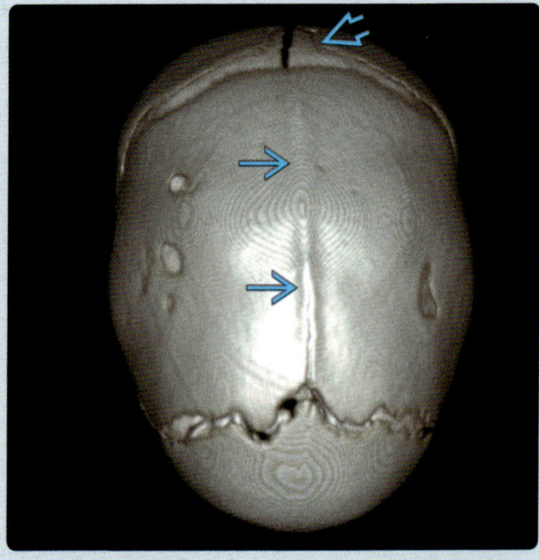

(Left) *Axial NECT in bone windows of a 3-week-old girl with dolichocephaly demonstrates classic AP elongation of the skull with a shortened transverse dimension. Note that the metopic ➔, coronal ➔, & lambdoid ➔ sutures are patent.* **(Right)** *Vertex 3D skull reformatted CT in the same patient demonstrates osseous fusion ➔ & ridging of the sagittal suture. Note that the anterior fontanel ➔ is patent. The sagittal suture does not normally fuse until ~ 22 years of age.*

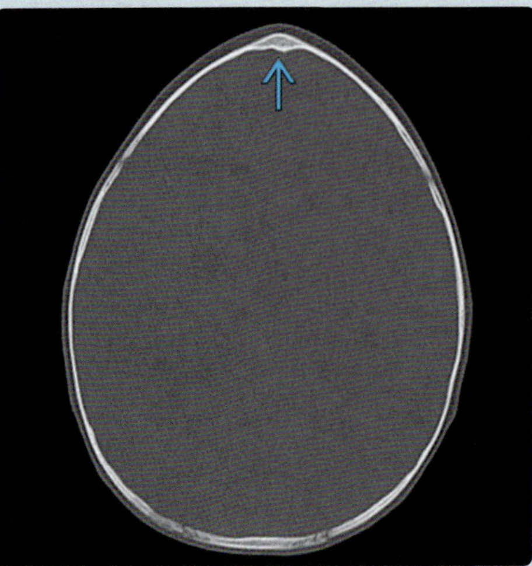

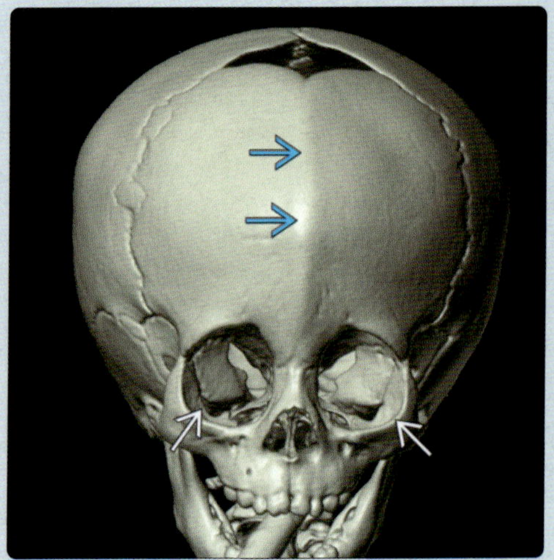

(Left) *Axial NECT in bone windows of a 6-month-old boy with trigonocephaly shows anterior pointing of the calvarium & osseous fusion of the metopic suture ➔. The metopic suture typically fuses in the first 3-9 months of life but not with the abnormal ridging seen here.* **(Right)** *Anterior 3D skull reformatted CT in the same patient demonstrates anterior ridging of the fused metopic suture ➔. There is associated hypotelorism ➔.*

TERMINOLOGY

Synonyms

- Craniosynostosis, craniostenosis, sutural synostosis, premature sutural fusion

Definitions

- Premature fusion of 1 or more cranial sutures, often resulting in abnormal cranial morphology &/or size
- Can be primary or secondary
  - Primary: Underlying genetic abnormality; can be nonsyndromic (most common) or syndromic
    - Nonsyndromic (~ 85%): Usually sporadic
      - Simple or single-suture synostosis (~ 75-80%): Typically normal development, intelligence, & intracranial pressure (ICP)
      - Multisuture nonsyndromic (~ 20-25%): If > 2 sutures involved, high incidence of ↑ ICP, cerebellar tonsillar herniation, & developmental delay
    - Syndromic (~ 15%): > 200 associated syndromes; high incidence of other associated anomalies & developmental delay
      - Precise classification is difficult due to considerable overlap; patients with same gene mutations can have different phenotypic manifestations
  - Secondary: From external causes
    - Intrauterine skull compression (especially in oligohydramnios)
    - Teratogens: Phenytoin, valproic acid, retinoic acid
    - Lack of normal brain growth
    - Shunt induced
    - Metabolic disorders: Rickets, hyperthyroidism, lysosomal storage disorders

IMAGING

General Features

- Best diagnostic clue
  - Abnormal head shape &/or size
- Size
  - Part or all of suture may be fused, 1 or multiple sutures may be involved
- Morphology
  - Classic imaging appearance: Calvarial (& facial) dysmorphology based on suture(s) involved
    - Dolichocephaly (scaphocephaly): ↑ AP elongation, ↓ transverse dimension, frontal bossing → sagittal synostosis
    - Trigonocephaly: Anterior pointing of frontal bone, compensatory posterior widening, hypotelorism → metopic synostosis
    - Plagiocephaly: Calvarial asymmetry
      - Unilateral anterior plagiocephaly: Ipsilateral upturned orbit or "harlequin eye," ipsilateral forehead flattening, contralateral frontal bossing → unilateral coronal synostosis
      - Unilateral posterior plagiocephaly: Ipsilateral occipital flattening → unilateral lambdoid synostosis
    - Brachycephaly: ↑ transverse dimension, ↓ AP → bicoronal synostosis
    - Turricephaly (oxycephaly, acrocephaly): Upward growth of brain through enlarged anterior fontanelle ("towering skull"), disproportionately enlarged frontal horns of lateral ventricles, small skull base & posterior fossa → bilateral coronal, bilateral lambdoid, & sagittal synostosis
      - Conflicting literature as to whether turricephaly & oxycephaly are same or distinct entities
    - Kleeblattschädel (cloverleaf skull): Expansion of membranous bone between sutures, shallow orbits → sagittal & bilateral coronal ± bilateral lambdoid synostosis
    - Unclassified: Other combinations of sutural synostoses

Radiographic Findings

- Skull: Dense suture; "bone bridge," inner table scalloping
  - Can be useful screening tool
- Extremities: Many anomalies described, some specific
  - Apert: Hand/foot syndactyly
  - Pfeiffer: Wide "stub" thumbs
  - Saethre-Chotzen: Duplicated distal phalanx, cone-shaped hallux epiphysis
  - Muenke-type mutations: Calcaneocuboid fusion
  - Crouzon: Hands/feet normal

CT Findings

- Fibrous or bony "bridging" ± sutural ridging
- Head shape determined by involved suture(s)

MR Findings

- Syndromic: Abnormal head shape ± cerebellar tonsillar ectopia, hydrocephalus, agenesis of corpus callosum
- Nonsyndromic: Abnormal head shape; brain is usually normal
- ± congenital venous drainage anomalies
- Postoperative dural venous occlusion

Ultrasonographic Findings

- Fetal: Diagnosis suggested by calvarial dysmorphology, loss of normal sutural hypoechogenicity
- Post natal: Focused high-resolution linear transducer can determine suture patency; may be used in surgical planning

Imaging Recommendations

- Best imaging tool
  - Low-dose CT with 3D reconstructions best for evaluating relationship between sutural fusion & calvarial dysmorphology
  - MR for brain abnormalities

DIFFERENTIAL DIAGNOSIS

Positional Plagiocephaly or Molding

- Sutures normal
- Normal infants: Marked ↑ in incidence after 1994 pediatric "back to sleep" campaign
  - Parallelogram skull on axial images, ipsilateral anterior ear displacement
- Hypotonic infant: Lies on back → posterior flattening
- Premature infant: Lies on side → dolichocephaly

PATHOLOGY

General Features

- Etiology
  - Normal sutures permit skull growth perpendicular to long axis
    - Order of fusion: Metopic (3-9 months) > sagittal (~ 22 years) > coronal (~ 24 years) > lambdoid (~ 26 years) > squamosal (~ 60 years)
    - Sutures are often visible after head reaches adult size; normal head growth stops within 1st decade of life
  - Premature upregulation of growth factors signaling sutural fusion → anomalous skull base development, craniostenosis
    - Transforming growth factor (TGF) & fibroblast growth factor/receptor (FGF/FGFR) mutations are expressed in face, skull base, & limb buds
  - ↓ growth of 1 suture is compensated by ↑ growth of other sutures
    - Skull growth ↓ perpendicular & ↑ parallel to fused suture → abnormal head shape
- Genetics
  - Single sutural & nonsyndromic synostoses are believed to be caused by genetic abnormality
    - Recent identification of mutations in isolated sagittal, metopic, & unilateral coronal synostosis
    - Gene expression is often suture specific
  - Syndromic synostoses are usually autosomal dominant
    - *FGFR1* (Pfeiffer syndrome)
    - *FGFR2* (Apert, Pfeiffer, Crouzon, Jackson-Weiss)
    - *FGFR3* (Muenke, Crouzon)
    - *TWIST1* (Saethre-Chotzen syndrome)
    - *MSX2* (Boston-type craniosynostosis)
- Associated abnormalities
  - Limb anomalies: Syndactyly & polysyndactyly (30%), deficiencies (22%)
  - Neurologic abnormalities/complications
    - ↑ ICP: Mechanical brain distortion, hydrocephalus, dural & collateral venous outflow obstruction at skull base
    - Tonsillar herniation ± syringohydromyelia
    - Exophthalmos, visual loss, intellectual disabilities (secondary to ↑ ICP)

Gross Pathologic & Surgical Features

- Fibrous or osseous "bridging," ridging, or "beaking" along suture

Microscopic Features

- ↑ osteoblastic cell differentiation/maturation

CLINICAL ISSUES

Presentation

- Most common signs/symptoms
  - Asymmetric face/cranium, ↓ head growth
  - Affected patients with more severe abnormalities often present at birth
- Other signs/symptoms
  - Extremity anomalies, developmental delay
- Clinical profile
  - Craniofacial asymmetry ± extremity anomalies
  - More common in twins, perhaps related to mechanical forces

Demographics

- Age
  - Usually present at birth or in infancy
- Epidemiology
  - Overall: 1:2,500
  - Sagittal (55-60%), coronal (20-30%), plagiocephaly (5-10%), metopic (1-2%)
  - Isolated sagittal synostosis: 60% is nonsyndromic

Natural History & Prognosis

- Single suture → cosmetic only or secondary mandibular/maxillary deformities (suture dependent)
- Multiple sutures → cosmetic with secondary mandibular/maxillary deformities, ↑ ICP, ↓ cerebral blood flow; airway/aural/visual compromise
  - Craniofacial deformity is socially stigmatizing
- Nonsyndromic → typically normal cognitive & motor development
- Syndromic ± midline brain anomalies → developmental delay

Treatment

- Mild deformity or positional molding
  - Aggressive physiotherapy, head repositioning, orthotic headband/helmet therapy
- Moderate to severe deformity
  - Surgical cranial vault reconstruction or cranial vault distraction osteogenesis

DIAGNOSTIC CHECKLIST

Consider

- Nonsyndromic does not mean nongenetic: Single suture synostoses is also governed by genes
- Venous drainage anomalies are important in surgical planning (typically multisutural synostosis)

Image Interpretation Pearls

- 3D skull & maximum intensity projection (MIP) reformats from CT can be helpful, particularly in early or partial sutural fusion
- In patients with shunt, microcephaly, or abnormal bone mineralization → think of secondary craniosynostosis

SELECTED REFERENCES

1. Okamoto T et al: Cranial suture measurement by 2-point method in ultrasound screening of craniosynostosis. Plast Reconstr Surg Glob Open. 7(5):e2225, 2019
2. Barkovich MJ et al: Congenital malformations of the brain and skull. In Barkovich AJ et al: Pediatric Neuroimaging. 6th ed. Wolters Kleuwer. 592-7, 2018
3. Ginat DT et al: CT imaging findings after craniosynostosis reconstructive surgery. Pediatr Neurosurg. 53(4):215-21, 2018
4. Blaser SI et al: Skull base development and craniosynostosis. Pediatr Radiol. 45 Suppl 3:S485-96, 2015
5. Governale LS: Craniosynostosis. Pediatr Neurol. 53(5):394-401, 2015
6. Idriz S et al: CT of normal developmental and variant anatomy of the pediatric skull: distinguishing trauma from normality. Radiographics. 35(5):1585-601, 2015
7. Derderian C et al: Syndromic craniosynostosis. Semin Plast Surg. 26(2):64-75, 2012
8. Garza RM et al: Nonsyndromic craniosynostosis. Semin Plast Surg. 26(2):53-63, 2012

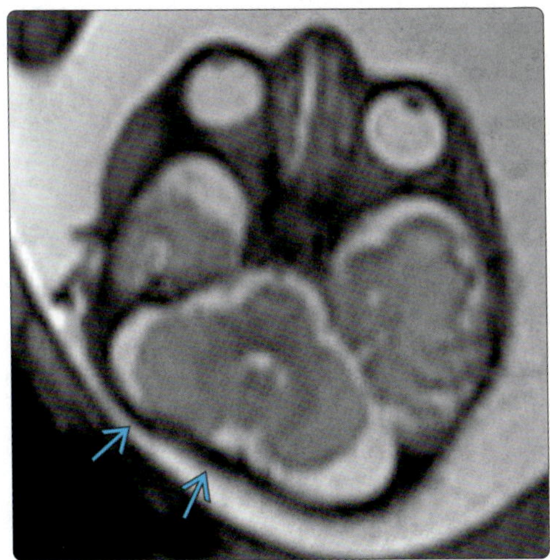

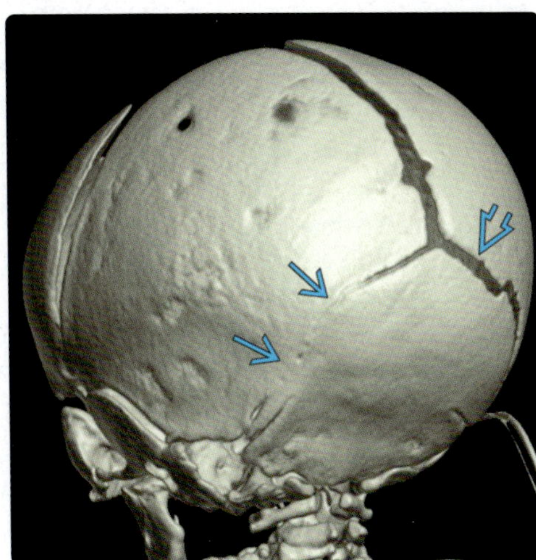

(Left) *Axial T2 MR SSFSE of a 35-weeks gestational age male fetus with right pulmonary agenesis shows flattening of the left occipital calvarium ➔, raising the possibility of unilateral lambdoid suture synostosis.* **(Right)** *Left posterior oblique 3D skull reformatted CT from the same patient at 1 month of age confirms partial osseous fusion of the left lambdoid suture ➔. Note the patent right lambdoid suture ➔.*

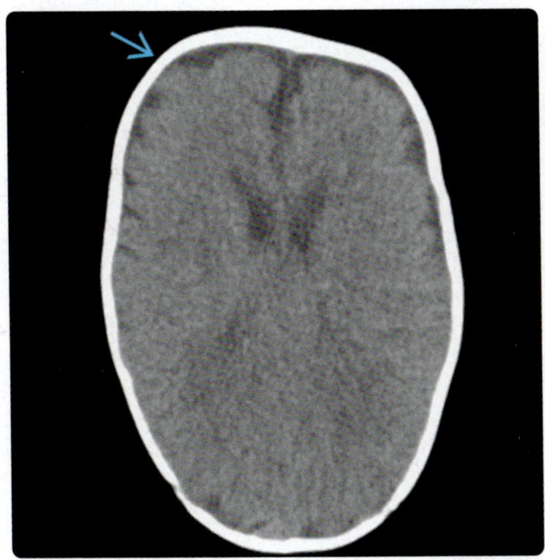

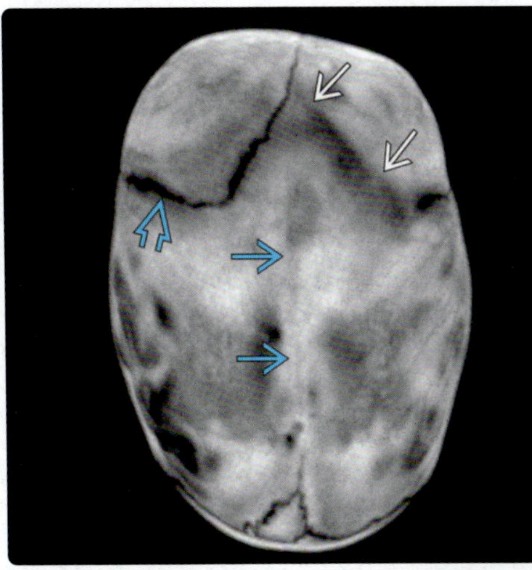

(Left) *Axial NECT in brain windows in a 2-month-old boy evaluated for scaphocephaly shows additional anterior bulging of the right frontal calvarium ➔ or plagiocephaly.* **(Right)** *Maximum intensity projection (MIP) CT from the same patient demonstrates osseous fusion of the sagittal suture ➔ & partial fusion of the left coronal suture ➔. The right coronal suture remains open ➔.*

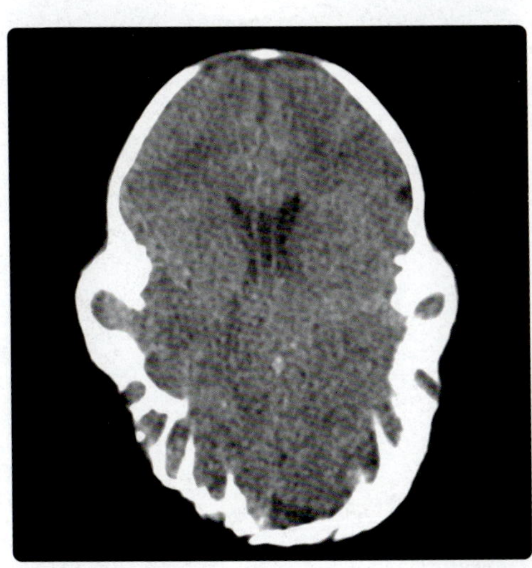

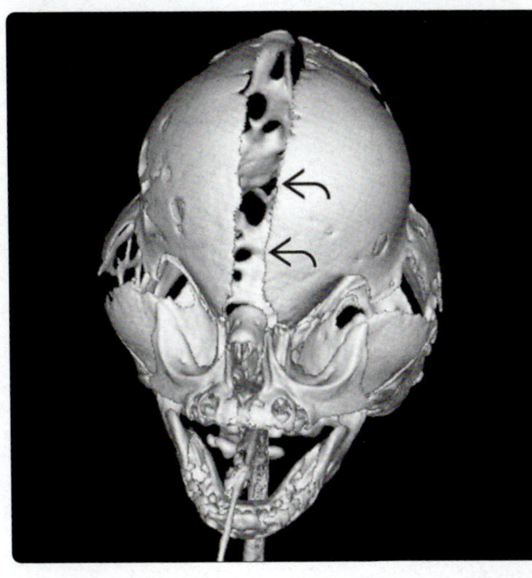

(Left) *Axial NECT in a 1-day-old infant with Carpenter syndrome reveals marked irregularity of the calvarium. The intracranial compartment is small, producing brain compression with effacement of the posterior convexity sulci & bitemporal protrusion in a cloverleaf or Kleeblattschädel appearance.* **(Right)** *Anterior 3D skull reformatted CT in the same patient shows a very wide metopic suture ➔ with bilateral "harlequin eyes" & a small face due to premature closure of the bilateral coronal & squamosal sutures.*

CSF Shunts and Complications

KEY FACTS

TERMINOLOGY

- Shunt malfunction comprises wide spectrum of potential complications associated with CSF diversion, mainly undershunting → acute hydrocephalus

IMAGING

- Undershunting is most common: ↑ ventricular size, periventricular edema, extraaxial CSF space effacement, hindbrain herniation; widening of sutures in infants
- Overshunting: Largely clinical diagnosis; look for intracranial hypotension, slit-like ventricles, subdural fluid collections
- Additional complications: Shunt infection, intraparenchymal hemorrhages (neonates), abdominal pseudocyst

TOP DIFFERENTIAL DIAGNOSES

- Shunt failure with normal or stable ventricular size
  - Seen in up to 1/3 of patients with shunt malfunction
- Progressive cerebral volume loss in presence of shunt
  - ↑ size of ventricles & extraaxial CSF spaces

CLINICAL ISSUES

- Since patients with shunts often have impaired ventricular compliance, shunt malfunction requiring emergent revision may be present even when ventricles are normal or stable in size (i.e., diagnosis may be clinically based)
- Infants: Bulging fontanelle, ↑ head circumference, irritability, lethargy
- Older children/adults: Headache, vomiting, lethargy, seizure, neurocognitive symptoms

DIAGNOSTIC CHECKLIST

- Comparison to prior imaging studies is essential as patients with shunts often have abnormal ventricular size & morphology at baseline
  - Must understand clinical scenario from time that prior imaging was obtained
- Subtle changes in ventricular & extraaxial CSF space size can have significant clinical implications

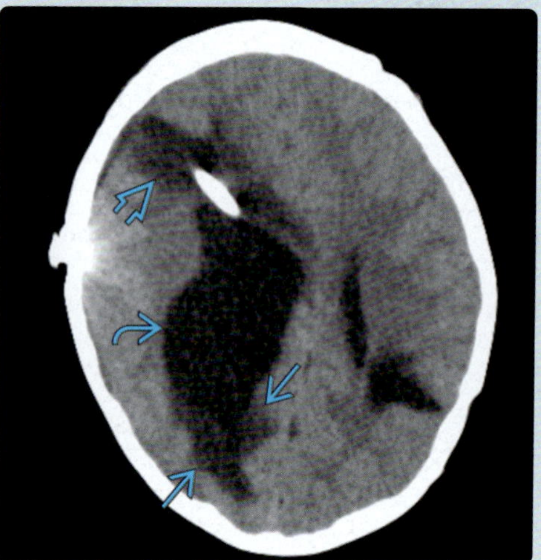

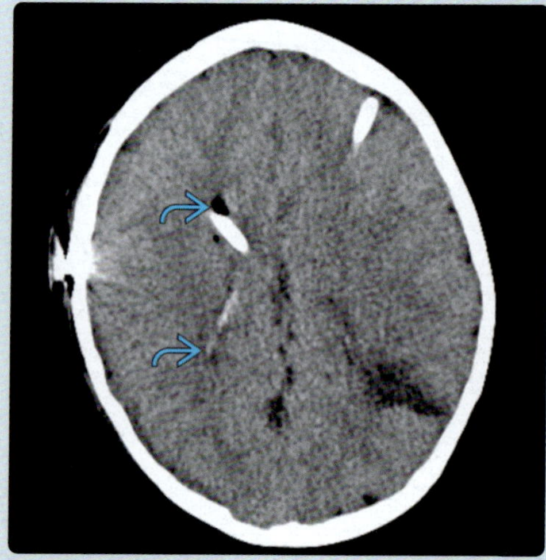

(Left) *Axial NECT of the brain in a 4-year-old with Chiari 2 malformation & evidence of acute shunt malfunction shows significant interval ↑ in size of the right lateral ventricle ➔ with new periventricular hypodensity ➔ & hypodensity surrounding the shunt ➔, consistent with acute hydrocephalus.* **(Right)** *Axial NECT in the same patient 1 month earlier (immediately after shunt placement) shows a nearly slit-like right lateral ventricle ➔.*

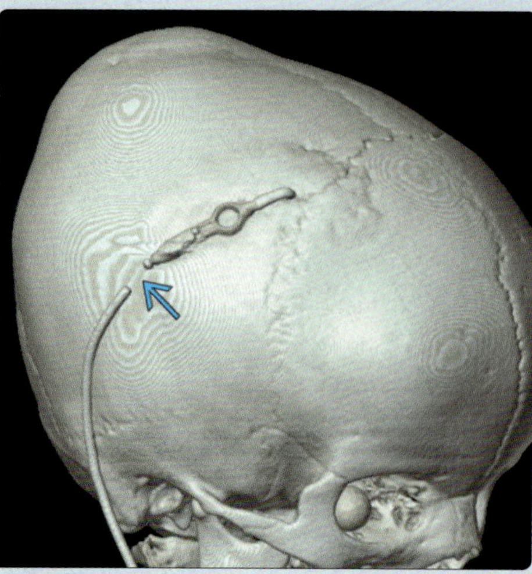

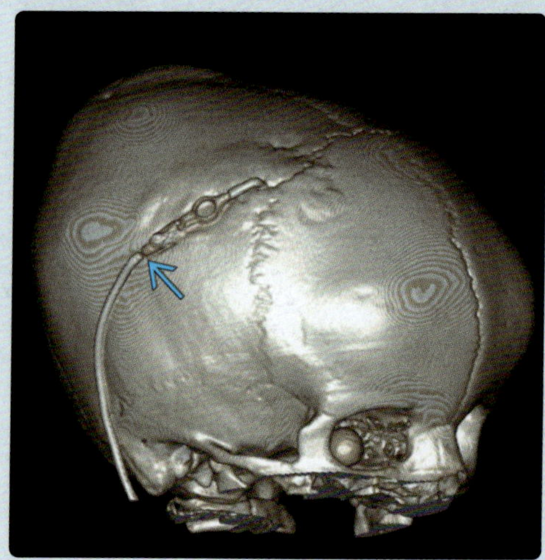

(Left) *Oblique lateral 3D NECT skull reformat in an 8-year-old with Dandy-Walker malformation & shunted hydrocephalus presenting with concern for shunt malfunction shows focal separation ➔ of the peritoneal shunt catheter tubing from the shunt valve.* **(Right)** *Similar 3D NECT skull reformat performed 1 month earlier in the same patient shows a normal connection ➔ between the shunt catheter tubing & shunt valve. This is a common location for shunt disconnection.*

TERMINOLOGY

Abbreviations

- Shunt types: Ventriculoperitoneal (VP), ventriculoatrial (VA), ventriculopleural (VPL), lumboperitoneal (LP), externalized (draining outside body)
- Endoscopic 3r ventriculostomy (ETV)

Definitions

- Complications related to CSF diversion
  - Undershunting: Inadequate CSF drainage → ↑ intraventricular pressure → acute hydrocephalus
    - Can be secondary to shunt blockage or breakage (usually at sites of connection)
  - Overshunting can → intracranial hypotension
  - Subdural collections: Most often occur in severe hydrocephalus with early CSF overshunting
  - Infection: Usually from colonization of skin flora; also from distal end infection (such as bowel perforation) or hematogenous seeding
  - Relative catheter shortening related to patient growth
  - CSF egress around shunt
  - Craniocerebral disproportion: Chronic CSF shunting → lack of normal skull growth
  - Abdominal complications: Ascites, pseudocyst formation, viscus perforation, intestinal obstruction, granulomatous reaction
  - Multifocal intraparenchymal hemorrhages
    - Unique to infants, especially preterm

IMAGING

General Features

- Best diagnostic clue
  - Undershunting: Findings of acute hydrocephalus include ↑ ventricular size, periventricular edema, empty sella, dilated optic nerve sheaths (papilledema), depressed floor of 3rd ventricle, acute herniation, effacement of extraaxial CSF spaces over cerebral convexities; sutural widening in infants
- Location
  - Shunt components: Ventriculostomy catheter, ± reservoir (for CSF sampling or acutely relieving pressure), unidirectional valve (usually in scalp), & distal drainage catheter (usually peritoneal)
    - Programmable magnetic valves are MR compatible but must almost always be reset after MR exam
  - Tip of ventriculostomy catheter should ideally be within ventricles without contact of choroid plexus; frontal & occipital horns are preferred locations
    - Catheter has many sideholes; if tip has gone beyond ventricle, any sideholes remaining in ventricular system may result in adequate drainage
- Size
  - Ventricular size is relative; enlargement may indicate shunt failure in 1 patient vs. stable finding in another
    - Chronically shunted patients have ↓ ventricular compliance; small changes in ventricle size may be clinically significant
    - Up to 1/3 of patients with shunt failure will not have supportive imaging findings, leaving clinical presentation as key to diagnosis in many cases
- Morphology
  - Ventricular morphology varies greatly in patients based on underlying brain malformation, presence of prior brain injury, & how long patient has been shunted

Radiographic Findings

- Evaluate shunt catheter system integrity
  - Separation at connection points (most common), catheter breakage, migration
  - Distal catheter may retract out of abdomen if significant somatic growth has occurred since shunt placement
- Programmable shunt valve settings are often assessed using radiography or fluoroscopy
  - Can refer to individual manufacturer's guidelines for setting interpretation

CT Findings

- NECT
  - Evaluation of size & morphology of ventricles & extraaxial CSF spaces
  - High spatial resolution is ideal for evaluation of shunt catheter/tubing integrity
    - 3D skull reformats can be helpful in evaluating extracranial course of tubing
  - Periventricular hypodensity may reflect interstitial edema in acute hydrocephalus
    - Without prior studies, this can be difficult to differentiate from gliosis
- Intraventricular contrast injection through shunt + NECT→ identifies failure of contrast to disperse throughout CSF (ventricular isolation, which requires additional catheter placement)

MR Findings

- T1, T2, FLAIR
  - Periventricular T2-/FLAIR hyperintense signal in acute hydrocephalus
  - Midline structures in hydrocephalus
    - Upward bowing & thinning of corpus callosum
    - Anterior displacement of lamina terminalis
    - Depression of floor of 3rd ventricle
- T2-SSFSE/HASTE
  - Fast MR protocol can be performed to evaluate ventricular size without radiation or sedation

Ultrasonographic Findings

- Grayscale ultrasound
  - Head US: Useful in neonates for serial assessment of ventricular size (but requires open fontanelle)
  - Abdominal US: May identify localized collection (pseudocyst) restricting egress of CSF from catheter tip

Imaging Recommendations

- Best imaging tool
  - Brain NECT to assess for acute ventricular size change & catheter integrity
  - Nonsedated fast MR protocols (HASTE, SSFSE) to avoid cumulative radiation exposure & sedation
  - In neonatal period, US, MR, & CT may be used interchangeably; in conjunction with open sutures, this may create confusing assessment
    - Coronal US parameters correlate well with axial, coronal, or volumetric MR data

- Frontal occipital horn ratio (FOHR)
- Frontal temporal horn ratio (FTHR)

- Protocol advice
  - Brain CT or MR to evaluate ventricle size
  - 3D CT skull reformats to evaluate shunt course
  - Plain film shunt series to identify distal mechanical shunt fracture or disconnection

DIFFERENTIAL DIAGNOSIS

Shunt Failure With Normal or Stable Ventricle Size

- Seen in up to 1/3 of patients with shunt malfunction
- Diagnosis on clinical grounds

Progressive Cerebral Volume Loss in Presence of Shunt

- ↑ size of ventricles & extraaxial CSF spaces
- No periventricular edema
- Diagnosis is ultimately clinical

PATHOLOGY

General Features

- Etiology
  - CSF shunt establishes accessory drainage pathway to bypass obstructed natural CSF flow pathways
    - Restores or maintains normal ICP
  - Each shunt, valve, & device carries its own complications
    - All types → material degradation/fatigue, mechanical stress (especially craniocervical junction, inferior ribs)
    - VP → abdominal complications (CSF pseudocyst, ascites, bowel perforation)
    - VPL → symptomatic pleural effusion
    - VA → shunt nephritis, cor pulmonale, pulmonary embolus
    - LP → arachnoiditis, cerebellar tonsillar herniation, high catheter migration rate
    - ETV: Establishes alternate route of CSF egress from 3rd ventricle to suprasellar cistern; requires no residual internal device
      - ~ 5-10% complication rate (e.g., hemorrhage, hypothalamic injury, etc.)
      - 10-50% failure rate depending on indication, most within 1-2 weeks
      - Overshunting not possible

CLINICAL ISSUES

Presentation

- Most common signs/symptoms
  - Children, adults: Headache, vomiting, lethargy, seizure; neuropsychologic, cognitive, or behavioral
  - Infants: Bulging fontanelle, ↑ head circumference, irritability, lethargy
- Clinical profile
  - Depends on underlying clinical diagnosis necessitating CSF diversion, number of previous shunts, complications

Demographics

- Age: Shunts are placed early in life for aqueductal stenosis, intraventricular hemorrhage (typically grades 3-4)
  - Need for CSF diversion in Chiari 2 may be ↓ with in utero repair of myelomeningocele
  - Shunts are placed in older children following trauma, meningitis, tumor

Natural History & Prognosis

- Acute shunt failure in shunt-dependent patient is life-threatening emergency
- Majority of shunts eventually fail; complication rate: 25-37%
  - ≤ 40% shunts fail in 1st year, 80% fail by 10 years
  - 50% of patients need multiple revisions with progressively shorter time intervals between each failure

Treatment

- Shunt revision
  - Replace intraventricular component/valve for proximal obstruction
  - Alter valve pressure setting/type if over- or undershunting
    - Programmable shunt valves permit transcutaneous adjustment of pressure setting
  - Lengthen distal shunt as child grows
- ETV to avoid indwelling shunt if blockage is distal to 3rd ventricle
  - Requires that suprasellar, interpeduncular, & prepontine cisterns are patent (which may not be true with recent/prior hemorrhage or meningitis)
- Laparoscopic or open abdominal procedure for distal obstruction related to CSF pseudocyst

DIAGNOSTIC CHECKLIST

Consider

- Unless there are overt imaging findings of acute hydrocephalus, shunt failure is clinical diagnosis ultimately
  - Significant number of patients with shunt failure have normal or stable ventricle size

Image Interpretation Pearls

- Comparison to priors is important as patients with shunts often have baseline abnormal ventricle size & morphology
  - Reviewing multiple prior exams (with awareness of clinical scenario at time of prior imaging, i.e., baseline vs. acute presentation for failure) can be helpful in understanding current imaging
- Subtle changes in ventricular & extraaxial CSF spaces can have significant clinical implications

Reporting Tips

- Be clear to exactly which prior studies you are comparing current exam
- Rapidly communicate clear acute shunt failure

SELECTED REFERENCES

1. Nagaraj UD et al: Imaging diagnosis of ventriculomegaly: fetal, neonatal, and pediatric. Childs Nerv Syst. 36(8):1669-79, 2020
2. Radhakrishnan R et al: Frontal occipital and frontal temporal horn ratios: comparison and validation of head ultrasound-derived indexes with MRI and ventricular volumes in infantile ventriculomegaly. AJR Am J Roentgenol. 213(4):925-31, 2019
3. Hanak BW et al: Cerebrospinal fluid shunting complications in children. Pediatr Neurosurg. 52(6):381-400, 2017
4. Rinker EK et al: CSF shunt complications: what the abdominal imager needs to know. Abdom Imaging. 40(6):2030-40, 2015
5. Sivaganesan A et al: Neuroimaging of ventriculoperitoneal shunt complications in children. Pediatr Radiol. 42(9):1029-46, 2012
6. Lollis SS et al: Programmable CSF shunt valves: radiographic identification and interpretation. AJNR Am J Neuroradiol. 31(7):1343-6, 2010

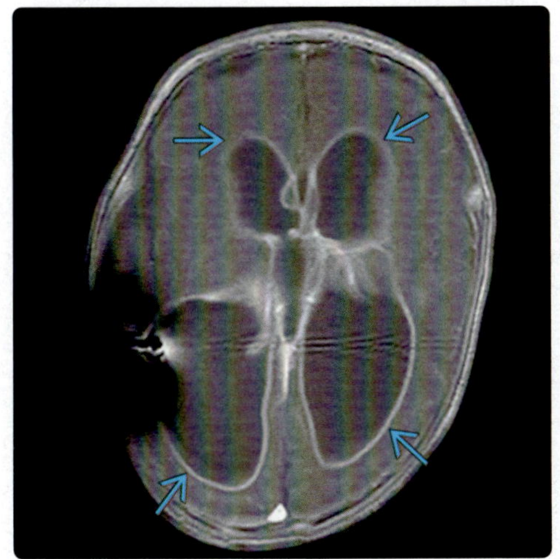

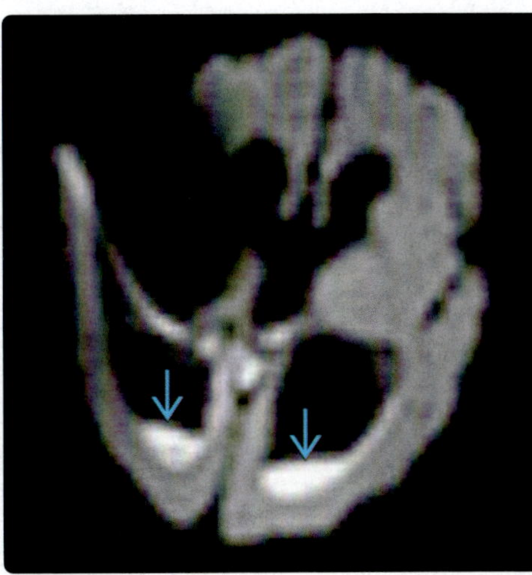

(Left) *Axial T1 C+ FS MR in a 4-month-old girl with shunted hydrocephalus & persistent seizures demonstrates diffuse ependymal thickening & enhancement ⇨, consistent with ventriculitis.* **(Right)** *Axial DWI MR in the same patient demonstrates diffusion restriction of the layering debris ⇨ in the dependent portions of the ventricles, consistent with layering purulent material in this patient with ventriculitis, an uncommon but serious shunt complication.*

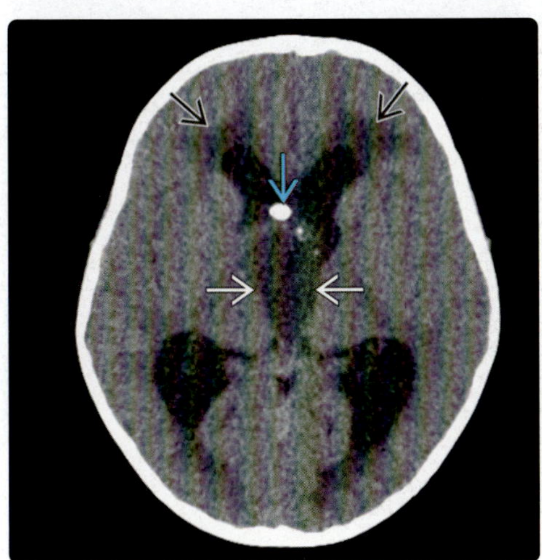

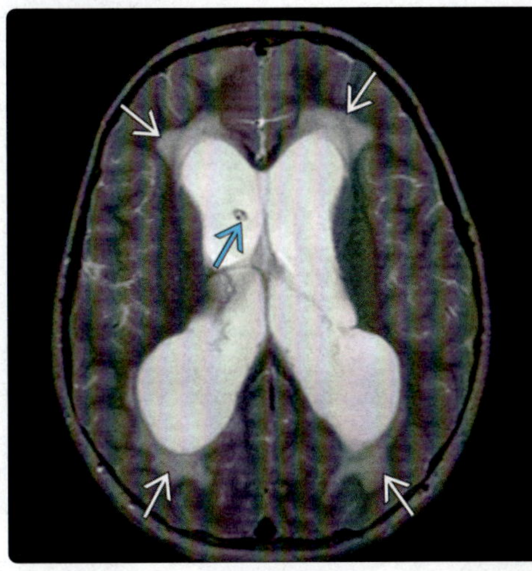

(Left) *Axial NECT in an 8-year-old with a suprasellar pilocytic astrocytoma & shunting ⇨ for hydrocephalus shows the mass expanding the 3rd ventricle ➡. There is lateral ventriculomegaly with periventricular edema ⇨.* **(Right)** *Axial T2 MR in the same patient demonstrates the shunt in the ventricle ⇨ with hyperintense periventricular edema ➡, consistent with uncompensated acute hydrocephalus. Periventricular edema may take some time to resolve, even after adequate shunting.*

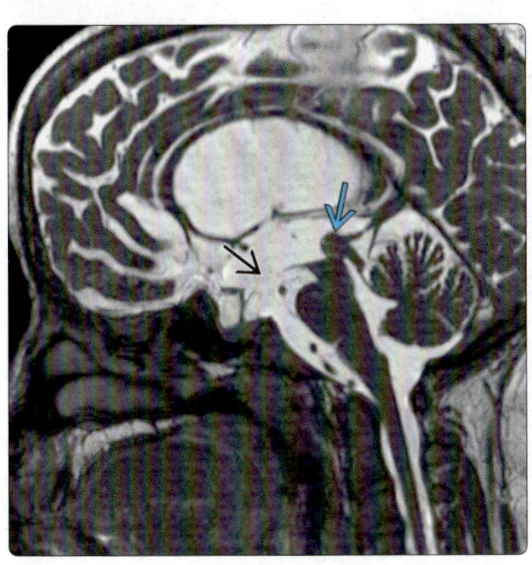

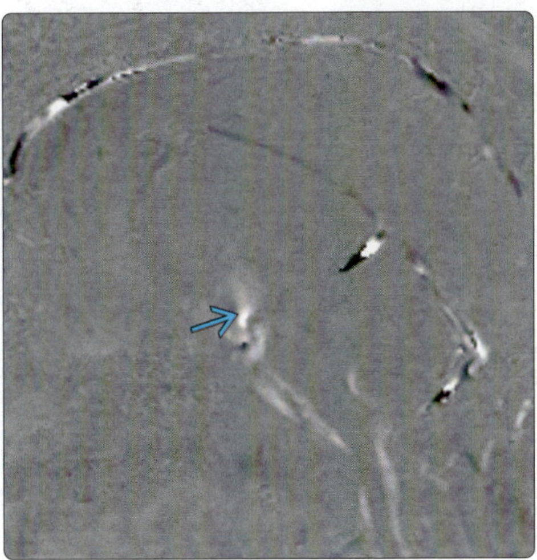

(Left) *Sagittal 3D FIESTA MR in a 13-year-old girl with a tectal plate glioma ⇨ treated with an endoscopic 3rd ventriculostomy ⇨ confirms a patent defect in the floor of the 3rd ventricle.* **(Right)** *Sagittal phase-contrast CSF flow study in the same patient demonstrates a dephasing jet through the ventriculostomy site ⇨, confirming its patency. Approximately 10-50% of 3rd ventriculostomies fail depending on the indication, most within weeks of the procedure.*

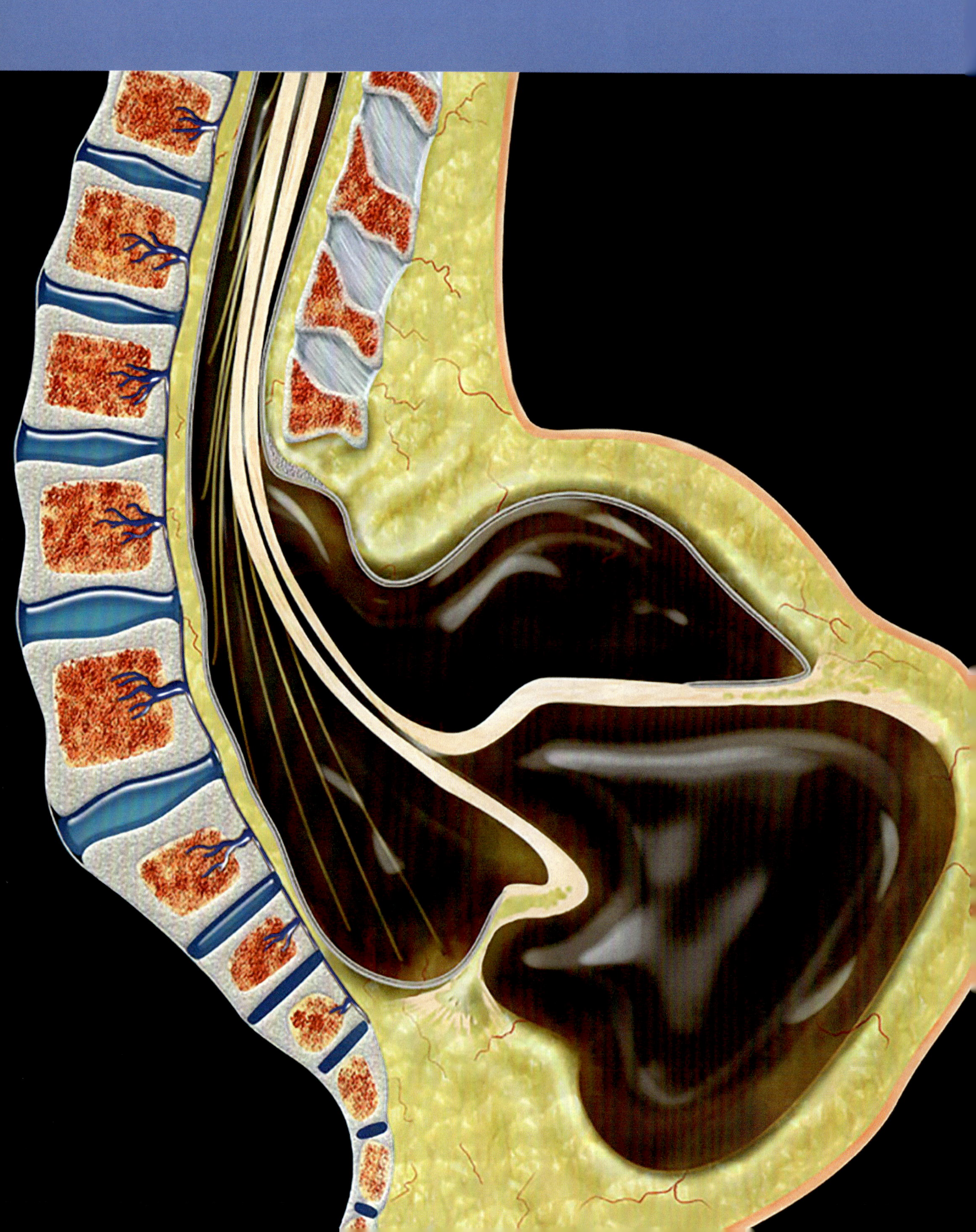

SECTION 8

Spine

Pathology-based Imaging Issues

In the newborn, the spine is most commonly imaged when a cutaneous lesion, such as a hemangioma or hairy patch, overlies the lumbosacral spine & implies the presence of an underlying spinal abnormality. Other findings on physical exam prompting investigation include a subcutaneous fatty mass, forked gluteal crease, or atypical dimple (above the gluteal crease). Within the first 4 months of life, US excels at imaging the spinal cord, CSF, & nerve roots, allowing for detection of a low-lying conus medullaris or intraspinal mass. Additionally, it has the advantage of requiring no sedation in the young infant. After ~ 4-6 months of age, too much of the pediatric vertebral cartilage has ossified to allow an adequate acoustic window into the spine. US can also provide vital real-time information in the operating suite to guide resection of intramedullary tumors & access syrinx cavities.

Conventional radiographs are fast, well tolerated, & relatively inexpensive but provide limited information for most pediatric spinal pathology. When combined with a good-quality clinical exam, radiographs are often sufficient for trauma evaluations. However, the negative predictive value of radiographs is low, so when clinical suspicion is high or if the clinical exam is positive or limited, further evaluation with CT &/or MR is imperative.

Speed, accessibility, & high bony detail make CT ideal for the initial evaluation of spinal trauma, but MR is essential for the assessment of neural & ligamentous injury. For chronic back pain in the older child, spondylolysis is a commonly encountered pathology that is often more confidently evaluated by CT, especially in combination with nuclear medicine SPECT. Primary osseous lesions can sometimes be more accurately characterized by investigation of their appearance on CT. Modern CT scanners allow for the rapid construction of multiplanar & volume-rendered images, which can be invaluable in the demonstration of pathology. High-quality CT images of the spine are routinely created from abdominal & thoracic CT acquisitions; therefore, dedicated CT imaging of the spine is typically not necessary if these studies have been performed.

MR provides the most complete & accurate assessment of congenital, inflammatory, & neoplastic disease of the spine. For the latter 2 categories, the administration of IV contrast is essential, but it rarely provides additional insight in congenital malformations. It is important to recognize that orthopedic stabilization devices may cause marked susceptibility artifact on MR, severely hampering the ability to evaluate the spine after surgery. This should not prevent the use of MR in evaluation of the postoperative instrumented spine; however, in many cases, the key features needed to make an accurate diagnosis can still be discerned despite the presence of marked image distortion.

Imaging Protocols

There is a temptation to always increase spatial resolution when performing medical imaging. This ignores the fact that increasing spatial resolution comes at the cost of decrease in signal-to-noise ratio. It is key to strike a balance between the best spatial resolution & image quality, so that the radiologist can not only see the lesion, but also confidently characterize it.

To that end, it can be counterproductive to image the pediatric spine with exceedingly small fields of view (FOVs). In neonates, you may achieve the best imaging quality with a single sagittal FOV, whereas 2 or even 3 overlapping FOVs are appropriate in older children. T2 should be the mainstay of most spine imaging protocols, providing the best assessment of both the spinal cord & the normal pediatric intervertebral disc. Fluid-sensitive sequences (such as STIR or T2 FS) diminish the signal of normal fat that may interfere with the assessment of pathologic fluid in fat-containing tissues; these sequences are essential for the detection of marrow & soft tissue edema in cases of trauma &/or pain. Precontrast spin-echo-based T1 provides an excellent assessment of normal bone marrow as well as any fat-containing intraspinal pathology. Postcontrast T1 should be performed with fat-saturation techniques whenever possible. High spatial resolution 3D sequences, such as CISS, T2 DRIVE, or FIESTA, are very helpful in the detection of smaller lesions & of arachnoid webs & adhesions. DWI of the spine is of most benefit in assessing for abscess & inclusion cysts (dermoid/epidermoid). The utility of DWI in the evaluation of subarachnoid tumor is still in evolution.

Embryology

In order to confidently & accurately diagnose congenital spinal abnormalities, it is necessary to have a working understanding of spinal embryology. Congenital spinal malformations can be classified into neural tube defects, split-cord or notochord malformations, & abnormalities of the caudal cell mass. Neural tube defects result from abnormalities in closure of the neural tube (neurulation), which occurs between 17-27 days of gestation. Failure of the neural ectoderm to separate from the cutaneous ectoderm will result in an open neural tube defect, which can be large in the case of a myelocele or myelomeningocele or small in the case of a dorsal dermal sinus. If disjunction occurs but is complicated by inclusion of mesoderm within the neural tube (perhaps a result of premature separation), a lipomatous malformation (lipomyelocele or lipomyelocystocele) will result. If the notochord splits during migration from the Hensen node (perhaps due to an adhesion of the ectoderm & endoderm), a split cord malformation, such as a diastematomyelia or neurenteric cyst, is the consequence. Finally, if there is a disruption of the normal canalization & retrogressive differentiation of the caudal cell mass, distal lesions, such as a terminal myelocystocele or syndrome of caudal regression, will develop. The nomenclature for these congenital lesions is confusing & often based on observations & assumptions that are no longer valid. Recognizing this, the neuroradiologist should take great care to identify & describe all the salient characteristics of the malformation, rather than assuming a diagnosis & adjusting the interpretation to fit.

Selected References

1. Behbahani M et al: Cutaneous stigmata of the spine: a review of indications for imaging and referral. Pediatr Clin North Am. 68(4):895-913, 2021
2. Colafati GS et al: The pediatric spine. Semin Musculoskelet Radiol. 25(1):137-54, 2021
3. Jea A et al: Cervical spine injury in children and adolescents. Pediatr Clin North Am. 68(4):875-94, 2021
4. McAllister AS et al: Emergent imaging of pediatric cervical spine trauma. Radiographics. 39(4):1126-42, 2019
5. Orman G et al: Ultrasound to evaluate neonatal spinal dysraphism: a first-line alternative to CT and MRI. J Neuroimaging. 29(5):553-64, 2019
6. Alvarado E et al: Pediatric spinal ultrasound: neonatal and intraoperative applications. Semin Ultrasound CT MR. 38(2):126-42, 2017
7. Rossi A et al: Diagnostic approach to pediatric spine disorders. Magn Reson Imaging Clin N Am. 24(3):621-44, 2016

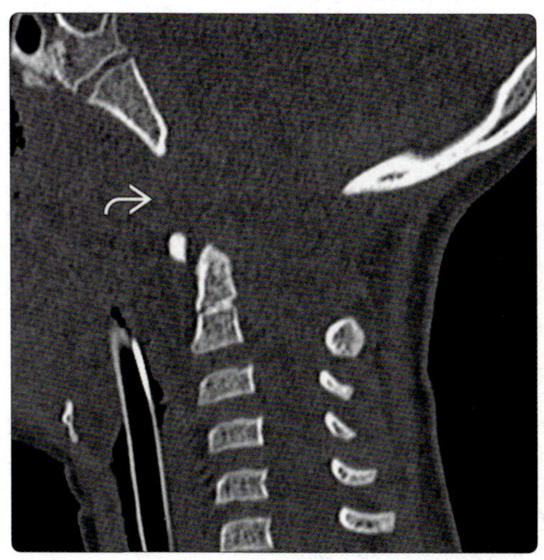

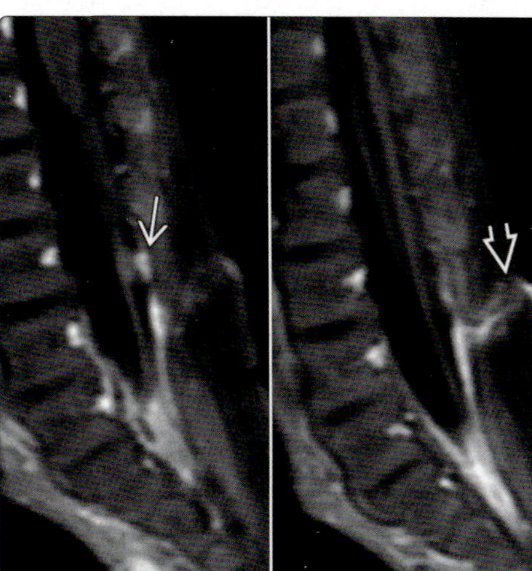

(Left) *Sagittally reconstructed CT of the craniocervical junction in a 5-year-old ejected from the car after a motor vehicle accident shows abnormal widening of the atlantooccipital articulation ➲, reflecting complete disruption of the tectorial membrane & other stabilizing ligaments.* **(Right)** *Sagittal T1 C+ FS MR images in an infant with a midline dimple above the gluteal crease (which should raise concern for a dermal sinus) show infection extending along the sinus ➡ into the lumbar canal ➡.*

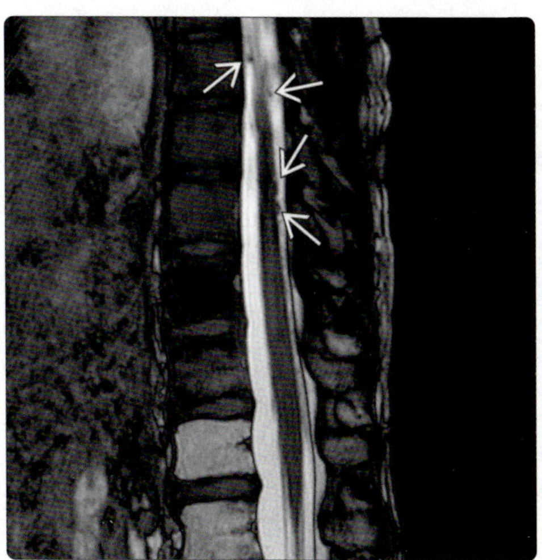

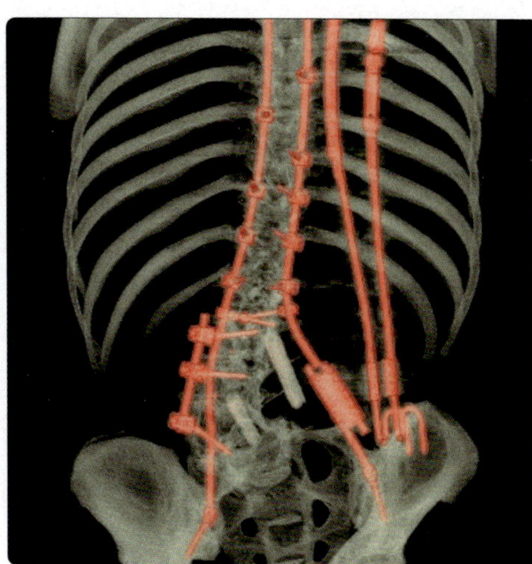

(Left) *Sagittal 3D SSFP MR can be very helpful in detecting small, nonenhancing drop metastases ➡, as in this teenager with ependymoma.* **(Right)** *Coronal oblique bone CT with volume-rendered 3D reformatting clearly shows the relationship of multiple orthopedic devices (posterior spinal fusion rods, growing rods, & transpedicular screws) to the bony skeleton in this 11-year-old with neurofibromatosis type 1 & dural ectasia. 3D reconstructions can be very valuable in surgical planning.*

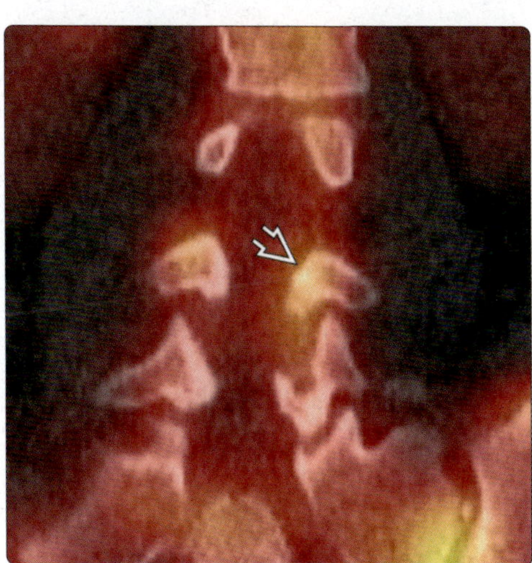

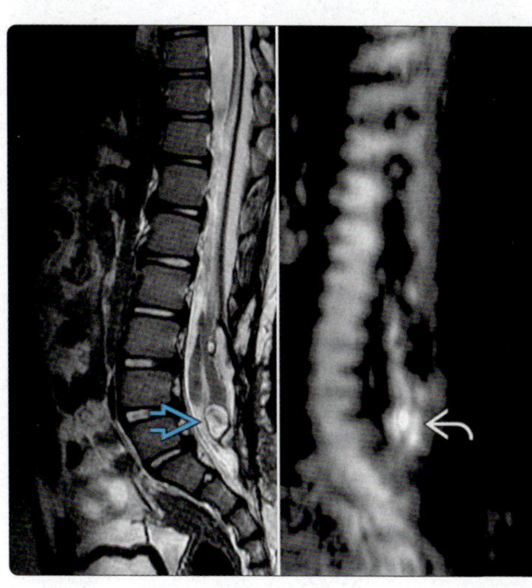

(Left) *Coronal fused SPECT bone scan shows pars interarticularis defects & confirms reactive bony changes ➡ as a source of back pain.* **(Right)** *Sagittal T2 MR (left) in a teen with a Chiari 2 malformation shows a cystic lesion ➡ at the site of a prior lumbar myelomeningocele repair. The lesion has markedly restricted diffusion on DWI ➲, confirming the diagnosis of epidermoid inclusion cyst. Recent advances have made diffusion a reasonable & useful tool in spinal imaging.*

Myelomeningocele

KEY FACTS

TERMINOLOGY

- Myelomeningocele (MMC) & myelocele (MC) comprise spectrum of open (not skin-covered) spinal dysraphisms
- MMC: Neural placode outside of spinal canal with measurable sac
- MC: Neural placode flush with skin surface or inside spinal canal

IMAGING

- Fetal US/MR: Lumbosacral dysraphism ± thin-walled MMC sac + intracranial findings of Chiari 2 (lemon sign, banana sign, ± ventriculomegaly)
- Postnatal spine imaging typically only performed after repair: Expect soft tissue covering of defect
  - Posterior osseous dysraphic defect & elongation of spinal cord persist
  - Neural placode (distal, nonneurulated segment of cord) inserts onto dorsal aspect of distal thecal sac

TOP DIFFERENTIAL DIAGNOSES

- Closed (skin-covered) spinal dysraphism
- Postoperative pseudomeningocele

CLINICAL ISSUES

- Most common neurologic deficits: Lower extremities, bowel & bladder dysfunction
- ~ 80-85% have hydrocephalus requiring CSF diversion, though lower incidence reported after fetal repair
- Mortality: 10-30% die before adulthood
  - Brainstem/cerebellar dysfunction or shunt malfunction

DIAGNOSTIC CHECKLIST

- Most common spinal cause of delayed neurologic deterioration: Cord retethering (clinical diagnosis)
  - Spine MR (± brain imaging) to look for other causes
- For postnatal spine imaging, check clinical history to confirm history of open spinal dysraphism
  - MMC vs. MC on prenatal imaging only

(Left) *Longitudinal US of the spine in a 20-weeks-gestation fetus shows absence of posterior lumbosacral spinal elements & a measurable sac extending beyond the expected contours of the skin, consistent with a myelomeningocele (MMC)* ➡. **(Right)** *Sagittal 2D SSFP MR in the same fetus, now at 21-weeks gestation, shows the lumbosacral MMC* ➡*. There is a small posterior fossa, caudal cerebellar herniation* ➡*, & absence of the normal 4th ventricle, consistent with Chiari 2 malformation.*

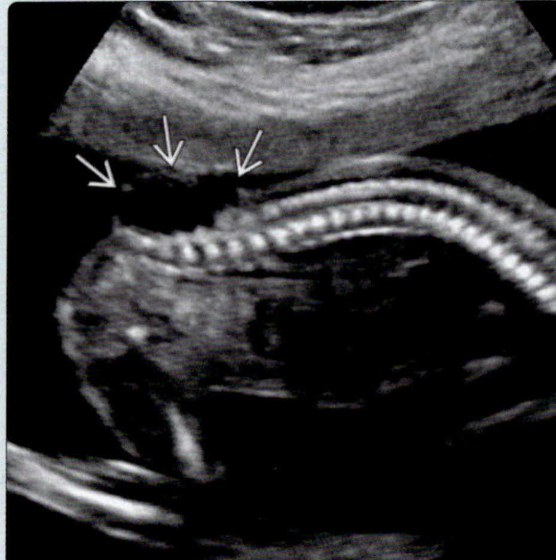

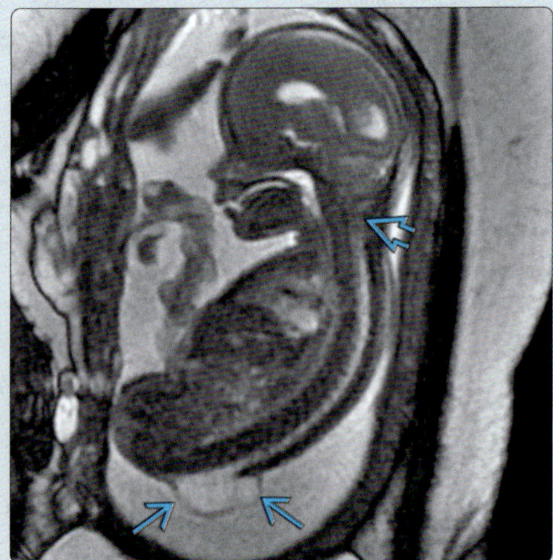

(Left) *Axial 2D SSFP MR in the lumbosacral spine from the same fetus demonstrates the neural placode* ➡ *outside of the open spinal canal* ➡*, consistent with an MMC.* **(Right)** *Sagittal T1 MR in the same patient at 10 months of age (status post-MMC closure) shows an expected skin-covered, postoperative appearance. The neural placode is attached to the dorsal thecal sac at the repair site* ➡*, which is a typical finding.*

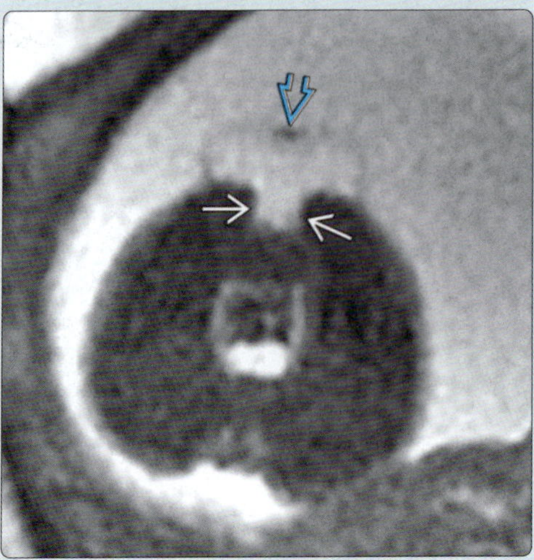

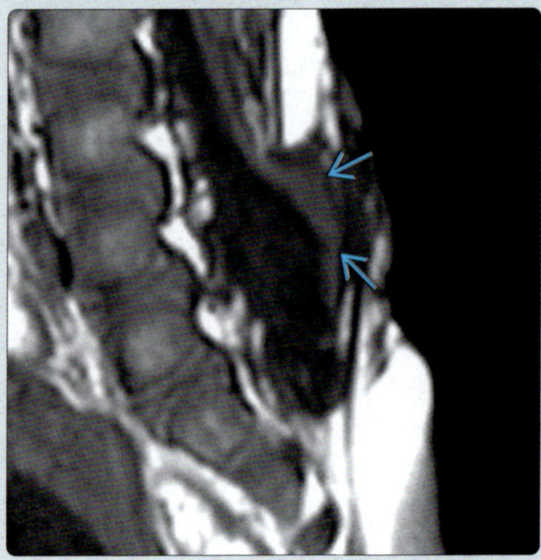

TERMINOLOGY

Definitions

- Myelomeningocele (MMC): Open (lacking skin covering) spinal dysraphism in which neural placode (exposed flattened end of elongated spinal cord) protrudes as sac beyond skin surface dorsal to spinal canal
- Myelocele (MC): Open spinal dysraphism with neural placode flush with skin surface or in spinal canal (no sac)
- Some authors refer to all open spinal dysraphisms as MMC (as MMC & MC fall along same pathologic spectrum)

IMAGING

General Features

- Best diagnostic clue
  - Absent posterior osseous elements, distorted low-lying spinal cord/roots, postoperative skin closure changes
    - Rarely imaged before repair in postnatal period due to infection risk
  - > 80% have significant hindbrain herniation in setting of Chiari 2 malformation

MR Findings

- Fetal MR
  - Abnormal elongation of spinal cord with neural placode extending into osseous dysraphism ± MMC sac
  - Intracranial findings of Chiari 2 malformation
- Postnatal MR: T1, T2
  - Postoperative soft tissue changes of MMC closure
  - Elongation of spinal cord extending to flat neural placode adherent to posterior thecal sac
    - Loss of normal posterior epidural fat at level of defect
  - Postoperative complications
    - Syringohydromyelia
    - Spinal cord compression by dermoid/epidermoid or arachnoid cyst
    - Constricting dural ring
    - Cord ischemia from vascular compromise
  - Associated anomalies: Split cord malformation (31-46%), dorsal dermal sinus, segmentation anomalies, caudal agenesis

DIFFERENTIAL DIAGNOSIS

Closed (Occult) Spinal Dysraphism

- Skin-covered osseous defect

Postoperative Pseudomeningocele

- History & clinical exam allow for differentiation

PATHOLOGY

General Features

- Etiology
  - Failure of neural tube closure in 3rd-gestational week
    - Due to lack of expression of specific receptors on surface of neuroectodermal cells
    - Likely multifactorial: Folate deficiency, toxins, genetics
  - Neurologic deficits are worsened by chronic mechanical injury & amniotic fluid exposure (chemical trauma)

CLINICAL ISSUES

Presentation

- Most common signs/symptoms
  - Clinically obvious at birth: Exposed neural placode, usually leaking CSF
  - Dysfunction of bowel, bladder, & lower extremities
    - Higher level spine defect correlates with greater motor & somatosensory deficits
- Other signs/symptoms
  - ~ 80-85% of those that undergo postnatal repair have hydrocephalus requiring CSF diversion, though lower incidence is reported with in utero repair

Natural History & Prognosis

- Stable postoperative motor deficit in majority (~ 73%)
  - Neurologic deterioration suggests complication
- ~ 2/3 have normal intelligence, ~ 23% have ≥ 1 seizure
- Bladder, bowel, & sexual dysfunction
  - ~ 80% are bladder continent (most with catheterization)
  - ~ 38% require bowel regimen
- Lower extremity dysfunction
- Mortality: 10-30% die before adulthood
  - Majority die during infancy & early childhood from brainstem/cerebellar dysfunction
  - 2nd peak in early adulthood from shunt malfunction

Treatment

- MMC closure < 48 hours after delivery to stabilize neurologic deficits & prevent infection
- In utero surgical repair: ↓ need for shunting, ↓ Chiari 2 findings; may improve neurologic function
- Subsequent management of postoperative complications
  - Cord untethering, CSF diversion

DIAGNOSTIC CHECKLIST

Consider

- Open spinal dysraphisms are rarely imaged before repair postnatally
- Differentiation between MMC vs. MC is on prenatal imaging & has implications for fetal surgical approach
- Hindbrain herniation is seen in majority of open spinal dysraphisms after postnatal repair but not prenatal repair
- After repair, it cannot always be determined what type of spinal dysraphism was repaired (even open vs. closed spinal dysraphism) → must be correlated with clinical history

Image Interpretation Pearls

- Cord retethering is clinical diagnosis of exclusion as neural placode will always appear attached to operative site
  - Imaging is used to look for other complications causing symptoms, such as syrinx, arachnoid cyst, dermoid/epidermoid cyst

SELECTED REFERENCES

1. Nagaraj UD et al: Imaging of open spinal dysraphisms in the era of prenatal surgery. Pediatr Radiol. 50(13):1988-98, 2020
2. Nagaraj UD et al: Myelomeningocele versus myelocele on fetal MR images: are there differences in brain findings? AJR Am J Roentgenol. 211(6):1376-80, 2018
3. Nagaraj UD et al: Spinal imaging findings of open spinal dysraphisms on fetal and postnatal MRI. AJNR Am J Neuroradiol. 39(10):1947-52, 2018

Lipomyelomeningocele

KEY FACTS

TERMINOLOGY

- Subtype of closed (skin-covered) spinal dysraphism characterized by lipoma extending through dorsal defect
  - Neural placode of elongated spinal cord attaches to lipomatous tissue that is continuous with dorsal subcutaneous fat through spinal dysraphic defect, forming placode-lipoma interface
  - Lipomyelomeningocele/lipomyelocele (LMMC/LMC) spectrum: Placode-lipoma interface can be within (LMC) or protrude outside (LMMC) spinal canal

IMAGING

- Elongated spinal cord ends in neural placode attached dorsally to lipomatous tissue
  - ± subarachnoid space expansion around neural placode
- ± syrinx, split cord malformation, segmentation anomalies, caudal agenesis (group 2)
- Anorectal & GU tract malformations in 5-10%

TOP DIFFERENTIAL DIAGNOSES

- Other closed spinal dysraphisms
  - With subcutaneous mass: Meningocele, terminal myelocystocele
  - Without subcutaneous mass: Intradural lipoma, dorsal dermal sinus
- Open spinal dysraphisms: Myelomeningocele, myelocele
- Sacrococcygeal teratoma

DIAGNOSTIC CHECKLIST

- Terminology is not uniformly adhered to in general clinical practice; precise anatomic descriptions involving placode-lipoma interface may be most helpful
- Check surgical history; accurate characterization of any spinal dysraphism is made prior to surgery
- LMMC/LMC spectrum can coexist with other closed spinal dysraphisms
- Careful evaluation for associated anomalies

(Left) *Graphic of a lumbar lipomyelomeningocele (LMMC) shows elongation of the spinal cord into a fatty mass with the placode-lipoma interface ➡ located outside the spinal canal due to the posterior spinal dysraphism.* **(Right)** *Sagittal US in a newborn shows an elongated, nondependent spinal cord ➡ attached to echogenic lipomatous tissue ➡. The mass extends dorsally through dysraphic posterior elements, but the placode-lipoma interface ➡ remains in the spinal canal, consistent with a lipomyelocele (LMC).*

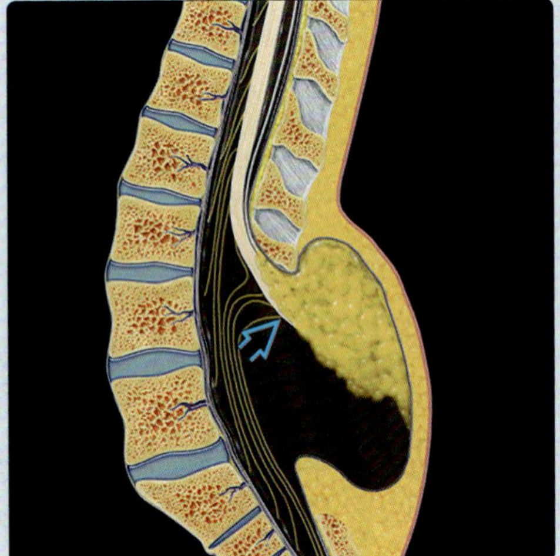

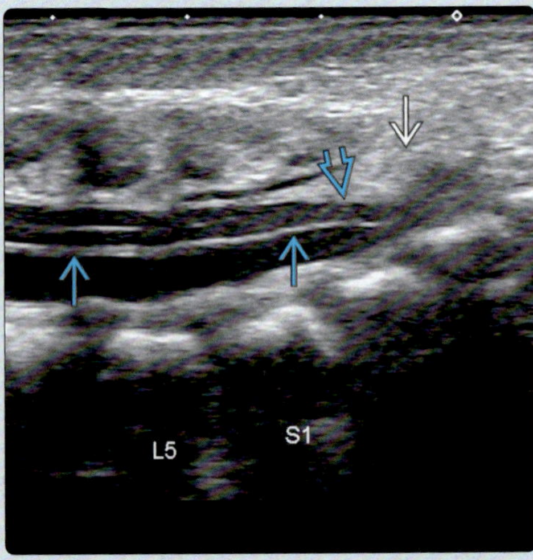

(Left) *Sagittal T1 MR of an 11-month-old with a LMMC/LMC lesion shows a low-lying conus attached to lipomatous tissue ➡ in direct communication with expanded subcutaneous fat through a spinal dysraphic defect.* **(Right)** *Sagittal T1 MR of an LMMC in a newborn shows a low-lying conus ➡ with the placode-lipoma interface ➡ extending dorsally through the deficient posterior elements. Associated sacral hypogenesis & coccygeal aplasia are noted ➡, consistent with group 2 caudal agenesis.*

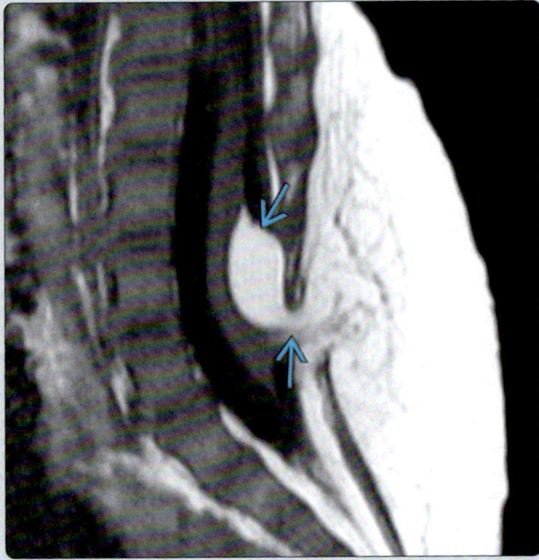

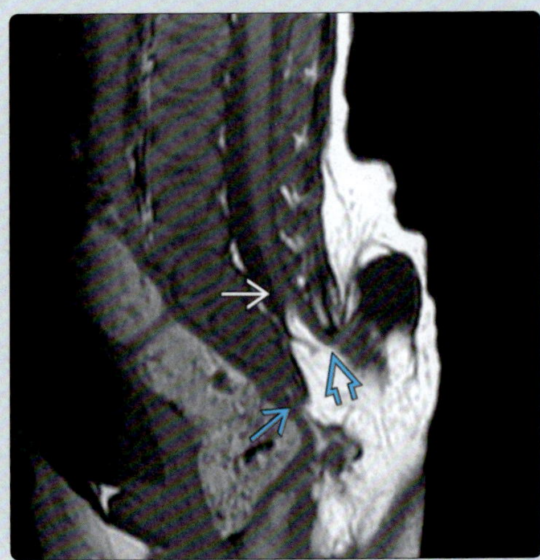

KEY FACTS

TERMINOLOGY

- Midline/paramidline subcutaneous sinus tract extending from skin surface toward spinal canal
- Located anywhere along neuraxis, from cranium to intergluteal cleft; most common location (~ 70%) is lumbosacral region above intergluteal cleft

IMAGING

- Linear, midline/paramidline, sagittal T1-hypointense tract in subcutaneous tissues
- Terminates anywhere from subcutaneous tissues (blind ending) to spine (epidural, intradural/intrathecal, or even intramedullary)
- ± (epi-)dermoid cysts along tract (~ 50%)
  - DWI or thin-section fluid-sensitive sequences are helpful for intrathecal mass visualization
- ± tethered cord with low-lying conus medullaris, intradural lipoma, or split cord malformation

TOP DIFFERENTIAL DIAGNOSES

- Coccygeal pit
- Pilonidal sinus/cyst
- (Epi-)dermoid without sinus tract
- Limited dorsal myeloschisis
- Lipomyelomeningocele (or other closed dysraphisms)

PATHOLOGY

- Closed spinal dysraphism due to incomplete disjunction of cutaneous & neural ectoderm at 3- to 8-weeks gestation

CLINICAL ISSUES

- Presentations include
  - Asymptomatic (incidentally noted skin dimple)
  - Infection (meningitis, abscess)
  - Neurologic deficits from cord tethering or compression
- Dorsal dermal sinus typically requires excision of entire tract
  - Intraspinal extension may be occult on imaging (necessitating operative exploration of dura)

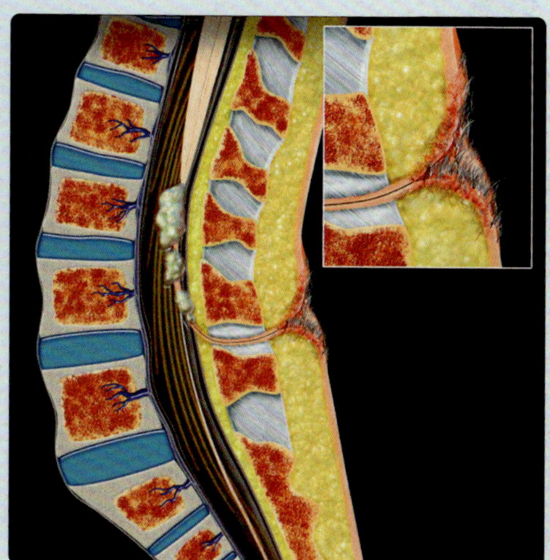

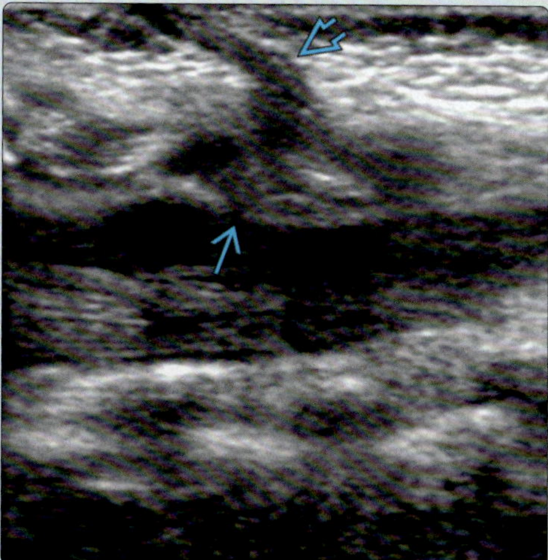

(Left) *Sagittal graphic shows a dermal sinus extending from the skin surface into the spinal canal to terminate with epidermoid cysts at the conus medullaris. In this case, the sinus opening is marked by a skin dimple with a hairy tuft & capillary stain.* **(Right)** *Sagittal ultrasound of the spine in an infant with a cutaneous lumbar dimple demonstrates a hypoechoic dorsal dermal sinus tract ⇨ in the subcutaneous tissues. A dural defect ⇨ confirms communication of the tract with the thecal sac & subarachnoid space.*

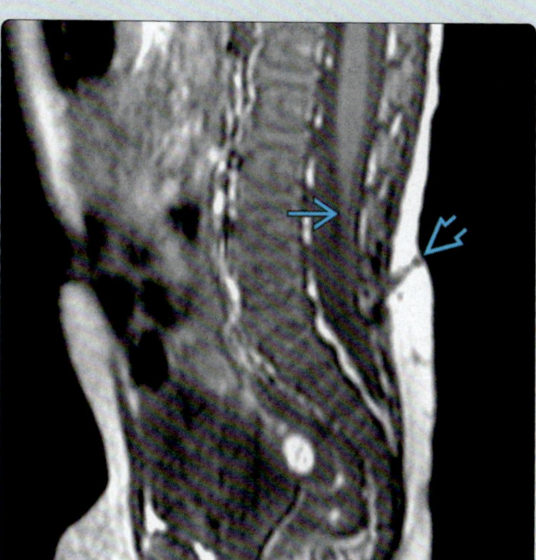

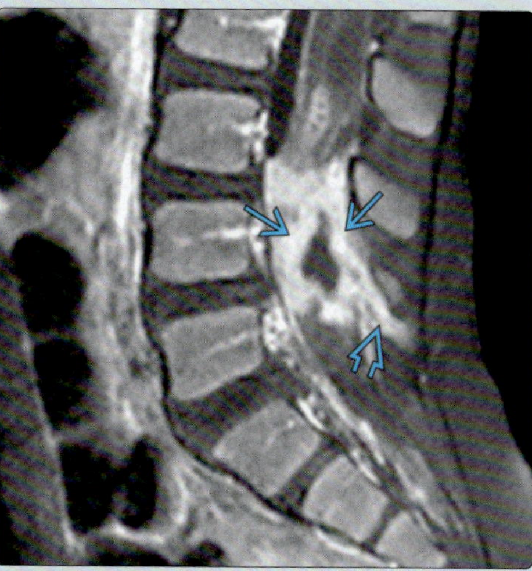

(Left) *Sagittal T1 MR in the same patient shows a hypointense dorsal dermal sinus tract ⇨ in the subcutaneous tissues. The conus medullaris ⇨ is low-lying at the L4 level. No associated intraspinal mass or cyst is identified.* **(Right)** *Sagittal T1 C+ FS MR in the same patient at 3 years of age demonstrates the interval development of a rim-enhancing intraspinal abscess ⇨. Note that there is also enhancement along the dorsal dermal sinus tract ⇨ as it enters the spinal canal.*

Caudal Regression

KEY FACTS

TERMINOLOGY

- Sacral agenesis, caudal agenesis, caudal dysplasia, caudal dysgenesis

IMAGING

- Congenital absence of portion of caudal spine, frequently in conjunction with spinal cord malformations
- Spectrum ranges in severity from isolated coccygeal aplasia to complete lumbosacral (& even lower thoracic) spine agenesis
- 2 main types
  - Group 1: High (L1 or higher), blunted distal spinal cord
    - "Double-bundle" nerve roots
    - More severe distal osseous anomalies
  - Group 2: Tapered, low-lying distal cord
    - Other signs of cord tethering: ↓ nerve root movement, intradural lipoma, thick filum
    - Less severe osseous anomalies
- Coexisting anorectal & genitourinary anomalies are common (group 1 > group 2)

TOP DIFFERENTIAL DIAGNOSES

- Tethered spinal cord
- Other closed spinal dysraphisms
- Occult intrasacral meningocele
- Currarino triad

CLINICAL ISSUES

- ~ 200x more common in infants of diabetic mothers
- Clinical spectrum from normal to severely impaired
- Group 2 patients are more likely to require neurosurgical intervention (cord detethering) than group 1
- Usually sporadic but can be seen in various syndromes
  - OEIS, VACTERL, Currarino triad

DIAGNOSTIC CHECKLIST

- Look for caudal spine anomalies in patients with genitourinary &/or anorectal malformations

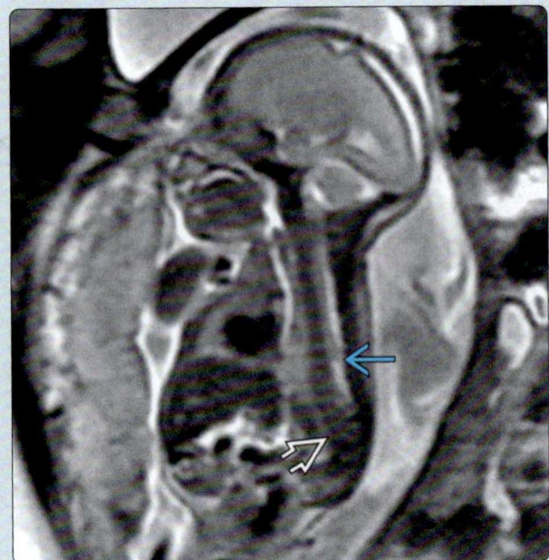

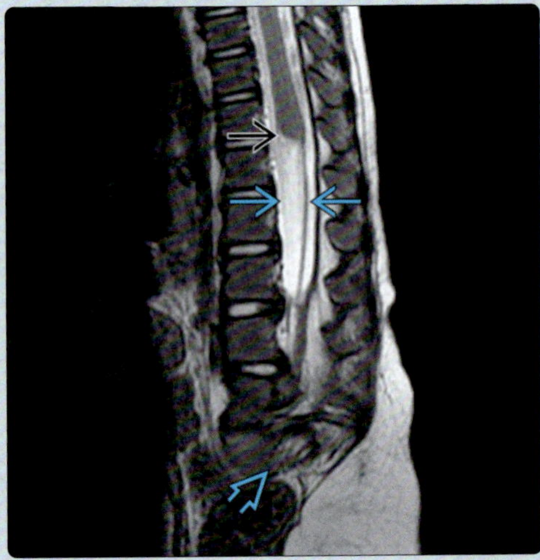

(Left) *Sagittal T2 SSFSE MR of a 24-weeks-gestation fetus with group 1 caudal regression shows absence of the sacrum with lumbar spine hypoplasia ➡ & a high, blunted conus ➡ terminating at the midthoracic spine. This fetus also had bilateral clubfeet (not shown).* **(Right)** *Sagittal T2 MR in an infant with group 1 caudal regression shows complete absence of the sacrum ➡, a blunted, wedge-shaped conus ➡, & a double-bundle appearance of the spinal nerve roots ➡ clumped anteriorly & posteriorly.*

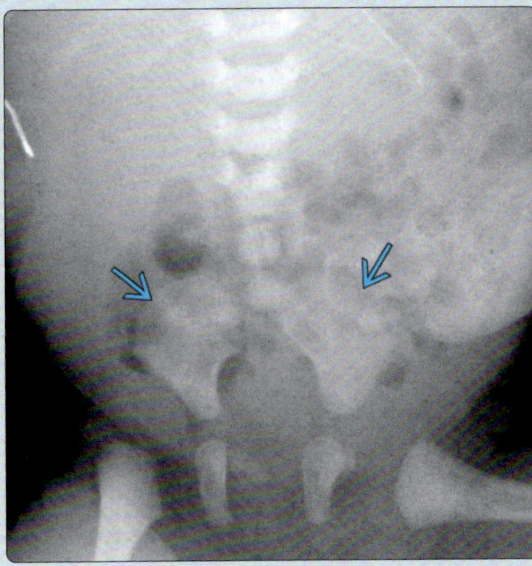

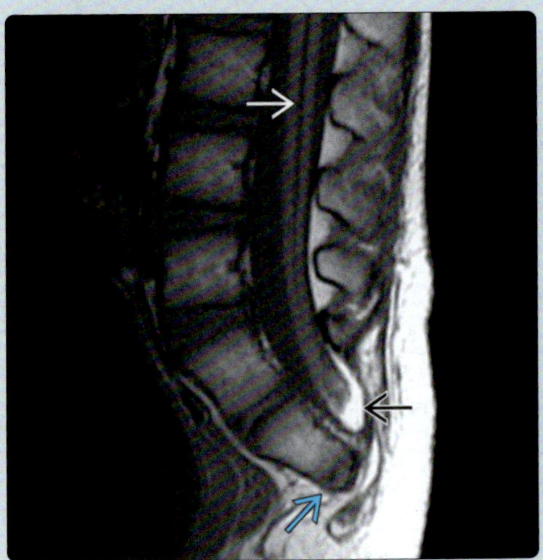

(Left) *AP radiograph in a newborn with group 1 caudal regression shows absence of the sacrum & medialization of the hypoplastic iliac bones ➡. There is also hypoplasia of L3-L5.* **(Right)** *Sagittal T1 MR in a 5-year-old patient with group 2 caudal regression shows absence of the lower sacrum & coccyx ➡ with elongation of the spinal cord (which terminates in an intradural lipoma ➡). Note the mild dilation of the central canal diffusely ➡. Group 2 is suggested by less severe osseus aplasia & an elongated tethered cord.*

Split Cord Malformation

KEY FACTS

TERMINOLOGY

- Traditional terms diastematomyelia & diplomyelia are out of favor as these entities remain difficult to differentiate

IMAGING

- Split cord malformation (SCM): Sagittal division of spinal cord into 2 hemicords
  - Hemicords have variable symmetry & may or may not unite below cleft
- Divided into 2 types
  - Type I SCM: 2 separate dural tubes, usually with bony/cartilaginous cleft
  - Type II SCM: Single dural sac, usually with thin, separating fibrous band
- Location is most commonly thoracolumbar (> 85%)
- Radiographs detect septum in < 50% of cases, may show widening of interpediculate distances
- ~ 85% of cases are associated with other spinal anomalies
  - Open or closed spinal dysraphisms
  - Hydromyelia, lipoma, dermal sinus, (epi-)dermoid, tethering adhesions (meningocele manqué)
  - Segmentation anomalies, kyphoscoliosis

PATHOLOGY

- Believed to be result of splitting of notochord/neural plate around abnormal adhesion between ectoderm & endoderm during gastrulation

CLINICAL ISSUES

- Usually presents in early childhood
  - Cutaneous stigmata on back in > 50%
    - Hypertrichosis (hairy patch) is most common
  - Progressive kyphoscoliosis in older children & adults
  - Orthopedic foot problems (~ 50%)
  - Bladder & bowel dysfunction
- Prophylactic surgery to prevent symptom progression, especially type I SCM
  - Resection of spur, lysis of adhesions, detethering

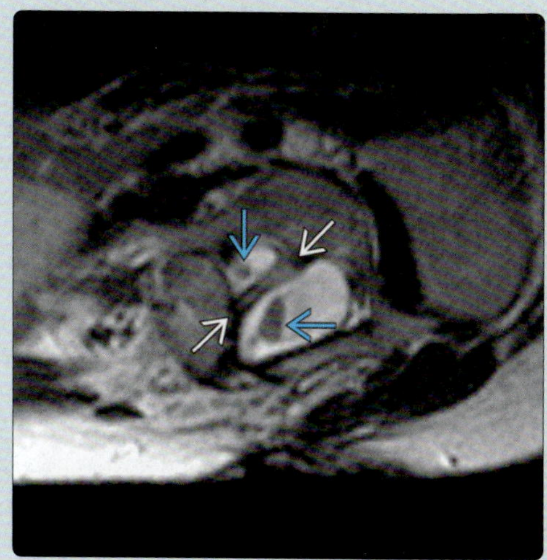

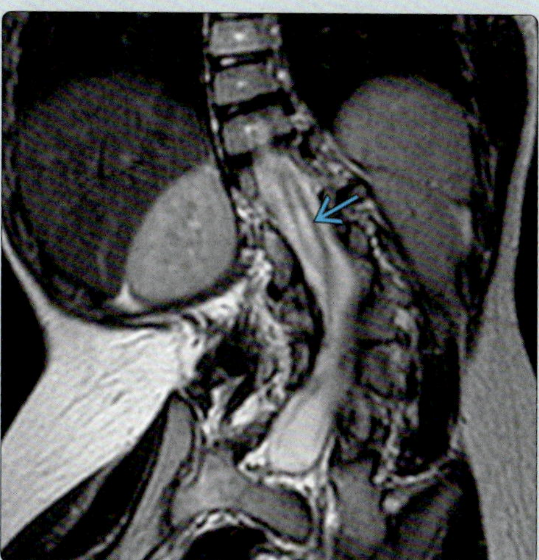

(Left) *Axial T2 MR in a 6-year-old girl with a type I split cord malformation (SCM) at the level of the midlumbar spine demonstrates 2 hemicords ⇒ within dural sacs that are separated by a bony spur ➡. The hemicords are asymmetric in size.* **(Right)** *Coronal T2 MR in the same patient demonstrates a spinal cord syrinx ⇒ above the level of the SCM. There is also marked left apex scoliosis. Associated abnormalities of the spinal cord (e.g., syrinx) & osseus spine (e.g., segmentation anomalies) are commonly seen with SCMs.*

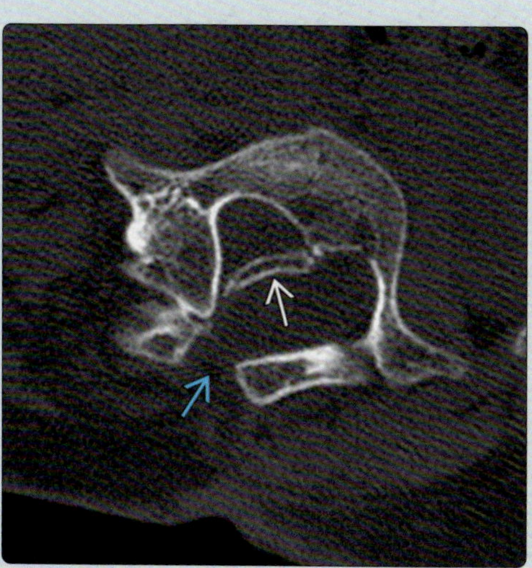

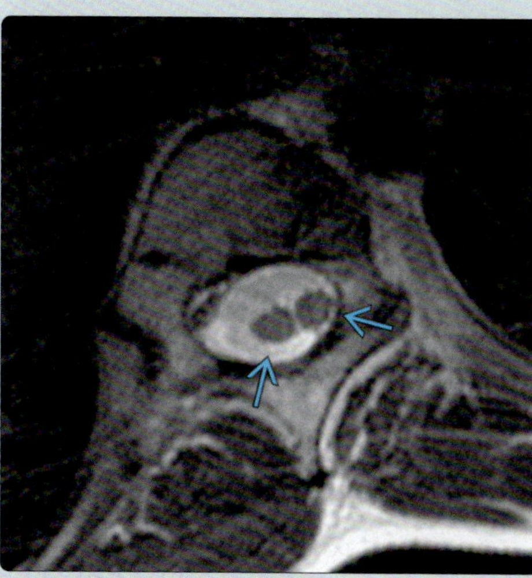

(Left) *Axial bone CT in the same patient with a type I SCM at the level of the midlumbar spine more clearly delineates the bony septum ➡ separating the 2 dural sacs. Also note the associated dorsal spinal dysraphism ⇒, a common finding that is present in up to 85% of SCMs.* **(Right)** *Axial T2 MR in a 10-year-old with congenital scoliosis & clinical signs of tethered cord shows 2 separate hemicords ⇒ of equal size within a single dural sac. Note the lack of a bony or fibrous septum in this type II SCM.*

Terminal Myelocystocele

KEY FACTS

IMAGING

- Closed (skin-covered) spinal dysraphism with bulging subcutaneous cystic mass
- Hydromyelic, low-lying spinal cord extends through osseous defect of lumbosacral spine into sac & attaches to subcutaneous fat
  - "Trumpet flaring" of distal cord
- ± T1-hyperintense lipoma or fatty thickening of sac wall (lipomyelocystocele), holocord syrinx, Chiari/hindbrain herniation (unlike other closed spinal dysraphisms)
- 3D SSFP MR images are helpful in diagnosis & delineating margins of terminal myelocystocele

TOP DIFFERENTIAL DIAGNOSES

- Meningocele
- Lipomyelomeningocele
- Other closed spinal dysraphisms
- Sacrococcygeal teratoma

PATHOLOGY

- Exact etiology is unclear; may be due to anomaly of caudal cell mass during secondary neurulation
- Associated malformations: OEIS [omphalocele, exstrophy (bladder/cloaca), imperforate anus, spinal anomalies], caudal agenesis (group 2), hindbrain herniation (not as common as seen in open spinal dysraphisms)

CLINICAL ISSUES

- Presents at birth with lumbosacral skin-covered mass
- Can have rapid neurologic deterioration early in life, more so than other closed spinal dysraphisms
- Early neurosurgical intervention is recommended

DIAGNOSTIC CHECKLIST

- Early diagnosis & surgery → best chance for normal neurological outcome
- Nonneurological prognosis is largely linked to severity of associated anomalies

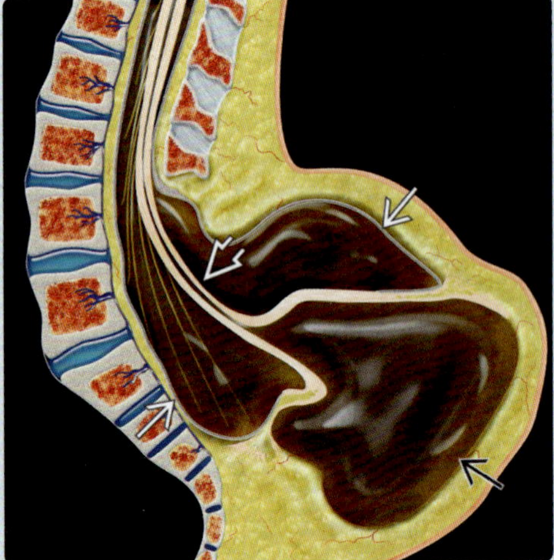

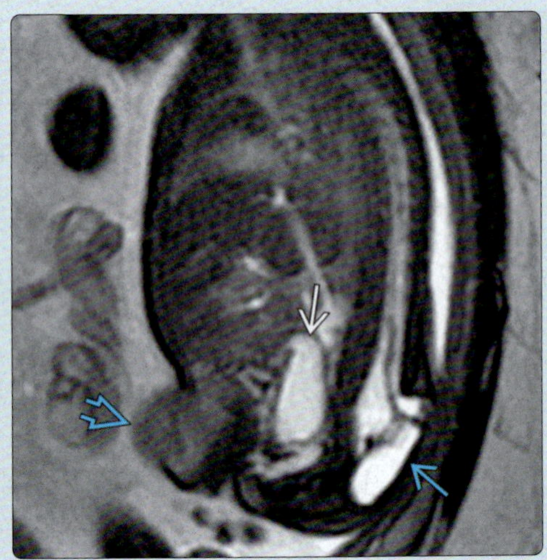

(Left) *Sagittal graphic displays a closed (skin-covered) dysraphism with a low-lying, hydromyelic spinal cord ➡ piercing an expanded subarachnoid space (meningocele ➡) & terminating in a myelocystocele ➡, which is in continuity with the central canal of the spinal cord.* **(Right)** *Sagittal SSFP MR of a fetus at 28-weeks-gestational age demonstrates a terminal myelocystocele ➡. There are additional findings of the OEIS complex, including a low omphalocele ➡ & a cloacal malformation ➡.*

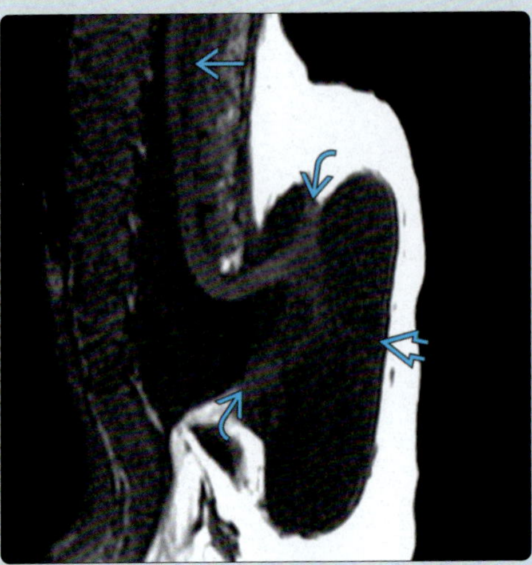

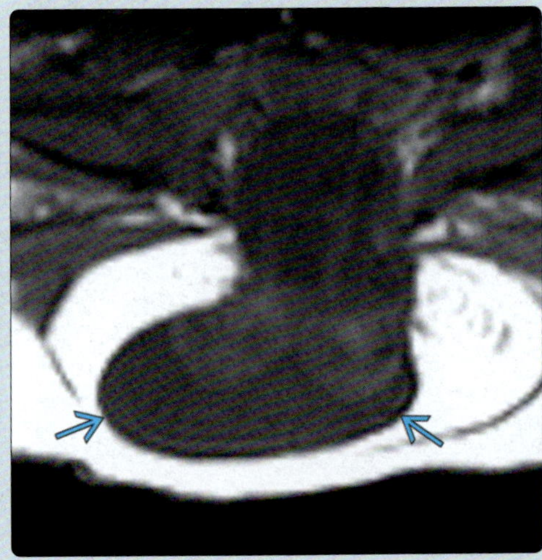

(Left) *Postnatal T1 MR in the same patient 11 weeks after delivery confirms the presence of a skin-covered terminal myelocystocele with splaying of the neural elements ➡ around a fluid collection ➡ that does not communicate with the surrounding subarachnoid space. There is also syringohydromyelia ➡.* **(Right)** *Axial T1 MR in the same patient shows the terminal myelocystocele ➡ located superficial & posterior to the spinal dysraphism. The terminal myelocystocele is covered by skin & fat.*

Neurenteric Cyst

KEY FACTS

TERMINOLOGY

- Cyst along neuraxis is lined with mucin-secreting cuboidal or columnar epithelium resembling alimentary tract
  - Derived from displaced endodermal tissue
- Synonyms: Enteric, enterogenous, or endodermal cyst

IMAGING

- Cyst along neuraxis (intraspinal/paraspinal) ± vertebral anomalies
  - Associated bony abnormalities in most cases
- Most are intradural extramedullary simple, unilocular cysts ventral to spinal cord
- Can be associated with other closed spinal dysraphisms
- ± associated fistulae & mediastinal/abdominal cysts

TOP DIFFERENTIAL DIAGNOSES

- Arachnoid cyst
- (Epi-)dermoid cyst
- Anterior spinal meningocele

PATHOLOGY

- Enteric & spinal structures are connected through persistent neurenteric canal (a.k.a. canal of Kovalevsky)
- Subgroup of split notochord syndrome spectrum
  - Sporadic or syndromic (Klippel-Feil, VACTERL, OEIS)
  - Associated with vertebral anomalies, split cord malformation, lipoma, dermal sinus tract, & tethered spinal cord

CLINICAL ISSUES

- Some are asymptomatic but most show progressive neurologic deterioration
- Best treatment (not always possible): Complete excision

DIAGNOSTIC CHECKLIST

- Location, size of cyst, degree of cord compression, & severity of associated anomalies determine prognosis
- Look for associated mediastinal or abdominal cysts, connecting fistulae, or vertebral anomalies

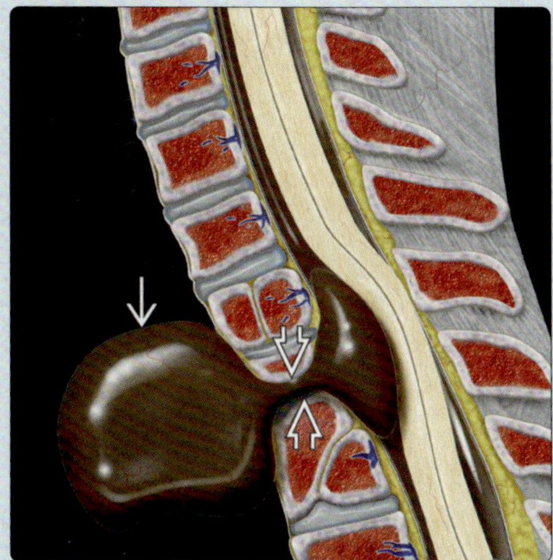

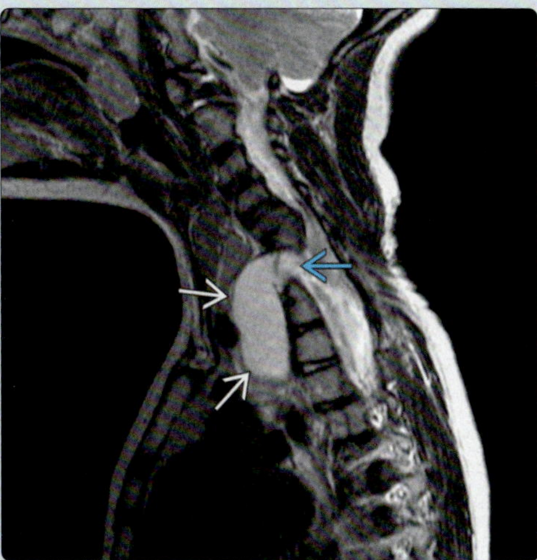

(Left) *Sagittal graphic shows a large mediastinal enteric cyst ➡ extending into the ventral spinal canal through a persistent neurenteric canal (a.k.a. canal of Kovalevsky) ⇨. There is dorsal displacement & compression of the thoracic spinal cord. Associated bony abnormalities are present in most cases.* **(Right)** *Sagittal T2 MR of a 3-year-old boy with a remote history of a high-spinal dysraphism repair shows a ventral dysraphic defect ⇨ of the lower cervical spine associated with a cyst in the paraspinal soft tissues ➡.*

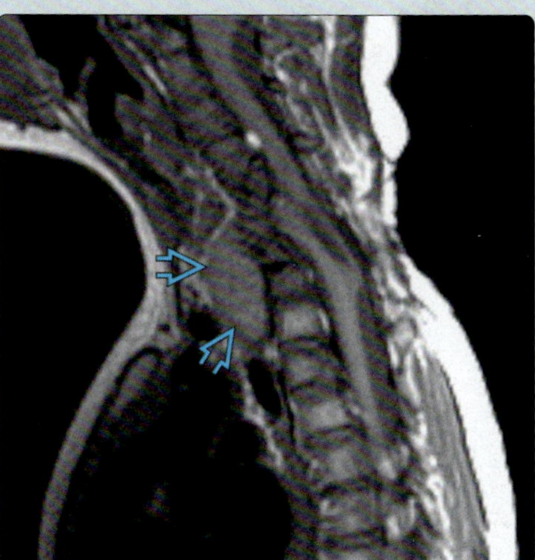

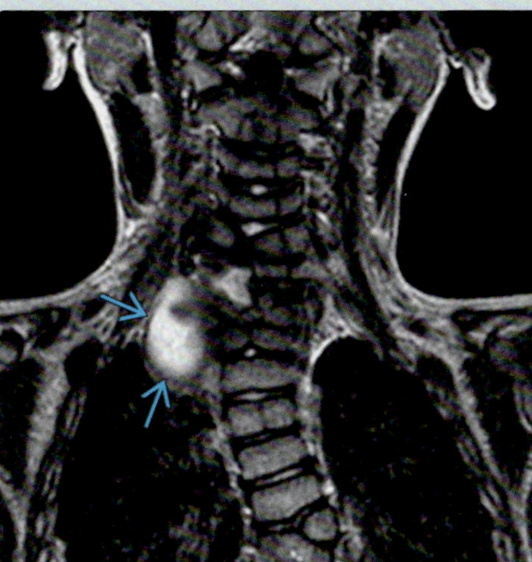

(Left) *Sagittal T1 MR in the same patient shows intermediate signal in the paraspinal cyst ⇨, hyperintense to CSF, making a neurenteric cyst the leading consideration. This was confirmed on pathology after resection.* **(Right)** *Coronal T2 MR in the same patient demonstrates the right paraspinal neurenteric cyst ⇨ with multiple adjacent segmentation anomalies at the cervicothoracic junction.*

KEY FACTS

TERMINOLOGY

- Hydromyelia: Cystic dilation of spinal cord central canal
- Syringomyelia: Cystic spinal cord cavity not contiguous with central canal

IMAGING

- Overlap between incidental (nonprogressive) & pathologic central canal dilation
- Incidental/nonprogressive central canal dilation may be up to 4 mm
  - True syrinx is associated with cord expansion
- Extent & morphology are best demonstrated on T2
  - Axial plane is most reliable for diameter measurement
- Volumetric/3D sequences may demonstrate adhesions
- Give contrast to look for underlying lesion if atypical features are present
  - Not needed in vast majority of cases

PATHOLOGY

- Central canal of spinal cord transmits CSF in rostral direction toward obex
- Lesions obstructing both central canal & subarachnoid space (SAS) → syrinx
  - Tumor, inflammation
  - Chiari malformation
- Congenital anomalies (frequent in children)
  - Chiari 1 malformation (not always congenital)
    - 10-15% of children with Chiari 1 present with syrinx
    - Combination of scoliosis + Chiari 1 is associated with larger cavities
  - Chiari 2 malformation

CLINICAL ISSUES

- Those associated with underlying malformations (Chiari 1 or 2, tethering lesions) are more likely to progress
- Suboccipital decompression can reverse/resolve syrinx associated with Chiari malformations

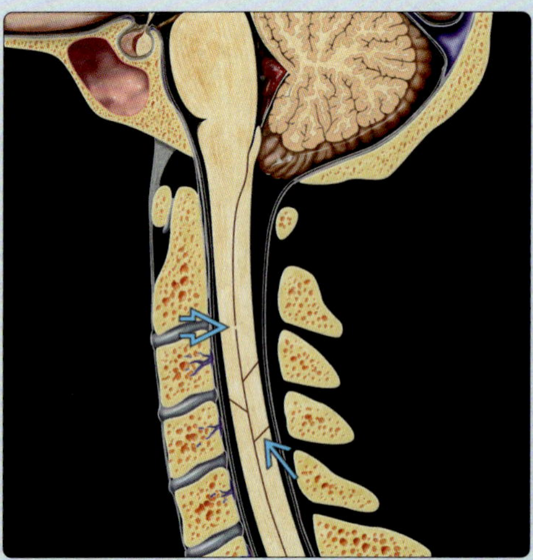

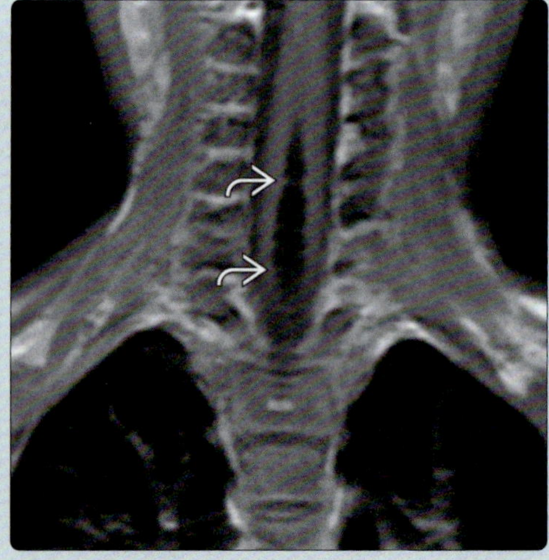

(Left) *Sagittal graphic shows that the normal central canal has multiple small obstructions* ➡ *but also small channels* ➡ *that lead from the central canal to the subarachnoid space. As a result, CSF flow must be impeded in both compartments for a syrinx to develop. Small obstructions may serve the same function as venous valves in the lower extremities, directing CSF flow cephalad to the obex.* **(Right)** *Coronal T1 MR shows resulting pseudohaustrations* ➡ *in a syrinx.*

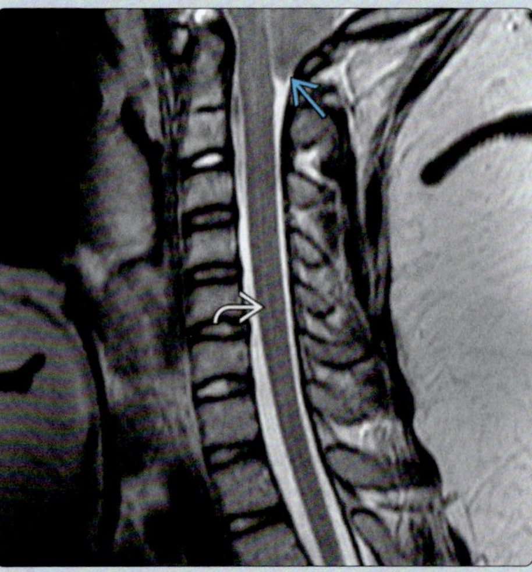

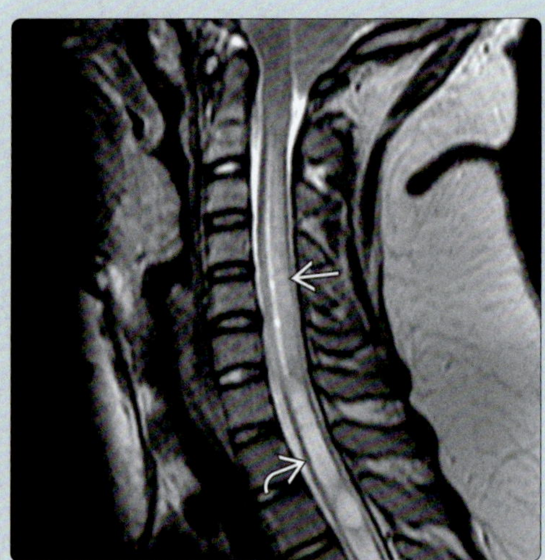

(Left) *Sagittal T2 MR in a teenager with a Chiari 1 malformation* ➡ *of the craniocervical junction shows that the central canal* ➡ *is barely visible.* **(Right)** *Sagittal T2 MR obtained 14 months later in the same patient because of right arm pain when sneezing shows development of a syrinx at the cervicothoracic junction* ➡ *with dilation of the central canal cephalad & extensive presyrinx edema in the cervical cord* ➡*. Subsequent suboccipital decompression resulted in complete resolution of the syrinx.*

TERMINOLOGY

Definitions

- Hydromyelia: Cystic dilation of spinal cord central canal
- Syringomyelia: Cystic spinal cord cavity not contiguous with central canal
- Syringohydromyelia: Features of both syringomyelia & hydromyelia
- Syringobulbia: Extension of syrinx/cavity into brainstem
- "Presyrinx" state: Reversible spinal cord edema produced by alterations in CSF flow dynamics

IMAGING

General Features

- Location
  - Intramedullary spinal cord
  - Typically centrally located on axial images
    - Off-midline location is of ↑ concern for neoplastic, traumatic, or inflammatory etiology
  - Thoracic > cervicothoracic > cervical
- Size
  - Cavity diameter: Small → markedly dilated
    - Overlap between incidental (nonprogressive) & pathologic, central canal dilation
      - Incidental/nonprogressive central canal dilation may be up to 4 mm
      - True syrinx is associated with cord expansion
  - Cavity length: Ranges from short segment (1 or 2 levels) to holocord
- Morphology
  - CSF-filled cavity in spinal cord
    - May have flow artifact (seen in larger lesions)
    - May be septated & lobulated or smooth & simple

MR Findings

- T2WI
  - Hyperintense, cystic, intramedullary cavity ± adjacent gliosis, myelomalacia
  - ± flow artifact with poorly defined, heterogeneously hypointense signal throughout larger cavities
  - ± adhesions on 3D/volumetric sequences
- T1WI C+
  - Simple syrinx does not enhance; enhancement suggests inflammatory or neoplastic lesion

Imaging Recommendations

- Protocol advice
  - Extent & morphology are best demonstrated on T2
    - Axial plane is most reliable for diameter measurement
  - Volumetric/3D sequences may demonstrate adhesions
  - Give contrast to look for underlying lesion if atypical features are present
    - Not needed in vast majority of cases

PATHOLOGY

General Features

- Etiology
  - Central canal of spinal cord transmits CSF in rostral direction toward obex
    - Normal canal has multiple sites of obstruction/adhesion/collapse (↑ with age)
      - May function like valves in venous system
    - Multiple microscopic channels lead from canal to subarachnoid space (SAS)
      - Similar to perivascular spaces in brain
      - Allow CSF to be driven into canal from SAS
    - Lesions obstructing both central canal & SAS → syrinx
      - Tumor, inflammation
      - Chiari malformation
    - Posttraumatic or postinflammatory myelomalacia can also cause cavitation
      - Analogous to porencephaly in brain
- Associated abnormalities
  - Congenital anomalies (frequent in children)
    - Chiari 1 malformation (not always congenital)
      - 10-15% of children with Chiari 1 present with syrinx
      - May develop syrinx over time
      - Combination of scoliosis + Chiari 1 is associated with larger cavities
    - Chiari 2 malformation
  - Scoliosis
  - Tumors
    - Up to 45% of primary spinal cord tumors have syrinx at presentation
      - More common in adults than children

CLINICAL ISSUES

Presentation

- Distal upper extremity weakness, gait instability
- Cloak-like pain & temperature sensory loss
  - Shock-like pain with Valsalva (sneezing)
- May be asymptomatic

Natural History & Prognosis

- Variable; dependent on underlying etiology
  - Those associated with underlying malformations (Chiari 1 or 2, tethering lesions) are more likely to progress

Treatment

- Suboccipital decompression can reverse/resolve syrinx associated with Chiari malformations

DIAGNOSTIC CHECKLIST

Image Interpretation Pearls

- Do not label central canal of 1- to 2-mm diameter as syrinx
- Simple syringomyelia does not require contrast
  - Give contrast for associated cord signal abnormalities, complex morphology, focal mass, or off-midline location

SELECTED REFERENCES

1. Kurzbuch AR et al: Iatrogenic syringomyelia postcranial surgery in pediatric patients: systematic review and illustrative case. Childs Nerv Syst. 37(9):2879-90, 2021
2. Heiss JD et al: Origin of syrinx fluid in syringomyelia: a physiological study. Neurosurgery. 84(2):457-68, 2019
3. Holly LT et al: Chiari malformation and syringomyelia. J Neurosurg Spine. 31(5):619-28, 2019
4. Jones BV: Cord cystic cavities: syringomyelia and prominent central canal. Semin Ultrasound CT MR. 38(2):98-104, 2017
5. Rodriguez A et al: Management of idiopathic pediatric syringohydromyelia. J Neurosurg Pediatr. 16(4):452-7, 2015

KEY FACTS

IMAGING

- Best clue: Low-lying conus medullaris
  - May have thickened filum terminale ± fatty infiltration or lipomatous mass
  - Accompanied by clinical signs & symptoms of tethering
    - Lower extremity weakness, spasticity, & ↓ sensation; abnormal gait; bladder dysfunction
- General imaging features
  - Conus below L2-L3 disc level
  - May appear taut or directly apposed to dorsal thecal sac
    - Lack of conus motion with CSF pulsations
    - Lack of dependent ventral shift of conus when prone
  - Filum > 2 mm thick (at L5-S1 on axial/transverse images)
    - ± echogenic (US) or T1 (MR) bright fatty mass at conus
    - ± bony/soft tissue dysraphism
- Ultrasound to screen infants (< 6 months old) at ↑ risk of spinal anomalies (as suggested by certain cutaneous stigmata or associated systemic anomalies)
- MR to define underlying anomalies for surgical planning in symptomatic patients

PATHOLOGY

- Cutaneous stigmata in up to 50%
  - Hairy patch, hemangioma, skin tag, atypical dimple
- Tethering also found in clinically apparent open & closed spinal dysraphisms
- Tethered filum is histologically abnormal
  - ↑ connective tissue with dense collagen fibers, hyalinization, & dilated capillaries

CLINICAL ISSUES

- Tethered cord syndrome: Clinical diagnosis; imaging in specific screening circumstances or to detect associated anomalies for surgical planning
- Symptomatic presentation is most common during rapid growth (4-8 years of age & adolescent growth spurt)
- Majority show improvement or stabilization of neurologic deficits following surgical untethering

(Left) *Sagittal 3D SSFP MR in a 6-month-old with bilateral clubfeet & multiple segmentation anomalies ➡ shows a taut & thickened filum terminale ➡ tethering the conus medullaris, which terminates at the level of L3.* **(Right)** *Sagittal T2 MR in a 4-year-old with a sacral dimple shows an intradural lipoma tethering the conus medullaris at the level of L3. Note the chemical shift artifact ➡ at the junction of the lipoma & the conus.*

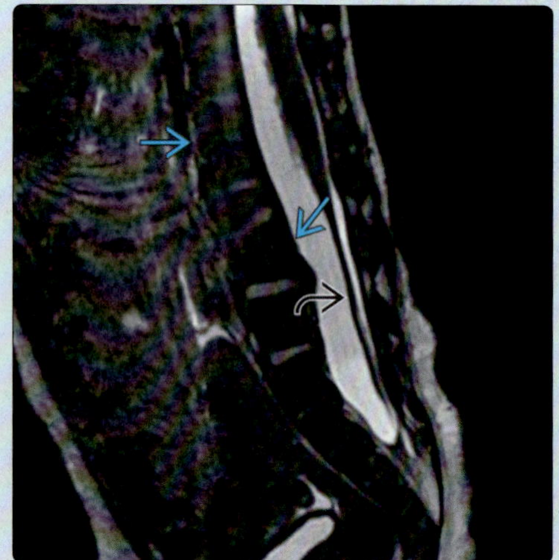

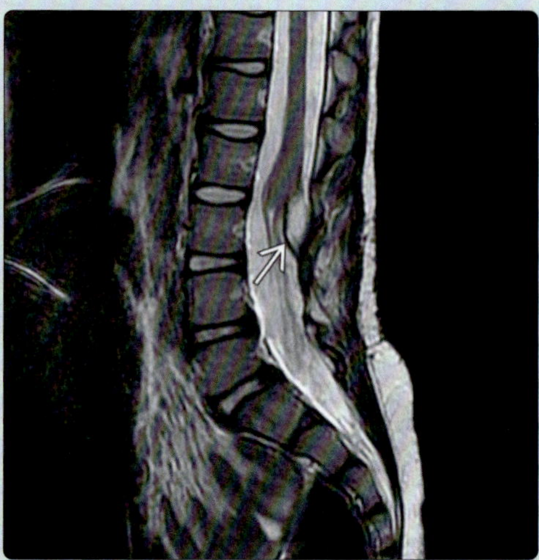

(Left) *Sagittal T1 MR in an 18-month-old with motor delay, ↑ lower extremity tone, & plantar flexion shows fatty infiltration of the filum terminale ➡ (filar fibrolipoma), which is adherent to the dorsal aspect of the lumbar canal.* **(Right)** *Sagittal T1 MR in the same patient after surgical tethered cord release shows the slightly retracted distal limb of the sectioned filum ➡, now fallen away from the dorsal canal.*

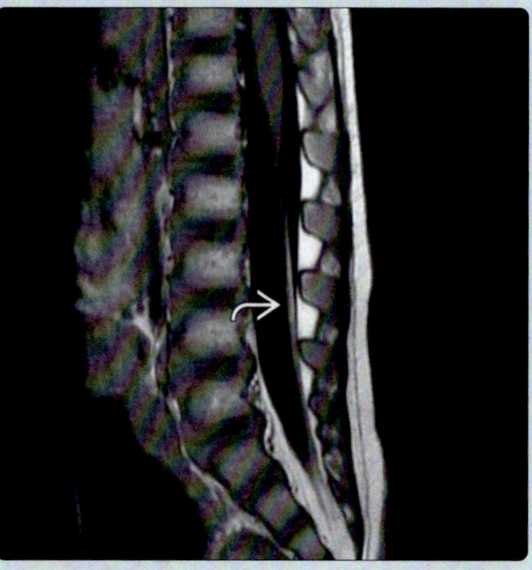

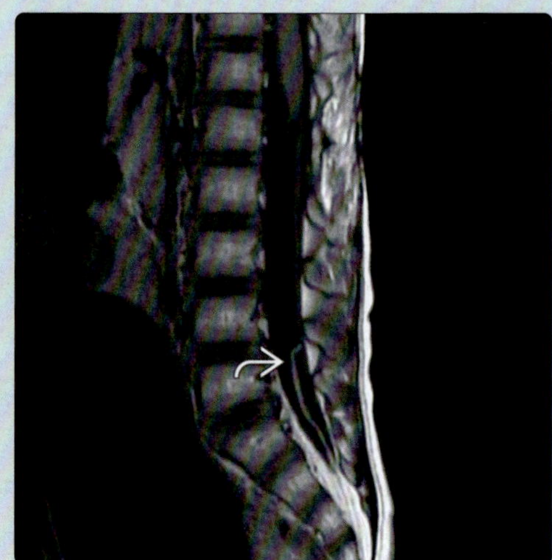

KEY FACTS

TERMINOLOGY

- 2016 WHO CNS tumor classification designation
- Low-grade glioneuronal tumor that presents with diffuse leptomeningeal dissemination

IMAGING

- Best clue: Diffuse leptomeningeal neoplastic disease without identifiable primary tumor
- Hydrocephalus in ~ 30%
- Location: 73% intracranial, 62% intraspinal
- Leptomeningeal thickening & enhancement
- ± leptomeningeal nonenhancing cystic foci
- ± nonenhancing intramedullary spinal lesions
- Best imaging: MR with contrast of entire neuraxis

TOP DIFFERENTIAL DIAGNOSES

- Chronic infection
  - Tuberculosis
  - Neurocysticercosis (especially racemose type)
- Leptomeningeal metastatic disease
- Vascular disease (e.g., Sturge-Weber syndrome)
- Neurosarcoidosis
- Neurocutaneous melanosis

PATHOLOGY

- Low-grade neoplasm of neuronal & glial populations with propensity for leptomeningeal dissemination
- Commonly show *BRAF* mutations

CLINICAL ISSUES

- Headache, seizures, cranial nerve dysfunction
- Variable prognosis with typical slow tumor growth
- No optimal evidence-based treatment strategy

DIAGNOSTIC CHECKLIST

- Consider in young patient with diffuse leptomeningeal disease, no primary tumor, & no clinical signs of infection

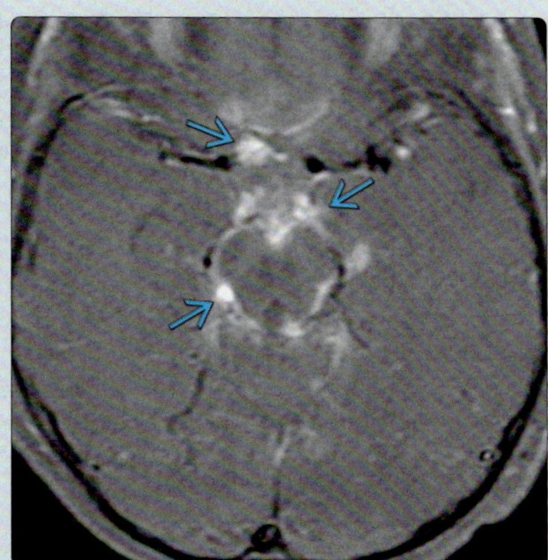

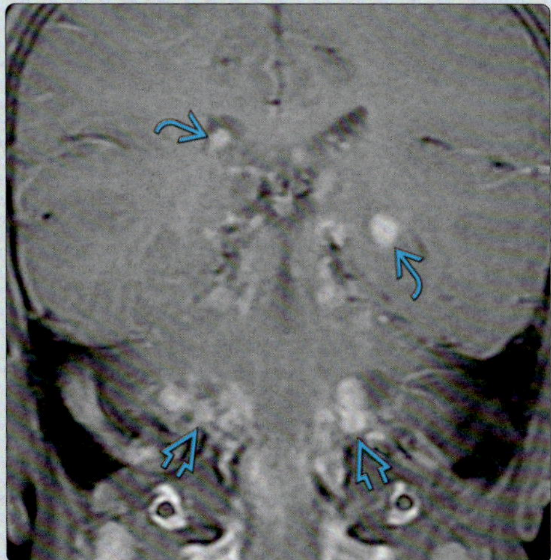

(Left) *Axial T1 C+ FS MR in a 6-year-old who presented years earlier with hydrocephalus of unknown etiology, later diagnosed with diffuse leptomeningeal glioneuronal tumor (DLGNT), shows extensive leptomeningeal enhancement & nodularity ➡ in the basilar cisterns, which is the most common area of intracranial involvement in DLGNT.* **(Right)** *Coronal T1 C+ FS MR in the same patient shows the heaviest burden of leptomeningeal disease in the inferior cerebellar regions ➡ with intraventricular disease ➡ as well.*

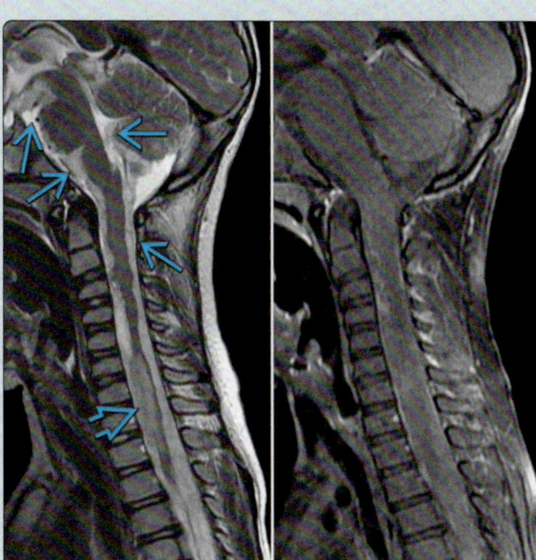

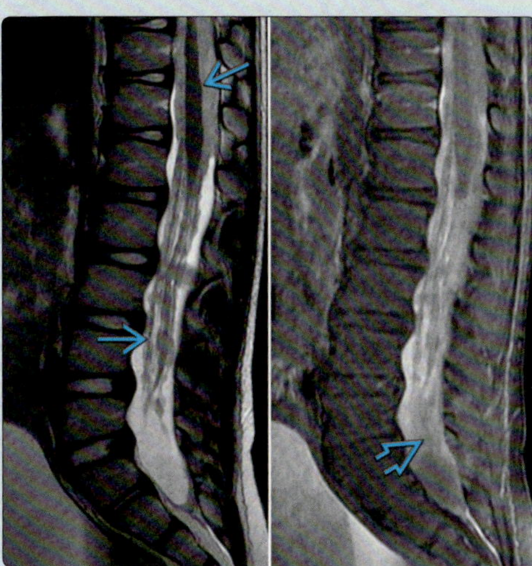

(Left) *Sagittal T2 (left) & T1 C+ FS (right) MR images in a 5-year-old with headaches & abnormal gait show extensive leptomeningeal disease ➡ within the posterior fossa & spine. Also note the sizable intramedullary lesion ➡ at the cervicothoracic junction, a finding seen in ~ 20% of DLGNT cases.* **(Right)** *Sagittal T2 (left) & T1 C+ FS (right) MR images in the same patient show disease ➡ along the distal cord & cauda equina. In cases of DLGNT with large tumor burden, contrast may leak into the thecal sac ➡, as in this case.*

Spinal Cord Ependymoma

KEY FACTS

TERMINOLOGY

- Spinal cord neoplasm arising from ependymal cells

IMAGING

- Heterogeneous, intramedullary spinal cord mass
- Cervicothoracic, filum/conus
  - Most are intramedullary
  - Myxopapillary tumors are found at conus medullaris & arising from filum terminale
- Heterogeneous but mostly hyperintense on T2
  - Hemorrhage & cysts are common

TOP DIFFERENTIAL DIAGNOSES

- Astrocytoma
  - Less heterogeneous than ependymoma
  - Indistinct margins
- Cavernous malformation
- Hemangioblastoma

PATHOLOGY

- Most are WHO grade 2
  - 4 subtypes: Cellular, papillary, clear cell, tanycytic
- Myxopapillary are WHO grade 1
- Rare WHO grade 3: Anaplastic ependymoma
  - *MYCN* amplification is associated with anaplastic features, aggressive clinical behavior
- At least 1/3 of those with NF2 will eventually develop spinal cord ependymoma

CLINICAL ISSUES

- Neck or back pain, progressive paraparesis, paresthesias
- 2nd most common primary spinal cord tumor in children
- Prognosis of grade 1 & 2 tumors is largely dependent upon extent of resection
  - Most series report 5- & 10-year survival rates of 50-100% following combination of both surgery & postoperative radiation treatment

(Left) *Sagittal T2 MR in a 16-year-old with 2 weeks of back pain after minor trauma shows a complex hemorrhagic mass ➡ at the base of the cauda equina, consistent with the eventual histologic diagnosis of myxopapillary ependymoma.* **(Right)** *Sagittal T1 C+ FS MR in a teenager with NF2 shows a bilobed enhancing intramedullary mass, confirmed to be an ependymoma (grade 2). Any intramedullary cord tumor in NF2 is presumed to be an ependymoma, & they are diagnosed in at least 1/3 of those with NF2.*

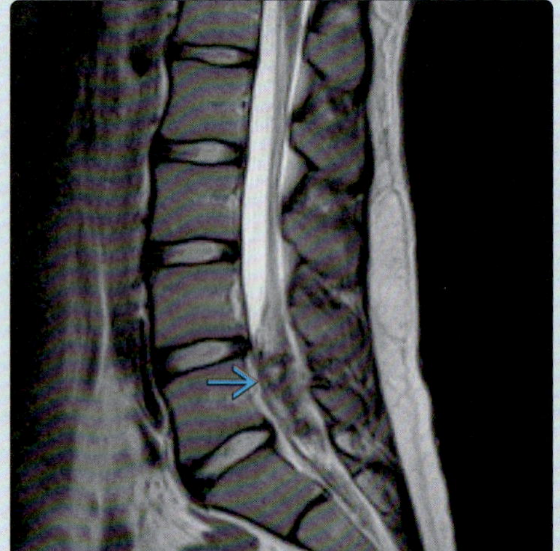

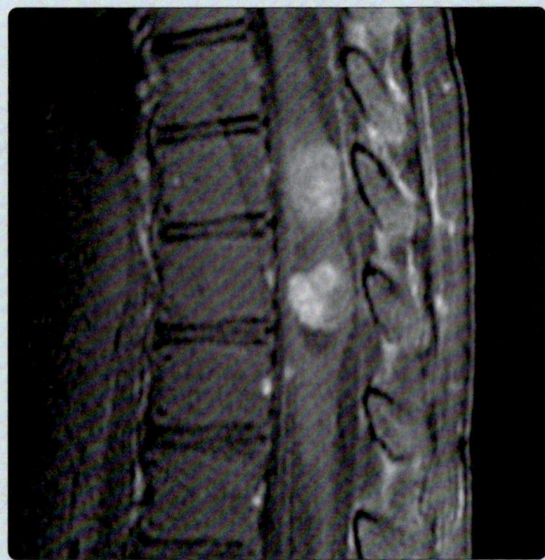

(Left) *Sagittal T2 MR in a 13-year-old presenting with neck/back pain & subsequent gait abnormalities shows a well-defined, exophytic tumor ➡ at the cervicothoracic junction, with internal cysts.* **(Right)** *Sagittal T1 C+ FS MR in the same patient shows diffuse & heterogeneous enhancement of the tumor ➡, which was an anaplastic ependymoma (grade 3) at surgery. Most spinal ependymomas are grade 1 or 2 lesions; higher grades are seen in < 10% of cases.*

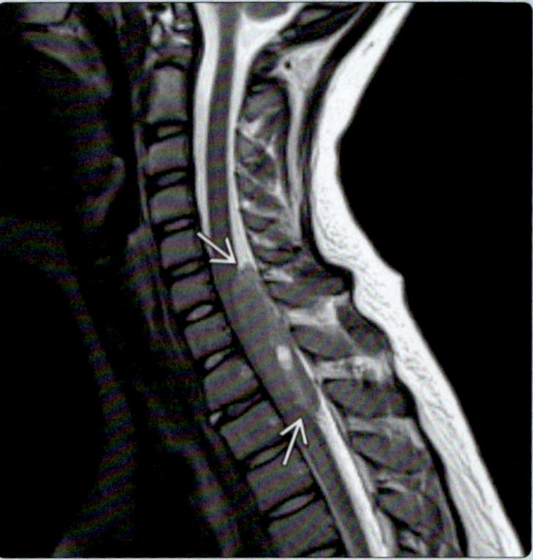

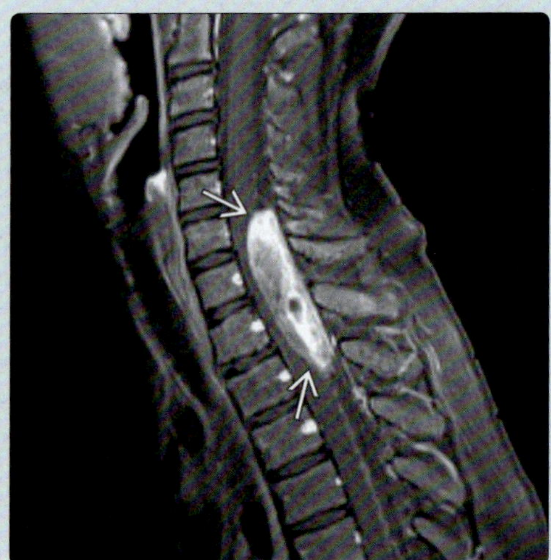

TERMINOLOGY

Definitions

- Spinal cord neoplasm arising from ependymal cells

IMAGING

General Features

- Best diagnostic clue
  - Heterogeneous, intramedullary spinal cord mass
- Location
  - Cervicothoracic, filum/conus
  - Most are intramedullary
    - Myxopapillary tumors are found at conus medullaris, arising from filum terminale
      - More frequent in adults
- Morphology
  - Well circumscribed
  - May have exophytic component
- Typical MR features
  - Isointense to hypointense on T1
  - Heterogeneous but mostly hyperintense on T2
    - May have cystic foci
      - May be within tumor, at rostral & caudal margins, or due to reactive syrinx
  - Hemorrhagic foci in or at margins of tumor
  - Heterogeneous enhancement

Imaging Recommendations

- Best imaging tool
  - Sagittal & axial T2 & T1 C+

DIFFERENTIAL DIAGNOSIS

Astrocytoma

- Most common primary cord neoplasm in children
- Less heterogeneous than ependymoma
  - Hemorrhage & cysts are less common
- Often larger, can be holocord
- Indistinct margins

Cavernous Malformation

- Focal hemorrhagic lesion
- Little or no enhancement
- Rare below cervical cord

Hemangioblastoma

- Older patients
- 1/3 with von Hippel-Lindau disease
- Cyst with enhancing, highly vascular nodule
  - Flow voids may be present

Multiple Sclerosis

- Often multifocal; 90% have brain lesions
- Lesions are more often peripheral, posterolateral
- Typically < 2 vertebral segments in length
- < 1/2 cross-sectional area of cord involved on axial images

Idiopathic Transverse Myelitis

- Cord expansion is less pronounced
- Less well defined
- Diagnosis of exclusion

Cord Infarction

- Sudden onset of symptoms
- Central gray matter is typically involved

Cord Contusion

- History of trauma

PATHOLOGY

General Features

- Genetics
  - Different from intracranial ependymoma

Staging, Grading, & Classification

- Most are WHO grade 2
- Myxopapillary are WHO grade 1
- Rare WHO grade 3: Anaplastic ependymoma

Microscopic Features

- Arises from ependymal cells of central canal
- 4 subtypes (grade 2): Cellular, papillary, clear cell, tanycytic
  - Cellular is most common intramedullary tumor subtype
  - *MYCN* amplification is associated with anaplastic features, aggressive clinical behavior
  - H3K27me3 may predict better prognosis

CLINICAL ISSUES

Presentation

- Neck or back pain, progressive paraparesis, paresthesias
- Delay in diagnosis is due to slow growth

Demographics

- Epidemiology
  - 2nd most common primary spinal cord tumor in children
  - 30% of all ependymomas are spinal
  - At least 1/3 of those with neurofibromatosis type 2 (NF2) will eventually develop spinal cord ependymoma

Treatment

- Prognosis of grade 1 & 2 tumors is largely dependent upon extent of resection
  - Gross total resection in > 85% of cases
- Radiation for subtotal resection, grade 3, or recurrent disease
- Chemotherapy for failed surgery & radiotherapy
- Most series report 5- & 10-year survival rates of 50-100% following combination of both surgery & postoperative radiation treatment

SELECTED REFERENCES

1. Han Z et al: Prognostic value of H3K27me3 in children with ependymoma. Pediatr Blood Cancer. 67(3):e28121, 2020
2. Abdallah A et al: Long-term surgical resection outcomes of pediatric myxopapillary ependymoma: experience of two centers and brief literature review. World Neurosurg. 136:e245-61, 2019
3. Swanson AA et al: Spinal cord ependymomas with MYCN amplification show aggressive clinical behavior. J Neuropathol Exp Neurol. 78(9):791-7, 2019
4. Celano E et al: Spinal cord ependymoma: a review of the literature and case series of ten patients. J Neurooncol. 128(3):377-86, 2016
5. Plotkin SR et al: Spinal ependymomas in neurofibromatosis Type 2: a retrospective analysis of 55 patients. J Neurosurg Spine. 14(4):543-7, 2011

Spinal Cord Astrocytoma

KEY FACTS

IMAGING

- Cervical > thoracic > lumbar locations
- Oblong, fusiform expansion of cord
  - 40% have tumor cysts or syringohydromyelia
- Variable enhancement
  - Pilocytic tumors (WHO grade 1) typically enhance avidly
  - Diffuse astrocytomas (WHO grade 2) typically have minimal, if any, enhancement

TOP DIFFERENTIAL DIAGNOSES

- Transverse myelitis
  - Similar imaging features
- Ganglioglioma
  - Similar imaging features
- Ependymoma
  - Less common in children than adults
- Multiple sclerosis
  - Short-segment lesions involving < 1/2 of cord cross section

PATHOLOGY

- 75-80% are low grade
  - Pilocytic astrocytoma = WHO grade 1
    - Rosenthal fibers
  - Diffuse astrocytoma = WHO grade 2
    - ↑ cellularity, variable atypia/mitoses
- 20-25% are high grade
  - Anaplastic astrocytomas = WHO grade 3
    - Dispersed anaplasia
  - Glioblastoma = WHO grade 4
    - Microvascular proliferation & palisading necrosis
  - Diffuse midline glioma = WHO grade 4
    - K27M mutation in histone 3

CLINICAL ISSUES

- Most common spinal cord tumor in children
- Survival varies with tumor histology/grade & degree of tumor resection; 80% 5-year survival for low grade

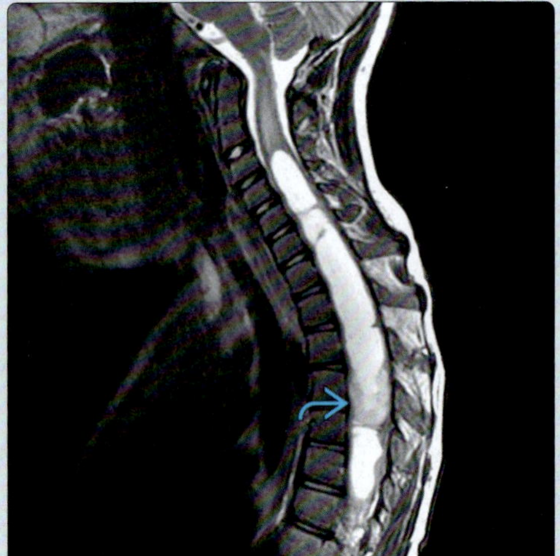

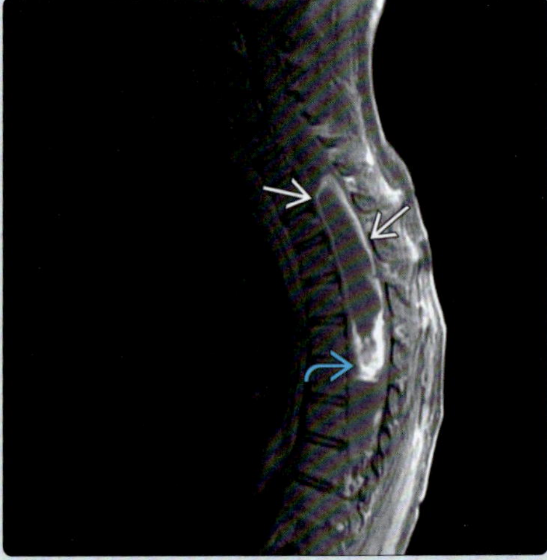

(Left) *Sagittal T2 MR in an 11-year-old with back pain & scoliosis shows a complex, intramedullary cyst in the cervicothoracic cord. Note the solid tissue ➲ at the caudal aspect of the lesion.* **(Right)** *Sagittal T1 C+ FS MR in the same patient demonstrates avid enhancement of the solid portions of the lesion ➲ as well as the walls of the cyst ➡. Surgery confirmed a pilocytic astrocytoma (WHO grade 1).*

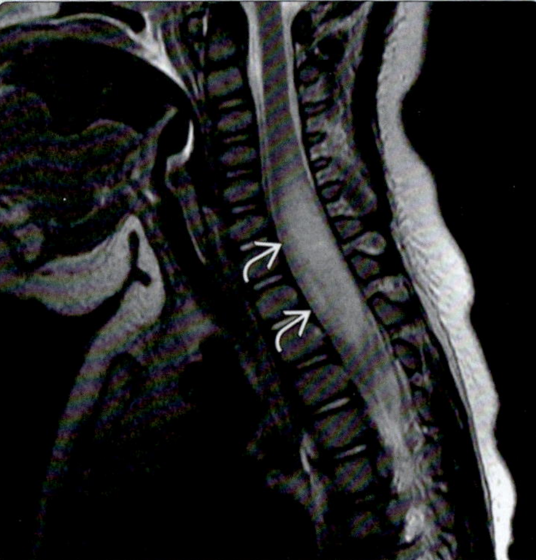

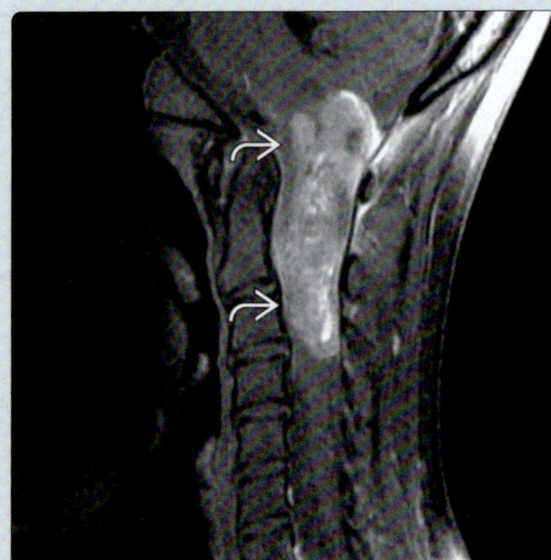

(Left) *Sagittal T2 MR in an infant initially treated for transverse myelitis at 6 months of age shows a residual, expansile, hyperintense mass ➲ of the cervicothoracic cord, shown to be a WHO grade 3 anaplastic astrocytoma upon biopsy.* **(Right)** *Sagittal T1 C+ FS MR in a 13-year-old who had 3 weeks of vomiting & headache followed by arm weakness shows a heterogeneously enhancing tumor ➲ extending from the cervicomedullary junction into the cord. Glioblastoma (WHO grade 4) was found at biopsy.*

TERMINOLOGY

Definitions

- Primary intramedullary neoplasm of spinal cord originating from astrocytes

IMAGING

General Features

- Location
  - Cervical > thoracic > lumbar
- Morphology
  - Oblong, fusiform expansion of cord
- Typical MR features
  - Up to 40% have tumor cysts or syringohydromyelia
  - Solid portion is hypo-/isointense on T1, hyperintense on T2; rarely hemorrhagic
  - Variable enhancement
    - Pilocytic tumors (WHO grade 1) typically enhance avidly
    - Diffuse astrocytomas (WHO grade 2) typically have minimal, if any, enhancement
  - Diffusion
    - Facilitated diffusion (↑ ADC values) if low grade
    - Restricted diffusion (↓ ADC values) if high grade

DIFFERENTIAL DIAGNOSIS

Transverse Myelitis

- Similar imaging features; absent or mild enhancement

Ganglioglioma

- Similar imaging features

Ependymoma

- Less common in children than adults
- Sharply delineated tumor, often with hemorrhage
  - May present as superficial siderosis

Multiple Sclerosis

- Short-segment lesions involving < 1/2 of cord cross section
- Predominantly in dorsal aspect of cord

Cord Infarct

- Central gray matter involvement is typical, may involve entire cord cross section

PATHOLOGY

General Features

- Associated abnormalities
  - Some ↑ risk with neurofibromatosis type 1 & 2 (NF1, NF2); ependymoma & extramedullary tumors are more common in NF2

Staging, Grading, & Classification

- 75-80% low grade
  - Pilocytic astrocytoma = WHO grade 1
  - Diffuse astrocytoma = WHO grade 2
- 20-25% high grade
  - Anaplastic astrocytomas = WHO grade 3
  - Glioblastoma = WHO grade 4
  - Diffuse midline glioma = WHO grade 4

Microscopic Features

- Pilocytic astrocytoma
  - Rosenthal fibers
  - Glomeruloid/hyalinized vessels
  - Low prevalence of nuclear atypia/mitoses
- Diffuse astrocytoma
  - ↑ cellularity, variable atypia/mitoses
  - Parenchymal infiltration
- Anaplastic astrocytoma
  - Dispersed anaplasia
  - Significant proliferative activity
- Glioblastoma
  - Highly cellular & heterogeneous
  - Microvascular proliferation & palisading necrosis
- Diffuse midline glioma
  - K27M mutation in histone 3
  - Resembles diffuse astrocytoma microscopically but far more infiltrative & aggressive

CLINICAL ISSUES

Presentation

- Scoliosis, pain, myelopathy, muscle wasting

Demographics

- Most common spinal cord tumor in children
  - 30-35% of intraspinal neoplasms in children
  - 60% of primary spinal cord tumors in children
  - Higher-grade lesions are much less frequent in children

Natural History & Prognosis

- Most are slow growing
- Survival varies with tumor histology/grade & degree of tumor resection
  - 80% 5-year survival for low grade

Treatment

- Gross total resection is goal in pilocytic & low-grade tumors
  - Definitive treatment for pilocytic tumors
  - Intraoperative evoked potentials are helpful for maximal resection without damaging normal tissue
  - Intraoperative US can show extent of tumor vs. syrinx

DIAGNOSTIC CHECKLIST

Consider

- Remember inflammatory lesions in differential

Image Interpretation Pearls

- Image entire spinal cord
- Subtotal surgical resection may be unimpressive on imaging
  - Residual lesion "fills in" resection cavity

SELECTED REFERENCES

1. Perwein T et al: High frequency of disease progression in pediatric spinal cord low-grade glioma (LGG): management strategies and results from the German LGG study group. Neuro Oncol. 23(7):1148-62, 2021
2. Carey SS et al: Evaluating pediatric spinal low-grade gliomas: a 30-year retrospective analysis. J Neurooncol. 145(3):519-29, 2019
3. She DJ et al: MR imaging features of spinal pilocytic astrocytoma. BMC Med Imaging. 19(1):5, 2019
4. Aboian MS et al: Imaging characteristics of pediatric diffuse midline gliomas with histone H3 K27M mutation. AJNR Am J Neuroradiol. 38(4):795-800, 2017

Sacrococcygeal Teratoma

KEY FACTS

TERMINOLOGY

- Teratomas are made up of various parenchymal cell types from > 1 germ layer, usually all 3
- Sacrococcygeal teratoma (SCT) arises from coccyx, potentially grows both internally & externally
- Both benign & malignant (17%) varieties occur

IMAGING

- Always has presacral component; exophytic extension is more common than internal growth
- Heterogeneous, mixed solid & cystic masses
  - Ca^{2+}, fat, hemorrhage, cysts, various soft tissues in mass
  - Solid components may show moderate to high vascularity
- MR is best for identifying intraspinal extension

PATHOLOGY

- Malignant characteristics ↑ with age, type IV
- Currarino triad: Presacral mass (anterior meningocele or SCT), anorectal malformation, sacral anomalies
- American Academy of Pediatrics Surgical Section classification
  - Type I (47%): Primarily external in location
  - Type II (34%): Dumbbell, pelvic & external components
  - Type III (9%): Primarily located within abdomen/pelvis
  - Type IV (10%): Entirely internal, no external component

CLINICAL ISSUES

- Prognosis is variable: Fetal SCT can be quite vascular & grow rapidly → hydrops, intratumoral hemorrhage, rupture → demise
  - Hydrops before 30-weeks gestation > 90% mortality
  - Large tumors have > 25% perinatal mortality
- Excellent prognosis for patients with benign tumors & complete surgical resection
- Complete surgical resection must include coccyx
- 5-15% risk of recurrence

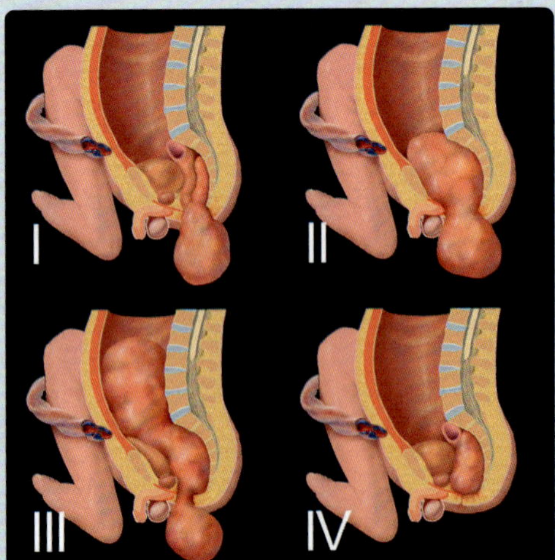

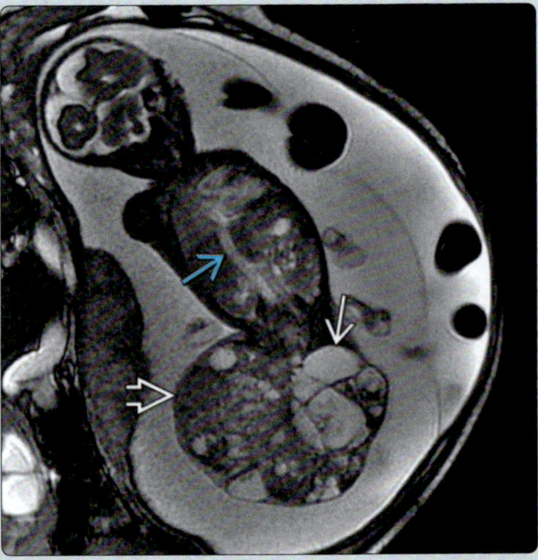

(Left) *Graphic shows the AAP tumor classification scheme: Type I is primarily exophytic, type II has equivalent-size internal & external masses, type III has a larger intraabdominal component, & type IV is entirely internal.* **(Right)** *Coronal SSFP MR of a twin gestation shows a fetus with a large, predominantly exophytic mass extending from the perineum. Note the solid & cystic areas within the mass. The inferior vena cava is prominent due to the amount of blood flow coursing through this tumor. However, no hydrops is seen.*

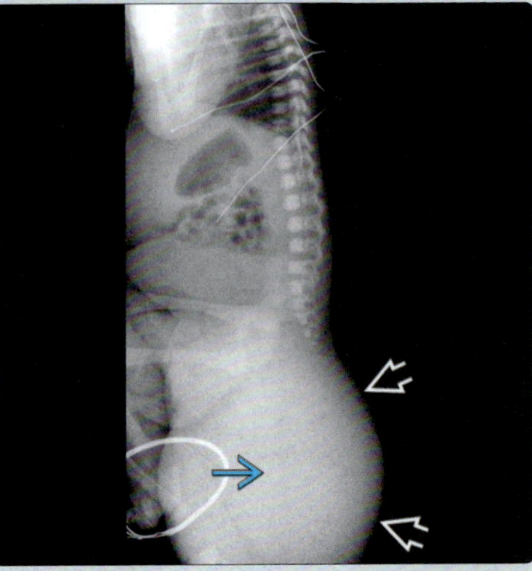

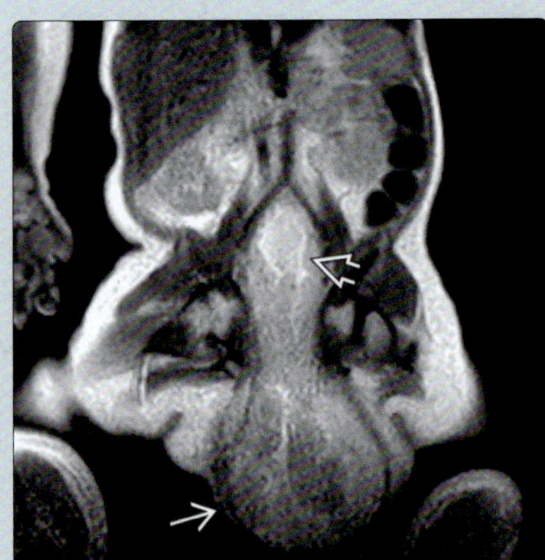

(Left) *Lateral radiograph shows a newborn infant with a large, exophytic mass extending from the sacrum & coccygeal region. A few Ca^{2+} are visible within the mass, typical of a sacrococcygeal teratoma (SCT).* **(Right)** *Coronal T2 MR in a newborn infant shows a heterogeneous, solid mass protruding externally with dumbbell extension internally, splaying the aortic bifurcation in this case of a type II SCT.*

TERMINOLOGY

Abbreviations

- Sacrococcygeal teratoma (SCT)

Synonyms

- Teratoma, germ cell tumor of coccyx

Definitions

- Teratomas are made up of various parenchymal cell types from > 1 germ layer, usually all 3
  - Tumors may contain hair, teeth, cartilage, & fat, among other tissues
- SCT arises from pluripotential cells at caudal tip of notochord (coccyx)
- Can grow both internally & externally (with latter being more common)
- Both benign & malignant varieties exist

IMAGING

General Features

- Best diagnostic clue
  - Large, solid, cystic, or mixed mass with exophytic perineal/buttock component & relatively small presacral component
  - May see Ca^{2+}, bone, fat, fluid levels, various soft tissues in mass
- Location
  - Origin from coccyx, but growth can occur in any direction
    - Presacral components are always present
  - Look for intraspinal extension
- Size
  - Ranges from small to massive in volume, potentially exceeding fetal weight
- Morphology
  - External components tend to be round &/or lobulated
  - Bilobed or dumbbell shape is often seen with large internal & external components
    - Lesion narrows passing through pelvis

Radiographic Findings

- Large mass extending outside infant
- Ca^{2+} may be present

Fluoroscopic Findings

- Type IV SCT may be found incidentally during fluoroscopy studies for constipation or voiding problems
- Patients rarely have long-term sequela of bladder outlet obstruction

CT Findings

- NECT
  - Demonstrates fatty components, Ca^{2+}, & fluid levels
  - Heterogeneous mass wrapped around coccyx but typically without bony destruction
- CECT
  - Variable enhancement pattern in solid & cystic components

Ultrasonographic Findings

- Grayscale ultrasound
  - Ultrasound may be limited due to large size & internal Ca^{2+}
  - Heterogeneous echotexture mass
    - Ca^{2+} & fat cause highly echogenic foci while cystic areas are hypo- to anechoic
    - Numerous interfaces are typically present in lesion
- Color Doppler
  - Solid components may show moderate to high vascularity
  - Arterial steal may be seen in nearby vessels to supply tumor

MR Findings

- Heterogeneous, similar to CT
- Fat is best confirmed on T1 ± FS
- Variable enhancement; does not predict malignancy
- Best study for identifying intraspinal extension (rare)

Nuclear Medicine Findings

- PET
  - Used more often in evaluation of malignant recurrence than in initial diagnosis

Imaging Recommendations

- Best imaging tool
  - Prenatal sonography is most common initial diagnostic modality
  - Prenatal or postnatal MR to determine full extent of mass & aid surgical planning

DIFFERENTIAL DIAGNOSIS

Pelvic Rhabdomyosarcoma

- Solid mass without Ca^{2+}, fat, or substantial cysts (usually)

Neuroblastoma

- May arise in pelvis at organ of Zuckerkandl
- Solid mass with Ca^{2+} & vascular encasement

Myelocystocele

- Skin-covered dorsal dysraphism
- Elongated spinal cord with dilated central canal & meninges ("cyst within cyst")

Other Intrapelvic Masses

- Consider Burkitt lymphoma, ovarian tumors, lymphatic malformation, hematometrocolpos

PATHOLOGY

General Features

- Etiology
  - Probably results from rests of pluripotential cells at caudal end of notochord/spine
- Genetics
  - Not inherited
    - Except Currarino type, which is autosomal dominant mutation in *MNX1* gene
  - Familial tendency is reported, prompting some to recommend screening asymptomatic siblings
- Associated abnormalities
  - 10% of SCTs are associated with other congenital anomalies

- Primarily defects of hindgut & cloacal region, which exceeds baseline rate of 2.5% expected in general population
- SCT is 2nd most common lesion after anterior meningocele in familial disorder of Currarino
  - Autosomal dominant triad of presacral mass, partial sacral agenesis, & anorectal defects
- Malignant characteristics ↑ with
  - Age at diagnosis
  - Internal subtype (type IV is worst)
  - Male sex
  - Presence of necrosis or hemorrhage
- α-fetoprotein is often elevated

Staging, Grading, & Classification

- American Academy of Pediatrics (AAP) Surgical Section classification
  - Type I (47%)
    - Primarily external in location
  - Type II (34%)
    - Dumbbell shape, equal internal/external components
  - Type III (9%)
    - Primarily located within abdomen/pelvis
  - Type IV (10%)
    - Entirely internal, no external component visible

Gross Pathologic & Surgical Features

- Typical of all teratomas: Multiple tissue types in varying stages of maturation & differentiation
- Solid & cystic components are common

Microscopic Features

- Tumors can be mature or immature
- Only 17% of SCTs have malignant features

CLINICAL ISSUES

Presentation

- Most common signs/symptoms
  - Frequently diagnosed in utero
    - Large fetal tumors require C-section delivery or in utero surgical intervention (open fetal surgery, radiofrequency or thermal ablation of tumor)
  - Most others are diagnosed within 1st few days of life
    - Exophytic masses are easily diagnosed clinically
  - Type IV lesions can present in childhood with urinary retention, bowel issues, Ca^{2+} on scoliosis study, etc.
  - Arteriovenous shunting in tumor → high-output cardiac failure
- Other signs/symptoms
  - In utero complications: Fetal SCT can be quite vascular & grow rapidly → hydrops, intratumoral hemorrhage, or rupture → fetal demise
    - Hydrops before 30-weeks gestation: > 90% mortality rate
      - Solid masses are more likely to develop hydrops
      - Doppler parameters may help predict hydrops
    - Maternal mirror syndrome (preeclampsia) may develop

Demographics

- Age
  - Typically diagnosed in fetus or newborn
  - Delayed diagnoses are possible in childhood, rarely in adults
- Epidemiology
  - Prevalence: 1 in 14,000 (Sweden) to 40,000 births

Natural History & Prognosis

- Prognosis is excellent in patients with benign tumors resected after birth
  - Gait abnormalities & early arthrosis are reported with extensive pelvic muscle resection
  - Rarely long-term bladder & bowel issues
- 5-15% risk of recurrence
  - Intraoperative tumor spillage & incomplete resection ↑ risk
- Masses diagnosed after 1st birthday & located only internally have higher malignant potential
  - Prognosis is variable in malignant tumors
  - Serum α-fetoprotein is useful tumor marker postoperatively
- Malignant components may be found at presentation or at time of recurrence
  - Yolk sac tumor is most common
  - Embryonal carcinoma is 2nd most common
  - With intensive chemotherapy, 5-year relapse-free survival rate is reported 76-90%
- Study from Netherlands showed normal fertility in adult female survivors

Treatment

- Complete surgical resection to include coccyx
- Benign tumors do not require additional therapy
- Malignant tumors are treated with chemotherapy (platinum-based agents) & radiation
- Consideration of in utero intervention with development of early hydrops; must weigh benefits with risks of prematurity

SELECTED REFERENCES

1. Seilern Und Aspang J et al: Sacrococcygeal teratoma with intraspinal extension: a case series and review of literature. J Pediatr Surg. 55(10):2022-5, 2020
2. Baumgarten HD et al: Preemptive delivery and immediate resection for fetuses with high-risk sacrococcygeal teratomas. Fetal Diagn Ther. 45(3):137-44, 2019
3. Gebb JS et al: High tumor volume to fetal weight ratio is associated with worse fetal outcomes and increased maternal risk in fetuses with sacrococcygeal teratoma. Fetal Diagn Ther. 45(2):94-101, 2019
4. Ladenhauf HN et al: Sacrococcygeal teratoma presenting with vaginal discharge and polyp in an infant. J Pediatr Adolesc Gynecol. 31(3):318-20, 2018
5. Lee SM et al: Antenatal prediction of neonatal survival in sacrococcygeal teratoma. J Ultrasound Med. 37(8):2003-9, 2018
6. Wessell A et al: Surgical treatment of a type IV cystic sacrococcygeal teratoma with intraspinal extension utilizing a posterior-anterior-posterior approach: a case report. Childs Nerv Syst. 34(5):977-82, 2018
7. Yoon HM et al: Sacrococcygeal teratomas in newborns: a comprehensive review for the radiologists. Acta Radiol. 59(2):236-46, 2018
8. Hambraeus M et al: Sacrococcygeal teratoma: a population-based study of incidence and prenatal prognostic factors. J Pediatr Surg. 51(3):481-5, 2016
9. Adekola H et al: The clinical relevance of fetal MRI in the diagnosis of type IV cystic sacrococcygeal teratoma–a review. Fetal Pediatr Pathol. 34(1):31-43, 2015
10. Dirix M et al: Malignant transformation in sacrococcygeal teratoma and in presacral teratoma associated with Currarino syndrome: a comparative study. J Pediatr Surg. 50(3):462-4, 2015

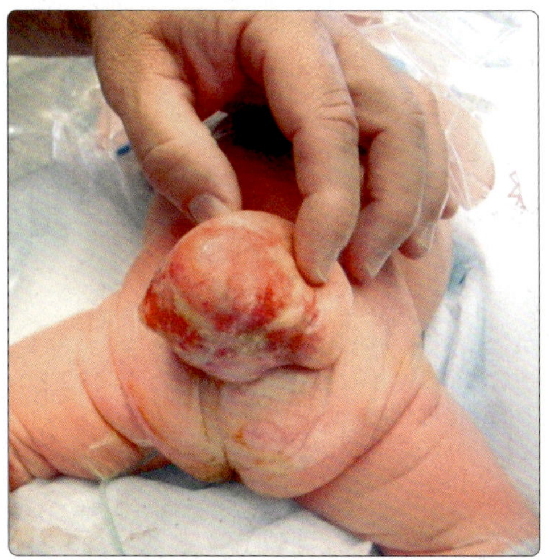

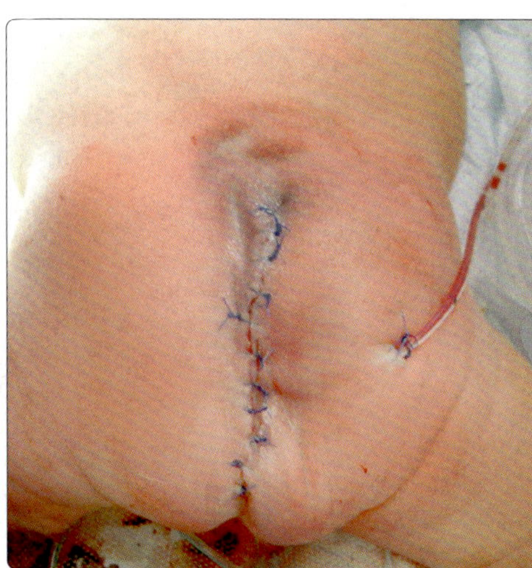

(Left) *Clinical photograph shows an infant prior to resection of a type I SCT. Cross-sectional imaging is helpful to delineate the intrapelvic/intraabdominal extent of tumor & develop an appropriate surgical plan.* **(Right)** *Clinical photograph shows the immediate postoperative appearance of the buttocks following SCT resection. After several months, the gluteal crease & buttocks assumed a nearly normal appearance.*

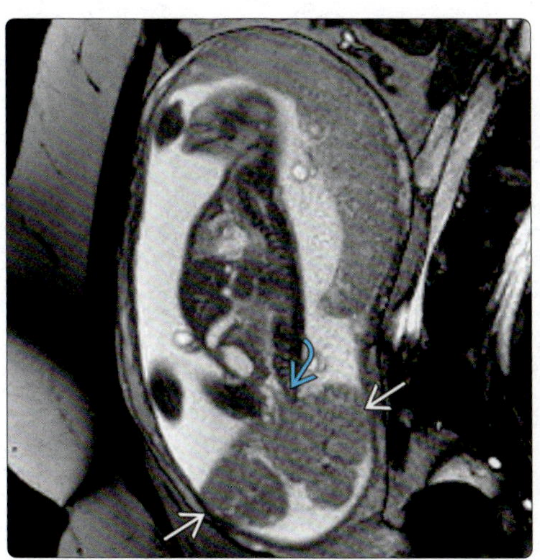

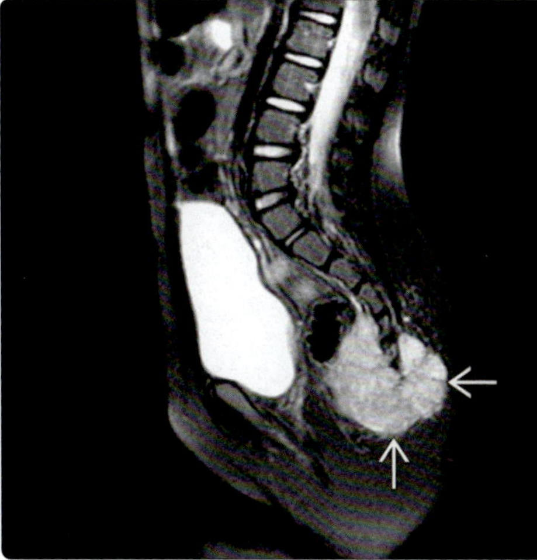

(Left) *Sagittal SSFP MR of a fetus shows a primarily solid, lobulated, & exophytic mass ➔ extending out of the pelvis with only a small intrapelvic component abutting the coccyx ➜, consistent with a type I SCT.* **(Right)** *Sagittal T2 FS MR in a 3-year-old boy (who was imaged for the changing appearance of his sacral dimple with firmness to palpation of the area) shows a high signal intensity solid mass ➔ surrounding the coccyx but not reaching the skin surface, a type IV SCT.*

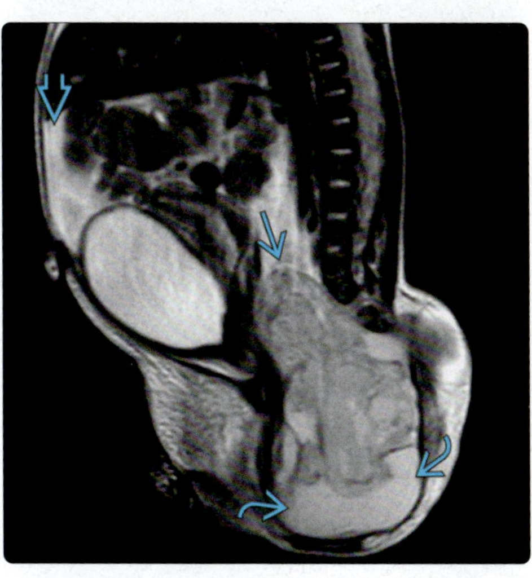

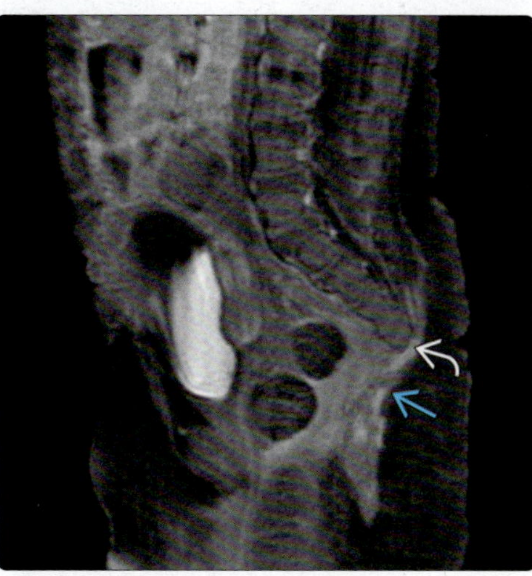

(Left) *Sagittal T2 MR in a newborn shows a dumbbell-shaped, mixed solid & cystic, high signal intensity mass extending from the lower abdomen ➔ into the external component ➜. Note the elevation & dilation of the urinary bladder. The ascites ➔ was secondary to hydrops at delivery.* **(Right)** *Sagittal T1 C+ FS MR in the same patient 6 months after complete surgical resection of the mature type II SCT shows minimal postsurgical changes in the pelvis ➔ & truncated sacrum (minus the coccyx) ➜.*

Discitis/Osteomyelitis

KEY FACTS

TERMINOLOGY

- Bacterial infection of intervertebral disc & adjacent vertebrae

IMAGING

- Disc-centered process: Disc space narrowing & adjacent endplate irregularity in young children
  - Lumbosacral (75%) > thoracic > cervical spine
- Early: MR is most sensitive & specific modality
  - Abnormal disc signal & enhancement
  - Ill-defined abnormal marrow signal & enhancement of adjacent vertebral bodies
  - Paraspinal & epidural phlegmon or abscess
- Subacute: Endplate destruction/erosion
- Chronic: ↑ bone density ± vertebral fusion with healing

TOP DIFFERENTIAL DIAGNOSES

- Langerhans cell histiocytosis
- Chronic recurrent multifocal osteomyelitis (CRMO)
- Spinal metastases
- Tuberculous vertebral osteomyelitis
- Degenerative endplate changes

PATHOLOGY

- Hematogenous spread to vascularized disc or subchondral vertebral growth plate in children
- *Staphylococcus aureus* is most common pathogen
  - Consider *Kingella kingae* in young children

CLINICAL ISSUES

- Peak age: 6 months to 4 years
- Variable & nonspecific symptoms
  - May delay diagnosis for weeks in children
- Elevated ESR, CRP, WBC
- Treat early with empiric IV antibiotics until causative organism is identified

(Left) *Midline sagittal T1 C+ FS MR in a 7-month-old shows poor definition & abnormal enhancement of the L2-L3 disc space ➡. Patchy abnormal enhancement is also noted in the marrow of the adjoining vertebral bodies. No drainable collection is identified within the adjacent paraspinal soft tissues or epidural space.* **(Right)** *Axial T2 MR in the same patient shows abnormal thickening & poorly defined fluid signal in the anterior & lateral paraspinal soft tissues ↪ in this patient with spondylodiscitis.*

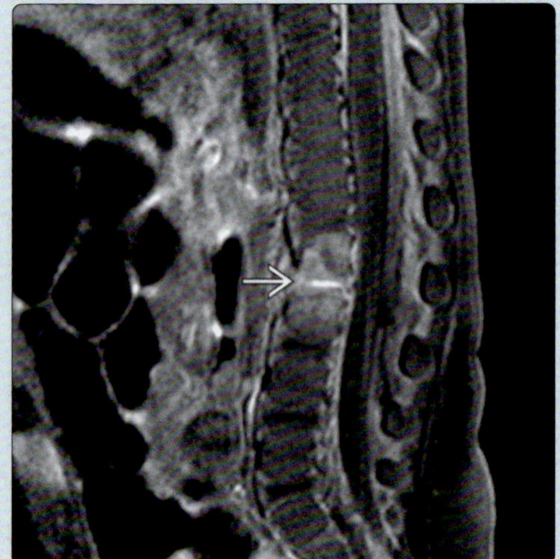

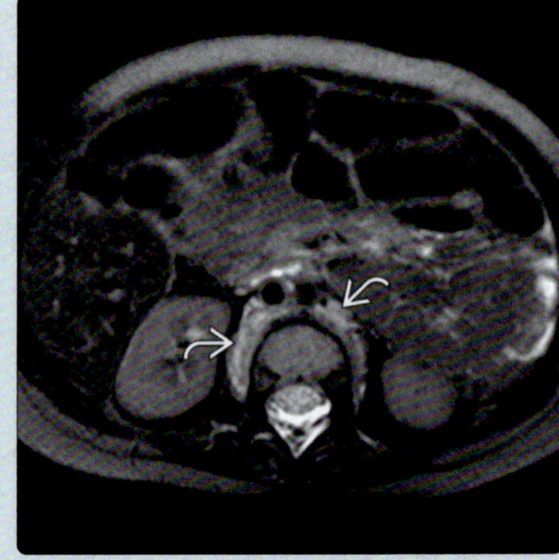

(Left) *Lateral radiograph (left) shows L4-L5 disc space narrowing ➡ & endplate irregularity in this 1-year-old with back pain. Sagittal SPECT bone scan (right) confirms abnormal uptake ➡ in the vertebral bodies, typical of spondylodiscitis.* **(Right)** *Sagittal STIR (left) & T1 C+ FS (right) MR images in a 2-year-old show disc space narrowing ➡ & enhancement ➡ with abnormal signal/enhancement of the L4-L5 vertebral marrow. Enhancing soft tissue in the epidural space ↪ is due to contiguous inflammation.*

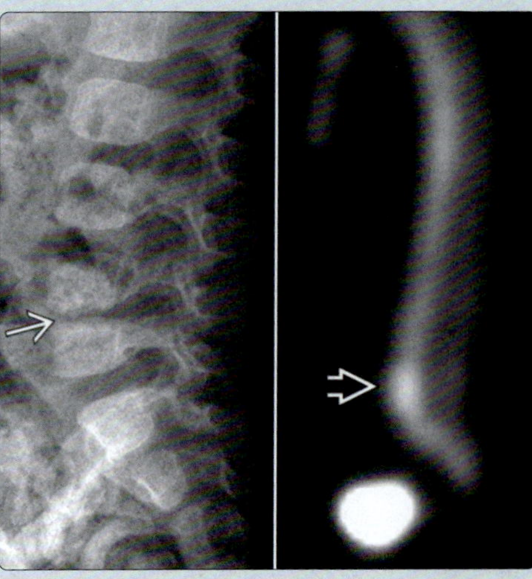

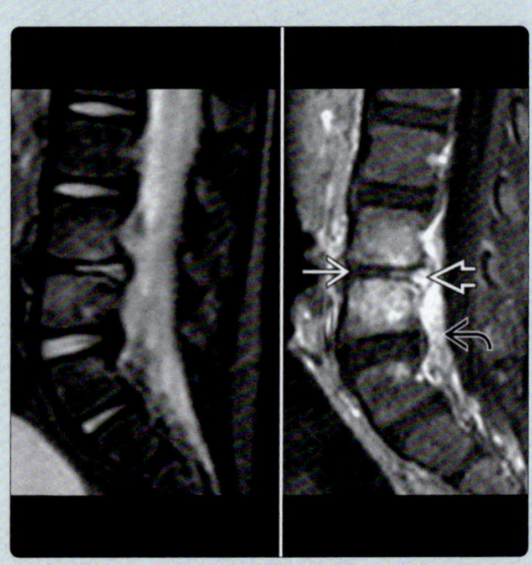

TERMINOLOGY

Definitions

- Bacterial suppurative infection of intervertebral disc & adjacent vertebrae

IMAGING

Radiographic Findings

- Negative up to 2-8 weeks after onset of symptoms
- Initial endplate & vertebral osteolysis
- Loss of intervening disc space height
- ↑ bone density ± intervertebral fusion with successful treatment
- Total vertebral destruction/collapse with treatment delay/failure

MR Findings

- Abnormal disc space
  - Loss of normal disc height, signal, & morphology
  - T1 hypointense, variable T2 signal intensity
  - Diffuse or rim enhancement with contrast
- Vertebral marrow signal abnormality abutting disc
  - T1 hypointense
  - Poorly defined ↑ fluid signal, most conspicuous on T2 FS or STIR images
  - Typically enhances with contrast unless necrotic
- Paraspinal & epidural phlegmon or abscess
  - Thickened T2-/STIR hyperintense tissues
  - Poorly defined fluid signal & stranding of fat
  - Diffuse enhancement vs. rim-enhancing collections
    - Abscess will restrict diffusion
- Follow-up: No single MR finding predicts clinical status
  - Abnormal imaging persists for months, does not necessarily equate residual/recurrent infection
  - Further bony destruction or new fluid collection can direct tissue sampling (if needed to direct treatment)

Nuclear Medicine Findings

- Bone scan
  - Tc-99m scan shows ↑ activity about affected disc space in all phases

Imaging Recommendations

- Best imaging tool
  - Targeted MR provides excellent diagnostic detail
  - Nuclear medicine bone scan or whole-body MR can localize nonspecific signs & symptoms
- Protocol advice
  - STIR or FS T2 MR for marrow & soft tissue involvement
  - T1 C+ FS MR to evaluate for drainable paraspinal & epidural fluid collections

DIFFERENTIAL DIAGNOSIS

Langerhans Cell Histiocytosis

- Enhancing marrow lesion ± lytic destruction, enhancing soft tissue mass; spares disc
- Single level vs. noncontiguous multifocal involvement
- Collapse of vertebra → vertebra plana

Chronic Recurrent Multifocal Osteomyelitis

- Autoimmune inflammatory disorder of bone
- Little disc involvement

Spinal Metastases

- Rare in children → neuroblastoma, leukemia
- Marrow abnormalities with disc space preservation
- Discrete or ill-defined vertebral lesions
- Noncontiguous vertebral involvement

Tuberculous Vertebral Osteomyelitis

- Usually centered in vertebral body rather than disc
- Midthoracic or thoracolumbar > lumbar or cervical
- Large dissecting paraspinal abscesses out of proportion to vertebral involvement
- Much more common in developing nations

Degenerative Changes

- Rare in children
- Normal marrow ± vertebral endplate preservation

PATHOLOGY

General Features

- Etiology
  - Pathophysiology
    - Intervertebral disc & adjacent vertebral growth plates are highly vascularized in young children
    - Hematogenous seeding of intervertebral disc/subchondral bone is most common source
      - Lumbosacral (75%) > thoracic > cervical spine
  - Most common pathogen: *Staphylococcus aureus*

CLINICAL ISSUES

Presentation

- Clinical profile
  - Peak age range: 6 months to 4 years
  - Clinical symptoms are variable & nonspecific in children
    - Difficulty walking, back/hip pain, fever (< 50%), irritability
  - Elevated ESR, CRP
    - WBC is often normal (~ 60%)

Treatment

- Early empiric IV antibiotics, broad-spectrum coverage until causative pathogen is isolated
- Organism-specific parenteral antibiotics for 6-8 weeks
- Spinal immobilization with bracing for 6-12 weeks
- CT-guided or open biopsy may be indicated if blood cultures are negative & conservative treatment fails
- Surgery is rarely indicated except in advanced infection

SELECTED REFERENCES

1. Afshari FT et al: Paediatric spondylodiscitis: a 10-year single institution experience in management and clinical outcomes. Childs Nerv Syst. 36(5):1049-54, 2020
2. Dayer R et al: Spinal infections in children: a multicentre retrospective study. Bone Joint J. 100-B(4):542-8, 2018
3. Mohanty CB et al: Pediatric spinal infections-a review of non-tuberculous infections. Childs Nerv Syst. 34(10):1947-56, 2018
4. Tyagi R: Spinal infections in children: a review. J Orthop. 13(4):254-8, 2016

KEY FACTS

TERMINOLOGY

- Acute inflammatory pathologies of spinal cord, not secondary to other CNS inflammatory or demyelinating disease
  - Transverse myelitis (TM)
  - Acute flaccid myelitis (AFM)
  - Guillain-Barré syndrome (GBS)
  - Paralytic poliomyelitis

IMAGING

- TM: Diffuse cord swelling & abnormal signal > 2 vertebral segments in length
- AFM: Abnormal T2 hyperintensity in cord gray matter, often asymmetric
- GBS: Symmetric prominent enhancement of ventral nerve roots in cauda equina
- Poliomyelitis: Abnormal T2 hyperintensity in anterior horn cells

TOP DIFFERENTIAL DIAGNOSES

- Spinal cord astrocytoma
- Neuromyelitis optica
- Multiple sclerosis

PATHOLOGY

- TM: Many cases are associated with antimyelin oligodendrocyte glycoprotein (MOG) antibodies
  - COVID-19 can manifest as TM
- AFM: Majority are attributable to infection with enterovirus D68
- GBS: *Campylobacter jejuni* is most common preceding infection
  - Another CNS manifestation of pediatric COVID-19 infection
- Poliomyelitis: Caused by poliovirus, but West Nile virus can cause identical clinical syndrome

(Left) *Sagittal T2 MR in a 14-month-old who developed progressive upper then lower extremity weakness followed by respiratory failure shows diffuse swelling & hyperintensity of the entire cervical & upper thoracic cord ➡, characteristic of transverse myelitis.* **(Right)** *Sagittal T2 MR of the same patient 8 years later shows severe atrophy of the entire cord ➡. Approximately 25% of transverse myelitis cases will have permanent disability, with little or no recovery of function.*

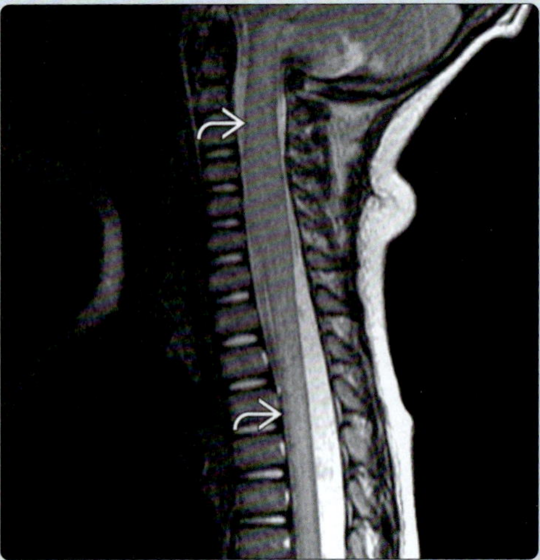

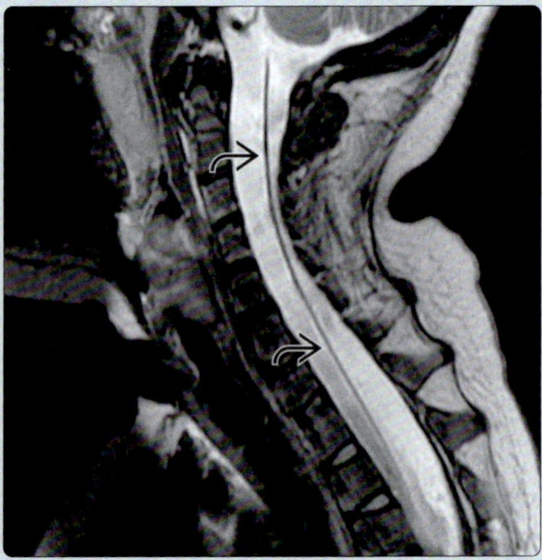

(Left) *Axial T2 MR in a 4-year-old with left upper extremity weakness & cerebellar ataxia after a febrile illness shows abnormal hyperintense signal in the central gray matter of the cervical cord ➡, especially the anterior horn cells, due to acute flaccid myelitis associated with enterovirus infection.* **(Right)** *Sagittal T2 MR in a teenager with West Nile myelitis who presented with fevers, bilateral lower extremity weakness, & urinary incontinence shows mild swelling & abnormal gray matter signal ➡ in the distal cord & conus.*

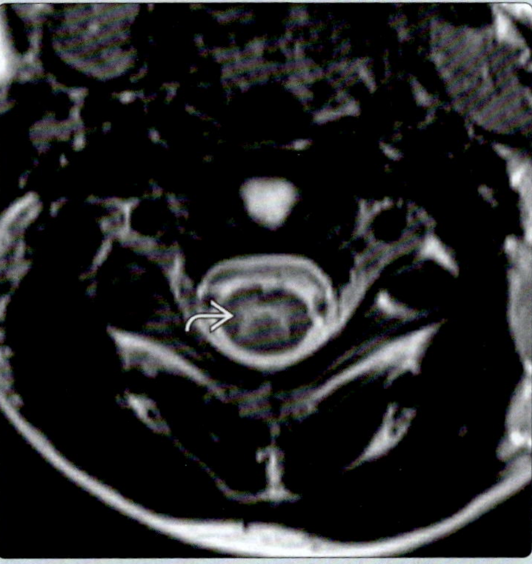

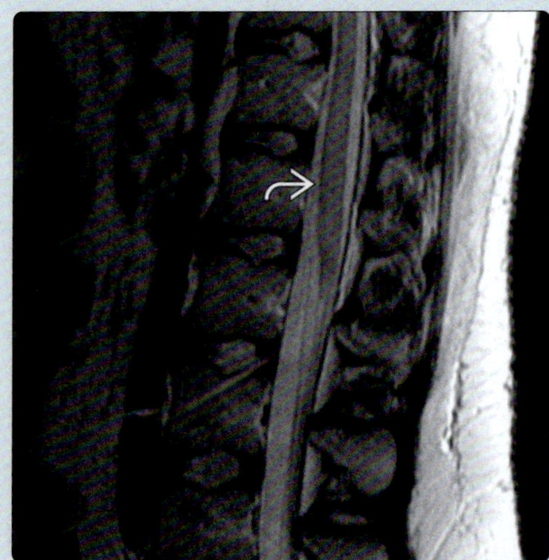

TERMINOLOGY

Definitions

- Acute inflammatory pathologies of spinal cord, not secondary to other CNS inflammatory or demyelinating disease
  - Transverse myelitis (TM)
  - Acute flaccid myelitis (AFM)
  - Guillain-Barré syndrome (GBS)
  - Paralytic poliomyelitis

IMAGING

General Features

- Best diagnostic clue
  - TM: Diffuse cord swelling & abnormal signal > 2 vertebral segments in length
  - AFM: Abnormal T2 hyperintensity in cord gray matter, often asymmetric
  - GBS: Symmetric prominent enhancement of ventral nerve roots in cauda equina
  - Poliomyelitis: Abnormal T2 hyperintensity in anterior horn cells
- Location
  - TM: Thoracic > cervical
  - AFM: Cervical > thoracic
  - GBS: Conus & cauda equina
  - Poliomyelitis: Cervical > thoracic
- Size
  - Cord involvement in TM & AFM is typically lengthy, covering 3 or more vertebral levels [longitudinally extensive TM (LETM)]

DIFFERENTIAL DIAGNOSIS

Spinal Cord Astrocytoma

- Homogeneous cord expansion
- Diffuse or nodular contrast enhancement

Neuromyelitis Optica

- LETM (> 3 vertebral segments) in central cord + optic nerve enhancement
- CSF with aquaporin 4-specific antibodies

Multiple Sclerosis

- Peripheral lesions ± central enhancement
- < 2 vertebral segments in length
- < 1/2 of cross-sectional area of cord
- 90% have intracranial lesions

PATHOLOGY

General Features

- Etiology
  - TM, AFM, & GBS are clinical syndromes, not diagnoses per se
    - Combinations of signs & symptoms
    - Variety of etiologies
  - TM: Many cases are associated with antimyelin oligodendrocyte glycoprotein (MOG) antibodies
    - COVID-19 can manifest as TM
  - AFM: Majority are attributable to infection with enterovirus D68
  - GBS: *Campylobacter jejuni* is most common preceding infection
    - Another CNS manifestation of pediatric COVID-19 infection
  - Poliomyelitis: Caused by poliovirus, but West Nile virus can cause identical clinical syndrome

CLINICAL ISSUES

Presentation

- Most common signs/symptoms
  - TM: Sensory, motor, or autonomic dysfunction attributable to spinal cord, typically bilateral
  - AFM: Extremity weakness/paralysis following febrile illness, often asymmetric
  - GBS: Ascending weakness, 2-4 weeks after illness or immunization

Demographics

- Epidemiology
  - TM incidence: 2 per 500,000 population
    - 4.6 new cases of idiopathic acute TM per 1 million people per year in USA
    - 1,200 new cases per year in USA
    - Late winter through spring
  - AFM: 0.71 per million in patients ≤ 21 years old
    - Late summer through fall
  - GBS: 0.5-1.5 cases per 100,000 < 18 years old
    - Rare < 2 years of age

Natural History & Prognosis

- TM: Rule of 3s
  - 1/3 have good to complete recovery
  - 1/3 have fair recovery
    - Residual spasticity & urinary dysfunction
  - 1/3 have poor recovery
    - Persistent complete deficits
- AFM: < 10% recover completely
- GBS: 20% have persistent significant deficits

DIAGNOSTIC CHECKLIST

Image Interpretation Pearls

- Evaluate brain/orbits to exclude neuromyelitis optica, MS
- Document reduced swelling by imaging
  - Persistent cord enlargement suggests neoplasm (astrocytoma)

SELECTED REFERENCES

1. Caress JB et al: COVID-19-associated Guillain-Barré syndrome: the early pandemic experience. Muscle Nerve. 62(4):485-91, 2020
2. Chhabda S et al: Relapsing demyelinating syndromes in children: a practical review of neuroradiological mimics. Front Neurol. 11:627, 2020
3. Kaur H et al: Transverse myelitis in a child with COVID-19. Pediatr Neurol. 112:5-6, 2020
4. Bulut E et al: MRI predictors of recurrence and outcome after acute transverse myelitis of unidentified etiology. AJNR Am J Neuroradiol. 40(8):1427-32, 2019
5. Christy A et al: Acute flaccid myelitis associated with enterovirus D68: a review. J Child Neurol. 34(9):511-6, 2019
6. Grill MF: Infectious myelopathies. Continuum (Minneap Minn). 24(2, Spinal Cord Disorders):441-73, 2018

Craniocervical Junction Injuries

KEY FACTS

TERMINOLOGY

- Traumatic injury to upper cervical region: Occiput to C2

IMAGING

- Normal measurements in adults may not translate to children due to dynamic skeletal changes in early life
- Radiography: Initial screening test for most children
  - > 20% of cervical fractures are missed by radiography alone
  - 10% of craniocervical junction (CCJ) fractures are shown by CT, not radiography
- CT: Asymmetry & ↑ joint space measurements
- CT: Look for retroclival hematoma & perimedullary hemorrhage
- MR: T2 for ligament integrity & cord edema
- MR: STIR for bone marrow & soft tissue edema
- MR: SWI/T2* GRE for cord hemorrhage
- MRA: Vertebral artery injury may be associated with CCJ injuries; often clinically occult

TOP DIFFERENTIAL DIAGNOSES

- Os odontoideum
- Nontraumatic ligamentous instability
- Congenital fusion & segmentation anomalies

CLINICAL ISSUES

- Motor vehicle accidents, abusive head trauma, sports-related injuries, & falls
  - Higher mortality rate than adults
- Injury at CCJ is most common in 1st decade
  - Disproportionate head size, ligamentous laxity, & immature muscles may contribute
- Neurologic status at presentation predicts outcome

DIAGNOSTIC CHECKLIST

- Include C1-C2 on all head trauma CT studies
- MR in patients with normal radiographs/CT who continue to have neurologic symptoms
- STIR & MRA on all cervical spine trauma MR studies

(Left) *Coronal bone CT in a 9-year-old girl after an MVA shows ↑ of the condyle-C1 intervals (CCIs) ➡ as well as lateral mass intervals (LMIs) ⇨, consistent with severe atlantooccipital dissociation (AOD) & atlantoaxial dissociation (AAD).* **(Right)** *Sagittal STIR MR in the same patient shows disruption of the tectorial membrane ➡ & transection of the posterior atlantooccipital ligament ⇨. The spinal cord shows hyperintense signal (likely contusion) ➡ as well as a few foci of low signal ⇨ (possibly hemorrhage).*

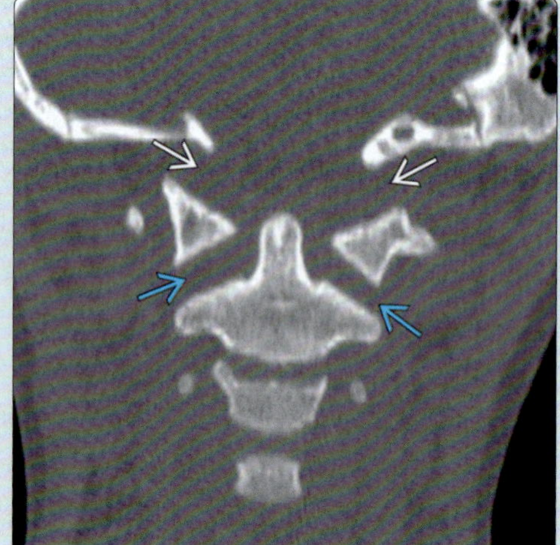

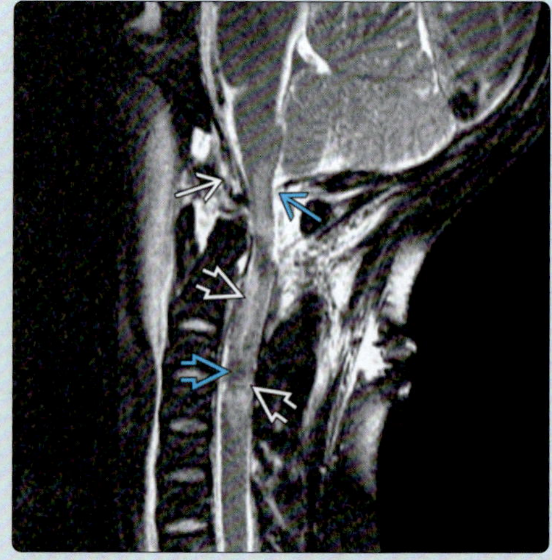

(Left) *Axial NECT in a 7-year-old boy involved in an MVA shows a retroclival epidural hematoma ⇨. Such a finding should prompt imaging investigation for craniocervical injury.* **(Right)** *Coronal STIR MR in the same patient shows effusions ⇨ in the bilateral occipital condyle-C1 & atlantoaxial joints as well as disruption of the left transverse ligament ⇨. Also note the extension of fluid ➡ beyond the left OC-C1 joint capsule, consistent with capsular rupture. These findings are consistent with AOD.*

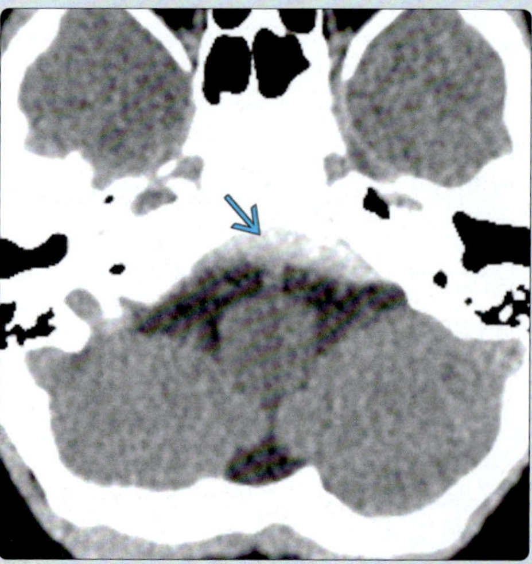

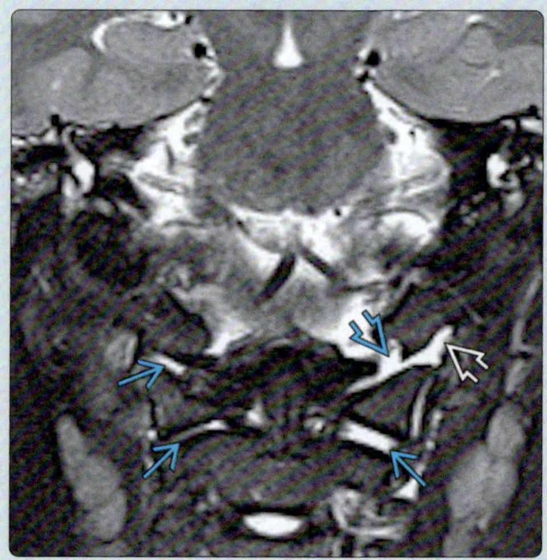

TERMINOLOGY

Definitions

- Craniocervical junction (CCJ) injuries: Traumatic injury to upper cervical region: Occiput to C2
  - Much more common in 1st decade than in teens/adults

Types of Pediatric Craniocervical Junction Injuries

- Atlantooccipital dissociation (AOD)
- Atlantoaxial dissociation (AAD)
- Jefferson fracture (C1 ring)
- Odontoid (C2) fracture
- Hangman's (C2) fracture
- Atlantoaxial rotatory fixation (AARF)
- Spinal cord injury without radiographic abnormality (SCIWORA)

IMAGING

General Features

- Best diagnostic clue
  - Abnormal alignment, joint space widening, abnormal fluid collection, or fracture involving occiput to C2
- Size
  - Numerous normal measurements have been proposed as signs of CCJ injury
  - **Key point**: Most measurements have been shown to be helpful in severe injuries but insensitive for mild to moderate injuries
  - **Key point**: Normal measurements in children change significantly with age & normal osseous development
  - **Occipital condyle-C1 interval (CCI) > 4 mm → AOD**
    - Found to be superior (most sensitive & specific) to all other measures for diagnosis of AOD but still insensitive to mild/moderate injury
    - Requires averaging multiple CCI measurements
    - Normal CCI varies with age; largest (> 2 mm) at 2-4 years, smallest (< 1 mm) after late teenage years
    - Normal CCI joint is wider medially in young children, so single medial measurement > 4 mm will lead to false-positives
      - Avoid measuring in occipital condyle notch to avoid false-positives
  - **Powers ratio > 1.0 → AOD**
    - Powers ratio is calculated as BC/OA
      - BC: Basion to posterior C1 arch
      - OA: Opisthion to anterior C1 arch
    - Difficult to calculate in very young patients due to incomplete C1 ring ossification
  - **Basion-dens interval (BDI) > 1.2 cm or < 0 → AOD**
    - ↓ with age as dens ossifies
    - May cause false-positive in very young patients
  - **Interspinous ratio > 2.5 → AOD, AAD, or C2 dens fracture**
    - Interspinous ratio = C1-C2:C2-C3
  - **Lateral atlantodental space > 5-mm asymmetry → C1 ring fracture**
    - Some asymmetry is normal with head rotation/angulation
  - **Atlantodental interval > 6 mm → AAD**
    - Mean: ~ 2 mm in children
  - **Lateral mass interval (LMI) > 5 mm → AAD**
    - ↓ with age (mean: ~ 3 mm in children, ~ 1 mm in adults)

Radiographic Findings

- Prevertebral soft tissue thickening is often seen in severe CCJ injuries but is often absent in mild to moderate injuries
- AOD
  - Severe: ↑ CCI, Powers ratio > 1, abnormal BDI, ↑ interspinous ratio
  - Mild to moderate: Typically normal radiographs
- AAD
  - Severe: ↑ joint space; ± joint space asymmetry on frontal view
  - Mild to moderate: Typically normal radiographs
- Jefferson (C1 ring) fracture
  - Lateral displacement of C1 lateral mass in relation to C2 lateral mass on AP/open-mouth views
    - Highly specific sign, especially when bilateral
  - Lateral atlantodental space > 5-mm asymmetry
    - Usually due to positioning/rotation rather than fracture
    - Often leads to false-positive radiograph interpretation
- Odontoid (C2) fracture
  - Type 1, 2, or 3 based upon level of fracture
  - Typically occurs at C2 synchondroses in younger children
  - When severe, will lead to abnormal alignment at CCJ
- Hangman's (C2) fracture
  - Fracture of pars interarticularis on lateral radiographs
  - ± anterolisthesis of C2 on C3
- Rotation injuries & torticollis
  - Rotation of mandible over upper cervical spine on lateral view

CT Findings

- AOD
  - Abnormal measurements (especially CCI) & asymmetry
  - Retroclival hematoma
  - Perimedullary hemorrhage
- AAD
  - ↑ LMI ± asymmetric LMI
  - ↑ asymmetric distance between C1 & C2 lateral masses
- C1 & C2 fractures are clearly delineated
  - > 20% of cervical fractures are missed by radiography alone
  - 10% of CCJ fractures are shown by CT & not radiography
  - Sagittal & coronal reformats are essential
- Rotation injuries & torticollis
  - 3D reconstruction is ideal for rotational injuries
  - Dynamic CT for fixed atlantoaxial rotatory subluxation
    - Axial images through C1-C2 in neutral position & with maximal voluntary rotation in each direction
    - Measure degree of rotation of C1 relative to C2
    - If no significant change in C1/C2 relationship with rotation → fixed rotatory subluxation
- CTA if plane of injury affects vessel course

MR Findings

- T1WI
  - Helpful in identifying blood products

- Fat saturation to differentiate blood from fat in soft tissues
- Can identify vessel dissection
- T2WI
  - Best sequence for cord edema
    - Axial & sagittal to confirm subtle cases
  - Best conventional sequence for ligament integrity
    - Challenging in very young patients due to CSF flow artifact
- STIR
  - Best sequence for bone marrow & soft tissue edema
- 3D SSFP (CISS, FIESTA)
  - High spatial resolution with near-complete CSF flow artifact suppression
  - Ideal for detection of intraspinal nerve root avulsion
  - Ideal for ligamentous injury at CCJ
- DWI
  - ADC values correlate with severity of spinal cord injury & can predict cavity formation
- SWI/T2* GRE
  - Detects blood products in cord
- MRA
  - Key adjunct in cervical spine injuries
  - Vertebral artery injury in up to 25% of adults with cervical spine trauma; may be clinically occult

Imaging Recommendations

- Best imaging tool
  - Imaging algorithm is based upon ability to clinically clear cervical spine
  - Radiographs: Initial screening test in most children
  - NECT with reformats: Further evaluation of abnormal radiographs, high-risk mechanism, or persistent clinical symptoms in face of normal radiographs
  - Head/neck CTA: Fastest evaluation for any concern of vascular injury
  - MR + MRA: Optimal evaluation of ligamentous, spinal cord, & vascular injury
- Protocol advice
  - Include through C2 on all trauma head CT studies
  - Perform MR when clinical symptoms or subtle CT clues are present (even when CCJ measurements are normal on CT)

DIFFERENTIAL DIAGNOSIS

Os Odontoideum

- Result of aberrant embryogenesis vs. fracture through odontoid synchondrosis prior to fusion (5-6 years)
  - Can be source of instability
  - More common in children with skeletal dysplasias
- Ossiculum terminale → nonfusion of distal ossification center
  - Smaller & without clinical significance

Nontraumatic Ligamentous Instability

- Abnormal laxity of ligaments stabilizing C1-C2
- Grisel syndrome → atlantoaxial instability associated with inflammation in adjacent soft tissues
- Down syndrome → laxity of transverse ligament
  - 10-20% incidence

Congenital Fusion & Segmentation Anomalies

- C1-occiput, C1-C2
- Klippel-Feil spectrum

PATHOLOGY

General Features

- Etiology
  - Mechanism: Motor vehicle accidents (MVAs) are most common in young children
    - Also seen with falls & abusive head trauma
    - Sports-related injuries predominate in 2nd decade

CLINICAL ISSUES

Presentation

- Most common signs/symptoms
  - AOD
    - Many die prior to reaching medical care
    - > 1/2 have cardiorespiratory arrest
    - 25-30% are neurologically intact at presentation
  - Jefferson (C1) fracture
    - Axial loading injury (e.g., diving into shallow pool)
  - Odontoid & hangman's fractures
    - Flexion or extension with distraction (usually MVA)
  - Rotational injuries
    - Present with painful torticollis

Demographics

- Age
  - 0-9 years: High incidence of upper cervical spine injury compared to adolescents & adults
    - Disproportionate head size, ligamentous laxity, & immature muscles have all been postulated as causes

Natural History & Prognosis

- Neurologic status at presentation is best predictor of outcome
  - Intact or incomplete injury → likely good outcome
  - Complete loss of function at level of injury → poor chance of recovery
- Spinal cord hemorrhage → worse potential for recovery

Treatment

- Support of impaired systemic function
- Stabilization of spine to prevent further injury
- Internal or external surgical stabilization
  - May impair ability to assess with MR
- Emergent decompression of spinal cord impingement
- Administration of steroids for acute spinal cord injury is controversial

SELECTED REFERENCES

1. Beckmann NM et al: Accuracy of craniocervical measurements on CT for identifying partial or complete craniocervical ligament injuries in pediatric patients. Skeletal Radiol. 50(1):159-69, 2021
2. Fiester P et al: Pediatric retroclival epidural hematoma in the acute trauma setting: a sign of tectorial membrane stripping injury. AJR Am J Roentgenol. 216(6):1641-8, 2021
3. Beckmann NM et al: Epidemiology and imaging classification of pediatric cervical spine injuries: 12-year experience at a level 1 trauma center. AJR Am J Roentgenol. 214(6):1359-68, 2020
4. McAllister AS et al: Emergent imaging of pediatric cervical spine trauma. Radiographics. 39(4):1126-42, 2019

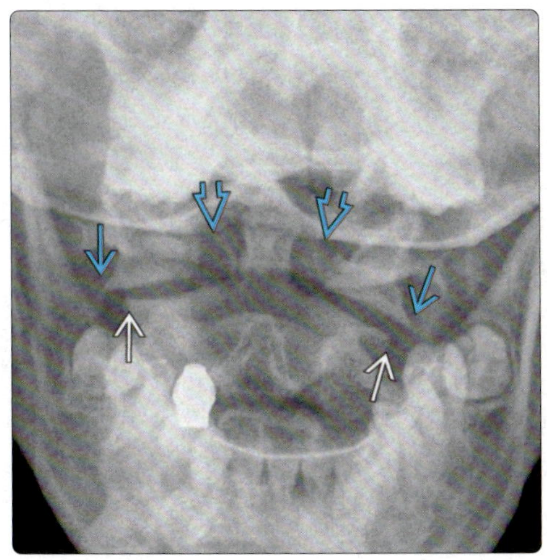

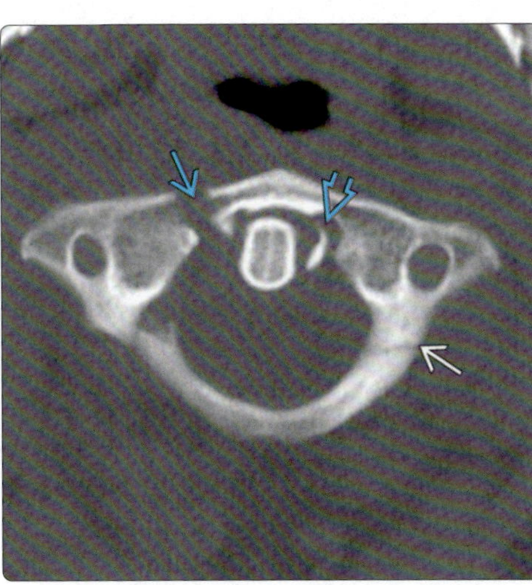

(Left) *Frontal open-mouth radiograph in a 17-year-old girl who fell while performing a back flip shows the C1 lateral masses* ➙ *extending lateral to the C2 lateral masses* ➙ *as well as widening of the lateral atlantodental spaces* ➙*, consistent with a Jefferson fracture.* **(Right)** *Axial NECT in the same patient shows a displaced fracture of the right anterior arch of C1* ➙*, a nondisplaced fracture of the left posterior arch of C1* ➙*, & a posterior cortical avulsion fracture of the left anterior arch of C1* ➙*.*

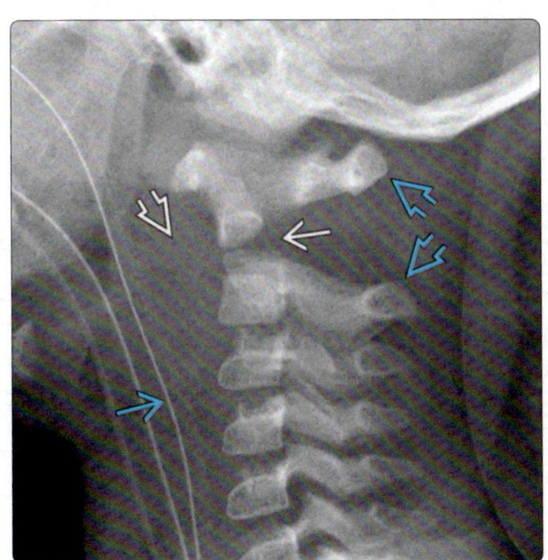

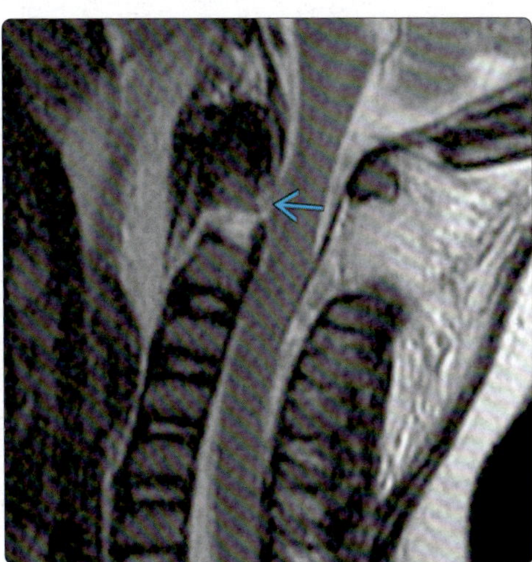

(Left) *Lateral radiograph in a 2-year-old girl in an MVA shows a displaced fracture* ➙ *of the odontoid at the synchondrosis, separating the odontoid & C2 body. Also note the extensive prevertebral soft tissue swelling* ➙ *with displacement of the nasoenteric tube* ➙ *as well as widening of the C1-C2 interspinous distance* ➙*.* **(Right)** *Sagittal T2 MR in the same patient shows disruption of the posterior longitudinal ligament* ➙*, a commonly associated injury in the setting of an odontoid fracture.*

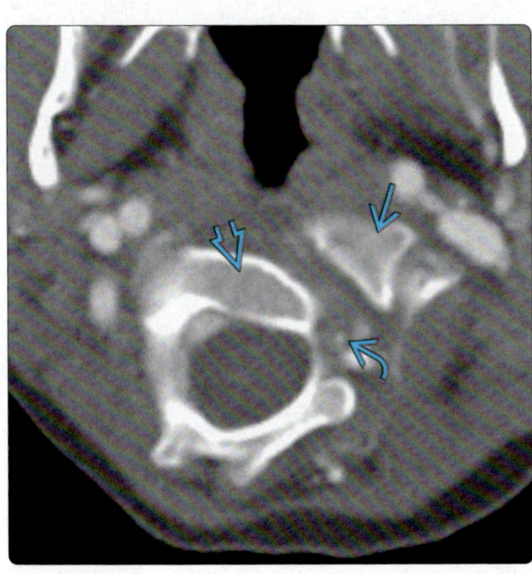

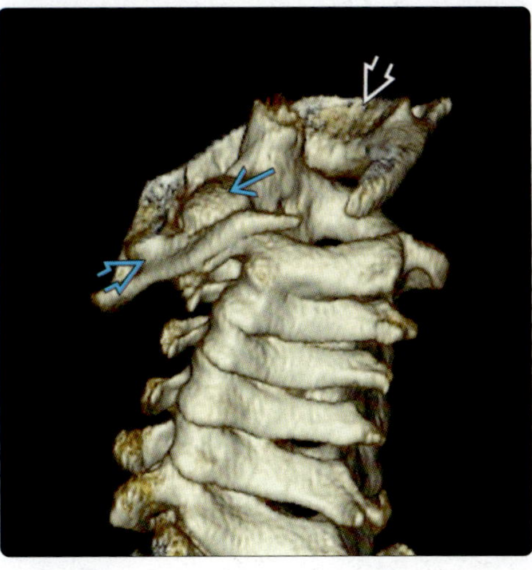

(Left) *Axial CTA in a 5-year-old with torticollis shows the left lateral mass of C1* ➙ *rotated anterior to the body of C2* ➙*, consistent with atlantoaxial rotatory subluxation. The left vertebral artery* ➙ *is extremely small due to dissection related to the subluxation.* **(Right)** *Posterior oblique 3D surface rendering in the same CT shows the left C1 lateral mass* ➙ *dislocated & rotated anterior to the left C2 lateral mass* ➙*. The right C1 lateral mass* ➙ *is rotated superior & posterior to the right C2 lateral mass.*

Chance Fracture

KEY FACTS

TERMINOLOGY

- Synonyms: Flexion-distraction injury, seat belt fracture
- Definition: Compression injury of anterior column of spine with distraction of middle & posterior columns
  - Anterior column: Anterior longitudinal ligament, anterior 1/2 of vertebral body, anterior anulus fibrosis
  - Middle column: Posterior longitudinal ligament, posterior 1/2 of vertebral body, posterior anulus fibrosis
  - Posterior column: Posterior neural arch, facet joint capsular ligaments, ligamentum flavum, inter- & supraspinous ligaments
- May be completely osseous, ligamentous (rare "Chance equivalent"), or mixed (most frequent)
- Extension across 3 columns may invoke osseous & soft tissue structures at multiple adjacent levels

IMAGING

- 78% occur between T12-L2
- Wedging of anterior vertebral body
- Posterior bony & ligamentous distraction injuries result in
  - Focal kyphosis
  - Wide splitting of pedicles & laminae on AP view
  - Separation of facet joints with ↑ interspinous distance
  - Artifactual ↑ in radiolucency of vertebral body on AP radiograph secondary to splayed spinous processes
- Vertebral marrow edema & posterior ligamentous disruptions are best seen on STIR or T2 FS MR

CLINICAL ISSUES

- Classic history: Motor vehicle accident with lap belt restraint & cutaneous seat belt sign over abdomen
  - ~ 80% have significant abdominal injuries
    - Bowel/mesentery (most common), aorta

DIAGNOSTIC CHECKLIST

- Crucial to create sagittal & coronal bone reformatted images from abdominal CT exams in trauma patients

(Left) *AP chest radiograph of a teenager injured in a motor vehicle accident while wearing a seat belt shows a horizontal lucency splitting the T12 pedicles ➡ with widening of the costovertebral joints ➡, indicative of a Chance fracture.* **(Right)** *Sagittal (left) & coronal (right) bone windowed CECT images in the same patient show anterior wedging of the T12 vertebral body ➡ with a horizontal fracture plane splitting the posterior elements ➡. Note the splaying/distraction of the T12 spinous process fragments ➡.*

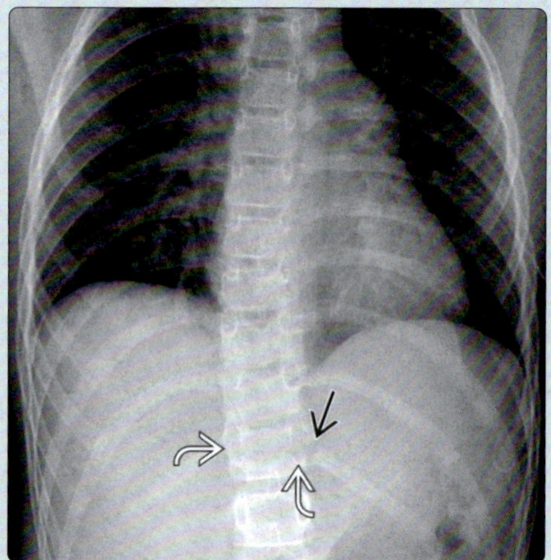

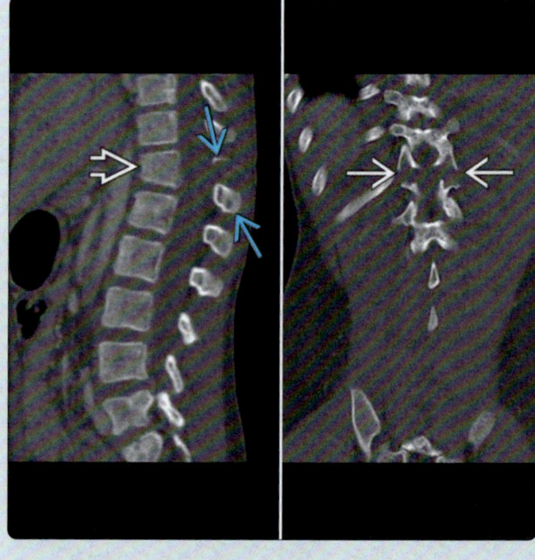

(Left) *3D posterior oblique CT images in the same patient clearly show the horizontal splitting & distraction of the T12 posterior elements ➡, characteristic of the posterior column injury in a Chance fracture.* **(Right)** *Sagittal T2 MR in a 7-year-old with a primarily ligamentous injury shows mild anterior wedging of the L2 vertebra ➡ with disruption of the ligamentum flavum ➡ & interspinous ligaments ➡ resulting in splaying of the L1 & L2 posterior elements ➡.*

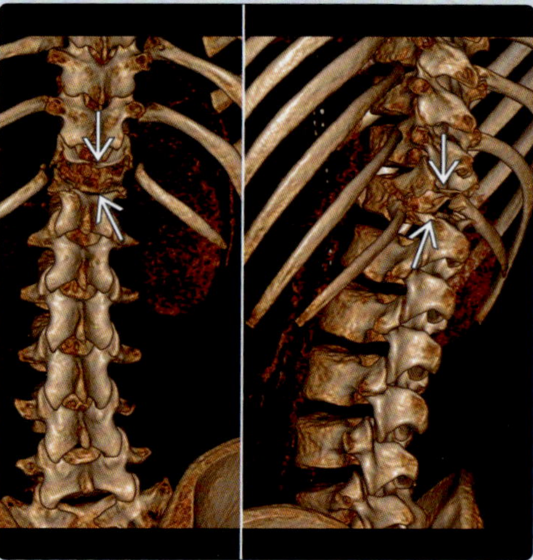

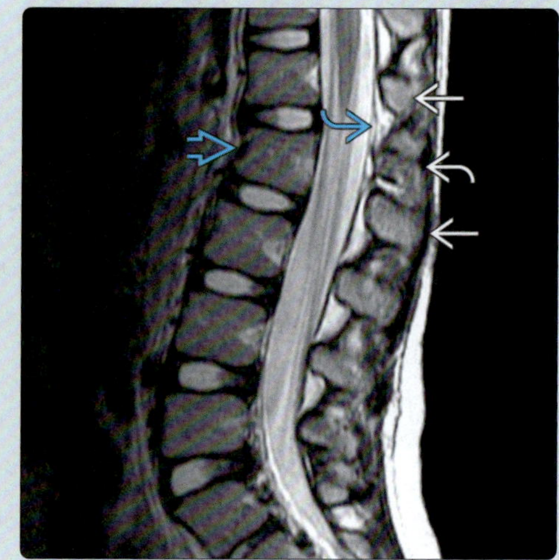

TERMINOLOGY

Synonyms

- Flexion-distraction injury, seat belt fracture

Definitions

- Compression injury of anterior column of spine with distraction of middle & posterior columns
  - Anterior column: Anterior longitudinal ligament (ALL), anterior 1/2 of vertebral body, anterior anulus fibrosis
  - Middle column: Posterior longitudinal ligament, posterior 1/2 of vertebral body, posterior anulus fibrosis
  - Posterior column: Posterior neural arch, facet joint capsular ligaments, ligamentum flavum, inter- & supraspinous ligaments

IMAGING

General Features

- Location
  - Usually occurs at T11-L3; 78% occur between T12-L2
  - May have anterior column injury at 1 level with posterior column injury (fracture &/or soft tissue disruption) at adjacent level

Radiographic Findings

- Wedging of anterior vertebral body with focal kyphosis
  - ± sclerotic transverse fracture line due to trabecular impaction
  - Vertebral body height loss is often > 40-50%
- Bony & ligamentous injuries to posterior column
  - Splitting of pedicles & laminae on AP view
  - Empty body sign on AP view: Artifactual ↑ in radiolucency of vertebral body secondary to splayed spinous processes
  - Separation of facet joints with ↑ interspinous distance
- No subluxation of vertebral body

CT Findings

- Vertebral body fracture may be comminuted
  - May have mild retropulsion of posterior cortex
- Transversely oriented posterior element fracture &/or posterior ligamentous injury
  - ↑ interspinous distance
  - Separation of facet joints: Naked facet sign

MR Findings

- Varying degrees of marrow edema (poorly defined ↑ T2/STIR signal intensity) surrounding fracture plane
  - May be seen in multiple adjacent vertebral bodies with radiographically occult fractures/contusions
- Low-signal ALL is not discontinuous
  - May be partially stripped from vertebral attachment
- Posterior element fractures are difficult to see if splaying is absent
- Low-signal interspinous & supraspinous ligaments are often disrupted by high fluid signal
- Poorly defined fluid in surrounding soft tissues

Imaging Recommendations

- Best imaging tool
  - CT scan
    - Data is typically acquired as part of abdominal CECT
  - MR is indicated to investigate neurologic deficit, ligamentous injuries

DIFFERENTIAL DIAGNOSIS

Distraction Injury

- Vertebral body displacement & ALL disruption distinguish from Chance fracture

Traumatic Compression Fracture

- No posterior element fracture

Burst Fracture

- Also involves posterior vertebral body cortex
- Vertically oriented fractures of posterior elements

PATHOLOGY

General Features

- Etiology
  - Typical setting: Motor vehicle accident or fall
  - Classic pattern: Lap seat belt without shoulder strap
    - Seat belt, in high position, serves as fulcrum anterior to vertebral column → compression of anterior column + distraction of posterior column
    - Up to 40% have 3-point restraint (not just lap belt), typically incorrectly positioned
- Associated abnormalities
  - Up to 80% of children with cutaneous seat belt sign have significant abdominal injuries
    - Bowel/mesentery (most common)
      - Look for unexplained mesenteric & peritoneal fluid with focal bowel wall thickening/dilation (± free air)
    - Aorta > solid organs

CLINICAL ISSUES

Presentation

- Traumatic back pain ± neurologic injury
- Seat belt sign of transverse low abdominal wall contusion/injury → up to 50% will have spine injuries

DIAGNOSTIC CHECKLIST

Image Interpretation Pearls

- Radiographic recognition is essential → prompts further evaluation for abdominal injury
- Search for spine injury on sagittal & coronal reformats from abdominal CT exams in trauma patients
  - Especially with clinical evidence of lap belt injury

SELECTED REFERENCES

1. Compagnon R et al: Epidemiology of spinal fractures in children: cross-sectional study. Orthop Traumatol Surg Res. 106(7):1245-9, 2020
2. Eberhardt CS et al: The seatbelt syndrome-do we have a chance? A report of 3 cases with review of literature. Pediatr Emerg Care. 32(5):318-22, 2016
3. Arkader A et al: Pediatric Chance fractures: a multicenter perspective. J Pediatr Orthop. 31(7):741-4, 2011
4. Mulpuri K et al: The spectrum of abdominal injuries associated with chance fractures in pediatric patients. Eur J Pediatr Surg. 17(5):322-7, 2007
5. Bernstein MP et al: Chance-type fractures of the thoracolumbar spine: imaging analysis in 53 patients. AJR Am J Roentgenol. 187(4):859-68, 2006
6. Groves CJ et al: Chance-type flexion-distraction injuries in the thoracolumbar spine: MR imaging characteristics. Radiology. 236(2):601-8, 2005

Spondylolysis and Spondylolisthesis

KEY FACTS

TERMINOLOGY

- Spondylolysis: Defect/break in pars interarticularis
  - Repetitive microtrauma is likely etiology
- Spondylolisthesis: Spondylolysis + anterior slippage of vertebra in relation to vertebra below

IMAGING

- Bone CT
  - Linear lucency or defect in pars interarticularis
    - Sagittal or oblique sagittal reformatted imaging is vital
  - Incomplete ring sign on axial imaging ± distraction
    - May simulate "extra" or double facet joints
    - May be confused with facet joint
      - Lysis is located anterior to facet joint
      - Lysis is more transverse in orientation on axial images compared to more oblique facet joint
      - Facet joint is smooth, while lysis typically is irregular/fragmented
  - Spondylolisthesis & foraminal narrowing on sagittal reformatted images
  - Secondary finding of sclerosis &/or hypertrophy of contralateral pedicle & lamina
  - May be insensitive to early stress injury (edema with microtrabecular fracture)
- SPECT bone scan imaging is helpful for diagnosis
  - Intense focal uptake in posterior elements, unilateral or bilateral
  - Triangular pattern of uptake on sagittal images
  - Remote or healed may be occult (normal)
- SPECT/CT: Confirms diagnosis with anatomy & physiology
- MR for lysis: Adjust spine protocol toward musculoskeletal system by adding STIR/T2 FS (↑ conspicuity of marrow & soft tissue edema)

CLINICAL ISSUES

- 40% incidence in children with lower back pain
  - L5: 85%; L4: 5-15%; rarely higher

(Left) *Lateral radiograph in a 15-year-old female basketball player with back pain shows a linear lucency at the L3 pars interarticularis ➡. There is no anterior subluxation of L3 relative to L4 to suggest spondylolisthesis.* **(Right)** *Axial STIR MR in the same patient shows irregular low signal intensity pars interarticularis defects ➡ bilaterally at L3 with adjacent marrow ➡ & soft tissue ➡ edema.*

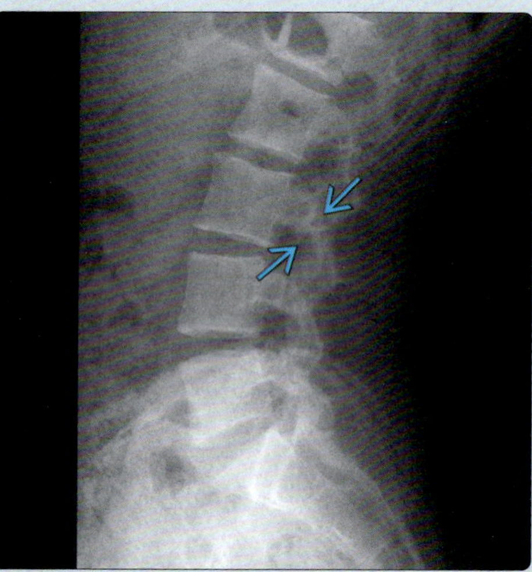

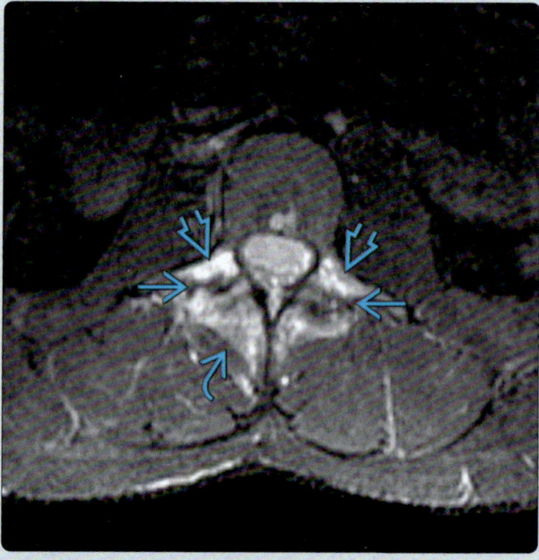

(Left) *Coronal SPECT bone scan in a 15-year-old who presents with lower back pain shows asymmetric uptake ➡ in the posterior elements of L5, R > L. NECT images (not shown) demonstrated right L5 spondylolysis with reactive stress changes at the left L5 pars interarticularis.* **(Right)** *Axial NECT in a 14-year-old girl who presents with severe left flank pain for a renal stone evaluation shows an incomplete osseous ring with bilateral distracted pars interarticularis defects ➡ at L5.*

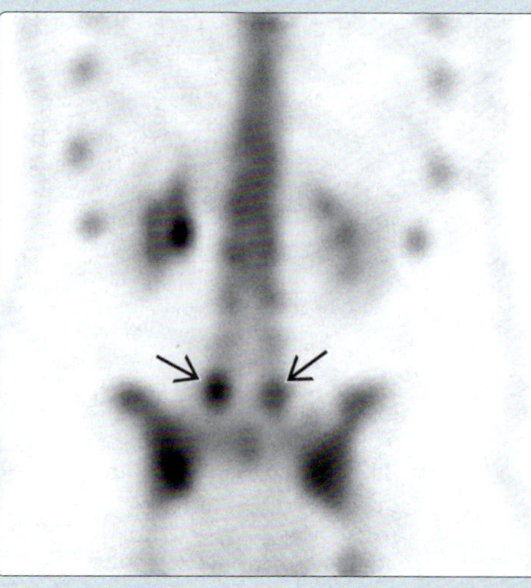

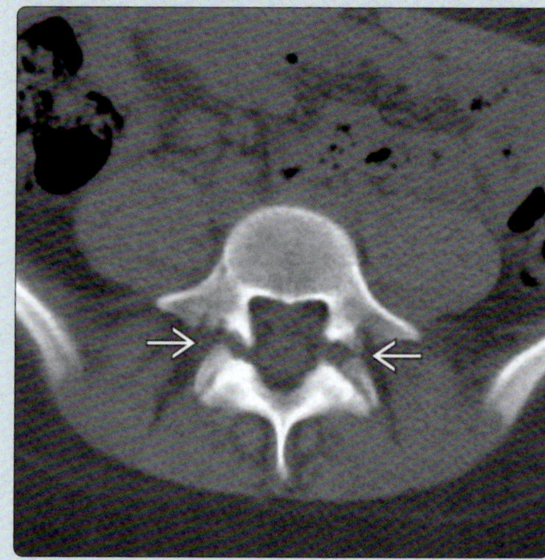

TERMINOLOGY

Synonyms

- Lysis, isthmic spondylolysis

Definitions

- Spondylolysis: Defect/break in pars interarticularis
- Spondylolisthesis: Spondylolysis + anterior slippage of vertebral body in relation to vertebra below

IMAGING

General Features

- Location
  - L5: 85%; L4: 5-15%; rarely above
  - Cervical spine location is usually congenital
  - 10-15% are unilateral

Radiographic Findings

- Classic: Break in neck of "Scotty dog" (pars interarticularis defect on oblique views of standing lumbar spine)
  - ± anterolisthesis
  - Positive predictive value of 57%

CT Findings

- Bone CT: Lucent defect of pars interarticularis
  - Sagittal or oblique sagittal reformatted images are vital
  - Incomplete ring sign on axial imaging ± distraction
- High sensitivity with multiplanar reformats but often overlooked on abdominal/pelvic studies obtained for other reasons

MR Findings

- T1: Discontinuity (sagittal images best), ↓ signal in pars interarticularis
- T2: ↓ signal in pars interarticularis (reactive sclerosis), ↑ signal in pars interarticularis (marrow edema)
- STIR/T2 FS: ↑ conspicuity of surrounding marrow & soft tissue edema, suggesting spondylolysis at classic location even if fracture not seen
- MR for lysis: Sensitivity: 57-86%; specificity: 81-82%
- Additional sequences that may ↑ sensitivity
  - 3D GRE T1: Volumetric, thin slices
  - Ultrashort TE (UTE) or zero TE (ZTE): Improved visualization of cortical bone

Nuclear Medicine Findings

- ↑ uptake is best seen on SPECT bone scan
- Can be fused with bone CT

Imaging Recommendations

- Best imaging tool
  - Radiographs first
  - If source of back pain is not clear, consider MR
    - Include STIR or T2 FS for marrow & soft tissue edema
  - Targeted helical/volumetric bone CT with multiplanar reformats
  - Bone scan SPECT/CT is better than SPECT alone
    - Anatomic & physiologic confirmation
    - Helps differentiate completed lysis vs. uptake from stress changes

PATHOLOGY

General Features

- Etiology
  - Believed to be caused by repetitive microtrauma, particularly hyperextension → stress fracture
  - Common associated activities: Gymnastics, tennis, baseball, weightlifting, wrestling, cricket, & football at young age
- Associated abnormalities
  - Spondylolisthesis (50%), scoliosis, Scheuermann disease, spina bifida occulta

CLINICAL ISSUES

Presentation

- Most common signs/symptoms
  - Asymptomatic (80%)
  - 40% incidence in children with lower back pain (LBP)
- Other signs/symptoms
  - Tight hamstring muscles
    - Waddling gait secondary to tight hamstring muscles
  - Back spasms or radiating pain
  - Chronic LBP in older children & adults
  - Back pain exacerbated by rigorous activities
  - Radiculopathy & cauda equina syndrome in lysis with high-grade spondylolisthesis

Demographics

- Epidemiology
  - Incidence: 3-10%
  - ↑ incidence in competitive athletes, especially males

Treatment

- Mainly conservative first; surgical if conservative treatment fails or subluxation progresses

DIAGNOSTIC CHECKLIST

Image Interpretation Pearls

- Typical bone scan findings with normal radiographs or bone CT suggest stress reaction or early spondylolysis

SELECTED REFERENCES

1. Chung CC et al: Lumbosacral spondylolysis and spondylolisthesis. Clin Sports Med. 40(3):471-90, 2021
2. Berger RG et al: Spondylolysis 2019 update. Curr Opin Pediatr. 31(1):61-8, 2019
3. Finkenstaedt T et al: Ultrashort time-to-echo magnetic resonance imaging at 3 T for the detection of spondylolysis in cadaveric spines: comparison with CT. Invest Radiol. 54(1):32-8, 2019
4. Lemoine T et al: The prevalence of lumbar spondylolysis in young children: a retrospective analysis using CT. Eur Spine J. 27(5):1067-72, 2018
5. Trout AT et al: Spondylolysis and beyond: value of SPECT/CT in evaluation of low back pain in children and young adults. Radiographics. 35(3):819-34, 2015

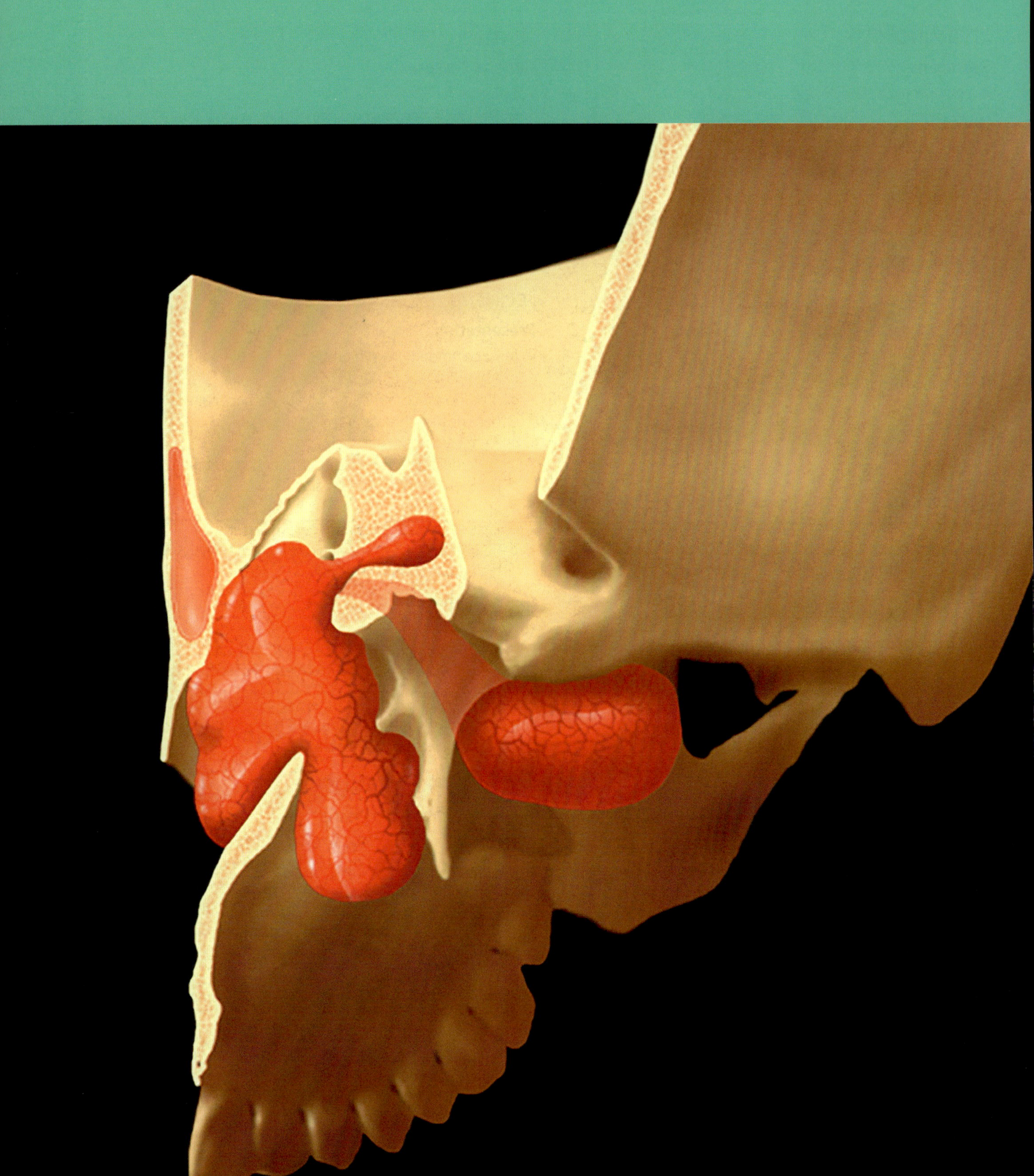

SECTION 9

Head and Neck

Summary Thoughts: Congenital Cystic Neck Masses

Palpable masses are a common indication for imaging the pediatric head & neck (H&N). Most are congenital or inflammatory in children; only 5% of childhood neoplasms occur in the H&N (excluding the brain). The most common extrathyroid, nonneoplastic solid neck masses in children are related to inflammatory disease & do not require imaging unless there is concern for deep neck infection or abscess. The most common cystic masses in the pediatric H&N are congenital lesions secondary to abnormal embryogenesis involving the thyroglossal duct (TGD), the branchial apparatus, or the vascular endothelium. TGD cysts (TGDCs) account for 70-90% of all congenital neck abnormalities in children. The most common branchial apparatus lesion is the 2nd branchial cleft or apparatus cyst (BCC/BAC), & lymphatic malformations are the most common vascular malformations in the H&N.

Whenever a cystic neck mass is encountered on a pediatric imaging study, a very reasonable differential diagnosis can be made based on its location (midline, paramidline, or lateral, as well as location relative to carotid sheath), imaging appearance (simple cyst, complicated cyst, enhancement, ± solid component), & clinical presentation (present since birth or acute onset, ± clinical evidence of infection).

Terminology

A TGDC or tract is an anomalous remnant of the TGD that completely involutes during normal development. Cysts are located anywhere from the midline posterior tongue at the foramen cecum to the thyroid bed in the lower neck.

Branchial apparatus anomalies can be cysts, sinus tracts, or fistulae. Cysts are fluid filled with well-defined walls secondary to the failure of obliteration of a branchial cleft or pouch. Sinus tracts are congenital tracts with 1 opening, either externally to the skin surface (or external auditory canal) or internally to the pharynx (2nd branchial cleft), superolateral hypopharynx (3rd branchial cleft), or pyriform sinus (4th or 3rd branchial pouch). Fistulae are congenital tracts with 2 openings (1 internally & 1 externally) secondary to failure of obliteration of the branchial cleft & pouch.

Imaging Techniques & Indications

US, CT, & MR are all reasonable options for the initial imaging of neck masses in children. Modality choice depends on the clinical presentation, the referring clinical service, & the modalities available at the time. For instance, if there is concern that a child with cellulitis & cervical adenitis has a drainable abscess deep to a palpable neck mass, US may be very helpful in determining the presence of underlying drainable fluid. Likewise, if a child is thought to have a TGDC, US is the imaging modality of choice to evaluate the suspected TGDC & prove the presence of a normal-appearing thyroid gland in the lower neck. US is also the modality of choice in patients with suspected infantile hemangioma, as color Doppler findings can be quite characteristic. However, CECT is the initial imaging modality of choice to evaluate the total extent of disease in children with suspected deep neck infection & to assess for a possible underlying pyriform sinus tract in children with left-sided neck abscesses that involve the left thyroid lobe.

In children not presenting with signs & symptoms of infection, CT or MR may be used as the initial imaging modality. The choice of which modality may depend on the need for sedation/anesthesia, which is usually required for MR in children under 5 or 6 years of age. MR is the preferred imaging modality for children with suspected vascular malformations due to its excellent soft tissue contrast resolution, variety of methods of interrogation, & lack of limitations regarding depth.

Embryology

The thyroid gland migrates from the foramen cecum at the midline posterior tongue to the paramidline location in the lower neck via the path of the TGD. The TGD normally involutes during the 5th or 6th week of gestation. However, remnant epithelium anywhere along the tract may persist & form a TGDC. As the TGD diverticulum descends caudally, it passes along the anterior surface of the developing hyoid bone; therefore, remnants may be found anterior to the preepiglottic space of the larynx.

Branchial apparatus structures develop between the 4th & 6th week of gestation & consist of 6 pairs of mesodermal arches separated by 5 paired endodermal pouches internally & 5 paired ectodermal clefts externally. During the 6th week of gestation, the 2nd branchial arch overgrows the 3rd & 4th branchial arches, resulting in a combined 2nd, 3rd, & 4th branchial cleft, termed the "cervical sinus of His." Anomalies of the branchial apparatus include cysts, sinus tracts, & fistulae. The most common lesions for which imaging is indicated are BCCs/BACs, & most of these are related to anomalous development of a branchial cleft. However, a few are related to anomalous development of a branchial pouch.

The location of the lesion is the best clue to the origin of a branchial apparatus anomaly. First BCCs account for ~ 8% of all branchial anomalies. They are located in or around the external auditory canal, ear lobe, or parotid gland & may extend inferiorly to the angle of the mandible. Second BCCs account for up to 95% of all branchial apparatus anomalies & are subclassified by location using the Bailey system: Type I cysts are located deep to the platysma muscle/anterior to the sternocleidomastoid (SCM) muscle; type II cysts are posterior to the submandibular gland/anterior to the SCM (& are the most common); type III cysts protrude between the external & internal carotid arteries; & type IV cysts are directly adjacent to the pharyngeal wall (thought to be a remnant of the 2nd pouch). Fistulas are rare; however, a 2nd branchial apparatus fistula is occasionally identified with an internal opening at the level of the pharynx & an external skin opening anterior to the lower aspect of the SCM.

Third BCCs are rare & located in the posterior compartment of the upper neck or anterior compartment of the lower neck. Third pharyngeal pouch remnants are more common than cleft remnants & are related to descent of the thymic primordium from the lateral margins of the pharynx to the upper anterior mediastinum (via the thymopharyngeal duct) during the 6th-9th weeks of gestation. If the duct does not undergo normal involution, a cervical thymic cyst may form that is in close association with the anterior margin of the carotid sheath. The cyst formation is from interactions between the endodermal primordia & neural crest cells during normal thymic development & migration. Histologically, Hassall corpuscles will be identifiable within the cyst wall. Ectopic foci of solid thymic tissue may also be deposited along the remnant duct.

Types of Congenital Cystic Neck Masses

Types of Congenital Cystic Neck Masses
Thyroglossal Duct Lesions
Thyroglossal duct cyst: Tongue base to thyroid bed; embedded in strap muscles when infrahyoid
Ectopic thyroid tissue: Lingual location is most common
Branchial Apparatus Lesions
1st branchial cleft cyst (type I): Located anterior, inferior, or posterior to external auditory canal
1st branchial cleft cyst (type II): Located in or adjacent to parotid gland; may extend inferiorly to angle of mandible
2nd branchial cleft cyst: Most common location is posterior to submandibular gland, lateral to carotid space, & anteromedial to SCM muscle
3rd branchial cleft cyst: Posterior cervical space in upper neck or anterior to SCM in lower neck
3rd branchial pouch remnant → thymopharyngeal duct cyst or ectopic thymus: Along course from pharynx to upper mediastinum
4th branchial pouch remnant → pyriform sinus tract: Patients present with left-sided abscess involving thyroid gland
Vascular Malformations
Venous malformation: Patchy, gradual enhancement; phleboliths are common; ± fluid-fluid levels
Lymphatic malformation: Multilocular cyst ± fluid-fluid levels; rim/septal enhancement
Venolymphatic malformation: Mixed enhancing venous & nonenhancing lymphatic components

SCM = sternocleidomastoid.

Pyriform sinus tracts, or rarely fistulae, represent a unique congenital anomaly of the 4th (or 3rd) pharyngeal pouch. This lesion should be suspected in any child presenting with neck infection involving the left thyroid lobe. The inflammation can frequently be traced superiorly to an asymmetric pyriform sinus apex. A postbarium swallow CT study is frequently helpful to define the barium-filled tract extending from the pyriform sinus to the anterior lower neck.

Vascular malformations are congenital malformations of endothelial development that can be divided into simple or combined lesions with combined lesions containing 2 or more vessel types in 1 lesion. Simple lesions can be divided based on the predominant endothelial characteristics of the lesion into capillary malformations, lymphatic malformations, venous malformations, arteriovenous malformations, & arteriovenous fistulae. The most common vascular malformations identified in the H&N are lymphatic, venous, & combined venolymphatic lesions.

Imaging Anatomy

Recognizing the defined location of a congenital abnormality, particularly congenital cysts, is key to arriving at the correct diagnosis or differential diagnosis. TGD remnants may be in the form of cysts or solid ectopic thyroid tissue anywhere from the midline tongue base to the infrahyoid paramidline thyroid bed. First BCCs are in or around the external auditory canal or parotid gland. Second BCCs are most commonly posteromedial to the submandibular gland & anteromedial to the SCM. Cysts in the posterior triangle of the upper neck may be 3rd BCCs or lymphatic malformations. Cysts along the lower anterior margin of the SCM may be from the 2nd or 3rd branchial cleft or may be lymphatic malformations. Cysts or solid masses in close association with the carotid sheath along the tract of the thymopharyngeal duct (from the angle of the mandible to the upper mediastinum) should raise the question of cervical thymic cyst or ectopic thymus.

Differential Diagnosis

Thyroglossal Duct Lesions

- TGDC: Tongue base to thyroid bed
- Ectopic thyroid: Lingual thyroid is most common

Branchial Apparatus Lesions

- 1st BCC: Type I cysts lie anterior, inferior, or posterior to external auditory canal
- 1st BCC: Type II cysts in superficial, parotid, or parapharyngeal space may extend as low as posterior submandibular space
- 2nd BCC: Most common posterolateral to submandibular gland, lateral to carotid space, & anteromedial to SCM
- 3rd BCC: Posterior cervical space of upper neck or along anterior border of SCM in mid- & lower neck
- 3rd branchial pouch remnant: Thymopharyngeal duct cyst or ectopic thymus
- 4th branchial pouch remnant: Pyriform sinus tract → recurrent thyroiditis or thyroid abscess, usually left sided; recent literature suggests this may be 3rd branchial pouch remnant

Vascular Malformations

- Venous malformations: Patchy, gradual enhancement; ± fluid-fluid levels & phleboliths
- Lymphatic malformations: Classically multilocular & transspatial with fluid-fluid levels & minimal rim/septal enhancement
- Venolymphatic malformations: Nonenhancing lymphatic & enhancing venous elements ± phleboliths

Selected References

1. Tokarz E et al: Proposed ultrasound algorithm to differentiate thyroglossal duct and dermoid cysts. Int J Pediatr Otorhinolaryngol. 142:110624, 2021
2. Corvino A et al: Thyroglossal duct cysts and site-specific differential diagnoses: imaging findings with emphasis on ultrasound assessment. J Ultrasound. 23(2):139-49, 2020
3. Buch K et al: MR imaging evaluation of pediatric neck masses: review and update. Magn Reson Imaging Clin N Am. 27(2):173-99, 2019
4. Merrow AC et al: 2014 revised classification of vascular lesions from the International Society for the Study of Vascular Anomalies: radiologic-pathologic update. Radiographics. 36(5):1494-516, 2016
5. Ibrahim M et al: Congenital cystic lesions of the head and neck. Neuroimaging Clin N Am. 21(3):621-39, viii, 2011
6. Thomas B et al: Revisiting imaging features and the embryologic basis of third and fourth branchial anomalies. AJNR Am J Neuroradiol. 31(4):755-60, 2010

(Left) *Anterior graphic of a 6-week embryo shows the 2nd branchial arch growing inferiorly over the 3rd & 4th arches, resulting in the cervical sinus of His that combines the 2nd, 3rd, & 4th branchial clefts (BCs). Note that the thymopharyngeal duct is a remnant of the 3rd branchial pouch.* **(Right)** *Oblique graphic shows the tract of a type I 1st BC anomaly from the medial bony external auditory canal (EAC) toward the retroauricular area. The tract of a type II 1st BC anomaly connects the EAC to the angle of the mandible.*

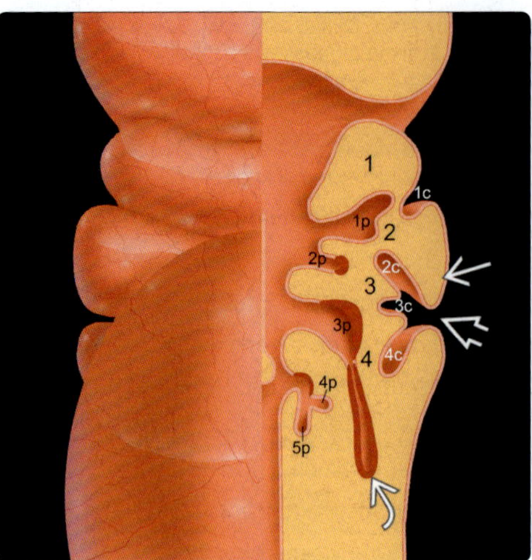

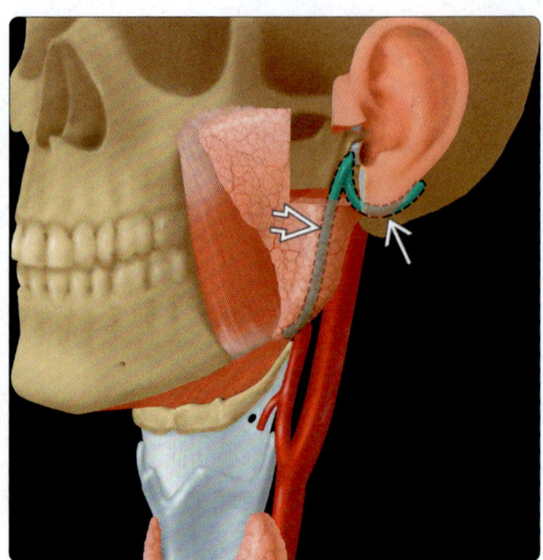

(Left) *Oblique graphic of the tract of a 2nd BC fistula shows a proximal opening in the faucial tonsil & a distal opening in the anterior supraclavicular neck.* **(Right)** *Oblique graphic illustrates the tract of a 3rd BC anomaly extending from the cephalad aspect of the lateral hypopharynx to the supraclavicular anterior neck skin.*

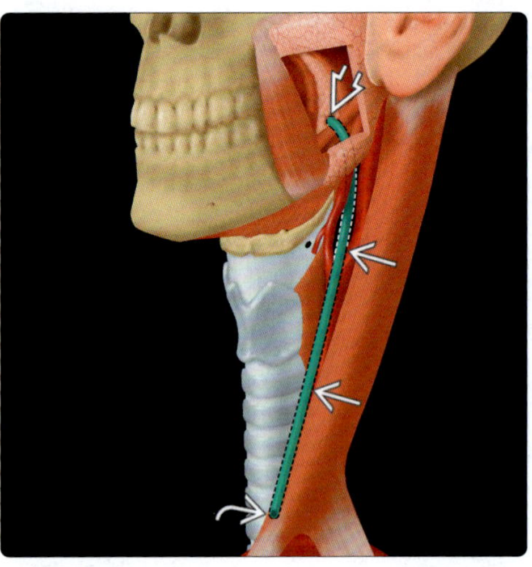

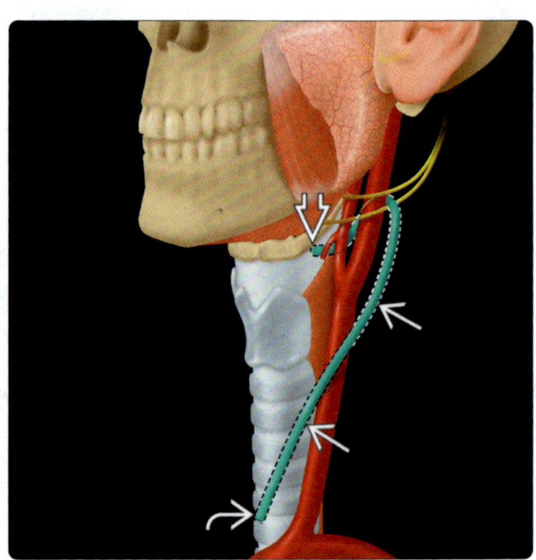

(Left) *Anterior graphic shows both thymopharyngeal duct tracts extending from the lateral hypopharyngeal area to the location of the normal lobes of the thymus in the superior mediastinum.* **(Right)** *Oblique graphic of the neck shows the tract of a 4th BC anomaly extending from the hypopharynx to the location of the left thyroid lobe. This relationship explains why this lesion often presents with thyroiditis.*

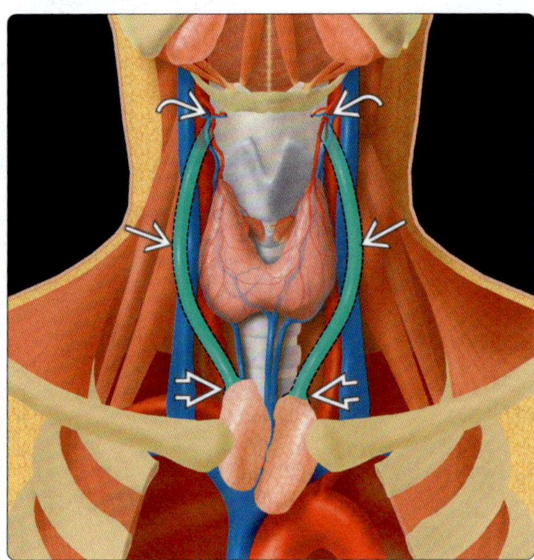

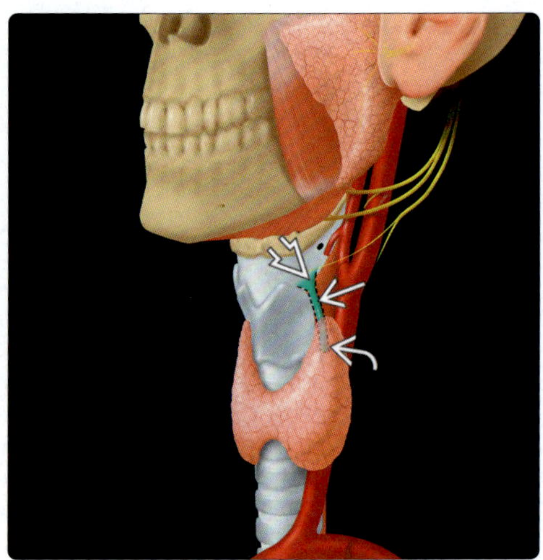

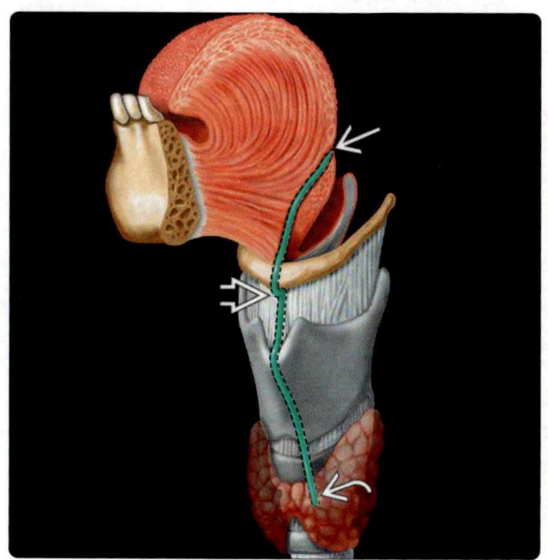

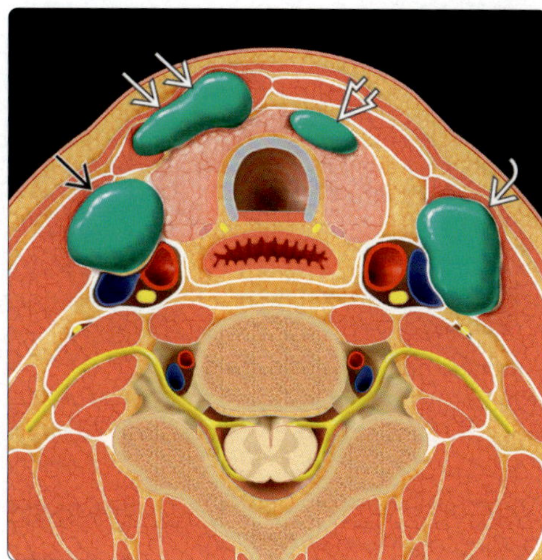

(Left) *Oblique graphic illustrates the tract of the thyroglossal duct descending from the foramen cecum ➡ (at the tongue base) to the midline hyoid bone ➡ before tracking off midline to the thyroid lobe ➡.* **(Right)** *Axial graphic demonstrates the locations of 4 major congenital cystic lesions of the head & neck. Shown here are the infrahyoid 2nd & 3rd BC cysts ➡, the infrahyoid thyroglossal duct cyst ➡, the cervical thymic cysts ➡, & the 4th branchial apparatus sinus tracts ➡.*

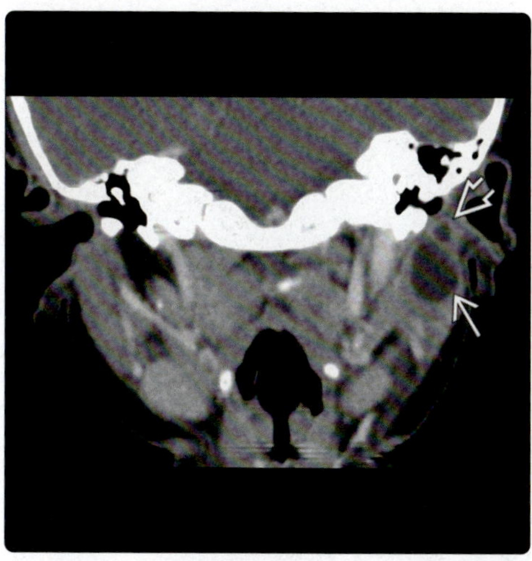

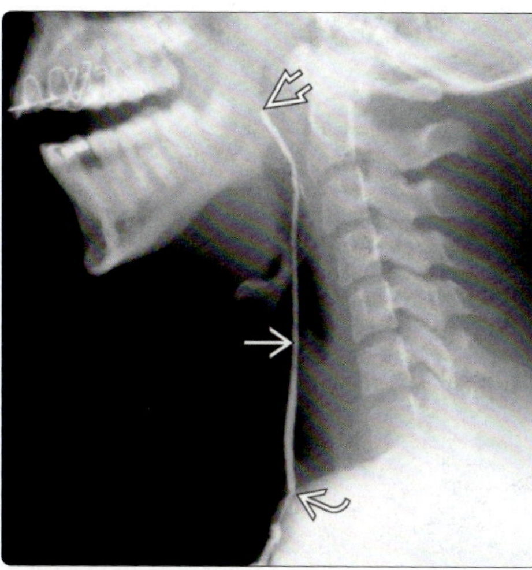

(Left) *Coronal CECT shows a bilobed, cystic mass, the largest portion ➡ lying within the left parotid gland & the smaller portion ➡ extending toward the junction of the cartilaginous & osseous EAC, typical of a 1st BC cyst.* **(Right)** *Lipiodol fistulagram of a 2nd BC fistula ➡ shows the proximal opening into the lateral oropharynx ➡ & the distal opening in the anterior supraclavicular neck ➡.*

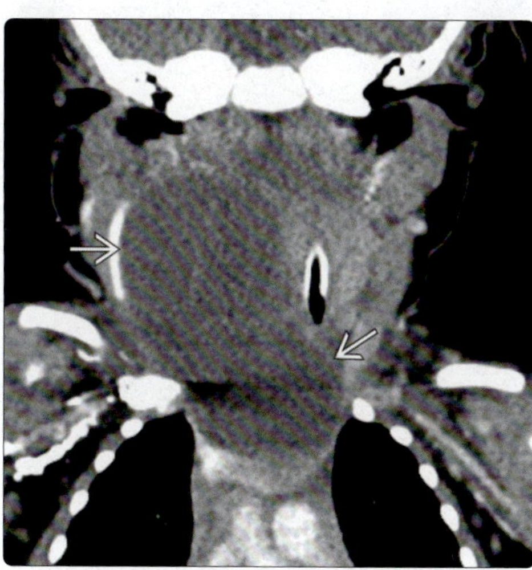

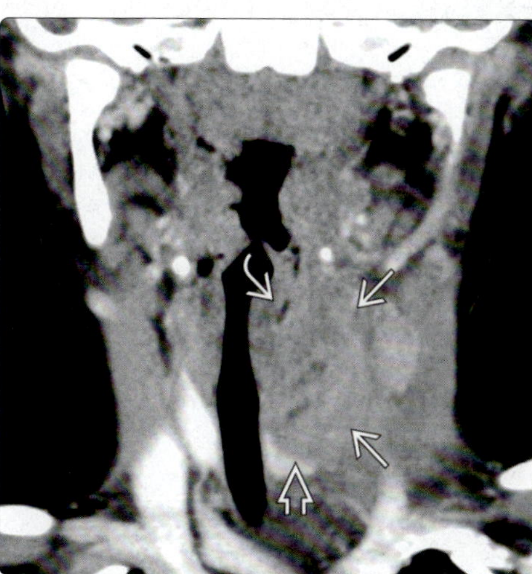

(Left) *Coronal CECT in a 4-month-old shows the typical appearance of a 3rd branchial pouch remnant cervical thymic cyst extending from the anterior neck to the mediastinum ➡.* **(Right)** *Coronal CECT in a 4-year-old boy shows a phlegmonous mass ➡ in the left neck involving the left thyroid lobe ➡. There is a tract of inflammation ➡ coursing toward the left pyriform sinus, consistent with an inflamed 4th (or 3rd) branchial sinus tract.*

KEY FACTS

TERMINOLOGY

- Defective embryogenesis of anterior neuropore
- Results in any mixture of dermoid cyst, epidermoid cyst, &/or sinus tract in frontonasal region

IMAGING

- Midline location, anywhere from nasal tip to anterior skull base at foramen cecum
- MR
  - T2: Fluid-signal tract in septum from nasal dorsum to skull base (sinus)
  - T1: Focal low-signal (epidermoid or nonfatty dermoid) or high-signal (dermoid) mass between tip of nose & apex of crista galli
- CT
  - Bifid crista galli with large foramen cecum
  - Fluid-attenuation tract (sinus)/cyst (epidermoid) or fat-containing mass (dermoid)
    - From nasal dorsum to skull base within nasal septum

TOP DIFFERENTIAL DIAGNOSES

- Yellow marrow in crista galli
- Unossified foramen cecum
- Frontoethmoidal cephalocele
- Nasal glioma (nasal glial heterotopia/cerebral heterotopia)

PATHOLOGY

- Intracranial extension of nasal dermal sinus (NDS) in 20%
  - May rarely lead to meningitis
- Associated craniofacial anomalies in 15%

CLINICAL ISSUES

- Nasoglabellar mass (30%)
- Pit (± protruding hair) on skin of nasal bridge at osteocartilaginous nasal junction

DIAGNOSTIC CHECKLIST

- Nasoglabellar mass or pit on nose leads clinician to search for NDS with intracranial extension

(Left) *Lateral graphic depicts a nasal dermal sinus with 2 dermoids. An extracranial dermoid is present just deep to a cutaneous nasal pit ➡. An intracranial dermoid ➡ splits a bifid crista galli ➡.* **(Right)** *Sagittal NECT in an 8-year-old with known midline anomalies shows a fat-lined nasal dermal sinus ➡ deep to the nasal bones. The sinus leads to a large fat- & fluid-attenuation dermoid ➡. There is a wide foramen cecum ➡ with fatty foci ➡ extending along the falx. Agenesis of the corpus callosum ➡ is also noted.*

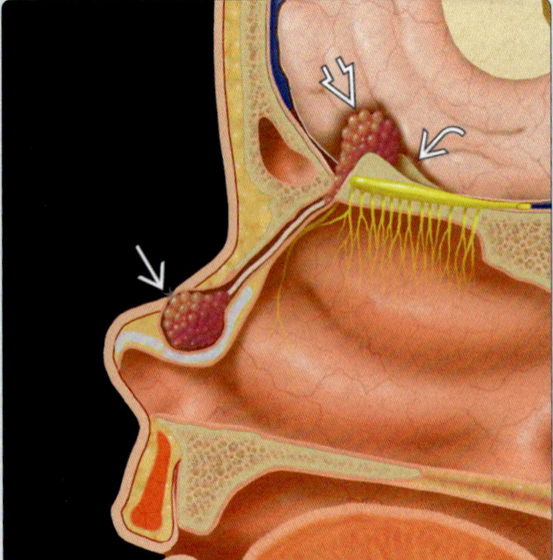

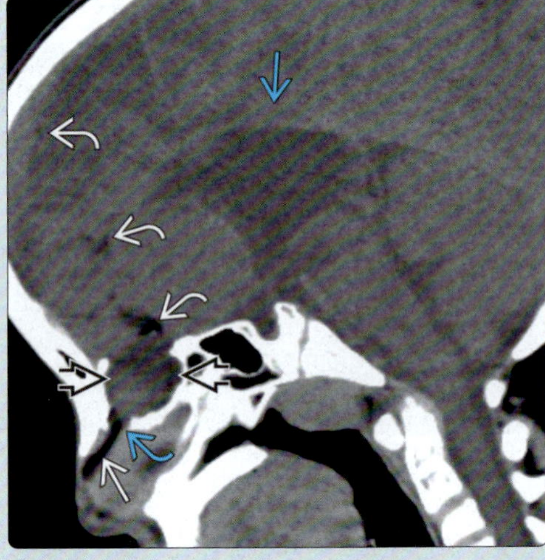

(Left) *Coronal bone CT in the same patient shows the bony nasal septum split ➡ by a large fat & fluid-attenuation dermoid.* **(Right)** *Sagittal T1 MR in the same patient shows the fat-lined nasal dermal sinus ➡, large mixed signal intensity dermoid ➡, & falcine foci of fat ➡ (consistent with intracranial extension & rupture). Agenesis of the corpus callosum ➡ is again noted. The dermoid was ultimately resected. Note that the size & extent of findings in this case is greater than typically seen.*

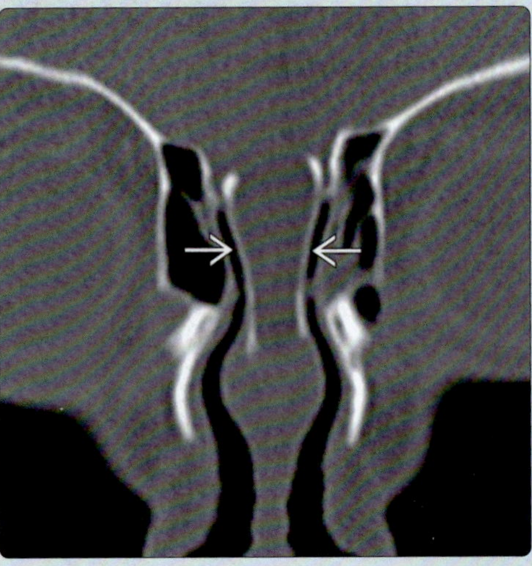

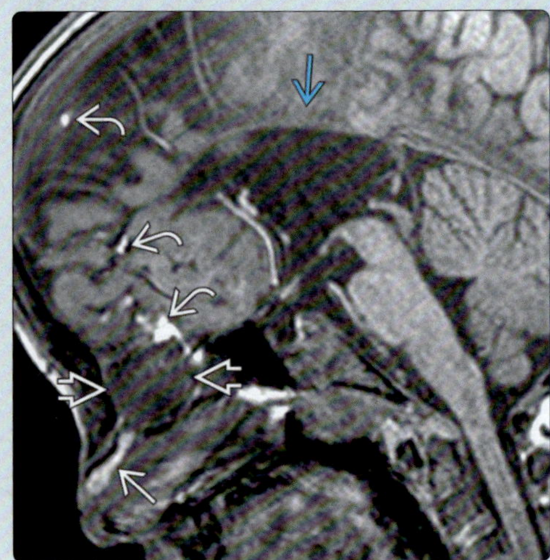

TERMINOLOGY

Abbreviations

- Nasal dermal sinus (NDS)

Synonyms

- Nasal dermoid, nasal dermal cyst, anterior neuropore anomaly

Definitions

- Defective embryogenesis of anterior neuropore
- Results in any mixture of dermoid cyst, epidermoid cyst, &/or sinus tract in frontonasal region

IMAGING

General Features

- Best diagnostic clue
  - CT
    - Bifid crista galli with large foramen cecum
    - Fluid-attenuation tract (sinus)/cyst (epidermoid) or fat-containing mass (dermoid)
      - From nasal dorsum to skull base within nasal septum
  - MR
    - Fluid-signal tract in septum from nasal dorsum to skull base (sinus)
    - Focal T1 low-signal (epidermoid) or high-signal (dermoid) between tip of nose & apex of crista galli
- Location
  - Midline lesion anywhere from nasal tip to anterior skull base at foramen cecum
- Size
  - 5 mm to 2 cm for dermoid/epidermoid
- Morphology
  - Ovoid mass ± tubular sinus tract

CT Findings

- Bone CT
  - Focal tract (sinus) or mass (dermoid or epidermoid) anywhere from nasal bridge to crista galli
    - Fluid-density tract = sinus
    - Fluid-density mass = epidermoid
    - Fat-density mass = dermoid
  - Large foramen cecum with bifid or deformed crista galli or cribriform plate suggests intracranial extension
    - Caution: Anterior skull base ossification is widely variable in 1st few years of life
    - Wide foramen cecum alone is not strong indicator of intracranial extension; correlate with MR

MR Findings

- T1WI
  - ↓ signal tract = sinus
  - ↑ signal mass = dermoid (with ↓ signal on fat-suppressed images)
  - ↓ signal mass = epidermoid or dermoid without fat
- T2WI
  - ↑ signal in sinus, epidermoid, or dermoid
  - Coronal plane shows septal lesions to best advantage
- DWI
  - ↑ signal = epidermoid usually, dermoid rarely
  - Susceptibility artifacts at skull base may obscure signal from epidermoid

Imaging Recommendations

- Best imaging tool
  - MR is more sensitive for delineating sinus tract & detecting intracranial extension
    - MR characterizes epidermoid/dermoid lesions better
  - Bone CT is optimal for identifying skull base defect & crista galli deformity
- Protocol advice
  - Imaging "sweet spot" is small & anterior
    - Focus imaging from tip of nose to back of crista galli
    - Inferior end of axial imaging is hard palate
    - Contrast helps with infectious complications or consideration of other differential diagnoses
      - Not for primary dermoid/epidermoid diagnosis
  - CT
    - Thin-section (1-2 mm) bone & soft tissue images
  - MR
    - Sagittal plane displays course of sinus tract from nasal dorsum to skull base
    - Fat-suppressed T1 images confirm presence of fat in dermoids
    - DWI raises sensitivity for lesion
    - 3D T2/SSFP sequences, such as CISS, FIESTA, or SPACE
      - May demonstrate sinus tract, intracranial continuity, & associated tiny epidermoid/dermoid

DIFFERENTIAL DIAGNOSIS

Yellow Marrow in Crista Galli

- No nasoglabellar mass or pit on nose
- CT & MR are otherwise normal

Unossified Foramen Cecum

- Cartilaginous small midline bone "defect" lying between frontal & ethmoid bones, just anterior to crista galli of ethmoid
- ~ 4-mm diameter at birth
- Foramen cecum ossification usually completes by 2 years
  - Sometimes delayed until 5 years
- Crista galli is not deformed or bifid

Frontoethmoidal Cephalocele

- Bone dehiscence is typically larger, involving broader area of midline cribriform plate or frontal bone
- Direct extension of meninges & subarachnoid space ± brain in cephalocele on sagittal MR

Nasal Glioma

- Solid mass of dysplastic glial tissue separated from brain by subarachnoid space & meninges
- Preferred terms: Nasal glial heterotopia, nasal cerebral heterotopia
- Most commonly projects extranasally onto paramedian bridge of nose
- Less commonly lies intranasal along anterior nasal septum, off midline

PATHOLOGY

General Features

- Etiology
  - Anterior neuropore anomaly: General term for anomalous anterior neuropore regression; 3 main types
    - NDS
    - Nasal glioma (preferred term: Nasal glial/cerebral heterotopia)
    - Frontoethmoidal (sincipital) cephalocele
  - Embryology-anatomy: Development of anterior neuropore in 4th-gestational week
    - Dural stalk passes from area of future foramen cecum to area of osteocartilaginous nasal junction
      - Later regresses completely
    - Failure of involution may leave neuroectodermal remnants along tract of dural stalk
    - Results in dermoid or epidermoid alone or in association with NDS tract
- Associated abnormalities
  - Intracranial extension of NDS is seen in 20%
  - Craniofacial anomalies is seen in 15%

Gross Pathologic & Surgical Features

- Sinus = tract can be followed through bones
- Epidermoid = well-defined cyst; dermoid = lobular, well-defined mass

Microscopic Features

- Sinus = midline epithelial-lined tract
- Epidermoid cyst contains desquamated epithelium
- Dermoid cyst contains epithelium, keratin debris, skin adnexa

CLINICAL ISSUES

Presentation

- Most common signs/symptoms
  - Nasoglabellar mass (30%)
  - Pit on skin of nasal bridge at osteocartilaginous nasal junction
    - ± protruding hair
- Other signs/symptoms
  - Intermittent discharge of sebaceous material from pit
  - < 50% have broadening of nasal root & bridge
  - Nasal sinus tract rarely leads to recurrent meningitis
- Clinical profile
  - Child (mean age: 32 months) with nasal pit ± nasoglabellar mass
  - Rarely presents in adult population
    - Meningitis may be 1st problem leading to diagnosis

Demographics

- Age
  - Newborn to 5 years old
- Sex
  - Male patients with dermal sinus are more likely to have intracranial extension
- Epidemiology
  - Congenital midline nasal lesions are rare (1 in 20,000-40,000 births)
    - Nasal dermoid is most common

Natural History & Prognosis

- Isolated problem when surgical correction is successful
- Untreated patients have nasal bridge broadening ± recurrent meningitis

Treatment

- 80% require extracranial excision only
  - Local procedure to remove pit
  - Any associated dermoid or epidermoid is simultaneously removed from nasal bridge
    - Open rhinoplasty vs. transnasal endoscopic excision
- 20% undergo combined extracranial & intracranial resection
  - Biorbitofrontal nasal craniotomy approach
    - Dermoid or epidermoid removed along with involved dura & crista galli
    - Primary closure of surgical margins of dura
  - Midline approach via keyhole frontal craniotomy has been recently described → less blood loss & shorter hospital stay

DIAGNOSTIC CHECKLIST

Consider

- Nasoglabellar mass or pit on nose leads clinician in search of NDS with intracranial extension
- Focused thin-section MR is key to radiologic diagnosis
  - Axial coverage from cephalad margin of crista galli to hard palate
  - Coronal coverage from tip of nose to posterior aspect of crista galli
- Some surgeons prefer to add bone CT if NDS with intracranial extension is found on MR

Image Interpretation Pearls

- If dermal sinus tract reaches dura of anterior cranial fossa, crista galli will be bifid with large foramen cecum
- If foramen cecum is large but crista galli is not bifid & tract is not seen, foramen cecum is normal & not yet closed
  - Foramen cecum may not close before age of 5 years
  - Do not overcall "large foramen cecum" or unnecessary craniotomy may result
  - Repeat imaging in 6-12 months to confirm foramen cecum closure may be acceptable in difficult cases

SELECTED REFERENCES

1. Kotowski M et al: Radiological diagnostics in nasal dermoids: pitfalls, predictive values and literature analysis. Int J Pediatr Otorhinolaryngol. 149:110842, 2021
2. Purnell CA et al: Nasal dermoid cysts with intracranial extension: avoiding coronal incision through midline exposure and nasal bone osteotomy. J Neurosurg Pediatr. 1-7, 2019
3. Ray CN et al: Infected nasal dermoid cyst/sinus tract presenting with bilateral subperiosteal supraorbital abscesses: the midline nasal tuft of hair, an overlooked finding. Ophthalmic Plast Reconstr Surg. 34(1):e31-4, 2018
4. Rodriguez DP et al: Masses of the nose, nasal cavity, and nasopharynx in children. Radiographics. 37(6):1704-30, 2017
5. Gnagi SH et al: Nasal obstruction in newborns. Pediatr Clin North Am. 60(4):903-22, 2013
6. Valencia MP et al: Congenital and acquired lesions of the nasal septum: a practical guide for differential diagnosis. Radiographics. 28(1):205-24; quiz 326, 2008
7. Hedlund G: Congenital frontonasal masses: developmental anatomy, malformations, and MR imaging. Pediatr Radiol. 36(7):647-62; quiz 726-7, 2006

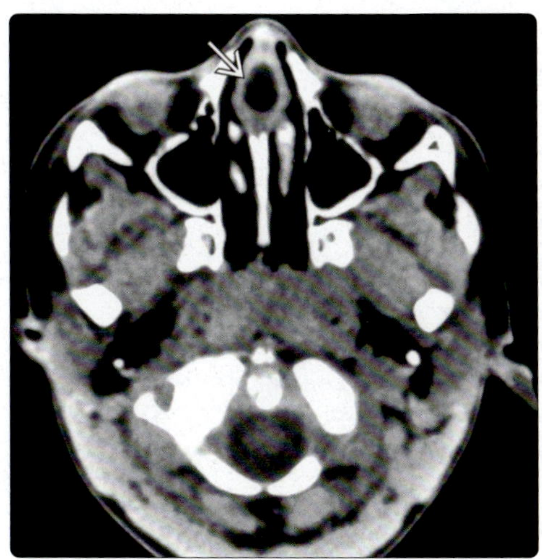

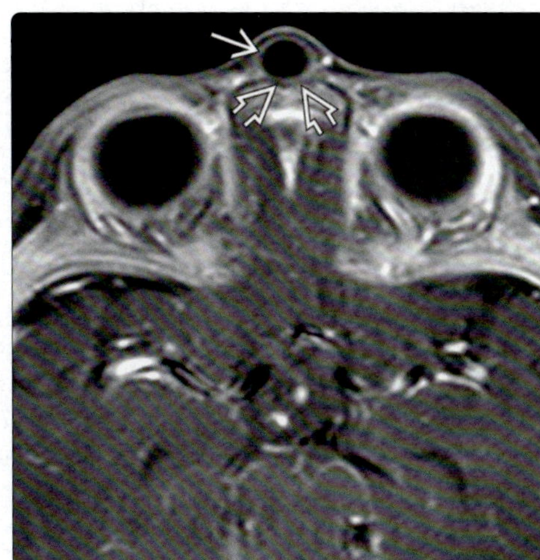

(Left) *Axial NECT demonstrates a characteristic low-attenuation dermoid* ➡ *centered in the cartilaginous portion of the nasal septum. The mass is slightly higher in attenuation than adjacent fat.* **(Right)** *Axial T1 C+ FS MR in a 4-month-old infant with a glabellar mass demonstrates a nonenhancing, fluid-signal intensity dermoid cyst* ➡ *with mild remodeling of the underlying nasal bones* ➡*. Although dermoid cysts may contain fat, the majority of them do not.*

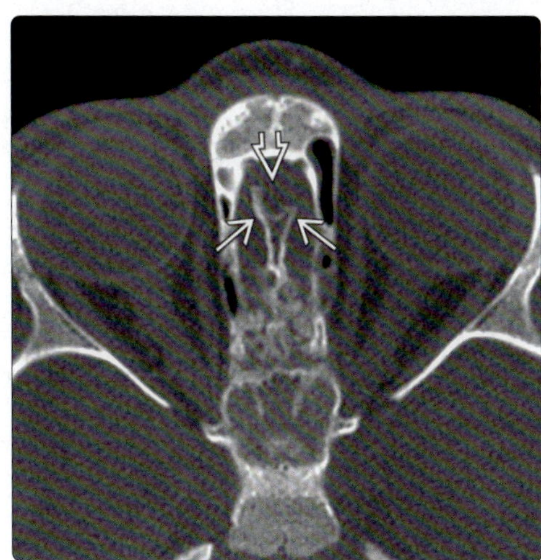

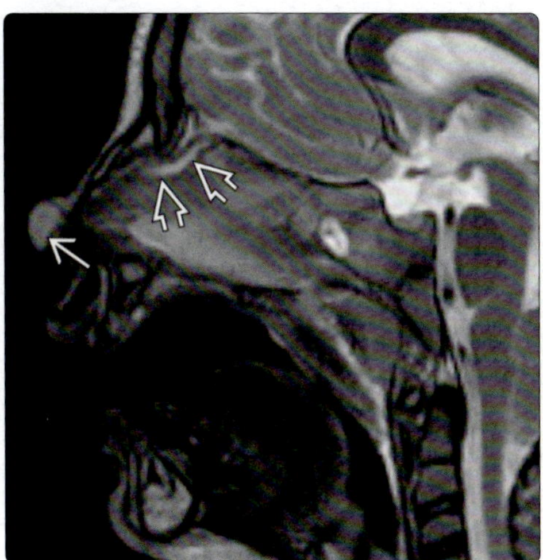

(Left) *Axial bone CT demonstrates a bifid crista galli* ➡ *surrounding an intracranial dermoid* ➡ *at a persistently large foramen cecum.* **(Right)** *Sagittal T2 MR in a 1-year-old with a mass at the tip of his nose shows an ovoid, hyperintense mass* ➡ *& a tubular lesion* ➡ *traversing the nasal septum to the foramen cecum without intracranial extension. At the level of the foramen cecum, the lesion demonstrated diffusion restriction (not shown), typical of a dermoid.*

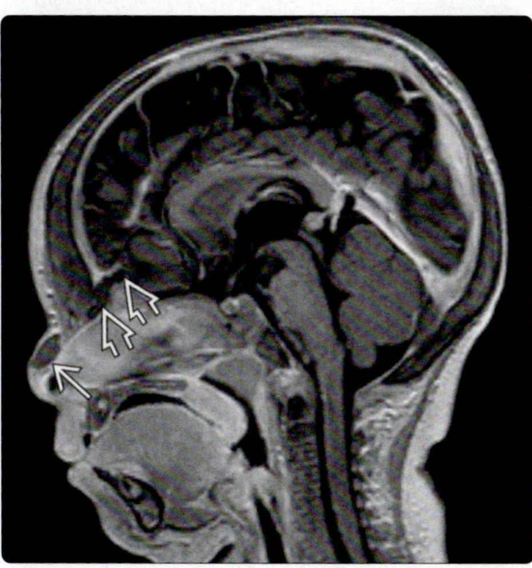

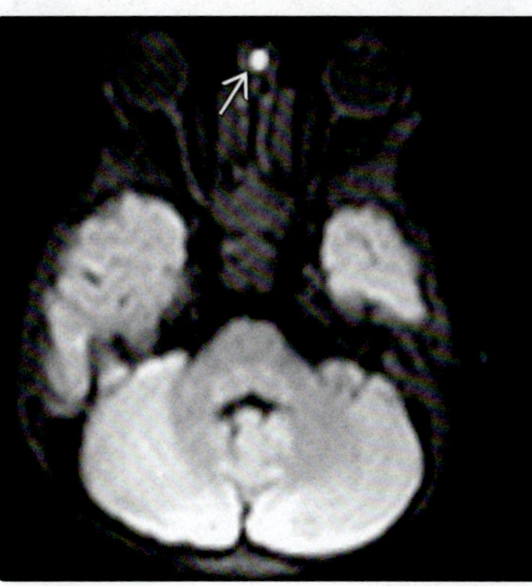

(Left) *Sagittal T1 C+ MR in a 1-year-old with a nasal dorsum mass shows the subcutaneous, nonenhancing midline mass* ➡ *with a fluid-filled lesion extending to the foramen cecum* ➡*, imaging characteristics consistent with dermoid or epidermoid cysts.* **(Right)** *Axial DWI MR in the same patient demonstrates restricted diffusion in the lesion at the level of the foramen cecum* ➡*, typical of a dermoid cyst.*

Juvenile Angiofibroma

KEY FACTS

TERMINOLOGY

- Benign, vascular, nonencapsulated, locally invasive mass originating in nasal cavity

IMAGING

- Centered in posterior nasal cavity arising at sphenopalatine foramen; extends into nasopharynx, sphenoid sinus, pterygopalatine fossa, masticator space, orbit, skull base
- CT findings in juvenile angiofibroma (JAF)
  - Heterogeneous vs. diffuse, avid enhancement
  - Bone remodeling & destruction
    - Posterior wall of maxillary sinus bowed anteriorly
    - ± skull base invasion, intracranial extension
- MR findings in JAF
  - Tubular signal voids on spin echo-based sequences due to fast flow in enlarged vessels
  - Intense enhancement, diffuse or heterogeneous
- Angiography is typically performed at time of preoperative embolization; shows tumor blush
  - Most common feeding artery: Internal maxillary branch of external carotid artery

TOP DIFFERENTIAL DIAGNOSES

- Rhabdomyosarcoma
- Childhood nasopharyngeal carcinoma
- Antrochoanal polyp
- Esthesioneuroblastoma

CLINICAL ISSUES

- Occurs almost exclusively in adolescent males
- Unilateral nasal obstruction (90%), epistaxis (60%)
- Preferred treatment: Complete surgical resection using preoperative embolization to ↓ blood loss
  - ± adjuvant radiation therapy after surgery or as primary treatment in some cases

DIAGNOSTIC CHECKLIST

- Look for JAF extension into surrounding structures
- Consider other diagnoses (or genetic testing) in females

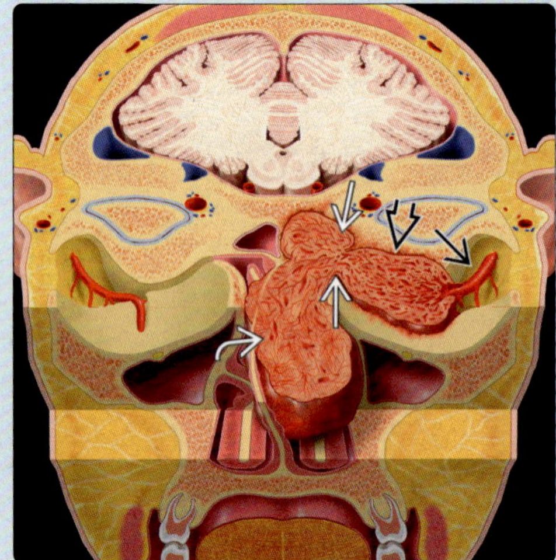

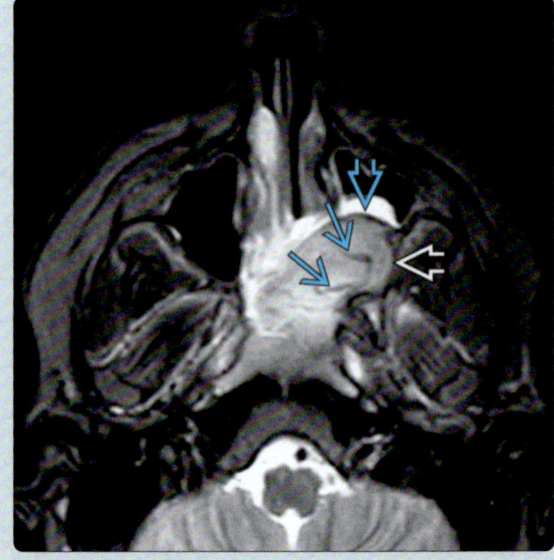

(Left) *Tiered graphic shows the classic features & location of a juvenile angiofibroma (JAF). The site of origin is the sphenopalatine foramen (SPF) ➔ with extension into the pterygopalatine fossa (PPF) ➔ & nasal cavity ➔. The internal maxillary artery ➔ is the dominant feeding vessel of this vascular mass.* **(Right)** *Axial STIR MR in a teenager shows a well-defined mass with intralesional flow voids ➔ widening the left PPF, deviating the posterior wall of the maxillary sinus ➔, & extending into the left infratemporal fossa ➔.*

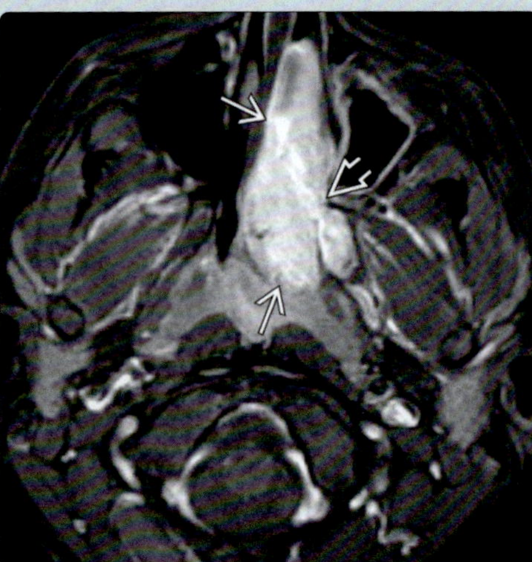

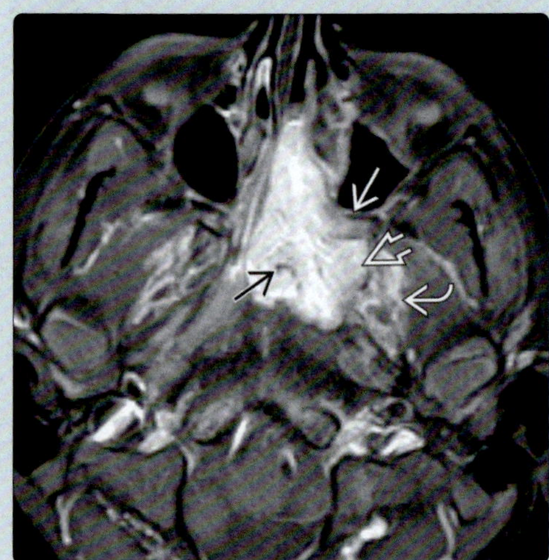

(Left) *Axial T1 C+ FS MR in a 15-year-old boy with nasal obstruction shows an enhancing JAF ➔ filling the left nasal cavity & extending into the nasopharynx. The presumed site of origin is the SPF ➔.* **(Right)** *Axial T1 C+ FS MR in the same patient shows a few intralesional, high-flow vessels ➔ with extension of the JAF into the widened PPF ➔. There is destruction of the left pterygoid ➔ with extension of the mass into the masticator space ➔.*

TERMINOLOGY

Abbreviations

- Juvenile angiofibroma (JAF)

Synonyms

- Juvenile nasopharyngeal angiofibroma (JNA); fibromatous or angiofibromatous hamartoma
  - JAF of nasal cavity is more correct terminology
  - JNA is commonly used term, but tumor begins in nasal cavity, not in nasopharynx

Definitions

- Benign, vascular, nonencapsulated, locally invasive nasal cavity mass

IMAGING

General Features

- Best diagnostic clue
  - Intensely enhancing soft tissue mass originating at sphenopalatine foramen (SPF) in adolescent boy
- Location
  - Centered in posterior wall of nasal cavity off midline, at margin of SPF
    - SPF is medial opening of pterygopalatine fossa (PPF) into superior meatus of nose
    - Extends more anteriorly into nasal cavity, posteriorly into nasopharynx, & laterally into PPF
      - Penetrates PPF early (90%) with involvement of upper medial pterygoid lamina
    - Sphenoid sinus extension (60%)
    - May extend into maxillary (43%) & ethmoid sinuses (35%), masticator space, inferior orbital fissure
    - 5-20% extend into middle cranial fossa via vidian canal or foramen rotundum
  - Extranasopharyngeal angiofibroma: Entity showing pathologic findings of JAF but with other differences
    - Located at nasal septum, turbinate, etc.
    - M:F 2.1:1.0; mean age: 28.7 years
    - Mainly nasal obstruction; epistaxis in 25% only
    - Female sex or normal vascularity does not exclude
- Size
  - Usually 2-6 cm but may become massive
- Morphology
  - Lobular, usually well-circumscribed mass
    - Large lesions have infiltrating margins

Radiographic Findings

- Lateral skull radiograph shows anterior displacement of posterior wall of maxillary antrum
  - Called antral sign, bow sign, or Holman-Miller sign
  - Nonspecific sign denoting any slow-growing mass
- Associated with nasal cavity opacification
- ± nasal cavity/nasopharyngeal soft tissue mass

CT Findings

- CECT
  - Heterogeneous vs. diffuse, avid enhancement of soft tissue mass in nasal cavity originating near SPF
  - Frequent extension into adjacent nasopharynx & PPF
  - ± opacified sphenoid sinus (obstructed, nonenhancing secretions vs. enhancing tumor infiltration)
  - ± intracranial & rare orbital extension
- Bone CT
  - Bone remodeling ± destruction
    - Antral sign is nonspecific
    - Ipsilateral nasal cavity & PPF are enlarged
    - ± skull base invasion; pterygoid lamina erosion is specific
- CTA
  - Enlarged, ipsilateral external carotid artery (ECA) & internal maxillary artery (IMAX)

MR Findings

- T1WI
  - Heterogeneous, intermediate signal
  - Signal voids represent flow in enlarged vessels
- T2WI
  - Heterogeneous, intermediate- to high-signal mass
  - Punctate & serpentine flow voids within tumor
- T1WI C+
  - Intense enhancement ± flow voids
- T1WI C+ FS
  - Coronal plane shows cavernous sinus, sphenoid sinus, or skull base extension
- MRA
  - Enlarged ipsilateral ECA & IMAX artery
  - Lesional vessels may be too small to evaluate with MRA

Angiographic Findings

- Conventional angiography is typically performed at time of preoperative embolization
- Intense capillary tumor blush is fed by enlarged feeding vessels from ECA
  - Most common feeding vessels: IMAX & ascending pharyngeal arteries from ECA
  - With skull base or cavernous sinus extension, internal carotid artery (ICA) supply is common
  - ± supply from contralateral ECA branches

Imaging Recommendations

- Best imaging tool
  - Maxillofacial bone-only NECT in axial & coronal planes for evaluating bone remodeling vs. destruction
  - Postcontrast MR is optimal for mapping lesion extent & determining vascularity
  - Catheter angiography of both ECA & ICA
    - Often in conjunction with embolization therapy
    - Helps plan surgery & ↓ intraoperative blood loss
- Protocol advice
  - Maxillofacial MR with T1 C+ FS in axial & coronal planes
    - Multiplanar imaging for evaluating extension into sphenoid sinus, orbit, skull base
  - Precontrast T1 without fat suppression is vital in evaluating infiltration of normal fat in PPF & adjacent bone
  - CECT may be helpful for evaluating residual disease in postoperative period

DIFFERENTIAL DIAGNOSIS

Rhabdomyosarcoma

- Intermediate to mildly high T2 signal mass with variable enhancement (often mild to moderate) & restricted diffusion, ± bone destruction
- Can arise in many locations (not necessarily nasal cavity)
- Rarely penetrates SPF into PPF

Childhood Nasopharyngeal Carcinoma

- Mostly EBV-related, undifferentiated carcinoma
- Invasive mass of lateral nasopharynx
- Mild to moderate enhancement
- 90% with nodal metastases, usually diagnosed at advanced stage

Antrochoanal Polyp

- Maxillary antrum is opacified
- Homogeneous mass herniates into anterior nasal cavity, then nasopharynx; PPF is not involved
- Peripheral enhancement only

Encephalocele

- Nasoethmoidal type presents as intranasal mass
- Connection to intracranial cavity **is** seen on imaging
- No enhancement
- Usually more anterior in position

Esthesioneuroblastoma

- 1st incidence peaks in 2nd decade; F > M
- Presenting symptoms are same as JAF
- Nasal cavity mass near cribriform plate
- Cystic intracranial components are characteristic

PATHOLOGY

General Features

- Etiology
    - Source of fibrovascular tissue of JAF is not known
    - Best current hypothesis: Primitive mesenchyme of SPF is source of JAF

Staging, Grading, & Classification

- Staging systems are based on tumor size (< or > 6 cm), invasion to PPF anterior &/or posterior to pterygoid plates, & skull base/intracranial invasion

Gross Pathologic & Surgical Features

- Reddish-purple, compressible, mucosa-covered mass
- Cut surface has spongy appearance

Microscopic Features

- Unencapsulated, highly vascular polypoid mass of angiomatous tissue in fibrous stroma
- Myofibroblast thought to be cell of origin
- ± estrogen, testosterone, or progesterone receptors

CLINICAL ISSUES

Presentation

- Most common signs/symptoms
    - Unilateral nasal obstruction (90%), epistaxis (60%)
- Other signs/symptoms
    - Nasal voice, nasal discharge, anosmia, pain or swelling in cheek, proptosis, serous otitis media

Demographics

- Age range: 10-25 years reported
    - Average age at onset: 15 years
- Sex: Almost exclusively occurs in male patients
    - If found in female, may have genetic mosaicism
- Epidemiology: 0.5% of all head & neck neoplasms

Natural History & Prognosis

- May rarely spontaneously regress
- Local recurrence rate with surgery: 6-24%
    - Local recurrence is more common with large lesions (> 6 cm), intracranial spread, previous treatment

Treatment

- Preferred: Complete surgical resection using preoperative embolization to ↓ blood loss
    - Biopsy in outpatient setting should be avoided due to risk of hemorrhage
- Multiple surgical approaches
    - Open resection (midface degloving) vs. endoscopic removal ± laser assistance
        - Endoscopic resection is associated with ↓ bleeding & shorter hospital stay
- Radiation therapy (RT)
    - Adjuvant to surgery for unresectable intracranial disease & cavernous sinus involvement
        - 78% control rates are reported
    - RT is used alone for cure in some institutions
    - Used with caution in young patients due to potential to induce malignancies
- Hormonal therapy (estrogen) is controversial
    - Not routine as complete tumor regression is not achieved
    - Feminization side effects are undesirable in adolescent male

DIAGNOSTIC CHECKLIST

Consider

- JAF in adolescent male patient with epistaxis & enhancing posterior nasal cavity mass
- Consider other diagnoses (or genetic testing) in females

Image Interpretation Pearls

- Evaluate JAF extension into surrounding structures
    - Orbit, infratemporal fossa, sphenoid sinus, & skull base
    - Failure to identify subtle deep growth will result in incomplete surgical resection

SELECTED REFERENCES

1. Scholfield DW et al: Midfacial degloving for juvenile angiofibroma: a case-series of 21 adult males: An alternative to the endoscopic approach and when it should be considered. Clin Otolaryngol. 46(3):659-64, 2020
2. Schreiber A et al: Early postoperative magnetic resonance in the diagnosis of persistent juvenile angiofibroma. Laryngoscope. 131(8):E2436-41, 2020
3. Windfuhr JP et al: Extranasopharyngeal angiofibroma revisited. Clin Otolaryngol. 43(1):199-222, 2018
4. Rodriguez DP et al: Masses of the nose, nasal cavity, and nasopharynx in children. Radiographics. 37(6):1704-30, 2017
5. Schmalbach CE et al: Managing vascular tumors—open approaches. Otolaryngol Clin North Am. 49(3):777-90, 2016

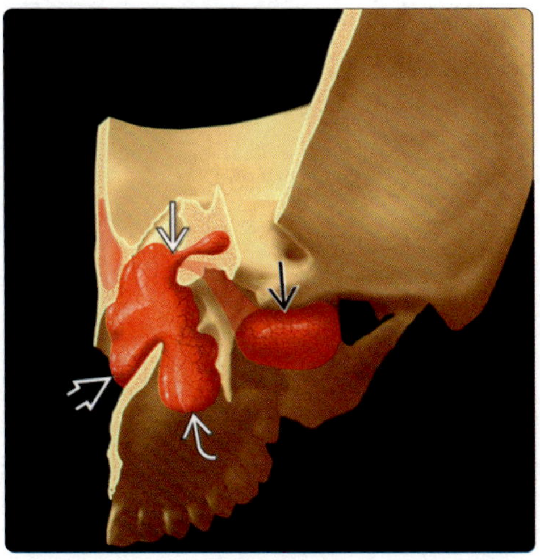

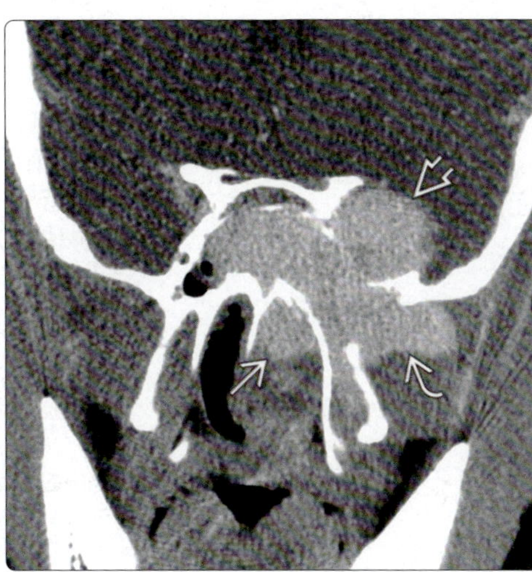

(Left) *Posterior oblique sagittal graphic shows the spread patterns of a JAF. The lesion originates at the SPF ➡ & extends into the nasal cavity ➡, nasopharynx/oropharynx ➡, & infratemporal fossa ➡.* **(Right)** *Coronal CECT shows a large JAF extending into the nasopharynx ➡, infratemporal fossa ➡, & middle cranial fossa ➡. The sphenoid sinus is replaced by the tumor. As seen in this case, the JAF classically shows avid enhancement.*

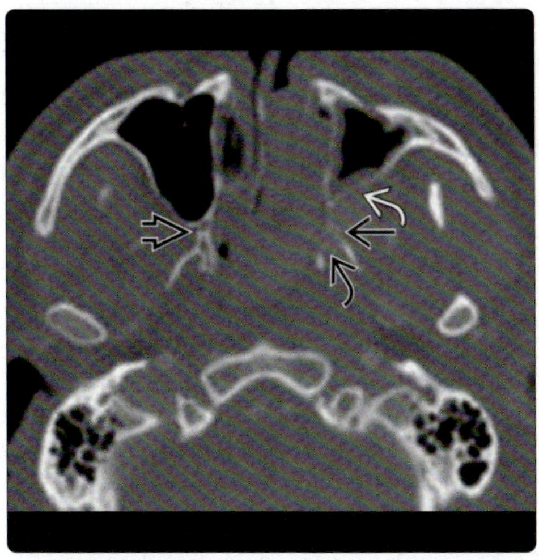

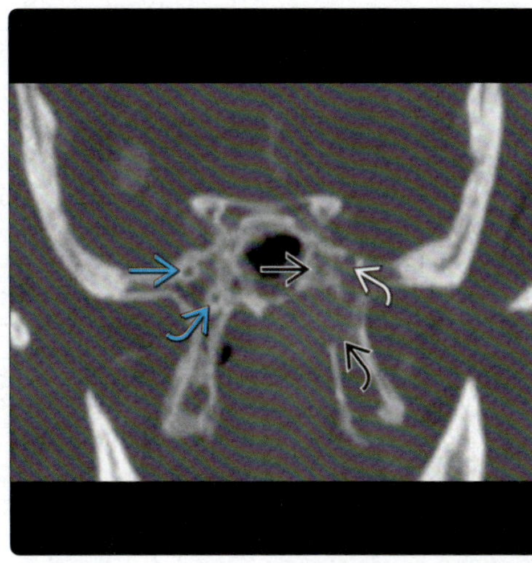

(Left) *Axial CECT in bone windows shows anterior bowing of the left maxillary sinus posterior wall ➡ & erosion of left medial pterygoid plate ➡ & pterygoid process ➡ by a JAF in the nasal cavity, nasopharynx, & PPF. Note the normal right PPF ➡ & pterygoid.* **(Right)** *Coronal CECT in bone windows in the same patient shows the left pterygoid erosions ➡. The left vidian canal (VC) ➡ is invaded by the JAF, & the margin of the left foramen rotundum (FR) ➡ shows fine erosions. Note the normal right VC ➡ & FR ➡.*

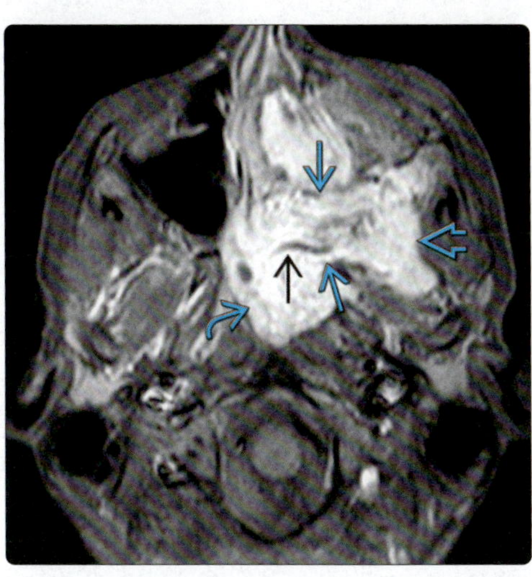

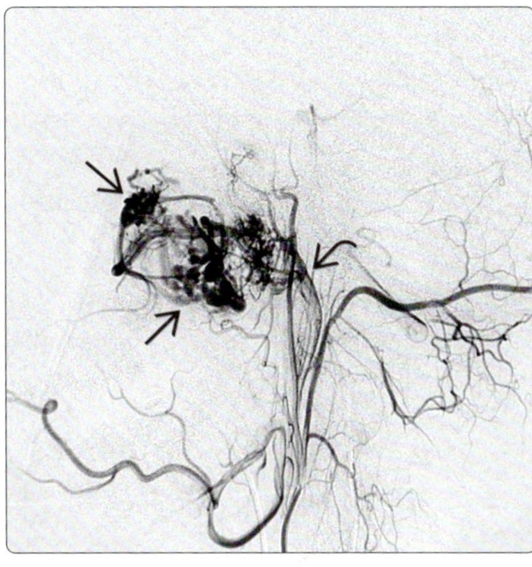

(Left) *Axial T1 C+ FS MR shows avid enhancement throughout a JAF. The mass is centered at the SPF ➡ & extends laterally into the masticator space ➡ & medially into the nasopharynx ➡. Several serpiginous flow voids ➡ are noted in the mass, consistent with enlarged feeding vessels.* **(Right)** *Lateral DSA from an external carotid artery injection shows areas of dense tumor blush ➡ within a JAF prior to embolization. As is typical, the main arterial feeding vessel for this JAF is the internal maxillary artery ➡.*

Acute Rhinosinusitis

KEY FACTS

TERMINOLOGY

- Pediatric acute rhinosinusitis (ARS): Sinonasal inflammation lasting < 12 weeks with sudden onset of symptoms
  - ≥ 2 of nasal congestion/obstruction, discolored nasal discharge, or cough
- Classified into acute bacterial rhinosinusitis (ABRS) vs. viral (VRS) based on clinical presentation

IMAGING

- ARS is clinical diagnosis & imaging is rarely necessary
- Radiography: Mucosal thickening, complete opacification, air-fluid level
- NECT: Can suggest ARS but lacks specificity & should not be performed routinely for diagnosis
  - May be considered to evaluate complications or if diagnosis remains uncertain on clinical grounds
  - Best sign = air-fluid level (nonspecific) ± bubbly secretions with mucosal thickening
  - Most common in ethmoid & maxillary sinuses
  - Often shows asymmetric sinus involvement
- CECT/MR: Indicated for suspected complications

TOP DIFFERENTIAL DIAGNOSES

- Pseudofluid level from large maxillary polyp/cyst
- Posttraumatic blood level
- Postobstructive noninfected secretions

PATHOLOGY

- Most cases follow viral upper respiratory infection

CLINICAL ISSUES

- Purulent nasal drainage, nasal obstruction, & facial pain, pressure, fullness
- VRS: Signs/symptoms last < 10 days, do not progress
- ABRS: Signs/symptoms fail to improve within 10 days **or** worsen within 10 days after initial improvement
- ABRS complications are rare but important to identify
  - Orbital cellulitis, subperiosteal abscess, meningitis, subdural empyema, brain abscess, venous thrombosis

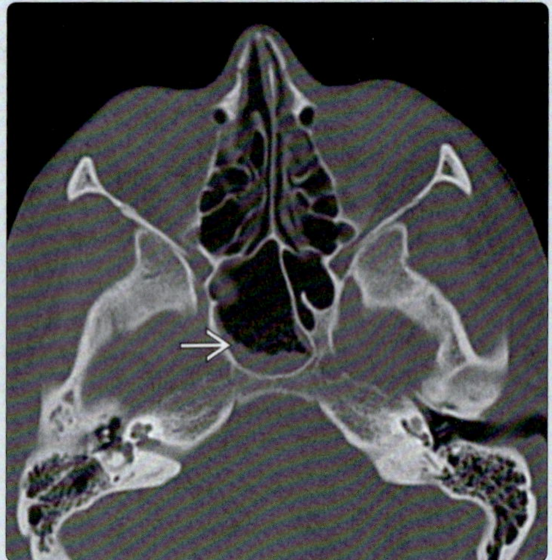

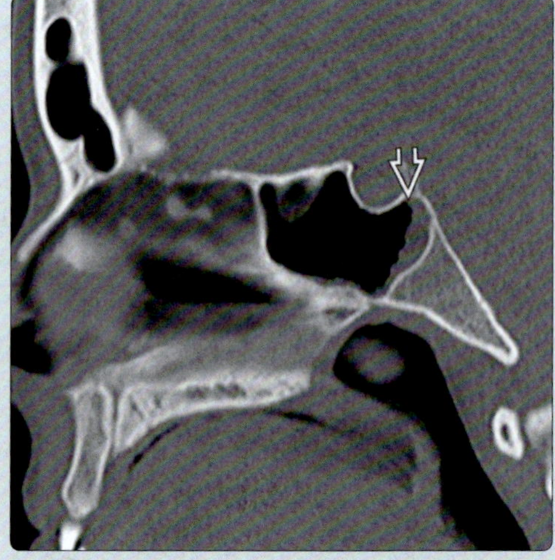

(Left) *Axial NECT in a patient with headache, fever, & purulent nasal discharge shows a bubbly air-fluid level ➔ in the right sphenoid sinus, corroborating a clinical history of acute bacterial rhinosinusitis (ABRS).* **(Right)** *Sagittal reconstruction NECT in the same patient delineates a frothy air-fluid level ➔, which layers dependently in the sphenoid sinus.*

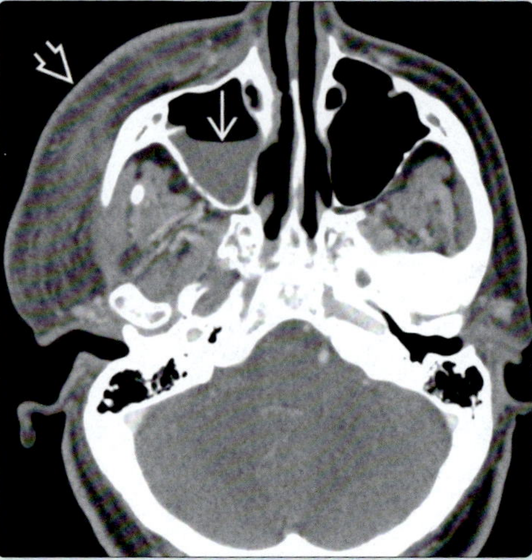

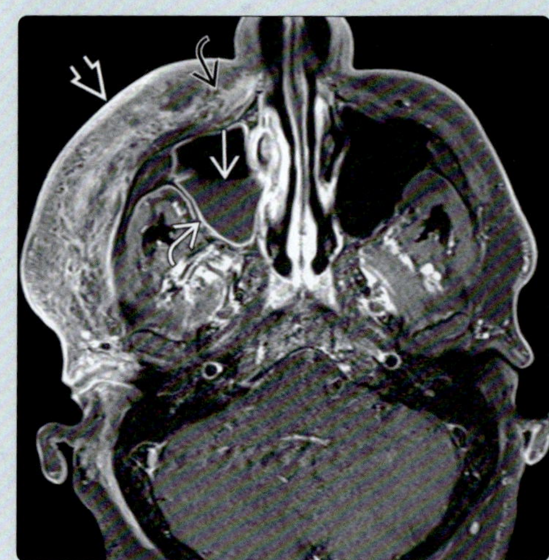

(Left) *Axial CECT in a patient with ABRS complicated by facial cellulitis shows a right maxillary sinus air-fluid level ➔ as well as skin thickening & subcutaneous edema of the right cheek ➔.* **(Right)** *Axial T1 C+ FS MR in the same patient shows circumferential mucosal thickening ➔ of the right maxillary sinus with an air-fluid level ➔. MR better delineates complications, including diffuse right facial cellulitis with skin thickening ➔, subcutaneous edema, & thickening of the superficial musculoaponeurotic system ➔.*

TERMINOLOGY

Abbreviations

- Acute rhinosinusitis (ARS)
- Acute bacterial rhinosinusitis (ABRS)
- Viral rhinosinusitis (VRS)

Definitions

- Adult ARS: Sinonasal inflammation lasting < 4 weeks & demonstrating sudden onset of symptoms
  - Symptoms: **Both** nasal congestion/obstruction **or** nasal discharge & facial pain/pressure **or** reduced smell
- Pediatric ARS: Sinonasal inflammation lasting < 12 weeks & demonstrating sudden onset of symptoms
  - Symptoms: 2 or more of nasal congestion/obstruction, discolored nasal discharge, or cough
- ARS is clinical diagnosis, which does not require imaging or endoscopy to make initial diagnosis
  - Image to assess for complications, surgical planning, or unclear clinical diagnosis (uncommon)
- Classified into VRS vs. ABRS based on clinical presentation

IMAGING

General Features

- Best diagnostic clue
  - Imaging findings are imperfect & lack specificity → need appropriate clinical history
  - Air-fluid level (nonspecific) ± bubbly/frothy secretions within sinus with mucosal thickening
- Location
  - Ethmoid & maxillary sinuses are most common, typically asymmetric

Radiographic Findings

- Mucosal thickening, complete opacification, air-fluid levels

CT Findings

- NECT
  - Air-fluid level, bubbly- or frothy-appearing secretions
    - Air-fluid level is nonspecific & can also be seen with recent sinus irrigation
  - Moderate mucosal thickening, generally > 1 cm in sinus cavity, ostium, or nasal cavity
  - May see polypoid inflammatory tissue obstructing drainage pathways
- CECT
  - Indicated when orbital or intracranial complications are suspected clinically
  - Inflamed sinus mucosa enhances but thin, linear soft tissue deep to mucosa does not
    - Central secretions do not enhance
  - Invasive fungal sinusitis (in immunocompromised host) is suggested by
    - Induration of perimaxillary fat
    - Nonenhancement of mucosa
- Bone CT
  - Bone destruction is not typical for acute infection
    - If present, suspect aggressive invasive sinus infection or neoplasm
  - Osteoneogenesis with sinus wall sclerosis & thickening usually indicates chronic inflammation

MR Findings

- T1WI
  - Mucosal thickening is isointense to soft tissue
  - Air-fluid level
  - Hyperintense secretions if chronic sinusitis is present
- T2WI
  - Thickened edematous mucosa, especially in maxillary & ethmoids
  - Air-fluid level
    - Anterior ethmoid cells are generally too small for discrete fluid level
  - Low signal intensity secretions if proteinaceous or chronic
- T1WI C+
  - Enhancing mucosa lines sinus cavity
  - Central secretions do not enhance

Imaging Recommendations

- Best imaging tool
  - ARS is clinical diagnosis
  - Radiographic findings are nonspecific
    - Not recommended in evaluation of acute disease
  - CT: Consider only if evaluating for complications, failed medical therapy, alternative diagnoses, or surgical candidacy
    - NECT delineates anatomic variants prior to endoscopic sinus surgery
    - CECT is indicated with concern for complications
  - MR is superior for evaluating orbital or intracranial complications, invasive fungal disease, neoplasm
- Protocol advice
  - Bone CT
    - Axial ≤ 1-mm slice thickness with coronal & sagittal reconstructions to evaluate drainage pathways
  - MR
    - Multiplanar T1 & T2 sequences are necessary
    - T1 C+ FS & DWI are best for intracranial/orbital complications

DIFFERENTIAL DIAGNOSIS

Pseudofluid Level

- Mucus retention cyst mimics air-fluid level
- Rounded contour with incomplete fluid level

Posttraumatic Blood Level

- Clinical history of recent facial injury
- ↑ attenuation of layering fluid (blood)
- Associated sinus wall fractures

Postobstructive Secretions

- Lesion obstructs sinus drainage pathway, resulting in noninfected trapped sinus cavity fluid
- MR differentiates tumor from obstructed secretions
  - Neoplasm is generally of ↓ SI on T2 compared to hyperintense secretions & frequently hypoenhancing relative to sinonasal mucosa

PATHOLOGY

General Features

- Etiology

- ABRS uncommonly follows VRS (0.5-2.0% of cases) in adults but more commonly follows upper respiratory infection (URI) in children (4-7%)
  - URI (typically viral) → mucosal swelling → sinus outflow obstruction → static secretions in sinus → infection
  - Viral symptoms usually improve in 7-10 days
  - Symptoms > 10 days or worsening after 5-7 days suggest bacterial superinfection
    - Common organisms: *Streptococcus pneumonia*, *Haemophilus influenzae*, *Moraxella catarrhalis*
- Odontogenic rhinosinusitis: Apical periodontitis with dehiscence or transosseous spread of infection into maxillary sinus
  - Likely underdiagnosed (reported prevalence of 10-15% but may be as high as 45%)

- Genetics
  - Cystic fibrosis (autosomal recessive disorder) predisposes to rhinosinusitis & polyps
- Associated abnormalities
  - Structural abnormalities may narrow drainage pathways
    - Anatomic variants of septum, uncinate process, middle turbinate, frontal recess, ethmoid sinuses
    - Polyps, either isolated or associated with allergic sinusitis with diffuse polyposis
    - Benign or malignant neoplasms
  - Predisposing systemic disorders: Allergies, immunoglobulin deficiency, immotile cilia syndrome, cystic fibrosis, vitamin D deficiency

CLINICAL ISSUES

Presentation

- Most common signs/symptoms
  - Cardinal signs/symptoms of ARS: < 4 weeks of purulent nasal drainage & obstruction, facial pain, or pressure
    - VRS: Signs/symptoms last < 10 days, do not progress
    - ABRS: Signs/symptoms fail to improve within 10 days or worsen within 10 days after initial improvement
- Other signs/symptoms
  - Fever, cough, malaise, hyposmia, anosmia, dental pain, ear pressure/fullness
    - Facial/dental pain predicts ABRS, but location correlates poorly with site of involvement
- Clinical profile
  - Nasal discharge & obstruction following viral URI lasting < 4 weeks (adult) or < 12 weeks (child)
  - Laboratory results
    - Nasal/nasopharynx cultures poorly correlate with sinus cultures, do not differentiate ABRS from VRS
    - Endoscopic middle meatus aspiration is more specific but generally not necessary in uncomplicated ARS

Demographics

- Age
  - Children & adults
    - Typically follows viral URI in children
- Epidemiology
  - Sinonasal inflammatory disease is ubiquitous
  - Rhinosinusitis affects nearly 31 million patients in USA annually
  - VRS & ARS often follow/coexist with common cold

Natural History & Prognosis

- VRS is usually self-limited
- ABRS may resolve without antibiotics
- ABRS course may be shortened by medical therapy, surgical drainage, & possibly saline irrigation
- If ABRS is untreated, complications rarely ensue
  - Orbital cellulitis, subperiosteal abscess, meningitis, subdural empyema, brain abscess, venous sinus thrombosis

Treatment

- Medical therapy
  - Antibiotics (in uncomplicated cases with worsening after 7 days, earlier if extenuating circumstances)
  - Intranasal corticosteroids
  - Topical saline irrigation (adjunct to antibiotics for ABRS)
- Surgical therapy
  - More often performed for chronic rhinosinusitis
  - Drainage procedures performed in acute disease (frontal & sphenoid) to prevent development of complications

DIAGNOSTIC CHECKLIST

Consider

- Bone CT for suspected alternative diagnoses, failed therapy, complications, or surgical candidate
  - Acquire ≤ 1-mm axial slices with coronal & sagittal reformations
- CT limitations
  - Cannot differentiate viral from bacterial disease
  - High incidence of sinus mucosal abnormalities in asymptomatic patients

Image Interpretation Pearls

- Air-fluid level is not always present & not highly specific
- In correct clinical setting, even severe mucosal thickening can indicate ABRS
- Normal nasal mucosal cycle may be impossible to distinguish from ARS mucosal thickening
- Look for signs of invasive fungal sinusitis in immunocompromised patient

SELECTED REFERENCES

1. Martins M et al: Management of post-septal complications of acute rhinosinusitis in children: a 14-year experience in a tertiary hospital. Int J Pediatr Otorhinolaryngol. 151:110925, 2021
2. Velasquez N et al: Clinical and radiologic characterization of frontal sinusitis in the pediatric population. Ann Otol Rhinol Laryngol. 130(8):923-8, 2021
3. Blanco CH et al: Management of complicated pediatric rhinosinusitis in the COVID-19 era. Am J Otolaryngol. 41(6):102746, 2020
4. Frerichs N et al: Rhinosinusitis and the role of imaging. Cleve Clin J Med. 87(8):485-92, 2020
5. Harreld JH et al: The use of imaging to identify immunocompromised children requiring biopsy for invasive fungal rhinosinusitis. Pediatr Blood Cancer. 67(11):e28676, 2020
6. Orlandi RR et al: International Consensus Statement on rhinology and allergy: rhinosinusitis. Int Forum Allergy Rhinol. 11(3):213-739, 2020
7. Orman G et al: Imaging of paranasal sinus infections in children: a review. J Neuroimaging. 30(5):572-86, 2020
8. Expert Panel on Neurologic Imaging et al: ACR Appropriateness Criteria® sinonasal disease. J Am Coll Radiol. 14(11S):S550-9, 2017
9. Dankbaar JW et al: Imaging findings of the orbital and intracranial complications of acute bacterial rhinosinusitis. Insights Imaging. 6(5):509-18, 2015
10. Joshi VM et al: Imaging in sinonasal inflammatory disease. Neuroimaging Clin N Am. 25(4):549-68, 2015

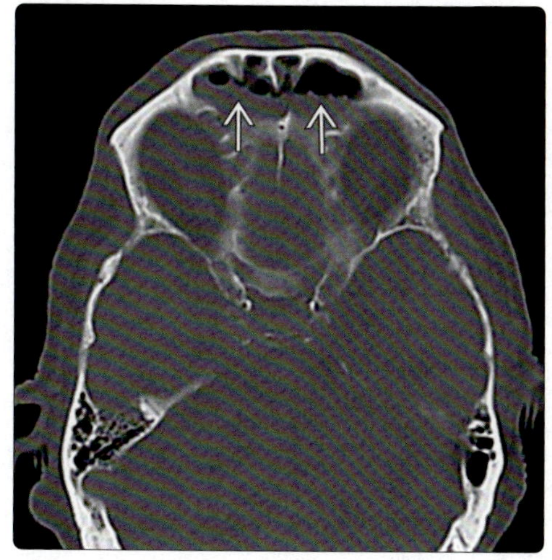

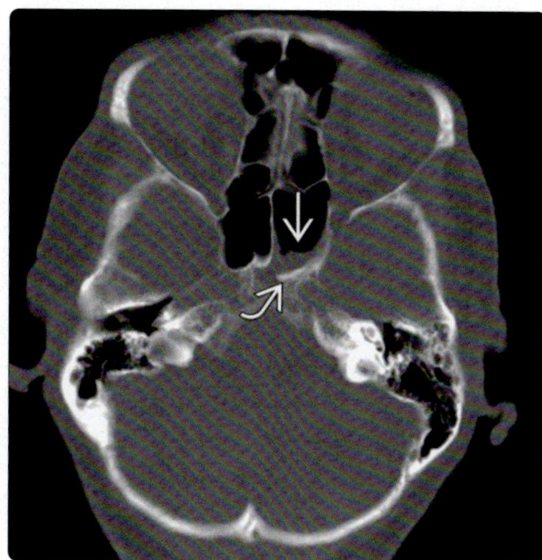

(Left) *Axial NECT performed for headache & fever reveals frothy air-fluid levels ➡ in both frontal sinuses. Although ABRS is a clinical diagnosis, imaging may be performed to rule out suspected complications.* **(Right)** *Axial NECT in patient with a clinical diagnosis of ABRS demonstrates an air-fluid level ➡ in the left sphenoid sinus. Note osteoneogenesis ↪, or a sclerotic sinus wall, suggesting chronic sinus inflammatory disease, as well as an acute ABRS component.*

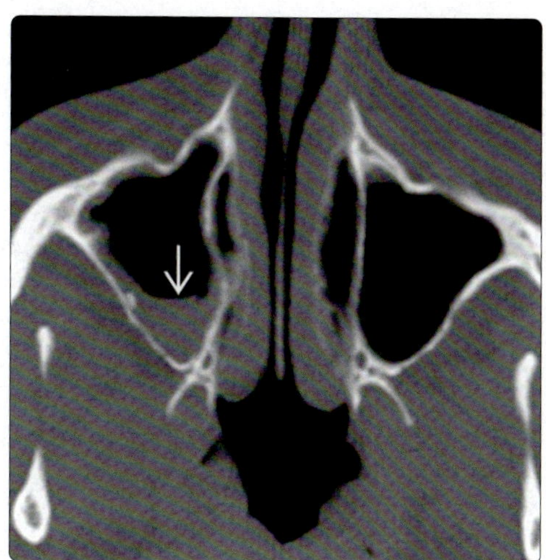

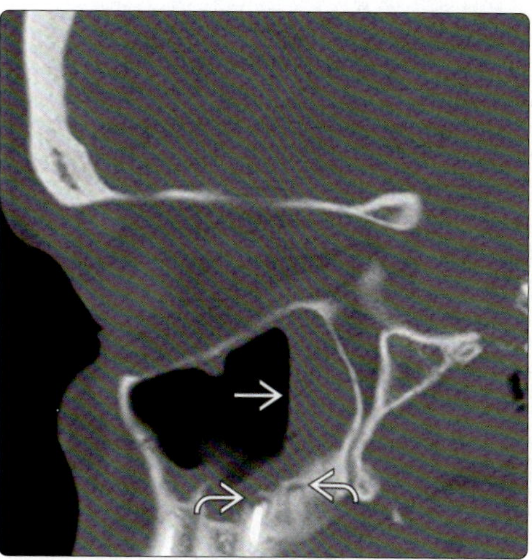

(Left) *Axial NECT in a patient with facial pain & purulent nasal discharge shows a partially opacified right maxillary sinus with bubbly air-fluid level ➡, consistent with clinical history of acute rhinosinusitis (ARS).* **(Right)** *Sagittal NECT reconstruction in a patient with clinical ARS shows corroborating air-fluid level ➡ in the maxillary sinus. Careful inspection reveals periapical lucencies of the maxillary teeth ↪, an easily overlooked finding that may contribute an odontogenic component to the maxillary sinusitis.*

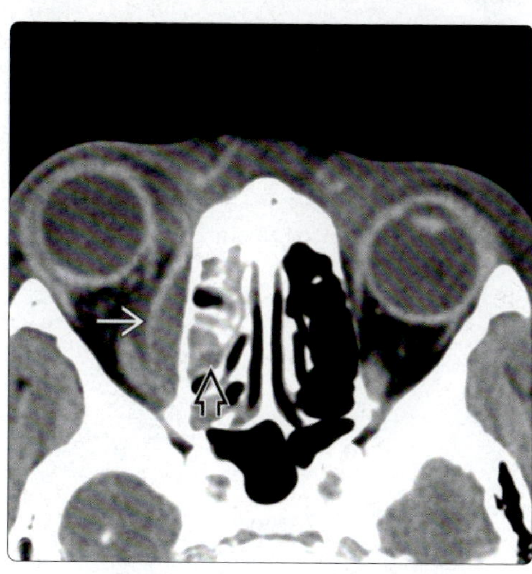

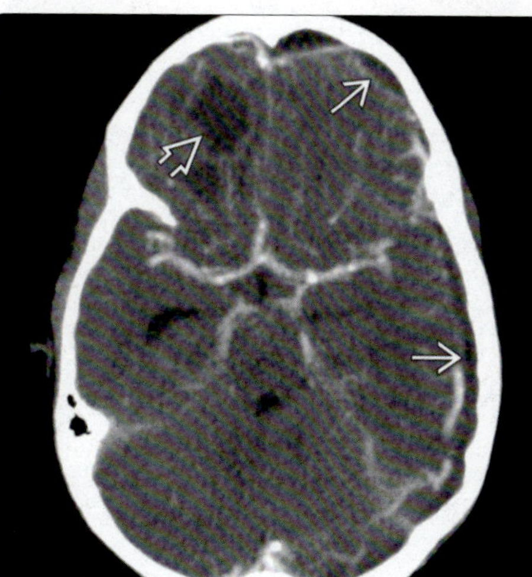

(Left) *Axial CECT in a child shows right ethmoid sinusitis ⇨ complicated by postseptal orbital cellulitis with a medial orbital subperiosteal abscess ➡. Orbital disease may be the initial presentation of sinusitis in children.* **(Right)** *Axial CECT in a 5-year-old with fever & COVID-19 positive serology who developed right-sided weakness shows a large left subdural empyema ➡ & right frontal lobe abscess ➡ as a complications of ABRS (not shown).*

Orbital Cellulitis

KEY FACTS

TERMINOLOGY

- Preseptal cellulitis: Infection anterior to orbital septum
- Postseptal cellulitis: Infection posterior to orbital septum
- Orbital septum: Periosteal reflection of bony orbit → upper lid levator aponeurosis & lower lid tarsal plate

IMAGING

- Thickening & edema of orbital/periorbital soft tissues
- Preseptal cellulitis: Limited to anterior tissues
- Postseptal cellulitis
  - Low-attenuation, rim-enhancing collection
    - Drainable subperiosteal abscess (SPA) in majority
    - 20% without drainable abscess (phlegmon)
  - Associated myositis is common with swollen extraocular muscles, ± abnormal enhancement
  - ± thrombosed superior ophthalmic vein
- ± extraorbital complications of sinusitis
  - Frontal osteomyelitis, meningitis, subdural/epidural effusion or empyema, cerebritis, parenchymal abscess

TOP DIFFERENTIAL DIAGNOSES

- Idiopathic orbital inflammation
- Langerhans cell histiocytosis
- Orbital soft tissue or osseous neoplasm
  - Rhabdomyosarcoma
  - Metastatic neuroblastoma
- Orbital vascular anomaly
  - Infantile hemangioma
  - Venous malformation

PATHOLOGY

- Preseptal/periorbital cellulitis: Typically due to trauma (skin infection, insect bites, etc.)
- Postseptal cellulitis: Most common cause is sinusitis

CLINICAL ISSUES

- Treatment: Intravenous antibiotics ± sinus drainage procedures, SPA drainage

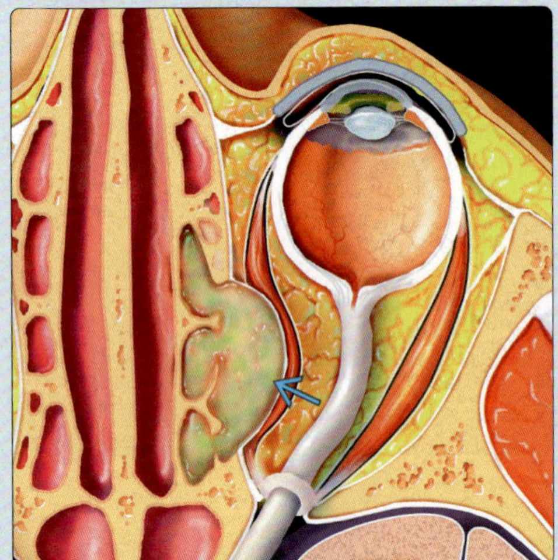

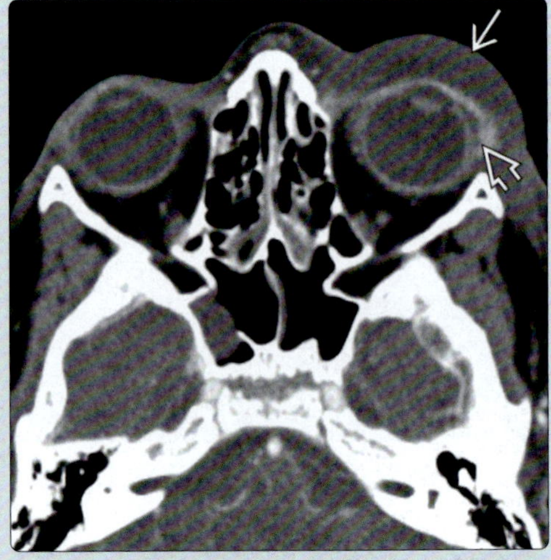

(Left) *Axial graphic shows the spread of infection from the ethmoid sinuses through the lamina papyracea into the medial orbit, resulting in a subperiosteal abscess (SPA)* ⇨ *that places the optic nerve at risk.* **(Right)** *Axial CECT in a 7-year-old with neutropenia & left eyelid swelling demonstrates marked preseptal periorbital soft tissue edema* ➡. *There is a low-attenuation crescent with rim enhancement marginating the anterolateral globe* ➡, *consistent with chemosis. The postseptal orbit is normal.*

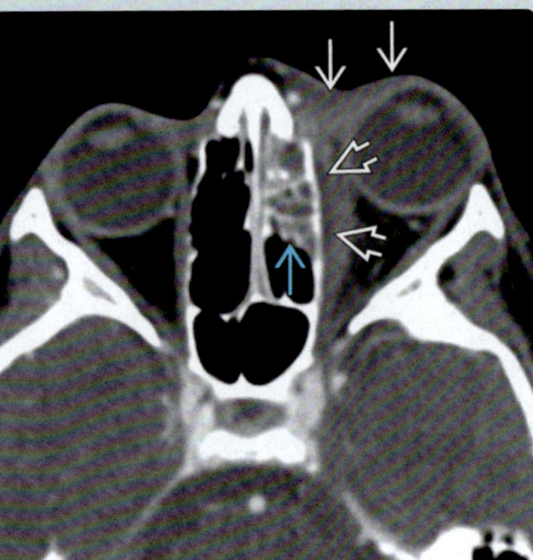

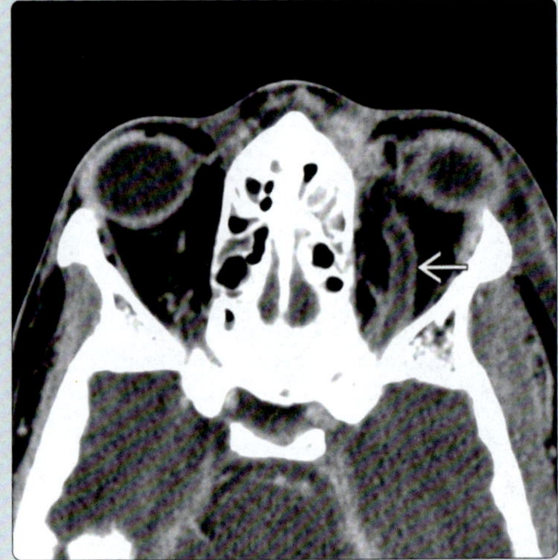

(Left) *Axial CECT in a 6-year-old boy demonstrates moderate preseptal cellulitis* ➡, *a medial subperiosteal fluid collection* ➡ *deviating the left medial rectus muscle, & ipsilateral left ethmoid sinus disease* ⇨, *which is the typical cause of postseptal inflammation. There is also mild associated proptosis.* **(Right)** *Axial CECT shows diffuse enlargement & lack of central enhancement in a thrombosed left superior ophthalmic vein* ➡. *There is associated ethmoid sinus disease with preseptal & postseptal orbital cellulitis.*

TERMINOLOGY

Definitions

- Preseptal cellulitis: Inflammation anterior to orbital septum
- Postseptal cellulitis: Inflammation posterior to orbital septum
- Orbital septum: Periosteal reflection bony orbit → upper lid levator aponeurosis & lower lid tarsal plate

IMAGING

General Features

- Best diagnostic clue
  - Thickening & edema of periorbital &/or orbital soft tissues = cellulitis
  - Low-attenuation, rim-enhancing subperiosteal collection in medial or superior orbit
    - Drainable subperiosteal abscess (SPA) in majority
    - Phlegmon in 20% without drainable abscess
- Location
  - Preseptal: Disease limited to periorbital soft tissues, anterior to orbital septum
  - Postseptal: Disease posterior to orbital septum
    - Intraconal: Within cone formed by extraocular muscles (EOMs)
    - Extraconal: Between bony orbit & EOMs
    - Subperiosteal: Between bony orbit & orbital periosteum
    - Associated myositis is common
      - □ Swollen EOMs ± abnormal enhancement
  - ± extraorbital complications of sinusitis
    - Frontal osteomyelitis, meningitis, subdural/epidural effusion or empyema, cerebritis, parenchymal abscess

CT Findings

- CECT
  - Infiltration of periorbital &/or intraorbital fat with poorly defined diffuse mild enhancement
  - ± focal elongated/lentiform rim-enhancing SPA or intraorbital abscess
    - Medial > > superior orbit
    - ± foci of gas in abscess
  - ± EOM enlargement due to myositis; EOM deviation by inflammatory collections
  - ± enlarged, centrally nonenhancing superior ophthalmic vein due to thrombosis
  - Careful review of anterior & middle cranial fossae for fluid collection or findings of parenchymal edema

MR Findings

- T1: Hypointense infiltration of normal fat
- T2 FS: Heterogeneous hyperintensity of fat ± fluid in focal collection
- DWI: Restricted diffusion suggests abscess
- T1 C+ FS: Heterogeneous enhancement of inflamed tissues ± rim-enhancing SPA

Imaging Recommendations

- Best imaging tool
  - CECT: Axial & coronal reformatted images
  - MR with contrast: Best for evaluation of intracranial complications of sinusitis

DIFFERENTIAL DIAGNOSIS

Idiopathic Orbital Inflammation

- Acute to subacute orbital pain, swelling, restricted motion, diplopia, proptosis, & impaired vision
- Poorly marginated, mass-like enhancing soft tissue involving any region of orbit
  - Unilateral or bilateral

Langerhans Cell Histiocytosis

- Classic punched-out round or geographic lytic bone lesion
- Bone lesion is often filled with homogeneously enhancing soft tissue mass ± intra- & extracranial extension

Orbital Neoplasm

- Variably enhancing mass originating in bone or soft tissues
- Bone-centered lesions (primary or metastatic) show aggressive permeative destruction & periosteal reaction, particularly in superolateral orbit
  - Metastatic neuroblastoma: Perpendicular radiating spicules of new bone; may show mild osseous expansion
- Soft tissue neoplasms are often well-defined without surrounding edema

Orbital Vascular Anomaly

- Infantile hemangioma
  - Well-circumscribed, lobular, diffusely enhancing mass
  - Superficial lesions typically show characteristic cutaneous features (raised red "strawberry mark")
    - Appear in 1st days-weeks of life with rapid growth prior to gradual involution
- Venous malformation
  - Infiltrative pre- &/or postseptal fluid signal lesion with septated mass-like components &/or tubular channels
  - ± fluid-fluid levels, low-signal thrombi, patchy gradual enhancement
  - ± bluish skin discoloration that bulges with Valsalva
    - Present at birth
    - May ↑ at puberty/pregnancy or with thrombosis

PATHOLOGY

General Features

- Etiology
  - Most common causes of preseptal or periorbital cellulitis
    - Trauma (skin infection, insect bites, foreign body), sinusitis, & primary bacteremia (< 36 months of age)
  - Most common cause of postseptal cellulitis: Sinusitis
    - Up to 3% of sinusitis patients develop cellulitis (most common complication)
      - □ May precede signs & symptoms of sinusitis
      - □ Usually secondary to ethmoiditis
    - Spread of sinus infection to orbit
      - □ Direct extension via thin bone with acquired dehiscence &/or normal foramina in lamina papyracea
      - □ Valveless venous system (diploic veins of Breschet) connects orbital circulation with ethmoid, frontal, & maxillary sinus circulation
    - Occasional underlying cause of sinusitis
      - □ Antrochoanal polyp
      - □ Sinonasal foreign body

- Odontogenic sinusitis
- Other causes: Nasolacrimal duct mucocele or dacryocystocele may lead to periorbital cellulitis; retinoblastoma rarely presents as periorbital cellulitis
- Associated abnormalities
  - Superior ophthalmic vein &/or cavernous sinus thrombosis
    - Expanded with central heterogeneous or nonenhancing thrombus
  - Frontal osteomyelitis (Pott puffy tumor)
    - Forehead cellulitis, phlegmon ± subgaleal abscess
    - Frontal bone lytic lesion may be difficult to detect
  - Meningitis
    - ± abnormal meningeal contrast enhancement
      - Absence of enhancement does not exclude meningitis with clinical suspicion
  - Effusions
    - Epidural (lenticular) or subdural (crescentic) fluid collections without rim enhancement or restricted diffusion
  - Empyema
    - Epidural (lenticular) or subdural (crescentic) collection of pus
    - Usually shows peripheral dural enhancement
    - Restricted diffusion on MR (↑ signal on DWI with ↓ signal on ADC map)
  - Cerebritis
    - Amorphous parenchymal edema without rim-enhancing collection
  - Brain abscess
    - Round or ovoid collection of pus within brain
    - Ring-enhancing wall may be thicker superficially; ± low T2 signal rim on MR
    - Hyperintense DWI, hypointense ADC on MR

Staging, Grading, & Classification

- Chandler classification: Orbital complications of sinusitis
  - Preseptal cellulitis
    - Inflammation anterior to orbital septum
    - Eyelid edema
    - No tenderness, visual loss, or impaired EOM motility (ophthalmoplegia)
  - Orbital cellulitis without abscess
    - Diffuse postseptal edema of orbital fat
  - Orbital cellulitis with SPA
    - ± proptosis, impaired vision, or ophthalmoplegia
  - Orbital cellulitis with abscess in orbital fat
    - Usually severe proptosis, ↓ vision, & ophthalmoplegia
  - Cavernous sinus thrombosis secondary to orbital phlebitis: Unilateral or bilateral

CLINICAL ISSUES

Presentation

- Most common signs/symptoms
  - Depends on degree of inflammation
    - Fever, eyelid swelling, erythema, tenderness, chemosis, proptosis, ophthalmoplegia resulting in diplopia, ↓ visual acuity
- Other signs/symptoms
  - Cranial nerve palsies (III-VI) with cavernous sinus thrombosis
  - Seizures, mental status changes with intracranial complications

Demographics

- 50% of affected children < 4 years of age

Natural History & Prognosis

- Excellent with appropriate treatment
- Rare cause of blindness if untreated

Treatment

- Medical management: Intravenous antibiotics
- Surgical management
  - Chandler classification + imaging characteristics ↑ ability to predict surgical need
  - SPA: Not absolute surgical indication
    - Younger children may only require antibiotics with more aggressive surgical drainage in older children
    - Emergent surgery if visual disturbance develops from optic nerve or retinal compromise
  - Drainage of orbital fat abscess
  - Sinus drainage procedures
  - Intracranial empyema is classically considered surgical emergency, particularly with neurologic signs/symptoms
    - Collection may resolve with antibiotics

DIAGNOSTIC CHECKLIST

Consider

- Imaging indications: CECT
  - Impairment in visual acuity or ophthalmoplegia
  - No improvement or worsening of symptoms on appropriate antibiotics
  - Severe eyelid edema prohibiting evaluation of vision & EOM motility
- Imaging indications: MR with contrast
  - Suspected intracranial complications
    - Fluid collection is presumed infected if neurologic symptoms (seizure, altered mental status) are present
    - Clinical & CT findings may dictate operative intervention before MR

Image Interpretation Pearls

- Distinguishing SPA from phlegmon may be difficult
- Cavernous sinus thrombosis may be subtle
- Look for underlying cause of sinusitis & extraorbital complications

SELECTED REFERENCES

1. Nagaraj UD et al: Imaging of orbital infectious and inflammatory disease in children. Pediatr Radiol. 51(7):1149-61, 2021
2. Santos JC et al: Pediatric preseptal and orbital cellulitis: a 10-year experience. Int J Pediatr Otorhinolaryngol. 120:82-8, 2019
3. Jabarin B et al: Indicators for imaging in periorbital cellulitis secondary to rhinosinusitis. Eur Arch Otorhinolaryngol. 275(4):943-8, 2018
4. Wong SJ et al: Management of pediatric orbital cellulitis: a systematic review. Int J Pediatr Otorhinolaryngol. 110:123-9, 2018
5. Le TD et al: The effect of adding orbital computed tomography findings to the Chandler criteria for classifying pediatric orbital cellulitis in predicting which patients will require surgical intervention. J AAPOS. 18(3):271-7, 2014

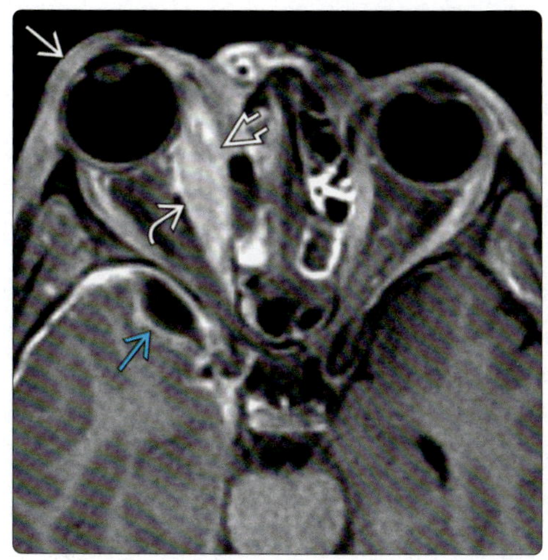

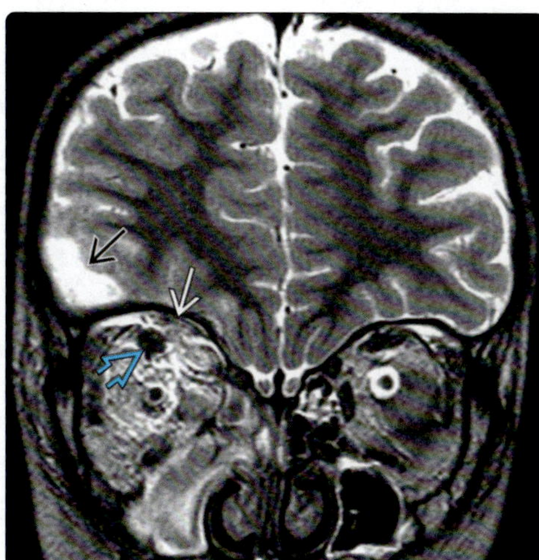

(Left) *Axial T1 C+ FS MR in a 5-year-old with right proptosis & seizures shows ethmoid sinus disease, preseptal orbital cellulitis ➡, medial extraconal postseptal phlegmon ➡ with an enlarged medial rectus muscle ➡, & a middle cranial fossa epidural abscess ➡.* **(Right)** *Coronal T2 MR in the same child shows additional extraconal disease in the superior right orbit ➡ with inferior displacement of the superior rectus muscle complex ➡. There is an extraaxial fluid collection in the right anterior cranial fossa ➡.*

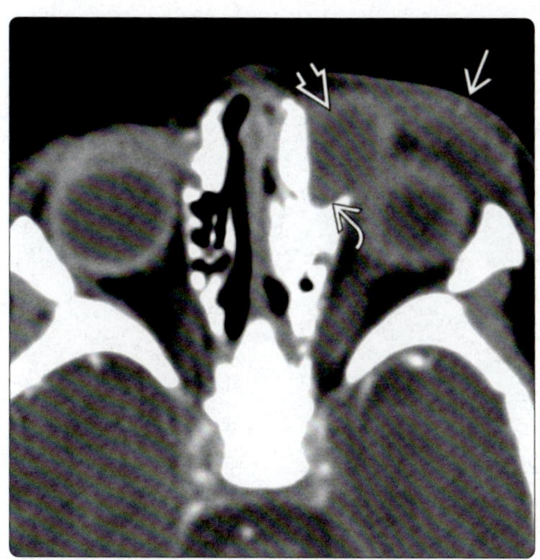

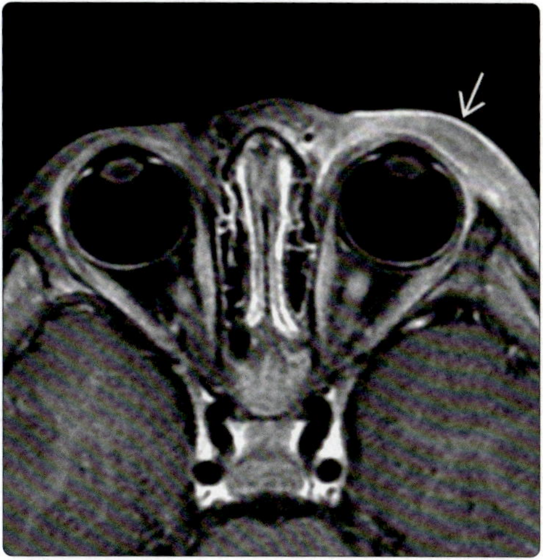

(Left) *Axial CECT in a 9-day-old presenting with eye swelling shows left preseptal orbital edema ➡ in the setting of a nasolacrimal duct mucocele. The lacrimal sac ➡ & lacrimal fossa/proximal canal ➡ are enlarged. There was an associated distal intranasal component to the mucocele (not shown).* **(Right)** *Axial T1 C+ FS MR in a 7 year old imaged for follow-up of an intracranial abnormality demonstrates new, unsuspected left preseptal cellulitis ➡. In this case, the cellulitis was secondary to a bee sting 1 day prior.*

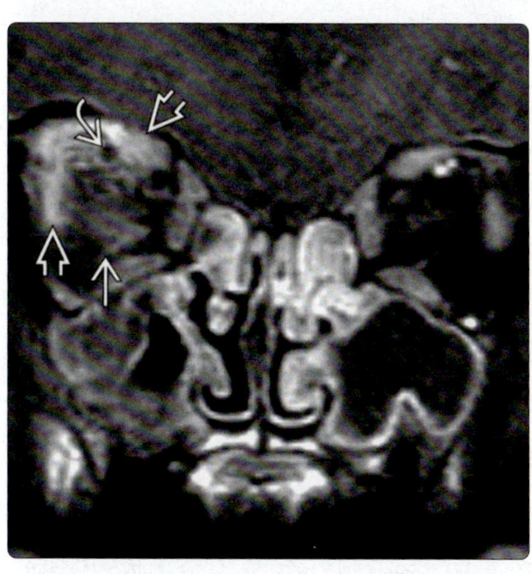

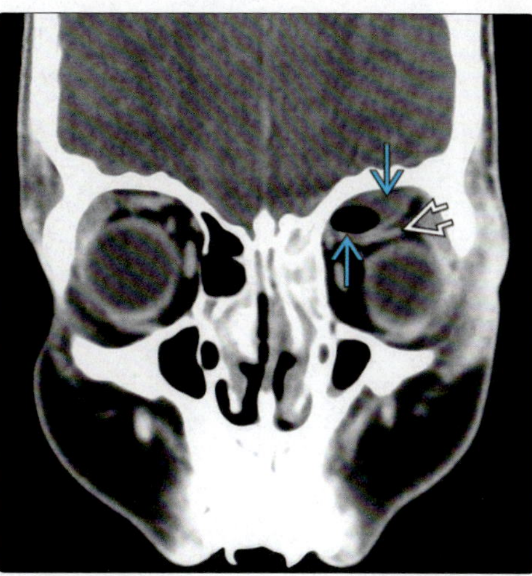

(Left) *Coronal T1 C+ FS MR in a child with extensive sinusitis shows hazy ↑ enhancement of the right intraconal fat ➡, thickening of the superior & lateral rectus muscles ➡ (consistent with myositis), & enlargement of a nonenhancing superior ophthalmic vein ➡, consistent with thrombosis.* **(Right)** *Coronal CECT in a child with left ethmoid sinusitis shows an ipsilateral superior orbital gas-containing SPA ➡. The left superior rectus muscle complex ➡ & globe are deviated inferiorly.*

KEY FACTS

TERMINOLOGY

- Retinoblastoma (RB): Malignant primary retinal neoplasm
- Trilateral/quadrilateral RB: Bilateral ocular RB + pineal tumor ± suprasellar tumor

IMAGING

- Unilateral in 60%, bilateral in 40%
- Trilateral or quadrilateral disease is rare
- Extraocular extension in < 10%: Poor prognosis
- CT: Ca^{2+} in > 90%
- MR: Assess extent of intraocular tumor + presence of optic nerve, orbital, &/or intracranial involvement
  - T1: Mild hyperintensity
  - T2: Moderate to marked hypointensity
  - T1 C+: Moderate to marked heterogeneous enhancement

TOP DIFFERENTIAL DIAGNOSES

- Persistent hyperplastic primary vitreous
- Coats disease
- Retinopathy of prematurity
- Orbital toxocariasis

PATHOLOGY

- Primitive neuroectodermal tumor
- Sporadic (nongermline) *RB1* mutation: Most are unilateral
- Inherited (germline) *RB1* mutation: Multilateral > unilateral
  - ↑ risk of 2nd remote malignancy

CLINICAL ISSUES

- Most common intraocular tumor of childhood
- Leukocoria in 50-60%
- 90-95% are diagnosed by age 5 years

DIAGNOSTIC CHECKLIST

- Calcified intraocular mass in child: RB until proven otherwise

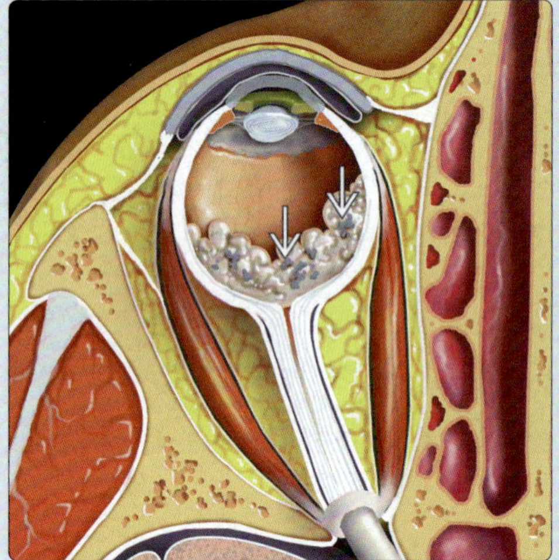

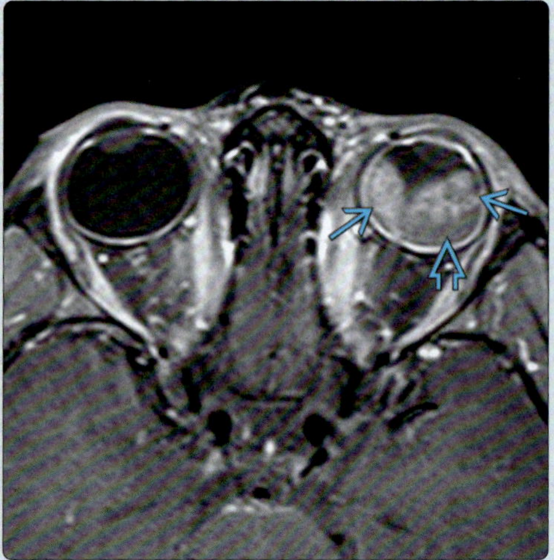

(Left) *Axial graphic depicts a retinoblastoma (RB) with lobulated tumor extending through the limiting membrane into the vitreous. Characteristic punctate Ca^{2+} ➔ are shown.* **(Right)** *Axial T1 C+ FS MR in a 3-year-old with leukocoria demonstrates a large, moderately enhancing, bilobed left RB ➔. Mild ↓ signal intensity posteriorly ➔ represents subretinal fluid secondary to retinal detachment.*

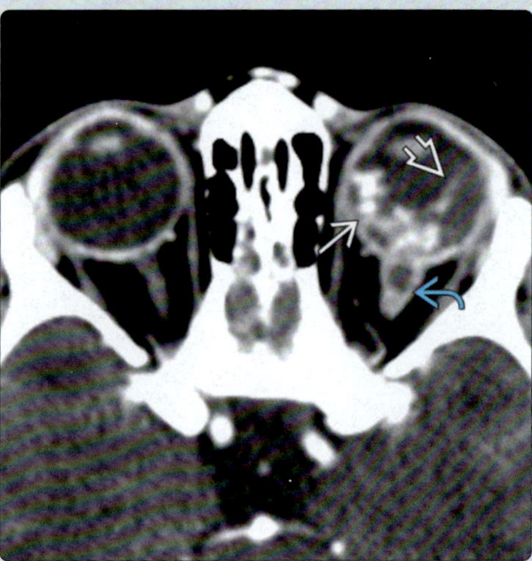

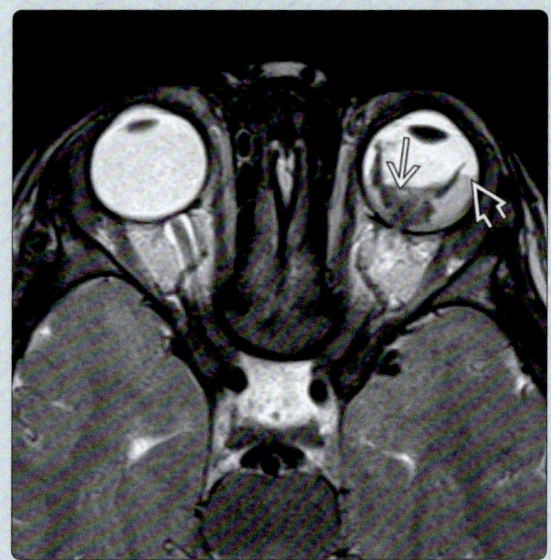

(Left) *Axial CECT in a 3-year-old with leukocoria shows a partially calcified RB ➔ in the left globe with a focus of retinal detachment &/or noncalcified subretinal tumor at the temporal aspect of the globe ➔. There is also postlaminar optic nerve/sheath invasion ➔.* **(Right)** *Axial T2 MR in the same child shows hypointensity ➔ in the calcified portions of the ocular mass with a lateral subretinal fluid level ➔ secondary to retinal detachment.*

TERMINOLOGY

Abbreviations

- Retinoblastoma (RB)

Definitions

- Malignant primary retinal neoplasm
- Trilateral RB: Bilateral ocular tumors + midline intracranial neuroblastic tumor, typically pineal
- Quadrilateral/tetralateral RB: Bilateral disease + pineal & suprasellar tumors

IMAGING

General Features

- Best diagnostic clue
  - Intraocular, calcified mass in young child
  - Diagnosed typically with ophthalmoscopy & ultrasound
    - MR for tumor mapping & prognostication
- Location
  - Unilateral in 60%, bilateral in 40%
  - Trilateral or quadrilateral disease is rare
  - Extraocular extension in < 10%
    - Spreads along scleral vessels into orbit & along optic nerve to subarachnoid space
  - Predictors for metastatic disease: Involvement of optic nerve, choroid, anterior chamber, or orbit
    - Anterior chamber enhancement reflects neoangiogenesis → associated with more aggressive tumor behavior
  - Role of MR imaging
    - Exclude pseudoneoplastic lesions
    - Assess intraocular (choroid, sclera, prelaminar optic nerve), extraocular (postlaminar optic nerve, orbital), & intracranial (pineal, parasellar, metastatic) involvement
- Morphology
  - Irregular & heterogeneous mass within normal or small globe
- Growth patterns
  - Endophytic form (45%)
    - Inward protrusion into vitreous
    - Associated with vitreous seeding
  - Exophytic form (45%)
    - Outward growth into subretinal space, typically with hemispherical configuration
    - Associated retinal detachment & subretinal exudate
  - Mixed endophytic & exophytic (10%)
  - Diffuse infiltrating form (rare, older children)
    - Plaque-like growth along retina; often no Ca^{2+}
    - Simulates inflammatory or other conditions

CT Findings

- Punctate, coarse or finely speckled Ca^{2+} (> 90-95%)
- Moderate to marked heterogeneous enhancement

MR Findings

- T1: Variable, mildly hyperintense (relative to vitreous)
- T2: Moderate to marked hypointensity (vs. vitreous)
  - Helps distinguish from hyperintense lesions (e.g., persistent hyperplastic primary vitreous, Coats disease)
  - Best to identify subretinal fluid ± vitreous hemorrhage
- T1 C+: Moderate to marked heterogeneous enhancement
  - Best to assess extent of intraocular disease & presence of optic nerve or extraocular invasion
    - Choroidal invasion: Localized thickening & heterogeneous contrast enhancement near tumor
    - Scleral invasion: Interruption in thin, hypointense zone surrounding enhancing choroid
    - Optic nerve invasion: Thickening of optic disc (prelaminar), enhancement of nerve (postlaminar)
- Imaging of orbital prosthesis
  - Fibrovascularization secures prosthesis & provides surface for muscular attachment
    - Progressive ↓ T2 signal & ↑ peripheral enhancement

Ultrasonographic Findings

- A-scan: Highly reflective spikes at Ca^{2+}
- B-scan: Echogenic, irregular mass with focal shadows

Imaging Recommendations

- Best imaging tool
  - MR: T1 C+ FS & T2 are best for tumor mapping
  - CT: Intraocular Ca^{2+} is relatively specific in child
- Protocol advice
  - Include whole brain to assess for intracranial disease

DIFFERENTIAL DIAGNOSIS

Persistent Hyperplastic Primary Vitreous

- Small globe, hyperdense tissue, no Ca^{2+}
- Hyperintense on T2 MR with enhancing retrolental stalk

Coats Disease

- Normal-sized globe, hyperdense exudate, rare Ca^{2+}
- Hyperintense on T1 & T2 MR

Retinopathy of Prematurity

- Retrolental fibroplasia; associated with excess oxygen & premature retinal vessels
- Bilateral, small globes; hyperdense tissue, Ca^{2+} if advanced

Retinal Astrocytic Hamartoma

- Rare lesion often associated with tuberous sclerosis; ± Ca^{2+}

Toxocariasis

- Uveoscleral enhancement with no Ca^{2+} in acute phase
- Moderately enhancing retinal nodule
- Intravitreal membranes & retinal detachment

Other Causes of Leukocoria

- Retinal detachment
  - Subretinal hemorrhage, retinal folds
- Choroidal osteoma, choroidal angioma
- Retinal dysplasia

PATHOLOGY

General Features

- Etiology
  - Primitive neuroectodermal tumor
  - Sporadic (nongermline): 60% of RB
    - Spontaneous somatic mutation or deletion of both copies of *RB1* in retinoblasts
    - Majority (85%) of unilateral disease

- Inherited (germline): 40% of RB
  - Germline mutation or deletion of 1 copy of *RB1* + spontaneous mutation of other copy
  - Essentially all bilateral & multilateral disease
    - Minority (15%) of unilateral disease
  - Autosomal dominant with 90% penetrance
  - Positive family history in 5-10%
  - New germline mutations in 30-35%
- Genetics
  - *RB1* gene (chromosome 13q14) codes for pRB tumor suppressor protein
    - Lack of both *RB1* alleles in embryonic retinoblasts leads to absence of pRB, resulting in malignancy
  - Somatic mosaicism in 10-20% of RB patients
- Associated abnormalities
  - ↑ risk of 2nd malignancy in germline disease
    - Sarcoma, melanoma, CNS tumors, epithelial tumors (lung, bladder, breast)
    - 20-30% in nonirradiated patients
    - 50-60% in irradiated patients
    - Occurs within 30 years; average 10-13 years
  - 13q deletion syndrome: RB + multiple organ anomalies

Staging, Grading, & Classification

- Reese-Ellsworth classification
  - Groups 1-5
  - Based on size, location, & multifocality
  - More useful in radiation therapy management
- International (Murphree) classification of retinoblastoma
  - Groups A-E
  - Based on size, retinal location, subretinal or vitreous seeding, & several specific prognostic features
  - More useful in chemotherapy management

Microscopic Features

- Small round cells, scant cytoplasm, & large nuclei
- Flexner-Wintersteiner rosettes & fleurettes

CLINICAL ISSUES

Presentation

- Most common signs/symptoms
  - Leukocoria in 50-60%
- Other signs/symptoms
  - Severe vision loss
  - Strabismus with macular involvement or retinal detachment
  - Proptosis with significant orbital disease
  - Rubeosis iridis (redness of iris secondary to neovascularization) correlates with anterior chamber enhancement on MR
  - Inflammatory signs in 10%
  - Less common: Anisocoria, heterochromia, glaucoma, cataract, nystagmus

Demographics

- Age
  - Average age of RB diagnosis: 18 months
    - Unilateral: 24 months; bilateral: 13 months
    - Earlier with family history & routine screening
  - 90-95% are diagnosed by age 5 years
- Epidemiology
  - Most common intraocular tumor of childhood
  - Incidence of 1:17,000 live births (↑ in past 60 years)
  - 3% of cancers in children < 15 years old
  - 1% of cancer deaths; 5% of childhood blindness

Natural History & Prognosis

- Degree of nerve involvement correlates with survival
  - Superficial or no invasion: 90%
  - Invasion to lamina cribrosa (prelaminar): 70%
  - Invasion beyond lamina cribrosa (postlaminar): 60%
  - Involvement at surgical margin: 20%
- Poor prognosis for extraocular disease
  - < 10% 5-year disease-free survival
- Poor prognosis for trilateral disease or CSF spread
  - < 24-month survival

Treatment

- > 95% of children with RB in USA are cured with modern techniques
  - Maintaining eye & vision remains problematic
- Therapy is based on tumor volume & localization, intraocular tumor extent, & extraocular stage of disease
- Enucleation: Used in advanced disease with no chance of preserving useful vision
- External beam radiation therapy: Bulky tumors with seeding
  - Unfavorable complications (e.g., arrested bone growth, radiation-induced tumors)
- Chemotherapy ("chemoreduction"): Currently favored 1st-line therapy for lower grade intraocular tumors
  - Intraarterial & intravitreous chemotherapy are gaining traction with high globe salvage rates
    - Limits need for systemic chemotherapy, external radiation, & enucleation
- Plaque radiotherapy: Locally directed I-125 or other isotope
  - Selected solitary or small tumors
- Cryotherapy: Primary local treatment small anterior tumors
- Photocoagulation: Primary local treatment of small posterior tumors

DIAGNOSTIC CHECKLIST

Image Interpretation Pearls

- Calcified intraocular mass in child: RB until proven otherwise
- Assess for intraocular & extraocular spread
- Check for intracranial trilateral or quadrilateral disease in pineal & suprasellar regions

SELECTED REFERENCES

1. Li Z et al: Diagnosis of postlaminar optic nerve invasion in retinoblastoma with MRI features. J Magn Reson Imaging. 51(4):1045-52, 2020
2. Chen Q et al: Comparison between intravenous chemotherapy and intra-arterial chemotherapy for retinoblastoma: a meta-analysis. BMC Cancer. 18(1):486, 2018
3. Wyse E et al: A review of the literature for intra-arterial chemotherapy used to treat retinoblastoma. Pediatr Radiol. 46(9):1223-33, 2016
4. Learned KO et al: Imaging of the postoperative orbit. Neuroimaging Clin N Am. 25(3):457-76, 2015

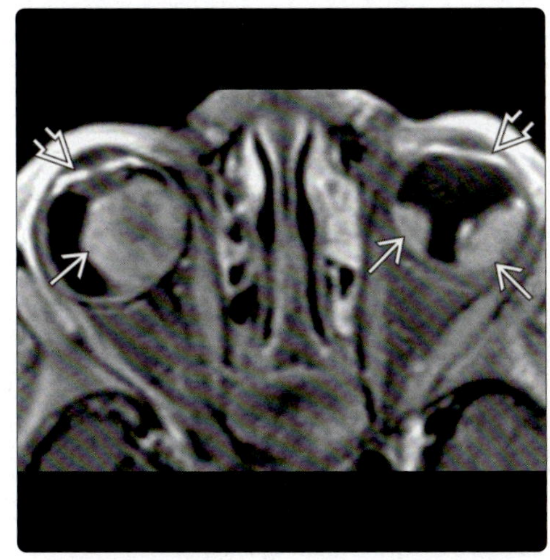

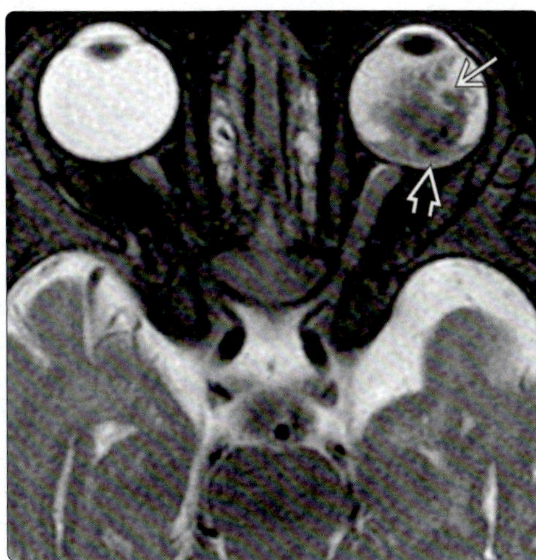

(Left) *Axial T1 C+ FS MR shows bulky, enhancing intraocular masses ➡ compatible with bilateral RB. Note the prominent enhancement of each iris ➡. Anterior segment enhancement is associated with more aggressive tumor behavior.* **(Right)** *Axial T2 FS MR reveals a lobular, hypointense mass filling much of the vitreous compartment of the left globe ➡. Note the posterior fluid level ➡ indicating vitreous hemorrhage associated with an endophytic form of RB.*

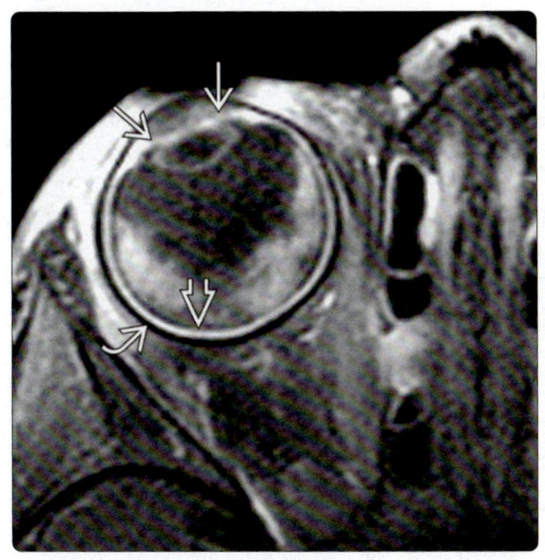

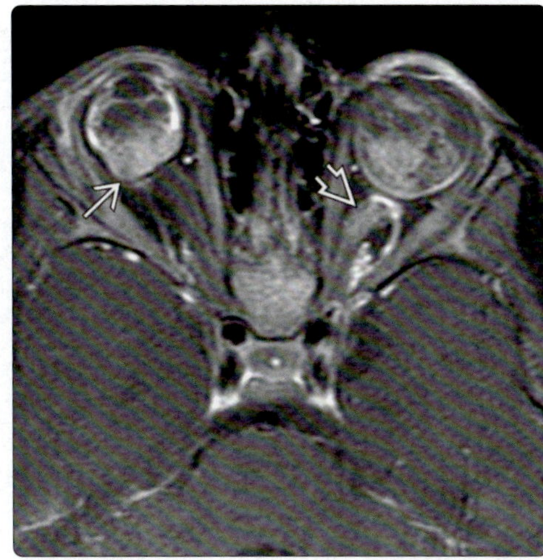

(Left) *Axial T1 C+ FS MR shows a moderately enhancing RB associated with prominent anterior segment enhancement ➡. Note the intact thin lines of enhancing choroid ➡ & hypointense sclera ➡, indicating absence of invasion.* **(Right)** *Axial T1 C+ FS MR shows interruption of linear hypointensity posteriorly with focal contour abnormality ➡, indicating scleral invasion by RB on the right. The left postlaminar optic nerve demonstrates asymmetric enlargement & enhancement ➡, consistent with tumor extension.*

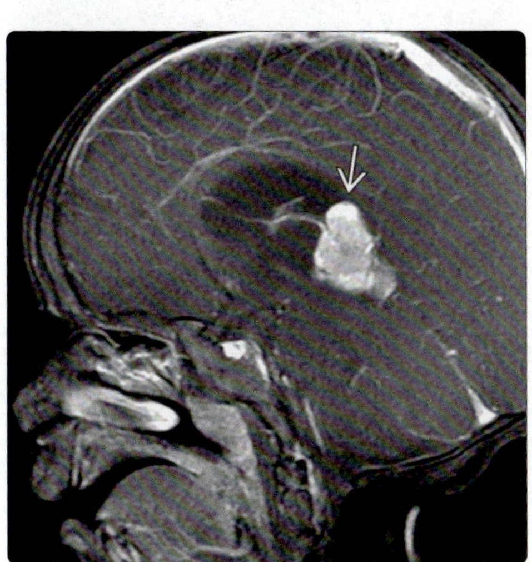

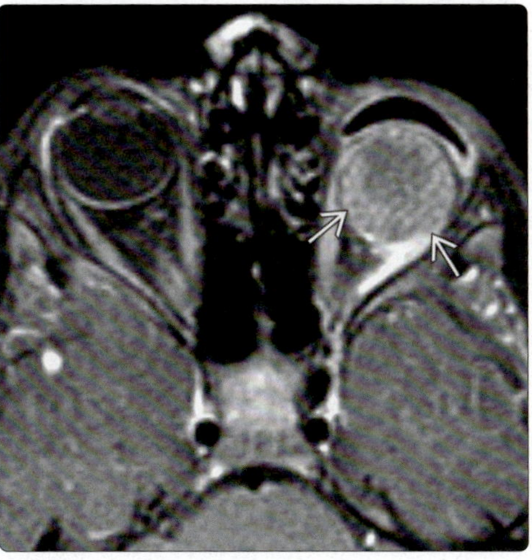

(Left) *Sagittal T1 C+ FS MR in a 3-year-old with bilateral RB demonstrates a lobulated, enhancing mass ➡ in the region of the pineal gland. This mass was proven to represent pineoblastoma/PNET, typical of trilateral RB.* **(Right)** *Axial T1 C+ FS MR in a child after left globe enucleation for treatment of a large RB shows the hydroxyapatite intraorbital component with a well-defined, spherical prosthesis ➡. There is typical moderate, heterogeneous postcontrast enhancement secondary to fibrovascular tissue infiltration.*

Congenital Auricle Malformations

KEY FACTS

TERMINOLOGY

- Congenital aural dysplasia (CAD): Congenital external ear malformation
- Outer ear: Auricle (pinna) & external auditory canal (EAC)
- Microtia: Congenital malformation with underdeveloped, misshapen auricle

IMAGING

- Small, malformed, ± low-set pinna
- EAC stenosis/atresia & middle ear (ME)/ossicular anomalies
- Degree of microtia correlates with degree of EAC stenosis/atresia & ME anomalies

TOP DIFFERENTIAL DIAGNOSES

- Syndromes with auricle malformations
  - Treacher Collins syndrome
  - Hemifacial microsomia
  - Branchiootorenal syndrome
  - CHARGE syndrome

PATHOLOGY

- Weerda classification of auricular dysplasia
  - 1st-degree dysplasia: Macrotia, prominent ear, pocket ear, absence of upper helix, absence of tragus, clefts, lobular deformities, & cup ear types I & II
  - 2nd-degree dysplasia: Cup ear type III, miniear
  - 3rd-degree dysplasia: Auricular remnant with no recognizable structures of normal auricle
- Minor microtia: 1st & 2nd degree
  - Associated with EAC stenosis
- Major microtia: 3rd degree
  - Associated with EAC atresia (75%)
- Associated temporal bone abnormalities
  - EAC stenosis or atresia & malformed ossicles
  - ± ↓ ME & mastoid pneumatization
  - 1/3 with CAD have inner ear malformations
  - Anomalous CNVII canal ± oval window anomaly
  - Congenital or acquired ME cholesteatoma

(Left) *Frontal 3D soft tissue surface-rendered NECT reformation in a 3-year-old girl with hemifacial microsomia demonstrates a right-sided 2nd-degree microtia, a small right mandible, & a normal left pinna.* **(Right)** *Frontal 3D soft tissue surface-rendered NECT reformation in a child with Treacher Collins syndrome shows bilateral 3rd-degree microtia, downward-slanting palpebral fissures, & symmetric micrognathia.*

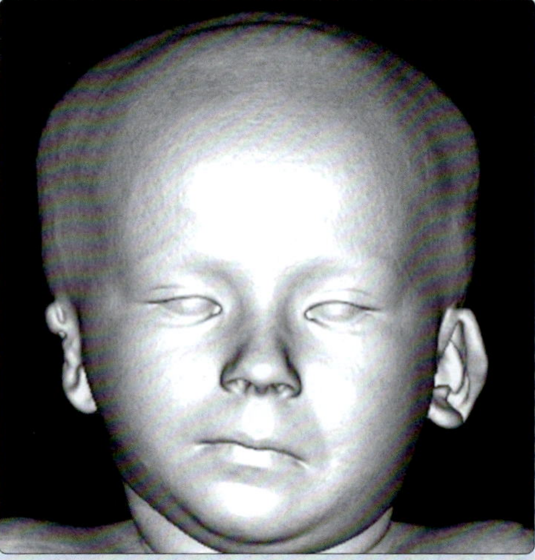

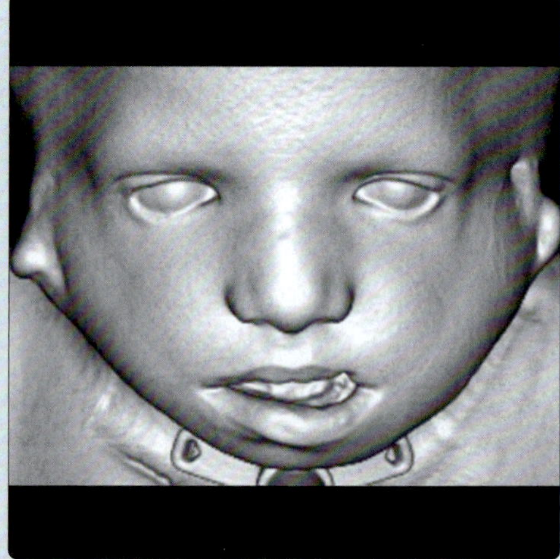

(Left) *Lateral 3D soft tissue surface-rendered NECT reformation shows a moderately deformed right pinna (2nd-degree malformation) in a 10-month-old with right congenital external & middle ear malformation.* **(Right)** *Coronal CT images of the temporal bones in the same patient show the atretic right EAC ➡. The deformed right malleus & incus ➡ are fused to the lateral epitympanic cavity, & the middle ear cavity is underdeveloped. The normal left temporal bone is shown for comparison.*

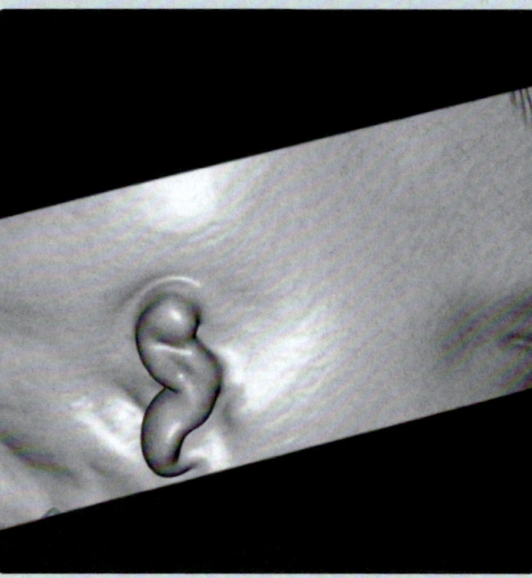

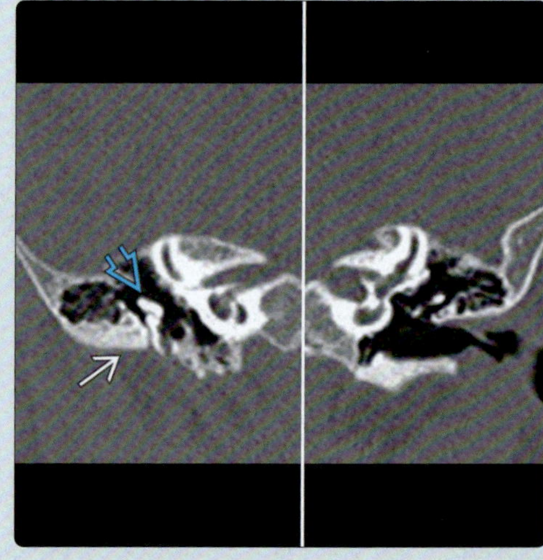

TERMINOLOGY

Synonyms

- Congenital aural dysplasia: Congenital external ear malformation
- Outer ear: Auricle & external auditory canal (EAC)
- Auricle: Pinna

Definitions

- Microtia: Congenital malformation with underdeveloped & misshapen auricle
- Anotia: Absent auricle

IMAGING

General Features

- Best diagnostic clue
  - Small, malformed, ± low-set pinna
    - Associated EAC stenosis/atresia, middle ear (ME) & ossicular malformation
  - Degree of microtia correlates with degree of EAC stenosis/atresia & ME anomalies
- Location
  - Auricle, EAC, ME, ± inner ear (IE)
  - R > L (60:40); 1/3 of cases are bilateral

CT Findings

- Bone CT
  - Identifies congenital external & ME malformation (CEMEM)
  - 3D soft tissue reconstruction demonstrates microtia

Imaging Recommendations

- Best imaging tool
  - Temporal bone CT with multiplanar & 3D reconstruction

DIFFERENTIAL DIAGNOSIS

Syndromes With Auricle Malformations

- Treacher Collins syndrome
- Hemifacial microsomia
- Branchiootorenal syndrome
- Pierre Robin sequence
- CHARGE syndrome

PATHOLOGY

General Features

- Etiology
  - CEMEM is secondary to anomalous 1st & 2nd branchial arch development during 1st trimester
  - Genetic or teratogenic insult
- Associated abnormalities
  - < 30% of CEMEM have IE malformations
  - Up to 30% of CEMEM have syndromic etiology
  - ↓ ME & mastoid pneumatization in 25% of minor & 66% of major microtia
  - Abnormal course of CNVII canal ± oval window atresia
  - Congenital or acquired cholesteatoma lies behind atretic plate in up to 10% of patients with CEMEM
  - Micrognathia with low-set pinna in syndromic cases

Staging, Grading, & Classification

- Weerda classification of auricular dysplasia
  - Minor microtia
    - 1st-degree dysplasia: Macrotia, prominent ear, pocket ear, absence of upper helix, absence of tragus, clefts, lobular deformities, & cup ear types I & II
    - 2nd-degree dysplasia: Cup ear type III, miniear
      - ± low, anterior position of pinnae
      - 75% of minor microtia patients have EAC stenosis
  - Major microtia
    - 3rd-degree dysplasia: Auricular remnant with no recognizable structures of normal auricle
      - Includes anotia
      - Severely dysplastic ears are frequently anterior & inferior in position secondary to incomplete embryologic ascent in neck
      - 75% of patients with major microtia have EAC atresia; remainder have EAC stenosis

CLINICAL ISSUES

Presentation

- Most common signs/symptoms
  - Microtia or anotia & stenotic/absent EAC
  - Conductive or mixed hearing loss
- Other signs/symptoms
  - Micrognathia: Unilateral (hemifacial microsomia) or bilateral (Treacher Collins) with low-set pinna

Demographics

- Overall incidence of CEMEM: 1/3,300-10,000 live births

Treatment

- Complicated surgical correction of pinna
  - Autogenous rib construction: 2 or more stages
    - More durable, less prone to infection
  - Alloplastic porous high-density polyethylene reconstruction: 2 stages
    - More aesthetic, less morbidity, & can be done at younger age
- ± drilling of new EAC &/or ossicle reconstruction

DIAGNOSTIC CHECKLIST

Image Interpretation Pearls

- Degree of microtia correlates with underdevelopment of EAC, ME, & mastoid air cells
- Look for erosive opacity due to associated cholesteatoma

SELECTED REFERENCES

1. Nada A et al: Cross-sectional imaging evaluation of congenital temporal bone anomalies: what each radiologist should know. Curr Probl Diagn Radiol. 50(5):716-24, 2021
2. Zhang TY et al: International Consensus Recommendations on Microtia, Aural Atresia and Functional Ear Reconstruction. J Int Adv Otol. 15(2):204-208, 2019
3. Bartel-Friedrich S: Congenital auricular malformations: description of anomalies and syndromes. Facial Plast Surg. 31(6):567-80, 2015
4. Cabin JA et al: Microtia reconstruction: autologous rib and alloplast techniques. Facial Plast Surg Clin North Am. 22(4):623-38, 2014
5. Casale G et al: Acquired ear canal cholesteatoma in congenital aural atresia/stenosis. Otol Neurotol. 35(8):1474-9, 2014
6. Nadaraja GS et al: Hearing outcomes of atresia surgery versus osseointegrated bone conduction device in patients with congenital aural atresia: a systematic review. Otol Neurotol. 34(8):1394-9, 2013

Large Vestibular Aqueduct

KEY FACTS

TERMINOLOGY

- Large vestibular aqueduct (LVA): Bony VA houses large endolymphatic sac (ES) & duct (ED)
- Incomplete partition type II (IP-II): Between middle & apical cochlear turns; often seen with LVA
- IP-II + LVA + minimally dilated vestibule: Mondini deformity

IMAGING

- Axial CT: Midpoint of VA (between posterior labyrinth & operculum) > 1.5 mm
- MR: Enlarged ES & ED
- Cochlea: Abnormal in ~ 75% of LVA cases
    - Absent interscalar septum between middle & apical turns with deficient modiolus (IP-II) → enlarged scala vestibuli
- 2nd interscalar ridge notch angle ↑ & depth ↓
- Vestibule: Normal or minimally enlarged

TOP DIFFERENTIAL DIAGNOSES

- Cystic cochleovestibular malformation (IP-I)
- Cochlear hypoplasia
- CHARGE syndrome (funnel-shaped LVA)
- Branchiootorenal syndrome (funnel-shaped LVA)

PATHOLOGY

- *SLC26A4* mutations in ~ 50% of LVA patients
    - Pendred syndrome: Sensorineural hearing loss (SNHL) + thyroid organification defect ± goiter

CLINICAL ISSUES

- Most common imaging abnormality in pediatric SNHL
- Bilateral anomaly (most); initially normal hearing
    - Progressive/fluctuating SNHL due to high pulsating CSF pressure or head trauma
- Avoid contact sports & try to prevent head trauma
- Hearing aid first, cochlear implantation later
    - Cochlear nerve is present in IP-II

(Left) *Left inner ear graphic shows large endolymphatic sac (ES) epidural ➡ & intraosseous ➡ components. The cochlea is malformed with absent septation between middle & apical turns, which appear bulbous ➡.* **(Right)** *Axial bone CT in a 15-year-old boy with sensorineural hearing loss (SNHL) shows a large vestibular aqueduct (LVA) ➡. The modiolus is defective toward the apex & present at the base ➡. Note that the scalar chambers are asymmetric (anterior scala vestibuli > posterior scala tympani) ➡.*

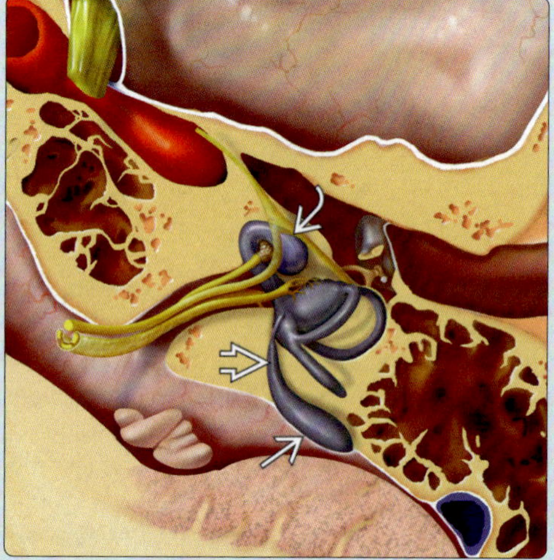

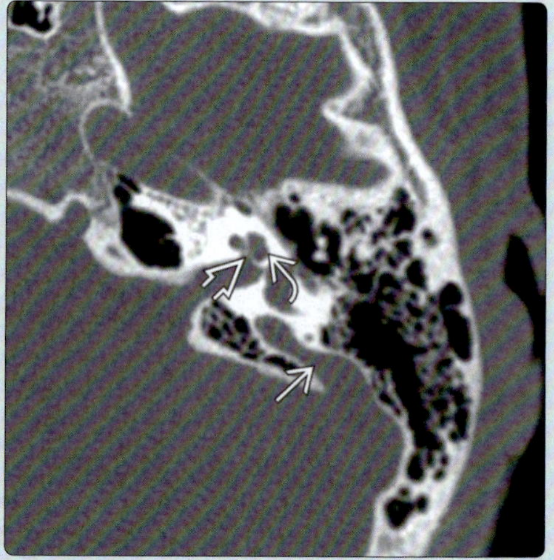

(Left) *Axial bone CT in a 17-year-old girl with Pendred syndrome shows a LVA ➡ & absent septation between the middle & apical cochlear turns ➡ with a deficient modiolus ➡. This is typical of incomplete partition type II (IP-II), which results in a baseball cap-shaped cochlea.* **(Right)** *Axial T2 MR in a 12-year-old girl with right SNHL shows a large endolymphatic sac anomaly (LESA) ➡ & typical IP-II cochlear anomaly. Note deficiency of the ISS, resulting in plump cochlear middle & apical turns ➡, resembling a baseball cap.*

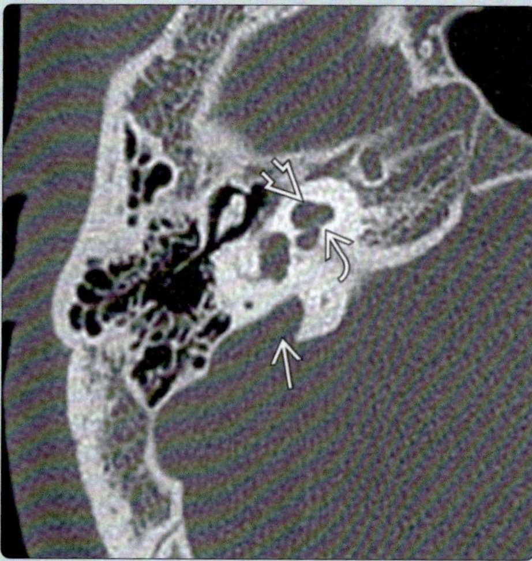

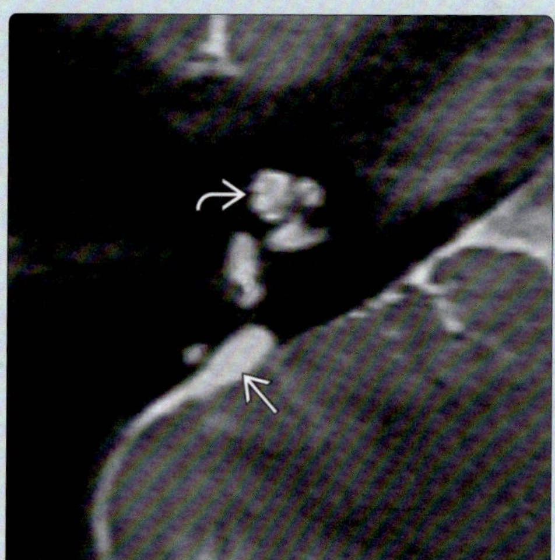

TERMINOLOGY

Abbreviations

- Large vestibular aqueduct (LVA)

Synonyms

- Large endolymphatic sac anomaly (LESA): T2/SSFP MR term
- Enlarged vestibular aqueduct (EVA): CT term
- Mondini deformity (historic terminology): LVA + minimally dilated vestibule + incomplete partition type II (IP-II)

Definitions

- LVA: Enlarged, bony VA houses large endolymphatic sac (ES) & duct (ED)
  - Associated with variable cochlear malformation
- IP-II: Deficient modiolus & interscalar septum (ISS) between middle & apical cochlear turns, + LVA
  - IP-II has normal cochlear external dimensions
    - Not correct to call IP-II if cochlea has 1.5 turns
    - Term "cochlea with 1.5 turns" should be used only for cochlear hypoplasia (CH)

IMAGING

General Features

- Best diagnostic clue
  - CT: EVA ± IP-II; 3D T2/SSFP MR: LESA ± IP-II
- Size
  - Valvassori criteria: Vertical & axial VA width > 1.5 mm at midpoint of labyrinth & operculum (most accepted)
  - Additional criteria in literature
    - Cincinnati criteria: LVA ≥ 1 mm at midpoint (more sensitive), ± ≥ 2 mm at operculum on axial images
    - Pöschl 45° oblique plane: 0.8 mm at midpoint is borderline enlarged

CT Findings

- Bone CT
  - LVA: May scallop posterior margin of petrous bone
  - Cochlea: Abnormal on CT in ~ 75% of LVA cases
    - Normal or deficient ISS between plump apical & middle turns (IP-II); normal basal turn
      - Results in baseball cap appearance of cochlea
    - Asymmetric scalar chambers: Anterior > posterior
    - Deficient (typical), absent, or normal modiolus
  - Vestibule: Normal or minimally enlarged
  - Semicircular canals (SCCs): Normal or mildly dilated
    - Reduced size of lateral SCC bone island with enlargement of lateral SCC may be seen in IP-II
  - Middle ear space & ossicles: Normal

MR Findings

- 3D T2 SPACE or 3D SSFP (FIESTA, CISS or equivalent)
  - ES & ED: Enlarged, variable hyperintense signal
  - Cochlea: Deficient ISS between plump apical & middle turns (IP-II); normal in LVA only
  - Interscalar R2 notch angle > 114° & depth ≤ 0.31 mm suggests IP-II & scala communis
  - In IP-II, 2nd part of ISS bulges anteriorly due to enlarged scala vestibuli in 3D T2 MR

DIFFERENTIAL DIAGNOSIS

Cystic Cochleovestibular Malformation (IP-I)

- Cystic cochlea & vestibule without internal structure

Cochlear Hypoplasia

- Small cochlea; usually < 2 turns

CHARGE Syndrome

- Funnel-shaped LVA, small vestibule, & small/absent SCC
- Cochlear nerve canal stenosis/atresia & thickened modiolus; occasional CH

Branchiootorenal Syndrome

- Funnel-shaped LVA, tapered basal turn, & small offset middle & apical turns

High-Riding Jugular Bulb

- Communicates with jugular foramen, not vestibule

PATHOLOGY

General Features

- Genetics
  - *SLC26A4* mutations (*PDS* gene, chromosome 7)
    - ~ 50% of LVA patients have *SLC26A4* mutations
  - Syndromic deafness: Pendred syndrome
    - Sensorineural hearing loss (SNHL) + thyroid organification defect ± goiter
    - Autosomal recessive; biallelic *SLC26A4* mutation; ~ 10% of hereditary deafness

CLINICAL ISSUES

Presentation

- Most common signs/symptoms
  - SNHL (or MHL due to "3rd window" effect)
    - Bilateral or unilateral
    - Fluctuating or progressive course
    - SNHL precipitated by minor head trauma
- Other signs/symptoms
  - Tinnitus, vertigo, dizziness
  - Pendred syndrome: Hypothyroidism in ~ 50%, ± goiter in adolescence

Treatment

- Avoid contact sports & try to prevent head trauma
- Hearing aid first, cochlear implantation later in IP-II
  - Cochlear nerve is present in IP-II

SELECTED REFERENCES

1. O'Brien WT , Sr et al: Nonsyndromic congenital causes of sensorineural hearing loss in children: an illustrative review. AJR Am J Roentgenol. 1-8, 2021
2. Ginat DT: Imaging findings in syndromes with temporal bone abnormalities. Neuroimaging Clin N Am. 29(1):117-28, 2019
3. Booth TN et al: Evaluation of the normal cochlear second interscalar ridge angle and depth on 3D T2-weighted images: a tool for the diagnosis of scala communis and incomplete partition type II. AJNR Am J Neuroradiol. 39(5):923-7, 2018
4. Sennaroğlu L et al: Classification and current management of inner ear malformations. Balkan Med J. 34(5):397-411, 2017
5. Boston M et al: The large vestibular aqueduct: a new definition based on audiologic and computed tomography correlation. Otolaryngol Head Neck Surg. 136(6):972-7, 2007

Congenital Cholesteatoma

KEY FACTS

TERMINOLOGY

- Congenital cholesteatoma (CCh): Benign mass secondary to epithelial rests of embryonal origin
- CCh most commonly occurs in middle ear (ME), behind intact tympanic membrane (TM) in patient without history of surgery, chronic otitis media (COM), or otorrhea

IMAGING

- Majority are in ME (CCh-ME)
  - Anterosuperior tympanic cavity near eustachian tube or stapes is most common
  - Posterior epitympanum at tympanic isthmus
  - Other sites include EAC, petrous apex, & mastoid
- Temporal bone CT findings
  - Small, well-circumscribed ME lesion medial to ossicles
  - Large mass may erode ossicles, ME wall, lateral semicircular canal, or tegmen tympani
- MR findings: Peripherally enhancing ME mass with diffusion restriction in larger lesions

TOP DIFFERENTIAL DIAGNOSES

- Acquired cholesteatoma
- Rhabdomyosarcoma
- Langerhans cell histiocytosis
- Glomus tympanicum paraganglioma
- ME cholesterol granuloma

CLINICAL ISSUES

- Avascular pearly white ME mass behind intact TM without prior history of inflammation or trauma
- Unilateral conductive hearing loss in 30%
- Large ME lesions can obstruct eustachian tube → ME effusion & infection
- Complete surgical extirpation = treatment of choice

DIAGNOSTIC CHECKLIST

- Child with ME mass medial to ossicles, normal mastoid aeration, & no history of COM = CCh-ME

(Left) *Coronal graphic shows a congenital cholesteatoma (CCh) involving the middle ear (ME) cavity. Note that the lesion has extended medially to the ossicles ➡ as it engulfs the entire ossicular chain. The tympanic membrane (TM) is intact, a typical finding in congenital lesions, as opposed to acquired cholesteatomas (which are associated with TM perforation).* **(Right)** *Axial bone CT in a 3-year-old child without a history of chronic otitis media shows a typical round, well-circumscribed CCh ➡ anteromedial to the malleus manubrium.*

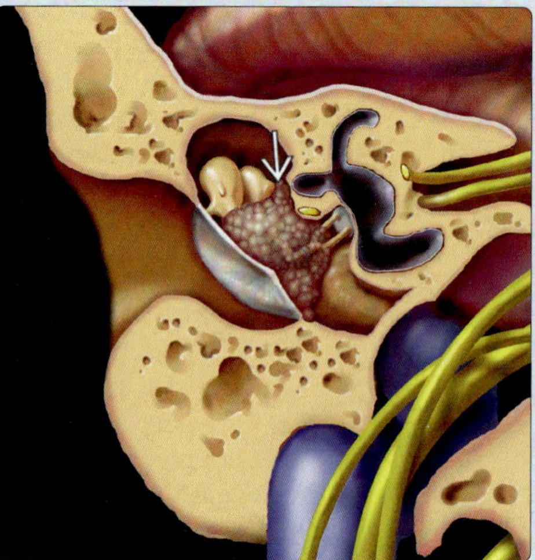

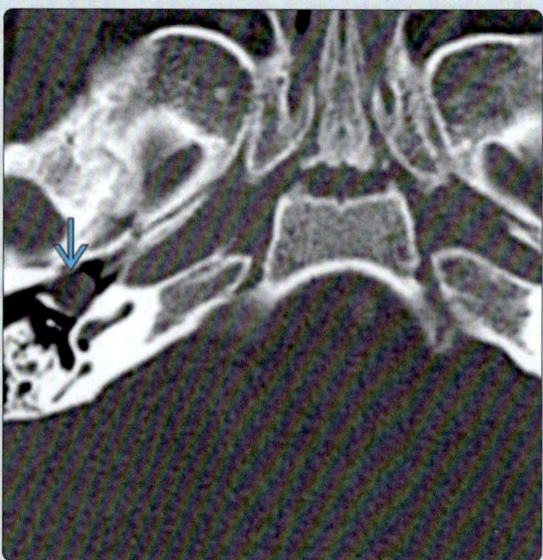

(Left) *Axial T2 MR in the same patient shows the CCh as an intermediate signal intensity, well-defined ME mass ➡ anterolateral to the basal turn ➡ of the right cochlea.* **(Right)** *Axial T1 C+ FS MR in the same patient shows the centrally nonenhancing CCh with a thin rim of peripheral enhancement ➡ adjacent to the cochlea ➡. This is a typical appearance & location for a CCh.*

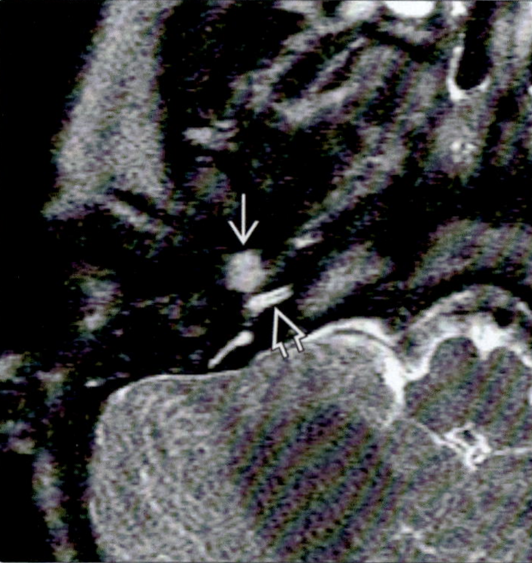

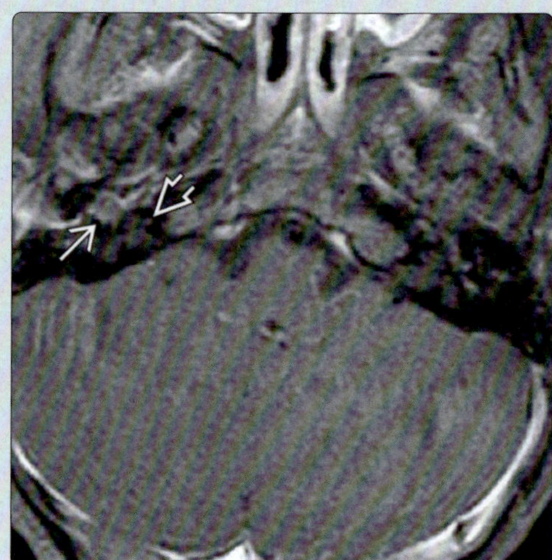

TERMINOLOGY

Synonyms

- Primary cholesteatoma, epidermoid

Definitions

- Congenital cholesteatoma (CCh): Benign mass secondary to epithelial rests of embryonal origin
- Most commonly occurs in middle ear (ME), behind intact tympanic membrane (TM) in patient without history of surgery, chronic otitis media, or otorrhea

IMAGING

General Features

- Best diagnostic clue
  - Smooth, well-circumscribed ME mass ± ossicular erosions
- Location
  - Majority in ME (CCh-ME)
  - Other locations: External auditory canal (EAC), mastoid, petrous apex, cerebellopontine angle, facial nerve canal, incudostapedial joint

CT Findings

- Bone CT
  - Appearance depends on size of lesion & location
  - Small CCh-ME: Well-circumscribed lesion
  - Large CCh-ME: Mass may erode ossicles, ME wall, lateral semicircular canal, or tegmen tympani [similar to acquired cholesteatoma (ACh)]
    - Bone erosion < ACh; occurs late in disease
    - Long process of incus & stapes superstructure are most commonly destroyed ossicles
    - If aditus ad antrum is occluded, mastoid air cells opacify with retained secretions
  - Petrous apex CCh: Expansile mass with smooth bone remodeling/erosion
    - May become very large before discovered
  - Mastoid CCh: Expansile mass with smooth bone erosion; may exit mastoid into EAC, parotid space, carotid space
  - EAC CCh: Rare; ↑ with EAC malformations

MR Findings

- T1: Iso- to hypointense mass
- T2: Intermediate signal intensity mass
  - Larger ME lesions → aditus ad antrum obstruction → high-signal retained secretions in mastoid air cells
- DWI: Larger lesions demonstrate diffusion restriction
- T1 C+: Peripherally enhancing ME mass
  - CCh-ME shows nonenhancing material surrounded by thin, subtle rim enhancement

DIFFERENTIAL DIAGNOSIS

Acquired Cholesteatoma Acquired Cholesteatoma

- Pars flaccida-ACh
- Pars tensa-ACh

Rhabdomyosarcoma

- Destructive mass in petrous apex, ME, or mastoid

Langerhans Cell Histiocytosis

- Enhancing soft tissue mass with bone destruction

Glomus Tympanicum Paraganglioma

- Pulsatile, vascular mass behind TM
- Enhancing mass on cochlear promontory; no bone erosion
- Unusual in pediatric & adolescent patients

Middle Ear Cholesterol Granuloma

- ME mass with high signal intensity on T1 MR

Facial Nerve Schwannoma

- Enlarged bony facial nerve canal

PATHOLOGY

General Features

- Etiology
  - 2 principal theories of CCh-ME
    - Congenital ectodermal rest in ME cavity left behind at time of neural tube closure
    - Lack of regression of epidermoid formation
      - Epidermoid formation: Point of epithelial transformation between tympanic cavity & eustachian tube
- Associated abnormalities
  - EAC atresia may have associated CCh of ME or EAC

Staging, Grading, & Classification

- CCh-ME staging system
  - Stage 1: Single quadrant; no ossicular involvement or mastoid extension
  - Stage 2: Multiple quadrants; no ossicular involvement or mastoid extension
  - Stage 3: Ossicular involvement; no mastoid extension
  - Stage 4: Mastoid extension

CLINICAL ISSUES

Presentation

- Most common signs/symptoms
  - Avascular pearly white ME mass behind intact TM without prior history of inflammation or trauma

Demographics

- Age
  - Average age of presentation or detection
    - Anterior or anterosuperior: 4 years
    - Posterosuperior & mesotympanum: 12 years
    - Attic & mastoid antrum: 20 years or older
- Epidemiology
  - 2-5% of temporal bone cholesteatomas are congenital

Natural History & Prognosis

- CCh-ME: Smaller anterior lesions have better outcome with complete surgical resection
- Large lesions or posterior epitympanic CCh have recurrence rates as high as 20%

SELECTED REFERENCES

1. McCabe R et al: The endoscopic management of congenital cholesteatoma. Otolaryngol Clin North Am. 54(1):111-23, 2021
2. Hao J et al: The significance of staging in the treatment of congenital cholesteatoma in children. Ear Nose Throat J. 145561320933965, 2020
3. Juliano AF et al: Imaging review of the temporal bone: part II. Traumatic, postoperative, and noninflammatory nonneoplastic conditions. Radiology. 276(3):655-72, 2015

Acquired Cholesteatoma

KEY FACTS

TERMINOLOGY

- Secondary or acquired cholesteatoma (ACh)
  - Tympanic membrane (TM) retraction or perforation → accumulation of stratified squamous epithelial cells in middle ear (ME) → mass-like keratin ball
- Pars flaccida cholesteatoma (PFCh): 80%
- Pars tensa cholesteatoma (PTCh): 15%
  - Sinus cholesteatoma = PTCh in sinus tympani

IMAGING

- Nonenhancing ME soft tissue mass + ossicular erosion
  - PFCh: In Prussak space with scutum erosion
    - ± tegmen tympani, lateral semicircular canal, facial nerve canal, or sigmoid sinus plate dehiscence
  - PTCh: In posterior mesotympanum medial to ossicles
    - ± ossicular erosion, involvement of sinus tympani, facial recess, aditus ad antrum, or mastoid
- Restricts diffusion on DWI MR
- Associated granulation tissue or scar may enhance
- Best modalities
  - Noncontrast bone CT: Axial & coronal
    - Ossicular & adjacent bone evaluation
  - Coronal T1 C+ FS MR
    - Suspected intracranial extension/infection

TOP DIFFERENTIAL DIAGNOSES

- Chronic otitis media
- Congenital cholesteatoma
- Acute coalescent otomastoiditis with abscess
- Langerhans cell histiocytosis
- Rhabdomyosarcoma

CLINICAL ISSUES

- Recurrent or chronic ME infections with TM perforation or retraction pocket
- Conductive hearing loss
- Affects children & adults
  - Unusual in children < 4 years of age

(Left) *Coronal graphic shows a large acquired cholesteatoma of the pars flaccida (PF). Complications include erosion of the ossicles & lateral semicircular canal (SCC) ➡ + thinning of the tegmen tympani ➡.* **(Right)** *Coronal bone CT in a 7-year-old patient shows a large middle ear mass filling the upper mesotympanum with opacification of the epitympanum & Prussak space ➡, blunting of the scutum ➡, & near-complete erosion of the ossicles ➡, typical of a PF cholesteatoma (PFCh).*

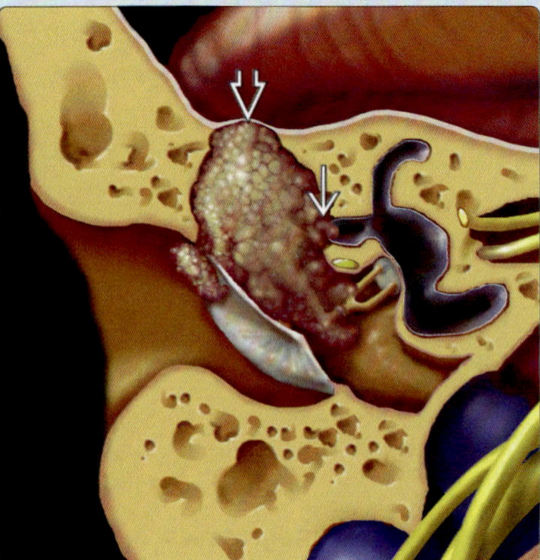

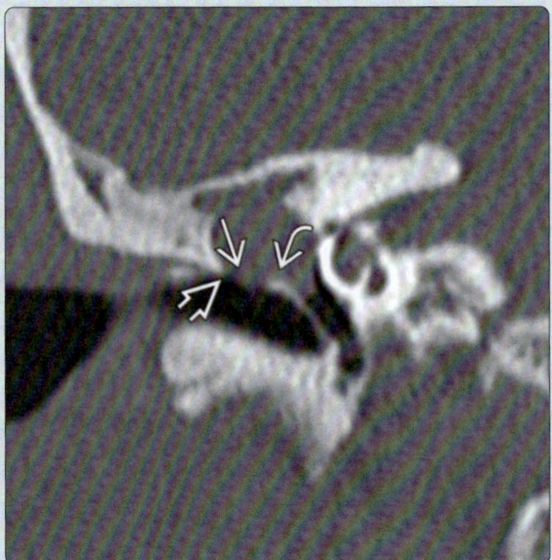

(Left) *Coronal bone CT in a 10-year-old patient with chronic right otitis media & otorrhea shows a large PFCh ➡ nearly filling the mesotympanum & epitympanum. The demineralized/partially eroded ossicles ➡ are deviated inferior & medial.* **(Right)** *Axial bone CT in the same patient demonstrates focal dehiscence of the right lateral SCC ➡ compared to the normal covering of the left lateral SCC ➡. Also note the underdevelopment of the right mastoid air cells relative to the left, a common finding in chronic inflammatory disease.*

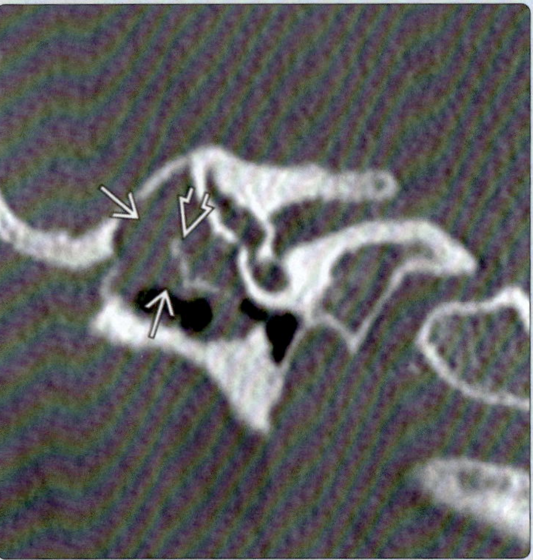

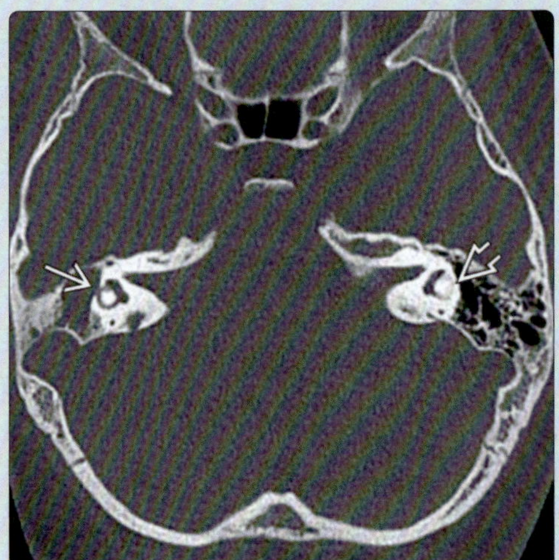

TERMINOLOGY

Definitions

- Secondary or acquired cholesteatoma (ACh): Stratified squamous epithelium-lined sac filled with exfoliated keratin debris in middle ear (ME)
  - Attic or Prussak space ACh = pars flaccida cholesteatoma (PFCh)
  - Pars tensa ACh (PTCh) lies in posterior mesotympanum, medial to ossicles
- Due to abnormal migration of ectoderm in external auditory canal (EAC) spontaneously or 2° to surgery/trauma

IMAGING

General Features

- Location
  - PFCh: 80% of all cholesteatomas
    - 2° to tympanic membrane (TM) perforation or retraction pocket in anterior superior pars flaccida portion of TM (also called Shrapnell membrane)
  - PTCh: 15% of all cholesteatomas
    - Secondary to TM perforation or retraction pocket in inferior pars tensa portion of TM

CT Findings

- Bone CT
  - PFCh: Soft tissue mass in Prussak space, lateral to malleus head; scutum erosion is characteristic
    - Ossicular erosion in 70%: Most commonly involves incus long process; less commonly involves incus body & malleus head
    - ± posterolateral extension to aditus ad antrum & mastoid antrum or inferiorly to posterior ME recesses
    - May also erode lateral semicircular canal, facial nerve canal, tegmen tympani, &/or sigmoid sinus plate
  - PTCh: Erosive mass in posterior mesotympanum medial to ossicles
    - ± sinus tympani, facial recess, aditus ad antrum, &/or mastoid involvement
    - Ossicular erosion is common (90%): Especially at medial aspect of incus long process, stapes suprastructure, & malleus manubrium
  - EACCh: Soft tissue mass with scalloping of EAC ± bone flecks

MR Findings

- ↓ T1, mildly ↑ T2 (< trapped secretions) ME mass
- PFCh & PTCh do not enhance; ± rim-enhancement of EACCh
- Associated granulation tissue or scar may enhance
- If tegmen tympani is dehiscent, coronal may show dural enhancement adjacent to bony defect
- ± cephalocele, intracranial extension or infection
- Restricted diffusion on DWI

Imaging Recommendations

- Noncontrast bone CT: Axial & coronal
- Coronal T1 C+ MR is useful adjunct when cephalocele, intracranial extension, or intracranial infection is suspected
- Nonecho planar DWI MR can help detect ACh amidst chronic inflammation

DIFFERENTIAL DIAGNOSIS

Chronic Otitis Media

- Soft tissue/fluid density may be indistinguishable from ACh on CT
- Erosions favor ACh but may be seen with chronic inflammation (especially at distal incus)

Congenital Cholesteatoma

- Well-defined ME mass behind intact TM, medial to ossicles
- Osseous erosion is similar to ACh if large
- Usually lacks history of recurrent infection or TM perforation

Acute Coalescent Otomastoiditis With Abscess

- Fever, periauricular erythema, pain, fluctuance
- Rim-enhancing fluid collection adjacent to opacified mastoid air cells = intracranial or extracranial abscess

Langerhans Cell Histiocytosis

- Enhancing mass + mastoid > petrous apex bone destruction

Rhabdomyosarcoma

- Soft tissue mass with variable contrast enhancement + petrous apex > mastoid permeative bone destruction

PATHOLOGY

General Features

- Etiology
  - TM retraction or perforation → accumulation of stratified squamous epithelial cells in ME → mass-like keratin ball

CLINICAL ISSUES

Presentation

- Most common signs/symptoms
  - Recurrent or chronic ME infections with TM perforation or retraction pocket
  - Conductive hearing loss (CHL)
  - ME mass with TM perforation on otoscopy

Demographics

- Unusual in children < 4 years of age

Treatment

- Surgical excision, mastoidectomy, & ossicular chain reconstruction if needed

DIAGNOSTIC CHECKLIST

Image Interpretation Pearls

- When ME & mastoid are opacified, difficult to differentiate effusion from ACh
- Presence of ossicular erosion favors ACh (but may rarely occur in noncholesteatomatous chronic otitis media)

SELECTED REFERENCES

1. Fischer N et al: MRI of middle ear cholesteatoma: the importance of observer reliance from diffusion sequences. J Neuroimaging. ePub, 2021
2. Campion T et al: Imaging of temporal bone inflammations in children: a pictorial review. Neuroradiology. 61(9):959-70, 2019
3. Shekdar KV et al: Imaging of pediatric hearing loss. Neuroimaging Clin N Am. 29(1):103-15, 2019

KEY FACTS

TERMINOLOGY

- Acute coalescent (or confluent) otomastoiditis (ACOM)
- Definition: Acute middle ear-mastoid infection with progressive bony resorption & demineralization due to intramastoid empyema

IMAGING

- Bone CT findings
  - Opacified mastoid cells
  - Erosion of mastoid cortex ± trabecula (confluent mastoiditis)
- Contrast-enhanced CT or MR findings
  - Subperiosteal abscess: Periauricular fluid collection
  - Bezold abscess: Walled-off pus in & around sternocleidomastoid muscle
  - Middle cranial fossa abscess (epidural or temporal lobe abscess)
  - Posterior fossa abscess (epidural or cerebellar abscess)
  - Dural sinus thrombosis: Adjacent venous filling defect

TOP DIFFERENTIAL DIAGNOSES

- Acquired cholesteatoma
- Apical petrositis
- Langerhans cell histiocytosis
- Rhabdomyosarcoma

PATHOLOGY

- Common pathophysiology
  - Granulation tissue or cholesteatoma blocks aditus ad antrum & prevents mastoid air cell drainage
- Less common pathophysiology
  - Mastoid cortex remains intact with septic thrombophlebitis of emissary veins seeding periosteum

CLINICAL ISSUES

- Young child with 1 day to 1 week history of otalgia, posterior auricular swelling, fever, & otorrhea
- Identify associated complications → appropriate treatment

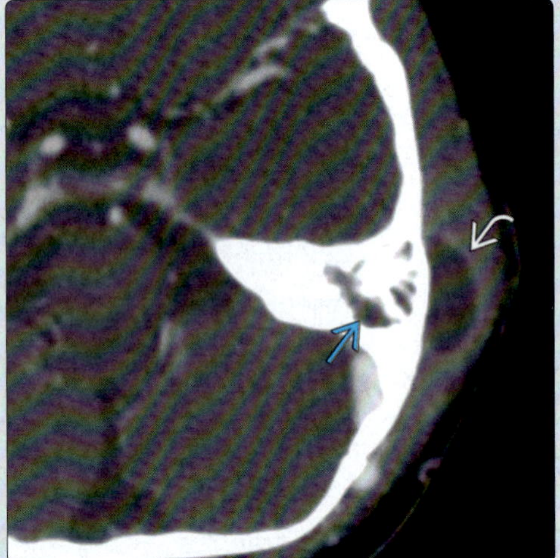

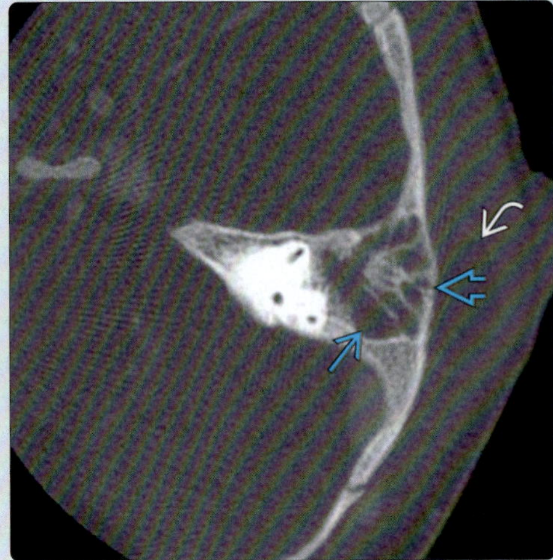

(Left) *Axial CECT in an 8-month-old girl shows a rim-enhancing fluid collection ➡ superficial to opacified left mastoid air cells ➡, consistent with a subperiosteal abscess. There is edema of the surrounding soft tissues.* **(Right)** *Axial bone CT in the same patient shows opacification of the mastoid air cells ➡ without septal destruction. Subtle bony dehiscence ➡ is suggested deep to the abscess ➡. However, bony destruction need not be present to establish a diagnosis of acute mastoiditis.*

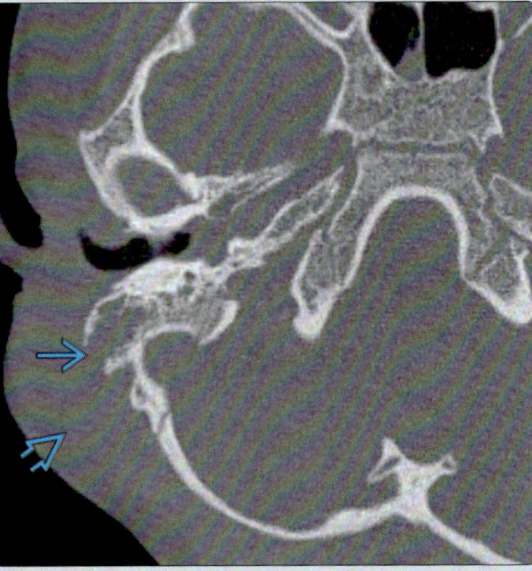

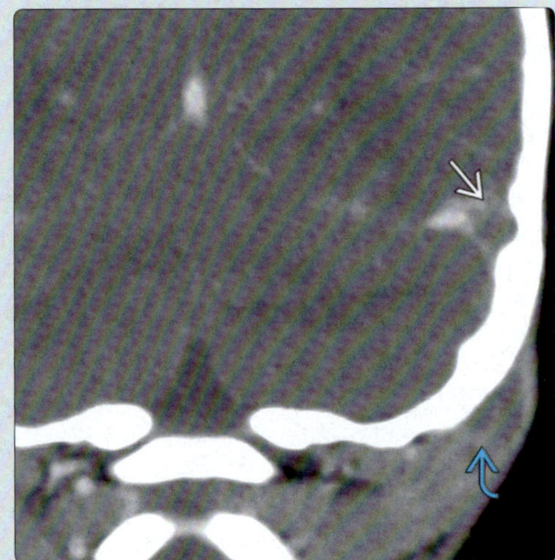

(Left) *Axial bone CT in a 3-year-old shows bony dehiscence ➡ of the posterolateral wall of the mastoid with overlying soft tissue swelling ➡. Acute otomastoiditis may be diagnosed with or without bony dehiscence. Overlying soft tissue inflammation is very common.* **(Right)** *Coronal CECT venogram in a 4-year-old shows an empty delta sign ➡ with lack of contrast opacification in the left transverse sinus secondary to acute otomastoiditis. Note the subperiosteal abscess ➡ inferior to the left mastoid.*

TERMINOLOGY

Synonyms

- Coalescent (or confluent) otomastoiditis with abscess

Definitions

- Acute mastoiditis (AM): Active infection in mastoid without destruction of mastoid septations or cortex
- Acute otitis media (AOM): Acute middle ear-mastoid infection with progressive bony resorption & demineralization due to intramastoid empyema
- Acute coalescent (or confluent) otomastoiditis (ACOM) + abscess: Coalescent mastoiditis with resultant intracranial or extracranial abscess

IMAGING

General Features

- Best diagnostic clue
  - Rim-enhancing fluid collection adjacent to opacified mastoid cells with eroded cortex
- Location
  - Abscess location depends on direction of mastoid cortical dehiscence
    - Lateral mastoid wall
      - Postauricular abscess (cortical bone is thin here)
      - Pre- or periauricular abscess
    - Inferior mastoid wall
      - Mastoid tip → Bezold abscess
      - Other inferior mastoid cortical dehiscence → transspatial abscess
    - Tegmen mastoideum → temporal lobe abscess
    - Medial mastoid wall → epidural or cerebellar abscess

CT Findings

- CECT
  - Subperiosteal abscess
    - Periauricular fluid collection
      - Thick, enhancing lateral wall represents inflamed periosteum
  - Bezold abscess
    - Walled-off pus in & around sternocleidomastoid muscle
  - Middle cranial fossa abscess (epidural or temporal lobe abscess)
    - Epidural or intratemporal lobe rim-enhancing fluid
  - Posterior fossa abscess (epidural or cerebellar abscess)
    - Epidural or intracerebellar rim-enhancing fluid
  - Dural sinus thrombosis (DST)
    - Filling defect within venous sinus
- Bone CT
  - Middle ear & mastoid opacification
  - Variable trabecular & cortical erosions (confluent disease)
  - Subtle to obvious cortical dehiscence deep to abscess
    - Lateral mastoid cortex → subperiosteal abscess
    - Mastoid tip cortex → Bezold abscess
    - Tegmen mastoideum cortex → epidural or temporal lobe abscess
    - Medial mastoid cortex → epidural or cerebellar abscess

MR Findings

- T2WI
  - High signal fills middle ear & mastoid
    - Complete opacification is more common in children (90%)
  - High signal fluid in epidural or parenchymal abscess
- DWI
  - Restricted diffusion in abscess
- T1WI C+
  - Variable enhancement of middle ear & mastoid
    - More common in children (90%)
  - Perimastoid dural enhancement
    - More common in children (80%)
  - Rim-enhancing pus in subperiosteal, epidural, or brain parenchymal abscess
    - Subperiosteal abscess is more common in children (50%)
  - 3D volumetric gradient-echo T1 C+ imaging allows optimal detection of venous sinus thrombosis
- MRV
  - May show DST
    - Focus of diminished or absent vascular signal on flow-sensitive sequences

Imaging Recommendations

- Best imaging tool
  - Temporal bone CT defines bony changes (confluence, cortical dehiscence)
    - CECT will define most infectious complications
  - Enhanced temporal bone MR is more sensitive for intracranial complications (DST, meningitis, subdural empyema, abscess)
- Protocol advice
  - Thin-section SE T1 MR with FS gives best evaluation of bone
  - 3D gradient-echo T1 C+ allows optimal delineation of epidural abscess & venous sinus thrombosis
  - Non-EPI DWI techniques ↓ susceptibility artifact from bone & air in skull base

DIFFERENTIAL DIAGNOSIS

Acquired Cholesteatoma

- Clinical: Retraction or rupture of tympanic membrane; may be superinfected
- Imaging: CT shows erosive mass with poor enhancement
- May lead to ACOM & associated complications
- Important to identify underlying cholesteatoma as it may alter surgical management strategy

Apical Petrositis

- Clinical: CNIV palsy, retroauricular pain, AOM
- Imaging: CT shows coalescent changes in petrous apex
  - T1 C+ MR shows enhancing meninges & focal, walled-off fluid in petrous apex
- Usually no associated intracranial abscess

Langerhans Cell Histiocytosis

- Clinical: Child with draining ear & periauricular mass
- Imaging: Extensive, often bilateral, mastoid destruction with homogeneously enhancing soft tissue

- Look for additional lesions (e.g., punched-out, well-defined lytic calvarial lesions)

Rhabdomyosarcoma

- Clinical: Neurologic deficits common, including CNVII palsy
- Imaging: CT shows extensive bone lysis & permeation, intracranial extension
  - T1 C+ MR shows variably enhancing soft tissue mass emanating from middle ear

PATHOLOGY

General Features

- Etiology
  - Inflammation, granulation tissue, or cholesteatoma block aditus ad antrum & prevent mastoid air cell drainage
  - Local hyperemia-acidosis creates enzymatic resorption of trabeculae (confluent mastoiditis)
  - Subtle or obvious cortical dehiscence conveys infection into adjacent tissues
  - Less common pathophysiology: Mastoid cortex remains intact with septic thrombophlebitis of emissary veins seeding periosteum
- Macewen triangle
  - Surgical access point to mastoid antrum at posterosuperior EAC
  - Weak bone, loose periosteum allow breakout of infection in postauricular location

Gross Pathologic & Surgical Features

- Pus in mastoid, adjacent abscess cavity
- Granulation tissue or cholesteatoma is occasionally identified in middle ear-mastoid

Microscopic Features

- *Streptococcus* species is most common
- Polymicrobial aerobes & anaerobes are less common

CLINICAL ISSUES

Presentation

- Most common signs/symptoms
  - Otalgia (ear pain)
  - Other signs/symptoms
    - Fever
    - Otorrhea (ear drainage)
    - Postauricular pain & swelling
    - Lateralized auricle (ear pushed outward by abscess)
    - Conductive > sensorineural hearing loss
    - ↑ WBC, ↑ ESR
- Clinical profile
  - Young child with 1 day to 1 week history of otalgia, postauricular swelling, fever, & otorrhea
  - 35-70% of patients have received antibiotics for AOM
  - Postauricular edema (Griesinger sign) is common in uncomplicated acute mastoiditis (85%)
    - Enhancing fluid collection confirms subperiosteal abscess

Demographics

- Age
  - Infants & young children
  - Older age group is typical when ACOM results from acquired cholesteatoma
- Epidemiology
  - 46% of children have > 2 episodes of AOM by age 3
  - 0.24% of patients with AOM develop ACOM

Natural History & Prognosis

- Isolated extracranial subperiosteal abscess
  - Excellent prognosis with prompt therapy
  - Worse if prior incomplete antibiotic therapy, virulent organism, or immunocompromised host
- Intracranial abscess (temporal lobe is most common)
  - Worse prognosis, particularly with concomitant complications
    - Venous sinus thrombosis
    - Epidural abscess or subdural empyema

Treatment

- Intravenous antibiotics ± tympanocentesis with myringotomy tube placement
- Surgical treatment
  - I&D of extracranial subperiosteal abscess
  - Simple mastoidectomy is typically reserved for patients that fail initial conservative management
  - Radical mastoidectomy if cholesteatoma is present

DIAGNOSTIC CHECKLIST

Consider

- Look for other complications of ACOM
  - Temporal bone findings (T1 C+ MR)
    - Facial nerve paralysis: Enhancing CNVII
    - Labyrinthitis: Enhancement within membranous labyrinth
    - Apical petrositis: Enhancing apical air cells on MR
  - Intracranial findings (T1 C+ MR)
    - Epidural or brain abscess
    - Subdural empyema, meningitis ± DST

SELECTED REFERENCES

1. Cassano P et al: Acute mastoiditis in children. Acta Biomed. 91(1-S):54-59, 2020
2. Stern Shavit S et al: Surgical intervention for acute mastoiditis: 10 years experience in a tertiary children hospital. Eur Arch Otorhinolaryngol. 276(11):3051-6, 2019
3. Marom T et al: Acute mastoiditis in children: necessity and timing of imaging. Pediatr Infect Dis J. 35(1):30-4, 2016
4. Saat R et al: MR Imaging features of acute mastoiditis and their clinical relevance. AJNR Am J Neuroradiol. 36(2):361-7, 2015
5. Chesney J et al: What is the best practice for acute mastoiditis in children? Laryngoscope. 124(5):1057-8, 2014
6. Minks DP et al: Acute mastoiditis–the role of radiology. Clin Radiol. 68(4):397-405, 2013
7. Chien JH et al: Mastoiditis diagnosed by clinical symptoms and imaging studies in children: disease spectrum and evolving diagnostic challenges. J Microbiol Immunol Infect. 45(5):377-81, 2012
8. Luntz M et al: Acute mastoiditis: the role of imaging for identifying intracranial complications. Laryngoscope. 122(12):2813-7, 2012
9. Tamir S et al: Shifting trends: mastoiditis from a surgical to a medical disease. Am J Otolaryngol. 31(6):467-71, 2010
10. Zevallos JP et al: Advanced pediatric mastoiditis with and without intracranial complications. Laryngoscope. 119(8):1610-5, 2009

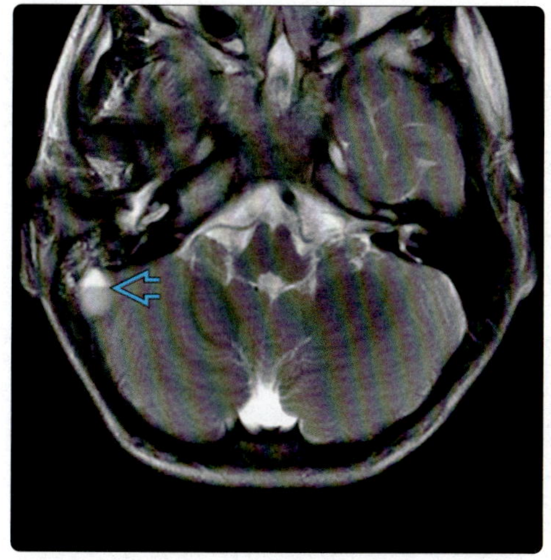

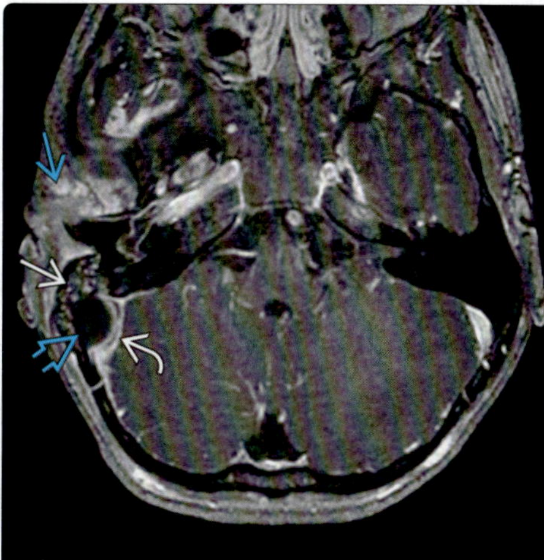

(Left) *Axial T2 MR in a 7-year-old boy with acute mastoiditis shows an epidural abscess in the right jugular fossa. Note the internal fluid-fluid level ⇨, which is most frequently due to blood products.* **(Right)** *Axial T1 C+ FS 3D SPGR MR in the same patient shows enhancement of the right mastoid air cells ➡ with right periauricular soft tissue swelling ⇨. There is an epidural abscess ⇨ in the right sigmoid fossa. The dura is medially displaced with narrowing & thrombosis of the right sigmoid sinus ➡.*

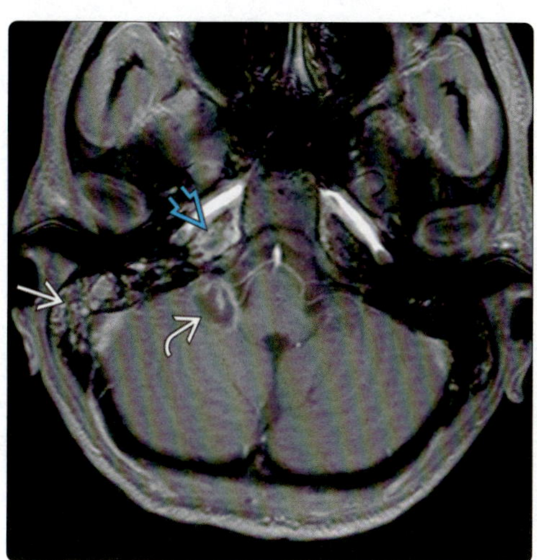

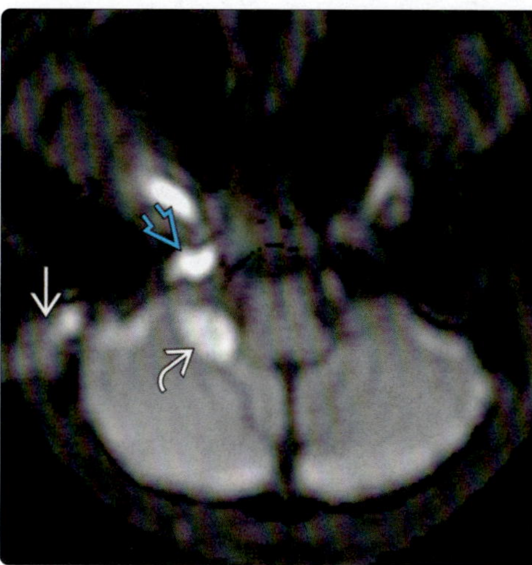

(Left) *Axial T1 C+ FS MR in a 14-year-old boy with right acute otomastoiditis & petrous apicitis shows extensive mastoid ➡ & petrous apex ⇨ enhancement with an intraparenchymal abscess involving the right cerebellar flocculus ➡.* **(Right)** *Axial DWI MR in the same patient demonstrates restricted diffusion in the right mastoid ➡ & petrous apex ⇨ as well as the right flocculus intraparenchymal abscess ➡. DWI can be a helpful sequence in determining the full extent of purulent material in acute otomastoiditis.*

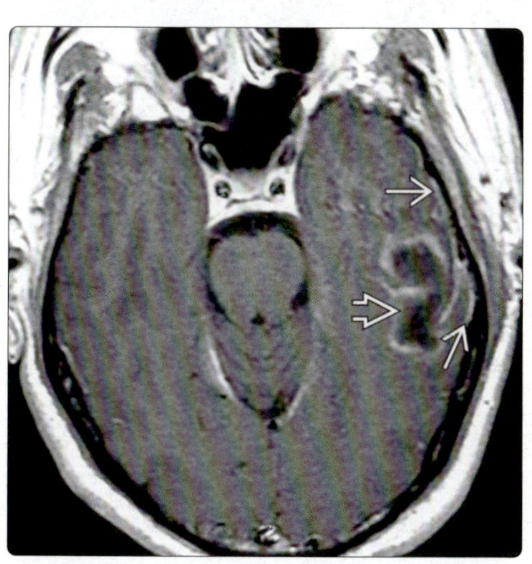

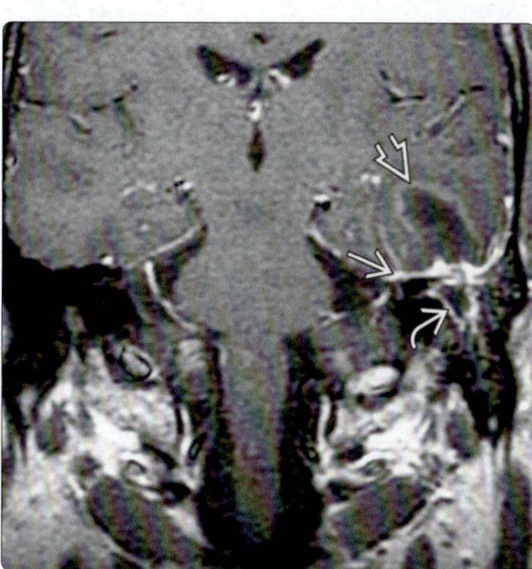

(Left) *Axial T1 C+ FS MR in an adult with ↓ consciousness & fever demonstrates a bilobed, rim-enhancing temporal lobe abscess ➡ along with meningeal enhancement ➡, consistent with meningitis.* **(Right)** *Coronal T1 C+ MR in the same patient reveals the source of infection to be acute otomastoiditis with extension of infection from the mastoid ➡ to the temporal lobe ➡ across the tegmen tympani. Associated meningitis ➡ is again noted.*

CHARGE Syndrome

KEY FACTS

TERMINOLOGY

- CHARGE
  - **C**oloboma
  - **H**eart anomaly
  - **A**tresia of choanae
  - **R**estriction: Mental & somatic development
  - **G**enital hypoplasia
  - **E**ar abnormalities
- Major signs: Coloboma, choanal atresia, semicircular canal (SCC) hypoplasia/aplasia, cranial nerve (CN) involvement
- Minor signs: Hindbrain, external/middle ear, cardiac/esophageal malformations, hypothalamo-hypophyseal dysfunction, intellectual disability

IMAGING

- Choanal atresia, coloboma (variable), cleft lip/palate
- Hypoplastic vestibule & hypoplastic/absent SCC
- Mildly flattened apical ± middle turns + thickened modiolus or single cochlear turn/hypoplasia
- Stenotic/atretic cochlear nerve canal
- Stenotic/atretic oval window ± overlying anomalous tympanic segment of CNVII
- Large emissary veins, hypoplasia of basiocciput, basilar invagination, & vertebral anomalies
- Hypoplastic pons, uplifted vermis ± cerebellar malformation
- CN hypoplasia/aplasia (mainly CNI, CNVII, & CNVIII)

TOP DIFFERENTIAL DIAGNOSES

- VACTERL association
- Kallmann syndrome
- Branchiootorenal syndrome

PATHOLOGY

- *CHD7* mutation in 60-90%
- Highly predictive of CHARGE: Cup-shaped pinna, agenesis/hypoplasia of SCC, arrhinencephaly

(Left) *Axial T2 MR in a 3-year-old girl with multiple congenital anomalies & a CHD7 gene mutation reveals bilateral colobomas near the optic nerve insertions onto the globes ➔.* **(Right)** *Axial bone CT in the same child shows right-sided, predominantly osseous choanal atresia ➔ with a fluid level within the nasal cavity ➔. This combination of findings should raise the question of CHARGE syndrome & alert the imager to closely assess the temporal bones & skull base for additional abnormalities.*

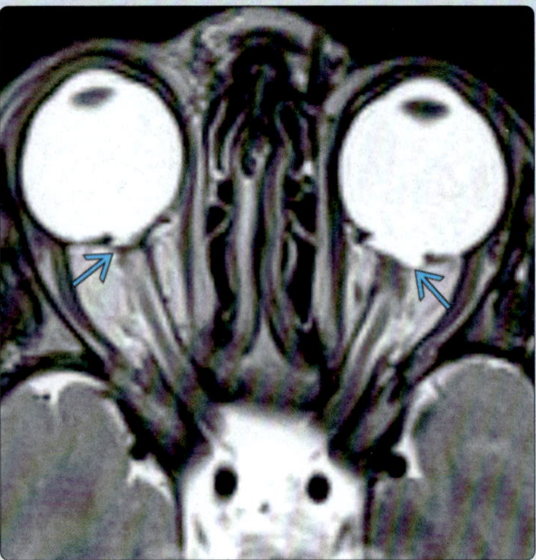

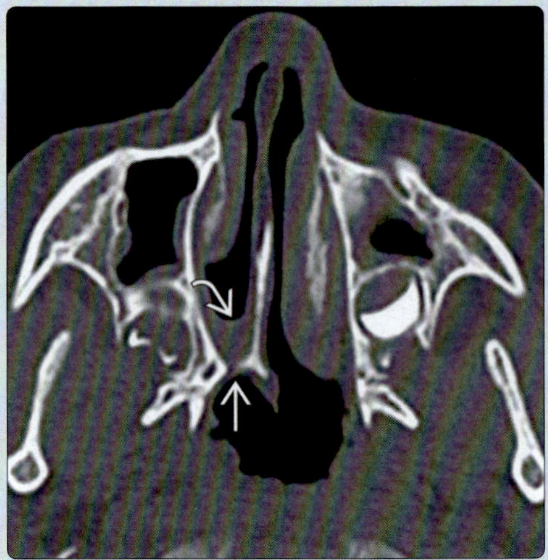

(Left) *Axial bone CT in the same child with CHARGE syndrome reveals a hypoplastic vestibule ➔ with absence of the semicircular canals (SCCs). The cochlea is hypoplastic with prominence of the modiolus ➔ & narrowing of the cochlear nerve canal ➔, suggesting cochlear nerve deficiency. Dysmorphic ossicles are partially visualized ➔.* **(Right)** *Coronal T2 MR in the same child shows absent left ➔ & diminutive right ➔ olfactory bulbs.*

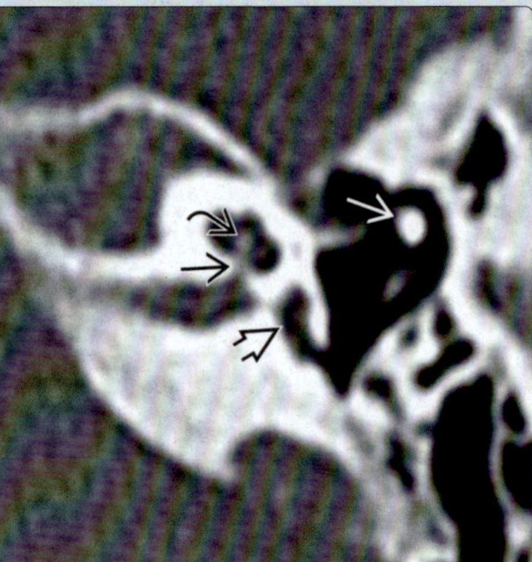

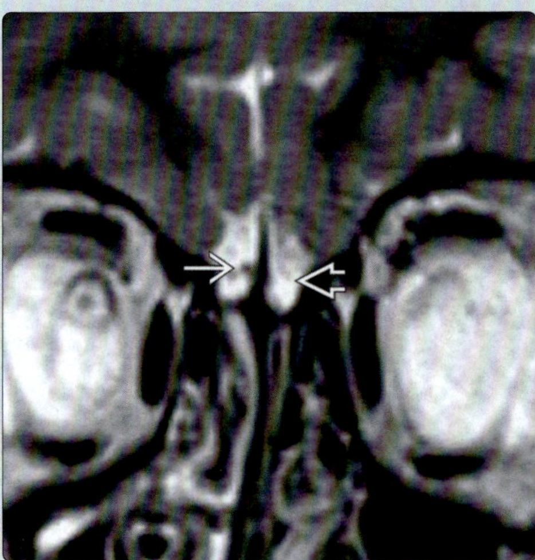

KEY FACTS

TERMINOLOGY

- Branchiootorenal syndrome (BOR): Autosomal dominant
  - Deafness & ear anomalies
  - Branchial anomalies/preauricular pits
  - Renal abnormalities

IMAGING

- Neck: Branchial cleft cyst/fistula
- Temporal bone CT findings
  - Dilated eustachian tubes
  - External ear: Variable stenosis/atresia
  - Middle ear: Dysmorphic; fused, malformed ossicles
  - Cochlea: Tapered basal turn, hypoplastic & offset middle/apical turns
  - Semicircular canal anomalies
  - Dilated, bulbous vestibular aqueduct
  - Flared internal auditory canal; anomalous CNVII canal
- Abdominal ultrasound/CT/MR findings: Renal cysts, dysplasia, agenesis
- Variable, asymmetric micrognathia

TOP DIFFERENTIAL DIAGNOSES

- Branchiootic syndrome
  - Normal kidneys; BOR genetic overlap
- Otofaciocervical syndrome: BOR genetic overlap
- Congenital nonsyndromic external ear & middle ear malformation

PATHOLOGY

- BOR 1: 8q13.3 locus, *EYA1* gene mutation
- BOR 2: 19q13.3 locus, *SIX5* mutation

CLINICAL ISSUES

- Clinical presentation
  - Hearing loss (sensorineural, conductive, or mixed): ~ 98%
  - Preauricular tag, pit: ~ 84%
  - Branchial anomalies: ~ 70%
  - Renal anomalies: ~ 40%

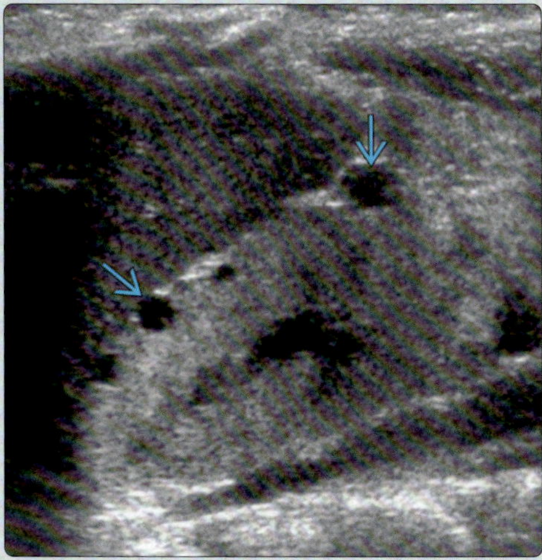

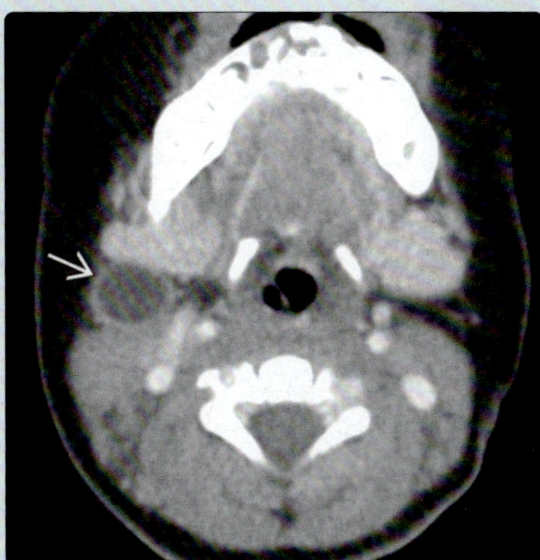

(Left) *Longitudinal ultrasound in a 4-month-old boy presenting with Potter syndrome shows a solitary, echogenic left kidney with numerous peripheral cysts ➡. This patient with branchiootorenal syndrome (BOR) also had a branchial cleft cyst & microtia.* **(Right)** *Axial CECT in a 5-month-old boy with preauricular pits & a family history of renal & ear anomalies shows a hypodense, rim-enhancing, cystic lesion ➡, consistent with a 2nd branchial cleft cyst. The patient also had ear anomalies characteristic of BOR.*

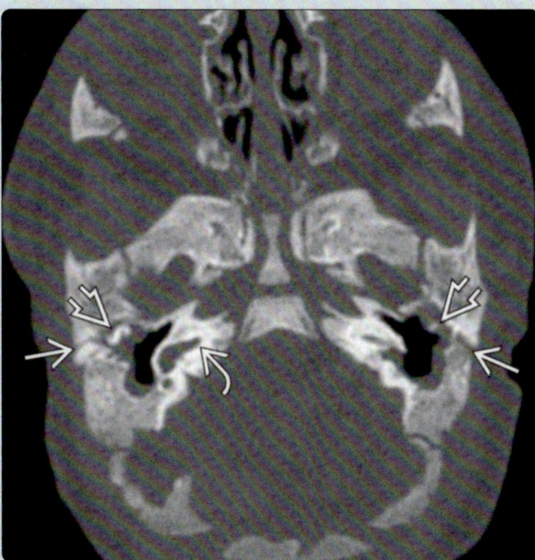

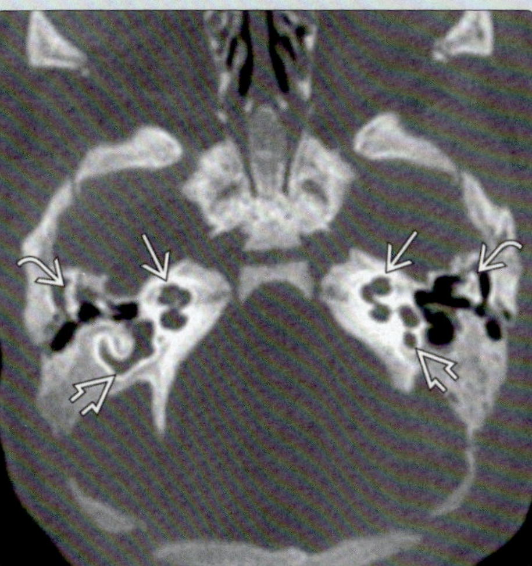

(Left) *Axial bone CT in the same patient imaged at 10 days of age (to evaluate microtia) shows bilateral external auditory canal (EAC) atresia ➡. The ossicles are malformed, fused, & laterally located ➡. Note the tapered basal turn of the right cochlea ➡.* **(Right)** *Axial bone CT in the same patient shows unwound or offset hypoplastic middle & apical cochlear turns ➡ & deficiency of the right cochlear modiolus. The posterior semicircular canals (SCCs) ➡ & ossicles ➡ are malformed. The CT findings are characteristic of BOR.*

Treacher Collins Syndrome

KEY FACTS

TERMINOLOGY

- Treacher Collins syndrome (TCS)
- Nager syndrome: TCS + limb anomalies
- Craniofacial malformation: Downslanting palpebral fissures, micrognathia, zygomatic & malar hypoplasia, microtia/anotia, ± limb defects

IMAGING

- Temporal bone findings
  - EAC: Stenosis/atresia, small/absent tympanic plate
  - ↓/absent mastoid pneumatization
  - Hypoplastic/atretic middle ear space
  - Malformed or absent ossicles ± fixation
  - Oval window stenosis/atresia
  - Facial nerve canal anomalies/dehiscence
  - Normal or malformed cochlea (flattened turns)
  - Normal or malformed lateral SCC ± vestibule
- Relatively symmetric micrognathia, zygomatic/malar hypoplasia
- Coloboma, hypoplastic muscles of mastication, absent or hypoplastic parotid glands

TOP DIFFERENTIAL DIAGNOSES

- Bilateral facial microsomia
- Nonsyndromic congenital external & middle ear malformation
- Branchiootorenal syndrome

PATHOLOGY

- Autosomal dominant > > recessive, phenotypic variability & genetic heterogeneity, "ribosomopathy"
- TCS: *TCOF1*, *POLR1D*, & *POLR1C* gene mutations
- Nager syndrome: *SF3B4* gene mutation

CLINICAL ISSUES

- Airway obstruction, deafness
- Treatment: Airway support, reconstructive surgery, hearing aids, developmental support

(Left) *Lateral 3D soft tissue surface-rendered CT in an infant with Nager syndrome shows micrognathia, malar flattening, mildly low-set ears, & external auditory meatus atresia.* **(Right)** *Lateral 3D bone CT in the same infant with Nager syndrome shows micrognathia with an obtuse mandibular angle & marked hypoplasia of the neck & condyle of the mandible. There is hypoplasia of the midface & zygomatic complex with absence of the zygomatic arch. There is also EAC atresia.*

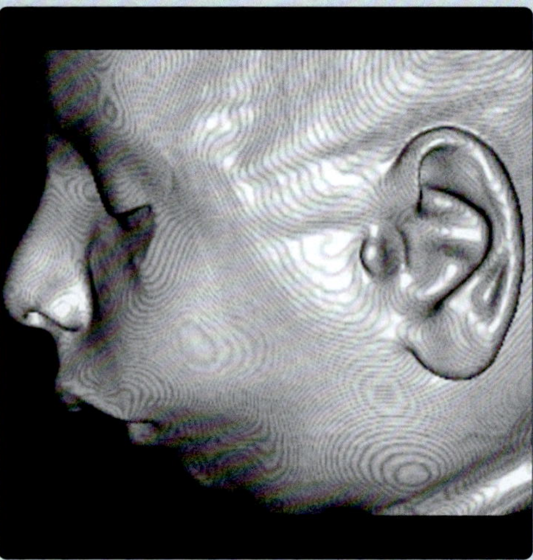

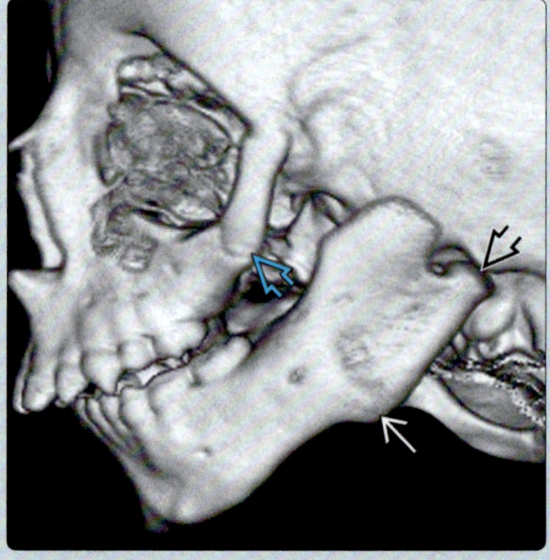

(Left) *Axial bone CT in a 13-year-old girl with Treacher Collins syndrome (TCS) shows zygomatic complex hypoplasia with posteriorly slanted maxillae, absent zygomatic arches, & hypoplastic mandibular condyles. Note the EAC atresia, absent mastoid pneumatization, & an enlarged mastoid emissary vein.* **(Right)** *Axial soft tissue NECT in a 1-year-old with TCS shows bilateral mandibular hypoplasia, EAC atresia, microtia with hypoplastic muscles of mastication, & aplasia of the parotid glands.*

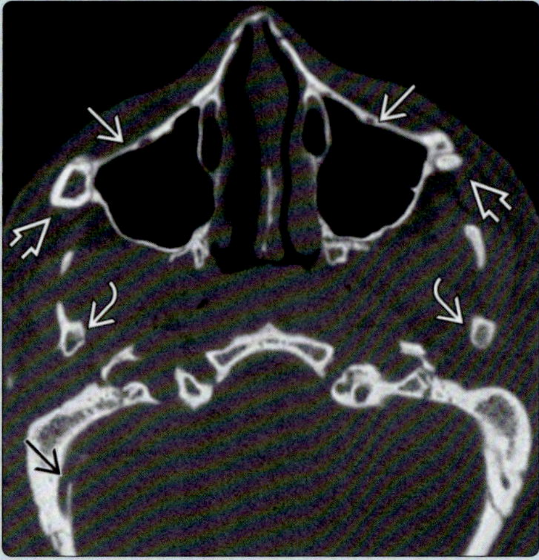

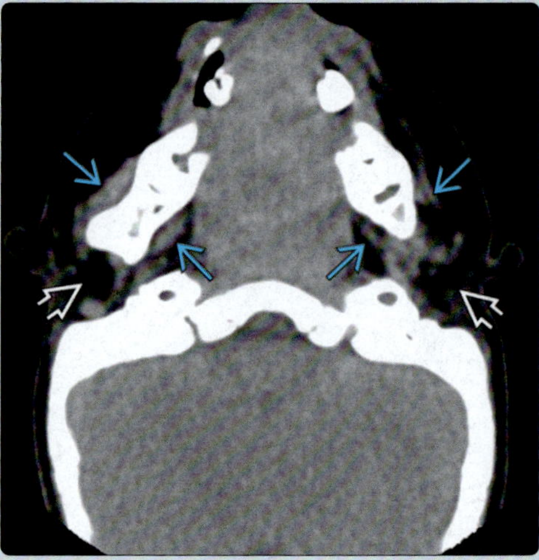

KEY FACTS

TERMINOLOGY

- Pierre Robin sequence (PRS) triad: Micrognathia, glossoptosis, airway obstruction

IMAGING

- Micrognathia: Bilateral, usually symmetric
- Glossoptosis: Elevated, posteriorly displaced tongue
- Posterior, U-shaped cleft palate
- Additional features depend on syndromic etiology
- Temporal bone
  - EAC: Normal, stenotic (e.g., Stickler syndrome), or atretic [e.g., Treacher Collins syndrome (TCS), Nager syndrome]
  - Middle ear & mastoid: Normal or hypoplastic ± opacification
  - Ossicles: Normal, mildly malformed [e.g., stapes in velocardiofacial syndrome (VCFS)], or severely malformed ± fixation (e.g., TCS)
  - Inner ear: Normal or malformed (e.g., small semicircular canal bone island/anlage anomaly in VCFS & TCS)

TOP DIFFERENTIAL DIAGNOSES

- Stickler & related syndromes (18% of PRS)
- VCFS (~ 7% of PRS)
- TCS (~ 5% of PRS)

PATHOLOGY

- Primary micrognathia → glossoptosis → failure of palatal shelf elevation & fusion
- Collagen (*COL*) gene mutations: Stickler syndrome
- 22q11.2 deletion: VCFS

CLINICAL ISSUES

- Feeding & breathing difficulties, failure to thrive
- Stickler: Progressive myopia, joint degeneration
- VCFS: Cardiac anomalies, adenoidal hypoplasia, velopharyngeal insufficiency, medial deviation of cervical internal carotid arteries, learning difficulties
- TCS: Malar flattening, downslanting palpebral fissures, coloboma

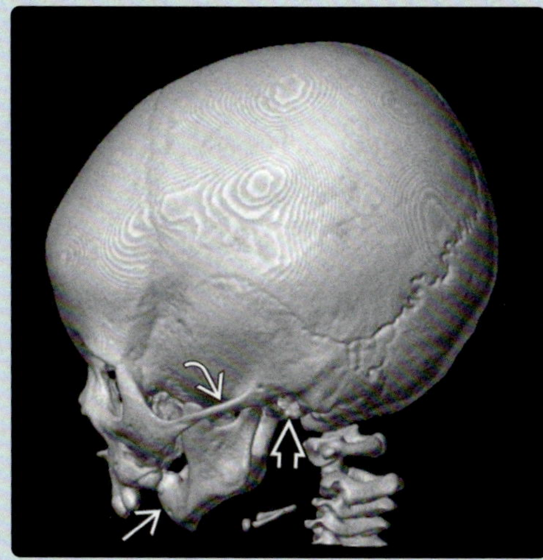

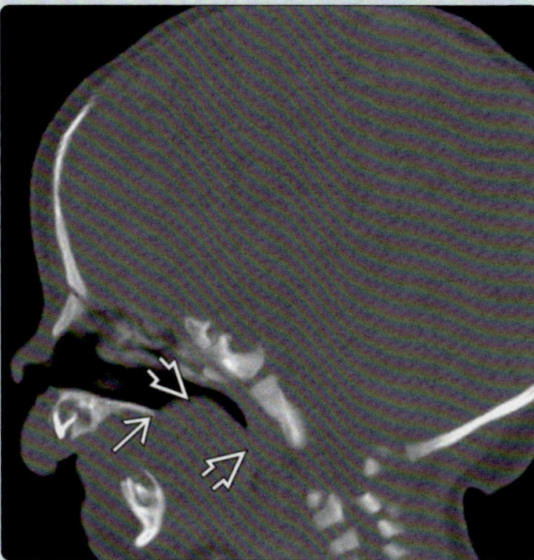

(Left) *Lateral 3D surface-rendered CT in a 1-year-old with Pierre Robin sequence (PRS) shows significant symmetric micrognathia ➡ with a normal external auditory canal ➡ & zygomatic arch ➡.* **(Right)** *Sagittal bone CT reconstruction in a 3-week-old with PRS reveals a shortened hard palate ➡ & glossoptosis (abnormal downward or backward displacement of tongue) ➡. The tongue, which protrudes above & behind the palate, obstructs the oropharynx, resulting in difficulty with breathing & feeding.*

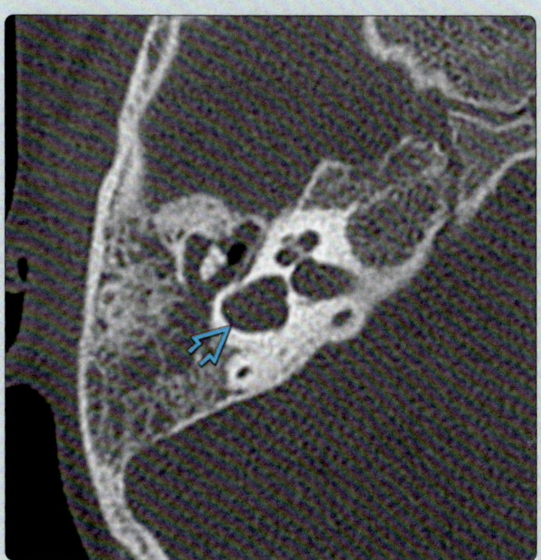

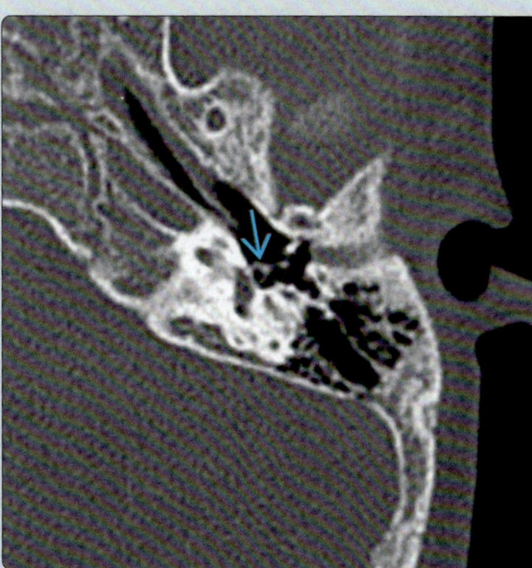

(Left) *Axial bone CT in a 5-year-old with velocardiofacial syndrome (VCFS) shows an anlage anomaly where the lateral semicircular canal (SCC) & vestibule form a single globular space without a bone island ➡. There is diffuse opacification of the middle ear space & mastoid air cells.* **(Right)** *Axial bone CT in a 7-year-old with VCFS & hearing loss shows mild thickening of anterior crus of the stapes ➡ & mildly reduced mastoid pneumatization. A more cephalad image (not shown) demonstrated a slightly small lateral SCC bone island.*

Thyroglossal Duct Cyst

KEY FACTS

TERMINOLOGY

- Thyroglossal duct cyst (TGDC): Cystic remnant of embryologic thyroglossal duct (TGD)

IMAGING

- Best diagnostic clue: Round or ovoid midline suprahyoid or midline/paramidline infrahyoid cystic neck mass
- Suprahyoid neck: ~ 20-25%, typically midline
- At hyoid bone: ~ 50%
- Infrahyoid neck: ~ 25%, midline or paramidline
  - Embedded in strap muscles: Claw sign
- ± wall enhancement, soft tissue stranding if infected

TOP DIFFERENTIAL DIAGNOSES

- Dermoid or epidermoid
- Lingual thyroid
- Lymphatic malformation
- 4th branchial apparatus anomaly
- Cervical thymic cyst

PATHOLOGY

- Failure of involution of TGD + persistent secretion of epithelial cells lining duct → TGDC
- Lies anywhere along TGD route of thyroid anlage descent from foramen cecum at tongue base to thyroid bed in infrahyoid neck

CLINICAL ISSUES

- Most common congenital neck lesion
- Treatment: Sistrunk procedure (excision of cyst, tract, & midline hyoid bone) → ↓ recurrences

DIAGNOSTIC CHECKLIST

- Relationship to hyoid bone important to note: Suprahyoid, hyoid, or infrahyoid in location
- Nodularity or Ca^{2+} can suggest associated thyroid carcinoma
- Confirm normal thyroid by ultrasound prior to TGDC or lingual thyroid resection

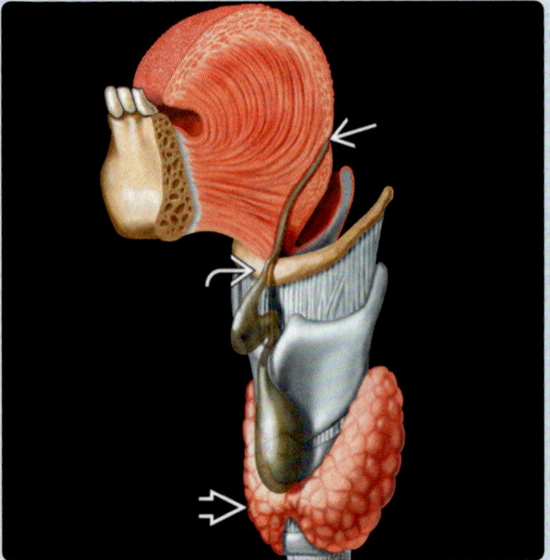

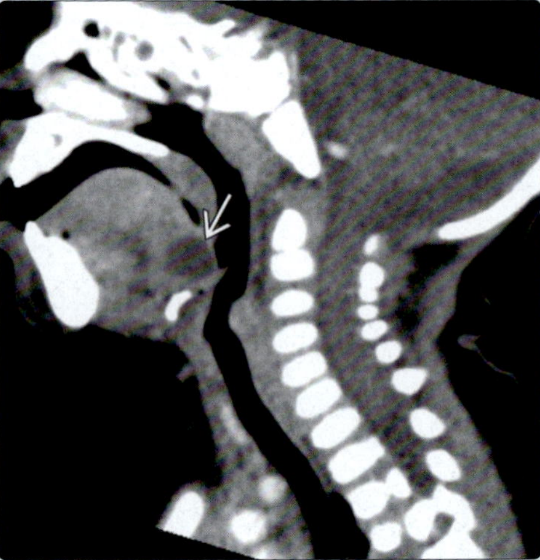

(Left) *Sagittal oblique graphic shows the potential sites of a thyroglossal duct cyst (TGDC) from the foramen cecum ➡ to the thyroid bed ⇨. Note the close relationship of the midportion of the hyoid bone ↪ to this pathway. A cyst can occur anywhere along this tract.* **(Right)** *Sagittal CECT in a young child shows a well-defined, cystic-appearing mass ➡ at the midline base of the tongue. This mass was incidentally found on a CT performed to evaluate the extent of a deep neck infection (not shown). A TGDC was proven upon resection.*

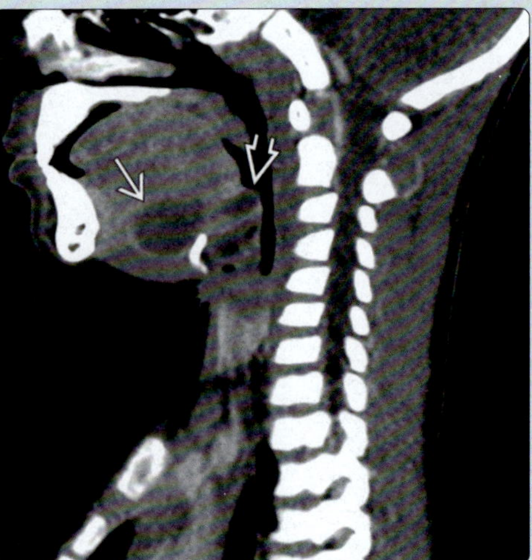

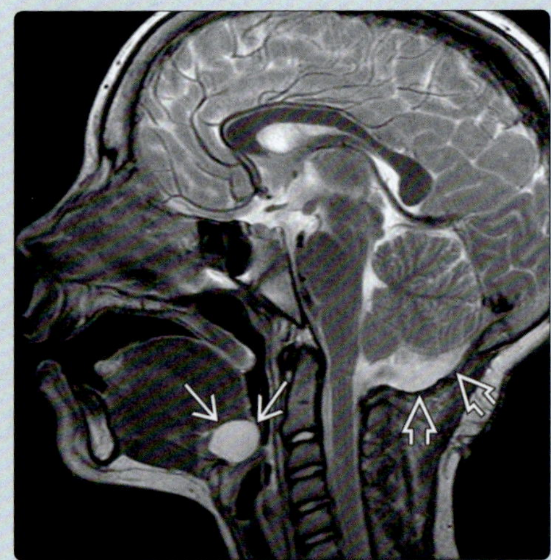

(Left) *Sagittal CECT in a child with sore throat & difficulty swallowing shows a lobulated, rim-enhancing, fluid-attenuation mass ➡ in the midline sublingual space with a small, posterior extension at the tongue base ⇨. Histologically, this proved to be an inflamed TGDC.* **(Right)** *Sagittal T2 MR incidentally shows a well-defined, hyperintense TGDC ➡ in the midline base of the tongue (at the level of the foramen cecum) in a patient imaged after posterior fossa decompression ⇨ for treatment of Chiari 1.*

TERMINOLOGY

Synonyms

- Thyroglossal duct cyst (TGDC)
- Thyroglossal duct (TGD) remnant

Definitions

- Remnant of embryologic TGD found between foramen cecum at tongue base & thyroid bed in infrahyoid neck

IMAGING

General Features

- Best diagnostic clue
  - Anterior midline suprahyoid or midline/paramidline infrahyoid cystic neck mass
- Location
  - Suprahyoid neck: ~ 20-25%, typically midline
    - Base of tongue or within posterior floor of mouth
  - At hyoid bone: ~ 50%
    - Usually abutting anterior hyoid bone
    - May project into preepiglottic space
  - Infrahyoid neck: ~ 25%, midline or paramidline, embedded in strap muscles
    - Further inferior TGDC is more likely to be off midline
- Size
  - Variable, usually 2-4 cm
- Morphology
  - Round or ovoid cyst
  - More likely to be irregular in shape, elongated toward tongue base, & have ill-defined margins vs. dermoid

Ultrasonographic Findings

- Anechoic or hypoechoic midline neck mass
- Internal heterogeneity, septations, & solid components are more likely in TGDC than dermoid
  - SIST score (favors TGDC over dermoid): Septations + irregular walls + solid components = TGDC
- Synchronous movement with hyoid bone
- Elongation toward tongue base
- Must image lower neck to prove presence of normal-appearing bilobed thyroid

CT Findings

- CECT
  - Low-attenuation, cystic midline neck mass with thin rim of peripheral enhancement
    - ± wall enhancement, soft tissue stranding if infected
    - Occasional septations
  - Paramidline infrahyoid TGDC embedded in strap muscles may show claw sign
  - < 1% contain associated thyroid carcinoma (usually papillary carcinoma)
    - Solid eccentric mass, often with Ca^{2+}, within cyst
    - May only be microscopic & not identifiable prospectively with imaging
    - Majority occur in adults but may occur in teenagers
      - Youngest reported: 10 years old

MR Findings

- T1WI
  - Usually hypointense; hyperintense if proteinaceous fluid
- T2WI
  - Hyperintense, often homogeneous
- DWI
  - Mean ADC values of ~ 2.2×10^{-3} mm^2/s
- T1WI C+
  - Nonenhancing cyst
    - Rim enhancement if infected

Imaging Recommendations

- Ultrasound can suggest TGDC vs. other lesions & confirm normal thyroid
- Nuclear scintigraphy is helpful if ectopic thyroid is suspected

DIFFERENTIAL DIAGNOSIS

Dermoid or Epidermoid

- Dermoid: Fat, fluid, or mixed
  - ADC ~ 1.54×10^{-3} mm^2/s
- Epidermoid: Fluid
- More likely to be in subcutaneous fat
- Floor of mouth & suprasternal notch are classic locations

Lingual Thyroid

- Most common location of ectopic thyroid
- In 75% of patients, lingual thyroid is only functioning thyroid tissue
- May expand rapidly during puberty
- Solid, round, hyperattenuating mass in base of tongue on NECT; avid enhancement on CECT
- Variable T1 & T2 signal, variable contrast enhancement on MR

Lymphatic Malformation

- Classic appearance: Multilocular & transspatial
- Microcystic or macrocystic
- Fluid-fluid levels are common secondary to hemorrhage
- Thin rim & septal enhancement unless infected, microcystic, or part of combined venolymphatic malformation

4th Branchial Apparatus Anomaly

- May present with recurrent thyroiditis
- Majority are sinus tracts from apex of left pyriform sinus to lower neck → abscess in or adjacent to left thyroid lobe
- May be 4th (or 3rd) pharyngeal pouch remnant

Cervical Thymic Cyst

- Congenital cyst, anywhere along thymopharyngeal duct from pyriform sinus to anterior mediastinum
  - May be bilobed with waist at thoracic inlet
- L > R
- Close association with carotid sheath
  - May splay carotid artery & jugular vein, particularly near skull base
- May be combined solid thymic tissue & cyst

Mixed Laryngocele

- Off-midline, fluid- or air- & fluid-containing mass
- Traces back to laryngeal origin
- Not embedded within strap muscles

Delphian Chain Necrotic Node

- Can be difficult to differentiate from infected TGDC

- Rare in children

PATHOLOGY

General Features

- Genetics
  - Thyroid developmental anomalies often occur in same family
- Associated abnormalities
  - Thyroid agenesis, ectopia, or pyramidal lobe
  - Occasionally associated with carcinoma
    - Most common: Papillary carcinoma within TGDC
- Embryology/anatomy
  - TGD originates near foramen cecum at posterior 3rd of tongue
  - Thyroid anlage arises at base of tongue → descends around or through hyoid bone → descends along strap muscles → final position in thyroid bed, anterior to thyroid cartilage or cricoid cartilage
  - At 5- to 6-gestational weeks, TGD usually involutes
    - Foramen cecum & pyramidal thyroid lobe may be left as normal remnants
  - Failure of TGD involution with persistent secretory activity of epithelial cells lining duct → TGDC
  - TGDC or ectopic thyroid tissue may occur anywhere along TGD
  - At autopsy > 7% of population will have TGD remnant somewhere along course of tract

Gross Pathologic & Surgical Features

- Smooth, benign-appearing cyst with tract to hyoid bone ± foramen cecum

Microscopic Features

- Cyst is lined by respiratory or squamous epithelium
- Small deposits of thyroid tissue with colloid are commonly associated
- ± thyroid carcinoma (papillary carcinoma is most common)

CLINICAL ISSUES

Presentation

- Most common signs/symptoms
  - Midline or paramidline doughy, compressible, painless neck mass in child or young adult
  - Cyst elevates when tongue protrudes if TGDC is located around hyoid bone
- Other signs/symptoms
  - Recurrent midline neck mass with upper respiratory tract infections or trauma
  - ± multiple prior incision & drainage procedures for neck abscess
  - Rarely, lingual TGDC may lead to airway obstruction in infants
  - Small lesion may be recognized as incidental finding on brain MR
    - Majority are at base of tongue

Demographics

- Age
  - < 10 years at presentation (up to 90%)
- Epidemiology
  - Most common congenital neck lesion
    - Up to 90% of nonodontogenic congenital cysts

Natural History & Prognosis

- Recurrent, intermittent swelling of mass, usually following minor upper respiratory infection
- Rapidly enlarging mass suggests either infection or differentiated thyroid carcinoma (< 1%)
  - 85% papillary carcinoma

Treatment

- Complete surgical resection: Sistrunk procedure ↓ recurrence rate from 50% to < 4%
  - Tract to foramen cecum is dissected free
  - Entire cyst & midline portion of hyoid bone are resected
    - Even if imaging shows no obvious connection to hyoid bone
    - Exception: Low infrahyoid neck TGDC
  - Prognosis is excellent with complete surgical resection
- Isolated lingual TGDC may be treated endoscopically
- Recurrences (from incomplete resection) are often complicated & lateral
  - ↑ risk of recurrence in patients with postoperative infection
- Increasing reports of successful sclerotherapy

DIAGNOSTIC CHECKLIST

Consider

- Relationship to hyoid bone is important to note
  - Suprahyoid, hyoid, or infrahyoid in location
- Nodularity or Ca^{2+} can suggest associated thyroid carcinoma
- Image thyroid bed with ultrasound to confirm presence of normal thyroid gland prior to TGDC or lingual thyroid excision

SELECTED REFERENCES

1. Lee E et al: Efficacy of ethanol ablation as a treatment of benign head and neck cystic lesions. Am J Otolaryngol. 42(6):103082, 2021
2. Tokarz E et al: Proposed ultrasound algorithm to differentiate thyroglossal duct and dermoid cysts. Int J Pediatr Otorhinolaryngol. 142:110624, 2021
3. Abdel Razek AAK et al: Differentiation of sublingual thyroglossal duct cyst from midline dermoid cyst with diffusion weighted imaging. Int J Pediatr Otorhinolaryngol. 126:109623, 2019
4. Chang KV et al: Thyroglossal duct cyst: dynamic ultrasound evaluation and sonoanatomy revisited. Med Ultrason. 21(1):99-100, 2019
5. Devine CM et al: Preoperative ultrasound for the diagnosis of thyroglossal duct cysts: a validation study. Int J Pediatr Otorhinolaryngol. 122:89-92, 2019
6. Lekkerkerker I et al: Pediatric thyroglossal duct cysts: post-operative complications. Int J Pediatr Otorhinolaryngol. 124:14-17, 2019
7. Liaw J et al: Primary papillary thyroid cancer of a thyroglossal duct cyst. Ear Nose Throat J. 98(3):136-8, 2019
8. Patel S et al: Thyroglossal duct pathology and mimics. Insights Imaging. 10(1):12, 2019
9. Pitner H et al: Diagnostic accuracy of midline pediatric neck masses. Otolaryngol Head Neck Surg. 160(6):1111-7, 2019
10. Bansal AG et al: US of pediatric superficial masses of the head and neck. Radiographics. 38(4):1239-63, 2018
11. Choi HI et al: Ultrasonographic features differentiating thyroglossal duct cysts from dermoid cysts. Ultrasonography. 37(1):71-77, 2018
12. Oyewumi M et al: Ultrasound to differentiate thyroglossal duct cysts and dermoid cysts in children. Laryngoscope. 125(4):998-1003, 2015
13. Koch BL: Cystic malformations of the neck in children. Pediatr Radiol. 35(5):463-77, 2005

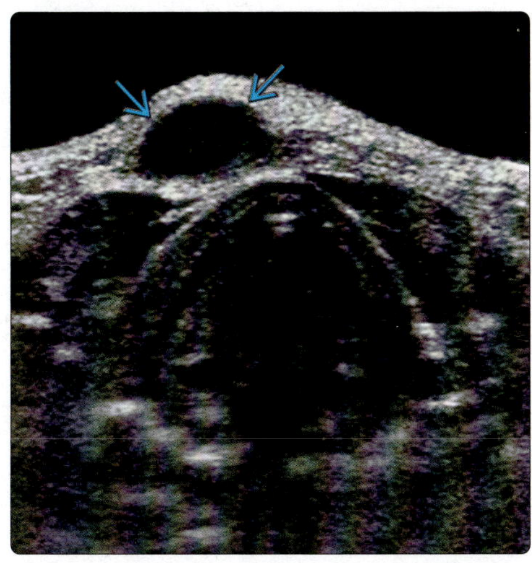

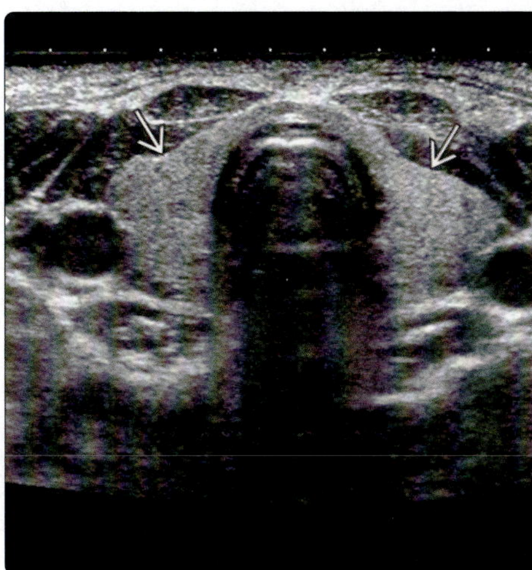

(Left) *Transverse US of the anterior neck shows a well-defined, subcutaneous, right paramidline, hypoechoic mass ➔ ventral to the strap muscles. This lesion was surgically removed & confirmed to be a TGDC.* **(Right)** *Transverse US in a child with a suspected TGDC (not shown) demonstrates a normal-appearing, bilobed thyroid ➔ at the expected location in the lower anterior midline neck. It is important to document the presence of normal thyroid tissue in all patients imaged for the work-up of a TGDC.*

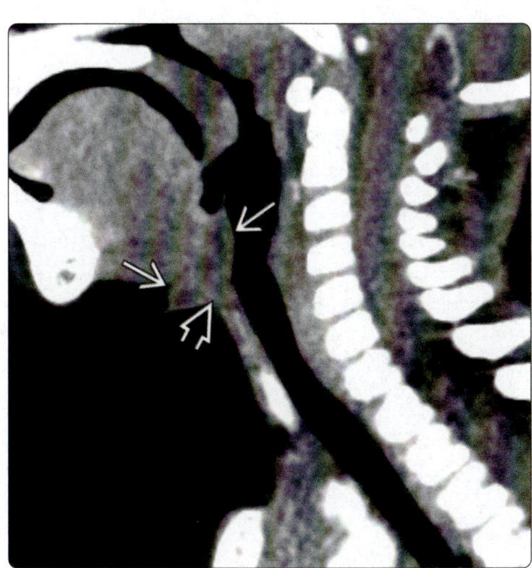

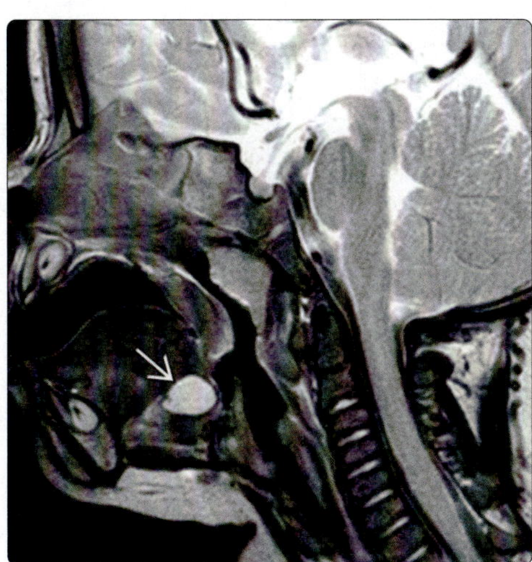

(Left) *Sagittal CECT in a child with a proven recurrence of a TGDC demonstrates a lobulated, heterogeneous mass ➔ in the midline suprahyoid neck. By imaging, this is indistinguishable from a postsurgical collection. Note the absence of a midline hyoid bone ➔, consistent with a prior Sistrunk procedure.* **(Right)** *Sagittal T2 MR in a child undergoing brain imaging for the work-up of seizures shows an incidental, well-defined, hyperintense mass ➔ at the midline tongue base, subsequently proven to be a TGDC.*

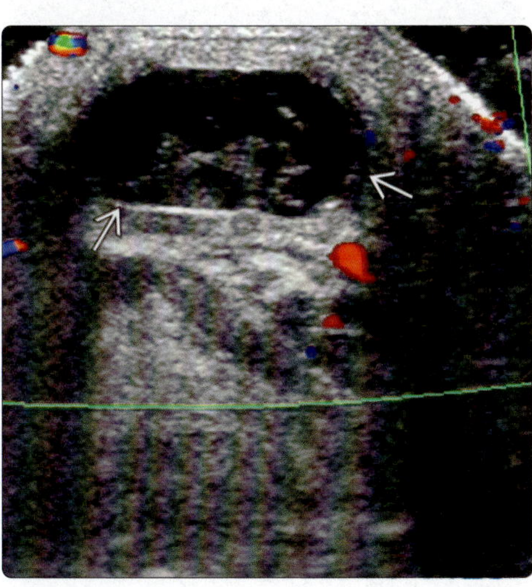

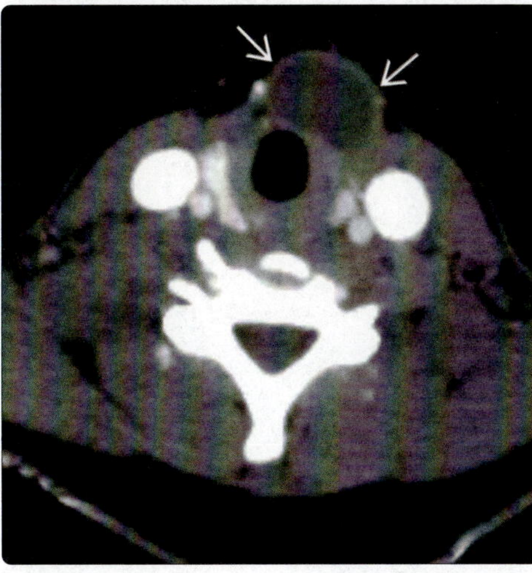

(Left) *Transverse color Doppler US in a child with the new onset of a paramidline anterior left neck mass shows a heterogeneously hypoechoic lesion ➔ with internal echoes. No internal vascularity is seen. Histologically, the lesion proved to be an uncomplicated TGDC.* **(Right)** *Axial CECT of the neck in a teenager with the new onset of a neck mass demonstrates a low-attenuation infrahyoid mass ➔ embedded within the left strap muscle, typical of a TGDC.*

Branchial Cleft Anomalies

KEY FACTS

TERMINOLOGY

- Branchial cleft cyst, branchial apparatus cyst (BAC), branchial apparatus anomaly (BAA)
- Anomaly/remnant of embryologic endodermal pouch, mesodermal arch, or ectodermal cleft
  - May be cyst, fistula, or sinus tract

IMAGING

- Well-defined, smooth-walled unilocular cyst of face/neck
  - ± wall thickening, enhancement, & septation with surrounding edema if infected
- Location
  - 1st BAC: Periauricular, in or adjacent to parotid
  - 2nd BAC (most common): Anterior to sternocleidomastoid muscle, posterior to submandibular gland, lateral to carotid sheath
  - 3rd BAC: Posterior triangle in upper neck or anterior triangle in lower neck
  - Cervical thymic cyst: Anywhere along thymopharyngeal duct from lateral hypopharynx to location of normal lobes of thymus in superior mediastinum
  - 4th BAA: Typically sinus tract or fistula extending from apex of pyriform sinus to anterior lower neck, usually in or adjacent to left thyroid lobe

TOP DIFFERENTIAL DIAGNOSES

- Suppurative lymph node or abscess
- Thyroglossal duct cyst
- Lymphatic malformation
- Dermoid & epidermoid

CLINICAL ISSUES

- Typical presentations include soft, painless mass vs. recurrent infections or drainage
  - 1st BAC: ± otorrhea or recurrent parotid abscess
  - 4th BAA: ± left thyroid lobe abscess
- Treatment requires complete surgical excision of cyst & associated fistula or sinus tract, if present

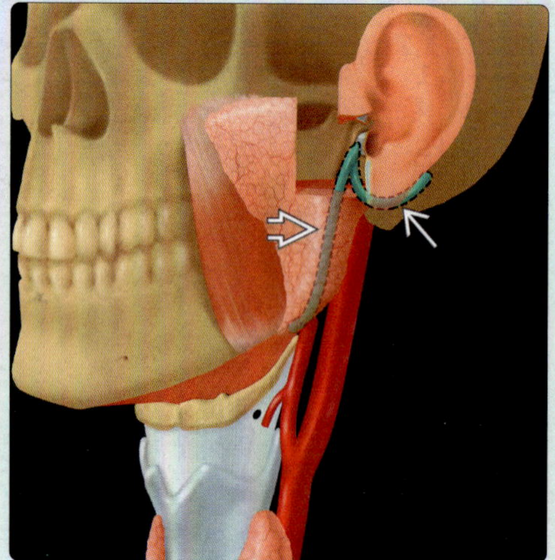
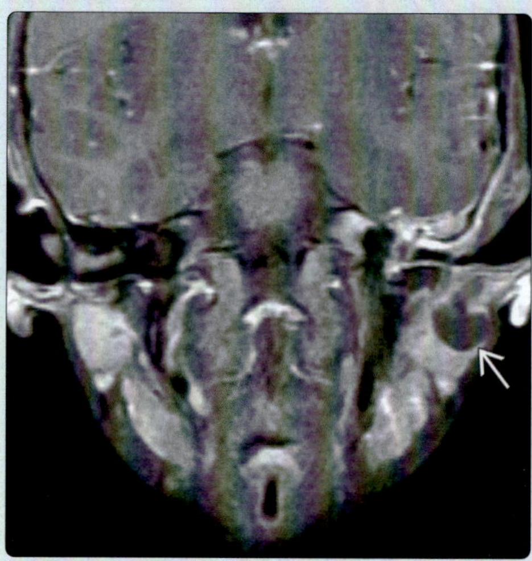

(Left) *Oblique graphic shows the 2 forms of a 1st branchial apparatus cyst (BAC). A type 1 1st BAC ➡ courses from the medial bony external auditory canal (EAC) toward the retroauricular area. The tract of a type 2 first BAC ➡ connects the EAC to the angle of the mandible.* **(Right)** *Coronal T1 C+ FS MR in a 3-year-old patient with a 1st BAC shows a lobulated, nonenhancing periparotid cyst ➡ extending toward the junction of the cartilaginous & bony EAC.*

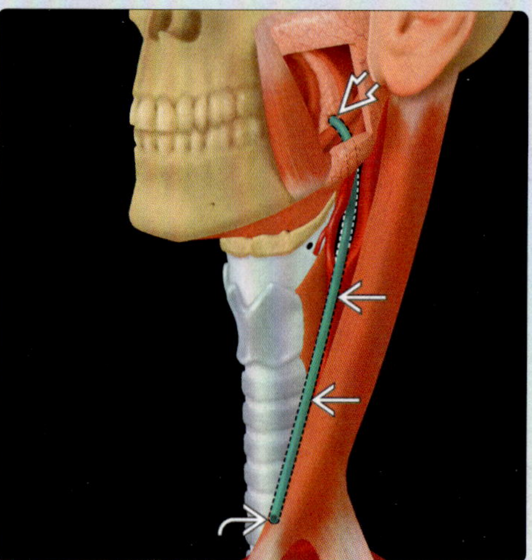
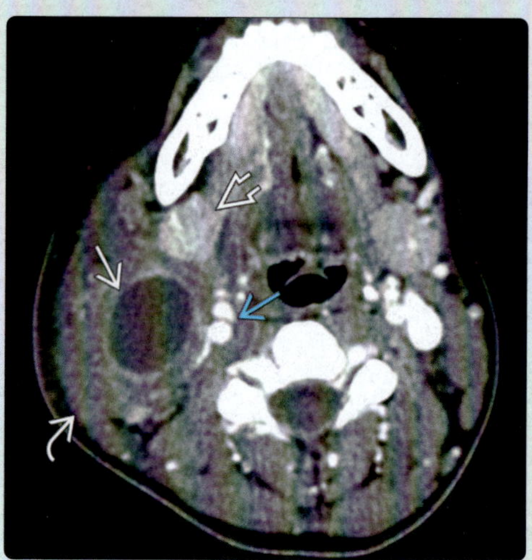

(Left) *Oblique graphic of the tract of a 2nd BAC ➡ shows a proximal opening ➡ in the faucial tonsil & a distal opening in the anterior supraclavicular neck ➡.* **(Right)** *Axial CECT in a teenager with an enlarging mass shows a cystic-appearing lesion ➡ in the typical location of a 2nd BAC (dorsal to the submandibular gland ➡, anterior to the SCM ➡, & lateral to the carotid sheath vessels ➡). Note the thick, irregular rim & adjacent soft tissue edema, consistent with superimposed infection & cellulitis/myositis.*

TERMINOLOGY

Synonyms

- Branchial cleft cyst, branchial apparatus cyst (BAC), branchial apparatus anomaly (BAA)

Definitions

- Anomaly/remnant of embryologic endodermal pouch, mesodermal arch, or ectodermal cleft
- May be cyst, fistula, or sinus tract

IMAGING

General Features

- Best diagnostic clue
  - Well-defined, smooth-walled cyst (types 1-3)
    - ± surrounding edema/enhancement if infected
  - Left thyroid lobe abscess: Suspect pyriform sinus fistula or sinus tract (type 4)
    - CT after barium swallow best identifies sinus tract or fistula
- Location
  - 1st BAC
    - Periauricular (type 1)
    - Periparotid (type 2): May extend to angle of mandible
  - 2nd BAC (95%): 4 locations based on Bailey classification
    - Deep to platysma (type 1): Rare
    - Anterior to sternocleidomastoid (SCM) muscle, posterior to submandibular gland, lateral to carotid sheath (type 2): Most common
    - Protrude between internal carotid artery & external carotid artery (type 3)
    - Adjacent to lateral pharyngeal wall (type 4, probably remnant of 2nd pharyngeal pouch)
  - 3rd BAC
    - Posterior triangle in upper neck, anterior triangle in lower neck
  - Cervical thymic cyst
    - 3rd pharyngeal pouch remnant: Thymopharyngeal duct remnant from lateral hypopharynx to location of normal lobes of thymus in superior mediastinum
    - ± solid ectopic thymus along same tract
    - Remnants may be mixed cystic & solid
  - 4th BAA
    - Sinus tract or fistula extending from apex of pyriform sinus to anterior lower neck, usually adjacent to left thyroid lobe
    - 4th pharyngeal pouch remnant (or recent literature suggests 3rd pouch remnant)
- Size
  - Variable from small to several cm
- Morphology
  - Most BACs are well defined, unilocular, & round or ovoid

CT Findings

- CECT
  - Low-density cyst with nonenhancing wall in typical location
    - If infected: Thickened, enhancing wall with surrounding cellulitis
  - Pyriform sinus fistula (extends to skin surface) or sinus tract (does not extend to skin surface)
    - Abscess in or adjacent to left thyroid lobe
    - May only show subtle inflammation around apex of pyriform sinus
    - Sinus tract or fistula is best demonstrated on neck CT obtained immediately after swallowing oral contrast

MR Findings

- Without infection: Thin-walled, fluid-filled cyst
- If infected: Thick wall with variable signal intensity of fluid + surrounding cellulitis
- Ideal to demonstrate small sinus tract or fistula associated with type 1 BAC

Ultrasonographic Findings

- Thin-walled, hypoechoic cyst ± mobile internal echoes
- Remnant ectopic thymus shows characteristic "dot & dash" echoes in otherwise hypoechoic thymic tissue

Imaging Recommendations

- Best imaging tool
  - Ultrasound is helpful to confirm cystic nature & location
    - May not show total extent of lesion
  - MR is best to evaluate suspected 1st BAC
  - CECT in acute setting (typically infected cyst)
- Protocol advice
  - Suspected 1st BAC: Cover periauricular tissues through angle of mandible
    - MR best identifies associated fistula or sinus tract
    - Coronal images help evaluate relationship to external auditory canal (EAC)
  - Suspected 2nd or 3rd BACs: Image entire neck to upper mediastinum
  - Suspected pyriform sinus fistula or sinus tract: Helpful to image after swallowing oral contrast

DIFFERENTIAL DIAGNOSIS

Suppurative Lymph Nodes

- Thick, enhancing nodal wall with central hypoattenuation/hypoechogenicity = nodal necrosis/intranodal abscess
- Edema in surrounding fat (cellulitis)
- ± thickening of muscles (myositis)
- Associated nonsuppurative adenopathy
- Nontuberculous mycobacterial adenitis lacks surrounding inflammatory change

Abscess

- Conglomeration of suppurative nodes or rupture of node → extranodal abscess
- Superficial: Anterior or posterior cervical or submandibular spaces (SMSs)
- Deep: Retropharyngeal, parapharyngeal, or tonsillar; may grow rapidly → airway compromise ± mediastinal extension
- If anterior to left thyroid lobe, think of 4th BAA
- Exclude dental infection & salivary gland calculus as cause of head & neck infection

Thyroglossal Duct Cyst

- Remnant of thyroglossal duct, anywhere from foramen cecum/base of tongue to thyroid bed in infrahyoid neck
- Cyst with minimal rim enhancement

- Location: 50% at hyoid, up to 25% suprahyoid, up to 25% infrahyoid
  - Suprahyoid lesions are usually midline
  - Infrahyoid may be off midline, embedded in strap muscles
- ± nodularity or Ca^{2+} if associated thyroid carcinoma (usually adults)

Lymphatic Malformation

- Congenital slow-flow vascular malformation composed of variably-sized abnormal lymphatic channels
- Often multilocular transspatial mass
  - Thin rim/septal enhancement; ↑ enhancement if infected, microcystic, or combined with venous malformation
- Present at birth, grows commensurate with child; rapid growth from hemorrhage or hormonal stimulation
  - Hemorrhage → internal debris or fluid-fluid levels

Ranula

- Simple: Postinflammatory retention cyst with epithelial lining; arises in sublingual gland (or minor salivary gland) in sublingual space (SLS)
  - Well-defined, elongated cyst in SLS
- Diving: Ruptures out of SLS into SMS
  - Cyst in both SLS & SMS
  - May see "tail" if SLS component is collapsed

Dermoid & Epidermoid

- Dermoid: Epithelial & dermal elements
- Epidermoid: Epithelial elements only
- Well-defined cyst filled with fluid = dermoid or epidermoid
- Well-defined cyst with fatty material, mixed fluid ± Ca^{2+} = dermoid
- Diffusion restriction on DWI = dermoid or epidermoid

PATHOLOGY

General Features

- Associated abnormalities
  - Bilateral branchial apparatus fistulas/cysts & preauricular tag or pit are associated with branchiootorenal syndrome
    - Autosomal dominant inheritance
    - Profound mixed hearing loss: Cochlear & semicircular canal malformations, stapes fixation
    - Renal anomalies: Cysts, dysplasia, agenesis
    - Patulous eustachian tubes

CLINICAL ISSUES

Presentation

- Most common signs/symptoms
  - Soft, painless, compressible mass
  - Fever & cellulitis with superimposed infection or pyriform sinus fistula (or sinus tract)
  - Drainage at skin opening if fistula is present
- Other signs/symptoms
  - Large thymic cysts may lead to airway compromise in neonates

Natural History & Prognosis

- If not recognized & treated, 1st BAC may present with recurrent otorrhea or parotid abscess
- If not recognized & completely excised, 4th BAA/BAC anomalies may present with recurrent thyroiditis

Treatment

- Complete surgical excision of cyst & associated fistula or sinus tract, if present
  - Proximity of facial nerve to cyst puts nerve at risk during surgical excision of 1st BACs
  - Large cervical thymic cysts may require otolaryngology & thoracic surgery

DIAGNOSTIC CHECKLIST

Consider

- 1st BAC if cyst is in or around EAC or parotid gland
  - May present with otorrhea or recurrent parotid gland abscess
- 2nd BAC if cyst is anterior to SCM, posterior to submandibular gland, & lateral to carotid sheath
- Thymic cyst if cystic mass extends from neck to superior mediastinum &/or associated with anterior carotid sheath
- Pyriform sinus fistula or sinus tract if abscess is identified in or adjacent to left thyroid lobe

Image Interpretation Pearls

- If "abscess" is seen in typical location, think of infected preexisting BAC/BAA
- If patient is > 30 years of age, consider cystic nodal metastasis in differential diagnoses of 2nd or 3rd BAC

SELECTED REFERENCES

1. Pupić-Bakrač J et al: Branchial cleft anomalies: hybrid "branchial inclusion" theory. Eur Arch Otorhinolaryngol. 278(7):2593-601, 2021
2. Kang B et al: Congenital midline cervical cleft: an easily misdiagnosed disease. Arch Craniofac Surg. 21(6):372-5, 2020
3. King J et al: Computed tomography findings of complete branchial cleft fistula. Ear Nose Throat J. ePub, 2020
4. Li WX et al: Surgical treatment of fourth branchial apparatus anomalies: a case series study. J Otolaryngol Head Neck Surg. 49(1):79, 2020
5. Liu H et al: Clinical Manifestations, diagnosis, and management of first branchial cleft fistula/sinus: a case series and literature review. J Oral Maxillofac Surg. 78(5):749-61, 2020
6. Liu W et al: Clinical analysis of type ii first branchial cleft anomalies in children. Laryngoscope. 131(4):916-20, 2020
7. Magdy EA et al: Unusual isolated parapharyngeal second branchial cleft cyst: a case report and literature review. Case Rep Otolaryngol. 2020:8814071, 2020
8. Maksimoski M et al: Combination surgical procedure for fourth branchial anomalies: operative technique and outcomes. Ann Otol Rhinol Laryngol. 3489420971674, 2020
9. Rossi ME et al: Fourth branchial anomalies: predictive factors of therapeutic success. J Pediatr Surg. 54(8):1702-7, 2019
10. Adams A et al: Branchial cleft anomalies: a pictorial review of embryological development and spectrum of imaging findings. Insights Imaging. 7(1):69-76, 2016
11. Shinn JR et al: First branchial cleft anomalies: otologic manifestations and treatment outcomes. Otolaryngol Head Neck Surg. 152(3):506-12, 2015
12. Goff CJ et al: Current management of congenital branchial cleft cysts, sinuses, and fistulae. Curr Opin Otolaryngol Head Neck Surg. 20(6):533-9, 2012
13. Thomas B et al: Revisiting imaging features and the embryologic basis of third and fourth branchial anomalies. AJNR Am J Neuroradiol. 31(4):755-60, 2010
14. Koch BL: Cystic malformations of the neck in children. Pediatr Radiol. 35(5):463-77, 2005
15. Mukherji SK et al: Imaging of congenital anomalies of the branchial apparatus. Neuroimaging Clin N Am. 10(1):75-93, viii, 2000

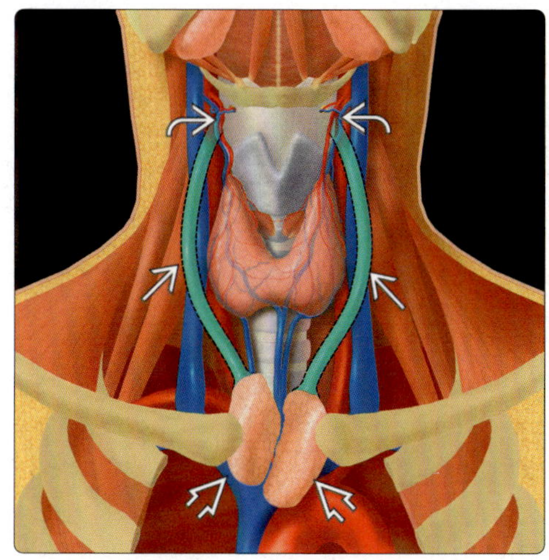

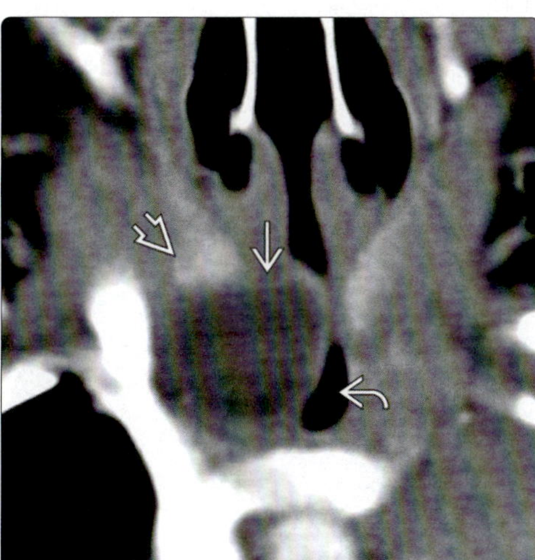

(Left) *Coronal graphic shows both thymopharyngeal duct tracts ➡ extending from the lateral hypopharyngeal area ↗ to the location of the normal lobes of the thymus ⇨ in the superior mediastinum. The thymopharyngeal tracts are remnants of the 3rd branchial pouch.* **(Right)** *Coronal CECT in an infant with respiratory distress shows a thymic cyst ➡ inferior to the right thyroid lobe ⇨, deviating & compressing the trachea ↗.*

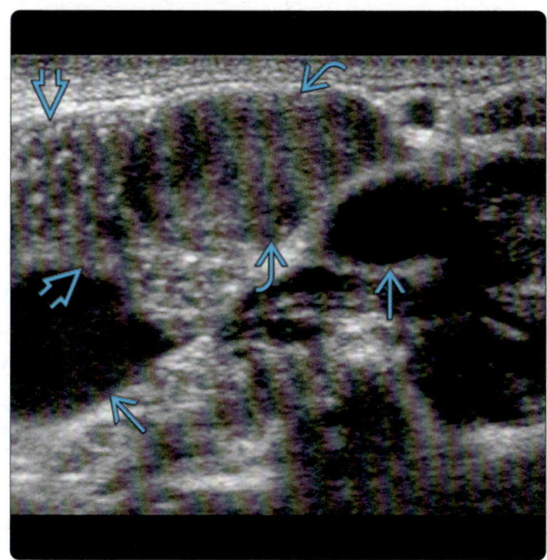

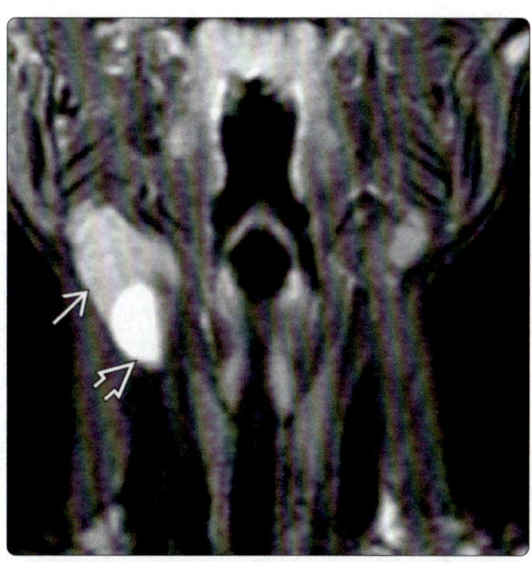

(Left) *Transverse ultrasound in a 7-year-old demonstrates a mixed cystic & solid thymic remnant splaying the carotid sheath vessels ➡. The lateral component demonstrates the "dot & dash" echogenicity typical of thymus ⇨ while the medial component is cystic (showing mobile intraluminal echoes ↗ on real-time imaging).* **(Right)** *Coronal T2 FS MR in the same patient shows a mixed solid ➡ & cystic ⇨ thymic remnant, the solid portion of which was isointense to intrathoracic thymus on all sequences (not shown).*

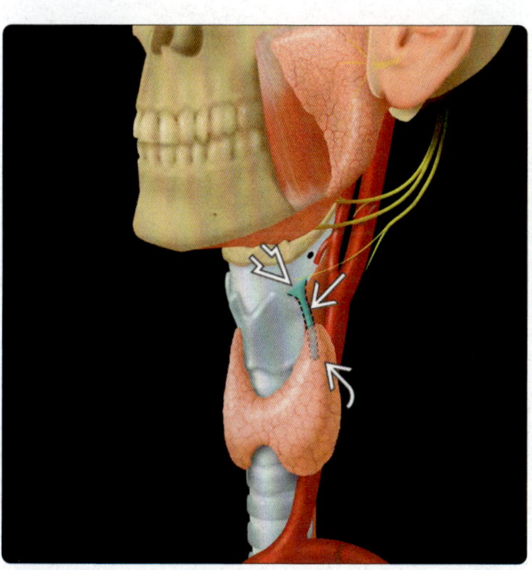

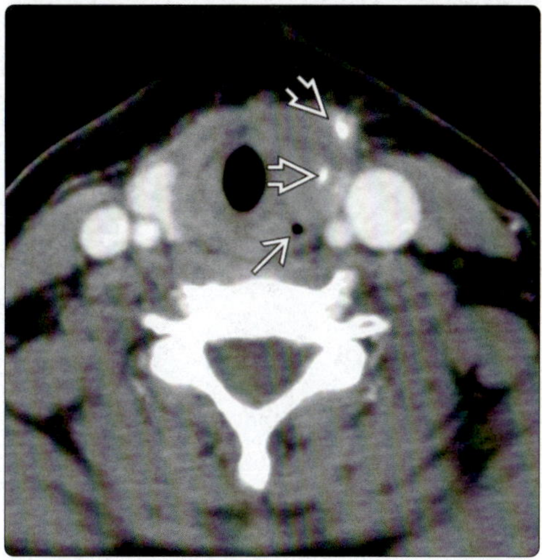

(Left) *Oblique graphic of the neck shows the tract of a 4th BAA ⇨ extending from the hypopharynx ➡ to the location of the left thyroid lobe ↗. This explains why this lesion often presents with thyroiditis/abscess.* **(Right)** *Axial CECT in a child with a recurrent draining 4th BAA fistula was obtained after a barium swallow study. Air is in the proximal fistulous tract ➡ just below the left pyriform sinus. Barium is in the tract extending anteriorly through the strap muscles ⇨. Barium was also noted at a skin opening (not shown).*

KEY FACTS

TERMINOLOGY

- Acute inflammation of parotid gland
  - Bacterial: Localized bacterial infection ± abscess
  - Viral: Usually from systemic viral infection
  - Calculus-induced: Ductal obstruction by sialolith
  - Autoimmune: Acute episode of chronic disease
  - Juvenile recurrent parotitis (JRP): Intermittent idiopathic episodes of parotid inflammation

IMAGING

- Typical appearance: ↑ size & enhancement of parotid ± stranding of surrounding fat; parotid retains normal shape
- Bacterial parotitis: Typically unilateral
  - Periparotid cellulitis/stranding is common
  - Intra- or periparotid abscess may occur
- Viral parotitis: Typically bilateral
  - Clinical diagnosis; imaging rarely required
- Calculus-induced parotitis: Typically unilateral
  - Large duct with intraluminal stone
- Autoimmune parotitis: Typically bilateral
  - Diagnosed with serum markers
  - Sialography for chronic complications
- JRP: Often unilateral clinically with bilateral imaging abnormalities
  - Normal main duct with dilated intraglandular branches (sialectasis)

TOP DIFFERENTIAL DIAGNOSES

- Infected 1st branchial cleft anomaly
- Parotid infantile hemangioma
- Salivary gland neoplasms
- Parotid sialosis
- Benign lymphoepithelial lesions of HIV

DIAGNOSTIC CHECKLIST

- Reimage if mass persists after resolution of infection (to exclude underlying branchial cleft cyst or malignancy)
- Sialography for recurrent disease to assess complications

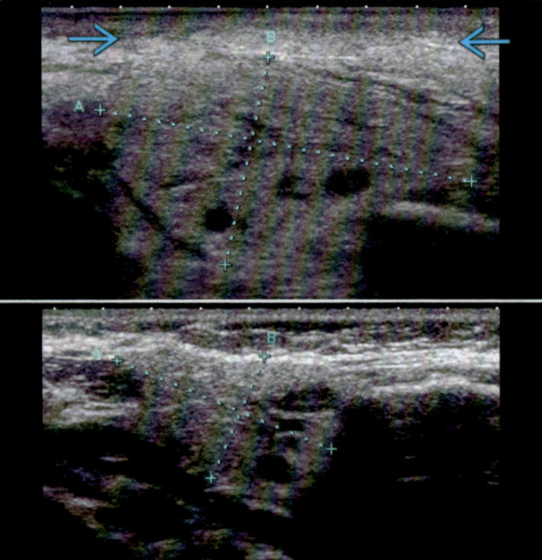

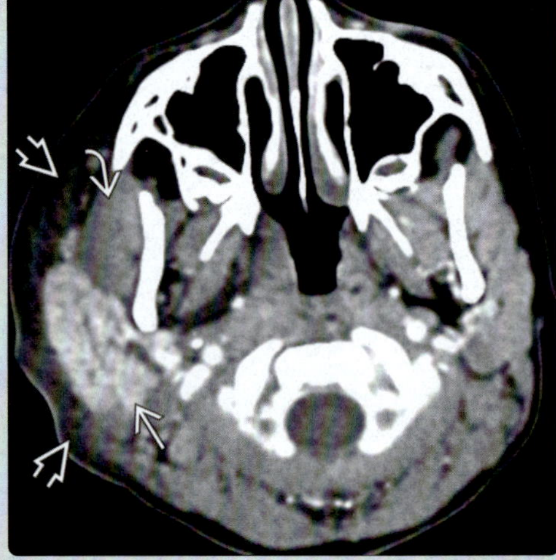

(Left) *Transverse US of the right (upper) & left (lower) parotid glands (denoted by calipers) in a toddler with right facial swelling shows normal size & echogenicity of the left parotid gland & overlying soft tissues. The right parotid gland is enlarged & mildly heterogeneous with induration of the overlying soft tissues ➡, typical of parotitis.* **(Right)** *Axial CECT shows diffuse, asymmetric enlargement & enhancement of the right parotid gland ➡ with associated facial cellulitis ➡ & myositis ➡ due to acute bacterial parotitis.*

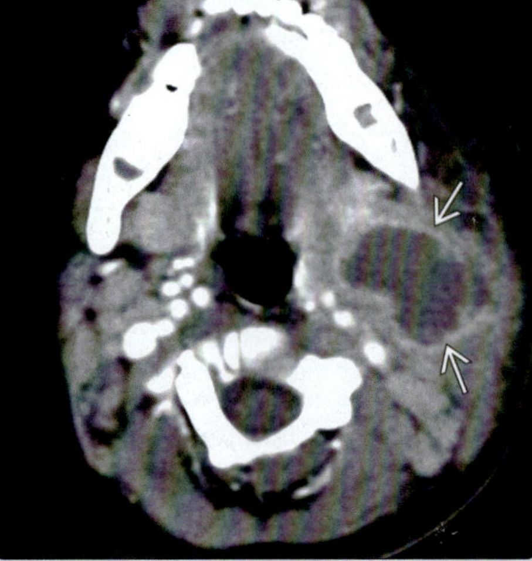

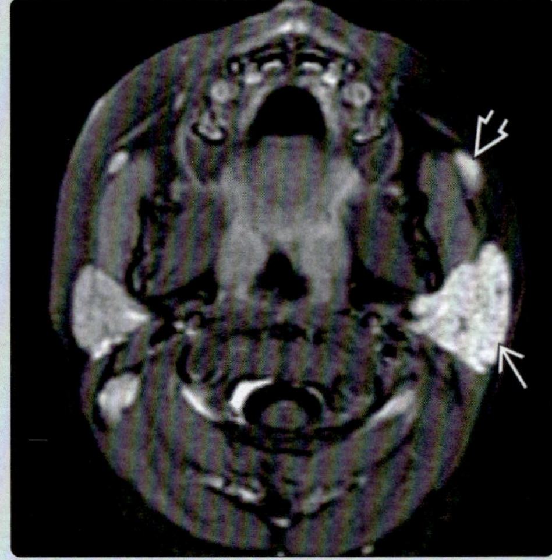

(Left) *Axial CECT shows a low-density, rim-enhancing collection ➡ replacing the left parotid gland. There is substantial surrounding fat stranding. These findings are consistent with an abscess complicating acute bacterial parotitis.* **(Right)** *Axial T1 C+ FS MR in a child with recurrent parotitis shows an enlarged, asymmetrically enhancing left parotid gland ➡ without significant cellulitis. Note the moderate enhancement in the ipsilateral accessory glandular tissue as well ➡.*

TERMINOLOGY

Synonyms

- Acute sialadenitis

Definitions

- Acute inflammation of parotid gland
  - Bacterial: Localized infection ± abscess
  - Viral: Usually from systemic viral infection
  - Calculus-induced: Ductal obstruction by sialolith
  - Autoimmune: Acute episodes of chronic disease
  - Juvenile recurrent parotitis (JRP) or chronic recurrent parotitis of childhood: Intermittent idiopathic episodes of parotid inflammation

IMAGING

General Features

- Best diagnostic clue
  - Enlarged parotid(s) with surrounding fat stranding
- Location
  - Bacterial: Usually unilateral
  - Viral: 75% bilateral; ± submandibular &/or sublingual gland involvement
    - Rare cases of COVID-19 parotitis, often unilateral
  - Calculus-induced: Unilateral
  - Autoimmune: Usually bilateral
  - Juvenile recurrent: Unilateral or asymmetric clinical presentations with bilateral imaging findings
- Morphology
  - Entire gland is usually involved (but can be focal); parotid retains normal triangular configuration

CT Findings

- CECT
  - Bacterial: Enlarged, diffusely enhancing parotid
    - Inflammatory stranding of surrounding fat
    - Rim enhancement of low-density abscess (if present)
  - Viral: Enlarged parotids with mild enhancement
  - Calculus-induced: Calcified stone; dilated parotid duct with enhancing walls; otherwise like bacterial
  - Autoimmune: Less stranding of surrounding fat; may have ductal dilation if longstanding disease

MR Findings

- T2WI
  - Diffuse moderately high signal ± focal areas of fluid signal (microabscesses or dilated ducts)
- T1WI C+
  - Enlarged parotid gland with diffuse, moderate enhancement; abscesses: Rim-enhancing fluid collections
- MR sialography (3D SSFP)
  - Exquisite for demonstrating cysts or dilated ducts
  - JRP: Normal main duct with dilated intraglandular branches (sialectasis)

Ultrasonographic Findings

- Enlarged, hypoechoic, heterogeneous gland
- Numerous small, hypoechoic lesions bilaterally in JRP
- Echogenic calculi with posterior acoustic shadowing ± dilated, hypoechoic duct
- Focal hypoechoic collection suggests abscess formation

Other Modality Findings

- Sialography is contraindicated in acute suppurative parotitis
  - Useful in evaluating recurrent disease & complications

Imaging Recommendations

- Best imaging tool
  - Bacterial & calculus-induced inflammation: CECT is best for detection of stone or abscess
  - Viral: Typically diagnosed clinically; imaging rarely required
  - Autoimmune disease: Diagnosed with serum markers
    - Sialography for chronic complications
  - JRP: MR sialography or conventional sialogram

DIFFERENTIAL DIAGNOSIS

Infected 1st Branchial Cleft Anomaly

- 1st branchial cleft cyst lies in or adjacent to parotid gland
- Superinfection presents as parotid abscess

Parotid Infantile Hemangioma

- Diffusely expanded, hypervascular, & homogeneously hyperenhancing parotid; normal surrounding soft tissues
- Presents with swelling in 1st few weeks to months of life

Salivary Gland Neoplasms

- Firm focal or infiltrative mass without hyperenhancement

Parotid Sialosis

- Bilateral prolonged, painless, soft parotid (& occasionally submandibular) gland enlargement

Benign Lymphoepithelial Lesions of HIV

- Bilateral, heterogeneous parotids, ± cystic & solid lesions
- Prominent Waldeyer ring & cervical nodes

CLINICAL ISSUES

Presentation

- Most common signs/symptoms
  - Bacterial: Sudden onset of parotid pain & swelling
  - Viral: Prodromal symptoms of headaches, malaise, myalgia followed by parotid pain, earache, trismus
  - Calculus-induced: Recurrent episodes of swollen, painful gland, usually related to eating
  - Autoimmune: Recurrent episodes of swollen, painful gland + dry mouth; JRP: Recurrent episodes ± fever, malaise

Demographics

- Age
  - Viral: Most < 15 years; peak age: 5-9 years
  - JRP: Usually begins by 5 years; resolves by ages 10-15
  - Bacterial: > 50 years or neonates

SELECTED REFERENCES

1. Ekemen Keles Y et al: Acute parotitis in a 4-year-old in association with COVID-19. J Paediatr Child Health. 57(6):958-9, 2021
2. Tucci FM et al: Juvenile recurrent parotitis: diagnostic and therapeutic effectiveness of sialography. Retrospective study on 110 children. Int J Pediatr Otorhinolaryngol. 124:179-84, 2019
3. Inarejos Clemente EJ et al: Imaging evaluation of pediatric parotid gland abnormalities. Radiographics. 38(5):1552-75, 2018
4. Guerin JB et al: Pediatric parotid region lesions: an imaging review. Neurographics. 8(6):294-312, 2018

Infantile Hemangioma, Cervicofacial

KEY FACTS

TERMINOLOGY

- Benign vascular neoplasm of proliferating endothelial cells; **not** vascular malformation

IMAGING

- Ultrasound + Doppler
  - Soft subcutaneous mass with patchy ↑ echogenicity
  - High vessel density (> 5/cm²) with low resistance arterial waveforms but no arteriovenous shunting
- Contrast-enhanced CT/MR
  - Well-defined mass with diffuse & intense enhancement during proliferative phase
  - High-flow vessels in/adjacent to mass during proliferation
  - ↓ size with ↑ fatty replacement during involuting phase

TOP DIFFERENTIAL DIAGNOSES

- Congenital hemangioma
- Venous malformation
- Arteriovenous malformation
- Soft tissue sarcoma
- Plexiform neurofibroma

PATHOLOGY

- GLUT-1(+) in all phases of growth & regression
- In contrast to GLUT-1(-) congenital hemangioma

CLINICAL ISSUES

- Typically inapparent at birth → appears in 1st few weeks of life → grows rapidly for months → spontaneously involutes over years
  - Typically warm, soft, raised reddish or strawberry-like cutaneous lesion
- Majority do not require treatment; propranolol is 1st-line therapy in setting of ulceration or vital structure compromise (e.g., airway or orbit)
- If age, clinical/imaging appearance, or growth history are atypical for infantile hemangioma, biopsy is recommended

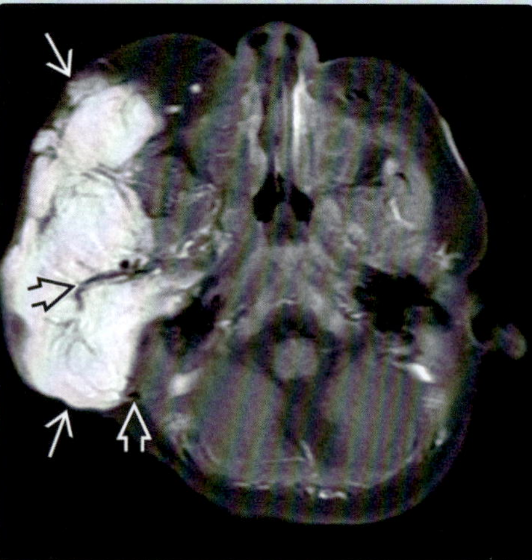

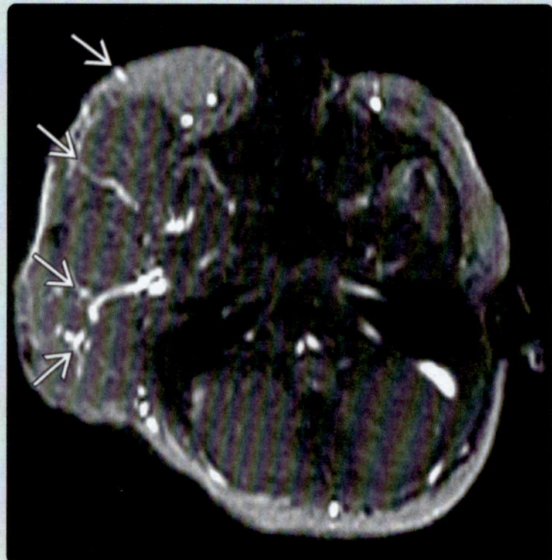

(Left) *Axial T1 C+ FS MR in a 5-month-old shows a large, lobulated, intensely enhancing lesion ➡ infiltrating the massively enlarged right parotid gland. Note the prominent intralesional ⇨ & perilesional ➡ flow voids typical of an infantile hemangioma (IH).* **(Right)** *Axial 2D SPGR flow-sensitive MR sequence in the same patient shows the typical appearance of multiple high-flow vessels ➡ within & adjacent to the primary parotid IH.*

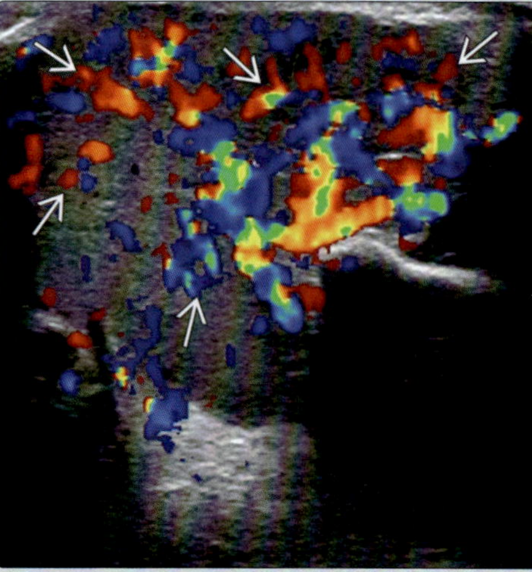

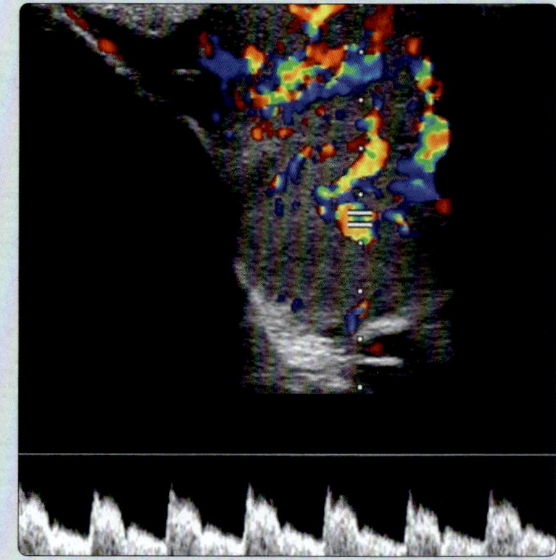

(Left) *Transverse color Doppler ultrasound in a 1-month-old child shows a lobular lesion replacing & expanding the parotid gland. Note the high vessel density ➡, typical of a proliferating IH.* **(Right)** *Transverse color Doppler spectral tracing through the lesion in the same patient demonstrates low-resistance arterial waveforms, typical of a proliferating IH. The waveforms will develop a high-resistance pattern during involution, & there will be a ↓ in vessel density.*

TERMINOLOGY

Synonyms

- Capillary hemangioma
- Widespread misuse of term "hemangioma" in literature; infantile hemangioma (IH) is different entity from
  - Congenital hemangioma, spindle cell hemangioma, epithelioid hemangioma, lobular capillary hemangioma (pyogenic granuloma): All benign but different vascular neoplasms
  - Hemangioendothelioma: Higher grade vascular neoplasm
  - Cavernous hemangioma, vertebral body hemangioma, & synovial hemangioma: Venous malformations

Definitions

- IH: Benign vascular neoplasm (not malformation) of proliferating endothelial cells
  - Most common soft tissue tumor of infancy
- **Not** vascular malformation
- 2018 revised classification by International Society for Study of Vascular Anomalies (ISSVA) retains 2 main categories
  - Vascular tumors: True neoplasms with cellular proliferation; generally grow out of proportion to patient
  - Vascular malformation: Congenital errors of vessel development; generally grow commensurate with patient

IMAGING

General Features

- Best diagnostic clue
  - During proliferative phase: Lobular, well-defined mass with intense, diffuse enhancement + high-flow vessels in/adjacent to mass
  - During involuting phase: ↓ size, vascularity, & enhancement with progressive fatty replacement
- Location
  - 60% occur in head & neck
    - Any space: Parotid space, orbit, nasal cavity, subglottic airway, face, neck, rarely intracranial
      - When intracranial &/or multiple, consider PHACE(S) association
      - Typically not deep/intramuscular (in absence of syndrome)
- Size
  - Depends on phase of growth & regression; predictable clinical course
    - Proliferative phase: Rapid growth beginning days-weeks after birth & continuing 6-24 months
    - Involuting phase: Gradual regression over next several years
    - Involuted phase: Relatively small, residual lesion
- Morphology
  - Majority: Isolated, focal, well-circumscribed, lobulated lesions in subcutaneous tissues
    - Tend to displace/efface rather than encase normal structures
  - Occasionally multiple, transspatial, or deep
    - May be part of PHACE(S) association
      - **P**osterior fossa malformations (cerebellar hypoplasia is most common)
      - **H**emangioma (infantile) of face & neck, typically segmental or midline; can involve deep tissues
      - **A**rterial stenosis, occlusion, aneurysm, hypoplasia, agenesis, aberrant origin
      - **C**ardiovascular defects (aortic coarctation/aneurysm/dysplasia, aberrant subclavian artery ± vascular ring)
      - **E**ye abnormalities (coloboma, morning glory disc anomaly, optic nerve hypoplasia, peripapillary staphyloma, microphthalmia, cataract, sclerocornea)
      - **S**upraumbilical raphe & sternal clefts/defects
- Ultrasonographic findings
  - Grayscale
    - Soft lobular mass with variable echogenicity & few macroscopic vessels; ↑ echogenicity during involution
  - Color/spectral Doppler
    - High vessel density (> 5 vessels/cm^2); high systolic Doppler shift (> 2 kHz) & low resistive indices in arteries without arterialized veins (to suggest shunting) during proliferation
    - Mean venous peak velocities are not elevated
  - ↓ vessel density, ↑ resistive indices during involution
- CECT
  - Well-circumscribed lobulated mass with diffuse & intense contrast enhancement during proliferation
    - Prominent vessels in/adjacent to mass
    - No internal Ca^{2+} or surrounding edema
  - Progressive fatty infiltration of mass + ↓ size during involution
- MR
  - T1: Isointense to muscle in proliferation; hyperintense from fatty replacement during involution
  - T2: Mildly hyperintense relative to muscle
  - T2 FS/STIR: At least moderately hyperintense relative to muscle (but not fluid signal intensity) during proliferation; hypointense to muscle (follows fat) during involution
  - GRE: High-flow vessels in/adjacent to mass in proliferation
    - Corresponding serpiginous flow voids in/adjacent to mass on SE/FSE sequences
  - DWI: ADC values are higher in IHs vs. pediatric soft tissue malignancies
    - IH: ~ 1.3-1.6 x 10^{-3} mm^2/sec
    - Sarcomas: ~ 0.7-1.2 x 10^{-3} mm^2/sec
  - Perfusion/ASL: Markedly hyperintense during proliferation
  - T1 C+ FS: Intense uniform contrast enhancement in proliferation
  - MRA: Stenosis, occlusion, agenesis, or aneurysm of craniocervical vessels in PHACE(S) association

Imaging Recommendations

- No imaging is necessary in majority of patients due to characteristic cutaneous appearance & timeframe
- Best imaging tool depends on indications

- To establish diagnosis with atypical history, appearance, or clinical behavior of lesion: US with spectral Doppler if relatively superficial
  - Deeper lesions may not have classic cutaneous appearance
- To define deep extension of lesion with implications for compromise of vital structures (e.g., orbit & airway): MR
- To evaluate for suspected PHACE(S) association (e.g., large segmental facial IH): MR

DIFFERENTIAL DIAGNOSIS

Congenital Hemangioma (RICH/NICH/PICH)

- Present at birth or on prenatal imaging; does not proliferate after birth
  - Rapidly involuting congenital hemangioma (RICH): Involutes by 3-14 months
  - Noninvoluting congenital hemangioma (NICH)
  - Partially involuting congenital hemangioma (PICH)
- Solid, heterogeneous, less well-defined mass ± Ca^{2+}, hemorrhage, necrosis
- Glucose transporter 1 (GLUT-1) negative on histology

Venous Malformation

- Congenital vascular malformation composed of large venous lakes
- Fluid signal intensity throughout mass; ± fluid-fluid levels, phleboliths
- Gradual patchy fill-in with contrast

Arteriovenous Malformation

- Congenital high-flow vascular malformation
- Arteriovenous shunting through tangle of feeding arteries & large draining veins
  - ± other soft tissue components

Soft Tissue Sarcoma

- Solid or mixed cystic/solid mass, typically firm
- Variable enhancement ± osseous erosion
- Variable internal vascularity but typically << IH
- Typically restricts diffusion (lower ADC values)
- Fat is highly unlikely

Plexiform Neurofibroma

- Infiltrative lobulated masses with target appearance in cross section
- Transspatial involvement ± poorly defined margins
- Additional stigmata of neurofibromatosis type 1

PATHOLOGY

Microscopic Features

- Prominent endothelial cells forming small vascular channels during proliferation; flat endothelial cells + fibrofatty replacement during involution

Immunohistochemical Features

- GLUT-1 positive during all phases of proliferation & regression

CLINICAL ISSUES

Presentation

- Most common signs/symptoms
  - Growing superficial soft tissue mass in young infant, typically with warm, soft, raised reddish or strawberry-like cutaneous discoloration
  - Deeper lesions may show bluish skin discoloration secondary to prominent draining veins
- Other signs/symptoms
  - Ulceration of overlying skin
  - Airway obstruction from airway involvement
  - Proptosis from orbital lesion
  - Associated abnormalities in PHACE(S) association

Demographics

- Age
  - Median at presentation: 2 weeks; majority by 1-3 months
    - Typically inapparent at birth
    - Up to 1/3 are nascent at birth (i.e., pale or erythematous macule, telangiectasia, pseudoecchymotic patch or red spot)
- Epidemiology
  - Most common head & neck tumor in infants
  - 1-2% of neonates; 12% by 1 year of age
  - ↑ in preterm infants & low birth weight infants
    - Up to 30% of infants weighing < 1 kg
- Ethnicity
  - Most frequent in White patients
- Sex: F > M (1.5-4:1)

Natural History & Prognosis

- Gradual spontaneous regression
  - 90% resolve by 9 years of age
- Large & segmental facial hemangiomas have ↑ incidence of complications if not treated

Treatment

- Majority do not require treatment
- Treatment indications
  - Compromise of vital structures (e.g., optic nerve compression or airway obstruction)
  - Significant skin ulceration
- Treatment options
  - Oral propranolol (β-blocker) is now primary therapy (instead of oral steroids) due to low side effect profile
  - Less common: Intralesional steroids, laser, rarely surgical excision

SELECTED REFERENCES

1. Maldonado FR et al: Quantitative characterization of extraocular orbital lesions in children using diffusion-weighted imaging. Pediatr Radiol. 51(1):119-27, 2021
2. Gong X et al: Conventional ultrasonography and elastography for the diagnosis of congenital and infantile hemangiomas. J Dermatol. 47(5):527-33, 2020
3. Saito M et al: Usefulness of diffusion-weighted magnetic resonance imaging using apparent diffusion coefficient values for diagnosis of infantile hemangioma. J Comput Assist Tomogr. 43(4):563-7, 2019
4. ISSVA Classification of Vascular Anomalies. Published April 2014. Updated May 2018. Accessed March 28, 2020. https://www.issva.org/UserFiles/file/ISSVA-Classification-2018.pdf
5. Johnson CM et al: Clinical and sonographic features of pediatric soft-tissue vascular anomalies part 1: classification, sonographic approach and vascular tumors. Pediatr Radiol. 47(9):1184-95, 2017
6. Mamlouk MD et al: Arterial spin-labeled perfusion for vascular anomalies in the pediatric head and neck. Clin Imaging. 40(5):1040-6, 2016
7. Merrow AC et al: 2014 Revised classification of vascular lesions from the International Society for the Study of Vascular Anomalies: radiologic-pathologic update. Radiographics. 36(5):1494-516, 2016

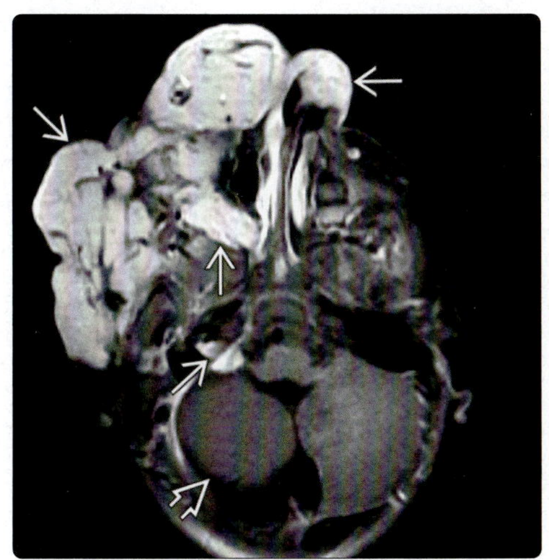

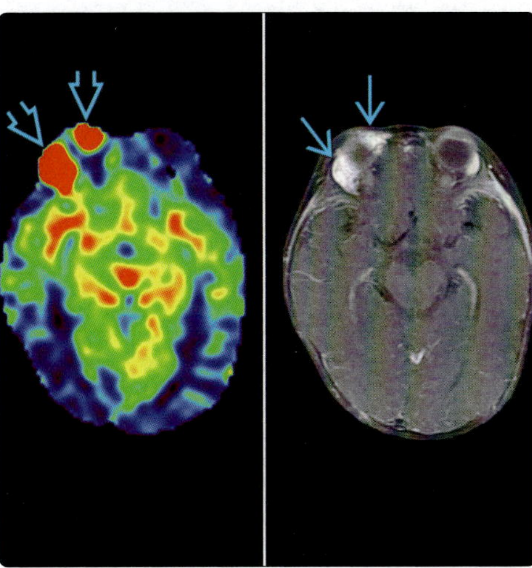

(Left) *Axial T1 C+ FS MR in a 4-month-old girl with PHACE(S) association demonstrates multiple enhancing hemangiomas* ➔ *in the right parotid space, right posterior-inferior orbit, right cheek, nose, & right internal auditory canal (IAC)/cerebellopontine angle (CPA). Also note the ipsilateral right cerebellar hemisphere hypoplasia* ⇨. **(Right)** *Axial arterial spin-labeled (ASL) (left) & T1 C+ FS (right) MR images in a 6-week-old show markedly ↑ perfusion* ⇨ *& uniform enhancement* ➔ *of a periorbital & intraorbital IH.*

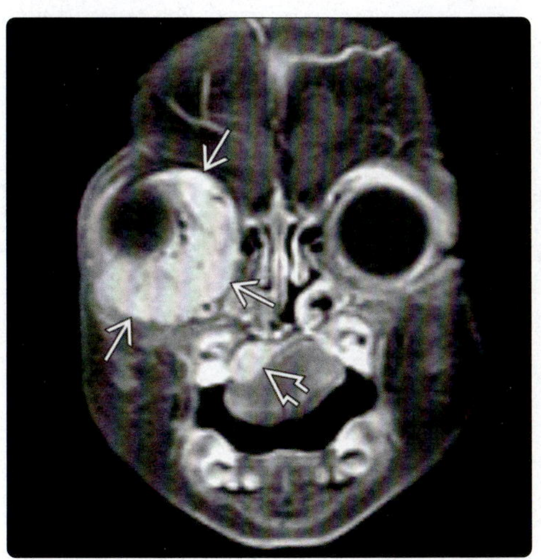

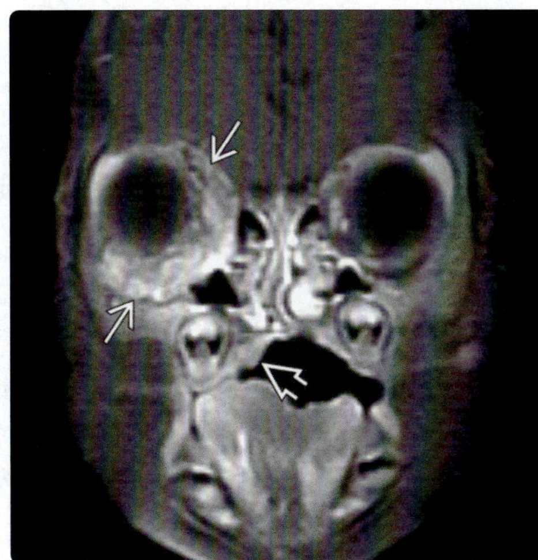

(Left) *Coronal T1 C+ FS MR in a 2-month-old shows a large, intensely enhancing IH involving the right intraconal & extraconal orbit* ➔. *There is a 2nd lesion involving the right palate* ⇨. **(Right)** *Coronal T1 C+ FS MR in the same patient after 6 months of propranolol therapy (which was instituted to prevent orbital complications) shows interval regression of the orbital* ➔ *& palatal* ⇨ *lesions. In a patient with multiple IHs, consider PHACE(S) association.*

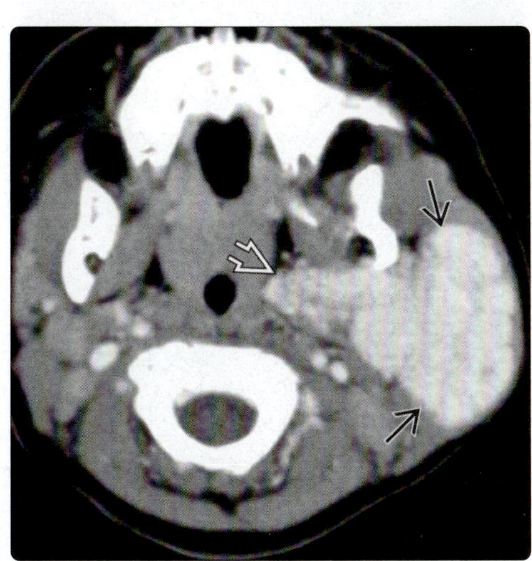

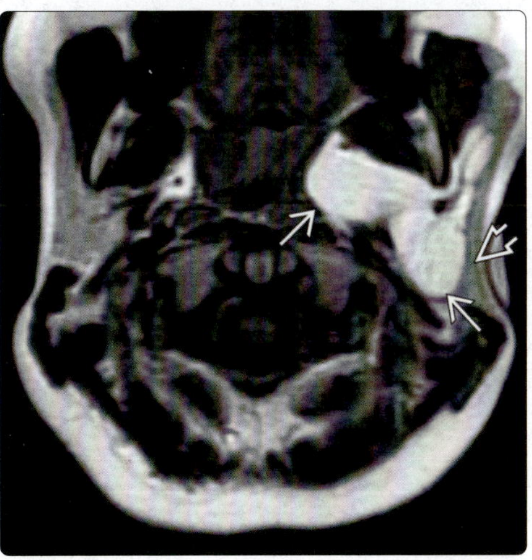

(Left) *Axial CECT in a 1-year-old girl demonstrates intense homogeneous enhancement of a very large IH replacing the entire superficial* ➔ *& deep* ⇨ *lobes of the left parotid gland.* **(Right)** *Axial T1 MR in the same child 8 years later shows interval size ↓ & diffuse fatty replacement* ➔ *of the left parotid IH. Note the thin sliver of overlying normal-appearing, superficial parotid gland tissue* ⇨.

KEY FACTS

TERMINOLOGY

- Rhabdomyosarcoma (RMS): Most common childhood soft tissue sarcoma

IMAGING

- Up to 40% occur in H&N
  - Orbital, parameningeal, other sites
- MR is best to
  - Characterize solid soft tissue mass
    - Often intermediate signal on T2 FS or STIR
    - Variable contrast enhancement
    - Typically restrict diffusion
  - Evaluate intracranial spread (requires contrast)
- CT is best to look for bone destruction or remodeling
- Neck imaging for cervical metastatic adenopathy
  - PET/CT may improve staging & treatment evaluation

TOP DIFFERENTIAL DIAGNOSES

- Infantile hemangioma
- Slow-flow vascular malformations
- Fibromatosis colli
- Metastatic neuroblastoma
- Langerhans cell histiocytosis
- Juvenile angiofibroma
- Nasopharyngeal carcinoma
- Non-Hodgkin & Hodgkin lymphoma
- Plexiform neurofibroma

PATHOLOGY

- 3 histologic subtypes
  - Embryonal RMS: Most common; young children
  - Alveolar RMS: 2nd most common; 15-25 years of age
  - Pleomorphic RMS: Least common; 40-60 years of age

CLINICAL ISSUES

- Presentation: 70% < 12 years of age, 40% < 5 years
- Treatment: Surgery, chemotherapy, ± radiation therapy

(Left) *Coronal CECT in an 8-year-old shows a nonspecific, mildly heterogeneous extraconal mass ➡ in the inferior & inferomedial left orbit without bone destruction.* **(Right)** *Coronal T1 C+ FS MR in the same child shows a heterogeneously enhancing mass ➡ with an atypical appearance for a hematoma, hemangioma, or vascular malformation. Biopsy confirmed an embryonal rhabdomyosarcoma. The absence of bone destruction does not exclude rhabdomyosarcoma (RMS).*

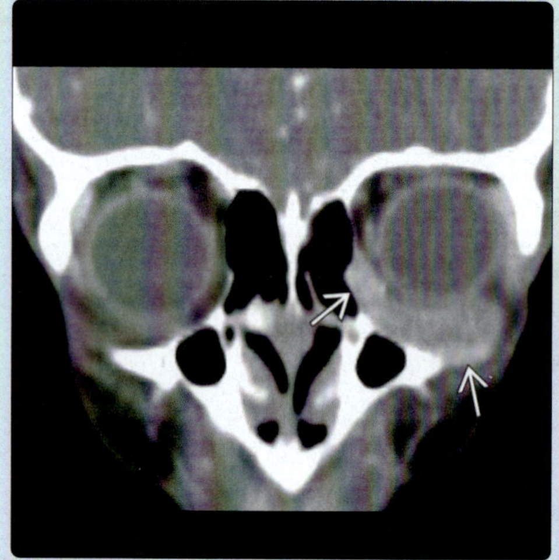

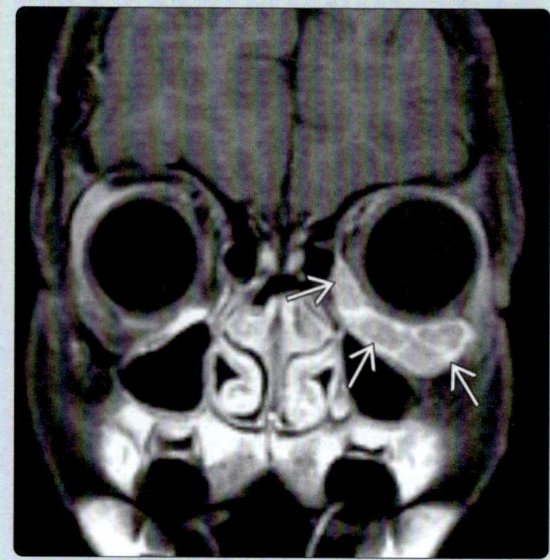

(Left) *Axial T1 C+ FS MR in a 15-month-old boy with intermittent epistaxis & swelling of the left nasal ala demonstrates a heterogeneously enhancing left intranasal/nasal alar mass ➡ obstructing the left nasal cavity.* **(Right)** *Axial STIR MR in the same patient demonstrates primarily intermediate signal intensity throughout the mass ➡ with the exception of a small cystic/necrotic region anteriorly ⇨. Subsequent biopsy revealed an alveolar RMS.*

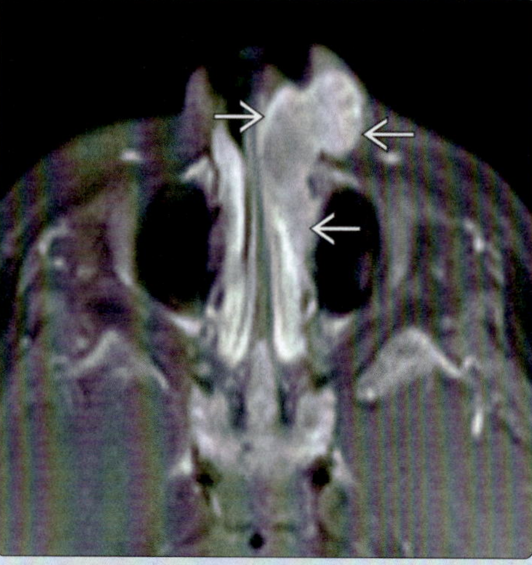

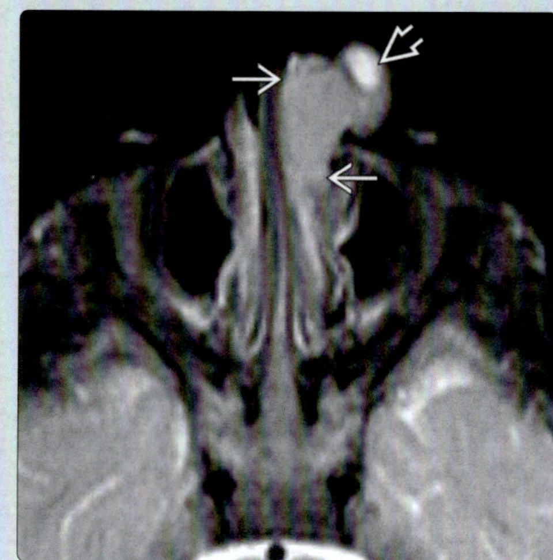

TERMINOLOGY

Definitions

- Rhabdomyosarcoma (RMS): Malignant neoplasm of rhabdomyoblasts
  - Most common childhood soft tissue sarcoma

IMAGING

General Features

- Best diagnostic clue
  - Solid soft tissue mass with variable enhancement
- Location
  - Up to 40% occur in head & neck, including orbit, parameningeal sites, neck/face soft tissues, nasal cavity
    - Parameningeal sites: Middle ear, paranasal sinus, nasal cavity, nasopharynx, masticator space, pterygopalatine fossa, parapharyngeal space
      - Intracranial extension in up to 55%
      - Temporal bone involvement: Petrous apex & middle ear > mastoid
    - Orbit
    - All other head & neck sites: Scalp, cheek, parotid, oral cavity, larynx, oropharynx, hypopharynx, thyroid/parathyroid
- Size
  - Variable; may present earlier in orbit due to confined space → early proptosis

Ultrasonographic Findings

- Solid, firm mass with variable internal vascularity
- May show bone destruction in superficial masses

CT Findings

- Invasive soft tissue mass with variable enhancement
- Osseous erosion is common but not seen in all cases

MR Findings

- Isointense T1, hyperintense T2 signal relative to muscle
  - Not "fluid bright" unless necrotic/cystic components
- Variable contrast enhancement, often mild to moderate
  - Diffuse, intense enhancement is atypical
- Often restricts diffusion
  - ADC values range from ~ $0.5\text{-}1.3 \times 10^{-3}/mm^2$
- ASL: Variable, but ↑ perfusion argues against benign low-flow vascular malformations

Nuclear Medicine Findings

- PET/CT
  - Hypermetabolic
    - May improve staging & posttreatment evaluation

Imaging Recommendations

- Best imaging tool
  - CT to evaluate osseous erosion
  - MR is best for soft tissue mass characterization
  - MR to evaluate perineural & intracranial spread of parameningeal RMS
    - Thickening & enhancement of nerves, leptomeninges
  - MR to distinguish between sinonasal tumor & obstructive/inflammatory disease
- Protocol advice
  - T2 FS or STIR MR: ↑ tumor conspicuity
  - Coronal T1 C+ FS MR: Detect intracranial extension
  - DWI MR: ADC values can help separate cellular tumor from benign vascular anomaly
  - Axial & coronal thin-section bone CT: Osseous erosion
  - Image neck: Rule out cervical metastatic adenopathy

DIFFERENTIAL DIAGNOSIS

Infantile Hemangioma

- Benign vascular neoplasm in infants, often with characteristic cutaneous involvement
- Intensely enhancing round or lobulated mass with high-flow vessels during proliferative phase
- ASL MR shows markedly ↑ perfusion
- ADC MR values typically range from ~ $1.3\text{-}1.6 \times 10^{-3}/mm^2$
- No bone destruction
- Fatty infiltration during involuting phase

Slow-Flow Vascular Malformation

- May be well defined or extensive/infiltrative
- Fluid signal contents ± layering blood products, retracted clots, or phleboliths (in venous type)
- Venous type shows gradual patchy enhancement; lymphatic macrocystic type shows thin septal enhancement
- ADC values typically range from ~ $2.0\text{-}2.6 \times 10^{-3}/mm^2$
- ASL MR will not show ↑ perfusion

Fibromatosis Colli

- Benign, self-limited, heterogeneous mass within & expanding midportion of sternocleidomastoid muscle in young infant with torticollis

Metastatic Neuroblastoma

- Most cervical disease is due to metastatic adenopathy rather than primary lesion
- Metastatic disease to skull/skull base is frequently bilateral: Enhancing masses surround aggressive osseous permeation/expansion with radiating spicules of new bone

Langerhans Cell Histiocytosis

- Enhancing soft tissue mass filling sharply marginated punched-out lytic bone lesion
- Temporal bone: Mastoid > petrous apex & middle ear

Juvenile Angiofibroma

- Highly vascular mass causing nasal obstruction &/or epistaxis in adolescent males
- Intensely enhancing lesion with bone destruction & internal high-flow vessels
- Originates at sphenopalatine foramen on lateral nasal wall
- Often involves nasal cavity, nasopharynx, skull base, masticator space ± orbit, sinus, intracranial extension

Nasopharyngeal Carcinoma

- Nasopharyngeal mass in 2nd decade of life
- Variable contrast enhancement
- Central skull base erosion, widening of petroclival fissure, extension to pterygopalatine fossa + masticator & parapharyngeal spaces
- Unilateral or bilateral cervical & lateral retropharyngeal adenopathy

Non-Hodgkin Lymphoma

- Non-Hodgkin lymphoma & Hodgkin lymphoma imaging findings are similar; difficult to differentiate
- Large, nonnecrotic nodes are typical
- Sinonasal, orbital, or nasopharyngeal NHL may cause osseous erosion

Plexiform Neurofibroma

- Benign peripheral nerve sheath tumor in neurofibromatosis type 1
- Lobulated masses with peripherally ↑ T2 signal & centrally ↓ T2 signal (target sign)
- Bone remodeling, typically without destruction

PATHOLOGY

General Features

- Etiology
  - Originates from primitive mesenchymal cells committed to skeletal muscle differentiation (rhabdomyoblasts)
- Genetics
  - ↑ incidence in children with *TP53* tumor suppressor gene mutation
  - Most embryonal RMS has loss of heterozygosity at 11p15 locus
  - Alveolar RMS: 50% have *FOX01* to *PAX3* (or *PAX7*) gene fusion
    - *PAX3-FKHR* gene fusion has better prognosis
- Associated abnormalities
  - ↑ incidence of embryonal RMS in Noonan syndrome
    - Hematologic malignancies & neuroblastoma are also seen
  - Rarely associated with neurofibromatosis type 1, Li-Fraumeni, & Beckwith-Wiedemann syndromes
  - Rarely associated with hereditary retinoblastoma
  - May occur as radiation-induced 2nd primary neoplasm

Staging, Grading, & Classification

- Soft Tissue Sarcoma Committee of Children's Oncology Group
  - Group I: Localized tumor completely resected
  - Group II: Gross total resection with microscopic residual
  - Group III: Incomplete resection with gross residual
  - Group IV: Distant metastases
- TNM: Tumor site, size, local invasion, lymph nodes, distant metastases

Microscopic Features

- 3 histologic subtypes
  - Embryonal RMS: Most common (> 50% of all RMS)
    - Occurs in younger children
    - 70-90% occur in head & neck or GU tract
    - Botryoid RMS: Gross appearance like cluster of grapes, typically in patients 2-5 years of age
      - 75% arise in vagina, prostate, or bladder
      - 25% in head/neck or bile ducts
  - Alveolar RMS: 2nd most common
    - Usually occurs in patients 15-25 years of age
    - Most common in extremities & trunk
  - Anaplastic RMS (also called pleomorphic): Least common
    - Usually in adults 40-60 years of age; rarely < 15 years
    - Most arise in extremities; rarely in head & neck

CLINICAL ISSUES

Presentation

- Most common signs/symptoms
  - Symptoms are variable, depend on location
    - Orbit: Mass, proptosis, ↓ vision
    - Sinonasal: Nasal obstruction, epistaxis; may present late with soft tissue facial mass
    - Temporal bone: Postauricular or external auditory canal mass, otitis media, CNVII palsy
    - Neck: Mass, pain, rarely airway compromise

Demographics

- Age
  - 70% < 12 years of age; 40% < 5 years of age
- Ethnicity
  - More common in White patients

Natural History & Prognosis

- Variable; depends on location & cell type
  - Orbit: Best prognosis (80-90% disease-free survival)
  - Parameningeal: Worst prognosis (40-50% disease-free survival)
  - Embryonal & pleomorphic: Better prognosis than alveolar RMS
    - Alveolar RMS without gene fusion: Prognosis is similar to embryonal RMS

Treatment

- Surgical debulking, chemotherapy, ± radiation therapy
- Research ongoing in proton therapy, immunotherapy, & vaccination
- Sentinel node biopsy may improve treatment stratification

DIAGNOSTIC CHECKLIST

Consider

- Not always associated with bone destruction
  - Beware of enhancing soft tissue mass without bone destruction; may simulate infantile hemangioma (IH)
    - IH is almost always found in 1st year of life; RMS is more common beyond 12 months
    - IH is typically soft/compressible while RMS is more likely firm
    - IH demonstrates high density of low-resistance arterial vessels on color Doppler
    - IH enhances more intensely & homogeneously
    - IH has higher ADC values on DWI MR

SELECTED REFERENCES

1. Maldonado FR et al: Quantitative characterization of extraocular orbital lesions in children using diffusion-weighted imaging. Pediatr Radiol. 51(1):119-27, 2021
2. Jawad N et al: The clinical and radiologic features of paediatric rhabdomyosarcoma. Pediatr Radiol. 49(11):1516-23, 2019
3. Kim JK et al: Patterns of radiotherapy use and outcomes in head and neck soft-tissue sarcoma in a national cohort. Laryngoscope. 130(1):120-7, 2019
4. Häußler SM et al: Head and neck rhabdomyosarcoma in children: a 20-year retrospective study at a tertiary referral center. J Cancer Res Clin Oncol. 144(2):371-9, 2018
5. Chevallier KM et al: Differentiating pediatric rhabdomyosarcoma and Langerhans cell histiocytosis of the temporal bone by imaging appearance. AJNR Am J Neuroradiol. 37(6):1185-9, 2016

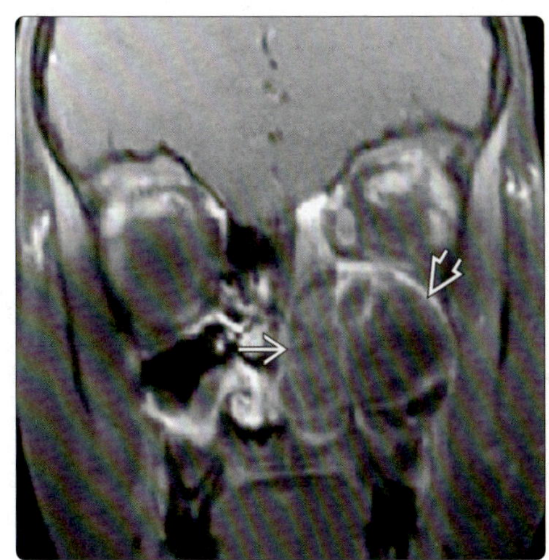

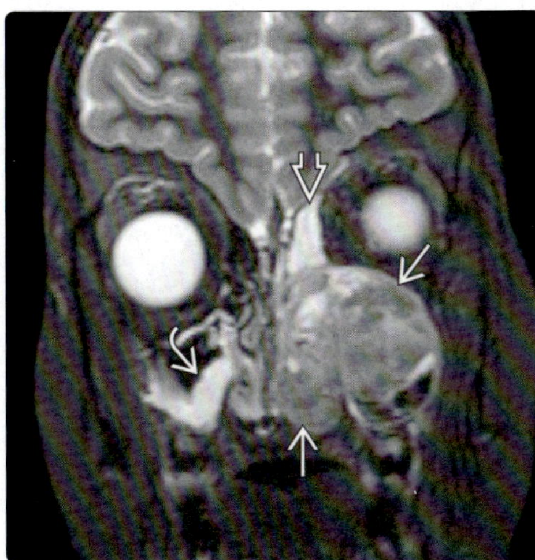

(Left) *Coronal T1 C+ FS MR shows a heterogeneously enhancing left nasal RMS* ➡ *with expansion of the left maxillary sinus* ➡. *Some component of the disease in the left maxillary sinus could represent inflammation rather than tumor.* **(Right)** *Coronal STIR MR in the same patient better differentiates the tumor* ➡ *filling the expanded left maxillary sinus & nasal cavity from hyperintense, inflammatory mucosal disease in the left ethmoid* ➡ *& right maxillary* ➡ *sinuses.*

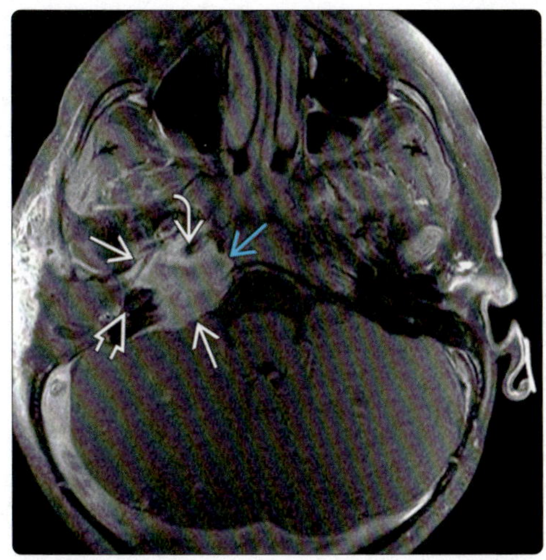

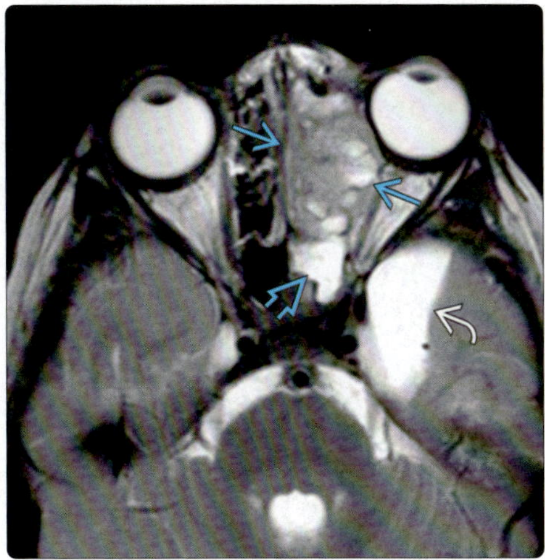

(Left) *Axial T1 C+ FS MR demonstrates a moderately enhancing RMS* ➡ *destroying the right petrous apex & otic capsule bone adjacent to the cochlea* ➡ *& extending along margins of the internal carotid artery* ➡ *into the clivus* ➡. **(Right)** *Axial T2 MR in a 5-year-old with left proptosis & palpable cervical adenopathy demonstrates a mixed-intensity alveolar RMS* ➡ *as compared to the hyperintense sphenoid sinus inflammatory disease* ➡ *& incidental middle cranial fossa arachnoid cyst* ➡.

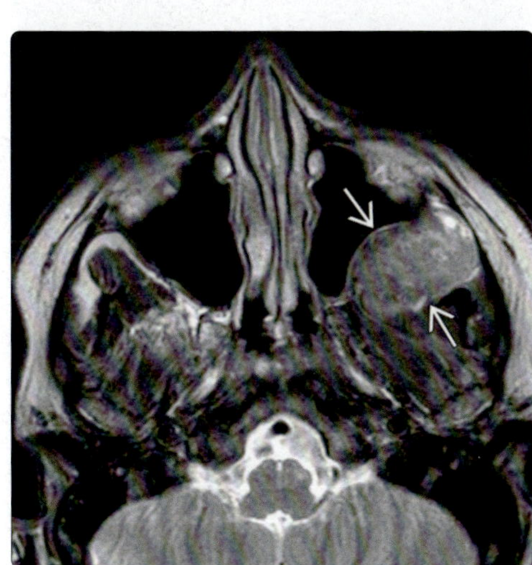

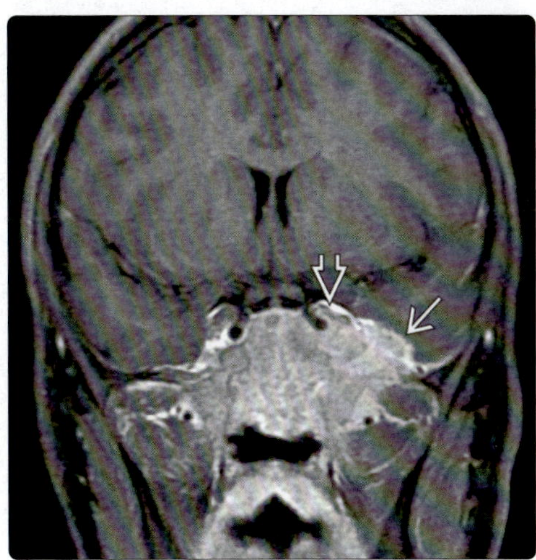

(Left) *Axial T2 MR in a 21-year-old with an embryonal RMS shows anterior bowing of the left maxillary sinus posterior wall by a heterogeneous, mildly hypointense left infratemporal fossa mass* ➡, *consistent with a highly cellular RMS. Although it is relatively hypointense without FS, it is hyperintense relative to skeletal muscle, typical of RMS.* **(Right)** *Coronal T1 C+ FS MR shows an extensive left skull base RMS with left middle cranial fossa extension (displacing the left temporal lobe* ➡*) & invasion of the left cavernous sinus* ➡.

KEY FACTS

TERMINOLOGY

- Benign fibrosis of sternocleidomastoid (SCM) muscle
- Most common cervical "mass" of infancy
- Postulated to be due to birth trauma, peripartum injury, in utero compartment syndrome, or maldevelopment

IMAGING

- Often diagnosed clinically without imaging
- Ultrasound is modality of choice if imaging is required
- Process is entirely intramuscular (contained within SCM) without local invasion or inflammatory changes
- Fusiform expansion of central SCM muscle
  - Thick & short compared to contralateral SCM
- Variable heterogeneity of lesion
  - Ranges from nearly homogeneous to markedly heterogeneous on ultrasound/CECT/MR
- Variable internal vascularity within/about mass
- No associated adenopathy, Ca^{2+}, extramuscular edema, intrasubstance hemorrhage, or fluid collection
- Fascial planes around SCM are preserved

TOP DIFFERENTIAL DIAGNOSES

- Cervical lymphadenopathy
- Infantile hemangioma
- Cervical teratoma
- Congenital neuroblastoma
- Rhabdomyosarcoma
- Branchial cleft anomalies
- Lymphatic malformation
- Cervical extension of mediastinal thymus
- Spinal fusion anomalies

CLINICAL ISSUES

- Painless, palpable mass with torticollis
- Contralateral occipital flattening (plagiocephaly) is common
- Peak presentation at 24 days old
- Self-limited, usually resolves completely by 6 months of age with conservative treatment/physical therapy

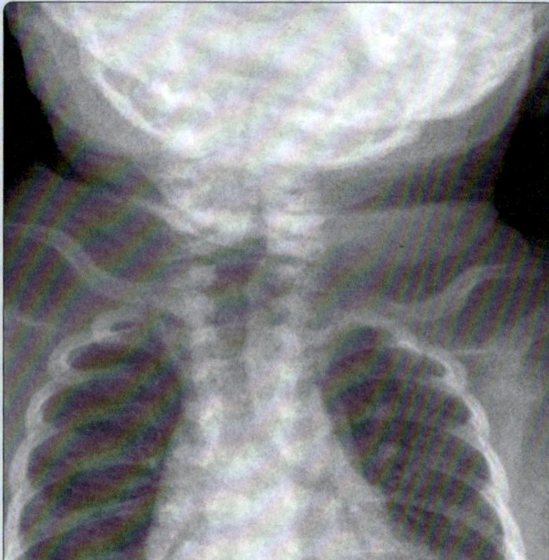

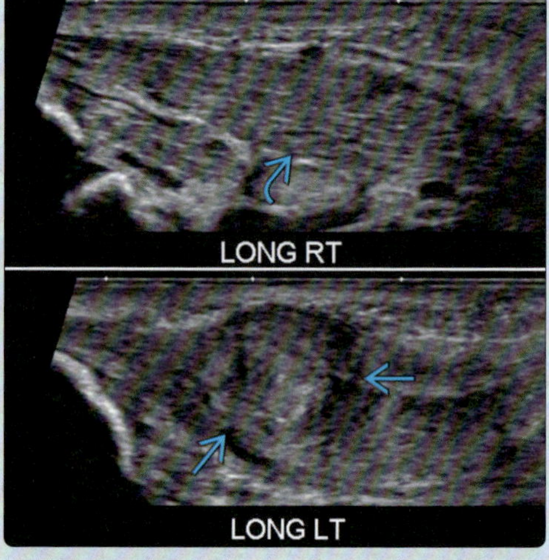

(Left) *AP radiograph of the neck shows mild torticollis with the left ear closer to the left shoulder & the chin slightly turned away. No bony anomalies are seen to explain this neck positioning in this infant with fibromatosis colli. Mild buckling of the trachea at the thoracic inlet is normal in young infants.* **(Right)** *Split-screen longitudinal US images in a 24-day-old boy with torticollis show a focally enlarged left sternocleidomastoid (SCM) muscle ➡ compared to the right ➡, typical of fibromatosis colli.*

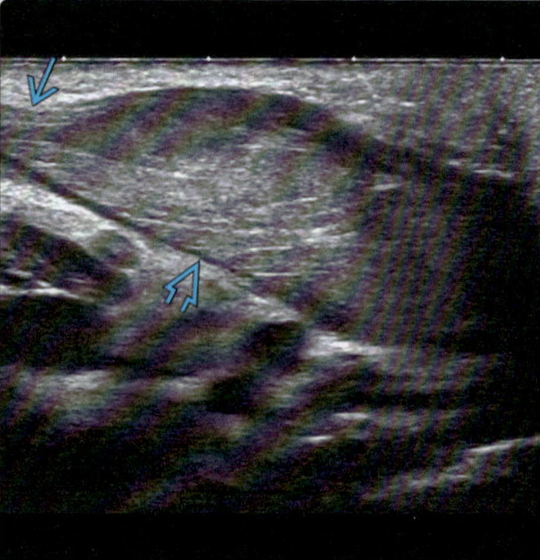

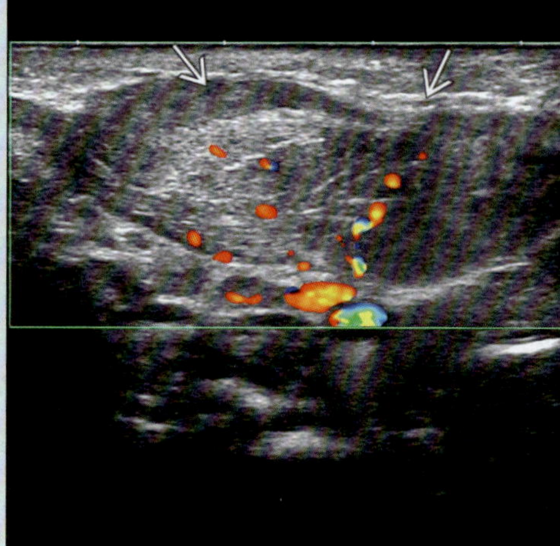

(Left) *Orienting the US transducer along the long axis of the SCM optimally shows the mildly heterogeneous enlargement/expansion of the muscle belly with normal SCM proximal tapering ➡ & sharp, distinct borders ➡ with adjacent tissues.* **(Right)** *Longitudinal US with color Doppler shows that the enlarged SCM muscle has mildly ↑ blood flow ➡ & slightly ↑ heterogeneous echotexture centrally.*

TERMINOLOGY

Synonyms

- Sternocleidomastoid (SCM) pseudotumor, SCM tumor of infancy, congenital muscular torticollis, neonatal torticollis, pseudotumor of infancy

Definitions

- Most common cervical "mass" of infancy
- Benign fibrosis of SCM muscle
- Postulated to be due to birth trauma, peripartum injury, in utero compartment syndrome, or maldevelopment
- Torticollis ("wryneck"): Persistent twisting of neck such that ear on affected side is positioned lower & more midline than normal
  - When bony causes of torticollis have been excluded, consider fibrosis of SCM muscle

IMAGING

General Features

- Best diagnostic clue
  - Focal thickening & fibrosis of sternal or clavicular head of SCM muscle
  - Process is entirely intramuscular without local invasion or inflammatory changes
- Location
  - Middle or lower 1/3 of SCM muscle belly
  - Sternal & clavicular muscle bundles are affected equally often
  - Unilateral: Equal frequency of right vs. left
- Size
  - 1-3 cm in length
  - May ↑ in size in first 2-3 months of life
- Morphology
  - Focal, heterogeneous to homogeneous expansion of SCM muscle, distorting normal muscle architecture
  - SCM tapers to normal thickness proximal & distal to lesion
  - Affected SCM is mildly shorter than contralateral side
  - No extramuscular extension, surrounding inflammatory changes, or adenopathy

Radiographic Findings

- Cervical spine radiographs may be obtained to exclude bony abnormality, causing torticollis
  - Hemivertebrae or omovertebral bones: Congenital bony anomalies not related to fibromatosis colli
- May see nonspecific, unilateral soft tissue fullness or "mass"
- Virtually never calcifies
  - If Ca^{2+} is seen, consider neuroblastoma & teratoma

Ultrasonographic Findings

- Grayscale ultrasound
  - Focal mass mildly or moderately expanding SCM muscle belly
  - Loss of normal muscle architecture
  - Variable echogenicity of mass; may be homogeneous or heterogeneous
  - Affected SCM is shorter & thicker than contralateral side
    - Comparison with asymptomatic side is useful
    - Extended field-of-view imaging is useful to show entire length of SCM
  - Fascial planes surrounding SCM are preserved
  - No associated adenopathy, Ca^{2+}, extramuscular edema, intrasubstance hemorrhage, or fluid collection
  - Lack of extramuscular involvement excludes other differential diagnoses
- Color Doppler
  - Variable hyperemia in acute phase
  - May see diminished blood flow in quiescent/fibrotic phase

CT Findings

- Focal thickening/expansion of unilateral SCM muscle
  - Variable enhancement & heterogeneity
- No associated adenopathy or regional inflammatory changes

MR Findings

- T1WI
  - Fusiform enlargement of affected SCM
  - Variable signal intensity
    - Usually isointense to hypointense compared to normal muscle
- T2WI FS/STIR
  - Heterogeneous intramuscular mass; affected SCM is overall hyperintense to other muscles
    - Hypointense zones are probably due to evolving fibrosis
- T1WI C+ FS
  - Affected muscle enhances heterogeneously

Imaging Recommendations

- Best imaging tool
  - Often diagnosed clinically without imaging
  - Ultrasound is modality of choice if imaging is required
    - No ionizing radiation or sedation
    - Clearly localizes mass within SCM muscle
  - MR is reserved for atypical cases
    - Best for determining extent of alternate malignant diagnoses
      - ▫ Intracranial extension (in rhabdomyosarcoma)
      - ▫ Intraspinal extension (in neuroblastoma)
  - CT is best modality for showing cortical bony abnormalities of alternate diagnoses
    - Erosion, destruction, remodeling, vertebral segmentation anomalies, or congenital scoliosis
- Protocol advice
  - Regardless of imaging modality, none of these findings should be seen with fibromatosis colli
    - Involvement of tissues outside SCM muscle
    - Ca^{2+} or cystic change
    - Lymphadenopathy
    - Airway compression
    - Vascular encasement
    - Bone involvement
    - Intracranial/intraspinal extension
    - Other neck masses

DIFFERENTIAL DIAGNOSIS

Cervical Lymphadenopathy

- Nodes are typically discrete & easily recognizable but may appear mass-like when enlarged & confluent
- Adenopathy is more likely to have lobulated contour than smooth, spindle shape of SCM

Infantile Hemangioma

- Rapidly growing, benign, vascular neoplasm presenting as soft mass weeks to months after birth, ultimately regressing over years
- Characteristic Doppler ultrasound appearance: > 5 vessels/cm^2, shows numerous low-resistance arterial waveforms

Cervical Teratoma

- Congenital mixed solid & cystic mass, often large
- Typically contains Ca^{2+}
- May present with airway or feeding difficulties

Congenital Neuroblastoma

- Arises from paraspinal sympathetic ganglia outside SCM
- May displace &/or encase vessels
- Look for Ca^{2+}, intraspinal extension, & bony erosion

Rhabdomyosarcoma

- Solid mass outside SCM, typically in older children
- Variable enhancement & vascularity

Branchial Cleft Anomalies

- Unilocular cyst adjacent to SCM

Lymphatic Malformation

- Compressible multicystic congenital mass, often with deep infiltration & extension across midline

Cervical Extension of Mediastinal Thymus

- Look for contiguity with mediastinal thymic tissue
- Characteristic dot & dash appearance on ultrasound

Spinal Fusion Anomalies

- Torticollis with cervical scoliosis due to hemivertebra, fused vertebra, bony bar, omovertebral body, etc.

PATHOLOGY

General Features

- Etiology
  - Uncertain: Probably response to perinatal injury, partial muscle tear, or intramuscular hematoma

Gross Pathologic & Surgical Features

- Seldom resected
- Fine-needle aspirates are more common than excisional specimens
- Firm, spindle-shaped thickening of muscle without transmuscular inflammation

Microscopic Features

- Bland-appearing fibroblasts & degenerative, atrophic skeletal muscle in clean background
- Collagen is always present
- Occasional giant cells & parallel clusters of fibroblasts

CLINICAL ISSUES

Presentation

- Most common signs/symptoms
  - Painless, palpable mass with torticollis
  - Contralateral occipital flattening (plagiocephaly) is common
  - History of breech presentation &/or "difficult" vaginal birth is common but not mandatory
- Other signs/symptoms
  - If severe or persistent, may result in limited range of motion at neck &/or facial asymmetry

Demographics

- Age
  - Newborn infants
  - Peak presentation at 24 days old
  - Classically noticed < 8 weeks of age but may worsen in first 2-3 months of life
- Sex
  - Males affected slightly more often than females
- Epidemiology
  - Occurs with 0.4% of live births
  - Associated with breech presentation & birth dystocia

Natural History & Prognosis

- Self-limited, usually resolves completely by 6 months of age
- Occasional cases recur or flare during periods of rapid somatic growth

Treatment

- Physical therapy to encourage full range of motion → "stretch" SCM
- 90% have full recovery with conservative treatment &/or physiotherapy
- Surgery is only indicated in unusual cases when craniofacial asymmetry or refractory torticollis persists after 1 year

SELECTED REFERENCES

1. Agarwal H et al: Non-malignant fibroblastic/myofibroblastic tumors in pediatric age group: clues and pitfalls to the cytological diagnosis. Cytopathology. 31(2):115-21, 2020
2. Navarro OM: Pearls and pitfalls in the imaging of soft-tissue masses in children. Semin Ultrasound CT MR. 41(5):498-512, 2020
3. Caprio MG et al: Paediatric neck ultrasonography: a pictorial essay. J Ultrasound. 22(2):215-26, 2019
4. Xiong Z et al: Unique finding in congenital muscular torticollis: clinic screening on the neck of one day old neonate and ultrasonographic imaging from birth through 3 years of follow-up. Medicine (Baltimore). 98(11):e14794, 2019
5. Bansal AG et al: US of pediatric superficial masses of the head and neck. Radiographics. 38(4):1239-63, 2018
6. Sargar KM et al: Pediatric fibroblastic and myofibroblastic tumors: a pictorial review. Radiographics. 36(4):1195-214, 2016
7. Wojcicki KM et al: Fibromatosis colli spuriously presenting as a retropharyngeal mass on cervical spine radiographs. Intern Emerg Med. 11(2):277-9, 2015
8. Ainsworth KE et al: Congenital infantile fibrosarcoma: review of imaging features. Pediatr Radiol. 44(9):1124-9, 2014
9. Lowry KC et al: The presentation and management of fibromatosis colli. Ear Nose Throat J. 89(9):E4-8, 2010
10. Murphey MD et al: From the archives of the AFIP: musculoskeletal fibromatoses: radiologic-pathologic correlation. Radiographics. 29(7):2143-73, 2009
11. Ekinci S et al: Infantile fibromatosis of the sternocleidomastoid muscle mimicking muscular torticollis. J Pediatr Surg. 39(9):1424-5, 2004

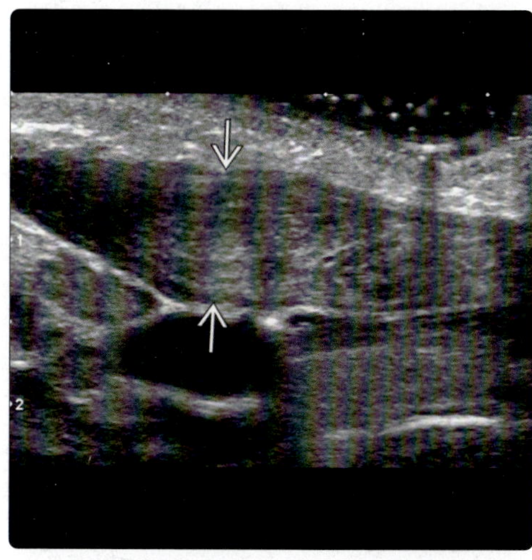

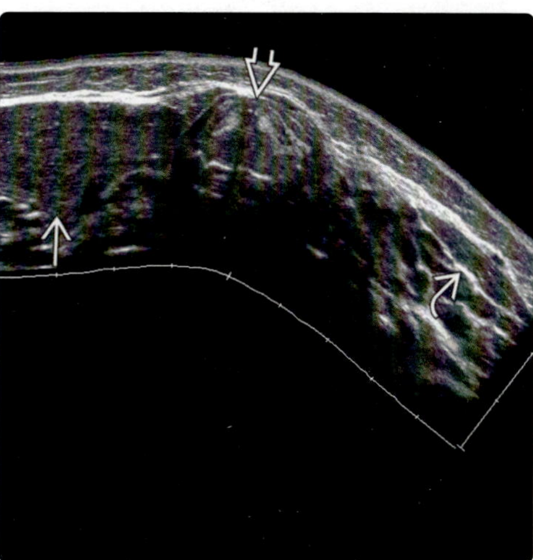

(Left) *Longitudinal US in a 1-month-old infant shows ↑ size & echotexture of the SCM ➡, consistent with fibromatosis colli. Note that the fat & facial planes around the muscle are preserved.* **(Right)** *Transverse extended field-of-view US across the neck in an infant with torticollis illustrates the enlargement of the right SCM ➡ as compared to the left ➡. The trachea is seen in the midline at the level of the vocal cords ➡.*

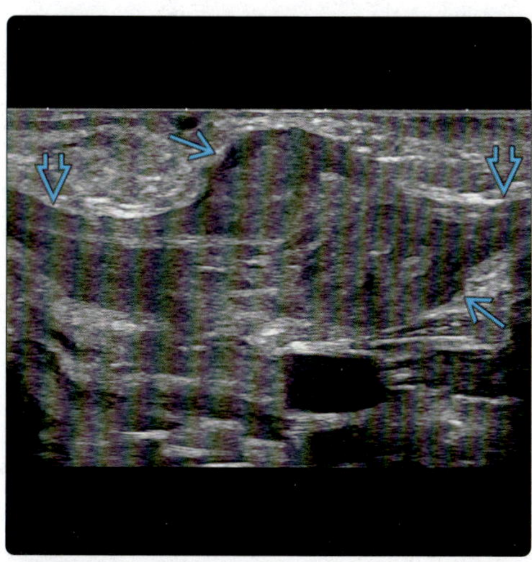

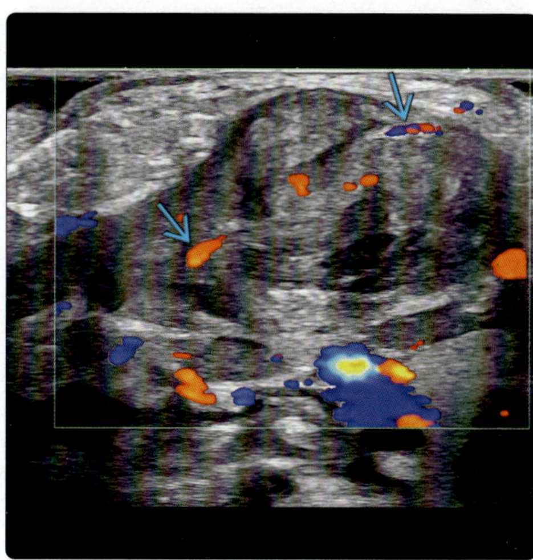

(Left) *Longitudinal US in a 28-day-old girl shows focal enlargement of both the sternal & clavicular bundles ➡ of the SCM in this patient with fibromatosis colli. Note the normal proximal & distal tapering of the muscle ➡.* **(Right)** *Longitudinal color Doppler US in the same patient shows normal to minimally ↑ blood flow ➡ in affected portions of the muscle.*

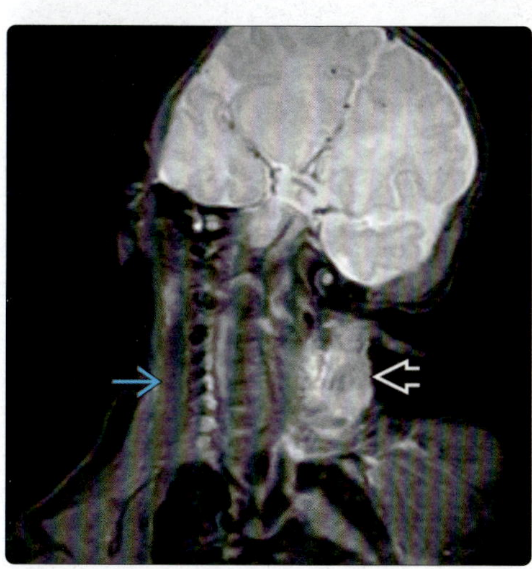

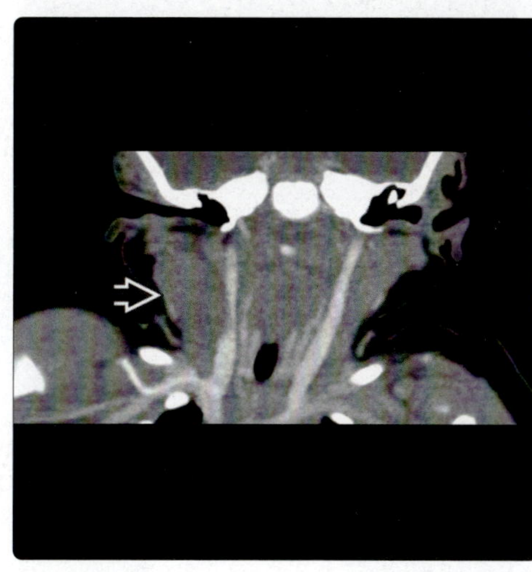

(Left) *Coronal STIR MR in an infant with obvious torticollis shows heterogeneously ↑ signal intensity & thickness of the left SCM ➡, consistent with fibromatosis colli. Note the normal right SCM ➡.* **(Right)** *Coronal CECT in an infant with facial anomalies shows homogeneous thickening of the right SCM ➡, which lies just superficial to the jugular & carotid vessels. Fibromatosis colli can appear much more heterogeneous than this.*

Suppurative Adenitis

KEY FACTS

TERMINOLOGY

- Pus formation within nodes from bacterial infection
- Synonyms: Adenitis, lymphadenitis, intranodal abscess

IMAGING

- Enlarged node(s) with internal fluid & surrounding inflammation (cellulitis)
  - Most often jugulodigastric, submandibular, or retropharyngeal
- Loss of normal nodal architecture & internal vascularity/enhancement
- Conglomeration of necrotic nodes progressing to abscess shows marked heterogeneity of irregular collection
  - Well-defined, enhancing/hyperemic wall
  - Complex hypoechoic/nonenhancing center
- US is useful to confirm true liquefaction with drainable pus
  - Swirling internal debris upon compression
- CECT best defines deep extent & complications
  - Lemierre syndrome (venous thrombophlebitis), internal carotid artery spasm or pseudoaneurysm, airway compression, mediastinal extension

TOP DIFFERENTIAL DIAGNOSES

- Nontuberculous *Mycobacterium* adenopathy
- Tuberculous adenopathy
- 2nd branchial cleft anomaly
- Rhabdomyosarcoma
- Lymphoma
- Lymphatic malformation
- Fibromatosis colli

PATHOLOGY

- *Staphylococcus* & *Streptococcus*: Most frequent organisms

DIAGNOSTIC CHECKLIST

- Look for primary infectious source on images
  - Pharyngitis, dental infection, salivary gland calculi

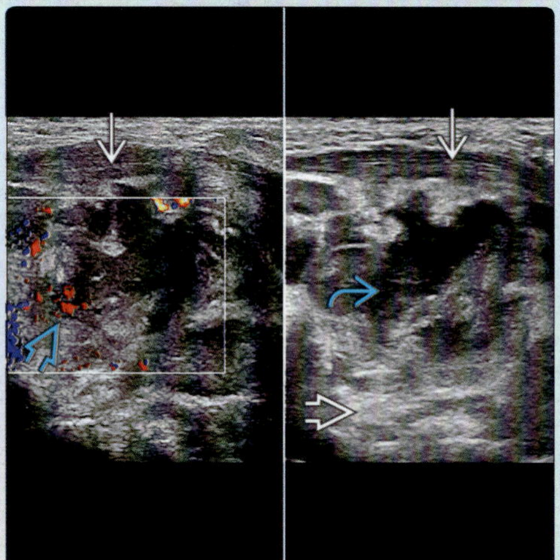
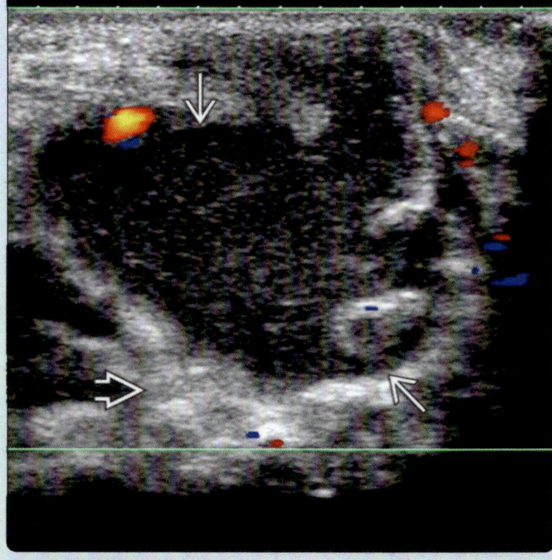

(Left) *Transverse (left) & long (right) Doppler & grayscale US images of an infant with suppurative adenitis show a heterogeneous conglomeration of level II nodes ➡ with internal debris ➡, posterior acoustic enhancement ➡, & peripheral hyperemia ➡.* **(Right)** *Transverse Doppler US in a 6-year-old with fever & a tender neck mass shows an irregular hypoechoic abscess ➡ with posterior acoustic enhancement ➡ & no internal vascularity. Swirling of debris upon compression can help confirm drainability.*

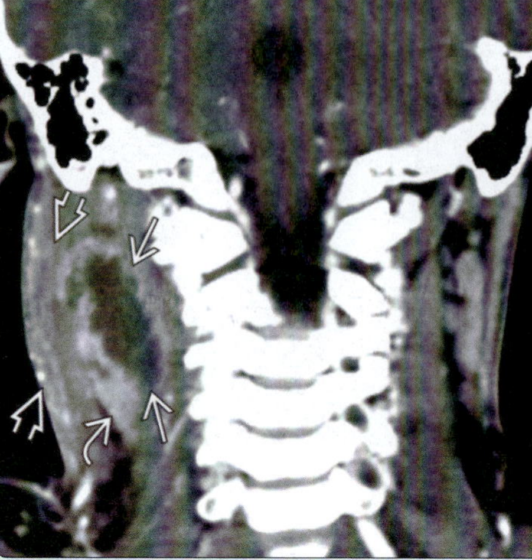
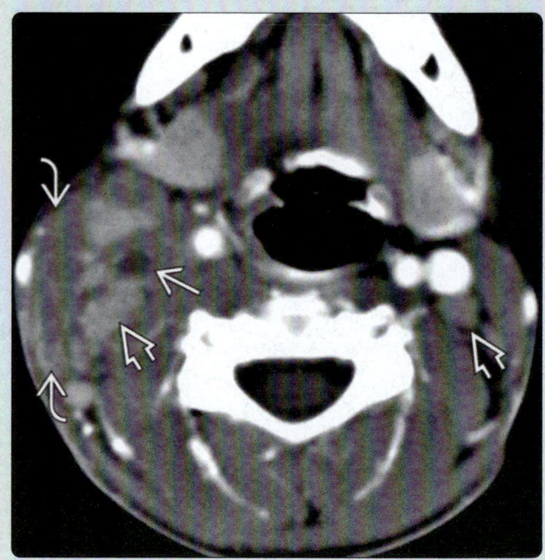

(Left) *Coronal CECT in a 6-year-old with fever & a fluctuant neck mass shows an irregular, rim-enhancing abscess ➡ with overlying myositis/cellulitis ➡ & an adjacent nonsuppurative lymph node ➡.* **(Right)** *More inferior axial CECT in the same child shows a round focus of nonenhancement, representing a segmental clot ➡ in the right internal jugular vein, consistent with Lemierre syndrome. Note the R > L nonsuppurative nodes ➡ as well as the overlying myositis/cellulitis ➡.*

TERMINOLOGY

Synonyms

- Adenitis, acute lymphadenitis, intranodal abscess

Definitions

- Pus formation within nodes from bacterial infection

IMAGING

General Features

- Best diagnostic clue
  - Enlarged node(s) with internal fluid & surrounding inflammation (cellulitis)
- Location
  - Any nodal groups of head/neck
    - Most often: Jugulodigastric, submandibular, retropharyngeal
  - May be unilateral or bilateral
- Size
  - Enlarged single node or conglomeration of nodes
    - Often in 1- to 4-cm range
- Morphology
  - Ovoid to round, large node with central necrosis
  - Margins are often poorly defined
  - Additional adjacent solid or suppurative nodes are typically present

Ultrasonographic Findings

- Early adenitis may show enlarged ovoid foci with retained nodal architecture & hyperemia
- Loss of architecture & internal vascularity occurs with necrosis
  - Central ↓ echogenicity with ↑ through transmission
- Conglomeration of necrotic nodes progressing to abscess shows marked heterogeneity of irregular collection
  - Liquefied pus: Swirling internal debris with compression
  - ↑ peripheral vascularity
    - Very low-resistance & pulsatility indices

CT Findings

- CECT
  - Enhancing nodal wall with central hypoattenuation/lack of enhancement
  - Stranding/edema of surrounding tissues = cellulitis
  - With progression to abscess → irregular, ill-defined, peripherally enhancing, low-attenuation collection
    - Caveat: Well-defined, low-attenuation collection with rim enhancement is not necessarily pathognomonic for drainable pus → consider US
      - Represents nondrainable phlegmon in ~ 20%
  - ± myositis, Lemierre syndrome (venous thrombophlebitis), deviation of carotid sheath vessels, internal carotid artery spasm or pseudoaneurysm, retropharyngeal soft tissue edema, mass effect on airway, mediastinal extension

MR Findings

- T1WI
  - Node with central low signal intensity
  - Dampening of normal high signal intensity of surrounding fat
- STIR/T2WI FS
  - Node with diffuse or central high signal intensity
  - Edema of surrounding soft tissues
- DWI
  - Complimentary to routine pulse sequences
  - Suppurative, necrotic nodes have reduced diffusivity (bright DWI, dark ADC signal)
    - May show higher DWI & lower ADC signal relative to metastatic necrotic nodes
      - Optimal ADC thresholds remain undefined
- T1WI C+ FS
  - Marked peripheral enhancement with poorly defined margin
  - Absent central enhancement

Nuclear Medicine Findings

- PET
  - Nonspecific ↑ FDG uptake
  - Abscess shows central ↓ FDG uptake

Imaging Recommendations

- Best imaging tool
  - Ultrasound to determine phlegmon vs. abscess & guide aspiration
    - May be difficult to determine deep relationships
  - CECT is best for deep neck infections
    - Determines epicenter & total extent for aspiration or surgical planning

DIFFERENTIAL DIAGNOSIS

Nontuberculous *Mycobacterium* Adenopathy

- Asymmetric, enlarged nodes with adjacent necrotic, ring-enhancing masses
- Minimal or absent subcutaneous fat stranding
- Purified protein derivative (PPD) skin test is weakly reactive in ~ 55%
- Usually ≤ 5 years of age

Tuberculous Adenopathy

- Painless low jugular & posterior cervical low-density nodes
- Ca^{2+} may be present
- Strongly reactive PPD skin test, positive interferon gamma release assay
- Systemically unwell if active pulmonary infection

2nd Branchial Cleft Anomaly

- Solitary unilocular cyst, posterior to submandibular gland
  - Anterior to sternocleidomastoid (SCM), posterolateral to carotid sheath
- Mimics suppurative node, particularly if inflamed

Rhabdomyosarcoma

- Solid, firm soft tissue neoplasm of children (typically beyond infancy) occurring in many head/neck locations
- Typically lacks surrounding edema
- ± bone destruction

Lymphoma

- Multifocal, solid, enhancing nodes, often of bilateral neck & chest
- ± enlargement of tonsillar tissue

Lymphatic Malformation

- Congenital, multicystic mass with thin rim & septations
- Variable internal echogenicity due to internal hemorrhage
- No significant internal vascularity
- Often infiltrative & transspatial, may be bilateral

Fibromatosis Colli

- Self-limited, benign reactive mass within SCM muscle of young infants, likely due to birth trauma
  - Usually appears within 2 weeks of delivery, regresses by 8 months
  - Associated torticollis in up to 30%
- Expands SCM focally or diffusely
- Ranges from homogeneous to very heterogeneous on ultrasound, CECT, & MR
  - Heterogeneous contrast enhancement is common
  - SCM muscle may be edematous surrounding mass, but further soft tissue edema is not typical
  - No adenopathy

PATHOLOGY

General Features

- Etiology
  - Primary head/neck infection: Pharyngitis, salivary gland ductal calculus, dental decay ± mandibular osteomyelitis
    - Adjacent lymph nodes enlarge 2° to pathogen: Reactive nodes
    - Intranodal exudate forms, containing protein-rich fluid with dead neutrophils (pus): Suppurative nodes
    - If untreated or incorrectly treated, suppurative nodes rupture → interstitial pus walled-off by immune system → extranodal abscess in soft tissues
  - Reactive nodes from viral pathogen may have 2° bacterial superinfection, creating suppurative nodes

Microscopic Features

- Acute inflammatory cell infiltrate in necrotic background
  - Presence of neutrophils & macrophages
  - Negative staining for acid-fast bacilli
- *Staphylococcus* & *Streptococcus* are most frequent organisms
  - ↑ incidence of MRSA
- Pediatric infections show clustering of organisms by age
  - Infants < 1 year: *Staphylococcus aureus*, group B *Streptococcus*
  - Children 1-4 years: *S. aureus*, group A β-hemolytic *Streptococcus*, atypical mycobacteria
  - 5-15 years: Anaerobic bacteria, toxoplasmosis, cat-scratch disease, tuberculosis
- Dental infections: Typically polymicrobial, predominantly anaerobic

CLINICAL ISSUES

Presentation

- Most common signs/symptoms
  - Painful neck mass
    - Overlying skin is often warm, erythematous
  - Fever, poor oral intake
  - Elevated WBC & ESR
- Other signs/symptoms
  - Symptoms referable to primary source of infection
    - Pharyngeal/laryngeal infection: Drooling, respiratory distress
    - Peritonsillar infection: Trismus
    - Retropharyngeal or paravertebral infection: Neck stiffness, torticollis
- Clinical profile
  - Young patient presents with acute/subacute onset of tender neck mass & fever
- Clinical predictors of drainable suppurative adenitis in children
  - Absence of pharyngitis, WBC > 15,000/mm³, age ≤ 3 years, anterior cervical chain, largest palpable diameter > 3 cm, prior antibiotic treatment ≥ 24 hours

Demographics

- Age
  - Most commonly seen in pediatric & young adult population
  - Odontogenic neck infections: Adults > > children

Natural History & Prognosis

- Conglomeration of suppurative nodes or rupture of node → abscess formation
  - Superficial neck abscesses: Anterior or posterior cervical space, submandibular space
  - Deep neck abscesses: Retropharyngeal or parapharyngeal space
    - Deep space abscesses can rapidly progress with airway compromise

Treatment

- Small suppurative nodes & primary infection → antibiotics
- Large suppurative nodes, abscesses, or poor response to antibiotics → incision & drainage
  - CT & US-guided aspiration for minimally invasive management
- Nodes from atypical mycobacteria → excision to prevent recurrence or fistula/sinus tract

DIAGNOSTIC CHECKLIST

Consider

- Nontuberculous mycobacterial adenitis if no significant inflammatory changes

Image Interpretation Pearls

- Look for primary infectious source on images
  - Pharyngitis, dental infection, salivary gland calculi
- Evaluate airway for compromise with any neck infection
  - More problematic in deep infections
- Evaluate vascular structures for thrombophlebitis

SELECTED REFERENCES

1. Park JE et al: Cervical lymphadenopathy in children: a diagnostic tree analysis model based on ultrasonographic and clinical findings. Eur Radiol. 30(8):4475-85, 2020
2. Matos R et al: Unilateral acute cervical lymphadenitis in children: can we predict the need for surgery? Int J Pediatr Otorhinolaryngol. 127:109655, 2019
3. Kimia AA et al: Predictors of a drainable suppurative adenitis among children presenting with cervical adenopathy. Am J Emerg Med. 37(1):109-13, 2018
4. Eisenmenger LB et al: Imaging of head and neck lymph nodes. Radiol Clin North Am. 53(1):115-32, 2015

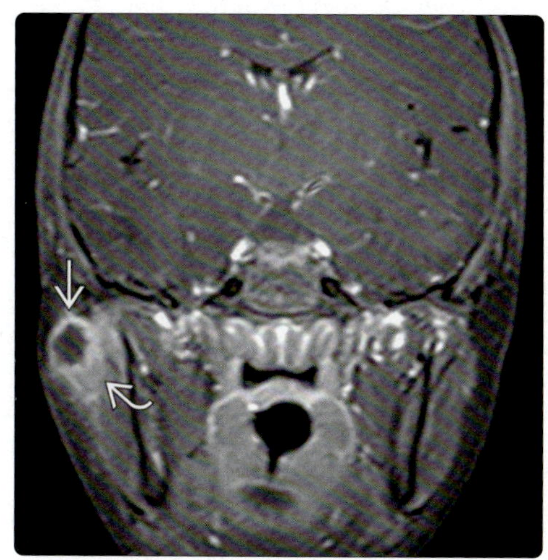

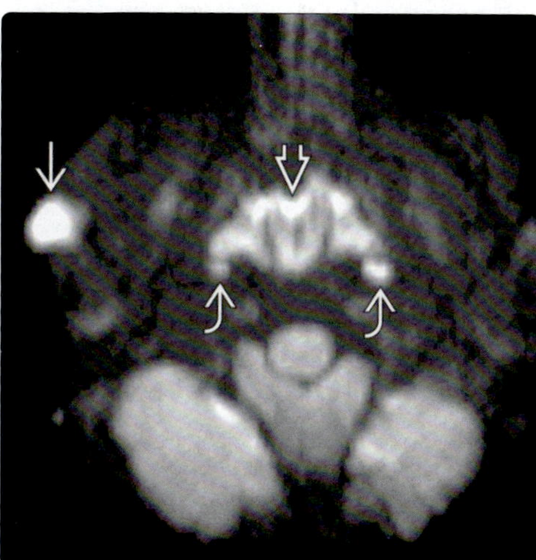

(Left) *Coronal T1 C+ FS MR in an 8-year-old boy with right cheek swelling shows a peripherally enhancing, centrally necrotic intraparotid mass* ➡ *with adjacent inflammatory stranding* ➡*. Fine-needle aspiration revealed suppurative adenitis.* **(Right)** *Axial DWI MR in the same patient shows the parotid mass* ➡ *to have centrally reduced diffusivity, typical of suppurative adenitis. Note the reactive enlargement of the nasopharyngeal lymphoid tissue* ➡ *& reactive retropharyngeal lymph nodes* ➡*.*

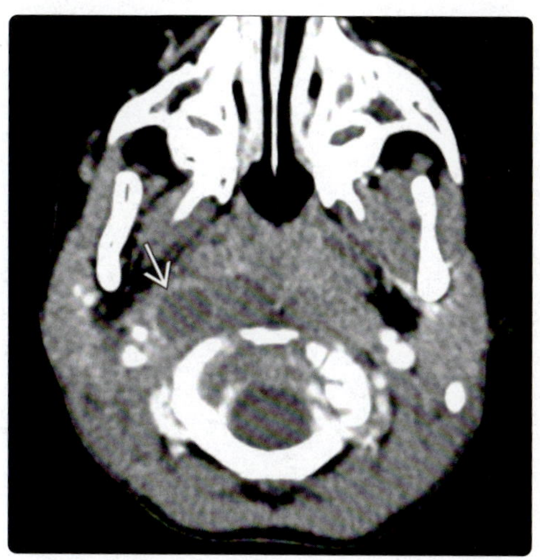

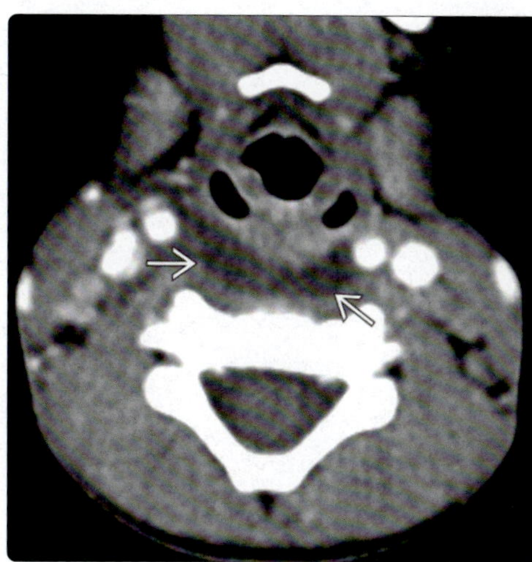

(Left) *Axial CECT in a child with fever & sore throat shows an enlarged, low-attenuation right lateral retropharyngeal lymph node with partial rim enhancement* ➡*, consistent with early purulence or phlegmon. Note the deviation of the right carotid sheath vessels, which are minimally ↓ in caliber compared to the left.* **(Right)** *Axial CECT in the same child demonstrates a poorly defined, prevertebral fluid collection* ➡ *with concave anterior margin & no rim enhancement, consistent with soft tissue edema rather than abscess.*

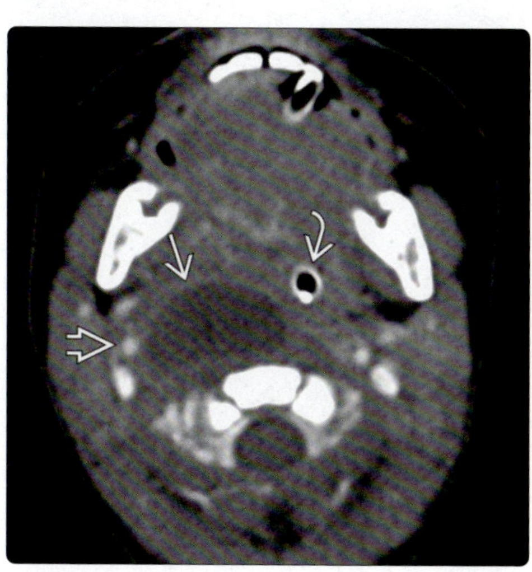

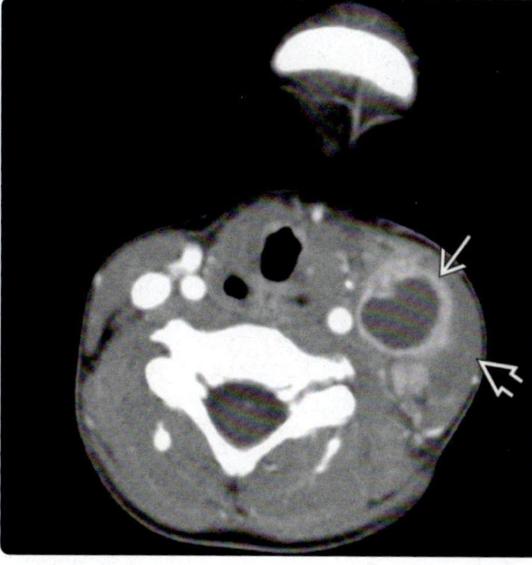

(Left) *Axial CECT in a 1-year-old shows a right lateral retropharyngeal low-attenuation abscess with peripheral enhancement* ➡*, secondary to suppurative adenitis. Note the mass effect on the carotid sheath* ➡ *& endotracheal tube* ➡*.* **(Right)** *Axial CECT in a child with left neck abscess secondary to a suppurative lymph node shows a well-defined, low-attenuation mass with diffuse, thick peripheral enhancement* ➡ *deep to the anterior aspect of the edematous left sternocleidomastoid muscle* ➡*.*

INDEX

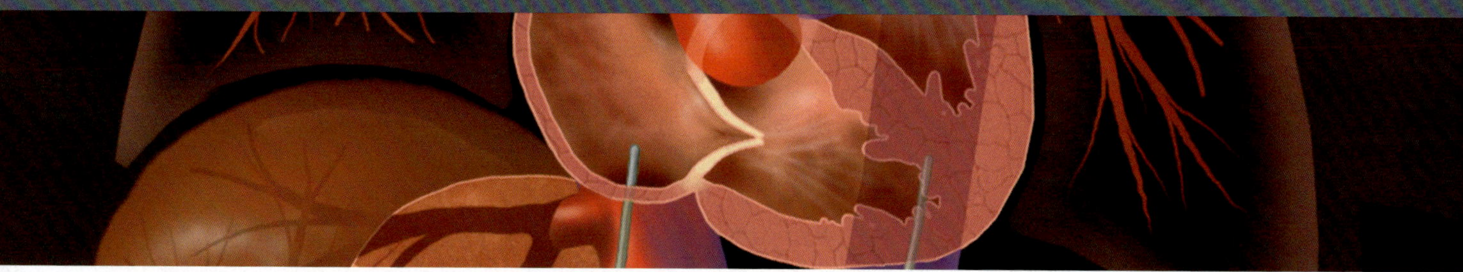

A

INDEX

INDEX

INDEX

INDEX

INDEX

B

INDEX

INDEX

INDEX

C

INDEX

INDEX

INDEX

INDEX

INDEX

INDEX

INDEX

D

INDEX

E

INDEX

F

INDEX

INDEX

G

INDEX

INDEX

H

INDEX

INDEX

INDEX

INDEX

I

INDEX

INDEX

INDEX

J

K

L

INDEX

INDEX

INDEX

M

INDEX

INDEX

INDEX

N

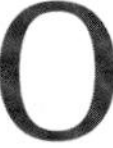

INDEX

P

INDEX

R

S

INDEX

INDEX

INDEX

INDEX

T

U

V

INDEX

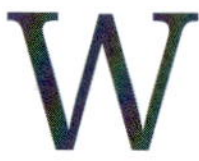

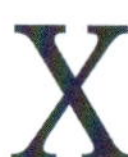

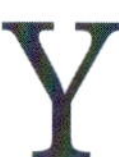

Z